Veterinary Anesthesia and Analgesia

Veterinary Anesthesia and Analgesia

The Sixth Edition of Lumb and Jones

Edited by

Leigh Lamont, DVM, MS, DACVAA
Department of Companion Animals, Atlantic Veterinary College, University of Prince Edward Island
Charlottetown, Prince Edward Island, Canada

Kurt Grimm, DVM, MS, PhD, DACVAA, DACVCP
Veterinary Specialists Services, PC
Conifer, Colorado, USA

Sheilah Robertson, BVMS (Hons), CertVA, PhD, DACVAA, DECVAA, DACAW, DECAWBM (AWSEL), FRCVS
Lap of Love Veterinary Hospice Inc.
Lutz, Florida, USA

Lydia Love, DVM, DACVAA
Department of Molecular Biomedical Sciences, College of Veterinary Medicine, North Carolina State University
Raleigh, North Carolina, USA

Carrie Schroeder, DVM, DACVAA
Department of Surgical Sciences, School of Veterinary Medicine, University of Wisconsin
Madison, Wisconsin, USA

WILEY Blackwell

Copyright © 2024 by John Wiley & Sons, Inc. All rights reserved.

Published by John Wiley & Sons, Inc., Hoboken, New Jersey.
Published simultaneously in Canada.

No part of this publication may be reproduced, stored in a retrieval system, or transmitted in any form or by any means, electronic, mechanical, photocopying, recording, scanning, or otherwise, except as permitted under Section 107 or 108 of the 1976 United States Copyright Act, without either the prior written permission of the Publisher, or authorization through payment of the appropriate per-copy fee to the Copyright Clearance Center, Inc., 222 Rosewood Drive, Danvers, MA 01923, (978) 750-8400, fax (978) 750-4470, or on the web at www.copyright.com. Requests to the Publisher for permission should be addressed to the Permissions Department, John Wiley & Sons, Inc., 111 River Street, Hoboken, NJ 07030, (201) 748-6011, fax (201) 748-6008, or online at http://www.wiley.com/go/permission.

Trademarks: Wiley and the Wiley logo are trademarks or registered trademarks of John Wiley & Sons, Inc. and/or its affiliates in the United States and other countries and may not be used without written permission. All other trademarks are the property of their respective owners. John Wiley & Sons, Inc. is not associated with any product or vendor mentioned in this book.

Limit of Liability/Disclaimer of Warranty: While the publisher and author have used their best efforts in preparing this book, they make no representations or warranties with respect to the accuracy or completeness of the contents of this book and specifically disclaim any implied warranties of merchantability or fitness for a particular purpose. No warranty may be created or extended by sales representatives or written sales materials. The advice and strategies contained herein may not be suitable for your situation. You should consult with a professional where appropriate. Further, readers should be aware that websites listed in this work may have changed or disappeared between when this work was written and when it is read. Neither the publisher nor authors shall be liable for any loss of profit or any other commercial damages, including but not limited to special, incidental, consequential, or other damages.

For general information on our other products and services or for technical support, please contact our Customer Care Department within the United States at (800) 762-2974, outside the United States at (317) 572-3993 or fax (317) 572-4002.

Wiley also publishes its books in a variety of electronic formats. Some content that appears in print may not be available in electronic formats. For more information about Wiley products, visit our web site at www.wiley.com.

Library of Congress Cataloging-in-Publication Data applied for
[HB ISBN: 9781119830276]

Cover Design: Wiley
Front Cover Images: Tortoise: Courtesy of Carrie Schroeder, Cow: © Clara Bastian/Getty Images, Dog & Horse: Courtesy of Leigh Lamont, Cat: Courtesy of Sheilah Robertson, Piglet: © Byrdyak/Getty Images, Cockatoo: © tracielouise/Getty Images,
Back Cover Images: Cat: Courtesy of Sheilah Robertson, Goat: © michelangeloop/Getty Images, Dog: Courtesy of Kurt Grimm, Horse: Courtesy of Carrie Schroeder, Cat: Courtesy of Lydia Love, Rabbit: © Brina Bunt/Getty Images, Dog: Courtesy of Sheilah Robertson

Set in 9/11pt Minionpro by Straive, Pondicherry, India

Printed in Singapore
M WEP312827 270924

Dedication

The sixth edition of this text is dedicated to the many people who support and make up the specialty of veterinary anesthesia and analgesia and, specifically, the membership of the American College of Veterinary Anesthesia and Analgesia. Without their contributions and guidance, this book would not be possible, and without their participation in disseminating and implementing the knowledge contained in this book, it would be without purpose.

Contents

List of Contributors, ix

Foreword, xiii

Preface, xiv

About the Companion Website, xv

Section 1: General Topics

1 Overview, History, and Current Issues in Veterinary Anesthesia and Analgesia, 3
William J. Tranquilli, Kurt A. Grimm and Leigh A. Lamont

2 Anesthetic Risk and Informed Consent, 10
Dave C. Brodbelt, Derek Flaherty and Glenn R. Pettifer

3 Introduction to Patient Safety, 24
Matt McMillan and Daniel S.J. Pang

4 Safety Considerations for Laser and Radiographic Procedures and Magnetic Resonance Imaging, 40
Julie A. Smith and Carrie Davis

5 Anesthetic Emergencies, Resuscitation, and Adverse Events, 54
Erik H. Hofmeister

6 Anesthesia Equipment, 74
Craig A.E. Mosley

7 Infection Prevention and Control in Anesthesia, 142
Raphaël Vézina Audette and Stephen D. Cole

8 Euthanasia and Humane Killing, 152
Robert E. Meyer

Section 2: Patient Monitoring

9 Biomedical Engineering, 169
Catherine M. Creighton and Nadja Johnson Bressan

10 Anesthetic Depth Monitoring and Electroencephalography, 176
Christopher L. Norkus

11 Electrocardiography, 187
Kyle J. Bartholomew

12 Blood Pressure Monitoring, 197
Odette O

13 Cardiac Output Measurement, 210
Alessio Vigani

14 Monitoring Ventilation, 220
Jessica D. Briley, Kate M. Bailey and Lydia Love

15 Monitoring Oxygenation, 231
Chiara Adami

16 Anesthetic Gas Monitoring, 240
Rebecca C. Reader

17 Perioperative Thermoregulation and Heat Balance, 246
Kurt A. Grimm

18 Point-of-Care Ultrasound in Anesthesia, 254
Søren R. Boysen and Daniel S.J. Pang

Section 3: Pharmacology

19 General Pharmacology of Anesthetic and Analgesic Drugs, 283
Ted Whittem, Thierry Beths and Sébastien H. Bauquier

20 Anticholinergics, 314
Phillip Lerche

21 Adrenergic Agents, 319
Jo C. Murrell

22 Sedatives and Tranquilizers, 333
Catherine M. Creighton and Leigh A. Lamont

23 Opioids, 355
Bradley T. Simon and Ignacio Lizarraga

24 Non-Steroidal Anti-Inflammatory Drugs, 398
Mark G. Papich

25 Anesthetic and Analgesic Adjunctive Drugs, 420
Daniel S.J. Pang

26 Neuromuscular Blockade, 448
Manuel Martin-Flores

27 Injectable Anesthetics, 462
Stephanie M. Hamilton

28 Inhalation Anesthetics, 489
Eugene P. Steffey, Robert J. Brosnan and Khursheed R. Mama

29 Local Anesthetics, 526
Eva Rioja Garcia

Section 4: Body Fluids and Fluid Therapy

30 Acid–Base Physiology, 555
Peter D. Constable and William W. Muir

31 Treatment of Coagulation and Platelet Disorders, 574
Benjamin M. Brainard

32 Clinical Pharmacology and Administration of Fluid, Electrolyte, and Blood Component Solutions, 580
Amandeep S. Chohan and Elizabeth B. Davidow

Section 5: Physiology and Anesthetic Management

33 Cardiovascular Physiology, 615
William W. Muir

34 Anesthesia for Cardiopulmonary Bypass, 667
Khursheed R. Mama

35 Cardiac Pacemakers and Anesthesia, 674
Barret J. Bulmer

36 Pathophysiology and Anesthetic Management of Patients with Cardiovascular Disease, 680
Sandra Z. Perkowski and Mark A. Oyama

37 Respiratory Physiology and Pathophysiology, 697
Carolyn L. Kerr and Francisco J. Teixeira-Neto

38 Oxygen Therapy, Mechanical Ventilation, and Anesthetic Management of Patients with Respiratory Disease, 750
Francisco J. Teixeira-Neto and Carolyn L. Kerr

39 Physiology, Pathophysiology, and Anesthetic Management of Patients with Neurologic Disease, 822
Tatiana H. Ferreira and Starr Cameron

40 Physiology, Pathophysiology, and Anesthetic Management of Patients with Hepatic Disease, 847
Vaidehi V. Paranjape and Fernando Garcia-Pereira

41 Physiology, Pathophysiology, and Anesthetic Management of Patients with Gastrointestinal Disease, 862
Jennifer G. Adams

42 Physiology, Pathophysiology, and Anesthetic Management of Patients with Endocrine Disease, 891
Renata S. Costa, Teela Jones and Thomas K. Graves

43 Physiology, Pathophysiology, and Anesthetic Management of Patients with Renal Disease, 922
Stuart C. Clark-Price and Julie R. Fischer

44 Anesthetic Considerations for Renal Replacement Therapy, 944
Rebecca A. Johnson

45 Anesthetic Considerations During Pregnancy and for the Newborn, 955
Marc R. Raffe and Elizabeth Goudie-DeAngelis

Section 6: Nociception and Pain

46 Physiology and Pathophysiology of Pain, 971
Kate L. White

47 Recognition and Quantification of Acute and Chronic Pain, 996
Jo C. Murrell

48 Clinical Management and Pharmacologic Treatment of Pain, 1010
Carolyn M. McKune

49 Non-Pharmacologic Management of Pain, 1023
Bonnie D. Wright

Section 7: Comparative Anesthesia and Analgesia

50 Comparative Anesthesia and Analgesia – Dogs and Cats, 1029
Peter J. Pascoe and Bruno H. Pypendop

51 Comparative Anesthesia and Analgesia – Community Medicine Settings, 1041
Emily McCobb

52 Comparative Anesthesia and Analgesia – Horses, 1048
Lori A. Bidwell

53 Comparative Anesthesia and Analgesia – Ruminants and Swine, 1052
HuiChu Lin

54 Comparative Anesthesia and Analgesia – Laboratory Animals, 1065
Henri G.M.J. Bertrand and Aurélie A. Thomas

55 Comparative Immobilization and Anesthesia – Free-Ranging Terrestrial Mammals, 1077
Nigel Caulkett and Jon M. Arnemo

56 Comparative Anesthesia and Analgesia – Marine Mammals, 1091
Julie A. Balko and James E. Bailey

57 Comparative Anesthesia and Analgesia – Reptiles, Amphibians, and Fishes, 1110
Sathya K. Chinnadurai and Cornelia I. Mosley

58 Comparative Anesthesia and Analgesia – Birds, 1127
John W. Ludders and David Sanchez-Migallon Guzman

Section 8: Anesthesia and Analgesia for Domestic Species

59 Dogs and Cats, 1157
Carolina H. Riccó Pereira and Phillip Lerche

60 Canine and Feline Local Anesthetic and Analgesic Techniques, 1166
Raphaël Vézina Audette, Alexander C.S. Thomson, Ciara A. Barr, Luis Campoy, Matt Read and Santiago Peralta

61 Horses, 1205
Regula Bettschart-Wolfensberger

62 Horses with Colic, 1217
Ludovica Chiavaccini and Lauren R. Duffee

63 Equine Local Anesthetic and Analgesic Techniques, 1235
Rachael E. Carpenter and Christopher R. Byron

64 Ruminants, 1262
Chiara E. Hampton and Thomas W. Riebold

65 Swine, 1285
Lais M. Malavasi

66 Ruminant and Swine Local Anesthetic and Analgesic Techniques, 1301
Alexander Valverde

Section 9: Anesthesia and Analgesia for Selected Patients

67 Ophthalmic Patients, 1327
Vaidehi V. Paranjape and Luisito S. Pablo

68 Neonatal and Pediatric Patients, 1348
Emily McCobb and Sheilah A. Robertson

69 Aging Patients, 1354
Sheilah A. Robertson and Kirk A. Muñoz

70 Cancer Patients, 1363
Timothy M. Fan and Stephanie Keating

71 Osteoarthritis Patients, 1377
Steven C. Budsberg and Whitney D. Hinson

Index, 1390

List of Contributors

Chiara Adami, DMV, PhD, DACVAA, DECVAA, FRCVS
Department of Veterinary Medicine, Cambridge Veterinary School
University of Cambridge
Madingley Road, Cambridge, UK

Jennifer G. Adams, DVM, DACVIM (LAIM), DACVAA
Hull, Georgia, USA

Jon M. Arnemo, DVM, PhD, DECZM
Inland Norway University of Applied Sciences
Campus Evenstad, Norway and
Swedish University of Agricultural Sciences
Umeå, Sweden

James E. Bailey, DVM, MS, DACVAA
Innovative Veterinary Medicine, Inc.
Ponte Vedra, Florida, USA

Kate M. Bailey, DVM, DACVAA
United Veterinary Care and
College of Veterinary Medicine, North Carolina State University (Adjunct)
Raleigh, North Carolina, USA

Julie A. Balko, VMD, DACVAA
Department of Molecular Biomedical Sciences, College of Veterinary Medicine
North Carolina State University
Raleigh, North Carolina, USA

Ciara A. Barr, VMD, DACVAA
Department of Clinical Sciences and Advanced Medicine
School of Veterinary Medicine, University of Pennsylvania
Philadelphia, Pennsylvania, USA

Kyle J. Bartholomew, DVM, DACVAA
Department of Surgical Sciences, School of Veterinary Medicine
University of Wisconsin
Madison, Wisconsin, USA

Sébastien H. Bauquier, DMV, IPSAV, MANZCVS, DACVAA, PhD
Melbourne Veterinary School, University of Melbourne
Werribee, Victoria, Australia and
Southpaws Specialty, Emergency and Referral Hospital
Malvern East, Victoria, Australia

Henri G.M.J. Bertrand, DVM, PhD, CertLAM, DECLAM, MRCVS
Agenda Veterinary Services
Kingston Upon Hull
East Riding of Yorkshire, UK

Thierry Beths, DVM, Cert VA, CVA, MSc, MRCVS, PhD
Melbourne Veterinary School, University of Melbourne and
Greencross Veterinary Hospital
Werribee, Victoria, Australia

Regula Bettschart-Wolfensberger, Prof. Dr. med. vet., PhD, DECVAA
Department of Diagnostics and Clinical Sciences, Vetsuisse Faculty
University of Zürich
Zürich, Switzerland

Lori A. Bidwell, DVM, DACVAA
East-West Equine Sports Medicine
Lexington, Kentucky, USA

Søren R. Boysen, DVM, DACVECC
Faculty of Veterinary Medicine, University of Calgary
Calgary, Alberta, Canada

Benjamin M. Brainard, VMD, DACVAA, DACVECC
Department of Small Animal Medicine and Surgery
College of Veterinary Medicine, University of Georgia
Athens, Georgia, USA

Jessica D. Briley, DVM, DACVAA
Department of Molecular Biomedical Sciences, College of Veterinary Medicine
North Carolina State University
Raleigh, North Carolina, USA

Dave C. Brodbelt, MA, VetMB, PhD, DVA, DECVAA, FRCVS
Veterinary Epidemiology, Economics and Public Health Group
Department of Pathobiology and Population Sciences, Royal Veterinary College
Hatfield, Herts, UK

Robert J. Brosnan, DVM, PhD, DACVAA
Department of Surgical and Radiological Sciences, School of Veterinary Medicine
University of California–Davis
Davis, California, USA

Steven C. Budsberg, DVM, MS, DACVS
Department of Small Animal Medicine and Surgery
College of Veterinary Medicine, University of Georgia
Athens, Georgia, USA

Barret J. Bulmer, DVM, MS, DACVIM (Cardiology)
Tufts Veterinary Emergency Treatment and Specialties
Walpole, Massachusetts, USA

Christopher R. Byron, DVM, MS, DACVS
Department of Large Animal Clinical Sciences
Virginia-Maryland College of Veterinary Medicine, Virginia Tech University
Blacksburg, Virginia, USA

Starr Cameron, BVetMed, MS, DACVIM (Neurology)
Department of Medical Sciences, School of Veterinary Medicine
University of Wisconsin
Madison, Wisconsin, USA

Luis Campoy, LV, CertVA, DECVAA, MRCVS
Department of Clinical Sciences, College of Veterinary Medicine
Cornell University
Ithaca, New York, USA

Rachael E. Carpenter, DVM
Department of Small Animal Clinical Sciences
Virginia-Maryland College of Veterinary Medicine, Virginia Tech University
Blacksburg, Virginia, USA

Nigel Caulkett, DVM, MVetSc, DACVAA
Faculty of Veterinary Medicine, University of Calgary
Calgary, Alberta, Canada

Ludovica Chiavaccini, DVM, DES, MS, DACVAA
Department of Comparative, Diagnostic and Population Medicine
College of Veterinary Medicine, University of Florida
Gainesville, Florida, USA

Sathya K. Chinnadurai, DVM, MS, DACZM, DACVAA, DACAW
Chicago Zoological Society/Brookfield Zoo
Brookfield, Illinois, USA

Amandeep S. Chohan, BVSc & AH, MVSc, MS, DACVAA
Department of Surgical and Radiological Sciences
School of Veterinary Medicine, University of California–Davis
Davis, California, USA

Stuart C. Clark-Price, DVM, MS, EMBA, DACVIM (LAIM), DACVAA
Department of Clinical Sciences, College of Veterinary Medicine
Auburn University
Auburn, Alabama, USA

Stephen D. Cole, VMD, MS, DACVM (Bacteriology/Mycology, Immunology, Virology)
Clinical Infectious Disease Laboratory, Department of Pathobiology
School of Veterinary Medicine, University of Pennsylvania
Philadelphia, Pennsylvania, USA

Peter D. Constable, BVSc, MS, PhD
College of Veterinary Medicine
University of Illinois at Urbana–Champaign
Urbana, Illinois, USA

Catherine M. Creighton, DVM, MSc, DACVAA
Department of Companion Animals, Atlantic Veterinary College
University of Prince Edward Island
Charlottetown, Prince Edward Island, Canada

Elizabeth B. Davidow, DVM, DACVECC
Timberline Veterinary Emergency and Specialty
Seattle, Washington, USA

Carrie Davis, DVM, DACVAA
MedVet Dallas Emergency Veterinary and Specialty Care
Dallas, Texas, USA

Lauren R. Duffee, VMD, DACVAA, CVA
Massachusetts Veterinary Referral Hospital
Woburn, Massachusetts, USA

Timothy M. Fan, DVM, PhD, DACVIM (SAIM, Oncology)
Department of Veterinary Clinical Medicine, College of Veterinary Medicine
University of Illinois at Urbana–Champaign
Urbana, Illinois, USA

Tatiana H. Ferreira, DVM, MSc, PhD, DACVAA
Department of Surgical Sciences, School of Veterinary Medicine
University of Wisconsin
Madison, Wisconsin, USA

Julie R. Fischer, DVM, DACVIM (SAIM)
Veterinary Specialty Hospital of North County (Ethos Veterinary Health)
San Marcos, California, USA

Derek Flaherty, BVMS, DVA, DECVAA, MRCA, FRCVS
Southern Counties Veterinary Specialists
Ringwood, Hampshire, UK

Fernando Garcia-Pereira, DVM, MS, DACVAA
Pet Urgent Response and Emergency
Jacksonville, Florida, USA

Thomas K. Graves, DVM, MS, PhD, DACVIM (SAIM)
Professor and Dean Emeritus, College of Veterinary Medicine
Midwestern University
Glendale, Arizona, USA

Elizabeth Goudie-DeAngelis, DVM, MS, DACVAA
Tristate Veterinary Anesthesia, PLLC
White Plains, New York, USA

Kurt A. Grimm, DVM, MS, PhD, DACVAA, DACVCP
Veterinary Specialist Services, PC
Conifer, Colorado, USA

Stephanie M. Hamilton, DVM, MSc, DACVAA
Department of Companion Animals, Atlantic Veterinary College
University of Prince Edward Island
Charlottetown, Prince Edward Island, Canada

Chiara E. Hampton, DVM, MS, DACVAA
Large Animal Clinical Sciences, College of Veterinary Medicine
University of Tennessee
Knoxville, Tennessee, USA

Whitney D. Hinson, DVM, MS, DACVS (SA)
Department of Small Animal Medicine and Surgery
College of Veterinary Medicine, University of Georgia
Athens, Georgia, USA

Erik H. Hofmeister, DVM, DACVAA, DECVAA, MA, MS
Department of Clinical Sciences, College of Veterinary Medicine
Auburn University
Auburn, Alabama, USA

Rebecca A. Johnson, DVM, MS, PhD, DACVAA
Department of Surgical Sciences, School of Veterinary Medicine
University of Wisconsin
Madison, Wisconsin, USA

Nadja Johnson Bressan, PhD
Faculty of Sustainable Design Engineering, University of Prince Edward Island
Charlottetown, Prince Edward Island, Canada

Teela Jones, DVM, MVetSc, DACVAA
Summit Veterinary Referral Center
Tacoma, Washington, USA

Stephanie Keating, DVM, DVSc, DACVAA
Department of Veterinary Clinical Medicine, College of Veterinary Medicine
University of Illinois at Urbana-Champaign
Urbana, Illinois, USA

Carolyn L. Kerr, DVM, DVSc, PhD, MScCH(HPTE), DACVAA
Department of Clinical Studies, Ontario Veterinary College
University of Guelph
Guelph, Ontario, Canada

Leigh A. Lamont, DVM, MS, DACVAA
Department of Companion Animals, Atlantic Veterinary College
University of Prince Edward Island
Charlottetown, Prince Edward Island, Canada

Phillip Lerche, BVSc, PhD, DACVAA
Department of Veterinary Clinical Sciences, College of Veterinary Medicine
The Ohio State University
Columbus, Ohio, USA

HuiChu Lin, DVM, MS, DACVAA
Department of Clinical Sciences, College of Veterinary Medicine
Auburn University
Auburn, Alabama, USA

Ignacio Lizarraga, MVZ, MVSc, PhD
AgResearch Limited
Grasslands Research Centre
Palmerston North, New Zealand

Lydia Love, DVM, DACVAA
Department of Molecular Biomedical Sciences, College of Veterinary Medicine
North Carolina State University
Raleigh, North Carolina, USA

John W. Ludders, DVM, DACVAA
Emeritus Professor, Department of Clinical Sciences
College of Veterinary Medicine, Cornell University
Ithaca, New York, USA

Matt McMillan, BVM&S, DECVAA, MRCVS
The Ralph Veterinary Referral Centre
Marlow, Buckinghamshire, UK

Lais M. Malavasi, DVM, MS, PhD
Department of Veterinary Clinical Sciences, College of Veterinary Medicine
Washington State University
Pullman, Washington, USA

Khursheed R. Mama, DVM, DACVAA
Department of Clinical Sciences
College of Veterinary Medicine and Biomedical Sciences, Colorado State University
Fort Collins, Colorado, USA

Manuel Martin-Flores, MV, DACVAA
Department of Clinical Sciences, College of Veterinary Medicine
Cornell University
Ithaca, New York, USA

Emily McCobb, DVM, MS, DACVAA
Department of Clinical Sciences, Cummings School of Veterinary Medicine
Tufts University
North Grafton, Massachusetts, USA

Carolyn M. McKune, DVM, DACVAA
Mythos Veterinary, LLC
Gainesville, Florida, USA

Robert E. Meyer, DVM, DACVAA
Professor Emeritus, Department of Clinical Sciences
College of Veterinary Medicine, Mississippi State University
Mississippi State, Mississippi, USA

Cornelia I. Mosley, DrMedVet, DACVAA, CVA
Elanco Animal Health
Mississauga, Ontario, Canada

Craig A.E. Mosley, DVM, MSc, DACVAA
VCA Canada, 404 Veterinary Emergency and Referral Hospital
Newmarket, Ontario, Canada

William W. Muir, DVM, PhD, DACVAA, DACVECC
Gillespie College of Veterinary Medicine (LMU-CVM)
Lincoln Memorial University
Harrogate, Tennessee, USA

Jo C. Murrell, BVSc (Hons), PhD, DECVAA, MRCVS
Bristol Veterinary Specialists
Severn Beach, Bristol, UK

Kirk A. Muñoz, DVM (Hons), MRCVS, MSc, DACVAA, cVMA
Department of Veterinary Clinical Sciences, College of Veterinary Medicine
The Ohio State University
Columbus, Ohio, USA

Christopher L. Norkus, DVM, DACVAA, CVPP, DACVECC
Allegheny Veterinary Emergency Trauma and Specialty (AVETS) Center
Monroeville, Pennsylvania, USA

Odette O, DVM, DACVAA
SAGE Veterinary Centers, a member of Ethos Animal Health
Dublin, California, USA

Mark A. Oyama, DVM, MSCE, DACVIM (Cardiology)
Department of Clinical Sciences and Advanced Medicine
School of Veterinary Medicine, University of Pennsylvania
Philadelphia, Pennsylvania, USA

Luisito S. Pablo, DVM, MS, DACVAA
Department of Comparative, Diagnostic, and Population Medicine
College of Veterinary Medicine, University of Florida
Gainesville, Florida, USA

Daniel S.J. Pang, BVSc, MSc, PhD, DACVAA, DECVAA, FRCVS
Faculty of Veterinary Medicine, University of Calgary
Calgary, Alberta, Canada and
Faculty of Veterinary Medicine, Université de Montréal
Saint-Hyacinthe, Québec, Canada

Mark G. Papich, DVM, MS, DACVCP
Department of Molecular Biomedical Sciences, College of Veterinary Medicine
North Carolina State University
Raleigh, North Carolina, USA

Peter J. Pascoe, BVSc, DVA, DACVAA, DECVAA, FRCVS
Emeritus Professor, Department of Surgical and Radiological Sciences
School of Veterinary Medicine, University of California-Davis
Davis, California, USA

Santiago Peralta, DVM, DAVDC, FF-AVDC-OMFS
Department of Clinical Sciences, College of Veterinary Medicine
Cornell University
Ithaca, New York, USA

Sandra Z. Perkowski, VMD, PhD, CVMA, DACVAA
BluePearl Specialty and Emergency Pet Hospital
Malvern, Pennsylvania, USA

Glenn R. Pettifer, BA (Hons), BSc, DVM, DVSc
College of Dental Hygienists of Ontario
Toronto, Ontario, Canada

Vaidehi V. Paranjape, BVSc & AH, MVSc, MS, DACVAA
Department of Small Animal Clinical Sciences
Virginia-Maryland College of Veterinary Medicine, Virginia Tech University
Blacksburg, Virginia, USA

Bruno H. Pypendop, DrMedVet, DrVetSci, DACVAA
Department of Surgical and Radiological Sciences
School of Veterinary Medicine, University of California–Davis
Davis, California, USA

Marc R. Raffe, DVM, MS, MBA, DACVAA, DACVECC
Veterinary Anesthesia and Critical Care Associates, LLC
St. Paul, Minnesota, USA

Matt Read, DVM, MVSc, DACVAA
MedVet Columbus
Worthington, Ohio, USA

Rebecca C. Reader, BA, DVM, DACVAA
MSPCA/Angell Animal Medical Center
Boston, Massachusetts, USA

Carolina H. Riccó Pereira, MV, MS, DACVAA
Department of Veterinary Clinical Sciences, College of Veterinary Medicine
The Ohio State University
Columbus, Ohio, USA

Thomas W. Riebold, DVM, DACVAA
Department of Clinical Sciences, College of Veterinary Medicine
Oregon State University
Corvallis, Oregon, USA

Eva Rioja Garcia, Lic Vet, DVSc, PhD, DACVAA, DECVAA, MRCVS
Optivet Referrals
Havant, Hampshire, UK

Sheilah A. Robertson, BVMS (Hons), CertVA, PhD, DACVAA, DECVAA, DACAW, DECAWBM (AWSEL), FRCVS
Lap of Love Veterinary Hospice Inc.
Lutz, Florida, USA

Renata Sampaio Costa, DVM, MPhil, GradDipEd, MANZCVS, DACVAA
Section of Anaesthesia and Analgesia, School of Veterinary Medicine
Murdoch University
Murdoch, Western Australia, Australia

David Sanchez-Migallon Guzman, LV, MS, DECZM (Avian, Small Mammal), DACZM
Department of Medicine and Epidemiology
School of Veterinary Medicine, University of California–Davis
Davis, California, USA

Carrie A. Schroeder, DVM, DACVAA
Department of Surgical Sciences, School of Veterinary Medicine
University of Wisconsin
Madison, Wisconsin, USA

Bradley T. Simon, DVM, MSc, DACVAA
Department of Small Animal Clinical Sciences
College of Veterinary Medicine and Biomedical Sciences, Texas A&M University
College Station, Texas, USA and
Veterinary Dentistry Specialists
Katy, Texas, USA

Julie A. Smith, DVM, DACVAA
MedVet Vancouver Emergency Veterinary and Specialty Care
Vancouver, Washington, USA

Eugene P. Steffey, VMD, PhD DACVAA, DECVAA (retired)
Emeritus Professor, Department of Surgical and Radiological Sciences
School of Veterinary Medicine, University of California–Davis
Davis, California, USA

Francisco J. Teixeira-Neto, MV, MSc, PhD, TEAV CBAV
Faculdade de Medicina Veterinária e Zootecnia
Universidade Estadual Paulista (UNESP)
Botucatu, Brazil

Aurelie A. Thomas, DVM, PhD, DECAWBM (AWSEL), MRCVS
Clinical Pharmacology and Safety Sciences
AstraZeneca
Cambridge, UK

Alexander C.S. Thomson, DVM, DACVAA
City University of Hong Kong Veterinary Medical Centre
Hong Kong SAR, China

William J. Tranquilli, BS(Ed), DVM, MS, DACVAA
Professor Emeritus, Department of Veterinary Clinical Medicine
College of Veterinary Medicine, University of Illinois at Urbana-Champaign
Urbana, Illinois, USA

Alexander Valverde, DVM, DVSc, DACVAA
Department of Clinical Studies, Ontario Veterinary College
University of Guelph
Guelph, Ontario, Canada

Raphaël Vézina Audette, DVM, MSc, CVA, DACVAA
Portland Veterinary Emergency and Specialty Care
Portland, Maine, USA

Alessio Vigani, DVM, PhD, DACVAA, DACVECC, DECVECC
Department of Small Animals, Faculty of Veterinary Medicine
University of Zürich
Zürich, Switzerland

Kate L. White, MA, VetMB, PhD, DVA, DECVAA, FRCVS
School of Veterinary Medicine and Science
University of Nottingham
Nottingham, UK

Ted Whittem, BVSc, PhD, DACVCP, FANZCVS, GAICD
College of Public Health, Medical and Veterinary Sciences
James Cook University
Townsville, Queensland, Australia

Bonnie D. Wright, DVM, DACVAA
MistralVet
Johnstown, Colorado, USA

Foreword

The extensively referenced content, important additions, and timely revisions of the sixth edition of *Veterinary Anesthesia and Analgesia* provide an impressive documentation of the basic and applied clinical science essential to the safe delivery of animal anesthesia and pain management. As such, this text continues to be the most comprehensive source of information for students, scientists, practitioners, and specialists alike. The sixth edition, once again, successfully chronicles the vital role that anesthesia and analgesia play in modern-day veterinary medicine.

As a previous editor of the third, fourth, and fifth editions of this text, and in memory of the three signees who penned the foreword to the fifth edition, Dr. William Lumb, Dr. Wynn Jones, and Dr. John Thurmon, I wish to acknowledge the efforts of the contributors, 104 in all, with special thanks to Dr. Lamont, Dr. Grimm, Dr. Robertson, Dr. Love, and Dr. Schroeder for assuming the editorship of such a large endeavor. Now, in the third decade of the 21st century, the publication of *Veterinary Anesthesia and Analgesia: The Sixth Edition of Lumb and Jones* continues to highlight the importance, significance, and necessity of continually improving animal anesthesia and analgesia. With their combined efforts, the contributing authors and editors have admirably upheld this text's long-standing reputation as an indispensable resource in advancing and improving animal care and the human animal bond.

William J. Tranquilli

Preface

The first edition of *Veterinary Anesthesia* was published in 1973, and the second edition followed in 1984. The third through fifth editions (*Lumb and Jones' Veterinary Anesthesia*, *Lumb and Jones' Veterinary Anesthesia and Analgesia*, and *Veterinary Anesthesia and Analgesia, the Fifth Edition of Lumb and Jones*) followed in 1996, 2007, and 2015, respectively. Now, in its 51st year, a sixth edition of this text is available with both editorial and content contributions from many new participants.

The sixth edition represents a generational change within the specialty of anesthesia and analgesia. Most of the early members of the Association of Veterinary Anaesthetists (AVA), the American College of Veterinary Anesthesia and Analgesia (ACVAA), and the European College of Veterinary Anaesthesia and Analgesia (ECVAA) have retired from clinical practice, and some are unfortunately no longer with us. However, as the membership of these specialty organizations continues to grow, and the demand for trained board-certified specialists in veterinary anesthesia and analgesia continues to outpace the supply, it is truly an exciting time to be a veterinary anesthesiologist. It is for those joining our specialty that this book is written, and we have intentionally tried to incorporate as many new voices as possible in the writing and editing of this text. It is our hope that the new generation will pick up the baton of advancing veterinary anesthesia, and continue to develop new ideas, disseminate new information, and carry on traditions such as *Lumb and Jones*.

We would like to personally thank our families and co-workers for allowing us the time necessary to complete this work, and the staff at Wiley for their ongoing support and encouragement.

Leigh A. Lamont
Kurt A. Grimm
Sheilah A. Robertson
Lydia Love
Carrie A. Schroeder

About the Companion Website

Don't forget to visit the companion website for this book:

www.wiley.com/go/lamont/anesthesia 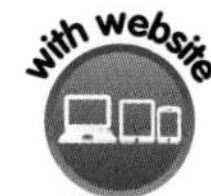

There you will find valuable materials, including:

- Videos

SECTION 1

General Topics

1 Overview, History, and Current Issues in Veterinary Anesthesia and Analgesia

William J. Tranquilli[1], Kurt A. Grimm[2] and Leigh A. Lamont[3]

[1] Professor Emeritus, Department of Veterinary Clinical Medicine, College of Veterinary Medicine, University of Illinois at Urbana–Champaign, Urbana, Illinois, USA

[2] Veterinary Specialists Services, PC, Conifer, Colorado, USA

[3] Department of Companion Animals, Atlantic Veterinary College, University of Prince Edward Island, Charlottetown, Prince Edward Island, Canada

Chapter contents

Overview, 3
- Terminology, 3

History of veterinary anesthesia, 4
- Early milestones, 5
- Conceptualizing depth of anesthesia, 5
- Evolution of veterinary anesthesia as a specialty, 6
- *Anesthesiologist* defined, 7

Current issues in veterinary anesthesia and analgesia, 7
- Environmental impact of anesthesia, 7
- Impact of the opioid epidemic on veterinary anesthesia, 8
- Emerging role of technology, 8

References, 9

Overview

Veterinary anesthesia continues to evolve as a science and specialty within the veterinary profession. The major drivers of change are advances in medical technology, development of evidence-based guidelines for patient care, and socioeconomic and demographic changes in countries where animals serve evolving roles. One thing that remains certain is that veterinary anesthesiologists will continue to be advocates for patient safety, humane care, and quality of life and serve as frontline educators for best practices in anesthesia, analgesia, and pain management.

Proper use of anesthetics, sedatives, and analgesics can alleviate pain, create amnesia, and produce muscle relaxation essential for safe and humane patient care [1]. Important uses include facilitation of immobilization for various diagnostic, surgical, and therapeutic procedures; safe transportation of wild and exotic animals; and euthanasia and the humane slaughter of food animals. Anesthesia, sedation, and analgesic drug administration are not without significant patient risk and are not recommended for trivial reasons. The continued development of better techniques and drugs along with continuing efforts to educate veterinary care providers has minimized the overall risk of anesthesia and pain alleviation in an ever-increasing and more sophisticated patient care environment. Any discussion with the animal-owning public, such as that occurring with owners when obtaining informed consent, requires the use of proper terminology and clear communication to convey the issues central to the safe delivery of veterinary anesthesia and pain therapy.

Terminology

The term *anesthesia*, derived from the Greek term *anaisthaesia*, meaning "insensibility," is used to describe the loss of sensation to the entire body or a specific portion of it. Anesthesia is induced by drugs that depress the activity of nervous tissue locally, regionally, or within the central nervous system (CNS). From a pharmacological viewpoint, there has been a significant redefining of the term *general anesthesia* [2], and both central nervous stimulants and depressants can be useful general anesthetics [3].

Management of pain in patients involves the use of drugs that are often called *analgesics*. The term is derived from *an*, which implies "negative" or "without," and *alges(is)*, meaning "pain" [4]. Clinical management of pain often results in varying degrees of effectiveness that represent states of hypoalgesia or decreased sensation of pain. It is important to understand that the administration of an analgesic drug does not necessarily create the state of analgesia.

The diverse uses for anesthesia (as it relates to immobilization, muscle relaxation, and antinociception) and the requirements peculiar to species, age, and disease state necessitate the use of a variety of drugs, drug combinations, and methods. Throughout this text and elsewhere, various terms are used to describe the effects of anesthetic drugs, pain-inhibiting drugs, and various techniques and routes of administration. Commonly used terms are defined below, and the reader is referred to other chapters for more details where appropriate.

Veterinary Anesthesia and Analgesia: The Sixth Edition of Lumb and Jones. Edited by Leigh Lamont, Kurt Grimm, Sheilah Robertson, Lydia Love and Carrie Schroeder.
© 2024 John Wiley & Sons, Inc. Published 2024 by John Wiley & Sons, Inc.
Companion website: www.wiley.com/go/lamont/anesthesia

Analgesia is the absence of pain in response to stimulation, which would normally be painful. The term is generally reserved for describing lack of pain in a conscious patient [5].

Acupuncture is a system of therapy using long, fine needles to induce hypoalgesia. Additional modalities of acupuncture point stimulation have been utilized, including mechanical and electrical stimulation. See Chapter 49.

Balanced anesthesia is achieved by the simultaneous use of multiple drugs and techniques. Different drugs contribute variably to specific components of the anesthetic state: amnesia, antinociception, muscle relaxation, and alteration of autonomic reflexes.

Dissociative anesthesia is induced by drugs (e.g., ketamine) that dissociate the thalamocortic and limbic systems. This form of anesthesia is characterized by a cataleptoid state, in which eyes remain open and swallowing reflexes remain intact. Skeletal muscle hypertonus persists unless a strong sedative or peripheral or central muscle relaxant is co-administered. See Chapter 27.

Electronarcosis, *electroanesthesia*, or *electrosleep* refers to the passage of electrical currents through the cerebrum to induce deep narcosis. Even though there have been successful studies, this form of anesthesia has never gained popularity and is rarely used in veterinary practice. Electronarcosis should not be confused with the inhumane practice of electroimmobilization.

General anesthesia is drug-induced unconsciousness that is characterized by controlled but reversible depression of the CNS and perception. In this state, the patient is not arousable by noxious stimulation. Sensory, motor, and autonomic reflex functions are attenuated to varying degrees, depending upon the specific drug(s) and technique(s) used.

Hypnosis is a condition of artificially induced sleep, or a trance resembling sleep, resulting from moderate depression of the CNS from which the patient is readily aroused.

Hypothermia refers to a decrease in body temperature, induced either locally or generally, to supplement insensitivity and decrease anesthetic drug requirements and reduce metabolic needs. It is primarily used in neonates or in patients undergoing cardiovascular surgery. See Chapter 34.

Inhalation or inhalant anesthesia refers to the practice of administering anesthetic gases or vapors via inhalation in combination with oxygen. See Chapter 28.

Injectable anesthesia refers to the practice of administering anesthetic solutions via intravenous, intramuscular, or subcutaneous injection. Other injectable routes include intraperitoneal and intrathoracic but, except for some laboratory animal species, these are not generally recommended. See Chapters 27 and 54.

Local and regional analgesia/anesthesia refers to loss of sensation, notably pain, in a particular area or region of the body, usually defined by the pattern of innervation of the affected nerve(s). Anesthetic drug may be applied topically or injected locally into or around the surgical site (variably referred to as "field block," "incisional block," or "infiltrative block"), perineurally around peripheral nerve(s), between fascial planes, or neuraxially (into the epidural or subarachnoid space). See Chapters 60, 63, and 66.

Narcosis is a drug-induced state of deep sleep from which the patient cannot be easily aroused. Narcosis may or may not be accompanied by antinociception, depending on the techniques and drugs used.

Nociception is the neural (physiologic) process of encoding noxious stimuli [5] that underlies the conscious perception of pain. Nociception does not require consciousness and can continue unabated during general anesthesia if techniques that interrupt or inhibit the transduction, transmission, and modulation of nociceptive stimuli are not utilized.

Oral (enteral) or rectal administration routes may be used to administer certain anesthetic or analgesic agents. There is often a greater degree of interspecies and interindividual variability in the dose–response relationship of orally administered drugs due to differences in absorption and first-pass hepatic metabolism.

Pain is an unpleasant sensory and emotional experience associated with, or resembling that associated with, actual or potential tissue damage [5]. See Chapter 46.

Sedation is a state characterized by CNS depression accompanied by drowsiness and some degree of centrally induced relaxation. The patient is generally unaware of its surroundings but can become aroused and is responsive to noxious stimulation. Sedatives are not recommended to immobilize a patient when painful stimuli are likely to occur (e.g., surgery). See Chapter 22.

Surgical general anesthesia is the state/plane of anesthesia that provides unconsciousness, amnesia, muscle relaxation, and hypoalgesia sufficient for painless surgery.

Total intravenous anesthesia (TIVA), *partial intravenous anesthesia (PIVA)*, and *targeted controlled infusion (TCI)* describe anesthetic techniques that utilize intravenous infusion of one or more drugs to produce a suitable anesthetic state. Automated infusion systems are available that allow the input of patient parameters and pharmacokinetic information for specific drugs and allow the anesthesiologist to target a predetermined plasma drug concentration (TCI).

Tranquilization results in behavioral change wherein anxiety is relieved and the patient becomes relaxed but remains aware of its surroundings. Tranquilizers are drugs that result in tranquilization when administered; however, many prefer to use the term "anxiolytic" or "anti-anxiety" when describing drugs that decrease anxiety and induce relaxation. See Chapter 22.

Transcutaneous electrical nerve stimulation (TENS, TNS, or TES) is a technique that induces local analgesia by low-intensity, high-frequency electrical stimulation of the skin through surface electrodes. TENS has many similarities to electroacupuncture. See Chapter 49.

Twilight anesthesia is a state of heavy sedation where the patient is still conscious, but cooperative, and has limited or no recall (amnesia). This technique is popular for outpatient anesthesia in human medicine for diagnostic procedures and for minor surgical procedures when combined with local anesthetics and additional analgesic drugs. *Twilight anesthesia* is a term in common use by laypeople to connote heavy sedation and does not refer to a specific anesthetic procedure or technique.

History of veterinary anesthesia

While there are accounts in both ancient western and eastern historical texts chronicling various drugs and techniques used to achieve insensibility in humans and animals, little appears in the formal literature until the 19th century. Not surprisingly, the history of human and veterinary anesthesia is tightly interwoven, and the early timeline includes contributions from chemists, physicians, dentists, and veterinarians alike. Other authors have chronicled the early history and evolution of veterinary anesthesia at various points over the past 65 years, and a number of interesting reviews are available elsewhere for readers looking for more detail [6–14]. By taking the time to reflect on the history of our specialty, we are better able to appreciate its continued evolution.

Early milestones

In 1800, Humphrey Davy administered nitrous oxide to a guinea pig and suggested that it may have anesthetic properties. Twenty-four years later, Henry Hickman demonstrated that pain associated with surgery in dogs could be alleviated by inhaling a mixture of nitrous oxide and carbon dioxide. He reasoned that the latter increased the rate and depth of breathing, thus enhancing the effects of nitrous oxide. Much later, in the early 1990s, studies confirmed that unconsciousness could be induced in 30–40 seconds in piglets breathing carbon dioxide (50%) in oxygen (50%) [15].

It was not until 1842 that diethyl ether was used for human anesthesia, and within a year of William Morton's famous public demonstration of "etherization" at Massachusetts General Hospital in 1846, others began using ether to produce unconsciousness in animals. The Boston physician, Charles Thomas Jackson, was among the first to publish his findings about the use of ether in animals in 1853 [16]. In 1844, a dentist from Connecticut named Horace Wells rediscovered the anesthetic properties of nitrous oxide and recognized its potential for dental practice. While his work was neglected for a number of years, nitrous oxide was ultimately introduced to human anesthesia in 1862.

Chloroform was discovered by Justus Liebig in 1831, and in 1847, Marie Jean Pierre Flourens used it to induce anesthesia in animals. Around this time, British physician George H. Dadd had immigrated to the United States and begun practicing veterinary medicine where he routinely employed general anesthesia in his animal patients. He was one of the first veterinarians in the United States to advocate for the humane treatment of animals, including the use of anesthesia in veterinary surgery, and he vigorously promoted the application of sound scientific principles to the practice of veterinary medicine [17].

In 1875, Oré published the first monograph on intravenous anesthesia using chloral hydrate and, three years later, Humbert described its use in horses. Pirogoff was the first to attempt rectal anesthesia with chloral hydrate in 1847, and intraperitoneal injection was first described in 1892 in France. Thus, by the end of the 19th century, various routes of anesthetic administration had been identified, and rudimentary investigations into the safety and efficacy of multiple anesthetics had been undertaken.

After the initial isolation of cocaine by Albert Niemann in Germany in 1860, Anrep suggested the possibility of using cocaine as a local anesthetic in 1878. In 1884, Koller used cocaine for local anesthesia of the eye, and Halsted described cocaine regional anesthesia a year later. Its use was subsequently popularized by Frederick Hobday, an English veterinarian. In 1885, James Leonard Corning was credited for using cocaine for spinal anesthesia in dogs. From his description, however, it would appear that he induced epidural anesthesia. In 1898, August Bier induced true spinal anesthesia in animals and then in himself and an assistant [18].

While local infiltration was first popularized by Reclus in 1890 and Schleich in 1892, conduction regional anesthesia had been earlier introduced by Halsted and Hall in New York in 1884. These techniques increased in popularity with the discovery of local anesthetics less toxic than cocaine. Local anesthetics were used by Cuille and Sendrail in 1901 in France to induce subarachnoid anesthesia in horses, cattle, and dogs. That same year, Cathelin reported epidural anesthesia in dogs, but it remained for Retzgen, Benesch, and Brook to utilize this technique in larger species during the 1920s. Although paralumbar anesthesia was employed in humans by Sellheim in 1909, it was not until the 1940s that Farquharson and Formston applied this technique in cattle. Despite all these promising advances in the latter half of the 19th century, and presumably due in large part to many unfavorable side effects, general anesthesia was not broadly adopted by the veterinary profession until well into the 20th century. Unfortunately, a "heavy hand," without analgesia/anesthesia or even sedation, was the stock-in-trade of many "large animal" practicing veterinarians well into the latter half of the 20th century.

Although diethyl ether and chloroform were utilized in pets in the early part of the 20th century, general anesthesia was not widely accepted until the discovery of barbiturates in the late 1920s, in particular, the introduction of pentobarbital in 1930 and thiopental in 1934. Because of rough, prolonged recoveries, the acceptance of barbiturate general anesthesia in larger species was delayed until phenothiazines were introduced by Charpentier in France in 1950.

General anesthesia of large farm animals was further advanced by the discovery of fluorinated hydrocarbons and the development of "large animal" inhalant anesthetic equipment. Since the 1970s, the introduction of newer classes of drugs together with techniques for their safe co-administration (e.g., phenothiazines, benzodiazepines, α_2-adrenergic receptor agonists, opioids, guaifenesin, and dissociatives) has further advanced the safety and utility of anesthesia for both large and small animal species [8].

The modern era of veterinary anesthesia began during the last three decades of the 20th century facilitated by the establishment of anesthesia specialty colleges within North America and Europe. Stated organizational missions were the improvement of patient safety and the development of new techniques and knowledge paralleling the advances made in human anesthesia. These organizations promoted new drug development and techniques with clinical utility in a variety of species and individual patient pathologies. In addition, an emphasis on patient monitoring for improved safety led to the adaptation of technologies such as pulse oximetry, capnography, and blood pressure measurement, which are now considered standard. The veterinary anesthesiologist's value as a member of the patient care team has led to their increased presence in private veterinary practice. The need for more sophisticated approaches to anesthesia care continues to grow with an increasing patient age demographic and medical and surgical advances. This demand will continue to expand the anesthesiologist's importance beyond the traditional roles of university instructor and pharmaceutical researcher. Demand has also been bolstered by the veterinary profession's quest to improve patient quality of life through better pain management. Many anesthesiologists have become leaders in pain management through their continued research and the creation of evidence-based species-specific pain assessment scales and therapeutic guidelines.

Conceptualizing depth of anesthesia

During the early years of ether administration to human and veterinary patients alike, the assessment of anesthetic depth was a learned skill, appreciated most fully by individuals with much experience and the courage to learn from trial and error. John Snow was the first physician to attempt to classify the depth of anesthesia based on observation of the patient [19]. Teaching new anesthetists how much anesthetic to administer required close oversight by an experienced individual.

Dr. Arthur Guedel, a physician from Indianapolis, Indiana, serving in the First World War, was tasked with training orderlies and nurses to administer diethyl ether to wounded soldiers. To facilitate this, he developed guidelines summarized on a wall chart that could be used by anesthetists to gauge the depth of anesthesia.

While Guedel's original observations were made in human patients anesthetized with ether, they were subsequently adapted for use with newer inhalant anesthetics. Modern anesthetic techniques seldom utilize inhalants alone, and the incorporation of other drugs (notably antimuscarinics and dissociative anesthetics) greatly influences the reflexive and autonomic responses, making Guedel's classification less relevant. Greater reliance on the monitoring of physiologic parameters, such as blood pressure, respiration, and neuromuscular tone evolved over time, and the use of processed electroencephalographic (EEG) signals (i.e., "depth-of-anesthesia" devices) has become increasingly common in human anesthesia. Nevertheless, despite the incorporation of new monitoring modalities, the anesthetist should continue to have a solid understanding of changing physical signs with anesthetic depth. Thus, Guedel's early observational classification will likely continue to have some relevancy. For more information on the physical signs relating to anesthetic depth, as well as EEG-derived indices of CNS activity, the reader is referred to Chapter 10.

Evolution of veterinary anesthesia as a specialty

In North America, during the late 1960s and early 1970s, a small group of physician anesthesiologists made it possible for a number of future diplomates of the American College of Veterinary Anesthesiologists (ACVA), now the American College of Veterinary Anesthesia and Analgesia (ACVAA), to participate in their training programs and to learn about the development of new anesthetic drugs and techniques. Among these physicians were Robert Dripps, University of Pennsylvania; Arthur Keats, Baylor University; Mort Shulman and Max Sadolv, University of Illinois; and Edmond I. Eger, University of California Medical College. During this same period, E. Wynn Jones (Oklahoma State University) and William Lumb (Colorado State University) were making significant contributions to the field of veterinary anesthesiology. Jerry Gillespie had made significant contributions through his work on the respiratory function of anesthetized horses and William Muir was reporting on the cardiopulmonary effects of anesthetic drugs in various species.

Even though there were many dedicated faculty within North American veterinary colleges and research laboratories, it was not until 1970 that a major effort was made to organize a stand-alone specialty. Initially, the American Society of Veterinary Anesthesia (ASVA) was established, and membership was open to all individuals working in the veterinary profession who had an interest in veterinary anesthesiology. In 1970, the first organizational meeting was held in conjunction with the American Veterinary Medical Association (AVMA) to coordinate the efforts and interests of all those wishing to develop the specialty of veterinary anesthesiology. Their primary goal was to improve anesthetic techniques and to disseminate knowledge whenever and wherever possible. Charles Short was elected the first President of the new society. Of major emphasis was the selection of individuals to speak at the ASVA and other scientific and educational meetings. As the ASVA developed, publication of original research and review articles seemed in order. Bruce Heath accepted editorial responsibilities for manuscripts submitted for the ASVA journal. In 1971, John Thurmon chaired the Ad Hoc Committee to establish the ACVA. Based on guidelines defined by the AVMA for new specialty colleges, the Ad Hoc Committee defined the requirements for ACVA founding charter diplomates, which included 10 years of active service in the specialty, significant publication in the discipline, intensive training, and either being a recognized head of an anesthesiology program or spending the majority of one's professional time devoted to anesthesia or a closely related subject area. Seven members of the ASVA were found to meet these qualifications and became the founding diplomates of the ACVA.

Between 1970 and 1975, the constitution and bylaws were drafted and formalized. In 1975, the AVMA Council on Education recommended preliminary approval of the ACVA, and it was confirmed by the AVMA House of Delegates that same year. Of importance throughout this process were the insights and efforts of William Lumb and E. Wynn Jones. They greatly assisted in the establishment of the ACVA because of their sincere interest in the sound principles of veterinary anesthesiology. During this same period, several didactic texts had been published further establishing anesthesia as a stand-alone discipline within veterinary medicine. The first edition of this text, *Lumb and Jones' Veterinary Anesthesia*, was published in 1973, *Clinical Veterinary Anesthesia*, edited by Charles Short, was published in 1974, and the *Textbook of Veterinary Anesthesia*, edited by Larry Soma, was published in 1971.

During the late 1970s, many of the founding diplomates established residency training programs in their respective veterinary colleges. From 1975 to 1980, the ACVA developed continuing education programs, programs in self-improvement, and guidelines for testing and certification of new diplomates. Along with residency training programs, anesthesiology faculty positions were created in a number of universities across North America. In 1980, an effort headed by the then president Eugene Steffey sought and achieved the full accreditation of the ACVA by the AVMA.

During the past 50 years, a number of organizations outside North America have promoted and contributed greatly to the advancement of veterinary anesthesia. They include the Association of Veterinary Anaesthetists of Great Britain and Ireland (AVA) and the Veterinary Anesthesia and Surgery Association in Japan. These associations, along with the ACVA, were instrumental in organizing the first International Congress of Veterinary Anesthesiology with its stated objective of globally advancing the field of veterinary anesthesiology. The first International Congress was held in Cambridge, England, in 1982 and has been held continually on a triannual basis around the world and on nearly every continent.

During the latter decades of the 20th century, anesthesiologists in the United Kingdom had established the Association of Veterinary Anaesthetists and awarded the Diploma of Veterinary Anaesthesia to those with advanced specialty training. Later, interest in board specialization became increasingly evident in the United Kingdom and many European countries, resulting in the establishment of the European College of Veterinary Anaesthesiologists (ECVA). In order to better recognize the central role anesthesiologists have in providing and advancing pain management, both the ECVA and the ACVA sought and were granted approval to incorporate the word "analgesia" into their names. Thus, the colleges were renamed the European College of Veterinary Anaesthesia and Analgesia (ECVAA) and the American College of Veterinary Anesthesia and Analgesia (ACVAA). Currently, a number of veterinary anesthesiologists are boarded by both the ACVAA and the ECVAA. Both the organizations recognize the legitimacy of either credential, allowing residency training programs supervised by ACVAA Diplomates to qualify candidates to sit the ECVAA Board Examination and vice versa. Interested readers are referred elsewhere for further information concerning the early history of both veterinary [6–14] and human [20–22] anesthesia.

The establishment of the ACVAA and the ECVAA helped to advance veterinary anesthesia and pain management on a global scale through promotion of quality research and dissemination of knowledge via scientific meetings and peer-reviewed publications. The ACVAA and the AVA have their own official scientific publication, the *Journal of Veterinary Anaesthesia and Analgesia*, which also serves as the official publication of the ECVAA and the International Veterinary Academy of Pain Management (IVAPM).

During the early 2000s, in an effort to improve outreach to practitioners interested in humane care and to increase pain management awareness, the IVAPM was initially conceived at an annual Veterinary Midwest Anesthesia and Analgesia Conference Scientific Meeting. The IVAPM's stated mission was to advance the multidisciplinary approach to pain management and was supported by an ongoing academic–pharmaceutical industry partnership, the Companion Animal Pain Management Consortium, led by ACVAA Diplomates Charles Short, William Tranquilli, and James Gaynor. The first president-elect of the IVAPM was the then current president of the ACVA, Peter Hellyer. In 2017, the North American Veterinary Anesthesia Society (NAVAS) was incorporated to improve ACVAA Diplomate continuing education outreach in coordination with private and public partners that share a common goal of advancing quality anesthesia and analgesia care. Alleviating animal pain and suffering is an increasingly important and defining issue for 21st century veterinary medicine. Today, anesthesiologists, practitioners, veterinary technicians, research and industry veterinarians, and animal scientists alike are working collaboratively through organizations such as the ACVAA, ECVAA, IVAPM, AVA, AVTAA (Academy of Veterinary Technicians in Anesthesia and Analgesia), and NAVAS to improve our knowledge and coordinate educational programs.

Anesthesiologist defined

A *boarded anesthesiologist* is a veterinarian who has been certified by either the ACVAA or ECVAA. The term *anesthetist* has more variable meaning because in some European countries, an anesthetist is equivalent to an anesthesiologist. In North America, however, anesthetist refers to a person who administers anesthetics but is not a physician or veterinarian (board-certified or otherwise). A veterinary anesthesiologist has completed a rigorous training program under the supervision of either ACVAA or ECVAA Diplomates and has passed a veterinary certifying anesthesia and analgesia specialty examination (i.e., either the ACVAA or ECVAA Certifying Board Examination). Board-certified anesthesiologists are considered experts at assessment and mitigation of anesthetic risks, delivery of anesthetic and analgesic drugs, maintenance and monitoring of physiologic well-being in anesthetized patients, and provision of the highest levels of perioperative patient care, including pain management, across a wide array of species and medical circumstances [23].

Current issues in veterinary anesthesia and analgesia

Environmental impact of anesthesia

Concerns about potential adverse effects associated with the use of anesthetic drugs fall into three general categories: (1) patient-experienced adverse drug reactions (ADRs); (2) occupational exposure experienced by anesthesia care providers; and (3) environmental impacts of inhalation anesthetics.

Regarding the first category, while the definition of an ADR remains largely unchanged over the past 50 years, the classification systems and nomenclature used to describe such reactions change frequently. Specific patient-experienced ADRs are discussed in other areas of this text, and reviews of ADRs as they relate to anesthesia are available elsewhere [24,25]. Regarding the second category of adverse effects, anesthesia care providers may be sporadically and acutely exposed to both injectable and inhalant anesthetics via accidental needle penetration or drug spillage. This highlights the importance of staff training and implementation of health and safety standard operating procedures to minimize the risk of exposure in the first place and reduce negative outcomes in the event an exposure occurs. In addition, chronic workplace exposure to low levels of inhalant anesthetic agents (waste anesthetic gases) has been a concern since their use began. Although studied repeatedly, questions still exist about the relative risk of inhalant anesthetic toxicity and their potential to cause infertility, miscarriage, cancer, and other chronic health problems. Part of the difficulty in determining safe levels of exposure is related to the apparently low incidence of adverse effects and the potentially long lag period between exposure and expression of toxicity. Usually, the question is approached through large epidemiological studies of healthcare providers that are administering anesthetics. This introduces many confounders such as provider age, agents in use, co-existing health problems, and measurement of actual provider exposure, which may make interpretation and generalization of results problematic. Further information on occupational exposure to waste anesthetic gases is available in Chapter 28.

The third type of anesthetic adverse effect is environmental. Historically, drug development and clinical use of anesthetic agents did not consider the resources consumed to produce drugs or their ultimate fate once eliminated by the patient. Nitrous oxide and the chlorine- or bromine-containing halogenated inhalants (i.e., isoflurane and halothane) are both greenhouse gases and ozone depleters [26]. While the other halogenated agents that lack chlorine or bromine (i.e., sevoflurane and desflurane) do not catalytically destroy ozone, they remain important greenhouse gases as trace amounts in the atmosphere absorb and reduce outgoing infrared thermal energy and contribute to global warming [27]. Of the inhalant anesthetics in clinical use, desflurane is responsible for the largest greenhouse gas emissions during its atmospheric lifecycle. On a MAC-hour basis, desflurane's emissions are approximately 15 times that of isoflurane and 20 times that of sevoflurane. The concurrent use of nitrous oxide to facilitate delivery of inhalant anesthetics further increases emissions. Further information on the environmental impact of inhalation anesthetics is available in Chapter 28.

As the most widely used injectable anesthetic, propofol's impact on greenhouse gas emissions is much smaller, by nearly four orders of magnitude, than that of desflurane or nitrous oxide. Greenhouse gas emissions associated with propofol and many other injectable anesthetic drugs are primarily related to the production and consumption of fossil fuels needed to manufacture and deliver the drugs [28]. Although the contribution of volatile anesthetics to total greenhouse gas emissions remains relatively small (0.1%) compared to that of carbon dioxide (82%), it is still important to consider the long-term, cumulative impact of inhaled anesthetics on climate change and pursue strategies to minimize the introduction of these agents into the environment [27]. Increasingly, anesthesia professional organizations as well as governmental and intergovernmental bodies are moving from knowledge to action to address environmental stewardship and greenhouse gas mitigation [29].

Impact of the opioid epidemic on veterinary anesthesia

According to the United States Centers for Disease Control and Prevention, the number of drug overdose deaths in the United States increased by nearly 30% from 2019 to 2020 and has quintupled since 1999 [30]. Three waves of opioid overdose deaths are recognized. The first wave began in the late 1990s corresponding with the development of extended-release formulations of potent opioid medications (e.g., Oxycontin® and Vicodin®) coupled with aggressive marketing to physicians and significant increases in opioid prescribing activity. The second wave began in 2010 and was associated with a rapid increase in overdose deaths involving the illicit opioid, heroin. The third wave began in 2013 with significant increases in deaths involving synthetic opioids, particularly those involving illicitly manufactured fentanyl. In the United States and elsewhere, the market for illicit fentanyl continues to change and the drug is now commonly found in combination with heroin, counterfeit pills, cocaine, and other drugs particularly relevant to veterinarians including xylazine and ketamine.

As licensed prescribers of controlled substances, veterinarians have an important role to play in combating the opioid epidemic. As researchers, policymakers, and public health professionals struggle to identify and implement strategies to mitigate misuse and abuse of opioids, veterinarians are increasingly feeling the impacts of this public health crisis [31,32]. Despite the overuse and abuse of opioids in humans, veterinarians paradoxically have found themselves facing shortages of opioids for legitimate clinical use. Reasons for this are not always readily apparent but may be related to institution of production limits by some regulatory bodies on opioids approved for humans, as well as tightening of bureaucratic regulations.

In addition to drug shortages, veterinarians are confronting increasing and rapidly evolving legal restrictions and requirements around the management of controlled drugs. In the United States, for example, numerous states now mandate continuing education relating to opioids for veterinarians applying for or renewing licensure. Media reports involving drug-seeking individuals turning to veterinary practices have resulted in increased scrutiny on the profession [33], and a number of jurisdictions have introduced legislation requiring veterinarians to participate in prescription drug monitoring programs (PDMPs) [34]. The AVMA has expressed support for veterinary continuing education programs addressing the judicious use, compliance, security, and prescribing of opioids, but it does not support mandatory controlled drug electronic prescribing systems or veterinary practitioner participation in PDMPs [35].

In a concerning new development, xylazine has been increasingly identified as an adulterant in illicit preparations of heroin and fentanyl in the United States and Canada. This trend has more recently expanded to other jurisdictions including the United Kingdom and Europe. As xylazine's effects are obviously not reversed by opioid antagonists, and because α_2-adrenergic receptor antagonists have not been available to first responders, illicit xylazine is implicated as a cause of increased overdose deaths [36,37]. The United States federal government has recently identified the combination of illicit fentanyl and xylazine as an "emerging threat" [38] and has proposed federal legislation to combat diversion of xylazine from veterinary sources. This may have significant implications, especially for those veterinarians in large animal practice. More information is available elsewhere on these regulatory changes within the United States, as well as the position statement from the AVMA, which supports the legislation while highlighting the need for continued veterinary access to this critically important drug [39].

Finally, veterinarians are also impacted by diversion of controlled drugs both by individuals working within a veterinary practice as well as those not affiliated with the practice (e.g., drug-seeking clients and outright drug theft). "Vet shopping" refers to the practice of soliciting multiple veterinarians under false pretenses to obtain prescriptions for controlled drugs [31,34]. In general, the best way for veterinarians to protect themselves, their staff, and their clients is to: (1) remain up-to-date and follow all regulations (both regional and federal) regarding the prescription of controlled substances in their jurisdiction; (2) exercise extreme caution when prescribing and dispensing opioids to clients for at-home pain medication and provide education on safe storage and disposal of their pet's medications; (3) embrace opioid-sparing techniques for in-hospital pain management where appropriate; (4) recognize the signs of opioid intoxication in pets and know how to treat it; and (5) recognize the signs of opioid abuse in clients and colleagues [40]. Additional resources to assist veterinarians in navigating the opioid epidemic are available from a number of national veterinary organizations such as the AVMA [41]. Further information on the opioid crisis is available in Chapter 23.

Emerging role of technology

The role of technology in human healthcare has expanded exponentially over the last two decades beginning with the transition to electronic health records and spawning the development of an entirely new subspecialty within anesthesia known as "anesthesia informatics." Collaboration between motivated anesthesiologists and software developers resulted in commercial Anesthesia Information Management Systems (AIMS) that are now used in both community hospitals and referral centers [42]. The ongoing need to adapt and optimize these sophisticated systems means that "anesthesiologist-informaticists" will likely play an increasing role in electronic anesthesia records, perioperative computerized decision-making support, and virtual patient care [43].

In veterinary medicine, the transition from paper to electronic management systems is underway and software has now evolved from primarily practice management tools (i.e., scheduling, inventory, billing, etc.) to capturing most aspects of the patient's medical record. While veterinary-specific anesthetic monitoring technology has made considerable advances, technology to capture and record that information has, until recently, lagged behind [42]. Several veterinary-specific anesthesia electronic medical record (AEMR) applications are available including the SurgiVet™ Advisor® Veterinary Data Logger (Smiths Medical), the SmartFlow® Patient Workflow Anesthetic Sheet (IDEXX Laboratories), and the Veterinary Digital Anesthesia Record, VetDAR® (Dimple Hill Software). Further information about each of these products, as well as the advantages and disadvantages of AEMRs more generally, is available elsewhere [42,44]. As these applications become more widely used in primary care veterinary practice, new opportunities for veterinary anesthesiologists to expand their scope of practice have emerged through both synchronous and asynchronous teleconsulting services. In the near future, it seems likely that an alternative care model may evolve whereby veterinary anesthesiologists are able to remotely monitor patients and consult from afar using cloud-based technologies [44].

Another emerging technology in veterinary anesthesia involves the use of simulation as an education and training tool. While simulation has been used in pre-clinical medical training for decades, development of applications for veterinary medicine, specifically anesthesia, is more recent. At least one veterinary simulation program is commercially available (Stage III Veterinary Education Simulation software, WholeLogic Inc.), and it is reportedly used by several veterinary medical colleges as part of their anesthesia curriculum [45]. A number of recent publications indicate that veterinary anesthesia simulation-based training has the potential to enhance cognitive and affective outcomes and better prepare students for patient care experiences [46–48].

References

1 Short CE. The management of animal pain: where have we been, where are we now, and where are we going? *Vet J* 2003; **165**: 101–103.

2 Heavner JE. Veterinary anesthesia update. *J Am Vet Med Assoc* 1983; **182**: 30.

3 Winters WD, Ferrer AT, Guzman-Flores C. The cataleptic state induced by ketamine: a review of the neuropharmacology of anesthesia. *Neuropharmacology* 1972; **11**: 303–315.

4 Askitopoulou H, Ramoutsaki IA, Konsolaki E. Analgesia and anesthesia: etymology and literary history of related Greek words. *Anesth Analg* 2000; **91**(2): 486–491.

5 International Association for the Study of Pain. *IASP Terminology*. https://www.iasp-pain.org/resources/terminology (accessed June 2023).

6 Hall LW. Anesthesiology. In: Brandly CA, Jungherr EL, eds. *Advances in Veterinary Science*, 3rd edn. New York, NY: Academic Press, 1957; 1–32.

7 Smithcors JF. The early use of anaesthesia in veterinary practice. *Brit Vet J* 1957; **113**: 284–291.

8 Stevenson DE. The evolution of veterinary anaesthesia. *Brit Vet J* 1963; **119**: 477–483.

9 Wright JG. Anaesthesia in animals: a review. *Vet Rec* 1964; **76**: 710–713.

10 Westhues M, Fritsch R. Introduction: history of general anaesthesia. In: Westhues M, Fritsch R, eds. *Animal Anaesthesia*, 1st English edn. Philadelphia, PA: Lippincott, 1965; xiii–xxi.

11 Smithcors JF. History of veterinary anesthesia. In: Soma LR, ed. *Textbook of Veterinary Aanesthesia*, 1st edn. Baltimore, MD: Williams & Wilkins, 1971; 1–23.

12 Weaver BMQ. The history of veterinary anesthesia. *Vet Hist* 1988; **5**: 43–57.

13 Jones RS. A history of veterinary anaesthesia. *An Vet Murcia* 2002; **18**: 7–15.

14 Steffey E. A history of veterinary anesthesia. In: Eger E II, Saidman L, Westhorpe R, eds. *The Wondrous Story of Anesthesia*. New York, NY: Springer, 2014.

15 Thurmon JC, Benson GJ. Anesthesia in ruminants and swine. In: Howard JL, ed. *Current Veterinary Therapy*, vol. **3**. Philadelphia, PA: WB Saunders, 1993; 58–76.

16 Jackson CT. Etherization of Animals. *Report of the Commissioner of Patients for the Year of 1853*. Washington, DC: Beverly Tucker, Senate Printer, 1853; 59.

17 Dadd GH. *The Modern Horse Doctor*. Boston, MA: JP Jewett, 1854.

18 Keys TE. The development of anesthesia. *Anesthesiology* 1942; **3**: 11–23.

19 Snow J. *On the Inhalation of the Vapor of Ether in Surgical Operations*. London, UK: Churchill, 1847.

20 Clark AJ. Aspects of the history of anesthetics. *Br Med J* 1938; **ii**: 1029.

21 Lee JA. *A Synopsis of Anesthesia*, 4th edn. Baltimore, MD: Williams & Wilkins, 1959.

22 Miller RD. *Anesthesia*, 2nd edn. New York, NY: Churchill Livingstone, 1986.

23 American College of Veterinary Anesthesia and Analgesia. website. https://acvaa.org (accessed June 2023).

24 Patton K, Borshoff DC. Adverse drug reactions. *Anaesthesia* 2018; **73**(Suppl 1): 76–84.

25 Cook TM, Harper NJN, Farmer L, *et al*. Anaesthesia, surgery, and life-threatening allergic reactions: protocol and methods of the 6th National Audit Project (NAP6) of the Royal College of Anaesthetists. *Br J Anaesth* 2018; **121**(1): 124–133.

26 Langbein T, Sonntag H, Trapp D, *et al*. Volatile anaesthetics and the atmosphere: atmospheric lifetimes and atmospheric effects of halothane, enflurane, isoflurane, desflurane and sevoflurane. *Br J Anaesth* 1999; **82**(1): 66–73.

27 Varughese S, Ahmed R. Environmental and occupational considerations of anesthesia: a narrative review and update. *Anesth Analg* 2021; **133**(4): 826–835.

28 Sherman J, Le C, Lamers V, *et al*. Life cycle greenhouse gas emissions of anesthetic drugs. *Anesth Analg* 2012; **114**(5): 1086–1090.

29 Devlin-Hegedus JA, McGain F, Harris RD, *et al*. Action guidance for addressing pollution from inhalational anaesthetics. *Anaesthesia* 2022; **77**(9): 1023–1029.

30 United States Centers for Disease Control and Prevention (CDC). *Understanding the Opioid Overdose Epidemic*. https://www.cdc.gov/opioids/basics/epidemic.html (accessed June 2023).

31 Mason DS, Tenney L, Hellyer PW, *et al*. Prescription opioid epidemic: do veterinarians have a dog in the fight? *Am J Public Health* 2018; **108**(9): 1162–1163.

32 Kogan L, Hellyer P, Rishniw M, *et al*. The US opioid epidemic and its impact on US general practice veterinarians. *Front Vet Sci* 2019; **6**: 222.

33 Hendricks B, Rudisill T, Pesarsick J, *et al*. Prescription drug monitoring program policy reform: human and veterinary practitioner prescribing in West Virginia, 2008–2020. *J Public Health Policy* 2021; **42**(2): 249–257.

34 Anand A, Hosanagar A. Drug misuse in the veterinary setting: an under-recognized avenue. *Curr Psychiatry Rep* 2021; **23**(2): 3.

35 The American Veterinary Medical Association (AVMA). *The Veterinary Profession's Role in Addressing the Opioid Epidemic*. https://www.avma.org/resources-tools/avma-policies/veterinary-professions-role-addressing-opioid-epidemic (accessed June 2023).

36 Ball NS, Knable BM, Relich TA, *et al*. Xylazine poisoning: a systematic review. *Clin Toxicol (Phila)* 2022; **60**(8): 892–901.

37 Ayub S, Parnia S, Poddar K, *et al*. Xylazine in the opioid epidemic: a systematic review of case reports and clinical implications. *Cureus* 2023; **15**(3): e36864.

38 United States Federal Government White House Briefing. *Biden-Harris Administration Designates Fentanyl Combined with Xylazine as an Emerging Threat to the United States*. https://www.whitehouse.gov/ondcp/briefing-room/2023/04/12/biden-harris-administration-designates-fentanyl-combined-with-xylazine-as-an-emerging-threat-to-the-united-states (accessed June 2023).

39 The American Veterinary Medical Association (AVMA). *AVMA Endorses US Federal Legislation to Address Illicit Xylazine*. https://www.avma.org/blog/avma-endorses-federal-legislation-address-illicit-xylazine (accessed June 2023).

40 United States Food and Drug Administration (FDA). *The Opioid Epidemic: What Veterinarians Need to Know*. https://www.fda.gov/animal-veterinary/resources-you/opioid-epidemic-what-veterinarians-need-know (accessed June 2023).

41 The American Veterinary Medical Association (AVMA). *Webinars to Help Veterinarians Navigate Opioid Epidemic*. https://www.avma.org/news/avma-webinars-help-veterinarians-navigate-opioid-epidemic (accessed June 2023).

42 Riebold T. Anesthetic records. In: Cooley KG, Johnson RA, eds. *Veterinary Anesthetic and Monitoring Equipment*, Hoboken, NJ: John Wiley and Sons, 2018; 323–333.

43 Lee R, Hitt J, Hobika GG, *et al*. The case for the anesthesiologist-informaticist. *JMIR Perioper Med* 2022; **5**(1): e32738.

44 Mitek A. Anesthesiologists in the ether: technology and telemedicine in anesthesiology. *Vet Clin North Am Small Anim Pract* 2022; **52**(5): 1099–1107.

45 WholeLogic Inc. *Stage III Veterinary Education Simulation website*. https://wholelogic.com (accessed June 2023).

46 Jones JL, Rinehart J, Spiegel JJ, *et al*. Teaching tip: development of veterinary anesthesia simulations for pre-clinical training: design, implementation, and evaluation based on student perspectives. *J Vet Med Educ* 2018; **45**(2): 232–240.

47 Jones JL, Rinehart J, Englar RE. The effect of simulation training in anesthesia on student operational performance and patient safety. *J Vet Med Educ* 2019; **46**(2): 205–213.

48 Noyes JA, Keegan RD, Carbonneau KJ, *et al*. Evaluating a multimodal clinical anesthesia course integrated into an existing veterinary curriculum. *Simul Healthc* 2021; **16**(3): 177–184.

2 Anesthetic Risk and Informed Consent

Dave C. Brodbelt[1], Derek Flaherty[2] and Glenn R. Pettifer[3]

[1] Veterinary Epidemiology, Economics and Public Health Group, Department of Pathobiology and Population Sciences, Royal Veterinary College, Hatfield, Herts, UK

[2] Southern Counties Veterinary Specialists, Ringwood, Hampshire, UK

[3] College of Dental Hygienists of Ontario, Toronto, Ontario, Canada

Chapter contents

Assessing anesthetic risk, 10
Preoperative patient risk assessment, 10
Morbidity and mortality, 13
Small animal anesthesia morbidity, 13
Large animal anesthesia morbidity, 14
Small animal anesthetic mortality, 14
Large animal anesthetic mortality, 18
Informed consent, 20
References, 21

Assessing anesthetic risk

Perioperative assessment of anesthetic risk is a valuable exercise in order to minimize complications and optimize anesthetic safety. A number of studies have been published in relation to anesthetic morbidity and mortality in both small and large animals. Based on this evidence, improved recognition of the risks of anesthesia and those patients that require the greatest care and preoperative management could help improve standards of veterinary anesthesia and patient outcome. For more information on related topics, the reader is referred to Chapters 3 and 5.

Preoperative patient risk assessment

Patient health assessment

The preoperative assessment of an animal's health status is valuable to acknowledge preanesthetic risks, to identify management priorities, and to advise clients appropriately prior to anesthesia and surgery. Health status has been consistently reported to be associated with anesthetic death in humans and in the spectrum of species commonly seen in veterinary anesthesia. Increased American Society of Anesthesiologists (ASA) physical status grade [1,2] (see Table 2.1) has been associated with an increased risk of death in a number of anesthetic studies in small animals [3–14], horses [15–18], and humans [19–39].

Anesthetic agents cause cardiopulmonary depression, and the presence of concurrent pathology involving the major body systems is likely to predispose to greater anesthetic-induced physiologic disturbance [40]. Pre-existing cardiopulmonary pathology is particularly relevant in the immediate preoperative period, as anesthetic-related mortality is likely to involve respiratory or cardiovascular compromise, and most anesthetics depress one or both systems at clinical levels of anesthesia [40].

Hematologic and biochemical abnormalities may also be a significant consideration. In particular, anemia will reduce oxygen-carrying capacity and predispose to hypoxia, and hypoproteinemia has been theorized to increase the response of the patient to highly protein-bound drugs and result in relative overdose [40]. Renal disease is also important, particularly if dehydration or uremia is present, as under these conditions, the renal system will have a lower tolerance to anesthesia and the patient may be more sensitive to some anesthetics and perioperative drugs such as non-steroidal anti-inflammatory agents. Neurologic disease may be relevant with respect to the occurrence of postoperative seizures, increased sensitivity to anesthetics, and when cardiopulmonary function is affected, e.g., medullary pathology can depress ventilation and cardiovascular function. Additionally, liver and endocrine disease may influence the response to anesthesia, with diabetes mellitus and potential intraoperative cellular changes in glucose concentrations being particularly relevant [41].

Hence, some form of physical health status assessment is an important preanesthetic consideration. Most frequently, ASA grade [1,2] has been utilized for this purpose, and there is some evidence that this can identify patients at increased risk of mortality until 24–72 h postanesthesia [42]. However, the repeatability and agreement between observers of such scoring systems have been questioned, and evidence suggests that interobserver agreement in ASA health status classification is poor in veterinary anesthesia [43]. Other assessment systems exist in human medicine, including the Acute Physiology and Chronic Health Evaluation (APACHE),

Veterinary Anesthesia and Analgesia: The Sixth Edition of Lumb and Jones. Edited by Leigh Lamont, Kurt Grimm, Sheilah Robertson, Lydia Love and Carrie Schroeder.
© 2024 John Wiley & Sons, Inc. Published 2024 by John Wiley & Sons, Inc.
Companion website: www.wiley.com/go/lamont/anesthesia

Table 2.1 Classification of physical status[a].

Category	Physical status	Possible examples of this category
1	Normal healthy patients	No discernible disease, e.g., animals scheduled for elective ovariohysterectomy, or castration
2	Patients with mild systemic disease	Skin tumor, fracture without shock, uncomplicated hernia, or compensated cardiac disease (e.g., stage B1 mitral valve disease)
3	Patients with severe systemic disease	Moderate anemia or hypovolemia, moderate renal or hepatic dysfunction
4	Patients with severe systemic disease that is a constant threat to life	Sepsis, marked hyperkalemia (e.g., urinary obstruction), end-stage organ disease (e.g., renal, hepatic, or cardiac), marked hypovolemia, or severe anemia
5	Moribund patients not expected to survive 24 h without the operation	Massive trauma

[a]This classification is the same as that adopted by the American Society of Anesthesiologists.

the Physiological and Operative Severity Score for the enUmeration of Mortality and Morbidity (POSSUM), and, in pediatric practice, the Neurological, Airway, Respiratory, Cardiovascular and Other (NARCO) score, and all were observed to predict perioperative risk [44–46]. However, these systems are complex, require more time to complete, and have yet to be evaluated for agreement between observers in a veterinary context. Hence, at present, there appears to be little consensus as to the optimal method of patient health status assessment for consistent and efficient classification across observers, and caution should be exercised in overinterpreting individual health status assessments. Nonetheless, there is a body of evidence that highlights that sicker patients are more likely to die perioperatively, and therefore, some form of preoperative patient assessment would be advisable to distinguish sick from healthy patients, to identify those at greater risk, and to manage patients appropriately in order to try to minimize risk prior to, during, and after anesthesia.

Preanesthetic blood testing

Given the fact that organ dysfunction and various pathologic conditions such as anemia or hypoproteinemia may contribute to increased anesthetic morbidity or mortality, it would seem sensible to make every effort to detect these prior to general anesthesia. For this reason, routine preanesthetic blood screening is commonly recommended by many veterinary practitioners and, indeed, some anesthesia specialists. However, although there is no doubt that prior biochemical and hematologic analyses are of definite value in certain patient groups, the question remains as to whether their use can be justified for every patient, in particular healthy animals undergoing elective procedures.

An internet search for "Preanesthetic blood screening in animals" (www.google.com, accessed July 2022) returned over 18 million hits, of which a substantial proportion appeared to be veterinary practices each detailing their reasons and prices for carrying out such a procedure; interestingly, the search term returned virtually no scientific papers relating to the practice. In addition, as with much information to be found on the internet, many of the relevant web pages providing advice on the subject were written by people with no apparent scientific background or credentials for discussing such a topic, with the majority of these being pet owner discussion forums. Although there may be no genuine scientific or clinical background behind these types of discussion groups, they almost certainly help perpetuate the need for ubiquitous preanesthetic blood testing, but given that many veterinary professionals also recommend its routine use, it obviously cannot all be dependent on owner perceptions. So, is there actually a sound rationale upon which the need for preanesthetic biochemical and hematologic sampling is based?

There are numerous studies in human anesthesia now questioning the necessity for preanesthetic laboratory testing in healthy patients [47–49], with each of these demonstrating that, for subjects with no demonstrable abnormalities on the basis of history and clinical examination, there appears to be no reduction in perianesthetic complications if prior blood sampling has been carried out. The United Kingdom (UK) National Institute for Health and Care Excellence (NICE) gathers evidence from a variety of sources and then produces recommendations for human clinicians for various medical and surgical interventions. In terms of preanesthetic blood testing, NICE subdivides its recommendations based on both the age of the patient and the grade of surgery the subject is undergoing (minor, intermediate, or major/complex). Based on this system, NICE does not recommend preanesthetic biochemical or hematological screening for ASA 1 or 2 human patients undergoing minor or intermediate grades of surgery, although assessment of renal function should be considered in ASA 2 subjects having intermediate surgery if they have some predisposition to development of possible acute kidney injury; in other words, unless the patient is sick, preanesthetic blood tests would only be recommended for humans undergoing major/complex surgery. Unsurprisingly, NICE does suggest considering preanesthetic blood screening for ASA 3–5 patients undergoing intermediate or major procedures [50].

As a result of the NICE recommendations, the guidelines of the Association of Anaesthetists of Great Britain and Ireland (AAGBI) [51] for human anesthesia conclude: "Routine preoperative investigations are expensive, labor intensive, and of questionable value, especially as they may contribute to morbidity or cause additional delays due to spurious results."

Aside from the issue of erroneous results impacting on the efficiency of case throughput, it is also important to remember that the reference ranges established for most laboratory tests incorporate only approximately 95% of the population, i.e., around one in 20 animals that are perfectly healthy will return laboratory results that are outside a "normal" range, which may then lead to further unnecessary investigations being carried out, in addition to delaying the planned procedure; the more tests that are run, the greater the likelihood of this occurring. Hence, it is important to carefully interpret test results obtained and to view them as part of the overall assessment of the patient.

The AAGBI also takes the view that history and examination performed by appropriately trained and competent personnel remain the most efficient and accurate way of initially detecting significant morbidity: "Thus, it is important that, where preanesthetic blood screening is carried out, it is seen as an adjunct to a full clinical examination, rather than an alternative." While this is undoubtedly the case in both veterinary and human anesthesia, the results from human studies relating to preanesthetic blood screening of healthy patients may not be directly applicable to animals. This is because the majority of humans are both cognitive and verbal and are able to self-report health issues. Veterinary clinicians, on the other hand, obtain the relevant health information by proxy (from the owner), which may mean that important details are not identified. Thus, it is possible that a higher incidence of abnormalities may be detected on preanesthetic screening of animals than has been reported for humans.

Given that the consensus opinion from human anesthesia seems to be that preanesthetic blood sampling appears to be justifiable only in sicker patients, and that healthy individuals undergoing elective procedures do not benefit from this practice, what recommendations should be put in place for veterinary anesthesia? There appear to be only a small number of studies relating to the validity of routine preanesthetic blood screening in animals [52]. Toews and Campbell [53] performed a complete blood count in 102 horses undergoing cryptorchidectomy and then determined whether any abnormalities detected impacted on the risk of surgical complications. They found that 55 animals had results outside the reference range for at least one hematologic parameter, but there was no correlation between those demonstrating abnormal values and the likelihood of either intra- or postoperative surgical complications, nor did these abnormalities dictate alterations in patient management. Alef *et al.* [54] analyzed results from over 1500 dogs undergoing anesthesia at the University of Leipzig and reported that if no potential issues were identified in either the animal's history or clinical examination, "the changes revealed by preoperative screening were usually of little clinical relevance and did not prompt major changes to the anesthetic technique." They concluded that preanesthetic blood screening is, therefore, unlikely to yield additional important information in most cases. However, the same study also documented that of those dogs where the history and clinical examination would not normally have resulted in preanesthetic laboratory testing being performed at their institution (equivalent to 84% of the dogs recruited), 8% demonstrated biochemical or hematologic abnormalities that would have reclassified them as a higher ASA status, even if this may not necessarily have altered the anesthetic protocol. In addition, they also identified that surgery would have been postponed due to the laboratory findings in 0.8% of these dogs where preanesthetic blood screening would not usually have been performed, while 1.5% would have received additional preanesthetic therapy. Although the authors concluded that only 0.2% of dogs in the study would have required an alteration to their proposed anesthetic protocol based on the biochemical or hematologic results, the implication that undiagnosed pathology may be detected prior to anesthesia using "routine" screening may have implications for whether the owner decides to proceed with anesthesia/surgery and may also alter the expected prognosis for the animal. Thus, from this study, despite the fact that preanesthetic biochemical and hematologic testing may not necessarily alter how the subsequent anesthetic would actually be performed in most animals, it may, in reality, be the deciding factor as to whether the procedure goes ahead. Davies and Kawaguchi [55] conducted a retrospective study of almost 800 dogs and cats of varying ASA status which underwent preanesthetic blood screening at a UK veterinary group practice and showed that 97% of cats and 95% of dogs had at least one result from the screening panel that was outside the reference interval (although not necessarily clinically significant). Almost 1% of cases had problems identified by the preanesthetic blood results that were not evident from the history or physical examination, while 4% of dogs and 9% of cats had their anesthetic protocol altered based on abnormalities in the blood work, although these cases were being anesthetized by first opinion practitioners rather than specialist anesthesiologists. A more recent study by Mitchell *et al.* [52], which presented five Diplomates of the American College of Veterinary Anesthesia and Analgesia with the medical records from 100 randomly selected previously presented cases, subsequently followed by the relevant results from preanesthetic blood screening tests for these animals, resulted in a change in the proposed anesthetic protocol in 79% of patients, based on abnormalities in the blood results. Of note is that 64% of changes were made by only one of the anesthesiologists, which suggests that there may be significant variability in whether alterations in certain preanesthetic tests are considered clinically relevant even between specialists.

While it is often said that "old age is not a disease," it might be intuitive to assume that older patients may require more intensive preanesthetic screening compared to those who are younger. However, with the exception of recommending a preanesthetic electrocardiogram (ECG) in patients greater than 65 years old undergoing major/complex surgery, NICE does not differentiate the requirements for preanesthetic assessment based on age alone, i.e., they do not suggest blood testing older patients of ASA 1 or 2 undergoing minor or intermediate procedures unless there are certain comorbidities (e.g., diabetes mellitus and cardiovascular or renal disease). In animals, Joubert [56] assessed whether hematologic and biochemical analyses were of value in geriatric dogs (> 7 years of age) presented for anesthesia. Of the 101 dogs recruited to the study, 30 new diagnoses (e.g., neoplasia and hyperadrenocorticism) were made on the basis of the blood sample, with 13 animals not undergoing general anesthesia as a result of the new diagnosis. However, similar to the conclusions of the study by Alef *et al.* [54], Joubert [56] suggested that although preanesthetic screening had revealed the presence of subclinical disease in almost 30% of the dogs in the study, and that screening of geriatric patients is important, "the value of screening before anesthesia is perhaps more questionable in terms of anesthetic practice, but it is an appropriate time to perform such an evaluation." In other words, although preanesthetic blood testing may be of value in uncovering undiagnosed pathology in geriatric patients, there was little evidence that what was detected would actually impact either how the subsequent anesthetic was managed, or the overall outcome from it. However, this study did identify that over 10% of the dogs had their anesthesia canceled due solely to the findings of the preanesthetic blood screening, which is obviously of significance.

Interestingly, and somewhat in contrast to the previous studies, work within the Confidential Enquiry into Perioperative Small Animal Fatalities (CEPSAF) highlighted a reduction in risk when preoperative blood work was performed in higher ASA grade patients. CEPSAF was a multicenter study undertaken in the UK between 2002 and 2004 and involved over 100 practices and data from approximately 200,000 dogs and cats [7]. When analyzing risk factors for anesthetic death in sick dogs (ASA grade 3–5), having a preoperative blood test was associated with reduced odds of death, particularly in ASA grade 4–5 dogs [57]. This association was not detected in the overall analyses where ASA grade 1–5 dogs were considered together or in cats but does suggest that preoperative biochemistry and hematology are most likely to be merited in the sicker animals that are anesthetized.

Thus, based on the evidence from human anesthesia, and from a smaller number of published veterinary studies, there would appear to be negligible benefit to apparently healthy animals (ASA 1 or 2, regardless of age) of biochemical or hematologic screening prior to anesthesia in terms of either anesthetic risk reduction or alteration of the anesthetic protocol; however, given that a significant percentage of animals may have the procedure canceled based on the results of these tests (due either to a worsened prognosis or the need for further treatment prior to anesthesia), this may counterbalance the preceding argument. Overall, the requirement for preanesthetic blood screening in healthy animals is likely to remain a contentious issue, with valid arguments both for and against.

The situation in animals that are ASA 3 or greater, however, is probably more clear-cut with the published veterinary studies providing some justification that preanesthetic screening may be of value in terms of potentially altering anesthetic management and outcome.

Aside from the impact (or lack thereof) that preanesthetic screening may have on the subsequent conduct of anesthesia and ultimate outcome for veterinary patients, there is perhaps another factor that may require consideration, namely that of potential litigation. It seems that an increasing number of clients are willing (sometimes overly so) to point the finger of blame at the veterinarian when things go wrong in relation to anesthesia, even when in many cases this may be completely unjustified. Hence, the genuine reason why many veterinary practices carry out routine preanesthetic screening may have more to do with covering one's back rather than providing the ability to alter anesthetic management suitably if abnormalities are actually detected. It is impossible to say what the legal system may make of a healthy animal undergoing an elective procedure that dies during anesthesia where no preoperative blood sampling had been performed, but based on the recommendations from human anesthesia and the lack of evidence of any benefit in the few veterinary studies that have been carried out, it would appear difficult for them to state that preanesthetic biochemical or hematologic screening is a basic standard of care. Given that there is a more limited evidence base for sicker animals, it may be considered wise to perform preanesthetic screening in patients of ASA 3 or above, from both standard of care and litigation points of view.

Morbidity and mortality

Non-fatal complications tend to occur more frequently than mortal events, although they have been less often documented in the veterinary literature. Reported small animal morbidity risks range from 2% to 10% [4,5,10,58]. Work in small and large animal anesthesia has acknowledged the difficulty of ensuring consistent detection and recording of morbid events in the practice setting [3,4,59,60]. Small animal practice standards of monitoring of anesthesia can be superficial [61–63] and, unless a given complication results in obvious patient disturbance, it may go unnoticed. Hence, in considering morbid complications, only major events, most likely to be consistently observed, that could contribute substantial physiologic disturbance and that could have the greatest impact on a patient (other than death) will be discussed here.

Small animal anesthesia morbidity

Small animal anesthesia morbidity studies have most frequently been veterinary teaching hospital based, with a few primary practice-based studies also reporting major non-fatal complications [3–5,10,58,62,64]. Conditions consistently described include respiratory, cardiovascular, renal, gastrointestinal, thermoregulatory, and neurologic complications.

Respiratory complications were observed in 0.54% of dog and 0.34% of cat anesthetics in a study of practitioners in Ontario, Canada, and included respiratory depression or apnea, respiratory distress, and difficulty with intubation (although the definitions of these were not stated) [4]. In a veterinary teaching hospital setting, similar respiratory complications were observed, but more often. Hypoventilation and hypercapnia (defined as a partial pressure of arterial carbon dioxide or end-tidal carbon dioxide > 55 mmHg) were reported in 1.3% and 0.15% of dogs and cats undergoing anesthesia, respectively. Hypoxemia (partial pressure of arterial oxygen < 60 mmHg or hemoglobin arterial oxygen saturation < 90%) was reported in 0.5% of dogs, and occasionally, airway compromise was also noted [58]. In a Spanish veterinary school hospital, hypoventilation (defined as minute ventilation < 100 mL/kg/min) was observed in over 60% and hypoxemia (defined as SpO_2 < 90%) in 16% of anesthetized dogs [65].

Cardiovascular compromise in small animals included the development of cardiac arrhythmias, notably bradycardia in 0.62% and 0.14% of dog and cat anesthetics in a primary practice setting, respectively, although bradycardia was classified as < 60 beats/min and irregular or < 50 beats/min and regular for both dogs and cats [4]. In contrast, in a teaching hospital setting, the most frequently recorded cardiovascular complications were hypotension (defined as systolic arterial pressure < 80 mmHg or mean arterial pressure < 60 mmHg and observed in 7% and 8.5% of dogs and cats, respectively), and cardiac arrhythmias (2.5% and 1.8% of dog and cats, respectively) [58]. Hosgood and Scholl [5,10] reported similar levels of arrhythmias in a teaching hospital environment, with 4% of dogs and 3.6% of cats exhibiting cardiac arrhythmias. The arrhythmias recorded included premature ventricular contractions, sick sinus syndrome, second-degree atrioventricular block, and ventricular tachycardia. Bradycardia (heart rate < 50 beats/min) was reported in approximately 36% and hypotension (mean arterial blood pressure < 60 mmHg, or systolic arterial blood pressure < 90 mmHg) in nearly 38% of dogs anesthetized at a veterinary school hospital in Spain [65].

Regurgitation was the most frequently documented perioperative gastrointestinal complication. The risk of regurgitation in dogs without pre-existing predisposing disease has been reported in some studies to be between 0.42% and 0.74% [66–68], whereas another report documented a substantially greater risk of regurgitation (5.5%) [69]. In a more recent study of geriatric dogs undergoing anesthesia, the risk of postoperative regurgitation was estimated to be 1.9% [70]. The variation in frequency across these studies likely reflects differences in procedures performed, premedication and anesthetic drugs and doses used, and the dog populations studied. The risk of gastroesophageal reflux, which may result in substantial esophageal mucosa injury, has been reported at a much higher level of 16–17% and even up to 27–60%, again depending on the animals studied and anesthetic drugs administered, suggesting that the risk of mucosal injury may be much greater than the proportion of patients where regurgitation is observed [66,67,69,71,72].

Hypothermia, when temperature is monitored, is a particularly common complication. In a veterinary teaching hospital study, 85% of dogs had a temperature recorded perioperatively of less than 37.3 °C and 51% of cats had a body temperature less than 35.0 °C during or after anesthesia [5,10]. Work in a veterinary university hospital in Spain highlighted perioperative hypothermia in over 70% of cats and 32% of dogs (body temperature < 36.5 °C) [64,73], and in a recent intervention study, perioperative hypothermia (body temperature < 36.0 °C) was observed in 36% of dogs and cats under routine perioperative management [74].

Poor recoveries have also been documented, often recorded as prolonged return to consciousness, and these were seen in 0.14–0.18% of dog and cat anesthetics in one study [4]. A smaller number of dogs and cats exhibited complications including excitement in recovery, collapse, prolonged hypothermia, reduced consciousness after an apparently normal recovery, and renal failure [4].

Further, occasional case reports of perioperative blindness have been published, but there are limited data on the frequency of this complication relative to the number of animals anesthetized [75,76]. Interestingly, the use of a mouth gag was reported in 16 of 20 cats observed with postanesthetic cortical blindness, although data relating to a comparative proportion of cats where the use of a mouth gag was observed but that had no evidence of blindness were not available, limiting the ability to conclude an association between the use of a gag or a procedure and the development of blindness [76]. Feline cortical blindness and possible etiology are discussed in more detail in Chapter 50.

Large animal anesthesia morbidity

A range of non-fatal complications has been reported, although information on their frequency in general equine populations is limited. Cardiovascular compromise, as reported in small animal anesthesia, is a major consideration in equine anesthesia. Hypotension and brady- and tachyarrhythmias have been described. In particular, second-degree atrioventricular block, atrial fibrillation, and ventricular premature contractions have all been reported [77]. Respiratory morbid complications have centered on hypoventilation, hypercapnia, and hypoxemia, and these have frequently been reported as potential complications of equine anesthesia [77,78]. In a more recent single-center study undertaken in France in 2019, cardiovascular and respiratory complications remained important perioperative considerations, representing 36% of all non-fatal complications [18].

In contrast to small animals, horses appear to demonstrate a wider range of postoperative complications, including fractures and soft tissue injury, myopathy, neuropathy, and myelopathy, with many resulting in death or euthanasia [77]. There are limited data on the frequency of these events in larger multicenter studies when non-fatal, although evidence of these complications resulting in mortality highlights their importance. Fractures have been reported intermittently and have often resulted in euthanasia. In the Confidential Enquiry into Perioperative Equine Fatalities (CEPEF), a multicenter prospective study of complications in equine anesthesia, fractures were estimated to be the cause of 25% of anesthetic deaths, myopathy 7%, and central nervous system complications 5.5% [60]. Similarly, in a single-center study in Kentucky in the United States (US), fractures were the cause of 19% of deaths or reason for euthanasia, and neuropathy and myopathy were the cause of 7% [79]. In the French single-center study, neuromuscular complications were the most common non-fatal event, accounting for 47% of non-fatal complications, and included evidence of neuropathy, myopathy, and wounds [18].

Other complications reported included postanesthetic colic, which in a multicenter study in the UK was estimated at approximately 5% of all anesthetized horses [80]. Two single-center studies reported that a similar number of horses (approximately 8–10%) developed colic within 7 days of general anesthesia [81,82], while in another single-center study, the incidence of postanesthetic colic for adult horses anesthetized for elective, non-abdominal procedures was estimated at 2.5% [83].

Small animal anesthetic mortality

Risk of anesthetic death

Mortality, in contrast to morbidity, has been reported extensively in the veterinary literature. In small animal anesthesia, the risk of death has been documented over the last 75 years [84], and trends in the reduction of risk over time have been reported (see Table 2.2). Referral-center- and university-based studies have generally reported higher death risks, potentially due to the nature of their patients and procedures, whereas practice-based studies tended to reflect healthier populations and simpler procedures. Direct comparison of risks of death between studies has been limited by a number of factors, including variations in study case definitions, study populations, and procedures performed.

Table 2.2 Summary risks of anesthetic death in dogs and cats published in primary practice, referral practice, and institutional studies.

Location [Reference]	Year(s)	Institution or practice	Risk of anesthetic death (%)	
			Dog	Cat
Angell Memorial AH, Boston, US [85]	1946–50	Institution	0.26	0.36
CSU, Colorado, US [86]	1955–57	Institution	1.08	1.79
Wheatridge AH, Colorado, US [86]	1960–69	Institution	0.23	0.40
Univ. Missouri VH, Missouri, US [86]	1968–69	Institution	0.8	0.53
CSU, Colorado, US [87]	1979–81	Institution	0.43	0.26
CSU, Colorado, US [58]	1993–94	Institution	0.43	0.35
LSU, Louisiana, US[a] [5,10]	1995–96	Institution	1.49	5.80
RVC, London, UK [6]	1999–2002	Institution	0.58	–
Scotland, UK [90]	1975	Primary practice	–	0.31
Vermont, US [91]	1989	Primary practice	0.11	0.06
UK [3]	1984–86	Primary practice	0.23	0.29
Ontario, Canada [4]	1993	Primary practice	0.11	0.10
Finland [92]	1993	Primary practice	0.13 in small animals	
South Africa [62]	1999	Primary practice	0.08 in dogs and cats	
UK [7]	2002–04	Primary practice	0.17	0.24
Spain [11]	2007–08	Primary practice	1.39 in dogs and cats	
France [12]	2008–10	Referral practice	1.35 in dogs and cats	
France [88]	2010–2011	Referral practice	0.8 in dogs and cats	
Japan [89]	2010–2011	Referral practice	0.65	–
US [13]	2010–2013	Primary practice	0.05	0.11
UK [14]	2010–2013	Primary practice	0.10	–
US [93]	2010–2016	Primary practice (spay-neuter clinic)	0.009	0.05

CSU, Colorado State University; AH, Animal Hospital; VH, Veterinary Hospital; LSU, Louisiana State University; RVC, Royal Veterinary College; US, United States; UK, United Kingdom.
[a] All reported perioperative deaths, not just anesthetic-related mortality.

Initial institution-based studies from the US documented a wide range of relatively high risks of mortality. An early study at the Angell Memorial Animal Hospital in Boston, Massachusetts published risks of anesthetic death of 0.26% in dogs, 0.36% in cats, and 5% in other species [85]. Colorado State University reported higher risks of 1.08% in dogs and 1.79% in cats between 1955 and 1957 [86], and the Wheatridge Animal Hospital in Colorado reported anesthetic death risks of 0.23% in dogs and 0.40% in cats between 1960 and 1969 [86]. At a similar time, the University of Missouri Veterinary Hospital reported mortality risks of 0.8% in dogs and 0.53% in cats [86]. More recent referral-center studies have reported lower risks of mortality, suggesting that outcomes have improved. Further work at Colorado State University documented risks of 0.43% in dogs and 0.26% in cats between 1979 and 1981 and 0.43% in dogs and 0.35% in cats between 1993 and 1994 [58,87]. Louisiana State University reported higher risks of perioperative death of 1.49% of dogs and 5.80% of cats at their institution between 1995 and 1996, although this related to all deaths, not just anesthetic-related mortality [5,10]. Work at the Royal Veterinary College in the UK reported an anesthetic-related mortality risk of 0.58% in dogs between 1999 and 2002 [6]. A subsequent single-center referral practice study in France estimated the risk of anesthetic death in dogs and cats combined at 1.4% between 2008 and 2010 [12], decreasing to 0.8% between 2010 and 2011 [88]. Consistent with the later dates of this work, a referral practice study from Japan estimated the risk between 2010 and 2011 at 0.65% in dogs [89]. Based on the more recent work described above, the risk of anesthetic-related death in the referral setting would appear to be of the order of 0.25–0.60% in dogs and cats.

Work undertaken in small animal primary practice has generally documented lower risks of mortality than referral and veterinary university hospital–based studies. An early practice-based study evaluated feline mortality in Scotland and published a risk of death of 0.31% in cats [90]. This was followed by a further survey of small animal anesthetic practice, undertaken in Vermont in the US, which reported the risk of death to be 0.11% and 0.06% in dogs and cats, respectively [91]. A similar study was undertaken in Finland in 1993 and reported a risk of death of 0.13% in small animals in general [92]. A retrospective study evaluated mortality in a South African practice population in 1999 and estimated a mortality risk of 0.08% in dogs and cats [62]. A private veterinary clinic in France reported an overall risk of anesthetic death of 1.35% but only 0.12% for healthy patients (ASA 1–2) [12]. The health status of the patients anesthetized in these studies was not always recorded, although it was likely to reflect relatively healthy animals consistent with the generally lower risks reported.

The first prospective multicenter cohort study of small animal practice complications was undertaken between 1984 and 1986 in the UK [3]. Fifty-three practices were recruited, 41,881 anesthetics were recorded, and anesthetic risks of death of 0.23% in dogs and 0.29% in cats were reported. For healthy patients (ASA grades 1–2; Table 2.1), the risk of death risk was 0.12% in dogs and 0.18% in cats, whereas in ill patients (ASA grades 3–5; Table 2.1), over 3% of dogs and cats died perioperatively. Perioperative deaths in healthy patients (ASA 1–2), occurring during or shortly after surgery, were considered primarily due to anesthesia unless an obvious surgical cause was present, whereas in sick patients (ASA 3–5), all deaths independent of cause were reported. This was followed by a further prospective multicenter cohort study of anesthetic mortality in small animal veterinary practices in Ontario, Canada [4]. During the 6-month study period, 8087 dogs and 8702 cats were anesthetized and 0.11% of dogs and 0.10% of cats had cardiac arrests and died. For healthy animals (ASA 1–2), the risks were 0.067% in dogs and 0.048% in cats, whereas for sick patients (ASA 3–5), 0.46% of dogs and 0.92% of cats died of a cardiac arrest. Only perioperative deaths within an unspecified follow-up period resulting from cardiac arrest were included.

The largest multicenter, small-animal-practice-based study, the Confidential Enquiry into Perioperative Small Animal Fatalities (CEPSAF), was undertaken in the UK between 2002 and 2004, and 98,036 anesthetics and sedations were recorded in dogs and 79,178 in cats, across 117 participating centers [7]. *Anesthetic-* and *sedation-related death* was defined as perioperative death within 48 h of termination of the procedure, except where death was due solely to inoperable surgical or pre-existing medical conditions (i.e., anesthesia and sedation could not be reasonably excluded from contributing to the death). The risk of anesthetic and sedation-related death was approximately 0.17% in dogs and 0.24% in cats (Tables 2.2 and 2.3). In healthy patients (ASA 1–2), the risks were 0.05% and 0.11% in dogs and cats, respectively, whereas in sick patients (ASA 3–5), over 1% of dogs and cats died.

Other small animal species were also evaluated within CEPSAF. Rabbits were the third most commonly anesthetized species

Table 2.3 Anesthetic- and sedation-related risk of death in small animals in CEPSAF.

Species	Number of anesthetic- and sedation-related deaths	Number of anesthetized and sedated patients	Risk of anesthetic-related death (%) (95% confidence interval, %)
Dog	163	98,036	0.17 (0.14–0.19)
Cat	189	79,178	0.24 (0.20–0.27)
Rabbit	114	8209	1.39 (1.14–1.64)
Guinea Pig	49	1288	3.80 (2.76–4.85)
Hamsters	9	246	3.66 (1.69–6.83)
Chinchilla	11	334	3.29 (1.38–5.21)
Rat	8	398	2.01 (0.87–3.92)

CEPSAF, Confidential Enquiry into Perioperative Small Animal Fatalities.
Source: Adapted from Brodbelt *et al.* [7].

in practice, but the risk of anesthetic-related death was substantially higher, with 0.73% of healthy rabbits and 7.37% of sick rabbits dying. The risks in other small animal species were also high, between 1% and 4% (Table 2.3). These risks are comparable to subsequent work. In a single-center study in the UK based on 185 rabbits being anesthetized between 2009 and 2016, the risk of death was 4.8% [94]. Similarly, one of the few studies to evaluate the risk of anesthetic death in birds reported an anesthetic-related risk of 3.9% [95].

Subsequently, a further prospective study was undertaken within 39 Spanish veterinary clinics between 2007 and 2008 and recorded data from 2012 anesthetics. *Anesthetic death* was defined as perioperative death within 24 h of the procedure, and a risk of death of 1.29% overall was reported, with risks in healthy dogs and cats of 0.33% and in sick animals 4.06% [11]. Two further multicenter primary practice studies have followed, one in the US and one in the UK, that evaluated the risk of death between 2010 and 2013. Both studies utilized electronic health record data from participating practices. The US study, reporting on 822 practices within a large corporate group, defined *anesthetic death* as death where anesthesia could not be reasonably ruled out as contributing to the death [13]. They estimated the risks of death within 7 days of anesthesia from an anesthetized population of just over 4 million dogs and 1 million cats at 0.05% and 0.11%, respectively. In the UK study, *anesthetic death* was defined similarly to the previous study, and from a population of over 150,000 dogs, the risk within 48 h was 0.10% [14]. For neuter procedures, the UK study estimated a risk of anesthetic death, in just under 90,000 dogs, at 0.006% within 48 h of the procedure. This was comparable to a subsequent single-center high-volume clinic in the US which neutered over 40,000 dogs and 70,000 cats between 2010 and 2016 and reported risks of anesthetic death at 0.009% in dogs and 0.05% in cats [93].

In summary, estimates of anesthetic death risks in primary practice are of the order of 0.05–0.25%, although in some circumstances, this may be higher, with the risk in healthy dogs and cats being approximately 0.05–0.20% and in sick dogs and cats 1–4% [3,4,7,11,12,62,91]. Cats appeared to be at greater risk of death than dogs in some work [3,7], and rabbits and other companion animal species appeared to be at even higher risk where studied [7,94,95]. In referral institutions, mortality ranged from 0.30% to 0.60% in dogs and cats [5–7,10,58].

Causes of anesthetic death

The physiologic cause of many anesthetic deaths may be multifactorial, although cardiovascular and respiratory complications represent the primary causes of many perioperative deaths reported.

Other causes reported include gastrointestinal, neurological, and hepatic- or renal-related deaths. Cardiac arrest has been reported to result from cardiac arrhythmias associated with increased circulating catecholamines, myocardial hypoxia, specific anesthetic agents, pre-existing pathology, specific procedures (e.g., vagal traction and enucleation), and myocardial depression due to relative anesthetic overdose [40,96]. Between 30% and 70% of deaths resulted from relative anesthetic overdose and myocardial depression, cardiac arrhythmias or circulatory failure, and hypovolemia in a number of studies [3–5,62,87]. Halothane, ether, and thiobarbiturate anesthesia were frequently associated with anesthetic overdose in earlier work [3,91]. Dogs more frequently had cardiovascular complications than cats in one study, and high-risk patients were the most likely patients to die from circulatory failure, often when hypovolemic [3].

Respiratory complications represented the other main cause of anesthetic-related death. Respiratory complications were an underlying cause of death in 30–40% of dogs and about 40–50% of cats [3,4,87]. Problems related to endotracheal intubation and respiratory obstruction represented the majority of feline respiratory causes of death [3,4]. In dogs, complications with endotracheal intubation and respiratory failure were equally reported, although in brachycephalic dogs, respiratory obstruction was the principal cause of respiratory complications [3,4,91].

In small animal anesthesia, causes other than respiratory and cardiovascular complications have infrequently been reported, but have included postoperative renal failure, iliac thrombosis in cats, aspiration of gastric contents, anaphylactic reactions, failure to regain consciousness, and unknown causes [3,4,62,91]. The unknown causes, often arising when patients were not being closely watched, represented approximately 5–20% of patients.

Timing of death

The timing of anesthetic deaths has varied, with more recent studies increasingly highlighting the postoperative period. Albrecht and Blakely [85] reported in an early study only one death during induction and one during recovery, with the remainder of the deaths occurring during maintenance of anesthesia. In contrast, work at Colorado State University in the 1950s reported that of 36 dog and cat deaths, 17% occurred during induction, 22% during maintenance, and interestingly the majority (61%) during recovery [86]. However, later work at Colorado (1979–1981) reported mostly intraoperative deaths [87], and work there in the 1990s reported that only approximately 25% of dogs and cats died during recovery, with the rest dying during anesthesia [58]. Other referral institutions reported differing high-risk periods; Hosgood and Scholl [5,10] documented that 9 of 14 (61%) deaths in dogs and 4 of 7 (57%) in cats occurred postoperatively, and more recently, a multicenter referral practice study from Japan reported that over 80% of deaths occurred postoperatively [89].

In the primary practice setting, only the larger studies quantified the timing of fatalities. Clarke and Hall [3] reported deaths occurring principally during anesthesia. In dogs, 22% died on induction of anesthesia, 55% during maintenance, and 18% in recovery, whereas in cats, 30% died during induction, 39% during anesthesia, and 31% during recovery. Similarly, in the study in Ontario, Canada [4], most dogs and cats died during anesthesia (6/9 dogs and 7/8 cats) and only 33% and 13% of dogs and cats, respectively, died postoperatively (3/9 dogs and 1/8 cats). More recently, CEPSAF highlighted the postoperative period as the most common time for dogs, cats, and rabbits to die [7]. Over 60% of cats and rabbits and nearly 50% of dogs died during this time period (see Table 2.4).

Table 2.4 Timing of death in dogs, cats, and rabbits in CEPSAF.

Timing of death	Dogs	Cats	Rabbits
After premedication	1 (1%)	2 (1%)	0
Induction of anesthesia	9 (6%)	14 (8%)	6 (6%)
Maintenance of anesthesia	68 (46%)	53 (30%)	29 (30%)
Postoperative death[a]	70 (47%)	106 (61%)	62 (64%)
0–3 h postoperative	31	66	26
3–6 h postoperative	11	9	7
6–12 h postoperative	12	7	13
12–24 h postoperative	13	12	9
24–48 h postoperative	3	10	3
Unknown time	0	2	4
Total[b]	148 (100%)	175 (100%)	97 (100%)

CEPSAF, Confidential Enquiry into Perioperative Small Animal Fatalities.
[a] Postoperative deaths were additionally categorized by time after anesthesia. Shown as number (% of cases).
[b] Only deaths where detailed information on time of death was available were included here.
Source: Brodbelt *et al.* [7], with permission of Elsevier.

Notably, most of these postoperative deaths occurred within 3 h of termination of the procedure, suggesting that increased vigilance, particularly in the early postoperative period, could reduce the risk of death. Subsequent to this study, work in Spain further highlighted the postoperative period with over 75% of dogs dying after anesthesia in this multipractice study [11].

These findings are supported by the most recent large-scale primary practice studies from the US and the UK. The US study reporting on over 4 million dog and 1 million cat anesthetic events identified over 50% of cat and 70% of dog deaths occurred either soon after anesthesia or after discharge [13]. In the UK study from a population of 150,000 dogs undergoing anesthetic events, of the 218 deaths recorded, more than 75% died after anesthesia [14]. Similarly, in a US study from a high-volume neutering practice, over 60% of cat deaths (21/34) and 100% of dog deaths (4/4) occurred postoperatively [93]. Hence, the postoperative period is increasingly recognized as a high-risk time and close monitoring and patient management until full recovery is recommended.

Risk factors for anesthetic death

Early institution-based studies suggested contributory factors without providing in-depth analysis of risk factors [85,86]. The use of specific drugs was associated with higher mortality in dogs and cats, and trauma patients, neutering procedures, certain breeds including brachycephalic, terrier, and spaniel breeds in dogs were frequently represented among the fatalities [85–87]. Old age and poor health status were associated with increased odds of mortality in dogs and poor health status only in cats in a subsequent referral-based study [5,10]. Work at the Royal Veterinary College also reported poor health status as increasing odds and additionally premedication with acepromazine being associated with reduced odds of death in dogs [6]. Although they identified important risk factors, all of these studies were single-center referral studies with small sample sizes and limited abilities to detect more than a small number of major risk factors.

Early practice-based work was also limited in its ability to evaluate risk factors. Dodman [90] identified a trend to reduced risk with thiopental (thiopentone)–halothane anesthesia relative to other drugs in feline anesthetic practice at that time. In a later study, Dodman and Lamb [91] identified high risk with xylazine administration and for brachycephalic breeds, although in both of these studies, quantification of risk factors was limited. Clarke and Hall identified a number of risk factors for anesthetic death in healthy dogs and cats [3]. Higher risks were seen with administration of the α_2-adrenergic receptor agonist xylazine and reduced risk with premedication with atropine or acepromazine. In cats, endotracheal intubation, induction of anesthesia with a volatile agent, thiopental, methohexital (methohexitone), ketamine, halothane, ether, and nitrous oxide use were also associated with higher risks of death and administration of alfaxalone–alfadolone (Saffan®) with lower risks, although statistical comparisons were not made. In dogs, Pekingese were the most commonly reported breed to die. Administration of xylazine was associated with higher risk of death, whereas halothane and thiopental use was associated with lower death risks. The Ontario study identified similar risk factors with xylazine administration and sick patients (ASA 3–5) being at increased odds of cardiac arrest in dogs, whereas in cats, sick patients (ASA 3–5) were at greater risk, while the presence of a technician monitoring anesthesia reduced the risk [4]. A study at a single center in France also highlighted increased risk with poor health status [12], and this was supported by a multicenter study in Spain [11].

More recently, in CEPSAF, within larger study populations, a number of risk factors were evaluated within multivariable regression models for cats and dogs [8,9]. In cats, increasing ASA grade, procedural urgency, major versus minor intended procedures, increasing age, extremes of weight, endotracheal intubation, and the use of fluid therapy were associated with increased odds of anesthetic- and sedation-related death (Table 2.5) [8]. Pulse and pulse oximetry monitoring were associated with a reduction in odds. In dogs, poorer health status (based on ASA grade), greater procedural urgency, major versus minor intended procedures, old age, and low weight were associated with anesthetic-related death. Additionally, increasing duration of the procedure and the anesthetic induction and maintenance combination used were associated with increased odds of anesthetic-related death. Maintenance with halothane after induction of anesthesia with an injectable anesthetic agent and dogs undergoing total inhalational anesthesia were both associated with an approximately sixfold increase in odds compared with isoflurane maintenance after induction of anesthesia with an injectable anesthetic agent [9].

The association between patient health status (ASA grade) and anesthetic-related death was repeatedly documented in many of the studies described above [3–12,14] and has been reviewed within a systematic review [42]. Pre-existing pathology may reduce the therapeutic index of administered anesthetics, predispose to cardiopulmonary depression, and depress other physiologic functions significantly. Additionally, in CEPSAF, procedural urgency was associated with increased odds of death [8,9]. This finding was supported by a later multicenter primary practice study, where non-elective and urgent procedures were at a substantially elevated risk [13]. Interestingly, in the US practice study, lack of evidence of a preanesthetic physical examination was associated with substantially increased odds in dogs [13]. Hence, greater attention to preoperative assessment and stabilization of the patient prior to the procedure could substantially reduce fatalities.

Increased risk with increasing age, independent of patient physical status (ASA grade), have been identified as an important risk factor, but not all small animal studies have reported this [5,8,9]. The most recent US and UK primary practice studies did, however, support this finding, and in particular, in the recent UK study, dogs over 9 years were more than 12 times more likely to die than those between 0.5 and 1.5 years of age [13,14]. Old patients may be more susceptible to the depressant effects of anesthetics, to hypothermia via impaired thermoregulatory mechanisms, and to prolonged recovery due to tendencies to reduced metabolic function and hypothermia [97–99].

Increased odds of death reported for small dogs and cats in CEPSAF [8,9] were consistent with work in pediatric anesthesia [100]. Smaller patients could be more prone to drug overdose, to hypothermia, and to perioperative management difficulties (e.g., intravenous catheter placement and endotracheal intubation). Increased risk with increasing weight seen in cats within CEPSAF likely reflected,

Table 2.5 Multivariable model of risk factors for anesthetic- and sedation-related death in cats in CEPSAF.

Risk factor	Categories	Odds ratio[a]	95% Confidence interval (%)	*P* value
Health status (ASA grade[b])	ASA 4–5 versus ASA 3 versus ASA 1–2 (trend[c])	3.2	2.0–5.0	< 0.001
Urgency of procedure	Emergent versus urgent versus scheduled (trend[c])	1.6	1.0–2.5	0.050
Intended procedure	Minor procedure	1		
	Major procedure	2.7	1.4–5.4	0.005
Age	0–0.5 years	0.4	0.1–2.4	0.058
	0.5–5 years	1		
	5–12 years	1.7	0.9–3.0	
	12 years and older	2.1	1.1–3.9	
Weight	0–2 kg	15.7	2.9–83.6	
	2–6 kg	1		
	6 kg and above	2.8	1.1–7.4	
	Unknown	1.1	0.2–5.5	0.002
Endotracheal (ET) intubation	No ET tube	1		
	ET tube	1.9	1.0–3.7	0.042
Pulse assessment and use of pulse oximeter	None	1		
	Pulse assessed only	0.3	0.2–0.6	
	Pulse oximeter used only	0.2	0.1–0.5	
	Pulse and pulse oximeter	0.2	0.1–0.4	< 0.001
Perioperative intravenous (IV) fluid administration	No fluids given	1		
	IV catheter used only	0.7	0.2–2.5	
	IV fluids given	3.9	2.2–7.1	< 0.001

CEPSAF, Confidential Enquiry into Perioperative Small Animal Fatalities; ASA, American Society of Anesthesiologists.
[a] Odds ratios greater than 1.0 indicate increased odds whereas odds ratios less than 1.0 indicate reduced odds of anesthetic-related death.
[b] ASA grade definitions: ASA 1–2, healthy/moderate disease only; ASA 3, severe disease limiting activity; ASA 4–5, life-threatening disease.
[c] Trend represents the odds ratio for a one-category increase in the risk factor.
Source: Adapted from Brodbelt *et al.* [8].

at least in part, risks associated with obesity, and this was supported by the recent US practice study where increased body weight was associated with increased odds of death [8,13].

The association of breed with anesthetic death for dogs was inconclusive in CEPSAF. There was a tendency toward a breed association in CEPSAF, but after adjusting for weight, this association dropped out. This suggested that a major aspect of the risk associated with breed could be related to animal size [9]. In earlier work, increased complications were observed with brachycephalic and terrier breeds, though the ability to demonstrate statistical associations was limited due to small study sample sizes [3,4,86]. The more recent UK study did explore breed as a risk factor. In the latter, only Rottweilers and West Highland White terriers were identified as at increased risk of death compared to crossbred dogs [14]. However, evaluating breed as a risk factor remains challenging due to most studies having limited power to evaluate individual breed types. A recent US study evaluated perioperative complications for a group of brachycephalic compared to non-brachycephalic dogs and identified increased risk of both intraoperative and postoperative complications, though no deaths were reported [101]. A subsequent US university hospital study explored further the risks of anesthetic death in brachycephalic and non-brachycephalic breeds and identified anesthetic death risks of 3.9% (9 deaths), 0.9% (2 deaths), and 0% in English Bulldogs, other brachycephalic dogs, and non-brachycephalic dogs, respectively [102]. The study suggested an increased risk in Bulldogs but was underpowered to identify a statistical difference. Nonetheless, given the increasing evidence of perioperative complications and predisposition to specific pathology types, caution with the anesthesia of these breeds may be advisable.

Increasing risk for patients presenting for major procedures, as documented in CEPSAF [8,9], was consistent with work in equine anesthesia [16,60]. This association was supported by the more recent UK primary practice study, where less complex surgery, neuter surgery in particular, was associated with lower risk [14]. More complex and invasive procedures were likely to impose greater stress on patient physiology, and when assessing patient risk prior to anesthesia, assessment of the procedure's complexity should be considered. Increasing duration, in addition to type of procedure, was associated with increased risk in dogs in CEPSAF [9]. More recently, longer duration was also associated with increased hospitalization cost in a single-center institutional study and in another single-center study, increased risk of gastroesophageal reflux, suggesting complication rates are likely to be higher for longer procedures [72,103]. Longer procedures could expose the patient to extended periods of physiologic compromise, increased hypothermia and fluid loss, slower recovery, and could be expected to predispose to greater risk to a range of complications [40]. The previously unreported association of increased risk of death associated with fluid therapy administration in cats in CEPSAF was surprising [8]. Although this may have reflected in part residual confounding, a component of the increased odds may have been related to excessive administration of fluids and fluid overload. Careful fluid administration and monitoring are recommended in cats, although further work is needed to confirm this observation.

The reduction in odds of anesthetic-related death with pulse and pulse oximetry monitoring in cats in CEPSAF has not been reported previously in small animals [8]. Theoretical analyses in human anesthesia support these findings and have suggested that pulse oximetry would have detected 40–82% of reported perioperative incidents, and when combined with capnography, this increases to 88–93% [104–106]. Further, the recent US primary practice study identified the lack of use of pulse oximetry as a risk factor for anesthetic death in cats [13]. These associations suggest that some form of assessment of cardiovascular function (pulse quality and rate) and respiratory function (oxygen saturation and end-tidal CO_2) may be important in minimizing mortality.

The role of specific anesthetic drugs in anesthetic death has been evaluated in a number of small animal studies. The premedication administered was a risk factor in a number of studies in dogs and cats [3,4,6]. Early work had identified acepromazine as being associated with reduced odds of death [3,6] and major morbid complications [4], compared with no premedication, whereas the α_2-adrenergic receptor agonist xylazine was associated with increased odds of death [3,4]. In CEPSAF, although there were trends to reduced odds with the administration of acepromazine, after adjustment for major confounders, this was not a major factor in dogs or cats. Further, when evaluating premedication with the α_2-adrenergic receptor agonist medetomidine, no increased odds of death was detected [8,9]. Xylazine has been found to reduce the threshold to catecholamine-induced arrhythmias under halothane anesthesia [107,108] whereas medetomidine did not [109]. This difference, combined with a greater awareness of the physiologic effects and a better understanding of the optimal method of administration of α_2-adrenergic receptor agonists, may be the basis of a lack of increased risk with medetomidine compared with acepromazine observed in CEPSAF.

The specific induction agent used did not appear important in CEPSAF, in contrast to the tendency for increased risk with the use of thiopental and ketamine and lower risk with alfaxalone–alfadolone (Saffan®) in cats and thiopental in dogs in the previous UK study [3,8,9]. The lack of a consistent difference in risks with different induction agents likely reflects that the effect of induction agent was small. The maintenance agent used, however, was relevant to dogs in CEPSAF, and isoflurane appeared to be associated with reduced odds compared with halothane after induction of anesthesia with an injectable anesthetic agent. This is supported by clinical studies indicating that, although isoflurane induces greater respiratory depression and vasodilation than halothane, it is associated with less direct myocardial depression and less sensitization of the heart to catecholamine-induced arrhythmias, and on balance would appear to cause less overall cardiovascular depression [110–119]. Further work evaluating the risks with other inhalational agents would be merited.

In summary, several studies have critically evaluated risk factors for death [3–14]. Commonly reported risk factors for death included poor health status, old age, poor monitoring, endotracheal intubation in cats, and possible breed associations in dogs [4–6, 8–10,13,14]. Additionally, CEPSAF and subsequent studies identified a number of further risk factors including major procedures, urgent and non-elective anesthesia, and longer duration procedures as being associated with increased risk; while in cats, the monitoring of anesthesia with pulse oximetry was associated with reduced odds of death [8,9,13,14]. Awareness of these risk factors can aid veterinarians in preoperatively identifying those patients at greatest risk of mortality and instituting appropriate perioperative management practices to reduce mortality.

Large animal anesthetic mortality

Risk of anesthetic death

Work in large animals has concentrated on equine anesthetic complications. Earlier studies focused principally on referral institution populations, and death risks were most frequently divided into elective and emergency populations, with the latter principally representing acute abdominal or colic surgery. Mitchell [120] conducted a retrospective study at the Royal (Dick) Vet School in the UK between 1962 and 1968; 473 horses were anesthetized, and seven deaths occurred (1.47%). Short, at the University of Missouri in the US, reported a smaller retrospective study of 125 horses anesthetized, with no deaths [86]. Heath reported an overall single clinic perioperative equine mortality risk, between 1968 and 1970, at Colorado State University of 4.35% (13 deaths out of 295 anesthetics) [86]. The anesthetic death risk decreased to 1.69% when only anesthetic-related deaths were considered. In a follow-up study at Colorado State University, a reduced overall death risk of 1.18% was reported [87]. Many of these fatalities were due to horses undergoing emergency gastrointestinal surgery that were high-risk patients, and all of these studies were limited by their small sample size and could only reflect approximate estimates of the frequency of death.

Tevick [121] retrospectively identified a single clinic equine perioperative mortality risk of 2.70% over a 17-year period, but this was reduced to 0.8% when due to anesthesia alone. The majority of these deaths occurred within 24 h of anesthesia. Gastrointestinal surgery represented the major operation type in those that died, and the majority of these patients were deemed high-risk cases. Further single-center reports concentrated on specific hospital populations. Evaluating horses undergoing colic surgery, Trim *et al.* [122] conducted a single clinic retrospective survey and found a perioperative death risk of 12.5% within 3 days of anesthesia and 20% within 16 days. In contrast, Young and Taylor excluded gastrointestinal surgery and reported a lower single clinic death risk over a 7-year period of 0.68% [123,124]. Subsequently, the Liverpool Veterinary School in the UK reported mortality risks for both elective and emergency procedures in a retrospective single clinic study [125,126]. Of 2276 anesthetics, 1279 were classified as elective and 995 as emergency procedures. Horses were followed until discharged. Of the elective cases, eight died where anesthesia and surgery contributed to the death (0.63%), whereas one (0.078%) died solely due to anesthesia [125]. For non-colic emergencies, the surgical/anesthetic death risk was 2%, and for colic surgeries, it was 4.35% [126]. The overall surgical/anesthetic death risk for elective and emergency procedures was 2%. Subsequent to this, Bidwell *et al.* [79] reported reduced risks at another single center in Kentucky in the US. Of 17,961 horses anesthetized at the clinic between 1997 and 2001, 0.12% died with deaths classified as directly related to anesthesia and 0.24% died or were euthanized within 7 days. Two more recent single-center studies, one from France and one from the UK, reported updated risks of death. In the French study, based on 1161 horses anesthetized between 2012 and 2016, the overall anesthesia mortality rate was 1.4%, and for non-colic procedures, it was 0.96%, while in the UK study based on 1416 horses anesthetized between 2010 and 2013, anesthesia-related mortality was 1.1% for all cases, 0.9% for elective cases, and 1.6% for colic surgery [17,18]. These estimates were generally lower than earlier work, though were likely to reflect, at least in part, differences in populations studied and duration of procedures (most procedures were less than 1 h). All of these reports were single-center studies, the precision of some of their estimates was likely to be limited by their sample sizes, and the risks were highly specific to the populations anesthetized.

The first prospective multicenter perioperative cohort study of equine anesthesia, the Confidential Enquiry into Perioperative Equine Fatalities (CEPEF), was undertaken in the UK between 1991 and 1997 [59,60]. Of a total of 41,824 horses anesthetized, 39,025 were alive and 785 were dead 7 days postoperatively, giving a death risk of 1.89% [60]. When emergency abdominal surgery and delivery of foals were excluded, the death risk decreased to 0.90% [60]. This was followed by CEPEF 3, a randomized controlled trial of 8242 horses comparing isoflurane with halothane anesthesia [16]. Although representing maintenance of anesthesia with inhalation agents only, they reported similar risks to their previous work. An overall death risk of 1.61% was reported in horses, but when colic and other emergency surgery were excluded, a risk of approximately 0.9% was reported. In both of these studies, *perioperative death* was defined as unexpected death or euthanasia for perioperative complications within 7 days of anesthesia. Subsequent to these studies, a further phase, CEPEF 4, conducted via internet-based data collection, has been undertaken, and based on data from 8656 procedures, the study reported a reduced overall mortality risk of 1.0%; 3.4% for colic surgery and 0.6% for non-colic procedures [127].

In summary, overall anesthetic death risks of approximately 1.0–1.5%, decreasing among non-emergency horses to approximately 0.9–0.6, have been reported [16,17,59,60,79,123–125,127]. Emergency anesthetics had a death risk of nearer 3.5% or above [59,60,122,126].

Causes of anesthetic death

In equine anesthesia, cardiac arrest and cardiovascular collapse were major causes of death, resulting in 20–50% of all reported deaths [59,60,121,123–127]. Respiratory complications, in contrast, were infrequently reported. Although Tevik [121] did not distinguish respiratory from cardiovascular causes, which when combined accounted for all ten anesthetic deaths described, other studies have reported less than 25% of all deaths as resulting from respiratory compromise [59,60,123–126]. Johnston *et al.* [59,60] documented that only 4% of deaths resulted from respiratory problems.

Non-cardiopulmonary causes have been reported as the cause of death or euthanasia in up to 77% of all equine fatalities [16,59,60,121,123–126]. Johnston *et al.* [59,60] attributed death in 55% of all cases to fractures on recovery, postoperative myopathy, and abdominal complications such as sepsis and colitis. Young and Taylor [124] reported deaths due to postoperative myopathy and fractures in seven of nine deaths, whereas Bidwell *et al.* [79] reported fractures and myopathy as the basis of over 50% of anesthetic deaths at their center. More recent single-center studies have supported this, with myopathy and fractures representing 50–70% of anesthetic deaths [18]. Following on from CEPEF 1 and 2, CEPEF 4 reported just over 42% of non-colic anesthetic deaths were due to fractures on recovery and spinal cord malacia [127]. Rarely have horses been reported to be found dead or dying of unknown cause, perhaps because horses are more closely observed on recovery than many small animal patients. Johnston *et al.* classified only 5% of equine fatalities as found dead [60].

Timing of anesthetic death

Consistent with work in small animals, recent work in equine anesthesia has also highlighted the postoperative period as a major period of risk. Johnston *et al.* [59,60] reported over 44% of deaths as postoperative events. Young and Taylor [124] reported postoperative fatalities in seven of nine deaths. In another single clinic study, over 50% of 22 deaths classified as related to anesthesia occurred postoperatively [79]. In the two recent single-center studies of 14 and 16 anesthetic deaths reported, 88 to 100% were seen to occur during recovery [17,18]. Similarly, in CEPEF 4, of 35 non-colic anesthetic deaths reported, over 85% occurred postoperatively [127]. Hence, although intraoperative concerns remain important, close attention to the postoperative period is also merited in equine anesthesia.

Risk factors for anesthetic death

A number of single-center retrospective studies identified risk factors associated with perioperative complications in horses. In studies undertaken at Colorado State University, anesthetic overdose was considered a major cause of death or euthanasia, and many fatalities were associated with emergency gastrointestinal surgery and high-risk status [86,87]. Tevick [121] identified gastrointestinal surgery as the principal operation type in those horses that died, and the majority of these were deemed high-risk cases. Among horses undergoing acute emergency abdominal surgery, long duration of anesthesia and intraoperative hypotension were associated with increased risk of death in a further single-center retrospective study [122]. When factors were evaluated in non-colic horses, similar risk factors were identified [123,124].

Intraoperative fluids and inotropic support were associated with reduced risk of fatal myopathy, whereas long procedures and old age were associated with increased risk of death or myopathy. Subsequent work evaluated both elective and emergency procedures in a further retrospective single clinic study [125,126]. High ASA grade in the elective cases (e.g., elective exploratory laparotomy for colic) was associated with increased risk of death, and among emergency patients, acute abdominal surgery (i.e., colic surgery) was associated with increased risk.

The prospective multicenter cohort undertaken by Johnston *et al.* [59,60] evaluated risk factors more thoroughly in a large population of anesthetized horses. They identified anesthesia of pregnant mares, foals, horses undergoing abdominal surgery, orthopedic cases requiring internal fixation, long operation time, positioning in dorsal recumbency, lack of sedation, and the use of xylazine as a premedicant with increased risk. Acepromazine premedication and total intravenous anesthesia were associated with reduced risk. The subsequent phase of the work, a randomized clinical trial of isoflurane and halothane for maintenance of anesthesia, reported similar findings [16]. In general, no difference in outcome between the two inhalant anesthetics was found, but in horses aged 2–5 years, isoflurane was associated with reduced odds. In both treatment groups, increased risk was seen with orthopedic and emergency abdominal surgery, whereas reduced risk occurred with monitoring of blood pressure, and with ear, nose, and throat, and urogenital surgery.

The CEPEF multicenter work has been uniquely powered and able to quantify specific risk factors and drug associations [16,59,60], but the patterns are similar to those reported in the other equine studies. Subsequent work has also highlighted similar trends, though has been based on smaller sample sizes limiting detailed risk factor analyses. Dugdale *et al.* in the UK [17] reported univariable associations of ASA physical status, dorsal recumbency, anesthetic maintenance agent, colic surgery, and duration as all being associated with mortality. Similarly, Laurenza [18] in their single-center French study, identified, in a multivariable model, ASA physical status and procedure as associated with mortality and additionally horse weight, surgeon experience, and the use of dobutamine as statistically significant risk factors.

The work in equine anesthesia indicates risk factors similar to those published in other species. In particular, emergency, abdominal, and orthopedic surgery, longer operations, and poor health status were commonly reported factors associated with death. In addition, risks associated with specific anesthetic agents have been addressed with CEPEF 1 and 2, in particular highlighting a number of associations. Further work is merited to build on these in the multicenter setting.

Informed consent

Informed client consent is the ethical and legal foundation upon which healthcare professionals deliver care and service. In addition to furnishing the anesthesia provider with information that informs available risk management strategies that may be assigned to treatments or interventions, knowledge and communication of perianesthetic risk is an essential component in the process of informed owner consent. In conversation with the anesthesia provider, an owner presented with an evidence-informed assessment of the significant risks associated with a proposed procedure for their animal is guided to a point of decision-making where they can consent to accept the risk or refuse consent because of perceived unmitigable risk. This process of obtaining informed owner consent or refusal involves a conversation between the owner and the anesthesia provider centering on a discussion of relevant and significant risks. At a time where information of varied credibility is readily accessible by the public, animal owners can seek out anesthesia care with existing conceptions of anesthesia-related risk. The possibility of such preconceptions indicates the heightened need for a discussion of risk with the client.

The legal underpinnings of an informed consent conversation generally require that consent be obtained from the owner of an animal that is being treated, an authorized representative of the owner, a valid substitute decision-maker, someone who holds a valid power of attorney for property, a representative of an organization that is legally qualified to make treatment decisions for the animal, or, at the very least, someone who the care provider determines is acting in the interest of the animal. How these elements are defined and enacted will vary from jurisdiction to jurisdiction. In conjunction with determining whether an individual is legally qualified to make the necessary treatment decisions, before entering into an informed consent conversation, the care provider will also need to formulate an opinion about the decision-maker's capacity to make an informed decision based on such factors as cognitive ability or health literacy.

Included in an informed consent discussion will be an acknowledgment of the extra-label use of drugs, if any. The process of veterinary anesthesia frequently involves the extra-label use of drugs of which the client should be informed. In many cases, the extra-label use of a drug is associated with low-level risk, and consent for such use of each drug is impractical. Rather, a blanket acknowledgment and brief discussion of the well-documented, low-level risk of extra-label use of these drugs can be made. In instances where extra-label use is not associated with significant precedence and the unknown risks may be more significant, informed consent for the specific use of this particular drug should be obtained.

With the expansion of multicentric clinical research in veterinary medicine, clinical anesthesia providers may be faced with the additional task of gathering informed consent from clients whose animals are candidates for enrollment in clinical investigations. In this realm, in addition to providing the owner with the ability to provide, refuse, or withdraw consent at any time, the informed consent conversation must be structured so that the owner's agency in providing consent is maintained and hierarchical imbalances that reduce an owner's agency are minimized [128].

Clients and animal owners operate under varied perceptions regarding the role of the veterinary anesthesiologist in the delivery of anesthesia care. Hence, an informed consent discussion should include an outline of the roles of the various individuals who will be involved in the delivery of anesthesia during a particular procedure. It may be that a certified anesthesia specialist (Diploma in Veterinary Anaesthesia [DVA], Diplomate of the European College of Veterinary Anaesthesia and Analgesia [DECVAA], or Diplomate of the American College of Veterinary Anesthesia and Analgesia [DACVAA]) is involved in the prescribing of a suitable anesthesia protocol and supervises the subsequent delivery of anesthesia care. Specific delivery of that care may be delegated to a non-veterinarian who may be a certified technician or nurse specialist or generalist.

Models for the delivery of anesthesia care are numerous. Proper informed client consent will include a discussion that leads to client understanding and acceptance of the model employed. In this, the client holds the very reasonable expectation of knowing who will be providing the anesthesia care and monitoring. Informed consent documentation can be as simple as the notation in the case record of the elements of the process that were discussed with the client. In cases where the associated risks of the procedure are more substantial, a prepared consent form may assist in structuring the informed consent conversation in a systematic way that affords consideration of all of the attendant, significant risks. Although the use of a signed consent form may serve to highlight the existence of real and substantial risk, the use of such a form does not negate the need for a frank and informed discussion with an owner in a manner that not only involves the one-way transfer of information to the client but also creates the space necessary for a provider–client dialogue in which the client is provided with the opportunity to ask questions and receive and understand the answers to those questions. This dialogue is central to the process of informed consent.

In summary, much improvement in small and large animal anesthesia has occurred over the last 50 years. Risks have reduced and standards of care have improved substantially, and a clearer understanding of factors associated with these complications has aided further improvements. Additionally, the successful communication of these risks to owners and clients is central to the professional provision of safe anesthesia and the maintenance of realistic owner expectations. Ongoing evaluation of risks and risk factors is merited to sustain and further improve veterinary anesthesia.

References

1 Anon. New classification of physical status. *Anesthesiology* 1963; **24**: 111.

2 American Society of Anesthesiologist ASA. *ASA Physical Status Classification. Park Ridge,* IL: American Society of Anesthesiologists (last amended December 13, 2020).

3 Clarke KW, Hall LW. A survey of anaesthesia in small animal practice: AVA/BSAVA report. *J Vet Anaesth* 1990; **17**: 4–10.

4 Dyson DH, Maxie MG, Schnurr D. Morbidity and mortality associated with anesthetic management in small animal veterinary practice in Ontario. *J Am Anim Hosp Assoc* 1998; **34**(4): 325–335.

5 Hosgood G, Scholl DT. Evaluation of age as a risk factor for perianesthetic morbidity and mortality in the dog. *J Vet Emerg Crit Care* 1998; **8**(3): 222–236.

6 Brodbelt DC, Hammond RA, Tuminaro D, *et al.* Risk factors for anaesthetic-related death in referred dogs. *Vet Rec* 2006; **158**(16): 563–564.

7 Brodbelt DC, Blissitt KJ, Hammond RA, *et al.* The risk of death: the Confidential Enquiry into Perioperative Small Animal Fatalities (CEPSAF). *Vet Anaesth Analg* 2008; **35**(5): 365–373.

8 Brodbelt DC, Pfeifer DU, Young L, *et al.* Risk factors for anaesthetic-related death in cats: results from the Confidential Enquiry into Perioperative Small Animal Fatalities (CEPSAF). *Br J Anaesth* 2007; **99**(5): 617–623.

9 Brodbelt DC, Pfeiffer DU, Young LE, *et al.* Results of the confidential enquiry into perioperative small animal fatalities regarding risk factors for anesthetic-related death in dogs. *J Am Vet Med Assoc* 2008; **233**(7): 1096–1104.

10 Hosgood G, Scholl DT. Evaluation of age and American Society of Anesthesiologists (ASA) physical status as risk factors for perianesthetic morbidity and mortality in the cat. *J Vet Emerg Crit Care* 2002; **12**(1): 9–15.

11 Gil L, Redondo JI. Canine anaesthetic death in Spain: a multicentre prospective cohort study of 2012 cases. *Vet Anaesth Analg* 2013; **40**(6): e57–e67.

12 Bille C, Auvigne V, Libermann S, *et al.* Risk of anaesthetic mortality in dogs and cats: an observational cohort study of 3546 cases. *Vet Anaesth Analg* 2012; **39**(1): 59–68.

13 Matthews NS, Mohn TJ, Yang M, *et al.* Factors associated with anesthetic-related death in dogs and cats in primary care veterinary hospitals. *J Am Vet Med Assoc* 2017; **250**(6): 655–665.

14 Shoop-Worrall SJ, O'Neill DG, Viscasillas J, *et al.* Mortality related to general anaesthesia and sedation in dogs under UK primary veterinary care. *Vet Anaesth Analg* 2022; **49**(5): 433–442.

15 Eastment JK, Johnston GM, Taylor PM, *et al.* Is isoflurane safer than halothane in equine anesthesia? Results from a multicentre randomised controlled trial. Proceedings of the Society of Veterinary Epidemiology and Preventative Medicine, Cambridge, UK, 4th April, 2002.

16 Johnston GM, Eastment JK, Taylor PM, *et al.* Is isoflurane safer than halothane in equine anaesthesia? Results from a prospective multicentre randomised controlled trial. *Equine Vet J* 2004; **36**(1): 64–71.

17 Dugdale AH, Obhrai J, Cripps PJ. Twenty years later: a single-centre, repeat retrospective analysis of equine perioperative mortality and investigation of recovery quality. *Vet Anaesth Analg* 2016; **43**(2): 171–178.

18 Laurenza C, Ansart L, Portier K. Risk factors of anesthesia-related mortality and morbidity in one equine hospital: a retrospective study on 1,161 cases undergoing elective or emergency surgeries. *Front Vet Sci* 2019; **6**: 514.

19 Marx GF, Mateo CV, Orkin LR. Computer analysis of postanesthetic deaths. *Anesthesiology* 1973; **39**(1): 54–58.

20 Hovi-Viander M. Death associated with anaesthesia in Finland. *Br J Anaesth* 1980; **52**(5): 483–489.

21 Lunn JN, Mushin WW. Mortality associated with anaesthesia. *Anaesthesia* 1982; **37**(8): 856.

22 Pottecher T, Tiret L, Desmonts JM, *et al.* Cardiac arrest related to anaesthesia: a prospective survey in France (1978–1982). *Eur J Anaesthesiol* 1984; **1**(4): 305–318.

23 Tiret L, Desmonts JM, Hatton F, *et al.* Complications associated with anaesthesia—a prospective survey in France. *Can Anaesth Soc J* 1986; **33**(3 Pt 1): 336–344.

24 Buck N, Devlin HB, Lunn JN. *The Report of a Confidential Enquiry into Perioperative Deaths 1987.* London, UK: Nuffield Provincial Hospitals Trust, The King's Fund, 1988.

25 Cohen MM, Duncan PG, Tate RB. Does anesthesia contribute to operative mortality? *J Am Med Assoc* 1988; **260**(19): 2859–2863.

26 Forrest JB, Cahalan MK, Rehder K, *et al.* Multicenter study of general anesthesia. *II. Results. Anesthesiology* 1990; **72**(2): 262–268.

27 NCEPOD. NCEPOD and perioperative deaths of children. *Lancet* 1990; **335**(8704): 1498–1500.

28 Pedersen T, Eliasen K, Henriksen E. A prospective study of mortality associated with anaesthesia and surgery: risk indicators of mortality in hospital. *Acta Anaesthesiol Scand* 1990; **34**(3): 176–182.

29 Forrest JB, Rehder K, Cahalan MK, *et al.* Multicenter study of general anesthesia. III. Predictors of severe perioperative adverse outcomes. *Anesthesiology* 1992; **76**(1): 3–15.

30 Pedersen T. Complications and death following anaesthesia. A prospective study with special reference to the influence of patient-, anaesthesia-, and surgery-related risk factors. *Dan Med Bull* 1994; **41**(3): 319–331.

31 Warden JC, Borton CL, Horan BF. Mortality associated with anaesthesia in New South Wales, 1984–1990. *Med J Aust* 1994; **161**(10): 585–593.

32 Tikkanen J, Hovi-Viander M. Death associated with anaesthesia and surgery in Finland in 1986 compared to 1975. *Acta Anaesthesiol Scand* 1995; **39**(2): 262–267.

33 McKenzie AG. Mortality associated with anaesthesia at Zimbabwean teaching hospitals. *S Afr Med J* 1996; **86**(4): 338–342.

34 Warden JC, Horan BF. Deaths attributed to anaesthesia in New South Wales, 1984–1990. *Anaesth Intensive Care* 1996; **24**(1): 66–73.

35 Wolters U, Wolf T, Stutzer H, *et al.* ASA classification and perioperative variables as predictors of postoperative outcome. *Br J Anaesth* 1996; **77**(2): 217–222.

36 Biboulet P, Aubus P, Dubourdieu J, *et al.* Fatal and non fatal cardiac arrest related to anesthesia. *Can J Anaesth* 2001; **48**(4): 326–332.

37 Morita K, Kawashima Y, Irita K, *et al.* Perioperative mortality and morbidity in 1999 with a special reference to age in 466 certified training hospitals of Japanese Society of Anesthesiologists-report of Committee on Operating Room Safety of Japanese Society of Anesthesiologists. *Masui* 2001; **50**(8): 909–921.

38 Donati A, Ruzzi M, Adrario E, *et al.* A new and feasible model for predicting operative risk. *Br J Anaesth* 2004; **93**(3): 393–399.
39 Hopkins TJ, Raghunathan K, Barbeito A, *et al.* Associations between ASA Physical Status and postoperative mortality at 48 h: a contemporary dataset analysis compared to a historical cohort. *Perioper Med (Lond)* 2016; **5**: 29.
40 Clarke KW, Hall LW, Trim CM. *Veterinary Anaesthesia.* 11th edn. London, UK: WB Saunders, 2014; 561.
41 Johnson CB. Endocrine disease. In: Seymour C, Gleed RD, eds. *Manual of Small Animal Anaesthesia and Analgesia.* Cheltenham, UK: BSAVA, 1999; 223–230.
42 Portier K, Ida KK. The ASA Physical Status Classification: what is the evidence for recommending its use in veterinary anesthesia? A systematic review. *Front Vet Sci* 2018; **5**: 204.
43 McMillan M, Brearley J. Assessment of the variation in American Society of Anesthesiologists [corrected] Physical Status Classification assignment in small animal anaesthesia. *Vet Anaesth Analg* 2013; **40**(3): 229–236.
44 Knaus WA, Draper EA, Wagner DP, *et al.* APACHE II: a severity of disease classification system. *Crit Care Med* 1985; **13**(10): 818–829.
45 Neary WD, Heather BP, Earnshaw JJ. The Physiological and Operative Severity Score for the enUmeration of Mortality and morbidity (POSSUM). *Br J Surg* 2003; **90**(2): 157–165.
46 Malviya S, Voepel-Lewis T, Chiravuri SD, *et al.* Does an objective system-based approach improve assessment of perioperative risk in children? A preliminary evaluation of the 'NARCO'. *Br J Anaesth* 2011; **106**(3): 352–358.
47 Schein OD, Katz J, Bass EB, *et al.* The value of routine preoperative medical testing before cataract surgery. Study of Medical Testing for Cataract Surgery. *N Engl J Med* 2000; **342**(3): 168–175.
48 Chung F, Yuan H, Yin L, *et al.* Elimination of preoperative testing in ambulatory surgery. *Anesth Analg* 2009; **108**(2): 467–475.
49 Benarroch-Gampel J, Sheffield KM, Duncan CB, *et al.* Preoperative laboratory testing in patients undergoing elective, low-risk ambulatory surgery. *Ann Surg* 2012; **256**(3): 518–528.
50 National Guideline Centre (UK). *Preoperative Tests (Update): Routine Preoperative Tests for Elective Surgery.* London, UK: National Institute for Health and Care Excellence (NICE), April 2016.
51 Association of Anaesthetists of Great Britain and Ireland (AAGBI) Safety Guideline 2. *Pre-Operative Assessment and Patient Preparation: The Role of the Anaesthetist.* London, UK: AAGBI, January 2010.
52 Mitchell K, Barletta M, Quandt J, *et al.* Effect of routine pre-anesthetic laboratory screening on pre-operative anesthesia-related decision-making in healthy dogs. *Can Vet J* 2018; **59**(7): 773–778.
53 Toews AR, Campbell JR. Influence of preoperative complete blood cell counts on surgical outcomes in healthy horses: 102 cases (1986–1996). *J Am Vet Med Assoc* 1997; **211**(7): 887–888.
54 Alef M, von Praun F, Oechtering G. Is routine pre-anaesthetic haematological and biochemical screening justified in dogs? *Vet Anaesth Analg* 2008; **35**(2): 132–140.
55 Davies M, Kawaguchi S. Pregeneral anaesthetic blood screening of dogs and cats attending a UK practice. *Vet Rec* 2014; **174**(20): 506.
56 Joubert KE. Pre-anaesthetic screening of geriatric dogs. *J S Afr Vet Assoc* 2007; **78**(1): 31–35.
57 Brodbelt DC. *The Confidential Enquiry into Perioperative Small Animal Fatalities.* London, UK: London University, 2006.
58 Gaynor JS, Dunlop CI, Wagner AE, *et al.* Complications and mortality associated with anesthesia in dogs and cats. *J Am Anim Hosp Assoc* 1999; **35**(1): 13–17.
59 Johnston GM, Taylor PM, Holmes MA, *et al.* Confidential Enquiry of Perioperative Equine Fatalities (CEPEF-1): preliminary results. *Equine Vet J* 1995; **27**(3): 193–200.
60 Johnston GM, Eastment JK, Wood JLN, *et al.* Confidential Enquiry of Perioperative Equine Fatalities (CEPEF): mortality results of Phases 1 and 2. *Vet Anaesth Analg* 2002; **29**(4): 159–170.
61 Wagner AE, Hellyer PW. Survey of anesthesia techniques and concerns in private veterinary practice. *J Am Vet Med Assoc* 2000; **217**(11): 1652–1657.
62 Joubert KE. Routine veterinary anaesthetic management practice in South Africa. *J S Afr Vet Assoc* 2000; **71**(3): 166–172.
63 Nicholson A, Watson A. Survey on small animal anaesthesia. *Aust Vet J* 2001; **79**(9): 613–619.
64 Redondo JI, Suesta P, Serra I, *et al.* Retrospective study of the prevalence of postanaesthetic hypothermia in dogs. *Vet Rec* 2012; **171**(15): 374.
65 Redondo JI, Rubio M, Soler G, *et al.* Normal values and incidence of cardiorespiratory complications in dogs during general anaesthesia. A review of 1281 cases. *J Vet Med A Physiol Pathol Clin Med* 2007; **54**(9): 470–477.
66 Galatos AD, Raptopoulos D. Gastro-oesophageal reflux during anaesthesia in the dog: the effect of age, positioning and type of surgical procedure. *Vet Rec* 1995; **137**(20): 513–516.
67 Galatos AD, Raptopoulos D. Gastro-oesophageal reflux during anaesthesia in the dog: the effect of preoperative fasting and premedication. *Vet Rec* 1995; **137**(19): 479–483.
68 Lamata C, Loughton V, Jones M, *et al.* The risk of passive regurgitation during general anaesthesia in a population of referred dogs in the UK. *Vet Anaesth Analg* 2012; **39**(3): 266–274.
69 Wilson DV, Evans AT, Miller R. Effects of preanesthetic administration of morphine on gastroesophageal reflux and regurgitation during anesthesia in dogs. *Am J Vet Res* 2005; **66**(3): 386–390.
70 Moyer AL, McKee TS, Bergman PJ, *et al.* Low incidence of postoperative nausea, vomiting, regurgitation, and aspiration pneumonia in geriatric dogs receiving maropitant, famotidine, and fentanyl as part of an anesthesia protocol. *J Am Vet Med Assoc* 2021; **260**(S1): S46–S51.
71 Wilson DV, Boruta DT, Evans AT. Influence of halothane, isoflurane, and sevoflurane on gastroesophageal reflux during anesthesia in dogs. *Am J Vet Res* 2006; **67**(11): 1821–1825.
72 Torrente C, Vigueras I, Manzanilla EG, *et al.* Prevalence of and risk factors for intraoperative gastroesophageal reflux and postanesthetic vomiting and diarrhea in dogs undergoing general anesthesia. *J Vet Emerg Crit Care (San Antonio)* 2017; **27**(4): 397–408.
73 Redondo JI, Suesta P, Gil L, *et al.* Retrospective study of the prevalence of postanaesthetic hypothermia in cats. *Vet Rec* 2012; **170**(8): 206.
74 Rodriguez-Diaz JM, Hayes GM, Boesch J, *et al.* Decreased incidence of perioperative inadvertent hypothermia and faster anesthesia recovery with increased environmental temperature: a nonrandomized controlled study. *Vet Surg* 2020; **49**(2): 256–264.
75 Jurk IR, Thibodeau MS, Whitney K, *et al.* Acute vision loss after general anesthesia in a cat. *Vet Ophthalmol* 2001; **4**(2): 155–158.
76 Stiles J, Weil AB, Packer RA, *et al.* Post-anesthetic cortical blindness in cats: twenty cases. *Vet J* 2012; **193**(2): 367–373.
77 Wagner AE. Complications in equine anesthesia. *Vet Clin North Am Equine Pract* 2008; **24**(3): 735–752.
78 Taylor PM, Clarke KW. *Handbook of Equine Anaesthesia.* Edinburgh, UK: WB Saunders Company Ltd, 1999.
79 Bidwell LA, Bramlage LR, Rood WA. Equine perioperative fatalities associated with general anaesthesia at a private practice-a retrospective case series. *Vet Anaesth Analg* 2007; **34**(1): 23–30.
80 Senior JM, Pinchbeck GL, Allister R, *et al.* Post anaesthetic colic in horses: a preventable complication? *Equine Vet J* 2006; **38**(5): 479–484.
81 Nelson BB, Lordan EE, Hassel DM. Risk factors associated with gastrointestinal dysfunction in horses undergoing elective procedures under general anaesthesia. *Equine Vet J Suppl* 2013; **45**: 8–14.
82 Jago RC, Corletto F, Wright IM. Peri-anaesthetic complications in an equine referral hospital: risk factors for post anaesthetic colic. *Equine Vet J* 2015; **47**(6): 635–640.
83 Bailey PA, Hague BA, Davis M, *et al.* Incidence of post-anesthetic colic in non-fasted adult equine patients. *Can Vet J* 2016; **57**(12): 1263–1266.
84 Jones RS. Comparative mortality in anaesthesia. *Br J Anaesth* 2001; **87**(6): 813–815.
85 Albrecht DT, Blakely CL. Anesthetic mortality: a five-year survey of the records of the Angell Memorial Animal Hospital. *J Am Vet Med Assoc* 1951; **119**(897): 429–433.
86 Lumb WV, Jones EW. *Veterinary Anesthesia.* Philadelphia, PA: Lea and Febiger, 1973.
87 Lumb WV, Jones EW. *Veterinary Anesthesia*, 2nd edn. Philadelphia, PA: Lea and Febiger, 1984.
88 Bille C, Auvigne V, Bomassi E, *et al.* An evidence-based medicine approach to small animal anaesthetic mortality in a referral practice: the influence of initiating three recommendations on subsequent anaesthetic deaths. *Vet Anaesth Analg* 2014; **41**(3): 249–258.
89 Itami T, Aida H, Asakawa M, *et al.* Association between preoperative characteristics and risk of anaesthesia-related death in dogs in small-animal referral hospitals in Japan. *Vet Anaesth Analg* 2017; **44**(3): 461–472.
90 Dodman NH. Feline anaesthesia survey. *J Small Anim Pract* 1977; **18**(10): 653–658.
91 Dodman NH, Lamb LA. Survey of small animal anesthetic practice in Vermont. *J Am Anim Hosp Assoc* 1992; **28**: 439–444.
92 Rintasalo J, Vainio O. A survey on anaesthetic practice in Finnish veterinary clinics. *Suomen Elainlaakarilehti* 1995; **101**(9): 541–544.
93 Levy JK, Bard KM, Tucker SJ, *et al.* Perioperative mortality in cats and dogs undergoing spay or castration at a high-volume clinic. *Vet J* 2017; **224**:11–15.
94 Lee HW, Machin H, Adami C. Peri-anaesthetic mortality and nonfatal gastrointestinal complications in pet rabbits: a retrospective study on 210 cases. *Vet Anaesth Analg* 2018; **45**(4): 520–528.
95 Dobbs P, Moittié S, Liptovszky M. Avian anaesthesia related mortality and the associated risk factors in a UK zoological collection. *Vet Anaesth Analg* 2021; **48**(6): 922–929.
96 Hall LW, Taylor PM. *Anaesthesia of the Cat*, 1st edn. London, UK: Bailliere Tindall, 1994.

97 Meyer RE. Geriatric patients. In: Seymour C, Gleed RD, eds. *Manual of Small Animal Anaesthesia and Analgesia*, 2nd edn. Cheltenham, UK: BSAVA, 1999; 253–256.
98 Waterman AE. Maintenance of body temperature during anaesthesia. *J Vet Anaesth* 1981; **9**: 73–85.
99 Dhupa N. Hypothermia in dogs and cats. *Compend Contin Educ Vet* 1995; **17**(1): 61–68.
100 Campling EA, Devlin HB, Lunn JN. *The Report of the National Confidential Enquiry into Perioperative Deaths 1989*. London, UK: Nuffield Provincial Hospitals Trust, The King's Fund, 1990.
101 Gruenheid M, Aarnes TK, McLoughlin MA, *et al.* Risk of anesthesia-related complications in brachycephalic dogs. *J Am Vet Med Assoc* 2018; **253**(3): 301–306.
102 Oda A, Wang WH, Hampton AK, *et al.* Perianesthetic mortality in English Bulldogs: a retrospective analysis in 2010–2017. *BMC Vet Res* 2022; **18**(1): 198.
103 Smith MD, Barletta M, Young CN, *et al.* Retrospective study of intra-anesthetic predictors of prolonged hospitalization, increased cost of care and mortality for canine patients at a veterinary teaching hospital. *Vet Anaesth Analg* 2017; **44**(6): 1321–1331.
104 Webb RK, Van der Walt JH, Runciman WB, *et al.* The Australian Incident Monitoring Study. Which monitor? An analysis of 2000 incident reports. *Anaesth Intensive Care* 1993; **21**(5): 529–542.
105 Tinker JH, Dull DL, Caplan RA, *et al.* Role of monitoring devices in prevention of anesthetic mishaps: a closed claims analysis. *Anesthesiology* 1989; **71**(4): 541–546.
106 Eichhorn JH, Cooper JB, Cullen DJ, *et al.* Standards for patient monitoring during anesthesia at Harvard Medical School. *J Am Med Assoc* 1986; **256**(8):1017–1020.
107 Muir WW, Werner LL, Hamlin RL. Effects of xylazine and acetylpromazine upon induced ventricular fibrillation in dogs anesthetised with thiamylal and halothane. *Am J Vet Res* 1975; **36**(9): 1299–1303.
108 Tranquilli WJ, Thurmon JC, Benson GJ, *et al.* Alterations in the Arrhythmogenic Dose of Epinephrine (ADE) following xylazine administration to halothane-anesthetised dogs. *J Vet Pharmacol Ther* 1986; **9**(2): 198–203.
109 Pettifer GR, Dyson DH, McDonnell WN. An evaluation of the influence of medetomidine hydrochloride and atipamizole hydrochloride on the arrhythmogenic dose of epinephrine in dogs during halothane anaesthesia. *Can J Vet Res* 1996; **60**(1): 1–6.
110 Tranquilli WJ, Thurmon JC, Benson GJ. Alterations in epinephrine-induced arrhythmias after xylazine and subsequent yohimbine administration in isoflurane-anesthetised dogs. *Am J Vet Res* 1988; **49**(7): 1072–1075.
111 Hellebrekers LJ. Comparison of isoflurane and halothane as inhalation anaesthetics in the dog. *Vet Q* 1986; **8**(3): 183–188.
112 Lemke KA, Tranquilli WJ, Thurmon JC, *et al.* Alterations in the arrhythmogenic dose of epinephrine following xylazine or medetomidine administration to isoflurane-anesthetised dogs. *Am J Vet Res* 1993; **54**(12): 2139–2145.
113 Hikasa Y, Okabe C, Takase K, *et al.* Ventricular arrhythmogenic dose of adrenaline during sevoflurane, isoflurane and halothane anaesthesia either with or without ketamine or thiopentone in cats. *Res Vet Sci* 1996; **60**(2): 134–137.
114 Hikasa Y, Ohe N, Takase K, *et al.* Cardiopulmonary effects of sevoflurane in cats: comparison with isoflurane, halothane and enflurane. *Res Vet Sci* 1997; **63**(3): 205–210.
115 Steffey EP, Howland MA. Isoflurane potency in the dog and cat. *Am J Vet Res* 1977; **38**(11): 1833–1836.
116 Steffey EP, Gillespie JR, Berry JD, *et al.* Circulatory effects of halothane and halothane-nitrous oxide anesthesia in the dog: spontaneous ventilation. *Am J Vet Res* 1975; **36**(2): 197–200.
117 Joas TA, Stevens WC. Comparison of the arrhythmic dose of epinephrine during forane, halothane and fluroxene anesthesia in dogs. *Anesthesiology* 1971; **35**(1): 48–53.
118 Hodgson DS, Dunlop CI, Chapman PL, *et al.* Cardiopulmonary effects of anesthesia induced and maintained with isoflurane in cats. *Am J Vet Res* 1998; **59**(2): 182–185.
119 Grandy JL, Hodgson DS, Dunlop CI, *et al.* Cardiopulmonary effects of halothane anesthesia in cats. *Am J Vet Res* 1989; **50**(10): 1729–1732.
120 Mitchell B. Equine anaesthesia: an assessment of techniques used in clinical practice. *Equine Vet J* 1969; **1**(6): 261–275.
121 Tevik A. The role of anesthesia in surgical mortality. *Nordisk Vetinarmedecin* 1983; **35**(4): 175–179.
122 Trim CM, Adams JG, Cowgill LM, *et al.* A retrospective survey of anaesthesia in horses with colic. *Equine Vet J Suppl* 1989; **7**: 84–90.
123 Young SS, Taylor PM. Factors leading to serious anaesthetic-related problems in equine anaesthesia. *J Vet Anaesth* 1990; **17**: 59.
124 Young SS, Taylor PM. Factors influencing the outcome of equine anaesthesia: a review of 1,314 cases. *Equine Vet J* 1993; **25**(2): 147–151.
125 Mee AM, Cripps PJ, Jones RS. A retrospective study of mortality associated with general anaesthesia in horses: elective procedures. *Vet Rec* 1998; **142**(11): 275–276.
126 Mee AM, Cripps PJ, Jones RS. A retrospective study of mortality associated with general anaesthesia in horses: emergency procedures. *Vet Rec* 1998; **142**(12): 307–309.
127 Gozalo-Marcilla M, Bettschart-Wolfensberger R, Johnston M, *et al.* data collection for the fourth multicentre Confidential Enquiry into Perioperative Equine Fatalities (CEPEF4) Study: new technology and preliminary results. *Animals (Basel)* 2021; **11**(9): 2549.
128 Moore SA, O'Kell A, Borghese H, *et al.* A CTSA One Health Alliance guidance on institutional review of veterinary clinical studies. *BMC Vet Res* 2021; **17**(1): 83.

3 Introduction to Patient Safety

Matt McMillan[1] **and Daniel S.J. Pang**[2]
[1] The Ralph Veterinary Referral Centre, Marlow, Buckinghamshire, UK
[2] Faculty of Veterinary Medicine, University of Calgary, Calgary, Alberta, Canada and
Faculty of Veterinary Medicine, Université de Montréal, Saint-Hyacinthe, Québec, Canada

Chapter contents

Introduction, 24
Nomenclature and terminology, 24
The risk of harm from healthcare, 24
Why things go wrong: Human error and the system, 25
The "process" of anesthesia, 26
Reason's Swiss cheese model, 27
Human factors, 27
Non-technical skills, 27
Organizational culture, 27
Blame and no-blame cultures, 28
Just culture, 28
Learning culture, 28
Safety I versus Safety II, 28
Assessing organizational safety culture, 28
Data gathering techniques, 28
Incident reporting systems, 29
Interviews, 29
Morbidity and mortality conferences, 29
Analysis techniques, 30
Root cause analysis, 30
Human Factors analysis techniques, 30
Patient safety evidence in anesthesia, 30
Patient safety interventions, 33
Checklists, 33
Other cognitive aids, 34
Communication tools: briefings, debriefings, and patient hand-offs, 35
Simulation-based training, 36
Engineering solutions, 36
Methods for reducing medication error, 36
Assessment of patient safety interventions, 37
Useful resources, 37
References, 37

Introduction

Not all harm to patients comes from illness and injury, some comes through healthcare itself. The World Health Organization (WHO) defines *patient safety* as "the reduction of risk of unnecessary harm associated with healthcare to an acceptable minimum" [1]. In this definition, "harm" encompasses a range of undesirable outcomes for the patient including disease, injury, pain, suffering, disability, and death [2]. "Unnecessary" implies that this harm was preventable, suggesting that it was iatrogenic in origin, caused by error, accident, or neglect rather than being "necessary" to treat the disease (e.g., trauma caused by surgery). Patient safety focuses on the prevention of error and accidental injury in healthcare.

Anesthesiologists have always been leaders in patient safety, perhaps because anesthesia itself has little to no therapeutic value and due to the immediacy of consequences of an error in anesthetic care [3]. These factors tend to make anesthetists risk averse and safety conscious. This chapter introduces patient safety science with special emphasis on safety during the perianesthetic period.

Nomenclature and terminology

The terminology around patient safety can be imprecise, compromising understanding of the subject and the literature [1]. Although there is no universally recognized nomenclature for safety in veterinary medicine, the WHO's World Alliance for Patient Safety developed a set of key terms which we have adapted and expanded for veterinary purposes and will use throughout this chapter for clarity and consistency (Box 3.1).

The risk of harm from healthcare

The most cited estimate of deaths from human healthcare-associated harm is the Institute of Medicine 2000 report "To Err is Human: Building a Safer Healthcare System" that describes an incidence of 44,000–98,000 deaths annually in the United States (US) [4]. This is now considered a gross underestimation with more recent studies estimating that between 200,000 and 400,000 patients a year die from preventable healthcare-associated harm in the US

Veterinary Anesthesia and Analgesia: The Sixth Edition of Lumb and Jones. Edited by Leigh Lamont, Kurt Grimm, Sheilah Robertson, Lydia Love and Carrie Schroeder.
© 2024 John Wiley & Sons, Inc. Published 2024 by John Wiley & Sons, Inc.
Companion website: www.wiley.com/go/lamont/anesthesia

Box 3.1 Common definitions based upon the list of preferred terms and definitions for key concepts adapted from the WHO's International Classification for Patient Safety.

Patient safety: the reduction of risk of unnecessary harm associated with healthcare to an acceptable minimum

Healthcare-associated harm: harm arising from or associated with plans or actions taken during the provision of healthcare rather than an underlying disease or injury

Patient safety incident: an event, hazard, or circumstance that could have resulted or did result in unnecessary harm to a patient

Event: something that happens to or involves a patient

Hazard: a circumstance, agent, or action with the potential to cause harm

Circumstance: a situation or factor that may influence an event, agent, or person

Near miss: an incident that did not reach the patient

No harm incident: an incident that reached the patient but did not result in discernible harm

Harmful incident (accident; adverse event): an incident that resulted in harm to a patient

Error: failure to carry out a planned action as intended or application of an incorrect plan. Includes slips, lapses, and mistakes

Slip: a memory failure, includes omitting planned items, losing place in a process, and forgetting intentions

Lapse: a failure of attention, includes omission, intrusion, reversal, misordering, and mistiming e.g., forgetting to open an adjustable pressure-limiting valve

Mistake: a rule- or knowledge-based error. Rule-based mistakes include the misapplication of a good rule or the application of a bad rule. Knowledge-based mistakes are many and varied

Violation: deliberate deviation from an operating procedure, standard, or rule. These can be routine, exceptional, or sabotage

Contributing factor: a circumstance, action, or influence that is thought to have played a part in the origin or development of an incident or to increase the risk of an incident

Mitigating factor: an action or circumstance that prevents or moderates the progression of an incident toward harming a patient

***System:** a set of interdependent elements interacting to achieve a common goal. In medicine, it relates to a healthcare organization's operational methods, processes, or infrastructure

Source: Adapted from Runciman *et al.* [1].
*Adapted from other sources.

alone [5,6]. This makes healthcare the third leading cause of death in the US, behind heart disease and cancer [5]. The risk of serious non-fatal healthcare-associated harm has been estimated to be between 10- and 20-fold greater [6].

In veterinary medicine, information on the incidence of veterinary healthcare-associated harm is limited. There are some clues in studies investigating perianesthetic fatality. In 1990, Clarke and Hall suggested that 70% of anesthetic deaths had an element of error and that many animals died while not under "close supervision" [7]. In a large prospective study of small animal anesthetics in 2008, Brodbelt *et al.* reported that a significant proportion of veterinary patients did not receive basic monitoring, and the risk of death was four to five times greater when an animal's pulses were not monitored [8]. Many of the reported deaths were in healthy animals, suggesting that they could have been preventable through the implementation of simple monitoring techniques.

Looking beyond fatality, safety incidents in veterinary anesthesia occur regularly; studies suggest a rate of between 3.7% and 5.1% in 4140 and 3379 anesthetics, respectively [9,10]. Common safety incidents reported by Hofmeister *et al.* included medication error (wrong drug, wrong dose, wrong route, and inaccurate labeling), adjustable pressure-limiting (APL) (i.e., pop-off) valves left closed, airway complications (including esophageal intubation), and intravenous catheter failures [9]. One case of a wrong site locoregional anesthetic technique and another of wrong site arterial catheter placement were also reported. McMillan *et al.* cited medication error, equipment failure, oxygen pipeline failure, and APL valve mismanagement as the most commonly reported safety incidents [10]. The minority of these incidents (6.3%) were near misses, 20.7% were no harm incidents, and the remainder were harmful incidents (73.0%).

In a wider view of veterinary healthcare, Wallis *et al.* analyzed safety incidents reported over a 3-year period in three veterinary hospitals [11]. Safety incidents occurred in 0.4–0.8% of hospital visits with approximately 54% being medication errors. Medication errors involved "wrong dose" (57.8%), "wrong drug" (18%), "wrong time" (12.2%), "wrong route" (5.8%), and "wrong patient" (3.8%), although the exact proportions varied between hospitals. Communication errors made up 30% of incidents and involved a mixture of source (missing information/incomplete information), transmission (illegible handwriting, inappropriate manner for transmitting information), and receiver (information forgotten or incorrectly interpreted). Other insights can be identified from examining professional litigation cases and closed claims analysis. Oxtoby *et al.* retrospectively reviewed records of claims made to a veterinary indemnity insurer in the United Kingdom [12]. Identifiable errors were present in 45% of records with the leading causes being cognitive limitation (55%), lack of technical skill or knowledge (15%), and communication (5%). Each of these studies is likely to only reflect a small fraction of the actual incidence of veterinary patient safety incidents and healthcare-associated harm [13].

Why things go wrong: Human error and the system

Discussion of patient safety must include the thorny issues of human error and human performance. Human error can be identified in incident investigations in all walks of life, including healthcare. It would be simple to assume that people are the problem that needs to be fixed. However, human error cannot be eliminated [4].

Modern views of safety consider that human error is a consequence of the conditions in which an accident occurred, not a cause of the incident. It is inevitable that accident investigations will find fault with human performance since humans are at the sharp end of processes in most industries, that is, people perform or control the task(s), make the decisions, and form the last line of defense. However, human performance is influenced by working conditions and is, therefore, systematically linked to the features of the tasks, tools, and environment of their work. Describing human error

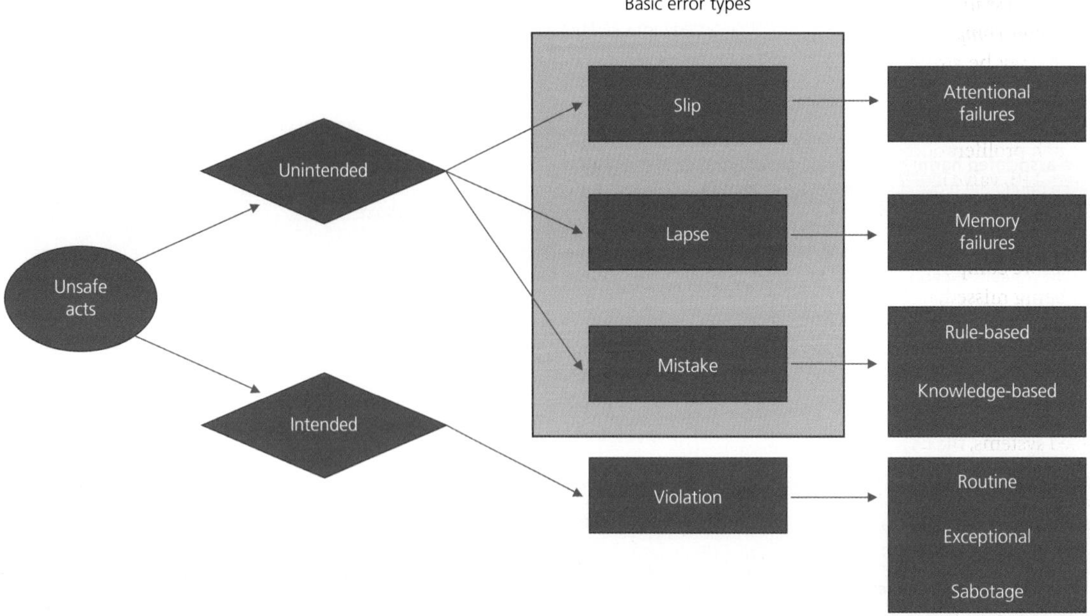

Figure 3.1 Reason's taxonomy of human error (1991). Source: Adapted from Reason [14]. See Box 3.1 for current definitions.

helps us to understand how and why it occurs. The psychologist James Reason developed a taxonomy that remains the foundation for describing types of human error today (Fig. 3.1) [14].

The "process" of anesthesia

Understanding human error requires us to learn about system vulnerabilities, resource constraints, pressures, and contradictions and understand how processes fail or succeed. There are several elements that make healthcare, in particular, anesthesia, susceptible to, and the people working within these areas prone to, error. Anesthesia requires the administration of rapidly acting drugs with significant physiological effects, the monitoring of patients in a vulnerable physiological state using advanced electronics, and the performance of highly technical procedures in a dynamic, unpredictable environment characterized by intense time pressure and high stakes. This situation may be further compounded by a concurrent teaching requirement. Gaba [15] and Reason [16] have discussed these factors at length, and their findings are summarized in Box 3.2.

Box 3.2 The characteristics of work for the anesthesiologist

- Uncertain, dynamic environments
- Multiple sources of concurrent information (i.e., many data streams)
- Shifting, ill-defined, or competing goals
- The need to maintain an up to date "mental model" of an often rapidly changing situation
- Reliance upon indirect or inferred indications
- Ill-structured problems
- Actions having immediate and multiple consequences
- Moments of intense time stress interleaved with long periods of routine activity
- Sophisticated technologies with many redundancies
- Complex and sometimes confusing human–machine interfaces
- High stakes (e.g., life and death)
- Multiple players with differing priorities (e.g., surgeon, internist, and anesthetist)
- A working environment highly influenced by group norms (including expected behaviors and hierarchies) and organizational culture

Source: Adapted from Gaba [15]; Reason [16].

Models for the development of safety incidents in high-risk, complex industrial activities such as nuclear power have been adapted to model anesthetic processes. "Normal Accident Theory," as described by Perrow in 1984, outlines two system attributes that commonly contribute to accidents: (1) the complexity of interactions between system components and (2) the tightness of coupling between these components [17].

A task or process is said to have complex interactions if there are many alternative and interrelated subtasks at any point in its completion. The more complex a system's interactions, the more likely it is that something will go wrong as the consequence of interactions cannot always be predicted. Gaba *et al.* subsequently expanded on Perrow's theory to outline how three different types of complexity (intrinsic, uncertainty, and proliferation) contribute to incidents in anesthesia [18].

Intrinsic complexity occurs due to the interconnected action of a multitude of individual agents within a system or process. The body can be considered an intrinsically complex system; huge numbers of cells and organs interact in a multitude of intricate ways, using a vast array of signals. In such a system, altering one component can have a knock-on effect on other components, with dynamic and unpredictable consequences.

Uncertainty complexity occurs when cause and effect relationships are not always clear and are difficult to predict. Anesthesia is easily achieved by drug administration; however, the pharmacological, physiological, and pathophysiological interactions that occur are often poorly understood. In addition, devices used for measurement and monitoring the effect of these interactions can be imprecise and inaccurate, often have low signal-to-noise ratios, and are prone to error. Prediction of drug effects is based upon our knowledge of what a drug does in the general population, but the effect on a given individual cannot be predicted with certainty. Nor are we able to measure all affected parameters or predict all potential consequences; we only ever have a partial picture of what is happening.

Finally, if a process involves many components and tasks, this can cause *proliferation complexity*. Although a process and individual steps within it may be simple, the components and tasks may be interconnected in a complex fashion. For example, they may have to be performed in a precise order or at specific times for the process to succeed. Such proliferation is what can lead to lapses such as failing to open an APL valve in a breathing system following a machine leak check. The task is simple, but, because it is one task of many which need to be performed before anesthesia, it is easily forgotten. As more and more components are added to a system, the chance of one of them being missed, or failing, increases. Indeed, anesthetists typically add proliferation complexity to a case to help combat uncertainty; using multiple electronic monitoring devices, each of which has a risk of error, imprecision, and failure [18].

Coupling refers to the way components in a system are linked. In tightly coupled systems, the change in state or function of one component directly affects other components within a short period of time. Tightly coupled systems result in more accidents because even minor errors can become problematic before they can be corrected. In loosely coupled systems, there is redundancy or temporal lag built in the system allowing components to function normally despite changes in other components. The interaction of numerous homeostatic mechanisms means that physiology is inherently loosely coupled. Body systems have intrinsic buffers, which allow normal functioning in a variety of conditions; for example, renal blood flow and glomerular filtration rate are kept stable through a range of perfusion pressures. However, the redundancy and buffer mechanisms responsible for this loose coupling are hindered by the anesthetic process making components more tightly coupled. This has the effect of transferring responsibility for monitoring and maintaining an adequate state of health to the anesthetist, aided by technology and pharmaceuticals.

Reason's Swiss cheese model

The psychologist James Reason considers complex systems to contain fundamental elements that must work together harmoniously if efficient and safe operations are to occur [14]. This requires certain preconditions to be met, such as well-maintained and functional equipment, and individuals with appropriate training, skills, and experience. Hazards are prevented from causing harm by a series of barriers, safeguards, and defenses. Some rely on people, while others are engineered into the system (e.g., alarms). In an ideal world, each layer would be intact; however, in reality, each has unintended weaknesses. These failings degrade the integrity of the system leading to vulnerabilities within different layers like holes in a slice of Swiss cheese. Unlike in Swiss cheese, these holes are continually opening, shutting, and shifting their location as conditions in the system change. The presence of holes in any single "slice" does not normally cause an incident or bad outcome. However, when the holes within these layers momentarily align, they allow an error to proceed through the layers of a system to reach the patient (Fig. 3.2).

Human factors

Human Factors (HF), sometimes referred to as "ergonomics," is a scientific discipline concerned with understanding interactions between people and the other elements of a system. Applying HF approaches in healthcare can enhance the way it is delivered and received. HF views people as a vital component of any system and that their abilities and limitations must be considered when attempting to improve system performance. The basic principle of HF is to analyze tasks, systems, or processes to understand the limitations put upon the humans within them. In essence, this can be achieved through asking: Can this team/person reliably and safely perform these tasks, with this training and information, using this equipment, in this environment, with these constraints and pressures, to the required standard? Through understanding human limitations and how humans process information, workplaces, tasks, and equipment can be designed and engineered to allow for variability in human performance, making it easier for frontline workers to do their job safely and effectively.

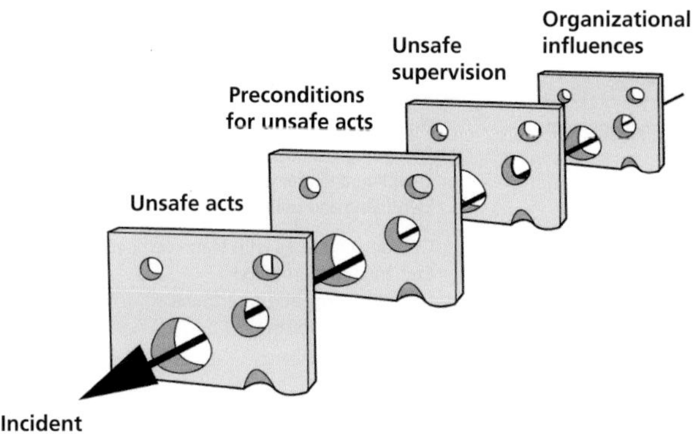

Figure 3.2 Reason's Swiss cheese model of incident causation. Additional terms in this figure are described in the Human Factors analysis section (Fig. 3.4 and Table 3.6). Source: Adapted from Pang [19].

Non-technical skills

One area that the HF approach has highlighted is the importance of non-technical skills. These are skills individuals use to perform their work that lie outside of the traditional medical competencies of knowledge and technical skills. Non-technical skills are cognitive, social, and personal management skills necessary for an individual to perform a role, task, or job safely and effectively [20]. They include situation awareness, decision-making, task management, teamwork, leadership, communication, and the management of stress and fatigue.

Until recently, little attention has been given to these competencies in medical professions. One of the early proponents of non-technical skills in anesthesiology were Howard *et al.*, who developed an "Anesthesia Crisis Resource Management (ACRM)" training course with the aim of introducing anesthesiologists to principles of dynamic decision-making, human performance, and the development of countermeasures aimed at combating and reducing error [21]. More recently, the "Anaesthetists' Non-Technical Skills (ANTS)" behavioral marker system was developed following collaboration between anesthesiologists and psychologists [20]. Task analysis was used to define the critical non-technical skills required for a safely functioning anesthetist, and an assessment scale was developed for ANTS training and observations in operating rooms or simulation settings (Table 3.1). Such training and observation rarely occur in the veterinary sector, but it is likely that non-technical skills are similarly important for veterinary anesthesia.

Organizational culture

Organizational culture is the collective beliefs, perceptions, and values shared between individuals in a workplace and how these are manifested in their work. Organizational culture sets the tone of the workplace by affecting the conditions, pressures, constraints, and expectations put upon individuals and the tasks they perform.

Table 3.1 Anesthetist non-technical skills.

Category	Elements
Task management	Planning and preparing Prioritizing Providing and maintaining standards Identifying and utilizing resources
Team working	Coordinating tasks with team members Exchanging information Using authority and assertiveness Assessing capabilities Supporting others
Situation awareness	Gathering information Recognizing and understanding Anticipating
Decision-making	Identifying options Balancing risks and selecting options Re-evaluating

Source: Adapted from Flin *et al.* [20].

Informally, culture represents "how things are done around here." Safety culture is those aspects of organizational culture that affect increasing or decreasing risk. Safety culture can be thought of as a "leading indicator" in the assessment of patient safety, as opposed to a "lagging indicator" (e.g., morbidity and mortality). Several organizational culture types are widely discussed in the literature and warrant examination.

Blame and no-blame cultures

A blame culture is one where incidents are blamed on individuals making errors despite those individuals having little or no control over the conditions in which the error occurred [22]. It leads to norms and attitudes characterized by an unwillingness to take risks or accept responsibility for mistakes because of a fear of criticism or repercussions. Blame culture cultivates distrust and fear, with people tending to blame each other to avoid being blamed themselves. This can result in few new ideas and a lack of personal initiative because people do not want to risk being wrong. Safety incidents tend to stay unreported, and investigations tend to be brief, finding culpability in frontline workers. Such cultures tend to evolve in hierarchical, rule-, and compliance-based systems but where the work is highly variable, such as healthcare.

A no-blame culture is in essence the opposite: a culture in which individuals are not held accountable for their actions. This should encourage people to report errors and provide an environment where innovation is encouraged [23]. However, a no-blame culture is neither feasible nor desirable. Most people desire some level of accountability when a safety incident occurs, and individuals should take ownership of their decisions and actions and be accountable for being part of any solution [23].

Just culture

A just culture is one in which individuals are not punished for human errors if their actions, decisions, or omissions were appropriate to their experience and training, but where negligence, willful violations, and destructive acts are not tolerated [24]. Unlike a no-blame culture, there is accountability; individuals are accountable for reporting incidents and organizations are accountable for implementing appropriate corrective actions to improve the system and reduce the risk of recurrence of incidents [23].

If staff members perceive that their reports are treated fairly and lead to positive change, and that people who willfully violate safety rules and take unnecessary risks are held accountable, the willingness to report will increase. This encourages reporting and investigation of incidents and improves safety.

Learning culture

Learning culture is concerned with the sustainability of learning from failure through the reporting and analysis of errors and incidents and the implementation of systems level interventions. It requires an atmosphere of psychological safety, that is, a supportive work environment in which team members believe that they can question existing practices, express their concerns, or dissent, and admit mistakes without suffering ridicule or punishment [25]. It requires open communication between all levels of staff within an organization, a flattening of hierarchy, and transparency in incident management.

Senge [26] has described five disciplines which together make a learning culture: (1) self-mastery, (2) shared mental models, (3) shared vision, (4) team learning, and (5) systems thinking [27]. Self-mastery involves realistic thinking about one's abilities. Shared mental models require team members to have a common understanding of the task being performed and of the involved teamwork, whereas a shared vision means all team members are working toward the same goal. Team learning represents a situation where all team members are continuously learning from each other and their successes and failures. Systems thinking, on the other hand, is an attempt to understand the way the system works and how this influences the behavior and performance of individuals working within it.

Safety I versus Safety II

Modern views of safety consider that people bring the innovation, creativity, flexibility, and resilience required for processes to succeed in systems with huge variation [28]. People can adjust what they do to match the conditions in which they work [28]. It can be argued that everyday performance variability provides the adaptations that are needed to respond to varying conditions and is the reason why systems are generally successful. Humans can consequently be seen as a resource necessary for system flexibility and resilience rather than a cause of the problem. Safety I can be viewed as the approach to safety, which concentrates on avoiding things going wrong. Safety II focuses on how things go right under varying conditions, exploring all possible outcomes to understand how flexibility in a system allows success. This concept is still in its infancy within medicine; however, it may give a better overall view of performance within the healthcare system [29].

Assessing organizational safety culture

Assessing safety culture can reveal potential issues in communication, teamwork, resources, and management strategies, delineating areas for targeted improvement efforts. Several validated measurement scales have been developed to assess safety culture in human healthcare organizations. One of these, the "Safety Attitudes Questionnaire" [30], has been modified for use in veterinary medicine. The resultant "Nottingham Veterinary Safety Culture Survey" was developed for use in veterinary practices within the United Kingdom and was subsequently further adapted for use in the US [31,32].

Data gathering techniques

Improving safety relies on the accurate identification of risks to safety. Data can be gathered using numerous techniques with the most common being incident reporting systems, interviews, and morbidity and mortality conferences (M&MCs). To generate the best possible account of the incident, it is common to use more than one approach.

Incident reporting systems

One of the main sources of information about patient safety has come from the systematic collection and analysis of incident reports. Moreover, incident reporting is central to the development of a learning culture, wherein errors are discussed, and systems analysis is applied to improve outcomes. There is also considerable value in reporting near misses and no harm incidents since they are harbingers of potential patient harm. To capture a range of different perspectives and build a more complete picture of an incident, information should be collected from all involved. Often, it is more junior team members (e.g., interns), animal health technicians, and support staff who are most exposed to weaknesses and flaws within a system.

Early reporting is important. As time passes after an incident, memories fade, bias creeps in, and an incident may never be reported as caregivers move on to other tasks. In the view of the authors, reporting should be completed within 12–48 h of an incident occurring, with harmful incidents reported toward the shorter end of this range (by the end of the workday is a good rule of thumb).

Information collected on incidents should focus on creating an account of events, describing the "5 Ws": "Who" (was involved), "What" (happened), "When" (the incident happened), "Where" (it happened), and "Why" (and how it happened).

Existing reporting systems in human medicine are effectively voluntary, with perhaps the exception of harmful incidents when there is a stronger expectation of reporting. While voluntary reporting systems have their drawbacks, they can be highly effective when properly designed and administered. Importantly, the success of any system is predicated upon its acceptance and use by caregivers. Several concepts to voluntary reporting system design facilitate their adoption and usefulness for incident analysis. These are confidentiality, ease of use, accessibility, independent analysis, and release of findings [33,34].

Confidentiality means individuals should be able to report incidents without the risk of personal or professional consequences [35]. Confidentiality should not be confused with anonymity. While anonymity confers further protection to those reporting, it removes the ability to follow up a report with the individual involved. To fully understand a reported incident, particularly when attempting to collate multiple reports of the same incident or simply to clarify circumstances, some degree of follow-up is often necessary. Also, under the protection of anonymity, there may be the tendency to use reporting systems as a means of personal attack or to vent frustrations with aspects of the system (e.g., supervisors and administration) drawing focus away from a more complete report of the incident.

Reporting systems must be easy to use, including clear language, use of checkboxes for some data entry, automatic field population, minimal mandatory fields, and a section for a narrative description of events. The latter is important in gathering an account of the incident [36]. The use of open questions encourages descriptions from the reporter's perspective.

Reporting systems must be easily accessible to all healthcare workers. Online reporting systems should be easy to find and preferably accessed through a "single click," from computers in and out of the hospital network. There remains an argument for offering a paper-based system in combination with a secure drop-off box for staff members that do not have private access to computers.

To reduce bias, reports should be analyzed by independent investigators not involved in the incident. Releasing the findings of investigations, as well as a general report of types and outcomes of incidents reported, "closes the loop," building faith in the system. This demonstrates that reports are taken seriously and acted upon and allows caregivers to be involved in any changes introduced by providing a period for comment. When an incident reveals significant system weaknesses that are likely to cause further incidents, it is critical that this information can be shared quickly and widely using multiple means (e.g., team meetings, email alerts, website notifications, and notice boards).

Voluntary reporting systems are limited by the quality of material collected and the extent to which they are representative of all incidents. Material collected is largely determined by the design of the reporting system. It is widely recognized that voluntary reports underestimate the true incidence of safety incidents [13]. However, if users understand the role and importance of submitting reports, the types of incidents to report, in combination with a reporting system that is easy to access and use, and can do so without fear of repercussion, uptake is likely to be improved. Education can be provided (e.g., as part of orientation for new employees) and reinforced within the system (e.g., regularly releasing findings emphasizes the value of reporting). There are a huge number of incident reporting systems in medicine with one of the first being the "Australian Incident Monitoring System (AIMS)" [36]. There are far fewer incident reporting systems in veterinary medicine, most being developed using digital forms and cloud-based software [11,37].

Interviews

A senior member of the clinical team who was not involved with the incident may interview individuals involved in an incident. The primary advantage to one-on-one interviews is the opportunity to elicit responses without the potential for pressure from discussing an incident in a group environment. However, this advantage is countered by several important disadvantages including the inherent power dynamic of the interview process and the potential to create significant bias through the format and scope of the questioning. The use of structured or semi-structured interview techniques, such as critical incident technique, and the use of open, non-accusatory language can help reduce this bias.

Morbidity and mortality conferences

Morbidity and mortality conferences (M&MCs) can promote learning from incidents and drive improvements in patient safety [38]. However, despite being in existence for well over 50 years, it is unclear to what extent they take place in veterinary medicine [39]. Conceptually, M&MCs can serve as a forum for collaborative review and investigation of incidents without fear of negative personal or professional consequences. When done well, M&MCs represent an opportunity to improve patient safety and maximize learning from an incident through open reflection and discussion [40–44].

In human medicine, M&MCs have successfully driven improved outcomes in patient care and management, including improving safety culture and care quality and reducing mortality and malpractice claims [45]. For M&MCs to fulfill their potential, key considerations are case selection, duration and frequency, roles of moderator and presenter, presentation format, incident analysis technique, and outcome and follow-up.

All cases of mortality resulting from error or potential error should be reviewed through an M&MC. In larger clinics/hospitals, where the number of cases presenting exceeds the capacity to review cases in a timely manner, it may be necessary to screen and select cases for M&MCs. This can be based on the number of systemic factors implicated, the number of future patients that may benefit, and educational value. Screening can be performed as part of the voluntary reporting system process.

Duration of M&MCs varies widely, from 20 to over 60 min, probably reflecting time available in many instances, as well as case complexity [40–42]. Similarly, the frequency of M&MCs is variable though once monthly is commonly reported in the literature [38]. There is a case to be made for having a regular schedule to emphasize that M&MCs are a normal and accepted part of clinical governance, rather than special events reflecting personal failings. Cases selected for M&MCs should be presented as soon as possible as a timely acknowledgment of the incident and to maximize the likelihood of collecting all pertinent information.

Moderators set the tone of M&MCs and must be familiar with the M&MC format, have a good understanding of analysis techniques, have sufficient experience and expertise to guide the presenter and audience, and be respected by the attendees [40,46,47]. Cases should be presented by someone directly involved as they are best placed to present the events and answer questions. The presenter can be a senior or junior team member. It is helpful to have senior members intermittently present to show their investment in the process and to demonstrate to junior/new team members the expected format and standard. Involvement of junior members as presenters is invaluable as an educational tool for critical evaluation of case management and in maintaining a just and learning culture. Audiences for M&MCs should reflect the personnel of the clinic (i.e., all members of staff should be invited). Attendance by senior team members shows support for the process and helps create a positive, productive discussion [39]. A multidisciplinary audience can enrich the discussion by bringing different perspectives and disseminate lessons learned more widely [39].

Standardized presentation formats help ensure that information is presented in a systematic, organized way, minimizing the risk of bias [39,41,42,48]. One such model is the "Situation, Background, Assessment, Recommendation (SBAR)" format (Table 3.2), a structured method for efficiently transferring information [41,42]. This method has been effectively used when information is being passed between personnel who occupy different positions in a hierarchy (e.g., senior clinician and intern) [49,50].

Table 3.2 Situation, Background, Assessment, Recommendations (SBAR) format for morbidity and mortality conferences (M&MCs).

SBAR component	Elements
Situation: brief statement of problem	Diagnosis at admission, statement of procedure, and patient safety incident
Background: clinical information pertinent to adverse event	History, indication for procedure, diagnostic studies, procedural details timeline of care, description of incident (recognition, management, outcome)
Assessment and analysis: evaluation of adverse event (what and why)	What: sequence of events Why: analysis, using preferred methodology*
Review of the literature: evidence-based practice	Relevant literature
Recommendations: prevention of recurrence	Identify how event could have been prevented or better managed Identify learning outcomes and recommendations

Source: Adapted from Pang *et al.* [38].
* See text for different analysis methods.

Analysis techniques

Analysis of patient safety incidents has three goals: to explain what happened, identify the roles and contributions of associated factors, and identify means to prevent similar incidents. Historically, the focus on investigating a safety incident begins and ends with what happened, with limited consideration of why it happened. This rarely brings effective change into the system and invariably results in the person(s) closest to the event shouldering the responsibility and blame. Modern investigation analysis techniques have moved away from a person-based ("blame and shame") approach to a structured-system-based (Human Factors) approach. While there are numerous analytical frameworks available, those used in human healthcare are largely based on the work of the psychologist, James Reason [14].

Root cause analysis

Root cause analysis (RCA) is a generic term used to describe a range of techniques which aim to identify problems and then work toward establishing the problem's root cause(s). A common misconception of RCA springs from the word "cause" appearing as singular, leading to the belief that a problem results from a single cause, whereas multiple causes are almost always involved, particularly in healthcare [51]. The simplest RCA method is the "five whys" technique, which involves asking "why?" five times, with each question following on from the previous answer to identify root causes of a problem. However, this technique promotes linear thinking, in that other contributing factors may be overlooked. Consequently, such techniques have now been replaced with more structured techniques, which ensure that the entire system is considered within the analysis.

Human Factors analysis techniques

Modern incident analysis techniques involve investigating the role of the entire system in the evolution of an incident. The "London Protocol" is a model of healthcare incident evolution based upon Reason's accident model and Human Factors approaches (Fig. 3.3) [52,53]. Reason's "unsafe acts" are termed "care delivery problems" and are affected by contributory factors, which can be classified into patient, task, individual team, work environment, and organizational/cultural levels. The framework provides a systematic and conceptually driven approach to accident investigation and to risk assessment in healthcare.

Another system commonly used for incident analysis in healthcare is the "Human Factors Analysis and Classification System (HFACS)" (Fig. 3.4). This system, based on Reason's model and developed for the investigation of aviation accidents [54], has been adapted to the healthcare setting [51,55]. Used correctly, this approach is believed to have the "potential to identify actionable systemic causes of error, focus specific performance improvement efforts, and ultimately improve patient safety" [51].

A fishbone diagram can be used as a visual representation of an analysis and an accessible entry into a system-based approach for incident investigation (Fig. 3.5) [34,38,56].

Patient safety evidence in anesthesia

Cooper *et al.*'s study of anesthetic "mishaps" was the first to really examine the causes of anesthetic safety incidents beyond the patient and inherent risk of anesthetic drugs [57]. Through structured interviews, it was established that human error was involved in 82% of the 359 investigated incidents, but many other associated factors

Contributing factors
Care delivery problems
Work environment
Team
Individual
Task/technology
Patient
Organization
culture
management
Unsafe acts
Errors
Slips
Lapses
Mistakes
Violations
Accident
Latent error
Error and violation producing conditions
Active failures

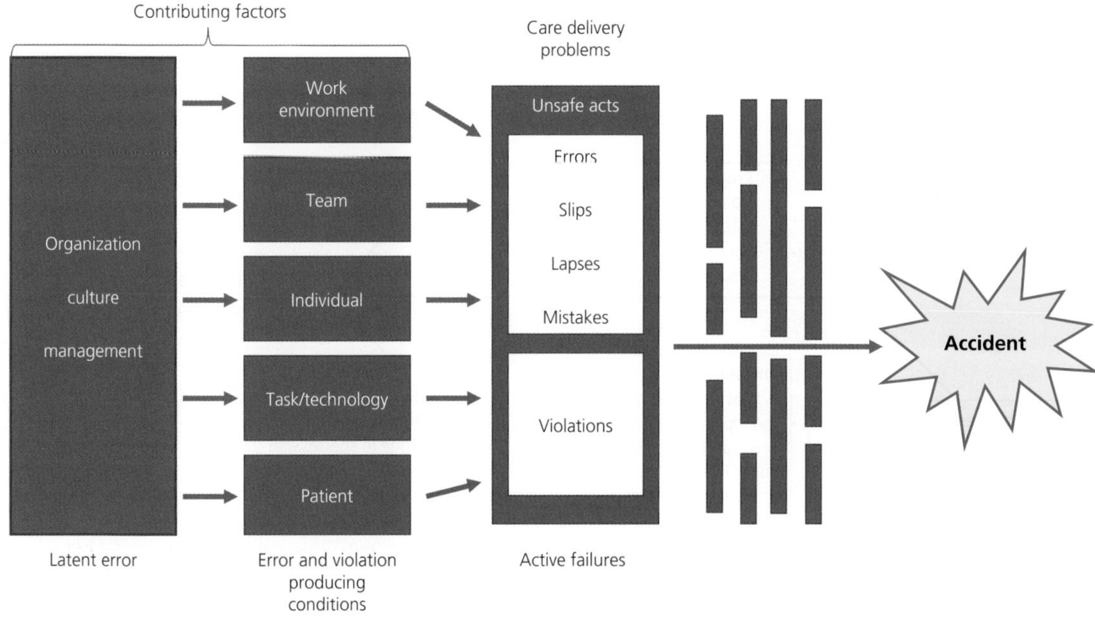

Figure 3.3 Vincent's model of accident causation in healthcare. Source: Adapted from Vincent *et al.* [52].

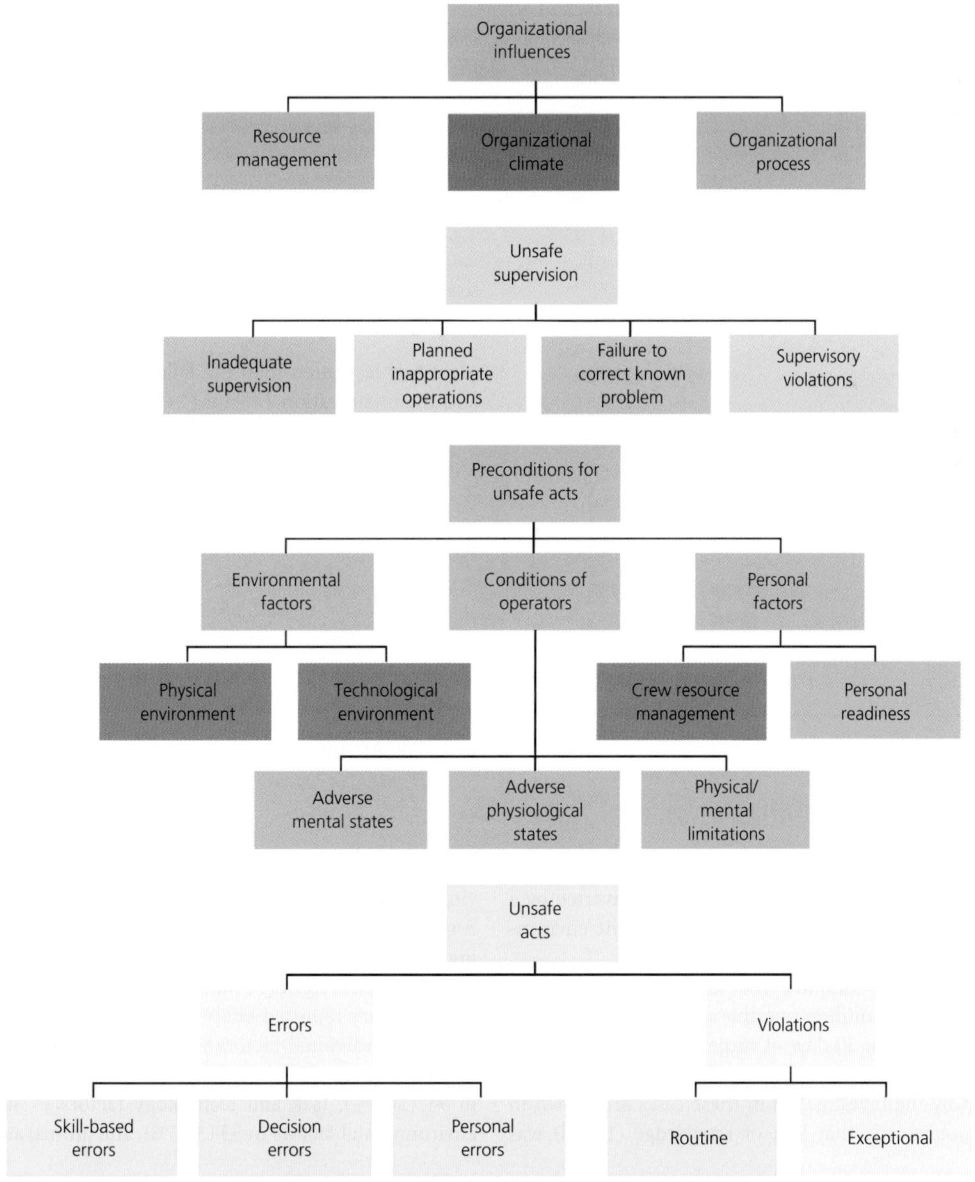

Organizational influences
Resource management
Organizational climate
Organizational process
Unsafe supervision
Inadequate supervision
Planned inappropriate operations
Failure to correct known problem
Supervisory violations
Preconditions for unsafe acts
Environmental factors
Conditions of operators
Personal factors
Physical environment
Technological environment
Crew resource management
Personal readiness
Adverse mental states
Adverse physiological states
Physical/ mental limitations
Unsafe acts
Errors
Violations
Skill-based errors
Decision errors
Personal errors
Routine
Exceptional

Figure 3.4 Human Factors Analysis and Classification System components. Source: Adapted from Pang [19].

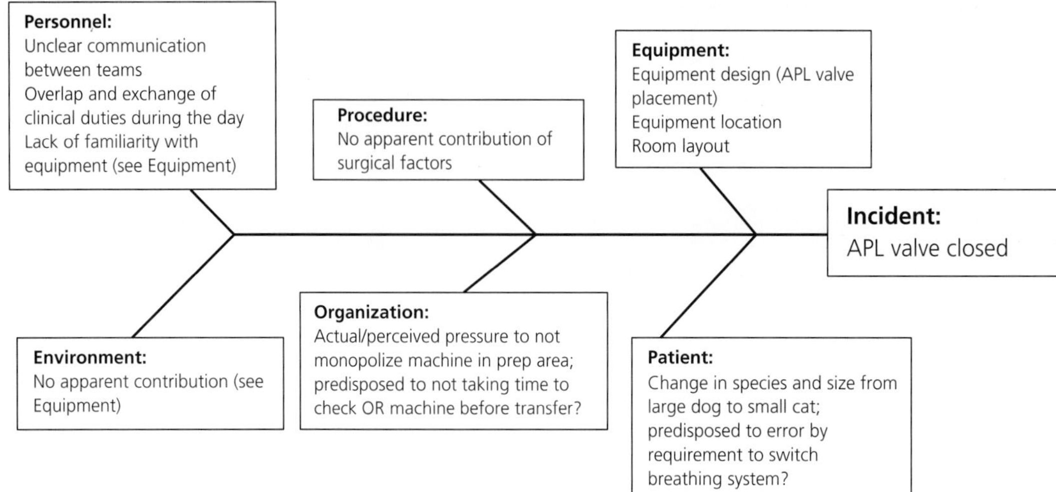

Figure 3.5 Example of a fishbone diagram made during an investigation of a closed APL valve. Source: Pang *et al.* [56], with permission of John Wiley & Sons.

Table 3.3 Factors involved in 359 anesthetic "mishaps" as identified through the critical incident technique.

Contributing factor	Relative frequency
Inadequate total experience	21.4%
Inadequate familiarity with equipment/device	12.5%
Poor communication with team, lab, etc.	7.5%
Haste	7.2%
Inattention/carelessness	7.2%
Fatigue	6.7%
Excessive dependency on other personnel	6.7%
Failure to perform a normal check	6.1%
Training or experience – other factors	6.1%
Supervisor not present enough	5.0%
Environment or colleagues – other factors	5.0%
Visual field restricted	4.7%
Mental or physical – other factors	4.5%
Inadequate familiarity with surgical procedure	3.9%
Distraction	3.6%
Poor labeling of controls, drugs, etc.	3.3%
Supervision – other factors	3.3%
Situation precluded normal precautions	2.8%
Inadequate familiarity with anesthetic technique	2.8%
Teaching activity under way	2.5%
Apprehension	2.2%
Emergency case	1.7%
Demanding or difficult case	1.7%
Boredom	1.4%
Nature of activity/other factors	1.4%
Insufficient preparation	0.8%
Slow procedure	0.8%
Other	0.8%

Source: Adapted from Cooper *et al.* [57].

were also identified (Table 3.3). Interestingly, many of the incidents were considered "representative of the kinds of error that residents are considered prone to commit in the training process" and "that most of the errors and associated outcomes could be averted by a more structured approach to preparing residents for the environments into which they are often suddenly immersed."

The first "Confidential Enquiry into Perioperative Deaths" reviewed just over half a million anesthetics and reported 4034 perioperative deaths within 30 days of surgery, 410 of which were considered associated with anesthetic management [58]. The factors identified by the investigators in these cases are shown in Table 3.4. It is noteworthy that lack of knowledge (15.1%) was identified less often than the failure to apply knowledge (75.1%), and the organizational factor (24.9%), such as lack of appropriate staffing levels, was the third most common factor identified.

Table 3.4 Factors identified as being associated with anesthetic deaths in the Confidential Enquiry into Perioperative Deaths.

Contributing factor	Relative frequency
Failure to apply knowledge	75.1%
Lack of care	30.0%
Failure of organization	24.9%
Lack of experience	23.7%
Lack of knowledge	15.1%
Drug effect	9.5%
Failure of equipment	1.7%
Other	2.7%

Source: Adapted from Buck *et al.* [58].

Runciman *et al.* published analysis of the first 2000 incidents to be reported through the "Australian Incident Monitoring System (AIMS)" (Table 3.5) [59]. Factors associated with the wider system were identified as contributing to 26% of incidents, and this increased to 81% if human behavior was included in the system. Interestingly, the system was considered a mitigating factor in 56% of incidents, and systems-based corrective strategies were suggested as solutions in 65%.

Neuhaus *et al.* applied the HFACS to 50 anesthetic incidents reported to a single center's incident reporting system. Investigations revealed 81 unsafe acts, 113 preconditions for unsafe acts, 39 instances of unsafe leadership, and 22 organizational influences [54]. Errors were identified 64 times and most commonly these were decision-based errors, followed by skills-based errors and, less commonly, perceptual-based errors. There were also 17 violations identified, most of which were considered as exceptional. A mean of 5.1 factors from the HFACS were identified as contributing to each incident (Table 3.6).

Data from veterinary anesthesia literature are limited. From 163 voluntary reported safety incidents analyzed using the London Protocol, individual factors were identified in 123 (70.7%), team factors in 108 (62.1%), organizational and management factors in 94 (54.0%), task and technology factors in 80 (46.0%), work environmental factors in 53 (30.5%), and animal and owner factors

Table 3.5 Contributing factors identified in the first 2000 incidents reported to the Australian Incident Monitoring System (AIMS).

Contributing factor	Relative frequency
Error of judgment	16%
Failure to check equipment	13%
Fault of technique	13%
Other factors	13%
Other equipment problem	13%
Inattention	12%
Haste	12%
Inexperience	11%
Communication problem	9%
Inadequate pre-operative assessment	7%
Monitor problem	6%
Inadequate pre-operative preparation	4%
Unfamiliar environment or equipment	4%
Inadequate assistance	3%
Fatigue	3%
Drug label	3%
Other stress	2%
Lack of facility	2%
Staff change	1%
Illness	1%

Source: Adapted from Runciman *et al.* [59].

Table 3.6 Contributing factors identified in 50 anesthetic incidents through the application of the Human Factors Analysis Classification System (HFACS).

HFACS category	HFACS contributing factor	Relative frequency (%)
Organizational influences	Resource management	6%
	Organizational climate	20%
	Organizational process	18%
Supervision	Inadequate leadership	8%
	Inappropriate planned operation	44%
	Failure to correct problem	14%
	Leadership violation	12%
Preconditions for unsafe acts	Physical environment	22%
	Technical environment	52%
	Operator mental state	18%
	Operator physiological state	4%
	Operator chronic performance limitation	8%
	Communication, coordination, planning	64%
	Fitness for duty	0%
Unsafe acts	Error, skills-based	36%
	Error, decision-based	82%
	Error, perceptual	10%
	Violation, routine	12%
	Violation, exceptional	22%

Source: Adapted from Neuhaus *et al.* [54].

in 36 (20.7%) incidents [10]. Importantly, factors from team, work environmental, and organizational and management categories were identified concurrently in 89.4% of incidents where individual factors were involved. The 14 most commonly identified contributing factors are reported in Table 3.7.

Patient safety interventions

Patient safety interventions should be aimed at specific system weaknesses identified during analysis of incidents and processes. There are, however, several general patient safety interventions, which have become universally accepted, such as cognitive aids (including checklists and algorithms), communication tools, simulation-based training, and engineering solutions.

Table 3.7 The 14 most common contributing factors identified following the systems analysis of 163 veterinary anesthesia patient safety incidents.

Systems category	Contributing factor	Relative frequency (%)
Patient and owner	Animal condition	30%
Task and technology	Failure to follow SOP	51%
	Equipment check	28%
Individual	Decision-making	65%
	Experience	44%
	Health, stress, fatigue	28%
	Task management	24%
Team	Supervision	48%
	Written communication	38%
	Verbal communication	33%
Work environmental	Distraction	42%
Organizational	Staffing level	53%
	Poor scheduling	32%
	Culture and priorities	28%

Source: Adapted from McMillan and Lehnus [10].

Checklists

Checklists are an organized list of action items or criteria that a user can record as present/absent as each item is considered or completed [60]. Fundamentally, the purpose of a checklist is to reduce error and improve performance [60]. A checklist achieves this by reinforcing accepted safety practices and fostering communication and teamwork, reducing the risk of error, and improving patient outcomes [61–64].

Much of the literature on checklists use comes from aviation, reflecting its early acknowledgment of the relationships between humans and complex systems. In aviation, checklists are a standard part of flight protocol; not completing checklists, or completing a checklist from memory, are considered violations [65]. By comparison, the widespread use of checklists is relatively recent in medicine but has been shown to be highly effective. This is exemplified by two well-known examples: the "Keystone Intensive Care Unit (ICU) Project" and the "Surgical Safety Checklist (SSC)" [61,62]. In the "Keystone ICU Project," catheter-related bloodstream infections were reduced from a mean baseline rate of 7.7 infections per 1000 catheter days to 1.4 infections per 1000 catheter days at 16–18 months after the introduction of a simple five-point checklist. These improvements were sustained over 5 years of follow-up, with estimated savings of $2–3 billion annually, and prevention of 30,000–60,000 deaths [62,63]. The introduction of the "SSC" in a diverse patient population from eight hospitals in eight countries, representing both high- and low-income settings, reduced mortality within 30 days of non-cardiac surgery from 1.5% to 0.8% and the overall complication rate (including surgical site infections, sepsis, and pneumonia, among others) from 11.0% to 7.0% [61]. The positive outcomes from this study led to its adoption by the WHO, its use in over 120 countries, representing 90% of the world's population, and over 230 million surgeries per year. The checklist comprises three sections: "sign in" (before induction of anesthesia), "time out" (before skin incision), and "sign out" (before patient leaves operating room), with five to seven checklist items per section [66]. The mechanisms underlying the improvements achieved were "likely multifactorial," reflecting both systems and behavioral changes [61]. These can be described in terms of technical and adaptive (cultural) aspects. Technical aspects encompass education and evaluation, and adaptive aspects encompass engagement and execution [62,63,66,67]. All must be considered for a checklist to be successful in design and implementation [63].

Table 3.8 Considerations when modifying the World Health Organization's Surgical Safety Checklist (SSC).

Focused	Keep the checklist concise, focused on critical items and those not checked by other means. Limit of five to nine items per checklist section.
Brief	No more than 1 min to complete each section. Longer checklists risk impeding the flow of care.
Actionable	Each listed item must link to a specific, unambiguous action to avoid confusion as to what should be done.
Verbal	Promoting verbal interactions among team members is a core component. The checklist is likely to be less successful if limited to a written instrument.
Collaborative	Considered modifications should be collaborative, involving representatives from groups involved in its use. This contributes to promoting "ownership" of the checklist.
Tested	Any modified checklist should be tested in a limited setting before wider adoption. Testing may include, a simulation, over single day, and by a single team.
Integrated	The checklist is not intended to be comprehensive and modification to integrate into existing safety processes is encouraged provided brevity and simplicity are not sacrificed. Integration could reflect specific procedure requirements.

Source: Adapted from WHO [66].

The WHO encourages SSC modification by local teams, provided that safety steps are not removed, and checklist modification is supported by the finding that meaningful improvements can be achieved without completing all of the original 19 checklist items [61]. Table 3.8 outlines modification considerations.

It is important to recognize that the SSC has not been universally successful. A major reason for failures when attempting to adopt checklists is underestimating the importance of adaptive components while focusing on technical components [67–70]. Of these, technical barriers are generally easier to overcome and may include provision of key equipment to facilitate checklist item completion and recognizing that checklists can be modified to reflect local conditions (e.g., redundancy with other safety checks). Cultural barriers are common in human medicine, with evidence that they exist in veterinary medicine [60,67,69,70]. There can be a tendency to feel that checklists infringe on clinical judgment and autonomy, reflect weakness by not relying on memory to perform tasks, and reflect a lack of knowledge or skill [60,67]. There can also be reluctance to accept direction to adopt checklists without discussion from administrators or those less actively involved in clinical practice [67,70]. Recognizing and addressing these potential barriers was an important part of the success of the "Keystone ICU Project" and the "SSC." Unfortunately, steps taken to overcome these barriers were not emphasized in the SSC report, which probably explains some of the challenges encountered by others in attempting its adoption [60,69]. Specific instructions on how to introduce and implement the WHO SSC have been published [66].

While it appears that versions of the SSC are in use in veterinary medicine, published reports are limited and results mixed [69,71]. Contrasting the reports of Bergström *et al.* [71] and Menoud *et al.* [69] is instructive in the context of technical and adaptive (cultural) barriers. In both cases, the WHO SSC was adapted for local use; however, the methods underlying adaptation were not described by Bergström *et al.*, while a Delphi method was used by the anesthesia team in Menoud *et al.* The length of the resulting checklist was comparable in each case (23 and 24 items). In the Bergström *et al.* study, checklist use was restricted to surgical procedures whereas in the Menoud *et al.* study, the checklist could be used for any anesthetic procedure. Bergström *et al.* provided oral instruction and practical training in checklist use over a 2-week period before implementation with a specified individual responsible for checklist completion. By contrast, Menoud *et al.* reported that an investigator was available to assist users but did not describe a formal instruction or training process. Bergström *et al.* focused on outcome measures as a marker of checklist impact, finding a greater number of complications in the pre-checklist group (52 complications identified in 300 dogs and cats) compared with the post-checklist group (15 complications identified in 220 dogs and cats). No process audit to track checklist use or compliance was reported. Menoud *et al.* performed two process audits by direct observation of procedures. The first (n = 69 anesthetized cases) found that the checklist was used in 32% of cases, not printed for use in 41% of cases, and printed but not used in 27% of cases. The second audit (n = 64 anesthetized cases) found that the checklist was printed for all cases and used in 45%, with no significant difference in use between audits. Menoud *et al.* concluded that difficulties faced in checklist use reflected a failure to designate someone responsible for managing the checklist, a lack of printed copies of the checklist, and attempting to apply the checklist to cases that underwent anesthesia but not surgery. Overall, they described the situation as one in which "users did not feel involved" and identified that introduction of the checklist could have been better managed [69].

An "Anaesthetic Safety Checklist" was produced by the Association of Veterinary Anaesthetists in 2014 and is freely available through the association website [72]. Fig. 3.6 shows the checklist used during the spay-neuter teaching laboratory at the University of Calgary. Hofmeister *et al.* quantified the incidence of APL valves unintentionally closed and esophageal intubations over approximately 1 year [9]. A focused checklist (added as checkboxes on the anesthesia record) was designed to address these two items, which resulted in a decrease in incidence for both over the subsequent year: APL valve closures from 20 to 5 occurrences; and esophageal intubations from 16 to 4 occurrences [9].

Other cognitive aids

There are many other cognitive aids that can be used to improve human performance and safety. Evidence for their use in settings outside of medicine is compelling and has led to much interest especially in acute medicine, surgery, and anesthesia [73]. Their use in emergency situations has perhaps received the most attention as it appears that failure to adhere to best clinical practice often occurs when time for decision-making is limited [74]. Many cognitive aids have been developed for emergency situations ranging from single-treatment algorithms and drug charts to large sets of checklists and cognitive aids grouped together in a "crisis manual."

Some of the earliest cognitive aids developed and put to widespread use were cardiopulmonary resuscitation (CPR) algorithms. In CPR, adherence to Advanced Cardiovascular Life Support protocols is associated with increased patient survival, whereas non-compliance and omissions of indicated steps are associated with decreased survival [75]. Error rates during CPR may be halved by using cognitive aids, at least in a high-fidelity simulator setting, suggesting that the use of cognitive aids may have significant effects on outcomes [76].

The Reassessment Campaign on Veterinary Resuscitation (RECOVER) developed a set of consensus guidelines for veterinary CPR alongside cognitive aids encompassing a CPR algorithm, a post-cardiac arrest care algorithm, and a quick reference chart of CPR drugs and doses [77]. Little evidence has been published as to the success of these guidelines to date; however, it appears the guidelines have changed CPR practices [78], although they still vary

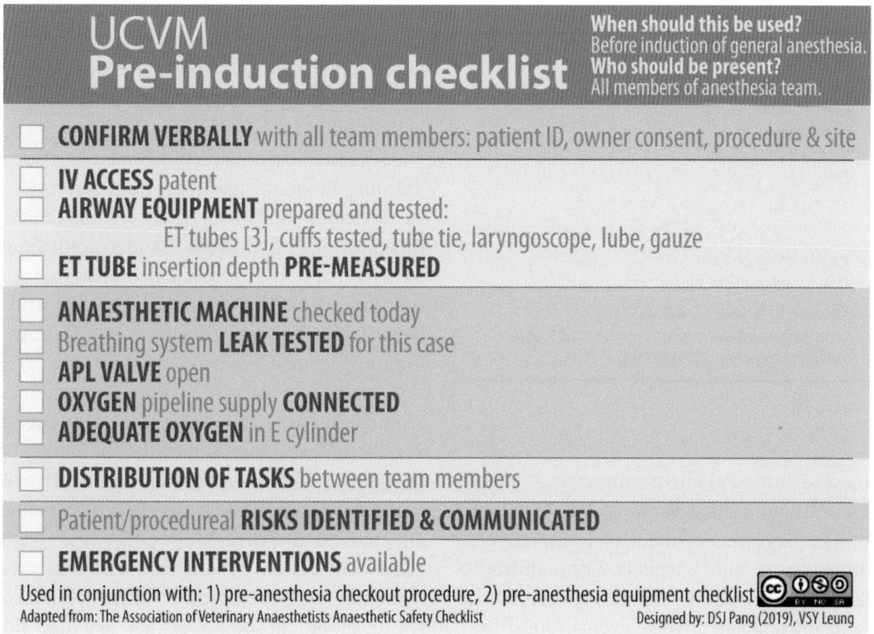

UCVM
Pre-induction checklist

When should this be used?
Before induction of general anesthesia.
Who should be present?
All members of anesthesia team.

- ☐ **CONFIRM VERBALLY** with all team members: patient ID, owner consent, procedure & site
- ☐ **IV ACCESS** patent
- ☐ **AIRWAY EQUIPMENT** prepared and tested:
  ET tubes [3], cuffs tested, tube tie, laryngoscope, lube, gauze
- ☐ **ET TUBE** insertion depth **PRE-MEASURED**
- ☐ **ANAESTHETIC MACHINE** checked today
- ☐ Breathing system **LEAK TESTED** for this case
- ☐ **APL VALVE** open
- ☐ **OXYGEN** pipeline supply **CONNECTED**
- ☐ **ADEQUATE OXYGEN** in E cylinder
- ☐ **DISTRIBUTION OF TASKS** between team members
- ☐ Patient/procedureal **RISKS IDENTIFIED & COMMUNICATED**
- ☐ **EMERGENCY INTERVENTIONS** available

Used in conjunction with: 1) pre-anesthesia checkout procedure, 2) pre-anesthesia equipment checklist
CC BY NC SA
Adapted from: The Association of Veterinary Anaesthetists Anaesthetic Safety Checklist
Designed by: DSJ Pang (2019), VSY Leung

Figure 3.6 Pre-induction checklist in use at the Faculty of Veterinary Medicine, University of Calgary. Source: Dr. Daniel Pang, with permission.

considerably [79]. One study of 141 dogs suffering cardiac arrest demonstrated that dogs resuscitated using the RECOVER guidelines and cognitive aids had better outcomes than dogs resuscitated using traditional CPR procedures, with improved return to spontaneous circulation (43% versus 17%) and higher survival rates (5% versus 0%) [80].

Several crisis manuals have now been developed for use in human anesthesia and surgery. Based upon information from the "Australian Incident Monitoring System (AIMS)," Runciman *et al.* developed a set of 24 crisis algorithms for managing anesthetic crises [81]. It is claimed that 60% of 4000 incidents reported to AIMS would be addressed in 40–60 s using the manual [81]. In a pilot trial of a surgical crisis manual developed by collaboration between medical and aviation experts, two surgical teams were exposed to eight crisis simulations, four with and four without the checklist [82]. Manual use led to a sixfold reduction in failure to perform critical steps and tasks [82]. Later, 17 operating room teams were exposed to 106 surgical crisis simulations. All teams performed better when using the manual and there was almost a 75% reduction in omissions of critical steps during crisis management [83].

Box 3.3 Strategies for safe and effective postoperative handovers consistently identified in the literature.

- Prepare monitor, alarms, equipment, and fluids before patient arrival
- Complete urgent care tasks before the verbal handover
- Set aside time for handover communication. Avoid performing other tasks during this time and, conversely, limit conversations while performing tasks
- Use the "sterile cockpit": only patient-specific conversation or urgent clinical interruptions can occur during the handover
- All relevant members of the operating room and postoperative receiving teams should be present during the handover
- Only one care provider should speak at a time, with minimal distractions and interruptions
- Provide an opportunity to ask questions and voice concerns
- Document the handover
- Use supporting documentation, e.g., lab test results, anesthesia chart
- Use structured checklists to guide communication and ensure completeness of information. Use forms or reference cards as reminders
- Use protocols to standardize processes
- Provide formal team or handover training

Source: Adapted from Segall *et al.* [85].

Communication tools: briefings, debriefings, and patient hand-offs

Communication is a significant component of perioperative checklists such as the WHO SSC, and in many organizations, the surgical "time-out" has developed into a miniature pre-procedural briefing. A recent study including over 8000 surgical procedures investigated outcomes before and after the introduction of a structured intraoperative briefing and found that mortality, unplanned re-operations, and prolonged hospital stays were all reduced [84].

A point of weakness for transfer of critical patient-related information is during hand-offs (handovers) [85,86]. Hand-offs occur whenever a transfer and acceptance of patient care responsibility between two caregivers or teams is required, for example, when a patient is moved from the operating theater to the recovery suite or ward. Effective hand-offs require passing safety-critical and patient-specific information from one caregiver to another and are key in facilitating the continuity and safety of the patient's care. Unstable recovering patients, competing demands upon caregivers, multitasking, and time limitations make postanesthetic hand-offs particularly vulnerable to error [86]. Such errors lead to fragmented postoperative care, delays in treatment and diagnosis, and cause significant patient harm [86]. A systematic review of the literature identified broad strategies to reduce risk around postanesthetic hand-offs which are summarized in Box 3.3 [85].

Numerous standardized postanesthetic hand-off communication tools have been suggested and studied in the literature. Currently, the system with the most evidence is "IPASS," which was developed from descriptions of best practice hand-off techniques cited in the literature [87,88]. The IPASS technique involves five

Table 3.9 Elements of the IPASS mnemonic hand-off system.

I	Illness severity	Stable, unstable, etc.
P	Patient summary	Summary statement Events leading up to admission Hospital course Ongoing assessment Plan
A	Action list	"To do" list Timeline of actions and who needs to perform them
S	Situation awareness and contingency planning	What's going on now Plan for what might happen in the future
S	Synthesis by receiver	Receiver summarizes what was heard Queries any unclear information/asks questions Restates key actions/"to do" task

Source: Adapted from Starmer *et al.* [87].

discussion points: I: Illness severity; P: Patient summary; A: Action list; S: Situation awareness and contingency planning; and S: Synthesis by receiver (Table 3.9). The largest assessment of IPASS covered over 10000 hospital admissions in nine hospitals. Through implementation of the IPASS system, there were significant decreases in medical errors (23%) and preventable adverse events (30%) [89]. Other systems for standardized hand-off communication exist and include the "Situation, Background, Assessment, Recommendation (SBAR)" and "Post-Anesthesia Team Handover (PATH)." Both these systems have been shown to improve hand-offs and reduce safety incidents; however, good-quality evidence on their overall effect on outcomes is limited [90,91].

Simulation-based training

Simulation is an immersive and interactive educational tool used to replace or amplify real experiences. It provides an opportunity for individuals to be trained together in a supportive learning environment where they can perform clinical tasks and processes without the risk of harming patients. Anesthesia was one of the first medical specialties to embrace simulation-based training and its role in the education of anesthetists in human medicine grows from year to year. The most obvious use for simulation in training is learning and improving the performance of technical skills. If well designed, with robust assessment and feedback mechanisms, technical skill training in simulation suites is highly effective and leads to large and sustainable improvements in skill acquisition and hastens the transition from novice to expert [92].

However, greater safety improvements can perhaps be made through simulations designed to encourage the development of non-technical skills, highlighting how aspects of work, such as teamwork and communication, can affect individual performance and outcomes. It may also help develop these skills in individuals and teams and lead to improved performance and clinical outcomes [92,93]. One of the first simulation-based training methods developed in anesthesia was the "Anesthesia Crisis Resource Management (ACRM)" course [21]. A catalog of 62 anesthetic critical incidents formed the basis of simulations designed to test a participant's dynamic decision-making and teamworking. Participants performed a pre- and post-ARCM course test on aspects of crisis management and the management of critical incidents. Residents scored considerably higher after participation in the course, though there was no improvement in the scores of experienced anesthetists. A review of the impact of crisis resource management simulation-based training in interdisciplinary teams found positive outcomes in all but two of the 12 studies included [94]. Significant improvements were documented in team behaviors in the workplace, including teamwork, staff attitudes toward patient safety, situational awareness, and workload management. A subset of these studies demonstrated sustained reductions in adverse patient outcomes [94].

Simulation training methods such as "Patient Safety Medical Team Training Program" and the "Team Strategies and Tools to Enhance Performance and Patient Safety (TeamSTEPPS®)" allow hospitals and organizations to provide standardized simulation-based training packages, which have been demonstrated to significantly improve outcomes including surgical morbidity and mortality [92]. More specifically, for anesthesia, the "Vital Anaesthesia Simulation Training" course has been demonstrated to improve non-technical skills scores of anesthetists in low-income human hospital settings [95]. Simulation-based training is also recommended for situations such as CPR and weaning from cardiopulmonary bypass [92].

A 2022 review investigating the effectiveness of veterinary simulators versus traditional instruction concluded simulators can be effective to improve knowledge- and technical-skill-based outcomes but did not identify any evidence investigating the effect of simulators on non-technical skills or clinical outcomes [96]. Despite the development some years ago of a high-fidelity veterinary simulator, little evidence has been published on the effect this has had on trainee performance [97]. Simulation does not appear to play any part in veterinary residency training programs currently, despite significant evidence from human medicine suggesting benefit.

Engineering solutions

Mechanisms that force users to perform tasks in a certain way or link easily forgotten tasks with tasks highly likely to be completed can be used to reduce error. For example, to limit the risk of delivering a hypoxic gas mixture, nitrous oxide and oxygen flowmeters can be physically linked, meaning that if oxygen flow rate was reduced, the nitrous oxide flow would also decrease, maintaining a minimum ratio of gases. Another solution is to tightly couple tasks, for example, when throat packs/gauzes are placed in orofacial surgery or dentistry, tying the throat pack to endotracheal tube can ensure that the pack will be removed at the time of extubation if not done beforehand.

Methods for reducing medication error

Medication errors can occur at any point of the medication management process, which involves prescribing, transcribing, dispensing, administering, and monitoring. Systematic countermeasures have been recommended to decrease the number of drug errors in anesthesia; however, surprisingly, few have been well studied. Recommendations include reading the labels of any drug ampule or syringe carefully before a drug is drawn up or injected; the standardization and optimization of legibility and contents of medication labels; always labeling syringes; formal standardized organization of drug drawers and workspaces; and checking of labels by a second person (double-checking) before a drug is drawn up or administered [98,99]. Although such interventions would appear foolproof, medication errors still occur regularly, and evidence for each of these recommendations is weak. For example, there is insufficient evidence that the implementation of double-checking is associated with lower rates of medication error or reduced harm [100]. Indeed, in busy modern clinical settings, whether double-checking policies warrant the considerable resource investments required to enforce them has yet to be determined [101]. In the veterinary sector, Hofmeister *et al.* introduced a read-out-loud protocol before administering medication under anesthesia, and although the incidence of medication error rate reduced from 1.2% of anesthetics to 0.7%, it is notable that the risk was not eliminated [9]. Whether or not this improvement was sustained has also not been reported. Drug labeling and color coding is another commonly used method to reduce the chance of drug error, and an international standard exists for labeling syringes used during anesthesia: ISO 26825 [102]. However, a substantial proportion of errors occur after labeling [102]. The conclusion that can be made from this is that medication errors will continue to occur, probably because routine violations of policies intended to reduce medication errors are required to help manage the pressures inherent in clinical work ("to get work done"). Nonetheless, the listed methods are considered best practice and are, therefore, recommended.

Assessment of patient safety interventions

While it is tempting to suppose that any intervention or control measure aimed at improving patient safety should work, it must not be assumed that they will automatically result in improvement. In fact, it is not only possible for control measures to fail to improve patient safety, but any improvement may be unsustainable and may even lead to migrating risk to other parts of the process, or the introduction of obstacles to effective performance [103]. To evaluate the impact of introduced changes, a system for monitoring, such as clinical audit, is needed.

Clinical audit facilitates an objective evaluation of performance, including assessing the impact of introduced changes against explicit criteria, with the goal of achieving improvement in service or care [104,105]. In human medicine, clinical audit is widely recognized as a standard of care [62,106,107]. The procedure of clinical audit involves measuring an outcome (outcome audit) or process (process audit), comparing findings to available current evidence or "best practice," and then implementing changes to improve the quality of care [107,108]. Importantly, the audit process is cyclical and does not end once changes are introduced but continues to evaluate the impact of these changes. Clinical audits are more likely to be successful if they are focused and if simple changes can be introduced. Doing this does not guarantee a favorable outcome but makes it easier to understand the impact on a system, reasons for failure, and plan future steps.

Several models of clinical audit are available; all of them are cyclical in nature emphasizing that clinical audit should seek to drive continuous improvement. For example, the "Model for Improvement" [107,108] employs three preparatory questions linked to the four phases of the "Plan," "Do," "Study," "Act" (PDSA) cycle (Fig. 3.7).

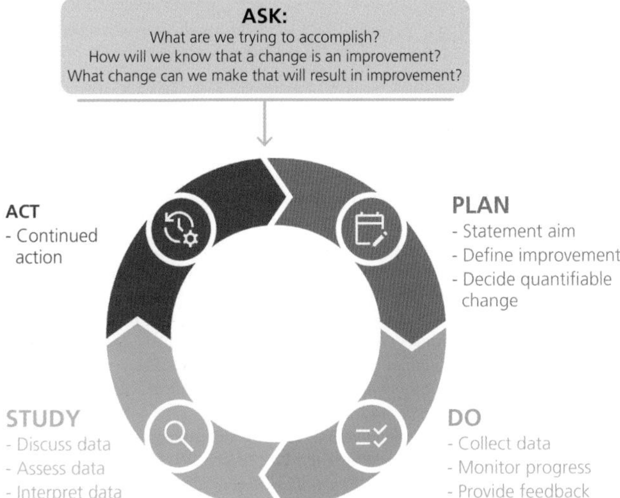

Figure 3.7 Preparatory questions and clinical audit cycle. Source: Adapted from Langley *et al.* [109].

Useful resources

- The Joint Commission (US) – https://www.jointcommission.org/resources/patient-safety-topics/
- Veterans Affairs (US) – https://www.patientsafety.va.gov
- National Health Service (UK) – https://www.england.nhs.uk/patient-safety/the-nhs-patient-safety-strategy/
- Institute for Safe Medication Practices (Canada) – https://www.ismp-canada.org/index.htm
- Canadian Patient Safety Institute – https://www.patientsafetyinstitute.ca/en/toolsresources/Pages/default.aspx\
- WHO patient safety – https://www.who.int/teams/integrated-health-services/patient-safety/research/safe-surgery
- Association of Veterinary Anaesthetists checklist – https://ava.eu.com/resources/checklists/
- TeamSTEPPS – https://www.ahrq.gov/teamstepps/instructor/index.html
- Anesthesia Patient Safety Foundation – https://www.apsf.org

References

1 Runciman W, Hibbert P, Thomson R, *et al.* Towards an international classification for patient safety: key concepts and terms. *Int J Qual Health Care* 2009; **21**(1): 18–26.
2 Catchpole K, Bell MD, Johnson S. Safety in anaesthesia: a study of 12606 reported incidents from the UK National Reporting and Learning System. *Anaesthesia* 2008; **63**(4): 340–346.
3 Gaba DM. Anaesthesiology as a model for patient safety in health care. *BMJ* 2000; **320**(7237): 785–788.
4 Institute of Medicine (US) Committee on Quality of Health Care in America. In: Kohn LT, Corrigan JM, Donaldson MS, eds. *To Err is Human: building a Safer Health System.* Washington, DC: National Academies Press (US), 2000.
5 Makary MA, Daniel M. Medical error-the third leading cause of death in the US. *BMJ* 2016; **353**: i2139.
6 James JT. A new evidence-based estimate of patient harms associated with hospital care. *J Patient Saf* 2013; **9**(3): 122–128.
7 Clarke KW, Hall LW. A survey of anaesthesia in small animal practice: AVA/BSAVA report. *Vet Anaesth Analg* 1990; **17**: 4–10.
8 Brodbelt DC, Blissitt KJ, Hammond RA, *et al.* The risk of death: the confidential enquiry into perioperative small animal fatalities. *Vet Anaesth Analg* 2008; **35**(5): 365–373.
9 Hofmeister EH, Quandt J, Braun C, *et al.* Development implementation and impact of simple patient safety interventions in a university teaching hospital. *Vet Anaesth Analg* 2014; **41**(3): 243–248.
10 McMillan MW, Lehnus KS. Systems analysis of voluntary reported anaesthetic safety incidents occurring in a university teaching hospital. *Vet Anaesth Analg* 2018; **45**(1): 3–12.
11 Wallis J, Fletcher D, Bentley A, *et al.* Medical errors cause harm in veterinary hospitals. *Front Vet Sci* 2019; **6**: 12.
12 Oxtoby C, Ferguson E, White K, *et al.* We need to talk about error: causes and types of error in veterinary practice. *Vet Rec* 2015; **177**(17): 438.
13 Garrouste-Orgeas M, Philippart F, Bruel C, *et al.* Overview of medical errors and adverse events. *Ann Intensive Care* 2012; **2**(1): 2.
14 Reason J. *Human Error.* Cambridge, UK: Cambridge University Press, 1991.
15 Gaba DM. Human error in dynamic medical domains. In: Bogner MS, ed. *Human Error in Medicine.* Hillsdale, NJ: Lawrence Erlbaum Associates, 1994.
16 Reason J. Safety in the operating theatre – Part 2: human error and organisational failure. *Qual Saf Health Care* 2005; **14**(1): 56–60.
17 Perrow C. *Normal Accidents: Living with High-Risk Technologies.* New York, NY: Basic Books, 1984.

18 Gaba DM, Maxwell M, DeAnda A. Anesthetic mishaps: breaking the chain of accident evolution. *Anesthesiology* 1987; **66**(5): 670–676.

19 Pang D. Accident and error management. In: Clark-Price S, Mama K, eds. *Equine Anesthesia and Co-Existing Disease*. Hoboken, NJ: Wiley-Blackwell, 2022: 352–384.

20 Flin R, Patey R, Glavin R, *et al.* Anaesthetists' non-technical skills. *Br J Anaesth* 2010; **105**(1): 38–44.

21 Howard SK, Gaba DM, Fish KJ, *et al.* Anesthesia crisis resource management training: teaching anesthesiologists to handle critical incidents. *Aviat Space Environ Med* 1992; **63**(9): 763–770.

22 Khatri N, Brown GD, Hicks LL. From a blame culture to a just culture in health care. *Health Care Manage Rev* 2009; **34**(4): 312–322.

23 Dekker SWA. Just culture: who gets to draw the line? *Cogn Tech Work* 2009; **11**(3): 177–185.

24 Eurocontrol Performance Review Commission. *Report on Legal and Cultural Issues in Relation to ATM Safety Occurrence Reporting in Europe: Outcome of a Survey Conducted by the Performance Review Unit in 2005–2006*. Brussels, Belgium: Eurocontrol, 2006.

25 Tucker AL, Nembhard IM, Edmondson AC. Implementing new practices: an empirical study of organizational learning in hospital intensive care units. *Manage Sci* 2007; **53**(6): 894–907.

26 Senge PM. *The Fifth Discipline: The Art and Practice of the Learning Organization*. New York, NY: Doubleday, 1990.

27 Stinson L, Pearson D, Lucas B. Developing a learning culture: twelve tips for individuals, teams and organizations. *Med Teach* 2006; **28**(4): 309–312.

28 Hollnagel E. Safety I and safety II. *The Past and Future of Safety Management*. Boca Raton, FL: CRC Press, 2014.

29 Hollnagel E, Wears RL, Braithwaite J. *From Safety-I to Safety-II: A White Paper. The Resilient Health Care Net. Published simultaneously by the University of Southern*. Denmark, University of Florida, USA, and Macquarie University, Australia, 2015.

30 Sexton JB, Helmreich RL, Neilands TB, *et al.* The safety attitudes questionnaire: psychometric properties, benchmarking data, and emerging research. *BMC Health Serv Res* 2006; **6**: 44.

31 Oxtoby C, Mossop L, White K, *et al.* Safety culture: the Nottingham Veterinary Safety Culture Survey (NVSCS). *Vet Rec* 2017; **180**(19): 472.

32 Love LC, Hedgpeth MW, Robertson JB, *et al.* Assessment of safety culture at a veterinary teaching hospital in the United States. *Front Vet Sci* 2021; **8**: 638764.

33 Dutton RP. Improving safety through incident reporting. *Curr Anesth Rep* 2014; **4**: 181–190.

34 Ludders JW, McMillan M. *Errors in Veterinary Anesthesia*, 1st edn. Ames, IA: Wiley-Blackwell, 2017.

35 Cooper JB. Is voluntary reporting of critical events effective for quality assurance? *Anesthesiology* 1996; **85**(5): 961–964.

36 Runciman WB. Lessons from the Australian Patient Safety Foundation: setting up a national patient safety surveillance system – is this the right model? *Qual Saf Health Care* 2002; **11**(3): 246–251.

37 Schortz L, Mossop L, Bergström A, *et al.* Type and impact of clinical incidents identified by a voluntary reporting system covering 130 small animal practices in mainland Europe. *Vet Rec* 2022; **191**(2): e1629.

38 Pang DSJ, Rouseau-Blass F, Pang JM. Morbidity and mortality conferences: a mini review and illustrated application in veterinary medicine. *Front Vet Sci* 2018; **5**: 43.

39 Orlander JD, Barber TW, Fincke BG. The morbidity and mortality conference: the delicate nature of learning from error. *Acad Med* 2002; **77**(10): 1001–1006.

40 Calder LA, Kwok ESH, Cwinn AA, *et al.* Enhancing the quality of morbidity and mortality rounds: the Ottawa M&M model. *Acad Emerg Med* 2014; **21**(3): 314–321.

41 Mitchell EL, Lee DY, Arora S, *et al.* SBAR M&M: a feasible reliable and valid tool to assess the quality of surgical morbidity and mortality conference presentations. *Am J Surg* 2012; **203**(1): 26–31.

42 Mitchell EL, Lee DY, Arora S, *et al.* Improving the quality of the surgical morbidity and mortality conference: a prospective intervention study. *Acad Med* 2013; **88**(6): 824–830.

43 Nimptsch U, Mansky T. Quality measurement combined with peer review improved German in-hospital mortality rates for four diseases. *Health Aff (Millwood)* 2013; **32**(9): 1616–1623.

44 Szekendi MK, Barnard C, Creamer J, *et al.* Using patient safety morbidity and mortality conferences to promote transparency and a culture of safety. *Jt Comm J Qual Patient Saf* 2010; **36**(1): 3–9.

45 Kirschenbaum L, Kurtz S, Astiz M. Improved clinical outcomes combining house staff self-assessment with an audit-based quality improvement program. *J Gen Intern Med* 2010; **25**(10): 1078–1082.

46 Joseph CW, Garrubba ML, Melder AM. Informing best practice for conducting morbidity and mortality reviews: a literature review. *Aust Health Rev* 2018; **42**(3): 248–257.

47 Prince JM, Vallabhaneni R, Zenati MS, *et al.* Increased interactive format for Morbidity & Mortality conference improves educational value and enhances confidence. *J Surg Educ* 2007; **64**(5): 266–272.

48 Aboumatar HJ, Blackledge CG, Dickson C, *et al.* A descriptive study of morbidity and mortality conferences and their conformity to medical incident analysis models: results of the morbidity and mortality conference improvement study, phase 1. *Am J Med Qual* 2007; **22**(4): 232–238.

49 De Meester K, Verspuy M, Monsieurs KG, *et al.* SBAR improves nurse-physician communication and reduces unexpected death: a pre and post intervention study. *Resuscitation* 2013; **84**(9): 1192–1196.

50 Leonard M, Graham S, Bonacum D. The human factor: the critical importance of effective teamwork and communication in providing safe care. *Qual Saf Health Care* 2004; **13**(Suppl 1): i85–i90.

51 Diller T, Helmrich G, Dunning S, *et al.* The Human Factors Analysis Classification System (HFACS) applied to health care. *Am J Med Qual* 2014; **29**(3): 181–190.

52 Vincent C, Taylor-Adams S, Stanhope N. Framework for analysing risk and safety in clinical medicine. *BMJ* 1998; **316**(7138): 1154–1157.

53 Vincent C, Taylor-Adams S, Chapman EJ, *et al.* How to investigate and analyse clinical incidents: clinical risk unit and association of litigation and risk management protocol. *BMJ* 2000; **320**(7237): 777–781.

54 Neuhaus C, Huck M, Hofmann G, *et al.* Applying the human factors analysis and classification system to critical incident reports in anaesthesiology. *Acta Anaesthesiol Scand* 2018; **62**(10): 1403–1411.

55 El-Bardissi AW, Wiegmann DA, Dearani JA, *et al.* Application of the human factors analysis and classification system methodology to the cardiovascular surgery operating room. *Ann Thorac Surg* 2007; **83**(4): 1412–1419.

56 Pang J, Yates E, Pang DSJ. A closed 'pop-off' valve and patient safety incident: a human factors approach to understanding error. *Vet Rec Case Rep* 2021; **9**(4): e189.

57 Cooper JB, Newbower RS, Long CD, *et al.* Preventable anesthesia mishaps: a study of human factors. *Anesthesiology* 1978; **49**(6): 399–406.

58 Buck N, Devlin HB, Lunn JN. *The Report of a Confidential Enquiry into Perioperative Deaths 1987*. London, UK: Nuffield Provincial Hospitals Trust, The King's Fund, 1988.

59 Runciman WB, Webb RK, Lee R, *et al.* The Australian Incident Monitoring Study. System failure: an analysis of 2000 incident reports. *Anaesth Intensive Care* 1993; **21**(5): 684–695.

60 Hales BM, Pronovost PJ. The checklist – a tool for error management and performance improvement. *J Crit Care* 2006; **21**(3): 231–235.

61 Haynes AB, Weiser TG, Berry WR, *et al.* A surgical safety checklist to reduce morbidity and mortality in a global population. *N Engl J Med* 2009; **360**(5): 491–499.

62 Pronovost P, Needham D, Berenholtz S, *et al.* An intervention to decrease catheter-related bloodstream infections in the ICU. *N Engl J Med* 2006; **355**(26): 2725–2732.

63 Pronovost P. Interventions to decrease catheter-related bloodstream infections in the ICU: the Keystone Intensive Care Unit Project. *Am J Infect Control* 2008; **36**(10): S171e1–e5.

64 Sexton JB, Thomas EJ, Helmreich RL. Error stress and teamwork in medicine and aviation: cross sectional surveys. *BMJ* 2000; **320**(7237): 745–749.

65 Helmreich RL. On error management: lessons from aviation. *BMJ* 2000; **320**(7237): 781–785.

66 World Health Organization (WHO) Surgical Safety Checklist (SSC) – Implementation Manual 2009. https://www.who.int/publications/i/item/9789241598590 (accessed March 2022.)

67 Bosk CL, Dixon-Woods M, Goeschel CA, *et al.* Reality check for checklists. *Lancet* 2009; **374**(9688): 444–445.

68 Haynes AB, Weiser TG, Berry WR, *et al.* Safe Surgery Saves Lives Study Group. Changes in safety attitude and relationship to decreased postoperative morbidity and mortality following implementation of a checklist-based surgical safety intervention. *BMJ Qual Saf* 2011; **20**(1): 102–107.

69 Menoud G, Axiak Flammer S, Spadavecchia C, *et al.* Development and implementation of a perianesthetic safety checklist in a veterinary university small animal teaching hospital. *Front Vet Sci* 2018; **5**: 60.

70 Pickering SP, Robertson ER, Griffin D, *et al.* Compliance and use of the World Health Organization checklist in UK operating theatres. *Br J Surg* 2013; **100**(2): 1664–1670.

71 Bergström A, Dimopoulou M, Eldh M. Reduction of surgical complications in dogs and cats by the use of a surgical safety checklist. *Vet Surg* 2016; **45**(5): 571–576.

72 Association of Veterinary Anaesthetists (AVA) Anaesthetic Safety Checklist. https://ava.eu.com/resources/checklists/ (accessed March 2022).

73 Marshall S. The use of cognitive aids during emergencies in anesthesia: a review of the literature. *Anesth Analg* 2013; **117**(5): 1162–1171.

74 Hepner DL, Arriaga AF, Cooper JB, *et al.* Operating room crisis checklists and emergency manuals. *Anesthesiology* 2017; **127**(2): 384–392.

75 McEvoy MD, Field LC, Moore HE, *et al.* The effect of adherence to ACLS protocols on survival of event in the setting of in-hospital cardiac arrest. *Resuscitation* 2014; **85**(1): 82–87.

76 Hall C, Robertson D, Rolfe M, *et al.* Do cognitive aids reduce error rates in resuscitation team performance? Trial of Emergency Medicine Protocols in Simulation Training (TEMPIST) in Australia. *Hum Resour Health* 2020; **18**(1): 1.

77 Fletcher DJ, Boller M, Brainard BM, *et al.* RECOVER evidence and knowledge gap analysis on veterinary CPR. Part 7: clinical guidelines. *J Vet Emerg Crit Care (San Antonio)* 2012; **22**(Suppl 1): S102–S131.

78 Donaldson L, Stevenson MA, Fletcher DJ, *et al.* Differences in the clinical practice of small animal CPR before and after the release of the RECOVER guidelines: results from two electronic surveys (2008 and 2017) in the United States and Canada. *J Vet Emerg Crit Care (San Antonio)* 2020; **30**(6): 615–631.

79 Gillespie Í, Fletcher DJ, Stevenson MA, *et al.* The compliance of current small animal CPR practice with RECOVER guidelines: an internet-based survey. *Front Vet Sci* 2019; **6**: 181.

80 Kawase K, Ujiie H, Takaki M, *et al.* Clinical outcome of canine cardiopulmonary resuscitation following the RECOVER clinical guidelines at a Japanese night-time animal hospital. *J Vet Med Sci* 2018; **80**(3): 518–525.

81 Runciman WB, Kluger MT, Morris RW, *et al.* Crisis management during anaesthesia: the development of an anaesthetic crisis management manual. *Qual Saf Health Care* 2005; **14**(3): e1.

82 Ziewacz JE, Arriaga AF, Bader AM, *et al.* Crisis checklists for the operating room: development and pilot testing. *J Am Coll Surg* 2011; **213**(2): 212–217.e10.

83 Arriaga AF, Bader AM, Wong JM, *et al.* Simulation-based trial of surgical-crisis checklists. *N Engl J Med* 2013; **368**(3): 246–253.

84 Tschan F, Keller S, Semmer NK, *et al.* Effects of structured intraoperative briefings on patient outcomes: multicentre before-and-after study. *Br J Surg* 2021; **109**(1): 136–144.

85 Segall N, Bonifacio AS, Schroeder RA, *et al.* Can we make postoperative patient handovers safer? A systematic review of the literature. *Anesth Analg* 2012; **115**(1): 102–115.

86 Abraham J, Meng A, Tripathy S, *et al.* Systematic review and meta-analysis of interventions for operating room to intensive care unit handoffs. *BMJ Qual Saf* 2021; **30**(6): 513–524.

87 Starmer AJ, Spector ND, Srivastava R, *et al.* I-PASS, a mnemonic to standardize verbal handoffs. *Pediatrics* 2012; **129**(2): 201–204.

88 Shahian D. I-PASS handover system: a decade of evidence demands action. *BMJ Qual Saf* 2021; **30**(10): 769–774.

89 Starmer AJ, O'Toole JK, Rosenbluth G, *et al.* Development implementation and dissemination of the I-PASS handoff curriculum: A multisite educational intervention to improve patient handoffs. *Acad Med* 2014; **89**(6): 876–884.

90 Müller M, Jürgens J, Redaèlli M, *et al.* Impact of the communication and patient hand-off tool SBAR on patient safety: a systematic review. *BMJ Open* 2018; **8**(8): e022202.

91 Jaulin F, Lopes T, Martin F. Standardised handover process with checklist improves quality and safety of care in the postanaesthesia care unit: the Postanaesthesia Team Handover trial. *Br J Anaesth* 2021; **127**(6): 962–970.

92 Higham H, Baxendale B. To err is human: use of simulation to enhance training and patient safety in anaesthesia. *Br J Anaesth* 2017; **119**(suppl 1): i106–i114.

93 Rall M, Dieckmann P. Simulation and patient safety: the use of simulation to enhance patient safety on a systems level. *Curr Anaesth Crit Care* 2005; **16**(5): 273–281.

94 Fung L, Boet S, Bould MD, *et al.* Impact of crisis resource management simulation-based training for interprofessional and interdisciplinary teams: a systematic review. *J Interprof Care* 2015; **29**(5): 433–444.

95 Mossenson AI, Bailey JG, Whynot S, *et al.* Qualities of effective vital anaesthesia simulation training facilitators delivering simulation-based education in resource-limited settings. *Anesth Analg* 2021; **133**(1): 215–225.

96 Noyes JA, Carbonneau KJ, Matthew SM. Comparative effectiveness of training with simulators versus traditional instruction in veterinary education: meta-analysis and systematic review. *J Vet Med Educ* 2022; **49**(1): 25–38.

97 Fletcher DJ, Militello R, Schoeffler GL, *et al.* Development and evaluation of a high-fidelity canine patient simulator for veterinary clinical training. *J Vet Med Educ* 2012; **39**(1): 7–12.

98 Jensen LS, Merry AF, Webster CS, *et al.* Evidence-based strategies for preventing drug administration errors during anaesthesia. *Anaesthesia* 2004; **59**(5): 493–504.

99 Merry AF, Anderson BJ. Medication errors – new approaches to prevention. *Paediatri Anaesth* 2011; **21**(7): 743–753.

100 Koyama AK, Maddox CS, Li L, *et al.* Effectiveness of double checking to reduce medication administration errors: a systematic review. *BMJ Qual Saf* 2020; **29**(7): 595–603.

101 Westbrook JI, Li L, Raban MZ, *et al.* Associations between double-checking and medication administration errors: a direct observational study of paediatric inpatients. *BMJ Qual Saf* 2021; **30**(4): 320–330.

102 Merry AF, Shipp DH, Lowinger JS. The contribution of labelling to safe medication administration in anaesthetic practice. *Best Pract Res Clin Anaesthesiol* 2011; **25**(2): 145–159.

103 Peerally MF, Carr S, Waring J, *et al.* The problem with root cause analysis. *BMJ Qual Saf* 2017; **26**(5): 417–422.

104 Mosedale P. Introducing clinical audit to veterinary practice. *In Pract* 1998; **20**: 40–42.

105 Rose N, Toews L, Pang DS. A systematic review of clinical audit in companion animal veterinary medicine. *BMC Vet Res* 2016; **12**: 40.

106 Patel NK, Sarraf KM, Joseph S, *et al.* Implementing the National Hip Fracture Database: an audit of care. *Injury* 2013; **44**(12): 1934–1939.

107 Colvin JR, Peden CJ. *Raising the Standard: A Compendium of Audit Recipes for Continuous Quality Improvement in Anaesthesia*, 3rd edn. London, UK: The Royal College of Anaesthetists, 2012.

108 Burgess R. *New Principles of Best Practice in Clinical Audit*, 2nd edn. Abingdon, UK: Radcliffe Publishing, 2011.

109 Langley GJ, Moen RD, Nolan KM, *et al.* *The Improvement Guide. A Practical Approach to Enhancing Organizational Performance*, 2nd edn. San Francisco, CA: Jossey-Bass, 2009.

4 Safety Considerations for Laser and Radiographic Procedures and Magnetic Resonance Imaging

Julie A. Smith[1] **and Carrie Davis**[2]

[1] MedVet Vancouver Emergency Veterinary and Specialty Care, Vancouver, Washington, USA

[2] MedVet Dallas Emergency Veterinary and Specialty Care, Dallas, Texas, USA

Chapter contents

Introduction, 40
Laser, 40
Laser beam hazard and safety, 40
Laser fire hazard and safety, 41
Anesthetic considerations for laser surgery, 41
Non-beam hazards and safety, 42
Radiography, 42
Ionizing radiation hazards and safety, 42
Anesthetic considerations for radiography, 43
Remote facilities, 45
Magnetic resonance imaging, 46
Strong static magnetic field, 46
Gradient magnetic fields, 49
Radiofrequency fields, 49
Cryogens, 49
Anesthetic management considerations, 50
Sedation versus general anesthesia, 50
Patient monitoring, 51
Standing equine MRI, 52
Gadolinium-based contrast agents, 52
Emergency procedures, 52
Personnel considerations, 52
References, 52

Introduction

Anesthesia is often required for patients undergoing procedures that incorporate the use of devices that could present a danger to the patient or the anesthetist. This chapter will focus on how to ensure a safe environment for both the anesthetist and the patient during the use of lasers and for diagnostic imaging procedures using radiation or high-strength magnetic fields.

Laser

The word "laser" is an acronym for Light Amplification by Stimulated Emission of Radiation. Surgical lasers produce an intense beam of pulsed or continuous invisible infrared light (radiation) that can be hazardous [1–3]. Laser devices are classified and labeled by the manufacturer according to their potential to cause biological damage. The classifications range from Class 1, the safest, to Class 4, the most hazardous. Wavelength, output power, and tissue exposure time are parameters used to categorize lasers and determine which precautions are necessary [4]. The most common lasers utilized in veterinary procedures have high emission levels and are listed in Class 3b or Class 4. The American National Standards Institute's Z136.3 document provides guidance for the safe operation of lasers in healthcare facilities, including veterinary hospitals [5–6]. The primary hazard associated with Class 3b and Class 4 lasers is related to accidental exposure to laser emissions.

Laser beam hazard and safety

Exposure may occur directly from the laser beam, or when the beam is reflected from a polished surface, metal instruments, or other objects. Reflected laser beams are unaltered and contain the same energy as the direct beam. Backscattering can also occur as the energy partially reflects on impact with tissue. The energy reflected in backscatter is less than the direct or reflected beam but may still have a damaging effect on staff and equipment. The Nd:YAG and the Argon laser are known to produce significant backscatter. The parts of the body at greatest risk are the eyes and skin.

The eye is extremely sensitive to laser radiation and can be permanently damaged from direct, diffuse, or reflected beams. Even brief or partial exposures can instantaneously damage the cornea, lens, or retina [1–3]. The extent of ocular damage is determined by the laser irradiance, exposure duration, and beam size. Infrared radiation is invisible; therefore, it is possible for eye damage to occur without awareness that an exposure has occurred. Since the eye cannot detect the invisible beam, it does not respond with a blink reflex or by averting the eye from the beam. Laser-induced

Veterinary Anesthesia and Analgesia: The Sixth Edition of Lumb and Jones. Edited by Leigh Lamont, Kurt Grimm, Sheilah Robertson, Lydia Love and Carrie Schroeder.
© 2024 John Wiley & Sons, Inc. Published 2024 by John Wiley & Sons, Inc.
Companion website: www.wiley.com/go/lamont/anesthesia

Box 4.1 Guidelines for eye protection during laser use.

- ALWAYS wear appropriate protective eyewear (glasses or goggles) whenever lasers are in use.
- Prescription eyewear, sunglasses, or contact lenses DO NOT protect eyes from laser beam.
- The wavelength number on protective eyewear should match the laser being used.
- Optical density (OD) number on protective eyewear should match, or be greater than, manufacturer recommendations for laser in use.
- Eye protection should fit snugly around the nose and have side and top guards.
- NEVER look directly at the laser or into the laser output port even when wearing eye protection.
- Protect glasses/goggles by returning them to their case or cover when not in use. Scratched, cracked, discolored, or loose lenses may allow injury to the eye.

Source: OSHA [1]; Lasers in Veterinary Practice [3].

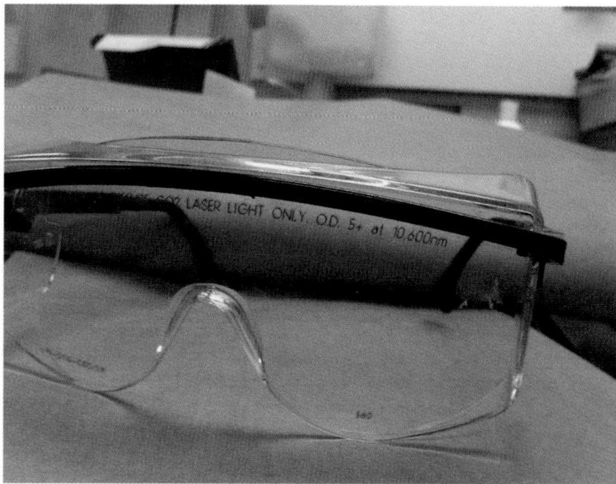

Figure 4.1 Protective eyewear performance characteristics are recommended by the manufacturer in the laser operation manual. The optical density (OD) and wavelength (nm) for which the protective eyewear is rated is imprinted directly on the glasses. Source: Dr. Kendall Taney, DAVDC, Center for Veterinary Dentistry and Oral Surgery, Gaithersburg, MD, with permission.

Table 4.1 Most common surgical lasers used in veterinary medicine. Common types of lasers used in veterinary procedures are listed along with their wavelengths and optical density number necessary for proper eye protection.

Laser type	Wavelength (nanometers)	Optical density (OD) number
Carbon dioxide	10,600	6+
Nd:YAG	1064	6+
Ho:YAG	2100	4+
Diode laser	810, 980	5+
KTP	532	6+
Argon	488, 514	6+

Source: Adapted from OSHA [1].

eye injury can occur in one or both eyes and may be temporary or permanent [3].

All persons within the operating area are at risk of eye injury, so it is critical for the anesthesia provider to take precautions and to use protective eyewear (Box 4.1). The United States Occupational Safety and Health Administration (OSHA) requires the use of eye protection for personnel in the presence of lasers that may result in eye injury [1]. Protective eyewear styles look similar but are not all the same. Options are based on the type of laser in use and rated for the specified wavelength range. Eyewear is also rated for its optical density, which is its ability to reduce the beam power. The optical density protection level is unique to each laser (Table 4.1) and will be recommended by the manufacturer in the laser operation manual. The wavelength and optical density for which the protective eyewear is rated can be found imprinted directly on the glasses (Fig. 4.1). It is important to observe warning signs in areas where lasers are in use and not enter without eye protection to prevent inadvertent exposure.

Eye protection is also important for the patient. The patient's eyes should be protected from direct or scattered laser beam by making sure that the eyelids are closed or protected by drapes. Pet eye protection goggles are available in a variety of sizes that are suitable for use with lasers classified as OD 6+ with wavelengths between 800 and 1100 nm.

Skin damage from exposure to the direct laser beam is possible for personnel who are very close to the procedure site. The severity of skin damage depends on the total energy deposited and penetration depth of the laser beam. Injuries range from a mild erythematous reaction to a severe burn. Drapes are effective protection for patients, and skin protection is usually not necessary for personnel in the laser use area because the energy density decreases rapidly beyond the focal point [2,3].

Laser fire hazard and safety

The direct or reflected beam of a high-emission Class 3b or Class 4 laser can ignite combustible materials and is a fire risk. Devastating operating room fires and combustion of the endotracheal tube (ETT) leading to fire in the trachea and lower airways are described in human medicine [7,8]. There is a single report documenting fire occurring during laser surgery in veterinary patients. It describes the ignition of the area around the face mask during inhalation anesthesia in two pet rodents, a mouse and a hamster, during cutaneous mass removal with a diode laser. The fire resulted in life-threatening burns on the face, head, and upper body of both rodents. Only one animal survived [9].

Anesthetic considerations for laser surgery

General anesthesia with inhalant anesthetics and high concentrations of oxygen are commonly used for immobilization during laser procedures. Anesthesia may be delivered through an ETT or by face mask depending on the species and situation. Lasers are frequently utilized for procedures in the oral cavity and close to the airway in veterinary patients where intubation is necessary to ensure proper ventilatory support [10,11]. Commonly used ETTs made of polyvinyl chloride (PVC), red rubber, and silicone are combustible [7,12]. The intense heat of the laser can burn through the ETT in seconds and cause a fire when the beam encounters the oxygen-enriched gas inside the tube [13].

Metal, copper-shielded, and insulated ETTs designed for use with laser procedures are commercially available and are the standard of care in human anesthesia care. However, these tubes are expensive, bulky, and not universally safe for all types of lasers, nor are they available in sizes suitable for horses or very small patients [7,14].

A latex red rubber ETT, tightly wrapped with spirally overlapping loops of self-adhesive non-reflective aluminum or copper tape, was reported as safe or safer than commercially available stainless

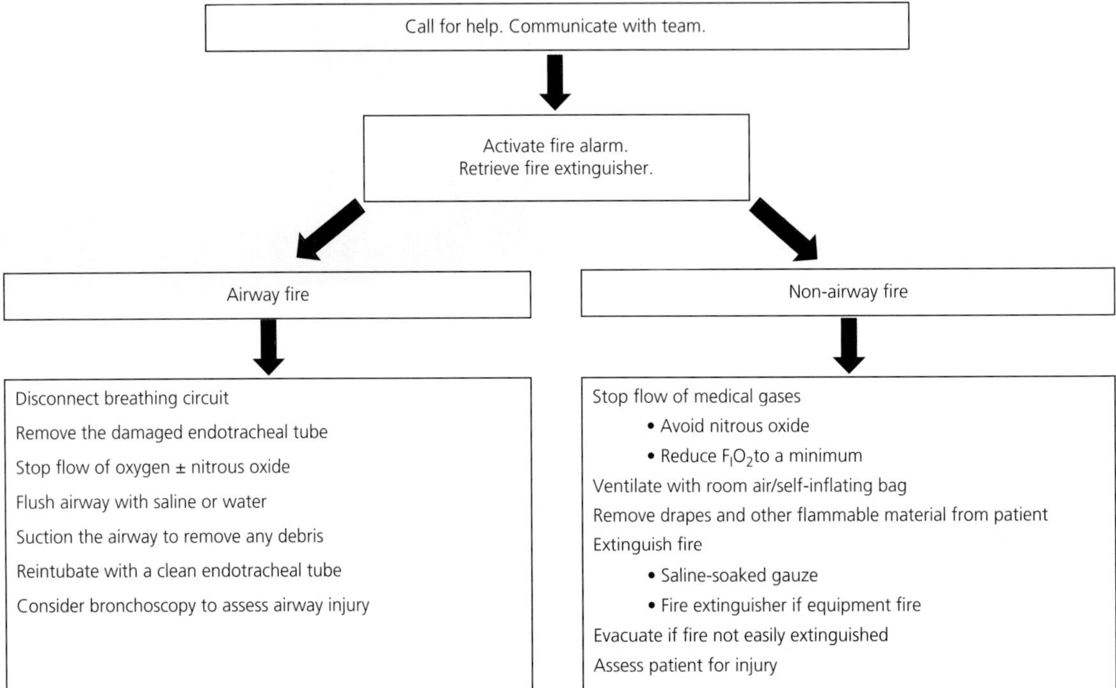

Figure 4.2 Crisis checklist in the event of an airway or operating room fire during laser surgery.

steel or insulated ETTs for use with CO_2 and Nd-YAG lasers [7,14–18]. Wrapping the ETT increases the external diameter and makes the surface potentially more irritating to delicate tracheal tissue. Tape can come loose from the wrapped ETT, and it is necessary to carefully examine the tube following extubation to ensure that none of the tape came off in the trachea [2,7,11,14,16]. A simple and effective method for protecting the ETT from combustion is to cover it with a thick layer of saline-soaked sponges [7,19]. Keep the sponges moist throughout the procedure to dissipate heat from any inadvertent exposure from the laser beam. Count sponges before and after placement to ensure that all sponges have been removed from the oropharynx prior to recovery.

The ETT cuff and pilot tubing are also susceptible to damage during laser surgery [2,7]. Inadvertent deflation of the cuff will allow leakage of high oxygen concentration and anesthetic gases into the oral cavity and around the head of the patient. Fire may result if the enriched oxygen gas contacts the laser beam. Protecting the pilot tube with saline-soaked gauze sponges and using saline instead of air to fill the cuff will dissipate heat and maintain patency of the cuff. Adding a dye, such as new methylene blue, to the saline used to inflate the cuff may indicate if the pilot tube is compromised [2,7,19].

When the use of a face mask to deliver inhalant anesthesia in high concentrations of oxygen cannot be avoided, efforts should be made to fit the mask tightly around the face or head of the patient, use the lowest flow rates possible, and provide a physical barrier to prevent oxygen-enriched gases from encountering the laser beam.

The risk of fire hazard during laser procedures can be minimized by choosing injectable anesthesia techniques, allowing spontaneous ventilation with room air or, in the case of laryngeal surgery, placing the ETT nasotracheally or through a tracheostomy [2,10,11]. Inspired oxygen concentrations may be lowered by mixing with medical gas if available. Nitrous oxide should be avoided. It may be necessary to remove the ETT and the oxygen source temporarily at several points during a procedure to facilitate safe access to the laryngeal area. To further reduce risk, avoid the use of flammable antiseptic solutions, drying agents, oil-based lubricants or ointments, or flammable plastics whenever lasers are being used [2,7,20]. Fig. 4.2 is a crisis checklist of emergent measures if an airway or operating room fire occurs. Emergency procedures should be determined in advance and practiced by all potential participants.

Non-beam hazards and safety

Laser–tissue interactions produce a plume of smoke that may contain bacterial and viral particles as small as 0.1–0.3 μm and potentially toxic gases, some of which may be carcinogens. Bronchospasm from bronchial irritation, alveolar edema, interstitial pneumonia, and diffuse pulmonary atelectasis are potential consequences of inhaled laser smoke [2,3].

Air evacuation systems are used to reduce pollution of the workspace and prevent inhalation and alveolar exposure of personnel in the laser-designated area. Laser filtration surgical face masks are available for added protection. Standard surgical masks alone do not provide adequate protection during laser procedures [3]. Patients who are intubated and connected to an anesthesia machine are not at risk for inhaling laser smoke. However, precautions should be taken for non-intubated patients to prevent inhalation exposure and potential pulmonary injury.

Radiography

Plain radiography, contrast studies, fluoroscopy, computed tomography (CT), and radiation therapy (RT) all incorporate the use of ionizing radiation.

Ionizing radiation hazards and safety

Ionizing radiation exposure is potentially hazardous and causes injury at the cellular level by transferring high levels of energy into atoms and molecules such as DNA, RNA, and other cellular proteins, damaging chemical bonds, and altering the electrical charge to create free radicals or ions [21–24].

Sensitivity to ionizing radiation is highest in the most actively replicating cells of the skin, bone marrow, small intestine, and reproductive cells. Developing embryos are particularly sensitive to the effects of ionizing radiation. Slow growing nerve and muscle cells are the most resistant to radiation damage [21–24].

Effects from the exposure to ionizing radiation may appear promptly or be delayed, depending on the type and duration of exposure. Effects resulting from chronic exposure to low levels of radiation are most relevant to veterinary anesthesia providers. Chronic radiation exposure is associated with an increased incidence of cataracts, squamous cell carcinoma, leukemia, and premature aging [21–25].

Regulations require that personnel limit the level of radiation exposure to "as low as reasonably achievable" (ALARA). This can be achieved by increasing distance from the source, using shielding, and minimizing the number of images and length of time of procedures.

The primary source of personnel occupational exposure is from X-rays that bounce off or scatter from objects in the path of the primary beam. The patient is the major source of scatter radiation. The amount of potential exposure from scatter radiation is directly related to the proximity of personnel to the source of the ionizing radiation and decreases rapidly with increased separation from the source. The best way to reduce exposure is to temporarily leave the radiology suite and view the patient from the doorway or through leaded glass when the machine is in use. When leaving the room is not possible, standing at least 3 feet away from the patient during X-ray use and wearing a protective lead apron are advised [22,25]. An anesthesia provider may not be able to move away from the patient when involved with positioning patients for radiographs or during fluoroscopy and other special procedures. When this is the case, avoid direct beam exposure and avoid leaning over the patient during imaging. When in close proximity to the source of radiation, protective attire should include a lead apron, thyroid shield, and gloves. A wrap-around lead apron is recommended for situations that may result in a high level of radiation exposure such as fluoroscopy to provide additional protection. Consider wearing protective goggles if a lot of time is spent in the radiology suite. It is important to note that lead-lined protective apparel is not designed to provide protection from direct beam exposure [22].

The risk of potential radiation exposure is increased with CT and RT due to higher levels of radiation involved in the procedures. During these procedures, it is safest for the anesthetist to leave the side of the patient and stand behind a portable barrier, move into the control room, or leave the room altogether. It is important to monitor cumulative radiation exposure by wearing a radiation exposure badge or dosimeter [22,23,25]. Each individual is provided with their own personal badge to wear at all times during participation in radiographic procedures, and badges should not be worn outside of the radiology suite. It is recommended that radiation badges be positioned at the neckline on the outside of the protective lead apron. Radiation levels are evaluated at scheduled intervals.

Pregnant workers should avoid exposure to radiation as much as possible, especially during the first 16 weeks of pregnancy, when the most rapid cell division occurs. It is important to inform management as soon as pregnancy is suspected so that arrangements can be made to only assign the anesthetist to situations that do not involve radiation. Incorporating the safety precautions of decreasing time of exposure, increasing distance from the source, and using shielding as much as possible will reduce exposure. Wearing two aprons or adding a flap to protect the fetus will increase protection. A separate radiation dosimeter, worn at the waistline under the apron(s), is recommended to monitor fetal exposure. Self-reading dosimeters are available that provide real-time measurements to further assure protection. The gestational radiation limit is 10% of the normal limit for radiation workers.

Anesthetic considerations for radiography

Radiology suites are rarely designed with the provision of anesthesia in mind. Therefore, in order to provide optimal anesthesia support for every patient during radiology procedures, communication with radiology personnel is critical. It is important to understand the procedure being done, the contrast agents to be administered, the route and rate of contrast administration, and the estimated duration of the procedure. The signalment and temperament of the patient, the underlying disease process, accessibility of positioning devices, familiarity with the procedure being done, anesthetic drug and equipment availability, and amount of assistance are all factors to consider.

Standard radiographs may be obtained easily with positioning devices without chemical restraint when the patient is cooperative. However, not all patients are cooperative and sedation will facilitate good positioning and reduce the need for repeat X-ray exposure for both patients and personnel. Longer duration procedures or those that may be invasive or painful (e.g., certain contrast studies and fluoroscopy) are best done using sedation or general anesthesia. The anesthetist must ensure access to the patient for monitoring and provision of thermoregulatory support, both of which must be achieved without interfering with the imaging procedure or risking radiation exposure.

Patients immobilized for radiographic procedures, even when not intubated or under general anesthesia, should be monitored closely and continuously. Monitoring should, at the very least, consist of direct observation of respiratory rate and effort, evaluation of mucous membrane color, palpation of pulse quality and rate, and the use of pulse oximetry and non-invasive blood pressure. Select monitors with easy-to-read screens, large numbers, and visual alarms that can be easily seen in a dimly lit radiology suite from behind a screen or through an observation window. A source of supplemental oxygen should be available at all times. Be prepared to supplement sedation, intubate, support ventilation, induce general anesthesia, or perform rescue procedures when necessary. Position the anesthesia machine and monitors, so they can be easily observed from outside the room or with a video camera. Controlled ventilation is advisable for ensuring adequate ventilation and consistent inhalant anesthesia delivery in patients during procedures such as fluoroscopy, CT, and RT when the anesthetist must leave the room.

CT uses high levels of radiation to obtain cross-sectional images and requires a motionless subject for best results. The imaging time varies depending on the type of CT being used (i.e., 1-slice versus 64-slice). While the actual imaging time may be short, the time to position the patient and evaluate the study can be much longer. Patients experiencing pain may not be willing to lie still or allow positioning with sedation alone. Even slight movement during the scan can result in motion artifacts that interfere with the quality of the images and their diagnostic value. If this occurs, the scan will have to be repeated, which increases the overall anesthesia time and the amount of radiation exposure for the patient.

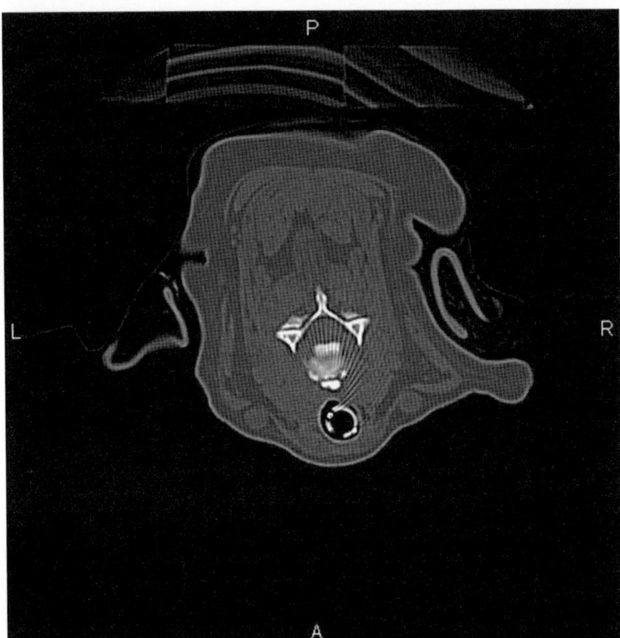

Figure 4.3 Cross-sectional CT image of a dog's neck and trachea showing artifact created by the radio-opaque markers embedded in the wall of many common endotracheal tubes. The artifacts are the white lines radiating outward from the markers in the tube wall situated within the trachea.

The radio-opaque stripe in most commonly used ETTs that makes the tube clearly visible on radiographs causes an artifact on CT images. These artifacts may interfere with the diagnostic value of images of the neck and head (Fig. 4.3). ETTs without the X-ray opaque stripe are available and should be considered when the ETT will be in the area being imaged. Additionally, armored ETTs (reinforced by metal coils) should be avoided if the tube will be included in the imaging area to avoid artifact and the need for repeated scanning.

During CT imaging, the presence of metal objects, such as electrocardiogram (ECG) clips and lead wires, in the scan field can lead to severe streaking artifacts that can obscure or simulate pathology. To avoid interfering with image acquisition, keep ECG leads, other monitoring cables, and any metal-containing item outside the anatomic scan field whenever possible. Valuable cardiac rhythm information is obtainable even when ECG leads are placed at nontraditional sites, such as the paws, ears, neck, etc. It may be necessary to disconnect one of the ECG leads temporarily in order to avoid creating artifacts on the images. Collars, halters, horseshoes, nail fragments, or other metal objects should be removed from the patient if they are included in the area being imaged.

During CT examination, the patient table will move in and out of the bore of the scanner. The anesthesia delivery hoses must be long enough to move with the patient during imaging without becoming kinked or disconnected. Monitoring cables and fluid administration lines should be positioned so that they will not get caught under the moving table or disconnected from the patient.

Thoracic CT imaging, particularly of the lungs, is best done immediately following induction to minimize atelectasis. Maintaining the patient in sternal recumbency may decrease positional atelectasis [personal communication: Ian D. Robertson, College of Veterinary Medicine, North Carolina State University]. Some thoracic studies may require apnea or breath-hold maneuvers to alleviate motion from chest expansion during ventilation. A brief period of apnea may be induced with hypnotic agents (propofol or alfaxalone) or by hyperventilation. Some facilities employ jet ventilation combined with total intravenous anesthesia (TIVA) to avoid respiratory motion. If lung aeration is required, the anesthetist can manually hold the lungs in inspiration during scanning or perform an alveolar recruitment maneuver. In this situation, the anesthetist should wear a protective apron, thyroid shield, and goggles while tucked behind a mobile shield. Alternatively, an anesthetic machine equipped with a positive end-expiratory pressure (PEEP) valve or a closed adjustable pressure-limiting (pop-off) valve with oxygen flow turned off may allow the anesthetist to temporarily depart the scanning room. Caution is advised with this method and strict, constant attentiveness is necessary to avoid catastrophic barotrauma.

RT uses a high dose of ionizing radiation delivered precisely by a direct beam into tumor tissue. The total treatment dose is divided into multiple sessions that are spread out over days or weeks. Patients must be motionless and positioned exactly the same for each treatment to prevent damage to surrounding healthy tissue. A variety of devices are used to aid in positioning patients depending on the location of the area being imaged. Certain positioning devices may interfere with anesthetic and monitoring equipment or influence placement of the intravenous (IV) catheter. Effective and safe anesthetic patient management depends on familiarity with the procedure and the specific device being used. All personnel must leave the room for several minutes during treatment. Patients can be observed from outside the room using a video camera(s), preferably with sound, positioned to provide a clear view of the patient monitor, the anesthesia machine, and the patient. The treatment session can be paused if patient movement or problems are detected.

General anesthesia is recommended for horses and other large animals during selected radiographic studies and CT scanning to provide the necessary immobility to obtain diagnostic images quickly and safely. Inadequately immobilized large animals may cause damage to the equipment or injury to themselves. Ropes and positioning pads should be available, and physical effort is required to move the table and patient. Horses with neurologic disease may present a higher risk to staff and themselves, particularly during induction and recovery.

Standing sedated CT of the equine head or distal limbs is an option at some facilities. Although the risk of general anesthesia is eliminated, a sedated neurologic or orthopedically unsound horse may fall and injure itself, staff, or equipment. Consequently, nonslip flooring is advised, and the handler should have an escape route planned. Additionally, a handler may remain horse-side and that individual should be positioned as far as possible from the radiation source behind a mobile shield and wear an apron, thyroid shield, and goggles. Sandbags, a rope halter, and a V-shaped trough to aid positioning, in addition to ear plugs and a blindfold to limit patient stimulation, may permit the assistant more distance from the radiation source.

Radiographic myelography of equids presents several challenges for the anesthetist in addition to radiation safety techniques. The study should be performed quickly to reduce recumbency time and limit time-dependent reabsorption and dilution of contrast media that may limit the study's diagnostic value. Horses presenting for myelography may have neurologic deficits, including ataxia, resulting in additional danger to the animal and staff throughout induction and recovery. Adverse reactions associated with anesthesia or myelographic technique that present danger to staff and patient, such as generalized or focal seizures, may occur during the procedure or at recovery. The anesthetist should be prepared to provide medical management or to re-anesthetize patients when indicated. Multiple position changes of equine patients require manpower and efficient coordination with all services involved. When spinal compression is suspected, careful manipulation of the patient is crucial to avoid exacerbation of any dynamic component to the compression. Constant vigilance to protect the eye, IV catheter, fluid line, anesthetic, and monitoring equipment while ensuring ETT safety and patency are essential. Positional changes and disconnection of the breathing circuit may result in personnel exposure to inhalant anesthetic. Attention to limb positioning and padding and support are essential. Radiolucent cushions should be available to aid neck positioning for image acquisitions to avoid repeat imaging. Inadequate padding under the patient when placed on the floor or myelogram table may increase the risk of developing myopathy or peripheral neuropathy.

Radiocontrast agents

Radiocontrast agents are used to improve the visibility of certain structures during radiography and CT. The most common contrast agents used for radiographic procedures are iodine- and barium-based preparations [26]. Barium compounds, used for gastrointestinal studies and given orally, do not usually require general anesthesia in companion animals, but it may be necessary for uncooperative, untamed, or exotic species. Prevention of barium aspiration is a critical part of anesthesia management during gastrointestinal studies, as it can cause serious health effects, ranging from pneumonia to death [26]. Protection of the airway with an appropriately sized ETT and inflated cuff and thorough inspection of the back of the mouth prior to extubation for any signs of barium regurgitation are important. If aspiration of barium is suspected, a thoracic radiograph will be able to identify barium in the lower airways and pulmonary parenchyma. The ETT should not be removed until the patient is awake enough to swallow and cough. Consideration can be given to leaving air in the ETT cuff during extubation in case of unobserved leakage of barium into the trachea proximal to the inflated cuff, though this must be weighed against the risk of potential laryngeal damage.

Iodine-based solutions can be administered orally, intravenously, intraluminally, or into the subarachnoid space. Adverse side effects are infrequent and depend on the site of administration and the type of contrast media used. Contrast reactions are related to the osmolality, molecular size, and complexity of the agent used. Effects range from minor physiological alterations to bronchospasm, renal insufficiency, and life-threatening anaphylaxis [26].

Contrast induced nephropathy is a poorly understood condition that is increasingly reported in people with pre-existing renal insufficiency and diabetes [26,27]. Studies in dehydrated dogs have shown reductions in renal blood flow and glomerular filtration rate following parenteral administration of hypertonic contrast media. Prior to administration of contrast agents, evaluate renal and hydration status, correct hypotension, and communicate any abnormalities to the radiologist to prevent possible renal impairment [personal communication: Ian D. Robertson, College of Veterinary Medicine, North Carolina State University]. Reduction in renal function due to contrast agents can usually be reversed with correction of hypotension and rehydration [27].

Myelography is a contrast study using plain radiography or CT scanning, consisting of a subarachnoid injection of a water-soluble, non-ionic contrast media either in either the lumbar area or cerebellomedullary cistern. This is an invasive and stimulating procedure, and the patient must be adequately anesthetized prior to the insertion of the needle. Patient movement can result in spinal cord damage or a non-diagnostic study. Side effects following subarachnoid injection depend on the agent selected, the site of administration, and needle placement. They include tachycardia, bradycardia, vomiting, seizures, and cardiac arrest [28,29]. Asystole that responded to anticholinergic administration was reported in one dog immediately after a cisternal injection of iohexol during a myelogram [30]. Postmyelographic side effects have become less frequent with the development of newer contrast agents. If an adverse reaction occurs, treatment is palliative and supportive. In addition to ensuring an adequate airway and providing oxygen and hemodynamic support, the anesthetist may need to manage anaphylaxis and bronchospasm with antihistamines, epinephrine, glucocorticoids, bronchodilators, vasopressors, or anticholinergics.

Extravasation of contrast agents may lead to local tissue damage. The severity of the effects caused by perivascular injection depends on the osmolality of the contrast agent and the volume injected and can range from mild swelling and erythema to ulceration and necrosis [26]. Some radiographic studies require the rapid injection of the contrast agent by hand injection or using a rapid injector pump at flow rates of 0.5–5 mL/s. Large volumes of contrast can be injected subcutaneously if the catheter is not properly placed. Box 4.2 lists steps to reduce the risk of extravasation as well as methods to treat accidental perivascular delivery of a contrast agent.

Remote facilities

Radiology facilities are often separated from the anesthesia induction area, sometimes on a different floor or in a separate building. Advance planning for transportation to and from the facility, including consideration of monitoring and anesthesia maintenance during transfer, is critical for patient safety. In addition to diligent planning, practice drills for emergent situations in sites distant from the anesthesia area are recommended. In facilities where a rapid return to the anesthesia or intensive care area is not practical, rescue drugs and equipment will need to be transported with the patient or in place in the radiology suite.

Box 4.2 Prevention and treatment of perivascular injection of radiocontrast agents.

Prevention

- Always inject contrast agents through an intravenous catheter.
- Use the largest bore catheter possible (> 20 gauge is best).
- Do not use peripheral central venous catheters for power injection.
- Check catheter patency prior to injection.
- Warm contrast media to decrease viscosity and resistance to injection.
- Inspect the area around the catheter immediately following injection.

Treatment

- Early recognition of catheter failure is the best way to prevent serious side effects.
- Apply a cold compress to areas of perivascular injection.
- Infiltrate the area with saline to dilute radiocontrast agent and aid with absorption.
- With extravasation of large volumes, hyaluronidase may be added to further increase absorption.
- Provide symptomatic therapy.

Source: ACR [26]; Belzunegui *et al.* [31]; Wang *et al.* [32]; Miles *et al.* [33].

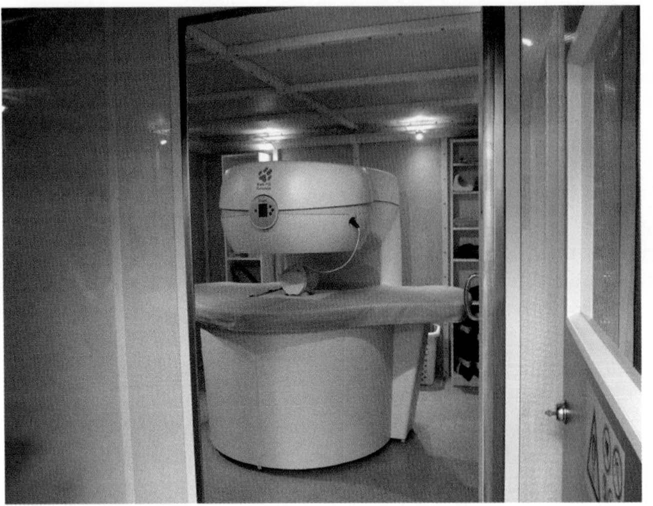

(A)

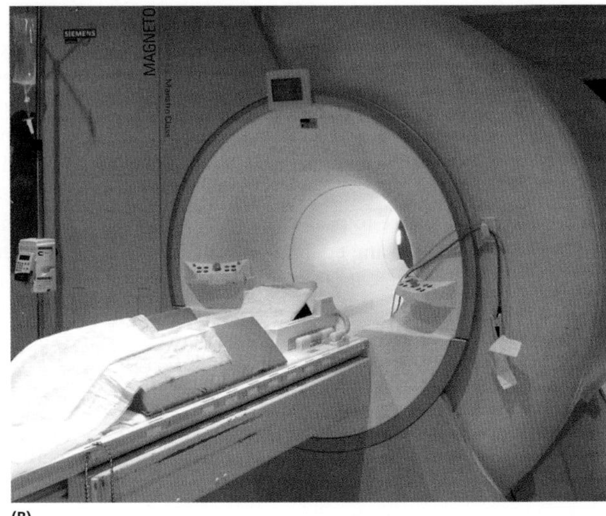

(B)

Figure 4.4 **A.** Low-field 0.2-T, open style magnet. **B.** High-field 1.5-T, closed style magnet.

Magnetic resonance imaging

Magnetic resonance imaging (MRI) utilizes a powerful static magnetic field, several weaker, rapidly changing, gradient magnetic fields, and high-frequency electromagnetic (radiofrequency [RF]) waves. The image is generated when protons strongly aligned to the static magnetic field are perturbed by RF pulses, releasing energy as they relax back into alignment. The energy released is detected by the scanner and transformed into an image.

Strong static magnetic field

The main component of an MRI system is the magnet. MRI systems are classified by the basic shape (e.g., open or closed) and the way the magnetic field is generated (e.g., by permanent magnet material or by currents in superconducting coils) [34]. The magnetic field is measured in tesla (T) units. Permanent magnets have low field strengths, less than 1.0 T, and have an open configuration. Superconducting magnets have high field strengths and a closed cylindrical shape (Fig. 4.4). The clinically functional strengths are 1.0 T, 1.5 T, and 3.0 T. Stronger systems, 4.0 T, 7.0 T, and 9.4 T, are being evaluated for practical safety and health implications [34–42]. Higher strengths are used for MRI research. The RF transmitter/receiver used to transfer energy into the tissue and capture the energy released from the tissue is called an "RF coil." The most common types are body and local or surface coils. The body coil is part of the scanner, whereas surface coils are placed over or wrapped around the body part being scanned (Fig. 4.5).

The resonance energy emitted from the patient is very weak, and any other sources of RF noise cause artifacts and interfere with the acquisition of clear images. Suites designed for MRI acquisition are shielded from external sources of RF energy by lining the walls with copper sheeting or by a metal Faraday cage around the scanner. A safety line is typically marked around the magnet indicating the "5-gauss line," which is the point at which the stagnant magnetic field strength is higher than 5 gauss or 0.5 mT. Beyond the 5-gauss line, all ferromagnetic objects are strictly prohibited (Fig. 4.6). Electrical devices produce RF waves and must be kept outside the 5-gauss line and the MRI room unless they are internally shielded and have been tested and designated as MRI safe or MRI conditional (see below). Penetration panels containing waveguides that filter stray RF can be built into the shielding to allow the passage of plastic anesthetic delivery hoses, sampling tubing, fiber-optic pulse oximetry cables, and non-conducting materials into the MRI room (Fig. 4.7) [42–44].

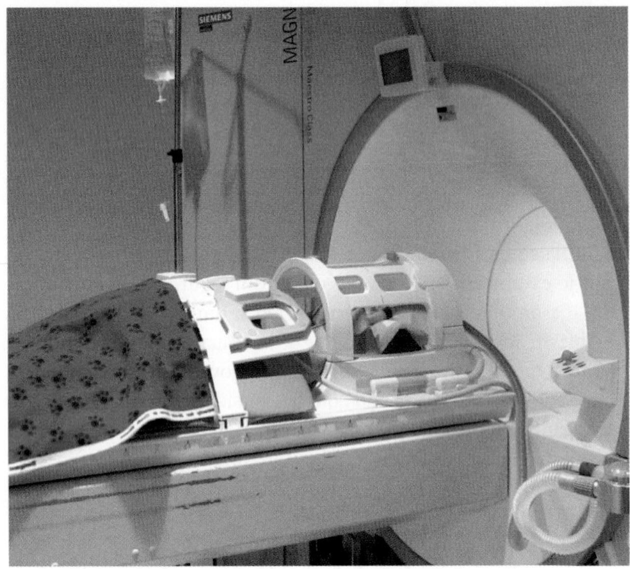

Figure 4.5 Dog positioned under radiofrequency transmitter/receiver coils for imaging of the head and neck prior to being moved into the bore of the MRI scanner.

The MRI environment presents hazards for both staff and patients, including ferromagnetic projectiles due to the displacement force of the static electromagnetic field, high-level acoustic noise, and systemic and localized heating. The magnetic field is always present (i.e., always "on") even when not scanning a patient. The field extends outside the bore of the magnet in all directions and is one of the major hazards of the magnetic resonance (MR) scanner. The extent of this "fringe" or stray field depends on the strength and shielding of the magnet. The magnet vendor provides each facility with a map of the fringe fields for onsite safety (Fig. 4.6). This invisible field is weakest at the outside edge and increases in strength as it approaches the scanner. It is critical to be familiar with the location of the 5-gauss line, as the magnetic strength increases

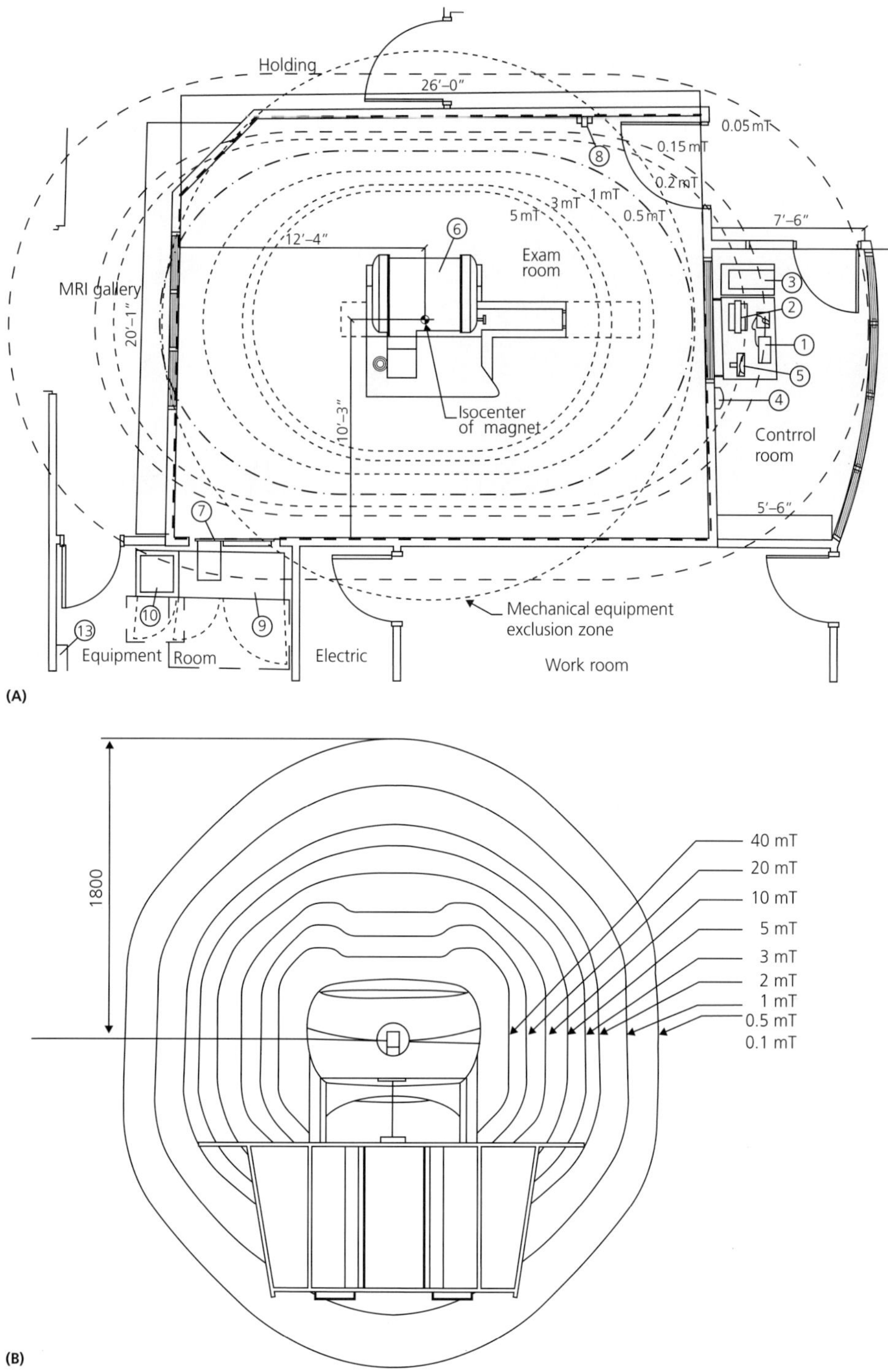

Figure 4.6 The magnetic field extends outside the bore of the magnet and is always present. The extent of this "fringe" or stray field depends on the strength and shielding of the magnet. **A.** A detailed map of fringe fields for a 1.5-T high-field magnet. Access is restricted inside the 5-gauss (0.5 mT) line, which, in this facility, actually extends beyond the wall of the room in one area. The fringe fields extend the same distance in all directions, above and below the magnet room. **B.** Diagram of fringe fields for a 0.2-T low-field magnet.

rapidly beyond this point, causing accidents and medical device malfunction. The 5-gauss line designates the perimeter of the MRI safety zone, inside which access is restricted to MRI safety trained personnel, MRI safety screened patients, and MRI designated safe or conditional devices (Box 4.3). The closer to the magnet, the stronger the attraction to ferromagnetic objects, causing them to become projectiles and causing serious injury to anyone in their path. The "missile" or "projectile" effect is the most significant hazard to personnel and patients when working in a magnetic environment. The larger the object, the faster it will be pulled into the magnet and the more difficult it is to remove. Removal may require interruption of the magnetic field and lead to expensive restoration of the magnetic field, costly equipment damage, and loss of revenue [42–44]. All ferromagnetic objects must be removed from

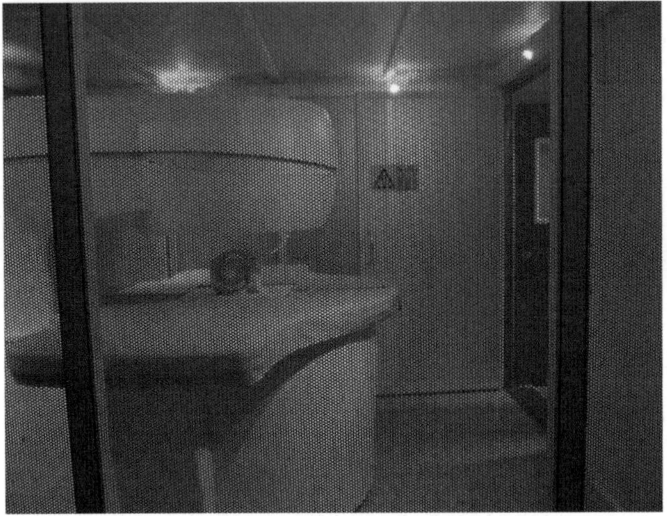
(A)

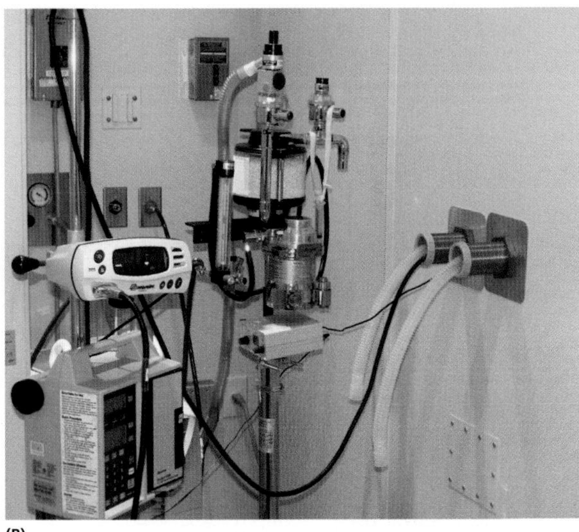
(B)

Figure 4.7 **A.** A low-field magnet inside a metal Faraday cage. **B.** Waveguide radiofrequency filters in one of the panels of the same Faraday cage. Non-compatible equipment (the anesthesia machine, pulse oximeter, and fluid pump) is kept outside the 5-gauss line and the magnet room and compatible hoses and cables are passed through the waveguide to the patient.

Box 4.3 Safety screening guidelines for access to the MRI safety zone.

Personnel

- Inform ALL personnel that the **MAGNET IS ALWAYS ON.**
- Provide an MRI safety course for all anesthesia personnel. Make it mandatory and verify compliance.
- Restrict access to the MRI safety zone to individuals who have completed the MRI safety course.
- Be prepared for an anesthetic emergency. Establish and practice an emergency action plan.
- Routinely update and review safety information and emergency procedures.
- Screen any personnel who will be providing patient care in the MRI suite for insulin pump, pacemaker, aneurysm clip, ocular metal, hearing aid, cochlear implant, metal piercings, recent surgery, etc.
- Pregnant personnel are not at risk in the MRI safety zone but should not remain in the MRI room during imaging.
- Be vigilant to prevent any ferromagnetic objects from being inadvertently brought into the MRI safety zone (stethoscopes, laryngoscopes, medical instruments, clippers, oxygen tanks, etc.).

Equipment

- Only equipment labeled conditional for the strength of the magnet in use should be taken into the MRI safety zone. Any other equipment must be tested and labeled as safe by the designated Safety Officer, MR technologist, and/or magnet engineer prior to entering the area.
- MRI-unsafe equipment located close to the MRI safety zone must be conspicuously labeled *"unsafe for MRI"* to prevent inadvertent transfer into the scan room.
- Screen any equipment that leaves the MRI area when it returns, as ferromagnetic items may have been placed on it.
- Ferromagnetic devices used inside the MRI safety zone must be positioned outside the 5-gauss line and physically secured with plastic or rope ties, non-magnetic bolts, or a weighted base system. Conspicuously label the device *"unsafe for MRI"* and mark the position of the 5-gauss line on the floor.

Patient

- Prior to entering the MRI safety zone, obtain a complete history and carefully screen patients for the presence of metal implants. Pacemakers, microchips, orthopedic implants, bullets or shrapnel, gold beads, ingested gravel or other metallic/magnetic substances in the gastrointestinal tract may pose a hazard for the patient or interfere with image acquisition.
- Remove collars, harnesses, halters, nose rings, hair clips, and any other items containing metal.
- Determine if the patient is ambulatory. Have a plan for getting large non-ambulatory patients into the facility/induction area.
- Transdermal patches (fentanyl and others) may contain aluminum that can heat up and cause skin irritation or burns. If the patch is located in the region being scanned, consider removing the patch prior to imaging and replacing it following the scan.
- Have available a non-ferromagnetic gurney, stretcher, or table to transport heavy patients into the MRI safety zone.
- Carefully inspect any attached medical devices for metal parts or needles (urine collection systems, triple lumen catheters, infusion pumps, etc.).
- Remove towels, blankets, and other items from around the patient before entering the MRI safety zone. Ferromagnetic items may be hidden under blankets and become missiles when they get close to the magnet.

Equine checklist

- Remove shoes and clean all feet. Cover or wrap feet not being imaged.
- Verify the region to be imaged. When imaging feet, radiograph before taking into the MRI safety zone to ensure that there are no metal pieces in the hoof.
- Confirm availability of MRI-safe table and scan time.
- Review table orientation and pad configuration prior to anesthesia.
- Place urinary catheter prior to entering the MRI Safety Zone to prevent contamination of and potential damage to the MRI scanner.
- Coordinate MRI safety trained personnel to assist with moving the patient into the MRI safety zone, to assist with positioning, and later to assist with moving the patient into recovery.
- Designate a system to identify MRI safety trained personnel (hats, shirts, etc.) to prevent inadvertent inclusion of an untrained volunteer.
- Keep scan time as short as possible (not to exceed 90 min).

personnel entering the MRI suite, including badges, phones, and hair pins, as well as from patients (e.g., horseshoes).

In the bore of the magnet, where the magnetic field is the strongest, implanted, non-spherical, metallic objects such as aneurysm clips will torque or rotate as they attempt to align with the magnetic field. The induced rotation may cause the object to move in such a way as to tear vital structures [42–45]. Other implanted materials such as microchips, intravascular coils and stents, and vascular clamps can be safely imaged 6 weeks following placement once adequate scarring has occurred [42]. Personnel and patients should be screened for ferromagnetic implants by the appointed Magnetic Resonance Safety Officer or healthcare professional.

Transdermal patches (e.g., fentanyl and others) can contain aluminum or other metallic substances that could cause skin burns if exposed to an RF field. Second-degree burns have been reported in humans due to transdermal patches [42]. A warning about this hazard was issued by the United States Food and Drug Administration (FDA), and removal of transdermal patches prior to imaging is recommended [46,47].

Medical devices are tested and labeled safe, conditional, or unsafe for use in a strong magnetic field using the American Society for Testing and Materials International classifications and icons [42]:

MRI Safe: Items made from materials considered safe in an MRI environment, such as glass, plastic, silicone, etc. and devices that have been tested and are considered safe for the patient and the individuals working in specific MR environments.

MRI Conditional: Depending on the specific MR environment, objects may or may not be safe for the patient or personnel working with them. There are eight subcategories in this classification. MRI safety of a particular device or implant can be found at the manufacturer's website or at www.mrisafety.com.

MRI Unsafe: Magnetic or metallic items known to pose hazards in all MRI environments to a patient or other individual. There are two subcategories in this classification depending on the type and degree of risk. It should be noted that the default magnetic field used to categorize devices is 1.5 T.

No substantial or harmful biological effects have been reported in patients or MRI technologists following short-term exposures to static magnetic fields up to 9.4 T [42], although transient symptoms such as vertigo or nausea are sometimes reported. Anesthesia is required to provide the necessary immobility for veterinary patients during MRI, and it is often the same individual providing anesthesia support, leading to repeated and prolonged exposure to static magnetic fields. There are no current studies regarding prolonged, chronic exposure to date. The use of MRI during interventional procedures and surgery in humans is becoming more common, leading to increased exposure for the patient, anesthetist, surgeon, and other hospital personnel [48]. Until more evidence is available regarding these effects, personnel providing anesthesia should take precautions to limit the overall time in the MRI room.

Gradient magnetic fields

Gradients, or time-varying magnetic fields, are created by weaker magnets located within the primary magnet. Gradients are switched on and off many times per second producing variations in the magnetic field that allow image slices to be formed. Gradient switching induces electrical currents, and conscious human patients have reported nerve stimulation or tingling during sequences using gradients. Safety standards have been installed in MR systems to protect patients from any potential hazard or injury [42].

Gradient switching is also the source of the "clanging" noise heard during MRI. The level of acoustic noise depends on the scan sequence and magnet strength. Noise levels range from 103–115 decibels (dB) for a 1.5-T magnet and 126–131 dB for a 3.0-T system [42,48]. The FDA and The International Electrotechnical Commission limit permissible sound levels to 99 dB with hearing protection in place. The OSHA and the Department of Health in the United Kingdom recommend a maximum noise exposure of 85 dB over an 8-h period [42,49]. To prevent temporary or permanent hearing damage from exposure to high noise levels, personnel in the MRI room during scanning should wear hearing protection. The best protection is provided by disposable or reusable ear plugs with a noise reduction rating (NRR) of 30–33 dB or close-fitting headphones with NRR ratings from 20–30 dB. Optimal protection depends on how the ear plugs fit. Combining ear plugs and headphones will improve protection by 5–10 dB [42].

While hearing protection was not traditionally used for veterinary patients during MR imaging, it is becoming more common and is routine at the authors' facility. The increased noise levels in the stronger magnets and extended scan times in clinical and research settings are reasons to consider using methods to reduce noise exposure [50]. Noise reduction may also allow lighter planes of anesthesia [51]. Isoflurane anesthesia has a protective effect on noise-induced hearing loss in mice [52,53]. Testing the hearing of veterinary patients during and after MR imaging to assess effectiveness of hearing protection devices is problematic, and there are currently no published studies on this subject. Hearing protection is commercially available for dogs and cats and has been tested to be safe during MRI [54], but the level of noise reduction has not been determined.

Radiofrequency fields

Radiofrequency (RF) radiation is pulsed into tissue, eliciting the release of energy or a resonance signal from tissue for image construction. The majority of the RF energy is transformed into heat within the patient's tissues and can elevate body temperature [42,49], especially in large dogs and when scan times are long. The stronger the magnet, the more RF energy is required (3.0 T > 1.5 T). The specific absorption rate (SAR) of the RF radiation is measured throughout the scan to prevent systemic thermal overload. The SAR is strictly limited by the MR scanner software based on guidelines established by the FDA and is calculated based on the weight of the patient. When potential overheating is detected, imaging will be interrupted by the system to allow more time between sequences and limit SAR [42,49].

Most MRI-related imaging injury reports in humans are related to RF burns resulting from the electrical currents induced in conductive materials such as ECG cables used during imaging. Cables placed against a patient's bare skin or that are looped can create a voltage strong enough to cause a burn that may require skin grafting [42,55]. To prevent the possibility of burns, take care to make sure that all cables run straight, do not contain loops, and are in parallel to the bore of the magnet. Insulate cables from areas of non-haired skin and only use MRI conditional devices tested for the strength of magnet.

Cryogens

Superconducting high-field-strength magnets generate a large amount of energy and heat and must be encased in supercooled liquefied gas or cryogens, usually liquid helium. If the system malfunctions and the temperature of the helium rises, enormous pressures can build up and cause an explosion called a "boiling liquid expanding vapor explosion" (BLEVE) or "quench." When this happens, the magnetic field is lost. Rooms designed for MRI are equipped with large vent pipes for the evacuation of the helium vapor if a quench occurs. A quench rarely happens spontaneously but can be manually triggered in the event of a fire in the magnet room or other life-threatening situation requiring termination of the magnetic field, such as someone being crushed against the MRI scanner by a large ferromagnetic object [56].

If the vent pipe fails to contain the helium vapor, a cloud of vapor will enter the MRI room. This vapor is still very cold and can cause frostbite and asphyxiation due to displacement of oxygen in the room. In the event of a quench, the room should be evacuated immediately. As the magnet could have a high-voltage electrical charge, care should be taken to avoid any physical contact with it when exiting. The patient should not be moved until the air in the room has returned to normal. Emergency and rescue personnel should not rush into the room as the magnetic field takes time to dissipate. Anesthesia providers should become familiar with and adhere to the quench protocol in place for the facility where they are working.

Anesthetic management considerations

For MR imaging, patients are placed on a long table, positioned in devices to prevent motion, covered with RF coils and insulating blankets, and then moved into the center of the bore of the MRI scanner (Fig. 4.5). Patients are difficult to visualize, and access is limited, especially in smaller patients. Like most anesthetic management, planning is key to success, particularly when anesthetizing a horse for MRI. Designation of staff roles throughout preparation and positioning due to the physical effort required and time-sensitive nature of equine recumbency is necessary to produce high-quality images in a safe and efficient manner.

The region being evaluated is imaged in different planes using sequences that are adjusted and repeated to optimize tissue visualization. These images are compared and used to localize lesions. Patients must be in the exact same position for every sequence. Positioning devices, such as sandbags or foam cushions, are used to support the patient and prevent leaning or moving out of position. Horses' limbs may be supported with wood stands and pads with their feet tied and, depending on the area of interest, pulled tightly and secured to the wall to aid positioning and prevent motion. Moldable bean bags and other types of positioning devices are used in patients when RT or imaging of the same region is planned, so that the exact same position can be replicated. These devices may interfere with monitoring or IV access, so it is critical to be familiar with the scan being performed and the equipment that will be used so that plans can be made in advance to place IV catheters and monitoring leads where they will be the most accessible during imaging. Urinary catheters are recommended in all horses that are visible and accessible for easy troubleshooting to prevent catastrophic urine leakage into the MRI unit or a safety hazard to personnel due to urine spillage on the floor. Additional extension lines and injection ports may be required for easy administration of fluids, contrast agents, and any other medications during scanning. The table can be moved out of the bore for injections, but it is best to not move the table or patient until the scan is complete.

A routine MRI scan can take 20–60 min depending on the strength of the magnet, the region being imaged, and the pathology discovered. It may be necessary to add additional image sequences or even another scan region that could double the overall anesthesia time. Plan ahead for this possibility and have additional sedatives, anesthetic agents, fluids, oxygen tanks, and other medications available. This is particularly critical when the MRI room is located outside the main anesthesia area, in a separate building, adjacent trailer, or other remote location. Large animal patients may have to be transported some distance from the induction area, and later back to the recovery area, so additional sedatives or injectable anesthetics may be required during transport.

Many small animal patients needing an MRI are non-ambulatory and require transport to and from the MRI suite. The safest option is a magnet-safe gurney or stretcher that can be used for transport from the holding area into the MRI safety zone. MRI-safe gurneys that are designed for humans work well, especially for large breed dogs or other patients up to 150 kg in weight. Heavy patients can be transferred directly onto the MRI table, which aids in keeping their spines supported during repositioning and requires fewer personnel to move them. Some magnets are equipped with a detachable table for transporting patients into and out of the room. Moving heavy, non-ambulatory patients into small MRI facilities, such as those located in trailers, requires additional personnel and an MRI-safe stretcher or other method.

Sedation versus general anesthesia

Regardless of whether sedation or general anesthesia is chosen, comprehensive vital sign monitoring is essential for adequate patient care during scanning. The authors recommend intubation with the ability to control ventilation to not only maintain a stable plane of anesthesia but prevent respiratory motion rendering non-diagnostic images. However, light or no sedation at all may be preferred for obtunded yet stable patients for short scans. Monitoring can be more challenging when the patient is not intubated or not anesthetized, and the vibration and loud noises may cause unexpected arousal, necessitating additional imaging and prolonging the process. It is recommended that someone stay in the magnet room to visually monitor sedated patients during scanning to observe respirations and palpate pulses as electronic monitors may be unreliable. Be prepared to intubate and support ventilation or switch to general anesthesia in the event there is respiratory depression or compromise, if the patient will not lie still, or if scanning time is extended. Additional ETTs, a resuscitation bag (e.g., Ambu® bag), and an oxygen source should be immediately available (see below).

General anesthesia, either injectable or inhalant, provides more reliable immobility and vital sign monitoring. Injectable protocols allow intubation for the provision of oxygen and ventilatory support, as well as the use of capnography. TIVA administered by repeated IV bolus injections or continuous infusion may be indicated for certain patient conditions or when an MRI-safe anesthesia machine and vaporizer are not available. Anesthetic infusions can be administered using a magnet-safe fluid or syringe pump or an inline fluid regulator. The infusion rate should be closely monitored when inline regulators are used for the delivery of anesthetic agents to prevent potentially fatal overdoses [57]. When MRI-safe equipment is not available, tubing can be passed through a waveguide to the patient from a pump located outside the MRI room (Fig. 4.7). Make sure the catheter is patent and secure, along with any connections, and the line is long enough before moving the patient into the bore of the magnet. Disconnection or a non-patent catheter will result in arousal, motion, and potential injury to the patient and the scanner.

A light plane of anesthesia is usually adequate to prevent movement during the scan. However, if the patient is too light and moves before the scan is completed, the sequence will have to be repeated, increasing anesthesia time. Even small amounts of body motion due to respiratory effort can interfere with some sequences. Controlled ventilation, manual or mechanical, can minimize this motion. Some sensitive, short (30–45 s) sequences are run using the "breath-hold/apnea" technique to eliminate all respiratory motion. Adequate anesthetic depth and monitoring are essential

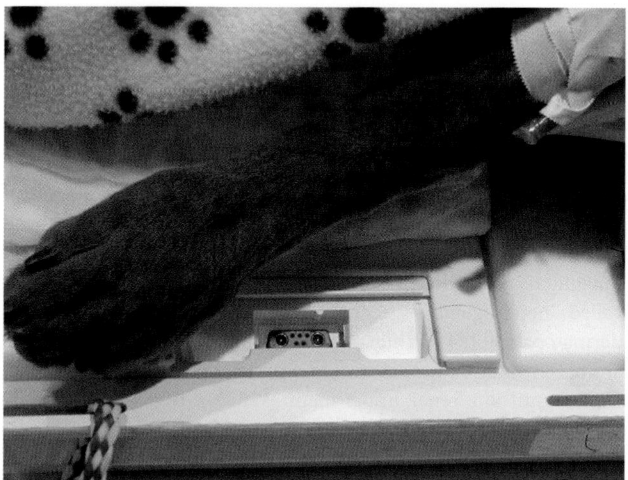

Figure 4.8 Location of a radiofrequency coil connection in the MRI table adjacent to the IV catheter in a dog anesthetized and positioned for an MRI scan. Such connections should be protected with absorbent, water-proof pads to prevent fluid damage.

in equine patients to prevent catastrophic damage to MRI equipment and the patient if the animal becomes light and thrashes within the bore.

Receiver coils plug into connections located in the MRI table. Precautions should be taken to protect these connections from any organic fluids (urine, blood, or feces) as well as leakage from the IV catheter to prevent a short circuit and the need for costly replacement (Fig. 4.8).

Inhalation anesthesia requires equipment and an oxygen source that is MRI conditional for the specific magnet strength being used. Oxygen can be piped into the room or MRI-safe aluminum tanks can be used. Non-compatible anesthesia machines can be used outside the room with long hoses passed through waveguides or, if used inside the MR room, positioned outside the 5-gauss line and secured to the wall or floor to prevent movement toward the magnet. Delivery hoses need to be long enough to reach the patient when they are moved inside the bore of the magnet and to accommodate any additional movement of the table. Coaxial delivery systems are commercially available up to 108 inches in length, or corrugated tubing can be cut to the desired length and attached to a Y-piece. Extra-long delivery hoses should be kept out of traffic areas to prevent disconnection, kinking, or obstruction of the tubing [57]. The pilot tube of the ETT may contain a small amount of metal that will cause an artifact on the images if it is in the scan field.

Ventilators can improve patient management and image quality by providing ventilatory support, a consistent plane of anesthesia, and control of respiratory motion. The ability to control ventilation is especially important for patients with pre-existing respiratory depression and those with suspected elevated intracranial pressure who require careful control of carbon dioxide concentrations.

To prevent potential hazards, the MRI-compatible anesthesia machine should be dedicated for use in the MRI room and remain within the MRI safety zone at all times. Metallic objects or other MRI-unsafe items may be placed on anesthetic machines when out of the area and accidentally brought into the room when the machine is returned. An additional anesthesia machine, conspicuously labeled MRI-unsafe, can be kept outside the MRI safety zone for induction, recovery, transport, and/or rescue procedures.

Patient monitoring

The monitoring standard and capability in an MRI facility should be comparable to the surgical suite or any other area where general anesthesia is performed. Ordinary monitoring equipment and accessories are not designed for use in the MRI environment as the RF fields can adversely affect their operation. The dangers associated with using monitors and/or monitoring probes and cables not confirmed safe for use inside the 5-gauss line include possible projectile hazard, patient burns, and degradation of the images. Available MRI-safe vital sign monitors are designed for use in humans but are easily adaptable for use in veterinary patients. Compared to standard monitoring systems, they are quite expensive. There are increasing numbers of affordable, refurbished MRI-safe monitors available for purchase due to constant upgrading of human systems. It should not be assumed that a monitor is safe for use with a 1.5-T magnet will be safe with a 3.0-T magnet. The anesthetist should check with the manufacturer before taking equipment into a new magnetic environment and be familiar with the location of the 5-gauss line.

Some MRI-safe monitoring systems are composed of a main monitor station with one or more wireless remote units so that anesthesia providers can monitor the patient when in the room as well as when outside the MRI room. If there is only one main monitor, the anesthetist may have to stay in the room for the entire procedure or the monitor can be positioned such that it can be visualized through a window or door or via a camera from outside the magnet room. Horses should be monitored constantly and directly to prevent disastrous consequences associated with sudden arousal. Monitors that are not safe for use in the MRI environment can be located outside the MRI safety zone with MRI-safe cables passed through waveguides to the patient. Long cables should be positioned outside of the work area to prevent damage, disconnection, or personnel injury. As gradient noise makes it difficult to hear alarms, monitors that have large, easy-to-see, colored flashing alarms are recommended. The alarm volume can be set to high, and the unit placed in a location where it can be easily visualized.

Gradient magnetic fields and radiofrequencies can interfere with the ECG, making it unreadable during many sequences. Newer MRI-safe monitoring systems have filters to help eliminate the interference. The appearance of the T wave or ST segment of the ECG complex may be elevated due to superimposed voltages generated by aortic blood flow in a magnetic field [56]. Voltages and currents generated during scanning can cause thermal injuries in tissues that contact conducting cables. There are reports of burns requiring skin grafts that resulted from a non-insulated ECG cable and a non-compatible pulse oximeter probe in people [49]. Burns can be prevented by keeping the cables away from the patient and making sure the cables are parallel to the bore of the magnet, do not overlap, or contain any loops. Newer monitors designed for MRI use have short wireless ECG cables to eliminate this hazard.

Carbon graphite ECG electrodes are recommended for use during MRI. Graphite patches work best with direct skin contact so shaving is required in most veterinary patients. When a dysrhythmia is suspected, the scan can be stopped so that the rhythm can be evaluated.

Fiber-optic pulse oximetry is MRI safe and is available in a variety of probe styles. The use of hard-wired pulse oximeters in the magnetic environment will result in unreliable readings, image degradation, and possibly patient burn injuries [49].

Capnography with sidestream sampling technology and extra-long sampling lines connected to a monitor inside or outside the magnet room is utilized during MR imaging.

Both invasive and non-invasive arterial blood pressure monitoring can be used during MR imaging. Non-invasive oscillometric blood pressure is available on MRI-safe monitoring systems, and the air-filled hoses are not hazardous. When monitoring arterial blood pressure invasively using an arterial catheter and transducer, keep the transducer outside the bore of the magnet to reduce vibration interference.

Hypothermia is a concern as MRI rooms can be very cold. Heat loss during scanning can be minimized by covering or wrapping the patient with fleece blankets or insulating material and requesting the MRI technologist to turn off the fan inside the bore of the magnet. External heat sources may be cautiously used, such as warmed fluid or rice bags, as long as they are insulated from direct contact with the patient. Snap or click instant heat sources are MRI safe, but there is a small metal button inside that will cause an artifact on the images if it is in the area being scanned. These devices should be used with caution as they get extremely hot immediately after activation and can cause serious burns if they are in direct contact with the patient. There are no commercially available electrical warming systems specifically designed for use in an MRI room. Circulating hot water blankets have been used safely but must be approved by the safety officer before they can be taken into the room. The water in the blanket will be visible on the scan if it is in the region being imaged and will create an artifact. If this is a concern, the blanket can be removed for certain sequences.

Hyperthermia may also be a concern during prolonged imaging in high-field-strength magnets, especially in large patients. Body temperature fluctuations can be assessed during MRI using a digital thermometer, a fiber-optic temperature probe, or a modified standard esophageal temperature probe. Skin surface temperature technology is unreliable in both human and veterinary patients [42,58].

Standing equine MRI

Standing, sedated low-field MRI (0.27 T) is available for horses. Despite the low field strength, the same safety precautions are advised as with high-field MRI; however, shoes need only be removed from the foot that is being imaged and the halter may remain in place. Standing MRI eliminates the need for and risks of general anesthesia but requires motionless imaging, challenging the anesthetist to appropriately titrate sedation and analgesia to maintain a steady, securely standing patient and avoid non-diagnostic images or injury. Furthermore, local blocks administered to the limb being imaged in an effort to assist weight bearing may induce artifact and contribute to non-diagnostic images. The authors advise consulting with radiology prior to making such decisions. Equipment for MRI should be protected by a handler at the head of the horse to avoid damage to the coil and floor level MRI unit secondary to horse hooves or urination. Monitoring should be employed at the same standard as any standing sedated procedure including, at a minimum, monitoring of heart rate, rhythm, and respiration.

Gadolinium-based contrast agents

Gadolinium-based contrast agents (GBCAs) are used to enhance the visibility of pathology for MRI studies. Gadolinium is a paramagnetic metal that is highly toxic in its natural state as it blocks physiologic pathways that rely on calcium. When gadolinium is chelated with a large organic molecule to form a stable complex, it is considered safe. The chelated compound has improved water solubility and is excreted predominantly unchanged by the kidneys [59]. The most common adverse effects observed in dogs and cats receiving a gadolinium chelate are bradycardia, tachycardia, hypotension, and hypertension [60–62]. Mild to severe anaphylactoid reactions have been reported in dogs. Dogs with a history of atopy may be more likely to have an adverse reaction [63]. An anaphylactoid reaction may be difficult to detect during MR imaging due to limited patient access and the effects of anesthesia. After administration of a GBCA, the patient should be closely monitored for any sudden changes in hemodynamic status or other signs of anaphylaxis. In people with acute kidney injury or advanced chronic kidney disease, administration of certain GBCAs for MR imaging has been linked to a rare but life-threatening skin disorder called "nephrogenic systemic fibrosis" or "nephrogenic fibrosing dermatopathy" [64]. While this condition has not been reported in animals, it may be best to avoid administering GBCAs to patients with significant renal impairment. While GBCAs are typically administered IV, they can be administered intramuscularly if IV access is unavailable. Contrast enhanced MRI is not commonly performed in horses.

Emergency procedures

Patients in the bore of the magnet are difficult to access during an emergency. An emergency plan specific to the facility being used should be designed in advance and practiced periodically. In the case of an emergency, support staff and emergency personnel should not run into the MRI room. Designate an area outside the MRI safety zone where patient assessment and rescue procedures can be conducted. The designated area should ideally have an anesthesia machine, patient monitor, emergency drugs, additional IV catheters and fluids, ETTs, laryngoscope, suction, and other relevant supplies. In the event of a cardiopulmonary arrest or other serious adverse event, the anesthetist should call for assistance, discontinue anesthesia, and signal to the technologist to stop the scan and move the table out of the bore of the magnet. The anesthetist can then assess the patient and initiate CPR, if indicated, while moving the patient from the MRI room to the predesignated area for resuscitation.

Personnel considerations

Powerful, invisible hazards make working in an MRI environment extremely hazardous. Prior to entering the MRI area, personnel must be carefully screened and made familiar with the safety guidelines associated with working in an MRI environment to prevent serious and life-threatening accidents. There are no reports of MR-related accidents in the veterinary literature though in human medicine accidents tend to be underreported [43]. Careful planning and continuous communication between all involved personnel is vital to ensure a safe work environment and a successful anesthetic event.

References

1 United States Department of Labor, Occupational Safety and Health Administration (OSHA) Technical Manual (OTM), Section III, Chapter 6. www.osha.gov/dts/osta/otm/otm_iii/otm_iii_6.html (accessed August 2023).
2 Hermens JM, Bennett MJ, Hirshman CA. Anesthesia for laser surgery. *Anesth Analg* 1983; **62**: 218–229.
3 *Lasers in Veterinary Practice: Safe Use Guidelines*. Version 2. Vancouver, BC: British Columbia Centre for Disease Control, 2011.
4 Laser Standards and Classifications. Rockwell Laser Industries. www.rli.com/resources/articles/classification.aspx (accessed August 2023).
5 American National Standards Institute (ANSI). *Safe Use of Lasers in Health Care*. ANSI Z136.3. Orlando, FL: Laser Institute of America, 2011.
6 Burns K. Laser guidelines encompass veterinarians. *JAVMA* 2012; **240**(7): 779.
7 Dorsh JA, Dorsch SE. Operating room fires and personnel injuries related to sources of ignition. In: Dorsch JA, Dorsch SE, eds. *Understanding Anesthesia Equipment*, 5th edn. Baltimore, MD: Lippincott, Williams and Wilkins, 2008: 907–928.

8 Stouffer DJ. Fires during surgery: two fatal incidents in Los Angeles. *J Burn Care Rehabil* 1992; **13**: 456–457.

9 Collarile T, DiGirolamo N, Nardini G, *et al.* Fire ignition during laser surgery in pet rodents. *BMC Vet Res* 2012; **8**: 177.

10 Driessen B, Zarucco L, Nann LE, *et al.* Hazards associated with laser surgery in the airway of the horse: implications for the anesthetic management. In: Steffey EP, ed. *Recent Advances in Anesthetic Management of Large Domestic Animals*. Ithaca, NY: International Veterinary Information Service, 2003. www.ivis.org

11 Quandt JE. Airway management. In: Greene SA, ed. *Veterinary Anesthesia and Pain Management Secrets*. Philadelphia, PA: Hanley and Belfus, 2002: 1–13.

12 Lai HC, Juang SE, Liu TJ, *et al.* Fires of endotracheal tubes of three different materials during carbon dioxide laser surgery. *Acta Anaesthesiol Sin* 2002; **40**(1): 47–51.

13 Steinberg TA. Combustion testing of non-metallic materials in ambient and oxygen-enriched atmospheres. In: Royals WT, Chou TC, Steinberg TA, eds. *Flammability and Sensitivity of Materials in Oxygen-Enriched Atmospheres*, vol. **8**. West Conshohocken, PA: American Society for Testing and Materials (ASTM), 1997: 370–384.

14 Dorsh JA, Dorsch SE. Tracheal tubes and associated equipment. In: Dorsch JA, Dorsch SE, eds. *Understanding Anesthesia Equipment*, 5th edn. Baltimore, MD: Lippincott, Williams and Wilkins, 2008: 561–628.

15 Mitchel B, Sosis MB. What is the safest endotracheal tube for Nd-YAG laser surgery? A comparative study. *Anesth Analg* 1989; **69**: 8024.

16 Sosis MB, Braverman B. Evaluation of foil coverings for protecting plastic endotracheal tubes from the potassium-titanyl-phosphate laser. *Anesth Analg* 1993; **77**(3): 589–591.

17 Mitchel B, Sosis MB, Braverman B, *et al.* Evaluation of a new laser-resistant fabric and copper foil-wrapped endotracheal tube. *Laryngoscope* 1996; **106**(7): 842–844.

18 Fried MP, Mallampati SR, Liu FC, *et al.* Laser resistant stainless steel endotracheal tube: experimental and clinical evaluation. *Lasers Surg Med* 1991; **11**(3): 301–306.

19 Sosis MB. Saline soaked pledgets prevent carbon dioxide laser-induced endotracheal tube cuff ignition. *J Clin Anesth* 1995; **7**(5): 395–397.

20 American Society of Anesthesiologists (ASA) Task Force on Operating Room Fires. Practice advisory for the prevention and management of operating room fires. An updated report. *Anesthesiology* 2013; **118**(2): 271–290.

21 National Research Council (NRC); Committee to Assess Health Risks from Exposure to Low Levels of Ionizing Radiation. *Health Risks from Exposure to Low Levels of Ionizing Radiation*. Washington, DC: National Academies Press, 2006.

22 California Veterinary Medical Board. *Radiation Safety Relating to Veterinary Medicine and Animal Health Technology in California*. Sacramento, CA: California Veterinary Medical Board, 2012.

23 *Radiation Protection Guidance for Hospital Staff*. Stanford, CA: Environmental Health and Safety, Stanford University, 2012.

24 Australian Radiation Protection and Nuclear Safety Agency (ARPANSA). *Radiation Protection in Veterinary Medicine. Code of Practice and Safety Guide, Radiation Protection Series Pub. No. 17*. Yallambie, Australia: Australian Radiation Protection and Nuclear Safety Agency, 2009.

25 Marcus A. Glowing risk: anesthesiologists' exposure to radiation on the job. *Anesthesiology News* 2009; **35**(10): 1–5.

26 American College of Radiology (ACR); Committee on Drugs and Contrast Media. *ACR Manual on Contrast Media, Version 9*. Reston, VA: American College of Radiology, 2013.

27 Katzberg RW. Contrast medium-induced nephrotoxicity: which pathway? *Radiology* 2005; **235**: 752–755.

28 Paithanpagare YM, Tank PH, Mankad MY, *et al.* Myelography in dogs. *Vet World* 2008; **1**(5): 152–154.

29 Roux FA, Deschamps JY. Inadvertent intrathecal administration of ionic contrast medium to a dog. *Vet Radiol Ultrasound* 2007; **48**(5): 414–417.

30 Carroll GL, Keene BW, Forrest LJ. Asystole associated with iohexol myelography in a dog. *Vet Radiol Ultrasound* 1997; **38**(4): 284–287.

31 Belzunegui T, Louis CJ, Torrededia L, *et al.* Extravasation of radiographic contrast material and compartment syndrome in the hand: a case report. *Scand J Trauma Resus Emerg Med* 2011; **19**: 9.

32 Wang CL, Cohan RH, Ellis JH, *et al.* Frequency, management and outcome of extravasation of nonionic iodinated contrast medium in 69,657 intravenous injections. *Radiology* 2007; **243**(1): 80–87.

33 Miles SG, Rasmussen JF, Litwiller T, *et al.* Safe use of an intravenous power injector for CT: experience and protocol. *Radiology* 1990; **176**(1): 69–70.

34 Overweg J. *MRI Main Field Magnets*. Hamburg, Germany: Philips Research. www.mri-q.com/uploads/3/4/5/7/34572113/main_field_magnets_ismrm2006.pdf (accessed August 2023).

35 Schenck JF, Dumoulin CL, Redington RW, *et al.* Human exposure to 4.0-Tesla magnetic fields in a whole-body scanner. *Med Phys* 1992; **19**(4): 1089–1098.

36 Theysohn JM, Maderwald S, Kraff O, *et al.* Subjective acceptance of 7 Tesla MRI for human imaging. *MAGMA* 2008; **21**(1–2): 63–72.

37 van Nierop LE, Slottje P, Kingma H, *et al.* MRI-related static magnetic stray fields and postural body sway: a double-blind randomized crossover study. *Magn Reson Med* 2013; **70**(1): 232–240.

38 van Nierop LE, Slottje P, van Zandvoort MJ, *et al.* Effects of magnetic stray fields from a 7 Tesla MRI scanner on neurocognition: a double-blind randomised crossover study. *Occup Environ Med* 2012; **69**(10): 759–766.

39 Elbel GK, Kalisch R, Czisch M, *et al.* Design and importance of continuous physiologic monitoring for fMRI in rats at 7T and first results with the novel anesthetic sevoflurane. In: *Proceedings of the 8th International Society for Magnetic Resonance in Medicine*. 2000; **2**: 928.

40 Okada T, Fujimoto K, Fushimi Y, *et al.* Neuroimaging at 7 Tesla: a pictorial narrative review. *Quant Imaging Med Surg* 2022; **12**(6): 3406–3435.

41 Schmierer K, Parkes HG, So PW, *et al.* High field (9.4 Tesla) magnetic resonance imaging of cortical grey matter lesions in multiple sclerosis. *Brain* 2010; **133**(Pt 3): 858–867.

42 Shellock FG. *Reference Manual for Magnetic Resonance Safety, Implants, and Devices*. Los Angeles, CA: Biomedical Research Publishing Group, 2013.

43 Kanal E, Barkovich AJ, Bell C, *et al.* ACR guidance document on MR safe practices: 2013. *J Magn Reson Imaging* 2013; **37**: 501–530.

44 Capizzani R. Magnetic Resonance Imaging Hazards and Safety Guidelines. Strategic Outcomes Practice, Technical Advisory Bulletin, 2009. www.koppdevelopment.com/articels/Willis%20MRI_Safety.pdf (accessed August 2023).

45 Klucznik RP. Placement of a ferromagnetic intracerebral aneurysm clip in a magnetic field with a fatal outcome. *Radiology* 1993; **187**: 855–856.

46 Kuehn BM. FDA warning: remove drug patches before MRI to prevent burns to skin. *JAMA* 2009; **301**(13): 1328.

47 JAVMA News. Some metal-backed drug patches lack warning about MRI burn risk. *J Am Vet Med Assoc* 2009; **235**(1): 16.

48 Hattori Y, Fukatsu H, Ishigaki T. Measurement and evaluation of the acoustic noise of a 3 Tesla MR scanner. *Nagoya J Med Sci* 2007; **69**: 23–28.

49 Jerrolds J, Keene S. MRI safety at 3T versus 1.5T. *Internet J World Health Soc Polit [Internet]* 2009; **6**(1). www.koppdevelopment.com/articels/MRI%20Safety%20at%203T%20VS%201-5T.pdf (accessed August 2023).

50 Lauer AM, El-Sharkawy AM, Kraitchman DL, *et al.* MRI acoustic noise can harm experimental and companion animals. *J Magn Reson Imaging* 2012; **36**(3): 743–747.

51 Oguriu M, Orhan ME, Cinar S, *et al.* Effect of headphones on sevoflurane requirement for MRI. *Pediatr Radiol* 2012; **42**: 1432–1436.

52 Chung JW, Ahn JH, Kim JY, *et al.* The effect of isoflurane, halothane and pentobarbital on noise-induced hearing loss in mice. *Anesth Analg* 2007; **6**: 1404–1408.

53 Kim JU, Lee HJ, Kang HH, *et al.* Protective effect of isoflurane anaesthesia on noise-induced hearing loss in mice. *Laryngoscope* 2005; **115**: 1996–1999.

54 Baker M. Evaluation of MR safety of a set of canine ear defenders (MuttMuffs®) at 1T. *Radiography* 2013; **19**(4): 339–342.

55 Medical Device Safety Reports. Thermal injuries and patient monitoring during MRI studies. *Health Devices* 1991; **20**(9): 362–363.

56 Menon DK, Peden CJ, Hall AS, *et al.* Magnetic resonance for the anaesthetist. Part I: physical principles, applications, safety aspects. *Anaesthesia* 1992; **47**(3): 240–255.

57 Kempen PM. Stand nearby in the MRI. Anesthesia Patient Safety Foundation (APSF). *Newsletter* 2005; **20**(2): 32–36. www.apsf.org/article/stand-near-by-in-the-mri (accessed August 2023).

58 Nasr VG, Schumann R, Bonney I, *et al.* Performance validation of a modified magnetic resonance imaging-compatible temperature probe in children. *Anesth Analg* 2012; **114**(6): 1230–1234.

59 Hao D, Ai T, Goerner F, *et al.* MRI contrast agents: basic chemistry and safety. *J Magn Reson Imaging* 2012; **36**(5): 1060–1071.

60 Pollard RE, Puchalski SM, Pascoe PJ. Hemodynamic and serum biochemical alterations associated with intravenous administration of three types of contrast media in anesthetized dogs. *Am J Vet Res* 2008; **69**(10): 1268–1273.

61 Pollard RE, Puchalski SM, Pascoe PJ. Hemodynamic and serum biochemical alterations associated with intravenous administration of three types of contrast media in anesthetized cats. *Am J Vet Res* 2008; **69**(10): 1274–1278.

62 Mair AR, Woolley J, Martinez M. Cardiovascular effects of intravenous gadolinium administration to anaesthetized dogs undergoing magnetic resonance imaging. *Vet Anaesth Analg* 2010; **37**(4): 337–341.

63 Girard NM, Leece EA. Suspected anaphylactoid reaction following intravenous administration of a gadolinium-based contrast agent in three dogs undergoing magnetic resonance imaging. *Vet Anaesth Analg* 2010; **37**(4): 352–356.

64 Woolen SA, Shankar PR, Gagnier JJ, *et al.* Risk of nephrogenic systemic fibrosis in patients with stage 4 or 5 chronic kidney disease receiving a group II gadolinium-based contrast agent: a systematic review and meta-analysis. *JAMA Intern Med* 2020; **180**(2): 223–230.

5 Anesthetic Emergencies, Resuscitation, and Adverse Events

Erik H. Hofmeister
Department of Clinical Sciences, College of Veterinary Medicine, Auburn University, Auburn, Alabama, USA

Chapter contents

Introduction, 54
Cardiopulmonary arrest, 55
  Basic life support, 55
  Advanced life support, 58
  Monitoring, 59
Cardiovascular complications, 60
  Hypotension, 60
  Hemorrhage, 60
  Cardiac dysrhythmias, 61
  Anaphylaxis, 61
Respiratory complications, 61
  Respiratory depression and apnea, 61
  Hypoxemia, 62
  Airway obstruction, 62
  Bronchospasm, 63
  Accidental extubation, 63
  Iatrogenic tracheal injury, 64
  Acute or undiagnosed pneumothorax, 64
  Pulmonary aspiration, 64
  Volutrauma and barotrauma, 65
  Wooden chest syndrome, 65
  Airway fire, 65
Anesthetic drug-related complications, 65
  Medical error resulting in overdose, 65
  Patient arousal, 66
Anesthetic equipment-related complications, 66
  Adjustable pressure-limiting valve closure or malfunction, 66
  Oxygen supply failure, 67
  Breathing system malfunction, 67
  Vaporizer-related complications, 67
Other complications, 67
  Gastroesophageal reflux and regurgitation, 67
  Ruminal tympany, 67
  Cerebral herniation, 67
  Hyperkalemia, 68
  Hypo- or hyperthermia, 68
  Myoclonus, 68
  Postanesthetic complications, 68
  Personnel injury, 70
Post-critical event debriefing, 70
References, 71

Introduction

An *adverse event* during anesthesia is defined as an event that may result in patient harm and may be due to the effects of anesthetic drugs, the patient's condition, the diagnostic or therapeutic procedure being conducted, or human error. These events are often emergencies due to the narrow therapeutic margins of drugs used to induce anesthesia, the co-opting of normal homeostatic mechanisms, and the manipulation of highly sensitive key organ systems such as the circulatory, respiratory, and neurologic systems. Rapid intervention is often needed before such an event leads to an adverse patient outcome.

Rates of adverse events differ among species, country, and across published studies. For example, the risk of death across species ranges from 1 in 2000 for dogs to 1 in 29 for birds [1,2]. The timeframe of what constitutes an anesthetic-related adverse event varies, ranging from an occurrence during anesthesia to any event occurring within seven days of anesthesia. Further information is available in Chapter 2.

The consequences of adverse events range from minimal to substantial. For example, a short episode of myoclonus during anesthesia is unlikely to affect a patient's long-term welfare, whereas gastroesophageal reflux leading to esophageal stricture will have significant negative effects on patient well-being. Death is often considered to be the worst possible outcome, although significant morbidity and suffering may arguably be worse in some cases.

Adverse events can be categorized according to a variety of criteria. These include the frequency or rate of occurrence, the severity of consequences to the patient, the organ system involved, and/or the causative circumstances. It is impractical to use frequency and severity to categorize adverse events as they are not always known in veterinary medicine. Organ system designations may not capture all adverse events, such as drug overdose or machine error.

Veterinary Anesthesia and Analgesia: The Sixth Edition of Lumb and Jones. Edited by Leigh Lamont, Kurt Grimm, Sheilah Robertson, Lydia Love and Carrie Schroeder.
© 2024 John Wiley & Sons, Inc. Published 2024 by John Wiley & Sons, Inc.
Companion website: www.wiley.com/go/lamont/anesthesia

Therefore, a causative circumstances framework will be used in this chapter, broadly considering that cardiovascular or respiratory events may be caused by a wide variety of circumstances.

The anesthetist should be prepared to rapidly identify and manage adverse events. A lack of awareness of any of these complications will almost certainly impair identification of the problem. Typically, when faced with a problem, people use cognitive shortcuts to determine if the scenario matches a pattern they have seen previously [3]. If it is not a pattern with which they are familiar, higher order cognitive processing, which is complex and time-consuming, must be employed. Because of the rapid intervention required for many anesthetic emergencies, familiarity with them so that pattern recognition can be employed in problem-solving is essential. Awareness of these events and understanding how to identify and manage them is a requirement for developing expertise in veterinary anesthesia.

Cardiopulmonary arrest

Cardiopulmonary arrest (CPA) describes the acute cessation of cardiac mechanical function with concurrent apnea [4] resulting in termination of oxygen delivery to tissues and death if not addressed rapidly. A variety of pathologic arrhythmias are associated with CPA, with treatment varying among them. The goal of cardiopulmonary resuscitation (CPR) is to provide effective blood flow to the heart and brain to facilitate return of spontaneous circulation (ROSC). CPR involves basic life support (BLS), which encompasses the initial steps taken in the face of CPA, and advanced life support (ALS), which involves drug therapy and more elaborate and specific treatments and monitoring during CPR. Postresuscitation care is an essential component of CPR, as merely succeeding to achieve ROSC does not guarantee successful patient discharge from the hospital [5].

CPR has overwhelmingly poor outcomes in both human and veterinary medicine. Reported rates of initial ROSC in dogs and cats are 17–58% and 21–57%, respectively [5–7]. Unfortunately, after CPR, the overall survival-to-discharge rates drop to 4–7% in dogs, 3–19% in cats, and 1.2% in exotic species [5–8] for all cases. The rates of ROSC and discharge are unknown in horses, although anecdotally the prognosis for foals is better than adult horses [9]. Successful ROSC and discharge after CPA in adult horses are sufficiently rare to warrant publication as case reports [10].

The prognosis for anesthetized small animals is notably higher, with 25–50% of patients having CPA under anesthesia surviving to discharge [5,6]. This difference may be due to the fact that CPA under anesthesia may be precipitated by human errors, rather than the severity of patient disease [11]. In addition, anesthetized patients usually have venous access established, are intubated and breathing enriched oxygen rather than room air, and are being monitored continuously, facilitating more rapid recognition of CPA [6].

In spite of the grave prognosis for CPR after CPA, one study reported that veterinary clients believe the rate of discharge after CPA to be 39% and do not believe that there is a difference in discharge rate between patients who suffer CPA while under anesthesia versus those not under anesthesia [12]. Most clients indicated that they want to discuss CPR with their veterinarian, and most want the veterinarian to make the decision to resuscitate [12]. This may explain why the euthanasia rate following ROSC is so high [7], as clients may not appreciate the low chance of discharge, the costs associated, or had an opportunity to discuss CPA/CPR with their veterinarian in advance. Given the risk of arrest during anesthesia, the likelihood of successful discharge, and client misinformation, it behooves the anesthesia team to communicate with the client about CPA before anesthetizing a patient.

Increased time from CPA to initiating CPR and duration of CPR decreases the likelihood of ROSC [5,6]. To ensure the highest chance of success, hospital staff should be prepared and trained to respond to the crisis quickly and efficiently. Training has been shown to improve adoption of activities that benefit CPR efforts [13]. During treatment of an arrest, the veterinarian in charge will usually take a central role coordinating the resuscitation procedures (i.e., running the code). It is important that the anesthesia team is well trained in current CPR procedures [14]. Regardless of initial training, there is always time-related decay of skills. Refresher training and mock CPR simulation every 6 months are recommended [4]. The necessary emergency drugs and equipment should be organized in one place (e.g., crash cart) and should be adequately stocked, regularly audited, and placed in a readily accessible area. This should include supplies for venous access, airway management, and initial pharmacological therapy. It is also wise to have a surgical kit for emergency thoracotomy, tracheostomy, and venous dissection available. Equipment failures during CPR were commonly cited as a deficiency in one veterinary study [15]. Therefore, regular testing and resupply of the crash cart should be conducted.

In 2012, the Reassessment Campaign on Veterinary Resuscitation (RECOVER) was organized to develop comprehensive, evidence-based CPR guidelines for veterinary medicine. It was a collaborative initiative involving Diplomates of the American College of Veterinary Anesthesia and Analgesia (ACVAA) and the American College of Veterinary Emergency and Critical Care (ACVECC) who systematically evaluated the published evidence relevant to small animal CPR and generated CPR guidelines (Fig. 5.1) [16,17]. Implementation of the RECOVER guidelines has been associated with an improved outcome in one study [18] but not in another [7]. Regardless, all hospital staff involved in CPR, particularly anesthesia and emergency staff, should be aware of these guidelines. One study indicated that, while specialists are aware of the guidelines, many general practitioners are not [19]. This suggests an education gap, which should be closed through the veterinary education curriculum and continuing education programs.

Basic life support

Basic life support (BLS) is the foundation for all modern CPR. It consists of recognition of CPA, initiation of chest compressions, management of the airway, and assisted ventilation [20]. Studies have shown that the quality of BLS performed is directly related to ROSC and survival rate; thus, early and sustained chest compressions are recommended [20]. When multiple trained rescuers are available, initiation of chest compressions and efforts to secure the airway can occur simultaneously, and subsequent ventilation can be delivered concurrent with chest compressions.

Chest compressions

Chest compressions should begin as soon as possible to facilitate effective blood flow to the heart and brain. Quality compressions with effective recoil are essential to optimize blood flow [20]. Chest compressions should be performed continuously without interruption by each resuscitator until a change in personnel is indicated to maintain compression quality.

A compression rate of *at least* 100 per minute should be sustained. Use of a mental metronome (such as a song with a beat per minute rhythm of 100) improves the accuracy of chest compression rates in veterinary students [21] and could be a valuable aid in CPR

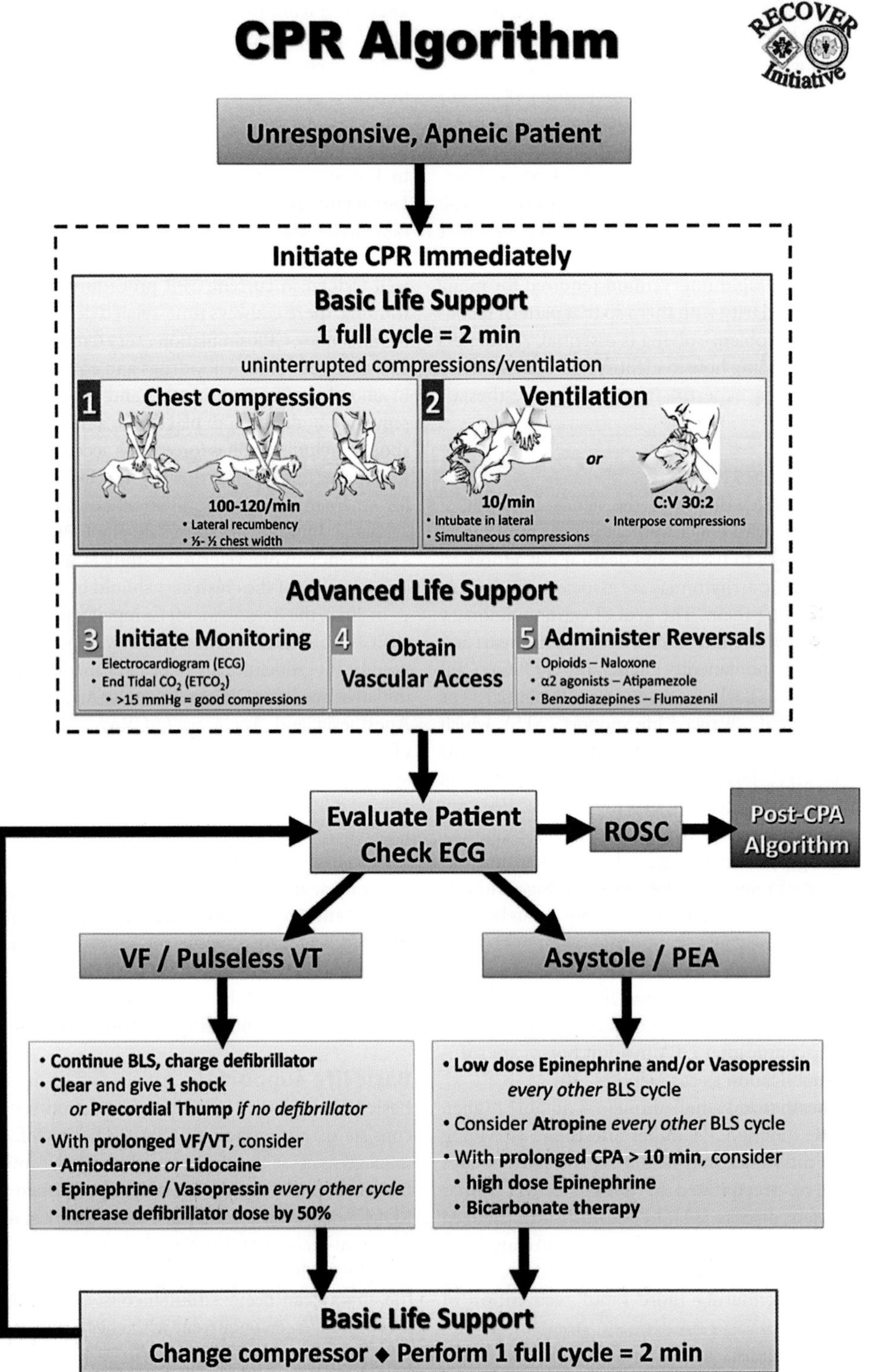

Figure 5.1 RECOVER CPR Algorithm. This algorithm summarizes clinical guidelines most relevant to the patient presenting acutely in CPA. The box surrounded by the gray dashed line contains, in order, the initial BLS and ALS actions to be taken when a patient is diagnosed with CPA: (1) administration of chest compressions, (2) ventilation support, (3) initiation of ECG and $P_{ET}CO_2$ monitoring, (4) obtaining vascular access for drug administration, and (5) administration of reversal agents if any anesthetic/sedative agents have been administered. The algorithm then enters a loop of 2-min cycles of CPR with brief pauses between to rotate compressors, to evaluate the patient for signs of ROSC, and to evaluate the ECG for a rhythm diagnosis. Patients in PEA or asystole should be treated with vasopressors and, potentially, anticholinergic drugs. These drugs should be administered no more often than every other cycle of CPR. Patients in VF or pulseless VT should be electrically defibrillated if a defibrillator is available or mechanically defibrillated with a precordial thump if an electrical defibrillator is not available. Immediately after defibrillation, another 2-min cycle of BLS should be started immediately. BLS, basic life support; CPA, cardiopulmonary arrest; CPR, cardiopulmonary resuscitation; C:V, compression-to-ventilation ratio; $ETCO_2$, end-tidal carbon dioxide; PEA, pulseless electrical activity; ROSC, return of spontaneous circulation; VF, ventricular fibrillation; VT, ventricular tachycardia. Source: Fletcher *et al.* [17], with permission.

team training. Myocardial blood flow is determined by the *coronary perfusion pressure* (C_oPP), defined as the difference between aortic diastolic and right atrial diastolic pressures:

$$C_oPP = ADP - RADP$$

where ADP is aortic diastolic pressure and RADP is right atrial diastolic pressure. Cerebral blood flow correlates with cerebral perfusion pressure (C_EPP):

$$C_EPP = MAP - ICP$$

where MAP is the mean arterial pressure and ICP is intracranial pressure. Therefore, interventions that increase diastolic or mean arterial pressures or decrease RADP and/or ICP are beneficial to patients undergoing CPR.

Cerebral blood flow in healthy animals is maintained at a fairly constant level when cerebral perfusion pressure is between 50 and 150 mmHg. During cardiac arrest, autoregulation of cerebral perfusion is disrupted and cerebral blood flow becomes linearly related to perfusion pressure. Optimizing the patient's hemodynamic status during CPR is essential to minimize the risk of adverse cardiac and neurologic outcomes [22]. Chest compressions in animals should be performed by compressing the chest by one-third to one-half of its width, with a greater depth of compression being associated with improved aortic pressures [20]. An appropriate chest compression technique also improves the pressure gradient between the aorta in diastole and the right atrium, which augments coronary perfusion and increases the probability of ROSC [20].

There are two theories that explain the mechanism of forward blood flow with chest compressions: the *thoracic pump theory* and the *cardiac pump theory*. The thoracic pump describes movement of blood out of the thoracic cavity due to changes in intrathoracic pressure (IttP). This mechanism is thought to be important in animals with a body weight over 15 kg [20]. The cardiac pump describes movement of blood out of the heart due to direct, mechanical compression of the heart by the thoracic wall [20]. After release of the compression, both the thoracic cavity and the heart itself recoil (i.e., chest recoil) during the decompression phase. The decompression phase is critical to successful ROSC as this is when the heart fills with blood, which facilitates effective stroke volume [20]. If the chest is not allowed to recoil fully, IttP remains positive, which decreases venous return to the heart and, hence, stroke volume [20].

As noted above, continuous administration of chest compressions with minimal interruption is essential. Even short pauses to evaluate the electrocardiogram (ECG), for example, decrease the aortic pressure and reduce the likelihood of successful ROSC. CPR should be performed in a 2-min cycle, with a resuscitator doing chest compressions for the full 2 min before exchanging with a different resuscitator. Performing high-quality chest compressions is fatiguing, requiring regular exchange of resuscitators to maintain compression effectiveness [20]. If the same resuscitator performs chest compressions for an extended period of time (e.g., 5 min), the number of correct chest compressions delivered has been shown to decrease [20].

In cats and small dogs, two-handed compression over the heart or one-handed compression around the base of the heart may be used. In larger dogs, two-handed compression over the heart (for keel-chested dogs) or over the widest part of the thorax (for round-chested dogs) is recommended [4]. Two-handed compression can also be used in foals. In adult horses, using the knees or sitting intermittently on the thorax may be used [10]. Chest compressions, as well as other manipulations associated with CPR, can cause pulmonary hemorrhage and liver fractures [23]. After ROSC, the patient should be evaluated for trauma, including ultrasound of the thoracic and abdominal cavity, and any damage appropriately addressed.

If multiple rescuers are present, interposed abdominal compression (IAC)-CPR can be performed where conventional chest compressions are combined with abdominal compressions delivered during the relaxation phase. While interposed abdominal compression has been shown to improve venous return and hemodynamic values in animal CPR models [20], in an actual clinical setting, it has been associated with a lower likelihood of success [24]. Attempting to synchronize abdominal and chest compressions while maintaining a fast compression rate may actually impair chest compressions, and this may explain why the beneficial effects in the laboratory do not translate to clinical CPA cases.

Open-chest CPR is recommended in cases where closed-chest CPR is ineffective or in cases of elevated IttP such as pleural space disease, pericardial disease, severe abdominal distension, or flail chest. With closed-chest compressions, the cardiac output generated is only 20–30% of normal. Performing a thoracotomy for open-chest CPR will not only increase cardiac output but also provides an opportunity to occlude the descending aorta, which redirects blood flow to essential organs (i.e., brain and heart). Concern about infection risk is often cited as a cause for delay in initiating open-chest CPR, but one human study found this risk to be very low [25]. The exact surgical approach through the thoracic wall does not need to be perfect, as either the fourth or fifth intercostal space has been found to be acceptable in dogs [26].

Breathing

Securing the airway and providing adequate ventilation is essential during CPR [20]. The most expedient technique for accomplishing this is usually via orotracheal intubation. If prompt orotracheal intubation is not possible (e.g., for out-of-hospital arrest), ventilation via a face mask or mouth-to-nose can be performed; however, these techniques are associated with significantly lower PaO_2 values and higher $PaCO_2$ values than those achieved with orotracheal intubation [27]. In people, even experienced personnel have only an 82% first-time intubation success rate during CPR [28]. Intubation should be confirmed by direct laryngoscopy or, if impractical, by auscultation of air movement in the lungs, observation of chest wall movement, or condensation within the endotracheal tube [29].

After the airway has been secured, the patient should be ventilated manually with the maximal available inspired oxygen concentration (i.e., F_IO_2~1.0). Although current guidelines suggest a ventilation rate of 10 breaths/min without interruption of chest compressions [20], a ventilation rate as low as one breath every 30 compressions (i.e., 3 breaths/min) is effective at maintaining oxygen and carbon dioxide at appropriate levels while minimizing detrimental effects on compression mechanics [30]. A full breath should be delivered in approximately 1 s with a 10 mL/kg tidal volume. A prolonged inspiratory time subjects the patient to a high IttP for an extended period, which decreases venous return, increases right ventricular afterload, and decreases left ventricular distensibility [31].

Advanced life support

Advanced life support (ALS) involves drug therapy, more elaborate and specific treatments (e.g., correction of electrolyte disturbances), and defibrillation when indicated [32].

Pharmacologic therapy

Pharmacologic therapy has been shown to improve outcomes in CPA (Table 5.1). Some drugs are indicated in most instances of CPA (e.g., epinephrine), whereas the decision to administer others depends on patient-specific factors (e.g., administering calcium to a patient with profound hypocalcemia). Drugs should be given by the route that facilitates the most rapid delivery to the heart. The order of preference for drug administration routes in CPR is: (1) central venous line, (2) forelimb intravenous catheter, (3) any other peripheral intravenous catheter, (4) intraosseous catheter, and (5) intratracheal delivery (for epinephrine, vasopressin, or atropine only). If epinephrine, atropine, or vasopressin is given by the intratracheal route, the dose should be increased (by 10-fold in the case of epinephrine), and it should be delivered via a long catheter (e.g., red rubber) advanced to the level of the carina [32].

Vasopressors are widely employed during veterinary CPA events to increase aortic pressures by increasing systemic vascular resistance and directing more of the intravascular volume from the peripheral circulation to the central compartment [32]. Both epinephrine and vasopressin are reasonable choices for all types of cardiac arrest. At the correct dosage, epinephrine exerts its critical vasoconstrictor effects by acting on vascular α-adrenergic receptors. Epinephrine's β-adrenergic effects (i.e., inotropy and chronotropy) are less important and may actually lead to detrimental increases in myocardial oxygen consumption once ROSC is achieved [32]. Vasopressin is a non-catecholamine vasopressor that acts on V_1 receptors in peripheral vessels while decreasing cellular hyperpolarization and increasing intracellular calcium concentration. In a study in dogs, similar outcomes were obtained with vasopressin and epinephrine [33]. A high dose (0.1 mg/kg) of epinephrine is no longer recommended for CPR.

Table 5.1 Pharmacotherapy during cardiopulmonary resuscitation (CPR).

Drug	Dose regimen	Comments
Epinephrine	0.01 mg/kg IV every 3–5 min	Use acceptable in most cases of CPA; causes peripheral vasoconstriction and increased aortic pressure
Vasopressin	0.8 IU/kg IV every 5 min	Use acceptable in most cases of CPA; causes peripheral vasoconstriction and increased aortic pressure
Corticosteroid	1 mg/kg IV prednisone equivalent	Use acceptable in most cases of CPA
Atropine	0.05 mg/kg IV every 5 min	Routine use is not recommended but is acceptable
Lidocaine	2 mg/kg IV	Routine use is not recommended but may be used in shock-resistant VT or VF
Amiodarone	5 mg/kg IV	Routine use is not recommended but may be used in shock-resistant VT or VF
Sodium bicarbonate	1 mEq/kg IV	Routine use is not recommended but may be used in prolonged CPA or CPA due to severe hyperkalemia or severe metabolic acidosis
Calcium gluconate	50 mg/kg IV	Routine use is not recommended but may be used in CPA due to calcium channel blocker overdose, severe hypocalcemia, or severe hyperkalemia

IV, intravenous; VT, ventricular tachycardia; VF, ventricular fibrillation; CPA, cardiopulmonary arrest.

For animals with high vagal tone (e.g., vomiting, ileus) and subsequent bradycardia/asystole, the use of atropine is reasonable [32]. Evidence supporting atropine's routine use in CPR is sparse, but, as it has not been associated with worse outcomes, such use is considered acceptable.

Although now-outdated recommendations did not support the routine use of corticosteroids, a systematic review in people provides evidence for the value of steroids in CPR [34]. This is consistent with a study in veterinary medicine, which documented a beneficial effect of steroids [5]. Potential beneficial effects of corticosteroids in CPA may be a result of counteracting relative adrenal insufficiency in patients with longstanding critical disease [35], counteracting impairment of adrenal function as a result of CPA, exerting anti-inflammatory effects, improving cardiovascular function, or blunting a catecholamine surge [34].

Lidocaine administration may be associated with vasodilation and a reduction in cardiac output. In pulseless ventricular tachycardia (VT) and ventricular fibrillation (VF), early and rapid defibrillation is advised. In dogs with shock-resistant VT or VF, amiodarone is preferred over lidocaine, although hypotension and anaphylactic reactions have been reported in this species following amiodarone administration [32].

The routine use of sodium bicarbonate during CPR is not recommended [32]. Bicarbonate administration may cause paradoxical cerebral acidosis, hyperosmolarity, and decreased catecholamine effectiveness. Bicarbonate use may be considered in prolonged CPA (i.e., greater than 10–15 min) or for CPA due to severe hyperkalemia or severe metabolic acidosis.

The routine use of calcium during CPR is not recommended [32]. The use of calcium may be considered for CPA due to calcium channel blocker overdose, severe hypocalcemia, or severe hyperkalemia. Calcium administration may cause cellular apoptosis with impaired neurological outcome and myocardial damage.

Fluid therapy is essential if CPA was caused by hypovolemia or hemorrhage. However, in euvolemic patients, aggressive fluid therapy may be detrimental due to decreased tissue blood flow caused by compromised tissue perfusion pressures [36]. In one study in euvolemic dogs with induced CPA, 11 mL/kg of either Lactated Ringer's solution or whole blood increased cardiac output but decreased both coronary and cerebral perfusion because of the disproportionate increase in RADP compared to ADP [37].

Defibrillation

In the face of ventricular fibrillation (VF), chest compressions should be initiated to circulate oxygenated blood to the myocardium before attempting electrical conversion with defibrillation. A hypoxic myocardium is unlikely to be successfully defibrillated. It is particularly important to initiate chest compressions before defibrillation if there is a delay between identification of CPA and administration of defibrillation. Immediately after a defibrillation attempt, chest compressions should be resumed for another full CPR cycle. Electrical defibrillation should start at 2–5 J/kg. If unsuccessful, a 2-min cycle of CPR should proceed; then, defibrillation attempted with a 50% increase in energy. This cycle, with concomitant increases in energy, continues until the rhythm changes (e.g., asystole develops) or ROSC is achieved.

Anesthesia-related CPA and CPR

If anesthesia-related CPA is due to drug overdose, reversal agents should be administered if available. Agents such as naloxone, flumazenil, and atipamezole should be administered in the case of opioid, benzodiazepine, or α_2-adrenergic receptor agonist overdose, respectively. All inhalant anesthetics cause myocardial depression, and their use should be terminated during CPR. Lipid rescue may be considered in animals with CPA due to local anesthetic overdose (see Chapter 29). If CPA occurs during an abdominal surgery, consideration should be given to performing open-chest CPR by accessing the heart through the diaphragm.

Adjunctive CPR techniques and devices

Several devices have been invented and tested to improve cardiac output during CPR. There are adjunctive CPR devices that actively decompress the chest during the expansion phase after delivery of a compression, devices that automate chest compressions, and devices that increase negative IttP during chest recoil to facilitate venous return (i.e., the impedance threshold device or ITD). Although the ITD has been shown to be beneficial in improving carotid blood flow and coronary perfusion in dogs undergoing CPR [22], there is currently no compelling evidence that any of these devices improve outcomes in people or animals [38].

Monitoring

Accurate and rapid identification of patients experiencing CPA is essential to ensure prompt initiation of CPR efforts, which directly impacts outcome. Monitoring the effectiveness of CPR efforts during CPR is critical to ensure that hemodynamic and respiratory goals are being met. Monitoring also provides important patient prognostic information and should guide postresuscitation planning and care.

Identifying CPA

Animals often experience agonal gasps or apnea as a prelude to CPA [5]. Other indications include collapse, a fixed gaze, lack of a palpable pulse, loss of an audible signal from a Doppler device (usually in an anesthetized patient), a rapid decrease in end-tidal carbon dioxide tension ($P_{ET}CO_2$) (in an anesthetized, intubated patient), observation of a characteristic arrhythmia on ECG, hypoventilation, and/or seizures. If CPA is suspected, the patient should be rapidly evaluated by auscultation of heart sounds. Seeking a peripheral pulse via palpation or placement of a Doppler probe delays the start of treatment and is not recommended to identify CPA [29].

The loss of sound from a preplaced Doppler device may precede CPA and should be investigated immediately [29]. Valuable time to initiate CPR efforts should not, however, be lost by checking the Doppler device or readjusting the probe. Other causes of a lost Doppler signal (e.g., a closed adjustable pressure-limiting [APL] valve) should also be investigated. In anesthetized, intubated patients, a rapid decrease in $P_{ET}CO_2$ can indicate a precipitous drop in cardiac output preceding cardiac arrest [29]. Observation of an abrupt decline in $P_{ET}CO_2$ should be taken as a strong indicator of actual or impending CPA, and the patient should be assessed immediately.

Monitoring during CPR

Once BLS steps have been initiated, ECG leads should be attached to identify if a treatable arrhythmia (e.g., bradycardia, ventricular fibrillation) is present. Continued ECG monitoring is warranted as patients may transition to a treatable arrhythmia during CPR efforts. The ECG can be checked during the change-over in personnel performing compressions every 2 min. Ceasing chest compressions more regularly to check the ECG rhythm is not recommended [29]. $P_{ET}CO_2$ monitoring should be instituted as it has a proven association with CPR outcomes [39]. $P_{ET}CO_2$ is a non-invasive surrogate for cerebral perfusion pressure and values ≥ 18 mmHg between 3 and 8 min after starting CPR is a sensitive predictor for ROSC [39]. If CPR efforts are not generating adequate $P_{ET}CO_2$ values, changes may need to be made (e.g., change personnel performing chest compressions and/or convert to thoracotomy for open-chest CPR).

Continued monitoring of ventilation parameters should include ensuring thoracic wall movements are occurring, respiratory rate is not exceeding 10 breaths/min, inspiratory time is 1 s, and inspiratory pressure is not excessive [29]. The respiratory rate, in particular, is often higher than is recommended even with experienced personnel. Venous blood gas monitoring can be used to inform the likelihood of ROSC and provide information about tissue perfusion and electrolytes (e.g., hypocalcemia), which may require targeted treatment.

During and after CPR, oxygenation goals are to maintain a PaO_2 of 80–100 mmHg or a saturation of 94–98%. Long-term hyperoxemia (i.e., PaO_2 > 100 mmHg) is undesirable as it can cause oxygen free-radical formation. After ROSC, hypoventilation is a common complication due to respiratory muscle weakness or poor responsiveness of the brainstem to CO_2 levels. A target $PaCO_2$ of 32–40 mmHg is desired and can be achieved with mechanical ventilation if the patient is not able to adequately ventilate spontaneously.

Postresuscitation care

Following ROSC, numerous body systems suffer injury secondary to interrupted blood flow and subsequent ischemia-reperfusion injury [40]. This constellation of problems is referred to as "postcardiac arrest syndrome" and includes damage to the brain, kidneys, and heart, as well as derangements of coagulation. Following the development of postcardiac arrest syndrome, other large-system inflammatory conditions, such as systemic inflammatory response syndrome (SIRS) and acute respiratory distress syndrome (ARDS) can develop. Ischemia-reperfusion in the brain leads to mitochondrial dysfunction, excitotoxicity, altered phospholipids, oxidative stress, increased lactate, endoplasmic reticulum stress, and inflammation [41]. Mortality (i.e., second arrest) is very common in the first 24 h after resuscitation [6].

Postcardiac arrest care should be intensive with diligent patient monitoring. Continuous or serial monitoring of the ECG, arterial oxygenation (SpO_2), body temperature, blood glucose, and systemic blood pressure should be instituted, as well as serial physical examinations and assessment of neurologic status [29]. Therapeutic protocols are based on hemodynamic optimization, cerebral protection, and therapeutic hypothermia [40].

Hemodynamic optimization aims to maintain blood pressure and, therefore, cerebral perfusion pressure. Numerous studies have found an association between arterial blood pressure and outcome in people [42–44]; however, the "optimal" blood pressure following ROSC has not been clearly defined. Targeting a mean arterial blood pressure (MAP) in the range of 70–80 mmHg with the use of inotropes and vasopressors seems to be associated with improved outcomes.

Cerebral protection can be facilitated by the use of a variety of pharmacologic interventions. Corticosteroids seem to offer some benefit, potentially due to relative adrenal insufficiency following CPA [41]. Numerous other interventions that target specific pathways of cerebral ischemia-reperfusion-induced dysfunction are being investigated, but evidence supporting their clinical use is lacking. Mannitol is often used to minimize cerebral edema following ROSC, but the evidence for its use is not particularly compelling. Therapeutic hypothermia has been used in people for decades, and there is strong evidence for its routine inclusion in postresuscitation care [45]. Beneficial effects of therapeutic hypothermia include reductions in cerebral oxygen requirement, brain metabolic demand, excitatory neurotransmitters, inflammatory cytokines, and free radicals, along with inhibition of neuronal cell apoptosis [41]. Potential complications include patient discomfort, longer tissue healing time, and coagulopathy. It appears that early application of even mild hypothermia (e.g., 36 °C/97 °F) is beneficial in the postresuscitation period and avoidance of hyperthermia is associated with improved survival in people.

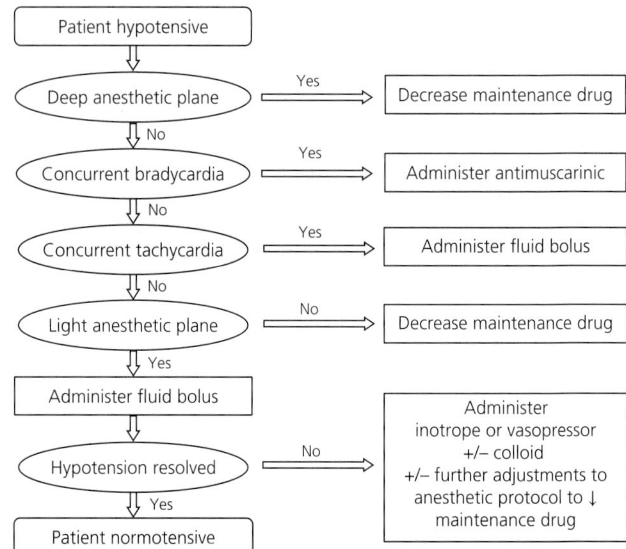

Figure 5.2 Clinical approach to hypotension. Note that other considerations, such as pre-existing cardiac disease, concurrent drug administration, blood volume status, and concurrent non-cardiac disease, may affect this generic approach.

Cardiovascular complications

The anesthetic complications involving the cardiovascular system discussed below are obviously not mutually exclusive and may occur alongside, or as a result of, many of the other complications presented in this chapter.

Hypotension

Hypotension has been reported to occur in 7–59% of anesthetized small animal patients [46–48]. The incidence in other species is also high, at 79% for rabbits [49] and 55% for horses [50]. While this complication occurs commonly in anesthetized animals, especially those anesthetized with inhalant agents, effective anticipation, recognition, and management means that it infrequently develops into a true anesthetic emergency. Pre-existing conditions associated with hemodynamic instability, surgical manipulations (e.g., compression of the vena cava), and various drugs can all precipitate or exacerbate significant hypotension and may present challenges for the anesthetist.

The adverse effects of hypotension are related to both its severity and duration. Relatively mild hypotension may be tolerated for some time, whereas profound hypotension for even 15 min may result in clinically significant morbidity. Classically, it is believed that maintaining a MAP over 60 mmHg maintains visceral organ perfusion [51,52], a MAP over 70 mmHg maintains muscle perfusion in large animals (e.g., adult horses) [53], and a diastolic arterial pressure (DAP) over 40 mmHg maintains myocardial perfusion [54]. Consciousness typically requires a systolic arterial pressure (SAP) over 50 mmHg [55].

Blood pressure is directly dependent on cardiac output and systemic vascular resistance (SVR). Cardiac output, in turn, depends on heart rate and stroke volume with the major determinants of stroke volume being preload, contractility, and afterload. Therefore, hypotension results from alterations to, or abnormalities of, any of these five variables (i.e., preload, contractility, afterload, heart rate, and SVR), and management of hypotension is directed at manipulating one or more of these. Continuous monitoring of blood pressure is indicated in any patient undergoing general anesthesia. Direct arterial blood pressure monitoring is indicated in all large animal cases anesthetized with inhalant anesthetics as well as any patients with the potential for hemodynamic instability during anesthesia. Monitoring blood pressure has been associated with a lower risk of cardiac-related mortality in horses [56].

A simple flowchart outlining the clinical approach to hypotension is presented in Fig. 5.2. Note that other considerations, such as pre-existing cardiac disease, concurrent drug administration, blood volume status, and concurrent non-cardiac disease may affect this simple approach. Further information is provided in Chapters 12, 32, 33, and 36.

Hemorrhage

Acute blood loss has two significant impacts on oxygen delivery to tissues: decreased preload and decreased hemoglobin concentration. Hemorrhage prior to or during anesthesia increases the risk of hemodynamic instability. Patients who have suffered hemorrhage prior to anesthesia should be stabilized if at all possible before the start of anesthesia. Those with severe ongoing hemorrhage requiring immediate surgical intervention should be aggressively treated during the preanesthetic period and throughout the maintenance phase of anesthesia.

In dogs undergoing anesthesia and surgery, the volume of hemorrhage has been associated with increased cost of care, with each mL of blood loss contributing $2 to the cost [57]. In dogs undergoing thoracic surgery, intraoperative blood product use (presumably due to hemorrhage) was associated with a 4.4-fold increase in the likelihood of postanesthetic death [58]. Similarly, in dogs undergoing emergency abdominal surgery, blood product use increased the risk of death by sevenfold [59]. These studies support the practice of hemodynamic stabilization prior to anesthesia whenever possible and highlight the negative impacts of acute intraoperative hemorrhage on patient outcomes.

The indications for treating hemorrhage include absolute blood volume loss, increased base excess or lactate, and changes in cardiovascular parameters associated with hemorrhage including relative increases in heart rate and decreases in systolic blood pressure (i.e., the shock index; HR/SAP). For absolute blood volume loss, treatment is recommended once estimated blood loss approaches 20% of total blood volume, or approximately 17 mL/kg in the dog [60]. Direct observation of intraoperative blood loss during the surgical procedure facilitates estimation of the volume lost and should be closely monitored. A base excess > 6.6 or a lactate > 5.0 mmol/L may indicate the need for treatment. In the awake dog, a shock index (HR/SAP) > 1.0 may be a more sensitive and specific indicator of 18% blood volume loss than heart rate or blood pressure alone [61]. General anesthesia may complicate interpretation of variables typically associated with the need to treat hemorrhage. For example, inhalant-induced hypotension and concurrent tachycardia due to intense surgical stimulation may make clinical decision-making more challenging. Volume replacement may consist of crystalloids, colloids, and/or blood products, and should be initiated as early as possible after recognition of blood loss. Further information is available in Chapter 32.

Cardiac dysrhythmias

The incidence of clinically significant cardiac dysrhythmias in healthy dogs under anesthesia is as high as 18% [62]. Cardiac dysrhythmias have the potential to decrease cardiac output by affecting diastolic filling (and hence venous return), contractility, and/or heart rate. They also have the potential to increase myocardial work by increasing heart rate above physiologic levels. Many arrhythmias occur in the absence of cardiac disease and may be precipitated by anesthesia, but most are clinically insignificant. However, the appearance of some arrhythmias under anesthesia may be more serious and warrant prompt recognition and intervention (e.g., atrial fibrillation and third-degree atrioventricular block). Specific treatment of an arrhythmia is generally undertaken if cardiac output is adversely affected or if increased myocardial work is putting excessive stress on the heart. Impacts on cardiac output are typically inferred based on arterial blood pressure measurement, although clinical signs such as syncope in a conscious patient may also indicate insufficient cardiac output. Increases in myocardial work caused by a tachyarrhythmia may be particularly problematic in patients with diastolic cardiac dysfunction (e.g., hypertrophic cardiomyopathy). Treatment is aimed at correcting the underlying cause of the arrhythmia (e.g., placement of a pacemaker in a patient with third-degree atrioventricular block) and/or pharmacologic manipulation of cardiac conduction. Further information is available in Chapters 11, 35, and 36.

Anaphylaxis

While uncommon, anaphylactic or anaphylactoid reactions may occur in the perianesthetic period and constitute adverse events. True anaphylaxis is a type I hypersensitivity reaction caused by rapid immunoglobulin E (IgE)-mediated interactions. Anaphylactoid reactions mimic anaphylaxis but are not caused by IgE. Both types of reactions cause release of substances by mast cells and basophils, primarily histamine. This results in a variety of effects, including pruritus, urticaria, hypotension, tachycardia, bronchospasm, and vomiting and diarrhea. Anaphylactic reactions can be caused by the patient encountering an antigen, which triggers anaphylaxis or by pharmacologic substances. Topical cleansing agents, antibiotics, radiographic contrast agents, and atracurium are common culprits in an anesthetic setting. In addition to symptomatic treatment to support cardiorespiratory function, epinephrine can be given IM at 0.01 mg/kg.

Respiratory complications

Many of the respiratory complications discussed below overlap and have cause-and-effect relationships with one another. For example, hypoxemia is a common sequela to many of the complications listed but general considerations for hypoxemia are also presented in its own section.

Respiratory depression and apnea

Respiratory depression (i.e., hypoventilation) is defined as inadequate CO_2 elimination that is detected as an increase in the partial pressure of arterial carbon dioxide ($PaCO_2$) or end-tidal carbon dioxide ($P_{ET}CO_2$). It is important to recognize that significant hypoventilation may occur in the face of a "normal" respiratory rate with few other associated clinical signs; thus, the only way to reliably identify hypoventilation is to measure CO_2. Although hypoventilation (i.e., $P_{ET}CO_2$ > 45 mmHg) is relatively common, severe hypoventilation (i.e., $P_{ET}CO_2$ > 60 mmHg) is relatively uncommon with one large-scale retrospective canine study reporting it in ~ 9% of patients [47]. Apnea refers to the complete absence of breathing and is the extreme endpoint on the spectrum of respiratory depression. While it can occur at any point during the perianesthetic period, apnea immediately following induction of anesthesia is common, depending on the anesthetic protocol and administration technique, with reported incidence rates in dogs as high as 75% [63]. Respiratory depression/apnea as an anesthetic complication spans a continuum ranging from mild hypercapnia, which may require no intervention, to apnea which requires immediate endotracheal intubation (if not already done) and ventilatory support.

In addition to the direct effects of hypercapnia (e.g., respiratory acidosis, tachycardia, etc.), hypoventilation induces indirect effects including the potential for hypoxemia and impaired uptake of inhalant anesthetics. Acidosis can disrupt enzyme systems, decreasing cardiac contractility, and reducing the effectiveness of certain drugs (e.g., inotropes) [64,65]. Hypercapnia can also precipitate arrhythmias, hypertension, hypoxemia, narcosis, and vasodilation with subsequent hypotension and increased intracranial pressure (ICP) [66].

The risk of hypoventilation producing hypoxemia depends on the inspired oxygen concentration (F_IO_2). With an F_IO_2 of 1.0, $P_{ET}CO_2$ would need to be > 500 mmHg to lower PaO_2 below 60 mmHg. This scenario is not clinically likely. However, with an F_IO_2 of 0.21 (i.e., a patient breathing room air), hypoventilation resulting in a $P_{ET}CO_2$ of ~70 mmHg will cause hypoxemia. Profound hypercapnia exerts a MAC-sparing effect starting at ~ 94 mmHg and linearly decreases MAC until it reaches 240 mmHg, at which point CO_2 achieves anesthesia alone [66].

By extension, the time to onset of hypoxemia due to apnea is also dependent on F_IO_2. In dogs preoxygenated with 88% oxygen for 3 min and then induced with propofol (causing subsequent apnea), SpO_2 values remained above 90% for an average of almost 5 min, compared with dogs without preoxygenation where SpO_2 values fell below 90% by 70 s [67]. Thus, provision of enriched oxygen immediately before induction of anesthesia will delay the onset of hypoxemia due to apnea or profound hypoventilation compared to inspiration of room air.

Inhalant anesthetics move down a series of partial pressure gradients from the anesthetic circuit to the alveoli and back for uptake and elimination. During apnea or profoundly decreased ventilation, uptake and elimination of the inhalant anesthetic may be impaired [68]. This is particularly relevant shortly after induction, when the combined effects of premedications, induction agents, and rising inhalant concentrations predispose to respiratory depression and apnea at the exact time when respiration is most crucial for inhalant uptake.

Indications to treat respiratory depression and apnea depend on the clinical scenario. In most cases, where a patient is breathing spontaneously but $P_{ET}CO_2$ is elevated, it is appropriate to first assess anesthetic depth and decrease the inhalant anesthetic concentration, if possible, as this often resolves hypercapnia. Mild to moderate elevations in $P_{ET}CO_2$ are often not treated with positive-pressure ventilation and some clinicians rely on modest hypercapnia to support blood pressure and cardiac output. If a patient is apneic and/or hypoxemic and/or not ventilating sufficiently for inhalant uptake and maintenance of an appropriate plane of anesthesia, positive-pressure ventilation is indicated. In certain high-risk patients (e.g., those with increased ICP), or if hypercapnia is severe or associated with other adverse effects (e.g., arrhythmia, tachycardia), positive-pressure ventilation is warranted. Further information is available in Chapters 14, 15, 37, and 38.

Hypoxemia

Hypoxemia refers to inadequate oxygen levels in arterial blood and often occurs without noticeable cyanosis. It is a common sequela to many of the other airway-related, pulmonary, or equipment-related complications discussed in this chapter and poses significant risks to the patient if unrecognized. Adverse effects associated with hypoxemia include lactic acidosis, pathologic arrhythmias, and cardiac, muscular, renal, and neurologic damage that may culminate in cardiac arrest. Certain species (e.g., horses), breeds (e.g., brachycephalic dogs), and patients with pre-existing disease conditions are predisposed to development of hypoxemia during anesthesia. In general, the risk of hypoxemia is much greater in anesthetized animals that are breathing room air versus those that are intubated and breathing enriched oxygen; however, routine monitoring of oxygenation is recommended for all patients. Detection of hypoxemia is via arterial blood gas analysis (decreased PaO_2) or, most commonly, via pulse oximetry (decreased SpO_2). Monitoring will facilitate early detection, investigation, and treatment, which will vary depending on the underlying cause and clinical scenario. Therapies may include increasing the F_IO_2, securing/clearing the airway, instituting various ventilation strategies, addressing an underlying condition, etc. Further information is available in Chapters 14, 15, 37, and 38.

Airway obstruction

Complete obstruction of the upper airway is an anesthetic emergency and, if not promptly addressed, may result in hypoxemia and subsequent cardiac arrest. Partial airway obstruction may also lead to serious adverse effects depending on how much of the airway lumen is occluded. Negative-pressure pulmonary edema may occur as a result of upper airway obstruction. This often manifests as foamy discharge from the airway and should be treated with diuretics and oxygen supplementation. There are a number of scenarios associated with airway obstruction that may occur at various clinical time points including at induction (i.e., a difficult or failed intubation), during maintenance, or at recovery. Being aware of different airway obstruction scenarios and associated risk factors will ensure the anesthetist is well prepared to prevent obstruction in the first place or to rapidly recognize it and intervene if it occurs.

Induction

The inability to successfully secure the airway at the outset of anesthesia, most often via endotracheal intubation, can result in a catastrophic emergency if not dealt with promptly. There is a great deal of jargon used in the human literature to describe these scenarios with terms like "difficult airway," "failed airway," "cannot intubate/cannot ventilate" (CICV), "cannot intubate/cannot oxygenate" (CICO), and "complete ventilation failure" (CVF) all in use. In some cases, a difficult intubation is anticipated, so a plan to manage the case can be made in advance. In other cases, a difficult intubation may arise unexpectedly, so having a variety of equipment and supplies immediately available is crucial.

In general, cats are considered to be more challenging to intubate than dogs and, like swine, they are prone to laryngospasm particularly in response to glottic stimulation. Consequently, it is common practice to prophylactically administer topical lidocaine to the arytenoid cartilages prior to attempting intubation to prevent laryngospasm. This should be done at least 45 s before stimulating the airway [69]. For cats, or other species where even routine intubation may be challenging (e.g., pigs, camelids, rabbits, and mice), it is important to have a range of endotracheal tubes, laryngoscopes, and other intubation aids readily available.

Conditions that predispose to difficult intubation include anatomic pathology (e.g., abnormalities associated with brachycephalic airway syndrome including elongated soft palate, and laryngeal collapse), oropharyngeal, laryngeal, tracheal, or retrobulbar masses (e.g., neoplasia, abscess, and foreign body), and any pathology limiting opening of the mouth (e.g., fractures, temporomandibular disease, oral pain, and other head and neck trauma). It is essential that patients at risk of a difficult intubation are thoroughly assessed prior to anesthesia and an airway management plan crafted. Such patients should be preoxygenated with 100% oxygen delivered by face mask (i.e., not "flow-by") for at least 5 min to prevent or delay the onset of hypoxemia [70]. Multiple options to facilitate intubation should be prepared, including laryngoscopes, a video laryngoscope if available, devices for manipulating oral structures (e.g., cotton tipped applicators, tongue depressors, etc.), a stylet, a bougie, supraglottic airway devices if available (e.g., laryngeal mask, v-gel), supplies to perform alternative airway approaches (e.g., pharyngostomy, retrograde intubation) and/or emergency surgical access (e.g., tracheostomy, cricothyrotomy), and a method to provide oxygen if intubation is not successful. The patient's neck should be clipped and prepared in the event surgical airway access becomes necessary. If orotracheal intubation cannot be attained, oxygen can be supplied via needle tracheostomy by percutaneously introducing a needle into the trachea via the cricothyroid cartilage and connecting it to an oxygen supply. If the patient's oral aperture is too small to visualize the arytenoids, it may be possible to expand it by layering tongue depressors horizontally between the incisors to sequentially enlarge it. In some cases, induction drugs that are less likely to cause significant respiratory depression and apnea (e.g., ketamine, tiletamine–zolazepam) may be preferred over drugs which are more likely to induce apnea (e.g., propofol, alfaxalone). Use of a laryngeal mask airway or another blind insertion airway device may be preferable to endotracheal intubation in cases where the arytenoids cannot be visualized [71].

When a difficult intubation arises unexpectedly during anesthetic induction and the patient has not been preoxygenated, oxygen should be supplied by flow-by or, if the patient is breathing spontaneously, by face mask to maintain hemoglobin saturation. It may be prudent to recover spontaneously breathing patients (assuming oxygenation remains adequate), re-evaluate the patient, and create a different anesthetic and airway management plan. If the patient is apneic, every effort should be made to rapidly intubate the trachea. The most experienced individual should attempt intubation and additional personnel should be summoned to collect the supplies outlined above for a difficult intubation. The decision to transition to emergency surgical airway access should be based on procedural and patient status criteria [72]. Multiple unsuccessful attempts at orotracheal intubation by an experienced veterinarian in a patient that is rapidly desaturating and/or apneic should signal the need to immediately proceed with a surgical approach.

Maintenance

Airway obstruction in an intubated patient during the maintenance phase of anesthesia may arise if the endotracheal tube becomes occluded or compressed. Potential causes include foreign material (e.g., mucus plugs, especially with small diameter endotracheal tubes), kinking of the endotracheal tube, overinflation of the cuff leading to compression of the tube lumen, asymmetric cuff inflation leading to obstruction of the bevel end of the tube, and external compression or obstruction between the tube and the breathing system. Procedures which hyperflex the atlanto-occipital joint (e.g., cerebral spinal fluid collection and ocular procedures) are particularly prone to causing a kinked endotracheal tube [73]. Obstruction of the endotracheal tube may be identified by observation of increased respiratory effort, thoracic excursions without effective air movement (e.g., breathing bag not moving), or by changes to or loss of the capnographic waveform. Attempts to provide positive-pressure ventilation are met with resistance and the patient's thoracic movement does not match the pressure being delivered. Spirometry may be helpful to diagnose an occluded endotracheal tube [74]. Recognition of an occluded endotracheal tube requires prompt intervention. Patient positioning should be checked and modified to address a kinked tube, cuff inflation should be evaluated, and other external compressions or obstructions removed. If the tube is potentially occluded with mucus, a stylet or catheter can be introduced to clear the lumen. If that fails to resolve the obstruction, the endotracheal tube may need to be exchanged.

Inadvertent endobronchial intubation (i.e., advancement of the endotracheal tube beyond the thoracic inlet and into a mainstem bronchus) is possible if tube length is excessive. This may occur with initial tube placement at induction, or when a tube that was correctly placed initially moves distally, most often with changes in patient positioning. Endobronchial intubation results in atelectasis and impaired oxygenation in the non-intubated lung. Healthy patients are usually able to compensate for this if the F_IO_2 is ~ 1.0 and hypoxemia may not result. Mechanical ventilation may predispose to volutrauma in the intubated lung. This complication is best prevented by determining the correct endotracheal tube length for the patient, cutting it to the correct size, and confirming correct placement by auscultating breath sounds on both sides of the chest.

Recovery

If airway obstruction occurs after extubation, it may make reintubation difficult or impossible. Using a delayed extubation technique, where the patient is extubated only once they are lifting their head and have regained normal muscle tone, may decrease the likelihood of obstruction occurring after extubation in certain high-risk patients (e.g., brachycephalic dogs). Patients with a potentially compromised airway should be carefully monitored after extubation and preparations should be in place to reintubate in the face of respiratory difficulties. If the patient appears stable and the airway remains patent after extubation, placement in a high F_IO_2 environment for several hours may help reduce the work of breathing, ensure adequate alveolar oxygen concentrations, and improve the chance of a successful recovery.

In cats, their small size and susceptibility to laryngospasm may increase the risk of airway trauma during intubation, which may manifest as airway obstruction at recovery. Similarly, in horses, laryngospasm/laryngeal dysfunction associated with intubation may also precipitate acute, catastrophic airway obstruction at recovery. In addition to partial airway obstruction due to nasopharyngeal congestion (routinely treated with topical phenylephrine), complete airway obstruction may occur in horses due to physical blockade of the nostrils (e.g., in the corner of a recovery stall). In cases of complete airway obstruction, the horse may thrash violently as hypoxemia causes significant distress. Unconsciousness may result, and negative-pressure pulmonary edema may occur [75]. Orotracheal intubation may not be successful in such cases, and an emergency tracheostomy is indicated if an airway cannot be rapidly established.

Bronchospasm

Bronchospasm may result from airway irritation or stimulation (e.g., endotracheal intubation in at-risk patients), anaphylactic reactions, underlying disease (e.g., asthma), or drugs (e.g., non-selective β-adrenergic blockers). In general, anesthetic maintenance with isoflurane or sevoflurane is usually well tolerated in patients with reactive airways as these agents promote bronchial relaxation.

Bronchospasm narrows the small airways and increases resistance to ventilation. In the most severe cases, this may progress to apnea and acute desaturation. In patients with pre-existing risk factors, bronchospasm should be suspected if a change in pulmonary resistance is noted (e.g., it becomes more difficult to provide positive-pressure ventilation), with or without an accompanying decrease in SpO_2. Changes to the capnographic waveform (i.e., the characteristic "shark fin" or "saw tooth" pattern) indicating uneven alveolar emptying, as well as increased peak airway pressures during mechanical ventilation, are typically observed. In some patients, wheezes may be appreciated on thoracic auscultation. Examination of pressure–volume loops created by spirometry will aid the diagnosis of changes in resistance and compliance. In the event of a change in pulmonary resistance, acute airway obstruction or pneumothorax should also be considered as rule-outs and investigated. Any underlying conditions that may precipitate bronchospasm should be treated if possible (e.g., epinephrine administration for an anaphylactic reaction). Symptomatic treatment of bronchospasm involves administration of bronchodilators (e.g., aminophylline, terbutaline, and albuterol) and positive-pressure ventilation with 100% oxygen.

Accidental extubation

Unexpected intraoperative extubation is particularly problematic if the patient was difficult to intubate initially, if patient positioning is not conducive to reintubation, and when extubation is not immediately recognized due to surgical drape coverings or other obstructions. An unexpected extubation means the airway is unprotected and the patient is not receiving oxygen or inhalant anesthesia. Creation of an oxygen-rich pocket under the surgical drapes due to an unexpected and unobserved extubation can precipitate a fire [76].

Determining if extubation has happened can be challenging if it is unobserved. Routine, continuous use of capnography is the best tool to detect accidental extubation as the patient's capnographic waveform will be lost with complete tube displacement or modified with partial displacement. Failure to observe breathing bag excursions or one-way valve movements (in a rebreathing circuit), a sudden decrease in resistance when providing positive-pressure ventilation, and/or detection of inhalant agent odor may indicate that an extubation has occurred. If the patient is being maintained with an inhalant agent and extubation is not promptly recognized, decreases in SpO_2 may be noted and anesthetic depth will lighten, potentially resulting in patient movement.

If patient movement is noted, restraint and deepening of the anesthetic plane with a rapid-acting injectable agent is required prior to attempting reintubation. Assistance is typically required, and additional injectable drugs should be available if reintubation is challenging. If extubation is recognized promptly, it may be possible to reintubate the patient without interrupting the ongoing procedure. If, however, intubation is not possible with the patient in the current position, the procedure may need to be paused and the patient repositioned. A bougie (endotracheal tube introducer) may be particularly useful for intubation in unusual positions, as it is often easier to introduce into the airway than an endotracheal tube. In the event that a patient with a difficult airway becomes unexpectedly extubated, a rapid transition to surgical airway access (e.g., a tracheostomy) is essential if orotracheal intubation cannot be quickly achieved.

Iatrogenic tracheal injury

A tracheal tear can occur when excessive force or torque is applied to the trachea or larynx. Cats are particularly sensitive to tracheal tears sustained during anesthesia [77–79]. Overinflation of the endotracheal tube cuff, changing body position with the patient's endotracheal tube connected to the anesthetic circuit, and forceful intubation are the most common causes of tracheal tears. Clinical signs associated with a tracheal tear include subcutaneous emphysema in the cervical region (which may be substantial), pneumomediastinum, and/or pneumothorax. If a tracheal tear is suspected under anesthesia, the patient should be managed without positive-pressure ventilation and pneumothorax may need to be treated via thoracocentesis. If possible, the procedure should be stopped so the patient can recover from anesthesia. Tracheostomy or bronchoscopy may be performed to confirm the diagnosis, although a tear is not always visible. Most tracheal tears typically heal without any active surgical intervention.

Acute or undiagnosed pneumothorax

While other types of pleural space disease (e.g., pleural effusion) may have adverse impacts under anesthesia, acute pneumothorax may manifest unexpectedly and has the potential to be life-threatening, especially if it develops into tension pneumothorax. Pneumothorax may arise because of a procedure (e.g., cranial abdominal or diaphragmatic surgery), excessive airway pressure (e.g., closed APL valve or incorrect ventilator settings), trauma to the airways, or the presence of abnormal pulmonary structures (e.g., bullae) [80]. The diagnosis is one of exclusion, as initial changes in vital signs (cardiorespiratory decompensation and difficulty with ventilation) are non-specific, and other causes of such changes (e.g., airway obstruction, bronchospasm, and endobronchial intubation) occur more commonly and must be ruled out. Increased pulmonary resistance is not a reliable indicator of pneumothorax [80]. It may be difficult to appreciate local clinical signs (e.g., diminished breath sounds) in the anesthetized patient without full access to the thorax, and other diagnostics (e.g., thoracic radiography) may not be available intraoperatively. If the patient's condition warrants immediate intervention, bilateral thoracocentesis should be performed even if the diagnosis has not been confirmed. Discontinuing positive-pressure ventilation may be warranted if there is suspicion that the air entered the thoracic cavity from the airways (e.g., ruptured pulmonary bulla) with or without progression to a tension pneumothorax.

Pulmonary aspiration

Aspiration of foreign material, most often gastric contents, into the trachea and lungs can precipitate airway obstruction, bronchospasm, and/or pneumonia. In rare cases, the endotracheal tube itself may be aspirated, for example, in a horse recovering with the tube in place, or in a small animal patient that bites the tube prior to extubation and inhales part of it. This clearly constitutes an anesthetic emergency and requires immediate intervention to clear the airway. In small animal patients, the risk of endotracheal tube aspiration can be minimized by recovering patients slowly in a controlled environment. If they do regain consciousness suddenly and begin biting the endotracheal tube, the mouth should be held closed until extubation is possible. If recovering a horse with the endotracheal tube in place, ensuring the tube is well secured and intervening to extubate in the event the tube is displaced from the interdental space will prevent it being bitten. Alternatively, maintaining the airway with a nasotracheal tube in recovery will prevent any risk of the tube being bitten.

Brachycephalic patients, patients with laryngeal dysfunction (e.g., laryngeal paralysis), esophageal dysfunction (e.g., megaesophagus), neurologic disease, and those undergoing upper airway surgeries may be at higher risk for developing aspiration pneumonia [81]. Regurgitation of gastric contents during or after anesthesia puts the patient at a higher risk for developing pneumonia [81]. Development of aspiration pneumonia may progress to respiratory failure resulting in death or, due to expense of treatment and/or poor prognosis, euthanasia may be elected [82]. In dogs, a large-scale retrospective multicenter study reported the incidence of postanesthetic aspiration pneumonia to range between 0.04% and 0.26% [81]. The rate is unknown in cats, but in one study, 40% of the cats diagnosed with aspiration pneumonia had undergone recent anesthesia [83].

Diagnosis of pulmonary aspiration may be made if regurgitated material is visualized in the oropharynx and the airway is unprotected. Even in anesthetized patients that are intubated, regurgitated fluid may pass by an inadequately inflated endotracheal tube cuff and enter the lungs, and this may not be recognized until days later when pneumonia develops [81]. Aspiration pneumonia is typically diagnosed on the basis of thoracic radiographs and physical examination.

Ensuring that the oropharynx is cleared of debris and that there are no small objects near the patient's mouth during recovery will reduce the risk of aspiration. If there is concern that fluid may remain in the trachea proximal to an inflated endotracheal tube cuff, extubation is sometimes performed with the cuff partially inflated to remove excess fluid. One study involving canine cadavers found that extubation with an inflated high-pressure low-volume endotracheal tube cuff reduced but did not completely eliminate intratracheal fluid [84]. This study did not evaluate potential adverse effects of this practice such as damage to the tracheal wall or larynx.

Reducing the risk of regurgitation and postanesthetic aspiration pneumonia is possible, but complicated. In the study by Ovbey *et al.*, the incidence of aspiration pneumonia in dogs varied considerably depending on the institution [81]. It was speculated that this may be related to different anesthetic practices, but it was unclear what those differences were. In another study involving dogs undergoing anesthesia for radiation treatment, procedural changes including decreasing the use of anticholinergics and pure μ-opioid receptor agonists, minimizing changes in body position, prophylactically treating nausea, maintaining the endotracheal tube cuff inflated until immediately before extubation, and improved aseptic handling of equipment used for endotracheal intubation reduced the incidence of postanesthetic aspiration pneumonia from 13% to 1.3% [85]. Thus, taking steps to reduce the risk of gastroesophageal reflux (GER) and regurgitation seems warranted, particularly in high-risk patients.

Volutrauma and barotrauma

Pulmonary volutrauma and/or barotrauma may occur as a result of equipment maloperation (i.e., a closed APL valve as discussed in the equipment section) or associated with positive-pressure ventilation (in humans, this is often referred to as "ventilator-associated lung injury" or "ventilator-induced lung injury"). Excessively high airway pressures (barotrauma) and/or volume overexpansion (volutrauma) can directly damage the lung leading to extra-alveolar air accumulation (potentially pneumothorax) as well as pulmonary edema and hemorrhage. The consequences of damage induced by positive-pressure ventilation may not be appreciated during the course of anesthesia as it takes time for the inflammatory response to develop in the lower airways. Frank hemorrhage or fluid within the endotracheal tube, changes to pulmonary compliance or resistance, and evidence of ventilation–perfusion mismatch may be observed. If pulmonary damage due to positive-pressure ventilation is suspected, adjustments to the ventilation strategy should be made with relatively low peak inspiratory pressure indicated in these cases [86]. Barotrauma and volutrauma are best prevented by avoiding excessive airway pressures and volumes in the first place. In patients with atelectasis, a recruitment maneuver with addition of positive end-expired pressure (PEEP) may be preferable to avoid delivering large volumes and pressures over a long period of time.

In patients with chronic atelectasis (e.g., a congenital pericardial-peritoneal diaphragmatic hernia or other chronic pleural space disease), even modest increases in positive airway pressure may precipitate re-expansion pulmonary edema and hypoxemia. This is a rare phenomenon in people [87], and the incidence in animals is unknown. Shear forces exerted by positive-pressure ventilation are thought to initiate an inflammatory response that increases vascular permeability and causes microvascular damage resulting in edema. Every effort should be made to prevent re-expansion pulmonary edema in patients with chronic lung collapse by using relatively low inspiratory pressures and volumes and allowing the lung to re-expand gradually over time. If re-expansion pulmonary edema occurs, it can be treated with diuretics, oxygen supplementation, and supportive care.

Wooden chest syndrome

Chest wall rigidity (wooden chest syndrome) is observed when a patient's intercostal muscles and diaphragm become rigid, significantly impairing ventilation. The phenomenon is associated with the use of fentanyl and its analogues and has been reported in people [88]. There are no reports of wooden chest syndrome in the veterinary literature, although it has been noted anecdotally in dogs receiving fentanyl. Clinical signs are consistent with a rigid thoracic cavity including failure of the chest wall to expand, higher than expected inspiratory airway pressures, and ventilatory failure in patients breathing spontaneously or being mechanically ventilated. In the face of these clinical events, it is important to distinguish possible chest wall rigidity due to fentanyl from more common causes of inability to ventilate or abrupt changes to thoracic compliance, such as bronchospasm, acute airway obstruction, and pneumothorax. If these more common causes are ruled out, chest wall rigidity due to fentanyl may be considered, and a neuromuscular blocking agent may be administered to decrease skeletal muscle tone and facilitate positive-pressure ventilation [88]. Reversal with naloxone alone does not resolve chest wall rigidity in people, although changing to a different opioid for continued surgery may be warranted.

Airway fire

Airway fire is a rarely reported but devastating complication in human anesthesia and, despite the increasing use of laser therapy in veterinary medicine there are very few reports in the veterinary literature [89]. Heat, fuel, and an oxidizer can occur together in the operating room, so it is important to be careful when cautery or laser energy is used around the endotracheal tube or other source of oxygen [90]. In patients that are not intubated (e.g., small exotics), care must be taken to ensure that an oxygen-rich environment does not occur in proximity to an ignition source [76].

The risk of a fire can be minimized by using an endotracheal tube not made of hydrocarbons (e.g., steel), ensuring that the cuff is properly inflated, filling the cuff with dye-colored water (to visualize if it has been damaged during the procedure), using less than 100% oxygen (i.e., an F_IO_2 of 33% by mixing with medical air), avoiding nitrous oxide, and packing the area around the surgical site with wet gauze. Simply wrapping an endotracheal tube in reflective foil may be insufficient to protect it from laser energy. In the event of a fire, it should be extinguished as quickly as possible using water, a fire extinguisher or, if neither of those are available, suffocation. The source of oxygen should be discontinued and physically removed from the fire. Extubation of the patient is not always the correct course of action but is recommended if the patient does not have a difficult airway that would complicate reintubation. In the event of a larger fire, the oxygen source should be removed entirely (e.g., the oxygen supply line shut down) and personnel evacuated. Additional information is available in Chapter 4.

Anesthetic drug-related complications

Medical error resulting in overdose

Medical errors present a significant problem in human medicine and are estimated to be the third leading cause of death in the United States [91]. In one veterinary teaching hospital, drug errors were the most common type of error reported [92]. The events that lead to a drug error are complex and are examined in Chapter 3. Drugs may be inadvertently given at the wrong dose, to the wrong patient, by the wrong route, at the wrong time, or the wrong drug may be given [92]. In the face of a drug error, the most immediate step is to try to withdraw as much drug as possible from the patient (i.e., for intravenously administered drugs, aspirate any drug remaining in the catheter). The next step is to determine if the overdose constitutes a risk to the patient and, if so, take steps to minimize patient harm.

Certain drugs used in veterinary anesthesia (e.g., opioids, benzodiazepines, α_2-adrenergic receptor agonists, and dissociatives) have relatively wide therapeutic margins and, depending on the magnitude of the overdose, may not constitute a threat to patient safety. Other drugs (e.g., propofol and bupivacaine) have narrower therapeutic margins, and overdose may have more serious adverse consequences. The patient's physiologic parameters should be evaluated and monitored following an overdose to determine if there is any clinically relevant impairment. If not, the procedure may proceed cautiously. If the patient is adversely affected by the drug overdose, administration of a specific antagonist is warranted if one is available. For local anesthetic toxicity, a lipid emulsion provides a depot for the drug to enter and minimizes systemic local anesthetic effects [93]. Overdose with a non-steroidal anti-inflammatory drug may be treated with plasmapheresis [94]. Excessive sedation caused by acepromazine may be managed with doxapram [95]. Further information about specific anesthetic, analgesic, and antagonist drugs is available in the relevant pharmacology chapters. Symptomatic support, including maintenance of body temperature, fluid administration, and cardiorespiratory support, may be necessary to give the patient time to clear the drug. The patient's status should be evaluated after treatment and, if possible, a delay in the procedure may be necessary if the patient's status is still unknown or unstable.

Patient arousal

Acute arousal is usually the result of human error (i.e., underdosing, inattention, judgment errors, or other knowledge gaps related to injectable drugs, inhalant agents, or anesthetic machine operation) and requires immediate intervention. Patient arousal and movement can result in injury to personnel, injury to the patient, prolongation of the procedure for which the patient was anesthetized, and damage to equipment. Significant movement in anesthetized large animals (e.g., adult horses) can have potentially devastating consequences. Underdosing during inhalant anesthesia may arise due to an inadequate fresh gas flow rate (e.g., flowmeter not turned on, compressed gas cylinder empty, and oxygen supply line disconnected), a vaporizer that is empty or not turned on, a tubing disconnection, and/or ineffective ventilation. In the face of movement during inhalant anesthesia, the patient should be restrained and then rapidly reanesthetized. Administration of an injectable agent is typically used for this purpose, but in some cases, delivery of a high oxygen flow rate and vaporizer setting may be employed. Once the patient's anesthetic plane has been stabilized, a thorough investigation into the cause of acute arousal must be undertaken, including evaluation of the anesthetic machine, and corrective action taken to prevent re-occurrence.

Anesthetic equipment-related complications

The reader is directed to Chapter 6 for further details about equipment function.

Adjustable pressure-limiting valve closure or malfunction

Occlusion of the adjustable pressure-limiting (APL) (i.e., pop-off) valve or exhaust tubing can result in a buildup of pressure within the anesthetic circuit and is a common anesthetic-related adverse incident [96]. An activated charcoal canister (e.g., F/air canister) placed on the ground preventing outflow of gases can also cause pressure to build up. Once the volume capacity of the breathing system has been reached (i.e., once the elastic limits of the breathing bag are exceeded), pressure in the breathing circuit climbs rapidly. This increasing pressure may result in airway injury (i.e., volutrauma, pneumothorax), and compromised venous return decreases cardiac output and may precipitate cardiovascular collapse and arrest if not addressed in time. Loss of a palpable peripheral pulse may be appreciated as the pressure in the breathing circuit is building. If excessive pressure has accumulated, it must be rapidly relieved by opening the APL valve or, if occlusion or dysfunction of the valve is suspected, disconnecting the circuit at any location. Prevention of inadvertent APL valve closure can be minimized by confirming its function and status during preanesthetic testing of the breathing circuit, having a second individual routinely pressure-check the circuit [96], using an APL valve with a momentary closure function either built-in or added to facilitate manual intermittent positive-pressure ventilation (Fig. 5.3A), and incorporating a pressure-relief valve in the anesthetic circuit (Fig. 5.3B).

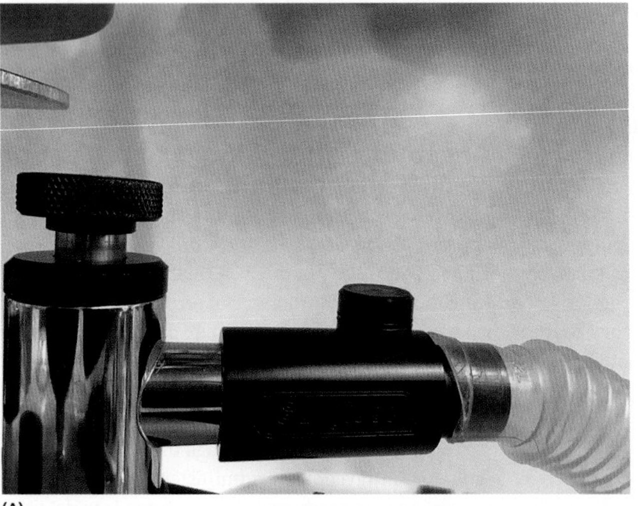
(A)

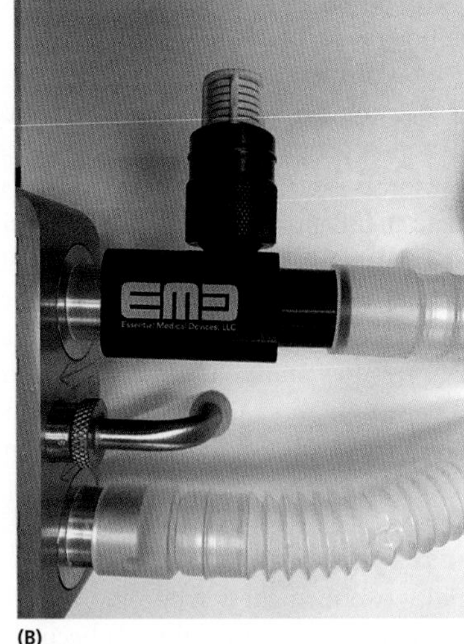

(B)

Figure 5.3 **A.** Addition of a momentary closure valve adjacent to a standard adjustable pressure-limiting (APL) valve in a small animal breathing circuit. This momentary closure function facilitates intermittent positive-pressure ventilation while minimizing the risk of the APL valve being inadvertently left closed. **B.** Addition of a pressure-relief valve to a standard small animal breathing circuit. This device will vent excess gases into the environment at a preset pressure in the event the APL valve is left closed and prevent pressure being transferred to the patient's airway. Source: Dr. Erik Hofmeister, with permission.

Oxygen supply failure

An empty oxygen tank or failure of the oxygen supply line results in no fresh gas flow to carry inhalant anesthetic to the patient and, potentially, a hypoxic mix of inspiratory gases. Failure of the flowmeter indicator to register gas flow, patient arousal and movement during inhalant anesthesia, and decreases in hemoglobin saturation (SpO_2) may all indicate an oxygen supply problem. It is important to realize that the flowmeter may initially register some oxygen flow if an oxygen tank was turned on to pressurize the line between the tank and flowmeter and then subsequently turned off. Therefore, the amount of oxygen remaining in the tank should always be confirmed by observing the tank pressure gauge prior to use. In the event of oxygen supply failure, with no readily available remedy (e.g., all available oxygen tanks empty), anesthesia may be maintained with total intravenous anesthesia, with the understanding that an F_IO_2 of 0.21 may predispose to hypoxemia.

Breathing system malfunction

A variety of accidents can occur involving the anesthetic breathing system. The carbon dioxide absorbent may be exhausted but the canister may not show an obvious color change due to channeling of gases through the interior of the cylinder. The inner tube in a coaxial breathing circuit (e.g., Bain or F-piece) may become twisted and occlude inspiratory flow [97]. In-circuit filters may become saturated with moisture and cause an obstruction [98]. A tear may occur in coaxial circuits leading to rebreathing of CO_2 [99]. One-way valves may become stuck or warped in rebreathing circuits, resulting in rebreathing of CO_2. When the anesthetist is faced with a confounding problem that could possibly be related to the anesthetic machine, changing machines and breathing circuits may be warranted until a thorough investigation of the original machine can be undertaken.

Vaporizer-related complications

In addition to the vaporizer being empty or not turned on which will lead to underdosing and patient arousal, the vaporizer may be filled with the incorrect anesthetic agent, may be tipped, or may not be secured to the manifold properly. Each vaporizer is designed to function with a specific inhalant anesthetic, as the saturated vapor pressure (SVP) of each inhalant is unique. Filling an isoflurane vaporizer (SVP 240 mmHg) with sevoflurane (SVP 160 mmHg) will result in underdosing, and filling a sevoflurane vaporizer with isoflurane will result in overdosing. If a vaporizer is tipped from the horizontal plane (e.g., if a machine falls over), the channel may fill with inhalant, resulting in a substantial overdose of the inhalant agent. If the vaporizer is not secured to the manifold, the circuit may pass a leak test but a leak will exist between the flowmeter and the common gas outlet. Use of an anesthetic agent analyzer to measure inspired inhalant concentrations may facilitate diagnosis of a vaporizer malfunction.

Other complications

Gastroesophageal reflux and regurgitation

Gastroesophageal reflux (GER) is the phenomenon of fluid passively moving from the stomach into the esophagus and, potentially, into the oropharynx. It is estimated to happen in a significant number of dogs under anesthesia with a reported incidence rate as high as 88% in one study [100]. GER also occurs in cats, though less often than in dogs, with rates up to 33% in one study [101]. Esophageal reflux is a risk factor for aspiration and can cause esophageal stricture formation [102,103]. Regurgitation into the oropharynx is associated with a fourfold increased risk of developing pneumonia after anesthesia [81]. While the exact incidence of esophageal stricture formation postanesthesia is unknown it appears to be rare. However, it is a potentially catastrophic adverse anesthetic event, which can have a significant impact on the patient's and client's quality of life [102,103].

Once GER has occurred, there are several treatment approaches to minimize potential damage to the esophagus. Although none of the treatments have documented an impact on the development of esophagitis, esophageal strictures, or aspiration pneumonia, it is expected that removing as much refluxate as possible and neutralizing any acidic or basic elements in the refluxate would minimize damage to the esophagus. In anesthetized dogs with persistent acidic esophageal pH despite repeated cycles of suctioning, lavaging with tap water, and further suctioning, the instillation of 20 mL of 4.2% sodium bicarbonate into the distal esophagus was effective in increasing esophageal pH [104]. A subsequent study indicated that the lavage with water may be an unnecessary step and suggested sole treatment with 4.2% sodium bicarbonate at 0.6 mL/kg after suctioning was sufficient [105]. Further information on GER is available in Chapters 2 and 41.

Ruminal tympany

In ruminants, distension of the rumen (i.e., bloat) due to inability of gas to escape through the esophagus may complicate anesthesia and increase the risk of regurgitation. Development of bloat compresses the diaphragm, decreases functional residual capacity, and causes respiratory compromise. Significant bloat may limit venous return and impair cardiac output. Appropriate fasting (i.e., 24–48 h) reduces the risk of bloat in adult ruminants. Passing a stomach tube via the esophagus into the rumen will help prevent bloat in patients that have not been fasted. In the event that bloat develops during a procedure, a stomach tube can be passed to relieve the pressure. If a stomach tube cannot be passed, possibly due to excess pressure at the cardiac sphincter, transcutaneous decompression (similar to trocharization in dogs with gastric dilatation-volvulus) can be performed. Further information is available in Chapters 53 and 64.

Cerebral herniation

Cerebral herniation describes the displacement of brain structures across anatomical boundaries within the calvarium (e.g., brainstem protruding through the foramen magnum). During anesthesia, abrupt increases in intracranial pressure (ICP) precipitated by intubation, hypercapnia, hypertension, hypoxemia, jugular occlusion, changes in head elevation, and/or exacerbation of intracranial disease (e.g., hemorrhage, swelling) increase the risk of cerebral herniation in at-risk patients. Cerebral herniation may stimulate a Cushing reflex, apnea, cardiovascular collapse, and/or failure to recover from anesthesia. A Cushing reflex manifests as an acute increase in arterial blood pressure and a reflex bradycardia in an attempt to maintain cerebral perfusion in the face of an increased ICP [106]. In at-risk patients, the risk of cerebral herniation may be reduced by maintaining $PaCO_2$ (or $P_{ET}CO_2$) in the low normal range (e.g., 32 mmHg), keeping the head elevated, avoiding jugular occlusion and hypoxemia, and potentially considering propofol rather than an inhalant for maintenance of anesthesia [107]. If cerebral herniation is suspected, the patient can be hyperventilated (target $P_{ET}CO_2$ of 25 mmHg), and mannitol (0.5–1 g/kg IV over 10 min) and/or hypertonic saline (2–4 mL/kg IV over 10 min) can be administered. Prednisone (1 mg/kg IV) may help reduce inflammation. Patients with acute cerebral herniation have a grave prognosis and failure to recover from anesthesia is not an unexpected outcome. Further information is available in Chapter 39.

Hyperkalemia

Development of acute hyperkalemia during general anesthesia in a patient with normal serum potassium prior to anesthesia is a rare but potentially life-threatening complication. In dogs and cats, while there have been reports of intraoperative hyperkalemia, and a definitive cause has not been identified, dexmedetomidine use has been implicated as a risk factor [108,109]. Horses diagnosed with or suspected to have hyperkalemic periodic paralysis may be at an increased risk of developing hyperkalemia under anesthesia [110]. Hyperkalemia may be identified by changes to the ECG, notably bradycardia (which is often resistant to treatment with antimuscarinics), absent P waves, and tented T waves [108,109]. Horses may exhibit muscle fasciculations [110]. Typical treatments for hyperkalemia that reduce the risk of fatal arrhythmias (e.g., calcium gluconate) and lower serum potassium concentrations (e.g., insulin, dextrose, and sodium bicarbonate) are indicated [109]. Hyperkalemia identified prior to anesthesia (e.g., due to urethral obstruction or uroperitoneum) should be corrected before induction of anesthesia if at all possible. Further information is available in Chapter 43.

Hypo- or hyperthermia

Hypothermia is a common event under anesthesia in dogs and cats, affecting up to 89% of dogs [111,112] and 98% of cats [113]. Dogs and cats with an American Society of Anesthesiologists (ASA) status of III or more are at increased risk of developing intraoperative hypothermia [114]. Other risk factors identified in dogs include body weight < 6 kg, receiving an α_2-adrenergic receptor agonist, receiving an opioid, having an anesthetic episode lasting > 1 h, having surgery for an orthopedic or neurologic condition, or undergoing an MRI [112]. A variety of strategies have been investigated to minimize intraoperative hypothermia, and the reader is directed to Chapter 17 for more information. Once hypothermia develops, active warming strategies (e.g., forced warm air and resistive polymer heating) are indicated although there is a lag period between implementation of active warming and changes to core temperature [115].

Hyperthermia during general anesthesia is much less common than hypothermia, affecting only 3–9% of dogs [111,112] and 1% of cats [113]. Hyperthermia during anesthetic maintenance is often iatrogenic, due to excessive warming, particularly in small patients. Postanesthetic hyperthermia has been documented in up to 47% of cats within 24 h [116]. It is associated largely with opioid administration [117], although cats receiving only medetomidine and either ketamine or propofol can also develop hyperthermia [118]. Postanesthetic hyperthermia in cats is typically self-limiting [117]; however, if the temperature is excessively high, naloxone 0.01 mg/kg IM or IV can be administered. Body temperature often rapidly returns to normal following opioid reversal. Further information is available in Chapter 17.

Malignant hyperthermia

The phenomenon of malignant hyperthermia is characterized by a rapid increase in body temperature caused by skeletal muscle contraction. This contraction is caused by an abnormal, excessive influx of calcium from the sarcoplasmic reticulum due to a defective calcium channel, most commonly the ryanodine receptor (RyR1). This abnormal influx is most commonly induced by anesthetic drugs, notably halogenated inhalant anesthetic agents (not gases such as nitrous oxide and xenon) and succinylcholine. Other triggers, such as stress and exercise, may rarely precipitate malignant hyperthermia. While malignant hyperthermia is extremely rare overall and is less common with modern inhalant anesthetics [119], it has been documented in dogs [120], cats [121], and horses [122] using isoflurane or sevoflurane. Pigs are the most commonly affected species and have been used as an animal model for the disease for decades [123]. Further information about malignant hyperthermia in pigs is available in Chapters 53 and 65.

Clinical signs of malignant hyperthermia vary by species and can manifest from induction through to recovery. Typically, evidence of a hypermetabolic syndrome predominates, particularly increased $P_{ET}CO_2$, heart rate, arrhythmias, and body temperature [120]. Muscle rigidity, changes to skin color due to vasodilation, metabolic acidosis, hyperkalemia, rhabdomyolysis, sweating, and disseminated intravascular coagulation can also occur [123]. Because the treatment for malignant hyperthermia is specific to that diagnosis, it is important to distinguish it from other hypermetabolic causes, such as hyperthermia [124], sepsis/endotoxemia [120], or thyrotoxicosis [125]. Any patient exhibiting an abrupt increase in $P_{ET}CO_2$ or body temperature should be considered for malignant hyperthermia. If suspected, inhalant anesthetics should be discontinued, the patient changed to a "clean" machine and circuit without recent inhalant exposure, and anesthesia maintained with an injectable protocol (e.g., propofol infusion). The specific treatment for malignant hyperthermia is the calcium channel blocker dantrolene at 2 mg/kg IV with additional doses as required up to 10 mg/kg IV. Because dantrolene is rarely available at most veterinary hospitals, symptomatic treatment and other calcium channel blockers may be used but are rarely successful [120–122]. Symptomatic treatment may include administration of sympatholytics (e.g., β-adrenergic blockers), insulin and dextrose to treat hyperkalemia, procainamide, neuromuscular blocking agents, hyperventilation, active cooling, and fluid support. Lidocaine and exogenous calcium administration may worsen the outcome [120]. Without acute dantrolene treatment, malignant hyperthermia is typically fatal [120–122].

Myoclonus

Myoclonus is the rhythmic contraction of skeletal muscles and can range from a small single-muscle tick to a whole-body contraction that resembles a seizure. In people, the electroencephalogram (EEG) of patients experiencing anesthesia drug-related myoclonus is not typical of seizure activity; therefore, myoclonus appears to be distinct from a seizure [126]. Myoclonus has been reported in dogs administered etomidate [127], epidural morphine [128], propofol [129], and ketamine [130]. Administering additional drugs, such as propofol or benzodiazepines, does not reliably stop the myoclonus [127,129], but pretreatment with an opioid or benzodiazepine may reduce the incidence [127,131]. Myoclonus occurring after induction typically subsides if no additional treatment is given and does not seem to be associated with adverse clinical effects for the patient [130].

Postanesthetic complications

Prolonged anesthetic recovery

The time to recover from anesthesia depends on the species, the drugs used and their route of administration, the duration of anesthesia, and patient characteristics [132,133]. In small animal patients, the time from termination of inhalant anesthesia to extubation of the patient is usually expected to be less than 30 min [134]. In equine patients in a university teaching hospital setting, the time from inhalant anesthesia termination to standing is typically expected to be less than 60 min [133]. If the patient's recovery exceeds these times (or those defined by the institution), it may be considered prolonged. A prolonged recovery may indicate physiologic disturbances, which must be corrected and is, therefore, a potential anesthetic emergency.

Common differential diagnoses for a prolonged recovery include hypothermia, hypotension, hemorrhage, hepatic incompetence, renal dysfunction, hypoglycemia, neurologic disease, hypocalcemia, and drug overdose. The potential for prolonged anesthetic recovery should be anticipated in patients where preanesthetic patient evaluation indicates hepatic incompetence (e.g., liver failure), renal dysfunction, and/or neurologic disease and their anesthetic protocols should be adjusted accordingly. In patients experiencing a prolonged recovery that was not expected, their physiologic status should be thoroughly evaluated, specifically temperature, blood glucose, ionized calcium, blood pressure, and packed cell volume if hemorrhage from a surgical procedure (e.g., postoperative ovariohysterectomy) is a possibility. Any physiologic derangements should be corrected. If no physiologic abnormalities are identified, a relative drug overdose should be considered, even if the drug dose was apparently appropriate for the patient. Opioids may be reversed with low-dose naloxone (0.01 mg/kg IV) and benzodiazepines with flumazenil (0.01 mg/kg IV). α_2-Adrenergic receptor agonists may be reversed with atipamezole, tolazoline, or yohimbine. Excessive sedation due to acepromazine may be treated with doxapram (1.25 mg/kg IV). In exceptional circumstances, recovery from inhalant anesthesia may be expedited with doxapram [135] or physostigmine [136]. If drug effects have been reversed and recovery still has not progressed, persistent neurologic dysfunction, possibly due to intraoperative hypotension, hypoperfusion, and hypoxia, should be considered. Administration of corticosteroids, mannitol, and/or hypertonic saline may be indicated if there is concern for increased ICP secondary to the patient's disease or suspected cerebral hypoxia.

Patient injury during recovery

Injuries may be incurred by patients during recovery from anesthesia. In small animals, thrashing body motions may cause trauma to the head and limbs, necessitating further medical care (e.g., wound care, fracture repair, and dental extraction). In horses, fractures sustained during recovery account for up to 64% of all anesthesia-related fatalities [137]. In addition to appropriate analgesia, sedation prior to recovery, particularly in patients expected to be anxious or aggressive, may help minimize the risk of injury. In an emergency situation where an animal is thrashing and may injure itself, serious consideration must also be given to the risk of injury to personnel. In a survey, up to 43% of equine hospitals reported injury to personnel in recovery, and most respondents felt those assisting with equine recovery were at greater risk of personal injury [138]. In small animal patients experiencing violent recoveries, the use of physical restraint aids where possible (e.g., leash, wooden board, and rabies pole) should be considered to minimize the risk to personnel and facilitate administration of injectable IM sedation (e.g., dexmedetomidine, ketamine, and/or tiletamine–zolazepam). In adult equine cases, there is little a single individual can do for the thrashing patient in recovery. Often the anesthetist must wait until the patient becomes calm enough to approach and handle and this may be due to exhaustion or asphyxiation and loss of consciousness. Once the equine patient can be handled, sedation and analgesia may be warranted. If the equine patient is unconscious due to airway obstruction, a tracheostomy should be rapidly performed and drugs readied to maintain the patient in an anesthetized or sedated state until an airway is re-established and the patient is stabilized.

Postanesthetic blindness

Postanesthetic blindness can occur due to decreases in cerebral perfusion during anesthesia or occlusion of the maxillary artery, particularly in cats. Cats suffering from hypoxia due to cardiac arrest or profound hypotension can develop cortical blindness [139]. Blindness may also be caused by decreased maxillary artery blood flow due to mouth gag placement for dental, oral, or endoscopic procedures [140,141]. Cortical blindness may be permanent, or vision may return with time [140]. Avoiding the use of spring-loaded mouth gags and minimizing any gag opening to 30 mm or less should prevent occlusion of the maxillary artery in cats [142]. As blindness is diagnosed after the hypoxic event has already occurred and the patient has recovered from anesthesia, therapeutic intervention is not possible and prevention remains the best course of action.

Postanesthetic neuropathy, rhabdomyolysis, or myelomalacia

Large animals, particularly horses, undergoing general anesthesia may experience complications related to nerve, muscle or, rarely, spinal cord damage that become apparent during recovery. Further information on these complications is available in the Chapters 52 and 61.

Rhabdomyolysis (i.e., postanesthetic myopathy) in horses occurs due to decreased perfusion of large muscles and subsequent reperfusion injury combined with increased muscle compartment pressure [143]. It can result in lameness, poor recovery quality, fracture, death, euthanasia, renal failure due to myoglobinuria, and/or failure to recover from anesthesia [137,144]. Postoperative rhabdomyolysis is one of the most common causes of morbidity and mortality associated with anesthesia in the horse, accounting for 7% of deaths [144] and 31% of non-fatal complications [56]. Prolonged duration of anesthesia, hypotension, and lateral recumbency are risk factors for the development of rhabdomyolysis [56]. The risk of developing rhabdomyolysis can be reduced by minimizing the duration of anesthesia, maintenance of MAP > 70 mmHg, provision of IV fluids, ensuring adequate padding and positioning, and avoiding excess strain on muscles [145]. Horses that develop rhabdomyolysis may have difficulty standing in recovery, exhibit lameness once standing, have swollen or hard muscles, and display signs of pain such as shaking, sweating, tachycardia, and/or tachypnea [146]. If rhabdomyolysis is suspected, the presence of myoglobinuria and/or a significantly elevated creatine kinase will support the diagnosis. Treatment in the acute phase is supportive and consists of appropriate analgesia (e.g., α_2-adrenergic receptor agonists, butorphanol, lidocaine infusion), aggressive fluid support, anti-inflammatory drugs (e.g., flunixin meglumine or corticosteroids), and physical therapy such as massage or water cooling.

Postanesthetic neuropathy in horses occurs due to pressure on peripheral nerves, which causes varying degrees of impairment. Although it is rarely reported to cause fatality, it may co-occur with rhabdomyolysis, which may mask the influence of neuropathy [147]. Neuropathy may impact recovery quality and postoperative morbidity, leading to prolonged recovery or euthanasia [148,149]. Facial nerve injury may result from the halter exerting pressure on superficial nerves which manifests as facial asymmetry [150]. Distal limb peripheral nerve injury can result from direct pressure exerted by poorly positioned poles or other pressure points and may lead to inability to extend the hoof. Radial nerve paralysis can occur in laterally recumbent horses and lead to a dropped shoulder and inability to extend the hoof [151]. Obturator nerve injury impacting anesthetic recovery associated with parturition and dystocia has been reported [147]. Bilateral femoral nerve paralysis has been associated with caudal extension of the hindlimbs in dorsally recumbent horses, but unilateral and bilateral pelvic limb neuropathies have been reported with various body positions in both dependent and non-dependent limbs [148,149,152]. The diagnosis of neuropathy is often made by exclusion of other possible causes of prolonged or difficult recovery, particularly rhabdomyolysis [149]. Steps to minimize the risk of neuropathy are similar to those taken to minimize the risk of rhabdomyolysis and include sufficient padding, avoiding pressure points, maintaining adequate blood flow, minimizing anesthesia duration, and pulling the dependent forelimb forward in laterally recumbent horses to minimize pressure on the radial nerve [149]. If neuropathy occurs, there are few options for acute treatment beyond anti-inflammatory drugs and physical therapy. Physical means of support (e.g., a sling, supporting bandages) may be necessary if the horse is unable to stand without assistance. The degree of damage is unknown at the time of injury and can range from neuropraxia (temporary loss of nerve conduction), to axonotmesis (significant axonal damage), to neurotmesis (complete transection of the nerve) [151]. Because the prognosis is dependent on the time required to recover nerve function, re-examination is warranted to assess the patient's progress [150]. Patients that have rapid resolution of signs likely had a mild injury (neuropraxia), whereas those that have permanent loss of function likely had complete disruption of the nerve fiber (neurotmesis) [148].

Myelomalacia is a softening of the spinal cord, which leads to catastrophic failure of spinal conducting pathways, resulting in paralysis. It is a rare but devastating complication in horses undergoing anesthesia [153]. Horses developing myelomalacia will be unable to stand in recovery, may adopt a dog-sitting posture due to paraplegia, and will lack anal tone and hind limb function [153]. The absence of anal tone, tail tone, and withdrawal reflexes help to distinguish it from bilateral femoral nerve paralysis. Myelomalacia most commonly occurs in horses that were in dorsal recumbency during anesthesia and seems to happen more commonly in draft breeds (e.g., Fresian, Morgan, and Percheron) [153]. Other risk factors have not been identified. There is no known prevention for the development of myelomalacia, and treatment has been unrewarding with a 100% fatality rate [153]. Any horse that has abnormal hind limb function following anesthesia should be assessed for the possibility of myelomalacia, and it should be distinguished from rhabdomyolysis and neuropathy, both of which may have more favorable outcomes.

Personnel injury

Injury to personnel around an anesthetic event can result in a crisis, which compounds or complicates patient welfare. If personnel are injured, resources need to be diverted to caring for them, which makes it more challenging to care for patients effectively. Injured personnel are also unable to care for their patients, so personnel safety should always be paramount in any veterinary setting. The breadth of patient types encountered in anesthetic practice means that the anesthetist may be faced with aggressive, wild, and/or venomous species, which can all pose a significant threat to human safety. Veterinary technicians working with more than six different species reported a twofold greater risk of injury than those working with less than four species [154]. Animals account for the majority of accidents veterinarians encounter, up to 66% [155,156]. Veterinary staff members tend to underestimate the risk of injury relative to an expert panel, indicating that risks exist which staff do not perceive as such (e.g., handling an animal in recovery) [156]. Bites from dogs accounted for 35% of the injuries associated with anesthetic procedures [157]. In one study, no survey respondents who reported being bitten in the previous year had been engaged in anesthesia activities, whereas 4% of those who did not report being bitten were engaged in an anesthesia procedure, suggesting that anesthesia activities may be safer than other activities [158]. This may be due to the ability of veterinary anesthesia staff to use sedatives, which contributes to a lower overall injury risk compared with non-veterinary workers such as groomers [159].

Risk to personnel should always be assessed, particularly in circumstances where control of the environment is limited. This is essential in field situations or in situations where the setting is suboptimal (e.g., managing a horse recumbent in a trailer). A plan should be prepared so that every individual knows their role, what the steps of the anesthesia event will include and in what order, and what to do if a problem occurs. Use of remote immobilization is often preferred if an animal cannot be approached safely. Aggressive or dangerous patients limited to a confined space (e.g., stall, corral, or carrier) may be sedated with a blowgun, a spring-loaded syringe pole, or a CO_2-powered pistol. Drug combinations involving α_2-adrenergic receptor agonists (e.g., dexmedetomidine, detomidine, romifidine, or xylazine) and dissociatives (e.g., ketamine or tiletamine) are typically used for pharmacologic restraint in domestic species, and ultrapotent opioids are often used in non-domestic species. Animals that can be physically restrained (i.e., squeeze cage, rabies pole, or capture net) may be able to be injected by hand.

In the event of an injury to personnel, it is the anesthetist's role to ensure continued personnel safety and patient management. An individual should be designated to care for the injured person so that the anesthetist can supervise management of the patient and environment. Once the injured person is receiving care, avoiding further personnel injury should be the most important priority. In some cases, this priority may have to temporarily supersede patient welfare (e.g., releasing a thrashing cat to avoid being bitten or leaving an enclosed space with a horse having a difficult recovery). Once personnel safety has been established, the patient should be attended to, and appropriate care provided. Sedation of the patient may be required to avoid further injury to personnel or the animal.

Post-critical event debriefing

Anesthetic emergencies often occur rapidly, threaten patient well-being and survival, and depend on the intervention of the anesthesia team for a successful outcome. All of these variables can place significant emotional strain on care providers. This may manifest as stress, burnout, anxiety, a feeling of helplessness, and/or depression [160]. In one study in human medical care providers, almost half of those who answered a trauma screening questionnaire reported one to five symptoms of psychological trauma [160]. Providers who did not have a debriefing event reported a higher incidence of post-traumatic stress disorder symptoms than those who did have a debriefing [160].

One study in veterinary medicine documented that debriefing occurred in ~ 60% of CPR events [15]. Most survey respondents indicated that a post-event debriefing tool improved team performance. The most commonly cited points for improvement included equipment issues, need for clinical standards, and medication errors being made. Applications of checklists, training, and proper organization and preparation of equipment should be considered for any anesthetic emergency that is likely to arise [14,15,96].

References

1 Matthews NS, Mohn TJ, Yang M, *et al.* Factors associated with anesthetic-related death in dogs and cats in primary care veterinary hospitals. *J Am Vet Med Assoc* 2017; **250**(6): 655–665.

2 Seamon AB, Hofmeister EH, Divers SJ. Outcome following inhalation anesthesia in birds at a veterinary referral hospital: 352 cases (2004–2014). *J Am Vet Med Assoc* 2017; **251**(7): 814–817.

3 Reason J. *Human Error*, 1st edn. Cambridge, UK: Cambridge University Press, 1990.

4 Boller M, Fletcher DJ. Update on cardiopulmonary resuscitation in small animals. *Vet Clin North Am Small Anim Pract* 2020; **50**(6): 1183–1202.

5 Hofmeister EH, Brainard BM, Egger CM, *et al.* Prognostic indicators for dogs and cats with cardiopulmonary arrest treated by cardiopulmonary cerebral resuscitation at a university teaching hospital. *J Am Vet Med Assoc* 2009; **235**(1): 50–57.

6 McIntyre RL, Hopper K, Epstein SE. Assessment of cardiopulmonary resuscitation in 121 dogs and 30 cats at a university teaching hospital (2009–2012). *J Vet Emerg Crit Care* 2014; **24**(6): 693–704.

7 Hoehne SN, Hopper K, Epstein SE. Prospective evaluation of cardiopulmonary resuscitation performed in dogs and cats according to the RECOVER guidelines. Part 2: patient outcomes and CPR practice since guideline implementation. *Front Vet Sci* 2019; **6**: 439.

8 Onuma M, Kondo H, Ono S, *et al.* Retrospective investigation of cardiopulmonary resuscitation outcome in 146 exotic animals. *J Vet Med Sci* 2017; **79**(9): 1611–1614.

9 Jokisalo JM, Corley KT. CPR in the neonatal foal: has RECOVER changed our approach? *Vet Clin North Am Equine Pract* 2014; **30**(2): 301–316.

10 Conde Ruiz C, Junot S. Successful cardiopulmonary resuscitation in a sevoflurane anaesthetized horse that suffered cardiac arrest at recovery. *Front Vet Sci* 2018; **5**: 138.

11 Hofmeister EH, Reed RA, Barletta M, *et al.* Critical incident technique analysis applied to perianesthetic cardiac arrests at a university teaching hospital. *Vet Anaesth Analg* 2018; **45**(3): 345–350.

12 Oberholtzer JA, Hofmeister EH. Perception of small animal cardiopulmonary resuscitation of owners presenting to a small animal teaching clinic including a large first opinion service. *J Vet Emerg Crit Care* 2020; **30**(4): 411–417.

13 Holmes AC, Clark L. Changes in adherence to cardiopulmonary resuscitation guidelines in a single referral center from January 2009 to June 2013 and assessment of factors contributing to the observed changes. *J Vet Emerg Crit Care* 2015; **25**(6): 801–804.

14 McMichael M, Herring J, Fletcher DJ, *et al.* RECOVER evidence and knowledge gap analysis on veterinary CPR. Part 2: preparedness and prevention. *J Vet Emerg Crit Care* 2012; **22**(Suppl 1): S13–S25.

15 Timothy CL, Brown AJ, Thomas EK. Implementation of a postarrest debriefing tool in a veterinary university hospital. *J Vet Emerg Crit Care* 2021; **31**(6): 718–726.

16 Boller M, Fletcher DJ. RECOVER evidence and knowledge gap analysis on veterinary CPR. Part 1: evidence analysis and consensus process: collaborative path toward small animal CPR guidelines. *J Vet Emerg Crit Care* 2012; **22**(Suppl 1): S4–S12.

17 Fletcher DJ, Boller M, Brainard BM, *et al.* RECOVER evidence and knowledge gap analysis on veterinary CPR. Part 7: clinical guidelines. *J Vet Emerg Crit Care* 2012; **22**(Suppl 1): S102–S131.

18 Kawase K, Ujiie H, Takaki M, *et al.* Clinical outcome of canine cardiopulmonary resuscitation following the RECOVER clinical guidelines at a Japanese nighttime animal hospital. *J Vet Med Sci* 2018; **80**(3): 518–525.

19 Gillespie Í, Fletcher DJ, Stevenson MA, *et al.* The compliance of current small animal CPR practice with RECOVER guidelines: an internet-based survey. *Front Vet Sci* 2019; **6**: 181.

20 Hopper K, Epstein SE, Fletcher DJ, *et al.* RECOVER evidence and knowledge gap analysis on veterinary CPR. Part 3: basic life support. *J Vet Emerg Crit Care* 2012; **22**(Suppl 1): S26–S43.

21 Kneba EJ, Humm KR. The use of mental metronomes during simulated cardiopulmonary resuscitation training. *J Vet Emerg Crit Care* 2020; **30**(1): 92–96.

22 Buckley GJ, Shih A, Garcia-Pereira FL, *et al.* The effect of using an impedance threshold device on hemodynamic parameters during cardiopulmonary resuscitation in dogs. *J Vet Emerg Crit Care* 2012; **22**(4): 435–440.

23 Quesada J, Londoño L, Buckley GJ, *et al.* Retrospective study of gross and histopathologic lesions associated with closed chest cardiopulmonary resuscitation in dogs. *J Small Anim Pract* 2021; **62**(9): 750–755.

24 Hofmeister EH, Brainard BM, Egger CM, *et al.* Additional variables identified as significant return of spontaneous circulation in cardiac arrest and resuscitation. *J Am Vet Med Assoc* 2013; **243**(4): 480.

25 Anthi A, Tzelepis GE, Alivizatos P, *et al.* Unexpected cardiac arrest after cardiac surgery: incidence, predisposing causes, and outcome of open chest cardiopulmonary resuscitation. *Chest* 1998; **113**(1): 15–19.

26 Warang AM, Mann FA, Middleton JR, *et al.* Comparison of left fourth and fifth intercostal space thoracotomy for open-chest cardiopulmonary resuscitation in dogs. *J Vet Emerg Crit Care* 2021; **31**(3): 331–339.

27 Hopper K, Rezende ML, Borchers A, *et al.* Efficacy of manual ventilation techniques during cardiopulmonary resuscitation in dogs. *Front Vet Sci* 2018; **5**: 239.

28 Kim SY, Park SO, Kim JW, *et al.* How much experience do rescuers require to achieve successful tracheal intubation during cardiopulmonary resuscitation? *Resuscitation* 2018; **133**: 187–192.

29 Brainard BM, Boller M, Fletcher DJ, *et al.* RECOVER evidence and knowledge gap analysis on veterinary CPR. Part 5: monitoring. *J Vet Emerg Crit Care* 2012; **22**(Suppl 1): S65–S84.

30 Cha KC, Kim YW, Kim TH, *et al.* Comparison between 30:1 and 30:2 compression-to-ventilation ratios for cardiopulmonary resuscitation: are two ventilations necessary? *Acad Emerg Med* 2015; **22**(11): 1261–1266.

31 Cournand A, Motley HL. Physiological studies of the effects of intermittent positive pressure breathing on cardiac output in man. *Am J Physiol* 1948; **152**(1):162–174.

32 Rozanski EA, Rush JE, Buckley GJ, *et al.* RECOVER evidence and knowledge gap analysis on veterinary CPR. Part 4: advanced life support. *J Vet Emerg Crit Care* 2012; **22**(Suppl 1): S44–S64.

33 Buckley GJ, Rozanski EA, Rush JE. Randomized, blinded comparison of epinephrine and vasopressin for treatment of naturally occurring cardiopulmonary arrest in dogs. *J Vet Intern Med* 2011; **25**(6): 1334–1340.

34 Wongtanasarasin W, Krintratun S. Clinical benefits of corticosteroid administration during adult cardiopulmonary resuscitation: a systemic review and meta-analysis. *World J Crit Care Med* 2021; **10**(5): 290–300.

35 Creedon JM. Controversies surrounding critical illness-related corticosteroid insufficiency in animals. *J Vet Emerg Crit Care* 2015; **25**(1): 107–112.

36 Fletcher DJ, Boller M. Fluid therapy during cardiopulmonary resuscitation. *Front Vet Sci* 2021; **7**: 625361.

37 Voorhees WD III, Ralston SH, Kougias C, *et al.* Fluid loading with whole blood or ringer's lactate solution during CPR in dogs. *Resuscitation* 1987; **15**(2): 113–123.

38 Panchal AR, Bartos JA, Cabañas JG, *et al.* Part 3: adult basic and advanced life support: 2020 American Heart Association guidelines for cardiopulmonary resuscitation and emergency cardiovascular care. *Circulation* 2020; **142**(16 Suppl 2): S366–S468.

39 Hogen T, Cole SG, Drobatz KJ. Evaluation of end-tidal carbon dioxide as a predictor of return of spontaneous circulation in dogs and cats undergoing cardiopulmonary resuscitation. *J Vet Emerg Crit Care* 2018; **28**(5): 398–407.

40 Smarick SD, Haskins SC, Boller M, *et al.* RECOVER evidence and knowledge gap analysis on veterinary CPR. Part 6: post-cardiac arrest care. *J Vet Emerg Crit Care* 2012; **22**(Suppl 1): S85–S101.

41 Choudhary RC, Shoaib M, Sohnen S, *et al.* Pharmacological approach for neuroprotection after cardiac arrest–a narrative review of current therapies and future neuroprotective cocktail. *Front Med* 2021; **8**: 636651.

42 Ai HB, Jiang EL, Yu JH, *et al.* Mean arterial pressure is associated with the neurological function in patients who survived after cardiopulmonary resuscitation: a retrospective cohort study. *Clin Cardiol* 2020; **43**(11): 1286–1293.

43 Ameloot K, Meex I, Genbrugge C, *et al.* Hemodynamic targets during therapeutic hypothermia after cardiac arrest: a prospective observational study. *Resuscitation* 2015; **91**: 56–62.

44 Annoni F, Dell'Anna AM, Franchi F, *et al.* The impact of diastolic blood pressure values on the neurological outcome of cardiac arrest patients. *Resuscitation* 2018; **130**: 167–173.

45 Tahsili-Fahadan P, Farrokh S, Geocadin RG. Hypothermia and brain inflammation after cardiac arrest. *Brain Circ* 2018; **4**(1): 1–13.

46 Gaynor JS, Dunlop CI, Wagner AE, *et al.* Complications and mortality associated with anesthesia in dogs and cats. *J Am Anim Hosp Assoc* 1999; **35**(1): 13–17.
47 Redondo JI, Rubio M, Soler G, *et al.* Normal values and incidence of cardiorespiratory complications in dogs during general anaesthesia. A review of 1281 cases. *J Vet Med A Physiol Pathol Clin Med* 2007; **54**(9): 470–477.
48 Dixon A, Fauber AE. Effect of anesthesia-associated hypotension on neurologic outcome in dogs undergoing hemilaminectomy because of acute, severe thoracolumbar intervertebral disk herniation: 56 cases (2007–2013). *J Am Vet Med Assoc* 2017; **250**(4): 417–423.
49 Harvey L, Knowles T, Murison PJ. Comparison of direct and Doppler arterial blood pressure measurements in rabbits during isoflurane anaesthesia. *Vet Anaesth Analg* 2012; **39**(2): 174–184.
50 Donaldson LL. Retrospective assessment of dobutamine therapy for hypotension in anesthetized horses. *Vet Surg* 1988; **17**(1): 53–57.
51 Bromage PR. Effect of induced vascular hypotension on the liver; alterations in appearance and consistence. *Lancet* 1952; **2**(6723): 10–12.
52 Langård O, Holdaas H, Eide I, *et al.* Conditions for humoral alpha-adrenoceptor stimulation of renin release in anaesthetized dogs. *Scand J Clin Lab Invest* 1981; **41**(6): 527–534.
53 Richey MT, Holland MS, McGrath CJ, *et al.* Equine post-anesthetic lameness. A retrospective study. *Vet Surg* 1990; **19**(5): 392–397.
54 Bellamy RF. Diastolic coronary artery pressure-flow relations in the dog. *Circ Res* 1978; **43**(1): 92–101.
55 Wayne HH. Syncope. Physiological considerations and an analysis of the clinical characteristics in 510 patients. *Am J Med* 1961; **30**: 418–438.
56 Johnston GM, Eastment JK, Taylor PM, *et al.* Is isoflurane safer than halothane in equine anaesthesia? Results from a prospective multicentre randomised controlled trial. *Equine Vet J* 2004; **36**(1): 64–71.
57 Smith MD, Barletta M, Young CN, *et al.* Retrospective study of intra-anesthetic predictors of prolonged hospitalization, increased cost of care and mortality for canine patients at a veterinary teaching hospital. *Vet Anaesth Analg* 2017; **44**(6): 1321–1331.
58 Robinson R, Chang YM, Seymour CJ, *et al.* Predictors of outcome in dogs undergoing thoracic surgery (2002–2011). *Vet Anaesth Analg* 2014; **41**(3): 259–268.
59 Fages A, Soler C, Fernández-Salesa N, *et al.* Perioperative outcome in dogs undergoing emergency abdominal surgery: a retrospective study on 82 cases (2018–2020). *Vet Sci* 2021; **8**(10): 209.
60 Edwards T, Parker J, Palmer L, *et al.* Transfusion for the Military Working Dog. https://jts.amedd.army.mil/assets/docs/cpgs/Transfusion_in_Military_Working_Dog_10_Dec_2019_ID77.pdf (accessed August 2022).
61 McGowan EE, Marryott K, Drobatz KJ, *et al.* Evaluation of the use of shock index in identifying acute blood loss in healthy blood donor dogs. *J Vet Emerg Crit Care* 2017; **27**(5): 524–531.
62 Duerr FM, Carr AP, Duke T, *et al.* Prevalence of perioperative arrhythmias in 50 young, healthy dogs. *Can Vet J* 2007; **48**(2): 169–177.
63 Bigby SE, Beths T, Bauquier S, *et al.* Postinduction apnoea in dogs premedicated with acepromazine or dexmedetomidine and anaesthetized with alfaxalone or propofol. *Vet Anaesth Analg* 2017; **44**(5): 1007–1015.
64 Walley KR, Lewis TH, Wood LD. Acute respiratory acidosis decreases left ventricular contractility but increases cardiac output in dogs. *Circ Res* 1990; **67**(3): 628–635.
65 Hagiya K, Takahashi H, Isaka Y, *et al.* Influence of acidosis on cardiotonic effects of colforsin and epinephrine: a dose-response study. *J Cardiothorac Vasc Anesth* 2013; **27**(5): 925–932.
66 Eisle JH, Eger EI II, Muallem M. Narcotic properties of carbon dioxide in the dog. *Anesthesiology* 1967; **28**: 856–865.
67 McNally EM, Robertson SA, Pablo LS. Comparison of time to desaturation between preoxygenated and nonpreoxygenated dogs following sedation with acepromazine maleate and morphine and induction of anesthesia with propofol. *Am J Vet Res* 2009; **70**(11): 1333–1338.
68 Lin CY. Uptake of anaesthetic gases and vapours. *Anaesth Intensive Care* 1994; **22**(4): 363–373.
69 Jones TL, Boyer K, Chapman K, *et al.* Evaluation of the time to desensitization of the larynx of cats following topical lidocaine application. *J Feline Med Surg* 2021; **23**(6): 563–567.
70 Ambros B, Carrozzo MV, Jones T. Desaturation times between dogs preoxygenated via face mask or flow-by technique before induction of anesthesia. *Vet Anaesth Analg* 2018; **45**(4): 452–458.
71 James T, Lane M, Crowe D, *et al.* A blind insertion airway device in dogs as an alternative to traditional endotracheal intubation. *Vet J* 2015; **203**(2): 187–191.
72 Hardjo S, Goodwin W, Haworth MD, *et al.* A proposed guideline for performance of emergency surgical airways in small animals: analysis of five unsuccessfully managed cannot intubate, cannot oxygenate cases. *Vet Sci* 2022; **9**(2): 39.
73 Campoy L, Hughes JM, McAllister H, *et al.* Kinking of endotracheal tubes during maxima flexion of the atlanto-occipital joint in dogs. *J Small Anim Pract* 2003; **44**(1): 3–7.
74 Calice I, Moens Y. Modern spirometry supports anesthetic management in small animal clinical practice: a case series. *J Am Anim Hosp Assoc* 2016; **52**(5): 305–311.
75 Tute AS, Wilkins PA, Gleed RD, *et al.* Negative pressure pulmonary edema as a post-anesthetic complication associated with upper airway obstruction in a horse. *Vet Surg* 1996; **25**(6): 519–523.
76 Barker SJ, Polson JS. Fire in the operating room: a case report and laboratory study. *Anesth Analg* 2001; **93**(4): 960–965.
77 Bauer MD, Clark-Price SC, McFadden MS. Anesthesia case of the month. *J Am Vet Med Assoc* 2009; **234**(12): 1539–1541.
78 Hardie EM, Spodnick GJ, Gilson SD, *et al.* Tracheal rupture in cats: 16 cases (1983–1998). *J Am Vet Med Assoc* 1999; **214**(4): 508–512.
79 Mitchell SL, McCarthy R, Rudloff E, *et al.* Tracheal rupture associated with intubation in cats: 20 cases (1996–1998). *J Am Vet Med Assoc* 2000; **216**(10): 1592–1595.
80 Harvey L, Murison PJ, Fews D, *et al.* Fatal post-anaesthetic pneumothorax in a dog. *Vet Anaesth Analg* 2010; **37**(1): 83–84.
81 Ovbey DH, Wilson DV, Bednarski RM, *et al.* Prevalence and risk factors for canine post-anesthetic aspiration pneumonia (1999–2009): a multicenter study. *Vet Anaesth Analg* 2014; **41**(2): 127–136.
82 Posner LP, Mariani CL, Swanson C, *et al.* Perianesthetic morbidity and mortality in dogs undergoing cervical and thoracolumbar spinal surgery. *Vet Anaesth Analg* 2014; **41**(2): 137–144.
83 Levy N, Ballegeer E, Koenigshof A. Clinical and radiographic findings in cats with aspiration pneumonia: retrospective evaluation of 28 cases. *J Small Anim Pract* 2019; **60**(6): 356–360.
84 Vance A, Hofmeister EH, Laas C, *et al.* The effects of extubation with an inflated versus deflated endotracheal tube cuff on endotracheal fluid volume in the dog. *Vet Anaesth Analg* 2011; **38**(3): 203–207.
85 Baetge C, Cummings KJ, Deveau M. Reduced risk of pneumonia after changes in anesthetic procedures for dogs receiving repeated anesthesia for radiation treatment. *Vet Radiol Ultrasound* 2019; **60**(2): 241–245.
86 Serpa Neto A, Schultz MJ, Gama de Abreu M. Intraoperative ventilation strategies to prevent postoperative pulmonary complications: systematic review, meta-analysis, and trial sequential analysis. *Best Pract Res Clin Anaesthesiol* 2015; **29**(3): 331–340.
87 Echevarria C, Twomey D, Dunning J, *et al.* Does re-expansion pulmonary oedema exist? *Interact Cardiovasc Thorac Surg* 2008; **7**(3): 485–489.
88 Pergolizzi JV Jr, Webster LR, Vortsman E, *et al.* Wooden Chest syndrome: the atypical pharmacology of fentanyl overdose. *J Clin Pharm Ther* 2021; **46**(6): 1505–1508.
89 Collarile T, Di Girolamo N, Nardini G, *et al.* Fire ignition during laser surgery in pet rodents. *BMC Vet Res* 2012; **8**: 177.
90 Akhtar N, Ansar F, Baig MS, *et al.* Airway fires during surgery: management and prevention. *J Anaesthesiol Clin Pharmacol* 2016; **32**(1): 109–111.
91 Makary MA, Daniel M. Medical error-the third leading cause of death in the US. *BMJ* 2016; **353**: i2139.
92 Wallis J, Fletcher D, Bentley A, *et al.* Medical errors cause harm in veterinary hospitals. *Front Vet Sci* 2019; **6**: 12.
93 Fettiplace MR, McCabe DJ. Lipid emulsion improves survival in animal models of local anesthetic toxicity: a meta-analysis. *Clin Toxicol* 2017; **55**(7): 617–623.
94 Rosenthal MG, Labato MA. Use of therapeutic plasma exchange to treat nonsteroidal anti-inflammatory drug overdose in dogs. *J Vet Intern Med* 2019; **33**(2): 596–602.
95 Zapata M, Hofmeister EH. Refinement of the dose of doxapram to counteract the sedative effects of acepromazine in dogs. *J Small Anim Pract* 2013; **54**(8): 405–408.
96 Hofmeister EH, Quandt J, Braun C, *et al.* Development, implementation and impact of simple patient safety interventions in a university teaching hospital. *Vet Anaesth Analg* 2014; **41**(3): 243–248.
97 Quandt JE. Anesthesia case of the month. Severe twist in the inner tube of the coaxial breathing circuit, resulting in obstruction of the inspiratory limb of the circuit. *J Am Vet Med Assoc* 2005; **227**(12): 1902–1904.
98 McNally E. Anesthesia case of the month. Expiratory obstruction. *J Am Vet Med Assoc* 2009; **234**(10): 1267–1269.
99 Carter JE, Nordaune JL, Pienschke EC, *et al.* Anesthesia case of the month. Capnogram obtained from a 5-month-old 4.4-kg (9.68-lb) sexually intact female Yorkshire Terrier mix undergoing elective ovariohysterectomy. *J Am Vet Med Assoc* 2012; **241**(11): 1441–1443.
100 Lambertini C, Pietra M, Galiazzo G, *et al.* Incidence of gastroesophageal reflux in dogs undergoing orthopaedic surgery or endoscopic evaluation of the upper gastrointestinal tract. *Vet Sci* 2020; **7**(4): 144.
101 Garcia RS, Belafsky PC, Della Maggiore A, *et al.* Prevalence of gastroesophageal reflux in cats during anesthesia and effect of omeprazole on gastric pH. *J Vet Intern Med* 2017; **31**(3): 734–742.
102 Bissett SA, Davis J, Subler K, *et al.* Risk factors and outcome of bougienage for treatment of benign esophageal strictures in dogs and cats: 28 cases (1995–2004). *J Am Vet Med Assoc* 2009; **235**(7): 844–850.

103 Adami C, Di Palma S, Gendron K, *et al.* Severe esophageal injuries occurring after general anesthesia in two cats: case report and literature review. *J Am Anim Hosp Assoc* 2011; **47**(6): 436–442.
104 Wilson DV, Evans AT. The effect of topical treatment on esophageal pH during acid reflux in dogs. *Vet Anaesth Analg* 2007; **34**(5): 339–343.
105 Allison A, Italiano M, Robinson R. Comparison of two topical treatments of gastro-oesophageal regurgitation in dogs during general anaesthesia. *Vet Anaesth Analg* 2020; **47**(5): 672–675.
106 Her J, Yanke AB, Gerken K, *et al.* Retrospective evaluation of the relationship between admission variables and brain herniation in dogs (2010–2019): 54 cases. *J Vet Emerg Crit Care* 2022; **32**(1): 50–57.
107 Chui J, Mariappan R, Mehta J, *et al.* Comparison of propofol and volatile agents for maintenance of anesthesia during elective craniotomy procedures: systematic review and meta-analysis. *Can J Anaesth* 2014; **61**(4): 347–356.
108 Jones SJ, Mama KR, Brock NK, *et al.* Hyperkalemia during general anesthesia in two Greyhounds. *J Am Vet Med Assoc* 2019; **254**(11): 1329–1334.
109 Tissotti T, Sanchez A, Nickell J, *et al.* Retrospective evaluation of acute hyperkalemia of unknown origin during general anesthesia in dogs. *Vet Anaesth Analg* 2023; **50**(2): 129–135.
110 Pang DS, Panizzi L, Paterson JM. Successful treatment of hyperkalaemic periodic paralysis in a horse during isoflurane anaesthesia. *Vet Anaesth Analg* 2011; **38**(2): 113–120.
111 Redondo JI, Suesta P, Serra I, *et al.* Retrospective study of the prevalence of postanaesthetic hypothermia in dogs. *Vet Rec* 2012; **171**(15): 374.
112 Clark-Price SC, Fischer BL, Kirwin KL, *et al.* Multicenter study to investigate factors associated with change in rectal temperature during anesthesia in dogs. *J Am Vet Med Assoc* 2021; **258**(1): 64–71.
113 Redondo JI, Suesta P, Gil L, *et al.* Retrospective study of the prevalence of postanaesthetic hypothermia in cats. *Vet Rec* 2012; **170**(8): 206.
114 Portier K, Ida KK. The ASA physical status classification: what is the evidence for recommending its use in veterinary anesthesia? A systematic review. *Front Vet Sci* 2018; **5**: 204.
115 Rodriguez-Diaz JM, Hayes GM, Boesch J, *et al.* Decreased incidence of perioperative inadvertent hypothermia and faster anesthesia recovery with increased environmental temperature: a nonrandomized controlled study. *Vet Surg* 2020; **49**(2): 256–264.
116 Niedfeldt RL, Robertson SA. Postanesthetic hyperthermia in cats: a retrospective comparison between hydromorphone and buprenorphine. *Vet Anaesth Analg* 2006; **33**(6): 381–389.
117 Posner LP, Pavuk AA, Rokshar JL, *et al.* Effects of opioids and anesthetic drugs on body temperature in cats. *Vet Anaesth Analg* 2010; **37**(1): 35–43.
118 Posner LP, Gleed RD, Erb HN, *et al.* Post-anesthetic hyperthermia in cats. *Vet Anaesth Analg* 2007; **34**(1): 40–47.
119 Wedel DJ, Gammel SA, Milde JH, *et al.* Delayed onset of malignant hyperthermia induced by isoflurane and desflurane compared with halothane in susceptible swine. *Anesthesiology* 1993; **78**(6): 1138–1144.
120 Chohan AS, Greene SA. Anesthesia case of the month. Malignant hyperthermia. *J Am Vet Med Assoc* 2011; **239**(7): 936–940.
121 Thomson SM, Burton CA, Armitage-Chan EA. Intra-operative hyperthermia in a cat with a fatal outcome. *Vet Anaesth Analg* 2014; **41**(3): 290–296.
122 Aleman M, Nieto JE, Magdesian KG. Malignant hyperthermia associated with ryanodine receptor 1 (C7360G) mutation in Quarter Horses. *J Vet Intern Med* 2009; **23**(2): 329–334.
123 Rosenberg H, Pollock N, Schiemann A, *et al.* Malignant hyperthermia: a review. *Orphanet J Rare Dis* 2015; **10**: 93.
124 Hofmeister EH, Hernandez-Divers SJ. Anesthesia case of the month. Tachycardia. *J Am Vet Med Assoc* 2005; **227**(5): 718–720.
125 Merkle JE, Boudreaux B, Langohr I, *et al.* Thyroid storm in a dog secondary to thyroid carcinoma. *J Vet Emerg Crit Care* 2021; **31**(3): 428–431.
126 Doenicke AW, Roizen MF, Kugler J, *et al.* Reducing myoclonus after etomidate. *Anesthesiology* 1999; **90**(1): 113–119.
127 Muir WW III, Mason DE. Side effects of etomidate in dogs. *J Am Vet Med Assoc* 1989; **194**(10): 1430–1434.
128 Iff I, Valeskini K, Mosing M. Severe pruritus and myoclonus following intrathecal morphine administration in a dog. *Can Vet J* 2012; **53**(9): 983–986.
129 Cattai A, Rabozzi R, Natale V, *et al.* The incidence of spontaneous movements (myoclonus) in dogs undergoing total intravenous anaesthesia with propofol. *Vet Anaesth Analg* 2015; **42**(1): 93–98.
130 Hellyer PW, Freeman LC, Hubbell JA. Induction of anesthesia with diazepam-ketamine and midazolam-ketamine in greyhounds. *Vet Surg* 1991; **20**(2): 143–147.
131 Jones TL, Calbay R, da Cunha AF, *et al.* Descriptive assessment of adverse events associated with midazolam-etomidate versus saline-etomidate in healthy hydromorphone premedicated dogs. *J Small Anim Pract* 2021; **62**(6): 437–441.
132 Kleine S, Hofmeister E, Egan K. Multivariable analysis of anesthetic factors associated with time to extubation in dogs. *Res Vet Sci* 2014; **97**(3): 592–596.
133 Voulgaris DA, Hofmeister EH. Multivariate analysis of factors associated with post-anesthetic times to standing in isoflurane-anesthetized horses: 381 cases. *Vet Anaesth Analg* 2009; **36**(5): 414–420.
134 Bennett RC, Fancy SP, Walsh CM, *et al.* Comparison of sevoflurane and isoflurane in dogs anaesthetised for clinical surgical or diagnostic procedures. *J Small Anim Pract* 2008; **49**(8): 392–397.
135 Robertson GS, MacGregor DM, Jones CJ. Evaluation of doxapram for arousal from general anaesthesia in outpatients. *Br J Anaesth* 1977; **49**(2): 133–140.
136 Wiese AJ, Brosnan RJ, Barter LS. Effects of acetylcholinesterase inhibition on quality of recovery from isoflurane-induced anesthesia in horses. *Am J Vet Res* 2014; **75**(3): 223–230.
137 Dugdale AH, Taylor PM. Equine anaesthesia-associated mortality: where are we now? *Vet Anaesth Analg* 2016; **43**(3): 242–255.
138 de Miguel Garcia C, Campoy L, Parry S, *et al.* Questionnaire on the process of recovering horses from general anesthesia and associated personnel injury in equine practice. *Vet Anaesth Analg* 2021; **48**(2): 223–229.
139 Jurk IR, Thibodeau MS, Whitney K, *et al.* Acute vision loss after general anesthesia in a cat. *Vet Ophthalmol* 2001; **4**(2): 155–158.
140 Stiles J, Weil AB, Packer RA, *et al.* Post-anesthetic cortical blindness in cats: twenty cases. *Vet J* 2012; **193**(2): 367–373.
141 Barton-Lamb AL, Martin-Flores M, Scrivani PV, *et al.* Evaluation of maxillary arterial blood flow in anesthetized cats with the mouth closed and open. *Vet J* 2013; **196**(3): 325–331.
142 Martin-Flores M, Scrivani PV, Loew E, *et al.* Maximal and submaximal mouth opening with mouth gags in cats: implications for maxillary artery blood flow. *Vet J* 2014; **200**(1): 60–64.
143 Raisis AL. Skeletal muscle blood flow in anaesthetized horses. Part II: effects of anaesthetics and vasoactive agents. *Vet Anaesth Analg* 2005; **32**(6): 331–337.
144 Johnston GM, Eastment JK, Wood J, *et al.* The confidential enquiry into perioperative equine fatalities (CEPEF): mortality results of Phases 1 and 2. *Vet Anaesth Analg* 2002; **29**(4): 159–170.
145 Duke T, Filzek U, Read MR, *et al.* Clinical observations surrounding an increased incidence of postanesthetic myopathy in halothane-anesthetized horses. *Vet Anaesth Analg* 2006; **33**(2): 122–127.
146 Trim CM, Mason J. Post-anaesthetic forelimb lameness in horses. *Equine Vet J* 1973; **5**(2): 71–76.
147 Bidwell LA, Bramlage LR, Rood WA. Equine perioperative fatalities associated with general anaesthesia at a private practice--a retrospective case series. *Vet Anaesth Analg* 2007; **34**(1): 23–30.
148 Dyson S, Taylor P, Whitwell K. Femoral nerve paralysis after general anaesthesia. *Equine Vet J* 1988; **20**(5): 376–380.
149 Mirra A, Klopfenstein Bregger MD, Levionnois OL. Suspicion of postanesthetic femoral paralysis of the non-dependent limb in a horse. *Front Vet Sci* 2018; **5**: 12.
150 Boorman S, Scherrer NM, Stefanovski D, *et al.* Facial nerve paralysis in 64 equids: clinical variables, diagnosis, and outcome. *J Vet Intern Med* 2020; **34**(3): 1308–1320.
151 Emond AL, Bertoni L, Seignour M, *et al.* Peripheral neuropathy of a forelimb in horses: 27 cases (2000–2013). *J Am Vet Med Assoc* 2016; **249**(10): 1187–1195.
152 Moreno KL, Scallan EM, Friedeck WO, *et al.* Transient pelvic limb neuropathy following proximal metatarsal and tarsal magnetic resonance imaging in seven horses. *Equine Vet J* 2020; *52*(3): 359–363.
153 Ragle C, Baetge C, Yiannikouris S, *et al.* Development of equine post anaesthetic myelopathy: thirty cases (1979–2010). *Equine Vet Educ* 2011; **23**(12): 630–635.
154 Nordgren LD, Gerberich SG, Alexander BH, *et al.* Evaluation of factors associated with work-related injuries to veterinary technicians certified in Minnesota. *J Am Vet Med Assoc* 2014; **245**(4): 425–433.
155 Nienhaus A, Skudlik C, Seidler A. Work-related accidents and occupational diseases in veterinarians and their staff. *Int Arch Occup Environ Health* 2005; **78**(3): 230–238.
156 Weaver DR, Newman LS, Lezotte DC, *et al.* Perceptions regarding workplace hazards at a veterinary teaching hospital. *J Am Vet Med Assoc* 2010; **237**(1): 93–100.
157 Lucas M, Day L, Shirangi A, *et al.* Significant injuries in Australian veterinarians and use of safety precautions. *Occup Med (Lond)* 2009; **59**(5): 327–333.
158 Drobatz KJ, Smith G. Evaluation of risk factors for bite wounds inflicted on caregivers by dogs and cats in a veterinary teaching hospital. *J Am Vet Med Assoc* 2003; **223**(3): 312–316.
159 Fowler H, Adams D, Bonauto D, *et al.* Work-related injuries to animal care workers, Washington 2007–2011. *Am J Ind Med* 2016; **59**(3): 236–244.
160 Spencer SA, Nolan JP, Osborn M, *et al.* The presence of psychological trauma symptoms in resuscitation providers and an exploration of debriefing practices. *Resuscitation* 2019; **142**: 175–181.

6 Anesthesia Equipment

Craig A.E. Mosley
VCA Canada, 404 Veterinary Emergency and Referral Hospital, Newmarket, Ontario, Canada

Chapter contents

Introduction, 74
Safety and design, 75
Introduction to airway management and support equipment, 75
Endotracheal tubes, lung isolation devices, supraglottic airway devices, laryngoscopes, intubation aids, and techniques, 75
  Endotracheal tubes, 75
  Endotracheal tubes for isolating one lung, 78
  Supraglottic airway devices, 82
  Laryngoscopes, 83
  Intubation aids and techniques, 84
  Nasotracheal intubation, 84
  Wire- or tube-guided techniques, 84
  Endoscope-guided technique, 85
  Endotracheal tube exchangers, 86
  Retrograde intubation, 86
  Tracheostomy, 86
  Lateral pharyngotomy, 87
Techniques of oxygen administration, 87
  Mask delivery, 87
  Nasal insufflation, 89
  Tracheal insufflation, 90
  Oxygen cages, 90
  Oxygen toxicity, 91
Introduction to anesthetic machines and breathing circuits, 91
Medical gas supply, 91
  Medical gas safety, 92
  Pressure-reducing valve (regulator), 94
  Pressure gauges, 94
The modern anesthetic machine, 94
  Gas flow within the anesthetic machine, 94
  Flowmeters, 96
  Vaporizers, 97
  Descriptions of vaporizers common in veterinary medicine, 99
  Maintenance of vaporizers, 103
  Use of the wrong anesthetic in an agent-specific vaporizer, 103
  Oxygen flush valve, 104
  Common gas outlet, 104
Breathing systems, 105
  Rebreathing (circle) system, 106
  Non-rebreathing systems, 111
Waste gas scavenge system, 112
  Routine anesthesia machine checkout procedure, 113
Anesthesia ventilators, 113
  Classification, 114
  Introduction to single- and dual-circuit ventilators, 117
  Single-circuit piston-driven ventilators, 117
  Single-circuit compressed gas-powered ventilators, 118
  Dual-circuit ventilators, 119
  Control of ventilator driving gas, 122
  Factors that affect delivered tidal volume, 122
  Alarms, 122
  Proper ventilator setup and monitoring, 123
  Selected ventilator models, 123
Respiratory assist devices, 139
  Manual resuscitators, 139
  Demand valves, 139
Acknowledgment, 139
References, 140

Introduction

The delivery and maintenance of safe anesthesia have become increasingly dependent upon mechanical and electrical equipment. It is necessary for the anesthetist to have a thorough understanding of equipment function and common failures as well as potential patient and personnel risks before use for routine patient care. Anesthesia equipment includes various airway support products, oxygen delivery devices, anesthetic machines, scavenge systems, ventilators, and many configurations of patient monitors and other support products. The products available to the veterinary anesthetist include nearly any human-patient product that can be adapted for use in veterinary anesthesia, regularly produced items specifically for the veterinary market, and many limited-production and/or custom products that may only be occasionally available. There are several excellent textbooks devoted to describing in great detail the anesthetic equipment available for use in human anesthesia [1–3] and, although not entirely applicable to veterinary anesthesia, much of the equipment used is the same (i.e., vaporizers, laryngoscopes, endotracheal tubes, some anesthetic machines) or is a modification of human products. As such, it would be impossible

Veterinary Anesthesia and Analgesia: The Sixth Edition of Lumb and Jones. Edited by Leigh Lamont, Kurt Grimm, Sheilah Robertson, Lydia Love and Carrie Schroeder.
© 2024 John Wiley & Sons, Inc. Published 2024 by John Wiley & Sons, Inc.
Companion website: www.wiley.com/go/lamont/anesthesia

to discuss all of the anesthetic-related equipment and products available today in a single chapter. More recently, a veterinary-specific anesthetic equipment textbook has been published which details the anesthetic and monitoring equipment frequently used in veterinary medicine [4]. This chapter intends to provide the reader with the operating principles and a practical working overview of common anesthetic-related products (i.e., endotracheal tubes, intubating aids, etc.), the anesthetic machine, vaporizers, breathing circuits, and ventilators. In addition, there are products that have been designed specifically for veterinary use, which are described in more detail here.

Safety and design

Since at least 1976, human anesthetic breathing circuits (i.e., circle system) and anesthesia machines sold in North America must meet both mandated and voluntary regulations established by the United States Food and Drug Administration (FDA) (Medical Device Amendments-1976, Good Manufacturing Practices-1978, and Mandatory Device reporting-1984) and organizations such as the International Organization for Standardization (ISO 5358-198a), American Society for Testing and Materials (ASTM F1850), and the Canadian Standards Association (CSA). Many of these standards are currently under re-review with updates anticipated. Anesthetic machines designed for veterinary use are not required to meet any specific design or safety standards beyond those associated with basic hazards to the operator (i.e., electrical safety requirements). Safety features are often added on an ad hoc basis and there are no requirements for demonstrating equipment efficacy. Ideally, some safety features, such as airway pressure alarms, should be integral to the design of the anesthetic machine. The inclusion of some of these safety systems on anesthetic machines may help eliminate preventable anesthetic accidents. However, until safety and design standards are adopted by the manufacturers of veterinary anesthetic equipment, there will remain equipment options of varying quality, efficacy, and safety available for delivering inhalant anesthetics to veterinary patients. Ancillary and support equipment for veterinary patients, including patient monitors and ventilators, are similarly devoid of required efficacy and safety testing. Fortunately, most reputable manufacturers and distributors readily provide the specifications, accuracy, and any available efficacy data for their designs. Regardless of the presence of standards, it will always be incumbent upon the veterinary anesthetist to understand thoroughly the function, principles of operation, and use of all anesthetic-related pieces of equipment and to ensure that the machine or piece of equipment is designed suitably well to accomplish its functions safely.

Introduction to airway management and support equipment

Airway management and support are vital for the safe delivery of anesthesia. Most, if not all, anesthetics cause respiratory depression at doses suitable for anesthesia. In addition, relaxation and/or loss of airway reflexes make the patient more prone to upper airway obstruction. Both of these factors put the anesthetized patient at higher risk for the development of hypoxia. Additionally, the inhalant anesthetics require delivery to the lungs while minimizing environmental and personnel exposure to waste anesthetic gases. For these reasons, airway management and support are critical aspects of properly performed inhalant general anesthesia.

Endotracheal tubes, lung isolation devices, supraglottic airway devices, laryngoscopes, intubation aids, and techniques

Endotracheal tubes

Endotracheal tubes are commonly used to maintain an airway in anesthetized patients. Supraglottic airway devices (SGADs) have also been evaluated in a number of domestic species and may be suitable alternatives in some instances [5–9]. A properly placed endotracheal tube or SGAD with a properly inflated cuff provides a patent airway, facilitates positive-pressure ventilation, protects the lungs from aspiration of fluids, and prevents contamination of the work environment with waste anesthetic gases. Occasionally, it is desirable to limit airway management to one lung field (i.e., thoracoscopy), and specially designed equipment is available to accomplish this task in dogs.

There are many styles and types of endotracheal tubes available that can be used in veterinary medicine. Most are manufactured for humans but can also be used in most small animal patients. There are some veterinary-specific products available for patients requiring tube sizes larger and smaller than those available for human use. Endotracheal tubes manufactured for human patients must have various markings and abbreviations directly on the tube describing the tube's characteristics as well as interval markings to measure the depth of insertion. The markings may include the manufacturer, internal diameter (ID), outer diameter (OD), and length of the tube, as well as codes indicating tissue toxicity or implantation testing (e.g., F29) (Fig. 6.1). There is no requirement for similar markings on tubes manufactured solely for veterinary use, but it is common for them to minimally list tube diameters and lengths. Endotracheal tubes are often sized according to their internal diameters. For example, a size 6.0 endotracheal tube refers to a tube with an internal diameter of 6 mm. Some tubes manufactured specifically for the veterinary market have their sizes indicated using the French gauge/catheter scale, and this should, but may not always, reflect the internal size of the tube. The outer diameter for any given tube size may vary depending upon the construction of the tube. Endotracheal tubes having thicker walls will have greater differences between the internal and outer diameters. This can become important when selecting tubes for very small patients. Very thick-walled tubes will effectively reduce the internal airway diameter compared with a thin-walled tube as ultimately, the size of the endotracheal tube that can be placed in a patient is limited by the outer diameter of the tube and not the inner diameter. However, very thin-walled soft tubes are susceptible to obstruction by external compression or kinking (Fig. 6.2).

Common endotracheal tube materials include polyvinyl chloride, silicone, or red rubber. Clear endotracheal tubes are generally preferred so that they can be inspected visually for the presence of mucus or blood intraoperatively, or debris within the tube lumen after cleaning. Generally, the largest size of an endotracheal tube that will fit without causing trauma in the patient's trachea should be used. Although various "rules-of-thumb" for selecting tube size exist, it is probably easiest to estimate the most appropriate tube size by palpating the individual patient's cervical trachea. The tube should not extend distally beyond the thoracic inlet and ideally should not extend rostrally beyond the patient's incisors, as any additional tube length extending beyond the patient's incisors will increase mechanical deadspace. If the endotracheal tube is too long, and further insertion would lead to the possibility of endobronchial intubation, the machine end can be cut, and the endotracheal tube connector reinserted.

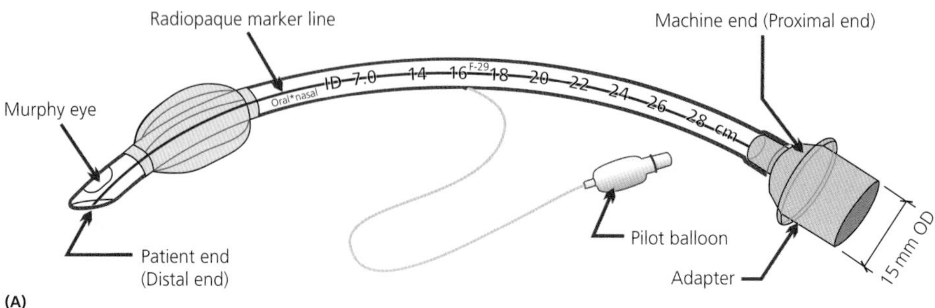

(A)

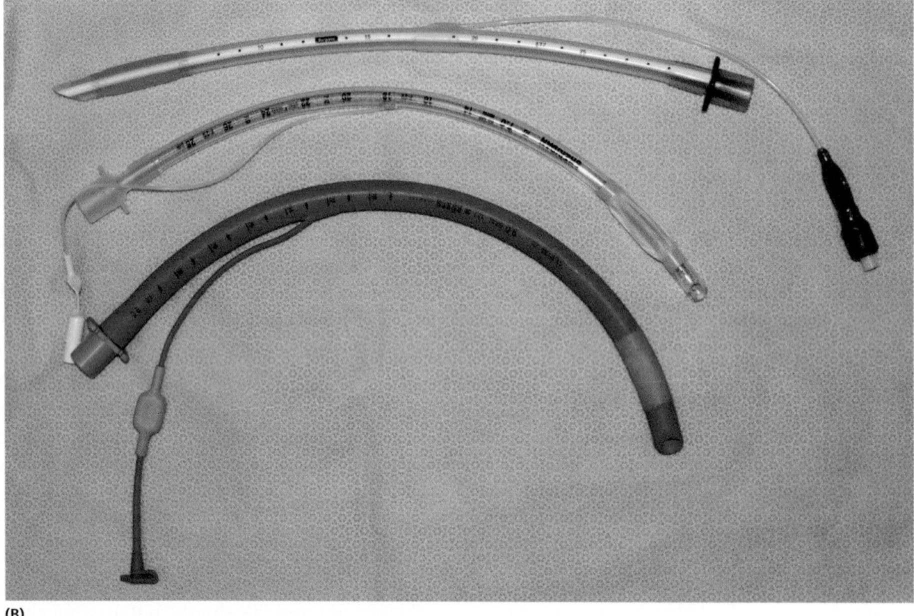

(B)

Figure 6.1 **A.** Most endotracheal tubes have common design features as shown here; however, the specific design and materials can vary among the various manufacturers. **B.** Tubes can be made of silicone, polyvinyl chloride, and red rubber (top to bottom). Source: Dr. Craig Mosley, with permission.

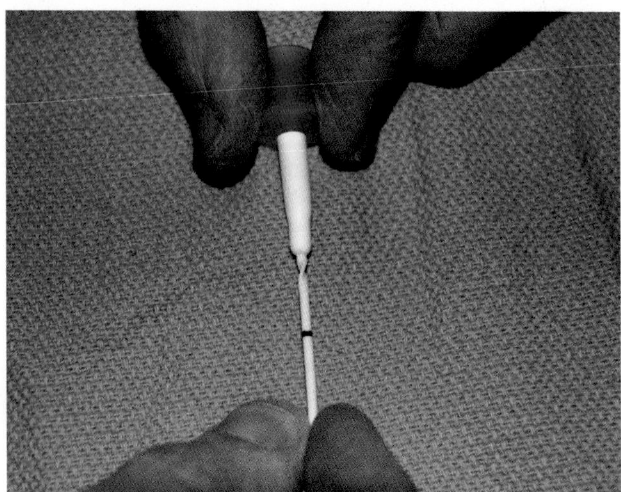

Figure 6.2 Very thin-walled endotracheal tubes are prone to occlusion from external compression or twisting. Continual evaluation of the endotracheal tube for patency is required when thin pliable walled endotracheal tubes are used. Source: Dr. Craig Mosley, with permission.

The most commonly used type of endotracheal tube in both large and small animals is the cuffed Murphy-type tube shown in Fig. 6.1. Cole-type and guarded (spiral embedded, armored) tubes are also occasionally used in veterinary medicine. Cole tubes are uncuffed and have a smaller diameter at the patient (distal) end relative to the machine (proximal) end. The distal smaller diameter portion of the tube is inserted into the trachea to a point where the shoulder contacts the larynx, forming a seal. However, Cole tubes will not produce the same degree of airway security as a standard cuffed tube and are normally used only in very small patients for short-term intubation (see Fig. 6.3). Guarded tubes incorporate a metal or nylon spiral-wound reinforcing wire into the endotracheal tube wall that helps prevent tube collapse and occlusion (Fig. 6.4). Guarded tubes are useful in situations where the tube is likely to be compressed or kinked, such as procedures requiring extreme flexion of the head and neck (e.g., cervical cerebrospinal fluid collection and ophthalmic procedures) or those that involve compression of the trachea (e.g., tracheal retraction during the ventral approach to the cervical spinal cord).

The machine end of the tube contains the endotracheal tube connector. The most proximal portion of the connector used for small

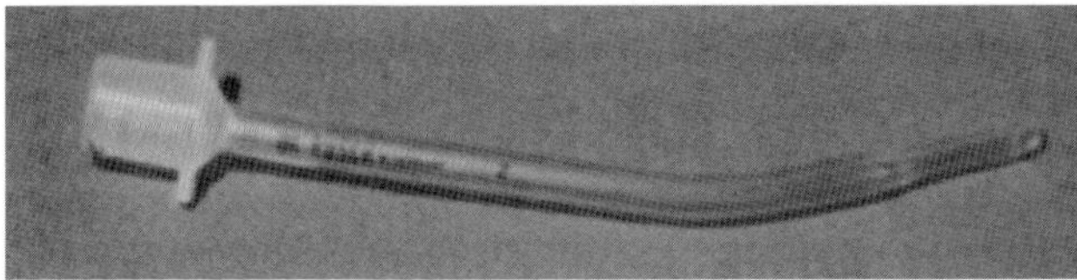

Figure 6.3 Cole endotracheal tube demonstrating the tapered shoulder used to position the tube in the larynx forming a seal. Note that the tube does not have a cuff or pilot balloon.

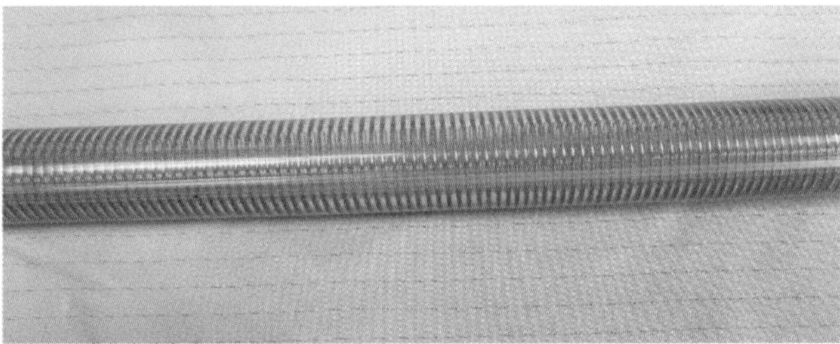

(A)

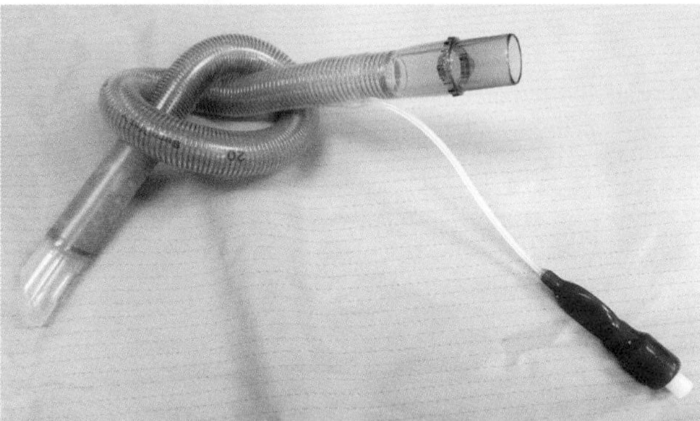

(B)

Figure 6.4 A. Guarded endotracheal tube with a metal or nylon spiral reinforcing wire. B. This spiral wire prevents collapse if the tube is bent or folded. Source: Dr. Craig Mosley, with permission.

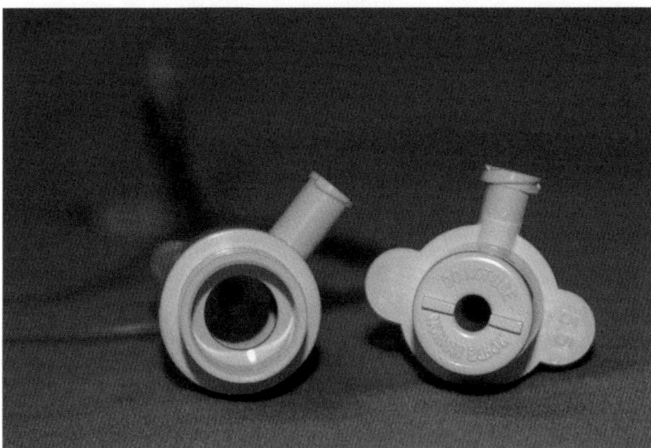

Figure 6.5 Two endotracheal tube adapters that incorporate a gas sampling port. Note the internal diameter (volume) of the pediatric design on the right. This type of design can help improve the accuracy of side-stream end-tidal gas sampling in smaller patients. Source: Dr. Craig Mosley, with permission.

animals and human patients is a uniform size (15 mm OD) facilitating universal connection to all standard anesthetic circuits. Tubes designed for use in large animals typically have larger connectors, which include metal-type and funnel-type connectors. The distal (patient) end of the connector varies in size according to the diameter of the endotracheal tube. Endotracheal tube adapters may also incorporate gas sampling ports (Fig. 6.5). These are particularly useful in small patients where minimizing equipment deadspace can be important and may improve the accuracy of gas sampling in smaller patients where non-rebreathing systems are often used.

Endotracheal tubes designed for large animals are normally manufactured with a silicone funnel adapter attached (Fig. 6.6) that is designed to fit over the large animal Y-piece (54 mm OD). There are also stainless-steel Bivona endotracheal tube adapters (22 OD) that are designed to fit the Bivona insert sometimes found on large animal Y-pieces.

The patient (distal) end of the endotracheal tube is normally beveled. Murphy-type tubes have a hole in the endotracheal tube wall opposite the bevel, referred to as a "Murphy eye" or "Murphy hole" (see Fig. 6.1A). The purpose of the hole is to provide an alternative route for gas flow should the beveled opening become occluded. Endotracheal tubes that lack a Murphy eye are referred to as Magill-type tubes. Most endotracheal tube sizes can be found without an inflatable cuff, although the use of cuffed tubes provides a more reliable airway. Tubes lacking cuffs tend to be very small diameter tubes where the addition of a cuff may not be possible or will limit the maximum diameter tube that can be used in a patient. The cuff is located on the machine-end side of the Murphy eye for cuffed tubes, and can be a low-volume, high-pressure or high-volume, low-pressure design (Fig. 6.7). In general, high-volume, low-pressure cuffs are preferred to minimize the risk of ischemic tracheal injury that may result from excessive cuff pressure against the tracheal wall. When a properly fitting endotracheal tube with a high-volume, low-pressure cuff is used, the pressure exerted by the cuff on the tracheal wall is similar to the intracuff pressure. This allows for a better estimation of the pressure on the tracheal wall exerted by the cuff. When using a low-volume, high-pressure cuffed endotracheal tube, the intracuff pressure does not reflect the pressure on the tracheal wall but rather the pressure created by the elastic recoil of the cuff, making estimates of pressure exerted by the cuff on the tracheal wall difficult. Tracheal wall pressures exceeding 48 cmH_2O may impede capillary blood flow, potentially causing ischemic tracheal damage, and pressure below 18 mmHg may increase the risk of aspiration [10]. There are also several cases of tracheal rupture or disruption reported in veterinary medicine leading to pneumothorax, pneumomediastinum, and/or subcutaneous emphysema [11].

A reliable method for ensuring that cuff pressures are within the recommended range is to use a cuff monitor to inflate high-volume, low-pressure cuffs. A cuff monitor is essentially a low-pressure manometer similar to those used for Doppler blood pressure measurement that is attached to the pilot balloon of the cuff and provides a measure of intracuff pressure. As noted above, these devices are only useful when using appropriately sized high-volume, low-pressure cuffs. If high-pressure cuffs are used or if the endotracheal tube is markedly undersized for the patient, the measured cuff pressure may not accurately reflect the pressure exerted on the tracheal wall. Other commercially available cuff inflation guides are available for the human market and can be adapted to veterinary use (Fig. 6.8). Alternatively, it is more common to use a leak test or the minimal occlusive volume (MOV)

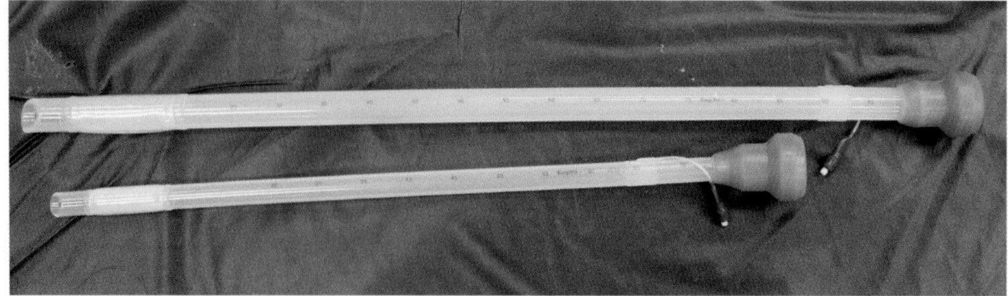

Figure 6.6 Two endotracheal tubes used for large animal anesthesia. These tubes are typically silicone and are commonly manufactured with a silicone funnel adapter that is compatible with the Y-piece of most large animal anesthetic breathing circuits. Source: Dr. Craig Mosley, with permission.

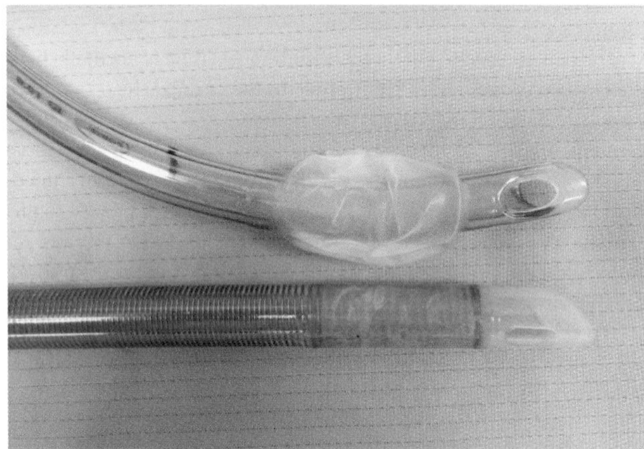

Figure 6.7 The upper endotracheal tube has a high-volume, low-pressure cuff, whereas the lower endotracheal tube shows an example of a low-volume, high-pressure cuff. Note the bulkiness that can be associated with the high-volume, low-pressure cuff compared with the low-volume, high-pressure cuff. The bulkiness associated with some cuffs can limit the endotracheal tube size, which can be problematic in very small patients. However, high-volume, low-pressure cuffs may help reduce tracheal damage resulting from cuff overinflation. Source: Dr. Craig Mosley, with permission.

technique, performed by inflating the cuff until a leak is no longer audible while maintaining airway pressures of 20–30 cmH_2O. Recently two commercially available syringe devices specifically designed for endotracheal tube cuff inflation have been evaluated for use in veterinary medicine that may help reduce the incidence of improperly inflated cuffs compared to MOV [12]. The pilot balloon used for inflating the endotracheal tube cuff is connected to the cuff via a channel incorporated into the endotracheal tube and normally includes a syringe-activated self-sealing valve system. However, there are also valveless pilot balloons that do not self-seal and require occlusion using either a clamp or plug.

An uncuffed self-sealing endotracheal tube (Safe-Seal™, Innovative Animal Products, Rochester, MN, USA, 55901) has been introduced into the veterinary market. The tube is designed with a series of flexible circumferential flanges at the patient end of the endotracheal tube that deform to the contours of the trachea, forming a seal against the tracheal wall eliminating the need to inflate a cuff (Fig. 6.9). There are currently no independent research studies evaluating the effectiveness of this tube for use in veterinary anesthesia. It is available with only a limited number of internal tube diameters and differs from a conventional endotracheal tube in that it has no Murphy eye or inflatable cuff.

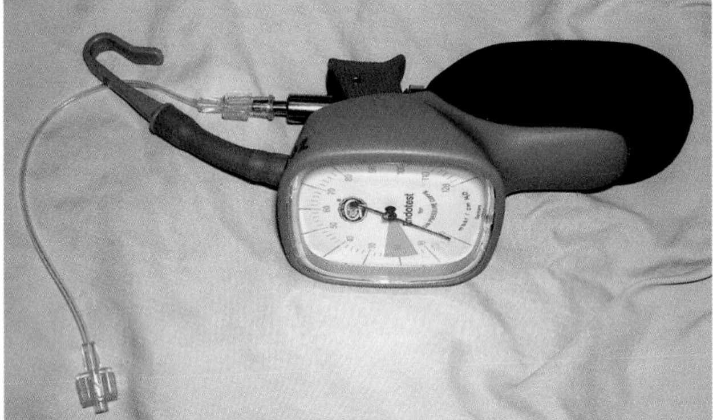

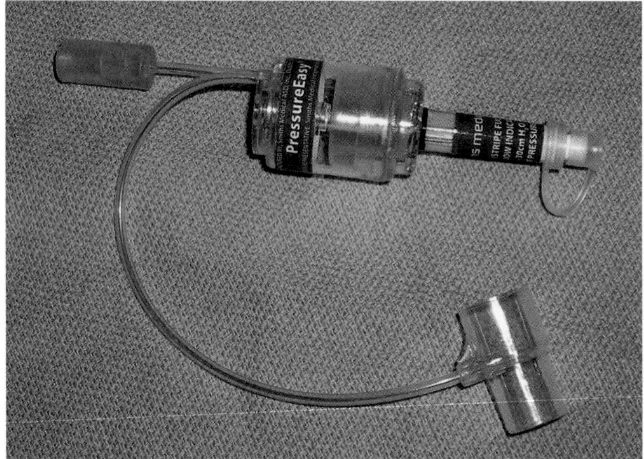

Figure 6.8 Examples of endotracheal tube inflation guides or pressure monitoring devices. These devices can be used to evaluate intracuff pressures and may help avoid tracheal injury secondary to excessive tracheal wall pressures. Several styles are available. Source: Dr. Craig Mosley, with permission.

Endotracheal tubes for isolating one lung

In addition to the endotracheal tubes described above, there are tubes specially designed for isolating or ventilating one lung. Indications for the use of these tubes include improving surgical conditions for various thoracic procedures (i.e., thoracoscopy), the control of contamination or hemorrhage, and use in circumstances where unilateral pathology exists. There are generally three methods of isolating or ventilating a single lung: a double-lumen tube (DLT), a bronchial blocker, or by using a long, standard endotracheal tube as an endobronchial tube.

Endobronchial intubation for single lung ventilation or isolation is probably the least desirable option as it provides less direct control for making changes in the non-intubated lung. However, it does not require specialized equipment, apart from a sufficiently long endotracheal tube, and is relatively easy to perform. Endobronchial intubation has been used in dogs successfully and may be an alternative when DLTs and bronchial blockers are not available [13,14].

DLTs tend to be the preferred option in human medicine. All commercially available DLTs have been designed specifically for human patients and have been adapted for use in dogs. There have been several types evaluated in a range of dog sizes and breeds [15–18]. DLTs consist of two single-lumen tubes bonded together and are available as right- or left-sided tubes (Fig. 6.10), where right and left designate which mainstem bronchus the tube is designed to fit.

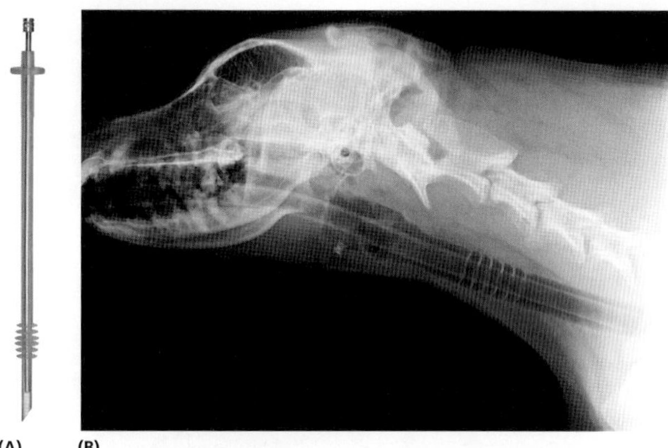

Figure 6.9 **A.** Example of a self-sealing endotracheal tube that lacks an inflatable cuff and instead relies on a series of soft flexible flanges to provide airway security. **B.** Lateral radiograph illustrating placement of a self-sealing endotracheal tube. Source: Dr. Craig Mosley, with permission.

Most DLTs are designed with an angled distal tip to facilitate placement into either the right or left bronchus. The three most commonly available styles of DLTs are the Robertshaw, Carlens, and White. The tubes have two elliptical cuffs: one occludes the trachea and the other occludes the bronchus (Fig. 6.11). The bronchial cuff and pilot balloon are normally colored blue for differentiation from the tracheal cuff.

The bronchial cuffs of right-sided tubes vary in shape and design in order to facilitate ventilation of the upper right lung lobe in humans. The use of right-sided tubes can introduce greater placement uncertainty and failures when used in dogs as the right cranial lung lobe bronchus of the dog branches more proximally than in humans; consequently, the bronchial cuff may occlude the bronchus or failure to completely isolate the hemithorax may occur. In general, left-sided tubes are most often used and can be used effectively for both right- and left-sided procedures. Even if proximal clamping or transection of the left mainstem bronchus is required, the left-sided tube can simply be withdrawn into the trachea so the distal bronchial portion of the tube does not interfere with clamping. The internal lumen of the tracheal portion of the tube is oval or D-shaped, and the sizes are designated using the French scale, ranging from 26 to 41 Fr. The reduced lumen size will increase resistance to breathing compared to an appropriately sized standard single lumen tube, but this is overcome by the frequent use of intermittent positive-pressure ventilation (IPPV) in these cases. DLTs allow the anesthetist to ventilate each lung field independently of the other or both lung fields together without replacing or moving the tube, but it does require disconnection and reconnection of the anesthetic circuit to the appropriate endotracheal tube adapter (bronchial or tracheal) or both by using a Y-piece adapter (Fig. 6.12).

The ability to ventilate selectively either or both lung fields is a distinct advantage over bronchial blocking systems or endobronchial intubation when surgical conditions require operating on both sides of the chest. However, the available sizes typically limit

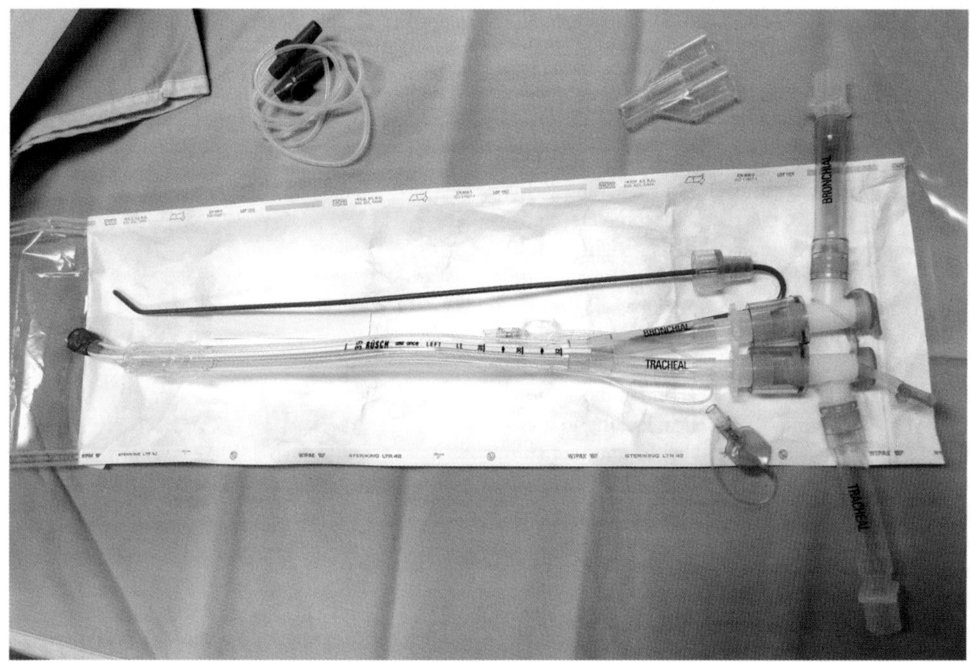

Figure 6.10 An example of a left-sided Robertshaw double-lumen endotracheal tube. DLTs can be used to ventilate selectively one or both lung fields in appropriately sized dogs. Source: Dr. Craig Mosley, with permission.

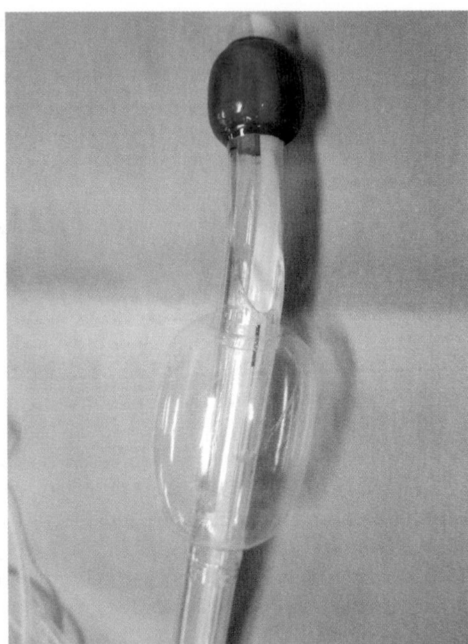

Figure 6.11 A closer image demonstrating the distal end of a left-sided Robertshaw double-lumen endotracheal tube. Note the angle of the distal end of the tube and the two cuffs. The more distal blue cuff is the bronchial cuff. This tube is designed to facilitate placement into the left mainstem bronchus. Source: Dr. Craig Mosley, with permission.

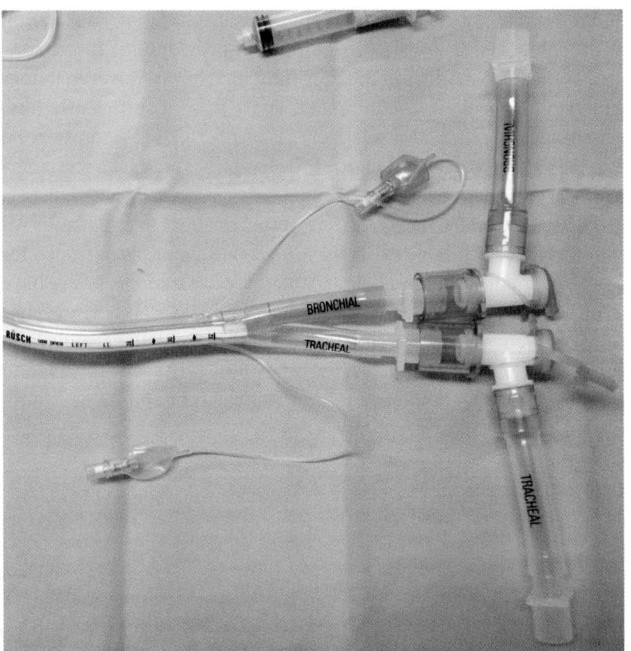

(A)

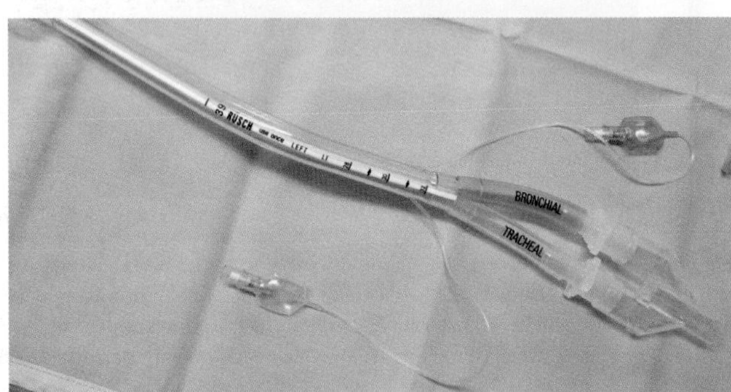

(B)

Figure 6.12 Double-lumen tubes (DLTs) can be used to ventilate (or collapse) each lung field independently or can ventilate both lung fields simultaneously. **A.** Adapter configuration required for independent lung field ventilation (or collapse). **B.** Use of a Y-adapter to facilitate simultaneous ventilation of both lung fields. Note the blue pilot balloon cuff and the blue tubing corresponding to the bronchial portion of the tube. Source: Dr. Craig Mosley, with permission.

the use of DLTs to dogs between 5 and 20 kg. Some DLTs (Carlens and White) also incorporate a carinal hook designed to aid in the proper placement of the tube and prevent movement after positioning. In veterinary patients, this modification may actually hinder rather than facilitate correct tube placement [15]. Additional care should also be taken when placing DLTs with a carinal hook to ensure that it does not catch on any tissues or structures when introducing the tube into the trachea. For this reason, the Robertshaw left-sided DLT is probably the most versatile type for use in dogs. In veterinary patients, the correct placement of a DLT is generally confirmed by direct visualization using a small-diameter bronchoscope. A thoracoscopic-assisted technique has also been described [15]. Correct and complete placement is further confirmed by ventilating both the right and left lung fields while auscultating for lung sounds. Correct and complete placement should ventilate all intended lung fields (i.e., right or left) without ventilating any lung fields on the contralateral side. Although blind placement is possible using some tubes, it is associated with a relatively high failure to achieve correct and complete tube placement [15]. Small movements of the tube and/or the patient may disrupt correct and complete placement and occasionally bronchial cuffs will prolapse into the trachea, leading to complete airway obstruction. Vigilance is required by the anesthetist to recognize and correct any positional problems should they occur (e.g., deflation of bronchial cuff).

Bronchial blockers represent another system for facilitating one-lung isolation or ventilation in dogs (Fig. 6.13) [14,16,19–22]. In human anesthesia, they are often used when patient size precludes the use of a DLT or when anatomic abnormalities or differences are present that may preclude optimal tube fit. The fact that they are very adaptable for use over a wider range of patient sizes and are not as anatomically specific as DLTs are distinct advantages of using

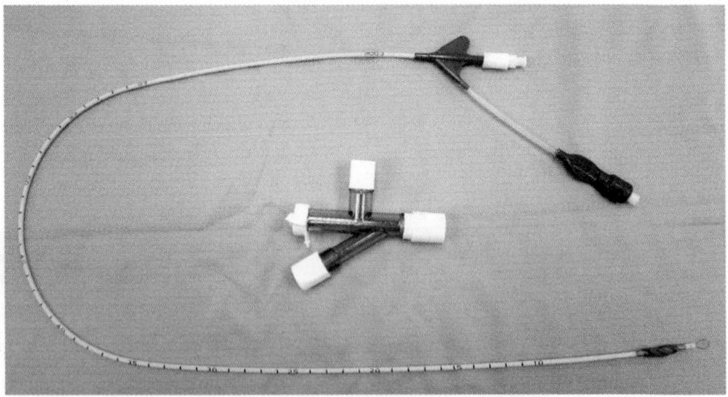

Figure 6.13 An example of a bronchial blocking system commonly used in veterinary medicine. The system consists of a bronchial blocker (balloon-tipped catheter) and a swivel adapter allowing for coaxial placement of the blocker. Source: Dr. Craig Mosley, with permission.

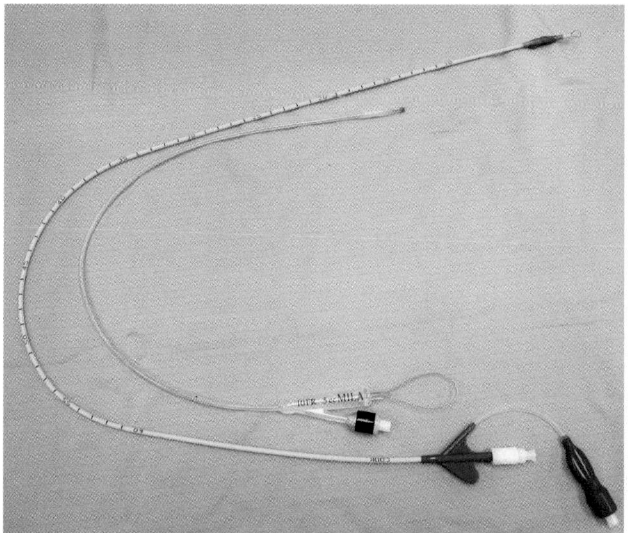

Figure 6.14 The yellow (or outermost) catheter with the obvious pilot balloon is specifically designed for use as a bronchial blocker. The inner shorter catheter is a balloon-tipped Foley catheter. Although Foley catheters are not designed for use as bronchial blockers, they have been placed alongside endotracheal tubes and used successfully for bronchial blockade, but they are not as simple to use or place as a purpose-designed bronchial blocker. Source: Dr. Craig Mosley, with permission.

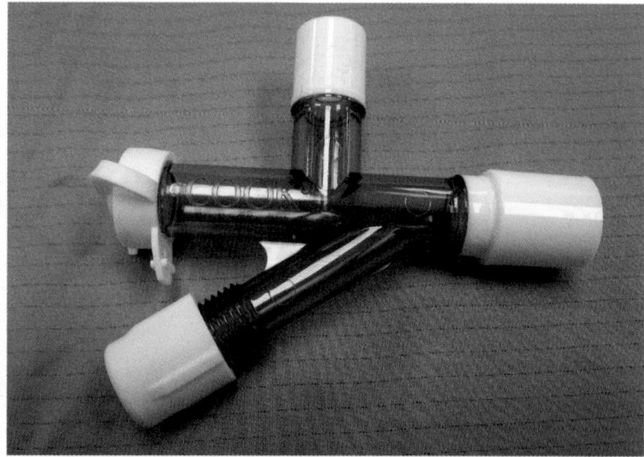

Figure 6.15 An example of the airway adapter supplied with the Arndt Endobronchial Blocker™ (Cook Medical, Bloomington, IN, USA). The adapter is placed between the endotracheal tube adapter and the breathing circuit. The port to the right attaches to the endotracheal tube adapter; the ports moving clockwise include the bronchial port (with an annular compression fitting), a bronchoscope port, and the patient circuit port. Source: Dr. Craig Mosley, with permission.

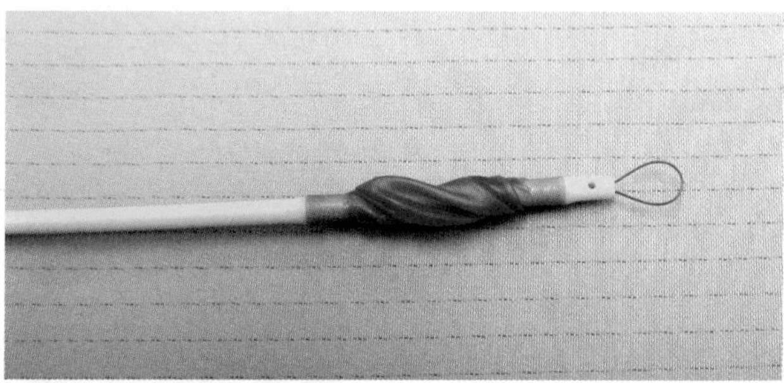

Figure 6.16 The distal end of an Arndt Endobronchial Blocker™ (Cook Medical, Bloomington, IN, USA) showing the wire loop used to facilitate proper placement using a bronchoscope. Source: Dr. Craig Mosley, with permission.

bronchial blockers in veterinary anesthesia. However, independent lung ventilation is not possible without withdrawing and replacing the bronchial blocker in the contralateral bronchus.

Bronchial blockers are essentially long catheters, tipped with an elliptical or round inflatable cuff or balloon (Fig. 6.14). The cuffs and pilot balloons of most purpose-designed bronchial blockers are blue to differentiate them from those of the endotracheal tube. Foley or balloon-type catheters used as bronchial blockers obviously do not follow this color scheme. Bronchial blockers can be used coaxially or in parallel with a standard endotracheal tube. Various swivel adapters are supplied with commercially available bronchial blockers to facilitate coaxial use. The swivel adapters connect to the endotracheal tube adapter and have ports for passing the bronchial blocker, a bronchoscope, and a connector for the anesthetic circuit (Fig. 6.15).

The ports are designed in a way to prevent leakage and to secure the bronchial blocker once it is in place. There is also a commercially available human coaxial product (Univent® tube, Teleflex Inc., Limerick, PA, USA) that incorporates the bronchial blocker in a channel running in the lumen of the endotracheal tube. However, the length of the bronchial blocker is limited and may not be sufficiently long for larger patients. A balloon catheter (Fogarty or Foley catheter) can also be used as a bronchial blocker placed in parallel with the endotracheal tube or coaxially with a custom adapter solution (see Fig. 6.14).

Bronchial blockers require fiber-optic-assisted direct visualization for correct placement. One of the unique features of bronchial blockers over DLTs is that they can be used to isolate a single lung lobe in addition to the entire hemithorax. The bronchial blocker can be directed into the bronchus to be blocked by directly manipulating the proximal portion of the bronchial blocker or by placing a guide wire into the bronchus to be blocked and sliding the bronchial blocker over the guide wire. One bronchial blocker (Ardnt Endobronchial Blocker™, Cook Medical, Bloomington, IN, USA) has a small wire loop exiting the distal end of the blocker (Fig. 6.16). The loop can be used to facilitate placement by sliding the loop over the end of the bronchoscope. Once correct placement has been achieved, the balloon or cuff can be inflated, precluding ventilation of that lung region. The lung is then allowed to collapse by opening the bronchial blocker catheter channel. The open channel can be used for continuous positive airway pressure (CPAP) application, oxygen insufflation, and/or suctioning. The placement of the bronchial blocker in the right bronchus can be challenging owing to the proximal branching of the cranial lung lobe. Prolapse of a bronchial blocker into the trachea can lead to complete airway obstruction; this is most likely to occur when placed proximally in the bronchus and/or if the tube and bronchial blocker assembly are withdrawn inadvertently when moving or manipulating the patient.

Another bronchial blocker (Rüsch® EZ-Blocker® endobronchial blocker, Teleflex Inc., Limerick, PA, USA) consists of paired of "bonded" blockers in a single tube that bifurcate at the distal tip (Fig 6.17). This design can ease placement by allowing the

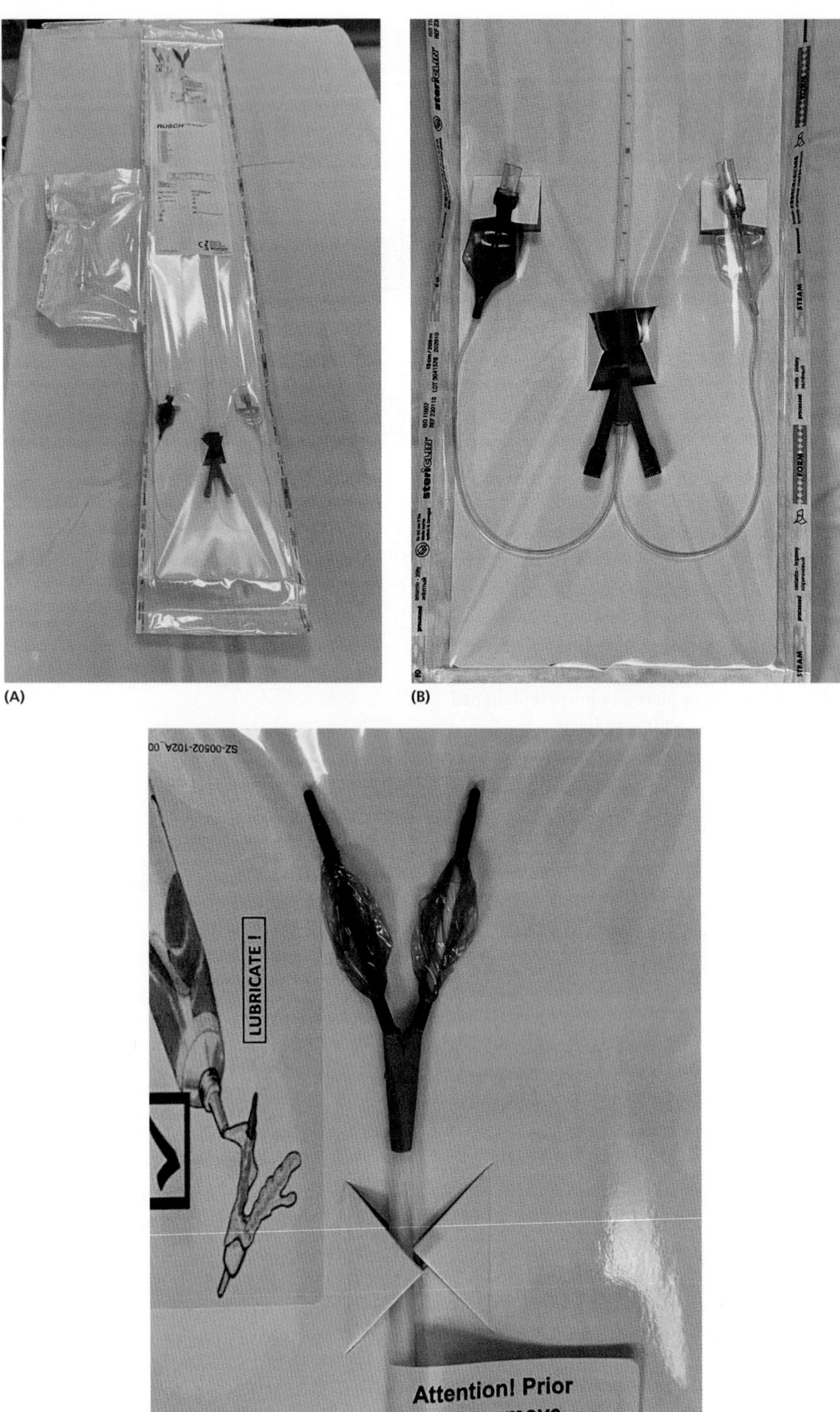

Figure 6.17 **A.** The Rüsch® EZ-Blocker® is a dual-lumen endobronchial blocker. **B.** Proximal end showing two inflatable cuffs/pilot balloons. **C.** Integrated distal bifurcation that can conveniently straddle the patient's carina when placed. The system comes with a multiport adapter that connects between the patient endotracheal tube and anesthetic breathing circuit. Source: Dr. Craig Mosley, with permission.

bifurcation to more intuitively straddle the carina with a blocker tip in both the right and left mainstem bronchus allowing for right or left blockade. However, the EZ-Blocker® cannot be used to isolate single lung lobes and, similar to other techniques, it remains difficult to collapse the right hemithorax due to the proximal branching of the right cranial lung lobe [21,22].

Supraglottic airway devices

Supraglottic airway devices (SGADs), also commonly referred to as "laryngeal mask airways" (LMAs), are becoming increasingly popular for veterinary use. There are a large number of products available that were designed for humans that have been adapted for veterinary use. However, these products have been optimized

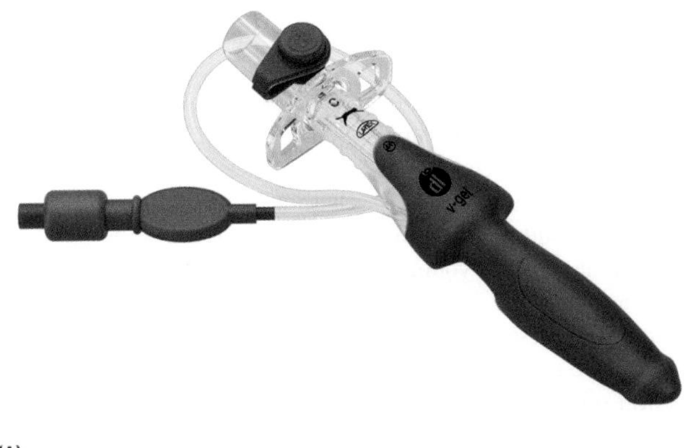

(A)

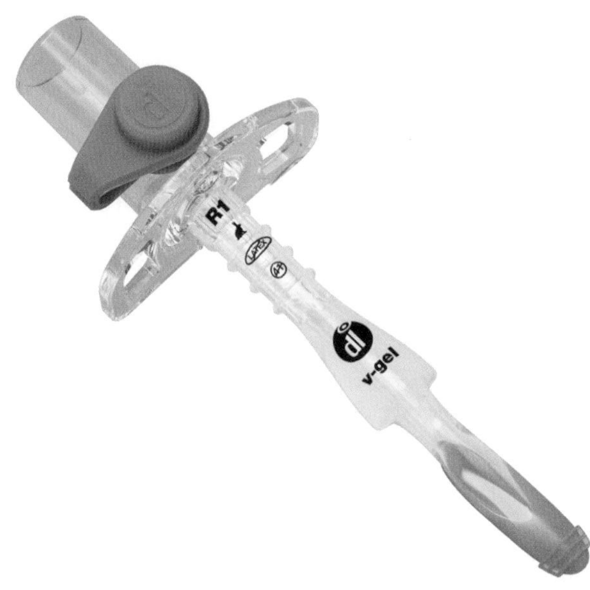

(B)

Figure 6.18 Veterinary-specific laryngeal masks (v-gel®) designed for use in **A.** cats and **B.** rabbits. These masks can be used as alternatives to tracheal intubation and may be easier to place than endotracheal tubes in some species. Source: Docsinnovent Ltd, London, UK; reproduced with permission.

specifically for the orolaryngeal/pharyngeal anatomy of humans and may not conform well to the varied anatomy, patient size, species, and breeds commonly encountered in veterinary medicine. Appropriate use of these products is important as inappropriate SGAD and/or patient selection may lead to placement difficulties/failures, damage to tissues of the oropharyngeal region, and/or improper protection and patency of the airway. There are several veterinary-specific SGADs that have been introduced (dog, cat, and rabbit v-gel®, Docsinnovent Ltd, London, UK) designed for use in dogs, cats, and rabbits (Fig. 6.18).

SGADs represent an alternative to endotracheal intubation for maintenance of a patent airway and there is some evidence that they may be simpler and faster to place than endotracheal tubes in some species [5,23,24]. There is also some evidence that less anesthetic is required for the placement of an SGAD compared with an endotracheal tube [25]. SGADs do not require the use of a laryngoscope for placement and do not enter the larynx or trachea. A typical device consists of a tube, similar to an endotracheal tube, connected to an elliptical mask that has an inflatable outer edge. When placed and inflated correctly, they form a seal around the glottis. The criteria for correct SGAD placement have been described for various species and should be reviewed prior to using these devices. Properly placed and inflated SGADs are not associated with greater leakage of anesthetic gases compared with endotracheal tubes and positive-pressure ventilation using an SGAD has been successfully performed and evaluated in several veterinary species [5–9,26–28]. The use of SGADs is relatively uncommon in veterinary medicine but as their use increases and further large prospective studies are completed, additional advantages and disadvantages related to relatively rare events (e.g., gastroesophageal reflux and subsequent aspiration, significant post-extubation airway irritation) may be detected.

Laryngoscopes

Laryngoscopes consist of a handle and lighted blade and are used to aid tracheal intubation and oropharyngeal evaluation during intubation. Unfortunately, laryngoscopes are often considered an optional piece of anesthetic-related equipment, but their proper use can be vital for successful intubation in some patients (e.g., brachycephalics and patients with laryngeal/oral trauma). Regardless of the absolute need for laryngoscope-assisted intubation, their use is recommended for all intubations to ensure that the anesthetist maintains the motor skills and coordination to use a laryngoscope properly while permitting a cursory oropharyngeal evaluation.

There are several styles and types of laryngoscopes and blades available. Some laryngoscopes have a fixed blade (i.e., one blade type and size) and may be made of plastic, whereas others are designed for use with multiple blade sizes and styles of blades and are made of stainless steel. Because there is such a range of patient sizes and different oral cavity configurations in veterinary medicine, the option to use multiple blades is a significant advantage when selecting a laryngoscope. The handle may also vary in size and, although this rarely impacts the functional use of the laryngoscope, a smaller handle may be more comfortable and easier to manipulate for some anesthetists, particularly when used for intubating very small patients. The handles are usually specific for either fiber-optic or bulb-in-blade illumination, although there are some handles that can accept either type of blade illumination system. There is no clear advantage of one lighting system over the other.

There are two main types of blades that are used in veterinary medicine, the MacIntosh and the Miller blade. Both come in a wide range of sizes (000–5). The MacIntosh is a curved blade with a prominent vertical flange, whereas the Miller is a straight blade with a less prominent vertical flange; both are suitable for intubation of most patients and the decision to use one over the other is often determined by personal preference (Fig. 6.19). However, the prominent flange of the MacIntosh blade can potentially interfere with laryngeal visualization when used for intubating veterinary patients (see below). In addition to the standard-sized blades available in human medicine, extremely long (~300 mm) Miller-style blades (useful for intubating swine, camelids, sheep, and goats) are also available.

Interestingly, the majority of human-designed laryngoscope blades and endotracheal tubes are designed for the anesthetist to use their right hand to pass the endotracheal tube while their left hand holds the laryngoscope. The endotracheal tube bevel faces the left when viewing the tube from the concave aspect and the laryngoscope blade flange is normally on the right side of the blade when

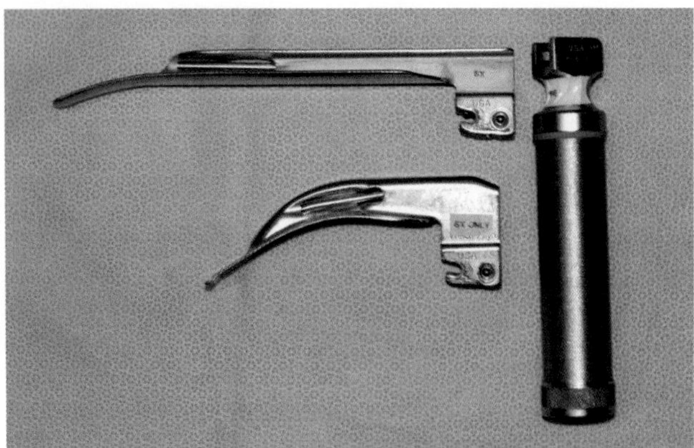

Figure 6.19 Laryngoscope handle with Miller (upper) and Macintosh (lower) blades. Note the more prominent vertical flange on the MacIntosh blade. This flange may impair visualization of the larynx when intubating a patient in sternal recumbency using the right hand. Source: Dr. Craig Mosley, with permission.

viewing the blade from the top. This configuration provides optimal visualization of the larynx when intubating a patient in the supine position (dorsal recumbency) where the laryngoscope is held with the blade in a downward position (inverted) and the endotracheal tube is held with the concave surface directed upwards. However, most veterinary patients are intubated in sternal recumbency where the flange of the laryngoscope, when held in the left hand, can obscure visualization and the bevel of the endotracheal tube will do little to improve visualization when held in the right hand. There are left-handed MacIntosh blades available that may be more appropriate for routine intubation in veterinary species as these blades place the flange on the left side of the blade, improving visualization of the laryngeal area when the laryngoscope is held in the left hand in an upright position. Since the Miller blade's flange is far less prominent, there is no real need for a left-handed design.

Intubation aids and techniques

Orotracheal intubation of most veterinary patients does not require any special equipment beyond the use of a laryngoscope and a familiarity with normal patient anatomy. However, there are circumstances and situations resulting from anatomic features, pathology, or trauma that make oral endotracheal intubation difficult or impossible. It is important that the veterinary anesthetist be familiar with and prepared to use alternative techniques to obtain a patent airway. The following sections present some of the options available, the associated equipment required, and descriptions of the techniques in general terms. For more specific details, the reader should consult species-specific chapters in this book or other species-specific veterinary anesthesia references [29].

Nasotracheal intubation

Nasotracheal intubation is a useful technique for procedures involving the oral cavity where a standard orotracheal tube may preclude or limit optimal surgical or diagnostic access or it can be used for procedures in sedated conscious animals that will not tolerate an orotracheal tube but require oxygen supplementation and support. Nasotracheal intubation can also be safely used for the administration of inhalant anesthetics for inducing anesthesia in some animals (foals and calves) [30,31]. The technique for nasotracheal intubation has been described in foals, calves, horses, camelids, rabbits, and a kangaroo but has certainly been performed and not reported in many other animal species [30–34].

The characteristics of an ideal nasotracheal tube include a tube with minimal curvature and a suitable length to extend distally beyond the larynx. The tube should be made of inert material (e.g., silicone rubber) and have relatively thin walls for maximum internal diameter, although this may increase the risk of tube compression or kinking. Low-volume, high-pressure cuffs are typically less bulky and may be less traumatic during placement, but high-volume, low-pressure cuffs may be best for longer periods of anesthesia. Tube size will be dependent upon species and patient size but will often be smaller than an appropriately sized orotracheal tube. The smaller internal diameter can increase resistance to gas flow and may be a problem for some spontaneously breathing patients.

Nasotracheal intubation involves passage of a properly sized endotracheal tube through the nostril, nasal meatus, and larynx, and into the trachea. Lidocaine-containing gel can facilitate placement and provide lubrication for the tube. It should be applied to the nostril and rostral portion of the nasal passage before advancing the tube in awake or sedated animals. A sterile water-soluble lubricant without lidocaine is appropriate for anesthetized patients. The tube should be passed gently and may require some rotation and redirection in order to facilitate passage between nasal conchae. Nasal hemorrhage or other tissue damage occasionally occurs during this procedure, particularly if excessive force or an excessively large tube is used relative to the nasal passages or if the tube is passed into the incorrect nasal meatus. In general, the patient's head and neck should be extended to facilitate passage of the tube from the nasopharynx into the trachea. However, species differences may necessitate alternative positioning or further manipulation of the head, neck, and laryngeal positions.

Air should move freely through a correctly placed tube during spontaneous ventilation. Confirmation of correct tube placement can be readily, and initially, assessed by using a bulb syringe adapted to the end of the nasotracheal tube. Once the tube is in place, the bulb can be squeezed and attached to the tube; if it readily expands, this suggests the tube is an airway, and if the bulb fails to expand, it is likely that the tube has entered the esophagus (Fig. 6.20). Further confirmation of correct tube placement using auscultation of lung sounds during manual ventilation and/or capnography waveform appearance should be used for definitive confirmation.

Extubation following nasotracheal intubation should be done carefully. After deflation of the cuff, the tube should be withdrawn slowly and deliberately, with the patient's head restrained to avoid any sudden, jerky motions. Rapid, rough extubation may cause nasal hemorrhage.

Wire- or tube-guided techniques

Wire- or tube-guided techniques are sometimes used when direct visualization of the laryngeal opening is not possible or obscured. This is commonly a result of species-specific anatomic features (e.g., rabbits and brachycephalic breeds) and patient size relative to available equipment. For example, the laryngoscope may be too small to be effective in a cow, and manual palpation and guide tube placement using a small-diameter tube is frequently used to facilitate passage of the desired endotracheal tube; in very small patients, the presence of both the laryngoscope and the endotracheal tube may obscure visualization and a thin wire can be initially placed to facilitate intubation [35].

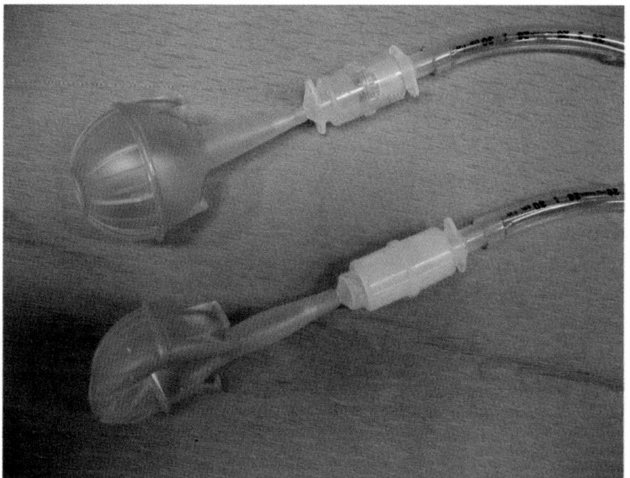

Figure 6.20 A suction bulb adapted to the end of an endotracheal tube can be used for the rapid assessment of correct endotracheal intubation. The bulb is deflated and attached to the tube using an appropriately sized adapter. If the endotracheal tube is in the trachea, the bulb should immediately reinflate. If the endotracheal tube is in the esophagus, the bulb will not generally reinflate. This technique provides a rapid assessment of proper intubation when direct visualization is not possible (i.e., nasotracheal intubation) but should always be used in conjunction with additional methods of confirming proper endotracheal intubation (i.e., observation of capnography waveform or auscultation of lung sounds during manual ventilation). Source: Dr. Thomas Riebold, College of Veterinary Medicine, Oregon State University, Corvallis, OR, USA; reproduced with permission of Dr. Riebold.

In some patients, trauma or other pathological conditions (nasopharyngeal polyp or mass) may obscure the laryngeal opening with only a small portion visible. In these circumstances, the placement of a small-diameter tube or a wire can be used as a guide for placement of a properly sized endotracheal tube (Fig. 6.21). The technique involves using a guide (wire or tube) with a smaller outer diameter than the internal diameter of the intended endotracheal tube. It should also be sufficiently long to allow complete intubation (about half the distance from the cricoid cartilage to the thoracic inlet) while still allowing the tube to be placed over the guide leaving a portion of the guide available for the operator to hold while advancing the tube (Fig. 6.22). The tube or wire should be blunt-ended so as not to damage the trachea or associated structures. The wire guides associated with some intravenous catheters (e.g., multiple-lumen jugular catheters) are blunt-ended and make excellent wire guides for some small patients. The guide is first appropriately placed and then the endotracheal tube is fed over the guide and through the laryngeal opening blindly; occasionally, slight rotation of the tube is required, and passing the tube through the larynx during inspiration when the arytenoids are fully abducted helps facilitate smooth passage. The guide is then removed, and the tube secured into place.

Endoscope-guided technique

Laryngoscopy with a flexible or rigid endoscope can be useful for assisting intubation in patients with abnormal anatomy or disease processes involving the pharynx, head, or neck. It is also often used in patients that can be challenging to intubate using direct visualization (e.g., pygmy rabbits and other small mammals). Depending

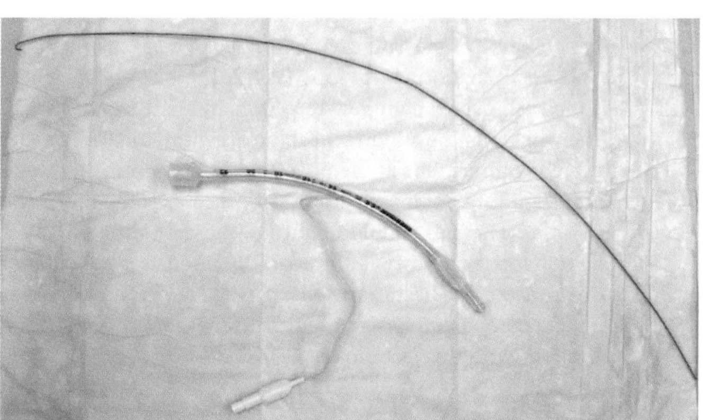

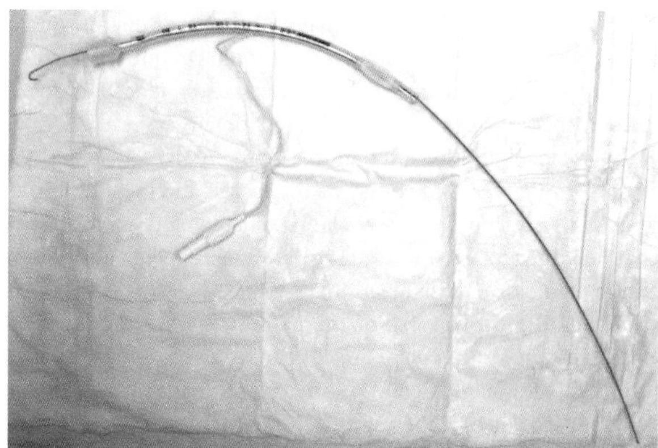

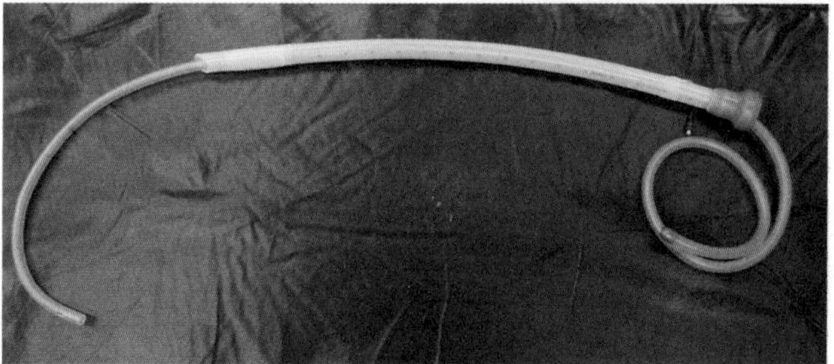

Figure 6.21 Examples of various guide wires and tube combinations used for guided endotracheal intubation. A wire or tube guide that is smaller and typically easier to place than the appropriately sized endotracheal tube is first placed in the trachea. The endotracheal tube is then fed over the guide, normally without further visualization. Once endotracheal intubation has been achieved, the guide is removed. Source: Dr. Craig Mosley, with permission.

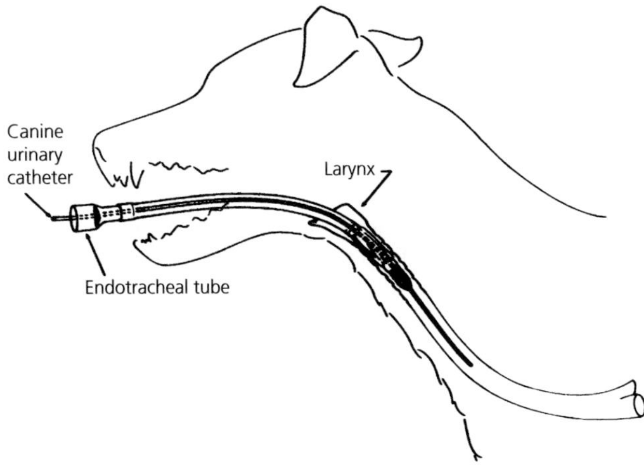

Figure 6.22 Diagram illustrating the passage of an endotracheal tube into the trachea of a dog using a guide device (urinary catheter). Source: Hartsfield [37], with permission.

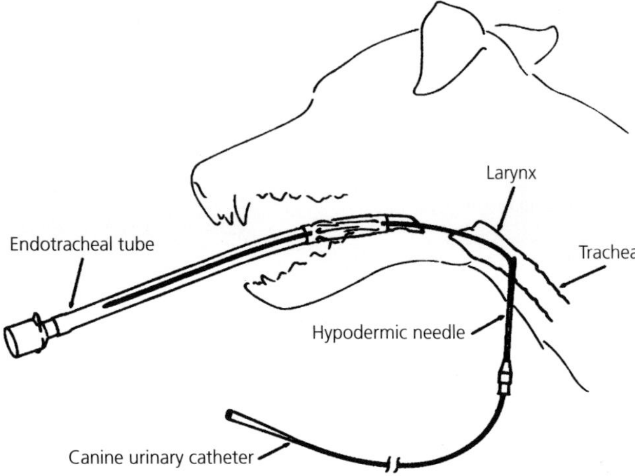

Figure 6.23 Illustration of intubation using a retrograde guide device in a dog. Catheter guide wires or other blunt-ended wires are optimal for this procedure owing to their small diameter. This technique should be reserved for cases that cannot be intubated by other methods. Source: Hartsfield [37], with permission.

on the species and the specific conditions, the endoscope can be placed inside the endotracheal tube to guide intubation directly or passed orally beside the endotracheal tube to guide correct placement visually. Rabbits and other small mammals are frequently intubated using this technique [36]. When appropriate, endoscopes can also be used to facilitate nasotracheal intubation. This technique can be particularly advantageous in horses (and other large animals) with abnormal oropharyngeal, laryngeal, and/or nasal anatomy where direct visualization using a laryngoscope is virtually impossible without specialized custom equipment.

Endotracheal tube exchangers

Changing endotracheal tubes during a surgical or diagnostic procedure in an anesthetized animal is occasionally required due to a failing cuff or when an alternative tube size or length is required. Patients that are positioned and draped for surgery are generally not situated "normally" for intubation. Changing the tube using a wire- or tube-guided technique may be the easiest and most efficient way to accomplish the procedure. However, in many instances, using good technique and a high-quality laryngoscope will allow for intubation using direct visualization.

Depending on the size of the patient, standard commercially available human tube exchangers can be used. Alternatively, any tubing or wire of sufficient diameter and length can be used; for example, stomach tubes and catheter wire guides. To change endotracheal tubes, the guide (tube or wire) is inserted through the original endotracheal tube to the area of the midcervical trachea. It should be noted that if the patient is being maintained under anesthesia using an inhalant anesthetic, it should be discontinued during tube exchange. Depending on the duration required to exchange the tube, the patient's anesthetic depth may become very light, and additional intravenous anesthetic and a means to administer it should be readily available. Next, the endotracheal tube cuff is deflated, and the endotracheal tube is pulled over the guide without removing the guide from the trachea. Then, the new endotracheal tube is maneuvered through the larynx and into the trachea by using the guide to direct its passage. The cuff of the new tube is inflated to protect the airway, and the new tube is secured in the manner appropriate for the specific species.

Retrograde intubation

If direct visualization of at least a portion of the glottis is impossible, retrograde intubation may be performed. Retrograde intubation has been evaluated as an alternative technique for endotracheal intubation in South America camelids and mice [38,39], and a cadaveric study has been performed in rabbits [40]. The technique essentially involves passing a needle through the skin of the ventral neck and into the trachea between upper tracheal rings. In human patients, the needle is passed through the cricothyroid membrane. A guidewire is then maneuvered through the needle rostrally into the larynx, pharynx, and oral cavity until it can be used as a guide for passage of an endotracheal tube (Fig. 6.23). The endotracheal tube is then fed over the guidewire and manipulated into the larynx. After the tip of the endotracheal tube is within the larynx, the needle and the guide tube are removed, and the endotracheal tube is manipulated into its final position with the cuffed end near the thoracic inlet. The cuff should be located caudal to the puncture site of the hypodermic needle to avoid forcing gases subcutaneously or into the mediastinum during positive-pressure ventilation. Subcutaneous emphysema and pneumothorax are possible complications with this technique.

Tracheostomy

A temporary tracheostomy can be performed for airway management during anesthesia. However, as it is invasive, it is typically reserved for those patients where oro- or nasotracheal intubation is not possible even with guided assistance, owing to anatomy, pathology, or surgical procedures. Occasionally a tracheostomy may be recommended to facilitate a surgical procedure involving the oropharynx although, if appropriate, a pharyngostomy tube may be a more desirable alternative in these cases. Tracheostomy tube placement may also be used when there is a reasonable expectation that the patient will require an ongoing tracheostomy following the anesthetic procedure (e.g., incomplete resection of laryngeal tumor, brachycephalic airway surgery) [41,42]. Occasionally patients may present to anesthesia with an emergency tracheostomy already present as the result of acute upper airway obstruction.

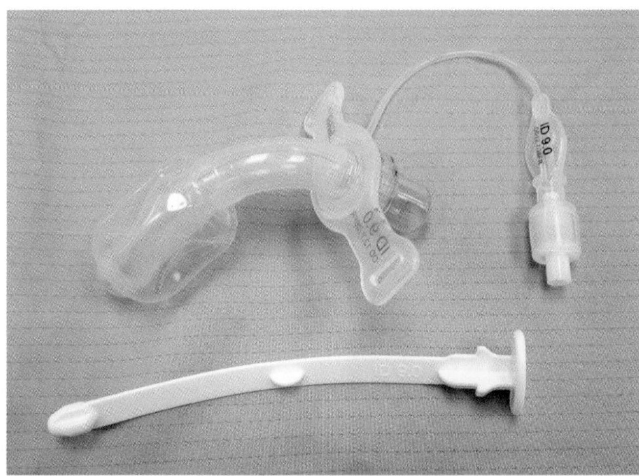

Figure 6.24 An example of a cuffed tracheostomy tube with an inner stylet to ease placement. Some tubes are also designed with a removal inner tube to facilitate cleaning of the tube. Source: Dr. Craig Mosley, with permission.

Intubation via a tracheostomy is relatively simple to perform but may be complicated in patients with very small-diameter tracheas or those with very thickened and calcified tracheal rings (e.g., some brachycephalics). A standard endotracheal tube or tracheostomy tube can be used for intubation; however, care should be taken when using a standard-length endotracheal tube as endobronchial intubation can easily result. Tracheostomy tubes are generally short with a pronounced curvature in the tube and an inner stylet to ease placement (Fig. 6.24). The curvature also allows the tube to be secured flatly to the patient's neck and tubes are normally fitted with a standard 15 mm endotracheal tube adapter, inflatable cuffs, and pilot balloons, although many of the smaller-sized tubes will be uncuffed. Some tracheostomy tubes also have an inner removable cannula to facilitate cleaning and longer-term maintenance of tracheostomy tubes in patients. Care of the tube is very important. Neglected tubes that are not cleaned regularly can be obstructed by mucus that dries within the lumen of the tube.

Tracheostomy has been associated with infection, granulomas, tracheal stricture, cartilage damage, hemorrhage, pneumothorax, subcutaneous emphysema, tracheocutaneous or tracheoesophageal fistula, aspiration, dysphagia, and tracheal malacia; hence tracheostomy should not be considered an innocuous procedure. The specific techniques, indications, and outcomes have been reviewed in cattle, horses, dogs, and cats [43–47].

Lateral pharyngotomy

A lateral pharyngotomy is an alternative to a tracheostomy and is suitable for facilitating surgical procedures of the mandible, maxilla, or oral cavity (Fig. 6.25). The use of a pharyngotomy provides improved visualization within the operative field during oropharyngeal surgery and normal dental occlusion to aid in the proper reduction of mandibular or maxillary fractures. It is also a potentially less invasive alternative to a tracheostomy when oral or nasal airway management is undesirable or unfeasible for facilitating a surgical procedure.

This technique has been described in detail elsewhere [48]. The basics of tube placement involve passage of a correctly sized, cuffed endotracheal tube and making a routine skin incision caudal to the angle of the mandible. Then, hemostats are bluntly passed through the skin incision into the caudal part of the pharynx. After the endotracheal tube adapter has been removed, the adapter end of the tube is grasped and pulled from the pharynx, through the subcutaneous tissue, and through the skin incision. The endotracheal tube adapter is replaced, and the tube is reconnected to the breathing system for maintenance. A correctly placed tube should be secured to the skin with several sutures and/or tape.

Techniques of oxygen administration

Supplemental oxygen is used in anesthetized and critically ill patients to increase the partial pressure of oxygen in arterial blood (PaO_2) and to promote the delivery of oxygen to the tissues. When a patient is breathing room air, values for PaO_2 that are less than 80 mmHg indicate the potential for hypoxemia. Any patient in respiratory distress or those likely to experience hypoxia in the perianesthetic period (e.g., brachycephalic breeds) should be provided supplemental oxygen. If the PaO_2 decreases to less than 60 mmHg, the need for supplemental oxygen is indicated. It is also important to recall that both hemoglobin and tissue perfusion play fundamental roles in ensuring sufficient delivery of oxygen to tissues and when indicated red blood cell transfusions and/or cardiovascular support may be required in addition to providing supplemental oxygen to prevent cellular hypoxia.

The fraction of oxygen in inspired gases (F_IO_2) plays a significant role in establishing the PaO_2. As a rule, the PaO_2 value should be approximately five times the F_IO_2 value if there are no major abnormalities in the matching of pulmonary ventilation and perfusion. Supplemental oxygen can be an effective way of correcting hypoxemia in animals with diffusion abnormalities, ventilation-perfusion mismatching, and/or hypoventilation. In addition to oxygen supplementation, the specific underlying condition(s) contributing to hypoxemia should be addressed when possible. Supplemental oxygen may not significantly improve PaO_2 in patients with substantial right to left vascular shunts (pulmonary or cardiac shunts).

Several techniques can be used to administer oxygen to anesthetized and ill patients. The effectiveness of oxygen supplementation is assessed by evaluation of the patient's clinical responses (e.g., improvement in mucous membrane color and character of ventilation), by measuring the F_IO_2, and by monitoring of PaO_2, arterial oxygen saturation (SaO_2), and saturation of peripheral oxygen (SpO_2). Although PaO_2 and SaO_2 data are reliable, they require periodic arterial blood sampling and the use of a blood gas analyzer. The SpO_2 can be conveniently measured by pulse oximetry. Pulse oximetry is a practical method for non-invasive, moment-to-moment estimation of the saturation of hemoglobin with oxygen in anesthetized, recovering, and ill patients [49–56]. Various techniques for supplementing oxygen to patients are outlined below and Table 6.1 summarizes the approximate F_IO_2 obtained using each of the commonly available techniques in dogs and cats.

Mask delivery

Masks for delivery of oxygen to veterinary patients are useful for preoxygenation immediately before induction of anesthesia and for conscious patients experiencing respiratory distress. The use of masks for oxygenation requires constant attention, and some patients will not accept a mask unless they are sedated. Both factors limit the effectiveness of masks in conscious patients. Indeed, some patients object to a mask so vigorously that the increase in oxygen consumption associated with restraint may nullify the benefits of a greater F_IO_2. If the oxygen mask is attached to an anesthetic breathing circuit, the circuit should be flushed in order to reduce

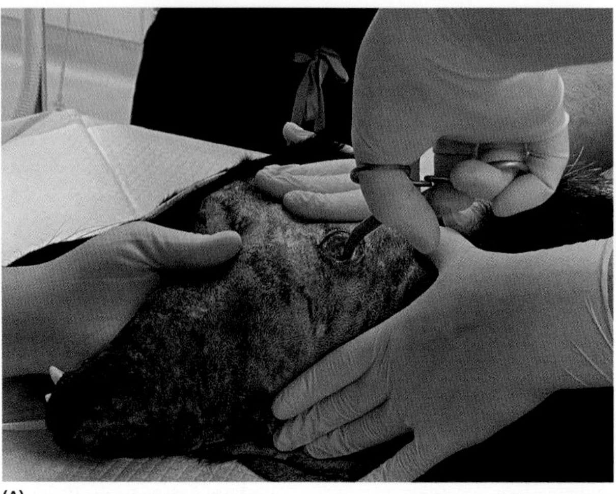

(A)

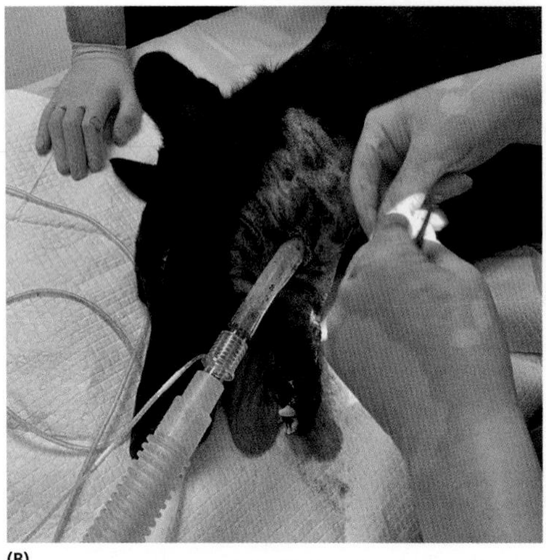

(B)

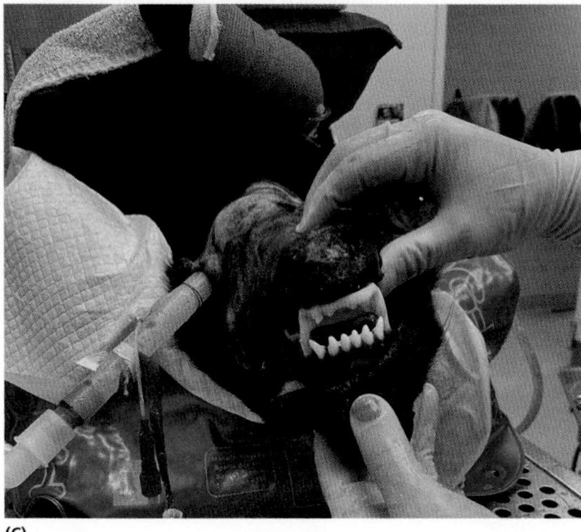

(C)

Figure 6.25 An endotracheal tube placed by external pharyngostomy in a dog to facilitate oropharyngeal surgery. **A.** The machine end of the endotracheal tube is grasped via the pharyngostomy incision. **B.** The machine end of the endotracheal tube is exteriorized and sutured to the surrounding tissues. **C.** Completed tube placement distal to the left mandibular ramus demonstrating ability to assess proper dental occlusion in orofacial surgeries. Source: Dr. Craig Mosley, with permission.

Table 6.1 Approximate F_IO_2 values obtained from various oxygen supplementation techniques for dogs and cats[a].

Technique	Approximate F_IO_2 obtainable (%)	Flow rate
Flow by oxygen	25–40	0.5–5 L/min
Face mask	35–60	2–8 L/min
Nasal insufflation	30–70	100–150 mL/kg/min
Tracheal insufflation	40–60	50 mL/kg/min
Oxygen cages	25–50	Variable

[a] These values are not applicable for all veterinary species during all circumstances and will be flow rate and respiratory character (rate and depth) dependent.

anesthetic odors and potentially improve compliance, but this is variably useful.

The flow rates generally recommended for increasing F_IO_2 when using masks are variable among species. For example, flow rates of 10–15 L/min of supplemental oxygen have been recommended to increase the inspired oxygen concentration to approximately 35–60% in adult horses, although supporting studies are lacking, and nasal and tracheal insufflation represent better, more practical options in larger patients. Flow rates for smaller patients, including dogs and cats, usually range from 2 to 8 L/min to produce inspired oxygen concentrations of 30–60% [57], although specific supporting studies are lacking. There is also increasing interest in the use of high-flow oxygen therapy in veterinary medicine [58]. With a tight-fitting mask, higher flow rates of oxygen tend to produce greater F_IO_2 values and less rebreathing of expired carbon dioxide.

Tight-fitting masks should be used with a breathing system (anesthetic circuit or manual resuscitation bag) with a reservoir that can meet the patient's tidal volume demands or with a vented or valved mask allowing entrainment of air from outside the mask. As an example, a dog with a tidal volume of 300 mL and an inspiratory time of 1 s has a peak inspiratory gas flow of approximately 18 L/min, which exceeds the practical flow rate for oxygen during masking. High inspiratory flow rates can be accommodated if the mask is attached to an anesthetic breathing system with a reservoir bag or a mask fitted to a manual resuscitation bag. In addition, an appropriate breathing system has an overflow that prevents the buildup of excessive pressure with a tight-fitting mask. Alternatively, a loose-fitting mask that allows room air to be entrained can be used, but entrained room air will reduce inspired F_IO_2 associated with supplemental oxygen delivery.

Face masks for oxygen supplementation in veterinary patients are readily available (Fig. 6.26). Most consist of a clear plastic cone fitted with a black rubber diaphragm that can improve fit and sealing around a patient's face. Unless they are sedated or otherwise minimally responsive, most conscious patients rarely accept snug-fitting face masks. Although face masks designed specifically for very small patients are available (Fig. 6.27), it is not uncommon to use a plastic syringe case, latex glove, and endotracheal tube adapter to "custom" design a face mask (Fig. 6.28). Traffic cones have been adapted and fitted to pigs for delivery of inhalant anesthetics.

Nasal insufflation

Insufflation involves the delivery of oxygen into the patient's airway at relatively high flow rates; the patient inspires oxygen and room air, the relative proportions of each being determined primarily by the oxygen flow rate and the rate of gas flow during inspiration. Insufflation can be accomplished by a variety of methods. For horses recovering from anesthesia, oxygen may be delivered from a flowmeter through a delivery tube and into an appropriately sized insufflation tube in the horse's nasal cavity or trachea. Appropriately sized endotracheal tubes or large animal stomach tubes are often used as nasal tubes. Intact stomach tubes are sufficiently long that they may also be used for tracheal insufflation if advanced through the nasal cavity and into the trachea. For most conscious patients, oxygen is insufflated through a nasal catheter, the tip of which is positioned in the nasopharynx. The catheter is usually made of soft rubber, and the tube should have several fenestrations to minimize jetting lesions from developing in the nasopharyngeal mucosa. For awake patients, instilling 2% lidocaine (or lidocaine gel) or 0.5% proparacaine into the nasal passage with the patient's head and neck extended and held upward may facilitate passage of the tube. Placement involves insertion of a suitable-sized insufflation catheter into the nasal passage and the nasopharynx, the distance being approximately the same as from the tip of the nose to the medial canthus of the eye. Specifically designed nasal insufflation catheters (with multiple fenestrations) are available or they can be made from feeding tubes or other soft non-reactive tubing and adapted to the

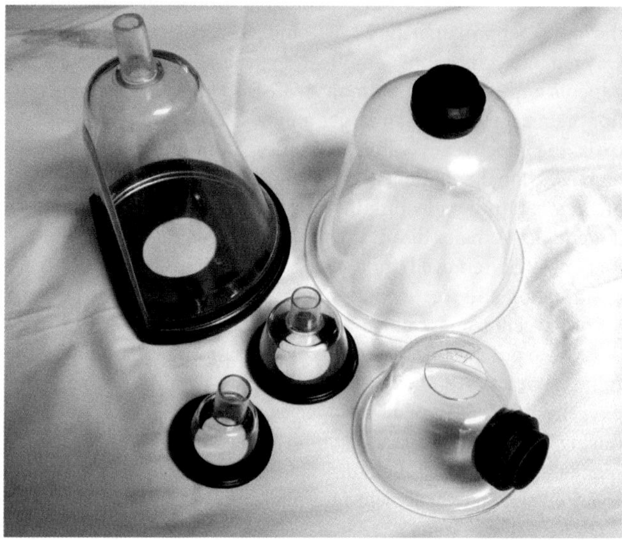

Figure 6.26 Commercial face masks are available in many styles and sizes. A face mask should be chosen to minimize the potential for rebreathing of exhaled gases (i.e., snug fitting), especially when used with the rubber diaphragm in place. Source: Dr. Craig Mosley, with permission.

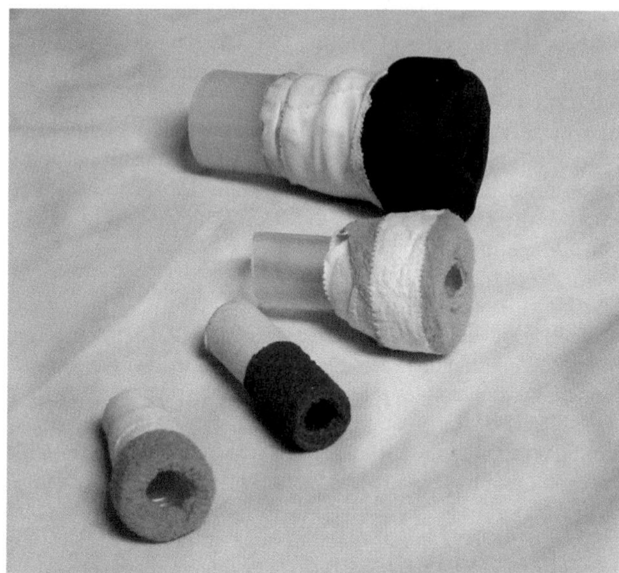

Figure 6.28 Face masks can be fashioned from syringe cases and rubber gloves are often made for use in very small patients. Source: Dr. Craig Mosley, with permission.

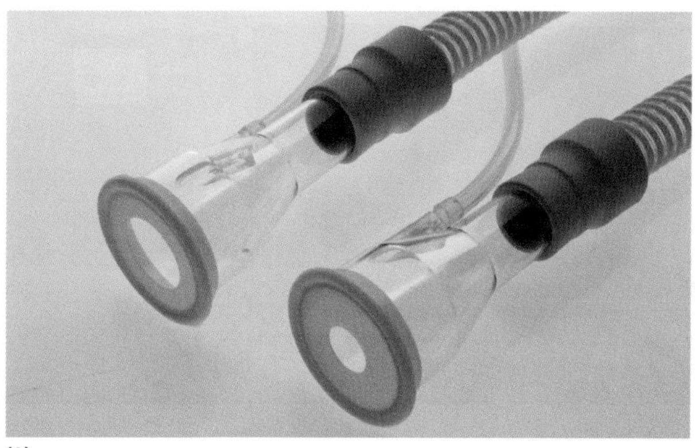

(A)

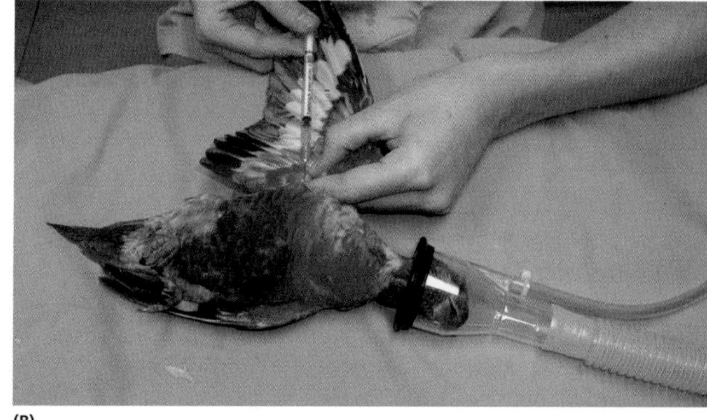

(B)

Figure 6.27 Commercial face masks designed specifically for use with very small patients. **A.** The masks are available with two sizes of interchangeable diaphragms. **B.** Use of the face mask in a small avian patient. Source: Advanced Anesthesia Specialists, Phoenix, AZ, USA; with permission.

oxygen delivery line. The external portion of the catheter is secured to the patient's head with tissue adhesive, tape, and/or sutures or staples. A flexible length of tubing supplies oxygen from a flowmeter and allows the patient some freedom for movement in a cage or stall. Changing the catheter to the opposite nasal passage every 1–2 days has been recommended to prevent pressure necrosis, jet lesions, and accumulation of mucus [59]. Humidification of the oxygen is also advisable if the need for insufflation will be for more than a short period of time.

The flow-rate requirements for oxygen during insufflation vary depending on a number of factors, with the patient's ventilation character and the desired F_IO_2 being two of the most important. Following anesthesia, adult horses require a minimum of 15 L/min of oxygen flow to improve the PaO_2 in arterial blood, and proportionally lower flows (e.g., 5 L/min) are suitable for smaller horses, foals, and calves [60–63]. In small animals, flow rates of 1–7 L/min are typically used for the administration of nasal oxygen. Approximate flow rates for dogs and cats to achieve rather specific ranges of F_IO_2 have been suggested but monitoring of SpO_2 or PaO_2 should ultimately guide flow rate adjustment [64]. In dogs, various flow rates of 100% oxygen administered intranasally were studied, and flow rates of 50, 100, 150, and 200 mL/kg/min produced inspired oxygen concentrations measured at the tracheal bifurcation of 28, 37, 40, and 47, respectively [59]. To prevent mucosal drying with prolonged insufflation, oxygen should be flowed through a bubble-type humidifier. Frequently, bilateral nasal insufflation catheters are placed and can be expected to improve the maximum achievable F_IO_2, achieving up to 80% at 200 mL/kg/min [65].

Tracheal insufflation

Tracheal insufflation can be achieved via nasotracheal or transtracheal oxygen administration. These techniques are useful for patients suffering from conditions causing upper airway obstruction.

Nasotracheal insufflation is achieved by passing a catheter through the nares into the trachea. In conscious animals, this process is normally performed after instilling a topical local anesthetic (lidocaine, proparacaine) into the nose and using a lubricant containing a local anesthetic (lidocaine gel). To facilitate tube placement into the trachea rather than the esophagus, the neck should be extended. Conscious patients will frequently cough as the catheter enters the larynx; coughing can be reduced by instilling a small amount of topical lidocaine through the nasotracheal tube on to the laryngeal area. Proper nasotracheal tube placement can be assessed by demonstrating a lack of negative pressure when air is evacuated from the tube/catheter. Air can be evacuated by attaching an appropriately sized syringe or compressed suction bulb to the catheter. If negative pressure is detected while evacuating air from the tube, this suggests that the tube is not in the trachea and may have been swallowed by the patient and is in the esophagus. Two-view radiographs may also be used to help confirm proper tube placement.

A transtracheal catheter can be placed percutaneously into the trachea through the cricothyroid membrane or between tracheal rings near the larynx and can be used to insufflate oxygen in a compromised patient. Intratracheal administration of 100% oxygen has been evaluated in dogs, and flow rates of 10, 25, 50, 100, 150, 200, and 250 mL/kg/min produced inspired oxygen concentrations at the tracheal bifurcation of 25, 32, 47, 67, 70, 78, and 86%, respectively [64]. The technique for tracheal insufflation has been described for small animals [64]. The catheter should be placed aseptically, be of the over-the-needle type, be relatively large bore, have several smooth fenestrations to prevent jet lesions, and ultimately be positioned with the tip near the carina. Oxygen should be humidified, and flow rates should approximate those used for nasal insufflation.

Oxygen cages

Oxygen cages (Fig. 6.29) specifically designed for small animals are commercially available, but expensive. These cages regulate oxygen flow, control humidity and temperature, and eliminate carbon dioxide from exhaled gases. Most oxygen cages are capable of producing oxygen concentrations between 30 and 60% but the flow rates required can be as high as 15 L/min [66]. However, there is considerable variability in design and efficacy among many commercially available products. There is also considerable variation in the time required to obtain the desired oxygen concentration, usually 30–45 min [66]. Factors that will influence this lag time include internal volume of the cage, air tightness of the cage, and how often the cage is opened. For small animals, flow rates of oxygen, cage temperature, and cage humidity have been recommended to be less than 10 L/min (but this will depend greatly on overall efficiency of the cage), approximately 22 °C, and 40–50%, respectively [67]. Oxygen concentrations of 30–40% generally are adequate for patients with moderate pulmonary disease [68]. Oxygen cages are not practical for horses or larger animals and, even in smaller animals, the effectiveness of an oxygen cage diminishes as body size increases. Smaller patients can be managed easily in oxygen cages, but temperature and humidity are more difficult to control with larger dogs. A major disadvantage of an oxygen cage is that the animal must be removed from the cage (or the doors opened) for examination and treatment, requiring the patient to breathe room air or oxygen by mask during this period.

Prior to purchasing an oxygen cage, it is important to understand fully its operation and oxygen requirements. Significant amounts of oxygen can be consumed by oxygen cages that are poorly sealed and during frequent openings of the cage for patient treatments and management. In these circumstances, the oxygen consumption required can quickly deplete a hospital's oxygen reserves.

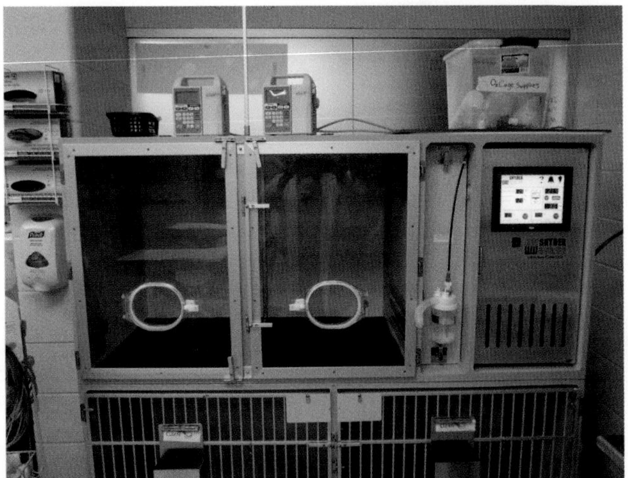

Figure 6.29 Commercial oxygen cages are available that can precisely control the oxygen concentration within the cage and remove exhaled CO_2. Many frequently also incorporate humidity and temperature controls (heating and cooling). Source: Dr. Craig Mosley, with permission.

Comparatively, oxygen cages are a relatively inefficient method of oxygen supplementation but can be extremely useful for managing specific patients. Oxygen cages are best reserved for short-term immediate supplementation of oxygen to smaller patients in respiratory distress. Clinically, some dogs and cats with serious ventilatory compromise respond very well to an oxygen-enriched environment as initial therapy; the increase in F_IO_2 is associated with decreased ventilatory effort, and the patient stabilizes and becomes more manageable prior to further examination and treatment. Nasal insufflation is a far more effective and efficient method of oxygen supplementation in most circumstances, particularly those requiring longer-term supplementation, even for smaller dogs and cats.

Oxygen toxicity

Oxygen toxicity develops with prolonged exposure to high oxygen concentrations, leading to deterioration of pulmonary function. Initial effects are endothelial damage, destruction of alveolar cells, and increasing microvascular permeability, leading to edema, hemorrhage, and congestion [57]. Later stages of toxicity are associated with alveolar type II and fibroblast proliferation resulting in fibrosis [57]. The length of time that a patient's PaO_2 is elevated may be more predictive of oxygen toxicity than the duration of exposure to a high F_IO_2 [69]. There is significant species and individual variability in susceptibility to oxygen toxicity [69]. In veterinary patients, the following guidelines are recommended: (1) use a PaO_2 of 70 mmHg as an endpoint of O_2 therapy; (2) use the lowest F_IO_2 possible to achieve a PaO_2 of 70 mmHg; and (3) do not use an F_IO_2 greater than 0.6 for longer than 24 h if possible [57].

Introduction anesthetic machines and breathing circuits

Inhalant anesthesia forms the foundation of most modern anesthetic protocols in veterinary medicine. The administration of potent inhaled anesthetics requires specific delivery techniques. The anesthetic machine permits the delivery of a precise yet variable combination of inhalant anesthetic and oxygen. The basic components and functions of all anesthetic machines are similar but significant design differences exist among them. Machines can be very simple, for example, those used for mobile applications, to very complex anesthetic workstations with built-in ventilators, monitors, and safety systems (Fig. 6.30). Regardless of the complexity of the design, all anesthetic machines share common components: (1) a source of oxygen, (2) a regulator for oxygen (this may be part of the gas supply system), (3) a flowmeter for oxygen, and (4) a vaporizer. If additional gases are used (e.g., nitrous oxide), there will also be a source, regulator, and flowmeter for each gas that generally parallels the path of oxygen with some exceptions (e.g., oxygen flush valve). The basic anesthetic machine is then used in conjunction with a breathing circuit and anesthetic waste gas scavenge system for delivery of anesthetic to and from the patient.

Medical gas supply

Anesthetic machines ideally have two gas supplies, one from small, high-pressure tanks attached directly to the machine and a second source often originating from a hospital's central pipeline supply. The small tanks mounted directly to the anesthesia machine are normally intended to be used as back-up or reserve gas sources should the pipeline malfunction or for working in an area without

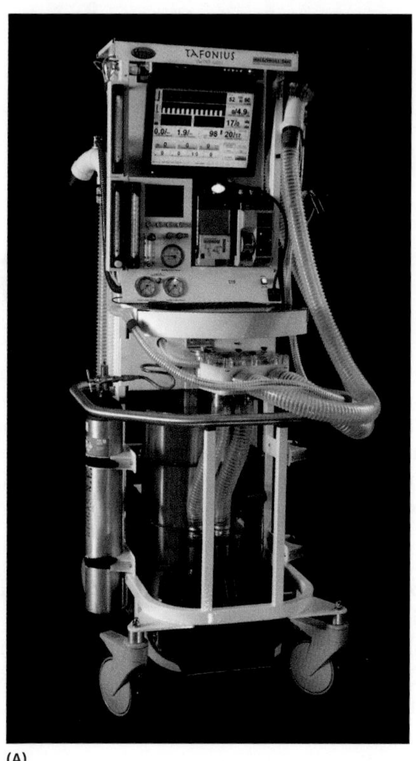

(A)

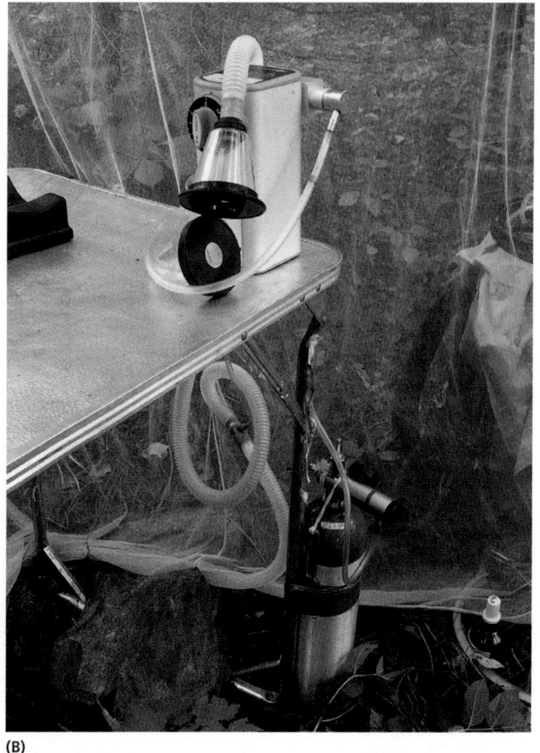

(B)

Figure 6.30 Anesthetic machines for veterinary use can vary considerably in their complexity and sophistication. **A.** Complete veterinary anesthetic workstation for large animal use. **B.** Portable anesthetic system for field use. Both systems provide all the components necessary for the controlled delivery of inhalant anesthetics. Source: part **A.**, Hallowell EMC, Pittsfield, MA, USA; reproduced with permission. Source: Part **B.**, Dr. Craig Mosley, with permission.

Table 6.2 Characteristics of medical gas cylinders.

Size	Gas	Gas symbol	Color code (US)	Color code (ISO)	Capacity and pressure (at 70 °F)	Empty cylinder weight (pounds)
E	Oxygen	O_2	Green	White	660 L 1900 psi	14
E	Nitrous oxide	N_2O	Blue	Blue	1590 L 745 psi	14
G	Nitrous oxide	N_2O	Blue	Blue	13,800 L 745 psi	97
H	Oxygen	O_2	Green	White	6900 L 2200 psi	119
H	Nitrous oxide	N_2O	Blue	Blue	15,800 L 745 psi	119

ISO, International Organization for Standardization; psi, pounds per square inch.
Source: Adapted from Dorsch and Dorsch [2].

access to the pipeline. Oxygen is by far the most commonly used medical gas during veterinary anesthesia, with nitrous oxide being used in conjunction with oxygen as an adjunct carrier gas for inhalants much less frequently. Most medical gases are normally stored under high pressure in gas cylinders of various sizes or in low-pressure insulated cryogenic liquid bulk tanks. The characteristics (e.g., working pressure) and capacity of the gas cylinders vary with the type of gas they contain (see Table 6.2). Alternatively, oxygen concentrators can be used to supply a hospital with its oxygen requirements in circumstances where obtaining and storing tanks is inconvenient, impossible, or prohibitively expensive (e.g., remote communities). Most oxygen concentrators use a system of absorbing nitrogen from air to produce gas with an oxygen concentration between 90 and 96%. Small, integrated, single-machine oxygen concentrating units have been made available in the veterinary market (Pureline™, Supera Anesthesia Innovations, Clackamas, OR, USA) (Fig. 6.31).

Most modern veterinary facilities will have some form of central gas supply and pipeline distribution system delivering medical gases to various work sites. The complexity of these systems can vary significantly, from a small bank of large (G or H) cylinders and a regulator to more complex systems consisting of multiple large liquid oxygen tanks, automatic manifolds, regulators, alarms, and banks of large high-pressure cylinders for back up (Fig. 6.32). The size and complexity of the gas distribution system will depend upon the gas needs, the area of required gas distribution, and the number of work sites required. Proper installation of large gas distribution systems is essential for safety and efficacy. All gas installations should be installed and properly evaluated by those with expertise in this area prior to using them to deliver gas to patients.

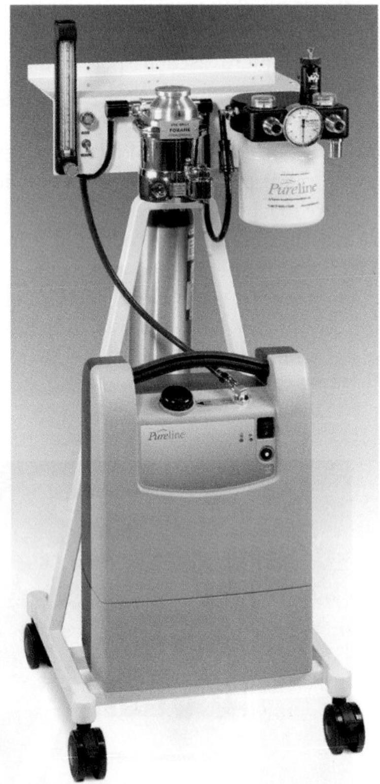

Figure 6.31 Small, quiet, portable oxygen concentrators are becoming increasingly available as an alternative to using refillable compressed gas tanks. This figure depicts an anesthesia machine with a built-in oxygen concentrator. The oxygen concentrator is located in the case on the bottom of the machine. Source: Supera Anesthesia Innovations, Clackamas, OR, USA; reproduced with permission.

Medical gas safety

There are several international (ASTM), national, and local documents related to the safe use, transport, and storage of pressurized gases. There are also standards surrounding the installation of medical gas piping systems and some of these provisions have been incorporated into hospital accreditation requirements in veterinary medicine. However, the specific guidelines can vary significantly among jurisdictions and regions. There have been several well-documented medical accidents related to the inappropriate use of medical gases in humans, but the incidence of such accidents seems to be decreasing [70,71]. The reduction of such accidents is likely due in large part to better monitoring and maintenance of gas delivery systems. Consequently, there are several safety systems that have been developed to help reduce and eliminate these problems. For example, all anesthetic equipment has a gas-specific non-interchangeable connector that is part of the base unit (anesthetic machine, ventilator). These connectors, diameter index safety system (DISS), pin index safety system (PISS), and quick connector are described below.

Color coding

Gas cylinders and gas lines are commonly color-coded to avoid improper use, but color-coding systems can vary among countries. For example, oxygen is colored white in Canada and green in

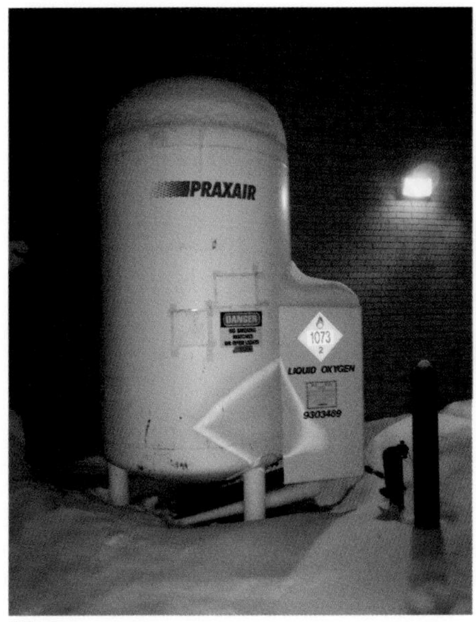

(A)

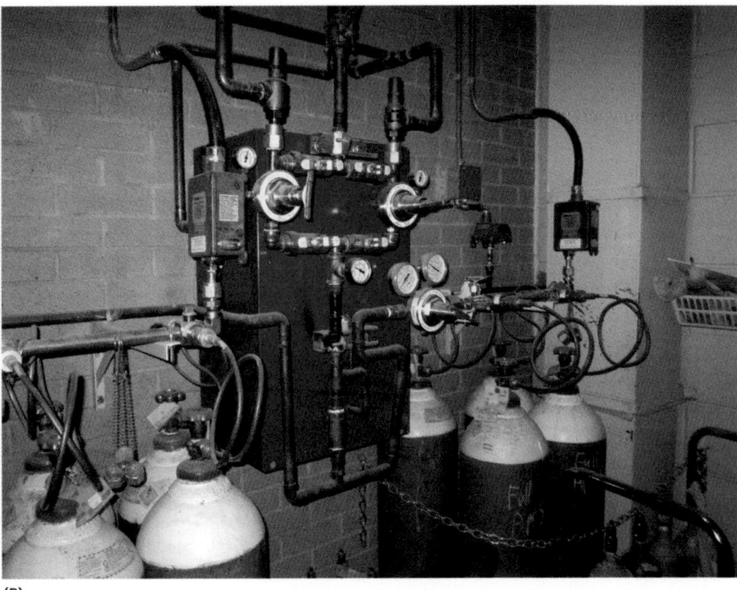

(B)

Figure 6.32 Bulk oxygen requirements for larger hospitals are frequently met using either **A.** large liquid oxygen tanks or **B.** banks of compressed gas tanks. Both of these systems are normally designed with a backup supply should the main supply fail or become depleted. Source: Dr. Craig Mosley, with permission.

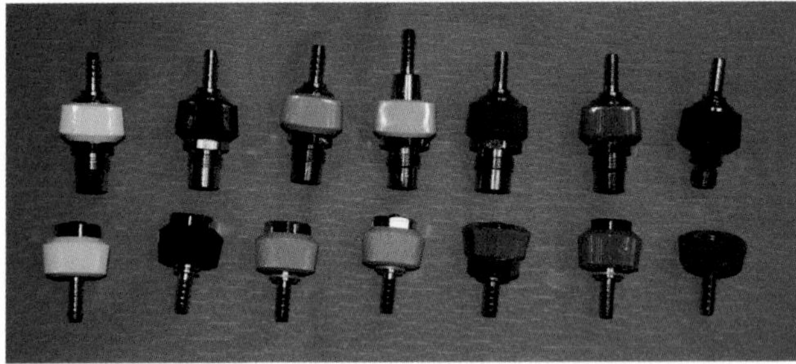

Figure 6.33 The diameter index safety system (DISS) uses a gas-specific non-interchangeable thread pattern to avoid incorrect gas delivery. Gases are also color-coded as apparent in the figure. Source: Dr. Thomas Riebold, College of Veterinary Medicine, Oregon State University, Corvallis, OR, USA; reproduced with permission of Dr. Riebold.

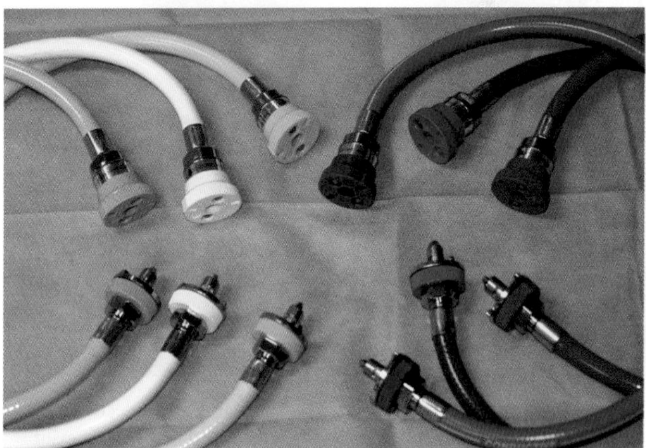

Figure 6.34 Proprietary quick-connect gas couplings are available to ease frequent connecting and disconnecting of gas lines. These systems, such as the Ohmeda system pictured here, are manufacturer-specific and are incompatible among various manufacturers. Source: Dr. Thomas Riebold, College of Veterinary Medicine, Oregon State University, Corvallis, OR, USA; reproduced with permission of Dr. Riebold.

the United States. In addition to color coding, all tanks have a labeling scheme consisting of various shaped labels, key words, and colors that are all used to identify hazards associated with the gas they contain. Most tanks originating from gas supply facilities normally have perforated tags (full, in use, empty) to track the cylinder's use status.

Diameter index safety system

The diameter index safety system (DISS) is a non-interchangeable gas-specific threaded connection system (Fig. 6.33). DISS is the gas connection used almost universally by all equipment and cylinder manufactures for the connection of medical gases.

Quick connectors

There are many proprietary (manufacturer-specific) quick-connect systems that have been developed. These are standardized within a manufacturer but are not generally compatible with the quick-connect systems of another manufacturer (Fig. 6.34). These systems facilitate rapid connecting and disconnecting of gas hoses and may be useful in situations where frequent connects and disconnects are required (e.g., multipurpose work areas).

Pin index safety system

The pin index safety system (PISS) uses gas-specific pin patterns that only allow connections between the appropriate cylinder yokes and small gas cylinders (E size). The PISS is commonly found on the yokes mounted on anesthesia machines and some cylinder-specific regulators/flowmeters (Fig. 6.35).

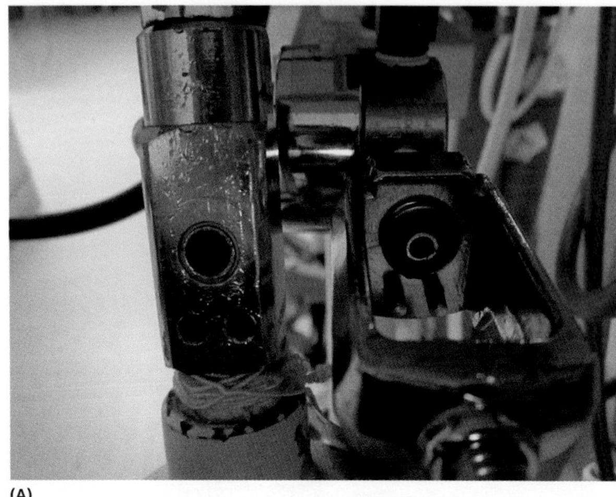
(A)

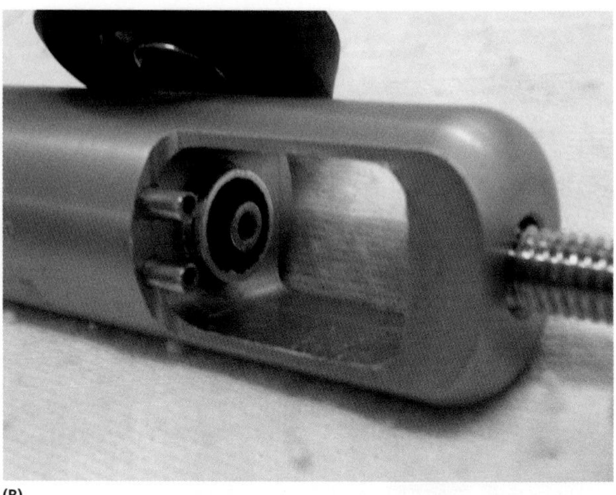
(B)

Figure 6.35 The pin index safety system (PISS) uses a series of gas-specific pin positions on the yolk that correspond to similarly positioned pin receiver ports on the tank. **A.** The PISS typical of the cylinder yolk of an anesthesia machine. **B.** The PISS being used on a combination regulator/flowmeter for the delivery of oxygen. Source: Dr. Craig Mosley, with permission.

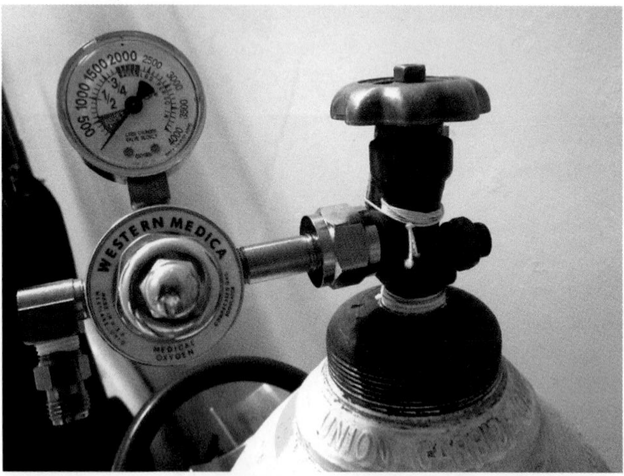

Figure 6.36 Pressure-reducing valves/regulators are used to decrease the pressure of the gas in a compressed gas cylinder down to a lower pressure, sometimes referred to as the "working pressure," normally 40–55psi. These valves maintain a constant pressure delivery from the gas supply and help prevent fluctuations associated with gas depletion and use. Source: Dr. Craig Mosley, with permission.

Pressure-reducing valve (regulator)

The pressure-reducing valve (regulator) is a key component required to bring the high pressures of gas cylinders down to a more reasonable and safe working pressure (i.e., 40–55 psi). Regulators also reduce or prevent fluctuations in pressure as the tank empties. Regulators are normally found wherever a high-pressure gas cylinder is in use (e.g., gas pipelines, cylinder connected directly to machine) (see Fig. 6.36). The regulators used for pipelines are normally adjustable whereas those on most anesthesia machines are set by the manufacturer. The ASTM standard requires that regulators on anesthesia machines be set to use pipeline gases preferentially before using gas from the backup cylinder on the anesthesia machine. However, since neither pipeline systems nor veterinary anesthesia machines are required to meet ASTM standards, it is not uncommon for machines to draw from the reserve or backup tank preferentially rather than the pipeline. This problem can be avoided by ensuring that the pipeline pressure is set approximately 5 psi higher than the anesthesia machine's regulator for the reserve oxygen cylinder.

Pressure gauges

Pressure gauges are commonly used to measure cylinder pressures, pipeline pressures, anesthetic machine working pressures, and pressures within the breathing system. Cylinder, pipeline, and anesthetic machine working pressures are normally expressed in pounds per square inch (psi) or kilopascals (kPa), whereas the pressures within the breathing system of the anesthetic machine are normally expressed in centimeters of water (cmH_2O) (Fig. 6.37). The gauge measuring the pressure of the breathing system is often also referred to as a "pressure manometer." The information provided by these gauges is vital for safe operation of anesthesia equipment.

The modern anesthetic machine

Gas flow within the anesthetic machine

The basic anesthesia delivery apparatus is made up from a series of parts that work collectively to deliver inhalant anesthetics safely and support breathing. These components include: the carrier gas delivery system (normally oxygen), the vaporizer, the breathing circuit, and the waste gas scavenge system. Perhaps the simplest way to describe an anesthetic machine is to describe the components in order of the flow of gas through the machine, from source to patient. However, prior to describing these components, it is important to recognize that the pressures of gas vary at different locations in an anesthesia machine and knowledge of these pressures facilitates the evaluation and safe operation of these machines. There are high-, intermediate-, and low-pressure areas. The high-pressure area accepts gases at cylinder pressure and reduces and regulates the pressure; this area includes gas cylinders, hanger yokes, yoke blocks, high-pressure hoses, pressure gauges, and regulators, with the pressure being as high as 2200 psi. The intermediate-pressure area accepts gases from the central pipeline or from the regulators on the anesthesia machine and conducts them to the flush valve and flowmeters; this area includes pipeline

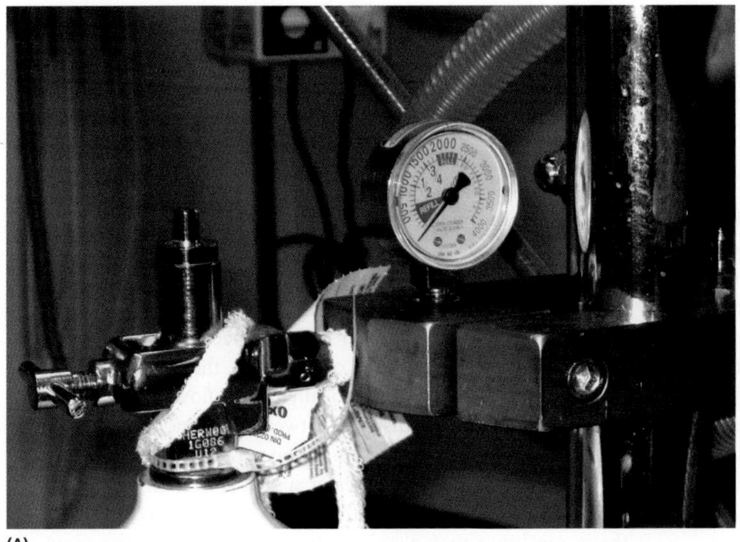

(A)

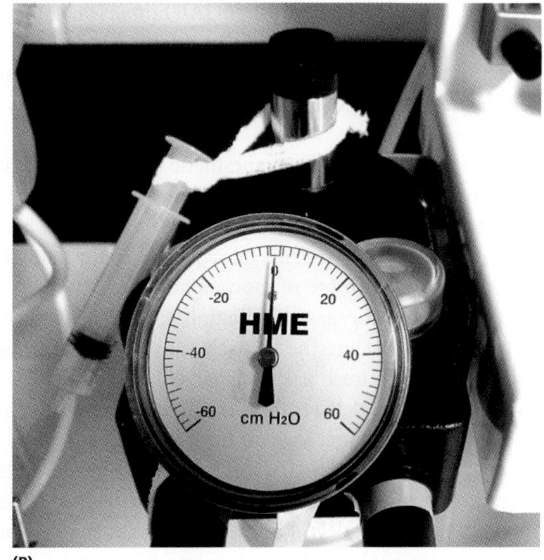

(B)

Figure 6.37 Pressure gauges are used to measure pressure in gas cylinders, anesthetic machines, and breathing systems. **A.** Pressure gauge associated with a compressed oxygen tank, measured in pounds per square inch (psi). **B.** Pressure gauge found commonly on most anesthetic breathing circuits. Note that the pressure in the breathing circuit is measured in cmH_2O. Source: Dr. Craig Mosley, with permission.

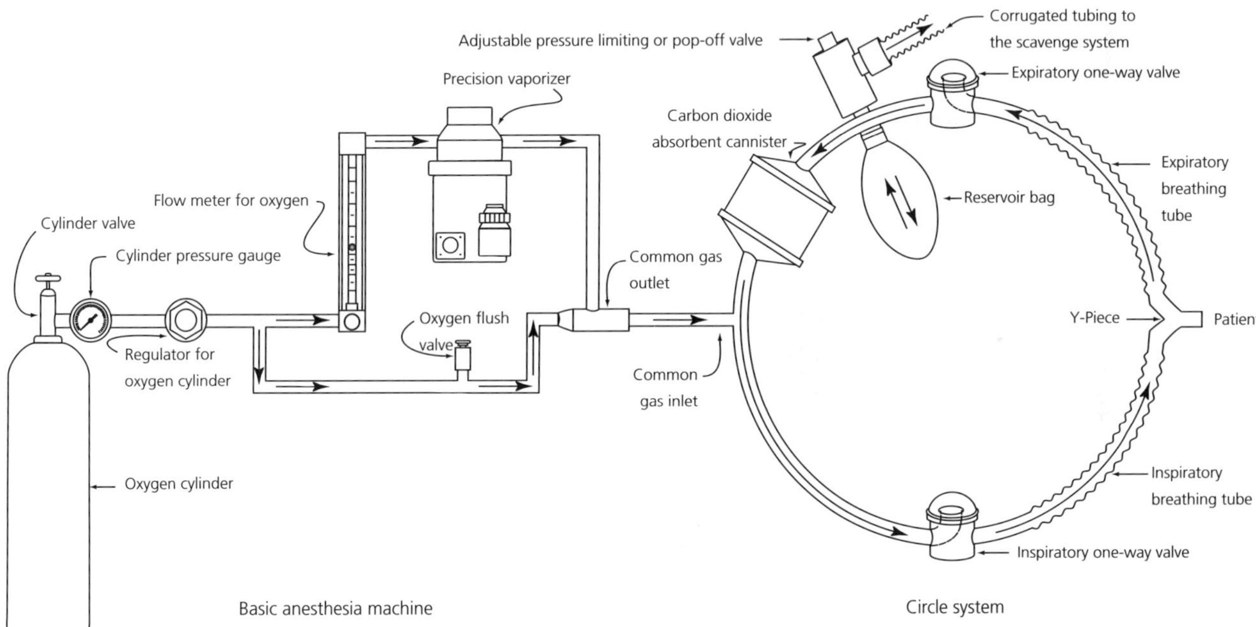

Figure 6.38 Diagram of the basic anesthetic machine and circle breathing system. The exact positions of the various components and specific features can vary markedly among manufacturers. Source: Dr. Kath Klassen, Douglas College, New Westminster, BC, Canada; reproduced with permission of Dr. Klassen.

inlets, power outlets for ventilators, conduits from pipeline inlets to flowmeters, and conduits from regulators to flowmeters, the flowmeter assembly, and the oxygen-flush apparatus. The pressure usually ranges from 40 to 55 psi. The low-pressure area consists of the conduits and components between the flowmeter and the common gas outlet; this area includes vaporizers, piping from the flowmeters to the vaporizer, conduit from the vaporizer to the common gas outlet, and the breathing system. The pressure in the low-pressure area is close to ambient pressure. Pressures within the low-pressure area can vary depending upon how the system is being used (e.g., positive-pressure ventilation) but should generally never exceed 30 cmH_2O as these pressures are transmitted directly to the patient's lungs (see Fig. 6.38).

Occasionally in veterinary medicine, multiple medical gases (e.g., oxygen, air, and nitrous oxide) are used with the anesthetic machine. However, 100% oxygen is normally the only gas used to deliver anesthesia and power anesthetic equipment (e.g., ventilators) in veterinary medicine. If the reader plans to use multiple gases for delivering anesthesia, it is their responsibility to understand fully the implications of the usage (indications and contraindications) and to ensure that the anesthetic equipment is properly designed and monitored to prevent the possibility of delivering a hypoxic gas mixture to the patient. All human machines must have a proportioning system associated with the oxygen flow and oxygen concentration monitors to ensure that a hypoxic gas mixture cannot be delivered; this is not generally the case with veterinary anesthesia machines.

The flow of gas within an anesthetic machine may take multiple routes once it enters the intermediate pressure areas of the machine. Minimally, gas must be delivered to the flowmeter, where it is then directed to the vaporizer and subsequently to the patient. However, in addition to this route of movement, there may be several more routes available for gas distribution in the anesthesia machine. Normally, on most anesthesia machines intermediate pressure gas is also diverted to a fresh gas flush valve that bypasses the flowmeter and vaporizer and delivers fresh gas directly to the breathing circuit. There are circumstances where flush valves may not be present or are unavailable on veterinary anesthesia machines. Additionally, gas from the intermediate pressure area may be diverted to one or more auxiliary oxygen outlets that may be used as the driving gas for a built-in or external ventilator or an external oxygen flowmeter.

Flowmeters

Flowmeters control the rate of gas delivery to the low-pressure area of the anesthetic machine and determine the fresh gas flow (FGF) to the anesthetic circuit. There must be a separate flowmeter for each gas type used with the anesthetic machine (Fig. 6.39). The type of breathing system used, the volume of the breathing circuit, and the size of the patient are all factors that influence the FGF rate.

There are several flowmeter designs available, but most are based on a tapered gas tube with a movable float. The gas normally flows into the bottom of the tube and out at the top. The tube is narrower at the bottom and wider at the top, so as the float moves up the tube more gas can flow around the float, producing higher flow rates (Fig. 6.40) The amount of gas entering the tube is controlled by a flow-control knob that adjusts a needle valve. A float indicates the gas flow on a calibrated scale. The gas flow rates are normally expressed in mL/min or L/min. The spatial distance between vertical markings on the flowmeter does not necessarily correspond to equal changes in flow rate. In other words, the distance between 0 and 1000 mL as measured vertically on the flowmeter may not be the same as the vertical distance between 1000 and 2000 mL. This is similar to the spatial separation of the percentages found on many vaporizers where there is a greater spatial allocation on the dial for normal working percentages than for those rarely used. Some anesthetic machines may also have two flowmeters for the same gas placed in series for allowing even greater precision at lower gas flow rates (Fig. 6.41).

Flowmeters are gas-specific and calibrated at 760 mmHg and 20 °C; accuracy may be affected if they are used under conditions significantly different from calibration, although this is rarely significant for routine clinical use. Flowmeters are also calibrated as a unit (flow tube, scale, and float) and therefore if any one of these fail it is best to replace the whole unit. Gasket, flow-control dial/knob, and/or washer replacement or repair are unlikely to affect accuracy but should only be performed by individuals familiar with flowmeter design and operation. The flow-control knob on contemporary human anesthesia machines must conform to ASTM standards. For example, the oxygen flow-control knob must be uniquely shaped, and it must be on the right-most side of the flowmeter bank downstream of all other gases. These design considerations are important for minimizing the accidental delivery of hypoxic gas mixtures.

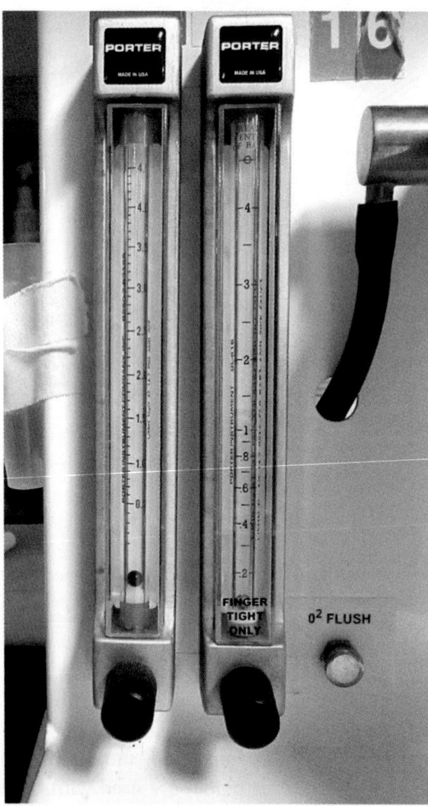

Figure 6.39 Two flowmeters arranged in parallel on an anesthetic machine with nitrous oxide (blue) on the left and oxygen (green) on the right. Flowmeters on human anesthesia machines must conform to specific positioning (i.e., oxygen right-most flowmeter) and control-knob dimension (i.e., oxygen is furled and protrudes out furthest); this is not the case for flowmeters on anesthetic machines designed solely for veterinary use. Source: Dr. Craig Mosley, with permission.

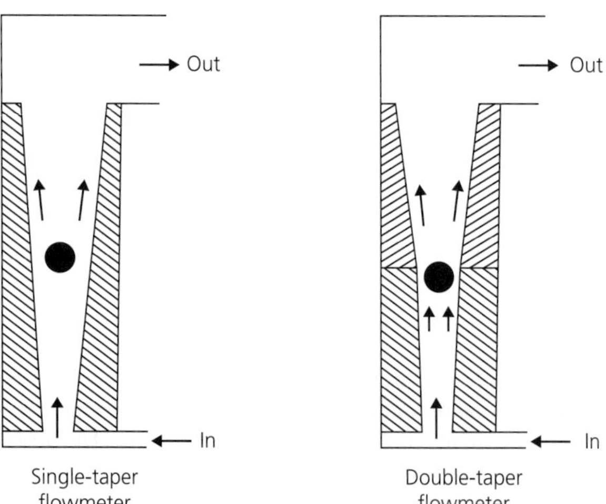

Figure 6.40 Diagram of a flowmeter illustrating gas flow from bottom to top with single and double tapers. As the flow indicator (bobbin, ball, or spindle) rises, flow increases because the orifice size increases. The double taper allows increased accuracy at the lower end of the tube while accurately metering higher flows from the top. Source: Hartsfield [72]; reproduced with permission.

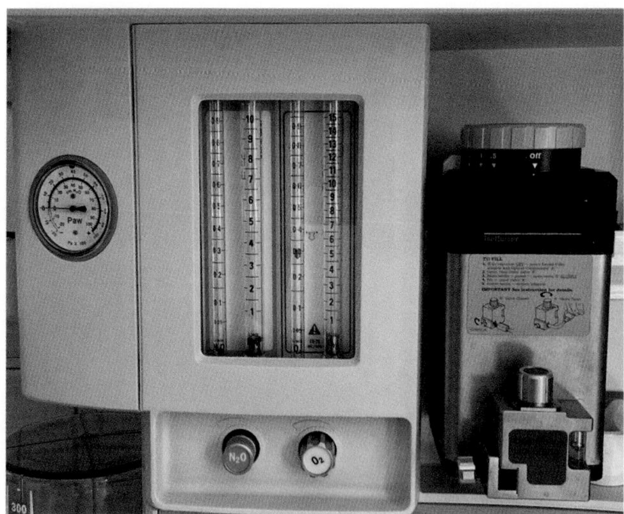

Figure 6.41 An example of multiple flowmeters being used on a single anesthetic machine designed for human use. Note the positioning of the flowmeters and shape of the control knobs. Also note that the nitrous oxide and oxygen flowmeters are dual-stage flowmeters in series allowing for increased precision of gas delivery. Source: Dr. Craig Mosley, with permission.

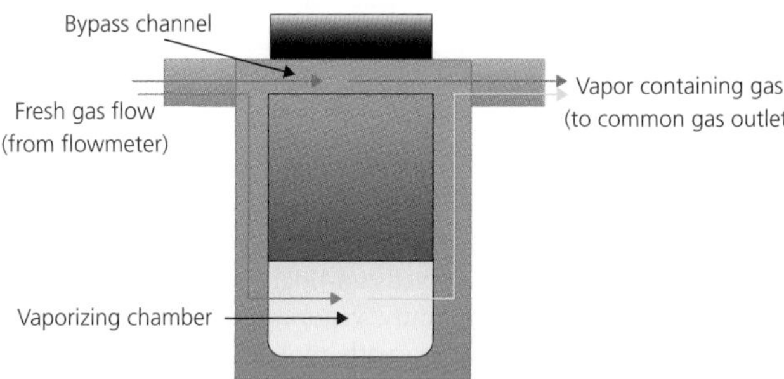

Figure 6.42 Schematic of a generic variable-bypass vaporizer demonstrating the splitting of the fresh gas flow to the vaporizing chamber and bypass channel. The splitting ratio and vapor pressure of the volatile anesthetic will determine the final percent output from the vaporizer. Source: Dr. Craig Mosley, with permission.

Vaporizers

Vaporizers change liquid anesthetic into vapor and meter the amount of vapor leaving the vaporizer. Most modern vaporizers are agent-specific, concentration-calibrated, variable-bypass, flow-over with wick, out-of-circuit, and high-resistance (or plenum) vaporizers that are compensated for temperature, flow, and back-pressure. Non-precision, low-resistance, in-circuit vaporizers are rarely found in veterinary medicine and, without accurate inspired inhalant concentration monitoring, these vaporizers would seem to pose unnecessary risks during anesthesia. Consequently, their use is discouraged unless used in conjunction with inhalant anesthetic agent monitoring. Most modern vaporizers work by splitting the carrier gas to flow into the vaporizing chamber (where it picks up anesthetic vapor) or to the bypass channel where it does not (Fig. 6.42). The ratio of the amount of gas that picks up inhalant to the gas that bypasses the inhalant, along with the vapor pressure of the volatile anesthetic, will determine the final concentration of the gas leaving the vaporizer. The output from the vaporizer is expressed as a concentration (e.g., volume percent) of vapor in the gas leaving the vaporizer.

Temperature, flow, and pressure are all factors that can potentially alter vaporizer output. The mechanisms for temperature, flow, and pressure compensation vary among vaporizer manufacturers and models. In general, most modern precision compensated vaporizers will maintain consistent output at flows between 0.5 and 10 L/min, temperatures between 15 and 35 °C, and pressure changes associated with positive-pressure ventilation and the use of the flush valve.

Temperature compensation

Temperature compensation is achieved by using materials for vaporizer construction that supply and conduct heat efficiently, promoting greater thermostability. In addition, most vaporizers have mechanical, and a few have electrical circuit-driven, thermocompensation systems. These vaporizers compensate for temperature changes by altering the splitting ratio so that a greater or lesser amount of gas is conducted through the vaporizing chamber as the temperature changes during use. In mechanical systems, as the vaporizer cools, the thermal element restricts gas flow to the bypass chamber, causing more carrier gas to enter the vaporizing chamber. The opposite will occur if the vaporizer becomes too warm. The exact thermocompensation systems vary among manufacturers but the thermal element is normally a heat-sensitive metal(s) that will reliably expand and contract when subjected to temperature changes.

Flow rate compensation

Changes in gas flow rate through the vaporizer can potentially lead to changes in the output. For example, if the flow is excessively high, complete saturation of the gas moving through the vaporizing chamber may not occur, leading to a reduction in output. Flow rate compensation is achieved by ensuring reliable and consistent saturation of all gas flowing through the vaporization chamber by using a series of wicks, baffles, and spiral tracks to facilitate liquid gas vaporization. These techniques are used to increase the surface area of the carrier gas–liquid interface, ensuring that all the gas exiting the vaporization chamber is fully saturated. All properly functioning modern vaporizers have very predictable outputs within a clinically useful range of gas flow rates (0.5–10 L/min).

Back-pressure compensation

Back-pressure on the vaporizer can occur during intermittent positive-pressure ventilation (IPPV) or with the use of the flush valve, and this effect can increase vaporizer output if compensation mechanisms are not in place. There are a number of ways in which the effects of back-pressure are minimized in modern vaporizers. One is to reduce the size of the vaporizing chamber relative to the bypass chamber. Another option is to use a long, spiral, or small-diameter tube connecting the vaporizer chamber to the bypass channel. Both will reduce the amount of pressurized gas reaching the vaporizing chamber. The use of one-way check valves immediately upstream from the vaporizer can also prevent the effects of back-pressure and they are incorporated into some machines. One-way check valves are also sometimes used downstream of the flush valve (upstream of the vaporizer) to prevent back-pressure associated with use of the flush valve.

Operational considerations

There are many vaporizers available for use in veterinary anesthesia, but most are based on three main styles of vaporizers: the Ohmeda Tec, the Dräger Vapor, and the Penlon Sigma series.

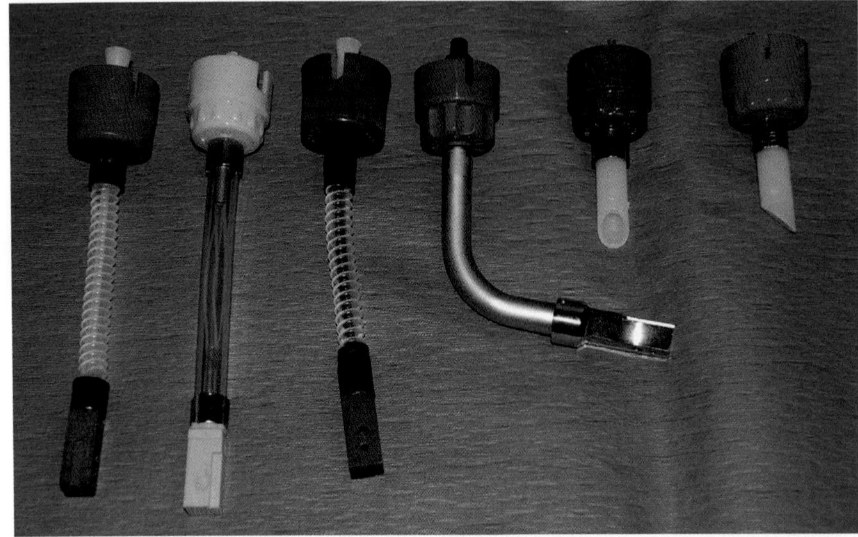

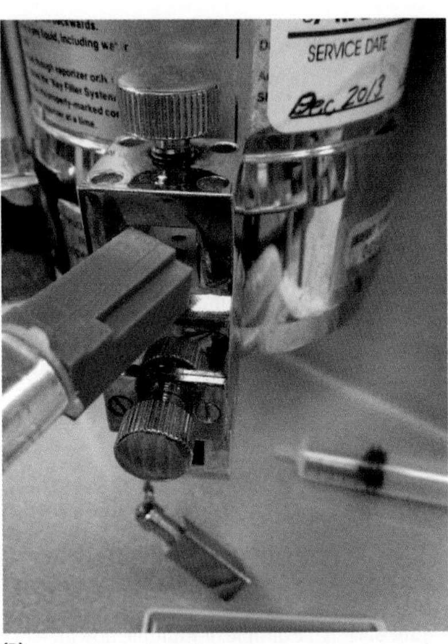

(A) (B)

Figure 6.43 Many vaporizers are filled using agent-specific filler keys represented by the four fillers located on the left in **A.** The keys are indexed to both the bottle and vaporizer (**B.**) and prevent inadvertent filling of a vaporizer with the wrong anesthetic agent. There are also many vaporizers that are not equipped with a keyed filler port and instead use a standard screw-topped filler port. Filling of these vaporizers is best performed using an inhalant-specific filler spout (second right-most in **A.**). These are indexed to a specific agent bottle but not the vaporizer. Source: part **A.**, Dr. Thomas Riebold, College of Veterinary Medicine, Oregon State University, Corvallis, OR, USA; reproduced with permission of Dr. Riebold. Source: part **B.**, Dr. Craig Mosley, with permission.

The primary differences among vaporizer series include capacity of the vaporization chamber (larger chambers allow longer times between fillings, particularly useful for large animal applications), susceptibility to alterations in output due to tipping (rarely a consideration under normal circumstances), and mounting options. All are very accurate and well designed; the use of one over another is often more about personal preference and availability than performance differences.

Most vaporizers are mechanical devices requiring no external power to function normally. However, due to the unique vapor properties of desflurane, this agent requires a specially designed electronic heated vaporizer to ensure consistent output. Despite the need for external power, most desflurane vaporizers function much like standard variable-bypass vaporizers, although technically they are classified as measured-flow vaporizers (see the description of the Tec 6 vaporizer below). There are also electronic vaporizers available for use in both humans (Aladin™ and Aladin2™ cassette vaporizer, GE Healthcare) and veterinary anesthesia (Vetland EX3000 Electronic Vaporization System). These vaporizers function as variable-bypass vaporizers but the splitting ratio of the carrier gas is determined electronically rather than mechanically. Since the system is electronic, various manufacturers and user alarm settings can be incorporated. For example, the vaporizer may alert the user if unusually high concentrations of anesthetic are being delivered from the vaporizer or if the vaporizer setting has not been altered within a specified time period, potentially avoiding inadvertent anesthetic overdose (e.g., the vaporizer output is momentarily increased and the user forgets to reduce the setting). Although electronic systems arguably provide additional information that may be valuable to the anesthetist, they may also be more prone to problems and damage related to the fact they rely on properly operating electronics to function. More recently, target-controlled inhalation anesthesia, also called "end-tidal-driven anesthetic delivery," has become available in some countries on newer anesthetic machines (e.g., Aisys CS2, Anesthesia Delivery System with Et Control, GE Healthcare). These systems allow the anesthetist to select a target end-tidal inhalant concentration and use the sampled end-tidal readings and computer processing to effectively optimize vaporizer output and FGF to achieve efficient inhalant delivery with minimal waste anesthetic gas (i.e., closed FGF rates) and oxygen use. These systems help the user safely and easily utilize low FGF rates; thereby, reducing costs, waste, and environmental contamination [73,74].

Vaporizers can be filled using a standard screw-capped filler port or an agent-specific keyed filler port. Keyed filler ports are intended to prevent inadvertent filling of a vaporizer with the wrong anesthetic agent (Fig. 6.43). Most modern vaporizers are extremely dependable and durable, requiring very little routine maintenance and care. However, maintenance and care should be performed according to the manufacturer's recommendations and only by a qualified technician.

Vaporizers are generally mounted on what is referred to as the "back bar," which simply refers to the rail or mounting system used to hold vaporizers on the machine. Most veterinary vaporizers use cage-mount systems for securing the vaporizer to the back bar; this system uses 23 mm taper push fittings (inlet and outlet, female and male) to attach the vaporizer to the gas delivery system, and the vaporizer is bolted directly to the back bar (Fig. 6.44). The tapered fittings are often referred to as "vaporizer caps," "adapters," or "elbows."

There are also several proprietary mounting bracket systems that allow vaporizers to be easily removed; for example, the GE Healthcare Ohmeda Selectatec and the Dräger Interlock, with the former being significantly more popular. The Selectatec mount consists of two vertically situated male valve ports, with an accessory pin and locking recess located between the inlet and outlet ports (Fig. 6.45). Selectatec-compatible vaporizers have two female ports with a recessed assembly to receive the accessory pin. The

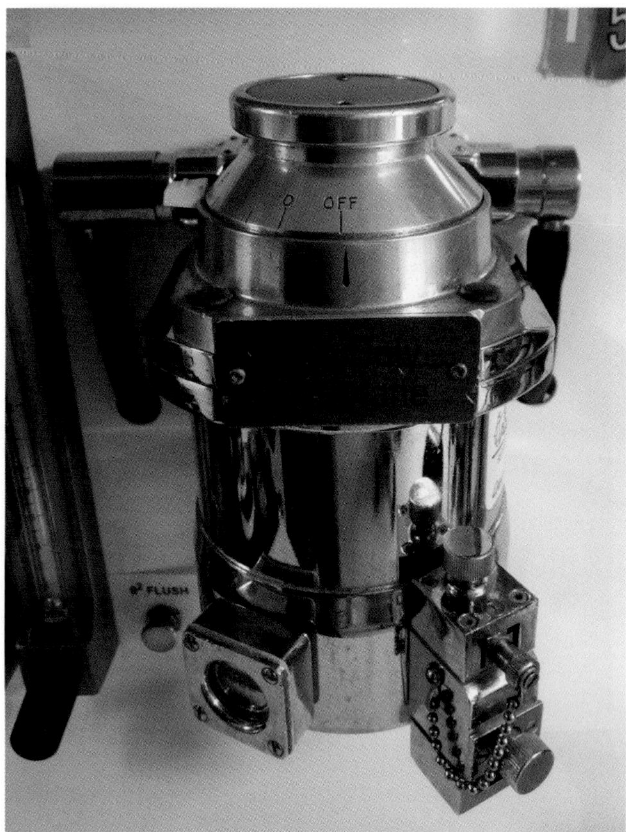

Figure 6.44 An example of a typical cagemount vaporizer with tapered push fittings for delivery of gas to and from the vaporizer. Source: Dr. Craig Mosley, with permission.

vaporizer is lowered on to the male valve ports and then locked into place using the locking knob located on the top of the vaporizer. The O-rings on the male valve ports ensure a gas-tight seal between the vaporizer and the Selectatec mount. Loss or deformation of these rings can lead to leaks between the vaporizer and the mount. The vaporizer cannot be turned on unless it is locked in place on the mount. When the vaporizer is turned on (Tec 4, 5, 6, 7), a retractable spindle depresses the ball valve in the male valve ports, allowing gas to flow from the vaporizer to the anesthetic machine. Tec 4 and above vaporizer models also incorporate a safety interlock system (vaporizer exclusion/isolation) that uses a horizontal push rod system that ensures that only one vaporizer can be used at a time when multiple vaporizers are mounted in series on a Selectatec mount. The Dräger Interlock mount system is very similar to the Selectatec mount and also includes a safety interlink system; however, the dimensions are unique, meaning that each system can only be used with a vaporizer compatible with the individual mounting system. Most vaporizers are available in models compatible with the Selectatec mounting system.

Descriptions of vaporizers common in veterinary medicine

The vaporizers described here are those most commonly used in veterinary anesthesia. Earlier vaporizers no longer being manufactured may still be in use and some have been described in earlier editions of this book and elsewhere [75,76].

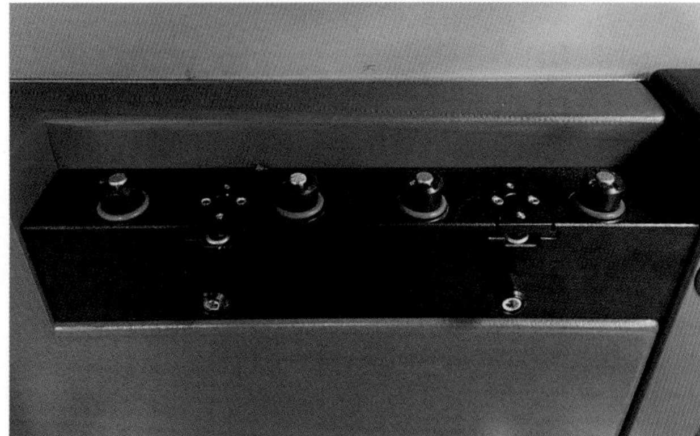

Figure 6.45 A Selectatec mounting bar for Tec-style vaporizers. This mounting system is convenient for quick placement and removal of vaporizers. The vertical male ports deliver gas to and from the vaporizer; the pin between the two ports is the locking system used to mount the vaporizer The vaporizer must be locked in place before the control dial can be turned on. Source: Dr. Craig Mosley, with permission.

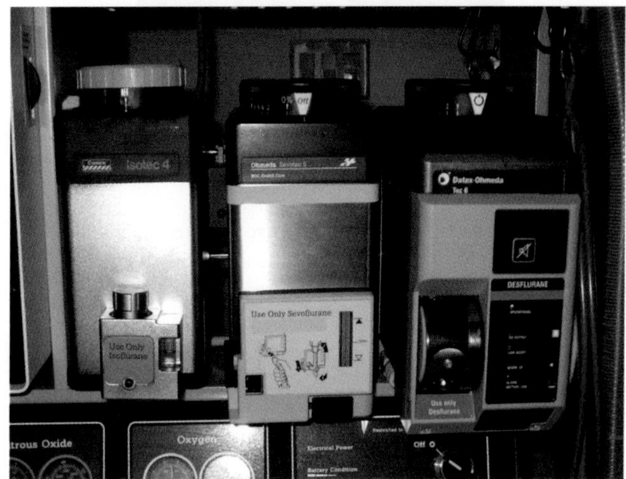

Figure 6.46 A machine mounted with several of the Ohmeda/Datex-Ohmeda Tec series of vaporizers. From the left: the Tec 4, Tec 5, and Tec 6 vaporizers. Source: Dr. Craig Mosley, with permission.

Ohmeda/Datex-Ohmeda/GE Healthcare Tec vaporizers

Tec vaporizers specifically designed for halothane or isoflurane vaporization, particularly the Fluotec Mark 3 and Isotec 3, are commonly used in veterinary anesthesia and are described in more detail below. They are considered reliable and are temperature, flow, and back-pressure compensated under normal operating conditions. The Fluotec Mark 3 predecessor, the Fluotec Mark 2, is no longer being manufactured but may still be available as used equipment and may still be found in some veterinary practices [75]. It was associated with relatively poor performance characteristics and replacement with more accurate and reliable units should be considered. Tec 4, 5, 6, and 7 vaporizers have superseded the Tec 3 vaporizers for use with contemporary human anesthesia machines [2]. The Tec 4 was only available for the delivery of isoflurane and the Tec 6 is a desflurane-specific model (Fig. 6.46). The Tec 5 series is available for delivery of enflurane, halothane, isoflurane, and sevoflurane and has been replaced by the more recent Tec 7 series of vaporizers (Fig. 6.47). These vaporizers are

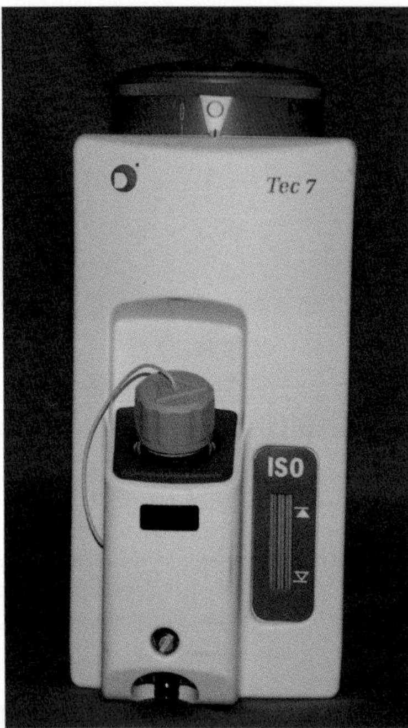

Figure 6.47 A Datex-Ohmeda/GE Healthcare Tec 7 isoflurane-specific vaporizer. The Tec 7 series is the latest variable-bypass plenum vaporizer series offered by Datex-Ohmeda/GE Healthcare. Source: Dr. Thomas Riebold, College of Veterinary Medicine, Oregon State University, Corvallis, OR, USA; reproduced with permission of Dr. Riebold.

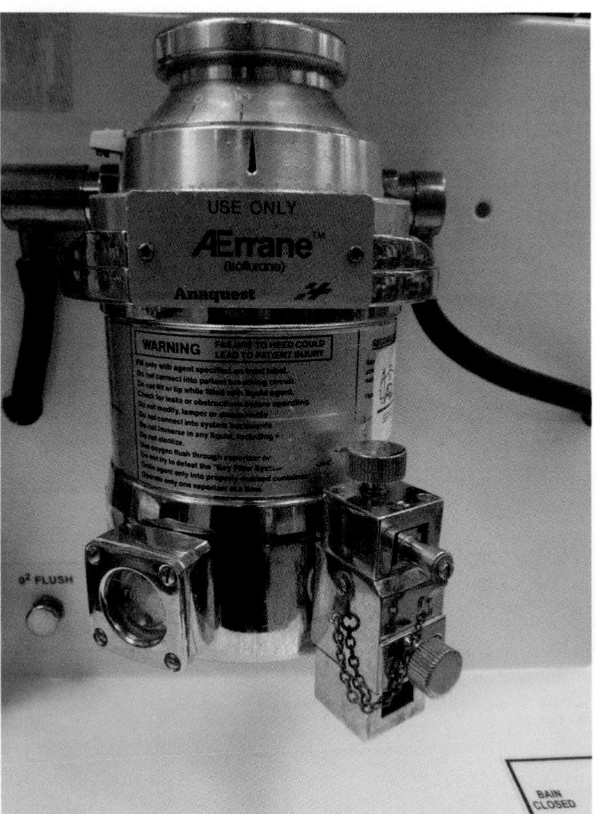

Figure 6.48 An example of a Tec 3 style isoflurane-specific vaporizer. This style of vaporizer is very common in many veterinary practices. Source: Dr. Craig Mosley, with permission.

becoming increasingly common for use in veterinary anesthesia and various publications and specific operating manuals offer information about their use and performance [1].

Tec 3 vaporizers

These vaporizers are classified as variable-bypass, flow-over with wick, automatic thermocompensation, agent-specific, high-resistance, and back-pressure compensated [68]. The Tec 3 model includes the Fluotec Mark 3, the Pentec Mark 2, and the Isotec 3 vaporizers (Fig. 6.48). As the Fluotec and Pentec were specific for halothane and methoxyflurane, respectively, and these inhalants are no longer marketed, it is unlikely that these vaporizers have clinical applicability in veterinary practice today. The Tec 3 (Isotec 3) vaporizer is temperature compensated with a bimetallic, temperature-sensitive element associated with the vaporization chamber. Output from the Tec 3 vaporizer is nearly linear over the range of concentrations and flow rates that would typically be selected for veterinary patients (250 mL/min–6 L/min). Back-pressure compensation is accomplished in the internal design of the vaporizer with a long tube leading to the vaporization chamber, an expansion area in the tube, and exclusion of wicks from the area of the vaporization chamber near the inlet [76].

Tec 4 and 5 vaporizers

These vaporizers are classified as variable-bypass, flow-over with wick, automatic thermocompensation, agent-specific, high-resistance, and back-pressure compensated [76]. The vaporizer's main design features over earlier models are associated with its obligatory use with a Selectatec mounting system. The Tec 4 was the earliest version of these vaporizers and was only available for isoflurane delivery (Fig. 6.49). The Tec 5 is available for the delivery of enflurane, halothane, isoflurane, and sevoflurane and

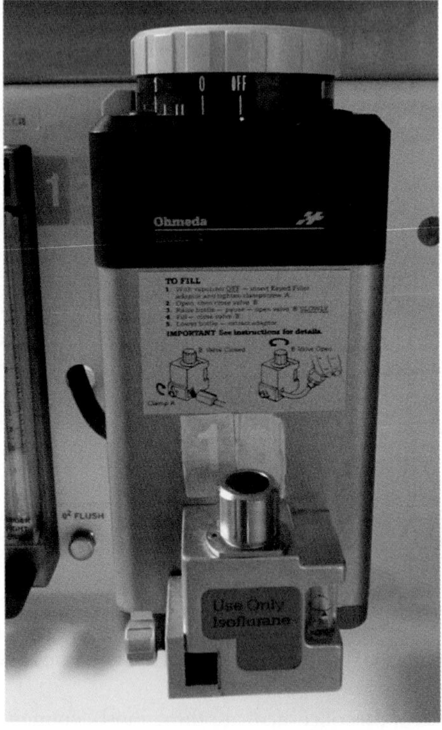

Figure 6.49 The Ohmeda Tec 4 (IsoTec) was the first vaporizer designed for use with the Selectatec mounting system and was only available for the delivery of isoflurane. Source: Dr. Craig Mosley, with permission.

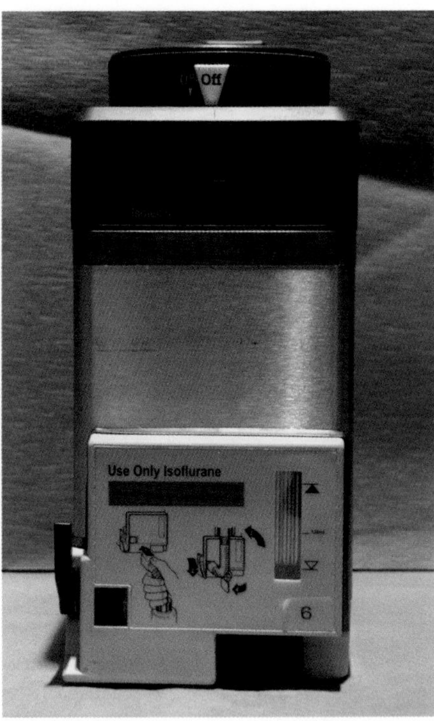

Figure 6.50 The Tec 5 series of vaporizers included enflurane-, halothane-, isoflurane-, and sevoflurane-specific models. The Tec 5 model also incorporated an interlock safety system that prevents multiple vaporizers from being turned on when mounted in series. Source: Dr. Thomas Riebold, College of Veterinary Medicine, Oregon State University, Corvallis, OR, USA; reproduced with permission of Dr. Riebold.

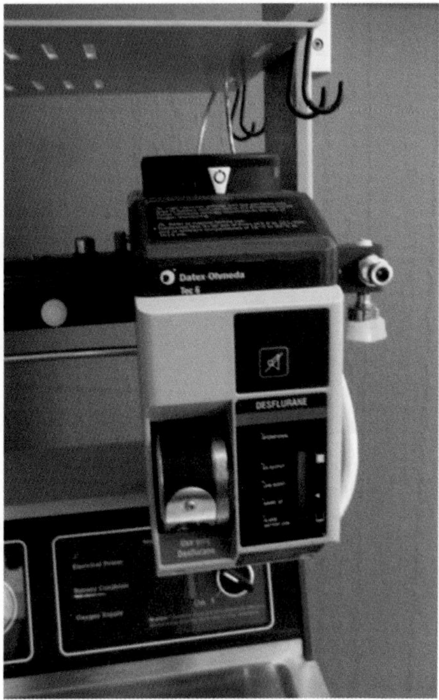

Figure 6.51 The Datex-Ohmeda Tec 6 vaporizer is a desflurane-specific model incorporating a heated vaporizing chamber. The Tec 6 Plus from Datex-Ohmeda/GE Healthcare is the latest available in this vaporizer series. Source: Dr. Craig Mosley, with permission.

can be found in either a key- or funnel-filled configuration (Fig. 6.50). When the dial is turned to “0” and the flowmeter is activated, all of the gas bypasses the vaporizer through the Selectatec mount rather than passing through the vaporizer’s bypass channel. Only when the vaporizer is turned from “0” will the gas enter the vaporizer. Temperature compensation is accomplished through a bimetallic strip located in the bypass channel; as the temperature decreases, less gas is allowed through the bypass channel so that relatively more gas passes through the vaporizing chamber. Tec 5 vaporizers also feature a safety interlock system (vaporizer isolation/exclusion system), activated when multiple vaporizers are mounted in series.

Tec 6

The Tec 6 vaporizer is designed for use only with desflurane (Fig. 6.51). Owing to its relatively low potency and low boiling point (near room temperature), desflurane liquid requires heating to ensure complete and stable vaporization of the liquid and accurate vaporizer output. The vaporizer is classified as a measured-flow vaporizer, automatic thermocompensation, agent-specific, high-resistance (see below), and back-pressure compensated. The vaporizer uses electronics to indicate its operational status, the level of agent, to control the pressure balance (between the diluent/bypass gas and the vaporized inhalant), to heat the liquid desflurane, and to charge the backup battery. The vaporizer can only be turned on once the electronics determine it to be operable. The heaters in the agent sump heat the desflurane to 39 °C, producing saturated desflurane at a vapor pressure of approximately 1500 mmHg in the reservoir.

When the vaporizer is turned on, the valve is opened and the pressurized vapor moves to a pressure regulator that reduces the pressure to that normally found in a high-resistance (plenum) vaporizer (10–20 cmH_2O). The desflurane vapor then moves to a variable restrictor controlled by the concentration selection dial, where it is added to the carrier gas leaving the vaporizer. The fresh gas (carrier gas) flow into the vaporizer passes through a fixed restrictor that increases its pressure to that normally found in a high-resistance (plenum) vaporizer. Two independent pressure sensors in the pathway detect pressure changes and instruct the pressure regulator to change the desflurane pressure (and flow) proportionately so as to maintain the set vapor concentration. For example, if the FGF rate is increased, the pressure created by the carrier gas moving through the fixed restrictor will increase. This will then instruct the desflurane pressure (and flow) to increase proportionately, maintaining the vaporizer output despite changes in carrier gas flow. If the readings from the two sensors are not similar, the vaporizer will shut off the vaporizing chamber, initiating an alarm. The filler port accepts only the specific filler nozzle associated with the desflurane bottle.

Dräger vapor vaporizers: Vapor 19.1

Dräger Vapor 19.1 series vaporizers are commonly found in veterinary medicine. An interlock-compatible model is also available, the Vapor 19.3 series. The Vapor 19.1 probably first became popular in veterinary anesthesia for large animal applications (Fig. 6.52). The Vapor 19.1 had a significantly larger inhalant reservoir capacity relative to the standard Tec 3 and 4 vaporizers commonly used at the time (although extended capacity Tec 3 models were also produced). The larger inhalant reservoir is well suited to the increased inhalant demands associated with

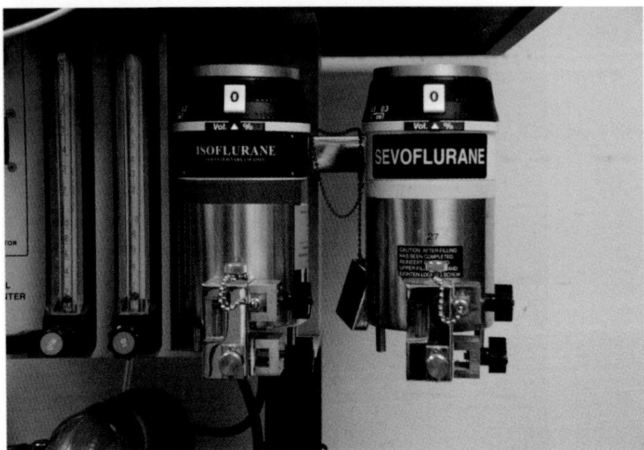

Figure 6.52 Isoflurane and sevoflurane Dräger Vapor 19.1 vaporizers mounted on a large animal anesthesia machine. These vaporizers probably first became popular for use in veterinary medicine for providing large animal anesthesia owing to their relatively large inhalant reservoir, requiring less filling during a case. Source: Dr. Thomas Riebold, College of Veterinary Medicine, Oregon State University, Corvallis, OR, USA; reproduced with permission of Dr. Riebold.

large animal inhalant anesthesia and reduced the likelihood of needing to refill the vaporizer in the middle of a case. The Vapor 19.1 series vaporizers are classified as variable-bypass, flow-over with wick, automatic thermocompensation, high-resistance, agent-specific, and pressure compensated [76]. Specific vaporizers are available for sevoflurane, isoflurane, enflurane, and halothane administration. Temperature compensation is automatic with a temperature compensator. The temperature compensator makes use of the thermal characteristics of two different materials to expand or contract the bypass channel, decreasing or increasing the amount of gas passing through the vaporization chamber. Pressure compensation is accomplished by the presence of a long spiral inlet tube to the vaporization chamber [2]. This vaporizer is accurate from 0.3 to 15 L/min of FGF at the lower settings on the control dial, but complete saturation may not occur at higher settings with higher flows. The vaporizer is designed for operation (temperature compensation) in the range 10–40 °C [2]. Dräger also produces desflurane-specific vaporizers, the D Vapor and the DIVA, which are additional examples of measure flow vaporizers, similar to the Tec 6.

Penlon Sigma Delta vaporizers

Penlon Sigma Delta vaporizers are another type of vaporizer occasionally used in veterinary medicine. The Sigma Delta vaporizer (Fig. 6.53) is classified as variable-bypass, flow-over with wick, temperature compensated, high-resistance, agent-specific, and vaporizer-out-of-circuit (VOC) [76]. Specific vaporizers are available for sevoflurane, isoflurane, enflurane, and halothane administration. Penlon also produces a desflurane vaporizer, the Sigma Alpha. Temperature compensation is through a thermostat in the bypass channel. The operating temperature is between 15 and 35 °C and the temperature-compensating mechanism reacts slowly, requiring 1–2 h to compensate for changes in room temperature. This vaporizer is accurate from 0.2 to 15 L/min of FGF at all dial settings, with only slightly decreased output at lower settings and slightly increased output at higher settings when using very low flow rates.

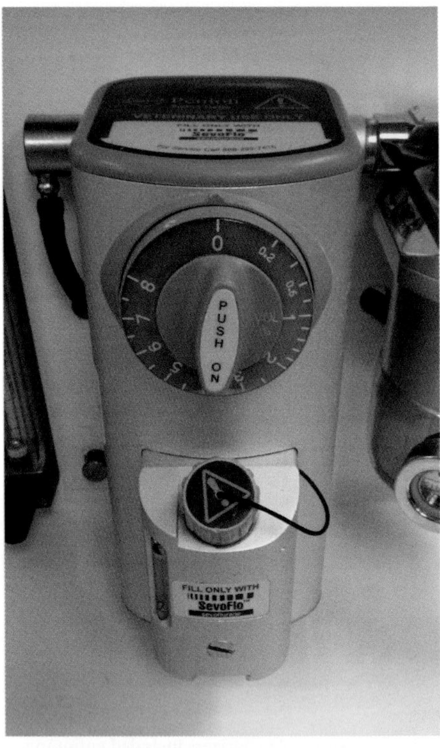

Figure 6.53 A sevoflurane-specific Penlon Sigma Delta vaporizer. The Sigma Delta is also available for the delivery of enflurane, halothane, and isoflurane. Source: Dr. Craig Mosley, with permission.

Ohio calibrated vaporizer

This vaporizer (Fig. 6.54) has been available for veterinary use and was commonly employed on human anesthesia machines for many years. It is no longer being manufactured but is still readily found being redistributed through veterinary equipment companies. It is classified as variable-bypass, flow-over with wick, automatically temperature compensated, agent-specific, VOC, and high-resistance [76]. Specific units were manufactured for isoflurane, halothane, and sevoflurane administration. These vaporizers were designed for accuracy at FGFs between 0.3 and 10 L/min, and temperature compensation occurs between 16 and 32 °C. Tilting these vaporizers up to 20° while in use or up to 45° when not in use does not cause problems. Greater tipping of the vaporizer may cause delivery of high concentrations. Between paper wicks, the vaporizer has plastic spacers that may react with enflurane or isoflurane to cause discoloration of the liquid anesthetic, apparently without significant consequences [76].

Measured-flow vaporizers

Verni-Trol and Copper Kettles are flowmeter-controlled vaporizers that were once popular for use in anesthesia of human patients [76]. Although these vaporizers are no longer being manufactured, are not covered by the ASTM standards for anesthesia equipment, and are rarely found in clinical use (or otherwise), a description of their operation may be instructive for those wanting an alternative explanation of vaporizer function. Historically they are also important as they were the first devices to permit precise vaporization of liquid anesthetics and served as the precursors to today's modern variable-bypass vaporizers.

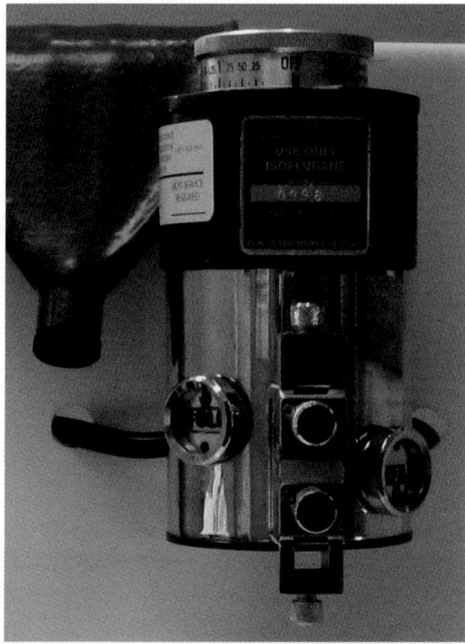

Figure 6.54 An isoflurane-specific Ohio vaporizer. It has also been manufactured for the delivery of halothane and sevoflurane. Source: Dr. Craig Mosley, with permission.

These flowmeter-controlled vaporizers are classified as measured-flow, bubble-through, high-resistance, VOC, temperature compensated (thermally stable with manual flow adjustments based on temperature of the liquid anesthetic), and multipurpose. They have been classified as saturation vaporizers. These vaporizers are constructed of copper (Copper Kettle) or silicon bronze (Verni-Trol) for thermostability. Back-pressure compensation mechanisms are present on later production models and can be fitted on older models (e.g., check valves). Since these vaporizers are multipurpose or universal, they can accurately vaporize halothane, isoflurane, sevoflurane, or methoxyflurane, and should be clearly labeled for the agent in use.

With measured-flow vaporizers, manual adjustments of flow rates are required to account for variations in total gas flow, day-to-day changes in temperature, and changes in liquid temperature during use, especially with high FGF rates. In most cases, a calculator wheel is supplied with each vaporizer for determining proper flow rates. The user selects the total FGF, the desired % output, and the temperature of the inhalant, and the calculator will determine the flowrate through the vaporizer to achieve the desired output. Anesthesia machines with measured-flow vaporizers have two oxygen flowmeters. One flowmeter routes all of its oxygen through the vaporization chamber, where it is fully saturated with anesthetic; the other flowmeter supplies oxygen that bypasses the vaporizer and supplies oxygen to meet the patient's requirements. By manually altering the ratio of gas going to the vaporizer to that bypassing the vaporizer, precise concentrations of anesthetic could be delivered to the patient. Both gas sources combine at a mixing valve to achieve the proper anesthetic concentration before gases enter the breathing system. Modern agent-specific variable-bypass vaporizers simply eliminated the need to determine and adjust these ratios manually. Further details concerning the use of measured-flow vaporizers can be found in earlier editions of this book [75].

Maintenance of vaporizers

Vaporizers are generally extremely robust and reliable but do require maintenance. In general, the best policy is to follow the manufacturer's guidelines for care and servicing. Recommendations vary but, regardless of the maintenance schedule, servicing should be performed on a vaporizer if, based on the responses of patients, the dialed anesthetic concentration is suspected to be erroneous, or if any of the components of the vaporizer function improperly (e.g., the control dial is difficult to adjust). Servicing as recommended by the manufacturer often includes an evaluation of operation, cleaning, changing of filters, replacement of worn parts, and recalibration. Halothane and methoxyflurane contain preservatives (thymol and butylated hydroxytoluene, respectively) that are not highly volatile and therefore collect in the vaporization chambers and on the wicks, potentially affecting anesthetic output. These vaporizers should be periodically drained to remove most of these preservatives. Vaporizers should not be overfilled or tipped significantly once filled. They should also be drained before removal from the anesthesia machine for service. In the past, flushing a vaporizer with diethyl ether to dissolve preservatives that collect within it has been recommended. Owing to the flammability and explosiveness of diethyl ether, and the common use of 100% oxygen as a carrier gas, this is no longer recommended. Flushing the vaporizer does not eliminate the need for regular service by a certified vaporizer technician.

Use of the wrong anesthetic in an agent-specific vaporizer

Using an agent-specific vaporizer for an anesthetic for which the vaporizer is not calibrated is problematic, especially if the introduction of an anesthetic is unintentional (i.e., the operator does not realize the mistake). Lower than indicated anesthetic output is expected if an anesthetic with a lower vapor pressure is placed in a vaporizer designed for a drug with a higher vapor pressure (e.g., sevoflurane used in an isoflurane vaporizer). Conversely, a highly volatile anesthetic used in an agent-specific vaporizer designed for a drug with a lower vapor pressure is likely to produce a high, potentially lethal concentration. The differential potencies of the drugs in question would be expected to affect the depth of anesthesia in either situation.

During the introduction of isoflurane into veterinary anesthesia, it was commonly administered with agent-specific halothane vaporizers that were relabeled, but not recalibrated for isoflurane. Because the vapor pressures of halothane and isoflurane are similar (e.g., 243 and 240 mmHg at 20 °C, respectively), the output was not expected to differ greatly from the control-dial setting. Indeed, halothane vaporizers produce concentrations of isoflurane that are reasonably close to the dial setting for halothane [77]. Nevertheless, current manufacturer recommendations are against the use of isoflurane in halothane-specific vaporizers and vice versa [78]. Depending on the vaporizer and conditions of operation, isoflurane in a halothane vaporizer may produce 25–50% more vapor than expected, and halothane in an isoflurane-specific vaporizer usually delivers a concentration that is lower than expected [78]. If isoflurane is to be used in an agent-specific halothane vaporizer, the vaporizer should be serviced and completely recalibrated for isoflurane. Complete calibration implies that the vaporizer has been tested for accuracy with an anesthetic-gas analyzer at various carrier gas flow rates and various temperatures to assure reliable function.

Oxygen flush valve

Oxygen flush valves are found on most, but not all, veterinary anesthetic machines. There is no convention regarding location, size, or design of the flush valve in veterinary medicine and they vary dramatically (e.g., button, toggle, or switch) (Fig. 6.55). Flush valves on human anesthetic machines must be a recessed button type and easily accessible on the front of the machine. Flush valves are designed to rapidly deliver large volumes of non-anesthetic-containing gas to the patient breathing circuit in emergency situations. The flow originates downstream of the regulator within the intermediate pressure area of the anesthetic machine (~50 psi) and bypasses the flowmeter and vaporizer, delivering gas at rates ranging between 35 and 75 L/min to the patient circuit. To avoid over-pressuring the patient circuit, the flush valve should not be used, or be used very cautiously, with non-rebreathing circuits, circuits attached to mechanical ventilators, and circuits with very low volumes (e.g., pediatric circle systems) as pressures within the breathing circuit may temporarily rise, creating dangerously high pressures to the patient's lungs. The adjustable pressure-limiting (APL) valve should be fully open at all times to help prevent over-pressurizing the breathing circuit.

Common gas outlet

The common gas outlet leads from the anesthetic machine to the breathing circuit (Fig. 6.56). Gas reaching the common gas outlet has traveled from the gas supply (cylinder or pipeline), through the regulator, flowmeter, and vaporizer. The gas flowing from the common gas outlet normally delivers the anesthetic and carrier gas(es) to the patient circuit at the concentration and flow rate determined by the vaporizer setting and flowmeter flow rate. However, the concentration of inhalant gas from the common gas outlet is not usually equivalent to the gas concentration inhaled by the patient when using

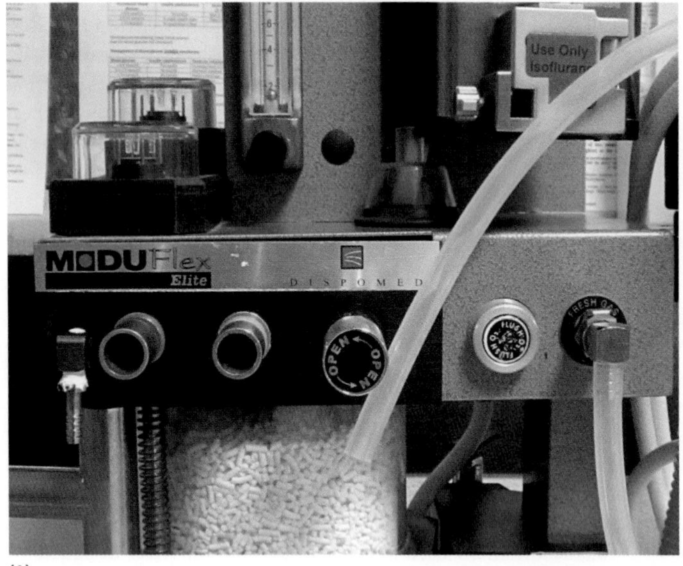

(A)

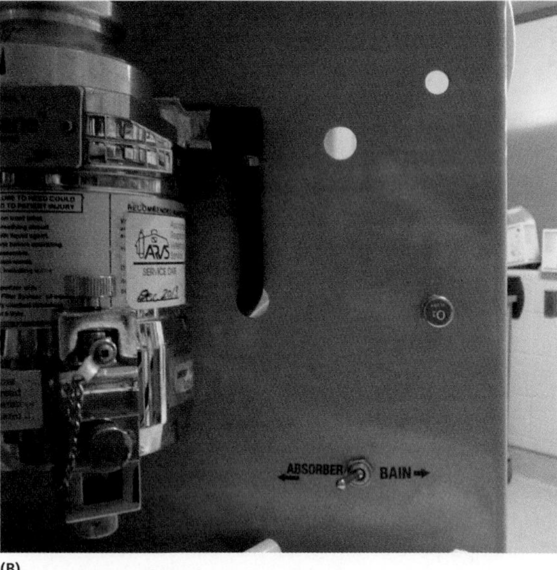

(B)

Figure 6.55 Examples of various flush valve buttons on anesthetic machines. **A.** The oxygen flush button is recessed in a protective collar to prevent inadvertent activation if bumped. **B.** Many oxygen flush buttons are relatively small and are unprotected from accidental activation. Source: Dr. Craig Mosley, with permission.

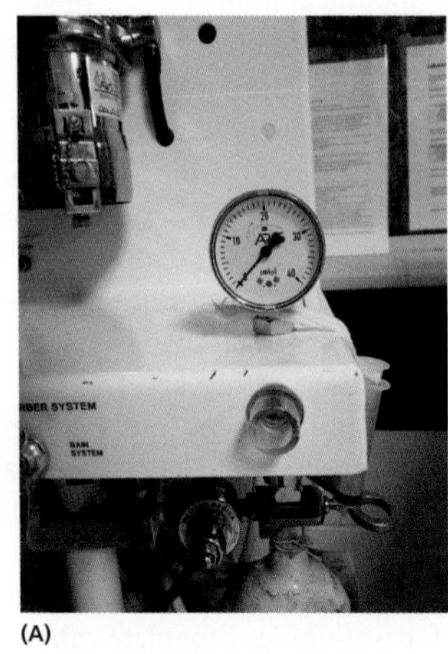

(A)

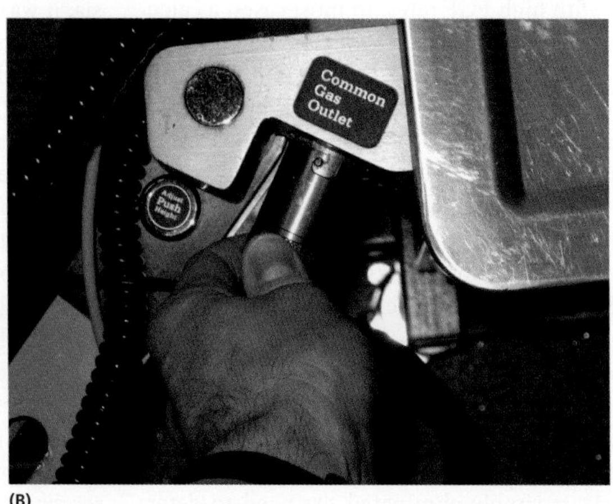

(B)

Figure 6.56 Common gas outlets deliver gas from the anesthetic machine to the patient breathing circuit. **A.** Push-type taper connections are common in veterinary medicine. **B.** Locking common gas outlets is standard on human anesthesia machines. Locking systems will help prevent inadvertent disconnection of the gas supply from the machine to the breathing circuit. Source: Dr. Craig Mosley, with permission.

rebreathing circuits, particularly when using low flow rates, due to dilution of incoming gases with those already in the patient circuit. The exact configuration of the common gas outlet varies among manufacturers, but it is normally a taper 15 mm ID port. Human anesthesia machines must have a locking mechanism in place to prevent inadvertent disconnection from the machine (Fig. 6.56), but this is not a requirement in veterinary medicine. However, at least one company designs their fresh gas outlet with a quick-connect system to prevent inadvertent disconnections (Fig. 6.57).

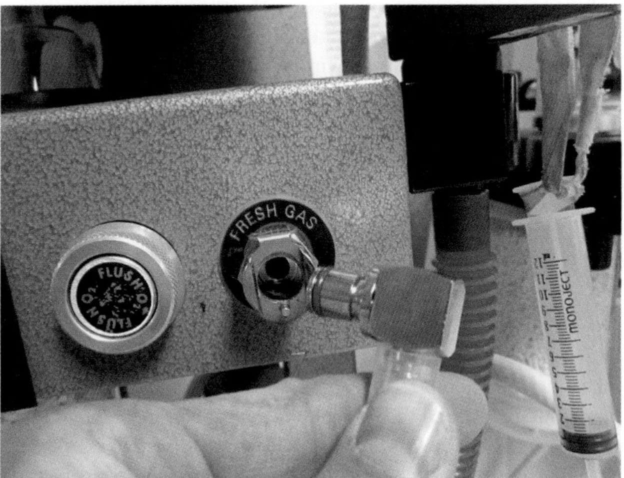

Figure 6.57 A quick-connect/disconnect system used for the common gas outlet on a machine designed for veterinary use can be a safety feature preventing inadvertent disconnections between the patient circuit and the anesthesia machine. Source: Dr. Craig Mosley, with permission.

Breathing systems

Although some parts of the breathing system are built into anesthesia machines (e.g., the circle system carbon dioxide absorbent canister), breathing systems are considered separately from the actual anesthesia machine (i.e., components upstream of the fresh gas outlet). This is a convenient way to discuss breathing systems in veterinary medicine as on any single anesthetic machine the breathing system may be frequently changed depending upon the needs of the patient or the circumstances in which anesthetic is delivered (Fig. 6.58). The primary purposes of the breathing system are to direct oxygen to the patient, deliver anesthetic gas to the patient, remove carbon dioxide from inhaled breaths (or prevent significant rebreathing of carbon dioxide), and provide a means of controlling/supporting ventilation.

Breathing systems have been classified using numerous schemes with little uniformity or consensus of nomenclature (i.e., open, semi-open, and semi-closed). For this reason, it is suggested that these terms be abandoned and rather a description of the flow rates and breathing system (e.g., circle system and Mapleson D system) are all that is needed. For clarity, it is easiest to classify the breathing circuits into one of two groups: those designed for rebreathing of exhaled gases that contain a means to absorb carbon dioxide (rebreathing or partial rebreathing system) and those designed to be used under circumstances of minimal to no rebreathing that do not contain a means to absorb carbon dioxide (non-rebreathing systems). Some have argued that this classification is somewhat of a misnomer since, depending upon the specific system used and the FGF rates used, a rebreathing system may have minimal rebreathing occurring (i.e., excessively high FGFs) or a non-rebreathing system may not completely prevent rebreathing (i.e., inadequate/low FGF). To help circumvent this debate, it has been suggested that in addition to describing the design of the breathing circuit, the FGF

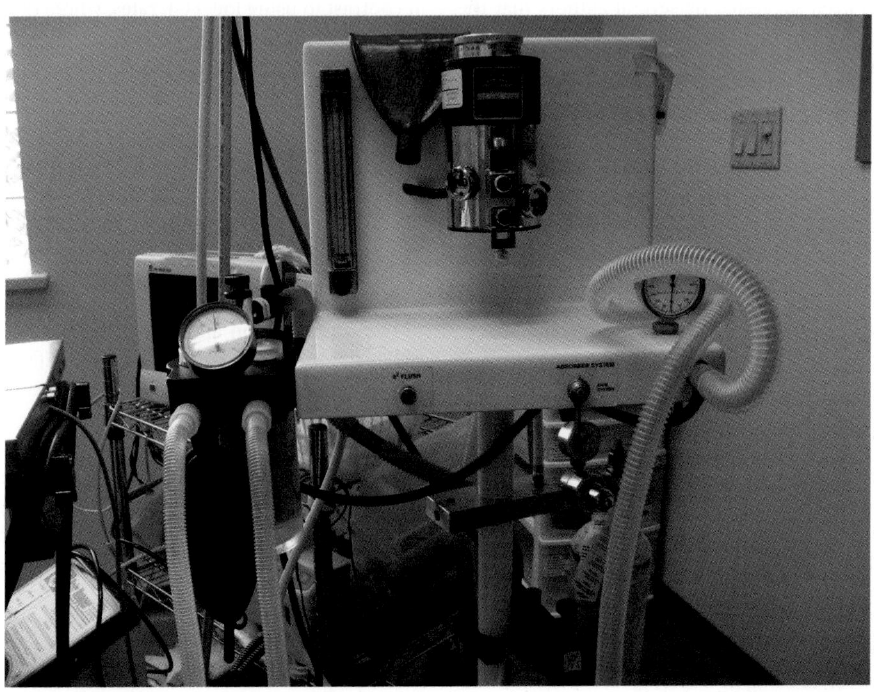

Figure 6.58 An example of an anesthetic machine mounted with both circle (left) and Bain (right) breathing circuits. Changing gas flow between the circuits is achieved through use of a switch handle located on the lower right front of the machine. There is no obvious common gas outlet on this machine as it is integrated into the breathing circuit toggle switch. Source: Dr. Craig Mosley, with permission.

rate should be provided to describe fully how the system is being used [79]. The FGF rate should be expressed in mL/kg/min in veterinary medicine owing to the vast range of patient sizes encountered. Additionally, the degree of rebreathing with breathing circuits can be affected by other factors such as the equipment deadspace and the patient's respiratory pattern. Breathing systems have intentionally been designed to function as rebreathing (contain means to absorb carbon dioxide) or non-rebreathing systems (no means to absorb carbon dioxide) and should be used in the manner for which they were originally intended. Another way to classify or describe breathing systems is by their means of preventing CO_2 rebreathing. A non-rebreathing system is entirely flow dependent for the prevention of rebreathing of CO_2, whereas a rebreathing system is flow independent, in that regardless of the FGF rate there should be no rebreathing as long as all components of the system (one-way valves, CO_2 absorber) are functioning properly.

Rebreathing (circle) system

The circle system is the most commonly used rebreathing system and will be the only one described here, although other types of rebreathing systems have been used (e.g., to-and-fro). Descriptions of these rarely used systems can be found in earlier editions of this book [75]. The circle system is designed to produce a unidirectional flow of gas through the system and has a means of absorbing carbon dioxide from exhaled gases and its ability to remove CO_2 is independent of the FGF rate. The components of the circle system include a fresh gas inlet, inspiratory one-way valve, breathing tubes, expiratory one-way valve, APL valve, reservoir bag, and carbon dioxide absorber (see Fig. 6.38).

The FGFs used with a circle system determine the amount of rebreathing; full rebreathing (closed), partial rebreathing (semi-closed or low flow), and minimal rebreathing. Historically, many terms have been applied to describe the amount of rebreathing, but there is no universally accepted standard or description of these terms. However, it has been suggested by several authors that the use of the terms "open," "semi-open," and "semi-closed" should be dropped to avoid confusion [80].

Full (complete) rebreathing system

This describes a circle system using flow rates equal to, or nearing, the metabolic oxygen consumption of the patient, between 3 and 14 mL/kg/min. This is sometimes also described as a closed system, but it may be best to avoid using such terms to avoid confusion. Note that in a "closed system," the APL is not normally closed, as it could create a potentially dangerous situation (increasing pressure within the patient circuit) should FGF rates exceed metabolic oxygen requirements.

Partial rebreathing system

This generally describes a circle system using a flow rate greater than metabolic oxygen consumption (e.g., 20 mL/kg/min) but less than that required to prevent rebreathing. Since this is a very large range, it is often divided arbitrarily into low flow (20–50 mL/kg/min), mid ("so-so") flow (50–100 mL/kg/min), and high flow (100–200 mL/kg/min), although this is not a universally accepted description.

Non-(minimal) rebreathing system

This describes a circle system using flow rates greater than 200 mL/kg/min (flow rates that would normally not be used in most circumstances). Such unusually high flow rates may result when circle systems are used for maintenance of anesthesia in very small patients (< 5 kg) with flow rates of 1000 mL/min or greater. Frequently in veterinary medicine, it is suggested that flow rates below 1000 mL/min should not be used. Although this recommendation may be clinically useful for preventing some anesthetic delivery errors, most modern anesthetic systems (i.e., vaporizers) continue to function optimally down to flow rates of 200–500 mL/min. With the availability of low-volume, low-deadspace pediatric and neonatal circle systems, coupled with improved patient monitoring (pulse oximetry and end-tidal carbon dioxide), it is common to use circle systems with partial rebreathing flow rates (i.e., < 1000 mL/min) in small patients (< 5 kg).

It is most economical in terms of both oxygen and inhalant anesthetic use to employ low flow rates when possible. Lower flow rates are also associated with less environmental contamination by halogenated hydrocarbons (all commonly available inhaled anesthetics) and marginally improved maintenance of body temperature. However, lower flow rates are also associated with decreased anesthetic gas delivery (unless higher vaporizer settings are utilized). Additionally, when low carrier gas flows are used (relative to the volume of the circuit), the time required to change the anesthetic concentration within the circuit significantly increases.

Most inhalant anesthetics are delivered initially using relatively high FGF rates (e.g., 50–100 mL/kg/min for dogs) to facilitate rapid increases in the inspired inhalant concentration within the breathing system and to replace the anesthetic vapor that is dissolving into patient tissues during the initial uptake period of inhalant anesthesia delivery. The flow rates are then decreased (e.g., to 20–50 mL/kg/min for dogs) after the initial uptake period (e.g., the first 10–20 min) to economize on gas use and waste. The initial and maintenance recommended flow rates (mL/kg/min) often used clinically tend to be much higher in smaller patients (e.g., cats) relative to larger patients (e.g., horses). Using higher flow rates ensures that the patient's inspired gas concentration is more reflective of the concentration of anesthetic gas delivered from the vaporizer. This is in contrast to using low FGF rates, where the inspired patient anesthetic concentration will not necessarily reflect the vaporizer concentration of gas until nearing equilibration. The use of anesthetic agent analyzers to monitor inspired and expired anesthetic partial pressures greatly facilitates decision-making with respect to vaporizer settings and timing changes in gas flows when using lower carrier gas flows. The interaction between the vaporizer output, circuit volume, patient size, and flow rate is often an unfamiliar and difficult concept to grasp. Equating anesthetic delivery to a constant rate infusion of an intravenous drug is perhaps a more familiar comparison for understanding inhalant anesthetic delivery.

The configuration and features of available circle systems vary somewhat depending upon the manufacturer, but in general, a common pattern of gas flow is followed through the fresh gas inlet, the inspiratory one-way valve, the inspiratory and expiratory breathing tubes (into and out of patient), the expiratory one-way valve, the APL valve, the reservoir bag, and the carbon dioxide absorbing canister back to the fresh gas inlet (Fig. 6.59). Some circle systems may also have additional incorporated features such as a switch to automatically engage the mechanical ventilator and oxygen sensor ports (Fig. 6.60).

Fresh gas inlet

The fresh gas inlet is the site of gas delivery to the circle system from the common gas outlet of the anesthetic machine. The fresh gas inlet is normally found after the carbon dioxide absorber and before the inspiratory one-way valve.

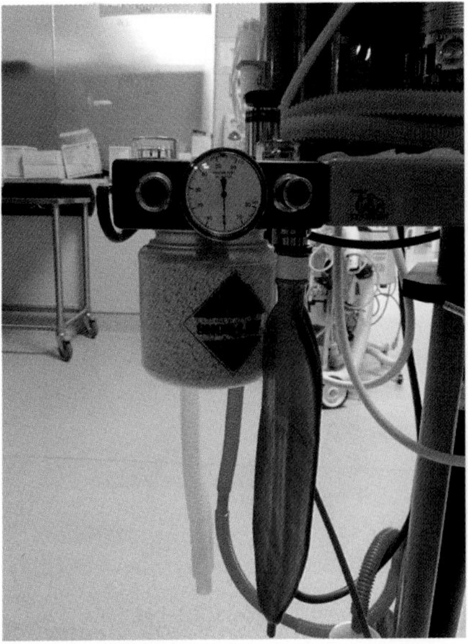

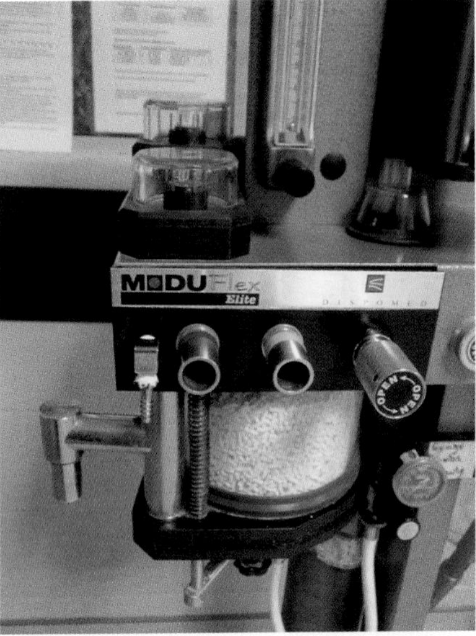

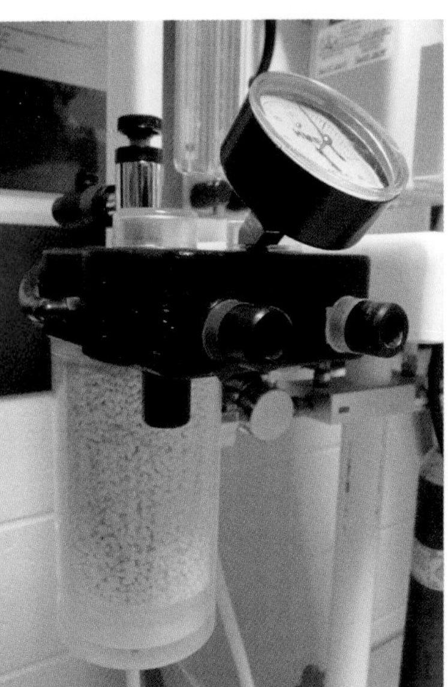

Figure 6.59 Examples of various circle rebreathing circuits used in veterinary medicine. The degree of integration into the anesthetic machine and added details vary markedly among manufacturers but the essential features and functions are similar. Source: Dr. Craig Mosley, with permission.

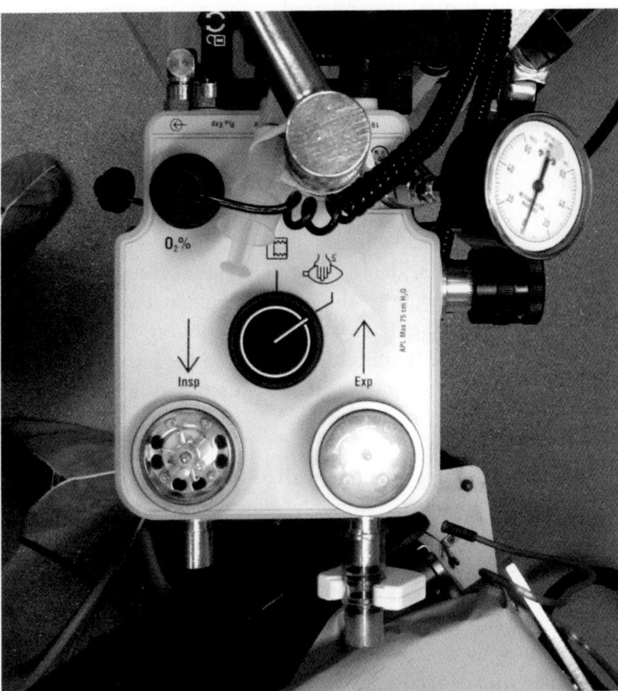

Figure 6.60 An example of a circle breathing system on an anesthetic machine with a built-in ventilator that uses a switch to engage the ventilator circuit. This can minimize the potential for misconnections, disconnections, or kinked hoses during ventilator set up. Source: Dr. Craig Mosley, with permission.

Inspiratory one-way valve

During inspiration, the inspiratory one-way valve opens, allowing gas to move from the fresh gas inlet and reservoir bag past through the one-way inspiratory valve into the inspiratory limb of the breathing circuit. These valves normally consist of a clear dome (for direct visualization of valve function), a light-weight valve, and a valve housing (valve seat and valve guides). The valves are normally accessible for cleaning and repair through a removable cover. During expiration, the inspiratory valve is closed, preventing exhaled gas from entering the inspiratory limb of the breathing circuit, and forcing it into the expiratory limb of the breathing circuit. At least one system (Matrx® circle system, Midmark Animal Health, Versailles, OH, USA) also incorporates a negative-pressure relief valve, providing an alternative path of gas flow (room air) to the patient should the inspiratory valve become stuck in the closed position (Fig. 6.61).

Breathing circuit tubing

The most basic breathing circuit is made up of a corrugated plastic or rubber inspiratory and expiratory limbs. The corrugated tubing helps prevent kinking and allows for some expansion if the breathing circuit is subjected to compression or traction. The two breathing limbs are connected via a Y-piece that connects to the endotracheal tube or facemask. There are also various coaxial designs that place the inspiratory limb within the expiratory limb of the breathing circuit. Coaxial systems reduce the bulk associated with the breathing system and (at least theoretically) facilitate warming the inspired gases by the expired gases. The Universal F-circuit (a coaxial breathing system) is designed to function with standard circle systems (e.g., 22 mm OD connectors of the circle system). Most breathing circuits are adapted for use with all circle systems as the fitting diameters are standardized. However, there is a proprietary coaxial circuit available that utilizes non-standard-sized circle system connectors requiring the use of a proprietary circle system (Moduflex Coaxial Breathing Circuit, Dispomed, Joliette, QC, Canada). There are also several sizes of breathing circuits available that vary in length, diameter, volume, and the amount of deadspace to meet various anesthetic requirements. Pediatric and neonatal rebreathing circuits are normally low-volume and low-deadspace systems, allowing them to function optimally in small patients (i.e., those with small tidal volumes) (Fig. 6.62).

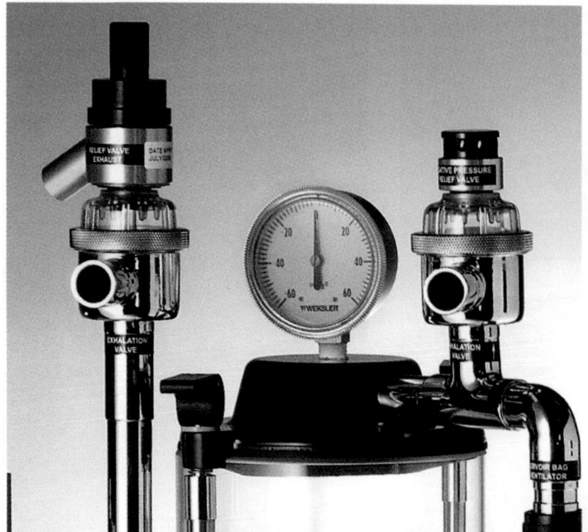

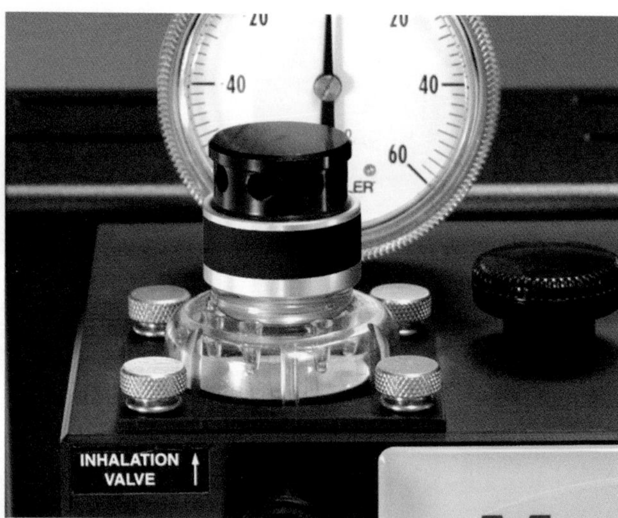

Figure 6.61 Examples of negative-pressure relief valves that are incorporated into some circle systems. Should the inspiratory valve become occluded or stuck, the negative-pressure relief valve is activated, allowing the patient in inhale air from the room.

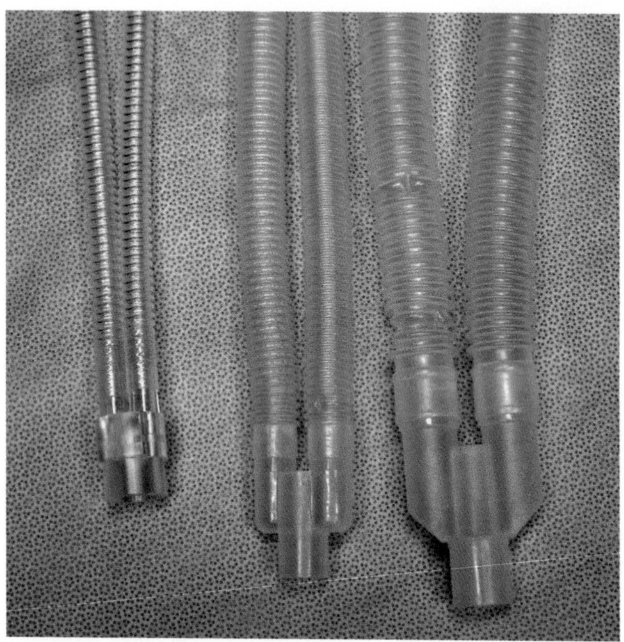

Figure 6.62 The Y-piece of three different-sized circle system circuits demonstrating the difference in deadspace. Circle system circuits are commonly available in neonatal/pediatric and adult configurations (middle and right, respectively). The system on the left is a veterinary-specific circuit designed specifically for very small patients and has minimal deadspace associated with its use. Source: Dr. Craig Mosley, with permission.

Expiratory one-way valve

The expiratory one-way valve functions together with the inspiratory one-way valve, closing upon inspiration and opening during expiration. This valve helps direct gas into the expiratory limb of the breathing system, through the expiratory valve, and into the reservoir bag.

Reservoir bag

The reservoir bag is also referred to as a "breathing bag" or "rebreathing bag". The purpose of the reservoir bag is to provide a compliant reservoir of gas that can rapidly change volume with the patient's expiration and inspiration. It is commonly recommended that the reservoir bag has a volume that is approximately 5–10 times the patient's normal tidal volume (10–20 mL/kg) or roughly equivalent to the patient's minute volume. Ultimately, the reservoir bag should be large enough to provide a reasonably sized reservoir of gas but not so large that it becomes difficult to observe movements of the bag associated with breathing. In addition, a very large reservoir bag will contribute to the overall functional volume of the rebreathing system (i.e., circle system), contributing to slower rates of change in anesthetic concentration within the breathing system when the vaporizer output is altered. This would not be the case when using a non-rebreathing system.

Adjustable pressure-limiting valve

The APL valve is also commonly referred to as the "overflow," "pop-off," or "pressure relief valve." The APL valve is a safety valve allowing excess gas to escape from the patient circuit. If the valve is functioning properly, gas should escape if system pressures exceed 1–3 cmH_2O. Normally, it should be left fully open at all times unless positive-pressure ventilation is being used, and then it should be immediately reopened when ventilation ceases to prevent excessive pressure from building in the patient circuit. The APL valve is partially closed in some instances to prevent collapse of the reservoir bag due to the negative pressure/vacuum from the scavenge system. Although this can remedy the situation, it is strongly discouraged as it can lead to partial or full closure of the valve, leading to excessive pressure building up in the patient circuit. If the reservoir bag continually collapses under normal use, this indicates the need to adjust the central vacuum/scavenge system and or the need to incorporate a properly functioning scavenge interface to offset this effect.

Several manufacturers market products that allow intermittent closure of the APL system. These devices allow temporary closure of outflow to the scavenge system when a button or the valve itself

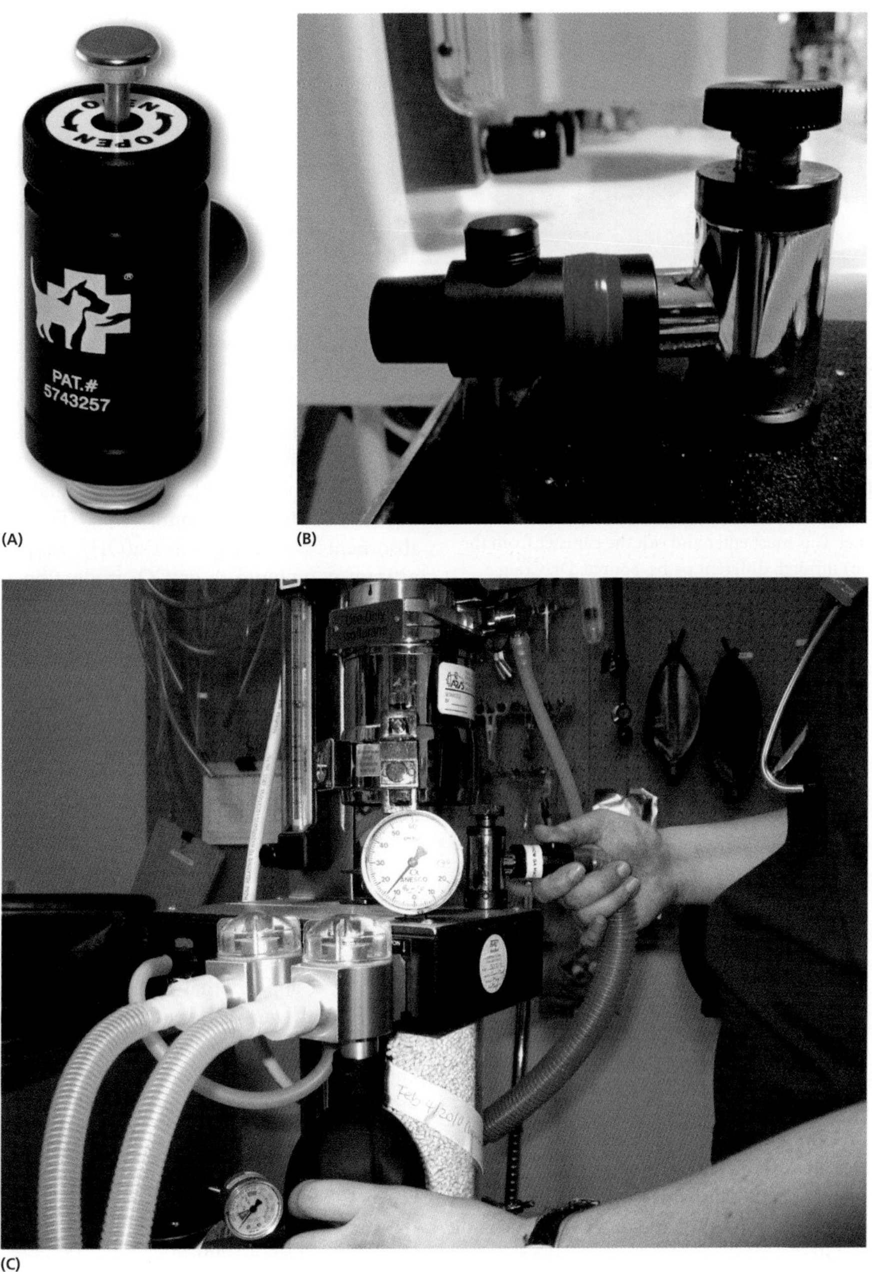

Figure 6.63 **A.** An example of a momentary closure valve built into the adjustable pressure-limiting (APL) valve. **B.** Momentary closure valve that can be added to any standard APL valve. **C.** Demonstration of the use of a momentary occlusion valve to deliver a breath to a patient. Source: part **A.**, Supera Anesthesia Innovations, Clackamas, OR, USA; with permission. Source: Parts **B.** and **C.**, Dr. Craig Mosley, with permission.

is depressed. These momentary closure systems are built directly into some APL valves or can be added to currently used APL valves (Fig. 6.63). These are extremely valuable additions to the APL valve system and help to prevent excessive pressure associated with an inadvertently closed APL valve that can lead to patient barotrauma or death. They also greatly facilitate the ease and safety of manual IPPV.

Carbon dioxide absorber

The carbon dioxide absorber contains the chemical absorbent for removing carbon dioxide from exhaled gases. There are many types (dual canister, disposable, etc.) and sizes of carbon dioxide absorbers available (Fig. 6.64). All contain some type of screen to prevent absorbent granules from entering the breathing circuit and most contain a baffling system to prevent channeling of gases within the absorber canister. However, despite the screens, the absorbent granules and/or dust will occasionally enter the breathing circuit. This is probably most commonly encountered in large animal systems, where relatively high peak flows of gas (associated with inspiration and expiration) are more common. Gas flow patterns within canisters vary considerably, but canister design normally attempts to ensure optimal and efficient absorbent use.

It is frequently suggested in veterinary medicine that the absorber canister must be twice the patient's tidal volume to ensure complete absorption of carbon dioxide, but there seems to be little evidence to support this statement. Most large animal machine canisters rarely

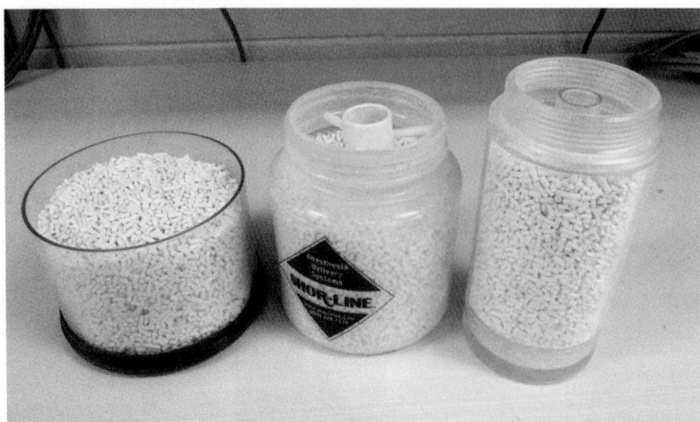

Figure 6.64 Three different absorber canisters. The canister on the far left is a bulk flow-through type canister where the exhaled gas from the patient circuit enters one side (i.e., top) of the canister and exits the other (i.e., bottom) upon inspiration. The two canisters on the right utilize a conducting tube to direct the exhaled or inhaled gases in a predictable pattern through the canister. Gas must enter and exit the canister from the same opening (i.e., the top) through different paths. Source: Dr. Craig Mosley, with permission.

have a volume equal to twice the patient's tidal volume and may in fact have a volume less than the patient's tidal volume. Moreover, many carbon dioxide absorbers used in human anesthetic machines have volumes less than the patient's tidal volume. Smaller canisters are often preferred to ensure more frequent changing of the absorbent, lessening the likelihood that toxic byproducts will be produced by desiccated absorbent. However, the relative efficiency of absorption (i.e., the carbon dioxide load absorbed when an absorbent appears exhausted) may improve with larger carbon dioxide absorbers [4]. Smaller carbon dioxide absorbers will reduce the internal volume of the breathing circuit, leading to vaporizer concentration changes being reflected more rapidly in the inspired gas concentration, but will require more frequent absorbent changes.

Carbon dioxide absorbents

The basic chemistry of carbon dioxide (CO_2) absorbents relies on an exothermic reaction combining CO_2 with calcium hydroxide ($Ca(OH)_2$) to form calcium carbonate ($CaCO_3$) and water (H_2O). Strong bases such as the metal hydroxides, sodium hydroxide (NaOH), potassium hydroxide (KOH), and barium hydroxide (BaOH), are added as catalysts to enhance the speed of the reaction and to increase the capacity to absorb CO_2. Absorbent brands are largely distinguished by the type and relative concentrations (3–20%) of strong bases (metal hydroxides) added to the $Ca(OH)_2$. There is also at least one absorbent, Amsorb® Plus (Armstrong Medical, Londonderry, UK) that contains no strong base.

The general chemical reaction when the strong base NaOH is present as the catalyst is as follows.

$$CO_2 + H_2O \rightleftharpoons H_2CO_3 \tag{6.1}$$

$$H_2CO_3 + 2NaOH \rightarrow Na_2CO_3 + 2H_2O + \text{energy} \tag{6.2}$$

$$Na_2CO_3 + Ca(OH)_2 \rightarrow CaCO_3 + 2NaOH \tag{6.3}$$

The general chemical reaction when no strong base (metal hydroxide) is added. The general chemical reaction when no strong base (metal hydroxide) is added is as follows:

$$CO_2 + H_2O \rightleftharpoons H_2CO_3 \tag{6.1}$$

$$H_2CO_3 + Ca(OH)_2 \rightarrow CaCO_3 + 2H_2O + \text{energy} \tag{6.4}$$

It is important to note that moisture is essential to the reaction allowing gaseous CO_2 to form carbonic acid (H_2CO_3) (eqn 6.1) so that it can react with $Ca(OH)_2$.

With the introduction of sevoflurane and desflurane in the early 1990s, it was discovered that both of these agents had the capacity to interact with CO_2 absorbents. Sevoflurane was found to interact and produce compound A, which was shown to be nephrotoxic in rats. Although compound A from sevoflurane use was never, and has never, been reported to cause a clinical problem in humans [81,82], many labels have nonetheless adopted the recommendation to maintain a minimum FGF of 2 L/min, thereby making its use in low-flow anesthesia unfeasible as per label guidelines. Desflurane was found to produce unacceptably high carbon monoxide (CO) concentrations, particularly in the presence of desiccated absorbents, so the general recommendation made was to use fresh absorbents (i.e., change them often) and use flow rates greater than 2–3 L/min [83,84]. Again, this makes using desflurane in a low-flow environment controversial. Further study identified that absorbents containing only $Ca(OH)_2$ were not associated with significant compound A or CO production leading to speculation that it is the added catalyst or strong base that leads to the production of undesirable byproducts [85]. However, the absorptive capacity of $Ca(OH)_2$ only absorbents (Amsorb®, Armstrong Medical, Londonberry, UK) was found to be 15–50% lower than those containing a strong base [85,86]. However, by adding small amounts of calcium chloride (2.0–3.5%) and calcium sulfate (0.6–1.5%) to the formulation, these limitations have been largely overcome by helping to increase CO_2 absorptive capacity and speeding the absorptive reaction [87]. Many current absorbents are either strong base free (Amsorb® Plus, Armstrong Medical, Londonberry, UK) with no risk for the production of toxic byproducts or they limit the amount of strong base (typically NaOH) to less than 3% to minimize the potential for the production of toxic byproducts. However, it appears that optimally those with concentrations of NaOH less than 2% (Sodasorb® LF, Molecular Products, Louisville, CO, USA; Drägersorb Free and Drägersorb 800, Dräger Medical, Lubeck, Germany; Medisorb, CareFusion, Helsinki, Finland) are preferred to avoid risks associated with compound A and CO production. The use of KOH and BaOH as catalysts seems increasingly uncommon in most commercially available products. There is also a newer product using solid absorbent technology (SpiraLith® Ca, Micropore Inc, Elkton, USA), where the $Ca(OH)_2$ is embedded on a solid polymer producing a non-granular dust-free product. However, this product is only available for use with modern human anesthetic machines with swappable absorbent canisters.

When in continuous use, the absorbents may appear exhausted (i.e., indicator color change) before the absorption capacity of the granules is exceeded. Granules normally turn from white to purple or pink as they become exhausted depending upon the indicator used. Ethyl violet (purple) and phenolphthalein (red) are pH-sensitive indicators commonly added to the granules to help identify absorbent exhaustion. The color change should not be used as the only indicator of absorbent exhaustion. It is common for absorbent that has changed color to turn back to white if allowed to stand unused for several hours. Fresh absorbent is normally easily crumbled under pressure, whereas used absorbent becomes hard (calcium carbonate). Additionally, since the reaction of carbon dioxide absorption produces heat and moisture, the activity of the absorbent may be evaluated by looking for evidence of both heat and moisture development within the canister. Also, where available, capnography can be used to detect absorbent exhaustion. The rate of absorbent exhaustion will be determined by the size of the patient (CO_2 production) and the rate of FGF (mL/kg/min). Absorbent exhaustion will occur faster in larger patients and when low FGF rates are used. The absorbent canister should be filled carefully to avoid overfilling, packing granules in the canister, and spilling granules into the breathing system.

Non-rebreathing systems

Non-rebreathing systems are characterized by the absence of unidirectional valves and a carbon dioxide absorber. Rather than relying on carbon dioxide absorption for removal of CO_2, these systems depend on high FGF rates to flush CO_2 from the circuit, dependent on the FGF rate. Non-rebreathing systems are normally reserved for patients under 10 kg as they are far less economical in larger patients owing to the use of high FGF rates required to prevent rebreathing of CO_2. Recommended flow rates to minimize the rebreathing of expired CO_2 range from 130 to 300 mL/kg/min, although values as high as 600 mL/kg/min have been recommended. The wide range of recommended flow rates is the result of the fact that in addition to the FGF rate, the patient's intrinsic respiratory pattern will influence if rebreathing occurs (discussed later).

Non-rebreathing systems have historically been recommended, somewhat arbitrarily, for use in all patients less than 5 kg, citing lower resistance during breathing, less equipment deadspace, and smaller total circuit volume. However, by using newer pediatric, neonatal, and small patient-specific rebreathing circuits, many of the advantages normally associated with non-rebreathing systems are negated and it is possible to maintain patients less than 5 kg safely using rebreathing systems provided that the patient's tidal volume is adequate to actuate the unidirectional valves. Small patient-specific circuits generally have no more, and in some cases less, deadspace and total volume than standard non-rebreathing systems (Fig. 6.62). Resistance to breathing is often cited as a reason for selecting non-rebreathing systems over circle systems, as the valves and carbon dioxide absorbent can increase the work of breathing. This is a highly over used and simplified concept as the relationship of resistance to work of breathing is complex and multifactorial with inspiratory/expiratory rates, FGFs, and endotracheal tube diameter and length all playing roles in the overall resistance to a patient breathing. Many studies make resistance claims simply by measuring the resistance of a given breathing system at the circuit adapter but in reality patients are not inspiring directly from the circuit but rather the distal end of the endotracheal tube attached to the circuit. In practice, it is actually the size of the endotracheal tube that is the major factor in determining resistance to breathing [88]. Hence, the resistance to breathing argument for selecting a non-rebreathing system over a rebreathing is largely unfounded and unsubstantiated.

There is no generally accepted or agreed upon minimum patient size for using a rebreathing system among anesthesiologists. The minimum patient size generally ranges between 3 and 7 kg, although individual anesthetists may choose patient sizes outside this range depending upon equipment, monitoring available (e.g., capnography for evaluation of rebreathing), and intended ventilation mode (spontaneous versus controlled).

Although the Mapleson system for classification of anesthetic breathing circuits was once popular, it has little relevance for today's commonly used non-rebreathing circuits, and diagrams are included here only for reference (Fig. 6.65 and Table 6.3). Although there are often three or more non-rebreathing systems commonly described for use in veterinary medicine in North America, all are nearly functionally identical and based on two of the six historically described Mapleson systems: D and F (see Fig. 6.66).

The non-rebreathing system includes a fresh gas-conducting hose, patient connection, exhalation-conducting tubing (normally corrugated), excess gas venting system, and a reservoir bag. All commonly used systems have the FGF entering near the patient connection and rely on the fresh gas inflow (flow dependent) to

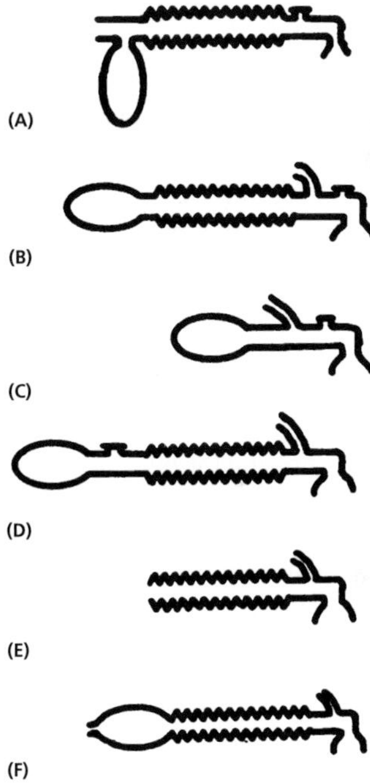

Figure 6.65 Diagrams of each of the historically described Mapleson breathing systems (**A** through **F**). Refer to Table 6.3 for characteristics of each system. Source: Rayburn [89]; reproduced with permission of the American Society of Anesthesiologists.

Table 6.3 Characteristics of the Mapleson breathing systems.

Class	Fresh gas inlet	Overflow location	Presence of a reservoir	Corrugated tubing	Example system
A	Near the reservoir	Near the patient	Yes	Yes	Magill
B	Near the patient	Near the patient	Yes	Yes	[a]
C	Near the patient	Near the patient	Yes	No	[a]
D	Near the patient	Away from the patient[b]	Yes	Yes	[a]
MD[c]	Near the patient	Away from the patient	Yes	Yes	Bain
E	Near the patient	Away from the patient	No	Yes	T-piece
F	Near the patient	Away from the patient[b]	Yes	Yes	Jackson-Rees

[a] No system in this classification is commonly used in veterinary anesthesia.
[b] The overflow may be located between the reservoir and the corrugated tubing of the system.
[c] MD, modified Mapleson D system.

displace the CO_2-containing expired breath down a variable length of conducting tubing toward the reservoir bag and ultimately into the scavenge system. High FGFs are necessary to help minimize the rebreathing of expired gases.

During the expiratory pause, the high FGF from the fresh gas-conducting tube pushes the exhaled gas from the previous expiration down the exhalation-conducting tube away from the patient toward the reservoir bag. When the patient inspires, it inspires gas coming from both the fresh gas-conducting tube and the exhalation-conducting tube. Under normal circumstances (i.e., patient with a normal respiratory pattern and inspiratory flow rate), the majority of the inspired breath normally comes from the exhalation-conducting tube. In some circumstances (i.e., patients with unusual respiratory patterns), a patient may rebreathe exhaled gases despite seemingly sufficient FGFs. For example, a patient breathing rapidly may not have an expiratory pause of sufficient duration for CO_2 to be washed distal enough from the patient end of the tube to prevent rebreathing, particularly if a sufficiently large breath is taken. End-tidal carbon dioxide monitoring can be useful in determining if adequate FGFs are being used to minimize rebreathing.

The Bain and the Modified Jackson-Rees systems are probably the names most commonly applied to non-rebreathing systems, but they do not adequately describe the systems as they are frequently used in veterinary medicine. Neither system is a specifically defined system in that they are not always reliably configured in the same manner. Based on the historical descriptions of these circuits, the Bain circuit (based on a Mapleson D system) would have an APL valve proximal to the reservoir bag, whereas the Modified Jackson-Rees (based on a Mapleson F system) would have a pinch or stopcock valve located distal to the reservoir bag. However, both breathing systems can be adapted for use with a mounting block and various reservoir bag and venting system combinations, making strict classification nearly impossible. Essentially, the main difference between how the two systems function clinically is that one is a coaxial design (Bain) and the other is not (Modified Jackson-Rees). Perhaps a less confusing and consistent way to classify the commonly used non-rebreathing circuits in veterinary medicine would be based on the configuration of the conducting tubing (i.e., coaxial or non-coaxial), location of scavenge system (i.e., proximal or distal to the reservoir bag), and method of scavenging (APL valve, pinch valve, or stopcock type valve).

The coaxial design of the Bain system reduces the overall bulk and provides a method to potentially warm the cold-inspired gases. Mounting blocks are convenient methods for arranging non-rebreathing systems by providing fixed connection points for the breathing circuit, reservoir bag, and scavenge tubing (Fig. 6.67). The use of a mounting block minimizes the potential for misconnections, disconnections, or kinked hoses. The fixed positioning relative to the anesthetic machine also allows the anesthetist to assess readily the integrity of all connections.

Non-rebreathing systems used without a mounting block can be placed anywhere in the anesthetic work area and run the risk of being covered by drapes hanging off surgical tables or being pulled or caught by moving legs or equipment in the operating room, all increasing the possibility of anesthetic complications. Most mounting blocks also have a pressure manometer built into the system, which is an invaluable addition enabling the user to monitor and assess changes in airway pressure. Most non-rebreathing systems sold to veterinarians are not configured with a pressure manometer as part of the standard system, which, along with high FGFs and relatively small circuit volumes, exposes patients to the potential for accidental barotrauma. One solution to overcome this problem if a mounting block with manometer is not available is to purchase disposable pressure manometers designed for use with a resuscitation bag. These can be easily placed within all non-rebreathing systems, used many times over, and are an inexpensive method of evaluating airway pressures (Fig. 6.68). Alternatively, high patient pressure alarms are available that can be inserted into the system between the patient and the valve used to isolate the breathing system from the scavenge system.

Waste gas scavenge system

The scavenge system directs waste gases from the anesthetic breathing circuit out of the immediate workspace and into the atmosphere. Ideally, the scavenge system includes the APL valve, an interface, and a waste gas elimination system (Fig. 6.69), although it is important to note that these components may not be found as part of all scavenge systems. Many systems in use consist of a hose connected to the APL valve (or other breathing circuit outlet) to a vent leading outside the immediate work area. The waste gas elimination system may be either an active or a passive system. A passive system does not use negative pressure (e.g., it opens to atmospheric pressure), whereas an active system uses a slight vacuum. The type of waste gas elimination system will determine the need and type of waste gas interface required. Passive waste gas systems may use an activated charcoal canister to absorb halogenated anesthetics or they may divert the waste anesthetic gases through a short conduit outside the work environment directly to the atmosphere.

Negative-pressure scavenge (vacuum) systems are increasingly being used in veterinary medicine. They may be part of a surgical vacuum (suction) system, stand-alone vacuum, fan/blower system, or other design since there are no specific standards regarding these systems. All negative-pressure scavenge systems require some type of scavenge interface to operate properly and prevent the patient airway from experiencing a vacuum. Ideally, waste gas scavenge interfaces should have means of managing both excessive positive and negative pressure, a reservoir system to accommodate rapid changes in waste gas delivery to the scavenge system, and a means of inactivating any halogenated gas that escapes the scavenge system (Fig. 6.70). Most scavenge interfaces fail to meet all these specifications under all the variable circumstances encountered during use (e.g., high negative-pressure scavenge systems, pressure alterations within the vacuum system, and marked alterations in the rate of waste gases exhausted to the scavenge system), but most perform adequately under normal operating conditions.

Low negative-pressure scavenge systems (blower or fan systems) work well with most scavenge interfaces. These systems are often dedicated to waste gas scavenge and may be centrally located or located at the machine itself. These are often blower- or fan-driven systems that do not maintain a steady evacuation rate (negative pressure) at all times and in all locations. Several factors, such as the number of sites they serve, the diameter of vacuum conduit, the distance from the blower or fan, and the number of sites being used, can affect evacuation rates at any given location. Higher-negative-pressure scavenge systems are most commonly found in larger facilities with centrally located medical vacuum systems and the active scavenge system works off the same negative-pressure system as used for medical suction. Although it is often seen as more convenient and cost-effective to use the same vacuum system for all functions in the hospital, there are some unique challenges associated with this type of installation. Since these systems are under a

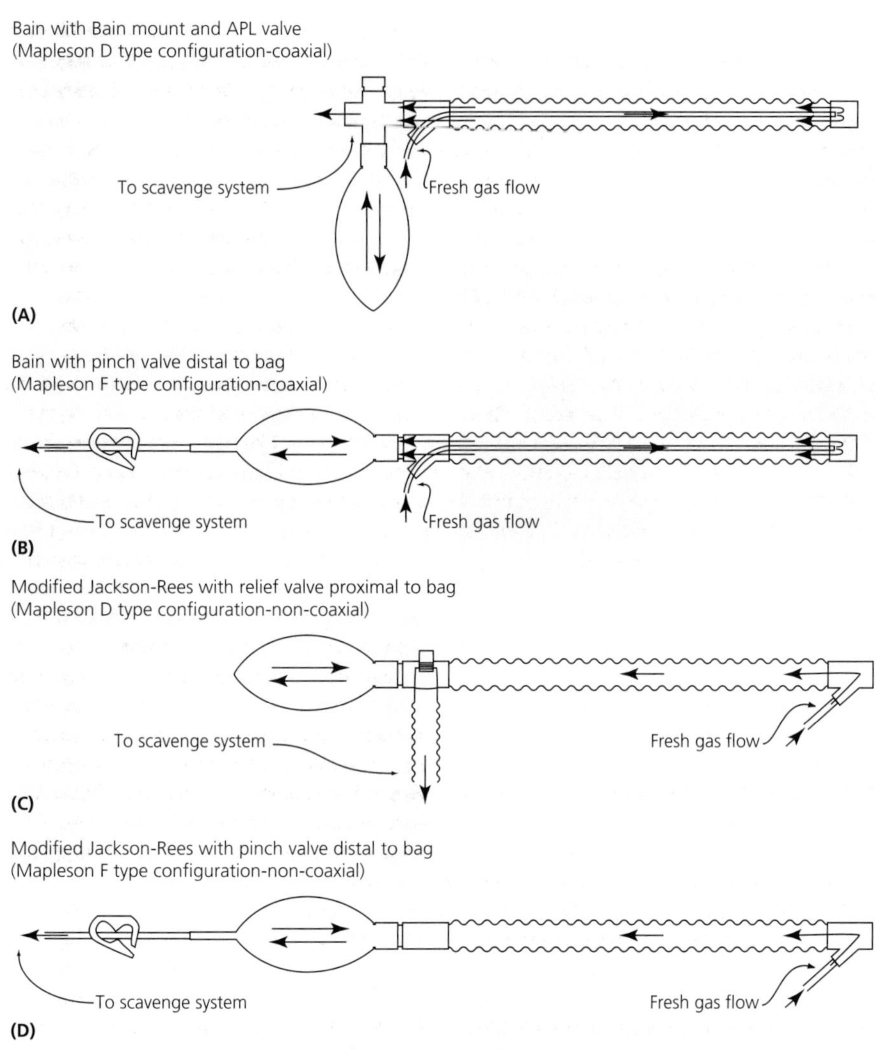

Figure 6.66 Diagrams of the Mapleson-type systems used most commonly as the foundation for modern non-rebreathing systems. Most modern non-rebreathing systems are modifications of the Mapleson classification and can no longer be strictly classified as one type or the other. For example, the Bain circuit is a coaxial system based on the Mapleson D classification, but it can be configured with the exhaust gas exiting prior to the reservoir bag as shown in **A.** (like Mapleson D), or after the reservoir bag as shown in **B.** (like Mapleson F). The Jackson-Rees circuit is a non-coaxial system that can be configured similarly with the exhaust gas exiting before the reservoir bag as shown in **C.** (like Mapleson D), or after the reservoir bag as shown in **D.** (like Mapleson F). Source: Dr. Kath Klassen, Douglas College, New Westminster, Canada; reproduced with permission of Dr. Klassen.

significant amount of negative pressure relative to that needed for scavenging, they require adjustable scavenge interfaces to regulate the level of suction at the scavenge interface and frequent minor adjustments to prevent the collapse of the reservoir bag of the breathing system. Regardless of the type of scavenge system used, canisters of activated charcoal should be available for situations where other modes of waste anesthetic gas scavenge are not available (e.g., when moving patients attached to the anesthetic machine, or when working in areas without scavenging facilities).

Routine anesthesia machine checkout procedure

Routine evaluation of the anesthetic machine and associated systems prior to and throughout the anesthetic period should be part of every anesthetist's standard operating procedures (SOP). Historically, equipment failures appear to have been a relatively common cause of anesthetic-related morbidity and mortality [2]. However, with improvements in technology and monitoring and the adoption of universal safety standards for human anesthetic equipment, complications related to equipment malfunctions have been reduced. Preanesthetic equipment checkout recommendations for human anesthetic equipment have been developed in conjunction with regulatory, industry, and anesthesia personnel and have been published in many countries. Unfortunately, there is no generally recognized standard for preanesthetic checkout recommendations in veterinary medicine. However, an excellent checklist for veterinary anesthetists developed by Hartsfield has been proposed that is based on the United States FDA's Center for Devices and Radiological Health "Anesthesia Apparatus Checkout Recommendations" [75,90]. Table 6.4 presents a modified summary of the checklist proposed by Hartsfield.

Anesthesia ventilators

The anesthesia ventilator is designed to provide patient ventilation in the perianesthetic period. Most anesthesia ventilators lack the sophistication of control and function found in intensive care unit

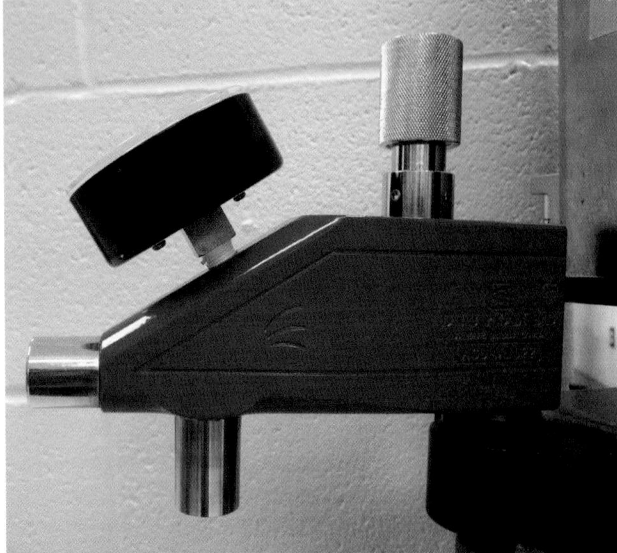

Figure 6.67 A mounting block (sometimes also referred to as a "Bain mount" although not exclusive for use with Bain circuits only) provides fixed connection points for the non-rebreathing circuit, the reservoir bag, and scavenge tubing. Most also incorporate an adjustable pressure-limiting (APL) valve and pressure gauge. Source: Dr. Craig Mosley, with permission.

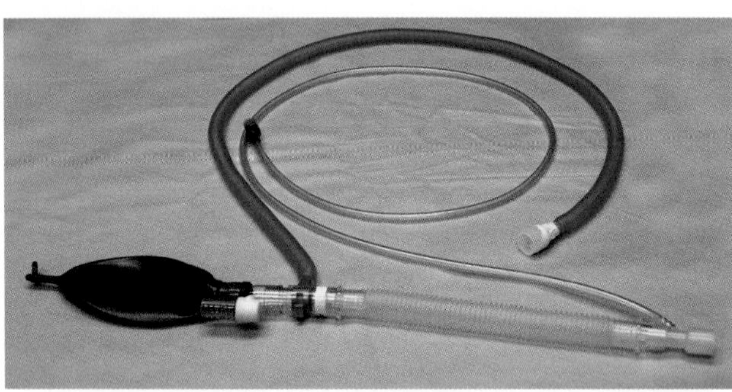

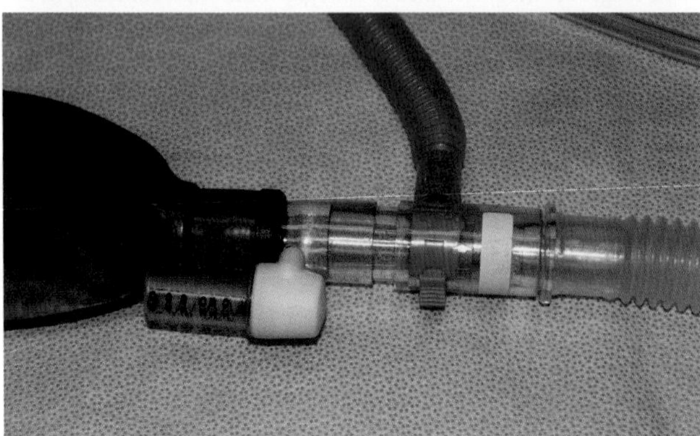

Figure 6.68 An example of a disposable resuscitation bag manometer that can be adapted for use with most non-rebreathing systems. The presence of the manometer will allow the anesthetist to evaluate better the airway pressures within the breathing system. Source: Dr. Craig Mosley, with permission.

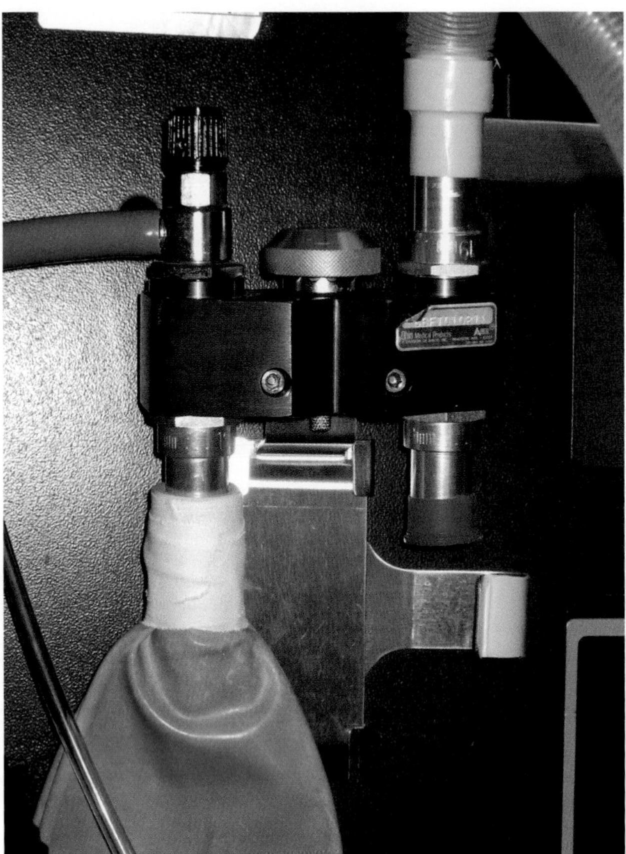

Figure 6.69 An adjustable scavenge interface with both positive- and negative-pressure relief functions. These types of interfaces work well with active scavenge systems. Source: Dr. Craig Mosley, with permission.

(ICU) ventilators and work best when used to ventilate patients with relatively normal lung function and simple ventilation needs. However, some human- and veterinary-specific anesthesia ventilators now offer features and performance rivaling those of a basic ICU ventilator. In North America, anesthesia ventilators designed for use in humans are subject to a series of international and national standards, whereas ventilators designed for the veterinary market are under no obligation to meet any similar design standards. Once again this makes it imperative that the veterinary anesthetist not only fully understands the physiological and practical implications of ventilator use but is also intimately familiar with the design, function, and troubleshooting of any ventilator used.

Classification

Ventilators are variably classified by a number of different criteria describing their design and control. Unfortunately, there are several inconsistencies in the use of the terminology and their definitions. There is also no generally accepted consensus as to how to classify anesthesia ventilators and some ventilators simply cannot be adequately described using current classification schemes. For example, some modern human anesthesia ventilators are sophisticated processor-controlled machines capable of multiple ventilation modes and deliver similar performance to ICU ventilators, hence they are not easily classified using current criteria. The most commonly used criteria used to describe or classify ventilators include the major control variable, the type of power source, the drive mechanism, the cycling mechanism, and the type of bellows.

Major control variable

Most ventilators are described as pressure- or volume-controlled ventilators. This refers to the target, preset, or limiting variable used to determine the tidal volume delivered by the ventilator. In a

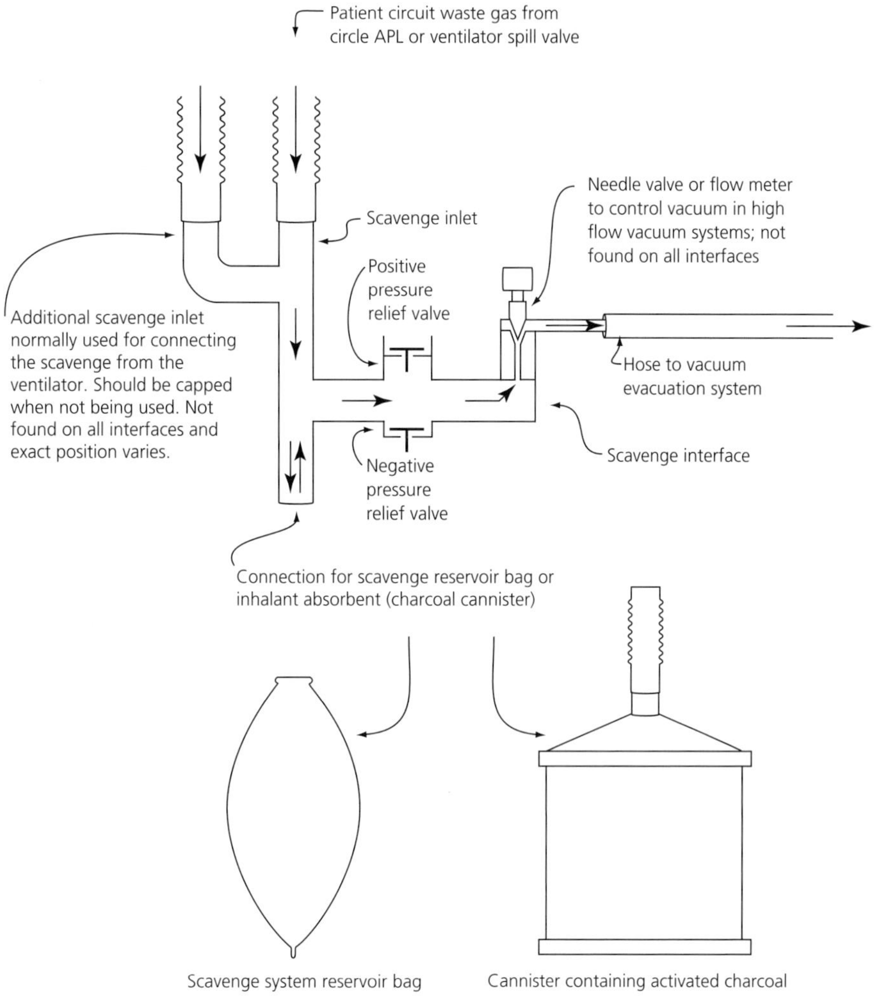

Figure 6.70 Diagram of a scavenge interface. The exact configurations of commercially available scavenge interfaces vary considerably and may not contain all the components shown. Source: Dr. Kath Klassen, Douglas College, New Westminster, Canada; reproduced with permission of Dr. Klassen.

volume-limited ventilator, the tidal volume is predetermined and will be delivered regardless of the associated pressures required to do so. This is not a precisely accurate statement as many ventilators (anesthetic machines/circuits) have built-in pressure relief or alarm systems that will activate and limit the volume delivered if excessively high airway pressures are reached. Additionally, changes in circuit and patient compliance will alter the actual tidal volume delivered to the patient compared with the apparent tidal volume set on the ventilator (see the later section, Factors that affect delivered tidal volume). This effect is normally negligible, as sustained significant changes in system or patient respiratory compliance are unlikely during a routine case. With a pressure-limited ventilator, a peak inspiratory pressure preset is used to limit the tidal volume delivered to the patient. The delivered volume can be affected by changes in patient respiratory or circuit compliance/resistance, inspiratory flow rates, leaks, inspiratory time, and the location of the pressure sensor.

Power source

The power source typically refers to what is required to operate a mechanical ventilator. It may be compressed gas, electricity, or both. Although not generally accepted, it may be more useful to classify ventilators based on what actually powers positive-pressure ventilation: compressed gas or an electronically controlled piston. Although historically many ventilators did not contain sophisticated microprocessors requiring electricity and required only compressed gas to function, most modern ventilators have some electrical components regardless of what actually produces positive-pressure ventilation. The drive mechanism normally refers more specifically to how positive-pressure ventilation is actually produced.

Drive mechanism/circuit

Either compressed gas or an electronically driven mechanical device, such as a piston, can drive ventilators. Ventilators using compressed gas for power are normally referred to as "dual-circuit ventilators," as they have two gas circuits, one containing gas to power the ventilator and the other containing gas being delivered to the patient. Ventilators that do not use gas to power ventilation are referred to as "single-circuit ventilators." There is also at least one commercially available ventilator design that uses compressed gas as its power source but contains neither a bellows nor a piston and is technically a single-circuit ventilator, the Penlon Nuffield 200 (Penlon Ltd, Abingdon, UK). However, this ventilator can also be combined with a bellows canister system ("bag in a box"), creating

Table 6.4 Ensuring that all equipment is properly functioning is a crucial step that should be performed prior to initiating anesthesia. The proposed equipment checkout recommendations are based on the United States FDA's Center for Devices and Radiological Health "Anesthesia Apparatus Checkout Recommendations."

Veterinary Anesthesia Apparatus Checkout Recommendations*

This anesthesia checkout list does not replace the experience of a knowledgeable operator continuously monitoring the anesthetic equipment. All parts of the anesthesia machine and breathing system should be present, properly functioning, free of defects, and correctly connected. This checklist includes the assessment of automated ventilators and patient monitors if they are present.

High-pressure system

Central gas supplies (oxygen, nitrous oxide, and air) should be adequate in quantity and pressure. The central pipeline pressure should not fluctuate and should remain at its preset level (normally about 50 psi) when flowmeters on the anesthesia machine are adjusted to a 3–5 L/min flow rate.

Portable gas supplies (oxygen cylinders on the anesthesia machine) should be adequate in quantity and pressure. These cylinders should be evaluated for leaks. With the flowmeter off and the cylinder valve open, there should be no audible leaks or decrease in cylinder pressure over time (i.e., 10 min).

Low-pressure system

Test the flowmeters of each gas. With the flow control off, the float should rest on the bottom of the glass tube. Adjust the flowmeter throughout its full range, the float should move smoothly with no sticking or erratic movements.

Vaporizers should be filled, filler caps tightened, and the control dial in the off position. The inlet and outlet connections should be in place and secure.

Leak test the low-pressure system.

a. Attach a "suction bulb" to the common gas outlet.
b. Squeeze the bulb until fully collapsed.
c. Verify the bulb stays fully collapsed for at least 10 s.
d. Open each vaporizer one at a time, if more than two vaporizers, and repeat steps (b) and (c) with each vaporizer.

Scavenge system

Ensure proper connection between the scavenge system and the APL valve.

Adjust the waste gas vacuum flow, if possible, to meet the needs of the individual case.

With the APL fully open and the patient port occluded.

a. Allow the scavenge reservoir back to fully collapse and verify that the circuit pressure gauge reads about zero.
b. With the oxygen flush valve activated, allow the scavenge reservoir bag to distend fully and then verify that the circuit pressure gauge reads less than 10 cmH_2O.

If the scavenge system involves a charcoal canister, the quality of the charcoal absorbent should be assessed.

Breathing system

Rebreathing (circle) system

Ensure the selected circuit and reservoir bag size are appropriate for the patient.

Check the breathing system is complete, undamaged, and unobstructed.

Verify that the carbon dioxide absorbent is adequate.

Perform a leak test of the breathing system.

a. Set all gas flows to zero (or minimum).
b. Close the APL valve and occlude the Y-piece.
c. Pressurize the breathing system using the flush valve to a pressure of about 30 cmH_2O.
d. Ensure the pressure remains fixed for at least 10 s. Alternatively, the leak rate required to maintain at 30 cmH_2O should be less than 300 mL/min.
e. Open the APL and ensure the pressure decreases appropriately.

Non-rebreathing system

Ensure the selected circuit and reservoir bag size are appropriate for the patient.

Check the breathing system is complete, undamaged, and unobstructed.

Perform a leak test of the breathing system.

a. Set all gas flows to zero (or minimum).
b. Close the APL valve and occlude the patient port.
c. Pressurize the breathing system using the flush valve to a pressure of about 30 cmH_2O. If there is no pressure gauge associated with the breathing system, the reservoir bag should remain fully distended with no loss of pressure.
d. For Bain systems (coaxial Mapleson D), the integrity of the inner tube should be evaluated. With the flowmeter set to 1 L/min, the inner tube should be briefly occluded, and the float of the flowmeter should fall to near zero.
e. Open the APL valve and ensure the pressure decreases appropriately.

Ventilator

Place a second reservoir bag on the patient circuit, appropriate for the size of the patient.

Set the appropriate ventilator parameters for the patient.

Connect the ventilator as directed by the manufacturer and fill the bellows and reservoir bag using the flush valve.

Turn the ventilator on and ensure adequate tidal volumes are delivered and that during expiration the bellows fill completely.

Check for the proper action of the unidirectional valves of the circle, if applicable.

Manipulate ventilation parameters to ensure all are functioning normally.

Turn off the ventilator and disconnect as directed by the manufacturer.

Monitors

Ensure all cables and connectors are present.

Ensure all alarms are appropriately set.

* Owing to the significant variability and lack of standards among veterinary anesthesia equipment, not all checkout procedures will apply to all anesthetic machines.

a dual-circuit ventilator. The lack of physical barrier in this design can potentially allow mixing of gas from the circuit used to power the ventilator with gas from the patient circuit. However, the clinical significance of mixing is minimal provided that FGF rates are suitable to ensure non-rebreathing. Any mixing between ventilator driving gas and patient circuit gas should only involve the exhaled patient gas being moved through the breathing circuit destined for evacuation and collection into the scavenge system.

Cycling mechanism

"Cycling mechanism" is a term that is used to describe how a ventilator cycles from inspiration to expiration and back. It is probably also the term used most inconsistently. The cycling in most ventilators is determined by a timing mechanism, although in at least one commonly used ventilator (Bird Mark series ventilators), pressure rather than time can be used to cycle the ventilator. An electronic microprocessor or a fluid logic unit can control the timing mechanism. Electronic timing mechanisms dominate current ventilators, although some fluid logic control systems are still produced. Before the advent of readily available microprocessors and electronics, fluid logic control was popular and can be found on many older ventilators still in use today (e.g., Air-Shields, Ohio V5A, and Metomatic). Electronic microprocessor units essentially open and close valves allowing gas to drive the ventilator or, in the case of a piston design, they activate movement of the piston. Fluid logic units work through use of compressed gas, normally at a constant pressure, to activate timing valves for inspiration and expiration. The amount of gas needed to activate these timing valves and hence inspiratory and expiratory times can be altered by increasing or decreasing the flow of gas into the timing valve, producing shorter or longer activation times. Ultimately, these valves are opened and closed by changes in gas pressure within the timing valves and it is likely this fact that has led to some confusion and misuse of terminology. Although pressure changes are used to activate the inspiratory and expiratory timers, these ventilators are strictly still time cycled with pressure being used to produce predictable fluid timers. The term "pressure cycled" should be reserved for those ventilators where pressure within the patient circuit is responsible for cycling the ventilator. The Bird Mark series of ventilators can be pressure cycled. The timing for inspiration in these ventilators is a function of the duration of time required to attain a specific pressure within the patient circuit during positive-pressure ventilation. The cycling duration can be modified by gas flow rates driving the ventilator and changes in patient lung compliance. When using these ventilators, the inspiration will continue until a specific pressure threshold is achieved regardless of the time required to achieve the pressure. The term "volume cycled" has been applied to anesthesia ventilators; however, timing mechanisms are generally the foundation of these ventilators and the term "volume cycled" should be reserved for describing a specific mode of ventilation normally possible only using an ICU-type ventilator and some advanced anesthesia ventilators equipped with spirometry and microprocessors capable of compensating for tidal volume changes caused by changes in lung and circuit compliance. The use of the terms "pressure cycled" and "volume cycled" should not be confused with the terms "pressure limited" and "volume limited," which are used to describe the principal factors that limit the tidal volume delivered to a patient. In essence, all time-cycled ventilators are volume limited, and only pressure-cycled ventilators are pressure-limited.

Bellows

If a ventilator has a bellows, they can be classified as ascending or descending. This terminology refers to the direction of the bellows during expiration and often creates confusion. The terms "standing" and "hanging" are perhaps more intuitive and are used to describe the ascending and descending bellows configuration, respectively. This then refers to the position of the bellows during the expiratory pause or prior to the initiation of ventilation.

Introduction to single- and dual-circuit ventilators

Most anesthesia ventilators used in veterinary medicine are electronically time-cycled ventilators and can be classified as either a dual-circuit gas-driven ventilator or single-circuit piston-driven ventilator. However, there are at least two compressed gas-powered ventilators that can be used as both dual- and single-circuit ventilators, depending upon how they are configured. They will be discussed separately later (see Single-circuit compressed gas-powered ventilators). It is important to note that the use of the term "single-circuit ventilator" by itself can be misleading. Historically, it has been used to describe ventilators using two gases (ventilator driving gas and patient circuit gas) that operate within a single circuit (i.e., there is no physical barrier between the gases). In this situation, there is the possibility of ventilator driving gas mixing with gas in the patient circuit. It is therefore more descriptive to include the terms "piston-driven" or "compressed gas–driven" when using the term "single circuit" to describe veterinary ventilators.

The anesthesia ventilator normally replaces the reservoir bag and APL valve of the anesthesia machine with a bellows (or piston chamber) and spill valve (i.e., dump or relief valve), respectively, but even here, there are exceptions in ventilator design and use. One manufacturer's design does not replace the reservoir bag and APL valve of the anesthetic machine but instead it is simply added to the patient circuit (Merlin, Vetronic Services, Abbotskerswell, Devon, UK).

Single-circuit piston-driven ventilators

Piston-driven ventilators use electronically controlled pistons to compress gas in the breathing circuit. The use of an electronically controlled piston eliminates the need for a second circuit (i.e., the driving gas), and this typically enables the ventilator to deliver tidal volumes more precisely since it will not be influenced by the presence of a compressible driving gas. Piston-driven ventilators are also more efficient in terms of gas use since additional gas is not required to drive the ventilator and they are normally controlled by sophisticated electronics that can provide more advanced modes of ventilation and cycling options. Electrical power is used to raise and lower the piston using a servomotor and ball screw assembly (linear actuator). Piston-driven ventilators can offer the user a very wide range of sophisticated ventilation options typically unavailable using common dual-circuit ventilators.

Each piston-driven ventilator is unique in its specific design, but most will share some of the following features: a cylinder, piston, linear actuator, rolling diaphragms, and positive/negative-pressure relief valves. The exact configuration of each component and mechanism for facilitating expiration and spontaneous breathing will vary among manufacturers. The Tafonius large animal anesthetic workstation ventilator (Hallowell EMC, Pittsfield, MA, USA) is a veterinary-specific piston-driven ventilator and will be used as an example for describing the operation of a piston-driven anesthetic ventilator. Descriptions of other piston-driven ventilators designed for human use such as the Dräger Apollo, Divan, or Fabius GS ventilator are available elsewhere [91].

There are two rolling diaphragms that seal the piston of the Tafonius ventilator to prevent mixing of ambient and patient circuit gas (Fig. 6.71). The lower diaphragm seals the breathing gas below the piston in the breathing system. The upper diaphragm seals the upper side of the lower diaphragm from ambient air, creating a space between the two diaphragms. A vacuum is applied to this space that holds the two diaphragms tightly against the piston and cylinder walls. As the piston is actuated, it moves downward and the space below the lower diaphragm decreases, forcing gas into the patient's lungs; at the end of inspiration the patient exhales and the piston rises. During controlled ventilation, the piston drives the inspiration according to the ventilator settings. When the patient expires, the piston moves in response to the measured airway pressure, measured at the patient Y-piece. When the airway pressure increases by 0.5 cmH_2O, the piston is moved up enough to bring the airway pressure back to zero. This correction is made every 5 ms

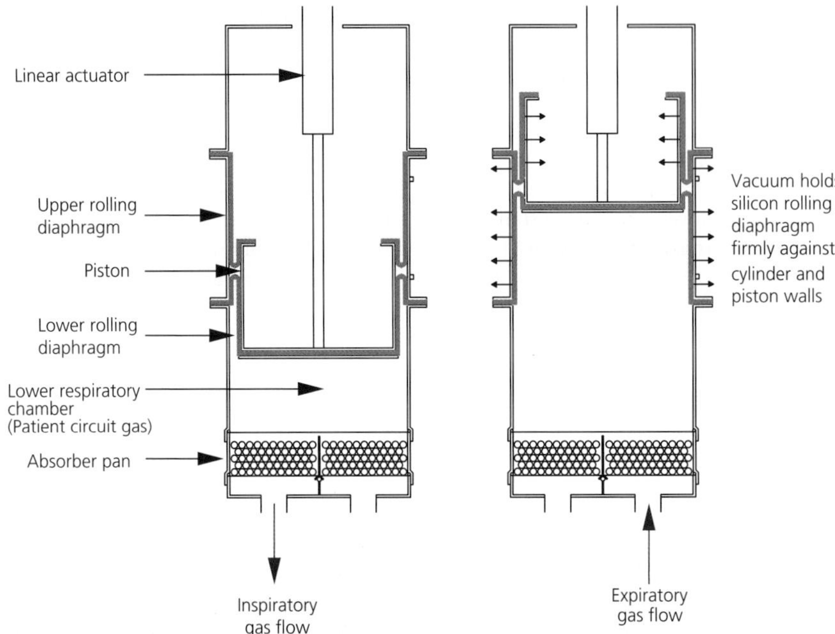

Figure 6.71 Configuration of a piston-driven ventilator (Tafonius rolling diaphragm system) during inspiration (left) and expiration (right), demonstrating various features and general principles of operation. Source: Hallowell EMC, Pittsfield, MA, USA; modified with permission.

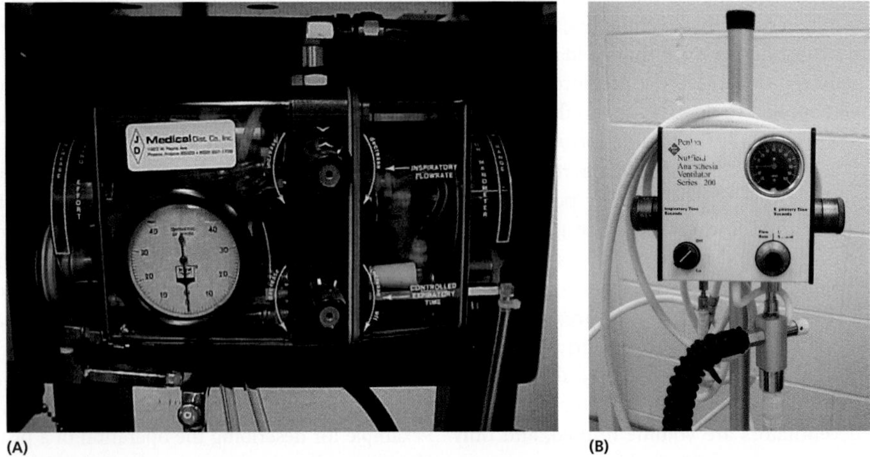

Figure 6.72 Examples of compressed gas-powered ventilators. **A.** Bird respirator. **B.** Penlon Nuffield 200 ventilator. They can be used as single- and dual-circuit ventilators, although the latter configuration is by far the most commonly used and most intuitive configuration. The patient valve, located on the bottom of the Penlon Nuffield ventilator, acts as a connection point for the ventilator drive gas controlled by the control unit, the conducting hose to the patient circuit (black corrugated tube), and the spill valve to the scavenge. Drive gas is delivered to this valve during inspiration pushing gas toward the patient. During expiration, the valve opens allowing excess gas to spill into the scavenge system. Source: Dr. Craig Mosley, with permission.

(200 times/s). This ensures that, unless desired, there is no resistance to exhalation (i.e., positive end-expiratory pressure [PEEP]).

Most standard standing bellows will have mandatory PEEP (2–4 cmH_2O) due to the design of the ventilator spill valve that is required to compensate for the weight of the bellows. During spontaneous breathing, the piston moves both upwards (expiration) and downwards (inspiration) in response to changes in measured airway pressure, ensuring that the airway pressure is maintained near zero. Expiration will occur as noted above, while conversely during inspiration when the airway pressure decreases by 0.5 cmH_2O, the piston will move down enough to bring the airway pressure back to zero. Electronic positive and negative relief valves are located at the scavenge manifold to protect against excessive positive or negative pressure within the patient circuit.

Single-circuit compressed gas-powered ventilators

There are at least two compressed gas-powered ventilators available in veterinary anesthesia that can be configured as single-circuit ventilators: Bird Mark series ventilators and Penlon Nuffield 200 ventilators (Fig. 6.72). When used as a single-circuit ventilator, there is no physical barrier between the gas that drives ventilation and the gas in the patient circuit. However, these ventilators do have two separate gas "circuits," the ventilator driving gas and the patient circuit gas, hence the use of the term "single circuit" is slightly misleading. The patient gas and the ventilator driving gas simply move within (or share) the same continuous circuit, with no physical barrier between the ventilator drive gas and the patient gas. Hence, they operate within a single physically uninterrupted gas circuit. It is important to note that the Bird Mark respirator and Penlon Nuffield 200 are commonly used as dual-circuit ventilators by combining them with bellows in a canister ("bag in a box"), as described later. A gas-powered single-circuit ventilator should only be used with non-rebreathing flow rates (and non-rebreathing circuits Mapleson D or F) to prevent contamination of the patient circuit with ventilator drive gas. As non-rebreathing flow rates are required, these types of ventilator configurations are best suited for use in smaller patients, although it is possible to ventilate larger patients requiring tidal volumes of approximately 1000 mL, but the efficiency of gas (oxygen and inhalant) consumption required is markedly reduced.

The Penlon Nuffield 200 ventilator is marketed and described as a single-circuit ventilator (see Fig. 6.72B). The ventilator is connected to the bag mount of the circuit by a long, corrugated tube that acts as a "reservoir," replacing the reservoir bag. The ventilator drive gas moves "to and from" the patient through this tube. The patient's exhaled gases will also move through this tube and will be scavenged from a so-called "patient" valve. The patient valve acts as a spill valve, allowing all excess gas – the drive gas from the ventilator, exhaled gas from the patient, and any excess FGF – to leave the system. The ventilator drive gas and the patient gas move within the same circuit without any physical separation, hence the term "single circuit." During inspiration, the patient valve closes, forcing the ventilatordriving gas into the "reservoir" tube, compressing the circuit gas back toward the patient, leading to inspiration. During the expiratory pause, the patient valve opens, allowing the ventilator driving gas to exit the system immediately as the pressure within the circuit drops back to zero. This gas is followed by the exhaled gas of the patient being pushed away from the patient as a result of the non-rebreathing FGF being delivered to the patient circuit. The FGF rate must be sufficiently high to prevent rebreathing of expired gases (i.e., a volume of fresh gas greater than or matching the patient's tidal volume must be delivered to the circuit during each respiratory cycle in order to minimize rebreathing of CO_2). The tidal volume is created by the combined effect of the volume of drive gas delivered by the ventilator and the volume of FGF entering the circuit during inspiration.

Dual-circuit ventilators

Dual-circuit ventilators have a physical separation between the ventilator driving gas and the patient circuit gas. Dual-circuit ventilators comprises the bellows assembly and the control mechanism for the drive gas. The control mechanism is normally an electronic microprocessor in most modern ventilators, but some older ventilators used fluid logic units to control the drive gas. The bellows assembly replaces the reservoir bag and APL valve and comprises the following components: bellows, housing, housing exhaust valve, spill valve, and ventilator hose connection (Fig. 6.73).

The primary circuit is continuous with the patient circuit and consists of the bellows and the spill valve. The second circuit contains the driving gas used to compress the bellows. The breathing circuit and the driving gas circuit are not connected or continuous; the bellows acts as a compliant barrier between these two circuits. Drive gas is allowed into the bellows housing for a specific period of time and delivered at a specified rate; during this time, the housing exhaust valve is closed, causing compression of the bellows and closing the spill valve. This forces gas inside the bellows to move toward the patient's lungs, expanding the chest. During expiration, the driving gas is discontinued (the housing pressure and consequently the patient circuit pressure drop) and the gas in the bellows housing is allowed to escape from an exhaust valve, allowing the patient to exhale passively into the bellows. The spill valve reopens, allowing excess FGF from the patient circuit to escape, preventing pressure from building up within the patient circuit. Although there are specific design differences in the way these functions are accomplished among dual-circuit ventilators, the general principles are similar.

Bellows configuration

The bellows is an accordion-like device attached to either the top or bottom of the bellows assembly. Anesthesia ventilators can be configured with ascending (standing) or descending (hanging) bellows (Fig. 6.74). The terms "ascending" and "descending" refer to the direction in which the bellows moves during exhalation and have been used historically to describe the orientation of the bellows. However, it is becoming increasingly common to replace these terms with "standing" (ascending) or "hanging" (descending) to describe the position of the bellows during the expiratory pause; this is often considered a more intuitive description of the configuration of the bellows. The vast majority of modern ventilators use a standing (ascending) bellows configuration where the bellows moves toward the base of the ventilator during inspiration and expand upward during exhalation. The tidal volume may be set by adjusting the inspiratory time and/or flow rate, or by a plate or other limiting device that limits the upward excursion of the bellows (see Fig. 6.73).

The spill valves on ventilators with standing bellows normally pose slight resistance (2–4 cmH_2O) to opening, thus creating slight PEEP in the system. This is to counteract the tendency of the bellows to collapse due to their weight and elastic nature. In the case of very large and heavy bellows, this may have the effect of producing a clinically relevant amount of PEEP. In some cases, this may be considered desirable, but at least one manufacturer has developed a method to overcome this PEEP effect by providing the option of applying a slight vacuum to the interior of the bellows housing. A desirable feature of the standing bellows configuration is that should a leak occur in the breathing system, the bellows will fail to expand fully and progressively collapse during the expiratory pause. A leak can be readily detected by an observant anesthetist.

The hanging (descending) bellows is attached to the top of the ventilator assembly and is compressed upwards during inspiration. During exhalation, the bellows descends passively, facilitated by a weight placed in the dependent portion of the bellows. As the bellows descends, it can cause a slight negative pressure in the bellows and breathing system. If a leak or disconnection develops in the breathing system, the weight of the bellows will cause the bellow to expand normally, drawing extraneous gases into the breathing system through the leak or a negative-pressure relief valve. During the subsequent inspiration, not only will the gas in the breathing circuit be diluted by the non-anesthetic-containing gases, but all or some of the inspiration will be lost through the leak. Leaks (particularly large leaks) in the breathing system are not as readily identified by visually assessing the bellows using this type of ventilator configuration compared with the standing configuration, hence its infrequent use in modern designs. However, it is possible

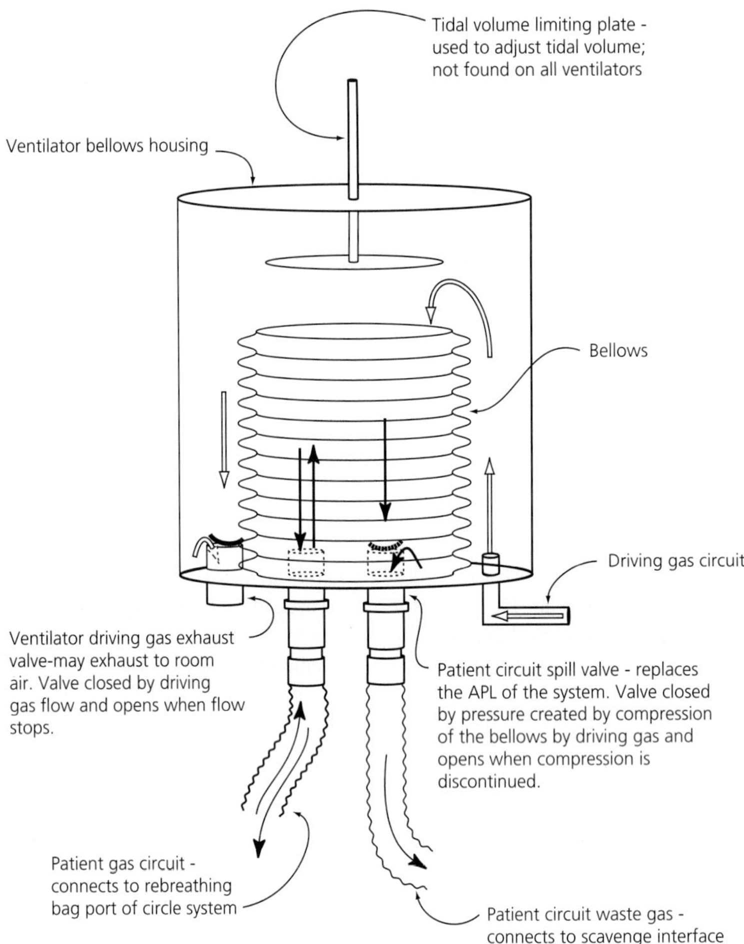

Figure 6.73 Schematic diagram of a generic dual-circuit ventilator demonstrating the gas flows within the ventilator during inspiration and expiration. Note that the exact position and design of the various components vary among manufacturers. Source: Dr. Kath Klassen, Douglas College, New Westminster, Canada; reproduced with permission of Dr. Klassen.

to detect small leaks that are made more significant by high pressure. For example, a small leak between the endotracheal tube cuff and the trachea of the patient will become much more significant as the airway pressures associated with IPPV rise; this will direct some of the tidal volume intended for the patient into the room. Upon exhalation, a volume of gas inadequate to replace the volume lost from the bellows during inspiration will be expelled from the animal's lungs. The bellows will then attempt to fall but will do so more slowly if the rate of aspiration of room air through a small leak (and volume contributed to the system via the FGF) is less than that required for the bellows to fall normally. The result will be a bellows that falls very slowly or does not fall completely before the next inspiration occurs. This effect is most commonly recognized during ventilation of large patients where the leak is often relatively small (and is increased with positive pressure), the tidal volume is relatively large, and the FGFs are low relative to the patient's tidal volume.

There is at least one unique dual-circuit ventilator (Anesthesia WorkStation, Hallowell EMC, Pittsfield, MA, USA) designed specifically for patients requiring tidal volumes of less than 100 mL that replaces the bellows with a floating disc (Fig. 6.75). The floating disc separates the patient breathing circuit and driving gas circuit. In this configuration, the driving gas and the patient circuit do not come into contact with one another, but they do move back and forth across the same surface of the ventilation tube. This configuration requires very precise machining of both the ventilation tube and the floating disc to ensure that gas remains separated within their respective circuits and that the disc moves freely without significant resistance.

Bellows housing

A housing made of clear plastic that allows observation of bellows movement by the anesthetist surrounds the bellows. The housing is sealed and can be pressurized during ventilator cycling, causing compression of the bellows. A scale is normally present on the side of the bellows indicating the approximate tidal volume delivered. However, this volume is usually not precisely equivalent to the actual tidal volume received by the patient (see Factors Affecting Tidal Volume below).

Exhaust valve

The exhaust valve allows communication between the inside of the bellows housing and the external atmosphere on pneumatically driven ventilators (i.e., those that use compressed gases to compress

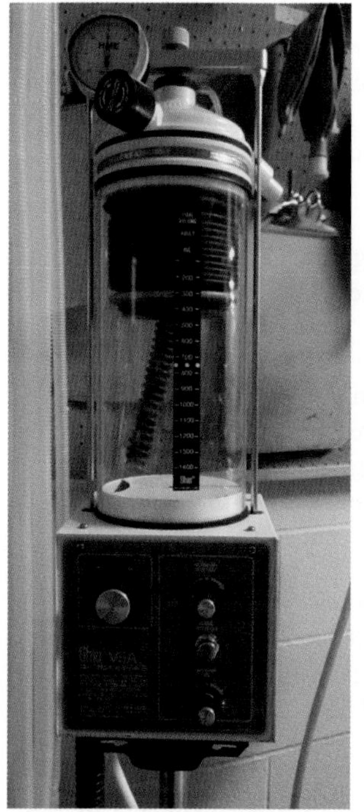
(A)

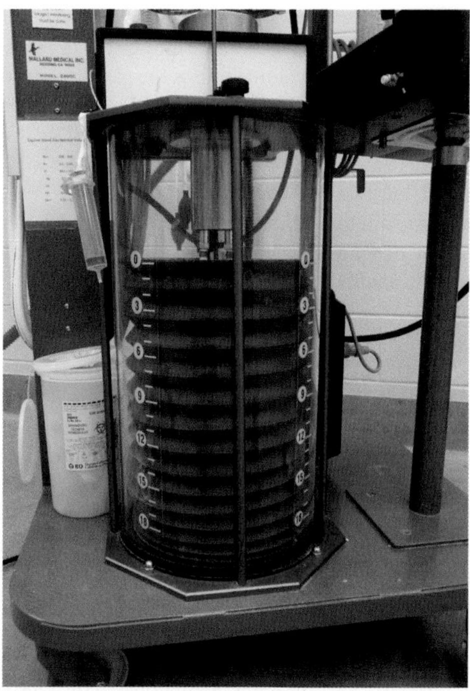
(B)

Figure 6.74 **A.** The Ohio V5A anesthesia ventilator is an example of a descending or hanging bellows configuration. A weight is used in the most dependent portion of the bellows to facilitate descent of the bellows during exhalation; this may also lead to a failure to recognize a disconnection or leak as the bellows will appear to move appropriately regardless of whether it is connected to a patient. **B.** The bellows of the Mallard 2800 large animal anesthesia ventilator is an example of an ascending or standing bellows configuration. Standing or ascending bellows normally produces slight positive pressure during the expiratory pause. Source: Dr. Craig Mosley, with permission.

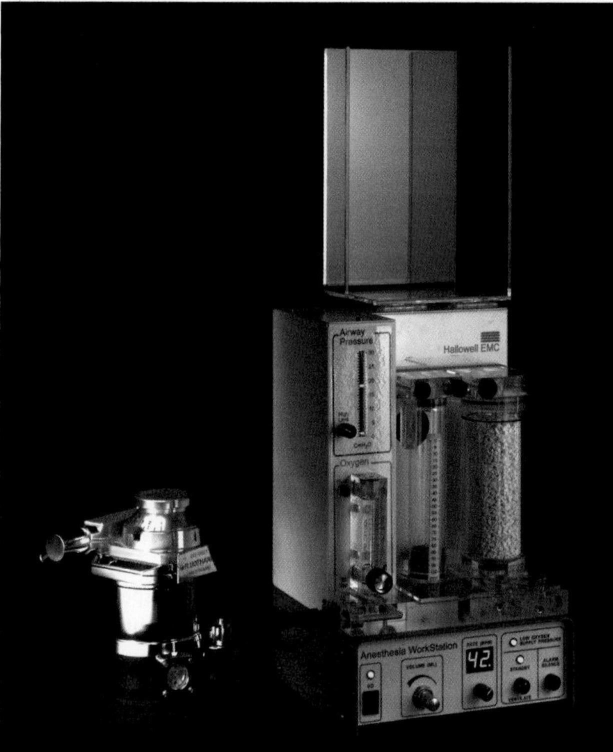

Figure 6.75 The Hallowell Anesthesia WorkStation (AWS) is a ventilator and circle breathing system designed specifically for very small animal patients (those between 150 g and 7 kg). The system features a unique ventilator that utilizes a floating puck, rather than a bellows, to separate the ventilator drive gas from the patient breathing circuit. The circle system is also optimized for very small patients with a low volume (circuit and absorbent canister) and a nearly zero deadspace Y-piece. Source: Hallowell EMC, Pittsfield, MA, USA; reproduced with permission.

the bellows). During inspiration, the exhaust valve is closed, allowing the driving gas to build pressure within the housing. During exhalation, the exhaust valve opens (and driving gas delivery stops), allowing the pressure to drop and the bellows to re-expand. Piston-driven ventilators have no need for an exhaust valve.

Spill valve

The spill valve replaces the function of the anesthetic machine's APL valve (which is still present but closed or otherwise isolated during mechanical ventilation) and is sometimes also referred to as a "vent valve," "dump valve," "overflow valve," "expired gas outlet," "pop-off valve," "relief valve," or "pressure relief valve." The valve is used to direct excess fresh gas from the breathing circuit into the scavenge system during the expiratory pause. During the ventilator's inspiratory cycle, the valve is closed to prevent escape of gas into the scavenge system and allow positive pressure to develop in the breathing circuit. This is similar to closing the APL valve in order to deliver a manual breath using the reservoir bag. With a standing bellows configuration, the spill valve normally has a minimal opening pressure of between 2 and 4 cmH_2O to offset the downward force created by the weight of the bellows. This allows the bellows to fill completely during exhalation. The spill valve is normally controlled pneumatically in ventilators using gas to compress the bellows, but in the case of piston-driven ventilators, it may be opened and closed electronically.

Ventilator hose connection

The ventilator hose connection is a standard-sized outlet (22 mm male conical fitting) normally found on the back of the ventilator bellows assembly. A length of standard-sized corrugated tubing is used between the ventilator hose connection and the machine's fitting that normally holds the reservoir bag. On anesthetic machines with built-in ventilators, this connection is often accomplished through the use of a switch or dial that automatically reconfigures the breathing system to the ventilator while isolating the APL valve, thereby minimizing the potential for misconnections, disconnections, or kinked hoses.

Control of ventilator driving gas

The driving gas supplied to the ventilator is normally under intermediate pressure (40–55 psi) and is delivered at a specified flow rate for a specific period of time to produce a volume of gas sufficient to compress the bellows and ventilate the patient's lungs. The driving gas is typically 100% oxygen and is used because it is usually readily available and to minimize the potential for reducing the oxygen concentration of the breathing circuit should a leak develop between the two ventilator circuits (breathing and driving gas circuit).

The driving gas flow to the ventilator is normally controlled electronically with dials labeled to adjust three fundamental variables: the duration of time driving gas is allowed into the bellows housing (inspiratory time), the rate at which the driving gas flows into the bellows housing (inspiratory flow rate), and the pause between inhalations (expiratory time). By manipulating these three variables, the more commonly described variables, respiratory frequency (f), tidal volume (V_t), and the inspiratory-to-expiratory ratio (I:E), can be controlled. Fluid logic-controlled ventilators are slightly less intuitive to operate but essentially, through manipulations related to pressure thresholds, flow rates, and time, the same variables can be controlled.

Factors that affect delivered tidal volume

Unless mechanisms for compensation are built into the anesthesia ventilator, various factors can affect the actual tidal volume delivered to the patient. Under most circumstances, and by using proper monitoring and setup procedures, these factors are insignificant.

Fresh gas flow

Although many modern human anesthesia ventilators compensate for changes in FGF, most veterinary ventilators do not. The electronics of most veterinary anesthesia ventilators are designed to deliver a set amount of driving gas regardless of the actual compression of the bellows. During inspiration, the FGF will continue into the patient circuit, contributing to the patient's actual tidal volume. Increasing the FGF or prolonging the inspiratory time will lead to larger tidal volumes. Although this effect may be insignificant in most patients, it can become significant in very small patients where a FGF of 1000 mL/min will contribute roughly 17 mL/s of gas to the patient's tidal volume during inspiration.

Compliance and compression volumes

Changes in compliance of the breathing system can be accompanied by changes in the tidal volume of gas delivered to the patient. Increases in the compliance of a breathing system can be accompanied by decreases in the patient tidal volume, as more of the delivered gas volume is expended expanding the breathing components. In addition, changes in airway pressures associated with ventilation and/or changes in lung compliance may alter the actual tidal volume of gas that the patient receives as gas volume is compressible when subjected to increasing pressures.

Leaks

Leaks within the system (e.g., around the endotracheal tube) will impact the delivered tidal volume, as some gas will escape through these leaks, leading to a reduction in the delivered tidal volume. Although side-stream airway gas monitors are not considered leaks, they do aspirate a small volume of gas from the breathing system (50–250 mL/min or 0.8–4 mL/s) that may marginally reduce tidal volume unless the gas is reintroduced as it leaves the monitor. This effect is normally negligible but may be significant in patients requiring extremely small tidal volumes (i.e., < 50 mL).

Alarms

There are no standard alarm configurations for veterinary anesthesia ventilators. Some of the more commonly found alarms are described below.

Low driving gas pressure alarm

This alarm is sometimes also referred to as the "low-pressure alarm" and will detect when the driving gas pressure falls below a preset value (i.e., 35 psi). A drop in driving gas pressure below a certain level may lead to a decrease in delivered tidal volume.

Airway pressure alarms

Both high and low airway pressure alarms are available on some ventilators. These are important to help protect a patient from barotrauma (high airway pressure) and help detect leaks or disconnects (low airway pressure). The alarm settings may be preset by the manufacturer or adjusted by the user. Occasionally, preset alarms are not compatible with the ventilation requirements in some patients. For example, a minimum airway pressure alarm set at 6 cmH_2O may exceed the maximum airway pressures used when ventilating very small patients with extremely compliant chests (e.g., kittens, puppies, reptiles, and birds).

Determinants of tidal volume

One of the principal risks associated with mechanical ventilation is inadvertent volutrauma or barotrauma to the patient's lungs if ventilator settings are improperly set. Fortunately, most of these errors are unlikely to be catastrophic as the vigilant anesthetist should, at minimum, immediately recognize such errors, or better, adopt the standard use of high airway pressure alarms on all anesthetic machines. The tidal volume on most pneumatically driven ventilators is limited (or determined) by the flow rate of gas entering the bellows housing and the duration of time that this gas is allowed to enter the bellows. Some ventilators will also use mechanical limiting devices to restrict movement of the bellows, thus effectively limiting the tidal volume that can be delivered regardless of changes in inspiratory flow rate and times (Mallard 2400V, Mallard Medical, Redding, CA, USA, and Dräger Large Animal Ventilator). One common recommendation when initiating mechanical ventilation in a patient is to start with low tidal volume settings and increase these based on monitored parameters once the ventilation is initiated. This is an especially important consideration if no mechanical volume-limiting device is present on the ventilator.

Tidal volume on most ventilators is controlled by dials variously labeled inspiratory flow rate, tidal volume, or minute volume and will be impacted by inspiratory time, I:E ratio, and respiratory rate. It is important to review the settings prior to the initiation of ventilation and to be fully aware of how changes in any one parameter may affect others. For example, if the respiratory rate is reduced on some ventilators, the inspiratory time will automatically be increased to reflect the new respiratory rate and to preserve the preset I:E ratio, leading to an increase in tidal volume (i.e., the inspiratory flow rate remains the same but the duration of inspiration increases).

Table 6.5 Guideline parameters for initiating intermittent positive-pressure ventilation in small animal patients and horses[a].

Patient	Respiratory rate (breaths/min)	Tidal volume (mL/kg)	Inspiratory pressure (cmH_2O)	I:E ratio
Small animal	10–15	10–20	10–15	1:2
Equine	6–8	10–20	10–25	1:3–1:4

[a] It is important to recognize that these are only guidelines and that specific settings can vary significantly among patients depending upon patient factors, such as breed, body condition, and disease. Additionally, ventilator limitations may influence the specific parameters attainable (e.g., minimum inspiratory flow limits). Ultimately, the adequacy of ventilation is best evaluated individually in each patient using capnography and/or blood gas analysis.

Proper ventilator setup and monitoring

Prior to using an anesthesia ventilator, it is important for the anesthetist to clearly determine the desired ventilator settings. Typical settings used for small and large animal patients are listed in Table 6.5. The anesthetist should have a solid understanding of the indications, contraindications, and physiology of IPPV prior to initiating ventilation. In addition, the anesthetist should ensure that they are familiar with all the features and proper operation of the ventilator they are using by reviewing the manufacturer's instructions. Improper use of positive-pressure ventilation equipment can lead to unnecessary morbidity and mortality. The following steps are intended as a general overview of ventilator setup and may not be applicable for all ventilators, patients, and circumstances.

1 Ensure power is available to the ventilator; most ventilators will require a source of compressed gas and an electrical supply.
2 Connect the scavenge hose from the ventilator to a scavenge system. Many scavenge interfaces have two scavenging ports, one for the anesthetic machine and the other for a ventilator.
3 Empty the reservoir bag into the scavenge system, remove the reservoir bag, and connect the ventilator breathing hose to the reservoir bag mount. Close the APL valve. Some machines with built-in ventilators do not require removal of the reservoir bag and closure of the APL valve; instead, a switch or dial is used to isolate the reservoir bag and APL valve from the ventilator.
4 Allow the bellows to fill. This can be facilitated by momentarily increasing the FGF rate. The flush valve should not be used for this purpose unless the FGF cannot be suitably increased to fill the bellows in a relatively rapid fashion (e.g., large animal ventilator).
5 Initiate ventilation based on the predetermined ventilation parameters. It is generally best to start with tidal volumes at the lower end of the typical range to avoid barotrauma or volutrauma. Under all circumstances, it is vital to immediately, and then routinely, evaluate the peak airway pressures and other monitored parameters (e.g., end-tidal CO_2, arterial blood gas analysis, and arterial blood pressure) to assess the adequacy of ventilator settings.

Selected ventilator models

Although not all-inclusive, the following discussion describes ventilators that are appropriate for veterinary patients. Some of these ventilators were designed specifically to support anesthetized veterinary patients, whereas others were designed for human use but are applicable to veterinary patients or can be modified for veterinary use. The classification, principles of operation, and other points about the general function of each ventilator are included. Before operating a ventilator, the user should consult the operating manuals and follow all pre-use evaluation procedures recommended by the manufacturer.

Dräger Small Animal Ventilator

This ventilator was marketed as an optional component for the Dräger Narkovet 2 Anesthesia Machine and was available on a mobile stand (universal pole) specifically designed for the ventilator. Currently, the ventilator is not being manufactured, but these ventilators remain in use for veterinary anesthesia. The small animal ventilator (SAV) is classified as double-circuit, time-cycled, with an ascending (standing) bellows; it is pneumatically powered and has fluidic circuitry. The pressure of the driving gas should be between 40 and 60 psi. The controls include a power ("on–off") switch, a tidal volume adjustment rod to set the attached plate within the bellows housing to the selected tidal volume (200–1600 mL), a frequency control knob (10–30 breaths/min), and an inspiratory flow knob to control the rate of flow into the bellows housing to deliver the breath. The inspiratory flow knob is normally set so that the bellows is fully compressed at the end of the inspiratory phase; however, the bellows should not be deformed at the end of inspiration. Deformation of the bellows at the end of inspiration may indicate an increase in tidal volume by as much as 100 mL. The inspiratory flow control setting affects the peak inspiratory pressure that is achieved and the inspiratory time. Higher inspiratory flows produce shorter inspiratory times and tend to produce higher peak inspiratory pressures. The ratio of inspiratory to expiratory time phase is preset to 1:2. The ventilator spill valve behind the bellows chamber compensates for the continuous entry of fresh gases into the breathing system. Because the ventilator uses an ascending bellows, the effect of gravity on the bellows maintains a PEEP of approximately 2 cmH_2O.

Before using the ventilator, the proper connections to the gas supply and scavenge system should be made, and the appropriate pre-use checkout procedures should be performed for all equipment. Assuming the anesthesia machine, breathing system, and ventilator are functional, the following is a reasonable step-by-step approach to the operation of this ventilator with a circle breathing system:

1 The tidal volume adjustment rod is set appropriately for the patient.
2 Corrugated tubing from the ventilator's breathing-hose terminal is connected to the circle system's reservoir bag mount.
3 The circle system's APL valve (adjustable pressure-limiting or pop-off valve) is closed.
4 The frequency of ventilation is adjusted to approximate the desired number of breaths per minute.
5 The ventilator's power switch is turned on.
6 The inspiratory flow control knob is adjusted to produce the desired inspiratory time to deliver the preset tidal volume.
7 The frequency of ventilation and inspiratory flow may need to be readjusted to achieve the desired rate of breathing and inspiratory time.

Engler ADS 1000 and 2000 Veterinary Anesthesia Delivery System and critical care ventilator

This microprocessor-controlled ventilator is marketed for use with a vaporizer or for patients not requiring an inhalant anesthetic (e.g., critical care patients). The ventilator–anesthesia system functions as a non-rebreathing circuit (unidirectional circuit), does not incorporate a bellows assembly or piston canister, and does not include a canister for chemical absorbent to eliminate carbon dioxide. It is not intended for connection to another breathing system.

This ventilator fits into the single-circuit class and is powered electrically and pneumatically. However, it is different in its function from both piston-driven and compressed gas-powered single-circuit ventilators. The ventilator only delivers gas intermittently to the patient (i.e., during inspiration) and, if used with a vaporizer, the ventilation drive gas moves through the vaporizer. In most other ventilation systems, gas flow to the vaporizer is independent of drive gas flow delivered by the ventilator and continuous. There is no possibility for rebreathing and the gas flow is unidirectional. According to the operating manual, the ventilator must be supplied with oxygen at a pressure of 50 (normal mode) or 5 (laboratory/low-flow mode) psi for the display to report the minute volume per kilogram of body weight accurately. When in laboratory mode, only tidal volume is reported. When used in normal mode, the ventilator's microprocessor will determine (estimate) the values for the various ventilatory parameters to be provided based on the patient's body weight. However, it is important to note that the preselected values may not optimally ventilate all patients and manual adjustments of ventilator parameters based on blood gas analysis and/or end-tidal CO_2 values should be used to ensure proper patient ventilation. The manufacturer's specifications suggest the ADS 2000 is capable of ventilating patients weighing less than 1 kg and as much as 68 kg. The ventilator is also capable of operating in an assist ventilation mode, delivering a breath each time the patient attempts to inspire spontaneously. The sensitivity of this feature is manually controlled by the user. The Engler ADS 2000 features updated electronics and microprocessors but is functionally the same as the Engler ADS 1000.

This ventilator acts as a non-rebreathing circuit, leading to excessive oxygen and inhalant anesthetic consumption when used in larger patients, particularly those over 10 kg. It is also important to note that the gas flow rates required to produce the tidal volumes required for larger patients may fall outside the recommended flow rates (200 mL/min to 15 L/min) for most vaporizers. For example, to produce a tidal volume of 600 mL using a 2-s inspiratory time will require the ventilator to deliver gas at a rate of 300 mL/s or 18 L/min to achieve the desired tidal volume. There is also some concern about the accuracy of vaporizer output resulting from the intermittent nature of carrier gas delivery to the vaporizer. When using this ventilator with a vaporizer, it is probably best to ensure that ventilator flow rates fall within those recommended by the vaporizer manufacturer to ensure accurate output.

The front panel of the ventilator has the following controls and components: power switch, mask-mode switch, set-run switch, weight-selection buttons, fill-hold button, breath button, display for various ventilatory parameters with adjustments for these parameters below the display, two ports for attachment of corrugated breathing tubes, and a gas sampling input port (this port was absent on earlier ADS 1000 models).

Before attempting to use the ventilator, the operator should read the manual supplied by the manufacturer and be very familiar with how ventilatory parameters can be modified manually, as the preset values may not be optimal for individual patients. The following is a summary of the manufacturer's guidelines for operating the ventilator, but is not intended to replace or supplant the manual supplied for the ventilator:

1 Connect the green oxygen hose on the back of the ventilator to an oxygen source (50 or 5 psi).
2 Attach the circle system tubes to the breathing-circuit ports on the front of the ventilator.
3 Connect the scavenge-out port on the back of the ventilator to the hospital scavenge system.
4 Connect the electric cord to an electric outlet.
5 Attach the vaporizer connectors to the appropriate ports on the back of the ventilator.
6 Attach the gas sampling line to the appropriate circuit adapter and gas sampling port on the ventilator.
7 Allow the ventilator to complete the self-diagnostic test described in the operator's manual. The test will help to determine failure of the safety pop-off valve, inadequate oxygen supply, and the presence of leaks.
8 After diagnostics are complete, the mask function should be off, and the set-run switch should be in the set position. The display will then show settings for a 20 kg patient (flow rate of 24 L/min, 9 breaths/min, peak inspiratory pressure of 15 cmH_2O, and the assist mode in the off position).
9 Using the weight-up or weight-down button, enter the correct weight of the patient in kilograms into the display, and the ventilator will automatically set the ventilatory parameters based on the patient's weight. Ventilation will be completely controlled (the default setting for assist is off).

Once these steps have been completed, the patient should be anesthetized and intubated with a cuffed endotracheal tube. The Y-piece connecting the breathing tubes should be attached to the endotracheal tube connector and the vaporizer should be set appropriately. The ventilator's set-run switch should be set to run. Controlled ventilation should begin.

Vetronics SAV03 and SAV04 small animal ventilator (exotic animal ventilator)

This microprocessor-controlled and pressure-cycled ventilator was designed for use in small animals (Fig 6.76). The manufacturer recommends its use in patients no larger than 12 kg, though it is most ideally suited for patients less than 5 kg due to the high oxygen flow rates and volumes of inhalant anesthetic required to operate it. The SAV04 is functionally the same as the SAV03 with upgraded alarms (e.g., patient disconnect, overpressure, apnea, valve disconnect, or failure).

This ventilator would be classified as a single-circuit, pressure-cycled, electronically powered ventilator with no bellows or piston. Technically, the tidal volume is driven/created pneumatically using the anesthetic machine's FGF and controlled electronically. In essence, the ventilator acts as a mechanical thumb, momentarily occluding the exhaust port causing the FGF to raise pressure within the patient circuit initiating inspiration. The ventilator consists of a control unit for setting respiratory parameters and a valve block/assembly unit that is inserted into the patient circuit. The valve block acts as part of the breathing circuit and functions as a non-rebreathing system (T-piece arrangement). There are three configurations described by the manufacturer: standard configuration, extension kit configuration (moves the valve block away from the patient's endotracheal tube), and low deadspace configuration. Regardless of the configuration, the functional aspects of the unit remain basically the same.

The valve unit contains a solenoid that opens and closes the exhaust port of the valve block (T-piece) based on the pressure settings designated by the user. The control unit has the following controls: power switch, IPPV (on/off) switch, target pressure dial, and expiratory time dial. The LED screen will display values for target

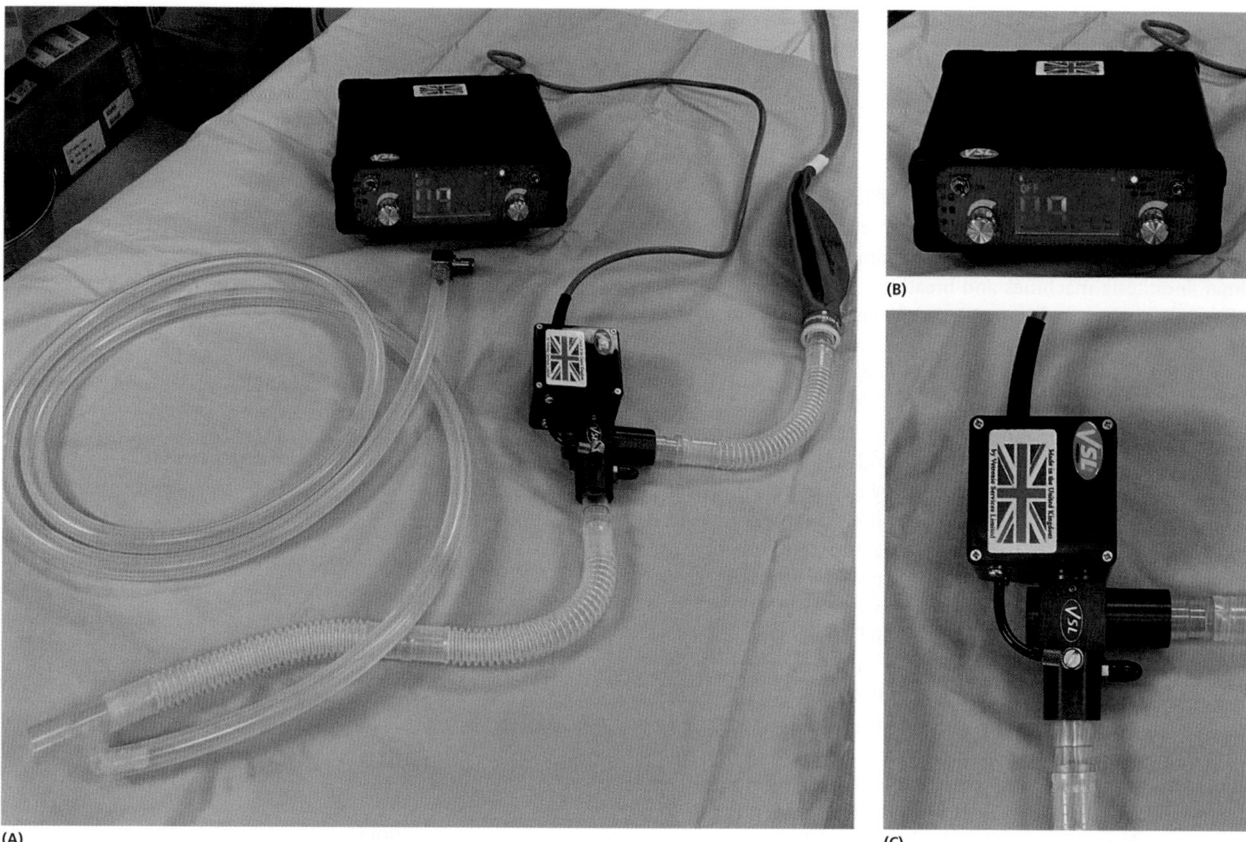

Figure 6.76 **A.** The Vetronics SAV04 small animal ventilator is unique in that it uses a valve to occlude the patient circuit exhaust port functionally closing the circuit allowing the machine's fresh gas flow to build pressure initiating inspiration in the patient. Due to the limitations of using fresh gas flow rate to create tidal volume, it is best reserved for use in patients less than 5 kg. **B.** The ventilator control unit. **C.** The valve block which is connected within a modified non-rebreathing patient circuit. Source: Dr. Craig Mosley, with permission.

pressure, airway pressure, IPPV status (on/off), alarm notifications, the set expiratory time, measured inspiratory time, and measured respiratory rate. The ventilation characteristics will be determined by the user settings for target airway pressure and expiratory time. The ventilator tidal volume is determined by the target airway pressure, while the inspiratory time and respiratory rate will be largely influenced by the FGF rate and the set expiratory time. In other words, a shorter set expiratory time will tend to increase respiratory rate as will a higher FGF rate (reducing the time required to reach target pressure). The ventilatory cycle operates in the following manner: the control unit occludes the exhaust port to initiate inspiration; inspiration will continue until the target pressure is reached as measured by a sensor in the valve block/assembly; once this pressure is obtained, exhalation is initiated by opening the exhaust port allowing the exhaled and ongoing FGF to escape the patient circuit; once the set expiratory time is reached, the inspiratory cycle is again initiated. It is important to note that this ventilator relies solely on the FGF rate from the anesthetic machine to create a tidal volume. For example, if the target tidal volume is 50 mL and the desired inspiratory time is 2 s, a FGF rate of 25 mL/s or 1.5 L/min will be required. Due to its inability to effectively ventilate larger patients and its mode of limiting tidal volume (pressure), this ventilator is most often used by those working with birds, reptiles, and other small mammals. Despite the manufacturer's recommendations that it can be used in patients weighing up to 12 kg, it is probably most suitable for use in patients less than 5 kg, as the high FGFs required make it very inefficient in terms of oxygen and inhalant anesthetic use in larger patients.

Before attempting to use the ventilator, the operator should carefully read the manual supplied by the manufacturer and be very familiar with the concept of occlusion-initiated ventilation (i.e., using the machine FGF to achieve a tidal volume), as this is an unusual means of achieving ventilation. The following is a summary of the manufacturer's guidelines for operating the ventilator, but is not intended to replace or supplant the manual supplied for the ventilator:

1 Connect the power supply and valve unit to the ventilator control assembly.
2 Set IPPV to off.
3 Set the target airway pressure and expiratory time based on the individual needs of the patient.
4 Assemble the breathing system in the desired configuration: standard, extended, or low deadspace. Note that a hose from the common gas outlet is required to connect to the inlet port of the valve block with a reservoir bag and scavenge on the exhaust port; the patient's endotracheal tube or extension tubing will be connected to the patient port of the valve block.

5 Set IPPV to on and carefully evaluate the adequacy of ventilation. Recall the complex interactions among FGF rate, expiratory time, desired tidal volume, and target airway pressure.
6 If required, adjust target pressure, expiratory time, and/or FGF rate to obtain optimal ventilation.

Hallowell EMC 2000, 2002 and 2002 PRO, and Matrx/Midmark 3000/3002 PRO anesthesia ventilators

These ventilators (Fig. 6.77) were designed for use with standard small animal anesthesia machines and breathing systems (rebreathing/circle and non-rebreathing circuits). The connections to the breathing system, scavenge system, and driving gas are located on the back of the unit. The Matrx 3000 model (now the Midmark 3002 PRO) is basically the Hallowell EMC 2002 PRO model ventilator produced for Matrx/Midmark. The 2002 PRO model has essentially replaced the 2002 and 2000 models, but many of these earlier models are still in use. The primary difference between the three models is changes made to the volume control valve. The initial model 2000 had a single valve adjustment for all tidal volumes, this made fine adjustments for smaller patients more difficult due to the limited sensitivity of the control dial. The 2002 model added a fine volume control dial that had much greater sensitivity when adjusting tidal volumes in small patients, while still retaining the original volume control dial for adjusting tidal volume in larger patients. The 2002 PRO further refined volume control with a dual control system that allows for very fine tidal volume adjustments with the first couple of turns of the volume dial with the remainder producing flow changes more suitable for larger tidal volumes. In other words, the volume dial acts as a two-stage volume adjustment with small tidal volumes and fine adjustments at the lower volume settings, and more course adjustments in the larger tidal volume range. This ventilator is classified as double-circuit and time-cycled with an ascending (standing) bellows and is electrically powered. The ventilator is pneumatically driven and electronically controlled by an electrically activated solenoid valve that allows gas pressure to be supplied to the volume control during the inspiratory phase of the ventilatory cycle. The ventilator's power switch is incorporated into the respiratory-rate control. The pressure of the driving-gas supply (either oxygen, nitrogen, or compressed conditioned air) should be regulated between 30 and 60 psi. High pressure is necessary only for high inspiratory flow rates in larger patients.

The control modules of the EMC 2000, 2002, and 2002 PRO model ventilators have the following adjustable components: the on–off switch, a respiratory rate control knob, a volume control knob (was labeled inspiratory flow on most Model 2002 ventilators), an inspiratory hold push button, and a maximum working pressure limit (MWPL) selector. The 2002 model also has a fine inspiratory flow adjustment dial (see Fig. 6.77). The ratio of inspiratory to expiratory time phase is preset at 1:2. However, this ventilator is available with an optional adjustable I:E ratio in the range of 1:1.5–1:4, enabling users greater flexibility in selecting ventilatory parameters. The inspiratory flow control is a variable orifice-metering valve that regulates the driving-gas flow. The inspiratory flow control is used to set tidal volume. It regulates the inspiratory flow rate directly, and a higher inspiratory flow rate at any given respiratory rate will produce a greater tidal volume. The inspiratory hold push button interrupts the ventilatory cycle and prevents discharge of gas from the bellows housing until the button is released or the MWPL is reached. The MWPL is measured in the patient circuit using a coupling placed in the patient circuit extending to a pressure transducer in the ventilator. The MWPL can be set between 10 and 60 cmH_2O. If the MWPL is reached at any time, the inspiratory phase of ventilation is terminated, an alarm sounds, and exhalation is allowed. Low breathing system pressure will be detected if the pressure at the end of inspiration is less than 5 cmH_2O; a red warning light will illuminate and an alarm will sound, indicating the possibility of a disconnection of the patient circuit from the ventilator.

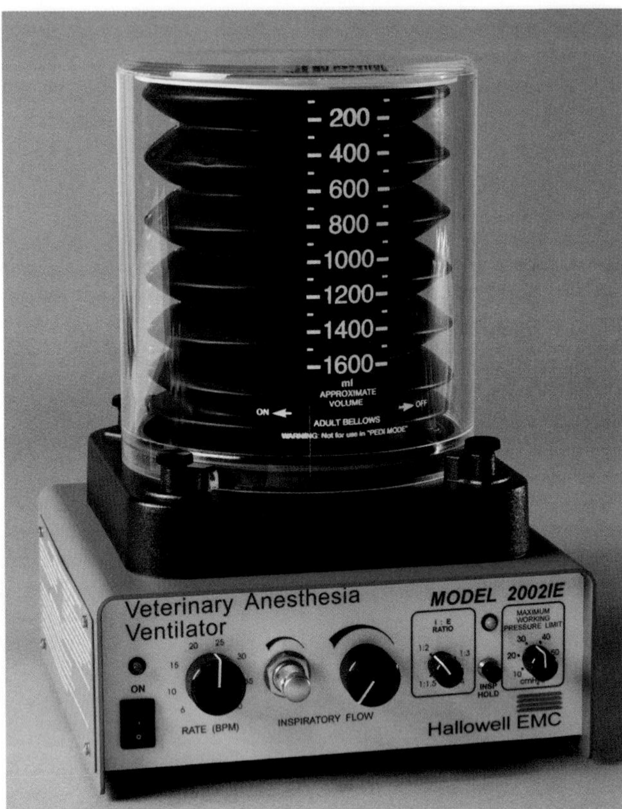

Figure 6.77 The Hallowell 2002 ventilator features a fine inspiratory flow dial, improving its ability to deliver more precise tidal volumes. It is also available with or without an adjustable I:E ratio. Source: Hallowell EMC, Pittsfield, MA, USA; reproduced with permission.

Three sizes of interchangeable bellows and bellows housings are available to enable various sizes of patients to be ventilated effectively (Fig. 6.78). With the proper bellows, the manufacturer indicates that tidal volumes as small as 20 mL and as large as 3 L can be delivered and that the patient can effectively breathe spontaneously from the bellows when the ventilator is not in operation. The ventilator spill valve compensates for the continuous entry of fresh gas into the breathing system, and the resistance of the spill valve creates a PEEP of 2–3 cmH_2O.

Before using the ventilator, connections to the gas supply and scavenge system should be made and the appropriate pre-use checkout procedures followed. Assuming proper functioning of the anesthesia machine, breathing system, and ventilator, the following is a reasonable operational approach for this ventilator with a circle breathing system:

1 The MWPL selector is set to the desired maximum pressure (safety limit), and the pressure coupler is connected to the breathing system according to the manufacturer's recommendations.

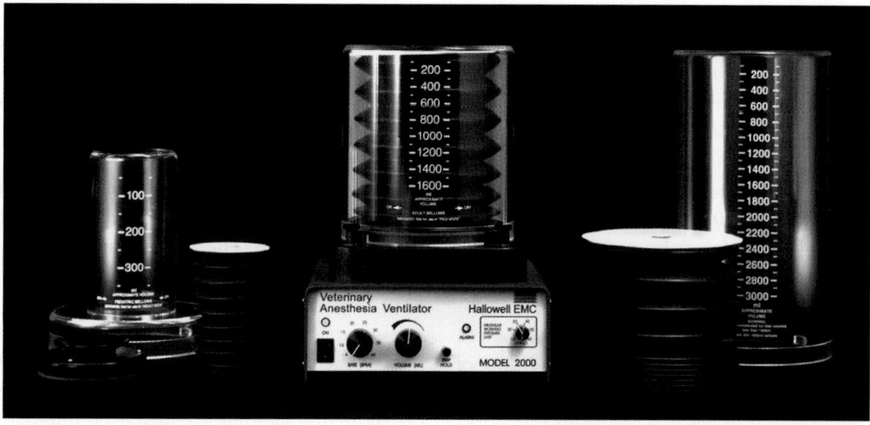

Figure 6.78 Many ventilators are available with different sizes of interchangeable bellows. This feature is convenient when ventilating patients requiring markedly different tidal volumes, but the bellows does not generally change the overall function of the ventilator (i.e., a small bellows does not mean that smaller tidal volumes can be achieved with the ventilator, it simply provides more precision in estimating tidal volume from movement of the bellows; the minimum tidal volume will be determined by the inspiratory flow rate and inspiratory time). Source: Hallowell EMC, Pittsfield, MA, USA; reproduced with permission.

2 Corrugated tubing from the ventilator's breathing system connector is attached to the circle system's reservoir bag mount, and the ventilator is attached to the scavenge system.
3 The circle system's pop-off (APL) valve is closed.
4 The ventilator's volume control is adjusted to the minimum setting.
5 The ventilator's power-rate switch is turned on and the desired frequency of ventilation is set.
6 The volume control knob (inspiratory flow on Model 2002) is adjusted to produce a flow of gas during inspiration that produces the desired tidal volume and/or peak inspiratory pressure.

Mallard Medical Model 2400V anesthesia ventilator

This ventilator was originally designed to allow continuous mechanical ventilation of anesthetized pediatric and adult human patients. It is sold to veterinarians as a stand-alone unit for use with a breathing system and anesthesia machine (Fig. 6.79). Classified as a double-circuit ventilator, it has electric power and is pneumatically driven. The ventilator is controlled by a microprocessor, and the manufacturer describes the ventilator as electronically time cycled and volume limited. The tidal volume is selected by limiting the upward expansion of the bellows by use of a bellows expansion limiting device. Tidal volume is adjusted by moving a cylinder and plate within the bellows housing to coincide with the desired setting in milliliters. The cylinder within the bellows housing is secured by a control knob (nut) located on the top center of the housing. This ventilator employs an ascending (standing) bellows. The bellows is pneumatically driven, and the ventilator operates at a driving gas pressure of 50 ± 10 psi.

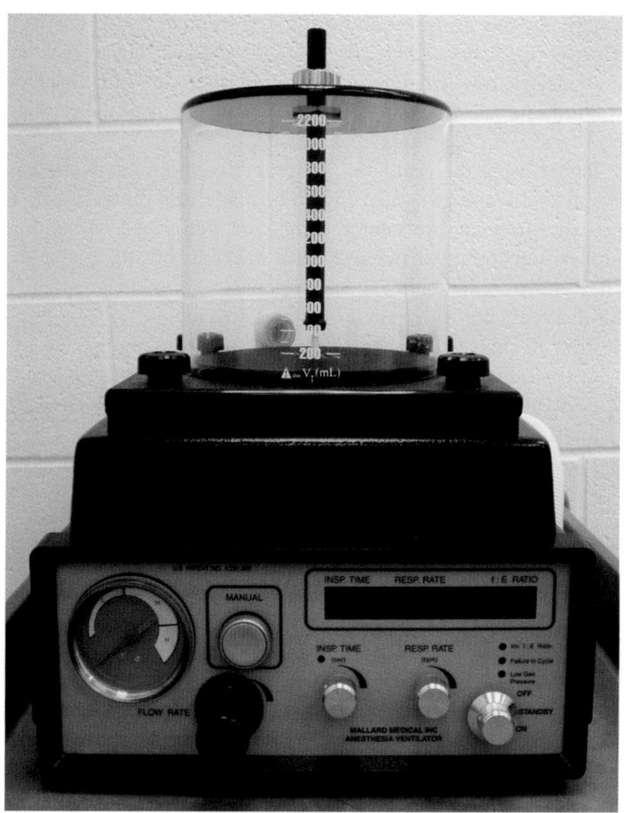

Figure 6.79 The Mallard 2400V anesthesia ventilator. The ventilator can be volume limited through the use of an adjustable bellows limiting device, or alternatively, the volume can be limited through changes in the driving gas flow rate. Source: Dr. Craig Mosley, with permission.

The controls are positioned on a console, which is located below the bellows housing. A master on-standby-off switch is present in the right lower corner of the console's front panel; the standby mode allows preselection of respiratory rate and inspiratory time (see Fig. 6.79). The I:E ratio is computed from these settings and displayed digitally on LED displays before mechanical ventilation is initiated. Respiratory rate and inspiratory time are controlled by ten-turn potentiometers to allow selection of 2–80 breaths/min (respiratory rate) and 0.1–3.0 s (inspiratory time), respectively. The I:E ratio display shows the relationship of inspiratory time to expiratory time, giving inspiratory time a value of 1. A black control knob located in the lower left portion of the front panel allows adjustment of inspiratory flow rate (10–100 L/min), and a display gauge near the control knob indicates whether the flow being used is low, medium, or high. The flow rate is normally adjusted to ensure complete compression of the bellows at the end of inspiration. If the flow rate is set higher than needed, it will produce a rapid time to peak inspiration volume and an inspiratory hold. A green push button is located in the front center portion of the control console; this button activates inspiration as long as the button is pushed in. This button can be used to maintain mechanical ventilation in the event of a power failure and can be used to sigh the patient.

Two sizes of bellows are available: the adult bellows provides tidal volumes, ranging from 200 to 2200 mL, and the pediatric bellows from 50 to 300 mL. An exhalation valve assembly is located on the back of the control console. This valve is closed pneumatically during the inspiratory phase of ventilation and opens automatically during the expiratory phase. Excess gas from the patient circuit also exits through this valve to prevent the buildup of pressure. The post (19 mm) of this valve should be attached to a scavenge system for elimination of waste gases from the working environment. With an ascending bellows, PEEP (usually 2–3 cmH_2O) will be present. In addition, PEEP of up to 20 cmH_2O can be added to the system with the control knob of the optional PEEP valve. Also, an adjustable overpressure spill valve within the console is preset to 80 cmH_2O, and this limits the maximum pressure that can be developed in the patient breathing circuit. Externally, this pressure can be adjusted from 20 to 100 cmH_2O. This ventilator has audible alarms if the ventilator fails to cycle or if an electric power failure occurs. In addition, the LED displays will indicate selection of an inverse I:E ratio, failure of the ventilator to cycle, and low supply-gas pressure (< 30 psi).

Before using the ventilator, the proper connections to the gas supply and scavenge system should be made, and the appropriate pre-use checkout procedures should be performed. Assuming proper functioning of the anesthesia machine, breathing system, and ventilator, the following is a reasonable operational approach for this ventilator with a circle breathing system:

1 Prior to clinical applications, refer to the operating manual for instructions and conduct performance verification procedures.
2 Select the appropriate control settings for the tidal volume by limiting the upward expansion of the bellows.
3 Place the master switch in the standby mode and dial the desired settings for the respiratory rate and the inspiratory time, based on the patient's needs.
4 Set the inspiratory flow control to the desired rate of flow, low, medium, or high, depending on the needs of the patient.
5 Connect the corrugated tubing from the ventilator's bellows to the circle system's reservoir bag mount and attach the ventilator to the scavenge system.
6 Close the circle system's pop-off (APL) valve.
7 Set the master switch to the on position.
8 The ventilator should cycle according to the selected settings, and only minor adjustments should be necessary (e.g., slight alterations of inspiratory time).

Ohio V5A ventilator

This ventilator is shown in Fig. 6.74A. This unit was produced for human use and is capable of delivering tidal volumes in the range 20–1400 mL. This ventilator is no longer produced but is still available. The Metomatic, a small animal-specific model, produced by Ohio Medical Products, is also no longer produced, although it may still be found in some veterinary practices and has been described elsewhere [75]. The Metomatic and the V5A are very similar in overall design, although the Metomatic offered an assist mode for ventilation and could be set to limit the tidal volume based on pressure. Arguably the Metomatic offered more features for precisely controlling ventilation but is perhaps less intuitive for those less familiar with IPPV. The V5A is classified as a double-circuit and time-cycled ventilator with fluidic circuitry and a descending (hanging) bellows. The ventilator is powered and driven pneumatically and will function properly with an oxygen supply pressure to 40–75 psi.

Controls for this ventilator are as follows: power (on–off) switch, inspiratory flow rate control, expiratory time control, and a manual inspiration button. There is also a dial on the side of the ventilator canister used to control tidal volume by limiting descent of the bellows (Fig. 6.80). The power switch controls a valve that supplies pneumatic power to the ventilator. The tidal volume control dial adjusts the bellows from 0 to 1400 mL (20–300 mL pediatric bellows). The inspiratory flow rate control regulates the rate of delivery of gas to the ventilator canister compressing the bellows during inspiration and is adjustable from 6 to 100 L/min. It should be set to deliver the complete tidal volume from the bellows over a reasonable period of time, normally 1–2 s. The expiratory time control adjusts the time between the end of one inspiratory phase of respiration and the beginning of the next and can be varied from 1 to 10 s; essentially, it is a setting for respiratory rate, although rate is influenced to some extent by other controls (e.g., inspiratory time). The manual inspiration push button allows the initiation of inspiration at any point during the respiratory cycle by depressing and immediately releasing the button. If the push button is depressed and held, inspiration will be initiated, and the bellows will remain at the

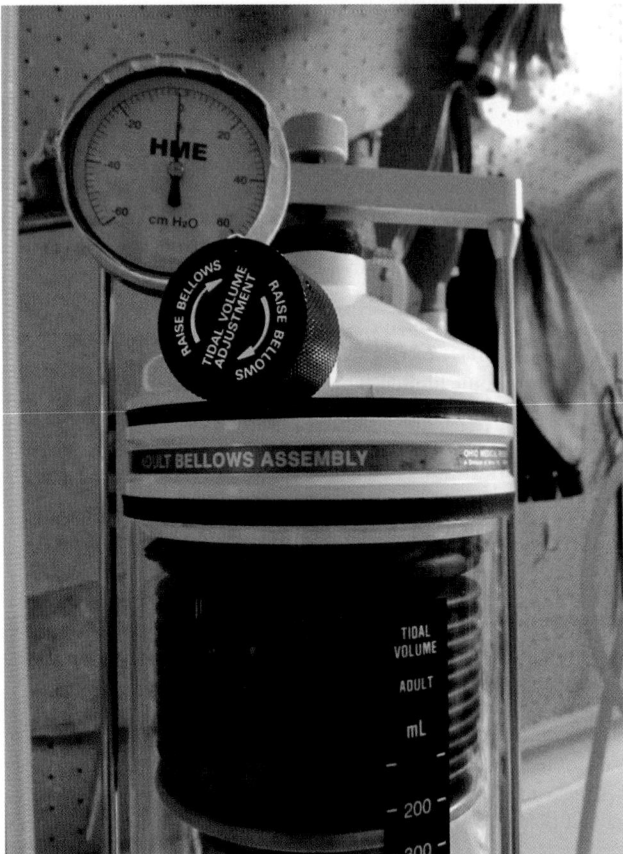

Figure 6.80 The tidal volume delivered to a patient using a "hanging" bellows ventilator is often controlled by using an adjustable dial that limits the descent of the bellows. Source: Dr. Craig Mosley, with permission.

end-inspiratory position until the button is released. The ventilator is also equipped with a low airway pressure alarm. This is a useful feature as a leak is not easily detected through observation of the ventilator bellows in a descending/hanging configuration. The ventilator provides a spill valve (pop-off valve) to allow the escape of excess gases that are delivered to the patient circuit. Generally, the pressure in the patient circuit returns to zero at the end of expiration, since a descending bellows is employed.

Before using the ventilator, the proper connections to the gas supply and scavenge system should be made, and the appropriate pre-use checkout procedures should be performed. Assuming that the anesthesia machine, breathing system, and ventilator are functional, the following is a step-by-step approach to the operation of the ventilator with a circle breathing system:

1 Select the desired tidal volume.
2 Set the inspiratory flow rate control to a mid-range setting. After the ventilator is in use, this control will be reset to deliver the tidal volume in approximately 1–2 s.
3 Set the expiratory time control to a mid-range setting. This control should be reset to allow the appropriate frequency of ventilation and desired I:E ratio after the ventilator is in use.
4 Connect the corrugated tube from the ventilator's bellows to the circle system's reservoir bag port.
5 Close the pop-off (APL) valve of the breathing system.
6 Turn the power switch on.
7 Observe the character and rate of ventilation and refine the adjustments of the various controls. Usually, inspiratory flow rate is adjusted first, followed by frequency or expiratory time.

Ohmeda 7000 and 7800 series electronic anesthesia ventilators

The Ohmeda 7000 and 7800 series ventilators are double-circuit human anesthesia ventilators with a pneumatically driven ascending/standing bellows (Fig. 6.81). The 7000 ventilator is electronically controlled with a preset minute volume, whereas the 7800 is electronically controlled with a preset tidal volume, which may be a specific advantage (as discussed below).

Both ventilators can be fitted with either an adult or a pediatric bellows, and they have been used extensively in human anesthesia [1,91]. These ventilators are available to purchase used and are readily applicable to small animal anesthesia. The scale on the bellows housing ranges from 100 to 1600 mL on the adult bellows and from 0 to 300 mL on the pediatric bellows. The bellows assembly exhaust port is 19 mm OD, the connection to the anesthesia machine is 22 mm, and there is a high-pressure (50 psi) DISS fitting for an oxygen line for the driving gas circuit. The driving gas supply is oxygen at 50 psi, which is reduced to 38 psi by a precision regulator within the ventilator. During the expiratory phase, gas from the patient circuit (flow from the anesthesia machine) enters the bellows. The ventilator spill opens when the bellows is fully distended and a pressure of 2.5 cmH_2O has been exceeded; excess gas from the patient circuit is vented into the scavenge system. The controls and specific details of each model series are discussed separately below.

The 7000 series control module (see Fig. 6.81A) has six controls, namely the minute volume dial (2–30 L/min with the adult bellows and 2–12 L/min with the pediatric bellows), the respiratory rate dial (6–40 breaths/min), the I:E ratio dial (1:1–1:3), power (on–off)

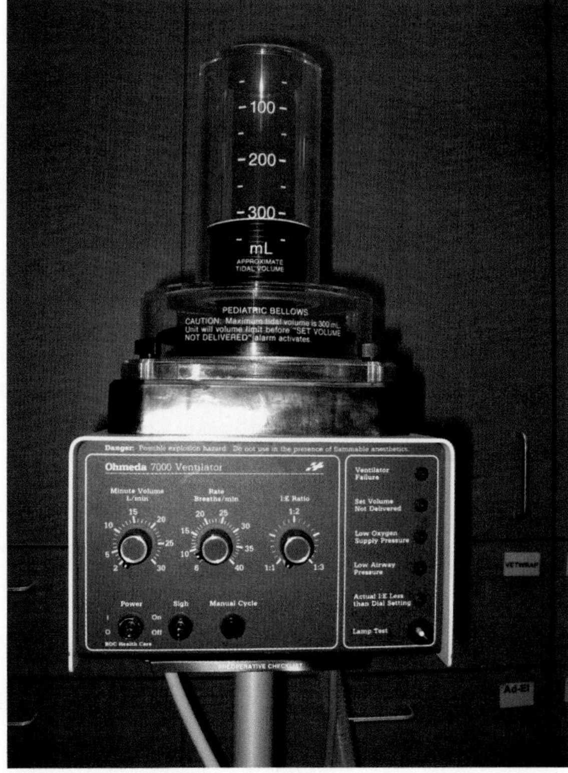

(A)

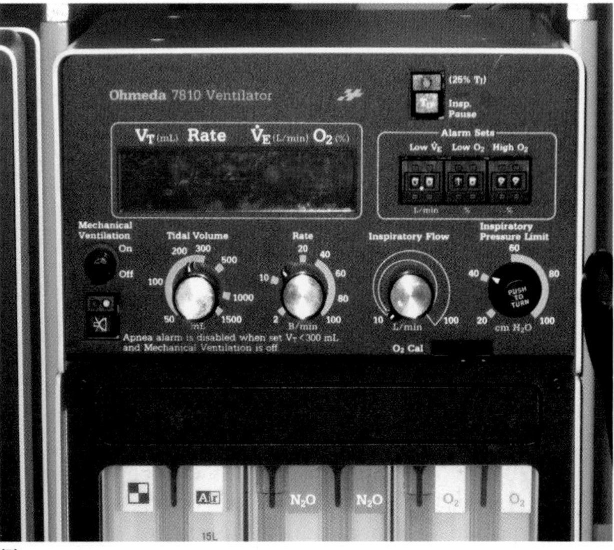

(B)

Figure 6.81 **A.** An Ohmeda 7000 series stand-alone ventilator. **B.** A built-in Ohmeda 7800 series (Model 7810 shown) showing the control panel. The Ohmeda 7800 provides greater functionality with built-in adjustable alarm parameters. Both of these ventilators are designed for use in humans but work well for most veterinary patients. Source: Dr. Craig Mosley, with permission.

switch, the sigh switch (to provide a "sigh" equal to 150% of the tidal volume once every 64 breaths), and a manual cycle button (used to initiate inspiration manually only during the expiratory phase). The controls for ventilation (minute volume, respiratory rate, and I:E ratio) are not interactive. If minute volume is increased and the rate held constant, the tidal volume will increase. Hence changing the minute volume is normally used to change the patient's tidal volume, although it is important to recognize that changing the respiratory rate can also change the tidal volume. If the respiratory rate is decreased while the minute volume is held constant, the tidal volume will increase. Inappropriate use of any ventilator without proper regard for how changes in one parameter may affect ancillary variables can be potentially dangerous for the patient (i.e., cause volutrauma or barotrauma).

The 7800 series represents an evolution of the 7000 series providing additional functionality, built-in alarms, and more intuitive control (see Fig. 6.81B). The respiratory parameters and the inspired oxygen concentration are displayed on a liquid crystal screen. There is a ventilation (on–off) toggle switch, alarm silence button (silences alarms for 30 s), tidal volume dial (50–1500 mL), respiratory rate dial (2–100 breaths/min), an inspiratory flow dial (10–100 L/min), an inspiratory pressure limit dial (20–100 cmH_2O; sustained alarm is 50% of set limit), an inspiratory pause switch (25% of inspiratory time), and a main power (on–off) toggle switch. There are also input plugins for an oxygen sensor (measuring percent inspired oxygen) and spirometer (measuring actual volume exhaled). There are three sets of toggle wheels for alarm settings: low minute ventilation, low oxygen concentration, and high oxygen concentration. The controls for ventilation (tidal volume, respiratory rate, and inspiratory flow rate) are not interactive. However, unlike the 7000 series, only changes to the tidal volume dial will result in changes in the tidal volume being delivered to the patient, which makes it less likely that an inadvertently large tidal volume will be delivered. Changing each of the ventilation controls (tidal volume, respiratory rate, and inspiratory flow rate) will alter its associated ventilator variable but will only lead to ancillary changes in the I:E ratio rather than delivered tidal volume. Normally, the ventilator is set by selecting the desired tidal volume and respiratory rate, with the inspiratory flow rate being used to select an appropriate I:E ratio.

The manufacturer recommends a bellows assembly leak test. With the ventilator attached to a circle breathing system with the breathing system's APL valve closed, the Y-piece occluded, all FGF off, and the bellows filled from the anesthesia machine's oxygen flush valve, the bellows should drop no more than 100 mL/min. If a significant leak is present, the ventilator should not be used until the leak has been sealed. If the anesthesia machine, breathing system, and ventilator are all in proper working order, as indicated by pre-use checkout procedures, the following guidelines are appropriate for use of the ventilator:

1 Properly connect the electric and pneumatic power sources for the ventilator.
2 For 7000 series ventilators, set the desired values for minute volume, respiratory rate (frequency), and I:E ratio. For 7800 series ventilators, set the desired values for tidal volume, respiratory rate, and I:E ratio (normally done by adjusting inspiratory flow rate). The alarm settings should be appropriately set.
3 Make the appropriate connections from the ventilator bellows to the circle system's reservoir bag port and to the scavenge system.
4 Close the pop-off (APL) valve of the circle system.
5 Make sure that the bellows is completely filled with oxygen-anesthetic mixture.
6 Switch the power control to on.
7 Make final adjustments to minute volume and respiratory rate to meet the needs of the patient.

ICU Medical (formerly Smith Medical/Surgivet) SAV 2500

This ventilator (Fig. 6.82) was designed for use with standard small animal anesthesia machines and breathing systems (circle and non-rebreathing circuits). This ventilator is classified as double-circuit and time cycled with an ascending (standing) bellows; it is pneumatically driven and electrically controlled. The pressure of the driving gas supply (oxygen, nitrogen, or compressed conditioned air) should be regulated between 50 and 55 psi.

The control module for the SAV 2500 ventilator has the following adjustable components located on the front of the ventilator control unit: the on–off switch, inspiratory time dial, breaths per minute, and inspiratory flow. A transport breath button (pneumatic manual) and an adjustable pressure relief valve are located on the back of the base or control unit. The on–off switch initiates IPPV, the inspiratory time dial adjusts the time allowed for inspiration, and the breaths per minute dial is used to set the number of respiratory cycles that the ventilator will deliver over time. An appropriate I:E ratio is obtained by adjusting the inspiratory time relative to the number of breaths per minute. The inspiratory flow determines the rate at which gas is delivered to the bellows housing during the inspiratory time and hence the compression of the bellows; it is essentially used to set the tidal volume. However, like many other ventilators, these dials are independent of one another, and changes in one will independently affect various respiratory parameters.

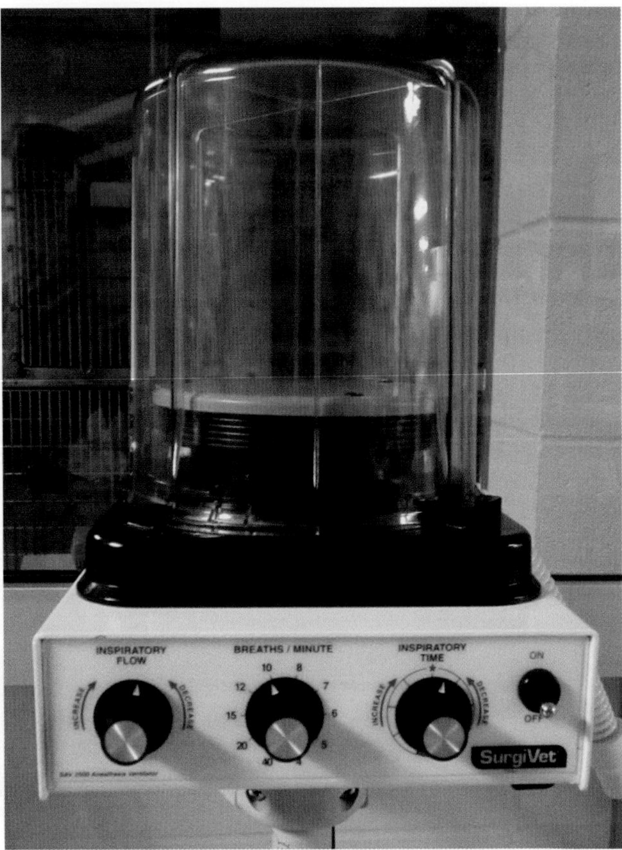

Figure 6.82 The Surgivet SAV 2500 showing the various control dials used to set respiratory parameters. Source: Dr. Craig Mosley, with permission.

For example, increasing inspiratory time or inspiratory flow rate will both increase tidal volume. Adjusting the breaths per minute will not alter tidal volume but will affect the I:E ratio. Changes should be made carefully with all ventilators and an immediate reassessment of ventilator parameters (tidal volume, peak airway pressures, and I:E ratio) should be made following all adjustments.

The transport button is pneumatically operated and can be used to ventilate a patient should electrical power be interrupted or temporarily unavailable. When the button is depressed, it delivers gas into the bellows housing, compressing the bellows until the button is released or when it exceeds the pressure relief valve limits. This button can be activated at any point during the ventilator cycle, making it possible to deliver "stacked" breaths (potentially leading to the delivery of an excessively large breath). The adjustable pressure relief valve adapted between the driving gas port of the control unit and the bellows housing limits the maximum pressure that can be generated by the driving gas helping to eliminate the possibility of patient barotrauma. The valve when closed will open at 60 cmH_2O (±5 cmH_2O) but can be adjusted to open at incrementally lower pressures down to almost 0 cmH_2O. Three sizes of interchangeable bellows (300, 1500, and 3000 mL) are available to facilitate ventilation in various sizes of patients. The ventilator spill valve compensates for the continuous entry of fresh gas into the breathing system, and the resistance of the spill valve creates a PEEP of 2–3 cmH_2O. An MRI-compatible ventilator model (SAV 2550) is also available, but it differs considerably from the SAV 2500 and is not discussed here.

Before using the ventilator, connections to the gas supply and scavenge system should be made, and the appropriate pre-use checkout procedures followed. Assuming proper functioning of the anesthesia machine, breathing system, and ventilator, the following is a reasonable operational approach for this ventilator with a circle breathing system:

1 The adjustable pressure relief valve can be set to open at the desired level. Although this is not absolutely necessary, setting it to a reasonable opening pressure (30–40 cmH_2O) can help minimize the risk of accidental ventilator-induced barotrauma.
2 Corrugated tubing from the ventilator's breathing system connector is attached to the circle system's reservoir bag mount, and the ventilator is attached to the scavenge system.
3 The circle system's pop-off (APL) valve is closed.
4 The ventilator's breaths per minute dial is set to the desired frequency.
5 The ventilator's inspiratory time is set. When the dial is turned to the 12 o'clock position (marked by an asterisk), the inspiratory time will be approximately 1 s.
6 The inspiratory flow dial should be set to a low setting initially to avoid delivering an inadvertently large tidal volume to the patient and the ventilator should be switched on. The inspiratory flow control dial is adjusted to produce a flow of gas during inspiration that produces the desired tidal volume and/or peak inspiratory pressure.
7 Make final adjustments to inspiratory flow rate, inspiratory time, and breaths per minute to meet the needs of the patient.

Penlon AV-S ventilator

The Penlon AV-S (Fig. 6.83) is a ventilator designed for human use that has recently seen uptake in some veterinary markets. This is probably owing to its ability to function both as a stand-alone and built-in ventilator, with integrated anesthesia ventilators becoming increasingly common in many modern anesthetic workstations.

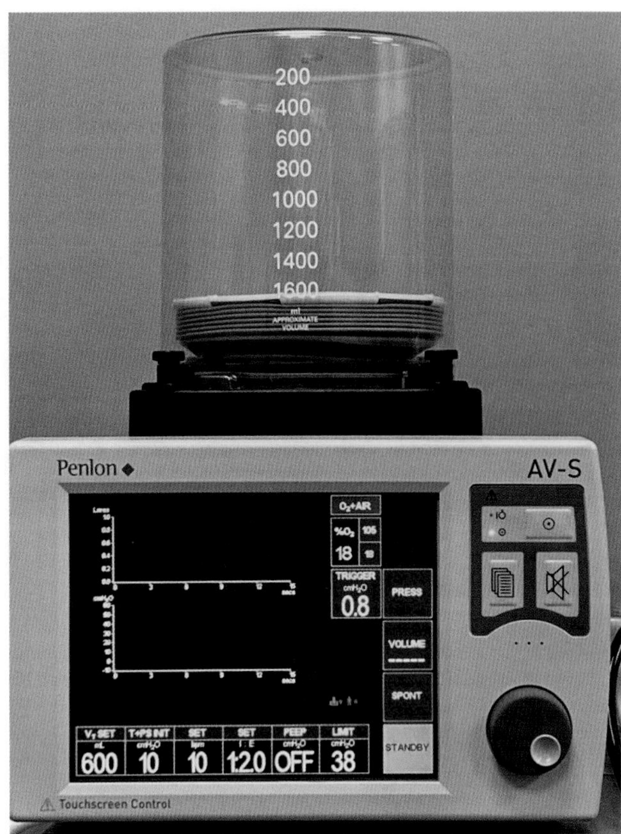

Figure 6.83 The Penlon AV-S is a full-featured anesthetic ventilator that can be cycled by either volume or pressure. It also has options to include spirometry and a circuit oxygen monitor and multiple ventilation modes not found on most traditional anesthetic ventilators (e.g., synchronized intermittent mandatory ventilation, pressure supported, and synchronized mandatory minute ventilation). Source: Dr. Craig Mosley, with permission.

This ventilator is classified as double-circuit, volume or pressure cycled, with an ascending (standing) bellows; it is pneumatically driven and electrically controlled. The Penlon AV-S is a fully featured anesthetic ventilator that can be cycled by either volume or pressure providing the anesthetist with greater flexibility compared to many standard anesthetic ventilators, which normally only offer a single cycling mode (volume or pressure). The ventilator has options to include spirometry and a circuit oxygen monitor and can be configured with multiple ventilation assist modes (e.g., synchronized intermittent mandatory ventilation, pressure supported, and synchronized mandatory minute ventilation). The spirometry units are frequently incorporated into the design of human anesthetic machines using this ventilator but when buying it as a stand-alone unit they need to be connected externally to the inspiratory and expiratory limb of the circle system (Fig. 6.84). Due to the overwhelming number of features, ventilation modes, and waveform display options, a complete description of its features is beyond the scope of this text.

The control module for the AV-S consists of an intuitive touch screen, a multifunction dial/button, and several shortcut buttons (e.g., feature menus, alarm mute, and power on/off). The spirometry and oxygen sensors are situated within the patient breathing system and connect back to the main control unit. With the spirometry module active, the display provides the user feedback regarding set versus measured tidal volume and can display multiple

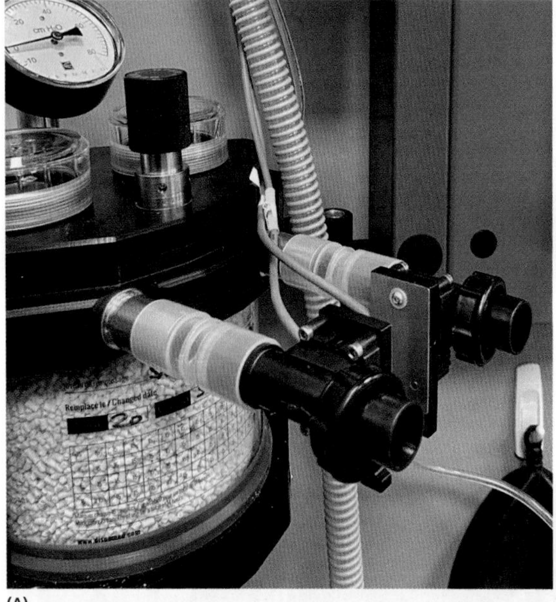

(A)

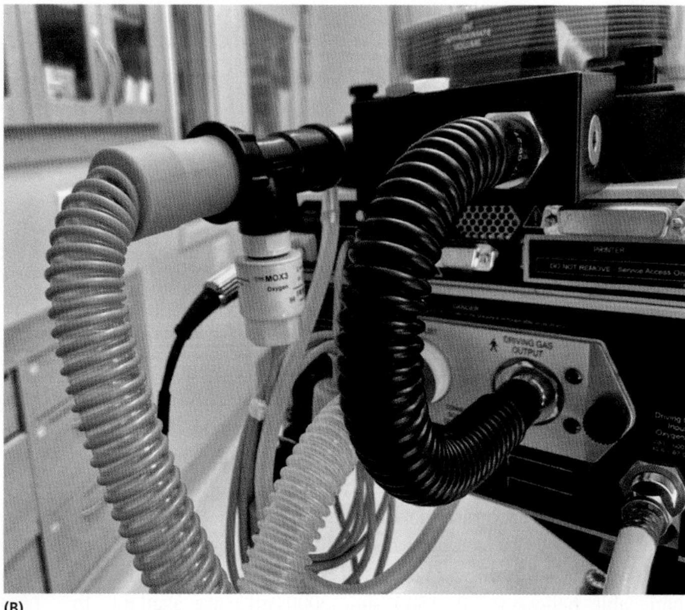

(B)

Figure 6.84 The spirometry module and oxygen monitor used with the Penlon AV-S ventilator require external connection within the patient circuit. **A.** The spirometry units are connected to their respective inspiratory and expiratory limbs of the circle. **B.** The oxygen sensor can be placed in any convenient location that is continuous with the patient circuit. The external location of the spirometry modules makes them prone to damage, so extra care must be taken not to break or disconnect them. Source: Dr. Craig Mosley, with permission.

waveforms (e.g., pressure versus time, volume versus time, and pressure versus volume). The maximum and mean airway pressures are also displayed. In addition to the multiple ventilation modes already mentioned, the ventilator can also provide PEEP during ventilation. The ventilator has preconfigured (or user defined) default adult and pediatric ventilation settings. The standard operating modes are standby, spontaneous ventilation, volume-cycled ventilation, and pressure-cycled ventilation; each of the operating modes is associated with a specific set of features and user display information. Depending upon the method chosen for cycling (pressure versus volume), various parameters are made available for adjustment by the user. The Penlon AV-S can be used with both rebreathing and non-rebreathing systems; however, it is easiest to use without spirometry on non-rebreathing systems, since the spirometry sensors are normally connected to the inspiratory and expiratory limbs of a circle system. While this does limit some of the functionality and features of the ventilator, it can nonetheless perform adequately under non-rebreathing conditions.

Before using the ventilator, it is imperative that the user has read and understands the information in the manufacturer's user guide. Although the ventilator is intuitively safe and relatively straightforward to use for those familiar with both pressure and volume-cycled ventilation, it is important the user familiarizes themselves with the numerous options and features should issues or questions arise during operation. Prior to using the ventilator, connections to the gas supply and scavenge system should be made and the appropriate pre-use checkout procedures followed. Assuming proper functioning of the anesthesia machine, breathing system, and ventilator, the following is a reasonable operational approach for this ventilator with a circle breathing system in volume-cycled mode:

1 Leave the ventilator in standby mode while setting ventilation parameters; the patient can still breathe normally in this mode, but no values will be reported or measured.
2 Connect the ventilator's breathing system tubing to the circle system's reservoir bag mount.
3 The circle system's pop-off (APL) valve is closed.
4 Set the target tidal volume (10–20 mL/kg), respiratory rate (10–15 breaths/min), and I:E ratio (1:2) and PEEP, if desired.
5 Set the pressure limit value, this will be the maximum airway pressure the ventilator will allow to be produced.
6 A similar process is followed for pressure-cycled ventilation but rather than setting a target tidal volume, a target airway pressure is set.

Vetronics Merlin small animal ventilator

The Merlin is a computer-controlled SAV designed specifically for small animal practice (Fig. 6.85). It is capable of delivering tidal volumes from 1 to 800 mL. The Merlin differs from most other commonly used veterinary ventilators in that it is piston-driven and can be computer-controlled. The ventilator is classified as single-circuit and electronically time, pressure, or volume cycled with a piston drive mechanism using a ventilator chamber; it is electrically powered and driven, and computer-controlled. The actual ventilation delivery system works similarly to a large syringe controlled precisely by a computer or microprocessor. The ventilator is capable of providing both controlled and assisted modes of ventilation. The ventilator can be configured for use with both rebreathing and non-rebreathing systems and does not require a separate gas supply, it only uses gas from the patient circuit and the electronically controlled piston to produce ventilation. In order to function properly when used with a non-rebreathing circuit, it is necessary to ensure that anesthetic machine FGF rates slightly exceed the minute ventilation delivered by the ventilator.

The ventilator control panel includes (see Fig. 6.85) flow rate/volume control (0.1–25 L/min or 1–800 mL), inspiratory time control (0.1–9.1 s), expiratory time control (0.1–9.1 s), maximum

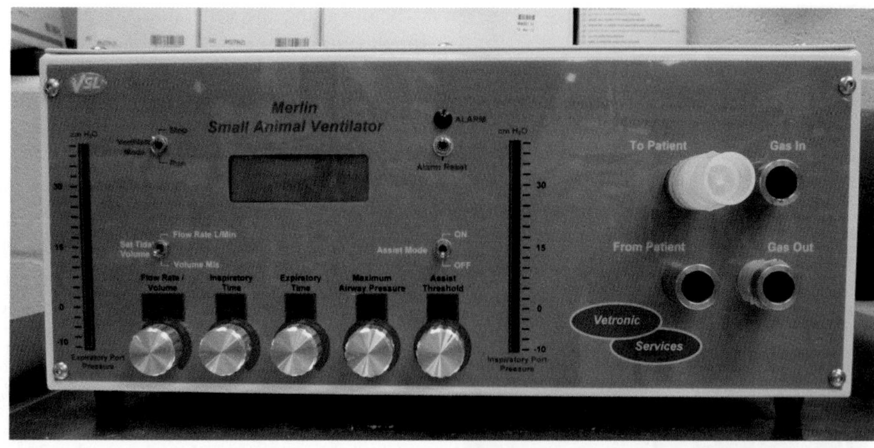

Figure 6.85 The front of the Merlin small animal ventilator showing its various control dials and connection points to the breathing circuit. It is important to note that for proper operation, a one-way valve must always be in place on the "To Patient" port. Source: Dr. Craig Mosley, with permission.

airway pressure (1–60 cmH_2O), assist threshold (−1 to −10 cmH_2O), ventilate mode switch (run-stop), and tidal volume set switch (volume or flow rate). Through the use of the various controls, the ventilator can be set to deliver a tidal volume limited by volume, time, or pressure variables. The volume-limited control mode is generally the easiest and most intuitive for most anesthetists. However, the ability to use it as a pressure-limited ventilator and in assist mode may be useful under specific circumstances. The front panel also contains a liquid crystal display screen that shows the following: tidal volume, minute volume, I:E ratio, respiratory rate, measured airway pressure, measured system compliance, and causes of alarm conditions. There are also two pressure monitors that show airway pressures in the inspiratory and expiratory limbs of the anesthetic circuit. There are four standard 22 mm stainless-steel tapered fittings to connect the breathing system to the ventilator labeled gas-in, gas-out, patient gas delivery, and patient gas exhaust. A non-return one-way valve must also be placed in the inspiratory limb to ensure unidirectional gas flow.

It is important to be completely familiar with the operation and limitations of any piece of anesthetic equipment prior to using it with a patient. If the anesthesia machine, breathing system, and ventilator are all in proper working order as indicated by pre-use checkout procedures and the ventilator is being used in volume-limited control mode, the following guidelines are appropriate for use of the ventilator:

1 Properly connect the electric power sources for the ventilator.
2 Ensure the ventilator is in stop mode, tidal volume is in volume mode, and the assist setting is off.
3 Set the desired tidal volume (10–20 mL/kg), inspiratory time (1–2 s), expiratory time (1–4 s), and maximum airway pressure (20–30 cmH_2O). It is not necessary to set the assist threshold unless this mode is being used.
4 Make the appropriate connections from the ventilator to the anesthetic machine and patient as described by the manufacturer. This includes placement of the one-way non-return valve on the patient inspiratory limb. The reservoir bag should remain in place and the adjustable pressure-limiting (APL) valve (pop-off valve) should NOT be closed.
5 Switch the ventilator to run mode.
6 Make final adjustments to tidal volume, inspiratory time, and expiratory time to meet the needs of the patient.

Dräger Large Animal Anesthesia Ventilator

This ventilator was included as a part of the Narkovet-E Large Animal Anesthesia Machine; the entire system is called the "Narkovet-E Large Animal Anesthesia Control Center." The ventilator was not marketed as a stand-alone unit for large animal anesthesia. Although they are no longer being manufactured, some of these ventilator–anesthesia machine combinations remain in use in veterinary hospitals. The ventilator is powered pneumatically, generally at a pressure of 50 psi. It is classed as double-circuit, tidal volume preset, time cycled, and pneumatically driven with a descending/hanging bellows, and it uses fluidic circuitry. The controls include an on–off switch, a tidal volume control with a scale of 4–15 L on the bellows housing, a frequency control (6–18 breaths/min), and a flow control knob that determines inspiratory flow (a combination of flow and maximum pressure being delivered to the bellows compartment); the manufacturer recommends that the flow setting be adjusted so that the bellows always reaches the upper stop. The I:E ratio of 1:2 is preset.

Before using the ventilator, the proper connections to the gas supply and scavenge system should be made, and the appropriate pre-use checkout procedures should be performed. The instruction manual for ventilators includes a standard pre-use check for the ventilator. The following is a logical approach to the operation of the ventilator with a circle breathing system:

1 Connect the compressed gas supply hose to the ventilator.
2 Adjust the tidal volume control to the appropriate setting for the patient and ensure that the self-locking mechanism is engaged to prevent inadvertent movement of the bellows stop plate during use.
3 Attach the corrugated breathing hose from the bellows to the reservoir bag port of the circle system.
4 Close the pop-off (APL) valve on the circle system.
5 Turn the power switch on.
6 Adjust the frequency control knob to the desired respiratory rate.
7 Adjust the flow control knob so that the bellows reaches the upper stop at end inspiration. If the bellows does not return to its original position during expiration (usually indicative of a leak in the patient circuit), the bellows can be filled by using a higher flow from the oxygen flowmeter, and the leak should be corrected.

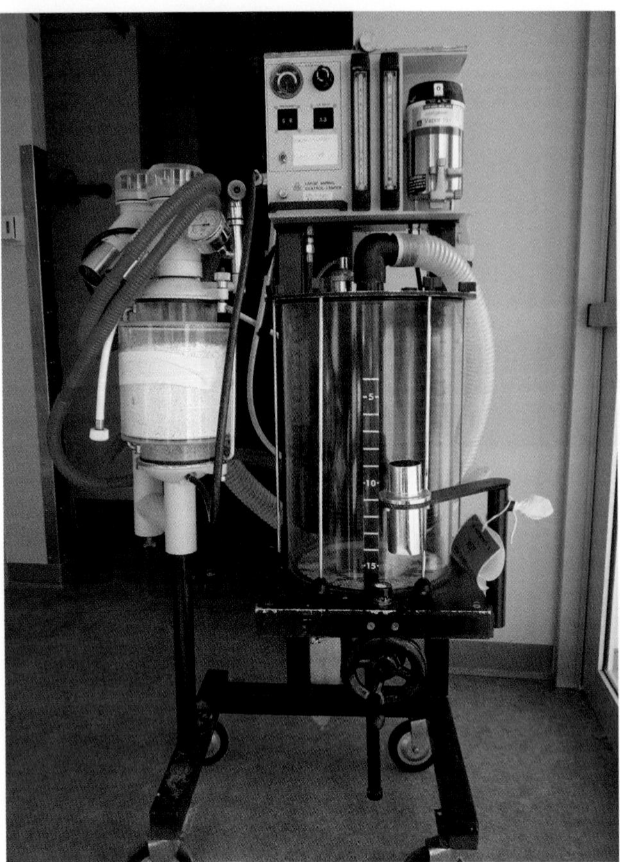

Figure 6.86 The Dräger Narkovet-E Electronic Large Animal Control Center: the bellows and bellows housing with markings for tidal volume (4–15 L), the corrugated breathing hose from the bellows to the circle system (behind the bellows housing), and the self-locking knob or wheel (bottom center) for selection of tidal volume. The controls are located above the bellows on the left. Source: Dr. Craig Mosley, with permission.

Narkovet-E Electronic Large Animal Control Center

This is a combination of Dräger's Narkovet E-2 Large Animal Anesthesia System (anesthesia machine and circle breathing system) with a Dräger AV-E ventilator (Fig. 6.86). The ventilator is not available as a stand-alone unit for large animals and is no longer being manufactured by Dräger, but machines are still in use. There is also at least one manufacturer (Vetland Medical, Louisville, KY, USA) that uses a reconfigured Dräger AV-E ventilator as part of its large animal workstation (LAS-4000). The ventilator is classified as double-circuit, tidal volume preset, and time cycled, with a descending bellows. The ventilator is electronically controlled and pneumatically driven. It is powered electrically and pneumatically (40–60 psi with oxygen, but air is an option). The controls include an on–off switch, a self-locking knob located below the bellows assembly to control the tidal volume (4–15 L), a thumbwheel controller-indicator switch to adjust the respiratory rate (frequency control from 1 to 30 breaths/min), a flow control setting to determine the inspiratory flow rate, and the I:E control (a thumbwheel indicator-controller to adjust the I:E ratio in increments of 0.5 from 1:1 to 1:4.5). The manufacturer recommends that the flow control knob be adjusted so that the bellows always reaches the upper stop of inspiration. The ventilator provides for controlled ventilation; assisted ventilation is not an option.

Before using the ventilator, the proper connections to the gas supply and scavenge system should be made, and the appropriate pre-use checkout procedures should be performed. The instruction manual for the ventilator includes a standard pre-use checklist. The following is a step-by-step approach to the operation of the ventilator with a circle breathing system:

1 Connect the gas supply (oxygen hose) to the anesthesia machine and ventilator.
2 Adjust the tidal volume control to the appropriate setting for the patient and ensure that the self-locking mechanism is engaged to prevent inadvertent movement of the bellows stop plate.
3 Select the desired frequency of ventilation.
4 Select the desired I:E ratio.
5 Attach the corrugated breathing hose from the bellows to the reservoir bag port of the circle system.
6 Close the pop-off (APL) valve on the circle system.
7 Turn the power supply switch on.
8 Adjust the flow control knob so that the bellows reaches the upper stop at end inspiration. If the bellows does not return to its original location during expiration, it can be filled by increasing the flow from the oxygen flowmeter.

Mallard Medical Rachel Model 2800 series anesthesia ventilator

This ventilator (Fig. 6.87) is a microprocessor-based, electronic control system used to control ventilation in large animals being maintained on circle breathing systems. The 2800 series has been upgraded since its initial introduction. The earlier Models 2800A and 2800B of the series are still widely used in veterinary practice; the most recent Model 2800C features updated electronics and display and an optional air flowmeter for controlling F_IO_2, and the bellows is reduced from 21 to 18 L, but it retains all the performance of the earlier models and is functionally very similar. The ventilator is currently available as part of a complete large animal anesthetic machine and circle system breathing circuit. The stand for the ventilator and the bellows is designed for the attachment of a circle breathing system and two vaporizers for inhalant anesthetics, and it has shelves to accommodate physiological monitoring devices. The ventilator is classified as dual-circuit and time-cycled, and it is pneumatically driven and electronically controlled with an ascending (standing) bellows configuration.

Most of the functional considerations for the Model 2800C are similar to those for the Model 2400V used for small animal applications. The control console for the 2800C is located above the bellows housing instead of below the housing as it is in the 2400V, and LED displays are employed as they are in the 2400V. The ventilator is controlled by a microprocessor, but the pneumatics have been modified for generation of greater inspiratory flow rates, which are adjustable from 10 to 600 L/min. The control dials include flow rate (10–660 L/min), inspiratory time, and respiratory rate (2–15 breaths/min), as well as a power switch (off-on-standby) and a manual ventilation button. The tidal volume is controlled by adjusting the flow rate dial until the desired tidal volume is obtained (read from the bellows canister) and the I:E ratio is calculated based on the selected inspiratory time and respiratory rate. The manual ventilation button will deliver the selected flow rate to compress the bellows as long as it is depressed and will operate even in circumstances where power is unavailable. The bellows (18 or 21 L) is standing and ascends during expiration. Like other ventilators with standing bellows, the Model 2800C produces PEEP. This is a result of the above atmospheric pressure required to activate (open) the

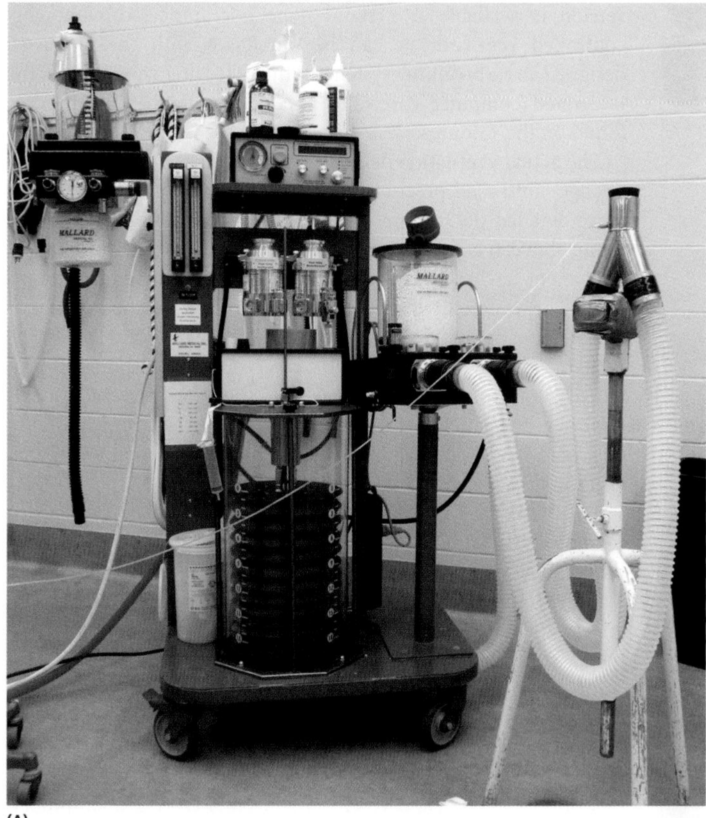

(A)

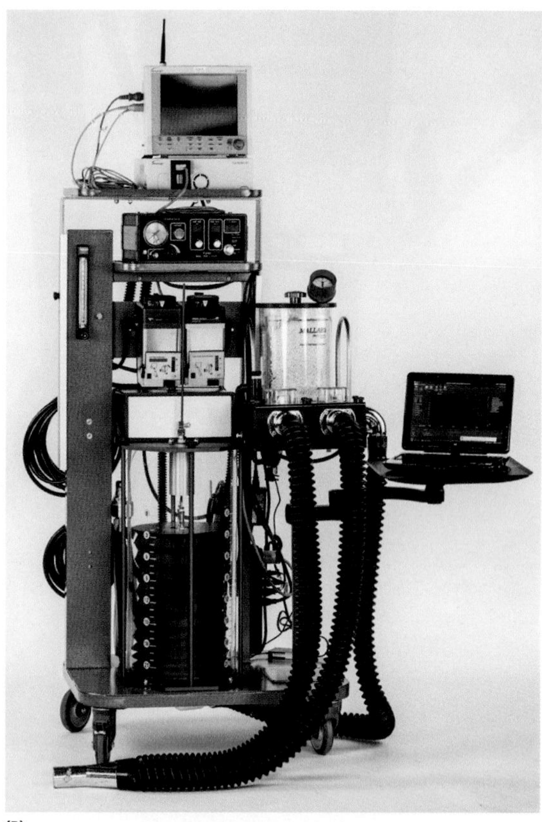
(B)

Figure 6.87 The Mallard 2800 large animal anesthetic machine and ventilator is available with an optional small animal circuit and ventilator, mounted on the top left of the machine (shown in **A.**). The ventilator uses the same control system as the large animal ventilator. The Mallard 2800 is also available in many custom configurations as shown in **B.** Source: Part **A.**, Dr. Craig Mosley, with permission. Source: Part **B.**, Dr. Ron E. Mandsager, College of Veterinary Medicine, Oregon State University, Veterinary Teaching Hospital, Corvallis, OR, USA; reproduced with permission of Dr. Mandsager.

spill valve(s) in order to offset the effect of gravity due to the weight of the bellows. The spill valves of the 2800C are unique in that they are a pair of spring-activated valves located on the top of the bellows and are activated to open only once the bellows reaches maximum ascension and the pin in the top of the spill valves is depressed, opening the valves (Fig. 6.88). The gas exiting the spill valves is then exhausted into a hollow cylinder located at the top of the bellows housing and removed. The pressure to activate the spill valves, resulting in PEEP, is between 4 and 6 cmH_2O. The amount of PEEP can also be controlled by a pneumatic vacuum pump on the 2800C; the pump creates negative pressure between the bellows and the bellows housing during the expiratory phase of ventilation and functions to reduce the level of PEEP according to the adjustments made by the operator. An ambient end-expiratory pressure may be achieved, although activation of this function is rarely needed and indeed the PEEP provided by the ventilator may even be beneficial. The patient is often allowed to breathe spontaneously through the bellows, even if the ventilator is off or in standby mode as the work of breathing is not significantly increased; this avoids the need to use a reservoir bag and disconnect and reconnect should ventilation be required. The hosing from the bellows to the circle system can be removed, facilitating drainage of moisture from the machine. There is also a "holding" assembly located on the top of the bellows that can be used to hold the bellows fully inflated when not in use to facilitate drying of the bellows. An MRI-compatible model is also available.

Before using the ventilator, the proper connections to the gas and electric power supplies and the scavenge system should be made, and the appropriate pre-use checkout procedures should be performed for all equipment. The following is a reasonable operational approach for the Model 2800C ventilator with a circle breathing system:

1 Place the master switch in the standby mode and dial the desired settings for respiratory rate and inspiratory time, according to the patient's needs.
2 Set the inspiratory flow control to the desired rate of flow – low, medium, or high – depending on the patient's needs; it is generally best to start at the low or medium rate to ensure excessive tidal volumes are not inadvertently administered.
3 Connect the corrugated tubing from the ventilator's bellows to the circle system's reservoir bag mount and the ventilator exhalation port to the scavenge system. Close the circle system's pop-off (APL) valve and release the ventilator's bellows. Ensure that the bellows is fully inflated and positioned at zero. Under normal use circumstances, the ventilator often remains continuously connected to the breathing circuit for convenience during a case as the patient can breathe through the bellows in this standing/ascending configuration without any additional effort.
4 Turn the master switch on, and inspiration should begin.
5 If the bellows does not return to zero, this may suggest a leak in the system; the bellows can be filled by turning up the flowmeter or alternatively by using the flush valve, and the leak should be

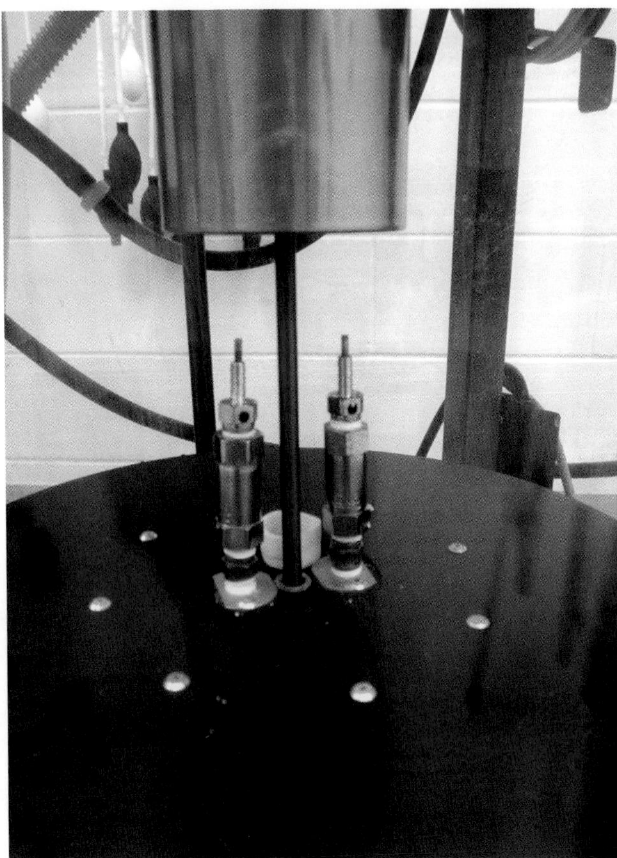

Figure 6.88 The ventilator spill valves of the Mallard Model 2800 are situated on the top of the bellows (spindle-shaped stainless-steel fixtures on top of the bellows) within the ventilator canister. When the bellows reaches full ascent, a pin in the top of the spill valve is depressed, allowing excess gas flow to escape. Note the stainless-steel cylinder (above the spill valves) in the top of the bellows housing into which the excess gas is evacuated. Source: Dr. Craig Mosley, with permission.

identified and corrected. If the flush valve is used to fill the bellows, the anesthetic concentration in the breathing circuit will be reduced.

6 The flow rate, inspiratory time, and respiratory rate can then be further adjusted to produce the appropriate ventilator parameters for the patient.
7 Finally, if desired, the PEEP control can be adjusted to set the desired end-expiratory pressure.

Hallowell Tafonius and Tafonius Junior

The Tafonius ventilator is a microprocessor/computer-controlled large animal ventilator designed specifically for large animal practice (Fig. 6.89). The Tafonius ventilator differs from most other commonly used veterinary ventilators in that it is piston-driven and can be computer-controlled, allowing for precise and customizable control of ventilator patterns and modes of ventilation. The ventilator is classified as single-circuit and electronically timed, volume cycled with a piston drive mechanism using a ventilator chamber; it is electrically powered and driven, and microprocessor/computer controlled. The ventilator is available in several configurations; the Tafonius is a complete anesthetic workstation (including a circle anesthetic system, complete patient monitoring module, ventilator, and integrated computer controller), while the Tafonius Junior version is available as a stand-alone microprocessor/computer-controlled ventilator or can be purchased with the Hallowell designed circle breathing system. Both of the latter versions lack the integrated computer controller and patient monitoring module found on the Tafonius.

The actual ventilation delivery system works similarly to a large syringe controlled precisely by a computer or microprocessor. A more detailed description of the piston drive mechanism can be found above. It is important to note that similar to other ventilators, the patient can breathe spontaneously while connected to the ventilator. The piston in the ventilator will move instantaneously as required to maintain an airway pressure near 0 cmH_2O at the patient circuit Y-piece. Although a reservoir bag attachment is provided, it is not necessary to use it if spontaneous ventilation is desired in the patient. As the ventilator requires electronic power to operate, there is an integrated battery and battery monitoring system should a power failure occur.

The ventilator is capable of providing both controlled and assisted modes of ventilation. Control of the ventilator is accomplished via the ventilator's auxiliary computer/microprocessor (Tafonius and Tafonius Junior) or via the integrated computer running the Tafonius system software found on the standard (complete) Tafonius anesthetic workstation. With appropriate programming, the integrated computer and Tafonius software could be used to customize ventilator control to produce nearly limitless breathing patterns. Primary ventilator control is achieved by altering the following parameters: tidal volume (0.1–20 L), respiratory rate (1–20 breaths/min), inspiratory time (0.5–4.0 s), and MWPL (10–80 cmH_2O). The microprocessor will automatically determine expiratory time and inspiratory flow rate based on these preset parameters within the limits of the equipment (maximum inspiratory flow rate is 900 L/min and minimum expiratory time is 0.5 s). Other ventilation controls include user-defined assist mode and CPAP/PEEP. There is also a dump valve button that functions as an electronic pop-off or spill valve found on conventional ventilators and a buffer volume button used to determine the size of the "virtual" reservoir bag. A detailed operational description of this ventilator is beyond the scope of this discussion as it will depend on the specific ventilator configuration being used (Tafonius or Tafonius Junior) and whether the ventilator is being controlled using the auxiliary ventilator control panel or the integrated computer system running the Tafonius software. However, ease of use of the ventilator is very comparable to that of other ventilators.

Before using the ventilator, the proper connections to the gas and electric power supplies and the scavenge system should be made. It is necessary for the Tafonius ventilators to perform an automatic start-up checkout procedure that calibrates the pressure transducers, initializes the piston, and leak tests the machine. The results of this self-test will be displayed on the auxiliary control screen and/or the integrated computer.

ICU Medical (formerly Surgivet) DHV1000 large animal ventilator

This large animal-specific ventilator can be purchased as a stand-alone ventilator compatible for use with any standard large animal anesthesia machine or purchased as part of a complete anesthesia workstation (LDS 3000 Large Animal Anesthesia Machine) (Fig. 6.90). The ventilator is classified as dual-circuit, tidal volume preset/limited, and time cycled and is pneumatically driven and electronically controlled with a descending/hanging bellows configuration.

The controls on the control module include power switch (on–off), respiratory rate dial, inspiratory time dial, flow dial

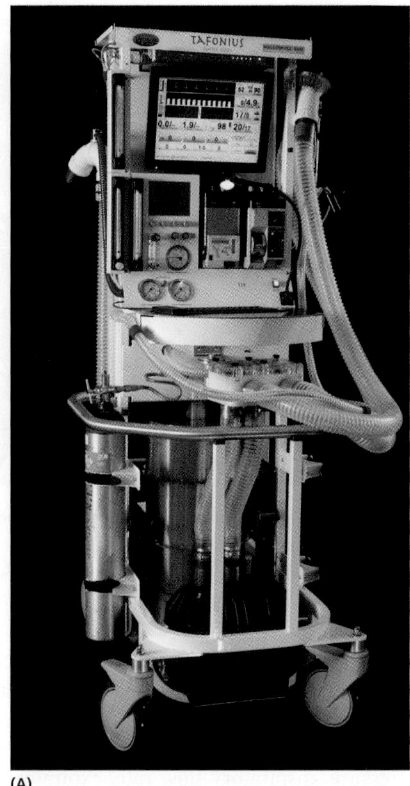

(A)

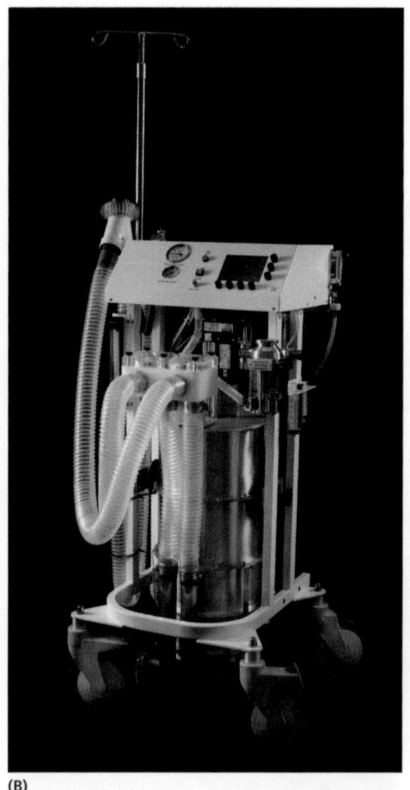
(B)

Figure 6.89 **A.** The Tafonius and **B.** the Tafonuis Junior are microprocessors/computer-controlled piston-driven large animal ventilators. The ventilator is available in a stand-alone configuration (Tafonius Junior) or with an integrated large animal anesthetic machine and patient monitoring system (Tafonius). Source: Hallowell EMC, Pittsfield, MA, USA; reproduced with permission.

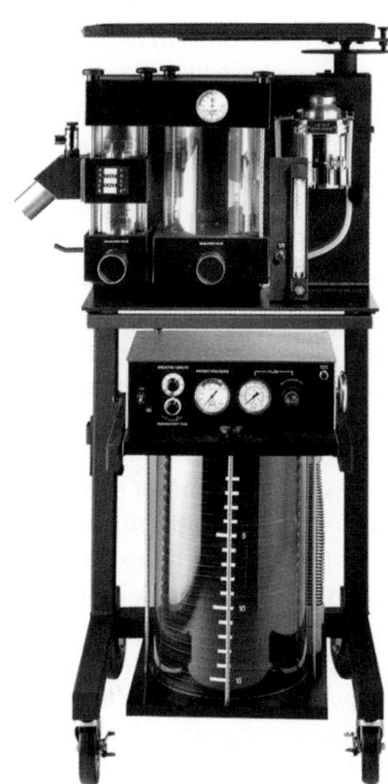

Figure 6.90 The ICU Medical (formerly Surgivet) DHV 1000 large animal ventilator can be purchased alone or as part of a complete large animal workstation as shown here. In this configuration, the ventilator unit is mounted on the machine cart below the large animal circle. Source: Smith Medical, Norwell, MA, USA; reproduced with permission.

(inspiratory gas flow), and a manual ventilation button. There is also a turn wheel located on the side of the control module used to adjust the maximum descent of the bellows.

Before using the ventilator, the proper connections to the gas supply and scavenge system should be made, and the appropriate pre-use checkout procedures should be performed. The instruction manual for the ventilator includes a standard pre-use checklist. The following is a step-by-step approach to the operation of the ventilator with a circle breathing system:

1 Connect the gas supply (oxygen hose) to the anesthesia machine and ventilator.
2 Adjust the tidal volume control wheel to the appropriate setting for the patient.
3 Select the desired respiratory rate.
4 Select the desired inspiratory time.
5 Attach the corrugated breathing hose from the bellows to the reservoir bag port of the circle system.
6 Close the pop-off (APL) valve on the circle system.
7 Turn the power supply switch on.
8 Adjust the flow control knob so that the bellows reaches the upper stop at end inspiration.
9 The flow rate, inspiratory time, and respiratory rate can then be further adjusted to produce the appropriate ventilator parameters for the patient.

Bird Mark respirator-driven ventilators

The Bird Mark 7 respirator was one of the first systems used to drive and control both small and large animal ventilators (so-called "bag-in-a-barrel" ventilators) and is still being used today (Fig. 6.91). The

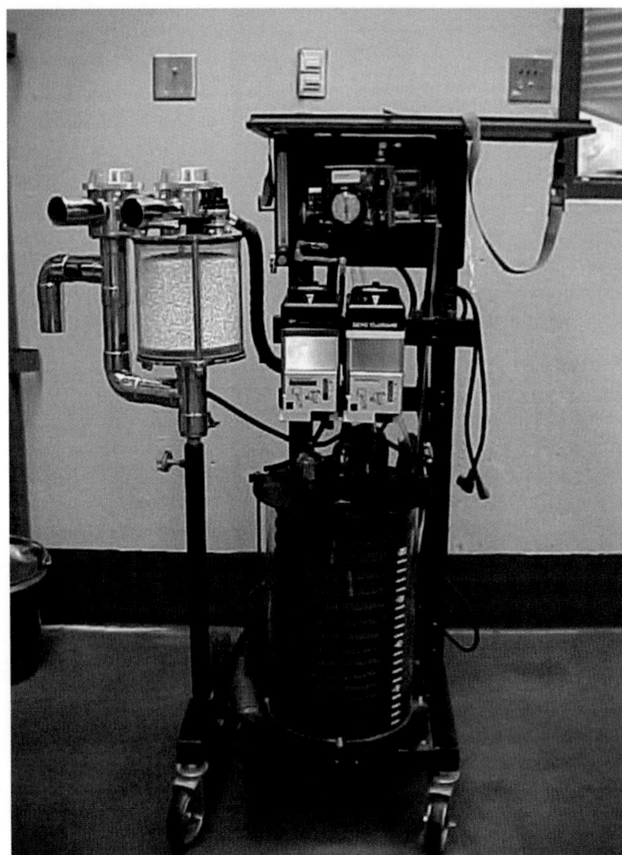

Figure 6.91 An example of a Bird Mark 7 respirator being used as the controller of a large animal anesthesia ventilator. Source: Dr. Thomas Riebold, College of Veterinary Medicine, Oregon State University, Corvallis, OR, USA; reproduced with permission of Dr. Riebold.

Bird Mark 7 was originally developed as a single-circuit respirator for humans and was not designed principally as an anesthetic ventilator; however, by applying the respirator function to a bag or bellows in a "box or barrel," a dual-circuit ventilator is created.

Uniquely, Bird respirator-driven ventilators can be used in control, assist, or assist-control modes and have the capability of limiting tidal volume based on airway pressure. This differs from most contemporary ventilators that only offer control modes of ventilation and tend to limit tidal volume based on the volume of gas delivered. Bird Mark 7 respirators are used to control and drive both JD Medical's LAV-2000 and LAV-3000 series large animal ventilators. Although other Bird respirator-driven ventilators are not discussed here, the general principles of operation are similar, although the design details may vary significantly.

The JD Medical LAV-3000 is a stand-alone ventilator that can be used with any large animal anesthetic machine and the LAV-2000 is an integrated ventilator and anesthesia machine available in several predesigned and custom configurations. The LAVC-2000 and LAVC-3000 systems can be converted to a 5 L system for use in foals by adding a 5000 mL bellows and a canister (bellows housing) insert. A modified Mark 7 respirator drives the bellows in the ventilator system. When the system is operating, the Bird ventilator supplies gas to pressurize the space between the bellows and the bellows housing (canister) to force the bellows in an upward motion delivering gases from the bellows, through the interface hose, to the breathing system. The LAVC-2000 and LAVC-3000 are classified as

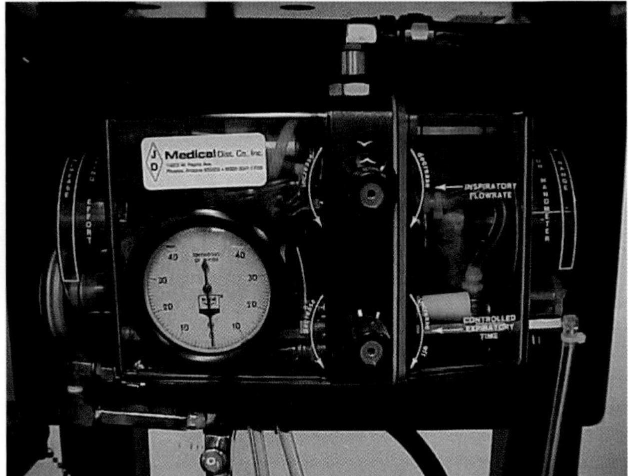

Figure 6.92 A Bird Mark 7 respirator showing the various controls used to control a ventilator. Source: Dr. Thomas Riebold, College of Veterinary Medicine, Oregon State University, Corvallis, OR, USA; reproduced with permission of Dr. Riebold.

dual-circuit, pressure limited, and time cycled, and are pneumatically controlled and driven with a descending/hanging bellows configuration.

The controls on a Bird Mark 7 (Fig 6.92) include inspiratory pressure, inspiratory flow rate, expiratory time (apnea control), and inspiratory sensitivity. In addition, a manometer, a hand timer (push–pull mechanism) used to manually initiate/end respiration, and a DISS connector for the source of pneumatic power are features of the ventilator. With the modified Bird Mark 7, inspiratory pressure can be varied from 5 to 65 cm H_2O, inspiratory sensitivity from −0.5 to −5 cm H_2O, expiratory time from 5 to 15 s, and inspiratory flow from 0 to over 450 L/min. The pneumatic power source should be delivered to the inlet of the ventilator at 50 psi. The bellows can deliver a tidal volume of up to 20 L. Inspiration can be started or stopped by the use of a hand timer. The Bird Mark 7 is a pressure-cycled ventilator unless the push–pull manual cycling rod is pulled out, which causes the ventilator to be time cycled.

Before using the Model LAV-3000 ventilator for controlling ventilation during anesthesia, the power supply and scavenge system should be connected, and the appropriate pre-use checkout procedures should be performed for all equipment. The following is a reasonable operational approach for the ventilator with a circle breathing system in the control mode:

1 Set the inspiratory sensitivity control to a high setting to minimize the possibility of patient-initiated ventilation.
2 Set the inspiratory pressure control to the range 20–30 cmH_2O and readjust the setting to achieve the desired tidal volume after steps 5 and 6 have been completed.
3 Connect the corrugated hose (interface hose) from the bellows to the reservoir bag port of the circle system.
4 Close the pop-off (APL) valve of the circle system. Then, the bellows may need to be filled by increasing the flow of oxygen to the patient circuit (oxygen flowmeter on the anesthesia machine).
5 Turn the inspiratory flow control on to start the ventilator and set the flow control to deliver a tidal volume in approximately 1.5–3.0 s.
6 Set the expiratory time control to establish a respiratory rate appropriate for the patient, often 7–10 breaths/min.

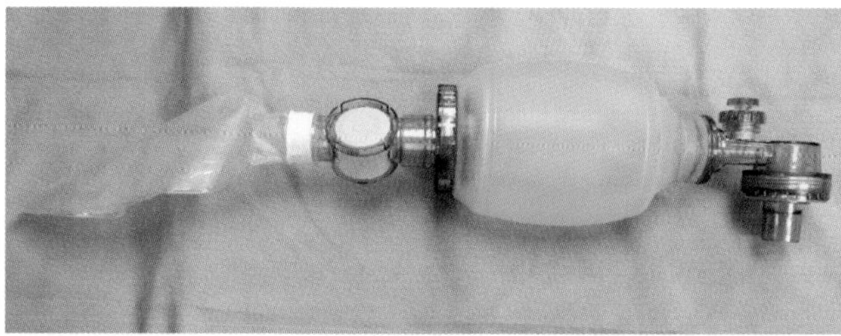

Figure 6.93 An example of a resuscitation bag suitable for use in veterinary medicine. This bag also has an expandable reservoir (left of image) to serve as a reservoir of enriched gas if being used with supplemental oxygen. However, it is important to note that resuscitation bags do not require supplemental gas delivery for use. Source: Dr. Craig Mosley, with permission.

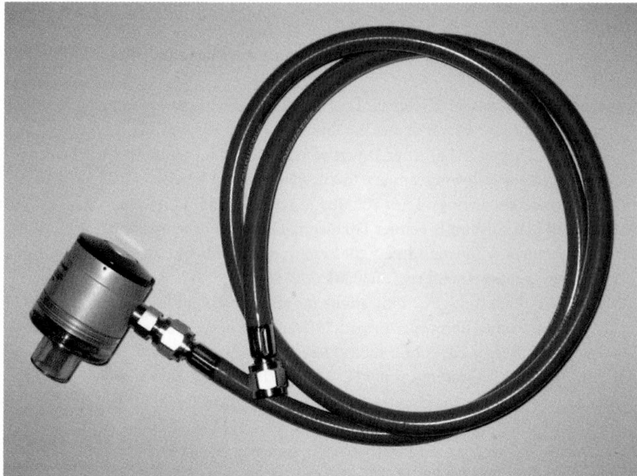

Figure 6.94 A demand valve is an oxygen delivery system that can be used to perform manual intermittent positive-pressure ventilation. Source: Dr. Craig Mosley, with permission.

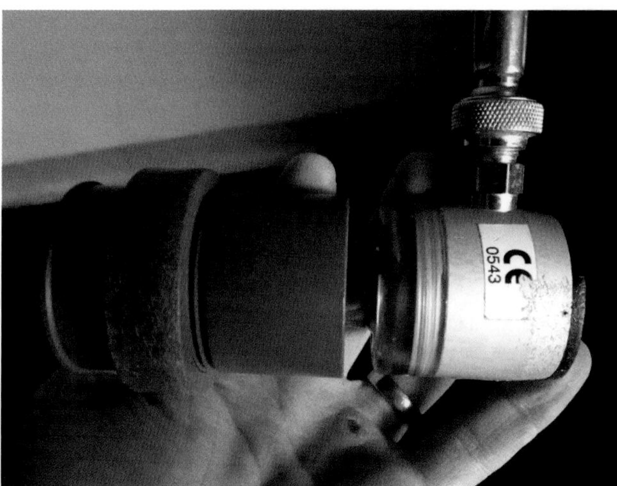

Figure 6.95 Demand valves are normally designed to fit standard endotracheal tube adapters. Large animal-specific adapters are normally required for use with the funnel-type (shown), or 22 mm OD stainless-steel adapters normally associated with large animal endotracheal tubes. Source: Dr. Craig Mosley, with permission.

7 For final settings, the operator should understand that there are interactions between the controls on a Bird ventilator (e.g., changing inspiratory flow may affect respiratory rate and vice versa).

Respiratory assist devices

Several types and brands of respiratory assist devices are available. Some are completely manual in operation (resuscitation bags with one-way valves) and some use compressed gas (oxygen) to assist ventilation (demand valves). The mechanics of these devices have been reviewed [2].

Manual resuscitators

A manual resuscitator is appropriate for the application of IPPV to small veterinary patients. Several brands of resuscitators are available. The basic components of a manual resuscitator are a compressible self-expanding bag, a bag refill valve, and a non-rebreathing valve. Some resuscitators can be attached to a source of oxygen to enrich the oxygen content of inspired gases (Fig. 6.93). Manual resuscitators can be fitted with a reservoir to serve as a source of oxygen when the oxygen flow to the resuscitator does not meet the filling demands of the resuscitator.

Demand valves

A demand valve can be used to deliver IPPV (Fig. 6.94). The demand valve is set to deliver oxygen when the patient begins to inspire (creating slight negative pressure, activating gas delivery) until exhalation starts or until a certain preset pressure is reached. Expiration is passive through the valve outlet. The outlet may be restrictive to expiration in large patients. The device can be disconnected from the endotracheal tube after inspiration to decrease the resistance to exhalation. A demand valve can be triggered manually to deliver oxygen to the patient as long as the activation button is held down or until the preset pressure limit is reached. Alternately compressing and releasing the control button allows application of IPPV. A demand valve with the capacity for a high inspiratory flow rate is most desirable for use in large animals; demand valves generating low inspiratory flows will cause an excessively long inspiratory time in patients requiring a large tidal volume.

Demand valves are available from various manufacturers. Most will deliver a maximum flow rate of approximately 160 L/min at 50 psi, though they are also available low-flow models (40 L/min), so it is best to confirm prior to purchase. The high-flow models are most suitable for large animal veterinary applications. The Hudson demand valve has been described for use in horses but is no longer readily available [92]. It delivers approximately 200 L/min if the oxygen supply pressure is 50 psi and more than 275 L/min if the supply pressure is 80 psi. Demand valves are normally designed to accept a standard endotracheal tube connector (15 mm OD) and a standard face mask (22 mm OD), although various adapters are available in veterinary medicine for large animal endotracheal tube adapters (funnel-type and stainless-steel 22 mm OD adapters) (Fig. 6.95).

Acknowledgment

The author and editors wish to thank Dr. Sandee Hartsfield for allowing use of some of his material from previous editions of this text in the preparation of this chapter. Portions of this chapter have also been reproduced in the text, *Veterinary Anesthetic and Monitoring Equipment*.

References

1 Dorsch JA, Dorsch SE. *A Practical Approach to Anesthesia Equipment*. Philadelphia, PA: Wolters Kluwer/Lippincott Williams & Wilkins Health, 2010.

2 Dorsch JA, Dorsch SE. *Understanding Anesthesia Equipment*, 5th edn. New York, NY: Lippincott Williams & Wilkins, 2008.

3 Davey AJ, Diba A. *Ward's Anaesthetic Equipment*, 6th edn. Philadelphia, PA: Saunders, 2012.

4 Cooley KG, Johnson RA. *Veterinary Anesthetic and Monitoring Equipment*, Hoboken, NJ: Wiley-Blackwell, 2018.

5 Fulkerson PJ, Gustafson SB. Use of laryngeal mask airway compared to endotracheal tube with positive-pressure ventilation in anesthetized swine. *Vet Anaesth Analg* 2007; **34**: 284–288.

6 Wenger S, Müllhaupt D, Ohlerth S, *et al.* Experimental evaluation of four airway devices in anaesthetized New Zealand White rabbits. *Vet Anaesth Analg* 2017; **44**: 529–537.

7 Prasse SA, Schrack J, Wenger S, *et al.* Clinical evaluation of the v-gel supraglottic airway device in comparison with a classical laryngeal mask and endotracheal intubation in cats during spontaneous and controlled mechanical ventilation. *Vet Anaesth Analg* 2016; **43**: 55–62.

8 Wiederstein I, Moens YP. Guidelines and criteria for the placement of laryngeal mask airways in dogs. *Vet Anaesth Analg* 2008; **35**: 374–382.

9 Huckins GL, Doss GA, Ferreira TH. Evaluation of supraglottic airway device use during inhalation anesthesia in healthy African pygmy hedgehogs (*Atelerix albiventris*). *Vet Anaesth Analg* 2021; **48**: 517–523.

10 Stewart SL, Secrest JA, Norwood BR, *et al.* A comparison of endotracheal tube cuff pressures using estimation techniques and direct intracuff measurement. *AANA J* 2003; **71**: 443–447.

11 Mitchell SL, McCarthy R, Rudloff E, *et al.* Tracheal rupture associated with intubation in cats: 20 cases (1996–1998). *J Am Vet Med Assoc* 2000; **216**: 1592–1595.

12 Hung WC, Ko JC, Weil AB, *et al.* Evaluation of endotracheal tube cuff pressure and the use of the three cuff inflation syringe devices in dogs. *Front Vet Sci* 2020; **6**: 39.

13 Jackson J, Richter KP, Launer DP. Thoracoscopic partial pericardiectomy in 13 dogs. *J Vet Intern Med* 1999; **13**: 529–533.

14 Radlinsky MG, Mason DE, Biller DS, *et al.* Thoracoscopic visualization and ligation of the thoracic duct in dogs. *Vet Surg* 2002; **31**: 138–146.

15 Mayhew PD, Culp WT, Pascoe PJ, *et al.* Evaluation of blind thoracoscopic-assisted placement of three double-lumen endobronchial tube designs for one-lung ventilation in dogs. *Vet Surg* 2012; **41**: 664–670.

16 Cantwell SL, Duke T, Walsh PJ, *et al.* One-lung versus two-lung ventilation in the closed-chest anesthetized dog: a comparison of cardiopulmonary parameters. *Vet Surg* 2000; **29**: 365–373.

17 Adami C, Axiak S, Rytz U, *et al.* Alternating one lung ventilation using a double lumen endobronchial tube and providing CPAP to the non-ventilated lung in a dog. *Vet Anaesth Analg* 2011; **38**: 70–76.

18 Mayhew KN, Mayhew PD, Sorrell-Raschi L, *et al.* Thoracoscopic subphrenic pericardectomy using double-lumen endobronchial intubation for alternating one-lung ventilation. *Vet Surg* 2009; **38**: 961–966.

19 Bauquier SH, Culp WT, Lin RC, *et al.* One-lung ventilation using a wire-guided endobronchial blocker for thoracoscopic pericardial fenestration in a dog. *Can Vet J* 2010; **51**: 1135–1138.

20 Lansdowne JL, Monnet E, Twedt DC, *et al.* Thoracoscopic lung lobectomy for treatment of lung tumors in dogs. *Vet Surg* 2005; **34**: 530–535.

21 Wang WH, Bernal SD, Mirra A, *et al.* Use of an "EZ-blocker" to facilitate thoracoscopic surgery in two dogs. *Vet Rec Case Rep* 2017; **5**: e000449.

22 Mayhew PD, Chohan A, Hardy BT, *et al.* Cadaveric evaluation of fluoroscopy-assisted placement of one-lung ventilation devices for video assisted thoracoscopic surgery in dogs. *Vet Surg* 2020; **49**(Suppl 1): 93–101.

23 Smith JC, Robertson LD, Auhll A, *et al.* Endotracheal tubes versus laryngeal mask airways in rabbit inhalation anesthesia: ease of use and waste gas emissions. *Contemp Top Lab Anim Sci* 2004; **43**: 22–25.

24 van Oostrom H, Krauss MW, Sap R. A comparison between the v-gel supraglottic airway device and the cuffed endotracheal tube for airway management in spontaneously breathing cats during isoflurane anaesthesia. *Vet Anaesth Analg* 2013; **40**: 265–271.

25 Wiederstein I, Auer U, Moens Y. Laryngeal mask airway insertion requires less propofol than endotracheal intubation in dogs. *Vet Anaesth Analg* 2006; **33**: 201–206.

26 Bateman L, Ludders JW, Gleed RD, *et al.* Comparison between facemask and laryngeal mask airway in rabbits during isoflurane anesthesia. *Vet Anaesth Analg* 2005; **32**: 280–288.

27 Johnson JA, Atkins AL, Heard DJ. Application of the laryngeal mask airway for anesthesia in three chimpanzees and one gibbon. *J Zoo Wildl Med* 2010; **41**: 535–537.

28 Cerveny SN, D'Agostino JJ, Davis MR, *et al.* Comparison of laryngeal mask airway use with endotracheal intubation during anesthesia of western lowland gorillas (*Gorilla gorilla gorilla*). *J Zoo Wildl Med* 2012; **43**: 759–767.

29 West G, Heard DJ, Caulkett N. *Zoo Animal and Wildlife Immobilization and Anesthesia*. Ames, IA: Blackwell Publishing, 2007; 718.

30 Read MR, Read EK, Duke T, *et al.* Cardiopulmonary effects and induction and recovery characteristics of isoflurane and sevoflurane in foals. *J Am Vet Med Assoc* 2002; **221**: 393–398.

31 Quandt JE, Robinson EP. Nasotracheal intubation in calves. *J Am Vet Med Assoc* 1996; **209**: 967–968.

32 Bauquier SH, Golder FJ. Extended anaesthesia and nasotracheal intubation of a red kangaroo (*Macropus rufus*). *Aust Vet J* 2010; **88**: 449–450.

33 Riebold TW, Engel HN, Grubb TL, *et al.* Orotracheal and nasotracheal intubation in llamas. *J Am Vet Med Assoc* 1994; **204**: 779–783.

34 Stephens Devalle JM. Successful management of rabbit anesthesia through the use of nasotracheal intubation. *J Am Assoc Lab Anim Sci* 2009; **48**: 166–170.

35 Hamacher J, Arras M, Bootz F, *et al.* Microscopic wire guide-based orotracheal mouse intubation: description, evaluation and comparison with transillumination. *Lab Anim* 2008; **42**: 222–230.

36 Johnson DH. Endoscopic intubation of exotic companion mammals. *Vet Clin North Am Exot Anim Pract* 2010; **13**: 273–289.

37 Hartsfield SM. Alternate methods of endotracheal intubation in small animals with emphasis on patients with oropharyngeal pathology. *Tex Vet Med J* 1985; **47**: 25.

38 Byers SR, Cary JA, Farnsworth KD. Comparison of endotracheal intubation techniques in llamas. *Can Vet J* 2009; **50**: 745–749.

39 Zhao X, Wu N, Zhou J, *et al.* A technique for retrograde intubation in mice. *Lab Anim* 2006; **35**: 39–42.

40 Corleta O, Habazettl H, Kreimeier U, *et al.* Modified retrograde orotracheal intubation techniques for airway access in rabbits. *Eur Surg Res* 1992; **24**: 129–132.

41 Worth DB, Grimes JA, Jiménez DA, *et al.* Risk factors for temporary tracheostomy tube placement following surgery to alleviate signs of brachycephalic obstructive airway syndrome in dogs. *J Am Vet Med Assoc* 2018; **253**: 1158–1163.

42 Stordalen MB, Silveira F, Fenner JVH, *et al.* Outcome of temporary tracheostomy tube placement following surgery for brachycephalic obstructive airway syndrome in 42 dogs. *J Small Anim Pract* 2020; **61**: 292–299.

43 Chesen AB, Rakestraw PC. Indications for and short- and long-term outcome of permanent tracheostomy performed in standing horses: 82 cases (1995–2005). *J Am Vet Med Assoc* 2008; **232**: 1352–1356.

44 Hedlund CS. Tracheostomy. *Probl Vet Med* 1991; **3**: 198–209.

45 McClure SR, Taylor TS, Honnas CM, *et al.* Permanent tracheostomy in standing horses: technique and results. *Vet Surg* 1995; **24**: 231–234.

46 Nichols S. Tracheotomy and tracheostomy tube placement in cattle. *Vet Clin North Am Food Anim Pract* 2008; **24**: 307–317.

47 Nicholson I, Baines S. Complications associated with temporary tracheostomy tubes in 42 dogs (1998 to 2007). *J Small Anim Pract* 2012; **53**: 108–114.

48 Smith MM. Pharyngostomy endotracheal tube. *J Vet Dent* 2004; **21**: 191–194.

49 Huss BT, Anderson MA, Branson KR, *et al.* Evaluation of pulse oximeter probes and probe placement in healthy dogs. *J Am Anim Hosp Assoc* 1995; **31**: 9–14.

50 Jacobson JD, Miller MW, Matthews NS, *et al.* Evaluation of accuracy of pulse oximetry in dogs. *Am J Vet Res* 1992; **53**: 537–540.

51 Chaffin MK, Matthews NS, Cohen ND, *et al.* Evaluation of pulse oximetry in anaesthetised foals using multiple combinations of transducer type and transducer attachment site. *Equine Vet J* 1996; **28**: 437–445.

52 Koenig J, McDonell W, Valverde A. Accuracy of pulse oximetry and capnography in healthy and compromised horses during spontaneous and controlled ventilation. *Can J Vet Res* 2003; **67**: 169–174.

53 Matthews NS, Hartsfield SM, Sanders EA, *et al.* Evaluation of pulse oximetry in horses surgically treated for colic. *Equine Vet J* 1994; **26**: 114–116.

54 Nishimura R, Kim H, Matsunaga S, *et al.* Evaluation of pulse oximetry in anesthetized dogs. *J Vet Med Sci* 1991; **53**: 1117–1118.

55 Quinn CT, Raisis AL, Musk GC. Evaluation of Masimo signal extraction technology pulse oximetry in anaesthetized pregnant sheep. *Vet Anaesth Analg* 2013; **40**: 149–156.

56 Wong DM, Alcott CJ, Wang C, *et al.* Agreement between arterial partial pressure of carbon dioxide and saturation of hemoglobin with oxygen values obtained by direct arterial blood measurements versus noninvasive methods in conscious healthy and ill foals. *J Am Vet Med Assoc* 2011; **239**: 1341–1347.

57 Manning AM. Oxygen therapy and toxicity. *Vet Clin North Am Small Anim Pract* 2002; **32**: 1005–1020.

58 Hopper K, Powell LL. Advanced oxygen therapy for the small animal patient – high-flow oxygen therapy and mechanical ventilation. *Vet Clin North Am Small Anim Pract* 2022; **52**: 689–705.

59 Fitzpatrick RK, Crowe DT. Nasal oxygen administration in dogs and cats: experimental and clinical investigations. *J Am Anim Hosp Assoc* 1986; **22**: 293–300.

60 Wilson DV, Schott HC, Robinson NE, *et al.* Response to nasopharyngeal oxygen administration in horses with lung disease. *Equine Vet J* 2006; **38**: 219–223.

61 Stewart JH, Rose RJ, Barko AM. Response to oxygen administration in foals: effect of age, duration and method of administration on arterial blood gas values. *Equine Vet J* 1984; **16**: 329–331.
62 Rose RJ, Hodgson DR, Leadon DP, *et al.* Effect of intranasal oxygen administration on arterial blood gas and acid base parameters in spontaneously delivered, term induced and induced premature foals. *Res Vet Sci* 1983; **34**: 159–162.
63 Bleul UT, Bircher BM, Kahn WK. Effect of intranasal oxygen administration on blood gas variables and outcome in neonatal calves with respiratory distress syndrome: 20 cases (2004–2006). *J Am Vet Med Assoc* 2008; **233**: 289–293.
64 Mann FA, Wagner-Mann C, Allert JA, *et al.* Comparison of intranasal and intratracheal oxygen administration in healthy awake dogs. *Am J Vet Res* 1992; **53**: 856–860.
65 Dunphy ED, Mann FA, Dodam JR, *et al.* Comparison of unilateral versus bilateral nasal catheters for oxygen administration in dogs. *J Vet Emerg Crit Care* 2002; **12**: 213–294.
66 Crowe DT. Oxygen therapy. In: Bonagura JD, Twedt DC, Hawkins EC, eds. *Kirk's Current Veterinary Therapy XIV*. St. Louis, MO: Saunders Elsevier, 2009; 596–602.
67 Court MH. Respiratory support of the critically ill small animal patient. In: Murtaugh RJ, Kaplan PM, eds. *Veterinary Emergency and Critical Care Medicine*. St. Louis, MO: Mosby, 1992; 575.
68 Fairman NB. Evaluation of pulse oximetry as a continuous monitoring technique in critically ill dogs in the small animal intensive care unit. *J Vet Emerg Crit Care* 1992; **2**: 50–56.
69 Lumb AB. Hyperoxia and oxygen toxicity. In: Lumb AB, ed. *Nunn's Applied Respiratory Physiology*, 7th edn. Edinburgh: Churchill Livingstone Elsevier, 2010; 377–390.
70 Caplan RA, Vistica MF, Posner KL, *et al.* Adverse anesthetic outcomes arising from gas delivery equipment: a closed claims analysis. *Anesthesiology* 1997; **87**: 741–748.
71 Mehta SP, Eisenkraft JB, Posner KL, *et al.* Patient injuries from anesthesia gas delivery equipment: a closed claims update. *Anesthesiology* 2013; **119**: 788–795.
72 Hartsfield SM. Machines and breathing systems for administration of inhalation anesthetics. In: Short CE, ed. *Principles and Practices of Veterinary Anesthesia*. Baltimore: Williams & Wilkins, 1987: 395.
73 Singaravelu S, Barclay P. Automated control of end-tidal inhalation anaesthetic concentration using the GE Aisys Carestation™. *Br J Anaesth* 2013; **110**: 561–566.
74 Tay S, Weinberg L, Peyton P, *et al.* Financial and environmental costs of manual versus automated control of end-tidal gas concentrations. *Anaesth Intensive Care* 2013; **41**: 95–101.
75 Hartsfield SM. Anesthetic machines and breathing systems. In: Tranquilli WJ, Thurmon JC, Grimm KA, eds. *Lumb and Jones' Veterinary Anesthesia and Analgesia*, 4th edn. Ames, IA: Blackwell Publishing, 2007; 453–494.
76 Dorsch JA, Dorsch SE. *Understanding Anesthesia Equipment*, 4th edn. Baltimore, MD: Lippincott Williams & Wilkins, 1999.
77 Steffey EP, Woliner MJ, Howland D. Accuracy of isoflurane delivery by halothane-specific vaporizers. *Am J Vet Res* 1983; **44**: 1072–1078.
78 Dorsch JA, Dorsch SE. *Understanding Anesthesia Equipment: Construction, Care, and Complications*, 3rd edn. Baltimore, MD: Williams & Wilkins, 1994.
79 Hamilton WK. Nomenclature of inhalation anesthetic systems. *Anesthesiology* 1964; **25**: 3–5.
80 Dorsch JA, Dorsch SE. The breathing system: general principles, common components, and classifications. In: Dorsch JA, Dorsch SE, eds. *Understanding Anesthesia Equipment*, 5th edn. New York, NY: Lippincott Williams & Wilkins, 2008; 191–208.
81 Baum JA, Woehlck HJ. Interaction of inhalational anaesthetics with CO_2 absorbents. *Best Pract Res Clin Anaesthesiol* 2003: **17**: 63–76.
82 Feldman JM, Hendrickx J, Kennedy RR. Carbon dioxide absorption during inhalation anesthesia: a modern practice. *Anesth Analg* 2021: **132**: 993–1002.
83 Fang ZX, Eger EI II, Laster MJ, *et al.* Carbon monoxide production from degradation of desflurane, enflurane, isoflurane, halothane, and sevoflurane by soda lime and Baralyme. *Anesth Analg* 1995; **80**: 1187–1193.
84 Kharasch ED, Powers KM, Artru AA. Comparison of Amsorb, sodalime, and Baralyme degradation of volatile anesthetics and formation of carbon monoxide and compound A in swine *in vivo*. *Anesthesiology* 2002; **96**: 172–182.
85 Murray JM, Renfrew CW, Bedi A, *et al.* Amsorb: a new carbon dioxide absorbent for use in anesthetic breathing systems. *Anesthesiology* 1999; **95**: 750–755.
86 Higuchi H, Adachi Y, Arimura S, *et al.* The carbon dioxide absorption capacity of Amsorb is half that of soda lime. *Anesth Analg* 2001; **93**: 221–225.
87 Kobayashi S, Bito H, Morita K, *et al.* Amsorb Plus and Drägersorb Free, two new-generation carbon dioxide absorbents that produce a low compound A concentration while providing sufficient CO_2 absorption capacity in simulated sevoflurane anesthesia. *J Anesth* 2004; **18**: 277–281.
88 Shandro J. Resistance to gas flow in the "new" anaesthesia circuits: a comparative study. *Can Anaesth Soc J* 1981; **29**: 387–390.
89 Rayburn RL. *Pediatric anesthesia circuits. Annual Refresher Course Lecture 117*. Washington, DC, 1981.
90 Hartsfield SM. Anesthesia equipment. In: Carroll GL, ed. *Small Animal Anesthesia and Analgesia*. Ames, IA: Blackwell Publishing, 2008; 3–24.
91 Dorsch JA, Dorsch SE. Anesthesia ventilators. In: Dorsch JA, Dorsch SE, eds. *Understanding Anesthetic Equipment*, 5th edn. New York, NY: Lippincott Williams & Wilkins, 2008; 310–372.
92 Riebold TW, Evans AT, Robinson NE. Evaluation of the demand valve for resuscitation of horses. *J Am Vet Med Assoc* 1980; **176**: 623–626.

7 Infection Prevention and Control in Anesthesia

Raphaël Vézina Audette[1] and Stephen D. Cole[2]

[1] Portland Veterinary Emergency and Specialty Care, Portland, Maine, USA

[2] Clinical Infectious Disease Laboratory, Department of Pathobiology, School of Veterinary Medicine, University of Pennsylvania, Philadelphia, Pennsylvania, USA

Chapter contents

Introduction, 142
Postoperative infections, 142
Infection control and prevention, 143
Important tools and steps for perianesthetic infection control, 143
Perioperative checklists, 143
Hand hygiene, 144
Attire, 144
Reprocessing of anesthetic and surgical equipment, 144
Laryngoscopes and mouth rinse plungers, 145
Endotracheal tubes, 145
Monitoring equipment, 145
Intravenous catheters, 146
Breathing circuits and ventilators, 146
Preparation of the surgical site and maintenance of the sterile field, 146
Risk factors associated with postoperative infections, 146
Patient-specific risk factors, 146
Iatrogenic factors, 147
Environmental factors, 147
Patient care and drug administration considerations, 147
Bandages and dressings, 147
Lubricants, 148
Anesthetics and analgesics, 148
References, 149

Introduction

Veterinary patients that undergo anesthesia face a genuine risk of infection, even when well-established preventative measures are precisely executed. Postoperative infections in domestic animals (dogs, cats, and horses) may manifest in various ways ranging from skin and soft tissue infections involving the surgical site, to osteomyelitis, pneumonia, urinary tract infection, and catheter-associated complications. Postoperative infections often result from a combination of several factors, including patient immunosuppression, disease, concomitant drug administration, breach of aseptic technique, prolonged procedures, prolonged recumbency, insufficient infection prevention measures, and postoperative surgical site management. The use of antimicrobial drugs perioperatively can impact host susceptibility to nosocomial infections but must be weighed against the risks of antibiotic resistance. This chapter explores the relationship between general anesthesia and perioperative infections and discusses the vital role anesthetists play in the prevention of nosocomial infections.

Postoperative infections

Skin and soft tissue infections at incision sites are the most common postsurgical infections among all veterinary species. Mild infections are easily managed but severe infections can progress to abscessation, cellulitis, and systemic disease or compromise surgical wounds leading to dehiscence. Bacteria of the genus *Staphylococcus* are the most common bacteria associated with incisional infections [1,2]. *Staphylococcus pseudintermedius,* which is part of the normal skin and oral cavity flora of dogs and cats, is the most common species associated with small animal incisional infections. Infection caused by this organism may originate from the patient itself or contaminated fomites. In contrast, *Staphylococcus aureus* is not considered normal flora of most dogs and cats (although it is more common in cats than dogs) and infections caused by *S. aureus* are most likely from an anthropogenic source (e.g., surgeon, anesthetist, and care staff) as it commonly constitutes a part of the cutaneous and respiratory flora in humans [3]. In horses, methicillin-resistant *S. aureus* (MRSA) postsurgical infection is much more common as a result of horse-adapted strains [4]. Enteric organisms (i.e., *Escherichia coli* and *Klebsiella pneumoniae*) have been reported to be more common in incisional infections following abdominal surgery [5]. Rates of postsurgical infection vary between procedures, facilities, and surgeons. Table 7.1 illustrates the variability of reported rates among common procedures for dogs, cats, and horses. Surgical wounds can be characterized as clean, clean-contaminated, contaminated, or dirty (infected) (see Box 7.1 for definitions). Infection rates for procedures characterized as clean may be lower than those characterized as contaminated or dirty.

Veterinary Anesthesia and Analgesia: The Sixth Edition of Lumb and Jones. Edited by Leigh Lamont, Kurt Grimm, Sheilah Robertson, Lydia Love and Carrie Schroeder.
© 2024 John Wiley & Sons, Inc. Published 2024 by John Wiley & Sons, Inc.
Companion website: www.wiley.com/go/lamont/anesthesia

Table 7.1 Wound classifications and associated infection rates in dogs and horses.

Procedure	Wound classification	Dogs	Horses	References
Ovariohysterectomy	Clean	1.3–5.7%	NA	[6]
Castration	Clean	2.0–3.4%	2.2–3.6%	[6–8]
Enterotomy or gastrotomy	Clean-contaminated	7.0–19.9%	19–40.4%	[5,9–11]
Orthopedic surgery	Clean	5.4–6.6%	3.7–14.2%	[12–15]
Cystotomy	Clean-contaminated	0.0–3.0%	NA	[16,17]

Box 7.1 Wound classification descriptions.

Clean: incision must not enter the respiratory, gastrointestinal, or urogenital tracts and there must not be a break in sterile technique. No inflammation or infection should be present at the surgical site (e.g., splenectomy and tibial plateau leveling osteotomy).

Clean-contaminated: incision is made into the respiratory, gastrointestinal, or urogenital tract with no inflammation or infection present (e.g., intestinal foreign body removal and cystotomy).

Contaminated: break in sterile technique during the procedure OR gastrointestinal tract spillage is present OR an incision is made into a site where acute, non-purulent inflammation is present. Traumatic wounds between 12 and 24 h typically fall into this category.

Dirty (infected): viscera perforated prior to or during the procedure OR when acute purulent inflammation is present during the operation. Prolonged traumatic wounds or wounds contaminated with feces or environmental debris often fall into this category (e.g., laparotomy for septic peritonitis and ovariohysterectomy for pyometra).

Infection control and prevention

All veterinarians must practice infection prevention to uphold their professional oath to protect animal health and welfare and to promote public health. The American Animal Hospital Association (AAHA) has described a hierarchy of controls for veterinary facilities, and this is shown in an adapted illustration (Fig. 7.1) [18]. The hierarchy ranks the following types of control (from most to least effective): elimination controls, engineering controls, administrative controls, and personal protective equipment (PPE). Elimination controls are the most effective, but often the most difficult to implement. Elimination controls remove or prevent the entry of a threat of infection (i.e., a pathogen) completely. Engineering controls are aspects of hospital design and setup that remove hazards or improve compliance with infection prevention procedures. Administrative controls are the policies and procedures focused on infection prevention. PPE includes the use of specialized attire or equipment to limit the spread of pathogens and is considered the least effective of these controls because it is the most dependent on human factors such as compliance and education. However, PPE is still a critical piece of an infection prevention program, but it cannot be the sole tool. Specific examples of controls relevant to the veterinary anesthesia team are highlighted in Fig. 7.1.

The success of an infection control program is dependent on the people participating in it. It is critical that veterinary anesthetists are champions of a facility's efforts to implement and use infection prevention strategies. Beyond the delivery of anesthesia and analgesia and ensuring a safe recovery from anesthesia, the anesthesia team is concerned with preoperative patient evaluation, including the identification of factors that may impact patient outcomes. It is fundamental to have a thorough understanding of factors that may influence patient safety and anesthetic risk, including nosocomial infections, so that risks can be mitigated, and patient safety improved [19]. Training is key to success but should not stand alone without some form of audit and feedback. For example, personnel responsible for reprocessing equipment should be trained at least annually with updates on procedures conducted when necessary. A review process should also be in place. Audit and feedback should never be punitive but viewed as an opportunity to demonstrate proficiency and identify areas for improvement.

Important tools and steps for perianesthetic infection control

Perioperative checklists

The preoperative patient preparation area and operating rooms (ORs) are high-task-density environments where omission of any critical steps risks severely compromising patient outcomes. Successfully getting a patient through surgery requires the meticulous orchestration of completion of each task in the correct fashion and order. Carrying out a wide variety of procedures, each with specific steps that must be remembered and executed properly,

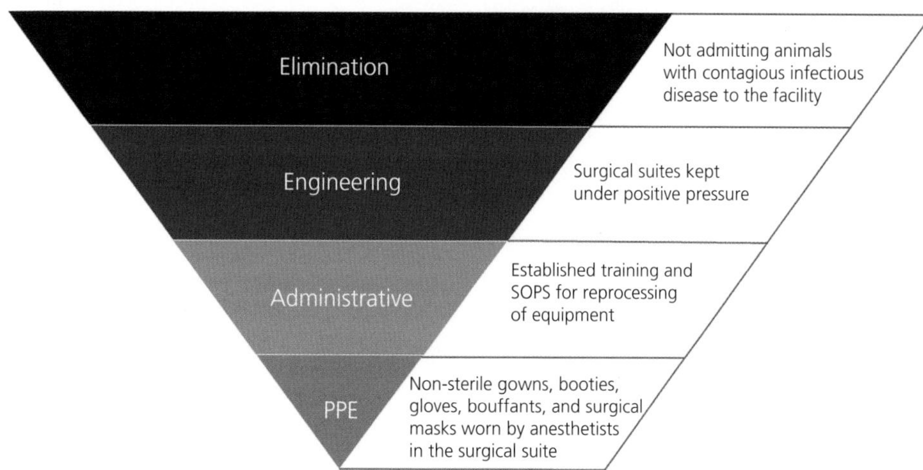

Figure 7.1 Hierarchy of infection controls. PPE, personal protective equipment; SOP, standard operating procedures.

is paramount to ensure patient safety. Observance of evidence-based perioperative guidelines, particularly antimicrobial use, has been described in veterinary medicine albeit in a limited number of publications [20,21]. The use of surgical checklists in human hospitals has been adopted globally and has contributed to a significant improvement in perioperative outcomes [22]. In veterinary medicine, the implementation of surgical checklists has also been studied, specifically relating to critical outcomes, including infection and mortality. In one study carried out in a private practice referral center, the implementation of a surgical checklist reduced the risk of incisional infections in dogs undergoing exploratory laparotomy for gastrointestinal foreign body obstructions [11]. Another study from a different academic institution determined that surgical checklist implementation decreased surgical complications such as missed perioperative antibiotic doses and operations at the wrong surgical site, decreased the rate of unexpected return to the OR, and improved implementation of safety measures; however, it did not affect morbidity or mortality rates or the incidence of incisional infections during the study [23].

Hand hygiene

Frequent hand hygiene is the single most important action that an individual can take to protect their patients' and their own health. Wearing gloves is never a substitute for hand hygiene. For hands without visible soiling, the use of alcohol-based hand sanitizers is considered an effective approach. Important exceptions include when working with patients known to be infected with non-enveloped viruses (e.g., canine parvovirus and equine rotavirus), fungal pathogens (e.g., dermatophytes), or spore-forming bacteria (e.g., *Clostridium spp.*). Handwashing with soap and water is the best strategy in cases of these pathogens or for people with visibly soiled hands. Box 7.2 describes best practices for the execution of hand hygiene. Auditing of hand hygiene practices allows for the identification of barriers to implementing hand hygiene (e.g., too few hand sanitizer stations) and it has been shown to be effective at improving compliance in veterinary facilities. For anesthetists that do not work within the sterile field, the use of routine hand hygiene strategies in combination with clean, non-sterile gloves for most procedures suffices. Handwashing or disinfection should always be performed before and after putting on gloves. Specialized and extensive hand hygiene, colloquially described as "scrubbing in," should be performed by all surgeons and other professionals whose hands will enter a sterile field during a surgical procedure.

Box 7.2 Considerations for specific hand hygiene techniques.

Alcohol-based hand sanitizer

- Only use if hands are not visibly soiled.
- Use enough to cover all surfaces of hands.
- Hands should remain wet for approximately 20 s if an adequate amount was used.
- Commonly missed sites include between fingers, thumbs, and fingertips.

Handwashing with soap and water

- Should be performed for specific pathogens of concern or for visibly dirty hands.
- Wet hands, removing as much debris as possible prior to application of soap.
- Apply soap and lather hands, including backs of hands and under fingernails.
- Scrub hands for at least 20 s.
- Rinse hands under clean running water.
- Dry hands with a clean towel or air dry.

Attire

Outside of the surgical suite the anesthetist should wear clean scrubs in patient care areas. Long hair should be tied back, and stethoscopes and lanyards should not dangle as they can act as fomites. Personnel should change into and out of scrubs when entering and leaving the facility, respectively, and always change when visibly soiled. Clean laboratory coats or water-resistant aprons are appropriate for protecting scrubs when performing procedures where extensive direct contact with animals (e.g., during physical restraint or when clipping hair) or biological materials will occur. Laboratory coats should never be worn outside of the hospital or inside a surgical suite. It is best practice to have work-dedicated footwear. In cases of animals with zoonotic or highly transmissible diseases, additional PPE including coveralls, gowns, face shields/masks, and shoe covers ("booties") should be considered on a case-by-case basis.

Inside the surgical suite, additional PPE is needed in addition to clean scrubs. For individuals not entering the sterile field, bouffant/surgical caps, face masks, non-sterile gowns, non-sterile gloves, and shoe covers have all been recommended. Surgeons and others entering the sterile field should use sterile gowns and gloves; in some cases, two pairs of gloves are worn ("double gloved"). Protective eyewear should be used particularly for contaminated and dirty (infected) wounds and for procedures involving irrigation.

Reprocessing of anesthetic and surgical equipment

Sterilization and disinfection are both processes used to allow for the safe reuse of medical devices and equipment (also known as "reprocessing"). Cleaning refers to the act of removing visible soilage from the surface of an object and is a critical first step that must be completed prior to disinfection or sterilization. Disinfection reduces or eliminates most (if not all) pathogenic microbes on the surfaces of inanimate objects with the important exception of bacterial or fungal spores. Sterilization, however, kills all microbial life, including spores. Whether a device needs to be cleaned and either disinfected or sterilized prior to reuse is based on the Spaulding classification system, which classifies devices as critical, semicritical, or noncritical [24]. Table 7.2 defines these classifications and

Table 7.2 Spaulding's classification of medical devices.

Class	Definition	Example(s)	Sterilization versus disinfection
Critical	Devices that contact or enter sterile tissues or bloodstream	Surgical instruments (i.e., forceps and scalpels), implants, biopsy tools	Sterilization
Semicritical	Devices that come into contact with mucous membranes but do not enter sterile tissues or the blood stream	Laryngoscope blades, endoscopes	Sterilization or high-level disinfection
Noncritical	Devices that come into contact with patient skin but not mucous membranes. Some devices that may not come in direct contact with patients may also require disinfection between patients	Laryngoscope handles, stethoscopes, blood pressure cuffs	Low- to intermediate-level disinfection

provides examples of devices used by anesthetists or surgeons. Reprocessing instructions for medical devices can be found within the manufacturer's instructions for use (MIFU).

Disinfection is primarily achieved with the use of liquid chemicals called "disinfectants." Disinfectants can be further categorized as low-level (kills vegetative bacteria, some viruses, and some fungi), intermediate-level (kills vegetative bacteria, most viruses, and most fungi and mycobacteria), or high-level (kills all microbial life, except for large numbers of spores). Some high-level disinfectants (e.g., 2% glutaraldehyde) can be considered chemical sterilants if used with prolonged exposure times (3–12 h). The efficacy of disinfectants is dependent on the removal of all organic materials prior to use along with appropriate wet contact time and proper dilution (if required). The MIFU should always be followed exactly when using a disinfectant and any deviation may lead to incomplete efficacy. Certain devices such as thermometers and ultrasound probes can be used with specially designed plastic covers, which may decrease their need for high-level disinfection following use. Some facilities designate certain devices (i.e., thermometers) that would need frequent disinfection for use with a single patient throughout their stay before discarding or sending home with the patient.

Sterilization is achieved by the use of an autoclave (steam with high heat under pressure), dry heat sterilizer, or ethylene oxide gas. Hydrogen peroxide liquid plasma and chemical sterilants may also be used. Sterility assurance monitoring (SAM) should be performed to ensure adequate processes are in place. A good SAM program always includes adequate documentation of results. SAM should include a multimodal approach to testing that includes biological indicator testing, chemical indicator testing, and mechanical monitoring. Biological indicator tests are the only tests that assure sterilization by assessing the killing of spore-forming organisms (e.g., *Bacillus* spp. or *Geobacillus* spp.) and are typically performed weekly. Chemical indicator testing involves chemical changes when the correct physical conditions are met that lead to a color change in an indicator (e.g., lead carbonate to lead (II) oxide). Chemical indicator tests should be included for each package of instruments to be sterilized (external indicators such as autoclave tape can also be used). Mechanical monitoring should follow guidelines from the sterilizer's manufacturer but often includes checking a variety of parameters on instrument gauges, screens, or printouts. Chemical indicator testing and mechanical monitoring do not ensure sterilization was achieved, but they can be used to detect procedural errors such as incorrect packaging or overloading. Common reasons for failure of sterilization include incorrect operation, incorrect settings, improper loading or overloading, and excessive packing. Certain medical devices are labeled as "single-use," which implies they cannot be reused [24].

Laryngoscopes and mouth rinse plungers

Laryngoscopes are considered an essential instrument to perform safe and atraumatic orotracheal intubation in cats and dogs [25]. Laryngoscopes, because they are expected to encounter a patient's mucosal surface, are considered semicritical devices according to Spaulding's classification and thus require, at a minimum, high-level disinfection between uses in different patients. Though no reports of hospital-acquired infections involving laryngoscopes exist in companion animals, disinfection protocols should be followed. Anecdotal reports of an epidemic of respiratory infectious disease in horses associated with the use of a mouth rinse plunger to flush the mouth prior to orotracheal intubation illustrate the necessity to ensure high-level decontamination in semicritical items. In one North American study, respiratory pathogens such as equine herpes virus 1 and 4 (EHV-1, EHV-4), equine influenza virus (EIV), equine rhinitis B virus (ERBV), and/or MRSA were detected in 22% of healthy horses presented for routine dental care [26]. These pathogens can be reasonably expected to contaminate the tip-of-mouth rinse plungers or bite blocks and orotracheal tubes.

Endotracheal tubes

Endotracheal tubes (ETTs) and laryngeal masks offer ways to maintain airway patency in veterinary patients during general anesthesia or deep sedation. Additionally, they are indispensable for the protection of a patient's airways against the potentially lethal risk of aspiration pneumonia. In 2018, an outbreak of carbapenem-resistant *E. coli* was linked to reuse of ETTs at a veterinary teaching hospital [27]. Most commercially available ETTs are labeled as single-use only. In the context of veterinary anesthesia, it may not be economically feasible to use a new ETT for each patient at all facilities. However, since ETTs encounter a patient's mucosal surface, they are deemed semicritical devices according to Spaulding's classification, and thus require high-level disinfection. While these devices are widely reused in the veterinary field [28], best practices for sterilization or disinfection have not been established. Crawford and Weese studied the efficacy of various disinfection strategies for ETTs against *in vitro* inoculated *Streptococcus zooepidemicus* and *Bordetella bronchiseptica* [29]. Although soaking in chlorhexidine gluconate or accelerated hydrogen peroxide solutions significantly reduced growth on direct and enrichment cultures compared to water or triclosan-containing soap solutions, high-level disinfection was not achieved with either method. A recent study evaluated the efficacy of four different protocols for ETT disinfection and found no difference in bacterial growth following cleaning of the ETT with either a water scrub, detergent scrub, detergent scrub and chlorhexidine gluconate soak, or detergent scrub and bleach soak all of which yielded significant bacterial growth [28]. Reprocessing single-use items may affect the integrity and efficacy of the device. For example, a study of ETT sterilization demonstrated that the physical integrity of the ETT cuff may become compromised following glutaraldehyde or ethylene oxide sterilization. If a facility chooses to reuse ETTs or other single-use devices against the MIFU, then they must include these factors in their risk assessment for the patient.

Monitoring equipment

Minimum standard monitoring equipment for patients under general anesthesia in veterinary medicine includes electrocardiography (ECG), pulse oximetry, capnography, and temperature probes [25]. Many different configurations exist for each instrument and the anatomical site on which they are used on patients will dictate the need for levels of disinfection or sterilization. For example, though rarely used in everyday practice, intravascular thermistors for measurement of core body temperature would be considered a critical device and thus require sterilization before use, whereas esophageal thermometers are considered semicritical and may only require high-level decontamination between patients. If rectal thermometers are in use, appropriate hygiene measures such as the use of plastic sleeves and high-level disinfection between patients are recommended. For this reason, instruments that do not represent an increased level of invasiveness may be preferred; for example, surface ECG monitors require low-level decontamination of leads applied to intact skin, compared to esophageal ECG leads, which require a higher level of decontamination.

Intravenous catheters

Catheters used for vascular cannulation are considered critical items. As such, they must only be used when sterile. Prior to the placement of vascular catheters, sterile preparation of the placement site by removing hair with clippers followed by the use of an antiseptic solution can prevent infectious complications [30,31]. For placement of peripheral intravenous (IV) catheters, a clean technique may suffice as long as appropriate hand hygiene is observed [32]. The current trend in human medicine is to remove IV catheters only when clinical signs of inflammation are observed. Commonly reported risk factors for infectious catheter complications in humans include the type of catheter used, blood sampling through the catheter, the type of IV infusate administered, the duration the catheter was in place, and the catheter location. A recent prospective study evaluated these proposed risk factors in cats and dogs in a private referral practice intensive care unit and did not identify any of them as being associated with an increased risk of a positive bacterial culture from the catheter tip [33]. In cats and dogs, one study suggested that a dwell time greater than 72 h was not associated with an increased risk of IV catheter contamination [34], whereas others reported increased rates of infections after a period of as little as 36 h [35]. An association between lack of experience and risk of catheter infection has been reported in dogs [36]. Concurrent corticosteroid therapy and the presence of phlebitis were also positively associated with a positive catheter tip culture [36].

Breathing circuits and ventilators

A prospective evaluation of microbial contamination of anesthesia breathing circuits used in the context of canine anesthesia demonstrated that in the absence of a biofilm, the environmental contaminants that colonize the breathing circuits are likely of low pathogenicity and short viability [37]. Evidence from simulation experiments supports the notion that anesthesia machines can be contaminated by bacterial pathogens, and that heat and moisture exchange filters can effectively prevent bacterial contamination [38]. Further, they demonstrated that volatile anesthetics (halothane) and carbon dioxide absorbents (soda lime) did not provide any demonstrable bactericidal action. Uncertainty remains about whether viral pathogens can contaminate an anesthesia breathing circuit after use in a sick animal shedding respiratory viruses, which would then be transferred to subsequent patients. Factors involved in the potential transfer of pathogens from corrugated tubing to a patient's airways are ill-defined. Bacterial filters may not be efficient against viral pathogens and, as such, it is recommended to discard breathing circuits when a risk for viral cross-contamination exists.

Preparation of the surgical site and maintenance of the sterile field

As part of the presurgical evaluation, close attention should be paid to the skin. If there is evidence of cutaneous infections (e.g., bacterial pyoderma and dermatophytosis) therapy should be initiated and the surgery rescheduled after clinical resolution. For emergent surgeries, antimicrobial therapy should encompass the suspected pathogens. A swab for bacterial culture and susceptibility can be collected for submission prior to antibiotic administration to guide postoperative care.

Skin cannot be sterilized or disinfected but antiseptic chemicals can be used to decrease the overall microbial burden of the skin. While protocols may vary, the effective and efficient preparation of the surgical site is a critical part of the aseptic technique. It has been demonstrated that prolonged time from clipping to incision is associated with an increased incidence of postsurgical infection [39,40]. After induction of anesthesia, hair on the surgery site should be clipped with electric clippers leaving a sufficient border around the intended incision site. Use of a size 10 blade over a size 40 blade has been advocated as it results in less irritation and lower numbers of colony-forming units (CFUs) [31]. Shaving should not be done as it is traumatic to the skin and is associated with higher rates of infection. Care should be used to avoid cross-contamination of patients with clipper blades. The next step after clipping is to remove gross organic material from the skin (cleaning) with a surgical scrub containing a detergent. Gauze swabs are used to scrub the skin in a concentric pattern away from the intended surgical site. Following an initial scrub, surgical sites are then rinsed with 70% alcohol, which doubles as an additional bacterial kill and removes the detergent. The final step is to use a surgical antiseptic (e.g., chlorhexidine gluconate or povidone-iodine). Box 7.3 addresses the preparation of the epidural injection site.

Box 7.3 Recommended steps for preparation of an epidural injection site.

- After induction of anesthesia, clip the surgery site with electric clippers fitted with a disinfected size 10 blade, leaving a sufficient border around the intended puncture site.
- After clipping, examine the skin overlying the lumbosacral junction for evidence of pyoderma or suspicious neoplastic lesions, as these would constitute contraindications for epidural injections.
- Wearing examination gloves, remove gross organic material from the skin (cleaning) with a surgical scrub containing a detergent (chlorhexidine scrub) and gauze swabs to scrub the skin in a concentric pattern moving away from the intended epidural puncture site.
- Rinse the site with 70% alcohol to remove the detergent. Alcohol-soaked cotton balls should be avoided as they can leave microscopic fibers that may be dragged into the epidural space with the needle.

Proper use of antiseptic solutions is more important than which type of solution is used. The MIFU should always be followed for appropriate dilution and contact time. Chlorhexidine gluconate may provide several advantages over povidone-iodine because it has longer residual activity and a shorter required contact time [41]. It is important to note that diluted antiseptics can become contaminated with environmental organisms such as *Pseudomonas aeruginosa* and *Serratia marcescens*, which can ultimately lead to severe incisional infections. Solutions should be made fresh from concentrates for each patient and discarded once used.

Risk factors associated with postoperative infections

Patient-specific risk factors

Patient-specific factors associated with increased risks of incisional infections have been investigated in veterinary patients. Conflicting reports in the literature stem from high variability in methods used to study perioperative infection risks and, at times, a lack of agreement between authors on basic definitions of surgical site complications. Despite these challenges, several studies have highlighted the role of specific patient-related factors in the development of incisional infections. The classification of surgical wounds based on the degree of contamination correlates well with the development of incisional infections, but alone, its predictive value for the development of incisional infections is only of moderate value highlighting the multifactorial nature of perioperative infection risk and the need to account for other patient-related factors [6].

The immune system can be compromised by a number of concurrent diseases. In cats and dogs, hypothyroidism, hyperthyroidism, hyperadrenocorticism, and diabetes mellitus have all been associated with an increased risk of developing incisional infections [42,43]. Stress also notably affects the immune system and may adversely impact wound healing [44,45]. Whether direct immunosuppression or glucocorticoid-induced hyperglycemia or a combination of both factors is responsible is unknown, as both have independently been implicated as risk factors for incisional infections [46]. The American Society of Anesthesiologists (ASA) status of patients undergoing surgery is associated with an increased risk of incisional infections [6]. Other patient-specific factors have been implicated in the development of infection and/or inflammatory surgical site complications such as obesity [6,47–49]. According to a multi-institution retrospective study, higher body mass index may increase the risk for the development of incisional complications in horses following emergency ventral midline celiotomy [50].

Veterinary patients often engage in behaviors that promote incisional infections such as licking their wounds, defecating in cages or stalls, and rubbing or scratching painful body parts. Adequate protection of a surgical site by means of appropriate perioperative antibiotherapy, topical antibiotic ointments and bandages, hand hygiene, use of single-use gloves during patient care, and e-collars may be relevant considerations to help reduce incisional infections [46,51], though they are no substitute for adequate husbandry practices and thorough pain control. It is the role of the anesthetist to discuss the presence of risk factors with the other members of a pet's healthcare team and ensure that owners can make informed decisions while consenting to elective surgeries and anesthesia. In the context of elective procedures, the opportunity to treat endocrinopathies and thus reduce the ASA status of a patient must be considered in light of the potential increase in perioperative morbidity and costs [46,52].

Iatrogenic factors

Human factors are considered important contributors to the development of perioperative infections; for example, a statistically significant association between the number of people present in an OR and the development of surgical site complications has been reported [6]. Since this variable was correlated with ASA status, it is unknown whether the number of people in an OR is causally related to incisional infections or whether it is merely reflective of the increased task density and need for more staff to care for sicker animals. Human traffic in and out of an operating suite can contribute to environmental contamination and should be kept to a minimum [53].

Surgical duration has been described as a strong predictor of incisional infections [6,13,54]. A retrospective study assessing risk factors associated with incisional infections in dogs undergoing tibial tuberosity advancement surgery suggests that the duration of surgery and anesthesia significantly increases the risk of infection [13], describing that for every minute increase in surgery and anesthesia time, the likelihood of developing an incisional infection increased by seven and four percent, respectively. A prospective clinical study on 100 client-owned dogs investigated associations between multiple perioperative factors and incisional infections and found no association between surgical duration, among many other factors, and the incidence of perioperative infections [1,27]. Their results conflict with other studies that found a relationship between incisional infections and duration of anesthesia and surgery. Further, the authors found that despite a high frequency of intraoperative bacterial contamination, incisional infection rates remain remarkably low. Whether increased incisional infections rates seen with longer surgical duration are directly related to time or are also confounded by other factors, such as a surgeon's experience level or the complexity of a procedure, remains unclear. For example, increasing surgeon experience has been associated with lower levels of inflammatory C-reactive protein but not cortisol in bitches undergoing ovariohysterectomy, suggesting that novice surgeons may lack the tissue handling skills to limit surgery-induced tissue inflammation but that the surgical stress response occurs regardless [55].

Environmental factors

Pathogens may become airborne in the operative room and may lead to contamination of surgical fields and potentially be a source of nosocomial infections [56]. Surgical site infections have multifactorial etiologies and poor OR air quality may be one of many factors to consider. OR personnel are considered the primary source of airborne bacteria [57]. Contamination of ORs with pathogenic bacteria originating from ventilation ducts and air handling systems leading to incisional infections has been reported [58]. Although laminar airflow systems have been promoted for use in operating theaters, the ideal ventilation design in ORs remains a subject of controversy [59–61]. It is likely that the nature of the filtration technology employed itself would be of greater significance than the mode of ventilation in optimizing OR air quality [62]. It is reasonable to assume that factors that increase air contamination such as increased number of personnel in the OR, traffic through the OR door, disruption of the positive pressure environment, and suboptimal ventilation may increase the risks of surgical field contamination. Items present in the OR, including forced warm air devices, may disrupt air flow if misused [63] and possibly lead to increased risks of incisional infections [64], though there is currently no evidence that forced-air warming devices are associated with an increased risk of incisional infections [65,66]. The benefit of maintaining normothermia or at least preventing severe hypothermia likely outweighs the potential risk associated with the use of forced-air warmers. Due to the association between intraoperative hypothermia and wound infections, it has been proposed that maintaining an OR temperature at 24 °C (75 °F) may be beneficial [67].

Outside of the surgical suite, working surfaces in veterinary hospitals represent a reservoir for microorganisms if disinfection protocols are not observed or if surgical wounds are not adequately protected [51]. Gurneys, and surgical and radiology tables frequently encounter patients and surgical sites and have been implicated in the transmission of methicillin-resistant *S. pseudintermedius* (MRSP) in companion animals [68,69]. A prospective clinical trial evaluating intraoperative surgeon and patient bacterial contamination during clean orthopedic surgeries and the relationship with surgical site infection in dogs found no relationship between surgical site infection and either surgeon or patient bacterial contamination [1]. The authors suggest that many surgical site infections are likely contracted postoperatively as intraoperative bacterial isolates were of low pathogenicity compared to those obtained from gurneys or radiology tables.

Patient care and drug administration considerations

Bandages and dressings

The protective value of bandages and dressings likely varies between procedures. While one might expect the presence of wound dressings and bandages to help protect against wound infections by providing a physical barrier against contaminated hospital surfaces, results of a prospective evaluation of wound dressings on incisional infection rates in dogs undergoing a clean orthopedic surgical procedure with implants (tibial plateau leveling osteotomy [TPLO]) demonstrated no advantage over control dogs with no dressings [49]. The use of antibacterial agents such as silver-based dressings or dialkylcarbamoylchloride (DACC)-coated postoperative dressings may provide additional protection [70,71], but veterinary studies evaluating their efficacy are lacking. In horses, the risk of infection after celiotomy for treatment of colic is lower for incisions covered with sterile towels or polyhexamethylene biguanide-impregnated dressings secured with sutures than when incisions were covered with gauze secured with iodine-impregnated adhesive drapes [72]. Whether the use of topical antibiotics applied to surgical wounds in clean and clean-contaminated surgeries reduces the risk of infection warrants further studies in veterinary medicine. This particular practice appears to yield no benefit in humans according to a recent systemic review and meta-analysis [73].

Lubricants

Anesthetics and opioids disrupt lacrimal function and ophthalmic lubricants are often used to prevent corneal ulcers perioperatively. In dogs, evidence suggests that corneal abrasions and ulcers still occur in roughly 20% and 0.5% of cases under general anesthesia, respectively [74]. In horses, 17.6% of cases developed corneal abrasions after undergoing anesthesia [75]. The potential for contamination of multidose formulations of ophthalmic products used by the ophthalmology service of a teaching veterinary hospital was evaluated and no significant bacterial contamination was found, suggesting that when used for up to two weeks and stored according to the manufacturer's recommendations, these products were safe and unlikely to cause ophthalmic infections [76]. Scarabelli *et al.* later found that in equine practice, ophthalmic preparations were rarely contaminated with bacteria (5.8%) and cross-contamination was never observed. They also found no incidence of corneal ulcers, but corneal abrasions were present in 17.6% of horses studied [75].

Anesthetics and analgesics

Opioids

Surgical pain associated with tissue inflammation and negative affective states have profound adverse impacts on the immune system. The activation of the hypothalamic–pituitary–adrenal axis and the production and release of neuroendocrine factors, including catecholamines and cortisol represent the underlying mechanism for the adverse immunomodulatory effects of pain. Though opioids have profound analgesic effects, recent preclinical studies have provided somewhat incriminating yet mixed evidence toward immunomodulatory effects of opioids on both the innate and the adaptive branches of the immune system. Cellular players of the immune system such as natural killer cells, macrophages, lymphocytes, and granulocytes all express μ-opioid receptors on their surface, and activation of the downstream intracellular signaling cascade that results from the receptor's interaction with μ-opioid agonists may lead to impaired immune function [77]. Putative immunosuppressive effects of opioids may affect clinical outcomes as suggested by studies in human patients treated with opioids preoperatively showing a greater risk for incisional infections following surgery [78,79].

Propofol

Propofol is a phenol derivative hypnotic agent and is available as a lipid-based emulsion that does not contain antimicrobials or preservatives. It is frequently administered as an IV injection for the induction of anesthesia or as an infusion for the maintenance of general anesthesia. In its original form, propofol can sustain rapid bacterial growth and according to the United States Center for Disease Control and Prevention has been linked to iatrogenic bacterial infections, including sepsis and incisional infections. Contamination of stopcocks on IV lines where propofol is injected has also been demonstrated [80]. A retrospective investigation of the association between propofol and postoperative wound infection rates determined that small animal patients (cats and dogs) induced with preservative-free propofol had an increased risk compared to patients in which general anesthesia was induced with different drugs [81]. Although formulations that contain preservatives are now readily available to veterinary practitioners, there remains a risk of contamination if appropriate hygiene and time-stamping measures are not observed to prevent contamination. Tomihari compared the effects of propofol and isoflurane in dogs anesthetized for a period of 2 h without undergoing surgery to tease out the potential immunosuppressive effect of surgery. This study reported that propofol had a lesser impact than inhaled anesthetics on both cellular and humoral immune systems [82]. Lymphocyte populations decreased less following propofol anesthesia compared to isoflurane anesthesia, and cytokine mRNA expression was less influenced by propofol than it was by inhaled anesthetics. Another study investigating risk factors associated with incisional infections in canine patients undergoing a lateral fabellotibial suture for cranial cruciate ligament rupture reported that induction with propofol posed a significant risk [48].

Volatile anesthetics

Maintenance of general anesthesia with inhaled anesthetics was found to inhibit the cytotoxic activity of natural killer cells in dogs [83]. Further, maintenance of anesthesia with isoflurane leads to a greater decrease in lymphocyte counts than total intravenous anesthesia (TIVA) with propofol [82]. Simeonova *et al.* compared the effects of inhaled anesthesia and epidural anesthesia on peripheral blood mononuclear cells and found that both anesthetic techniques induced a significant yet transient reduction in circulating lymphocytes in dogs [84]. Whether inhaled anesthetics are associated with a worsening of perioperative outcomes compared with TIVA or locoregional techniques remains to be determined. The impact of anesthetic techniques on clinical outcomes is multifactorial and interplay between a myriad of cellular receptors targeted by common anesthetics complicates the interpretation of currently available clinical data. Large-scale prospective controlled clinical trials are necessary to elucidate the contributions of individual components of anesthetic and analgesic regimens to clinical outcomes.

Locoregional and neuraxial anesthesia

Great care must be taken to limit the risk of infections associated with locoregional anesthesia techniques. Neuraxial blocks require that preservative-free drugs be used to avoid potential catastrophic neurotoxic effects on the spinal cord. It is advisable to ensure optimal hand hygiene and use a sterile technique, including aseptic skin preparation and the use of sterile gloves while performing epidural injections or placement of epidural catheters to minimize the risks of discospondylitis or epidural abscess formation [85]. Locoregional anesthesia techniques have been shown to block the surgical stress response in veterinary patients. Despite this beneficial effect, lidocaine epidural anesthesia in dogs has not shown an improved survival of peripheral blood mononuclear cells compared to dogs anesthetized with halothane, suggesting that epidural anesthesia has similar adverse immunoinhibitory effects as volatile anesthetics [84]. The use of epidural catheters for the provision of postoperative analgesia in the canine outpatient setting was reported to be associated with minor self-limiting complications such as urinary retention and fecal incontinence, and no evidence of infection was reported [86]. The use of ultrasound guidance to perform locoregional blocks adds a consideration for the potential for ultrasound probes to act as fomites.

Antimicrobials

Judicious antimicrobial prescribing practices can limit the emergence of antimicrobial resistance, which is among the most complex and urgent problems in veterinary medicine and public health. Antimicrobials should not be used in lieu of the infection prevention strategies and antisepsis techniques described throughout this chapter. Therapeutic use of antimicrobials is obviously indicated when performing surgery in the presence of infection (e.g., pyometra and septic abdomen). Antimicrobials can also be used prophylactically for contaminated procedures (e.g., wound repair) or clean-contaminated procedures (e.g., enterotomy). Given the low risk of incisional infections for clean procedures performed on healthy animals, the use of prophylactic administration of an antimicrobial is often discouraged, except in cases where indwelling medical devices will be used (e.g., implants). However, recent studies do not support postoperative antimicrobial therapy in clean orthopedic surgeries in dogs [13], including TPLO procedures [87,88]. The decision to prescribe antimicrobials prophylactically, perioperatively, and/or postoperatively should account for the overall health status of the patient, concurrent medications, and the extent of wound contamination (clean versus dirty or contaminated). For instance, a canine retrospective study described a very low incidence of major postoperative incisional infections (0.6%) in dogs undergoing hemilaminectomies without concurrent use of perioperative antibiotics [89]. However, minor complications occurred in 9.1% of cases that did not require treatment. Further, 30% of cases enrolled were excluded from the study, due in part to postoperative suspected or confirmed urinary tract infections, scrotal and preputial dermatitis, and suspected aspiration pneumonia.

In patients where antimicrobial prophylaxis is deemed necessary, treatment should be initiated before surgery and, in the name of antimicrobial stewardship, the duration should be as short as possible [20]. The goal of surgical prophylaxis is to reach bactericidal concentrations of an antimicrobial at the surgical site prior to contamination with bacteria. The selection of which antimicrobial to use during a procedure (either prophylactically or therapeutically) is multifactorial, but it should always be effective, and ideally bactericidal, against the confirmed, suspected, or most likely bacteria to be encountered. For example, if surgical wounds are made only in the skin, then a drug targeting *Staphylococcus* (e.g., cefazolin) would be a rational choice. Special consideration should be made for dogs with a history of methicillin-resistant *Staphylococcus* spp. infection as this organism is resistant to all veterinary beta-lactams. It has been suggested that for a procedure where the gastrointestinal tract is entered, broad-spectrum antimicrobials targeting anaerobes and gram-negative bacteria (e.g., cefoxitin and amikacin/ampicillin) may increase the odds of therapeutic success. Antimicrobials should not be highly protein-bound (e.g., cefovecin) given their low tissue concentrations compared to weakly bound drugs (e.g., cefazolin). Most antimicrobials complete their distribution into tissues within 30–60 min of administration; therefore, doses of most antimicrobials used prophylactically should be administered in the period immediately prior to initiating the surgery [90,91]. For time-dependent drugs (e.g., beta-lactams), the rate at which an antimicrobial is eliminated (most commonly by the kidney) is the most important factor for the administration of subsequent doses. Cefazolin, which is commonly used perioperatively in small companion animal medicine, has a relatively short elimination half-life of 1 h in dogs and should be re-dosed during procedures lasting longer than 2 h. Although recommendations vary slightly, a common regimen for prophylactic cefazolin in dogs is to give an initial dose of 20–22 mg/kg approximately 30–60 min before the procedure starts and then re-dose every 90–120 min until the procedure ends [90,91].

References

1 Andrade N, Schmiedt CW, Cornell K, *et al.* Survey of intraoperative bacterial contamination in dogs undergoing elective orthopedic surgery. *Vet Surg* 2016; **45**(2): 214–222.

2 Gallagher AD, Mertens WD. Implant removal rate from infection after tibial plateau leveling osteotomy in dogs. *Vet Surg* 2012; **41**(6): 705–711.

3 Hanselman BA, Kruth SA, Rousseau J, *et al.* Methicillin-resistant *Staphylococcus aureus* colonization in veterinary personnel. *Emerg Infect Dis* 2006; **12**(12): 1933–1938.

4 Cuny C, Witte W. MRSA in equine hospitals and its significance for infections in humans. *Vet Microbiol* 2017; **200**: 59–64.

5 Williams RW, Cole S, Holt DE. Microorganisms associated with incisional infections after gastrointestinal surgery in dogs and cats. *Vet Surg* 2020; **49**(7): 1301–1306.

6 Eugster S, Schawalder P, Gaschen F, *et al.* A prospective study of postoperative surgical site infections in dogs and cats. *Vet Surg* 2004; **33**(5): 542–550.

7 Hodgson C, Pinchbeck G. A prospective multicentre survey of complications associated with equine castration to facilitate clinical audit. *Equine Vet J* 2019; **51**(4): 435–439.

8 Kilcoyne I, Watson JL, Kass PH, *et al.* Incidence, management, and outcome of complications of castration in equids: 324 cases (1998–2008). *J Am Vet Med Assoc* 2013; **242**(6): 820–825.

9 Isgren CM, Salem SE, Archer DC, *et al.* Risk factors for surgical site infection following laparotomy: effect of season and perioperative variables and reporting of bacterial isolates in 287 horses. *Equine Vet J* 2017; **49**(1): 39–44.

10 Costa-Farré C, Prades M, Ribera T, *et al.* Does intraoperative low arterial partial pressure of oxygen increase the risk of surgical site infection following emergency exploratory laparotomy in horses? *Vet J* 2014; **200**(1): 175–180.

11 Launcelott ZA, Lustgarten J, Sung J, *et al.* Effects of a surgical checklist on decreasing incisional infections following foreign body removal from the gastrointestinal tract in dogs. *Can Vet J* 2019; **60**(1): 67–72.

12 Fitzpatrick N, Solano MA. Predictive variables for complications after TPLO with stifle inspection by arthrotomy in 1000 consecutive dogs. *Vet Surg* 2010; **39**(4): 460–474.

13 Yap FW, Calvo I, Smith KD, *et al.* Perioperative risk factors for surgical site infection in tibial tuberosity advancement: 224 stifles. *Vet Comp Orthop Traumatol* 2015; **28**(3): 199–206.

14 Curtiss AL, Stefanovski D, Richardson DW. Surgical site infection associated with equine orthopedic internal fixation: 155 cases (2008–2016). *Vet Surg* 2019; **48**(5): 685–693.

15 Daniels A, Pezzanite LM, Griffenhagen GM, *et al.* Evaluation of factors associated with surgical site infection in equine proximal interphalangeal joint arthrodesis: 54 cases (2010–2019). *Vet Med Sci* 2022; **8**(4): 1478–1488.

16 Appel S, Otto SJ, Weese JS. Cystotomy practices and complications among general small animal practitioners in Ontario, *Canada. Can Vet J* 2012; **53**(3): 303–310.

17 Grant DC, Harper TA, Werre SR. Frequency of incomplete urolith removal, complications, and diagnostic imaging following cystotomy for removal of uroliths from the lower urinary tract in dogs: 128 cases (1994–2006). *J Am Vet Med Assoc* 2010; **236**(7): 763–766.

18 Stull JW, Bjorvik E, Bub J, *et al.* 2018 AAHA Infection control, prevention, and biosecurity guidelines. *J Am Anim Hosp Assoc* 2018; **54**(6): 297–326.

19 Sharma A, Fernandez PG, Rowlands JP, *et al.* Perioperative infection transmission: the role of the anesthesia provider in infection control and healthcare-associated infections. *Curr Anesthesiol Rep* 2020; **10**(3): 233–241.

20 Weese JS, Halling KB. Perioperative administration of antimicrobials associated with elective surgery for cranial cruciate ligament rupture in dogs: 83 cases (2003–2005). *J Am Vet Med Assoc* 2006; **229**(1): 92–95.

21 Dallap Schaer BL, Linton JK, Aceto H. Antimicrobial use in horses undergoing colic surgery. *J Vet Intern Med* 2012; **26**(6): 1449–1456.

22 Fudickar A, Horle K, Wiltfang J, *et al.* The effect of the WHO Surgical Safety Checklist on complication rate and communication. *Dtsch Arztebl Int* 2012; **109**(42): 695–701.

23 Thieman Mankin KM, Jeffery ND, Kerwin SC. The impact of a surgical checklist on surgical outcomes in an academic institution. *Vet Surg* 2021; **50**(4): 848–857.

24 Josephs-Spaulding J, Singh OV. Medical device sterilization and reprocessing in the era of multidrug-resistant (MDR) bacteria: issues and regulatory concepts. *Front Med Technol* 2020; **2**: 587352.

25 Grubb T, Sager J, Gaynor JS, *et al.* 2020 AAHA Anesthesia and monitoring guidelines for dogs and cats. *J Am Anim Hosp Assoc* 2020; **56**(2): 59–82.

26 Pusterla N, Rice M, Henry T, *et al.* Investigation of the shedding of selected respiratory pathogens in healthy horses presented for routine dental care. *J Vet Dent* 2020; **37**(2): 88–93.

27 Lavigne SH, Cole SD, Daidone C, *et al.* Risk factors for the acquisition of a $bla_{\text{NDM-5}}$ Carbapenem-resistant *Escherichia coli* in a veterinary hospital. *J Am Anim Hosp Assoc* 2021; **57**(3).

28 Marquis CR, Gull T, Dodam J, *et al.* Comparison of four endotracheal tube cleaning protocols in anesthetized dogs. *J Am Vet Med Assoc* 2023; **261**(3): 336–341.

29 Crawford S, Weese JS. Efficacy of endotracheal tube disinfection strategies for elimination of *Streptococcus zooepidemicus* and *Bordetella bronchiseptica*. *J Am Vet Med Assoc* 2015; **247**(9): 1033–1036.

30 Burrows CF. Inadequate skin preparation as a cause of intravenous catheter-related infection in the dog. *J Am Vet Med Assoc* 1982; **180**(7): 747–749.

31 Messiaen Y, MacLellan JD, Pelsue DH. Evaluation of the number of colony forming units on the skin of dogs after clipping the hair with two sizes of clipper blades. *Am J Vet Res* 2019; **80**(9): 862–867.

32 Hughes D, Beal MW. Emergency vascular access. *Vet Clin North Am Small Anim Pract* 2000; **30**(3): 491–507.

33 Marsh-Ng ML, Burney DP, Garcia J. Surveillance of infections associated with intravenous catheters in dogs and cats in an intensive care unit. *J Am Anim Hosp Assoc* 2007; **43**(1): 13–20.

34 Mathews KA, Brooks MJ, Vaillant AE. A prospective study of intravenous catheter contamination. *J Vet Emerg Crit Care* 1996; **6**(1): 33–43.

35 Crisi PE, De Santis F, Aste G, *et al.* Inflammatory, mechanical and infectious complications associated with peripheral intravenous catheters in dogs and cats: a risk factor analysis. *Vet Sci* 2022; **9**(3): 118.

36 Guzman Ramos PJ, Fernandez Perez C, Ayllon Santiago T, *et al.* Incidence of and associated factors for bacterial colonization of intravenous catheters removed from dogs in response to clinical complications. *J Vet Intern Med* 2018; **32**(3): 1084–1091.

37 Pelligand L, Hammond R, Rycroft A. An investigation of the bacterial contamination of small animal breathing systems during routine use. *Vet Anaesth Analg* 2007; **34**(3): 190–199.

38 Leijten DT, Rejger VS, Mouton RP. Bacterial contamination and the effect of filters in anaesthetic circuits in a simulated patient model. *J Hosp Infect* 1992; **21**(1): 51–60.

39 Brown DC, Conzemius MG, Shofer F, *et al.* Epidemiologic evaluation of postoperative wound infections in dogs and cats. *J Am Vet Med Assoc* 1997; **210**(9): 1302–1306.

40 Mayhew PD, Freeman L, Kwan T, *et al.* Comparison of surgical site infection rates in clean and clean-contaminated wounds in dogs and cats after minimally invasive versus open surgery: 179 cases (2007–2008). *J Am Vet Med Assoc* 2012; **240**(2): 193–198.

41 Kulkarni AP, Awode RM. A prospective randomised trial to compare the efficacy of povidone-iodine 10% and chlorhexidine 2% for skin disinfection. *Indian J Anaesth* 2013; **57**(3): 270–275.

42 Nicholson M, Beal M, Shofer F, *et al.* Epidemiologic evaluation of postoperative wound infection in clean-contaminated wounds: a retrospective study of 239 dogs and cats. *Vet Surg* 2002; **31**(6): 577–581.

43 Sappenfield E, Jamieson DJ, Kourtis AP. Pregnancy and susceptibility to infectious diseases. *Infect Dis Obstet Gynecol* 2013; **2013**: 752852.

44 Godbout JP, Glaser R. Stress-induced immune dysregulation: implications for wound healing, infectious disease and cancer. *J Neuroimmune Pharmacol* 2006; **1**(4): 421–427.

45 Hekman JP, Karas AZ, Sharp CR. Psychogenic stress in hospitalized dogs: Cross species comparisons, implications for health care, and the challenges of evaluation. *Animals (Basel)* 2014; **4**(2): 331–347.

46 Espinel-Ruperez J, Martin-Rios MD, Salazar V, *et al.* Incidence of surgical site infection in dogs undergoing soft tissue surgery: risk factors and economic impact. *Vet Rec Open* 2019; **6**(1): e000233.

47 Spare P, Ljungvall I, Ljungvall K, *et al.* Evaluation of postoperative complications after mastectomy performed without perioperative antimicrobial prophylaxis in dogs. *Acta Vet Scand* 2021; **63**(1): 35.

48 Cox T, Maddox TW, Pettitt R, *et al.* Investigation of variables associated with surgical site infection following the management of canine cranial cruciate ligament rupture with a lateral fabellotibial suture. *Vet Comp Orthop Traumatol* 2020; **33**(6): 409–416.

49 Giannetto JJ, Aktay SA. Prospective evaluation of surgical wound dressings and the incidence of surgical site infections in dogs undergoing a tibial plateau levelling osteotomy. *Vet Comp Orthop Traumatol* 2019; **32**(1): 18–25.

50 Hill JA, Tyma JF, Hayes GM, *et al.* Higher body mass index may increase the risk for the development of incisional complications in horses following emergency ventral midline celiotomy. *Equine Vet J* 2020; **52**(6): 799–804.

51 Stine SL, Odum SM, Mertens WD. Protocol changes to reduce implant-associated infection rate after tibial plateau leveling osteotomy: 703 dogs, 811 TPLO (2006–2014). *Vet Surg* 2018; **47**(4): 481–489.

52 Nicoll C, Singh A, Weese JS. Economic impact of tibial plateau leveling osteotomy surgical site infection in dogs. *Vet Surg* 2014; **43**(8): 899–902.

53 Alexander JW, Van Sweringen H, Vanoss K, *et al.* Surveillance of bacterial colonization in operating rooms. *Surg Infect (Larchmt)* 2013; **14**(4): 345–351.

54 Stetter J, Boge GS, Grönlund U, *et al.* Risk factors for surgical site infection associated with clean surgical procedures in dogs. *Res Vet Sci* 2021; **136**: 616–621.

55 Michelsen J, Heller J, Wills F, *et al.* Effect of surgeon experience on postoperative plasma cortisol and C-reactive protein concentrations after ovariohysterectomy in the dog: a randomised trial. *Aust Vet J* 2012; **90**(12): 474–478.

56 Harper TA, Bridgewater S, Brown L, *et al.* Bioaerosol sampling for airborne bacteria in a small animal veterinary teaching hospital. *Infect Ecol Epidemiol* 2013; 3.

57 Sadrizadeh S, Aganovic A, Bogdan A, *et al.* A systematic review of operating room ventilation. *J Build Eng* 2021; **40**: 102693.

58 Fox BC, Chamberlin L, Kulich P, *et al.* Heavy contamination of operating room air by Penicillium species: identification of the source and attempts at decontamination. *Am J Infect Control* 1990; **18**(5): 300–306.

59 Bischoff P, Kubilay NZ, Allegranzi B, *et al.* Effect of laminar airflow ventilation on surgical site infections: a systematic review and meta-analysis. *Lancet Infect Dis* 2017; **17**(5): 553–561.

60 Surial B, Atkinson A, Kulpmann R, *et al.* Better operating room ventilation as determined by a novel ventilation index is associated with lower rates of surgical site infections. *Ann Surg* 2022; **276**(5): e353–e360.

61 Aganovic A, Cao G, Fecer T, *et al.* Ventilation design conditions associated with airborne bacteria levels within the wound area during surgical procedures: a systematic review. *J Hosp Infect* 2021; **113**: 85–95.

62 Dai R, Liu S, Li Q, *et al.* A systematic review and meta-analysis of indoor bioaerosols in hospitals: the influence of heating, ventilation, and air conditioning. *PLoS One* 2021; **16**(12): e0259996.

63 Dasari KB, Albrecht M, Harper M. Effect of forced-air warming on the performance of operating theatre laminar flow ventilation. *Anaesthesia* 2012; **67**(3): 244–249.

64 Lange VR. Forced air contamination risk in the OR. *Ann Med Surg (Lond)* 2022; **73**: 102976.

65 Ackermann W, Fan Q, Parekh AJ, *et al.* Forced-air warming and resistive heating devices. Updated perspectives on safety and surgical site infections. *Front Surg* 2018; **5**: 64.

66 Wood AM, Moss C, Keenan A, *et al.* Infection control hazards associated with the use of forced-air warming in operating theatres. *J Hosp Infect* 2014; **88**(3): 132–140.

67 Rodriguez-Diaz JM, Hayes GM, Boesch J, *et al.* Decreased incidence of perioperative inadvertent hypothermia and faster anesthesia recovery with increased environmental temperature: a nonrandomized controlled study. *Vet Surg* 2020; **49**(2): 256–264.

68 van Duijkeren E, Kamphuis M, van der Mije IC, *et al.* Transmission of methicillin-resistant *Staphylococcus pseudintermedius* between infected dogs and cats and contact pets, humans and the environment in households and veterinary clinics. *Vet Microbiol* 2011; **150**(3–4): 338–343.

69 Shoen HRC, Rose SJ, Ramsey SA, *et al.* Analysis of Staphylococcus infections in a veterinary teaching hospital from 2012 to 2015. *Comp Immunol Microbiol Infect Dis* 2019; **66**: 101332.

70 Totty JP, Hitchman LH, Cai PL, *et al.* A pilot feasibility randomised clinical trial comparing dialkylcarbamoylchloride-coated dressings versus standard care for the primary prevention of surgical site infection. *Int Wound J* 2019; **16**(4): 883–890.

71 Lawrie K, Waldauf P, Balaz P, *et al.* Silver-based dressings in the prevention of the incisional surgical site infection: a prospective multicenter observational controlled trial. *Surg Infect (Larchmt)* 2022; **23**(7): 682–690.

72 Kilcoyne I, Dechant JE, Kass PH, *et al.* Evaluation of the risk of incisional infection in horses following application of protective dressings after exploratory celiotomy for treatment of colic. *J Am Vet Med Assoc* 2019; **254**(12): 1441–1447.

73 Chen PJ, Hua YM, Toh HS, *et al.* Topical antibiotic prophylaxis for surgical wound infections in clean and clean-contaminated surgery: a systematic review and meta-analysis. *BJS Open* 2021; **5**(6): zrab125.

74 Dawson C, Sanchez RF. A prospective study of the prevalence of corneal surface disease in dogs receiving prophylactic topical lubrication under general anesthesia. *Vet Ophthalmol* 2016; **19**(2): 124–129.

75 Scarabelli S, Timofte D, Malalana F, *et al.* Corneal abrasion and microbial contamination in horses following general anaesthesia for non-ocular surgery. *Vet Anaesth Analg* 2018; **45**(3): 278–284.

76 Betbeze CM, Stiles J, Krohne SG. Assessment of bacterial contamination of three multidose ophthalmic solutions. *Vet Ophthalmol* 2007; **10**(2): 81–83.

77 Perry JA, Douglas H. Immunomodulatory effects of surgery, pain, and opioids in cancer patients. *Vet Clin North Am Small Anim Pract* 2019; **49**(6): 981–991.

78 Inagi T, Suzuki M, Osumi M, *et al.* Remifentanil-based anaesthesia increases the incidence of postoperative surgical site infection. *J Hosp Infect* 2015; **89**(1): 61–68.

79 Hassan Z, Nisiewicz MJ, Ueland W, *et al.* Preoperative opioid use and incidence of surgical site infection after repair of ventral and incisional hernias. *Surgery* 2020; **168**(5): 921–925.

80 Cole DC, Baslanti TO, Gravenstein NL, *et al.* Leaving more than your fingerprint on the intravenous line: a prospective study on propofol anesthesia and implications of stopcock contamination. *Anesth Analg* 2015; **120**(4): 861–867.

81 Heldmann E, Brown DC, Shofer F. The association of propofol usage with postoperative wound infection rate in clean wounds: a retrospective study. *Vet Surg* 1999; **28**(4): 256–259.

82 Tomihari M, Nishihara A, Shimada T, *et al.* A comparison of the immunological effects of propofol and isoflurane for maintenance of anesthesia in healthy dogs. *J Vet Med Sci* 2015; **77**(10): 1227–1233.

83 Miyata T, Kodama T, Honma R, *et al.* Influence of general anesthesia with isoflurane following propofol-induction on natural killer cell cytotoxic activities of peripheral blood lymphocytes in dogs. *J Vet Med Sci* 2013; **75**(7): 917–921.

84 Simeonova GP, Slavov E, Usunov R, *et al.* Increased apoptosis of peripheral blood mononuclear cells (PBMC) during general and epidural anaesthesia in dogs. *Vet Res Commun* 2008; **32**(8): 619–626.

85 Remedios AM, Wagner R, Caulkett NA, *et al.* Epidural abscess and discospondylitis in a dog after administration of a lumbosacral epidural analgesic. *Can Vet J* 1996; **37**(2): 106–107.

86 Phillips LR, McAbee KP, Stephenson N, *et al.* Evaluation of complications and feasibility of indwelling epidural catheter use for postoperative pain control in dogs in the home environment. *N Z Vet J* 2015; **63**(2): 86–91.

87 Budsberg SC, Torres BT, Sandberg GS. Efficacy of postoperative antibiotic use after tibial plateau leveling osteotomy in dogs: a systematic review. *Vet Surg* 2021; **50**(4): 729–739.

88 Spencer DD, Daye RM. A prospective, randomized, double-blinded, placebo-controlled clinical study on postoperative antibiotherapy in 150 arthroscopy-assisted tibial plateau leveling osteotomies in dogs. *Vet Surg* 2018; **47**(8): E79–E87.

89 Dyall BAR, Schmökel HG. Surgical site infection rate after hemilaminectomy and laminectomy in dogs without perioperative antibiotic therapy. *Vet Comp Orthop Traumatol* 2018; **31**(3): 202–213.

90 Boothe DM, Boothe HW, Jr. Antimicrobial considerations in the perioperative patient. *Vet Clin North Am Small Anim Pract* 2015; **45**(3): 585–608.

91 Howe LM, Boothe HW, Jr. Antimicrobial use in the surgical patient. *Vet Clin North Am Small Anim Pract* 2006; **36**(5): 1049–1060, vi.

8 Euthanasia and Humane Killing

Robert E. Meyer
Professor Emeritus, Department of Clinical Sciences, College of Veterinary Medicine, Mississippi State University, Mississippi, USA

Chapter contents

Introduction, 152
Terminology, 153
  Euthanasia, 153
  Humane slaughter, 153
  Depopulation, 154
Pain and consciousness, 154
Mechanisms of action, 155
Evaluating animal distress, 156
Choice of killing method relative to onset of unconsciousness, 158
Fetal sentience and euthanasia, 160
Low atmospheric pressure stunning, 160
Foam depopulation, 161
Agent purity and euthanasia, 161
Euthanasia in the clinical setting, 162
References, 162

Introduction

Anesthesiology and the intentional killing of animals at first glance seem to have diametrically opposed goals. The former is concerned with maintaining life, whereas the latter takes it; indeed, the act of performing euthanasia can be both physically and emotionally difficult for animal workers, caretakers, and veterinarians because of this perceived conflict [1,2]. However, the humane treatment of animals has increasingly become a subject of public debate and discussion, and a conservative and humane approach to the intentional killing of any creature is warranted, justifiable, and expected by society. As veterinarians, we take an oath on entry to the profession "… to use my scientific knowledge and skills for the benefit of society through the protection of animal health and welfare, the prevention and relief of animal suffering, the conservation of livestock resources …" [3]; further, we are reminded that our moral duty is to the welfare of animals under our care [4,5]. Therefore, whether for welfare concerns, food and fiber production, or in response to natural or man-made disasters, our duty as compassionate veterinarians is to minimize or eliminate animal pain, anxiety, and distress. Viewed in this context, veterinary anesthetists and anesthesiologists are uniquely positioned to contribute meaningfully to matters pertaining to the humane taking of animal life.

Determining the humaneness of euthanasia, slaughter, or depopulation methods can be difficult because as humans we can never fully know or understand the subjective experiences of animals during loss of consciousness. This problem has vexed veterinary medicine since 1847 when, after administering the then newly described ether anesthetic to dogs and cats, the eminent British veterinarian Edward Mayhew concluded [6]:

> The results of these trials are not calculated to inspire any very sanguine hopes. We cannot tell whether the cries emitted are evidence of pain or not; but they are suggestive of agony to the listener, and, without testimony to the contrary, must be regarded as evidence of suffering. The process, therefore, is not calculated to attain the object for which in veterinary practice it would be most generally employed, namely, to relieve the owner from the impression that his animal was subjected to torture. In another light, it is not likely to be of much practical utility.

One of the defining characteristics in humans undergoing anesthesia is feeling as if one is having an "out-of-body experience," suggesting a disconnection between one's sense of self and one's awareness of time and space [7]. Although we cannot know for certain the subjective experiences of animals, one can speculate that similar feelings of disorientation may contribute to apparent signs of animal distress observed during anesthesia. Fortunately, the development of anesthesia methods for animals continued despite Dr. Mayhew's initial misgivings.

Determining the humaneness of killing methods depends on our ability to assess pain and consciousness within the contexts of method and application. Events such as vocalization, paddling, or convulsions are often interpreted as unequivocal evidence of animal suffering. Although unpleasant to observe, such events have much less effect on animal welfare when they occur after loss of consciousness.

Veterinary Anesthesia and Analgesia: The Sixth Edition of Lumb and Jones. Edited by Leigh Lamont, Kurt Grimm, Sheilah Robertson, Lydia Love and Carrie Schroeder.
© 2024 John Wiley & Sons, Inc. Published 2024 by John Wiley & Sons, Inc.
Companion website: www.wiley.com/go/lamont/anesthesia

The purpose of this chapter is to review the mechanisms and methods used for the intentional taking of animal life, including during the fetal stage, within the contexts of pain perception and consciousness. Recently described novel methods of low atmospheric pressure stunning and foam depopulation for poultry are described, in addition to considerations on agent purity requirements for humane killing. For a more detailed overview of euthanasia, including recommendations and procedures for specific species, readers are strongly encouraged to consult the most recent guidelines issued by the American Veterinary Medical Association (AVMA) [8], the Canadian Council on Animal Care (CCAC) [9], and the World Organisation for Animal Health (WOAH, formerly OIE) [10].

Terminology

A notable update in the 2020 AVMA Euthanasia Guidelines is the clarification of the difference between sedation and anesthesia. *Sedation* is defined as "a state of CNS depression in which the animal is awake but calm, and with sufficient stimuli may be aroused." *General anesthesia* is defined as "a method used to produce unconsciousness." Anesthetized animals are not arousable by noxious stimuli. This distinction is important in that several common techniques (e.g., placement of intraosseous cannulas, intraorgan or intracardiac injections, intrathecal lidocaine, and use of saturated potassium (K^+) or magnesium (Mg^+) solutions) are considered acceptable only when performed on anesthetized or fully unconscious animals.

Euthanasia

Euthanasia (derived from the Greek *eu* + *thanatos*, or "good death") generally refers to the goal of ending the life of an individual animal in a way that minimizes or eliminates pain and distress. Currently, the term is applied to situations where death is induced in a manner, that is, (1) in accord with an animal's interests and/or because it is a matter of welfare (humane disposition); and (2) where humane techniques are applied to induce the most rapid, painless, and distress-free death possible. Hence, for an act of intentional killing to be considered euthanasia, both humane disposition and humane techniques must be considered together [8]. Euthanasia is not a substitute for poor veterinary care and should never be considered as the "easy way out" or as a means to justify questionable management decisions. Rather, euthanasia provides a humane and responsible solution to improve animal welfare by alleviating animal suffering.

There is debate as to whether the term *euthanasia* appropriately describes the killing of some animals at the end of biological experiments and of unwanted shelter animals; extensive discussion regarding these issues can be found in papers by McMillan [11] and Pavlovik *et al.* [12]. For a more extensive review of the moral and ethical considerations of euthanasia, including the decision processes, the reader is directed to the 2020 AVMA Guidelines on Euthanasia [8].

Within the 2020 AVMA Euthanasia Guidelines, methods are classified as *Acceptable*, *Acceptable with Conditions*, and *Unacceptable*; similar terminology is applied to euthanasia methods throughout this chapter:

- *Acceptable* methods are those that consistently produce a humane death when used alone or as the sole means of producing death.
- *Acceptable with Conditions* methods are those techniques that may require certain conditions to be met to produce humane death consistently, may have greater potential for operator error or to be a safety hazard, are not well documented in the scientific literature, or may require a secondary method to ensure death. Methods "acceptable with conditions" are equivalent to "acceptable methods" when all criteria for application of a method can be met.
- *Unacceptable* methods and techniques are those deemed inhumane under any conditions or pose a substantial risk to the human applying the technique. Examples include, but are not necessarily limited to:
  - Certain anesthetic agents and adjuncts, such as chloral hydrate, chloroform, diethyl ether, neuromuscular blocking agents in conscious vertebrate animals (includes nicotine; also magnesium sulfate ($MgSO_4$), potassium chloride (KCl), and all depolarizing and non-depolarizing curariform agents).
  - Certain chemicals, such as cyanide, formaldehyde, household products and solvents, cleaning products and disinfectants, pesticides, and strychnine.
  - Certain physical methods, such as air embolism, burning, rapid decompression, drowning, exsanguination, hypothermia, manually applied blunt force trauma to the head (exceptions apply), non-penetrating captive bolts (exceptions apply), rapid freezing (exceptions apply), smothering, and thoracic compression.
- Adjunctive methods are procedures and practices that should not be used as a sole or primary method, but which can be used in conjunction with acceptable methods to bring about humane death following initial loss of consciousness. Examples include, but are not necessarily limited to:
  - Exsanguination, pithing, intravenous or intracardiac $MgSO_4$ or KCl, or creating a pneumothorax.

The following criteria were used in the 2020 AVMA Guidelines on Euthanasia to evaluate methods used to take the life of animals intentionally:

- Ability to induce loss of consciousness and death with a minimum of pain and distress.
- Time required to induce loss of consciousness.
- Reliability.
- Safety of personnel.
- Irreversibility.
- Compatibility with intended animal use and purpose.
- Documented emotional effect on observers or operators.
- Compatibility with subsequent evaluation, examination, or use of tissue.
- Drug availability and human abuse potential.
- Compatibility with species, age, and health status.
- Ability to maintain equipment in proper working order.
- Safety for predators or scavengers should the carcass be consumed.
- Legal requirements.
- Environmental impacts of the method or carcass disposition.

Humane slaughter

Humane slaughter refers to processes and methods employed to intentionally kill animals raised for food, fur, or fiber production [13,14]. The term applies both to individual animals killed on-farm and to commercial production processes. From a welfare perspective, the term is inclusive of the transport and handling of an animal, the methods employed to induce unconsciousness, the period until unconsciousness is verified, and the time of death when the animal is ready for entry into the food chain. This means that efforts must be made to minimize and, where possible, eliminate distress, pain, suffering, or anxiety associated with the entire process of bringing that animal to slaughter. Although some humane slaughter methods may employ euthanasia techniques, not all humane slaughter methods meet the criteria required to be considered euthanasia.

In addition to animal welfare concerns, important considerations with regard to humane slaughter processes include public health and safety, food safety and quality, environmental and economic sustainability, production adequacy and sustainability, occupational health and impact on the labor force, international animal welfare and trade standards, and religious and cultural aspects. In the United States, methods for humane slaughter are federally codified for cattle, calves, horses, mules, sheep, and swine by the 1958 Humane Slaughter (HS) Act and the 1978 Humane Methods of Livestock Slaughter Act (Pub. L. 85-765; 7 USC 1901 *et seq.*) (Pub. L. 85-765, Sec. 1, Aug. 27, 1958, 72 Stat. 862; Pub. L. 85-765, §2, Aug. 27, 1958, 72 Stat. 862; Pub. L. 95-445, §5(a), Oct. 10, 1978, 92 Stat. 1069) [15]. Although methods for the humane slaughter of poultry, fish, and rabbits are not specifically included in the 1958 and 1978 Acts, similar considerations should be applied to these species [13,14].

Depopulation

Depopulation is defined as the rapid destruction of large numbers of animals in response to emergencies, such as the control of catastrophic infectious diseases, or exigent situations caused by natural or man-made disasters [16]. As defined by the AVMA in the 2019 Guidelines, the term applies to methods by which large numbers of animals must be destroyed quickly and efficiently with as much consideration given to the welfare of the animals as practicable, but where the circumstances and tasks facing those performing the depopulation are understood to be extenuating [16].

The AVMA classification of depopulation methods differs from terminology used for euthanasia; methods are classified as *Preferred*, *Permitted in Constrained Circumstances*, and *Not Recommended*.

- *Preferred* methods are recommended preferentially when circumstances allow implementation.
- *Permitted in constrained circumstances* methods are to be utilized *ONLY* when circumstances constrain the ability to reasonably implement a preferred method.
- *Not recommended* methods are to be utilized *ONLY* when the circumstances preclude the reasonable implementation of any of the preferred methods or those permitted in constrained circumstances *AND* when the risk of doing nothing is deemed likely to have a reasonable chance of resulting in significantly more animal suffering than the proposed depopulation technique.

Depopulation is especially problematic from a welfare standpoint owing to several factors, including the sheer number of animals potentially involved, the need for rapid and decisive responses to limit disease spread or economic damage, and the potential for extenuating circumstances limiting availability or deployment of supplies, equipment, and personnel. This combination of factors can lead to consideration of expedient solutions of questionable humaneness. For example, in large confinement production facilities, loss of system ventilation, whether by intentional or accidental means, will eventually result in animal death; a process called "Ventilation Shutdown Plus" has been described for both swine and poultry depopulation [17,18]. Although application of mass depopulation methods may result in the same ultimate outcome, it is our duty as compassionate veterinarians to develop and employ methods that minimize animal suffering under these adverse circumstances. As with humane slaughter methods, depopulation may employ euthanasia techniques, but not all depopulation methods may meet the criteria to be considered euthanasia.

Further, application of any recommended killing method must be performed in accord with applicable national, regional, or local laws governing drug acquisition and storage, occupational safety, and methods used for euthanasia and disposal of animals, with special attention to individual species requirements where possible. If drugs have been used, careful consideration must be given to appropriate carcass disposal and steps should be taken to avoid environmental contamination or harm to other animals [8].

Selection of the most appropriate killing method for a particular situation will depend on several factors, including the species and number of animals involved, available means for animal handling and restraint, the skill and proficiency of personnel, and the methods and equipment available. Information in the scientific literature and available from practical experience focuses primarily on domesticated animals, but the same general considerations can be applied to all species. Inevitably, there will be less-than-perfect situations in which "acceptable/preferred" methods or "acceptable with conditions/permitted in constrained circumstances" methods may not be possible; judgments on the suitability of the best method or agent under the circumstances will be necessary. It should be noted that any useful and potentially humane killing method can become inhumane through poor technique, improper application, or lack of strict adherence to specified conditions and contingencies.

Pain and consciousness

Euthanasia, humane slaughter, and depopulation methods initially produce unconsciousness through three basic mechanisms: (1) direct depression of neurons necessary for life functions; (2) hypoxia; and (3) physical disruption of brain activity. Death follows as the circulatory and respiratory centers fail, or as hypoxia or reduced pH renders intracellular processes non-functional. However, loss of consciousness occurs at substantially different rates, such that the suitability of any particular agent or method depends on whether an animal experiences pain or distress prior to loss of consciousness.

Pain is defined as a conscious perception. Pain is subjective in the sense that individuals can differ in their perceptions of intensity and also in their physical and behavioral responses. The International Association for the Study of Pain (IASP) describes *pain* as "an unpleasant sensory and emotional experience associated with, or resembling that associated with, actual or potential tissue damage." This most recent IASP definition also includes contextual notes, several of which are relevant to this discussion: (1) pain is always a personal experience that is influenced to varying degrees by biological, psychological, and social factors; (2) pain and nociception are different phenomena; pain cannot be inferred solely from activity in sensory neurons; and (3) verbal description is only one of several behaviors to express pain; inability to communicate does not negate the possibility that a human or a nonhuman animal experiences pain [19].

Based on mammalian models, the perception of pain requires nerve impulses from peripheral nociceptors to reach an awake, functioning cerebral cortex and associated subcortical brain structures. Impulses from peripheral nociceptors are conducted by primary afferent fibers to either the spinal cord or the brainstem and two general sets of neural networks. Reflex withdrawal and flexion in response to nociceptive input are mediated at the spinal level, while ascending nociceptive pathways carry impulses to the reticular formation, hypothalamus, thalamus, and cerebral cortex (somatosensory cortex and limbic system) for conscious sensory processing and spatial localization. This distinction is important, in that movements observed in response to nociception can be due to spinally mediated reflex activity (unconscious), cerebral cortical and subcortical processing (conscious), or a combination of the two. Consequently, the choice of specific killing agent or method is less critical if it is to be used on an animal that is already anesthetized or rendered unconscious, provided that the animal does not regain consciousness prior to death.

Although the perception of pain requires a conscious experience, defining consciousness, and therefore the ability to perceive pain, across many species is difficult. *Amnesia*, defined as loss of memory function in which old memories cannot be remembered or new memories cannot be formed, is a defining characteristic of anesthesia, in that with sufficient quantities, all anesthetics are capable of producing a state of amnesia where new memories cannot be formed [7]. *Unconsciousness*, defined as loss of individual awareness, occurs when the brain's ability to integrate information is blocked or disrupted. Anesthetics produce unconsciousness either by preventing integration (blocking interactions among specialized brain regions) or by reducing information (shrinking the number of activity patterns available to cortical networks) received by the cerebral cortex or equivalent structure or structures. Further, the abrupt loss of consciousness that occurs at a critical concentration of anesthetic implies that the integrated workings of the interconnected neural states underlying consciousness may collapse nonlinearly [20,21].

In humans, onset of *anesthetic-induced unconsciousness* has been functionally defined by loss of appropriate response to verbal command; in animals, *loss of consciousness* is functionally defined by loss of the righting reflex (LORR), also called "loss of position" (LOP) [22–24]. This definition, introduced with the discovery of general anesthesia over 160 years ago, is still useful because it is an easily observable, integrated whole-animal response that is applicable to a wide variety of species. Although surrogate measures of brain activity such as an electroencephalogram or functional magnetic resonance imaging (fMRI) are often applied in this context, these methods cannot yet provide definitive answers as to onset of either human or animal unconsciousness; limitations of these methods for this purpose are reviewed later in the section evaluating animal distress. The usefulness of LORR/LOP as an easily observable proxy for loss of animal consciousness has been reinforced in studies where a reduction in alpha:delta (α:δ) brain wave ratios was found to coincide with LOP in chickens [25,26].

Vocalization or physical movement observed during application of humane killing methods is often interpreted as unequivocal evidence of consciousness. While purposeful escape behaviors should not be observed during the transition to unconsciousness, human and animal studies confirm that amnesia is produced and conscious awareness is blocked at less than half the anesthetic concentration required to abolish physical movement [23]. Once consciousness is lost, subsequent activities such as seizures, vocalization, reflex struggling, breath holding, and tachypnea can be attributed to the "excitement" phase or anesthesia stage 2 which, by definition, lasts from loss of consciousness to the onset of a regular breathing pattern [27,28]. Hence, vocalization and non-purposeful movements observed following LORR/LOP are not necessarily signs of conscious perception by an animal.

Previously, it was thought that finfish, amphibians, reptiles, and invertebrates lacked the anatomic structures necessary to perceive pain as we understand it in birds and mammals. However, most invertebrates respond to noxious stimuli and many have endogenous opioids [29], and there is increasing taxa-specific evidence of the efficacy of analgesics to minimize the impact of noxious stimuli on amphibians and reptiles [30,31]. Suggestions that fish responses to pain merely represent simple reflexes [32] have been refuted by studies demonstrating differing forebrain and midbrain electrical activity in response to nociceptor stimulation [33,34]; further, finfish exhibit learning and memory consolidation when taught to avoid noxious stimuli [35]. Based on the above considerations, killing methods that "result in rapid loss of consciousness" and "minimize pain and distress" should be strived for, even in those species where it is difficult to determine that these criteria have been met.

Mechanisms of action

Physical methods (e.g., gunshot, captive bolt, cerebral electrocution, blunt force trauma, and maceration) produce instantaneous unconsciousness by destroying, or rendering non-functional, brain regions responsible for cortical integration; death quickly follows when the midbrain centers controlling respiration and cardiac activity fail. Signs of effective stun and onset of unconsciousness have been reviewed in the context of slaughter. In cattle, sheep, and pigs, signs include immediate collapse (LORR/LOP) and a several-second period of tetanic spasm, followed by slow hind limb movements of increasing frequency [36–40]. However, there is significant species variability in this response. The corneal reflex will be absent.

Signs of effective electrocution are loss of righting reflex, loss of eye blink and moving object tracking, extension of the limbs, opisthotonos, downward rotation of the eyeballs, and tonic (rigid) spasm changing to clonic (paddling) spasm, with eventual muscle flaccidity. The corneal reflex will be absent. Although generalized seizures may be observed following effective application of physical methods, these most often follow loss of consciousness. Physical methods are inexpensive, humane, and painless if performed properly, and leave no drug residues in the carcass. Furthermore, animals presumably experience less fear and anxiety with methods that require little preparatory handling. However, as noted in the section, choice of killing method relative to onset of unconsciousness, physical methods usually require more direct physical proximity with the animals to be euthanized, which can be both offensive and upsetting for the operator. Physical disruption methods are often followed by adjunctive methods such as exsanguination or pithing to ensure death.

Decapitation and cervical dislocation as physical methods of humane killing require separate comments. Electrical activity in the brain can persist for up to 30 s following these methods [41–44]; interpretation of the significance of this activity is controversial [45]. As discussed in the section evaluating animal distress, brain electrical activity cannot yet provide definitive answers as to the precise onset of unconsciousness. Other studies [46–50] indicate such activity does not imply the ability to perceive pain and conclude that loss of consciousness develops rapidly.

Anesthetics and carbon dioxide (CO_2) inhalation initially produce loss of consciousness through direct depression of the cortical neural system; death subsequently occurs due to respiratory or cardiovascular failure associated with agent overdose. Acute hypercapnia (defined as > 5% atmospheric CO_2) rapidly reduces intracellular pH, producing unconsciousness and a reversible anesthetic state characterized by reduction of both basal and evoked neural activities [51–54] and inhibits central *N*-methyl-D-aspartate (NMDA) receptors [55]. In contrast to inert gas killing methods, exposure to CO_2 does not rely on the induction of hypoxia to cause unconsciousness and death and can kill over a wide range of concentrations [56].

Hypoxia is commonly achieved by displacing oxygen; this can be achieved through exposure to high concentrations of inert gases, such as nitrogen (N) or argon (Ar). To be effective, O_2 levels of < 2% must be achieved and maintained, as re-establishment of a concentration of O_2 of 6% or greater prior to death will allow immediate recovery [56–59]. Carbon monoxide (CO) binds avidly to hemoglobin and produces hypoxemia by blocking uptake of oxygen within red blood cells. Exsanguination is another method of inducing hypoxemia, albeit indirectly, to ensure death in already unconscious or moribund animals. Low atmospheric pressure stunning of poultry (LAPS) represents a refinement in producing hypoxia (see the section low atmospheric pressure stunning). Whether a hypoxia-based method is classified as stunning or killing depends on the amount of time the animal remains in the modified atmosphere; killing methods eliminate the concern that animals may regain consciousness. Hypoxia-based methods are not appropriate for those species or stages of development that are tolerant to prolonged periods of hypoxemia.

Nitrous oxide (N_2O) is not a potent anesthetic in animals. The effective dose for N_2O is above 100 vol %; therefore, it cannot be used alone in any species at normal atmospheric pressure without producing hypoxia prior to respiratory or cardiac arrest. In humans, the minimum alveolar concentration (MAC) (defined as the median effective dose preventing purposeful movement; see Chapter 28) for N_2O is 104%; its potency in other species is less than half that in humans (i.e., approximately 200%). By comparison, the MAC for isoflurane is approximately 1.4%. Up to 70% N_2O can be added to an inhaled fluorocarbon anesthetic-oxygen vapor to speed the onset of unconsciousness through the "second gas effect." However, owing to its reduced potency in animals, N_2O will only reduce the fluorocarbon anesthetic MAC by 20–30%, or about half that expected in humans [60]. The combination of CO_2 with N_2O, administered at a displacement rate of 20 and 60% of the chamber volume per minute, produced LORR in C57Bl/6 and CD1 mice 10.3% faster than CO_2 alone (N_2O–CO_2, 96.7 ± 7.9 (mean ± SD) s; CO_2, 108.7 ± 9.4 (mean ± SD) s), and may represent a refinement over the use of CO_2 alone [61].

A gradual displacement rate between 30 and 70% of the container volume per minute is currently recommended for administration of CO_2 for euthanasia [8]. The build-up, or wash-in, of gases within enclosed spaces, is an exponential process dependent on chamber volume and gas displacement rate, such that time to loss of consciousness, and eventually death, will be a function of the time constant for that container [62]. The time constant can be calculated as the chamber volume divided by the gas displacement rate [62]. When starting from a gas concentration near zero, one time constant is required to reach a washed-in gas concentration of 63% such that a gas volume displacement rate of 20%/min represents a time constant of 5 min (1 divided by 0.2). Thus, applying any vapor or gas at a displacement rate of 20% of the container volume per minute will result in an exponential rise to 63% of the wash-in gas concentration within 5 min for a container of any size [62,63].

The application of inhaled gases into enclosed spaces can be further refined to meet specific inflow rates, delivery points, and optimal gas concentration profiles through use of computational fluid dynamic (CFD) modeling. Gas distribution and temperature within containers can be modeled in three dimensions using CFD software running inside desktop computer-aided design (CAD) systems. CFD simulation has proved to be a very powerful tool for modeling transient gas concentrations during gas wash-in and wash-out. It has further reduced the need for time- and labor-intensive experimental testing of many design alternatives for on-farm depopulation methods without the need for extensive experimental testing [64].

Loss of consciousness, as LORR/LOP, should always precede loss of muscle movement. However, as with the physical killing methods, some animals may exhibit motor activity or convulsions following loss of consciousness with anesthetics or with hypoxia-based methods. Indeed, anesthesia, coma, and generalized seizures all represent a loss of consciousness where both arousal and awareness in humans are low or absent [65]. Characteristic signs of effective neural depression are similar to those observed with physical methods or with deep levels of anesthesia, including LORR/LOP, loss of eye blink and corneal reflexes, and muscle flaccidity. Inhaled and hypoxia-based methods require a number of conditions and contingencies for their proper and appropriate use, such that they are currently classified as "acceptable with conditions" in the 2020 AVMA Guidelines [8].

Agents and methods that prevent movement through muscle paralysis without inhibiting or disrupting the cerebral cortex or equivalent structures (e.g., succinylcholine, strychnine, curare, nicotine, and potassium or magnesium salts) are not acceptable as sole agents for humane killing of vertebrates because they result in conscious perception of distress and pain prior to death. In contrast, magnesium salts are considered to be acceptable as the sole agent for euthanasia in many invertebrates owing to the absence of evidence for cerebral activity in some members of these taxa [66,67]; further, there is evidence that the magnesium ion acts centrally to suppress neural activity of cephalopods [68]. Magnesium chloride is effective on moon jellyfish and sea stars without the adverse side effects noted with KCl and MgSO4 [69,70].

In summary, the cerebral cortex or equivalent structure(s) and associated subcortical structures must be functional for conscious perception of pain to occur. If the cerebral cortex is non-functional because of neuronal depression, hypoxia, or physical disruption, pain is not experienced. Although distressing to observers, reflex motor activity or physical signs occurring following loss of consciousness, as defined by LORR/LOP, is not perceived by the animal as pain or distress. Given that we are limited to applying humane killing methods based on these three basic mechanisms, efforts should be directed toward education of involved personnel and toward achieving technical proficiency and refinement in the application of currently approved methods [71].

Evaluating animal distress

Stress and the resulting responses have been divided into three phases [72]. Eustress results when harmless stimuli initiate adaptive responses that are beneficial to the animal. Neutral stress results when the animal's response to stimuli causes neither harmful nor beneficial effects to the animal. Distress results when an animal's response to stimuli interferes with its well-being and comfort [73]. Distress may be created by the conditions prior to application of stunning or killing methods (e.g., transport conditions, environment, or restraint), or by the conditions under which methods are applied (e.g., gradual gas/vapor displacement or immersion) [74]. Simply placing Sprague–Dawley rats into an unfamiliar exposure chamber containing room air produces arousal, if not distress [75]. Pigs are social animals and prefer not to be isolated from one another; consequently, moving them to the CO_2 stunning box in groups, rather than lining them up single file as needed for electric stunning, improves voluntary forward movement, reduces handling stress, and reduces electric prod use [76]. While gradual-fill inhaled methods may be less stressful than more rapid displacements for certain species in some circumstances [77], this may not be true for all species under all circumstances [8]. Distress may manifest behaviorally (e.g., overt escape behaviors, approach-avoidance preferences (aversion)), or physiologically (e.g., changes in heart rate, sympathetic nervous system activity, hypothalamic–pituitary axis activity), such that a "one size fits all" approach cannot be easily applied to evaluate killing methods or determine specific species applications.

Both sympathetic nervous system (SNS) and hypothalamic–pituitary–adrenal axis (HPAA) activation are well accepted as stress response markers. However, it has been suggested that responses to systemic stressors associated with immediate survival, such as hypoxia and hypercapnia, are likely directly relayed from brainstem nuclei and are not associated with higher-order CNS processing and conscious experiences [78]. Marked increases in circulating catecholamines, glucagon, insulin, lactate, and free fatty acids have been reported in porcine experimental models where brain death is induced following induction of general anesthesia [79–81]. Forslid and Augustinsson reported that concentrations of norepinephrine and lactate increased 1 min after exposure of pigs to CO_2 [82]. Borovsky *et al.* found an increase in norepinephrine in rats following 30 s of exposure to 100% CO_2 [83]. Similarly, Reed *et al.* exposed rats to 20–25 s of CO_2, which was sufficient to render them recumbent, unconscious, and unresponsive, and observed tenfold increases in vasopressin and oxytocin concentrations [84]. Hypothalamic vasopressin-containing neurons are similarly activated in response to CO_2 exposure in both awake and anesthetized rats [85]. In pigs undergoing euthanasia with physical methods resulting in immediate unconsciousness (e.g., captive bolt; two-point electrocution) or inhaled methods where onset of unconsciousness is delayed (CO_2; 70% N_2–30% CO_2), cortisol levels were observed to be similar, whereas plasma norepinephrine and lactate were similarly increased in all groups [86]; although all gases and mixtures induced open-mouthed breathing prior to loss of righting reflex, the mean latency to onset of open-mouth breathing and subsequent loss of righting reflex was substantially longer with 70% N_2–30% CO_2 than with CO_2 alone. The fact that levels of stress hormones observed were similar with both physical and inhaled methods illustrates the difficulty in differentiating conscious from unconscious distress where interpretation is complicated by continued exposure during the period between loss of consciousness and death.

Behavioral assessment (e.g., purposeful escape behaviors; open-mouth breathing) and aversion testing have been used to subjectively evaluate inhaled killing methods in several species; these methods have recently been reviewed [8]. *Aversion*, defined as a desire to avoid or retreat from a stimulus, is usually determined using approach-avoidance studies, where the strength of avoidance to a particular situation or condition is determined by the animal's choice to forego a desirable reward. This quantitative feature makes aversion a powerful tool for behavior studies. However, it is important to note that although aversion is a measure of preference and may imply unpleasantness, aversion itself does not necessarily indicate pain or distress; further, approach-avoidance tests fail to distinguish adequately between aversion and distress, which is the inability to respond appropriately (either behaviorally or physiologically) to a stressor [74]. In addition, agents identified as being less aversive (e.g., Ar or N_2 gas mixtures) can still produce overt and extended signs of behavioral distress (e.g., open-mouth breathing) prior to loss of consciousness under certain conditions of administration (e.g., gradual displacement application) [86].

Measurements of brain electrical function, such as the electroencephalogram (EEG), bispectral analysis (BIS™), and visual and auditory evoked potentials, have been used to quantify the unconscious state. In humans, the issue is intraoperative awareness under anesthesia; in animals, the problem is procedural humaneness relative to onset of unconsciousness. The problem is even more complex in animals where we cannot question them directly and must infer from their actions and responses [87].

Brain electrical activity is acknowledged to be limited for this purpose, especially when trying to conflate electrical activity with a complex process such as consciousness. EEG is not a direct measure of consciousness – it measures brain electrical activity, and while that activity changes with levels of consciousness, EEG cannot provide definitive answers as to onset of unconsciousness using the current state of the art. Although consciousness must vanish at some level between behavioral unresponsiveness and the induction of a flat EEG (indicating the cessation of the brain's electrical activity and brain death), current EEG-based brain function monitors are limited in their ability to indicate directly the presence or absence of unconsciousness, especially around the transition point [20,88]; also, it is not always clear which EEG patterns are indicators of activation by stress or pain [89]. A 2012 editorial in a human anesthesiology journal neatly sums up the issues [90]:

> The electroencephalogram has been the Holy Grail of anesthetic depth monitoring for more than half a century but has fallen on hard times lately, largely because the focus of the dialog changed from electroencephalogram as a monitor of "depth" to one of intraoperative awareness ... consciousness and intraoperative awareness are neurobiologically exceedingly complex phenomena. This makes these states difficult to capture or evaluate with electroencephalography, no matter the parameter or sophistication of the processing algorithm. Recent studies examining the efficacy of the electroencephalogram bispectral index for minimizing the risk of intraoperative awareness confirm as much.

Although loss of visual evoked potentials (VEPs) is associated with brain death, visual cortex neurons remain responsive to flash stimulation under desflurane anesthesia [91], and reduction in flash-induced gamma (γ) oscillations in rat visual cortex is not a unitary correlate of anesthetic-induced unconsciousness [92]. Large interindividual variations in auditory evoked potentials (AEPs) and BIS analysis make it impossible to discriminate subtle changes in clinical state of consciousness in real time during propofol anesthesia [93].

Similarly, blood oxygen level-dependent (BOLD) MRI is a multifactorial surrogate for cerebral blood flow or cerebral blood volume, both of which are actual measures of neural activity. Although a BOLD MRI response is generally a good surrogate measure of neuronal activity, it is based on hemodynamic changes, which may not reflect actual neural activity patterns, especially during anesthesia or under pharmacological challenge; rather, observed effects may be directly due to drug effects, or indirectly through changes in autonomic activity, blood pressure, cardiac output, or respiration [94,95]. In contrast, imaging of cerebral blood flow using positron emission tomography (PET) has been used in human volunteers during manipulation of consciousness with anesthetics combined with response to verbal command [21]; application of this method to explore the transition between the conscious and unconsciousness state in animals will be difficult.

Choice of killing method relative to onset of unconsciousness

The suitability of any particular agent or method for humane killing depends largely on whether distress and/or pain are experienced prior to loss of consciousness. While a "gentle" death that takes longer is generally preferable to a rapid but more distressing death [89], in some species and under some circumstances, the most humane and pragmatic option may require the use of less-than-ideal agents or conditions resulting in rapid unconsciousness with few or no outward signs of distress [8]. Any perceived distress or discomfort associated with a specific killing method occurring prior to loss of consciousness must therefore be weighed against adverse welfare that may occur due to handling or restraining procedures [56].

People are disturbed less by the euthanasia process when they feel distanced from the physical act of euthanasia or when animals exhibit little or no movement. As noted previously, reflex and convulsive motor activities can be particularly unsettling, such that choice of stunning or killing method is substantially influenced by the perceptions and preferences of those individuals to whom the task has been charged. For example, laboratory technicians reported they felt more comfortable using inhaled methods, where they were more dissociated from the animals' death than directly killing the animal with cervical dislocation [96]. Focus groups of North Carolina swine farm managers preferred methods "where you give a shot and the animal goes to sleep," even when those methods prolonged time to death, over captive bolt and blunt force cranial trauma [97]. Injectable and inhaled killing methods can provide that distance, which may partially explain their widespread usage for this purpose.

Killing methods where unconsciousness is delayed have the potential to affect animal welfare adversely. With inhalational methods, onset of unconsciousness relies on a critical concentration of gases or vapors within the alveoli and blood for effect; similarly, onset of unconsciousness following administration of injectable agents is dependent on achieving an effective concentration at the site of action. This depends on the properties of the agent and route of administration; loss of consciousness can be relatively quick following direct injection into the circulatory system whereas injectable agent administration by non-intravenous routes can delay the process. Accordingly, both inhaled methods and non-intravenous administration of barbiturate acid derivatives are currently classified as "acceptable with conditions" [8].

Interestingly, more than 40% of human children aged 2–10 years display distress behaviors during sevoflurane induction, with 17% displaying significant distress and more than 30% physically resisting during induction [98]. Fear in children undergoing anesthesia may be due to odor, feel of the mask, or a true phobia of the mask [99]. That anesthetic agents can produce distress and aversion in humans, raises concerns for their use in animals, in that the United States Government Principles for the Utilization and Care of Vertebrate Animals Used in Testing, Research, and Training state: "Unless the contrary is established, investigators should consider that procedures that cause pain or distress in human beings may cause pain or distress in other animals" [100]. Despite evidence of distress and aversion, anesthesia continues to be clinically administered to both humans and animals because the benefits associated with use greatly outweigh any distress and/or aversion the agents themselves may cause.

An intravenous (IV) overdose of a barbiturate acid derivative, such as pentobarbital or secobarbital, is currently recommended for euthanasia of companion animals [8]. These agents are no longer commonly used veterinary anesthetics, and few veterinarians today have had clinical experience of using them outside the context of euthanasia. Onset of unconsciousness with IV administration of pentobarbital or secobarbital usually occurs within 30–60 s [101]; however, maximal depth of anesthesia may not be attained for 1 min or longer [102]. It is important to understand that overdoses of these agents are utilized to ensure death and do not result in faster induction times. Pentobarbital inductions are quiet in most cases; however, struggling, excitement, and/or vocalization are occasionally observed, with the recommendation to hold the animal firmly as the head begins to fall to help avoid provoking an excitement phase during induction [103]. The 2020 AVMA Guidelines state "pre-euthanasia sedation or general anesthesia should be provided whenever practicable" [8].

Non-intravenous administration of barbiturates is currently categorized as "acceptable with conditions" when IV access would be distressful, dangerous, or impractical due to animal size or behavioral considerations [8]. Administration by the intraperitoneal (IP) route is noted to produce a slow induction of anesthesia with excitement and vocalization, unpredictable levels of anesthesia, and damage to viscera in both dogs and cats [103]. In adult male Crl:CD(BR) rats, IP administration of 40 and 50 mg/kg pentobarbital produced loss of righting in 4.7 ± 1.4 and 3.5 ± 1.4 min, respectively (mean ± SEM) [104]; similar findings were reported in male and female Wistar U:WU(Cpb) rats [105]. Cats from an animal shelter administered 346.6 mg/kg pentobarbital and 17.7 mg/kg lidocaine intrahepatically while conscious showed incoordination in 27 s and recumbency in 67 s [106]. Although time to loss of consciousness in cats receiving IP pentobarbital was not reported, incoordination and recumbency were stated to be "significantly prolonged," with 25% of cats in the IP group and 9% of cats in the intrahepatic group showing at least 30 s of what was characterized as anesthesia Stage 1 and 2 excitement [106]. As both pentobarbital and secobarbital are highly alkaline, with a pH of ~ 10, IP administration is associated with significant peritoneal irritation and pain, evidenced by upregulation in spinal *c-fos* expression following administration of pentobarbital, even with the addition of the local anesthetic lidocaine [107].

When a gas or vapor is first introduced into a large air-filled confined space using gradual displacement methods, animals are not immediately exposed to conditions known to be aversive or painful. Time between onset of signs of distress and LOP with inhaled methods depends on the agent and displacement rate. Generally, loss of consciousness will be more rapid if animals are initially exposed to a high concentration of an inhaled agent. For example, the mean induction time for neonatal pigs is 90 s when exposed to 5% isoflurane [108] and 120 s for 5% halothane [109]. For many agents and species, however, forced exposure to high inhalant concentrations can be aversive and distressing, such that gradual exposure may be the most pragmatic and humane option.

Flecknell *et al.* reported violent struggling accompanied by apnea and bradycardia in rabbits administered isoflurane, halothane, and sevoflurane by mask or induction chamber, and concluded that these agents were aversive and should be avoided whenever possible [110]. Leach *et al.* found inhaled anesthetic vapors to be associated with some degree of aversion in laboratory rodents, with increasing aversion noted as concentration increased; halothane was least aversive for rats, and halothane and enflurane were least aversive for mice [111–113]. Makowska and Weary also reported halothane and isoflurane to be aversive to male Wistar rats, but less so than CO_2 [114].

Carbon monoxide is reported to be aversive to laboratory rats, but not as aversive as CO_2 [115]. Carbon monoxide produces LOP at a concentration of approximately 5% in male Wistar rats; however, mean time to LOP varies with CO displacement rate (104 s at 3% volume displacement rate; 64 s at 6% volume displacement rate; 53 s at 7% volume displacement rate) [115]; for comparison, a 10% CO atmosphere could be achieved within 30 s with administration of 100% CO at a volume displacement rate equivalent to 20% of the chamber volume per minute.

Aversion to the inert gases argon (Ar) and nitrogen (N_2) depends largely on species and conditions of administration [8]. Hypoxia resulting from exposure to these gases is aversive to rats, mice, and mink. In contrast, these gases appear not to be directly aversive to poultry, and the resulting hypoxia appears to be non-aversive or only mildly aversive. Similarly, Ar or N_2 gas mixtures do not appear to be directly aversive to pigs and seem to reduce, but not eliminate, behavioral responses to hypoxia [59]. However, based on the wash-in and wash-out exponential functions, gradual displacement administration of inert gases results in prolonged exposure to hypoxic conditions and can produce overt signs of behavioral distress, such as open-mouth breathing, for an extended period prior to loss of consciousness in laboratory rodents [75,77], pigs [86], and poultry [116]. Nitrogen-containing high-expansion foams are effective in purging air from containers and create stable anoxic conditions. Poultry immersed in high-expansion N_2-filled foam rapidly become ataxic, with loss of posture and vigorous wing flapping characteristic of anoxic death [117]. Pigs avoid putting their heads and snouts into the foam when foam levels become high and demonstrate escape attempts through the test box lid when foam covers their heads [118].

Distress during CO_2 exposure has been examined using behavioral assessment and aversion testing [8]. Variability in behavioral responses to CO_2 has been reported for rats and mice [74,77,119–125], pigs [57,59,126–129], and poultry [130–139]. Although signs of distress have been reported in animals in some studies, other researchers have not consistently observed these effects. This may be due to variations in gas administration and exposure methods, handling issues, types of behaviors assessed, and animal species and strains tested. Fossorial (burrowing) species appear to be more resistant to hypoxia and hypercarbia than terrestrial-dwelling species, making it difficult to generalize [140].

Using preference and approach-avoidance testing, rats, and mice show aversion to CO_2 concentrations sufficient to induce unconsciousness [112,113] and are willing to forego a palatable food reward to avoid exposure to CO_2 concentrations of approximately 15% and higher [114,141] after up to 24 h of food deprivation [142]. Mink will avoid a chamber containing a desirable novel object when it contains 100% CO_2 [143]. In contrast to other species, a large proportion of chickens and turkeys will enter a chamber containing moderate concentrations of CO_2 (60%) to gain access to food or social contact [135,137,139]. Following incapacitation and prior to loss of consciousness, birds in these studies show behaviors such as open-beak breathing and head shaking; these behaviors, however, may not be associated with distress because birds do not withdraw from CO_2 when these behaviors occur [133]. Exposure to CO_2 concentrations up to 30% does not appear to be aversive to pigs, as Duroc and Large White pigs, when given a choice, will tolerate 30% CO_2 to gain access to a food reward [57,127]. Hence it appears that birds and pigs are more willing than rodents and mink to tolerate CO_2 at concentrations sufficient to induce LORR/LOP.

Carbon dioxide exposure using gradual fill methods is less likely to cause pain due to nociceptor activation by carbonic acid prior to onset of unconsciousness, such that a CO_2 displacement rate between 30 and 70% of the chamber volume per minute is currently recommended for euthanasia [8,9]. When administered at these rates, unconsciousness occurs prior to exposure to CO_2 levels known to produce nociceptor stimulation [74,77]. In humans, rats, and cats, nociceptors begin to respond at CO_2 concentrations of approximately 40% [144–147]. Humans report that discomfort begins between 30 and 50% CO_2 and intensifies to overt pain with higher concentrations [148–150]. In rodents, distress begins at approximately 15% CO_2 concentration and lasts to onset of unconsciousness approximately 30 s later. Unconsciousness occurs within 106 s at a CO_2 concentration of approximately 30% with a CO_2 displacement rate equivalent to 17–20% of the chamber volume [125,141,150,151]. A slower 10%/min displacement increases time to onset of unconsciousness to 156 s at a CO_2 concentration of 21% [77]. When CO_2 is administered to neonatal pigs at 20% of the chamber volume per minute, unconsciousness (loss of righting reflex) occurs within 80 ± 15 s (mean ± SEM) at a CO_2 concentration of approximately 22% [86]. The CO_2 concentrations required to produce LOP for broilers, layers, turkeys, and ducks are 19.0, 19.9, 19.3, and 23.8%, respectively [131].

Genetics may play a role in CO_2 response variability. Panic disorder in humans is genetically linked to enhanced sensitivity to CO_2 [152]. The fear network, comprising the hippocampus, the medial prefrontal cortex, and the amygdala and its brainstem projections, appears to be abnormally sensitive to CO_2 in these patients [153]. The genetic background of some pigs, especially excitable lines such as the Hampshire and German Landrace, has been associated with animals that react poorly to CO_2 stunning, whereas calmer genetic lines combining the Yorkshire or Dutch Landrace conformations show much milder reactions [154]. Given a choice, Duroc and Large White pigs will tolerate 30% CO_2 to gain access to a food reward but will forego the reward to avoid exposure to 90% CO_2, even after a 24-h period of food deprivation [57,127]. A shock with an electric prod, however, is more aversive to Landrace × Large White pigs than inhaling 60 or 90% CO_2, with pigs inhaling 60% CO_2 willing to re-enter the crate containing CO_2 [126]. Jongman *et al.* linked variation in pig responses to CO_2 with pre-stunning lairage issues and animal handling [155]. Until further research is conducted, one can conclude that exposure to high levels of CO_2 may be humane for certain genetic lines of pigs and stressful for others [154].

Studies have found regions of the mouse amygdala associated with fear behavior to contain acid-sensing ion channels (ASIC) sensitive to elevated CO_2 [156]. Fear behaviors and aversion in response to CO_2 exposure were reduced in mice in which the ASIC receptors were eliminated or inhibited, suggesting that aversive responses to CO_2 in rodents, and potentially other species, are mediated in part by an innate fear response. Further studies defining the presence of ASIC and their role in CO_2-induced fear in other rodent strains, and also other animal species, are warranted.

The practice of immersion in a container prefilled with 100% CO_2 is now considered "unacceptable" for euthanasia [8,9]. However, a distinction must be made between immersion, where conscious animals are placed directly into a high concentration of a gas or vapor within a container, and commercial controlled atmosphere stunning (CAS) processes as employed for the stunning of poultry and swine. Unlike immersion, animals experience their introduction into CAS atmospheres gradually; this can be through physical transport at a controlled rate into a contained stunning atmosphere gradient, through controlled introduction of stunning gases into an enclosed space, or by controlled reduction of atmospheric pressure to produce hypoxia. Sequential combinations (so-called "two-step" or "multi-phase" processes) may utilize one gas or a gas mixture to induce unconsciousness prior to exposure to a different gas mixture or higher gas concentration. Animal transport or introduction rate may be slow or relatively quick, depending on the process, gases utilized, and the specific species. Further, denser than air gases such as CO_2 layer into defined gradients within an enclosed space [157]. Thus, animals are not immediately exposed to conditions known to be aversive or painful with CAS. The design of commercial CAS systems is described in the 2016 AVMA Humane Slaughter guidelines and has been reviewed by Grandin and Cockram [14].

Uncertainty exists as to the usefulness and feasibility of substituting inhaled anesthetic agents for CO_2 with respect to animal welfare and human health and safety [8,85]; in these types of studies, perception bias is a possible confounder [158]. Inhaled halocarbon anesthetics have been proposed as alternatives to CO_2 for rodent euthanasia [89,114,115,159] and the Canadian Council on Animal Care (CCAC) has adopted this position when feasible [9]. However, inhaled anesthetics are known to produce varying degrees of aversion in rodents [111–114,159–162]; inhaled anesthetics are noted to produce aversion, distress, and escape behaviors during anesthetic induction in other animal species [110] and humans [98,99]. Isoflurane anesthesia administered prior to CO_2 euthanasia increased adverse behavioral signs of distress and c-*fos* expression in the brains of female CD1 mice [74]. Consistent with the principles governing wash-in and wash-out of gases within closed containers, five of ten isoflurane-anesthetized mice showed signs of recovery of consciousness when CO_2 was added to the container [74]. Premedication with acepromazine or midazolam prior to exposure to CO_2 administered at a 20%/min displacement rate did not significantly alter observed behaviors but did induce significantly higher c-*fos* expression [74]. Premedication with 20 mg/kg zolazepam–tiletamine in cream cheese produced mild sedation and reduced the aversiveness of CO_2 euthanasia in mice [163]. Large amounts of inhaled anesthetics are absorbed and significant amounts remain in the body for days, even after apparent recovery [164], making these agents unsuitable for euthanasia of food-producing animals.

Fetal sentience and euthanasia

Fetal sentience during euthanasia of pregnant animals and ovariohysterectomy of pregnant dogs and cats has been extensively reviewed by Mellor *et al.* [165–168] and White [169]. Concerns about fetal suffering during humane slaughter of pregnant animals or ovariohysterectomy of pregnant dogs and cats may arise, at least in part, because of observation of fetal body and respiratory movements. However, these movements are a part of normal fetal physiology in utero and should not, in and of themselves, be a cause for welfare concerns. Although the term "fetal distress" has been used in the past, it is not meant to indicate or imply conscious emotional distress, awareness, or conscious suffering and is currently considered to be imprecise and non-specific in this context [169].

In an extensive review of fetal physiology and pain perception, Mellor and Diesch [165] asserted that "an animal must be both sentient and conscious for suffering to occur"; in other words, the animal must have adequate neural development for sensory perception or sentience and must also be in an awake conscious state. All mammalian embryos or fetuses studied to date remain in an unconscious state throughout pregnancy and birth [166]. This occurs in some species due to exceptional neurological immaturity (e.g., certain marsupials) or moderate neurological immaturity (e.g., cats, dogs, rabbits, rats, and mice). In those species which are neurologically mature at birth (e.g., cattle, deer, goats, sheep, horses, and guinea pigs), initial neurological immaturity is combined with in utero neuro-inhibitors. These neuro-inhibitors are unique to prenatal life and include adenosine (a potent promoter of sleep and/or unconsciousness), allopregnanolone and pregnanolone (neuroactive steroids with well-established anesthetic, sedative/hypnotic, and analgesic effects, synthesized by the fetal brain), and prostaglandin-D_2 (a potent sleep-inducing agent, synthesized by the fetal brain). Consciousness occurs within minutes or hours following birth in these species largely due to the combined effect of decreasing neuro-inhibition and the onset of strong neuro-activation. Further, an isoelectric EEG, which is incompatible with consciousness, rapidly appears after cessation of placental oxygen supply. Thus, embryos and fetuses cannot consciously experience sensations or feelings such as breathlessness or pain, and cannot suffer while dying *in utero* after the death of the dam, whatever the cause of her death. A rather similar, but qualified, conclusion has been drawn in avian species where EEG activity suggestive of the potential for pain perception may not occur until > 80% incubation in avian species [8,170].

Low atmospheric pressure stunning

Low atmospheric pressure stunning (LAPS) is a method for stunning poultry prior to humane slaughter. LAPS was added to the EU Directive 2018/723 (amendment to 1099/2009) in May 2018 and is listed in the USDA Food Safety and Inspection Service New Technology Table (07-NT-0289-N-A, August 2021; www.fsis.usda.gov/sites/default/files/media_file/2020-09/new-technologies-table.pdf, accessed May 2022). Unconsciousness occurs following a controlled and gradual reduction of barometric pressure due to hypoxia [171–173]. A significant advantage of LAPS over electrical stunning and "live-dump" controlled atmosphere stunning (CAS) using gas is elimination of welfare issues associated with dumping live birds onto the conveyor line and eliminating the need to handle live birds manually.

Rapid decompression is currently deemed "unacceptable" for euthanasia [8]. LAPS is not rapid decompression, but rather negative atmospheric pressure applied gradually over time, typically over 1 min in broilers, which results in an acute hypoxic state not unlike being in an unpressurized airplane at altitude. Maximum observed negative pressure during commercial broiler LAPS corresponds to an estimated atmospheric pressure of 160 mmHg and inspired partial pressure of oxygen of 33 mmHg [173]. Thus, LAPS PO_2 at maximum negative pressure is equivalent to a 4% dry oxygen atmosphere at sea level (33 mmHg/760 mmHg). For comparison, the atmospheric pressure (P_B) on top of Mount Everest (elevation approximately 29,000 feet) is 225 mmHg and the PO_2 is 47 mmHg; at 40,000 feet, P_B is 141 mmHg and PO_2 is 30 mmHg.

Rapid decompression can cause both pain and distress through expansion of gases present in enclosed spaces [174]. In the case of birds, however, gases are unlikely to be trapped in the lungs or abdomen during LAPS and are therefore unlikely to become a source of abdominal distention, due to the unique anatomic structure of the avian respiratory system. Avian lungs are open at both ends, rigid, attached to the ribs, and do not change in size during ventilation. Attached to the lungs are nine air sacs that fill all spaces within the thoracic and abdominal cavities. Because birds lack a diaphragm, they move air in and out during sternal movement using the intercostal and abdominal muscles; air movement is simultaneous and continuous with no passive or relaxed period. Hence, it is unlikely that significant amounts of gas can be trapped within the avian lungs or abdomen unless the trachea is blocked for some reason [175]. In contrast to reports of hemorrhagic lesions in the lungs, brain, and heart of animals undergoing rapid decompression, no such lesions were observed in birds undergoing LAPS [172]. Corticosterone concentrations in LAPS stunned broilers were nearly half the levels observed in electrically stunned birds [172].

During commercial operation, birds undergoing LAPS remain within palletized shipping cages. Following the LAPS cycle, the palletized cages containing unconscious birds are moved to the dumping station and moved by conveyor belt to the shackling area prior to entry to the processing line. LAPS target pressures for broilers are achieved within 1 min from the start of the LAPS cycle and maintained for 4 min and 40 s to assure that recovery to consciousness does not occur prior to exsanguination [172]. Time to first coordinated animal movement was 58.7 ± 3.0 s (mean ± SEM), with "light-headedness" (defined as time from first head movement to first wing flap) noted within 69.3 ± 6.4 s; LOP occurred within 64.9 ± 6.1 s (mean ± SEM). Wing and leg paddling was infrequent, lasting 15.1 ± 1.1 s (mean ± SEM) following LOP. Neither mandibulation (movements of the beak as if the bird was responding to sensations in the mouth) nor deep open-bill breathing was observed in LAPS birds; bill breathing and mandibulation are commonly reported during controlled atmosphere stunning with various gas mixtures [176]. Based on EEG studies, increasing slow (δ) wave activity consistent with a gradual loss of consciousness occurs within 10 s of the start of the LAPS cycle, peaking between 30 and 40 s and coincident with LOP and first brief movements [177]. The same group also determined that heart rate decreases over time during LAPS, implying minimal additional SNS stimulation, and concluded that LAPS is a humane approach that can potentially improve the welfare of poultry at slaughter by inducing unconsciousness without distress, eliminating live shackling, and ensuring that every bird is adequately stunned before exsanguination [177]. LAPS is currently considered a humane method of euthanasia of male layer chicks [178,179].

LAPS has been proposed as a more humane alternative to CO_2 stunning in pigs [180] and for euthanasia of mice [181]. While considered a promising euthanasia method for mice, it is not considered a humane alternative to CO_2 for preslaughter stunning of swine [182].

Foam depopulation

Foam depopulation methods were initially developed as an alternative to modified atmosphere depopulation methods for floor-raised poultry [183]. Advantages of foam over other depopulation methods include reduced overall time required to depopulate farms, reduced number of workers required and their potential exposure to zoonotic diseases, less physical activity while wearing personal protective equipment, suppression of airborne particulates, enhancement of carcass disposal using in-house composting, and greater flexibility of use in various style poultry houses, including those structurally damaged [184].

Foam depopulation uses medium- or high-expansion foam-generating equipment to create a blanket of water-based foam to cover the animals. Most current foam depopulation equipment uses compressed or ambient air to create the bubbles. Immersion in the foam produces rapid airway blockage and occlusion, resulting in death by suffocation. Water-based foam requires less time to death than CO_2 gas, with similar pretreatment and post-mortem corticosterone levels [183]. Based on cessation of EEG activity, water-based foam was as consistent as CO_2 gas, and more consistent than a 70% Ar–30% CO_2 gas mix [185]; EEG cessation time with ambient air-foam was not statistically different from that for CO_2-filled foam [183]. Foam is also an effective depopulation tool for chukar partridges, quail, ducks, and turkeys [186].

Water-based foam depopulation for poultry was conditionally approved in 2006 by the United States Department of Agriculture Animal and Plant Health Service (USDA APHIS). The use of foam is not an AVMA-approved method of euthanasia [8], but the AVMA has issued policy statements indicating that it "supports the use of water-based foam as a method of mass depopulation in accord with the conditions and performance standards outlined by the USDA APHIS" [16]. The use of foam is conditionally approved for situations in which animals are: (1) infected with a potentially zoonotic disease; (2) experiencing an outbreak of a rapidly spreading infectious disease that cannot be easily contained; or (3) housed in structurally unsound buildings.

Raj *et al.* [187] raised animal welfare concerns because water-based foam filled with ambient air produces airway occlusion, a form of suffocation; they proposed increasing bubble size as a means to reduce airway occlusion in addition to incorporating an inert gas in the foam to produce unconsciousness prior to death. Gerritzen *et al.* evaluated responses of broilers, ducks, and turkeys to CO_2-filled foam and N_2-filled foam [188]. Exposure of poultry to CO_2-filled foam resulted in an earlier induction of a transitional state of the EEG than when exposed to N_2-filled foam; the effect of CO_2 on consciousness started before the birds were submerged. After submersion, there was no difference in reduction of conscious state between CO_2- and N_2-filled foam, and it was concluded that the anoxic effects of both gas-filled foams were comparable and acceptable, with the warning that birds submerged under the leading edge of the foam with a height less than 80 cm are likely to be at risk of compromised welfare in the event of technical failure of the foam system. High-expansion nitrogen-filled foam is currently being investigated as a means to perform pig and poultry welfare culls [16,188–190].

Agent purity and euthanasia

The Office for Laboratory Animal Welfare (OLAW) and the USDA provide guidance on the use of nonpharmaceutical-grade substances. Both OLAW and USDA agree that pharmaceutical-grade chemicals and other substances, when available, must be used to avoid toxicity or side-effects that may threaten the health and welfare of vertebrate animals or interfere with the interpretation of research results. However, the decision to use nonpharmaceutical-grade substances rests with the Institutional Animal Care Committee [191]. OLAW, together with USDA and the International Association for the Assessment and Accreditation of Laboratory Animal Care (AAALAC), offers guidance on this issue [192]. Basically, the highest-grade-equivalent chemical reagent should be used if no equivalent veterinary or human drug is available for experimental use.

In the case of inhaled gases, industrial or food grades may be of similar or higher purity than medical grades. The federal government technical and USP specifications for CO_2 are detailed in BB-C-101D [193]. Grade A CO_2 is defined by BB-C-101D as conforming to the requirements of the United States Pharmacopeia/ National Formulary (USP/NF), whereas Grade B CO_2 is defined as having purity of no less than 99.5 vol %. Grade A gases are manufactured under certified Good Manufacturing Practices (cGMP) as defined by federal statute 21 CFR 211.84 and meet the applicable specifications of the USP/NF, which include a certificate of analysis, validated analytical procedures, lot number assignment, traceability, and recall procedures [194]. Industrial-grade gases generally do not have these cGMP attributes. Users wishing to substitute Grade B or industrial-grade gases will need to confirm with their gas supplier that product purity is equivalent to or greater than the corresponding medical or Grade A product.

Euthanasia in the clinical setting

Barbiturates and barbituric acid derivatives (e.g., sodium pentobarbital, secobarbital, and pentobarbital combination products), administered IV, are considered acceptable for euthanasia of conscious animals [8]. These agents can preferably be administered following sedation or general anesthesia or administered as the sole agent. With the exception of intramuscular delivery of select injectable anesthetics (e.g., an α_2-adrenergic receptor agonist combined with ketamine), the subcutaneous, intramuscular, intrapulmonary, and intrathecal routes of administration are unacceptable for administration of injectable euthanasia agents in awake and conscious animals because of the limited information available regarding their effectiveness and the high probability of pain associated with injection [8].

When IV access would be distressful, dangerous, or impractical (e.g., small patient sizes such as puppies, kittens, small dogs and cats, rodents, non-domestic species, or behavioral considerations for some small exotic mammals and feral domestic animals), barbiturates may be conditionally administered intraperitoneal (e.g., sodium pentobarbital, secobarbital; not pentobarbital combination products as these have only been approved for IV and intracardiac administration). Administration by the IP route has potential for peritoneal irritation and pain and, as noted previously, results in delayed loss of consciousness; hence this route is considered "acceptable with conditions" by the AVMA [8]. In unconscious or anesthetized animals, intra-organ injections (e.g., intraosseous, intracardiac, intrahepatic, intrasplenic, and intrarenal) may be used as an alternative. Intra-organ injections may speed the rate of barbiturate uptake over standard IP injections and, when an owner is present, this approach may be preferred over the IP route [8].

Apparent resistance to pentobarbital or delay of expected effect is sometimes seen clinically. Reduced venous return (e.g., dehydration, hemorrhage, and sepsis) or low cardiac output (e.g., heart failure) will predictably delay circulation time and subsequent onset of injectable agents. Animals treated for epilepsy are anecdotally reported to be more resistant to pentobarbital; this may be due to down-regulation of GABA receptors and upregulation of NMDA receptors [195].

Proper carcass disposal is important. Animals euthanized with barbiturates create risks for scavengers and other animals that may consume portions of the animal's remains [196,197]. Pentobarbital is resistant to chemical breakdown and may still be detectable 1 year after composting [198]. Lead poisoning due to exposed or poorly buried carcasses of gunshot animals is a serious issue for scavengers [197].

Intrathecal lidocaine has been proposed as a humane euthanasia method for horses, sheep, and goats [199] and produces brain death prior to cardiac death in horses [200]. The method poses a low risk for toxicity of carnivores and scavengers [201].

Injectable anesthetic overdose (e.g., combination of ketamine and an α_2-adrenergic receptor agonist given IV, IP, or IM, or propofol given IV) is acceptable for euthanasia when animal size, restraint requirements, or other circumstances indicate that these drugs are the best option. Assurance of death is paramount and may require a second step (e.g., a barbiturate, or additional doses of the anesthetic), or use of an acceptable adjunctive method (e.g., gunshot; penetrating captive bolt; exsanguination; potassium chloride, 1–2 mmol/kg, 75–150 mg/kg, or 1–2 mEq/kg, administered IV or IC) [8]. Potassium chloride or a saturated magnesium sulfate solution can only be used adjunctively to euthanize unconscious animals (defined as unresponsive to noxious stimuli) or under general anesthesia [8].

Production shortages in 2021 led to a dilemma for those practices needing pentobarbital for animal euthanasia. The background to the shortage and the responses by veterinary medical groups, laboratory research institutions, and the animal sheltering industry was documented by Cooney and Titcomb [202]. An alternative method to conserve pentobarbital by combining induction of a deep state of general anesthesia followed by one-half the usual amount of pentobarbital was advocated by the AVMA [203].

Alternatives to barbiturates for euthanasia include T-61 and Tributame™. T-61 is acceptable as an agent of euthanasia, provided that it is administered appropriately by trained individuals. Slow IV injection is necessary to avoid muscular paralysis prior to unconsciousness. Administration of T-61 by routes other than IV is unacceptable [8]. T-61 is not currently being manufactured in the United States but is obtainable from Canada. Tributame™, although not currently in production in the United States, is also an acceptable euthanasia drug for dogs provided that it is administered IV by an appropriately trained individual at recommended dosages and proper injection rates. If barbiturates are not available, its extra-label use in cats may be considered; however, adverse reactions, such as agonal breathing, have been reported and the current United States Food and Drug Administration (FDA) approved Tributame™ label recommends against its use in cats. Routes of Tributame™ administration other than IV injection are not acceptable [8].

References

1 Arluke A. Trapped in a guilt cage. *New Sci Publ* **1992**; 134(1815): 33–35.
2 Whiting TL, Marion CR. Perpetration-induced traumatic stress – a risk for veterinarians involved in the destruction of healthy animals. *Can Vet J* 2011; **52**(7): 794–796.
3 American Veterinary Medical Association. Veterinarian's Oath. www.avma.org/resources-tools/avma-policies/veterinarians-oath (accessed April 2022).
4 Rollin BE. The use and abuse of Aesculapian authority in veterinary medicine. *J Am Vet Med Assoc* 2002; **220**(8): 1144–1149.
5 Rollin BE. Euthanasia and the quality of life. *J Am Vet Med Assoc* 2006; **228**(7): 1014–1016.
6 Carter HE. Historical cases. *J Small Anim Pract* 1984; **25**(1): 31–35.
7 Alkire MT. General anesthesia. In: Banks WP, ed. *Encyclopedia of Consciousness*. Oxford, UK: Elsevier/Academic Press, 2009: 296–313.
8 American Veterinary Medical Association. AVMA Guidelines for the Euthanasia of Animals: 2020 Edition. www.avma.org/sites/default/files/2020-02/Guidelines-on-Euthanasia-2020.pdf (accessed April 2022).
9 Canadian Council on Animal Care. CCAC Guidelines on: Euthanasia of Animals Used in Science, 2010. www.ccac.ca/Documents/Standards/Guidelines/Euthanasia.pdf (accessed April 2022).
10 World Organisation for Animal Health (WOAH founded as OIE). Development of Animal Welfare Standards. www.woah.org/en/what-we-do/animal-health-and-welfare/animal-welfare/development-of-animal-welfare-standards (accessed April 2022).

11 McMillan FD. Rethinking euthanasia: death as an unintentional outcome. *J Am Vet Med Assoc* 2001; **219**(9): 1204–1206.

12 Pavlovic D, Spassov A, Lehmann C. Euthanasia: in defense of a good, ancient word. *J Clinic Res Bioeth* 2011; **2**: 1000105.

13 Leary SL, American Veterinary Medical Association. AVMA Guidelines for the Humane Slaughter: 2016 Edition. www.avma.org/KB/Resources/Reference/Animal Welfare/Documents/Humane-Slaughter-Guidelines.pdf?utm_source=email-optin&utm_medium=aw-focus-1608&utm_campaign=humane-endings&utm_term=link&utm_content=humane-slaughter-guidelines (accessed April 2022).

14 Grandin T, Cockram M, eds. *The Slaughter of Farmed Animals: Practical Ways of Enhancing Animal Welfare.* Boston, MA: CABI, 2020.

15 United States Code. 7 USC Chapter 48 – Humane Methods of Livestock Slaughter. www.govinfo.gov/content/pkg/USCODE-2017-title7/html/USCODE-2017-title7-chap48-sec1901.htm (accessed April 2022).

16 Leary SL, American Veterinary Medical Association. AVMA Guidelines for the Depopulation of Animals: 2019 Edition. www.avma.org/sites/default/files/resources/AVMA-Guidelines-for-the-Depopulation-of-Animals.pdf (accessed April 2022).

17 Baysinger A, Senn M, Gebhardt J, *et al.* A case study of ventilation shutdown with the addition of high temperature and humidity for depopulation of pigs. *J Am Vet Med Assoc* 2021; **259**(4): 415–424.

18 Eberle-Krish KN, Martin MP, Malheiros RD, *et al.* Evaluation of ventilation shutdown in a multi-level caged system. *J Appl Poult Res* 2018; **27**(4): 555–563.

19 International Association for the Study of Pain. IASP Terms. www.iasp-pain.org/resources/terminology (accessed April 2022).

20 Alkire MT, Hudetz AG, Tononi G. Consciousness and anesthesia. *Science* 2008; **322**(5903): 876–880.

21 Långsjö JW, Alkire MT, Kaskinoro K, *et al.* Returning from oblivion: imaging the neural core of consciousness. *J Neurosci* 2012; **32**(14): 4935–4943.

22 Hendrickx JF, Eger EI II, Sonner JM, *et al.* Is synergy the rule? A review of anesthetic interactions producing hypnosis and immobility. *Anesth Analg* 2008; **107**(2): 494–506.

23 Antognini JF, Barter L, Carstens E. Overview: movement as an index of anesthetic depth in humans and experimental animals. *Comp Med* 2005; **55**(5): 413–418.

24 Zeller W, Mettler D, Schatzmann U. Untersuchungen zur Betäubung des Schlachtgeflügels mit Kohlendioxid. *Fleischwirtschaft* 1988; **68**: 1308–1312 (as cited in Raj ABM, Gregory NG. Effect of rate of induction of carbon dioxide anaesthesia on the time of onset of unconsciousness and convulsions. *Res Vet Sci* 1990; **49**(3): 360–363).

25 McKeegan DEF, Sparks NHC, Sandilands V, *et al.* Physiological responses of laying hens during whole-house killing with carbon dioxide. *Br Poult Sci* 2011; **52**(6): 645–657.

26 Benson ER, Alphin RL, Rankin MK, *et al.* Evaluation of EEG based determination of unconsciousness vs. loss of posture in broilers. *Res Vet Sci* 2012; **93**(2): 960–964.

27 Tranquilli WJ, Grimm KA. Introduction: use, definitions, history, concepts, classification, and considerations for general anesthesia. In: Grimm KA, Lamont LA, Tranquilli WJ, *et al.*, eds. *Veterinary Anesthesia and Analgesia*, 5th edn. Ames, IA: John Wiley and Sons, 2015: 3–10.

28 Erhardt W, Ring C, Kraft H, *et al.* CO_2 stunning of swine for slaughter from the anesthesiological viewpoint. *Dtsch Tierarztl Wochenschr* 1989; **96**(3): 92–99.

29 Dyakonova VE. Role of opioid peptides in behavior of invertebrates. *J Evol Biochem Physiol* 2001; **37**(4): 335–347.

30 Sladky KK, Kinney ME, Johnson SM. Analgesic efficacy of butorphanol and morphine in bearded dragons and corn snakes. *J Am Vet Med Assoc* 2008; **233**(2): 267–273.

31 Baker BB, Sladky KK, Johnson SM. Evaluation of the analgesic effects of oral and subcutaneous tramadol administration in red eared slider turtles. *J Am Vet Med Assoc* 2011; **238**(2): 220–227.

32 Rose JD. The neurobehavioral nature of fishes and the question of awareness and pain. *Rev Fish Sci* 2002; **10**: 1–38.

33 Nordgreen J, Horsberg TE, Ranheim B, *et al.* Somatosensory evoked potentials in the telencephalon of Atlantic salmon (*Salmo salar*) following galvanic stimulation of the tail. *J Comp Physiol A Neuroethol Sens Neural Behav Physiol* 2007; **193**(12): 1235–1242.

34 Dunlop R, Laming P. Mechanoreceptive and nociceptive responses in the central nervous system of goldfish (*Carassius auratus*) and trout (*Oncorhynchus mykiss*). *J Pain* 2005; **6**(9): 561–568.

35 Braithwaite VA. Cognitive ability in fish. *Fish Physiol* 2006; **24**: 1–37.

36 Verhoeven MTW, Gerritzen MA, Hellebrekers LJ, *et al.* Indicators used in livestock to assess unconsciousness after stunning: a review. *Animals* 2015; **9**(2): 320–330.

37 Verhoeven MTW, Gerritzen MA, Kluivers-Poodt M, *et al.* Validation of behavioural indicators used to assess unconsciousness in sheep. *Res Vet Sci* 2015; **101**: 144–153.

38 Verhoeven M, Gerritzen M, Velarde A, *et al.* Time to loss of consciousness and its relation to behavior in slaughter pigs during stunning with 80 or 95% carbon dioxide. *Front Vet Sci* 2016; **3**: 38.

39 Terlouw C, Bourguet C, Deiss V. Consciousness, unconsciousness and death in the context of slaughter. Part I. Neurobiological mechanisms underlying stunning and killing. *Meat Sci* 2016; **118**: 133–146.

40 Terlouw C, Bourguet C, Deiss V. Consciousness, unconsciousness and death in the context of slaughter. Part II. Evaluation methods. *Meat Sci* 2016; **118**: 147–156.

41 Cartner SC, Barlow SC, Ness TJ. Loss of cortical function in mice after decapitation, cervical dislocation, potassium chloride injection, and CO_2 inhalation. *Comp Med* 2007; **57**(6): 570–573.

42 Close B, Banister K, Baumans V, *et al.* Recommendations for euthanasia of experimental animals: Part 1. DGXI of the European Commission. *Lab Anim* 1996; **30**(4): 293–316.

43 Close B, Banister K, Baumans V, *et al.* Recommendations for euthanasia of experimental animals: Part 2. DGXI of the European Commission. *Lab Anim* 1997; **31**(1): 1–32.

44 Gregory NG, Wotton SB. Effect of slaughter on the spontaneous and evoked activity of the brain. *Br Poult Sci* 1986; **27**(2): 195–205.

45 Bates G. Humane issues surrounding decapitation reconsidered. *J Am Vet Med Assoc* 2010; **237**(9): 1024–1026.

46 Holson RR. Euthanasia by decapitation: evidence that this technique produces prompt, painless unconsciousness in laboratory rodents. *Neurotoxicol Teratol* 1992; **14**(4): 253–257.

47 Derr RF. Pain perception in decapitated rat brain. *Life Sci* 1991; **49**(19): 1399–1402.

48 Vanderwolf CH, Buzak DP, Cain RK, *et al.* Neocortical and hippocampal electrical activity following decapitation in the rat. *Brain Res* 1988; **451**(1–2): 340–344.

49 Mikeska JA, Klemm WR. EEG evaluation of humaneness of asphyxia and decapitation euthanasia of the laboratory rat. *Lab Anim Sci* 1975; **25**(2): 175–179.

50 van Rijn CM, Krijnen H, Menting-Hermeling S, *et al.* Decapitation in rats: latency to unconsciousness and the 'wave of death'. *PLoS ONE* 2011; **6**(1): e16514

51 Martoft L, Lomholt L, Kolthoff C, *et al.* Effects of CO_2 anaesthesia on central nervous system activity in swine. *Lab Anim* 2002; **36**(2): 115–126.

52 Raj ABM, Johnson SP, Wotton SB, *et al.* Welfare implications of gas stunning pigs: 3. the time to loss of somatosensory evoked potentials and spontaneous electrocorticogram of pigs during exposure to gases. *Vet J* 1997; **153**(3): 329–339.

53 Ring C, Erhardt W, Kraft H, *et al.* CO_2 anaesthesia of slaughter pigs. *Fleischwirtschaft* 1988; **68**(11): 1304–1307.

54 Forslid A. Transient neocortical, hippocampal, and amygdaloid EEG silence induced by one minute inhalation of high CO_2 concentration in swine. *Acta Physiol Scand* 1987; **130**(1): 1–10.

55 Brosnan RJ, Pham TL. Carbon dioxide negatively modulates N-methyl-D-aspartate receptors. *Br J Anaesth* 2008; **101**(5): 673–679.

56 Raj M. Humane killing of nonhuman animals for disease control purposes. *J Appl Anim Welf Sci* 2008; **11**(2): 112–124.

57 Raj ABM, Gregory NG. Welfare implications of the gas stunning of pigs: 1. Determination of aversion to the initial inhalation of carbon dioxide or argon. *Anim Welf* 1995; **4**(4): 273–280.

58 Raj ABM. Behaviour of pigs exposed to mixtures of gases and the time required to stun and kill them: welfare implications. *Vet Rec* 1999; **144**(7): 165–168.

59 Dalmau A, Rodriguez P, Llonch P, *et al.* Stunning pigs with different gas mixtures: aversion in pigs. *Anim Welf* 2010; **19**(3): 325–333.

60 Steffey EP, Mama KR. Inhalation anesthetics. In: Grimm KA, Lamont LA, Tranquilli WJ, *et al.*, eds. *Veterinary Anesthesia and Analgesia*, 5th edn. Ames, IA: John Wiley and Sons, 2015: 311–312.

61 Thomas AA, Flecknell PA, Golledge HD. Combining nitrous oxide with carbon dioxide decreases the time to loss of consciousness during euthanasia in mice – refinement of animal welfare? *PLoS ONE* 2012; **7**(3): e32290.

62 Meyer RE, Morrow WEM. Carbon dioxide for emergency on-farm euthanasia of swine. *J Swine Health Prod* 2005; **13**(4): 210–217.

63 Meyer RE. Principles of carbon dioxide displacement. *Lab Anim* 2008; **37**(6): 241–242.

64 Stikeleather L, Morrow W, Meyer R, *et al.* Evaluation of CO_2 application requirements for on-farm mass depopulation of swine in a disease emergency. *Agriculture* 2013; **3**(4): 599–612.

65 Cavanna AE, Shah S, Eddy CM, *et al.* Consciousness: a neurological perspective. *Behav Neurol* 2011; **24**(1): 107–116.

66 Reilly JS. *Euthanasia of Animals Used for Scientific Purposes.* Adelaide, SA: Australia and New Zealand Council for the Care of Animals in Research and Teaching, Department of Environmental Biology, Adelaide University, 2001.

67 Murray MJ. Euthanasia. In: Lewbart GA, ed. *Invertebrate Medicine.* Ames, IA: Blackwell Publishing, 2006: 303–304.

68 Messenger JB, Nixon M, Ryan KP. Magnesium chloride as an anaesthetic for cephalopods. *Comp Biochem Physiol C Comp Pharmacol Toxicol* 1985; **82**(1): 203–205.

69 Doerr M, Stoskopf MK. Evaluation of euthanasia of Moon Jellyfish (*Aurelia Aurita*) using simple salt solutions. *J Zoo Wildl Med* 2019; **50**(1): 123–126.

70 Wahltinez SJ, Kroll KJ, Nunamaker EA, *et al.* Practical euthanasia method for common sea stars (*Asterias rubens*) that allows for high-quality RNA sampling. *Animals* 2021; **11**(7): 1847.

71 Meyer RE, Morrow WEM. Euthanasia. In: Rollin BE, Benson GJ, eds. *Improving the Well-being of Farm Animals: Maximizing Welfare and Minimizing Pain and Suffering*. Ames, IA: Blackwell Publishing, 2004: 351–362.

72 Breazile JE, Kitchell RL. Euthanasia for laboratory animals. *Fed Proc* 1969; **28**(4): 1577–1579.

73 McMillan FD. Comfort as the primary goal in veterinary medical practice. *J Am Vet Med Assoc* 1998; **212**(9): 1370–1374.

74 Valentine H, Williams WO, Maurer KJ. Sedation or inhalant anesthesia before euthanasia with CO_2 does not reduce behavioral or physiologic signs of pain and stress in mice. *J Am Assoc Lab Anim Sci* 2012; **51**(1): 50–57.

75 Sharp J, Azar T, Lawson D. Comparison of carbon dioxide, argon, and nitrogen for inducing unconsciousness or euthanasia of rats. *J Am Assoc Lab Anim Sci* 2006; **45**(2): 21–25.

76 Barton-Gade P, Christensen L. Transportation and pre-stun handling: CO_2-systems. In: *Proceedings of the Veterinary Congress*, Helsinki, Finland, November 19-27th, 2002: 19–27.

77 Burkholder TH, Niel L, Weed JL, *et al.* Comparison of carbon dioxide and argon euthanasia: effects on behavior, heart rate, and respiratory lesions in rats. *J Am Assoc Lab Anim Sci* 2010; **49**(4): 448–453.

78 Herman JP, Cullinan WE. Neurocircuitry of stress: central control of the hypothalamo-pituitary-adrenocortical axis. *Trends Neurosci* 1997; **20**(2): 78–84.

79 Barklin A, Larsson A, Vestergaard C, *et al.* Does brain death induce a pro-inflammatory response at the organ level in a porcine model? *Acta Anaesthesiol Scand* 2008; **52**(5): 621–627.

80 Chiari P, Hadour G, Michel P, *et al.* Biphasic response after brain death induction: prominent part of catecholamines release in this phenomenon. *J Heart Lung Transplant* 2000; **19**(7): 675–682.

81 Licker M, Schweizer A, Hohn L, *et al.* Haemodynamic and metabolic changes induced by repeated episodes of hypoxia in pigs. *Acta Anaesthesiol Scand* 1998; **42**(8): 957–965.

82 Forslid A, Augustinsson O. Acidosis, hypoxia and stress hormone release in response to one minute inhalation of 80% CO_2 in swine. *Acta Physiol Scand* 1988; **132**(2): 222–231.

83 Borovsky V, Herman M, Dunphy G, *et al.* CO_2 asphyxia increases plasma norepinephrine in rats via sympathetic nerves. *Am J Physiol* 1998; **274**(1): R19–R22.

84 Reed B, Varon J, Chait BT, *et al.* Carbon dioxide-induced anesthesia results in a rapid increase in plasma levels of vasopressin. *Endocrinology* 2009; **150**(6): 2934–2939.

85 Kc P, Haxhiu MA, Trouth CO, *et al.* CO_2-induced c-Fos expression in hypothalamic vasopressin containing neurons. *Resp Physiol* 2002; **129**(3): 289–296.

86 Meyer RE, Whitley JT, Morrow WE, *et al.* Effect of physical and inhaled euthanasia methods on hormonal measures of stress in pigs. *J Swine Health Prod* 2013; **21**(5): 261–269.

87 Meyer RE. Physiologic measures of animal stress during transitional states of consciousness. *Animals* 2015; **5**(3): 702–716.

88 Mashour GA, Orser BA, Avidan MS. Intraoperative awareness – from neurobiology to clinical practice. *Anesthesiology* 2011; **114**(5): 1218–1233.

89 Hawkins P, Playle L, Golledge H, *et al.* Newcastle consensus meeting on carbon dioxide euthanasia of laboratory animals. *Anim Technol Welf* 2006; **5**(3): 125.

90 Crosby G, Culley D. Processed electroencephalogram and depth of anesthesia: window to nowhere or into the brain? *Anesthesiology* 2012; **116**(2): 235–237.

91 Hudetz AG, Vizuete JA, Imas OA. Desflurane selectively suppresses long latency cortical neuronal response to flash in the rat. *Anesthesiology* 2009; **111**(2): 231–239.

92 Imas OA, Ropella KM, Ward BD, *et al.* Volatile anesthetics enhance flash-induced gamma oscillations in rat visual cortex. *Anesthesiology* 2005; **102**(5): 937–947.

93 Barr G, Anderson RE, Jakobsson JG. A study of bispectral analysis and auditory evoked potential indices during propofol-induced hypnosis in volunteers: the effect of an episode of wakefulness on explicit and implicit memory. *Anaesthesia* 2001; **56**(9): 888–893.

94 Baudelet C, Gallez B. Effect of anesthesia on the signal intensity in tumors using BOLD-MRI: comparison with flow measurements by laser Doppler flowmetry and oxygen measurements by luminescence-based probes. *Magn Reson Imaging* 2004; **2297**: 905–912.

95 Steward CA, Marsden CA, Prior MJW, *et al.* Methodological considerations in rat brain BOLD contrast pharmacological MRI. *Psychopharmacology* 2005; **180**(4): 687–704.

96 Arluke A. Uneasiness among laboratory technicians. *Occup Med* 1999; **14**(2): 305–316.

97 Matthis JS. *Selected Employee Attributes and Perceptions Regarding Methods and Animal Welfare Concerns Associated with Swine Euthanasia*. Dissertation submitted to the Graduate Faculty of North Carolina State University in partial fulfillment of the requirements for the degree of Doctor of Education, Occupational Education, Raleigh, NC, 2004.

98 Chorney JM, Kain ZN. Behavioral analysis of children's response to induction of anesthesia. *Anesth Analg* 2009; **109**(5): 1434–1440.

99 Przybylo HJ, Tarbell SE, Stevenson GW. Mask fear in children presenting for anesthesia: aversion, phobia, or both? *Paediatr Anaesth* 2005; **15**(5): 366–370.

100 National Institutes of Health, Office of Laboratory Animal Welfare. Interagency Research Animal Committee. US Government Principles for the Utilization and Care of Vertebrate Animals Used in Testing, Research and Training, 2015. https://olaw.nih.gov/policies-laws/gov-principles.htm (accessed April 20, 2022).

101 Branson KR. Injectable and alternative anesthetic techniques. In: Tranquilli WJ, Thurmon JC, Grimm KA, eds. *Veterinary Anesthesia and Analgesia*, 4th edn. Ames, IA: Blackwell Publishing, 2007: 273–299.

102 Price HL. The pharmacodynamics of thiobarbiturates. In: Soma LR, ed. *Textbook of Veterinary Anesthesiology*. Baltimore, MD: Williams & Wilkins, 1971: 105–110.

103 Hall LW, Clarke KW. Anaesthesia of the dog. In: Hall LW, Clarke KW, eds. *Veterinary Anaesthesia*, 8th edn. London, UK: Baillière Tindall, 1983: 305–340.

104 Field KJ, While WJ, Lang CM. Anaesthetic effects of chloral hydrate, pentobarbitone and urethane in adult male rats. *Lab Anim* 1993; **27**(3): 258–269.

105 Haberham ZL, van den Brom WE, Venker-van Haagen AJ, *et al.* EEG evaluation of reflex testing as assessment of depth of pentobarbital anaesthesia in the rat. *Lab Anim* 1999; **33**(1): 47–57.

106 Grier RL, Schaffer CB. Evaluation of intraperitoneal and intrahepatic administration of a euthanasia agent in animal shelter cats. *J Am Vet Med Assoc* 1990; **197**(12): 1611–1615.

107 Svendsen O, Kok L, Lauritzen B. Nociception after intraperitoneal injection of a sodium pentobarbitone formulation with and without lidocaine in rats quantified by expression of neuronal c-Fos in the spinal cord – a preliminary study. *Lab Anim* 2007; **41**(2): 197–203.

108 Walker B, Jäggin N, Doherr M, *et al.* Inhalation anaesthesia for castration of newborn piglets: experiences with isoflurane and isoflurane/NO. *J Vet Med A Physiol Pathol Clin Med* 2004; **51**(3): 150–154.

109 Jäggin N, Kohler I, Blum J, *et al.* Die Kastration von neugeborenen Ferkeln unter Halothananästhesie. *Prakt Tierarzt* 2001; **8**(12): 1054–1061.

110 Flecknell PA, Roughan JV, Hedenqvist P. Induction of anaesthesia with sevoflurane and isoflurane in the rabbit. *Lab Anim* 1999; **33**(1): 41–46.

111 Leach MC, Bowell VA, Allan TF, *et al.* Measurement of aversion to determine humane methods of anaesthesia and euthanasia. *Anim Welf* 2004; **13**(S1): S77–S86.

112 Leach MC, Bowell VA, Allan TF, *et al.* Aversion to gaseous euthanasia agents in rats and mice. *Comp Med* 2002; **52**(3): 249–257.

113 Leach MC, Bowell VA, Allan TF, *et al.* Degrees of aversion shown by rats and mice to different concentrations of inhalational anaesthetics. *Vet Rec* 2002; **150**(26): 808–815.

114 Makowska LJ, Weary DM. Rat aversion to induction with inhaled anaesthetics. *Appl Anim Behav Sci* 2009; **119**(3–4): 229–235.

115 Makowska IJ, Weary DM. Rat aversion to carbon monoxide. *Appl Anim Behav Sci* 2009; **121**(2): 148–151.

116 Webster AB, Collett SR. A mobile modified-atmosphere killing system for small flock depopulation. *J Appl Poult Res* 2012; **21**(1): 131–144.

117 McKeegan DEF, Reimert HGM, Hindle VA, *et al.* Physiological and behavioral responses of poultry exposed to gas-filled high expansion foam. *Poult Sci* 2013; **92**(5): 1145–1154.

118 Lindahl C, Sindhøj E, Brattlund Hellgren R, *et al.* Responses of pigs to stunning with nitrogen filled high-expansion foam. *Animals* 2020; **10**(12): 2210.

119 Niel L, Weary DM. Behavioural responses of rats to gradual-fill carbon dioxide euthanasia and reduced oxygen concentrations. *Appl Anim Behav Sci* 2006; **100**(3–4): 295–308.

120 Hackbarth H, Kuppers N, Bohnet W. Euthanasia of rats with carbon dioxide – animal welfare aspects. *Lab Anim* 2000; **34**(1): 91–96.

121 Smith W, Harrap SB. Behavioural and cardiovascular responses of rats to euthanasia using carbon dioxide gas. *Lab Anim* 1997; **31**(4): 337–346.

122 Coenen AML, Drinkenburg W, Hoenderken R, *et al.* Carbon dioxide euthanasia in rats: oxygen supplementation minimizes signs of agitation and asphyxia. *Lab Anim* 1995; **29**(3): 262–268.

123 Blackshaw JK, Fenwick DC, Beattie AW, *et al.* The behavior of chickens, mice and rats during euthanasia with chloroform, carbon dioxide and ether. *Lab Anim* 1988; **22**(1): 67–75.

124 Britt DP. The humaneness of carbon dioxide as an agent of euthanasia for laboratory rodents. In: *Euthanasia of Unwanted, Injured or Diseased Animals or for Educational or Scientific Purposes. Proceedings of a Symposium Organized by Universities Federation for Animal Welfare in Association with Humane Slaughter Association, Zoological Society of London*, 19th September 1986. Potters Bar: Universities Federation for Animal Welfare, 1987: 19–31.

125 Hornett TD, Haynes AR. Comparison of carbon dioxide/air mixture and nitrogen/air mixture for the euthanasia of rodents. Design of a system for inhalation euthanasia. *Anim Technol* 1984; **35**: 93–99.

126 Jongman EC, Barnett JL, Hemsworth PH. The aversiveness of carbon dioxide stunning in pigs and a comparison of the CO_2 stunner crate vs. the V-restrainer. *Appl Anim Behav Sci* 2000; **67**(1–2): 67–76.

127 Raj ABM, Gregory NG. Welfare implications of the gas stunning of pigs 2. Stress of induction of anaesthesia. *Anim Welf* 1996; **5**(1): 71–78.

128 Troeger K, Woltersdorf W. Gas anesthesia of slaughter pigs. 1. Stunning experiments under laboratory conditions with fat pigs of known halothane reaction type – meat quality, animal protection. *Fleischwirtschaft* 1991; **71**(2): 1063–1068.

129 Dodman NH. Observations on use of Wernberg dip-lift carbon dioxide apparatus for pre-slaughter anesthesia of pigs. *Br Vet J* 1977; **133**(1): 71–80.

130 Gerritzen M, Lambooij B, Reimert H, *et al.* A note on behaviour of poultry exposed to increasing carbon dioxide concentrations. *Appl Anim Behav Sci* 2007; **108**(1–2): 179–185.

131 Gerritzen MS, Lambooij E, Reimert HG, *et al.* Susceptibility of duck and turkey to severe hypercapnic hypoxia. *Poult Sci* 2006; **85**(6): 1055–1061.

132 McKeegan DEF, McIntyre JA, Demmers TGM, *et al.* Physiological and behavioural responses of broilers to controlled atmosphere stunning: implications for welfare. *Anim Welf* 2007; **16**(4): 409–426.

133 McKeegan DEF, McIntyre J, Demmers TGM, *et al.* Behavioural responses of broiler chickens during acute exposure to gaseous stimulation. *Appl Anim Behav Sci* 2006; **99**(3–4): 271–286.

134 Webster AB, Fletcher DL. Reaction of laying hens and broilers to different gases used for stunning poultry. *Poult Sci* 2001; **80**(9): 1371–1377.

135 Webster AB, Fletcher DL. Assessment of the aversion of hens to different gas atmospheres using an approach-avoidance test. *Appl Anim Behav Sci* 2004; **88**(3–4): 275–287.

136 Abeyesinghe SM, McKeegan DEF, McLeman MA, *et al.* Controlled atmosphere stunning of broiler chickens. I. Effects on behaviour, physiology and meat quality in a pilot scale system at a processing plant. *Br Poult Sci* 2007; **48**(4): 406–423.

137 Gerritzen MA, Lambooij E, Hillebrand SJW, *et al.* Behavioral responses of broilers to different gaseous atmospheres. *Poult Sci* 2000; **79**(6): 928–933.

138 Lambooij E, Gerritzen MA, Engel B, *et al.* Behavioural responses during exposure of broiler chickens to different gas mixtures. *Appl Anim Behav Sci* 1999; **62**(2–3): 255–265.

139 Raj ABM. Aversive reactions of turkeys to argon, carbon dioxide and a mixture of carbon dioxide and argon. *Vet Rec* 1996; **138**(24): 592–593.

140 Sprenger RJ, Kim AB, Dzal YA, *et al.* Comparison of the CO_2 ventilatory response through development in three rodent species: effect of fossoriality. *Respir Physiol Neurobiol* 2019; **264**: 19–27.

141 Niel L, Weary DM. Rats avoid exposure to carbon dioxide and argon. *Appl Anim Behav Sci* 2007; **107**(1–2): 100–109.

142 Kirkden RD, Niel L, Stewart SA, *et al.* Gas killing of rats: the effect of supplemental oxygen on aversion to carbon dioxide. *Anim Welf* 2008; **17**(1): 79–87.

143 Cooper J, Mason G, Raj M. Determination of the aversion of farmed mink (*Mustela vison*) to carbon dioxide. *Vet Rec* 1998; **143**(13): 359–361.

144 Chen XJ, Gallar J, Pozo MA, *et al.* CO_2 stimulation of the cornea – a comparison between human sensation and nerve activity in polymodal nociceptive afferents of the cat. *Eur J Neurosci* 1995; **7**(6): 1154–1163.

145 Peppel P, Anton F. Responses of rat medullary dorsal horn neurons following intranasal noxious chemical stimulation – effects of stimulus intensity, duration and interstimulus interval. *J Neurophysiol* 1993; **70**(6): 2260–2275.

146 Thurauf N, Hummel T, Kettenmann B, *et al.* Nociceptive and reflexive responses recorded from the human nasal mucosa. *Brain Res* 1993; **629**(2): 293–299.

147 Anton F, Peppel P, Euchner I, *et al.* Noxious chemical stimulation – responses of rat trigeminal brain stem neurons to CO_2 pulses applied to the nasal mucosa. *Neurosci Lett* 1991; **123**(2): 208–211.

148 Feng YW, Simpson TL. Nociceptive sensation and sensitivity evoked from human cornea and conjunctiva stimulated by CO_2. *Invest Ophthalmol Vis Sci* 2003; **44**(2): 529–532.

149 Thurauf N, Gunther M, Pauli E, *et al.* Sensitivity of the negative mucosal potential to the trigeminal target stimulus CO_2. *Brain Res* 2002; **942**(1–2): 79–86.

150 Danneman PJ, Stein S, Walshaw SO. Humane and practical implications of using carbon dioxide mixed with oxygen for anesthesia or euthanasia of rats. *Lab Anim Sci* 1997; **47**(4): 376–385.

151 Hewett TA, Kovacs MS, Artwohl JE, *et al.* A comparison of euthanasia methods in rats, using carbon dioxide in prefilled and fixed flow-rate filled chambers. *Lab Anim Sci* 1993; **43**(6): 579–582.

152 Battaglia M, Ogliari A, Harris J, *et al.* A genetic study of the acute anxious response to carbon dioxide stimulation in man. *J Psychiatr Res* 2007; **41**(11): 906–917.

153 Nardi AE, Freire RC, Zin WA. Panic disorder and control of breathing. *Respir Physiol Neurobiol* 2009; **167**(1): 133–143.

154 Grandin T, Cockram M, eds. *The Slaughter of Farmed Animals: Practical Ways of Enhancing Animal Welfare*. Boston, MA: CABI, 2020: 226–239.

155 Jongman EC, Woodhouse R, Rice M, *et al.* Pre-slaughter factors linked to variation in responses to carbon dioxide gas stunning in pig abattoirs. *Animal* 2021; **15**(2): 100134.

156 Ziemann AE, Allen JE, Dahdaleh NS, *et al.* The amygdala is a chemosensor that detects carbon dioxide and acidosis to elicit fear behavior. *Cell* 2009; **139**(5): 1012–1021.

157 Dalmau A, Llonch P, Rodriguez P, *et al.* Stunning pigs with different gas mixtures: gas stability. *Anim Welf* 2010; **19**(3): 315–323.

158 Baker BA, Hickman DL. Bias in rating of rodent distress during anesthesia induction for anesthesia compared with euthanasia. *J Am Assoc Lab Anim Sci* 2018; **57**(2): 143–156.

159 Wong D, Makowska IJ, Weary DM. Rat aversion to isoflurane versus carbon dioxide. *Biol Lett* 2013; **9**(1): 20121000.

160 Frost K, Shah M, Leung VSY, *et al.* Aversion to desflurane and isoflurane in Sprague–Dawley rats (*Rattus Norvegicus*). *Animals* 2020; **10**(6): 950.

161 Guedes SR, Valentim AM, Antunes LM. Mice aversion to sevoflurane, isoflurane and carbon dioxide using an approach-avoidance task. *Appl Anim Behav Sci* 2017; **189**: 91–97.

162 Kulkarni S, Hickman D. Isoflurane and carbon dioxide elicit similar behavioral responses in rats. *Animals* 2020; **10**(8): 1431.

163 Rodriguez-Sanchez R, Barnaby E, Améndola L, *et al.* Voluntary oral ingestion of a sedative prior to euthanasia with CO_2: behavioural responses of mice. *Animals* 2021; **11**(10): 2879.

164 Lockwood G. Theoretical context-sensitive elimination times for inhalational anaesthetics. *Br J Anaesth* 2010; **104**(5): 648–655.

165 Mellor DJ, Diesch TJ. Onset of sentience: the potential for suffering in fetal and newborn farm animals. *Appl Anim Behav Sci* 2006; **100**(1–2): 48–57.

166 Mellor DJ. Galloping colts, fetal feelings, and reassuring regulations: putting animal-welfare science into practice. *J Vet Med Educ* 2010; **37**(1): 94–100.

167 Mellor DJ, Diesch TJ, Johnson CB. Should mammalian fetuses be excluded from regulations protecting animals during experiments? *Proceedings of the 7th World Congress on Alternatives and Animal Use in the Life Sciences*, 2009. *ALTEX* 2010; **27**(Special Issue): 199–202.

168 Mellor DJ, Diesch TJ, Johnson CB. When do mammalian young become sentient? *Proceedings of the 7th World Congress on Alternatives and Animal Use in the Life Sciences*, 2009. *ALTEX* 2010; **27**(Special Issue): 275–280.

169 White SC. Prevention of fetal suffering during ovariohysterectomy of pregnant animals. *J Am Vet Med Assoc* 2012; **240**(10): 1160–1163.

170 Mellor DJ, Diesch TJ. Birth and hatching: key events in the onset of awareness in the lamb and chick. *N Z Vet J* 2007; **55**(5): 51–60.

171 Purswell JL, Thaxton JP, Branton SL. Identifying process variables for a low atmospheric pressure stunning–killing system. *J Appl Poult Res* 2007; **16**(4): 509–513.

172 Vizzier-Thaxton Y, Christensen KD, Schilling MW, *et al.* A new humane method of stunning broilers using low atmospheric pressure. *J Appl Poult Res* 2010; **19**(4): 341–348.

173 More S, Bicout D, Bøtner A, *et al.* Low atmospheric pressure system for stunning broiler chickens. *EFSA J* 2017; **15**(12): e05056.

174 Booth NH. Effect of rapid decompression and associated hypoxic phenomena in euthanasia of animals: a review. *J Am Vet Med Assoc* 1978; **173**(3): 308–314.

175 Fedde MR. Relationship of structure and function of the avian respiratory system to disease susceptibility. *Poult Sci* 1998; **77**(8): 1130–1138.

176 Coenen AML, Lankhaar J, Lowe JC, *et al.* Remote monitoring of electroencephalogram, electrocardiogram, and behavior during controlled atmosphere stunning in broilers: implications for welfare. *Poult Sci* 2009; **88**(1): 10–19.

177 McKeegan DE, Sandercock DA, Gerritzen MA. Physiological responses to low atmospheric pressure stunning and the implications for welfare. *Poult Sci* 2013; **92**(4): 858–868.

178 Wang X, Zhao D, Milby AC, *et al.* Evaluation of euthanasia methods on behavioral and physiological responses of newly hatched male layer chicks. *Animals* 2021; **11**(6): 1802.

179 Gurung S, White D, Archer G, *et al.* Evaluation of alternative euthanasia methods of neonatal chickens. *Animals* 2018; **8**(3): 37.

180 Bouwsema JA, Lines JA. Could low atmospheric pressure stunning (LAPS) be suitable for pig slaughter? A review of available information. *Anim Welf* 2019; **28**(4): 421–432.

181 Clarkson JM, McKeegan DEF, Sparrey J, *et al.* Determining candidate hypobaric hypoxia profiles for humane killing of laboratory mice. *Front Vet Sci* 2022; **9**: 834478.

182 McKeegan DEF, Martin J, Baxter EM. LAPS in pigs is not a humane alternative to stunning with carbon dioxide. *Meat Hyg* 2020; **180**: 20–22.

183 Benson E, Malone GW, Alphin RL, *et al.* Foam-based mass emergency depopulation of floor-reared meat-type poultry operations. *Poult Sci* 2007; **86**(2): 219–224.

184 Malone B, Benson E, Alphin B, *et al.* Methods of mass depopulation for poultry flocks with highly infectious disease. In: *Proceedings to ANECA Symposium on Emerging Diseases*, Queretaro, Mexico, November 2007.

185 Alphin RL, Rankin MK, Johnson KJ, *et al.* Comparison of water-based foam and inert-gas mass emergency depopulation methods. *Avian Dis* 2010; **54**(1 suppl): 757–762.

186 Benson ER, Alphin RL, Dawson MD, *et al.* Use of water-based foam to depopulate ducks and other species. *Poult Sci* 2009; **88**(5): 904–910.

187 Raj ABM, Smith C, Hickman G. Novel method for killing poultry in houses with dry foam created using nitrogen. *Vet Rec* 2008; **162**(22): 722–723.

188 Gerritzen MA, Reimert HGM, Hindle VA, *et al.* Welfare Assessment of Gas-Filled Foam as an Agent for Killing Poultry, Wageningen UR Livestock Research Report 399, 2010. www.library.wur.nl/WebQuery/wurpubs/403154 (accessed June 6, 2022).

189 McKeegan DEF, Reimert HGM, Hindle VA, *et al.* Physiological and behavioral responses of poultry exposed to gas-filled high expansion foam. *Poult Sci* 2013; **92**(5): 1145–1154.

190 Lorbach JN, Campler MR, Youngblood B, *et al.* Comparison of gaseous and water-based medium-expansion foam depopulation methods in cull sows. *Animals* 2021; (**11**): 3179.

191 National Institutes of Health, Office of Laboratory Animal Welfare. Frequently Asked Questions (FAQs): PHS Policy on Humane Care and Use of Laboratory Animals. https://olaw.nih.gov/faqs#/guidance/faqs?anchor=question50361 (accessed June 2022).

192 National Institutes of Health, Office of Laboratory Animal Welfare. Regulatory Considerations for Using Pharmaceutical Products in Research Involving Laboratory Animals. https://olaw.nih.gov/education/educational-resources/webinar-2015-06-04.htm (accessed June 2022).

193 General Services Administration. Metric BB-C-101D, Federal Specification Carbon Dioxide (CO_2): Technical and USP. www.everyspec.com/FED_SPECS/B/BB-C-101D_31791/(accessed April 2022).

194 Linde. VERISEQ® Pharmaceutical Grade Gases. Carbon Dioxide, 2022. http://hiq.linde-gas.com/en/images/VERISEQ_CarbonDioxide_tcm899-92234.pdf (accessed April 2022).

195 Sánchez Fernández I, Goodkin HP, Scott RC. Pathophysiology of convulsive status epilepticus. *Seizure* 2019; **68**: 16–21.

196 Kaiser AM, McFarland W, Siemion RS, *et al.* Secondary pentobarbital poisoning in two dogs: a cautionary tale. *J Vet Diagn Invest* 2010; **22**(4): 632–634.

197 Kelly TR, Johnson CK. Lead exposure in free-flying turkey vultures is associated with big game hunting in California. *PLoS ONE* 2011; **6**(4): e15350.

198 Payne J, Farris R, Parker G, *et al.* Quantification of sodium pentobarbital residues from equine mortality compost piles. *J Anim Sci* 2015; **93**(4): 1824–1829.

199 Zolhavarieh SM, Nourian AR, Sadeghi-nasab A. A new method for on-farm euthanasia with animal welfare considerations. *Iran J Vet Surg* 2011; **6**(12): 55–64.

200 Aleman M, Davis E, Williams DC, *et al.* Electrophysiologic study of a method of euthanasia using intrathecal lidocaine hydrochloride administered during intravenous anesthesia in horses. *J Vet Intern Med* 2015; **29**(6): 1676–1682.

201 Aleman M, Davis E, Knych H, *et al.* Drug residues after intravenous anesthesia and intrathecal lidocaine hydrochloride euthanasia in horses. *J Vet Intern Med* 2016; **30**(4): 1322–1326.

202 Cooney K, Titcombe L. Lessons and recommendations from a pentobarbital shortage: US and Canada 2021. *Animals* 2022; **12**(3): 365.

203 Conserving Pentobarbital in Times of Shortage. An Option to Consider for Small Companion Animals. American Veterinary Medical Association, 2021. www.avma.org/blog/conserving-pentobarbital-times-shortage (accessed April 2022).

SECTION 2

Patient Monitoring

9 Biomedical Engineering

Catherine M. Creighton[1] and Nadja Johnson Bressan[2]

[1]Department of Companion Animals, Atlantic Veterinary College, University of Prince Edward Island, Charlottetown, Prince Edward Island, Canada

[2]Faculty of Sustainable Design Engineering, University of Prince Edward Island, Charlottetown, Prince Edward Island, Canada

Chapter contents

Introduction, 169
History of biomedical engineering, 169
Subdisciplines of biomedical engineering, 170
Biomedical instrumentation systems, 170
Biomedical data, 171
Biomedical data and time series analysis, 171
Biomedical engineering milestones in anesthesia, 172
Stethoscopes, 172
Endotracheal tubes, laryngoscopes, and inhalant anesthetic delivery, 172
Anesthetic conserving device, 172
Pulse oximetry, 172
Evolution of monitoring equipment and guidelines, 173
Contemporary biomedical engineering applications in anesthesia, 173
Drug delivery systems, 173
Ultrasound-guided nerve blocks, 173
Models and simulators in anesthesia, 174
Biomedical engineering in veterinary medicine, 174
References, 174

Introduction

Collaboration between veterinarians and biomedical engineers is becoming increasingly common and serves to advance the field of veterinary medicine in general, and veterinary anesthesiology in particular. Veterinarians and biomedical engineers have similar scientific knowledge, and their skill sets tend to complement each other. This chapter provides a brief introduction to the discipline of biomedical engineering and highlights ways in which biomedical engineers have contributed to and continue to facilitate progress in veterinary anesthesia.

History of biomedical engineering

Biomedical engineering is a specialized field that applies engineering and physics theories to improve human health by producing tools, devices, and processes [1]. The field of biomedical engineering is not new; in fact, the first mention of a biomedical device in the historical record appears in 950 BC. The Greville Chester toe, a prosthetic big toe made of wood and leather, was found in a mummy in Egypt in 1800 [2]. The development of the field of biomedical engineering intensified between World War I and II when researchers across the globe started experimenting with biophysics and biomedical applications. The Oswalt Institute for Physics in Medicine in Frankfurt, Germany, was the first laboratory to offer formal training in biomedical engineering in 1921. The first North American biomedical engineering program, the Drexel-Presbyterian Hospital Program at the University of Pennsylvania, was established in 1959 as a master's degree for engineers to obtain knowledge of medical science and for life scientists to gain knowledge of physical science [3–5].

A number of scientists have played key roles in laying the foundation of what would later become biomedical engineering. One of these was Luigi Galvani, an Italian physician and physicist in the 18th century [6]. At that time, Galvani practiced surgery and became interested in the therapeutic application of electricity, known as "medical electricity." This field of research explored the effects of electricity on the human body and the use of electricity for treating diseases. Galvani's experiments with dead frog limbs that were exposed and connected to metal wires inserted across the vertebral canal tested the hypothesis that body movements were generated and controlled by a particular type of force. Galvani named this force "animal electricity." He hypothesized that the brain secreted "a fluid" flowing through the nerves, stimulating the muscle fibers [7]. Galvani's experiments laid the groundwork for the field of electrophysiology and formed the foundation for electromagnetic treatments currently used in medicine.

In the 19th century, a Dutch engineer named Alexander Muirhead connected a Thomson siphon recorder (designed to record transatlantic signals) to a patient's wrist and, for the first time, recorded cardiac electrical activity at St. Bartholomew's Hospital in London. The idea of converting an electrical signal into variations of a physical quantity was the fundamental principle utilized by Willem Einthoven in 1903 when he invented the electrocardiogram. Einthoven measured the electrical variance between leads to draw a projection of the heart dipole potential [8,9].

Veterinary Anesthesia and Analgesia: The Sixth Edition of Lumb and Jones. Edited by Leigh Lamont, Kurt Grimm, Sheilah Robertson, Lydia Love and Carrie Schroeder.
© 2024 John Wiley & Sons, Inc. Published 2024 by John Wiley & Sons, Inc.
Companion website: www.wiley.com/go/lamont/anesthesia

The interdisciplinary nature of biomedical engineering is the signature of this scientific field that merges concepts, theories, and methods of engineering, physics, and biological science to solve challenges in human medicine. Shortly after World War II, this novel field brought together physicians, biologists, physicists, and engineers with common interests to share knowledge and ideas. This organization evolved over time and was formalized as the Engineering in Medicine and Biology Society (EMBS), which is now the world's largest international society of biomedical engineers.

Subdisciplines of biomedical engineering

This cooperation between engineering and medical disciplines to develop knowledge, interventions, procedures, processes, and technologies has resulted in the creation of a wide range of subdisciplines within biomedical engineering including the following:

Bioinformatics utilizes computational methods and resources to develop methods to understand biological data, and acquire, store, analyze, and disseminate biological knowledge. The process of analyzing and interpreting biological data is referred to as "computational biology" [10].

Bioinstrumentation employs electronics, computer sciences, and physics to develop devices and tools to measure, evaluate, and treat biological systems [11].

Biomechanics applies principles of physics and mechanics to biological systems to understand the forces impacting system functionality within their environments [12]. A clinical example of this subdiscipline is the biomechanical analysis of the aorta for the estimation of vascular pathologies [13].

Biomechatronics uses principles of mechatronics engineering, namely the synergistic combination of electronics, mechanics, control systems, and informatics to interact, enhance, or apply to human biology [14]. The pacemaker is an example of electronics, mechanics, and control applied to the human body.

Biomimetics utilizes the principles of nature and natural behaviors to design and apply concepts that may benefit science, engineering, and medicine [15]. Swarm robotics is an example of this discipline that is based on the behavior of flocks of birds or schools of fish applied to robots to solve challenges in agriculture, defense, construction, or environmental monitoring [16].

Bionanotechnology employs near-atomic scale technology to produce new structures, materials, and devices relevant to medical or biological challenges. Bionanotechnology has been used for drug delivery for the past 30 years, revolutionizing fabrication and manufacturing, and improving efficiency and therapeutics [17].

Clinical engineering utilizes medical technology to optimize healthcare delivery [18].

Bioprocess applies chemical and biological principles to design and develop equipment and processes for manufacturing [19]. A novel bioprocess application is space bioprocess engineering, which creates and manages biologically driven technologies that support human life during space missions [20].

Neuroengineering utilizes engineering techniques to understand, repair, replace, or enhance neural systems [21]. An example of this discipline is deep brain stimulation (DBS), which is the application of a pacemaker that stimulates areas of the brain to treat different conditions ranging from Parkinson's disease to severe depression [22].

Rehabilitation engineering uses engineering principles to design and develop technological solutions to assist individuals with disabilities and aid the recovery of physical and cognitive functions lost due to injury or disease [23]. An example of this is electromyographical-based adaptive assist-as-needed controllers for patients who are recovering after a stroke [24].

Tissue engineering uses engineering, material, and biochemical methods to restore, maintain, improve, or replace different types of biological tissues [25].

Biomedical instrumentation systems

Historically, the development of sensors and devices was the origin of the collaboration between engineering and medicine, with the invention of sensors, transducers, devices, machines, and systems. The main challenge originally faced by scientists was to understand the biomedical data acquired by their instruments. Due to the complexity of biomedical data, sensors and transducers used in medical fields are not used as stand-alone components, as they would be in industry. To solve this challenge, biomedical sensors, and transducers were incorporated into instrumentation systems to accomplish the goal of measuring the target signal. An *instrumentation system* was defined by Eren and Fung as a "collection of instruments used to measure, monitor, and control a process" [26] (Fig. 9.1).

A biomedical instrumentation system (BIS) (Fig. 9.2) introduces additional components that a traditional instrumentation system does not have, such as "calibration." Calibration is a component that adjusts all the other system components according to the patient, environmental conditions, and health status, thereby establishing a certain linearity between output and input. A fundamental component of a BIS is the control or feedback component, collecting physiological data and stimulating a response from the "measurand." An example of biofeedback would be a ventilator that fires to replicate a particular respiratory pattern in response to readings of pulse oximetry and end-tidal carbon dioxide. Another important component of a BIS is the "bioelectric amplifier." Due to the small amplitudes and low frequencies of biological signals (in the order of mV to μV and mA to nA), any bioelectric potential to be measured and recorded in the body must be amplified. Bioelectrical amplifiers increase the physiological or neural electrical signal from its source to a greater output signal to be sampled by diverse sources [27].

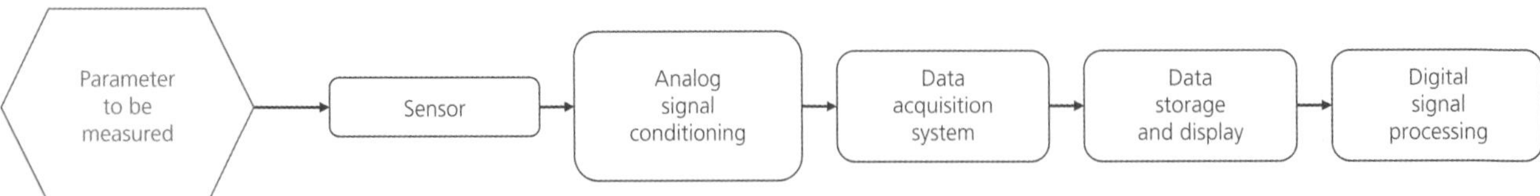

Figure 9.1 Basic components of an instrumentation system in engineering.

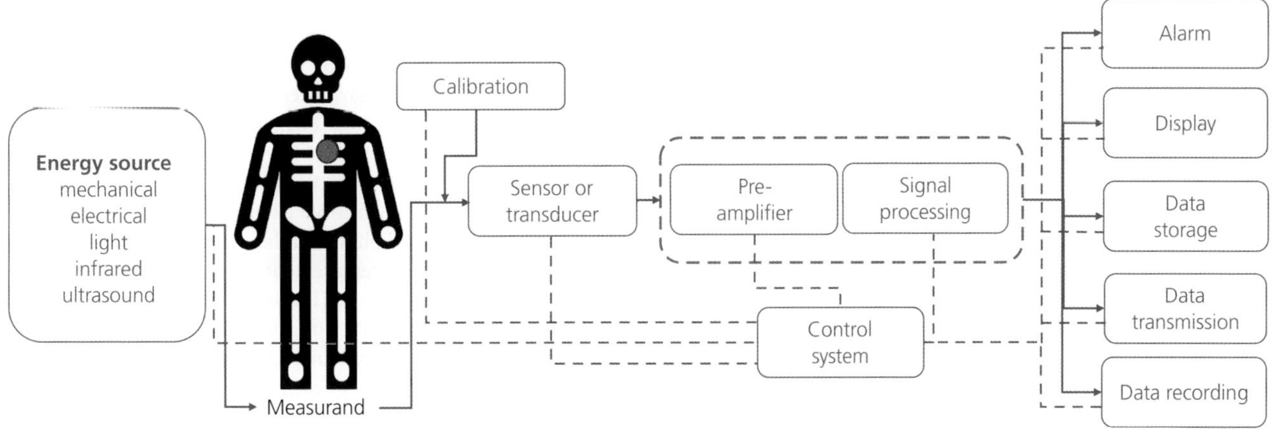

Figure 9.2 Diagrammatic representation of a biomedical instrumentation system (BIS). Biomedical instrumentation systems are more complex and introduce additional components including (1) calibration to adjust other system components according to patient and environmental factors; (2) a control or feedback system to collect physiologic data and stimulate a response from the patient ("measurand"); and (3) bioelectric amplification to increase the signal from its source to produce a greater output.

Biomedical data

After collecting data through a BIS, the next logical step is to clean and structure the data before analysis. An implicit step that is often overlooked, however, involves assessing and understanding the structure and behavior of the data. This step is fundamental if the data set is to be correctly analyzed and generate useful information.

Some biological data present linear behavior, with a constant rate of change, such as the amount of guanine and cytosine in each DNA molecule [28]. Most physiological and neurological data, on the other hand, present complex nonlinear dynamic systems behavior. Nonlinear systems are characterized by the relationship between variables where the increment change in one variable reflects a nonproportional change in another variable, while the complexity of the system can be explained as the concomitant interaction among several variables within the system. Examples of complex nonlinear dynamic systems include heart rate variability, the electrocardiogram, the electroencephalogram, and pulmonary oxygen uptake dynamics.

Quantifying this behavior in physiological, neurological, and pathological data has been used for detection, diagnosis, treatment, and proactive monitoring with the goal of improving treatment and patient outcomes [29]. Another characteristic of this type of data is its structure; because biomedical data is collected over time it is characterized as a "time series." In contrast to discrete data points, a time series is a collection of points over time, with underlying behavior and patterns. The challenges in analyzing this data reside in the presence of noise, quantization of effects, the lengths of the available "good" data, tuning or calibration parameters, and health status [30].

Biomedical data and time series analysis

To analyze a time series biomedical data set, specialized algorithms have been developed that enable measurement of the complexity of the time series through automation of parameters, machine learning techniques, and artificial intelligence methods. Before deciding on the analysis methodology, one must understand what patterns to explore, and this requires an understanding of the four main components of a time series [31]:

1 *Trend* – shows the tendency of the data to increase or decrease. "Trend" refers to the average, long-term, and smooth tendency of the data. A time series over several hours can present different trends at different periods.
2 *Seasonal* – the data variation due to predetermined patterns.
3 *Cyclical* – the repetitive movement of the data over time defining the seasonal patterns.
4 *Irregular* – the movement of the data that cannot be explained by cyclical movements. Often it presents different sampling rates between sequences. This component provides information on non-seasonal patterns.

Identifying the components of the data set supports design of the algorithm to analyze the data; knowing if the data is stationary or non-stationary guides the scientist to determine what method to use to measure its performance, accuracy, and precision. A stationary time series is characterized by a constant mean and variance, while a non-stationary time series presents statistical properties depending on time.

Once the physiological, neurological, and pathological data has been reviewed and characterized based on time series and complexity, then analysis methodology can be explored such as autoregressive integrated moving average (ARIMA) models, seasonal autoregressive integrated moving average (SARIMA) models, vector autoregression (VAR) models, and beyond. Choosing the method to analyze the biomedical time series is intrinsically related to the type of signal (physiological, neurological, and pathological), its energy source (electrical, mechanical, frequency, image, and sound), and the period to be considered.

Using the right metrics to evaluate the performance, accuracy, and precision of the model is as relevant as the method used to analyze the time series. However, just like the methodology for time series analysis, there are numerous choices to measure the performance of the data. Several of the most common performance measures utilized by biomedical engineers are presented below:

1 *R-Squared* – compares the stationary part of the model to a simple mean model. A high value of R^2 suggests that the model's variance is similar to the true values, and a low R^2 suggests the values are not related. Defined by:

$$R^2 = 1 - \frac{SS_{\text{res}}}{SS_{\text{tot}}}$$

2 *Mean Absolute Error (MAE)* – represents the average of the absolute difference between estimated and true values. The lower the

MAE value, the better the model; a value of zero indicates that the forecast is error-free. Defined by:

$$MAE = \frac{\Sigma_{i=1}^{n} |y_i - x_i|}{n}$$

3 *Mean Absolute Percentage Error (MAPE)* – represents the proportion of the average absolute difference between projected and true values divided by the true value. Like MAE, the lower the value, the better the model. Defined by:

$$MAPE = \frac{100}{n} \Sigma_{t=1}^{n} \left| \frac{A_t - F_t}{A_t} \right|$$

4 *Mean Squared Error (MSE)* – represents the average of the error squares. This measure penalizes large errors or outliers more than minor errors due to the square term. The closer MSE is to zero, the better. Defined by:

$$MSE = \frac{1}{n} \Sigma_{i=1}^{n} \left(Y_i - \hat{Y}_i\right)^2$$

5 *Root Mean Squared Error (RMSE)* – represents the square root of mean square error. This is an extension of MSE. This statistic is likewise always positive, with lower values indicating higher performance. Defined by:

$$RMSE = \sqrt{\frac{1}{n} \Sigma_{i=1}^{n} \left(Y_i - \hat{Y}_i\right)^2}$$

Understanding the biomedical data collected, structuring it in time series, and modeling and analyzing the performance enables the researcher to successfully implement evidence-based practices. However, it is vital that future predictions prioritize the contextualization in which the data is immersed and quantify the impact of this context in signal analyses.

Biomedical engineering milestones in anesthesia

The word "anesthesia" has been used since ancient Greek times, appearing in the Hippocratic collection of medical texts to describe a loss of consciousness and sensation [32]. Pain is also well described throughout ancient and modern historical texts and was generally accepted as a necessary component of disease or injury treatment. Following the first public demonstration of the use of ether vapor to relieve surgical pain in 1846 [33,34], the use of ether and chloroform spread rapidly as did reports of anesthetic deaths and questions of safety. In 1848, a 15-year-old girl suffered cardiac arrest during chloroform anesthesia for removal of a toenail [35], tragically highlighting the potential risks associated with anesthesia. Advances in asepsis along with the discovery of new drugs and techniques spearheaded rapid expansion in the fields of anesthesia and analgesia, an increased appreciation of patient safety (discussed further in Chapter 3), and the development of new equipment and monitoring techniques. Biomedical engineering has played a crucial role in fostering anesthesia safety culture and the following section highlights a few selected examples of important milestones.

Stethoscopes

Development of anesthesia-related equipment is usually driven by a need to better obtain accurate patient information. Breath sounds were initially auscultated simply by placing an ear on the person's thorax, until it was discovered in 1816 that a rolled piece of paper placed on the chest wall resulted in much clearer, more audible breath and heart sounds [36]. The first binaural stethoscope was invented in 1851, and today many variations exist. Recent advances in stethoscope technology have been made through collaboration of physicians with biomedical engineers; in 1999, Dr. Richard Deslauriers from the University of Toronto worked with engineers from the Bose Corporation to design and produce a recording stethoscope capable of blocking out external sounds. More recently, biomedical engineers and physicians have been designing and testing a possible stethoscope replacement: a foam pad that can simultaneously auscultate 14 chest wall locations with very good accuracy, being able to identify specific lung sounds such as crackles and high- or low-pitched wheezes. In 2022, a paper was published in The Lancet, describing a deep learning system applied to single-lead ECGs obtained using an ECG-enabled stethoscope [37]. This work would not have been possible without collaboration between physicians and biomedical engineers.

Endotracheal tubes, laryngoscopes, and inhalant anesthetic delivery

The use of endotracheal tubes began not long after the introduction of ether and chloroform as inhaled anesthetics [34]. The use of endotracheal tubes prompted the development of a handheld laryngoscope. Equipment designed to deliver inhalant anesthetics and remove carbon dioxide followed. This necessitated supplementation with additional gases such as air, oxygen, or nitrous oxide [38]. These gases required compression, storage, and transport, which needed to be cost-effective and safe, stimulating the development of new technologies. Between 1939 and 1960, John Henry Blease, an English engineer by trade without formal training, collaborated with anesthetists to improve anesthetic machines, eventually receiving 19 patents for his work [39]. This collaborative work added manifold technology, valves, temperature compensation, one-way valves, and an oxygen flowmeter to anesthetic machines, while also enabling carbon dioxide absorption. Their anesthetic machine, called the "all-purpose Alfo-Blease," was commercially available by 1944. In 1945, Blease designed a pulmonary ventilator which his anesthetist collaborators successfully tested on patients. One anesthetist recorded pneumographs to show that Blease's ventilator could produce a respiratory pattern very similar to spontaneous respiration, while patients were anesthetized with cyclopropane.

Anesthetic conserving device

More recently, physicians and biomedical engineers worked together to design the anesthetic conserving device (AnaConDa®, Sedana Medical, Danderyd, Sweden) to deliver isoflurane or sevoflurane using any non-rebreathing mechanical ventilator [40]. As of 2017, over 2,300,000 AnaConDa's have been used in hospitals, mostly to sedate mechanically ventilated patients in intensive care units. The device replaces the heat and moisture exchanger of the ventilator circuit, fitting between the Y-piece and the endotracheal tube. The AnaConDa reduces drug use and sedation costs by allowing reuse of 90% of administered drugs while also humidifying the fresh gas flow provided to the patient.

Pulse oximetry

The use of pulse oximetry is vital to ensure the safety of sedated and anesthetized patients. Oximetry, the measurement of oxygen saturation, can be traced back to Johann Lambert who, in 1760, formulated the law stating that absorbance of a material sample is directly proportional to its thickness [41]. A polymath who was interested in mathematics, physics, philosophy, astronomy, and map projections, Lambert might very well have been a biomedical engineer today. A Japanese bioengineer named Takuo Aoyagi was an integral part of the development of the first commercial pulse oximeter in 1974. Aoyagi realized that the pulsatile nature of blood flow through tissues could allow oxygen saturation to be measured. The Nellcor Company was founded in 1981 by an anesthesiologist and two engineers. In 1983, they introduced the Nellcor N-100 at the American Society of Anesthesiology (ASA) annual meeting and in a publication in the journal Anesthesiology describing the reliability of pulse oximetry. Pulse oximeters became so widely used that the ASA adopted pulse oximetry as a monitoring standard in 1986. A review paper published in 1989 evaluating closed malpractice claims found that when pulse oximetry and capnometry were used together, 93% of preventable anesthetic mishaps may have been averted [42].

Evolution of monitoring equipment and guidelines

As the use of anesthesia and sedation became more widespread and was performed on higher-risk patients, monitoring became more important to ensure patient safety. Minimum technical standards for monitoring anesthetized or sedated human patients were established by the ASA in 1985 and are periodically updated [43–45]. These guidelines include recommendations for supervision by an anesthetist during sedation or anesthesia, specific monitoring required for sedation, anesthesia, and transport of patients, the use of an anesthetic record with integration into the hospital's electronic health record system, and availability of additional equipment as needed. Minimum monitoring required in all cases includes pulse oximetry (SpO_2) with plethysmography, non-invasive blood pressure (NIBP), electrocardiography (ECG), and temperature [44]. If anesthesia is induced, monitoring of inspired and expired oxygen as well as waveform capnography is added. Other monitoring, such as inspired and end-tidal inhalant concentration, spirometry, neuromuscular activity, and processed electroencephalography (EEG) are recommended depending on circumstances. In veterinary anesthesia, similar guidelines exist for monitoring dogs, cats, and horses during anesthesia, and updates are published periodically [46,47]. The most recent recommendations for monitoring dogs and cats include the use of human senses to monitor the cardiorespiratory systems, as well as the use of SpO_2, end-tidal carbon dioxide ($P_{ET}CO_2$), NIBP, ECG, and body temperature. Monitoring guidelines for horses during inhalant anesthesia are similar, with the additional recommendations of invasive blood pressure monitoring and periodic analysis of arterial blood gases.

In human medicine, the institution of these guidelines and the resulting advancements in the field of anesthesia patient monitoring are partly responsible for a reduction of anesthesia-related mortality from 1 in 3000 in 1985 to 1 in 300,000 in 1996 [43]. As of 2021, anesthesia-related mortality in human ASA I and II patients is so low that it has not been quantified, but is estimated to be 1 in 400,000 or less. In veterinary medicine, large-scale studies are challenging, and retrospective studies determining overall mortality rates in healthy and ill populations are infrequent. Despite the considerable advances in anesthetic monitoring and the establishment of monitoring guidelines, it is not immediately apparent that anesthesia-related mortality rates have decreased significantly in dogs, cats, and horses. Current overall mortality rates in these species are 0.17%, 0.24%, and 1.1%, respectively [48–50]. It seems that as comprehensive perianesthetic monitoring of patients continues to advance through improved monitoring equipment and training of personnel, overall mortality rates in veterinary medicine should decline as they have in human medicine. Much of the monitoring equipment used in veterinary medicine is human-specific and has been adapted for veterinary use. Biomedical engineers are the logical resource for veterinarians to collaborate with to design and manufacture purpose-built, economically viable equipment for veterinary medicine, with the goal of improving anesthetic safety.

Commonly used monitoring equipment is typically user-friendly and designed to be used by healthcare workers who do not have specialized training in engineering. In human medicine, anesthetists are accustomed to recognizing a gap in their ability to monitor a specific body system or identifying a piece of anesthesia equipment that is lacking, and asking how this can be rectified. Veterinary anesthetists, on the other hand, are more often reaching out to their biomedical engineer colleagues to help design and test equipment with a specific veterinary purpose or application.

Contemporary biomedical engineering applications in anesthesia

A thorough review of contemporary biomedical engineering applications in clinical anesthesia is beyond the scope of this chapter. The following are just a few select examples with relevance to both human and veterinary anesthesia.

Drug delivery systems

Intravenous drugs have historically been administered as a bolus using a handheld syringe and needle or by constant rate infusion using a syringe pump. Target-controlled infusions (TCI) provide automatic adjustments to the infusion rate to maintain a specific plasma concentration of drug [51,52]. When using a TCI device, the clinician enters a desired target concentration, and the computer calculates the amount of drug required to achieve the programmed concentration and directs the syringe pump to administer the calculated boluses and infusion rates. TCI systems consist of a syringe pump connected to a computer that has been programmed with a model of the specific drug's pharmacokinetics as well as the patient's characteristics. This programming allows the computer to calculate tissue drug concentrations almost continuously and determine the required infusion rates to achieve the desired target concentration. The clinician can rapidly change the desired target concentration, as dictated by the clinical situation. Many anesthetists are not adept at computer programming and modeling, whereas most biomedical engineers are. This represents another example of the potential for members of these two specialties to work together to improve the delivery of anesthesia in the perioperative period.

Ultrasound-guided nerve blocks

Multimodal analgesia is achieved by using combinations of analgesic drugs to target multiple nociceptive receptors and transmission pathways and provides superior analgesia while reducing the incidence of side effects [53]. Regional anesthesia is often a component of multimodal analgesia. For regional anesthesia to be effective, local anesthetic drug must be deposited near the target nerve. Nerves may be located by palpation of landmarks and blind needle insertion, use of an electrical nerve stimulator, use of ultrasound guidance, or by a combination of techniques [54,55] (see Chapter 60). Ultrasound guidance allows direct visualization of the needle tip as it is placed close to the target nerve, increasing the chance of a successful block while minimizing the chance of iatrogenic damage to the nerve or other structures.

Clinicians who intend to use ultrasound to perform regional techniques need to become proficient in using the ultrasound probe and machine, and in interpreting the two-dimensional image provided. Three-dimensional ultrasound has been evaluated and may allow more accurate needle placement and better visualization of local anesthetic spread [56].

A robotic-assisted ultrasound-guided system called "Magellan" has been developed for performing regional anesthesia [57]. The Magellan system is composed of a joystick, a robotic arm, and a software control system. With the Magellan system, once the nerve is located using ultrasound, the anesthetist performs the block using the joystick located in a separate control center equipped with enhanced video imaging of the nerve block site. A single study of sciatic nerve blocks performed in 13 patients showed a 100% success rate with a total procedure time of 3–4 min.

Models and simulators in anesthesia

Models are used in anesthesia to help understand the complex physiologic and pharmacologic processes involved [58]. Computer-based modeling allows in-depth study of a topic with reduced reliance on animals, contributing to the principle of "reduction, replacement, refinement." In 1969, an article was published in the Journal of the American Medical Association discussing "Sim One," a computer-controlled manikin designed to help teach manual skills to medical students, interns, and residents [59]. This model was designed to resemble a living human, with realistic respiration and the ability to be mechanically ventilated, palpable peripheral pulses, and appropriate responses to the administration of anesthetic and vasopressor drugs. The authors suggested that using simulators in the training of healthcare workers would shorten effective education time, save faculty time, and produce more skilled graduates.

Veterinary anesthesia educators have also been working to reduce the use of live animals in teaching, recognizing ethical and safety concerns associated with live animal use in preclinical laboratories. At the same time, student learning and knowledge need to be sufficient for students to be successful in clinical rotations and after graduation. Using models in place of live animals in preclinical anesthesia labs allows veterinary students to learn critical anesthesia-related skills and build confidence without risk to a live patient [60]. Veterinary anesthesia simulators facilitate student learning by using real anesthesia machines and monitors, thereby creating realistic veterinary anesthesia environments. Simulator design focuses on anesthesia administration and patient monitoring during clinical scenarios, requiring students to interpret data, and provide interventions as they apply knowledge and problem-solving skills. Training models facilitate practice of a range of clinical skills including catheter placement, induction, endotracheal intubation, drug and fluid administration, ventilation, and maintenance of and recovery from anesthesia. Anesthesia monitoring equipment is linked with the simulator, allowing students to see changes in physiologic parameters of their "patient" in real-time. The immediate "patient" response to student inputs provides an interactive element that enhances student learning and understanding. Scenario content incorporates routine anesthesia skills and events, including commonly encountered complications; scenarios are designed to be specific to individual course content and learning outcomes. Simulations are followed by a debrief facilitated by anesthesia faculty to provide students with opportunities to reflect on their performance and to ask questions.

Models are also used in research settings to model pulmonary gas exchange or test and evaluate new equipment without the need for animal testing [61]. Modeling in research is typically done by a multidisciplinary team, to take advantage of each team member's area of expertise [58]. Biomedical engineers are a logical choice when veterinarians are looking for research collaborators in this realm as they are well suited to design models or simulations and are accustomed to working with other specialists.

Biomedical engineering in veterinary medicine

Though inhaled ether was used in domestic animals soon after it was introduced in people, it was not until many years later that the specialty of veterinary anesthesia was formally recognized with the foundation of the Association of Veterinary Anaesthetists [62], and the American College of Veterinary Anesthesiologists (see Chapter 1). Collaboration with other specialist veterinarians as well as with experts outside the field of veterinary medicine is an important way in which advances in anesthesia and analgesia are made. An example of this collaboration is the new and evolving field of "veterinary medicine engineering" which implements engineering technology to solve equipment and monitoring challenges that exist in veterinary medicine. In fact, a textbook dedicated to this topic, An *Introduction to Veterinary Medicine Engineering*, was published in 2023 that highlights the potential for collaborative design and application of technology to improve animal welfare and advance science [63].

References

1 Dow JW. The Bio-medical engineer. *Ire Trans Bio Med Electronics BME* 1961; **8**(4): 223–225.

2 Finch JL, Heath GH, David AR, *et al.* Biomechanical assessment of two artificial big toe restorations from ancient Egypt and their significance to the history of prosthetics. *Am Acad Orthotists Prosthetists* 2012; **24**(4): 181–191.

3 He B, Baird R, Butera R, *et al.* Grand challenges in interfacing engineering with life sciences and medicine. *IEEE Trans Biomed Eng* 2013; **60**(3): 589–598.

4 Karagozoglu B. Biomedical engineering: education, research and challenges. In: *Proceedings of the International Conference on Technological Advances in Electrical, Electronics and Computer Engineering (TAEECE)*. Konya, Turkey: IEEE, 2013: 430–436.

5 Valentinuzzi M. Why Study the history of BME, science, and technology? *IEEE Pulse* 2011; **2**(1): 45–47.

6 Bresadola M. Medicine and science in the life of Luigi Galvani (1737–1798). *Brain Res Bull* 1998; **46**(5): 367–380.

7 Piccolino M. Animal electricity and the birth of electrophysiology: the legacy of Luigi Galvani. *Brain Res Bull* 1998; **46**(5): 381–407.

8 Xiong Z, Nash MP, Cheng E, *et al.* ECG signal classification for the detection of cardiac arrhythmias using a convolutional recurrent neural network. *Physiol Meas* 2018; **39**(9): 094006.

9 Feher J. Diffusion. *In: Quantitative Human Physiology*, 2nd edn. London, UK: Elsevier, 2017: 75–86.

10 Gauthier J, Vincent AT, Charette SJ, *et al.* A brief history of bioinformatics. *Brief Bioinform* 2019; **20**(6): 1981–1996.

11 Yamakoshi K. In the spotlight: bioinstrumentation. *IEEE Rev Biomed Eng* 2009; **2**: 2–5.

12 Innocenti B. Biomechanics: a fundamental tool with a long history (and even longer future!). *Muscles Ligaments Tendons J* 2018; **7**(4): 491–492.

13 Bäck M, Gasser TC, Michel JB, *et al.* Biomechanical factors in the biology of aortic wall and aortic valve diseases. *Cardiovasc Res* 2013; **99**(2): 232–241.

14 Li Z, Yang C, Burdet E. Guest editorial: an overview of biomedical robotics and bio-mechatronics systems and applications. *IEEE Trans Syst Man Cybern Syst* 2016; **46**(7): 869–874.

15 Bhushan B. Biomimetics: lessons from nature – an overview. *Philos Trans A Math Phys Eng Sci* **2009**; 367(1893): 1445–1486.

16 Tan Y, Zheng Z. Research advance in swarm robotics. *Def Technol* 2013; **9**(1): 18–39.

17 Park K. Nanotechnology: what it can do for drug delivery. *J Control Release* 2007; **120**(1–2): 1–3.

18 Grimes SL. The future of clinical engineering: the challenge of change. *IEEE Eng Med Biol Mag* 2003; **22**(2): 91–99.
19 Abt V, Barz T, Cruz-Bournazou MN, *et al.* Model-based tools for optimal experiments in bioprocess engineering. *Curr Opin Chem Eng* 2018; **22**: 244–252.
20 Berliner AJ, Lipsky I, Ho D, *et al.* Space bioprocess engineering on the horizon. *Comms Eng* 2022; **1**(13). www.nature.com/articles/s44172-022-00012-9 (accessed August 2023).
21 Prochazka A. Neurophysiology and neural engineering: a review. *J Neurophysiol* 2017; **118**(2): 1292–1309.
22 Montgomery EB Jr., Gale JT. Mechanisms of action of deep brain stimulation (DBS). *Neurosci Biobehav Rev* 2008; **32**(3): 388–407.
23 Cooper RA, Cooper R. Rehabilitation Engineering: a perspective on the past 40-years and thoughts for the future. *Med Eng Phys* 2019; **72**: 3–12.
24 Arantes AR, Bressan N, McGibbon C. A comprehensive analysis of a novel real-time adaptive assist-as-needed controller for robot-assisted rehabilitation for stroke patients. *Res Sq* [Preprint] 2021. doi.org/10.21203/rs.3.rs-139605/v1
25 Ikada Y. Challenges in tissue engineering. *J R Soc Interface* 2006; **3**(10): 589–601.
26 Eren H, Fung C. *Instrumentation systems. In: Electrical Engineering, vol. II.* Abu Dhabi, UAE: UNESCO Encyclopedia of Life Support Systems, 2003.
27 Zhou G, Wang Y, Cui L. Biomedical sensor, device and measurement systems [Internet]. *Advances in Bioengineering.* InTech, 2015. doi.org/10.5772/59941
28 Oprzeska-Zingrebe EA. Molecular dynamics simulations for the study of interaction between non-canonical DNA structures and biochemically relevant co-solutes. Dissertation, 2023. doi.org/10.18419/opus-13417
29 Sterman JD. Learning in and about complex systems. *Syst Dyn Rev* 1994; **10**(2–3): 291–330.
30 Kuntzelman K, Jack Rhodes L, Harrington LN, *et al.* A practical comparison of algorithms for the measurement of multiscale entropy in neural time series data. *Brain Cogn* 2018; **123**: 126–135.
31 Danilov DL. Principal components in time series forecast. *J Comput Graph Stat* 1997; **6**(1): 112–121.
32 Astyrakaki E, Papaioannou A, Askitopoulou H. References to anesthesia, pain, and analgesia in the Hippocratic Collection. *Anesth Analg* 2010; **110**(1): 188–194.
33 Chaturvedi R, Gogna RL Retd. Ether day: an intriguing history. *Med J Armed Forces India* 2011; **67**(4): 306–308.
34 Robinson DH, Toledo AH. Historical development of modern anesthesia. *J Invest Surg* 2012; **25**(3): 141–149.
35 Methangkool E, Cole DJ, Cannesson M. Progress in patient safety in anesthesia. *JAMA* 2020; **324**(24): 2485–2486.
36 Choudry M, Stead TS, Mangal RK, *et al.* The history and evolution of the stethoscope. *Cureus* 2022; **14**(8): e28171.
37 Bachtiger P, Petri CF, Scott FE, *et al.* Point-of-care screening for heart failure with reduced ejection fraction using artificial intelligence during ECG-enabled stethoscope examination in London, UK: a prospective, observational, multicentre study. *Lancet Digit Health* 2022; **4**(2): e117–e125.
38 Strätling MWM. The history of "modern" anesthesia technology – A critical reappraisal: Part I: key criteria of "modern" anesthesia: technology and professionalism definitions, backgrounds and a short introduction to a changing evidence-base. *J Anesth Hist* 2020; **6**(3): 101–109.
39 McKenzie AG. The inventions of John Blease. *Br J Anaesth* 2000; **85**(6): 928–935.
40 Farrell R, Oomen G, Carey P. A technical review of the history, development and performance of the anaesthetic conserving device "AnaConDa" for delivering volatile anaesthetic in intensive and post-operative critical care. *J Clin Monit Comput* 2018; **32**(4): 595–604.
41 Van Meter A, Williams U, Zavala A, *et al.* Beat to beat: a measured look at the history of pulse oximetry. *J Anesth Hist* 2017; **3**(1): 24–26.
42 Tinker JH, Dull DL, Caplan RA, *et al.* Role of monitoring devices in prevention of anesthetic mishaps: a closed claims analysis. *Anesthesiology* 1989; **71**(4): 541–546.
43 Pandya AN, Majid SZ, Desai MS. The origins, evolution, and spread of anesthesia monitoring standards: from Boston to across the world. *Anesth Analg* 2021; **132**(3): 890–898.
44 Klein AA, Meek T, Allcock E, *et al.* Recommendations for standards of monitoring during anaesthesia and recovery 2021: guideline from the Association of Anaesthetists. *Anaesthesia* 2021; **76**(9): 1212–1223.
45 Deng Y, Navarro JC, Markan S. Advances in anesthesia monitoring. *Oral Maxillofac Surg Clin North Am* 2019; **31**(4): 611–619.
46 Grubb T, Sager J, Gaynor JS, *et al.* 2020 AAHA Anesthesia and Monitoring Guidelines for dogs and cats. *J Am Anim Hosp Assoc* 2020; **56**(2): 59–82.
47 Martinez EA, Wagner AE, Driessen B, *et al.* Guidelines for Anesthesia in Horses. American College of Veterinary Anesthesia and Analgesia (ACVAA) Equine Standards Committee. www.acvaa.org/wp-content/uploads/2019/05/Guidelines-for-Anesthesia-in-Horses.pdf (accessed August 2023).
48 Brodbelt DC, Pfeiffer DU, Young LE, *et al.* Results of the confidential enquiry into perioperative small animal fatalities regarding risk factors for anesthetic-related death in dogs. *J Am Vet Med Assoc* 2008; **233**(7): 1096–1104.
49 Brodbelt D. Feline anesthetic deaths in veterinary practice. *Top Companion Anim Med* 2010; **25**(4): 189–194.
50 Dugdale AH, Obhrai J, Cripps PJ. Twenty years later: a single-centre, repeat retrospective analysis of equine perioperative mortality and investigation of recovery quality. *Vet Anaesth Analg* 2016; **43**(2): 171–178.
51 van den Nieuwenhuyzen MC, Engbers FH, Vuyk J, *et al.* Target-controlled infusion systems: role in anaesthesia and analgesia. *Clin Pharmacokinet* 2000; **38**(2): 181–190.
52 Struys MM, De Smet T, Glen JI, *et al.* The history of target-controlled infusion. *Anesth Analg* 2016; **122**(1): 56–69.
53 Beverly A, Kaye AD, Ljungqvist O, *et al.* Essential elements of multimodal analgesia in enhanced recovery after surgery (ERAS) guidelines. *Anesthesiol Clin* 2017; **35**(2): e115–e143.
54 Mariano ER, Marshall ZJ, Urman RD, *et al.* Ultrasound and its evolution in perioperative regional anesthesia and analgesia. *Best Pract Res Clin Anaesthesiol* 2014; **28**(1): 29–39.
55 Comolli J, d'Ovidio D, Adami C, *et al.* Technological advances in exotic pet anesthesia and analgesia. *Vet Clin North Am Exot Anim Pract* 2019; **22**(3): 419–439.
56 Sen S, Ge M, Prabhakar A, *et al.* Recent technological advancements in regional anesthesia. *Best Pract Res Clin Anaesthesiol* 2019; **33**(4): 499–505.
57 Hemmerling TM, Taddei R, Wehbe M, *et al.* Technical communication: first robotic ultrasound-guided nerve blocks in humans using the Magellan system. *Anesth Analg* 2013; **116**(2): 491–494.
58 Beneken JE, van Oostrom JH. Modeling in anesthesia. *J Clin Monit Comput* 1998; **14**(1): 57–67.
59 Denson JS, Abrahamson S. A computer-controlled patient simulator. *JAMA* 1969; **208**(3): 504–508.
60 Jones JL, Rinehart J, Spiegel JJ, *et al.* Teaching tip: development of veterinary anesthesia simulations for pre-clinical training: design, implementation, and evaluation based on student perspectives. *J Vet Med Educ* 2018; **45**(2): 232–240.
61 Loughlin PJ, Bowes WA, Westenskow DR. An oil-based model of inhalation anesthetic uptake and elimination. *Anesthesiology* 1989; **71**(2): 278–282.
62 Jones RS. Association of Veterinary Anaesthetists – the beginnings. *Vet Anaesth Analg* 2014; **41**(5): 443–444.
63 Bressan NJ, Creighton CM. *An Introduction to Veterinary Medicine Engineering.* Cham, Switzerland: Springer Nature, 2023.

10 Anesthetic Depth Monitoring and Electroencephalography

Christopher L. Norkus
Allegheny Veterinary Emergency Trauma and Specialty (AVETS) Center, Monroeville, Pennsylvania, USA

Chapter contents

Introduction, 176
Minimum alveolar concentration, 176
Physical signs of anesthetic depth, 177
Stage 1, 178
Stage 2, 178
Stage 3, 179
Stage 4, 179
Electrophysiologic monitoring, 179
Depth-of-anesthesia devices, 180
The Bispectral Index™, 180
Spectral entropy, 182
Patient state index, 183
Cerebral state monitor, 183
Narcotrend® index, 183
Index of consciousness, 183
Auditory evoked potentials, 183
Clinical utility of depth-of-anesthesia devices, 184
References, 184

Introduction

Consciousness can be defined as explicit awareness. Awareness implies that the brain is in an aroused state and that the patient has perceptual qualities of an experience. Within the central nervous system, the brain stem, pons, thalamic nuclei, and cortex with their connecting neural pathways are the anatomic sites that contribute to the state of consciousness (Fig. 10.1). The American Society of Anesthesiologists (ASA) currently defines general anesthesia as "a drug-induced loss of consciousness during which patients are not arousable, even by painful stimulation" [1]. In effect, general anesthesia is thought to be a medically induced, reversible loss of consciousness. The traditional goals of successful general anesthesia include reversible unconsciousness, amnesia, analgesia, skeletal muscle relaxation resulting in immobility, and autonomic stability to maintain physiologic homeostasis. These goals are correlated with distinct sites within the central nervous system (CNS). For example, amnesia is associated with the limbic system, unconsciousness is associated with the interaction between the cerebral cortex and the thalamus, and immobility and analgesia are associated with the spinal cord [2].

Anesthetic depth is defined as the drug-induced probability of nonresponse to stimulation, calibrated against the strength of the stimulus and the difficulty of suppressing the response. Clinically, anesthetic depth is seen as the degree to which the CNS, predominantly the cortex, is depressed by a general anesthetic agent. Broadly speaking, this depends on the concentration of anesthetic agents within the brain, the magnitude of environmental stimulation (i.e., degree of surgical stimulus), and concurrent CNS depressant effects such as hypothermia, hypercarbia, or hypotension.

One of the current challenges in modern medicine is monitoring the depth of general anesthesia. This, along with measuring unconsciousness and recognizing awareness, is especially challenging in nonverbal veterinary species. Accurate assessment of the depth of anesthesia contributes to tailoring drug administration to the individual patient. Patient underdosing resulting in inadequate general anesthesia depth may lead to arousal or movement of the patient, which could be dangerous or even deadly to veterinary staff (e.g., horses kicking and large carnivores biting), exaggerated autonomic responses (e.g., arrhythmias, tachycardia, and hypertension), and intraoperative awareness with recall. Presently in humans, the incidence of perianesthetic awareness is approximately 0.1%, with this number increasing in cardiac surgery, cesarean section, and high-risk patients [3–7]. The incidence of perianesthetic awareness in veterinary species remains unknown. Patient overdosing resulting in excessive general anesthetic depth may result in prolonged patient recovery, increased postanesthetic complications, and patient death.

Minimum alveolar concentration

Effect-site concentration is the concentration of a drug at the site of its biological activity; for example, the brain with general anesthetics. Effect-site concentration is proportional to the pharmacological

Veterinary Anesthesia and Analgesia: The Sixth Edition of Lumb and Jones. Edited by Leigh Lamont, Kurt Grimm, Sheilah Robertson, Lydia Love and Carrie Schroeder.
© 2024 John Wiley & Sons, Inc. Published 2024 by John Wiley & Sons, Inc.
Companion website: www.wiley.com/go/lamont/anesthesia

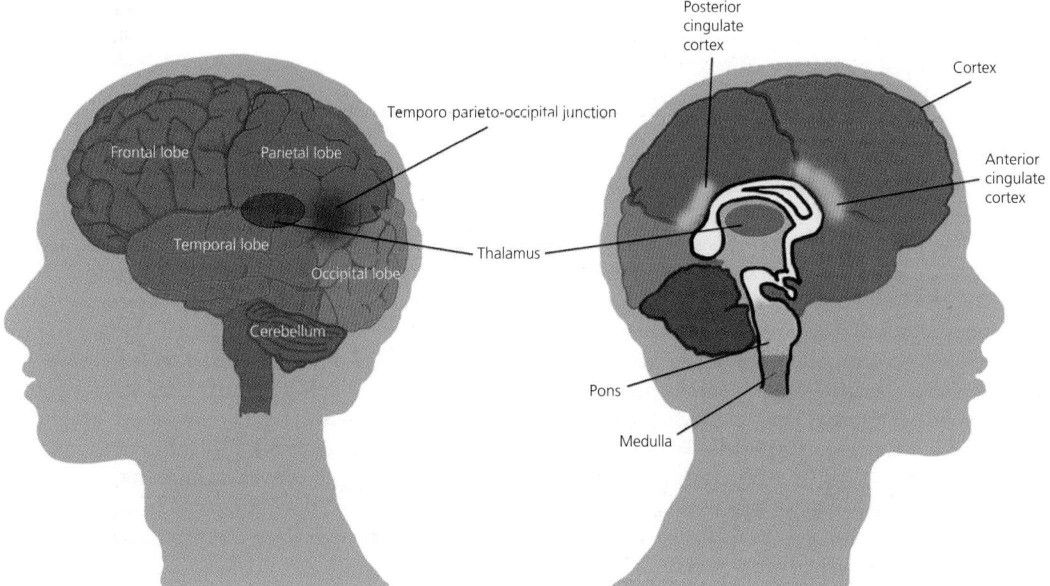

Figure 10.1 Key regions in the central nervous system that contribute to a patient's state of consciousness. Source: Dr. Christopher Norkus with illustration by Kyna Kozak, with permission.

effect, whereas measurement of solely plasma concentration may not be. Unfortunately, rapidly measuring effect-site concentration within the clinical anesthesia setting is not feasible at this time. In 1965, Eger introduced the concept of minimum alveolar concentration (MAC), and it has since been used as the standard measure of potency for volatile anesthetic agents. It is defined as the concentration of inhaled anesthetic within the alveoli at which 50% of subjects do not move in response to a noxious stimulus. In humans, this noxious stimulus is considered a surgical incision; however, in animals, this is often a noxious but non-surgical stimulus such as tail clamp. MAC creates a unifying principle for inhaled anesthetics as inhaled concentration can be associated with a given response and is reproducible across various anesthetic agents. For example, administration of 0.25 MAC (MAC-amnesia) will produce amnesia in humans, whereas 0.3–0.5 MAC (MAC-awake) of a volatile anesthetic agent is needed to produce unconsciousness or return to awakening [8–10]. The end-tidal concentration of inhaled anesthetic agents at which 50% of patients can be intubated smoothly is known as "MAC for endotracheal intubation" (MAC-EI).

Administration of 1 MAC (MAC) of a volatile anesthetic prevents movement in response to a surgical or otherwise noxious stimulus in 50% of subjects. Considering normal distribution, MAC represents only a single point on the dose-response curve and can be seen as equivalent to a median effective dose (ED_{50}). Therefore, an individual patient may require more or less inhalant anesthetic than MAC. Assuming a standard deviation of MAC to be 10% and following the properties of a normal distribution, immobility would be expected to be achieved in 68% of patients at 1.1 MAC, 95% of patients at 1.2 MAC, and 99.7% at 1.3 MAC [10]. Administration of 1.5 MAC (MAC-BAR) of a volatile anesthetic blunts autonomic responses to surgical incision in 50% of human patients. The autonomic responses commonly used to define MAC-BAR include changes in pupil dilation, heart rate, and blood pressure [9].

Clinically, these multiples of MAC may be useful to roughly gauge anesthetic depth and titrate anesthetics. For example, the use of MAC may result in an inadequate or light plane of general anesthesia, while 1.5 MAC would represent a deep plane of general anesthesia for many patients. There are, however, numerous limitations to relying solely on this approach. Numerous factors can alter MAC. MAC can be increased in the face of hyperthermia, hyperthyroidism, young age, and concurrent medications that raise circulating central catecholamines (e.g., ephedrine, monoamine oxidase inhibitors, and amphetamine intoxication). MAC can be reduced by factors such as hypothermia, severe hypotension, advanced age, concurrent use of other CNS depressants (e.g., opioids, dexmedetomidine, and ketamine), pregnancy, and severe hypoxemia. Additional pharmacogenetic factors such as red hair in humans have been shown to alter MAC as well as anesthetic recovery time [11,12]. MAC values vary widely between species, and it is quite possible that similar genotypic or phenotypic differences exist across different animal breeds and species.

The degree of noxious stimulus in question may also be variable and, depending on the procedure, may extend beyond a single skin incision, which defines MAC. Predicting end-tidal inhalant concentration may be impossible without the use of anesthetic gas monitoring equipment, which is often not available outside of veterinary specialty or academic practice settings. Lastly and most notably, volatile anesthetic concentrations are measured as expired end-tidal concentrations, which may not accurately reflect what anesthetic concentration reaches the brain. Similarly, with the use of total intravenous anesthesia (TIVA), target-controlled infusions (TCI) can be utilized to predict plasma concentrations. These approaches predict drug concentration and not necessarily drug effect. As a result, MAC, its multiples, and plasma concentrations should not be relied upon to be the sole determinant of anesthetic depth.

Physical signs of anesthetic depth

Physician Dr. Arthur Guedel served in the United States Army during the First World War and was stationed in France where he was responsible for overseeing up to six hospitals at one time.

As part of this oversight, he was tasked to train orderlies and nurses to administer diethyl ether to wounded soldiers returning from the battlefield. Guedel developed guidelines using a wall chart that could be used by anesthetists to gauge the depth of anesthesia (Fig. 10.2) [13]. While Guedel's original observations were made in human patients anesthetized with diethyl ether, they were subsequently adapted for use with other hypnotic agents and ultimately applied for use in animals.

Guedel described four progressive stages of anesthesia beginning at its initial administration and ending at near death. Within stage 3 (surgical anesthesia), sub-classifications of light, medium, and deep anesthesia planes were described. These planes of anesthesia represented the progressive CNS depression that could be observed while a patient was within a surgical depth of anesthesia. Modern balanced anesthetic and multimodal analgesia techniques utilize numerous agents, which may confound Guedel's classification system, originally developed for use with the single agent diethyl ether. For example, the use of anticholinergics might result in alterations to patient heart rate, while the use of a dissociative agent such as ketamine might impact eyeball position, ocular reflexes, and general muscle tone. This has necessitated a greater reliance on additional patient monitoring parameters, including blood pressure, respiration, and neuromuscular tone, and created a continued interest in depth-of-anesthesia devices based upon electroencephalographic monitoring of CNS activity. Nevertheless, despite the incorporation of many new monitoring modalities in practice, the veterinary anesthetist should continue to have a strong understanding of the correlation of changing physical signs and their relationship to anesthetic depth progression.

Stage 1

Stage 1 is considered the stage of voluntary movement and is defined as lasting from initial drug administration to loss of patient consciousness. Some analgesia may be present in the deeper phases of this stage. Excited, apprehensive animals may struggle. Respirations may become irregular, or increase, and the patient may voluntarily hold their breath for brief periods. A catecholamine release results in a strong, rapid heartbeat, increased patient blood pressure, and pupillary dilation. Cardiac arrhythmias may be observed during this stage. Salivation is frequent in some species, and urination or defecation may occasionally occur. Muscle tone remains and patients retain a normal eye position and palpebral and corneal reflex. Patients during this phase retain a pedal reflex and react strongly to surgical manipulation. With the approach of stage 2, animals become progressively ataxic, lose their ability to stand or right themselves, and assume lateral recumbency.

Stage 2

Stage 2 is considered the stage of delirium or involuntary movement. It is commonly clinically referred to as the "excitement phase." By definition, this stage lasts from loss of consciousness to the onset of a regular pattern of breathing. Patients may exhibit breath-holding, tachypnea, and hyperventilation. They may retain muscle tone. Continued catecholamine release causes an increased heart

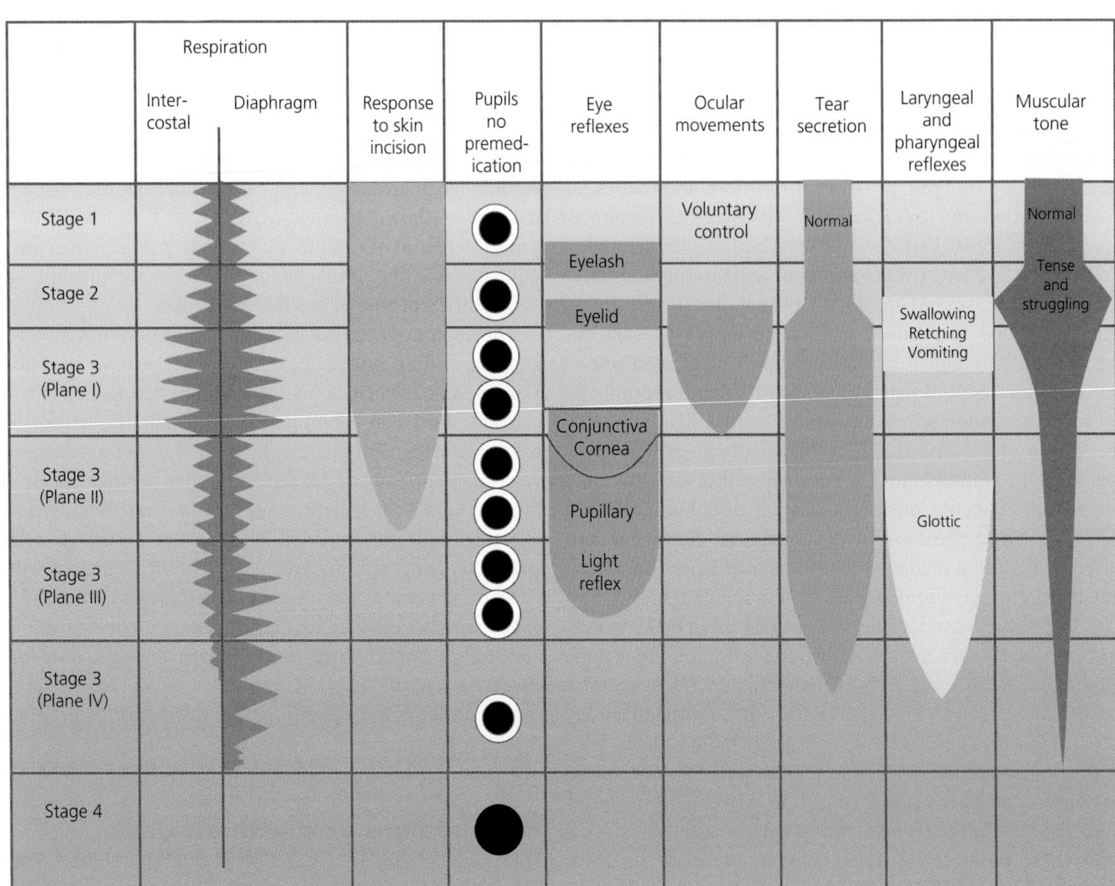

Figure 10.2 Characteristics of the stages of general anesthesia. Source: Dr. Christopher Norkus with illustration by Kyna Kozak, with permission.

rate and increased blood pressure. Arrhythmias may occur and the patient's pupils remain dilated. Palpebral and corneal reflexes remain brisk. Nystagmus commonly occurs in horses. During this stage, animals may briefly vocalize. In some species, especially ruminants and cats, salivation may occur. In some species, including dogs, cats, and goats, vomiting may be seen. The larynx of cats and pigs is very sensitive at this stage, and premature stimulation with an endotracheal tube may easily result in laryngospasm. Patients during this phase retain a pedal reflex and react strongly to surgical manipulation.

Stage 3

Stage 3 is considered the stage of surgical anesthesia. It is characterized by unconsciousness with progressive depression of reflexes. This stage is the targeted anesthetic level for procedures requiring general anesthesia. Muscle relaxation develops and ventilation becomes slow and regular. Vomiting and swallowing reflexes are lost. In humans, this stage has been further divided into planes I–IV for finer differentiation. Others have suggested the simpler classification of light (plane I), medium (plane II), and deep (plane III) planes are more appropriate.

Light anesthesia persists until eyeball movement ceases. Medium anesthesia is characterized by progressive intercostal paralysis, and deep anesthesia by diaphragmatic respiration. A medium depth of anesthesia has traditionally been considered a light to medium plane of surgical anesthesia (stage 3, plane II), characterized by stable respiration and pulse rate, abolished laryngeal reflexes, an absent palpebral reflex, a strong corneal reflex, and adequate muscle relaxation with absent response to surgical stimulation. Deep surgical anesthesia (stage 3, plane III) is characterized by decreased intercostal muscle function and tidal volume, increased respiration rate, profound muscle relaxation, diaphragmatic breathing, a weak corneal reflex, and a centered and dilated pupil.

Patients in stage 3 have their heart rates return to normal ranges and may experience progressive bradycardia. Blood pressure normalizes and begins to decrease as anesthetic depth is deepened. The frequency of arrhythmias decreases. Patients in light planes of anesthesia may react to surgical manipulation and have a pedal reflex, while these traits are lost in medium-to-deeper planes. In general, patients will progressively lose jaw tone and limb muscle tone, although this can vary depending on species and patient age. For example, young dogs may have minimal jaw tone even at light anesthesia planes, while other species such as ruminants and swine may maintain a high degree of jaw tone even at deep planes. Eyeball position will also vary depending on the species. In dogs and cats, for example, the globe will rotate to a ventromedial orientation. In other species such as horses, however, the globe will remain centrally oriented. In ruminants, the globe may rotate ventrally in light and medium anesthesia planes showing only the sclera and then returning centrally during deep anesthesia planes.

Stage 4

Stage 4 is that of extreme CNS depression and overdose. In this phase, cardiopulmonary function fails. The patient may exhibit marked hypotension, weak pulses, bradycardia or transient tachycardia, prolonged capillary refill time, and other cardiac arrhythmias. Patients will hypoventilate and respiration itself may cease or become irregular. Pupils will acutely dilate. All reflexes are blunted, and muscle tone is absent. The corneal reflex ceases. In dogs and cats, the eyeball position will rotate to a central position. In this stage, death quickly occurs unless immediate resuscitative steps are taken, including lessening the patient's anesthesia depth.

Electrophysiologic monitoring

Electroencephalography is the recording of spontaneous electrical brain activity from scalp electrodes [14–16]. Traditionally, these electrodes are placed at standard positions according to the International 10–20 system [14,16,17]. The electrical signals obtained from the surface of the scalp represent the summation of neuronal activity within the cerebral cortex, and result from excitatory and inhibitory postsynaptic potentials (PSPs) in large pyramidal neurons located in the lower layers, such as layer V, of the cerebral cortex [14,18–20]. The EEG amplitude and frequency are influenced by afferent inputs from sensory-specific thalamic nuclei serving as gates between peripheral receptors and the cortex, and by epicenters within the cerebral cortex [21].

In 1934, Hans Berger proposed that the appearance of α waves in the EEG may represent cerebrocortical events associated with consciousness in the awake man [22]. It is believed that EEG activity associated with consciousness is generated from pacemaker neurons within the ascending reticular activating system (ARAS), and then mediated and modulated through thalamic connections [19,21,23–25]. These pacemaker neurons oscillate in the frequency range of 8–12 Hz and synchronize the excitability of cells in the thalamocortical pathways. Small cerebrocortical areas appear to also act as epicenters from which α activity spreads through cortical neuronal networks, generating the α rhythm that dominates the resting EEG. In the awake state, consciousness is maintained by a circulating activity among the ARAS, intralaminar nuclei, and the cerebral cortex [21]. Additional sensory stimulation will cause cortical arousal that is characterized by the desynchronization of α oscillators with the appearance of a faster rhythm in the β frequency range (12–25 Hz) [21,25–28]. The term "desynchronization" is characterized by a shift in the EEG pattern from high-voltage, slow-wave activity to low-voltage, fast-wave activity [19,23,29].

As early as 1937, Gibbs and colleagues reported that anesthetic agents altered electroencephalogram (EEG) activity from low-voltage fast waves to high-voltage slow waves and proposed that the EEG could be used clinically to measure the effects of anesthesia [30]. In 1959, Martin and colleagues first described hypnotic general anesthetics as producing a biphasic EEG effect [31]. They observed that during light anesthesia, there was EEG desynchronization, which changed to progressive synchronization, slowing, and increased amplitude as anesthesia deepened (Fig. 10.3A–C). With further increases in anesthetic depth, the EEG displayed burst suppression and lengthening periods of EEG silence (Fig. 10.3D). Furthermore, a topographic distributional change from occipital lobe dominance to frontal lobe dominance was observed.

More specifically, the EEG frequency bands utilized for assessment of anesthetic depth are the δ (0–4 Hz), θ (4–8 Hz), α (8–13 Hz), and β (13–30 Hz) bands [32,33]. During induction and maintenance of anesthesia, there is a progressive decrease in EEG frequency content characterized by a shift from a low-voltage, fast-wave pattern to a high-voltage, slow-wave pattern [34–37]. As anesthetic depth increases, the predominant EEG pattern is characterized by a decrease in β activity and a concomitant increase in both α and δ activity [38]. As anesthesia deepens further, EEG activity in the θ and δ frequency bands appears initially in centroposterior regions with subsequent anterior spread [39]. Lastly, very deep

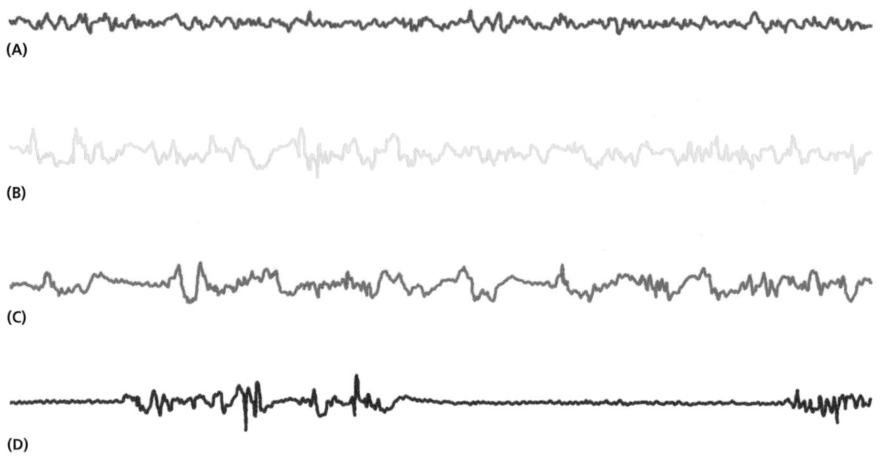

Figure 10.3 During induction and maintenance of anesthesia, there is a progressive decrease in EEG frequency content slowing, which will be characterized by a shift from a low-voltage, fast-wave pattern to a high-voltage, slow-wave pattern (**A–C**). Deep levels of general anesthesia are indicated by flat periods interspersed with a burst suppression pattern, followed by a complete loss of electrical discharge known as isoelectricity or electrical silence (**D**). Source: Dr. Christopher Norkus with illustration by Kyna Kozak, with permission.

levels of general anesthesia are first indicated by flat periods interspersed with periods of α and β activity, known as a "burst suppression pattern," followed by a complete loss of electrical discharge known as "isoelectricity" or "electrical silence" [35,36,40]. Upon reducing the dose of the anesthetic agent, these patterns reverse, and lighter levels of anesthesia are indicated again by a decrease in amplitude and an increase in frequency content.

Depth-of-anesthesia devices

Today we recognize the EEG as a continuous non-invasive indicator of cerebral cortical function in awake and unconscious patients alike. The EEG is thought to be a potential measure of anesthetic depth because it represents cortical electrical activity derived from summated inhibitory and excitatory postsynaptic activity resulting from subcortical events, including those that pass through subcortical thalamic nuclei. Additionally, the degree of measured EEG activity is associated with cerebral blood flow and metabolism, which can be altered by anesthetic drugs and surgical stimulation. Noxious stimulation during inadequate anesthesia ascends the reticular activating system (RAS) of the brainstem and results in EEG activation. These EEG changes vary with individual anesthetics and with the nature of the noxious stimulation. Clinical assessment of raw EEG signals to assess anesthetic depth is challenging to learn, subjective to interpret, and influenced by confounders such as electrical interferences. For these reasons, computer analysis techniques have been utilized to distill the EEG into a condensed, easy-to-interpret format known as the "processed" EEG which, in turn, may be useful in assessing general trends in clinical anesthetic depth.

Shortly before the turn of the last century, Aspect Medical Systems undertook research efforts to develop the EEG as a general measurement of anesthetic depth and developed the first depth-of-anesthesia device. Their original EEG monitor, known as the "Bispectral Index™" (BIS™) monitoring system, quantitates the effect of hypnotic anesthetics on the human brain. Several other competitors have manufactured similar depth-of-anesthesia devices over the past three decades based upon this general technology. While the details of each company's algorithms often remain proprietary, these devices and their development share several common principles. These devices present a continuous EEG parameter, or index, that usually ranges from an awake non-anesthetic drug-influenced state (value of 100) to isoelectricity or electrical silence (value of 0). These devices then use multiple EEG signal-processing approaches to capture incremental information. Clinically relevant data (e.g., response to verbal commands, plasma drug concentration, and recall) is then gathered from a large population of human subjects, and advanced multivariate statistical analysis is used to correlate the index value with the clinically relevant measure. Cumulatively, these monitoring devices generally display progressively decreasing index values from 100 to 0, which reflect a progressive increase in anesthetic depth and provide a framework for the titration of anesthetic agents.

The Bispectral Index™

The Bispectral Index (BIS™) is a proprietary EEG parameter developed by Aspect Medical Systems. The United States Food and Drug Administration approved the commercial use of the device to monitor the effect of anesthetics on the brain in 1996. A self-adhesive index sensor is placed on the patient's forehead. This sensor then obtains live raw EEG signals and transmits them to a BIS monitor via an interface cable. The BIS monitor then displays real-time EEG as well as a dimensionless BIS value for interpretation. In humans, BIS values between 40 and 60 represent adequate general anesthesia for surgery with values below 40 representing a deep or over-anesthetized state (Fig. 10.4).

In humans, however, numerous limitations influence the reliability of the BIS. The BIS appears strongly influenced by the anesthetic technique. Certain anesthetics such as ketamine and nitrous oxide may actually increase BIS values [41,42]. The BIS may also be influenced by patient age. In children under 6 months of age, emergence and recovery measures were unaffected by BIS titration; children between the ages of 6 months and 3 years also showed no differences in anesthetic use or recovery measures when BIS was compared to standard practice monitoring [43]. This may be due to differences in brain maturation and synapse formation resulting in differences in the EEG in this population. Hypothermic human patients show a wide variation in BIS values as body temperature decreases. Specifically, BIS appears to decrease by 1.12 units for each degree Celsius reduction in body temperature [44]. Interference with other

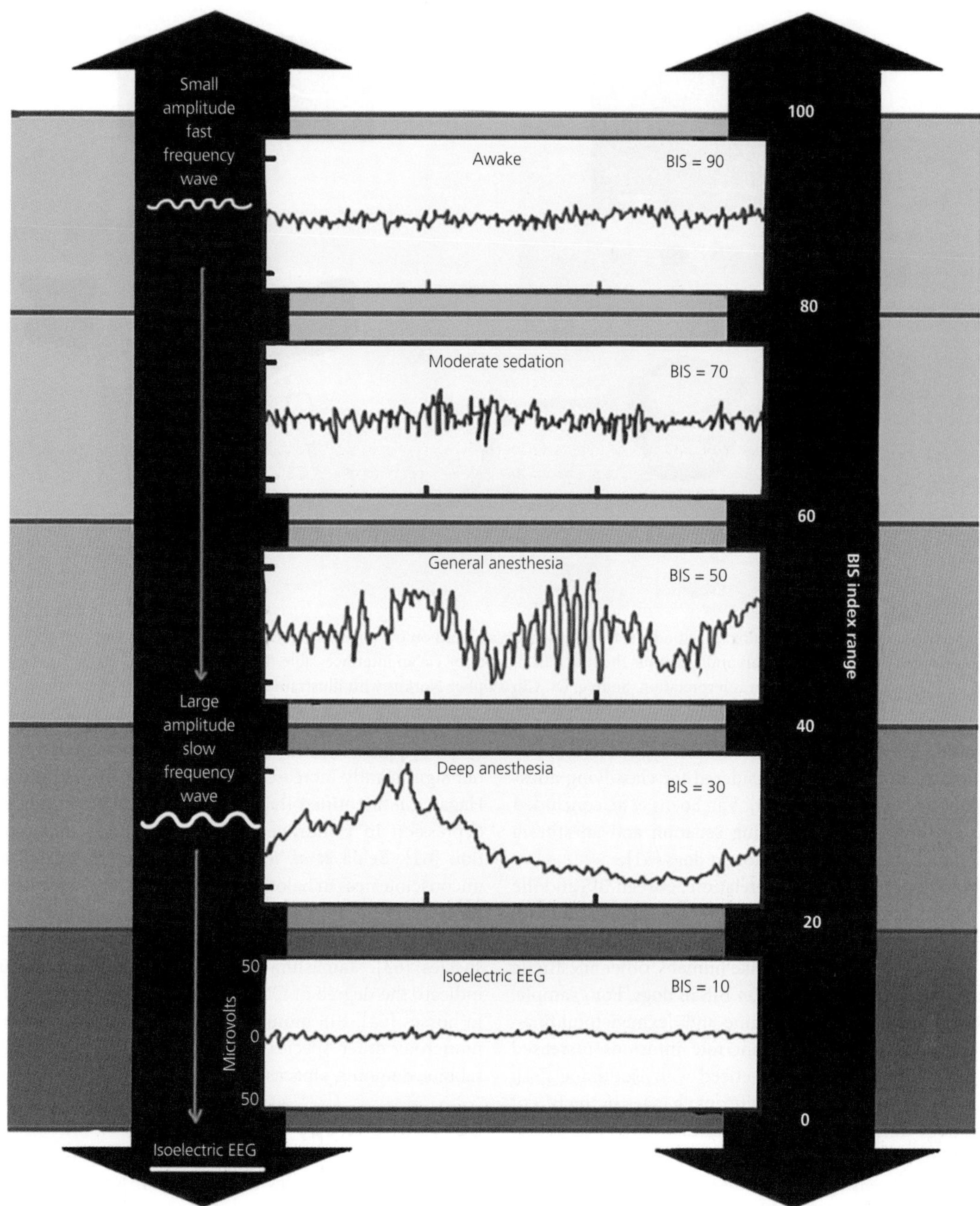

Figure 10.4 Bispectral Index™ aids the anesthetist by providing a numeral value between 0 (indicating EEG suppression) to 100 (fully conscious). Source: Dr. Christopher Norkus with illustration by Kyna Kozak, with permission.

medical devices such as electrosurgical cautery can cause EEG artifacts and thereby influence BIS reliability [45]. Lastly, neurologic impairment can markedly alter the ability of the BIS to acutely monitor the depth of anesthesia. Patients within this population generally have lower pre-existing BIS values [46].

The BIS has been evaluated in veterinary anesthesiology with conflicting results and interpretations of clinical utility (Fig. 10.5). Bleijenberg *et al.* evaluated 65 dogs undergoing anesthesia for surgery. Individual BIS values measured at light and surgical levels of anesthesia overlapped considerably. The authors concluded that BIS values and clinical depth of anesthesia had low specificity, sensitivity, and predictive values, and thus the use of BIS as a sole method to determine anesthetic depth in dogs was imprudent [47]. Campagnol *et al.* evaluated the correlation between BIS and end-tidal isoflurane concentration and also compared the use of three different BIS sensor positions in dogs. They proposed that frontal-temporal sensor positioning provided a better correlation with isoflurane depth of anesthesia in dogs compared to the other sensor configurations tested [48]. Additionally, their work suggested that BIS values might not reflect changes in depth of isoflurane anesthesia in the absence of noxious stimulation [48]. Previous work also identified that the use of subdermal needle electrodes was a reliable and practical alternative to the use of patch electrodes for the measurement of BIS in dogs [49]. The work of Ubiali *et al.*

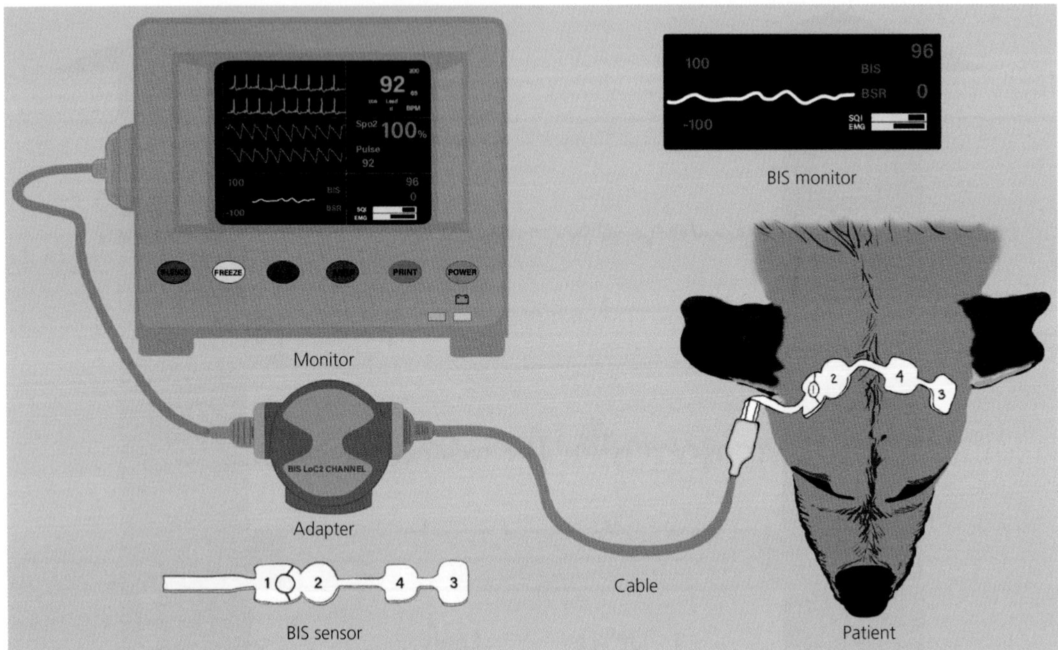

Figure 10.5 Bispectral Index™ usage in the dog. A self-adhesive index sensor is placed on the patient's forehead in the frontal–temporal position. This sensor then obtains live raw EEG signals and transmits them to a BIS™ monitor via an interface cable. The BIS monitor then displaces real-time EEG as well as a dimensionless BIS value for interpretation. Source: Dr. Christopher Norkus with illustration by Kyna Kozak, with permission.

in dogs evaluating BIS during propofol infusion suggested that BIS values for humans should not be considered for classifying anesthetic and hypnotic depths in dogs [50]. Van Soens *et al.* concluded that BIS was of limited use in titrating sedation and anesthesia during transcranial magnetic stimulation in dogs [51].

Other work in dogs has shown a correlation between BIS and the expired anesthetic fraction in halothane, isoflurane, and sevoflurane-anesthetized dogs [52]. An increase in propofol infusion rates appears to decrease BIS in dogs [53]. Like humans, other anesthetic agents appear to have variable effects on BIS in dogs. For example, the use of morphine–lidocaine–ketamine and dexmedetomidine–morphine–lidocaine–ketamine constant rate infusions increased BIS values in six healthy dogs anesthetized with isoflurane [54]. Morphine did not cause clinically significant changes in the BIS of unstimulated dogs during isoflurane anesthesia [55]. Atracurium also appeared to have minimal clinical effect on the BIS in anesthetized dogs [56]. BIS levels appear to be lower in puppies than in adults at the same alveolar concentration of sevoflurane [57]. Lastly, in 31 dogs with altered levels of consciousness, Saenubol *et al.* identified a significant correlation between modified Glasgow coma scale (MGCS) scores and BIS values, suggesting that BIS values could also be used as an alternative to MGCS monitoring in the veterinary intensive care unit, and like in humans with neurologic disease, might be influenced by other CNS factors beyond anesthetic depth [58].

Less data is available in other animal species. Values of BIS are inversely and linearly related to end-tidal sevoflurane and isoflurane concentrations in anesthetized cats [59,60]. In horses, BIS values were measured at multiple stages of sevoflurane anesthesia in five thoroughbred horses anesthetized with guaifenesin and thiopental following premedication with xylazine. BIS values were lower during anesthesia than in awake or sedated horses; however, no significant difference between BIS values was recorded at end-tidal sevoflurane concentrations of 2.8% and 3.5% [61]. During the recovery phase, the BIS values gradually increased over time but did not significantly increase until the horses showed movement [61]. Haga *et al.* identified that BIS was an imprecise indicator of CNS depression in isoflurane-anesthetized horses undergoing castration [62]. Belda *et al.* found that BIS approximated the level of unconsciousness in halothane and sevoflurane-anesthetized horses; however, it did not predict intraoperative movement, which would be a major shortcoming associated with BIS monitoring in this species [63]. Yamashita *et al.* also identified that BIS did not indicate the degree of CNS depression during propofol anesthesia in horses [64]. BIS monitoring has additionally been evaluated in numerous other species, including goats, sheep, pigs, cows, elk, rabbits, dolphins, alpacas, and chickens [65–73].

Spectral entropy

In chemistry, entropy is used as a measure of how the energy of atoms and molecules becomes more spread out in a process. For example, as a substance changes from a solid to a liquid, the mobility and potential for interactions among atoms increases and, consequently, so does its entropy. Mathematician Claude E. Shannon applied these concepts in 1948 to information theory and proposed that entropy could describe the complexity, irregularity, or unpredictability of a signal [74]. For example, a pure sinusoidal wave would have no entropy because of its regular and predictable nature, whereas a wave containing hugely variable frequencies would have a high entropy. As EEGs exhibit chaotic and non-linear behavior, it followed that entropy could be applied to their interpretation.

The GE Healthcare Entropy™ Module was released in 2003 as an index of anesthetic depth and is available as part of some Datex multiparameter monitors. The device uses a similar self-adhesive frontotemporal sensor as the BIS which connects to a monitor via an interface cable. In humans, facial electromyography (EMG) has a frequency range (> 20 Hz) that overlaps with that of the EEG (0.8–32 Hz). The facial EMG changes with levels of consciousness and the use of neuromuscular blocking agents. The device assesses two indices: State Entropy (SE) and Response Entropy (RE). SE is computed from the EEG in the 0.8–32 Hz range and is thought to encompass mainly the hypnotic elements of the EEG. RE, on the other hand, is computed from EEG signals in the 0.8–47 Hz range, which includes elements from the facial EMG. When EMG activity is low, SE and RE should be identical. However, with arousal and an increase in facial EMG, RE should increase [75].

Data in humans would suggest that the GE Healthcare Entropy Module produces results comparable to that of BIS when tested with intravenous and inhaled anesthetics [76–78]. The monitor displays the SE, RE, a raw EEG, as well as other monitored variables. The displayed SE range is 0 (no EEG activity) to 91 (full awake) and the RE range is 0–100. Numbers close to 100 mean that the patient is conscious, and numbers close to 0 denote very deep anesthesia. The manufacturer recommends that an SE between 40 and 60 is appropriate for general anesthesia and that values outside this range may require a dosing adjustment. In horses undergoing isoflurane and medetomidine general anesthesia, SE values of 27.4 ± 4.8 and RE values of 35.1 ± 7.1 were present during a surgical plane of anesthesia. There appeared to be a poor correlation between this technique and BIS [79]. Morgaz *et al.* evaluated entropy in sevoflurane-anesthetized dogs. Their work concluded that RE and RE-SE differences were not adequate indicators of antinociception, and SE and RE were unable to detect deep planes of anesthesia in dogs, although they were able to distinguish the awake and unconscious states [80].

Patient state index

The patient state index (PSI) uses time, frequency, phase information, and spatial information from the EEG to assess anesthetic depth via a multivariate algorithm [81]. A self-adhesive five-lead bilateral frontotemporal sensor is used. A PSI value of 25–50 is considered adequate for surgical anesthesia in humans. The index is shown as the current value as well as the patient's trend, which is color-coded to indicate whether the anesthetic depth is "too light," "too deep," or "just right." Data investigating or validating the use of PSI in veterinary species is lacking.

Cerebral state monitor

The cerebral state monitor (CSM) is a handheld portable device that analyses the frequency content of the EEG signal. The energy of the EEG is evaluated in specific frequency bands. These are used to define two energy ratios called *alpha* (α) and *beta* (β). Both of these show a shift in energy content from the higher to the lower frequencies during anesthesia. The relationship between these quantities is also analyzed as a separate parameter (β-α). Lastly, the monitor evaluates the amount of instantaneous burst suppression (BS) in each 30-s period of the EEG. This measurement quantifies the amount of "silent" or "flat" EEG periods characteristic of the deepest levels of hypnosis. These four parameters are used as input to a fuzzy logic classifier system that calculates the cerebral state index (CSI). The CSI ranges from 0 (no EEG activity) to 100 (awake state). Values between 40 and 60 are considered adequate for surgical anesthesia in humans. Bollen and Saxtorph evaluated CSM in dogs sedated with medetomidine undergoing dental scaling. Undisturbed sedated dogs had a median CSI value of 43. During dental scaling, CSI values increased to awake ranges with a median value of 99. The authors concluded CSM to be a promising method for monitoring the degree of sedation and hypnosis [82]. In other work in dogs, while increasing doses of propofol showed a correlation to CSI, no correlation was found between clinical depth of anesthesia during propofol induction [83,84]. Bollen *et al.* found good agreement between depth of anesthesia and CSI in propofol–fentanyl-infused pigs [85].

Narcotrend® index

In 1937, Loomis and colleagues categorized the EEG during sleep into characteristic patterns, which were assigned stages ranging from A to E [86]. The Narcotrend® monitor by MonitorTechnik was developed by anesthesiologists and engineers at the University Medical School of Hannover in Germany. The system takes raw EEG and, after artifact detection, uses a multivariate statistical algorithm to categorize patients into six stages, ranging from A (awake) to F (isoelectricity/burst suppression), and 14 substages to facilitate greater precision in monitoring anesthesia depth [87]. In humans, the Narcotrend index appears to correlate well with BIS analysis. Narcotrend stages D or E appear equivalent to BIS values between 65 and 40, indicating appropriate surgical anesthetic depth. The Narcotrend monitor is unique in that it uses standard electrocardiography electrodes rather than a proprietary electrode sensor. Limited data is available on the use of the Narcotrend index in veterinary anesthesia. In cats, the Narcotrend index correlated to increasing isoflurane MAC multiples, but its reliability decreased with the addition of dexmedetomidine [88].

Index of consciousness

The index of consciousness (IoC) is a depth-of-anesthesia device derived from a combination of symbolic dynamics, β-ratio, and EEG suppression rate [89]. IoC ranges from 0 to 99, where 99 indicates an awake patient, 80 is associated with sedation, the range 40–60 is defined as the state recommended for surgical anesthesia, and 0 indicates isoelectric EEG. IoC shows a considerable time delay before the correct index is displayed, which may limit the device's clinical utility [89].

Auditory evoked potentials

Auditory evoked potentials (AEPs) are electrical potentials evoked in the auditory pathway in response to sound stimuli [90]. To generate an AEP, an auditory stimulus is repeatedly delivered to a patient, and the EEG periods that immediately follow each stimulus are averaged. This eliminates the non-stimulus–related portions of the EEG and retains the specific evoked potential periods. These potentials are then divided into several sections based on the anatomical area of their origin and the time elapsed since the auditory stimulus. The middle latency auditory evoked potential (MLAEP), 40 and 60 ms after stimulation, represents neural activity within the thalamus and primary auditory cortex and has been used in humans to reflect the degree of CNS depression in response to anesthetics, and therefore general anesthetic depth [90]. One such newer device is the aepEXplus™ made by Medical Device Management, Essex, UK. These devices produce a dimensionless index known as the "A-line autoregressive index" (AAI) between 0 and 100 with which depth of anesthesia can be gauged.

In humans, AEP monitoring appears to correlate well with other depth-of-anesthetic devices and may be preferred over BIS when ketamine is used [91]. The use of AEP has also been evaluated in animal species. AEPs were found to correlate with end-tidal isoflurane concentrations and the administration of thiopental in dogs [92,93]. Additional work in dogs premedicated with acepromazine and morphine and anesthetized with thiopental and halothane found that indices generated from AEP also showed a good correlation with anesthetic depth assessed by a trained anesthetist [94]. Other work in dogs found that AEPs were not statistically correlated with magnetic motor evoked potentials in dogs undergoing transcranial magnetic stimulation and were of limited use in titrating anesthesia in this population [51]. AEPs were also not found to be effective in monitoring anesthetic depth in sevoflurane-anesthetized dogs [95].

Clinical utility of depth-of-anesthesia devices

The depth-of-anesthesia devices previously discussed primarily aim to measure the effect of injectable and inhaled hypnotic agents on the EEG. However, numerous drugs are often administered to patients as part of a balanced anesthesia technique and to achieve multimodal analgesia. Not all agents impact the EEG in the same way. Many drugs such as midazolam, dexmedetomidine, propofol, etomidate, thiopental, isoflurane, sevoflurane, and desflurane are thought to decrease BIS and other depth-of-anesthesia device indices in humans. However, low concentrations of opioids, the use of neuromuscular blocking agents, and nitrous oxide, do not appear to consistently change the BIS response during propofol or inhaled anesthesia. As discussed earlier in the chapter, agents such as ketamine and nitrous oxide may even increase BIS depending on dose [24,41]. Other agents administered during the perianesthetic period that affect the sympathetic nervous system may further influence depth-of-anesthesia devices. Administration of esmolol has been shown to markedly decrease BIS in propofol and alfentanil-infused humans, while sympathomimetics such as epinephrine increase arousal and BIS values [96,97]. These drug idiosyncrasies can easily create an inaccurate assessment of anesthetic depth and necessitate careful individual patient interpretation. Other factors such as patient age, hypothermia, pre-existing neurologic disease, and electrical interference from nearby medical devices may further influence and confound depth-of-anesthesia devices [43–45].

Is there a clear benefit to using depth-of-anesthesia devices? A 2017 systematic review and meta-analysis in humans found that the use of BIS monitoring reduced time to extubation, to attain orientation in time and place, and to discharge from both the operating room and postanesthetic care unit. The risk of nausea and vomiting after surgery also was reduced by 12%. A 3% reduction in the risk of cognitive impairment postoperatively at 3 months and a 6% reduction in the risk of postoperative delirium were also identified. Additionally, the risk of intraoperative recall was also reduced by 1% [98]. Despite these benefits, a 2004 meta-analysis also identified that the cost savings from reduced drug costs and time in the early recovery period were offset by the cost of the depth-of-anesthesia device itself and the cost of the monitoring electrodes [99].

The routine application of depth-of-anesthesia devices in animals is questionable since their algorithms are based on data collected in humans. March and Muir reviewed the use of BIS in animal species and suggested that interspecies differences in the EEG features associated with different hypnotic and amnesic states may affect the correlation between BIS values and depth of anesthesia [100]. To further complicate the picture, there currently is no consensus in human or veterinary anesthesiology on how to validate depth-of-anesthesia devices or even how best to determine depth of anesthesia. The absence of such "gold standards" limits the present-day anesthesiologist's ability to compare or judge future technologies [101]. In 2014, Schneider *et al.* performed a "head-to-head" comparison in humans between electroencephalogram-based monitoring (BIS), standard parameter-based monitoring (heart rate, blood pressure, end-tidal anesthetic concentration, and propofol concentration), or both strategies together, which were used to calculate an anesthesia multimodal index of consciousness (AMIC) [102]. Their work concluded that the use of the AMIC, including integration of both standard monitoring and electroencephalographic parameters more precisely reflected the depth-of-anesthesia compared to BIS or standard monitoring alone. Ultimately, if depth-of-anesthesia devices are to be used in veterinary anesthesia, they should be used cautiously and only in combination with other modalities such as Guedel's physical signs of anesthetic depth, inhalant anesthetic concentrations, and injectable drug plasma concentrations, and not used as the sole mechanism of determining anesthetic depth.

References

1 American Society of Anesthesiologists Committee on Quality Management and Departmental Administration. Continuum of depth of sedation: definition of general anesthesia and levels of sedation/analgesia. Position statement last amended on October 23, 2019. www.asahq.org/standards-and-practice-parameters/statement-on-continuum-of-depth-of-sedation-definition-of-general-anesthesia-and-levels-of-sedation-analgesia (accessed June 2023).

2 Mashour GA. Integrating the science of consciousness and anesthesia. *Anesth Analg* 2006; **103**: 975–982.

3 Sandin RH, Enlund G, Samuelsson P, *et al.* Awareness during anaesthesia: a prospective study. *Lancet* 2000; **355**: 707–711.

4 Myles PS, Leslie K, McNeil J, *et al.* Bispectral Index monitoring to prevent awareness during anesthesia: the B-Aware randomized controlled trial. *Lancet* 2004; **363**: 1757–1763.

5 Sebel PS, Bowdle TA, Ghoneim MM, *et al.* The incidence of awareness during anesthesia: a multicenter United States study. *Anesth Analg* 2004; **99**: 833–839.

6 Rungreungvanich M, Lekprasert V, Sirinan C, *et al.* An analysis of intraoperative recall of awareness in Thai Anesthesia Incidents Study (Thai Study). *J Med Assoc Thai* 2005; **88**: S95–S101.

7 Ghoneim MM, Block RI. Learning and memory during general anaesthesia, an update. *Anaesthesiology* 1997; **87**: 387.

8 Chortkoff B, Eger EI, Crankshaw DP, *et al.* Concentrations of desflurane and propofol that suppress response to command in humans. *Anest Analg* 1995; **81**: 737–743.

9 Eger EI. Age, minimum alveolar anesthetic concentration, and minimum alveolar anesthetic concentration-awake. *Anesth Analg* 2001; **93**(4): 947–953.

10 Aranake A, Mashour GA, Avidan MS. Minimum alveolar concentration: ongoing relevance and clinical utility. *Anaesthesia* 2013; **68**(5): 512–522.

11 Sessler DI. Red hair and anesthetic requirement. *Can J Anesth* 2015; **62**: 333–337.

12 Liem EB, Lin CM, Suleman MI, *et al.* Anesthetic requirement is increased in redheads. *Anesthesiology* 2004; **101**(2): 279–283.

13 Guedel AE. Third stage ether anesthesia: a sub-classification regarding the significance of the position and movements of the eyeball. *Pa Med J* 1921; **24**: 375–380.

14 Gugino LD, Aglio LS, Yli-Hankala A. Monitoring the electroencephalogram during bypass procedures. *Semin Cardiothorac Vasc Anesth* 2004; **8**: 61–83.

15 Angel A. Central neuronal pathways and the process of anaesthesia. *Br J Anaesth* 1993; **71**: 148–163.

16 Noachtar S, Binnie C, Ebersole J, *et al.* A glossary of terms most commonly used by clinical electroencephalographers and proposal for the report form for the EEG findings. *Klin Neurophysiol* 2004; **35**: 5–21.

17 Jasper HH. Report of the committee on methods of clinical examination in electroencephalography. *Electroencephalogr Clin Neurophysiol* 1957; **10**: 370–375.

18 Tooley MA, Grant LJ, Davies AR. A microprocessor based instrument for the spectral analysis of the EEG in anaesthesia. *Clin Phys Physiol Meas* 1984; **5**: 303–311.

19 Prince DA, Shanzer S. Effects of anesthetic upon the EEG response to reticular stimulation. Patterns of slow synchrony. *Electroencephalogr Clin Neurophysiol* 1966; **21**: 578–588.

20 Rampil IJ. A primer for EEG signal processing in anesthesia. *Anesthesiology* 1998; **89**: 980–1002.

21 John ER, Prichep LS. The anesthetic cascade: a theory of how anesthesia suppresses consciousness. *Anesthesiology* 2005; **102**: 447–471.

22 Berger H. Über das elektroenzephalogramm des menschen. *Achte mitteilung. Arch Psychiat* 1934; **101**: 452–469.

23 Moruzzi G, Magoun HW. Brain stem reticular formation and activation of the EEG. *Electroencephalogr Clin Neurophysiol* 1949; **1**: 455–473.

24 Arduini A, Arduini MG. Effect of drugs and metabolic alterations on brainstem arousal mechanism. *J Pharmacol Exp Ther* 1954; **110**: 76–85.

25 Skinner JE, Lindsley DB. Electrophysiological and behavioral effects of blockade of the nonspecific thalamo-cortical system. *Brain Res* 1967; **6**: 95–118.
26 Hughes JR, John ER. Conventional and quantitative electroencephalography in psychiatry. *J Neuropsychiatry Clin Neurosci* 1999; **11**: 190–208.
27 John ER. A field theory of consciousness. *Conscious Cogn* 2001; **10**: 184–213.
28 John ER, Prichep LS, Knox W, *et al.* Invariant reversible QEEG effects of anesthetics. *Conscious Cogn* 2001; **10**: 165–183.
29 Kaada BR, Thomas F, Alnaes E, *et al.* EEG synchronization induced by high frequency midbrain reticular stimulation in anesthetized cats. *Electroencephalogr Clin Neurophysiol* 1967; **22**: 220–230.
30 Gibbs FA, Gibbs EL, Lennox WG. Effect on the electroencephalogram of certain drugs which influence nervous activity. *Arch Intern Med (Chic)* 1937; **60**(1): 154–166.
31 Martin JT, Faulconer A, Bickford RG. Electroencephalography in anesthesiology. *Anesthesiology* 1959; **20**(3): 359–376.
32 Kaieda R, Todd MM, Warner DS. The effects of anesthetics and PaCO2 on the cerebrovascular, metabolic, and electroencephalographic responses to nitrous oxide in the rabbit. *Anesth Analg* 1989; **68**: 135–143.
33 Schwender D, Daunderer M, Mulzer S, *et al.* Spectral edge frequency of the electroencephalogram to monitor 'depth' of anaesthesia with isoflurane or propofol. *Br J Anaesth* 1996; **77**: 179–184.
34 Eger EI II, Stevens WC, Cromwell TH. The electroencephalogram in man anesthetized with forane. *Anesthesiology* 1971; **35**: 504–508.
35 Kiersey DK, Bickford RG, Faulconer A Jr. Electro-encephalographic patterns produced by thiopental sodium during surgical operations: description and classification. *Br J Anaesth* 1951; **23**: 141–152.
36 Clark DL, Rosner BS. Neurophysiologic effects of general anesthetics. I. The electroencephalogram and sensory evoked responses in man. *Anesthesiology* 1973; **38**: 564–582.
37 Keifer JC, Baghdoyan HA, Lydic R. Pontine cholinergic mechanisms modulate the cortical electroencephalographic spindles of halothane anesthesia. *Anesthesiology* 1996; **84**: 945–954.
38 Feshchenko VA, Veselis RA, Reinsel RA. Propofol-induced alpha rhythm. *Neuropsychobiology* 2004; **50**: 257–266.
39 Gugino LD, Chabot RJ, Prichep LS, *et al.* Quantitative EEG changes associated with loss and return of consciousness in healthy adult volunteers anaesthetized with propofol or sevoflurane. *Br J Anaesth* 2001; **87**: 421–428.
40 Newberg LA, Milde JH, Michenfelder JD. The cerebral metabolic effects of isoflurane at and above concentrations that suppress cortical electrical activity. *Anesthesiology* 1983; **59**: 23–28.
41 Hans P, Dewandre PY, Brichant JF, *et al.* Comparative effects of ketamine on Bispectral Index and spectral entropy of the electroencephalogram under sevoflurane anaesthesia. *Br J Anaesth* 2005; **94**(3): 336–340.
42 Mishra RK, Mahajan C, Prabhakar H, *et al.* Effect of nitrous oxide on Bispectral Index values at equi-minimum alveolar concentrations of sevoflurane and desflurane. *Indian J Anaesth* 2017; **61**(6): 482–485.
43 Bannister CF, Brosius KK, Sigl JC, *et al.* The effect of Bispectral Index monitoring on anesthetic use and recovery in children anesthetized with sevoflurane in nitrous oxide. *Anesth Analg* 2001; **92**(4): 877–881.
44 Doi M, Gajraj RJ, Mantzaridis H, *et al.* Effects of cardiopulmonary bypass and hypothermia on electroencephalographic variables. *Anaesthesia* 1997; **52**(11): 1048–1055.
45 Chan MT, Ho SS, Gin T. Performance of the Bispectral Index during electrocautery. *J Neurosurg Anesthesiol* 2012; **24**(1): 9–13.
46 Johansen J, Sebel P. Develop and clinical application of electroencephalographic bispectrum monitoring. *Anesthesiology* 2000; **93**: 1336–1344.
47 Bleijenberg EH, van Oostrom H, Akkerdaas LC, *et al.* Bispectral Index and the clinically evaluated anaesthetic depth in dogs. *Vet Anaesth Analg* 2011; **38**(6): 536–543.
48 Campagnol D, Teixeira Neto FJ, Monteiro ER, *et al.* Use of Bispectral Index to monitor depth of anesthesia in isoflurane-anesthetized dogs. *Am J Vet Res* 2007; **68**(12): 1300–1307.
49 Greene SA, Benson GJ, Tranquilli WJ, *et al.* Relationship of canine Bispectral Index to multiples of sevoflurane minimal alveolar concentration, using patch or subdermal electrodes. *Comp Med* 2002; **52**(5): 424–428.
50 Ubiali MLC, Meirelles GP, Vilani JM, *et al.* Evaluation of the anesthetic depth and Bispectral Index during propofol sequential target-controlled infusion in dogs. *Vet World* 2022; **15**(3): 537–542.
51 Van Soens I, Struys MM, Polis IE, *et al.* Effects of sedative and hypnotic drug combinations on transcranial magnetic motor evoked potential, Bispectral Index and ARX-derived auditory evoked potential index in dogs. *Vet J* 2009; **181**(2): 163–170.
52 de Mattos-Junior E, Ito KC, Conti-Patara A, *et al.* Bispectral monitoring in dogs subjected to ovariohysterectomy and anesthetized with halothane, isoflurane or sevoflurane. *Vet Anaesth Analg* 2011; **38**(5): 475–483.
53 Lopes PC, Nunes N, Paula DP, *et al.* Bispectral Index in dogs at three intravenous infusion rates of propofol. *Vet Anaesth Analg* 2008; **35**(3): 228–231.
54 Ebner LS, Lerche P, Bednarski RM, *et al.* Effect of dexmedetomidine, morphine–lidocaine–ketamine, and dexmedetomidine–morphine–lidocaine–ketamine constant rate infusions on the minimum alveolar concentration of isoflurane and Bispectral Index in dogs. *Am J Vet Res* 2013; **74**(7): 963–970.
55 Henao-Guerrero PN, McMurphy R, Kukanich B, *et al.* Effect of morphine on the Bispectral Index during isoflurane anesthesia in dogs. *Vet Anaesth Analg* 2009; **36**(2): 133–143.
56 Belda E, Laredo FG, Lucas X, *et al.* The effects of atracurium on Bispectral Index (BIS) values in dogs anaesthetized with isoflurane. *Vet J* 2012; **192**(2): 189–192.
57 Morgaz J, Granados MM, Domínguez JM, *et al.* Relationship of Bispectral Index to hemodynamic variables and alveolar concentration multiples of sevoflurane in puppies. *Res Vet Sci* 2009; **86**(3): 508–513.
58 Saenubol P, Akatvipat A, Pleumsamran A, *et al.* Correlation between Bispectral Index value and modified Glasgow coma scale score in dogs with altered level of consciousness. *J Vet Emerg Crit Care (San Antonio)* 2021; **31**(1): 52–58.
59 Lamont LA, Greene SA, Grimm KA, *et al.* Relationship of Bispectral Index to minimum alveolar concentration multiples of sevoflurane in cats. *Am J Vet Res* 2004; **65**(1): 93–98.
60 March PA, Muir WW. Use of the Bispectral Index as a monitor of anesthetic depth in cats anesthetized with isoflurane. *Am J Vet Res* 2003; **64**(12): 1534–1541.
61 Tokushige H, Kakizaki M, Ode H, *et al.* Validation of the Bispectral Index as an indicator of anesthetic depth in Thoroughbred horses anesthetized with sevoflurane. *J Equine Sci* 2016; **27**(4): 169–173.
62 Haga HA, Dolvik NI. Evaluation of the Bispectral Index as an indicator of degree of central nervous system depression in isoflurane-anesthetized horses. *Am J Vet Res* 2002; **63**(3): 438–442.
63 Belda E, Blissitt KJ, Duncan JC, *et al.* The Bispectral Index during recovery from halothane and sevoflurane anaesthesia in horses. *Vet Anaesth Analg* 2010; **37**(1): 25–34.
64 Yamashita K, Akashi N, Kataymaa Y, *et al.* Evaluation of Bispectral Index (BIS) as an indicator of central nervous system depression in horses anesthetized with propofol. *J Vet Med Sci* 2009; **71**(11): 1465–1471.
65 Antognini JF, Wang XW, Carstens E. Isoflurane anaesthetic depth in goats monitored using the Bispectral Index of the electroencephalogram. *Vet Res Commun* 2000; **24**(6): 361–370.
66 Martín-Cancho MF, Lima JR, Luis L, *et al.* Bispectral Index, spectral edge frequency 95%, and median frequency recorded for various concentrations of isoflurane and sevoflurane in pigs. *Am J Vet Res* 2003; **64**(7): 866–873.
67 Deschk M, Wagatsuma JT, Araújo MA, *et al.* Continuous infusion of propofol in calves: Bispectral Index and hemodynamic effects. *Vet Anaesth Analg* 2016; **43**(3): 309–315.
68 Martín-Cancho MF, Lima JR, Luis L, *et al.* Relationship of Bispectral Index values, haemodynamic changes and recovery times during sevoflurane or propofol anaesthesia in rabbits. *Lab Anim* 2006; **40**(1): 28–42.
69 Howard RS, Finneran JJ, Ridgway SH. Bispectral Index monitoring of unihemispheric effects in dolphins. *Anesth Analg* 2006; **103**(3): 626–632.
70 Garcia-Pereira FL, Greene SA, Keegan RD, *et al.* Effects of intravenous butorphanol on cardiopulmonary function in isoflurane-anesthetized alpacas. *Vet Anaesth Analg* 2007; **34**(4): 269–274.
71 Martin-Jurado O, Vogt R, Kutter AP, *et al.* Effect of inhalation of isoflurane at end-tidal concentrations greater than, equal to, and less than the minimum anesthetic concentration on Bispectral Index in chickens. *Am J Vet Res* 2008; **69**(10): 1254–1261.
72 Litscher G. Ten years evidence-based high-tech acupuncture. Part 3: a short review of animal experiments. *Evid Based Complement Alternat Med* 2010; **7**(2): 151–155.
73 Kreeger TJ, Huizenga M, Hansen C, *et al.* Sufentanil and xylazine immobilization of Rocky Mountain elk. *J Wildl Dis* 2011; **47**(3): 638–642.
74 Shannon CE. A mathematical theory of communication. *Bell Syst Tech J* 1948; **27**: 379–423, 623–656.
75 Viertiö-Oja H, Maja V, Särkelä M, *et al.* Description of the Entropy algorithm as applied in the Datex-Ohmeda S/5 Entropy Module. *Acta Anaesthesiol Scand* 2004; **48**(2): 154–161.
76 Ellerkmann RK, Soehle M, Alves TM, *et al.* Spectral entropy and Bispectral Index as measures of the electroencephalographic effects of propofol. *Anesth Analg* 2006; **102**(5): 1456–1462.
77 Ellerkmann RK, Liermann VM, Alves TM, *et al.* Spectral entropy and Bispectral Index as measures of the electroencephalographic effects of sevoflurane. *Anesthesiology* 2004; **101**(6): 1275–1282.
78 Vakkuri A, Yli-Hankala A, Talja P, *et al.* Time-frequency balanced spectral entropy as a measure of anesthetic drug effect in central nervous system during sevoflurane, propofol, and thiopental anesthesia. *Acta Anaesthesiol Scand* 2004; **48**(2): 145–153.

79 Navarrete-Calvo R, Morgaz J, Gómez-Villamandos RJ, *et al.* Comparison of Bispectral Index and spectral entropy during isoflurane and medetomidine general anaesthesia in horses. *Equine Vet J* 2020; **52**(5): 678–684.

80 Morgaz J, Granados MM, Domínguez JM, *et al.* Evaluation of spectral entropy to measure anaesthetic depth and antinociception in sevoflurane-anaesthetised Beagle dogs. *Vet J* 2011; **188**(3): 352–355.

81 Drover D, Ortega HR. Patient state index. *Best Pract Res Clin Anaesthesiol* 2006; **20**(1):121–128.

82 Bollen, PJ, Saxtorph, H. Cerebral state monitoring in Beagle dogs sedated with medetomidine. *Vet Anaesth Analg* 2006; **33**: 237–240.

83 Ribeiro LM, Ferreira DA, Bressan NM, *et al.* Brain monitoring in dogs using the cerebral state index during the induction of anesthesia via target-controlled infusion of propofol. *Res Vet Sci* 2008; **85**: 227–232.

84 Ribeiro LM, Ferreira DA, Bras S, *et al.* Correlation between clinical signs of depth of anaesthesia and cerebral state index responses in dogs during induction of anaesthesia with propofol. *Res Vet Sci* 2009; **87**: 287–291.

85 Bollen PJ, Nielsen BJ, Toft P. Influence of endotoxin-induced sepsis on the requirements of propofol–fentanyl infusion rate in pigs. *Basic Clin Pharmacol Toxicol* 2007; **101**(3): 192–196.

86 Loomis, AL, Harvey EN, Hobart GA. Cerebral states during sleep, as studied by human brain potentials. *J Exper Psych* 1937; **21**(2): 127–144.

87 Schultz B, Grouven U, Schultz A. Automatic classification algorithms of the EEG monitor Narcotrend for routinely recorded EEG data from general anaesthesia: a validation study. *Biomed Tech* 2002; **47**: 9–13.

88 Raue JF, Tünsmeyer J, Kästner SBR. Effects of isoflurane, remifentanil and dexmedetomidine on selected EEG parameters derived from a Narcotrend Monitor before and after nociceptive stimulation at different MAC multiples in cats. *BMC Vet Res* 2020; **16**(1): 332.

89 Kreuzer M, Zanner R, Pilge S, *et al.* Time delay of monitors of the hypnotic component of anesthesia: analysis of state entropy and index of consciousness. *Anesth Analg* 2012; **115**(2): 315–319.

90 Kurita T, Doi M, Katoh T, *et al.* Auditory evoked potential index predicts the depth of sedation and movement in response to skin incision during sevoflurane anesthesia. *Anesthesiology* 2001; **95**(2): 364–370.

91 Matsushita S, Oda S, Otaki K, *et al.* Change in auditory evoked potential index and Bispectral Index during induction of anesthesia with anesthetic drugs. *J Clin Monit Comput* 2015 Oct; **29**(5): 621–626.

92 Pypendop B, Poncelet L, Verstegen J. Use of midlatency auditory-evoked potentials as indicator of unconsciousness in the dog: characterisation of the effects of acepromazine-thiopentone, medetomidine-thiopentone and medetomidine-butorphanol-midazolam combinations. *Res Vet Sci* 1999; **67**(1): 35–39.

93 Joubert KE. Does the A-line ARX-Index provide a reasonable assessment of anaesthetic depth in dogs undergoing routine surgery? *J S Afr Vet Assoc* 2004; **75**(3): 110–115.

94 Joubert KE. Preliminary assessment of the AAI Index during isoflurane anaesthesia in dogs undergoing clinical procedures. *J S Afr Vet Assoc* 2009; **80**(3): 185–187.

95 Murrell JC, de Groot HN, Psatha E, *et al.* Investigation of changes in the middle latency auditory evoked potential during anesthesia with sevoflurane in dogs. *Am J Vet Res* 2005; **66**(7): 1156–1161.

96 Johansen JW. Esmolol promotes electroencephalographic burst suppression during propofol/alfentanil anesthesia. *Anesth Analg* 2001; **93**(6): 1526–1531.

97 Andrzejowski J, Sleigh JW, Johnson IA, *et al.* The effect of intravenous epinephrine on the Bispectral Index and sedation. *Anaesthesia* 2000; **55**(8): 761–763.

98 Oliveira CR, Bernardo WM, Nunes VM. Benefit of general anesthesia monitored by Bispectral Index compared with monitoring guided only by clinical parameters. Systematic review and meta-analysis. *Braz J Anesthesiol* 2017; **67**(1): 72–84.

99 Liu SS. Effects of Bispectral Index monitoring on ambulatory anesthesia: a meta-analysis of randomized controlled trials and a cost analysis. *Anesthesiology* 2004; **101**(2): 311–315.

100 March PA, Muir WW. Bispectral analysis of the electroencephalogram: a review of its development and use in anesthesia. *Vet Anaesth Analg* 2005; **32**: 241–255.

101 Heyse B, Van Ooteghem B, Wyler B, *et al.* Comparison of contemporary EEG derived depth of anesthesia monitors with a 5 step validation process. *Acta Anaesthesiol Belg* 2009; **60**(1): 19–33.

102 Schneider G, Jordan D, Schwarz G, *et al.* European Multicenter EEGAEP Anesthesia Monitoring Study Group and Research Group Knowledge-based Signal Processing. Monitoring depth of anesthesia utilizing a combination of electroencephalographic and standard measures. *Anesthesiology* 2014; **120**(4): 819–828.

11 Electrocardiography

Kyle J. Bartholomew
Department of Surgical Sciences, School of Veterinary Medicine, University of Wisconsin, Madison, Wisconsin, USA

Chapter contents

Introduction, 187
Electrical potentials and the lead system, 187
  Einthoven's triangle, 188
  Bipolar, unipolar, and precordial leads, 188
The ECG complex, 189
Evaluating an ECG, 190
  Heart rate calculation, 190
  Rhythm evaluation, 191
  Mean electrical axis, 191
Species-specific variations, 192
  Canine, 192
  Feline, 192
  Equine, 192
ECG equipment, 194
  Artifacts and filters, 194
Effect of anesthesia, 195
References, 195

Introduction

An electrocardiogram (ECG) is the graphical representation of the cardiac electrical activity recorded over time. The ECG allows the anesthetist to evaluate the heart rate and rhythm and, when evaluated in combination with blood pressure and other indicators of tissue perfusion and cardiac output, allows for an assessment of the cardiovascular status of the patient. Many disease states may lead to the development of arrhythmias (e.g., electrolyte disturbances, diseases of splanchnic viscera, paraneoplastic diseases, etc.), and some anesthetic drugs can increase the risk of spontaneous arrhythmias in otherwise healthy animals [1–4]. Due to the widespread availability of this technology, ECG monitoring should be considered for any patient undergoing anesthesia, even for short-duration or routine procedures.

A normal ECG is easily recognizable and represents the electrical activity of the heart. However, to understand why and how an abnormal rhythm may develop, it is important to understand the basic physics behind the ECG as well as the minor species differences. It is also important to understand the limitations of an ECG and how to differentiate common artifacts from true arrhythmias.

Electrical potentials and the lead system

There are many different systems available that can obtain an ECG; the underlying principles remain fairly constant between machines. Understanding the basics of electrocardiography requires integration of multiple concepts including generation of the cardiac action potential, the equivalent dipole theory, and the lead system. The cardiac action potential is covered in detail elsewhere (see Chapter 33). What follows is a brief description of the equivalent dipole theory, cardiac vectors, and the lead system.

The equivalent dipole theory states that the heart can be approximated to a dipole (i.e., it is equivalent to a dipole when measured); the force that is generated has a direction and magnitude and can be represented as a vector [5,6]. A dipole is a pair of electrical charges of equal and opposite polarity that are separated by a distance. The electrical potential generated can be measured with a galvanometer, which consists of two exploring electrodes placed on each side of the system. The electrical potential measured by the galvanometer is dependent on the intensity of the electrical force generated, the distance the electrodes from the dipole, and the position of the electrodes relative to the orientation of the dipole. Depolarization of the myocardium generates electrical forces of varying magnitudes and directions; this electrical activity can be thought of as vectors of electrical activation. Electrical activity occurring simultaneously creates a summation vector. The magnitude of these vectors is detected on the body surface, depending on the site of the exploring electrode and the direction of the vector. The electrode placed on a line parallel to the direction of the vector will be able to record the maximum amplitude of that activity [6].

When several exploring electrodes are attached on the surface of the patient, it is possible to record the magnitude and direction of

Veterinary Anesthesia and Analgesia: The Sixth Edition of Lumb and Jones. Edited by Leigh Lamont, Kurt Grimm, Sheilah Robertson, Lydia Love and Carrie Schroeder.
© 2024 John Wiley & Sons, Inc. Published 2024 by John Wiley & Sons, Inc.
Companion website: www.wiley.com/go/lamont/anesthesia

these cardiac vectors. The ECG records the electric potential (in mV, on the y axis) over time (in seconds, on the x axis) between a point on the body surface and an indifferent (or reference) electrode or between two recording electrodes. The lines joining these electrodes form what we refer to as "leads" along which the cardiac vectors are measured [6]. Leads may be defined as unipolar or bipolar. If the potential is recorded between an electrode on the body surface (exploring electrode) and an indifferent (or reference) electrode, the leads are unipolar. If the difference is recorded between two recording electrodes, the leads are bipolar.

The voltage change recorded by the leads is displayed graphically. Each electrical wave is defined by its amplitude, polarity, and duration. When the cardiac depolarization vector is parallel to the lead, the wave is of maximum amplitude; a depolarization vector perpendicular to the lead produces a wave of minimal amplitude. Typically, a vector directed toward the positive electrode is represented as a positive wave and a vector directed toward the negative electrode is represented as a negative wave.

Einthoven's triangle

Due to the directionality of an ECG, the direction of electrical activity can be "seen" from different directions depending on the leads used. A diagnostic ECG may be capable of up to 12 viewpoints in two planes: frontal and transverse. Clinically, the frontal plane is most commonly used.

Electrodes placed on the right forelimb, left forelimb, and left hindlimb make up an arrangement known as "Einthoven's triangle," named after Willem Einthoven, a Dutch doctor who is credited with developing the first apparatus utilized to detect electrical activity of the heart. The three potential differences created by this arrangement are called leads I, II, and III (Fig. 11.1). It has been suggested that this naming convention is largely historical, based on Einthoven's original description, rather than any intrinsic meaning [7].

Bipolar, unipolar, and precordial leads

Leads I, II, and III are referred to as the "standard bipolar leads" because they measure between two points of the electrodes (Fig. 11.1). Lead I measures the potential difference between the right and left forelimb with the left considered positive. Lead II, the most common lead used clinically, is between the right forelimb and left hindlimb with the hindlimb considered positive. Lead III is between the left forelimb and left hindlimb with the hindlimb considered positive [7].

As bipolar leads (and lead II specifically) are the primary leads utilized in perianesthetic monitoring, they will be the focus of the rest of the chapter; however, the other diagnostic leads are briefly discussed below. Because a lead is, by nature, the potential difference between two points, the theoretical number of leads that could exist is nearly limitless. Cardiologists commonly use other lead systems, such as the modified orthogonal lead system, and the descriptions provided below should by no means be considered exhaustive, only a summary of common configurations that may be used in the perianesthetic period [6].

The unipolar leads are created by comparing the three electrodes to a reference voltage created by the monitor, known as "Wilson's central terminal." The signal between the three electrodes and the reference (Wilson's central terminal) are known as aVL (left forelimb), aVR (right forelimb), and aVF (left hindlimb). These are also known as the "augmented limb leads," and they allow for a slightly different angle of evaluation in the frontal plane [7].

The unipolar precordial leads are based on a similar concept: six additional electrodes can be placed on the thorax near the heart and are compared to a reference electrode (Wilson's central terminal).

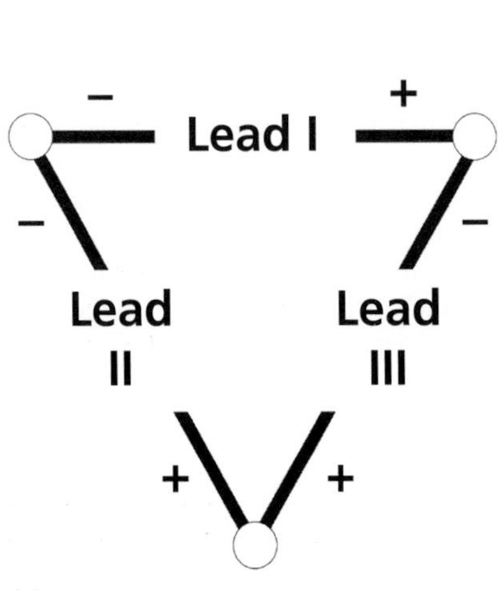

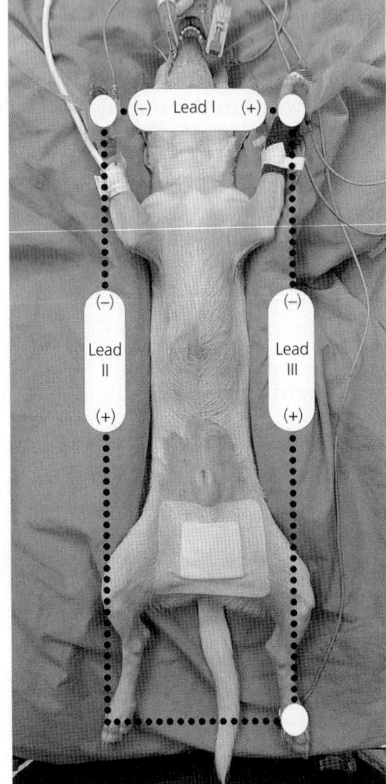

Figure 11.1 **A.** Einthoven's Triangle, the basic schematic for the modern bipolar lead system. **B.** Standard bipolar lead placement in a dog, used on most small domestic species; the white lead (RA) is placed on the right forelimb, the black lead (LA) is placed on the left forelimb, and the red lead (LL) is placed on the left hindlimb. Source: Dr. Kyle Bartholomew, with permission.

These leads (V1–V6) provide information in the transverse plane rather than the frontal plane like other leads. The precordial system is used with some frequency in human patients; however, it is less commonly used in veterinary medicine during the perianesthetic period.

In small animals, a multilead ECG may be used to generate targeted information about chamber enlargement, and lead II is used predominantly to monitor patients intraoperatively. In horses, however, it has been suggested that a multilead ECG is of less value because of the extensive branching of the Purkinje system in the ventricles. In these cases, a single-lead system is typically sufficient to optimize the signal along the direction of the maximal deflection of the electrical impulse generated within the heart. To accomplish this, the electrodes are placed parallel to this impulse in what is often referred to as the "base-apex lead" (Fig. 11.2) [8]. Although there is some debate as to whether the base-apex lead is the most effective lead for diagnostic evaluation of the horse, it is currently the most well established [9]. It has also been suggested that the base-apex lead arrangement accentuates the P wave of the equine ECG [10]. This arrangement historically uses the lead I setting with the negative (−) electrode (right forelimb/RA/white) placed over the jugular furrow or near the manubrium. The positive (+) electrode (left forelimb/LL/black) may be placed over the left apex of the heart, on the left side of the chest at the level of the olecranon or at the xiphoid. The ground electrode (left hindlimb/LL/red) may be attached to either side of the neck. Some portable ECG monitors utilize only two electrodes, which can be used to generate a single lead; the lead that is generated (I, II, or III) depends on where the electrodes are placed.

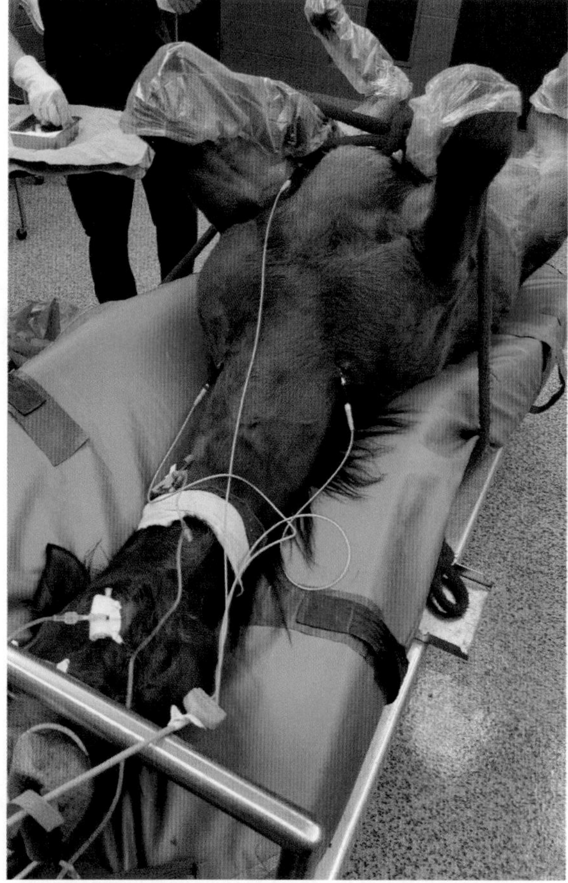

Figure 11.2 Base-apex lead arrangement in a horse: bipolar lead I is used with the right forelimb (RA/white) electrode placed over the jugular furrow, the left forelimb (LA/black) electrode placed on the left side of the chest just caudal to the forelimb, and ground electrode (left hindlimb/LL/red) is attached to either side of the neck. Source: Dr. Kyle Bartholomew, with permission.

It is also important to note that many systems available in North America use a standard color-coding system of right forelimb or RA (white), left forelimb or LA (black), and left hindlimb or LL (red). This color scheme is not always the same as that used internationally [11].

The ECG complex

The ECG complex is a representation of the electrical activity occurring in the myocardium during a single cardiac cycle, from cell depolarization at the beginning of the cycle to the cell repolarization at the end of the cycle. Different terminology may be used by different sources to discuss these concepts, but terms used here are wave, segment, and interval. A "wave" represents an electrical event in the myocardium and is represented as a deflection above or below baseline. A segment is a line joining two waves, and an interval is the time (or graphical distance) between two events. The primary deflections in an ECG are the P wave, the Q, R, and S waves (often referred to as the "QRS complex"), and the T wave (Fig. 11.3) [12].

In a normal heart, the cardiac cycle begins at the sinoatrial (SA) node, a small group of cells located in the right atrium that act as the dominant pacemaker of the heart. This event is not represented by a wave on the ECG due to the small number of cells that make up the SA node and, therefore, the very small amount of voltage this event produces. However, immediately following SA node activation, a wave of depolarization travels across the atria facilitated by the atrial conduction system, including Bachmann's bundle [13]. The depolarization of the atria is represented by the P wave on the ECG. As the wave of depolarization sweeps across the atria, it eventually reaches the atrioventricular (AV) node. The wave of depolarization propagates through the AV node and along the

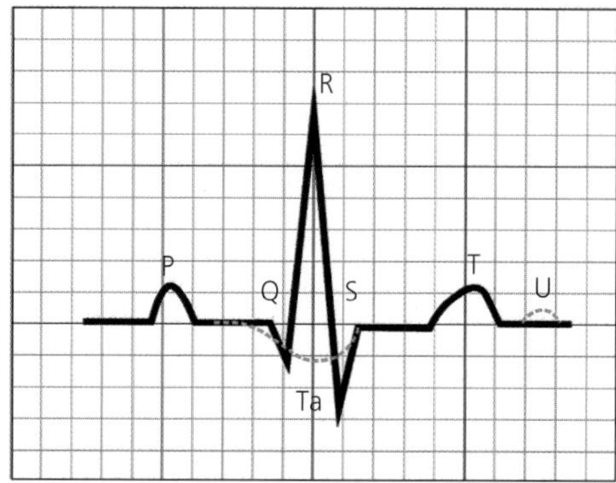

Figure 11.3 An example of the classic ECG recording; the P wave represents atrial depolarization and the QRS complex represents ventricular depolarization. The T wave represents ventricular repolarization. The blue dotted structures are rarely appreciated, the U wave is theorized to originate from late repolarization of the mid-myocardial cells or Purkinje cells and may be seen in patients who are bradycardic or suffering from hypokalemia; the Ta wave represents atrial repolarization and is rarely seen because its occurrence during the QRS complex obscures it. Source: Dr. Kyle Bartholomew, with permission.

bundle of His before following the right and left bundle branches and, finally, through the Purkinje network on its way to the contractile cardiac myocytes. The time it takes for the wave of depolarization to propagate from the atria through the ventricular conduction system is represented by the PQ (also referred to as PR) interval and is defined as the time from the onset of the P wave to the onset of the QRS complex [12]. The extensive Purkinje network spreads the impulse to the contractile cardiac myocytes starting at the apex of the heart and begins the formation of the QRS complex (i.e., the three waves representing ventricular depolarization: Q, R, and S). It should be noted that most individuals refer to the complex that represents ventricular depolarization as the QRS, regardless of whether the complex contains a distinct Q, R, and S wave. Mechanical contraction of the myocardium follows electrical depolarization. After depolarization, repolarization of the ventricles follows to reestablish the cellular electrical potential that allows for the next electrical depolarization and mechanical contraction. The electrical repolarization of the ventricle is represented as the T wave on the ECG. The atria also experience repolarization which is sometimes represented as the Ta wave on the ECG; however, this wave normally occurs during the depolarization of the ventricles (i.e., the QRS complex) and, therefore, is obscured due to the larger electrical potential of ventricular depolarization. The ST segment, defined as the segment between the end of the QRS complex (sometimes referred to as the J point) and the T wave, corresponds to ventricular systole during which the membrane potential of ventricular myocytes is equal and is, therefore, normally represented as a horizontal line [12]. The J wave and U wave are two underappreciated waves that may represent early and late ventricular repolarization, respectively. In humans, the J wave may be appreciated in a normal heart but can also appear as result of hypothermia, hypercalcemia, or myocardial ischemia [14,15]. The U wave, theorized to originate from repolarization of the mid-myocardial cells (M cells) or Purkinje cells, may be seen in patients who are bradycardic or suffer from hypokalemia [15].

The line that occurs between the end of the T wave and the beginning of the next P wave is generally called "baseline" or the "isoelectric line" and is associated with the absence of electrical activity. This becomes important when considering the pauses that occur during a single cardiac depolarization and the time between the cardiac cycles.

Evaluating an ECG

Evaluation of an ECG during anesthesia can give valuable information about the patient's heart rate and can lead to early recognition of dysrhythmias that could become pathologic if left untreated. However, perianesthetic ECG interpretation may come with limitations, such as patient positioning, limited sites for electrode placement, and operating room artifacts. Therefore, ECG tracings recorded as part of continuous anesthetic monitoring may not meet all the recommendations for standardization associated with a fully diagnostic ECG. Regardless, there is still crucially important information that may be obtained from perianesthetic ECG monitoring.

When evaluating the ECG, it is important to note that the horizontal axis of an ECG printout (also referred to as a strip or tracing) is time in seconds while the vertical axis is voltage, displayed in millivolts (mV). It is also important to note the underlying paper or sweep speed, the rate at which the ECG paper or screen travels while the ECG is being traced, commonly 25 mm/s or 50 mm/s. At a faster paper speed (50 mm/s), each small box (1 mm) on the horizontal axis represents 0.02 s and the ECG complex will appear wider. At a slower speed (25 mm/s), each small box represents 0.04 s, and the ECG complex will appear narrower comparatively.

Heart rate calculation

The ECG can be used as a source for determining the patient's heart rate; however, it can be susceptible to artifact and interference, which may make automated heart rate calculation by the monitor less accurate. There are multiple methods available to manually calculate a heart rate from a printed ECG. The simplest, albeit least accurate, way to calculate the heart rate is to determine the number of R waves within 3 s and multiply by 20 to obtain beats per minute (Fig. 11.4) [16].

A more useful method, especially in patients with an irregular rhythm, is calculation of an "instantaneous" heart rate using only one R-R interval, defined as the distance between two sequential R waves of the QRS complex. This method requires knowledge of the underlying paper or sweep speed. The R-R interval can be counted in terms of small boxes (mm); the number of boxes counted can then be multiplied by s/mm (0.02 for 50 mm/s paper speed and 0.04 for 25 mm/s paper speed) to obtain the amount of time (seconds) per beat. To convert this into beats per minute, simply divide 60 (s/min) by the number of seconds per beat. For example, an R-R interval that was counted to be 18 small boxes at a paper speed of 25 mm/s would be:

$$18 \text{ mm} \times 0.04 \text{ mm/s} = 0.72 \text{ s per R-R interval; and}$$

$$60 \text{ s/min} \div 0.72 \text{ s per interval} = 83.3 \text{ beats/min}$$

The instantaneous heart rate would be 83 beats/min. An alternative, and arguably easier method, is to divide the number of mm per minute by the number of mm between beats (R-R interval) to obtain beats per minute (Fig. 11.4). For a 25-mm/s paper speed,

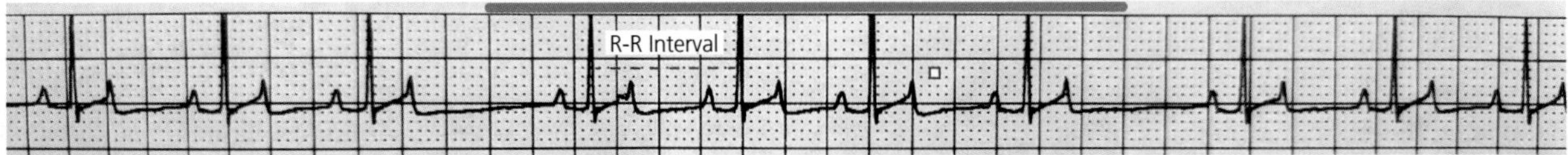

Figure 11.4 At the commonly used paper speed of 25 mm/s, 1 mm (small red outlined box) equals 0.04 s. At this speed, the blue line (75 mm) represents roughly 3 s (3/0.04 = 75) or roughly the length of a ballpoint pen. The number of complexes that occur during this period can be multiplied by 20 to roughly estimate the beats per minute (3 s × 20 = 60 s). The number of complexes that occur under the blue line is 4, so in this example, the heart rate would be approximately 80 beats/min (4 × 20 = 80). Another method of determining heart rate, particularly useful in patients with irregular rhythms like the one seen here, is to count the R-R interval in millimeters and divide this number into 1500 (where 1500 is the number of mm per minute at 25 mm/s paper speed). In this example, the R-R interval is ~18 mm and (1500/18 = 83.3); therefore, the heart rate is estimated to be 83 beats/min. This second method is often referred to as the "instantaneous heart rate" method. Source: Dr. Kyle Bartholomew, with permission.

there are 1500 mm/min, and for 50 mm/s, there are 3000 mm/min. In the previous example, this would mean:

$$1500 \text{ mm/min} \div 18 \text{ mm R-R interval} = 83.3 \text{ beats/min}$$

Rhythm evaluation

There are many approaches to systematically evaluate an ECG, but many of them follow the same general pattern: evaluate the heart rate, recognize the presence of all the normal waves that make up the ECG complex, and evaluate if there are any beats that do not belong. A simplified algorithm can be found in Box 11.1 and is described below. An algorithm such as this is not meant to diagnose a specific condition; rather, it is to be used to help guide localization of where an issue might be arising. For example, if the QRS morphology is abnormal, one should consider that ventricular conduction may be abnormal, but it is up to the user to determine what the specific problem is and how to appropriately act.

First, determine heart rate as previously described. Then, determine if the ventricular and atrial rates match. Normally, there is a fixed interval between the P waves and QRS complexes (PQ interval); however, in some cases, the ventricular rate (R-R interval) may not match the atrial rate (P-P interval), and a separate heart rate assessment may be needed for atrial and ventricular rates in some circumstances. Next, assess if every P wave has an associated QRS omplex. Normally, there is a fixed relationship of one P wave preceding every QRS complex, while ectopic (or abnormal) QRS complexes often originate without a preceding atrial depolarization. Premature complexes occur before the next anticipated sinus beat, while escape complexes generally occur significantly later than the next expected sinus beat. Next, determine if every QRS complex has an associated P wave. In normal sinus rhythm and sinus arrhythmia, there will be a P wave preceding every QRS complex, and the interval between the P waves and QRS complexes will be consistent. However, in some instances, the electrical impulse is blocked at the AV node or His–Purkinje system, preventing propagation and depolarization of the ventricles (e.g., AV block). Finally, determine if the QRS complexes appear supraventricular or ventricular. In dogs and cats, if the electrical impulse originates from the sinus node, atrial myocardium, or AV node, the QRS complex will generally be tall, upright, and narrow, otherwise referred to as "supraventricular" [16]. If the electrical impulse originates from the ventricle, the QRS complex will be wide and abnormal in appearance (sometimes used synonymously with the term "ventricular") because it does not utilize the normal His–Purkinje system [17–19].

Systematic assessment of the ECG by this method will allow for a rapid and accurate diagnosis of heart rate and rhythm. A dysrhythmia (also often referred to as arrhythmia) denotes an irregularity in the cardiac rhythm. In-depth discussions of the diagnosis of dysrhythmias along with underlying mechanisms and treatments are covered elsewhere [13]. In short, dysrhythmias are often characterized by the anatomic place of origin, rate, and/or regularity. Supraventricular arrhythmias arise from the atria or AV node, while ventricular arrhythmias arise from the ventricles. When dysrhythmias originate from the AV node, they are sometimes more specifically classified as junctional. When further characterized by rate, slow rates are referred to as bradyarrhythmias (e.g., sinus bradycardia, AV block, and sinus arrest), while rapid rates are referred to as tachyarrhythmias (e.g., sinus tachycardia, ventricular tachycardia, and supraventricular tachycardia). Common arrhythmias that occur at normal rates are respiratory sinus arrhythmia, and accelerated idioventricular rhythm. Dysrhythmias may also be classified according to their regularity. For example, fibrillation is an irregular, chaotic rhythm (e.g., atrial fibrillation), while tachycardia is a regular (non-irregular) rhythm [17]. Once the rate and rhythm are characterized, further decisions on alterations of anesthetic management or treatment course can be made as needed.

Box 11.1 Systematic approach for ECG evaluation.

1. Determine heart rate
2. Determine if the ventricular and atrial rates match
   The P-P interval and R-R interval normally match
3. Determine if every P wave has an associated QRS complex
   All P waves are normally followed by a QRS complex
4. Determine if every QRS complex has an associated P wave
   All QRS complexes are normally preceded by a P wave
5. Determine if the QRS complexes appear supraventricular or ventricular
   In dogs and cats, supraventricular complexes are tall, upright, and narrow while ventricular complexes are wide and abnormal

Mean electrical axis

The mean electrical axis (MEA) refers to the direction and orientation of ventricular depolarization and refers solely to the QRS complex. It may be thought of as the average vector of ventricular depolarization. Even though MEA can be measured in any plane, its characterization for ventricular evaluation occurs mainly in the frontal plane using a hexaxial reference system, a graphical arrangement of the three bipolar and three unipolar leads together [12]. The MEA may be determined to identify the presence of ventricular dilatation or hypertrophy and to detect intraventricular conduction defects. For example, in a normal heart, the left ventricle is the dominant ventricle; therefore, the normal MEA is generally to the left. However, if there is significant right ventricular hypertrophy, the MEA will be shifted to the right.

It is important to note that MEA is not only related to the mass that is being depolarized but also to the timing of the myocardial depolarization. Variations in MEA can occur due to abnormalities in the direction, magnitude, and timing of myocardial depolarization and may indicate hypertrophy of cardiac tissue or a conduction disturbance [12].

In describing the MEA, a degree system is used with 0° directed to the left, 90° directed down, and 180° directed to the right (Fig. 11.5). The MEA in the normal dog lies between 40° and 100°; in the cat, the MEA is more variable, from 0° to 160°. The MEA is typically determined by using the six standard ECG leads (three bipolar and three unipolar) and may be calculated by several different methods. First, if there is a lead with an isoelectric QRS complex (i.e., the deflection of the R and S complexes are equivalent), the MEA lies on the axis perpendicular to the isoelectric lead. If the net QRS amplitude is positive on that perpendicular lead (i.e., the deflection of the R complex is greater than that of the S), then the MEA points toward the positive pole. If the net QRS amplitude is negative on that perpendicular lead (i.e., the deflection if the R complex is less than that of the S), then the MEA points toward the negative pole. A slightly more cumbersome but more accurate method involves plotting the net amplitude of the QRS complex of leads I and aVF and the intersection will provide the vector equal to the MEA. The MEA can also be estimated (i.e., right versus left) simply by assessing the net deflection in lead I. If the net deflection of the QRS in lead I is positive, then the MEA lies to the left, and if the net deflection of the QRS in lead I is negative, then the MEA lies to the right [17].

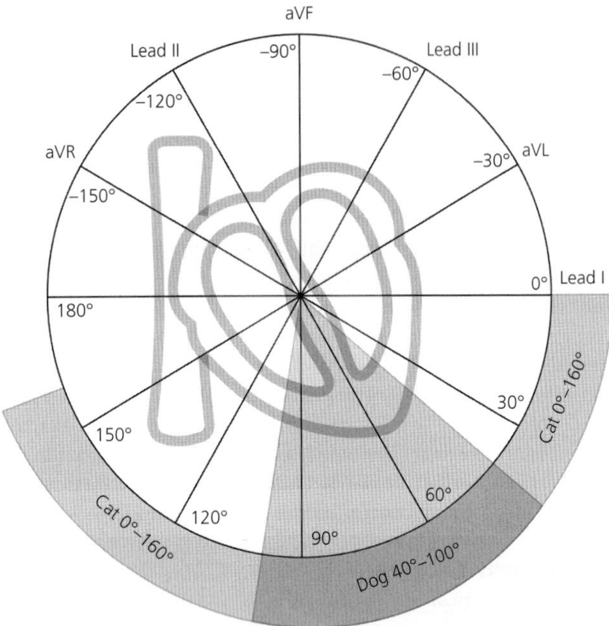

Figure 11.5 Mean electrical axis (MEA) is typically determined in the frontal plane by combining the three bipolar and three unipolar leads. There are many techniques for calculating MEA that range in accuracy and clinical usefulness. A classic way to determine MEA involves summation of net deflections of the QRS complex from different leads. Lead I can be used to quickly determine if the MEA lies to the left or right: if the net deflection of the QRS complex is positive in lead I, the MEA lies to the left; if the net deflection of the QRS complex is negative in lead I, the MEA lies to the right. The normal MEA is 40–100° in dogs and 0–160° in cats. Deviations in MEA can be caused by chamber enlargement or conduction disturbances. Source: Dr. Kyle Bartholomew, with permission.

Regardless of technique, it is important to note that consistency in technique may be important. For instance, there have been discussions comparing calculation of MEA using both the base-apex lead and alternative lead positioning systems in equine patients [9,20]. Although the focus of these studies has been on which system is the most clinically useful for determination of abnormalities, one thing is made clear by these investigations – the methodology used to determine the MEA can significantly change the established normal. Care must be taken to ensure comparisons are made between measurements obtained using the same standards [9,17,20].

Species-specific variations

There is an obvious difference in the morphology of the QRS complex between certain species that can be appreciated by even the most novice observer (Fig. 11.6). In some veterinary species, the normal QRS complex has a largely positive deflection from baseline in lead II. These include dogs, cats, primates, rats, and many other domestic mammals. In other veterinary species, namely horses, pigs, and ruminants, the QRS complex has a largely negative deflection in lead II, as well as in the more commonly used base-apex lead for horses. The basis for this was initially suggested by Hamlin and Smith in 1965 who proposed that species in their first category (category A; dogs, cats, and primates) had three "fronts" or vectors of depolarization during the classic QRS complex, while species in their second category (category B; horses, pigs, and ruminants) had only two fronts of depolarization (Fig. 11.7). In category B species, more general penetration of the Purkinje fibers into the epicardium results in a single burst of depolarization and simultaneous excitation of the majority of the mass in both ventricles [21]. In comparison, Purkinje fibers in category A species are distributed mainly in the subendocardial layer, leading to the classically recognized pattern of ventricular depolarization [21].

More deeply penetrating and diffuse Purkinje fiber distribution, similar to category B species, have also been recognized in other species including whales, dolphins, and birds [22]. It is important for anesthetists to be aware that these differences exist to avoid mistaking a normal QRS complex in a category B species with an ectopic ventricular beat in a category A species, as this could impact clinical case management. For example, avian species commonly have negatively deflected QRS complexes and rates exceeding 200–300 beats/min; this morphology may appear similar to ventricular tachycardia in other species, which could lead to misdiagnosis that would significantly change anesthetic management of the patient (Fig. 11.6D).

Canine

The normal heart rate of an adult dog is between 60 and 160 beats/min and, in addition to a normal sinus rhythm, healthy adult dogs may have a prominent respiratory sinus arrhythmia that is characterized by cyclic variations in heart rate approximately synchronous with the phase of respiration and the accompanying fluctuations in vagal tone [23,24]. The rate appears to accelerate during inspiration and decelerate during expiration, and the effect begins to diminish at higher heart rates. In dogs, the parasympathetic nervous system has pronounced effects on the modulation of heart rate [25]. It has been hypothesized that an increase in heart rate during inspiration increases cardiac output and, therefore, pulmonary perfusion during a period with increased lung volume, and this subsequently improves ventilation–perfusion ratios [26].

Normal P wave morphology and timing may vary from cycle to cycle in some dogs; this cyclic variation is a characteristic often referred to as a "wandering pacemaker" and is due to changes in the site of impulse origin within the sinus node and/or changes in the exit pathway from the sinus node [24].

Feline

The normal heart rate of cats can vary significantly from roughly 120–240 beats/min, although, anecdotally, it is uncommon to identify a cat with a heart rate near the lower end of the range in a hospital setting. Unlike dogs, respiratory sinus arrhythmia is uncommon in healthy adult cats in a hospital setting, but it has been recognized when recordings of heart rate and rhythm were generated remotely in cats at home [24,27].

Feline ECGs can be difficult to interpret due to their high heart rates and the low voltage of their ECG complexes detected by the surface electrodes (Fig. 11.6A). Lower voltage potentials lead to smaller amplitudes on an ECG, and this increases the likelihood of artifacts and interference, which complicates interpretation. This complication applies to most small animals including small mammals and birds.

Equine

Much like the dog, the underlying heart rate and rhythm of horses are heavily influenced by parasympathetic tone at rest. Cardiac arrhythmias due to high vagal tone (e.g., sinus arrhythmia, sinus block, sinus arrest, sinus bradycardia, wandering pacemaker,

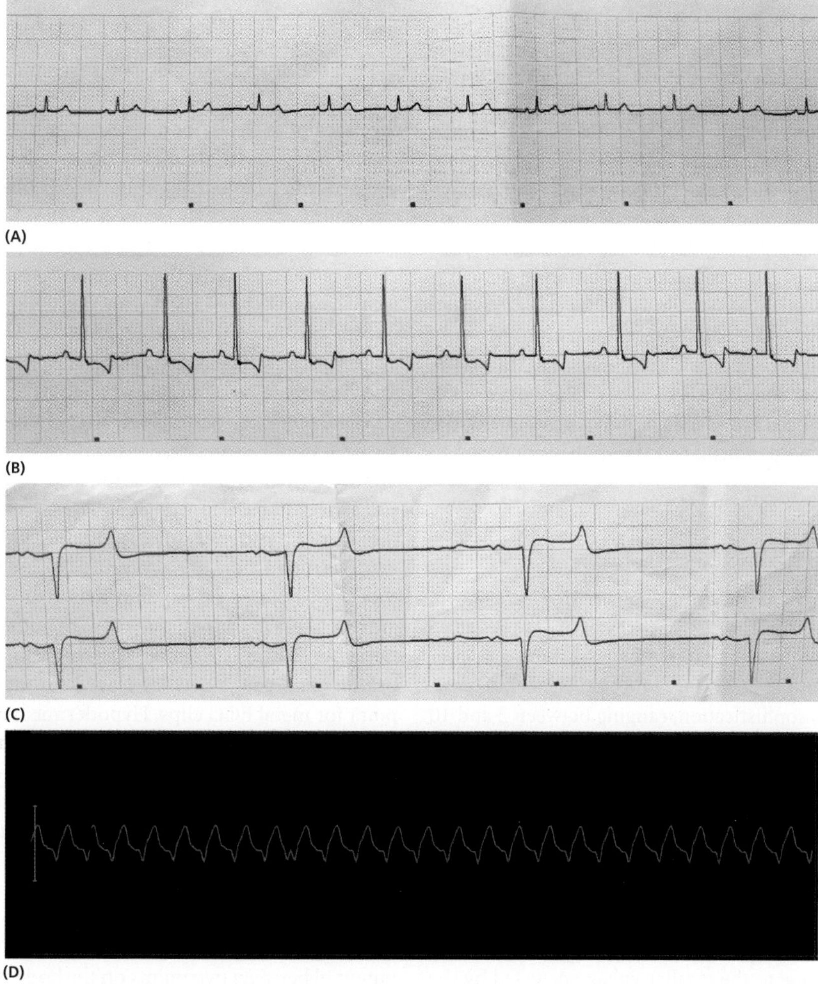

Figure 11.6 ECGs from four domestic species: **A.** feline, **B.** canine, **C.** equine, and **D.** avian. Note that the equine QRS complex morphology is largely negative in lead II and that the avian complex morphology is negative and wide, making it possible for individuals unfamiliar with ECG morphology in these patients to incorrectly assume that they are experiencing an inappropriate ventricular rhythm. Source: Dr. Kyle Bartholomew, with permission.

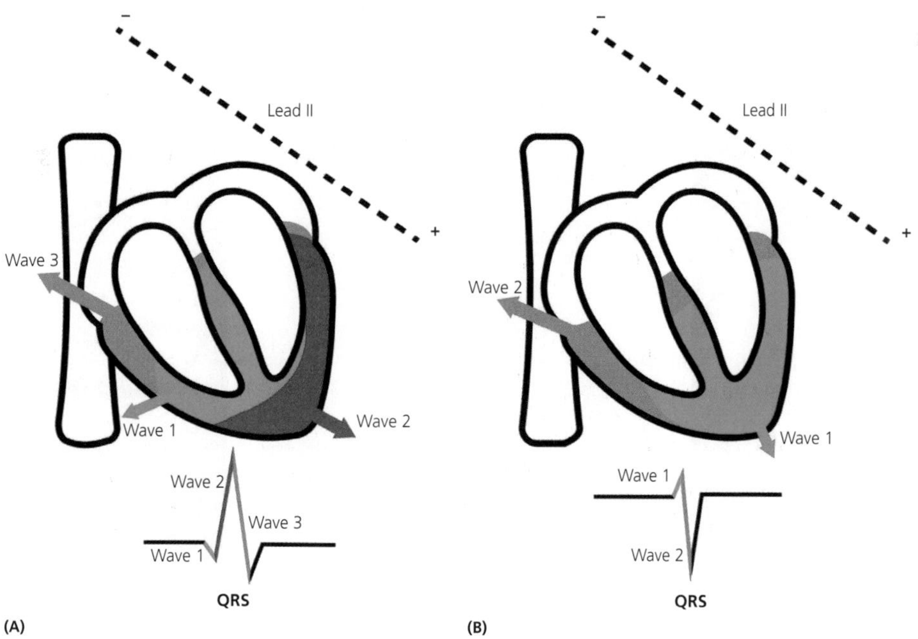

Figure 11.7 Schematic representations of sagittal heart views based on Hamlin and Smith's explanation of the differences between two categories (A and B) of ventricular myocardial depolarization and resulting variations in QRS complex morphology [21]. **A.** Species belonging to category A (e.g., dogs, cats, and primates) generally exhibit three "fronts" or waves of depolarization (represented by the three colored waves) resulting from largely subendocardial Purkinje fiber distribution. **B.** Species belonging to category B (e.g., horses, ruminants, and pigs) undergo depolarization in two waves (represented by two colored waves) resulting from Purkinje fibers penetrating the epicardium. Thus, distinctive differences in QRS morphologies in Lead II are noted in these different categories. Source: Dr. Kyle Bartholomew, with permission.

first-degree AV block, and second-degree AV block) may be found in resting, healthy horses and, in many cases, are considered normal and generally do not require therapy [28].

As mentioned earlier, there are differing opinions regarding the optimal technique for performing equine electrocardiography. The most common methodology among veterinary anesthetists in North America appears to be the base-apex lead system; however, utilization of the Dubois lead positioning system has been suggested [9]. This includes a 12-lead rather than two-lead system and is thought to compensate for the limitations of using the frontal plane in horses. As opposed to humans, for whom the majority of the lead placement systems have been developed, the orientation of the long axis (and axis of depolarization) of the equine heart tends to be perpendicular to the spine as opposed to parallel to it [20].

ECG equipment

The most basic modern ECG machines consist of electrodes, a screen to display waveforms, and a microprocessor to make evaluations, calculations, and adjustments; some may also have a printer to create physical copies of the ECG (Fig. 11.8). ECG machines can vary significantly in their sophistication, ranging between 2 and 10 electrodes capable of many different leads. As the ECG is a graphical representation of voltage over time, many monitors allow alteration of the scale on both the x axis (time, mm per second) and the y axis (voltage, mV). Common time intervals are 25 and 50 mm/s. Some monitors will automatically scale the y axis (voltage) to optimize the image; increasing the scale may allow the user to evaluate the waveform but will also make artifacts more prominent. For example, the ECG complex of a cat often appears significantly smaller than that of dog due to the smaller voltage detected by the ECG surface electrodes (Fig. 11.6A) [17].

Small, portable, single-lead ECG monitors are also available (Fig. 11.8B). These units often have just two electrodes and, while they are not as useful for diagnostic purposes, they can be useful for monitoring sedated or anesthetized patients in remote locations or areas in which larger equipment may be impractical. Cardiac telemetry monitors can also be used to monitor the ECG of a patient from a short distance such as a cage or stall without the need for cables connected to the display. Smartphone-based ECG monitoring units have also been used with success for monitoring of patients outside the hospital setting [29].

ECG electrode cables also come with a variety of different attachments for attaching to a patient (Fig. 11.8C). Metal "alligator" clips are often less desirable during prolonged sedation or anesthesia because they can cause discomfort or focal tissue ischemia and often require alcohol or electrode gel to improve the ECG signal. Care should be taken when applying alcohol to ECG electrodes on the skin of a patient immediately prior to defibrillation due to the risk of combustion [30]. Alternatives include adhesive ECG pads that can be placed on any non-haired or shaved skin surface; these are less likely to cause tissue damage but may still cause skin irritation upon removal. Another alternative for very small animals is the use of small-gauge needles placed through the skin as an anchor point for metal ECG clips. Hypodermic needles are often used, and metal clips may be attached to the needle after it is passed through the skin; the ends of the needle can be covered with rubber or the needle cap to reduce the likelihood of an inadvertent needle puncture. Commercially available specialized ECG needles are also available.

Artifacts and filters

The ECG is designed to detect very subtle changes in the electrical potential between two points on the body. This means that the ECG is also predisposed to outside influence in the form of "artifacts" or

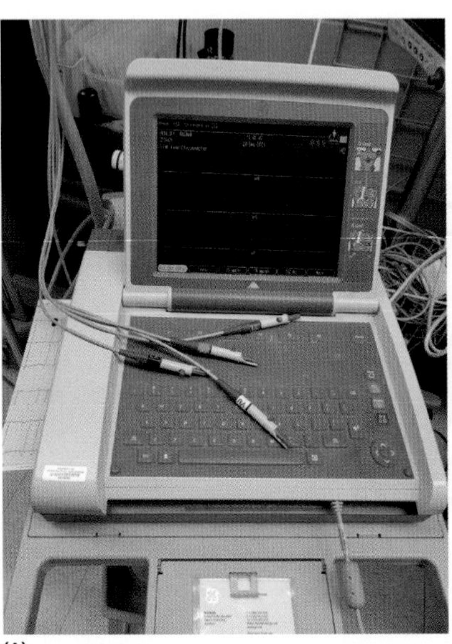
(A)

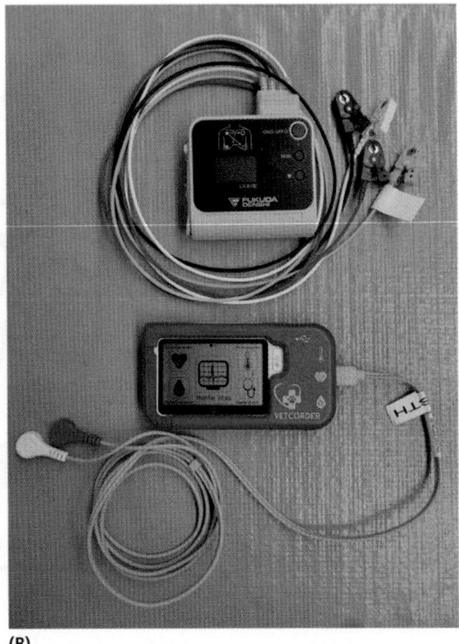

(B)

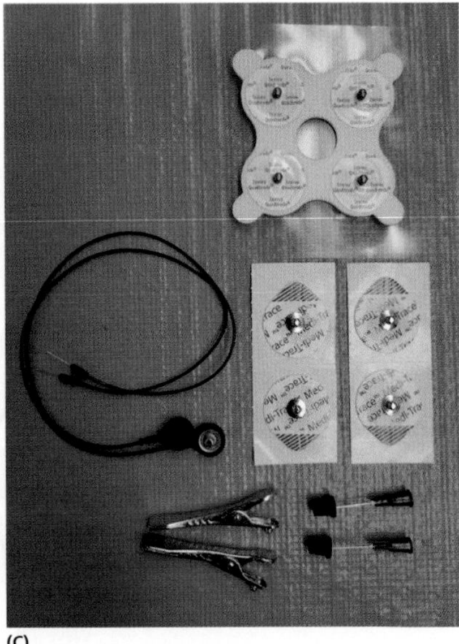
(C)

Figure 11.8 Available ECG machines vary in shape, size, and complexity. **A.** Standalone ECG machine complete with electrode clips, a monitor, and a printer. **B.** Portable ECG machines with small screens to monitor the ECG which are also capable of transmitting data wirelessly to larger more centralized monitors. **C.** Methods to attach ECG electrodes to patients for monitoring include clips, electrode-compatible adhesive pads, and needles. Specialized needles with built in ECG compatibility are available; alternatively, hypodermic needles can be inserted into the patient's skin, clipped onto electrodes and covered with rubber caps for personnel safety. Source: Dr. Kyle Bartholomew, with permission.

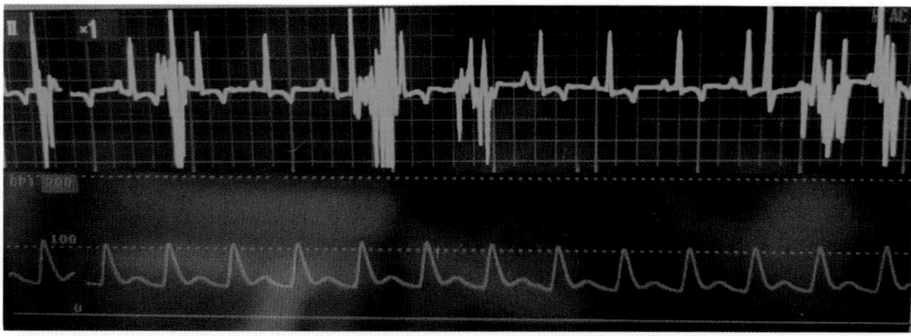

Figure 11.9 An example of ECG interference caused by electrocautery during surgery. Note the tall and rapid deviations from baseline, without disruption of the regular underlying current. Below the ECG is an arterial pressure tracing from the same dog, showing consistent pulsatile blood flow that would be unlikely to occur in the face of significant ectopy. Source: Dr. Kyle Bartholomew, with permission.

electrical noise; these can occur in both the low- and high-frequency ranges [11]. Almost all the modern ECG monitors have filters built into their design to remove these artifacts prior to displaying them on the screen or printout. Modern ECG machines employ what is referred to as a "bandpass filter," a filter that allows signal frequencies within a specific range to be displayed while removing electrical activity above and below this frequency. Bandpass filters have two components: the low-pass filter and the high-pass filter. The low-pass filter (or high-frequency filter) allows signals with a lower frequency than the cutoff frequency to be transmitted, while those with a higher frequency are attenuated. A high-pass filter (or low-frequency filter) does the opposite, attenuating signals with frequencies lower than the cutoff value.

Examples of low-frequency artifacts include respiration or patient movement. Some monitors not designed for use in veterinary medicine have a low-frequency filter setting of 0.5 Hz (30 beats/min), and some horses and reptiles may have heart rates that reasonably fall below this threshold, creating challenges in monitor interpretation [11,31].

High-frequency artifacts can be caused by muscle fasciculations, shivering, and, importantly, 60-cycle (Hz) electromagnetic interference from electrical equipment in the perioperative area. Most modern ECG machines include an additional notch filter to specifically attenuate artifacts within the 60-Hz frequency range. This may help limit the interference from surrounding electrical equipment. Types of electrical equipment that can commonly lead to artifacts include MRIs, flexible bronchoscopes or endoscopes, nerve stimulators, and, in some situations, cell phones [11].

Electrosurgery units are another potential source of ECG artifacts (Fig. 11.9). Electrosurgery units based on the concept of creating heat using a flow of electrical current through a small area of tissue can lead to changes in the ECG waveform that can be both overt and subtle [32,33]. Care must be taken to ensure that the patient is properly grounded, as there have been incidences of burns associated with electrosurgery units and ECG electrodes where grounding has been inadequate [34]. There is at least one documented case of severe esophageal burns caused by an esophageal ECG probe in a dog where grounding became inadequate during surgery [35].

Effect of anesthesia

The ECG is a useful diagnostic tool for monitoring patients undergoing sedation and anesthesia. It is especially important for patients with comorbidities that put them at risk for development of dysrhythmias, as well as for healthy patients whose risk of dysrhythmias may increase with anesthetic medications. Dysrhythmias may occur under anesthesia in the absence of underlying cardiac disease. In a study of 50 healthy young dogs undergoing elective procedures, 26 out of 50 had at least one instance of second-degree AV block, 22 out of 50 had ventricular premature contractions, and 2 out of 50 experienced ventricular tachycardia perioperatively; however, some of these dogs were anesthetized with halothane, which is known to sensitize the heart to certain arrhythmias [36–38]. In a study of 49 healthy cats without structural heart disease undergoing inhalant anesthesia with isoflurane or sevoflurane, 5 cats had at least one ventricular premature complex throughout the anesthetic period [4]. It has been suggested that healthy horses without underlying cardiac disease may have a prevalence of dysrhythmias as great as 25%, even when awake [28], with some of the most common arrhythmias being first and second-degree AV block. Horses undergoing inhalant anesthesia for colic and non-colic procedures had high incidences of arrhythmias postoperatively, exceeding 75% in both groups [39]. The causes of these cardiac rhythm disturbances under anesthesia are addressed elsewhere, but an understanding of the equipment used, the common artifacts encountered, and the species differences that occur can help the anesthetist differentiate a normal ECG from a life-threatening dysrhythmia and allow appropriate intervention and educated decision-making regarding patient care.

References

1 Kamibayashi T, Hayashi Y, Sumikawa K, *et al.* Enhancement by propofol of epinephrine-induced arrhythmias in dogs. *Anesthesiology* 1991; **75**: 1035–1040.

2 Hubbell JA, Muir WW, Bednarski RM, *et al.* Change of inhalation anesthetic agents for management of ventricular premature depolarizations in anesthetized cats and dogs. *J Am Vet Med Assoc* 1984; **185**: 643–646.

3 Alibhai HI, Clarke KW, Lee YH, *et al.* Cardiopulmonary effects of combinations of medetomidine hydrochloride and atropine sulphate in dogs. *Vet Rec* 1996; **138**:11–13.

4 Maney J, Durham H, Cavanaugh S, *et al.* Incidence of ventricular arrhythmias in healthy cats under general anesthesia: a pilot study. *Vet Anaesth Analg* 2019; **46**: 831 e11.

5 Geselowitz DB. Dipole theory in electrocardiography. *Am J Cardiol* 1964; **14**: 301–306.

6 Santilli RN, Moïse S, Pariaut R, *et al.* Principles of electrocardiography. In: Santilli RN, Moïse S, Pariaut R, *et al.*, eds. *Electrocardiography of the Dog and Cat: Diagnosis of Arrhythmias*, 2nd edn. Milano, Italy: Edra S.p.A, 2018: 37–51.

7 Middleton B, Phillips J, Thomas R, *et al.* Electrocardiography, pacing and difibrillation. In: Middleton B, Phillips J, Thomas R, Stacey S, eds. *Physics in Anaesthesia*. Oxfordshire, UK: Scion Publishing Ltd, 2012: 253–268.

8 Kimberly M, McGurrin J. Investigation of cardiac arrythmias. In: Sprayberry KA, Robinson NE, eds. *Robinson's Current Therapy in Equine Medicine*, 7th edn. Philadelphia, PA: W.B. Saunders, 2015: 506–509.

9 da Costa CF, Samesima N, Pastore CA. Cardiac mean electrical axis in thoroughbreds – standardization by the Dubois lead positioning system. *PLoS One* 2017; **12**: e0169619.

10 Schwarzwald CC, Bonagura JD, Muir WW. The cardiovascular system. In: Muir WW, Hubbell JAE, eds. *Equine Anesthesia: Monitoring and Emergency Therapy*, 2nd edn. St Louis, MO: Saunders Elsevier, 2009: 37–100.

11 Schroeder B, Mark, J, Barbeito A. Cardiovascular monitoring. In: Gropper MA, Miller RD, Eriksson LI, *et al.*, eds. *Miller's Anesthesia*. 9th edn. Philadelphia, PA: Elsevier Health Sciences, 2019: 1146–1193.

12 Santilli RN, Moïse S, Pariaut R, *et al.* Formation and interpretation of the electrocardiographic waves. In: Santilli RN, Moïse S, Pariaut R, *et al.*, eds. *Electrocardiography of the Dog and Cat: Diagnosis of Arrhythmias*, 2nd edn. Milan, Italy: Edra S.p.A, 2018: 52–89.

13 Dolber PC, Spach MS. Structure of canine Bachmann's bundle related to propagation of excitation. *Am J Physiol* 1989; **257**: H1446–H1457.

14 Shinde R, Shinde S, Makhale C, *et al.* Occurrence of "J waves" in 12-lead ECG as a marker of acute ischemia and their cellular basis. *Pacing Clin Electrophysiol* 2007; **30**: 817–819.

15 Hlaing T, DiMino T, Kowey PR, *et al.* ECG repolarization waves: their genesis and clinical implications. *Ann Noninvasive Electrocardiol* 2005; **10**: 211–223.

16 Santilli RN, Moïse S, Pariaut R, *et al.* Supraventricular beats and rhythms. In: Santilli RN, Moïse S, Pariaut R, *et al.*, eds. *Electrocardiography of the Dog and Cat: Diagnosis of Arrhythmias*, 2nd edn. Milan, Italy: Edra S.p.A, 2018: 145–159.

17 Tilley LP, Smith FWK. Electrocardiography. In: Tilly LP, Smith FWK, Oyama MA, Sleeper MM, eds. *Manual of Canine and Feline Cardiology*, 4th edn. St Louis, MO: Saunders Elsevier, 2008: 49–77.

18 Bulmer B. Interpreting ECGs with confidence: part 1. *NAVC Clinician's Brief* 2012: 32–35.

19 Willis R. Electrocardiography. In: Willis R, Oliveira P, Mavropoulou A, eds. *Guide to Canine and Feline Electrocardiography*. Hoboken, NJ: John Wiley & Sons, 2018: 35–56.

20 Hesselkilde EM, Isaksen JL, Petersen BV, *et al.* A novel approach for obtaining 12-lead electrocardiograms in horses. *J Vet Intern Med* 2021; **35**: 521–531.

21 Hamlin RL, Smith CR. Categorization of common domestic mammals based upon their ventricular activation process. *Ann NY Acad Sci* 1965; **127**: 195–203.

22 Ohkawa SI. Distribution of Purkinje cells in hearts of human and various animals. *J Arrhythm* 2008; **24**:177–179.

23 Hamlin RL, Smith CR, Smetzer DL. Sinus arrhythmia in the dog. *Am J Physiol* 1966; **210**: 321–328.

24 Santilli RN, Moïse S, Pariaut R, *et al.* Normal sinus rhythms. In: Santilli RN, Moïse S, Pariaut R, *et al.*, eds. *Electrocardiography of the Dog and Cat: Diagnosis of Arrhythmias*, 2nd edn. Milan, Italy: Edra S.p.A, 2018: 90–100.

25 Mace SE, Levy MN. Autonomic nervous control of heart rate: sympathetic-parasympathetic interactions and age related differences. *Cardiovasc Res* 1983; **17**: 547–552.

26 Hayano J, Yasuma F, Okada A, *et al.* Respiratory sinus arrhythmia: a phenomenon improving pulmonary gas exchange and circulatory efficiency. *Circulation* 1996; **94**: 842–847.

27 Ware WA. Twenty-four-hour ambulatory electrocardiography in normal cats. *J Vet Intern Med* 1999; **13**: 175–180.

28 McGuirk SM, Muir WW. Diagnosis and treatment of cardiac arrhythmias. *Vet Clin North Am Equine Pract* 1985; **1**: 353–370.

29 Vezzosi T, Tognetti R, Buralli C, *et al.* Home monitoring of heart rate and heart rhythm with a smartphone-based ECG in dogs. *Vet Rec* 2019; **184**: 96.

30 Cole SG, Drobatz KJ. Cardiopulmonary resuscitation. In: Tilly LP, Smith FWK, Oyama MA, Sleeper MM, eds. *Manual of Canine and Feline Cardiography*, 4th edn. St Louis, MO: Saunders Elsevier, 2008: 333–341.

31 Van Steenkiste G, van Loon G, Crevecoeur G. Transfer learning in ECG classification from human to horse using a novel parallel neural network architecture. *Sci Rep* 2020; **10**: 1–2.

32 Naik BN, Luthra A, Dwivedi A, *et al.* Artifactual ECG changes induced by electrocautery in a patient with coronary artery disease. *J Electrocardiol* 2017; **50**: 531–533.

33 Knight BP, Pelosi F, Michaud GF, *et al.* Clinical consequences of electrocardiographic artifact mimicking ventricular tachycardia. *N Engl J Med* 1999; **341**: 1270–1274.

34 Finlay B, Couchie D, Boyce L, *et al.* Electrosurgery burns resulting from use of miniature ECG electrodes. *Anesthesiology* 1974; **41**: 263–272.

35 Burgess RC, Freeman LJ, Jennings RN, *et al.* An alternative pathway electrosurgical unit injury in a dog. *Vet Surg* 2011; **40**: 509–514.

36 Duerr FM, Carr AP, Duke T, *et al.* Prevalence of perioperative arrhythmias in 50 young, healthy dogs. *Can Vet J* 2007; **48**: 169–177.

37 Day TK, Muir WW. Effects of halothane, enflurane, and isoflurane on supraventricular and ventricular rate in dogs with complete atrioventricular block. *Vet Surg* 1994; **23**: 206–212.

38 Hashimoto K, Hashimoto K. The mechanism of sensitization of the ventricle to epinephrine by halothane. *Am Heart J* 1972; **83**: 652–658.

39 Morgan RA, Raftery AG, Cripps P, *et al.* The prevalence and nature of cardiac arrhythmias in horses following general anaesthesia and surgery. *Acta Vet Scand* 2011; **53**: 1–8.

12 Blood Pressure Monitoring

Odette O
SAGE Veterinary Centers, a member of Ethos Animal Health, Dublin, California, USA

Chapter contents

Introduction, 197
Blood pressure determinants and definitions, 197
  Mean arterial pressure, 197
Normal ranges of blood pressure, 198
Autoregulation of blood pressure, 198
Invasive blood pressure measurement, 199
  Components for invasive blood pressure measurement, 200
  Physics of invasive blood pressure monitoring systems, 201
  Arterial catheter placement and maintenance, 202
Non-invasive blood pressure measurement, 202
  Doppler ultrasonographic blood pressure measurement, 202
  Oscillometric blood pressure measurement, 203
  High-definition oscillometric blood pressure measurement, 204
Central venous pressure measurement, 204
Indices of fluid responsiveness, 205
  Pulse pressure variation and systolic pressure variation, 205
  Plethysmography variability index, 207
Plethysmography and photoplethysmography, 207
Continued challenges with blood pressure measurement, 207
References, 208

Introduction

Blood pressure (BP) is a vital sign that is relatively easy to measure in most veterinary patients. Perfusion of organs and tissues is vital in delivering oxygen and nutrients as well as removing metabolic byproducts. While the measurement of BP does not directly measure perfusion, pressure is required to bring blood to tissues and vital organs including the heart, brain, and kidneys. Trauma and surgical interventions may cause hemodynamic shifts, while the administration of sedation and general anesthesia results in alterations in cardiac function and vasomotor tone, thereby affecting BP (Box 12.1). BP monitoring should be a part of the care and management of all patients undergoing sedation and anesthesia, as outlined in both the American Animal Hospital Association and American College of Veterinary Anesthesia and Analgesia monitoring guidelines [1,2].

Blood pressure determinants and definitions

BP measurement is traditionally expressed as a series of three values: systolic arterial pressure (SAP), diastolic arterial pressure (DAP), and mean arterial pressure (MAP), each with their own importance in patient assessment. SAP is the pressure exerted by blood against the arterial walls during systole of the cardiac cycle. DAP represents the amount of pressure that blood exerts on the arterial walls during cardiac relaxation (diastole). MAP is of great importance in anesthetized patients, as it determines perfusion pressure in the tissues and is directly influenced by cardiac output (CO) and systemic vascular resistance (SVR). Conversely, pulse pressure (PP) is simply the difference between SAP and DAP and does not indicate appropriate tissue perfusion. Since most sedative and anesthetic agents affect vasomotor tone, digital pulse palpation should not be used as a substitute for accurate measurement of BP in anesthetized patients.

Mean arterial pressure

MAP represents the area under the arterial pressure/time curve divided by the cardiac cycle duration. Modern invasive blood pressure measurement systems accurately calculate MAP based on analysis of the arterial waveform, while most non-invasive oscillometric systems measure MAP as the greatest cuff pressure amplitude variation. In addition, MAP may be roughly estimated by the following formula, though this equation has a number of limitations:

$$\text{MAP} = \text{DAP} + 1/3\left(\text{SAP} - \text{DAP}\right)$$

Factors that influence MAP include CO and SVR:

$$\text{MAP} = \text{CO} \times \text{SVR}$$

Cardiac output

CO is a product of heart rate (HR) and stroke volume (SV):

$$\text{CO} = \text{HR} \times \text{SV}$$

Veterinary Anesthesia and Analgesia: The Sixth Edition of Lumb and Jones. Edited by Leigh Lamont, Kurt Grimm, Sheilah Robertson, Lydia Love and Carrie Schroeder.
© 2024 John Wiley & Sons, Inc. Published 2024 by John Wiley & Sons, Inc.
Companion website: www.wiley.com/go/lamont/anesthesia

Box 12.1 Common causes of perianesthetic hypotension.

Hypovolemia
- Ongoing losses
- Incurred losses

Shock
- Septic shock
- Hypovolemic shock

Sedative/anesthetic drugs
Patient positioning
Use of positive-pressure ventilation
Epidural anesthesia with local anesthetics

Box 12.2 Patient factors that lead to an increased risk of secondary hypertension.

Common canine comorbidities	**Drugs**
Renal disease	Glucocorticoids
Hyperadrenocorticism	Mineralocorticoids
Diabetes mellitus	Erythropoiesis-stimulating agents
Pheochromocytoma	Phenylpropanolamine
Common feline comorbidities	Toceranib phosphate
Renal disease	
Hyperthyroidism	

A more in-depth discussion of CO may be found in elsewhere in this text (Chapter 33). Briefly, HR is influenced by chronotropy, lusitropy, and dromotropy, whereas SV is influenced by volume (inotropy, preload, and total blood volume) in addition to afterload. Chronotropy defines the physiologic timing of HR. Lusitropy is the period of cardiac relaxation that occurs during diastole when cardiac myocytes have a decreased level of cytosolic calcium, as opposed to inotropy when increased calcium uptake causes positive contractile effects in the cardiac myocytes. Dromotropy is the actual conduction of an impulse, usually through the AV node, which in turn influences HR.

Systemic vascular resistance

SVR, also known as "total peripheral resistance," is influenced by vascular size ($1/\infty$) and blood viscosity and is defined by the amount of force that the vasculature system exerts on circulating blood, excluding pulmonary circulation. SVR influences BP via three factors: vessel length, vessel diameter, and the viscosity of the blood [3]. Alterations in vessel diameter have an enormous effect on vessel flow, as defined by the Hagen–Poiseuille equation, whereby a reduction of vessel diameter by 1/2 decreases flow to only 1/16th of the original flow:

$$\Delta P = Q8L\eta/\pi r^4$$

where ΔP is the pressure difference between the two ends of the vessel, Q is the volumetric flow rate, L is the length of vessel, η is the dynamic viscosity, r^4 is the vessel radius to the fourth power, and $8/\pi$ is a constant of proportionality.

Normal ranges of blood pressure

A consensus statement by the American College of Veterinary Internal Medicine (ACVIM) details guidelines for the identification, evaluation, and management of systemic hypertension in dogs and cats [4]. This statement cites difficulty in determining a single value or range acceptable for all cats and dogs and that normal ranges of BP will vary by species and patient factors, including temperament, age, breed, body condition, and sex. Measurement technique and location will also affect the values obtained. Numerous studies have attempted to investigate and define normal ranges of BP in various species with variable results. In general, prehypertension is defined as SAP 140–150 mmHg, hypertension that may lead to potential target organ damage as SAP > 160–179 mmHg, and severe hypertension as SAP > 180 mmHg.

Difficulties in defining a universally acceptable range of BP emphasize the importance of obtaining baseline BP values in patients prior to an anesthetic event, especially if concerns exist for target organ damage and/or underlying risk factors are identified (Box 12.2).

Hypotension-related morbidity and mortality is difficult to determine and most likely depends on a number of individual factors. In a study of over 30,000 humans undergoing non-cardiac surgery, hypotension (defined as MAP < 55 mmHg) for as little as 1–5 min was associated with increased risk of acute kidney injury [5]. While large-scale trials in veterinary medicine are lacking, the importance of maintaining perfusion during anesthesia should nonetheless be prioritized. For instance, use of excessive levels of inhalant leads to a significant decrease in SVR and a relative hypovolemia [6]. Hypotension is one of the most common complications of anesthesia and can have serious consequences if left unmanaged [1]. In horses, postanesthetic myopathy is a complex and potentially fatal consequence of inadequate tissue perfusion pressure during anesthesia. Multiple studies in horses have demonstrated increased risk of complications when MAP < 60 mmHg [7,8]; as such, common practice is to ensure that MAP is greater than 70 mmHg at all times [9]. Current information indicates that, although maintenance of MAP is important, maintaining global perfusion without increasing SVR should be prioritized, and vasoactive support agents should be selected accordingly [10].

Autoregulation of blood pressure

The ability of organs to maintain a relatively constant blood flow despite changes in perfusion pressure is known as "autoregulation." Organs perform this task intrinsically via three main mechanisms [11]. Metabolic regulation of blood flow occurs when changes in metabolism result in the release of vasodilatory substances such as adenosine, carbon dioxide, and lactic acid. An example of such metabolic regulation would be the vasodilation that occurs in muscle beds in response to hypoxia. Myogenic (pressure-dependent) mechanisms autoregulate blood flow via smooth muscle-lined vessels; increased pressure within the vessels leads to vasoconstriction, and decreased pressure is followed by vasodilation in smaller arteries and arterioles. Myogenic regulation of blood flow is observed in renal tissues. Shear-stress-dependent (endothelial) mechanisms regulate blood flow via the endothelial release of vasoactive factors such as nitric oxide and prostacyclin, causing vasodilation of smooth muscle-lined vessels, as well as endothelin, which modulates vasoconstriction [12]. Such regulation may be observed in brain and cardiac tissue.

Organs that demonstrate the greatest ability for autoregulation of blood flow include the brain, heart, and kidneys. The brain maintains autoregulation largely by metabolic means along with myogenic and endothelial responses. Recall that cerebral perfusion pressure (CPP) is the difference between MAP and intracranial pressure (ICP); it is critical to maintain constant CPP and cerebral blood flow (see Chapter 39). In humans, cerebral perfusion is autoregulated within an MAP range of 60–160 mmHg, where, in the dog, autoregulation of cerebral perfusion has been reported to occur with the MAP range of 70–140 mmHg [13,14]. In the kidneys, autoregulation of blood flow protects them from injury due to fluctuations of arterial BP and maintains the perfusion necessary to meet metabolic needs. Myogenic mechanisms of autoregulation allow for maintenance of constant renal blood flow (RBF) within the MAP range of 90–150 mmHg in rats, 70–130 mmHg in humans, and 40–100 mmHg in dogs [15,16]. Interestingly, RBF and glomerular filtration rate are maintained independently of renal perfusion pressure (RPP) via intrarenal autoregulatory mechanisms in the defined range of 80–180 mmHg in humans [17]. This safeguard is provided by a combination of myogenic and tubuloglomerular feedback that buffers transmission of changes in RPP to the capillaries of the glomeruli, protecting them from potential barotrauma while preserving renal function.

During anesthetic events, the maintenance of systemic BP within ranges of autoregulation ensures consistent blood flow to the vital organs, including the kidneys, heart, and brain. Various studies in differing species and physiologic states demonstrate slight differences in ranges, so one recommended approach is to maintain BP within 20% of measured baseline BP taken prior to arrival in the operating room [18].

Invasive blood pressure measurement

Invasive blood pressure (IBP) monitoring is considered the gold standard for BP measurement in anesthetized veterinary patients and allows for continuous, beat-by-beat assessment of BP and pulse waveform analysis. As this technique requires catheterization of an artery (thus the name "invasive"), it also facilitates sampling for arterial blood gas analysis. The term "direct" BP measurement is sometimes also used to describe this method; however, almost all IBP systems incorporate a transducer (see below) to convert the kinetic energy produced by changes in arterial pressure into electrical energy. SAP and DAP are directly measured with this technique, and MAP is calculated as the area under the arterial waveform over the cardiac cycle (Fig. 12.1). Careful setup and specialized equipment are needed to obtain the graphical display of the arterial pressure waveform and the numeric values; accuracy relies upon factors including the arterial catheter, the saline-filled tubing connecting the catheter to the transducer, the transducer itself, and the electrical components.

Patients where IBP monitoring should be considered for perioperative care include those where continuous monitoring of BP and/or repeated arterial blood gas/electrolyte sampling is necessary. These include high-risk surgical and critically ill patients with anticipated rapid changes in hemodynamic status. Patients with comorbidities such as cardiac, pulmonary, or renal disease, significant risk of hemorrhage, and/or those receiving vasoactive substances (e.g., inotropes, vasopressors) should also be considered for IBP monitoring.

Disadvantages of this technique include the cost or availability of advanced monitoring equipment and the need to catheterize a peripheral artery as well as potential risk of local pain, hemorrhage, hematoma formation, infection at the catheterization site, embolism, or ischemia/thrombosis (Fig. 12.2). A retrospective study examining the catheterization sites of 267 dogs and cats found loss of palpable pulse postoperatively in 22.3% of animals without evidence of associated tissue ischemia [19]. Care should always be

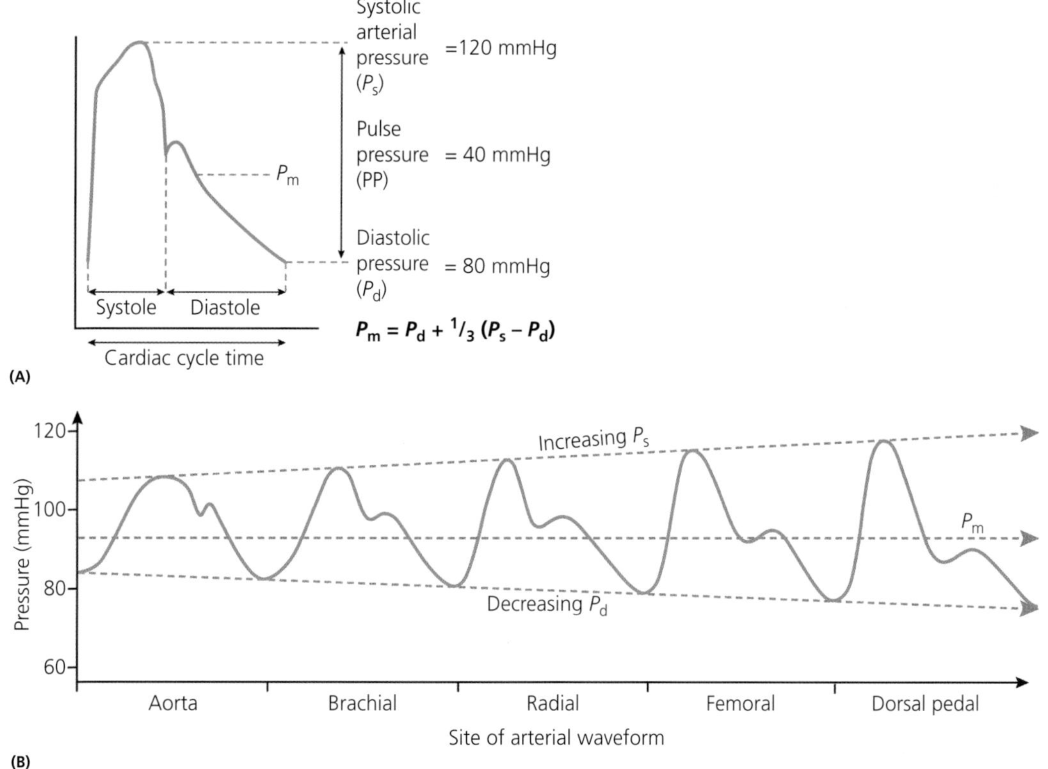

Figure 12.1 **A.** Mean arterial pressure (P_m) represents the area under the arterial blood pressure curve divided by the duration of the cardiac cycle. It can be estimated by adding one-third of the difference between the systolic arterial pressure (P_s) and diastolic arterial pressure (P_d) to P_d. P_s minus P_d is the pulse pressure (PP). **B.** P_s increases and P_m and P_d decrease with decreasing arterial diameter.

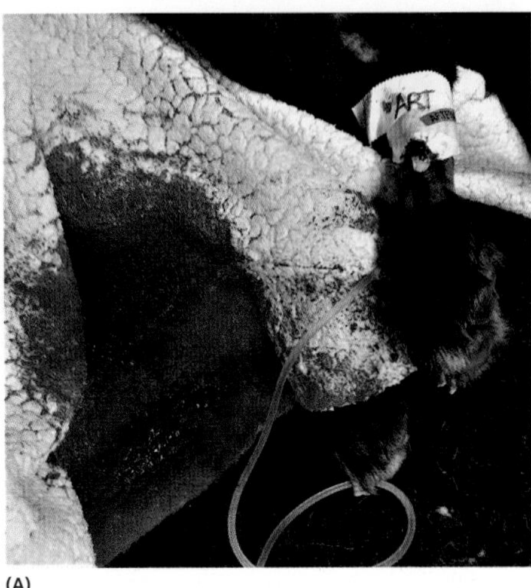

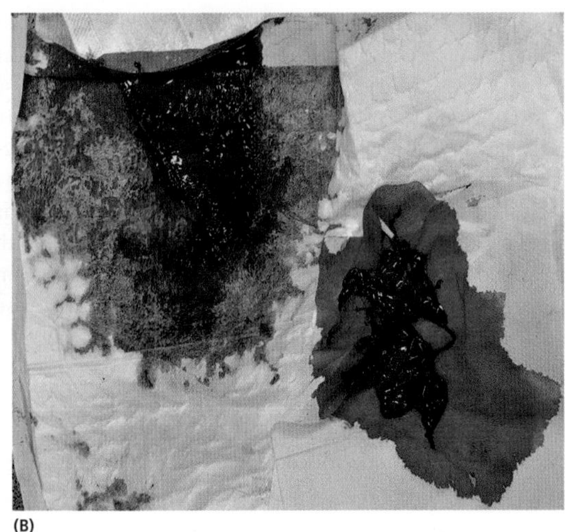

(A) (B)

Figure 12.2 **A.** Hemorrhage from displaced injection cap on a 22 gauge arterial catheter. The patient became tachycardic (> 180 bpm) and hypotensive (MAP < 60 mmHg). **B.** Blood loss was estimated to be 350 mL before disconnection was identified. Source: Dr. Odette O, with permission.

taken to avoid potential complications. Arterial catheters should be clearly labeled to avoid inadvertent administration of drugs and/or other substances into this catheter. Postoperative care and management of arterial catheters in hemodynamically stable patients include the recommendation for its removal as soon as possible with the placement of a temporary pressure wrap. For additional blood gas sampling, the push–pull technique has been described from venous catheters in order to minimize blood loss, which is an especially important consideration for very small patients. This method was described using 20 gauge catheters placed in the cephalic vein of dogs. An empty 3-mL syringe was used to aspirate 1.2 mL of blood from the intravenous (IV) catheter, then this blood was immediately pushed back into the catheter. This process is repeated three times. Finally, a new empty syringe is used to draw 1 mL of blood for immediate analysis. The IV catheter was then flushed with approximately 1 mL of saline [20]. It is important to note that this technique was utilized in venous catheters and has not been assessed in arterial catheters.

Components for invasive blood pressure measurement

While the use of an aneroid manometer alone has been described [21], standard IBP components typically include (1) an intra-arterial catheter, (2) fluid-filled, non-compliant tubing, (3) a pressure transducer, and (4) signal conditioning and monitoring software. For peripheral arterial catheterization, a standard over-the-needle catheter that is kink-resistant, biologically inert, and incompressible is used most often. The saline-filled tubing forms a continuous, non-compressible column of fluid producing "hydraulic coupling" between the arterial circulation and the transducer. In the clinical setting, most modern disposable IBP transducers are resistive devices that convert the mechanical (kinetic) energy arising from arterial pressure changes to changes in electrical resistance and ultimately an output voltage. Ohm's law provides a useful framework for understanding how this system works:

$$R = P / I$$

where R is the resistance (measured in ohms, Ω), P is the potential or voltage (measured in volts, V), and I is the current (measured in amperes, A). An ohm (Ω) is the basic unit of electrical resistance and, as defined by Ohm's law, a resistance of 1 Ω allows 1 A of current to flow under the influence of 1 V of potential. Resistance-type transducers are based on the principle that resistance of a wire (i.e., resistor) changes when it is subjected to "strain." Resistance increases as the wire is put under tension (i.e., as it is stretched and becomes longer and thinner) and decreases as it is subjected to compression (i.e., as it becomes shorter and wider) [22].

Most modern commercial BP transducers utilize four strain gauges (resistors) that are bonded to a movable diaphragm and arranged in a Wheatstone bridge circuit. Mechanical pressure variations associated with arterial pulsations physically deform the diaphragm, which creates tension in two of the strain gauges and simultaneous compression of the other two. These strain changes lead to variations in electrical resistance and, because the Wheatstone bridge is very sensitive to small changes in resistance, the bridge becomes unbalanced, and the potential difference (i.e., voltage) generated is proportional to the pressure applied [23]. The resulting raw electrical signal output from the galvanometer is processed, amplified, and converted to values that are displayed graphically and numerically by the monitor [24]. The Wheatstone bridge also compensates for any temperature changes as all four strain gauges are affected equally.

Transducer setup and priming of pressure tubing

The transducer must be connected to the arterial catheter via a length of non-compliant pressure tubing primed with normal saline to create a continuous non-compressible fluid column. For most accurate results, the length of tubing and the number of stopcocks should be minimized. In most cases, the tubing packaged with commercial transducers is appropriate. Transducers may be connected to a pressurized bag of saline (with or without heparin added) to facilitate continuous flush of the catheter, or they may be intermittently flushed to maintain patency (see arterial catheter maintenance below).

Leveling the transducer

It is convention to place the arterial BP transducer at the level of the aortic root or base of the right atrium (RA) to ensure a common reference standard and accurate interpretation of IBP

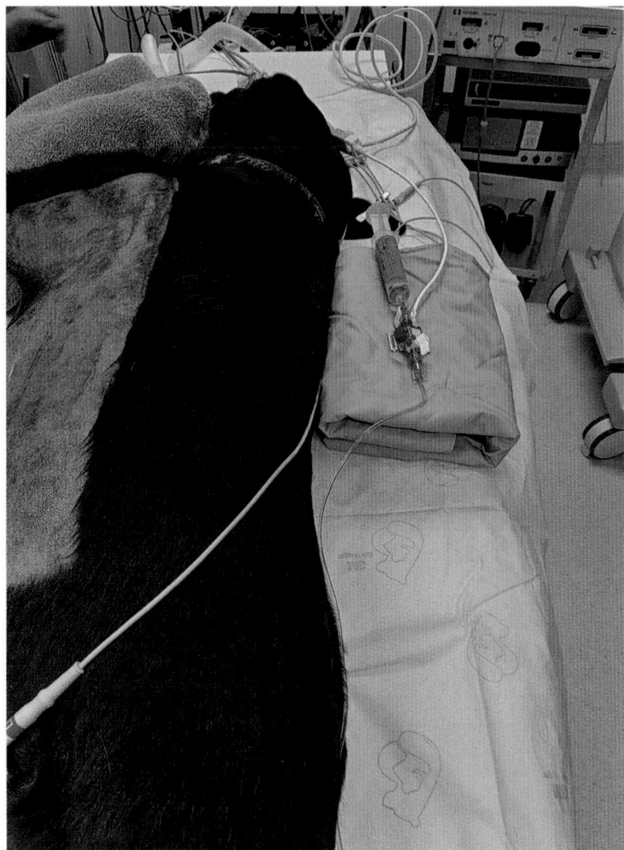

Figure 12.3 Invasive blood pressure setup. The transducer is positioned at the level of the right atrium and zeroed to atmospheric pressure. Note the open-ended (red) injection caps, which aid in maintenance of hygiene. Source: Dr. Odette O, with permission.

measurements (Fig. 12.3). Positioning the transducer below that level results in artifactually high pressures, whereas positioning it above that level results in artifactually low pressures. For every 10 cm that the transducer is positioned below the RA, the system will reportedly add 7.4 mmHg to displayed pressures, and vice versa [25].

Zeroing the transducer

While the processes of zeroing and leveling the IBP transducer tend to occur together in most clinical scenarios, they are actually different processes. Zeroing exposes the transducer to atmospheric pressure via an open air–fluid interface while leveling (as described above) assigns this zero-reference point to a specific position relative to the patient's body (i.e., the RA).

To zero the transducer, thus eliminating the effects of atmospheric pressure, the stopcock is turned "off" to the patient, the system is opened to atmospheric pressure (i.e., the non-vented cap from the stopcock is temporarily removed after opening it to room air), and the monitor's zeroing function is activated. Once the system has been zeroed, the stopcock can then be turned off to the atmosphere and an arterial waveform should appear on the monitor [25]. While zeroing does not necessarily have to be performed with the transducer positioned at the level of the patient's RA (as atmospheric pressure does not vary with these modest positional changes), rezeroing should be performed sporadically (i.e., several times per day) as both the transducer and atmospheric pressure will gradually drift away from the calibration point over time.

Physics of invasive blood pressure monitoring systems

Natural frequency and resonance

The IBP monitoring system (i.e., catheter, fluid-filled tubing, transducer, and electronics) is characterized as an underdamped, second-order dynamic system [24]. The fluid column between the artery and the transducer can be described as a simple harmonic oscillator that, when displaced by a heartbeat, begins to oscillate. In a frictionless system, the oscillations would continue indefinitely at the system's *natural frequency*; however, in a clinical patient, friction causes the system to oscillate briefly after a single displacement (i.e., one heartbeat) and then come to rest. This is analogous to a tennis ball dropped from a height that bounces several times before coming to rest on the ground [24].

The complex arterial pressure waveform is composed of one fundamental waveform (the first harmonic), which is equal to the pulse rate, and numerous other higher frequency/lower amplitude waveforms (second harmonic, third harmonic, etc.) that are multiples of the fundamental frequency. The IBP waveform is ultimately created by Fourier analysis, which sums the various sine waves of differing amplitudes and frequencies into a single complex waveform.

If the natural frequency of the IBP system (i.e., the frequency at which it freely oscillates) is close to the frequency of any of the harmonics, the system will *resonate* leading to amplification of the signal and falsely wide and tall waveform peaks. Consequently, the IBP system should have the highest possible natural frequency (preferably above the eighth harmonic frequency) to minimize resonance distortion, especially in patients with faster HRs and steeper systolic upstrokes. As an example, a cat with a HR of 180 beats per minute (bpm) (i.e., 3 Hz) would require a system with a natural frequency greater than 24 Hz. A number of variables influence natural frequency including the radius and length of the tubing, the elasticity of the system, and the density of the fluid. By (1) shortening the length of the pressure tubing, (2) increasing the diameter of the pressure tubing, (3) using non-compliant pressure tubing, and (4) using a low-density fluid to fill the system (i.e., saline), the system's elasticity is decreased and its natural frequency is increased [24]. Conversely, the presence of air bubbles in the system will increase elasticity and decrease the natural frequency.

Dynamic response testing and damping

The *dynamic response* of the IBP system to pulse pressure oscillations from the cardiac cycle is determined by the balance of natural frequency (discussed earlier) and damping of the system. Damping is defined as the frictional forces that oppose the oscillations and result in decreased wave amplitude. It is described by the *damping coefficient* and, like natural frequency, is influenced by the diameter and length of the catheter and tubing. A damping coefficient of approximately 0.7 is considered optimal [24]. Over- and under-damping will affect the waveform and accurate measurement of IBP (Fig. 12.4). A dynamic pressure response test or "fast flush test" can be used to help identify damping issues. To perform this test, high pressure (> 300 mmHg) is rapidly introduced to the catheter from the continuous flush device for 1–2 s and then abruptly stopped. A square waveform is produced and information is derived by observing the oscillation pattern as the pressure returns to baseline (Fig. 12.5). Upon termination of the flush, the waveform should return to baseline within one to two oscillations, neither being

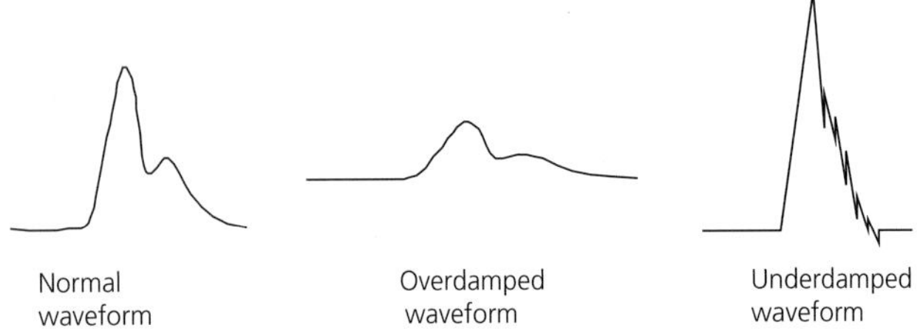

Figure 12.4 Normal, overdamped, and underdamped arterial pressure waveforms.

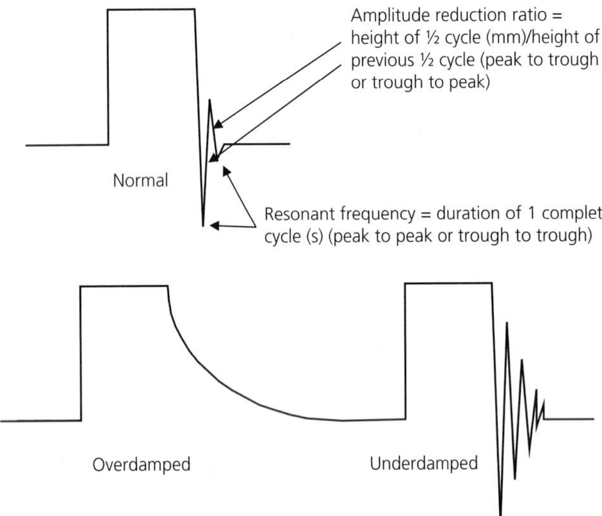

Figure 12.5 Dynamic pressure response test. A dynamic pressure response test is used to determine the resonant frequency and amplitude reduction ratio of a measuring system. A high pressure is applied to the measuring system while it is attached to the patient (usually with the continuous flush device). Sudden release of this pressure results in return of oscillations while the waveform returns to baseline. In a system with optimal damping, one to two positive and one to two negative oscillations should be observed before the waveform returns to baseline.

greater than 1/3 the height of the previous oscillation. A waveform with a dicrotic notch should return thereafter. Absence of this feature indicates an overdamped waveform. The presence of many oscillations after the square wave indicated underdamping [26]. A smaller gauge catheter has a higher damping coefficient and is more likely to be overdamped than a larger gauge catheter. Other factors leading to an overdamped BP waveform include air bubbles, catheter obstruction (i.e., clot or kinking of catheter), pressure tubing that is overly compliant or long, and/or the use of too many stopcocks. Overdamping causes an underestimation of SAP, while DAP may either be accurate or overestimated [26]. Underdamping results in an overestimation of SAP and underestimation of DAP. MAP is the parameter least affected by system damping [25]. Recent literature recommends the use of IBP MAP instead of SAP in humans for interventional decisions while in the perioperative period [27].

Arterial catheter placement and maintenance

Common sites for arterial cannulation in small animals include the dorsal pedal/metatarsal, palmar digital/metacarpal, radial, and coccygeal arteries; the femoral, brachial, and lingual arteries may

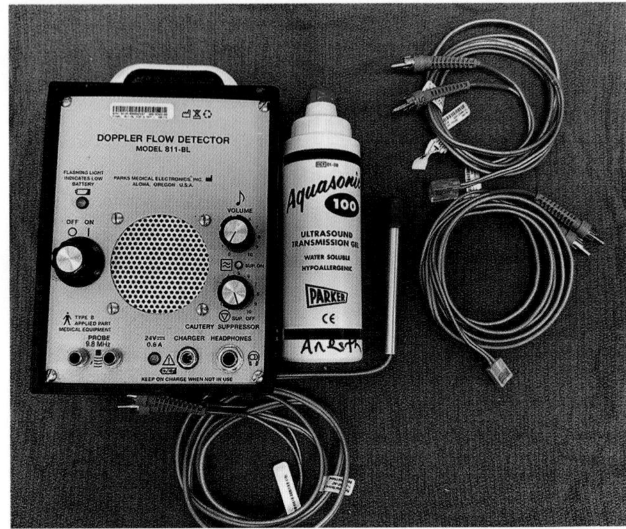

Figure 12.6 Parks Doppler unit. Source: Dr. Carrie Schroeder, with permission.

also be used. In large animals, common sites include the auricular artery in cattle and branches of the facial or metatarsal artery in equids. The location of catheter placement affects values obtained (Fig. 12.1B), so different peripheral sites should not be used interchangeably for comparative results in patients [28–31].

Catheter size varies from 24 to 22 gauge in very small patients, 22 to 20 gauge in medium and large dogs, and 20 to 18 gauge in large animals. Special care should always be taken to minimize the risk of intravascular catheter infections and guidelines in both human and veterinary medicine include staff education and training, hand hygiene, use of aseptic technique, and proper skin preparation as well as daily care after placement [32,33]. Indwelling arterial catheters require constant or intermittent flushing to remain patent. Heparinized saline is often used at various concentrations, but caution should be used in very small patients due to the risk of clinical effects with doses starting at 150 U/kg [34]. Recent studies have shown 0.9% sodium chloride to be as effective as heparinized saline for maintaining catheter patency [35,36].

Non-invasive blood pressure measurement

Doppler ultrasonographic blood pressure measurement

Doppler ultrasonography is an indirect, non-invasive method of measuring BP (NIBP). The equipment necessary for this technique includes a non-directional transcutaneous Doppler unit, probe, sphygmomanometer, inflatable cuffs of various sizes, and ultrasonic coupling gel (Fig. 12.6). A small 8.0–9.9 MHz ultrasound probe is placed over a shaved peripheral artery with ultrasonic coupling gel. The probe contains piezoelectric crystals, traditionally composed of quartz and more recently of polarized ceramics. A 10-mm beam of ultrasound wave contacts the artery at about 15° from perpendicular [37]. The waves generated from contact of the ceramics with pulsatile red blood cells within the peripheral artery result in deformation of the piezoelectric elements. As defined by the piezoelectric effect, deformation converts mechanical energy into electrical energy to receive the wave; then, realignment of the ceramics changes electrical energy back to mechanical energy, thereby creating sound waves; in other words, movement of red blood cells results in a change in pitch of the reflected sound waves [38]. Flat probes are designed to be taped into place for repeated use, while other shapes may be used for periodic pulse amplification. An amplifier connected to this probe intensifies the audible sound via a built-in speaker or headphones [37].

Common peripheral arteries used for Doppler BP measurement include the palmar metacarpal, plantar metatarsal, dorsal pedal, and coccygeal. An inflatable cuff is placed proximal to the Doppler probe. The cuff should have a width measuring approximately 30–40% of the circumference of the limb; alternatively, the measurement guide provided by the manufacturer may be used. A sphygmomanometer is then attached and rapidly inflated until occlusion of the artery occurs, as demonstrated by loss of the audible signal, and then inflated an additional 20–30 mmHg. The cuff is then deflated slowly until a return of the audible signal (known as "Korotkoff sounds") occurs. The sphygmomanometer pressure correlating to return of the first Korotkoff sound is widely accepted as SAP in most species. While changes in the character of the Korotkoff sounds may be appreciated as the cuff is deflated, DAP is not reliably estimated by this method, so calculation of MAP is not possible using this method of BP measurement. In cats, Doppler NIBP measurement tends to underestimate BP when compared to invasive femoral artery measurements, with Doppler SAP +14 mmHg more closely representing invasive femoral SAP values [39]. Nonetheless, it should be noted that in dogs < 5 kg, Doppler BP most closely reflects SAP and was found to be highly specific in predicting hypotension in anesthetized small dogs [40].

The advantages of Doppler NIBP measurement include that it is non-invasive, inexpensive, portable, provides real-time audible pulse sounds, and is easy to use in a variety of species. Disadvantages of this technique include that the cuff must be inflated manually, only a single value is provided for BP, and that electrical interference from other equipment (e.g., electrocautery) may result in excessive noise.

Oscillometric blood pressure measurement

Oscillometric BP measurement technology has been commercially available since the 1970s and remains popular today. The reasons for its popularity across a variety of species include ease of use, minimal equipment requirements, and automation. With many device options on the market, a multiorganizational universal standard for validation of this equipment for use in human patients was set in 2018 [41].

In general, this is a *counterpressure* measurement technique whereby the arterial pulse produces changes in the volume of a limb, which can be transmitted to and detected as changes in pressure within a cuff encircling the limb. An inflatable cuff is placed over the artery of a limb or the tail and attached with tubing to a monitor containing a microprocessor and pressure sensor (transducer) and, in some monitors, an amplifier and filter. The tongue has also recently been reported for use in canine patients, with MAP meeting ACVIM and American Association for Medical Instruments criteria for a wide range of pressures. However, it should be noted that SAP accuracy and precision was poor, only meeting ACVIM criteria during states of hypotension [42]. Identical to Doppler NIBP measurement, the cuff should have a width measuring approximately 30–40% of the circumference of the limb or the measurement guide provided by the manufacturer should be used (Fig. 12.7).

Oscillometric devices inflate the cuff to a pressure approximately 20–30 mmHg above that needed to obstruct blood flow and then slowly deflate it using either continuous linear or nonlinear (step-deflation) methods. Automatic cuff deflation allows for the gradual return of arterial blood flow and the corresponding changes in cuff pressure amplitudes (i.e., oscillations) persist until inflation pressure is released and blood flow returns to normal. The monitor records this series of cuff pressure amplitudes (i.e., absent, increasing to a maximum, then decreasing until absent) and analyses them. Microprocessors with various proprietary empirical algorithms then determine values for SAP, MAP, and DAP. All oscillometric NIBP monitors make use of these proprietary algorithms, making comparison between monitors from different manufacturers a challenge. There are no current regulatory standards governing how these systems obtain cuff pressure amplitudes and determine BP. The result is that accuracy, validation as compared to IBP, agreement among monitors, as well as repeatability remains a challenge in human and veterinary medicine alike. In addition, there are also no current reliable instruments to test the accuracy of these various algorithms or their performance, leaving the consumer to rely heavily on the manufacturers for quality assurance and on publications that attempt to establish formulas to illuminate details [43,44].

The MAP is considered the most valid pressure value provided by oscillometric NIBP systems, with SAP and DAP being calculated via manufacturer-specific proprietary algorithms [43]. Three

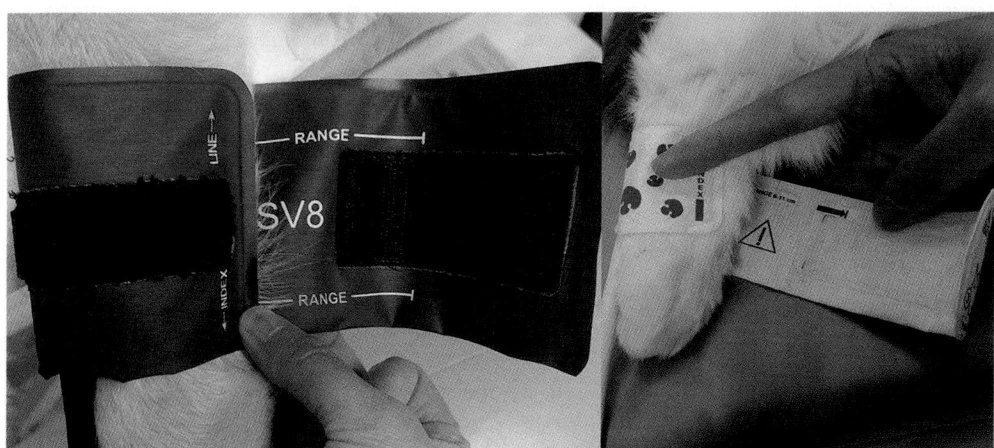

Figure 12.7 Blood pressure cuff width should be 30–40% of the limb circumference for accurate measurement. To use the range guidance, roll the edge of the cuff around the limb, where the index line falls within the range guide when secured onto the limb of use. Source: Dr. Odette O, with permission.

of the most popular empirical techniques include the maximum amplitude, derivative, and fixed-ratio algorithms. The maximum amplitude algorithm compares cuff pressure amplitudes to determine the point of maximal (peak) oscillations, which is measured as the MAP. There are various published methods for determining SAP and DAP based on the ratio of oscillation amplitudes, and different investigators have proposed different set points or ratios for SAP and DAP [43,45]. To add to this confusion, there is at least one study that has called into question the widely held assertion that the formula for the maximum amplitude algorithm represents MAP. Instead, they suggest that this algorithm actually estimates a weighted average of SAP and DAP where weighting is determined by arterial compliance curve widths [44]. Regarding the other techniques, the derivative algorithm estimates DAP and SAP from the slope of the oscillogram, while with the fixed-ratio algorithm estimates DAP and SAP as population-based fractions of their peak values. This last algorithm is prone to amplifying error, resulting in inaccurate BP measurements [44].

SunTech Medical, Inc. created the NIBP technology that is incorporated into many of the commonly used veterinary multiparameter monitors today, including the Digicare, DRE Veterinary, Midmark, Nonin, Smiths Medical (Surgivet), and Vmed Technology, in addition to human-based products such as the Masimo Root®. This manufacturer also produces a veterinary-specific line of standalone NIBP monitors reported to function at pulse rates of 25–300 bpm in small animals and 15–150 bpm in horses. These monitors measure SAP, MAP, and DAP at ranges of 40–265, 27–222, and 20–200 mmHg, respectively. The system uses a default inflation pressure of 180 mmHg, with subsequent inflations set at SAP +30 mmHg with a minimum inflation pressure of 120 mmHg. These monitors use nonlinear (stepwise) deflation for increased tolerance to motion and MAP determination based on their proprietary maximum amplitude and SAP and DAP calculation algorithms. The veterinary models also have reference ranges, changes in gain based on differing pulse volumes based on patient size, and internal manufacturer validation designed from specific animal populations, including small animals and horses [personal communication: P. Matsumura, SunTech Medical; September 7, 2021]

Limitations to accurate performance of the oscillometric method of BP measurement include situations of reduced blood flow, poor cuff sizing, patient movement/shivering, extremes of patient size, severe hypotension/hypertension, and cardiac arrhythmias. The uneven pulse waveforms created by arrhythmias result in an inaccurate MAP and subsequent SAP/DAP determinations. Oscillometric NIBP measurement is also intermittent, with lag time varying based on user settings.

High-definition oscillometric blood pressure measurement

High-definition oscillometry (HDO) is a non-invasive means of BP measurement that uses an HDO device with a 32-bit processor in conjunction with a computer or tablet, enabling real-time visualization of the pulse waveform during cuff inflation/deflation and assessment of validation through recognition of artifacts [46]. Gain is a feature unique to HDO. The system can optimize gain (amplify signal) and deflation rates to read low BPs and complete readings often within 8–15 s. The HDO permits a scan bandwidth of 16,000 Hz compared to an input of 50/60 Hz used in standard oscillometric devices. The system in units such as the HDO Vet MD PRO utilizes linear deflation and a veterinary-specific algorithm that enables measurement of SAP, MAP, and DAP. Coccygeal artery assessment is recommended, so tail base cuff placement is necessary, though the antebrachium can also be used in patients where coccygeal access is not possible. Software enables in-depth pulse wave analysis for users to assess functional parameters including SV, SVR, and SV variance. In anesthetized canine patients, HDO BP measurement has been shown to meet ACVIM consensus panel validation criteria for MAP and DAP but not SAP, where it was found to be unreliable in hypotensive dogs [47]. In awake cats, this BP technique met the criteria for SAP, but underestimated DAP [48].

Central venous pressure measurement

Central venous pressure (CVP) measures the hydrostatic pressure of the intrathoracic vena cava, as a close reflection of right atrial pressure (RAP) [49]. Traditionally, this modality has been considered an indirect indicator of intravascular volume and fluid responsiveness in veterinary patients. Although alternative means of measurement of CO, perfusion, and volume status exist, CVP measurement is still utilized in veterinary medicine due to its practicality, low cost, and relative ease of use. Lack of consistent and repeatable reference ranges for CVP across species, however, introduces challenges when it comes to interpretation of these values in veterinary medicine. CVP is actually a measure of intravascular pressure in relation to atmospheric pressure, whereas true RAP and right ventricular (RV) pressure (used as surrogates of left ventricular (LV) end-diastolic volume and cardiac preload) are transmural pressures. The complex relationship between CVP, CO, and the vascular system further complicates interpretation, despite values themselves being relatively easy to obtain [50]. In addition, the nonlinear nature of the Frank–Starling curve along with factors causing changes in cardiac and pulmonary compliance results in circumstances where pressure does not correlate well with volume status [51]. Consequently, CVP has fallen out of favor in human medicine in a number of situations, including guidance of fluid resuscitation in septic shock [52], while others still encourage its use with a clear understanding of the caveats [53]. Current veterinary publications on this topic remain inconclusive.

CVP should not be used as a single static measurement to make clinical decisions. Instead, it should be considered as part of a clinical picture, in conjunction with repeated readings and assessments of trends in the individual patient of interest, along with use of clinical values such as HR, arterial BP, lactate trends, and pulse quality for assessing patient hydration and perfusion status. In horses, increased lactate in combination with decreased CVP was noted in subjects experiencing blood loss despite insignificant changes in HR and venous blood gas values [54].

Patients that present with concerns related to their volume status and/or overhydration are potential candidates for CVP measurement as part of an overall clinical assessment. These patients may include high-risk anesthesia patients with shock or ongoing hemorrhage requiring large volume resuscitation and those with significant renal or cardiac disease. Catheterization of the vena cava is necessary for the measurement of CVP. The external jugular vein is most often used in veterinary medicine, due to its size, easy accessibility, and ability to maintain hygiene. Radiographic confirmation of correct placement should verify that the tip of the catheter is located at the entry to the RA. A catheter originating in the lateral saphenous vein (dogs) or medial saphenous vein (cats) may also be used; however, the catheter must be advanced into the thoracic vena cava at the level of the RA for accurate CVP measurement. It should be noted that peripheral venous pressure was poorly correlated with CVP in dogs and cats with stable cardiovascular status [55]. Various central line kits, both veterinary and non-veterinary, are commercially available. The use of prepackaged kits permits sterile placement of these catheters using the modified Seldinger technique and has been found to increase procedural quality through decreased technical errors and time required [56]. With appropriate care, these catheters may safely remain in place for multiple days.

The normal reference range for CVP is 0–10 centimeters of water (cmH_2O), more commonly 0–5 cmH_2O [49]. Depending on the technique used for measurement, millimeters of mercury (mmHg) can be converted to cmH_2O using a conversion factor of 1.36 (i.e., 1 mmHg = 1.36 cmH_2O). In the absence of other complicating factors, patients demonstrating negative values should be assessed for hypovolemia, while those in the range of 0–5 cmH_2O may be considered euvolemic, and those with values trending beyond 7–10 cmH_2O may be at increased risk for hypervolemia. These values are more helpful when considering the response to fluid challenges, rather than single-point determinations about volume status since many factors alter interpretation. For instance, the absence of a decrease in CVP that is normally observed during inspiration in fluid responsive patients (known as "Kussmaul's sign") may indicate concern for fluid intolerance [49,51].

Two methods may be utilized for the measurement of CVP. Readings should be performed in a consistent manner with the patient in the same body position for all measurements, the system leveled at the RA, and values taken at end-expiration. Historically, a water column setup was used, reflecting the common units used for CVP measurement, cmH_2O. This system offers the advantages of being low cost and requiring minimal equipment (i.e., a central line kit, ruler, IV pole, non-compliant tubing, three-way stopcock, and fluids). However, challenges with this setup include the need to manually level the zero point of the water manometer at the level of patient's RA and the lack of a waveform for analysis. Alternatively, an electronic pressure transducer system may be used to measure CVP. The setup is identical to that used for IBP measurement, as described previously. Benefits to use of this system include constant, real-time monitoring, and the production of a waveform for analysis (Fig. 12.8). Values from these electronic systems may be expressed in mmHg, depending on the manufacturer and monitor settings.

The decision to perform CVP monitoring should be made with a risk/benefit analysis. Aside from the limitations in accurately assessing vascular volume status and fluid responsiveness, there has been much controversy regarding its ability to predict morbidity and mortality in human medicine and its use and interpretation in veterinary medicine should be viewed with caution [51–53]. Highly skilled personnel are needed for both placement and maintenance of a central line as well as interpretation of the results. Potential immediate risks associated with jugular catheter placement are cardiac arrhythmias (most commonly atrial or ventricular premature contractions if a guide wire or catheter is advanced into the heart), hemorrhage, hematoma, air embolus, thrombus, pneumomediastinum, pneumothorax, hemothorax, tracheal trauma, and inadvertent carotid artery puncture [57]. Longer-term concerns include catheter-associated infection, recurrent laryngeal nerve damage, and jugular vein stenosis or occlusion. Contraindications to this approach include patients with concerns for increased intracranial pressure (ICP), coagulopathies, and those at increased risk of thromboembolic events. As such, current recommendations in veterinary medicine are to use CVP trends for additional data to assess patient needs, but central venous access should not be undertaken solely for this purpose [58].

Indices of fluid responsiveness

Pulse pressure variation and systolic pressure variation

The circulatory effects in dogs provided intermittent positive-pressure ventilation (IPPV) were first measured almost 60 years ago, with the cause of these effects attributed to the effect of intrathoracic pressure on venous return [59]. Since then, many studies have noted the variation in the arterial pressure waveform during IPPV and demonstrated that in mechanically ventilated patients, under certain circumstances, this physical sign can be an accurate predictor of fluid responsiveness. Pulse pressure variation (PPV) is a

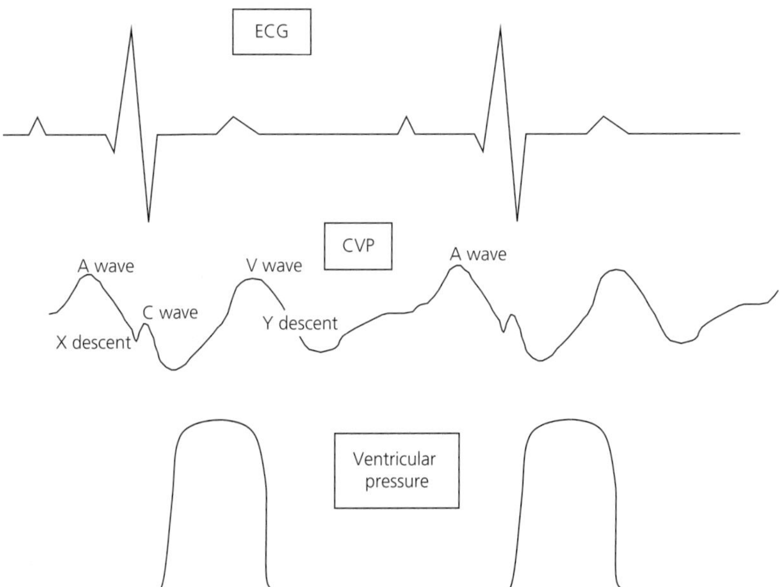

Figure 12.8 Central venous pressure (CVP) tracing and waveform. Note the features of the CVP waveform throughout the cardiac cycle: A wave represents right atrial contraction, seen after ECG P wave but prior to QRS; C wave reflects the tricuspid valve being pushed up into the atrium during ventricular contraction (note: this wave may or may not be evident); X descent reflects right atrial relaxation; V wave reflects rapid atrial filling with plateau; and Y descent reflects ventricular relaxation and early ventricular filling.

measure of the difference between systolic and diastolic pressures during IPPV inspiratory and expiratory phases.

In-depth reviews of the physiologic changes that occur during mechanical ventilation may be found elsewhere [60]. In short, increased pleural pressure due to positive-pressure ventilation compresses the vena cava and increases RAP, resulting in decreased venous return. In turn, decreased RA preload decreases RV output and pulmonary artery blood flow. Finally, LV filling and, thereby, output are decreased. Three additional mechanisms may cause respiratory variation via alteration of LV SV during the inspiratory phase of IPPV: (1) RV ejection is impeded by increased RV afterload resulting from increases in alveolar pressure that exceed increases in pleural pressure; (2) the increase in alveolar pressure relative to pleural pressure also sends blood from the alveolar capillaries toward the left side of the heart, resulting in increased LV preload; and (3) LV afterload is decreased via the reduction in thoracic blood volume resulting from increased systolic extracardiac pressure along with decreased systolic intracardiac pressure from the positive pleural pressure. In summary, during the IPPV inspiratory phase, RV preload is decreased, while RV afterload is increased; and LV preload is increased, while LV afterload is decreased. The RV output decrease is then translated a few beats later to the left heart. The main determinant of respiratory variation in PP is the variation in LV SV.

In general, hypovolemic patients demonstrate greater respiratory variations in SV and arterial pressure for four main reasons: (1) the vena cava is more collapsible during hypovolemia; (2) an underfilled RA during hypovolemia will be more sensitive to the transmission of pleural pressure during inspiration; (3) the effect of inspiration on RV afterload is more significant during hypovolemia where West's zone 1 (pulmonary arterial pressure < alveolar pressure) and/or West's zone II (pulmonary venous pressure < alveolar pressure) conditions are likely met; and (4) during hypovolemia, both left and right ventricles are more likely functioning on the steep portion of the Frank–Starling curve where there is a greater sensitivity to preload changes than if operating on the flatter portion of the curve (Fig. 12.9).

Thus, during hypovolemic conditions, patients demonstrate greater respiratory variation in PP. When these waveforms are displayed on patient-side monitors, they can be a valuable tool in assessing fluid responsiveness during IPPV. Waveform variation requires quantification for true utility since monitors variably record arterial waveform at differing speeds and scales. Analysis of these waveforms has been described by various methods including systolic pressure variation (SPV), which is the difference between maximum and minimum SAP over a single respiratory cycle. Assessment of systolic reference pressure at the end-expiratory pause then allows differentiation between inspiratory increase and expiratory decrease. When PPV was first described in critically ill patients in 1978, SPV > 10 mmHg was observed in hypovolemic patients with SPV < 10 mmHg seen in normo- and hypervolemic patients [61]. Alternatively, there is a different calculation with the aim of monitoring changes in LV SV where respiratory variation in arterial PP is quantified by determining the difference between maximum and minimum PPs during one mechanical breath with the mean of the two values expressed as a percentage [62]:

$$\Delta PP(\%) = 100 \times (PP_{max} - PP_{min}) / [(PP_{max} + PP_{min})/2]$$

Since the inspiratory increase in LV SV itself has minimal effect on respiratory variation, another proposed method uses PP measured at the end-expiratory pause as the reference PP to measure the expiratory decrease in arterial PP [63].

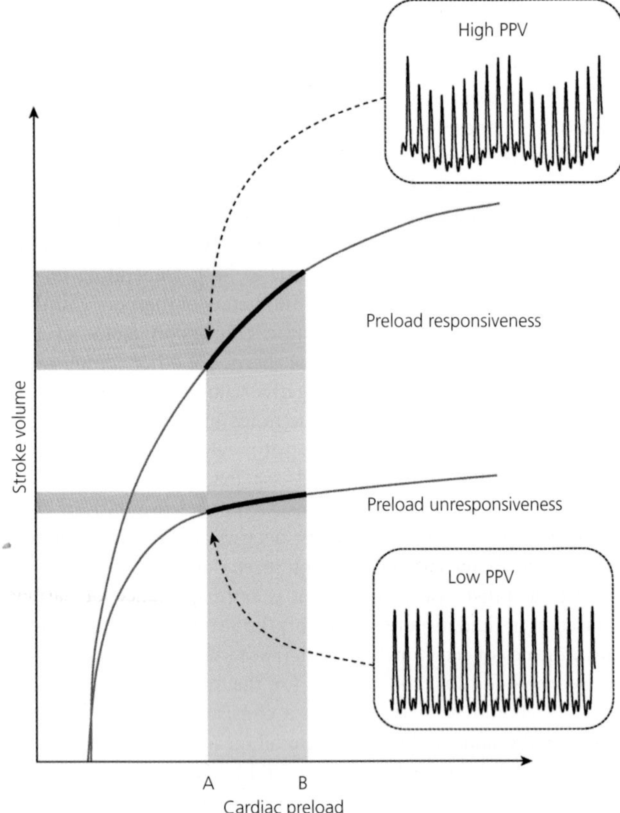

Figure 12.9 Frank-Starling relationship, preload responsiveness, and pulse pressure variation (PPV). When the heart is operating on the steep part of the Frank-Starling relationship (top), an increase in cardiac preload (from A to B) results in an increase in stroke volume (preload or fluid responsiveness). When the heart is operating on the plateau of the Frank-Starling relationship (bottom), the same increase in cardiac preload (from A to B) does not result in a significant increase in stroke volume (preload or fluid unresponsiveness). While cardiac preload itself (however it is measured) cannot predict fluid responsiveness/unresponsiveness, PPV is a valuable tool to predict a patient's response to fluid therapy. Source: Teboul *et al.* [64], reprinted with permission of the American Thoracic Society.

The clinical usefulness of PPV includes the ability to provide a dynamic assessment of fluid volume status and cardiac preload, and prediction of hemodynamic response to volume expansion. In human medicine, PPV fluid response has only been validated specifically in mechanically ventilated deeply sedated or anesthetized patients, so careful application is warranted.

In patients receiving positive-pressure ventilation while IBP is being measured, PPV may be utilized using a capable monitor to predict volume responsiveness. SV depends on preload, afterload, and cardiac contractility and, as this parameter is dynamic, fluid responsiveness is defined by the rising portion of the Frank–Starling curve (Fig. 12.9) [64]. Preload contributes to CO (i.e., increases in preload result in increased SV) up to maximum point in fluid responsive patients. Fluid responsiveness decreases significantly in patients on the plateau portion of the curve (i.e., further increases in preload are not associated with proportional increases in SV). In summary, patients demonstrating greater PPV during positive-pressure ventilation are considered preload/fluid responsive, while those showing only minimal PPV are less likely to increase SV in response to fluid therapy. A meta-analysis of the effectiveness of using dynamic parameters such as PPV for providing goal-directed fluid therapy in human surgical patients found that this approach decreased postoperative morbidity and decreased intensive care unit length of stay [65].

PPV has been found to be useful in predicting fluid responsiveness in isoflurane-anesthetized, mechanically ventilated dogs [66–68]. In one study, SPV was found to be even more accurate than PPV in predicting fluid responsiveness in mechanically ventilated isoflurane-anesthetized dogs and may provide another useful tool in assessing fluid responsiveness using an automated algorithm [69]. Overall, PPV values > 7–16% predict fluid responsiveness in canine patients under inhalant anesthesia receiving IPPV [66,68,70,71]. In veterinary medicine, the usefulness of PPV for assessing fluid status has also been examined in a number of other species including horses [72], pigs [73–75], and rabbits [76,77].

It should be noted that many factors influence PPV and SPV, including current volume status, resuscitation fluid type and volume, ventilator settings, chest wall compliance, intra-abdominal pressure, venous vasomotor tone, and the presence of cardiac abnormalities making direct comparisons from these studies difficult. Nevertheless, a number of veterinary studies have shown the utility in using this clinical tool to help predict fluid responsiveness [58] and encourage the use of this parameter to guide fluid therapy over previous conventional methods [78].

Other methods described with some success in measuring respiratory variation on LV SV include computerized pulse contour analysis using a modified Wesseling algorithm and Doppler measurement of aortic blood flow. It should be noted that the plethysmographic waveform from a pulse oximeter has been shown to have some correlation with arterial pressure variations in mechanically ventilated patients but has been associated with inaccuracies in several publications (see below).

Plethysmography variability index

The plethysmography (or pleth) variability index (PVI) is an algorithm built into specific pulse oximeters that has been shown to be effective in predicting fluid responsiveness in anesthetized, mechanically ventilated canine patients [66,67,79]. During IPPV, RV SV is minimal at end-inspiration due to the reduction in venous return during this phase. As a result, LV preload and SV subsequently decrease and are minimal at end-expiration. Changes in the pulse waveform amplitude during the respiratory cycle are detected and measured during mechanical ventilation. The magnitude of this variation is proportional to the likelihood that a patient will increase SV when their preload is augmented via a fluid bolus [64]. With this non-invasive, dynamic index, larger variations in waveform amplitude predict preload dependence and, thus, greater fluid responsiveness. PVI and PPV were found to be considerably more accurate than CVP in predicting fluid responsiveness in mechanically ventilated, isoflurane-anesthetized canines [66]. Depending on the study, PVI values greater than or equal to approximately 13% may indicate fluid responsiveness.

Plethysmography and photoplethysmography

Pulse oximeters with a plethysmographic display may be utilized to estimate BP in veterinary patients with the use of an inflatable occlusive cuff [80]. The method described uses a pulse oximeter probe placed distally on the tongue of a canine subject with an occlusive cuff placed proximally. The cuff is inflated slowly until the plethysmographic pulsatile waveform disappears. The highest value maintaining a visible waveform is an estimation of SAP. Several factors including patient size, vasoconstriction, and compromised CO limit the accuracy and utility of this method. However, it may be useful for monitoring trends of SAP under certain circumstances.

Photoplethysmography (PPG) is a specific monitoring method that provides information including HR, SpO_2, and NIBP developed using principles of infrared light emitted from an LED source on a small probe passing through a tissue bed where the light is altered by blood flow. PPG alone may estimate BP via blood volume pulsations in peripheral tissue beds without use of an inflatable cuff. PPG does not measure actual BP; rather, units utilize a microprocessor that employs an algorithm based on waveform analysis and theoretical models to estimate BP [81].

To date, veterinary-specific monitors are not widely available in North America, limiting this technique to patient sizes where human-based probes may be utilized, most commonly a finger probe. In addition to its use on the lingual site, the use of PPG on the tail and metacarpus has been reported in dogs and on the digit of cats (with limitations) [82]. Technology using PPG in combination with oscillometry to measure BP indirectly has become available in veterinary medicine in Japan, using the BP100D Fukuda ME. This device has demonstrated close correlation with invasive techniques in cats [83].

For humans, wearable devices have been examined using the PPG method as a cuffless, continuous means of non-invasive BP measurement. The most common site of measurement is the finger, but other locations that have been assessed include the toes, forehead, and wrist. Future functionality of this technology may increase in veterinary medicine as use increases in humans at various anatomical sites, making sensors of shapes and different sizes more readily available. However, the overall accuracy of this methodology still warrants further investigation [84].

Increasingly, technology is integrated into patient-side monitors that use PPG with waveform assessment parameters. PPG technology may be used to estimate arterial waveform and fluid responsiveness in humans [85]. Despite the questions that remain regarding the accuracy of plethysmography and PPG for BP estimation itself, important patient information is still provided by perfusion waveforms that are generated.

Continued challenges with blood pressure measurement

Acceptable BP values under anesthesia depend on multiple patient factors, including age, species, comorbidities, and level of consciousness. Even when an acceptable range is established, validating BP measurements across different species, anatomic locations, and methodologies introduces additional challenges. Countless publications in veterinary medicine compare values obtained in different species, during different patient states (e.g., conscious versus anesthetized), using different monitors, all with varying reliability. Even with the gold standard of IBP, values may differ significantly within the same patient based on the site selected. It is important to keep in mind that all methods have inherent limitations, and translation of data across sites, species, conditions, and technologies is not recommended. Values obtained by any method should be interpreted in the context of the overall clinical picture for an individual patient with the goal of optimizing management.

References

1 Grubb T, Sager J, Gaynor JS, *et al.* 2020 AAHA anesthesia and monitoring guidelines for dogs and cats. *J Am Anim Hosp Assoc* 2020; **56**(2): 59–82.

2 American College of Veterinary Anesthesia and Analgesia. Guidelines and Position Statement Documents: Small Animal Monitoring Guidelines. www.acvaa.org/veterinarians/guidelines (accessed December 2022).

3 Trammel JE, Sapra A. Physiology, systemic vascular resistance. In: StatPearls [Internet]. *Treasure Island*, FL: StatPearls Publishing LLC, 2022.

4 Acierno MJ, Brown S, Coleman AE, *et al.* ACVIM consensus statement: guidelines for the identification, evaluation, and management of systemic hypertension in dogs and cats. *J Vet Intern Med* 2018; **32**(6): 1803–1822.

5 Walsh M, Devereaux PJ, Garg AX, *et al.* Relationship between intraoperative mean arterial pressure and clinical outcomes after noncardiac surgery: toward an empirical definition of hypotension. *Anesthesiology* 2013; **119**(3): 507–515.

6 Portier K, Ida KK. Editorial: anesthetic risk and complications in veterinary medicine. *Front Vet Sci* 2020; **7**: 397.

7 Grandy JL, Steffey EP, Hodgson DS, *et al.* Arterial hypotension and the development of postanesthetic myopathy in halothane-anesthetized horses. *Am J Vet Res* 1987; **48**(2): 192–197.

8 Lindsay WA, Robinson GM, Brunson DB, *et al.* Induction of equine postanesthetic myositis after halothane-induced hypotension. *Am J Vet Res* 1989; **50**(3): 404–410.

9 Duke T, Filzek U, Read MR, *et al.* Clinical observations surrounding an increased incidence of postanesthetic myopathy in halothane-anesthetized horses. *Vet Anaesth Analg* 2006; **33**(2): 122–127.

10 Raisis AL. Skeletal muscle blood flow in anaesthetized horses. Part II: effects of anaesthetics and vasoactive agents. *Vet Anaesth Analg* 2005; **32**(6): 331–337.

11 Carlson BE, Arciero JC, Secomb TW. Theoretical model of blood flow autoregulation: roles of myogenic, shear-dependent, and metabolic responses. *Am J Physiol Heart Circ Physiol* 2008; **295**(4): H1572–H1579.

12 Koller A, Sun D, Kaley G. Role of shear stress and endothelial prostaglandins in flow- and viscosity-induced dilation of arterioles *in vitro*. *Circ Res* 1993; **72**(6): 1276–1284.

13 Armstead WM. Cerebral blood flow autoregulation and dysautoregulation. *Anesthesiol Clin* 2016; **34**(3): 465–477.

14 Rothe CF, Nash FD, Thompson DE. Patterns in autoregulation of renal blood flow in the dog. *Am J Physiol* 1971 Jun; **220**(6): 1621–1626.

15 Burke M, Pabbidi MR, Farley J, *et al.* Molecular mechanisms of renal blood flow autoregulation. *Curr Vasc Pharmacol* 2014; **12**(6): 845–858.

16 Berthold H, Münter K, Just A, *et al.* Contribution of endothelin to renal vascular tone and autoregulation in the conscious dog. *Am J Physiol* 1999; **276**(3): F417–F424.

17 Carlström M, Wilcox CS, Arendshorst WJ. Renal autoregulation in health and disease. *Physiol Rev* 2015; **95**(2): 405–511.

18 Ard JL, Kendale S. Searching for a baseline blood pressure: a comparison of blood pressure at three different care points. *J Clin Neurosci* 2016; **34**: 59–62.

19 Trim CM, Hofmeister EH, Quandt JE, *et al.* A survey of the use of arterial catheters in anesthetized dogs and cats: 267 cases. *J Vet Emerg Crit Care (San Antonio)* 2017; **27**(1): 89–95.

20 Barr CA, Gianotti G, Graffeo CE, *et al.* Effect of blood collection by the push-pull technique from an indwelling catheter versus direct venipuncture on venous blood gas values before and after administration of alfaxalone or propofol in dogs. *J Am Vet Med Assoc* 2017; **251**(10): 1166–1174.

21 Tao KM, Sokha S, Yuan HB. Sphygmomanometer for invasive blood pressure monitoring in a medical mission. *Anesthesiology* 2019; **130**(2): 312.

22 Davis PD. Electricity. In: Davis PD, Kenny GNC, eds. *Basic Physics and Measurement in Anesthesia*, 5th edn. Edinburgh, UK: Butterworth-Heinemann, 2003: 149.

23 Davis PD.Blood pressure measurement. In: Davis PD, Kenny GNC, eds. *Basic Physics and Measurement in Anesthesia*, 5th edn. Edinburgh, UK: Butterworth-Heinemann, 2003: 187.

24 Moxham IM. Physics of invasive blood pressure monitoring. *S Afr J Anaesth Analg* 2014; **9**(1): 33–38.

25 Saugel B, Kouz K, Meidert AS, *et al.* How to measure blood pressure using an arterial catheter: a systematic 5-step approach. *Crit Care* 2020; **24**(1): 172.

26 Gardner RM. Direct blood pressure measurement--dynamic response requirements. *Anesthesiology* 1981; **54**(3): 227–236.

27 Lam S, Liu H, Jian Z, *et al.* Intraoperative invasive blood pressure monitoring and the potential pitfalls of invasively measured systolic blood pressure. *Cureus* 2021; **13**(8): e17610.

28 Monteiro ER, Campagnol D, Bajotto GC, *et al.* Effects of 8 hemodynamic conditions on direct blood pressure values obtained simultaneously from the carotid, femoral and dorsal pedal arteries in dogs. *J Vet Cardiol* 2013; **15**(4): 263–270.

29 Acierno MJ, Domingues ME, Ramos SJ, *et al.* Comparison of directly measured arterial blood pressure at various anatomic locations in anesthetized dogs. *Am J Vet Res* 2015; **76**(3): 266–271.

30 Wilson KA, Raisis AL, Drynan EA, *et al.* Agreement between invasive blood pressure measured centrally and peripherally in anaesthetized horses. *Vet Anaesth Analg* 2018; **45**(4): 467–476.

31 Wilson KAT, Raisis AL, Drynan EA, *et al.* Agreement between invasive blood pressures measured in three peripheral arteries in anaesthetized horses under clinical conditions. *Vet Anaesth Analg* 2018; **45**(3): 338–344.

32 Centers for Disease Control and Prevention. Summary of Recommendations: Guidelines for the Prevention of Intravascular Catheter-Related Infections (Edited 2017). www.cdc.gov/infectioncontrol/guidelines/bsi/recommendations.html (accessed December 2022).

33 American Animal Hospital Association. AAHA Guidelines, Protocols: Placement and Maintenance of Peripheral Intravenous Catheters to Prevent Infection. www.aaha.org/aaha-guidelines/infection-control-configuration/protocols/intravenous-catheter-placement-and-maintenance2 (accessed December 2022).

34 Helmond SE, Polzin DJ, Armstrong PJ, *et al.* Treatment of immune-mediated hemolytic anemia with individually adjusted heparin dosing in dogs. *J Vet Intern Med* 2010; **24**(3): 597–605.

35 Vose J, Odunayo A, Price JM, *et al.* Comparison of heparinized saline and 0.9% sodium chloride for maintaining central venous catheter patency in healthy dogs. *Peer J* 2019; **7**: e7072.

36 Sasaki K, Paredes GP, Shiga T. Heparinized saline solution vs. saline solution (0.9% sodium chloride) for the maintenance of dorsal pedal arterial catheter patency in dogs undergoing general anesthesia: a pilot study. *Front Vet Sci* 2020; **7**: 428.

37 811-B Doppler Flow Detector Operating / Service Manual. *Parks Medical Electronics, Inc.* Aloha, OR, USA. www.parksmed.com/products/non-directional-dopplers (accessed December 2022).

38 Jiao P, Egbe K-JI, Xie Y, *et al.* Piezoelectric sensing techniques in structural health monitoring: a state-of-the-art review. *Sensors* 2020; **20**(13): 3730.

39 Grandy JL, Dunlop CI, Hodgson DS, *et al.* Evaluation of the Doppler ultrasonic method of measuring systolic arterial blood pressure in cats. *Am J Vet Res* 1992; **53**(7): 1166–1169.

40 Kennedy MJ, Barletta M. Agreement between Doppler and invasive blood pressure monitoring in anesthetized dogs weighing <5 kg. *J Am Anim Hosp Assoc* 2015; **51**(5): 300–305.

41 Stergiou GS, Alpert B, Mieke S, *et al.* A universal standard for the validation of blood pressure measuring devices: Association for the Advancement of Medical Instrumentation/European Society of Hypertension/International Organization for Standardization (AAMI/ESH/ISO) collaboration statement. *J Hypertens* 2018; **36**(3): 472–478.

42 Kim D, Kim H, Shin D, *et al.* Evaluation of the tongue for oscillometric measurement of arterial pressure in anesthetized Beagle dogs. *Vet Anaesth Analg* 2022; **49**(2): 149–155.

43 Jilek J, Fukushima T. Oscillometric blood pressure measurement: the methodology, some observations, and suggestions. *Biomed Instrum Technol* 2005; **39**(3): 237–241.

44 Chandrasekhar A, Yavarimanesh M, Hahn JO, *et al.* Formulas to explain popular oscillometric blood pressure estimation algorithms. *Front Physiol* 2019; **10**: 1415.

45 Geddes LA. Characterization of the oscillometric method for measuring indirect blood pressure. *Ann Biomed Eng* 1982; **10**: 271–280.

46 HDO Vet BP Monitor Specifications. www.vethdo.com (accessed December 2022).

47 Seliškar A, Zrimšek P, Sredenšek J, *et al.* Comparison of high definition oscillometric and Doppler ultrasound devices with invasive blood pressure in anaesthetized dogs. *Vet Anaesth Analg* 2013; **40**(1): 21–27.

48 Martel E, Egner B, Brown SA, *et al.* Comparison of high-definition oscillometry – a non-invasive technology for arterial blood pressure measurement – with a direct invasive method using radio-telemetry in awake healthy cats. *J Feline Med Surg* 2013; **15**(12): 1104–1113.

49 de Laforcade AM, Rozanski EA. Central venous pressure and arterial blood pressure measurements. *Vet Clin North Am Small Anim Pract* 2001; **31**(6): 1163–1174.

50 Reems MM, Aumann M. Central venous pressure: principles, measurement, and interpretation. *Compend Contin Educ Vet* 2012; **34**: E1–E10.

51 Hutchinson KM, Shaw SP. A review of central venous pressure and its reliability as a hemodynamic monitoring tool in veterinary medicine. *Top Companion Anim Med* 2016; **31**(3): 109–121.

52 Sasai T, Tokioka H, Fukushima T, *et al.* Reliability of central venous pressure to assess left ventricular preload for fluid resuscitation in patients with septic shock. *J Intensive Care* 2014; **2**(1): 58.

53 De Backer D, Vincent JL. Should we measure the central venous pressure to guide fluid management? Ten answers to 10 questions. *Crit Care* 2018; **22**(1): 43.

54 Magdesian KG, Fielding CL, Rhodes DM, *et al.* Changes in central venous pressure and blood lactate concentration in response to acute blood loss in horses. *J Am Vet Med Assoc* 2006; **229**(9): 1458–1462.

55 Chow RS, Kass PH, Haskins SC. Evaluation of peripheral and central venous pressure in awake dogs and cats. *Am J Vet Res* 2006; **67**(12): 1987–1991.

56 Fenik Y, Celebi N, Wagner R, *et al.* Prepackaged central line kits reduce procedural mistakes during central line insertion: a randomized controlled prospective trial. *BMC Med Educ* 2013; **13**: 60.

57 Kornbau C, Lee KC, Hughes GD, *et al.* Central line complications. *Int J Crit Illn Inj Sci* 2015; **5**(3): 170–178.

58 Boysen SR, Gommeren K. Assessment of volume status and fluid responsiveness in small animals. *Front Vet Sci* 2021; **8**: 630643.

59 Morgan BC, Martin WE, Hornbein TF, *et al.* Hemodynamic effects of intermittent positive pressure ventilation. *Anesthesiology* 1966; **27**: 584–590.

60 Michard F. Changes in arterial pressure during mechanical ventilation. *Anesthesiology* 2005; **103**(2): 419–428.

61 Rick JJ, Burke SS. Respirator [sic] paradox. *South Med J* 1978; **71**: 1376–1378.

62 Michard F, Chemla D, Richard C, *et al.* Clinical use of respiratory changes in arterial pulse pressure to monitor the hemodynamic effects of PEEP. *Am J Respir Crit Care Med* 1999; **159**: 935–939.

63 Morelot-Panzini C, Lefort Y, Derenne JP, *et al.* Simplified method to measure respiratory-related changes in arterial pulse pressure in patients receiving mechanical ventilation. *Chest* 2003; **124**: 665–670.

64 Teboul JL, Monnet X, Chemla D, *et al.* Arterial pulse pressure variation with mechanical ventilation. *Am J Respir Crit Care Med* 2019; **199**(1): 22–31.

65 Benes J, Giglio M, Brienza N, *et al.* The effects of goal-directed fluid therapy based on dynamic parameters on post-surgical outcome: a meta-analysis of randomized controlled trials. *Crit Care* 2014; **18**(5): 584.

66 Sano H, Seo J, Wightman P, *et al.* Evaluation of pulse pressure variation and pleth variability index to predict fluid responsiveness in mechanically ventilated isoflurane-anesthetized dogs. *J Vet Emerg Crit Care (San Antonio)* 2018; **28**(4): 301–309.

67 Klein AV, Teixeira-Neto FJ, Garofalo NA, *et al.* Changes in pulse pressure variation and plethysmographic variability index caused by hypotension-inducing hemorrhage followed by volume replacement in isoflurane-anesthetized dogs. *Am J Vet Res* 2016; **77**(3): 280–287.

68 Fantoni DT, Ida KK, Gimenes AM, *et al.* Pulse pressure variation as a guide for volume expansion in dogs undergoing orthopedic surgery. *Vet Anaesth Analg* 2017; **44**(4): 710–718.

69 Dalmagro TL, Teixeira-Neto FJ, Celeita-Rodríguez N, *et al.* Comparison between pulse pressure variation and systolic pressure variation measured from a peripheral artery for accurately predicting fluid responsiveness in mechanically ventilated dogs. *Vet Anaesth Analg* 2021; **48**(4): 501–508.

70 Endo Y, Tamura J, Ishizuka T, *et al.* Stroke volume variation (SVV) and pulse pressure variation (PPV) as indicators of fluid responsiveness in sevoflurane anesthetized mechanically ventilated euvolemic dogs. *J Vet Med Sci* 2017; **79**(8): 1437–1445.

71 Celeita-Rodríguez N, Teixeira-Neto FJ, Garofalo NA, *et al.* Comparison of the diagnostic accuracy of dynamic and static preload indexes to predict fluid responsiveness in mechanically ventilated, isoflurane anesthetized dogs. *Vet Anaesth Analg* 2019; **46**(3): 276–288.

72 Fielding CL, Stolba DN. Pulse pressure variation and systolic pressure variation in horses undergoing general anesthesia. *J Vet Emerg Crit Care (San Antonio)* 2012; **22**(3): 372–375.

73 Behem CR, Graessler MF, Friedheim T, *et al.* The use of pulse pressure variation for predicting impairment of microcirculatory blood flow. *Sci Rep* 2021; **11**(1): 9215.

74 Oshiro AH, Otsuki DA, Hamaji MW, *et al.* Pulse pressure variation and stroke volume variation under different inhaled concentrations of isoflurane, sevoflurane and desflurane in pigs undergoing hemorrhage. *Clinics (Sao Paulo)* 2015; **70**(12): 804–809.

75 Jacques D, Bendjelid K, Duperret S, *et al.* Pulse pressure variation and stroke volume variation during increased intra-abdominal pressure: an experimental study. *Crit Care* 2011; **15**(1): R33.

76 Westphal GA, Gonçalves AR, Bedin A, *et al.* Vasodilation increases pulse pressure variation, mimicking hypovolemic status in rabbits. *Clinics (Sao Paulo)* 2010; **65**(2): 189–194.

77 Fonseca EB, Otsuki DA, Fantoni DT, *et al.* Comparative study of pressure- and volume-controlled ventilation on pulse pressure variation in a model of hypovolaemia in rabbits. *Eur J Anaesthesiol* 2008; **25**(5): 388–394.

78 Araos J, Kenny JS, Rousseau-Blass F, *et al.* Dynamic prediction of fluid responsiveness during positive pressure ventilation: a review of the physiology underlying heart-lung interactions and a critical interpretation. *Vet Anaesth Analg* 2020; **47**(1): 3–14.

79 Endo Y, Kawase K, Miyasho T, *et al.* Plethysmography variability index for prediction of fluid responsiveness during graded haemorrhage and transfusion in sevoflurane-anaesthetized mechanically ventilated dogs. *Vet Anaesth Analg* 2017; **44**(6): 1303–1312.

80 Dyson DH. Indirect measurement of blood pressure using a pulse oximeter in isoflurane anesthetized dogs. *J Vet Emerg Crit Care (San Antonio)* 2007; **17**: 135–142.

81 Xing X, Ma Z, Zhang M, *et al.* An unobtrusive and calibration-free blood pressure estimation method using photoplethysmography and biometrics. *Sci Rep* 2019; **9**: 8611.

82 Cugmas B, Štruc E, Spigulis J. Photoplethysmography in dogs and cats: a selection of alternative measurement sites for a pet monitor. *Physiol Meas* 2019; **40**(1): 01NT02.

83 Heishima Y, Hori Y, Chikazawa S, *et al.* Indirect arterial blood pressure measurement in healthy anesthetized cats using a device that combines oscillometry with photoplethysmography. *J Vet Med Sci* 2016; **78**(7): 1179–1182.

84 Hosanee M, Chan G, Welykholowa K, *et al.* Cuffless single-site photoplethysmography for blood pressure monitoring. *J Clin Med* 2020; **9**(3): 723.

85 Bartels K, Thiele RH. Advances in photoplethysmography: beyond arterial oxygen saturation. *Can J Anaesth* 2015; **62**(12): 1313–1328.

13 Cardiac Output Measurement

Alessio Vigani
Department of Small Animals, Faculty of Veterinary Medicine, University of Zürich, Zürich, Switzerland

Chapter contents

Introduction, 210
Basic principles of cardiac output monitoring, 211
History of cardiac output measurement, 211
Techniques of determination of cardiac output, 212
  The Fick principle, 212
  Pulmonary artery catheter thermodilution, 212
  Transpulmonary thermodilution and ultrasound indicator dilution, 214
  Lithium dilution, 214
  Arterial waveform analysis, 215
  Echocardiography and echo-Doppler, 215
  Thoracic bioimpedance and bioreactance, 216
  Standard capnography as indicator of cardiac output, 217
References, 217

Introduction

Cardiac output is the volume of blood ejected from each of the ventricles per minute, usually reported in L/min, and is the product of the heart rate and stroke volume. Cardiac index is the cardiac output referenced to the body surface area or body weight of the patient and is expressed in L/min/m^2 or L/min/kg, respectively (Table 13.1). Cardiac output is determined by five primary variables: heart rate, rhythm, preload, contractility, and afterload [1].

Cardiac output summarizes in one single value the contribution of the cardiovascular system to global oxygen delivery from the heart to the body. It, therefore, appears reasonable to monitor cardiac output in the assessment of cardiovascular insufficiency in any critical patient undergoing anesthesia. Unfortunately, no definitive studies have shown that the determination of cardiac output or its changes in response to therapy is superior to standard hemodynamic monitoring in terms of outcome [2]. In fact, there is lack of evidence of improved outcomes in acutely ill patients with use of any specific monitoring device, not only cardiac output monitors [3]. Moreover, cardiac output should not be evaluated as a sole variable in a clinical setting. For instance, if metabolic rate is increased or blood flow distribution is abnormal in septic patients, they often have a normal or even increased cardiac output and may still be in circulatory failure [4].

This raises the question: why do we measure cardiac output? There is clear evidence that persistence of a low cardiac output state has significant detrimental effects on organ perfusion and oxygenation [5]. In critically ill human patients, a low cardiac output with sustained unresponsiveness to therapy has been associated with a high mortality rate [6]. Thus, at least in some specific patients, the measurement of cardiac output may represent a supplemental aid to assess the adequacy of therapy and to guide targeted therapeutic interventions (e.g., goal-directed fluid therapy) [2]. More specifically, in a hypotensive patient, whenever the clinical signs are difficult to interpret or the cause of hypotension is not obvious and likely multifactorial (including anesthetic drug effects), the use of cardiac output monitoring should be considered. In this regard, estimation of cardiac output is a useful tool for patient management during anesthesia.

Measuring cardiac output is advantageous in monitoring anesthetic-related hemodynamic changes as well as assessing effectiveness of resuscitation in trauma and critically ill patients [7]. Monitoring the extent of the relative changes in cardiac output, for example, following fluid resuscitation in hypovolemic patients, allows the anesthetist to assess the effectiveness of the intervention and to separate fluid responders from non-responders [8–10]. In different scenarios, following patient trends in cardiac output rather than blood pressure, such as during dobutamine or a nitroprusside infusion, gives more meaningful information as to the hemodynamic response to therapy [11].

Importantly, the determination of absolute values of cardiac output is often less important than following trends. The assessment of relative changes in cardiac output following challenge of the cardiovascular system with fluid loading or medications is referred to as "functional cardiac output monitoring" [12]. Once it is determined that assessing cardiac output may be indicated for a given circumstance, then it is also important that its measurement is accurate enough to identify clinically relevant changes in response to therapy. An acute increase in cardiac output of 20–25% is usually

Veterinary Anesthesia and Analgesia: The Sixth Edition of Lumb and Jones. Edited by Leigh Lamont, Kurt Grimm, Sheilah Robertson, Lydia Love and Carrie Schroeder.
© 2024 John Wiley & Sons, Inc. Published 2024 by John Wiley & Sons, Inc.
Companion website: www.wiley.com/go/lamont/anesthesia

Table 13.1 Examples of typical cardiac output indices reported in veterinary species.

Species	Stroke volume index (mL/kg/beat)	Heart rate (beats/min)	Cardiac index (mL/min/kg)
Cat	0.90–1.0	180	160–180
Cattle	0.7–0.8	60	35–50
Dog	1.6–1.9	120	190–230
Goat	1.1–1.3	80	85–100
Horse	2.6–3.0	45	115–135
Mouse	1.5–1.8	400	600–720
Rabbit	0.4–0.6	250	100–150
Rat	1–1.2	300	300–360
Sheep	0.7–0.9	80	55–70
Swine	1.2–1.4	100	120–140

accepted as a clinically relevant positive response because such a change corresponds to the limit of accuracy of current measuring techniques [13].

The ideal cardiac output monitoring technique would provide accurate, interpretable, and reproducible measurements, be user-friendly, and be readily available. The ideal device should also be safe for the patient, operator independent, provide a rapid response time, and be cost effective. Ultimately, the results obtained should be clinically relevant to guide therapy. To be useful in the management of hemodynamically unstable patients, the technique should allow cardiac output to be measured rapidly and repetitively [14]. At present, there is no available device that meets all these criteria.

Basic principles of cardiac output monitoring

Veterinary anesthesiologists now have an increasing number of techniques and measuring devices available to assess cardiac output. Each technique has its own strengths and limitations [15,16]. As for the selection of monitoring systems for any other physiologic parameter, the following general principles can serve as guidelines to determine the most suitable cardiac output monitoring technique for use in a particular setting.

No hemodynamic monitoring technique can improve outcome by itself and estimating cardiac output is not an exception. Three fundamental conditions must be met for hemodynamic monitoring to positively affect outcome: (1) the results obtained must be of clinical relevance to the patient; (2) the obtained data must be sufficiently accurate and precise to trigger a therapeutic intervention; and (3) the therapeutic intervention must improve outcome. If the information obtained is inaccurate, or interpreted or applied incorrectly, the resultant intervention is unlikely to improve the patient's condition and may potentially be detrimental [3,13].

The choice of monitoring system depends on the patient (species and size) and often on the devices and expertise available at a specific hospital or institution. The expertise and familiarity of the operator represents a critical factor in obtaining reliable results with many cardiac output monitoring devices. A typical example of high operator dependency is represented by echocardiography compared to other automatic devices that consistently produce results with low interoperator variability [13].

As with any other monitored parameter, it is critical to integrate cardiac output data with other physiologic variables from multiple sources. The patient's blood pressure is important complementary information. A low cardiac output in a hypotensive patient will likely indicate hypovolemia or decreased cardiac function, whereas a high cardiac output in a hypotensive patient would suggest decreased systemic vascular resistance [12].

In the clinical setting, cardiac output is estimated, not measured [16]. The only technique that allows its user to directly measure cardiac output is electromagnetic flowmetry, which requires the surgical implantation of a flow probe circumferentially on the main pulmonary artery. This technique is considered the gold standard in the research setting, but it is, for obvious reasons, impractical for clinical applications [17]. All values from bedside techniques are estimates of cardiac output based on assumptions and algorithms. Because of this estimation, comparison of results from different techniques often produces relatively poor agreement and significant bias [16]. In humans, the invasive pulmonary artery catheter (PAC) thermodilution technique is generally considered as the "reference" standard for clinical purposes but has its own limitations [8]. A measurement obtained by a less invasive technique may be preferable if it can be obtained more rapidly and easily, even if it is slightly less accurate. In veterinary medicine, an example of this is the utilization of the lithium dilution cardiac output technique as a suitable reference method in horses for comparison of other cardiac output monitoring devices [15,18–20].

Non-invasiveness of the technique should not be the priority. Although obviously preferable, being non-invasive is not always possible and may even be counterproductive. For instance, the real advantage of echocardiography over other cardiac output techniques is not its non-invasiveness but the peculiarity of providing a direct evaluation of cardiac function [21,22]. A completely non-invasive technique such as bioimpedance, despite reliability in healthy human individuals, has proved inconsistent when applied to critically ill patients or when used in other species [13,23].

History of cardiac output measurement

The first technique for calculation of cardiac output was described by Adolph Fick in 1870. Fick described the calculation of cardiac output from the measurement of the oxygen content of arterial and mixed venous blood as well as oxygen consumption [24]. The Fick technique requires catheterization of the pulmonary artery for mixed venous blood sampling. This was first performed experimentally in live dogs in 1886 by Grehant and Quinquaud [25], and then by Zuntz and Hagemann in a horse in 1898 [26]. Its clinical use in humans did not occur for almost another 50 years. Measurement of oxygen consumption has always represented a significant challenge, and this remains a major limitation of the Fick technique [27]. For this reason, the use of estimates of oxygen consumption was introduced, and the method was referred to as the "modified Fick technique." The Fick technique became the standard for the measurement of cardiac output until the development of dye dilution techniques.

The dye dilution technique of cardiac output determination is based on the independent work of Stewart and Hamilton in the late nineteenth and early twentieth centuries [28]. The equation they derived allowed for the estimation of cardiac output by knowing the amount of an injected indicator and calculating the area under its dilution curve measured downstream. Dye dilution techniques were repeatedly shown to be as reliable as the Fick technique and of better suitability in the clinical setting [29–31]. Thus, dye dilution rapidly became the "accepted method of reference" for cardiac output measurement [32].

Thermodilution, first described by Fegler in 1954, uses heat as an indicator and relies on the same principles of dye dilution [33]. The landmark article on right heart catheterization with a balloon-tipped catheter by Swan *et al.* in 1970 [34] finally set the stage for the widespread clinical use of cardiac output monitoring [35]. Since then, the accuracy of thermodilution-based cardiac output measurements has been assessed by hundreds of studies. Interestingly, all of these studies share a common major limitation – the lack of a gold standard for comparison. Over time, PAC-based thermodilution showed good agreement with direct Fick calculations and dye dilution techniques in a wide range of clinical conditions, and this, combined with the relative ease of insertion of PACs in humans, has made this technique the clinical "gold standard" for comparison for all new cardiac output monitors [32,36,37].

Despite the widespread use of PAC thermodilution, many studies have questioned the effectiveness and safety of this technology [38–43]. This has driven the recent interest in the development of alternative technologies that can measure cardiac output less invasively [44–46].

Techniques of determination of cardiac output

The development and validation of new technologies to measure cardiac output has potential applications in both veterinary clinical and research settings. Many of the techniques described in this chapter are currently in use or will eventually be suitable for use in veterinary medicine.

The Fick principle

Cardiac output can be elegantly estimated by using the Fick principle. The technique is based on the law of conservation of mass [27]. The principle states that over a given time period, the quantity of O_2 or CO_2 entering or leaving the lungs is equal to the quantity of the gas taken up or expelled by the blood flowing in the pulmonary circulation. In mathematical terms, the Fick principle-derived cardiac output equals the patient's oxygen uptake (VO_2) divided by the difference between arterial and mixed venous oxygen content ($CaO_2 - C\bar{v}O_2$) [47]:

$$\text{Cardiac output} = \frac{VO_2}{CaO_2 - C\bar{v}O_2}$$

This relationship is true only in the absence of any cardiopulmonary shunting [47]. Determining cardiac output using the "direct Fick method" requires catheterization of both a peripheral artery and the main pulmonary artery for arterial and mixed venous blood sampling, respectively [27]. The measurement of VO_2 also requires accurate collection and analysis of exhaled gases or determination via closed-circuit techniques. The measurement of VO_2 is the most problematic step of the direct Fick method that has ultimately limited its use for clinical purposes [47].

Indirect techniques based on the Fick principle (also known as the "partial rebreathing technique") have been developed to eliminate the need for pulmonary artery catheterization and invasive blood gas sampling. The technique utilizes elimination of carbon dioxide (CO_2) rather than uptake of oxygen [48] and involves intermittent periods of partial rebreathing to allow minimally invasive estimation of arterial and mixed venous CO_2 content. The monitor consists of a carbon dioxide sensor, a disposable airflow sensor connected to a closed loop system, and a pulse oximeter. Arterial and mixed venous CO_2 content is estimated from measurements of end-tidal CO_2 partial pressure ($P_{ET}CO_2$) during normal breathing and rebreathing maneuvers. VCO_2 is calculated from minute ventilation and its carbon dioxide content. The arterial carbon dioxide content ($CaCO_2$) is estimated from end-tidal carbon dioxide during periods of ventilation. Intermittent phases of partial rebreathing allow estimation of mixed venous CO_2 partial pressure ($P\bar{v}CO_2$), from which CO_2 content ($C\bar{v}CO_2$) is calculated. As the patient rebreathes, the level of $P_{ET}CO_2$ rises to a plateau corresponding to the partial pressure of CO_2 in the blood entering the lungs (or mixed venous blood). At this equilibrium point, the CO_2 elimination from the lungs approaches zero, and the partial pressure of CO_2 in the end-pulmonary capillary blood (mixed venous blood) can be assumed equal to $P_{ET}CO_2$ [49].

Each cardiac output determination requires about 4 min. Every 3 min, a rebreathing valve that prevents normal volumes of CO_2 from being eliminated is activated, and the patient's inhaled and exhaled gases are diverted through the loop for 50 s [48]. As a result, the elimination of CO_2 drops and the concentration of CO_2 in the pulmonary artery increases. It is assumed that cardiac output remains unchanged under normal (N) and rebreathing conditions (R). To compensate for the presence of shunted blood, cardiopulmonary shunting is estimated by use of pulse oximetry and FiO_2 [49]. The general equation that forms the basis of this technique is:

$$\text{Cardiac output} = \frac{VCO_2N - VCO_2R}{\left(C\bar{v}CO_2N - CaCO_2N\right) - \left(C\bar{v}CO_2R - CaCO_2R\right)}$$

where VCO_2, $C\bar{v}CO_2$, and $CaCO_2$ are CO_2 consumption, mixed venous CO_2 content, and arterial CO_2 content, respectively.

Because the diffusion rate of carbon dioxide is 20 times higher than that of oxygen, it is assumed that no difference in venous CO_2 ($C\bar{v}CO_2$) will occur, whether under normal or rebreathing conditions. Hence, the above equation is simplified as:

$$\text{Cardiac output} = \frac{VCO_2N - VCO_2R}{\left(CaCO_2N - CaCO_2R\right)}$$

The partial CO_2 rebreathing (indirect Fick) technique for cardiac output estimation has shown sufficient reliability for clinical application in adult and pediatric human patients [50–52]; however, its accuracy in critical patients has been questioned [53]. One such device (the NICO® monitor, Novametrix Medical Systems) has been tested in veterinary species including dogs and horses, but more modern technologies are available [53–55]. The need for endotracheal intubation and mechanical ventilation limits the use of this device to the intraoperative period. Furthermore, the need for constant CO_2 elimination precludes use during spontaneous breathing in small animals due to tidal volume variability [55]. In validation studies in humans and in dogs, a tidal volume of 12 mL/kg produced cardiac output determinations that correlated well with measurements obtained by both thermodilution and lithium dilution techniques [55,56].

Pulmonary artery catheter thermodilution

The traditional intermittent thermodilution technique uses a bolus of ice-cold sterile saline as an indicator that is injected into the right atrium via a PAC (Swan-Ganz catheter). The change over time in temperature of the blood in the main pulmonary artery is then used to calculate cardiac output [36].

A saline bolus of known volume and temperature is injected into the right atrium via the proximal port of a Swan-Ganz catheter [57,58]. The saline solution can be cooled in ice or injected at room temperature and can be administered in a volume of either

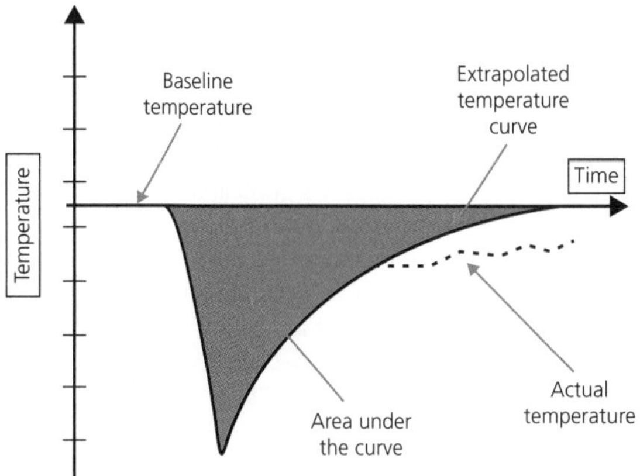

Figure 13.1 Graphical representation of the dilution curve for pulmonary artery catheter (PAC) thermodilution-derived cardiac output.

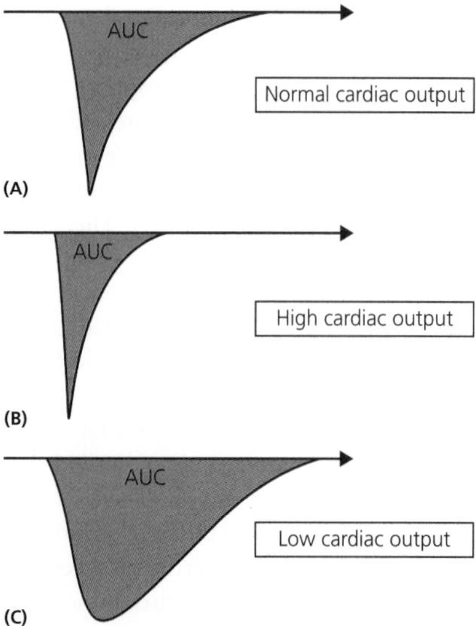

Figure 13.2 Graphical representation of cardiac output thermodilution curves. **A.** Normal cardiac output. **B.** High cardiac output. **C.** Low cardiac output. Note the inverse relationship between the area under the curve (AUC) and cardiac output.

5 or 10 mL. As a general rule, higher volumes and lower temperatures produce the most accurate results. The saline mixes with the blood as it passes through the right ventricle and the pulmonary artery, thus decreasing the temperature of the blood. The blood temperature changes are detected by a thermistor at the distal end of the catheter, which lies within the main pulmonary artery, and a computer acquires the thermodilution curve over time (Fig. 13.1) [33]. The cardiac output computer then calculates flow (cardiac output from the right ventricle) using the acquired blood temperature information, and the starting temperature and volume of the injected saline bolus. The injection is normally repeated at least twice and the measurements averaged. Because cardiac output changes during the respiratory cycle, it is important to inject the saline during a consistent phase of respiration; conventionally, this is done at the end of expiration [37].

As with all of the indicator-dilution methods, the measurement of thermodilution cardiac output is based on the Stewart–Hamilton equation:

$$\text{Cardiac output} = \frac{\text{Volume of indicator} \times \left(\text{Temp}_{\text{patient}} - \text{Temp}_{\text{indicator}}\right)}{\int \Delta\text{Temp}\, dt}$$

The denominator in the formula is a mathematical integration defined by the integral sign $\int$, while ΔTemp is the gradient in temperature and represents the integral in the function. dt indicates that time (t) is the variable of integration. The domain of the integration is from $t = 0$ to $t = \infty$. The function is then defined as the area under the curve bounded by the graph of ΔTemp, the time axis, and the vertical lines $t = 0$ and $x = \infty$. The temperature curve does not actually return to baseline because of recirculation; the computer accounts for this in the calculation of the area under the curve by extrapolating the projected return to baseline of the temperature.

Cardiac output is inversely proportional to $\int \Delta\text{Temp}\, dt$; therefore, when cardiac output is high, the indicator crosses the temperature sensor quickly, producing a small area under the ΔTemp curve. Conversely, when cardiac output is low, the bolus of cold saline diffuses in the right ventricle and pulmonary artery over a relatively long time, causing the area under the temperature versus time curve to be larger (Fig. 13.2).

A modification of the original Swan-Ganz catheter includes a proximal thermal coil to warm blood in the cranial vena cava. The changes in blood temperature are then detected at the PAC's distal end using a thermistor. This method allows the continuous estimation of cardiac output, with the displayed values representing the average value of repeated determinations over the previous 10 min [58,59]. The use of averaged values of cardiac output corrects the inaccuracy of thermodilution associated with possible arrhythmias. The main disadvantage of this method is not being able to produce real-time values, thus limiting its usefulness in rapidly recognizing cardiac output changes in hemodynamically unstable patients.

Pulmonary artery catheterization allows simultaneous measurements of other hemodynamic parameters in addition to cardiac output, including pulmonary artery pressures, right-sided and left-sided filling pressures, and mixed venous oxygen saturation ($S\bar{v}O_2$) [37].

There are some important sources of error with thermodilution measurements that must be considered. If the volume injected is lower than that entered into the computer, the detected area under the curve (AUC) will be artificially small and the calculated cardiac output will be falsely high. Further, if the temperature of the injected saline is colder than expected (e.g., using iced rather than room temperature saline), the temperature change will be artificially large and the estimated cardiac output will be erroneously low [38].

Significant complications have been associated with the use of PACs, and several reports have described the intrinsic risk of morbidity and mortality [39–43]. The "PAC Man" study in human patients recorded complications in 10% of insertions. The most common complications were arrhythmias, heart block, rupture of the right heart or pulmonary artery, thromboembolism, pulmonary infarction, valvular damage, and endocarditis. Similar endocardial and valvular lesions were also described in horses following PAC placement [60]. Therefore, the use of the PAC should be restricted only to selected patients where the benefit of its use may substantially outweigh the risks. Current recommendations in humans limit the use of PACs to patients with severe right ventricular failure and those requiring intensive monitoring of pulmonary vascular resistance during vasodilator therapy. Moreover, the use of PACs and PAC thermodilution necessitate appropriate training as placement errors and misinterpretation of data are common.

In veterinary patients, there is limited experience with clinical use of PACs and PAC thermodilution, and the technique has been largely limited to research settings [61–64]. This is mainly due to the invasiveness and the difficulty of placing and maintaining the catheter in the appropriate location. In addition, the PACs available on the market are specifically sized and designed for use in humans and, as such, are often inadequate for direct use in other species due to morphological differences. In small dogs (less than 5 kg) and cats, for example, a standard PAC designed for adult human use advanced into the main pulmonary artery would likely have the proximal port located in the jugular vein. The injection of the indicator in this location, rather than in the right atrium, will create loss and delayed mixing with significant error in the estimation of cardiac output. The opposite scenario occurs in horses where adult human PACs are too short. The proximal opening would then be located in the right ventricle, instead of its proper place in the right atrium, significantly altering the estimation of cardiac output. However, pediatric human PACS and custom-designed PACs of appropriate size for various veterinary species have been used for research purposes.

Transpulmonary thermodilution and ultrasound indicator dilution

The basic principles of PAC thermodilution also apply to newer cardiac output monitoring systems that do not require the use of an actual pulmonary arterial catheter. Examples of these systems are the PiCCO® (Pulsion Medical Systems) and COstatus® (Transonic; no longer commercially available) that allow cardiac output to be estimated using central venous and arterial catheters only [65,66]. The Stewart–Hamilton equation is still the basis for estimating cardiac output using these systems. The PiCCO® system is based on transpulmonary thermodilution for cardiac output determination and requires dedicated femoral artery access for measurements. PiCCO® estimates cardiac output using central venous injections of ice-cold intravenous fluid as an indicator and measuring the changes over time in temperature by an arterial thermistor-tipped catheter placed in the femoral artery [65].

The COstatus® monitor is no longer manufactured but is a system that is still utilized in the scientific literature [66]. This monitor estimates cardiac output by using ultrasound technology to measure changes in the ultrasound velocity of blood following an injection of a small saline bolus (0.5–1 mL/kg) warmed to body temperature (37 °C). To obtain measurements, a roller pump circulates blood through a disposable extracorporeal arteriovenous (AV) loop interposed between the peripheral arterial catheter and the distal lumen of the central venous catheter. Two reusable sensors that measure changes in blood ultrasound velocity and blood flow in the AV loop are clamped onto the arterial and venous limbs of the loop. The venous sensor detects the injection of saline and records the time and volume of injection. The arterial sensor then measures the changes in concentration of saline in the blood as a dilution and records the indicator travel time through the cardiopulmonary system. Stroke volume is then derived from the dilution curves obtained [67].

The agreement of cardiac output values measured using transpulmonary and ultrasound indicator-dilution techniques with those measured using PAC thermodilution was shown to be adequate for clinical use in humans [68–71]. Moreover, both technologies provide volumetric variables in addition to cardiac output, such as global end-diastolic volume and measurements of extravascular lung water. These variables have been utilized as indicators of fluid responsiveness with promising results [72,73].

PiCCO® and COstatus® appear significantly more practical and user-friendly than PAC thermodilution. In addition, they do not require any specific customization for use in veterinary species. COstatus® has been shown to be accurate and safe in very small patients [70]. All of these factors may allow a wider use of these systems in veterinary medicine, especially in small animals, when compared to PAC thermodilution [74,75].

Lithium dilution

The lithium dilution technique is an example of dye dilution cardiac output monitoring, based on intravascular injection of a minute amount of an isotonic lithium chloride (0.002–0.004 mmol/kg) solution used as an indicator [76]. These lithium doses are too small to exert any pharmacological or toxic effects. The lithium concentration in the blood is derived by a lithium-selective electrode connected to a peripheral arterial catheter. An advantage of the lithium indicator-dilution cardiac output technique is that no central venous line is necessary for the injection of the indicator, which can be given via a regular peripheral line [77]. The lithium concentration over time curve is recorded by withdrawing blood (4.5 mL/min) through a special disposable sensor, attached to the patient's arterial line. The voltage signal across the lithium-selective membrane is converted to a lithium concentration by a computer. Cardiac output is then calculated according to the following equation [76]:

$$\text{Cardiac output} = \frac{\text{LiCl} \times 60}{\text{AUC} \times (1 - \text{PCV})}$$

In this equation, LiCl is the lithium chloride dose expressed in mmol, AUC is the area under the primary dilution curve, and PCV is the packed cell volume. A correction for PCV is necessary to transform plasma flow into total blood flow because lithium is distributed only in the plasma. The lithium dilution technique has been shown to be at least as accurate as PAC thermodilution, but with the advantages of being simple to set up and operate. In addition, the system conveniently uses catheters likely to be already in place in a critically ill patient. The system requires some familiarity to set up but is relatively quick and user-friendly. Similar to thermodilution, the lithium dilution technique performs poorly in the presence of tachyarrhythmias [76].

The LiDCO™ system (Masimo Corporation) has now become widely used in veterinary medicine in both clinical and research settings. Good agreement with PAC thermodilution was demonstrated in dogs, cats, and horses, with the advantage of being less invasive, less expensive, and more user-friendly [78–81]. In pigs, lithium dilution performed even better than PAC thermodilution when compared to electromagnetic flowmetry. In this study, cardiac output measured by lithium dilution, using a central venous catheter for injection, showed better agreement with electromagnetic flowmetry than PAC thermodilution [82]. Notably, although correlation studies of the LiDCO™ system with electromagnetic flowmetry (direct measurement of cardiac output) are lacking in many veterinary species, LiDCO™ is often arbitrarily used in research settings as a reference for comparison of other cardiac output monitoring systems [15,18–20,83,84]. This approach may potentially lead to inaccurate conclusions.

The main disadvantage of lithium dilution is the blood loss associated with withdrawal of arterial blood for the determination of lithium concentration. Although the loss associated with a single measurement is minimal, sampling-induced reductions in blood volume should be considered when multiple determinations are made in small animal patients.

Arterial waveform analysis

Arterial pressure waveform analysis allows the continuous determination of cardiac output [85]. In addition to the intermittent dilution cardiac output measurement discussed above, the PiCCO® and LiDCO™ systems are also integrated with arterial pressure waveform analysis functions [59,86]. PiCCO® uses arterial pulse contour analysis, whereas LiDCO™ uses pulse power analysis for the beat-to-beat estimation of cardiac output [87]. Both methods require calibration before measurement of cardiac output based on the assumption that stroke volume is equal to the sum of systolic and diastolic flows, which are proportional to systolic and diastolic areas in the arterial pressure waveform (Fig. 13.3). The PiCCO® system uses transpulmonary thermodilution for the calibration procedure, whereas LiDCO™ is calibrated using lithium dilution [88]. Repeated calibrations of the arterial pulse contour analysis systems are required in order to obtain adequate estimations of cardiac output. Recalibration is also needed whenever there is a change in vasomotor tone or any other significant change in the patient's clinical condition [89,90].

Other cardiac output devices based on arterial waveform analysis, such as the FloTrac (Edwards Lifesciences), are available. These devices reportedly do not require baseline calibration and calculate SV empirically [91]. However, the accuracy and precision of these methods have been questioned by many investigators [90,92]. Moreover, arterial pulse contour analysis is highly prone to technical difficulties related to damping and resonance within the measurement system [93]. For these reasons, further investigation of arterial waveform analysis techniques in different species and clinical scenarios is needed to define indications and recommendations for clinical use.

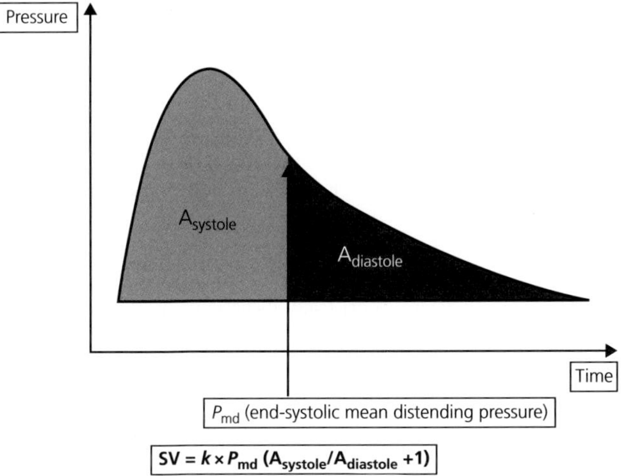

Figure 13.3 Arterial waveform analysis. Components of the arterial waveform used in the "area under the curve" method. Stroke volume (SV) is the sum of systolic and diastolic flows, which are proportional to their respective areas ($A_{systole}$ and $A_{diastole}$) under the arterial pressure curve. P_{md} is the increment in mean arterial pressure at the end of systole and is used for calculating diastolic flow; k is the calibration factor and is measured by calibrating against a known stroke volume, for example using transpulmonary thermodilution. Once k is known, beat-to-beat stroke volume can be calculated.

Echocardiography and echo-Doppler

Cardiac output can be determined with echocardiography using non-Doppler or Doppler-based methods [94,95]. A great advantage of echocardiography over other monitoring techniques is the large amount of hemodynamic information obtained beyond just cardiac output. Cardiac contractility and chamber filling can be rapidly assessed, and valves and pericardium can be directly visualized [21].

Non-Doppler techniques are based on approximate volumetric reconstructions of the left ventricular chamber. The most common method is based on Simpson's rule, wherein the left ventricle is divided into a series of disks stacked from base to apex. Two orthogonal planes are needed to construct the disks, and left ventricular volume is calculated by summing the approximated volumes of the individual disks. SV is calculated by determining the difference in volume between diastole and systole [94]. The time-consuming nature of the non-Doppler technique can make cardiac output estimation inadequate for a rapid assessment in emergency situations. Difficulty with endocardial border definition also can produce largely inaccurate results. For these reasons, non-Doppler techniques are rarely used for clinical purposes.

When an ultrasound beam is directed along the aorta, part of the ultrasound signal is reflected back by red blood cells moving at a different frequency. The resultant shift in the signal's frequency, referred to as the "Doppler effect," is used to determine the flow velocity. This represents the basic principle behind echo-Doppler cardiac output determination. Echo-Doppler cardiac output monitoring may be performed either transthoracically or transesophageally [96,97].

The determination of cardiac output begins with measurement of the cross-sectional area (CSA) of the left ventricular outflow tract (LVOT). The reason for choosing this location is that the cross section of the LVOT is essentially a circle and its area can be easily determined as πr^2. CSA can also be more accurately measured by tracing the boundary of the LVOT (Fig. 13.4A).

Following the CSA determination, a sample volume for pulsed wave Doppler is placed at the location where area was determined. In small animals, the subcostal echocardiographic view is recommended for this assessment. Subcostal views of the heart can be obtained with the patient in right- or left-sided recumbency and are relatively easy to obtain. These views usually are three- or four-chambered (left ventricle, portions of the right ventricle or atrium, portions of the left atrium, and LVOT with aorta) and allow the operator to obtain near perfect parallel alignment of the Doppler cursor with the LVOT. The pulsed wave Doppler window can be placed just below the aortic valve plane, and this view provides good flow tracings and accurate measurements. A profile of velocity over time is generated by this Doppler interrogation using the following formula:

$$V = \frac{f_d c}{2 f_i \cos\theta}$$

where V is the erythrocyte velocity, f_d is the Doppler shift, c represents the velocity of the ultrasound wave, f_i is the ultrasound frequency, and θ is the angle at which the ultrasound waves penetrate the vessel.

The tracing of the boundary of the velocity profile allows for the determination of its integral over time. The velocity time integral

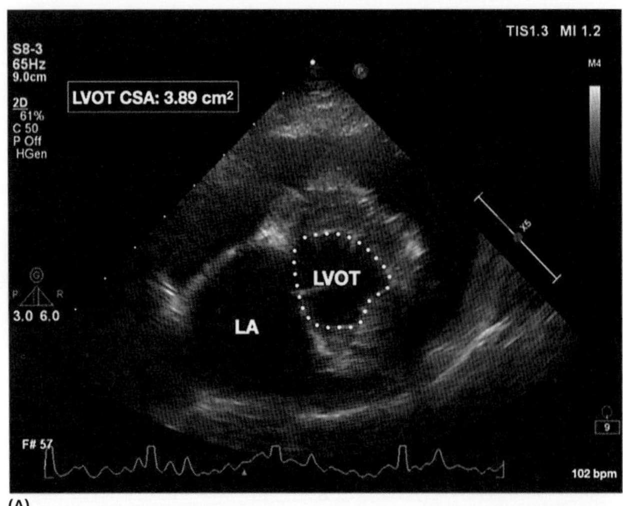

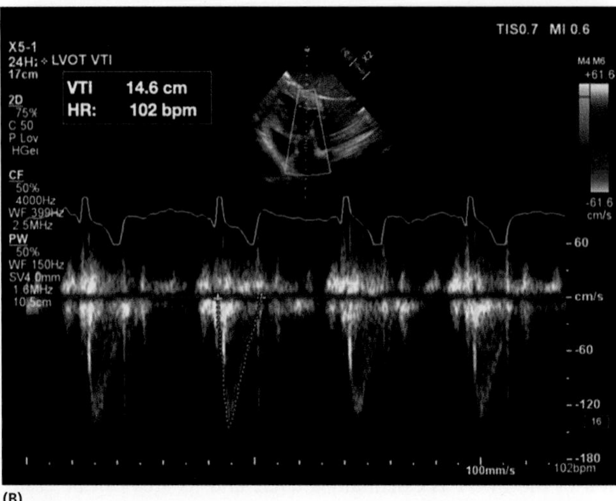

Figure 13.4 Transthoracic echo-Doppler estimation of cardiac output in a 27-kg dog. **A.** Short axis view for determination of cross-sectional area (CSA) of the left ventricular outflow tract (LVOT). The dotted white line represents the tracing of the boundary of the LVOT. LA, left atrium. **B.** Transhepatic view of the LVOT. A pulsed wave Doppler window is placed just below the aortic valve plane to obtain flow tracings and calculation of the velocity time integral (VTI) of the LVOT. HR, heart rate. Cardiac output is calculated as the product of the VTI times CSA times HR. This patient's estimated cardiac output is 5.792 L/min.

(VTI) essentially represents the distance that blood travels during one beat and is referred to as "stroke distance." Multiplying VTI by the cross-sectional area (CSA) of the LVOT yields SV; this multiplied by heart rate (HR) determines cardiac output (Fig. 13.4B):

$$\text{Cardiac output} = \text{HR} \times \text{CSA} \times \text{VTI}$$

This technique requires knowledge and skills to avoid pitfalls and to recognize inaccurate results [98]. Overall, Doppler-based cardiac output determination appears to be an acceptable alternative to thermodilution for clinical purposes, if performed correctly [99,100]. Important factors that can significantly affect accuracy are image quality, sample site, angle of insonation, the velocity signal-to-noise ratio, the possibility of measuring the diameter of the LVOT, and the shape of the aortic valve.

A described complication associated with the use of esophageal probes is esophageal injury. Transesophageal echocardiography probes are large and generate a certain degree of heat and, thus, are not suited for continuous cardiac output assessment; additionally, small patient size may limit probe placement [101,102].

In the past, echocardiography instrumentation and expertise were rarely available to veterinary anesthesiologists and were solely the domain of veterinary cardiologists. With the increasing availability of portable patient-side ultrasonography and point-of-care ultrasound, such limitations no longer exist (see Chapter 18). There is significant evidence supporting the accuracy and practical applicability of echocardiography for cardiac output determination in many veterinary species, which will likely result in a wider array of use for clinical purposes [103–106].

Thoracic bioimpedance and bioreactance

Bioimpedance uses changes in conductivity of a high-frequency, low-magnitude alternating current passing across the thorax to derive SV [107]. The changes in electrical conductivity are produced by variations in intrathoracic blood flow during each cardiac cycle. A series of ECG-type electrodes are placed on the thorax and neck. A small, non-painful current is passed between the electrodes and the changes in voltage, also termed "bioimpedance," is measured. The value of bioimpedance is converted to SV using mathematical algorithms. Several patented algorithms based on different mathematical models of the thorax have been described [108,109]. Stroke volume (SV) is generally calculated using the following formula:

$$\text{Stroke volume} = \rho \times \frac{L^2}{Z_0^2} \times \left(\frac{\mathrm{d}Z}{\mathrm{d}t}\right)_{max} \times VET$$

where ρ is the resistivity of blood, L is the mean distance between the inner electrodes (the thoracic length), VET is the ventricular ejection time, $(\mathrm{d}Z/\mathrm{d}t)_{max}$ is the maximum value of the first derivative during systole, and Z_0 is the basal thoracic impedance. Bioimpedance provides real-time estimation of SV and cardiac output, along with measures of thoracic fluid content, left ventricular ejection time, systemic vascular resistance, and left cardiac work index [108].

Bioreactance has been developed from the bioimpedance technique but measures changes in frequency of electrical currents, rather than voltage, potentially making it less prone to noise-derived errors [110]. Both techniques are non-invasive and can be applied quickly. However, the biggest concern with these techniques is the accuracy and precision of the measurements. Physiological studies in healthy humans showed good reliability of the results, but this was not consistent in critically ill patients, particularly in the presence of pulmonary edema and/or pleural effusion. In addition, electrical interference may also occur from other anesthesia monitoring devices connected to the patient [111–113].

Little or no evidence exists on the accuracy and reliability of these techniques in veterinary species [114,115]. Therefore, bioimpedance and bioreactance cardiac output determination should not be considered as a valid and reproducible method at present. A shortcoming of both bioimpedance and bioreactance mathematical models is the approximation of the shape of the chest as a cylinder or a cone for stroke volume determination. These represent oversimplifications of the electrical events occurring inside the thorax during the cardiac cycle and are sources of technique inaccuracy. It seems unlikely that the algorithms designed for human patients would be sufficiently accurate for use in various veterinary species.

Standard capnography as an indicator of cardiac output

A simple and practical indicator of cardiac output in any anesthetized patient is end-tidal carbon dioxide ($P_{ET}CO_2$) measured by capnography. $P_{ET}CO_2$ is determined by CO_2 production (VCO_2), alveolar ventilation, and pulmonary perfusion. Assuming stable conditions of patient minute ventilation and body temperature, and in absence of airway obstruction or extra-metabolic sources of CO_2 (e.g., laparoscopic surgery or sodium bicarbonate administration), a sudden change in $P_{ET}CO_2$ has been shown to reflect a proportional alteration in cardiac output [116,117]. Studies on preload optimization have demonstrated that percentage changes in $P_{ET}CO_2$ induced by intravascular volume expansion linearly reflect percentage increases in cardiac output [118].

In practical terms, the simultaneous decrease in systemic blood pressure and $P_{ET}CO_2$ in an anesthetized patient (with constant minute ventilation) may reflect a primary reduction in cardiac output. In such conditions, if sinus rhythm and normal HR are confirmed, therapeutic interventions should focus on optimization of preload and myocardial contractility to support SV.

In contrast, a decrease in blood pressure with no reduction in $P_{ET}CO_2$ suggests a decrease in systemic vascular resistances rather than a decrease in cardiac output, indicating that vasopressor therapy is the most appropriate intervention to correct the hypotension.

In clinical scenarios of drastically decreased blood flow such as hemorrhagic shock or impending cardiac arrest, the correlation between changes in $P_{ET}CO_2$ and cardiac output is no longer linear. In cases where oxygen consumption becomes supply dependent (critical O_2 delivery), the drop in $P_{ET}CO_2$ is also accompanied by a decrease in VCO_2. In dogs, it was demonstrated that the relationship between percentage changes in $P_{ET}CO_2$ and cardiac output during hemorrhagic shock is best determined by the following logarithmic function:

$$y = 3.3617 \ln(x) + 31.854$$

where y represents cardiac index (mL/min/kg) and x represents $P_{ET}CO_2$ (mmHg). This implies that the greatest decrease in $P_{ET}CO_2$ occurs at the lowest cardiac output [119].

References

1 Hall JE, Hall ME. Cardiac output, venous return, and their regulation. In: Hall JE, Hall ME, eds. *Guyton and Hall Textbook of Medical Physiology*, 14th edn. Philadelphia, PA: Elsevier, 2021: 245–258.

2 Della Rocca G, Pompei L. Goal-directed therapy in anesthesia: any clinical impact or just a fashion? *Minerva Anestesiol* 2011; **77**(5): 545–553.

3 Ospina-Tascon GA, Cordioli RL, Vincent JL. What type of monitoring has been shown to improve outcomes in acutely ill patients? *Intensive Care Med* 2008; **34**: 800–820.

4 Kehlet H, Bundgaard-Nielsen M. Goal-directed perioperative fluid management: why, when, and how? *Anesthesiol* 2009; **110**: 453–455.

5 Pinsky MR. Why measure cardiac output? *Crit Care* 2003; **7**(2): 114–116.

6 Pinsky MR. Hemodynamic evaluation and monitoring in the ICU. *Chest* 2007; **132**: 2020–2029.

7 Bilovski RN, Rivers EP, Horst HM. Targeted resuscitation strategies after injury. *Curr Opin Crit Care* 2004; **10**: 529–538.

8 Monnet X, Lai C. Which haemodynamic monitoring should we choose for critically ill patients with acute circulatory failure? *Curr Opin Crit Care* 2023; **29**(3): 275–280.

9 Rex S, Brose S, Metzelder S, *et al.* Prediction of fluid responsiveness in patients during cardiac surgery. *Br J Anaesth* 2004; **93**: 782–788.

10 Reuter DA, Geopfert MS, Goresch T, *et al.* Assessing fluid responsiveness during open chest conditions. *Br J Anaesth* 2005; **94**: 318–323.

11 García X, Mateu L, Maynar J, *et al.* Estimating cardiac output. Utility in the clinical practice. Available invasive and non-invasive monitoring. *Med Intensiva* 2011; **35**(9): 552–561.

12 Pinsky MR, Payen D. Functional hemodynamic monitoring. *Crit Care* 2005; **9**: 566–572.

13 Vincent JL, Rhodes A, Perel A, *et al.* Clinical review: update on hemodynamic monitoring – a consensus of 16. *Critical Care* 2011; **15**: 229.

14 Geerts BF, Aarts LP, Jansen JR. Methods in pharmacology: measurement of cardiac output. *Br J Clin Pharmacol* 2011; **71**(3): 316–330.

15 Corley KTT, Donaldson LL, Durando MM, *et al.* Cardiac output technologies with special reference to the horse. *J Vet Intern Med* 2003; **17**: 262–272.

16 Pugsley J, Lerner AB. Cardiac output monitoring: is there a gold standard and how do the newer technologies compare? *Semin Cardiothorac Vasc Anesth* 2010; **14**: 274–282.

17 Tabrizchi R, Iida N. Electromagnetic blood flow measurements. In: Moore J, Zouridakis G, eds. *Biomedical Technology and Devices Handbook*. New York, NY: CRC Press LLC, 2003.

18 Shih A, Giguère S, Sanchez LC, *et al.* Determination of cardiac output in neonatal foals by ultrasound velocity dilution and its comparison to the lithium dilution method. *J Vet Emerg Crit Care* 2009; **19**(5): 438–443.

19 Valverde A, Giguère S, Morey TE, *et al.* Comparison of noninvasive cardiac output measured by use of partial carbon dioxide rebreathing or the lithium dilution method in anesthetized foals. *Am J Vet Res* 2007; **68**(2): 141–147.

20 Shih AC. Cardiac monitoring in horses. *Vet Clin North Am Equine Pract* 2019; **35**(1): 205–215.

21 Mantovani MM, Fantoni DR, Gimenes AM, *et al.* Clinical monitoring of cardiac output assessed by transoesophageal echocardiography in anaesthetized dogs: a comparison with the thermodilution technique. *BMC Vet Res* 2017; **13**(1): 325.

22 Rozental O, Thalappillil R, White RS, *et al.* To Swan or not to Swan: indications, alternatives, and future directions. *J Cardiothoracic Vasc Anesth* 2021; **35**(2): 600–615.

23 Silver MA, Cianci P, Brennan S, *et al.* Evaluation of impedance cardiography as an alternative to pulmonary artery catheterization in critically ill patients. *Congest Heart Fail* 2004; **10**: 17–21.

24 Fick A. Ueber die Messung des Blutquantums in den Herzventrikeln. *Sitzber Physik Med Ges Wurzburg* 1870; **36**(2): 290–291.

25 Grehant H, Quinquaud CE. Recherches experimentales sur la mesure du volume de sang qui traverse les poumons en un temps donne. *Compt Rend Sci Soc Biol* 1886; **30**: 159.

26 Zuntz N, Hagemann O. Untersuchungen uber den Stoffwechsel des Pferdes bei Ruhe und Arbeit. *Landwirtschaftl Jahrb Z Wiss Land-wirtschaft* 1898; **27**(3): 1–450.

27 Laszlo G. Respiratory measurements of cardiac output: from elegant idea to useful test. *J Appl Physiol* 2004; **96**: 428–437.

28 Stewart GN. Researches on the circulation time and on the influences which affect it. IV. The output of the heart. *Physiol* 1897; **22**: 159–183.

29 Hamilton WF, Riley RL, Attyah AM, *et al.* Comparison of the Fick and dye injection methods of measuring the cardiac output in man. *Amer J Physiol* 1948; **153**: 309.

30 Werko L, Lagexlof H, Bucht H, *et al.* Comparison of Fick and Hamilton methods for determination of cardiac output in man. *Scand J Clin Lab Invest* 1949; **1**: 109.

31 Miller DE, Gleason WL, McIntosh HD. A comparison of the cardiac output determination by the Fick method and dye dilution method using indocyanine green dye and a cuvette densitometer. *J Lab Clin Med* 1962; **59**: 345.

32 Venkataraman K, De Guzman MF, Khan AH. Cardiac output measurement: a comparison of direct Fick, dye dilution and thermodilution methods in stable and acutely ill patients. *J Nation Med Assoc* 1976; **68**(4): 281–284.

33 Fegler G. Measurement of cardiac output in anesthetized animals by a thermodilution method. *Quart J Exp Physiol* 1954; **39**: 153.

34 Swan HJ, Ganz W, Forrester J, *et al.* Catheterization of the heart in man with use of a flow-directed balloon-tipped catheter. *N Engl J Med* 1970; **283**: 447–453.

35 Ganz W, Donoso R, Marcus HS, *et al.* A new technique for measurement of cardiac output by thermodilution in man. *Am J Cardiol* 1971; **27**: 392–396.

36 Weisel RD, Berger RL, Hectman HB. Measurement of cardiac output by thermodilution. *N Engl J Med* 1975; **292**: 682.

37 Reuter DA, Huang C, Edrich T, *et al.* Cardiac output monitoring using indicator-dilution techniques: basics, limits, and perspectives. *Anesth Analg* 2010; **110**(3): 799–811.

38 Tournadre JP, Chassard D, Muchada R. Overestimation of low cardiac output measured by thermodilution. *Brit J Anaesth* 1997; **79**: 514–516.

39 Harvey S, Harrison DA, Singer M, *et al.* Assessment of the clinical effectiveness of pulmonary artery catheters in management of patients in intensive care (PAC Man): a randomised controlled trial. *Lancet* 2005; **366**: 472–477.

40 Shah MR, Hasselblad V, Stevenson LW, *et al.* Impact of the pulmonary artery catheter in critically ill patients: meta-analysis of randomized clinical trials. *JAMA* 2005; **294**(13): 1664–1670.

41 Coonors AF Jr., Speroff T, Dawson NV, *et al.* The effectiveness of right heart catheterization in the initial care of critically ill patients, SUPPORT Investigators. *JAMA* 1996; **276**: 889–897.

42 Polanczyk CA, Rohde LE, Goldman L, *et al.* Right heart catheterization and cardiac complications in patients undergoing noncardiac surgery. *J Am Med Assoc* 2001; **286**: 309–314.

43 Elliott CG, Zimmerman GA, Clemmer TP. Complications of pulmonary artery catheterization in the care of critically ill patients. *A prospective study. Chest* 1979; **76**: 647–652.

44 Cholley BP, Payen D. Noninvasive technique for measurements of cardiac output. *Curr Opin Crit Care* 2005; **11**: 424–429.

45 Parmley CL, Pousman RM. Noninvasive cardiac output monitoring. *Curr Opin Anaesthesiol* 2002; **15**: 675–680.

46 Botero M, Labato EB. Advances in noninvasive cardiac output monitoring: an update. *J Cardiothorac Vasc Anaesth* 2001; **15**: 631–640.

47 Haryadi DG, Orr JA, Kuck K, *et al.* Partial CO_2 rebreathing indirect Fick technique for non-invasive measurement of cardiac output. *J Clin Monit Comput* 2000; **16**(5–6): 361–374.

48 Jaffe MB. Partial CO_2 rebreathing cardiac output – operating principles of the NICO system. *J Clin Monit Comput* 1999; **15**: 387–401.

49 Haryadi DG, Orr JA, Kuck K, *et al.* Partial CO_2 rebreathing indirect Fick technique for non-invasive measurement of cardiac output. *J Clin Monit Comput* 2000; **16**: 361–374.

50 van Heerden PV, Baker S, Lim SI, *et al.* Clinical evaluation of the Non-Invasive Cardiac Output (NICO) monitor in the intensive care unit. *Anaesth Intensive Care* 2000; **28**: 427–430.

51 Levy RJ, Chivacci RM, Nicolson SC, *et al.* An evaluation of a noninvasive cardiac output measurement using partial carbon dioxide rebreathing in children. *Anesth Analg* 2004; **99**: 1642–1647.

52 Nilsson LB, Eldrup N, Berthelsen PG. Lack of agreement between thermodilution and carbon dioxide-rebreathing cardiac output. *Acta Anaesthesiol Scand* 2001; **45**: 680–685.

53 Giguère S, Bucki E, Adin DB, *et al.* Cardiac output measurement by partial carbon dioxide rebreathing, 2-dimensional echocardiography, and lithium-dilution method in anesthetized neonatal foals. *J Vet Intern Med* 2005; **19**(5): 737–743.

54 Gedeon A, Krill P, Kristensen J, *et al.* Noninvasive cardiac output determined with a new method based on gas exchange measurements and carbon dioxide rebreathing: a study in animals/pigs. *J Clin Monit* 1992; **8**(4): 267–278.

55 Gunkel CI, Valverde A, Morey TE, *et al.* Comparison of non-invasive cardiac output measurement by partial carbon dioxide rebreathing with the lithium dilution method in anesthetized dogs. *J Vet Emerg Crit Care* 2004; **14**(3): 187–195.

56 Berton C, Cholley B. Equipment review: new techniques for cardiac output measurement – oesophageal Doppler, Fick principle using carbon dioxide and pulse contour analysis. *Crit Care* 2002; **6**: 216–221.

57 Forrester JS, Ganz W, Diamond G, *et al.* Thermodilution cardiac output determination with a single flow directed catheter. *Am Heart J* 1972; **83**: 306.

58 Mathews L, Singh RK. Swan Ganz catheter in haemodynamic monitoring. *J Anaesth Clin Pharmacol* 2006; **22**: 335–345.

59 Della Rocca G, Costa MG, Pompei L, *et al.* Continuous and intermittent cardiac output measurement: pulmonary artery catheter versus aortic transpulmonary technique. *Br J Anaesth* 2002; **88**: 350–356.

60 Schlipf JW, Dunlop CI, Getzy DM, *et al.* Lesions associated with cardiac catheterization and thermodilution cardiac output determination in horses. In: *Proceedings of the 5th International Congress of Veterinary Anesthesia*, 1994: 71–72.

61 Muir WW, Skarda RT, Milne DW. Estimation of cardiac output in the horse by thermodilution techniques. *Am J Vet Res* 1976; **37**: 697–700.

62 Mizuno Y, Aida H, Hara H, *et al.* Comparison of methods of cardiac output measurements determined by dye dilution, pulsed Doppler echocardiography and thermodilution in horses. *J Vet Med Sci* 1994; **56**: 1–5.

63 Hendriks FFA, Schipperheyn JJ, Quanjer PH. Thermal dilution measurement of cardiac output in dogs using an analog computer. *Basic Res Cardiol* 1978; **73**: 459–468.

64 Dyson DH, McDonell WN, Horne JA. Accuracy of thermodilution measurement of cardiac output in low flows applicable to feline and small canine patients. *Can J Comp Med* 1984; **48**: 425–427.

65 Messina A, Alicino V, Cecconi M. Transpulmonary thermodilution. *Curr Opin Crit Care* 2023; **29**(3): 223–230.

66 Paranjape VV, Shih AC, Garcia-Pereira FL, *et al.* Transpulmonary ultrasound dilution is an acceptable technique for cardiac output measurement in anesthetized pigs. *Am J Vet Res* 2022; **83**(6): ajvr.21.11.0189.

67 de Boode WP, van Heijst AF, Hopman JC, *et al.* Application of the ultrasound dilution technology for cardiac output measurement: cerebral and systemic hemodynamic consequences in a juvenile animal model. *Pediatr Crit Care Med* 2010; **11**(5): 616–623.

68 Della Rocca G, Costa MG, Coccia C, *et al.* Cardiac output monitoring: aortic transpulmonary thermodilution and pulse contour analysis agree with standard thermodilution methods in patients undergoing lung transplantation. *Can J Anaesth* 2003; **50**: 707–711.

69 Sakka SG, Reinhart K, Meier-Hellmann A. Comparison of pulmonary artery and arterial thermodilution cardiac output in critically ill patients. *Intensive Care Med* 1999; **25**: 843–846.

70 de Boode WP, van Heijst AF, Hopman JC, *et al.* Cardiac output measurement using an ultrasound dilution method: a validation study in ventilated piglets. *Pediatr Crit Care Med* 2010; **11**(1): 103–108.

71 Ballestero Y, Urbano J, López-Herce J, *et al.* Pulmonary arterial thermodilution, femoral arterial thermodilution and bioreactance cardiac output monitoring in a pediatric hemorrhagic hypovolemic shock model. *Resusc* 2012; **83**: 125–129.

72 Vigani A, Shih A, Queiroz P, *et al.* Quantitative response of volumetric variables measured by a new ultrasound dilution method in a juvenile model of hemorrhagic shock and resuscitation. *Resusc* 2012; **83**(8): 1031–1037.

73 Paranjape VV, Henao-Guerrero N, Menciotti G, *et al.* Volumetric evaluation of fluid responsiveness using a modified passive leg raise maneuver during experimental induction and correction of hypovolemia in anesthetized dogs. *Vet Anaesh Analg* 2023; **50**(3): 211–219.

74 Shih A, Maisenbacher HW, Bandt C, *et al.* Assessment of cardiac output measurement in dogs by transpulmonary pulse contour analysis. *J Vet Emerg Crit Care* 2011; **21**(4): 321–327.

75 Shih A, Giguère S, Vigani A, *et al.* Determination of cardiac output by ultrasound velocity dilution in normovolemia and hypovolemia in dogs. *Vet Anaesth Analg* 2011; **38**(4): 279–285.

76 Linton RA, Band DM, Haire KM. A new method in measuring cardiac output in man using lithium dilution. *Br J Anaesth* 1993; **71**: 262–266.

77 Mason DJ, O'Grady M, Woods JP, *et al.* Comparison of a central and a peripheral (cephalic vein) injection site for the measurement of cardiac output using the lithium-dilution cardiac output technique in anesthetized dogs. *Can J Vet Res* 2002; **66**(3): 207–210.

78 Mason DJ, O'Grady M, Woods JP, *et al.* Assessment of lithium dilution cardiac output as a technique for measurement of cardiac output in dogs. *Am J Vet Res* 2001; **62**(8): 1255–1261.

79 Beaulieu KE, Kerr CL, McDonell WN. Evaluation of a lithium dilution cardiac output technique as a method for measurement of cardiac output in anesthetized cats. *Am J Vet Res* 2005; **66**(9): 1639–1645.

80 Linton RA, Young LE, Marlin DJ, *et al.* Cardiac output measured by lithium dilution, thermodilution, and transesophageal Doppler echocardiography in anesthetized horses. *Am J Vet Res* 2000; **61**(7): 731–737.

81 Corley KT, Donaldson LL, Furr MO. Comparison of lithium dilution and thermodilution cardiac output measurements in anaesthetised neonatal foals. *Equine Vet J* 2002; **34**(6): 598–601.

82 Kurita T, Morita K, Kato S, *et al.* Comparison of the accuracy of the lithium dilution technique with the thermodilution technique for measurement of cardiac output. *Br J Anaesth* 1997; **79**: 770–775.

83 Corley KT, Donaldson LL, Furr MO. Comparison of lithium dilution and thermodilution cardiac output measurements in anaesthetised neonatal foals. *Equine Vet J* 2002; **34**(6): 598–601.

84 Schauvliege S, Van den Eede A, Duchateau L, *et al.* Comparison between lithium dilution and pulse contour analysis techniques for cardiac output measurement in isoflurane anaesthetized ponies: influence of different inotropic drugs. *Vet Anaesth Analg* 2009; **36**(3):197–208.

85 Saugel B, Kouz K, Scheeren TWL, *et al.* Cardiac output estimation using pulse wave analysis – physiology, algorithms, and technologies: a narrative review. *Br J Anaesth* 2021; **126**(1): 67–76.

86 Jonas MM, Tanser SJ. Lithium dilution measurement of cardiac output and arterial pulse waveform analysis: an indicator dilution calibrated beat-by-beat system for continuous estimation of cardiac output. *Curr Opin Crit Care* 2002; **8**(3): 257–261.

87 Thiele RH, Durieux ME. Arterial waveform analysis for the anesthesiologist: past, present, and future concepts. *Anesth Analg* 2011; **113**(4): 766–776.

88 Ambrisko TD, Coppens P, Kabes R, *et al.* Lithium dilution, pulse power analysis, and continuous thermodilution cardiac output measurements compared with bolus thermodilution in anaesthetized ponies. *Br J Anaesth* 2012; **109**(6): 864–869.

89 Rhodes A, Sunderland R. Arterial pulse power analysis, the LiDCO™ plus system. In: Pinsky MR, Pyen D, eds. *Functional Hemodynamics*. Berlin: Springer Verlag, 2005: 183–192.

90 Takei T, Kumagai M, Suzuki M, *et al.* Accuracy of cardiac output measured by fourth-generation FloTrac and LiDCOrapid, and their characteristics regarding systemic vascular resistance in patients undergoing cardiac surgery. *J Cardiothorac Vasc Anesth* 2023; **37**(7): 1143–1151.

91 Manecke GR Jr., Auger WR. Cardiac output determination from the arterial pressure wave: clinical testing of novel algorithm that does not require calibration. *J Cardiothorac Vasc Anaesth* 2007; **21**: 3–7.

92 Compton FD, Zukunft B, Hoffmann C, *et al.* Performance of a minimally invasive uncalibrated cardiac output monitoring system (Flotrac/Vigileo) in haemodynamically unstable patients. *Br J Anaesth* 2008; **100**(4): 451–456.

93 Singer M, Allen MJ, Webb AR, *et al.* Effects of alterations in left ventricular filling, contractility and systemic vascular resistance on the ascending aortic blood velocity waveform of normal subjects. *Crit Care Med* 1991; **19**: 1138–1145.
94 Uehara Y, Koga M, Takahashi M. Determination of cardiac output by echocardiography. *J Vet Med Sci* 1995; **57**(3): 401–407.
95 Madan AK, UyBarreta VV, Aliabadi-Wahle S, *et al.* Esophageal Doppler ultrasound monitor versus pulmonary artery catheter in the hemodynamic management of critically ill surgical patients. *J Trauma* 1999; **46**: 607–612.
96 Josephs SA. The use of current hemodynamic monitors and echocardiography in resuscitation of the critically ill or injured patient. *Int Anesthesiol Clin* 2007; **45**(3): 31–59.
97 Gouveia V, Marcelino P, Reuter DA. The role of transesophageal echocardiography in the intraoperative period. *Curr Cardiol Rev* 2011; **7**(3): 184–196.
98 Lefrant JY, Bruelle P, Aya AG, *et al.* Training is required to improve the reliability of esophageal Doppler to measure cardiac output in critically ill patients. *Intensive Care Med* 1998; **24**: 347–352.
99 Chew MS, Poelaert J. Accuracy and repeatability of pediatric cardiac output measurement using Doppler: 20-year review of literature. *Intensive Care Med* 2003; **29**: 1889–1894.
100 Perrino AC Jr., Harris SN, Luther MA. Intraoperative determination of cardiac output using multiplane transesophageal echocardiography: a comparison to thermodilution. *Anesthesiology* 1998; **89**: 350–357.
101 Urbanowicz JH, Kernoff RS, Oppenheim G, *et al.* Transesophageal echocardiography and its potential for esophageal damage. *Anesthesiol* 1990; **72**(1): 40–43.
102 Stoner CH, Saunders AB, Heseltine JC, *et al.* Prospective evaluation of complications associated with transesophageal echocardiography in dogs with congenital heart disease. *J Vet Int Med* 2022; **36**(2): 406–416.
103 Blissit KJ, Young LE, Jones RS, *et al.* Measurement of cardiac output in standing horses by Doppler echocardiography and thermodilution. *Equine vet J* 1997; **29**(1): 18–25.
104 Young LE, Blissit KJ, Bartram DH, *et al.* Measurement of cardiac output by transoesophageal Doppler echocardiography in anaesthetized horses: comparison with thermodilution. *Br J Anaesth* 1996; **77**: 773–780.
105 Lopes PC, Sousa MG, Camacho AA, *et al.* Comparison between two methods for cardiac output measurement in propofol-anesthetized dogs: thermodilution and Doppler. *Vet Anaesth Analg* 2010; **37**(5): 401–408.
106 Haskings EM, Eissa M, Allard RV, *et al.* Point-of-care ultrasound use in emergencies: what every anaesthetist should know. *Anesthesia* 2023; **78**(1): 105–118.
107 Kubicek WG, Karnegis JN, Patterson RP, *et al.* Development and evaluation of an impedance cardiac output system. *Aerosp Med* 1966; **37**: 1208–1212.
108 Bernstein DP. Continuous non-invasive real time monitoring of stroke volume and cardiac output by thoracic electrical bioimpedance. *Crit Care Med* 1986; **14**: 898–903.
109 Van De Water JM, Miller TW. Impedance cardiography: the next vital sign technology. *Chest* 2003; **123**: 2028–2033.
110 Heerdt PM, Wagner CL, DeMais M, *et al.* Noninvasive cardiac output monitoring with bioreactance as an alternative to invasive instrumentation for preclinical drug evaluation in beagles. *J Pharm Toxicol Meth* 2011; **64**: 111–118.
111 Albert N, Hail M, Li J, *et al.* Equivalence of bioimpedance and thermodilution methods in measuring cardiac output in patients with advanced, decompensated chronic heart failure hospitalized in critical care. *J Am J Crit Care* 2004; **13**: 469–479.
112 Sagemam WS, Riffenburgh RH, Spiess BD. Equivalence of bioimpedance and thermodilution in measuring cardiac index after cardiac surgery. *J Cardiothorac Vasc Anaesth* 2002; **1691**: 8–14.
113 Yung GL, Fedullo PF, Kinninger K, *et al.* Comparison of impedance cardiography to direct Fick and thermodilution cardiac output determination in pulmonary arterial hypertension. *Congest Heart Fail* 2004; **10**: 7–10.
114 Tibballs J, Hochmann M, Osborne A, *et al.* Accuracy of the BoMED NCCOM3 bioimpedance cardiac output monitor during induced hypotension: an experimental study in dogs. *Anaesth Intensive Care* 1992; **20**(3): 326–331.
115 Yamashita K, Ueyama Y, Miyoshi K, *et al.* Minimally invasive determination of cardiac output by transthoracic bioimpedance, partial carbon dioxide rebreathing, and transesophageal Doppler echocardiography in beagle dogs. *J Vet Med Sci* 2007; **69**(1): 43–47.
116 Shibutani K, Muraoka M, Shirasaki S, *et al.* Do changes in end-tidal pCO2 quantitatively reflect changes in cardiac output? *Anesth Analg* 1994; **79**: 829–833.
117 Wahba RW, Tessler MJ, Kleiman SJ. Changes in pCO2 with acute changes in cardiac index. *Can J Anaesth* 1996; **43**: 243–245.
118 Lakhal K, Nay MA, Kamel T, *et al.* Change in end-tidal carbon dioxide outperforms other surrogates for change in cardiac output during fluid challenge. *Br J Anaesth* 2017; **118**(3): 355–362.
119 Dubin A, Murias G, Estenssoro E, *et al.* End-tidal CO2 pressure determinants during hemorrhagic shock. *Intensive Care Med* 2000; **26**(11): 1619–1623.

14 Monitoring Ventilation

Jessica D. Briley[1], Kate M. Bailey[2] and Lydia Love[1]

[1] Department of Molecular Biomedical Sciences, College of Veterinary Medicine, North Carolina State University, Raleigh, North Carolina, USA

[2] United Veterinary Care, and College of Veterinary Medicine, North Carolina State University (Adjunct), Raleigh, North Carolina, USA

Chapter contents

Introduction, 220
Physiology of aerobic respiration, 220
  Carbon dioxide and acid–base implications, 221
Importance of monitoring ventilation, 221
  Monitoring standards, 221
Physical methods of monitoring ventilation, 222
Apnea monitors, 222
Quantitative monitoring of carbon dioxide, 222
  Methods of carbon dioxide measurement, 223
Time-based capnography, 224
  The normal capnogram, 224
  Abnormal capnograms, 225
  Specific clinical indications and uses of time-based capnography, 225
  Species considerations, 227
Volumetric capnography, 228
References, 228

Introduction

Since William Thomas Green Morton's demonstration of ether use in 1846, the delivery of anesthesia and the monitoring of anesthetized patients have undergone significant transformation [1]. Today, vigilant perianesthetic care necessitates the assessment of cardiovascular, ventilatory, and metabolic status. Among these, monitoring ventilation plays a role in providing crucial patient- and equipment-related information. During anesthesia, the patient's ability to maintain proper ventilation may be compromised by anesthetic and analgesic drugs, muscle relaxation, and changes in respiratory drive. Monitoring ventilation allows assessment of carbon dioxide production, delivery to the lungs, and elimination via gas exchange, thereby preventing complications and ensuring patient well-being [2,3]. It is imperative for an anesthetist to understand the physiologic principles of ventilation and various assessment methods to ensure patient safety and optimize anesthesia delivery.

Physiology of aerobic respiration

Although occasionally used interchangeably, ventilation and respiration can be viewed as two separate physiologic functions. *Ventilation* refers to the movement of gases, specifically oxygen and carbon dioxide (CO_2), in and out of the alveoli in the lungs. *Respiration* refers to the cellular utilization of oxygen in the process of generating energy in the form of adenosine triphosphate (ATP). In aerobic respiration, glycolysis of carbohydrates occurs in the cytoplasm in the presence of oxygen. Pyruvate moves into mitochondria and enters the tricarboxylic acid (TCA) cycle after conversion to acetyl-CoA (Fig. 14.1). The final step in aerobic respiration is oxidative phosphorylation, including the electron transport chain and the process of chemiosmosis.

This series of reactions generates ATP, which is the primary source of energy for cells. For efficient aerobic respiration to occur, there must be an adequate supply of glucose and oxygen-rich blood to the mitochondria in the tissues. Carbon dioxide is generated as a by-product of aerobic respiration. The partial pressure of carbon dioxide (PCO_2) is highest within the mitochondria, from which it passes through the cytoplasm to the blood, and then is carried to the lungs for excretion. Carriage of CO_2 within the blood occurs primarily as bicarbonate, as a dissociation product from the buffering of CO_2 with water to form carbonic acid, and, to a lesser extent, as carbamino compounds bound to hemoglobin and plasma proteins or dissolved gas (see Chapter 37). Once delivered to the lungs, alveolar ventilation allows for gas exchange between the alveoli and circulation resulting in the acquisition of oxygen and expiration of CO_2. Alveolar CO_2 (P_ACO_2) is directly proportional to the amount of CO_2 produced by metabolism (VCO_2) and subsequently delivered to the lungs and inversely proportional to alveolar ventilation (V_A):

$$P_ACO_2 = \frac{VCO_2 \times 0.863}{V_A}$$

The constant 0.863 accounts for dissimilar units. Given the relationship between ventilation and perfusion, monitoring CO_2 in the respiratory gases provides the anesthetist with important information about metabolism, cardiac output, and ventilation.

Veterinary Anesthesia and Analgesia: The Sixth Edition of Lumb and Jones. Edited by Leigh Lamont, Kurt Grimm, Sheilah Robertson, Lydia Love and Carrie Schroeder.
© 2024 John Wiley & Sons, Inc. Published 2024 by John Wiley & Sons, Inc.
Companion website: www.wiley.com/go/lamont/anesthesia

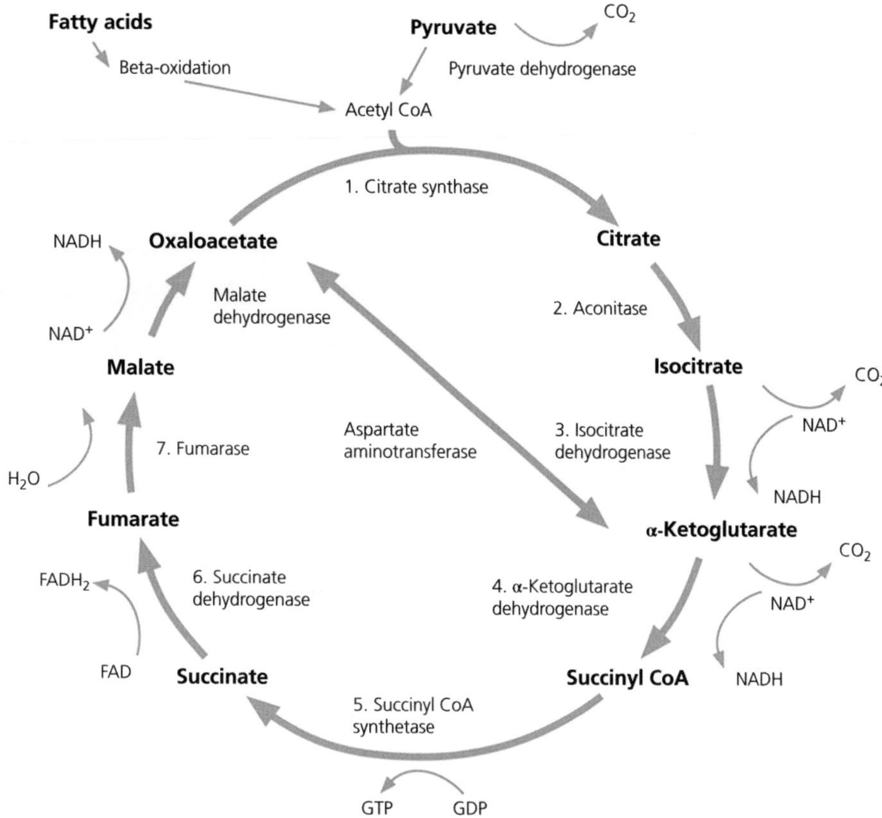

Figure 14.1 The tricarboxylic acid (TCA) cycle is the foundation of cellular energy generation. In the cytoplasm, glycolysis of carbohydrates creates pyruvate. Pyruvate enters the TCA cycle in the mitochondrial matrix after conversion to acetyl-Coenzyme A (acetyl-CoA) by pyruvate dehydrogenase (PDH). Each oxidative step in the TCA cycle reduces a coenzyme (nicotinamide adenine dinucleotide [NADH] or flavin adenine dinucleotide [$FADH_2$]). These reduced coenzymes participate in the electron transport chain, creating the majority of ATP production. FAD, flavin adenine dinucleotide; $FADH_2$, flavin adenine dinucleotide (reduced); GDP, guanosine diphosphate; GTP, guanosine triphosphate; NAD^+, nicotinamide adenine dinucleotide; NADH, nicotinamide adenine dinucleotide (reduced). Source: Borkum [4], with permission.

Carbon dioxide and acid–base implications

Carbon dioxide and its equilibration between the intracellular and extracellular environments are critical to acid–base homeostasis and can provide valuable information about respiratory status and compensatory mechanisms. The concentration of CO_2 in the blood is directly related to the regulation of pH. Increased levels of CO_2 result in higher carbonic acid (H_2CO_3) formation and thus the generation of H^+ ions, leading to a decrease in blood pH (acidemia) and a compensatory increase in blood bicarbonate (HCO_3^-) concentration. Conversely, decreased CO_2 levels reduce carbonic acid formation, resulting in an increase in blood pH (alkalemia) and compensatory decrease in blood HCO_3^-. Respiratory alkalemia (hypocapnia) and acidemia (hypercapnia) result in rapid equilibration between the extra- and intracellular fluids, causing more dramatic shifts in pH during these conditions when compared to metabolic acidemia or alkalemia [5].

There are many potential physiologic consequences of hypercapnic acidemia including catecholamine release (may lead to tachyarrhythmias), increased cardiac output, electrolyte shifts (e.g., hyperkalemia), rightward shift of the oxygen–hemoglobin dissociation curve, and cerebral vasodilation [6–8]. In the face of severe hypercapnia (> 80 mmHg), central nervous system signs including narcosis and coma can occur [9,10]. When decreases in the arterial partial pressure of CO_2 ($PaCO_2$) result in pH greater than 7.6, the physiologic consequences may include cerebral and myocardial vasoconstriction with resulting decreases in blood flow, decreased cardiac output, leftward shift of the oxygen–hemoglobin dissociation curve, hypokalemia, and predisposition to arrhythmias [11].

Importance of monitoring ventilation

Perianesthetic mortality trends appear to be decreasing in veterinary patients over time, though remain significantly higher than in humans [12–23]. Given the wide array of physiologic consequences of ventilatory derangements, early detection of respiratory events through advanced monitoring, including capnography, allows for timely intervention and enhanced patient safety throughout the perioperative period [24–27].

Monitoring standards

The American College of Veterinary Anesthesia and Analgesia (ACVAA) published its stance on anesthetic monitoring of small animal patients in 2009 [28]. Within those recommendations, multiple ventilation monitoring techniques are mentioned, including subjective measurements, such as visualization of chest wall expansion or movement of an attached reservoir bag, and thoracic auscultation via external or esophageal stethoscope, or the use of an audible respiratory monitor. These techniques indicate a binary endpoint (i.e., absence or presence) and do not allow for objective measurements, as they do not provide a carbon dioxide value. Partial pressure of end-tidal carbon dioxide ($P_{ET}CO_2$) with a capnograph or blood gas analysis to obtain $PaCO_2$ or partial pressure of venous carbon dioxide ($PvCO_2$) are the major objective monitoring methods for ventilation. The use of spirometry is mentioned for measurement of tidal volume and investigation of respiratory mechanics, and while this is an objective measurement, it does not provide partial pressure of carbon dioxide. The subjective measurements are considered essential or required by the ACVAA. Capnography is recommended, and blood gas analysis recommended as needed on a patient-specific basis. The Small Animal Monitoring Guidelines are in the process of being updated as of 2023.

The American Society of Anesthesiologists (ASA) has dictated since 1989 that any procedure in which endotracheal intubation or laryngeal mask airway is used requires the use of capnometry, capnography, or mass spectroscopy to quantify expired carbon dioxide. The requirement for quantitative monitoring of carbon dioxide was extended to sedated patients in 2010 [29]. It is recommended that alarms associated with abnormal carbon dioxide are audible in the operating room. A closed claims analysis at the end of the last century determined that of respiratory events, including inadequate ventilation, esophageal intubation, and difficult airway, 72% could have been prevented using better respiratory monitoring, and specifically, that the combination of pulse oximetry and capnography could have prevented > 90% of claims for inadequate ventilation and esophageal intubation [2].

The value of capnography in veterinary anesthesia and critical care settings is such that its use should be encouraged in primary care practice settings and an expectation in a specialty or tertiary care setting.

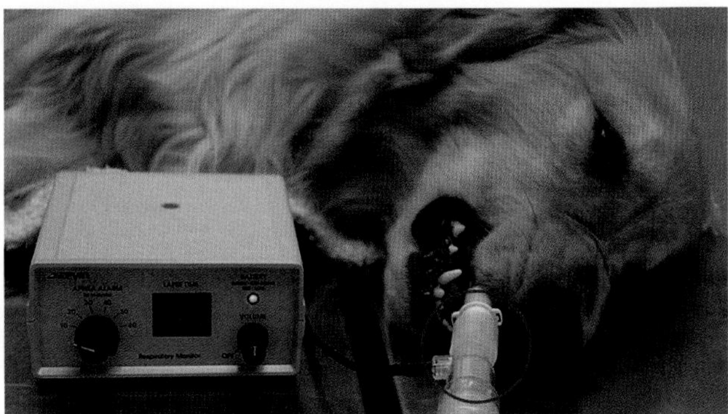

Figure 14.2 A digital apnea alert device attached to the endotracheal tube. The red circle highlights the airway adapter, which is connected to the digital display. An audible signal indicates air flow across the sensor with each breath and the apnea alarm can be adjusted to be 10–60 s in duration. Source: Thomas and Lerche [30].

Table 14.1 Definitions associated with the various forms of carbon dioxide measurement during ventilation.

Capnometry	The measurement of the partial pressure of carbon dioxide in respiratory gas
Capnometer	A diagnostic tool that measures the partial pressure of carbon dioxide in respiratory gas
Capnogram	A cyclical waveform of respiratory gas carbon dioxide plotted against time or expired volume
Capnography	The continuous analysis and recording of the measurement of the partial pressure of carbon dioxide in respiratory gases over time or expired volume
Capnograph	The instrument that analyzes CO_2 in respiratory gases and displays a capnogram

Physical methods of monitoring ventilation

The most accessible methods to monitor ventilation are the subjective assessment of breathing by visualization and auscultation of all lung fields and the trachea with a stethoscope. These methods should be included in every preanesthetic assessment, should accompany other monitoring techniques throughout the anesthetic event, including the recovery period, and should be utilized diagnostically in the event of a respiratory complication. Additionally, auscultation of lung sounds bilaterally directly after intubation is a highly recommended technique to confirm appropriate endotracheal tube (ETT) placement and aid in early diagnosis of endobronchial or esophageal intubation.

The lung sounds, as well as respiratory rate, effort, and quality, can indicate various causes for a change in ventilation. For example, a patient with a fixed airway obstruction will tend toward a decreased respiratory rate with a longer inspiratory phase. A patient with an alveolar disease or pleural space disease will often experience an increase in respiratory effort and could have increased (e.g., crackles in pneumonia) or decreased (e.g., absence due to pleural fluid) lung sounds. Respiratory disease may negatively impact ventilation; anesthetic management requirements of specific respiratory conditions vary and are discussed in Chapter 38.

Apnea monitors

Apnea monitors are simple respiratory monitoring tools that have been used historically in veterinary medicine and persist in some practice settings. Apnea monitors attach to the circuit between the distal end of the ETT and the patient end of the breathing circuit. The major information gained from an apnea monitor is the presence of inhalation/exhalation and a respiratory rate. Their design can be as simple as a low-profile plastic attachment that creates a "whistle" noise during the breathing cycle. They also come in a more sophisticated design with a circuit attachment and separate digital display that alerts the user with an audible and visual respiratory "beep" with each breath, displays the time between breaths, and provides an alarm that is triggered by a preset apnea duration (Fig. 14.2). Most models are equipped with battery power, making them highly portable. These monitors give a binary response (i.e., movement of gas or not) but do not provide any information about the effectiveness of respiratory efforts. In addition, like any adapter between the ETT and the breathing circuit, they add mechanical deadspace.

Quantitative monitoring of carbon dioxide

The use of quantified carbon dioxide as a monitoring tool in general anesthesia has multiple merits and can be accomplished in several forms (Table 14.1). In addition to the ability to provide information about metabolism, lung perfusion, and adequacy of ventilation, detection of carbon dioxide in respiratory gases can indicate integrity of the ETT and breathing circuit. Continuous CO_2 monitoring provides real-time data and allows for immediate detection of changes in ventilation and prompt intervention. It is primarily used to confirm ventilatory status (including respiratory rate, $P_{ET}CO_2$, and inhaled CO_2 [P_ICO_2]). Importantly, capnometry/capnography is the most reliable primary method for identifying whether an endotracheal tube is correctly placed within the airway instead of the esophagus.

Capnometry/capnography can also be instrumental in detecting life threatening cardiorespiratory complications. For example, the rapid decline in $P_{ET}CO_2$ as detected by a capnograph may be the first and only reliable indicator of cardiopulmonary arrest in the anesthetized patient, as detailed below.

Methods of carbon dioxide measurement

Like other forms of patient monitoring in veterinary medicine, the implementation of CO_2 measurement requires equipment that meets specific criteria to ensure its regular use and effectiveness. It is important for monitoring equipment to be affordable and readily available. Cost-effective options enable wider accessibility, allowing veterinary professionals to incorporate CO_2 monitoring into their standard protocols. Equipment should be easy to use and should not require extensive training or complex setup procedures. Additionally, lightweight, portable, and durable equipment offers flexibility for the rigors of daily use and enables monitoring in different areas of the veterinary hospital or during transport. In the case of monitoring ventilation, equipment should be ideal for the properties of CO_2 and be able to distinguish it among other gases that are present with minimal interference.

Blood gas analysis

The gold standard for determination of $PaCO_2$ is arterial blood gas analysis. An arterial sample is obtained either via puncture or from an indwelling catheter into a preheparinized syringe. Air bubbles are expelled, and the sample should be analyzed within 30 min or stored on ice. Both laboratory-based and patient-side blood gas analyzers are available that utilize a glass electrode covered with a CO_2 permeable membrane (the Severinghaus electrode) to ascertain CO_2 concentrations. Carbon dioxide from the blood sample diffuses across the membrane into a bicarbonate solution. Carbonic acid is created and devolves into H^+ and HCO_3^-. The generation of H^+ ions, and therefore pH, is logarithmically related to the concentration of CO_2 in the sample, creating a voltage difference between the glass electrode and the reference electrode [31].

Disadvantages of arterial blood gas analysis include intermittent sampling and the need to puncture an artery. In addition, the required equipment may not be available in all veterinary clinical settings.

Chemical detection (colorimetry)

Chemical detection is based on the principle that when CO_2 is combined with water, carbonic acid is formed, which then dissociates into hydrogen ions and bicarbonate. In turn, the pH is decreased, and this change acts as a surrogate marker for detection of CO_2 when using a pH-sensitive indicator. These devices typically house a color changing, pH-sensitive indicator within a clear window, which can be connected to standard endotracheal tube and breathing circuit components. For each device, a chart will reference which color change correlates with a range of CO_2 measurements. Though the measurements are not precise, they have proven to be successful at detection of endotracheal intubation, prediction of return of spontaneous circulation in resuscitation, and monitoring of ventilation for many hours where quantitative methods are not available [32–34]. Advantages for this type of device include its light weight and low cost. Disadvantages include generation of semiquantitative results, conditional interpretation of color change, short-term usability, and added resistance to flow.

Infrared spectroscopy

The widely used technology that possesses a majority of the aforementioned qualities is infrared (IR) spectroscopy. IR spectroscopy involves the analysis of the interaction between IR radiation and asymmetric, polyatomic molecules at distinct spectra. Homogeneous molecules, such as oxygen, do not absorb IR radiation, and techniques for oxygen measurement are discussed in Chapter 15. IR radiation consists of a range of wavelengths that fall between the visible and microwave regions of the electromagnetic spectrum. When a sample is exposed to IR radiation, the molecules within the sample absorb energy at specific frequencies that are characteristic of the chemical bonds present. The wavelength at which CO_2 has the strongest absorption band is approximately 4.3 µm, which allows reasonable discrimination from other molecules that also absorb IR radiation and are commonly found in an expired breath (i.e., inhalant anesthetics). Notably, two molecules with IR absorption bands close to CO_2 that may cause cross-interference are water vapor and nitrous oxide (N_2O).

Once the absorption of IR radiation by CO_2 in a sample of expired breath is measured, the principles of the Beer–Lambert law are applied:

$$A = \varepsilon lc$$

where A is the absorbance, ε is the molecular absorption coefficient, l is the length of the optical path, and c is the molecular concentration. Absorption of IR radiation at the specified wavelength is proportional to the concentration of the molecule (CO_2) being measured. When the absorbance is compared to a known standard, the amount of CO_2 present in respiratory gases can be quantified as a partial pressure (representative of the number of molecules present) or converted to a percent concentration (expressed as a proportion of the total).

The essential elements for IR spectroscopy include: a source of IR radiation, a sample cell, and a photodetector [35]. IR capnographs may use an optical filter to transmit only the desired wavelength (nondispersive) or may separate the wavelengths spatially with prisms or diffraction (dispersive). Nondispersive IR spectroscopy is most commonly in use as it is more efficient.

Infrared radiation source

In general, IR radiation sources may be considered broad- or narrowband. One example of a broadband source is a heated element known as a "blackbody emitter." In this case, filters are utilized to eliminate IR that is outside the desired range, and the constant source is mechanically chopped by a spinning wheel. The spinning wheel alternately blocks and allows the IR radiation to pass through to the sample or detector. This chopping action creates a time-varying signal, which is important for separating the desired IR signal from any background noise or interference. Multigas analyzers employ several specific narrowband filters to allow for the measurement of halogenated agents along with CO_2 and may also include integrated technology for measurement of oxygen.

An example of a narrowband IR source is laser-based molecular correlation spectroscopy, or Microstream technology. This uses a unique approach to emit a band of IR radiation that is highly precise for CO_2. In Microstream technology, a glass electrode that contains several gases, including nitrogen and CO_2, is exposed to a radio frequency voltage. Consequently, the nitrogen molecules experience excitation and their interaction with CO_2 causes excitation of those molecules. When CO_2 returns to its resting state, it emits radiation, which is used as the narrow spectrum IR source. This IR source is then electronically modulated in order to allow sampling every 25 ms.

Ultimately, the IR light is transmitted through the sample chamber, and the filtered and modulated signal reaches a detector where the intensity is measured, processed, and directed to the user interface where it is displayed.

Problems with infrared spectroscopy

The IR absorption band for CO_2 lies between two strong water vapor absorption bands, and water vapor can interfere with CO_2 measurement in several ways. When exhaled breath passes through the respiratory system, it picks up water vapor, which can significantly contribute to the total gas volume. Water vapor can condense at the sample cell, where it will absorb IR radiation, leading to a falsely increased CO_2 reading. Heating of sensors, water traps, absorbent filters, and specialized permeable (e.g., Nafion) tubing are a few solutions utilized to limit this interference. In sidestream/diverting monitors (see below), the cooling of the sampled gas will affect the concentration of water vapor and lead to slight overestimation of $P_{ET}CO_2$ [36]. Water vapor and secretions can also cause full or partial occlusion of sampling lines leading to altered measurements or even no measurement at all.

Another phenomenon known as "collision broadening" causes apparent increases in CO_2 due to the molecular interaction with gases such as N_2O and O_2, which can result in widened absorption spectra.

Mainstream capnometry/capnography

Mainstream (non-diverting) CO_2 devices utilize IR technology with the sensor placed between the patient and the breathing system. The sample cell (cuvette) functions as the airway adapter and the IR source and detector are all housed within the sensor. The transmitted signal may be displayed directly on the sensor housing, or a cable may be used to connect to an external monitor. Advantages to mainstream devices include rapid response times, higher accuracy with small tidal volumes and faster respiratory rates, no need to separately scavenge sampled gases, and no waste of inhalant agents. Disadvantages to mainstream devices include added weight and mechanical deadspace to airway with limited adaptability, susceptibility to damage, and secretions on the windows of the cuvette causing interference with readings. Many of the noted disadvantages to mainstream technology are historical and have been minimized with contemporary solid-state technology [35,37].

Sidestream capnometry/capnography

Sidestream (diverting) CO_2 devices use a variety of airway adapters attached to a long sampling line to connect to the sample cell housed within a distant monitor. Samples are constantly aspirated at variable rates (typically 50–200 mL/min). A combination of water permeable tubing, filters, and water traps may be used to limit water vapor contamination. Advantages to sidestream devices include the lightweight nature of the ETT adapter, potential to minimize deadspace by connecting sampling tubing directly to a specialized ETT adapter, the protected status of the sensor within the monitor housing, and the ability to monitor $P_{ET}CO_2$ in non-intubated patients with nasal catheters. Disadvantages include delay time (based on sampling rate), the need for rerouting of sampled gas (scavenged or returned to circuit), and the potential for issues with the sampling line or water trap devices (e.g., leaks, kinks, or occlusions) [38].

Raman spectroscopy

Historically, another form of spectroscopy has been used that takes advantage of the phenomenon called "Raman scatter." In this technology, a high-intensity argon laser is applied to a gas sample. The laser causes excitation of the molecules within the sample, creating an altered energy state. When the molecules return to their stable state, energy is emitted in a signature specific to that molecule, known as "Raman scatter radiation." It provides a fingerprint-like spectrum that represents the specific vibrational and rotational modes of the molecules present. This technology is not currently used in clinical settings for capnometry as smaller, lighter, and less expensive technology has prevailed [39].

Mass spectrometry

Mass spectrometry measures components of a gas mixture based on their mass and charge. A sample is drawn into a vacuum chamber where it is exposed to an electron beam. The ionized fragments are then accelerated by an electrical field and separated by a magnetic field. Detectors are then able to measure individual components of the sample. While mass spectrometry remains a valuable analytical tool for research and specialized applications, the size, complexity, and cost limitations make it impractical for routine patient monitoring in clinical settings. More accessible and cost-effective technologies are currently preferred for continuous patient monitoring, especially in veterinary medicine [40,41].

Transcutaneous measurement

Transcutaneous measurement of carbon dioxide ($P_{TC}CO_2$) is a non-invasive method used to measure CO_2 by placing heated electrochemical sensors on the skin. The technique relies on the principle that CO_2 can diffuse through the skin, allowing its measurement at the skin surface. As in arterial blood gas analysis, a Severinghaus electrode is used to assess CO_2 concentrations. While $P_{TC}CO_2$ measurement could be particularly useful in situations involving non-intubated patients, or where frequent blood sampling is impractical or stressful, there remain many limitations to its use in veterinary clinical practice. In rabbits, it was demonstrated that $P_{TC}CO_2$ was able to reasonably approximate $PaCO_2$ [42]. However, in cats [43], sheep [44], and dogs [44,45], $P_{TC}CO_2$ consistently overestimates $PaCO_2$ and cannot be used as a reliable surrogate. Development of optical detection technology may offer an alternative to electrochemical-based means in the future [46].

Time-based capnography

A capnogram wave is most commonly plotted as CO_2 partial pressure in millimeters of mercury (mmHg) against time. In this format, there are four phases to the capnogram, one that represents inhalation and three that represent phases of exhalation. Of note, there is still disagreement within the literature as to the correct labeling system in phase number for the capnogram. While the numbering system might vary, the actual phase of inhalation or exhalation represented by the component of the graphical image remains the same.

The normal capnogram

A normal time capnogram, as described below, is shown in Fig. 14.3.

Phase 0 = inspiratory phase or inspiratory downstroke. Represented by a rapid downswing in expiratory CO_2 partial

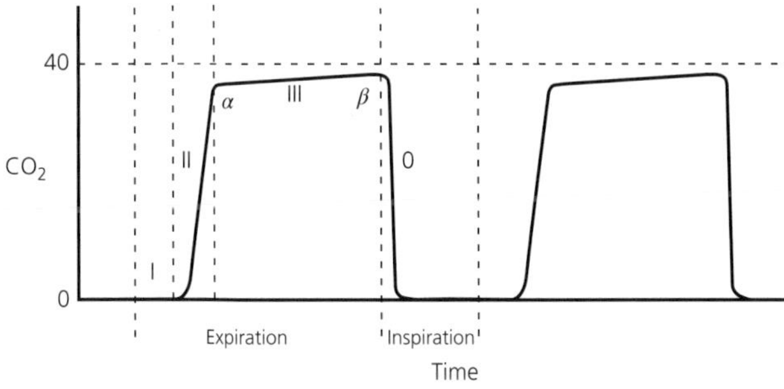

Figure 14.3 The normal time-based capnogram. Expiration is divided into phases I (CO_2-free deadspace gas), II (a mixture of deadspace and alveolar gas), and III (alveolar gas) and inspiration is represented by phase 0. The α angle represents the transition to CO_2-rich alveolar gas and the β angle marks the transition to inspiration.

pressure. In a normal waveform, the CO_2 partial pressure rapidly reaches zero.

Phase I = respiratory baseline. It marks the start of expiration and represents emptying of anatomic deadspace, which is CO_2 free.

Phase II = expiratory upstroke. Continued exhalation of a mixture of alveolar gas and deadspace gas from the conducting airways. The expired CO_2 partial pressure rapidly increases.

Phase III = the alveolar plateau. Continued exhalation of alveolar gas creates a gradually elevating line due to uneven alveolar emptying. The peak of the plateau represents the $P_{ET}CO_2$ at the end of the exhaled tidal volume.

Alpha (α) angle = the transition from phase II to III. In normal states, this angle should be approximately 100°. The α angle represents the transition from airway gas to alveolar gas.

Beta (β) angle = the transition from phase III to phase 0. In normal states, it should be approximately 90°. It is at this point in the capnogram waveform that a $P_{ET}CO_2$ value is measured.

Abnormal capnograms

In the process of critically evaluating a capnogram waveform, there are multiple pieces of information to gather, all of which lead to a clinical picture of respiratory status: (1) respiratory rate and consistency of rate; (2) $P_{ET}CO_2$ value; and (3) waveform appearance. A change in respiratory rate or a change in the consistency of the respiratory rate provides information related to anesthetic depth, nociceptive signaling, or brainstem status or pathology, among other states. Capnography is a powerful tool in helping to estimate, with good accuracy in healthy patients, the $PaCO_2$; however, $P_{ET}CO_2$ typically underestimates $PaCO_2$ by approximately 1–7 mmHg in small animals, and this underestimation may be greater in large animals during general anesthesia. This is due to two major factors: the presence of a constant anatomic deadspace and the concentration gradient of CO_2 between the pulmonary capillary and alveolus. There are abnormal states that can lead to a larger gradient between $PaCO_2$ and $P_{ET}CO_2$, and those will be discussed briefly later [47,48].

As a surrogate of $PaCO_2$, $P_{ET}CO_2$ reliably provides information on the status of metabolism, pulmonary perfusion (and therefore cardiac output), and ventilation, as described above. In addition, a change in $P_{ET}CO_2$ can provide information about the integrity and function of anesthesia equipment, including the breathing circuit and ETT, and, when combined with interpretation of the capnogram waveform, can provide a targeted focus for intervention. Examples of waveforms commonly encountered in veterinary clinical practice are presented in Fig. 14.4.

Specific clinical indications and uses of time-based capnography

The continuous and real-time measurement of $P_{ET}CO_2$ provides important insight into respiratory and metabolic status. While capnography is always useful for monitoring clinical status, it is also a critical tool in certain disease processes and case presentations.

Differential diagnosis of hypoxemia

A major strength of the quantitative measurement of $P_{ET}CO_2$ is the ability to detect clinical situations that may lead to hypoxemia as well as to focus the differential diagnosis for hypoxemia when it has occurred. For example, a capnogram with an obtuse α angle ("shark swimming to the left") indicates an obstruction to exhalation that could be due to upper airway (partial endotracheal tube obstruction or kinking) or lower airway (severe bronchospasm) issues (Fig. 14.4B). Another example is the absence of a waveform that could indicate apnea, esophageal intubation, complete airway obstruction, or disconnection of the patient from the anesthesia circuit. A capnogram with an elevated baseline can point to rebreathing of carbon dioxide, which indicates equipment issues with clearance of exhaled CO_2, including a dysfunctional one-way valve in the breathing circuit, an exhausted carbon dioxide absorbent canister, a significant amount of mechanical deadspace, or insufficient oxygen flow rate in a non-rebreathing circuit, many of which could lead to a hypoxemic gas mixture if left unattended (Fig. 14.4D).

Intracranial disease

In patients at risk for elevated intracranial pressure, it is crucial that cerebral blood flow is maintained in a normal range. Carbon dioxide partial pressure has a significant and linear effect on cerebral vascular reactivity and tone, causing cerebral vasodilation as local CO_2 partial pressure increases, and cerebral vasoconstriction as it decreases [49]. In these patients, identification of a normal arterial to expired carbon dioxide [$P(a\text{-}ET)CO_2$] gradient via blood gas analysis, followed by continuous monitoring of capnography, is imperative. Maintenance of $PaCO_2$ at or slightly below a normal partial pressure (35–40 mmHg) will significantly reduce the likelihood of brain herniation, an irreversible and devastating patient outcome [50]. Information related to anesthetic management of patients with intracranial disease is available in Chapter 39.

Acid–base derangements

In patients that are suffering from diseases that predispose them to acidemia, the close monitoring and maintenance of $PaCO_2$ is imperative to focused care. An increase in $PaCO_2$ causes a decrease in pH as discussed earlier, and therefore, hypoventilation precipitated by anesthesia may add to a pre-existing metabolic acidemia. Additionally, many patients that have a chronic metabolic acid–base disorder will have enlisted respiratory compensation as a mechanism to maintain favorable physiologic status. As a non-invasive estimate of $PaCO_2$, $P_{ET}CO_2$ can be utilized to avoid compounding an acid–base abnormality.

Hyper- and hypokalemia

An increase in CO_2 leads to an increase in H^+ concentration in the blood. Hydrogen ions are exchanged across the cell membrane for potassium ions (K^+) in the cell to maintain electroneutrality, leading to an increase in serum K^+ concentrations. The result is a precipitous increase in K^+ in the blood, which can have multiple negative consequences that will quickly and significantly affect patient outcome,

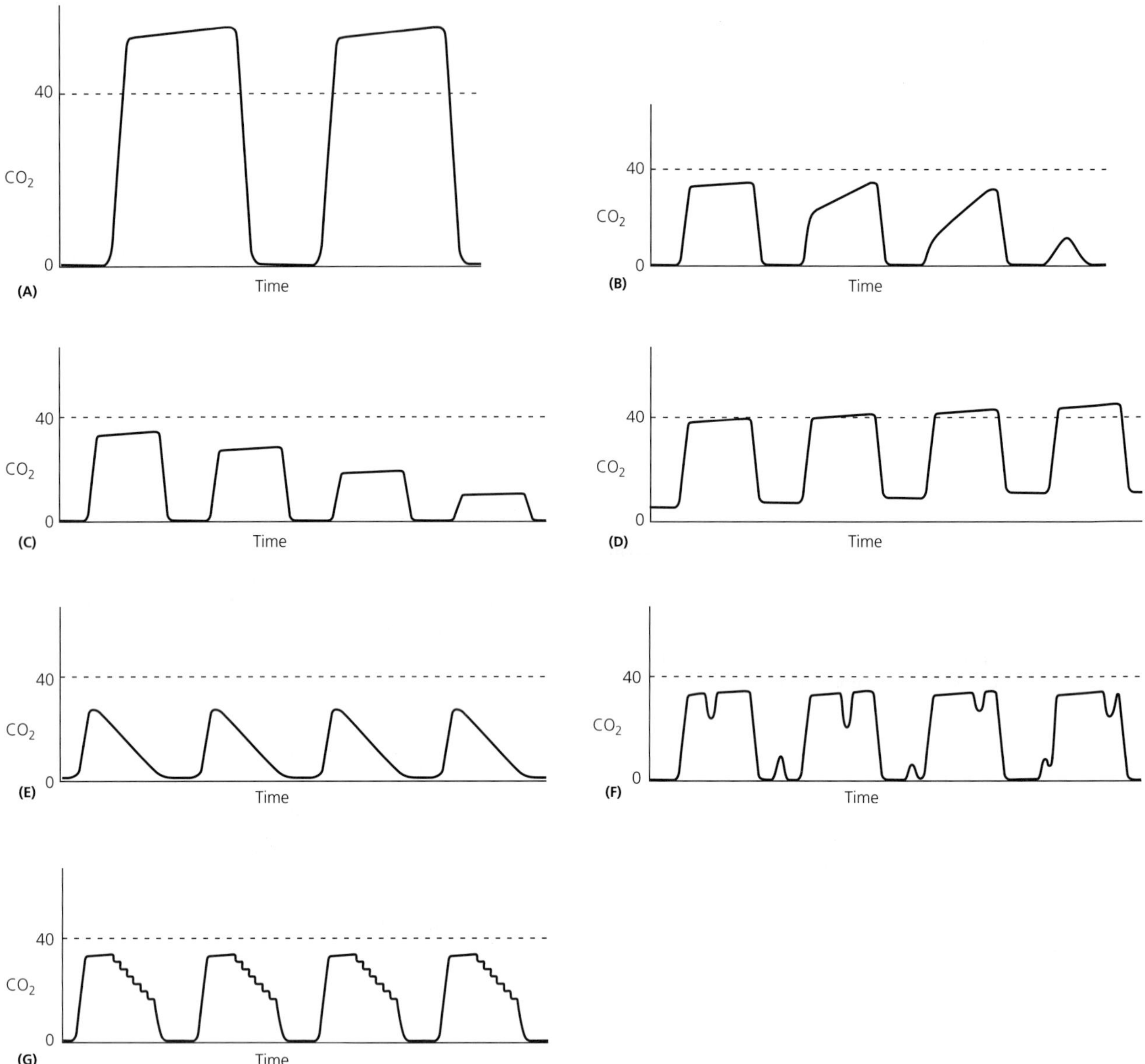

Figure 14.4 Variations in the normal capnogram. **A.** A normally shaped capnogram with an elevated plateau is indicative of hypoventilation. **B.** Obstruction to exhalation results in an obtuse α angle and may be due to upper airway (e.g., a kinked endotracheal tube) or lower airway (e.g., bronchoconstriction) issues **C.** A rapid reduction in the alveolar plateau to near zero in the absence of a change in ventilation indicates poor pulmonary perfusion or cardiovascular collapse. **D.** Properly functioning anesthetic equipment will prevent the rebreathing of CO_2 which is indicated by a capnogram with a baseline that does not return to zero. **E.** An obtuse β angle indicates dilution of $P_{ET}CO_2$ with CO_2 free gas and may be due to a high sampling rate, a leak around the endotracheal tube cuff, or high fresh gas flows in a non-rebreathing circuit. **F.** Spontaneous ventilatory efforts during mechanical ventilation are indicated by interruptions in the normal capnogram waveform. When a decrease in CO_2 concentrations is noted during phase III, it is traditionally known as a "curare cleft." **G.** Cardiogenic oscillations included an obtuse β angle accompanied by oscillations in the downstroke. Occurring more frequently at slow respiratory rates, these are thought to be due to mixing of inspired and expired gas in the trachea due to the mechanical activity of the nearby heart.

including cardiac arrhythmias, hypotension, and cardiopulmonary arrest. Maintenance of $PaCO_2$ at the patient's established normal level is important in patients that are at a risk for becoming hyperkalemic and hyperventilation can be considered if hyperkalemia develops during anesthesia. Commonly, diseases that cause hyperkalemia also cause metabolic acidemia, and these two problems should be considered simultaneously during creation of the anesthetic management plan. Hyperventilation, on the other hand, leads to hypokalemia, which can also precipitate arrhythmias as well as muscle weakness [51–53].

Difficult airway and lower airway disease

During routine, emergent, and difficult endotracheal intubation scenarios, capnography can be an important tool for verifying correct placement of the ETT. Confirmation that the ETT is properly positioned in the trachea rather than the esophagus will reduce the risk of complications related to misplacement [2]. Furthermore, changes in the capnogram, as outlined in the capnogram section above, may indicate developing or worsening airway obstruction and can demonstrate response to interventions (e.g., bronchodilator therapy).

Cardiopulmonary arrest

The capnograph is arguably the most useful monitor during cardiopulmonary arrest (CPA) and resuscitation, as it reflects pulmonary perfusion, and therefore cardiac output, in real time. It is non-invasive, easy to connect, and does not require any adjustment. Cardiopulmonary resuscitation (CPR) scenarios result in a degree of patient movement that creates significant artifacts for almost all other monitoring equipment, while the capnograph suffers little to no artifact due to thoracic compressions [54,55].

The $P_{ET}CO_2$ is related to cardiac output both in normal scenarios and during a CPR event. It can help to determine the quality of ongoing chest compressions or internal cardiac massage because the amount of blood returning to the lungs will largely determine the amount of CO_2 delivered to the lungs. For the same reason, capnography will be the first monitor to reliably convey if the patient has experienced cessation of blood flow and therefore CPA, and it is also extremely useful in identifying return of spontaneous circulation (ROSC) quickly. Finally, capnography is a powerful prognostic tool during the CPR event. Hofmeister *et al.* found that in instances where $P_{ET}CO_2$ was measured during CPR, dogs experiencing sustained $P_{ET}CO_2 > 15$ mmHg during a CPR event had an 86% chance of ROSC, while patients who did not sustain a $P_{ET}CO_2 > 15$ mmHg had a 94% chance of non-survival [56].

Cardiac output measurement

As mentioned above, $P_{ET}CO_2$ is directly related to cardiac output due to the fact that the cardiovascular system is circular, and therefore, almost the entire cardiac output passes through the lungs. This means the $P_{ET}CO_2$ sampled at the end of the endotracheal tube is correlated with cardiac output if metabolism and ventilation are held constant. Due to this correlation, $P_{ET}CO_2$ can be used to effectively measure trends in cardiac output, if not the exact value. It can be argued that clinically, knowing trends in cardiac output as opposed to the exact amount is more valuable, because the relative change in cardiac output in response to intervention might change patient outcome.

The relationship between carbon dioxide and cardiac output can be used to non-invasively measure cardiac output via the indirect Fick method. This is based on the Fick principle, which states that the quantity of gas (oxygen or CO_2) delivered to or taken away from the lungs is equal to the amount of gas absorbed by the pulmonary circulation or diffused from circulation to the alveoli and respiratory bronchioles. While the Fick principle-derived cardiac output measurement method relies on oxygen uptake by the patient, which can be difficult to measure, the indirect Fick method relies on partial rebreathing of carbon dioxide. The Non-Invasive Cardiac Output (NICO®) monitor is a piece of equipment that creates periods of partial rebreathing to estimate arterial and mixed venous CO_2 partial pressures based on $P_{ET}CO_2$ [57]. It is attached to the circuit in between the endotracheal tube and the circle system. Unfortunately, this monitor can only be used for patients with a tidal volume of 200 mL or more [58,59]. Cardiac output monitoring is covered in detail in Chapter 13.

Nasal catheter

The use of CO_2 measurement for veterinary patients can be critical in patients that are not intubated and where continuous blood sampling is not ideal. Use of a nasal catheter for the measurement of $P_{ET}CO_2$ has been investigated in dogs and foals [60–62], and displays reasonable correlation with paired CO_2 values. While correlation is better for those patients who are not simultaneously receiving oxygen therapy through the catheter, correlation was acceptable in both scenarios. More importantly, these results were clinically relevant and indicate that nasal catheters might be used to measure $P_{ET}CO_2$ non-invasively in patients pre- and postoperatively and in critical care settings.

Species considerations

While mammalian respiratory anatomy and function share similarities across species, there are variations that reflect adaptations to size, environment, and physiological needs. Furthermore, the adaptations of non-mammalian species warrant consideration, but do not preclude the use of capnography in these animals. It is important to remember that the rationale for use of non-invasive $P_{ET}CO_2$ monitoring in veterinary medicine is the assumption that it will correlate closely with $PaCO_2$ and, therefore, be a good surrogate for ventilatory adequacy.

Dogs and cats

There is reasonable evidence in anesthetized dogs with a closed chest that $P_{ET}CO_2$ correlates well with $PaCO_2$ in a variety of different ventilation modes [63–66]. However, during thoracotomy, $P_{ET}CO_2$ was found not to be a reliable indicator of $PaCO_2$ and, thus, adequacy of ventilation [66]. There is little published information examining the differences in $P_{ET}CO_2$ and $PaCO_2$ in cats. In one study that included six ventilated cats, the authors found that $P_{ET}CO_2$ was generally lower than $PaCO_2$ and was a good predictor of hypoventilation, but direct arterial sampling for the measurement of $PaCO_2$ was still recommended [67].

Horses

Measurement of $P_{ET}CO_2$ in horses is primarily focused on sidestream monitoring in anesthetized horses, but it has been shown that there is a relatively small difference in $P(a\text{-}ET)CO_2$ in horses that are standing and healthy [68]. In anesthetized and recumbent horses and ponies, there can be significant changes in ventilation–perfusion (V/Q) matching resulting in wide variation in $P(a\text{-}ET)CO_2$, although differences are improved when controlled ventilation is instituted compared to spontaneous ventilation [69–74]. Capnometry has significant limitations in the anesthetized horse unless it is paired with blood gas analysis.

Birds and reptiles

The significant anatomic and physiologic differences in non-mammalian respiratory systems are discussed elsewhere (Chapters 57 and 58). Notably, in birds, gas flow is unidirectional and gas exchange occurs through a cross-current mechanism. This adaptation can result in a negative $P(a\text{-}ET)CO_2$ gradient. In mechanically ventilated African Gray Parrots (*Psittacus erithacus*), a strong correlation was found between $P_{ET}CO_2$ and $PaCO_2$, with $P_{ET}CO_2$ consistently overestimating $PaCO_2$ by about 5 mmHg [75]. In anesthetized raptors, correlation between $P_{ET}CO_2$ and $PaCO_2$ was seen, but agreement varied with high, low, and normal $P_{ET}CO_2$ values [76]. During air sac insufflation in chickens, $P_{ET}CO_2$ often exceeded $PaCO_2$, but there was not a strong correlation between the two [77]. Finally, a study in anesthetized Amazon parrots (*Amazona ventralis*) also found that $P_{ET}CO_2$ overestimated $PaCO_2$ during spontaneous ventilation, but this difference reversed over time with mechanical ventilation [78].

In reptiles, the adaptation of intracardiac shunting may have a significant impact on the interpretation of capnometry. In a study of anesthetized and ventilated green iguanas (*Iguana iguana*), differences in the $P(a\text{-}ET)CO_2$ gradient were relatively minimal, but as time passed, this difference significantly increased [79].

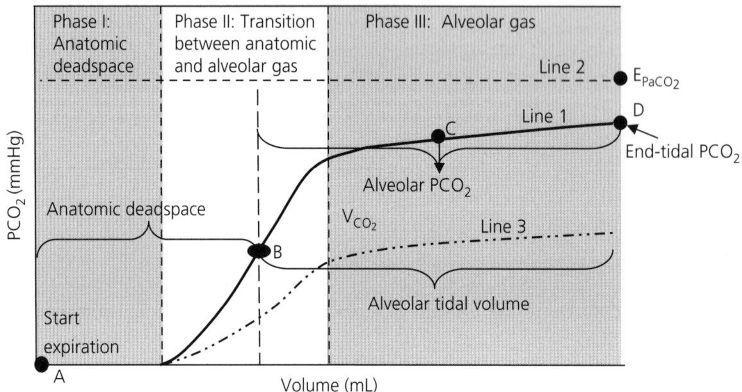

Figure 14.5 Volumetric capnography. The capnogram displays the expired CO_2 as a function of volume; the analyzer resets itself after each inspiration and inspiratory PCO_2 is not visible. Expiration begins at the black dot in the lower left-hand corner of the figure (A) and the first gas exhaled is that of airway deadspace (phase I). The sloping line of phase II (Line 1) represents a mixture of airway deadspace and alveolar gases. The phase III plateau (Line 1) represents alveolar gases and often continues to escalate until the end of the breath. End-tidal PCO_2 is the highest PCO_2 at the end of the breath (D). $PaCO_2$ (measured separately) is usually 3–6 mmHg higher than $P_{ET}CO_2$. The horizontal dashed line (Line 2) at the level of $PaCO_2$ is the theoretical $P_{ET}CO_2$ (E) if there were no airway or alveolar deadspace. Airway deadspace can be estimated as the expired volume at which the PCO_2 is half-way between zero (at the beginning of phase II) and the shoulder of the plateau (at the end of phase II) (B). The area under the curve of Line 1 represents the volume of carbon dioxide expelled during that breath (V_{CO_2}), derived from integrating volume and CO_2 over time. The area above the curve of Line 1, to the left of the mid-phase II vertical line (B), and below Line 2 represents airway deadspace. The area above the curve and to the right of the mid-phase II vertical line (B), and below Line 2 represents alveolar deadspace (high V/Q) and atelectasis (0 V/Q). Mixed-expired PCO_2 ($P_{ME}CO_2$) is calculated as V_{CO_2}/tidal volume. Average alveolar PCO_2 ($P_{av_{alveolar}}CO_2$) is the PCO_2 on the horizontal axis of Line 1, midway between the phase II vertical line and the endpoint of the breath (C). Physiologic deadspace (%) is calculated by the Bohr equation ($PaCO_2 - P_{ME}CO_2$)/($PaCO_2 - P_ICO_2$), where P_ICO_2 = inspired PCO_2. Airway deadspace (%) can be calculated as either ($P_{av_{alveolar}}CO_2 - P_{ME}CO_2$)/($P_{av_{alveolar}}CO_2 - P_ICO_2$) or ($P_{ET}CO_2 - P_{ME}CO_2$)/($P_{ET}CO_2 - P_ICO_2$). Alveolar deadspace (%) is calculated as physiologic deadspace − airway deadspace. Physiologic, airway, and alveolar deadspaces (mL) are calculated as physiologic, airway, or alveolar deadspace (%) × tidal volume.

Volumetric capnography

Volumetric capnography (VCap) plots exhaled CO_2 against expired volume, allowing for the determination of physiologic deadspace (the sum of anatomic and alveolar deadspace), effective alveolar tidal volume, and volume of CO_2 eliminated per breath [80] (Fig. 14.5). Volumetric capnograms have a similar waveform as time-based capnograms, excluding the inspiratory segment. Phase I of the volume capnogram starts at zero as the first gas exhaled is from airway (anatomic) deadspace and is free of CO_2. The slope at phase II rises sharply as a mixture of gas from the anatomic deadspace and alveoli is exhaled. The slope at phase III is determined by the distribution of ventilation and perfusion within the alveoli and usually escalates until the end of the breath. The area under the curve of this capnogram is the amount of carbon dioxide exhaled within a tidal volume. The point-of-care ability to ascertain deadspace and investigate V/Q abnormalities provides valuable information about the effectiveness of ventilation. It can better focus treatment of hypoxemia or impending hypoxemia, revealing whether the problem is primarily a ventilation or a deadspace issue [81–83]. Due to its ability to quantify pulmonary perfusion, and therefore cardiac output, this is a useful non-invasive tool for anesthetized patients [84]. To date, the use of Vcap in veterinary species of interest has been mostly limited to research settings [85–87].

References

1 Chaturvedi R, Gogna RL. Ether day: an intriguing history. *Med J Armed Forces India* 2011; **67**(4): 306–308.
2 Caplan RA, Posner KL, Ward RJ, *et al.* Adverse respiratory events in anesthesia: a closed claims analysis. *Anesthesiology* 1990; **72**(5): 828–833.
3 Gelb AW, Morris WW, Johnson W, *et al.* World Health Organization-World Federation of Societies of Anaesthesiologists (WHO-WFSA) international standards for a safe practice of anesthesia. *Can J Anesth* 2018; **65**(6): 698–708.
4 Borkum JM. The tricarboxylic acid cycle as a central regulator of the rate of aging: implications for metabolic interventions. *Adv Biol (Weinh)* 2023; **7**(7): e2300095.
5 Cohen JJ, Brackett NC Jr., Schwartz WB. The nature of the carbon dioxide titration curve in the normal dog. *J Clin Invest* 1964; **43**(5): 777–786.
6 Cullen DJ, Eger EI. Cardiovascular effects of carbon dioxide in man. *Anesthesiology* 1974; **41**(4): 345–348.
7 Grubb RL, Raichle ME, Eichling JO, *et al.* The effects of changes in $PaCO_2$ cerebral blood volume, blood flow, and vascular mean transit time. *Stroke* 1974; **5**(5): 630–639.
8 Yoon S, Zuccarello M, Rapoport R. pCO2 and pH regulation of cerebral blood flow. *Front Physiol* 2012; **3**: 365.
9 Brosnan RJ, Eger EI, Laster MJ, *et al.* Anesthetic properties of carbon dioxide in the rat. *Anesth Analg* 2007; **105**(1): 103–106.
10 van der Schrier R, van Velzen M, Roozekrans M, *et al.* Carbon dioxide tolerability and toxicity in rat and man: a translational study. *Front Toxicol* 2022: 4.
11 Laffey JG, Kavanagh BP. Hypocapnia. *N Engl J Med* 2002; **347**(1): 43–53.
12 Bidwell LA, Bramlage LR, Rood WA. Equine perioperative fatalities associated with general anaesthesia at a private practice – a retrospective case series. *Vet Anaesth Analg* 2007; **34**(1): 23–30.
13 Brodbelt DC, Blissitt KJ, Hammond RA, *et al.* The risk of death: the confidential enquiry into perioperative small animal fatalities. *Vet Anaesth Analgesia* 2008; **35**(5): 365–373.
14 Dugdale AH, Taylor PM. Equine anaesthesia-associated mortality: where are we now? *Vet Anaesth Analg* 2016; **43**(3): 242–255.
15 Laurenza C, Ansart Lè, Portier K. Risk factors of anesthesia-related mortality and morbidity in one equine hospital: a retrospective study on 1,161 cases undergoing elective or emergency surgeries. *Front Vet Sci* 2020; **6**: 514.
16 Deutsch J, Taylor PM. Mortality and morbidity in equine anaesthesia. *Equine Vet Educ* 2022; **34**(3): 152–168.
17 Morrison JA, Spofford N, Yang M, *et al.* Development and implementation of veterinary anesthesia medical quality standards for primary care. *Vet Anaesth Analg* 2022; **49**(3): 233–242.
18 Shoop-Worrall SJ, O'Neill DG, Viscasillas J, *et al.* Mortality related to general anaesthesia and sedation in dogs under UK primary veterinary care. *Vet Anaesth Analg* 2022; **49**(5): 433–442.
19 Steen J, Romano M, Portela DA, *et al.* A single-cohort retrospective analysis of factors associated with morbidity and mortality in 193 anesthetized domestic goats. *Vet Anaesth Analg* 2023; **50**(3): 245–254.

20 Li G, Warner M, Lang BH, *et al.* Epidemiology of anesthesia-related mortality in the United States, 1999–2005. *Anesthesiology* 2009; **110**(4): 759–765.

21 Gottschalk A, Van Aken H, Zenz M, *et al.* Is anesthesia dangerous? *Dtsch Arztebl Int* 2011; **108**(27): 469–474.

22 Pollard RJ, Hopkins T, Smith CT, *et al.* Perianesthetic and anesthesia-related mortality in a southeastern United States population: a longitudinal review of a prospectively collected quality assurance data base. *Anesth Analg* 2018; **127**(3): 730–735.

23 Lim G. What is new in obstetric anesthesia in 2020: a focus on research priorities for maternal morbidity, mortality, and postpartum health. *Int J Obst Anesth* 2022; **51**: 103568.

24 Saunders R, Struys MMRF, Pollock RF, *et al.* Patient safety during procedural sedation using capnography monitoring: a systematic review and meta-analysis. *BMJ Open* 2017; **7**(6): e013402.

25 Wollner E, Nourian MM, Booth W, *et al.* Impact of capnography on patient safety in high- and low-income settings: a scoping review. *Br J Anaesth* 2020; **125**(1): e88–e103.

26 Khanna AK, Bergese SD, Jungquist CR, *et al.* Prediction of opioid-induced respiratory depression on inpatient wards using continuous capnography and oximetry: an international prospective, observational trial. *Anesth Analg* 2020; **131**(4): 1012–1024.

27 Stites M, Surprise J, McNiel J, *et al.* Continuous capnography reduces the incidence of opioid-induced respiratory rescue by hospital rapid resuscitation team. *J Patient Saf* 2021; **17**(6): e557–e561.

28 American College of Veterinary Anesthesia and Analgesia (ACVAA). Recommendations for Monitoring Anesthetized Veterinary Patients, 2009. www.acvaa.org/wp-content/uploads/2019/05/Small-Animal-Monitoring-Guidlines.pdf (accessed July 2023).

29 American Society of Anesthesiologists (ASA). Standards for Basic Anesthetic Monitoring, 2020. www.asahq.org/standards-and-practice-parameters/standards-for-basic-anesthetic-monitoring (accessed July 2023).

30 Thomas J, Lerche P. Anesthetic monitoring. In: Thomas J, Lerche P, eds. *Anesthesia and Analgesia for Veterinary Technicians*, 5th edn. St. Louis, MO: Elsevier, 2017: 195.

31 Severinghaus JW, Freeman Bradley A. Electrodes for blood pO_2 and pCO_2 determination. *J Appl Physiol* 1958; **13**(3): 515–520.

32 Hayden SR, Sciammarella J, Viccellio P, *et al.* Colorimetric end-tidal CO_2 detector for verification of endotracheal tube placement in out-of-hospital cardiac arrest. *Acad Emerg Med* 1995; **2**(6): 499–502.

33 Nakatani K, Yukioka H, Fujimori M, *et al.* Utility of colorimetric end-tidal carbon dioxide detector for monitoring during prehospital cardiopulmonary resuscitation. *Am J Emerg Med* 1999; **17**(2): 203–206.

34 Sakles JC, Ross C, Kovacs G. Preventing unrecognized esophageal intubation in the emergency department. *J Am Coll Emerg Physicians Open* 2023; **4**(3): e12951.

35 Jaffe MB. Respiratory gas analysis-technical aspects. *Anesth Analg* 2018; **126**(3): 839–845.

36 Fletcher R, Werner O, Nordström L, *et al.* Sources of error and their correction in the measurement of carbon dioxide elimination using the Siemens-Elema CO_2 Analyzer. *Br J Anaesth* 1983; **55**(2): 177–185.

37 Neto FJT, Carregaro AB, Mannarino R, *et al.* Comparison of a sidestream capnograph and a mainstream capnograph in mechanically ventilated dogs. *J Am Vet Med Assoc* 2002; **221**(11): 1582–1585.

38 Weingarten M. Respiratory monitoring of carbon dioxide and oxygen: a ten-year perspective. *J Clin Monit* 1990; **6**(3): 217–225.

39 Lockwood GG, Landon MJ, Chakrabarti MK, *et al.* The Ohmeda Rascal II. A new gas analyser for anaesthetic use. *Anaesthesia* 1994; **49**(1): 44–53.

40 Grévisse P, Delcambre Y, Picart P, *et al.* Turning the mass-spectrometer into an easy to handle clinical instrument for routine multipatient surveillance of respiratory and anesthetic gases during anesthesia. *Acta Anaesthesiol Belg* 1987; **38**(1): 37–43.

41 Turner PG, Dugdale A, Young IS, *et al.* Portable mass spectrometry for measurement of anaesthetic agents and methane in respiratory gases. *Vet J* 2008; **177**(1): 36–44.

42 Barter LS, Hopper K. Transcutaneous monitor approximates $PaCO(_2)$ but not $PaO(_2)$ in anesthetized rabbits. *Vet Anaesth Analg* 2011; **38**(6): 568–575.

43 Mann FA, Wagner-Mann C, Branson KR. Transcutaneous oxygen and carbon dioxide monitoring in normal cats. *J Vet Emerg Crit Care* 1997; **7**(2): 99–109.

44 Vogt R, Rohling R, Kästner S. Evaluation of a combined transcutaneous carbon dioxide pressure and pulse oximetry sensor in adult sheep and dogs. *Am J Vet Res* 2007; **68**(3): 265–270.

45 Holowaychuk MK, Fujita H, Bersenas AME. Evaluation of a transcutaneous blood gas monitoring system in critically ill dogs. *J Vet Emerg Crit Care* 2014; **24**(5): 545–553.

46 Eberhard P. The design, use, and results of transcutaneous carbon dioxide analysis: current and future directions. *Anesth Analg* 2007; **105**(6 Suppl): S48–S52.

47 Choudhury M, Kiran U, Choudhary SK, *et al.* Arterial-to-end-tidal carbon dioxide tension difference in children with congenital heart disease. *J Cardiothorac Vasc Anesth* 2006; **20**(2): 196–201.

48 Heneghan CPH, Scallan MJH, Branthwaite MA. End-tidal carbon dioxide during thoracotomy. *Anaesthesia* 1981; **36**(11): 1017–1021.

49 Carr JMJR, Caldwell HG, Ainslie PN. Cerebral blood flow, cerebrovascular reactivity and their influence on ventilatory sensitivity. *Exp Physiol* 2021; **106**(7): 1425–1448.

50 Greene SA. Anesthesia for patients with neurologic disease. *Top Companion Anim Med* 2010; **25**(2): 83–86.

51 Edwards R, Winnie AP, Ramamurthy S. Acute hypocapneic hypokalemia: an iatrogenic anesthetic complication. *Anesth Analg* 1977; **56**(6): 786–792.

52 Hassan H, Gjessing J, Tomlin PJ. Hypercapnia and hyperkalaemia. *Anaesthesia* 1979; **34**(9): 897–899.

53 Muir WW III, Wagner AE, Buchanan C. Effects of acute hyperventilation on serum potassium in the dog. *Vet Surg* 1990; **19**(1): 83–87.

54 Fletcher DJ, Boller M, Brainard BM, *et al.* RECOVER evidence and knowledge gap analysis on veterinary CPR. Part 7: clinical guidelines. *J Vet Emerg Crit Care* 2012; **22**(Suppl 1): S102–S131.

55 Hamrick JL, Hamrick JT, Lee JK, *et al.* Efficacy of chest compressions directed by end-tidal CO_2 feedback in a pediatric resuscitation model of basic life support. *J Am Heart Assoc* 2014; **3**(2): e000450.

56 Hofmeister EH, Brainard BM, Egger CM, *et al.* Prognostic indicators for dogs and cats with cardiopulmonary arrest treated by cardiopulmonary cerebral resuscitation at a university teaching hospital. *J Am Vet Med Assoc* 2009; **235**(1): 50–57.

57 Haryadi DG, Orr JA, Kuck K, *et al.* Partial CO_2 rebreathing indirect Fick technique for non-invasive measurement of cardiac output. *J Clin Monit Comput* 2000; **16**(5–6): 361–374.

58 Van Heerden PV, Baker S, Lim SI, *et al.* Clinical evaluation of the Non-Invasive Cardiac Output (NICO) monitor in the intensive care unit. *Anaesth Intensive Care* 2000; **28**(4): 427–430.

59 Giguère S, Bucki E, Adin DB, *et al.* Cardiac output measurement by partial carbon dioxide rebreathing, 2-dimensional echocardiography, and lithium-dilution method in anesthetized neonatal foals. *J Vet Intern Med* 2005; **19**(5): 737–743.

60 Kelmer E, Scanson LC, Reed A, *et al.* Agreement between values for arterial and end-tidal partial pressures of carbon dioxide in spontaneously breathing, critically ill dogs. *J Am Vet Med Assoc* 2009; **235**(11): 1314–1318.

61 Wong DM, Alcott CJ, Wang C, *et al.* Agreement between arterial partial pressure of carbon dioxide and saturation of hemoglobin with oxygen values obtained by direct arterial blood measurements versus noninvasive methods in conscious healthy and ill foals. *J Am Vet Med Assoc* 2011; **239**(10): 1341–1347.

62 Pang D, Hethey J, Caulkett NA, *et al.* Partial pressure of end-tidal CO_2 sampled via an intranasal catheter as a substitute for partial pressure of arterial CO_2 in dogs. *J Vet Emerg Crit Care* 2007; **17**(2): 143–148.

63 Williams HM. Alveolar-arterial oxygen pressure gradient in normal dogs. *Am J Physiol* 1953; **173**(1): 77–81.

64 Hightower CE, Kiorpes AL, Butler HC, *et al.* End-tidal partial pressure of CO_2 as an estimate of arterial partial pressure of CO_2 during various ventilatory regimens in halothane-anesthetized dogs. *Am J Vet Res* 1980; **41**(4): 610–612.

65 Grosenbaugh DA, Muir WW III. Accuracy of noninvasive oxyhemoglobin saturation, end-tidal carbon dioxide concentration, and blood pressure monitoring during experimentally induced hypoxemia, hypotension, or hypertension in anesthetized dogs. *Am J Vet Res* 1998; **59**(2): 205–212.

66 Wagner AE, Gaynor JS, Dunlop CI, *et al.* Monitoring adequacy of ventilation by capnometry during thoracotomy in dogs. *J Am Vet Med Assoc* 1998; **212**(3): 377–379.

67 Hendricks JC, King LG. Practicality, usefulness, and limits of end-tidal carbon dioxide monitoring in critical small animal patients. *J Vet Emerg Crit Care* 1994; **4**(1): 29–39.

68 Littlejohn A, Mitchell B. Acid–base and blood gas studies in horses. I. A comparison of capillary and arterial blood samples for the estimation of acid–base values in horses. *Res Vet Sci* 1969; **10**(3): 260–262.

69 Meyer RE, Short CE. Arterial to end-tidal CO_2 tension and alveolar dead space in halothane- or isoflurane-anesthetized ponies. *Am J Vet Res* 1985; **46**(3): 597–599.

70 Cribb PH. Capnographic monitoring during anesthesia with controlled ventilation in the horse. *Vet Surg* 1988; **17**(1): 48–52.

71 Geiser DR, Rohrbach BW. Use of end-tidal CO_2 tension to predict arterial CO_2 values in isoflurane-anesthetized equine neonates. *Am J Vet Res* 1992; **53**(9): 1617–1621.

72 Neto FJ, Luna SP, Massone F, *et al.* The effect of changing the mode of ventilation on the arterial-to-end-tidal CO_2 difference and physiological dead space in laterally and dorsally recumbent horses during halothane anesthesia. *Vet Surg* 2000; **29**(2): 200–205.

73 Koenig J, McDonell W, Valverde A. Accuracy of pulse oximetry and capnography in healthy and compromised horses during spontaneous and controlled ventilation. *Can J Vet Res* 2003; **67**(3): 169–174.

74 Mosing M, Böhm SH, Rasis A, *et al.* Physiologic factors influencing the arterial-to-end-tidal CO_2 difference and the alveolar dead space fraction in spontaneously breathing anesthetised horses. *Front Vet Sci* 2018; **5**: 58.

75 Edling TM, Degernes LA, Flammer K, *et al.* Capnographic monitoring of anesthetized African grey parrots receiving intermittent positive pressure ventilation. *J Am Vet Med Assoc* 2001; **219**(12): 1714–1718.

76 Desmarchelier M, Rondenay Y, Fitzgerald G, *et al.* Monitoring of the ventilatory status of anesthetized birds of prey by using end-tidal carbon dioxide measured with a Microstream capnometer. *J Zoo Wildl Med* 2007; **38**(1): 1–6.
77 Paré M, Ludders JW, Erb HN. Association of partial pressure of carbon dioxide in expired gas and arterial blood at three different ventilation states in apneic chickens (*Gallus domesticus*) during air sac insufflation anesthesia. *Vet Anaesth Analg* 2013; **40**(3): 245–256.
78 Pettifer GR, Cornick-Seahorn J, Smith JA, *et al.* The comparative cardiopulmonary effects of spontaneous and controlled ventilation by using the Hallowell EMC Anesthesia WorkStation in Hispaniolan Amazon Parrots (*Amazona ventralis*). *J Avian Med Surg* 2002; **16**(4): 268–276.
79 Hernandez-Divers SM, Schumacher J, Stahl S, *et al.* Comparison of isoflurane and sevoflurane anesthesia after premedication with butorphanol in the green iguana (*Iguana iguana*). *J Zoo Wildl Med* 2005; **36**(2): 169–175.
80 Tusman G, Sipmann FS, Böhm SH. Rationale of dead space measurement by volumetric capnography. *Anesth Analg* 2012; **114**(4): 866–874.
81 Verscheure S, Massion PB, Verschuren F, *et al.* Volumetric capnography: lessons from the past and current clinical applications. *Crit Care* 2016; **20**(1): 184.
82 Sacks M, Mosing M. Volumetric capnography to diagnose venous air embolism in an anaesthetised horse. *Vet Anaesth Analg* 2017; **44**(1): 189–190.
83 Zhang L, Jin K, Sun F, *et al.* Assessment of a new volumetric capnography-derived parameter to reflect compression quality and to predict return of spontaneous circulation during cardiopulmonary resuscitation in a porcine model. *J Clin Monit Comput* 2022; **36**(1): 199–207.
84 Kremeier P, Böhm SH, Tusman G. Clinical use of volumetric capnography in mechanically ventilated patients. *J Clin Monit Comput* 2020; **34**(1): 7–16.
85 Bumbacher S, Schramel JP, Mosing M. Evaluation of three tidal volumes (10, 12 and 15 mL kg(-1)) in dogs for controlled mechanical ventilation assessed by volumetric capnography: a randomized clinical trial. *Vet Anaesth Analg* 2017; **44**(4): 775–784.
86 Mosing M, Auer U, MacFarlane P, *et al.* Regional ventilation distribution and dead space in anaesthetized horses treated with and without continuous positive airway pressure: novel insights by electrical impedance tomography and volumetric capnography. *Vet Anaesth Analg* 2018; **45**(1): 31–40.
87 Portela DA, Di Franco C, Chiavaccini L, *et al.* Effect of end-inspiratory pause on airway and physiological dead space in anesthetized horses. *Vet Anaesth Analg* 2023; **50**(4): 363–371.

15 Monitoring Oxygenation

Chiara Adami
Department of Veterinary Medicine, Cambridge Veterinary School, University of Cambridge, Madingley Road, Cambridge, UK

Chapter contents

Introduction, 231
Hypoxia versus hypoxemia, 231
  Alveolar gas equation, 232
Oxygen content, delivery, and consumption, 232
  Oxygen content, 232
  Oxygen delivery, 232
  Oxygen consumption, 232
  Oxygen extraction ratio, 232
Visual assessment of oxygenation, 232
Measuring oxygen partial pressure, 232
  Arterial blood gas analysis, 232
  Transcutaneous measurement of blood gases, 233
Measuring hemoglobin saturation with oxygen, 233
  CO-oximetry, 234
  Pulse oximetry, 234
Inspired and expired oxygen concentrations, 236
Near-infrared and Raman spectroscopy, 237
Other techniques, 238
  Continuous laser Doppler flowmetry, 238
  Mitochondrial redox state, 238
References, 238

Introduction

The goal of physiologic monitoring during anesthesia is to ensure an adequate oxygen supply to maintain mitochondrial aerobic metabolism and, ultimately, cellular function. Several techniques have been developed to monitor oxygenation for clinical and research purposes. Currently, there is no gold standard technique for monitoring oxygenation that combines quick response time, suitability for *in vivo* assessment, ease of use, inexpensiveness, and ability to evaluate local and regional tissue oxygenation. The available techniques provide information reflecting the status of the whole body, making them unsuitable to detect regional and local alterations until they are well established and may have resulted in irreversible organ damage. On the other hand, many techniques that specifically investigate oxygen concentrations at the cellular level are only applicable *in vitro*, on prepared isolated tissues, or are poorly applicable to the clinical setting due to cost of the equipment, difficulty of use, and limited experience in veterinary patients.

This chapter describes the techniques available for real-time monitoring of tissue oxygenation and metabolism in living animals, with a focus on the technical aspects, clinical use, and limitations.

Hypoxia versus hypoxemia

Although the terms *hypoxia* and *hypoxemia* are often used interchangeably, they are not the same (Table 15.1). Hypoxia is a condition in which the supply of oxygen to tissues fails to ensure normal cellular metabolism, whereas hypoxemia describes a state of low arterial oxygen tension (interchangeably referred to as "oxygen partial pressure"). Hypoxemia is a frequent cause of tissue hypoxia, but it is not the only one, with other major causes being anemia, histotoxicity, and reduced forward blood flow. The causes of hypoxemia are classified in various ways in the literature and include low inspired oxygen partial pressure, hypoventilation, and venous admixture. Venous admixture represents all the ways venous blood can move from the right to the left side of the circulation without being oxygenated, including low ventilation–perfusion (V/Q) ratios, anatomic or physiologic shunt, and diffusion impairment. Some authors will also include reduced venous oxygen content secondary to either low cardiac output or high oxygen extraction by the tissues (e.g., seizures) [1].

Alveolar gas equation

The alveolar gas equation allows the calculation of the expected partial pressure of oxygen in alveoli (P_AO_2) and, subsequently, the evaluation of pulmonary gas exchange. It is commonly written as

$$P_AO_2\,(\text{mmHg}) = F_IO_2\,(P_B - P_{H2O}) - (PaCO_2/R)$$

where F_IO_2 is the fraction of inspired oxygen (21% in room air), $P_B - P_{H2O}$ is the estimated barometric pressure minus the partial pressure of water in fully humidified inspired gas, $PaCO_2$ is the partial pressure of carbon dioxide in arterial blood, and R is the

Veterinary Anesthesia and Analgesia: The Sixth Edition of Lumb and Jones. Edited by Leigh Lamont, Kurt Grimm, Sheilah Robertson, Lydia Love and Carrie Schroeder.
© 2024 John Wiley & Sons, Inc. Published 2024 by John Wiley & Sons, Inc.
Companion website: www.wiley.com/go/lamont/anesthesia

Table 15.1 Comparison of the causes of tissue hypoxia (low oxygen concentrations in tissues) with causes of hypoxemia (low oxygen partial pressure in arterial blood).

Causes of hypoxia	Causes of hypoxemia
Hypoxemic hypoxia Low arterial oxygen tension	Decreased inspired oxygen partial pressure
Anemic hypoxia Low hemoglobin concentration	Hypoventilation
Stagnant/ischemic hypoxia Decreased perfusion	Venous admixture Areas of low V/Q Physiologic or anatomic shunt Diffusion impairment
Histotoxic hypoxia Inability of mitochondria to utilize delivered oxygen	

Venous admixture includes the various ways blood can move from the right to the left side of circulation without being oxygenated. V, ventilation; Q, perfusion. Areas of high V/Q do not cause venous admixture.

respiratory quotient. The respiratory quotient is an expression of the ratio of CO_2 elimination over O_2 uptake, and it varies slightly with diet and metabolic state but is typically estimated at 0.8. Knowledge of the expected P_AO_2 in comparison to the measured arterial partial pressure of oxygen (PaO_2) allows for the evaluation of pulmonary gas exchange.

Oxygen content, delivery, and consumption

The following equations are fundamental in the evaluation of oxygen transport and utilization.

Oxygen content

Oxygen content of arterial blood (CaO_2) is the total amount of oxygen in arterial blood and is calculated as follows:

$$CaO_2\ (mL/dL) = (1.34 \times Hb \times SaO_2) + (0.0031 \times PaO_2)$$

where Hb is the total hemoglobin concentration and SaO_2 is the arterial saturation of hemoglobin with oxygen (see discussion of functional versus fractional oxygen saturation below). The first term of the equation represents the amount of oxygen bound to hemoglobin, and the second term characterizes the quantity of oxygen dissolved in plasma. The vast majority of the oxygen in blood is carried by hemoglobin (~98%), whereas only a small amount is dissolved (~2%).

Oxygen delivery

Oxygen delivery ($\dot{D}O_2$) is the amount of oxygen delivered to the tissues each minute and is calculated as follows:

$$\dot{D}O_2\ (mL/minute) = CO \times CaO_2$$

where CO is cardiac output in L/min. It is important to note that adequate oxygen delivery is dependent on adequate cardiac output, hemoglobin concentration, and PaO_2. This calculation does not consider abnormal hemoglobin species such as methemoglobin or carboxyhemoglobin.

Oxygen consumption

Oxygen consumption ($\dot{V}O_2$) is the amount of oxygen used for metabolic processes per minute and is calculated via the Fick equation:

$$\dot{V}O_2\ (mL/min) = CO \times C(a - \bar{v})O_2$$

where $C(a-\bar{v})O_2$ is the difference between systemic arterial and mixed venous (i.e., pulmonary arterial) oxygen content. If both $\dot{D}O_2$ and $\dot{V}O_2$ are known, the oxygen extraction ratio can be calculated.

Oxygen extraction ratio

The oxygen extraction ratio (O_2ER) is simply $\dot{V}O_2$ divided by $\dot{D}O_2$:

$$O_2ER = \dot{V}O_2/\dot{D}O_2.$$

Causes of increased O_2ER include anything that increases oxygen consumption (e.g., seizures, hyperthermia, and sepsis) or decreases oxygen delivery (including hypoxemia and anemia). A low O_2ER is usually due to decreased oxygen consumption as caused by anesthesia, mechanical ventilation, and hypothermia. A major factor limiting routine clinical use of O_2ER is that it requires measurement of mixed venous O_2 via a pulmonary arterial catheter.

Visual assessment of oxygenation

Gray to blue mucous membrane discoloration (cyanosis) indicates the presence of deoxygenated blood in the observed tissue. The detection of cyanosis may be unreliable as a measure of tissue oxygenation, however, as it depends upon both the visual acuity of the observer and the local concentration of deoxygenated hemoglobin; moreover, it may be affected by lighting conditions [2]. A minimal concentration of deoxygenated hemoglobin (5 g/dL) is required to cause a degree of cyanosis sufficient to be detected visually [3]. Therefore, an anemic animal might be hypoxemic without showing cyanosis because the decreased hemoglobin concentration would be saturated with oxygen even in the presence of considerably reduced partial pressures of oxygen in the blood. Drug-induced peripheral vasoconstriction (e.g., as caused by α_2-adrenergic receptor agonists) can cause peripheral cyanosis. When peripheral blood flow slows down due to vasoconstriction, oxygen can diffuse into the tissues over a longer time (i.e., oxygen extraction increases), leaving more deoxygenated hemoglobin in the capillary bed [4].

Measuring oxygen partial pressure

The partial pressure of oxygen (PO_2) can be measured in a liquid (e.g., blood), a gas (e.g., inspired gas), or at the skin using technology based on the polarographic Clark electrode, which is composed of a silver anode, a platinum cathode, and a gas-permeable membrane through which oxygen molecules can diffuse freely. When a polarizing voltage is applied to the cathode, a current that is proportional to the partial pressure of oxygen is generated between the anode and the cathode, where oxygen is reduced. The following information focuses on the measurement of PO_2 in arterial blood, mixed venous blood, or diffusing through the skin. Measurement of oxygen in inspired and expired gas will be discussed in a separate section later in this chapter.

Arterial blood gas analysis

Analysis of arterial blood gases includes the measurement of partial pressures of oxygen and carbon dioxide in the arterial blood, reported in North America in mmHg. Partial pressures are often misinterpreted as a measure of how much oxygen and carbon dioxide are in the blood; however, instead, they indicate the pressure exerted by the dissolved, unbound molecules of each gas against the measuring electrode. The only parameter that quantifies the amount of oxygen in the blood, expressed as mL/dL, is the CaO_2, which is calculated from both SaO_2 and PaO_2 values as outlined above.

Arterial oxygen saturation of hemoglobin is a function of PaO_2, and their relationship is expressed by the oxygen–hemoglobin dissociation curve. Arterial blood gas analysis remains the most popular method for advanced monitoring of oxygenation in animals, with PaO_2, SaO_2, and the calculated alveolar–arterial (A-a) gradient used clinically to assess oxygenation. The A-a gradient is the measured arterial PO_2 (PaO_2) subtracted from the P_AO_2, calculated from the alveolar gas equation. A normal A-a gradient is less than 20 mmHg. As the A-a gradient widens during oxygen supplementation, the ratio of PaO_2 to fractional inspired oxygen (PaO_2/F_IO_2), also known as the "Horowitz index," may be calculated instead. At sea level, the normal PaO_2/F_IO_2 ratio is approximately 400–500; values below 400 suggest the presence of gas exchange abnormalities. The PaO_2/F_IO_2 ratio is a widely used clinical indicator of pulmonary function; nevertheless, its reliability is controversial. The main disadvantages of using the PaO_2/F_IO_2 ratio to guide clinical decisions are its dependence on barometric pressure and its inability to distinguish alveolar hypoventilation from other causes of hypoxemia, such as V/Q mismatch and shunt [5,6]. Moreover, the PaO_2/F_IO_2 ratio does not indicate CaO_2, which depends on hemoglobin concentration, nor does it provide information on oxygen delivery to tissues [5,6].

The biggest limitation of arterial blood gas analysis is its inability to detect regional or local changes in tissue oxygenation. The noncontinuous nature of monitoring and the costs associated with repeated testing also represent clinically relevant limitations. In addition, arterial blood gas analysis requires anaerobic sampling and either immediate analysis or special handling.

There are no unanimous guidelines with respect to the frequency of arterial blood sampling and analysis for proper monitoring of the oxygenation status in animals. In human patients undergoing thoracoscopy, it takes only 5, 10, or 20 min for the arterial partial pressure of oxygen to change by 10%, 20%, or 40% of its initial value, respectively [7]. This finding may suggest that frequent sampling would be necessary for prompt detection of severe changes in blood oxygenation in animals with compromised respiratory function. Another potential disadvantage of monitoring oxygenation through arterial blood gas analysis is the need for placing an indwelling arterial catheter to facilitate frequent blood sampling. Although this procedure is usually performed in animals with no or minor complications, hematoma formation, hemorrhage, vasculitis, and thrombus formation are possible sequelae. Moreover, obtaining arterial samples can be technically challenging in very small animals, and frequent blood sampling from small patients may result in iatrogenic anemia.

Mixed venous oxygen partial pressure

Mixed venous blood refers to blood in the pulmonary artery and is representative of venous blood from all organs and tissues. The partial pressure of oxygen in mixed venous blood ($P\bar{v}O_2$) reflects metabolic activity and oxygen consumption. The normal $P\bar{v}O_2$ while breathing room air is around 40 mmHg, corresponding to a saturation of around 70% (see discussion of mixed venous O_2 saturation below). The $P\bar{v}O_2$ can be used to calculate mixed venous O_2 content, $\dot{V}O_2$, and O_2ER; however, the measurement of $P\bar{v}O_2$ requires placement of a pulmonary arterial catheter. This procedure is rarely performed in veterinary patients and has fallen out of favor in critically ill human patients [8].

Transcutaneous measurement of blood gases

Transcutaneous blood gas monitoring systems are commercially available and have been used in dogs, sheep, mice, rats, and cats [9–12]. Blood gases diffusing through the skin can be detected and quantified by a sensor applied to the body surface. The digital sensors used to measure transcutaneous gases incorporate a Clark electrode for PO_2 measurement and a Severinghaus-type sensor to detect PCO_2. There are models that incorporate pulse oximetry instead of the Clark electrode [13]. The PCO_2 is measured from the pH of an electrolyte solution separated from the skin by a membrane that is highly permeable to CO_2; the changes in pH of the electrolyte solution are proportional to the logarithm of the changes in PCO_2. The sensor must be heated to 41 °C/105.8 °F prior to use to enhance local blood perfusion and CO_2 diffusion though the intact skin.

The main advantage of transcutaneous monitoring is that this technique is suitable for continuous and non-invasive monitoring of oxygenation and ventilation. It provides real-time information on partial pressures of oxygen and carbon dioxide, enabling clinicians to detect changes in respiratory status more quickly than with intermittent blood gas analysis. Moreover, its use avoids the drawbacks and costs associated with frequent arterial blood sample collection and analysis.

Transcutaneous blood gas monitoring is widely used in human medicine, especially in neonatal patients, to obtain non-invasive and continuous blood gas measurements during mechanical ventilation or procedures potentially resulting in impaired gas exchange, such as bronchoscopy and bronchial lavage [14]. Other applications include monitoring of respiratory function associated with sleep apnea or other conditions potentially resulting in hypoxemia and hypercapnia [15]. In the veterinary literature, however, information pertaining to transcutaneous blood gas monitoring is limited and seems to suggest that transcutaneous measurement of PCO_2 lacks accuracy [10–12,16–19]. In dogs, transcutaneous PCO_2 overestimated $PaCO_2$ by more than 10 mmHg; moreover, quick changes in $PaCO_2$ caused by alterations of the breathing pattern were detected by transcutaneous monitoring with a 6-min delay [12]. It was, therefore, concluded that, while transcutaneous PCO_2 monitoring might be useful for detecting changes or trends in $PaCO_2$, it was not sufficiently accurate to be used as a valid surrogate of $PaCO_2$. Very similar conclusions were drawn from a study conducted in rats, whereas in mice a good correlation was established between transcutaneous PCO_2 and $PaCO_2$ [10,11]. An experimental study conducted on anesthetized dogs demonstrated that decreases in cardiac output caused by iatrogenic hemorrhage resulted in less accurate PCO_2 readings; however, correlation with PaO_2 values improved after fluid resuscitation [16]. In critically ill dogs, the level of agreement between transcutaneous and arterial readings was lower than that reported in human patients, and the transcutaneous monitor consistently overestimated both PaO_2 and $PaCO_2$ [19]. In a slightly different application, some studies report the use of transcutaneous PCO_2 to evaluate skin graft viability in experimental dogs [17,18]. One study investigated the use of transcutaneous oxygen monitoring in Louisiana pine snakes [20].

Measuring hemoglobin saturation with oxygen

The percentage of hemoglobin saturated with oxygen is measured clinically either by CO-oximetry or pulse oximetry. It is important to note that these methodologies report slightly different values. A CO-oximeter can measure all forms of hemoglobin, including the abnormal forms that cannot bind oxygen: carboxyhemoglobin (COHb), methemoglobin (MetHb), and sulfhemoglobin (SulfHb). Consequently, CO-oximeters report the *fractional hemoglobin saturation* (FO_2Hb), that is, the percent of total hemoglobin that is saturated by oxygen:

$$FO_2Hb = O_2Hb/O_2Hb + HHb + COHb + MetHb + SulfHb$$

where O_2Hb represents hemoglobin bound to oxygen and HHb is reduced or deoxygenated hemoglobin. Pulse oximeters, on the other hand, generally cannot measure abnormal hemoglobins and, therefore, report *functional hemoglobin saturation* (SO_2), that is, the fraction of effective hemoglobin that is saturated by oxygen:

$$SO_2 = O_2Hb/O_2Hb + HHb.$$

In most patients, FO_2Hb and SO_2 will be very similar, with the SO_2 slightly higher as small amounts of COHb and MetHb exist in normal individuals. When significant concentrations of abnormal Hb exist, the FO_2Hb is the correct parameter to use in the calculation of CaO_2 and $\dot{D}O_2$.

Historically, the direct measurement of hemoglobin saturation with oxygen in blood was accomplished via the volumetric or manometric methods in which the volume of gas or the pressure exerted by that gas was directly measured. Modern methodology incorporates spectrophotometers that detect the absorbance of light by the molecules of interest. Moreover, pulse oximeters non-invasively measure hemoglobin saturation with oxygen using spectrophotometry. The following discussion will address both invasive and non-invasive techniques for SO_2 measurement.

CO-oximetry

CO-oximetry (also known as "hemoximetry") reports total Hb, saturation of arterial or venous Hb by oxygen, as well as concentrations of abnormal hemoglobins. CO-oximeters utilize spectrophotometry with multiple wavelengths of light. A blood sample placed in the machine is heated and hemolyzed. Light is fractionated and filtered, with specific wavelengths directed through the blood sample and onto photodiode sensors. According to the Beer–Lambert law, the absorbance of light of a specific wavelength is logarithmically related to the concentration of molecules in a solution that will absorb that wavelength. Most modern blood gas analyzers now have an integrated CO-oximeter such that the reported saturation is measured (i.e., FO_2Hb). Some older analyzers, however, do not have this capability, and the reported saturation may be calculated based on the measured PO_2 using an idealized oxygen–hemoglobin dissociation curve. If the resulting estimated saturation is used in various calculations of oxygenation (e.g., CaO_2 or $\dot{D}O_2$), clinically important error may be introduced.

Arterial hemoglobin saturation

Direct measurement of arterial hemoglobin saturation with oxygen (FaO_2Hb) is achieved with CO-oximetric analysis of a properly handled arterial blood sample. As described above, the CO-oximetric FaO_2Hb is the proportion of total hemoglobin that is oxygenated, as all species of hemoglobins are investigated.

Mixed venous hemoglobin saturation

Mixed venous oxygen saturation ($S\bar{v}O_2$), that is the saturation by oxygen of hemoglobin as measured in the pulmonary artery, can be used to assess the adequacy of systemic oxygen delivery versus consumption. While breathing room air, $S\bar{v}O_2$ in the healthy patient is expected to be between 65% and 80%. A low $S\bar{v}O_2$ indicates that $\dot{D}O_2$ is not meeting metabolic oxygen demands, helping to guide clinical decision-making in critically ill patients. Continuous measurement of $S\bar{v}O_2$ can be achieved with a fiberoptic catheter equipped with a CO-oximeter [21]. However, as previously mentioned, placement of pulmonary arterial catheters has fallen out of routine use in human medicine and is rarely performed in veterinary clinical practice. Blood obtained from the cranial vena cava may be used as a reasonable clinical surrogate of mixed venous blood to assess central venous oxygen saturation ($ScvO_2$) [22–24].

Jugular venous saturation ($SjvO_2$) is used mostly to monitor brain oxygenation. Venous samples can be obtained through an indwelling jugular catheter and analyzed intermittently; alternatively, for continuous monitoring of $SjvO_2$, the use of specific fiberoptic jugular catheters equipped with an oximeter is required.

Measured $SjvO_2$ is used to assess the balance between cerebral oxygen delivery and cerebral oxygen demand and is therefore used as an indirect marker of the cerebral metabolic rate of oxygen ($CMRO_2$). The therapeutic target for this purpose is generally to maintain $SjvO_2$ values greater than 50%. Increased oxygen supply or decreased oxygen demand will increase $SjvO_2$, whereas decreased supply and increased demand will have the opposite effect. Clinical scenarios that cause decreased $SjvO_2$ include generalized hypoxemia, local or systemic hypoperfusion, and increased cerebral metabolism or oxygen extraction resulting from conditions such as pyrexia and seizures [21,25]. In contrast, increased $SjvO_2$ may result from reduced cerebral metabolism, alteration in oxygen diffusion or extraction due to neuronal infarction or inflammation, or cerebral hyperemia.

The arteriovenous difference in oxygen ($AVDO_2$) can be extrapolated from SaO_2 and $SjvO_2$. It is postulated that, while $SjvO_2$ is accepted as a measure of oxygen delivery, $AVDO_2$ may better represent cerebral extraction of oxygen [26]. As a measure of oxygen extraction, low $AVDO_2$ may suggest the presence of neuronal infarction, with resulting metabolic derangement and mitochondrial injury.

On a balance of risk and benefit, $SjvO_2$ monitoring is considered a safe and valuable tool. However, it has several limitations. First, it relies on several assumptions, including static SaO_2, hemoglobin concentration, and hemoglobin dissociation over time. Second, it cannot be used to detect focal brain ischemia as the gained information rather reflects the generalized brain perfusion and oxygenation status. Finally, although placement and maintenance of central venous catheters is a relatively simple procedure in dogs and has been associated with a low incidence of life-threatening sequelae [27], puncture of the carotid artery, hematoma formation, infection, thrombosis, and raised intracranial pressure remain possible complications in animals as well as in humans. Pitfalls of measurements may result from positional changes of the head, microthrombi formation at tip of the catheter, and the necessity for frequent calibrations whenever fiberoptic catheters are used [21].

Pulse oximetry

Pulse oximetry is based on the principle that O_2Hb and HHb hemoglobin differentially absorb red and near-infrared light, with O_2Hb absorbing greater amounts of near-infrared light and lower amounts of red light than does HHb. This is consistent with clinical observation, as well-oxygenated blood, with its higher concentration of O_2Hb, appears bright red to the eye because it scatters more red light than does HHb. Traditional pulse oximeters emit two wavelengths of light, red light (at 660 nm), and near-infrared light (at 940 nm) from light-emitting diodes located in one arm of the probe [28]. The light that is transmitted through the tissues is then detected by a photodiode on the opposite arm of the probe (transmittance). In the case of reflectance probes, the sensing diode is placed next to the transmitting diode. The relative amount of red and infrared light absorbed are used to determine the proportion of hemoglobin bound to oxygen (SpO_2), based on the Beer–Lambert law which logarithmically correlates the concentration of a substance with the absorbance of transmitted light of a certain wavelength (Fig. 15.1). The signal is divided into an AC component (representative of greater light absorption during pulsatile arterial flow) and a DC component (the baseline light absorption by venous blood and tissue) (Fig. 15.2). The pulse oximeter analyzes the absorption of light by measuring the increase in light absorption due to the increase in arterial blood volume during systole, calculating an optical density ratio (R) using the following equation:

$$R = \frac{AC/DC\left(660\ \text{nm}\right)}{AC/DC\left(940\ \text{nm}\right)}$$

A manufacturer-specific algorithm is used to correlate R to SpO_2, which is expressed on the screen as a percentage. Many pulse oximeters display the photoplethysmograph, a waveform indicating the change in light absorption over time indicative of peripheral pulsatile blood flow. Useful information on the patient's cardiovascular performance can be gained from plethysmogram analysis [29].

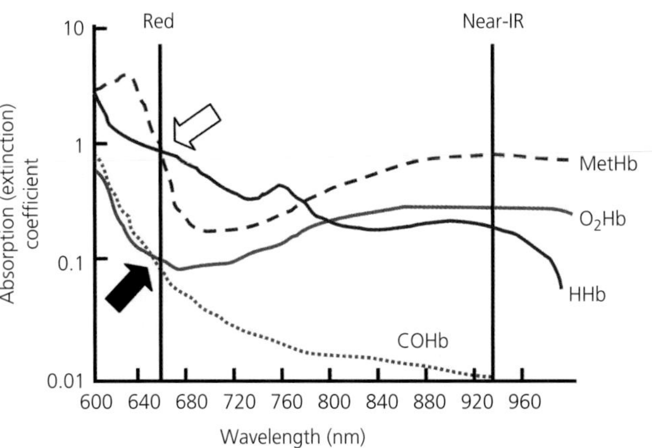

Figure 15.1 Absorption spectra for O_2Hb, HHb, COHb, and MetHb species. The absorption (extinction) coefficient of the four different Hb species is plotted as a function of the wavelength of the incident light. Note that COHb and O_2Hb absorb red light similarly (black arrow). In addition, red light absorbance of MetHb and HHb are nearly identical (white arrow), and that MetHb absorbs red and near-infrared light equally well. O_2Hb, oxyhemoglobin; HHb, deoxyhemoglobin; COHb, carboxyhemoglobin; MetHb; methemoglobin. Source: Chan *et al.* [32], with permission of Elsevier.

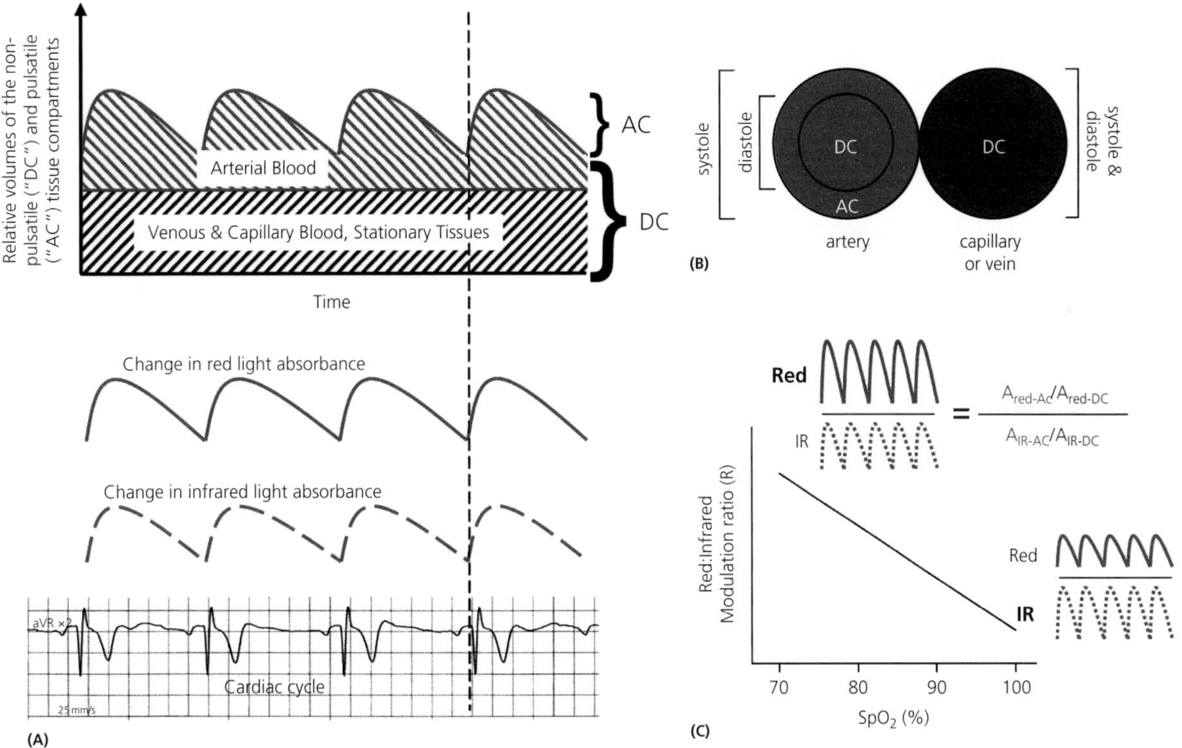

Figure 15.2 Schematic diagram of light absorbance by a pulse oximeter. **A.** In a patient with good cardiac function, the onset of cardiac systole (as denoted by the onset of the QRS complex) coincides with the increase in arterial blood volume. The amount of red and infrared (IR) light absorbed in the arterial compartment also rises and falls with systole and diastole, respectively, due to these changes in blood volume. The component that increases with systole is also known as the "pulsatile" or "alternating current" (AC) compartment and the component that does not change with the cardiac cycle is known as the "non-pulsatile" or "direct current" (DC) compartment. **B.** A cross-sectional diagram of an artery and a vein displaying the pulsatile (AC) and non-pulsatile (DC) compartments of the blood vessels. Note that only the artery has a pulsatile (AC) component. **C.** Diagram of a calibration (standard) curve of the Red:IR Modulation Ratio in relation to the SpO_2. Increased red light absorbance (increased R) is associated with increased deoxyhemoglobin, that is, lower SpO_2. Source: Chan *et al.* [32], with permission of Elsevier.

Pulse width correlates with the systemic vascular resistance, whereas systolic amplitude has been related to stroke volume and was found to be directly proportional to local vascular distensibility over a wide range of cardiac output values. Moreover, the position of the dicrotic notch is used as an indicator of systemic vascular resistance [30,31]. The plethysmographic variability index is a non-invasive dynamic indicator of fluid responsiveness based on heart–lung interactions over the respiratory cycle that some pulse oximeters display, and it is described in more detail in Chapter 12.

Many of its features, particularly ease of use, non-invasiveness, and the continuous nature of monitoring, have made pulse oximetry very popular in veterinary practice, and it has been a standard of basic anesthetic care in people since the 1980s. Despite its widespread use, however, several studies indicate that many general practitioners do not know the basic principles behind pulse oximetry technology, a knowledge that is fundamental to appreciate its limitations and to recognize erroneous readings [32,33].

In anesthetized animals, erroneous SpO_2 readings are commonly caused by poor peripheral perfusion, resulting from vasoactive drugs, hypotension, and hypothermia. Dysrhythmias, arterial compression caused by the sphygmomanometer cuff, and peripheral vascular disease can also affect the quality of pulse oximetry wave tracings [34–36]. Additionally, venous pulsations may result in falsely low SpO_2 readings because they cause venous O_2Hb saturation to be added to the signals coming from arterial blood [37]. Excessive movement becomes an issue mostly in non-anesthetized animals that require frequent or continuous assessment of their respiratory function. Another important limitation of pulse oximetry is that the PaO_2 is estimated from SpO_2 values based on the assumption that the relationship between the two variables is consistent with that described by the equation for the oxyhemoglobin dissociation curve. However, this may not be the case in anesthetized animals, in which alterations in pH, temperature, and partial pressure of carbon dioxide (PCO_2) are expected to shift the curve [38]. One study performed in critically ill dogs concluded that pulse oximetry sensitivity for the detection of hypoxemia was poor and that SpO_2 was not a clinically suitable surrogate for PaO_2, although the correlation between measured and predicted (based on SpO_2) PaO_2 values was higher in anesthetized and mechanically ventilated dogs compared to awake dogs [39]. Another group reported delayed detection of hypoxemia, defined as SpO_2 lower than 90%, following endotracheal tube cuff herniation in two dogs [40]. Finally, pulse oximetry may be a late indicator of respiratory impairment during oxygen supplementation, providing a false sense of security as SpO_2 as detected by pulse oximetry may remain within normal ranges despite a declining PaO_2 [41,42]. This is due to the sigmoid shape of the oxyhemoglobin dissociation curve, wherein saturation is nearly complete at PaO_2 values as low as 90–100 mmHg and increasing the PaO_2 above this level will no longer affect the SpO_2. Therefore, when SpO_2 is ≥ 97%, the PaO_2 could be anywhere between 90 and 600 mmHg [43,44].

Within the last couple of decades, more sophisticated, multi-wavelength pulse oximeter devices have become commercially available [45,46]. Besides providing non-invasive and continuous readings of SpO_2, pulse CO-oximetry allows the detection of COHb and MetHb, as well as evaluation of derived variables, including hemoglobin concentration, perfusion index, plethysmogram variability index, oxygen reserve index (ORI), non-invasive FO_2Hb, and CaO_2 [47]. One study conducted in dogs compared values of SpO_2, CaO_2, and hemoglobin concentration obtained from a pulse CO-oximeter with those measured invasively using a spectrophotometric-based blood gas analyzer and found that calibration of the device using a measured hemoglobin concentration was necessary to improve the accuracy and precision of pulse CO-oximetry when used to monitor hemoglobin [48]. In anesthetized pregnant sheep, Masimo pulse CO-oximetry was a useful and reliable tool for monitoring SpO_2 during phases of clinically significant cardiovascular and respiratory dysfunction [49]. The ORI is useful to assess the oxygenation status during oxygen supplementation and states of moderate hyperoxia (PaO_2 of approximately 100–200 mmHg), which represents a significant limitation for traditional pulse oximetry. As mentioned previously, supplemental oxygen administration increases the PaO_2 to values ranging from 100 to 600 mmHg, while SpO_2 reaches a maximum of 100% at a PaO_2 around 100 mmHg. Simultaneously, the venous oxygen saturation ($S\bar{v}O_2$) will progressively increase until the PaO_2 reaches about 200 mmHg, and it will stabilize at about 80%. The simultaneous evaluation of changes in PaO_2, SpO_2, and $S\bar{v}O_2$ over time is the basis for the ORI calculation, which results in a number ranging between 0 and 1 [44]. Decreases in ORI to near 0.24 may provide advanced indication of declining PaO_2 when SpO_2 is still > 98% [50].

Inspired and expired oxygen concentrations

Measurement of inspired oxygen concentrations in the anesthetic circuit, accompanied by a low concentration alarm, is required standard monitoring in human anesthesia care as it allows the detection of delivery of hypoxic gas mixtures. It is less commonly performed in veterinary anesthesia, however, due to associated expense and lack of training. Inspired and expired oxygen concentrations can be measured with paramagnetic, polarographic, and electrochemical oxygen analysis [51,52]. Infrared analysis cannot be used because oxygen is a nonpolar molecule. Most current oxygen analyzers employ paramagnetic analysis, which relies on the fact that unpaired electrons in the outer shell of an oxygen atom cause it to be attracted to the strongest part of an inhomogeneous magnetic field, whereas all other common respiratory gases move to the weakest part of it. Sampling and reference chambers separated by a pressure transducer are subjected to a switched electromagnetic field, and the resulting pressure difference is converted to a voltage that is directly proportional to the concentration of oxygen in the sample gas. Most of the commercially available paramagnetic analyzers are accurate and not affected by anesthetic gases, although the response time is limited by the maximal gas flow rate through the measuring cell [53].

Polarographic oxygen analysis, as described earlier in this chapter, is based on a modified, battery-powered Clark-type electrode [51]. Traditional electrochemical oxygen analyzers are based on the galvanic cell. Briefly, the oxygen sensor is composed of a membrane, a cathode, and an anode surrounded by an electrolyte solution. Oxygen diffuses through both the anode and membrane and reaches the cathode, where it is reduced, generating a current that is proportional to its partial pressure. While traditional electrochemical analyzers respond slowly to changes in oxygen and, therefore, are not suitable for measuring end-tidal oxygen concentrations, novel electrochemical imaging systems with integrated microelectrode arrays seem to offer an attractive means of measuring oxygen consumption rate in real time [52].

Measuring inspired and end-tidal oxygen concentrations may be used to estimate the level of oxygenation in the body and the effectiveness of ventilation. While a 4–5% difference between inspired and expired oxygen concentrations is considered normal, one study conducted in pigs found that a difference greater than 5% after having reached a steady state is a sensitive indicator of hypoventilation [54]. In this study, the decrease in oxygen end-tidal concentrations was promptly followed by a decrease in PaO_2, whereas changes in SpO_2 were not detectable until ventilation was decreased to 37% of the initial value. Moreover, studies conducted in humans determined that the difference between inspired and expired volumes of oxygen can be used as an estimate of the patient's oxygen consumption [55,56]. Low end-tidal oxygen levels are useful indicators of hypoventilation and low inspired oxygen concentrations can alert the anesthetist to inadequate fresh gas flow delivery and oxygen supply malfunctions [57].

Near-infrared and Raman spectroscopy

Near-infrared and Raman spectroscopy are used in human medicine for non-invasive continuous monitoring of regional tissue perfusion and oxygenation, and several studies demonstrate benefit in monitoring cerebral, intestinal, and renal perfusion to detect tissue ischemia and hypoxia [58,59]. These technologies share with pulse oximetry its basic principles, as both techniques are based on the differential light absorption of oxygenated and deoxygenated hemoglobin [60,61]. However, while pulse oximetry can only provide readings of the percentage of oxyhemoglobin in pulsatile blood, spectroscopy is capable of measuring oxyhemoglobin in non-pulsatile environments, such as the peripheral microcirculatory system. The "optical window" of near-infrared spectroscopy (NIRS) includes wavelengths of 650–950 nm. Light below 650 nm is too strongly absorbed by hemoglobin, whereas light above 950 nm is mostly absorbed by water. On the contrary, light in the near-infrared optical window can propagate relatively deeply, usually a few centimeters, into biological tissue, as absorption from water, hemoglobin, collagen, and proteins is negligible at these wavelengths. Instruments specifically developed for brain functional analysis use two (usually 780 and 830 nm) or more wavelengths [59,61–63]. Raman spectroscopy relies on the detection of a shift in frequency of light inelastically scattered following the excitation of a molecule of interest [64]. The fundamental differences between NIRS and Raman techniques lie in the nature of the molecular transitions taking place (change in molecular polarizability for Raman and dipole moment change for NIRS), in the type of monochromatic light used (within the near-infrared range for Raman and within the infrared range for NIRS), and in the strength of absorbance and transmittance (weaker for Raman compared to NIRS) [65]. Investigation into Raman spectroscopy for monitoring tissue oxygenation is mostly preclinical in nature, and no literature surrounding their use in veterinary patients exists.

Practical use of NIRS devices requires the user to switch on the light source, direct the emitted light into the tissue to be analyzed, and then measure the reflectance re-emerging from that tissue, a few centimeters distant from the light source. Engineering sophistication has led to the development of miniaturized spectrometers, making notable impact on the applicability of NIRS to the human clinical setting. There are a wide variety of commercially available devices in the market, with system complexity ranging from few sources and detectors, suitable to imaging small areas, to systems covering wider regions of the body. The sources and detectors can be placed directly onto the skin (Fig. 15.3) or, alternatively, the light can be guided to the target tissues through a system composed of optical fibers and receiving probes, to be applied to the area of interest. To reduce the running costs, most devices employ reusable sensors that can be disinfected.

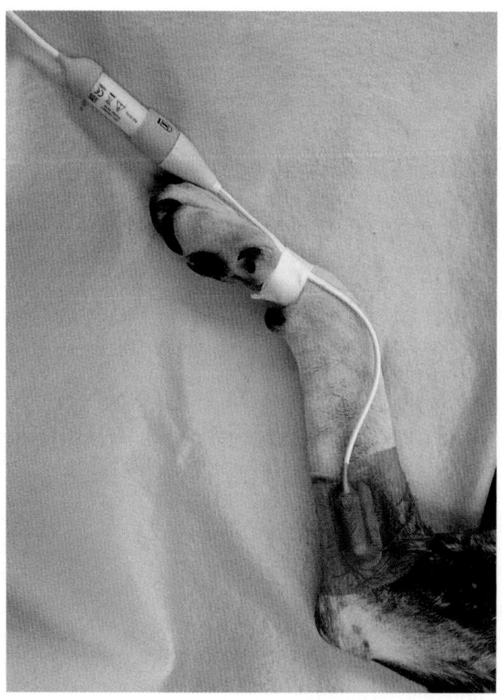

Figure 15.3 Near-infrared spectroscopy (NIRS) monitoring device placed on the forelimb of a dog. Source: Dr. Noah Pavlisko, with permission.

Variables measured by NIRS include local or regional hemoglobin oxygen saturation and the oxygenation/deoxygenation hemoglobin ratio, but also the oxygenated/deoxygenated myoglobin ratio in skeletal muscle [63]. Spectroscopy has been used to study a range of diverse conditions, including epilepsy, metabolic myopathy, and diabetes mellitus [63,66,67]. The most common clinical and experimental application of NIRS in humans remains the analysis of brain function and cerebral blood flow. Local cerebral blood flow typically increases as a result of enhanced neural activity; because blood flow increases more than cerebral oxygen extraction, during phases of increased cerebral metabolism, there is a localized rise in oxygen levels and, therefore, in oxygenated hemoglobin. Consequently, the ratio of oxygenated/deoxygenated hemoglobin is used to estimate neural activity [68].

The first report on the use of spectroscopy to assess oxygenation was conducted in cats [60]. Several more recent studies investigated the use of NIRS in both clinical and experimental dogs [69–75]. One study found that, in Chihuahuas, changes in cerebral oxygenation levels were associated with the administration of anesthetics [75]. Another investigation reported the use of near-infrared technology to monitor myocardial oxygenation during ischemic preconditioning [69], while other investigators used spectroscopy for monitoring of skin, subcutaneous tissue, and skeletal muscle oxygenation status [71,74]. In a study of dogs presented for acute hemorrhage, NIRS was able to differentiate those in a clinically determined state of shock from those without shock [76]; moreover, lower tissue oxygen saturation as determined by NIRS was associated with more severe shock in a different population of dogs [77].

Other techniques

Other techniques have been reported that may provide insight into hypoxia and oxygen debt. Currently, these methodologies are largely experimental in nature.

Continuous laser Doppler flowmetry

Laser Doppler flowmetry is based on light–tissue interaction and measures the amount of Doppler-shifted laser light reflected at a superficial level to determine microcirculatory flux of erythrocytes. Although it cannot be used to calculate absolute blood flow, the potential applications of this non-invasive and relatively inexpensive technique include qualitative evaluation of cutaneous, renal, and ocular/retinal blood flow, as well as assessment of the microcirculatory status of any potentially unhealthy tissues during intestinal, orthopedic, or plastic surgeries [78–80]. In humans, a correlation was demonstrated between decreased cutaneous microcirculatory flow and symptoms of ischemia of the lower extremities [81].

While laser Doppler flowmetry may be a useful measure to evaluate regional and local blood flow, its usefulness as a method to assess regional tissue oxygenation is debatable and relies on the assumption that systemic hypoxemia can be excluded. Another limitation is the potential for inaccurate readings in case of increased blood viscosity or administration of vasoactive drugs such as norepinephrine [82].

Mitochondrial redox state

The two pyridine nucleotides, nicotinamide adenine dinucleotide (NAD) and nicotinamide adenine dinucleotide phosphate (NADP), play a critical role in defining mitochondrial energy producing pathways. Ultimately, adenosine triphosphate (ATP) production is coupled to the energy released by the reduction of oxygen to water using electrons carried by the reduced form of NAD (NADH). The primary role of NADP is that of an electron donor in anabolic pathways, and most of this nucleotide is kept in a significantly reduced state in the cellular system. In contrast, NAD acts as an electron acceptor in catabolic pathways, which requires the NAD pool to be maintained in an oxidized state and the reduced/oxidized NAD ratio to be kept low. Impaired microvascular oxygen supply reduces oxidative phosphorylation and causes an increase in cellular NADH, which can be monitored and used as a reliable indicator of oxygen tissue supply and consumption.

Mitochondrial redox state assessment is mostly applied *in vitro* for the assessment of oxygenation in isolated tissues and cells [83,84]. Nevertheless, in the literature, there are examples of *in vivo* applications on various animal models [85–87]. Tissue concentrations of NADH have been monitored by high-resolution fluorescence microscopy in rat livers following hemorrhagic shock and resuscitation, suggesting that this parameter appropriately reflects the relation between local oxygen supply and demand in hepatic tissue *in vivo* [85]. Moreover, intracellular measurements of NADH concentrations by two-photon microscopy were used *in vivo* to monitor cerebral hypoxia and neuronal necrosis in rats after traumatic brain injury and hemorrhagic shock [87].

References

1 Bishop MJ, Cheney FW. Effects of pulmonary blood flow and mixed venous O2 tension on gas exchange in dogs. *Anesthesiology* 1983; **58**(2): 130–135.

2 Kelman GR, Nunn JF. Clinical recognition of hypoxaemia under fluorescent lamps. *Lancet* 1966; **1**(7452): 1400–1403.

3 Martin L, Khalil H. How much reduced hemoglobin is necessary to generate central cyanosis? *Chest* 1990; **97**(1): 182–185.

4 Sinclair MD. A review of the physiological effects of alpha2-agonists related to the clinical use of medetomidine in small animal practice. *Can Vet J* 2003; **44**(11): 885–897.

5 Gattinoni L, Busana M, Camporota L. Standardised PaO_2/FiO_2 ratio in COVID-19: added value or risky assumptions? *Eur J Intern Med* 2021; **92**: 31–33.

6 Rice TW, Wheeler AP, Bernard GR, *et al.* National Institutes of Health, National Heart, Lung, and Blood Institute ARDS Network. Comparison of the SpO_2/FIO_2 ratio and the PaO_2/FIO_2 ratio in patients with acute lung injury or ARDS. *Chest* 2007; **132**(2): 410–417.

7 Ganter MT, Schneider U, Heinzelmann M, *et al.* How often should we perform arterial blood gas analysis during thoracoscopic surgery? *J Clin Anesth* 2007; **19**(8): 569–575.

8 De Backer D, Vincent JL. The pulmonary artery catheter: is it still alive? *Curr Opin Crit Care* 2018; **24**(3): 204–208.

9 Schlaefke ME, Schaefer T, Kronberg H, *et al.* Transcutaneous monitoring as trigger for therapy of hypoxemia during sleep. *Adv Exp Med Biol* 1987; **220**: 95–100.

10 Stout RW, Cho DY, Gaunt SD, *et al.* Transcutaneous blood gas monitoring in the rat. *Comp Med* 2001; **51**(6): 524–533.

11 Sahbaie P, Modanlou S, Gharagozlou P, *et al.* Transcutaneous blood gas CO_2 monitoring of induced ventilatory depression in mice. *Anesth Analg* 2006; **103**(3): 620–625.

12 Vogt R, Rohling R, Kästner S. Evaluation of a combined transcutaneous carbon dioxide pressure and pulse oximetry sensor in adult sheep and dogs. *Am J Vet Res* 2007; **68**(3): 265–270.

13 Rohling R, Biro P. Clinical investigation of a new combined pulse oximetry and carbon dioxide tension sensor in adult anaesthesia. *J Clin Monit Comput* 1999; **15**: 23–27.

14 Sankaran D, Zeinali L, Iqbal S, *et al.* Non-invasive carbon dioxide monitoring in neonates: methods, benefits, and pitfalls. *J Perinatol* 2021; **41**(11): 2580–2589.

15 Sandberg KL, Brynjarsson H, Hjalmarson O. Transcutaneous blood gas monitoring during neonatal intensive care. *Acta Paediatr* 2011; **100**(5): 676–679.

16 Tremper KK, Waxman K, Shoemaker WC. Effects of hypoxia and shock on transcutaneous PO2 values in dogs. *Crit Care Med* 1979; **7**(12): 526–531.

17 Rochat MC, Pope ER, Payne JT, *et al.* Transcutaneous oxygen monitoring for predicting skin viability in dogs. *Am J Vet Res* 1993; **54**(3): 468–475.

18 Rochat MC, Payne JT, Pope ER, *et al.* Evaluation of skin viability in dogs, using transcutaneous carbon dioxide and sensor current monitoring. *Am J Vet Res* 1993; **54**(3): 476–480.

19 Holowaychuk MK, Fujita H, Bersenas AM. Evaluation of a transcutaneous blood gas monitoring system in critically ill dogs. *J Vet Emerg Crit Care* 2014; **24**(5): 545–553.

20 Cushing AC, Smith CK, Ramsay EC, *et al.* Transcutaneous oxygen monitoring in Louisiana pine snakes (*Pituophis ruthveni*). *J Zoo Wildl Med* 2020; **50**(4): 874–878.

21 Macmillan CS, Andrews PJ. Cerebrovenous oxygen saturation monitoring: practical considerations and clinical relevance. *Intensive Care Med* 2000; **26**: 1028–1036.

22 Hayes GM, Mathews K, Boston S, *et al.* Low central venous oxygen saturation is associated with increased mortality in critically ill dogs. *J Small Anim Pract* 2011; **52**(8): 433–440.

23 Young BC, Prittie JE, Fox P, *et al.* Decreased central venous oxygen saturation despite normalization of heart rate and blood pressure post shock resuscitation in sick dogs. *J Vet Emerg Crit Care* 2014; **24**(2): 154–161.

24 Walton RAL, Hansen B. Comparison of venous hemoglobin saturation measurements obtained by *in vivo* oximetry and calculated from blood gas analysis in critically ill dogs. *J Vet Emerg Crit Care* 2021; **31**(5): 578–584.

25 Rohlwink UK, Figaji AA. Methods of monitoring brain oxygenation. *Childs Nerv Syst* 2010; **26**(4): 453–464.

26 Stocchetti N, Canavesi K, Magnoni S, *et al.* Arterio-jugular difference of oxygen content and outcome after head injury. *Anesth Analg* 2004; **99**: 230–234.

27 Reminga CL, Silverstein DC, Drobatz KJ, *et al.* Evaluation of the placement and maintenance of central venous jugular catheters in critically ill dogs and cats. *J Vet Emerg Crit Care* 2018; **28**(3): 232–243.

28 Yoshiya I, Shimada Y, Tanaka K. Spectrophotometric monitoring of arterial oxygen saturation in the fingertip. *Med Biol Eng Comput* 1980; **18**: 27–32.

29 Elgendi M. On the analysis of fingertip photoplethysmogram signals. *Curr Cardiol Rev* 2012; **8**(1): 14–25.

30 Dorlas J, Nijboer J. Photo-electric plethysmography as a monitoring device in anaesthesia. *Application and interpretation. Br J Anaesth* 1985; **57**: 524–530.

31 Murray W, Foster P. The peripheral pulse wave: information overlooked. *J Clin Monit Comput* 1996; **12**: 365–377.

32 Chan ED, Chan MM, Chan MM. Pulse oximetry: understanding its basic principles facilitates appreciation of its limitations. *Respir Med* 2013; **107**(6): 789–799.

33 Stoneham MD, Saville GM, Wilson IH. Knowledge about pulse oximetry among medical and nursing staff. *Lancet* 1994; **344**: 1339–1342.

34 Ralston AC, Webb RK, Runciman WB. Potential errors in pulse oximetry. I. Pulse oximeter evaluation. *Anaesthesia* 1991; **46**(3): 202–206.

35 Webb RK, Ralston AC, Runciman WB. Potential errors in pulse oximetry. II. Effects of changes in saturation and signal quality. *Anaesthesia* 1991; **46**(3): 207–212.

36 Thawley V, Waddell LS. Pulse oximetry and capnometry. *Top Companion Anim Med* 2013; **28**(3): 124–128.

37 Mardirossian G, Schneider RE. Limitations of pulse oximetry. *Anesth Prog* 1992; **39**(6): 194–196.

38 Dempsey JA. With haemoglobin as with politics – should we shift right or left? *J Physiol* 2020; **598**(8): 1419–1420.

39 Farrell KS, Hopper K, Cagle LA, *et al.* Evaluation of pulse oximetry as a surrogate for PaO_2 in awake dogs breathing room air and anesthetized dogs on mechanical ventilation. *J Vet Emerg Crit Care* 2019; **29**(6): 622–629.

40 Bergadano A, Moens Y, Schatzmann U. Two cases of intraoperative herniation of the endotracheal tube cuff. *Schweiz Arch Tierheilkd* 2004; **146**(12): 565–569.

41 Nitzan M, Romem A, Koppel R. Pulse oximetry: fundamentals and technology update. *Med Devices (Auckl)* 2014; **8**(7): 231–239.

42 Pertzov B, Brachfeld E, Unterman A, *et al.* Significant delay in the detection of desaturation between finger transmittance and earlobe reflectance oximetry probes during fiberoptic bronchoscopy: analysis of 104 cases. *Lung* 2019; **197**(1): 67–72.

43 Martin ML. PaO_2, SaO_2 and Oxygen content. In: Percy C, ed. *All You Really Need to Know to Interpret Arterial Blood Gases*, 2nd edn. Philadelphia: Lippincott Willliams & Wilkins, 1999: 68–82.

44 Scheeren TWL, Belda FJ, Perel A. The oxygen reserve index (ORI): a new tool to monitor oxygen therapy. *J Clin Monit Comput* 2018; **32**(3): 379–389.

45 Goldman JM, Petterson MT, Kopotic RJ, *et al.* Masimo signal extraction pulse oximetry. *J Clin Monit Comput* 2000; **16**(7): 475–483.

46 Hiscock R, Kumar D, Simmons SW. Systematic review and meta-analysis of method comparison studies of Masimo pulse co-oximeters (Radical-7™ or Pronto-7™) and HemoCue® absorption spectrometers (B-Hemoglobin or 201+) with laboratory haemoglobin estimation. *Anaesth Intensive Care* 2015; **43**(3): 341–350.

47 Feiner JR, Bickler PE, Mannheimer PD. Accuracy of methemoglobin detection by pulse CO-oximetry during hypoxia. *Anesth Analg* 2010; **111**(1): 143–148.

48 Tayari H, Flaherty D, Yamaoka TT, *et al.* Assessment of pulse CO-oximetry technology after *in vivo* adjustment in anaesthetized dogs. *Vet Anaesth Analg* 2021; **48**(3): 297–304.

49 Quinn CT, Raisis AL, Musk GC. Evaluation of Masimo signal extraction technology pulse oximetry in anaesthetized pregnant sheep. *Vet Anaesth Analg* 2013; **40**(2): 149–156.

50 Fleming NW, Singh A, Lee L, *et al.* Oxygen reserve index: utility as an early warning for desaturation in high-risk surgical patients. *Anesth Analg* 2021; **132**(3): 770–776.

51 Burton GW. Measurement of inspired and expired oxygen and carbon dioxide. *Brit J Anaesth* 1969; **41**: 723.

52 Tedjo W, Obeidat Y, Catandi G, *et al.* Real-time analysis of oxygen gradient in oocyte respiration using a high-density microelectrode array. *Biosensors (Basel)* 2021; **11**(8): 256.

53 Hendrickx JF, van Zundert AA, de Wolf AM. Influence of the reference gas of paramagnetic oxygen analyzers on nitrogen concentrations during closed-circuit anesthesia. *J Clin Monit Comput* 1998; **14**(6): 381–384.

54 Linko K, Paloheimo M. Inspiratory end-tidal oxygen content difference: a sensitive indicator of hypoventilation. *Crit Care Med* 1989; **17**(4): 345–348.

55 Barnard JP, Sleigh JW. Breath-by-breath analysis of oxygen uptake using the Datex Ultima. *Br J Anaesth* 1995; **74**(2): 155–158.

56 Hill RW. Determination of oxygen consumption by use of the paramagnetic oxygen analyzer. *J Appl Physiol* 1972; **33**(2): 261–263.

57 Linko K, Paloheimo M. Monitoring of the inspired and end-tidal oxygen, carbon dioxide, and nitrous oxide concentrations: clinical applications during anesthesia and recovery. *J Clin Monit* 1989; **5**(3): 149–156.

58 Naulaers G, Meyns B, Miserez M, *et al.* Measurement of the liver tissue oxygenation by near-infrared spectroscopy. *Intensive Care Med* 2005; **31**(1): 138–141.

59 Sakudo A. Near-infrared spectroscopy for medical applications: current status and future perspectives. *Clin Chim Acta* 2016; **455**: 181–188.

60 Jobsis FF. Noninvasive, infrared monitoring of cerebral and myocardial oxygen sufficiency and circulatory parameters. *Science* 1977; **198**: 1264–1267.

61 Marin T, Moore J. Understanding near-infrared spectroscopy. *Adv Neonatal Care* 2011; **11**(6): 382–388.

62 Scholkmann F, Kleiser S, Metz AJ, *et al.* A review on continuous wave functional near-infrared spectroscopy and imaging instrumentation and methodology. *Neuroimage* 2014; **85**(1): 6–27.

63 Watanabe E, Nagahori Y, Mayanagi Y. Focus diagnosis of epilepsy using near-infrared spectroscopy. *Epilepsia* 2002; **43**(9): 50–55.

64 Stevens AR, Stickland CA, Harris G, *et al.* Raman spectroscopy as a neuromonitoring tool in traumatic brain injury: a systematic review and clinical perspectives. *Cells* 2022: **11**(7): 1227.

65 Wartewig S. *IR and Raman Spectroscopy: Fundamental Processing*. Weinheim, Germany: Wiley-VCH, 2003.

66 Bank W, Chance B. An oxidative defect in metabolic myopathies: diagnosis by non-invasive tissue oximetry. *Ann Neurol* 1994; **36**(6): 830–837.

67 Scheuermann-Freestone M, Madsen PL, Manners D, *et al.* Abnormal cardiac and skeletal muscle energy metabolism in patients with type 2 diabetes. *Circulation* 2003; **107**(24): 3040–3046.

68 Fox PT, Raichle ME. Focal physiological uncoupling of cerebral blood flow and oxidative metabolism during somatosensory stimulation in human subjects. *Proc Natl Acad Sci USA* 1986; **83**(4): 1140–1144.

69 Kawasuji M, Ikeda M, Sakakibara N, *et al.* Near infrared monitoring of myocardial oxygenation during ischemic preconditioning. *Ann Thorac Surg* 2000; **69**(6): 1806–1810.

70 Hall K, Greg B. Measurement of tissue oxygen saturation levels using portable near-infrared spectroscopy in clinically healthy dogs. *J Vet Emerg Crit Care* 2008; **18**: 594–600.

71 Engbers S, Boysen SR, Engbers J, *et al.* A comparison of tissue oxygen saturation measurements by 2 different near-infrared spectroscopy monitors in 21 healthy dogs. *J Vet Emerg Crit Care* 2014; **24**(5): 536–544.

72 Pavlisko ND, Henao-Guerrero N, Killos MB, *et al.* Evaluation of tissue oxygen saturation with near-infrared spectroscopy during experimental acute hemorrhagic shock and resuscitation in dogs. *Am J Vet Res* 2014; **75**(1): 48–53.

73 Pavlisko ND, Killos M, Henao-Guerrero N, *et al.* Evaluation of tissue hemoglobin saturation (StO2) using near-infrared spectroscopy during hypoxemia and hyperoxemia in Beagle dogs. *Vet Anaesth Analg* 2016; **43**(1):18–26.

74 Cugmas B, Plavec T, Bregar M, *et al.* Detection of canine skin and subcutaneous tumors by visible and near-infrared diffuse reflectance spectroscopy. *J Biomed Opt* 2015; **20**(3):037003.

75 Hiwatashi K, Doi K, Mizuno R, *et al.* Examiner's finger-mounted near-infrared spectroscopy is feasible to analyze cerebral and skeletal muscle oxygenation in conscious Chihuahuas. *J Biomed Opt* 2017; **22**(2): 26006.

76 Gray SL, Hall KE, Powell LL, *et al.* Tissue oxygen saturation in dogs with acute hemorrhage. *J Vet Emerg Crit Care* 2018; **28**(5): 408–414.

77 Berg AN, Conzemius MG, Evans RB, *et al.* Evaluation of tissue oxygen saturation in naturally occurring canine shock patients. *J Vet Emerg Crit Care* 2019; **29**(2): 149–153.

78 Schabauer AM, Rooke TW. Cutaneous laser Doppler flowmetry: applications and findings. *Mayo Clin Proc* 1994; **69**(6): 564–574.

79 Riva CE, Geiser M, Petrig BL. Ocular blood flow assessment using continuous laser Doppler flowmetry. *Acta Ophthalmol* 2010; **88**(6): 622–629.

80 Kouadio AA, Jordana F, Koffi NJ, *et al.* The use of laser Doppler flowmetry to evaluate oral soft tissue blood flow in humans: a review. *Arch Oral Biol* 2018; **86**: 58–71.

81 Kvernebo K, Slasgsvold CE, Stranden E, *et al.* Laser Doppler flowmetry in evaluation of lower limb resting skin circulation: a study in healthy controls and atherosclerotic patients. *Scand J Clin Lab Invest* 1988; **48**: 621–626.

82 Rajan V, Varghese B, van Leeuwen TG, *et al.* Review of methodological developments in laser Doppler flowmetry. *Lasers Med Sci* 2009; **24**(2): 269–283.

83 Blacker TS, Duchen MR. Investigating mitochondrial redox state using NADH and NADPH autofluorescence. *Free Radic Biol Med* 2016; **100**: 53–65.

84 Grossini E, Concina D, Rinaldi C, *et al.* Association between plasma redox state/mitochondria function and a flu-like syndrome/COVID-19 in the elderly admitted to a long-term care unit. *Front Physiol* 2021; **12**: 707587.

85 Vollmar B, Burkhardt M, Minor T, *et al.* High-resolution microscopic determination of hepatic NADH fluorescence for *in vivo* monitoring of tissue oxygenation during hemorrhagic shock and resuscitation. *Microvasc Res* 1997; **54**(2): 164–173.

86 Burger N, Logan A, Prime TA, *et al.* A sensitive mass spectrometric assay for mitochondrial CoQ pool redox state *in vivo*. *Free Radic Biol Med* 2020; **147**: 37–47.

87 Bragin DE, Bragina OA, Berliba L, *et al.* Addition of drag-reducing polymers to colloid resuscitation fluid enhances cerebral microcirculation and tissue oxygenation after traumatic brain injury complicated by hemorrhagic shock. *Adv Exp Med Biol* 2021; **1269**: 283–288.

16 Anesthetic Gas Monitoring

Rebecca C. Reader
MSPCA/Angell Animal Medical Center, Boston, Massachusetts, USA

Chapter contents

Introduction to respiratory gas monitoring, 240
Units of measurement, 240
  Partial pressure, 240
  Volume percent, 240
Monitors, 241
  Gas sampling systems, 241
Technologies used for respiratory gas analysis, 241
  Infrared analysis, 242
Historical technologies used for respiratory gas analysis, 243
  Mass spectrometry, 243
  Raman spectroscopy, 243
Applications of volatile agent monitoring, 244
References, 244

Introduction to respiratory gas monitoring

The ability to monitor anesthetic gases is incorporated into many multiparameter physiologic monitors. Respiratory gases of interest to the anesthesiologist include oxygen, carbon dioxide, and the volatile inhaled anesthetics. Information obtained from respiratory gas monitoring can be used as a teaching tool, to aid in the determination of minimum alveolar concentrations (MAC) in research settings, and to assist in monitoring patient anesthetic depth and safety. This chapter will discuss principles and technologies associated with the monitoring of volatile anesthetic agents; information pertaining to the monitoring of carbon dioxide and oxygen gas is discussed in Chapters 14 and 15, respectively.

Units of measurement

Respiratory gas monitors may report data as partial pressure, which is an absolute term, or volume percent (vol %), which is a ratio, and understanding the difference between these two values is important. Respired gases consist of molecules in constant motion. These molecules strike the walls of the respiratory tract or anesthesia delivery system and exert pressure against those walls. At a given temperature, the pressure exerted is proportional to the number of molecules present; that is, the greater the number of molecules present, the greater the pressure exerted [1,2].

Partial pressure

Dalton's law of partial pressure states that the total pressure exerted by a mixture of gases is equal to the arithmetic sum of the partial pressures of each gas in the mixture [1]. At sea level, the total sum of all gases in an anesthesia system is equal to 760 mmHg (i.e., the pressure is equivalent to the surrounding atmospheric pressure) [2]. With this information, it is possible to calculate the partial pressures of each gas in the mixture. For example, for a patient administered 2% isoflurane in 100% oxygen, the partial pressure of each respiratory gas is as follows:

$$\text{Partial pressure oxygen} = 0.98 \times 760\ \text{mmHg} = 744.8\ \text{mmHg}$$

$$\text{Partial pressure isoflurane} = 0.02 \times 760\ \text{mmHg} = 15.2\ \text{mmHg}$$

Thus, partial pressure quantifies the number of molecules of gas that are present in absolute terms, such as millimeters of mercury (mmHg). This method is used in infrared (IR) analysis of respiratory gases [2]. As described in detail below, gas molecules with two or more dissimilar atoms (carbon dioxide and inhaled anesthetics) absorb distinct wavelengths of IR radiation. In accordance with the Beer–Lambert law, the greater the number of molecules of gas present, the more radiation of that wavelength that will be absorbed [1]. Because the total amount of radiation of a specific wavelength that is absorbed is determined by the number of molecules present, and each molecule contributes to the total pressure of the system, IR analyzers can measure and report the partial pressure of the gas in question [2].

Volume percent

Volume percent (vol %) separates the molecular components of a gas mixture into individual portions, and is expressed as a ratio, or proportion of the gases in the mixture [2]. Using the previous example, two molecules of isoflurane would be present in a sample

Veterinary Anesthesia and Analgesia: The Sixth Edition of Lumb and Jones. Edited by Leigh Lamont, Kurt Grimm, Sheilah Robertson, Lydia Love and Carrie Schroeder.
© 2024 John Wiley & Sons, Inc. Published 2024 by John Wiley & Sons, Inc.
Companion website: www.wiley.com/go/lamont/anesthesia

containing 100 molecules, and isoflurane would represent 2% of the gas sample. This would be expressed as 2 vol %, or as a fractional concentration (0.02). This type of analysis is used with mass spectrometry. If the absolute pressure reading of the system is known, such as 760 mmHg at sea level, it is possible to convert the proportions to readings in mmHg:

$$\text{Isoflurane vol \%} = 2 \text{ vol \%} = 0.02 \times 760 \text{ mmHg} = 15.2 \text{ mmHg}$$

$$\text{Oxygen vol \%} = 98 \text{ vol \%} = 0.98 \times 760 \text{ mmHg} = 744.8 \text{ mmHg}$$

Monitors

Gas sampling systems

Monitors equipped to analyze respiratory gases must place the gas to be analyzed within proximity of the analyzer. This can be accomplished by bringing the sampled gas to the analyzer or by placing the analyzer in the path of the gas. Monitors that place the analyzer in the path of the gas are called *mainstream* or *non-diverting* monitors, as no gas is removed from the circuit for analysis. Monitors that sample gas from the airway and bring it to the analyzer are called *sidestream* or *diverting* monitors.

Anesthesia providers must be able to rapidly respond to changes in respiratory gas composition. As a result, it is important to understand the *total response time* of each sampling system. The total response time is typically sigmoid in shape (Fig. 16.1) and is made up of the system's transit time and rise time [2]. The *transit time* (or *lag time*) accounts for the delay that occurs as the gas sample travels to the analyzer. Transit time applies only to sidestream monitors, as there is no delay for the sample to reach the analyzer in mainstream monitors [2]. The response time of sidestream systems depends heavily on the inner diameter and length of the sampling line as well as the gas sampling rate. *Rise time* refers to the time it takes an analyzer to react to a change in gas concentration, and is generally defined as the time it takes the analyzer to move from 10% to 90%

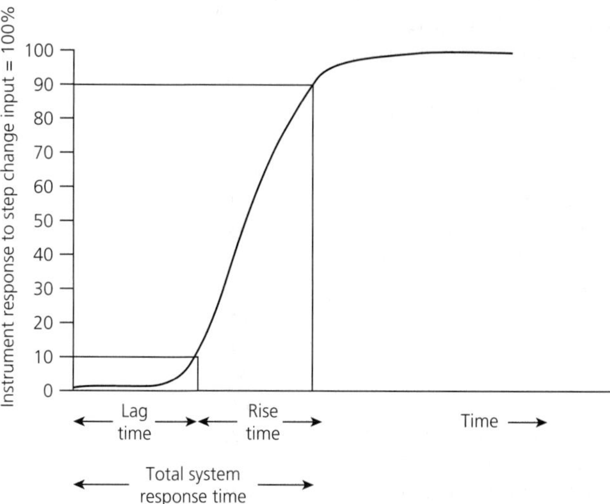

Figure 16.1 Total response time for a sidestream respiratory gas sampling system. The transit (lag) time reflects the delay that occurs as the gas sample travels to the analyzer and is generally defined as the time required to achieve 10% of the final gas concentration. Rise time refers to the time it takes an analyzer to react to a change in gas concentration and is typically defined as the time required to move from 10% to 90% after a sudden change in concentration. Source: Reproduced from Jaffe *et al.* [2], with permission of Elsevier.

of a sudden change in concentration [2]. For example, if an analyzer detected a change in carbon dioxide concentration from 0 mmHg to 50 mmHg, the rise time would be the time it took the monitor to report a change from 5 mmHg (10% of a 50 mmHg increase) to 45 mmHg (90% of the total increase).

Until recently, the only respiratory gases that could be analyzed using mainstream systems were carbon dioxide (using IR technology) and oxygen (using a fuel cell). However, mainstream multigas analysis is now available for carbon dioxide, oxygen, and potent volatile inhalant anesthetics [2,3]. Mainstream multigas analyzers require a special airway adapter that uses a miniaturized spinning filter wheel placed in the breathing system near the patient's airway. The adapters are designed to be lightweight and add only a small amount of deadspace to the patient circuit. Because the analyzer is located within the circuit, data is displayed in real time with minimal delay due to transit time for gas to reach the analyzer. Despite the lightweight design, when used with small patients, traditional mainstream adapters can be bulky, adding weight to the end of the endotracheal tube and contributing to mechanical deadspace. Some of the newer mainstream analyzers address this issue using "solid-state" design, which relies on electronic components instead of a spinning filter wheel, making the adapters more compact and less prone to breaking. Mainstream multigas monitors are also subject to interference from water vapor, secretions, and blood [2,4].

Sidestream monitors continuously aspirate gas from the breathing circuit and pump it through tubing to an analyzer within the main unit of the monitor [4]. Sampled gas must first pass through a filter or water trap prior to entering the analyzer. The sampling flow rates for these monitors range between 50 and 200 mL/min depending on the monitor and settings selected by the user. Sidestream analyzers have the advantage that all respiratory gases of interest can be measured simultaneously. Because the analyzer is located distant from the patient, the analyzer can be any size allowing for more versatility in monitoring capabilities. Disadvantages of sidestream analyzers typically involve problems with the sampling line, such as kinking or becoming clogged with secretions or water, or failure of the pump itself. There is also a short delay between sample collection and data display (typically < 3 s) as the respiratory gas is transported to the main unit of the monitor [2,4].

Erroneous readings can occur with sidestream monitors. Water droplets or respiratory secretions may be aspirated into the sample tubing, decreasing the accuracy of the system. At higher respiratory rates or with long sampling lines, several breaths from the patient may be present in the line, resulting in a lack of clear separation between breaths and a summation of data [2]. In small patients, if the fresh gas flow rates exceed the patient expiratory flow rate the sample obtained will be artificially low due to dilution with fresh gas. In very small patients, there is also the potential for the sampling flow rate of the monitor to exceed the patient's fresh gas flow rate, creating the potential for negative pressures within the breathing system [2].

Technologies used for respiratory gas analysis

There are many different manufacturers of anesthetic gas monitors, yet all rely on just a few technologies to perform respiratory gas analysis. The most common technology in use today relies on IR analysis to measure multiple gases such as carbon dioxide, nitrous oxide, and potent inhaled anesthetics.

Infrared analysis

Infrared (IR) spectroscopy is a measure of the vibrational frequency of atoms within a heteroatomic molecule. Molecules vibrate in multiple ways, with each distinct motion called a vibration "mode." Molecules with two atoms vibrate simply by moving closer together and farther apart. Molecules with three or more atoms can vibrate in more complex patterns. Molecules with more complex vibration modes are more likely to interact with electromagnetic radiation [1,2]. The IR spectrum consists of wavelengths between 0.40 μm and 40 μm. Asymmetrical molecules, including volatile anesthetics and nitrous oxide, absorb IR energy when their atoms rotate or vibrate asymmetrically. In contrast, nonpolar molecules such as oxygen do not absorb IR energy. Carbon dioxide is symmetrical and nonpolar but has three different vibration modes and develops a dipole moment when stretched and is therefore capable of absorbing IR energy [1].

The Beer–Lambert law states that when a light beam passes through a mixture containing a substance, which absorbs light at that wavelength, the intensity of the transmitted light decreases linearly with an increase in the concentration of the substance [1]. IR analyzers rely on the Beer–Lambert law to correlate the amount of IR energy absorbed with the number of molecules of gas present in a sample. The greater the number of molecules of gas present, the more radiation of that wavelength that will be absorbed resulting in decreased intensity of the transmitted light [1].

IR analyzers can be classified as *dispersive* or *non-dispersive*. A dispersive monitor passes IR radiation through a gas sample and then separates the radiation into component wavelengths. The component wavelengths are then ordered sequentially, and a plot of absorbance versus wavelength is constructed. The respiratory gas mixture to be analyzed will absorb one or more components of the radiation spectrum emitted. As long as the gases in the mixture have distinct absorption peaks, the composition of the mixture can be analyzed and quantified based on the amount of absorbance measured for each wavelength [2].

Non-dispersive monitors filter the radiation emitted and allow only bands of a specific wavelength to pass through the gas mixture. The wavelengths allowed to pass through the filter correspond to the absorption peak of the gas of interest. Most respiratory gas monitors in use today are non-dispersive and agent-specific, measuring each agent with a unique set of wavelengths selected by filters on the chopper wheel [2]. In doing so, it is possible for most analyzers to identify and quantify individual components in a mixture of gases. For example, carbon dioxide molecules have a peak absorption between 4.2 and 4.4 μm and nitrous oxide molecules absorb strongly between 4.4 and 4.6 μm. The potent volatile anesthetic agents absorb strongly at 3.3 μm and between 8 and 12 μm. Monitors that filter wavelengths between 3 and 5 μm and 8 and 12 μm can identify and quantify the amount of carbon dioxide, nitrous oxide, and volatile anesthetic in a respiratory gas mixture.

Basic components of an infrared analyzer

The basic components of an IR analyzer include a source of radiation, a narrow-band filter, a sample cell, and a detector that generates an output signal [2,4]. IR analyzers continuously focus IR light on a spinning chopper wheel. The source of IR radiation is a heated element called a "blackbody radiator," which absorbs all thermal energy and does not reflect light, thus appearing black [2,4]. As the radiator absorbs energy, it heats up and reemits that energy in the form of electromagnetic radiation. The blackbody radiator emits a broad IR spectrum, and the filters on the spinning chopper wheel in non-dispersive units are selected to allow only radiation of wavelengths that correspond to the peak absorption of the desired gas to pass through. The gas sample is pumped through the sampling chamber, and the filtered light is passed through the sampling chamber as well as a reference chamber. The light then hits a photosensitive detector, and the change in light levels hitting the detector produces an electric current (Fig. 16.2).

The detector can be made of a radiation-sensitive solid-state material, such as lead selenide; or a Luft cell, which is a chamber filled with gas that expands as the IR radiation enters the chamber and is absorbed [2,4]. The intensity of radiation reaching the detector is inversely related to the concentration of gas being measured (according to the Beer–Lambert law as previously described). The signal processor then converts the measured electrical currents from the detector to display the partial pressure of the gas.

Advantages of infrared analysis

IR analyzers are capable of measuring carbon dioxide, nitrous oxide, and the commonly used potent inhaled anesthetics. Most newer models can be incorporated into multiparameter monitors and are capable of detecting and quantifying anesthetic agents in a mixture of respiratory gases [5]. Additionally, many models are capable of measuring inspired and expired concentrations of gas [4]. IR analyzers do not alter anesthetic agents and the sampled gas can be returned to the breathing system for waste gas scavenging [4]. Most IR analyzers are highly accurate but tend to underestimate inspired concentrations and overestimate expired concentrations at high respiratory rates [6].

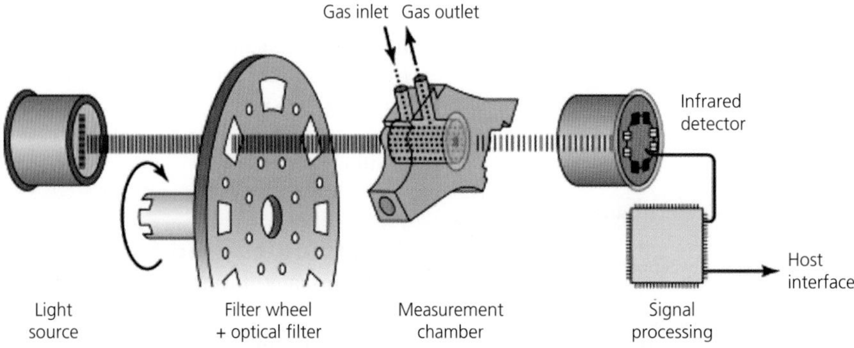

Figure 16.2 Diagram of an infrared analyzer with multiple filters on a spinning chopper wheel. Source: Reproduced from Jaffe *et al.* [2], with permission of Elsevier.

Disadvantages of infrared analysis

One main disadvantage of IR analysis is that the concentrations of nonpolar molecules such as oxygen and nitrogen cannot be measured [4]. Erroneous readings may result due to cross-interference, or the overlapping of absorption bands of some gases such as carbon dioxide and nitrous oxide. As mentioned previously, carbon dioxide molecules have a peak absorption between 4.2 and 4.4 μm and nitrous oxide molecules absorb strongly between 4.4 and 4.6 μm. The close absorption bands of these two gases may cause some analyzers to be inaccurate when high concentrations of nitrous oxide are present [2]. The use of narrow-band sources or narrow-band filters can reduce the impact of cross-interference [2].

Similarly, methane absorbs IR light at a wavelength of 3.3 μm, which overlaps with many of the volatile inhaled anesthetic agents. This can cause erroneously high readings of anesthetic agent concentrations with short IR wavelength analyzers (3.3 μm only), particularly in animals with a large intestinal fermentation compartment such as horses [7,8]. The impact of methane on measured end-tidal anesthetic concentrations is increased with the use of low fresh gas flow rates (due to the concentration of exhaled gases within the circuit), and in animals subjected to shorter fasting times (due to greater methane production from the gastrointestinal tract) [7]. As a result, it is recommended that the use of short IR wavelength analyzers be avoided in species that produce and excrete significant amounts of methane, particularly when accuracy is important [7].

Erroneous readings may also be caused by *collision broadening*, a phenomenon where the dipole moment of the gas to be analyzed is changed by collisions with other molecules in the gas mixture. Variations in the dipole moment result in the IR absorption band for that molecule being broadened, thus altering the absorption measurement for that molecule. For example, 10% nitrous oxide will result in a 1.0% increase in the measured carbon dioxide due to collision broadening. Many gas analyzers in use today automatically compensate for the effect of collision broadening if they measure the concentration of interfering gases [2].

Finally, since modern IR analyzers are non-dispersive and agent-specific, measuring each agent with a unique set of wavelengths selected by filters on the chopper wheel, it can be difficult to add new volatile agents for analysis as they come into use [2].

Historical technologies used for respiratory gas analysis

The majority of commercially available multigas anesthetic monitors use IR technology due to a variety of technical and economic reasons, including the ability to identify multiple agents, patient-side use, and lower cost. Occasionally, other technologies may be encountered in certain clinical settings, on the secondhand market, and in research environments.

Mass spectrometry

Mass spectrometry was one of the earliest forms of respiratory gas analysis, first used in human critical care in the 1970s followed by clinical use in anesthesia through the 1990s. A mass spectrometer is a machine that weighs charged atoms and molecules based on how far they travel when ionized in a vacuum and deflected by an electric or magnetic charge [9]. The mass spectrometer draws the sample gas into a low-pressure chamber. The gas sample is then passed into a second chamber at a pressure nearing that of a vacuum. In this second chamber, the molecules are ionized and then accelerated toward a cathode plate. A magnet or electromagnet then separates the ions based on mass and charge [9]. The mass spectrometer determines the composition of a respiratory gas sample by comparing how far the components travel against known values.

Traditionally, mass spectrometers are very large pieces of equipment and do not fit inside individual operating rooms. Instead, a central mass spectrometer is located in a remote room and connected to a monitor on top of the anesthesia machine with a sampling line. As a result, there is a significant time delay in receiving data updates on the operating room monitor, making these units clinically unwieldy. Mass spectrometers are also very complicated machines requiring a lot of downtime and are expensive to produce and maintain [9]. A portable unit has been described for use in horses but does not appear to be clinically available [8]. Interestingly, mass spectrometry has been used to quantify exhaled propofol concentrations, correlating to anesthetic depth [10]. At least one clinically available unit is currently marketed in Europe and is in human clinical trials in the United States (Edmon® – **E**xhaled **D**rug **Mon**itor, B. Braun) [11].

Raman spectroscopy

Raman spectroscopy uses light to create molecular vibrations and then analyzes light scattering to gain more information about a gas sample. The majority of the time, when light photons collide with a gas molecule they bounce off and their wavelength remains unchanged (Rayleigh scattering). Occasionally, photons lose energy to the molecule they strike, which alters the wavelength of the light. This alteration in wavelength is called the "Raman effect." Raman spectroscopy measures the difference in energy of scattered light to create a fingerprint for molecules, which is then used as a reference to analyze respiratory gas composition [2,12].

The components of a Raman spectrometer include a light source (laser), an optic filter, a spectrograph, and a computer analyzer. The laser focuses light molecules of the same wavelength on the gas sample to be analyzed. The optic filter only allows photons of Raman scattered wavelengths to pass through. The spectrograph then acts as a prism and guides photons in different directions based on wavelength. The detector then quantifies the Raman scattered light based on both wavelength and intensity of light, which is directly proportional to the number of photons of that wavelength [12]. Each molecule exhibits a specific change in energy (wavelength) in Raman scattered light, creating a unique fingerprint for that molecule [2].

Raman spectroscopy came into use in clinical anesthesia in the late 1980s, replacing mass spectrometry. Raman spectroscopy can be used to analyze carbon dioxide, oxygen, nitrogen, and potent volatile anesthetics. Monoatomic gases such as helium, xenon, and argon, which lack intramolecular bonds, do not exhibit Raman activity [2]. Raman spectrometers perform all the same functions as a mass spectrometer but in a much smaller machine, allowing for analyzers to be located within each individual operating room. Raman spectrometers also have a fast response time, can perform multigas analysis, and analysis does not result in degradation of the molecule under examination [9]. The Ohmeda Rascal II was a commonly used multigas analyzer that utilized Raman scattering to measure oxygen, nitrogen, carbon dioxide, nitrous oxide, and the volatile anesthetic agents (halothane, enflurane, isoflurane, sevoflurane, and desflurane) [13]. The Rascal II was compact, user friendly, and accurate over a wide range of respiratory gas concentrations [13]. Raman spectroscopy is no longer in use today as IR gas monitoring technology is less expensive to buy and maintain [2,12], although given the Rascal II's widespread use, one may still come across it in some settings.

Photoacoustic spectrometry

Photoacoustic spectrometry works much like IR analysis as described earlier [2]. An IR source emits a beam through a spinning chopper wheel that filters specific wavelengths of light corresponding to the desired gas to be analyzed. The light is absorbed by the gas sample, and when the excited molecules relax to the ground state the generation of thermal energy produces a sound wave with the same frequency [14]. A microphone converts gas vibration frequencies into electrical signals that are used to determine gas concentrations.

Photoacoustic spectrometry has the advantage over IR analysis in that a simple microphone detector can be used to measure the IR-absorbing gases [2] and no optical sensor is required [8]. The main drawback of photoacoustic spectrometry is that the device is sensitive to interference from loud noises and vibration [2].

Piezoelectric analysis

Piezoelectric analysis utilizes lipid-coated vibrating crystals to measure volatile anesthetic agents. When the crystals are exposed to a volatile anesthetic agent, the vapor is absorbed into the lipid coating. The resultant increase in mass of the lipid changes the vibration frequency of the crystal. Piezoelectric systems have two circuits: one with an uncoated reference crystal and one coated crystal. The difference in the electric signal generated from the two crystals is proportional to the concentration of vapor present in the gas sample [4].

The presence of water vapor and nitrous oxide may affect the accuracy of piezoelectric systems, but even so the accuracy of these systems is better than 0.1%. These systems have a fast response time and are capable of measuring both inspired and expired concentrations of respiratory gases. There is no need for waste gas scavenging with piezoelectric systems because the analysis does not alter anesthetic agents and the sampled gas can be returned to the breathing system [4].

Piezoelectric technology only has the capability to monitor a single agent at a time [9], and cannot measure oxygen, carbon dioxide, nitrogen, or nitrous oxide. Additionally, piezoelectric monitors cannot discriminate between agents – the agent to be analyzed must be selected on the monitor prior to use. If the wrong agent is selected, the results can be extremely inaccurate [2,9].

Refractometry

A refractometer shines beams of monochromatic light through two chambers, one containing the sample gas to be analyzed and the other containing air [4]. Vapor slows the velocity of light, so the portion of light passing through the chamber containing the sample gas will be delayed [4]. The beams are then recombined and form a pattern of light and dark bands [9]. The nature of these bands depends on the refractive index and concentration of the components in the gas sample [9], with refractivity being a nonlinear function of the partial pressure of the gas [4]. The position of the bands is viewed through an eyepiece, superimposed against a scale that indicates the vapor concentration [4]. In order to use this device, the refractivity number of the gas being analyzed must be known [4,5]. These monitors are impractical for breath-by-breath analysis and are more frequently used in research, to calibrate vaporizer output, or to measure environmental gas exposure [6,9,15].

Applications of volatile agent monitoring

Respiratory anesthetic gas monitoring has applications in both research and clinical settings. End-tidal inhalant partial pressure closely approximates alveolar inhalant partial pressure. With modern inhalant anesthetics of low solubility, these partial pressures quickly equilibrate with those of the central nervous system, reflecting the amount of drug delivered to the effect site. End-tidal inhalant monitoring is frequently used in research settings to determine the MAC of volatile anesthetics in different species [6]. Strictly speaking, the definition of *MAC* includes "concentration at sea level" and is therefore actually reflective of partial pressure rather than concentration.

There are also several clinical applications for respiratory anesthetic gas analysis, including monitoring the uptake and elimination of inhalant anesthetics by the patient, facilitating a safer, more targeted use of the vaporizer to reach desired end-tidal inhalant concentrations and therefore anesthetic depth. Comparing end-tidal agent concentrations to established MAC values may prevent accidental awareness under anesthesia, particularly in patients who have been administered a neuromuscular blocking agent [2]. A patient who has reached 75% of the MAC value for that agent may not yet be at a surgical plane of anesthesia but is very unlikely to experience awareness [16]. Of course, monitoring end-tidal agent concentrations should not be used as a replacement for other means of assessing anesthetic depth and the entire clinical picture should be evaluated. Respiratory anesthetic gas monitoring can also allow the anesthetist to titrate fresh gas flow and vaporizer settings more precisely. For example, one might use a high fresh gas flow rate at the beginning of anesthesia to ensure that the anesthetic gas concentration changes rapidly. Once the desired end-tidal concentration is achieved, the vaporizer and fresh gas flow can be adjusted to maintain the concentration at a steady level. The reverse can be done in recovery; the fresh gas flow rate may be increased to reduce the anesthetic gas concentrations in the system. This may also be useful for teaching purposes, demonstrating the relationship between agent concentration and the fresh gas flow rate [2]. In addition, respiratory gas monitors may detect the presence of incorrect or mixed anesthetic agents in a vaporizer, as well as contaminants. High- or low-concentration alarms may warn of vaporizer malfunction and can be used to potentially indicate the presence of an empty vaporizer (although this would be a very late method for recognizing the need to refill the vaporizer) or failure of the operator to turn on the vaporizer [2].

Respiratory anesthetic gas monitors can also be used to verify the calibration of vaporizers in use, a practice that is recommended at least once yearly or any time the vaporizer is disconnected from the anesthesia machine or otherwise jostled, tipped, or disturbed [2].

References

1 Pisano A. Light, air pollution and pulse oximetry: the Beer–Lambert Law. In: Pisano, A, ed. *Physics for Anesthesiologists: from Daily Life to the Operating Room*. Cham, Switzerland: Springer International, 2017: 117–125.

2 Jaffe MB, Eisenkraft JB, Orr J. Respiratory gas monitoring. In: Ehrenwerth J, Eisenkraft JB, Berry JM, eds. *Anesthesia Equipment: Principles and Applications*, 3rd edn. St. Louis, MO: Elsevier Health Sciences, 2021: 218–236.

3 Berggren M, Hosseini N, Nillson K, *et al.* Improved response time with a new miniaturized mainstream multigas monitor. *J Clin Monit Comput* 2009; **23**: 355–61.

4 Dorsch JA, Dorsch SE. Gas monitoring. In: Dorsch JA, Dorsch SE, eds. *Understanding Anesthesia Equipment*, 5th edn. Philadelphia, PA: Wolters Kluwer, Lippincott Williams & Wilkins, 2008.

5 Cheam EWS, Lockwood GG. The use of a portable refractometer to measure desflurane. *Anaesthesia* 1995; **50**(7): 607–610.
6 Rudolff AS, Moens YP, Driessen B, *et al.* Comparison of an infrared anaesthetic agent analyser (Datex-Ohmeda) with refractometry for measurement of isoflurane, sevoflurane and desflurane concentrations. *Vet Anaesth Analg* 2014; **41**(4): 386–392.
7 Dujardin CL, Gootjes P, Moens Y. Isoflurane measurement error using short wavelength infrared techniques in horses: influence of fresh gas flow and pre anaesthetic food deprivation. *Vet Anaesth Analg* 2005; **32**(2): 101–106.
8 Turner PG, Dugdale A, Young IS, *et al.* Portable mass spectrometry for measurement of anaesthetic agents and methane in respiratory gases. *Vet J* 2008; **177**(1): 36–44.
9 Langton JA, Hutton A. Respiratory gas analysis. *Contin Edu Anaesth Crit Care & Pain* 2009; **9**(1): 19–23.
10 Hornuss C, Praun S, Villinger J, *et al.* Real-time monitoring of propofol in expired air in humans undergoing total intravenous anesthesia. *Anesthesiology* 2007; **106**(4): 665–674.
11 United States National Library of Science, ClinicalTrials.gov. Comparison Between Propofol Concentration in Exhaled Breath and Blood Plasma Using the Exhaled Drug Monitor "Edmon" (ProDect). www.clinicaltrials.gov/ct2/show/NCT04586998 (accessed April 2022).
12 Mulvaney SP, Keating CD. Raman spectroscopy. *Anal Chem* 2000; **72**(12): 145–158.
13 Lockwood GG, Landon MJ, Chakrabarti MK, *et al.* The Ohmeda Rascall II. A new gas analyser for anaesthetic use. *Anaesthesia* 1994; **49**(1): 44–53.
14 Patimisco P, Scamarcio G, Tittel FK, *et al.* Quartz-enhanced photoacoustic spectroscopy: a review. *Sensors* 2014; **14**(4): 6165–6206.
15 Ambrisko TD, Klide AM. Comparison of use of an infrared anesthetic gas monitor and refractometry for measurement of anesthetic agent concentrations. *Am J Vet Res* 2011; **72**(10): 1299–1304.
16 Eger EI. Age, minimum alveolar anesthetic concentration, and minimum alveolar anesthetic concentration-awake. *Anesth Analg* 2001; **93**(4): 947–953.

17 Perioperative Thermoregulation and Heat Balance

Kurt A. Grimm
Veterinary Specialists Services, PC, Conifer, Colorado, USA

Chapter contents

Introduction, 246
Thermodynamics, 246
Thermoregulation, 246
Core-to-periphery gradient, 247
Mechanisms of heat transfer, 247
Active patient warming, 249
  Forced warm air units, 250
  Circulating warm water systems, 250
  Resistive polymer electric heating, 250
Hyperthermia, 250
Clinical significance of hypothermia, 251
Perianesthetic management of hypothermia, 251
References, 252

Introduction

Perianesthetic hypothermia, and less commonly hyperthermia, occurs in almost all patients undergoing anesthesia. Despite the common occurrence of body temperature changes, few anesthetists understand the complex patterns of heat transfer and the multitude of factors which influence the rate and extent to which it occurs. This chapter will address these factors, the techniques used to limit heat loss, and the impact of hypo- and hyperthermia on patient morbidity.

Thermodynamics

Thermodynamics is the study of the transfer of heat and work between systems. In biology, the thermodynamic laws can be applied to explain many phenomena, but of interest to the anesthetist is the analysis of the transfer of body heat, clinically measured as core body temperature, to the external environment. The reverse (e.g., heat transfer from the external environment to the patient) is also of interest since an understanding of the process will allow a safe and effective means of maintaining or increasing patient temperature during the perianesthetic period. The heat transfer and storage properties of materials which contact the patient are also important since they often present hazards in the form of potential sources of burns. Fortunately, a detailed knowledge of the application of the laws of thermodynamics is not necessary to understand heat balance; however, a general understanding of conservation of energy (the first law of thermodynamics) and the heat flow to establish an equilibrium between systems (the second law of thermodynamics) will be useful.

Thermoregulation

An organism possesses heat energy which is conveniently measured as body temperature. The total amount of heat energy is a function of the temperature and the mass of the patient, just as kinetic energy is a function of the velocity (speed) of an object and its mass. In most domestic mammalian species, the amount of heat energy (temperature) is relatively constant (homeothermic) despite continual metabolic heat production, and environmental heat gain and losses. The amount of body heat can be described using the terms *normothermia* (*euthermia*), *hypothermia*, and *hyperthermia*, which refer to normal, decreased, and increased amounts of body heat, respectively. Hyperthermia is an increase in temperature, but usually occurs in response to increased environmental temperature or altered thermoregulation. Pyrexia (i.e., fever) is similar in that it is an abnormal increase in temperature but it is due to an increase in the set-point, often related to immune response to pathogens. Hypothermia is the opposite condition and is most commonly associated with heat loss in excess to metabolic production or decreased thermoregulatory set-point, which delays shivering or other homeostatic mechanisms.

Measured temperature values corresponding to these different states depend on the species since the normal ranges of core body temperature can vary. Additionally, temperature can fluctuate with the time of day (or time of year for hibernating animals), hormonal influences, and activity levels, although these variations are usually minor compared to the changes induced by anesthesia. Additionally, some species (especially amphibians, reptiles, and some fish) are normally subject to significant environmental temperature

Veterinary Anesthesia and Analgesia: The Sixth Edition of Lumb and Jones. Edited by Leigh Lamont, Kurt Grimm, Sheilah Robertson, Lydia Love and Carrie Schroeder.
© 2024 John Wiley & Sons, Inc. Published 2024 by John Wiley & Sons, Inc.
Companion website: www.wiley.com/go/lamont/anesthesia

influences (poikilothermic), and definition of normal body temperature becomes problematic. Interestingly, the naked mole rat is the only known mammal to exhibit poikilothermic responses to environmental temperature changes as an adult [1].

Body temperature is sensed by temperature-responsive cells throughout the body. There are distinct populations of peripheral nerve endings (receptors) in the skin, which discharge when their thermal thresholds are reached. Most receptors appear to utilize ion channels that belong to the transient receptor potential (TRP) family of cation channels [2]. There are also visceral receptors which are found generally in the brain (especially the anterior hypothalamus and preoptic area), spinal cord, and abdominal structures such as the gastrointestinal tract and urinary bladder [2]. The afferent input to the central nervous system (CNS) is carried by different nerve fiber types (e.g., Aδ and C fibers) depending on whether the input is cold, hot, or noxious. These signals traverse ascending tracts of the spinal cord and eventually reach the hypothalamus where the signals are integrated and responses issued. Since local temperature can vary depending on the tissue type and metabolic activity, the thermal input to the CNS is a summary of multiple core and peripheral sensors. This "averaging" of temperature allows the body to maintain a narrow thermal set-point, which is associated with an interthreshold range (temperature variation where no compensatory responses [e.g., shivering, sweating, vasoconstriction, or vasodilation] occur) of approximately ± 0.2 °C (Fig. 17.1). Anesthetic drugs can alter thermoregulatory thresholds for compensatory responses, which is why perioperative patients often fail to shiver even though they are mildly hypothermic. The increase in the interthreshold range (approximate increased range of 3.5 °C) caused by drugs such as opioids, sedatives, and anesthetics is to some degree drug- and dose-dependent and reduces the patient's ability to tightly regulate core body temperature.

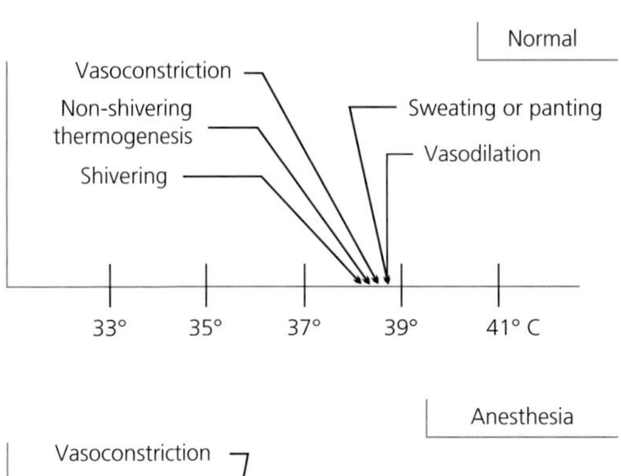

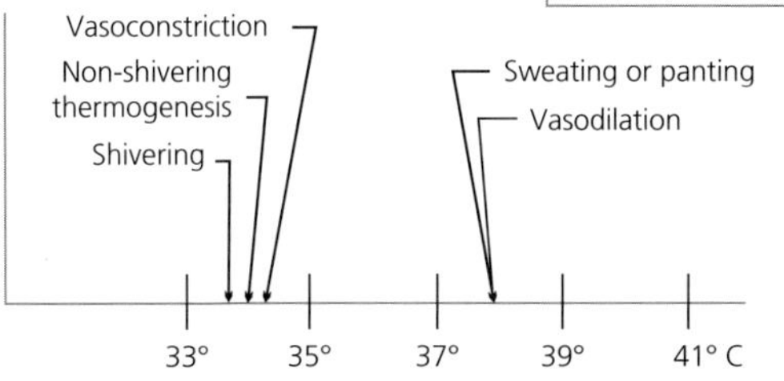

Figure 17.1 Thermoregulation is tightly controlled in healthy, unmedicated individuals. Many drugs used during the perianesthetic period (e.g., opioids and inhalant anesthetics) can alter the range over which compensatory responses to altered environmental and core body temperature occur.

Core-to-periphery gradient

It is important to understand that body heat is not uniformly distributed throughout the organism. For example, the core body temperature is often several degrees (2–4 °C) higher than skin temperature (Fig. 17.2) [3]. There is also significant longitudinal variation in temperature in the limbs, with the core-to-skin difference being greater the further the measurement is made from the trunk. This temperature gradient is maintained by the autonomic nervous system through mechanisms which regulate peripheral blood flow [4].

The majority of heat transfer between the core and periphery occurs via blood-borne convection (with some due to tissue-to-tissue conduction). Factors which influence the distribution of blood include arteriovenous anastomoses, cutaneous vasoconstriction or dilation, and countercurrent vascular heat exchange [3]. Sweating (in those species which possess this capability) and environmental temperature will also modify the redistribution of heat [3]. Additional mechanisms exist such as panting or shivering which can modify heat loss and gain, although these mechanisms more directly affect the core temperature rather than the skin-to-core temperature gradient.

Interestingly, in humans about 95% of metabolically generated heat is lost to the environment via transfer across the skin with only about 5% lost through the respiratory tract. This implies that heat conservation devices such as airway heat exchangers will have minimal influence on the rate of change of core temperature during anesthesia [5–7]. Since human skin and hair density is significantly different from that of many domestic species, the importance of cutaneous heat loss may vary, but in general it remains a major mechanism contributing to perianesthetic hypothermia.

The reason why it is important to understand the skin-to-core temperature gradient is that it helps explain why anesthetized patients undergo a rapid decrease in body temperature following administration of anesthetic drugs, especially those which cause profound peripheral vasodilation (e.g., acepromazine and inhalant anesthetics). Drugs which cause less peripheral vasodilation often result in a less rapid decrease in temperature (e.g., total intravenous anesthesia with propofol or following premedication with dexmedetomidine) [8,9].

Most of the clinical research into anesthesia-associated body temperature change has been performed with human subjects. It should be remembered that body size, and more specifically the surface area-to-mass ratio (alternatively the core-to-peripheral compartment ratio) can greatly influence the rate of change of core body temperature. The typical pattern of perianesthetic hypothermia has been described as having three phases: an initial rapid hypothermic phase, the linear decrease, and the plateau phase (Fig. 17.3)

Mechanisms of heat transfer

Heat energy that has reached the patient's body surface is transferred to the environment via four main mechanisms: radiation, conduction, convection, and evaporation. Radiation of heat is the electromagnetic (photon) transfer of infrared and far-infrared energy between surfaces [10]. It does not depend upon the temperature of the air around the patient, but does depend on the emissivity of the involved surfaces and their temperature difference (in °K) raised to the fourth power. Emissivity is an object's capacity to exchange heat, with a value of 1.0 being a perfect absorber of heat and 0 being a perfect reflector. Human skin has been described as

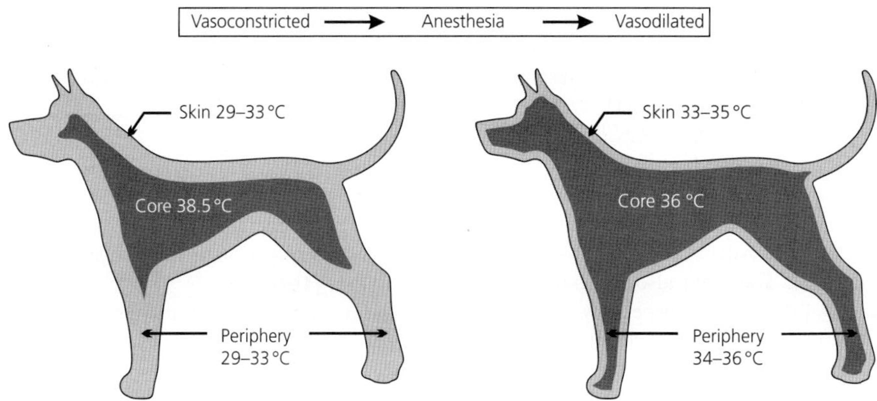

Figure 17.2 A temperature gradient normally exists between the skin surface and the body's core. The gradient is maintained by physiologic mechanisms such as peripheral vasoconstriction and altered blood flow distribution. Many anesthetics which cause indiscriminate vasodilation result in mixing of core and peripheral blood, leading to a lessening of the gradient and ultimately a decrease in core body temperature.

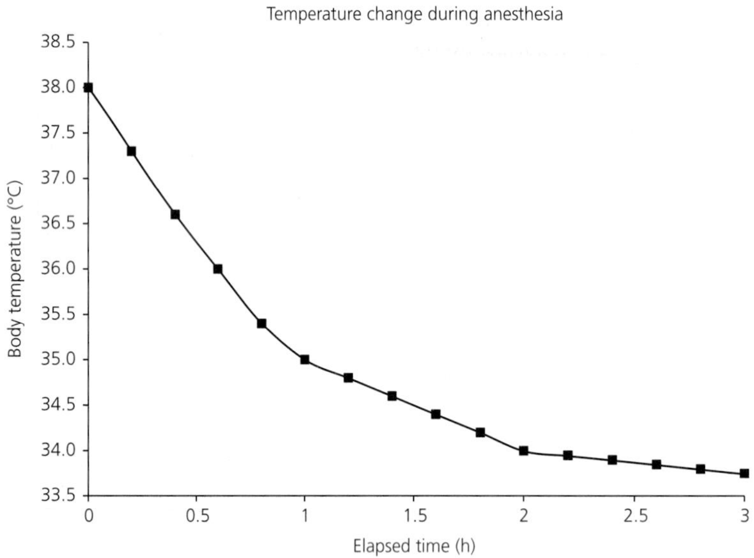

Figure 17.3 The hypothetical pattern of body temperature decrease during general anesthesia of a canine patient with minimal or no external heat support. During the first hour, core temperature usually decreases 1–1.5 °C. A second slower phase follows which represents less influence of core-skin blood redistribution and more dependence on environmental heat loss. Eventually, patients reach a psuedoequilibrium with the environment, and heat loss is minimal. Patients with a greater surface area-to-mass ratio (e.g., cats or small dogs) will experience faster changes while larger patients (e.g., horses) will experience slower changes. Use of supplemental heat sources in the perioperative period will tend to slow the rate of decrease in body temperature and elevate the minimum temperature reached. The surgical or diagnostic procedure being performed can also modify the rate of heat loss.

having an emissivity of 0.95 (regardless of pigmentation) for infrared light [3]. Radiation has been identified as the most important mechanism resulting in heat loss and perianesthetic hypothermia [3] and of note, it is not significantly inhibited by common methods used to limit patient hypothermia (e.g., cloth blankets, circulating water blankets, and forced warm air heaters).

Conduction and convection share a common theme in that heat energy flows from a warmer to a cooler surface. Conduction is usually direct transfer between two adjacent surfaces, whereas convection is facilitated via an intermediary (e.g., moving air or flowing liquid). Transfer of heat via conduction is proportional to the difference between two surface temperatures and can be inhibited by placing insulation between them. With convection, the movement of air ("wind chill") increases heat loss proportional to the square root of the air velocity. The use of an air-trapping sheet or blanket around the patient will limit airflow and thus reduce the effects of convection by about 30% [11,12]. Adding additional layers does little to reduce heat loss from convection, emphasizing the importance of decreasing airflow rather than focusing on the insulating capability of the cover. Using towels, pads, or circulating water blankets underneath the patient will act as a layer of insulation and limit direct transfer of heat via conduction.

One important species difference to consider when interpreting studies of heat loss in domestic mammals compared to human subjects is the insulating effect of fur on conduction and convection. Convection is generally regarded as the second most important cause of intraoperative heat loss in humans, but can become the most important in environments with high airflow.

Evaporation of liquids from the skin or body cavity surface results in patient heat loss due to the "donation" of heat energy required to vaporize the liquid. It is recognized that heat loss is greater with surgeries requiring large incisions and exposure of internal surfaces than with small incisions or non-invasive procedures. Evaporative losses can reach 50% of the total heat loss for smaller animal patients (rabbits) with large surgical fields [13], but are estimated to be less relative to skin loss with larger animals (swine) [14]. Another source of evaporative heat loss is associated with use of water- or alcohol-based solutions to prepare the surgical site. Heat loss has been suggested to be less with water-based solutions than with alcohol [15]. However, recent studies in cats and dogs have found little or no difference in temperature outcomes related to surgical preparation solutions [16,17]. Relative to other sources of heat loss, evaporative losses due to surgical site preparation tend to be small but, in some scenarios, may be significant.

Decreased core body temperature has long been associated with the intravenous administration of fluid therapy. The magnitude of this effect is a function of the temperature of the fluids being administered and their volume relative to the patient's body mass. When fluids are introduced at less than blood temperature, heat energy is transferred to the solution to increase the temperature until it reaches equilibrium with the patient's blood. Warming intravenous fluid can minimize this source of heat loss, but a medical fluid warming device should be used to avoid accidental overheating, which could result in blood protein and enzyme damage. Many commercial devices limit fluid temperature to 104 °F (40 °C), which is approximate to the blood temperature of a febrile patient. Important limitations of fluid warmers include the rate of fluid flow and distance they can be positioned from the patient. Many fluid warmers have a specified range of fluid flow rates where the fluid they output will be at or near the indicated temperature. If flow rates are too high, there is inadequate time to absorb heat and reach equilibrium with the warmer surface resulting in cooler than indicated fluid. If flow rates are too low, the fluid loses significant heat to room air on its way to the patient [18]. Long fluid lines positioned between the warmer and the patient will have a similar effect. Under clinical conditions, the amount of perianesthetic heat loss prevented by warming intravenous fluids is minor relative to other routes [19,20].

Active patient warming

Although patient heat loss cannot be completely prevented during anesthesia, several methods have succeeded in replacing heat losses or limiting their magnitude. The first phase of heat loss is the result primarily of the transfer of core heat to the periphery due to vasodilation (see Fig. 17.2). This phase is nearly impossible to prevent by application of an external heat source after induction. The most effective strategy is prewarming the skin and peripheral tissues to minimize the thermal gradient between the skin and the core so that once blood flow increases to the periphery, the heat energy required to re-establish equilibrium is minimal [21]. This strategy is employed on some human patients but has obvious limitations in veterinary patients. It is often impossible to restrain the patient to apply a warming device, but some species can be placed into warm ambient environments prior to induction. A major downside to this approach is that the patient will often respond by attempting to maintain a normal core temperature by panting, sweating, or other compensatory mechanisms.

Once anesthesia is induced, the focus is on limiting heat loss and maximizing safe heat supplementation. The use of blankets over the patient can reduce convective losses by approximately 30%, and placing insulation or circulating warm water blankets under all points where the patient contacts the surgery table or positioning devices will reduce conductive losses. However, the mainstay of limiting perianesthetic hypothermia is application of an external heat source (forced air unit, circulating warm water blanket, or resistive foam electrical unit).

Numerous methods to supply supplemental heat have been tried over the years by veterinarians during hospitalization or recovery from anesthesia. These have included using electric heating coils (e.g., farrowing heat pads), containers filled with warm water (e.g., latex gloves, bleach bottles, and IV fluid bags), and bags filled with various cereal grains which can be microwaved [22,23]. None of these methods should be used during anesthesia due to the relatively high potential for causing skin burns to patients [24]. Conscious patients are able to sense impending thermal injury and will usually move away from a dangerous heat source. They also alter their body position frequently to limit the exposure of one area to pressure or heat. These innate protective mechanisms are abolished by general anesthesia, placing responsibility for protecting the patient from burns on the anesthetist. A complicating factor is peripheral blood flow to the skin, since lower blood flow allows accumulation of heat energy at the skin surface, increasing the risk of thermal injury. Since the previously mentioned methods of heat supplementation were not designed for use in anesthetized patients, they can be hazardous. Their main limitation is the heat content of solids and liquids is great enough that if left in contact with skin for a prolonged period, there can be enough heat transfer to cause a burn.

Forced air units circumvent this problem because the heat content of air is low (unless a hair dryer is used instead of a patient warmer). By using large volumes of warm air (containing relatively little heat energy), the risk of injury is less. However, if an object made of metal, water, or plastic is in contact with both the warmed air and skin, there is a potential to concentrate the heat energy and cause a burn, especially if an appropriate forced warm air blanket is not used to distribute the airflow.

The use of circulating warm water blankets reduces the risk of thermal injury by limiting the water temperature and distributing the water flow to areas of the pad which are not under significant pressure. Pressure points created by patient contact with the underlying table or positioning devices can create local areas of relative skin hypoperfusion. This local decrease in blood flow allows heat to accumulate in the hypoperfused tissue, increasing the risk of a burn.

Inexpensive electric heating pads do not redistribute heat delivery away from areas of pressure and hypoperfusion which is why they should never be used on anesthetized or recovering patients. Resistive foam electric heating pads are available and designed for use in anesthetized patients. However, failure of the system design can allow patients to receive dangerous levels of heat energy under certain circumstances. Systems designed for anesthetized patients will be discussed in more detail below.

It should be apparent that the efficiency of heat transfer is directly related to the proportion of body surface which can be exposed to the external heat source. Also important is the surface area-to-mass ratio of the area being warmed. Heat loss (and gain) is usually greatest in areas with a large blood flow and low mass such as the limbs. The use of insulation (e.g., bubble wrap) around legs has been suggested to slow heat loss while application of heat to the limbs versus the trunk has been shown to result in more effective warming [25]. While dentistry patients may have 80–90% of their body surface covered, abdominal and thoracic surgery patients are often only covered 50% or less due to the need for surgical access. This fact, coupled with increased evaporative losses due to large incisions and body cavity exposure, can result in significant hypothermia in small patients.

Forced warm air units

Many different models of forced warm air heating units are available. These are distinctly different from other sources of forced warm air which may have historically been used on veterinary patients such as hair dryers. The heat output of the unit is a function of the air temperature and the airflow volume at the hose end. However, the efficacy of the system to warm patients is mainly a function of the design of the blanket [26]. Important considerations are that the blanket should have minimal temperature differences between the warmest and coolest areas and that the effectiveness is a function of the temperature difference between the patient and the blanket. Patient coverage by the blanket is also a critical factor. With this knowledge, it would seem ill-advised to save money by making blankets out of items such as pillowcases. Additionally, the use of a blanket is important for even distribution of heat. “Hosing” patients (aiming the blanket-end of the hose toward the patient) is inefficient and may result in overheating of plastic, metal, or other objects in direct contact with the patient’s skin. Forced air warming units and their blankets are engineered as a system and when utilized as such can be effective [27,28].

Circulating warm water systems

One of the older systems designed for use with anesthetized patients consists of a water reservoir/heater/pump unit and a replaceable blanket/pad [29]. Key features of the pump are the incorporation of electrical safety features, since water and electricity are in close proximity, and the ability to limit the temperature of the water delivered to the patient (usually around 104 °F [40 °C]). Most units can be attached to several sizes and shapes of blankets and have internal features to warn of low water levels. Blankets are available in many sizes and shapes which is useful to maximize the body contact area. Water circulates through the blanket in channels formed between the plastic layers. Occlusion of some of the channels by patient pressure results in shunting of flow around that area, reducing the risk of heat accumulation at pressure points.

While circulating warm water systems are generally less expensive than other systems designed for anesthetized patients, there are some drawbacks. Usually, the blanket is placed between the patient and the table. If more patient coverage is desired, additional blankets or units are needed. Also, failure or leakage of a blanket can result in drenching of the patient, causing significantly increased heat loss due to evaporation during transport and recovery. While circulating water blankets are more effective than no external heat support, they are usually less effective than forced warm air units [30]. Many anesthetists choose to use a circulating warm water blanket under the patient in combination with a forced warm air unit placed over or around the patient.

Resistive polymer electric heating

Resistive polymer heating systems (e.g., HotDog Patient Warming System, Augustine Biomedical + Design, Eden Prairie, MN; Inditherm, Inditherm plc, Rotherham, UK) differ from forced air and circulating warm water in that they are conductive rather than convective heat delivery devices. The major concern limiting the use of electric heating pads during anesthesia and recovery has been (and remains) the concern for thermal injury. Commercial systems typically incorporate spot sensors for monitoring patient/pad interface area temperature and provide alarms and electrical cutoffs if temperatures are out of the specified ranges. However, the sensors are not uniformly distributed and patient positioning may decrease their effectiveness. Additionally, if a foreign substance such as surgical irrigation fluid or urine is introduced between the pad and the patient the thermal conductivity of the system may increase and cause dangerous conditions leading to burns.

Pad construction consists of several layers composed of the polymer, padding, waterproofing, and a protective layer. The integrity of the pad construction appears to be important since moisture inside the pad can alter function and heat delivery characteristics of the system and has been associated with thermal injury to patients. Most systems include “pad expiration” dates in an attempt to encourage replacement of older pads in order to limit the risk of burns from damaged pad surfaces. However, variables other than age can influence the risk of damage such as heavy use, caustic or erosive cleaning agents, accidental puncture by sharp instruments or claws, and general environmental conditions. Regular pad inspection is encouraged to limit the risk of patient injury.

Advantages of this system include less concern for surgical site contamination due to airflow (forced warm air systems) [31], lower disposable costs (forced warm air and circulating warm water systems), quiet solid-state functioning, and a simple direct current electrical cord connection between the pad and the controller unit. Potential downsides to the system include a relatively large initial purchase price and concern for thermal injury when the pad is damaged without obvious external signs. Many users (especially for dental procedures) wrap the pad around the patient, but a safer approach may be to place the pad over the patient to limit pressure points. The effectiveness of resistive polymer heating has been compared to forced warm air and other methods. Generally, the resistive polymer system is similar or somewhat more effective [32–36]. However, the major limitation with heat transfer and patient temperature maintenance remains the amount of body surface which can contact the pad.

Hyperthermia

Hyperthermia is rare during anesthesia. When it does occur, it is usually due to iatrogenic causes (e.g., too much heat gain from warming devices), large heavy-coated animals undergoing diagnostic procedures associated with little heat loss (e.g., a Newfoundland dog undergoing magnetic resonance imaging), or metabolic derangement or disease (e.g., malignant hyperthermia or suspected serotonin syndrome). When recognized, hyperthermia should be evaluated as to the clinical significance and a differential list of causes should be formulated. Transient mild hyperthermia (up to 104 °F [40 °C]) is seldom a risk to the patient and usually responds to remedying the suspected cause (turn off or turn down the heat support). If hyperthermia is associated with other signs of hypermetabolism (increased end-tidal CO_2, metabolic acidosis, and hypoxia), malignant hyperthermia or some variant of hypermetabolic disease should be suspected and treated aggressively. Malignant hyperthermia has been reported in several species, including humans, cats, dogs, horses, and swine [37–48]. Similar hypermetabolic syndromes have also been reported during capture of free-ranging wildlife.

A confounding factor in diagnosing the cause of hyperthermia, especially in cats, is the association of opioid administration with perianesthetic hyperthermia [49,50]. This effect appears to be related to opioid-altered thermoregulation in the CNS. Most other companion animal species experience hypothermia perianesthetically following opioid administration, although there appear to be exceptions (e.g., Greyhounds) [38]. More detailed species-specific discussions of malignant hyperthermia appear elsewhere in this text.

Clinical significance of hypothermia

The first obstacle to a meaningful discussion of the significance of anesthetic-related hypothermia is defining at what patient temperature hypothermia occurs. Strictly speaking, it would be at any temperature below the patient's normal temperature. However, practical experience tells us that mild hypothermia is seldom associated with significant long-term complications; therefore, many choose to define *mild hypothermia* as a body temperature between the patient's normal euthermic temperature and approximately 96.8 °F (36 °C), the temperature below which risk of complications is thought to increase in most species. It should be apparent that decreasing body temperature is a continuum and the risk of adverse outcomes is usually multifactorial. Therefore, defining at what temperature hypothermia is significant depends on the individual patient and comorbidities present. In general, it can be assumed that the risk of adverse outcomes increases as body temperature decreases, but accurately predicting the breakpoints at which an individual patient will have complications is impossible.

Anesthesia-related hypothermia in veterinary medicine is very common. Usually, larger animals (equine and bovine species) will experience some degree of hypothermia, but the magnitude is usually small due to the large body mass-to-surface ratio, and potentially the high frequency of use of vasoconstricting α_2-adrenergic receptor agonists as preanesthetics. Even though hypothermia may be classified as mild, there are several studies which have associated hypothermia in horses with longer times to standing [28,51]. Smaller species, including dogs and cats, often have mild-to-moderate hypothermia, even when supplemental heat sources are used. However, the reported incidence varies greatly depending on what temperature is used to define its onset [52–56].

The incidence and magnitude of hypothermia are highly correlated with several non-temperature-dependent risk factors for postanesthetic complications, including anesthetic duration, American Society of Anesthesiologists (ASA) status, patient size, patient age, surgical site, and reason for surgery [57,58]. Common complications usually attributed to hypothermia include increased risk of anesthetic overdose [59], prolonged recovery from anesthesia [60], postoperative wound infection, impairment of coagulation [61,62], increased shivering and discomfort during recovery, increased blood viscosity, and cardiac complications, including arrhythmias and arrest [63]. While *in vitro* measures of coagulation and platelet function are temperature dependent and generally are impaired by hypothermia-associated temperatures, *in vivo* effects of hypothermia on coagulation can be variable depending on many patient and surgical factors.

Cardiac arrest is the most extreme example of increased mortality from hypothermia but does not usually occur until core temperature is below approximately 70 °F (20–23 °C) [63]. Other cardiovascular complications can occur at much higher body temperatures (e.g., hypotension, myocardial ischemia, and arrhythmias due to increased oxygen demands secondary to shivering in recovery), but are of greater concern in patients with pre-existing cardiac disease than in normal healthy patients.

Postoperative wound infections have been demonstrated to be more common when mild hypothermia occurs during anesthesia [64], but others have found little difference when studying the rate of infection in clean wounds and instead suggest surgery time is more important [65]. Proposed mechanisms include decreased peripheral tissue blood flow during recovery and decreased function of T cells and neutrophils [64]. However, other factors, especially surgery time, surgery location, underlying health of the patient, and anesthesia-associated hypoxemia (relatively common in horses), should also be considered since these also correlate with wound infection rates [66–68]. Controlled hypothermia can be protective for some patients. The decreased rate of cellular metabolism associated with hypothermia may be protective in some conditions such as neurologic disease [69–71], myocardial ischemia [63], and tissue hypoxia [72].

Perianesthetic management of hypothermia

No formal guidelines exist for the management of body temperature during anesthesia of veterinary patients. However, body temperature monitoring in the perioperative period is recommended in the American College of Veterinary Anesthesia and Analgesia Monitoring Guidelines so that "patients do not encounter serious deviations from normal body temperature" [73]. It should be appreciated that monitoring patient temperature does not alter heat balance changes associated with anesthesia. Application of appropriate external heat sources can alter, but seldom prevents, changes in temperature during the operative period unless patients can be in contact with the source over a large portion of their skin surface area and for a sufficient time to absorb adequate heat energy.

Management of patient temperature is a series of compromises made between the anesthetist, surgeon, and other personnel involved in the perioperative care of the patient. All anesthetists would like to have their patients wake up euthermic if possible since feeling cold can be uncomfortable. However, surgical, patient transport, and recovery logistics are often at odds with maintenance of euthermia. For example, dentistry patients can often be warmed by covering 80–90% of their skin surface area, and may be extubated at or near normal body temperature. However, a surgeon cannot gain access to the abdomen for an exploratory laparotomy with heating devices draped over the caudal half of the patient, so a significant decrease in heat transfer is mandated by surgical needs. Additionally, surgeons often expose abdominal contents during laparotomy, further decreasing patient heat balance through increased losses. Operating room temperature could be increased to minimize the temperature differential between the patient and environment but most surgeons prioritize their own comfort and keep operating room temperatures cool. Even with the limitations imposed by surgical needs, reasonable efforts should be made to apply effective means of heat supplementation to anesthetized patients, especially if the surgery is invasive or anesthesia time longer than a few minutes.

Since the majority (in some cases over 90%) of heat loss occurs through radiation, conduction, and convection of heat from the skin, focus should be placed on limiting these losses. Placing patients on insulating pads will slow conductive losses into the surgery table. Placing warming devices specifically designed for anesthetized patients over as much skin surface as reasonably possible will decrease the skin-to-environment temperature gradient and further slow or reverse loss. Placing one layer of material over or around the patient can limit air circulation and slow convective loss. Some have used radiant heat lamps over the patient to limit or reverse radiant heat loss (a significant proportion of overall loss) but this is not common practice and may be difficult to control.

Other methods of patient warming or heat loss prevention have been studied. In general, they are effective at addressing the intended mechanism, but often those mechanisms are relatively minor and do not have a major impact on overall heat loss. These include use of fluid warmers, airway humidifiers, and heaters [74], and additional insulation or blanket layers (e.g., bubble wrap on the feet). When considering the utility of these techniques, there should be thoughtful discussion about their effectiveness and potential to complicate or delay the anesthetic and surgical procedure.

Significant hypothermia in patients arriving in recovery is common, especially in small animal species after surgeries lasting 30 min or longer. The drugs used for premedication and anesthesia can significantly influence the observed body temperature decrease since vasoconstrictors (e.g., α_2-adrenergic receptor agonists) tend to limit cutaneous blood flow and heat transfer while vasodilators (e.g., acepromazine and inhalant anesthetics) tend to increase both [8,9]. While the amount of vasoconstriction or vasodilation can modify the rate at which heat is lost, they can also modify the rate at which externally applied supplemental heat sources can warm a patient in recovery. It can be more difficult to raise body temperature in an animal with profound peripheral vasoconstriction (due to normal response to hypothermia or pharmacologically induced). In some cases, it may be reasonable to administer an antagonist to the drugs responsible for delaying patient warming (e.g., α_2-adrenergic receptor antagonists or opioid antagonists) to help restore cutaneous blood flow and central thermoregulatory responses. However, this is not frequently done following major surgery due to the loss of sedative and analgesic actions following reversal. Additionally, rapid increases in oxygen demands will follow onset of shivering. If the patient cannot increase oxygen delivery (diminished cardiovascular function or anemia) or has marginal blood oxygenation (respiratory disease), rapid tissue hypoxia may follow.

While hypothermia has been associated with several postoperative complications (e.g., increased wound infections, decreased coagulation and hemostasis, etc.), it seldom represents a true anesthetic emergency, even when severe. Therefore, personnel should initially focus on critical parameters such as cardiovascular function (heart rate, blood pressure, and cardiac output) and pulmonary function (end-tidal CO_2, oxyhemoglobin saturation, and airway management) before addressing patient rewarming when patients present to recovery. Once the patient's vital functions are being monitored and supported, heat support can be applied. During the early recovery period when patients are unconscious or heavily sedated, the same concerns exist as during anesthesia with respect to placing heat sources not designed for anesthetized patients near or on the patient.

References

1 Daly TJ, Williams LA, Buffenstein R. Catecholaminergic innervation of interscapular brown adipose tissue in the naked mole-rat (*Heterocephalus glaber*). *J Anat* 1997; **190**: 321–326.

2 Morrison SF, Nakamura K. Central neural pathways for thermoregulation. *Front Biosci* 2011; **16**: 74–104.

3 Sessler DI. Perioperative heat balance. *Anesthesiology* 2000; **92**(2): 578–596.

4 Kurz A, Sessler DI, Christensen R, *et al.* Thermoregulatory vasoconstriction and perianesthetic heat transfer. *Acta Anaesthesiol Scand Suppl* 1996; **109**: 30–33.

5 Raffe MR, Martin FB. Effect of inspired air heat and humidification on anestheticinduced hypothermia in dogs. *Am J Vet Res* 1983; **44**(3): 455–458.

6 Hofmeister EH, Brainard BM, Braun C, *et al.* Effect of a heat and moisture exchanger on heat loss in isoflurane-anesthetized dogs undergoing single-limb orthopedic procedures. *J Am Vet Med Assoc* 2011; **239**(12): 1561–1565.

7 Goldberg ME, Epstein R, Rosenblum F, *et al.* Do heated humidifiers and heat and moisture exchangers prevent temperature drop during lower abdominal surgery? *J Clin Anesth* 1992; **4**(1): 16–20.

8 Vainionpää M, Salla K, Restitutti F, *et al.* Thermographic imaging of superficial temperature in dogs sedated with medetomidine and butorphanol with and without MK-467 (L-659'066). *Vet Anaesth Analg* 2013; **40**(2): 142–148.

9 Khenissi L, Covey-Crump G, Knowles TG, *et al.* Do heat and moisture exchangers in the anaesthesia breathing circuit preserve body temperature in dogs undergoing anaesthesia for magnetic resonance imaging? *Vet Anaesth Analg* 2017; **44**(3): 452–460.

10 Zarndt BS, Buchta JN, Garver LS, *et al.* Use of a far-infrared active warming device in guinea pigs (*Cavia porcellus*). *J Am Assoc Lab Anim Sci* 2015; **54**(6): 779–782.

11 Onozawa E, Azakami D, Seki S, *et al.* Effect of an insulation device in preventing hypothermia during magnetic resonance imaging examinations for dogs and cats under general anesthesia. *Animals (Basel)* 2021; **11**(8): 2378.

12 Sessler DI, McGuire J, Sessler AM. Perioperative thermal insulation. *Anesthesiology* 1991; **74**(5):875–879.

13 Roe CF. Effect of bowel exposure on body temperature during surgical operations. *Am J Surg* 1971; **122**(1): 13–15.

14 English MJ, Papenberg R, Farias E, *et al.* Heat loss in an animal experimental model. *J Trauma* 1991; **31**(1): 36–38.

15 Sessler DI, Sessler AM, Hudson S, Moayeri A. Heat loss during surgical skin preparation. *Anesthesiology* 1993; **78**(6): 1055–1064.

16 Isaza D, DiGangi BA, Isaza N, *et al.* Impact of surgical preparatory rinses with isopropyl alcohol or water on perioperative body temperature in pediatric female dogs and cats. *Vet Anaesth Analg* 2021; **48**(2): 198–204.

17 Kreisler RE, Douglas ML, Harder KN. Comparison of the effect of isopropyl alcohol and chlorhexidine solution rinses on body temperature of female cats undergoing sterilization surgery. *J Feline Med Surg* 2021; **23**(10): 875–882.

18 Jourdan G, Didier C, Chotard E, *et al.* Heated intravenous fluids alone fail to prevent hypothermia in cats under general anaesthesia. *J Feline Med Surg* 2017; **19**(12): 1249–1253.

19 Atayde IB, Franco LG, Silva MAM, *et al.* Fluid Heating System (SAF): effects on clinical and biochemistry parameters in dogs submitted to inhalatory anesthesia. *Acta Cirúrgica Bras Soc Bras Para Desenvolv Pesqui Em Cir* 2009; **24**(2): 144–149.

20 Chiang V, Hopper K, Mellema MS. In vitro evaluation of the efficacy of a veterinary dry heat fluid warmer. *J Vet Emerg Crit Care* 2011; **21**(6): 639–647.

21 Rufiange M, Leung VSY, Simpson K, *et al.* Pre-warming following premedication limits hypothermia before and during anesthesia in Sprague–Dawley rats (*Rattus norvegicus*). *Can J Vet Res* 2021; **85**(2): 106–111.

22 Dyson D, Stoate C. Combating hypothermia, including recommendations for the use of oat bags. *Can Vet J* 1997; **38**(8): 517–518.

23 Jirapaet K, Jirapaet V. Assessment of cereal-grain warming pad as a heat source for newborn transport. *J Med Assoc Thail Chotmaihet Thangphaet* 2005; **88**(Suppl 8): S203–S210.

24 Dunlop CI, Daunt DA, Haskins SC. Thermal burns in four dogs during anesthesia. *Vet Surg* 1989; **18**(3): 242–246.

25 Cabell LW, Perkowski SZ, Gregor T, *et al.* The effects of active peripheral skin warming on perioperative hypothermia in dogs. *Vet Surg* 1997; **26**(2): 79–85.

26 Bräuer A, Quintel M. Forced-air warming: technology, physical background and practical aspects. *Curr Opin Anaesthesiol* 2009; **22**(6): 769–774.

27 Machon RG, Raffe MR, Robinson EP. Warming with a forced air warming blanket minimizes anesthetic-induced hypothermia in cats. *Vet Surg* 1999; **28**(4): 301–310.

28 Tomasic M. Temporal changes in core body temperature in anesthetized adult horses. *Am J Vet Res* 1999; **60**(5): 556–562.

29 Evans AT, Sawyer DC, Krahwinkel DJ. Effect of a warm-water blanket on development of hypothermia during small animal surgery. *J Am Vet Med Assoc* 1973; **163**(2): 147–148.

30 Clark-Price SC, Dossin O, Jones KR, *et al.* Comparison of three different methods to prevent heat loss in healthy dogs undergoing 90 minutes of general anesthesia. *Vet Anaesth Analg* 2013; **40**(3): 280–284.

31 Dasari KB, Albrecht M, Harper M. Effect of forced-air warming on the performance of operating theatre laminar flow ventilation. *Anaesthesia* 2012; **67**(3): 244–249.

32 Kibanda JO, Gurney M. Comparison of two methods for the management of intraoperative hypothermia in dogs. *Vet Rec* 2012; **170**(15): 392.

33 HotDog Patient Warming. www.vetwarming.com (accessed April 2022).

34 Brandt S, Oguz R, Hüttner H, *et al.* Resistive-polymer versus forced-air warming: comparable efficacy in orthopedic patients. *Anesth Analg* 2010; **110**(3): 834–838.

35 Kimberger O, Held C, Stadelmann K, *et al.* Resistive polymer versus forced-air warming: comparable heat transfer and core rewarming rates in volunteers. *Anesth Analg* 2008; **107**(5): 1621–1626.

36 Hasegawa K, Negishi C, Nakagawa F, *et al.* The efficacy of carbon-fiber resistive-heating in prevention of core hypothermia during major abdominal surgery. *Masui* 2003; **52**(6): 636–641.

37 Chohan AS, Greene SA. Anesthesia case of the month. Malignant hyperthermia. *J Am Vet Med Assoc* 2011; **239**(7): 936–940.

38 Court MH. Anesthesia of the sighthound. *Clin Tech Small Anim Pract* 1999; **14**(1): 38–43.

39 Roberts MC, Mickelson JR, Patterson EE, *et al.* Autosomal dominant canine malignant hyperthermia is caused by a mutation in the gene encoding the skeletal muscle calcium release channel (RYR1). *Anesthesiology* 2001; **95**(3): 716–725.

40 Cosgrove SB, Eisele PH, Martucci RW, *et al.* Evaluation of greyhound susceptibility to malignant hyperthermia using halothane-succinylcholine anesthesia and caffeine-halothane muscle contractures. *Lab Anim Sci* 1992; **42**(5): 482–485.

41 Cornick JL, Seahorn TL, Hartsfield SM. Hyperthermia during isoflurane anaesthesia in a horse with suspected hyperkalaemic periodic paralysis. *Equine Vet J* 1994; **26**(6): 511–514.

42 De Jong RH, Heavner JE, Amory DW. Malignant hyperpyrexia in the cat. *Anesthesiology* 1974; **41**(6): 608–609.

43 Otto K. Malignant hyperthermia as a complication of anesthesia in the dog. *Tierärztl Prax* 1992; **20**(5): 519–522.

44 Kirmayer AH, Klide AM, Purvance JE. Malignant hyperthermia in a dog: case report and review of the syndrome. *J Am Vet Med Assoc* 1984; **185**(9): 978–982.

45 Bagshaw RJ, Cox RH, Knight DH, *et al.* Malignant hyperthermia in a Greyhound. *J Am Vet Med Assoc* 1978; **172**(1): 61–62.

46 Klein L, Ailes N, Fackelman GE, *et al.* Postanesthetic equine myopathy suggestive of malignant hyperthermia. *A case report. Vet Surg* 1989; **18**(6): 479–482.

47 Bellah JR, Robertson SA, Buergelt CD, *et al.* Suspected malignant hyperthermia after halothane anesthesia in a cat. *Vet Surg* 1989; **18**(6): 483–488.

48 Adami C, Axiak S, Raith K, *et al.* Unusual perianesthetic malignant hyperthermia in a dog. *J Am Vet Med Assoc* 2012; **240**(4): 450–453.

49 Posner LP, Gleed RD, Erb HN, *et al.* Post-anesthetic hyperthermia in cats. *Vet Anaesth Analg* 2007; **34**(1): 40–47.

50 Niedfeldt RL, Robertson SA. Postanesthetic hyperthermia in cats: a retrospective comparison between hydromorphone and buprenorphine. *Vet Anaesth Analg* 2006; **33**(6): 381–389.

51 Voulgaris DA, Hofmeister EH. Multivariate analysis of factors associated with postanesthetic times to standing in isoflurane-anesthetized horses: 381 cases. *Vet Anaesth Analg* 2009; **36**(5): 414–420.

52 Waterman A. Accidental hypothermia during anaesthesia in dogs and cats. *Vet Rec* 1975; **96**(14): 308–313.

53 Redondo JI, Suesta P, Gil L, *et al.* Retrospective study of the prevalence of postanaesthetic hypothermia in cats. *Vet Rec* 2012; **170**(8): 206.

54 Redondo JI, Suesta P, Serra I, *et al.* Retrospective study of the prevalence of postanaesthetic hypothermia in dogs. *Vet Rec* 2012; **171**(15): 374.

55 Redondo JI, Rubio M, Soler G, *et al.* Normal values and incidence of cardiorespiratory complications in dogs during general anaesthesia. A review of 1281 cases. *J Vet Med A Physiol Pathol Clin Med* 2007; **54**(9): 470–477.

56 Kennedy KC, Tamburello KR, Hardie RJ. Peri-operative morbidity associated with ovariohysterectomy performed as part of a third-year veterinary surgical-training program. *J Vet Med Educ* 2011; **38**(4): 408–413.

57 Brodbelt DC, Pfeiffer DU, Young LE, *et al.* Results of the confidential enquiry into perioperative small animal fatalities regarding risk factors for anesthetic-related death in dogs. *J Am Vet Med Assoc* 2008; **233**(7): 1096–1104.

58 Brodbelt DC, Blissitt KJ, Hammond RA, *et al.* The risk of death: the confidential enquiry into perioperative small animal fatalities. *Vet Anaesth Analg* 2008; **35**(5): 365–373.

59 Regan MJ, Eger EI II. Effect of hypothermia in dogs on anesthetizing and apneic doses of inhalation agents. Determination of the anesthetic index (Apnea/MAC). *Anesthesiology* 1967; **28**(4): 689–700.

60 Pottie RG, Dart CM, Perkins NR, *et al.* Effect of hypothermia on recovery from general anaesthesia in the dog. *Aust Vet J* 2007; **85**(4): 158–162.

61 Park KH, Lee KH, Kim H. Effect of hypothermia on coagulatory function and survival in Sprague–Dawley rats exposed to uncontrolled haemorrhagic shock. *Injury* 2013; **44**(1): 91–96.

62 Taggart R, Austin B, Hans E, *et al.* In vitro evaluation of the effect of hypothermia on coagulation in dogs via thromboelastography. *J Vet Emerg Crit Care* 2012; **22**(2): 219–224.

63 Fujiki M, Misumi K, Sakamoto H, *et al.* Circulatory arrest under hypothermic anesthesia using abdominal cavity cooling. *J Vet Med Sci* 1998; **60**(11): 1237–1242.

64 Putzu M, Casati A, Berti M, *et al.* Clinical complications, monitoring and management of perioperative mild hypothermia: anesthesiological features. *Acta BioMedica Atenei Parm* 2007; **78**(3): 163–169.

65 Beal MW, Brown DC, Shofer FS. The effects of perioperative hypothermia and the duration of anesthesia on postoperative wound infection rate in clean wounds: a retrospective study. *Vet Surg* 2000; **29**(2): 123–127.

66 Sturgeon C, Lamport AI, Lloyd DH, *et al.* Bacterial contamination of suction tips used during surgical procedures performed on dogs and cats. *Am J Vet Res* 2000; **61**(7): 779–783.

67 Brown DC, Conzemius MG, Shofer F, *et al.* Epidemiologic evaluation of postoperative wound infections in dogs and cats. *J Am Vet Med Assoc* 1997; **210**(9): 1302–1306.

68 Nicholson M, Beal M, Shofer F, *et al.* Epidemiologic evaluation of postoperative wound infection in clean-contaminated wounds: a retrospective study of 239 dogs and cats. *Vet Surg* 2002; **31**(6): 577–581.

69 Steen PA, Newberg L, Milde JH, *et al.* Hypothermia and barbiturates: individual and combined effects on canine cerebral oxygen consumption. *Anesthesiology* 1983; **58**(6): 527–532.

70 Wass CT, Lanier WL, Hofer RE, *et al.* Temperature changes of > or = 1 degree C alter functional neurologic outcome and histopathology in a canine model of complete cerebral ischemia. *Anesthesiology* 1995; **83**(2): 325–335.

71 Michenfelder JD, Milde JH. The relationship among canine brain temperature, metabolism, and function during hypothermia. *Anesthesiology* 1991; **75**(1): 130–136.

72 Ohta S, Yukioka T, Wada T, *et al.* Effect of mild hypothermia on the coefficient of oxygen delivery in hypoxemic dogs. *J Appl Physiol* 1995; **78**(6): 2095–2099.

73 ACVAA Small Animal Monitoring Guidelines. www.acvaa.org (accessed April 2022).

74 Kelly CK, Hodgson DS, McMurphy RM. Effect of anesthetic breathing circuit type on thermal loss in cats during inhalation anesthesia for ovariohysterectomy. *J Am Vet Med Assoc* 2012; **240**(11): 1296–1299.

18 Point-of-Care Ultrasound in Anesthesia

Søren R. Boysen[1] and Daniel S.J. Pang[2]
[1] Faculty of Veterinary Medicine, University of Calgary, Calgary, Alberta, Canada
[2] Faculty of Veterinary Medicine, University of Calgary, Calgary, Alberta, Canada and Faculty of Veterinary Medicine, Université de Montréal, Saint-Hyacinthe, Québec, Canada

Chapter contents

Introduction, 254
Perioperative POCUS, 254
General applications of POCUS, 255
Application of P-POCUS, 255
Equipment and patient preparation, 256
Airway assessment, 256
Endotracheal tube placement, 256
Pleural space and lung ultrasound, 256
Machine settings for PLUS, 257
Normal PLUS findings, 257
Abnormal PLUS findings, 261
Abdominal point-of-care ultrasound, 269
Gastric volume, 269
Urinary bladder volume, 271
Cardiac POCUS, 271
Cardiac POCUS windows and views, 272
Interpretation and integration of cardiac POCUS findings, 273
POCUS in cardiopulmonary resuscitation, 275
POCUS and monitoring fluid therapy, 277
Limitations, 277
References, 277

Introduction

In 2004, publication of the abdominal-focused assessment with sonography for trauma (FAST) exam in dogs suffering motor vehicular injury [1] was the first work in small animals to become more broadly known as *point-of-care ultrasound* (POCUS). Although the terms POCUS and FAST are often used interchangeably, they are not synonymous. FAST exams in both human and veterinary medicine were developed to, and still primarily focus on, the search for free fluid in body cavities and pneumothorax [1–6]. By contrast, POCUS is broader in scope; it incorporates all clinically driven real-time assessments that can be answered within minutes using ultrasonography [4,5]. More specifically, *POCUS* is defined as the acquisition, interpretation, and immediate clinical integration of ultrasonographic imaging performed patient-side by an attending clinician, not by a radiologist or cardiologist, with the goal of answering a focused question or series of questions rather than assessing all structures of an organ(s) [5]. To this end, it is best applied as a problem-based assessment based on Bayes' theorem of pretest probabilities, which enables the clinician to gather key pieces of information in real time to help narrow or determine a diagnosis, streamline care, guide ongoing management, and reduce cognitive errors [7,8]. The concept of POCUS as a focused ("limited" or "goal-directed") exam [9,10] is in contrast to sonography performed by an imaging specialist/cardiologist (Table 18.1). Finally, POCUS provides relevant information that is otherwise unattainable on physical examination alone and is therefore complementary to triage, physical examination, and other point-of-care diagnostic and clinical tests or findings; it does not replace them. Evidence in human medicine supports that POCUS can result in improved clinical decision-making [11,12], and when combined with other clinical findings, confirms the suspected clinical diagnosis in up to 50% of cases and supports a change in the initial diagnosis in 23% of cases [13].

Perioperative POCUS

With the exception of ultrasound-guided regional anesthesia and vascular access, POCUS is in its infancy in veterinary anesthesia. In contrast, POCUS is widely used in human anesthesia to answer specific questions in daily patient management, narrow differential diagnoses, and improve the safety of routine procedures [14–20] (Table 18.2). When compared to traditional assessment techniques, human studies suggest anesthesiologist-performed POCUS improves diagnostic accuracy of new pathologies as well as assessing the severity of known pathologies [21], and impacts perioperative management decisions [21–23]. Currently, perioperative POCUS (P-POCUS) is most widely used for cardiovascular evaluation [16,22,24,25], pulmonary/airway [23,26–28], and abdominal/gastric [29,30] examinations, although it can be used to augment almost all aspects of the physical exam (Table 18.2).

Veterinary Anesthesia and Analgesia: The Sixth Edition of Lumb and Jones. Edited by Leigh Lamont, Kurt Grimm, Sheilah Robertson, Lydia Love and Carrie Schroeder.
© 2024 John Wiley & Sons, Inc. Published 2024 by John Wiley & Sons, Inc.
Companion website: www.wiley.com/go/lamont/anesthesia

Table 18.1 Comparison of formal and point-of-care ultrasound.

Formal ultrasound	Point-of-care ultrasound
Consultative; assessing all organs, anatomy, and structures	Focused on key structures to answer specific clinical questions (often binary choice)
Often performed with nonspecific findings and when multiple or an open-ended list of differential diagnoses are possible	Often performed when specific signs are present and a high pretest probability of a specific diagnosis (es) is likely (Bayes' theorem)
Requires years of training	Requires minimal experience
Often takes > 30–60 min	Performed in < 5–10 min
Usually performed by specialists (cardiologists, radiologists)	Often performed by non-specialists (emergency clinicians, general practitioners)
Patients often stable	Patients often unstable
Patient taken to the machine	Machine taken to the patient
Patient scanned in lateral or dorsal recumbency	Patient scanned in the position they are most comfortable, rarely if ever dorsal recumbency
Fur is typically clipped	Fur is rarely clipped
Gel preferred as the coupling agent	Uses alcohol ± gel as the coupling agent

With growing evidence demonstrating the efficacy of anesthetist-performed POCUS, its uptake by human anesthesiology training programs is increasing. A 2017 survey reported 100% (13/13) of academic anesthesiology programs surveyed had some POCUS training as part of their residency training and 70–77% believed POCUS should be expanded beyond ultrasound-guided vascular access and nerve blocks, which are currently part of the National Curriculum for Canadian Anesthesia Residency [31]. Additional POCUS applications that respondents felt should be included in anesthesiology residency programs included lung ultrasound and vena cava assessment in 12, abdominal ultrasound in 8, gastric ultrasound in 4, airway ultrasound in 3, and optic nerve sheath diameter in 1 out of the 13 academic anesthesiology programs surveyed [31].

General applications of POCUS

The application of POCUS varies depending on the clinical setting (Fig. 18.1) [34]: (1) triage POCUS uses the minimum number of views possible to identify the most immediate life-threatening and critical conditions; (2) serial POCUS is applied to monitor progression or resolution of pathology and response to therapy; (3) systemic or multiorgan POCUS is performed in more stable patients (with or without specialist assistance) to detect asymptomatic conditions, new developments, and/or to ensure sonographically detectable problems have not arisen before undertaking procedures, anesthesia, or discharge/service transfer; and (4) interventional POCUS is used to reduce complications of procedures where applicable (Fig. 18.1). Which POCUS examination(s) to choose will also depend on the pretest probability of a problem being present [7,8].

Though it is rapid, repeatable, and associated with minimal risk, POCUS should never be completed at the risk of compromising patient safety. The decision to apply POCUS should always be dictated by the context of the clinical setting encountered. Only if the patient is sufficiently stable should multiorgan, systemic POCUS be performed. In unstable patients, the objective is to identify immediately life-threatening conditions with the minimum number of sonographic views possible, stabilize the patient, reassess the patient, and then decide if, and what, further point-of-care diagnostics, including POCUS are required.

Table 18.2 Common point-of-care applications in human anesthesiology [4,32,33], which should be applicable to veterinary medicine, although veterinary research is lacking for most applications.

Target system	Diagnostic applications
Airway	Endotracheal tube placement
Pleural space and lung ultrasound (PLUS)	Pleural space pathology a. Pneumothorax b. Pleural effusion
	Alveolar–interstitial syndromes (AIS) I. Increased B-lines a. Increased extravascular lung water (EVLW; i.e., "wet" lung causes) i. Cardiogenic edema ii. Fluid overload iii. Non-cardiogenic pulmonary edema iv. Acute respiratory distress syndrome (ARDS) v. Aspiration pneumonia vi. Contusions/hemorrhage b. Non-EVLW causes of increased B-lines (i.e., "dry" lung causes) i. Fibrosis/amyloidosis ii. Inflammatory cell infiltrates iii. Neoplastic cell infiltrates II. Lung consolidation a. Shred b. Nodule c. Wedge d. Translobar
	Atelectasis (can result in both increased B-lines and consolidation) Bilateral versus unilateral lung ventilation
Abdominal	Intra-abdominal free fluid (particularly useful when sudden clinical deterioration and hypotension occur) Gastric content and volume Inferior vena cava assessment for vascular volume status Bladder volume
Cardiac	Pericardial effusion Left atrial size Volume assessment Ventricular ± valvular function
Cardiac arrest	Reversible causes of arrest Presence of intrinsic cardiac activity
Hemodynamics and resuscitation	Volume status and response to fluid boluses
Eye	Intracranial hypertension, optic nerve sheath swelling
Ultrasound-guided interventions	Thoracocentesis, abdominocentesis, pericardiocentesis, cystocentesis, fine needle aspiration
Locoregional anesthesia	Nerve blocks
Vascular	Aortic dissection (not common in veterinary patients) Carotid artery
Physical examination assistance	Evaluation of: Trauma patients Abnormal pulmonary auscultation Respiratory distress Suspected volume overload and hypovolemia Hemodynamic instability/collapse/hypotension Decreased mentation Cardiac arrhythmias Pulsus paradoxus Cardiac murmurs

Application of P-POCUS

Use of POCUS is an active field of research, with new applications identified regularly; however, applications employed should be determined by an individual sonographer's proficiency. The American Society of Anesthesiologists (ASA) recently introduced a POCUS certification program with three primary applications (cardiac, lung, and abdominal ultrasound) and six secondary applications (airway, musculoskeletal/soft tissue, ocular, renal/

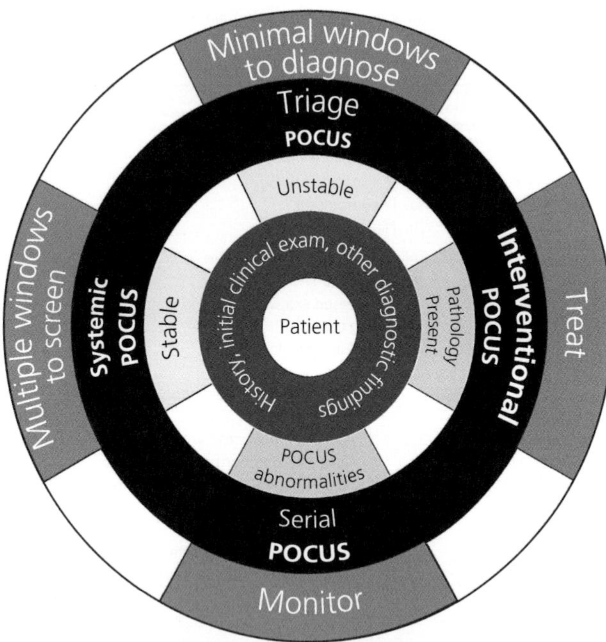

Figure 18.1 POCUS is patient centered and targeted. It is also integrative and has four general applications, which vary depending on the targeted objectives of the scan, the pretest probability of a problem being present (based on history, initial clinical exam, and other diagnostic findings), and the clinical setting encountered: (1) triage POCUS uses the minimum number of windows possible to identify the most immediate life-threatening and critical conditions; (2) serial POCUS is applied to monitor progression or resolution of any pathology, and response to therapy; (3) systemic or multiorgan POCUS uses multiple windows in more stable patients (with or without specialist assistance) to detect asymptomatic conditions, new developments, and/or to ensure sonographically detectable problems have not arisen prior to undertaking procedures, anesthesia, or discharge/service transfer; and (4) therapeutic POCUS is used to reduce complications of interventions where applicable. POCUS, point-of-care ultrasound. Source: Dr. Søren Boysen, with permission.

genitourinary, transcranial Doppler, and deep venous thrombosis) [4,32,33,35]. In principle, these suggested primary and secondary applications in human anesthesiology are applicable in veterinary anesthesia (Table 18.2). However, in veterinary medicine Doppler is not routinely used, musculoskeletal and soft tissue POCUS have not been studied, and optic nerve sheath diameter (ONSD) is only just starting to be investigated in small animals. A case series in dogs suffering trauma reports monitoring ONSD values serially in two dogs [36], and reference intervals have been reported in dogs and cats [37–40]. A single study in cats ($n = 57$) suggests an ONSD of 1–1.4 mm indicates the absence of intracranial hypertension (ICH), while a value > 1.5 mm is suggestive of ICH (based on seven cats with suspected ICH) [38]. These three POCUS applications will not be covered in this chapter, and nerve blocks and vascular access are addressed elsewhere in this textbook.

Equipment and patient preparation

An advantage of POCUS is the ability to bring the ultrasound machine to the patient, limiting interference with patient care and comfort. Although some authors prefer to restrain patients in a specific position to perform POCUS and FAST exams [3,41,42], there is minimal evidence to support this practice and increasing evidence that restraining cats and dogs in a particular position can increase patient anxiety and stress [43]. The authors advocate performing POCUS in the position in which the patient is most comfortable. Given patient position may be dictated by surgical or other procedures in anesthetized animals, it is particularly important that anesthesiologists become familiar performing POCUS with animals in different positions. However, sonographers must be aware that localization of some sonographically identifiable pathology will change with patient positioning (e.g., fluid falls and gas rises). Where the probe is situated on the patient should be modified to ensure the location of positionally dependent pathology is assessed. Although certain sonographic examinations are facilitated by specific ultrasound probes, in general, a 5 mHz (larger dogs) to 7 mHz (smaller dogs and cats) micro-convex probe and B-mode imaging are used for nearly all POCUS applications [1–3,42]. For vascular access and ultrasound-guided nerve blocks, a linear probe is generally preferred over a micro-convex probe, though the latter can still be used. To maintain efficiency, fur is not clipped but parted to provide access to the skin, and alcohol is used as the coupling agent, with or without gel [2,41]. In unstable patients where time is critical, the authors use only alcohol as the coupling agent. Caution is advised in some situations, as alcohol may cause radiographic artifact and poses a fire hazard if electrocautery, defibrillators, or laser devices are used following its application. In more stable patients, gel can be added to the probe head in addition to applying alcohol to the patient if image quality is suboptimal. Alternatively, fur can be clipped and ultrasound gel applied as the sole coupling agent at the probe–skin interface, particularly if image quality remains suboptimal [1].

Airway assessment

Assessment of the airway typically involves assessment of the cervical region for evaluation of correct endotracheal (ET) tube placement.

Endotracheal tube placement

A recent meta-analysis in human medicine documented a pooled sensitivity of 0.93 (95% CI: 0.86–0.96) and specificity of 0.97 (95% CI: 0.95–0.98) for identification of esophageal intubation using POCUS [44]. Although there is a lack of research in veterinary medicine, a small cadaveric study in dogs ($n = 6$) demonstrated sensitivity of 62–75% and specificity 38–62.5% for identification of esophageal intubation when the probe was placed on the ventral neck just caudal to the larynx near the jugular furrow, depending on the experience of the operator [45]. ET intubation is recognized by identifying the presence of only one hyperechoic curved line with distal reverberation artifact, created by the presence of air inside a correctly placed ET tube (Fig. 18.2). Esophageal intubation is recognized by the presence of two hyperechoic curved lines with distal reverberation artifact, created by the presence of air inside the trachea and air contained within an esophageally placed ET tube [45] (Fig. 18.2).

Pleural space and lung ultrasound

Pleural space and lung ultrasound (PLUS) is broadly used to search for: (1) two pleural space pathologies (pneumothorax and pleural effusion); (2) alveolar–interstitial syndromes (AIS) through identification of two abnormal sonographic lung findings (increased B-lines and lung consolidations; see abnormal PLUS findings

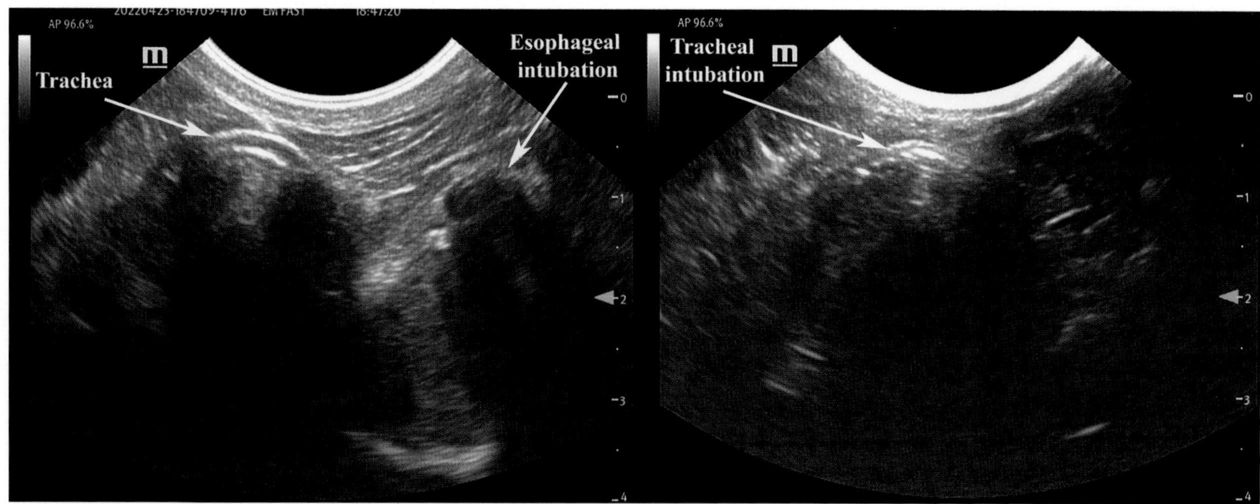

Figure 18.2 Labeled still ultrasound images of tracheal versus esophageal intubation. Right: Tracheal intubation where only one circular gas-filled structure (intubated trachea) with distal shadowing is visible. Left: With esophageal intubation, a second gas-filled structure with distal shadowing (air-filled endotracheal tube within the lumen of the esophagus) becomes visible in addition to the gas-filled trachea. Source: Dr. Søren Boysen, with permission.

below); and (3) to assess for evidence of endobronchial intubation (Table 18.2). Numerous pleura, pleural space, and lung ultrasound protocols have been described in human and veterinary medicine, all of which assess different percentages of pleura and lung surface area transthoracically, with or without inclusion of the subxiphoid window and assessment of the abdominal curtain sign (ACS) (see below for definitions) [36,42,46–51]. With the exception of thoracic FAST, which only assesses a single transthoracic lung site over each hemithorax, all veterinary protocols scan multiple lung regions bilaterally [36,42,46–49]. In human medicine, evidence suggests lung ultrasound protocols that evaluate more lung sites (12–28 sites versus 4–6 sites) have a higher sensitivity and specificity for detecting pathology, but take longer to perform [50,52]. The clinician must therefore balance the risk of missing pathology against the time required to perform sonographic examination. Including the subxiphoid window and ACS may identify pathology in dogs otherwise missed with traditional transthoracic protocols [1,42,46], and assessment of the ACS may allow earlier identification of pleural effusion in humans [51]. The lack of research comparing veterinary protocols makes translation of results between studies, and establishment of cutoff values to detect pleura and lung pathology, challenging. Where applicable, a summation of findings of veterinary studies published has been used to provide guidelines to differentiate normal from abnormal PLUS findings. Fortunately, understanding normal sonographic anatomy and physiology of the pleura, pleural space, and lung, factors that change normal findings, and where to look for pathology, should allow the operator to choose the most appropriate protocol within the clinical setting encountered. As a rule of thumb, conditions resulting in marked dyspnea are likely to be diffuse in nature [48,53], and PLUS should be limited to the minimal number of windows and shortest time possible to identify pathology (Figs. 18.1 and 18.3). Once stable, or in less dyspneic animals, more comprehensive scanning protocols can be used, particularly when very localized or focal pleura and lung pathology is suspected (e.g., isolated lung nodules). Depending on the clinical setting encountered, the authors currently use the PLUS protocol outlined in Fig. 18.3 to scan the dorsal, middle, and ventral thirds of the thorax, focusing on different sites depending on the pleural space and lung pathologies suspected (Video 18.1).

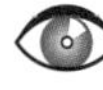

Machine settings for PLUS

To perform PLUS, adjust the machine depth setting (according to body condition) so the field of view in the ultrasound image extends to approximately 4–6 cm and the pleural line (P-line) is visible at the junction between the proximal and middle thirds of the window/field of view. Adjust the gain to maximize appearance of the thoracic wall, while also allowing any far-field image artifact to be visible (Fig. 18.4).

Normal PLUS findings

To help differentiate normal from abnormal PLUS findings, operators should become familiar with several PLUS lines and signs that can be identified in healthy animals and know how these lines and signs change in animals with suspected pathology. These include the BAT sign, P-line, lung sliding, lung pulse, A-lines, B-lines, and the ACS.

BAT sign

The BAT sign (i.e., gator sign) refers to the characteristic appearance of the P-line and adjacent ribs [42,54]. It is identified when the probe is positioned over lung, between and perpendicular to the ribs, with the indicator marker directed cranially (Fig. 18.4). If placed between and parallel to the ribs, only the P-line is seen, which is not interrupted by the ribs [54].

Using the BAT mnemonic – "ultrasound beams do not traverse Bone or Air with the probe Transverse to the ribs" – helps sonographers identify key anatomic structures and understand what is being visualized, as follows:

- Ultrasound beams cannot transmit beyond the proximal rib surface (PRS), which creates rib shadowing beneath the ribs. If rib shadows are identified, they can be traced proximally until they end at convex hyperechoic lines (PRS, "wings of the bat").
- Ultrasound beams cannot transmit beyond a soft tissue–air interface (99% of ultrasound beams are reflected from soft tissue–air/gas interfaces), which is present where parietal pleura (inside lining of the chest wall) contacts the visceral pleura (lung surface) and air-filled lung [55,56]. If the skin and soft

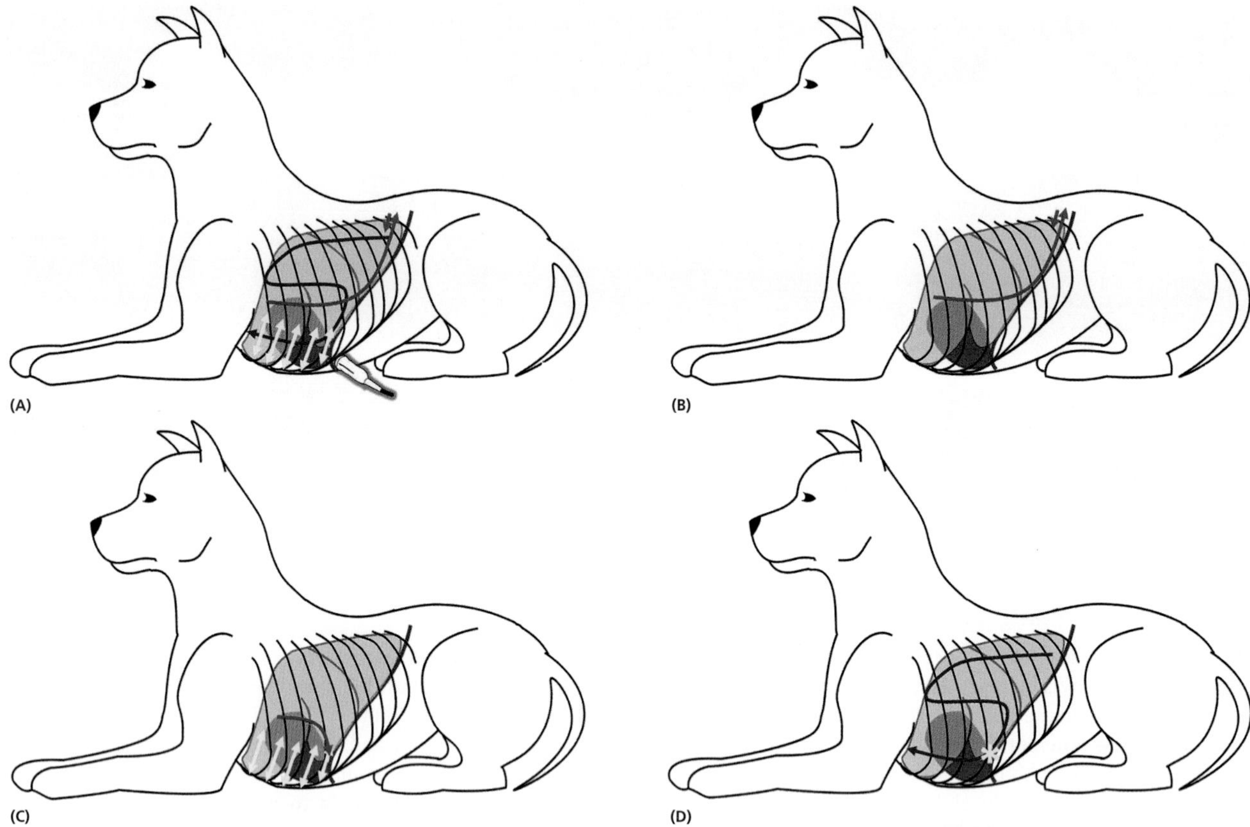

Figure 18.3 Schematic images of pleura and lung ultrasound (PLUS) to assess for pneumothorax, lung pathology, and pleural effusion using sonographically defined landmarks and lung borders with patients in a sternal or standing position. **A.** Combined comprehensive PLUS protocol often used in more stable patients to assess the pleura, pleural space, and lungs bilaterally. The subxiphoid site is also included (red highlighted probe) to assess the caudal lung and pleural space regions not otherwise accessible transthoracically. **B.** Abbreviated pleural space protocol to rapidly assess the abdominal curtain sign (ACS) and most gravity-independent sites for pneumothorax in respiratory-compromised patients. In the sternal or standing patient (shown), with the probe situated perpendicular to the ribs (probe indicator marker directed cranially), slide caudally from the starting point (just behind the front limb) until the ACS is identified, followed by sweeping the probe dorsally along the ACS until the hypaxial muscles are encountered (loss of the pleural line; curved red arrow). The probe is then swept ventrally off the hypaxial muscles until the pleural line reappears (the most gravity-independent site; short red arrow). If the patient is in lateral recumbency (not shown), the widest non-gravity region of the thorax and ACS are assessed. **C.** Abbreviated lung scanning protocol to rapidly assess multiple lung surface regions in the dorsal, middle, and ventral thirds of the thorax with the probe orientated perpendicular to the ribs using an S-shaped pattern (blue arrow) in respiratory-compromised patients. Lung pathology tends to be less affected by position than pleural space pathology, and the same lung ultrasound protocol can be used regardless of patient position, however, given some lung pathology can concentrate locally or regionally (e.g., aspiration pneumonia and positional atelectasis) different regions of the lung can be emphasized. At the pericardio-diaphragmatic (PD) window (yellow asterisk), the probe can be turned parallel to the ribs (see image D) or maintained in a perpendicular orientation to scan the ventral lung surfaces. Time permitting, the subxiphoid site can also be assessed (not shown). **D.** Abbreviated pleural space and lung ultrasound protocol to rapidly assess the most gravity-dependent pleural sites for pleural effusion and ventral lung pathology in respiratory-compromised patients. Identifying the PD window (red arrow) with the probe situated perpendicular to the ribs helps differentiate pleural and pericardial effusion. In the sternal or standing patient, the probe can be turned parallel to the ribs at the PD window (with the probe indicator marker directed dorsally) and slid ventrally until the sternal muscles fill 1/3 to 1/2 of the ultrasound image. This allows the most ventral pleural regions to be assessed for the presence of smaller volume pleural effusion. With the probe maintained in parallel orientation to the ribs, it can be slid both dorsally and ventrally within each intercostal space (yellow arrows) to assess both the ventral lung regions and the most ventral pleural space regions, respectively, from the ACS caudally to the thoracic inlet cranially. If the patient is in lateral recumbency, the widest gravity-dependent region of the thorax should be assessed for pleural effusion (not shown). Time permitting the subxiphoid site can also be included (not shown) (Video 18.1). Source: Adapted from Boysen *et al.* [46].

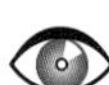

tissue structures of the chest wall are identified, they can be traced distally to where a horizontal concave hyperechoic line is visible just below the ribs and joining the rib shadows (the P-line, "body of the bat").

- If the BAT sign is identified, the proximal ribs and P-line are the last true structures the ultrasound beam encounters in healthy animals: everything beyond the PRS and P-line is artifact. Most pleura and lung pathology creates sonographically visible abnormalities originating from the P-line.

Pleural line

The pleural line (P-line) is the bright white line below the soft tissue structures of the thoracic wall (Fig. 18.4), and is either comprised of the parietal and visceral pleura when the lung apposes the chest wall, or is composed of only the parietal pleura when the lung is separated from the chest wall [54,57,58].

- The lung can be separated from the chest wall by space-occupying pathologies (pneumothorax, pleural effusion, diaphragmatic hernia, and pleural masses) [58].

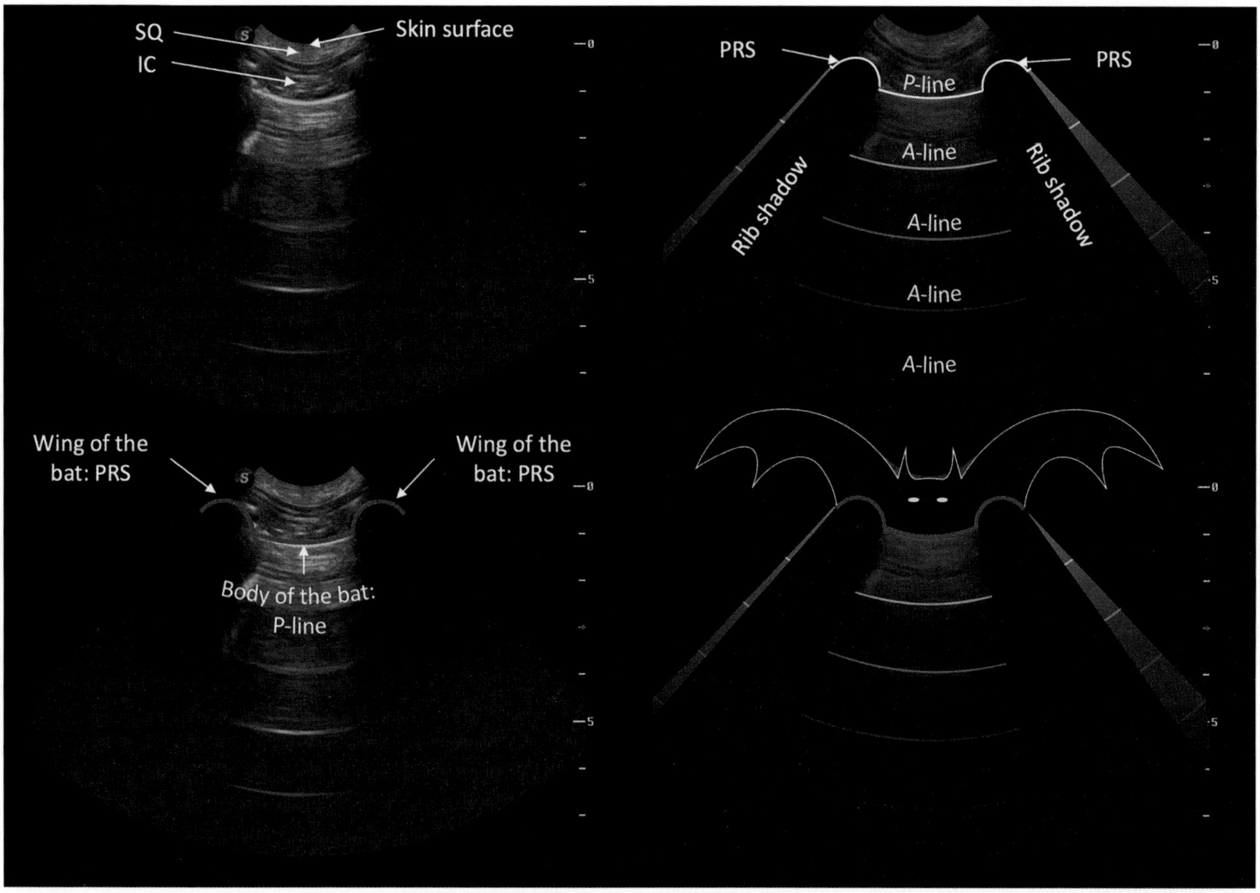

Figure 18.4 Labeled and unlabeled still and overlaid schematic images of the "BAT sign" and A-lines. The proximal rib surface (PRS) of two adjacent ribs forms the wings of the bat while the pleural line (P-line) forms the body of the bat when the probe is situated perpendicular to the ribs. The gain is adjusted based on the appearance of the thoracic wall (region above the pleural line) while also allowing A-lines to be visualized in the far field of the image. The depth is at 7 cm to allow far-field A-lines and B-lines (not shown) to be appreciated. The depth could be decreased in this example to put the pleural line at the junction between the proximal and middle thirds of the ultrasound image, which will make lung sliding easier to identify in real time. SQ, subcutaneous tissues; IC, intercostal muscles; PRS, proximal rib surface. Source: Dr. Søren Boysen, with permission.

- When the lung is separated from the chest wall by pleural effusion, the lung surface (visceral pleura) will be visible (fluid transmits ultrasound). The lung surface is not visible with pneumothorax (air inhibits the transmission of ultrasound beams).
- All pleural space pathology originates at the P-line.
- All sonographically detectable lung pathology originates from the lung surface (visceral pleura), which will be the P-line when lung is apposed to the chest wall, and distal to the P-line when the lung is visibly separated from the chest wall (e.g., pleural effusion).

Lung sliding (the glide sign)

Lung sliding is the to-and-fro shimmer that is visible at the P-line as a result of the visceral pleura sliding along the parietal pleura during lung inflation and deflation that occurs with the respiratory cycle [54,57,58] (Video 18.2).

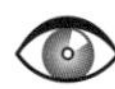

- Two criteria must be met for lung sliding to be visible: (1) the two pleura must be in apposition; (2) the patient must actively respire to cause the visceral pleura to slide across the parietal pleura [58].
- When visible, lung sliding makes space-occupying pleural space pathology very unlikely, particularly pneumothorax (100% specificity, negative predictive value 100%) [59,60], at the site the probe is positioned on the thorax [54,57,58].
- Lung sliding is lost when the pleura are separated or adhered to one another [54,58].
- Making the P-line appear "grainier" helps visualize lung sliding. This can be achieved by changing the angle the ultrasound beam strikes the P-line (from perpendicular), placing the probe over a single rib, decreasing the depth setting, and/or decreasing the gain setting. If the depth and gain are decreased to visualize lung sliding, they should be re-adjusted (increased) to look for B-lines, the curtain sign, and lung consolidations (see below).
- Lung sliding can be difficult to identify in patients with rapid shallow breathing patterns that result in minimal movement of the lung across the chest wall (e.g., tachypnea/hyperpnea, panting).
- Diagnostic sensitivity/specificity is improved by keeping the probe steady and only interpreting lung sliding when the patient is not moving (movement creates a false positive).

Lung pulse

The lung pulse refers to rhythmic movement of the visceral pleura, which is visible at the P-line, when cardiac vibrations transmit through motionless lung (as occurs in the lung bypassed during endobronchial intubation, see below) (Video 18.3). It confirms that the parietal and visceral pleura are in apposition to one another.

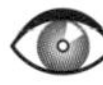

Therefore, the lung pulse has significant clinical implications as it can help rule out pneumothorax (see pneumothorax below) and may suggest endobronchial intubation or an obstructive bronchial foreign body when assessed in conjunction with lung sliding (see endobronchial intubation below) [61]. Note that the lung pulse is typically lost when lung sliding is present (lung sliding dominates the lung pulse), and when the visceral pleura are separated from the parietal pleura (e.g., pneumothorax, pleural effusion, and other space-occupying pleural space pathology) [58,61]. The lung pulse becomes more difficult to visualize in well-aerated lung tissue and in lung regions located distal to the heart [57,58]. In healthy dogs and cats, it is possible to identify the lung pulse during the respiratory pause between respirations, particularly when the probe is situated over the thorax and lung in proximity to the heart (Video 18.3).

A-lines

A-lines are a type of reverberation artifact appearing as hyperechoic (white) horizontal lines that run parallel and equidistant from the skin to the P-line below a soft tissue-to-air interface [54–58,59] (Fig. 18.4). They are created by the reflection of the ultrasound beam between two highly reflective surfaces: (1) the ultrasound probe and (2) the soft tissue–air interface at the P-line.

- The "A" in A-lines stands for air. A-lines are visible below the soft tissue–air interface created when air-filled lung contacts the chest wall, and when free gas occupies the pleural space (pneumothorax). It only requires a 2–3 mm depth of aerated lung to create a soft tissue–air interface. Therefore, lung pathology located more than 2–3 mm below the surface of aerated lung cannot be seen and only reverberation artifact and A-lines will be visualized [62].
- Although visualizing A-lines alone does not differentiate pneumothorax from air-filled lung, the combined identification of A-lines and lung sliding is a normal finding in healthy animals and suggests the lung surface, and likely underlying parenchymal lung tissue, is normal at that probe location, thus ruling out pneumothorax.

B-lines

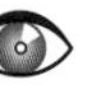

B-lines (Fig. 18.5) are a type of sonographic lung surface artifact that occur when there is decreased aerated lung (increased lung density) at the lung periphery (Video 18.4). Depending on the quantity identified at a single probe window and over an entire hemithorax, they may be a normal finding or may be representative of alveolar–interstitial pathology [63,64] (see increased B-lines below). In healthy individuals, they are believed to result from normal interlobar septa and/or regions with microatelectasis at the lung periphery [65]. They are defined by the following five criteria [54–56,58]: (1) vertical white/hyperechoic projections; (2) originating from the lung surface; (3) extending through the far field without fading; (4) swinging to-and-fro with lung sliding; and (5) often obliterating A-lines if present. If lung is in contact with the chest wall, B-lines originate at the P-line. Although 10–50% of healthy cats and dogs have isolated B-lines identified on PLUS, the majority of sonographically scannable lung surface will not contain B-lines [42,47,49,66–68]. If present, it is more common to see a single B-line at one to two locations on either hemithorax, or two B-lines at a single location when scanning the lung surfaces. Although rare, three B-lines have been reported at a single sonographic window of healthy cats and dogs [47,66]; however, the presence of three B-lines is rare and should not occur at multiple lung locations over the same hemithorax [47,66]. Finding more than two positive sites on either hemithorax, regardless of the number of B-lines at each site, should raise concern for underlying lung pathology [69]. Due to the variation in number of B-lines reported with different lung protocols in healthy animals, and the small number of studies in healthy dogs and cats reported to date, the clinical context must be considered when deciding if identified B-lines represent a normal finding or if lung pathology is likely (see increased B-lines below).

Abdominal curtain sign

The abdominal curtain sign (ACS) is a normal sonographic artifact of healthy animals that orientates the operator to the area of the thorax being viewed (caudolateral lung margin) and can be used to

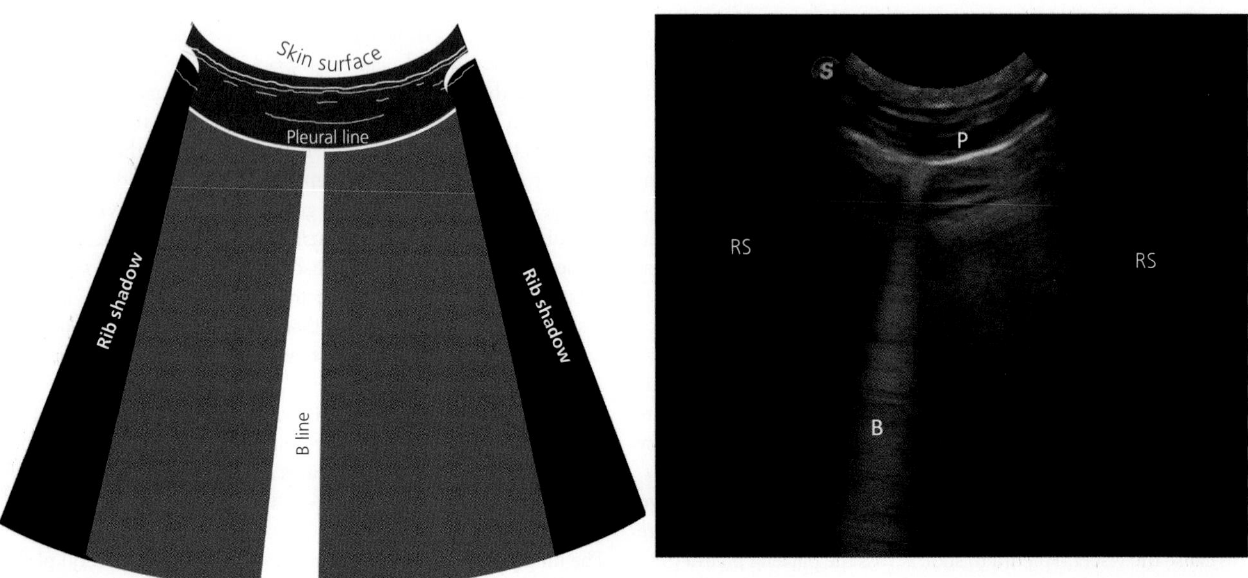

Figure 18.5 Schematic and still image of a single B-line originating at the lung surface from the pleural line when the lung is in contact with the chest wall. A single B-line can be a normal finding, although interpretation should always be within clinical context. RS, rib shadow; B, B-line; P, pleural line. Source: Dr. Søren Boysen, with permission.

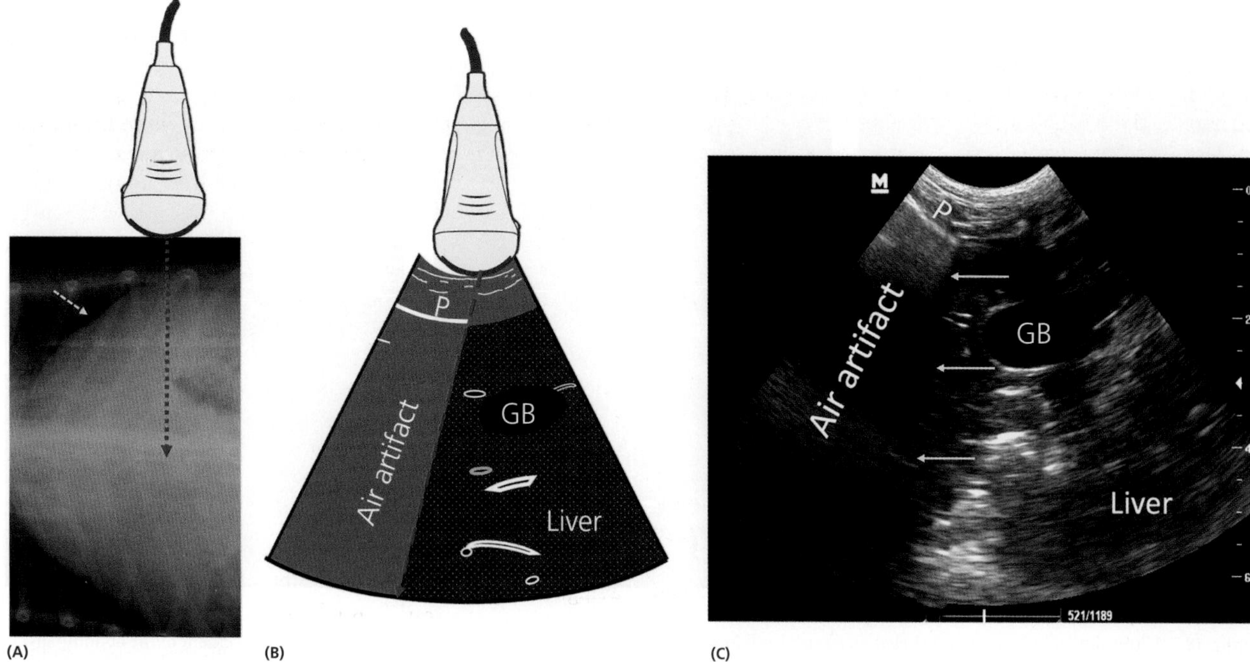

Figure 18.6 Radiographic, schematic, and still images of the location and sonographic appearance of a normal abdominal curtain sign (ACS) artifact. **A.** Thoracic radiograph of a dog showing the probe location to identify the ACS. The dotted red arrow represents the division where air-filled lung (left of arrow) overlies the soft tissue abdominal structures (right of arrow) at the costophrenic recess. The dotted white arrow shows the diaphragm curving away from the chest wall, which is not visible due to overlying air-filled lung. **B.** Schematic image showing ultrasonographic image with the probe positioned as shown in A. **C.** Still ultrasound image showing the normal vertical edge artifact (yellow arrows) of the ACS. P, pleural line; GB, gallbladder. Source: Dr. Søren Boysen, with permission.

identify pleural space (pneumothorax and pleural effusion) and lung (consolidation) pathology [51,58,70]. It is defined as the sharply demarcated vertical edge artifact that occurs along the caudolateral lung margins where air-filled lung overlies the diaphragm and soft tissues of the abdomen at the costophrenic recess [46,51,54,70]. The ACS is created by the combination of two factors: (1) the acoustic impedance mismatch between gas (air-filled lung) and adjacent soft tissue (abdominal structures) that casts the characteristic sharp vertical artifact at the interface between the two; and (2) the anatomical relationship of the thorax with the abdomen, resulting in the costophrenic recess covering parts of the cranial abdomen and the diaphragm, which abuts against air-filled lung cranially in healthy patients [46,51,54,58,70].

- When the ultrasound probe is positioned over both air-filled lung and soft tissue structures of the abdomen with the marker of the probe directed cranially, the cranial half of the image (lung) will not allow the ultrasound beam to extend past the P-line (A-lines often seen), while the caudal half of the image (soft tissue structures) transmits the beam, permitting soft tissue structures at that probe location to be visualized [58] (Fig. 18.6).
- During inspiration, the ACS and abdominal contents move caudally, and during expiration, the ACS and abdominal contents move cranially, in a synchronous manner [51,54,70] (Video 18.5). Do not confuse movement of the ACS with lung sliding (Fig. 18.7).

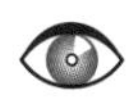

Abnormal PLUS findings

Ultrasound can only be used to interpret characteristics at the surface of a soft tissue–air interface because air/gas is a strong ultrasound beam reflector, making it difficult to visualize structures below the soft tissue–air interface. Therefore, pathology lying deep to the lung surface cannot be visualized. Fortunately, most (> 90%) alveolar–interstitial pathology (e.g., pulmonary edema, contusions, aspiration pneumonia, and fibrosis) results in B-lines and/or lung consolidations that are detectable at the lung surface with sonography [56,70] (Table 18.3).

Endobronchial tube placement

In human medicine, lung ultrasound has been used to diagnose endobronchial intubation with the advantage of being a rapid modality, compared to confirmation with thoracic radiography [61]. In humans, bronchial intubations occur in 5–15% of intended tracheal intubations in both pre-hospital and in-patient settings [71–75], and 6–25% of cases go unrecognized [71,76–78]. The consequences of single-lung intubation include suboptimal ventilation/oxygenation and barotrauma, which may result in pneumothorax and unilateral pulmonary edema [61,79]. The application of intended one-lung ventilation in small animals is well-established for the management of various underlying pathologies [80–83]. Although there are several techniques reported to confirm correct placement of one-lung devices in dogs and cats [82,84], the use of PLUS to assess bilateral versus unilateral lung intubation has not been studied, despite first being reported in human medicine in 2003 [61,85]. One-lung ventilation can be confirmed through detection of a lung pulse and the absence of lung sliding on the non-intubated side of the thorax. This contrasts with the presence of lung sliding (with or without a lung pulse) on the contralateral, intubated, side of the thorax (Fig.18.8). One-lung intubation is associated with atelectasis, which makes the lung pulse easier to visualize [57,58,61]. In contrast, endobronchial intubation is unlikely when bilateral lung sliding is present during respiration.

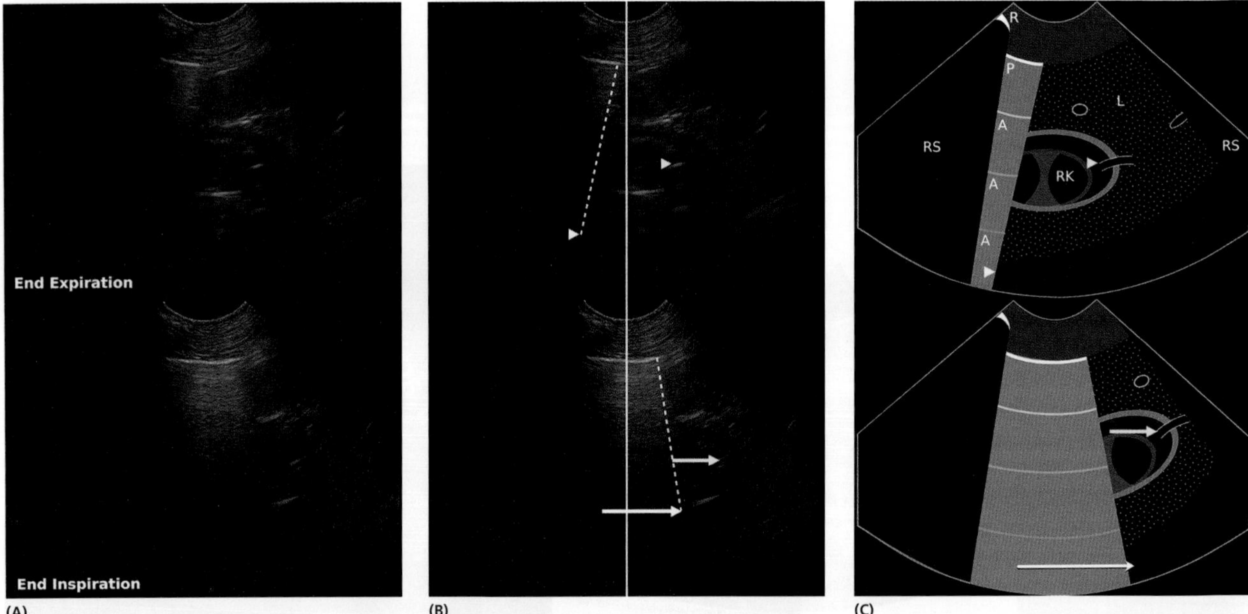

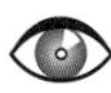

Figure 18.7 Ultrasound still images. **A.** Labeled ultrasound still images. **B.** and **C.** Schematic images showing the normal movement of the abdominal curtain sign during inspiration (bottom row) and expiration (top row). The ultrasound probe was positioned over the right paralumbar region at the level of the right kidney, over the liver, between the 11th and 12th intercostal spaces, and incorporates the air/soft tissue interface between the abdomen and the thorax, which appears as a vertical edge (abdominal curtain sign). The position of the abdominal curtain sign (white arrowhead) and abdominal contents (yellow arrowhead) at end-expiration are shown. During inspiration, the vertical edge of the curtain sign (vertical dotted white line) and the abdominal contents move caudally (white and yellow arrows, respectively). Although the curtain sign may move more than the abdominal contents, the two move in the same direction during the same phases of respiration. Dashed lines represent vertical edges (air/soft tissue interface). Solid line represents center of image; R, rib; RS, rib shadow; P, pleural line; A, A-line; L, liver; RK, right kidney; Arrow shows direction of movement of the vertical edge during inspiration (also see Video 18.5). Source: Boysen *et al.* [46], with permission from Frontiers Media S.A. / CC BY 4.0.

Table 18.3 Causes of diffuse and localized B-lines along with common history and clinical findings.

Multiple diffuse bilateral B-lines	Focal /unilateral/localized B-lines
Interstitial pneumonia or pneumonitis (e.g., lymphocytic interstitial pneumonitis, eosinophilic pneumonia, and drug reactions)	Focal pneumonia/pneumonitis, particularly aspiration: often a history of vomiting
Pulmonary edema – cardiogenic or non-cardiogenic: heart murmur common with cardiogenic causes, may have history of seizures, chewing an electrical cord, upper airway obstruction, or smoke inhalation	Pulmonary contusions: often a history of trauma
Diffuse parenchymal lung disease (e.g., pulmonary fibrosis)	Atelectasis: often a history of prolonged recumbency and/or anesthesia
Acute respiratory distress syndrome: may have spared lung regions	Pleural disease: interpret B-lines cautiously when pleural effusion is present as compression atelectasis can result in B-lines
	Neoplasia: often associated with sonographic areas of focal lung consolidation, particularly nodules

Pneumothorax

Human studies demonstrate a sensitivity and specificity of 87% and 97%, respectively, with lung ultrasound, and 28% and 100%, respectively, with thoracic radiography for identification of pneumothorax [86]. The clinical accuracy of ultrasound to diagnose pneumothorax in companion animals is unclear and determination of sensitivity and specificity is hindered by a failure to compare findings with accepted reference standards, and/or by the inclusion of only small case numbers [6,36,42,46,58,87–89]. For example, recent studies comparing the veterinary bedside lung ultrasound exam (VetBLUE) or TFAST protocols to computed tomography (CT) correctly identified pneumothorax in 3/7, 3/6, and 1/6 cases, respectively [6,87,89]. A well-controlled experimental study that induced small-volume pneumothorax (2–10 mL/kg of air) in dogs under anesthesia (n = 9) suggests lung ultrasound is more sensitive (89% versus 67%) and equally specific (89%) to radiographs compared with CT when multiple lung ultrasound criteria are combined to diagnose pneumothorax in dogs; however, translation of these findings to patients with naturally occurring and larger-volume pneumothorax in the clinical setting has not been performed [88]. There is even less information available regarding lung ultrasound to diagnose pneumothorax in cats, with only two small clinical studies that were combined with findings from dogs, neither of which reported any cats with confirmed pneumothorax [87,89]. The accuracy of ultrasound to diagnose pneumothorax likely depends on the experience of the sonographer, underlying pathology, patient positioning, scanning protocol, and criteria used to diagnose pneumothorax [36,42,78,87,89]. If the pleura is in contact, pneumothorax is ruled out. The following sonographic findings confirm the pleura is in apposition below the probe (Fig. 18.9): (1) detection of lung sliding and/or a lung pulse, and (2) detection of B-lines and/or lung consolidation (see below) arising from the P-line [58,88].

The absence of all these signs should prompt consideration of a pneumothorax (Video 18.6); however, lung sliding is not always easy to detect, the lung pulse may be lost with aerated lung or may not be visible distal to the heart, and B-lines and lung consolidation are often not seen in healthy animals. In human medicine the

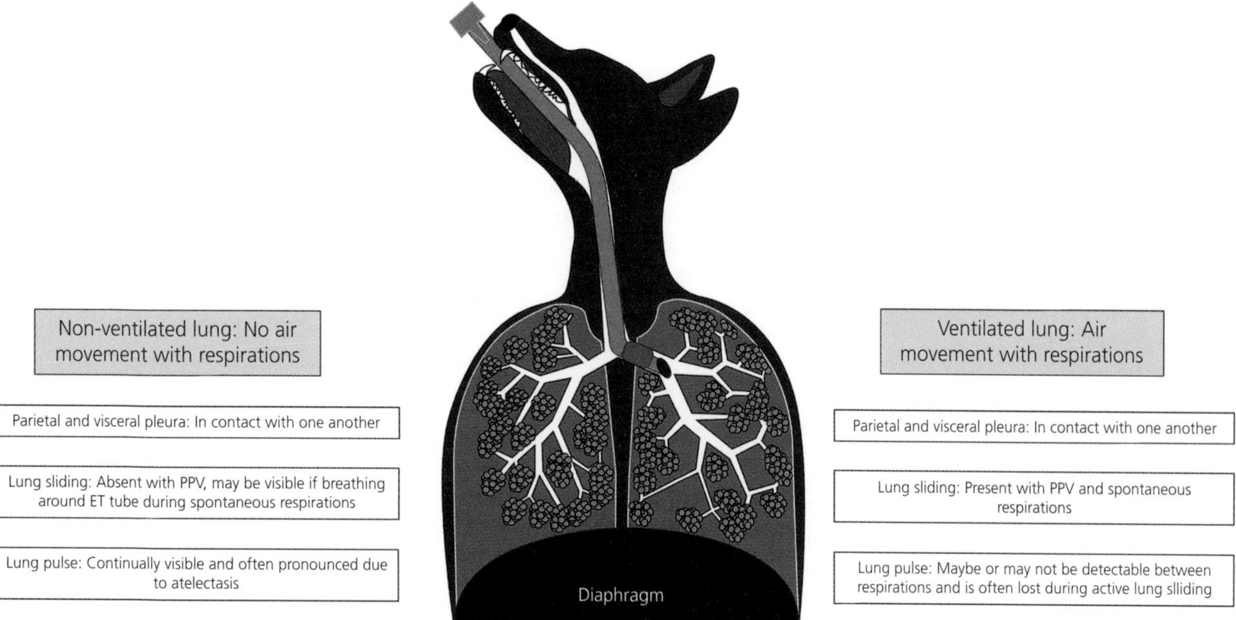

Figure 18.8 Schematic image depicting one-lung intubation and a comparison of the two hemithoraces with regards to the sonographic identification of the lung pulse and lung sliding during spontaneous and positive-pressure ventilation (PPV). ET, endotracheal. Source: Dr. Søren Boysen, with permission.

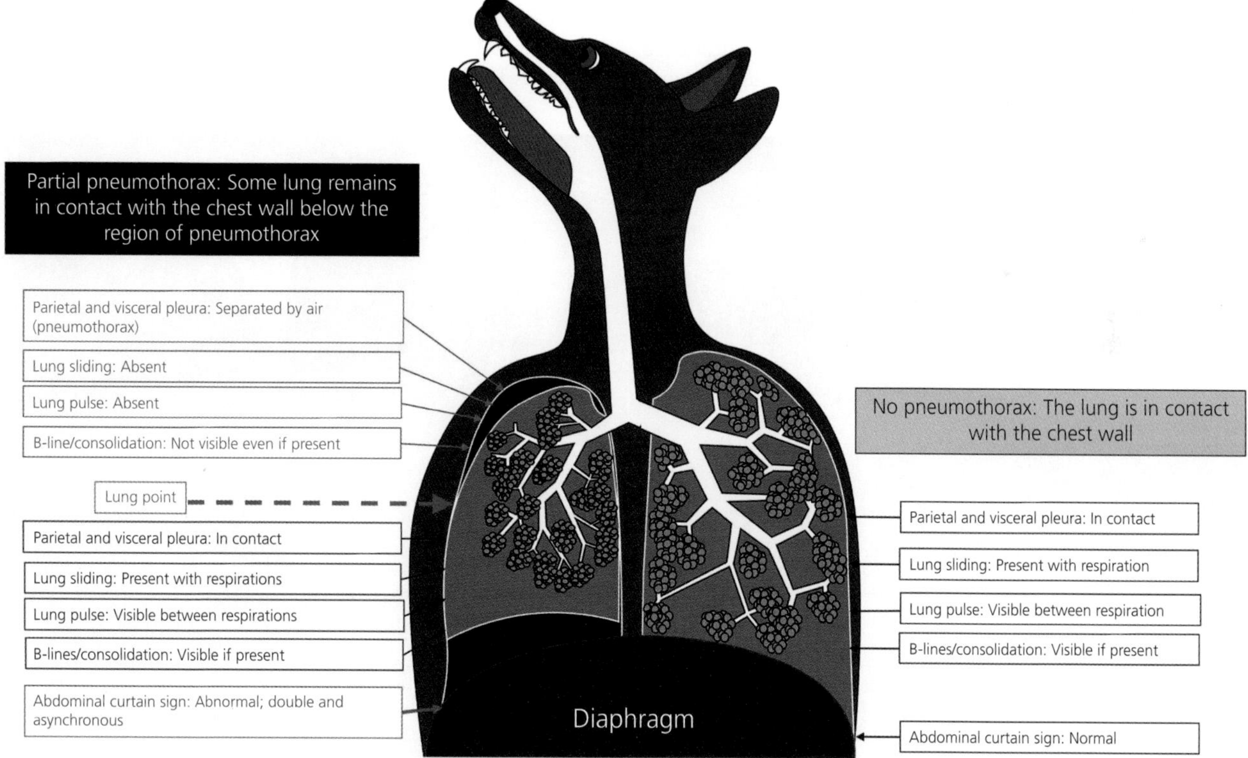

Figure 18.9 Schematic image of the sonographic finding on either side of the chest when a moderate unilateral pneumothorax is present (pneumothorax shown in black). Each arrow represents different sonographic findings when the probe is placed over an area where there is a pneumothorax, and where there is lung in contact with the chest wall. The location of the abdominal curtain sign (ACS) is also shown. A pneumothorax will often result in an abnormal ACS due to free pleural gas interacting with the costophrenic recess when it displaces the lung lobe cranially. With massive pneumothorax where lung fails to recontact the chest wall, there will not be a lung point and there will be an absence of B-lines/consolidation, lung pulse, and lung sliding over the entire hemithorax. Source: Dr. Søren Boysen, with permission.

positive predictive value of absent lung sliding for the detection of pneumothorax is 87% in the general population, falls to 56% in the critically ill, and to 27% in patients with respiratory failure [51,59,90,91]. If the history and clinical exam are supportive, thoracocentesis is indicated when lung sliding, lung pulse, and lung pathology are not visible, particularly when assessed at locations where free pleural gas is likely to accumulate (widest part of the thorax with a patient in lateral recumbency, caudodorsal site with a patient in sternal recumbency or standing). If the patient is sufficiently stable, the operator may increase the likelihood of diagnosing pneumothorax by finding the lung point (Video 18.7) and/or an abnormal ACS (Video 18.8) [46,58,88]. The lung point is the location within the thorax where the lung re-contacts the parietal pleura and creates an intermittent or partial glide sign within a section of the ultrasound image when the patient breathes [58,54]. The lung point is located by moving the probe from an area with no perceived lung sliding toward the hilus, where lung sliding reappears within a region of the ultrasound window [54,58]. In the standing or sternal patient, the probe is often moved from the caudodorsal lung regions toward the elbow. The lung point will not be seen if the lung fails to recontact the chest wall (massive/complete pneumothorax), and has an overall sensitivity of 66%, and a specificity of 100% in human patients [54]. An experimental study of anesthetized dogs demonstrated a sensitivity of 20% and 40% and specificity of 100% for the lung point to diagnose pneumothorax with volumes of 2 and 10 mL/kg of pleural air, respectively [88].

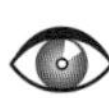

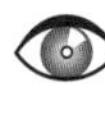

Abnormalities of the ACS identified with pneumothorax include asynchronous and double curtain signs [46]. The *asynchronous curtain sign* is defined as the cranial movement of the vertical edge artifact (created by free pleural gas versus air-filled lung overlying the diaphragm and soft tissue structures of the abdomen at the costophrenic recess) with concomitant caudal movement of abdominal contents during the inspiratory phase of the respiratory cycle, with the opposite movements occurring during expiration (Fig. 18.10; Video 18.8). This creates the appearance of the curtain sign and abdominal contents moving toward each other on inspiration and away from each other on expiration, the opposite of what is expected with a normal ACS.

The *double curtain sign* is defined as two parallel vertical abdominal edge artifacts visible in Figure 18.11 and Video 18.8. Of note, all three types of ACS (normal, double, and asynchronous) have been identified over each hemithorax in dogs with pneumothorax, with normal ACS visible in the ventral third of the thorax. However, these abnormal ACSs have only been described in dogs with mild to moderate degrees of pneumothorax, and extrapolation of these findings to larger-volume pneumothorax is unknown [46]. The accuracy of an abnormal ACS was not reported, and only six dogs have been investigated, suggesting further research regarding the use/presence of an abnormal ACS to diagnose pneumothorax is needed [46].

Pleural effusion

In human medicine, ultrasound has a sensitivity and specificity of 92–100% and 88–100% for the detection of pleural effusion, respectively, when compared to CT [34]. Similar to pneumothorax, the accuracy of diagnosing pleural effusion using POCUS in veterinary patients is variable and limited by a lack of controlled, prospective studies and small sample sizes [6,45,89]. Recent studies comparing VetBLUE and TFAST protocols to CT correctly identified pleural effusion in 2/3 and 3/6 cases, respectively [87,89]. Pleural effusion appears as hypoechoic accumulations between the thoracic wall,

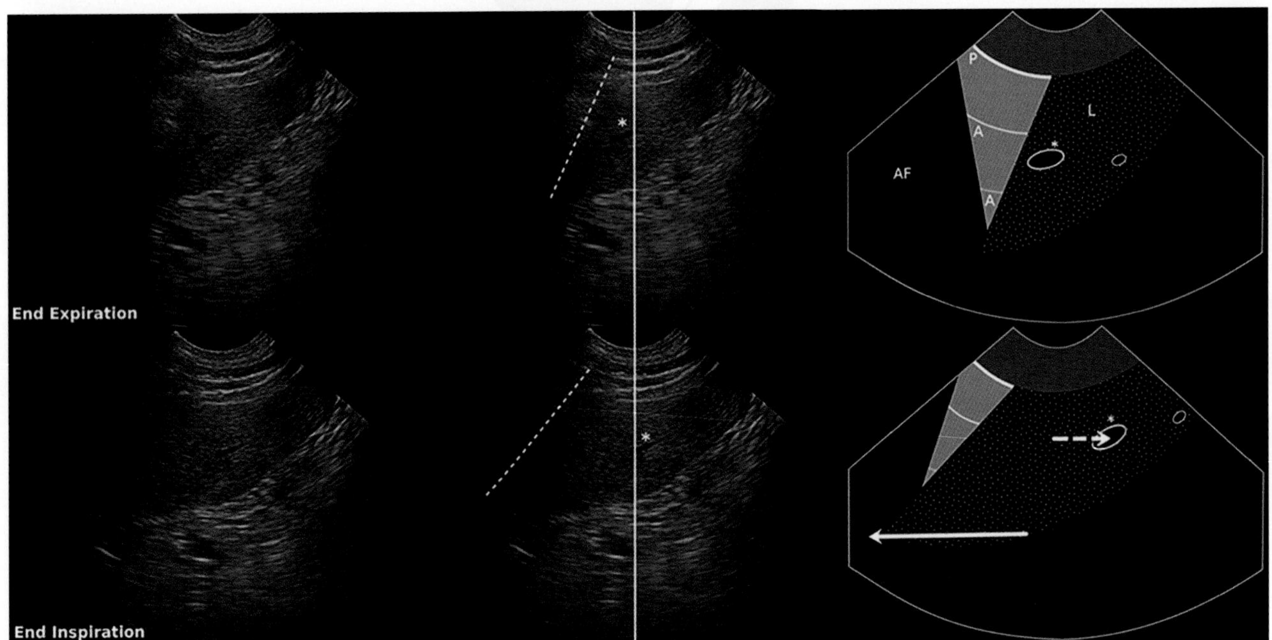

Figure 18.10 Still images and schematic of an asynchronous curtain sign at end-expiration (top row) and end-inspiration (bottom row). The ultrasound probe was positioned over the right paralumbar region just below the right kidney, over the liver, between the 9th and 10th intercostal spaces, and incorporates the air/soft tissue interface between the abdomen and the thorax, which appears as a vertical edge (curtain sign). During inspiration, the vertical edge of the curtain sign moves in the opposite direction (cranially) of the abdominal contents (caudally). Dashed lines represent vertical edges (air/soft tissue interface). Solid line represents center of image. P, pleural line; A, A-line; L, liver; asterisk "*", hepatic vessel. Solid arrow shows direction of movement of the vertical edge during inspiration. Dashed arrow shows direction of movement of the abdominal contents during inspiration. Length of arrow represents degree of movement relative to the image above (also see Video 18.8). Source: Boysen *et al.* [46], with permission from Frontiers Media S.A. / CC BY 4.0.

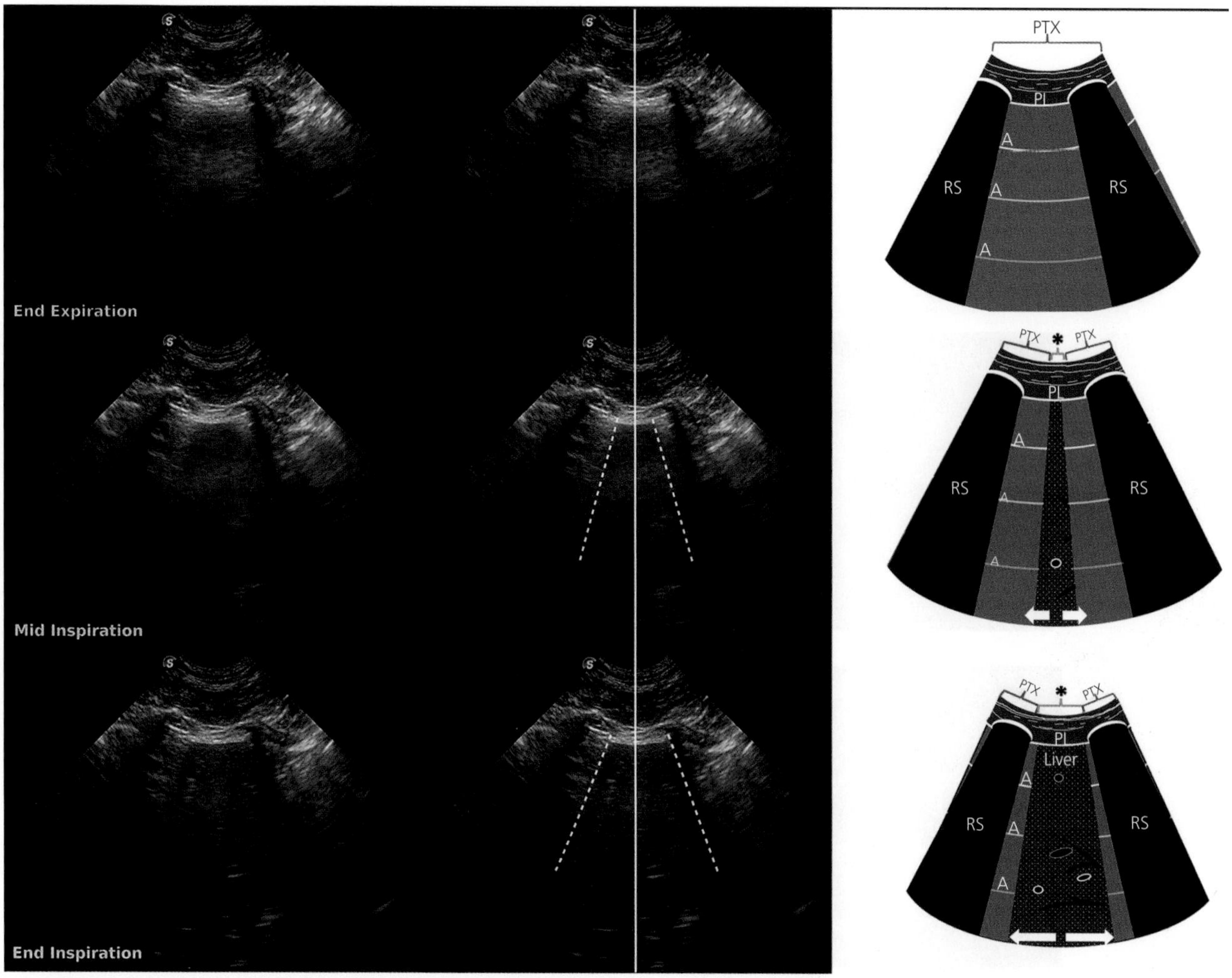

End Expiration

Mid Inspiration

End Inspiration

PTX

PTX ✱ PTX

PL

A

RS

Liver

Figure 18.11 Still images and schematic of a double curtain sign at end-expiration (top row), mid-inspiration (middle row), and end-inspiration (bottom row). The ultrasound probe is located over the liver, about halfway up the thorax, between the 7th and 8th intercostal spaces, over the air/soft tissue interface between the abdomen and the thorax. During inspiration, two vertical edges of the curtain sign are visible in the same sonographic window. The asterisk "*" represents a region where the probe is situated over the diaphragm and associated underlying soft tissue structures at the costophrenic recess. Dashed lines represent vertical edges (air/soft tissue interface). Solid line represents center of image. R, rib; RS, rib shadow; P, pleural line; A, A-line; L, liver. Arrows show movement of the vertical edges in opposite directions during inspiration in this example. Length of arrow represents degree of movement relative to the image above (also see Video 18.8). Source: Boysen *et al.* [46], with permission from Frontiers Media S.A. / CC BY 4.0.

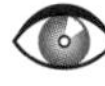

diaphragm, and lung surfaces. Its appearance varies with the cellularity and quantity of the effusion, probe location, patient positioning, and the presence of adhesions. In dogs and cats, pleural effusion is generally identified via transthoracic and subxiphoid windows. Locating the pericardio-diaphragmatic (PD) window transthoracically helps differentiate pleural effusion from pericardial effusion. The PD window is identified when the probe is positioned such that the heart and ACS or diaphragm are visible within the same sonographic window (Fig. 18.12).

With smaller volume effusions, fluid occupies the costophrenic angle/recess, causing minimal compressive atelectasis of the surrounding lung tissue. In this scenario, the dynamic motion of the air-filled lung expanding across the pleural effusion and soft tissue abdominal structures is still seen; however, the ACS does not overlap the costophrenic recess as much as in the absence of effusion [51,54]. The diaphragm can be seen curving away from the chest wall due to the presence of pleural effusion accumulating within the costophrenic recess [51,54]. As the quantity of effusion increases, the lung progressively covers less and less of the costophrenic recess, even uncovering it on inspiration, and the lungs may become atelectatic, appearing as floating tissue-like structures (termed the "jellyfish" sign in human medicine) [54,70,91]. In contrast to pleural effusion, pericardial effusion is contained and curves away from the diaphragm following the contour of the heart. To identify very small to scant volumes of pleural effusion that might not cause respiratory distress, but might be diagnostically important to sample and analyze, the most ventral pleural regions between the sternal muscles and the lung should be assessed from the diaphragm to the thoracic inlet, with the patient in a sternal or standing position (Fig. 18.13) [46]. The ventral pleural regions can be identified by placing the probe parallel to the ribs in the ventral third of the thorax and sliding the probe ventrally until the sternal muscles become visible within the ultrasound image (Fig. 18.13).

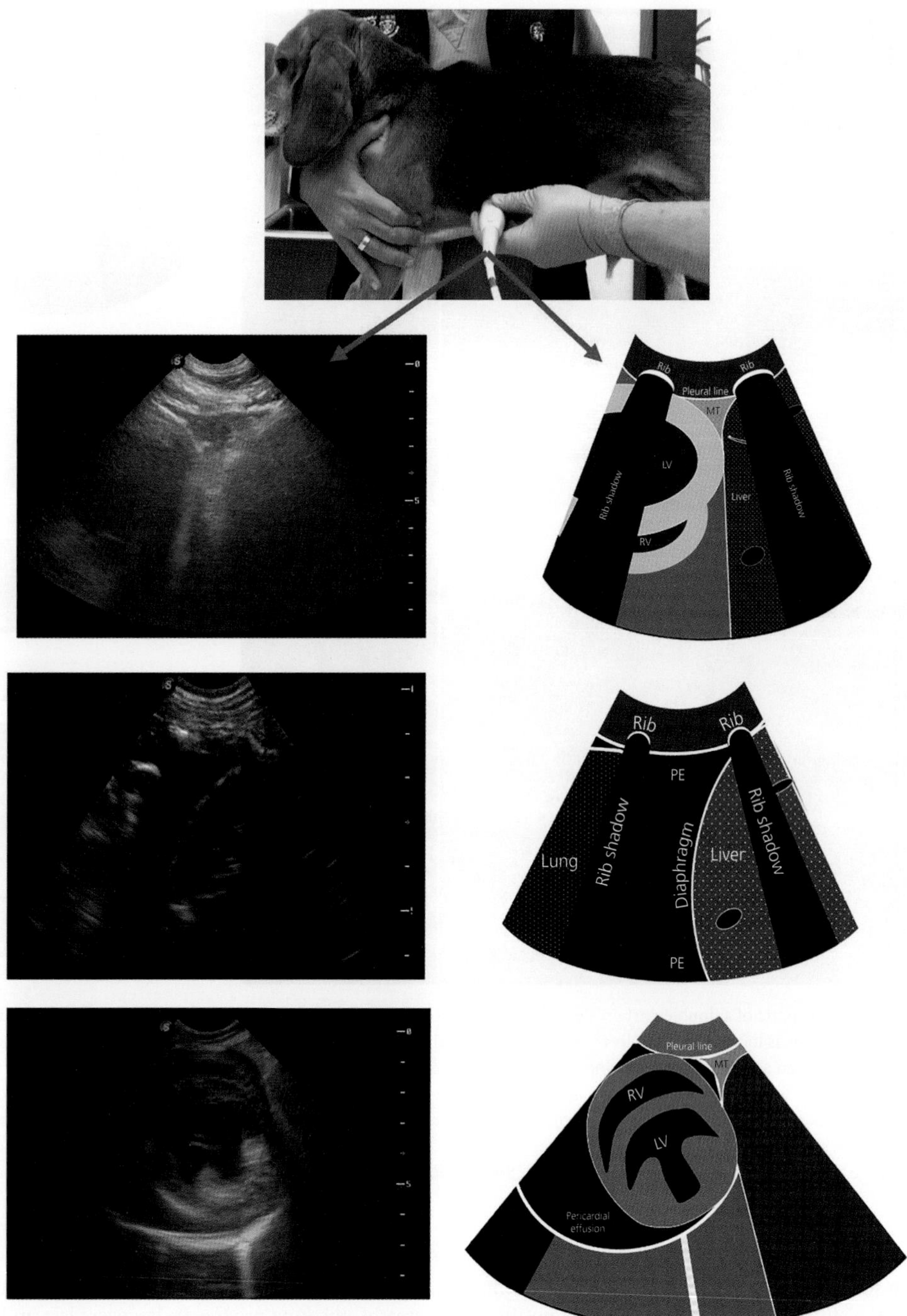

Figure 18.12 Photograph, still, and schematic images of the location, normal appearance, and abnormal findings identified at the pericardio-diaphragmatic (PD) window. (Top) Photograph of a dog demonstrating the location of the probe to find the PD window. (2nd row) Still (left) and schematic image (right) showing the normal appearance of the PD window when the heart and diaphragm are visible within the same image. (3rd row) Still (left) and schematic image (right) of pleural effusion. (4th row) Still (left) and schematic image (right) of pericardial effusion, which is easily differentiated from pleural effusion at this location. PE, pleural effusion; MT, mediastinal triangle; LV, left ventricle; RV, right ventricle. Source: Dr. Søren Boysen, with permission.

Increased B-lines

If > 3 B-lines are visible in a single sonographic window, alveolar interstitial syndrome (AIS) should be considered (Fig. 18.14) (Video 18.9). B-lines are a sensitive marker of injury and appear concurrent with loss of lung aeration; in some instances, before gas exchange deterioration [92]. B-lines are an early and sensitive finding of increased lung density [53,92–95]. In cases of pulmonary edema, their presence or absence may guide fluid administration [96,97]. It has been proposed that their appearance warrants fluid caution or restriction, particularly if serial monitoring is performed in patients receiving IV fluids. In contrast, B-lines disappear with successful treatment of pulmonary edema. Monitoring B-lines serially for progression or resolution may also help determine if B-lines are a normal variation or if true pathology is present.

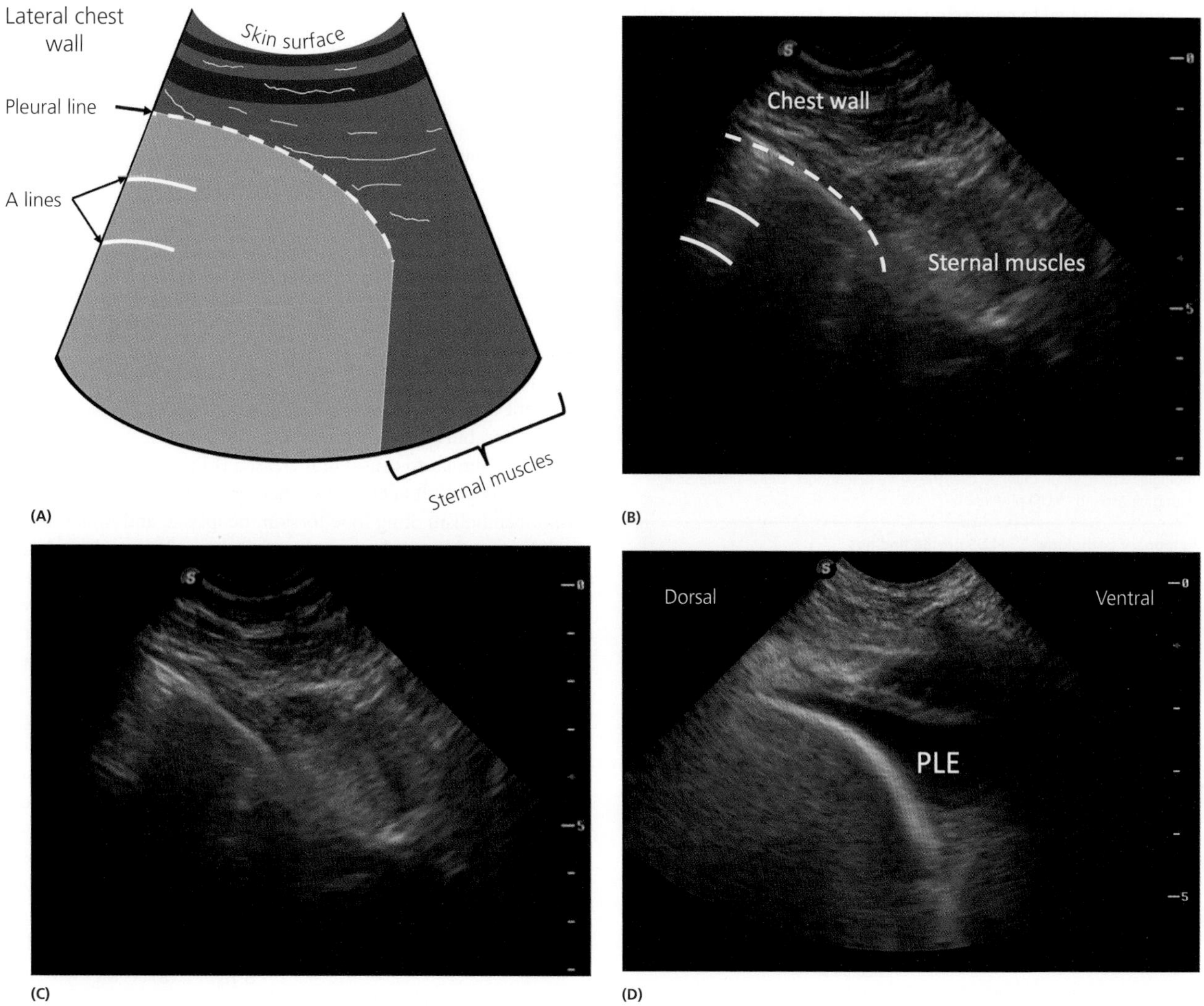

Figure 18.13 Schematic and still ultrasound images of the lung, pleura, and sternal muscle interfaces. **A–C.** Schematic, labeled still, and unlabeled still ultrasound image of a healthy patient. **D.** Labeled still image of pleural effusion (PLE) located ventrally between the sternal muscles and lung. Source: Dr. Søren Boysen, with permission.

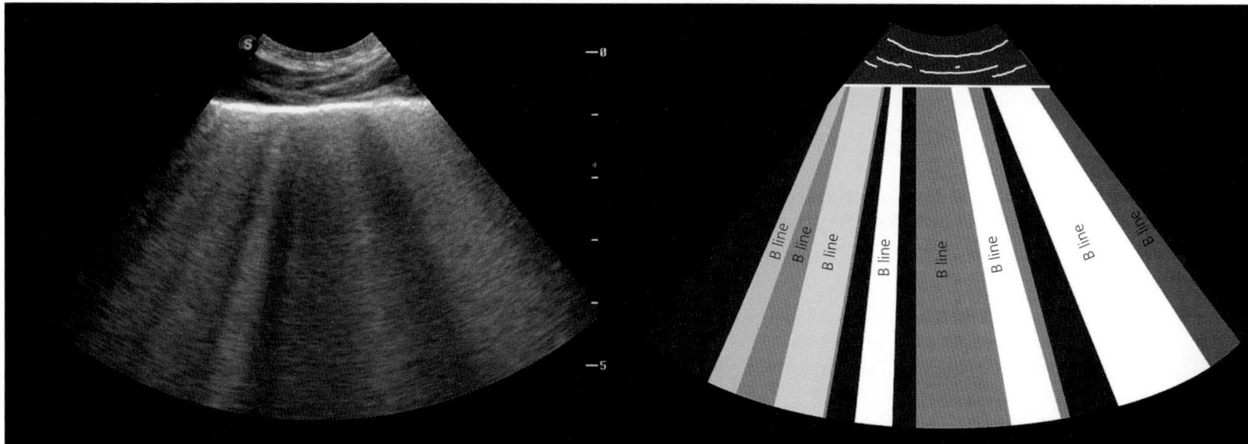

Figure 18.14 Increased to coalescing B-lines. Note the absence of ribs above the pleural line and the absence of rib shadows because the probe is orientated parallel and between two ribs. The finding of > 3 B-lines in any sonographic window is considered abnormal. Source: Dr. Søren Boysen, with permission.

Multiple individual to coalescing B-lines (> 3 per sonographic window, or > 2 positive sites on a hemithorax) should raise suspicion of increased lung density at the lung periphery [47,49,66], often referred to as "wet lung" [47,89]. "Wet lung" is, however, a misnomer; although increased extravascular lung water (EVLW) is the most common cause of increased B-lines, any process that increases lung density, including atelectasis, fibrosis, collagen, neoplastic cells, and inflammatory cells [54,64,92] can result in increased B-lines. Given atelectasis occurs in recumbent animals and patients undergoing general anesthesia, knowing the cause of increased B-lines is important, as therapy differs depending on the cause. History, concurrent diagnostic testing, and mapping the entire PLUS profile by scanning multiple lung regions bilaterally help determine the underlying cause (Table 18.4).

Table 18.4 Sonographic findings seen with different pleural space and lung pathologies which, when mapped over the entire hemithorax, create pleural space and lung ultrasound (PLUS) profiles.

Pulmonary pathology	PLUS profile findings (often combined with CVC and cardiac findings)
Pneumothorax	Absent lung sliding, lung pulse, B-lines, consolidation Lung point (often difficult to sonographically identify) Abnormal curtain signs (asynchronous/double) A-lines visible (parietal pleura reflection)
Pleural effusion	Absent lung sliding Visible separation of the parietal and visceral pleura (may need to extend depth if large pleural effusion is present) ± B-lines and consolidations arising from the lung surface, deep to pleural effusion ± "Jellyfish" sign
Pneumonia	Shred signs, translobar signs Thickened irregular pleura Subpleural consolidation Unilateral or bilateral B-lines Possible small-volume pleural effusion Reduced lung sliding due to consolidations in severe cases Dynamic air bronchograms ± Static air bronchograms ± Fluid bronchograms
Cardiogenic pulmonary edema and fluid overload	Widespread and bilateral B-lines Coalescing B-lines with increasing severity Normal lung sliding Possible bilateral effusion depending on the severity and species (e.g., more common in cats) *Enlarged left atrium present (LA:Ao often > 2:1) *CVC may be enlarged if right heart also affected Note: the absence of B-lines in the dyspneic patient rules out cardiogenic pulmonary edema – search for other causes of respiratory distress
Acute respiratory distress syndrome (ARDS)	Bilateral or unilateral B-lines Normal lung sliding Shred signs, translobar signs Mixed pattern with spared regions
Feline asthma	A-lines visible Reduced lung sliding with overinflation ± B-lines and consolidation, particularly if right middle lung lobe affected
Pulmonary embolism (PE)	Normal lung sliding ± Wedge sign *Right ventricular enlargement and a distended CVC may be seen with massive/submassive PE
Atelectasis	Partial and translobar consolidation B-lines often visible ± Static air bronchograms Absence of dynamic bronchograms Reduced lung volume – easy to detect with compressive atelectasis secondary to pleural effusion

CVC, caudal vena cava; LA:Ao, left atrial to aortic root ratio; PE, pulmonary embolism

Lung consolidation

Healthy lung comprises roughly 85–95 % air and 5–15 % non-aerated tissue [55,59,62,63,98]. A change in the ratio of aerated to non-aerated lung within 1–3 mm of the lung surface results in specific abnormal lung ultrasound findings, mainly increased B-lines and lung consolidation. When there is sufficient air within the lung tissue at its periphery (>10% lung aeration), the soft tissue–air interface at the P-line is maintained and the ultrasound beam is reflected from the lung surface, rendering the lung invisible [62]. In this situation, it is only possible to visualize lung pathology through interpretation of lung surface artifacts such as increased B-lines [55,59,62,63,98]. When the ratio of aerated to non-aerated lung tissue directly below the visceral pleura falls below 5–10% (i.e., 90% consolidation), the acoustic impedance between the thoracic wall and lung is decreased to a point the lung ultrasound beam is no longer reflected from the lung surface, but is instead transmitted through the underlying lung tissue [97]. Similar to causes of increased B-lines, lung consolidation can occur as a result of atelectasis, hemorrhage, bronchopneumonia, thromboembolism, lung lobe torsion, neoplasia, and inflammatory conditions such as pulmonary contusions and acute lung injury. Unlike B-lines, which can occasionally be normal and will increase with even mild increases in lung density, consolidation is always abnormal and only occurs when pathology is severe enough that the ultrasound beam can traverse lung tissue. Consolidation can be translobar (traversing the entire lung lobe from one surface to the other), or partial (partial thickness, where the consolidated region within the lobe encounters air-filled lung distal to the consolidated region) [59,70]. Although many pathologies can result in consolidation, most will result in three common ultrasonographic appearances (Table 18.5):

1 "Shred" sign – Partial lung consolidation. This occurs when there is a focal area of consolidated lung in apposition to underlying (deeper) air-filled lung. The boundary between consolidated and aerated lung appears "shredded" (fractal/shredded border). Often seen with inflammatory lung pathology (e.g., acute lung injury and aspiration pneumonia).
2 "Nodule" sign – Partial lung consolidation. Differs from the shred sign in that the distal border between the consolidation and aerated lung is often well-defined, smooth, and circular. The differential diagnoses for nodule signs are similar to those for

Table 18.5 Classification of lung consolidation and common differential diagnoses.

Partial consolidation	Ultrasound appearance	Differential diagnoses
Shred	Appears as if "chunks" removed from the lung creating echo-poor areas; junction from consolidated lung to aerated lung very irregular, hyperechoic, serrated, and blurred, creating a "shred-like" appearance similar to a "torn" or shredded piece of paper	Pneumonia Hemorrhage Inflammatory-associated increases in extravascular lung water (e.g., ARDS) Thromboembolic disease Neoplasia
Nodule	Smooth hypoechoic or moderately echogenic region; well delineated, often has semicircular, oval, to circular deep boundary	Fungal Primary or metastatic neoplasia Abscesses
Wedge	Wedge-shaped and often well delineated	Pulmonary thromboembolism Not specific and may result from other pathologies causing shred signs

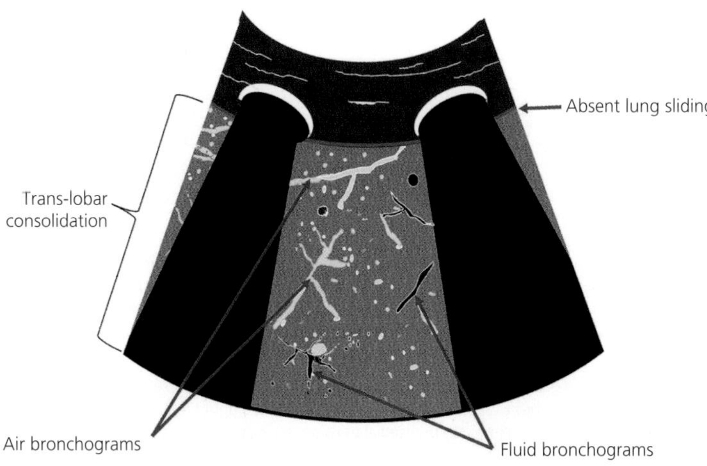

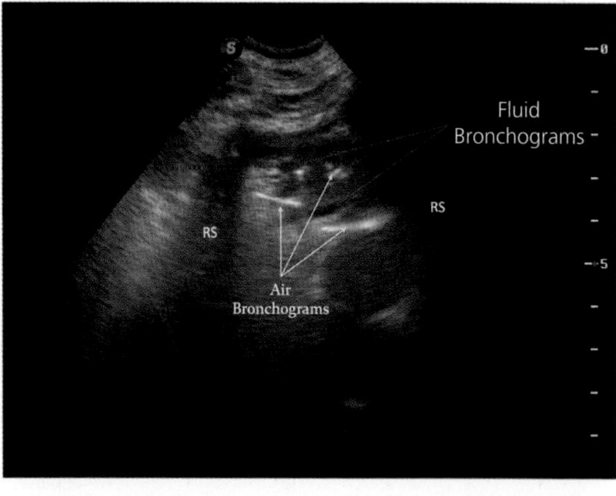

Figure 18.15 Schematic and still image of air bronchograms. White punctate and linear structures within consolidated lung represent bronchi that still contain air (air bronchograms) and black punctate and linear structures represent fluid filling the bronchi (fluid bronchograms). Note that lung sliding tends to be lost with consolidated lung as the soft tissue–air interface is lost. The still image shows mixed fluid and air bronchograms in the same pathologic lung region. Source: Dr. Søren Boysen, with permission.

radiographic nodules, with neoplasia and fungal disease being the more common causes.

3 "Hepatization" – Translobar lung consolidation. The entire width of lung lobe is filled with fluid, cells, or tissue, and/or contains no air (complete atelectasis), which creates a "tissue-like" pattern. The term "hepatization" is often used as the lung takes on a similar sonographic appearance to liver.

The "wedge" sign is reported in the human literature and is often associated with pulmonary thromboembolism when identified in patients with concurrent deep vein thrombosis. The wedge sign and its significance have not been well documented in small animals.

Air bronchograms

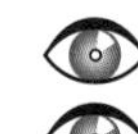

The sonographic appearance of lung consolidation, particularly shred and translobar consolidation, varies depending on whether the smaller airways contain air (air bronchogram, Fig. 18.15, Video 18.10) or are fluid-filled (fluid bronchogram, Fig. 18.15, Video 18.10) [99,100]. Air bronchograms appear as punctate or linear hyperechoic foci visible between the hyperechoic walls of bronchi [99,100]. Fluid bronchograms can be difficult to differentiate from pulmonary vessels, although some may have air visible in addition to fluid, which helps confirm their presence. Doppler imaging, in conjunction with breath holding, is used in human medicine to differentiate vessels and fluid bronchograms.

In veterinary patients, differentiation of the two is challenging as it can be difficult to obtain optimal views. It is possible to find mixed fluid and air bronchograms within the same consolidated region of lung or in different regions of the same lung lobe. In human medicine, air bronchograms help classify the type of consolidation and possibly the underlying cause. When bronchioles within consolidated lung remain patent, communicating with the large airways, changes in air movement (> 1 mm) with tidal volume can create visible movement of air within smaller airways [99,100]. This movement of air within the small airways creates a "shimmering" referred to as a "dynamic air bronchogram," and appears similar to the shimmer of lung sliding (Video 18.10). Dynamic air bronchograms are most often seen with pneumonia and inflammatory causes of lung consolidation. In contrast, static air bronchograms are often seen with atelectasis but can also be seen with inflammatory causes of lung consolidation, including acute respiratory distress syndrome (ARDS) and aspiration pneumonia. A complete lack of air bronchograms is suggestive of complete atelectasis, although severe pneumonia or lobar hemorrhage cannot be excluded.

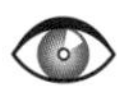

Abdominal point-of-care ultrasound

Veterinary abdominal point-of-care ultrasound (APOCUS) has expanded from the original FAST scan in trauma patients and searching for free abdominal fluid to become a clinical tool for the management and diagnosis of any patient with suspected abdominal pathology [1–3,101–112] (Table 18.6). Basic ultrasound knowledge of abdominal organ anatomy is essential; however, a detailed assessment of organs should be performed by a radiologist if abnormal parenchymal organ structure is detected [113–117]. Most veterinary APOCUS questions can be answered by assessing five windows of the abdomen, which is the authors' preferred general APOCUS approach (5-point APOCUS, Fig. 18.16). To answer questions rapidly, but thoroughly, at least two sonographic planes (short and long axis), with fanning and rocking probe movements should be performed at each window [1,2,87]. It is important to remember that APOCUS windows and regions assessed should be adapted based on the clinical setting encountered. For example, patient positioning can impact where some pathologies accumulate (fluid falls and gas rises), and APOCUS should be performed and adapted to patient positioning in order to maximize the chances of detecting pathology. The specific goal-directed questions and key organs to assess at each window are listed in Table 18.6 and illustrated in Fig. 18.16.

In human anesthesia, APOCUS has been used to look for free abdominal fluid, particularly in patients with sudden clinical deterioration, such as hypotension [116–118], to stratify patients at risk for pulmonary aspiration (through gastric volume assessment), and to monitor urinary bladder volume.

Gastric volume

Gastric APOCUS is applied in humans as a limited examination to assess gastric content (empty, anechoic "clear" fluid, hyperechoic "thick" fluid/solid), and volume, with the ultimate goal of assessing pulmonary aspiration risk [119–121]. The findings from gastric

Table 18.6 Clinically driven questions that can be answered in small animals with a 5-point abdominal POCUS (APOCUS) exam, scanning through multiple planes in both short- and long-axis orientations at each window.

APOCUS window	Clinically driven question(s) to answer	Interpretation	Clinical significance
All five sites	Pneumoperitoneum	Reverberation artifact not originating within the lumen of the gastrointestinal tract, enhanced peritoneal strip sign if free gas contacts the peritoneal lining; be sure to assess the most gravity-independent sites.	Pneumoperitoneum in patients who have not undergone laparotomy is abnormal and hollow organ rupture should be ruled out. Free gas reverberation artifact often obliterates structures below it.
	Free abdominal fluid	Free fluid appears as dark (anechoic or hypoechoic) triangles/sharp angles between organs and structures; be sure to thoroughly evaluate each site considering patient position and where fluid will accumulate.	Obtain fluid samples for in-house analysis (cytology, refractometer, parameters of sepsis or uroabdomen), which may dictate immediate interventions (surgery, antibiotics, transfusion, etc.). Consider sample submission to reference laboratory (cytology, culture) if indicated.
Subxiphoid	Gallbladder halo sign	Thickening of the normally very thin gallbladder wall that forms a classic striated white, black, white pattern due to edema of the gallbladder wall.	Nonspecific findings but in the unstable patient often seen with anaphylaxis, increased right atrial pressures (heart failure, pericardial effusion, fluid overload), and sepsis.
	Caudal vena cava (CVC) size and index	Assess for the cardiac pulse, overall size at end-expiration, as well as the change in diameter during the respiratory cycle.	A small CVC that fully collapses, or that changes more than 50% is often the result of hypovolemia. A distended CVC that loses the cardiac pulse and changes less than 25% suggests increased right atrial pressures, including fluid overload.
	Pericardial effusion	Identified beyond the diaphragm as contained anechoic fluid that curves away from the diaphragm and around the apex of the heart.	Confirms pericardial effusion and differentiates it from pleural effusion.
	Pleural effusion	Results in loss of mirror image artifact and appears as uncontained anechoic fluid that tracks along the diaphragm.	Confirms pleural effusion and differentiates it from pericardial effusion, although centesis and fluid analysis are required to determine the fluid type.
	Caudal lung pathology	B-lines and lung consolidation can be detected (if present) in the caudal lung lobes, which are not accessible transthoracically.	See increased B-lines and consolidations.
	Gastric motility	Peristaltic movement of ingesta within the lumen or propagation of a wave along the serosal surface.	Often assessed along with the duodenum and residual gastric contents to detect generalized ileus and decide the need for gastric suctioning and/or prokinetics. The mean number of peristaltic contractions of the stomach and proximal duodenum is 4–5 contractions per minute, although this decreases with fasting.
	Cardiac activity during cardiopulmonary resuscitation (CPR)	Assess the cardiac muscle for activity during the 10-s window when changing compressors – can detect ventricular fibrillations.	Presence or absence of sonographic cardiac activity during CPR is a strong predictor of outcome in human patients.
Umbilical	Splenic lesions/masses	Can detect splenic lesions through changes in echogenicity and structure.	The accuracy of APOCUS to detect splenic masses by non-specialists has not been assessed, and it is often not possible to sonographically determine if splenic lesions are malignant or benign using ultrasonography.
Right paralumbar	Retroperitoneal injury	Anechoic angles and triangles, or an anechoic rim surrounding the kidney, but not free in the abdominal space.	APOCUS only assesses a small, focused site of the retroperitoneal space surrounding the kidney and pathology can be missed.
	Renal pelvic dilation	Often easiest to assess in short-axis orientation.	Shows good diagnostic accuracy for ureteral obstruction in azotemic cats, although overlap with pyelonephritis exists.
	Duodenal motility	Normal motility is 3–5 contractions/min, although this decreases with fasting.	Absence of duodenal and gastric motility, in conjunction with residual gastric volume suggests generalized ileus. The presence of luminal content in the absence of gastrointestinal motility is a stronger indicator of ileus.
Left paralumbar	Retroperitoneal injury	Anechoic angles and triangles, or an anechoic rim surrounding the kidney, but not free in the abdominal space.	APOCUS only assesses a focused site of the retroperitoneal space surrounding the kidney and pathology can be missed.
	Renal pelvic dilation	Often easiest to assess in short-axis orientation.	Shows good diagnostic accuracy for ureteral obstruction in azotemic cats, although overlap with pyelonephritis exists.
Urinary bladder/ pelvic	Urinary bladder volume	Uses the formula for the calculation of the volume of a sphere: measurements in cm and answer in mL: L × W × D × 0.52.	More accurate when the urinary bladder is round, the probe is perpendicular to the urinary bladder at the widest diameter. Measuring the depth in long and short axes should be similar if the widest diameter is obtained in both planes. Although not 100% accurate, a lack of change in bladder volume despite appropriate IV fluid in a well-hydrated patient could be indicative of anuria or oliguria.
	Pyometra	Contained fluid-filled structures dorsal to the urinary bladder with thicker walls than the large intestine.	Accuracy of APOCUS by non-specialists has not been studied.
	Aortic thromboembolism in cats	Hypoechoic structures within the vessel lumen that can be confirmed with Doppler.	Accuracy of APOCUS by non-specialists has not been studied.

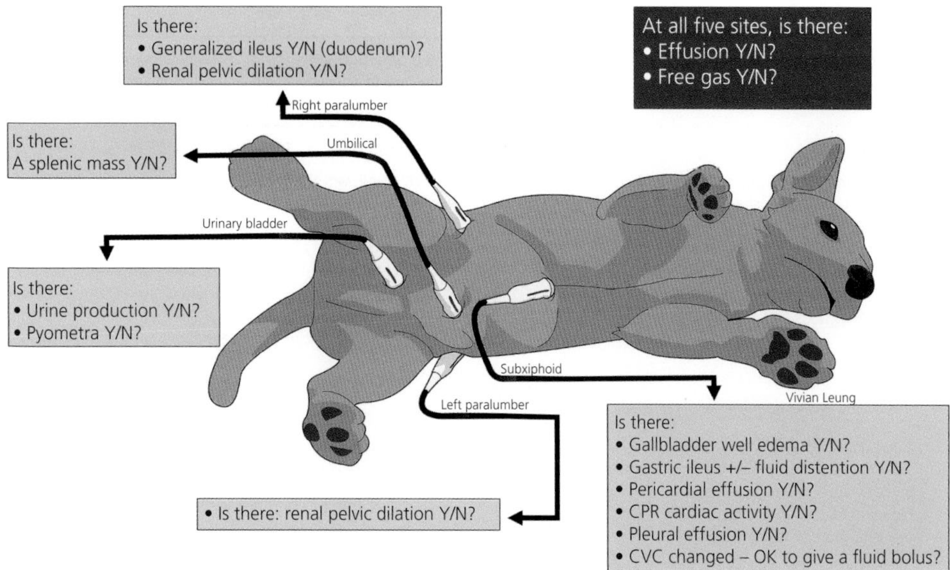

Figure 18.16 5-point abdominal point-of-care ultrasound (APOCUS) exam and the binary questions that have been evaluated at each site in small animals. The APOCUS exam should be completed in the position the patient is most comfortable (left lateral recumbency shown in this image). Depending on the question to answer and patient status, the probe is rocked and fanned through 45 degrees in both the short- and long-axis planes at all five sites. Consider the pretest probability of the pathology in question and then modify the protocol to increase the chance of detecting the specific pathology based on how the patient is positioned and where pathology is likely to accumulate (gas rises, fluid falls). CPR, cardiopulmonary resuscitation; CVC, caudal vena cava. Source: Dr. Vivian Leung, with permission.

APOCUS may help guide airway and/or anesthetic management in the acute care setting to reduce the risk of aspiration [19]. An empty stomach identified on APOCUS carries a low aspiration risk. In contrast, thick fluid content and particulate fluid of solid gastric content are associated with an increased risk of aspiration. In humans, a sonographically determined gastric volume of < 1.5 mL/kg is normal in fasted patients (baseline gastric secretions) and associated with a low aspiration risk. Conversely, volumes > 1.5 mL/kg are uncommon in fasted individuals, and suggest incomplete gastric emptying and possibly higher aspiration risk. Although a strict gastric volume threshold associated with aspiration risk is controversial, clinical data strongly suggest that volumes of up to 1.5 mL/kg are normal and safe in fasted humans [122–124]. A semiquantitative three-point grading system has also been developed in human anesthesiology to differentiate low from high gastric volume states and the risk of aspiration pneumonia [122–124]. Although gastrointestinal motility and emptying have been evaluated and used as a point-of-care assessment in small animals, the role of gastric POCUS to stratify aspiration risk in animals is unclear [103,125–128].

Urinary bladder volume

Urinary bladder volume calculation, and estimation of urine production, can help diagnose postoperative urinary retention and reduce postoperative urinary catheterization in human anesthesiology departments [129,130]. Sonographic urinary bladder volume estimation has been reported in veterinary medicine using both 2D and 3D ultrasound. A recent canine study suggests the formula $L \times W \times D \times 0.52$ may be the most accurate of the urinary volume formulas studied [131–133]. Urinary bladder volume calculation and a potential role in peri- and postoperative patient management of veterinary patients have not been reported despite the calculation of urinary bladder volume being easy to perform.

Cardiac POCUS

With cardiac POCUS (CPOCUS), the sonographer uses a specific imaging protocol (e.g., right parasternal short-axis left atrial to aortic root [LA:Ao] ratio) to answer a specific question or series of questions by interpreting views of one or a few preselected targets, with responses typically binary (present or absent). Although CPOCUS is less sensitive and specific than comprehensive echocardiography, it provides valuable information to supplement physiologic data and physical examination findings [134–137]. The American Society of Echocardiography has established guidelines for CPOCUS use by acute care providers [138,139]. In human anesthesiology, CPOCUS is useful for the acute assessment of gross cardiovascular function, assessment of causes of hemodynamic instability, and cardiac assessment during cardiac arrest [140–142]. It can also accurately detect a state of low cardiac preload and facilitates rapid, goal-directed fluid resuscitation [143,144]. More specifically, CPOCUS is used to qualitatively evaluate the size of the cardiac chambers, the thickness of the walls, ventricular function, intracardiac volume status, and the presence of pericardial effusion or air emboli [134,140,145,146]. Although clinical studies are lacking, most of these variables have also been evaluated with CPOCUS in companion animals (Table 18.7).

In addition, CPOCUS compliments PLUS in the evaluation of patients with respiratory distress (i.e., the finding of diffuse bilaterally increased B-lines should prompt CPOCUS evaluation to confirm or rule out cardiac causes of pulmonary edema). In contrast, the absence of B-lines in a patient with respiratory distress essentially rules out cardiac causes, and other respiratory pathologies should be considered. Finally, it is important to realize that CPOCUS has limited applications in human patients with congenital heart disease and subtle chronic pathology as it focuses on the identification of acute conditions (pericardial effusion and

Table 18.7 Cardiac POCUS windows, structures of interest, clinically driven (often binary response) questions to answer, and suggested guidelines for interpretation of findings.

Cardiac POCUS window	Anatomic structures assessed	Clinically driven question(s) to answer/physiology to assess	Clinical interpretation/most common causes
Right parasternal short-axis views			
Mushroom view	Papillary muscles just ventral to the mitral valve: assess left ventricular chamber size, contractility, and wall thickness. Less commonly, right ventricular size and ventricular septal flattening are assessed. Left ventricular contractility is reported to be 30–50% in dogs and 40–60% in cats.	1. Is the lumen enlarged with thin walls? 2. Is the lumen small with thick walls? 3. Is contractility increased or decreased? 4. Is the interventricular septum flat/deviated into the right ventricle?	Consider dilated cardiomyopathy if contractions are weak with an enlarged left atrium; consider volume overload if the heart is hyperkinetic with an enlarged left atrium. Consider hypertrophic cardiomyopathy if the left atrium is also enlarged; consider pseudohypertrophy if the left atrium is normal to small. Increased contractility can be seen with iatrogenic volume overload and hypertrophic cardiomyopathy.
Fish mouth view	Mitral valve	Not applicable	Landmark to identify correct mushroom and LA:Ao windows
Mercedes and the whale view	Heart base: left atrial to aortic root ratio (LA:Ao). Normal LA:Ao ratios should generally be between 1–1.5 in cats and dogs (slightly higher in cats). Can fit 2.5 aortic diameters into the left atrium of healthy cats.	1. Is the left atrium enlarged? 2. Is the left atrium small?	Congestive heart failure causing respiratory distress (increased B-lines) usually has an LA:Ao ≥ 2:1 in cats and dogs. Iatrogenic volume overload can also cause an enlarged left atrium. Hypovolemia should be suspected when the LA:Ao ≤ 1.
Right parasternal long-axis view			A subjective RV:LV ratio of > 1 is pathologic.
Subxiphoid view	Pericardial space: effusion appears sonographically as an anechoic space adjacent to cardiac structures. Sensitivity and specificity for detection of a pericardial effusion are high regardless of patient position. To avoid missing loculated pericardial effusion, multiple acoustic windows should be assessed.		Pericardial effusion appears as a circular accumulation of fluid adjacent to and surrounding the cardiac chambers, with the pericardial sac often being visualized as a hyperechoic (white) line on the side of the anechoic effusion opposite the cardiac structures. Be sure to extend the depth to visualize the entire heart. If it is unclear whether anechoic fluid accumulation is pericardial or pleural in origin assess the pericardio-diaphragmatic (PD) windows; parasternal transthoracic windows found on both the right and left side of the thorax (see PLUS). Pericardial effusion may be detected between the diaphragm and cardiac apex via the subxiphoid view

LA:Ao, left atrial to aortic root ratio; RV:LV, right ventricular to left ventricular ratio.

hypovolemia) and assessment of global myocardial function rather than detailed structural diagnostics or measurements [147]. This may limit its application in veterinary anesthesiology to identify the cause and significance of preanesthetic cardiac murmurs identified on physical examination, although research in this area is lacking. If left atrial (LA) enlargement, valve thickening, or subtle changes in wall thickness or contractility are noted, echocardiography performed by a cardiologist is recommended. Applications of veterinary CPOCUS are presented in Table 18.7.

Extensive quantitative calculations are not a goal of CPOCUS. When time and training allow, simple calculations can be performed, but are not necessary. In human and veterinary studies, a good correlation between visually estimated (qualitative) and formally measured (quantitative) cardiac parameters has been reported [148–151]. Although a phased array transducer is advantageous in obtaining echocardiographic images, CPOCUS is often performed using a micro-convex curvilinear transducer. Although M-mode recordings allow quantitative measurement of cardiac dimensions and analysis of motion patterns, most CPOCUS questions can be answered using B-mode alone.

Cardiac POCUS windows and views

CPOCUS incorporates right parasternal short-axis (Fig. 18.17) and long-axis views, the subxiphoid view, and occasionally, left-sided views. Acquiring all views is often unnecessary. For example, the LA:Ao ratio can still have diagnostic value, even if it is the only view obtained [151–153]. Furthermore, although left-sided views can be helpful in some situations (e.g., identification of intracardiac thrombi in cats), they are not required to answer most CPOCUS questions [154].

Right parasternal short-axis views

There are three key right parasternal short-axis views that can answer most CPOCUS questions (Fig. 18.18) [152,154,155]:

a. "Mushroom view" (Fig. 18.18A): A common view for estimating volume status and contractility at the left midventricular/papillary muscle region just below the mitral valve.

b. "Fish mouth view" (Fig. 18.18B): Obtained at the level of the mitral valve and serves as a landmark to obtain other views. Confidently identifying this view provides the reference point above (dorsal) and below (ventral) from which the two key views used to answer most CPOCUS questions can be found: the Mercedes and whale view, and the mushroom view, respectively.

c. "Mercedes and the whale view" (Fig. 18.18C): Allows assessment of the LA:Ao ratio.

Reference intervals vary slightly depending on where measurements are made, if the pulmonary artery is included, the ultrasound beam angle of insonation (i.e., the angle at which the ultrasound beam strikes the target organ or structure of interest, which may vary in laterally recumbent versus standing patients), and by the operator's skill level. In general, a normal LA:Ao ratio should be between 1–1.5 in cats and dogs [155–157]. There is a gray zone regarding LA:Ao ratio enlargement, with values ranging up to 1.7 in cats.

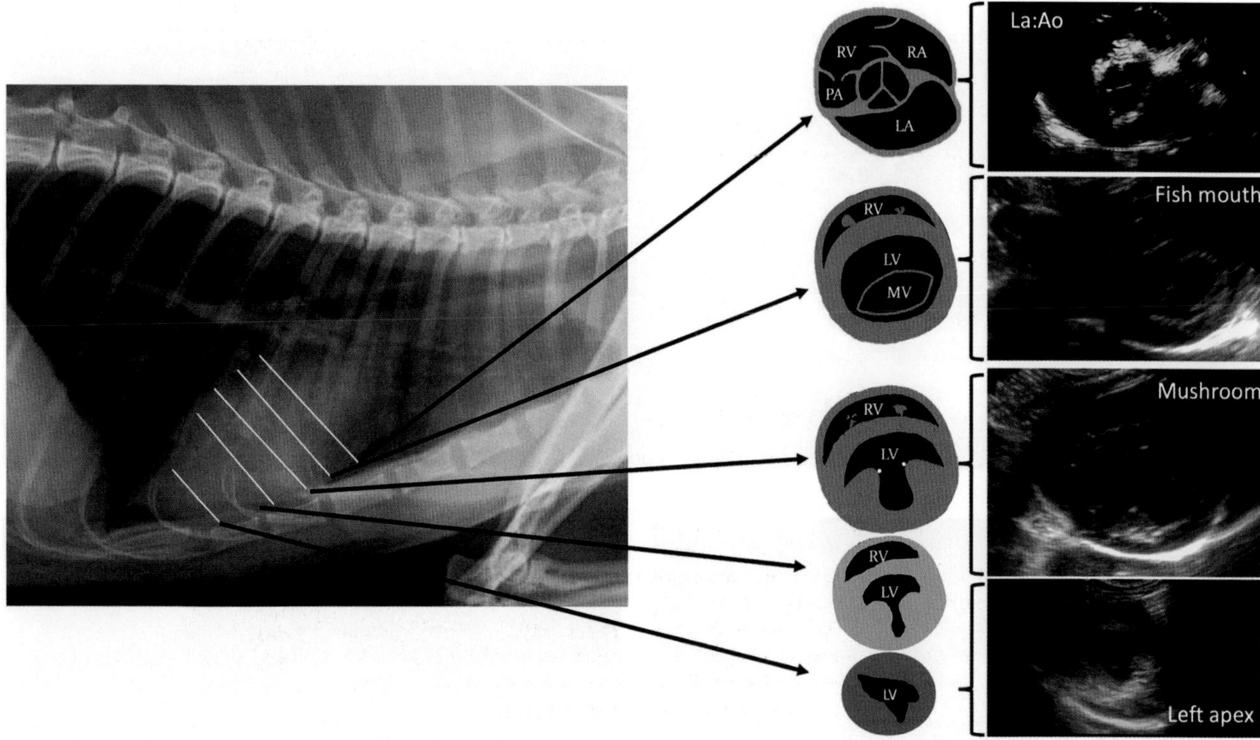

Figure 18.17 Radiographic, schematic, and still images of the different right parasternal short-axis views starting at the apex of the left ventricle and moving toward the heart base through the papillary muscle level, mitral valve, and finally the left atrial to aortic root (La:Ao). The corresponding cardiac still images are labeled: "left apex," "mushroom," "fish mouth," and "La:Ao," also referred to as the "Mercedes and the whale." The heart base image above the left atrial to aortic root is not shown in this figure. LA, left atrium; RA, right atrium; RV, right ventricle; PA, pulmonary artery; LV, left ventricle; MV, mitral valve. Source: Dr. Søren Boysen, with permission.

Right parasternal long-axis views

The four-chamber view is arguably the most common right parasternal long-axis view assessed during CPOCUS (Fig. 18.19). With this view the sonographer can subjectively evaluate the size of all cardiac chambers [152,158]; left atrium (LA), left ventricle (LV), right atrium (RA), and right ventricle (RV). The RA and the LA should be of similar size (1:1 ratio). The interatrial septum should lie in a relatively neutral position and not bulge into either atrium. The RV internal chamber diameter is approximately one-third that of the LV internal diameter. The free wall of the RV equals one-third to one-half the thickness of the LV free wall. The interventricular septum and the LV free wall are normally similar in thickness. Interpretation of changes in chamber size, wall thickness, and contractility in the right parasternal long-axis views are similar to changes in the right parasternal short-axis views.

The four-chamber view may be more sensitive for diagnosing cardiac tamponade compared to the short-axis views. Tamponade appears as a compression of the RA-free wall into the atrium, intermittently reducing atrial chamber size (RA wall compressed inwards during systole; Fig. 18.20). However, it should be kept in mind that tamponade is a clinical diagnosis and the finding of shock in a patient with identifiable pericardial effusion should prompt an increased index of suspicion for tamponade.

Subxiphoid view

The subxiphoid view provides a useful acoustic window into the caudal thorax, which can identify pericardial and/or pleural effusion and assess caudal lung regions not accessible transthoracically [1,159]. The caudal vena cava (CVC) can also be evaluated at this site (see below).

Interpretation and integration of cardiac POCUS findings

All CPOCUS findings should be interpreted in light of clinical examination and other POCUS findings.

Left atrial to aortic root ratio (LA:Ao)

Most patients presenting with respiratory distress secondary to congestive heart failure have LA:Ao ratios ≥ 2, well above upper reference limits [151,154,159]. If the LA is enlarged, it suggests increased LA volume and/or pressure, which is often associated with left-sided congestive heart failure or iatrogenic fluid overload. Alternatively, in cats (not yet studied in dogs), if > 3 times the area of the aorta can subjectively fit within the LA, the LA should be considered enlarged (Fig. 18.21) [152]. Using both of these methods in cats is a good way to help confirm if the LA is truly enlarged [154]. A small LA:Ao ($\leq$1:1) suggests pseudohypertrophy. Pseudohypertrophy results from hypovolemia and decreased ventricular filling, which causes decreased LA and LV chamber size, and the appearance of a thickened interventricular septum and ventricular free wall [160,161]. This resolves with restoration of effective circulating volume.

Left ventricular lumen size and function

The subjective identification of an enlarged LV lumen may suggest volume overload or conditions causing myocardial dysfunction (e.g., dilated cardiomyopathy) [154,155,158]. Both volume overload and dilated cardiomyopathy can cause an enlarged LA and increased B-lines on lung ultrasound. Assessing LV contractility is important for differentiating the two conditions (see below). The subjective finding of a decreased LV lumen size with thickened ventricular

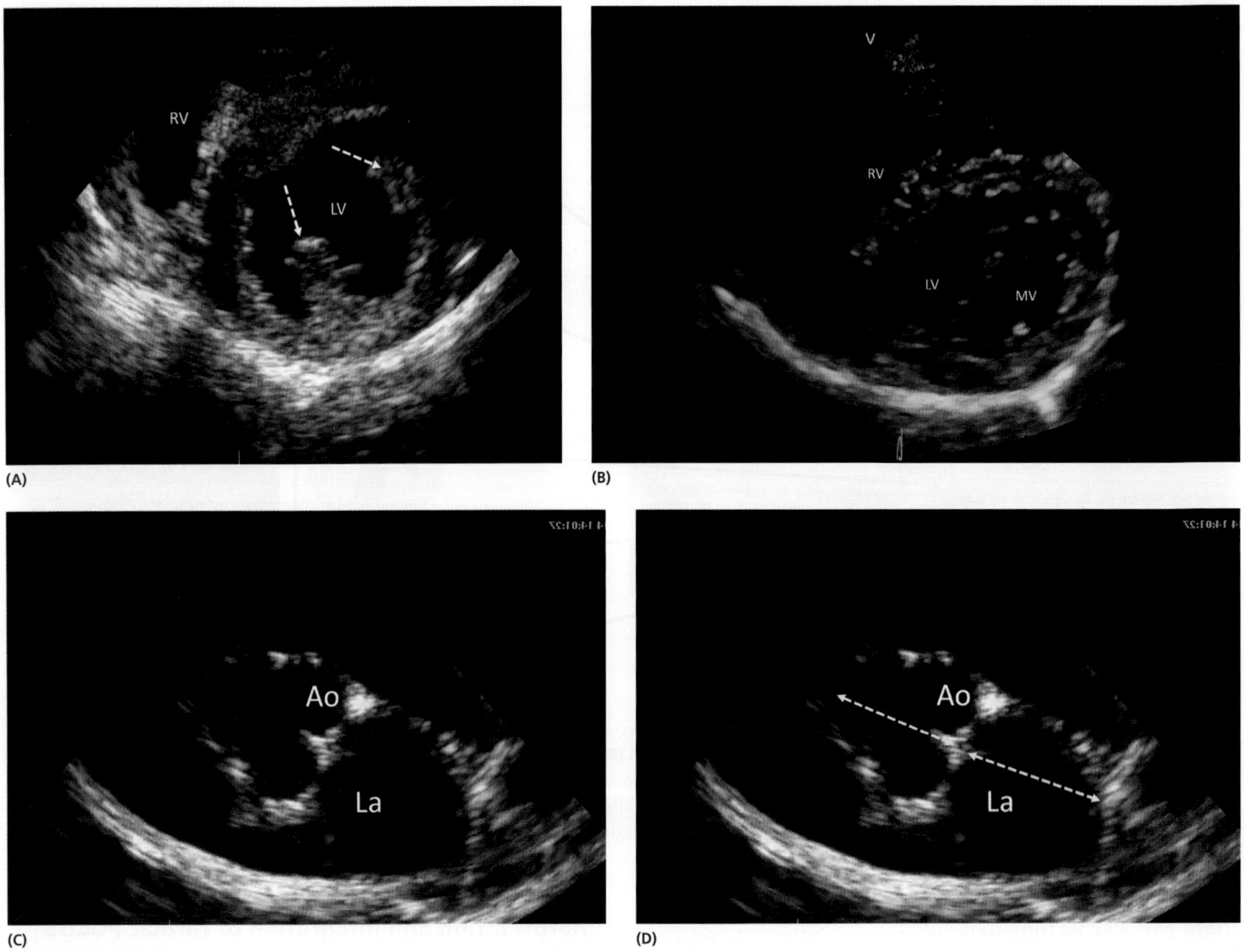

Figure 18.18 Two-dimensional short-axis view, right parasternal window showing still images of the three key views used to answer most cardiac POCUS questions. **A.** Mushroom view, often the first view obtained, which is located at the midventricular level where the papillary muscles are visible (white arrows). **B.** Fish mouth view, identified by slowly fanning the transducer dorsally from the mushroom view directing the ultrasound beams toward the base of the heart until the mitral valve (MV) becomes apparent within the left ventricular lumen (LV). **C.** Mercedes and the whale view, obtained by fanning the ultrasound beam toward the base of the heart from the mushroom/fish mouth view. Image contains a short-axis view of the left atrium-to-aortic root ratio (La:Ao). (La, "whale") and aortic root (Ao, "Mercedes"). **D.** Still image demonstrating the objective measurement of the La:Ao (yellow dotted arrows), although this measurement is often made subjectively during cardiac POCUS. IVS, interventricular septum; RV, right ventricle. Source: Lindsey Strang, RVT, VTS (ECC), with permission.

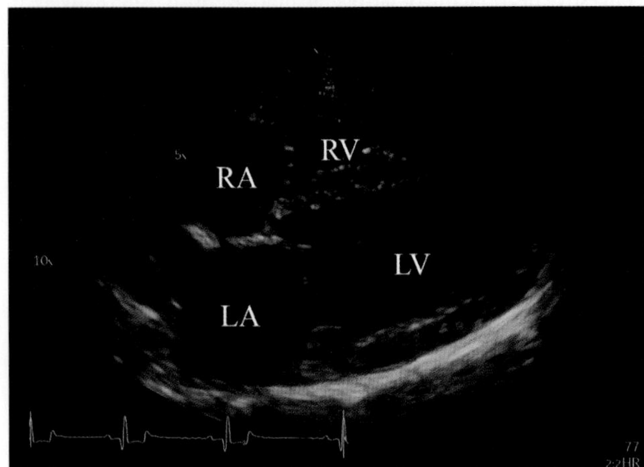

Figure 18.19 Two-dimensional long-axis view, right parasternal window four-chamber view of the heart showing the left ventricle (LV), left atrium (LA), right atrium (RA), and right ventricle (RV). Source: Lindsey Strang, RVT, VTS (ECC), with permission.

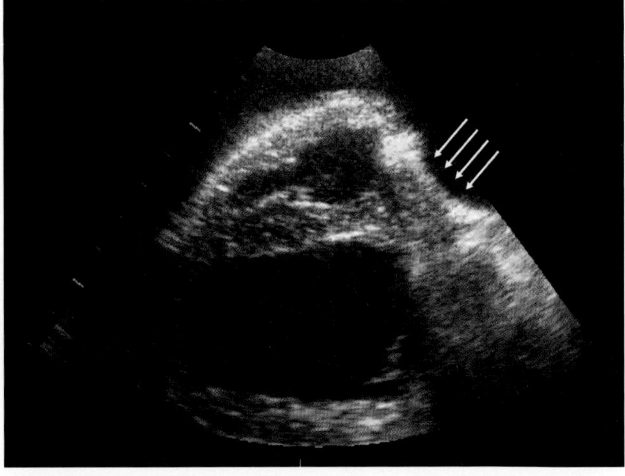

Figure 18.20 Tamponade secondary to pericardial effusion. The right atrium is collapsed and concave (white arrows). Source: Lindsey Strang, RVT, VTS (ECC), with permission.

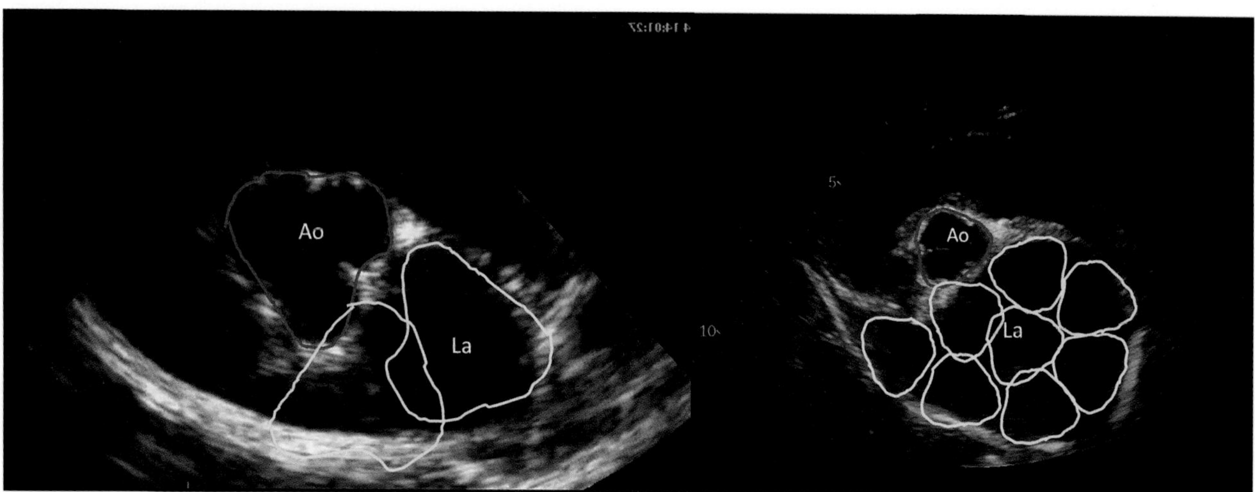

Figure 18.21 Still ultrasound images of a normal-sized left atrium (left) and a much-enlarged left atrium (right). In cats, the number of aortic areas that can fit within the left atrium can be used to subjectively decide if the left atrium is enlarged. The image on the left cannot fit more than 2.5 left aortic areas within the left atrium, while is possible to fit more than seven aortic areas within the left atrium in the image on the right. Source: Dr. Søren Boysen, with permission.

walls may suggest pseudohypertrophy secondary to volume depletion or true myocardial hypertrophy. To help differentiate pseudohypertrophy from hypertrophic cardiomyopathy, LA size should be evaluated: LA size is normal to small in patients with pseudohypertrophy and often enlarged in patients with cardiomyopathy. A loss of the visible ventricular chamber during systole, known as "ventricular chamber obliteration," may reflect severe hypovolemia due to markedly decreased ventricular filling pressures and potential impending cardiovascular collapse [33]. In the absence of systemic disease (e.g., hyperthyroidism, systemic hypertension, subaortic stenosis, and acromegaly), increased LV wall thickness is often associated with hypertrophic cardiomyopathy in cats but may also be seen with pseudohypertrophy in both dogs and cats.

Ventricular contractility can be subjectively assessed by estimating the relative change in size of the LV lumen during diastole and systole, which should be roughly 30–50% in dogs and 40–60% in cats. With practice, and by scanning healthy animals, a subjective evaluation of ventricular contraction is usually sufficient to determine if contractile abnormalities are present [154,158]. Hyperdynamic/increased contractile states can occur in hypervolemic patients (provided there is no concurrent myocardial dysfunction), high sympathetic drive states (e.g., stress), and in patients that have decreased afterload (e.g., arterial vasodilation) without myocardial dysfunction [33,134]. Decreased contractility can be seen with hypovolemia in the absence of myocardial dysfunction (due to decreased myocardial stretch), conditions associated with poor myocardial contractility (e.g., dilated cardiomyopathy or sepsis), and cases with increased afterload (e.g., severe arterial vasoconstriction) [33,134].

Flattening of the interventricular septum combined with an enlarged RV chamber, and/or increased RV wall thickness suggests increased RV pressures or volume [134,154]. These presentations arguably take more skill to identify and interpret. If this triad of right heart findings is present, causes of pulmonary arterial hypertension should be considered (e.g., heartworm disease), chronic bronchopulmonary disease (e.g., dynamic airway disease/obstruction, chronic bronchitis, or pulmonary fibrosis), and pulmonary thromboembolism [154].

Caudal vena cava assessment at the subxiphoid window

Although controversial in human medicine, the inferior vena cava (IVC) diameter and collapsibility index are often used in the clinical setting as a means of assessing volume status [33,134]. In dogs and cats, the CVC diameter (CVCd) and caudal vena cava collapsibility index (CVCCI) have been described at several POCUS windows, including the subxiphoid site (Fig. 18.22) [162,163]. This change in size of the CVC between inspiration and expiration is referred to as "CVC collapsibility" and is calculated as the CVCCI. The CVCCI expresses the change (%) in the diameter of the CVC during the respiratory cycle:

$$\text{CVCCI} = \text{CVCd max} - \text{CVCd min}/\,\text{CVCd max}$$

Although small animal research is limited, a small clinical study ($n = 27$) in spontaneously breathing dogs with compromised hemodynamics or tissue hypoperfusion suggested that CVCCI can accurately predict fluid responsiveness, although the authors also concluded that further research is necessary to assess generalizability of their results to a larger population [164]. An enlarged or distended CVC with less than a 20% change in the CVCCI suggests increased RA pressures, which may be secondary to hypervolemia, congestive heart disease, or cardiac tamponade (Fig. 18.22). Assessment of other cardiac POCUS findings should differentiate causes of an enlarged CVC (see above). In contrast, a thin collapsed CVC with no change in the CVCCI, or a change in the CVCCI of more than 50%, is suggestive of hypovolemia (Fig. 18.22). If increased RA pressures are suspected based on CVC assessment, other clinical parameters and POCUS examinations should be evaluated to determine the cause, particularly assessment of PLUS for lung edema and pleural effusion, as well as CPOCUS for volume status.

POCUS in cardiopulmonary resuscitation

CPOCUS may be helpful during cardiopulmonary resuscitation (CPR) to identify reversible causes of arrest and determine if mechanical cardiac activity is present, provided it does not interfere with CPR efforts [134,165]. With adequate training, images can be acquired during the 10-s pauses allotted for pulse checks

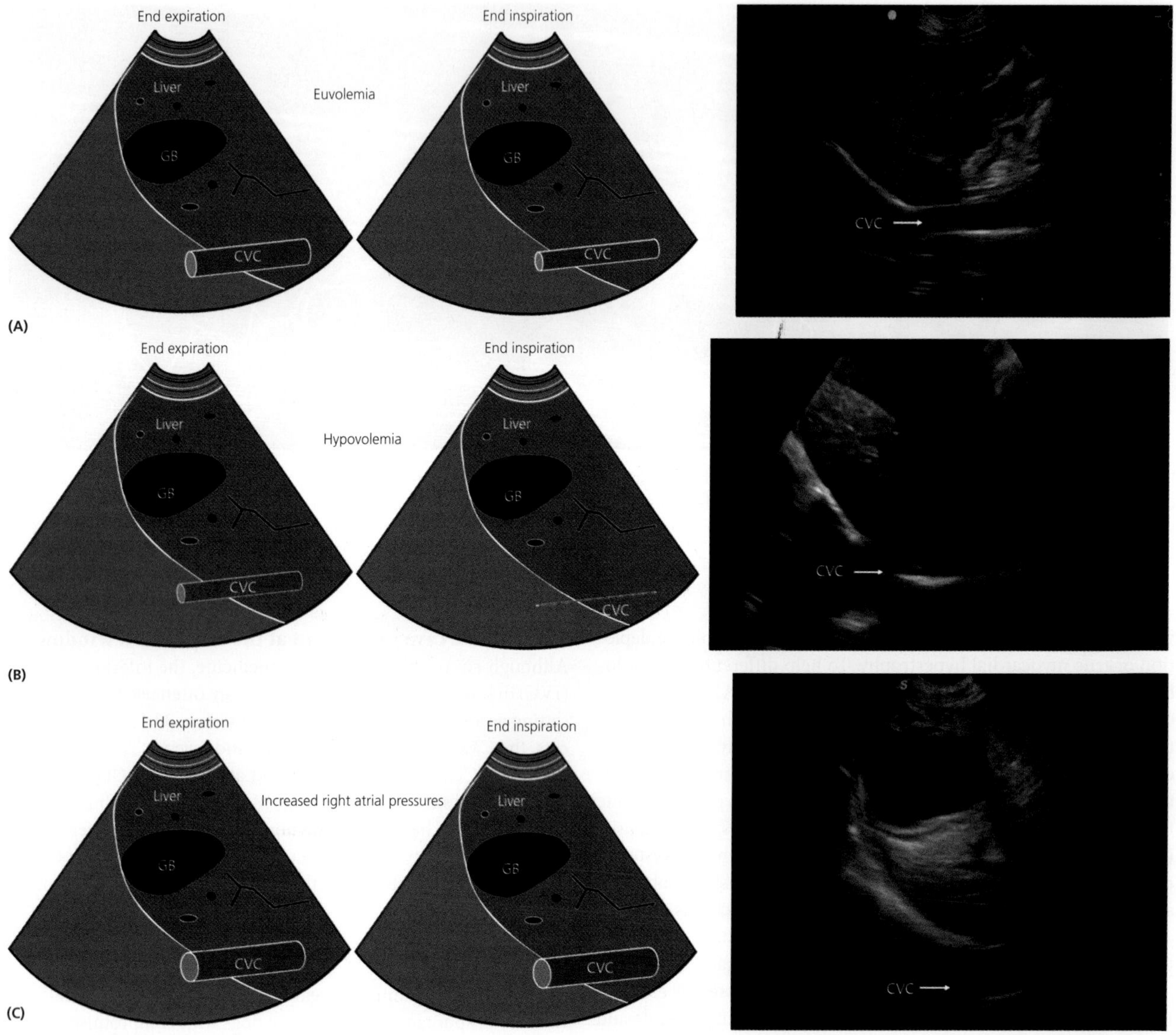

Figure 18.22 Schematic ultrasound images at end-expiration and end-inspiration, and still ultrasound images at end-inspiration. **A.** A euvolemic patient with a normal caudal vena cava (CVC). **B.** A hypovolemic patient with a "flat" CVC and subjectively narrow collapsibility index. Although a large CVC collapsibility index is suggestive of hypovolemia if the CVC is close to collapsed and very "flat," the change from flat to fully collapsed can be difficult to appreciate creating the impression of a small CVC collapsibility index. **C.** A patient with increased right atrial pressures and a "fat" CVC with almost no collapsibility index (in this case due to pericardial effusion (not visible). Also note there is gallbladder (GB) wall edema (halo sign) in this example, which is very common in patients with pericardial effusion. Source: Dr. Søren Boysen, with permission.

and to change CPR providers [165]. Given the portability of ultrasound, CPOCUS has been recommended as part of the code response in humans [165]. CPOCUS can predict survivability to hospital admission in patients presenting without a pulse. The subxiphoid view in humans has been used to detect cardiac activity during CPR. Any non-fibrillating motion in humans is associated with greater survival to hospital admission (23.5% versus 1.9%, respectively) [166]. The presence of cardiac motion on ultrasound has been shown to be the most important predictor of survivability when trauma patients present in pulseless electrical activity (PEA) (odds ratio 33.9) [167]. Although not reported in the veterinary literature, anecdotal evidence suggests the subxiphoid view can be used to assess the heart during active CPR in dogs and cats

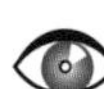

(Video 18.11). During human CPR, CPOCUS has been used to evaluate for cardiac standstill when deciding to stop CPR [134,165].

CPOCUS can also help guide early post-arrest management by allowing rapid assessment of reversible causes of arrest, including pericardial tamponade, hypovolemia, cardiogenic shock, RV failure (air emboli), and pneumothorax [134,168–170]. On return of spontaneous circulation following cardiac arrest, CPOCUS has been used to qualitatively assess LV systolic recovery over time [33,165]. However, the reasons for arrest identified on POCUS must be distinguished from non-arrest–related findings [171]. For example, visualized peritoneal fluid could be ascites, not acute hemorrhage; a pericardial effusion could be present without tamponade physiology; and right heart dilation may accumulate over the course of CPR without the presence of a massive pulmonary embolism [170,172,173]. Treatment of an erroneous diagnosis suggested by POCUS may result in iatrogenic injury or delayed identification of the true cause [171].

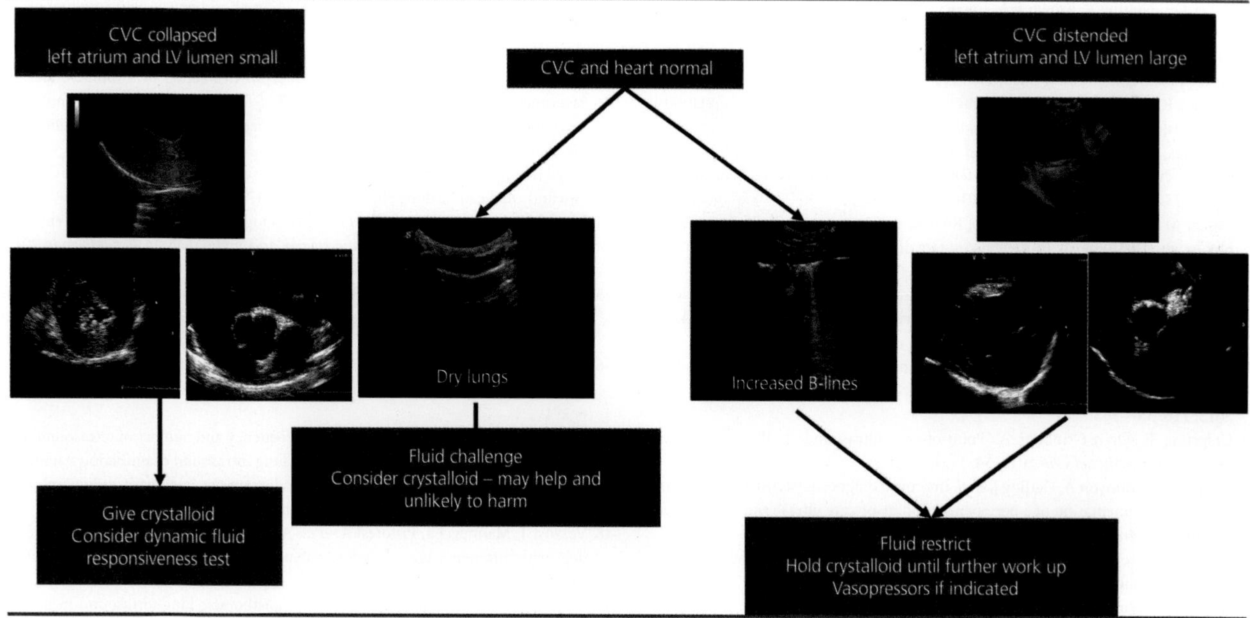

Figure 18.23 Point-of-care ultrasound fluid resuscitation guide. Adapted to veterinary medicine by the authors based on human point-of-care ultrasound fluid resuscitation guidelines [175]. LV, left ventricle; CVC, caudal vena cava. Source: Dr. Søren Boysen, with permission.

POCUS and monitoring fluid therapy

A combination of POCUS findings can be used to assess a patient's volume status and monitor response to fluid therapy (Fig. 18.23). Patients with a history of aggressive fluid therapy and combined CPOCUS findings of a hyperkinetic heart (increased fractional shortening), an enlarged LA, distended CVC, and increased B-lines on PLUS should prompt consideration of fluid overload. Because PLUS provides dynamic information, the change in B-line count can be used to monitor for the development of pulmonary edema secondary to fluid therapy, and the effectiveness of decongestive therapy in patients with congestive heart failure or fluid overload. PLUS provides a way to evaluate for lung congestion in patients before visible signs of congestion become apparent on physical examination [174]. Therefore, establishing a baseline PLUS profile, along with other baseline POCUS evaluations, particularly CVC respiratory variation, LA size, LV size, ventricular wall thickness, gallbladder wall thickness, and cavitary effusions in patients receiving intravenous fluid therapy is reasonable and allows serial evaluation over time.

Limitations

POCUS favors specificity over sensitivity, such that unambiguous findings provide information useful for patient care, while a negative POCUS exam does not exclude pathology, and any uncertainty or incidental findings outside the scope of POCUS should prompt consultation with an imaging specialist or cardiologist. Intraoperative access to the patient and patient positioning under anesthesia may limit the clinician's ability to obtain usable quality images that allow interpretation. Obese patients, very small patients, and patients with open body cavities may be difficult to image. Interpretation of POCUS examinations in patients with complex chronic heart disease and parenchymal organ changes is limited and should be approached with caution. There is a learning curve to POCUS and sonographers should know their limitations; some skills are easier to acquire than others. States of hypovolemia or severe dehydration may limit detection of effusion, and repeat POCUS examinations following fluid therapy are warranted. Finally, a lack of adequate training in indications, image acquisition, and interpretation may limit integration of POCUS into anesthesia practice.

References

1 Boysen SR, Rozanski EA, Tidwell AS, *et al.* Evaluation of a focused assessment with sonography for trauma protocol to detect free abdominal fluid in dogs involved in motor vehicle accidents. *J Am Vet Med Assoc* 2004; **225**(8): 1198–1204.
2 McMurray J, Boysen SR, Chalhoub S. Focused assessment with sonography for triage in non-trauma dogs and cats in the emergency and critical care setting. *J Vet Emerg Crit Care* 2016; (**1**): 64–73.
3 Lisciandro GR, Lagutchik MS, Mann KA, *et al.* Evaluation of an abdominal fluid scoring system determined using abdominal focused assessment with sonography for trauma in 101 dogs with motor vehicle trauma. *J Vet Emerg Crit Care* 2009; **19**(5): 426–437.
4 Meineri M, Bryson GL, Arellano R, *et al.* Core point-of-care ultrasound curriculum: what does every anesthesiologist need to know? *Can J Anaesth* 2018; **65**(4): 417–426.
5 Díaz-Gómez JL, Mayo PH, Koenig SJ. Point-of-care ultrasonography. *N Engl J Med* 2021; **385**(17): 1593–1602.
6 Sepuya RG, Dozeman ET, Prittie JE, *et al.* Comparing diagnostic findings and cost of whole body computed tomography to traditional diagnostic imaging in polytrauma patients. *J Vet Emerg Crit Care (San Antonio)* 2022; **32**(3): 334–340.
7 Shokoohi H, Duggan NM, Adhikari S, *et al.* Point-of-care ultrasound stewardship. *J Am Coll Emerg Physicians Open* 2020; **1**(6): 1326–1331.
8 Tanael M. Users' guide to point-of-care ultrasonography. *J Am Coll Emerg Physicians Open* 2020; **1**(6): 1777.
9 Moore CL, Copel JA. Point-of-care ultrasonography. *N Engl J Med* 2011; **364**(8): 749–757.
10 Ramsingh D, Bronshteyn YS, Haskins S, *et al.* Perioperative point-of-care ultrasound: from concept to application. *Anesthesiology* 2020; **132**(4): 908–916.
11 Patel MD, Horrow MM, Kamaya A, *et al.* Mapping the ultrasound landscape to define point-of-care ultrasound and diagnostic ultrasound: a proposal from the society of radiologists in ultrasound and ACR commission on ultrasound. *J Am Coll Radiol* 2021; **18**(1 Pt A): 42–52.
12 Riishede M, Laursen CB, Teglbjærg LS, *et al.* Diagnostic value of whole-body-focused ultrasonography in high-acuity patients in the emergency department: a prospective single-center cross-sectional study. *Ultrasound J* 2019; **11**(1): 11.

13 Baker DE, Nolting L, Brown HA. Impact of point-of-care ultrasound on the diagnosis and treatment of patients in rural Uganda. *Trop Doct* 2021; **51**: 291–296.
14 Chan VW, Perlas A, Rawson R, *et al.* Ultrasound-guided supraclavicular brachial plexus block. *Anesth Analg* 2003; **97**: 1514–1517.
15 Asheim P, Mostad U, Aadahl P. Ultrasound-guided central venous cannulation in infants and children. *Acta Anaesthesiol Scand* 2002; **46**: 390–392.
16 Adler AC, Greeley WJ, Conlin F, *et al.* Perioperative anesthesiology ultrasonographic evaluation (PAUSE): a guided approach to perioperative bedside ultrasound. *J Cardiothorac Vasc Anesth* 2016; **30**: 521–529.
17 Bøtker MT, Vang ML, Grofte T, *et al.* Routine pre-operative focused ultrasonography by anesthesiologists in patients undergoing urgent surgical procedures. *Acta Anaesthesiol Scand* 2014; **58**: 807–814.
18 Das SK, Choupoo NS, Haldar R, *et al.* Transtracheal ultrasound for verification of endotracheal tube placement: a systematic review and meta-analysis. *Can J Anesth* 2015; **62**: 413–423.
19 Perlas A, Mitsakakis N, Liu L, *et al.* Validation of a mathematical model for ultrasound assessment of gastric volume by gastroscopic examination. *Anesth Analg* 2013; **116**: 357–363.
20 Ursprung E, Oren-Grinberg A. Point-of-care ultrasound in the perioperative period. *Int Anesthesiol Clin* 2016; **54**: 1–21.
21 Ramsingh D, Runyon A, Gatling J, *et al.* Improved diagnostic accuracy of pathology with the implementation of a perioperative point-of-care ultrasound service: quality improvement initiative. *Reg Anesth Pain Med* 2020; **45**: 95–101.
22 Cowie B. Three years' experience of focused cardiovascular ultrasound in the perioperative period. *Anaesthesia* 2011; **66**: 268–273.
23 Ramsingh D, Rinehart J, Kain Z, *et al.* Impact assessment of perioperative point-of-care ultrasound training on anesthesiology residents. *Anesthesiology* 2015; **123**: 670–682.
24 Canty DJ, Royse CF, Kilpatrick D, *et al.* The impact of focused transthoracic echocardiography in the pre-operative clinic. *Anaesthesia* 2012; **67**: 618–625.
25 Zimmerman JM, Coker BJ. The nuts and bolts of performing focused cardiovascular ultrasound (focus). *Anesth Analg* 2017; **124**: 753–60.
26 Díaz-Gómez JL, Perez-Protto S, Hargrave J, *et al.* Impact of a focused transthoracic echocardiography training course for rescue applications among anesthesiology and critical care medicine practitioners: a prospective study. *J Cardiothorac Vasc Anesth* 2015; **29**:576–581.
27 Ford JW, Heiberg J, Brennan AP, *et al.* A pilot assessment of 3 point-of-care strategies for diagnosis of perioperative lung pathology. *Anesth Analg* 2017; **124**: 734–742.
28 Yao W, Zhou Y, Wang B, *et al.* Can mandibular condylar mobility sonography measurements predict difficult laryngoscopy? *Anesth Analg* 2017; **124**: 800–806.
29 Haskins SC, Desai NA, Fields KG, *et al.* Diagnosis of intraabdominal fluid extravasation after hip arthroscopy with point-of-care ultrasonography can identify patients at an increased risk for postoperative pain. *Anesth Analg* 2017; **124**: 791–799.
30 Perlas A, Van de Putte P, Van Houwe P, *et al.* I-AIM framework for point-of-care gastric ultrasound. *Br J Anaesth* 2016; **116**: 7–11.
31 Mok D, Schwarz SK, Rondi K. Point-of-care ultrasonography in Canadian anesthesiology residency programs: a national survey of program directors. *Can J Anesth* 2017; **64**: 1023–1026.
32 Meineri M, Arellano R, Bryson G, *et al.* Canadian recommendations for training and performance in basic perioperative point-of-care ultrasound: recommendations from a consensus of Canadian anesthesiology academic centres. *Can J Anaesth* 2021; **68**(3): 376–386.
33 Adler AC, Brown KA, Conlin FT, *et al.* Cardiac and lung point-of-care ultrasound in pediatric anesthesia and critical care medicine: uses, pitfalls, and future directions to optimize pediatric care. *Paediatr Anaesth* 2019; **29**(8): 790–798.
34 Soni NJ, Lucas BP. Diagnostic point-of-care ultrasound for hospitalists. *J Hosp Med* 2015; **10**(2): 120–124.
35 Heinz ER, Vincent A. Point-of-care ultrasound for the trauma anesthesiologist. *Curr Anesthesiol Rep* 2022; **20**: 1–9.
36 Armenise A, Boysen RS, Rudloff E, *et al.* Veterinary-focused assessment with sonography for trauma-airway, breathing, circulation, disability and exposure: a prospective observational study in 64 canine trauma patients. *J Small Anim Pract* 2019; **60**(3): 173–182.
37 Dupanloup A, Osinchuk S. Relationship between the ratio of optic nerve sheath diameter to eyeball transverse diameter and morphological characteristics of dogs. *Am J Vet Res* 2021; **82**(8): 667–675.
38 Evangelisti MA, Carta G, Burrai GP, *et al.* Repeatability of ultrasound examination of the optic nerve sheath diameter in the adult cat: comparison between healthy cats and cats suffering from presumed intracranial hypertension. *J Feline Med Surg* 2020; **22**(10): 959–965.
39 Smith JJ, Fletcher DJ, Cooley SD, *et al.* Transpalpebral ultrasonographic measurement of the optic nerve sheath diameter in healthy dogs. *J Vet Emerg Crit Care* 2018; **28**(1): 31–38.
40 Lee HC, Choi HJ, Choi MC, *et al.* Ultrasonographic measurement of optic nerve sheath diameter in normal dogs. *J Vet Sci* 2003; **4**(3): 265–268.
41 Lisciandro GR. Abdominal and thoracic focused assessment with sonography for trauma, triage, and monitoring in small animals. *J Vet Emerg Crit Care* 2011; **21**(2): 104–122.
42 Lisciandro GR, Lagutchik MS, Mann T, *et al.* Evaluation of a thoracic focused assessment with sonography for trauma (TFAST) protocol to detect pneumothorax and concurrent thoracic injury in 145 traumatized dogs. *J Vet Emerg Crit Care* 2008; **18**: 258–269.
43 Lloyd JKF. Minimising stress for patients in the veterinary hospital: why it is important and what can be done about it. *Vet Sci* 2017; **4**(2): 22.
44 Chou EH, Dickman E, Tsou PY, *et al.* Ultrasonography for confirmation of endotracheal tube placement: a systematic review and meta-analysis. *Resuscitation* 2015; **90**: 97–103.
45 Herreria-Bustillo VJ, Kuo KW, Burke PJ, *et al.* A pilot study evaluating the use of cervical ultrasound to confirm endotracheal intubation in dogs. *J Vet Emerg Crit Care* 2016; **26**(5): 654–658.
46 Boysen S, McMurray J, Gommeren K. Abnormal curtain signs identified with a novel lung ultrasound protocol in six dogs with pneumothorax. *Front Vet Sci* 2019; **6**: 291.
47 Lisciandro GR, Fosgate GT, Fulton RM. Frequency and number of ultrasound lung rockets (B-lines) using a regionally based lung ultrasound examination named vet BLUE (veterinary bedside lung ultrasound exam) in dogs with radiographically normal lung findings. *Vet Radiol Ultrasound* 2014; **55**(3): 315–322.
48 Vezzosi T, Mannucci T, Pistoresi A, *et al.* Assessment of lung ultrasound B-lines in dogs with different stages of chronic valvular heart disease. *J Vet Intern Med* 2017; **31**(3): 700–704.
49 Rademacher N, Pariaut R, Pate J, *et al.* Transthoracic lung ultrasound in normal dogs and dogs with cardiogenic pulmonary edema: a pilot study. *Vet Radiol Ultrasound* 2014; **55**(4): 447–452.
50 Buessler A, Chouihed T, Duarte K, *et al.* Accuracy of several lung ultrasound methods for the diagnosis of acute heart failure in the ED: a multicenter prospective study. *Chest* 2020; **157**(1): 99–110.
51 Lee FCY. The curtain sign in lung ultrasound. *J Med Ultrasound* 2017; **25**: 101–104.
52 Kok B, Schuit F, Lieveld A, *et al.* Comparing lung ultrasound: extensive versus short in COVID-19 (CLUES): a multicentre, observational study at the emergency department. *BMJ Open* 2021; **11**(9): e048795.
53 Ward JL, Lisciandro GR, Ware WA, *et al.* Ultrasonography findings in dogs with various underlying causes of cough. *J Am Vet Med Assoc* 2019; **255**(5): 574–583.
54 Bhoil R, Ahluwalia A, Chopra R, *et al.* Signs and lines in lung ultrasound. *J Ultrasound* 2021; **21**: e225–e233.
55 Miller A. Practical approach to lung ultrasound. *BJA Educ* 2016; **16**: 39–45.
56 Lichtenstein DA. Lung ultrasound in the critically ill. *Ann Intensive Care* 2014; **4**(1): 1.
57 Husain LF, Hagopian L, Wayman D, *et al.* Sonographic diagnosis of pneumothorax. *J Emerg Trauma Shock* 2012; **5**(1): 76–81.
58 Boysen SR. Lung ultrasonography for pneumothorax in dogs and cats. *Vet Clin North Am Small Anim Pract* 2021; **51**(6): 1153–1167.
59 Lichtenstein DA, Mezière GA. Relevance of lung ultrasound in the diagnosis of acute respiratory failure: the BLUE protocol. *Chest* 2008; **134**: 117–125.
60 Lichtenstein D, Menu Y. A bedside ultrasound sign ruling out pneumothorax in the critically ill: lung sliding. *Chest* 1995; **108**: 1345–1348.
61 Alerhand S, Tsung JW. Unmasking the lung pulse for detection of endobronchial intubation. *J Ultrasound Med* 2020; **39**(11): 2105–2109.
62 Soldati G, Sher S, Testa A. Lung and ultrasound: time to "reflect." *Eur Rev Med Pharmacol Sci* 2011; **15**(2): 223–227.
63 Picano E, Pellikka PA. Ultrasound of extravascular lung water: a new standard for pulmonary congestion. *Eur Heart J* 2016; **37**(27): 2097–2104.
64 Yu X, Zhai Z, Zhao Y, *et al.* Performance of lung ultrasound in detecting perioperative atelectasis after general anesthesia. *Ultrasound Med Biol* 2016; **42**(12): 2775–2784.
65 Goffi A, Kruisselbrink R, Volpicelli G. The sound of air: point-of-care lung ultrasound in perioperative medicine. *Can J Anaesth* 2018; **65**(4): 399–416.
66 Rigot M, Boysen S, Masseau I, *et al.* Evaluation of B-lines with two point-of-care lung ultrasound protocols in cats with radiographically normal lungs. *In press.*
67 Lisciandro GR, Fulton RM, Fosgate GT, *et al.* Frequency and number of B-lines using a regionally based lung ultrasound examination in cats with radiographically normal lungs compared to cats with left-sided congestive heart failure. *J Vet Emerg Crit Care* 2017; **27**(5): 499–505.
68 Martins A, Gouveia D, Cardoso A, *et al.* Incidence of Z, I and B-lines detected with point of care ultrasound in healthy shelter dogs. *J Vet Emerg Crit Care* 2019; **29**: S17–S39.
69 Volpicelli G, Elbarbary M, Blaivas M, *et al.* International Liaison Committee on Lung Ultrasound (ILC-LUS) for International Consensus Conference on Lung Ultrasound (ICC-LUS). International evidence-based recommendations for point-of-care lung ultrasound. *Intensive Care Med* 2012; **38**(4): 577–591.

70 Lee FCY. Lung ultrasound – a primary survey of the acutely dyspneic patient. *J Int Care* 2016; **4**: 57.

71 Bissinger U, Lenz G, Kuhn W. Unrecognized endobronchial intubation of emergency patients. *Ann Emerg Med* 1989; **18**: 853–855.

72 Kollef MH, Legare EJ, Damiano M. Endotracheal tube misplacement: incidence, risk factors, and impact of a quality improvement program. *South Med J* 1994; **87**: 248–254.

73 Geisser W, Maybauer DM, Wolff H, *et al.* Radiological validation of tracheal tube insertion depth in out-of-hospital and in-hospital emergency patients. *Anaesthesia* 2009; **64**: 973–977.

74 Wirtz DD, Ortiz C, Newman DH, *et al.* Unrecognized misplacement of endotracheal tubes by ground prehospital providers. *Prehosp Emerg Care* 2007; **11**: 213–218.

75 Timmermann A, Russo SG, Eich C, *et al.* The out-of-hospital esophageal and endobronchial intubations performed by emergency physicians. *Anesth Analg* 2007; **104**: 619–623.

76 Jones JH, Murphy MP, Dickson RL, *et al.* Emergency physician–verified out-of-hospital intubation: miss rates by paramedics. *Acad Emerg Med* 2004; **11**: 707–709.

77 Katz SH, Falk JL. Misplaced endotracheal tubes by paramedics in an urban emergency medical services system. *Ann Emerg Med* 2001; **37**: 32–37.

78 Jemmett ME, Kendal KM, Fourre MW, *et al.* Unrecognized misplacement of endotracheal tubes in a mixed urban to rural emergency medical services setting. *Acad Emerg Med* 2003; **10**: 961–965.

79 Kramer MR, Melzer E, Sprung CL. Unilateral pulmonary edema after intubation of the right mainstem bronchus. *Crit Care Med* 1989; **17**: 472–474.

80 Mosing M, Iff I, Moens Y. Endoscopic removal of a bronchial carcinoma in a dog using one-lung ventilation. *Vet Surg* 2008; **37**(3): 222–225.

81 Adami C, Axiak S, Rytz U, *et al.* Alternating one lung ventilation using a double lumen endobronchial tube and providing CPAP to the non-ventilated lung in a dog. *Vet Anaesth Analg* 2011; **38**(1): 70–76.

82 Mayhew PD, Culp WT, Pascoe PJ, *et al.* Evaluation of blind thoracoscopic-assisted placement of three double-lumen endobronchial tube designs for one-lung ventilation in dogs. *Vet Surg* 2012; **41**(6): 664–670.

83 Marvel SJ, Hafez A, Monnet E. Thoracoscopic treatment of persistent right aortic arch in dogs with and without one lung ventilation. *Vet Surg* 2022; **51**(Suppl 1): O107–O117.

84 Mayhew PD, Chohan A, Hardy BT, *et al.* Cadaveric evaluation of fluoroscopy-assisted placement of one-lung ventilation devices for video-assisted thoracoscopic surgery in dogs. *Vet Surg* 2020; **49**(Suppl 1): O93–O101.

85 Lichtenstein DA, Lascols N, Prin S, *et al.* The "lung pulse": an early ultrasound sign of complete atelectasis. *Intensive Care Med* 2003; **29**: 2187–2192.

86 Wilkerson RG, Stone MB. Sensitivity of bedside ultrasound and supine anteroposterior chest radiographs for the identification of pneumothorax after blunt trauma. *Acad Emerg Med* 2010; **17**(1): 11–17.

87 Walters AM, O'Brien MA, Selmic LE, *et al.* Evaluation of the agreement between focused assessment with sonography for trauma (AFAST/TFAST) and computed tomography in dogs and cats with recent trauma. *J Vet Emerg Crit Care* 2018; **28**(5): 429–435.

88 Hwang TS, Yoon YM, Jung DI, *et al.* Usefulness of transthoracic lung ultrasound for the diagnosis of mild pneumothorax. *J Vet Sci* 2018; **19**(5): 660–666.

89 Cole L, Pivetta M, Humm K. Diagnostic accuracy of a lung ultrasound protocol (Vet BLUE) for detection of pleural fluid, pneumothorax and lung pathology in dogs and cats. *J Small Anim Pract* 2021; **62**(3): 178–186.

90 Soldati G, Testa A, Sher S, *et al.* Occult traumatic pneumothorax: diagnostic accuracy of lung ultrasonography in the emergency department. *Chest* 2008, **133**: 204–211.

91 Lichtenstein DA. Pleural effusion and introduction to the lung ultrasound technique. In: Lichtenstein DA, ed. *General Ultrasound in the Critically Ill.* Berlin, Germany: Springer-Verlag, 2005: 96–104.

92 Acosta CM, Maidana GA, Jacovitti D, *et al.* Accuracy of transthoracic lung ultrasound for diagnosing anesthesia-induced atelectasis in children. *Anesthesiology* 2014; **120**: 1370–1379.

93 Dicker SA, Lisciandro GR, Newell SM, *et al.* Diagnosis of pulmonary contusions with point-of-care lung ultrasonography and thoracic radiography compared to thoracic computed tomography in dogs with motor vehicle trauma: 29 cases (2017–2018). *J Vet Emerg Crit Care* 2020; **30**(6): 638–646.

94 Rodrigues JN, Giraud L, Billen F, *et al.* Comparison of lung ultrasound, chest radiographs, C-reactive protein, and clinical findings in dogs treated for aspiration pneumonia. *J Vet Inter Med* 2022; **36**(2): 743–752.

95 Łobaczewski A, Czopowicz M, Moroz A, *et al.* Lung ultrasound for imaging of B-lines in dogs and cats-a prospective study investigating agreement between three types of transducers and the accuracy in diagnosing cardiogenic pulmonary edema, pneumonia and lung neoplasia. *Animals (Basel)* 2021; **11**(11): 3279.

96 Murphy SD, Ward JL, Viall AK, *et al.* Utility of point-of-care lung ultrasound for monitoring cardiogenic pulmonary edema in dogs. *J Vet Intern Med* 2021; **35**(1): 68–77.

97 Cereda M, Xin Y, Goffi A, *et al.* Imaging the injured lung: mechanisms of action and clinical use. *Anesthesiology* 2019; **131**(3): 716–749.

98 Lichtenstein DA. Current misconceptions in lung ultrasound: a short guide for experts. *Chest* 2019; **156**(1): 21–25.

99 Sperandeo M, Filabozzi P, Varriale A, *et al.* Role of thoracic ultrasound in the assessment of pleural and pulmonary diseases. *J Ultrasound* 2008; **11**(2): 39–46.

100 Dietrich CF, Mathis G, Cui XW, *et al.* Ultrasound of the pleurae and lungs. *Ultrasound Med Biol* 2015; **41**(2): 351–365.

101 Lamb CR, Dirrig H, Cortellini S. Comparison of ultrasonographic findings in cats with and without azotaemia. *J Feline Med Surg* 2018; **20**(10): 948–954.

102 Quantz JE, Miles MS, Reed AL, *et al.* Elevation of alanine transaminase and gallbladder wall abnormalities as biomarkers of anaphylaxis in canine hypersensitivity patients. *J Vet Emerg Crit Care* 2009; **19**(6): 536–544.

103 Sanderson JJ, Boysen SR, McMurray JM, *et al.* The effect of fasting on gastrointestinal motility in healthy dogs as assessed by sonography. *J Vet Emerg Crit Care* 2017; **27**(6): 645–650.

104 Cole LP, Mantis P, Humm K. Ultrasonographic findings in cats with acute kidney injury: a retrospective study. *J Feline Med Surg* 2019; **21**(6): 475–480.

105 Lamb CR, Cortellini S, Halfacree Z. Ultrasonography in the diagnosis and management of cats with ureteral obstruction. *J Feline Med Surg* 2018; **20**(1): 15–22.

106 Kim SY, Park KT, Yeon SC, *et al.* Accuracy of sonographic diagnosis of pneumoperitoneum using the enhanced peritoneal stripe sign in Beagle dogs. *J Vet Sci* 2014; **15**(2): 195–198.

107 Turner K, Boyd C, Stander N, *et al.* Clinical characteristics of two-hundred thirty-two dogs (2006–2018) treated for suspected anaphylaxis in Perth, *Western Australia. Aust Vet J* 2021; **99**(12): 505–512.

108 Cole L, Humm K, Dirrig H. Focused ultrasound examination of canine and feline emergency urinary tract disorders. *Vet Clin North Am Small Anim Pract* 2021; **51**(6): 1233–1248.

109 Fulton RM. Focused ultrasound of the fetus, female and male reproductive tracts, pregnancy, and dystocia in dogs and cats. *Vet Clin North Am Small Anim Pract* 2021; **51**(6): 1249–1265.

110 Mays E, Phillips K. Focused ultrasound of vascular system in dogs and cats-thromboembolic disease. *Vet Clin North Am Small Anim Pract* 2021; **51**(6): 1267–1282.

111 Birkbeck R, Greensmith T, Humm K. Haemoabdomen due to suspected anaphylaxis in four dogs. *Vet Rec Case Rep* 2019; **7**(1): e000734.

112 Caldwell DJ, Petras KE, Mattison BL. Spontaneous hemoperitoneum and anaphylactic shock associated with Hymenoptera envenomation in a dog. *J Vet Emerg Crit Care* 2018; **28**(5): 476–482.

113 Akgür FM, Aktuğ T, Olguner M, *et al.* Prospective study investigating routine usage of ultrasonography as the initial diagnostic modality for the evaluation of children sustaining blunt abdominal trauma. *J Trauma* 1997; **42**: 626–628.

114 Kameda T, Taniguchi N. Overview of point-of-care abdominal ultrasound in emergency and critical care. *J Intensive Care* 2016; **4**: 53.

115 Marin JR, Abo AM, Arroyo AC, *et al.* Pediatric emergency medicine point-of-care ultrasound: summary of the evidence. *Crit Ultrasound J* 2016; **8**: 16.

116 Singh Y, Tissot C, Fraga MV, *et al.* International evidence-based guidelines on Point of Care Ultrasound (POCUS) for critically ill neonates and children issued by the POCUS Working Group of the European Society of Paediatric and Neonatal Intensive Care (ESPNIC). *Crit Care* 2020; **24**(1): 65.

117 McGahan JP, Richards J, Gillen M. The focused abdominal sonography for trauma scan: pearls and pitfalls. *J Ultrasound Med* 2002; **21**: 789–800.

118 Pereira BM, Pereira RG, Wise R, *et al.* The role of point-of-care ultrasound in intra-abdominal hypertension management. *Anestezjologia Intensywna Terapia* 2017; **49**: 373–381.

119 Perlas A, Davis L, Khan M, *et al.* Gastric sonography in the fasted surgical patient: a prospective descriptive study. *Anesth Analg* 2011; **113**: 93–97.

120 Bouvet L, Mazoit JX, Chassard D, *et al.* Clinical assessment of the ultrasonographic measurement of antral area for estimating preoperative gastric content and volume. *Anesthesiology* 2011; **114**: 1086–1092.

121 Van de Putte P. Bedside gastric ultrasonography to guide anesthetic management in a nonfasted emergency patient. *J Clin Anesth* 2013; **25**: 165–166.

122 Hutchinson A, Maltby JR, Reid CR. Gastric fluid volume and pH in elective inpatients. Part I: coffee or orange juice versus overnight fast. *Can J Anaesth* 1988; **35**: 12–15.

123 Agarwal A, Chari P, Singh H. Fluid deprivation before operation: the effect of a small drink. *Anesthesia* 1989; **44**: 632–634.

124 Maltby JR, Lewis P, Martin A, *et al.* Gastric fluid volume and pH in elective patients following unrestricted oral fluid until three hours before surgery. *Can J Anaesth* 1991; **38**: 425–429.

125 Penninck DG, Nyland TG, Fisher PE, *et al.* Ultrasonography of the normal canine gastrointestinal tract. *Vet Radiol* 1989; **30**(6): 272–276.

126 Choi M, Seo M, Jung J, *et al.* Evaluation of canine gastric motility with ultrasonography. *J Vet Med Sci* 2002; **64**(1): 17–21.

127 Tsukamoto A, Ohno K, Tsukagoshi T, *et al.* Real-time ultrasonographic evaluation of canine gastric motility in the postprandial state. *J Vet Med Sci* 2011; **73**(9): 1133–1138.
128 Rutherford S, Gaschen F, Husnik R, *et al.* Ultrasonographic evaluation of the effects of azithromycin on antral motility and gastric emptying in healthy cats. *J Vet Intern Med* 2022; **36**(2): 508–514.
129 Ozturk NK, Kavakli AS. Use of bladder volume measurement assessed with ultrasound to predict postoperative urinary retention. *North Clin Istanb* 2017; **3**(3): 209–216.
130 Møller T, Engedal MS, Plum LM, *et al.* Reduced need for urinary bladder catheterization in the postanesthesia care unit after implementation of an evidence-based protocol: a prospective cohort comparison study. *Eur Urol Open Sci* 2021; **26**: 27–34.
131 Kendall A, Keenihan E, Kern ZT, *et al.* Three-dimensional bladder ultrasound for estimation of urine volume in dogs compared with traditional 2-dimensional ultrasound methods. *J Vet Intern Med* 2020; **34**(6): 2460–2467.
132 Atalan G, Barr FJ, Holt PE. Frequency of urination and ultrasonographic estimation of residual urine in normal and dysuric dogs. *Res Vet Sci* 1999; **67**(3): 295–299.
133 Lisciandro GR, Fosgate GT. Use of urinary bladder measurements from a point-of-care cysto-colic ultrasonographic view to estimate urinary bladder volume in dogs and cats. *J Vet Emerg Crit Care* 2017; **27**(6): 713–717.
134 Via G, Hussain A, Wells M, *et al.* International Liaison Committee on Focused Cardiac UltraSound (ILC-FoCUS); International Conference on Focused Cardiac UltraSound (IC-FoCUS). International evidence-based recommendations for focused cardiac ultrasound. *J Am Soc Echocardiogr* 2014; **27**: 683.
135 Martin LD, Howell EE, Ziegelstein RC, *et al.* Hand-carried ultrasound performed by hospitalists: does it improve the cardiac physical examination? *Am J Med* 2009; **122**: 35–41.
136 Kobal SL, Trento L, Baharami S, *et al.* Comparison of effectiveness of hand-carried ultrasound to bedside cardiovascular physical examination. *Am J Cardiol* 2005; **96**: 1002–1006.
137 McKiernan CA, Lieberman SA. Circulatory shock in children. *Pediatr Rev* 2016; **26**: 451–460.
138 Spencer KT, Kimura BJ, Korcarz CE, *et al.* Focused cardiac ultrasound: recommendations from the American Society of Echocardiography. *J Am Soc Echocardiogr* 2013; **26**: 567–581.
139 Labovitz AJ, Noble VE, Bierig M, *et al.* Focused cardiac ultrasound in the emergent setting: a consensus statement of the American Society of Echocardiography and American College of Emergency Physicians. *J Am Soc Echocardiogr* 2010; **23**: 1225–1230.
140 Marin JR, Lewiss RE. Point-of-care ultrasonography by pediatric emergency medicine physicians. *Pediatr Emerg Care* 2015; **31**: 525.
141 Sicari R, Galderisi M, Voigt JU, *et al.* The use of pocket-size imaging devices: a position statement of the European Association of Echocardiography. *Eur J Echocardiogr* 2011; **12**: 85–87.
142 Riera A, Weeks B, Emerson BL, *et al.* Evaluation of a focused cardiac ultrasound protocol in a pediatric emergency department. *Pediatr Emerg Care* 2021; **37**(4): 191–198.
143 EL-Nawawy AA, Abdelmohsen AM, Hassouna HM. Role of echocardiography in reducing shock reversal time in pediatric septic shock: a randomized controlled trial. *J Pediatr (Rio J)* 2018; **94**: 31–39.
144 Arnal LE, Stein F. Pediatric septic shock: why has mortality decreased? The utility of goal-directed therapy. *Semin Pediatr Infect Dis* 2003; **14**: 165–172.
145 Longjohn M, Wan J, Joshi V, *et al.* Point-of-care echocardiography by pediatric emergency physicians. *Pediatr Emerg Care* 2011; **27**: 693–696.
146 Zimmerman JM, Coker BJ. The nuts and bolts of performing Focused Cardiovascular Ultrasound (FoCUS). *Anesth Analg* 2017; **124**: 753–760.
147 Lai WW, Geva T, Shirali GS, *et al.*; Task Force of the Pediatric Council of the American Society of Echocardiography; Pediatric Council of the American Society of Echocardiography. Guidelines and standards for performance of a pediatric echocardiogram: a report from the Task Force of the Pediatric Council of the American Society of Echocardiography. *J Am Soc Echocardiogr* 2006; **19**: 1413–1430.
148 Rich S, Sheikh A, Gallastegui J, *et al.* Determination of left ventricular ejection fraction by visual estimation during real-time two-dimensional echocardiography. *Am Heart J* 1982; **104**: 603–606.
149 Hope MD, de la Pena E, Yang PC, *et al.* A visual approach for the accurate determination of echocardiographic left ventricular ejection fraction by medical students. *J Am Soc Echocardiogr* 2003; **16**: 824–831.
150 Mark DG, Ku BS, Carr BG, *et al.* Directed bedside transthoracic echocardiography: preferred cardiac window for left ventricular ejection fraction estimation in critically ill patients. *Am J Emerg Med* 2007; **25**: 894–900.
151 Ward JL, Lisciandro GR, Ware WA, *et al.* Evaluation of point-of-care thoracic ultrasound and NT-proBNP for the diagnosis of congestive heart failure in cats with respiratory distress. *J Vet Intern Med* 2018; **32**(5): 1530–1540.
152 Loughran KA, Rush JE, Rozanski EA, *et al.* The use of focused cardiac ultrasound to screen for occult heart disease in asymptomatic cats. *J Vet Intern Med* 2019; **33**: 1892–1901.
153 Janson CO, Hezzell MJ, Oyama MA, *et al.* Focused cardiac ultrasound and point of-care NT-proBNP assay in the emergency room for differentiation of cardiac and noncardiac causes of respiratory distress in cats. *J Vet Emerg Crit Care* 2020; **30**(4): 376–383.
154 Loughran K. Focused cardiac ultrasonography in cats. *Vet Clin North Am Small Anim Pract* 2021; **51**(6): 1183–1202.
155 Darnis E, Merveille AC, Desquilbet L, *et al.* Interobserver agreement between non-cardiologist veterinarians and a cardiologist after a 6-hour training course for echographic evaluation of basic echocardiographic parameters and caudal vena cava diameter in 15 healthy beagles. *J Vet Emerg Crit Care* 2019; **29**(5): 495–504.
156 Ware W. *Cardiovascular Disease in Small Animal Medicine*, 1st edn. London: Manson Publishing Ltd, 2011.
157 Boon JA. *Two Dimensional and M-Mode Echocardiography for the Small Animal Practitioner*. Jackson, WY: Teton NewMedia, 2002.
158 DeFrancesco TC, Ward JL. Focused canine cardiac ultrasound. *Vet Clin North Am Small Anim Pract* 2021; **51**(6): 1203–1216.
159 Lisciandro GR. The use of the diaphragmatico-hepatic (DH) views of the abdominal and thoracic focused assessment with sonography for triage (AFAST/TFAST) examinations for the detection of pericardial effusion in 24 dogs (2011–2012). *J Vet Emerg Crit Care* 2016; **26**(1): 125–131.
160 Campbell FE, Kittleson MD. The effect of hydration status on the echocardiographic measurements of normal cats. *J Vet Intern Med* 2007; **21**(5): 1008–1015.
161 Durkan SD, Rush J, Rozanski E, *et al.* Echocardiographic findings in dogs with hypovolemia. *Abstract J Vet Emerg Crit Care* 2005; **15**(s1): S1–S13.
162 Hultman TM, Boysen SR, Owen R, *et al.* Ultrasonographically derived caudal vena cava parameters acquired in a standing position and lateral recumbency in healthy, lightly sedated cats: a pilot study. *J Feline Med Surg* 2022; **24**(10): 1039–1045.
163 Darnis E, Boysen S, Merveille AC, *et al.* Establishment of reference values of the caudal vena cava by fast-ultrasonography through different views in healthy dogs. *J Vet Intern Med* 2018; **32**(4): 1308–1318.
164 Donati PA, Guevara JM, Ardiles V, *et al.* Caudal vena cava collapsibility index as a tool to predict fluid responsiveness in dogs. *J Vet Emerg Crit Care* 2020; **30**(6): 677–686.
165 Boretsky KR, Kantor DB, DiNardo JA, *et al.* Focused cardiac ultrasound in the pediatric perioperative setting. *Anesth Analg* 2019; **129**(4): 925–932.
166 Cureton EL, Yeung LY, Kwan RO, *et al.* The heart of the matter: utility of ultrasound of cardiac activity during traumatic arrest. *J Trauma Acute Care Surg* 2012; **73**(1): 102–110.
167 Tayal VS, Kline JA. Emergency echocardiography to detect pericardial effusion in patients in PEA and near-PEA states. *Resuscitation* 2003; **59**: 315–318.
168 Chardoli M, Heidari F, Rabiee H, *et al.* Echocardiography integrated ACLS protocol versus conventional cardiopulmonary resuscitation in patients with pulseless electrical activity cardiac arrest. *Chin J Traumatol* 2012; **15**: 284–287.
169 Tran A, Fernando SM, Rochwerg B, *et al.* Pre-arrest and intra-arrest prognostic factors associated with survival following traumatic out-of-hospital cardiac arrest – a systematic review and meta-analysis. *Resuscitation* 2020; **153**: 119–135.
170 Blanco P, Volpicelli G. Common pitfalls in point-of-care ultrasound: a practical guide for emergency and critical care physicians. *Crit Ultrasound J* 2016; **8**(1): 15.
171 Reynolds JC, Nicholson T, O'Neil B, *et al.* Advanced Life Support Task Force at the International Liaison Committee on Resuscitation ILCOR. Diagnostic test accuracy of point-of-care ultrasound during cardiopulmonary resuscitation to indicate the etiology of cardiac arrest: a systematic review. *Resuscitation* 2022; **172**: 54–63.
172 Querellou E, Leyral J, Brun C, *et al.* In and out-of-hospital cardiac arrest and echography: a review. *Ann Fr Anesth Reanim* 2009; **28**: 769–778.
173 Aagaard R, Granfeldt A, Bøtker MT, *et al.* The right ventricle is dilated during resuscitation from cardiac arrest caused by hypovolemia: a porcine ultrasound study. *Crit Care Med* 2017; **45**: e963–e970.
174 Mallamaci F, Benedetto FA, Tripepi R, *et al.* Detection of pulmonary congestion by chest ultrasound in dialysis patients. *JACC Cardiovasc Imaging* 2010; **3**(6): 586–594.
175 Lee CW, Kory PD, Arntfield RT. Development of a fluid resuscitation protocol using inferior vena cava and lung ultrasound. *J Crit Care* 2016; **31**(1): 96–100.

SECTION 3

Pharmacology

19 General Pharmacology of Anesthetic and Analgesic Drugs

Ted Whittem[1], Thierry Beths[2] and Sébastien H. Bauquier[3]

[1] College of Public Health, Medical and Veterinary Sciences, James Cook University, Townsville, Queensland, Australia

[2] Melbourne Veterinary School, University of Melbourne, and Greencross Veterinary Hospital, Werribee, Victoria, Australia

[3] Melbourne Veterinary School, University of Melbourne, Werribee, Victoria, Australia, and Southpaws Specialty, Emergency and Referral Hospital, Malvern East, Victoria, Australia

Chapter contents

Introduction, 283
Classical receptor theory, 283
  Affinity and activity of a ligand, 284
  Selectivity and specificity of a ligand, 284
  Assessment of the ligand–receptor interaction, 284
  Receptor agonists and antagonists: definition and examples, 284
Receptor state theory, 285
Receptor structure, 285
  Sodium ion channels, 285
  GABA receptors, 286
  AMPA and NMDA receptors, 286
  G-protein receptors – second messengers, 287
  Angiotensin-converting enzyme 2 – SARS-CoV-2 receptors, 287
Clinical evaluation of drug effects, 287
  Efficacy, potency, and concentration–response relationship, 288
  Effective dose, lethal dose, toxic dose, and therapeutic index, 288
Pharmacokinetics and pharmacodynamics, 290
  Fundamentals of pharmacodynamics, 290
  Fundamentals of pharmacokinetics, 290
  Half-life of elimination, 291
  Apparent volume of distribution, 291
  Total body clearance, 292
  Hepatic clearance, 292
  Renal clearance, 294
  Absorption, 294
  Bioavailability, 294
  Pharmacokinetics of inhalant anesthetic agents, 294
  Linear and nonlinear pharmacokinetics, 295
Experiments in pharmacokinetics, 295
  Preparation for the study, 295
  Experimental design and conduct, 296
  Data analysis – compartmental models, 296
  Data analysis – noncompartmental models, 298
  Data analysis in more complex models, 299
Constant rate therapy, 299
  Intermittent boluses, 299
  Continuous rate infusion, 299
Drug interactions, 305
  Physicochemical interactions, 305
  Pharmacokinetic interactions, 305
  Pharmacodynamic interactions, 306
Adverse drug reactions, 307
Drug metabolism, 307
  Phase I biotransformation, 308
  Phase II biotransformation or conjugation, 308
  Transport of metabolites (Phase III biotransformation), 308
  Isomers and stereoisomers, 309
  The effect of formulation, 309
References, 309

Introduction

Anesthesia and pain management are two branches of veterinary clinical medicine that inarguably are inextricably intertwined with clinical pharmacology. A thorough, deep, and workable understanding of the principles of clinical pharmacology is fundamental to successful clinical practice in these disciplines. The primary objective of this chapter is to introduce these fundamental pharmacological concepts as they relate to the practice of anesthesia, and to do so in sufficient detail to provide the basis for which sound clinical decisions can be made, even when specific evidence to support the decision is unavailable or unknown. This chapter also strives to provide the nascent anesthetic scientist with an elementary understanding of some of the commonly used research methods and tools for pharmacokinetic research in veterinary clinical pharmacology.

Classical receptor theory

To allow communication between organs and between cells, the body uses messengers or signals. The role of the biological receptors is to convert signals into different forms of stimuli that will induce a reaction from the cell or organ. The French scientist Claude Bernard (1813–1878) was the first to demonstrate the existence of circulating messengers allowing communication between different parts of the body [1]. This discovery was the prelude to the receptor theory.

A receptor is a component of a cell, usually a protein or glycoprotein, which interacts with the signaling messenger substance. Classically, the signaling messenger substance is called a "ligand." Ligands can be, for example, hormones or drugs. The combination of a drug–ligand with its receptor induces pharmacological effects; the initial effect is called the "action" of the drug, whereas

Veterinary Anesthesia and Analgesia: The Sixth Edition of Lumb and Jones. Edited by Leigh Lamont, Kurt Grimm, Sheilah Robertson, Lydia Love and Carrie Schroeder.
© 2024 John Wiley & Sons, Inc. Published 2024 by John Wiley & Sons, Inc.
Companion website: www.wiley.com/go/lamont/anesthesia

succeeding effects are called drug "effects" [2]. The relationship between a ligand and its receptor follows the law of mass-action:

$$[L]+[R]\underset{K_d}{\overset{K_a}{\rightleftharpoons}}[LR] \quad (19.1)$$

where

$$K_a = \frac{1}{K_d} = \frac{[LR]}{[L][R]}$$

where K_a is the rate constant of association of the ligand with the receptor, K_d is the rate constant of dissociation of the ligand with the receptor, [L] is the concentration of unbound ligand, [R] is the concentration of unbound receptor, and [LR] is the concentration of bound receptors.

Affinity and activity of a ligand

The affinity describes the relationship between a particular receptor and its ligand: from eqn 19.1, if the amount of ligand administered is just enough to occupy 50% of the receptors, then

$$[LR]=[R] \xrightarrow{yields} K_a = \frac{[R]}{[L][R]} \xrightarrow{yields} K_a = \frac{1}{[L]} \quad (19.2)$$

A high K_a (and a low K_d) implies that at equilibrium the number of unbound ligand molecules is low, showing a high affinity of the ligand for the receptor. Conversely, a low K_a (and a high K_d) indicates a poor affinity of the ligand for the receptor. However, a ligand can have a strong affinity to a receptor without producing an effect. The activity will describe the ability of a ligand to induce an action. For example, the mu (μ) and kappa (κ) opioid receptors are the main opioid receptors involved in opioid-modulation of pain. Buprenorphine is classified as a partial μ-opioid receptor agonist. It has a high affinity for the μ-opioid receptor and as a consequence its effects, although moderate, are difficult to antagonize [3]. Butorphanol is classified as an agonist–antagonist opioid [2]. It produces its effect by activating κ-opioid receptors and also binds to μ-opioid receptors. However, even though butorphanol has a strong affinity for μ-opioid receptors, it is unable to activate them and will cause no action from the association with those receptors.

Selectivity and specificity of a ligand

The selectivity of a ligand determines its capacity to produce a particular effect. A highly selective drug will only produce one effect through activity at only one class or subclass of receptor. Dopamine is a catecholamine that produces different cardiovascular effects at different doses; when given at a relatively low dose it will increase myocardial contractility (β-adrenergic receptor-mediated); however, when the dose is increased, dopamine will induce some peripheral vasoconstriction (α-adrenergic receptor-mediated). This lack of selectivity occurs because dopamine acts as a ligand at different subclasses of adrenergic receptors with varying affinity. In contrast, dobutamine is a more selective catecholamine (β-adrenergic receptor-mediated only) and its main effect will be to increase myocardial contractility without inducing major peripheral vasoconstriction [4].

The specificity of a ligand describes its capacity to associate with only one specific type of receptor. The effects of a highly specific ligand can be numerous but are due to only one type of receptor–ligand interaction. For example, atropine associates with one specific type of receptor even though these receptors are present in different tissues and the effects are diverse [5]. In comparison, inhalant anesthetics will interact with several different receptors to induce their broad effect, unconsciousness [6].

Assessment of the ligand–receptor interaction

It can be difficult to directly assess the interaction of a receptor with its ligand by observing the number of bound or unbound receptors or even by looking at drug action. As a consequence, investigators often measure the effects of the drugs to try to quantify the receptor occupancy. The effect of the drug is proportional to the concentration of ligand molecules available to bind, which is a function of the dose and method of administration of the ligand, physicochemical and pharmacokinetic properties of the ligand, and location of the receptor. Delays from dosing to onset of pharmacological effects are common and are often referred to as the "lag-time." The delays can be due to the relative difficulty of a ligand reaching the receptor (pharmacokinetics) or can be due to post-transduction delay (pharmacodynamics). For example, glucocorticoid receptors are nuclear receptors, which, when not bound to a ligand such as cortisol or another glucocorticoid, are located in the cytosol. Once activated by ligand binding, the glucocorticoid receptor–drug complex is actively transported into the nucleus where it induces the transcription of genes coding for anti-inflammatory proteins and inhibits the transcription of genes usually upregulated by inflammatory mediators [7]. In this case, the onset of activity is post-transduction and the long lag-time explains why glucocorticoids fail to show good results as emergency drugs.

Receptor agonists and antagonists: definition and examples

The term "agonist" comes from the Greek *agōnistēs* meaning "contestant" or "champion." An agonist ligand is a ligand that binds to the receptor and usually activates it the same way that endogenous molecules would. An agonist ligand can be a full agonist, fully activating the receptor, or a partial agonist that does not fully activate the receptor and therefore produces a less intense maximum effect (see below). It is unknown why some molecules work as full agonists and others work as partial agonists; however, the beginning of the explanation involves the receptor state concept (see below). For example, morphine and buprenorphine are full μ-opioid receptor agonists and partial μ-opioid receptor agonists, respectively. Accordingly, morphine can provide better analgesic effects than buprenorphine, even though buprenorphine's affinity for μ-opioid receptors is higher than that of morphine.

A ligand can also be classified as a neutral antagonist. In this case, the ligand will bind to the receptor but will be unable to activate it. No action following the association of the ligand with the receptor will be seen. This association is usually competitive but can also be noncompetitive. The competitive inhibition of the receptor can be overcome by administering a large enough amount of an agonist ligand, whereas the same action will have no effect if the inhibition is noncompetitive.

Reverse agonists are ligands that will activate the receptor but will induce opposite effects compared to the agonist ligands. Another way to see it is to consider that a receptor has a baseline agonist effect that is not nil, and the administration of the reverse agonist will decrease the baseline effect. The explanation of this phenomenon is based on the receptor state theory discussed below. If the agonist effect is to provide analgesia, the reverse agonist effect will be to increase the sensation of pain.

Flumazenil and Ro 19-4063 are examples of competitive neutral antagonist and reverse agonist, respectively. Mandema *et al.* studied the averaged concentration-EEG effect relationships of all individual rats that had received an intravenous bolus administration of midazolam, flumazenil, or Ro 19-4603. Midazolam was followed by a positive effect, whereas flumazenil and Ro 19-4063 were followed by neutral and negative effects, respectively [8].

Confusion between neutral antagonist and reverse agonist can occur when the baseline agonist effect is minimal. Also, the classification of agonist, partial agonist, neutral antagonist, and reverse agonist applies to a ligand in relation to a particular receptor, and the overall effect of a drug may be different from the effect expected from its action on a particular receptor. Although naloxone is a well-known opioid receptor antagonist, low doses of naloxone can induce analgesic effects. The mechanism by which an opioid antagonist can enhance the opioid agonist effect is unknown, although it could be explained by its effects on: increasing the release of endogenous ligands, upregulation of postsynaptic receptors, inhibiting counteraction by G_s proteins, uncoupling of filament A, and attenuating the increase in the expression of glial fibrillary acidic protein (GFAP) [9].

Receptor state theory

The classic receptor theory implies that the receptor is by default in a nonactivated form and needs an agonist ligand in order to be activated. Although the nonactivated receptor form represents most of the receptors, experiments have shown that without the presence of an agonist ligand, some receptors can exist in their activated form. The role of the ligand would then be not to activate the receptor but to stabilize the receptor's activated form. The two major implications of this theory are the existence of a baseline agonist effect for the receptor and the differentiation between antagonist drugs and inverse agonist drugs.

Receptor structure

Receptors are mainly multiprotein entities and so have four levels of structure. The primary structure is a linear sequence of amino acids, the secondary structure is a regular local substructure (α-helix or β-sheets), the tertiary structure is the three-dimensional structure of a single peptide molecule, and the quaternary structure is the combination of the multiple tertiary structures of different proteins linked together. All these levels of structure are of particular importance, as a ligand will have to fit with these four levels of structure to be able to associate with and activate the receptor.

The aim of this chapter is to illustrate the study of receptor structures using a few examples only of receptors that have a particular importance in the field of anesthesia. The discussion will be limited to some ion channels, G-protein receptors, and the angiotensin-converting enzyme 2 (ACE2) receptor.

Sodium ion channels

One key role of the sodium channel is to allow the genesis of action potentials [10]. Indeed, sodium channels are voltage-gated ion channels that conduct the sodium cation into the cell, generating an action potential. When the membrane potential equals the resting potential of the cell, the channels are closed. However, as the membrane potential increases, the conformation of the central pore of the channel changes, increasing sodium permeability and allowing influx of sodium ions and consequently initiating or propagating an action potential. This change of conformation is made possible by the presence of particular transmembrane-spanning segments (α-helices) called "voltage sensors."

The sodium channel is comprised of three peptide subunits: one α glycoprotein subunit and two accessory β subunits [10] (Fig. 19.1). The α subunit is composed of four homologous domains and each domain contains six transmembrane-spanning segments. The primary structure of one of these segments includes a high number of positively charged amino acids, and when the membrane potential

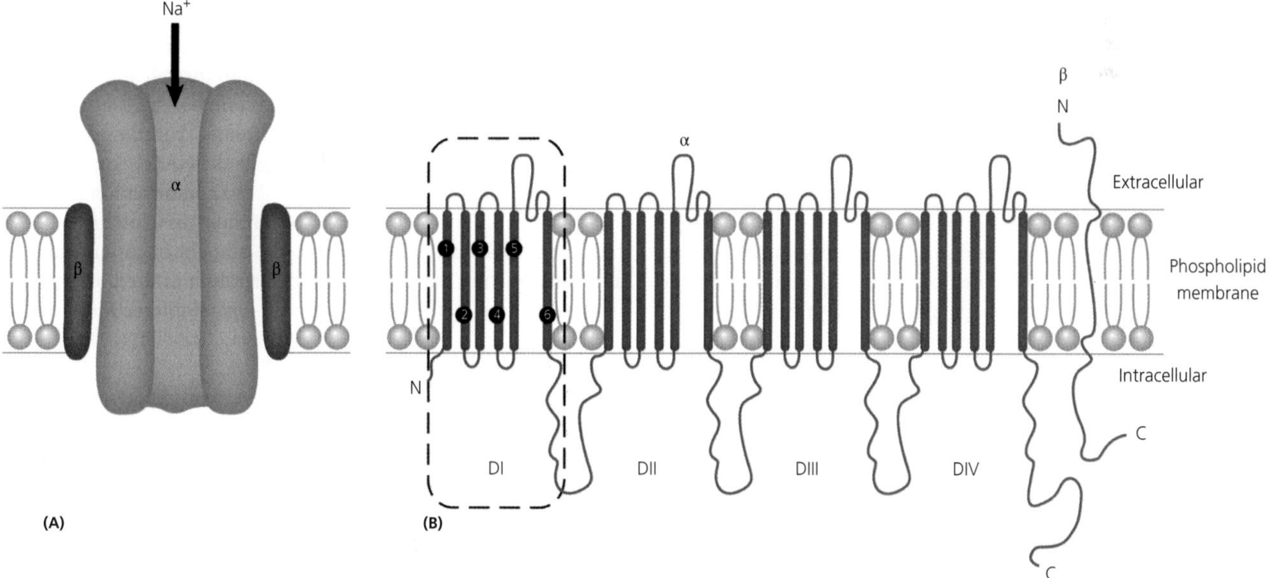

Figure 19.1 Structure of the sodium channel. **A.** Schematic of a sodium channel composed of one α subunit and two accessory β subunits. **B.** Schematic of the α glycoprotein subunit showing the four homologous domains (DI–DIV) containing six membrane-spanning segments numbered 1–6. The primary structure of segment 4 includes positively charged amino acids placed at every fourth position. When the membrane potential increases, the positively charged segments move toward the extracellular side of the membrane, changing the conformation of the channel, and allowing more sodium cations to enter the cell.

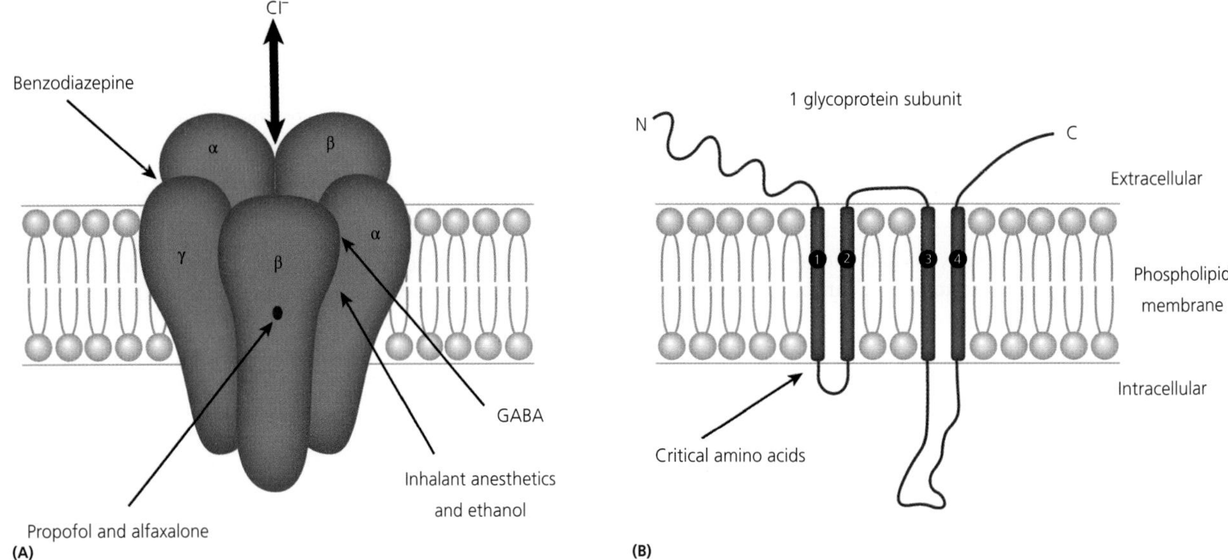

Figure 19.2 Structure of the $GABA_A$ receptor. **A.** Schematic of a $GABA_A$ receptor composed of two α, two β, and one γ subunits showing the binding site of the agonist GABA and of the allosteric modulators: benzodiazepines, inhalant anesthetics, ethanol, propofol, and alfaxalone. **B.** Schematic of one glycoprotein subunit showing the four membrane-spanning segments numbered 1–4.

increases, the positively charged segments move toward the extracellular side of the membrane changing the conformation of the channel. Although their mechanism of action is not completely understood, the local anesthetics work by blocking these channels, thus preventing the formation of action potentials.

GABA receptors

Activated by the neurotransmitter ligand γ-aminobutyric acid (GABA), the neuro-inhibitory GABA receptors ($GABA_A$ and $GABA_B$) are mainly present in the central nervous system in mammals. The $GABA_A$ (fast response) receptors are anion channels, whereas the $GABA_B$ (slow response) receptors are G-protein-coupled receptors. Of this ligand's receptor types, only the $GABA_A$ receptor will be addressed in this chapter.

$GABA_A$ receptors

The $GABA_A$ receptors are ligand-gated anion channels that allow the passage of chloride anions into the cell. The hyperpolarization of the neuron following activation of the receptor inhibits subsequent depolarization of the neuron, reducing central nervous system activity. GABA is the main agonist of this receptor. Most of the drugs used in anesthesia that bind to the $GABA_A$ receptor do not directly activate the receptor but induce an allosteric change (i.e., change of the quaternary structure) of the conformation of the receptor and are called "allosteric modulators." Barbiturates, benzodiazepines, propofol, etomidate, alfaxalone, inhalant anesthetics, and ethanol are examples of ligands that increase the efficiency of the receptor, allowing greater hyperpolarization of the neuron and are thus called "positive allosteric modulators" [11]. The benzodiazepine reversal agent flumazenil decreases the efficiency of the receptor and is therefore a negative allosteric modulator.

The $GABA_A$ receptor is a heteropentamer (five subunits) comprising α, β, and γ subunits, with many combinations of those subunits being possible [11]. Agonist and antagonist ligands and allosteric modulators bind to specific sites of these subunits as illustrated in Figure 19.2A. Also, each subunit has four transmembrane-spanning (α-helix) segments creating the chloride channel (Fig. 19.2B).

AMPA and NMDA receptors

The α-aminohydroxymethylisoxazolepropionic acid (AMPA) and *N*-methyl-D-aspartate (NMDA) receptors are both cation channels. Their endogenous agonist is glutamate [12] and they usually co-exist on the same postsynaptic membranes. Their interaction is thought to be one key element of central sensitization.

AMPA receptors

The AMPA receptor is a ligand-gated ionotropic receptor. This cation channel allows the entrance of Na^+ into the cell and the exit of K^+ from the cell. The AMPA receptor is composed of four subunits, with each subunit having four membrane-spanning segments, which create the cation channel [12]. Like the $GABA_A$ receptor, the association with an agonist ligand induces a conformational change allowing the channel to open. The amount of glutamate being released in the synapse will dictate the amount of cation transfer, and consequently the degree of depolarization of the postsynaptic neuron induced by the AMPA receptor–ligand interaction.

NMDA receptors

The NMDA receptor is both a ligand-gated and voltage-gated ionotropic receptor [12] (Fig. 19.3). This cation channel allows the entrance of Na^+ and Ca^{2+} into the cell, and the exit of K^+ out of the cell. In contrast to the AMPA receptor, a molecule of Mg^{2+} keeps the channel closed until a strong enough depolarization of the postsynaptic membrane occurs. Although weak activation of the AMPA receptor is not enough to activate the NMDA receptor, multiple or stronger activations of the AMPA receptor will induce a strong enough depolarization of the postsynaptic membrane to release the Mg^{2+} from inside the channel of the NMDA receptor.

Glutamate and aspartate are the main endogenous agonists for the NMDA receptor and glycine is a co-agonist required to

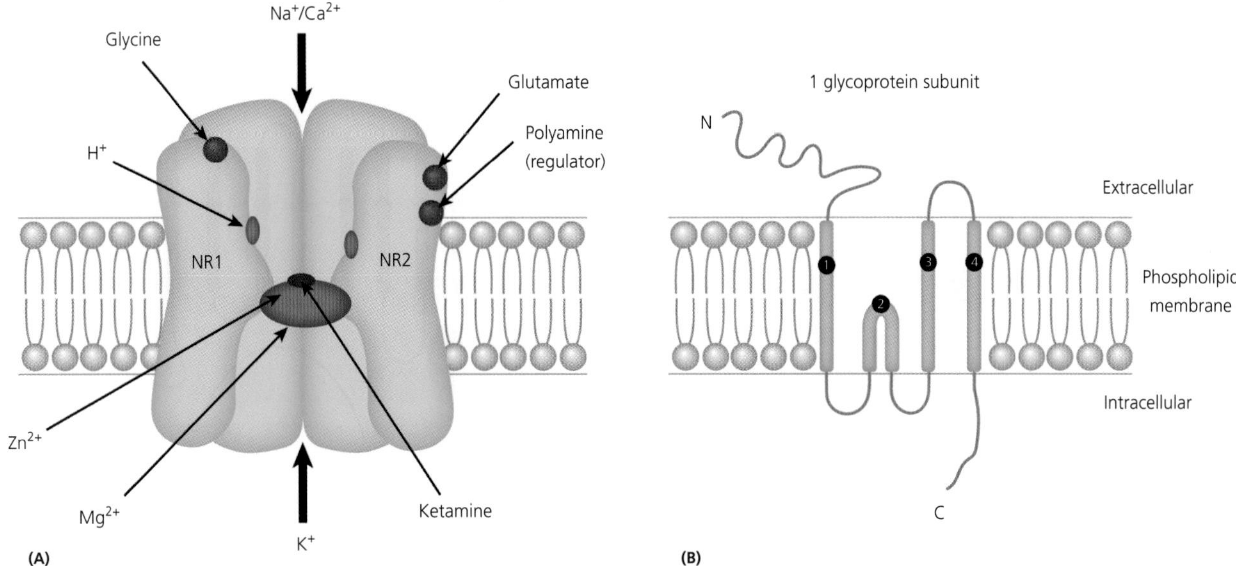

Figure 19.3 Structure of the NMDA receptor. **A.** Schematic of an NMDA receptor composed of four subunits (two NR1 subunits and two NR2 subunits) showing the binding site of the agonist glutamate, the co-agonist glycine, the antagonist ketamine, and the modulators zinc and copper. Other axillary subunits have also been described. **B.** Schematic of one glycoprotein subunit showing the four membrane-spanning segments numbered 1–4. It should be noted that segment numbered 2 does not cross the membrane but kinks back on itself toward the intracellular side of the membrane.

efficiently open the channel. NMDA is a partial agonist and amantidine, gabapentin, ketamine and phencyclidine derivatives, ethanol, xenon, nitrous oxide, and some opioids (methadone and tramadol) are NMDA receptor antagonists. Magnesium, sodium, calcium, potassium, zinc, and copper are modulators of the NMDA receptor.

G-protein receptors – second messengers

To transduce extracellular signals, some transmembrane receptors use intermediaries such as guanine nucleotide-binding proteins (G-proteins). A series of intracellular biochemical events (or second messengers) is initiated by the receptor–ligand interaction and ultimately leads to the observation of the clinical effect. Guanosine triphosphate (GTP) supplies the energy required by such complex G-protein receptors. These receptors are some of the most common and important receptors. The β-adrenergic receptor will be discussed as an example of a G-protein-coupled receptor.

β-Adrenergic receptors

There are three types of β-adrenergic receptors: β_1 found in the cardiac sarcolemma, β_2 found in the bronchial and vascular smooth muscle, and β_3 found in adipose tissue. The β-adrenergic receptors are linked to the adenylate cyclase (AC) enzyme system through the G-proteins and are activated by the endogenous β-adrenergic receptor agonists, epinephrine, and norepinephrine. The stimulatory G-protein (G_s or $G\alpha_s$), linked to the β-adrenergic receptor, is composed of α, β, and γ subunits and is located on the intracellular side of the cellular membrane. By default, the α subunit is associated with guanosine diphosphate (GDP), and the protein is considered switched off. However, interaction of the β-adrenergic receptor with norepinephrine or epinephrine changes its conformation allowing GTP to replace the GDP on the α-subunit, and the protein is switched on. The associated AC is stimulated, inducing the production of cyclic AMP (cAMP), which in turn activates protein kinase A (PKA) and numerous downstream enzymes (Fig. 19.4). The AC can also be inhibited by the inhibitory G-proteins (G_i or $G\alpha_i$), which have a similar mechanism of activation to G_s. Indeed, G_i is linked to a β_2-adrenergic receptor and is a likely mechanism of modulation.

Angiotensin-converting enzyme 2 – SARS-CoV-2 receptors

Most anesthesiologists are familiar with angiotensin-converting enzyme (ACE), which has an important role in blood pressure homeostasis through conversion of angiotensin I to angiotensin II – a potent vasoconstrictor within the renin–angiotensin–aldosterone system (RAAS). However, angiotensin-converting enzyme 2 (ACE2) plays a key balancing role in this system principally through generation of the vasodilator angiotensin-(1–7) from angiotensin II. More recently, the human ACE2 has been identified as an entry receptor for SARS-CoV-2 [13]. ACE2 is abundantly present in the lung and small intestinal epithelia and in most organs' arterial and venous endothelial cells and arterial smooth muscle cells [14]. It is a transmembrane monocarboxypeptidase zinc-containing metalloprotease receptor that binds to the spike proteins of SARS-CoV-2 and blocks it in place when the virus comes in contact with the respiratory epithelium [13,15]. Furthermore, cell surface proteases and lysosomal proteases will both activate SARS-CoV-2 entry [13]. The protease cuts the SARS-CoV-2 spike protein at a specific location, allowing the spike protein to remodel and insert itself into the epithelium cell's membrane. The spike protein then pulls the cell and virus membranes toward each other. After fusion, the viral RNA is transferred into the host cell.

Clinical evaluation of drug effects

To study pharmacodynamics, or the effects of a drug on the whole body, one can evaluate the efficacy, potency, concentration–response relationship, effective dose, lethal dose, and the therapeutic index. Although one general pharmacological principle remains – the more drug, the more effects (with effects being measured either within an

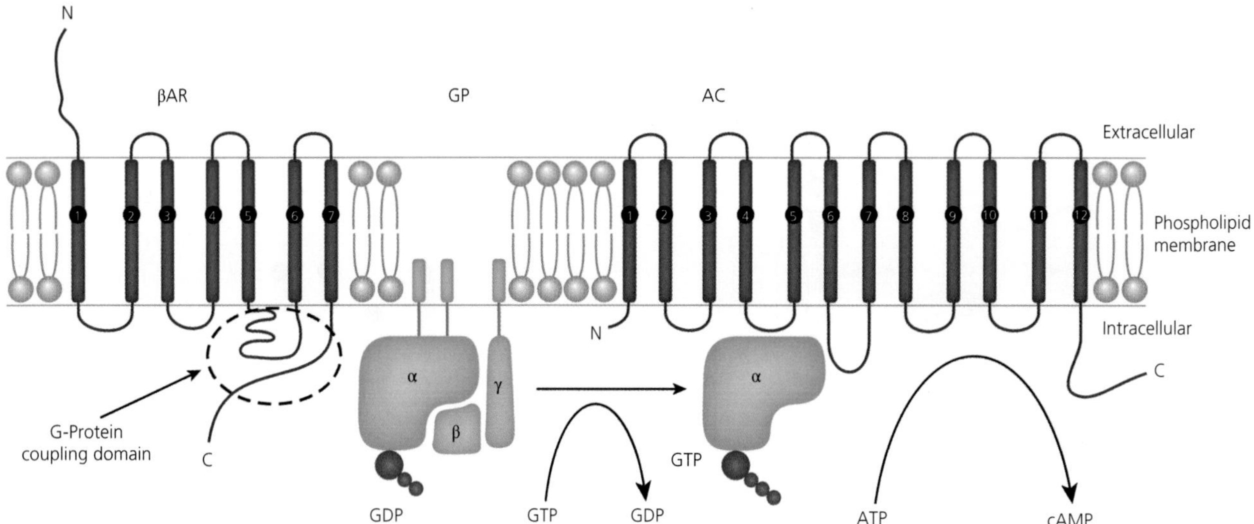

Figure 19.4 Illustration of the association between the β-adrenergic receptor (βAR), G-proteins (GP), and adenylate cyclase (AC). The βAR and AC glycoproteins are showing 7 and 12 membrane-spanning segments, respectively. The GP is composed of α, β, and γ subunits and is located on the intracellular side of the cellular membrane. The conformation of the βAR and the GP are closely linked together. When an agonist ligand binds to the βAR and changes its conformation, the α subunit of the GP also changes conformation, allowing a GTP (guanosine triphosphate) to bind instead of a GDP (guanosine diphosphate). The α subunit of the GP is switched on and will stimulate the AC, inducing the production of cAMP (cyclic AMP) from ATP (adenosine triphosphate).

individual or within a population) – the occurrences of U-shaped (or inverted U-shaped) dose–response curves are widely and independently observed phenomena [16]. "Hormesis" defines dose–response relationships characterized by stimulatory effects at low doses and inhibitory effects at higher doses, resulting in an inverted U-shaped dose–response curve. Naloxone is one example of this hormetic response (see above paragraph on receptor agonist and antagonist), and all receptors assessed to date display dose–response relationships with identifiable mechanisms regulated by agonist concentration gradients [16].

Efficacy, potency, and concentration–response relationship

Earlier in the chapter, it was described how the association of a ligand with a receptor follows the laws of mass-action (eqn 19.1). The total concentration of receptors [R_T] is equal to the sum of [LR] plus [R], and if [R] is replaced by [R_T] – [LR] in eqn 19.1, the relationship becomes:

$$\frac{1}{K_d} = \frac{[\mathrm{LR}]}{[\mathrm{L}]([\mathrm{R_T}]-[\mathrm{R}])} \tag{19.3}$$

which rearranges to:

$$\frac{[\mathrm{LR}]}{[\mathrm{R_T}]} = \frac{[\mathrm{L}]}{[\mathrm{L}]+K_d} \tag{19.4}$$

Also, knowing that the maximum efficacy (E_{max}) represents the maximal pharmacological effect of a drug or a ligand, and that the pharmacological effect (E) of the drug is directly proportional to the percentage of activated receptors [17], then eqn 19.4 becomes:

$$\frac{\mathrm{E}}{\mathrm{E_{max}}} = \frac{[\mathrm{L}]}{[\mathrm{L}]+K_d} \xrightarrow{\text{yields}} \mathrm{E} = \frac{\mathrm{E_{max}}[\mathrm{L}]}{K_d+[\mathrm{L}]} \tag{19.5}$$

This equation indicates a sigmoid relationship between the logarithm of the concentration of ligand and the effect (concentration–response relationship) and that in the absence of ligand, the effect approaches nil. However, the receptor state theory implies the existence of a baseline agonist effect (E_0) of the receptor, and this baseline effect is taken into consideration in Hill's equation:

$$\mathrm{E} = \frac{(\mathrm{E_{max}}-\mathrm{E_0})[\mathrm{L}]}{K_d+[\mathrm{L}]} \tag{19.6}$$

The concentration–response relationship is usually illustrated showing the effect as a function of the ligand's concentration (or other measure of exposure). The term "potency" characterizes the concentration of drug needed to obtain a pharmacological effect that equals 50% of E_{max}, that is, the EC_{50}. The lower the EC_{50}, the less drug that is needed to achieve the required effect and the higher the potency of the drug (Fig. 19.5).

Effective dose, lethal dose, toxic dose, and therapeutic index

The effective dose (ED_{50}) corresponds to the dose of drug necessary to induce the desired effect in 50% of the animals to which it is administered. Similarly, the lethal dose (LD_{50}) corresponds to the dose of drug necessary to induce death in 50% of the animals to which the drug is administered. In most human trials, the lethal dose is not established, and is replaced by the toxic dose (TD_{50}). The TD_{50} corresponds to the dose of drug necessary to induce toxic effects in 50% of the patients to whom it is administered. The therapeutic index is the ratio LD_{50}/ED_{50} or TD_{50}/ED_{50}. The higher the therapeutic index, the safer the drug is considered to be. However, the therapeutic index does not take into consideration the slope of the concentration–response curve. Two drugs, A and B, with the same therapeutic index and given at ED_{90} (the effective dose in 90% of the population) can induce a significantly different prevalence of side effects, and therefore the therapeutic index is not useful as a measure of a drug's clinical safety (Fig. 19.6).

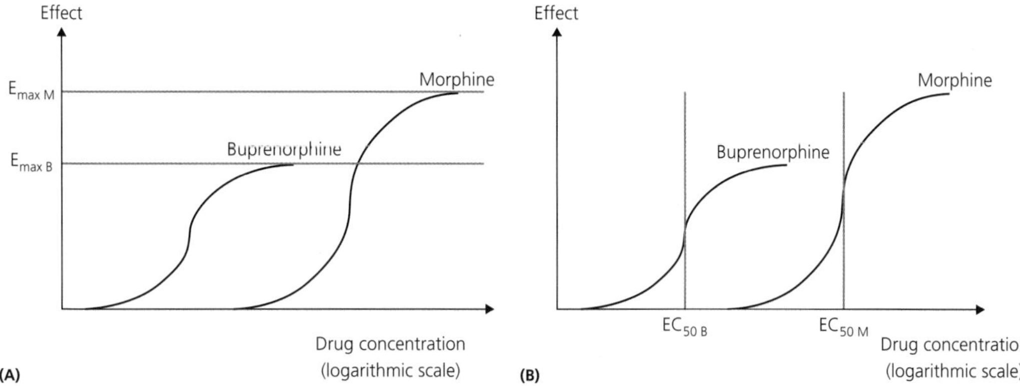

Figure 19.5 Illustration of the concentration–response relationships of the two opioids morphine and buprenorphine, the considered measured effect being analgesia. **A.** The maximal analgesic effect of buprenorphine ($E_{max\ B}$) is lower than that of morphine ($E_{max\ M}$). Indeed, morphine is a full μ-opioid receptor agonist, whereas buprenorphine is a partial μ-opioid receptor agonist. **B.** The concentration of drug needed to obtain a pharmacological effect that equals 50% of the maximal effect is lower for buprenorphine ($EC_{50\ B}$) than for morphine ($EC_{50\ M}$).

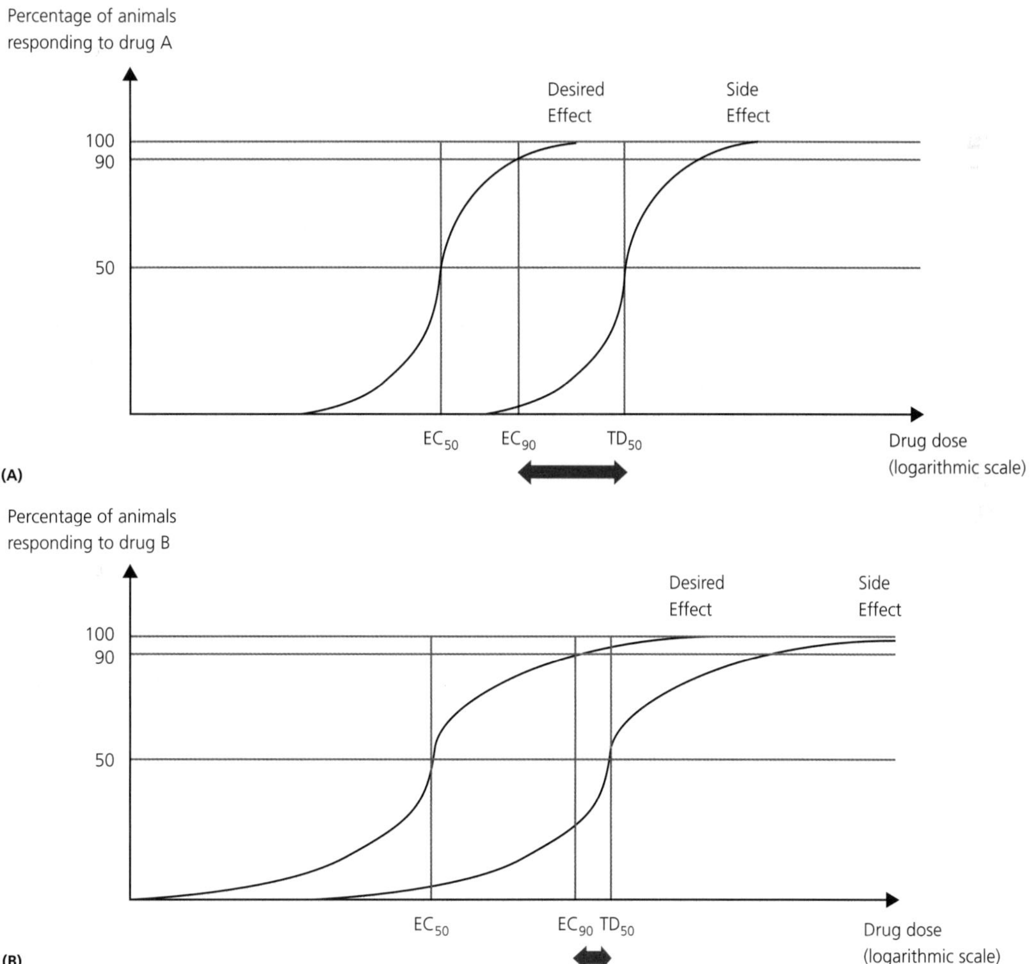

Figure 19.6 Illustration of the limitation of the therapeutic index to establish the safety profile of a drug. Drugs A and B have the same therapeutic index (ED_{50}/TD_{50}, the ratio of the effective dose in 50% of the population to the toxic dose in 50% of the population) but different dose–response curve slopes. **A.** The EC_{90} (effective dose in 90% of the population) of drug A is significantly different from the TD_{50}, implying that most of the population will benefit from drug A without encountering side effects. **B.** The EC_{90} of drug B is similar to the TD_{50}, implying that a large part of the population that benefits from drug B will encounter toxic effects.

It is fundamental to recognize that variability between the sensitivity of individuals to drug effects results in a range of doses that may be effective or toxic in some individuals, and not in others. It is less self-evident, but equally important, to recognize that between-occasion variability in response to a fixed dose exists within an individual. The sum of between-individual and between-occasion variability causes uncertainty in the dose–response correlation, necessitating attention to the individual response on each occasion of drug administration.

Pharmacokinetics and pharmacodynamics

When drugs are administered to animals two interactions are initiated. The animal's body initiates its actions on the drug; absorption, distribution, metabolism, and elimination (ADME). These processes are described by the discipline called "pharmacokinetics." At the same time, the drug initiates its actions on the body and this process is described by the discipline called "pharmacodynamics."

Fundamentals of pharmacodynamics

As discussed above, the interaction of free drug with its receptor stimulates the effect response by the organism. The association between receptor–drug concentration and response can differ between drugs, receptor systems, and occasions. As discussed above, the effect response is regarded as directly proportional to the ratio of the receptor–drug concentration and the total receptor concentration [17]. Experimental description of the effect response helps us to illustrate and understand the nature and extent of drug responses.

One of the purposes of drug effect response modeling is to allow one to make predictions of the outcome from clinical use of the drug. Consequently, a good pharmacodynamic model is one that closely describes the data and allows the development and evaluation of hypotheses about the drug's effect response at doses not directly tested. Several routine approaches are made to describe pharmacodynamic effect response data mathematically.

Where the effect response being measured is induced by a drug–receptor complex between 20 and 80% of maximal binding capacity at a single receptor class, then the effect response is often approximately log-linear in relation to drug concentration. Therefore, in the absence of a maximal effect being achieved, where E is the effect response measure, C is the drug concentration, and E_0 is a constant which represents baseline activity, the effect response measure can be approximated by a straight line:

$$E = m \ln C + E_0 \tag{19.7}$$

In single receptor systems where a maximal response is measured so that the effect response measure approaches an asymptote, the shape of the response curve may be described in the same form as for receptor binding (eqn 19.5). Where E_{max} is the maximum achievable response and EC_{50} is the concentration at which a response is achieved that equals 50% of the E_{max}, the effect response can sometimes be described as:

$$E = \frac{E_{max} C}{EC_{50} + C} \tag{19.8}$$

Sometimes, the relationship between drug concentration and effect response reflects changes in the sensitivity of the signaling pathway to the presence of the drug. This may be a function of biological processes such as receptor tachyphylaxis or may be unrelated to known processes. These cases are not well approximated by the E_{max} model shown above, but can often be better described by the following related equation, where h (the Hill coefficient) modifies the steepness of the effect response curve:

$$E = \frac{(E_{max} C)^h}{{EC_{50}}^h + C^h} \tag{19.9}$$

when $h = 1$, this equation reduces to the standard E_{max} model of eqn 19.8. For example, the dose–response curves illustrated in Fig. 19.6A versus Fig. 19.6B are examples of curves with the same E_{max} and EC_{50} but with different slopes, hence they would have differing values for h.

More complex models are needed for drugs, which achieve the measured effect response through multiple signaling pathways, and for effect responses, which are not objectively measured on continuous distributions. During the 1950s, Robins and Rall formulated the "free hormone hypothesis," which is now generally accepted to be true both for hormones and for drugs [18]. Robins and Rall presented a convincing argument that, where a hormone (or drug) is present in protein-bound and unbound (or free) forms in equilibrium, the activity of the drug or hormone at its site of action is proportional to the concentration of the free drug or free hormone in the plasma, irrespective of the total drug or hormone concentration. Based on the assumption that free drugs can diffuse readily to their sites of action, or that there are alternative facilitated or active processes that assist drugs to reach their site of action, the free hormone hypothesis allows the linkage of the plasma concentration to the drug's effect response. Consequently, to examine the degree, extent, and duration of drug effect, a drug's pharmacokinetics is usually sufficiently described by its disposition in blood, plasma, or serum.

Fundamentals of pharmacokinetics

Most pharmacokinetic processes within mammalian bodies occur as saturable processes (Michaelis-Menton kinetics): the speed at which a process occurs has an upper limit, which can be reached, at least in theory. However, we can simplify the mathematics for pharmacokinetics by assuming that processes occur either at constant rates (zero-order) or at rates constant in proportion to the concentration of administered drug (first-order). This simplification is usually acceptable because usually, the concentration range of drugs used is narrow.

Zero-order processes are those in which the change of drug concentration in a body fluid such as plasma or urine occurs at a constant rate, irrespective of the concentration of the drug present in that body fluid. Since this process is constant, the formula for a straight line can be used to describe the plasma drug disposition curve. Consequently, the equation for a zero-order elimination has the following form:

$$C(t) = C(0) - k_0 t \tag{19.10}$$

where $C(t)$ is the concentration of the drug in the sample at any time t and the zero-order elimination rate (k_0) is the slope of the curve when concentration is plotted as a function of time and is called the "zero-order rate equation." This is the equation for a straight line, that is, $y = b + mx$, where y is the concentration in the sample, $C(0)$ is the y-intercept when $x = 0$, and x is time.

Sometimes, drug delivery devices or formulations are designed purposefully to achieve zero-order delivery (constant rate delivery) to maintain a constant effect of the drug for a prolonged period. Constant rate delivery is discussed later in this chapter.

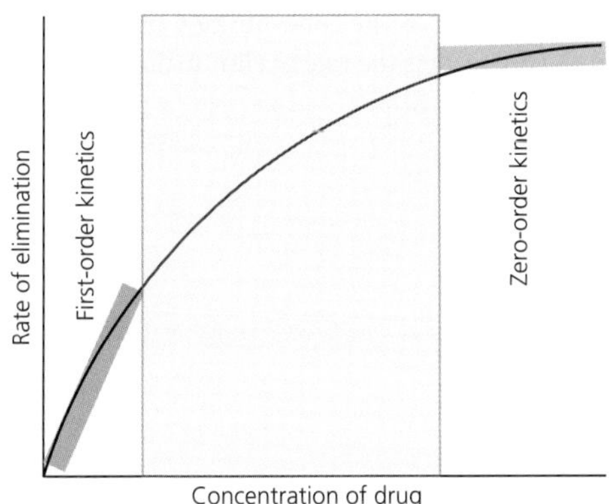

Figure 19.7 For most drugs, the elimination processes obey saturable kinetics, but at the concentrations used clinically most drugs approximate linear "first-order" pharmacokinetics because the elimination processes are not approaching saturation.

In contrast to zero-order processes, a first-order process is one where the rate of change in concentration of drug in a body fluid is proportional to the concentration of the drug in that fluid at that time. In this case, to describe the plasma drug disposition curve, an exponential function is appropriate, conforming to a straight line on a semi-logarithmic plot:

$$\ln C(t) = \ln C(0) - k_{el}t \quad (19.11)$$

where ln*(C)* is the natural logarithm of the concentration of drug in the sample at any time *t* and the first-order elimination rate constant (k_{el}) is the slope. This reduces to

$$C(t) = C(0)e^{-k_{el}t} \quad (19.12)$$

which is called the "first-order rate equation." Many drugs used in anesthesia and analgesia adhere to first-order pharmacokinetics with respect to their elimination from the body, and there are several drugs which are absorbed or eliminated by zero-order processes (Fig. 19.7).

Half-life of elimination

The plasma elimination half-life of a drug is the time interval needed for the plasma concentration to be reduced to 50% (half) of its initial value [19].

Drugs eliminated by zero-order kinetics have half-lives, which are a function of the initial plasma concentration of the drug at the beginning of the time interval. Therefore, plasma half-life is not constant for these drugs and consequently is of no clinical value.

In contrast, drugs eliminated by first-order kinetics have plasma elimination half-lives, which are fixed at a constant rate per unit time. The half-life is inversely proportional to the rate of elimination (k_{el}) as derived in the following sequence from the first-order rate equation:

$$\frac{1}{2}C(0) = C(0)e^{-k_{el}t_{1/2}} \quad (19.13)$$

$$\frac{1}{2} = e^{-k_{el}t_{1/2}} \quad (19.14)$$

$$\ln\left(\frac{1}{2}\right) = -k_{el}t_{1/2} \quad (19.15)$$

$$0.693 = k_{el}t_{1/2} \quad (19.16)$$

$$t_{1/2} = \frac{0.693}{k_{el}} \quad (19.17)$$

Superficially, the concept of elimination half-life appears easy to understand. However, this is a hybrid parameter and is influenced by many factors. Both metabolism and elimination commonly affect the elimination half-life of a drug. Some factors that affect the rate of metabolism of a drug include the species, the age, the gender, the bodyweight, disease states (especially cardiac, renal, and hepatic diseases), and drug interactions.

The time one must wait after administering a drug or changing a drug dose rate before attaining a new steady-state plasma concentration, or before attaining complete elimination of a drug, is a function solely of the half-life of that drug. If the fraction of drug that is eliminated is *FE* from the first-order rate equation, we can derive:

$$FE = 1 - e^{-k_{el}t} \quad (19.18)$$

For practical purposes in clinical veterinary practice, approximately 4–5 half-lives must pass before a change in dose achieves a new steady-state plasma concentration (at about 97% of total). Similarly, approximately 4–5 half-lives must pass after cessation of administration before all drug is effectively eliminated.

Apparent volume of distribution

The mass of drug in the body at any time is proportional to the concentration measured in the sample space (often the plasma) at any time and can be expressed as the following equality:

$$X_B = CV_d \quad (19.19)$$

where X_B is the mass of drug in the body and V_d is the proportionality constant. This proportionality constant V_d is known as the "apparent volume of distribution" [20]. The reason that the word "apparent" is used in the parameter is, although it has units of volume, it does not actually represent any particular physiological or anatomical space and cannot be attributed to any such space from any simple physiological or pharmacokinetic analysis.

It is clear that each sample space will have its own volume parameter, so in complex models, each "compartment" will have an individual volume, for example, the volume of the circulation is often referred to as the volume of the "central compartment" (V_c). The sum of all volumes, central and peripheral, is often referred to as the "volume of distribution at steady state" (V_{dss}). Understanding and having an estimate for volume parameters facilitates dose calculations, for example:

$$\text{loading dose} = C_{(\text{desired})}V_c \quad (19.20)$$

Just as there are several different volume parameters, there are also different methods to calculate them. It is important to understand that estimates of a volume parameter might be differently derived and therefore have different absolute values.

Particular volume parameters are better suited to particular uses; for example, the apparent volume of the central compartment (V_c) is usually used for calculating loading doses for rapidly acting or toxic drugs such as an induction dose of an anesthetic, whereas the apparent volume of distribution at steady state (V_{dss}) is often used for calculating constant rate infusions (CRIs) or repeated analgesic drug dosing regimens (see discussion below in the section on Constant rate therapy).

Within a species, the apparent volume of distribution varies from individual to individual. Individual factors which affect the volume of distribution include the state of hydration, the age and gender of the animal, the bodyweight and body composition (fat, muscle, and water ratios), the protein content of serum especially for protein-bound drugs, the presence of plasma expanders such as lipids after a meal, and drug interactions (rarely, due to competition for binding sites).

Total body clearance

Total body clearance is defined as the volume of blood from which drug is completely removed, per unit of time. It is commonly referred to simply as "clearance" (*Cl*) and the units for clearance are volume per time (e.g., mL/min or L/h) often normalized by body weight (e.g., mL/min/kg). *Cl* is a measure of the efficiency of drug elimination and is often directly compared or contrasted with cardiac output (CO) in the species under examination.

As *Cl* describes the relationship between the rate of excretion of a drug and its plasma concentration, if X_E is the mass of drug eliminated from the body and equals $-X_B$ if no further dose is administered, it can be described algebraically as follows:

$$Cl = \frac{-\frac{dX_B}{dt}}{C} \quad (19.21)$$

$$Cl = \frac{X_B k_{el}}{C} \quad (19.22)$$

However, we have already seen that $X_B = CV_d$ (eqn 19.19). Therefore, in this simplified example:

$$Cl = k_{el} V_d \quad (19.23)$$

Cl can thereby be understood as a function of both the volume of distribution and the concentration of drug present in the sample space. While this is demonstrated to be true for total body *Cl*, it is useful to foresee that this can be extrapolated to clearance from individual compartments in complicated multi-compartment systems.

Total body *Cl* is the sum of the clearance achieved by all mechanisms. Although some anesthetic drugs are cleared by the lungs, the most important two components are usually attributed to hepatic and renal clearance. Thus, total body *Cl* can be defined as follows:

$$Cl_{\text{Total body}} = Cl_H + Cl_R + Cl_{\text{other}} \quad (19.24)$$

where Cl_H and Cl_R are the clearances due to hepatic and renal mechanisms, respectively. Total body *Cl* is a very important pharmacokinetic parameter and must be comprehensively understood [21].

Hepatic clearance

Consider the flow diagram in Fig. 19.8, where Q_H is the rate of organ blood flow through the liver, C_A is the concentration of drug in the arterial blood, C_V is the concentration of drug in the venous blood, and $Q_H(C_A - C_V)$ is the rate of elimination by the liver.

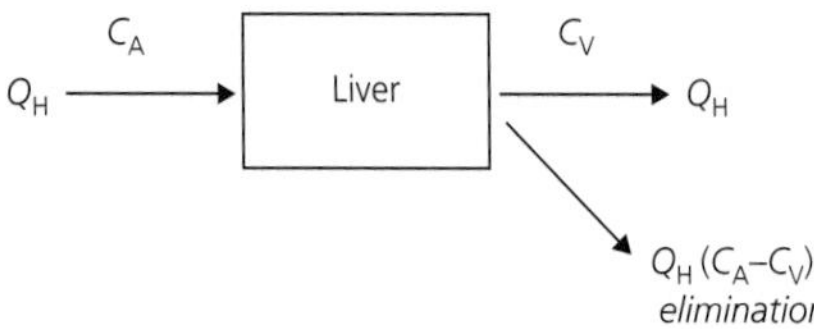

Figure 19.8 Hepatic clearance of drugs is estimated from hepatic blood flow (Q_H) and the concentration difference between the drug in the hepatic blood inflow (C_A) and outflow (C_V).

Then, since

$$Cl = \frac{\frac{dX_E}{dt}}{C} \quad (19.25)$$

$$Cl_H = \frac{\text{rate of elimination}}{C_A} \quad (19.26)$$

$$Cl_H = \frac{Q_H(C_A - C_V)}{C_A} \quad (19.27)$$

Now, since the fraction of drug removed from the blood on each pass of the blood through the liver is the extraction ratio (*ER*), it can be seen that:

$$ER = \frac{C_A - C_V}{C_A} \quad (19.28)$$

and hence by substitution:

$$Cl_H = Q_H ER \quad (19.29)$$

Because most body systems and processes are saturable, the liver in each individual animal has a maximum capacity for removing a drug from the blood when there are no blood flow constraints. This capacity for drug elimination by the combination of biotransformation and by excretion in the bile is a function of liver mass and of the amount and activity of the enzymes of drug metabolism that are present in that individual's hepatocytes. This maximum capacity for drug removal from the blood is the intrinsic ability of the liver to remove drug; the innate capacity of the liver to clear drug is known as its "intrinsic clearance" (Cl_I). An understanding of the concept of Cl_I allows us to redefine the *ER* in terms of Cl_I:

$$ER = \frac{Cl_I}{Q_H + Cl_I} \quad (19.30)$$

Therefore, by substitution:

$$Cl_H = \frac{Q_H Cl_I}{Q_H + Cl_I} \quad (19.31)$$

A corollary to the free hormone hypothesis is that the availability of a hormone or drug for binding to receptors or to enzymes of biotransformation is proportional to the free concentration. If *fu* is the fraction of drug not bound to plasma proteins (i.e., the free fraction) and Cl_I' is the Cl_I for free drug only, it can be seen that:

$$Cl_I = fu\, Cl_I' \quad (19.32)$$

For each drug in each individual, a relationship will exist between the intrinsic hepatic clearance and that animal's particular hepatic blood flow. This relationship between drugs is likely to be a continuum from one extreme, where Cl_I is very much less than hepatic blood flow to the other extreme, where hepatic Cl_I is very much greater than hepatic blood flow.

If Cl_I is very much less than hepatic blood flow, then Cl_I is not a significant contributor to the denominator in eqn 19.31 above.

Therefore, in this special case, where Cl_I is much less than hepatic blood flow, by cancellation it can be seen that:

$$Cl_H = Cl_I \tag{19.33}$$

Since intrinsic hepatic clearance is the product of the fraction unbound (*fu*) and the Cl_I for free drug only, it is clear that in this special case, hepatic clearance is proportional to the fraction of drug unbound [22]. It is with drugs for which this special set of conditions is true that alterations to plasma protein binding of the drug can significantly affect the rate of that drug's excretion. Similarly, for these drugs, induction of hepatic enzymes for biotransformation can have a large effect on their elimination rate, as discussed further below in this chapter.

Now let us consider the alternate case where the intrinsic hepatic clearance is very much greater than hepatic blood flow. In this case, it is the contribution of hepatic blood flow to the denominator of eqn 19.31 that is insignificant. Consequently, in this alternate special case:

$$Cl_H = Q_H \tag{19.34}$$

For drugs that conform to this set of special conditions, it is clear that alterations in hepatic blood flow will profoundly influence the rate of hepatic clearance. The elimination of such drugs will be dependent upon factors such as CO and normal structure and function of hepatic blood vessels. Anesthesiologists understand that many of the drugs used have significant effects on CO and regional blood flow and that surgical procedures and pathology can also lead to marked changes in hepatic blood flow. Therefore, the rate of elimination of many common anesthetic drugs can differ from that predicted due to changes in hepatic blood flow induced by the animal's pathophysiology or by the procedure itself.

It can be seen in Example 1 (Box 19.1) that doubling the intrinsic hepatic clearance for a high Cl_I drug resulted in an increase in the rate of hepatic clearance by a factor of only 1.09, whereas in Example 2 (Box 19.2) the doubling of the intrinsic hepatic clearance rate for a low intrinsic hepatic clearance drug has resulted in a doubling of its hepatic clearance.

Since the Cl_I is the product of the *fu* and the Cl_I for the unbound fraction (Cl_I'), an increase in Cl_I' can be caused either by increasing the displacement of the drug from binding sites and hence increasing the *fu*, or by inducing the activity or expression of enzymes of metabolism through enzyme induction. In the former case, changing the plasma protein binding would result in a change in the volume of distribution of the drug, whereas in the latter case, a change in the expression of enzymes on metabolism would result in a change in the excretion rate constant for the drug.

It is also notable that drugs with a high intrinsic hepatic clearance have consequently high *ER*s and therefore they have a low bioavailability (*F*) when administered by the oral route:

$$F = 1 - ER \tag{19.35}$$

This is known as the "first-pass effect" and is clinically a very real effect with some drugs when they are administered orally. The first-pass effect explains why certain drugs require markedly different dose rates when administered by oral versus parenteral routes (e.g., opioids).

In clinical anesthesiology, drug interactions are thought to cause alterations in hepatic clearance. Although there is little published evidence that such interactions are clinical realities, the clinician should be aware of which drugs have intrinsically high hepatic clearance and which drugs have intrinsically low hepatic clearance in order to correctly anticipate the need to adjust dose rates in cases where multiple drug protocols are being used. An additional point to consider is that many drugs have multiple mechanisms involved in the establishment of their plasma concentrations (e.g., hepatic biotransformation and redistribution as with propofol); therefore, the clinical impact of changes in hepatic clearance may not be as great as predicted.

Box 19.1 Example 1: high hepatic clearance drugs.

This example illustrates what the effect would be of doubling the intrinsic hepatic clearance rate of a drug where hepatic clearance is very much greater than hepatic blood flow.

$Cl_I >> Q_H$, e.g., propranolol
$Cl_I = 7.0\,\text{L/min}$
$Q_H = 1.5\,\text{L/min}$
$ER = 7/(7+1.5)$
$= 0.82$

$Cl_H = Q_H \times ER$
$= 1.5 \times 0.82$
$= 1.23\,\text{L/min}$

After enzyme induction:
$Cl_I = 14.0\,\text{L/min}$
$Q_H = 1.5\,\text{L/min}$
$ER = 14/(14+1.5)$
$= 0.9$

$Cl_H = Q_H \times ER$
$= 1.5 \times 0.9$
$= 1.35\,\text{L/min}$

Box 19.2 Example 2: low hepatic clearance drugs.

This example illustrates what the effect would be of doubling the intrinsic hepatic clearance rate of a drug where hepatic clearance is very much less than hepatic blood flow.

$Cl_I << Q_H$, e.g., theophylline
$Cl_I = 0.1\,\text{L/min}$
$Q_H = 1.5\,\text{L/min}$
$ER = 0.1/(0.1+1.5)$
$= 0.06$

$Cl_H = Q_H \times ER$
$= 1.5 \times 0.06$
$= 0.094\,\text{L/min}$

After enzyme induction:
$Cl_I = 0.2\,\text{L/min}$
$Q_H = 1.5\,\text{L/min}$
$ER = 0.2/(0.2+1.5)$
$= 0.12$

$Cl_H = Q_H \times ER$
$= 1.5 \times 0.12$
$= 0.18\,\text{L/min}$

Renal clearance

Renal clearance defines the relationship between the rate of change of the amount of drug in the urine and the plasma drug concentration. Algebraically, this can be expressed as follows:

$$Cl_R = \frac{\frac{dX_u}{dt}}{C} \quad (19.36)$$

where Cl_R is the renal clearance, X_u is the amount of drug in the urine, and C is the plasma concentration. It is important to note that the clearance of drug from the plasma by the kidneys is achieved by the summation of renal filtration and active renal tubular secretion of drug into the urinary ultrafiltrate. Renal clearance is diminished from this sum by any tubular resorption of drug that might occur. Where RF is the rate of renal filtration, RS is the rate of renal secretion, and RR is the rate of renal resorption:

$$Cl_R = \frac{RF}{C} + \frac{RS}{C} - \frac{RR}{C} \quad (19.37)$$

It should be noted that drugs bound to plasma proteins cannot be filtered because of the size-exclusion capability of the glomerulus. Therefore, the rate of renal filtration is a function of the glomerular filtration rate (GFR) and the plasma concentration of unbound drug. Where C_u is the concentration of unbound drug in the plasma:

$$RF = GFR \times C_u \quad (19.38)$$

Since

$$fu = \frac{C_u}{C} \quad (19.39)$$

$$RF = GFR \times fu \times C \quad (19.40)$$

Therefore, in the absence of renal secretion or resorption:

$$Cl_R = \frac{GFR \times fu \times C}{C} \quad (19.41)$$

$$Cl_R = GFR \times fu \quad (19.42)$$

It is obvious that if the fraction unbound is $fu = 1$ (i.e., if no drug is bound to plasma proteins) then the renal clearance of the drug equals the GFR. For practical purposes, this is accepted as true for the endogenous metabolite of muscle creatinine, for the inert carbohydrate xenobiotic inulin, and for the radiographic contrast agent iohexol, which allows their use for measuring renal filtration rate.

If renal clearance is greater than the product of the fu and the GFR, then renal secretion must be occurring. If renal clearance is less than the product of fu and the GFR, then renal resorption must be occurring.

Absorption

It is usually accepted that drugs formulated for standard delivery methods are absorbed by concentration-dependent processes that are linear (i.e., first-order processes). When drugs are administered by routes other than intravenously, the rate of absorption across membranes, which are barriers to entry is proportional to the difference in concentration across the membrane, the area of the membrane, and its permeability to the drug. Surface area can be manipulated, for example, by giving a dose in aliquots to multiple sites. The concentration of drug in the formulation will partially determine the steepness of the diffusion gradient for drug absorption (e.g., transdermal fentanyl solution). The concentration of the drug in the formulation may be altered by dilution prior to administration or after injection due to water movement as a function of an osmotic gradient. The rates of lymph and blood flow, CO, and factors controlling local blood flow can alter the concentration gradient. The proximity of an administration to impermeable boundaries such as fascial planes and fat is an important determinant of the rate of drug absorption and is to some extent controllable by appropriate choice of injection site. These factors can result in unexpected inefficacy or toxicity with high-potency drugs because of changes in the rate and extent of drug absorption.

A special case is that of constant rate intravenous infusions, and some transdermal patch delivery devices. In these cases, the administration of drug is achieved at a constant rate per unit time (i.e., it is zero-order). For zero-order delivery when elimination is first-order, the following equation approximates the predicted plasma concentration:

$$C(t) = \frac{k_0}{(V_d k_{el})(1 - e^{-k_{el}t})} \quad (19.43)$$

Now, since as time approaches infinity, e^{-kelt} approaches zero, so under this assumption the concentration at steady state (C_{ss}):

$$Css \cong \frac{k_0}{V_d k_{el}} \quad (19.44)$$

But we have seen earlier that

$$Cl = k_{el} V_d \quad (19.45)$$

Hence, by substitution and rearrangement we can determine that for a drug of known total body Cl, to maintain a target steady-state plasma concentration, the zero-order infusion rate (k_0) must equal the elimination rate and can be calculated:

$$k_0 = Css\,Cl = \text{elimination rate} \quad (19.46)$$

Bioavailability

The bioavailability (F) of a drug is the fraction of the dose given, which finds its way into the systemic circulation [23]. It should be noted that this is not necessarily equal to the fraction of the dose which is absorbed, since a drug might be absorbed (e.g., across the gastrointestinal lumen) but removed by metabolism from the portal blood by the liver or from the pulmonary blood by the lungs, before reaching the systemic circulation. Similarly, for topically applied drugs, the skin is an organ of drug metabolism and might biotransform a drug already absorbed before it reaches the circulation.

The bioavailability of a drug administered by a given route is calculated by comparing the total drug exposure of the dose compared to that achieved when the same dose is delivered intravenously. However, drugs administered by any route may be incompletely delivered to the systemic circulation. Even for simple intravenous injections, a drug may have bioavailability less than 100% if it is metabolized or excreted by the lungs.

Pharmacokinetics of inhalant anesthetic agents

The absorption, disposition, and fate of inhalant agents, like any agent administered to an animal, adhere to the principles of pharmacokinetics. However, both absorption and elimination of inhalational agents are mostly through the lungs and are therefore influenced by all the factors acting on their alveolar partial pressure (P_A). The role of the lungs causes inhalant agents to behave differently from injectable agents, seemingly counterintuitive for the clinician who is more familiar with IV pharmacokinetics. While the speed of induction will be proportional to the CO for the intravenous hypnotic agents, it will be inversely proportional for the inhalant due to the effect of the high CO on P_A. Similarly, an increase in blood solubility of the inhalant agent, will drive more drug from the alveoli into the blood, resulting in a decrease in the P_A and consequently in a decrease in the speed of induction. These factors are discussed in detail in Chapter 28.

Linear and nonlinear pharmacokinetics

When the behavior of a drug in the body obeys the principle of superposition, the pharmacokinetics are said to conform to a linear pharmacokinetic model. The principle of superposition states that the response to any combination of inputs must equal the sum of the responses when input separately. For pharmacokinetics, the input is the dose, and the response is the sample's drug concentration. The clinical effect of linear pharmacokinetics is that plasma drug concentrations achieved after changes in drug dose are predictable because, for example, the doubling of the dose would achieve twice the peak plasma concentration [24]. In contrast to drugs with zero-order pharmacokinetics, drugs that display first-order pharmacokinetics are usually approximated well by linear pharmacokinetic models.

Generally, having linear pharmacokinetics indicates that a drug behaves predictably; for example, in a stochastic system, each molecule of the drug introduced to the body moves through the system independently of all other molecules of the same drug introduced to the system, as well as any daughter molecules produced through metabolism [25]. Exceptions do occur and warrant careful clinical use. For example, the non-steroidal anti-inflammatory (NSAID) and analgesic drug phenylbutazone, in both the dog and the horse, appears to have linear pharmacokinetics because it has log-linear plasma drug concentration decay after any chosen dose. However, the primary metabolite oxphenbutazone interferes with its parent moiety's metabolism, hence this is a non-stochastic system. The result is that the elimination half-life is dose-dependent and therefore the pharmacokinetics of phenylbutazone in these species are nonlinear [26–28].

The application of clinical pharmacokinetics depends on the assumptions of linearity and superposition, assumptions which are violated for many drugs used in anesthesia and pain management. Nonlinearity may be due to changes wrought by the drug on its own absorption, distribution, metabolism, or elimination. Changes can be either immediate or delayed. It is no great challenge to identify examples of drugs used in the practice of anesthesia and analgesia, which create non-stochastic pharmacokinetics.

Experiments in pharmacokinetics

Background knowledge of the pharmacokinetics of a drug is necessary to enable the proper use of that drug in clinical cases. Therefore, with new drugs, or with older drugs used in new applications, it is important to adequately describe their pharmacokinetics in the target population. Systematic planning and execution of pharmacokinetic experiments (Box 19.3) will ensure informative results.

Box 19.3 Example 3: steps for planning and conducting pharmacokinetic experiments.

1. Conduct a pilot study OR choose a suitable PK model and determine parameter estimates from the literature with or without the use of inter-species allometry.
2. Determine the target plasma concentration.
3. Develop and validate the analytical assay.
4. Choose the dosing strategy: doses, frequency, formulation, routes of administration.
5. Choose the sampling strategy: sample space, sample frequency and volume, sample processing, and storage.
6. Choose the study design: consult a statistician if needed.
7. Conduct the study.
8. Analyze the results.
9. Review the results for plausibility and repeat steps 8 and 9 as many times as needed, changing methodology as needed to establish robustness of estimates.
10. Return to step 4 and repeat if your assumptions for step 1 were not realistic.

Preparation for the study

To plan the study properly, it is necessary to have a reasonable prediction of its outcome. Therefore, carrying out a pilot study is the foundation of a well-planned pharmacokinetic experiment. Predictions are needed of the approximate target plasma concentration, the likely elimination rate constant, the probability of linear pharmacokinetics, and the likelihood that the formulation might markedly affect the pharmacokinetics.

The approximate target plasma concentration needs to be known so that the analytical assay can be planned, developed, and validated. The assay must be capable of accurately measuring concentrations at least tenfold lower than the minimum effective concentration. It is important to have a validated assay prior to initiation of sample collection. Assay validation parameters that are minimally required include: the inter- and intra-day coefficients of variation at low and high concentrations, measures of linearity of the standard curve or curves (or statistical evaluation of nonlinear standard curves), robustness of the assay, especially between laboratory technicians and equipment (if different technicians and equipment are likely to be used), the stability of stock and standard solutions at storage temperatures, the stability of samples at −80 and possibly −20 °C and the extent of analyte recovery through the sample preparation process [29]. The minimum acceptable sample volume must be known, derived from the intersection of the analyte recovery and the expected minimum target concentration.

Traditionally, an assay's lower limit of quantification (LLOQ) was also defined, to address the loss of analytical precision at low concentrations: both drug regulators and analytical chemists still adhere to this tradition. All methods for setting an LLOQ are arbitrary, having been selected using criteria with no formal justification [30]. Furthermore, it has been clearly demonstrated that discarding data below an arbitrary LLOQ can mislead parameter estimation [31,32]. Therefore, pharmacokineticists in human and veterinary sciences have developed methods to incorporate all data [32–34]. The use of data below LLOQ is widely applied in nonlinear mixed effects (NLME) modeling, which is also called "population pharmacokinetics" (POP-PK) (see below) [35] as it is unbiased and minimizes information loss. It is wise to ensure that the analyst and the pharmacokineticist for a project consult on this issue.

The likely elimination rate constant, or elimination half-life, informs the experimental design. An accepted rule of thumb is that it is not possible to accurately predict the half-life of a drug unless several samples are collected over at least 2 to 3 half-lives. If sample collection is not sufficiently frequent and prolonged, or if the assay used is not sufficiently sensitive then the experiment can be compromised by this lack of planning. Where pilot data in the target species are unavailable, it is reasonable to use allometric scaling from data in other species in order to get suitable estimates for experimental design. Methods that can be used for this allometry are available [36] and there are examples of the use of such methods for pharmacokinetic studies in veterinary medicine [37].

Many drugs for anesthesia are quite lipophilic. Their lack of water solubility increases the need for biotransformation. Biotransformation processes are often saturable. Furthermore, most anesthetic drugs have been demonstrated to affect CO and regional tissue blood flow. Therefore, it is common that anesthetic drugs have nonlinear pharmacokinetics. The external validity of the planned experiment, that is, the ability to extrapolate its results to novel clinical situations, requires the experiment to demonstrate whether the drug behaves with linear pharmacokinetics. The simplest way to address this question in the first instance is to perform the experiment at multiple doses [38].

While the pharmacokinetics of an active moiety can be markedly influenced by the formulation excipients, this is generally not true for intravenous preparations. If the study is planned to evaluate a formulation that is to be administered by a route other than intravenous, then attention to the effect of formulation is needed. In order to completely describe the new formulation's pharmacokinetics, it is necessary to have access to the pharmacokinetics of the active moiety after intravenous administration. If these data are not available, then the study should be planned to include both the intravenous and the intended routes of administration.

Experimental design and conduct

The background understanding gained from the preparation for the study will determine the optimum study design. Study types that are commonly used include the naive pooled data set, the standard two-stage approach, a pharmacokinetic-pharmacodynamic (PK-PD) study, or a POP-PK approach [39]. The study type will influence the chosen experimental design. The naive pooled study type is the least desirable. In this study type, all the data from all the animals are pooled together for data analysis. Taking this approach loses the opportunity to develop an understanding of differences between animals within the population or of the variance within a population. Although suboptimal, naive pooled studies are sometimes necessary when each individual animal is only able to be sampled on one or two occasions. This restriction occurs when the sample volume is large relative to the circulating blood volume, where the act of sampling is likely to alter the pharmacokinetics at subsequent time points, or where the species to be evaluated is difficult to capture, handle, or restrain. Before planning a study of this type, the researcher should consider whether a population approach is possible, since if it is possible then it is likely to result in more useful outcomes.

Historically in veterinary science, the most frequently used study type is the standard two-stage (STS) approach. This approach is now falling out of favor, with most focus being placed on POP-PK approaches (see below). Usually, for an STS approach, a cohort is enrolled of similar individuals from the target population. After dosing, each individual is sampled at the same time points and on multiple occasions. After a suitable washout period, generally accepted to be longer than five half-lives of the drug, the cohort can be dosed again and similarly sampled so as to evaluate either the dose proportionality or the effect of a chosen manipulation on the drug's pharmacokinetics. Typical manipulations include changes in dose, presence or absence of concomitant medications, or modeled disease states. The data from each individual are analyzed independently and the resulting predicted variables are used to generate estimates for the mean variables in the population. Routine statistical comparisons can be made between the results before and after the manipulation. These statistical comparisons are enhanced by careful choice of experimental design, paying attention to randomization, balance, bias elimination, masking, and a priori decisions for statistical evaluation of the resulting data. Typically, these study designs lend themselves to statistical evaluation using general linear models with factors for dose, sequence, animal, period, sequence plus animal interactions, and other manipulations.

The PK-PD type of study is an embellishment of the STS approach. In PK-PD studies, data are collected to measure the drug concentration, and usually, at the same time points, samples or measurements are also taken to assess one or more effects of the drug. Ideally, the targeted effect outcome can be evaluated using a rigorous and objective measure. Alternatively, a surrogate variable can be used. Surrogate variables used for evaluation of efficacy include biological markers such as intermediate enzyme activities or second messenger concentrations. Once again, the data from each animal are analyzed independently and then combined to generate estimates for the population variables, but the nature of the data analysis differs in complexity from PK-only studies. Typically, PK-PD studies are used to evaluate the correlation between dose and effect, to better predict ideal doses, and to gain a better understanding of the drug effect on pathophysiologic processes. The data need to support the determination of the pharmacokinetic and statistical models as in an STS analysis, plus the superimposition of a model for the relationship between drug concentration and efficacy. Therefore, it is necessary to have "rich" data (i.e., a large number of sample time points per animal) in order to accurately estimate a larger number of variables.

The POP-PK approach is an excellent type of study to evaluate the pharmacokinetics of a drug in clinical cases. For this study type, a small number of samples, usually from 2–5, is taken from each case at times convenient for that case; preferably, animals are sampled at different times from one individual to another. In addition, data are collected from each case which describe covariates that are hypothesized to have potential to affect the pharmacokinetics of the drug. Generally, it is expected that 30–50 cases are needed to adequately describe the effect of each covariate. It is necessary to have access to a previous study, which adequately describes a suitable model for the pharmacokinetics of the drug. Alternatively, a small number of individual cases should be sampled sufficiently frequently to adequately describe the drug's pharmacokinetics. Often, the population modeling is performed on a subset of the available data and the resulting model is validated using the data that were excluded from model development. The POP-PK approach allows identification of those factors within the clinical population, which might markedly alter the pharmacokinetics, and hence also alter the efficacy or toxicity of the drug. Such knowledge allows for an appropriate evidence-based adaptation of clinical dosing regimens based on individual animal characteristics.

Data analysis – compartmental models

The availability of off-the-shelf pharmacokinetic analysis software, including purpose-written programs and spreadsheet plug-ins has all but eliminated the potential barrier (or energy of activation) needed to initiate pharmacokinetic data analysis. These programs allow the researcher to enter time and concentration data and, without further intellectual input, to obtain tables of pharmacokinetic variable estimates. The temptation to take this approach can result in the rejection of manuscripts from peer-reviewed publications. A skilled and systematic approach to the review, evaluation, and then analysis of pharmacokinetic data is necessary, since within this mathematical discipline, it is necessary to make subjective decisions and evaluate the legitimacy of assumptions. Evaluation of pharmacokinetic data requires the researcher to determine both the ideal pharmacokinetic structural model and the ideal statistical model needed to describe the data adequately.

Classical pharmacokinetic models include the one-, two-, and three-compartment mammillary models with first-order elimination only from the central compartment and administration only to the central compartment. Alternatively, noncompartmental modeling (sometimes erroneously referred to as "model-independent analysis") is often used. The purpose of any of these modeling approaches is to evaluate the data so as to derive estimates of pharmacokinetic variables. These estimates may then be used to predict outcomes. The accuracy of the predictions will depend on external validity of the modeling approach taken.

For one-, two-, and three-compartmental models, when plotted on semi-logarithmic axes, the data appear to draw one, two, or three straight lines, respectively. Referring to the first-order rate equation discussed earlier (eqn 19.12), a common representation of these models is as follows, with i as the number of compartments and k_i the slopes of the ith straight portion of the plasma concentration versus time curve. At this time, it is useful to begin to consider that all experiments include some imprecision, or variability, represented by ϵ:

$$C(t)=\sum_{i}\left(A_i e^{-k_i t}\right)+\varepsilon \tag{19.47}$$

For compartmental analysis of data, a typical first step is to plot the time and concentration data on semi-logarithmic axes. Working with the example of intravenous administration of alfaxalone to a Greyhound dog [40], the first step is to check that the data can be described by a single straight line. If so, that suggests that a one-compartment model is appropriate. In this case (Fig. 19.9), it is clear that a single straight line does not adequately describe these data. The line does not "fit to" the data and the residuals; in other words, the differences between the measured concentration *C(t)* and the concentration predicted for each time point are not randomly distributed around zero. Accordingly, for these data, we would choose to evaluate them next in a two-compartment model. This example shows that it is necessary to review each animal's data graphically in order to direct the modeling software toward an acceptable solution. Whether a correct choice has been made is subsequently confirmed by statistically comparing the output of the model parameters for a one- versus a two- (or more) compartment model, often using Akaike's Information Criterion (AIC) as the test statistic [41]. The process of fitting the best model to the data is iterative. We choose an objective criterion, such as the sum of the squares of the errors (SSE), and iterate in search for the solution that minimizes this criterion.

Having chosen the pharmacokinetic model for this example as:

$$C(t)=A_1 e^{-k_1 t}+A_2 e^{-k_2 t} \tag{19.48}$$

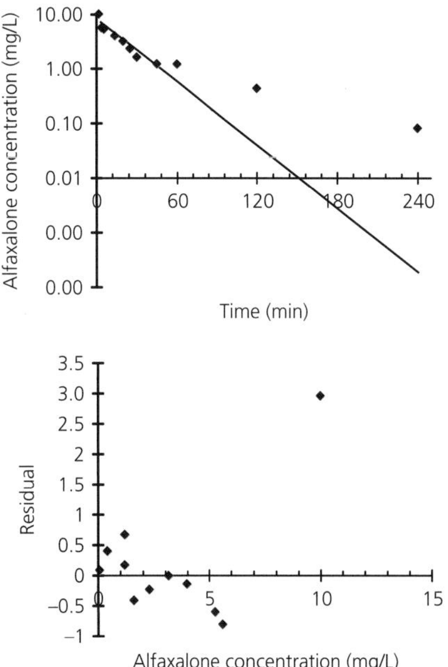

Figure 19.9 Plasma concentration versus time on semi-logarithmic axes and residuals versus concentration, after intravenous administration of 2 mg/kg alfaxalone to a Greyhound dog, showing failure to be approximated by a single straight line. Source: Adapted from Pasloske *et al.* [40].

we now must estimate the model's variables A_i and k_i. It should be noted that it is possible to parameterize compartmental models for intercepts and rates as described above using the first-order rate equation, or using the inter-compartmental rate micro-constants, or in terms of clearance and volume. Some authorities prefer the latter approach [42].

Some computer software requires manual input of initial estimates for model variables and some packages derive their own initial estimates. The choice of initial estimates can markedly affect the outcome of the model fitting. It is good practice to test your model for robustness to variation in the initial estimates. If different initial estimates yield different results, then the pharmacokinetic model or the statistical model may be unsuited to the data.

It is still premature to make the statistical comparison between models, because first a statistical model must be chosen for this process. The statistical model needs to describe the relationship between the dependent variable (usually, the plasma concentration) and the distribution of its estimates around the mean value (i.e., variance). A variety of variance models are used in pharmacokinetic analyses. Frequently, the SSE is not weighted if the distribution of the residuals is homoscedastic. If, however, an examination of residuals has a pattern or a nonrandom distribution and there is confidence that the pharmacokinetic model is sound, then the model for variance should be changed. The variance model can markedly impact the resulting parameter estimates. For example, the same alfaxalone data can be compared with the residuals unweighted or weighted.

For these data, the residuals are evenly scattered with the weighted SSE model, derived in this case by summing the products of each squared error and the reciprocal of its corresponding measured drug concentration (i.e., $1/y$) (Fig. 19.10). Having chosen the pharmacokinetic model and the model for variance, the next step in data analysis is to repeat the pharmacokinetic modeling for all animals, using the same chosen statistical model, and then statistically compare the fits using a test such as AIC. Note that the variance

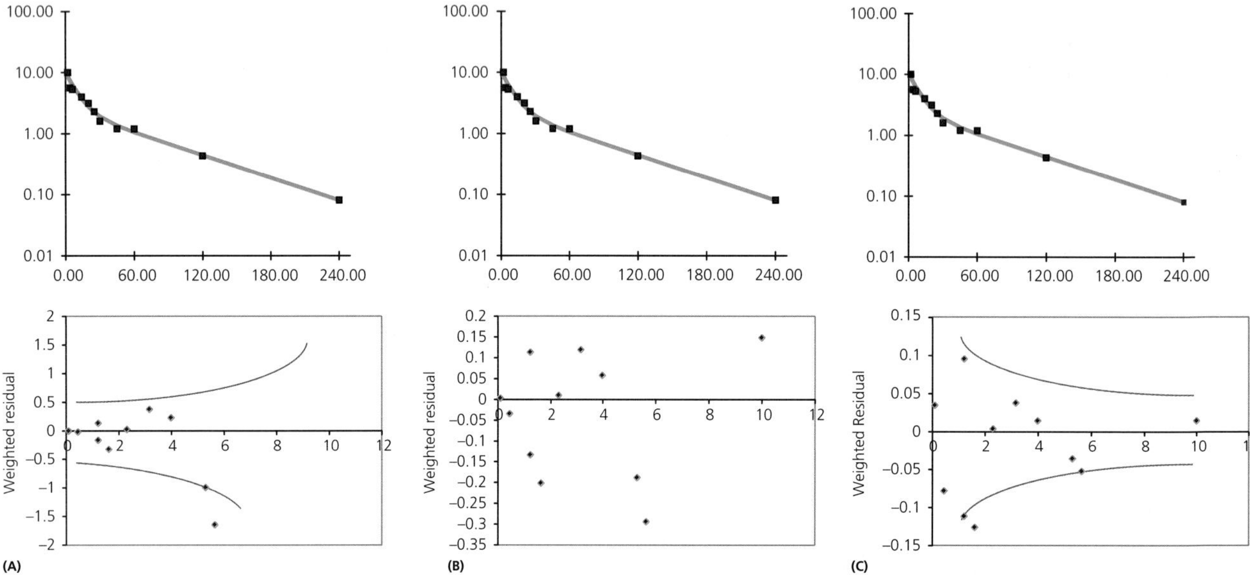

Figure 19.10 Plasma concentration versus time on semi-logarithmic axes and residuals versus concentration, after intravenous administration of 2 mg/kg alfaxalone to a Greyhound dog, fitted using a two-compartment model, showing the effect of changing the variance models on the distribution of residuals: weight[var(y)] = $1/y^z$, where **A.** $z = 0$, **B.** $z = 1$, and **C.** $z = 2$. Source: Adapted from Pasloske *et al.* [40].

model must be unchanged in order to evaluate the best-fitting pharmacokinetic structural model. Finally, one must review the model and evaluate its deficiencies. If necessary, the process must be repeated from the beginning to correct errors in experimental design, data collection, analysis, or interpretation [43].

Software for pharmacokinetic model fitting usually offers options to choose the mathematical approach, the "size" of the steps, and the number of iterations. Making the wrong decisions can result in inaccurate or imprecise parameter estimates. The three main mathematical approaches are those which directly compare the minimizing criterion either using random iterations to vary the parameter estimates (e.g., Monte Carlo) or using a simple step-wise approach (e.g., simplex), or "gradient" methods, which use either first- or second-order derivatives of the minimizing criterion (e.g., Gauss–Newton and Marquardt) [44]. Monte Carlo and simplex methods are robust to poor initial parameter estimates but tend to be slow and computer-intensive. With Monte Carlo approaches, care should be taken not to restrict the number of iterations greatly. For simplex methods, one should start with large step sizes and gradually reduce the step size through several runs of the minimization process, to avoid finding false solutions. The gradient methods tend to require good initial estimates in order to proceed, but they have high reliability at quickly finding the best solution, if they have had a good starting point. Data are often analyzed first with a simplex method, then the results of that analysis can be used as the initial estimates for a gradient method.

Data analysis – noncompartmental models

After planning and conducting a pharmacokinetic experiment for a compartmental modeling approach as described above, it is possible to analyze the data using a noncompartmental approach. This approach has the advantage of being applicable to both stochastic and non-stochastic pharmacokinetics and results in the calculation of volumes of distribution, clearance, and mean time parameters.

Generally, mean time parameters describe the average total time spent by molecules in a kinetic space after introduction to the kinetic space. The kinetic space is defined by the experimental design, where the samples are derived from the sample space and may represent homogeneous or heterogeneous kinetic spaces. A homogenous kinetic space is analogous to a single compartment in a compartmental model, whereas a heterogeneous kinetic space is likened to a grouping of multiple independent compartments of a complex compartmental model. This is an important concept to understand when interpreting the meaning of mean time parameters [25].

> **Box 19.4** Example 4: the linear trapezoidal rule.
>
> The area under the plasma concentration versus time curve can be estimated using the linear trapezoidal rule using the equation:
>
> $$AUC_{(0-\infty)} = \sum_{t=1}^{n}\left(\left\{\left[\frac{C(t)+C(t-1)}{2}\right]\left[t-(t-1)\right]\right\}+\frac{C(n)}{k_{el}}\right)$$
>
> The accuracy of this estimate depends upon the frequency and choice of sample time points, the lower limit of quantification of the assay, the terminal slope of the elimination curve (k_{el}), and the dimension of the excluded initial and estimated final triangles. Subtle changes to the equation are needed for non-intravenous data.
>
> Source: Gibaldi and Perrier [45].

The mathematics routinely used for the noncompartmental approach [45] are simpler than for compartmental modeling, although their derivation and hence ease of understanding are more opaque. It is important to note that many of the frequently used formulas rely on the same underlying assumption of linear pharmacokinetics [25]. The two most important calculated variables used for parameter estimation in noncompartmental analyses are the area under the concentration versus time curve from the time of introduction of the dose ($t = 0$) until infinity [AUC(0–∞)], and the area under the first moment of the concentration versus time curve from the time of dosing ($t = 0$) until infinity [AUMC(0–∞)]. These are usually calculated from the data using the linear or log-linear trapezoidal methods (Box 19.4) [46].

Errors in estimation of these variables result in misleading pharmacokinetic parameter estimates. The most common error in estimating AUC and AUMC is failing to define the pharmacokinetic curve for an adequate time period, resulting in a large portion of the total area being under the portion of the curve that is after the last quantified time point, that is, the portion of the curve which is extrapolated. As a rule of thumb, if the percent of the total area that was extrapolated is greater than 20%, then the experimental design is inadequate for this approach to data analysis. Parts of the experimental design that need to be re-evaluated in this case are the duration and frequency of sampling and the sensitivity of the assay.

Noncompartmental modeling can provide the same useful pharmacokinetic parameters that are used for dose calculation and for understanding the need for alterations to pharmacokinetics in diseased animals. There are differences of opinion as to whether the added complexity in data analysis for compartmental modeling provides great benefit over the arithmetically simpler noncompartmental approaches for generation of pharmacokinetic variable estimates.

Data analysis in more complex models

The examples discussed above are conveniently simple. However, there are many variations from these simple modeling approaches that can become necessary to describe data adequately. The compartmental models introduced above are used with an implicit understanding of their many assumptions. The implications of these assumptions are especially troubling to anesthesiologists. The most troubling of these assumptions is that there is assumed to be instantaneous mixing of the drug after introduction to a large, homogenous central compartment. Pharmacokinetic studies rarely include sample collection at less than 2 min after an intravenous dose because it has been demonstrated that complete mixing of a rapid intravenous bolus dose in the dog is delayed for approximately 1 min [47]. For intravenous general anesthesia, many of the important pharmacodynamic events are well underway or completed within 2 min, but the simple compartmental and noncompartmental models do not assist us to understand the rapid pharmacokinetics changes that drive these events. Physiologically based pharmacokinetic models (PBPK) make allowances for individual organ and tissue blood flow as a proportion of CO. Appropriate PBPK study designs allow determination of the *ER* for each organ of interest and the drug clearance achieved by that organ and estimation of organ or tissue drug concentration.

For example, the evaluation of propofol administration using PBPK models led to a better understanding of the effect of slow intravenous administration on the duration of anesthesia, markedly altering anesthetic practice and ultimately improving the quality of transition to a volatile anesthetic [48,49]. Finally, PBPK models allow understanding of the effect of drug recirculation on the arterial and venous drug concentrations, an understanding that is fundamental to modern intravenous anesthesia [47,50].

For drugs where there are multiple points of drug input, such as complex formulations with nonlinear absorption, data analysis that uses a deconvolution approach may be needed: the intravenous pharmacokinetics can be defined independently in each individual, and then progress to modeling of the absorption phases.

Delayed absorption or distribution can result in a lag between dosing and changes in concentration, or between appearance of drug in the sample space and its distribution to the site of action. This is frequently exemplified by NSAIDs. Modeling NSAIDs in PK-PD can require inclusion of lag-times in the models [51].

Using POP-PK allows the estimation of large numbers of model parameters and more careful characterization of the sources of variance. Purpose-written software with capabilities such as convolution and deconvolution, parametric and non-parametric nonlinear mixed effects modeling for data analysis is available but requires targeted training in its use. Pharmacokineticists with deep expertise in understanding and implementing such data analyses are increasingly turning to more code-driven advanced statistical software.

Constant rate therapy

Constant rate therapy is used when maintenance of a specific plasma concentration and its consequent effect is desired. Constant rate therapy is usually achieved intravenously, although constant rate release devices and systems are also available such as patches and slow-release injectable agents [52]. To produce a sustained drug plasma concentration, a constant rate of absorption is required. For simplicity, we will consider that such devices behave similarly to a constant rate IV infusion. To provide constant rate therapy and maintain constant plasma concentration using intravenous administration, two techniques are usually described [53]: intermittent bolus injection and continuous infusion. The aim of both these techniques is to administer drug at a rate equal to its clearance.

Intermittent boluses

Intermittent IV bolus administration is a very simple technique. The only equipment needed consists of an IV catheter and a syringe containing the agents (anesthetic, analgesic, etc.). After injection of the loading dose, the effect can be maintained by repeated injections. After each injection, the plasma drug concentration reaches a peak and then starts decreasing as a function of distribution and clearance. This decrease of plasma drug concentration will cause decreasing drug concentration at the effect site and reach a point where the effect will not be adequate (e.g., patient waking up and breakthrough pain), and a new bolus will be necessary for the desired effect to be re-established. With intermittent IV bolus administration, the drug plasma concentration tends to oscillate between peaks of relative excess and troughs of ineffective amounts (Fig. 19.11). In addition to the very poor consistency in the targeted effect, this technique can result in the administration of a large total drug dose and consequently can cause a slower and longer recovery from the effect [53,54].

Continuous rate infusion

By eliminating the peaks and troughs in plasma concentration that occur with the intermittent boluses technique, continuous infusion results in a better quality of effect and a decrease in the total drug dose delivered [53,54]. The cheapest but least accurate way to maintain a continuous infusion is to use a bag containing the chosen agent(s) and an administration set [53,55]. The flow rate can be adjusted by varying the radius of the infusion tubing using a "regulating" clamp (Fig. 19.12). The infusion rate can be calculated knowing the volume of each drop (e.g., 20 vs. 60 drops/mL), and counting the drip rate. In this system, the speed of infusion is gravity-dependent and depends also on the diameter and length of the connecting tube, the size of the drops, the size of the cannula, the viscosity of the agent, the height of the fluid, and the venous pressure of the patient. As the fluid decreases in the bag, the infusion rate decreases and needs readjusting.

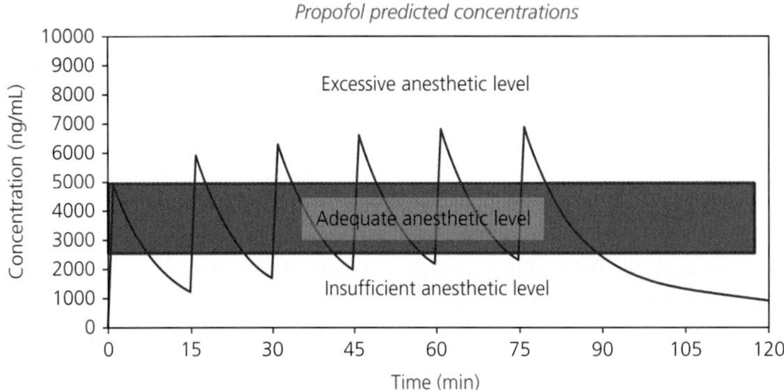

Figure 19.11 Simulated plasma concentration of propofol in the dog following repeated bolus (4 mg/kg) injections over time. Propofol is injected every 15 minutes. The shaded area represents the targeted effect area.

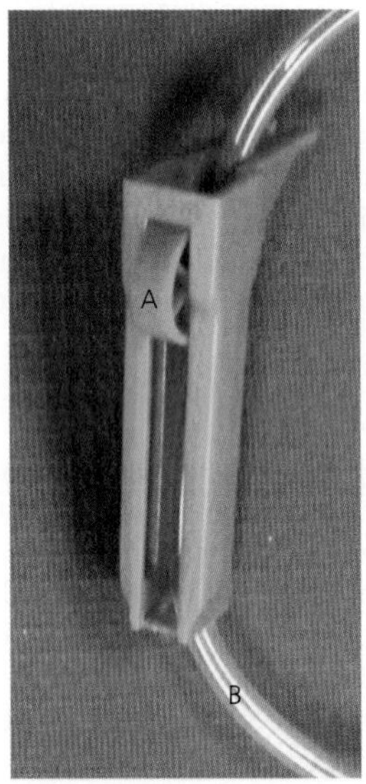

Figure 19.12 "Regulating" clamp used to modify the radius of the infusion tubing. The wheel (A) allows modification of the radius of the infusion tubing (B), allowing the speed of the infusion to be varied.

Infusion pumps and syringe drivers allow a more controlled continuous, accurate, and safer infusion [53,55]. Larger volume infusions will be accurately administered using an infusion pump while a syringe driver is more appropriate for smaller volumes at slower rates.

Potential hazards with infusion pumps and syringe drivers include a too rapid rate of infusion (administration set not properly clamped), failure of power (main and battery), infusion of air, and continued infusion, although cannula has become extravascular. Modern infusion devices are able to detect some of these faults, such as air in the system and line blockage. In addition, with syringe drivers, the clinician should also be aware that the position of the device is important. If positioned higher than the patient's heart, siphoning may occur due to the weight of the liquid [53], which will result in a larger volume of drug being administered than was programmed. To avoid this, the device must have protection against the syringe plunger moving faster than its motor-drive. Conversely, a syringe driver that is positioned lower than the vascular access port can result in less agent being infused than programmed, owing both to the back pressure from the venous bed and to the weight of the liquid. To avoid these hazards, infusion sets should incorporate a one-way valve system. Further, if the syringe driver is positioned vertically, the outlet should be placed downwards to avoid infusing bubbles formed by gas coming out of solution.

When choosing an infusion pump or a syringe driver, the clinician should consider the following: versatility (choice of bolus or infusion mode, internal calculator for choice of dosing scheme, choice of infusion rates, and possibility for using differently sized syringes, even from different manufacturers), lightweight, clear display of drug administered and infusion rate, a simple protocol for initiation or change of infusion rates, a digital interface for recordkeeping or external automated control, and alarms for tubing disconnect, high pressure, and the presence of bubbles in the tubing [53,56].

Continuous rate infusion can be classified as being either non-pharmacokinetic or pharmacokinetic dependent.

Non-pharmacokinetic-dependent infusion systems – constant rate infusion and rate-controlled infusion

When using a constant rate infusion (CRI), the clinician decides empirically on an infusion rate and maintains that rate for the whole procedure. Unfortunately, with such a system, the plasma drug concentration that is achieved is not controlled. Administration via CRI is not appropriate for drugs with relatively long elimination half-lives because the plasma drug concentration will be low at the beginning of the procedure and may not provide an adequate effect. Over time, as the mass of drug accumulates in the animal and the concentration increases, a more adequate effect is achieved. If the procedure is prolonged, the plasma drug concentration may reach the point at which undesired side effects occur (Fig. 19.13). To avoid the initial lack of effect, a loading dose may be administered immediately prior to beginning the CRI (Fig. 19.14). Unfortunately, in prolonged CRI therapy, monitoring for undesired clinical effects is the only practical approach available to alert the clinician to drug accumulation. Despite these shortcomings, CRI is a useful technique in some clinical settings, for example, the administration of morphine to dogs for analgesia or of ketamine in the triple drip anesthesia technique in horses.

To minimize drug accumulation and the consequent adverse effects, the clinician can change the drug infusion rate according to the observed needs of the patient. This technique (rate-controlled infusion [RCI]) can provide a much smoother anesthesia with lower total drug used, but frequent adjustments might sometimes be necessary to fine-tune the infusion to the patient's needs.

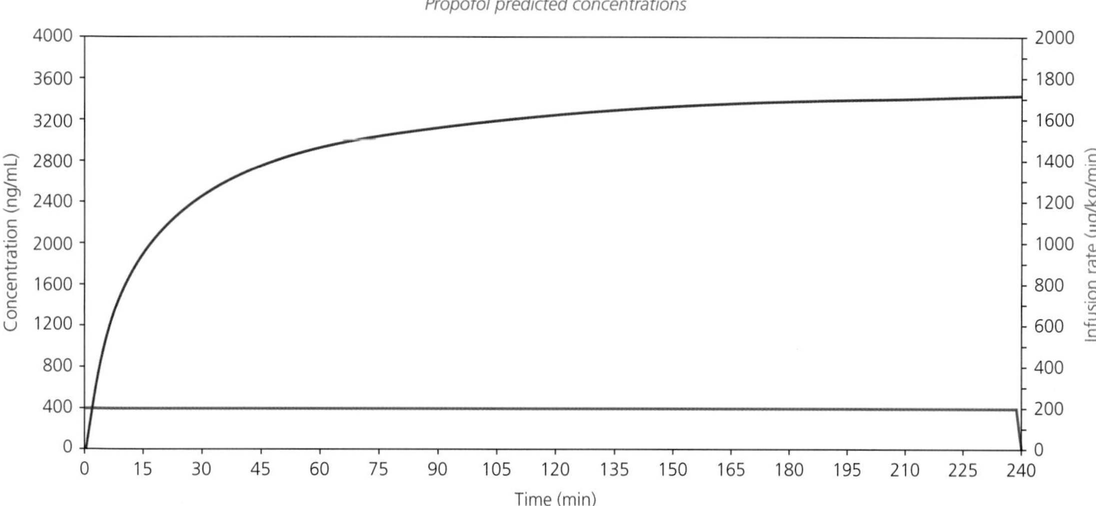

Figure 19.13 Simulated plasma concentration of propofol in the dog during a constant rate infusion over time, derived using the PK simulator PK-SIM (Specialised Data Systems, Jenkintown, PA, USA) and PK parameters of propofol. The blue line represents the predicted plasma concentration. The green line represents the infusion rate (200 µg/kg/min). The infusion rate can be based on empirical data or, as in this case, on pharmacokinetic data. Source: Adapted from Beths [55].

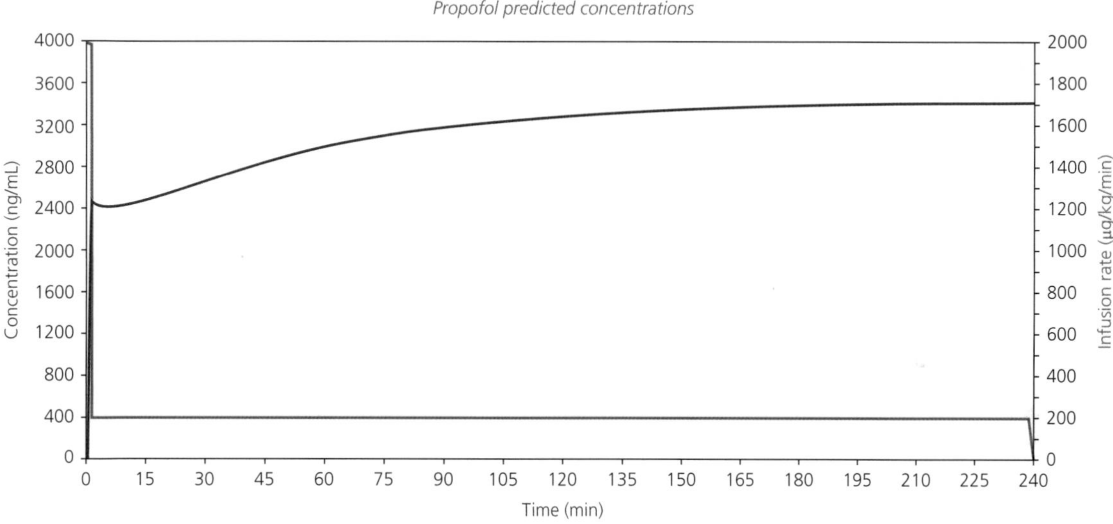

Figure 19.14 Simulated plasma concentration of propofol in the dog after a bolus injection followed by a constant rate infusion over time, derived using the PK simulator PK-SIM (Specialised Data Systems, Jenkintown, PA, USA) and PK parameters of propofol. The blue line represents the predicted plasma concentration. The green line represents the loading dose (2 mg/kg) and the following infusion rate (200 µg/kg/min). The bolus or loading dose and the infusion rate can be based on empirical data or, as in this case, on pharmacokinetic data. Source: Adapted from Beths [55].

Pharmacokinetic-dependent infusion systems

Knowing a specific agent's pharmacokinetics and its effective plasma concentration allows development of an infusion scheme, which targets the desired plasma drug concentration. The techniques for PK-dependent infusion can be either manually controlled using an RCI or a stepped infusion, or electronically controlled with the help of a computer adjusting the speed of infusion, that is, target-controlled infusion (TCI). The more reliant the technique is on pre-existing PK data, the more the achieved plasma drug concentration will depend on the quality and relevance of the PK model used and the similarities of the patient and the experimental subjects used for initial data collection. Therefore, deviations from the conditions in which the PK data were obtained may result in unexpected plasma drug concentrations. Deviations that should be considered include different species, breed, gender, age, disease state, and concurrent medications.

To maintain a constant targeted plasma drug concentration, that is, a steady-state plasma drug concentration (C_{ss}), the amount of drug infused must equal the amount of drug being eliminated. This can be expressed by the following equation:

$$\text{maintenance rate} = \text{elimination rate} \tag{19.49}$$

Assuming first-order elimination, the mass of drug eliminated per unit time (the elimination rate) will depend on the plasma drug concentration at steady state (C_{ss}) of the agent and the Cl (see eqn 19.46). Therefore, the necessary maintenance infusion rate (k_0) will depend on both the targeted drug plasma concentration at steady state (C_{ss}) and the drug's total body *Cl*. As observed with the non-PK dependent CRI (Fig. 19.13), it will take about 4 to 5 times the elimination half-life for the plasma drug concentration to approach its accumulation plateau. Of course, if an estimate of the V_c is available, a loading dose can also be calculated and administered before the start of the CRI to reach effective plasma concentration more rapidly (Fig. 19.14). The clinician must realize that although an effective targeted plasma concentration has been reached, it will still take 4–5 half-lives before reaching C_{ss} (Fig. 19.15).

To calculate the loading dose, there are two possible methods: either calculating the dose to fill the central compartment (V_c) or calculating the dose to fill the total distribution volume at steady state (V_{ss}). With the first method using V_c only, the plasma drug concentration obtained will be low while with the second method (V_{ss}), there will be an overshoot and an initial increased risk of side effects.

These simple approaches of applied PK are not always suitable for anesthesia or analgesia and more complex infusion strategies can better achieve the desired initial blood concentration. Ideal infusion schemes can be predicted using known PK parameters and a computer simulation program. The stepped infusion [57–59] consists of a series of CRIs aimed at reaching the targeted plasma drug concentration as rapidly as possible while neither under- nor overshooting (Fig. 19.16). Usually, using a small number of infusion steps helps to ensure a practical series.

With a stepped infusion, a fast initial infusion is administered to fill the V_c, followed by a maintenance infusion, which will be determined by the desired target or central compartment drug concentration and the drug's rate of clearance [58]. Unfortunately, like the CRI system, the stepped infusion system is very rigid and difficult to adapt to the clinical situation [53,60]. A low target will result in

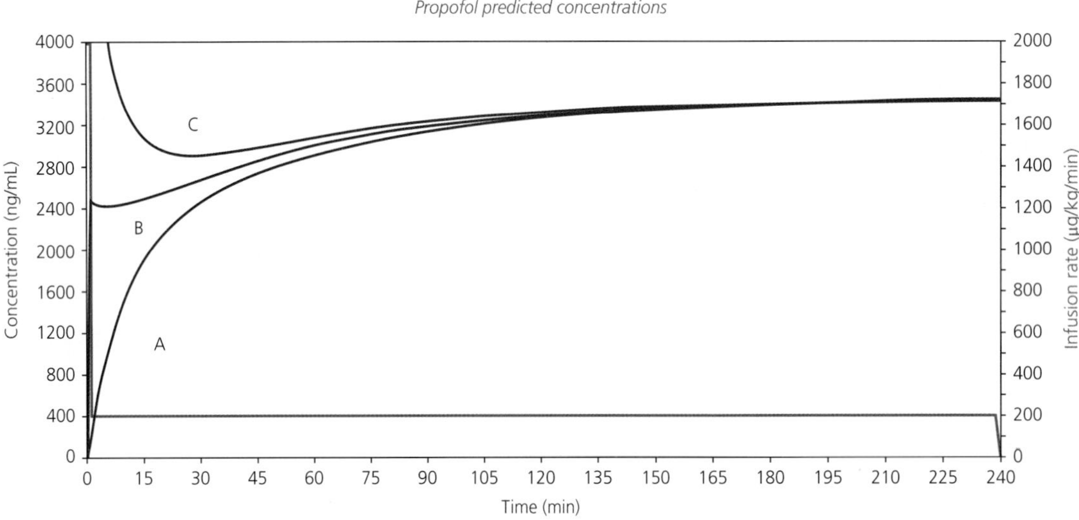

Figure 19.15 Simulated plasma concentration of propofol in the dog during a constant rate infusion over time (A) or preceded by a bolus of 2 mg/kg (B) and 4 mg/kg (C), derived using the PK simulator PK-SIM (Specialised Data Systems, Jenkintown, PA, USA) and PK parameters of propofol. The blue line represents the predicted plasma concentration. The green line represents the loading doses (2 and 4 mg/kg) and the following infusion rate (200 µg/kg/min). This graph shows that 3–4 half-lives are still necessary to reach the steady-state concentration (C_{ss}), without a loading dose preceding the CRI. The bolus or loading dose and the infusion rate can be based on empirical data or, as in this case, on pharmacokinetic data. Source: Adapted from Beths [55].

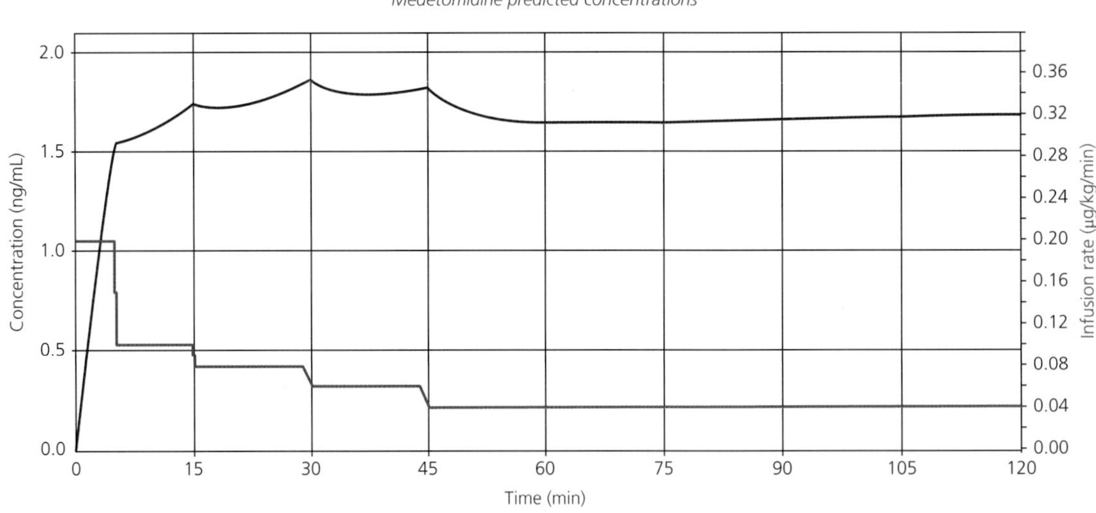

Figure 19.16 Five-step infusion (green line) of medetomidine in the dog with a target blood concentration of 1.7 ng/mL and the predicted plasma concentration of medetomidine (blue line), derived using the PK simulator PK-SIM (Specialised Data Systems, Jenkintown, PA, USA).

inadequate anesthesia while a high target will result in increased side effects (hypotension, apnea, and delayed recovery).

In 1968, Kruger-Thiemer described an infusion scheme known as "BET" – for Bolus (loading dose), Elimination (steady-state rate of infusion according to drug's elimination), and Transfer (exponentially decreasing rate to match the redistribution of drug from the central compartment to peripheral sites) [57]. In 1981, by interfacing a computer with an infusion pump, Schwilden demonstrated the clinical application of the BET infusion scheme [61]. The first drugs to be administered by this system were etomidate and alfentanil in 1983 [62]. The development of new pumps, computer systems, and infusion rate control algorithms to enable the anesthetist to vary the target plasma drug concentration followed [63]. The first TCI system was described by Schuttler *et al.* in 1988 [64]. It was only 8 years later, in 1996, that the first commercial TCI system for use with propofol in humans was launched [65,66].

The fundamental principles and development of the TCI system were described by Gray and Kenny [67] and Glen [66]. Succinctly, a TCI system is a computer programmed with a set of PK parameters (specific for a species and a drug) and coupled with a syringe driver. The computer pump control algorithm calculates the infusion rate that is necessary to achieve a blood target concentration. Once the target blood concentration is achieved, the computer will control the pump to maintain the blood target concentration.

The speed of infusion is calculated as follows:

$$\text{infusion rate} = C_t V_c \left(k_{10} + k_{12}e^{-k21t} + k_{13}e^{-k31t}\right) \quad (19.50)$$

where C_t is the targeted concentration, V_c is the volume of the central compartment, t is the time, and k_{10}, k_{12}, k_{21}, k_{13}, and k_{31} are the micro-constants describing the movement of the agent between the different compartments of the three-compartment model [68].

To begin, a bolus is calculated ($C_t \times V_c$) and administered. As illustrated by the equation, if the target is kept constant, the infusion rate will exponentially decrease over time to match the cumulative characteristic of the agent [69]. At any point, the clinician can choose to modify the target. An increase in target concentration will result in injection of a calculated bolus dose using the same equation as above ($V_c \times C_t$), but where C_t is the difference between the current C and the new C_t. It will then be followed by an exponentially decreasing infusion rate, which will be higher than the original infusion rate. Following a decrease in target concentration, the infusion will cease until the new target, as predicted by the computer, is reached. Thereafter, an exponentially decreasing infusion rate will resume, at a lower rate than previously [69]. Examples of these schemes are illustrated in Figs. 19.17 and 19.18.

The accuracy of a TCI system is dependent upon the PK variables that have been used to program the device. Consequently, the system must be validated before general use in clinical practice. The evaluation of the predictive performance of a TCI system is carried out by comparing the drug concentrations predicted by the system with the measured drug concentrations either in venous or arterial blood samples taken at various time points during anesthesia, over a range of target concentrations, according to a methodology which has been used by many authors [70–80]. This methodology is based on the calculation of the percentage prediction error (*PE%*) as the difference between measured and predicted values expressed as a percentage of the predicted value [74]:

$$PE\% = \frac{\text{measured concentration} - \text{predicted concentration}}{\text{predicted concentration}} \times 100 \quad (19.51)$$

Using values of *PE%* derived at each measurement point, a number of indices of performance in an individual subject are calculated. The median prediction error (*MDPE%*), provides a measure of bias to indicate whether measured concentrations are systematically above or below targeted values. The median absolute prediction error (*MDAPE%*) measures inaccuracy and gives information on the typical size of the difference between measured and targeted concentrations [78,81].

$$MDPE\% = \text{median}\left\{PE_{ij}, j = 1, \ldots, N_i\right\} \quad (19.52)$$

where N_i is the number of $|PE|$ values obtained for the ith subject, and

$$MDAPE\% = \left\{\left|PE_{ij}\right|, j = 1, \ldots, N_i\right\} \quad (19.53)$$

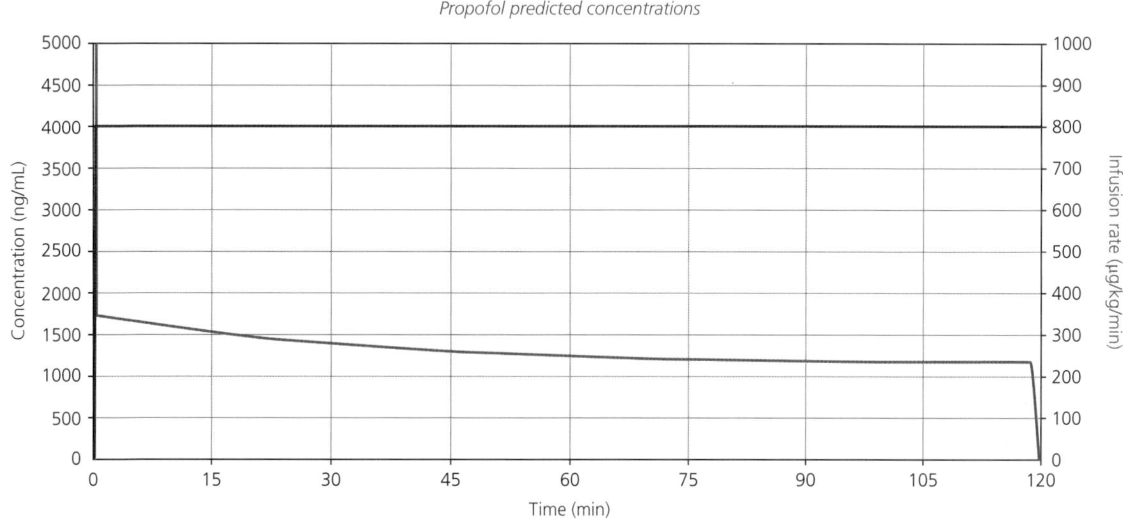

Figure 19.17 Simulated plasma concentration of propofol in the dog during a target-controlled infusion (TCI) over time, derived using the PK simulator PK-SIM (Specialised Data Systems, Jenkintown, PA, USA) and PK parameters of propofol. The blue line represents the plasma concentration with a propofol target of 4000 ng/mL. The green line represents the exponentially decreasing infusion rate. Source: Adapted from Beths [55].

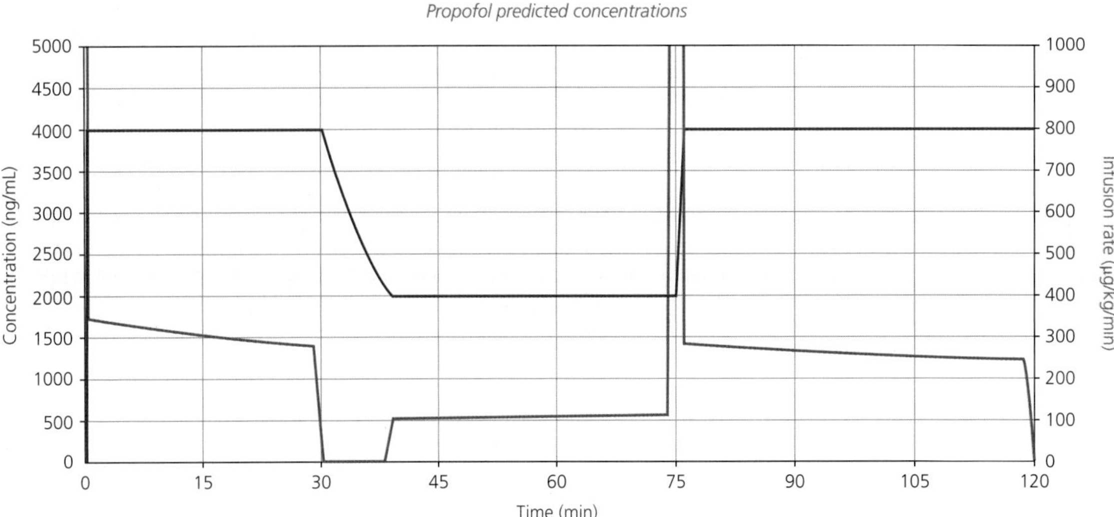

Figure 19.18 Simulated plasma concentration of propofol in the dog during a target-controlled infusion (TCI) over time, derived using the PK simulator PK-SIM (Specialised Data Systems, Jenkintown, PA, USA) and PK parameters of propofol. This graph simulates anesthesia where the clinician, 30 minutes after targeting a propofol plasma concentration (blue line) of 4000 ng/mL, decided to decrease the level of anesthesia with a new propofol plasma concentration of 2000 ng/mL. Then 45 minutes later, the anesthesia is deepened by the change to a new propofol plasma concentration (4000 ng/mL). The green line represents the exponentially decreasing infusion rate for the different plasma concentrations. Note that the infusion stopped at time 30 minutes, allowing the propofol plasma concentration to decrease from 4000 to 2000 ng/mL. Note the bolus injection given at 75 minutes when the propofol plasma concentration was once again changed to 4000 ng/mL. Source: Adapted from Beths [55].

Two other indices are wobble and divergence, both of which reflect time-related changes. Wobble measures the total intra-individual variability in performance error, and divergence describes any systematic time-related changes in measured concentrations away from or toward the targeted concentration. A positive value indicates a widening of the gap between the predicted and measured concentrations over time, while a negative value indicates that the measured concentrations converge on the predicted values. Information regarding how those can be calculated can be found elsewhere [73,78,81].

Although no reference values are reported for divergence or wobble, it has been suggested that the performance of a TCI system is clinically acceptable if the bias (*MDPE%*) is not greater than ±10–20% and the inaccuracy (*MDAPE%*) falls between 15% and 40% [69,73,76,82]. In veterinary medicine, such systems have been developed and validated for propofol in the dog [71,83], for alfentanil, propofol, and alfaxalone in the cat [84–88], for lidocaine, alfentanil, and detomidine in the horse [86,89,90], and for propofol in rabbits [91].

Context-sensitive half-time

Knowledge of the PK of an agent combined with a computer-driven infusion pump allows for a more precise infusion and easier titration to effect, which could result in quicker recovery. In fact, after cessation of the infusion, the duration of drug effect is more dependent on the PK of the agent than the method of administration [92]. Moreover, for most of the agents, the time to recovery increases with the duration of the infusion. This dependence comprises the concept of context-sensitive half-time (CSHT), wherein the context is the variation of the duration of the infusion [93,94]. The CSHT is the time from the end of the infusion necessary for the plasma's drug concentration to decrease by 50%. For most anesthetic agents, after a bolus injection, the duration of their clinical effect is mostly dependent on redistribution of the drug from the brain to other tissues. After infusion, however, the explanation of the mechanism for recovery from anesthesia varies [94]. Because most anesthetic drugs behave according to multiple compartmental pharmacokinetics, different explanations are needed for different durations of infusion. For short-term infusions, the CSHT will be quite dependent on redistribution (e.g., a short period of thiopental administration). For moderate infusion times, the CSHT will depend on both the drug's distribution and elimination. For long infusions where the peripheral compartments (tissues) are saturated, the CSHT will approach the true elimination half-life of the drug ($t_{1/2}$) [94].

The CSHTs for some drugs in cats have been described (Fig. 19.19). Drugs vary in their sensitivity to context; fentanyl is very context-sensitive, while remifentanil is context insensitive [95]. Regarding alfaxalone, although the infusion rate seems to have little effect on a 50% decrease in plasma concentration (CSHT), recovery from alfaxalone anesthesia may necessitate a decrease of the plasma concentration by 85–95%. In this case, the duration of alfaxalone infusion has a much more pronounced effect [87]. This is not specific to alfaxalone and other agents will be context sensitive for effect needing a decrease by 85–95% of the plasma concentration.

The CSHT is interesting in the clinical setting mostly if it corresponds to the dissipation of a specific observable drug effect (i.e., recovery of spontaneous breathing, recovery of the swallowing reflex, etc.). As this desired clinical effect can occur earlier or later than the 50% decrease in the concentration of the drug, investigators often provide the times needed for 20%, 50% (CSHT), and 80% decrements in drug concentration. The clinician is usually more interested in the drug concentration at the effect site than in the plasma [96].

A more general term, which was first described in humans for the recovery from opioids, is the context-sensitive effect-site "decrement" time in which the decrease in concentration is modeled specifically for the compartment of the effect site [68,97].

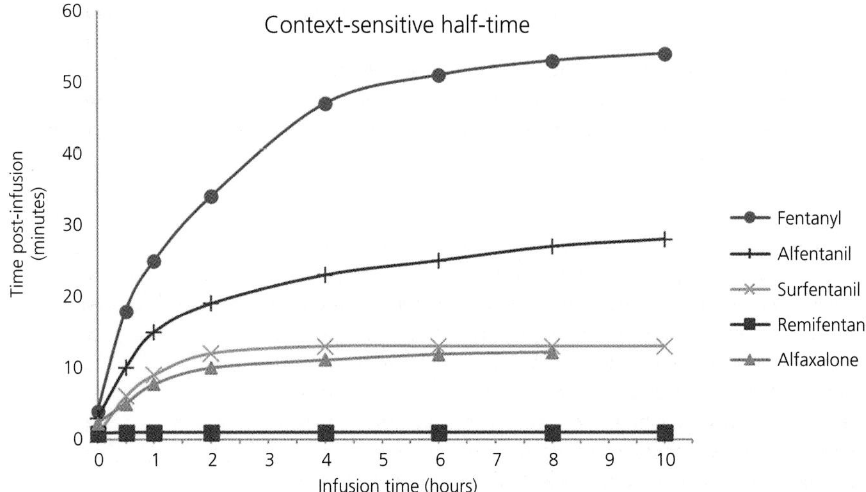

Figure 19.19 Context-sensitive half-time (CSHT) in cats for four opioids and alfaxalone after a bolus and infusion of different duration (0.5–10 hours). For the four opioids CSHT determination, cats were under isoflurane anesthesia. Source: Adapted from Pypendop *et al.* [87]; Pypendop [95].

This parameter allows the clinician to better determine when to stop an infusion (to enable awakening at the end of a surgery). To achieve this, the clinician needs to remember the decrease in concentration necessary for the recovery (percentage), the duration of the infusion (context), and the context-sensitive effect-site decrement time required for the necessary decrease [68].

In 2000, Struys *et al.* [98] compared a TCI system targeting plasma concentration versus a TCI system targeting the effect-site concentration. They concluded that targeting the effect-site compartment resulted in less variability and greater predictability in the time to loss of consciousness. They also observed that when targeting the effect site, the onset of drug effect was quicker and without adverse hemodynamic consequences. An effect-site PK parameter (k_{e0}) has been incorporated into human TCI systems to reflect the passage of the drug from the blood to the effect site [99]. The k_{e0} can be determined during an integrated PK/PD study [100]. Unfortunately, with this method, the k_{e0} value will be specific for this set of PK parameters and will result in poor predictions of the time course of drug effect if one wanted to use it with a different set of PK parameters [99,101]. To be able to link the k_{e0} from an integrated PK/PD study to PK parameters determined in another study, Minto *et al.* in 2003 introduced the time of maximum effect-site concentration (t_{peak}) [100]. Knowing the t_{peak} for a specific agent, the investigator can calculate the value of k_{e0} that accurately predicts t_{peak} when using the set of parameters of interest. With simulations for thiopentone, remifentanil, and propofol, Minto *et al.* showed that the k_{e0} determined through the t_{peak} method better approximated the time course of drug effect than the simple transfer of a k_{e0} value from one set of PK parameters to another. In 2008, Bras *et al.* using the t_{peak} method, determined the k_{e0} for propofol (0.7320 min^{-1}) and incorporated it to the TCI PK model from Beths *et al.* [71,102]. The usefulness of integrated PK/PD incorporating effect-site rate constants and time of maximum effect-site concentration has not yet been explored extensively in veterinary anesthesiology.

Drug interactions

Combinations of drugs may occasionally result in drug–drug interactions, which can be synergistic, antagonistic, or additive [103]. These interactions can be explained by three mechanisms: physicochemical, PK, and PD.

Physicochemical interactions

Physicochemical interactions usually occur when two incompatible drugs are mixed together *in vitro* (e.g., pH difference). The interaction can take several forms, including changes in physical stability of complex formulations, changes in solubility with precipitation, changes in chemical stability of active or excipient ingredients, adsorption onto delivery device surfaces, and chelation or chemical reactions such as reduction or oxidation. These *in vitro* interactions may be inconsistent between different formulations of the same active ingredients, so clinicians should not assume a combination, which is proven acceptable with particular brands of products will necessarily be equally acceptable with alternate product brands. Unless specific data are available as evidence that a particular combination is without interaction, *in vitro* mixtures should be avoided. Commonly known incompatibilities are tabulated in former editions of this book and are listed in most common formularies.

Pharmacokinetic interactions

Interactions during the different PK phases of absorption, distribution, elimination, or biotransformation are each possible. Some such interactions are used as a deliberate mechanism to alter drug action or duration, for example, the inclusion of epinephrine in formulations of lidocaine delays the systemic absorption of the lidocaine, prolonging its local action. Although drug interactions in distribution can occur as a function of their interaction at cell membrane transporters in peripheral tissues, these interactions are not described as having clinical relevance in anesthesia and analgesia. Alterations to plasma protein binding by competition between drugs for the same binding site were thought to be of clinical importance [104] but a more thorough understanding of clearance, as discussed above, has led to an understanding that displacement of drugs from protein binding does not markedly alter the unbound fraction in circulation, and therefore affects elimination rate more than efficacy [22]. Consequently, there is a need for many clinicians to "unlearn" the dogma that has been taught, of the potential for clinical toxicity from drug interactions through displacement from plasma protein binding sites by competition between concomitantly administered drugs.

Drug–drug interactions during biotransformation are generally more frequent [103] and can be of clinical significance depending on the hepatic Cl_I for each drug, as discussed earlier in this chapter. Hepatic drug metabolism can be studied *in vitro* or *in vivo*. *In vitro* studies on PK interactions are both time- and cost-effective. They offer the opportunity to investigate specific biotransformation pathways under strictly controlled conditions and to investigate the ability of a drug to alter the metabolism of other drugs. For these reasons, *in vitro* studies form part of the screening processes used by pharmaceutical companies in the selection of new drugs [105–107]. However, both *in vitro* and *in vivo* evidence for drug–drug interactions in metabolism should be interpreted with care, as there is a growing understanding of the extent of genetic polymorphism among individuals or breeds of the same species (e.g., reduced hepatic metabolism of butorphanol in certain dog breeds) and its impact on drug metabolism and toxicity [108,109]. The well-described sensitivity of the rough collies to ivermectin has been attributed to a frame-shift mutation within the multidrug resistance (MDR1) gene, which has now been discovered within several other related breeds of dogs [110–112]. However, the clinical relevance of this mutation in canine anesthesia has not been demonstrated. Further, it is not possible to extrapolate drug metabolism evidence between species as major differences exist in metabolic pathways and enzyme activities [113,114].

Elimination or clearance of a drug is also subject to drug–drug interactions. While inhibition of clearance would result in a rise of the drug concentration, possibly to toxic levels, increases in clearance would result in a decrease of the drug blood concentration and possibly lack of efficacy and/or therapeutic failure. Both the inhibition and the induction of drug clearance can affect either the cytochrome P450 isoenzymes (CYPs) (see Phase I metabolism) or the transporters (see Phase III metabolism). Clinically important interactions affecting elimination or clearance are rare.

In addition to those two types of clearance alteration, other causes have been described. Pharmacokinetic interaction can be mediated physiologically. For example, it has been well-documented that during CRI or TCI with drugs of high intrinsic hepatic clearance, increases in CO will result in decreases in plasma drug concentration, and consequent changes to efficacy and vice versa. This alteration in hepatic clearance related to change in CO has been demonstrated with propofol in humans, sheep, and pigs and likely occurs with many anesthetics and analgesics [48,115–119].

Pharmacodynamic interactions

Pharmacodynamic interactions result in the modification of the response of the body to one or more concomitantly administered drugs. These modifications can be due to mechanisms such as the alteration of the receptor sensitivity or affinity to one agent by the other. Alternatively, the production of additive or inhibitory effects can occur either through action at different effect sites or by actions through alternative receptor mechanisms. Interactions through PD mechanisms are common clinical realities, such as the sparing effect of opioids or α_2-adrenergic receptor agonists on the minimum alveolar concentration (MAC) values of inhalant agents or on propofol infusion doses. However, when considering clinically important drug–drug interrelationships, it is worth noting that interindividual PD variability frequently ranges between 300 and 400% and interindividual variance of PK can be in the order of 70–80% [120,121]. This interindividual PK and PD variability makes it difficult to identify an unexpected clinical occurrence as an unwanted drug interaction rather than simply a function of interindividual variability.

There are two major types of studies developed to assess PD interactions, either isobolographic analyses or response surface modeling techniques. Knowledge from studies using these methods permits dosing decisions designed to maximize or minimize an interaction. Interactions are often deleterious to clinical case management, but can also be beneficial (e.g., optimizing speed of induction of anesthesia, increasing hemodynamic stability at induction and during maintenance of anesthesia, decreasing time to awakening, optimizing spontaneous respiration, and minimizing the level of postoperative pain) [120,122,123].

Isobolographic analyses

Isobolographic studies evaluate the effects of different concentrations of two agents on a specific effect, such as loss of consciousness. Different dosing pair combinations resulting in the same effect are evaluated. An isobole can be constructed by drawing a line through those "iso-effective" combinations. A straight line called the "line of additivity" or "additive interaction" is drawn between the two concentrations for each single agent associated with the same effect (Fig. 19.20). Synergism is usually associated with a concave-up-shaped isobole, while infra-additivity is associated with a concave-down-shaped isobole. One of the main problems with this system is that the information is only in two dimensions and only gives the information for a specific effect level (i.e., EC_{50} or EC_{95}) [122].

Response surface analyses

To describe a more complete set of effect levels (EC_{01}–EC_{99}), a response surface is constructed using three-dimensional graphs that incorporate all the available isoboles for different levels of the effect (Fig. 19.21). In such a system, every single combination of the two drugs are points on a surface, the height of which is the drug effect of interest [124]. Different mathematical approaches have been described to produce the response surface [125,126]. It has been proposed that while the mathematical approach of Minto *et al.* is appropriate for the analysis of unimodal endpoints (loss of consciousness, return of consciousness), Bol *et al.*'s approach was better suited to analyze multimodal endpoint (adequacy of anesthesia which includes hypnotic and analgesic components) [127]. If one is studying the interaction between drugs that on their own do not produce the studied effect, other models have been proposed such as the Reduced Greco, Fixed C_{50O} Hierarchical, and Scaled C_{50O}

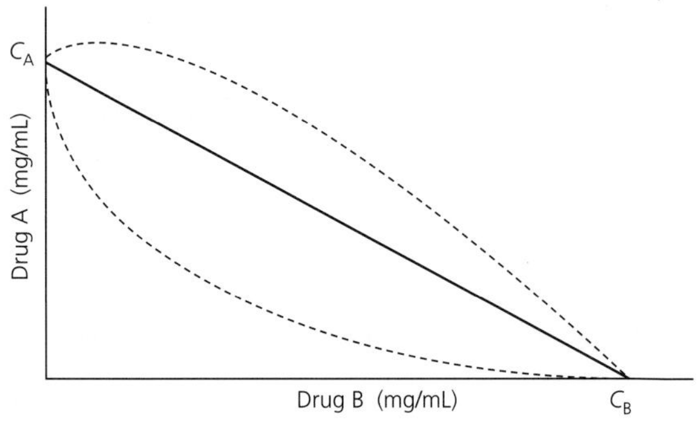

Figure 19.20 Example of an isobole for two agents, A and B, when given alone (CA and CB) and when given in combination to induce an effect such as endotracheal intubation. The isobole can take different shapes depending on the nature of the interaction between the two agents.

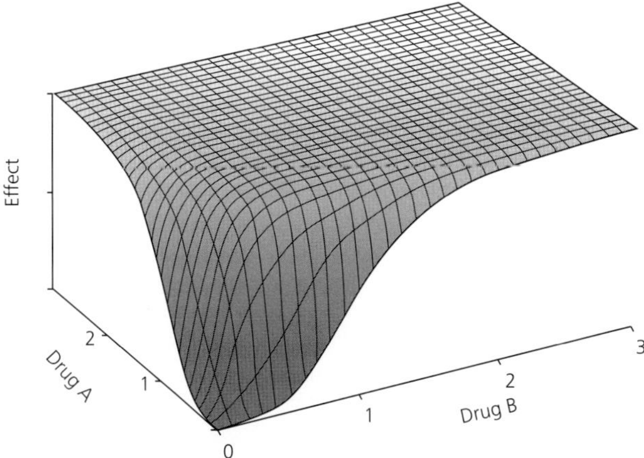

Figure 19.21 Modeling of a response (effect) surface between two hypothetical agents, Drug A and Drug B. Source: Adapted from Minto and Vuyk [122].

Hierarchical models [128]. To determine the optimal response, these models can be used in combination with PK data [129]. In humans, PK-PD modeling of propofol and different opioids has been used to maximize the use of both agents [123]. The PK-PD modeling determines the various optimal propofol-opioid concentrations associated with intraoperative adequacy of anesthesia and the most rapid return to consciousness thereafter. As expected, the optimal propofol concentration changes with both the opioid used and the length of infusion [120,123].

Adverse drug reactions

"Adverse drug reactions" (ADRs) and "adverse drug events" (ADEs) are collective terms which are each used to describe events that include both undesired effects and inefficacy, relative to the expected effects after drug administration [130,131]. Evaluation of ADEs divides them into several categories, although the categories are not exclusive: dose-related, non-dose-related, dose- and time-related, time-related, withdrawal, and unexpected inefficacy.

Population variability in drug-response blurs the boundary between ADEs that are non-dose-related (unexpected events) and dose-related (inefficacy and toxicity). Toxic events can occur at unexpectedly low doses in sensitive individuals. Apparent inefficacy can occur at labeled doses, when the labeled dose is established using population parameters such as the effective dose for a proportion of the population. For example, in some regulatory territories, the labeled dose of alfaxalone is its ED_{90} [132].

Drugs that induce physiological adaptation, receptor down regulation or tachyphylaxis, and enzyme induction or inhibition can result in time-related undesired effects. These effects can be either direct or caused by drug interactions, as previously discussed. Developing tolerance can result in the onset of inefficacy, or upon their withdrawal unexpected ADEs can occur because of the unmasking of the adapted physiological changes. Although such ADEs are rarely recognized in veterinary medicine, some drugs frequently used possess characteristics that lead to these time-related ADEs (e.g., adrenergic receptor agonists such as clenbuterol [133] and opiate analgesics) [134].

Voluntary reports of ADEs submitted through voluntary reporting schemes are likely to underestimate the true number of ADEs

Table 19.1 Chemical reactions usually associated with Phase I and Phase II metabolism.

Phase I	Phase II
Oxidation – involving CYP	Glucuronidation
Oxidation – other	Glycosidation
Reduction	Sulfation
Hydrolysis	Methylation
Hydration	Acetylation
Others:	Amino acid conjugation
Isomerization	Glutathione conjugation
Ring cyclization	Condensation
Dimerization	Fatty acid conjugation
Transamidation	
Decarboxylation	
Dethioacetylation	
N-Carboxylation	

CYP, Cytochrome P450.
Source: Adapted from Gibson and Skett [105].

that occur. Despite this likely underreporting large numbers of ADEs are reported each year. Within the drug classes of relevance to the practice of anesthesia and analgesia, the NSAIDs are the category of drugs about which ADEs are most frequently reported [131]. Relative to the number of doses used, voluntary reports of ADEs for anesthetic induction agents such as propofol, ketamine, and alfaxalone are relatively rare [135].

Regulatory agencies and drug manufacturers endeavor to assess each ADE and assign a causal probability classification. A commonly used causality classification is a categorical system that is subjectively based: certain, probable, possible, unlikely, and unassessable [130]. Some regulatory jurisdictions use a flowchart scoring system [136]. Drug products that receive a high number of "certain" or "probable" assessments are occasionally subject to regulatory review. For example, a high number of ADEs to an injectable propofol formulation in Australia in 2004 [137] resulted in a regulatory review with subsequent mandatory label changes warning of ADEs.

Drug metabolism

Metabolism of administered xenobiotics can result in their activation from ineffective prodrugs, transformation or modification of the extent or nature of their activity or can result in their detoxification and facilitate their excretion. Metabolism of drugs, or biotransformation, is classically described as occurring in two phases. A xenobiotic may be metabolized by either or both of these phases depending on the physicochemical properties of the drug and the species of animal. Phase I biotransformations aim to convert fat-soluble (lipophilic) compounds into water-soluble (hydrophilic) compounds ready for immediate renal clearance, or to add chemically reactive sites to a relatively chemically inert molecule so as to allow further biotransformation. Secondary biotransformation processes can be either further Phase I reactions or may be conjugation reactions. In general, conjugation reactions attach the exogenous compound covalently to a substrate, which both increases the molecular weight and the water solubility of the complex. Conjugation reactions collectively are called "Phase II reactions." The chemical reactions associated with Phases I and II are reported in Table 19.1 [138–157].

The water-soluble compounds formed during Phases I and II metabolism need to be transported out of the cells prior to excretion. Some excretion processes are also transcellular, requiring further transport across biological membranes. These transcellular transport processes have recently been labeled as a "third phase" or Phase III of the drug metabolism process [158]. Factors described as affecting drug metabolism include species, gender, genetics, age, hormone and disease status, drug–drug interactions, diet, and environment (i.e., nearly everything!) [159,160].

Phase I biotransformation

The bulk of the Phase I biotransformation reactions are performed by a family of enzymes called the cytochrome P450 isoenzymes (CYPs) which are found mostly in the liver, but also in the gastrointestinal tract, skin, brain, lung, kidney, and other tissues [161]. The CYPs are principally located on the endoplasmic reticulum of the metabolically active cells and are mainly responsible for oxidation, reduction, hydrolysis, and hydration reactions, which prepare xenobiotics for Phase II conjugation reactions.

The CYPs are hemoproteins that exhibit a spectral absorbance maximum at 450 nm when reduced and complexed with carbon monoxide. The general reaction catalyzed by the CYPs can be written as follows:

$$\mathrm{NADPH} + \mathrm{H}^+ + \mathrm{O}_2 + \mathrm{RH} \xrightarrow{\mathrm{CYP450}} \mathrm{NADP}^+ + \mathrm{H}_2\mathrm{O} + \mathrm{ROH} \quad (19.54)$$

where RH represents an oxidizable drug substrate and ROH its hydroxylated metabolite.

The CYP isoenzymes are a superfamily with a modern classification and nomenclature derived from gene cloning and sequencing [162]. The superfamily is divided into families which are themselves divided into subfamilies, depending on the percentage of their genome the CYPs have in common. The enzyme families are described by an Arabic number, the subfamilies by a capital letter, and a final Arabic number denotes individual enzymes. Many CYPs have been screened and identified in humans, mice, rats, and monkeys, and several are now known in dogs, including CYP 1A1, 1A2, 2B11,2E, 2C21, 2C41, 2D15, 3A12, and 3A26 [163,164]. In dogs, CYP 2B11 has been recognized as being responsible for propofol hydroxylation and also for the breed differences seen in propofol metabolism [165,166], whereas CYP3A seems to be the main contributor to medetomidine metabolism [150].

Induction and inhibition of drug metabolism can lead to drug–drug interactions. The CYP enzymes are most commonly responsible for the metabolism-based interactions [103] the pharmacokinetics of which have been discussed above in this chapter under hepatic clearance. Induction of enzyme activity results from several factors: increased synthesis, decreased degradation, activation of pre-existing components, or a combination of those three processes [105]. In dogs, phenobarbital increases the activity of CYPs 2B11, 2C21, and 3A26, rifampin induces CYP 3A26, and omeprazole induces CYP 1A2 [163]. In the rat, ketamine has been shown to induce propofol metabolism [167]. Four facts are of importance for the clinician to remember regarding enzyme induction: (1) induction is usually a slow process (days to weeks), (2) the effect on drug concentration can alter treatment outcomes, (3) clinical relevance is mostly confined to drugs with low intrinsic hepatic clearance, and (4) the process is usually reversible [168].

An inhibitor will result in a decrease in metabolic enzyme activity. Four main processes have been described, which cause CYP inhibition: competitive inhibition, noncompetitive inhibition, uncompetitive inhibition, and mechanism-based inhibition [169]. Inhibition of a biotransformation enzyme is mostly reversible in nature, but occasionally can be irreversible and lead to permanent loss of enzyme activity until new enzymes are synthetized [105]. Unlike induction, CYP inhibition is usually an immediate response. The clinical consequences of enzyme inhibition are usually higher plasma drug concentrations and/or prolonged elimination half-life, increasing the risk for accumulation and toxic effects. Table 19.2 contains a non-exhaustive list of veterinary anesthesia-related agents, which can inhibit CYP isoenzymes.

Table 19.2 Non-exhaustive list of anesthesia-related agents with CYP inhibitory activity in different species.

Drug	Species	Reference
Propofol	Human	[138–147]
	Rat	[148]
	Hamster	[138,141]
	Pig	
Medetomidine	Dog	[149–151]
	Rat	[149,151]
	Fish	[152,153]
Dexmedetomidine	Human	[154–156]
	Dog	[149]
	Rat	[149,157]
Levomedetomidine	Human	[155]
	Dog	[149]
	Rat	[149,157]
Atipamezole	Dog	[151]

Phase II biotransformation or conjugation

During this phase, endogenous and xenobiotic metabolites will be conjugated resulting in products of higher molecular weight and usually less activity than their substrates. The products of conjugation are excreted either by the bile, if they are of high molecular weight, or in the urine, if they are both of low molecular weight and high water solubility [162]. Although this phase is generally seen as enhancing the detoxification effect, in some cases, the conjugation may result in activated metabolites and increased toxicity [161].

Different mechanisms are involved in conjugation: glucuronidation, sulfation, methylation, acetylation, amino acid conjugation, glutathione conjugation, and fatty acid conjugation. Glucuronidation is quantitatively the most important form of conjugation for drugs and endogenous compounds in most species and can occur with alcohols, phenols, hydroxylamines, carboxylic acids, and so on. Glutathione is regarded as a protective compound in the body for the removal of potentially toxic electrophilic compounds such as epoxides, haloalkanes, nitroalkanes, alkenes, and aromatic halo- and nitro-compounds. Sulfation is a major metabolic pathway for phenols [170]. The enzymes that facilitate conjugation reactions belong to a superfamily of enzymes and include sulfotransferases (SULT), UDP-glucuronosyltransferases (UGT), and glutathione *S*-transferases (GST) [161].

Transport of metabolites (Phase III biotransformation)

Drug transporters can be found in numerous tissues (intestine, liver, kidney, and brain) and are involved in absorption, distribution, and excretion. They are usually transmembrane transporters, which may aid drug and drug–metabolite movement and they include P-glycoprotein (P-gp), organic anion transporting polypeptide 2 (OATP2), and multidrug resistance-associated protein (MRP). The MRP and the P-gp are called "ATP-binding cassette (ABC) transporters" as they utilize the energy from ATP to transport substrates across the cell membrane [161]. In the liver, these transporters are found on the canalicular membrane where they are involved in the biliary excretion of both parents' drugs and their metabolite, and the transporters are also found on the sinusoidal membrane where they are responsible for the uptake of drugs from the blood into the hepatocytes [171]. In the kidneys, the organic anion and cation transport systems are found on brush border and basolateral membranes of the tubular epithelial cells and are responsible for the secretion of drugs into the urine [161,171].

Just as for the CYPs, transporter activity can be increased or decreased and can play a role in drug absorption as well as drug elimination. For example, in humans, fruit juices are well-known inhibitors of organic anion transporters and result in reduced oral drug bioavailability. Also in humans, the hepatic and/or renal excretion of digoxin is altered by verapamil and quinidine, which are potent inhibitors of P-gp. The inhibition of P-gp results in increased plasma concentration of the cardiac glycoside [171–173].

Isomers and stereoisomers

Although labeled simply with the active drug's pharmacopeial name, many of the drug products commonly used contain more than one form of the active molecule. Drug molecules often are carbon-based entities, the majority of which have multiple structural molecular forms, called "isomers." Isomers can be either constitutional isomers or stereoisomers. Constitutional isomers are those with the same number and type of atoms, but where the connectivity between the atoms differs (e.g., propane versus cyclopropane). Stereoisomers occur either because of the inflexibility of carbon–carbon double bonds (*cis-trans* isomers), or because a carbon molecule may have four different covalently bonded moieties, thus creating one or more chirally active centers (enantiomers and diastereomers).

Constitutional isomers pose little practical clinical problem, as drug products rarely contain mixtures of such isomers. Similarly, because *cis-trans* isomers usually have major differences in affinity for drug receptors or metabolizing enzymes, products rarely have more than a minor contamination of the less active isomer. In contrast to non-chiral isomers, chirally active stereoisomers pose a major consideration for clinical pharmacology, pharmacokinetics, and anesthesia. There are two types of chiral stereoisomers, enantiomers and diastereomers. Enantiomers are chirally active stereoisomers, which have planar symmetry, that is, one form is the mirror image of the other. Where a molecule has two chirally active centers, there is a possibility of four isomers. Two of the possible pairings result in symmetry and are stereoisomers, but the other four pairing permutations do not have planar symmetry and are called "diastereomers." Products which contain a mixture of enantiomers are called "racemic mixtures."

For stereoisomers, there are two naming conventions, which do not necessarily align with one another. The *R–S* system of naming involves a deliberate orientation of the molecule in space, then reading the direction of descending atomic mass; clockwise is *R*, where *R* is from the Latin *rectus* = straight, and anticlockwise is *S*, where *S* is from the Latin *sinister* = left. Alternatively, if polarized light rotates to the right when passed through a solution of an enantiomer, then the enantiomer is designated as the dextrorotatory (+) isomer, while the image is its levorotatory (−) isomer. Many of the drugs used in anesthesia have chiral isomers and are marketed as racemic mixtures (e.g., thiopental, ketamine, carprofen, and ketoprofen). The mammalian body is a very chiral environment and enantiomers can have markedly different efficacy, potency, safety, and pharmacokinetics [174–178]. Sometimes these differences are exemplified or altered by unequal binding to albumin [179,180]. Further, for some drugs, the mammalian isomerase enzymes can convert isomers between forms, but for other enantiomers such enzyme isomerization is not achieved [181].

As techniques for manufacture of purified enantiomers become cheaper, products are likely to be marketed as pure enantiomers or non-racemic mixtures. These products may have different efficacy and toxicity profiles from their racemic look-alikes, and may require attention to different dosing regimens, (e.g., medetomidine versus dexmedetomidine).

The effect of formulation

Most of the drug products we commonly use are not labeled with information about their contents, other than the name and concentration of the active molecule. The drug products usually contain a far greater mass of other "ingredients" called "excipients." The excipients can have marked effects on drug efficacy and safety.

An example of formulation effects is illustrative of the need for clinical attention to formulation. The white-colored propofol is formulated as a stabilized emulsion using oil and emulsifiers to provide a useful formulation that maintains its physical stability for a suitable shelf life. However, aqueous solutions are preferred for intravenous use and therefore efforts have been made to formulate an aqueous solution of propofol. Several successful approaches have resulted in formulations, which appear initially to have similar properties to the pioneer milky emulsion [182,183]. However, aqueous microemulsion formulations have been marketed in several countries in which the solubilization was achieved using various polyethoxylated detergents. These aqueous preparations have resulted in reported ADRs such as anaphylaxis and increased pain on injection [184,185].

Just as isomerization can result in more than one form of the active drug's molecule, other variations of form for the active ingredient can markedly alter a drug's pharmacokinetics. Many oral drugs are dosed as compressed tablets. The active drug in the tablet may be the drug's free base or may be an ionic or organic salt. The drug may be in a dry amorphous form or may be crystals. Different salts and different crystal shapes can have markedly different solubilities causing large changes in bioavailability.

The preparation of a consistently performing, effective, and stable formulation is a high-level pharmaceutical skill. In most major global territories, the manufacturers of products are regulated by governing authorities, providing users with assurance that the product will perform as labeled. In contrast, the adoption of products sourced from unlicensed manufacturers, such as compounding pharmacies, may be problematic. Unlicensed manufacturers are of unknown skill and their processes and products are not evaluated, reviewed, or approved. In human and veterinary medicine, there are numerous examples of morbidity and mortality that are directly attributable to poor knowledge, lack of skill, or unsatisfactory processes of and by compounding pharmacies [186–188].

References

1 Bernard C. Analyse physiologique des proprietes des sytemes musculaire et nerveux au moyen du curare. *Compte Rendu des Siances de l'Academie des Sciences* 1856; **43**: 825.

2 Adams HR. *Veterinary Pharmacology and Therapeutics*, 8th edn. Ames, IA: Iowa State University Press, 2001: 1201.

3 Heit HA, Gourlay DL. Buprenorphine: new tricks with an old molecule for pain management. *Clin J Pain* 2008; **24**(2): 93–97.

4 Povoa P, Carneiro AH. Adrenergic support in septic shock: a critical review. *Hosp Pract (1995)* 2010; **38**(1): 62–73.

5 Goodman LS, Gilman A, Brunton LL. *Goodman & Gilman's Manual of Pharmacology and Therapeutics*. New York, NY: McGraw-Hill Medical, 2008: 1219.

6 Sonner JM, Antognini JF, Dutton RC, *et al.* Inhaled anesthetics and immobility: mechanisms, mysteries, and minimum alveolar anesthetic concentration. *Anesth Analg* 2003; **97**(3): 718–740.

7 Barnes PJ. Glucocorticosteroids: current and future directions. *Br J Pharmacol* 2011; **163**(1): 29–43.

8 Mandema JW, Kuck MT, Danhof M. Differences in intrinsic efficacy of benzodiazepines are reflected in their concentration-EEG effect relationship. *British J Pharmacol* 1992; **105**(1): 164–170.

9 Taylor R, Pergolizzi JV, Porreca F, *et al.* Opioid antagonists for pain. *Expert Opin Investig Drugs* 2013; **22**(4): 517–525.

10 Yu FH, Catterall WA. Overview of the voltage-gated sodium channel family. *Genome Biol* 2003; **4**(3): 207.

11 Johnston GA. GABAA receptor pharmacology. *Pharmacol Ther* 1996; **69**(3): 173–198.

12 Traynelis SF, Wollmuth LP, McBain CJ, *et al.* Glutamate receptor ion channels: structure, regulation, and function. *Pharmacol Rev* 2010; **62**(3): 405–496.

13 Shang J, Wan Y, Luo C, *et al.* Cell entry mechanisms of SARS-CoV-2. *Proc Natl Acad Sci USA* 2020; **117**(21): 11727–11734.

14 Hamming I, Timens W, Bulthuis ML, *et al.* Tissue distribution of ACE2 protein, the functional receptor for SARS coronavirus. A first step in understanding SARS pathogenesis. *J Pathol* 2004; **203**(2): 631–637.

15 Lubbe L, Cozier Gyles E, Oosthuizen D, *et al.* ACE2 and ACE: structure-based insights into mechanism, regulation and receptor recognition by SARS-CoV. *Clin Sci (London)* 2020; **134**(21): 2851–2871.

16 Calabrese EJ, Baldwin LA. U-shaped dose-responses in biology, toxicology, and public health. *Annu Rev Public Health* 2001; **22**: 15–33.

17 Ariens EJ. Affinity and intrinsic activity in the theory of competitive inhibition. I. Problems and theory. *Arch Int Pharmacodyn Ther* 1954; **99**(1): 32–49.

18 Robbins J, Rall JE. The interaction of thyroid hormones and protein in biological fluids. *Recent Prog Horm Res* 1957; **13**: 161–202.

19 Toutain PL, Bousquet-Melou A. Plasma terminal half-life. *J Vet Pharmacol Ther* 2004; **27**(6): 427–439.

20 Toutain PL, Bousquet-Melou A. Volumes of distribution. *J Vet Pharmacol Ther* 2004; **27**(6): 441–453.

21 Toutain PL, Bousquet-Melou A. Plasma clearance. *J Vet Pharmacol Ther* 2004; **27**(6): 415–425.

22 Toutain PL, Bousquet-Melou A. Free drug fraction vs free drug concentration: a matter of frequent confusion. *J Vet Pharmacol Ther* 2002; **25**(6): 460–463.

23 Toutain PL, Bousquet-Melou A. Bioavailability and its assessment. *J Vet Pharmacol Ther* 2004; **27**(6): 455–466.

24 Thron CD. Linearity and superposition in pharmacokinetics. *Pharmacol Rev* 1974; **26**(1): 3.

25 Veng-Pedersen P. Mean time parameters in pharmacokinetics. Definition, computation and clinical implications (Part 1). *Clin Pharmacokinet* 1989; **17**(5): 345–366.

26 Dayton PG, Cucinell SA, Weiss M, *et al.* Dose-dependence of drug plasma level decline in dogs. *J Pharmacol Exp Ther* 1967; **158**(2): 305–316.

27 Maylin GA. Disposition of phenylbutazone in the horse. In: *Proceedings of the 20th Convention of the Association of American Equine Practitioners. Association of American Equine Practitioners*; 1974.

28 Lees P, Taylor JBO, Higgins AJ, *et al.* Phenylbutazone and oxyphenbutazone distribution into tissue fluids in the horse. *J Vet Pharmacol Therap* 1986; **9**: 204–212.

29 Ng LL. Reviewer Guidance: Validation of Chromatographic Methods Washington DC: Food and Drug Administration: *Center for Drug Evaluation and Research*; 1994. http://www.fda.gov/downloads/Drugs/Guidances/UCM134409.pdf

30 Woodward A, Whittem T. The lower limit of quantification in pharmacokinetic analyses. *J Vet Pharmacol Therap* 2019; **42**(6): 585–587.

31 Beal SL. Ways to fit a PK model with some data below the quantification limit. *J Pharmacokinet Pharmacodyn* 2001; **28**(5): 481–504.

32 Keizer RJ, Jansen RS, Rosing H, *et al.* Incorporation of concentration data below the limit of quantification in population pharmacokinetic analyses. *Pharmacol Res Perspect* 2015; **3**(2): e00131.

33 Henri J, Jacques AM, Sanders P, *et al.* The present and future of withdrawal period calculations for milk in the European Union: dealing with data below the limit of quantification. *J Vet Pharmacol Ther* 2017; **40**(2): 116–122.

34 Jelliffe RW, Schumitzky A, Bayard D, *et al.* Describing assay precision-reciprocal of variance is correct, not CV percent: its use should significantly improve laboratory performance. *Ther Drug Monit* 2015; **37**(3): 389–394.

35 Yang S, Roger J. Evaluations of Bayesian and maximum likelihood methods in PK models with below-quantification-limit data. *Pharm Stat* 2010; **9**(4): 313–330.

36 Mordenti J. Man versus beast: pharmacokinetic scaling in mammals. *J Pharm Sci* 1986; **75**(11): 1028–1040.

37 Fiakpui NN, Hogan DF, Whittem T, *et al.* Dose determination of fondaparinux in healthy cats. *Am J Vet Res* 2012; **73**(4): 556–561.

38 Committee for Veterinary Medicinal Products. *Guidelines for the Conduct of Pharmacokinetic Studies in Target Animal Species*. London, UK: European Agency for the Evaluation of Medicinal Products, 2000.

39 Sheiner LB. The population approach to pharmacokinetic data analysis: rationale and standard data analysis methods. *Drug Metabol Rev* 1984; **15**(1–2): 153–171.

40 Pasloske K, Sauer B, Perkins N, *et al.* Plasma pharmacokinetics of alfaxalone in both premedicated and unpremedicated Greyhound dogs after single, intravenous administration of Alfaxan at a clinical dose. *J Vet Pharmacol Ther* 2009; **32**(5): 510–513.

41 Yamaoka K, Nakagawa T, Uno T. Application of Akaike's Information Criterion (AIC) in the evaluation of linear pharmacokinetic equations. *J Pharmacokin Biopharm* 1978; **6**(2): 165–175.

42 Sheiner LB, Beal SL. Evaluation of methods for estimating population pharmacokinetic parameters. III. Monoexponential model: routine clinical pharmacokinetic data. *J Pharmacokin Biopharm* 1983; **11**: 303–319.

43 Sheiner LB. Analysis of pharmacokinetic data using parametric models–1: regression models. *J Pharmacokin Biopharm* 1984; **12**(1): 93–117.

44 Sheiner LB. Analysis of pharmacokinetic data using parametric models. II. Point estimates of an individual's parameters. *J Pharmacokin Biopharm* 1985; **13**(5): 515–540.

45 Gibaldi M, Perrier D. Noncompartmental analysis based on statistical moment theory. In: Swarback J, ed. *Pharmacokinetics*, 2nd edn. New York, NY: Marcel Dekker, 1982: 409–417.

46 Purves RD. Optimum numerical integration methods for estimating area-under-the-curve (AUC) and area-under-the-moment-curve (AUMC). *J Pharmacokin Biopharm* 1992; **20**: 211–226.

47 Avram MJ, Krejcie TC, Niemann CU, *et al.* Isoflurane alters the recirculatory pharmacokinetics of physiologic markers. *Anesthesiology* 2000; **92**(6): 1757–1768.

48 Upton RN, Ludbrook GL. A model of the kinetics and dynamics of induction of anaesthesia in sheep: variable estimation for thiopental and comparison with propofol. *Br J Anaesth* 1999; **82**(6): 890–899.

49 Upton RN, Ludbrook GL. A physiological model of induction of anaesthesia with propofol in sheep. 1. Structure and estimation of variables. *Br J Anaesth* 1997; **79**(4): 497–504.

50 Krejcie TC, Avram MJ. Recirculatory pharmacokinetic modeling: what goes around, comes around. *Anesth Analg* 2012; **115**(2): 223–226.

51 Giraudel JM, Diquelou A, Laroute V, *et al.* Pharmacokinetic/pharmacodynamic modelling of NSAIDs in a model of reversible inflammation in the cat. *Br J Pharmacol* 2005; **146**(5): 642–653.

52 Rowland M, Tozer TN. Constant-rate therapy. In: Troy DB, ed. *Clinical Pharmacokinetics and Pharmacodynamics: Concepts and Applications*, 4th edn. Baltimore, MD: Lippincott Williams & Wilkins, 2011: 259–292.

53 Smith I, White PF. Intravenous anaesthesia delivery and monitoring systems. In: Hahn CEW, Adams AP, eds. *Total Intravenous Anaesthesia*. London, UK: BMJ Books, 1998: 98–127.

54 Padfield NL. Administration of intravenous anaesthesia/total intravenous anaesthesia. In: Tait M, ed. *Total Intravenous Anaesthesia*, 1st edn. London, UK: Butterworth Heinemann, 2000: 66–86.

55 Beths T. Total intravenous techniques for anaesthesia. *In Pract* 2007; **29**(7): 410–414.

56 Glass PS, Jacobs JR, Quill TJ. Intravenous drug delivery systems. In: Fragen RJ, ed. *Drug Infusions in Anesthesiology*. New York, NY: Raven Press, 1991: 23–62.

57 Kruger-Thiemer E. Continuous intravenous infusion and multicompartment accumulation. *Eur J Pharmacol* 1968; **4**(3): 317–324.

58 Wagner JG. A safe method for rapidly achieving plasma concentration plateaus. *Clin Pharmacol Ther* 1974; **16**(4): 691–700.

59 Miller DR. Intravenous infusion anaesthesia and delivery devices. *Can J Anaesth* 1994; **41**(7): 639–651.

60 Gepts E. Pharmacokinetic concepts for TCI anaesthesia. *Anaesthesia* 1998; **53**(Suppl 1): 4–12.

61 Schwilden H. A general method for calculating the dosage scheme in linear pharmacokinetics. *Eur J Clin Pharmacol* 1981; **20**(5): 379–386.

62 Schuttler J, Schwilden H, Stoekel H. Pharmacokinetics as applied to total intravenous anaesthesia. *Practical implications. Anaesthesia* 1983; **38**(Suppl): 53–56.

63 Alvis JM, Reves JG, Govier AV, *et al.* Computer-assisted continuous infusions of fentanyl during cardiac anesthesia: comparison with a manual method. *Anesthesiology* 1985; **63**(1): 41–49.

64 Schuttler J, Kloos S, Schwilden H, *et al.* Total intravenous anaesthesia with propofol and alfentanil by computer-assisted infusion. *Anaesthesia* 1988; **43**(Suppl): 2–7.

65 Milne SE, Kenny GN. Target controlled infusions. *Curr Anaesth Crit Care* 1998; **9**: 4.

66 Glen JB. The development and future of target controlled infusion. *Adv Exp Med Biol* 2003; **523**: 123–133.

67 Gray JM, Kenny GN. Development of the technology for 'Diprifusor' TCI systems. *Anaesthesia* 1998; **53**(Suppl 1): 22–27.

68 Glass SA, Shafer SL, Reves JG. Intravenous drug delivery systems. In: Krehling E, ed. *Miller's Anesthesia*, vol. **1**. Philadelphia, PA: Churchill Livingstone Elsevier, 2009: 825.

69 Egan TD. Target-controlled drug delivery: progress toward an intravenous "vaporizer" and automated anesthetic administration. *Anesthesiology* 2003; **99**(5): 1214–1219.

70 Short TG, Lim TA, Tam YH. Prospective evaluation of pharmacokinetic model-controlled infusion of propofol in adult patients. *Br J Anaesth* 1996; **76**(2): 313–315.

71 Beths T, Glen JB, Reid J, *et al.* Evaluation and optimisation of a target-controlled infusion system for administering propofol to dogs as part of a total intravenous anaesthetic technique during dental surgery. *Vet Rec* 2001; **148**(7): 198–203.

72 Oei-Lim VL, White M, Kalkman CJ, *et al.* Pharmacokinetics of propofol during conscious sedation using target-controlled infusion in anxious patients undergoing dental treatment. *Br J Anaesth* 1998; **80**(3): 324–331.

73 Swinhoe CF, Peacock JE, Glen JB, *et al.* Evaluation of the predictive performance of a 'Diprifusor' TCI system. *Anaesthesia* 1998; **53**(Suppl 1): 61–67.

74 Varvel JR. Measuring the predictive performance of computer-controlled infusion pumps. *J Pharmacokinet Biopharm* 2002; **20**(1): 31.

75 Slepchenko G, Simon N, Goubaux B, *et al.* Performance of target-controlled sufentanil infusion in obese patients. *Anesthesiology* 2003; **98**(1): 65–73.

76 Li YH, Xu JH, Yang JJ, *et al.* Predictive performance of 'Diprifusor' TCI system in patients during upper abdominal surgery under propofol/fentanyl anesthesia. *J Zhejiang Univ Sci B* 2005; **6**(1): 43–48.

77 Ko YP, Hsu YW, Hsu K, *et al.* Simulation analysis of the performance of target-controlled infusion of propofol in Chinese patients. *Acta Anaesthesiol Taiwan* 2007; **45**(3): 141–147.

78 Coetzee JF, Glen JB, Wium CA, *et al.* Pharmacokinetic model selection for target controlled infusions of propofol. Assessment of three parameter sets. *Anesthesiology* 1995; **82**(6): 1328–1345.

79 Vuyk J, Engbers FH, Burm AG, *et al.* Performance of computer-controlled infusion of propofol: an evaluation of five pharmacokinetic parameter sets. *Anesth Analg* 1995; **81**(6): 1275–1282.

80 Glen JB. The development of 'Diprifusor': a TCI system for propofol. *Anaesthesia* 1998; **53**(Suppl 1): 13–21.

81 Varvel JR, Donoho DL, Shafer SL. Measuring the predictive performance of computer-controlled infusion pumps. *J Pharmacokinet Biopharm* 1992; **20**(1): 63–94.

82 Glass PS. Pharmacokinetic basis of intravenous drug delivery. *Baill Clin Anaesth* 1991; **5**(3): 40.

83 Cattai A, Bizzotto R, Cagnardi P, *et al.* A pharmacokinetic model optimized by covariates for propofol target-controlled infusion in dogs. *Vet Anaesth Analg* 2019; **46**(5): 568–578.

84 Ilkiw JE, Pascoe PJ, Fisher LD. Effect of alfentanil on the minimum alveolar concentration of isoflurane in cats. *Am J Vet Res* 1997; **58**(11): 1274–1279.

85 Pypendop BH, Ilkiw JE. Assessment of the hemodynamic effects of lidocaine administered IV in isoflurane-anesthetized cats. *Am J Vet Res* 2005; **66**(4): 661–668.

86 Pypendop BH, Ilkiw JE, Robertson SA. Effects of intravenous administration of lidocaine on the thermal threshold in cats. *Am J Vet Res* 2006; **67**(1): 16–20.

87 Pypendop BH, Ranasinghe MG, Pasloske K. Pharmacokinetics of alfaxalone infusions, context-sensitive half-time and recovery times in male neutered cats. *Vet Anaesth Analg* 2018; **45**(5): 630–639.

88 Cattai A, Pilla T, Cagnardi P, *et al.* Evaluation and optimisation of propofol pharmacokinetic parameters in cats for target-controlled infusion. *Vet Rec* 2016; **178**(20): 503.

89 Pascoe PJ, Steffey EP, Black WD, *et al.* Evaluation of the effect of alfentanil on the minimum alveolar concentration of halothane in horses. *Am J Vet Res* 1993; **54**(8): 1327–1332.

90 Daunt DA, Dunlop CI, Chapman PL, *et al.* Cardiopulmonary and behavioral responses to computer-driven infusion of detomidine in standing horses. *Am J Vet Res* 1993; **54**(12): 2075–2082.

91 Chen JY, Yi M, Yao SL, *et al.* Propofol target-controlled infusion modeling in rabbits: pharmacokinetic and pharmacodynamic analysis. *J Huazhong Univ Sci Technolog Med Sci* 2016; **36**(3): 428–433.

92 Shafer SL, Varvel JR. Pharmacokinetics, pharmacodynamics, and rational opioid selection. *Anesthesiology* 1991; **74**(1): 53–63.

93 Lagneau F, Tod M, Marty J. Clinical applications of intravenous anaesthetics pharmacology: the example of hypnotics and opioids. *Ann Fr Anesth Reanim* 2004; **23**(10): 986–997.

94 Bailey JM. Context-sensitive half-times: what are they and how valuable are they in anaesthesiology? *Clin pharmacokinet* 2002; **41**(11): 793–799.

95 Pypendop BH. Context-sensitive half-times of fentanyl, alfentanil, sufentanil, and remifentanil in cats anesthetized with isoflurane obtained by pharmacokinetic simulation. *Presented at the 11th World Congress of Veterinary Anaesthesiology*, Cape Town, 2013.

96 Engbers F. Basic pharmacokinetic principles for intravenous anaesthesia. In: Vuyk J, Schraag S, eds. *Advances in Modelling and Clinical Applications of Intravenous Anaesthesia. Advances in Experimental Medicine and Biology*. New York, NY: Kluwer Academic/Plenum Publishers, 2003: 3–18.

97 Youngs EJ, Shafer SL. Pharmacokinetic parameters relevant to recovery from opioids. *Anesthesiology* 1994; **81**(4): 833–842.

98 Struys MM, De Smet T, Depoorter B, *et al.* Comparison of plasma compartment versus two methods for effect compartment-controlled target-controlled infusion for propofol. *Anesthesiology* 2000; **92**(2): 399–406.

99 Wakeling HG, Zimmerman JB, Howell S, *et al.* Targeting effect compartment or central compartment concentration of propofol: what predicts loss of consciousness? *Anesthesiology* 1999; **90**(1): 92–97.

100 Minto CF, Schnider TW, Gregg KM, *et al.* Using the time of maximum effect site concentration to combine pharmacokinetics and pharmacodynamics. *Anesthesiology* 2003; **99**(2): 324–333.

101 Gentry WB, Krejcie TC, Henthorn TK, *et al.* Effect of infusion rate on thiopental dose–response relationships. Assessment of a pharmacokinetic-pharmacodynamic model. *Anesthesiology* 1994; **81**(2): 316–324.

102 Bras S, Bressan N, Ribeiro L, *et al.* A step towards effect-site target-controlled infusion with propofol in dogs: a k(e0) for propofol. *J Vet Pharmacol Ther* 2009; **32**(2): 182–188.

103 Benet LZ, Kroetz DL, Sheiner LB. Pharmacokinetics. In: Molinoff PB, Ruddon RW, eds. *Goodman and Gilman's The Pharmacological Basis of Therapeutics*, 9th edn. New York, NY: The McGraw-Hill Company, 1996: 3–28.

104 Aarons L. Kinetics of drug–drug interactions. *Pharmacol Ther* 1981; **14**(3): 321–344.

105 Gibson GG, Skett P. Induction and inhibition of drug metabolism. In: Gibson GG, Skett P, eds. *Introduction to Drug Metabolism*, 3rd edn. Cheltenham, UK: Nelson Thornes, 2001: 87–118.

106 Lin JH, Lu AY. Inhibition and induction of cytochrome P450 and the clinical implications. *Clin Pharmacokinet* 1998; **35**(5): 361–390.

107 Venkatakrishnan K, von Moltke LL, Obach RS, *et al.* Drug metabolism and drug interactions: application and clinical value of in vitro models. *Curr Drug Metab* 2003; **4**(5): 423–459.

108 Funk-Keenan J, Sacco J, Wong YY, *et al.* Evaluation of polymorphisms in the sulfonamide detoxification genes CYB5A and CYB5R3 in dogs with sulfonamide hypersensitivity. *J Vet Intern Med* 2012; **26**(5): 1126–1133.

109 Paulson SK, Engel L, Reitz B, *et al.* Evidence for polymorphism in the canine metabolism of the cyclooxygenase 2 inhibitor, celecoxib. *Drug Metab Dispos* 1999; **27**(10): 1133–1142.

110 Gramer I, Leidolf R, Doring B, *et al.* Breed distribution of the nt230 (del4) MDR1 mutation in dogs. *Vet J* 2011; **189**(1): 67–71.

111 Geyer J, Doring B, Godoy JR, *et al.* Frequency of the nt230 (del4) MDR1 mutation in Collies and related dog breeds in Germany. *J Vet Pharmacol Ther* 2005; **28**(6): 545–551.

112 Mealey KL, Bentjen SA, Gay JM, *et al.* Ivermectin sensitivity in collies is associated with a deletion mutation of the mdr1 gene. *Pharmacogenetics* 2001; **11**(8): 727–733.

113 Fink-Gremmels J. Implications of hepatic cytochrome P450-related biotransformation processes in veterinary sciences. *Eur J Pharmacol* 2008; **585**(2–3): 502–509.

114 Sharer JE, Shipley LA, Vandenbranden MR, *et al.* Comparisons of phase I and phase II in vitro hepatic enzyme activities of human, dog, rhesus monkey, and cynomolgus monkey. *Drug Metab Dispos* 1995; **23**(11): 1231–1241.

115 Takizawa D, Hiraoka H, Nakamura K, *et al.* Influence of the prone position on propofol pharmacokinetics. *Anaesthesia* 2004; **59**(12): 1250–1251.

116 Takizawa D, Nishikawa K, Sato E, *et al.* A dopamine infusion decreases propofol concentration during epidural blockade under general anesthesia. *Can J Anaesth* 2005; **52**(5): 463–466.

117 Takizawa E, Ito N, Ishizeki J, *et al.* The effect of positive end-expiratory pressure ventilation on propofol concentrations during general anesthesia in humans. *Fundam Clin Pharmacol* 2006; **20**(5): 489–492.

118 Myburgh JA, Upton RN, Grant C, *et al.* Epinephrine, norepinephrine and dopamine infusions decrease propofol concentrations during continuous propofol infusion in an ovine model. *Intensive Care Med* 2001; **27**(1): 276–282.

119 Kurita T, Morita K, Kazama T, *et al.* Influence of cardiac output on plasma propofol concentrations during constant infusion in swine. *Anesthesiology* 2002; **96**(6): 1498–1503.

120 Lichtenbelt BJ, Mertens M, Vuyk J. Strategies to optimise propofol-opioid anaesthesia. *Clin Pharmacokinet* 2004; **43**(9): 577–593.

121 Vuyk J. TCI: supplementation and drug interactions. *Anaesthesia* 1998; **53**(Suppl 1): 35–41.

122 Minto C, Vuyk J. Response surface modelling of drug interactions. *Adv Exp Med Biol* 2003; **523**: 35–43.

123 Vuyk J. Clinical interpretation of pharmacokinetic and pharmacodynamic propofol-opioid interactions. *Acta Anaesthesiol Belg* 2001; **52**(4): 445–551.

124 Short TG, Ho TY, Minto CF, *et al.* Efficient trial design for eliciting a pharmacokinetic-pharmacodynamic model-based response surface describing the interaction between two intravenous anesthetic drugs. *Anesthesiology* 2002; **96**(2): 400–408.

125 Minto CF, Schnider TW, Short TG, *et al.* Response surface model for anesthetic drug interactions. *Anesthesiology* 2000; *92*(6): 1603–1616.

126 Bol CJ, Vogelaar JP, Tang JP, *et al.* Quantification of pharmacodynamic interactions between dexmedetomidine and midazolam in the rat. *J Pharmacol Exp Ther* 2000; **294**(1): 347–355.

127 Mertens MJ, Olofsen E, Engbers FH, *et al.* Propofol reduces perioperative remifentanil requirements in a synergistic manner: response surface modeling of perioperative remifentanil-propofol interactions. *Anesthesiology* 2003; **99**(2): 347–359.

128 Heyse B, Proost JH, Schumacher PM, *et al.* Sevoflurane remifentanil interaction: comparison of different response surface models. *Anesthesiology* 2012; **116**(2): 311–323.

129 Manyam SC, Gupta DK, Johnson KB, *et al.* Opioid-volatile anesthetic synergy: a response surface model with remifentanil and sevoflurane as prototypes. *Anesthesiology* 2006; **105**(2): 267–278.

130 Edwards IR, Aronson JK. Adverse drug reactions: definitions, diagnosis, and management. *Lancet* 2000; **356**(9237): 1255–1259.

131 Hampshire VA, Doddy FM, Post LO, *et al.* Adverse drug event reports at the United States Food and Drug Administration Center for Veterinary Medicine. *J Am Vet Med Assoc* 2004; **225**(4): 533–536.

132 Emmerich I, Ungemach F. Neue Arzneimittel für Kleintiere 2008. *Tierärztliche Praxis Kleintiere* 2009; **6**(2009).

133 Thompson JA, Eades SC, Chapman AM, *et al.* Effects of clenbuterol administration on serum biochemical, histologic, and echocardiographic measurements of muscle injury in exercising horses. *Am J Vet Res* 2012; **73**(6): 875–883.

134 Stanton-Hicks M, Wüst HJ, Koch U, *et al.* Experimental tachyphylaxis: development of a continuous epidural dog model. In: Wüst H, Stanton-Hicks M, eds. *New Aspects in Regional Anesthesia*, 4th edn. Berlin, Germany: Springer, 1986: 32–38.

135 APVMA. *Report of Adverse Experiences for Veterinary Medicines and Agricultural Chemicals, Calendar Year 2009.* Canberra, Australia: Australian Pesticides and Veterinary Medicines Authority, 2010.

136 Kramer MS, Leventhal JM, Hutchinson TA, *et al.* An algorithm for the operational assessment of adverse drug reactions: I. background, description, and instructions for use. *J Am Med Assoc* 1979; **242**(7): 623–632.

137 APVMA. *Report of Adverse Experiences, 2004 Calendar Year, Veterinary Medicines. Canberra, Australia: Australian Pesticides and Veterinary Medicines Authority*, 2005.

138 Janicki PK, James MF, Erskine WA. Propofol inhibits enzymatic degradation of alfentanil and sufentanil by isolated liver microsomes in vitro. *Br J Anaesth* 1992; **68**(3): 311–312.

139 Chen TL, Ueng TH, Chen SH, *et al.* Human cytochrome P450 mono-oxygenase system is suppressed by propofol. *Br J Anaesth* 1995; **74**(5): 558–562.

140 McKillop D, Wild MJ, Butters CJ, *et al.* Effects of propofol on human hepatic microsomal cytochrome P450 activities. *Xenobiotica* 1998; **28**(9): 845–853.

141 Lejus C, Fautrel A, Malledant Y, *et al.* Inhibition of cytochrome P450 2E1 by propofol in human and porcine liver microsomes. *Biochem Pharmacol* 2002; **64**(7): 1151–1156.

142 Inomata S, Nagashima A, Osaka Y, *et al.* Propofol inhibits lidocaine metabolism in human and rat liver microsomes. *J Anesth* 2003; **17**(4): 246–250.

143 Yang LQ, Yu WF, Cao YF, *et al.* Potential inhibition of cytochrome P450 3A4 by propofol in human primary hepatocytes. *World J Gastroenterol* 2003; **9**(9): 1959–1962.

144 Osaka Y, Inomata S, Tanaka E, *et al.* Effect of propofol on ropivacaine metabolism in human liver microsomes. *J Anesth* 2006; **20**(1): 60–63.

145 Baker MT, Chadam MV, Ronnenberg WC. Inhibitory effects of propofol on cytochrome P450 activities in rat hepatic microsomes. *Anesth Analg* 1993; **76**(4): 817–821.

146 Gemayel J, Geloen A, Mion F. Propofol-induced cytochrome P450 inhibition: an in vitro and in vivo study in rats. *Life Sci* 2001; **68**(26): 2957–2965.

147 Yamazaki H, Shimizu M, Nagashima T, *et al.* Rat cytochrome P450 2C11 in liver microsomes involved in oxidation of anesthetic agent propofol and deactivated by prior treatment with propofol. *Drug Metab Dispos* 2006; **34**(11): 1803–1805.

148 Chen TL, Wang MJ, Huang CH, *et al.* Difference between in vivo and in vitro effects of propofol on defluorination and metabolic activities of hamster hepatic cytochrome P450-dependent mono-oxygenases. *Br J Anaesth* 1995; **75**(4): 462–466.

149 Beths T, Glen JB, Reid J, *et al.* The inhibitory effect of medetomidine and its enantiomers on canine and rat liver microsomal propofol metabolism *'in vitro'. Presented at the World Congress of Veterinary Anaesthesiology, University of Tennessee*, September 2003.

150 Duhamel MC, Troncy E, Beaudry F. Metabolic stability and determination of cytochrome P450 isoenzymes' contribution to the metabolism of medetomidine in dog liver microsomes. *Biomed Chromatogr* 2010; **24**(8): 868–877.

151 Baratta MT, Zaya MJ, White JA, *et al.* Canine CYP2B11 metabolizes and is inhibited by anesthetic agents often co-administered in dogs. *J Vet Pharmacol Ther* 2010; **33**(1): 50–55.

152 Lennquist A, Celander MC, Forlin L. Effects of medetomidine on hepatic EROD activity in three species of fish. *Ecotoxicol Environ Saf* 2008; **69**(1): 74–79.

153 Lennquist A, Hilvarsson A, Forlin L. Responses in fish exposed to medetomidine, a new antifouling agent. *Mar Environ Res* 2010; **69**(Suppl): S43–S45.

154 Kharasch ED, Hill HF, Eddy AC. Influence of dexmedetomidine and clonidine on human liver microsomal alfentanil metabolism. *Anesthesiology* 1991; **75**(3): 520–524.

155 Kharasch ED, Herrmann S, Labroo R. Ketamine as a probe for medetomidine stereoisomer inhibition of human liver microsomal drug metabolism. *Anesthesiology* 1992; **77**(6): 1208–1214.

156 Rodrigues AD, Roberts EM. The in vitro interaction of dexmedetomidine with human liver microsomal cytochrome P4502D6 (CYP2D6). *Drug Metab Dispos* 1997; **25**(5): 651–655.

157 Pelkonen O, Puurunen J, Arvela P, *et al.* Comparative effects of medetomidine enantiomers on in vitro and in vivo microsomal drug metabolism. *Pharmacol Toxicol* 1991; **69**(3): 189–194.

158 Coleman MD. Drug biotransformational systems – origins and aims. In: Coleman MD, ed. *Human Drug Metabolism*, 2nd edn. Chichester, UK: Wiley-Blackwell, 2010: 13–22.

159 Gibson GG, Skett P. Factors affecting drug metabolism: internal factors. In: Gibson GG, Skett P, eds. *Introduction to Drug Metabolism*, 3rd edn. Cheltenham, UK: Nelson Thornes, 2001: 119–45.

160 Gibson GG, Skett P. Factors affecting drug metabolism: external factors. In: Gibson GG, Skett P, eds. *Introduction to Drug Metabolism*, 3rd edn. Cheltenham, UK: Nelson Thornes, 2001: 146–170.

161 Xu C, Li CY, Kong AN. Induction of phase I, II and III drug metabolism/transport by xenobiotics. *Arch Pharm Res* 2005; **28**(3): 249–268.

162 Chang GW, Kam PC. The physiological and pharmacological roles of cytochrome P450 isoenzymes. *Anaesthesia* 1999; **54**(1): 42–50.

163 Trepanier LA. Cytochrome P450 and its role in veterinary drug interactions. *Vet Clin North Am Small Anim Pract* 2006; **36**(5): 975–985.

164 Martignoni M, Groothuis GM, de Kanter R. Species differences between mouse, rat, dog, monkey and human CYP-mediated drug metabolism, inhibition and induction. *Expert Opin Drug Metab Toxicol* 2006; **2**(6): 875–894.

165 Court MH, Hay-Kraus BL, Hill DW, *et al.* Propofol hydroxylation by dog liver microsomes: assay development and dog breed differences. *Drug Metab Dispos* 1999; **27**(11): 1293–1299.

166 Hay Kraus BL, Greenblatt DJ, Venkatakrishnan K, *et al.* Evidence for propofol hydroxylation by cytochrome P4502B11 in canine liver microsomes: breed and gender differences. *Xenobiotica* 2000; **30**(6): 575–588.

167 Chan WH, Chen TL, Chen RM, *et al.* Propofol metabolism is enhanced after repetitive ketamine administration in rats: the role of cytochrome P-450 2B induction. *Br J Anaesth* 2006; **97**(3): 351–358.

168 Coleman MD. Induction of cytochrome P450 systems. In: Coleman MD, ed. *Human Drug Metabolism*, 2nd edn. Chichester, UK: Wiley-Blackwell, 2010: 65–92.

169 Coleman MD. Cytochrome P450 inhibition. In: Coleman MD, ed. *Human Drug Metabolism*, 2nd edn. Chichester, UK: Wiley-Blackwell, 2010: 93–124.

170 Gibson GG, Skett P. Pathways of drug metabolism. In: Gibson GG, Skett P, eds. *Introduction to Drug Metabolism*, 3rd edn. Cheltenham, UK: Nelson Thornes, 2001: 1–36.

171 Mizuno N, Niwa T, Yotsumoto Y, *et al.* Impact of drug transporter studies on drug discovery and development. *Pharmacol Rev* 2003; **55**(3): 425–461.

172 Hedman A, Angelin B, Arvidsson A, *et al.* Interactions in the renal and biliary elimination of digoxin: stereoselective difference between quinine and quinidine. *Clin Pharmacol Ther* 1990; **47**(1): 20–26.

173 Hedman A, Angelin B, Arvidsson A, *et al.* Digoxin-verapamil interaction: reduction of biliary but not renal digoxin clearance in humans. *Clin Pharmacol Ther* 1991; **49**(3): 256–262.

174 Mather LE, Duke CC, Ladd LA, *et al.* Direct cardiac effects of coronary site-directed thiopental and its enantiomers: a comparison to propofol in conscious sheep. *Anesthesiology* 2004; **101**(2): 354–364.

175 Larenza MP, Knobloch M, Landoni MF, *et al.* Stereoselective pharmacokinetics of ketamine and norketamine after racemic ketamine or S-ketamine administration in Shetland ponies sedated with xylazine. *Vet J* 2008; **177**(3): 432–435.

176 Larenza MP, Ringer SK, Kutter AP, *et al.* Evaluation of anesthesia recovery quality after low-dose racemic or S-ketamine infusions during anesthesia with isoflurane in horses. *Am J Vet Res* 2009; **70**(6): 710–718.

177 Lipscomb VJ, AliAbadi FS, Lees P, *et al.* Clinical efficacy and pharmacokinetics of carprofen in the treatment of dogs with osteoarthritis. *Vet Rec.* 2002; **150**(22): 684–689.

178 Arifah AK, Landoni MF, Frean SP, *et al.* Pharmacodynamics and pharmacokinetics of ketoprofen enantiomers in sheep. *Am J Vet Res* 2001; **62**(1): 77–86.

179 Lapicque F, Muller N, Payan E, *et al.* Protein binding and stereoselectivity of nonsteroidal anti-inflammatory drugs. *Clin Pharmacokinet* 1993; **25**(2): 115–123.

180 Rahman MH, Maruyama T, Okada T, *et al.* Study of interaction of carprofen and its enantiomers with human serum albumin-II. Stereoselective site-to-site displacement of carprofen by ibuprofen. *Biochem Pharmacol* 1993; **46**(10): 1733–1740.

181 Jamali F, Lovlin R, Aberg G. Bi-directional chiral inversion of ketoprofen in CD-1 mice. *Chirality* 1997; **9**(1): 29–31.
182 McIntosh MP, Rajewski RA. Comparative canine pharmacokinetics-pharmacodynamics of fospropofol disodium injection, propofol emulsion, and cyclodextrin-enabled propofol solution following bolus parenteral administration. *J Pharm Sci* 2012; **101**(9): 3547–3552.
183 Trapani G, Latrofa A, Franco M, *et al.* Inclusion complexation of propofol with 2-hydroxypropyl-beta-cyclodextrin. Physicochemical, nuclear magnetic resonance spectroscopic studies, and anesthetic properties in rat. *J Pharm Sci* 1998; **87**(4): 514–518.
184 Lee SJ, Kim SI, Jung BI, *et al.* Suspected anaphylactic reaction associated with microemulsion propofol during anesthesia induction. *J Korean Med Sci* 2012; **27**(7): 827–829.
185 Jung JA, Choi BM, Cho SH, *et al.* Effectiveness, safety, and pharmacokinetic and pharmacodynamic characteristics of microemulsion propofol in patients undergoing elective surgery under total intravenous anaesthesia. *Br J Anaesth* 2010; **104**(5): 563–576.
186 Desta B, Maldonado G, Reid H, *et al.* Acute selenium toxicosis in polo ponies. *J Vet Diagn Invest* 2011; **23**(3): 623–628.
187 Kairuz TE, Gargiulo D, Bunt C, *et al.* Quality, safety and efficacy in the 'off-label' use of medicines. *Curr Drug Saf* 2007; **2**: 89–95.
188 Gershman MD, Kennedy DJ, Noble-Wang J, *et al.* Multistate outbreak of Pseudomonas fluorescens bloodstream infection after exposure to contaminated heparinized saline flush prepared by a compounding pharmacy. *Clin Infect Dis* 2008; **47**(11): 1372–1379.

20 Anticholinergics

Phillip Lerche
Department of Veterinary Clinical Sciences, College of Veterinary Medicine, The Ohio State University, Columbus, Ohio, USA

Chapter contents

Introduction, 314
History, 314
General pharmacology, 314
Specific anticholinergic drugs, 316
B Atropine, 316
Glycopyrrolate, 317
Drug combinations, 317
References, 317

Introduction

Anticholinergic drugs are commonly used in veterinary anesthesia to treat and/or prevent anesthetic and preanesthetic bradycardia, decrease airway and salivary secretions, dilate the pupil, block vagally mediated reflexes (viscerovagal, oculocardiac, and Branham), and block the effects of parasympathomimetic drugs. Historically, inhalant anesthetics such as diethyl ether produced profound parasympathetic effects that resulted in hypersalivation and bradycardia. As such, anticholinergics were consistently used preoperatively to counteract these unwanted adverse effects. Modern inhalant anesthetics have lesser effects on the autonomic nervous system, making the indiscriminate use of anticholinergic drugs less popular. The administration of an anticholinergic drug as part of a patient's premedication should be based on a thorough knowledge of the drug's benefits and risks, taking into account the drugs to be co-administered, the patient's species, age, and disease status, and the procedure being performed.

History

Plants such as deadly nightshade (*Atropa belladonna*) (Fig. 20.1), henbane (*Hyoscyamus niger*), mandrake (*Mandragora officinalis*), and *Datura* species contain naturally occurring tropane alkaloids (atropine, hyoscyamine, and scopolamine) in concentrations that are potentially toxic to most species. For example, ingesting 3–5 nightshade berries may prove lethal to a person. Despite this risk, extracts from these plants have been used since ancient times for their anesthetic, mydriatic, antidiarrheal, and analgesic properties. In the 1830s, atropine was isolated from deadly nightshade, and in the 1880s hyoscine was isolated from henbane. These breakthroughs paved the way for a clearer understanding of how the autonomic nervous system functions and the eventual discovery of the neurotransmitter acetylcholine [1,2]. The anticholinergic preparations used in modern veterinary anesthesia have a relatively high margin of safety by comparison.

General pharmacology

Modern anticholinergics exert their effects by competitively antagonizing acetylcholine at postganglionic muscarinic cholinergic receptors in the parasympathetic nervous system. This has led some to prefer the use of the term *antimuscarinics* to differentiate the drugs that only act as antagonists at muscarinic receptors from some naturally occurring compounds that can non-specifically antagonize both muscarinic and nicotinic acetylcholine receptors. Muscarinic receptors have five subtypes, classified as M_1–M_5, based on the order in which they were cloned [3]. Intracellular signaling by activation of the different subtypes occurs via coupling to multiple G-proteins, with single receptor subtypes being capable of activating more than one G-protein in the same cell [4]. The muscarinic receptors can be placed into two groups based on the primary G-protein to which they couple: M_1, M_3, and M_5 couple with $G_{q/11}$-type proteins and have an excitatory action. M_2 and M_4 couple with $G_{i/o}$-type proteins which are inhibitory. There is also evidence that M_1, M_2, and M_3 receptors can cause actions via non-G-protein mechanisms, such as protein kinase [5]. In addition to being able to activate different G-proteins, the muscarinic receptor subtypes show a tissue-specific anatomic distribution, and physiologic response (Table 20.1) [6–10].

Atropine and glycopyrrolate, the anticholinergics most commonly used in veterinary anesthesia, are relatively unselective in their binding to muscarinic receptor subtypes. Different tissue types, however, appear to have different responses to clinically administered doses of these drugs (Table 20.2) [11]. Receptors in

Veterinary Anesthesia and Analgesia: The Sixth Edition of Lumb and Jones. Edited by Leigh Lamont, Kurt Grimm, Sheilah Robertson, Lydia Love and Carrie Schroeder.
© 2024 John Wiley & Sons, Inc. Published 2024 by John Wiley & Sons, Inc.
Companion website: www.wiley.com/go/lamont/anesthesia

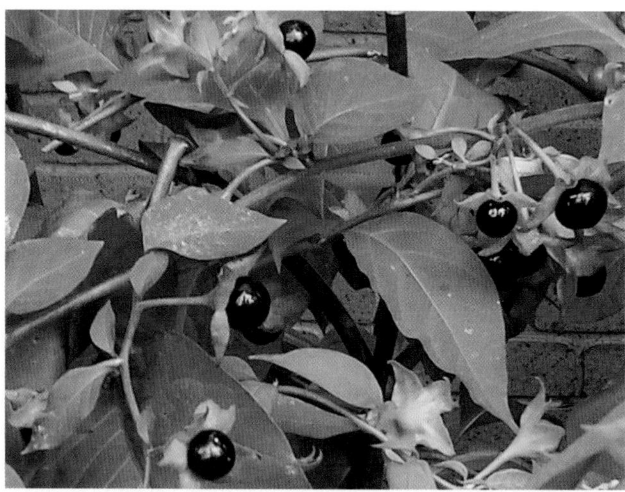

Figure 20.1 Deadly nightshade (*Atropa belladonna*) plant with berries.

Table 20.1 Muscarinic receptor subtypes, cellular response, tissue location, and physiologic responses in mammals.

Receptor	Cellular response	Tissue location	Physiologic response
M_1	Stimulation	CNS	Modulation of memory and learning Analgesia
		Cardiovascular	↑ Heart rate ↑ Inotropy Modulates vascular tone
		Gastrointestinal	↑ H^+ secretion in stomach ↑ Salivation
M_2	Inhibition	Lungs	Bronchoconstriction
		Cardiovascular	Bradycardia, atrioventricular block ↓ Inotropy Vasodilation
M_3	Stimulation	CNS	Insulin homeostasis Emesis
		Ocular	Mydriasis
		Airway smooth muscle	Bronchoconstriction ↑ Secretions
		Gastrointestinal	↑ H^+ secretion in stomach ↑ Salivation ↑ Peristalsis
M_4	Inhibition	CNS	Dopamine regulation Locomotion modulation
		Heart	Modulates high-voltage-activated Ca^{2+} channels Modulates K^+ channels
M_5	Stimulation	CNS	Specific action not fully elucidated

CNS, central nervous system; H^+, hydrogen ions.

Table 20.2 Comparison of clinical effects of systemically administered atropine and glycopyrrolate.

Drug	Antisialagogue effects	Heart rate increase	Smooth muscle relaxation	Ocular effects
Atropine	+	+ + +	+ +	++
Glycopyrrolate	+ +	+	+ +	0

salivary, cardiac, and bronchial tissues are more sensitive than those in the urinary and gastrointestinal tracts.

Anticholinergic effects in the heart are mediated by pre- and postsynaptic M_2 receptors located in the sinoatrial and atrioventricular nodes and also in the atrial myocardium. Systemic anticholinergic drug administration typically leads to an increase in sinus rate, acceleration of atrioventricular nodal conduction, and increased atrial contractility. The increase in heart rate may result in tachycardia and tachydysrhythmias, which may be unwanted, particularly if these changes result in decreased cardiac output (CO) or significantly increased myocardial oxygen consumption. Routine use of anticholinergics should be avoided in patients with hypertrophic or restrictive forms of cardiomyopathy.

Sometimes, worsening of bradycardia may occur immediately following anticholinergic administration. This paradoxical effect has been postulated to be due to more rapid blockade of presynaptic M_1 receptors that inhibit the negative feedback mechanism, resulting in a transient increase in acetylcholine release and further slowing of the heart rate [12]. When this occurs in the clinical setting, waiting a few minutes or repeating the dose of anticholinergic administered will typically induce blockade of postsynaptic M_2 receptors, resulting in the desired increase in heart rate.

Bronchodilation and reduced airway secretions via M_2 and M_3 receptor antagonism can decrease airway resistance and the likelihood of airway obstruction, but can contribute to hypoventilation and, theoretically, decreased arterial oxygen tension as a result of increased anatomic deadspace. This is unlikely to be clinically relevant when a patient is breathing 100% oxygen. Additionally, in many species, the viscosity of the airway secretions increases as the volume is decreased following anticholinergic administration, potentially offsetting any benefit with respect to reducing airway secretions.

In the eye, cholinergic fibers originating from cranial nerve III innervate the circular muscles (sphincter pupillae) of the iris that control pupil diameter, and also the ciliary muscle that controls the shape of the lens, facilitating accommodation. Topical application of anticholinergic drugs to the cornea blocks the action of acetylcholine at both of these sites and results in mydriasis and cycloplegia. This has been well documented for atropine in numerous species, including sheep, goats, cats, and horses [13–17], and for glycopyrrolate in rabbits [18]. Topical application of anticholinergic drugs has also been shown to acutely increase intraocular pressure (IOP) caused by drainage angle closure in cats [15], but not in sheep and horses [13,17]. These mixed findings have led some to suggest that this route of administration should be avoided in patients with pre-existing elevations of IOP or those predisposed to developing angle-closure glaucoma.

The potential to induce mydriatic and cycloplegic effects with systemic (i.e., either intravenous [IV] or intramuscular [IM]) administration of anticholinergics is lower than with topical administration and is probably drug and dose-dependent. Scopolamine, a drug rarely used in veterinary medicine, appears to have the most potent ocular effects when administered systemically, followed by atropine and finally glycopyrrolate. There are few data for any species to suggest that systemic administration of atropine or glycopyrrolate at clinically relevant doses for the treatment of reflex or drug-induced bradycardia would cause adverse effects in patients with glaucoma. Both drugs can, however, decrease tear production, resulting in corneal drying [19,20].

Anticholinergics that cross the blood–brain barrier, such as scopolamine and atropine, also have the potential to induce sedation and prolong anesthetic recovery when administered systemically via M_1 receptor antagonism. In the case of atropine, however, its sedative potential is negligible when clinically relevant doses are administered.

Anticholinergics (M_3) are effective antisialogogues in monogastrics. In ruminants, however, salivation is not inhibited completely; rather, the saliva becomes more viscous to the point where the thickened, ropy saliva may pose a risk of causing airway obstruction. Routine anticholinergic use is therefore not recommended in ruminants, with the exception of treating intraoperative bradycardia.

Although the dose of an anticholinergic required to decrease gastrointestinal motility via blockade of M_3 receptors is higher than that required to treat bradycardia, there is some risk of gastrointestinal ileus following administration. This may lead to symptoms of colic in horses, hence the routine use of anticholinergics is generally avoided in this species [21]. As with ruminants, anticholinergic use in horses should be reserved for treating intraoperative bradycardia. In monogastrics, anticholinergics have been shown to decrease lower esophageal sphincter function, which may lead to an increased risk of gastroesophageal reflux and associated complications such as aspiration pneumonia, esophagitis, and esophageal stricture [22].

Specific anticholinergic drugs

Atropine

Pharmacology

Atropine is a racemic mixture of *S*(−)-hyoscyamine and *R*(+)-hyoscyamine, with the *S*(−) isomer (previously designated as *levo* or *l*-) being responsible for the majority of the drug's activity. The atropine molecule has a lipid-soluble tertiary amine structure consisting of a tropic acid ester linked to an organic base (see Fig. 20.2), and it easily crosses the blood–brain and blood–placenta barriers [23].

Onset of action after IV and IM atropine administration is approximately 1 and 5 min, respectively, in dogs, with an increase in heart rate lasting for about 30 min [24]. Other body systems are generally affected for one to several hours, although mydriasis after topical administration can persist for up to 3 days.

The metabolism of atropine varies between species. Atropine is rapidly cleared by atropine esterase, which is present in the plasma, and hydrolyzes the parent compound to inactive tropic acid. Atropinase levels are not the same across animal species [25]. Rabbits can eat the leaves of the usually toxic deadly nightshade with impunity because they have the ability to metabolize atropine-like compounds rapidly via a plasma esterase, atropinase, which may render typical clinical doses ineffective. Not all rabbits possess large amounts of this enzyme, hence the full picture of how this species metabolizes atropine is yet to be elucidated [25]. In cats and rats, hepatic and renal esterases contribute to atropine's clearance from the plasma, while in dogs up to 90% may be excreted unchanged by the kidneys [26,27].

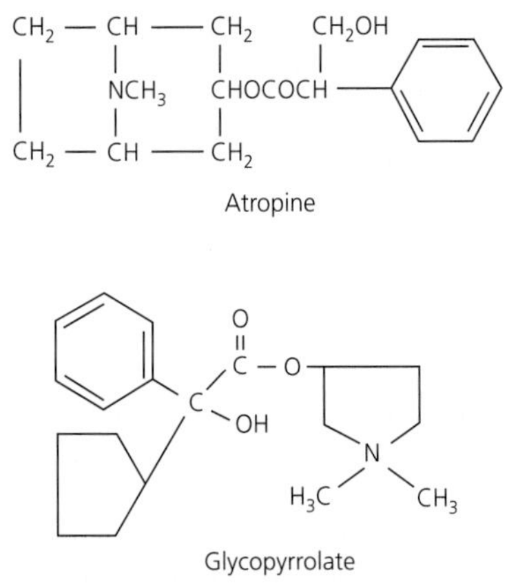

Figure 20.2 Chemical structures of muscarinic antagonists. Source: Adapted from Stoelting and Hillier [11], with permission.

Clinical use

Atropine is mostly used to prevent or treat bradycardia associated with anesthesia. IM and IV dosing are preferred over the subcutaneous route by most anesthesiologists in order to maximize absorption and minimize onset time.

Cardiac rhythm disturbances associated with atropine administration can be pronounced [28]. Transient bradycardia and second-degree atrioventricular block are common parasympathomimetic effects that tend to occur more frequently with administration of lower doses [29]. Evidence suggests that these paradoxical effects result from the initial blockade of presynaptic peripheral M_1 receptors that normally inhibit acetylcholine release. This causes a transient increase in acetylcholine prior to the onset of atropine-induced postsynaptic M_2 receptor blockade [12]. The resulting bradycardia (with or without atrioventricular block) typically resolves spontaneously with establishment of postsynaptic blockade, or upon administration of a supplemental dose of drug. In sheep, unexpected bradycardia has been reported after administration of a higher dose (0.08 mg/kg IV) of atropine [30]. It surprisingly resolved after administration of edrophonium, the reasons for which are not clear (see Table 20.3 for dose ranges).

Dose-dependent tachycardia is frequently observed following atropine administration [24]. The mean dose required to increase heart rate by 50% in conscious dogs was reported to be approximately 0.04 mg/kg IV [24]. Greater increases in heart rate may be observed in patients with high pre-existing vagal tone, a phenomenon called "excess tachycardia." In addition, occasional premature ventricular contractions have also been reported in dogs but are not necessarily proportional to the magnitude of tachycardia [29]. Although transient tachycardia is generally well tolerated in normal healthy veterinary patients, atropine should be used with caution in those who may be adversely impacted by tachycardia, such as patients with hypertrophic or restrictive forms of cardiomyopathy.

Atropine is commonly used prior to administration of cholinergic drugs such as neostigmine and edrophonium when reversing neuromuscular blockade (see Chapter 26). Additionally, atropine has historically been recommended during cardiopulmonary-cerebral resuscitation (CPCR). The role and effectiveness of atropine use in CPCR have been reviewed as part of the RECOVER initiative [31] (see Chapter 5). After a review of the literature, the authors found that atropine had neither a positive nor negative effect on whether patients had return of spontaneous circulation during CPCR. Atropine is, however, still considered useful in cases where cardiac arrest may be due to high vagal tone, and the RECOVER guidelines state that it can be administered after

Table 20.3 Dose ranges for atropine and glycopyrrolate IV or IM (mg/kg).

Animal	Atropine	Glycopyrrolate
Cats and dogs	0.02–0.04	0.005–0.01
Horses	0.02–0.04	0.0025–0.005
Ruminants	0.04–0.08	0.0025–0.005
Pigs	0.04–0.08	0.0025–0.005
Rabbits	—	0.01 IV, 0.1 IM

initiating basic life support when the underlying electrocardiogram shows asystole or pulseless electrical activity. Atropine can be delivered via the endotracheal tube at two to three times the usual IV dose if venous access has not been established prior to cardiopulmonary collapse.

Glycopyrrolate

Pharmacology

Glycopyrrolate is a synthetic quaternary ammonium compound that is poorly lipid soluble, making it difficult for the molecule to cross the blood–brain or blood–placenta barriers [23]. The molecule consists of a mandelic acid ester linked to an organic base (see Fig. 20.2). Glycopyrrolate has four times the potency of atropine.

The onset of action of glycopyrrolate is slightly slower than that of atropine, usually occurring within a few minutes. In people, the duration of action is similar to that of atropine but in conscious dogs, the cardiovascular effects lasted for approximately 1 h, which was longer than those associated with atropine [32]. Hepatic metabolism of glycopyrrolate has been demonstrated in mice and rats, as has limited biotransformation via the liver in dogs, with the main metabolite, M9, being inactive [33]. Glycopyrrolate is otherwise cleared from the plasma relatively rapidly, with most of it being excreted unchanged in the urine.

Whereas topical glycopyrrolate has been shown to readily induce persistent mydriasis and cycloplegia in rabbits [18], systemic administration of clinically relevant doses is reported to have minimal effects on ocular parameters in dogs [34,35].

In people, the purported benefit of glycopyrrolate over atropine is its improved cardiovascular parameters with less risk of tachycardia. This is not the case in dogs, where drug effects on the cardiovascular system are similar between the two anticholinergics [29].

The effect of glycopyrrolate on gastrointestinal motility has been evaluated in anesthetized dogs and horses. Motility was decreased for up to 30 min in dogs and the duration of decreased motility in horses was dose-dependent, lasting for over 6 h after a 0.005 mg/kg IV dose [36,37]. Development of colic postoperatively in horses is multifactorial and antimuscarinic drug administration may be a contributing factor. Of 17 horses that received glycopyrrolate intraoperatively, one subsequently showed signs of colic [38,39].

Clinical use

Glycopyrrolate is mostly used to treat or prevent bradycardia in the perioperative period. It can also be used to counteract the cholinergic effects when reversing neuromuscular blockade with a cholinergic drug such as neostigmine, and in some countries, the two drugs are combined in a single preparation for this purpose. It is not used as an emergency drug in CPCR when atropine is available owing to its longer onset time. See Table 20.3 for dose ranges.

Drug combinations

Anticholinergics are water soluble and have historically been used in premixed combinations of preanesthetic medications in small animal anesthesia such as "BAG" (butorphanol, acepromazine, and glycopyrrolate) and "superBAG" (buprenorphine, acepromazine, and glycopyrrolate). Anticholinergics are often selected to counteract the bradycardia associated with the use of α_2-adrenergic receptor agonists. Clinically, it is important to determine whether the bradycardia is a baroreceptor response to an increase in arterial blood pressure secondary to peripheral vasoconstriction, or is due to centrally mediated suppression of sympathetic output with accompanying low blood pressure. Increasing the heart rate in the face of arterial vasoconstriction has the potential to decrease CO further while significantly increasing myocardial oxygen consumption [40]. CO is usually not significantly improved when dogs are sedated with dexmedetomidine compared with dexmedetomidine and atropine. The routine use of atropine was not recommended by the authors owing to the detection of cardiac arrhythmias when atropine was co-administered and lack of any clear benefit [41]. Similarly, Monteiro *et al.* found no benefit in sedating cats with dexmedetomidine and atropine versus dexmedetomidine alone, although CO was not measured [42]. The rationale for use of an anticholinergic with an α_2-adrenergic receptor agonist when preceding general anesthesia (versus sedation) has yet to be critically evaluated.

Following the use of α_2-adrenergic receptor agonists, if the arterial blood pressure is low, administration of an anticholinergic may be considered to counter bradycardia and improve blood pressure. However, if bradycardia is secondary to decreased sympathetic nervous system activity, antagonism of parasympathetic influence on the sinus node may not cause improvement in heart rate. In those cases, administration of a sympathomimetic agent (e.g., ephedrine), or reversal of the α_2-adrenergic receptor agonist, may be beneficial.

It is important to consider that adverse effects of combinations of drugs may be additive. For example, anticholinergics, opioids, and α_2-adrenergic agonists can all decrease gastrointestinal activity. Although this does not preclude the use of anticholinergics as part of a preanesthetic medication, their use should not be indiscriminate and instead should be based on a risk-benefit analysis for the individual patient.

References

1 Lee MR. Solanaceae III: henbane, hags and Hawley Harvey Crippen. *J R Coll Physicians Edinb* 2006; **36**: 366–373.

2 Lee MR. Solanaceae IV: Atropa belladonna, deadly nightshade. *J R Coll Physicians Edinb* 2007; **37**: 77–84.

3 Caulfield MP, Birdsall NJM. International Union of Pharmacology. XVII. Classification of muscarinic acetylcholine receptors. *Pharmacol Rev* 1998; **50**: 279–290.

4 Karakiulakis G, Roth M. Muscarinic receptors and their antagonists in COPD: anti-inflammatory and antiremodeling effects. *Mediators Inflamm* 2012; **2012**: 409580.

5 Rosenblum K, Futter M, Jones M, *et al.* ERKI/II regulation by the muscarinic acetylcholine receptors in neurons. *J Neurosci* 2000; **20**: 977–985.

6 Eglen, RM. Overview of muscarinic receptor subtypes. In: Fryer AD, Christopoulos A, Nathanson NM, eds. *Muscarinic Receptors, Handbook of Experimental Pharmacology*. Berlin, Heidelberg: Springer, 2012; **208**: 3–28.

7 Saternos HC, Almarghalani DA, Gibson HM, *et al.* Distribution and function of the muscarinic receptor subtypes in the cardiovascular system. *Physiol Genom* 2018; **50**: 1–9.

8 Cuevas J, Adams DJ. M4 muscarinic receptor activation modulates calcium channel currents in rat intracardiac neurons. *J Neurophysiol* 1997; **78**: 1903–1912.

9 Croy CH, Chan WY, Castetter AM, *et al.* Characterization of PCS1055, a novel muscarinic M4 receptor antagonist. *Eur J Pharmacol* 2016; **782**: 70–76.

10 Raffa RB. The M5 muscarinic receptor as possible target for treatment of drug abuse. *J Clin Pharm Ther* 2009; **34**: 623–629.

11 Stoelting RK, Hillier SC. *Anticholinergic drugs. Pharmacology and Physiology in Anesthetic Practice*, 4th edn. Philadelphia, PA: Lippincott Williams & Wilkins, 2006: 266–275.

12 Wellstein A, Pitschner HF. Complex dose-response curves of atropine in man explained by different functions of M1- and M2-cholinoceptors. *Naunyn Schmiedebergs Arch Pharmacol* 1988; **338**: 19–27.

13 Ribeiro AP, Crivelaro RM, Teixeira PP, *et al.* Effects of different mydriatics on intraocular pressure, pupil diameter, and ruminal and intestinal motility in healthy sheep. *Vet Ophthalmol* 2014; **17**: 397–402.

14 Whelan NC, Castillo-Alcala FC, Lizarraga I. Efficacy of tropicamide, homatropine, cyclopentolate, atropine and hyoscine as mydriatics in Angora goats. *N Z Vet J* 2011; **59**: 328–331.

15 Stadtbäumer K, Frommlet F, Nell B. Effects of mydriatics on intraocular pressure and pupil size in the normal feline eye. *Vet Ophthalmol* 2006; **9**: 233–237.

16 Davis JL, Stewart T, Brazik E, *et al.* The effect of topical administration of atropine sulfate on the normal equine pupil: influence of age, breed and gender. *Vet Ophthalmol* 2003; **6**: 329–332.

17 Mughannam AJ, Buyukmihci NC, Kass PH. Effect of topical atropine on intraocular pressure and pupil diameter in the normal horse eye. *Vet Ophthalmol* 1999; **2**: 213–215.

18 Varsanno D, Rothamn S, Haas K, *et al.* The mydriatic effect of topical glycopyrrolate. *Graefes Arch Clin Exp Ophthalmol* 1996; **234**: 205–207.

19 Ludders JW, Heavner JE. Effect of atropine on tear formation in anesthetized dogs. *J Am Vet Med Assoc* 1979; **175**: 585–586.

20 Arnett BD, Brightman AH, Mussleman EE. Effect of atropine sulfate on tear production in the cat when used with ketamine hydrochloride and acetylpromazine maleate. *J Am Vet Med Assoc* 1984; **185**: 214–215.

21 Ducharme NG, Fubini SL. Gastrointestinal complications associated with the use of atropine in horses. *J Am Vet Med Assoc* 1983; **167**: 200–202.

22 Roush JK, Keene BW, Eicker SW, *et al.* Effects of atropine and glycopyrrolate on esophageal, gastric and tracheal pH in anesthetized dogs. *Vet Surg* 1990; **19**: 88–92.

23 Proakis AG, Harris GB. Comparative penetration of glycopyrrolate and atropine across the blood–brain and placental barriers in anesthetized dogs. *Anesthesiology* 1978; **48**: 339–344.

24 Hendrix PK, Robinson EP. Effects of a selective and a nonselective muscarinic cholinergic antagonist on heart rate and intestinal motility in dogs. *J Vet Pharmacol Ther* 1997; **20**: 387–395.

25 Harrison PK, Tattersall JE, Gosden E. The presence of atropinesterase activity in animal plasma. *Naunyn Schmiedebergs Arch Pharmacol* 2000; **373**: 230–236.

26 Godeaux J, Tønnsen M. Investigations into atropine metabolism in the animal organism. *Acta Pharm* 1949; **5**: 95–109.

27 Albanus L, Sundwall A, Vangbo B, *et al.* The fate of atropine in the dog. *Acta Pharmacol Toxicol* 1968; **26**: 571–582.

28 Muir WW. Effects of atropine on cardiac rate and rhythm in dogs. *J Am Vet Med Assoc* 1978; **172**: 917–921.

29 Richards DL, Clutton RE, Boyd C. Electrocardiographic findings following intravenous glycopyrrolate to sedated dogs: a comparison with atropine. *J Assoc Vet Anaesth* 1989; **16**: 46–50.

30 Clutton RE, Glasby MA. Cardiovascular and autonomic nervous effects of edrophonium and atropine combinations during neuromuscular blockade antagonism in sheep. *Vet Anaesth Analg* 2008; **35**: 191–200.

31 Fletcher D, Boller M, Brainard BM, *et al.* RECOVER evidence and knowledge gap analysis on veterinary CPR. Part 7: clinical guidelines. *J Vet Emerg Crit Care (San Antonio)* 2012; **22**(Suppl 1): S102–S131.

32 Lemke KA. Electrocardiographic and cardiopulmonary effects of intramuscular administration of glycopyrrolate and romifidine in conscious Beagle dogs. *Vet Anaesth Analg* 2001; **28**: 75–86.

33 Chabicovsky M, Winkler S, Soeberdt M, *et al.* Pharmacology, toxicology and clinical safety of glycopyrrolate. *Toxicol Appl Pharmacol* 2019; **370**: 154–169.

34 Frischmeyer KJ, Miller PE, Bellay Y, *et al.* Parenteral anticholinergics in dogs with normal and elevated intraocular pressure. *Vet Surg* 1993; **22**: 230–234.

35 Hall LW, Clarke KW, Trim CM. Principles of sedation, analgesia and premedication. In: Hall LW, Clarke KW, Trim CM, eds. *Veterinary Anaesthesia*, 10th edn. Philadelphia, PA: Saunders, 2000: 75–112.

36 Short CE, Paddleford RR, Cloyd GD. Glycopyrrolate for prevention of pulmonary complications during anesthesia. *Mod Vet Pract* 1974; **55**: 194–196.

37 Singh S, McDonell WN, Young SS, *et al.* The effect of glycopyrrolate on heart rate and intestinal motility in conscious horses. *J Vet Anaesth* 1997; **24**: 14–19.

38 Gonçalves S, Julliand V, Leblond A. Risk factors associated with colic in horses. *Vet Res* 2002; **33**: 641–652.

39 Dyson DH, Pascoe PJ, McDonell WN. Effects of intravenously administered glycopyrrolate in anesthetized horses. *Can Vet J* 1999; **40**: 29–32.

40 Lemke KA, Tranquilli WJ, Thurmon JC, *et al.* Hemodynamic effects of atropine and glycopyrrolate in isoflurane–xylazine-anesthetized dogs. *Vet Surg* 1993; **22**: 163–169.

41 Congdon JM, Marquez M, Niyom S, Boscan P. Evaluation of the sedative and cardiovascular effects of intramuscular administration of dexmedetomidine with and without concurrent atropine administration in dogs. *J Am Vet Med Assoc* 2011; **239**: 81–89.

42 Monteiro ER, Campagnol D, Parrilha LR, *et al.* Evaluation of cardiorespiratory effects of combinations of dexmedetomidine and atropine in cats. *J Feline Med Surg* 2009; **11**: 783–792.

21 Adrenergic Agents

Jo C. Murrell
Bristol Veterinary Specialists, Severn Beach, Bristol, UK

Chapter contents

Introduction, 319
Catecholamines and other adrenergic agonists, 319
Naturally occurring catecholamines, 319
Synthetic catecholamines, 322
α_1-Adrenergic receptor agonists, 324
α_2-Adrenergic receptor agonists, 325
β_2-Adrenergic receptor agonists, 325
Mixed α- and β-adrenergic receptor agonists, 326
Adrenergic receptor antagonists, 326
α_1-Adrenergic receptor antagonists, 326
α_2-Adrenergic receptor antagonists, 327
Non-selective α-adrenergic receptor antagonists, 327
β_1-Adrenergic receptor antagonists, 328
Non-selective β-adrenergic receptor antagonists, 329
References, 329

Introduction

Adrenergic agents are drugs that act on the sympathetic nervous system (SNS) and as such are widely used in veterinary anesthesia for the management of cardiorespiratory function. In order to understand the mechanism of action of the different drugs, it is important to have a thorough knowledge of the physiology of adrenergic receptors and the autonomic nervous system (further details are available in the neurologic disease chapter). Table 21.1 provides a brief overview of the distributions, effects, and mechanisms of action of adrenergic and dopaminergic receptors. This is useful to help predict the physiologic effects of the different drugs acting at these receptor types.

There are a number of different systems that can be used to classify adrenergic agents, for example, the receptor at which the drug exerts an effect, whether the drug is an agonist or antagonist at the receptor, or whether the drug is a naturally occurring or synthetic agent.

Classification of adrenergic agents can also be confusing because some agents act at more than one type of receptor (e.g., ephedrine is an agonist at both α- and β-adrenergic receptors), whereas others may act differentially at receptors depending on dose (e.g., dopamine is a β_1-adrenergic receptor agonist when administered at low doses, but at higher doses, α_1-agonist effects tend to predominate).

Adrenergic agents that are agonists at α_1-, β_1-, and β_2-adrenergic receptors are also classified as sympathomimetics because they cause stimulation or activation of the SNS. Drugs acting at dopamine receptors are also sympathomimetics and, therefore, are included in this chapter. Sympathomimetics can also be classified according to whether they have a direct effect at adrenergic receptors or whether they act indirectly by causing the release of norepinephrine. In contrast, antagonists at α- and β-adrenergic receptors are classified as sympatholytics because they reduce the level of activation of the SNS.

Catecholamines and other adrenergic agonists

The structure of sympathomimetics is based on a benzene ring with various amine side-chains attached at the C1 position. Where a hydroxyl group is present at the C3 and C4 positions, the agent is known as a "catecholamine" (because 3,4-dihydroxybenzene is otherwise known as "catechol"). In this chapter, the naturally occurring catecholamines are discussed first, followed by synthetic catecholamines and then other non-catecholamine synthetic adrenergic agents. The synthetic adrenergic agents are classified according to receptor type and whether they act as agonists or antagonists.

Naturally occurring catecholamines

Epinephrine

Epinephrine acts non-selectively and directly as an agonist at all of the adrenergic receptors (i.e., α_1, α_2, β_1, and β_2) (see Table 21.1). In veterinary anesthesia, epinephrine is principally used to support cardiovascular function during cardiopulmonary resuscitation.

Veterinary Anesthesia and Analgesia: The Sixth Edition of Lumb and Jones. Edited by Leigh Lamont, Kurt Grimm, Sheilah Robertson, Lydia Love and Carrie Schroeder.
© 2024 John Wiley & Sons, Inc. Published 2024 by John Wiley & Sons, Inc.
Companion website: www.wiley.com/go/lamont/anesthesia

Table 21.1 Adrenergic and dopaminergic receptor distributions, effects, and mechanisms of action.

Receptor	Subtype	Location	Effects when stimulated	Mechanism of action
Alpha (α)	1	Smooth muscle (blood vessels, bronchi, GI system, uterus, urinary system)	Contraction of smooth muscle, vasoconstriction	Excitatory G-protein-coupled receptor linked to PLC; receptor binding activates PLC, which increases intracellular IP_3 and leads to an increase in intracellular [Ca^{2+}]
	2	Throughout the CNS	Sedation, analgesia, attenuation of sympathetically mediated responses	Inhibitory G-protein-coupled receptor linked to AC; receptor binding reduces AC activity which leads to a decrease in intracellular [cAMP]
		Platelets	Platelet aggregation	
Beta (β)	1	Heart	Positive inotropic and chronotropic effects	Excitatory G-protein-coupled receptor linked to AC; receptor binding activates AC and leads to an increase in intracellular [cAMP]
	2	Smooth muscle (blood vessels, bronchi, GI system, uterus, urinary system)	Relaxation of smooth muscle, vasodilation	Excitatory G-protein-coupled receptor linked to AC; receptor binding activates AC and leads to an increase in intracellular [cAMP]; cAMP activates PKA and also increases Na^+-K^+ ATPase activity, causing hyperpolarization
		Heart	Positive inotropic and chronotropic effects (minor)	
	3	Adipose tissue	Lipolysis	Excitatory G-protein-coupled receptor linked to AC; receptor binding activates AC and leads to an increase in intracellular [cAMP]
Dopamine	1	Throughout the CNS	Modulates extrapyramidal activity	Excitatory G-protein-coupled receptor linked to AC; receptor binding activates AC and leads to an increase in intracellular [cAMP]
		Vascular smooth muscle, kidney, sympathetic ganglia, etc.	Vasodilation of renal and mesenteric vasculature	
	2	Throughout the CNS	Reduced pituitary hormone output	Inhibitory G-protein-coupled receptor linked to AC; receptor binding reduces AC activity, which leads to a decrease in intracellular [cAMP]
		Vascular smooth muscle, kidney, sympathetic ganglia, etc.	Inhibit further norepinephrine release	

GI, gastrointestinal; PLC, phospholipase C; IP_3, inositol triphosphate; AC, adenylate cyclase; cAMP, cyclic adenosine monophosphate; PKA, protein kinase A; CNS, central nervous system.

Epinephrine for systemic administration is available in vials and prefilled syringes at concentrations of 0.1 mg/mL (1:10,000) and 1 mg/mL (1:1000). It must be protected from light and, therefore, is presented in colored glass vials or prefilled syringes stored inside protective packaging. In animals, it is administered systemically by intravenous injection or via the airway during resuscitation (intratracheal administration), although for humans, epinephrine is also available in a metered aerosol preparation to treat swelling associated with upper airway obstruction due to its vasoconstrictive effects. Epinephrine is also formulated with local anesthetic solutions for infiltration at concentrations ranging from 1:200,000 to 1:80,000. Most formulations contain racemic epinephrine, although the *R*(−) isomer (levo-epinephrine) is the active form.

Cardiovascular system effects

The cardiovascular effects of epinephrine are dose dependent. Low doses of epinephrine administered by bolus (0.01 mg/kg IV) cause β_1- and β_2-adrenergic receptor agonist effects to predominate. The cardiac effects of β_1-adrenergic agonism result in increased cardiac output, myocardial oxygen consumption, coronary artery dilation, and a reduced threshold for arrhythmias. In low doses, peripheral β_2-adrenergic receptor agonist effects result in a decrease in diastolic blood pressure and peripheral vascular resistance. At high doses (0.1 mg/kg IV), α_1-adrenergic effects predominate, causing a marked rise in systemic vascular resistance.

Data describing the detailed cardiovascular effects of epinephrine in different species are sparse. However, in cats anesthetized with isoflurane, the cardiovascular effects of epinephrine infusion at dose rates of 0.125–2 μg/kg/min were dose dependent [1]. All infusion rates caused increases in packed cell volume (PCV) due to α_1-adrenergic-induced splenic contraction [2], arterial oxygen content, heart rate, cardiac index, and stroke volume index (SVI) [1]. Increases in SVI were greatest with infusion rates of 1 and 2 μg/kg/min. Mean arterial blood pressure increased at infusion rates of 0.5 μg/kg/min and higher. At the infusion rates tested, epinephrine was not associated with an increase in systemic vascular resistance, reflecting the predominant β-adrenergic effects at these lower dose rates. However, the increases in blood pressure and cardiac index were also associated with increased lactate concentrations and progressive metabolic acidosis. The cardiovascular effects of epinephrine waned after the end of the infusion and the majority of the parameters returned to preinfusion values 30 min later. Extravasation of epinephrine can cause tissue necrosis due to localized vasoconstriction; hence, care must be taken during intravenous administration.

Epinephrine, along with other catecholamines, is recognized to be proarrhythmogenic, causing a decrease in threshold for ventricular fibrillation and increased incidence of premature ventricular contractions and missed beats [3]. The precise mechanisms underlying the proarrhythmogenic effects of epinephrine are complex and are likely multifactorial [4]. Agonist effects at postsynaptic α_1-and β_1-adrenergic receptors on myocardial cells are implicated, in addition to activation of cardiac cholinergic reflexes [3].

Importantly, some anesthetic agents, notably halothane, are recognized to sensitize the myocardium to catecholamine-induced arrhythmias [5]. The proarrhythmogenic effects of epinephrine during halothane anesthesia have been documented in a wide range of species, including dogs [4], cats [6], horses [7], and swine [8]. Similar to the proarrhythmogenic effects of catecholamines in awake animals, the mechanisms are multiple and complex and are considered to involve α_1-adrenergic, β_1-adrenergic, and cholinergic receptors in the heart [3,4]. In comparison with halothane, isoflurane and sevoflurane do not sensitize the myocardium to epinephrine to any great extent [9,10].

The effects of other anesthetic agents, in combination with halothane, on the arrhythmogenic dose of epinephrine have also been investigated in a variety of species. Xylazine does not alter the arrhythmogenic dose of epinephrine in horses induced with thiopental and maintained with halothane [11]. Ketamine decreases the arrhythmogenic dose of epinephrine in halothane-anesthetized cats [12,13] and dogs [14].

Other effects

Epinephrine will produce a small increase in minute volume through its bronchodilator effects, which are β_2-adrenergic receptor mediated. Pulmonary vascular resistance is increased at higher dose rates reflecting agonism at pulmonary vascular α_1-adrenergic receptors [15].

Epinephrine has wide-ranging effects on metabolism that are dose dependent. Basal metabolic rate is increased, resulting in a slight increase in body temperature following administration [1]. Plasma glucose concentration is increased via multiple mechanisms, including inhibition of insulin secretion (an α_2- and β_2-adrenergic effect), glycogenolysis in liver and muscle (an α_1- and β_2-adrenergic effect), lipolysis (a β_2- and β_3-adrenergic effect), and gluconeogenesis (an α_1- and β_2-adrenergic effect). Serum potassium concentration will increase initially following epinephrine administration, followed by hypokalemia caused by increased uptake of potassium into cells (a β_2-effect).

Anesthetic requirement is related to the release of CNS catecholamines [16]; therefore, it would be predicted that epinephrine will increase the minimum alveolar concentration (MAC) of volatile agents. However, no effect of low-dose epinephrine on the MAC of halothane was reported in dogs [17].

Epinephrine causes the release of renin from the kidney through multiple mechanisms, including stimulation of intrarenal β_1- and β_2-adrenergic receptors in addition to extrarenal adrenergic receptors [18,19]. Renal blood flow is moderately decreased due to regional vasoconstriction.

Pharmacokinetics

Epinephrine has a very short half-life due to rapid metabolism, necessitating frequent redosing or administration by infusion for a prolonged effect. Following intravenous administration, epinephrine is rapidly metabolized by mitochondrial monoamine oxidase and catechol-*O*-methyltransferase within the liver, kidney, and circulation to inactive metabolites (3-methoxy-4-hydroxymandelic acid and metanephrine). The metabolites are conjugated with glucuronic acid or sulfates and excreted in the urine.

Norepinephrine

Norepinephrine acts as an agonist at α_1-, α_2-, and β_1-adrenergic receptors, with effects at α-adrenergic receptors predominating at clinically used dose rates (see Table 21.1). Norepinephrine is predominantly used during anesthesia to manage hypotension, particularly when caused by a reduction in systemic vascular resistance (i.e., vasodilation) due to sepsis or administration of volatile anesthetic agents.

Norepinephrine differs from epinephrine in the absence of a methyl group on the nitrogen atom. It is generally supplied as a 1 mg/mL solution in the form of the bitartrate salt with the preservative sodium metabisulfite.

Cardiovascular system effects

At very low dose rates (0.025 µg/kg/min), norepinephrine's β_1-adrenergic receptor-mediated effects predominate and are manifested as increases in heart rate and cardiac output and decreases in systemic vascular resistance [20]. At higher dose rates (greater than 0.5–1.5 µg/kg/min), norepinephrine causes dose-dependent increases in systolic, diastolic, and mean arterial blood pressures, cardiac output, and systemic and pulmonary vascular resistance [21–23]. Norepinephrine will also cause coronary vasodilation to promote increased coronary blood flow. Tachycardia is less likely when compared with administration of epinephrine. A recent study in healthy, isoflurane-anesthetized dogs, administered norepinephrine at doses ranging between 0.05 and 2 µg/kg/min and measured changes in blood pressure, cardiac index, and systemic vascular resistance. This study found that cardiac index and mean arterial blood pressure increased in a dose-dependent manner with infusion of norepinephrine with no significant differences in systemic vascular resistance, thereby concluding that, at the doses studied, norepinephrine does not cause excessive vasoconstriction that interferes with the systemic circulation [24].

Norepinephrine (0.3 and 1.0 µg/kg/min) was effective at improving cardiovascular function and maintaining splanchnic function in foals [22] and alpacas [23] with isoflurane-induced hypotension. At high doses, the increased systemic vascular resistance will ultimately reduce cardiac output and increase myocardial oxygen consumption due to the increase in afterload [25]. Extravasation of norepinephrine can cause tissue necrosis due to localized vasoconstriction; hence, care must be taken during intravenous administration. The arrhythmogenic effects of norepinephrine are similar to those of epinephrine.

Pharmacokinetics

Exogenously administered norepinephrine is metabolized similarly to epinephrine and has a short half-life. Unlike epinephrine, approximately 25% of administered norepinephrine is extracted from the circulation as it passes through the lung, where it is deactivated by monoamine oxidase and catechol-*O*-methyltransferase in the endothelial cells of the pulmonary microvasculature [26].

Dopamine

The receptor effects of dopamine are dose dependent. At low doses (1–2 µg/kg/min), effects on dopamine receptors (D_1 and D_2) predominate. As dose rates increase further, β_1- and β_2-adrenergic receptor effects predominate. Finally, α_1-adrenergic receptor effects are noted at infusion rates greater than 10 µg/kg/min (see Table 21.1). Dopamine will also stimulate the release of endogenous norepinephrine from presynaptic storage sites at adrenergic receptors to cause an endogenous sympathomimetic effect. Dopamine is predominantly used by continuous rate infusion to improve hemodynamic parameters.

Dopamine is available as an injectable preparation, typically as a 40 mg/mL dopamine hydrochloride solution. It contains the preservative sodium metabisulfite. Dopamine hydrochloride in 100 mL dextrose 5% is also commercially available in a range of concentrations from 0.8 to 6.4 mg/mL.

Cardiovascular system effects

At dose rates less than 10 µg/kg/min, the β_1-adrenergic effects of dopamine predominate, leading to increases in myocardial contractility, heart rate, cardiac output, and coronary blood flow. At dose rates greater than 10 µg/kg/min, α_1-adrenergic receptor agonist effects dominate, leading to increased systemic and pulmonary vascular resistance, venous return, and PCV due to splenic contraction. Tachycardia can occur at higher dose rates. A reduction in mean arterial blood pressure and cardiac output generally occurs after cessation of dopamine infusions, with return to preinfusion values within 30 min, leading to the recommendation that administration of dopamine be stopped in a stepwise manner [1].

The cardiovascular effects of dopamine given by continuous rate infusion have been studied in dogs, cats, and horses during volatile agent anesthesia. In dogs anesthetized with isoflurane, increasing infusion rates of dopamine from 3 to 20 μg/kg/min caused a dose-dependent increase in cardiac index and blood pressure, with increases in heart rate and systemic vascular resistance noted at dose rates greater than 7 μg/kg/min [27]. Doses less than 7 μg/kg/min were insufficient to support hemodynamic variables using the defined criteria (e.g., mean arterial blood pressure greater than 70 mmHg). At a dopamine infusion rate of 10 μg/kg/min and greater, there was a marked increase in systemic vascular resistance and a reduction in stroke volume, reflecting increased myocardial work associated with the increased afterload. This dose recommendation is supported by other studies investigating the dose-dependent effects of dopamine in dogs [28–31].

Similar dose-dependent effects have been reported in cats [1], with infusion rates around 10 μg/kg/min necessary to maintain mean arterial blood pressure above 70 mmHg in cats anesthetized with isoflurane. Wiese *et al.* [32] investigated the effects of a dopamine infusion on cardiovascular variables in cats with hypertrophic cardiomyopathy anesthetized with isoflurane. Dopamine infusion rates between 2.5 and 10 μg/kg/min increased heart rate, blood pressure, cardiac output, and oxygen delivery, while global oxygen consumption was reduced. However, all six cats in the study developed premature ventricular complexes, and the authors suggested that dopamine may have negatively impacted myocardial oxygen consumption, which was not measured, despite the observed increase in global oxygen delivery. A recent study investigated the effects of a dopamine continuous rate infusion on systemic vasodilation produced by infusions of vatinoxan and dexmedetomidine in isoflurane-anesthetized cats [33]. Even high doses of dopamine were insufficient to prevent hypotension caused by vatinoxan suggesting that dopamine had limited effects on systemic vascular resistance in this study. Hypotension has been documented in cats following the rapid termination of dopamine infusions, likely attributed to the rapid metabolism of dopamine [1]. It has been suggested that dopamine infusion rates be reduced in a stepwise manner to avoid rebound hypotension on abrupt termination of the infusion.

In horses, the effect of dopamine infusion for management of hypotension during volatile agent anesthesia has been widely investigated. A dopamine infusion rate of 5 μg/kg/min increases myocardial contractility and cardiac output with little effect on blood pressure [34–38]. This is attributed to a reduction in systemic vascular resistance caused by a decrease in smooth muscle vascular tone elicited by stimulation of D_1 and D_2 receptors [39] in the absence of α_1-adrenergic receptor agonist effects, which are only activated at higher doses. Continuous infusion rates of 1, 2, and 5 μg/kg/min dopamine in isoflurane-anesthetized horses were found to increase heart rate, stroke volume, and cardiac output while reducing mean arterial blood pressure and systemic vascular resistance in a dose-dependent manner [40]. Importantly, at these infusion rates, dopamine decreased microperfusion of the gastrointestinal tract.

Extravasation of dopamine can cause tissue necrosis due to localized vasoconstriction; therefore, care must be taken during intravenous administration. Dopamine has the potential to be proarrhythmogenic at higher doses (10 μg/kg/min or greater).

Other effects

Infusions of dopamine attenuate the response of the carotid body to hypoxemia [41]. Early studies suggested that at very low doses (less than 2 μg/kg/min), dopamine infusions had a renal-specific action, preferentially increasing renal blood flow and causing renal artery dilation, leading to a concomitant increase in urine output [42,43]. This was attributed to an effect of dopamine at renal D_1 and D_2 receptors. Consequently, in human patients, there was significant use of low-dose dopamine for the management of acute renal failure in the intensive care unit [44]. However, it is now recognized that increased urine output associated with dopamine administration is caused by improved hemodynamic function [45,46] in combination with inhibition of proximal tubular Na^+ reabsorption [47]. Dopamine will produce vasodilation in mesenteric vascular beds [48] mediated by D_1 receptor activation [49].

Pharmacokinetics

Dopamine has a short half-life of approximately 3 min and, therefore, is given by continuous rate infusion. Onset of action after the start of an infusion can be up to 5 min. Dopamine is metabolized via monoamine oxidase and catechol-*O*-methyltransferase in the liver, kidney, and plasma to inactive compounds that are excreted in the urine as sulfate and glucuronide conjugates. About 25% is converted to norepinephrine in sympathetic nerve terminals.

Synthetic catecholamines

Dobutamine

Dobutamine primarily stimulates β_1-adrenergic receptors but at higher dose rates (5–10 μg/kg/min) will also stimulate β_2- and α_1-adrenergic receptors. It does not exert an effect at α_2-adrenergic receptors. Dobutamine is principally used to augment low cardiac output states associated with reduced myocardial function. It is very commonly used in equine inhalant anesthesia to manage hypotension.

Dobutamine is a direct-acting synthetic catecholamine that is a derivative of isoproterenol. It is available in a range of concentrations from 12.5 to 50 mg/mL; the solution usually contains sodium metabisulfite as a preservative.

Cardiovascular system effects

The effects on the cardiovascular system are dose dependent and have been well described in cats, dogs, and horses. In halothane-anesthetized normotensive horses, very low-dose infusion of dobutamine for 30 min (0.5 μg/kg/min) increased systolic, diastolic, and mean arterial blood pressure but did not increase myocardial contractility or cardiac output; PCV was also increased [50]. Infusion rates of 4–5 μg/kg/min to halothane-anesthetized horses increased arterial blood pressure and cardiac output with minimal effects on heart rate and systemic vascular resistance [34,38,51]. Dancker *et al.* studied the cardiovascular effects of low-dose infusions of dobutamine in isoflurane-anesthetized horses (0.5, 1, and 3 μg/kg/min) and found dose-dependent increases in stroke volume and cardiac output and a reduction in systemic vascular resistance that was associated with increased microperfusion of the gastrointestinal tract [40]. Dobutamine at 10 μg/kg/min tends to increase systemic vascular resistance and heart rate, with increases in cardiac output at high doses attributed to both inotropic and chronotropic effects of the drug [34,38]. In comparison with dopamine, dopexamine, and phenylephrine, dobutamine has been shown to have a more consistent effect in increasing intramuscular blood flow in ponies anesthetized with halothane [38]. In conscious horses, dobutamine 2 μg/kg/min increased blood pressure and decreased heart rate without a concomitant statistically significant increase in cardiac output or systemic vascular resistance [52]. However, the authors proposed that a vasoconstrictive effect occurred, which was not detected in their analysis due to the small sample size.

In isoflurane-anesthetized dogs, dobutamine at doses up to 10 μg/kg/min had more limited effects on blood pressure, but caused increases in cardiac output, heart rate, and systemic vascular resistance [27,30]. The authors noted that owing to the limited effect of dobutamine on blood pressure, assessment of the effectiveness of dobutamine to improve hemodynamic function was challenging in the absence of cardiac output measurements. In a recent study, the effects of dobutamine infusions (2–12 μg/kg/min) on cardiovascular function in dogs anesthetized with different concentrations of isoflurane with experimentally induced mitral valve insufficiency were studied [53]. Dobutamine increased myocardial contractility, which was attenuated by isoflurane suggesting that dobutamine may be useful to manage poor cardiovascular function in dogs with mitral valve disease.

In cats, dobutamine at similar dose rates to those studied in dogs also had limited effects on blood pressure and increased heart rate [1]. Systemic vascular resistance decreased, reflecting the β_2-adrenergic receptor agonist effects of the drug causing peripheral vasodilation in skeletal muscle.

Like other catecholamines, dobutamine has the potential to be proarrhythmogenic at high doses (10 μg/kg/min or greater).

Pharmacokinetics

Dobutamine has a short half-life and is, therefore, administered by continuous rate infusion. It is predominantly metabolized via catechol-*O*-methyltransferase in the liver to inactive metabolites that are conjugated and excreted in the urine.

Dopexamine

Dopexamine is a potent stimulator of β_2-adrenergic receptors with weak agonist effects at β_1, D_1, and D_2 receptors. It has no effect on α_1-adrenergic receptors. Dopexamine inhibits the neuronal uptake of endogenous catecholamines. In human medicine, dopexamine is primarily used to improve cardiac output and mesenteric perfusion. The potential ability of dopexamine to protect hepatosplanchnic and renal blood flow has resulted in the recommendation of dopexamine over other positive inotropes such as dopamine and dobutamine for use in patients particularly at risk of poor splanchnic blood flow, although evidence to support this contention is lacking [54]. Dopexamine is available as a 10 mg/mL solution in 5 mL vials.

Cardiovascular system effects

Dopexamine has a positive inotropic effect via cardiac β_2-adrenergic receptors, although systemic blood pressure may fall due to β_2-receptor-mediated vasodilation of peripheral blood vessels, particularly in skeletal muscle. The reduction in systemic vascular resistance helps to promote an increase in cardiac output. The cardiovascular effects of dopexamine infusion at dose rates varying from 1 to 10 μg/kg/min have been investigated in horses anesthetized with halothane [38,55–57]. Low doses (1–2.5 μg/kg/min) increased blood pressure and cardiac output, but higher dose rates (at or above 5 μg/kg/min) were associated with tachycardia, cardiac arrhythmias, muscle twitching, and poor recoveries from anesthesia. Therefore, despite the positive hemodynamic effects of dopexamine, administration to support hemodynamic function during anesthesia in horses is not recommended.

There are a few reports on the investigation of the effects of dopexamine infusions in dogs; dopexamine increased cardiac output and heart rate in a dose-dependent manner [58,59], with one study indicating that the arrhythmogenic potential of dopexamine is lower than that of dopamine [60]. These studies evaluated infusion rates between 0.25 and 3.5 μg/kg/min. Despite the potential advantages of increased cardiac output with reduced systemic vascular resistance and, therefore, a more limited effect on myocardial oxygen consumption compared with other inotropes, dopexamine is not commonly used clinically in dogs.

Other effects

Dopexamine causes bronchodilation via β_2-adrenergic receptors. Blood flow to the gastrointestinal system and kidneys is increased due to increased cardiac output and reduced regional vascular resistance; there is a concomitant increase in urine output. The clinical benefit of selecting dopexamine over other inotropes in human patients where increased splanchnic perfusion is desirable has been debated [61].

Pharmacokinetics

Dopexamine has a short half-life and is rapidly metabolized by *O*-methylation and sulfation in the liver [62].

Isoproterenol (isoprenaline)

Isoproterenol is a very potent synthetic catecholamine that is an agonist at β_1- and β_2-adrenergic receptors. It has no α-adrenergic receptor effects. Isoproterenol is used to increase heart rate and myocardial contractility during anesthesia. In human medicine, isoproterenol may also be used to promote abnormal electrical activity of the heart during electrophysiological studies. Low doses of isoproterenol are used as a "test dose" to detect intravascular needle placement during epidural anesthesia in children. This is to prevent inadvertent intravascular injection of local anesthetics that may be associated with adverse effects [63]. There are very limited data on the clinical use of isoproterenol in animals.

Isoproterenol is typically available as a 0.2 mg/mL solution that contains sodium metabisulfite as a preservative. It should be protected from light.

Cardiovascular system effects

Stimulation of β_1-adrenergic receptors causes an increase in heart rate, myocardial contractility, and cardiac output [64]. Agonist effects at β_2-adrenergic receptors generally reduce systemic vascular resistance such that the mean arterial blood pressure falls. At higher infusion rates (2.5 μg/kg/min), myocardial oxygen delivery is likely to be compromised owing to the combined effects of increased heart rate reducing coronary filling time, while decreased systemic blood pressure reduces coronary perfusion [65]. However, a very low-dose infusion (0.1 μg/kg/min) of isoproterenol in dogs anesthetized with isoflurane increased cardiac output and heart rate while increasing myocardial blood flow such that adequate myocardial oxygenation was maintained [64]. This was attributed to metabolically driven vasodilation of coronary blood vessels rather than direct stimulation of coronary vasculature β_2-adrenergic receptors. Given these actions, the administration of a potent β_1/β_2-agonist such as isoproterenol to a low blood volume patient (e.g., hemorrhagic shock or severe dehydration) dependent upon intense compensatory vasoconstriction for coronary perfusion pressure is problematic and discouraged, unless and until blood and stroke volume can be restored. Isoproterenol has been used for its chronotropic effects in dogs with third-degree atrioventricular block or sick sinus syndrome.

Isoproterenol has well-characterized proarrhythmogenic effects through its effects on ion channel kinetics and promotion of intracellular calcium accumulation and tachycardia [66].

Other effects

Isoproterenol is a potent bronchodilator, increasing anatomic deadspace and thus ventilation–perfusion mismatching, which has the potential to cause systemic hypoxemia. It causes stimulation of the central nervous system and, therefore, can increase the level of arousal during general anesthesia [67]. Isoproterenol increases splanchnic and renal blood flow via selective vasodilation mediated by stimulation of β-adrenergic receptors [68].

Typical metabolic effects of β-adrenergic receptor stimulation are seen following isoproterenol administration, including increases in blood glucose and free fatty acid concentrations, and a decrease in serum potassium concentration caused by a shift of potassium into cells.

Pharmacokinetics

Isoproterenol has a short half-life. It is rapidly metabolized by catechol-*O*-methyltransferase in the liver, in addition to being excreted in the urine unchanged [69]. In addition, both isoproterenol and its metabolites may be excreted as conjugated sulfates in the urine.

α_1-Adrenergic receptor agonists

Phenylephrine

Phenylephrine is a direct-acting sympathomimetic amine with potent α_1-adrenergic receptor agonist effects, and therefore, it is often referred to as "vasopressor." It has no effect on β-adrenergic receptors. Phenylephrine is used systemically during anesthesia to increase systemic vascular resistance and, therefore, increase blood pressure. Phenylephrine can also be administered topically to mucosal surfaces to produce localized vasoconstriction and reduce edema or hemorrhage. In the horse, phenylephrine may be used in the medical management of nephrosplenic entrapment prior to rolling or laparoscopic surgical correction of the condition. The aim of phenylephrine administration is to reduce splenic size and, therefore, facilitate medical or surgical correction of the entrapment.

Phenylephrine is typically available for injection as a 10 mg/mL solution as the hydrochloride salt. However, phenylephrine is also present in some topical eye preparations and is a common ingredient in decongestants for use in people.

Cardiovascular system effects

Administered systemically, phenylephrine causes a dose-dependent increase in systemic vascular resistance and mean arterial blood pressure and a reflex reduction in heart rate. Cardiac output is usually minimally altered or may fall as a result of increased afterload combined with bradycardia. In horses, phenylephrine is typically infused intravenously at a rate of 1 μg/kg/min preceded by a 2 μg/kg loading dose [50,70] until the blood pressure is increased. The hemodynamic effects wane rapidly once the infusion is terminated. Systemic and pulmonary vascular resistances are increased, and there is a limited effect on cardiac output. Phenylephrine at dose rates between 0.25 and 2 μg/kg/min did not improve skeletal muscle blood flow in horses anesthetized with halothane [38,50]. Frederick *et al.* [71] reported five cases of severe phenylephrine-associated hemorrhage in aged horses. The phenylephrine was administered to facilitate management of nephrosplenic entrapment and the hemorrhage was attributed to secondary hypertension caused by increased systemic vascular resistance. The negative effects of phenylephrine on cardiac output and skeletal muscle blood flow suggest that phenylephrine should not be used to manage hypotension primarily caused by myocardial depression in anesthetized horses. Phenylephrine at 0.5, 1, and 3 μg/kg/min also decreased microvascular blood flow of the gastrointestinal tract in healthy isoflurane-anesthetized horses [40].

There are limited clinical data on the use of phenylephrine in dogs, but a few experimental studies have investigated the cardiovascular effects of infusion. A dose of at least 0.4 μg/kg/min was necessary to increase mean arterial blood pressure significantly in conscious dogs [72], followed by linear increases in blood pressure up to the maximum infusion rate evaluated of 4 μg/kg/min. A reduction in heart rate occurred at the lowest infusion rate tested (0.008 μg/kg/min), which was attributed to a vagally mediated reflex bradycardia [72]. Phenylephrine at 0.14 mg/kg was necessary to manage hypotension caused by acepromazine in halothane-anesthetized dogs [73].

The cardiovascular effects of phenylephrine have been studied in healthy cats anesthetized with isoflurane [1] and in cats with hypertrophic cardiomyopathy [32]. In healthy cats, infusion rates of 0.125–2 μg/kg/min were studied. Mean arterial blood pressure was significantly increased at infusion rates at and above 1 μg/kg/min, which was associated with increased systemic vascular resistance. Heart rate did not change as isoflurane likely obtunded baroreflex-mediated reflex activity. In contrast to horses, these infusion rates were associated with an increase in cardiac output; oxygen delivery was also increased, which was attributed to an increase in PCV and cardiac output. Phenylephrine infusion rates of 0.25–1 μg/kg/min were studied in cats with hypertrophic cardiomyopathy anesthetized with isoflurane [32]. Similar changes in heart rate and blood pressure to those observed in healthy cats were reported; there was no change in cardiac output, but oxygen delivery increased with no change in global oxygen consumption.

There is little evidence to suggest that phenylephrine is proarrhythmogenic when used clinically.

Other effects

Phenylephrine has no stimulatory effects on the central nervous system. Hepatic and renal blood flow are reduced, mediated by α_1-adrenergic receptor-induced vasoconstriction [74,75]. Phenylephrine will reduce uterine blood flow, and it is generally recommended to avoid administration during pregnancy due to potential adverse effects on fetal oxygen delivery [76].

Intranasal administration of phenylephrine to anesthetized horses prior to recovery from anesthesia is used to reduce nasal edema and the potential for upper airway obstruction [77].

Administration of 5 mL of 0.15% phenylephrine solution into each nostril approximately 50 min before extubation was sufficient to reduce nasal edema and significantly reduced the requirement for placement of a nasal tube during recovery in the majority of horses studied (20 horses) compared with a control group (20 horses). No adverse cardiovascular effects following administration were noted.

Topical eye drops containing 10% phenylephrine hydrochloride caused increased blood pressure in both anesthetized and conscious dogs [78,79].

Pharmacokinetics
Phenylephrine has a short half-life when administered intravenously. It is metabolized in the liver by monoamine oxidase.

Methoxamine

Methoxamine is a direct-acting sympathomimetic amine with specific α_1-adrenergic receptor agonist effects and is also classified as a vasopressor. The clinical effects of methoxamine are similar to those of phenylephrine; however, methoxamine is purported to have a longer duration of action, despite limited pharmacological data on systemically administered methoxamine in animals. Methoxamine is reported to predominantly cause vasoconstriction of arterioles, with little effect at capacitance vessels. In horses, a dose of 0.04 mg/kg IV approximately 5–10 min before induction of anesthesia did not modulate halothane-induced hypotension during the maintenance phase of anesthesia, with no effect on mean arterial blood pressure, heart rate, cardiac output, or central venous pressure [80]. However, experimental studies have demonstrated the cardiovascular effects of methoxamine in other species. Doses of methoxamine from 0.4 to 6.0 mg/kg in lambs caused an increase in cardiac output, attributed to stimulation of α_1-adrenergic receptors in the lamb myocardium [81]. In contrast, no positive inotropic action was reported in dogs [82,83], suggesting species-specific effects of methoxamine on the myocardium.

Methoxamine is available as a 20 mg/mL solution as the hydrochloride salt for intravenous injection.

α_2-Adrenergic receptor agonists

Dexmedetomidine, medetomidine, detomidine, xylazine, and romifidine

These agents are not classified as sympathomimetics, but they are used extensively in veterinary medicine for their excellent sedative and analgesic properties. Their other α_2-adrenergic receptor-mediated effects are considered, in most instances, to be adverse side effects. Further information on α_2-adrenergic receptor agonist pharmacology is available in Chapter 22.

β_2-Adrenergic receptor agonists

Clenbuterol, albuterol (salbutamol), and terbutaline

Clenbuterol, albuterol, and terbutaline are predominantly used for the management of bronchospasm in people with asthma. In veterinary medicine, they are used to treat bronchospasm in both awake and anesthetized animals. In addition, clenbuterol has been used illegally to increase the muscle mass and reduce the fat composition of carcasses of food-producing animals.

Clenbuterol has Marketing Authorization for administration to horses for the management of chronic obstructive pulmonary disease and is available as an injectable solution for administration intravenously, and also as syrup and granule preparations for oral administration. An injectable preparation is also licensed for administration to cattle to delay the onset of parturition by causing uterine relaxation. Albuterol and terbutaline are not licensed for administration to animals but are available as aerosol and oral preparations for the management of asthma in people.

Cardiovascular system effects
At high doses, this class of agents can also exert agonist effects at β_1-adrenergic receptors causing tachycardia, whereas at lower doses, decreases in blood pressure are noted due to β_2-adrenergic receptor-mediated vasodilation.

These agents are noted to be proarrhythmogenic as they shorten the refractory period of the atrioventricular node, slow ventricular conduction, and shorten the refractory period of the ventricular myocardium [84]. The arrhythmogenic effects are likely to be more pronounced during concurrent hypoxemia (e.g., caused by an increase in shunt fraction) or during hypokalemia.

Other effects
These agents stimulate Na^+-K^+ ATPase, leading to increased intracellular uptake of K^+ and hypokalemia. The blood glucose concentration typically increases. In the respiratory system, they cause relaxation of bronchial smooth muscle and reversal of hypoxic pulmonary vasoconstriction (see below).

Clenbuterol and albuterol have been evaluated in anesthetized horses for the management of hypoxemia. Data pertaining to the clinical effects of clenbuterol (IV) are conflicting. Early studies investigating clenbuterol at 0.8 and 2.4 mg/kg IV reported improved arterial oxygenation in horses anesthetized with halothane [85,86], with a prolonged duration of effect of up to 90 min. However, more recent studies have found no effect of clenbuterol on arterial oxygen concentrations at similar doses rates, or a potentiation of hypoxemia [38,87]. Potentiation of hypoxemia [87] was attributed to an increased shunt fraction associated with bronchodilation and a reduction in hypoxic pulmonary vasoconstriction. At these dose rates, clenbuterol caused hemodynamic effects consistent with β_2-adrenergic receptor stimulation, causing a small increase in heart rate and cardiac output that persisted for up to 30 min after administration and that was associated with a transient increase in muscle perfusion. Adverse effects of clenbuterol include profuse sweating and increased oxygen consumption associated with the sympathomimetic effects on cardiovascular function. Consequently, clenbuterol administered intravenously is not recommended as a treatment for hypoxemia in anesthetized horses.

Albuterol, administered via inhalation through the endotracheal tube, has been shown to improve arterial oxygenation in anesthetized horses, predominantly through a sympathomimetic effect on hemodynamic function. Robertson and Bailey [88] administered 2 μg/kg albuterol using a human metered dose inhaler, with the dose delivered over a number of consecutive breaths at the start of each inspiration. This treatment was administered to 81 horses during volatile agent anesthesia when PaO_2 decreased below 70 mmHg. The authors reported an almost twofold increase in PaO_2 within 20 min of administration, with no concurrent effects on heart rate or mean arterial blood pressure. Patschova *et al.* [89] investigated the effects of the same dose (2 μg/kg) administered via the endotracheal tube on arterial oxygen concentrations and hemodynamics in isoflurane-anesthetized horses. There was a significant increase in cardiac output 15 min after albuterol administration, persisting for the duration of the monitored period (60 min). There was a transient increase in heart rate, while mean arterial blood pressure was unchanged, which was attributed to a reduction in systemic vascular resistance mediated by β_2-adrenergic receptors. The PaO_2:F_IO_2 ratio improved, but to a lesser extent than reported by Robertson and Bailey [88] and coincided with the peak effect of albuterol on cardiac output. These data suggest that improvements in oxygenation following albuterol administration arise predominantly from the positive hemodynamic effects of the drug. Collectively, these studies support the use of inhaled albuterol to manage hypoxemia in anesthetized horses.

There are no clinical reports of administration of this class of drugs to dogs during anesthesia; however, a number of studies have investigated the efficacy of inhaled albuterol in the management of bronchospasm in cats [90–92]. Albuterol at 100 μg/kg, delivered via a face mask immediately prior to induction of anesthesia, was effective at reducing bronchoconstriction in response to bronchoalveolar lavage in both normal cats and cats with experimentally induced asthma [90]. This investigation did not monitor for concurrent cardiovascular effects of drug administration. Terbutaline is also used in cats for the management of bronchospasm during bronchoscopy and bronchoalveolar lavage, particularly in cats with asthma. A dose of 0.01 mg/kg IM or SC has a duration of action of about 4 h, with peak effects occurring approximately 15 min after administration [93].

Mixed α- and β-adrenergic receptor agonists

Ephedrine

Ephedrine has both direct and indirect sympathomimetic actions, acting as an agonist at α_1-, α_2-, β_1-, and β_2-adrenergic receptors. It also inhibits the action of monoamine oxidase on norepinephrine. Tachyphylaxis occurs with repeated dosing due to depletion of norepinephrine stores and therefore a reduction in the magnitude of indirect sympathomimetic effects [94].

Ephedrine is used in the management of hypotension during anesthesia. Its longer duration of action compared with many other vasopressors and inotropes allows the administration of an intravenous bolus to produce clinical effects, removing the necessity for administration of drugs by continuous rate infusion. Infusions can be more time consuming to prepare and, therefore, delay the initiation of vasopressor or inotropic therapy.

Ephedrine is available in a variety of formulations for human use as a decongestant. For use during anesthesia, a 30 or 50 mg/mL solution is typically used. There are at least four isomers of ephedrine, all of which show some activity in dogs and cats [95], although this may vary between species [96]; two of the isomers are termed "pseudoephedrine" and the other two "ephedrine." The commercially available medical preparation is (1*R* ,2*S*)(−)-ephedrine.

Cardiovascular system effects

Ephedrine increases cardiac output, heart rate, blood pressure, coronary blood flow, and myocardial oxygen consumption. In horses anesthetized with halothane, administration of ephedrine (0.06 mg/kg IV) caused an increase in cardiac output and mean arterial blood pressure, with minimal effect on systemic vascular resistance [97]. The increase in cardiac output was attributed to increased stroke volume rather than a chronotropic effect. The effect of ephedrine was detected at 10 min (the first measured time point) after administration and persisted for 45–60 min. In this study, there was a concurrent increase in PaO_2, attributed to the effect of increased cardiac output on pulmonary perfusion. A similar dose of ephedrine administered to halothane-anesthetized horses with blood pressures below 65 mmHg also caused an increase in mean arterial blood pressure, detected 5 min after administration [51]; heart rate was unchanged, and there was no significant increase in PCV.

In dogs, single doses of ephedrine have been evaluated for the management of isoflurane-induced hypotension during anesthesia [31,98]. Chen *et al.* [31] administered ephedrine at 0.2 mg/kg IV to dogs with a mean arterial blood pressure lower than 70 mmHg and documented increased cardiac output, stroke volume, blood pressure, and global oxygen delivery; however, these effects were very transient, with a duration of effect of approximately 5 min. A repeat dose of ephedrine given 10 min later was ineffective at improving any cardiovascular parameters, which was attributed to tachyphylaxis. These findings were similar to those in an earlier study by Wagner *et al.* [98], although they investigated three different doses of ephedrine and found a more sustained increase in hemodynamic parameters following a 0.25 mg/kg dose, persisting for up to 30 min after administration. In contrast to the effect of ephedrine in horses, PCV increased at the higher dose in dogs, and this was attributed to α-adrenergic-induced splenic contraction [99].

There are limited clinical data on the administration of ephedrine to cats. Egger *et al.* [100] reported the cardiovascular effects of ephedrine at 0.1 mg/kg IM in cats anesthetized with acepromazine, ketamine, and isoflurane. The ephedrine was given 10 min before induction of anesthesia and was noted to delay the onset of hypotension (defined as a systolic arterial blood pressure of less than 80 mmHg) until 25 min after induction of anesthesia, compared with cats administered saline. No other cardiovascular changes occurred; however, cardiovascular monitoring was less rigorous in this study compared with studies in dogs and horses.

As with other sympathomimetics, administration of ephedrine may promote cardiac arrhythmias.

Other effects

Ephedrine causes stimulation of the respiratory system and bronchodilation similar to other drugs with β_2-adrenergic receptor agonist activity [see clenbuterol in the section Clenbuterol, albuterol (salbutamol), and terbutaline for details].

Ephedrine reduces renal blood flow with an associated reduction in glomerular filtration rate, attributed to regional vasoconstriction following stimulation of α_1-adrenergic receptors [101].

Pharmacokinetics

The pharmacokinetics of ephedrine have been described in the dog [102]. It undergoes rapid *N*-demethylation to norephedrine, which also has vasopressor effects and is likely to contribute to the hemodynamic effects of ephedrine seen in this species. There are limited data available on the metabolism of ephedrine in cats or horses, but data in ponies suggest that ephedrine is also metabolized to norephedrine [103].

Metaraminol

Similar to ephedrine, metaraminol is a synthetic amine with both direct and indirect sympathomimetic effects that acts predominantly on α-adrenergic receptors with some β-adrenergic receptor activity. In contrast to ephedrine, owing to relatively greater effects at α_1-adrenergic receptors, its major cardiovascular action is to increase blood pressure through an increase in systemic vascular resistance; consequently, cardiac output often falls. Metaraminol is not commonly used in veterinary anesthesia.

Adrenergic receptor antagonists

Adrenergic receptor antagonists prevent the actions of sympathomimetic amines on adrenergic receptors and are, therefore, called "sympatholytics." This class of drug can be subdivided depending on whether a drug is an antagonist at α- or β-adrenergic receptors, and then further subdivided according to whether it is selective for the α_1, α_2, β_1, or β_2-subtype.

α_1-Adrenergic receptor antagonists

Prazosin

Prazosin, a quinazoline derivative, is a highly selective α_1-adrenergic receptor antagonist. It is used predominantly for the management of functional urethral obstruction in cats and dogs. Stimulation of

α_1-adrenergic receptors in the bladder neck and proximal urethra narrows the bladder outlet maintaining continence. Inappropriate contraction of the bladder neck or urethra during voiding prevents normal urine flow and is termed "functional urethral obstruction." Although prazosin is not used during the management of anesthesia, it is important to understand the physiological effects of the drug and their relevance to anesthesia because of the requirement to anesthetize dogs and cats that are receiving prazosin therapy. Prazosin is available in an oral preparation (0.5–2 mg tablets) and an injectable form. The oral preparation is used most commonly in animals.

Cardiovascular system effects

Prazosin produces vasodilation of arteries and veins and reduces systemic vascular resistance; this is associated with a reduction in blood pressure, with diastolic blood pressure being impacted most significantly. There is little or no reflex tachycardia, which is attributed to a reduction in central thoracic sympathetic outflow [104]. There are limited clinical data on the cardiovascular effects of oral prazosin in cats or dogs. In a small study of three dogs, prazosin 0.025 mg/kg administered intravenously caused a maximal reduction in blood pressure that occurred 10 min after administration, but did not cause clinical hypotension (i.e., mean arterial blood pressure less than 70 mmHg). However, anecdotally, clinical signs attributable to hypotension have been reported in cats receiving prazosin for functional urethral obstruction. Prazosin is recommended for administration every 8–12 h in cats and dogs for the management of functional urethral obstruction. Therefore, in order to reduce the likelihood of hypotension during anesthesia of animals receiving prazosin for this purpose, it is reasonable to recommend cessation of administration 12–24 h before induction of anesthesia. Prazosin may also be used in the management of hemodynamic function in patients with pheochromocytoma, although phenoxybenzamine is more commonly used for this purpose (see below).

Pharmacokinetics

The pharmacokinetics of oral and intravenous prazosin have been described in awake dogs and dogs anesthetized with sodium pentobarbital [105]. Orally, although well absorbed from the gastrointestinal tract, prazosin has a relatively low bioavailability (approximately 38%), with hepatic extraction contributing to a major proportion of the presystemic metabolism of the drug. Following intravenous administration, initial plasma concentrations decrease rapidly due to extensive tissue distribution. The major liver hepatic pathways were demethylation, amide hydrolysis, and *O*-glucuronidation [105,106]. Anesthesia had a minimal effect on the pharmacokinetics of prazosin; however, it is predicted that drug metabolism would be significantly slowed in animals with liver dysfunction. The pharmacokinetics of prazosin in cats have not been described.

α_2-Adrenergic receptor antagonists

Atipamezole, yohimbine, and tolazoline

In veterinary anesthesia, these agents are used for the reversal of sedation produced by α_2-adrenergic receptor agonists such as medetomidine and dexmedetomidine. Further information is available in Chapter 22.

Non-selective α-adrenergic receptor antagonists

Phentolamine

Phentolamine is a competitive non-selective α-adrenergic receptor blocker, with three times greater affinity for α_1- than α_2-adrenergic receptors. During anesthesia, phentolamine is used in the management of hypertensive crises due to excessive administration of sympathomimetics and pheochromocytoma, especially during tumor manipulation. In human dentistry, a preparation of phentolamine is available to reverse the effects of local anesthetic administration [107]. Vasodilation produced by α-adrenergic receptor blockade increases the systemic absorption of local anesthetics and therefore shortens the duration of sensory blockade. Phentolamine is also used in the management of pain associated with complex regional pain syndrome in people, although there are limited clinical data to support use in this context [108]. There are very limited published clinical data on the administration of phentolamine to companion animals. Phentolamine is available as a 10 mg/mL injectable preparation.

Blockade of postjunctional vascular α_1- and α_2-adrenergic receptors causes vasodilation and hypotension. Blockade of presynaptic α_2-adrenergic receptors facilitates norepinephrine release, leading to tachycardia and an increase in cardiac output. Pulmonary artery pressure is also reduced.

Phentolamine can cause an increase in insulin secretion, precipitating hypoglycemia; it is advisable to monitor blood glucose following administration. The drug is metabolized in the liver, with a short half-life following intravenous administration (approximately 20 min in people). There are no published data on the specific metabolic pathways of phentolamine in companion animals.

Phenoxybenzamine

Phenoxybenzamine is a long-acting, non-selective α-adrenergic receptor blocker, with greater affinity for α_1- than α_2-adrenergic receptors. Its effects are mediated by a reactive intermediate that forms a covalent bond and alkylates the α-adrenergic receptor, resulting in irreversible blockade. In addition to receptor blockade, phenoxybenzamine also inhibits neuronal and extraneuronal uptake of catecholamines.

In veterinary patients, phenoxybenzamine is most commonly used for the preoperative management of pheochromocytoma, administered orally. The aims of administration are to reverse chronic vasoconstriction due to increased circulating concentrations of epinephrine and norepinephrine that are produced by the tumor and thereby facilitate expansion of intravascular volume. The long duration of action of oral phenoxybenzamine allows twice daily dosing.

In people, preoperative stabilization of patients with pheochromocytoma with oral phenoxybenzamine significantly decreases mortality rates in the perioperative period [109]. Phenoxybenzamine is also used to control changes in heart rate and blood pressure during surgical tumor manipulation, where the irreversible nature of the adrenergic blockade results in greater efficacy compared with shorter acting competitive blockers such as phentolamine.

A retrospective study in dogs with pheochromocytoma [110] also found preoperative administration of phenoxybenzamine for a median period of 20 days before adrenalectomy also decreased mortality compared with untreated controls. The long duration of action can result in persistent hypotension following tumor removal; therefore, some anesthetists elect to stop administration of phenoxybenzamine 48 h prior to surgery. Phenoxybenzamine may also be used in the management of functional urethral obstruction in dogs and cats, where more limited effects on blood pressure are advantageous compared with treatment with prazosin [111]. Phenoxybenzamine is available as an oral and injectable preparation.

The cardiovascular effects of phenoxybenzamine are similar to those of phentolamine. Phenoxybenzamine does not prevent arrhythmias from occurring during adrenalectomy for pheochromocytoma removal as a result of tumor manipulation. In people, concurrent β-adrenergic blockade is sometimes instituted to control arrhythmias and reduce tachycardias resulting from β-adrenergic receptor stimulation [112]. The requirement for concurrent β-blockade depends on the tumor type and associated hormone secretion. In dogs with pheochromocytoma, oral doses of approximately 0.6 mg/kg every 12 h reduced mortality in the perioperative period [110]. Doses of 0.5 mg/kg twice daily have been recommended in cats.

A reduction in central nervous system sympathetic outflow as a result of adrenergic blockade can cause mild sedation in treated animals, although this is not normally of sufficient magnitude to cause clinically relevant effects.

Phenoxybenzamine is incompletely and variably absorbed from the gut of people, with an oral bioavailability of about 25%. It is reasonable to assume that this is also the case in monogastric animals. The drug is extensively metabolized in the liver and excreted in urine and bile. Although the plasma half-life is 24 h in people, the duration of action can be up to 3 days, reflecting the biologic requirement of new α-adrenergic receptor synthesis for effects to wane and eventually terminate.

β_1-Adrenergic receptor antagonists

General properties of β-adrenergic receptor antagonists are presented in Table 21.2. β-Adrenergic receptor antagonists (commonly termed "beta-blockers" or "β-blockers") are all competitive antagonists with varying degrees of selectivity for β_1- and β_2-adrenergic receptors. Some β-blockers have intrinsic sympathomimetic activity (ISA), resulting in a partial agonist effect at β_1, β_2, or both types of adrenergic receptors [113]. Membrane-stabilizing activity, similar to that of local anesthetics on the cardiac action potential, is also a feature of some β-adrenergic receptor antagonists, although concentrations greater than those achieved by therapeutic doses are usually required to elicit this effect.

The therapeutic usefulness of β-adrenergic receptor antagonists is mediated through their effect at β_1-adrenergic receptors, while concurrent effects at β_2-receptors are deemed undesirable. Atenolol and esmolol demonstrate β_1-adrenergic receptor selectivity, although at high doses antagonist effects at β_2-receptors also occur.

β-Adrenergic receptor antagonists that have ISA are able to stimulate these receptors and oppose the stimulating effects of catecholamines in a competitive way. Therefore, the balance between agonism and antagonism depends on the circulating level of catecholamines. β-Blockers with ISA are partial agonists at β-adrenergic receptors and elicit a submaximal response at full receptor occupancy. The presence of ISA results in less resting bradycardia and a smaller reduction in cardiac output than are observed with β-blockers without ISA [114]. In the long term, they may produce arterial vasodilation and increase arterial compliance, which is postulated to be beneficial in the management of hypertension in humans [114].

Table 21.2 Comparison of receptor selectivity, intrinsic sympathomimetic activity (ISA), and membrane-stabilizing activity of β-adrenergic receptor antagonists used in veterinary medicine.

Drug	β_1-receptor selectivity	Intrinsic sympathomimetic activity	Membrane-stabilizing activity
Atenolol	+	+	–
Esmolol	++	–	–
Metoprolol	++	–	+
Pindolol	–	++	+
Propranolol	–	–	++
Sotalol	–	–	–

In human medicine, β-adrenergic receptor antagonists are predominantly used in the treatment of hypertension, angina, and myocardial infarction. These drugs are also widely used in veterinary medicine, predominantly for the management of the hemodynamic and neuroendocrine consequences of cardiac disease, including the management of cardiac arrhythmias. Therefore, it is important to have a good understanding of the clinical pharmacology of β-adrenergic receptor antagonists in order to determine potential effects during anesthesia in animals receiving therapy. During anesthesia, β-blockers are predominantly used in the management of inappropriate tachycardia, where the increased heart rate is having a negative effect on hemodynamic function. They are also used in the perioperative management of pheochromocytomas to prevent reflex tachycardia associated with α-adrenergic blockade therapy, and to control arrhythmias and tachycardias associated with β-adrenergic receptor stimulation due to hormone secretion from the tumor.

β-Adrenergic receptor antagonists decrease the heart rate by reducing automaticity in the sinoatrial node and prolonging the conduction time in the atrioventricular node. A reduction in heart rate lengthens diastole and, therefore, can improve coronary perfusion and increase regional myocardial oxygen delivery. They are class II antiarrhythmic agents and are mainly used to treat arrhythmias associated with high circulating levels of catecholamines. At the same time, they have a negative inotropic effect, which decreases oxygen demand, thereby collectively improving the balance between myocardial oxygen supply and demand. Potential negative effects on cardiovascular function are a prolonged systolic ejection time, dilation of ventricles, and an increase in coronary vascular resistance due to the antagonism of coronary vasodilatory β_2-adrenergic receptors. In human patients with poor left ventricular function, β-blockade is recognized to be a risk factor for the development of cardiac failure [115].

β-Blockers control blood pressure [116] predominantly through a reduction in heart rate and cardiac output and also via inhibition of the renin–angiotensin system due to blockade of β_1-adrenergic receptors at the juxtaglomerular apparatus. A reduction in circulating angiotensin II will ameliorate vasoconstriction that also drives the secretion of aldosterone. However, when β-adrenergic blockers are administered acutely during anesthesia, the reductions in cardiac output and heart rate are the primary mechanisms responsible for decreased blood pressure.

High doses of all β-blockers, irrespective of selectivity for β_1-adrenergic receptors at clinical dose rates, will precipitate bronchospasm via blockade of β_2-adrenergic receptors in bronchioles, opposing tonic sympathetically mediated bronchodilation [117].

The metabolic effects of β-blockers are complex owing to the multiple pathways and organs involved in the regulation of blood glucose concentration. However, β-blockers can lead both to an increase in blood glucose concentration (through peripheral insulin resistance and decreased insulin secretion from pancreatic cells) and to a decrease in blood glucose concentration (by mitigating the normal increase that occurs during exercise). They can also have complex effects on lipid metabolism, resulting in increased plasma triglycerides [118].

Atenolol

Atenolol is a relatively cardioselective (i.e., β_1) adrenergic receptor antagonist that is available as tablet and syrup formulations for oral administration, and as an injectable preparation (0.5 mg/mL) for intravenous use. Although it is not widely administered during anesthesia, atenolol is prescribed to delay the onset of adverse sequelae in cats with hypertrophic cardiomyopathy and for the management of ventricular arrhythmias in cats and dogs; therefore, knowledge of atenolol pharmacology is important. It is worth noting that in human medicine, continuation of β-adrenergic blocker therapy is generally recommended in the perioperative period for patients with cardiac disease [119,120].

In cats, atenolol is well absorbed orally, with recommended clinical doses producing plasma concentrations that are within the therapeutic range within 1 h of oral administration, with effects that persist for up to 12 h, allowing twice daily dosing [121]. Twice daily dosing with atenolol, orally, is also recommended in dogs [122]. In people, atenolol is excreted unchanged in the urine, and effects are, therefore, more prolonged in patients with renal impairment; whether this is also the case in small animals is unknown.

Esmolol

Esmolol is highly selective for the β_1-adrenergic receptor and is very lipophilic, with a rapid onset and offset of action when given intravenously; therefore, it is the β-blocker of choice for use during anesthesia to control tachycardia, hypertension, and acute supraventricular tachycardia associated with inappropriate sympathetic nervous system activity. It is commonly given by infusion, using a controlled infusion apparatus in order to prevent overdose. In dogs and cats, a bolus dose of 2 μg/kg followed by an infusion of 50 μg/kg/min is generally recommended to decrease heart rate and systolic function [123,124]. A recent small retrospective study reported the use of esmolol for heart rate reduction in non-anesthetized dogs and cats. A median bolus dose of 330 μg/kg followed in most cases by a continuous rate infusion of 50 μg/kg/min was effective at reducing heart rate by 20% in 46% of animals [125]. Esmolol is rapidly metabolized by red blood cell esterases to an essentially inactive metabolite with a long half-life and methanol. It has no ISA or membrane-stabilizing properties.

Metoprolol

Metoprolol is also relatively selective for the β_1-adrenergic receptor and has no ISA. It is available as an oral tablet preparation and has been evaluated in the management of dogs with acquired cardiac disease [126]. Metoprolol is rapidly absorbed from the gut but undergoes very high first-pass metabolism, giving an oral bioavailability of approximately 50% across species [127,128]. The half-life of metoprolol is approximately 2 h in dogs [129], with twice daily dosing generally recommended. In humans, rats, dogs, and horses, metabolism is via oxidative pathways, with metoprolol and its metabolites excreted mainly in urine in an unconjugated form [128].

Non-selective β-adrenergic receptor antagonists

Pindolol

Pindolol is a non-selective β-adrenergic antagonist with intrinsic sympathomimetic and membrane-stabilizing properties that is also a serotonin receptor (5-$HT_{1A/1B}$) antagonist [130]. In addition to the typical cardiovascular effects of the drug, pindolol may potentiate analgesia provided by tramadol in dogs [131], presumably due to augmentation of serotonergic effects of tramadol by activation of the serotonergic modulatory system.

Propranolol

Propranolol is a non-selective β-adrenergic antagonist without ISA. It is available as a racemic mixture, although the *S*-isomer confers most of the therapeutic cardiac effects of the drug. The *R*-isomer prevents the peripheral conversion of thyroxine (T4) to triiodothyronine (T3) in people, although whether this effect is also present in animal species has not yet been determined. Propranolol is available as injectable and oral preparations; in animals, it is most commonly administered orally for the control of heart rate and hypertension prior to thyroidectomy in cats with hyperthyroidism, or as part of the presurgical management of animals with pheochromocytoma. Use of propranolol during anesthesia has been largely superseded by the availability of esmolol, which has greater selectivity for the β_1-adrenergic receptor. Propranolol is well absorbed through the gut, but has a very high first-pass hepatic metabolism in humans, dogs, rats, and cats [132,133]. The major metabolic pathways for propranolol also occur in the liver [133]. It is noteworthy that the metabolism of oral propranolol is prolonged in hyperthyroid compared with euthyroid cats [134], necessitating dosing adjustments.

Sotalol

Sotalol, in addition to being a non-selective β-adrenergic antagonist without ISA, is a class III antiarrhythmic and has potassium channel-blocking effects. It is most commonly used orally to treat ventricular tachyarrhythmias and has been shown to reduce the number of ventricular premature contractions in Boxer dogs with familial ventricular arrhythmias [122]. It is well absorbed from the gut when administered orally and is excreted largely unchanged in the urine; therefore, renal impairment will significantly reduce clearance. In dogs, the plasma half-life is approximately 4 h [135].

References

1 Pascoe PJ, Ilkiw JE, Pypendop BH. Effects of increasing infusion rates of dopamine, dobutamine, epinephrine, and phenylephrine in healthy anesthetized cats. *Am J Vet Res* 2006; **67**: 1491–1499.

2 Grassi-Kassisse DM, Faro R, Withrington PG, *et al.* Characterisation of functional endothelin receptors in the canine isolated perfused spleen. *Eur J Pharmacol* 1995; **282**: 57–63.

3 Igić R. Mechanism of epinephrine-induced dysrhythmias in rat involves local cholinergic activation. *Can J Physiol Pharmacol* 1996; **74**: 85–88.

4 Maze M, Smith CM. Identification of receptor mechanism mediating epinephrine-induced arrhythmias during halothane anesthesia in the dog. *Anesthesiology* 1983; **59**: 322–326.

5 Katz RL, Bigger JT Jr. Cardiac arrhythmias during anesthesia and operation. *Anesthesiology* 1970; **33**: 193–213.

6 Black GW, Clarke RS, Howard PJ, McCullough H. The cardiovascular effects of teflurane in the cat. *Br J Anaesth* 1969; **41**: 288–296.

7 Lees P, Tavernor WD. Influence of halothane and catecholamines on heart rate and rhythm in the horse. *Br J Pharmacol* 1970; **39**: 149–159.

8 Tranquilli WJ, Thurmon JC, Benson GJ. Halothane–catecholamine arrhythmias in swine (Sus scrofa). *Am J Vet Res* 1986; **47**: 2134–2137.

9 Hikasa Y, Okabe C, Takase K, *et al.* Ventricular arrhythmogenic dose of adrenaline during sevoflurane, isoflurane, and halothane anaesthesia either with or without ketamine or thiopentone in cats. *Res Vet Sci* 1996; **60**: 134–137.

10 Pettifer G, Dyson D, McDonell W. The arrhythmogenic dose of epinephrine in halothane and isoflurane anesthetized dogs: an assessment of repeatability. *Can J Vet Res* 1997; **61**: 221–226.

11 Gaynor JS, Bednarski RM, Muir WW III. Effect of xylazine on the arrhythmogenic dose of epinephrine in thiamylal/halothane-anesthetized horses. *Am J Vet Res* 1992; **53**: 2350–2354.

12 Bednarski RM, Majors LJ. Ketamine and the arrhythmogenic dose of epinephrine in cats anesthetized with halothane and isoflurane. *Am J Vet Res* 1986; **47**: 2122–2125.

13 Bednarski RM, Sams RA, Majors LJ, *et al.* Reduction of the ventricular arrhythmogenic dose of epinephrine by ketamine administration in halothane-anesthetized cats. *Am J Vet Res* 1988; **49**: 350–354.

14 Niiya S. The effect of ketamine on epinephrine-induced arrhythmias in dogs anesthetized with halothane–nitrous oxide. *Masui* 1990; **39**: 1652–1659.

15 Kaye AD, Hoover JM, Baber SR, *et al.* Effects of norepinephrine on alpha-subtype receptors in the feline pulmonary vascular bed. *Crit Care Med* 2004; **32**: 2300–2303.

16 Miller RD, Way WL, Eger EI II. The effects of alpha-methyldopa, reserpine, guanethidine, and iproniazid on minimum alveolar anesthetic requirement (MAC). *Anesthesiology* 1968; **29**: 1153–1158.

17 Steffey EP, Eger EI. The effect of seven vasopressors of halothane MAC in dogs. *Br J Anaesth* 1975; **47**: 435–438.

18 Johnson MD. Circulating epinephrine stimulates renin secretion in anesthetized dogs by activation of extrarenal adrenoceptors. *Am J Physiol* 1984; **246**: F676–F684.

19 Johnson MD, Whitener CJ, Sears TS. Epinephrine-induced renin secretion is not initiated by cardiac adrenoceptors. *Am J Physiol* 1988; **254**: E265–E271.

20 Laks M, Callis G, Swan HJ. Hemodynamic effects of low doses of norepinephrine in the conscious dog. *Am J Physiol* 1971; **220**: 171–173.

21 Melchior JC, Pinaud M, Blanloeil Y, *et al.* Hemodynamic effects of continuous norepinephrine infusion in dogs with and without hyperkinetic endotoxic shock. *Crit Care Med* 1987; **15**: 687–691.

22 Valverde A, Giguère S, Sanchez LC, *et al.* Effects of dobutamine, norepinephrine, and vasopressin on cardiovascular function in anesthetized neonatal foals with induced hypotension. *Am J Vet Res* 2006; **67**: 1730–1737.

23 Vincent CJ, Hawley AT, Rozanski EA, *et al.* Cardiopulmonary effects of dobutamine and norepinephrine infusion in healthy anesthetized alpacas. *Am J Vet Res* 2009; **70**: 1236–1242.

24 Kojima K, Ishizuka T, Sasaki N, *et al.* Cardiovascular effects of dose escalating of norepinephrine in healthy dogs anesthetized with isoflurane. *Vet Anaesth Analg* 2021; **48**: 654–662.

25 Bakker J, Vincent JL. Effects of norepinephrine and dobutamine on oxygen transport and consumption in a dog model of endotoxic shock. *Crit Care Med* 1993; **21**: 425–432.

26 Gillis CN, Pitt BR. The fate of circulating amines within the pulmonary circulation. *Annu Rev Physiol* 1982; **44**: 269–281.

27 Rosati M, Dyson DH, Sinclair MD, *et al.* Response of hypotensive dogs to dopamine hydrochloride and dobutamine hydrochloride during deep isoflurane anesthesia. *Am J Vet Res* 2007; **68**: 483–494.

28 Brooks HL, Stein PD, Matson JL, *et al.* Dopamine-induced alterations in coronary hemodynamics in dogs. *Circ Res* 1969; **24**: 699–704.

29 Scott A, Chakrabarti MK, Hall GM. Oxygen transport during dopamine infusion in dogs. *Br J Anaesth* 1979; **51**: 1011–1019.

30 Dyson DH, Sinclair MD. Impact of dopamine or dobutamine infusions on cardiovascular variables after rapid blood loss and volume replacement during isoflurane-induced anesthesia in dogs. *Am J Vet Res* 2006; **67**: 1121–1130.

31 Chen HC, Sinclair MD, Dyson DH. Use of ephedrine and dopamine in dogs for the management of hypotension in routine clinical cases under isoflurane anesthesia. *Vet Anaesth Analg* 2007; **34**: 301–311.

32 Wiese AJ, Barter LS, Ilkiw JE, *et al.* Cardiovascular and respiratory effects of incremental doses of dopamine and phenylephrine in the management of isoflurane-induced hypotension in cats with hypertrophic cardiomyopathy. *Am J Vet Res* 2012; **73**: 908–916.

33 Kobluk K, Pypendop BH. Effects of dopamine, norepinephrine or phenylephrine on the prevention of hypotension in isoflurane-anesthetized cats administered vatinoxan or vatinoxan and dexmedetomidine. *Vet Anaesth Analg* 2022; **49**: 54–64.

34 Swanson CR, Muir WW III, Bednarski RM, *et al.* Hemodynamic responses in halothane-anesthetized horses given infusions of dopamine or dobutamine. *Am J Vet Res* 1985; **46**: 365–370.

35 Trim CM, Moore JN, White NA. Cardiopulmonary effects of dopamine hydrochloride in anaesthetised horses. *Equine Vet J* 1985; **17**: 41–44.

36 Robertson SA, Malark JA, Steele CJ, *et al.* Metabolic, hormonal, and hemodynamic changes during dopamine infusions in halothane anesthetized horses. *Vet Surg* 1996; **25**: 88–97.

37 Young LE, Blissitt KJ, Clutton RE, *et al.* Haemodynamic effects of a sixty minute infusion of dopamine hydrochloride in horses anaesthetised with halothane. *Equine Vet J* 1998; **30**: 310–316.

38 Lee YH, Clarke KW, Alibhai HI, *et al.* Effects of dopamine, dobutamine, dopexamine, phenylephrine, and saline solution on intramuscular blood flow and other cardiopulmonary variables in halothane-anesthetized ponies. *Am J Vet Res* 1998; **59**: 1463–1472.

39 Lokhandwala MF, Jandhyala BS. The role of sympathetic nervous system in the vascular actions of dopamine. *J Pharmacol Exp Ther* 1979; **210**: 120–126.

40 Dancker C, Hopster K, Rohn K, *et al.* Effects of dobutamine, dopamine, phenylephrine and noradrenaline on systemic haemodynamics and intestinal perfusion in isoflurane anaesthetized horses. *Equine Vet J* 2018; **50**: 104–110.

41 Tatsumi K, Pickett CK, Weil JV. Decreased carotid body hypoxic sensitivity in chronic hypoxia: role of dopamine. *Respir Physiol* 1995; **101**: 47–57.

42 McNay JL, Mcdonald RH Jr, Goldberg LI. Direct renal vasodilatation produced by dopamine in the dog. *Circ Res* 1965; **16**: 510–517.

43 MacCannell KL, McNay JL, Meyer MB, *et al.* Dopamine in the treatment of hypotension and shock. *N Engl J Med* 1966; **275**: 1389–1398.

44 Karthik S, Lisbon A. Low-dose dopamine in the intensive care unit. *Semin Dial* 2006; **19**: 465–471.

45 Clark KL, Robertson MJ, Drew GM. Do renal tubular dopamine receptors mediate dopamine-induced diuresis in the anesthetized cat? *J Cardiovasc Pharmacol* 1991; **17**: 267–276.

46 Furukawa S, Nagashima Y, Hoshi K, *et al.* Effects of dopamine infusion on cardiac and renal blood flows in dogs. *J Vet Med Sci* 2002; **64**: 41–44.

47 Takemoto F, Cohen HT, Satoh T, *et al.* Dopamine inhibits Na/K-ATPase in single tubules and cultured cells from distal nephron. *Pflugers Arch* 1992; **421**: 302–306.

48 Clark BJ, Menninger K. Peripheral dopamine receptors. *Circ Res* 1980; **46**: I59–I63.

49 Voelckel WG, Lindner KH, Wenzel V, *et al.* Effect of small-dose dopamine on mesenteric blood flow and renal function in a pig model of cardiopulmonary resuscitation with vasopressin. *Anesth Analg* 1999; **89**: 1430–1436.

50 Raisis AL, Young LE, Blissitt KJ, *et al.* Effect of a 30-minute infusion of dobutamine hydrochloride on hind limb blood flow and hemodynamics in halothane-anesthetized horses. *Am J Vet Res* 2000; **61**: 1282–1288.

51 Hellyer PW, Wagner AE, Mama KR. The effects of dobutamine and ephedrine on packed cell volume, total protein, heart rate, and blood pressure in anaesthetized horses. *J Vet Pharmacol Ther* 1998; **21**: 497–499.

52 Meier M, Bettschart-Wolfensberger R, Schwarzwald CC, *et al.* Effects of dobutamine on cardiovascular function and oxygen delivery in standing horses. *J Vet Pharmacol Ther* 2020; **43**: 470–476.

53 Goya S, Wada T, Shimada K, *et al.* Dose-dependent effects of isoflurane and dobutamine on cardiovascular function in dogs with experimental mitral regurgitation. *Vet Anaesth Analg* 2018; **45**:432–442.

54 Renton MC, Snowden CP. Dopexamine and its role in the protection of hepatosplanchnic and renal perfusion in high-risk surgical and critically ill patients. *Br J Anaesth* 2005; **94**: 459–467.

55 Muir WW III. Inotropic mechanisms of dopexamine hydrochloride in horses. *Am J Vet Res* 1992; **53**: 1343–1346.

56 Muir WW III. Cardiovascular effects of dopexamine HCl in conscious and halothane-anaesthetised horses. *Equine Vet J Suppl* 1992; (**11**): 24–29.

57 Young LE, Blissitt KJ, Clutton RE, *et al.* Temporal effects of an infusion of dopexamine hydrochloride in horses anesthetized with halothane. *Am J Vet Res* 1997; **58**: 516–523.

58 Einstein R, Abdul-Hussein N, Wong TW, *et al.* Cardiovascular actions of dopexamine in anaesthetized and conscious dogs. *Br J Pharmacol* 1994; **111**: 199–204.

59 Scheeren TW, Arndt JO. Different response of oxygen consumption and cardiac output to various endogenous and synthetic catecholamines in awake dogs. *Crit Care Med* 2008; **28**: 3861–3868.

60 Neustein SM, Dimich I, Sampson I, *et al.* Arrhythmogenic potential of dopexamine hydrochloride during halothane anaesthesia in dogs. *Can J Anaesth* 1994; **41**: 542–546.

61 Asfar P, De Backer D, Meier-Hellmann A, *et al.* Clinical review: influence of vasoactive and other therapies on intestinal and hepatic circulations in patients with septic shock. *Crit Care* 2004; **8**: 170–179.

62 Gray PA, Jones T, Park GR. Blood concentrations of dopexamine in patients during and after orthotopic liver transplantation. *Br J Clin Pharmacol* 1994; **37**: 89–92.

63 Tobias JD. Caudal epidural block: a review of test dosing and recognition of systemic injection in children. *Anesth Analg* 2001; **93**: 1156–1161.

64 Crystal GJ, Salem MR. Beta-adrenergic stimulation restores oxygen extraction reserve during acute normovolemic hemodilution. *Anesth Analg* 2002; **95**: 851–857.

65 Sandusky GE, Means JR, Todd GC. Comparative cardiovascular toxicity in dogs given inotropic agents by continuous intravenous infusion. *Toxicol Pathol* 1990; **18**: 268–278.

66 Volders PG, Kulcśar A, Vos MA, *et al.* Similarities between early and delayed afterdepolarizations induced by isoproterenol in canine ventricular myocytes. *Cardiovasc Res* 1997; **34**: 348–359.

67 O'Neill DK, Aizer A, Linton P, *et al.* Isoproterenol infusion increases level of consciousness during catheter ablation of atrial fibrillation. *J Interv Card Electrophysiol* 2012; **34**: 137–142.

68 Zhang H, De Jongh R, De Backer D, *et al.* Effects of alpha- and beta-adrenergic stimulation on hepatosplanchnic perfusion and oxygen extraction in endotoxic shock. *Crit Care Med* 2001; **29**: 581–588.

69 Szefler SJ, Acara M. Isoproterenol excretion and metabolism in the isolated perfused rat kidney. *J Pharmacol Exp Ther* 1979; **210**: 295–300.

70 Linton RA, Young LE, Marlin DJ, *et al.* Cardiac output measured by lithium dilution, thermodilution, and transesophageal Doppler echocardiography in anesthetized horses. *Am J Vet Res* 2000; **61**: 731–737.

71 Frederick J, Giguère S, Butterworth K, *et al.* Severe phenylephrine-associated hemorrhage in five aged horses. *J Am Vet Med Assoc* 2010; **237**: 830–834.
72 Robinson JL. Effect of vasopressin and phenylephrine on arterial pressure and heart rate in conscious dogs. *Am J Physiol* 1986; **251**: H253–H260.
73 Ludders JW, Reitan JA, Martucci R, *et al.* Blood pressure response to phenylephrine infusion in halothane-anesthetized dogs given acetylpromazine maleate. *Am J Vet Res* 1983; **44**: 996–999.
74 Richardson PD, Withrington PG. The role of beta-adrenoceptors in the responses of the hepatic arterial vascular bed of the dog to phenylephrine, isoproterenol, noradrenaline and adrenaline. *Br J Pharmacol* 1977; **60**: 239–249.
75 Strandhoy JW, Wolff DW, Buckalew VM Jr. Renal alpha 1- and alpha 2-adrenoceptor mediated vasoconstriction in dogs. *J Hypertens Suppl* 1984; **2**: S151–S153.
76 Erkinaro T, Mäkikallio K, Kavasmaa T, *et al.* Effects of ephedrine and phenylephrine on uterine and placental circulations and fetal outcome following fetal hypoxaemia and epidural-induced hypotension in a sheep model. *Br J Anaesth* 2004; **93**: 825–832.
77 Lukasik VM, Gleed RD, Scarlett JM, *et al.* Intranasal phenylephrine reduces post anesthetic upper airway obstruction in horses. *Equine Vet J* 1997; **29**: 236–238.
78 Herring IP, Jacobson JD, Pickett JP. Cardiovascular effects of topical ophthalmic 10% phenylephrine in dogs. *Vet Ophthalmol* 2004; **7**: 41–46.
79 Martin-Flores M, Mercure-McKenzie TM, Campoy L, *et al.* Controlled retrospective study of the effects of eyedrops containing phenylephrine hydrochloride and scopolamine hydrobromide on mean arterial blood pressure in anesthetized dogs. *Am J Vet Res* 2010; **71**: 1407–1412.
80 Dyson DH, Pascoe PJ. Influence of preinduction methoxamine, lactated Ringer solution, or hypertonic saline solution infusion or postinduction dobutamine infusion on anesthetic-induced hypotension in horses. *Am J Vet Res* 1990; **51**: 17–21.
81 Lee JC, Fripp RR, Downing SE. Myocardial responses to alpha-adrenoceptor stimulation with methoxamine hydrochloride in lambs. *Am J Physiol* 1982; **242**: H405–H410.
82 Brewster WR, Osgood PF, Isaacs JP, *et al.* Haemodynamic effects of a pressor amine (methoxamine) with predominant vasoconstrictor activity. *Circ Res* 1960; **8**: 980–988.
83 Imai S, Shigei T, Hashimoto K. Cardiac actions of methoxamine with special reference to its antagonistic action to epinephrine. *Circ Res* 1961; **9**: 552–560.
84 Canepa-Anson R, Dawson JR, Frankl WS, *et al.* Beta 2 adrenoceptor agonists. Pharmacology, metabolic effects and arrhythmias. *Eur Heart J* 1982; (Suppl D): 129–134.
85 Gleed RD, Dobson A. Effect of clenbuterol on arterial oxygen tension in the anaesthetised horse. *Res Vet Sci* 1990; **48**: 331–337.
86 Keegan RD, Gleed RD, Sanders EA, *et al.* Treatment of low arterial oxygen tension in anesthetized horses with clenbuterol. *Vet Surg* 1991; **20**: 148–152.
87 Dodam JR, Moon RE, Olson NC, *et al.* Effects of clenbuterol hydrochloride on pulmonary gas exchange and hemodynamics in anesthetized horses. *Am J Vet Res* 1993; **54**: 776–782.
88 Robertson SA, Bailey JE. Aerosolized salbutamol (albuterol) improves PaO_2 in hypoxaemic anaesthetized horses – a prospective clinical trial in 81 horses. *Vet Anaesth Analg* 2002; **29**: 212–218.
89 Patschova M, Kabes R, Krisova S. The effects of inhalation salbutamol administration on systemic and pulmonary hemodynamic, pulmonary mechanics and oxygen balance during general anaesthesia in the horse. *Vet Med (Czech)* 2010; **55**: 445–456.
90 Kirschvink N, Leemans J, Delvaux F, *et al.* Bronchodilators in bronchoscopy-induced airflow limitation in allergen-sensitized cats. *J Vet Intern Med* 2005; **19**: 161–167.
91 Leemans J, Kirschvink N, Clercx C, *et al.* Functional response to inhaled salbutamol and/or ipratropium bromide in *Ascaris suum*-sensitised cats with allergen-induced bronchospasms. *Vet J* 2010; **186**: 76–83.
92 Leemans J, Kirschvink N, Bernaerts F, *et al.* Salmeterol or doxycycline do not inhibit acute bronchospasm and airway inflammation in cats with experimentally-induced asthma. *Vet J* 2012; **192**: 49–56.
93 Padrid P, Church DB. Drugs used in the management of respiratory diseases. In: Maddison J, Page SW, Church D, eds. *Small Animal Clinical Pharmacology*, 2nd edn. Edinburgh: Saunders Elsevier, 2008: 458–468.
94 Takasaki K, Urabe M, Yamamoto R. Tachyphylaxis of indirectly acting sympathomimetic amines. II. Recovery of tyramine tachyphylaxis and crossed tachyphylaxis between tyramine and other indirectly acting sympathomimetic amines in dogs. *Kurume Med J* 1972; **19**: 11–22.
95 Patil PN, Tye A, Lapidus JB. A pharmacological study of the ephedrine isomers. *J Pharmacol Exp Ther* 1965; **148**: 158–168.
96 Young R, Glennon RA. Discriminative stimulus properties of (–)-ephedrine. *Pharmacol Biochem Behav* 1998; **60**: 771–775.
97 Grandy JL, Hodgson DS, Dunlop CI, *et al.* Cardiopulmonary effects of ephedrine in halothane-anesthetized horses. *J Vet Pharmacol Ther* 1989; **12**: 389–396.
98 Wagner AE, Dunlop CI, Chapman PL. Effects of ephedrine on cardiovascular function and oxygen delivery in isoflurane-anesthetized dogs. *Am J Vet Res* 1993; **54**: 1917–1922.
99 Davies BN, Withrington PG. The actions of drugs on the smooth muscle of the capsule and blood vessels of the spleen. *Pharmacol Rev* 1973; **25**: 373–413.
100 Egger C, McCrackin MA, Hofmeister E, *et al.* Efficacy of preanesthetic intramuscular administration of ephedrine for prevention of anesthesia-induced hypotension in cats and dogs. *Can Vet J* 2009; **50**: 179–184.
101 Amorin RB, Braz JR, Castiglia YM, *et al.* Effects of ephedrine on cardiovascular and renal function of dogs anesthetized with sodium pentobarbital. *Rev Bras Anestesiol* 2002; **52**: 434–445.
102 Axelrod J. Studies on sympathomimetic amines I. The biotransformation and physiological disposition of l-ephedrine and l-norephedrine. *J Pharm Exp Ther* 1953; **109**: 62–73.
103 Nicholson JD. The metabolism of l-ephedrine in ponies. *Arch Int Pharmacodyn Ther* 1970; **188**: 375–386.
104 Ramage AG. The effect of prazosin, indoramin and phentolamine on sympathetic nerve activity. *Eur J Pharmacol* 1984; **106**: 507–513.
105 Rubin P, Yee YG, Anderson M, *et al.* Prazosin first-pass metabolism and hepatic extraction in the dog. *J Cardiovasc Pharmacol* 1979; **1**: 641–647.
106 Erve JC, Vashishtha SC, DeMaio W, *et al.* Metabolism of prazosin in rat, dog, and human liver microsomes and cryopreserved rat and human hepatocytes and characterization of metabolites by liquid chromatography/tandem mass spectrometry. *Drug Metab Dispos* 2007; **35**: 908–916.
107 Becker DE, Reed KL. Local anesthetics: review of pharmacological considerations. *Anesth Prog* 2012; **59**: 90–101.
108 Rowbotham MC. Pharmacologic management of complex regional pain syndrome. *Clin J Pain* 2006; **22**: 425–429.
109 Russell WJ, Metcalfe IR, Tonkin AL, *et al.* The preoperative management of phaeochromocytoma. *Anaesth Intensive Care* 1998; **26**: 196–200.
110 Herrera MA, Mehl ML, Kass PH, *et al.* Predictive factors and the effect of phenoxybenzamine on outcome in dogs undergoing adrenalectomy for pheochromocytoma. *J Vet Intern Med* 2008; **22**: 1333–1339.
111 Fischer JR, Lane IF, Cribb AE. Urethral pressure profile and hemodynamic effects of phenoxybenzamine and prazosin in non-sedated male beagle dogs. *Can J Vet Res* 2003; **67**: 30–38.
112 Myklejord DJ. Undiagnosed pheochromocytoma: the anesthesiologist nightmare. *Clin Med Res* 2004; **2**: 59–62.
113 Frishman WH, Saunders E. β-Adrenergic blockers. *J Clin Hypertens* 2011; **13**: 649–653.
114 Jaillon P. Relevance of intrinsic sympathomimetic activity for beta blockers. *Am J Cardiol* 1990; **66**: 21C–23C.
115 Ventura HO, Kalapura T. Beta-blocker therapy and severe heart failure: myth or reality? *Congest Heart Fail* 2003; **9**: 197–202.
116 Wiysonge CS, Bradley HA, Volmink J, *et al.* Beta-blockers for hypertension. *Cochrane Database Syst Rev* 2012; **(11)**: CD002003.
117 Foresi A, Cavigioli G, Signorelli G, *et al.* Is the use of beta-blockers in COPD still an unresolved dilemma? *Respiration* 2010; **80**: 177–187.
118 Fonseca VA. Effects of beta-blockers on glucose and lipid metabolism. *Curr Med Res Opin* 2010; **26**: 615–629.
119 Flynn BC, Vernick WJ, Ellis JE. β-Blockade in the perioperative management of the patient with cardiac disease undergoing non-cardiac surgery. *Br J Anaesth* 2011; **107**: 13–15.
120 Flier S, Buhre WF, van Klei WA. Cardioprotective effects of perioperative β-blockade in vascular surgery patients: fact or fiction? *Curr Opin Anaesthesiol* 2011; **24**: 104–110.
121 Khor KH, Campbell FE, Charles BG, *et al.* Comparative pharmacokinetics and pharmacodynamics of tablet, suspension and paste formulations of atenolol in cats. *J Vet Pharmacol Ther* 2012; **35**: 437–445.
122 Meurs KM, Spier AW, Wright NA, *et al.* Comparison of the effects of four antiarrhythmic treatments for familial ventricular arrhythmias in Boxers. *J Am Vet Med Assoc* 2002; **221**: 522–527.
123 Quon CY, Gorczynski RJ. Pharmacodynamics and onset of action of esmolol in anesthetized dogs. *J Pharmacol Exp Ther* 1986; **237**: 912–918.
124 Schober KE, Fuentes VL, Bonagura JD. Comparison between invasive hemodynamic measurements and noninvasive assessment of left ventricular diastolic function by use of Doppler echocardiography in healthy anesthetized cats. *Am J Vet Res* 2003; **64**: 93–103.
125 Verschoor-Kirss M, Rozanski E, Rush JE. Use of esmolol for control of tachycardia in 28 dogs and cats (2003–2020). *J Vet Emerg Crit Care (San Antonio)* 2022; **32**: 243–248.
126 Rush JE, Freeman LM, Hiler C, *et al.* Use of metoprolol in dogs with acquired cardiac disease. *J Vet Cardiol* 2002; **4**: 23–28.
127 Fang J, Semple HA, Song J. Determination of metoprolol and its four metabolites in dog plasma. *J Chromatogr B* 2004; **809**: 9–14.
128 Dumasia MC. In vivo biotransformation of metoprolol in the horse and on-column esterification of the aminocarboxylic acid metabolite by alcohols during

solid phase extraction using mixed mode columns. *J Pharm Biomed Anal* 2006; **40**: 75–81.
129 Regårdh CG, Ek L, Hoffmann KJ. Plasma levels and beta-blocking effect of alpha-hydroxymetoprolol – metabolite of metoprolol – in the dog. *J Pharmacokinet Biopharm* 1979; **7**: 471–479.
130 Romero L, Bel N, Artigas F, *et al.* Effect of pindolol on the function of pre- and postsynaptic 5-HT1A receptors: in vivo microdialysis and electrophysiological studies in the rat brain. *Neuropsychopharmacol* 1996; **15**: 349–360.
131 Kongara K, Chambers P, Johnson CB. Glomerular filtration rate after tramadol, parecoxib and pindolol following anaesthesia and analgesia in comparison with morphine in dogs. *Vet Anaesth Analg* 2009; **36**: 86–94.
132 Mills PC, Siebert GA, Roberts MS. A model to study intestinal and hepatic metabolism of propranolol in the dog. *J Vet Pharmacol Ther* 2004; **27**: 45–48.
133 Baughman TM, Talarico CL, Soglia JR. Evaluation of the metabolism of propranolol by linear ion trap technology in mouse, rat, dog, monkey, and human cryopreserved hepatocytes. *Rapid Commun Mass Spectrom* 2009; **23**: 2146–2150.
134 Jacobs G, Whittem T, Sams R, *et al.* Pharmacokinetics of propranolol in healthy cats during euthyroid and hyperthyroid states. *Am J Vet Res* 1997; **58**: 398–403.
135 Ishizaki T, Tawara K. Relationship between pharmacokinetics and pharmacodynamics of the beta adrenergic blocking drug sotalol in dogs. *J Pharmacol Exp Ther* 1979; **211**: 331–337.

22 Sedatives and Tranquilizers

Catherine M. Creighton and Leigh A. Lamont
Department of Companion Animals, Atlantic Veterinary College, University of Prince Edward Island, Charlottetown, Prince Edward Island, Canada

Chapter contents

Introduction, 333
Phenothiazines, 334
Acepromazine, 334
Butyrophenones, 335
Azaperone, 335
Benzodiazepines, 336
Diazepam, midazolam, and zolazepam, 336
Benzodiazepine antagonist, 338
Flumazenil, 338
α_2-Adrenergic receptor agonists, 338
Xylazine, detomidine, romifidine, medetomidine, and dexmedetomidine, 338
α_2-Adrenergic receptor antagonists, 344
Yohimbine, tolazoline, atipamezole, and vatinoxan, 344
Acknowledgement, 347
References, 347

Introduction

Sedatives and tranquilizers play an important role in day-to-day veterinary practice. The use of these medications as part of an anesthetic plan has many advantages, including, but not limited to, calming the patient, facilitating intravenous (IV) catheterization, providing analgesia, blunting sympathetic responses to surgical stimulation, reducing anesthetic requirements, and promoting smooth induction and recovery. The selection of drugs should be individualized to the patient. Species, age, patient temperament, pathologic processes, blood volume status, and so on should be considered when selecting drugs and doses.

The distinction between a tranquilizer and sedative is often nebulous due to species and dosing differences. For example, α_2-adrenergic receptor agonists are effective in both horses and cattle, but cattle may require one-tenth the horse dose to achieve a comparable level of sedation. Phenothiazines are efficacious in dogs and horses but not so in swine. These distinctions are discussed in this chapter and in chapters pertaining to techniques in different species.

In general, a tranquilizer induces a feeling of calm (anxiolysis). Sedatives, while reducing anxiety, also reduce the overall response to external stimuli. Analgesia is a feature of some sedatives but certainly not all. Clinical practice demonstrates that different species can vary widely in their response to a class of drug, and individuals within a species may also display variable effects. Terminology used varies depending on the source but, in this chapter, all the medications are termed "sedatives," knowing that effects will vary with species and dose.

There are a variety of classes of sedatives currently used in veterinary medicine. Phenothiazines, benzodiazepines, and α_2-adrenergic receptor agonists are among the most commonly used in domestic animals, and they are often combined with opioids and/or other injectable agents to produce variable states of calmness, sedation, and possibly analgesia depending on the medications used. In dogs and cats, increasing appreciation of the stress associated with veterinary visits has resulted in a significant increase in the use of off-label anti-anxiety medications such as gabapentin, trazodone, and melatonin in animals presenting as both out-patients and in-patients. In many cases, these animals also require sedation or general anesthesia while hospitalized for a variety of diagnostic or surgical procedures. Unfortunately, there is little evidence regarding the interactions of these drugs when they are combined with phenothiazines, benzodiazepines, α_2-adrenergic receptor agonists, injectable anesthetics, and inhalant anesthetics in dogs and cats. As a result, most decisions about sedative and anesthetic drug and dose selection in patients receiving gabapentin, trazodone, and melatonin are based on empirical observations of the animal's temperament and demeanor in the immediate preanesthetic period. More information about gabapentin and trazodone is available in Chapter 25.

Veterinary Anesthesia and Analgesia: The Sixth Edition of Lumb and Jones. Edited by Leigh Lamont, Kurt Grimm, Sheilah Robertson, Lydia Love and Carrie Schroeder.
© 2024 John Wiley & Sons, Inc. Published 2024 by John Wiley & Sons, Inc.
Companion website: www.wiley.com/go/lamont/anesthesia

Phenothiazines

In humans, phenothiazines have been used since the 1950s and were once the most widely used antipsychotic agents, prescribed to reduce symptoms in a wide variety of conditions including schizophrenia. They also have clinical applications for control of nausea and vomiting. Interestingly, while sedation is a well-recognized side effect of phenothiazines in people, most antipsychotic drugs cause unpleasant subjective effects in nonpsychotic individuals [1]. Extrapyramidal side-effects have been noted, typically with long-term use in humans or overdose in veterinary patients (tremor, coma/catalepsy, and rigidity). Phenothiazines exhibit activity at a wide variety of receptor systems both centrally and peripherally, including adrenergic, muscarinic, dopaminergic, serotonergic, and histaminergic.

Acepromazine

Mechanism of action and indications

The sedative effects of the phenothiazines are mediated primarily by blockade of dopamine receptors, specifically D_2 receptors. This pre- and postsynaptic G-protein-coupled receptor blockade leads to a decrease in cyclic adenosine monophosphate (cAMP) and adenylate cyclase activity, calcium conductance, and alterations in postsynaptic potassium conductance. Blockade of central α_1-adrenergic, muscarinic, and histaminic (H_1) receptors may also play a role in sedation. α_1-Adrenergic receptor antagonism mediates the decrease in blood pressure noted with this group of medications and may play a role in the decrease in thermoregulatory control (tendency toward poikilothermia), along with serotonin blockade.

Acepromazine has been among the most widely used sedatives in veterinary practice for many years and is labeled for use in small and large animals in many countries. It is generally reliable as a sedative when given parentally, often at doses lower than the label dose, but failure to sedate and/or arousal with stimulation is not uncommon. Muscle relaxation with acepromazine is reasonably good, and the drug has been used to counteract muscle rigidly associated with other agents, such as ketamine. Acepromazine has no inherent analgesic properties when administered alone and is frequently given in combination with opioids to produce *neuroleptanalgesia*, a state characterized by both sedation and analgesia. There is no antagonist available to reverse the clinical anti-dopaminergic effects of acepromazine.

Pharmacokinetics

Acepromazine is highly protein-bound with a large volume of distribution (V_d) [2]. Peak central nervous system (CNS) effects are usually noted 10–20 min after IV administration and 30–40 min after intramuscular (IM) administration [3]. It has a long duration of action with reported elimination half-lives of 3–5 h in the horse [2,4] and 7 h in the dog [5]. In the horse, acepromazine is metabolized extensively in the liver with urinary excretion of metabolites [6]. In dogs, bioavailability after oral administration is approximately 20% [5].

Pharmacodynamics

Cardiovascular system

The hemodynamic impact of acepromazine is variable, likely due to its diverse receptor interactions both centrally and peripherally. Acepromazine-induced blockade of vascular α_1-adrenergic receptors results in peripheral vasodilation and has been reported to decrease stroke volume, cardiac output, and arterial blood pressure by 20–30% in conscious dogs administered 0.1 mg/kg IV [7,8]. More recently, hemodynamic effects were studied in conscious dogs administered IV acepromazine incrementally to cumulative doses of 0.01, 0.025, 0.05, and 0.1 mg/kg. Maximal decreases in stroke index and mean arterial pressure of 16% and 17%, respectively, were reported, but there were no significant changes in systemic vascular resistance or heart rate. The authors attributed the reduction in arterial pressure to reduced myocardial contractility [9]. Conscious horses administered 0.1 mg/kg IV showed a 20–30% decrease in mean aortic pressure and a 10–15% decrease in cardiac output [10]. Mean arterial pressure measured at the tail (not corrected for height) was significantly reduced in standing horses receiving 0.1 mg/kg acepromazine [11]. Standing horses receiving 0.04 mg/kg acepromazine IV had lower facial artery pressures but no real change in digital palmar arterial flow compared with saline-treated horses [12].

Blood pressure can also be reduced in inhalant-anesthetized dogs and horses. Dogs anesthetized with halothane receiving acepromazine at 0.05, 0.125, and 0.25 mg/kg IV displayed reductions in mean arterial pressure of 2.3%, 9.4%, and 16.8%, respectively, that were attenuated by phenylephrine [13]. Dogs anesthetized with propofol and isoflurane receiving IV acepromazine incrementally to cumulative doses of 0.01, 0.025, 0.05, and 0.1 mg/kg had increases in cardiac index but no significant changes in stroke index, systolic, diastolic, or mean arterial pressure, or heart rate [14]. Systemic vascular resistance index, however, decreased by 25% in the dogs receiving 0.05 and 0.1 mg/kg IV cumulative doses. Halothane-anesthetized horses receiving IV acepromazine at 0.03 mg/kg showed a decrease in mean arterial blood pressure of up to 25% [15]. Clinical experience suggests that healthy animals premedicated with low, clinically applicable doses of acepromazine rarely display dramatic decreases in blood pressure during isoflurane or sevoflurane anesthesia; however, the drug's hypotensive effects may be potentiated in hemodynamically unstable patients or in those receiving epidural or spinal local anesthetics. While changes in heart rate are variable and typically not significant, mild reflex tachycardia has been noted in response to decreased systemic vascular resistance and arterial blood pressure [7,10]. Premedication with acepromazine will increase the dose of epinephrine required to induce a ventricular arrhythmia, likely due to α-adrenergic receptor blockade [16–18].

Respiratory system

Acepromazine administration has little effect on pulmonary function. Respiratory rates often decrease, but arterial partial pressure of carbon dioxide ($PaCO_2$) and pH are not typically affected because tidal volume is increased to maintain adequate minute ventilation [10,19]. Acepromazine has been shown to have no impact on respiratory rate and arterial blood gases in halothane-anesthetized horses [15]. Pretreatment with acepromazine (0.035 mg/kg IM) in horses that were subsequently sedated or anesthetized with romifidine, butorphanol, and tiletamine–zolazepam reduced the impact of intrapulmonary shunt and ventilation–perfusion mismatching [20].

Central nervous system

Acepromazine administration has a significant dose-dependent impact on inhalant anesthetic requirements. In dogs, acepromazine at 0.2 mg/kg reduced halothane requirement by 28% and isoflurane requirement by 48% [21]. In another study of dogs anesthetized with halothane, IM administration of acepromazine at 0.02 and 0.2 mg/kg reduced the minimum alveolar concentration (MAC) by

34% and 44%, respectively [22]. In ponies receiving 0.05 mg/kg acepromazine IV, halothane MAC was reduced by 37% [23]. These across-species MAC-sparing effects indicate that patients receiving acepromazine must be closely monitored during anesthesia and the delivery of inhalant anesthetics adjusted accordingly.

For many years, acepromazine administration was associated with seizure activity and was considered contraindicated in veterinary patients with seizure histories. This association dates back to a series of 1950's case reports and experimental studies involving electroencephalographic (EEG) changes induced by another phenothiazine, chlorpromazine, in rabbits and people [24]. A subsequent 1970 study went on to report that high-dose chlorpromazine altered EEG activity in epileptic dogs [25]. Since that time, however, several clinical studies have evaluated the effects of acepromazine in dogs with seizure histories [26,27], or undergoing procedures associated with increased seizure risk (e.g., myelography) [28], and found that acepromazine has no discernible effect on seizure frequency.

Other effects

Hematologic effects of acepromazine administration include decreased packed cell volume and potential effects on platelet aggregation. Hematocrit is reduced in some dogs and horses by 20–30% shortly after acepromazine administration as a result of splenic engorgement after α_1-adrenergic receptor blockade [2,3,12,29]. This effect can last several hours. Hemoglobin is similarly reduced by 14–22% in conscious dogs [9]. Evidence on the effects of acepromazine on platelet function in dogs is conflicting. One study demonstrated decreased platelet aggregation and altered coagulation times with acepromazine [30], while a subsequent thromboelastography study found no effect of acepromazine on platelet function [31].

Acepromazine has well-recognized antiemetic properties that are attributed to antagonism of dopamine receptors in the chemoreceptor trigger zone. In dogs, administration of acepromazine 15 min prior to a variety of opioids reduced the incidence of vomiting from 45% to 18% [32]; however, its efficacy as an antiemetic was less than that of the neurokinin-1 receptor antagonist, maropitant, prior to hydromorphone [33]. Lower esophageal sphincter tone and gastric emptying are reduced with acepromazine in dogs [34–36], but acepromazine with butorphanol was considered acceptable for restraint when performing upper gastrointestinal contrast studies in healthy dogs [36]. In horses, acepromazine administration is associated with similar effects on gastrointestinal motility [37,38]. In dogs, the combination of acepromazine–hydromorphone was less effective than dexmedetomidine–hydromorphone at reducing gastroesophageal reflux during anesthesia when compared to hydromorphone premedication alone [39].

Penile prolapse (priapism) in stallions has been associated with acepromazine administration [40,41]. A 2011 retrospective study by Driessen *et al.* showed that 2.4% of male horses developed penile prolapse lasting 1–4 h [41]. One stallion (0.02%) developed a prolapse lasting more than 12 h but less than 18 h. The incidence of permanent penile paralysis is extremely low but could be catastrophic in valuable breeding males. Glomerular filtration is maintained in dogs premedicated with acepromazine [42,43]. Acepromazine reduces urethral pressure in male cats anesthetized with halothane [44].

Acepromazine has antihistamine effects through its interactions at H_1 receptors and should not be used for intradermal skin testing in dogs when wheal size and induration is assessed [45].

Clinical considerations

For more detailed information on the clinical use of acepromazine in the perianesthetic period in specific species, the reader is directed to species-specific chapters elsewhere in this text.

Dogs and cats

In healthy dogs and cats, acepromazine is commonly administered, often in combination with an opioid, for sedation or prior to induction of general anesthesia at doses ranging from 0.01–0.1 mg/kg IM, subcutaneous (SC), or IV (with the lower end of the dose range typically suggested for the IV route of administration). Lower doses have also been used during recovery from anesthesia to counteract emergence delirium or reduce hospital-associated anxiety. In healthy dogs, the combination of acepromazine with an α_2-adrenergic receptor agonist (e.g., medetomidine and dexmedetomidine) prior to inhalant anesthesia has been investigated and, while effective, the combination does not appear to offer significant advantages [46–48].

There are anecdotal reports that dogs homozygous for the MDR1 (ABCB1) gene mutation, which results in non-functional P-glycoprotein, may show increased sensitivity to various sedative or analgesic drugs, including acepromazine. A small prospective study involving genotyped rough-coated collies showed that those with the homozygous MDR1 mutation tended to have increased and prolonged sedation scores after 0.04 mg/kg acepromazine IV compared to heterozygous or normal dogs [49], but the clinical significance in this and other susceptible breeds remains to be determined. For more information on canine and feline P-glycoprotein deficiency, the reader is referred elsewhere [50]. There have also been anecdotal reports of collapse and sudden death in Boxer dogs following acepromazine administration [51], though the underlying mechanism remains undefined. If this represents an enhanced vasovagal response, then use of a much-reduced dose and/or pretreatment with an anticholinergic may preempt or blunt these adverse effects.

Horses

In horses, acepromazine is administered during the pre- or postanesthetic periods, usually at doses ranging from 0.01–0.05 mg/kg IV. The use of acepromazine in the perianesthetic period has been associated with decreased risk of anesthetic morbidity and mortality [52]. An equine study found that acepromazine 0.02 mg/kg IV was similar to xylazine 0.3 mg/kg IV in its effects on unassisted recovery scores when administered after general anesthesia with isoflurane [53].

Pigs

Acepromazine is used infrequently for sedation in pigs and, when administered alone, its sedative effects in this species are generally considered to be inadequate. In pigs, high doses of acepromazine (1.1 and 1.65 mg/kg IM) have been shown to reduce the incidence of halothane-induced malignant hyperthermia in susceptible animals, while lower doses (0.55 mg/kg IM) only delay its onset [54].

Butyrophenones

Azaperone

Like the phenothiazines, butyrophenone derivatives (e.g., haloperidol) are considered first-generation antipsychotics in humans and have been used for this purpose since the 1950s. In veterinary medicine, this class of drugs is rarely used for sedation in dogs, cats, horses, and domestic cattle; however, the butyrophenone azaperone continues to have clinical applications in swine, zoo animals, and wildlife. Azaperone's mechanism of action, like acepromazine, involves antagonism of central dopaminergic (primarily D_2)

receptors. It also has a similar side effect profile, though with potentially less hypotension due to decreased affinity for vascular α_1-adrenergic receptors [1]. For more information on azaperone as a sedative in veterinary medicine, the reader is referred to species-specific chapters (Chapters 55, 64, and 65) elsewhere in this text.

Benzodiazepines

The benzodiazepines are sedative-hypnotic drugs that have been widely used in human and veterinary medicine for many years. The prototypical drug, diazepam (Valium®), was marketed in the 1960s for anxiety in people, and it became the top-selling pharmaceutical in the United States throughout the 1970s and early 1980s [55]. While there are over 50 benzodiazepine agents used in people and animals for their behavior modifying and anticonvulsant properties [51], only diazepam, midazolam, and zolazepam will be discussed here as they have primary indications in the perianesthetic period.

Benzodiazepines are considered controlled substances in many jurisdictions. In the United States, they are classified as Schedule IV drugs by the Drug Enforcement Administration.

Diazepam, midazolam, and zolazepam

Mechanism of action and indications

γ-aminobutyric acid (GABA) is the primary inhibitory neurotransmitter in the CNS [56]. The $GABA_A$ receptor is a heteropentameric ligand-gated (ionotropic) chloride channel assembled from a family of at least 19 subunits encoded by distinct genes, and these various subunit combinations give rise to numerous receptor subtypes [57]. Benzodiazepines augment GABA-mediated inhibitory transmission at all levels of the CNS through positive allosteric modulation of the $GABA_A$ receptor, resulting in increased chloride conductance and hyperpolarization of postsynaptic cell membranes [58]. The benzodiazepine recognition site on the $GABA_A$ receptor is located at the interface between the α and γ_2 subunits [59]. Barbiturates, ethanol, etomidate, and propofol also all modulate activity at $GABA_A$ receptors, and synergistic effects can result in significant CNS depression. As benzodiazepines enhance endogenous GABA binding to the receptor but lack direct agonist activity, these drugs are associated with a wide safety margin with regard to CNS depression.

While all benzodiazepines share a common chemical structure characterized by a benzene ring linked to a seven-membered diazepine ring, the response to benzodiazepines *in vivo* is multifactorial. Variations in receptor subunit configurations, their locations within the CNS, and a specific drug's affinity for these receptors, as well as lipid solubility and other pharmacokinetic parameters, all impact the clinical effect of a particular drug and dose. In addition, the discovery of the benzodiazepine-binding site on the $GABA_A$ receptor has long fueled speculation that the brain produces its own endogenous ligands for this site [60]. While a number of endogenous benzodiazepine ligands ("endozepines") have been identified [61–63], one in particular (variably called "diazepam-binding inhibitor" [DBI] and "acyl-CoA-binding protein" [ACBP]) has been shown to compete with diazepam for receptor occupation and may be involved in anxiety and mood disorders in humans [64].

Diazepam and midazolam are the most commonly used parenterally administered benzodiazepines in veterinary anesthesia, and their primary indications in the perianesthetic period include anxiolysis, sedation, and muscle relaxation. Their sedative effects, however, are species- and patient-dependent and tend to be mild. In healthy dogs, cats, and horses, they may induce paradoxical behavioral effects including vocalization, excitement, and dysphoria, while in neonatal, geriatric, or systemically ill patients, their sedative effects may be more reliable [51].

Zolazepam is a benzodiazepine that is only available in combination with the dissociative agent, tiletamine, and marketed to veterinarians as Telazol® and Zoletil®. Zolazepam metabolism varies significantly across species, impacting both the duration of effect and quality of recovery with tiletamine–zolazepam combinations. More information about tiletamine–zolazepam can be found in Chapters 27, 55, and 65.

Benzodiazepines do not affect nociceptive pathways and have no inherent analgesic properties. The effects of benzodiazepines are reversible with the specific antagonist, flumazenil.

Pharmacokinetics

Diazepam is highly lipid-soluble and is supplied for injection as a solution of an organic solvent including propylene glycol and ethanol. The formulation is viscous with a pH of 6.6–6.9 and may cause pain on injection. Uptake of diazepam after IM administration is erratic and unpredictable, and this route is not recommended [65]. Diazepam is light sensitive (i.e., undergoes photodegradation) and will bind to plastics if exposed to light for long periods [66,67]. In dogs, diazepam is rapidly absorbed from the gastrointestinal tract, with very high bioavailability, and is metabolized by hepatic microsomal enzymes via oxidative pathways [68,69].

In dogs, the elimination half-life of IV diazepam has been reported to range between 14–16 min (0.5 mg/kg) [70] and 3.2 h (2 mg/kg) [71]. The authors of the former study suggested that this disparity was a result of their lower administered dose or inadequate assay sensitivity such that the terminal phase of their concentration–time curve was not detectable. In dogs given 0.5 mg/kg IV, the active metabolites nordiazepam (also known as "desmethyldiazepam") and oxazepam appear rapidly and persist for longer than the parent compound, with elimination half-lives of 2.2–2.8 and 3.5–5.1 h, respectively [70]. In Greyhounds receiving diazepam at 0.5 mg/kg IV, terminal half-lives were 1.0 h for the parent drug, 2.4 h for nordiazepam, and 6.2 h for oxazepam, indicating that breed differences do exist [68].

Cats receiving very high IV doses of diazepam (5, 10, and 20 mg/kg) had an elimination half-life of approximately 5.5 h. About 50% of the diazepam is rapidly metabolized to nordiazepam, which has a half-life of 21 h in this species [72]. Cats have limited capacity to form glucuronide conjugates of diazepam and its metabolites, which can result in diazepam-induced liver injury with repeated dosing in this species [73].

Horses administered 0.05–0.4 mg/kg diazepam IV demonstrated a half-life of the parent drug ranging from 2.5–21.6 h. Nordiazepam and oxazepam were not detected in plasma but were present in urine, suggesting rapid excretion in this species [74].

Midazolam is the other benzodiazepine commonly administered to veterinary patients in the perianesthetic period. The drug has an open diazepine ring and is formulated at a pH of less than 4.0, which effectively stabilizes the diazepine ring and confers water solubility. On injection at physiologic pH, the diazepine ring closes, rendering the drug lipid-soluble and able to cross the blood–brain barrier rapidly to produce its central effects [75]. This unique chemical structure, along with the fact that midazolam does not contain propylene glycol as a vehicle, means that it does not cause pain on IV injection and is reliably absorbed after IM administration across species. Like diazepam, midazolam is sensitive to light and undergoes photodegradation; it is also extensively metabolized by hepatic microsomal enzymes [76].

In dogs, the elimination half-life of IV midazolam has been reported to range between 63 min (0.2 mg/kg) [77] and 77 min (0.5 mg/kg) [78]. Bioavailability following IM injection is reliable, ranging between 50% [77] and 90% [78]. Time to peak plasma concentration after IM administration of 0.2 or 0.5 mg/kg is 7.8 and 15 min, respectively [77,78]. Mucosal absorption after oral administration in dogs occurs in the oral cavity, esophagus, and stomach and is highly influenced by local pH [79]. The intranasal (IN) route of administration has been investigated in dogs, and both nasal drops and atomizer administration have been shown to be effective [80]. An IN gel formulation had a bioavailability of 70.4% in dogs [81]. Unlike diazepam, the rectal route of administration does not result in clinically useful plasma concentrations with midazolam, and this route is not recommended for acute seizure management [77]. Recent multicenter trials involving canine status epilepticus indicate that IN midazolam (administered via a mucosal atomizer) was superior to rectal diazepam [82] and comparable to IV midazolam for acute seizure management [83]; however, when the time required for IV catheter placement was taken into account, IN midazolam was considered the best option for controlling status epilepticus [83].

In cats administered midazolam at 0.3 mg/kg IV under sevoflurane anesthesia, the elimination half-life was 79 min, and peak plasma concentrations of the active metabolite 1-hydroxymidazolam were reached at 15 min after midazolam administration [84]. This study also reported high inter-individual variability in plasma concentrations of 1-hydroxymidazolam, which had a low clearance and persisted for longer compared to the parent drug. The combination of IN midazolam and ketamine has been evaluated in cats, and this route was associated with a similar onset, degree, and duration of sedation compared to IM administration and was well-tolerated by the cats [85].

In horses, the elimination half-life of IV midazolam has been reported to be 216 min (0.05 mg/kg) and 408 min (0.1 mg/kg), demonstrating dose-dependent kinetics [86].

Pharmacodynamics

Cardiovascular system

Benzodiazepines induce relatively minor cardiovascular changes across species. In healthy dogs, clinically relevant IV doses of diazepam and midazolam have minimal effects on cardiac output, stroke volume, systemic vascular resistance, and coronary arterial blood flow [87]. Similarly, in horses, heart rate, cardiac output, and mean pulmonary arterial, aortic, and right atrial pressures are unchanged after IV diazepam (0.05–0.4 mg/kg) [74]. Consequently, these drugs are commonly suggested for veterinary patients with cardiovascular disease [88,89]. In dogs, however, there is no evidence suggesting that the combination of a benzodiazepine with an induction agent (e.g., propofol or alfaxalone) improves cardiovascular function compared to the induction agent alone.

Respiratory system

The effects of benzodiazepines on pulmonary function are also minimal. Arterial blood gas values are unchanged in horses receiving IV diazepam (0.05–0.4 mg/kg) [74], and in swine receiving IV midazolam (0.1–1.0 mg/kg) [90]. At high doses, when combined with other CNS depressants, or when administered to patients with significant pulmonary disease, benzodiazepine-induced respiratory depression may be evident.

Central nervous system

Diazepam and midazolam modestly reduce injectable and inhalant anesthetic requirements when administered in the perianesthetic period. In healthy dogs, both diazepam and midazolam have been shown to reduce the induction dose requirements for propofol and alfaxalone, but the addition of the benzodiazepine does not necessarily improve cardiopulmonary stability over propofol or alfaxalone alone [91–94]. Inhalant-sparing effects have also been documented with diazepam (0.044 mg/kg IV) reducing halothane MAC by 29% in ponies [95] and the combination of diazepam-fentanyl reducing isoflurane MAC by 74% compared to 54% with fentanyl alone in dogs [96]. In isoflurane-anesthetized dogs, IV midazolam (loading dose and constant-rate infusion [CRI]) dose-dependently reduces MAC, but a ceiling effect is evident with maximal MAC reduction of approximately 30% [97].

Benzodiazepines produce muscle relaxation through inhibitory effects on polysynaptic reflexes and spinal internuncial transmission and, at very high doses, may depress skeletal neuromuscular junction transmission [98]. At clinical doses, they may cause muscle weakness and ataxia and, in some species, this may progress to recumbency. Benzodiazepines are frequently co-administered with dissociative agents (ketamine and tiletamine) to counteract muscle rigidity associated with these drugs.

Benzodiazepines have well-recognized anticonvulsant properties and are able to inhibit the development and spread of epileptiform electrical activity in the CNS [98]. In the case of diazepam, its active metabolites, nordiazepam and oxazepam, are associated with 25–33% less anticonvulsant activity than the parent drug [99]. They generally have a favorable profile with regard to cerebral perfusion, reducing cerebral oxygen consumption to a greater extent than cerebral blood flow [100].

Clinical considerations

Dogs and cats

In dogs and cats, diazepam and midazolam are commonly administered in the preanesthetic period, often in combination with opioids, or as co-induction agents with ketamine, propofol, or alfaxalone. In hemodynamically unstable small animal patients, the combination of a benzodiazepine and full μ-opioid receptor agonist may be used to induce general anesthesia. While midazolam is considered more potent than diazepam in humans, dose ranges in dogs and cats are similar (0.1–0.4 mg/kg IV), and the two drugs are often used interchangeably in the perianesthetic period. Anticonvulsant doses for both drugs tend to be higher (0.5–1.0 mg/kg IV). As discussed above, the IM route of administration is not recommended for diazepam due to pain and erratic absorption associated with the propylene glycol vehicle. The availability of multiple effective routes of administration for midazolam make it a more versatile option in the clinical setting. In general, the sedative effects of benzodiazepines in healthy dogs and cats are minimal and unreliable if not combined with other sedative-hypnotic agents. Paradoxical excitation characterized by restlessness, agitation, and vocalization is common as doses increase, especially in cats [78,101]. Behavioral disinhibition due to anxiolysis may even provoke aggressive behavior in some animals.

Horses

In adult horses, midazolam (0.5–0.1 mg/kg IV) alone produces minimal sedation but is associated with ataxia, weakness, postural sway, and agitation [86], making it unsuitable for procedures requiring standing sedation. In neonatal foals, however, the combination of an IV benzodiazepine with an opioid tends to produce reliable sedation but may be accompanied by weakness leading to recumbency. For induction of general anesthesia in adult horses sedated with an α_2-adrenergic receptor agonist, either diazepam or midazolam (0.05–0.1 mg/kg IV) is commonly co-administered with ketamine to enhance muscle relaxation, smooth induction, and facilitate endotracheal intubation. With commercial preparations of guaifenesin no longer available in many countries, midazolam has also been investigated as an alternative to guaifenesin for equine total intravenous anesthesia (TIVA). The infusion of midazolam–xylazine–ketamine after induction appears to be suitable for extending the duration of anesthesia for up to 1 h in horses [102].

Other species

In addition to dogs, cats, and horses, midazolam has been used in a wide variety of species including swine, goats, sheep, alpacas, ferrets, rabbits, guinea pigs, and birds [103–108]. In general, small ruminants, ferrets, rabbits, and birds tend to sedate reasonably well with benzodiazepines, often in combination with other drugs such as opioids, α_2-adrenergic receptor agonists, alfaxalone, and ketamine. The IN route of administration has been studied in rabbits [107] and various avian species [109,110].

Benzodiazepine antagonist

Flumazenil

Flumazenil is a competitive antagonist with a high affinity for the benzodiazepine recognition site on the $GABA_A$ receptor but no appreciable agonist activity at the site. As the drug is specific to the benzodiazepine-binding site on the receptor, it does not antagonize the CNS effects of other anesthetic agents interacting with the $GABA_A$ receptor such as propofol, alfaxalone, etomidate, and barbiturates. Flumazenil attenuates the CNS depressant effects of benzodiazepines and has been shown to reverse their EEG changes in dogs [111,112]. When administered in the absence of a benzodiazepine, the drug does not appear to induce appreciable CNS stimulation (e.g., agitation, excitement, and tachypnea) in veterinary species [51]. While flumazenil is thought to antagonize the effects of endogenous benzodiazepine-like substances (endozepines), which are elevated in human patients with hepatic encephalopathy, there is little evidence supporting its use for clinical management of hepatic encephalopathy in people [113].

As a conventional antagonist (as opposed to an inverse agonist that acts as a negative allosteric modulator of GABA receptor function), flumazenil appears devoid of direct cardiovascular, respiratory, or musculoskeletal effects but is effective in reversing benzodiazepine-induced changes in these systems. In humans, however, antagonism of benzodiazepine-induced respiratory depression may be less predictable [98].

There is little pharmacokinetic information available about flumazenil in veterinary species. Reversal of excessive benzodiazepine-induced sedation in the perianesthetic period may be accomplished in dogs with IV doses of 0.01–0.04 mg/kg, and in horses with IV doses of 0.01–0.02 mg/kg. Repeated doses may be necessary if sedation persists or if re-sedation is noted.

In humans, it is well recognized that flumazenil may precipitate abstinence syndrome in individuals that have developed physiologic dependence to chronic oral benzodiazepines. This phenomenon has been reported experimentally in dogs, though the doses of flumazenil studied were very high [114]. Furthermore, flumazenil may precipitate seizures and cardiac arrhythmias in humans that have ingested an overdose of benzodiazepines with tricyclic antidepressants. An experimental study involving dogs administered infusions of midazolam and amitriptyline that were suddenly reversed with flumazenil demonstrated the potential for convulsions and arrhythmias in this species [115]. For these reasons, flumazenil is not routinely recommended for the treatment of benzodiazepine or mixed drug overdose in humans but should be reserved for selected patients where the benefits of flumazenil administration outweigh the potential risks [116].

α_2-Adrenergic receptor agonists

Xylazine was discovered in 1962 as an antihypertensive agent by Farbenfabriken Bayer AG in Leverkusen, Germany, many years before its mechanism of action as an α_2-adrenergic receptor agonist was elucidated [117]. During early clinical trials in people, xylazine induced excessive CNS depression, and the drug was abandoned for human use and introduced to the veterinary market as a sedative, analgesic, and muscle relaxant [117]. Early reports of its use in animals began appearing in the late 1960s and early 1970s [118–122], and it soon became one of the most commonly administered sedatives in veterinary medicine, especially in large animals. It was not until 1981 that xylazine's CNS depressant effects were definitively attributed to its actions at central α_2-adrenergic receptors [123]. Over the next 40 years, that discovery would spearhead development of new, more specific veterinary α_2-adrenergic receptor agonists including detomidine, romifidine, and medetomidine/dexmedetomidine. Dexmedetomidine is also used in human patients for procedural sedation, ICU sedation in mechanically ventilated patients, and as an adjunct to general anesthesia.

While α_2-adrenergic receptor agonists have not historically been classified as controlled substances, concerns about illicit xylazine use as an emerging public health threat, coupled with the potential for diversion from veterinary channels, is leading to regulatory changes involving xylazine in several jurisdictions including in the United States and Canada.

Xylazine, detomidine, romifidine, medetomidine, and dexmedetomidine

Mechanism of action and indications

The clinically desired effects of these drugs (sedation, analgesia, and muscle relaxation) are a result of their interactions with α_2-adrenergic receptors located both pre- and postsynaptically in the CNS. In addition, α_2-adrenergic receptors are also widely distributed throughout peripheral tissues with pre- and postsynaptic receptors found in many organs and postsynaptic (extrajunctional) receptors located on vascular endothelium and on platelets. These peripheral receptors mediate many of the adverse effects associated with α_2-adrenergic receptor agonist administration in the clinical setting.

The α_2-adrenergic receptor is a G-protein-coupled receptor that has been recognized as four distinct subtypes: α_{2A}, α_{2B}, α_{2C}, and α_{2D}. The α_{2A} subtype was first discovered in human platelets and rabbit spleen, the α_{2B} subtype in rat lung and kidney, the α_{2C} subtype in opossum kidney, and the α_{2D} subtype in rat submaxillary gland and bovine pineal gland [124]. Because the α_{2A} and α_{2D} subtypes are structurally similar in mammalian species, they are now believed to be the same receptor but with differing pharmacologic profiles in humans, dogs, rabbits, pigs, and chickens (α_{2A}) versus rats, mice, and cattle (α_{2D}) [125,126]. To further complicate the nomenclature, a fourth non-mammalian receptor subtype, also called "α_{2D}," has also been identified in zebrafish [127]. Despite the potential for subtype-specific effects, the distinction is not clinically relevant as none of the currently available α_2-adrenergic receptor agonists or antagonists is subtype specific.

Agonist binding at all subtypes by endogenous ligands (norepinephrine, epinephrine) or exogenous α_2-adrenergic receptor agonists results in allosteric inhibition through $G_{i/o}$ leading to inhibition of adenylate cyclase activity and decreased cAMP concentrations. Subsequent inhibition of Ca^{2+} entry and activation of outward-opening K^+ channels result in membrane hyperpolarization and suppression of neuronal firing [128,129]. While inhibition of adenylate cyclase is considered the classic α_2-adrenergic receptor signaling pathway, other effector mechanisms also appear to play a role.

The α_{2A} and α_{2C} subtypes predominate in the CNS and are largely responsible for the sedative, analgesic, and sympatholytic effects of α_2-adrenergic receptor agonists [130]. The locus coeruleus in the medial dorsal pons is the major noradrenergic nucleus of the brain and contains dense populations of α_2-adrenergic receptors. Activation of presynaptic receptors here results in inhibition of norepinephrine release and reduced activity in ascending noradrenergic pathways, resulting in hypnosis and sedation [131,132]. Activation of this negative feedback loop may also produce reductions in heart rate and blood pressure and attenuation of the sympathetic stress response.

At the level of the spinal cord dorsal horn, stimulation of α_2-adrenergic receptors inhibits nociceptive neurons and reduces the release of norepinephrine and substance P. Although there is some evidence for supraspinal (i.e., descending modulation via the locus coeruleus) and peripheral sites of analgesic action, the spinal mechanism is thought to be responsible for most of the analgesia associated with α_2-adrenergic receptor agonists [132].

The α_{2B} subtype is located primarily on vascular smooth muscle and largely mediates vasoconstriction [132]. Some effects of α_2-adrenergic receptor stimulation do not appear to be mediated through G-protein coupling, such as inhibition of platelet aggregation.

In addition to their effects at α_2-adrenergic receptors, all α_2-adrenergic receptor agonists currently in clinical use also have some impact on α_1-adrenergic receptors and most also activate nonadrenergic imidazoline receptors (Table 22.1). Activation of vascular α_1-adrenergic receptors contributes to vasoconstriction and increased systemic vascular resistance, while activation of central α_1-adrenergic receptors has been associated with increased arousal, restlessness, vigilance, and locomotor activity in animals [133]. In theory, α_2-adrenergic receptor agonists that are less selective for α_2-adrenergic receptors may be more likely to cause adverse effects such as paradoxical excitement and locomotor activity. Of the commonly used α_2-adrenergic receptor agonists, xylazine has the lowest α_2:α_1 adrenergic receptor binding ratio (Table 22.1).

Table 22.1 α_2:α_1 adrenergic receptor selectivity and imidazoline activity for selected α_2-adrenergic receptor agonists and antagonists.

Drug	α_2:α_1 adrenergic receptor binding ratio	Imidazoline receptor activity
Agonists		
Xylazine	160:1	No[a]
Detomidine	260:1	Yes
Romifidine	340:1	Yes
Medetomidine	1620:1	Yes[a]
Dexmedetomidine	1620:1	Yes[a]
Antagonists		
Tolazoline	4:1	Yes
Yohimbine	40:1	No[a]
Atipamezole	8526:1	Yes[a]
Vatinoxan	105:1[b]	Yes[c]

[a] [136];
[b] [137];
[c] [138]

All of the α_2-adrenergic receptor agonists currently used in veterinary medicine, except for xylazine, have structural similarities to imidazoline and thus may also activate the various subtypes of imidazoline receptors (Table 22.1). Differentiating α_2-adrenergic versus imidazoline receptor-mediated effects is difficult and there appears to be considerable overlap. The I_1 receptor plays a role in cardiovascular regulation and has been implicated in modulation of sodium excretion and urine output, inhibition of catecholamine-induced arrhythmias, and possibly neuroprotective effects [134]. The I_2 receptor may be involved in control of central noradrenergic and hypothalamic–pituitary–adrenal axis activity, regulation of intestinal motility, and opioid-induced antinociception [134]. The I_3 receptor may play a role in insulin secretion and contribute to α_2-adrenergic agonist-induced hyperglycemia [135].

The α_2-adrenergic receptor agonists are used extensively in veterinary patients to provide chemical restraint, sedation, analgesia, and as adjuncts to general anesthesia. They are a versatile class of drugs and can be administered via a variety of routes including IV, IM, IV CRI, oral transmucosal (OTM), IN, neuraxial (epidural, spinal), and perineural. In some species, notably cats, α_2-adrenergic receptor agonists reliably induce vomiting and may be used as emetics.

Pharmacokinetics

In general, the onset of action of α_2-adrenergic receptor agonists after IV administration is rapid (within minutes), and peak effects are noted shortly thereafter. IM administration of α_2-adrenergic receptor agonists is typically associated with rapid absorption, but plasma concentrations show significant variation in the first 60 min following IM administration across species and between individuals of the same species. Differences in study design and pharmacokinetic methodology can further confound interpretation. While the SC route of administration has not historically been recommended due to concerns about poor absorption related to peripheral vasoconstriction, there is some evidence in humans [139,140] and horses [141] to suggest that the SC route may be effective and could be clinically useful. Other alternate routes of systemic administration such as OTM and IN have also been investigated for specific drugs. As the α_2-adrenergic receptor agonists are highly lipophilic, neuraxial (epidural, spinal) administration to enhance and prolong local anesthetic-induced regional anesthesia results in significant systemic absorption and is usually accompanied by dose-dependent CNS depression (sedation) and cardiovascular effects that are comparable to systemic α_2-adrenergic receptor agonist administration. Perineural administration to enhance and prolong local anesthetic-induced peripheral nerve blockade tends to be associated with lower plasma drug concentrations and possibly fewer systemic side effects.

For xylazine, pharmacokinetic parameters have been described in dogs, horses, cattle, and sheep by a two-compartment model [142]. In the same study, elimination half-lives after IV administration of varying species-specific doses ranged between 22 min in sheep and 50 min in horses. After IM administration, peak plasma concentrations were attained within 12–14 min in all species, but mean bioavailability was higher in dogs (74%) compared to horses (45%) and sheep (41%) [142]. In racing horses, the pharmacokinetics of xylazine have been re-evaluated more recently from a regulatory medicine perspective. After IV administration of 0.3–0.4 mg/kg xylazine, drug disposition was found to fit a three-compartment model with reported systemic clearances of 12.7 and 15.8 mL/min/kg, β half-lives of 2.79 and 3.53 h, and γ half-lives of 26 and 29.8 h [143,144]. Identification of this third compartment, and the associated prolonged γ half-lives, reflects increased sensitivity of the analytical methods used and may not be clinically relevant in the perianesthetic period. In conscious horses receiving xylazine at 0.5 mg/kg IV followed by a CRI of 1 mg/kg/h for 2, 4, and 6 h, plasma concentration–time curves were best described by a one-compartment model, and xylazine did not appear to accumulate in plasma or tissues with longer infusion periods [145]. In horses recovering from isoflurane anesthesia, a single IV dose of 0.2 mg/kg xylazine was associated with significantly slower plasma kinetics compared to a single IV dose of 0.875 μg/kg dexmedetomidine, but no differences in time to stand or recovery quality were observed [146]. The intraosseous route has also been shown to be effective for administration of xylazine in horses [147].

Regarding detomidine, pharmacokinetic studies in horses at IV doses ranging between 10 and 80 μg/kg suggest a two-compartment model with some evidence of dose-dependent elimination [148–150]. In resting horses, 40 μg/kg IV had a median half-life of 26 min, a volume of distribution of 585 mL/kg, and a median clearance of 15 mL/min/kg. After supramaximal exercise, these parameters increased to 46 min, 1296 mL/kg, and 20 min, respectively [150]. In another equine study, the mean elimination half-life of a 30 μg/kg dose was 26 min for the IV route of administration versus 53 min for the IM route [151]. In cattle, 80 μg/kg of detomidine IV or IM showed rapid absorption and distribution, with an elimination half-life of 1.3 h following the IV dose and 2.6 h following the IM dose [148].

Injectable detomidine has also been evaluated for OTM administration, and an oromucosal gel is marketed in some countries for use in horses. In horses, the mean bioavailability for the gel was 22% after sublingual administration of 40 μg/kg, compared with 38.2% following the same dose of injectable detomidine administered IM [152]. In addition to horses, OTM detomidine administration has been evaluated in other species including calves [153], dogs [154–156], ferrets [157], rabbits [158], and cats [159] with varying results. Though bioavailability with the OTM route of administration was lower, clinically relevant sedation was achieved in dogs, ferrets, and cats. In horses and alpacas, detomidine gel administered intravaginally resulted in clinically relevant sedation and bioavailabilities of 25% and 20%, respectively [160,161]. Detomidine has also been administered intranasally via a mucosal atomizer in sheep [162].

Romifidine administered at 80 μg/kg IV to horses resulted in plasma concentrations fitted to a two-compartment model with a prolonged elimination half-life of 135 min [163]. Administration of a lower dose (10 μg/kg IV) prior to exercise in horses confirmed the two-compartment model and the extended elimination half-life [164].

The pharmacokinetics of dexmedetomidine and racemic medetomidine (a mixture of both dexmedetomidine and levomedetomidine) are very similar in dogs [165]. All of the pharmacologic actions of medetomidine are due to the dextrorotatory isomer, which is isolated in dexmedetomidine. Administration of medetomidine at 40 μg/kg IV and dexmedetomidine at 20 and 10 μg/kg IV produced peak sedation at 10–20 min at plasma concentrations of 18.5, 14, and 5.5 ng/mL, respectively, in dogs. Terminal half-lives of 0.96, 0.78, and 0.66 h were reported [166]. Administration of levomedetomidine produced no apparent sedation or analgesia. Clearance of levomedetomidine was faster [166]. The pharmacokinetics of IM dexmedetomidine (10 μg/kg) administered to healthy dogs have been reported and show significant variations in individual plasma concentrations. In cats anesthetized with isoflurane and administered 10 μg/kg dexmedetomidine IV over 5 min, a mean terminal half-life of 198 min was reported [167]. In horses and ponies, IV dexmedetomidine or medetomidine results in rapid reductions in plasma drug concentrations with reported elimination half-lives ranging between 8 and 29 min depending on the study [168–170]. In horses recovering from isoflurane anesthesia, a single IV dose of 0.875 μg/kg dexmedetomidine was associated with significantly faster plasma kinetics compared to a single IV dose of 0.2 mg/kg xylazine, but no differences in time to stand or recovery quality were observed [146].

Similar to detomidine, OTM administration of injectable medetomidine and dexmedetomidine has been investigated in cats and dogs, and an oromucosal dexmedetomidine gel is also marketed for noise phobia in dogs in a number of countries. In cats, OTM medetomidine produced similar sedation compared to IM injection but took longer to achieve peak plasma concentrations (43 versus 21 min). Individual variation was suspected to be secondary to salivation and drug loss [171]. Dexmedetomidine has also been administered to cats using the OTM route, sometimes combined with buprenorphine [172–174]. In dogs, 20 μg/kg of dexmedetomidine administered OTM was compared to a 5 μg/kg IV dose. Despite a bioavailability of only 11.2%, OTM dexmedetomidine produced a similar degree of sedation and a prolonged duration of action compared to IV administration [175]. The OTM route has also been evaluated for a combination of dexmedetomidine and methadone in dogs [176].

IN dexmedetomidine has been evaluated for sedation in children and, more recently, in dogs and cats. In healthy Beagles, 20 μg/kg dexmedetomidine administered IN resulted in slower absorption and lower plasma concentrations at all time points compared to IM administration, despite clinically similar sedation effects [177]. Perineural administration of 0.5 μg/kg dexmedetomidine with levobupivacaine for inferior alveolar and infraorbital nerve blocks in anesthetized dogs resulted in lower plasma dexmedetomidine concentrations compared to IV administration [178].

In most species, dexmedetomidine appears to undergo hepatic metabolism to pharmacologically inactive metabolites by hydroxylation, oxidation, or conjugation. In human intensive care unit patients, where the drug is commonly used as a sedative, high inter-individual pharmacokinetic variability has been described with factors such as body size, hepatic impairment, plasma albumin, and cardiac output reported to influence pharmacokinetics.

Pharmacodynamics

Cardiovascular system

The α_2-adrenergic receptor agonists in current clinical use induce significant cardiovascular effects that are typically described as biphasic. Initially, activation of postsynaptic α_1- and α_{2B}-adrenergic receptors results in peripheral vasoconstriction, increased systemic vascular resistance, and increased arterial blood pressure. These peripheral changes induce a baroreceptor-mediated reflex bradycardia, which, while it may attenuate hypertension to some extent, results in significant reductions in cardiac output. While there is substantial variation depending on the drug, the dose, the route of administration, and the species, initial hemodynamic changes typically include bradycardia, with or without bradyarrhythmias, and hypertension. At the same time, activation of central presynaptic α_{2A}- and α_{2C}-adrenergic receptors results in reduced norepinephrine release and sympathetic outflow, which perpetuates bradycardia and the reduction in cardiac output. The net result of these secondary hemodynamic changes is usually bradycardia and hypotension.

At clinically relevant doses, α_2-adrenergic receptor agonists have been shown to decrease cardiac output in most species by greater than 50% [179–182]. This reduction in cardiac output is largely due to changes in cardiac loading conditions (increased systemic vascular resistance and bradycardia) rather than direct effects on myocardial contractility [183,184]. While these effects are often considered to be dose-dependent, even low bolus doses may induce adverse cardiovascular effects [179], and there seems to be a "ceiling effect" whereby higher doses do not necessarily worsen cardiovascular parameters [166]. It is important to note that the influence of other drugs administered concurrently (e.g., inhalant anesthetics) and the route of administration (e.g., IV bolus, versus IM, versus low-dose CRI) will also impact the magnitude of cardiovascular changes [185,186].

The reduction in cardiac output is not uniform across all tissue beds with blood flow redistributed away from nonessential regions such as skin, adipose tissue, skeletal muscle, and intestine, and is redirected to essential organs such as brain, heart, and kidneys [179,187]. α_2-Adrenergic receptor agonists do not adversely impact myocardial perfusion and may beneficially modulate coronary blood flow during myocardial ischemia [188,189].

The bradycardia induced by α_2-adrenergic receptor agonists can be significant and, in addition to sinus bradycardia, vagally mediated bradyarrhythmias such as first- and second-degree atrioventricular block are commonly observed in some species (dogs and horses) [190]. More serious bradyarrhythmias such as third-degree atrioventricular block and sinus arrest are rare. The less selective α_2-adrenergic receptor agonist, xylazine, has been shown to reduce the arrhythmogenic dose of epinephrine (ADE) in halothane- and isoflurane-anesthetized dogs [191,192]; however, the more selective agents (with less α_1-adrenergic receptor activity), such as detomidine, medetomidine, and dexmedetomidine, do not alter the ADE and may even have a protective effect against ventricular arrhythmias [193–195].

Routine administration of an anticholinergic to prevent or counteract bradycardia during the initial phase of α_2-adrenergic receptor agonist-mediated peripheral vasoconstriction is not recommended. While anticholinergic administration in the face of increased systemic vascular resistance may increase heart rate, cardiac output does not increase proportionally and other adverse effects have been documented including hypertension, increased myocardial oxygen consumption, and arrhythmias [190,196–198]. Once the initial increase in systemic vascular resistance begins to wane leaving the central sympatholytic effects to predominate, anticholinergic administration may be considered on a case-by-case basis to treat persistent bradycardia, especially if it is accompanied by hypotension.

Respiratory system

α_2-Adrenergic receptor agonists induce centrally mediated reductions in both respiratory rate and minute ventilation [199,200]; however, increases in arterial carbon dioxide tension ($PaCO_2$) and decreases in arterial oxygen tension (PaO_2) are not usually significant in most species [181,199–202]. Co-administration of α_2-adrenergic receptor agonists with other sedatives, opioids, or anesthetics may lead to more significant impairment of ventilatory drive predisposing to hypercapnia and possibly hypoxemia. In isoflurane-anesthetized mechanically ventilated dogs, however, a low-dose dexmedetomidine CRI (1 μg/kg/h IV), with or without a 1 μg/kg IV loading dose, actually improved oxygenation and respiratory system compliance, and reduced intrapulmonary shunt fraction and airway resistance [203]. In humans, dexmedetomidine is commonly used for sedation in patients requiring mechanical ventilation in intensive care settings.

Administration of α_2-adrenergic receptor agonists commonly causes mucous membranes to appear "muddy" or pale blue/gray as peripheral vasoconstriction slows blood flow in the periphery. The prolonged capillary transit time allows greater oxygen extraction, resulting in a greater amount of deoxygenated hemoglobin being present at the venous end of the capillary. This often exceeds the 5 mg/dL threshold of deoxygenated hemoglobin associated with the clinical observation of cyanosis. It should be appreciated that PaO_2 values in this situation are often normal or near normal; thus, the observation of cyanosis in this context has a different implication than when it is noted in patients with arterial hypoxemia due to pulmonary disease or severe hypoventilation.

Sheep are uniquely susceptible to hypoxemia following administration of α_2-adrenergic receptor agonists due to activation of pulmonary intravascular macrophages, which damage capillary endothelium and alveolar type I cells, leading to intra-alveolar hemorrhage and interstitial and pulmonary edema [204,205].

Central nervous system

α_2-Adrenergic receptor agonist-mediated sedation results from activation of α_2-adrenergic receptors in the locus coeruleus of the pons and the rostroventral lateral medulla (the primary areas for sympathetic outflow from the CNS). This reduces norepinephrine release, which diminishes arousal as the discharge frequency of tracts into the cortex slows.

Rigidity, seizures, and/or excitement have been noted following accidental intracarotid injection of xylazine in horses. Failure to sedate, or paradoxical excitement, can result when animals are excited, fearful, in pain, or otherwise stressed. These conditions result in high circulating catecholamine levels, which are difficult to overcome with α_2-adrenergic receptor agonist administration [190,206]. Animals that appear sedated may be suddenly aroused and display aggressive behavior if disturbed and may demonstrate increased sensitivity to sound and tactile stimulation [206]. Activation of central α_1-adrenergic receptors has been shown to functionally antagonize the hypnotic response to α_2-adrenergic receptor agonists [207], and α_1-adrenergic stimulation may contribute to some of these paradoxical behaviors, especially with less selective agents such as xylazine.

Analgesia results from agonist binding to pre- and postsynaptic α_2-adrenergic receptors at various points in nociceptive pathways including the substantia gelatinosa of the spinal cord dorsal horn and the locus coeruleus of the brainstem [208]. Afferent input into the dorsal horn from peripheral nociceptors continues but is modulated and dampened by decreases in norepinephrine and substance P release resulting from presynaptic α_2-adrenergic receptor binding. Postsynaptic α_2-adrenergic receptor binding in the dorsal horn and supraspinally results in neuronal hyperpolarization and inhibition of nociceptive neurons. Interaction with imidazoline receptors (specifically the I_2 receptor) may also play a role in α_2-adrenergic receptor agonist analgesia through modulation of opioid antinociception [134]. It has been noted that analgesic effects seem to be shorter-lived than sedative effects in a number of species, and plasma drug concentrations exceeding those associated with sedation may be required to produce antinociception [149].

While α_2-adrenergic receptors and opioid receptors share similar molecular machinery and are present in similar locations throughout the CNS, α_2-adrenergic receptor agonists and opioids have sufficiently different mechanisms of analgesia to result in synergism when co-administered. Co-administration with other analgesics such as local anesthetics and ketamine via a variety of routes (systemically, neuraxially, or in peripheral nerve blocks) is common in clinical practice. In humans, dexmedetomidine has been shown to significantly improve postoperative outcomes when used as part of an Enhanced Recovery After Surgery (ERAS) protocol and is recommended as part of a multimodal opioid-sparing approach [209].

The central effects of α_2-adrenergic receptor agonists (both sedative and analgesic) induce significant anesthetic-sparing effects when combined with injectable or inhalant anesthetics. Effects are dose-dependent and vary by drug, species, and route of administration, but α_2-adrenergic receptor agonist-induced reductions in anesthetic requirements of up to 90% have been reported [51,190]. This underscores the importance of titrating injectable and inhalant anesthetic doses to effect when combined with this potent class of drugs.

The effects of α_2-adrenergic receptor agonists on cerebral hemodynamics and intracranial pressure (ICP) have been studied experimentally in animals and clinically in humans with various types of neurologic disease. In isoflurane-anesthetized dogs, medetomidine did not change ICP [210], and dexmedetomidine reduced cerebral blood flow with no alteration in cerebral metabolic rate of oxygen [211]. In humans, these neuroprotective effects (i.e., reduced cerebral blood flow and ICP) have led to dexmedetomidine's use in neurosurgical patients and those with traumatic brain injury to provide sedation and lower opioid requirements [212]. In veterinary patients with neurologic disease, the decision to include an α_2-adrenergic receptor agonist in the anesthetic plan should be made on a case-by-case basis after considering the potential for respiratory depression when these drugs are combined with opioids and anesthetic agents, the significant hemodynamic effects, the potential for hyperglycemia, and the potential to induce vomiting and elevate ICP.

Thermoregulation is impaired in patients administered α_2-adrenergic receptor agonists due to CNS depression and reduced muscle activity. However, as these drugs cause peripheral vasoconstriction and redistribution of blood flow from the skin to the core, hypothermia may be less significant compared to drugs that cause peripheral vasodilation, such as acepromazine and inhalant anesthetics. Regardless, body temperature should be monitored, especially in small animals, and thermoregulatory support provided as needed.

The effects of α_2-adrenergic receptor agonists on pupil size vary by species with mydriasis reported in cats, rats, and rabbits, and either no change in pupil size or miosis reported in dogs. In most species, reductions in intraocular pressure have been reported, but this effect is less consistent in dogs. The potential for α_2-adrenergic receptor agonist-induced nausea and vomiting must be considered when planning to sedate or anesthetize small animal patients that may be adversely affected by fluctuations in intraocular pressure [190].

Gastrointestinal system

α_2-Adrenergic receptor agonists induce nausea and vomiting in dogs and cats through stimulation of the chemoreceptor trigger zone, which is in close proximity to the locus coeruleus [213–215]. Depending on the drug, dose, route of administration, and other drugs administered concurrently, α_2-adrenergic receptor agonists may induce vomiting in up to 90% of cats and 30% of dogs [51,190].

Gastrointestinal transit time is prolonged and gastric acid secretion, reticuloruminal contractions, and colonic motility are reduced with α_2-adrenergic receptor agonists [216–218]. These effects are reversible with α_2-adrenergic receptor antagonists confirming that effects on gastrointestinal motility are mediated by α_2-adrenergic receptors.

Genitourinary system

The diuretic effects of α_2-adrenergic receptor agonists are mediated through multiple mechanisms including reduced production or release of antidiuretic hormone (ADH) from the pituitary gland; inhibition of ADH activity on renal collecting tubules; and enhanced sodium excretion [219–222]. The renin–angiotensin–aldosterone system is also impacted directly through activation of renal α_2-adrenergic receptors and indirectly through α_2-adrenergic receptor agonist-induced hypertension, resulting in reduced renin secretion and enhanced diuresis [223]. α_2-Adrenergic receptor agonists also impact micturition resulting in decreased micturition pressure, urinary bladder capacity, micturition volume, and residual volume, and these effects appear to be mediated largely through central (spinal) mechanisms [224]. Clinically, the net result of these effects is that animals administered α_2-adrenergic receptor agonists tend to produce large volumes of dilute urine.

Myometrial tone and intrauterine pressure can increase with α_2-adrenergic receptor stimulation [225–229]; however, the clinical effects of α_2-adrenergic receptor agonist administration are not consistent, and there is considerable variation with different drugs, doses, routes of administration, timing within the reproductive cycle, and species. Classically, xylazine was reported to induce oxytocin-like contraction of the bovine uterus [225] and, based on anecdotal reports of premature labor and spontaneous abortions in heifers, its use in heavily pregnant cattle was cautioned despite minimal evidence implicating xylazine in these cases. Regarding the more specific α_2-adrenergic receptor agonists, detomidine (< 60 μg/kg IM in the cow and horse) [230,231] and medetomidine (< 20 μg/kg IV in the dog) [229] have been shown to decrease myometrial contractions. However, higher doses of medetomidine (40–60 μg/kg IV) did increase electrical activity of the pregnant canine uterus [229]. Fluctuations in circulating levels of steroid hormones throughout pregnancy may impact these changes with estrogen upregulating excitatory α-adrenergic receptors and progesterone upregulating inhibitory β-adrenergic receptors in the reproductive tract [229,232]. Overall, these reproductive effects, combined with potentially significant cardiovascular effects, suggest α_2-adrenergic receptor agonists should only be administered to near-term pregnant animals on a case-by-case basis after a risk-benefit analysis.

Other effects

Muscle relaxation is reliably produced through inhibition of α_2-adrenergic receptors at spinal cord interneurons and, like benzodiazepines, α_2-adrenergic receptor agonists are frequently co-administered with dissociative agents to counteract muscle rigidity. Involuntary muscle twitching (jactitations) has been reported in dogs, cats, and, occasionally, in horses but these effects tend to be self-limiting.

The neuroendocrine stress response is modulated by α_2-adrenergic receptor agonists. Studies involving various drugs (xylazine, medetomidine, and detomidine) consistently report decreased circulating catecholamine levels in dogs [233–236], horses [237], and cattle and sheep [238]. These reductions in epinephrine and norepinephrine levels are reversible by α_2-adrenergic receptor antagonists [236,238]. Effects on basal and induced cortisol levels in animals are more variable. Reduced cortisol concentrations have been reported after medetomidine or dexmedetomidine administration in dogs [233,235,239]. However, other studies in dogs [234,240], horses [237], and cattle and sheep [238] report no suppression of cortisol activity. In humans, a meta-analysis of over 4800 patients found that dexmedetomidine infusion during the perioperative period inhibited release of epinephrine, norepinephrine, and cortisol and concluded that the drug attenuated perioperative stress and inflammation and protected immune function in surgical patients [241].

Glucose regulation is also impacted by α_2-adrenergic receptor agonist administration. Elevations in serum glucose are primarily a result of activation of α_{2A}-adrenergic receptors in pancreatic β-cells suppressing insulin release, though stimulation of glucagon release by pancreatic α-cells promoting gluconeogenesis has also been suggested [242–244]. Transient hyperglycemia has been reported in horses and cattle after xylazine [245,246], and in dogs after medetomidine [236] and dexmedetomidine [240]. In dogs, hyperglycemic effects induced by medetomidine were reversed with the α_2-adrenergic receptor antagonists yohimbine and atipamezole [236], and hyperglycemia was prevented when dexmedetomidine was co-administered with the peripheral α_2-adrenergic receptor antagonist, vatinoxan (MK-467) [240]. Clinically, α_2-adrenergic receptor agonist-induced hyperglycemia does not typically exceed the renal threshold for glucose (~180 mg/dL) and is not associated with glucosuria [51].

Clinical considerations

A search of the veterinary literature reveals that α_2-adrenergic receptor agonists have been administered to virtually every species. For more detailed information on clinical use of these drugs in specific species, including doses, the reader is directed to species-specific chapters in this text and elsewhere. While differences in species sensitivity tend to be more significant for drugs that are less selective/less potent (i.e., xylazine) compared to those that are more selective/more potent agents (i.e., medetomidine, dexmedetomidine), the approximate ranking of species according to α_2-adrenergic receptor agonist sensitivity from most sensitive to least sensitive is: goats > sheep, cattle > camelids > horses, dogs, cats > pigs > small laboratory animals.

While α_2-adrenergic receptor agonists have not historically been classified as controlled substances, the regulatory considerations regarding these drugs, notably xylazine, are rapidly evolving. In North America, illicit fentanyl adulterated with xylazine has been identified as an emerging threat to human health, and some jurisdictions are moving to make xylazine a scheduled drug. The impact of these regulatory changes on large animal veterinarians remains to be seen.

Dogs and cats

While xylazine is approved for use in dogs and cats and was historically widely used in these species, the more selective and potent α_2-adrenergic receptor agonists, medetomidine (a racemic mixture of both levomedetomidine and dexmedetomidine) and dexmedetomidine (the pharmacologically active *S*(+)-enantiomer of medetomidine), have largely supplanted xylazine in small animals. Romifidine is also approved for use in dogs and cats in some countries.

The α_2-adrenergic receptor agonists have wide-ranging clinical applications in dogs and cats. Even with low doses, caution is advised in patients with cardiac disease (especially those with systolic dysfunction), bradyarrhythmias, dehydration, hypovolemia, or sepsis due to significant hemodynamic effects. Combination with other sedatives, analgesics, or anesthetics will exacerbate CNS, cardiovascular, and respiratory depressant effects, and diligent titration of both injectable and inhalant anesthetics is necessary even in healthy patients. As noted previously, stimulation may cause sudden arousal in an animal that is seemingly well sedated with an α_2-adrenergic receptor agonist. Common clinical applications are listed in Box 22.1.

Box 22.1 Common clinical applications of α_2-adrenergic receptor agonists in dogs and cats.

1. IV or IM administration, often in combination with an opioid, for sedation-analgesia to facilitate non-invasive or minimally invasive procedures.
2. IV or IM administration in the preanesthetic period, often in combination with an opioid, prior to induction with an IV injectable anesthetic.
3. IM administration in combination with IM opioids, benzodiazepines, ketamine, or alfaxalone to produce a state ranging from profound sedation to general anesthesia.
4. IV CRI as an adjunct to inhalant anesthesia for MAC reduction, often in combination with other agents such as opioids, lidocaine, or ketamine [247–249].
5. IV CRI for injectable maintenance of anesthesia (TIVA) in combination with other drugs such as opioids, propofol, alfaxalone, ketamine, and benzodiazepines [250–252].
6. Low-dose IV bolus administration for postanesthetic sedation-analgesia and management of emergence delirium at recovery.
7. IV CRI for sedation, analgesia, and anxiolysis postoperatively or in an intensive care setting [253,254].
8. Epidural anesthesia–analgesia, usually in combination with other agents such as local anesthetics, opioids, or ketamine [255–258].
9. Perineural administration in combination with a local anesthetic to prolong or enhance peripheral nerve blockade [178,259].
10. OTM or intranasal administration (detomidine injectable or gel, dexmedetomidine) for sedation and anxiolysis in dogs or cats where IV administration is not feasible or desirable [155,159,260].

Horses

Multiple α_2-adrenergic receptor agonists are approved for use in horses not destined for human consumption (xylazine, detomidine, and romifidine), and both medetomidine and dexmedetomidine have also been used off-label in this species. Approximate equipotent IV doses for equine sedation are 1 mg/kg xylazine ~ 40–80 μg/kg romifidine ~ 20–40 μg/kg detomidine ~ 5–10 μg/kg medetomidine (or 2.5–5 μg/kg dexmedetomidine) [261–263]. Duration of action varies by drug and dose, but in general, detomidine is associated with the longest duration, romfidine and medetomidine are intermediate, and xylazine has the shortest duration of action in horses [262,264,265]. It has been suggested that romifidine may be associated with less ataxia and lowering of the head when administered for standing sedation, but other α_2-adrenergic receptor agonists are commonly used for this purpose as well.

As in dogs and cats, the α_2-adrenergic receptor agonists have numerous clinical applications in horses listed below (Box 22.2).

Cattle

In the United States, no α_2-adrenergic receptor agonists are approved by the Food and Drug Administration for use in cattle, though xylazine is frequently used off-label. The Food Animal Residue Avoidance Database (FARAD) provides recommendations for extra-label drug use in cattle and withholding guidelines for

Box 22.2 Common clinical applications of α_2-adrenergic receptor agonists in horses.

1. IV bolus administration for standing sedation or chemical restraint, often in combination with an opioid.
2. IV bolus or CRI for management of visceral pain associated with colic [266].
3. IV CRI for standing procedures usually in combination with opioids and locoregional anesthesia to facilitate a variety of surgical procedures [267–270].
4. IV administration in the preanesthetic period, often in combination with an opioid, prior to induction with an IV injectable anesthetic.
5. IV CRI as an adjunct to inhalant anesthesia for MAC reduction and/or modification of recovery [271–274].
6. IV CRI for injectable maintenance of anesthesia (TIVA) in combination with other drugs (ketamine and guaifenesin in "Triple Drip" or other combinations) [275,276].
7. Low-dose IV bolus administration for postanesthetic sedation-analgesia to enhance recovery from inhalant anesthesia [146,277].
8. Epidural anesthesia–analgesia, usually in combination with other agents such as local anesthetics, opioids, or ketamine [278–280].
9. Perineural administration in combination with a local anesthetic to prolong or enhance peripheral nerve blockade [281].
10. OTM administration (detomidine injectable or gel) for sedation and anxiolysis in horses where IV administration is not feasible or desirable [152,282].

xylazine vary by dose and route of administration (24–120 h for milk and 4–10 days for meat) [283]. These recommendations reflect different xylazine labeling in other countries where the drug is approved in this species. Detomidine is approved for use in cattle in Europe with reported milk and meat withholding times varying between 12–72 h and 2–3 days, respectively.

Cattle are particularly sensitive to the CNS depressant effects of α_2-adrenergic receptor agonists, especially xylazine, and typically require approximately one-tenth of the equine dose to produce a comparable clinical response. It has been speculated that this may be due to differences in α_2-adrenergic receptor density or subtype pattern (i.e., $\alpha_{2A/D}$), but this has not been substantiated as a cause for their increased sensitivity to xylazine [284]. Differences in α_2-adrenergic receptor G-protein coupling efficiency induced by xylazine versus detomidine have been documented in bovine brain tissue, and it is possible that these molecular events further down the signaling cascade may contribute to the species differences in xylazine sensitivity noted clinically [284]. It has also been noted that certain breeds of cattle (Herefords, Brahmans) appear to be more sensitive to the effects of xylazine than others (Holsteins). The other more specific α_2-adrenergic receptor agonists (detomidine and dexmedetomidine) appear to be more potent in cattle with less interspecies variation, and clinical doses closer to those used in horses may be appropriate.

Common clinical applications for α_2-adrenergic receptor agonists in cattle are listed in Box 22.3.

Anesthetic recovery in cattle is typically uneventful and postanesthetic sedation is rarely indicated.

Sheep

α_2-Adrenergic receptor agonists are potent and effective sedative–analgesics in sheep and are often used in combination with other drugs for induction and maintenance of anesthesia similar to cattle. As noted in the respiratory system section, however, this class of drugs may induce hypoxemia in sheep due to activation of pulmonary intravascular macrophages leading to intra-alveolar hemorrhage and interstitial and pulmonary edema [204,205]. The magnitude of hypoxemia seems to be highly variable and dependent on breed-related factors, being most severe after IV injection during general anesthesia. In light of these factors, and because subclinical pulmonary disease is common in sheep, rapid IV injection of α_2-adrenergic receptor agonists in situations where provision of supplemental oxygen is not feasible should be avoided [285,286].

Box 22.3 Common clinical applications of α_2-adrenergic receptor agonists in cattle.

1. IV or IM administration for standing sedation or chemical restraint, often in combination with an opioid.
2. IV administration in the preanesthetic period, often in combination with an opioid, prior to induction with an IV injectable anesthetic.
3. IV CRI (very low "ruminant" dose) for injectable maintenance of anesthesia (TIVA) in combination with other drugs (ketamine and guaifenesin in "Triple Drip" or other combinations).
4. Epidural anesthesia–analgesia, usually in combination with other agents such as local anesthetics, opioids, or ketamine.

Pigs

α_2-Adrenergic receptor agonists are widely used in pigs, usually in combination with other agents such as dissociatives (ketamine or tiletamine in Telazol®), opioids, and benzodiazepines. Pigs tend to require higher doses of α_2-adrenergic receptor agonists compared to horses, dogs, and cats, and significantly higher doses compared to ruminants, especially for xylazine. Doses for the more selective/potent agents (dexmedetomidine and medetomidine) appear to be less variable.

α_2-Adrenergic receptor antagonists

The ability to pharmacologically antagonize the sedative, cardiovascular, or respiratory effects of α_2-adrenergic receptor agonists is considered a major advantage when using this class of drugs clinically in domestic animals as well as in zoo animals and free-ranging wildlife. There are four α_2-adrenergic receptor antagonists of current clinical interest in veterinary medicine: yohimbine, tolazoline, atipamezole, and vatinoxan. A fifth antagonist, idazoxan, has been reported to reverse xylazine in sheep [287] and calves [288], but is rarely used clinically.

Yohimbine was first extracted from the bark of the *Pausinystalia yohimbe* tree over 100 years ago and was the first α_2-adrenergic receptor antagonist used in veterinary medicine to reverse xylazine. Not long after, in the early 1980s, reports of tolazoline administration for xylazine reversal also began appearing in the veterinary literature.

Atipamezole was developed specifically to reverse the effects of medetomidine in dogs, and it was released to the veterinary market in 1996. Vatinoxan (previously known as "MK-467" and "L-659,066") has been studied since the early 1990s but has only recently garnered interest for clinical use in veterinary medicine. It has recently been marketed in combination with medetomidine in the veterinary product Zenalpha®.

Yohimbine, tolazoline, atipamezole, and vatinoxan

Mechanism of action and indications

Similar to the α_2-adrenergic receptor agonists, antagonists have unique α_2:α_1 adrenergic receptor selectivity ratios and, depending on their structure, variably bind to imidazoline receptors (Table 22.1).

These receptor binding characteristics impact an antagonist's clinical efficacy and side effect profile. Functionally, these drugs act as competitive antagonists at α_2-adrenergic receptors and, like the agonists, they have no subtype specificity. Differences in lipid solubility, however, impact how α_2-adrenergic receptor antagonists are distributed, and their clinical effects vary accordingly. Yohimbine, tolazoline, and atipamezole are widely distributed and affect both central and peripheral α_2-adrenergic receptors, while vatinoxan impacts peripheral α_2-adrenergic receptors only (see below).

Yohimbine shows minimal selectivity for the α_2-adrenergic receptor and lacks imidazoline receptor affinity. In addition to α-adrenergic antagonism, yohimbine also interacts with dopaminergic, serotonergic, and cholinergic receptors [289]. Tolazoline is a non-selective antagonist with comparable affinity at both α_2- and α_1-adrenergic receptors, as well as affinity at imidazoline receptors. Its interactions at histaminergic and cholinergic receptors may contribute to some of the side effects associated with clinical its use.

Atipamezole is by far the most specific α_2-adrenergic receptor antagonist with an α_2:α_1 binding ratio of over 8500:1. It has no significant effects at dopaminergic, serotonergic, histaminergic, or cholinergic receptors, and this specificity contributes to its favorable side effect profile compared to the less selective antagonists, yohimbine and tolazoline. Atipamezole's chemical structure includes an imidazoline ring, so it may interact with imidazoline receptors.

Vatinoxan is classified as a selective α_2-adrenergic receptor antagonist with an α_2:α_1 binding ratio of 105:1 [137] and potential imidazoline activity due to its chemical structure. Despite its lower α_2:α_1 selectivity ratio compared to atipamezole, a study in horses and sheep demonstrated no effect of vatinoxan on the cardiovascular response to the α_1-adrenergic receptor agonist, methoxamine, suggesting that vatinoxan has no clinically relevant effects at vascular α_1-adrenergic receptors [290]. Unlike the other three α_2-adrenergic receptor antagonists, which are highly lipophilic and readily penetrate the blood–brain barrier, vatinoxan is poorly lipid soluble and is effectively excluded from the CNS after systemic administration [137]. This feature, likely in combination with other factors such as molecular weight, degree of ionization, protein binding, or active transport efflux mechanisms, means that vatinoxan is able to selectively antagonize peripheral postsynaptic α_2-adrenergic receptors in vascular endothelium with minimal effects on supraspinal and spinal α_2-adrenergic receptors. These characteristics open the door to novel clinical applications for vatinoxan, which are discussed below.

Common clinical indications for antagonist administration include reversal of both central (i.e., sedation and cardiopulmonary depression) and/or peripheral (i.e., cardiovascular) effects mediated by α_2-adrenergic receptor agonists. It is important to remember that, for antagonists that cross the blood–brain barrier (yohimbine, tolazoline, atipamezole), reversal of α_2-adrenergic receptor-mediated spinal and supraspinal analgesia will also occur. In animals with sustained nociception administered atipamezole to reverse the effects of α_2-adrenergic receptor agonists, atipamezole increased pain-related responses by blocking norepinephrine-mediated inhibitory nociceptive pathways [291]. In addition to loss of analgesia, there is also potential for inducing excitation and adverse cardiovascular effects (vasodilation, hypotension, and tachycardia), so the decision to administer an α_2-adrenergic receptor antagonist should be made on a case-by-case basis. In some species and in certain clinical circumstances, it may be advantageous to administer a "full dose" of an α_2-adrenergic receptor antagonist but, in many situations, lower partial doses of antagonist are effective in antagonizing excessive sedation without reversing all sedative and analgesic effects and may be associated with fewer adverse effects.

Pharmacokinetics

In horses, IV yohimbine and tolazoline have been reported to have large volumes of distribution and are cleared slowly leading to prolonged terminal half-lives [292,293]. In dogs administered IM atipamezole, both absorption and elimination appear to be rapid, with the maximum plasma concentration occurring within 30 min and an elimination half-life of approximately 1 h [294].

Atipamezole has been shown to reduce the area under the curve of medetomidine in sedated dogs, demonstrating that administration of an α_2-adrenergic receptor antagonist can impact the pharmacokinetics of an agonist [294]. It was speculated that the increased clearance of medetomidine in the presence of atipamezole may result from restoration of hemodynamic function after atipamezole administration. Both atipamezole and medetomidine undergo hepatic metabolism by hydroxylation in dogs, but there is no evidence of direct metabolic interactions between these two drugs [294].

The pharmacokinetics of IV vatinoxan concentrations in isoflurane-anesthetized cats have been reported to fit a three-compartment model with a small volume of distribution and a low clearance [295]. Dexmedetomidine did not have a significant effect on plasma concentrations of vatinoxan in dogs or cats [296–298].

Other potential routes of administration have been reported for certain α_2-adrenergic receptor antagonists, including endotracheal administration of tolazoline in dogs [299], but this appears to have limited clinical relevance in veterinary medicine.

Pharmacodynamics

Cardiovascular system

When administered alone (without the influence of an α_2-adrenergic receptor agonist), α_2-adrenergic receptor antagonists typically cause minimal dose-dependent cardiovascular changes characterized by increased heart rate and decreased systemic vascular resistance [300].

In animals under the influence of an agonist, administration of an α_2-adrenergic receptor antagonist will partially reverse the cardiovascular effects induced by the agonist. In the case of vatinoxan, only those effects mediated by peripheral (vascular) α_2-adrenergic receptors will be impacted. Usually, this manifests as a return of systemic vascular resistance, arterial blood pressure, and heart rate toward pre-sedation values with a concomitant increase in cardiac output and resolution of bradyarrhythmias. A number of other factors, however, including the specific drug, the dose, the timing, and the route of administration will impact these cardiovascular effects. Rapid IV administration of an α_2-adrenergic receptor antagonist to a sedated patient with significantly increased systemic vascular resistance has been reported to cause vasodilation and marked hypotension, so caution is warranted with this route of administration.

Reversal of cardiovascular effects, however, is not complete even for drugs with high α_2-adrenergic receptor specificity. In dogs, reversal of medetomidine (20 μg/kg IM) with atipamezole (100 μg/kg IM) administered 30 min later failed to result in sustained decreases in systemic vascular resistance or increases in heart rate and cardiac index [301]. The hemodynamic effects of reversal may differ between sedated animals and those that are anesthetized, with inhalant anesthetics introducing the potential for significant arterial hypotension. In isoflurane-anesthetized cats administered dexmedetomidine (5 μg/kg IV), administration of atipamezole (25 μg/kg or 50 μg/kg IM) 5 min after dexmedetomidine was ineffective at increasing heart rate or cardiac output but was associated with transient but severe arterial hypotension [302].

Vatinoxan's cardiovascular effects have also been evaluated in the presence of medetomidine or dexmedetomidine, with or without the influence of an inhalant anesthetic in several species. In conscious dogs administered IM medetomidine or IV dexmedetomidine, vatinoxan attenuated but did not prevent α_2-adrenergic receptor agonist-induced hemodynamic effects including reductions in heart rate and cardiac index and increases in systemic vascular resistance and arterial blood pressure [303,304]. In isoflurane-anesthetized dogs administered dexmedetomidine (2.5 μg/kg IV) and vatinoxan (100 μg/kg IV), vatinoxan similarly attenuated dexmedetomidine-induced decreases in cardiac index and increases in systemic vascular resistance, but resulted in hypotension [305]. In this study, infusion of dobutamine or norepinephrine not only restored normotension but significantly improved cardiac index. In a clinical study in sevoflurane-anesthetized dogs administered medetomidine–butorphanol–vatinoxan, significant arterial hypotension requiring intervention was reported [306].

In conscious cats, co-administration of vatinoxan with dexmedetomidine attenuated dexmedetomidine-induced bradycardia [307,308], as well as reductions in cardiac index and increases in systemic vascular resistance [309]. Similar to dogs, the co-administration of vatinoxan with dexmedetomidine via target-controlled infusion in isoflurane-anesthetized cats attenuated dexmedetomidine-induced reductions in cardiac index and increases in systemic vascular resistance, but vasodilatory effects resulted in arterial hypotension [310–312]. Infusions of norepinephrine and phenylephrine, but not dopamine, were effective in preventing hypotension in dexmedetomidine–vatinoxan–isoflurane-anesthetized cats [312].

In standing horses administered medetomidine with and without vatinoxan (140 μg/kg IV) followed by medetomidine CRI, vatinoxan was associated with higher heart rates, lower systemic vascular resistance, lower arterial blood pressure, and higher cardiac index compared to medetomidine alone [313]. In horses anesthetized with isoflurane, co-administration of vatinoxan with infusions of either dexmedetomidine or medetomidine lowered systemic vascular resistance and improved indices of global and peripheral perfusion and oxygenation but increased the need for inotropic support of arterial blood pressure [314,315].

Respiratory system

While the respiratory depressant effects of the α_2-adrenergic receptor agonists are much less significant than their cardiovascular effects, reversal with an α_2-adrenergic receptor antagonist with CNS penetration is expected to return any changes in arterial blood gas parameters toward baseline in most species. As discussed previously, sheep are uniquely susceptible to pulmonary edema and hypoxemia with administration of α_2-adrenergic receptor agonists, notably xylazine [316]. In an experimental study, atipamezole was required in a significant number of sheep receiving xylazine, but not medetomidine, to counteract tachypnea and hypoxemia, but no discussion of the efficacy of atipamezole in reversing these pulmonary changes was provided [316].

Administration of vatinoxan (750 μg/kg IV) to sheep prior to xylazine (0.5 mg/kg IV) improved PaO_2 without impacting pulmonary histopathologic changes observed after euthanasia with pentobarbital, suggesting that further investigations are warranted [317]. In sevoflurane-anesthetized sheep, vatinoxan pretreatment prevented dexmedetomidine-induced bronchoconstriction, pulmonary edema, and arterial hypoxemia [318].

Central nervous system

Administration of an α_2-adrenergic receptor antagonist that readily penetrates the blood–brain barrier (yohimbine, tolazoline, or atipamezole) is expected to reverse the sedative–analgesic effects of an α_2-adrenergic receptor agonist. These effects have been studied for yohimbine [319–321], tolazoline [320,322,323], and atipamezole [322,324–327] in numerous species. Full reversal of all agonist-induced CNS depressant effects is not always attained, and reasons for this are multifactorial depending on the drug's selectivity for the α_2-adrenergic receptor (both the agonist and the antagonist), the dose administered (both the agonist and the antagonist), the timing after agonist administration, and the route of administration. In general, the sedative effects of the most selective α_2-adrenergic receptor agonists (medetomidine and dexmedetomidine) tend to be the most reliably reversed by the most selective α_2-adrenergic receptor antagonist (atipamezole).

In animals anesthetized with inhalant anesthetics, the MAC reduction effects induced by an α_2-adrenergic receptor agonist are also reversed by administration of an antagonist that penetrates the CNS [328,329], though the hemodynamic consequences of this practice caution against routine reversal of α_2-adrenergic receptor agonists in inhalant-anesthetized patients.

As vatinoxan does not enter the CNS, its effects on α_2-adrenergic receptor agonist-induced sedation are presumed to be minimal, and this appears to be the case in dogs [330–332]. Interestingly, in standing horses administered a medetomidine bolus (7 μg/kg IV) followed by a CRI, the addition of vatinoxan (140 μg/kg IV) to the medetomidine bolus slightly but significantly lowered sedation scores for the first 20 min, and the authors suggest that this could be a result of vatinoxan promoting distribution and clearance of medetomidine during the initial phase of the infusion [313]. Conversely, in sheep co-administered medetomidine (30 μg/kg IM) and vatinoxan (300 μg/kg IM), the addition of vatinoxan resulted in faster onset of more intense sedation compared to medetomidine alone [333].

The interactions between multiple antagonists (atipamezole and vatinoxan) are also of interest in the clinical setting. In conscious dogs sedated with IM medetomidine or medetomidine–vatinoxan, atipamezole reversed medetomidine-induced sedation more efficiently in vatinoxan-treated dogs and resulted in fewer cases of recurrent sedation [301]. Similar findings were reported in sheep where reversal of medetomidine-induced sedation with atipamezole was enhanced when medetomidine was co-administered with vatinoxan [333].

Due to its purported limited penetration of the CNS, the effects of vatinoxan on the MAC-sparing effects of α_2-adrenergic receptor agonists would be expected to be negligible; however, this may not be the case. In isoflurane-anesthetized cats, vatinoxan alone administered using a target-controlled infusion system increased isoflurane MAC, and significantly reduced the MAC-sparing effects of a dexmedetomidine target-controlled infusion [334]. Reasons for this are unclear, and the authors suggest that further studies are warranted to establish whether vatinoxan penetrates the blood–brain barrier in cats and the mechanism by which it increases inhalant anesthetic MAC.

Similarly, in sevoflurane-anesthetized dogs, vatinoxan administered alone as a loading dose followed by a CRI significantly and unexpectedly increased MAC at the highest vatinoxan infusion rate [335]. In a subsequent study, when vatinoxan was infused with dexmedetomidine in sevoflurane-anesthetized dogs, partial attenuation of dexmedetomidine's MAC-sparing effects was observed [336]. The authors propose that, because MAC is a measure of immobility that is largely mediated at the level of spinal cord rather than at supraspinal structures, it is likely that vatinoxan penetrates the spinal cord in concentrations sufficient to alter inhalant anesthetic requirements [336]. Further studies investigating the effects of both atipamezole and vatinoxan on inhalant anesthetic MAC seem warranted.

The analgesic effects of the α_2-adrenergic receptor agonists, as expected, are readily reversed by systemic administration of antagonists that readily cross the blood–brain barrier (yohimbine, tolazoline, and atipamezole) [337–339].

Vatinoxan, with its limited penetration of the CNS, would be expected to have minimal effects on systemic α_2-adrenergic receptor agonist-induced analgesia, but this may be an oversimplification. In dogs, co-administration of vatinoxan (250 μg/kg IV) with medetomidine (10 μg/kg IV) significantly attenuated racemic medetomidine-induced antinociception, which was accompanied by lower plasma concentrations of dexmedetomidine [340]. The authors attributed these effects to vatinoxan-induced alterations in medetomidine distribution and clearance, which could be ameliorated by administration of a higher dose of medetomidine when combined with vatinoxan [340]. Another canine study investigated this possibility and found that co-administration of vatinoxan did not significantly interfere with medetomidine-induced analgesia as long as plasma dexmedetomidine concentrations remained above the threshold needed for antinociception [341].

Other effects

In general, the other effects of α_2-adrenergic receptor agonists on gastrointestinal function [342], urine output [224,343], and glucose regulation [344] are largely reversed by administration of the "traditional" α_2-adrenergic receptor antagonists, yohimbine, tolazoline, and atipamezole.

The effects of vatinoxan on these parameters are less consistent. In conscious horses, co-administration of vatinoxan with detomidine, romifidine, or medetomidine attenuated the reduction in intestinal hypomotility induced by the α_2-adrenergic receptor agonist [313,345–347]. However, in isoflurane-anesthetized horses receiving a medetomidine IV bolus and CRI, IV vatinoxan did not influence the reduction in fecal output noted after anesthesia [315].

Unlike atipamezole, vatinoxan failed to show any detectable improvement in voiding parameters in mice administered dexmedetomidine [224]. In dogs, co-administration of vatinoxan with dexmedetomidine prevented significant dexmedetomidine-induced changes in plasma glucose, insulin, and lactate [240].

Clinical considerations

While atipamezole, the most selective α_2-adrenergic antagonist, has largely supplanted yohimbine and tolazoline for clinical use in small animals, the older, less selective antagonists are still used clinically in domestic cattle and free-ranging hoofstock, especially for reversal of xylazine. High IV doses of tolazoline in particular have been associated with adverse CNS effects (hyperesthesia and opisthotonos) in adult cattle, and very high IV doses induced serious CNS, cardiovascular, respiratory, and gastrointestinal side effects in calves. For these reasons, lower IV doses of tolazoline are recommended in cattle (or any species), or avoidance of the IV route except in emergency situations.

In all species, decisions about if, when, or how to reverse the effects of an α_2-adrenergic agonist should be made on a case-by-case basis after considering potential advantages and disadvantages. Potential disadvantages of α_2-adrenergic antagonist administration include CNS stimulation or excitation, loss of analgesia, and adverse cardiovascular effects such as vasodilation, hypotension, and tachycardia. In some species and in certain clinical circumstances, administration of a full "label" dose may be indicated, but, in many situations, a lower partial dose of antagonist is effective in reversing excessive or persistent sedation while retaining some sedative and analgesic effects and avoiding adverse side effects.

Vatinoxan, the peripherally acting α_2-adrenergic antagonist, has recently been approved in several countries in combination with racemic medetomidine for use as an IM sedative–analgesic in dogs, and a brief overview of this product is provided below.

Medetomidine–vatinoxan combination (Zenalpha®)

The combination of vatinoxan with medetomidine in Zenalpha® is purported to partially counteract the cardiovascular depressant effects of dexmedetomidine (the pharmacologically active enantiomer in medetomidine) while preserving dexmedetomidine's centrally mediated sedative and analgesic effects [348]. Each milliliter of Zenalpha® contains 0.5 mg medetomidine and 10 mg vatinoxan along with mannitol, citric acid monohydrate, methylparaben, and propylparaben. Label dosing recommendations are 1 mg medetomidine/m^2 body surface area, which corresponds to a 40 μg/kg medetomidine dose and an 800 μg/kg vatinoxan dose in a 20 kg dog. Approved indications include "clinical examinations, clinical procedures, and minor surgical procedures." In a field efficacy trial, dogs treated with Zenalpha® had a shorter time to onset of sedation, shorter duration of sedation, and less cardiovascular and respiratory depression with fewer adverse reactions compared to dogs in the control group receiving dexmedetomidine alone. Administration of IM atipamezole at the approved dose to reverse medetomidine results in reversal of Zenalpha®'s sedative and analgesic effects within 5–10 min [348].

Despite its more favorable safety profile, the label indicates that Zenalpha® is contraindicated in dogs with "cardiac disease, respiratory disease, shock, severe debilitation that have hypoglycemia or are at risk of developing hypoglycemia, or are stressed due to extreme heat, cold, or fatigue." It is not labeled for administration in combination with any other drugs; thus, its use in the perianesthetic period as a preanesthetic agent prior to an injectable and/or inhalant anesthetic constitutes extra-label use. The product has generated considerable interest, and numerous studies are emerging describing the use of this particular formulation in dogs, both on and off-label, in a variety of clinical situations. While numerous other extra-label uses in different species are also being investigated, it should be noted that the 1:20 ratio of medetomidine to vatinoxan in Zenalpha® may not be appropriate for other species (e.g., cats).

Acknowledgement

The authors would like to acknowledge Dr. David C. Rankin for his valuable work on the previous edition of this chapter.

References

1 DeBattista C. Antipsychotic agents and lithium. In: Katzung BG, Vanerah TW, eds. *Basic and Clinical Pharmacology*, 15th edn. New York, NY: McGraw Hill, 2021: 529.

2 Ballard S, Shults T, Kownacki AA, *et al.* The pharmacokinetics, pharmacological responses and behavioral effects of acepromazine in the horse. *J Vet Pharmacol Ther* 1982; **5**: 21–31.

3 Marroum PJ, Webb AI, Aeschbacher G, *et al.* Pharmacokinetics and pharmacodynamics of acepromazine in horses. *Am J Vet Res* 1994; **55**: 1428–1433.
4 Knych HK, Seminoff K, McKemie DS, *et al.* Pharmacokinetics, pharmacodynamics, and metabolism of acepromazine following intravenous, oral, and sublingual administration to exercised Thoroughbred horses. *J Vet Pharmacol Ther* 2018; **41**: 522–535.
5 Hashem A, Kietzmann M, Scherkl R. The pharmacokinetics and bioavailability of acepromazine in the plasma of dogs. *Dtsch Tierarztl Wochenschr* 1992; **99**: 396–398.
6 Dewey EA, Maylin GA, Ebel JG, *et al.* The metabolism of promazine and acetylpromazine in the horse. *Drug Metab Dispos* 1981; **9**: 30–36.
7 Coulter DB, Whelan SC, Wilson RC, *et al.* Determination of blood pressure by indirect methods in dogs given acetylpromazine maleate. *Cornell Vet* 1981; **71**: 75–84.
8 Stepien RL, Bonagura JD, Bednarski RM, *et al.* Cardiorespiratory effects of acepromazine maleate and buprenorphine hydrochloride in clinically normal dogs. *Am J Vet Res* 1983; **44**: 996–999.
9 Rangel JPP, Monteiro ER, Bitti FS, *et al.* Hemodynamic, respiratory and sedative effects of progressively increasing doses of acepromazine in conscious dogs. *Vet Anesth Analg* 2020; **47**: 447–453.
10 Muir WW, Skarda RT, Sheehan W. Hemodynamic and respiratory effects of a xylazine–acetylpromazine drug combination in horses. *Am J Vet Res* 1979; **40**: 1518–1522.
11 Pequito M, Amory H, Serteyn D, *et al.* Comparison of the sedative and hemodynamic effects of acepromazine and promethazine in the standing horse. *J Equine Vet Sci* 2012; **32**: 799–804.
12 Leise BS, Fugler LA, Stokes AM, *et al.* Effects of intramuscular administration of acepromazine on palmar digital blood flow, palmar digital arterial pressure, transverse facial arterial pressure, and packed cell volume in clinically healthy, conscious horses. *Vet Surg* 2007; **36**: 717–723.
13 Ludders JW, Reitan JA, Martucci R, *et al.* Blood pressure response to phenylephrine infusion in halothane anesthetized dogs given acetylpromazine maleate. *Am J Vet Res* 1983; **44**: 996–999.
14 Rangel JPP, Monteiro ER, Bitti FS, *et al.* Hemodynamic effects of incremental doses of acepromazine in isoflurane-anesthetized dogs. *Vet Anesth Analg* 2021; **48**: 167–173.
15 Steffey EP, Kelly AB, Farver TB, *et al.* Cardiovascular and respiratory effects of acetylpromazine and xylazine on halothane anesthetized horses. *J Vet Pharmacol Ther* 1985; **8**: 290–302.
16 Muir WW, Werner LL, Hamlin RL. Effects of xylazine and acetylpromazine upon induced ventricular fibrillation in dogs anesthetized with thiamylal and halothane. *Am J Vet Res* 1975; **36**: 1299–1303.
17 Dyson D, Pettifer G. Evaluation of the arrhythmogenicity of a low dose of acepromazine: comparison with xylazine. *Can J Vet Res* 1997; **61**: 241–245.
18 Lemke KA, Tranquilli WJ. Anesthetics, arrhythmias, and myocardial sensitization to epinephrine. *J Am Vet Med Assoc* 1994; **205**: 1679–1684.
19 Popovic NA, Mullane JF, Yhap EO. Effects of acetylpromazine maleate on certain cardiorespiratory responses in dogs. *Am J Vet Res* 1972; **33**: 1819–1824.
20 Marntell S, Nyman G, Funkquist P, *et al.* Effects of acepromazine on pulmonary gas exchange and circulation during sedation and dissociative anaesthesia in horses. *Vet Anaesth Analg* 2005; **32**: 83–93.
21 Webb AI, O'Brien JM. The effect of acepromazine maleate on the anesthetic potency of halothane and isoflurane. *J Am Anim Hosp Assoc* 1988; **24**: 609–613.
22 Heard DJ, Webb AI, Daniels RT. Effect of acepromazine on the anesthetic requirement of halothane in the dog. *Am J Vet Res* 1986; **47**: 2113–2115.
23 Doherty TJ, Geiser DR, Rohrback BW. Effect of acepromazine and butorphanol on halothane minimum alveolar concentration in ponies. *Equine Vet J* 1997; **29**: 374–376.
24 Fabisch W. The effect of chlorpromazine on the electroencephalogram of epileptic patients. *J Neurol Neurosurg Psychiat* 1957; **20**: 185.
25 Holliday TA, Cunningham JG, Gutnick MJ. Comparative clinical and electroencephalographic studies of canine epilepsy. *Epilepsia* 1970; **11**: 281–292.
26 Tobias KM, Marioni-Henry K, Wagner R. A retrospective study on the use of acepromazine maleate in dogs with seizures. *J Am Anim Hosp Assoc* 2006; **42**: 283–289.
27 McConnell J, Kirby R, Rudloff E. Administration of acepromazine maleate to 31 dogs with a history of seizures. *J Vet Emerg Crit Care* 2007; **17**: 262–267.
28 Drynan EA, Gray P, Raisis AL. Incidence of seizures associated with the use of acepromazine in dogs undergoing myelography. *J Vet Emerg Crit Care (San Antonio)* 2012; **22**: 262–266.
29 Lang SM, Eglen RM, Henry AC. Acetylpromazine administration: its effect on canine haematology. *Vet Rec* 1979; **105**: 397–398.
30 Barr SC, Ludders JW, Looney AL, *et al.* Platelet aggregation in dogs after sedation with acepromazine and atropine and during subsequent general anesthesia and surgery. *Am J Vet Res* 1992; 53: 2067–2070.
31 Conner BJ, Hanel RM, Hansen BD, *et al.* Effects of acepromazine maleate on platelet function assessed by use of adenosine diphosphate activated- and arachidonic acid- activated modified thromboelastography in healthy dogs. *Am J Vet Res* 2012; **73**: 595–601.
32 Valverde A, Cantwell S, Hernández J, *et al.* Effects of acepromazine on the incidence of vomiting associated with opioid administration in dogs. *Vet Anaesth Analg* 2004; **31**: 40–45.
33 Claude AK, Dedeaux A, Chiavaccini L, *et al.* Effects of maropitant citrate or acepromazine on the incidence of adverse events associated with hydromorphone premedication in dogs. *J Vet Intern Med* 2014; **28**: 1414–1417.
34 Strombeck DR, Harrold D. Effects of atropine, acepromazine, meperidine, and xylazine on gastroesophageal sphincter pressure in the dog. *Am J Vet Res* 1985; **46**: 963–965.
35 Hall JA, Magne ML, Twedt DC. Effect of acepromazine, diazepam, fentanyl–droperidol, and oxymorphone on gastroesophageal sphincter pressure in healthy dogs. *Am J Vet Res* 1987; **48**: 556–557.
36 Scrivani PV, Bednarski RM, Myer CW. Effects of acepromazine and butorphanol on positive-contrast upper gastrointestinal tract examination in dogs. *Am J Vet Res* 1998; **59**: 1227–1233.
37 Davies JV, Gerring EL. Effect of spasmolytic analgesic drugs on the motility patterns of the equine small intestine. *Res Vet Sci* 1983; **34**: 334–339.
38 Doherty TJ, Andrews FM, Provenza MK, *et al.* The effect of sedation on gastric emptying of a liquid marker in ponies. *Vet Surg* 1999; **28**: 375–379.
39 Costa RS, Wetmore LA, Stein A. Randomized, blinded, controlled clinical trial to assess gastroesophageal reflux and regurgitation in dogs undergoing general anesthesia after hydromorphone premedication with or without acepromazine or dexmedetomidine. *Am J Vet Res* 2021; **82**: 695–700.
40 Pearson H, Weaver BM. Priapism after sedation, neuroleptanalgesia, and anaesthesia in the horse. *Equine Vet J* 1979; **11**: 33–35.
41 Driessen B, Zarucco L, Kalir B, Bertolotti L. Contemporary use of acepromazine in the anaesthetic management of male horses and ponies: a retrospective study and opinion poll. *Equine Vet J* 2011; **43**: 88–98.
42 Bostrom I, Nyman G, Kampa N, *et al.* Effects of acepromazine on renal function in anesthetized dogs. *Am J Vet Res* 2003; **64**: 590–598.
43 Newell SM, Ko JC, Ginn PE, *et al.* Effects of three sedative protocols on glomerular filtration rate in clinically normal dogs. *Am J Vet Res* 1997; **58**: 446–450.
44 Marks SL, Straeter-Knowlen IM, Moore M, *et al.* Effects of acepromazine maleate and phenoxybenzamine on urethral pressure profiles of anesthetized, healthy, sexually intact male cats. *Am J Vet Res* 1996; **57**: 1497–1500.
45 Moriello KA, Eicker SW. Influence of sedative and anesthetic agents on intradermal skin test reactions in dogs. *Am J Vet Res* 1991; **52**: 1484–1498.
46 Kramer BM, Hector RC, Rezende ML, *et al.* Sedative and cardiopulmonary effects of intramuscular combinations of hydromorphone, acepromazine, dexmedetomidine, and glycopyrrolate followed by intravenous propofol and inhalant isoflurane anesthesia in healthy dogs. *Am J Vet Res* 2022; **83**: 22.06.0098.
47 Alvaides RK, Teixeira Neto FJ, Aguiar AJA, *et al.* Sedative and cardiorespiratory effects of acepromazine or atropine given before dexmedetomidine in dogs. *Vet Rec* 2008; **162**: 852–856.
48 Saponaro V, Crovace A, De Marzo L, *et al.* Echocardiographic evaluation of the cardiovascular effects of medetomidine, acepromazine and their combination in healthy dogs. *Res Vet Sci* 2013; **95**: 687–692.
49 Deshpande D, Hill KE, Mealey KL, *et al.* The effect of the canine ABCB1-1Δ on sedation after intravenous administration of acepromazine. *J Vet Intern Med* 2016; **30**: 636–641.
50 Mealey KL, Owens JG, Freeman E. Canine and feline P-glycoprotein deficiency: what we know and where we need to go. *J Vet Pharmacol Ther* 2023; **46**: 1–16.
51 Posner LP. Sedatives and tranquilizers. In: Riviere JE, Papich MG, eds. *Veterinary Pharmacology and Therapeutics*, 10th edn. Hoboken, NJ: Wiley Blackwell, 2018; 324–368.
52 Johnston GM, Eastment JK, Wood J, *et al.* The confidential enquiry into perioperative equine fatalities (CEPEF): mortality results of Phases 1 and 2. *Vet Anaesth Analg* 2002; **29**: 159–170.
53 Valverde A, Black B, Cribb NC, *et al.* Assessment of unassisted recovery from repeated general isoflurane anesthesia in horses following post-anesthetic administration of xylazine or acepromazine or a combination of xylazine and ketamine. *Vet Anesth Analg* 2013; **40**: 3–12.
54 McGrath CJ, Rempel WE, Addis PB, *et al.* Acepromazine and droperidol inhibition of halothane-induced malignant hyperthermia (porcine stress syndrome) in swine. *Am J Vet Res* 1981; **42**: 195–198.
55 Calcaterra NE, Barrow JC. Classics in chemical neuroscience: diazepam (valium). *ACS Chem Neurosci* 2014; **5**: 253–260.
56 Goodchild CS. GABA receptors and benzodiazepines. *Br J Anaesth* 1993; **71**: 127–133.
57 Engin E, Liu J, Uwe R. α2-containing $GABA_A$ receptors: a target for the development of novel treatment strategies for CNS disorders. *Pharmacol Ther* 2012; **136**: 142–152.

58 Everington EA, Gibbard AG, Swinny JD, *et al.* Molecular characterization of GABA-A receptor subunit diversity within major peripheral organs and their plasticity in response to early life psychosocial stress. *Front Mol Neurosc* 2018; **11**: 18.

59 Goetz T, Arslan A, Wisden W, *et al.* GABA(A) receptors: structure and function in the basal ganglia. *Prog Brain Res* 2007; **160**: 21–41.

60 Costa E, Guidotti A. Endogenous ligands for benzodiazepine recognition sites. *Biochem Pharmacol* 1985; **34**: 3399–3403.

61 Baraldi M, Avallone R, Corsi L, *et al.* Endogenous benzodiazepines. *Therapie* 2000; **55**: 143–146.

62 Cortelli P, Avallone R, Baraldi M, *et al.* Endozepines in recurrent stupor. *Sleep Med Rev* 2005; **9**: 477–487.

63 Ahboucha S, Gamrani H, Baker G. GABAergic neurosteroids: the 'endogenous benzodiazepines' of acute liver failure. *Neurochem Int* 2012; **60**: 707–714.

64 Tonon M-C, Vaudry H, Chuquet J, *et al.* Endozepines and their receptors: structure, functions and pathophysiological significance. *Pharmacol Ther* 2020; **208**: 1–56.

65 Abbara C, Rousseau JM, Turcant A, *et al.* Bioavailability of diazepam after intramuscular injection of its water-soluble prodrug alone or with atropine-pralidoxime in healthy volunteers. *Br J Pharmacol* 2009; **157**: 1390–1397.

66 Treleano A, Wolz G, Brandsch R, *et al.* Investigation into the adsorption of nitroglycerine and diazepam into PVC tubes and alternative tube materials during application. *Int J Pharm* 2009; **369**: 30–37.

67 Winsnes M, Jeffsson R, Sjoberg B. Diazepam absorption to infusion sets and plastic syringes. *Acta Anaesthesiol Scand* 1981; **25**: 93–96.

68 KuKanich B, Nauss JL. Pharmacokinetics of the cytochrome P-450 substrates phenytoin, theophylline, and diazepam in healthy Greyhound dogs. *Vet Pharm Ther* 2012; **35**: 275–281.

69 Shou M, Norcross R, Sandig G, *et al.* Substrate specificity and kinetic properties of seven heterologously expressed dog cytochromes p450. *Drug Metab Dispos* 2003; **31**: 1161–1169.

70 Papich MG, Alcorn J. Absorption of diazepam after its rectal administration in dogs. *Am J Vet Res* 1995; **56**: 1629–1636.

71 Löscher W, Frey HH. Pharmacokinetics of diazepam in the dog. *Arch Int Pharmacodyn Ther* 1981; **254**: 180–195.

72 Cotler S, Gustafson JH, Colburn WA. Pharmacokinetics of diazepam and nordiazepam in the cat. *J Pharm Sci* 1984; **73**: 348–351.

73 van Beusekom CD, van den Heuvel JJ, Koenderink JB, *et al.* Feline hepatic biotransformation of diazepam: differences between cats and dogs. *Res Vet Sci* 2015; **103**: 119–125.

74 Muir WW, Sams RA, Huffman RH, *et al.* Pharmacodynamic and pharmacokinetic properties of diazepam in horses. *Am J Vet Res* 1982; **43**: 1756–1762.

75 Kanto JH. Midazolam: the first water-soluble benzodiazepine. Pharmacology, pharmacokinetics and efficacy in insomnia and anesthesia. *Pharmacotherapy* 1985; **5**: 138–155.

76 KuKanich B, Hubin M. The pharmacokinetics of ketoconazole and its effects on the pharmacokinetics of midazolam and fentanyl in dogs. *J Vet Pharmacol Ther* 2010; **33**: 42–49.

77 Schwartz M, Muñana KR, Nettifee-Osborne JA, *et al.* The pharmacokinetics of midazolam after intravenous, intramuscular, and rectal administration in healthy dogs. *J Vet Pharmacol Ther* 2013; **36**: 471–477.

78 Court MH, Greenblatt DJ. Pharmacokinetics and preliminary observations of behavioral changes following administration of midazolam to dogs. *J Vet Pharm Ther* 1992; **15**: 343–350.

79 Zhang J, Niu S, Zhang H, Streisand JB. Oral mucosal absorption of midazolam in dogs is strongly pH dependent. *J Pharm Sci* 2002; **91**: 980–982.

80 Henry RJ, Ruano N, Casto D, *et al.* A pharmacokinetic study of midazolam in dogs: nasal drop vs. atomizer administration. *Pediatr Dent* 1998; **20**: 321–326.

81 Eagleson JS, Platt SR, Strong DL, *et al.* Bioavailability of a novel midazolam gel after intranasal administration in dogs. *Am J Vet Res* 2012; **73**: 539–545.

82 Charalambous M, Bhatti SFM, Van Ham L, *et al.* Intranasal midazolam versus rectal diazepam for the management of canine status epilepticus: a multicenter randomized parallel-group clinical trial. *J Vet Intern Med* 2017; **31**: 1149–1158.

83 Charalambous M, Volk HA, Tipold A, *et al.* Comparison of intranasal versus intravenous midazolam for management of status epilepticus in dogs: a multi-center randomized parallel group clinical study. *J Vet Intern Med* 2019; **33**: 2709–2717.

84 Dholakia U, Seddighi R, Cox SK, *et al.* Pharmacokinetics of midazolam in sevoflurane-anesthetized cats. *Vet Anesth Analg* 2020; **47**: 200–209.

85 Marjani M, Akbarinejad V, Bagheri M. Comparison of intranasal and intramuscular ketamine-midazolam combination in cats. *Vet Anesth Analg* 2015; **42**: 178–181.

86 Hubbell JAE, Kelly EM, Aarnes TK, *et al.* Pharmacokinetics of midazolam after intravenous administration to horses. *Equine Vet J* 2013; **45**: 721–725.

87 Jones DJ, Stehling LC, Zauder HL. Cardiovascular responses to diazepam and midazolam maleate in the dog. *Anesthesiology* 1979; **51**: 430–434.

88 Flacke JW, Davis LJ, Flacke WE, *et al.* Effects of fentanyl and diazepam in dogs deprived of autonomic tone. *Anesth Analg* 1985; **64**: 1053–1059.

89 Machado CG, Dyson DH, Mathews KA. Evaluation of induction by use of a combination of oxymorphone and diazepam or hydromorphone and diazepam and maintenance of anesthesia by use of isoflurane in dogs with experimentally induced hypovolemia. *Am J Vet Res* 2005; **66**: 1227–1237.

90 Smith AC, Zellner JL, Spinale FG, *et al.* Sedative and cardiovascular effects of midazolam in swine. *Lab Anim Sci* 1991; **41**: 157–161.

91 Robinson R, Borer-Weir K. A dose titration study into the effects of diazepam or midazolam on the propofol dose requirements for induction of general anaesthesia in client owned dogs, premedicated with methadone and acepromazine. *Vet Anesth Analg* 2013; **40**: 455–463.

92 Ko JC, Payton ME, White AG, *et al.* Effects of intravenous diazepam or microdose medetomidine on propofol induced sedation in dogs. *J Am Anim Hosp Assoc* 2006; **42**: 18–27.

93 Italiano M, Robinson R. Effect of benzodiazepines on the dose of alfaxalone needed for endotracheal intubation in healthy dogs. *Vet Anaesth Analg* 2018; **45**: 720–728.

94 Miller C, Hughes E, Gurney M. Co-induction of anaesthesia with alfaxalone and midazolam in dogs: a randomized, blinded clinical trial. *Vet Anaesth Analg* 2019; **46**: 613–619.

95 Matthews NS, Dollar NS, Shawley RV. Halothane sparing effect of benzodiazepines in ponies. *Cornell Vet* 1990; **80**: 259–265.

96 Hellyer PW, Mama KR, Shafford HL, *et al.* Effects of diazepam and flumazenil on minimum alveolar concentrations for dogs anesthetized with isoflurane or a combination of isoflurane and fentanyl. *Am J Vet Res* 2001; **62**: 555–560.

97 Seddighi R, Egger CM, Rohrbach BW, *et al.* The effect of midazolam on the end-tidal concentration of isoflurane necessary to prevent movement in dogs. *Vet Anaesth Analg* 2011; **38**: 195–202.

98 Trevor AJ. Sedative-hypnotic drugs. In: Katzung BG, Vanerah TW, eds. *Basic and Clinical Pharmacology*, 15th edn New York, NY: McGraw Hill, 2021: 395.

99 Bagley RS, Chen AV. Anticonvulsants. In: Peterson ME, Talcott PA, eds. *Small Animal Toxicology*, 3rd edn. St. Louis, MO: Elsevier-Saunders, 2013: 450.

100 Hoffman WE, Albrecht RF, Miletich DJ, *et al.* Cerebrovascular and cerebral metabolic effects of physostigmine, midazolam, and a benzodiazepine antagonist. *Anesth Analg* 1986; **65**: 639–644.

101 Ilkiw JE, Suter CM, Farver TB, *et al.* The behavior of healthy awake cats following intravenous and intramuscular administration of midazolam. *J Vet Pharmacol Ther* 1996; **19**: 205–216.

102 Aarnes TK, Lerche P, Bednarski RM, *et al.* Total intravenous anesthesia using a midazolam-ketamine-xylazine infusion in horses: 46 cases (2011–2014). *Can Vet J* 2018; **59**: 500–504.

103 Bustamante R, Valverde A. Determination of a sedative dose and influence of droperidol and midazolam on cardiovascular function in pigs. *Can J Vet Res* 1997; **61**: 246–250.

104 Dzikiti TB, Zeiler GE, Dzikiti LN, *et al.* The effects of midazolam and butorphanol, administered alone or combined, on the dose and quality of anaesthetic induction with alfaxalone in goats. *J S Afr Vet Assoc* 2014; **85**: 1047.

105 Simon BT, Scallan EM, O O, *et al.* Pharmacokinetics and pharmacodynamics of midazolam following intravenous and intramuscular administration to sheep. *Am J Vet Res* 2017; **78**: 539–549.

106 Aarnes TK, Fry PR, Hubbell JA, *et al.* Pharmacokinetics and pharmacodynamics of midazolam after intravenous and intramuscular administration in alpacas. *Am J Vet Res* 2013; **74**: 294–299.

107 Robertson SA, Eberhart S. Efficacy of the intranasal route for administration of anesthetic agents to adult rabbits. *Lab Anim Sci* 1994; **44**: 159–165.

108 Álvarez ER, Solé LV, de Carellán Mateo AG. Comparison of subcutaneous sedation with alfaxalone or alfaxalone-midazolam in pet guinea pigs (*Cavia porcellus*) of three different age groups. *J Am Vet Med Assoc* 2022; **260**: 1024–1030.

109 Mans C, Guzman DS, Lahner LL, *et al.* Sedation and physiologic response to manual restraint after intranasal administration of midazolam in Hispaniolan Amazon parrots (*Amazona ventralis*). *J Avian Med Surg* 2012; **26**: 130–139.

110 Schaffer DPH, de Araújo NLLC, Raposo ACS, *et al.* Sedative effects of intranasal midazolam administration in wild caught blue-fronted Amazon (*Amazona aestiva*) and orange-winged Amazon (*Amazona amazonica*) parrots. *J Avian Med Surg* 2017; **31**: 213–218.

111 Greene SA, Moore MP, Keegan RD, *et al.* Quantitative electroencephalography for measurement of central nervous system responses to diazepam and the benzodiazepine antagonist, flumazenil, in isoflurane-anaesthetized dogs. *J Vet Pharmacol Ther* 1992; **15**: 259–266.

112 Keegan RD, Greene SA, Moore MP, *et al.* Antagonism by flumazenil of midazolam-induced changes in quantitative electroencephalographic data from isoflurane-anesthetized dogs. *Am J Vet Res* 1993; **54**: 761–765.

113 Goh ET, Andersen ML, Morgan MY, *et al.* Flumazenil versus placebo or no intervention for people with cirrhosis and hepatic encephalopathy. *Cochrane Database Syst Rev* 2017; **7**: CD002798.

114 Martin WR, Sloan JW, Wala E. Precipitated abstinence in orally dosed benzodiazepine-dependent dogs. *J Pharmacol Exp Ther* 1990; **255**: 744–755.

115 Lheureux P, Vranckx M, Leduc D, *et al.* Flumazenil in mixed benzodiazepine/tricyclic antidepressant overdose: a placebo-controlled study in the dog. *Am J Emerg Med* 1992; **10**: 184–188.

116 An H, Godwin J. Flumazenil in benzodiazepine overdose. *CMAJ* 2016; **188**: E537.

117 Greene SA, Thurmon JC. Xylazine – a review of its pharmacology and use in veterinary medicine. *J Vet Pharmacol Ther* 1988; **11**: 295–313.

118 Clarke KW, Hall LW. "Xylazine" – a new sedative for horses and cattle. *Vet Rec* 1969; **85**: 512–517.

119 Kerr DD, Jones EW, Huggins K, *et al.* Sedative and other effects of xylazine given intravenously to horses. *Am J Vet Res* 1972; **33**: 525–532.

120 Klein L, Baetjer C. Preliminary report: xylazine and morphine sedation in the horse. *Vet Anesth* 1974; **2**: 2–4.

121 Antonaccio MJ, Robson RD, Kerwin L. Evidence for increased vagal tone and enhancement of baroreceptor reflex activity after xylazine (2-(2,6-dimethylphenylamino)-4-H-5,6-dihydro-1,3-thiazine) in anesthestized dogs. *Eur J Pharmacol* 1973; **23**: 311–316.

122 Moye RJ, Pailet A, Smith MW Jr. Clinical use of xylazine in dogs and cats. *Vet Med Small Anim Clin* 1973; **68**: 236.

123 Hsu WH. Xylazine-induced depression and its antagonism by alpha adrenergic blocking agents. *J Pharmacol Exp Ther* 1981; **218**: 188–192.

124 Bylund DB, Ray-Prenger C, Murphy TJ. Alpha-2A and alpha-2B adrenergic receptor subtypes: antagonist binding in tissues and cell lines containing only one subtype. *J Pharmacol Exp Ther* 1988; **245**: 600–607.

125 Bylund DB. Alpha-2 adrenoceptor subtypes: are more better? *Br J Pharmacol* 2005; **144**: 159–160.

126 Raczak-Gutknecht J, Frąckowiak T, Nasal A, *et al.* Are alpha-2D adrenoceptor subtypes involved in rat mydriasis evoked by new imidazoline derivatives: marsanidine and 7-methylmarsanidine? *Dose Response* 2017; **15**: 1559325817701213.

127 Ruuskanen JO, Xhaard H, Marjamäki A, *et al.* Identification of duplicated fourth alpha2-adrenergic receptor subtype by cloning and mapping of five receptor genes in zebrafish. *Mol Biol Evol* 2004; **21**: 14–28.

128 Ma D, Rajakumaraswamy N, Maze M. α_2-Adrenoceptor agonists: shedding light on neuroprotection? *Br Med Bull* 2005; **71**: 77–92.

129 Pichot C, Ghignone M, Quintin L. Dexmedetomidine and clonidine: from second- to first-line sedative agents in the critical care setting? *J Intensive Care Med* 2012; **27**: 219–237.

130 Buerkle H, Yaksh TL. Pharmacological evidence for different alpha 2-adrenergic receptor sites mediating analgesia and sedation in the rat. *Br J Anaesth* 1998; **81**: 208–215.

131 Carollo DS, Nossaman BD, Ramadhyani U. Dexmedetomidine: a review of clinical applications. *Curr Opin Anaesthesiol* 2008; **21**: 457–461.

132 Giovannitti JA Jr, Thoms SM, Crawford JJ. Alpha-2 adrenergic receptor agonists: a review of current clinical applications. *Anesth Prog* 2015; **62**: 313–319.

133 Puumala T, Riekkinen P Sr, Sirviö J. Modulation of vigilance and behavioral activation by alpha-1 adrenoceptors in the rat. *Pharmacol Biochem Behav* 1997; **56**: 705–712.

134 Bousquet P, Hudson A, García-Sevilla JA, *et al.* Imidazoline receptor system: the past, the present, and the future. *Pharmacol Rev* 2020; **72**: 50–79.

135 Li Y, Cheng KC, Asakawa A, *et al.* Activation of imidazoline-I3 receptors ameliorates pancreatic damage. *Clin Exp Pharmacol Physiol* 2015; **42**: 964–971.

136 Matsukawa T, Hikasa Y. Effects of imidazoline and nonimidazoline α-adrenoceptor agonists and antagonists, including xylazine, medetomidine, dexmedetomidine, yohimbine, and atipamezole, on aggregation of feline platelets. *Am J Vet Res* 2020; **81**: 159–171.

137 Clineschmidt BV, Pettibone DJ, Lotti VJ, *et al.* A peripherally acting alpha-2 adrenoceptor antagonist: L-659,066. *J Pharmacol Exp Ther* 1988; **245**: 32–40.

138 Pakkanen S. *Interaction of alpha$_2$-adrenoceptor agonists and vatinoxan, a peripherally acting alpha$_2$-adrenoceptor antagonist, in horses.* Academic Dissertation, University of Helsinki, 2019.

139 Uusalo P, Al-Ramahi D, Tilli I, *et al.* Subcutaneously administered dexmedetomidine is efficiently absorbed and is associated with attenuated cardiovascular effects in healthy volunteers. *Eur J Clin Pharmacol* 2018; **74**: 1047–1054.

140 Ashraf MW, Uusalo P, Scheinin M, *et al.* Population modelling of dexmedetomidine pharmacokinetics and haemodynamic effects after intravenous and subcutaneous administration. *Clin Pharmacokinet* 2020; **59**: 1467–1482.

141 Rabbogliatti V, Amari M, Brioschi FA, *et al.* Use of dexmedetomidine repeated subcutaneous administration for balanced anaesthesia in horses. *BMC Vet Res* 2022; **18**: 269.

142 Garcia-Villar R, Toutain PL, Alvinerie M, *et al.* The pharmacokinetics of xylazine hydrochloride: an interspecific study. *J Vet Pharmacol Ther* 1981; **4**: 87–92.

143 Knych HK, Stanley SD, McKemie DS, *et al.* Pharmacokinetic and pharmacodynamics of xylazine administered to exercised thoroughbred horses. *Drug Test Anal* 2017; **9**: 713–720.

144 Habershon-Butcher J, Cutler C, Viljanto M, *et al.* Re-evaluation of the pharmacokinetics of xylazine administered to Thoroughbred horses. *J Vet Pharmacol Ther* 2020; **43**: 6–12.

145 Hopster K, Soma LR, Li X, *et al.* Pharmacokinetics of xylazine after 2-, 4-, and 6-hr durations of continuous rate infusions in horses. *J Vet Pharmacol Ther* 2020; **43**: 557–564.

146 Guedes A, Knych H, Tucker L, *et al.* Pharmacokinetics and clinical effects of xylazine and dexmedetomidine in horses recovering from isoflurane anesthesia. *J Vet Pharmacol Ther* 2020; **43**: 369–376.

147 Santonastaso A, Hardy J, Cohen N, *et al.* Pharmacokinetics and pharmacodynamics of xylazine administered by the intravenous or intra-osseous route in adult horses. *J Vet Pharmacol Ther* 2014; **37**: 565–570.

148 Salonen JS, Vähä-Vahe T, Vainio O, *et al.* Single-dose pharmacokinetics of detomidine in the horse and cow. *J Vet Pharmacol Ther* 1989; **12**: 65–72.

149 Elfenbein JR, Sanchez LC, Robertson SA, *et al.* Effect of detomidine on visceral and somatic nociception and duodenal motility in conscious adult horses. *Vet Anaesth Analg* 2009; **36**: 162–172.

150 Hubbell JAE, Sams RA, Schmall LM, *et al.* Pharmacokinetics of detomidine administered to horses at rest and after maximal exercise. *Equine Vet J* 2009; **5**: 419–422.

151 Grimsrud KN, Mama KR, Thomasy SM, *et al.* Pharmacokinetics of detomidine and its metabolites following intravenous and intramuscular administration in horses. *Equine Vet J* 2009; **4**: 361–365.

152 Kaukinen H, Aspegren J, Hyyppa S, *et al.* Bioavailability of detomidine administered sublingually to horses as an oromucosal gel. *J Vet Pharm Ther* 2011; **34**: 76–81.

153 Hokkanen AH, Raekallio MR, Salla K, *et al.* Sublingual administration of detomidine to calves prior to disbudding: a comparison with the intravenous route. *Vet Anaesth Analg* 2014; **41**: 372–377.

154 Hopfensperger MJ, Messenger KM, Papich MG, *et al.* The use of oral transmucosal detomidine hydrochloride gel to facilitate handling in dogs. *J Vet Behav Clin Appl Res* 2013; **8**: 114–123.

155 Messenger KM, Hopfensperger M, Knych HK, *et al.* Pharmacokinetics of detomidine following intravenous or oral-transmucosal administration and sedative effects of the oral-transmucosal treatment in dogs. *Am J Vet Res* 2016; **77**: 413–420.

156 Kasten JI, Messenger KM, Campbell NB. Sedative and cardiopulmonary effects of buccally administered detomidine gel and reversal with atipamezole in dogs. *Am J Vet Res* 2018; **79**: 1253–1260.

157 Phillips BE, Harms CA, Messenger KM. Oral transmucosal detomidine gel for the sedation of the domestic ferret (*Mustela putorius furo*). *J Exot Pet Med* 2015; **24**: 446–454.

158 Williams MD, Long CT, Durrant JR, *et al.* Oral transmucosal detomidine gel in New Zealand white rabbits (*Oryctolagus cuniculus*). *J Am Assoc Lab Anim Sci* 2017; **56**: 436–442.

159 Smith P, Tolbert MK, Gould E, *et al.* Pharmacokinetics, sedation and hemodynamic changes following the administration of oral transmucosal detomidine gel in cats. *J Feline Med Surg* 2020; **22**: 1184–1190.

160 Seddighi R, Knych HK, Cox SK, *et al.* Evaluation of the sedative effects and pharmacokinetics of detomidine gel administered intravaginally to horses. *Vet Anaesth Analg* 2019; **46**: 772–779.

161 Chow NS, Seddighi R, Knych HK, *et al.* Sedative effects and pharmacokinetics of detomidine when administered intravenously and intravaginally as a gel in alpacas. *Vet Anaesth Analg* 2020; **47**: 773–780.

162 Tahmasbi T, Raisi A, Zakian A, *et al.* Comparing the effects of intravenous injection and intranasal atomisation of detomidine in sheep. *Vet Med Sci* 2023; **9**: 353–362.

163 Wojtasiak-Wypart M, Soma LR, Rudy JA, *et al.* Pharmacokinetic profile and pharmacodynamic effects of romifidine hydrochloride in the horse. *J Vet Pharmacol Ther* 2012; **35**: 478–488.

164 Knych HK, Stanley SD, McKemie DS, *et al.* Pharmacokinetics and selected pharmacodynamics of romifidine following low-dose intravenous administration in combination with exercise to quarter horses. *J Vet Pharmacol Ther* 2017; **40**: 569–574.

165 Levionnois OL, Barbarossa A, Bardhi A, *et al.* Enantiospecific pharmacokinetics of intravenous dexmedetomidine in beagles. *J Vet Pharmacol Ther* 2022; **45**: 366–372.

166 Kuusela E, Raekallio M, Anttila M, *et al.* Clinical effects and pharmacokinetics of medetomidine and its enantiomers in dogs. *J Vet Pharmcol Ther* 2000; **23**: 15–20.

167 Escobar A, Pypendop BH, Siao KT, *et al.* Pharmacokinetics of dexmedetomidine administered intravenously in isoflurane anesthetized cats. *Am J Vet Res* 2012; **73**: 285–289.

168 Rezende ML, Grimsrud KN, Stanley SD, *et al.* Pharmacokinetics and pharmacodynamics of intravenous dexmedetomidine in the horse. *J Vet Pharmacol Ther* 2015; **38**: 15–23.

169 Bettschart-Wolfensberger R, Freeman SL, Bowen IM, *et al.* Cardiopulmonary effects and pharmacokinetics of IV dexmedetomidine in ponies. *Equine Vet J* 2005; **37**: 60–64.
170 Grimsrud KN, Mama KR, Steffey EP, *et al.* Pharmacokinetics and pharmacodynamics of intravenous medetomidine in the horse. *Vet Anaesth Analg* 2012; **39**: 38–48.
171 Ansah OB, Raekallio M, Vainio O. Comparing oral and intramuscular administration of medetomidine in cats. *J Vet Anaesth* 1998; **25**: 41–46.
172 Slingsby LS, Taylor OM, Monroe T. Thermal antinociception after dexmedetomidine administration in cats: a comparison between intramuscular and oral transmucosal administration. *J Feline Med Surg* 2009; **11**: 829–834.
173 Santos LCP, Ludders JW, Erb HN, *et al.* Sedative and cardiorespiratory effects of dexmedetomidine and buprenorphine administered to cats via oral transmucosal or intramuscular routes. *Vet Anesth Analg* 2010; **37**: 417–424.
174 Porters N, Bosmans T, Debille M, *et al.* Sedative and antinociceptive effects of dexmedetomidine and buprenorphine after oral transmucosal or intramuscular administration in cats. *Vet Anaesth Analg* 2014; **41**: 90–96.
175 Dent BT, Aarnes TK, Wavreille VA, *et al.* Pharmacokinetics and pharmacodynamic effects of oral transmucosal and intravenous administration of dexmedetomidine in dogs. *Am J Vet Res* 2019; **80**: 969–975.
176 Gioeni D, Brioschi FA, Di Cesare F, *et al.* Oral transmucosal or intramuscular administration of dexmedetomidine-methadone combination in dogs: sedative and physiological effects. *Animals (Basel)* 2020; **10**: 2057.
177 Santangelo B, Harel M, Fourel I, *et al.* Intranasal dexmedetomidine in healthy beagles: an echocardiographic and pharmacokinetic/pharmacodynamic study. *Vet J* 2019; **251**: 105346.
178 Pavlica M, Kržan M, Nemec A, *et al.* Cardiopulmonary effects and pharmacokinetics of dexmedetomidine used as an adjunctive analgesic to regional anesthesia of the oral cavity with levobupivacaine in dogs. *Animals (Basel)* 2022; **12**: 1217.
179 Pypendop BH, Verstegen JP. Hemodynamic effects of medetomidine in the dog: a dose titration study. *Vet Surg* 1998; **27**: 612–622.
180 Pypendop BH, Verstegen JP. Cardiovascular effects of romifidine in dogs. *Am J Vet Res* 2001; **62**: 490–495.
181 Lamont LA, Bulmer BJ, Grimm KA, *et al.* Cardiopulmonary evaluation of the use of medetomidine hydrochloride in cats. *Am J Vet Res* 2001; **62**: 1745–1749.
182 Bueno AC, Cornick-Seahorn J, Seahorn TL, *et al.* Cardiopulmonary and sedative effects of intravenous administration of low doses of medetomidine and xylazine to adult horses. *Am J Vet Res* 1999; **60**: 1371–1376.
183 de Morais HS, Muir WW III. The effects of medetomidine on cardiac contractility in autonomically blocked dogs. *Vet Surg* 1995; **24**: 356–364.
184 Muir WW, Piper FS. Effect of xylazine on indices of myocardial contractility in the dog. *Am J Vet Res* 1977; **38**: 931–934.
185 Kaartinen J, Pang D, Moreau M, *et al.* Hemodynamic effects of an intravenous infusion of medetomidine at six different dose regimens in isoflurane-anesthetized dogs. *Vet Ther* 2010; **11**: E1–E16.
186 Hopster K, Wittenberg-Voges L, Kästner SBR. Xylazine infusion in isoflurane-anesthetized and ventilated healthy horses: effects on cardiovascular parameters and intestinal perfusion. *Can J Vet Res* 2017; **81**: 249–254.
187 Lawrence CJ, Prinzen FW, de Lange S. The effect of dexmedetomidine on nutrient organ blood flow. *Anesth Analg* 1996; **83**: 1160–1165.
188 Snapir A, Posti J, Kentala E, *et al.* Effects of low and high plasma concentrations of dexmedetomidine on myocardial perfusion and cardiac function in healthy male subjects. *Anesthesiology* 2006; **105**: 902–910.
189 Roekaerts PM, Prinzen FW, De Lange S. Beneficial effects of dexmedetomidine on ischaemic myocardium of anaesthetized dogs. *Br J Anaesth* 1996; **77**: 427–429.
190 Sinclair MD. A review of the physiological effects of alpha2-agonists related to the clinical use of medetomidine in small animal practice. *Can Vet J* 2003; **44**: 885–897.
191 Tranquilli WJ, Thurmon JC, Benson GJ, *et al.* Alteration in the Arrhythmogenic Dose of Epinephrine (ADE) following xylazine administration to halothane-anesthetized dogs. *J Vet Pharmacol Ther* 1986; **9**: 198–203.
192 Tranquilli WJ, Thurmon JC, Benson GJ. Alterations in epinephrine-induced arrhythmogenesis after xylazine and subsequent yohimbine administration in isoflurane-anesthetized dogs. *Am J Vet Res* 1988; **49**: 1072–1075.
193 Lemke KA, Tranquilli WJ, Thurmon JC, *et al.* Alterations in the arrhythmogenic dose of epinephrine after xylazine or medetomidine administration in halothane-anesthetized dogs. *Am J Vet Res* 1993; **54**: 2132–2138.
194 Lemke KA, Tranquilli WJ, Thurmon JC, *et al.* Alterations in the arrhythmogenic dose of epinephrine after xylazine or medetomidine administration in isoflurane-anesthetized dogs. *Am J Vet Res* 1993; **54**: 2139–2144.
195 Hayashi Y, Sumikawa K, Maze M, *et al.* Dexmedetomidine prevents epinephrine-induced arrhythmias through stimulation of central alpha 2 adrenoceptors in halothane-anesthetized dogs. *Anesthesiology* 1991; **75**: 113–117.
196 Short CE. Effects of anticholinergic treatment on the cardiac and respiratory systems in dogs sedated with medetomidine. *Vet Rec* 1991; **129**: 310–313.
197 Ko JC, Fox SM, Mandsager RE. Effects of preemptive atropine administration on incidence of medetomidine-induced bradycardia in dogs. *J Am Vet Med Assoc* 2001; **218**: 52–58.
198 Singh S, Young SS, McDonell WN, *et al.* Modification of cardiopulmonary and intestinal motility effects of xylazine with glycopyrrolate in horses. *Can J Vet Res* 1997; **61**: 99–107.
199 Bloor BC, Abdul-Rasool I, Temp J, *et al.* The effects of medetomidine, an α2-adrenergic agonist, on ventilatory drive in the dog. *Acta Vet Scand* 1989; (Suppl 85): 65–70.
200 Lerche P, Muir WW III. Effect of medetomidine on breathing and inspiratory neuromuscular drive in conscious dogs. *Am J Vet Res* 2004; **65**: 720–724.
201 Klide AM, Calderwood HW, Soma LR. Cardiopulmonary effects of xylazine in dogs. *Am J Vet Res* 1975; **36**: 931–935.
202 Selmi AL, Barbudo-Selmi GR, Moreira CF, *et al.* Evaluation of sedative and cardiorespiratory effects of romifidine and romifidine-butorphanol in cats. *J Am Vet Med Assoc* 2002; **221**: 506–510.
203 Di Bella C, Skouropoulou D, Stabile M, *et al.* Respiratory and hemodynamic effects of 2 protocols of low-dose infusion of dexmedetomidine in dogs under isoflurane anesthesia. *Can J Vet Res* 2020; **84**: 96–107.
204 Celly CS, McDonell WN, Young SS, *et al.* The comparative hypoxaemic effect of four alpha(2) adrenoceptor agonists (xylazine, romifidine, detomidine and medetomidine) in sheep. *J Vet Pharmacol Ther* 1997; **20**: 464–471.
205 Celly CS, Atwal OS, McDonell WN, *et al.* Histopathologic alterations induced in the lungs of sheep by use of alpha2-adrenergic receptor agonists. *Am J Vet Res* 1999; **60**: 154–161.
206 Clarke KW, England GCW. Medetomidine, a new sedative-analgesic for use in the dog and its reversal with atipamezole. *J Small Anim Pract* 1989; **30**: 343–348.
207 Guo TZ, Tinklenberg J, Oliker R, *et al.* Central alpha 1-adrenoceptor stimulation functionally antagonizes the hypnotic response to dexmedetomidine, an alpha 2-adrenoceptor agonist. *Anesthesiology* 1991; **75**: 252–256.
208 Yaksh TL. Pharmacology of spinal adrenergic systems which modulate spinal nociceptive processing. *Pharmacol Biochem Behav* 1985; **22**: 845–858.
209 Kaye AD, Chernobylsky DJ, Thakur P, *et al.* Dexmedetomidine in enhanced recovery after surgery (ERAS) protocols for postoperative pain. *Curr Pain Headache Rep* 2020; **24**: 21.
210 Keegan RD, Greene SA, Bagley RS, *et al.* Effects of medetomidine administration on intracranial pressure and cardiovascular variables of isoflurane anesthetized dogs. *Am J Vet Res* 1995; **56**: 193–198.
211 Zornow MH, Fleischer JE, Scheller MS, *et al.* Dexmedetomidine, an alpha 2-adrenergic agonist, decreases cerebral blood flow in the isoflurane-anesthetized dog. *Anesth Analg* 1990; **70**: 624–630.
212 Flower O, Hellings S. Sedation in traumatic brain injury. *Emerg Med Int* 2012; **2012**: 637171.
213 Colby ED, McCarthy LE, Borison HL. Emetic action of xylazine on the chemoreceptor trigger zone for vomiting in cats. *J Vet Pharmacol Therap* 1981; **4**: 93–96.
214 Hikasa Y, Ogasawara S, Takase K. Alpha adrenoceptor subtypes involved in the emetic action of dogs. *J Pharmacol Exp Ther* 1992; **261**: 746–754.
215 Lang IM, Sarna SK. The role of adrenergic receptors in the initiation of vomiting and its gastrointestinal motor correlates. *J Pharmacol Exp Ther* 1992; **263**: 395–403.
216 Ruckebusch Y, Allal C. Depression of reticulo-ruminal motor functions through the stimulation of α_2-adrenoceptors. *J Vet Pharmacol Ther* 1987; **10**: 1–10.
217 Rutkowski JA, Ross MW, Cullen K. Effects of xylazine and/or butorphanol or neostigmine on myoelectric activity of the cecum and right ventral colon in female ponies. *Am J Vet Res* 1989; **50**: 1096–1101.
218 Maugeri S, Ferrè JP, Intorre L, *et al.* Effects of medetomidine on intestinal and colonic motility in the dog. *J Vet Pharmacol Ther* 1994; **17**: 148–154.
219 Humphreys MH, Reid LA, Chou LYN. Suppression of antidiuretic hormone secretion by clonidine in the anesthetized dog. *Kidney Int* 1975; **7**: 405–412.
220 Reid IA, Nolan PL, Wolf JA, *et al.* Suppression of vasopressin secretion by clonidine: effect of alpha-adrenoceptor antagonists. *Endocrinology* 1979; **104**: 1403–1406.
221 Gellai M, Edwards RM. Mechanism of α_2-adrenoceptor agonist-induced diuresis. *Am J Physiol* 1988; **255**: 317–323.
222 Smyth DD, Unemura S, Pettinger WA. Alpha$_2$-adrenoceptor antagonism of vasopression-induced changes in sodium excretion. *Am J Physiol* 1985; **248**: 767–772.
223 Smyth D, Umemura S, Yang E, *et al.* Inhibition of renin release by alpha-adrenoceptor stimulation in the isolated perfused rat kidney. *Eur J Pharmacol* 1987; **140**: 33–38.
224 Aro E, Bastman S, Andersson KE, *et al.* Is there a peripheral site of action contributing to the voiding effects of α_2-adrenoceptor agonists and antagonists? *World J Urol* 2015; **33**: 433–440.
225 LeBlanc MM, Hubbell JA, Smith HC. The effects of xylazine hydrochloride on intrauterine pressure in the cow. *Theriogenology* 1984; **21**: 681–690.

226 Rexroad CE, Barb CR. Contractile response of the uterus of the estrous ewe to adrenergic stimulation. *Biol Reprod* 1978; **19**: 297–305.

227 Jansen CA, Lowe KC, Nathanielsz PW. The effects of xylazine on uterine activity, fetal, and maternal oxygenation, cardiovascular function and fetal breathing. *Am J Obstet Gynecol* 1984; **148**: 386–390.

228 Schatzmann U, Jossfck H, Starffer JL, *et al.* Effects of alpha 2-agonists on intrauterine pressure and sedation in horses: comparison between detomidine, romifidine, and xylazine. *Zentralbl Veterinarmed A* 1994; **41**: 523–529.

229 Jedruch J, Gajewski Z, Ratajska-Michalczak K. Uterine motor responses to an α2-adrenergic agonist medetomidine hydrochloride in the bitches during the end of gestation and the post-partum period. *Acta Vet Scand* 1989; **85**: 129–134.

230 Jedruch J, Gajewski Z. The effect of detomidine hydrochloride (Domosedan) on the electrical activity of the uterus in cows. *Acta Vet Scand* 1986; **82**: 189–192.

231 Jedruch J, Gajewski Z, Kuussaari J. The effect of detomidine hydrochloride on the electrical activity of uterus in pregnant mares. *Acta Vet Scand* 1988; **30**: 307–311.

232 Re G, Badino P, Odore R, *et al.* Identification of functional alpha-adrenoceptor subtypes in the bovine female genital tract during different phases of the oestrous cycle. *Vet Res Commun* 2002; **26**: 479–494.

233 Benson GJ, Grubb TL, Neff-Davis C, *et al.* Perioperative stress response in the dog: effect of pre-emptive administration of medetomidine. *Vet Surg* 2000; **29**: 85–91.

234 Ambrisko TD, Hikashi Y. Neurohormonal and metabolic effects of medetomidine compared with xylazine in beagle dogs. *Can J Vet Res* 2002; **6**: 42–49.

235 Vaisanen M, Raekallio M, Kuusela E, *et al.* Evaluation of the perioperative stress response in dogs administered medetomidine or acepromazine as part of the preanesthetic medication. *Am J Vet Res* 2002; **63**: 969–975.

236 Ambrisko TD, Hikashi Y. The antagonistic effects of atipamezole and yohimbine on stress-related neurohormonal and metabolic responses induced by medetomidine in dogs. *Can J Vet Res* 2003; **67**: 64–67.

237 Raekallio M, Vainio O, Scheinin M. Detomidine reduces the plasma catecholamine, but not cortisol concentrations in horses. *Zentralbl Veterinarmed A* 1991; **38**: 153–156.

238 Ranheim B, Horsberg TE, Søli NE, *et al.* The effects of medetomidine and its reversal with atipamezole on plasma glucose, cortisol and noradrenaline in cattle and sheep. *J Vet Pharmacol Ther* 2000; **23**: 379–387.

239 Maze M, Virtanen R, Daunt D, *et al.* Effects of dexmedetomidine, a novel imidazole sedative-anesthetic agent, on adrenal steroidogenesis: in vivo and in vitro studies. *Anesth Analg* 1991; **73**: 204–208.

240 Restitutti F, Raekallio M, Vainionpää M, *et al.* Plasma glucose, insulin, free fatty acids, lactate and cortisol concentrations in dexmedetomidine-sedated dogs with or without MK-467: a peripheral α-2 adrenoceptor antagonist. *Vet J* 2012; **193**: 481–485.

241 Wang K, Wu M, Xu J, *et al.* Effects of dexmedetomidine on perioperative stress, inflammation, and immune function: systematic review and meta-analysis. *Br J Anaesth* 2019; **123**: 777–794.

242 Brockman RP. Effect of xylazine on plasma glucose, glucagon and insulin concentrations in sheep. *Res Vet Science* 1981; **30**: 383–384.

243 Angel I, Langer SZ. Adrenergic induced hyperglycaemia in anaesthetised rats: involvement of peripheral α2-adrenoceptors. *Eur J Pharmacol* 1988; **154**: 191–196.

244 Niddam R, Angel I, Bidet S, *et al.* Pharmacological characterization of alpha-2 adrenergic receptor subtype involved in the release of insulin from isolated rat pancreatic islets. *J Pharmacol Exp Ther* 1990; **254**: 883–887.

245 Thurmon J, Steffey E, Zinkl J, *et al.* Xylazine causes transient dose-related hyperglycemia and increased urine volumes in mares. *Am J Vet Res* 1984; **45**: 224–227.

246 Hsu WH, Hummel SK. Xylazine-induced hyperglycemia in cattle: a possible involvement of alpha 2-adrenergic receptors regulating insulin release. *Endocrinology* 1981: **109**: 825–829.

247 Pascoe PJ, Raekallio M, Kuusela E, *et al.* Changes in the minimum alveolar concentration of isoflurane and some cardiopulmonary measurements during three continuous infusion rates of dexmedetomidine in dogs. *Vet Anaesth Analg* 2006; **33**: 97–103.

248 Pascoe PJ. The cardiopulmonary effects of dexmedetomidine infusions in dogs during isoflurane anesthesia. *Vet Anaesth Analg* 2015; **42**: 360–368.

249 Simon BT, Scallan EM, Coursey CD, *et al.* The clinical effects of a low dose dexmedetomidine constant rate infusion in isoflurane anesthetized cats. *Vet J* 2018; **234**: 55–60.

250 Quirós-Carmona S, Navarrete R, Domínguez JM, *et al.* A comparison of cardiopulmonary effects and anaesthetic requirements of two dexmedetomidine continuous rate infusions in alfaxalone-anaesthetized Greyhounds. *Vet Anaesth Analg* 2017; **44**: 228–236.

251 Sanches MC, Bessi WH, Rusch E, *et al.* Cardiopulmonary and propofol-sparing effects of dexmedetomidine in total intravenous anesthesia in cats undergoing ovariohysterectomy. *J Feline Med Surg* 2022; **24**: e490–e497.

252 Raffe MR. Total Intravenous anesthesia for the small animal critical patient. *Vet Clin North Am Small Anim Pract* 2020; **50**: 1433–1444.

253 Lin GY, Robben JH, Murrell JC, *et al.* Dexmedetomidine constant rate infusion for 24 hours during and after propofol or isoflurane anaesthesia in dogs. *Vet Anaesth Analg* 2008; **35**: 141–153.

254 Valtolina C, Robben JH, Uilenreef J, *et al.* Clinical evaluation of the efficacy and safety of a constant rate infusion of dexmedetomidine for postoperative pain management in dogs. *Vet Anaesth Analg* 2009; **36**: 369–383.

255 Campagnol D, Teixeira Neto FJ, Giordano T, *et al.* Effects of epidural administration of dexmedetomidine on the minimum alveolar concentration of isoflurane in dogs. *Am J Vet Res* 2007; **68**: 1308–1318.

256 O O, Smith LJ. A comparison of epidural analgesia provided by bupivacaine alone, bupivacaine + morphine, or bupivacaine + dexmedetomidine for pelvic orthopedic surgery in dogs. *Vet Anaesth Analg* 2013; **40**: 527–536.

257 Caramalac SM, Albuquerque VB, Oliveira AR, *et al.* Analgesic, cardiorespiratory effects and motor block characteristics of epidural levobupivacaine alone or in combination with methadone or dexmedetomidine in bitches undergoing unilateral total mastectomy. *An Acad Bras Cienc* 2022; **94**(suppl 3): e20210082.

258 Souza SS, Intelisano TR, De Biaggi CP, *et al.* Cardiopulmonary and isoflurane-sparing effects of epidural or intravenous infusion of dexmedetomidine in cats undergoing surgery with epidural lidocaine. *Vet Anaesth Analg* 2010; **37**: 106–115.

259 Lamont LA, Lemke KA. The effects of medetomidine on radial nerve blockade with mepivacaine in dogs. *Vet Anaesth Analg* 2008; **35**: 62–68.

260 Hommuang K, Sattasathuchana P, Thengchaisri N. Effects of intranasal and intramuscular dexmedetomidine in cats receiving total intravenous propofol anesthesia. *Vet World* 2022; **15**: 1706–1713.

261 England GC, Clarke KW, Goossens L. A comparison of the sedative effects of three α2-adrenoceptor agonists (romifidine, detomidine, and xylazine) in the horse. *J Vet Pharm Ther* 1992; **15**: 194–201.

262 Yamashita K, Muir WW III, Tsubakishita S, *et al.* Clinical comparison of xylazine and medetomidine for premedication of horses. *J Am Vet Med Assoc* 2002; **221**: 1144–1149.

263 Bryant CE, England GC, Clarke KW. Comparison of the sedative effects of medetomidine and xylazine in horses. *Vet Rec* 1991; **129**: 421–423.

264 Hamm D, Turchi P, Jöchle W. Sedative and analgesic effects of detomidine and romifidine in horses. *Vet Rec* 1995; **136**: 324–327.

265 Freeman SL, England GC. Investigation of romifidine and detomidine for the clinical sedation of horses. *Vet Rec* 2000; **147**: 507–511.

266 Valverde A. Alpha-2 agonists as pain therapy in horses. *Vet Clin North Am Equine Pract* 2010; **26**: 515–532.

267 Ringer SK, Portier K, Torgerson PR, *et al.* The effects of a loading dose followed by constant rate infusion of xylazine compared with romifidine on sedation, ataxia and response to stimuli in horses. *Vet Anaesth Analg* 2013; **40**: 157–165.

268 Pallarols NB, Lamuraglia R, Guglielminetti A, *et al.* Behavioral and cardiopulmonary effects of a constant rate infusion of remifentanil-xylazine for sedation in horses. *J Equine Vet Sci* 2020; **91**: 103111.

269 Gozalo-Marcilla M, Luna SP, Gasthuys F, *et al.* Clinical applicability of detomidine and methadone constant rate infusions for surgery in standing horses. *Vet Anaesth Analg* 2019; **46**: 325–334.

270 Hollis AR, Pascal M, Van Dijk J, *et al.* Behavioural and cardiovascular effects of medetomidine constant rate infusion compared with detomidine for standing sedation in horses. *Vet Anaesth Analg* 2020; **47**: 76–81.

271 Pöppel N, Hopster K, Geburek F, *et al.* Influence of ketamine or xylazine supplementation on isoflurane anaesthetized horses – a controlled clinical trial. *Vet Anaesth Analg* 2015; **42**: 30–38.

272 Menzies MP, Ringer SK, Conrot A, *et al.* Cardiopulmonary effects and anaesthesia recovery quality in horses anaesthetized with isoflurane and low-dose S-ketamine or medetomidine infusions. *Vet Anaesth Analg* 2016; **43**: 623–634.

273 Kälin I, Henze IS, Ringer SK, *et al.* Comparison of recovery quality following medetomidine versus xylazine balanced isoflurane anaesthesia in horses: a retrospective analysis. *Animals (Basel)* 2021; **11**: 2440.

274 Marcilla MG, Schauvliege S, Segaert S, *et al.* Influence of a constant rate infusion of dexmedetomidine on cardiopulmonary function and recovery quality in isoflurane anaesthetized horses. *Vet Anaesth Analg* 2012; **39**: 49–58.

275 Greene SA, Thurmon JC, Tranquilli WJ, *et al.* Cardiopulmonary effects of continuous intravenous infusion of guaifenesin, ketamine, and xylazine in ponies. *Am J Vet Res* 1986; **47**: 2364–2367.

276 Umar MA, Fukui S, Kawase K, *et al.* Cardiovascular effects of total intravenous anesthesia using ketamine-medetomidine-propofol (KMP-TIVA) in horses undergoing surgery. *J Vet Med Sci* 2015; **77**: 281–288.

277 Guedes AGP, Tearney CC, Cenani A, *et al.* Comparison between the effects of postanesthetic xylazine and dexmedetomidine on characteristics of recovery from sevoflurane anesthesia in horses. *Vet Anaesth Analg* 2017; **44**: 273–280.

278 Leblanc PH, Eberhart SW. Cardiopulmonary effects of epidurally administered xylazine in the horse. *Equine Vet J* 1990; **22**: 389–391.

279 Grubb TL, Riebold TW, Huber MJ. Comparison of lidocaine, xylazine, and xylazine/lidocaine for caudal epidural analgesia in horses. *J Am Vet Med Assoc* 1992; **201**: 1187–1190.

280 Robinson EP, Natalini CC. Epidural anesthesia and analgesia in horses. *Vet Clin North Am Equine Pract* 2002; **18**: 61–82, vi.

281 Nichols CL, Doherty TJ, Schumacher J, *et al.* Dexmedetomidine prolongs the duration of action of mepivacaine on anesthesia of the palmar digital nerves of horses. *Am J Vet Res* 2021; **83**: 114–118.

282 Dai F, Rausk J, Aspegren J, *et al.* Use of detomidine oromucosal gel for alleviation of acute anxiety and fear in horses: a pilot study. *Front Vet Sci* 2020; **7**: 573309.

283 United States Food Animal Residue Avoidance Database (FARAD) Withdrawal Interval Recommendations. http://www.farad.org/wdilookup/wdi_cattle.html (accessed April 2023).

284 Torneke K, Bergstrom U, Neil A. Interactions of xylazine and detomidine with α 2-adrenoceptors in brain tissue from cattle, swine and rats. *J Vet Pharmacol Ther* 2003; **26**: 205–211.

285 Kästner SB. A2-agonists in sheep: a review. *Vet Anaesth Analg* 2006; **33**: 79–96.

286 Kästner SB, Ohlerth S, Pospischil A, *et al.* Dexmedetomidine-induced pulmonary alterations in sheep. *Res Vet Sci* 2007; **83**: 217–226.

287 Hsu WH, Hanson CE, Hembrough FB, *et al.* Effects of idazoxan, tolazoline, and yohimbine on xylazine-induced respiratory changes and central nervous system depression in ewes. *Am J Vet Res* 1989; **50**: 1570–1573.

288 Doherty TJ, Ballinger JA, McDonell WN, *et al.* Antagonism of xylazine induced sedation by idazoxan in calves. *Can J Vet Res* 1987; **51**: 244–248.

289 Goldberg MR, Robertson D. Yohimbine: a pharmacological probe for study of the alpha 2-adrenoreceptor. *Pharmacol Rev* 1983; **35**: 143–180.

290 Bryant CE, Thompson J, Clarke KW. Characterisation of the cardiovascular pharmacology of medetomidine in the horse and sheep. *Res Vet Sci* 1998; **65**: 149–154.

291 Pertovaara A, Haapalinna A, Sirviö J, *et al.* Pharmacological properties, central nervous system effects, and potential therapeutic applications of atipamezole, a selective alpha2-adrenoceptor antagonist. *CNS Drug Rev* 2005; **11**: 273–288.

292 Dimaio Knych HK, Steffey EP, Stanley SD. Pharmacokinetics and pharmacodynamics of three intravenous doses of yohimbine in the horse. *J Vet Pharmacol Ther* 2011; **34**: 359–366.

293 Casbeer HC, Knych HK. Pharmacokinetics and pharmacodynamic effects of tolazoline following intravenous administration to horses. *Vet J* 2013; **196**: 504–509.

294 Salonen S, Vuorilehto L, Vainio O, *et al.* Atipamezole increases medetomidine clearance in the dog: an agonist-antagonist interaction. *J Vet Pharmacol Ther* 1995; *18*: 328–332.

295 Pypendop BH, Ahokoivu H, Honkavaara J. Pharmacokinetics of vatinoxan in male neutered cats anesthetized with isoflurane. *Vet Anaesth Analg* 2020; **47**: 70–75.

296 Honkavaara J, Restitutti F, Raekallio M, *et al.* Influence of MK-467, a peripherally acting α_2-adrenoceptor antagonist on the disposition of intravenous dexmedetomidine in dogs. *Drug Metab Dispos* 2012; **40**: 445–449.

297 Pypendop BH, Honkavaara J, Ilkiw JE. Pharmacokinetics of dexmedetomidine, MK-467, and their combination following intravenous administration in male cats. *J Vet Pharmacol Ther* 2016; **39**: 460–468.

298 Pypendop BH, Honkavaara J, Ilkiw JE. Pharmacokinetics of dexmedetomidine, MK-467 and their combination following intramuscular administration in male cats. *Vet Anaesth Analg* 2017; **44**: 823–831.

299 Paret G, Eyal O, Mayan H, *et al.* Endotracheal tolazoline: pharmacokinetics and pharmacodynamics in dogs. *Acta Paediatr* 1999; **88**: 1020–1023.

300 Pagel PS, Proctor LT, Devcic A, *et al.* A novel alpha 2-adrenoceptor antagonist attenuates the early, but preserves the late cardiovascular effects of intravenous dexmedetomidine in conscious dogs. *J Cardiothorac Vasc Anesth* 1998; **12**: 429–434.

301 Turunen H, Raekallio MR, Honkavaara J, *et al.* Cardiovascular and sedation reversal effects of intramuscular administration of atipamezole in dogs treated with medetomidine hydrochloride with or without the peripheral α_2-adrenergic receptor antagonist vatinoxan hydrochloride. *Am J Vet Res* 2019; **80**: 912–922.

302 Zatroch KK, Sakai DM, Parry S, *et al.* Evaluation of atipamezole as a treatment for dexmedetomidine-induced cardiovascular depression in anesthetized cats. *Am J Vet Res* 2019; **80**: 455–460.

303 Honkavaara JM, Restitutti F, Raekallio MR, *et al.* The effects of increasing doses of MK-467, a peripheral alpha(2)-adrenergic receptor antagonist, on the cardiopulmonary effects of intravenous dexmedetomidine in conscious dogs. *J Vet Pharmacol Ther* 2011; **34**: 332–337.

304 Restitutti F, Kaartinen MJ, Raekallio MR, *et al.* Plasma concentration and cardiovascular effects of intramuscular medetomidine combined with three doses of the peripheral alpha2-antagonist MK-467 in dogs. *Vet Anaesth Analg* 2017; **44**: 417–426.

305 Huuskonen V, Restitutti F, Raekallio M, *et al.* Cardiovascular effects of dobutamine, norepinephrine and phenylephrine in isoflurane-anaesthetized dogs administered dexmedetomidine-vatinoxan. *Vet Anaesth Analg* 2022; **49**: 546–555.

306 Salla KM, Turunen HA, Kallio-Kujala IJ, *et al.* Effects of vatinoxan in dogs premedicated with medetomidine and butorphanol followed by sevoflurane anaesthesia: a randomized clinical study. *Vet Anaesth Analg* 2022; **49**: 563–571.

307 Honkavaara J, Pypendop B, Ilkiw J. The impact of MK-467 on sedation, heart rate and arterial blood pressure after intramuscular coadministration with dexmedetomidine in conscious cats. *Vet Anaesth Analg* 2017; **44**: 811–822.

308 Honkavaara J, Pypendop B, Turunen H, *et al.* The effect of MK-467, a peripheral α2-adrenoceptor antagonist, on dexmedetomidine-induced sedation and bradycardia after intravenous administration in conscious cats. *Vet Anaesth Analg* 2017; **44**: 42–51.

309 Pypendop BH, Honkavaara J, Ilkiw JE. Cardiovascular effects of dexmedetomidine, with or without MK-467, following intravenous administration in cats. *Vet Anaesth Analg* 2017; **44**: 52–62.

310 Martin-Flores M, Sakai DM, Honkavaara J, *et al.* Hemodynamic effects of MK-467 following intravenous administration to isoflurane-anesthetized cats concurrently receiving dexmedetomidine. *Am J Vet Res* 2018; **79**: 711–717.

311 Jaegar AT, Pypendop BH, Ahokoivu H, *et al.* Cardiopulmonary effects of dexmedetomidine, with and without vatinoxan, in isoflurane-anesthetized cats. *Vet Anath Analg* 2019; **46**: 753–764.

312 Kobluk K, Pypendop BH. Effects of dopamine, norepinephrine or phenylephrine on the prevention of hypotension in isoflurane-anesthetized cats administered vatinoxan or vatinoxan and dexmedetomidine. *Vet Anaesth Analg* 2022; **49**: 54–64.

313 Tapio H, Raekallio MR, Mykkanen AK, *et al.* Effects of vatinoxan on cardiorespiratory function and gastrointestinal motility during constant-rate medetomidine infusion in standing horses. *Equine Vet J* 2019; **51**: 646–652.

314 Neudeck S, Twele L, Kopp V, *et al.* Pharmacodynamics and plasma concentrations of dexmedetomidine with or without vatinoxan as a constant-rate infusion in horses anaesthetized with isoflurane-A pilot study. *J Vet Pharmacol Ther* 2021; **44**: 754–765.

315 Tapio H, Raekallio MR, Mykkanen AK, *et al.* Effects of vatinoxan on cardiorespiratory function, fecal output and plasma drug concentrations in horses anesthetized with isoflurane and infusion of medetomidine. *Vet J* 2019; **251**: 105345.

316 Raisis AL, Hosgood GL, Crawford N, *et al.* Comparison of pulmonary function in isoflurane anaesthetized ventilated sheep (*Ovis aries*) following administration of intravenous xylazine versus medetomidine. *Lab Anim* 2021; **55**: 443–452.

317 Adam M, Lindén J, Raekallio M, *et al.* Effects of vatinoxan on xylazine-induced pulmonary alterations in sheep. *J Vet Pharmacol Ther* 2022; **45**: 117–125.

318 Adam M, Huuskonen V, Raekallio MR, *et al.* Cardiopulmonary effects of vatinoxan in sevoflurane-anaesthetised sheep receiving dexmedetomidine. *Vet J* 2018; **238**: 63–69.

319 Hatch RC, Kitzman JV, Zahner JM, *et al.* Antagonism of xylazine sedation with yohimbine, 4-aminopyridine, and doxapram in dogs. *Am J Vet Res* 1985; **46**: 371–375.

320 Kollias-Baker CA, Court MH, Williams LL. Influence of yohimbine and tolazoline on the cardiovascular, respiratory, and sedative effects of xylazine in the horse. *J Vet Pharmacol Ther* 1993; **16**: 350–358.

321 Guard CL, Schwark WS. Influence of yohimbine on xylazine-induced depression of central nervous, gastrointestinal and cardiovascular function in the calf. *Cornell Vet* 1984; **74**: 312–321.

322 Hubbell JA, Muir WW. Antagonism of detomidine sedation in the horse using intravenous tolazoline or atipamezole. *Equine Vet J* 2006; **38**: 238–241.

323 Powell JD, Denhart JW, Lloyd WE. Effectiveness of tolazoline in reversing xylazine-induced sedation in calves. *J Am Vet Med Assoc* 1998; **212**: 90–92.

324 Vainio O, Vähä-Vahe T. Reversal of medetomidine sedation by atipamezole in dogs. *J Vet Pharmacol Ther* 1990; **13**: 15–22.

325 Granholm M, McKusick BC, Westerholm FC, *et al.* Evaluation of the clinical efficacy and safety of dexmedetomidine or medetomidine in cats and their reversal with atipamezole. *Vet Anaesth Analg* 2006; **33**: 214–223.

326 Yamashita K, Yonezawa K, Izumisawa Y, *et al.* Antagonistic effects of atipamezole on medetomidine-induced sedation in horses. *J Vet Med Sci* 1996; **58**: 1049–1052.

327 Rioja E, Kerr CL, Enouri SS, *et al.* Sedative and cardiopulmonary effects of medetomidine hydrochloride and xylazine hydrochloride and their reversal with atipamezole hydrochloride in calves. *Am J Vet Res* 2008; **69**: 319–329.

328 Weitz JD, Foster SD, Waugaman WR, *et al.* Anesthetic and hemodynamic effects of dexmedetomidine during isoflurane anesthesia in a canine model. *Nurse Anesth* 1991; **2**: 19–27.

329 Ewing KK, Mohammed HO, Scarlett JM, *et al.* Reduction of isoflurane anesthetic requirement by medetomidine and its restoration by atipamezole in dogs. *Am J Vet Res* 1993; **54**: 294–299.

330 Honkavaara JM, Raekallio MR, Kuusela EK, *et al.* The effects of L-659,066, a peripheral $alpha_2$-adrenoceptor antagonist, on dexmedetomidine-induced sedation and bradycardia in dogs. *Vet Anaesth Analg* 2008; **35**: 409–413.

331 Restitutti F, Honkavaara JM, Raekallio MR, *et al.* Effects of different doses of L-659'066 on the bispectral index and clinical sedation in dogs treated with dexmedetomidine. *Vet Anaesth Analg* 2011; **38**: 415–422.

332 Rolfe NG, Kerr CL, McDonell WN. Cardiopulmonary and sedative effects of the peripheral α2-adrenoceptor antagonist MK 0467 administered intravenously or

intramuscularly concurrently with medetomidine in dogs. *Am J Vet Res* 2012; **73**: 587–594.

333 Adam M, Raekallio MR, Vainio OM. Sedative effects of intramuscular medetomidine with and without vatinoxan (MK-467), and its reversal with atipamezole in sheep. *Vet Anaesth Analg* 2018; **45**: 788–793.

334 Pypendop BH, Ahokoivu H, Honkavaara J. Effects of dexmedetomidine, with or without vatinoxan (MK-467), on minimum alveolar concentration of isoflurane in cats. *Vet Anaesth Analg* 2019; **46**: 443–451.

335 Hector RC, Rezende ML, Mama KR, *et al.* Effects of constant rate infusions of dexmedetomidine or MK-467 on the minimum alveolar concentration of sevoflurane in dogs. *Vet Anaesth Analg* 2017; **44**: 755–765.

336 Hector RC, Rezende ML, Mama KR, *et al.* Combined effects of dexmedetomidine and vatinoxan infusions of minimum alveolar concentration and cardiopulmonary function in sevoflurane-anesthetized dogs. *Vet Anaesth Analg* 2021; **48**: 314–323.

337 Siegenthaler J, Pleyers T, Raillard M, *et al.* Effect of medetomidine, dexmedetomidine, and their reversal with atipamezole on the nociceptive withdrawal reflex in beagles. *Animals (Basel)* 2020; **10**: 1240.

338 Skarda RT, Muir WW III. Influence of atipamezole on effects of midsacral subarachnoidally administered detomidine in mares. *Am J Vet Res* 1998; **59**: 468–477.

339 Skarda RT, Muir WW III. Effects of intravenously administered yohimbine on antinociceptive, cardiorespiratory, and postural changes induced by epidural administration of detomidine hydrochloride solution to healthy mares. *Am J Vet Res* 1999; **60**: 1262–1270.

340 Bennett RC, Salla KM, Raekallio MR, *et al.* Effects of MK-467 on the antinociceptive and sedative actions and pharmacokinetics of medetomidine in dogs. *J Vet Pharmacol Ther* 2016; **39**: 336–343.

341 Huuskonen V, Restitutti F, Honkavaara JM, *et al.* Investigation of the effects of vatinoxan on somatic and visceral antinociceptive efficacy of medetomidine in dogs. *Am J Vet Res* 2020; **81**: 299–308.

342 Hikasa Y, Takase K, Emi S, *et al.* Antagonistic effects of alpha-adrenoceptor blocking agents on reticuloruminal hypomotility induced by xylazine in cattle. *Can J Vet Res* 1988; **52**: 411–415.

343 Harada T, Constantinou CE. The effect of alpha 2 agonists and antagonists on the lower urinary tract of the rat. *J Urol* 1993; **149**: 159–164.

344 Hsu WH. Yohimbine increases plasma insulin concentrations and reverses xylazine-induced hypoinsulinemia in dogs. *Am J Vet Res* 1988; **49**: 242–244.

345 Vainionpää MH, Raekallio MR, Pakkanen SA, *et al.* Plasma drug concentrations and clinical effects of a peripheral alpha-2-adrenoceptor antagonist, MK-467, in horses sedated with detomidine. *Vet Anaesth Analg* 2013; **40**: 257–264.

346 Tapio HA, Raekallio MR, Mykkänen A, *et al.* Effects of MK-467 hydrochloride and hyoscine butylbromide on cardiorespiratory and gastrointestinal changes induced by detomidine hydrochloride in horses. *Am J Vet Res* 2018; **79**: 376–387.

347 de Vries A, Pakkanen SA, Raekallio MR, *et al.* Clinical effects and pharmacokinetic variables of romifidine and the peripheral α2 -adrenoceptor antagonist MK-467 in horses. *Vet Anaesth Analg* 2016; **43**: 599–610.

348 Dechra, Zenalpha® (medetomidine and vatinoxan hydrochlorides injection) Product Label. https://www.dechra-us.com/Files/Files/ProductDownloads/US/07IN-ZEN22002-0622-Zenalpha-Product-Insert-Final-1.pdf (accessed April 2023).

23 Opioids

Bradley T. Simon[1] and Ignacio Lizarraga[2]
[1]Department of Small Animal Clinical Sciences, College of Veterinary Medicine and Biomedical Sciences, Texas A&M University, College Station, Texas, USA, and Veterinary Dentistry Specialists, Katy, Texas, USA
[2]AgResearch Limited, Grasslands Research Centre, Palmerston North, New Zealand

Chapter contents

Introduction, 355
History of opioid use in veterinary practice, 355
Scheduling, 356
Opioid crisis in North America: veterinary shopping, diversion, and opioid misuse and abuse in veterinary practice, 356
Pharmacology, 358
Opioid receptors, 358
Pharmacokinetics, 360
Opioid tolerance, dependence, withdrawal, and opioid-induced hyperalgesia, 363
Clinical pharmacology, 364
Analgesia, 364
Sedation, euphoria, and dysphoria, 366
Cardiovascular system, 367
Respiratory system, 367
Gastrointestinal system, 367
Nervous system, 369
Renal system, 370
Antitussive effects, 371
Thermoregulatory effects, 371
Ophthalmic effects, 371
Immune system effects and effects on cancer metastasis, 371
Effects on inhalant anesthetic minimum alveolar concentration, 372
Traditional routes of administration, 373
Full opioid agonists, 373
Morphine, 373
Hydromorphone, 377
Methadone, 377
Oxymorphone, 378
Fentanyl, 378
Remifentanil, 380
Sufentanil, 380
Meperidine (pethidine), 380
Carfentanil, etorphine, alfentanil, and thiafentanil, 380
Hydrocodone, oxycodone, and codeine, 381
Partial opioid agonists, 381
Buprenorphine, 381
Mixed opioid agonist–antagonists, 382
Butorphanol, 382
Nalbuphine, 383
Opioid antagonists, 384
Naloxone, naltrexone, and methylnaltrexone, 384
Multitargeting molecules, 384
Tramadol, 384
Tapentadol, 385
References, 385

Introduction

Opiates are drugs derived from opium, which is the latex of unripe seed pods of *Papaver somniferum* that contains naturally occurring alkaloids. Opioids are not naturally occurring drugs; rather, they are partially or completely synthesized in the laboratory. Both opiates and opioids interact with opioid receptors. In this chapter, the term "opioid" will be used to refer to naturally occurring or synthetic drugs that interact with opioid receptors. Opioids are the prototypical analgesics, antitussives, and antidiarrheal drug class. The opioid receptor system has been identified in a variety of amphibians, fish, reptiles, birds, and mammals [1,2].

History of opioid use in veterinary practice

Humans have used opium (from *Papaver somniferum*) for its analgesic effects for more than 8000 years [3]. The earliest documented use of opium in domestic animals, attributed to Robert Boyle, dates to the 17th century. Boyle focused on opium as a poison and wrote: "*we have more than once given to a Dog, without much harming him, such a quantity of Opium, as would probably have suffic'd to have kill'd several Men*" [4]. In 1659, in collaboration with Christopher Wren, Boyle injected an infusion of opium into a superficial pelvic limb vein causing deep stupor to an experimental dog [5]. In 1664, Robert Hooke proposed a practical union between opiate narcosis and surgery [4]. At that time, opium had been used in combination with alcohol and

Veterinary Anesthesia and Analgesia: The Sixth Edition of Lumb and Jones. Edited by Leigh Lamont, Kurt Grimm, Sheilah Robertson, Lydia Love and Carrie Schroeder.
© 2024 John Wiley & Sons, Inc. Published 2024 by John Wiley & Sons, Inc.
Companion website: www.wiley.com/go/lamont/anesthesia

other ingredients to form various forms of laudanum, or tincture of opium. This became widely used to prepare patients for surgery until the discovery of effective anesthesia. Paregoric was a weaker preparation, named after the Greek word for "soothing" or "consoling" and included opium, honey, licorice root, camphor, aniseed, and wine [6]. Recognizing the limitations of opium for surgical anesthesia, James Moore reported in 1784 on opium's postoperative analgesic effects [6].

In 1805, Friedrich Wilhelm Adam Sertürner reported the isolation of an alkaline substance from opium, which he later named "morphium" [7]. Sertürner administered an aqueous alcoholic extraction of the salt to four dogs and a mouse. The dogs vomited, convulsed, and appeared sleepy, but did not sleep; one dog died [8]. Although these early studies did not provide evidence of morphine's analgesic effects, the isolation of morphine permitted accurate calculation of doses. The use of morphine became widespread following the development of the hypodermic needle and syringe in the 1850s.

In 1908, Frederick Hobday reported that morphine's effects varied considerably by animal species with cats and horses experiencing delirium and dogs experiencing narcosis, although a few displayed idiosyncratic reactions. He suggested a dose of 1/16th of a grain per pound of body weight to induce narcosis and analgesia in dogs [9]. In 1917, Howard Jay Milks reported that, other than in dogs, morphine had no value to relieve pain in veterinary animal species. However, he mentioned that two to five grains of morphine-induced sedation in horses and one-fifth to five grains had anesthetic-sparing effects in dogs [10].

A limiting factor for the use of morphine in veterinary medicine was its excitatory effects. In 1921, Fröhner reported excitement combined with sensory and motor depression in horses administered morphine at doses of 0.4, 0.75, 1.5, and 10 g [11]. Although body weight was not reported, these morphine doses are considerably higher than those recommended in contemporary equine practice. In 1937, Amadon and Craigie described minimal analgesia and excitement in pain-free horses administered morphine at doses of 0.2 and 0.5 mg/kg, respectively [12]. This may have prompted many to focus on the adverse effects rather than the analgesic actions of morphine and other opioids [13].

The increased use of opioids to provide analgesia in veterinary patients can be attributed to Yoxall who proposed that it was the veterinarian's duty to alleviate pain whenever it may occur [14]. Since then, many opioid drugs in a variety of dosage forms and routes of administration have been used in animal species of veterinary interest. These have included the intra-articular administration or intravenous regional limb perfusion of morphine to induce analgesia and prevent inflammation associated with orthopedic procedures in dogs and horses [15–19], the subcutaneous, intramuscular, intravenous, or intranasal administration of high-concentration injectable buprenorphine solutions for analgesic purposes in cats and dogs [20,21], the transdermal administration of fentanyl contained in patches in dogs, pigs, and sheep [22–25], the subcutaneous administration of extended-release buprenorphine solutions for analgesia in mice and rats [26,27], the transdermal administration of long-acting fentanyl and buprenorphine solutions for analgesia in cats and dogs [28,29], and the buccal transmucosal administration of buprenorphine gels for analgesia in dogs [30].

Scheduling

The 1971 Convention of Psychotropic Substances, a United Nations treaty, introduced control provisions for narcotics. These provisions aimed to prevent diversion and abuse by limiting the prescription and clinical use of controlled substances to licensed parties. Global jurisdictions introduced systems and agencies to comply with these provisions. Moreover, under federal, state, and local law (where appropriate), controlled drugs must be maintained in locked storage areas with use documented in a log subject to inspection. In the United States (US), the Controlled Substances Act places regulated substances into one of five schedules (I to V). Scheduling is based on the substance's medical use, potential for abuse, and safety or dependence liability. The abuse potential is a determinant in scheduling; Schedule I substances have a high potential for abuse and psychological and/or physical dependence, and Schedule V substances represent the least potential for abuse.

Opioid crisis in North America: veterinary shopping, diversion, and opioid misuse and abuse in veterinary practice

In the 19th and the early 20th centuries, the US experienced an opiate crisis involving over-the-counter opium, morphine, and heroin products, and the spread of opium dens. Consumer advocacy and legislation ended the over-the-counter sale of opiate products and outlawed opium dens [31]. The contemporary North American opioid crisis, also known as the "opioid epidemic," has been a decades-long crisis with three major upsurges. The first upsurge started in 1995 and involved a profit-driven increase in prescription opioids that were misleadingly marketed as safe and low-risk extended-release analgesics. The second upsurge began around 2010 when drug traffickers realized that people addicted to prescription opioids were a lucrative target for heroin. The third upsurge began around 2014 and has been characterized by illegal drug producers adding potent synthetic opioids to forged pharmaceutical pills, heroin, and stimulants [32].

Initial anecdotal evidence suggested [33], and more recent scientific evidence has confirmed [34–36], that veterinarians are a source for misused prescription opioids. An example of prescription opioid misuse is opioid diversion, which is the illegal distribution or abuse of a prescribed opioid or its use for purposes not intended by the prescriber. Some pet owners seek opioids from veterinarians for their own use and request opioids for their pets when they are not needed or recommended. Some have even intentionally made an animal ill, injured an animal, or made an animal seem ill or injured to obtain opioids [34]. Some may solicit opioid prescriptions from multiple veterinarians for the purpose of misuse, which is known as "vet shopping" [36,37]. In addition to clients, veterinary practice staff, including veterinarians, have been involved in opioid diversion [34,35]. Thus, opioid diversion could contribute to the growing opioid crisis, and veterinarians have a role in preventing opioid abuse and misuse.

A few studies have shed some light on the situation veterinarians in the US face regarding opioid diversion and vet shopping. In a study conducted in 2018 involving 697 general veterinarians practicing across the US, 63.5% of veterinarians expressed concerns for opioid diversion to pet owners and 24.7% to staff within the clinic [35]. Mason *et al.* reported in 2018 that out of 189 veterinarians practicing in Colorado, 73% had either fair, poor, or no veterinary medical school training on opioid abuse or misuse and 64% had not completed continuing education on best practices for prescribing opioids since entering practice. Opioid abuse prevention (81%), pain management guidelines (55%), and how to engage electronic resources (54%) were identified as continuing educational priorities. Thirty-six percent of respondents recommended improving prescription drug monitoring program (PDMP) guidelines and tutorials to help improve access and utilization [34]. A study including 14 veterinarians practicing in tri-state Appalachian counties (Tennessee, $n = 8$; Kentucky, $n = 4$; and Virginia, $n = 2$) found that 93% of respondents had heard of vet shopping, 57% had encountered vet shopping in their own practice, 86% indicated vet shopping was a problem in tri-state Appalachian counties, and 71% had received no training on prevention and/or management of vet shopping. Respondents mentioned more efficient communication with other veterinarians and medical professionals including pharmacists, a valid veterinary–client–patient relationship (VCPR), more education for themselves and/or their staff, better tracking of animal prescriptions through databases, and judicious use of opioid prescriptions as means to prevent and control vet shopping [36]. Enhanced curricular offerings, continuing education trainings, and workplace policies, practices, procedures, and monitoring may foster opioid stewardship among veterinarians and may mitigate the risks of opioid diversion by both staff and clients.

The implementation of mandatory PDMP enrollment for healthcare providers may deter opioid diversion and foster opioid stewardship [34,38]. As of April 30, 2021, and except for Missouri, all states and the District of Columbia had a PDMP in place. A total of 47 states had PDMP use mandates for any clinician before controlled substances may be prescribed. Of these, 37 states exempted veterinarians from mandates and 10 did not: Alaska, Connecticut, Indiana, Maine, Oklahoma, and West Virginia required veterinarians to check PDMP records of owners in some instances; and Arkansas, District of Columbia, Rhode Island, and South Carolina required veterinarians to check records of animals. None required veterinarians to check records of both owners and animals [37]. Although PDMP use mandates might improve controlled substances prescribing behaviors by veterinarians and deter opioid diversion, the benefits of these mandates should outweigh their costs and consider the impact of their implementation. For instance, time cost for veterinarians, incompatibility of PDMPs with veterinarians' electronic medical record systems, privacy concerns among animal owners, lack of linkages between animal and owner PDMP records in many states, possibility of multiple PDMP records for animals, scope and types of information available to veterinarians during a PDMP review, protocols to detect and report suspected cases of veterinary shopping, and regulations for interstate sharing of PDMP data from animals and owners must be considered [37]. In line with this, the American Veterinary Medical Association has lobbied that PDMPs not be implemented for veterinarians until further evidence and better systems are put in place.

Published information on the utility of PDMPs to identify potential vet shoppers is scarce. In a survey of 50 state PDMPs, Simpson concluded that less than 10 vet shoppers nationwide would be identified by PDMPs per year [39]. Using data collected between 2014 and 2019 from US retail and mail-order pharmacies, the number of potential vet shoppers with prescriptions from greater than four veterinarians during a year for opioid cough-and-cold medications increased from 150 in 2014 to 1348 in 2019; for opioid analgesics, this number peaked at 868 in 2016 before decreasing to 733 in 2019 [37] (Table 23.1).

The temporal distribution, use, prescription, and dispensation of opioids for animals has been investigated. Piper *et al.* analyzed data from approximately 200 registrants nationwide for distribution of Schedule II and III opioids to animals from 2006 to 2019 in US veterinary teaching institutions [40]. By weight, codeine was the predominant dispensed opioid with a peak of approximately 2200 g in 2017, which then decreased to 1200 g in 2019. Hydrocodone followed codeine with a maximum of 550 g in 2010, which declined to 160 g in 2011. Oxycodone went from 233 g in 2006 to less than 5 g in 2012, and meperidine reached 55 g in 2006 to then dropped to 10 g in 2019. The distribution of morphine, hydromorphone, and oxymorphone was relatively stable during 2006–2019. However, the distribution of methadone increased from approximately 9 g in 2006 to 155 g in 2019. The distribution of fentanyl analogs peaked at 380 mg for remifentanil in 2008, 50 mg for sufentanil in 2009, and 40 mg for alfentanil in 2013. By percentage of total morphine milligram equivalents (MME), the top seven Schedule II and III opioids distributed in 2019 were methadone (42.3%), fentanyl (35.4%), codeine (6.4%), hydromorphone (5%), morphine (4.5%), hydrocodone (4%), and buprenorphine (2.4%). Despite the highly variable

Table 23.1 Potential vet-shopping behavior[a] by US pet owners from 2014 to 2019.

Outcome	2014	2015	2016	2017	2018	2019
Number of patients with ≥ 1 veterinarian prescription						
Any controlled substance class	479,755	538,996	577,161	567,021	502,291	448,541
Opioid analgesics	241,391	274,935	290,809	275,612	229,485	184,364
Opioid cough-and-cold medications	49,164	59,902	72,907	82,865	90,786	101,749
Benzodiazepines	199,151	215,884	225,762	219,831	191,707	171,140
Number of patients linked to potential vet-shopping behavior						
Any controlled substance class[b]	935	1711	2192	2325	2520	2875
Opioid analgesics	401	662	868	850	815	733
Opioid cough-and-cold medications	150	453	677	839	1041	1348
Benzodiazepines	185	274	335	375	381	440
Prevalence (%) of potential vet-shopping behavior						
Any controlled substance class	0.19	0.32	0.38	0.41	0.50	0.64
Opioid analgesics	0.17	0.24	0.30	0.31	0.36	0.40
Opioid cough-and-cold medications	0.31	0.76	0.93	1.01	1.15	1.32
Benzodiazepines	0.09	0.13	0.15	0.17	0.20	0.26

[a] Defined as the occurrence of dispensed controlled substance prescriptions from ≥ 4 veterinarians during the year.

[b] The numbers in the second through fourth rows in this section do not add up to the number in the first row because (1) the second through fourth rows are not mutually exclusive (e.g., a patient could have opioid prescriptions from ≥ 4 veterinarians and benzodiazepine prescriptions from ≥ 4 veterinarians) and (2) some patients did not receive prescriptions for any given medication class from ≥ 4 veterinarians, but still received controlled substance prescriptions from ≥ 4 veterinarians (e.g., opioid prescriptions from two veterinarians and benzodiazepine prescriptions from two other veterinarians).

Source: Adapted from Chua *et al.* [37].

temporal pattern for individual opioids, a decline in hydrocodone use (which preceded its up-scheduling from Schedule III to II), a recent decline in codeine, a decline in fentanyl use from 2013, and a gradual increase in methadone distribution were evident. The overall use of opioids by MME was relatively stable from 2014 to 2019, with only a 5.7% reduction. A limitation of this study was the lack of information on the Schedule IV opioids tramadol and butorphanol.

Kogan *et al.* surveyed 697 veterinarians practicing in the US in 2018 and 97.8% used opioids in-clinic, 80.3% dispensed them, and 70.3% prescribed them [35]. Buprenorphine, butorphanol, hydromorphone, methadone, morphine, injectable fentanyl, and tramadol were the most frequently administered opioids in-clinic. Buprenorphine, tramadol, and hydrocodone were the most frequently dispensed opioids to clients, and tramadol, buprenorphine, and hydrocodone were the most frequently prescribed opioids to outside pharmacies. Overall, 99.7% of respondents used opioids in-clinic, dispensed, or prescribed them. Buprenorphine (96.0%), tramadol (90.8%), butorphanol (90.5%), hydromorphone (71.7%), hydrocodone (61.4%), morphine (44.5%), fentanyl patch (27.3%), fentanyl injectable (21.4%), methadone (10.9%), and oxymorphone (5.6%) were the most frequently mentioned opioids. The greater use of μ-opioid agonists in-clinic compared to prescribing or dispensing of these drugs may be due to concerns about injectable opioids leaving the clinic, lack of efficacy of oral μ-opioid receptor agonists in dogs and cats, and veterinarian concern over diversion of potent opioid drugs.

During 2007–2017, veterinarians practicing at a small animal veterinary teaching hospital prescribed a total of 1,051,836 tramadol tablets, 97,547 hydrocodone tablets, 38,939 codeine tablets, and 3153 fentanyl patches to dogs (73.0%), cats (22.5%), and exotic species (4.5%). Although prescribing of tramadol tablets and fentanyl patches decreased, overall MME use increased by 41.2%, whereas visits only increased by 12.8% over the study period. The large and increasing volume of opioids prescribed at this veterinary teaching hospital highlights parallel concerns about excessive opioid prescribing in humans [41]. Increasing opioid prescribing trends were also found in veterinary practices using pharmacies to fill pet medications and reporting to West Virginia's PDMP between January 2008 and June 2020. Veterinary practices reporting to West Virginia's PDMP ranged from 1 in 2008 to 61 in 2019. Sixty-nine veterinary practices submitted 7919 opioid prescriptions: 96.4% for tramadol, 1.4% for codeine, 1% for fentanyl, 1% for hydrocodone–acetaminophen, and 0.2% for morphine. Mandates in the PDMP and the introduction of tramadol as a controlled substance in 2014 may have contributed to the increasing trend in opioid prescribing [42].

Using IQVIA Longitudinal Prescription Datasets, which reports all prescriptions dispensed from 92% of US retail pharmacies and 70% of US mail-order pharmacies, a mean of 1,110,594 (standard deviation 104,109) controlled substance prescriptions from veterinarians were dispensed annually from 2014 through 2019. During this period, tramadol accounted for the highest share of opioid analgesic prescriptions (92.6%), followed by codeine (2.9%), and hydrocodone (1.9%). Opioid analgesic dispensing peaked in 2016 (290,809 prescriptions) before declining in 2019 (184,364 prescriptions). Hydrocodone products accounted for 99.6% of opioid cough-and-cold medication prescriptions, while codeine products accounted for the other 0.4%. Opioid cough-and-cold medication dispensing doubled between 2014 and 2019, from 106,663 to 211,960 prescriptions [37].

Veterinarians require opioids for the practice of modern veterinary medicine. However, opioids carry risks to both animal patients and humans. These risks must be carefully managed at the individual and system levels, and it should be recognized that both patients and their owners can be harmed by clinical decisions to prescribe or not to prescribe opioids. There are times when opioids are the best medical choice and ensuring that veterinarians can provide these drugs to their patients is critically important. Paradoxically, in the midst of an opioid crisis, veterinarians have struggled to obtain opioids for their patients and have relied on alternative multimodal analgesic and anesthetic plans, sometimes without opioids. In 2018, 83% and 59% of 697 veterinarians practicing in the US reported difficulties obtaining opioids for use in-clinic or to dispense to clients between May and October and in October alone, respectively. Conversely, 29% and 22% reported difficulties prescribing opioids to clients between May and October and in October alone, respectively. The most difficult opioids to obtain were hydromorphone, morphine, injectable fentanyl, oxymorphone, and methadone, all Schedule II drugs. The opioid shortage moderately or significantly affected the ability of 75% and 73% of veterinarians to provide optimal analgesia and anesthesia to their patients, respectively. Although only 11% of veterinarians canceled or postponed any procedures between May and October due to the opioid shortage, 45% discussed the opioid shortage with clients in situations where their pet required opioid treatment [35].

Although many believe that an opioid crisis could not happen outside the US, Canada has had a similar explosion of opioid prescribing and is facing an opioid epidemic. In both countries, more than 600,000 opioid overdose fatalities have been recorded since 1999 with a record peak in 2020: 70,168 deaths in the US and 6306 deaths Canada [32]. Furthermore, pharmaceutical companies based in the US are actively expanding opioid markets worldwide and are using tactics now banned domestically. This may partially explain the disproportionate distribution of controlled opioids with 21 countries consuming 89% of all controlled opioids between 2015 and 2017 and recent sharp increases in opioid prescribing in Australia, the Netherlands, Spain, Israel, Iceland, England, and Brazil [32,34,43].

A 2021 survey of veterinarians in the United Kingdom (UK) showed that 88.2% of respondents agreed with the statement "*some drugs prescribed by veterinary professionals are at risk of misuse.*" Of these, 29.9% had suspected a client of taking a drug prescribed to their animal, and 20.1% had suspected veterinary staff of taking a veterinary prescription medicine. The opioids tramadol, fentanyl (transdermal patch), buprenorphine, and codeine were in the top 10 drugs identified at risk of misuse by humans when prescribed by UK veterinarians [44]. Only 10.5% of respondents had received formal training regarding recognizing, preventing, or dealing with suspected drug misuse involving staff or clients, and 95.6% felt they would benefit from additional training or guidance [44]. Thus, veterinarians worldwide may be a source of prescription opioid misuse and training about this issue is required.

Pharmacology

Opioid receptors

The Nomenclature and Standards Committee of the International Union of Basic and Clinical Pharmacology approves the use of the well-established Greek symbol terminology for the three types of opioid receptors: μ, δ, and κ. Also approved are the symbols spelled out (mu, delta, and kappa), and the acronyms MOP, DOP, and KOP where OP stands for opioid peptide [45]. The genes encoding these receptors are the opioid receptor mu 1 (*OPRM1*), opioid receptor delta 1 (*OPRD1*), and opioid receptor kappa 1 (*OPRK1*), respectively [45]. The principal endogenous agonists are: (1) β endorphin (derived from proopiomelanocortin) for the μ-opioid receptor; (2) leucine- and methionine-enkephalin (derived from proenkephalin) for the δ-opioid receptor; and (3) big dynorphin and dynorphin A (derived from prodynorphin) for the κ-opioid receptor [45].

The nociceptin/orphanin FQ (N/OFQ) or nociceptin opioid peptide (NOP) receptor is the fourth member of the opioid receptor family, and it is activated by the peptide of the same name (i.e., N/OFQ). Despite sharing high structural homology with conventional opioid receptors, N/OFQ is considered opioid-related because it displays distinct pharmacology [45]. This receptor modulates various central processes including pain, learning and memory, emotional states, neuroendocrine control, food intake, and motor control [46]. Because no drugs interacting with this receptor are available for clinical use, it is beyond the scope of this chapter to discuss this receptor further.

Opioid receptor regulation

Opioid receptors belong to the family of G-protein-coupled receptors. Upon activation by an agonist, opioid receptors change their conformation causing the $G\alpha_{i/o}$ subunit to dissociate from the receptor and the Gβγ dimer. The guanosine triphosphate bound to the $G\alpha_{i/o}$ subunit is hydrolyzed to guanosine diphosphate rendering the $G\alpha_{i/o}$ subunit active, which, in turn, inhibits adenylate cyclase and cAMP-related pathways. Voltage-gated Ca^{2+} channels are inhibited through a $G\alpha_{i/o}$-GTP-tyrosine kinase pathway in a voltage-independent manner and by Gβγ dimers in a voltage-dependent manner. The Gβγ dimer also activates G-protein-coupled inwardly rectifying K^+ (GirK) channels [47]. This increases the membrane potential rendering the cell less susceptible to depolarization. If opioid receptor activation continues long term, Gβγ dimers recruit G-protein receptor kinase (GRK) to the receptor for phosphorylation. This changes receptor conformation allowing β-arrestin to dock and subsequently recruit the endocytosis machinery causing receptor internalization. Receptors are either recycled after some time to the cell membrane or transported to proteasomes and lysosomes for degradation. The latter causes receptor downregulation, which decreases the number of opioid receptors available for activation in the cell membrane. Thus, opioid receptors undergo homologous desensitization becoming less responsive to continuous or repeated sustained activation by opioid agonists, which may contribute to the development of tolerance. Interestingly, opioid receptor activation has been demonstrated to occur not only at the cell membrane, but within cytoplasmic compartments [48]. Receptor regulation and desensitization is dependent on cellular location, cell type, and agonist type.

The fact that different agonists produce different pharmacologic responses when acting at the same opioid receptor led to speculation that multiple subtypes of μ-, δ-, and κ-opioid receptors existed [49,50]. However, molecular cloning has failed to confirm the existence of such subtypes, and knockout of each of these receptors results in a loss of ligand binding and function associated with that receptor [50]. Instead, differences in response are mediated by rather more complex opioid receptor functions. These include spatiotemporal specificity in opioid receptor cellular signaling, ligand-directed biased signaling, positive and negative allosteric modulation of ligand binding and signaling, homo- and heterodimerization of different opioid receptors, and the existence of splice variants with different ligand specificity [51,52].

Alternative splicing of opioid receptor genes may contribute to interindividual variation in response to opioid treatment. Various single-nucleotide polymorphisms (SNPs) of the *OPRM1* gene have been identified in dogs [53,54]. Interestingly, the C-15A SNP, which had high prevalence in the Alaskan Malamute, Siberian Husky, and Labrador Retriever dogs that were studied, seems to play a role in opioid-induced dysphoria [53].

Opioid receptor localization

Opioid receptors are distributed throughout the body, including the brain, spinal cord, peripheral sensory nerve terminals, enteric neurons, genitourinary tract, synovial membranes, leukocytes, and blood vessels. Therefore, the activation of opioid receptors induces various effects (Table 23.2). The distribution of opioid receptors in key areas of pain transmission and modulation contributes to the analgesic effects of opioid agonists. However, μ- and κ-opioid receptor distribution in the brain differs by species [55], and μ-opioid receptor density in the spinal cord increases in chronic pain states [56]. Activation of opioid receptors in extravascular

Table 23.2 Physiological effects associated with stimulation of opioid receptor types.

μ-opioid receptor	κ-opioid receptor	δ-opioid receptor
Analgesia (supraspinal, spinal) Euphoria/sedation Miosis/mydriasis (species specific) Bradycardia Hypothermia/hyperthermia (species specific) Urinary retention Antidiuresis Reduced gastrointestinal motility Reduced gastrointestinal secretions Reduced biliary secretions Emesis/antiemesis Pyloric muscle spasm or relaxation Cough suppression Respiratory depression (decreased sensitivity of respiratory center to CO_2) Immunomodulation Physical dependence	Analgesia (supraspinal, spinal) Dysphoria/sedation Miosis/mydriasis (species specific) Diuresis (inhibition of antidiuretic hormone release) Reduced gastrointestinal motility Reduced gastrointestinal secretions	Analgesia (supraspinal, spinal) Reduced gastrointestinal motility (minimal) Urinary retention Respiratory depression Emesis Immunomodulation

leukocytes by exogenous opioids triggers secretion of endogenous opioid peptides from the immune cells contributing to the analgesic effect of exogenously administered opioid receptor agonists [57].

Opioid receptor–opioid drug interactions

Opioids can also be classified according to the receptor or receptors they interact with, as well as the effect elicited (e.g., concentration–response or dose–response relationship). Classically, a full agonist produces a dose-dependent increase in effect until maximum stimulation of the receptor is achieved (Fig. 23.1A). A partial agonist also produces a dose-dependent increase in effect, but plateaus at a maximal response that is less than that achieved with a full agonist (Fig. 23.1B).

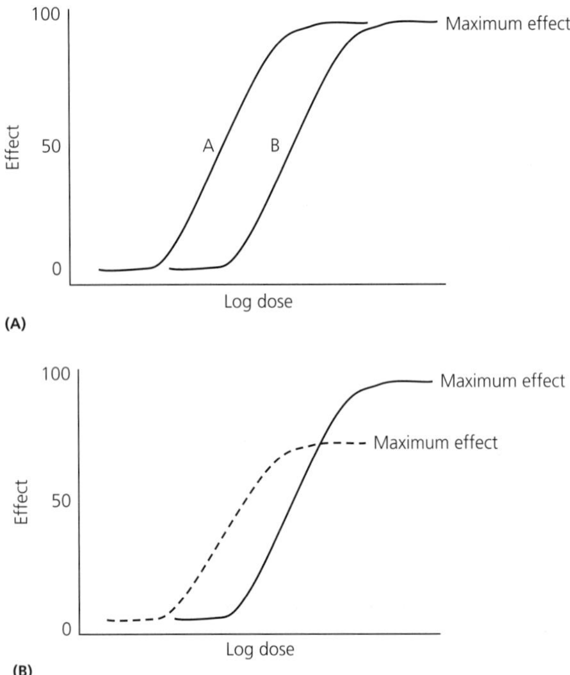

Figure 23.1 **A.** Dose–response curves for two opioids with equal efficacy but different potencies. This example could represent the full agonists morphine (line B) and fentanyl (line A). The dose of fentanyl needed to achieve a given effect is lower, but the maximum effect of both fentanyl and morphine will be similar. **B.** Dose–response curves for two opioids with different efficacies and potencies. This example could represent the full agonist morphine (solid line) and partial agonist buprenorphine (dashed line). Despite buprenorphine being a more potent drug with high affinity for opioid receptors, the maximum effect attained with morphine is greater.

An antagonist binds to a receptor with high affinity but produces no intrinsic effect and inhibits the binding of agonists (both endogenous and exogenous). Administration of an antagonist will, therefore, "reverse" the receptor-mediated effects of an agonist by inhibiting agonist binding and displacing previously bound agonist due to its greater affinity for the receptor. Most opioid receptor antagonists are considered competitive antagonists based on their lack of intrinsic activity and the fact that high concentrations of an agonist can overcome antagonism and still produce a maximum effect (i.e., the antagonist shifts the agonist's dose–response curve to the right). Administration of a partial agonist can act as an antagonist by partially reversing the effects of a full agonist (also shifting the dose–response curve to the right) and this approach may be preferred over an antagonist in certain situations (e.g., if maintenance of some analgesia is desired) [58].

The potency of an agonist describes the relative dose needed to elicit a response. For opioids, the response of interest is usually analgesia measured as a change in withdrawal latency or increased threshold to a noxious stimulus. For example, fentanyl is a more potent opioid than morphine, which means the dose of fentanyl (0.01 mg/kg) needed to produce an equivalent analgesic response to morphine (1 mg/kg) is lower (Fig. 23.1A). Note that potency does not describe duration of effect or efficacy. In the example of fentanyl (0.01 mg/kg) and morphine (1 mg/kg), both opioids produce equivalent maximum analgesic effects, but duration of analgesia is considerably shorter with fentanyl. While fentanyl and morphine can be equally efficacious analgesics since both are μ-opioid receptor agonists, the typical dose of morphine is 100-fold greater than that of fentanyl since it is less potent.

Pharmacokinetics

Pharmacokinetics can be defined simplistically as "what the body does to a drug," and it can be divided into absorption, distribution, metabolism, and excretion. These processes depend on the drug itself and its formulation, as well as the species, age, disease status, and other factors specific to the individual. By determining drug concentrations, usually in blood plasma, pharmacokinetic studies can estimate the rate and extent of drug absorption, the persistence of drug after a given dose, and sometimes the potential for drug interactions. Table 23.3 summarizes selected pharmacokinetic parameter estimates for commonly used opioids in domestic species.

Absorption

Absorption is the movement of a drug from its site of administration into the systemic circulation. Once in systemic circulation, the drug

Table 23.3 Selected pharmacokinetic parameters of some clinically relevant opioids in awake, healthy animals[a].

Opioid	Route	Dose (mg/kg)	$t_{½}$ (hours)	V_{dss} (L/kg)	*Cl* (mL/min/kg)	*F* (%)	Reference
Dog							
Buprenorphine[b]	IV or SC	0.12	16.05	6.36	5.7	131	[59]
Butorphanol	IM or SC	0.5	1.62	7.96	57.5		[60]
Fentanyl	IV	0.01	0.75 ± 0.14	4.94 ± 0.86	77.9 ± 22.3		[61]
Fentanyl	IV + CRI	0.01 + 0.01/h for 1 h	0.5 ± 0.4	4.77 ± 0.25	61.9 ± 4.6		[61]
Fentanyl	IV + CRI	0.01 + 0.01/h for 3 h	0.86 ± 0.59	4.38 ± 0.39	46.9 ± 7.5		[61]
Fentanyl	IV + CRI	0.01 + 0.01/h for 4 h	0.69 ± 0.54	4.04 ± 0.26	47.9 ± 16.4		[61]
Hydromorphone[c]	IV	0.1	0.63 (0.50–0.66)	4.1 (3.3–5.5)	112 (83.7–135.4)		[62]
Hydromorphone[c]	IV	0.5	1.03 (0.70–1.44)	4.7 (3.8–5.3)	55.1 (45–85)		[62]
Hydromorphone[c]	SC	0.1	0.67 (0.61–0.80)	3.1 (3–3.6)	58.6 (44–74.2)	185	[62]
Hydromorphone[c]	SC	0.5	1.06 (1.04–1.21)	3.3 (3.2–4.1)	35.3 (33.2–40.4)	164	[62]
Meperidine	IV	2	0.61 ± 0.01	3.14 ± 0.58	77 ± 8.28		[63]

Table 23.3 (Continued)

Opioid	Route	Dose (mg/kg)	$t_{½}$ (hours)	V_{dss} (L/kg)	Cl (mL/min/kg)	F (%)	Reference
Morphine	IV	0.5	1.58 (1.09–2.2)	7.2 (5.9–9.0)	85.2 (71.6–99.2)		[64]
Morphine	IM	1	1.36 (0.97–2.23)	6.8 (2.1–7.2)	91.2 (83.1–94.6)	119 (57.9–161)	[64]
Morphine	Rectal	2	1.1 (0.66–1.66)	6.1 (3.6–9.0)	88.4 (85.6–90.3)	16.5 (10.9–27.4)	[64]
Tapentadol	IV	50	0.86 ± 0.2	6.45 ± 0.44	87.8 ± 22.62		[65]
Tapentadol	PO	200	0.35 ± 0.15	35.07 ± 20.37	57.92 ± 13.52		[65]
Tramadol	IV	4	1.02 ± 0.2	1 ± 0.47	15.38 ± 7.67		[66]
Tramadol	IM	4	2.28 ± 0.85	0.29 ± 0.15	18.85 ± 2.43	92 ± 9	[66]
Tramadol	PO	10	1.1 (0.9–1.3)	23 (15.4–39.8)	245 (143.9–543.7)		[67]
Cat							
Buprenorphine	IV	0.01	6.9 ± 2.9	7.1 ± 3.2	16.7 ± 6.2		[68]
Buprenorphine	IM	0.01	6.3 ± 2.2	8.9 ± 5.9	23.6 ± 12.6		[68]
Buprenorphine[b]	IV, SC, OTM	0.12–0.24	12.3	7.89	16.33	94 SC, 23.6 OTM	[69]
Butorphanol	IM	0.4	6.28 ± 2.77	7.6 ± 6.28	12.92 ± 5.04		[70]
Butorphanol	OTM	0.4	5.23 ± 1.72	15.63 ± 5.7	25.35 ± 6.55	37.16 ± 14.95	[70]
Fentanyl	IV	0.00445–0.01116	2.35 ± 0.57	2.56 ± 0.32	19.83 ± 2.67		[71]
Meperidine	IM	5	3.6 ± 2.0	5.2 ± 2.1	20.1 ± 10.6		[68]
Morphine	IV	0.2	1.3 ± 0.3	2.6 ± 1.3	24.1 ± 10.3		[68]
Morphine	IM	0.2	1.6 ± 0.1	1.7 ± 0.8	13.9 ± 4.0		[68]
Remifentanil	IV CRI for 5 min	0.001	0.29 (0.09–15.34)	7.63 (2.28–76.04)	766 (408–1,473)		[72]
Tapentadol	IV	5	2.93 ± 0.86	8.79 ± 1.97	35.60 ± 7.05		[73]
Tapentadol	IM	5	2.28 ± 0.85	7.53 ± 2.95	37.85 ± 5.68	93.93 ± 9.91	[73]
Tapentadol	SC	5	2.05 ± 0.6	7.06 ± 2.10	40.13 ± 9.97	90.01 ± 6.52	[73]
Tramadol	IV	2	2.23 ± 0.3	1.6 ± 0.1	20.8 ± 3.2		[74]
Tramadol	PO	5.2	3.4 ± 0.13	3.7 ± 1.2	21.1 ± 3.0	93 ± 7	[74]
Horse							
Buprenorphine	IV	0.005	3.58 ± 3.92	3.01 ± 1.69	7.97 ± 5.16		[75]
Buprenorphine	IM	0.005	4.24 ± 1.04			65.22 ± 16.74	[75]
Buprenorphine[b]	SC	0.0025	3.41 ± 0.93	5.23 ± 0.78	18.3 ± 3.2		[76]
Buprenorphine[b]	SC	0.005	4.77 ± 1.79	7.06 ± 2.87	17.18 ± 2.78		[76]
Butorphanol	IV	0.1	5.9 ± 1.5	1.4 ± 0.3	11.5 ± 2.5		[77]
Codeine	PO	0.3	1.84 (1.00–3.90)				[78]
Codeine	PO	0.6	1.94 (1.06–4.59)				[78]
Codeine	PO	1.2	2.60 (1.66–5.32)				[78]
Hydromorphone	IV	0.04	0.57 ± 0.21	1.46 ± 0.32	74.0 ± 10.5		[79]
Hydromorphone	IV	0.04	0.32 ± 0.15	1.13 ± 0.31	79.0 ± 12.9		[80]
Hydromorphone	IM	0.04	0.45 ± 0.15			155–200	[80]
Hydromorphone	IV	0.08	0.69 ± 0.54	2.24 ± 0.95	92.7 ± 13.9		[79]
Morphine	IV	0.2	6.43 (4.11–10.2)	7.96 (4.75–10.5)	34.5 (26.8–39.6)		[81]
Morphine	IV	0.2	5.17 (3.22–19.4)	6.72 (4.36–11.9)	32.8 (26.4–40.8)		[78]
Morphine	IM	0.1	1.48	4.49	34.9		[82]
Tramadol	IV	2	1.37 ± 0.17	2.17 ± 0.52	26 ± 3		[83]
Tramadol	IM	2	1.53 ± 0.23			111 ± 39	[83]
Cattle							
Butorphanol	IV	0.25	82	4.18 ± 1.15	34.6 ± 7.7		[84]
Butorphanol	IV	0.25	82	4.18 ± 1.15	34.6 ± 7.7		[84]
Fentanyl	IV	0.005	12.7 (7.5–35.1)	24.8 (15.8–58.8)	33.3 (25.1–47.0)		[85]
Morphine	IV	0.5	1.18 ± 1.07	4.7 ± 3.0	37.3 ± 13.65		[86]
Morphine	IM	0.5	2.12 ± 0.82				[86]
Nalbuphine	IV	0.4	0.68 (0.53–0.79)	6.8 (4.9–8.9)	114 (104.3–129.7)		[87]
Sheep							
Buprenorphine	IV	0.01	1.75 (1.07–31.0)	8.04 (1.05–49.3)	56.5 (4.17–100.33)		[88]
Fentanyl	IV	0.0025	3.08 (2.2–3.36)	8.86 (5.55–15.04)	60.33 (41.83–89.83)		[89]
Morphine	IV CRI for 10 min	1	1.98 ± 0.30	6.38 ± 0.9	34.3 ± 8.5		[90]
Oxycodone	IV	0.1	0.64 (0.33–4.4)	1.8 (1.5–4.7)	5.2 (4.6–6.2)		[91]
Tramadol	IV	4	0.67 ± 0.42	3.27 ± 1.92	74.43 ± 24.5		[92]
Tramadol	IV	6	0.57 ± 0.12	4.29 ± 0.75	78.87 ± 58.48		[92]
Goat							
Butorphanol	IV	0.1	1.87 ± 1.49	1.27 ± 0.63	96 ± 24		[93]
Butorphanol	IM	0.1	2.75 ± 1.93			82 ± 41	[93]
Fentanyl	IV	0.0025	1.2 ± 0.78	1.51 ± 0.39	34.83 ± 10.33		[94]
Morphine	IV	0.4	2.67 ± 0.82	9.64 ± 6.18	121.25 ± 38.53		[95]
Morphine	IM	0.4	1.73 ± 0.30			144.6 ± 50.5	[95]
Morphine	SC	0.4	1.63 ± 0.17			131.9 ± 61.3	[95]
Tapentadol	IV	5	3.22 ± 3.27	4.39 ± 1.94	74.15 ± 18.9		[96]
Tapentadol	IM	5	1.29 ± 0.54			87.8 ± 35.6	[96]
Tramadol	IV	1	0.94 ± 0.34	2.48 ± 0.58	36.33 ± 3.83		[97]
Tramadol	PO	2	2.67 ± 0.54			30 ± 7	[97]

[a] $t_{½}$, elimination half-life; V_{dss}, volume of distribution at steady state; Cl, clearance; F, bioavailability; IV, intravenous; IM, intramuscular; SC, subcutaneous; CRI, constant rate infusion; PO, oral; OTM, oral transmucosal.

[a] Values are mean ± standard error or median and (range).

[b] High-concentration formulation (1.8 mg/mL).

[c] Values are median and (25th–75th percentiles).

is considered to be bioavailable. By definition, a drug that is administered intravenously (IV) bypasses absorption (i.e., it is already in the systemic circulation). Opioids are very lipophilic, which allows them to move easily across cell membranes. Generally, they are rapidly and extensively absorbed after intramuscular (IM) or subcutaneous (SC) administration. Differences in onset of action and duration of effect have been reported with SC administration of hydromorphone and the "traditional" 0.3 mg/mL formulation of buprenorphine in cats, with the SC route associated with shorter duration antinociception and analgesia compared to IM or IV routes [98,99]. However, certain controlled-release opioid formulations (e.g., sustained-release buprenorphine for SC administration) produce prolonged effects compared to readily absorbable formulations (e.g., "traditional" 0.3 mg/mL buprenorphine) [20]. After oral (PO) or rectal administration, opioids can move across membranes in the gastrointestinal tract and enter local capillaries and then travel to the portal vein and liver where they usually undergo extensive metabolism [100]. This is known as "first-pass metabolism" and renders the drug ineffective when administered at standard doses. The oral transmucosal (OTM) route bypasses first-pass metabolism, and some buprenorphine formulations have demonstrated high bioavailability with this route of administration [30,101].

Transdermal administration of specially formulated opioids can result in absorption across the stratum corneum. Transdermal fentanyl patches designed for humans have been used with some success in veterinary animal species [102]. A buprenorphine transdermal matrix patch has also been evaluated in cats and, while adequate plasma concentrations were obtained, no effect on thermal threshold was measured [103]. Limitations associated with transdermal patch delivery of opioids to animals such as adherence to animal skin, accurate dosing, and potential for misuse deter their use.

A novel transdermal buprenorphine formulation approved by the US Food and Drug Administration (FDA) results in plasma drug concentrations that persist for 7 days after a single administration in cats [104].

Regional or local opioid administration has been used to maximize therapeutic efficacy and minimize systemic adverse events. For instance, epidurally administered opioids are used to induce analgesia with minimal excitation in horses. Interestingly, morphine concentrations were higher in blood plasma than in the cerebrospinal fluid for 24 h after epidural administration and hysteresis, a delay in analgesia compared to peak drug concentration, of about 4 h occurred [105,106]. In a similar way, buprenorphine was detectable in the synovial fluid of inflamed radiocarpal joints of horses at high concentrations for up to 24 h after intra-articular administration, but only for up to 6 h and at low concentrations after IV administration; both routes of administration produced similar blood plasma drug concentrations [107].

Distribution

For a drug to induce its therapeutic effects, it needs to reach its site of action at effective drug concentrations. The central nervous system (CNS) is where opioids induce their analgesic, antitussive, and sedative effects. Although most opioids penetrate the CNS, not all induce CNS effects. The μ-opioid receptor agonist loperamide is actively excluded from the CNS and is sent back into the circulation by P-glycoprotein efflux pumps. Consequently, loperamide generally acts peripherally and is used as an antidiarrheal. However, dogs with non-functional P-glycoprotein due to homozygous mutation of the ABCB1-1Δ gene display CNS effects after loperamide administration [108]. Various opioids are substrates for P-glycoprotein and patients with homozygous or heterozygous ABCB1-1Δ gene mutation may have longer lasting and more intense effects than wild-type gene carriers [109]. Interestingly, morphine accumulated more in the brain than in blood plasma of near-term pregnant sheep (1.19 ratio) and premature lambs (1.89 ratio) suggesting lack of an efflux transporter across the blood–brain barrier in sheep [90]. In addition to the blood–brain barrier, opioids can be transported across other specialized barriers such as the placenta and subsequently enter the fetal circulation [90,91,110].

Opioids have large volumes of distribution, but there are differences between drugs (see Table 23.3). These differences are due to the biochemical characteristics of the drug and the relative organ blood supply. For instance, fentanyl (4.28 log P) is more than 1000-fold more lipophilic than morphine (1.07 log P) and distributes faster into and out of highly perfused tissues such as the CNS [111]. Therefore, after IV administration, fentanyl has a faster onset, but shorter duration of analgesia compared to morphine [112]. These differences in lipophilicity can be exploited when selecting an opioid for epidural administration, with less lipophilic opioids producing longer lasting analgesia compared to more lipophilic opioids when administered by this route [105,113].

When opioids are administered into or close to their intended site of action, such as with epidural or intra-articular administration, their therapeutic effects are terminated by absorption of the opioid into the local vasculature before they are metabolized and eliminated.

Metabolism

Opioids are extensively metabolized by the liver. Phase I reactions, which include oxidation (via the cytochrome P450 system), reduction, and hydrolysis, convert the parent drug to a more polar- or water-soluble molecule. Phase II reactions increase the water solubility of a molecule by conjugation of subgroups usually with glucuronate, acetate, or sulfate. Glucuronidation is the main metabolic pathway for opioids [78–80,114]. However, cats are deficient in this pathway and use conjugation with sulfate to metabolize morphine [115]. In contrast to humans, opioids have low oral and rectal bioavailability in animals due to extensive first-pass metabolism, usually rendering them ineffective when administered by these routes at standard doses [64,116]. Opioid metabolizing enzymes are also found in other tissues such as the intestine and the brain [117]. Differences in individual responses to opioids may be mediated by genetic polymorphisms in metabolizing enzymes [109].

In general, drug metabolites are less active than the parent drug; however, many opioid metabolites maintain some pharmacologic activity. In many species, for instance, morphine is conjugated with glucuronate to form morphine-3-glucuronide and morphine-6-glucuronide. Although morphine-6-glucuronide is regarded as the active metabolite, morphine-3-glucuronide may be active too, and interactions between these metabolites and the parent drug may contribute to the effects of morphine [81]. Tramadol is metabolized to its active *O*-desmethyltramadol metabolite [116]. Some opioids are pro-drugs and become active drugs after being metabolized. For example, hydrocodone is metabolized to the active compound hydromorphone and the less active norhydrocodone [79,80].

Some drugs induce or inhibit drug metabolizing enzymes and interactions between these drugs and opioids may have important clinical implications. After oral tramadol administration in dogs, for instance, the enzyme inhibitor fluconazole increased by more than 30-fold both tramadol and *O*-desmethyltramadol blood plasma and urine concentrations [118]. Similarly, the enzyme inhibitors ketoconazole and cimetidine increased mean oral tramadol bioavailability from 2.6% to 18.2% and 20.3% and mean maximum blood plasma concentration from 22.9 ng/mL to 109.9 ng/mL and 143.2 ng/mL, respectively [119]. On the other hand, in dogs, the enzyme inducer grapefruit juice decreased the maximum blood plasma tramadol concentration (C_{max}) (490 versus 270 ng/mL), delayed the time that C_{max} occurred (T_{max}) (1.33 versus 1.7 h), and decreased the area under the curve (AUC) (11,610 versus 5890 h·ng/mL) [120]. Also in this last study, *O*-desmethyltramadol C_{max} was increased (80 versus 130 ng/mL), T_{max} occurred faster (1.36 versus 0.86 h), and AUC was decreased (340 versus 160 h·ng/mL) [120].

Excretion

In general, very little of the opioid dose is excreted as the parent drug via the urine or feces. Opioid metabolites are often eliminated in the urine, but some can be eliminated in the feces by biliary secretion. Patients with hepatic or renal impairment may have altered opioid clearance and may require dose adjustments to avoid drug accumulation and the potential for adverse events [121].

Opioid tolerance, dependence, withdrawal, and opioid-induced hyperalgesia

Opioid agonists activate reward processes in the absence of significant pain and motivate repeated use of escalating doses of the drugs simply for pleasure. This alters the brain so that it functions more or less normally when the drugs are present and abnormally when they are not. Two clinically important results of this alteration are opioid tolerance and dependence. Opioid tolerance is the need to take higher dosages of drugs to achieve the same therapeutic effect. Opioid dependence is the need to use an opioid agonist to avoid a withdrawal syndrome. Opioid withdrawal symptoms, together with social and genetic effects, contribute to the development of opioid addiction. Opioid addicts require detoxification and pharmacological treatment, usually with methadone, levo-α-acetylmethadol, buprenorphine, or naltrexone, which must be accompanied by psychosocial therapy [122].

The exact mechanisms involved in the development of opioid tolerance and reward processes remain to be elucidated. However, opioid tolerance develops in the midbrain periaqueductal gray (PAG) and rostral ventral medulla descending system. Increased activation of adenylate cyclase in γ-aminobutyric acid (GABA) interneurons in the PAG results in protein kinase A-mediated phosphorylation of Ca^{2+} channels and, therefore, increased calcium conductance. The overall effect is increased GABA release and, therefore, stronger inhibition of PAG output neurons [123]. Opioid reward takes place in the mesolimbic dopamine system where opioid agonists generate signals in the ventral tegmental area that result in the release of dopamine in the nucleus accumbens inducing feelings of pleasure. Other areas of the brain create memories that associate these good feelings with the circumstances and environment in which they occur. These conditioned associations lead to the craving for drugs when the abuser reencounters those people, places, or things, and they drive abusers to seek out more drugs [122].

Opioid tolerance usually precedes opioid dependence, and it may be overcome by increasing the dose or administering a different opioid agonist (i.e., opioid rotation). However, increasing the dose increases the risk of opioid-induced adverse events. Opioid tolerance has been extensively studied in experimental pain-free dogs and cats (Table 23.4). Daily administration of 3 mg/kg of morphine to dogs initially induced sedation lasting up to 24 h, which gradually decreased in both degree and duration. Sedation was increased by increasing the dose, but within three weeks of starting treatment, morphine did not induce sedation despite the increased doses. Complete tolerance to morphine's emetic effects developed within 10 days [124]. Although the route of administration was not stated in this report, the dosage used was higher than the recommended morphine dosage for clinical use in dogs. SC administration of morphine at lower dose rates (twice a day for 7 days at 0.5 and 2.5 mg/kg or infused at 1–5 mg/kg/day for 8 days) induced faster tolerance development in dogs [125]. In cats, however, administration of high doses of morphine (1–4 mg/kg/day IV) for 7 days induced minimal tolerance [126]. Procedural details rather than species differences between dogs and cats may explain the differences in the development of tolerance. The cat study also suggests that tolerance can be prevented by large opioid doses. Cats exposed to rounds of increasing lower doses of morphine (1–2 mg/kg/day SC divided into morning and evening doses over 24 to 30 days) developed tolerance, which was overcome by increasing the morphine dose [127].

Opioid dependence, determined by appearance of withdrawal signs, was also reported in the abovementioned studies. One to two months after morphine (3 mg/kg/day) administration, dogs became irritable and fought frequently at the end of the 24-h administration, which was overcome by shortening the dosing interval or increasing the dose [124]. After ceasing morphine administration, 8 out of 10 dogs showed mild signs of opioid withdrawal characterized by rigidity with spastic gait, muscle twitching, retracted belly, sleepiness, salivation, diarrhea, and vomiting; one dog showed moderate signs which also included restlessness, piloerection, gnawing at objects, whining, hiccough, panting, and growling; and one dog showed marked signs which additionally included jerky respiration, and being irritable, belligerent, and very noisy. Maximal signs were seen three days after morphine withdrawal and all signs disappeared after 8–10 days. When morphine withdrawal was induced by nalorphine administration, seven, nine, and six dogs showed slight, moderate, and marked withdrawal signs,

Table 23.4 Effects of morphine on opioid-induced tolerance in dogs and cats.

Species	Route	Dose, frequency/duration	Comments	Reference
Dog	Not reported	3 mg/kg, daily	At 21 days post-administration sedation no longer observed At 10 days post-administration vomiting no longer observed	[124]
	SC	0.5 mg/kg and 2.5 mg/kg twice daily or infused at 1–5 mg/kg/day	Dogs developed opioid tolerance within 8 days of administration	[125]
Cat	IV	1–4 mg/kg/day	Minimal tolerance observed at 7 days of administration	[126]
	SC	1–2 mg/kg/day divided into morning and evening doses	Tolerance was developed by 24–30 days. Tolerance was overcome via increasing the morphine dose	[127]

IV, intravenous; SC, subcutaneous.

respectively. 1 h after nalorphine administration, excitement was observed, and 1 h later, it had disappeared [124]. Similarly, after one week of morphine administration and withdrawal precipitated by subcutaneous naloxone (1 mg/kg) administration, dogs showed signs of hyperactivity, biting, licking, grooming, digging, tremors, nausea, hyperthermia, mydriasis, and increased wakefulness [125]. In cats, whole body shakes, head shakes, urination (often in a standing position), miosis, and catatonic-like posturing resulted from naloxone (0.5 mg/kg IV)-precipitated withdrawal in cats maintained for 12 days on IV morphine (1–4 mg/kg/day) [126]. After being exposed to 24- to 30-day-rounds of increasing doses of morphine, cats slept most of the day and ate very little during a 2-day withdrawal period. This behavior was similar during a 2-week withdrawal period, with appetite and activity levels improving during the second week. Fatigue, muscle weakness, and pupillary constriction were noted during the first and second day of withdrawal periods. Mild muscle tremors were observed, especially early in the final withdrawal period [127]. Interestingly, plasma cortisol levels increased in these cats at the beginning of the withdrawal periods and decreased to baseline levels when morphine was administered again or 6 weeks after morphine withdrawal [127]. In another cat study, psychological dependence to opioids was demonstrated by self-administration of morphine [128]. Together, these studies suggest that opioid-dependent cats will self-medicate with opioids, if available, and that opioid withdrawal is stressful.

Repeated exposure to opioid agonists may cause an exacerbated pain state known as "opioid-induced hyperalgesia" (OIH). This phenomenon was described as early as 1870 [129]; however, the first prospective, controlled clinical trial demonstrating OIH was published in 2006 [130]. In this trial, participants suffering from lower back pain developed hyperalgesia, as assessed by a cold pressor test, after one month of oral morphine therapy [130]. The exact mechanisms by which OIH occurs are not fully understood but involve maladaptive plastic changes in opioid-responsive pain processing pathways. Some of these changes include: (1) activation of descending pain facilitation from the rostral ventromedial medulla by increased activity of cholecystokinin and "on-cell" firing which in turn activates spinal pathways to upregulate dynorphin and enhance spinal nociceptive inputs; (2) spinal glutaminergic systems, via sustained activation of *N*-methyl-D-aspartate receptors, which sensitize dorsal horn neurons to intensify pronociceptive ascending pathways; and (3) increased activity of catechol-*O*-methyltransferase with subsequent higher breakdown of dopamine and noradrenaline enhancing nociceptive responses [123,131]. Neuroimmune cell communication has also been implicated in OIH. Upregulation of P2X4-purinergic receptors in microglia and subsequent release of brain-derived neurotrophic factor activated tropomyosin receptor kinase B on spinal dorsal horn neurons, which downregulated potassium-chloride co-transporter KCC2, shifting GABA receptor activation from inhibitory to excitatory [132].

Few studies have investigated OIH in domestic animal species. Two studies demonstrated a κ-opioid-receptor-mediated pontine-medullary hyperalgesic system in dogs [133,134], and one study reported thermal hyperalgesia after morphine administration in cockerels [135]. Although naloxone reversed the development of hyperalgesia in these three studies, hyperalgesia was induced after a single systemic or local administration of an opioid agonist.

Opioid tolerance, dependence, withdrawal, or OIH has not yet been systematically assessed in veterinary clinical cases. However, these phenomena may not present practical concerns as opioids are mainly administered for acute uses and long-term use is not recommended for chronic pain control [136,137]. Furthermore, approved opioid medications in animals maintain clinical efficacy for up to 4 days after a single administration [104].

Clinical pharmacology

Analgesia

Opioid analgesics have been the cornerstone for perioperative pain management in veterinary medicine for several decades. A comprehensive understanding related to their molecular and cellular mechanism of action allows the clinician to maximize the efficacy of opioid analgesics and mitigate their unwanted adverse effects. Opioids, acting as endogenous (e.g., endorphins, enkephalins, dynorphins, endomorphins, and nociceptins) or exogenous (e.g., methadone, hydromorphone, morphine, etc.) ligands, bind to μ-, δ-, and κ-opioid receptors as well as nociceptin/orphanin FQ receptors producing a desired effect [138].

Opioid receptors are structurally classified as seven transmembrane G-protein-coupled receptors and are located at supraspinal (e.g., cortex, thalamus, hypothalamus, locus coeruleus, periaqueductal gray, amygdala, and cingulate gyrus), spinal (e.g., dorsal horn of the spinal cord), and peripheral tissue (e.g., dorsal root ganglia, peripheral nerve endings of sensory neurons, inflamed tissue, and immune cells) levels [139,140]. Binding of an exogenous or endogenous opioid ligand to opioid receptors results in a conformational change that allows intracellular coupling of G_i/G_o proteins to the C terminus of the opioid receptor (Fig. 23.2) [140]. This activation dissociates the trimeric receptor into several active subunits (Gα, Gβ, Gγ). The Gα subunit then binds to adenylate cyclase preventing the formation of cyclic adenosine monophosphate, an important secondary messenger associated with autonomic tone [138]. In addition, activation of Gα subunits open inwardly rectifying potassium channels (Kir3) resulting in an efflux of potassium ions. This effect hyperpolarizes the cell membrane, preventing neuronal excitation and/or the duration of the action potential. Gβ and Gγ subunits directly interact with voltage-gated calcium channels (VGCC) decreasing calcium influx via closure of pre- and postsynaptic calcium channels, thereby decreasing intracellular calcium concentrations. Within laminae I and II of the dorsal horn of the spinal cord, a reduction of calcium influx reduces the spinal release of glutamate and substance P [141]. Similar to the effect observed with Gα on Kir3 channels, the action potential duration and the release of pronociceptive neuropeptides is reduced [138,140]. In the PAG, binding of exogenous opioids or endogenous opioid peptides to opioid receptors inhibits GABAergic interneurons, activating descending inhibitory pathways that project to the dorsal horn of the spinal cord, thereby modulating transmission of the nociceptive impulse [142].

Stimulation of opioid receptors on peripheral terminals of primary afferent nerves associated with inflamed tissue can also induce potent antinociceptive effects [143–145]. Endogenous and exogenous opioids bind to opioid receptors synthesized in the dorsal root ganglia that are transported along intra-axonal microtubules to peripheral sensory neuron terminals. This results in inhibition of peripheral ion channels (e.g., transient receptor potential vanilloid-1 [TRPV1], hyperpolarization-activated cyclic nucleotide-gated [HCN], sodium, acid-sensing ion [ASIC] channels) and substance P [140]. Increased neuronal electrical activity and production of inflammatory cytokines associated with inflamed peripheral tissue stimulate mRNA and specific proteins to upregulate production of

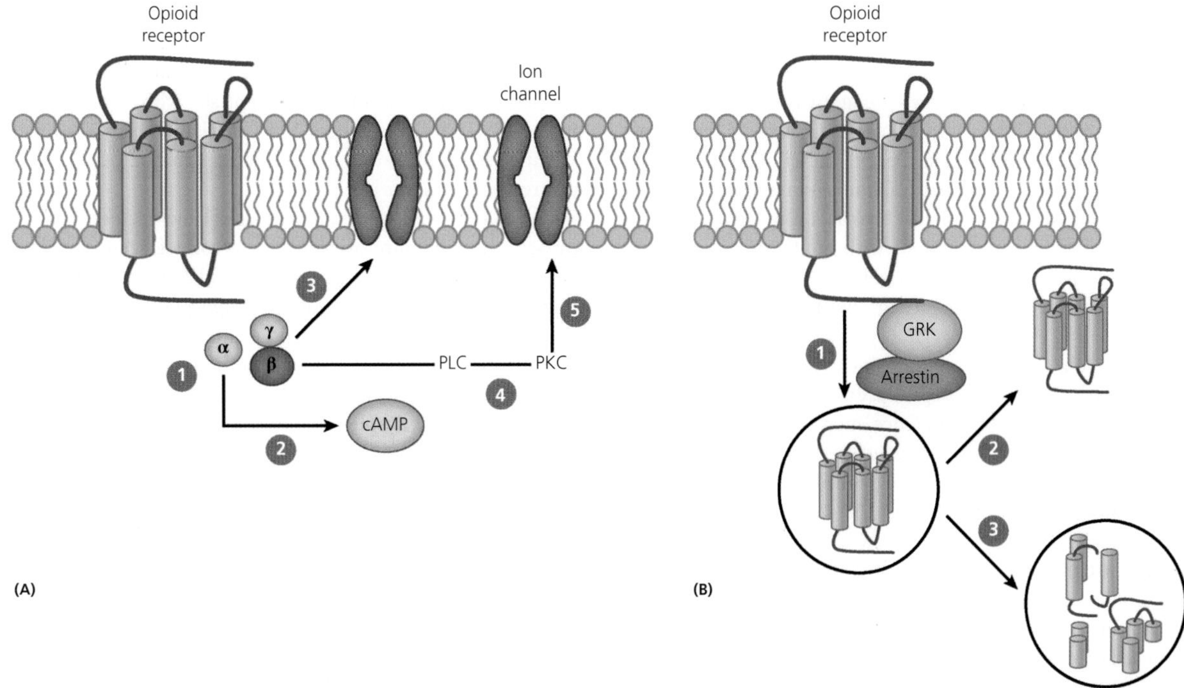

Figure 23.2 Opioid receptor signaling and recycling. **A.** Opioid receptor ligands induce a conformational change at the receptor that allows coupling of G-proteins to the receptor. The heterotrimeric G-protein dissociates into active Gα and Gβγ subunits, which can inhibit adenylate cyclase and reduce cAMP, decrease the conductance of voltage-gated Ca^{2+} channels, or open rectifying K^{+} channels. In addition, the phospholipase C (PLC)/phosphokinase C (PKC) pathways can be activated to modulate Ca^{2+} channel activity in the plasma membrane. **B.** Opioid receptor desensitization and trafficking is activated by G-protein-coupled receptor kinase (GRK). After arrestin binding, the receptor is in a desensitized state at the plasma membrane. Arrestin-bound receptors can then be internalized via a clathrin-dependent pathway, and either be recycled to the cell surface or degraded in lysosomes.
Source: Stein [140], Annual Reviews.

opioid receptors and induce differential regulation of opioid receptor types [140]. This has been observed more consistently with μ-opioid receptors [146]. Similar influences on opioid receptor expression are observed at sites of nerve injury and in tissues innerved by damaged nerves [147].

Opioid analgesics administered locally to inflamed tissues bind to peripheral opioid receptors and dampen excitatory impulses of sensory nerves similar to that observed at presynaptic opioid receptors in the spinal cord. Thus, peripheral analgesic effects are only produced when opioid agonists are administered to tissues that are inflamed or affected by nerve injury.

Multiple effective routes of administration contribute to the versatility of opioids as analgesics in a variety of clinical settings. This is largely a function of the diverse locations of opioid receptors within the neuroaxis, which allows for effective pain control when opioids are administered peripherally (intra-articular), neuraxially (intrathecal and epidural), systemically (IV, IM, SC, and OTM), or transdermally. Choosing the appropriate opioid for pain management depends on several patient-related and drug-specific considerations (Box 23.1). Opioids can be administered in combination with other perioperative agents to produce neuroleptanalgesia (e.g., a benzodiazepine or acepromazine with an opioid), and as part of multimodal analgesic protocols. Full μ-opioid receptor agonists are often preferred over partial or mixed agonists due to their efficacy in managing acute surgical pain. A higher fraction of opioid receptor occupancy is often required with partial agonists (i.e., buprenorphine) to achieve an analgesic response of equivalent magnitude when compared to full agonists. In most domestic

Box 23.1 Patient- and drug-related considerations when treating pain with opioid analgesics.

Patient-related considerations

Constipation or gastrointestinal ileus (particularly with large animal species)
Gastrointestinal reflux disease (e.g., hiatal hernia, gastrointestinal obstruction)
Brachycephalic patients (e.g., prone to gastrointestinal reflux, high vagal tone, respiratory obstruction which can be exacerbated by opioid analgesics)
Bradyarrhythmias (i.e., third-degree atrioventricular block, atrial standstill, sick sinus syndrome)
High vagal tone or procedures with potential for vagal stimulation (e.g., ophthalmic surgery or procedures adjacent to the carotid artery)
Increased intracranial pressure (exacerbated with emesis associated with hydromorphone and morphine)
Mast cell tumors (caution with IV morphine or meperidine administration)
Significant respiratory disease (e.g., $PaCO_2$ > 60mmHg)
Severity and duration of pain

Analgesic drug-related considerations

Duration of action
Magnitude of analgesia
Routes of administration available
Hospital versus outpatient setting
Chronicity of administration
Legal concerns
Opioid availability
Cost of opioid use in large animal species

species, full μ-opioid receptor agonists provide more profound analgesic effects when compared to partial agonists [148–150], while both full and partial agonists provide superior analgesia when compared to mixed agonist–antagonist agents [151–155]. This may not always be the case with certain species of birds; however, this remains controversial. Despite differences among full agonists, partial agonists, and mixed agonist–antagonists, all three mediate analgesia to some degree and partial or mixed agonists can provide effective therapy in patients with moderate or mild pain, respectively. It has been generally accepted that administration of a partial μ-opioid receptor agonist (e.g., buprenorphine) produces an analgesic ceiling effect [156]. However, the classic "bell-shaped" dose–response curve for buprenorphine reported in some early rodent studies has not been reproduced in more recent animal studies or in humans. Some evidence suggests this ceiling effect may be more relevant to non-analgesic effects, such as respiratory depression, rather than analgesia [157]. Similar findings may apply to other opioids such as butorphanol [158–160].

Sedation, euphoria, and dysphoria

Opioids induce dose-dependent sedation in most species [161]. When combined with acepromazine, the rank order of opioids based on sedative intensity in dogs was methadone (0.5 mg/kg) > morphine (0.5 mg/kg) > butorphanol (0.15 mg/kg) > nalbuphine (0.5 mg/kg) [162,163]. Butorphanol (0.2 mg/kg), when combined and administered IV with dexmedetomidine (2 μg/kg), had a faster onset and greater magnitude of sedation when compared to methadone (0.2 mg/kg) in dogs [163]. Sedation associated with opioid administration does not always correlate with analgesia; thus, the clinician must assess the patient for appropriate pain control. For example, in two human trials, morphine-induced sedation was a poor indicator of appropriate analgesia during IV titration [164] and did not ensure adequate pain relief postoperatively [165]. Opioid-based procedural sedation protocols (e.g., an opioid combined with an α_2-adrenergic receptor agonist [166]) used for blood donation or diagnostic imaging are generally safe with minimal negative effects on diagnostic findings in healthy dogs [167,168] and cats [169–172].

The mechanism of opioid-induced sedation is complex and not completely understood [173]. One theory is that opioids decrease sensory input and promote the probability of sleep [174]. Contrary to this theory, there is evidence that opioid administration disrupts the normal sleep–wake patterns by decreasing the amount of rapid eye movement (REM) sleep in animals [175,176]. Selectivity for the opioid receptor may also vary the influence on REM sleep. For example, intracerebroventricular administration of DAMGO, a selective μ-opioid receptor agonist, inhibited REM sleep, whereas DPDE and U50,488H (μ/δ- and κ-opioid receptor agonists, respectively) have minimal to no effect on REM cycles [176]. Spectral analysis of EEG recordings has been used to further understand the sedative effects of opioid receptor agonists when administered peripherally and centrally in animals. High-amplitude, low-frequency EEG recordings were observed in combination with a wide range of behaviors (e.g., stupor, immobility, catatonia, ataxia, increased locomotion, and hyperreactivity) [173]. Similar findings were observed in humans administered short-acting μ-opioid receptor agonists [173]. Evoked potentials have also been used to evaluate the effects of opioid receptor agonists in animals. In rats, small increases in amplitude and AUC of the cortical evoked potential were associated with morphine-induced sedation [177]. Morphine administered to human cancer patients resulted in a delayed response to an auditory stimulus when compared to those that did not receive opioids [178]. In contrast, the administration of morphine to relieve chronic non-malignant pain in humans resulted in enlarged evoked potentials with reduced reaction times [179,180]. Researchers from the latter study postulate that cognitive status improved because of the removal of pain as a mental stressor/distractor [179,180].

In addition to individual patient-related factors, species also impacts the reliability of opioids to produce sedation. Cats have been reported to exhibit euphoric and/or dysphoric behaviors following opioid administration. *Euphoria*, defined as rolling, kneading with forepaws, vocalizing, and purring, is evident following hydromorphone, butorphanol, methadone, and buprenorphine administration in cats [58,181]. Butorphanol has also been reported to cause dysphoria (i.e., vocalizing, pacing, and staring) in cats [182,183]. Both situations hinder the ability to appropriately restrain patients for intravenous catheterization and routine diagnostic procedures. Cats also exhibit unique behavioral effects with the administration of morphine. "Morphine mania" or "feline mania" is a dose-dependent (> 5–10 mg/kg) behavioral response characterized by behavioral excitation, motor agitation, and aggression [184,185]. Morphine administered to cats at 3 mg/kg intraperitoneally (still considerably higher than doses used clinically) resulted in three distinct behavioral stages: (1) the autonomic stage (0–15 min post-drug administration) characterized by vocalization, salivation, licking, swallowing, and vomiting; (2) the quiet stage (15–60 min post-drug administration) characterized by sitting, staring, mydriasis, and pricked pinnae; and (3) the head movement stage (30–60 min and decreasing within 5 h post-drug administration) characterized by sitting, arousal, discrete head movements that appear in response to visual-tracking, pouncing/avoidance paw movements, rocking, pivoting, and backing [186]. Minimal evidence of sleep, grooming, micturition, and defecation were noted during these stages [186]. Healthy dogs anesthetized with inhalant anesthetics and administered a μ-opioid receptor agonist (i.e., fentanyl or morphine) may also exhibit signs of dysphoria during the recovery period [187,188]. The administration of a 0.5 μg/kg dexmedetomidine bolus IV over 10 min immediately prior to extubation in dogs administered fentanyl infusions and inhalant anesthetics can reduce the incidence of opioid-induced dysphoria [189].

Horses also are reported to have excitatory responses following μ-opioid receptor agonist administration (Table 23.2) [190]. Dose-dependent increases in arousal and locomotor activity (i.e., foot stepping, spontaneous flexion of forelimbs, postural changes) are observed following 2.5, 5, and 10 μg/kg IV doses of fentanyl [191]. Excitation has also been observed following morphine, hydromorphone, pentazocine, meperidine, buprenorphine, and methadone administration in this species [13,192]. It has been suggested that opioid-induced locomotor enhancement in horses is due to opioid and dopamine receptor stimulation [191], as the locomotor effects of fentanyl and morphine can be antagonized by naloxone (0.015–0.02 mg/kg IV) and acepromazine (0.10–0.16 mg/kg IV) [193]. Conclusions pertaining to opioid-induced locomotion in horses include: (1) opioids induce eating behavior at low doses; (2) dose-dependent locomotor activity with incoordination is observed at high doses; (3) the median effective dose for morphine to result in increased locomotion is 0.91 mg/kg, which is significantly higher than doses used to produce analgesia; and (4) there is variability in behavioral responses in the horse population [194]. It is difficult to determine if activation of different opioid receptor types plays a role in opioid-induced excitation in horses. Butorphanol is reported to enhance locomotor activity associated with fentanyl administration [190]. However, yawning, ataxia, and staggering are more commonly observed following κ-opioid receptor agonist administration [195]. In the author's experience, butorphanol also results in head twitching following administration. In general, μ-opioid receptor agonists promote increased locomotion when compared to κ-opioid receptor agonists.

Cardiovascular system

Opioids increase parasympathetic tone and inhibit sympathetic tone leading to vagally mediated bradycardia and occasionally hypotension. Several predisposing risk factors may increase the likelihood of opioid-induced bradycardia. These include the administration of β-adrenergic blocking agents, calcium channel antagonists, α_2-adrenergic receptor agonists [196], inhalant anesthetics [197], muscle relaxants that lack parasympatholytic properties (e.g., vecuronium), high vagal tone (e.g., brachycephalic breeds) or various vagotonic physical stimuli (e.g., traction of ophthalmic muscles [198] or carotid massage [199]), high doses of opioids, and rapid IV bolus administration. Methadone's chemical structure resembles that of calcium blocking agents and results in functional L-type calcium channel blockade [200]. This is independent of its μ-opioid receptor effects [200] and, therefore, may potentiate bradycardia [201]. Meperidine exhibits a slightly different action than other opioids (e.g., increased heart rate) due to its anticholinergic effects [202]. Conversely, opioids have been reported to increase heart rate in horses at clinically relevant doses [79].

Opioids generally exhibit a dose-dependent effect on cardiac index (CI) that is associated with a reduction in heart rate (HR); however, this may be affected by species and the specific opioid administered. Morphine administered at 1 mg/kg IV to dogs resulted in a 26% and 19% reduction in HR and CI, respectively, at 120 min post-administration. Methadone resulted in more pronounced depressant effects on HR and CI in conscious dogs compared to morphine at similar doses (i.e., 0.5 mg/kg methadone reduced HR by 19–28% and CI by 17–27%; 1 mg/kg methadone reduced HR by 32–46% and CI by 24–52%) [203]. Alterations in systemic vascular resistance index (SVRI) vary among opioids. In general, administration of opioids (e.g., methadone and buprenorphine) has been reported to increase SVRI via increased vasopressin concentrations in anesthetized and conscious dogs [197,203]. Morphine, however, has been reported to decrease SVRI [203], and butorphanol has been reported to have limited effects [204]. Similarly, meperidine has been reported to reduce SVRI due to its direct smooth muscle relaxant effect and indirect histamine releasing effect [205].

Opioids have been reported to alter the electrocardiogram and these effects may be exacerbated during inhalant anesthesia [206]. For example, methadone and hydromorphone prolong the PR and QT intervals when administered at clinically relevant doses in dogs. Opioids disrupt the delayed rectifier potassium current resulting in reduction of potassium efflux. This effect prolongs the action potential and delays ventricular repolarization, thus prolonging the QT interval on the electrocardiogram [207]. Delays in the PR interval following opioid administration have been known to result in bradyarrhythmias such as second-degree atrioventricular (AV) block. The calcium blocking effects of methadone contribute to delayed depolarization of both the sinoatrial (SA) and AV nodal pacemaker cells [206]. Administration of an anticholinergic drug (e.g., glycopyrrolate or atropine) can be used to treat or prevent opioid-induced bradyarrhythmias [208].

Respiratory system

Opioids have been reported to exert their respiratory depressant effects at several supraspinal locations (Box 23.2) [209,210]. Opioid-induced ventilatory depression is a result of interactions with supraspinal μ-opioid receptors in the forebrain, superficial and deep brainstem tissue, and/or in the suprapontine tissue [209]. A large component of excitatory drive to the medullary rhythm generator (chemodrive) is routed through an area of the brain called the Parabrachial Nucleus/Kölliker-Fuse Complex and assists in determining respiratory rate, while tidal volume is dependent on direct output projections from the retrotrapezoid nucleus to the preBötzinger Complex neurons [210]. Opioids depress Parabrachial Nucleus/Kölliker-Fuse Complex activity in addition to acting at the nucleus of the solitary tract and the medullary raphe (Fig. 23.3) [210].

Clinically, opioids exert a dose-dependent respiratory depressant effect resulting in respiratory acidosis and increased arterial carbon dioxide tension ($PaCO_2$), with a resultant decrease in arterial oxygen tension (PaO_2) in patients that are breathing room air [211]. Pure μ-opioid receptor agonists [212,213] result in more significant depressant effects than partial [214] or mixed opioid agonists [215]. The magnitude of respiratory depression is directly correlated with the degree of sedation and/or analgesia produced [216]. Opioid overdose may limit the respiratory center's response to profound hypoxia and hypercapnia, thus requiring full or partial reversal with administration of naloxone or butorphanol, respectively [217–220]. While effects are considered mild in healthy individuals, with $PaCO_2$ and PaO_2 often remaining within clinically acceptable limits, opioids may pose more significant risks in patients with respiratory compromise [221]. Mild reductions in PaO_2 are a result of alveolar hypoventilation [212]. Elevations of $PaCO_2$ are related to reductions in respiratory rate more so than decreased minute volume; however, elevations in respiratory rate (e.g., panting) may be observed [211]. Despite the latter, $PaCO_2$ still remains elevated [211]. Opioid-induced apnea is characterized by arrest of the respiratory cycle during the expiratory phase (i.e., impaired respiratory rate control) rather than from a profound decrease in tidal volume [222–224].

Gastrointestinal system

Both peripheral and central mechanisms associated with μ-opioid receptor agonist stimulation may impair gastrointestinal motility or promote ileus. μ-Opioid receptors are present in the enteric nervous system and are distributed in the stomach (corpus and antrum), duodenum, jejunum, ileum, and proximal and distal colon [225]. Stimulation of these opioid receptors suppresses neuronal excitability via inhibition of Ca^{2+} channels, membrane hyperpolarization, and

Box 23.2 Supraspinal sites involved in μ-opioid receptor-mediated respiratory depression.

Carotid body
Nucleus tractus solitarii
Retrotrapezoid nucleus
Medullary raphe
Forebrain
Periaqueductal gray
Parabrachial Nucleus/Kölliker-Fuse Complex
PreBötzinger Complex
Premotor neurons
Phrenic motoneurons

Source: Adapted from Palkovic *et al.* [210].

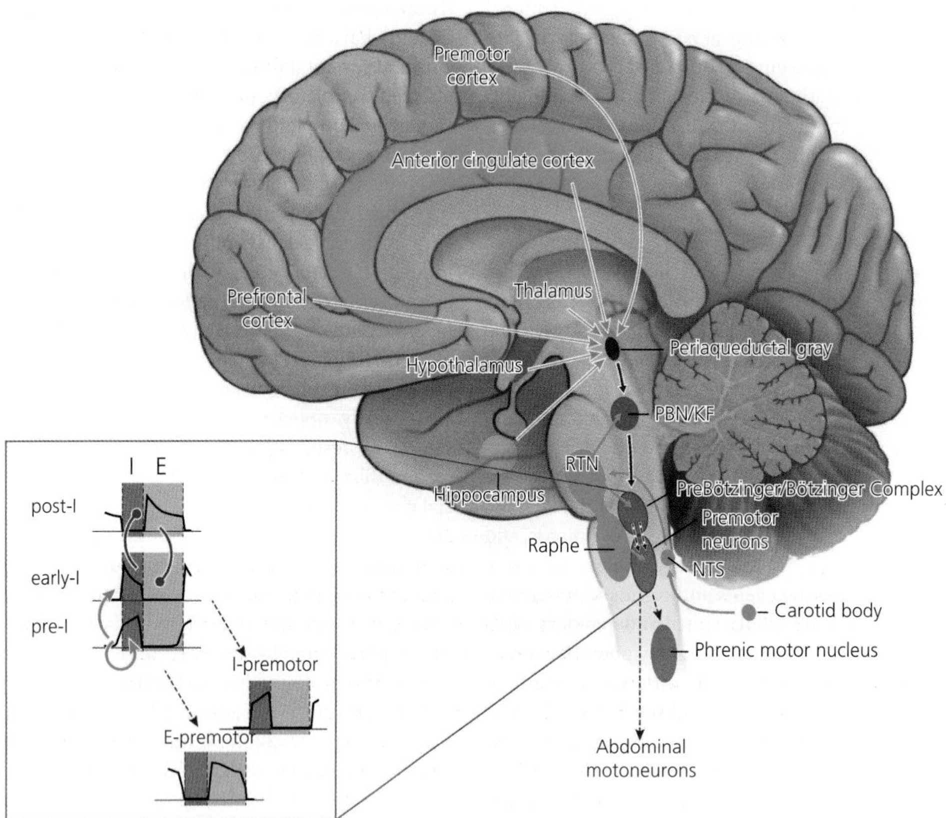

Figure 23.3 Excitatory connections within the respiratory control center and opioid effects. Tonic chemodrive (green solid arrows) is the main excitatory drive to the medullary rhythm generator. A large component of chemodrive is routed through the Parabrachial Nucleus/Kölliker-Fuse Complex (PBN/KF) to phase-switching neurons in the preBötzinger Complex and determines respiratory rate (dark blue solid arrow). Phasic inputs from the preBötzinger Complex activate inspiratory (I) and expiratory (E) premotor and motoneurons (blue dotted arrows). Respiratory motor output (tidal volume) depends on direct projections from the retrotrapezoid nucleus (RTN) to preBötzinger Complex neurons, premotor neurons, and motoneurons. The corticolimbic system contributes tonic drive to the medullary rhythm generator (light blue solid arrows). *Not shown:* direct projections from the motor cortex to phrenic motoneurons as a pathway to override automatic rhythm; projections from the hypothalamus and cerebellum to the medullary raphe, which may contribute to the state-dependency of respiratory activity. *Opioid effects:* Parabrachial Nucleus/Kölliker-Fuse Complex activity was depressed in all studies and at all opioid concentrations. Opioid-induced depression was also shown for the preBötzinger Complex, nucleus tractus solitarii (NTS), and the medullary raphe. Opioid-induced sedation suggests depression of forebrain inputs. Premotor neurons are only directly depressed at very high opioid concentrations. *Inset:* neuronal subtypes constituting the core of respiratory rhythm generation. Through mutual excitation, network activity of pre-inspiratory neurons (pre-I) in the preBötzinger Complex results in activation of early inspiratory (early-I) neurons (green arrows). Activity of these neurons is terminated through inhibition by postinspiratory neurons (post-I), which themselves are inhibited by early-I neurons during the inspiratory phase (red circles). Phasic excitation is relayed to inspiratory (I) and expiratory (E) premotor neurons. Source: Palkovic *et al.* [210], The American Physiological Society.

decreased cyclic adenosine monophosphate and protein kinase A activity [225]. The net effect is decreased excitatory neurotransmitter release (e.g., acetylcholine, vasoactive intestinal polypeptide, and substance P) from acetylcholine- or substance P-containing neurons [226,227]. Clinical effects lead to reductions in gastrointestinal motility, coordination, secretions, gastric emptying, and propulsive activity, as well as increases in pyloric and anal sphincter tone and constipation [225–227]. The effects of opioids on the large intestine are considered biphasic with initial stimulation of colonic motility leading to defecation shortly after administration followed by decreased colonic propulsive motility and secretions [64,187]. The route of administration may impact the magnitude of opioid-induced gastrointestinal effects. In horses, IV administration of morphine has been reported to result in more significant gastrointestinal stasis when compared to epidural morphine administration [228,229].

Opioid-induced vomiting is a result of δ-opioid receptor stimulation within the chemoreceptor trigger zone (CTZ) outside the blood–brain barrier [230], a circumventricular organ located on the floor of the fourth ventricle in the postrema medulla [231]. Opioids with lower lipid solubility, such as hydromorphone, morphine, and meperidine, initially stimulate δ-opioid receptors through fenestrated capillaries in the CTZ prior to crossing the blood–brain barrier where all opioids act at the medulla to inhibit the vomiting center (i.e., antiemetic effect) [230]. Thus, subsequent doses of opioid analgesic are less likely to result in vomiting compared to the initial dose [232]. Opioids that are highly lipophilic (i.e., fentanyl) penetrate the blood–brain barrier more rapidly and may inhibit vomiting [230,231]. Higher doses and/or concentrations of less lipophilic opioids (i.e., morphine and hydromorphone) may provide a more pronounced antiemetic effect [230,233]. For example, one study reported the incidences of morphine-associated vomiting in dogs administered IV doses of 0.3, 1, and 2 mg/kg were 100%, 60%, and 0%, respectively [230]. SC and IM routes of administration of morphine and/or hydromorphone result in higher incidences of vomiting when compared to the IV route in dogs [62,234,235].

Morphine may induce a similar or slightly increased frequency of vomiting compared to hydromorphone in dogs [234,236]. In cats, vomiting may occur regardless of route, but usually less often following IV administration. For example, vomiting has been reported in approximately 83% (5/6 cats) [98], 40% (4/10 cats) [237], and 0% (0/6 cats) [238] to 86% (6/7 cats) [239] of cats administered hydromorphone via the SC, IM, and IV routes, respectively. Methadone and oxymorphone generally produce fewer vomiting episodes when administered by similar routes compared to hydromorphone or morphine [240]. Vomiting may still be observed with methadone when administered via the OTM route to dogs [241]. In a study involving healthy dogs, meperidine (8.8 mg/kg IM) resulted in no episodes of vomiting, while morphine (0.66 mg/kg IM) resulted in a 50% incidence of vomiting [242]. Several studies have reported ways to reduce opioid-induced vomiting (Box 23.3) which include the use of acupuncture, maropitant, or acepromazine prior to hydromorphone or morphine administration [243–245].

Opioid administration has been reported to promote gastroesophageal reflux (GER) in anesthetized dogs [242,243,248,250,251]. Opioids potentiate GER via delayed gastric emptying, decreased lower esophageal sphincter tone, and reductions in gastroesophageal pressure [252–254]. Similar studies evaluating the effects of opioids on GER in anesthetized cats have not been performed; however, GER does occur in cats administered inhalant anesthetics [255]. Further discussion pertaining to GER frequency and species differences in dogs versus cats is beyond the scope of this chapter.

The effects of opioids on GER may be dose related. Morphine administered IM at 0.22 and 1.1 mg/kg resulted in a GER frequency of 50% and 60%, respectively, compared to 27% in isoflurane-anesthetized dogs that received a placebo [250]. Morphine combined with common premedication agents (e.g., dexmedetomidine, acepromazine, or midazolam) produced GER in 35–45% of inhalant-anesthetized dogs [256]. Meperidine, when administered IM, is associated with a lower incidence of GER when compared to IM morphine in anesthetized dogs (8/20 or 40% versus 11/20 or 55%), respectively [242]. The incidence of GER with hydromorphone was reported to be approximately 30–69% in anesthetized dogs [243,251]. Butorphanol may in fact result in the highest incidence of GER among opioids, but this is difficult to determine as it has not been studied as a sole agent. One study reported the incidence of GER in dogs receiving butorphanol with either dexmedetomidine or acepromazine to be 53.3% and 66.7%, respectively [256]. Maropitant has not been shown to be effective in reducing GER associated with opioids in dogs [243]. Esomeprazole (1 mg/kg IV) with cisapride (1 mg/kg IV) administered 12–18 h and 1–1.5 h before anesthetic induction can reduce the incidence of reflux events when compared to placebo (11% versus 38%, respectively) in isoflurane-anesthetized dogs administered SC hydromorphone for premedication and a fentanyl constant rate infusion (CRI) [257]. Metoclopramide administered at a high dose (bolus loading dose of 1.0 mg/kg IV, followed by CRI at 1.0 mg/kg/h) was associated with a 54% reduction in relative risk of developing GER in isoflurane-anesthetized dogs administered morphine as premedication [258]. Lower doses (0.4 mg/kg IV loading dose followed by 0.3 mg/kg/h) did not significantly affect the incidence of opioid-induced GER in a similar population [258].

Box 23.3 Strategies to reduce the incidence of perioperative opioid-induced vomiting.

- Acepromazine 0.05 mg/kg IM administered 15 min prior to opioid administration [234]
- Electroacupuncture at pericardium-6 applied 20 min prior to opioid administration [244]
- Electroacupuncture at pericardium-6, stomach-36, gallbladder-34, bladder-20, and bladder-21 applied 20 min prior to opioid administration [244]
- Acupuncture at pericardium-6 applied 30 min prior to opioid administration [246]
- Maropitant 1 mg/kg SC administered 15–30 min prior opioid administration [247]
- Maropitant 2–4 mg/kg PO administered 2 h prior to opioid administration [248]
- Maropitant 8 mg total dose PO administered 2–2.5 h prior to opioid administration in cats [249]

Nervous system

In general, opioids have minimal adverse effects on cerebral blood flow (CBF), intracranial pressure (ICP), and cerebral metabolic oxygen consumption in humans, dogs, and cats [259–263]. Average CBF, oxygen extraction, and oxygen consumption were not significantly affected following morphine administration in cats [259]. However, regional changes may exist in areas with dense populations of opioid receptors [259]. Decreased CBF and oxygen extraction were noted in the hypothalamus, and decreased oxygen extraction and consumption were noted in the thalamic region following IV morphine administration in cats [259].

Indices of cerebral perfusion were significantly decreased at 30 min following morphine administration when compared to baseline in the right frontal cortex, whereas the left parietal cortex and subcortical region showed significantly increased perfusion indices at 30 min post-morphine. No significant differences were noted for the other regions or at other time points [264]. Several studies have reported a decrease in CBF by up to 70% following systemic opioid administration in dogs [264–267]. Administration of morphine (1 mg/kg IV) also reduces spinal cord blood flow (SCBF) by similar amounts. Cerebral changes may be a result of decreases in metabolic oxygen demand and consumption as well as cerebral metabolic rate for glucose [265,266]. Morphine injected directly into the subarachnoid space was reported to have no effect on CBF and SCBF in dogs, which may indicate that the effects of opioids on cerebral hemodynamics are a result of their interaction with opioid receptors at supraspinal sites [265].

In cats, both decreased CBF [268] and no change in CBF [259] have been reported following opioid administration. Contrary to these findings, a study in cats found that CBF was significantly increased for approximately 20 min following sufentanil at doses of 10–200 μg/kg. Following this period, CBF gradually decreased below baseline levels at 60 min post-administration [269]. Increases in CBF appear to be a result of decreases in cerebrovascular resistance [269] and, based on these findings, sufentanil should be used with some degree of caution in patients with acute increases in ICP. However, an alternative may be remifentanil as it has been reported to be an effective and safe analgesic in human patients with traumatic brain injury [261].

While there is conflicting evidence regarding the effects of opioids on ICP, most animal studies suggest that their impact is minimal [266,269]. Remifentanil administered at 0.05 to 1.0 μg/kg followed by a CRI at 0.03–0.26 μg/kg/min decreased ICP with minimal effects on cerebral perfusion pressure (CPP) in human subjects [270]. Remifentanil and alfentanil both reduced ICP during low- (0.5 and 1.6 μg/kg/min, respectively) and high-dose (1 and 3.2 μg/kg/min, respectively) infusions in dogs anesthetized with 1.0% end-tidal isoflurane and 50% nitrous oxide in oxygen [267]. However, increases in ICP post-opioid infusion did occur during the recovery period. Sufentanil administration was reported to have little effect on ICP in adequately ventilated normal dogs and in dogs with elevated baseline ICP [271]. The use of fentanyl, sufentanil, and morphine at sedative doses in human subjects was well tolerated and did not result in changes in ICP. However, in another study, both fentanyl and sufentanil increased ICP in human head trauma patients [272].

Morphine may negatively impact recovery of neurologic function following acute spinal cord injury (SCI) (Fig. 23.4). The mechanisms mediating these effects can be classified as neuronal- or glial-mediated. Morphine's agonist effects at the κ-opioid receptor inhibit locomotor function by inducing central sensitization, enhancing excitatory amino acid levels and augmenting *N*-methyl-D-aspartate (NMDA) receptor-mediated neurotoxicity through reduced glutamate reuptake, and negatively impacting spinal plasticity [273]. Opioids have also been reported to enhance immune cell trafficking (e.g., increased glial cell expression of Toll-like receptors) and chemokine/cytokine activity, which can further increase pain and the development of neuronal apoptosis [273]. Several studies have evaluated the effects of morphine following SCI in rats [273–275]. Repeated morphine administration in rats significantly decreased the expression of neurons and glia following SCI when compared to vehicle controls [273,275]. The administration of morphine to rats also increased the size of the SCI lesion, delayed recovery of locomotor function post-SCI, and contributed to the development of opioid-induced hyperalgesia with subjects displaying increased reactivity to innocuous mechanical stimulation [273–275]. A one-time administration of morphine within the acute phase following SCI (< 24 h) also contributed to the development of neuropathic pain at three weeks post-injury [274]. To the authors' knowledge, only one study has evaluated the effects of fentanyl administration in dogs undergoing thoracolumbar spinal surgery for intervertebral disk herniation [276]. In this study, fentanyl had little impact on the recovery characteristics in dogs [276]; however, this could be attributed to the lack of κ-opioid receptor activity associated with fentanyl. Therefore, fentanyl could be a superior alternative to morphine in cases with SCI.

Renal system

Opioid analgesics have a dose-dependent effect on postoperative urinary retention [277,278], and can lead to increased bladder filling volume, increased micturition cycle duration, or a complete loss of the voiding phase via reduced coordination between external urethral sphincter activity and detrusor contractions [279]. μ-Opioid receptor agonists are responsible for decreasing the force of detrusor contractions and the sensation of fullness via decreasing afferent inputs from the urinary bladder to the spinal cord [280]. Naloxone or methylnaltrexone have both been shown to reverse these effects [281]. Opioids can also decrease electrolyte excretion and promote antidiuresis via μ-opioid receptor activation. In contrast to the μ-opioid receptor effects, κ-opioid receptor activation produces diuresis via suppressed release of arginine vasopressin (antidiuretic hormone) from the hypothalamus [282].

Epidural administration of opioid analgesics has been associated with the development of urinary retention in dogs [283–286] and cats [287,288]. Debate persists as to whether it occurs at a high enough incidence to determine its clinical relevance in these species [286,289], but it has been reported to be as high as 18% in dogs receiving epidural opioids during total hip replacement surgery [288,290]. Currently, data regarding the incidence of postoperative urinary retention after systemic opioid administration in other companion animal species are lacking [291]. When administered epidurally, methadone may have an opposite effect on the detrusor muscle by increasing its tone in dogs when compared to morphine [292]. Buprenorphine has been considered for epidural administration in veterinary species [113,293], as it may result

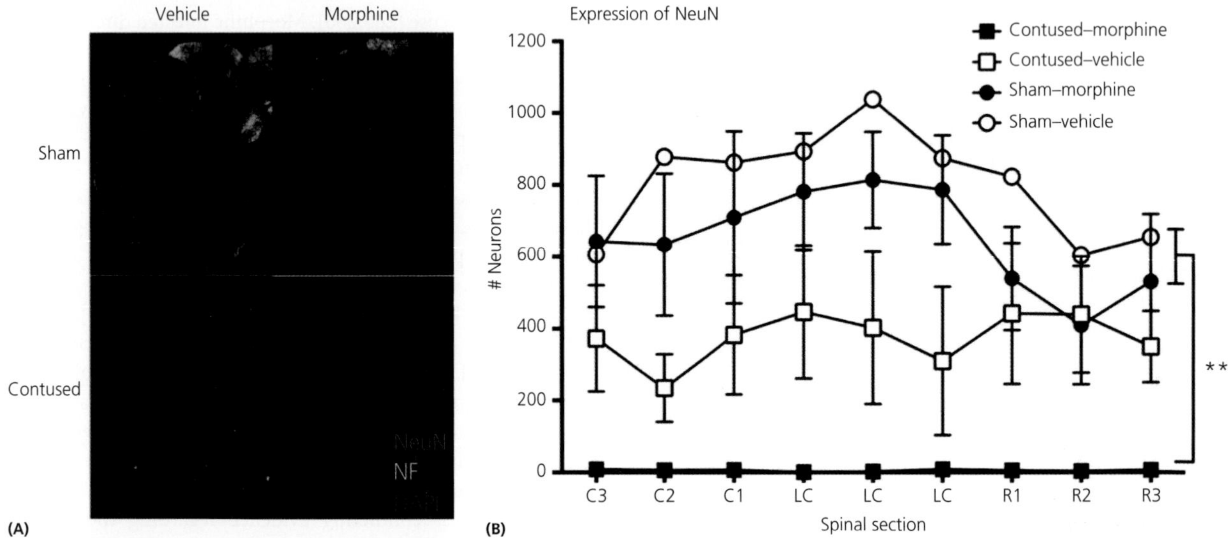

Figure 23.4 **A.** Representative images (4×) are shown depicting neuronal (NeuN and NF) expression in one-half of a spinal section, at the center of the lesion, for each treatment group of rats. Sham subjects are shown in the upper images; contused subjects in the lower images; panels on the left were treated with vehicle for seven days; panels on the right were treated with seven days of intravenous morphine. The contusion injury significantly decreased NeuN and NF expression at the center of the lesion, but when morphine was administered to the subjects with spinal cord injury (SCI) for seven days, there were virtually no neurons remaining at the injury site. **B.** There was a significant effect of SCI on NeuN expression at the center and rostral to the injury site, with less NeuN expression in the contused subjects. Morphine-treated subjects with SCI had significantly less NeuN expression, at the center and rostral to the injury site, than both sham control groups. $n = 3$; $^{**}p < 0.05$. Source: Hook *et al.* [275], with permission from Mary Ann Liebert, Inc.

in a lower incidence of urinary retention when compared to morphine [294]. However, data in humans suggest that urinary retention can occur with both full and partial μ-opioid receptor agonists [295–297]. Lastly, administration of opioids at the lumbosacral level is associated with a higher incidence of urinary retention compared to opioids administered at the thoracic level [280].

Antitussive effects

Butorphanol, methadone, hydrocodone, codeine, and morphine are effective antitussive agents against pathologically and experimentally induced cough in the dog [298,299]. The duration of antitussive effects associated with morphine and butorphanol are longer than that of codeine, lasting approximately 4 h when administered as compounded oral formulations [299]. Tramadol also has antitussive properties in cats [300]. Naloxone inhibits the antitussive effects of morphine, butorphanol, and codeine but not dextromethorphan [299]. The antitussive effects of opioids are mediated predominantly by μ- and κ-opioid receptors [301]. More recent evidence also suggests a potential role of δ-opioid receptor antagonism in the antitussive effects of this class of drugs [302].

Thermoregulatory effects

Opioid-induced hyperthermia has been reported in cats and can occur following the administration of hydromorphone, buprenorphine, butorphanol, meperidine, morphine, and transdermal fentanyl patches [303–307]. Opioid-induced hyperthermia (> 39.4 °C or 103 °F) is often self-limiting (e.g., < 4 h) [305] with body temperatures in the range of 40–41.1 °C (104–106 °F) [307]. However, temperatures exceeding 42.2 °C (108 °F) have been reported [303] and, in these situations, treatment with IV naloxone may be required. High-concentration buprenorphine administered at 0.24 mg/kg SC may predispose cats to greater risk of hyperthermia compared to morphine administered at 0.1 mg/kg SC [307]. Studies in rats suggest that opioids alter thermoregulation by raising the temperature set point that is controlled by the hypothalamus [308]. Horses may also exhibit transient mild increases in body temperature following administration of high-dose hydromorphone (0.08 mg/kg), but not after 0.02 and 0.04 mg/kg [79], and after transdermal fentanyl application [309]. However, clinically relevant changes in body temperature with opioid administration in horses do not routinely occur [310–312].

In contrast to the effects of opioids on feline thermoregulation, canine subjects may experience hypothermia following opioid administration [313–315]. It has been postulated that the mechanism associated with hypothermia following opioid administration in dogs is due to lowering of the thermoregulatory set point [315]. Other species have been investigated, and the effects of opioids on body temperature appear to be dependent on dose, route, and the opioid administered [316].

Ophthalmic effects

The administration of IV morphine can cause sustained miosis in dogs; however, topical ocular administration does not appear to produce similar effects. Morphine has excitatory effects on pupilloconstrictor neurons in the visceral nuclei of the oculomotor nuclear complex in subcortical regions causing pupillary constriction [317]. More recent findings in humans administered fentanyl suggest that opioids also may induce miosis by blocking the inhibitory input into the pupilloconstrictor nucleus, resulting in reduced pupillary reflex dilation [318]. In cats, mice, and rats, morphine results in mydriasis via inhibition of the preganglionic parasympathetic nucleus (central component) and disruption of the release of acetylcholine from parasympathetic fibers of the ciliary nerves of the iris (peripheral component) [319].

Immune system effects and effects on cancer metastasis

Opioids exhibit a broad effect on the body's immune system and in general inhibit cell-mediated and humoral immunity as well as interact with inflammatory cytokines including interleukin (IL)-1, IL-4, IL-6, and tumor necrosis factor [320–323]. Stimulation of μ-opioid receptors by morphine and fentanyl decreases the expression of Toll-like receptors on macrophages and suppresses natural killer (NK) cell function, respectively [324–326]. Morphine also may exhibit effects on tumor cells, modulating cell cycle, apoptosis, and angiogenesis (Fig. 23.5). Immune-mediated responses and the

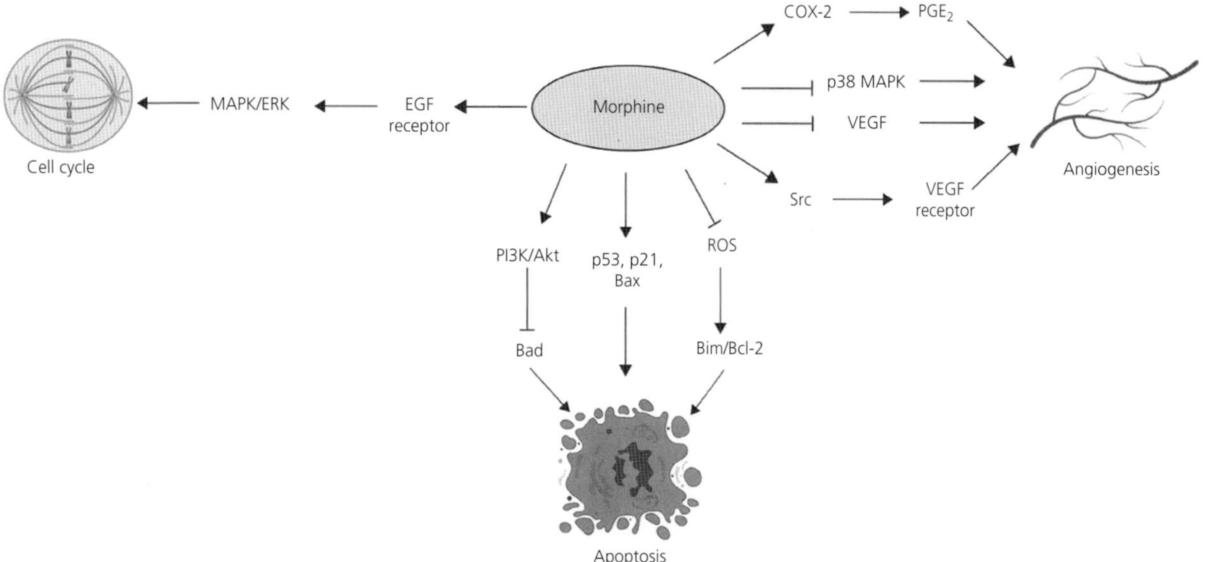

Figure 23.5 Mechanism of action of morphine on the tumor cell, modulating cell cycle, apoptosis, and angiogenesis. Source: Szczepaniak *et al.* [327], Springer Nature, CCBY 4.0, public domain.

effects of opioids on cancer cells are variable depending on the opioid and patient-related factors. This variation, along with the limited clinical trials in companion animals and contradictory conclusions indicating both positive and negative effects on cancer development and metastasis, makes it difficult to definitively determine clinical implications.

Effects on inhalant anesthetic minimum alveolar concentration

Dogs

The impact of opioids on inhalant anesthetic minimum alveolar concentration (MAC) requirements depends on the type and dose of opioid and the species. In general, opioid agonists reduce MAC via an indirect effect on neurons associated with modulation within the dorsal horn of the spinal cord in response to a noxious stimulus [328]. A thorough review on opioid MAC-sparing effects in dogs is available elsewhere [329] (Table 23.5). A CRI of morphine at 0.198 mg/kg/h can reduce end-tidal isoflurane concentrations by 48% with minimal hemodynamic effects (e.g., decreased HR) [330]. Extraordinarily high bolus doses of morphine (7 and 27 mg/kg) can reduce the MAC of enflurane by up to 67% [331]. More clinically relevant doses of morphine (0.5 and 2 mg/kg) result in MAC reduction of 17 and 34%, respectively. Oxymorphone, methadone, hydromorphone, and fentanyl all result in similar dose-dependent MAC-reducing effects in dogs [332,333]. Fentanyl and remifentanil CRIs of 0.2 μg/kg/min or greater can achieve MAC reductions

Table 23.5 Bolus doses, infusion rates, plasma concentration, and MAC effects in studies using pure μ-opioid agonists in dogs.

Drug	IV bolus dose (mg/kg)	Infusion rate (μg/kg/min)	Plasma concentration (ng/mL)	MAC effect (%)	Reference
Morphine	0.5	N/A	ND	↓ 17% (E)	[331]
	2	N/A		↓ 32%	
	7	N/A		↓ 63%	
	27	N/A		↓ 67%	
Morphine	2	N/A	295	↓ 50% (I)	[340]
Morphine	1	N/A	ND	↓ 34% (I)	[341]
Morphine	None	3.3	ND	↓ 48% (I)	[330]
Morphine	0.5	3.3	ND	↓ 25% (S)	[342]
Oxymorphone	0.05	N/A	ND	↓ 43% (I)	[332]
Hydromorphone	0.1	N/A	ND	↓ 48% (I)	[332]
Methadone	0.5	N/A	ND	↓ 35% (I)	[333]
	1			↓ 48%	
Methadone	0.5	N/A	ND	↓ 30% (I)	[343]
Meperidine	2.75	N/A	880[a]	↓ 48% (H)	[344]
	5.5		930	↓ 68%	
	11		1180	↓ 73%	
Fentanyl	0.015	0.05	3.1	↓ 33% (E)	[334]
	0.015	0.1	6.5	↓ 53%	
	0.03	0.2	11, 8.2[b]	↓ 57%, ↓ 56%	
	0.09	0.8	29	↓ 64%	
	0.27	3.2	99	↓ 66%	
Fentanyl	0.015	0.05	1	↓ 28% (E)	[345]
	0.045	0.2	3	↓ 44%	
Fentanyl	0.015	0.05	1	↓ 13% (E)	[346]
	0.045	0.2	4	↓ 40%	
Fentanyl	0.005	0.15	ND	↓ 35% (I)	[347]
Fentanyl	0.01	0.3	ND	↓ 53% (I)	[348]
Fentanyl (MAC_{NM})	0.015	0.1	3.25	↓ 39% (S)	[349]
Fentanyl (MAC_{NM})	0.0075	0.05	2.19	↓ 22% (S)	[350]
	0.015	0.1	5.13	↓ 35%	
	0.03	0.2	11.94	↓ 41%	
Fentanyl	0.005	0.15	ND	↓ 50% (I)	[351]
Fentanyl	33	0.2	6.2	↓ 42% (I)	[352]
	102	0.8	29.5	↓ 77%	
Remifentanil	None	0.055–5.5	10–15	Plateau at ↓ 63% (E)	[353]
Remifentanil	None	0.15	ND	↓ 43% (I)	[335]
		0.3		↓ 59%	
		0.6		↓ 66%	
		0.9		↓ 71%	
Alfentanil	0.0146	0.625	19	↓ 24% (E)	[354]
	0.0146	1.6	44	↓ 53%	
	0.072	8	223	↓ 69%	
	0.288	32	960	↓ 73%	
	0.720	80	2613	↓ 70%	
Sufentanil	0.0015	0.005	0.51	↓ 43% (E)	[355]
	0.003	0.015	0.92	↓ 57%	
	0.009	0.045	2.28	↓ 63%	
	0.120	0.405	17.43	↓ 67%	
	0.243	1.215	48.07	↓ 70%	

ND, not determined; N/A, not applicable; E, enflurane; S, sevoflurane; H, halothane; I, isoflurane.

[a] Blood for plasma concentrations not drawn at exact time of MAC determination. MAC reduction percentage and associated plasma concentrations derived by the authors from figures provided in the original manuscript.

[b] Two groups received this treatment.

Source: Reed and Doherty [329], with permission.

> 50% [334,335]. A one-time bolus of buprenorphine can reduce MAC by 25–35% and, due to its long duration of action, MAC reductions of 16% have been reported at 6 h following administration [336]. Butorphanol's effects on MAC are minimal (e.g., 8–15% reduction) at clinically relevant doses as are its effects on cardiopulmonary parameters [331,337]. Epidural morphine administration at 0.1 mg/kg reduced MAC of halothane from 1.04% to 0.60% following a supramaximal electrical stimulus applied to a pelvic limb [338]. Tramadol administered as an IV bolus of 1.5 mg/kg followed by a CRI of 1.3 mg/kg/h, or as an IV bolus of 3 mg/kg followed by 2.6 mg/kg/h resulted in MAC reductions of 26% and 36%, respectively [339].

Cats

Opioids produce less of a MAC-sparing effect in cats compared to dogs. Intravenous morphine at 1 mg/kg, butorphanol at 0.08 mg/kg and 0.8 mg/kg, and buprenorphine at 0.05 mg/kg produced reductions in isoflurane MAC of 28%, 19%, and 14%, respectively [356]. Morphine at 0.1 mg/kg and buprenorphine at 0.005 mg/kg did not produce clinically relevant reductions in MAC in cats [356]. Hydromorphone at 0.1 mg/kg IV produced an approximate 30% reduction in the MAC of sevoflurane [357]. Methadone at 0.3 mg/kg IV had a sevoflurane sparing effect of 25%, with sevoflurane concentrations returning to baseline concentrations at 156 min following administration [358]. Butorphanol at low (0.25 mg/kg IV bolus followed by 85 μg/kg/min for 20 min, then 43 μg/kg/min for 40 min, then 19 μg/kg/min), medium (double the low dose), and high doses (quadruple the low dose) dose-dependently reduced the MAC of isoflurane by 23%, 37%, and 68%, respectively [359]. Butorphanol administered IM at 0.2 mg/kg to cats resulted in a 15% reduction in isoflurane MAC [360]. Application of a fentanyl patch applied 24 h prior to testing and dosed at 25 and 50 μg/h produced reductions in isoflurane requirements of approximately 20% [361]. Remifentanil infusions between 0.25 and 1 μg/kg/min produced a reduction in isoflurane MAC between 23% and 29% and did not differ significantly between dosages [362]. Epidurally administered morphine at 0.1 mg/kg and buprenorphine at 0.012 mg/kg had minimal effect on the MAC of isoflurane in cats [363]. Tramadol administered PO at 8.6 to 11.6 mg/kg produced a significant 40% reduction in sevoflurane MAC [357]. The opioid receptor antagonist naltrexone had no effect on the MAC of isoflurane in cats [364].

Horses

The effects of opioids on MAC in horses are variable and can result in decreases or increases in inhalant requirements. For example, IV morphine at 0.25 mg/kg and 2.0 mg/kg produced alterations in MAC ranging from −20.2% to +28.3% and −18.9% to +56.2%, respectively [365]. Fentanyl CRI doses of approximately 0.36 and 3.5 μg/kg/h (equivalent to plasma concentrations of 0.72 and 8.43 ng/mL) had no significant effect on MAC in horses, but higher doses of 6–7 μg/kg/h (13.3 ng/mL) did reduce MAC by approximately 18% [366]. Contrary to these findings, other studies evaluating fentanyl concentrations of 16 ng/mL did not produce inhalant-sparing effects in horses [367]. Epidurally administered morphine at 0.1 mg/kg reduced MAC by approximately 15% [368]. Epidural butorphanol at 0.05 mg/kg had no MAC-sparing effects. Intravenous butorphanol at similar doses (0.022–0.05 mg/kg) also had no significant effect on the MAC of halothane [369]. Alfentanil CRIs at varying doses did not provide MAC-sparing effects in horses [370].

Traditional routes of administration

The route of opioid administration often influences the onset, magnitude, and duration of analgesia and therefore should be considered by the clinician prior to use [99,371,372]. Intravenous administration has been considered advantageous over other traditional routes (IM or SC) because of its rapid onset and rapid pain relief. In patients without an intravenous cannula, the SC route is often associated with less pain on injection than the IM or IV routes; however, it may not provide a similar magnitude of analgesia. For example, SC administration of hydromorphone or the standard concentration of buprenorphine (0.3 mg/mL) in cats provided significantly less analgesia when compared with the IM or IV routes [98,137]. Similarly, in dogs, buprenorphine (0.3 mg/mL) administered SC failed to provide clinical analgesia due to erratic drug absorption when compared to equivalent doses administered via IV and IM routes [372]. Therefore, it is generally recommended that most opioids be administered IV or IM, unless otherwise labeled specifically for SC administration.

Full opioid agonists

Morphine

Morphine, a natural alkaloid derived from the opium poppy *Papaver somniferum*, has a unique and rich history of more than 200 years and was first isolated in its pure state by Friedrich Wilhelm Adam Sertürner, a German pharmacist, who published his original report in 1805 and again in 1806 [373]. In the US, it is classified as a Schedule II narcotic under the Controlled Substances Act. Morphine has been studied and administered to dogs and cats since the late 1800s [374] and early 1900s [375–378] and continues to be administered today as a perioperative analgesic agent for moderate to severe pain. Morphine's versatility has contributed to its attractiveness in veterinary medicine as it can be administered parenterally [379], epidurally [113], intra-articularly [380], topically (e.g., cornea) [381], orally [382,383], as a CRI [187,384], or via nebulization [385]. However, there is limited evidence supporting the clinical utility of the topical and oral administration routes in most species.

Morphine, a phenanthrene (Table 23.6), is a weak base (pK_a 7.9) that is highly hydrophilic and poorly soluble in lipids at physiological pH (7.4). It is considered a full agonist at the μ-opioid receptor and, in humans and other species, maintains moderate binding affinity (K_i) for the μ-opioid receptor (approximately 1.16 nM) (Table 23.7) [386,387]. Morphine binds 3.4 times and 10 times more avidly to the μ-opioid receptor compared to the κ- and δ-opioid receptors, respectively [386,388–390]. Morphine's clinical effects are predominately due to its binding and activation at the μ-opioid receptor [391], with a higher binding affinity for the pharmacologically defined μ_1 subtype (analgesia) compared to the μ_2 subtype (respiratory depression, gastrointestinal side effects) [391,392]; though as discussed previously, molecular evidence for the existence of these different subtypes is lacking. Morphine also has the ability to bind to the nociceptin opioid peptide (N/OFQ or NOP), a G-protein-coupled receptor system that, on a cellular level, produces similar actions to classical opioid receptors [393].

Table 23.6 Opioid chemical structures.

Chemical class	Basic chemical structure	Examples
Phenanthrenes		Buprenorphine Codeine Hydrocodone Hydromorphone Morphine Nalbuphine Oxycodone
Morphinans		Butorphanol
Phenylpiperidines and piperidines	4-Phenylpiperidine Piperidine	Alfentanil Diphenoxylate Fentanyl Loperamide Meperidine Remifentanil Sufentanil
Phenylheptylamines		Methadone

Source: Chemical structures from the National Center for Biotechnology Information. PubChem Compound Summary for CID 995, Phenanthrene. https://pubchem.ncbi.nlm.nih.gov/compound/Phenanthrene; PubChem Compound Summary for CID 6857497, (–)-Morphinan. https://pubchem.ncbi.nlm.nih.gov/compound/6857497; PubChem Compound Summary for CID 69873, 4-Phenylpiperidine. https://pubchem.ncbi.nlm.nih.gov/compound/4-Phenylpiperidine; PubChem Compound Summary for CID 8082, Piperidine. https://pubchem.ncbi.nlm.nih.gov/compound/Piperidine; PubChem Compound Summary for CID 91495676, Diphenylheptylamine. https://pubchem.ncbi.nlm.nih.gov/compound/Diphenylheptylamine. (accessed September 2023).

Dogs

Following administration of morphine at 0.5 mg/kg IV, mean ± standard error values for half-life, apparent volume of distribution, and clearance were 1.16 ± 0.15 h, 4.55 ± 0.17 L/kg, and 62.46 ± 10.44 mL/min/kg, respectively [394]. Canine liver microsomal enzymes catalyze glucuronidation of morphine-3- and morphine-6-*O*-glucuronide at 10 times the rate of that observed in humans [395]; however, the active metabolite, morphine-6-glucuronide, cannot be detected in significant concentrations in canine plasma following IV or oral administration [394]. Based on plasma concentrations associated with analgesia in humans (> 25 ng/mL) and pharmacodynamic modeling using a von Frey device, it has been suggested that morphine should be administered IV every 2–4 h at 0.5–1.0 mg/kg in dogs (Table 23.8) [313,394,396]. Intramuscular administration of morphine at 1 mg/kg should be dosed at a frequency similar to IV administration [187] based on previous pharmacokinetic data in dogs where median plasma morphine concentrations remained > 20 ng/mL from 5–120 min following IM administration [64]. Bioavailability for IM morphine (119%; range 58–160%) is comparable to that of IV morphine (100%) in dogs; however, variability in absorption is higher with the IM route.

Table 23.7 Binding affinity (K_i) at the μ-opioid receptor for various opioids in humans.

Weak binders		Moderate binders		Strong binders	
Drug	K_i (nM)	Drug	K_i (nM)	Drug	K_i (nM)
Tramadol	12,486	Hydrocodone	41.58	Butorphanol	0.7622
Codeine	734.2	Oxycodone	25.87	Levorphanol	0.4194
Meperidine	450.1	Diphenoxylate	12.37	Oxymorphone	0.4055
Propoxyphene	120.2	Alfentanil	7.391	Hydromorphone	0.3654
Pentazocine	117.8	Methadone	3.378	Buprenorphine	0.2157
		Nalbuphine	2.118	Sufentanil	0.1380
		Fentanyl	1.346		
		Morphine	1.168		

Strong binders, $K_i < 1$ nM; moderate binders, $1 < K_i < 100$ nM; weak binders, $K_i > 100$ nM.
Source: Modified from Kilpatrick and Smith [386]; Volpe *et al*. [387].

Morphine infusion rates greater than 0.15 mg/kg/h are required to maintain plasma concentrations greater than 30 ng/mL [397]. At higher doses (0.34 mg/kg/h), steady-state plasma concentrations ranged from 93 to 180 ng/mL [313]. Terminal half-life was 38 ± 5 and 27 ± 14 min for high-dose (0.34 mg/kg/h) and low-dose (0.17 mg/kg/h) CRIs, respectively [313]. Sedation and analgesia were observed with both infusion rates; however, the magnitude of both appears to be dose-dependent [313]. Interestingly, consistent analgesia during the infusion rates was only reported at plasma concentrations greater than 100 ng/mL and not at concentrations less than 50 ng/mL [313]. The authors suggest this apparent lack of analgesia may be related to their study population (healthy dogs in an experimental setting) and the model of nociception used. Therefore, clinicians should always use validated pain assessment tools to ensure that analgesia is adequate.

Oral morphine, in any formulation, is not recommended as a sole analgesic due to its poor and highly variable absorption characteristics in dogs. Oral bioavailability following extended-release tablets at 1.6 ± 0.1 mg/kg is extremely low at 5% [394]. In a pharmacokinetic study comparing extended-release and conventional (immediate-release) morphine formulations administered at 15 mg PO, both produced similarly low bioavailabilities (15–17%) [382]. In addition, there was no prolonged effect on serum morphine concentrations with extended-release compared to immediate-release morphine [382]. Rectal morphine suppository administered at 1, 2, or 5 mg/kg produced similar bioavailability (16–24%) when compared to that of orally administered morphine [64].

Table 23.8 Authors' recommendations pertaining to dose, route, and frequency of administration for commonly used opioids in dogs, cats, and horses. In all clinical situations, dose and dosing intervals should be guided by use of validated pain assessment tools.

Drug	Dog	Cat	Horse
Morphine	0.3–1.0 mg/kg IM, IV q2–4 h 0.1–0.2 mg/kg/h IV CRI	0.2–0.4 mg/kg IM, IV q4–6 h 0.05–0.1 mg/kg/h IV CRI	0.05–0.3 mg/kg IM, IV q8 h 0.03 mg/kg/h IV CRI
Hydromorphone	0.05–0.2 mg/kg IM, IV q2–4 h 0.02–0.04 mg/kg/h IV CRI	0.025–0.1 mg/kg IM, IV q2–4 h 0.02–0.03 mg/kg/h IV CRI	0.01–0.04 mg/kg IM, IV q7–12 h
Oxymorphone	0.05–0.2 mg/kg IM, IV q4 h	0.025–0.1 mg/kg IM, IV q4–6 h	0.01–0.02 mg/kg IM, IV
Methadone	0.5–1 mg/kg IM, IV q3–4 h	0.3–0.5 mg/kg IM, IV q4 h	0.05–0.1 mg/kg IM, IV 0.05 mg/kg h IV CRI
Meperidine (pethidine)	3–5 mg/kg IM q1–2 h	3–5 mg/kg IM q1–2 h	1–2 mg/kg IM
Fentanyl (injectable)	2–10 µg/kg IV followed by 3–20 µg/kg/h IV CRI	1–10 µg/kg IV followed by 2–15 µg/kg/h IV CRI	2–4 µg/kg IM, IV q3–4 h 0.3–0.5 µg/kg/h IV CRI
Fentanyl (transdermal)	3–5 µg/kg applied as a patch q3 days	3–5 µg/kg applied as a patch or 1 x 25 µg/h patch per cat q5 days	3 x 100 µg/h patches per adult horse q36–48 h
Buprenorphine	0.01–0.02 mg/kg IV, IM, SC q6–8 h[a]	0.01–0.02 mg/kg IV, IM, SC, OTM q4–8 h[a] 0.24 mg/kg SC q24 h[b] 8–20 mg transdermal topical[c]	0.005–0.01 mg/kg IV, IM, SC[a]
Butorphanol	0.4 mg/kg IV, IM, SC q2–4 h 0.2 mg/kg IV followed by 0.2 mg/kg/h IV CRI	0.2–0.4 mg/kg IV, IM, SC q1–4 h	0.01–0.1 mg/kg IV, IM, SC q2–6 h 0.024 mg/kg/h IV CRI
Nalbuphine	0.25–1 mg/kg IV, IM, SC q2–4 h	0.1–0.25 mg/kg IV, IM, SC q2–4 h	
Tramadol	2–4 mg/kg IM, IV q4–8 h 4–10 mg/kg PO q4–6 h	2–4 mg/kg PO 6–12 h	
Tapentadol	5–10 mg/kg IV q8–12 h 10–30 mg/kg PO q12 h	5 mg/kg IV, IM, SC q4–8 h 5–10 mg/kg PO q8–12 h	

[a] 0.3 mg/mL injectable (approved for use in dogs and cats in some countries; approved for use in humans in the US)
[b] Simbadol®
[c] Zorbium®
IV, intravenous; IM, intramuscular; SC, subcutaneous; CRI, constant rate infusion; OTM, oral transmucosal; PO, oral.

In dogs, morphine is commonly administered during the perioperative period and can provide analgesia for thoracotomy [398], tumor removal [399], orthopedic [400], mastectomy [401], neutering [402], or laparotomy [187] procedures. Morphine analgesia has been reported in dogs with a variety of routes of administration (e.g., parenteral, epidural, intrathecal, intra-articular), as well as nontraditional techniques such as nebulization, topical application, and injection into acupoints (pharmacopuncture) [15,144,381,403–405]. However, the analgesic efficacy of morphine administered by nebulization or topical ocular application, as well as the extradural route via gel-foam remains questionable [381,406,407]. The effective dose (ED_{50}) of IV morphine in dogs is 0.71 mg/kg with an onset and duration of analgesia of 10 min and 2–4 h, respectively [396,397,408]. When administering morphine as a CRI in dogs, doses of 0.15 ± 0.02 mg/kg/h were required to maintain significant antinociception as assessed by von Frey thresholds [397]. Interestingly, it has been reported that the use of 0.5 mg/kg IV boluses may provide more consistent and effective analgesic plasma concentrations of morphine when compared to a CRI [397]. Epidurally or intrathecally administered morphine has provided long-lasting analgesia for up to 24 h following administration in dogs undergoing laparotomy, thoracotomy, and orthopedic procedures with minimal adverse effects.

Intravenous morphine provides moderate to marked dose-dependent sedation with an onset of 2–5 min, a peak effect at 15–30 min, and a duration of up to 2 h at higher doses (e.g., 1.0 mg/kg) [161,203]. The onset of action for sedation with IM morphine administration can take as long as 30 min [161]. Behavioral adverse effects are also dose-dependent and include dysphoria and vocalization following IV administration in dogs [203,235,313]. Dysphoria may occur less commonly in dogs administered morphine when compared to other opioids such as methadone [203,235].

Morphine reduces HR in dogs by 26% for up to 2 h following IV administration, with minimal negative changes in CI [203]. Dogs may experience a transient (< 10-min duration) elevation in mean arterial pressure 5 min following IV administration [203]. Morphine has very little effect on arterial pH, $PaCO_2$, and PaO_2 values [203]. Increases in minute ventilation via increased respiratory rate (e.g., panting) without effects on tidal volume are often observed following administration [203].

Morphine has been reported to cause systemic histamine release in dogs following IV administration [235]. Maximum plasma histamine concentrations reached 440 ng/mL and 589 ng/mL following 0.5 and 1.0 mg/kg of morphine, respectively [235]. Flushing of the skin is most notable at the higher dose within 1 min following administration. Cardiovascular parameters are minimally affected following these doses of morphine despite the release of histamine. In a previous study, hypotension was noted in one of five dogs at 2 and 5 min following 1.0 mg/kg morphine corresponding to histamine concentrations of 589 and 351 ng/mL, respectively [235]. Clinically used infusion doses result in insignificant cardiovascular effects associated with morphine-induced histamine release [235].

Following IM morphine administration, nausea and emesis have been reported in 30–80% and 50–75% of dogs, respectively [234,244,245,409]. The emetic effect of morphine generally occurs within 10 min following IM administration and time to cessation is approximately 1–3 min [234,244]. Salivation and defection are also commonly observed shortly after administration. Urinary retention, pruritis, myoclonus, and rarely priapism, have been noted following epidural or intrathecal morphine administration in dogs [284,285,410]. Priapism is self-resolving within 7–8 h following intrathecal morphine, but supportive interventions such as lubrication and massage are advised to minimize trauma to the penis. Urinary retention generally resolves within 24 h but has been reported to persist for 7 days following epidural morphine administration [283,286]. Manual expression of the urinary bladder is recommended if this happens. These side effects are more commonly observed with intrathecal administration and/or when using morphine with preservatives [284,286].

Cats

Morphine is effective in treating moderate to severe pain in cats and should be administered every 4–6 h at doses of 0.2–0.4 mg/kg [137,182,379,411]. Early studies using extremely high doses (> 5–10 mg/kg) resulted in neuroexcitatory behaviors consisting of excitement, motor agitation, and aggression (i.e., "feline mania" or "morphine mania"). At the time, these observations led to the erroneous conclusion that cats were poor subjects for future opioid investigations [184–186]. At clinically relevant doses (0.2 mg/kg), however, cats generally do not show signs of dysphoria, but rather euphoria (e.g., purring, kneading, rolling, and or affectionate behavior) or mild sedation, which can last up to 3 h following IM administration [182,412].

Similar to dogs, the half-life and apparent volume of distribution of morphine is 76.3 min and 2.6 L/kg, respectively, following a 0.2 mg/kg IV bolus in cats [68]. However, clearance is about half that of dogs at 24.1 mL/kg/min. Cats lack the enzyme UDP-glucuronosyltransferase 2B7 (UGT 2B7), which is responsible for the glucuronidation of morphine in humans [413]. This enzyme deficiency may contribute to the lack of metabolites produced following morphine biotransformation in cats [68]. To compensate for slow glucuronidation, morphine undergoes extensive sulfation in cats [115,413]. Like dogs, no detectable concentrations of morphine-3-glucuronide were noted following morphine administration in cats, and in one study, the metabolite morphine-6-glucuronide was detected in only 3 of 11 cats [68].

Horses

Morphine provides excellent analgesia in horses, but its use remains controversial due to the potential for gastrointestinal ileus, excitement, and increased locomotor activity [194,414,415]. The dramatic adverse effects published in earlier studies utilized morphine doses of 0.5–1.0 mg/kg and even up to 2.4 mg/kg [193,416]. For example, morphine sulfate at 0.5 mg/kg IV can produce muscle fasciculations, pawing, and pacing for 2–4 h post-administration [417,418]. In contrast, lower doses of morphine (0.05–0.1 mg/kg) may not induce any excitatory effects or only minimal, transient (< 5 min) pawing, head shaking, and circling [310,418]. Furthermore, in a clinical setting, preoperative doses of 0.1–0.2 mg/kg have not been shown to increase the incidence of postoperative gastrointestinal complications or produce excitement during the anesthetic recovery period [419–421]. The epidural route in particular (either lumbosacral or cervical) is associated with a very low risk of excitation when similar doses are administered [228,422,423].

Morphine administered at doses of 0.5 mg/kg and greater can result in reduced cecocolic motility that may be prolonged, lasting for up to 360 min [416,417,424]. A single lower dose of morphine at 0.05 mg/kg IV did not induce alterations in gut motility. Abdominal auscultation scores and the number of borborygmus events were reported to be decreased for up to 60 min following 0.05 and 0.1 mg/kg IM and 0.1 mg/kg IV [310]. Borborygmus frequency was also reduced at 120 min following the 0.1 mg/kg IV dose [310]. Mean weight of feces collected was not different for 48 h following administration of IM and IV doses of 0.05 and 0.1 mg/kg, and horses did not show evidence of colic [310]. Repeated morphine doses every 4 h of 0.1 mg/kg or higher can produce signs associated with colic in horses [417]. Despite the apparent dose-dependent effects on gastrointestinal motility reported when comparing low and high doses of morphine in horses, analgesia was not detected via thermal and electrical threshold testing [310,425]. Epidurally administered morphine at 0.1 mg/kg can provide long-lasting analgesia with minimal gastrointestinal or behavioral effects when compared to systemically administered morphine [105,229]; however, higher epidural doses may impact gastrointestinal motility [228].

A minimum of 0.1–0.2 mg/kg of IV morphine can provide analgesia in horses, with the higher dose producing a more consistent effect [423,426]. At these doses, antinociception can be provided from 120–240 min [423,426]. Horses produce both morphine-3-glucuronide and morphine-6-glucuronide following morphine administration, and these metabolites may contribute to sedation and thermal antinociceptive effects in this species [81,418]. Administration of these metabolites, rather than the parent compound, could prove beneficial during the perioperative period.

In one study, morphine administered as an IV bolus of 0.15 mg/kg follow by a CRI at 0.1 mg/kg/h provided analgesia in horses with carpal synovitis; however, increased HR, respiratory rate, and systolic blood pressure as well as decreased gut sounds were observed [427]. Another study using a similar dosing regimen did not significantly alter cardiopulmonary variables [428]. Infusion rates of 0.1–0.3 mg/kg/h can be used intraoperatively for pain management in horses undergoing general anesthesia and surgery with minimal negative consequences on recovery quality [429]. Similarly, two systematic reviews published in 2022 reported that morphine administration at clinically relevant doses has minimal effect on recovery in horses and in some instances can improve recovery quality [430,431]. Morphine (120 mg) administered intra-articularly also provides significant pain relief in horses with synovitis with few adverse effects [432]. Oral morphine has been recently studied in horses and is associated with fewer adverse behavioral effects. At doses of 0.2–0.8 mg/kg PO, it has a bioavailability of approximately 30% [433]. Additional studies are required to determine the analgesic benefit of orally administered morphine in this species. In donkeys, morphine at 0.1 and 0.5 mg/kg IV produced dose-dependent mechanical antinociceptive effects for 60 and 300 min, respectively, with minimal adverse effects [434].

Food and fiber animals

Opioids are not commonly utilized for pain management in farm animal species due to withdrawal times (i.e., the need to ensure no drugs are present in meat and milk) and the need for controlled substance record keeping [435]. Morphine provides dose-dependent thermal antinociception in cattle at doses as low as 0.15 mg/kg, increasing the thermal threshold by 10 °C. Increased locomotor activity is generally not observed in cattle at IV doses of 0.5 or 1.0 mg/kg [436]. Epidural morphine at 0.1 mg/kg can be a cost-effective technique to provide adequate analgesia in cows and pigs undergoing surgical procedures or experiencing acute pain [437–439].

Morphine administration has been recently evaluated in goats. When comparing morphine plasma concentrations to those associated with effective analgesia in humans (> 16 ng/mL) [440], morphine administered at 0.25 mg/kg IV to goats would be expected to provide a brief period of analgesia lasting approximately 30 min [95]. A higher dose of 0.4 mg/kg IV appears to provide little additional benefit. IM dosing at 0.25 and 0.4 mg/kg may provide analgesia for 1–3 and 3–4 h, respectively [95]. SC administration provided a similar duration of analgesia compared to IM doses of 0.25 mg/kg and 0.4 mg/kg, with durations of approximately 1–2 and 2–3 h, respectively [95].

In llamas, morphine had minimal cardiovascular effects and induced dose-dependent decreases in respiratory rate and increases in sedation and body temperature when administered at 0.05, 0.25, and 0.5 mg/kg IV [441]. Following administration of morphine at 0.5 mg/kg IM, bioavailability was 120% with a significantly longer mean terminal half-life (342 min) in llamas compared to both dogs (81 min) and cats (93 min) [441]. The metabolite morphine-6-glucuronide was infrequently detected and remained at concentrations < 40 ng/mL following 0.5 mg/kg IM and IV [441]. Morphine at 0.5 mg/kg IV may produce muscle tremors, hyperexcitability, and sedation lasting up to 1 h following administration in llamas [441]. Morphine can be dosed at 0.25 mg/kg IV every 4 h to produce analgesia in llamas [441].

Hydromorphone

Dogs and cats

Hydromorphone is a full μ-opioid receptor agonist that provides similar dose-dependent magnitude and duration of analgesia and sedation, with reduced histamine levels, compared to IV morphine [235,442,443]. It is 5–10 times more potent than morphine on a milligram basis with similar cardiopulmonary adverse effects. The duration of analgesia provided by IV hydromorphone at 0.1–0.2 mg/kg is at least 2 h with the potential to last up to 4 h in dogs and 4–8 h in cats [236,443]. Lower IV doses of 0.05 mg/kg hydromorphone provided a significantly shorter duration of analgesia (up to 80 min) in cats [442]. Following 0.1 mg/kg IM administration in cats, analgesia onset occurred in 15 min and duration of action was 345 min [183]. SC administration in cats resulted in a much slower onset to peak analgesic effect of (105 min) with a duration of action of 210 min [98]. The duration and magnitude of analgesia was less when hydromorphone was administered to cats 6 months of age compared to adult cats; therefore, it should be dosed more frequently in younger animals [237]. Liposomal encapsulated hydromorphone administered SC also provided long-lasting analgesia for up to 24 h in dogs undergoing limb amputation [444]. Repeated administration of hydromorphone within a 4-h period can result in excitation or prolonged anesthetic recovery [236]. Duration of sedation is up to 3 h following 0.2 mg/kg SC administration [213], but may be unreliable at lower doses in clinically healthy dogs [445]. When evaluating its analgesic efficacy as a CRI, 0.03 mg/kg/h can provide pain relief similar to fentanyl [446]. Hydromorphone has also been administered epidurally in cats, but its duration of analgesia is significantly shorter than that provided by epidural morphine (i.e., 5 h versus 24 h) [447].

Horses

In horses, hydromorphone administered at 0.02–0.08 mg/kg IV provides analgesia for up to 12 h [311]. Increases in respiratory rate, HR, and body temperature were also observed [311]. Hydromorphone 0.04 mg/kg IM was shown to have high bioavailability in horses (217%) and can provide similar duration and magnitude of analgesia when compared to IV administration [80]. Hydromorphone increased arterial pressure and decreased borborygmi without altering fecal output when administered at 0.025 and 0.05 mg/kg IV [448]. Reductions in borborygmi may persist for 90–120 min at these doses and routes [448]. Horses may experience excitement (e.g., pacing, vocalizing, rearing, and kicking) for 1–2 h following administration [80]. Hydromorphone administration was not shown to increase the incidence of postanesthetic signs of colic in horses [449]. Hydromorphone at 0.04 mg/kg IV may provide better analgesia in horses undergoing elective arthroscopy compared to butorphanol at 0.02 mg/kg IV [450].

Methadone

Dogs and cats

Methadone, a phenylheptylamine (Table 23.6), is a full μ-opioid receptor agonist that also has effects at monoamine and NMDA receptors. It is commonly used in the perioperative period in dogs and cats. It can be administered via a variety of routes; however, more variability in plasma concentrations was noted with the standard formulation when administered SC. Methadone produces more potent dose-dependent cardiovascular depressant effects on HR when compared to that of morphine (reductions of 32–46% with methadone versus 15–26% with morphine) [203]. Methadone may hinder the feasibility of gastroduodenoscopy when compared to butorphanol [203] and potentially should be avoided in non-painful patients undergoing these procedures. Vomiting is generally rare following methadone administration; however, it can still occur.

Methadone alone provides mild sedation in dogs, but they may occasionally whine [314]. When administered with acepromazine, it can provide dose-dependent sedation of greater magnitude than morphine–acepromazine or butorphanol–acepromazine [162,451]. Oral transmucosal methadone at 0.4 mg/kg in dogs can also provide sedative effects; however, sedation is less than that observed following IM administration of a similar dose [241].

Methadone possesses both opioid and monoamine effects (mediated by the levo- or R(−)-enantiomer) as well as NMDA antagonistic effects (mediated by the dextro- or *S*(+)-enantiomer) [452–454]. The latter could be beneficial in patients with chronic pain, hyperalgesia, and central sensitization [455]. In cats, methadone at 0.3 mg/kg IV and 0.6 mg/kg OTM produced antinociception for greater than 2 and 4 h, respectively [456]. IM methadone also provided a 4-h duration of antinociception [457]. Methadone can be administered as a CRI at 0.1 mg/kg/h in dogs and provided analgesia up to 2 h following its discontinuation [458]. Methadone also provides superior analgesia when compared to buprenorphine for dogs undergoing orthopedic and ovariohysterectomy procedures [149,459]. Similar findings were reported in cats undergoing neutering procedures [150]. Chloramphenicol and fluconazole act as enzyme inhibitors of CYP2B11 in dogs and can alter the pharmacokinetics of opioids [460]. The combination of methadone–fluconazole administered SC twice within a 6-h period was shown to provide safe and effective postoperative analgesia for up to 12–24 h following the second dose in dogs with minimal adverse effects [461]. In Greyhounds, the dose to maintain analgesic plasma concentrations of 40 ng/mL is 1.5–2 times higher than that observed in Beagle dogs [454]. Therefore, a dose of 1–1.5 mg/kg is recommended every 3–4 h in this breed [454].

Horses and ruminants

Methadone provides some sedation in horses, but less than that associated with butorphanol [462]. When administered as a sole agent to horses, dysphoria, euphoria, and spontaneous locomotor activity can be observed for up to 2 h post-administration [463]. This is particularly evident at a dose of 0.5 mg/kg [464]. When combined with detomidine, sedation and analgesia is enhanced, but there is a marked increase in ataxia [465]. The combination of methadone with detomidine may be a more suitable premedication to maintain cardiovascular stability (e.g., less depressant effects on blood pressure) than the combination of methadone and acepromazine [466]. Methadone also produces more pronounced antinociceptive effects when combined with detomidine than when combined with acepromazine [467]. Increases in blood pressure and respiratory rate and decreases in gut sounds are noted following methadone administration [427]. Methadone has little effect on arterial blood gas values in horses [463].

Methadone may be an effective analgesic addition when administered via parenteral or epidural routes to horses for standing procedures or for surgical procedures requiring general anesthesia [468,469]. Methadone was effective in providing analgesia for lipopolysaccharide-induced carpal synovitis when administered as a 0.25 mg/kg IV bolus followed by a CRI of 0.25 mg/kg/h [427]. Lower infusion rates (0.05 mg/kg/h) have also been used in combination with detomidine for standing procedures [470]. Inconsistent antinociceptive effects have been reported with doses of 0.2 mg/kg IV, with more reliable antinociception at 0.5 mg/kg [464]; however, negative behavioral side effects may be observed. Oral administration of the injectable and lipid nanocarrier formulations of methadone does not provide antinociception in horses [471]. Epidurally administered methadone (0.1 mg/kg) provides effective analgesia for up to 5 h with no appreciable side effects [468]. As with any analgesic intervention, horses should be monitored closely to ensure adequate pain relief when administering methadone.

Methadone at 0.3 mg/kg IV provides effective analgesia in small ruminant species and reduces autonomic responses associated with noxious stimuli [472]. Methadone can also be administered epidurally to sheep and cows for pain management [473,474]. Additional research pertaining to the use of methadone in ruminants would provide a better understanding of the drug's pharmacodynamic effects in these species.

Oxymorphone

Oxymorphone is approximately 10 times more potent than morphine and acts primarily at the μ-opioid receptor. Oxymorphone is metabolized mainly via conjugation, with small amounts excreted as intact drug or other metabolites in dogs. Its adverse effects are similar to those of other opioids (e.g., whining, panting, sedation, dysphoria, and bradycardia) and, though vomiting is rarely observed with IV administration, it can occur following SC administration [371]. Oxymorphone provides 90 min of antinociception following 0.2 mg/kg IM in dogs [475] and up to 5–6 h of clinical analgesia in dogs and cats following 0.05 mg/kg IV [476]. Like other full μ-opioid receptor agonists, oxymorphone provides more effective postoperative analgesia compared to butorphanol in dogs [477]. Oxymorphone did not demonstrate antinociceptive effects in cats when administered via the OTM route at 0.1 or 0.25 mg/kg due to its low bioavailability, which is approximately half that of OTM methadone (19% versus 44%) [238,478]. Pharmacokinetic data suggest a dose of 0.03 mg/kg followed by 0.02 mg/kg every 2 h would maintain therapeutic analgesic concentrations in cats. However, this will create high- but short-lived peak concentrations, which could predispose cats to transient adverse behavioral effects [479]. An alternative would be to administer a 0.005 mg/kg bolus followed by a CRI of 0.005 mg/kg/h [479]. Pharmacokinetic data in dogs recommend dosing at 0.1 mg/kg every 2–4 h or 0.006–0.012 mg/kg/h as a CRI [371]. Due to the associated costs, few reports exist regarding the use of oxymorphone in large animal species.

Fentanyl

Dogs and cats

Fentanyl is a highly protein-bound, lipophilic phenylpiperidine derivative (Table 23.6) with a rapid onset, short duration of action, and a potency 75–100 times greater than morphine. It is often administered as CRI due to its short duration of action which is attributed to its rapid redistribution from the central to the peripheral compartment following injection [61]. In humans, the context-sensitive half-time for fentanyl increases substantially following 3 h of administration which may contribute to cumulative effects [480]. This effect has not been reported in dogs following a 4-h infusion which makes fentanyl CRIs clinically useful for prolonged pain management in this species [61,351,481,482]. In dogs, fentanyl is rapidly absorbed following SC administration, and pharmacokinetics are comparable to the IV route of administration [483,484]. Significant pain occurs following subcutaneous injection, and the addition of 8.4% sodium bicarbonate to fentanyl (1:20 ratio) prior to injection abolishes discomfort [483]. Fentanyl does not induce vomiting in dogs [485] and may be associated with fewer adverse effects compared to morphine [486].

Fentanyl can produce sedation and recumbency in dogs and increased locomotor activity and euphoria in cats [487]. The latter effects are more commonly observed at doses > 20 μg/kg IV [487]. It was reported that 25% of healthy dogs undergoing orthopedic procedures administered a fentanyl CRI developed dysphoria following extubation [188]. The administration of a low bolus dose (0.5 μg/kg) of dexmedetomidine given slowly IV may improve recovery quality in dogs administered prolonged fentanyl CRIs (e.g., > 2 h) [189]. Fentanyl has been reported to cause "woody chest syndrome" in humans which results in reduced chest wall compliance and impaired ventilation [488]; however, similar findings have not been reported in dogs [489]. At high doses > 20 μg/kg IV, fentanyl can cause hypoventilation and cyanosis. Severe bradycardia and asystole have been reported following a 3 μg/kg IV bolus of fentanyl in two dogs [490].

Fentanyl provides adequate analgesia for acute pain management in dogs and cats [276,446,491,492]. In cats, a fentanyl CRI at 5 μg/kg/h produced significant thermal and mechanical antinociception that was short-lived following cessation of the infusion [493,494]. A lower infusion rate of 3 μg/kg/h, however, did not significantly increase thermal thresholds in cats [494].

Fentanyl can be administered via transdermal patch to provide postoperative pain relief for up to 72–96 h. In dogs, the recommended dose is approximately 4 μg/kg/h, and in cats greater than 2 kg, application of one 25-μg/h patch is recommended. Marked individual variability in drug absorption has been reported in both dogs and cats using reservoir (gel pouch) patches; however, higher bioavailability and less variability is observed in dogs compared to cats [71,495] (Fig. 23.6). Adverse effects are the same as those observed following parenteral administration. The thickness of the epidermis may delay the onset of action without disrupting peak plasma concentrations [496]. Body temperature also influences serum fentanyl concentration in cats [497]. In general, the onset of analgesia following application in dogs and cats is approximately

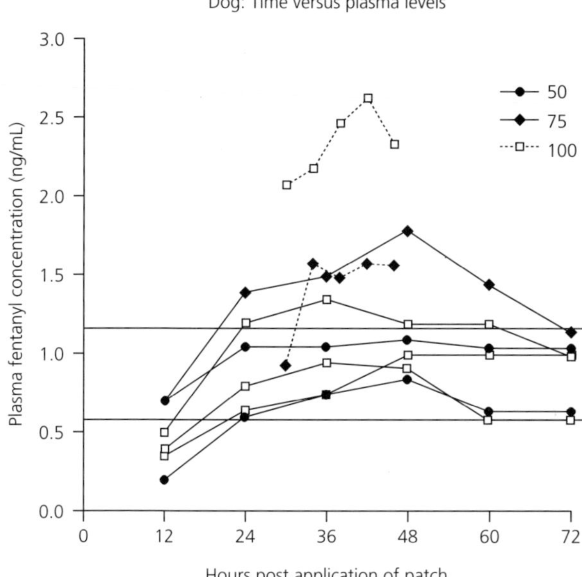

(A)

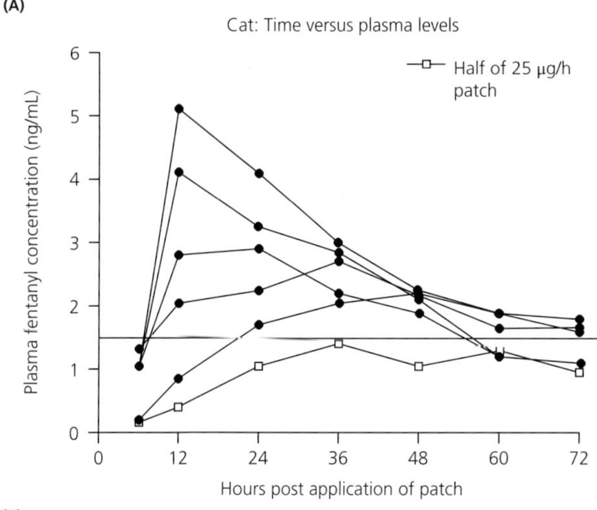

(B)

Figure 23.6 Fentanyl patch plasma concentrations in dogs and cats. **A.** Time versus fentanyl plasma concentrations in six groups of dogs. 50, 50-μg/h patch; 75, 75-μg/h patch; 100, 100-μg/h patch. Solid horizontal lines represent the minimum (0.6 ng/mL) and mean (1.18 ng/mL) plasma fentanyl concentrations consistent with analgesia. Dotted lines represent plasma concentrations from dogs where the fentanyl patch was placed on the caudal abdomen. **B.** Time versus fentanyl plasma concentration in six groups of cats. All cats received a 25-μg/h transdermal fentanyl patch (solid circles), but one group (open squares) was exposed to half of a 25-μg/h patch. The solid horizontal line represents a plasma fentanyl level of 1.56 ng/mL, which has been correlated to analgesia. Note that the cats given half of a 25-μg/h patch did not achieve plasma levels shown to be consistent with analgesia. Source: Hofmeister and Egger [498], American Animal Hospital Association.

24 and 7–12 h, respectively [498]. When transdermal fentanyl patches remain in contact with the skin, they can provide analgesia for up to 72 h; however, there is the potential for plasma fentanyl concentrations to fall below analgesic levels in cats by 72 h (Fig. 23.6B). Transdermal patches are generally safe, but accidental ingestion and exposure resulting in serious adverse effects have been reported in dogs, pigs, and children [499,500]. Treatment requires naloxone or naltrexone [500]; however, clinicians must be aware of the potential for renarcotization following administration of an antagonist. To minimize adverse effects and illegal use, the original formulation of a particular transdermal patch (Duragesic®) was modified, and the gel pouch containing a reservoir of liquid drug was replaced by a "drug-in-adhesive matrix" designed to minimize fentanyl leakage and potential for abuse (Duragesic® package insert 2014) [379]. After use, the FDA recommends promptly disposing of patches by folding them in half with the sticky sides together and then flushing them down a toilet [501]. The FDA recommends this method of disposal because a patch could be harmful and possibly fatal in a single dose if used by someone other than the individual for whom it is intended. It is recommended that patches not be placed in household trash cans where children or pets can have access. When prescribing transdermal fentanyl patches, veterinarians should be aware of potential complications, absorption variability, liability issues in the event of accidental human exposure through ingestion or contact, considerations for extra-label use during acute or intermittent postoperative pain, and potential adverse effects associated with their use [379].

Horses and food animals

Fentanyl at clinically relevant doses may not provide analgesia in horses and results in dose-dependent adverse behavioral effects (e.g., head and eye movement, fine muscle fasciculations, and shifting of forelimbs) [502]. A minimum dose of 10 μg/kg IV provided thermal antinociception in horses between 10 and 30 min [503]. This equates to minimum fentanyl plasma concentrations of 6.1–6.8 ng/mL, which is approximately six times what is required in dogs and cats [23,504]. Intravenous fentanyl is well tolerated in foals 1–6 weeks of age. Increased locomotor activity was observed in foals at doses of 8 and 16 μg/kg, while mild and heavy sedation was observed at 4 and 32 μg/kg, respectively [505]. Plasma concentrations associated with analgesia were comparable to those reported for adult horses; thus, the clinical utility of IV fentanyl in horses remains somewhat unclear at this time [505]. In sevoflurane-anesthetized piglets, intravenous fentanyl at 10 μg/kg produces transient and spontaneously resolving muscle tremors [506]. This could pose significant issues in specific research surgical settings. In isoflurane-anesthetized adult pigs, infusions of 5, 10, and 20 μg/kg/h also produced "shivering" [507].

Transdermal fentanyl patches have been used in horses for long-term analgesic therapy [508]. The onset of action is rapid with peak plasma fentanyl concentrations occurring 8–15 h post-application. Plasma concentrations are maintained between 1 and 3 ng/mL for up to 48 h [309]; bioavailability is high and reported to be approximately 96% [309]. Despite these advantages, peak concentrations did not exceed 3 ng/mL; therefore (based on a previous study), transdermal fentanyl may not provide adequate analgesia when administered as monotherapy.

Transdermal fentanyl application in goats produces variable plasma concentrations (0.83–16.69 ng/mL) with an onset of peak plasma concentrations similar to horses [94,509]. Sheep, however, demonstrated more stable plasma concentrations (0.62–2.73 ng/mL) with peak effects at 12 h following application [89]. Application of fentanyl patches to calves, even at doses as low as 1–2 μg/kg/h, resulted in neuroexcitation and tachycardia suggesting that caution is warranted [510]. In pigs, transdermal fentanyl is well tolerated and is potentially a better analgesic option than buprenorphine following surgical procedures [507].

Remifentanil

Remifentanil is a μ-opioid receptor agonist that is structurally similar to fentanyl (Table 23.6). It has an extremely short half-life (e.g., 6 min in dogs) and duration of action [511]. Remifentanil is metabolized via ester hydrolysis by nonspecific esterases in blood and tissues. This unique pharmacokinetic feature is attributed to its propanoic acid methyl ester linkage on the piperidine nitrogen [512]. Recovery from remifentanil is rapid regardless of dose and infusion duration, as the context-sensitive half-time remains unchanged at less than 5 min [512,513].

In cats, a minimum dose of 0.3 μg/kg/min may be required to prevent the generation of a motor response from an electrical noxious stimulus [514]. In a clinical study in isoflurane-anesthetized cats undergoing ovariohysterectomy, 0.4 μg/kg/min provided more appropriate analgesia when compared to 0.1 and 0.2 μg/kg/min infusion rates [515]. Species differences in the antinociceptive effects of remifentanil at the level of the spinal cord have been observed between dogs and cats. For example, remifentanil's inhibitory effect on nociceptive transmission at the spinal cord was shown to be less pronounced in cats compared to dogs [516]. Presumably, this is due to the differences in Aδ fiber distribution within the CNS, which may account for additional species-level differences in the antinociceptive effects of μ-opioid receptor agonists [516]. Remifentanil has been associated with acute opioid tolerance and opioid-induced hyperalgesia in rats, mice, and rabbits [517–519]. Evidence to support similar findings in dogs is lacking [520].

Remifentanil increases arginine vasopressin concentrations in anesthetized dogs [521]. As with other opioids, this may be a physiologic compensatory response to bradycardia-induced hypotension or result from direct stimulation of μ-opioid receptors in the neurohypophysis [522,523]. There are limited studies comparing the adverse effects associated with remifentanil and fentanyl in dogs and cats. A prospective randomized multicenter study in humans reported that the frequency of adverse effects was similar between remifentanil and fentanyl; however, hypotension occurred more commonly in patients receiving remifentanil [524]. Other clinical trials found similar results pertaining to blood pressure, but also reported lower HRs in patients administered remifentanil compared to fentanyl [525]. Remifentanil, however, may be a better alternative to fentanyl when early and frequent postoperative neural and motor function assessments are required [526]. Remifentanil has been used successfully as part of a multimodal protocol in a horse undergoing a 13-h surgical procedure [527]. It has also been used as part of an equine sedation protocol at 6 μg/kg/h in conjunction with a xylazine CRI [528]. In isoflurane-anesthetized horses also receiving dexmedetomidine, peak blood remifentanil concentrations occurred at 45–50 min after starting an IV remifentanil CRI at 6 μg/kg/h [529].

Sufentanil

Sufentanil is a highly lipid soluble μ-opioid receptor agonist that is 10–15 times more potent than fentanyl. It is a thienyl analogue of 4-anilinopiperidine (Table 23.6). In isoflurane-anesthetized cats, the clearance, volume of distribution, and terminal half-life of sufentanil is longer than that of fentanyl and alfentanil [530]. Like fentanyl, sufentanil has been administered for intraoperative analgesia and constitutes a good alternative during times of fentanyl shortages. Recovery quality in dogs undergoing ovariohysterectomy was significantly better in dogs administered a sufentanil infusion when compared to fentanyl, with comparable degrees of analgesia and respiratory depression [531]. Similar effects on recovery quality were reported when sufentanil was compared to fentanyl and administered in combination with lidocaine and ketamine in dogs undergoing total ear canal ablation and bulla osteotomy [532]. Recovery quality following general anesthesia in cats is similar between sufentanil and fentanyl [533]. Sufentanil can be combined with bupivacaine and administered epidurally in dogs and has been reported to provide a greater degree of analgesia in the postoperative period when compared to fentanyl and bupivacaine [534]. A novel long-lasting sufentanil formulation has been evaluated in dogs and can be administered intramuscularly for prolonged postoperative pain relief (e.g., approximately 24 h) [535]. Despite its antinociceptive effects, a high incidence of intraoperative respiratory and cardiovascular complications currently precludes use of this product in clinical scenarios [535]. Limited data are available regarding the use of sufentanil in large animal species.

Meperidine (pethidine)

Meperidine (pethidine) is a phenylpiperidine synthetic opioid (Table 23.6) and μ-opioid receptor agonist. Meperidine provides good but short-duration analgesia lasting approximately 60–90 min post-administration in dogs [536,537] and cats [538,539]. An active metabolite, normeperidine, is produced following metabolism by *N*-demethylation via hepatic cytochrome P450. Normeperidine is a CNS excitotoxic agent and can produce agitation, noise sensitization, and muscle twitching in dogs with inappropriate dosing [540]. Benzodiazepines, but not naloxone, are recommended to treat these adverse effects [540]. Meperidine possesses vagolytic properties at medium doses, but bradycardia is observed at very high doses due to its local anesthetic-like actions resulting in direct myocardial depression [541,542]. Tachycardia may also be a result of histamine release following IV administration. Meperidine's effects on HR do not attenuate dexmedetomidine-induced bradycardia [196]. Meperidine can induce pain during IM injection, which may be related to its acidic pH (3.5–6.0) [196]. Meperidine administered to conscious dogs at 10 mg/kg IV stimulates peripheral mast cells resulting an acute and transient period of vocalizing, flare reaction, scratching, hypersalivation, urination, defecation, and tachypnea [543]. It also can result in local edema and erythema due to cutaneous histamine release following IM injection [242]. Despite these local effects, meperidine generally does not result in clinically significant systemic histamine concentrations following IM administration [544].

Meperidine administered IV, SC, and IM at 1 mg/kg does not produce thermal antinociceptive effects in horses [311,545]. However, there may be some short-term analgesic benefit with alleviation of equine lameness at a dose of 1 mg/kg IM [546]. Meperidine can, however, provide long-lasting analgesia (240–300 min) with a quick onset (12 min) following caudal epidural administration with minimal sedation and ataxia and no adverse cardiopulmonary effects [547].

Carfentanil, etorphine, alfentanil, and thiafentanil

Carfentanil, a fentanyl analogue that is 20–30 times more potent than fentanyl and 10,000 times more potent than morphine, was approved for veterinary use in 1986 as an intramuscular large animal tranquilizer. In the US, veterinarians must receive authorization and be placed on an "Approved Carfentanil Users List" with special Drug Enforcement Agency (DEA) registration class approval. In Canada, carfentanil is considered a Schedule I substance, meaning that it serves no accepted medical use and has high abuse potential. Currently, its only approved use in humans is as a radiolabeled isotope, [11C]-carfentanil, to aid in mapping the μ-opioid receptor via positron emission tomography in research settings.

Veterinarians must handle carfentanil with extreme caution as very small quantities (0.01 mL) can be lethal. Accidental carfentanil intoxication in humans can lead to miosis, respiratory and CNS depression, and potentially death. It is best to handle highly potent opioids (i.e., thiafentanil, etorphine, and carfentanil) with at least two people present, to wear protective clothing, gloves, and a face shield, and have an opioid receptor antagonist (e.g., naloxone, naltrexone, or diprenorphine) readily available. The first confirmed human accidental overdose exposure associated with carfentanil occurred when a veterinarian accidentally splashed carfentanil citrate 1.5 mg and xylazine 50 mg from an immobilization dart into his eyes and mouth [548]. Despite irrigation, sedation occurred within 2 min and the subject was administered naltrexone 100 mg parenterally (supplied in the same package as carfentanil) prior to arrival at the hospital [548]. The veterinarian was discharged a day later after a complete recovery [548]. Etorphine and thiafentanil carry similar concerns and are discussed elsewhere (Chapter 55).

Hydrocodone, oxycodone, and codeine

Hydrocodone is a μ-opioid receptor agonist and undergoes *N*-demethylation and *N*-oxidation to norhydrocodone and *N*-oxide metabolites (major metabolites) as well as hydromorphone and hydromorphone glucuronide (minor metabolites) [549]. Hydrocodone is predominately used in dogs as an antitussive agent (0.22–0.5 mg/kg PO every 6–12 h) and exerts its antitussive properties via simulation of μ-opioid receptors on sensory nerve endings that initiate cough as well within the CNS [550]. Hydrocodone is often formulated with an anticholinergic drug (homatropine), nonsteroidal anti-inflammatory agent, or acetaminophen (paracetamol). The latter combination should not be used in cats because acetaminophen is toxic in this species. Codeine has also been used as an antitussive agent in dogs; however, sedation may be more prominent than with hydrocodone.

Previous studies evaluating oral administration of opioids such as hydrocodone and codeine have demonstrated low bioavailability, large individual variability, erratic gastrointestinal absorption, and limited analgesic effect, particularly in dogs [551–553]. One study, however, evaluating hydrocodone at 0.5 mg/kg PO in Greyhound dogs reported that plasma concentrations of the metabolite hydromorphone did exceed those previously reported to provide analgesia from 0.5 to 8 h [554]. A clinical trial compared the analgesic efficacy of oral extended-release hydrocodone (3.0 mg/kg) to firocoxib in dogs undergoing tibial plateau leveling osteotomy (TPLO) [555]. In this study, dogs administered hydrocodone had higher pain scores and lower limb function than dogs administered firocoxib. Similarly, pain relief was considered unacceptable in dogs administered hydrocodone–acetaminophen PO for TPLO surgery [556]. In dogs, differing metabolic and elimination pathways along with a more vigorous first-pass effect [557–560] may explain the lack of bioavailability and analgesic efficacy of these drugs compared to other species.

Codeine is classified as a μ-opioid receptor agonist and can be administered IV, IM, SC, PO, or as a CRI. Oral bioavailability of codeine is extremely low in dogs (4%) [551]. Metabolism of codeine generates many metabolites including morphine, codeine, and codeine-6-glucuronide [561]. Codeine at 1–3 mg/kg SC provides dose-dependent antinociceptive effects for 1–3 h based on the electrical dental pulp stimulation model in dogs [562]. While postoperative codeine at 2 mg/kg SC every 8 h for 24 h alone provided adequate analgesia in 6/9 (66%) dogs undergoing maxillectomy or mandibulectomy [563], pain assessment in this study involved numeric rating and simple descriptive scales rather than a validated multidimensional pain scale. In cats, codeine at 2 mg/kg PO failed to produce thermal antinociceptive effects [564]. Orally administered codeine in horses is rapidly metabolized to morphine, morphine-3-glucuronide, morphine-6-glucuronide, codeine-6-glucuronide, and norcodeine [565]. Plasma concentrations of morphine-6-glucuronide following codeine at 0.6 mg/kg PO were comparable to those following an analgesic dose of morphine in horses [81,565]. Codeine is generally well tolerated in horses but lacks the ability to provide antinociception when administered PO at doses of 0.3, 0.6, and 1.2 mg/kg [78].

More studies are required to prove the analgesic efficacy of these drugs in veterinary medicine. Due to the lack of evidence supporting clinical efficacy of orally administered codeine, oxycodone, or hydrocodone, the authors do not recommend their use as monotherapies for treatment of pain in dogs or cats [379].

Partial opioid agonists

Buprenorphine

Dogs and cats

Buprenorphine is a μ-opioid receptor partial agonist. It is available as a hydrochloride salt in various formulations approved for use in humans, cats, and dogs depending on the jurisdiction. In the US, in addition to the human 0.3 mg/mL preservative-free injectable solution (Buprenex®), two concentrated buprenorphine formulations are commercially available for use in cats for postoperative analgesia. One contains 1.8 mg/mL buprenorphine (Simbadol®) and is administered SC once daily for up to 72 h. The other formulation contains 20 mg/mL buprenorphine (Zorbium®) for single transdermal administration providing analgesia for up to 96 h. In Europe, Canada, and Australia, 0.3 mg/mL multidose injectable formulations are available for IM or IV administration and provide analgesia for 6–8 h in dogs [566] and 4–8 h in cats [20]. In the following discussion, if not specifically noted, statements pertain to the 0.3 mg/mL injectable formulation, which will be referred to as the "traditional" injectable formulation where applicable.

In dogs, premedication with buprenorphine (0.02 mg/kg IM) produces inferior postoperative analgesia compared to methadone (0.3 mg/kg IM) for ovariohysterectomy [149]. However, when administered IV as a CRI (0.015 mg/kg loading dose and 0.0025 mg/kg/h for 6 h), buprenorphine provides satisfactory postoperative analgesia for elective ovariectomy [567]. Buprenorphine transdermal patches (0.005–0.006 mg/kg/h applied 40 h before anesthesia) or IV buprenorphine (0.02 mg/kg administered 30 min before the induction of anesthesia and then every 6 h for 24 h) provided similar intra- and postoperative analgesia following unilateral mastectomy [566]. The addition of buprenorphine (0.1 mL of 0.3 mg/mL solution) to bupivacaine (0.3 mL of 5 mg/mL solution) for infraorbital nerve blocks enhanced the duration of analgesia in dogs with acute dental pain [568].

A commercially available concentrated buprenorphine solution (1.8 mg/mL, Simbadol®) has been investigated in dogs. Used as premedication at 0.02 mg/kg, it provided adequate postoperative analgesia following ovariohysterectomy when administered IV or IM, but not when administered SC [372]. The authors attributed this to erratic drug absorption after SC administration. However, a larger dosage (0.12 mg/kg IV, SC) in awake dogs demonstrated complete

SC absorption [59]. After intranasal or OTM administration at 0.03 mg/kg, buprenorphine bioavailability was 58% and 41%, respectively; and plasma drug concentrations associated with analgesia were maintained for up to 5 h [21]. Sedation, panting, whining, hypersalivation, ataxia, decreased rectal temperature, reduced appetite, and diarrhea have been observed in awake dogs [21,59]. These effects may limit the clinical utility of Simbadol® as an analgesic in dogs. A lipid encapsulated, extended-release buprenorphine formulation (0.2 mg/kg SC) provided sustained analgesic plasma drug concentrations and antinociception for up to 72 h [569].

In cats, the traditional formulation of buprenorphine administered at 0.02 mg/kg IM preoperatively did not provide postoperative pain relief after ovariohysterectomy; however, an additional buprenorphine dose administered during wound closure was associated with adequate analgesia [153]. Concurrent administration of meloxicam (0.2 mg/kg SC) or gabapentin (50 mg PO) also seemed to improve the analgesic effect of preoperative buprenorphine (0.02 mg/kg IM) for ovariohysterectomy [570]. Similarly, preoperative buprenorphine (0.02 mg/kg IM) in conjunction with intratesticular lidocaine block (2 mg/kg) and postoperative meloxicam (0.3 mg/kg SC) induced good postoperative analgesia after orchidectomy in cats [571]. Thus, repeated doses of the traditional (0.3 mg/mL) injectable formulation of buprenorphine or its use as part of a multimodal analgesic protocol is required to provide adequate postoperative analgesia after neutering in cats.

The need for outpatient pain control in cats has encouraged the investigation of alternative formulations and routes of administration for buprenorphine. For instance, both commercially available and compounded formulations of injectable buprenorphine are absorbed by the OTM route. However, individual variation in buprenorphine absorption and poor palatability associated with some formulations (those with preservatives) may preclude clinical utility of this route of administration [572,573]. The commercially available concentrated buprenorphine formulation (1.8 mg/mL; 0.24 mg/kg SC, Simbadol®) provided similar analgesia to the traditional injectable formulation (0.3 mg/mL; 0.02 mg/kg IM) following dental extractions [20]. The concentrated formulation has the advantage of longer lasting analgesia compared to the traditional formulation and, therefore, less frequent dosing and potential aversion to drug administration. However, the concentrated buprenorphine formulation produced a higher prevalence of postoperative hyperthermia than morphine (0.1 mg/kg SC) following ovariohysterectomy [307]. A single administration of a compounded liposomal encapsulated buprenorphine formulation (0.2 mg/kg SC) maintains putative analgesic drug concentrations for 96 h [574]. A novel transdermal buprenorphine formulation (20 mg/mL; Zorbium®) also provides 96 h of analgesia when applied topically to the cervical skin (8 mg to cats 1.2–3 kg, and 20 mg to cats > 3–7.5 kg) 1–2 h prior to both elective surgical reproductive sterilization and forelimb onychectomy [29].

Horses

In horses, preoperative buprenorphine (0.005 mg/kg IV) provides better intraoperative analgesia than butorphanol (0.025 mg/kg IV) [154], and a larger dose (0.01 mg/kg IV) induces effective postoperative analgesia for surgical castration [575]. Buprenorphine (0.0075 mg/kg IV) also induces good sedation for cheek tooth extraction [576]; however, postoperative locomotor stimulation may occur [154,576]. Attempts to induce long-lasting analgesia with a single administration of a compounded buprenorphine formulation (0.1 mg/kg SC or IM) failed due to the severity and duration of adverse gastrointestinal effects and behavioral excitation [577]. A single off-label administration of a commercially available concentrated buprenorphine formulation (1.8 mg/mL; 0.0025 and 0.005 mg/kg SC, Simbadol®) induced antinociception but only at the lower dose rate and for a duration comparable to that achieved with traditional concentration buprenorphine (0.3 mg/mL; 0.005–0.01 mg/kg IV) [76,575]. The gastrointestinal and behavioral adverse effects may preclude the use of doses greater than 0.005 mg/kg SC for the concentrated buprenorphine formulation. Alternative routes of administration have been explored in attempts to prolong the analgesic effects of buprenorphine. For instance, buprenorphine concentrations are detectable for at least 24 h in inflamed joints after a single intra-articular administration (0.005 mg/kg), but the chondrotoxic effects may preclude clinical use of this route of administration [107,578].

Mixed opioid agonist–antagonists

Butorphanol

Butorphanol is structurally classified as a morphinan (Table 23.6) and exhibits antagonist to partial agonist activity at μ-opioid receptors, and agonist activity at κ-opioid receptors. It is approved for use as an antitussive in dogs and an analgesic in cats and horses, but approval varies among countries. It is available as butorphanol tartrate and may be administered via IV (bolus and CRI), IM, SC, or PO routes. There are also reports of alternative routes of administration such as intravenous regional limb perfusion in horses [579] and intranasal administration in parrots and rabbits [580,581]. Butorphanol tablets, despite producing antitussive and mild sedative effects, have low oral bioavailability and do not induce effective analgesia. Extravascular parental administration may be painful on injection [582].

Dogs and cats

In dogs, butorphanol induces opioid effects measured as decreased rectal temperature following IV bolus (0.4 mg/kg), IV CRI (0.2 mg/kg IV followed by 0.2 mg/kg/h), and SC injection of butorphanol (0.8 mg/kg) with bicarbonate (forming a poorly-water-soluble suspension), but not after SC administration of butorphanol (0.4 mg/kg) alone [582]. Lower butorphanol doses may be used for sedation than those required for analgesia. Procedural sedation with butorphanol (0.4 mg/kg IV) allows easier and faster endoscopic duodenal intubation compared to methadone (0.3 mg/kg IV) [583]. When combined with dexmedetomidine (2 μg/kg IV), butorphanol (0.2 mg/kg IV) also induces rapid onset of deep sedation that facilitates positioning for radiographic examination [584]. When administered as premedication or immediately after completing surgery, butorphanol (0.4 mg/kg IV or IM) provides insufficient postoperative analgesia after ovariohysterectomy, laparotomy, or shoulder arthrotomy in dogs [477,585,586]. However, the criteria for rescue analgesia in the Gomes *et al.* study [585] was set below the validated intervention point for the scale used (i.e., Glasgow Composite Measure Pain Scale total score > 3.5/20 instead of > 5/20).

In cats, butorphanol (0.1–0.4 mg/kg IM) induces good quality sedation, but potentially inferior to that achieved with full μ-opioid receptor agonists [587]. Butorphanol also prevents vomiting and reduces the incidence and severity of nausea induced by dexmedetomidine [588,589]. Compared to buprenorphine (20 μg/kg IM), the incidence of vomiting is less with butorphanol [589]. Butorphanol (0.4 mg/kg IM) combined with medetomidine (15 μg/kg IM) for premedication failed to induce postoperative analgesia after ovariohysterectomy; even after adding another dose of butorphanol during wound closure [153]. In contrast, butorphanol (0.3 mg/kg IM) as part of a multimodal analgesic protocol with dexmedetomidine, lidocaine, and meloxicam provided effective postoperative analgesia after orchidectomy [571]. The requirement of isoflurane is also reduced with butorphanol compared with buprenorphine in cats [571], and butorphanol IV CRI dose-dependently reduced the MAC of isoflurane by 23–68% [359].

Horses

Administered alone to healthy, non-painful horses, butorphanol increases locomotor activity. Locomotion is prevented by pre-administering a sedative (e.g., an α_2-adrenergic receptor agonist) and/or a tranquilizer (e.g., acepromazine) [590]. Increased locomotion with butorphanol is not noted in newborn foals, but sedation and increased nursing is observed [591]. Mild sedation induced by a combination of butorphanol (0.01 mg/kg IV) and detomidine (0.01 mg/kg IV) does not affect the grade of laryngeal function in horses undergoing endoscopic examination of the upper respiratory tract [592]. When administered as part of a premedication protocol, butorphanol (0.02–0.1 mg/kg IV) induces acceptable postoperative analgesia in horses undergoing elective surgical procedures [155]. Acceptable postoperative analgesia is also achieved when butorphanol (0.02 mg/kg IV) is administered just before skin incision in horses undergoing elective arthroscopy [450]. However, premedication with detomidine (0.01 mg/kg IV) followed by butorphanol (0.1 mg/kg IV) may not provide adequate postoperative analgesia following castration in ponies [593].

Interactions with full opioid agonists

Butorphanol decreases some of the effects induced by μ-opioid receptor agonists while still inducing analgesia via μ- and κ-opioid receptor activation. Thus, butorphanol (0.2 mg/kg IV) decreases but still preserves some of the antinociception induced by hydromorphone (0.1 mg/kg) in cats [239]. Butorphanol (0.1–0.2 mg/kg IV) partially reverses oxymorphone-induced respiratory depression and bradycardia in the early postoperative period in dogs [218]. It also attenuates respiratory depression and decreases immobilizing effects induced by etorphine (0.1 mg/kg IM) in goats [594]. In the case of a prolonged recovery or relative μ-opioid receptor agonist overdose, titrating butorphanol IV to effect is recommended over bolus administration [218,239].

Nalbuphine

Nalbuphine is a κ-opioid receptor agonist and μ-opioid receptor antagonist. It remains the only narcotic analgesic not controlled under the Controlled Substances Act in the US. An injectable formulation containing nalbuphine hydrochloride at 10 or 20 mg/mL is approved for use in humans in the US. Nalbuphine alone induces sedation and analgesia in dogs, but both effects are less potent than with pure μ-opioid receptor agonists. Also, the sedation and analgesia may not be sufficient to perform some clinical procedures (e.g., clipping/prepping and catheterization) or alleviate some types of pain [595]. Both sedation and analgesia exhibit ceiling effects [596,597]. Deeper sedation is achieved when nalbuphine is administered in neuroleptanalgesic combinations with acepromazine or α_2-adrenergic receptor agonists [163,595,597]. However, nalbuphine (0.5 mg/kg or 1 mg/kg IV) combined with acepromazine failed to provide sufficient intra- or postoperative analgesia in dogs undergoing ovariohysterectomy (as was also the case for butorphanol and morphine in this study) [585]. Administration of IV nalbuphine (0.75 mg/kg) every 4 h or less or as a CRI has been recommended for postoperative analgesia in dogs [598]. Epidural nalbuphine administration (0.3–0.6 mg/kg) induces MAC-sparing effects and long-lasting postoperative analgesia and sedation [599]. However, data on the analgesic effects of nalbuphine CRI and the safety of epidural nalbuphine in dogs are lacking. Compounded nalbuphine applied topically to the cornea at 0.8–1% had no effect on pain scores in experimental dogs with surgically damaged corneas [600], or dogs undergoing phacoemulsification cataract surgery [601], or on corneal sensitivity in clinically normal horses [602]. Thus, topical ophthalmic nalbuphine cannot be recommended as an analgesic. Nalbuphine induces minimal cardiovascular changes in healthy dogs after IV bolus administration (1–2 mg/kg), after an IV loading dose (0.3 mg/kg IV) followed by a CRI (0.4 mg/kg/h), or after epidural administration (0.3–0.6 mg/kg) [597,599,603,604].

There is limited information on nalbuphine in other domestic animal species. For instance, mild sedation has been reported with a neuroleptanalgesic combination of nalbuphine (0.5 mg/kg IV or IM) and acepromazine (0.05 mg/kg IV or IM) in cats, and sedation was similar to that achieved with butorphanol (0.4 mg/kg IV or IM) and acepromazine [605]. Similarly, nalbuphine (0.15 mg/kg IM) is not inferior to butorphanol (0.15 mg/kg IM) when used in combination with dexmedetomidine and tiletamine–zolazepam for induction of anesthesia to perform gonadectomy in cats [606]. When administered as an IV premedication in horses, nalbuphine (0.75 mg/kg) combined with xylazine (1.1 mg/kg) alone or xylazine (0.5 mg/kg) and acepromazine (0.02 mg/kg) induced smoother inductions and recoveries from anesthesia, longer duration of anesthesia, and increased analgesia compared to xylazine alone (1.1 mg/kg) [607]. This is in contrast to another study that reported similar analgesia with xylazine alone (1.1 mg/kg IV) or combined with nalbuphine (0.75 mg/kg IV) in experimental horses during electrical stimulation of the dentine of a canine tooth [608]. Nalbuphine (0.4 mg/kg IV) reduced some pain-related behaviors but did not eliminate physiological signs of distress in calves after surgical castration [87]. Compared to ketamine alone (10 mg/kg IV), nalbuphine (0.5 mg/kg IV) combined with ketamine (5 mg/kg IV) induced smoother induction and recovery from anesthesia and better postoperative analgesia in goats [609]. Nalbuphine (1 mg/kg SC) induced sedation and analgesia without affecting cardiovascular function in sheep [610]. Further studies are required to determine the true clinical utility of nalbuphine in domestic animal species.

Measuring thermal nociceptive thresholds in Hispaniolan Amazon parrots, nalbuphine hydrochloride (12.5 mg/kg IM, but not 25 and 50 mg/kg IM) induced antinociception compared to saline control and all three doses induced antinociception for up to 3 h compared to baseline values. However, the two larger doses induced less antinociception than the lowest dose. This is consistent with a bell-shaped dose–response curve demonstrating a ceiling effect [611]. Antinociception for up to 12 h was obtained with nalbuphine decanoate (37.7 mg/kg IM) [612]. Differences in the duration of antinociception are due to differences in the pharmacokinetic profile of these two nalbuphine salts [613,614].

When nalbuphine is used concurrently with μ-opioid receptor agonists, both μ- and κ-opioid receptor-mediated analgesia may be achieved while decreasing the severity of μ-opioid receptor-mediated adverse events. This has been partially demonstrated in dogs where the administration of nalbuphine (0.3–1 mg/kg IV) decreased the degree of sedation induced by a combination of morphine (0.5 mg/kg IV) and acepromazine (0.05 mg/kg IV) [596], and decreased the adverse cardiovascular effects induced by fentanyl (50 μg/kg IV) [615]. Also, in goats, nalbuphine (0.8 mg/kg IV) decreased the level of immobilization but had minimal effects on the respiratory depressant effects induced by etorphine (0.1 mg/kg IM) [594].

Opioid antagonists

Naloxone, naltrexone, and methylnaltrexone

Naloxone is a short-acting opioid receptor antagonist that is rapidly absorbed after IV and IM administration. A dose of 0.04 mg/kg IV is recommended for opioid reversal during cardiopulmonary arrest in dogs and cats [616]. Intranasal naloxone (administered with an atomizer) is also an effective route in dogs, particularly for emergency use in working canines accidentally exposed to opioids [617,618]. The required dose of intranasal naloxone is four times higher than the IV dose, with an approximately 50% reduction in maximum plasma concentrations. Naloxone is often used to reverse the sedative effects associated with pure μ-opioid receptor agonists. Patients should be closely monitored as renarcotization may occur following IV and IM naloxone administration [217]. In dogs that received oxymorphone, this may occur within 20–40 and 40–70 min following IV and IM naloxone administration, respectively [619]. Similar findings were reported in cats 1 h following 0.04 mg/kg IV naloxone administration to reverse the effects of 0.1 mg/kg IV hydromorphone [239]. Studies have reported that rapid administration of IV naloxone can result in depressed mentation and blepharospasm [126,620]. The etiology of this adverse effect is yet to be determined but may be associated with acute opioid withdrawal [126,620], alterations in cerebral vascular tone [621], or systemic hypertension [622]. In humans, the administration of IV naloxone did not ablate the analgesic effect of epidural morphine [623]; however, it may reduce the effects of epidural morphine on urinary bladder function [624]. Naloxone also may attenuate some of the cardiovascular responses associated with shock. For example, naloxone administered at 0.04 mg/kg IV significantly lowered endotoxin-induced increases in right ventricular pressure and HR in horses [625].

Naltrexone is an opioid antagonist at μ-, κ-, and δ-opioid receptors. Naltrexone is often administered to reverse the sedative effects of carfentanil and etorphine in wildlife and zoo animals but would also be effective in reversing other opioids as well. The dose of naltrexone is 100 mg per 1 mg of carfentanil administered; typically, one-quarter of the dose is administered IV and the remainder is administered SC. Naltrexone's longer duration of action, at least twice that of naloxone in some species, makes it desirable in wildlife and zoo animals where repeat dosing may not be feasible. In dogs, however, the duration of action of naltrexone may not differ significantly from that of naloxone. Serum half-life during the elimination phase (mean ± SE) was reported to be 71.2 ± 8.9 min for naloxone and 85.1 ± 9.0 min for naltrexone in dogs [626]. Therefore, while naltrexone may be longer acting compared to naloxone in other species, its effects dissipate quickly in the dog [626]. In cats, naltrexone at 0.6 mg/kg IV should be administered every 60–120 min to reverse high-dose opioid agonists [627].

Methylnaltrexone is a quaternary derivative of naltrexone and is a selective peripherally-acting μ-opioid receptor antagonist [628]. Methylnaltrexone does not bind with δ-opioid receptors but binds μ-opioid receptors with an eightfold higher potency than κ-opioid receptors [629]. The addition of the methyl group forms a positively charged compound with greater polarity and lower lipid solubility compared to naltrexone [629]. At clinically relevant doses, methylnaltrexone is restricted from crossing the blood–brain barrier in animals. This property allows for reduced peripheral adverse effects while maintaining the central analgesic effects of opioid agonists. For example, methylnaltrexone can prevent or treat postoperative opioid-induced gastrointestinal ileus [630]. This could be of particular benefit in horses administered morphine [631,632]. Its effects on reducing the gastrointestinal effects associated with buprenorphine may be limited [633].

Multitargeting molecules

Tramadol

Between 2014 and 2019, tramadol was the most widely prescribed opioid by veterinarians in the US [37]. Tramadol is a racemic mixture of (+)-tramadol and (−)-tramadol. The positive enantiomer has low μ-opioid and α_2-adrenergic receptor affinity and inhibits neuronal serotonin reuptake. The negative enantiomer binds to α_2-adrenergic receptors and inhibits neuronal norepinephrine reuptake [634]. Tramadol is extensively metabolized by cytochrome P450 enzymes and the profile and extent are species- and individual-specific [634]. The metabolite *O*-desmethyltramadol, or M_1, has little intrinsic activity at μ-opioid receptors but has a 200-fold affinity compared to tramadol [634]. The opioid-mediated analgesic efficacy of tramadol relies on *O*-desmethyltramadol. The serotoninergic and noradrenergic effects of tramadol may also contribute to analgesia by augmenting descending inhibitory pathways. Tramadol is available in oral formulations in North America, Europe, and Oceania, and in injectable formulations in parts of Europe and Latin America.

Dogs produce very low concentrations of *O*-desmethyltramadol, and the clinical utility of tramadol has been questioned in this species. Tramadol (1–10 mg/kg IV) induces minimal, short-lived mechanical antinociception and no thermal antinociception [408,635]. A meta-analysis concluded low certainty of tramadol's analgesic evidence for postoperative pain management [636]. The need for rescue analgesia with tramadol is reduced compared to no treatment, placebo, codeine, buprenorphine, butorphanol, or nalbuphine, increased compared to methadone, and similar compared to morphine [636]. Administered before surgery, tramadol (3 mg/kg SC) induced postoperative analgesia similar to that of morphine (0.5 mg/kg IV) in dogs undergoing surgical neutering [402,637]. However, when administered postoperatively, tramadol (3 mg/kg IV every 4 h) induced insufficient analgesia following surgical tumor removal [399]. When administered during anesthesia, tramadol (1.5 mg/kg loading dose followed by 1.3 or 2.6 mg/kg/h CRI) had no meaningful sevoflurane MAC-sparing effect (5% and 8%) [638,639]. Thus, tramadol should be used judiciously in dogs and the potential for analgesic failure is high. Tramadol monotherapy is unlikely to have meaningful benefits for pain control in dogs.

Compared to carprofen (2.2 mg/kg PO every 12 h), tramadol (5 mg/kg PO every 8–12 h) provided less effective postoperative analgesia following enucleation in dogs [640]. It had no clinical benefit for dogs with osteoarthritis of the elbow or stifle [641]. Similarly, the combination of tramadol (4 mg/kg IV) and meloxicam (0.2 mg/kg IV) administered as premedication is not superior to meloxicam alone at inducing postoperative analgesia following surgical neutering [642]. Adequate analgesia for up to 30 days following TPLO is achieved with cimicoxib (2 mg/kg PO every 24 h) and tramadol (2 mg/kg PO every 12 h), but only cimicoxib improved limb function and range of motion and reduced the occurrence of hock edema [643]. Non-steroidal anti-inflammatory drugs seem to be superior to tramadol for inducing analgesia in dogs suffering from painful clinical conditions.

In cats, oral tramadol (0.5–4 mg/kg) induced dose-dependent thermal antinociception with doses of at least 2 mg/kg necessary to induce a significant analgesic effect, and doses of 4 mg/kg every 6 h associated with maintenance of a near maximal antinociceptive effect [644]. Preoperative oral tramadol (6 mg/kg) provides at least equivalent analgesia to that of IM tramadol (4 mg/kg), which in turn is more effective than IM meperidine (6 mg/kg) following ovariohysterectomy [645,646]. Oral tramadol (2 mg/kg PO every 12 h for 5 days) improves mobility and activity in geriatric cats with osteoarthritis but adverse effects were reported [647]. Although tramadol may be a useful drug for acute and chronic pain in cats, oral formulations are rarely palatable and induce profuse salivation and poor treatment compliance. This has led to exploration of alternative routes of administration in this species. Epidural administration of tramadol (1 mg/kg) plus lidocaine (2 mg/kg) induced better postoperative analgesia than either drug alone following orchidectomy [648]. A tramadol gel product (1.9–3.2 mg/kg) has been investigated for transdermal administration but plasma drug concentrations were low or undetectable [649].

Adverse effects have been reported after tramadol administration in cats and clinical signs include increased neuromuscular activity, tachycardia, fever, tachypnea, and agitation related to excessive levels of serotonin [650]. The risk of serotonin syndrome should be considered when serotonin antagonists and/or reuptake inhibitors (e.g., trazodone and fluoxetine), monoamine oxidase inhibitors (e.g., selegiline), or tricyclic antidepressants (e.g., amitriptyline and clomipramine) are co administered with tramadol.

In horses, IV bolus tramadol administration (2 mg/kg) induced no thermal antinociception [651], and a tramadol IV CRI (1 mg/kg bolus followed by 3 mg/kg/h) induced no mechanical antinociception [652]. However, tramadol co-infused with acetaminophen (6 g/h IV) induced mechanical antinociception 20 min after starting the infusion that persisted for 15 min after stopping the infusion [652]. Oral tramadol administration (5 mg/kg PO every 12 h for 1 week) produced minimal analgesia in horses with chronic laminitis, whereas co-administration of a subanesthetic dosage of ketamine (0.6 mg/kg/h IV for 6 h on each of the first 3 days of tramadol administration) induced immediate and lasting analgesia [653]. Intra-articular administration of tramadol (4 mg/mL) produced no postoperative analgesia following arthroscopic surgery [654]. Tramadol alone may not induce clinical analgesia in horses.

Tapentadol

Tapentadol has a dual mechanism of action as a μ-opioid receptor agonist and a norepinephrine reuptake inhibitor. Current investigations have focused on determining if tapentadol is an efficacious analgesic alternative in dogs and cats. Immediate and extended-release PO formulations are available in the US and Europe, and an injectable formulation is also available in Europe. After PO administration to dogs and cats, tapentadol undergoes extensive first-pass metabolism [65,655,656]. The major metabolite in dogs is tapentadol-*O*-glucuronide and in cats it is tapentadol-*O*-sulfate [655,656].

In dogs, IV (1.4 -6.8 mg/kg) but not PO (5.7–30 mg/kg) administration of tapentadol induced sedation, salivation, panting, ataxia, and diarrhea [65,408,655]. Thermal antinociception, similar to that of morphine (0.5–1.0 mg/kg IV), has been documented with tapentadol (4.6–6.8 mg/kg IV) [408]. Clinical cases of unilateral cranial cruciate ligament rupture improved in subjective (simple descriptive scale) but not objective (pressure sensitive walkway system) lameness evaluations at 4 h following tapentadol (30 mg/kg PO) administration [657]. However, in the latter study, the assessor was not blinded to treatment and no negative control group was included.

In cats, IV, IM, or SC administration of tapentadol (5 mg/kg) induced mild sedation, salivation, and panting, with the effects being less intense and of shorter duration following IM and SC administration. The bioavailability of IM and SC tapentadol is 94% and 90%, respectively [73]. Oral tapentadol (5.7 and 11.4 mg/kg) induced salivation and thermal antinociception with the higher dosage inducing a similar duration of antinociception as buprenorphine (0.02 mg/kg IM) and twice as long as the lower tapentadol dosage [658].

Although experimental studies indicate potential analgesic benefits of tapentadol in dogs and cats, more research is needed before any recommendations can be made regarding its use in clinical veterinary practice.

References

1 Dreborg S, Sundström G, Larsson TA, *et al.* Evolution of vertebrate opioid receptors. *Proc Natl Acad Sci USA* 2008; **105**(40): 15487–15492.

2 Stevens CW. The evolution of vertebrate opioid receptors. *Front Biosci (Landmark Ed)* 2009; **14**(4): 1247–1269.

3 Brook K, Bennett J, Desai SP. The chemical history of morphine: an 8000-year journey, from resin to *de-novo* synthesis. *J Anesth Hist* 2017; **3**(2): 50–55.

4 Dorrington KL, Poole W. The first intravenous anaesthetic: how well was it managed and its potential realized? *Br J Anaesth* 2013; **110**(1): 7–12.

5 Musser R, Krants JC. The friendship of Robert Boyle and Christopher Wren. *Bull Hist Med* 1939; **7**: 970–974.

6 Hamilton GR, Baskett TF. In the arms of Morpheus the development of morphine for postoperative pain relief. *Can J Anaesth* 2000; **47**(4): 367–374.

7 Jurna I. Sertürner and morphine--a historical vignette. *Schmerz* 2003; **17**(4): 280–283.

8 Clutton RE. An Anglocentric history of anaesthetics and analgesics in the refinement of animal experiments. *Animals (Basel)* 2020; **10**(10): 1933.

9 Hobday F. The value and use of morphia in canine surgery. *Vet J* 1908; **64**: 220–228.

10 Milks HJ. Opium-morphine. In: Milks HJ, ed. *Practical Veterinary Pharmacology and Therapeutics*. New York, NY: The Macmillan Company, 1917: 136–144.

11 Fröhner E. Morphinum hydrochloricum. Salzsaures morphium. In: Fröhner E, ed. *Lehrbuch der Arzneiverordnungslehre für Tierärzte*. Stuttgart, Germany: Verlag von Ferdin & Enke, 1921: 62–70.

12 Amadon RS, Craigie AH. The actions of morphine on the horse. Preliminary studies: diacetylmorphine (heroin), dihydrodesoxymorphine-D (desomorphine) and dihydroheterocodeine. *J Am Vet Med Assoc* 1937; **91**: 674–678.

13 Combie J, Dougherty J, Nugent E, *et al.* The pharmacology of narcotic analgesics in the horse. IV. Dose and time response relationships for behavioral responses to morphine. meperidine, pentazocine, anileridine, methadone, and hydromorphone. *J Equine Med Surg* 1979; **3**: 377–385.

14 Yoxall AT. Pain in small animals--its recognition and control. *J Small Anim Pract* 1978; **19**(8): 423–438.

15 Day TK, Pepper WT, Tobias TA, *et al.* Comparison of intra-articular and epidural morphine for analgesia following stifle arthrotomy in dogs. *Vet Surg* 1995; **24**(6): 522–530.

16 Sheehy JG, Hellyer PW, Sammonds GE, *et al.* Evaluation of opioid receptors in synovial membranes of horses. *Am J Vet Res* 2001; **62**(9): 1408–1412.

17 Lindegaard C, Gleerup KB, Thomsen MH, *et al.* Anti-inflammatory effects of intra-articular administration of morphine in horses with experimentally induced synovitis. *Am J Vet Res* 2010; **71**(1): 69–75.

18 Lindegaard C, Thomsen MH, Larsen S, *et al.* Analgesic efficacy of intra-articular morphine in experimentally induced radiocarpal synovitis in horses. *Vet Anaesth Analg* 2010; **37**(2): 171–185.

19 Hunter BG, Parker JE, Wehrman R, *et al.* Morphine synovial fluid concentrations after intravenous regional limb perfusion in standing horses. *Vet Surg* 2015; **44**(6): 679–686.
20 Watanabe R, Marcoux J, Evangelista MC, *et al.* The analgesic effects of buprenorphine (Vetergesic or Simbadol) in cats undergoing dental extractions: a randomized, blinded, clinical trial. *PLoS ONE* 2020; **15**(3): e0230079.
21 Enomoto H, Love L, Madsen M, *et al.* Pharmacokinetics of intravenous, oral transmucosal, and intranasal buprenorphine in healthy male dogs. *J Vet Pharmacol Ther* 2022; **45**(4): 358–365.
22 Kyles AE, Hardie EM, Hansen BD, *et al.* Comparison of transdermal fentanyl and intramuscular oxymorphone on post-operative behaviour after ovariohysterectomy in dogs. *Res Vet Sci* 1998; **65**(3): 245–251.
23 Robinson TM, Kruse-Elliott KT, Markel MD, *et al.* A comparison of transdermal fentanyl versus epidural morphine for analgesia in dogs undergoing major orthopedic surgery. *J Am Anim Hosp Assoc* 1999; **35**(2): 95–100.
24 Harvey-Clark CJ, Gilespie K, Riggs KW. Transdermal fentanyl compared with parenteral buprenorphine in post-surgical pain in swine: a case study. *Lab Anim* 2000; **34**(4): 386–398.
25 Christou C, Oliver RA, Rawlinson J, *et al.* Transdermal fentanyl and its use in ovine surgery. *Res Vet Sci* 2015; **100**: 252–256.
26 Carbone ET, Lindstrom KE, Diep S, *et al.* Duration of action of sustained-release buprenorphine in 2 strains of mice. *J Am Assoc Lab Anim Sci* 2012; **51**(6): 815–819.
27 Alamaw ED, Franco BD, Jampachaisri K, *et al.* Extended-release buprenorphine, an FDA-indexed analgesic, attenuates mechanical hypersensitivity in rats (*Rattus norvegicus*). *J Am Assoc Lab Anim Sci* 2022; **61**(1): 81–88.
28 Freise KJ, Linton DD, Newbound GC, *et al.* Population pharmacokinetics of transdermal fentanyl solution following a single dose administered prior to soft tissue and orthopedic surgery in dogs. *J Vet Pharmacol Ther* 2012; **35**(Suppl 2): 65–72.
29 Clark TP, Linton DD, Freise KJ, *et al.* Multicentered masked placebo-controlled phase 3 clinical study of an extended duration transdermal buprenorphine solution for post-operative pain in cats. *J Vet Pharmacol Ther* 2022; **45**(Suppl 1): S52–S66.
30 Krotscheck U, Boothe DM, Little AA, *et al.* Pharmacokinetics of buprenorphine in a sodium carboxymethylcellulose gel after buccal transmucosal administration in dogs. *Vet Ther* 2010; **11**(3): E1–E8.
31 Presley CC, Lindsley CW. DARK Classics in chemical neuroscience: opium, a historical perspective. *ACS Chem Neurosci* 2018; **9**(10): 2503–2518.
32 Humphreys K, Shover CL, Andrews CM, *et al.* Responding to the opioid crisis in North America and beyond: recommendations of the Stanford-Lancet Commission. *Lancet* 2022; **399**(10324): 555–604.
33 Russell C, Fischer B, Fidalgo TM. Sourcing of opioid analgesics for nonmedical use: are veterinarians the latest frontier? *J Opioid Manag* 2018; **14**(2): 77–79.
34 Mason DS, Tenney L, Hellyer PW, *et al.* Prescription opioid epidemic: do veterinarians have a dog in the fight? *Am J Public Health* 2018; **108**(9): 1162–1163.
35 Kogan L, Hellyer P, Rishniw M, *et al.* The US opioid epidemic and its impact on US general practice veterinarians. *Front Vet Sci* 2019; **6**: 222.
36 Patel FC, Raines JA, Kim RW, *et al.* Veterinarians' attitudes and practices regarding opioid-related vet shopping practices in tri-state Appalachian counties: an exploratory study. *BMC Vet Res* 2020; **16**(1): 210.
37 Chua KP, Perrone J, Redding LE, *et al.* Trends in the number of patients linked to potential vet-shopping behavior in the United States (2014–2019). *Am J Vet Res* 2022; **83**(2): 147–152.
38 Collins LK, Pande LJ, Chung DY, *et al.* Trends in the medical supply of fentanyl and fentanyl analogues: United States, 2006 to 2017. *Prev Med* 2019; **123**: 95–100.
39 Simpson RJ. Prescription drug monitoring programs: applying a one size fits all approach to human and veterinary medical professionals, custom tailoring is needed. *J Anim Environ Law* 2014; **5**: 1–43.
40 Piper BJ, McCall KL, Kogan LR, *et al.* Assessment of controlled substance distribution to U.S. veterinary teaching institutions from 2006 to 2019. *Front Vet Sci* 2020; **7**: 615646.
41 Clarke DL, Drobatz KJ, Korzekwa C, *et al.* Trends in opioid prescribing and dispensing by veterinarians in Pennsylvania. *JAMA Netw Open* 2019; **2**(1): e186950.
42 Hendricks B, Rudisill T, Pesarsick J, *et al.* Prescription drug monitoring program policy reform: human and veterinary practitioner prescribing in West Virginia, 2008–2020. *J Public Health Policy* 2021; **42**(2): 249–257.
43 Richards GC, Aronson JK, Mahtani KR, *et al.* Global, regional, and national consumption of controlled opioids: a cross-sectional study of 214 countries and non-metropolitan territories. *Br J Pain* 2022; **16**(1): 34–40.
44 Lehnus KS, Fordyce PS, McMillan MW. Electronic survey investigating UK veterinarians' perceptions of the potential for veterinary prescription medication misuse or abuse. *Vet Anaesth Analg* 2024; **51**(1): 16–25.
45 Alexander SP, Christopoulos A, Davenport AP, *et al.* The concise guide to pharmacology 2021/22: G protein-coupled receptors. *Br J Pharmacol* 2021; **178**(Suppl 1): S27–S156.
46 Toll L, Bruchas MR, Calo G, *et al.* Nociceptin/Orphanin FQ receptor structure, signaling, ligands, functions, and interactions with opioid systems. *Pharmacol Rev* 2016; **68**(2): 419–457.
47 Pan HL, Wu ZZ, Zhou HY, *et al.* Modulation of pain transmission by G-protein-coupled receptors. *Pharmacol Ther* 2008; **117**(1): 141–161.
48 Stoeber M, Jullié D, Lobingier BT, *et al.* A genetically encoded biosensor reveals location bias of opioid drug action. *Neuron* 2018; **98**(5): 963–976.
49 Zaki PA, Bilsky EJ, Vanderah TW, *et al.* Opioid receptor types and subtypes: the delta receptor as a model. *Annu Rev Pharmacol Toxicol* 1996; **36**: 379–401.
50 Dietis N, Rowbotham DJ, Lambert DG. Opioid receptor subtypes: fact or artifact? *Br J Anaesth* 2011; **107**(1): 8–18.
51 Cox BM, Christie MJ, Devi L, *et al.* Challenges for opioid receptor nomenclature: IUPHAR Review 9. *Br J Pharmacol* 2015; **172**(2): 317–323.
52 Valentino RJ, Volkow ND. Untangling the complexity of opioid receptor function. *Neuropsychopharmacol* 2018; **43**(13): 2514–2520.
53 Hawley AT, Wetmore LA. Identification of single nucleotide polymorphisms within exon 1 of the canine mu-opioid receptor gene. *Vet Anaesth Analg* 2010; **37**(1): 79–82.
54 Kubinyi E, Bence M, Koller D, *et al.* Oxytocin and opioid receptor gene polymorphisms associated with greeting behavior in dogs. *Front Psychol* 2017; **8**: 1520.
55 Hellyer PW, Bai L, Supon J, *et al.* Comparison of opioid and alpha-2 adrenergic receptor binding in horse and dog brain using radioligand autoradiography. *Vet Anaesth Analg* 2003; **30**(3): 172–182.
56 Brandt SA, Livingston A. Receptor changes in the spinal cord of sheep associated with exposure to chronic pain. *Pain* 1990; **42**(3): 323–329.
57 Celik M, Labuz D, Henning K, *et al.* Leukocyte opioid receptors mediate analgesia via Ca(2+)-regulated release of opioid peptides. *Brain Behav Immun* 2016; **57**: 227–242.
58 Simon BT, Steagall PV, Monteiro BP, *et al.* Antinociceptive effects of intravenous administration of hydromorphone hydrochloride alone or followed by buprenorphine hydrochloride or butorphanol tartrate to healthy conscious cats. *Am J Vet Res* 2016; **77**(3): 245–251.
59 Hansford J, Henao-Guerrero N, Machado ML, *et al.* Pharmacokinetics of a high-concentration formulation of buprenorphine (Simbadol) in male dogs. *Vet Anaesth Analg* 2021; **48**(4): 509–516.
60 Pfeffer M, Smyth RD, Pittman KA, *et al.* Pharmacokinetics of subcutaneous and intramuscular butorphanol in dogs. *J Pharm Sci* 1980; **69**(7): 801–803.
61 Sano T, Nishimura R, Kanazawa H, *et al.* Pharmacokinetics of fentanyl after single intravenous injection and constant rate infusion in dogs. *Vet Anaesth Analg* 2006; **33**(4): 266–273.
62 KuKanich B, Hogan BK, Krugner-Higby LA, *et al.* Pharmacokinetics of hydromorphone hydrochloride in healthy dogs. *Vet Anaesth Analg* 2008; **35**(3): 256–264.
63 Kalthum W, Waterman AE. The pharmacokinetics of intravenous pethidine HCl in dogs: normal and surgical cases. *J Vet Anaesth* 1988; **15**: 39–55.
64 Barnhart MD, Hubbell JA, Muir WW, *et al.* Pharmacokinetics, pharmacodynamics, and analgesic effects of morphine after rectal, intramuscular, and intravenous administration in dogs. *Am J Vet Res* 2000; **61**(1): 24–28.
65 Giorgi M, Meizler A, Mills PC. Pharmacokinetics of the novel atypical opioid tapentadol following oral and intravenous administration in dogs. *Vet J* 2012; **194**(3): 309–313.
66 Giorgi M, Del Carlo S, Łebkowska-Wieruszewska B, *et al.* Pharmacokinetics of tramadol and metabolites after injective administrations in dogs. *Pol J Vet Sci* 2010; **13**(4): 639–644.
67 Kukanich B, Papich MG. Pharmacokinetics and antinociceptive effects of oral tramadol hydrochloride administration in Greyhounds. *Am J Vet Res* 2011; **72**(2): 256–262.
68 Taylor PM, Robertson SA, Dixon MJ, *et al.* Morphine, pethidine and buprenorphine disposition in the cat. *J Vet Pharmacol Ther* 2001; **24**(6): 391–398.
69 Doodnaught GM, Monteiro BP, Benito J, *et al.* Pharmacokinetic and pharmacodynamic modelling after subcutaneous, intravenous and buccal administration of a high-concentration formulation of buprenorphine in conscious cats. *PLoS ONE* 2017; **12**(4): e0176443.
70 Wells SM, Glerum LE, Papich MG. Pharmacokinetics of butorphanol in cats after intramuscular and buccal transmucosal administration. *Am J Vet Res* 2008; **69**(12): 1548–1554.
71 Lee DD, Papich MG, Hardie EM. Comparison of pharmacokinetics of fentanyl after intravenous and transdermal administration in cats. *Am J Vet Res* 2000; **61**(6): 672–677.
72 Pypendop BH, Brosnan RJ, Siao KT, *et al.* Pharmacokinetics of remifentanil in conscious cats and cats anesthetized with isoflurane. *Am J Vet Res* 2008; **69**(4): 531–536.
73 Lee HK, Łebkowska-Wieruszewska B, Kim TW, *et al.* Pharmacokinetics of the novel atypical opioid tapentadol after intravenous, intramuscular and subcutaneous administration in cats. *Vet J* 2013; **198**(3): 620–624.
74 Pypendop BH, Ilkiw JE. Pharmacokinetics of tramadol, and its metabolite O-desmethyl-tramadol, in cats. *J Vet Pharmacol Ther* 2008; **31**(1): 52–59.
75 Davis JL, Messenger KM, LaFevers DH, *et al.* Pharmacokinetics of intravenous and intramuscular buprenorphine in the horse. *J Vet Pharmacol Ther* 2012; **35**(1): 52–58.

76 Flynn H, Cenani A, Brosnan RJ, *et al.* Pharmacokinetics and pharmacodynamics of a high concentration of buprenorphine (Simbadol) in conscious horses after subcutaneous administration. *Vet Anaesth Analg* 2021; **48**(4): 585–595.

77 Knych HK, Casbeer HC, McKemie DS, *et al.* Pharmacokinetics and pharmacodynamics of butorphanol following intravenous administration to the horse. *J Vet Pharmacol Ther* 2013; **36**(1): 21–30.

78 Knych HK, Stucker K, Gretler SR, *et al.* Pharmacokinetics, adverse effects and effects on thermal nociception following administration of three doses of codeine to horses. *BMC Vet Res* 2022; **18**(1): 196.

79 Reed R, Barletta M, Mitchell K, *et al.* The pharmacokinetics and pharmacodynamics of intravenous hydromorphone in horses. *Vet Anaesth Analg* 2019; **46**(3): 395–404.

80 Reed RA, Knych HK, Barletta M, *et al.* Pharmacokinetics and pharmacodynamics of hydromorphone after intravenous and intramuscular administration in horses. *Vet Anaesth Analg* 2020; **47**(2): 210–218.

81 Knych HK, Kanarr K, Fang Y, *et al.* Characterization of the pharmacokinetics, behavioral effects and effects on thermal nociception of morphine 6-glucuronide and morphine 3-glucuronide in horses. *Vet Anaesth Analg* 2022; **49**(6): 634–644.

82 Devine EP, KuKanich B, Beard WL. Pharmacokinetics of intramuscularly administered morphine in horses. *J Am Vet Med Assoc* 2013; **243**(1): 105–112.

83 Shilo Y, Britzi M, Eytan B, *et al.* Pharmacokinetics of tramadol in horses after intravenous, intramuscular and oral administration. *J Vet Pharmacol Ther* 2008; **31**(1): 60–65.

84 Court MH, Dodman NH, Levine HD, *et al.* Pharmacokinetics and milk residues of butorphanol in dairy cows after single intravenous administration. *J Vet Pharmacol Ther* 1992; **15**(1): 28–35.

85 Smith JS, Coetzee JF, Fisher IWG, *et al.* Pharmacokinetics of fentanyl citrate and norfentanyl in Holstein calves and effect of analytical performances on fentanyl parameter estimation. *J Vet Pharmacol Ther* 2018; **41**(4): 555–561.

86 Bussières G, Smith J, Cox S, *et al.* Pharmacokinetics of morphine and plasma concentrations of morphine-6-glucuronide after a single intravenous and intramuscular administration in the cow. *Vet Anaesth Analg* 2023; **50**(1): 107.e101.

87 Coetzee JF, Lechtenberg KF, Stock ML, *et al.* Pharmacokinetics and effect of intravenous nalbuphine in weaned Holstein calves after surgical castration. *J Vet Pharmacol Ther* 2014; **37**(2): 169–177.

88 Hakomäki H, Kokki H, Lehtonen M, *et al.* Pharmacokinetics of buprenorphine in pregnant sheep after intravenous injection. *Pharmacol Res Perspect* 2021; **9**(2): e00726.

89 Ahern BJ, Soma LR, Rudy JA, *et al.* Pharmacokinetics of fentanyl administered transdermally and intravenously in sheep. *Am J Vet Res* 2010; **71**(10): 1127–1132.

90 Bengtsson J, Ederoth P, Ley D, *et al.* The influence of age on the distribution of morphine and morphine-3-glucuronide across the blood–brain barrier in sheep. *Br J Pharmacol* 2009; **157**(6): 1085–1096.

91 Kinnunen M, Kokki H, Hautajärvi H, *et al.* Oxycodone pharmacokinetics and fetal exposure after intravenous or epidural administration to the ewe. *Acta Obstet Gynecol Scand* 2018; **97**(10): 1200–1205.

92 Bortolami E, Della Rocca G, Di Salvo A, *et al.* Pharmacokinetics and antinociceptive effects of tramadol and its metabolite O-desmethyltramadol following intravenous administration in sheep. *Vet J* 2015; **205**(3): 404–409.

93 Carroll GL, Boothe DM, Hartsfield SM, *et al.* Pharmacokinetics and selected behavioral responses to butorphanol and its metabolites in goats following intravenous and intramuscular administration. *Vet Anaesth Analg* 2001; **28**(4): 188–195.

94 Carroll GL, Hooper RN, Boothe DM, *et al.* Pharmacokinetics of fentanyl after intravenous and transdermal administration in goats. *Am J Vet Res* 1999; **60**(8): 986–991.

95 Gordon E, Dirikolu L, Liu CC, *et al.* Pharmacokinetic profiles of three dose rates of morphine sulfate following single intravenous, intramuscular, and subcutaneous administration in the goat. *J Vet Pharmacol Ther* 2022; **45**(1): 107–116.

96 Lavy E, Lee HK, Mabjeesh SJ, *et al.* Use of the novel atypical opioid tapentadol in goats (Capra hircus): pharmacokinetics after intravenous, and intramuscular administration. *J Vet Pharmacol Ther* 2014; **37**(5): 518–521.

97 de Sousa AB, Santos AC, Schramm SG, *et al.* Pharmacokinetics of tramadol and O-desmethyltramadol in goats after intravenous and oral administration. *J Vet Pharmacol Ther* 2008; **31**(1): 45–51.

98 Robertson SA, Wegner K, Lascelles BD. Antinociceptive and side-effects of hydromorphone after subcutaneous administration in cats. *J Feline Med Surg* 2009; **11**(2): 76–81.

99 Giordano T, Steagall PV, Ferreira TH, *et al.* Postoperative analgesic effects of intravenous, intramuscular, subcutaneous or oral transmucosal buprenorphine administered to cats undergoing ovariohysterectomy. *Vet Anaesth Analg* 2010; **37**(4): 357–366.

100 Kukanich B, Lascelles BD, Aman AM, *et al.* The effects of inhibiting cytochrome P450 3A, P-glycoprotein, and gastric acid secretion on the oral bioavailability of methadone in dogs. *J Vet Pharmacol Ther* 2005; **28**(5): 461–466.

101 Messenger KM, Davis JL, LaFevers DH, *et al.* Intravenous and sublingual buprenorphine in horses: pharmacokinetics and influence of sampling site. *Vet Anaesth Analg* 2011; **38**(4): 374–384.

102 Buchholz T, Hildebrand M, Heider A, *et al.* Transdermal fentanyl uptake at two different patch locations in Swiss White Alpine sheep. *Animals (Basel)* 2020; **10**(9): 1675.

103 Murrell JC, Robertson SA, Taylor PM, *et al.* Use of a transdermal matrix patch of buprenorphine in cats: preliminary pharmacokinetic and pharmacodynamic data. *Vet Rec* 2007; **160**(17): 578–583.

104 Freise KJ, Reinemeyer C, Warren K, *et al.* Single-dose pharmacokinetics and bioavailability of a novel extended duration transdermal buprenorphine solution in cats. *J Vet Pharmacol Ther* 2022; **45**(Suppl 1): S31–S39.

105 Natalini CC, Robinson EP. Evaluation of the analgesic effects of epidurally administered morphine, alfentanil, butorphanol, tramadol, and U50488H in horses. *Am J Vet Res* 2000; **61**(12): 1579–1586.

106 Natalini CC. Plasma and cerebrospinal fluid alfentanil, butorphanol, and morphine concentrations following caudal epidural administration in horses. *Ciência Rural* 2006; **36**: 1436–1443.

107 Castro-Cuellar G, Cremer J, Queiroz-Williams P, *et al.* Pharmacokinetics of intra-articular buprenorphine in horses with lipopolysaccharide-induced synovitis. *J Vet Pharmacol Ther* 2023; **46**(4): 229–237.

108 Long WM, Sinnott VB, Bracker K, *et al.* Use of 20% intravenous lipid emulsion for the treatment of loperamide toxicosis in a Collie homozygous for the ABCB1-1Δ mutation. *J Vet Emerg Crit Care (San Antonio)* 2017; **27**(3): 357–361.

109 Kongara K. Pharmacogenetics of opioid analgesics in dogs. *J Vet Pharmacol Ther* 2018; **41**(2): 195–204.

110 Golub MS, Eisele JH Jr., Anderson JH. Maternal-fetal distribution of morphine and alfentanil in near-term sheep and rhesus monkeys. *Dev Pharmacol Ther* 1986; **9**(1): 12–22.

111 Burns SM, Cunningham CW, Mercer SL. DARK classics in chemical neuroscience: fentanyl. *ACS Chem Neurosci* 2018; **9**(10): 2428–2437.

112 MacKenzie M, Zed PJ, Ensom MH. Opioid pharmacokinetics-pharmacodynamics: clinical implications in acute pain management in trauma. *Ann Pharmacother* 2016; **50**(3): 209–218.

113 Steagall PVM, Simon BT, Teixeira-Neto FJ, *et al.* An update on drugs used for lumbosacral epidural anesthesia and analgesia in dogs. *Front Vet Sci* 2017; **4**: 68.

114 Wu WN, McKown LA, Gauthier AD, *et al.* Metabolism of the analgesic drug, tramadol hydrochloride, in rat and dog. *Xenobiotica* 2001; **31**(7): 423–441.

115 Yeh SY, Chernov HI, Woods LA. Metabolism of morphine by cats. *J Pharm Sci* 1971; **60**(3): 469–471.

116 Giorgi M, Del Carlo S, Saccomanni G, *et al.* Pharmacokinetics of tramadol and its major metabolites following rectal and intravenous administration in dogs. *N Z Vet J* 2009; **57**(3): 146–152.

117 Richards J, Miksys S, Novalen M, *et al.* CYP2D in the brain impacts oral hydrocodone analgesia *in vivo*. *Neuropharmacol* 2022; **221**: 109291.

118 Perez Jimenez TE, Kukanich B, Joo H, *et al.* Oral coadministration of fluconazole with tramadol markedly increases plasma and urine concentrations of tramadol and the O-desmethyltramadol metabolite in healthy dogs. *Drug Metab Dispos* 2019; **47**(1): 15–25.

119 KuKanich B, KuKanich K, Black J. The effects of ketoconazole and cimetidine on the pharmacokinetics of oral tramadol in greyhound dogs. *J Vet Pharmacol Ther* 2017; **40**(6): e54–e61.

120 Giorgi M, MacCheroni M, Del Carlo S, *et al.* Effect of oral co-administration of frozen-dried grapefruit juice on pharmacokinetics of tramadol in dogs. *Iran J Vet Res* 2011; **12**: 8–15.

121 Dean M. Opioids in renal failure and dialysis patients. *J Pain Symptom Manage* 2004; **28**(5): 497–504.

122 Kosten TR, George TP. The neurobiology of opioid dependence: implications for treatment. *Sci Pract Perspect* 2002; **1**(1): 13–20.

123 Khan F, Mehan A. Addressing opioid tolerance and opioid-induced hypersensitivity: recent developments and future therapeutic strategies. *Pharmacol Res Perspect* 2021; **9**(3): e00789.

124 Anonymous. General behavior of dogs, rats and cats in morphine tolerance and withdrawal. *Acta Physiol Scand* 1963; **58**(s204): 30–38.

125 Yoshimura K, Horiuchi M, Konishi M, *et al.* Physical dependence on morphine induced in dogs via the use of miniosmotic pumps. *J Pharmacol Toxicol Methods* 1993; **30**(2): 85–95.

126 French ED, Vasquez SA, George R. Behavioral changes produced in the cat by acute and chronic morphine injection and naloxone precipitated withdrawal. *Eur J Pharmacol* 1979; **57**(4): 387–397.

127 Barr MC, Huitron-Resendiz S, Sanchez-Alavez M, *et al.* Escalating morphine exposures followed by withdrawal in feline immunodeficiency virus-infected cats: a model for HIV infection in chronic opiate abusers. *Drug Alcohol Depend* 2003; **72**(2): 141–149.

128 Kilbey MM, Ellinwood EH Jr. Self-administration of morphine in the cat. *Int J Addict* 1980; **15**(3): 447–460.

129 Albutt C. On the abuse of hypodermic injections of morphia. *Practitioner* 1870; **5**: 327–331.

130 Chu LF, Clark DJ, Angst MS. Opioid tolerance and hyperalgesia in chronic pain patients after one month of oral morphine therapy: a preliminary prospective study. *J Pain* 2006; **7**(1): 43–48.

131 Lee M, Silverman SM, Hansen H, *et al.* A comprehensive review of opioid-induced hyperalgesia. *Pain Physician* 2011; **14**(2): 145–161.

132 Ferrini F, Trang T, Mattioli TA, *et al.* Morphine hyperalgesia gated through microglia-mediated disruption of neuronal Cl^- homeostasis. *Nat Neurosci* 2013; **16**(2): 183–192.

133 Kamerling SG, Martin WR, Wu KM, *et al.* Medullary kappa hyperalgesic mechanisms II. The effects of ethylketazocine administered into the fourth cerebral ventricle of the conscious dog. *Life Sci* 1983; **33**(18): 1839–1843.

134 Wu KM, Martin WR, Kamerling SG, *et al.* Possible medullary kappa hyperalgesic mechanism. I. A new potential role for endogenous opioid peptides in pain perception. *Life Sci* 1983; **33**(18): 1831–1838.

135 Hughes RA. Codeine analgesic and morphine hyperalgesic effects on thermal nociception in domestic fowl. *Pharmacol Biochem Behav* 1990; **35**(3): 567–570.

136 Gruen ME, Lascelles BDX, Colleran E, *et al.* 2022 AAHA Pain management guidelines for dogs and cats. *J Am Anim Hosp Assoc* 2022; **58**(2): 55–76.

137 Steagall PV, Robertson S, Simon B, *et al.* 2022 ISFM Consensus guidelines on the management of acute pain in cats. *J Feline Med Surg* 2022; **24**(1): 4–30.

138 Finkel JC, Pukish J. Molecular biology of opioid analgesia and its clinical considerations. *Clin J Pain* 2019; **35**(6): 473–480.

139 Mansour A, Fox CA, Thompson RC, *et al.* mu-Opioid receptor mRNA expression in the rat CNS: comparison to mu-receptor binding. *Brain Res* 1994; **643**(1–2): 245–265.

140 Stein C. Opioid receptors. *Annu Rev Med* 2016; **67**: 433–451.

141 Go VL, Yaksh TL. Release of substance P from the cat spinal cord. *J Physiol* 1987; **391**: 141–167.

142 Fields H. State-dependent opioid control of pain. *Nat Rev Neurosci* 2004; **5**(7): 565–575.

143 Stein C. The control of pain in peripheral tissue by opioids. *N Engl J Med* 1995; **332**(25): 1685–1690.

144 Keates HL, Cramond T, Smith MT. Intraarticular and periarticular opioid binding in inflamed tissue in experimental canine arthritis. *Anesth Analg* 1999; **89**(2): 409–415.

145 Zollner C, Shaqura MA, Bopaiah CP, *et al.* Painful inflammation-induced increase in mu-opioid receptor binding and G-protein coupling in primary afferent neurons. *Mol Pharmacol* 2003; **64**(2): 202–210.

146 Busch-Dienstfertig M, Stein C. Opioid receptors and opioid peptide-producing leukocytes in inflammatory pain--basic and therapeutic aspects. *Brain Behav Immun* 2010; **24**(5): 683–694.

147 Machelska H. Dual peripheral actions of immune cells in neuropathic pain. *Arch Immunol Ther Exp (Warsz)* 2011; **59**(1): 11–24.

148 Potter JJ, MacFarlane PD, Love EJ, *et al.* Preliminary investigation comparing a detomidine continuous rate infusion combined with either morphine or buprenorphine for standing sedation in horses. *Vet Anaesth Analg* 2016; **43**(2): 189–194.

149 Shah MD, Yates D, Hunt J, *et al.* A comparison between methadone and buprenorphine for perioperative analgesia in dogs undergoing ovariohysterectomy. *J Small Anim Pract* 2018; **59**(9): 539–546.

150 Shah M, Yates D, Hunt J, *et al.* Comparison between methadone and buprenorphine within the QUAD protocol for perioperative analgesia in cats undergoing ovariohysterectomy. *J Feline Med Surg* 2019; **21**(8): 723–731.

151 Freitas GC, Carregaro AB, Gehrcke MI, *et al.* Epidural analgesia with morphine or buprenorphine in ponies with lipopolysaccharide (LPS)-induced carpal synovitis. *Can J Vet Res* 2011; **75**(2): 141–146.

152 Warne LN, Beths T, Holm M, *et al.* Comparison of perioperative analgesic efficacy between methadone and butorphanol in cats. *J Am Vet Med Assoc* 2013; **243**(6): 844–850.

153 Warne LN, Beths T, Holm M, *et al.* Evaluation of the perioperative analgesic efficacy of buprenorphine, compared with butorphanol, in cats. *J Am Vet Med Assoc* 2014; **245**(2): 195–202.

154 Rigotti C, De Vries A, Taylor PM. Buprenorphine provides better anaesthetic conditions than butorphanol for field castration in ponies: results of a randomised clinical trial. *Vet Rec* 2014; **175**(24): 623.

155 Taylor PM, Hoare HR, de Vries A, *et al.* A multicentre, prospective, randomised, blinded clinical trial to compare some perioperative effects of buprenorphine or butorphanol premedication before equine elective general anaesthesia and surgery. *Equine Vet J* 2016; **48**(4): 442–450.

156 Nielsen S, Rivas C, Demirkol A, *et al.* Effects of ascending buprenorphine doses on measures of experimental pain: a pilot study. *J Subst Abuse Treat* 2019; **104**: 128–134.

157 Dahan A, Yassen A, Romberg R, *et al.* Buprenorphine induces ceiling in respiratory depression but not in analgesia. *Br J Anaesth* 2006; **96**(5): 627–632.

158 Zola EM, McLeod DC. Comparative effects and analgesic efficacy of the agonist-antagonist opioids. *Drug Intell Clin Pharm* 1983; **17**(6): 411–417.

159 Pircio AW, Gylys JA, Cavanagh RL, *et al.* The pharmacology of butorphanol, a 3,14-dihydroxymorphinan narcotic antagonist analgesic. *Arch Int Pharmacodyn Ther* 1976; **220**(2): 231–257.

160 Talbert RL, Peters JI, Sorrells SC, *et al.* Respiratory effects of high-dose butorphanol. *Acute Care* 1988; **12**(Suppl 1): 47–56.

161 Monteiro ER, Rabello TA, Rangel JPP, *et al.* Effects of 3 morphine doses, in combination with acepromazine, on sedation and some physiological parameters in dogs. *Can J Vet Res* 2019; **83**(3): 235–240.

162 Monteiro ER, Junior AR, Assis HM, *et al.* Comparative study on the sedative effects of morphine, methadone, butorphanol or tramadol, in combination with acepromazine, in dogs. *Vet Anaesth Analg* 2009; **36**(1): 25–33.

163 Gomes VH, Oliveira RL, Marques JL, *et al.* Comparison of the sedative effects of nalbuphine and butorphanol, alone or in combination with acepromazine in dogs. *Vet Anaesth Analg* 2018; **45**(1): 68–72.

164 Paqueron X, Lumbroso A, Mergoni P, *et al.* Is morphine-induced sedation synonymous with analgesia during intravenous morphine titration? *Br J Anaesth* 2002; **89**(5): 697–701.

165 Lentschener C, Tostivint P, White PF, *et al.* Opioid-induced sedation in the postanesthesia care unit does not insure adequate pain relief: a case-control study. *Anesth Analg* 2007; **105**(4): 1143–1147.

166 Kellihan HB, Stepien RL, Hassen KM, *et al.* Sedative and echocardiographic effects of dexmedetomidine combined with butorphanol in healthy dogs. *J Vet Cardiol* 2015; **17**(4): 282–292.

167 Santarelli G, López JT, Del Palacio JF. Effects of a combination of acepromazine maleate and butorphanol tartrate on conventional and two-dimensional speckle tracking echocardiography in healthy dogs. *Am J Vet Res* 2017; **78**(2): 158–167.

168 Fernández Castañer J, Quirós Carmona S, Martínez Bernal C, *et al.* Sedation quality and cardiorespiratory, echocardiographic, radiographic and electrocardiographic effects of intramuscular alfaxalone and butorphanol in Spanish Greyhound dogs. *Animals (Basel)* 2023; **13**(18): 2937.

169 Ward JL, Schober KE, Fuentes VL, *et al.* Effects of sedation on echocardiographic variables of left atrial and left ventricular function in healthy cats. *J Feline Med Surg* 2012; **14**(10): 678–685.

170 Ribas T, Bublot I, Junot S, *et al.* Effects of intramuscular sedation with alfaxalone and butorphanol on echocardiographic measurements in healthy cats. *J Feline Med Surg* 2015; **17**(6): 530–536.

171 Reader RC, Barton BA, Abelson AL. Comparison of two intramuscular sedation protocols on sedation, recovery and ease of venipuncture for cats undergoing blood donation. *J Feline Med Surg* 2019; **21**(2): 95–102.

172 Reader RC, Yang VK, Babyak JM, *et al.* The effects of two intramuscular sedation protocols on echocardiographic variables in cats following sedation and blood donation. *J Vet Emerg Crit Care* 2021; **31**(2): 256–262.

173 Young-McCaughan S, Miaskowski C. Definition of and mechanism for opioid-induced sedation. *Pain Manag Nurs* 2001; **2**(3): 84–97.

174 Martin WR. Pharmacology of opioids. *Pharmacol Rev* 1983; **35**(4): 283–323.

175 Arankowsky-Sandoval G, Gold PE. Morphine-induced deficits in sleep patterns: attenuation by glucose. *Neurobiol Learn Mem* 1995; **64**(2): 133–138.

176 Cronin A, Keifer JC, Baghdoyan HA, *et al.* Opioid inhibition of rapid eye movement sleep by a specific mu receptor agonist. *Br J Anaesth* 1995; **74**(2): 188–192.

177 Danneman PJ. Cortical potentials evoked by tooth pulp stimulation differentiate between the analgesic and sedative effects of morphine in awake rats. *J Pharmacol Exp Ther* 1994; **269**(3): 1100–1106.

178 Banning A, Sjøgren P. Cerebral effects of long-term oral opioids in cancer patients measured by continuous reaction time. *Clin J Pain* 1990; **6**(2): 91–95.

179 Lorenz J, Beck H, Bromm B. Cognitive performance, mood and experimental pain before and during morphine-induced analgesia in patients with chronic non-malignant pain. *Pain* 1997; **73**(3): 369–375.

180 Lorenz J, Beck H, Bromm B. Differential changes of laser evoked potentials, late auditory evoked potentials and P300 under morphine in chronic pain patients. *Electroencephalogr Clin Neurophysiol* 1997; **104**(6): 514–521.

181 Moreno KL, Scallan EM, Monteiro BP, *et al.* The thermal antinociceptive effects of a high-concentration formulation of buprenorphine alone or followed by hydromorphone in conscious cats. *Vet Anaesth Analg* 2021; **48**(4): 570–576.

182 Robertson SA, Taylor PM, Lascelles BD, *et al.* Changes in thermal threshold response in eight cats after administration of buprenorphine, butorphanol and morphine. *Vet Rec* 2003; **153**(15): 462–465.

183 Lascelles BD, Robertson SA. Antinociceptive effects of hydromorphone, butorphanol, or the combination in cats. *J Vet Intern Med* 2004; **18**(2): 190–195.

184 Dhasmana KM, Dixit KS, Jaju BP, *et al.* Role of central dopaminergic receptors in manic response of cats to morphine. *Psychopharmacologia* 1972; **24**(3): 380–383.

185 Fertziger AP, Stein EA, Lynch JJ. Letter: suppression of morphine-induced mania in cats. *Psychopharmacologia* 1974; **36**(2): 185–187.

186 Villablanca JR, Harris CM, Burgess JW, *et al.* Reassessing morphine effects in cats: I. Specific behavioral responses in intact and unilaterally brain-lesioned animals. *Pharmacol Biochem Behav* 1984; **21**(6): 913–921.

187 Lucas AN, Firth AM, Anderson GA, *et al.* Comparison of the effects of morphine administered by constant-rate intravenous infusion or intermittent intramuscular injection in dogs. *J Am Vet Med Assoc* 2001; **218**(6): 884–891.

188 Becker WM, Mama KR, Rao S, *et al.* Prevalence of dysphoria after fentanyl in dogs undergoing stifle surgery. *Vet Surg* 2013; **42**(3): 302–307.

189 Jarosinski SK, Simon BT, Baetge CL, *et al.* The effects of prophylactic dexmedetomidine administration on general anesthesia recovery quality in healthy dogs anesthetized with sevoflurane and a fentanyl constant rate infusion undergoing elective orthopedic procedures. *Front Vet Sci* 2021; **8**: 722038.

190 Mama KR, Pascoe PJ, Steffey EP. Evaluation of the interaction of mu and kappa opioid agonists on locomotor behavior in the horse. *Can J Vet Res* 1993; **57**(2): 106–109.

191 Kamerling SG, DeQuick DJ, Weckman TJ, *et al.* Dose-related effects of fentanyl on autonomic and behavioral responses in performance horses. *Gen Pharmacol* 1985; **16**(3): 253–258.

192 Szöke MO, Blais D, Cuvelliez SG, *et al.* Effects of buprenorphine on cardiovascular and pulmonary function in clinically normal horses and horses with chronic obstructive pulmonary disease. *Am J Vet Res* 1998; **59**(10): 1287–1291.

193 Combie J, Shults T, Nugent EC, *et al.* Pharmacology of narcotic analgesics in the horse: selective blockade of narcotic-induced locomotor activity. *Am J Vet Res* 1981; **42**(5): 716–721.

194 Clutton RE. Opioid analgesia in horses. *Vet Clin North Am Equine Pract* 2010; **26**(3): 493–514.

195 Tobin T, Combie J, Miller JR, *et al.* The pharmacology of narcotic analgesics in the horse. II. Studies on the detection, pharmacokinetics, urinary clearance times and behavioral effects of pentazocine and fentanyl in the horse. *Irish Vet J* 1979; **33**: 169–176.

196 Grint NJ, Burford J, Dugdale AH. Does pethidine affect the cardiovascular and sedative effects of dexmedetomidine in dogs? *J Small Anim Pract* 2009; **50**(2): 62–66.

197 Garofalo NA, Teixeira-Neto FJ, Pereira CD, *et al.* Cardiorespiratory and neuroendocrine changes induced by methadone in conscious and in isoflurane anaesthetised dogs. *Vet J* 2012; **194**(3): 398–404.

198 Arnold RW, Jansen S, Seelig JC, *et al.* Anesthetic impacts on the oculocardiac reflex: evidence from a large, observational study. *Clin Ophthalmol* 2021; **15**: 973–981.

199 de Burgh Daly M, Korner PI, Angell-James JE, *et al.* Cardiovascular and respiratory effects of carotid body stimulation in the monkey. *Clin Exp Pharmacol Physiol* 1978; **5**(5): 511–524.

200 Lichtenwalner MR, Mencken T, Tully R, *et al.* False-positive immunochemical screen for methadone attributable to metabolites of verapamil. *Clin Chem* 1998; **44**(5): 1039–1041.

201 Yang JC, Shan J, Ng KF, *et al.* Morphine and methadone have different effects on calcium channel currents in neuroblastoma cells. *Brain Res* 2000; **870**(1–2): 199–203.

202 Latta KS, Ginsberg B, Barkin RL. Meperidine: a critical review. *Am J Ther* 2002; **9**(1): 53–68.

203 Maiante AA, Teixeira-Neto FJ, Beier SL, *et al.* Comparison of the cardio-respiratory effects of methadone and morphine in conscious dogs. *J Vet Pharmacol Ther* 2009; **32**(4): 317–328.

204 Greene SA, Hartsfield SM, Tyner CL. Cardiovascular effects of butorphanol in halothane-anesthetized dogs. *Am J Vet Res* 1990; **51**(8): 1276–1279.

205 Priano LL, Vatner SF. Generalized cardiovascular and regional hemodynamic effects of meperidine in conscious dogs. *Anesth Analg* 1981; **60**(9): 649–654.

206 Keating S, Fries R, Kling K, *et al.* Effect of methadone or hydromorphone on cardiac conductivity in dogs before and during sevoflurane anesthesia. *Front Vet Sci* 2020; **7**: 573706.

207 Lin C, Somberg T, Molnar J, *et al.* The effects of chiral isolates of methadone on the cardiac potassium channel IKr. *Cardiology* 2009; **113**(1): 59–65.

208 Stanley TH, Liu WS, Webster LR, *et al.* Haemodynamic effects of intravenous methadone anaesthesia in dogs. *Can Anaesth Soc J* 1980; **27**(1): 52–57.

209 Pelligrino DA, Peterson RD, Henderson SK, *et al.* Comparative ventilatory effects of intravenous versus fourth cerebroventricular infusions of morphine sulfate in the unanesthetized dog. *Anesthesiology* 1989; **71**(2): 250–259.

210 Palkovic B, Marchenko V, Zuperku EJ, *et al.* Multi-level regulation of opioid-induced respiratory depression. *Physiology (Bethesda)* 2020; **35**(6): 391–404.

211 Berg RJ, Orton EC. Pulmonary function in dogs after intercostal thoracotomy: comparison of morphine, oxymorphone, and selective intercostal nerve block. *Am J Vet Res* 1986; **47**(2): 471–474.

212 Campbell VL, Drobatz KJ, Perkowski SZ. Postoperative hypoxemia and hypercarbia in healthy dogs undergoing routine ovariohysterectomy or castration and receiving butorphanol or hydromorphone for analgesia. *J Am Vet Med Assoc* 2003; **222**(3): 330–336.

213 Wunsch LA, Schmidt BK, Krugner-Higby LA, *et al.* A comparison of the effects of hydromorphone HCl and a novel extended release hydromorphone on arterial blood gas values in conscious healthy dogs. *Res Vet Sci* 2010; **88**(1): 154–158.

214 Dahan A, van Lemmen M, Jansen S, *et al.* Buprenorphine: a treatment and cause of opioid-induced respiratory depression. *Br J Anaesth* 2022; **128**(3): 402–404.

215 Trim CM. Cardiopulmonary effects of butorphanol tartrate in dogs. *Am J Vet Res* 1983; **44**(2): 329–331.

216 Dahan A, Romberg R, Teppema L, *et al.* Simultaneous measurement and integrated analysis of analgesia and respiration after an intravenous morphine infusion. *Anesthesiology* 2004; **101**(5): 1201–1209.

217 Dyson DH, Doherty T, Anderson GI, *et al.* Reversal of oxymorphone sedation by naloxone, nalmefene, and butorphanol. *Vet Surg* 1990; **19**(5): 398–403.

218 McCrackin MA, Harvey RC, Sackman JE, *et al.* Butorphanol tartrate for partial reversal of oxymorphone-induced postoperative respiratory depression in the dog. *Vet Surg* 1994; **23**(1): 67–74.

219 Cashman JN, Dolin SJ. Respiratory and haemodynamic effects of acute postoperative pain management: evidence from published data. *Br J Anaesth* 2004; **93**(2): 212–223.

220 Lötsch J, Dudziak R, Freynhagen R, *et al.* Fatal respiratory depression after multiple intravenous morphine injections. *Clin Pharmacokinet* 2006; **45**(11): 1051–1060.

221 Quintavalla F, Spindler KP, Aldigeri R, *et al.* The effect of different opioids on acid-base balance and blood gas analysis in hospitalized dogs. *Front Vet Sci* 2022; **9**: 802186.

222 Lalley PM. Mu-opioid receptor agonist effects on medullary respiratory neurons in the cat: evidence for involvement in certain types of ventilatory disturbances. *Am J Physiol Regul Integr Comp Physiol* 2003; **285**(6): R1287–R1304.

223 Prkic I, Mustapic S, Radocaj T, *et al.* Pontine μ-opioid receptors mediate bradypnea caused by intravenous remifentanil infusions at clinically relevant concentrations in dogs. *J Neurophysiol* 2012; **108**(9): 2430–2441.

224 Saunders SE, Levitt ES. Kölliker-Fuse/Parabrachial complex mu opioid receptors contribute to fentanyl-induced apnea and respiratory rate depression. *Respir Physiol Neurobiol* 2020; **275**: 103388.

225 DeHaven-Hudkins DL, DeHaven RN, Little PJ, *et al.* The involvement of the mu-opioid receptor in gastrointestinal pathophysiology: therapeutic opportunities for antagonism at this receptor. *Pharmacol Ther* 2008; **117**(1): 162–187.

226 Kromer W. Endogenous and exogenous opioids in the control of gastrointestinal motility and secretion. *Pharmacol Rev* 1988; **40**(2): 121–162.

227 Wood JD, Galligan JJ. Function of opioids in the enteric nervous system. *Neurogastroenterol Motil* 2004; **16**(Suppl 2): 17–28.

228 Sano H, Martín-Flores M, Santos LC, *et al.* Effects of epidural morphine on gastrointestinal transit in unmedicated horses. *Vet Anaesth Analg* 2011; **38**(2): 121–126.

229 Martín-Flores M, Campoy L, Kinsley MA, *et al.* Analgesic and gastrointestinal effects of epidural morphine in horses after laparoscopic cryptorchidectomy under general anesthesia. *Vet Anaesth Analg* 2014; **41**(4): 430–437.

230 Blancquaert JP, Lefebvre RA, Willems JL. Emetic and antiemetic effects of opioids in the dog. *Eur J Pharmacol* 1986; **128**(3): 143–150.

231 Costello DJ, Borison HL. Naloxone antagonizes narcotic self blockade of emesis in the cat. *J Pharmacol Exp Ther* 1977; **203**(1): 222–230.

232 Stern LC, Palmisano MP. Frequency of vomiting during the postoperative period in hydromorphone-treated dogs undergoing orthopedic surgery. *J Am Vet Med Assoc* 2012; **241**(3): 344–347.

233 Barnes NM, Bunce KT, Naylor RJ, *et al.* The actions of fentanyl to inhibit drug-induced emesis. *Neuropharmacol* 1991; **30**(10): 1073–1083.

234 Valverde A, Cantwell S, Hernández J, *et al.* Effects of acepromazine on the incidence of vomiting associated with opioid administration in dogs. *Vet Anaesth Analg* 2004; **31**(1): 40–45.

235 Guedes AG, Papich MG, Rude EP, *et al.* Comparison of plasma histamine levels after intravenous administration of hydromorphone and morphine in dogs. *J Vet Pharmacol Ther* 2007; **30**(6): 516–522.

236 Pettifer G, Dyson D. Hydromorphone: a cost-effective alternative to the use of oxymorphone. *Can Vet J* 2000; **41**(2): 135–137.

237 Simon BT, Scallan EM, Monteiro BP, *et al.* The effects of aging on hydromorphone-induced thermal antinociception in healthy female cats. *Pain Rep* 2019; **4**(2): e722.

238 Pypendop BH, Shilo-Benjamini Y, Ilkiw JE. Effect of morphine, methadone, hydromorphone or oxymorphone on the thermal threshold, following intravenous or buccal administration to cats. *Vet Anaesth Analg* 2016; **43**(6): 635–642.

239 Simon BT, Scallan EM, Baetge CL, *et al.* The antinociceptive effects of intravenous administration of three doses of butorphanol tartrate or naloxone hydrochloride following hydromorphone hydrochloride to healthy conscious cats. *Vet Anaesth Analg* 2019; **46**(4): 538–547.

240 Ingvast-Larsson C, Holgersson A, Bondesson U, *et al.* Clinical pharmacology of methadone in dogs. *Vet Anaesth Analg* 2010; **37**(1): 48–56.

241 Gioeni D, Brioschi FA, Di Cesare F, *et al.* Oral transmucosal or intramuscular administration of dexmedetomidine-methadone combination in dogs: sedative and physiological effects. *Animals (Basel)* 2020; **10**(11): 2057.

242 Wilson DV, Tom Evans A, Mauer WA. Pre-anesthetic meperidine: associated vomiting and gastroesophageal reflux during the subsequent anesthetic in dogs. *Vet Anaesth Analg* 2007; **34**(1): 15–22.

243 Johnson RA. Maropitant prevented vomiting but not gastroesophageal reflux in anesthetized dogs premedicated with acepromazine-hydromorphone. *Vet Anaesth Analg* 2014; **41**(4): 406–410.

244 Koh RB, Isaza N, Xie H, *et al.* Effects of maropitant, acepromazine, and electroacupuncture on vomiting associated with administration of morphine in dogs. *J Am Vet Med Assoc* 2014; **244**(7): 820–829.

245 Lorenzutti AM, Martín-Flores M, Litterio NJ, *et al.* Evaluation of the antiemetic efficacy of maropitant in dogs medicated with morphine and acepromazine. *Vet Anaesth Analg* 2016; **43**(2): 195–198.

246 Scallan EM, Simon BT. The effects of acupuncture point Pericardium 6 on hydromorphone-induced nausea and vomiting in healthy dogs. *Vet Anaesth Analg* 2016; **43**(5): 495–501.

247 Hay Kraus BL. Effect of dosing interval on efficacy of maropitant for prevention of hydromorphone-induced vomiting and signs of nausea in dogs. *J Am Vet Med Assoc* 2014; **245**(9): 1015–1020.

248 Burke JE, Hess RS, Silverstein DC. Effectiveness of orally administered maropitant and ondansetron in preventing preoperative emesis and nausea in healthy dogs premedicated with a combination of hydromorphone, acepromazine, and glycopyrrolate. *J Am Vet Med Assoc* 2021; **260**(S1): S40–S45.

249 Martín-Flores M, Mastrocco A, Lorenzutti AM, *et al.* Maropitant administered orally 2-2.5 h prior to morphine and dexmedetomidine reduces the incidence of emesis in cats. *J Feline Med Surg* 2017; **19**(8): 876–879.

250 Wilson DV, Evans AT, Miller R. Effects of preanesthetic administration of morphine on gastroesophageal reflux and regurgitation during anesthesia in dogs. *Am J Vet Res* 2005; **66**(3): 386–390.

251 Costa RS, Wetmore LA, Stein A. Randomized, blinded, controlled clinical trial to assess gastroesophageal reflux and regurgitation in dogs undergoing general anesthesia after hydromorphone premedication with or without acepromazine or dexmedetomidine. *Am J Vet Res* 2021; **82**(9): 695–700.

252 Kostritsky-Pereira A, Woussen-Colle MC, De Graef J. Effects of morphine, enkephalins and naloxone on postprandial gastric acid secretion, gastric emptying and gastrin release in dogs. *Arch Int Physiol Biochim* 1984; **92**(1): 19–26.

253 Mittal RK, Frank EB, Lange RC, *et al.* Effects of morphine and naloxone on esophageal motility and gastric emptying in man. *Dig Dis Sci* 1986; **31**(9): 936–942.

254 Hall JA, Magne ML, Twedt DC. Effect of acepromazine, diazepam, fentanyl-droperidol, and oxymorphone on gastroesophageal sphincter pressure in healthy dogs. *Am J Vet Res* 1987; **48**(4): 556–557.

255 Garcia RS, Belafsky PC, Della Maggiore A, *et al.* Prevalence of gastroesophageal reflux in cats during anesthesia and effect of omeprazole on gastric pH. *J Vet Intern Med* 2017; **31**(3): 734–742.

256 Flouraki ES, Savvas I, Kazakos G, *et al.* The effect of premedication on the incidence of gastroesophageal reflux in 270 dogs undergoing general anesthesia. *Animals (Basel)* 2022; **12**(19): 2667.

257 Zacuto AC, Marks SL, Osborn J, *et al.* The influence of esomeprazole and cisapride on gastroesophageal reflux during anesthesia in dogs. *J Vet Intern Med* 2012; **26**(3): 518–525.

258 Wilson DV, Evans AT, Mauer WA. Influence of metoclopramide on gastroesophageal reflux in anesthetized dogs. *Am J Vet Res* 2006; **67**(1): 26–31.

259 Buchweitz E, Grandison L, Weiss HR. Effect of morphine on regional cerebral oxygen consumption and supply. *Brain Res* 1984; **291**(2): 301–308.

260 Werner C, Kochs E, Bause H, *et al.* Effects of sufentanil on cerebral hemodynamics and intracranial pressure in patients with brain injury. *Anesthesiology* 1995; **83**(4): 721–726.

261 Engelhard K, Reeker W, Kochs E, *et al.* Effect of remifentanil on intracranial pressure and cerebral blood flow velocity in patients with head trauma. *Acta Anaesthesiol Scand* 2004; **48**(4): 396–399.

262 Fodale V, Schifilliti D, Praticò C, *et al.* Remifentanil and the brain. *Acta Anaesthesiol Scand* 2008; **52**(3): 319–326.

263 Mitra S, Babadagli ME, Hatfield T, *et al.* Effect of fentanyl boluses on cerebral oxygenation and hemodynamics in preterm infants: a prospective observational study. *Neonatology* 2020; **117**(4): 480–487.

264 Adriaens A, Peremans K, Waelbers T, *et al.* The effect of morphine on regional cerebral blood flow measured by 99mTc-ECD SPECT in dogs. *PLoS ONE* 2014; **9**(10): e109680.

265 Matsumiya N, Dohi S. Effects of intravenous or subarachnoid morphine on cerebral and spinal cord hemodynamics and antagonism with naloxone in dogs. *Anesthesiology* 1983; **59**(3): 175–181.

266 Werner C, Hoffman WE, Baughman VL, *et al.* Effects of sufentanil on cerebral blood flow, cerebral blood flow velocity, and metabolism in dogs. *Anesth Analg* 1991; **72**(2): 177–181.

267 Hoffman WE, Cunningham F, James MK, *et al.* Effects of remifentanil, a new short-acting opioid, on cerebral blood flow, brain electrical activity, and intracranial pressure in dogs anesthetized with isoflurane and nitrous oxide. *Anesthesiology* 1993; **79**(1): 107–113.

268 Freeman J, Ingvar H. Effects of fentanyl on cerebral cortical blood flow and EEG in the cat. *Acta Anaesthesiol Scand* 1967; **11**(4): 381–391.

269 Milde LN, Milde JH, Gallagher WJ. Effects of sufentanil on cerebral circulation and metabolism in dogs. *Anesth Analg* 1990; **70**(2): 138–146.

270 Tipps LB, Coplin WM, Murry KR, *et al.* Safety and feasibility of continuous infusion of remifentanil in the neurosurgical intensive care unit. *Neurosurgery* 2000; **46**(3): 596–601.

271 Van Hemelrijck J, Mattheussen M, Wüsten R, *et al.* The effect of sufentanil on intracranial pressure (ICP) in anesthetized dogs. *Acta Anaesthesiol Belg* 1989; **40**(4): 239–245.

272 Sperry RJ, Bailey PL, Reichman MV, *et al.* Fentanyl and sufentanil increase intracranial pressure in head trauma patients. *Anesthesiology* 1992; **77**(3): 416–420.

273 Woller SA, Hook MA. Opioid administration following spinal cord injury: implications for pain and locomotor recovery. *Exp Neurol* 2013; **247**: 328–341.

274 Hook MA, Moreno G, Woller S, *et al.* Intrathecal morphine attenuates recovery of function after a spinal cord injury. *J Neurotrauma* 2009; **26**(5): 741–752.

275 Hook MA, Woller SA, Bancroft E, *et al.* Neurobiological effects of morphine after spinal cord injury. *J Neurotrauma* 2017; **34**(3): 632–644.

276 Lovell S, Simon B, Boudreau EC, *et al.* Randomized clinical trial comparing outcomes after fentanyl or ketamine-dexmedetomidine analgesia in thoracolumbar spinal surgery in dogs. *J Vet Intern Med* 2022; **36**(5): 1742–1751.

277 Marret E, Remy C, Bonnet F. Meta-analysis of epidural analgesia versus parenteral opioid analgesia after colorectal surgery. *Br J Surg* 2007; **94**(6): 665–673.

278 Choi S, Awad I. Maintaining micturition in the perioperative period: strategies to avoid urinary retention. *Curr Opin Anaesthesiol* 2013; **26**(3): 361–367.

279 von Siebenthal M, Schneider MP, Zheng S, *et al.* Effects of opioids and benzodiazepines on bladder function of awake restrained mice. *Am J Clin Exp Urol* 2021; **9**(6): 456–468.

280 Baldini G, Bagry H, Aprikian A, *et al.* Postoperative urinary retention: anesthetic and perioperative considerations. *Anesthesiology* 2009; **110**(5): 1139–1157.

281 Rosow CE, Gomery P, Chen TY, *et al.* Reversal of opioid-induced bladder dysfunction by intravenous naloxone and methylnaltrexone. *Clin Pharmacol Ther* 2007; **82**(1): 48–53.

282 Leander JD, Zerbe RL, Hart JC. Diuresis and suppression of vasopressin by kappa opioids: comparison with mu and delta opioids and clonidine. *J Pharmacol Exp Ther* 1985; **234**(2): 463–469.

283 Herperger LJ. Postoperative urinary retention in a dog following morphine with bupivacaine epidural analgesia. *Can Vet J* 1998; **39**(10): 650–652.

284 Kona-Boun JJ, Pibarot P, Quesnel A. Myoclonus and urinary retention following subarachnoid morphine injection in a dog. *Vet Anaesth Analg* 2003; **30**(4): 257–264.

285 Kalchofner Guerrero KS, Guerrero TG, Schweizer-Kölliker M, *et al.* Incidence of delayed hair re-growth, pruritus, and urinary retention after epidural anaesthesia in dogs. *Tierarztl Prax Ausg K Kleintiere Heimtiere* 2014; **42**(2): 94–100.

286 Peterson NW, Buote NJ, Bergman P. Effect of epidural analgesia with opioids on the prevalence of urinary retention in dogs undergoing surgery for cranial cruciate ligament rupture. *J Am Vet Med Assoc* 2014; **244**(8): 940–943.

287 Fujiyama M, Lavallée J, Lewis K, *et al.* Myoclonus and hypersensitivity of the hind limbs and tail with urinary retention following neuraxial administration of morphine in a cat. *Can Vet J* 2021; **62**(4): 389–392.

288 Troncy E, Junot S, Keroack S, *et al.* Results of preemptive epidural administration of morphine with or without bupivacaine in dogs and cats undergoing surgery: 265 cases (1997–1999). *J Am Vet Med Assoc* 2002; **221**(5): 666–672.

289 Arnholz M, Hungerbühler S, Weil C, *et al.* Comparison of ultrasound guided femoral and sciatic nerve block versus epidural anaesthesia for orthopaedic surgery in dogs. *Tierarztl Prax Ausg K Kleintiere Heimtiere* 2017; **45**(1): 5–14.

290 Viilmann I, Klöppel H, Wringe E, *et al.* Success rate and perioperative complications of lumbosacral extradural anaesthesia in dogs undergoing total hip replacement: a double-centre retrospective study. *Vet Comp Orthop Traumatol* 2022; **35**(2): 81–89.

291 Vasquez EJ, Kendall A, Musulin S, *et al.* Three-dimensional bladder ultrasound to measure daily urinary bladder volume in hospitalized dogs. *J Vet Intern Med* 2021; **35**(5): 2256–2262.

292 Drenger B, Magora F, Evron S, *et al.* The action of intrathecal morphine and methadone on the lower urinary tract in the dog. *J Urol* 1986; **135**(4): 852–855.

293 Smith LJ, Yu JK. A comparison of epidural buprenorphine with epidural morphine for postoperative analgesia following stifle surgery in dogs. *Vet Anaesth Analg* 2001; **28**(2): 87–96.

294 Drenger B, Magora F. Urodynamic studies after intrathecal fentanyl and buprenorphine in the dog. *Anesth Analg* 1989; **69**(3): 348–353.

295 Simpson KH, Madej TH, McDowell JM, *et al.* Comparison of extradural buprenorphine and extradural morphine after caesarean section. *Br J Anaesth* 1988; **60**(6): 627–631.

296 Edwards RT, McCormick-Deaton C, Hosanagar A. Acute urinary retention secondary to buprenorphine administration. *Am J Emerg Med* 2014; **32**(1): 109.e101–102.

297 Khan FA, Memon GA, Kamal RS. Effect of route of buprenorphine on recovery and postoperative analgesic requirement in paediatric patients. *Paediatr Anaesth* 2002; **12**(9): 786–790.

298 Rosiere CE, Winder CV, Wax J. Ammonia cough elicited through a tracheal side tube in unanesthetized dogs: comparative antitussive bioassay of four morphine derivatives and methadone in terms of ammonia thresholds. *J Pharmacol Exp Ther* 1956; **116**(3): 296–316.

299 Cavanagh RL, Gylys JA, Bierwagen ME. Antitussive properties of butorphanol. *Arch Int Pharmacodyn Ther* 1976; **220**(2): 258–268.

300 Nosáľová G, Strapková A, Korpás J. Relationship between the antitussic and analgesic activity of substances. *Acta Physiol Hung* 1991; **77**(2): 173–178.

301 Kamei J. Role of opioidergic and serotonergic mechanisms in cough and antitussives. *Pulm Pharmacol* 1996; **9**(5–6): 349–356.

302 Kamei J. Delta-opioid receptor antagonists as a new concept for central acting antitussive drugs. *Pulm Pharmacol Ther* 2002; **15**(3): 235–240.

303 Niedfeldt RL, Robertson SA. Postanesthetic hyperthermia in cats: a retrospective comparison between hydromorphone and buprenorphine. *Vet Anaesth Analg* 2006; **33**(6): 381–389.

304 Posner LP, Gleed RD, Erb HN, *et al.* Post-anesthetic hyperthermia in cats. *Vet Anaesth Analg* 2007; **34**(1): 40–47.

305 Posner LP, Pavuk AA, Rokshar JL, *et al.* Effects of opioids and anesthetic drugs on body temperature in cats. *Vet Anaesth Analg* 2010; **37**(1): 35–43.

306 Gellasch KL, Kruse-Elliott KT, Osmond CS, *et al.* Comparison of transdermal administration of fentanyl versus intramuscular administration of butorphanol for analgesia after onychectomy in cats. *J Am Vet Med Assoc* 2002; **220**(7): 1020–1024.

307 Martín-Flores M, Lorenzutti AM, Nugen SA, *et al.* High-dose buprenorphine results in a greater occurrence of postoperative hyperthermia than morphine in a randomized clinical trial in cats undergoing ovariohysterectomy. *Am J Vet Res* 2022; **83**(6): ajvr.21.11.0183.

308 Cox B, Ary M, Chesarek W, *et al.* Morphine hyperthermia in the rat: an action on the central thermostats. *Eur J Pharmacol* 1976; **36**(1): 33–39.

309 Maxwell LK, Thomasy SM, Slovis N, *et al.* Pharmacokinetics of fentanyl following intravenous and transdermal administration in horses. *Equine Vet J* 2003; **35**(5): 484–490.

310 Figueiredo JP, Muir WW, Sams R. Cardiorespiratory, gastrointestinal, and analgesic effects of morphine sulfate in conscious healthy horses. *Am J Vet Res* 2012; **73**(6): 799–808.

311 Hanafi AL, Reed RA, Trenholme HN, *et al.* Pharmacokinetics and pharmacodynamics of meperidine after intramuscular and subcutaneous administration in horses. *Vet Surg* 2021; **50**(2): 410–417.

312 Skrzypczak H, Reed R, Brainard B, *et al.* The pharmacokinetics of a fentanyl matrix patch applied at three different anatomical locations in horses. *Equine Vet J* 2022; **54**(1): 153–158.

313 Guedes AG, Papich MG, Rude EP, *et al.* Pharmacokinetics and physiological effects of two intravenous infusion rates of morphine in conscious dogs. *J Vet Pharmacol Ther* 2007; **30**(3): 224–233.

314 Monteiro ER, Figueroa CD, Choma JC, *et al.* Effects of methadone, alone or in combination with acepromazine or xylazine, on sedation and physiologic values in dogs. *Vet Anaesth Analg* 2008; **35**(6): 519–527.

315 Lee S, Lee A, Kim WH. Fentanyl-induced hypothermia in a dog. *Int J Appl Res Vet Med* 2021; **19**: 68–73.

316 Clark WG, Lipton JM. Changes in body temperature after administration of acetylcholine, histamine, morphine, prostaglandins and related agents: II. *Neurosci Biobehav Rev* 1985; **9**(3): 479–552.

317 Lee HK, Wang SC. Mechanism of morphine-induced miosis in the dog. *J Pharmacol Exp Ther* 1975; **192**(2): 415–431.

318 Larson MD. Mechanism of opioid-induced pupillary effects. *Clin Neurophysiol* 2008; **119**(6): 1358–1364.

319 Pickworth WB, Sharpe LG. Morphine-induced mydriasis and inhibition of pupillary light reflex and fluctuations in the cat. *J Pharmacol Exp Ther* 1985; **234**(3): 603–606.

320 Saurer TB, Ijames SG, Carrigan KA, *et al.* Neuroimmune mechanisms of opioid-mediated conditioned immunomodulation. *Brain Behav Immun* 2008; **22**(1): 89–97.

321 Kraus J. Regulation of mu-opioid receptors by cytokines. *Front Biosci (Schol Ed)* 2009; **1**(1): 164–170.

322 Gach K, Wyrębska A, Fichna J, *et al.* The role of morphine in regulation of cancer cell growth. *Naunyn Schmiedebergs Arch Pharmacol* 2011; **384**(3): 221–230.

323 Gong L, Qin Q, Zhou L, *et al.* Effects of fentanyl anesthesia and sufentanil anesthesia on regulatory T cells frequencies. *Int J Clin Exp Pathol* 2014; **7**(11): 7708–7716.

324 Franchi S, Moretti S, Castelli M, *et al.* Mu opioid receptor activation modulates Toll like receptor 4 in murine macrophages. *Brain Behav Immun* 2012; **26**(3): 480–488.

325 Heaney A, Buggy DJ. Can anaesthetic and analgesic techniques affect cancer recurrence or metastasis? *Br J Anaesth* 2012; **109**(Suppl 1): i17–i28.

326 Liang X, Liu R, Chen C, *et al.* Opioid system modulates the immune function: a review. *Transl Perioper Pain Med* 2016; **1**(1): 5–13.

327 Szczepaniak A, Fichna J, Zielińska M. Opioids in cancer development, progression and metastasis: Focus on colorectal cancer. *Curr Treat Options Oncol* 2020; **21**(1): 6.

328 Sonner JM, Antognini JF, Dutton RC, *et al.* Inhaled anesthetics and immobility: mechanisms, mysteries, and minimum alveolar anesthetic concentration. *Anesth Analg* 2003; **97**(3): 718–740.

329 Reed R, Doherty T. Minimum alveolar concentration: key concepts and a review of its pharmacological reduction in dogs. Part 2. *Res Vet Sci* 2018; **118**: 27–33.

330 Muir WW 3rd, Wiese AJ, March PA. Effects of morphine, lidocaine, ketamine, and morphine-lidocaine-ketamine drug combination on minimum alveolar concentration in dogs anesthetized with isoflurane. *Am J Vet Res* 2003; **64**(9): 1155–1160.

331 Murphy MR, Hug CC Jr. The enflurane sparing effect of morphine, butorphanol, and nalbuphine. *Anesthesiology* 1982; **57**(6): 489–492.

332 Machado CE, Dyson DH, Grant Maxie M. Effects of oxymorphone and hydromorphone on the minimum alveolar concentration of isoflurane in dogs. *Vet Anaesth Analg* 2006; **33**(1): 70–77.

333 Credie RG, Teixeira-Neto FJ, Ferreira TH, *et al.* Effects of methadone on the minimum alveolar concentration of isoflurane in dogs. *Vet Anaesth Analg* 2010; **37**(3): 240–249.

334 Murphy MR, Hug CC Jr. The anesthetic potency of fentanyl in terms of its reduction of enflurane MAC. *Anesthesiology* 1982; **57**(6): 485–488.

335 Monteiro ER, Teixeira-Neto FJ, Campagnol D, *et al.* Effects of remifentanil on the minimum alveolar concentration of isoflurane in dogs. *Am J Vet Res* 2010; **71**(2): 150–156.

336 Queiroz-Williams P, Egger CM, Qu W, *et al.* The effect of buprenorphine on isoflurane minimum alveolar concentration in dogs. *Vet Anaesth Analg* 2014; **41**: 312–318.

337 Ko JC, Lange DN, Mandsager RE, *et al.* Effects of butorphanol and carprofen on the minimal alveolar concentration of isoflurane in dogs. *J Am Vet Med Assoc* 2000; **217**(7): 1025–1028.

338 Valverde A, Dyson DH, McDonell WN. Epidural morphine reduces halothane MAC in the dog. *Can J Anaesth* 1989; **36**(6): 629–632.

339 Seddighi MR, Egger CM, Rohrbach BW, *et al.* Effects of tramadol on the minimum alveolar concentration of sevoflurane in dogs. *Vet Anaesth Analg* 2009; **36**(4): 334–340.

340 Steffey EP, Baggot JD, Eisele JH, *et al.* Morphine-isoflurane interaction in dogs, swine and rhesus monkeys. *J Vet Pharmacol Ther* 1994; **17**(3): 202–210.

341 Ko JC, Weil AB, Inoue T. Effects of carprofen and morphine on the minimum alveolar concentration of isoflurane in dogs. *J Am Anim Hosp Assoc* 2009; **45**(1): 19–23.

342 Mahidol C, Niyom S, Thitiyanaporn C, *et al.* Effects of continuous intravenous infusion of morphine and morphine-tramadol on the minimum alveolar concentration of sevoflurane and electroencephalographic entropy indices in dogs. *Vet Anaesth Analg* 2015; **42**(2): 182–186.

343 Campagnol D, Teixeira-Neto FJ, Peccinini RG, *et al.* Comparison of the effects of epidural or intravenous methadone on the minimum alveolar concentration of isoflurane in dogs. *Vet J* 2012; **192**(3): 311–315.

344 Steffey EP, Martucci R, Howland D, *et al.* Meperidine-halothane interaction in dogs. *Can Anaesth Soc J* 1977; **24**(4): 459–467.

345 Schwieger IM, Hall RI, Hug CC Jr. Less than additive antinociceptive interaction between midazolam and fentanyl in enflurane-anesthetized dogs. *Anesthesiology* 1991; **74**(6): 1060–1066.

346 Salmenperä MT, Szlam F, Hug CC Jr. Anesthetic and hemodynamic interactions of dexmedetomidine and fentanyl in dogs. *Anesthesiology* 1994; **80**(4): 837–846.

347 Ueyama Y, Lerche P, Eppler CM, *et al.* Effects of intravenous administration of perzinfotel, fentanyl, and a combination of both drugs on the minimum alveolar concentration of isoflurane in dogs. *Am J Vet Res* 2009; **70**(12): 1459–1464.

348 Hellyer PW, Mama KR, Shafford HL, *et al.* Effects of diazepam and flumazenil on minimum alveolar concentrations for dogs anesthetized with isoflurane or a combination of isoflurane and fentanyl. *Am J Vet Res* 2001; **62**(4): 555–560.

349 Suarez MA, Seddighi R, Egger CM, *et al.* Effect of fentanyl and lidocaine on the end-tidal sevoflurane concentration preventing motor movement in dogs. *Am J Vet Res* 2017; **78**(1): 12–16.

350 Reilly S, Seddighi R, Egger CM, *et al.* The effect of fentanyl on the end-tidal sevoflurane concentration needed to prevent motor movement in dogs. *Vet Anaesth Analg* 2013; **40**(3): 290–296.
351 Simões CR, Monteiro ER, Rangel JP, *et al.* Effects of a prolonged infusion of fentanyl, with or without atropine, on the minimum alveolar concentration of isoflurane in dogs. *Vet Anaesth Analg* 2016; **43**(2): 136–144.
352 Williamson EJ, Soares JHN, Pavlisko ND, *et al.* Isoflurane minimum alveolar concentration sparing effects of fentanyl in the dog. *Vet Anaesth Analg* 2017; **44**(4): 738–745.
353 Michelsen LG, Salmenperä M, Hug CC Jr., *et al.* Anesthetic potency of remifentanil in dogs. *Anesthesiology* 1996; **84**(4): 865–872.
354 Hall RI, Szlam F, Hug CC Jr. The enflurane-sparing effect of alfentanil in dogs. *Anesth Analg* 1987; **66**(12): 1287–1291.
355 Hall RI, Murphy MR, Hug CC Jr. The enflurane sparing effect of sufentanil in dogs. *Anesthesiology* 1987; **67**(4): 518–525.
356 Ilkiw JE, Pascoe PJ, Tripp LD. Effects of morphine, butorphanol, buprenorphine, and U50488H on the minimum alveolar concentration of isoflurane in cats. *Am J Vet Res* 2002; **63**(8): 1198–1202.
357 Ko JC, Abbo LA, Weil AB, *et al.* Effect of orally administered tramadol alone or with an intravenously administered opioid on minimum alveolar concentration of sevoflurane in cats. *J Am Vet Med Assoc* 2008; **232**(12): 1834–1840.
358 Ferreira TH, Steffey EP, Mama KR, *et al.* Determination of the sevoflurane sparing effect of methadone in cats. *Vet Anaesth Analg* 2011; **38**(4): 310–319.
359 Pypendop BH, Goich M, Shilo-Benjamini Y. Effect of intravenous butorphanol infusion on the minimum alveolar concentration of isoflurane in cats. *Vet Anaesth Analg* 2022; **49**(2): 165–172.
360 Zwijnenberg RJ, C LdR, Pollet RA, *et al.* Effects of perzinfotel, butorphanol tartrate, and a butorphanol-perzinfotel combination on the minimum alveolar concentration of isoflurane in cats. *Am J Vet Res* 2010; **71**(11): 1270–1276.
361 Yackey M, Ilkiw JE, Pascoe PJ, *et al.* Effect of transdermally administered fentanyl on the minimum alveolar concentration of isoflurane in cats. *Vet Anaesth Analg* 2004; **31**(3): 183–189.
362 Ferreira TH, Aguiar AJ, Valverde A, *et al.* Effect of remifentanil hydrochloride administered via constant rate infusion on the minimum alveolar concentration of isoflurane in cats. *Am J Vet Res* 2009; **70**(5): 581–588.
363 Pypendop BH, Pascoe PJ, Ilkiw JE. Effects of epidural administration of morphine and buprenorphine on the minimum alveolar concentration of isoflurane in cats. *Am J Vet Res* 2006; **67**(9): 1471–1475.
364 Brosnan RJ, Pypendop BH, Majewski-Tiedeken CR, *et al.* Naltrexone does not affect isoflurane minimum alveolar concentration in cats. *Vet Anaesth Analg* 2013; **40**(2): 225–228.
365 Steffey EP, Eisele JH, Baggot JD. Interactions of morphine and isoflurane in horses. *Am J Vet Res* 2003; **64**(2): 166–175.
366 Thomasy SM, Steffey EP, Mama KR, *et al.* The effects of i.v. fentanyl administration on the minimum alveolar concentration of isoflurane in horses. *Br J Anaesth* 2006; **97**(2): 232–237.
367 Knych HK, Steffey EP, Mama KR, *et al.* Effects of high plasma fentanyl concentrations on minimum alveolar concentration of isoflurane in horses. *Am J Vet Res* 2009; **70**(10): 1193–1200.
368 Doherty TJ, Geiser DR, Rohrbach BW. Effect of high volume epidural morphine, ketamine and butorphanol on halothane minimum alveolar concentration in ponies. *Equine Vet J* 1997; **29**(5): 370–373.
369 Doherty TJ, Geiser DR, Rohrbach BW. Effect of acepromazine and butorphanol on halothane minimum alveolar concentration in ponies. *Equine Vet J* 1997; **29**(5): 374–376.
370 Pascoe PJ, Steffey EP, Black WD, *et al.* Evaluation of the effect of alfentanil on the minimum alveolar concentration of halothane in horses. *Am J Vet Res* 1993; **54**(8): 1327–1332.
371 KuKanich B, Schmidt BK, Krugner-Higby LA, *et al.* Pharmacokinetics and behavioral effects of oxymorphone after intravenous and subcutaneous administration to healthy dogs. *J Vet Pharmacol Ther* 2008; **31**(6): 580–583.
372 Steagall PV, Ruel HLM, Yasuda T, *et al.* Pharmacokinetics and analgesic effects of intravenous, intramuscular or subcutaneous buprenorphine in dogs undergoing ovariohysterectomy: a randomized, prospective, masked, clinical trial. *BMC Vet Res* 2020; **16**(1): 154.
373 Wicks C, Hudlicky T, Rinner U. Morphine alkaloids: history, biology, and synthesis. *Alkaloids Chem Biol* 2021; **86**: 145–342.
374 McLaughlin JA. How much morphine can a dog stand? Can arsenic produce paralysis of the lower jaw? *J Comp Med Vet Arch* 1891; **12**(1): 30–31.
375 Cohn AE. The effect of morphin on the mechanism of the dog's heart after removal of one vagus nerve. *J Exp Med* 1913; **18**(6): 715–738.
376 Stewart GN, Rogoff JM. The influence of certain factors, especially emotional disturbances, on epinephrin content of the adrenals. *J Exp Med* 1916; **24**(6): 709–738.
377 Auer J, Kleiner IS. Morphine hyperglycemia in dogs with experimental pancreatic deficiency. *J Exp Med* 1918; **27**(1): 49–63.
378 Schmidt CF, Harer WB. The action of drugs on respiration : I. The morphine series. *J Exp Med* 1923; **37**(1): 47–67.
379 Simon BT, Steagall PV. The present and future of opioid analgesics in small animal practice. *J Vet Pharmacol Ther* 2017; **40**(4): 315–326.
380 Santos LC, de Moraes AN, Saito ME. Effects of intraarticular ropivacaine and morphine on lipopolysaccharide-induced synovitis in horses. *Vet Anaesth Analg* 2009; **36**(3): 280–286.
381 Thomson SM, Oliver JA, Gould DJ, *et al.* Preliminary investigations into the analgesic effects of topical ocular 1% morphine solution in dogs and cats. *Vet Anaesth Analg* 2013; **40**(6): 632–640.
382 Dohoo SE, Tasker RA. Pharmacokinetics of oral morphine sulfate in dogs: a comparison of sustained release and conventional formulations. *Can J Vet Res* 1997; **61**(4): 251–255.
383 Aragon CL, Read MR, Gaynor JS, *et al.* Pharmacokinetics of an immediate and extended release oral morphine formulation utilizing the spheroidal oral drug absorption system in dogs. *J Vet Pharmacol Ther* 2009; **32**(2): 129–136.
384 Gozalo-Marcilla M, Hopster K, Gasthuys F, *et al.* Minimum end-tidal sevoflurane concentration necessary to prevent movement during a constant rate infusion of morphine, or morphine plus dexmedetomidine in ponies. *Vet Anaesth Analg* 2014; **41**(2): 212–219.
385 Xu X, Wang X, Ge W, *et al.* The pharmacokinetics of inhaled morphine delivered by an ultrasonic nebulizer in ventilated dogs. *J Aerosol Med Pulm Drug Deliv* 2012; **25**(1): 41–46.
386 Kilpatrick GJ, Smith TW. Morphine-6-glucuronide: actions and mechanisms. *Med Res Rev* 2005; **25**(5): 521–544.
387 Volpe DA, McMahon Tobin GA, Mellon RD, *et al.* Uniform assessment and ranking of opioid μ receptor binding constants for selected opioid drugs. *Regul Toxicol Pharmacol* 2011; **59**(3): 385–390.
388 Porreca F, Mosberg HI, Hurst R, *et al.* Roles of mu, delta and kappa opioid receptors in spinal and supraspinal mediation of gastrointestinal transit effects and hot-plate analgesia in the mouse. *J Pharmacol Exp Ther* 1984; **230**(2): 341–348.
389 Zhang Q, Schäffer M, Elde R, *et al.* Effects of neurotoxins and hindpaw inflammation on opioid receptor immunoreactivities in dorsal root ganglia. *Neuroscience* 1998; **85**(1): 281–291.
390 Wang YH, Sun JF, Tao YM, *et al.* The role of kappa-opioid receptor activation in mediating antinociception and addiction. *Acta Pharmacol Sin* 2010; **31**(9): 1065–1070.
391 Sverrisdóttir E, Lund TM, Olesen AE, *et al.* A review of morphine and morphine-6-glucuronide's pharmacokinetic-pharmacodynamic relationships in experimental and clinical pain. *Eur J Pharm Sci* 2015; **74**: 45–62.
392 Kristensen K, Christensen CB, Christrup LL. The mu1, mu2, delta, kappa opioid receptor binding profiles of methadone stereoisomers and morphine. *Life Sci* 1995; **56**(2): Pl45–Pl50.
393 James A, Williams J. Basic opioid pharmacology – An update. *Br J Pain* 2020; **14**(2): 115–121.
394 KuKanich B, Lascelles BD, Papich MG. Pharmacokinetics of morphine and plasma concentrations of morphine-6-glucuronide following morphine administration to dogs. *J Vet Pharmacol Ther* 2005; **28**(4): 371–376.
395 King C, Finley B, Franklin R. The glucuronidation of morphine by dog liver microsomes: identification of morphine-6-O-glucuronide. *Drug Metab Dispos* 2000; **28**(6): 661–663.
396 KuKanich B, Lascelles BD, Papich MG. Assessment of a von Frey device for evaluation of the antinociceptive effects of morphine and its application in pharmacodynamic modeling of morphine in dogs. *Am J Vet Res* 2005; **66**(9): 1616–1622.
397 KuKanich B, Lascelles BD, Papich MG. Use of a von Frey device for evaluation of pharmacokinetics and pharmacodynamics of morphine after intravenous administration as an infusion or multiple doses in dogs. *Am J Vet Res* 2005; **66**(11): 1968–1974.
398 Thompson SE, Johnson JM. Analgesia in dogs after intercostal thoracotomy. A comparison of morphine, selective intercostal nerve block, and interpleural regional analgesia with bupivacaine. *Vet Surg* 1991; **20**(1): 73–77.
399 Gültekin Ç. Comparison of the analgesic effects of morphine and tramadol after tumor surgery in dogs. *Open Vet J* 2021; **11**(4): 613–618.
400 Lewis KA, Bednarski RM, Aarnes TK, *et al.* Postoperative comparison of four perioperative analgesia protocols in dogs undergoing stifle joint surgery. *J Am Vet Med Assoc* 2014; **244**(9): 1041–1046.
401 Minto BW, Rodrigues LC, Steagall PV, *et al.* Assessment of postoperative pain after unilateral mastectomy using two different surgical techniques in dogs. *Acta Vet Scand* 2013; **55**(1): 60.
402 Kongara K, Chambers JP, Johnson CB. Effects of tramadol, morphine or their combination in dogs undergoing ovariohysterectomy on peri-operative electroencephalographic responses and post-operative pain. *N Z Vet J* 2012; **60**(2): 129–135.

403 Abelson AL, Armitage-Chan E, Lindsey JC, *et al.* A comparison of epidural morphine with low dose bupivacaine versus epidural morphine alone on motor and respiratory function in dogs following splenectomy. *Vet Anaesth Analg* 2011; **38**(3): 213–223.

404 Luna SP, Martino ID, Lorena SE, *et al.* Acupuncture and pharmacopuncture are as effective as morphine or carprofen for postoperative analgesia in bitches undergoing ovariohysterectomy. *Acta Cir Bras* 2015; **30**(12): 831–837.

405 Dancker C, MacFarlane PD, Love EJ. The effect of neuraxial morphine on postoperative pain in dogs after extrahepatic portosystemic shunt attenuation. *Vet Anaesth Analg* 2020; **47**(1): 111–118.

406 Novello L, Corletto F, Rabozzi R, *et al.* Sparing effect of a low dose of intrathecal morphine on fentanyl requirements during spinal surgery: a preliminary clinical investigation in dogs. *Vet Surg* 2008; **37**(2): 153–160.

407 Barker JR, Clark-Price SC, Gordon-Evans WJ. Evaluation of topical epidural analgesia delivered in gelfoam for postoperative hemilaminectomy pain control. *Vet Surg* 2013; **42**(1): 79–84.

408 Kögel B, Terlinden R, Schneider J. Characterisation of tramadol, morphine and tapentadol in an acute pain model in Beagle dogs. *Vet Anaesth Analg* 2014; **41**(3): 297–304.

409 Lorenzutti AM, Martín-Flores M, Litterio NJ, *et al.* A comparison between maropitant and metoclopramide for the prevention of morphine-induced nausea and vomiting in dogs. *Can Vet J* 2017; **58**(1): 35–38.

410 Lardone E, Giaiot V, Franci P. A case of priapism following intrathecal morphine injection in a dog. *Open Vet J* 2022; **12**(5): 693–696.

411 Stanway GW, Taylor PM, Brodbelt DC. A preliminary investigation comparing pre-operative morphine and buprenorphine for postoperative analgesia and sedation in cats. *Vet Anaesth Analg* 2002; **29**(1): 29–35.

412 Steagall PV, Carnicelli P, Taylor PM, *et al.* Effects of subcutaneous methadone, morphine, buprenorphine or saline on thermal and pressure thresholds in cats. *J Vet Pharmacol Ther* 2006; **29**(6): 531–537.

413 Court MH. Feline drug metabolism and disposition: pharmacokinetic evidence for species differences and molecular mechanisms. *Vet Clin North Am Small Anim Pract* 2013; **43**(5): 1039–1054.

414 Muir WW. Pain: mechanisms and management in horses. *Vet Clin North Am Equine Pract* 2010; **26**(3): 467–480.

415 Robertson SA, Sanchez LC. Treatment of visceral pain in horses. *Vet Clin North Am Equine Pract* 2010; **26**(3): 603–617.

416 Roger T, Bardon T, Ruckebusch Y. Colonic motor responses in the pony: relevance of colonic stimulation by opiate antagonists. *Am J Vet Res* 1985; **46**(1): 31–35.

417 Boscan P, Van Hoogmoed LM, Farver TB, *et al.* Evaluation of the effects of the opioid agonist morphine on gastrointestinal tract function in horses. *Am J Vet Res* 2006; **67**(6): 992–997.

418 Hamamoto-Hardman BD, Steffey EP, Weiner D, *et al.* Pharmacokinetics and selected pharmacodynamics of morphine and its active metabolites in horses after intravenous administration of four doses. *J Vet Pharmacol Ther* 2019; **42**(4): 401–410.

419 Mircica E, Clutton RE, Kyles KW, *et al.* Problems associated with perioperative morphine in horses: a retrospective case analysis. *Vet Anaesth Analg* 2003; **30**(3): 147–155.

420 Love EJ, Lane JG, Murison PJ. Morphine administration in horses anaesthetized for upper respiratory tract surgery. *Vet Anaesth Analg* 2006; **33**(3): 179–188.

421 Clark L, Clutton RE, Blissitt KJ, *et al.* The effects of morphine on the recovery of horses from halothane anaesthesia. *Vet Anaesth Analg* 2008; **35**(1): 22–29.

422 Valverde A, Little CB, Dyson DH, *et al.* Use of epidural morphine to relieve pain in a horse. *Can Vet J* 1990; **31**(3): 211–212.

423 Hopster K, Watkins AR, Hurcombe SD. Comparison of cervical epidural morphine with intravenous morphine administration on antinociception in adult horses using thermal threshold testing. *Vet Anaesth Analg* 2022; **49**(4): 417–422.

424 Kohn CW, Muir WW 3rd. Selected aspects of the clinical pharmacology of visceral analgesics and gut motility modifying drugs in the horse. *J Vet Intern Med* 1988; **2**(2): 85–91.

425 Tessier C, Pitaud JP, Thorin C, *et al.* Systemic morphine administration causes gastric distention and hyperphagia in healthy horses. *Equine Vet J* 2019; **51**(5): 653–657.

426 Dönselmann Im Sande P, Hopster K, Kästner S. Effects of morphine, butorphanol and levomethadone in different doses on thermal nociceptive thresholds in horses. *Tierarztl Prax Ausg G Grosstiere Nutztiere* 2017; **45**(2): 98–106.

427 Carregaro AB, Freitas GC, Ribeiro MH, *et al.* Physiological and analgesic effects of continuous-rate infusion of morphine, butorphanol, tramadol or methadone in horses with lipopolysaccharide (LPS)-induced carpal synovitis. *BMC Vet Res* 2014; **10**: 966.

428 Clark L, Clutton RE, Blissitt KJ, *et al.* Effects of peri-operative morphine administration during halothane anaesthesia in horses. *Vet Anaesth Analg* 2005; **32**(1): 10–15.

429 Chesnel MA, Clutton RE. A comparison of two morphine doses on the quality of recovery from general anaesthesia in horses. *Res Vet Sci* 2013; **95**(3): 1195–1200.

430 Loomes K, Louro LF. Recovery of horses from general anaesthesia: a systematic review (2000–2020) of risk factors and influence of interventions during the recovery period. *Equine Vet J* 2022; **54**(2): 201–218.

431 Loomes K, Louro LF. Recovery of horses from general anaesthesia: a systematic review (2000–2020) of the influence of anaesthetic protocol on recovery quality. *Equine Vet J* 2022; **54**(2): 219–261.

432 van Loon JP, de Grauw JC, van Dierendonck M, *et al.* Intra-articular opioid analgesia is effective in reducing pain and inflammation in an equine LPS induced synovitis model. *Equine Vet J* 2010; **42**(5): 412–419.

433 Poth MKM, McKemie DS, Traynham M, *et al.* Concentrations, pharmacokinetics and selected pharmacodynamics of morphine and its active metabolites following oral administration to horses. *J Vet Pharmacol Ther* 2023; **46**(4): 238–249.

434 Maney JK, Dzikiti BT, Escobar A, *et al.* Morphine in donkeys: antinociceptive effect and preliminary pharmacokinetics. *Equine Vet J* 2023; **55**(6): 1086–1093.

435 Marchionatti E, Lardé H, Steagall PV. Opioid-induced adverse effects in a Holstein calf. *Vet Anaesth Analg* 2015; **42**(2): 229–230.

436 Machado Filho LC, Hurnik JF, Ewing KK. A thermal threshold assay to measure the nociceptive response to morphine sulphate in cattle. *Can J Vet Res* 1998; **62**(3): 218–223.

437 Fierheller EE, Caulkett NA, Bailey JV. A romifidine and morphine combination for epidural analgesia of the flank in cattle. *Can Vet J* 2004; **45**(11): 917–923.

438 Malavasi LM, Nyman G, Augustsson H, *et al.* Effects of epidural morphine and transdermal fentanyl analgesia on physiology and behaviour after abdominal surgery in pigs. *Lab Anim* 2006; **40**(1): 16–27.

439 Rialland P, Otis C, de Courval ML, *et al.* Assessing experimental visceral pain in dairy cattle: a pilot, prospective, blinded, randomized, and controlled study focusing on spinal pain proteomics. *J Dairy Sci* 2014; **97**(4): 2118–2134.

440 Dahlström B, Tamsen A, Paalzow L, *et al.* Patient-controlled analgesic therapy, Part IV: pharmacokinetics and analgesic plasma concentrations of morphine. *Clin Pharmacokinet* 1982; **7**(3): 266–279.

441 Uhrig SR, Papich MG, KuKanich B, *et al.* Pharmacokinetics and pharmacodynamics of morphine in llamas. *Am J Vet Res* 2007; **68**(1): 25–34.

442 Wegner K, Robertson SA. Dose-related thermal antinociceptive effects of intravenous hydromorphone in cats. *Vet Anaesth Analg* 2007; **34**(2): 132–138.

443 Guedes AG, Papich MG, Rude EP, *et al.* Pharmacokinetics and physiological effects of intravenous hydromorphone in conscious dogs. *J Vet Pharmacol Ther* 2008; **31**(4): 334–343.

444 Krugner-Higby L, Smith LJ, Schmidt B, *et al.* Postoperative analgesia provided by liposomal hydromorphone in client-owned dogs undergoing limb amputation. *J Am Anim Hosp Assoc* 2016; **52**(1): 13–21.

445 Hofmeister EH, Chandler MJ, Read MR. Effects of acepromazine, hydromorphone, or an acepromazine-hydromorphone combination on the degree of sedation in clinically normal dogs. *J Am Vet Med Assoc* 2010; **237**(10): 1155–1159.

446 Biello P, Bateman SW, Kerr CL. Comparison of fentanyl and hydromorphone constant rate infusions for pain management in dogs in an intensive care unit. *Vet Anaesth Analg* 2018; **45**(5): 673–683.

447 Ambros B, Steagall PV, Mantovani F, *et al.* Antinociceptive effects of epidural administration of hydromorphone in conscious cats. *Am J Vet Res* 2009; **70**(10): 1187–1192.

448 Martins FC, Keating SC, Clark-Price SC, *et al.* Pharmacokinetics and pharmacodynamics of hydromorphone hydrochloride in healthy horses. *Vet Anaesth Analg* 2020; **47**(4): 509–517.

449 Skrzypczak H, Reed R, Barletta M, *et al.* A retrospective evaluation of the effect of perianesthetic hydromorphone administration on the incidence of postanesthetic signs of colic in horses. *Vet Anaesth Analg* 2020; **47**(6): 757–762.

450 Reed R, Trenholme N, Skrzypczak H, *et al.* Comparison of hydromorphone and butorphanol for management of pain in equine patients undergoing elective arthroscopy: a randomized clinical trial. *Vet Anaesth Analg* 2022; **49**(5): 490–498.

451 Bitti FS, Campagnol D, Rangel JP, *et al.* Effects of three methadone doses combined with acepromazine on sedation and some cardiopulmonary variables in dogs. *Vet Anaesth Analg* 2017; **44**(2): 237–245.

452 Shimoyama N, Shimoyama M, Elliott KJ, *et al.* d-Methadone is antinociceptive in the rat formalin test. *J Pharmacol Exp Ther* 1997; **283**(2): 648–652.

453 Carpenter KJ, Chapman V, Dickenson AH. Neuronal inhibitory effects of methadone are predominantly opioid receptor mediated in the rat spinal cord *in vivo*. *Eur J Pain* 2000; **4**(1): 19–26.

454 KuKanich B, Borum SL. The disposition and behavioral effects of methadone in Greyhounds. *Vet Anaesth Analg* 2008; **35**(3): 242–248.

455 Salpeter SR, Buckley JS, Bruera E. The use of very-low-dose methadone for palliative pain control and the prevention of opioid hyperalgesia. *J Palliat Med* 2013; **16**(6): 616–622.

456 Ferreira TH, Rezende ML, Mama KR, *et al.* Plasma concentrations and behavioral, antinociceptive, and physiologic effects of methadone after intravenous and oral transmucosal administration in cats. *Am J Vet Res* 2011; **72**(6): 764–771.
457 Slingsby LS, Sear JW, Taylor PM, *et al.* Effect of intramuscular methadone on pharmacokinetic data and thermal and mechanical nociceptive thresholds in the cat. *J Feline Med Surg* 2016; **18**(11): 875–881.
458 Amon T, Kästner SBR, Kietzmann M, *et al.* Plasma levels of a methadone constant rate infusion and their corresponding effects on thermal and mechanical nociceptive thresholds in dogs. *BMC Vet Res* 2021; **17**(1): 35.
459 Hunt JR, Attenburrow PM, Slingsby LS, *et al.* Comparison of premedication with buprenorphine or methadone with meloxicam for postoperative analgesia in dogs undergoing orthopaedic surgery. *J Small Anim Pract* 2013; **54**(8): 418–424.
460 KuKanich B, KuKanich K. Chloramphenicol significantly affects the pharmacokinetics of oral methadone in Greyhound dogs. *Vet Anaesth Analg* 2015; **42**(6): 597–607.
461 Bieberly ZD, KuKanich B, KuKanich KS, *et al.* Long-acting injectable methadone (methadone-fluconazole) provides safe and effective postoperative analgesia in a randomized clinical trial for dogs undergoing soft tissue surgery. *Am J Vet Res* 2022; **83**(8): ajvr.22.01.0014.
462 Nannarone S, Giannettoni G, Laurenza C, *et al.* Methadone or butorphanol as pre-anaesthetic agents combined with romifidine in horses undergoing elective surgery: qualitative assessment of sedation and induction. *Animals (Basel)* 2021; **11**(9): 2572.
463 Muir WW, Skarda RT, Sheehan WC. Cardiopulmonary effects of narcotic agonists and a partial agonist in horses. *Am J Vet Res* 1978; **39**(10): 1632–1635.
464 de Oliveira FA, Pignaton W, Teixeira-Neto FJ, *et al.* Antinociceptive and behavioral effects of methadone alone or in combination with detomidine in conscious horses. *J Equine Vet Sci* 2014; **34**(3): 380–386.
465 Clarke KW, Paton BS. Combined use of detomidine with opiates in the horse. *Equine Vet J* 1988; **20**(5): 331–334.
466 Carregaro AB, Ueda GI, Censoni JB, *et al.* Effect of methadone combined with acepromazine or detomidine on sedation and dissociative anesthesia in healthy horses. *J Equine Vet Sci* 2020; **86**: 102908.
467 Lopes C, Luna SP, Rosa AC, *et al.* Antinociceptive effects of methadone combined with detomidine or acepromazine in horses. *Equine Vet J* 2016; **48**(5): 613–618.
468 Olbrich VH, Mosing M. A comparison of the analgesic effects of caudal epidural methadone and lidocaine in the horse. *Vet Anaesth Analg* 2003; **30**(3): 156–164.
469 Gozalo-Marcilla M, Luna SP, Crosignani N, *et al.* Sedative and antinociceptive effects of different combinations of detomidine and methadone in standing horses. *Vet Anaesth Analg* 2017; **44**(5): 1116–1127.
470 Gozalo-Marcilla M, de Oliveira AR, Fonseca MW, *et al.* Sedative and antinociceptive effects of different detomidine constant rate infusions, with or without methadone in standing horses. *Equine Vet J* 2019; **51**(4): 530–536.
471 Crosignani N, Luna SP, Dalla Costa T, *et al.* Pharmacokinetics and pharmacodynamics of the injectable formulation of methadone hydrochloride and methadone in lipid nanocarriers administered orally to horses. *J Vet Pharmacol Ther* 2017; **40**(4): 398–405.
472 Bellini L, De Benedictis GM. Effect of three opioid-based analgesic protocols on the perioperative autonomic-mediated cardiovascular response in sheep. *Lab Anim* 2019; **53**(5): 491–499.
473 Bergadano A, Moens Y, Schatzmann U. Continuous extradural analgesia in a cow with complex regional pain syndrome. *Vet Anaesth Analg* 2006; **33**(3): 189–192.
474 DeRossi R, Pagliosa RC, de Carvalho AQ, *et al.* Fentanyl and methadone used as adjuncts to bupivacaine for lumbosacral epidural analgesia in sheep. *Vet Rec* 2017; **180**(4): 96.
475 Barnhart MD, Hubbell JA, Muir WW. Evaluation of the analgesic properties of acepromazine maleate, oxymorphone, medetomidine and a combination of acepromazine-oxymorphone. *Vet Anaesth Analg* 2000; **27**(2): 89–96.
476 Bateman SW, Haldane S, Stephens JA. Comparison of the analgesic efficacy of hydromorphone and oxymorphone in dogs and cats: a randomized blinded study. *Vet Anaesth Analg* 2008; **35**(4): 341–347.
477 Mathews KA, Paley DM, Foster RA, *et al.* A comparison of ketorolac with flunixin, butorphanol, and oxymorphone in controlling postoperative pain in dogs. *Can Vet J* 1996; **37**(9): 557–567.
478 Pypendop BH, Ilkiw JE, Shilo-Benjamini Y. Bioavailability of morphine, methadone, hydromorphone, and oxymorphone following buccal administration in cats. *J Vet Pharmacol Ther* 2014; **37**(3): 295–300.
479 Siao KT, Pypendop BH, Stanley SD, *et al.* Pharmacokinetics of oxymorphone in cats. *J Vet Pharmacol Ther* 2011; **34**(6): 594–598.
480 Hughes MA, Glass PS, Jacobs JR. Context-sensitive half-time in multicompartment pharmacokinetic models for intravenous anesthetic drugs. *Anesthesiology* 1992; **76**(3): 334–341.
481 Murphy MR, Hug CC Jr., McClain DA. Dose-independent pharmacokinetics of fentanyl. *Anesthesiology* 1983; **59**(6): 537–540.
482 Iizuka T, Nishimura R. Context-sensitive half-time of fentanyl in dogs. *J Vet Med Sci* 2015; **77**(5): 615–617.
483 KuKanich B. Pharmacokinetics of subcutaneous fentanyl in Greyhounds. *Vet J* 2011; **190**(2): e140–e142.
484 KuKanich B, Allen P. Comparative pharmacokinetics of intravenous fentanyl and buprenorphine in healthy greyhound dogs. *J Vet Pharmacol Ther* 2014; **37**(6): 595–597.
485 Lefebvre RA, Willems JL, Bogaert MG. Gastric relaxation and vomiting by apomorphine, morphine and fentanyl in the conscious dog. *Eur J Pharmacol* 1981; **69**(2): 139–145.
486 Freye E, Schnitzler M, Schenk G. Opioid-induced respiratory depression and analgesia may be mediated by different subreceptors. *Pharm Res* 1991; **8**(2): 196–199.
487 Kamata M, Nagahama S, Kakishima K, *et al.* Comparison of behavioral effects of morphine and fentanyl in dogs and cats. *J Vet Med Sci* 2012; **74**(2): 231–234.
488 Çoruh B, Tonelli MR, Park DR. Fentanyl-induced chest wall rigidity. *Chest* 2013; **143**(4): 1145–1146.
489 Soares JH, Henao-Guerrero N, Pavlisko ND, *et al.* The effect of two doses of fentanyl on chest wall rigidity at equipotent doses of isoflurane in dogs. *Vet Anaesth Analg* 2019; **46**(3): 360–364.
490 Jang M, Son WG, Lee I. Fentanyl-induced asystole in two dogs. *J Small Anim Pract* 2015; **56**(6): 411–413.
491 Glerum LE, Egger CM, Allen SW, *et al.* Analgesic effect of the transdermal fentanyl patch during and after feline ovariohysterectomy. *Vet Surg* 2001; **30**(4): 351–358.
492 Gutierrez-Blanco E, Victoria-Mora JM, Ibancovichi-Camarillo JA, *et al.* Postoperative analgesic effects of either a constant rate infusion of fentanyl, lidocaine, ketamine, dexmedetomidine, or the combination lidocaine-ketamine-dexmedetomidine after ovariohysterectomy in dogs. *Vet Anaesth Analg* 2015; **42**(3): 309–318.
493 Ambros B, Alcorn J, Duke-Novakovski T, *et al.* Pharmacokinetics and pharmacodynamics of a constant rate infusion of fentanyl (5 µg/kg/h) in awake cats. *Am J Vet Res* 2014; **75**(8): 716–721.
494 Carrozzo MV, Alcorn J, Ambros B. Effects of two fentanyl constant rate infusions on thermal thresholds and plasma fentanyl concentrations in awake cats. *Vet Anaesth Analg* 2018; **45**(6): 831–838.
495 Kyles AE, Papich M, Hardie EM. Disposition of transdermally administered fentanyl in dogs. *Am J Vet Res* 1996; **57**(5): 715–719.
496 Schultheiss PJ, Morse BC, Baker WH. Evaluation of a transdermal fentanyl system in the dog. *Contemp Top Lab Anim Sci* 1995; **34**(5): 75–81.
497 Pettifer GR, Hosgood G. The effect of rectal temperature on perianesthetic serum concentrations of transdermally administered fentanyl in cats anesthetized with isoflurane. *Am J Vet Res* 2003; **64**(12): 1557–1561.
498 Hofmeister EH, Egger CM. Transdermal fentanyl patches in small animals. *J Am Anim Hosp Assoc* 2004; **40**(6): 468–478.
499 Schmiedt CW, Bjorling DE. Accidental prehension and suspected transmucosal or oral absorption of fentanyl from a transdermal patch in a dog. *Vet Anaesth Analg* 2007; **34**(1): 70–73.
500 Sredenšek J, Bošnjak M, Lampreht Tratar U, *et al.* Case Report: intoxication in a pig (*Sus scrofa domesticus*) after transdermal fentanyl patch ingestion. *Front Vet Sci* 2020; **7**: 611097.
501 FDA U. Accidental exposures to fentanyl patches continue to be deadly to children: U.S. Food and Drug Administration; 2023. Available from: https://www.fda.gov/consumers/consumer-updates/accidental-exposures-fentanyl-patches-continue-be-deadly-children
502 Sanchez LC, Robertson SA, Maxwell LK, *et al.* Effect of fentanyl on visceral and somatic nociception in conscious horses. *J Vet Intern Med* 2007; **21**(5): 1067–1075.
503 Echelmeyer J, Taylor PM, Hopster K, *et al.* Effect of fentanyl on thermal and mechanical nociceptive thresholds in horses and estimation of anti-nociceptive plasma concentration. *Vet J* 2019; **249**: 82–88.
504 Robertson SA, Taylor PM, Sear JW, *et al.* Relationship between plasma concentrations and analgesia after intravenous fentanyl and disposition after other routes of administration in cats. *J Vet Pharmacol Ther* 2005; **28**(1): 87–93.
505 Knych HK, Steffey EP, Casbeer HC, *et al.* Disposition, behavioural and physiological effects of escalating doses of intravenously administered fentanyl to young foals. *Equine Vet J* 2015; **47**(5): 592–598.
506 Ringer SK, Spielmann N, Weiss M, *et al.* Fentanyl bolus induces muscle tremors in sevoflurane-anaesthetized piglets. *Lab Anim* 2016; **50**(4): 312–314.
507 Goutchtat R, Chetboun M, Wiart JF, *et al.* Long-term analgesia following a single application of fentanyl transdermal solution in pigs. *Eur Surg Res* 2021; **62**(2): 115–120.
508 Thomasy SM, Slovis N, Maxwell LK, *et al.* Transdermal fentanyl combined with nonsteroidal anti-inflammatory drugs for analgesia in horses. *J Vet Intern Med* 2004; **18**(4): 550–554.

509 Burke MJ, Soma LR, Boston RC, *et al.* Evaluation of the analgesic and pharmacokinetic properties of transdermally administered fentanyl in goats. *J Vet Emerg Crit Care (San Antonio)* 2017; **27**(5): 539–547.

510 Smith JS, Mochel JP, Borts DJ, *et al.* Adverse reactions to fentanyl transdermal patches in calves: a preliminary clinical and pharmacokinetic study. *Vet Anaesth Analg* 2018; **45**(4): 575–580.

511 Hoke JF, Cunningham F, James MK, *et al.* Comparative pharmacokinetics and pharmacodynamics of remifentanil, its principle metabolite (GR90291) and alfentanil in dogs. *J Pharmacol Exp Ther* 1997; **281**(1): 226–232.

512 Westmoreland CL, Hoke JF, Sebel PS, *et al.* Pharmacokinetics of remifentanil (GI87084B) and its major metabolite (GI90291) in patients undergoing elective inpatient surgery. *Anesthesiology* 1993; **79**(5): 893–903.

513 Chism JP, Rickert DE. The pharmacokinetics and extra-hepatic clearance of remifentanil, a short acting opioid agonist, in male beagle dogs during constant rate infusions. *Drug Metab Dispos* 1996; **24**(1): 34–40.

514 Correa Mdo A, Aguiar AJ, Neto FJ, *et al.* Effects of remifentanil infusion regimens on cardiovascular function and responses to noxious stimulation in propofol-anesthetized cats. *Am J Vet Res* 2007; **68**(9): 932–940.

515 Machado ML, Soares JHN, Kuster de Albuquerque Gress MA, *et al.* Dose-finding study comparing three treatments of remifentanil in cats anesthetized with isoflurane undergoing ovariohysterectomy. *J Feline Med Surg* 2018; **20**(2): 164–171.

516 Nagakubo D, Muta K, Kamata M, *et al.* Effects of remifentanil on the noxiously stimulated somatosensory evoked potentials recorded at the spinal cord in dogs and cats. *Res Vet Sci* 2023; **158**: 13–16.

517 Hayashida M, Fukunaga A, Hanaoka K. Detection of acute tolerance to the analgesic and nonanalgesic effects of remifentanil infusion in a rabbit model. *Anesth Analg* 2003; **97**(5): 1347–1352.

518 Gómez de Segura IA, de la Vibora JB, Aguado D. Opioid tolerance blunts the reduction in the sevoflurane minimum alveolar concentration produced by remifentanil in the rat. *Anesthesiology* 2009; **110**(5): 1133–1138.

519 Aguado D, Bustamante R, Gómez de Segura IA. Toll-like receptor 4 deficient mice do not develop remifentanil-induced mechanical hyperalgesia: an experimental randomised animal study. *Eur J Anaesthesiol* 2018; **35**(7): 505–510.

520 Ruíz-López P, Navarrete-Calvo R, Morgaz J, *et al.* Determination of acute tolerance and hyperalgesia to remifentanil constant rate infusion in dogs undergoing sevoflurane anaesthesia. *Vet Anaesth Analg* 2020; 47(2): 183–190.

521 Akashi N, Murahata Y, Hosokawa M, *et al.* Cardiovascular and renal effects of constant rate infusions of remifentanil, dexmedetomidine and their combination in dogs anesthetized with sevoflurane. *J Vet Med Sci* 2021; **83**(2): 285–296.

522 Rockhold RW, Crofton JT, Wang BC, *et al.* Effect of intracarotid administration of morphine and naloxone on plasma vasopressin levels and blood pressure in the dog. *J Pharmacol Exp Ther* 1983; **224**(2): 386–390.

523 Hellebrekers LJ, van den Brom WE, Mol JA. Plasma arginine vasopressin response to intravenous methadone and naloxone in conscious dogs. *J Pharmacol Exp Ther* 1989; **248**(1): 329–333.

524 Joshi GP, Warner DS, Twersky RS, *et al.* A comparison of the remifentanil and fentanyl adverse effect profile in a multicenter phase IV study. *J Clin Anesth* 2002; **14**(7): 494–499.

525 Twersky RS, Jamerson B, Warner DS, *et al.* Hemodynamics and emergence profile of remifentanil versus fentanyl prospectively compared in a large population of surgical patients. *J Clin Anesth* 2001; **13**(6): 407–416.

526 Fleisher LA, Hogue S, Colopy M, *et al.* Does functional ability in the postoperative period differ between remifentanil- and fentanyl-based anesthesia? *J Clin Anesth* 2001; **13**(6): 401–406.

527 Benmansour P, Duke-Novakovski T. Prolonged anesthesia using sevoflurane, remifentanil and dexmedetomidine in a horse. *Vet Anaesth Analg* 2013; **40**(5): 521–526.

528 Pallarols NB, Lamuraglia R, Guglielminetti A, *et al.* Behavioral and cardiopulmonary effects of a constant rate infusion of remifentanil-xylazine for sedation in horses. *J Equine Vet Sci* 2020; **91**: 103111.

529 Benmansour P, Billinsky J, Duke-Novakovski T, *et al.* Blood concentrations of remifentanil during and after infusion in horses anesthetized with isoflurane and dexmedetomidine. *Res Vet Sci* 2016; **107**: 202–206.

530 Pypendop BH, Brosnan RJ, Majewski-Tiedeken CR, *et al.* Pharmacokinetics of fentanyl, alfentanil, and sufentanil in isoflurane-anesthetized cats. *J Vet Pharmacol Ther* 2014; **37**(1): 13–17.

531 Bufalari A, Di Meo A, Nannarone S, *et al.* Fentanyl or sufentanil continuous infusion during isoflurane anaesthesia in dogs: clinical experiences. *Vet Res Commun* 2007; **31**(Suppl 1): 277–280.

532 Van Wijnsberghe AS, Marolf V, Claeys S, *et al.* Effects of fentanyl-lidocaine-ketamine versus sufentanil-lidocaine-ketamine on the isoflurane requirements in dogs undergoing total ear canal ablation and lateral bulla osteotomy. *Vet Anaesth Analg* 2020; **47**(5): 595–603.

533 Mendes GM, Selmi AL. Use of a combination of propofol and fentanyl, alfentanil, or sufentanil for total intravenous anesthesia in cats. *J Am Vet Med Assoc* 2003; **223**(11): 1608–1613.

534 Almeida TF, Fantoni DT, Mastrocinque S, *et al.* Epidural anesthesia with bupivacaine, bupivacaine and fentanyl, or bupivacaine and sufentanil during intravenous administration of propofol for ovariohysterectomy in dogs. *J Am Vet Med Assoc* 2007; **230**(1): 45–51.

535 Slingsby LS, Murison PJ, Goossens L, *et al.* A comparison between pre-operative carprofen and a long-acting sufentanil formulation for analgesia after ovariohysterectomy in dogs. *Vet Anaesth Analg* 2006; **33**(5): 313–327.

536 Lascelles BD, Butterworth SJ, Waterman AE. Postoperative analgesic and sedative effects of carprofen and pethidine in dogs. *Vet Rec* 1994; **134**(8): 187–191.

537 Slingsby LS, Waterman-Pearson AE. Analgesic effects in dogs of carprofen and pethidine together compared with the effects of either drug alone. *Vet Rec* 2001; **148**(14): 441–444.

538 Slingsby LS, Waterman-Pearson AE. Comparison of pethidine, buprenorphine and ketoprofen for postoperative analgesia after ovariohysterectomy in the cat. *Vet Rec* 1998; **143**(7): 185–189.

539 Dixon MJ, Robertson SA, Taylor PM. A thermal threshold testing device for evaluation of analgesics in cats. *Res Vet Sci* 2002; **72**(3): 205–210.

540 Golder FJ, Wilson J, Larenza MP, *et al.* Suspected acute meperidine toxicity in a dog. *Vet Anaesth Analg* 2010; **37**(5): 471–477.

541 Avril G, Freye E. Effects of high doses of pethidine and fentanyl on hemodynamics in the dog. *Cah Anesthesiol* 1984; **32**(1): 15–19.

542 Jaffe RA, Rowe MA. A comparison of the local anesthetic effects of meperidine, fentanyl, and sufentanil on dorsal root axons. *Anesth Analg* 1996; **83**(4): 776–781.

543 Akcasu A, Yillar DO, Akkan AG, *et al.* The role of mast cells in the genesis of acute manifestations following the intravenous injection of meperidine in dogs. *J Basic Clin Physiol Pharmacol* 2009; **20**(1): 67–72.

544 Yang NY, Ko JC, Wang HC, *et al.* A preliminary study comparing the sedative, cardiorespiratory, and histaminic-releasing effects of intramuscular and intravenous administration of pethidine (meperidine) with midazolam in healthy cats. *Vet Anim Sci* 2021; **14**: 100218.

545 Hamamoto-Hardman BD, Steffey EP, McKemie DS, *et al.* Meperidine pharmacokinetics and effects on physiologic parameters and thermal threshold following intravenous administration of three doses to horses. *BMC Vet Res* 2020; **16**(1): 368.

546 Foreman JH, Ruemmler R. Efficacy of intramuscular meperidine hydrochloride versus placebo in experimental foot lameness in horses. *Equine Vet J Suppl* 2013; (**45**): 48–53.

547 Skarda RT, Muir WW 3rd. Analgesic, hemodynamic, and respiratory effects induced by caudal epidural administration of meperidine hydrochloride in mares. *Am J Vet Res* 2001; **62**(7): 1001–1007.

548 George AV, Lu JJ, Pisano MV, *et al.* Carfentanil--an ultra potent opioid. *Am J Emerg Med* 2010; **28**(4): 530–532.

549 Li AC, Chovan JP, Yu E, *et al.* Update on hydrocodone metabolites in rats and dogs aided with a semi-automatic software for metabolite identification Mass-MetaSite. *Xenobiotica* 2013; **43**(4): 390–398.

550 Hsieh BM, Beets AK. Coughing in small animal patients. *Front Vet Sci* 2019; **6**: 513.

551 KuKanich B. Pharmacokinetics of acetaminophen, codeine, and the codeine metabolites morphine and codeine-6-glucuronide in healthy Greyhound dogs. *J Vet Pharmacol Ther* 2010; **33**(1): 15–21.

552 Benitez ME, Roush JK, KuKanich B, *et al.* Pharmacokinetics of hydrocodone and tramadol administered for control of postoperative pain in dogs following tibial plateau leveling osteotomy. *Am J Vet Res* 2015; **76**(9): 763–770.

553 KuKanich B. Pharmacokinetics and pharmacodynamics of oral acetaminophen in combination with codeine in healthy Greyhound dogs. *J Vet Pharmacol Ther* 2016; **39**(5): 514–517.

554 KuKanich B, Spade J. Pharmacokinetics of hydrocodone and hydromorphone after oral hydrocodone in healthy Greyhound dogs. *Vet J* 2013; **196**(2): 266–268.

555 Heffernan AE, Katz EM, Sun Y, *et al.* Once daily oral extended-release hydrocodone as analgesia following tibial plateau leveling osteotomy in dogs. *Vet Surg* 2018; **47**(4): 516–523.

556 Benitez ME, Roush JK, McMurphy R, *et al.* Clinical efficacy of hydrocodone-acetaminophen and tramadol for control of postoperative pain in dogs following tibial plateau leveling osteotomy. *Am J Vet Res* 2015; **76**(9): 755–762.

557 Yeh SY, McQuinn RL, Gorodetzky CW. Biotransformation of morphine to dihydromorphinone and normorphine in the mouse, rat, rabbit, guinea pig, cat, dog, and monkey. *Drug Metab Dispos* 1977; **5**(4): 335–342.

558 Cone EJ, Darwin WD, Gorodetzky CW, *et al.* Comparative metabolism of hydrocodone in man, rat, guinea pig, rabbit, and dog. *Drug Metab Dispos* 1978; **6**(4): 488–493.

559 Cone EJ, Darwin WD, Gorodetzky CW. Comparative metabolism of codeine in man, rat, dog, guinea-pig and rabbit: identification of four new metabolites. *J Pharm Pharmacol* 1979; **31**(5): 314–317.

560 Garrett ER, Jackson AJ. Pharmacokinetics of morphine and its surrogates. III: morphine and morphine 3-monoglucuronide pharmacokinetics in the dog as a function of dose. *J Pharm Sci* 1979; **68**(6): 753–771.

561 Lötsch J, Skarke C, Schmidt H, *et al.* Evidence for morphine-independent central nervous opioid effects after administration of codeine: contribution of other codeine metabolites. *Clin Pharmacol Ther* 2006; **79**(1): 35–48.

562 Skingle M, Tyers MB. Further studies on opiate receptors that mediate antinoception: tooth pulp stimulation in the dog. *Br J Pharmacol* 1980; **70**(2): 323–327.

563 Martins TL, Kahvegian MA, Noel-Morgan J, *et al.* Comparison of the effects of tramadol, codeine, and ketoprofen alone or in combination on postoperative pain and on concentrations of blood glucose, serum cortisol, and serum interleukin-6 in dogs undergoing maxillectomy or mandibulectomy. *Am J Vet Res* 2010; **71**(9): 1019–1026.

564 Steagall PV, Monteiro BP, Lavoie AM, *et al.* Preliminary investigation of the thermal antinociceptive effects of codeine in cats. *J Feline Med Surg* 2015; **17**(12): 1061–1064.

565 Gretler SR, Finno CJ, McKemie DS, *et al.* Metabolism, pharmacokinetics and selected pharmacodynamic effects of codeine following a single oral administration to horses. *Vet Anaesth Analg* 2020; **47**(5): 694–704.

566 Galosi M, Troisi A, Toniolo P, *et al.* Comparison of the transdermal and intravenous administration of buprenorphine in the management of intra- and postoperative pain in dogs undergoing a unilateral mastectomy. *Animals (Basel)* 2022; **12**(24): 3468.

567 Barbarossa A, Rambaldi J, Giunti M, *et al.* Pharmacokinetics of buprenorphine following constant rate infusion for postoperative analgesia in dogs undergoing ovariectomy. *Vet Anaesth Analg* 2017; **44**(3): 435–443.

568 Snyder LB, Snyder CJ, Hetzel S. Effects of buprenorphine added to bupivacaine infraorbital nerve blocks on isoflurane minimum alveolar concentration using a model for acute dental/oral surgical pain in dogs. *J Vet Dent* 2016; **33**(2): 90–96.

569 Barletta M, Ostenkamp SM, Taylor AC, *et al.* The pharmacokinetics and analgesic effects of extended-release buprenorphine administered subcutaneously in healthy dogs. *J Vet Pharmacol Ther* 2018; **41**(4): 502–512.

570 Steagall PV, Benito J, Monteiro BP, *et al.* Analgesic effects of gabapentin and buprenorphine in cats undergoing ovariohysterectomy using two pain-scoring systems: a randomized clinical trial. *J Feline Med Surg* 2018; **20**(8): 741–748.

571 Moser KL, Hasiuk MM, Armstrong T, *et al.* A randomized clinical trial comparing butorphanol and buprenorphine within a multimodal analgesic protocol in cats undergoing orchiectomy. *J Feline Med Surg* 2020; **22**(8): 760–767.

572 Bortolami E, Slingsby L, Love EJ. Comparison of two formulations of buprenorphine in cats administered by the oral transmucosal route. *J Feline Med Surg* 2012; **14**(8): 534–539.

573 Gulledge BM, Messenger KM, Cornell KK, *et al.* Pharmacokinetic comparison of two buprenorphine formulations after buccal administration in healthy male cats. *J Feline Med Surg* 2018; **20**(4): 312–318.

574 Johnson RJ, Kerr CL, Enouri SS, *et al.* Pharmacokinetics of liposomal encapsulated buprenorphine suspension following subcutaneous administration to cats. *J Vet Pharmacol Ther* 2017; **40**(3): 256–269.

575 Love EJ, Taylor PM, Whay HR, *et al.* Postcastration analgesia in ponies using buprenorphine hydrochloride. *Vet Rec* 2013; **172**(24): 635.

576 Haunhorst FR, Hopster K, Schmicke M, *et al.* Clinical effect of buprenorphine or butorphanol, in combination with detomidine and diazepam, on sedation and postoperative pain after cheek tooth extraction in horses. *Can Vet J* 2022; **63**(1): 39–46.

577 Levionnois OL, Graubner C, Spadavecchia C. Colon constipation in horses after sustained-release buprenorphine administration. *Vet Anaesth Analg* 2018; **45**(6): 876–880.

578 Castro-Cuellar G, Cremer J, Liu CC, *et al.* Buprenorphine has a concentration-dependent cytotoxic effect on equine chondrocytes *in vitro*. *Am J Vet Res* 2023; **84**(3): ajvr.22.08.0143.

579 Crabtree NE, Mochal-King CA, Sloan PB, *et al.* Synovial butorphanol concentrations and mechanical nociceptive thresholds after intravenous regional limb perfusion in standing sedated horses. *Vet Surg* 2019; **48**(8): 1473–1482.

580 Conner CM, Hoppes SM, Stevens BJ, *et al.* Intranasal butorphanol and midazolam administered prior to intramuscular alfaxalone provides safe and effective sedation in Quaker parrots (Myiopsitta monachus). *Am J Vet Res* 2022; **83**(12): ajvr.22.08.0140.

581 Okur S, Yanmaz LE, Golgeli A, *et al.* Sedative and cardiopulmonary effects of intranasal butorphanol with midazolam or dexmedetomidine in New Zealand white rabbits. *Vet Rec* 2023; **193**(1): e2999.

582 Springfield D, KuKanich B, Gray M, *et al.* Dosing protocols to increase the efficacy of butorphanol in dogs. *J Vet Pharmacol Ther* 2022; **45**(6): 516–529.

583 McFadzean WJ, Hall EJ, van Oostrom H. Effect of premedication with butorphanol or methadone on ease of endoscopic duodenal intubation in dogs. *Vet Anaesth Analg* 2017; **44**(6): 1296–1302.

584 Trimble T, Bhalla RJ, Leece EA. Comparison of sedation in dogs: methadone or butorphanol in combination with dexmedetomidine intravenously. *Vet Anaesth Analg* 2018; **45**(5): 597–603.

585 Gomes VH, Barbosa DJ, Motta AS, *et al.* Evaluation of nalbuphine, butorphanol and morphine in dogs during ovariohysterectomy and on early postoperative pain. *Vet Anaesth Analg* 2020; **47**(6): 803–809.

586 Gültiken N, Gürler H, Yarım GF, *et al.* Antioxidant and analgesic potential of butorphanol in dogs undergoing ovariohysterectomy. *Theriogenology* 2022; **190**: 1–7.

587 Giannettoni G, Moretti G, Menchetti L, *et al.* Sedation quality of alfaxalone associated with butorphanol, methadone or pethidine in cats injected into the supraspinatus or the quadriceps muscle. *J Feline Med Surg* 2022; **24**(8): e269–e280.

588 Papastefanou AK, Galatos AD, Pappa E, *et al.* The effect of butorphanol on the incidence of dexmedetomidine-induced emesis in cats. *Vet Anaesth Analg* 2015; **42**(6): 608–613.

589 Bhalla RJ, Trimble TA, Leece EA, *et al.* Comparison of intramuscular butorphanol and buprenorphine combined with dexmedetomidine for sedation in cats. *J Feline Med Surg* 2018; **20**(4): 325–331.

590 Lizarraga I, Castillo-Alcala F. Sedative and mechanical hypoalgesic effects of butorphanol in xylazine-premedicated donkeys. *Equine Vet J* 2015; **47**(3): 308–312.

591 Arguedas MG, Hines MT, Papich MG, *et al.* Pharmacokinetics of butorphanol and evaluation of physiologic and behavioral effects after intravenous and intramuscular administration to neonatal foals. *J Vet Intern Med* 2008; **22**(6): 1417–1426.

592 Almonte H, Schumacher J, Johnson CR, *et al.* Effect of a combination of butorphanol and detomidine on endoscopic assessment of laryngeal function in Thoroughbred yearlings. *Vet Rec* 2022; **190**(9): e1483.

593 Love EJ, Taylor PM, Clark C, *et al.* Analgesic effect of butorphanol in ponies following castration. *Equine Vet J* 2009; **41**(6): 552–556.

594 Haw AJ, Meyer LC, Fuller A. Nalbuphine and butorphanol reverse opioid-induced respiratory depression but increase arousal in etorphine-immobilized goats (Capra hircus). *Vet Anaesth Analg* 2016; **43**(5): 539–548.

595 Lester PA, Gaynor JS, Hellyer PW, *et al.* The sedative and behavioral effects of nalbuphine in dogs. *Contemp Top Lab Anim Sci* 2003; **42**(4): 27–31.

596 Gomes VH, Barcellos MC, Lima VC, *et al.* Effect of three doses of nalbuphine on reversal of sedation and cardiopulmonary effects of morphine-acepromazine in healthy dogs. *Vet Anaesth Analg* 2019; **46**(4): 429–434.

597 Gomes VH, Marques JLR, Janiques Borré LDS, *et al.* Comparison of the sedative effects of three nalbuphine doses, alone or combined with acepromazine, in dogs. *Am J Vet Res* 2022; **83**(7): ajvr.21.12.0214.

598 Flecknell PA, Kirk AJ, Liles JH, *et al.* Post-operative analgesia following thoracotomy in the dog: an evaluation of the effects of bupivacaine intercostal nerve block and nalbuphine on respiratory function. *Lab Anim* 1991; **25**(4): 319–324.

599 Frazílio Fde O, DeRossi R, Jardim PH, *et al.* Effects of epidural nalbuphine on intraoperative isoflurane and postoperative analgesic requirements in dogs. *Acta Cir Bras* 2014; **29**(1): 38–46.

600 Clark JS, Bentley E, Smith LJ. Evaluation of topical nalbuphine or oral tramadol as analgesics for corneal pain in dogs: a pilot study. *Vet Ophthalmol* 2011; **14**(6): 358–364.

601 Lee CH, Lin SL, Chi TT, *et al.* Effect of topical administration of 0.8% nalbuphine on the cornea in dogs after phacoemulsification. *J Vet Med Sci* 2013; **75**(8): 1041–1047.

602 Wotman KL, Utter ME. Effect of treatment with a topical ophthalmic preparation of 1% nalbuphine solution on corneal sensitivity in clinically normal horses. *Am J Vet Res* 2010; **71**(2): 223–228.

603 Muhammad SA, Farooq AA, Khan A, *et al.* Anaesthetic efficacy of nalbuphine HCl alone and in-combination with propofol and ketamine HCL in dogs. *Pak J Life Soc Sci* 2004; **2**: 40–42.

604 Marques MG, Marques A, de Siqueira CE, *et al.* Conventional echocardiography and two-dimensional speckle tracking in healthy sevoflurane-anesthetized dogs undergoing continuous rate infusion of nalbuphine. *Vet Med Int* 2020; **2020**: 9278751.

605 Costa GP, Monteiro ER, Marques É J, *et al.* Sedative effects of acepromazine in combination with nalbuphine or butorphanol, intramuscularly or intravenously, in healthy cats: a randomized, blinded clinical trial. *J Feline Med Surg* 2021; **23**(6): 540–548.

606 Kreisler RE, Cornell HN, Smith VA, *et al.* Use of nalbuphine as a substitute for butorphanol in combination with dexmedetomidine and tiletamine/zolazepam: a randomized non-inferiority trial. *J Feline Med Surg* 2020; **22**(2): 100–107.

607 Kulkarni H, William BJ, George RS, *et al.* Analgesic and adjunct actions of nalbuphine hydrochloride in xylazine or xylazine and acepromazine premedicated horses. *Indian J Anim Res* 2015; **49**: 699–703.

608 Brunson DB, Majors LJ. Comparative analgesia of xylazine, xylazine/morphine, xylazine/butorphanol, and xylazine/nalbuphine in the horse, using dental dolorimetry. *Am J Vet Res* 1987; **48**(7): 1087–1091.

609 Abouelfetouh MM, Salah E, Liu L, *et al.* Immediate postoperative analgesia of nalbuphine-ketamine combination compared with ketamine alone in xylazine-sedated goats undergoing left flank laparotomy. *Animals (Basel)* 2022; **12**(4): 509.
610 O'Hair KC, Dodd KT, Phillips YY, *et al.* Cardiopulmonary effects of nalbuphine hydrochloride and butorphanol tartrate in sheep. *Lab Anim Sci* 1988; **38**(1): 58–61.
611 Sanchez-Migallon Guzman D, KuKanich B, Keuler NS, *et al.* Antinociceptive effects of nalbuphine hydrochloride in Hispaniolan Amazon parrots (*Amazona ventralis*). *Am J Vet Res* 2011; **72**(6): 736–740.
612 Sanchez-Migallon Guzman D, Braun JM, Steagall PV, *et al.* Antinociceptive effects of long-acting nalbuphine decanoate after intramuscular administration to Hispaniolan Amazon parrots (*Amazona ventralis*). *Am J Vet Res* 2013; **74**(2): 196–200.
613 Keller DL, Sanchez-Migallon Guzman D, Klauer JM, *et al.* Pharmacokinetics of nalbuphine hydrochloride after intravenous and intramuscular administration to Hispaniolan Amazon parrots (*Amazona ventralis*). *Am J Vet Res* 2011; **72**(6): 741–745.
614 Sanchez-Migallon Guzman D, KuKanich B, Heath TD, *et al.* Pharmacokinetics of long-acting nalbuphine decanoate after intramuscular administration to Hispaniolan Amazon parrots (*Amazona ventralis*). *Am J Vet Res* 2013; **74**(2): 191–195.
615 Mills CA, Flacke JW, Flacke WE, *et al.* Narcotic reversal in hypercapnic dogs: comparison of naloxone and nalbuphine. *Can J Anaesth* 1990; **37**(2): 238–244.
616 Fletcher DJ, Boller M, Brainard BM, *et al.* RECOVER evidence and knowledge gap analysis on veterinary CPR. Part 7: clinical guidelines. *J Vet Emerg Crit Care (San Antonio)* 2012; **22**(Suppl 1): S102–S131.
617 Palmer LE, Gautier A. Clinical update: the risk of opioid toxicity and naloxone use in operational K9s. *J Spec Oper Med* 2017; **17**(4): 86–92.
618 Wahler BM, Lerche P, Ricco Pereira CH, *et al.* Pharmacokinetics and pharmacodynamics of intranasal and intravenous naloxone hydrochloride administration in healthy dogs. *Am J Vet Res* 2019; **80**(7): 696–701.
619 Copland VS, Haskins SC, Patz J. Naloxone reversal of oxymorphone effects in dogs. *Am J Vet Res* 1989; **50**(11): 1854–1858.
620 Rzasa Lynn R, Galinkin JL. Naloxone dosage for opioid reversal: current evidence and clinical implications. *Ther Adv Drug Saf* 2018; **9**(1): 63–88.
621 Turner DM, Kassell NF, Sasaki T, *et al.* High dose naloxone produces cerebral vasodilation. *Neurosurgery* 1984; **15**(2): 192–197.
622 Levin ER, Sharp B, Drayer JI, *et al.* Severe hypertension induced by naloxone. *Am J Med Sci* 1985; **290**(2): 70–72.
623 Thind GS, Wells JC, Wilkes RG. The effects of continuous intravenous naloxone on epidural morphine analgesia. *Anaesthesia* 1986; **41**(6): 582–585.
624 Rawal N, Möllefors K, Axelsson K, *et al.* An experimental study of urodynamic effects of epidural morphine and of naloxone reversal. *Anesth Analg* 1983; **62**(7): 641–647.
625 Weld JM, Kamerling SG, Combie JD, *et al.* The effects of naloxone on endotoxic and hemorrhagic shock in horses. *Res Commun Chem Pathol Pharmacol* 1984; **44**(2): 227–238.
626 Pace NL, Parrish RG, Lieberman MM, *et al.* Pharmacokinetics of naloxone and naltrexone in the dog. *J Pharmacol Exp Ther* 1979; **208**(2): 254–256.
627 Pypendop BH, Brosnan RJ, Ilkiw JE. Use of naltrexone to antagonize high doses of remifentanil in cats: a dose-finding study. *Vet Anaesth Analg* 2011; **38**(6): 594–597.
628 Brown DR, Goldberg LI. The use of quaternary narcotic antagonists in opiate research. *Neuropharmacol* 1985; **24**(3): 181–191.
629 Chandrasekaran A, Tong Z, Li H, *et al.* Metabolism of intravenous methylnaltrexone in mice, rats, dogs, and humans. *Drug Metab Dispos* 2010; **38**(4): 606–616.
630 Beavers J, Orton L, Atchison L, *et al.* The efficacy and safety of methylnaltrexone for the treatment of postoperative ileus. *Am Surg* 2022; **88**(3): 409–413.
631 van Hoogmoed LM, Boscan PL. *In vitro* evaluation of the effect of the opioid antagonist N-methylnaltrexone on motility of the equine jejunum and pelvic flexure. *Equine Vet J* 2005; **37**(4): 325–328.
632 Boscan P, Van Hoogmoed LM, Pypendop BH, *et al.* Pharmacokinetics of the opioid antagonist N-methylnaltrexone and evaluation of its effects on gastrointestinal tract function in horses treated or not treated with morphine. *Am J Vet Res* 2006; **67**(6): 998–1004.
633 Martín-Flores M, Singh B, Walsh CA, *et al.* Effects of buprenorphine, methylnaltrexone, and their combination on gastrointestinal transit in healthy New Zealand White rabbits. *J Am Assoc Lab Anim Sci* 2017; **56**(2): 155–159.
634 Domínguez-Oliva A, Casas-Alvarado A, Miranda-Cortés AE, *et al.* Clinical pharmacology of tramadol and tapentadol, and their therapeutic efficacy in different models of acute and chronic pain in dogs and cats. *J Adv Vet Anim Res* 2021; **8**(3): 404–422.
635 Schütter AF, Tünsmeyer J, Kästner SBR. Influence of tramadol on acute thermal and mechanical cutaneous nociception in dogs. *Vet Anaesth Analg* 2017; **44**(2): 309–316.
636 Donati PA, Tarragona L, Franco JVA, *et al.* Efficacy of tramadol for postoperative pain management in dogs: systematic review and meta-analysis. *Vet Anaesth Analg* 2021; **48**(3): 283–296.
637 Kongara K, Chambers JP, Johnson CB, *et al.* Effects of tramadol or morphine in dogs undergoing castration on intra-operative electroencephalogram responses and post-operative pain. *N Z Vet J* 2013; **61**(6): 349–353.
638 Thengchaisri N, Mahidol C. Evaluating the effects of continuous intravenous infusions of tramadol and tramadol-lidocaine on sevoflurane minimum alveolar concentration (MAC) and entropy values in dogs. *J Vet Med Sci* 2019; **81**(5): 682–688.
639 El-Hawari SF, Oyama N, Koyama Y, *et al.* Sparing effect of tramadol, lidocaine, dexmedetomidine and their combination on the minimum alveolar concentration of sevoflurane in dogs. *J Vet Sci* 2022; **23**(4): e53.
640 Delgado C, Bentley E, Hetzel S, *et al.* Comparison of carprofen and tramadol for postoperative analgesia in dogs undergoing enucleation. *J Am Vet Med Assoc* 2014; **245**(12): 1375–1381.
641 Budsberg SC, Torres BT, Kleine SA, *et al.* Lack of effectiveness of tramadol hydrochloride for the treatment of pain and joint dysfunction in dogs with chronic osteoarthritis. *J Am Vet Med Assoc* 2018; **252**(4): 427–432.
642 Meunier NV, Panti A, Mazeri S, *et al.* Randomised trial of perioperative tramadol for canine sterilisation pain management. *Vet Rec* 2019; **185**(13): 406.
643 Piras LA, Mancusi D, Olimpo M, *et al.* Post-operative analgesia following TPLO surgery: a comparison between cimicoxib and tramadol. *Res Vet Sci* 2021; **136**: 351–359.
644 Pypendop BH, Siao KT, Ilkiw JE. Effects of tramadol hydrochloride on the thermal threshold in cats. *Am J Vet Res* 2009; **70**(12): 1465–1470.
645 Evangelista MC, Silva RA, Cardozo LB, *et al.* Comparison of preoperative tramadol and pethidine on postoperative pain in cats undergoing ovariohysterectomy. *BMC Vet Res* 2014; **10**: 252.
646 Bauquier SH. Randomised clinical trial comparing the perioperative analgesic efficacy of oral tramadol and intramuscular tramadol in cats. *J Feline Med Surg* 2022; **24**(8): 683–690.
647 Guedes AGP, Meadows JM, Pypendop BH, *et al.* Evaluation of tramadol for treatment of osteoarthritis in geriatric cats. *J Am Vet Med Assoc* 2018; **252**(5): 565–571.
648 Vullo C, Falcone A, Marino G, *et al.* Comparison between the effects of epidural lidocaine, tramadol, and lidocaine-tramadol on postoperative pain in cats undergoing elective orchiectomy. *Acta Vet Scand* 2023; **65**(1): 33.
649 Aldrich LA, Roush JK, KuKanich B. Plasma concentrations of tramadol after transdermal application of a single metered dose of a compounded tramadol gel to cats. *Am J Vet Res* 2021; **82**(10): 840–845.
650 Indrawirawan Y, McAlees T. Tramadol toxicity in a cat: case report and literature review of serotonin syndrome. *J Feline Med Surg* 2014; **16**(7): 572–578.
651 Dhanjal JK, Wilson DV, Robinson E, *et al.* Intravenous tramadol: effects, nociceptive properties, and pharmacokinetics in horses. *Vet Anaesth Analg* 2009; **36**(6): 581–590.
652 Tavanaeimanesh H, Azarnoosh A, Ashar FS, *et al.* Comparison of analgesic effects of a constant rate infusion of both tramadol and acetaminophen versus those of infusions of each individual drug in horses. *J Equine Vet Sci* 2018; **64**: 101–106.
653 Guedes AG, Matthews NS, Hood DM. Effect of ketamine hydrochloride on the analgesic effects of tramadol hydrochloride in horses with signs of chronic laminitis-associated pain. *Am J Vet Res* 2012; **73**(5): 610–619.
654 Di Salvo A, Chiaradia E, Della Rocca G, *et al.* Efficacy, chondrotoxicity and plasma concentrations of tramadol following intra-articular administration in horses undergoing arthroscopy: preliminary findings. *Vet Q* 2018; **38**(1): 129–137.
655 Howard J, Aarnes TK, Dyce J, *et al.* Pharmacokinetics and pharmacodynamics after oral administration of tapentadol hydrochloride in dogs. *Am J Vet Res* 2018; **79**(4): 367–375.
656 Lakritz J, Aarnes TK, Alva B, *et al.* Pharmacokinetics of oral tapentadol in cats. *J Vet Pharmacol Ther* 2024; **47**(1): 14–20.
657 Kieves NR, Howard J, Lerche P, *et al.* Effectiveness of tapentadol hydrochloride for treatment of orthopedic pain in dogs: a pilot study. *Can Vet J* 2020; **61**(3): 289–293.
658 Doodnaught GM, Evangelista MC, Steagall PVM. Thermal antinociception following oral administration of tapentadol in conscious cats. *Vet Anaesth Analg* 2017; **44**(2): 364–369.

24 Non-Steroidal Anti-Inflammatory Drugs

Mark G. Papich
Department of Molecular Biomedical Sciences, College of Veterinary Medicine, North Carolina State University, Raleigh, North Carolina, USA

Chapter contents

Introduction, 398
Mechanism of action, 398
Metabolism of arachidonic acid, 398
Other possible mechanisms of action, 404
COX-1 versus COX-2 inhibition, 404
Pharmacokinetic properties, 405
Stereoisomerism, 406
Pharmacokinetic-pharmacodynamic properties, 406
In vivo assessment of PK-PD models, 406
Unique features of non-traditional NSAIDs, 406
Grapiprant, 406
Acetaminophen (Paracetamol), 407
Dipyrone (Metamizole), 408
Adverse effects of NSAIDs, 408
Gastrointestinal injury, 408
Kidney injury related to NSAID administration, 410
Effects of NSAIDs on the liver, 411
Injury to cartilage, 412
Blood coagulation effects: platelet inhibition and thrombotic abnormalities, 412
Risks in people compared to animals, 412
Drug selection, 412
COX-2 inhibition as selection criterion, 412
Selection of NSAIDs for dogs, 413
Selection of NSAIDs for cats, 414
Selection of NSAIDs for horses, 414
NSAID selection for food animals, 415
References, 415

Introduction

Non-steroidal anti-inflammatory drugs (NSAIDs) are among the most important drugs used in all species of animals. They have the advantage of producing both analgesic and anti-inflammatory effects in animals. Because they are not controlled or scheduled drugs, they can be easily prescribed and dispensed. There are a variety of formulations and routes of administration to choose from that include oral tablets, oral caplets, oral liquids, chewable tablets, paste (for horses), oral transmucosal mist, transdermal, and injectable solutions for intravenous (IV) or subcutaneous (SC) administration (Table 24.1, Box 24.1).

This chapter will focus primarily on the most common drugs used in most countries, but the reader should appreciate that availability, registration, licensing, and approvals by regulatory authorities vary greatly around the world. There are drugs available in some countries that are not available in others and some older drugs on the market that have been replaced by newer approved animal drugs in some countries. Some older drugs for which new information has not been generated in many years (aspirin for example) will not be covered in this chapter, but details of their pharmacology may be found in previous editions of this and other older textbooks. Although this chapter focuses primarily on the major veterinary species of dogs, cats, horses, and cattle, the use of NSAIDs in other animals should not be overlooked. There has been extensive work in zoo and exotic species, particularly new work published in non-mammalian species. Surprising differences in both activity (e.g., cyclo-oxygenase [COX] activity) and pharmacokinetics exist among these other species. But it is beyond the scope of this chapter to address all the other animal species in which NSAIDs are administered; therefore, the reader is encouraged to consult species-specific publications for more guidance.

Information on the pharmacology of these agents has been provided by Lees [1] as well as many other authors [2–5]. Guidelines for clinical use in dogs [2,6–8], cats [7–11], horses [12], and food animals [13] are available in species-specific reviews. A description of the chemistry, mechanism of action, and clinical use of the coxib class of NSAIDs is also available [14,15]. Because these extensive and complete reviews are available, these details will be abbreviated for this chapter.

Mechanism of action

Metabolism of arachidonic acid

As shown in Fig. 24.1, arachidonic acid, a fatty acid consisting of 20 carbons, is released from cell membranes by the enzyme phospholipase A_2 (PLA_2). Arachidonic acid is the predominant fatty acid in animal cell membranes. The products of arachidonic acid biotransformation are referred to as "eicosanoids" because of their structure

Veterinary Anesthesia and Analgesia: The Sixth Edition of Lumb and Jones. Edited by Leigh Lamont, Kurt Grimm, Sheilah Robertson, Lydia Love and Carrie Schroeder.
© 2024 John Wiley & Sons, Inc. Published 2024 by John Wiley & Sons, Inc.
Companion website: www.wiley.com/go/lamont/anesthesia

Table 24.1 Classification and pharmacologic parameters for selected non-steroidal anti-inflammatory drugs commonly used in animals.

Drug	Chemical group and structure	COX-1 or COX-2 inhibitory	Half-life ($t_{1/2}$)	Apparent volume of distribution (V_d)[a]	Bioavailability (F%)[b]	Protein binding
Acetaminophen (Paracetamol)	Aminophenol	No significant COX activity	Dogs: 1–4 h (depending on the study) Cats: 0.6 h Horses: 2–5 h (depending on the study)	Dogs: 0.87–1.3 L/kg	Dogs: 44–100% (depending on the study)	
Carprofen	Propionic acid	Preferential for COX-2	*S*(+)-enantiomer Dogs: 11.7 h (100 mg IV bolus) and ~ 8 h (range 4.5–9.8 h, oral) Horses: 8–20 h (depending on the study) Cats: 20±16.6 h (range 9–49 h); and 10.7±5.17 h Calves: 37±2.4 h Cows: 30.7±2.3 h (43±2.3 h with mastitis)	Dogs: 0.14±0.02 L/kg Cats: 0.14±0.05 L/kg; and 0.25 L/kg Horses: 0.307±0.036 L/kg Calves: 0.163±0.002 L/kg Cows: 0.091±0.003 L/kg	Dogs: > 90% (oral)	Dogs: > 99%
Deracoxib	Coxib (diaryl substituted pyrazole)	Selective for COX-2	Dogs: 3 h (2–3 mg/kg IV) Cats: 7.9 h	Dogs: ~ 1.5 L/kg	Dogs: > 90% (2 mg/kg, oral)	Dogs: > 90%
Robenacoxib	Coxib	Selective for COX-2	Dogs: 0.63 and 1.1 h Cats: 1.49, 1.87, 0.84, and 0.78 h (depending on the study)	Dogs: 0.24 L/kg Cats: 0.13 and 0.19 L/kg (depending on the study)	Dogs: 84% (non-fed); 62% (fed) Cats: 49% (non-fed); 10% (fed)	Dogs: 98% Cats: 99.9%

(*Continued*)

Table 24.1 (Continued)

Drug	Chemical group and structure	COX-1 or COX-2 inhibitory	Half-life ($t_{1/2}$)	Apparent volume of distribution (V_d)[a]	Bioavailability (F%)[b]	Protein binding
Etodolac	Pyranocarboxylic acid 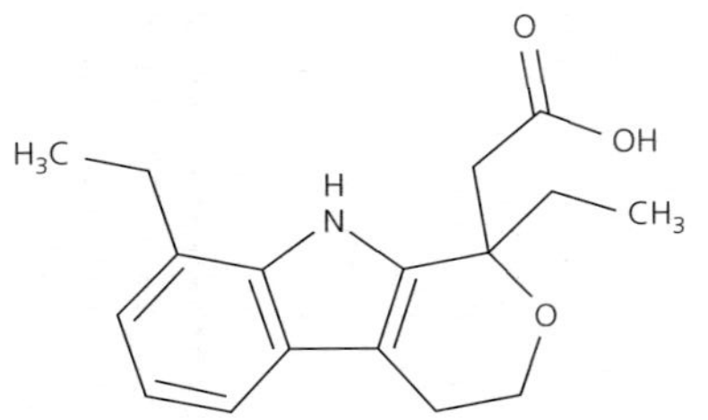	Non-selective for COX-2 or preferential for COX-2 (depending on the study)	Dogs: 7.66±2.05 h (oral, fasted); 11.98±5.52 h (oral, non-fasted); 9.7±0.97 h (IV) Horses: 2.85 h (mean)	Dogs: 1.14 L/kg Horses: 0.29±0.09 L/kg	Dogs: ~ 100% Horses: 77% (range 43–100%)	Dogs: > 95%
Firocoxib	Coxib 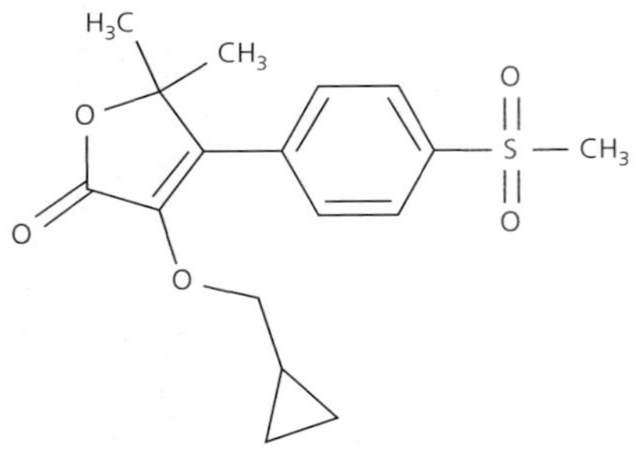	Selective for COX-2 (most highly selective of all the veterinary NSAIDs)	Dogs: 7.8 h Horses: ~ 30–40 h	Dogs: ~ 4.6 L/kg Horses: 1.7 L/kg	Dogs: ~ 38% Horses: 80–100%	Dogs: 96% Horses: > 97%
Grapiprant	Piprant 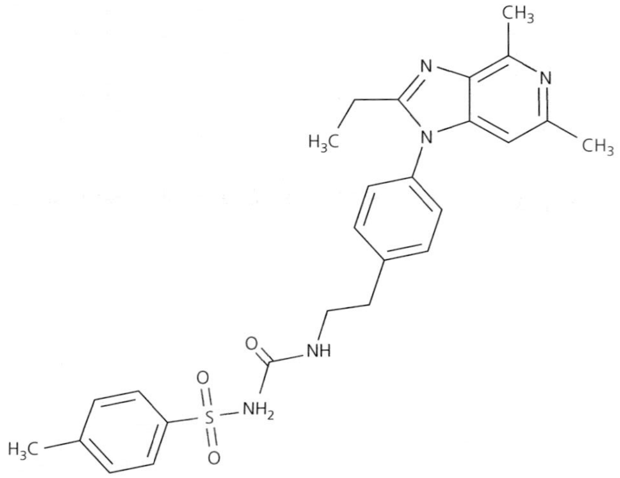	No COX activity; antagonist of the prostaglandin-E_2 (PGE_2) receptor 4 (EP4)	Dogs: 1.95–5.42 h Cats: 4.4 h Horses: 5.86 h	Dogs: 1.9 L/kg Cats: 0.92 L/kg	Dogs: 90% (higher in fasted) Cats: 40%	Dogs: 95%

Ketoprofen	Propionic acid 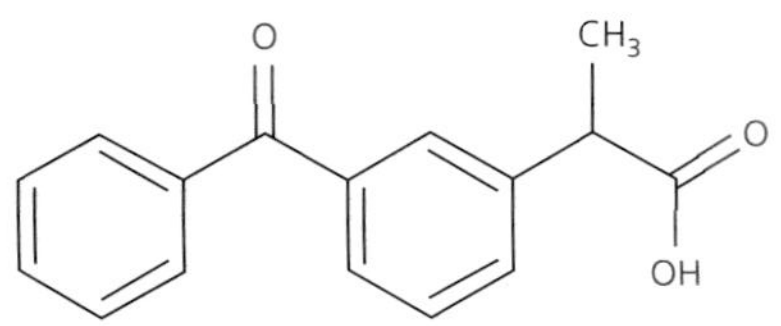	Non-selective for COX-2	*S*(+)-enantiomer Dogs: 1.65 ±0.48 h (oral) Cats: 1.5 h Horses: 1–7 h (depending on the study) Calves: 0.42–2.19 h (depending on study and age)	*S*(+)-enantiomer Dogs: 0.39±0.07 L/kg Horses: 0.14±0.02 L/kg and 0.22±0.08 L/kg Calves: 0.26±0.06 L/kg	Dogs, Cats: almost 100% Horses: 70–100%	Horses: 93%
Mavacoxib	Coxib 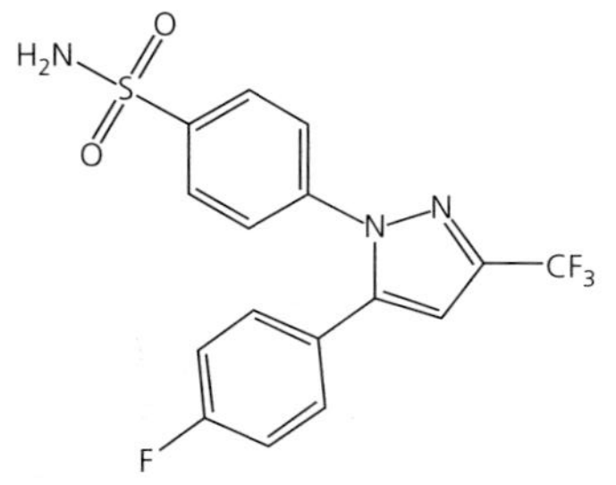	COX-2 selective	Dogs: 17 days median (range 8–39 days in Beagle dogs) and 39 days (in field trial dogs, with some dogs > 80 days)	Dogs: 1.6 L/kg	Dogs: 46.1% (fasted), 87.4% (fed); dose based on fed dogs	Dogs: 98%
Meloxicam	Enolic acid derivative (oxicam) 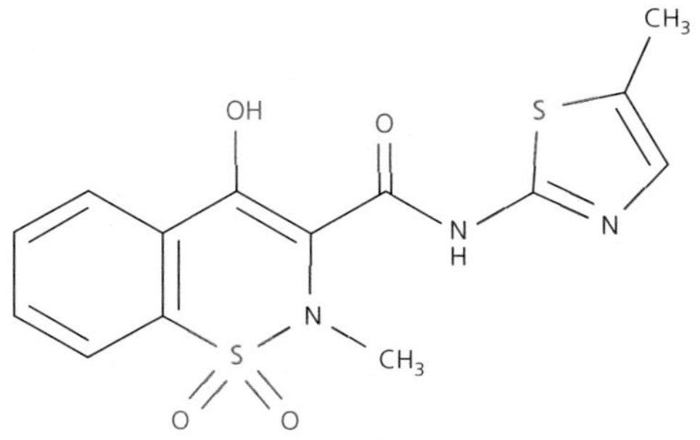	COX-2 preferential, but at high doses COX-2 specificity diminishes	Dogs: 24.0±26.2% h (IV), 23.7±30.0% h (oral) Cats: 26–37 h (depending on study) Horses: 5–12 h (depending on the study and formulation) Cattle: 20–30 h (depending on the study), 14.6 h (cows)	Dogs: ~ 0.32±20% L/kg ($V_{d\text{-}area}$) Horses: 0.23 and 0.12 L/kg (depending on study) Cats: 0.245 L/kg (V_d/F) Cattle: 0.194 L/kg	Dogs: 100% Horses: 75–100% Cattle: 100%	Dogs: 97% Horses: 98.5%
Phenylbutazone	Pyrazolone (pyrazolidinedione) 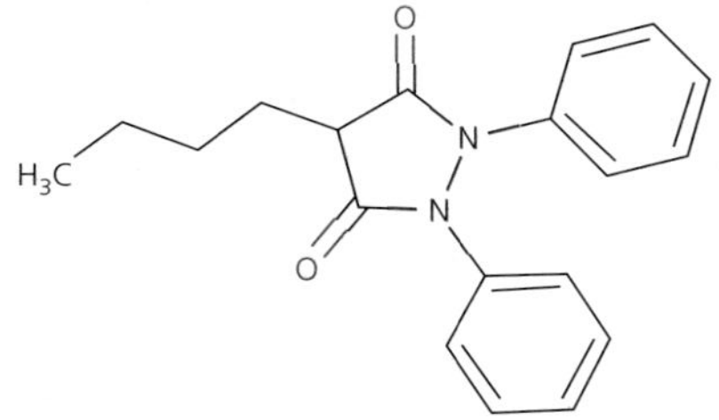	Non-selective for COX-2	Horses: 5 and up to 7 h (depending on the study) Calves: 53.4 h Bulls: 62 h Cows: 36–55 h (depending on the study) Dogs: 4–6 h	Cattle: 0.13–0.14 L/kg Horses: 0.14 L/kg	Cattle: 54–69% and 69–89% (depending on the study) Horses: 70% (delayed with feeding)	Horses: 99% Cattle: 93–98%

(*Continued*)

Table 24.1 (Continued)

Drug	Chemical group and structure	COX-1 or COX-2 inhibitory	Half-life ($t_{1/2}$)	Apparent volume of distribution (V_d)[a]	Bioavailability (F%)[b]	Protein binding
Flunixin	Anthranilic acid (pyridinecarboxylic acid) 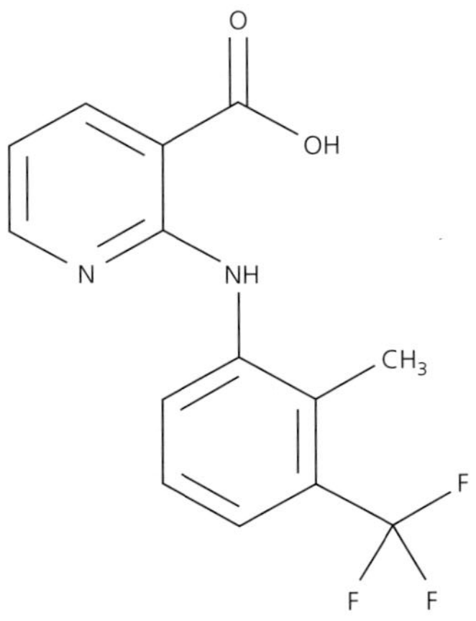	Non-selective for COX-2	Horses: 2–3 h (in most studies) Cows: 3–8 h (depending on the study) Dogs: 3.7 h Cats: 6.6 h	Horses: 0.15±0.04 L/kg Dogs: 0.18±0.08 L/kg Cats: 0.75 L/kg Cows: 0.42, 0.78, and 0.50 L/kg in different studies	Dogs: ~ 100% Horses: 72%	> 90% in all animals studied
Dipyrone (Metamizole)	Pyrazolone 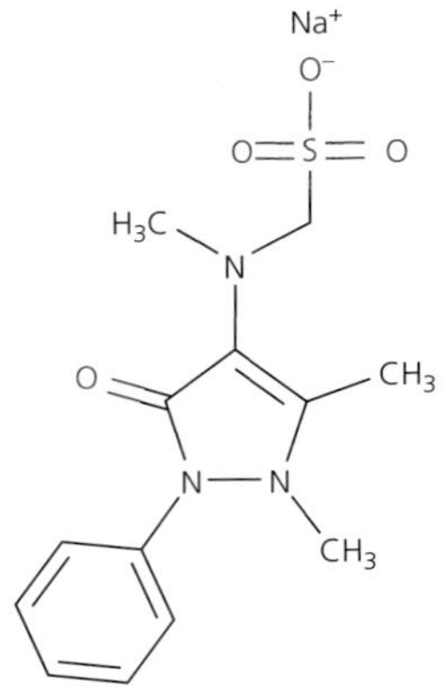	Mechanism uncertain; may inhibit COX-3 or act through other mechanisms	All values based on the major active metabolite. Horses: 3–6 h Dogs: 5–6 h Cats: 6–7 h	All values based on the major active metabolite. Horses: 1.4–1.6 L/kg Dogs: 5 L/kg Cats: 0.967 L/kg	All values based on the major active metabolite. Dogs: 100% Cats: 81%	Not reported

Pharmacokinetic parameters derived from references cited in the text.
[a] Apparent volume of distribution (V_d) for most drugs at steady state, unless otherwise noted.
[b] Percent bioavailability (F%) after oral administration.
Colored portions of the structural diagrams represent the reactive groups.

Box 24.1 NSAIDS that have been used in various species.

NSAIDs used in dogs
- Aspirin[a]
- Phenylbutazone[b]
- Carprofen (Rimadyl, and generic)[e]
- Etodolac (EtoGesic)[b]
- Meloxicam (Metacam, and generic)[e]
- Ketoprofen (Anafen)[d]
- Deracoxib (Deramaxx)
- Firocoxib (Previcox)
- Meclofenamic acid (Arquel)[b]
- Robenacoxib (Onsior)[e,g]
- Grapiprant (Galliprant)
- Tepoxalin (Zubrin)[b]
- Mavacoxib (Trocoxil)[f]
- Tolfenamic acid (Tolfedine)[d,e]
- Cimicoxib[f]

NSAIDs used in cats
- Aspirin[a]
- Meloxicam (Metacam)[c,e]
- Carprofen[e,f]
- Robenacoxib[e]
- Ketoprofen[d]
- Tolfenamic acid (Tolfedine)[d,e]

NSAIDs used in horses
- Aspirin[a]
- Flunixin meglumine
- Ketoprofen
- Phenylbutazone
- Meclofenamic acid[b]
- Meloxicam[f]

NSAIDs used in cattle
- Flunixin meglumine
- Ketoprofen
- Meloxicam[f]

NSAIDs used in pigs
- Ketoprofen[f]
- Meloxicam[f]

[a] Aspirin is not FDA-approved for dogs, cats, or horses, with the exception of a combination with methylprednisolone (Cortaba tablets, 0.5 mg of methylprednisolone and 300 mg of aspirin).
[b] Approved but not actively marketed.
[c] Approved for cats also as a single dose in the US, but for oral multiple doses in other countries.
[d] Approved in Canada and other countries for small animals but not in the US for small animals.
[e] Available as an injectable as well as oral formulation.
[f] Approved for this use in other countries, but not the US.
[g] Oral robenacoxib was withdrawn by the sponsor for dogs in the US.

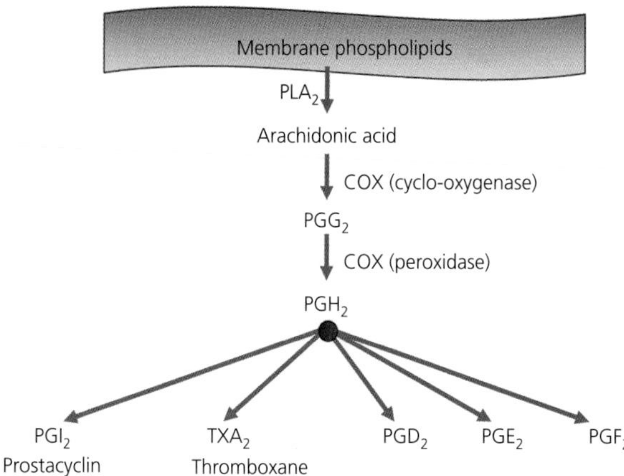

Figure 24.1 Membrane phospholipids are the source of arachidonic acid, the major eicosanoid in animals. Arachidonic acid is further metabolized by COX enzymes to the various prostaglandins (PGs), prostacyclin, and thromboxane to produce clinical, immunologic, and physiologic functions. The COX enzymes are the targets for non-steroidal anti-inflammatory drugs.

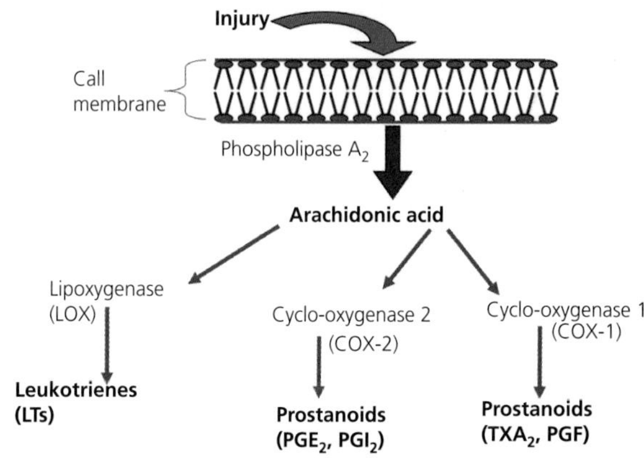

Figure 24.2 Metabolism of arachidonic acid products. The cell membrane generates arachidonic acid via de-esterification by the enzyme phospholipase A_2. Arachidonic acid is further metabolized by cyclo-oxygenase enzymes (COX-1 and COX-2) to the various prostaglandins (PGs), prostacyclin (PGI_2), and thromboxane (TXA_2) to produce clinical, immunologic, and physiologic functions. An alternative pathway is via the lipoxygenase enzyme (LOX), which produces the inflammatory leukotrienes (LTs). The COX enzymes are the targets for non-steroidal anti-inflammatory drugs, but do not ordinarily affect the LOX enzymes.

of 20 carbons (Greek *eikosi* = 20). Most arachidonic acid is recycled back to the cell membranes, but in the face of various stimuli, arachidonic acid may be acted upon by COX or lipoxygenase (LOX) enzymes to form various eicosanoids, which have a role in homeostasis and disease (Fig. 24.2). Prostanoids are specific eicosanoids that are further metabolized into the various prostaglandins (PGD_2, $PGF_{2\alpha}$, and PGE_2), prostacyclin (PGI_2), and thromboxane (TXA_2). These products act locally via G-protein-coupled receptors to generate inflammatory and immunological responses and are also responsible for important physiological functions. A group of LOX products, the leukotrienes, are also responsible for inflammation, but are not inhibited by the traditional drugs covered in this chapter and will not be further discussed.

The action of traditional NSAIDs is to inhibit COX enzymes and alter the formation of the prostanoids [16]. The significant development that improved the understanding of NSAIDs' mechanism of action occurred in the early 1990s when new details about the targets of these drugs emerged [17,18]. It was elucidated that there are two isoenzymes (isoforms) of COX (also known as "prostaglandin synthase") that are responsible for synthesis of prostaglandins. Prostaglandin synthase-1 (COX-1) is usually simplistically described as a constitutive enzyme expressed in tissues [17,18]. Prostaglandins, prostacyclin, and thromboxane synthesized by this enzyme are responsible for normal physiologic functions. Prostaglandin synthase-2 (COX-2), on the other hand, is inducible (upregulated) and synthesized by macrophages and inflammatory cells after stimulation by cytokines and other mediators of inflammation. In 2002, a third isoenzyme of COX was described [19,20]. The COX-3 enzyme is a splice variant from the COX-1 gene, which to date has only been identified in the canine brain, human brain, and heart [20]. It is hypothesized that the mechanism of action of acetaminophen (paracetamol) is by inhibition of COX-3 although this hypothesis predated the discovery of the COX-3 splicing variant [19,20]. Acetaminophen may have other mechanisms of action, as discussed later in this chapter.

An exception to this traditional view of COX enzyme inhibition by NSAIDs is the action of grapiprant, a new class of drugs that can technically be considered "non-steroidal anti-inflammatory drugs," but do not inhibit the COX enzyme. This agent will be discussed in more detail later in the chapter. Instead of inhibiting production of prostaglandins, it blocks the prostaglandin receptor. After inflammation is triggered and prostaglandins are synthesized, prostaglandin-E_2 (PGE_2) exerts its effects via four receptors (EP1-4). The EP4 receptor is responsible for some of the sensitization of sensory neurons and signs of inflammation. Although other receptors are activated during inflammation, the EP4 receptor has been identified as the primary receptor responsible for mediating pain and inflammation associated with osteoarthritis. One of the new "non-traditional" NSAIDs, also called "piprants," is grapiprant, which blocks this receptor.

The explanation of COX function described above is likely too simplistic. Both enzymes can participate in regulatory and homeostatic function, and both can produce pain and inflammation. The predominant enzyme reflects the tissue or cell type in which it is produced. For example, COX-1 is the dominant enzyme in platelets, and COX-2 is the dominant enzyme in inflammatory cells. In bone, COX-1 is expressed under normal conditions, but COX-2 is expressed during mechanical stress. Some COX-2 products are important for homeostatic function, and COX-1 products are involved in pain and inflammation. Prostaglandin synthesis is inherently higher in canine gastric mucosa than duodenal mucosa [21,22], but COX-2 production of prostaglandins can be upregulated in these tissues, responding to inflammatory stimuli to produce a protective and healing role [23]. COX-2 products are also important in normal renal function. COX-2 may be upregulated under conditions that may be stressful to the kidney, such as hypovolemia or severe hypotension [24,25].

Therefore, the perception that COX-2 is a "bad" enzyme and COX-1 is a "good" enzyme is too simplistic because we now understand that there is some overlap in the functions of these isoforms on organs [26]. Drugs that inhibit these enzymes (e.g., NSAIDs) can be effective and/or harmful regardless of whether they are selective or non-selective in their action on these enzymes. Nevertheless, some of the most recently developed NSAIDs have targeted COX-2 inhibition, so that COX-1 is spared as much as possible with the goal of producing analgesia and suppressing inflammation without inhibiting physiologically important prostanoids, particularly the COX-1 products in the gastrointestinal tract.

Other possible mechanisms of action

Although it is assumed that prostaglandin inhibition in both peripheral and nervous system (spinal and brain) tissues is the most important mechanism of action for most NSAIDs, there may be other mechanisms to explain some of their effects. These properties have not been accepted as a mechanism compared to prostaglandin inhibition but deserve some consideration. Some NSAIDs, including salicylates, may inhibit nuclear factor kappa-B (NF-κB), which promotes synthesis of other inflammatory mediators. There is not universal agreement on the mechanism of action of carprofen, which is the most commonly prescribed NSAID in dogs. Carprofen significantly inhibited PGE_2 (a biomarker for COX-2) directly at sites of inflammation in dogs, providing evidence that carprofen does indeed act on COX-2 [27]. Other evidence indicates that it inhibits prostaglandins *in vitro* [28], but carprofen did not show an *in vivo* antiprostaglandin effect in dogs [29,30]. In another study, the investigators were unable to show that carprofen inhibited either COX-1 or COX-2 [31], suggesting either a central mechanism of action or activity on other pathways.

In horses, similar questions have been raised [32] with a conclusion that the anti-inflammatory effects of carprofen in horses were not caused by COX inhibition. In another study in the same laboratory [33], they concluded that recommended doses of carprofen produce minimal inhibition of COX, and it is likely to achieve its therapeutic effects at least partially through other pathways, possibly including weak to moderate inhibition of 5-lipoxygenase and enzyme release. Other investigators [34] also concluded that there may be COX-independent mechanisms for some NSAIDs in the equine intestine.

COX-1 versus COX-2 inhibition

Selectivity of COX-2 versus COX-1 has been expressed as the COX-1:COX-2 inhibitory ratio. This ratio is derived from studies in which the inhibitory effect, usually expressed as the inhibitory concentration to inhibit 50% of activity (IC_{50}), is measured from stimulating cells that are capable of expressing products of these enzymes. In the whole blood assay, the source for COX-1 products (thromboxane or TXA_2) is platelets and the source of COX-2 products (PGE_2) is leukocytes. The ratio is expressed as COX-1 [IC_{50}]:COX-2 [IC_{50}], or simply COX-1:COX-2. The higher the value above 1.0, the greater the inhibitory action of the drug is for COX-2 compared to COX-1. There is subjective value placed on the magnitude of the ratio when considering the drug as "COX-1 sparing," "COX-2 specific," "COX-2 preferential," or "COX-2 selective." These terms have been used by other investigators [35], but the magnitude of the ratios that define these criteria has not been agreed upon. In reality, COX-2 selectivity is a continuous variable that does not easily allow a distinct definition of COX-2 selective or non-selective. These are relative definitions, rather than absolute categories of NSAIDs.

The drugs with the highest inhibitory ratios are the selective COX-2 inhibitors (based on *in vitro* assays for the COX-2 enzyme) often called the "coxibs" or "coxib class of NSAIDs." These drugs include the veterinary products firocoxib, deracoxib, robenacoxib, and mavacoxib and the human product celecoxib (other coxibs such as rofecoxib have been withdrawn from the human market because of adverse effects on the cardiovascular system in human patients). Carprofen and meloxicam can be considered somewhat COX-2 preferential. Ketoprofen is non-selective, and etodolac has been classified as somewhat preferential to non-selective, depending on the study referenced. Aspirin is highly COX-1 selective. Although the IC_{50} ratio is the normal convention used for determination of COX selectivity [4,5], some investigators have proposed that a higher inhibitory concentration ratio (e.g., IC_{80}) may be better for predicting clinical efficacy, because such a high degree of inhibition may be necessary for analgesia or anti-inflammatory effects [36].

Comparisons of COX-1 versus COX-2 inhibition of veterinary NSAIDs vary among the drugs, animal species, and study technique used [15,37]. For example, deracoxib is considered a highly selective COX-2 inhibitor based on an assay performed in purified enzymes [38]. In this study, the COX-1:COX-2 ratio was 1275, much higher than other drugs tested. But when tested using canine whole blood and compared to other NSAIDs, deracoxib had a ratio of only 12 [39]. In the same study, carprofen had a ratio of 6–7 and firocoxib had a ratio of 384–427 [39]. Although etodolac is no longer used in dogs, there was a tremendous difference between the canine and human COX-1:COX-2 ratio, with a value of 8.1 in humans but 0.52–0.53 in dogs [40].

In a study using canine enzyme systems, carprofen had a COX-1:COX-2 ratio of 129 [28], but in another study, using cell lines of another species (sheep and rodent), the ratio was 1.0 [16], and in a study using canine macrophages, the ratio was 1.75 [41]. Yet another study on carprofen showed a ratio of 5.3, which was 1000 times less potent in whole blood than in cell culture [42]. Large differences among animal species have been shown for carprofen [5,33], which may be attributed to effects of carprofen on human cells being relatively selective for COX-1, but for canine and feline cells, carprofen shows preferential activity against COX-2, and for equine cells, it is non-selective or slightly preferential for COX-2.

In view of the discrepancies among studies and techniques, it is generally accepted that the whole blood assay should be the gold standard for determining COX-1/COX-2 specificity because it most closely simulates the appropriate physiologic conditions [4,5,35,36,43]. The advantage of the whole blood assay is that it incorporates the components into the assay that normally occur in circulating blood, namely proteins, cells, platelets, and enzymes. These components are not present in isolated cells or enzyme systems used for some earlier assays. Because the NSAIDs are highly protein bound (as discussed below), this is particularly important as only a small fraction, the unbound fraction, is biologically active in blood. The whole blood assay measures COX-2 products (PGE_2) from stimulated leukocytes and COX-1 products (TXA_2) from stimulated platelets.

Pharmacokinetic properties

Pharmacokinetic parameter estimates for NSAIDs are available from a variety of research reports and the drug package inserts from sponsors. Some selected values are shown in Table 24.1 and are derived from a variety of sources. It is not possible to provide an exhaustive list of every study because there are hundreds of pharmacokinetic studies published for NSAIDs in animals. The common features possessed by the NSAIDs used in animals are worth noting. All have high protein binding (> 90%). Generally, all are well absorbed after oral administration and are weak acids that have high lipophilicity at physiologic tissue pH. The lipid/water partition coefficient, reported as the logarithm of the partition coefficient, or LogP, for these drugs is greater than or near 2.0. If the LogP for a medication is close to or above 2.0, diffusion across biologic membranes is favored (unless restricted by protein binding) and oral absorption is favored by high lipophilicity. Being weak acids, the lipophilicity (LogD) is highest at the low pH of the stomach and is lower, but still above 0.0, at the physiologic pH of 7.0. Meloxicam is an exception because the LogD is –0.75 at a pH of 7.0. Mavacoxib is another exception because it is a weak base.

Both lipophilicity and protein binding affect a drug's volume of distribution. The volume of distribution varies considerably among the NSAIDs (Table 24.1). For many drugs, high protein binding is associated with a small volume of distribution because protein binding decreases diffusion out of the extracellular compartment (e.g., plasma and extracellular fluid), but this is not a consistent feature of the NSAIDs. Carprofen and phenylbutazone have the lowest volume of distribution at 0.14 L/kg (lower than extracellular water volume), and most NSAIDs have volumes of distribution less than 1.0 L/kg. However, firocoxib, deracoxib, and etodolac all have volumes of distribution greater than 1.0 L/kg. Firocoxib has the highest volume of distribution (approximately 4.6 L/kg in dogs) [44], while it has the lowest lipophilicity (LogP 1.96). Interestingly, carprofen has one of the highest lipophilicity values among the NSAIDS (LogP of 3.79), but also has the lowest volume of distribution.

The estimated plasma half-life varies tremendously among the NSAIDs, and among species (Table 24.1). For example, in dogs, the half-life is < 1 h for robenacoxib, 1.6 h for ketoprofen, 3 h for deracoxib, and up to 24 h for meloxicam. Phenylbutazone ranges from 5–6 h in dogs and horses to over 50 h in cattle. Firocoxib has a half-life of 7.8 h in dogs, but 30 h or more in horses. Mavacoxib, an NSAID approved for dogs in Europe but not the United States (US), is unusual in that it has very low systemic clearance, resulting in a half-life in laboratory Beagles of 15.5–19.3 days [45]. However, in osteoarthritic dogs of other breeds, the half-life was highly variable with an average of 44 days but exceeding 80 days in some dogs [46].

Despite these differences, the half-life does not appear to influence dosing intervals. In other words, the canine-approved labels for these drugs generally state once-daily oral administration for osteoarthritis or soft tissue inflammation despite the disparate half-lives. Mavacoxib is a notable exception with initial dosing at a 14-day interval with subsequent doses given every 30 days [46].

One of the reasons why plasma drug pharmacokinetic parameters (e.g., half-life) may not predict the dose interval is because of a lag time between the tissue concentrations and blood concentrations, raising questions about the value of plasma or serum pharmacokinetics to predict dose and dose intervals. Even the drugs with short half-lives can be administered once daily because the tissue concentrations and inhibitory effects persist much longer. Protein binding has historically been used to explain the long persistence in tissues, but these drugs are bound in plasma as well as tissues, which challenges this assumption. The high lipophilicity of these drugs also may explain the long tissue half-lives because high lipophilicity favors intracellular distribution, which can serve as a reservoir for prolonged tissue levels. The concept of "ion trapping" has been used to explain the high concentrations of NSAIDs in tissues compared to plasma. However, this is a false application of this principle. NSAIDs generally have a low pK_a (weak acids); therefore, they are ionized in both plasma and tissue. The pH in tissues, even when inflamed, is generally not below the pK_a, making ion trapping unlikely because of the small differential between tissue and plasma pH, compared to the pK_a of many NSAIDs, which have a pK_a in the range of 4–5. In other words, the tissue pH does not fall below the pK_a of these NSAIDs for ion trapping to factor into the drug's distribution.

The NSAIDs are biotransformed by hepatic mechanisms, which is characteristic of lipophilic, poorly water-soluble compounds that have relatively low systemic clearance. Clearance values are not listed in Table 24.1, but all NSAIDs have clearance values of approximately 0.4 L/kg/h (6.67 mL/kg/min) or less. With liver blood flow being approximately 30 mL/kg/min in dogs [47], such a low value for these NSAIDs would qualify them as low clearance compounds. Mavacoxib is an extreme example with systemic clearance of only 0.0027 L/kg/h in Beagle dogs [45]. Similar properties are observed for the NSAIDs in other species in which the systemic clearance is much lower than liver blood flow. There are a few exceptions: systemic clearance of meloxicam in horses is approximately three to five times higher than in humans and three times higher than in dogs [48,49]. Robenacoxib has a clearance of approximately

9–12 mL/kg/min in cats [50,51] and 13 mL/kg/min in dogs [51,52], which is higher than the other NSAIDs, and it also has a correspondingly short half-life in each of these species.

Gastrointestinal absorption is generally high for the formulations approved for animals (above 90% and often close to 100%), but there are exceptions. Firocoxib and mavacoxib are unusual with only 38% and 46% oral bioavailability in dogs, respectively. Robenacoxib has unusually low bioavailability in cats that is significantly affected by feeding [51]. There are also lower values for oral absorption of some drugs in horses and cattle (Table 24.1).

Feeding may increase, inhibit, or delay absorption of concurrently administered NSAIDs. For example, feeding horses at the same time as oral phenylbutazone administration does not decrease absorption, but it is delayed significantly, presumably because of binding to materials in feed and release in the distal intestine [53]. Robenacoxib is highly affected by feeding with oral absorption of 10% in fed cats versus 49% in fasted cats [51,54] and 62% in fed dogs versus 84% in fasted dogs [51,52]. Mavacoxib (unique because it is a weak base instead of a weak acid) is affected in the opposite direction, with feeding increasing the oral absorption from 46% to 87% [45]. Meloxicam has good oral absorption and is only slightly affected by feeding in horses (Table 24.1).

Stereoisomerism

The propionic acid derivatives (carprofen and ketoprofen) exist as *R*(–) and *S*(+) chiral enantiomers. Chirality is important because each isomer may exhibit different pharmacokinetic and pharmacodynamic behavior. For example, the *S*(+)-enantiomer (eutomer) is most active (lowest IC_{50}) for prostaglandin inhibition for these two NSAIDs. Etodolac also exists as a chiral enantiomer, with the *S*(+)-isomer being more active. None of the other drugs listed in Table 24.1 have chiral enantiomers.

Pharmacokinetic-pharmacodynamic properties

The association between the drug's pharmacokinetics and action at the target site has been the focus of pharmacokinetic-pharmacodynamic (PK-PD) studies. If the plasma or serum pharmacokinetic properties can be compared to the pharmacodynamic studies that measure COX-1 and COX-2 inhibitory concentrations, or observations of clinical response, it allows investigators to use the estimated pharmacokinetic parameters of the drug to derive optimal and safe dosing for animals. These approaches have been used to evaluate various NSAIDs used in animals [4,5,55–57]. For example, this approach was used to characterize the dose for robenacoxib in dogs and cats [50,51,55–59] and was used to evaluate NSAIDs for horses [48,49].

This approach entails the use of a blood concentration corresponding to 80% inhibition of COX-2 (IC_{80}) to produce a therapeutic effect, and a 20% inhibition of COX-1 (IC_{20}) to avoid adverse effects. A value of 80% COX-2 inhibition is used to predict clinical effects because a drug concentration that inhibits the enzyme by only 50% may not be enough to produce a therapeutic effect. Using these inhibitory concentration values as targets, PK-PD modeling can be used to derive doses to attain optimal blood concentrations [36,60]. The doses derived are intended to be starting points from which other studies investigating clinical safety and effectiveness can be planned. For example, using the PK-PD modeling approach, investigators determined a dose of meloxicam of 0.17 mg/kg every 24 h in cats [56]. This dose of meloxicam deviates from doses derived from clinical studies because it is below the US Food and Drug Administration (FDA)-registered single dose (0.3 mg/kg) for cats [61] but higher than the chronic dose used clinically and registered in other countries, including Europe [62]. On the other hand, this approach correctly identified the optimum dose of 2 mg/kg of robenacoxib in cats [50,51,57,59,63] and dogs [51,64].

In vivo assessment of PK-PD models

Rather than using an *in vitro* assay such as the whole blood assay to measure COX inhibition as the pharmacodynamic surrogate marker for efficacy, another approach is to use an *in vivo* measure. An *in vivo* measure is more likely to reflect physiologic and pathologic conditions and predict clinical outcome. Several *in vivo* models have been used to test NSAIDs in animals, which are described in other reports [4,27]. A typical *in vivo* model involves inducing inflammation in a tissue cage and measuring the inhibition of the inflammatory response in relation to the drug concentration. Alternatively, the model may use an injection of an irritant into a joint followed by an observation of the response by measuring the degree of lameness produced, heat, and/or pain [39,49,50]. Values such as 50% inhibitory concentration (IC_{50}) can be estimated from the *in vivo* model as it was for the *in vitro* model and used to derive an effective dose. One example of this approach was used to derive a dose for meloxicam in cats. Inflammation was induced in experimental cats, and the response was matched to pharmacokinetic parameters for PK-PD modeling [55]. These investigators calculated a single dose of 0.25–0.3 mg/kg of meloxicam to produce optimum analgesic, anti-inflammatory, and antipyretic effects. This dose agrees with the dose derived from clinical trials that led to the current FDA-registered dose for cats in the US [61], but is higher than the dose used clinically by many practitioners. In a tissue study of carprofen in dogs [27], the investigators showed that carprofen persists in tissue sites much longer than in plasma. But, contrary to popular views, the concentration in the inflamed tissue was not different from healthy tissue. Carprofen significantly decreased PGE_2 in the inflamed tissue.

Unique features of non-traditional NSAIDs

The mechanisms of action described above do not apply to other agents used for acute and chronic pain in animals. Grapiprant is technically classified as an NSAID, but it does not inhibit the COX enzyme. Acetaminophen is often not listed with other NSAIDs because it does not have anti-inflammatory properties and the mechanism of action has yet to be fully identified. However, acetaminophen will be listed in this chapter because it is sometimes considered as an oral treatment option for dogs, and more recently for horses. Dipyrone (metamizole in some countries) is also listed in this chapter with the NSAIDs. It lacks significant anti-inflammatory effects, and the mechanism of action is not entirely understood. However, it has some COX inhibiting activity, is used in small animals for acute pain in some countries, and is approved for use in horses in the US.

Grapiprant

Grapiprant is a non-COX-inhibiting agent. Instead of inhibiting production of prostaglandins, it blocks the prostaglandin receptor. After inflammation is triggered and prostaglandins are synthesized, PGE_2 exerts its effects via four receptors (EP1-4). The EP4 receptor is responsible for some of the sensitization of sensory neurons and signs of inflammation. Although other receptors are activated during inflammation, the EP4 receptor has been identified as the primary receptor responsible for mediating pain and inflammation associated with osteoarthritis. In dogs, grapiprant has high binding affinity for the EP4 receptor and binds competitively at a single site [65,66]. The effective dose in dogs, based on PK-PD analysis, and extrapolation from laboratory animal models of pain, is 1.7 mg/kg [65], which is almost the same as the FDA-approved dose of 2 mg/kg once daily.

In a pivotal clinical study [67], grapiprant showed effectiveness comparable to traditional COX inhibiting drugs in dogs with naturally occurring osteoarthritis. In dogs with osteoarthritis, 48% were classified as treatment successes compared to 31.3% of placebo-treated dogs (131 dogs in each group). In studies in which grapiprant has been compared to other NSAIDs for treatment of acute pain, it did not perform as well. Compared to firocoxib in a model of acute pain [68], it was not as effective, and in dogs with experimentally induced synovitis, grapiprant was the least effective agent, compared to carprofen and another experimental drug [69]. In another study performed in dogs undergoing ovariohysterectomy surgery, there was no difference between carprofen and grapiprant using a validated scoring system for postsurgical pain [70]. However, these were acute pain models and may not indicate effects during chronic pain treatment.

Adverse reactions in dogs have been minimal and are typical as for traditional NSAIDs. These may include vomiting, diarrhea, and decreased appetite, which can be observed after administration of other NSAIDs. These events have been mild and usually transient. In a safety study with research dogs, they tolerated a dose equivalent to 30 mg/kg of the tablet for 9 months with adverse effects attributed to the gastrointestinal tract characterized as mild and infrequent [71].

The pharmacokinetics in cats were similar to dogs [72]. In a safety assessment for cats [73], it was safe at doses suggested for therapeutic use (similar dose as for dogs). However, clinical efficacy in cats has not been established.

Grapiprant has not been evaluated in horses, except for pharmacokinetic studies [74]. The plasma concentrations have been low, and it was concluded that it will likely require a higher dose than the canine dose of 2 mg/kg to achieve efficacy.

Acetaminophen (Paracetamol)

Acetaminophen has been administered alone or in combination with opiates (codeine, oxycodone, or hydrocodone). Acetaminophen should never be prescribed for cats because of the potential for severe toxicity [75]. However, it is safe in dogs, even when administered at high doses [75]. Acetaminophen has been considered when oral treatment is needed for dogs that are refractory to traditional NSAIDs alone or have adverse effects from NSAIDs. Acetaminophen has not produced renal or gastric injury in dogs when prescribed at 15 mg/kg orally, every 8–12 h. Evidence of toxicity was not observed in dogs until doses of 100 mg/kg were exceeded [75].

Although it produces mild analgesic effects, acetaminophen does not produce anti-inflammatory effects at clinically relevant doses [76,77]. A study in a canine surgery model that demonstrated anti-inflammatory effects used doses that are higher than recommended clinically [76]. On the other hand, when acetaminophen was administered at a dose of 15 mg/kg every 8 h to dogs, there were no differences between treatments when acetaminophen was compared to carprofen or meloxicam for analgesia in dogs after ovariohysterectomy surgery [78]. In experimental dogs with joint pain, acetaminophen combined with codeine was not as effective as oral carprofen [79]. There are no studies on the long-term use for osteoarthritis in dogs. In people, acetaminophen has not been effective (or minimally effective) for the treatment of osteoarthritis of the hip and knee [80].

Most of the experience with clinical use of acetaminophen in dogs has been anecdotal as an alternative to NSAIDs or opioids. It has been administered to dogs in combination with codeine, oxycodone, and hydrocodone, despite a lack of clinical studies on the effectiveness of these preparations. Codeine absorption is low in dogs, and there are no studies that demonstrate that it produces convincing analgesia.

The mechanism of acetaminophen's action is unknown, but there are a few proposed theories [81,82]. Although it has long been assumed that acetaminophen does not inhibit the COX enzyme, it may be a COX inhibitor but act in cells in which low concentrations of arachidonic acid are present [81]. The site of acetaminophen action may be the peroxidase enzyme component of prostaglandin-H_2 synthase [83]. Prostaglandin-H_2 synthase consists of both peroxidase and COX portions but is collectively referred to as "COX" in most papers. The target for traditional NSAIDs is the COX portion of prostaglandin-H_2 synthase. COX inhibition probably occurs at site-specific tissues, sparing the gastrointestinal mucosa, platelets, and kidneys, but acting centrally [20]. It may also be a selective COX-2 inhibitor in selected tissues [84].

Other evidence presented to support the analgesic efficacy of acetaminophen is that it appears to inhibit the COX-1 variant referred to as "COX-3" [19]. This action may be more prominent in dogs than in any other species. COX-3 effects occur in the brain without affecting prostaglandin synthesis at other sites in the body (e.g., kidney and gastrointestinal mucosa) that could potentially lead to adverse effects. Other non-traditional NSAIDs (dipyrone and phenacetin) also appear to inhibit COX-3. Because COX-3 may be responsible for pyrexia and mediating central pain, this may explain the efficacy of acetaminophen for the treatment of mild pain and fever reduction. On the other hand, in other review papers, the authors have not supported this mechanism for the action of acetaminophen [83,85,86], and other mechanisms discussed in this section may be more important.

There is some evidence that acetaminophen may affect inhibitory pain pathways involved in chronic pain and neuropathic pain syndromes. Descending inhibitory pain pathways are mediated by serotonin (5-HT_3). Acetaminophen can stimulate these inhibitory pain pathways, which can be blocked by serotonin antagonists [87]. This evidence suggests that acetaminophen may activate serotonin receptors responsible for modulating inhibitory pain pathways in experimental pain models.

A more recent theory for the action of acetaminophen is that the parent drug or a metabolite acts centrally as an activator of transient receptor potential vanilloid 1 (TRPV1) or TRPA receptors [81,82]. In rats, acetaminophen is deacetylated to its primary amine and is then conjugated with arachidonic acid in the brain and the spinal cord to form the potent TRPV1 agonist *N*-arachidonoylphenolamine (AM404). This action may play a role in some pain syndromes, but the relevance is undetermined for clinical use and has not been identified in dogs. However, this mechanism represents a possible overlap with the endogenous cannabinoid system.

Acetaminophen may have some potential for treating pain in dogs (and perhaps horses), but effective doses and blood concentrations are undetermined, and more work is needed before conclusions and recommendations can be made for animal use. One of the disadvantages of acetaminophen in dogs is that frequent dosing is needed because of the short half-life of slightly more than 1 h. Although 15 mg/kg every 8 h was used in some of the studies cited above, in Labrador Retriever dogs, a dose of 20 mg/kg every 6 h is needed to maintain drug concentrations in the therapeutic range that is considered effective in people [88]. Frequent dosing may be inconvenient for many pet owners. This was confirmed in another study in which they showed that even at a high dose of over 30 mg/kg, these effective concentrations were maintained for only 2 h [89].

The effects of acetaminophen in horses have recently been examined [90–94]. The pharmacokinetics are favorable with a half-life of approximately 3–5 h. Oral doses of 20 mg/kg every 12 h for 14 days were well tolerated, but the analgesic effects were not measured [92]. In horses with experimentally induced endotoxemia, it effectively reduced pyrexia, but effects on the outcome of clinical endotoxemia were not evaluated [93]. It also produced improvement in lameness scores in a model of mechanically induced lameness (30 mg/kg orally) [91], and after a single treatment of 20 mg/kg orally, acetaminophen produced a significant thermal antinociceptive effect. The clinical usefulness of acetaminophen in horses has not been established, but the authors of some of the studies listed above concluded that it is safe for administration to treat chronic lameness but may not be effective when used alone [94].

Despite favorable effects in people, dogs, and horses, acetaminophen should not be used in cats. The adverse effects are well documented in other feline references. It is well known that as little as one tablet can kill a cat, unless they are treated promptly with agents such as acetylcysteine that increase the clearance. The susceptibility in cats is related to two properties: (1) cats have poor ability to form a glucuronide metabolite of the toxic byproduct of acetaminophen (*N*-acetyl-*p*-benzoquinone imine [NAPQI]), and as this metabolite accumulates, it causes cellular injury; and (2) the injury to cats is an oxidative injury, both to the liver and red blood cells. Cats are particularly susceptible to red blood cell oxidative injury because the feline erythrocyte has eight sulfhydryl groups that can be oxidized (six more than other mammals). Red blood cell injury (Heinz body formation) and methemoglobinemia (chocolate brown color of the blood) are tell-tale observations if cats are administered toxic doses of acetaminophen.

Dipyrone (Metamizole)

Dipyrone is an older antipyretic/analgesic agent often grouped in the NSAID class. In many countries, it is known as "metamizole." It was once approved for use in people but removed in 1977 because of concern of bone marrow toxicity [95]. It was also banned for use in people in the United Kingdom, France, Sweden, Canada, Australia, and Norway. Therefore, if used in animals, it should be handled carefully to avoid unintended exposure. However, it is still approved for use in people in some European countries, Asia, and South America.

Although it has been listed as a non-steroidal anti-inflammatory drug with analgesic and anti-inflammatory properties like other NSAIDs, it has weak anti-inflammatory properties, and it is likely acting through other non-traditional mechanisms. Dipyrone appears to be neither a COX-1 nor COX-2 inhibitor but may inhibit PGE_2 synthesis through other mechanisms that reduce the oxidation states of COX-1 and COX-2 [96]; this action may be similar to that of acetaminophen. It is also unique from the traditional NSAIDs in that it acts through other mechanisms, most likely central inhibition of COX-3, much like the mechanism for acetaminophen [19,20]. Another proposed mechanism, in addition to what is described above, is that it activates the opioid system or the endogenous cannabinoid system (CB_1 receptor mediated effects).

Dipyrone is a pro-drug, metabolized to other structurally related pyrazolone compounds. The first reaction is nonenzymatic to convert dipyrone to the active form, 4-methyl-amino-antipyrene, which is responsible for analgesic and antipyretic effects. This metabolite can be further metabolized by cytochrome P450 enzymes to non-methylated and oxidized products.

Dipyrone is capable of blocking fever (pyrexia) through prostaglandin-dependent and independent mechanisms. In horses, it has long been considered an anti-spasmodic agent that is capable of relieving discomfort associated with some types of colic in horses. This mechanism may be through inhibited release of intracellular calcium.

The most common use for dipyrone has been in horses. Dipyrone is approved for IV use in horses under the trade name Zimeta®, but equine veterinarians have used compounded formulations for many years. The approved indication is to treat pyrexia at a dose of 30 mg/kg IV, twice daily for up to three days. Although the approved indication is for pyrexia, many equine veterinarians use it for other indications.

In the US, it has not been used in small animals, but this use is more common in countries where it is more readily available. In other countries, particularly South America, it is known as "metamizole" and used for perioperative analgesia. The most common dose in dogs is 25–50 mg/kg IV, intramuscular (IM), or SC, every 12 h. Most of the experience has been for short-term treatment (e.g., postoperative pain). Although human-label tablets are available in some countries, long-term oral treatment has not been reported for chronic pain in animals. There is not much known about the pharmacokinetics or effects from repeated doses.

In dogs, the pharmacokinetics of the parent drug and metabolites have been characterized [97]. The safety concerns expressed for people [95] have not been observed in veterinary species. Based on plasma concentrations of the active metabolite, analgesia is anticipated for approximately 12 h after administration in dogs [97]. In dogs, it provided superior postoperative analgesia compared to meloxicam and a control group (saline) at a dose of 25 mg/kg IV, but when combined with meloxicam, the analgesic effects were improved [98]. When different doses were compared in dogs [99], dipyrone provided sufficient postoperative analgesia without adverse effects after 2 days of administration. These investigators found that a dose of either 25 or 35 mg/kg was effective, but not a lower dose of 15 mg/kg.

In cats, the pharmacokinetics and analgesic effects have been characterized [100–102]. The dose in cats is the same as in dogs (25 mg/kg), although they have a slightly longer half-life (based on the major active metabolite). Dipyrone administration had significant COX-1 and COX-2 inhibiting activity in cats [100] and produced postoperative analgesia that was equivalent to meloxicam. Dipyrone (25 mg/kg at various intervals) was effective to manage postoperative pain in cats [101]; however, the cats also received tramadol, and the response was not better than tramadol alone. In these studies, except for some salivation and occasional vomiting from oral administration, no adverse effects were reported. In the analgesic studies [100,101], there were no hematological changes observed in treated cats.

Adverse effects of NSAIDs

Gastrointestinal injury

Among the adverse reactions caused by NSAIDs, gastrointestinal problems are the most frequent reason to discontinue NSAID therapy or consider alternative treatment. Gastrointestinal adverse events, including vomiting, diarrhea, inappetence, and ulceration, have been documented in the veterinary literature, primarily in dogs and horses but also for other species.

Gastrointestinal toxicity is likely caused by at least two mechanisms; direct irritation of the drug on the gastrointestinal mucosa and the result of prostaglandin inhibition [23,103–106]. Direct mucosal irritation occurs because acidic NSAIDs become more lipophilic in the acid milieu of the stomach and diffuse into the gastric mucosa cells, where they cause injury. Direct effects also occur in the intestine where NSAIDs within the lumen can directly injure the intestinal villi. Diagnostic techniques have previously focused on stomach injury, but with improved imaging and endoscopic methods available, it is apparent that the intestine is also an important site of direct injury [104–105]. Drugs that enter the lumen via the bile perhaps pose a higher risk for injury, which presents a greater problem for the NSAIDs that undergo enterohepatic recycling and produce high biliary concentrations. These effects may not result in perforation but may be an important cause of the nausea, vomiting, and diarrhea observed in animals following administration of NSAIDs.

Prostaglandins (along with other eicosanoid products such as lipoxins) have a cytoprotective effect on the gastrointestinal mucosa. Inhibition of prostaglandins by NSAIDs results in decreased cytoprotection, diminished blood flow, decreased synthesis of protective mucus, and inhibition of mucosal cell turnover and repair. This can lead to gastritis, enteritis, erosions, ulcers, and perforation. Because NSAIDs can also inhibit platelet function, injury to the gastrointestinal tract that causes bleeding can be exacerbated and result in significant blood loss. Serious complications have been observed with NSAID use in practically all animal species and are discussed with specific examples provided below.

Canine examples of gastrointestinal injury

The gastrointestinal effects of any NSAID can range from mild gastritis and vomiting to severe gastrointestinal ulceration, bleeding, and death. Vomiting, anorexia, nausea, and diarrhea are by far the most common events documented [37,107]. Coxibs (COX-2 selective agents) were not associated with fewer adverse effects than non-selective agents [107]. In people, both traditional NSAIDs and coxibs can increase the risk of upper gastrointestinal complications [108]. Gastrointestinal ulceration and perforation are rare but can be catastrophic. An examination of published reports of gastrointestinal injury related to administration of NSAIDs in animals indicates that the most (but not all) serious problems are caused by doses that are higher than recommended [109,110]. This is usually a result of accidental ingestion, administration of an incorrect dose, or using inaccurate body weight. Overdosage is studied prior to regulatory approval by administration of exaggerated doses (e.g., 5× or 10×) in target animal safety studies performed by pharmaceutical sponsors and results are available in Freedom of Information (FOI) documents. Some drugs may lose their COX-2 selectivity at high doses [104]. Dose-dependent toxicity was shown for etodolac; at the label dose, it was safe, but at higher doses (2.7× dose), it produced gastrointestinal lesions, and at the highest dose (5.3× dose), it caused death [111]. At high doses, meloxicam also produced gastrointestinal injury in dogs [110,112,113].

As with most NSAIDs, individual patients can have adverse effects at lower doses, and according to one report, the sponsors of meloxicam in Europe recommended reducing the original approved dose from 0.2 to 0.1 mg/kg because of some initial gastrointestinal problems [114].

Factors that may increase the risk of gastrointestinal injury include concurrent corticosteroid administration and/or concurrent gastrointestinal disease or injury. In people, there is now evidence that genetic variation may determine one's susceptibility to NSAIDs. Whether or not this is a factor in animals is undetermined but is presumed to be likely due to genetic diversity [115].

In the gastrointestinal tract of healthy dogs, COX-1 is the primary enzyme that produces prostaglandins (primarily PGE_2) [42]. COX-2 is normally present but is upregulated after exposure to an irritant [21]. Both COX-1 and COX-2 can be upregulated in the feline duodenum [116]. In the canine stomach, there is a relatively high level of COX-1-synthesized prostaglandins because of the requirement to protect the stomach from high shear forces and gastric acid and produce mucosal bicarbonate. Therefore, it is logical that inhibition of COX-1 in the stomach would increase the risk of gastric erosions and ulcers. In the duodenum, on the other hand, the prostaglandin requirement is lower because there is less acid, less requirement for mucosal bicarbonate (bicarbonate is secreted by the pancreas), and less shear force because of the trituration of food that has already occurred in the stomach. However, clinical observations show that the proximal duodenum is often the site of severe NSAID-associated perforating ulcers in dogs. Injury or insult to the duodenum induces COX-2 to produce protective and healing prostaglandins. If the COX-2-mediated prostaglandins are inhibited by NSAIDs, it may increase the risk of duodenal ulceration. This adverse event has been observed following treatment with deracoxib, one of the most selective COX-2 inhibitors in dogs [109]. Although most dogs in this report were predisposed to injury because of other factors, it appeared to be the administration of this selective COX-2 inhibitor that was the trigger for the duodenal injury.

Although there are several drugs available for use in dogs (Box 24.1), there is no evidence in the published literature of controlled clinical trials to show that one NSAID is noticeably safer for the gastrointestinal tract than another [37,107]. However, rarely are these agents compared to one another in prospective controlled studies. For example, in a study in which carprofen, meloxicam, and ketoprofen were compared in dogs using endoscopic evaluation after 7 and 28 days of administration, there was no statistical difference among the drugs with respect to development of gastroduodenal lesions [114]. In another study that compared the gastrointestinal effects of recommended doses of carprofen, etodolac, and aspirin on the canine stomach and duodenum for 28 days, etodolac and carprofen produced significantly fewer lesions than aspirin [117]. Lesion scores in the carprofen and etodolac groups were no different from administration of placebo.

Equine examples of gastrointestinal injury

The NSAIDs are the drugs most often prescribed to treat pain and inflammation in horses. As in other animals, gastric ulceration and intestinal injury have posed important limitations to their use. Gastric ulcers and related syndromes are a major health problem in horses, especially in performance horses and foals with stressful clinical illnesses.

Gastric and intestinal injury in horses is a multifactorial problem and NSAIDs are just one of the factors contributing to the problem [118]. Phenylbutazone-induced injury to the gastrointestinal tract of horses has been documented in the literature for at least 30 years, and details of these findings can be found in other publications [1,119–123]. As described earlier, adverse effects are associated with inhibition of protective prostaglandins in the stomach, coupled with high stress, exercise, and diet. The most severe ulcers in horses occur in the glandular mucosa, referred to as "equine glandular gastric disease" (EGGD). It was presumed that these ulcers are more likely the result of prostaglandin (PGE and/or PGI) inhibition by NSAIDs. However, there is debate on the role that NSAIDs have on this disease. Some studies have shown an association between phenylbutazone administration and EGGD [121,122], with non-selective agents producing more severe lesions than COX-2-specific inhibitors [121], but other research that has studied the effects of NSAIDs on the equine glandular mucosa and incidence of EGGD have not supported this association. Phenylbutazone can cause equine glandular lesions, but without reducing prostaglandins (PGE_2) in the mucosa [122].

Effects on the equine intestine have also been extensively studied. These effects have been documented, with effects of specific agents described [34,120–127]. Although NSAIDs are commonly used in the management of pain and endotoxemia associated with colic in the horse [12,123,128], the effects must be balanced against the association with adverse gastrointestinal effects, and inhibition of mucosal barrier healing. Flunixin meglumine, one of the agents most administered for this indication, decreases small intestine barrier function. When the equine intestine is exposed to flunixin, it inhibits recovery after intestinal ischemia and increases permeability to lipopolysaccharide. By contrast, experimental evidence suggests that those NSAIDs with anti-inflammatory effects either independent of COX inhibition or a COX-2-selective mode of action, such as firocoxib, may offer significant advantages over traditional NSAIDs [34,126,127].

Non-steroidal anti-inflammatory agents, particularly phenylbutazone, can also affect the equine colon, producing impaired intestinal barrier function and contributing to right dorsal colitis [120,123,129]. The pathophysiology is not completely understood, but it is known that phenylbutazone administration to horses can cause hypoalbuminemia, neutropenia, changes in blood flow to the right dorsal colon, alterations in luminal concentrations of volatile fatty acids, and microbial dysbiosis [120,123,129].

Gastrointestinal adaptation and chronic NSAID administration

One of the features consistent in clinical and basic research studies of NSAIDs is that animals may exhibit an initial adverse reaction to these agents, but tolerance often develops with continued administration. Indeed, there are accounts of dogs, cats, horses, and people that have survived on daily administration of NSAIDs for a majority of their lives. What accounts for this tolerance? The process of gastrointestinal adaptation involves many factors. Attenuation of gastric mucosal injury occurs after repeated exposure to aspirin [130]. Gastric adaptation may be attributed to enhanced production of growth factors, increased cell proliferation, and mucosal regeneration. These authors also argued that gastric adaptation was a long-lasting effect that produces increased resistance of the adapted mucosa to subsequent damage by ulcerogenic agents.

Most information and review papers on this topic deal primarily with laboratory rodents, but studies in dogs from many years ago [131–138] demonstrated adaptation to administration of aspirin. These reports showed that gastric lesions were observed in the first few days during aspirin treatment, but after 1–2 weeks of aspirin administration, the lesions resolved in the face of continued administration. The adaptation to aspirin in the dogs was accompanied by a rise in gastric blood flow, reduction in inflammatory cell infiltration, and an increase in mucosal cell regeneration and mucosal content of epidermal growth factor [133–138]. These observations are consistent with stimulation of a protective factor known as "aspirin-triggered lipoxin" (ATL) [136–138]. This factor is produced by acetylated COX-2 and inhibited by COX-2 inhibitors. Additional evidence for upregulation of COX-2 after mucosal injury was demonstrated in the duodenum of dogs [21]. COX-2 was increased in the duodenum of dogs after 3 days of administration of aspirin. These observations raise questions about the safety of selective COX-2 inhibiting NSAIDs in the face of intestinal injury. The phenomenon of adaptation related to chronic administration is not without controversy as other studies have failed to demonstrate gastric adaptation after aspirin administration to dogs. When dogs received aspirin at an unusually high dose of 25 mg/kg every 8 h, there was no evidence of adaptation, and lesions were as severe or worse on day 28 compared to earlier in the study [139].

Kidney injury related to NSAID administration

In the kidney, prostaglandins play an important role in modulating the tone of blood vessels and regulating salt and water balance. Renal injury caused by NSAIDs may limit the use of NSAIDs in patients that have renal compromise. Reported cases of toxicity usually are associated with high doses of NSAIDs or when there were other risk factors [140]. Renal injury occurs as a result of inhibition of renal prostaglandin synthesis. Animals with decreased renal perfusion caused by dehydration, anesthesia, shock, or pre-existing renal disease are at greater risk for NSAID-induced renal ischemia [25,140–142].

NSAIDs are not inherently nephrotoxic, but when the kidneys are compromised, NSAIDs can interfere with protective mechanisms [143]. In healthy animals, the kidneys are usually able to compensate for NSAID-associated effects. Kidney injury can be associated with co-existing clinical or occult renal compromise [144]. In the face of factors that produce renal compromise (e.g., dehydration, tubular dysfunction, electrolyte depletion, and hemodynamic changes associated with anesthesia), the kidney is dependent on COX-1 and COX-2 for prostaglandin synthesis to regulate water homeostasis, tubular function, and renal blood flow [145].

Acute kidney injury associated with NSAIDs is characterized by decreased renal perfusion, sodium and fluid retention, decreased tubular function, and azotemia. In people, pain in the kidney area is one of the characteristics of NSAID-induced kidney injury. One should not assume that NSAIDs that are more specific for the COX-2 enzyme are safer for the kidneys. Both COX-1 and COX-2 enzymes are involved in renal blood flow regulation and tubular function. Some of the prostaglandins that play an important role in salt and water regulation and hemodynamics in the kidney are synthesized by COX-2 enzymes [24,146]. Administration of a specific COX-2 inhibitor to salt-depleted people decreased renal blood flow, glomerular filtration rate, and electrolyte excretion [146]. Corticosteroids may also increase the risk of injury because it was shown that administration of prednisolone to dogs in combination with either meloxicam or ketoprofen has a potential for serious adverse effects on the kidneys as well as the gastrointestinal tract [147].

There is another form of analgesic nephropathy, usually caused by chronic use of acetaminophen (paracetamol) in people [148]. This syndrome has not been described in domestic animals.

NSAID effects on kidneys in dogs

Of the currently available NSAIDs for dogs, the effects of carprofen and meloxicam on renal function have been most extensively studied. Because these drugs are used perioperatively, investigations were performed to determine if there was any evidence of acute kidney injury, particularly in association with anesthesia. Based on these studies, the risk of kidney injury from these medications appears to be low. In one study, carprofen, ketorolac, and ketoprofen were examined in healthy dogs undergoing surgery, but without IV fluid administration. There were minor increases in renal tubular epithelial cells in urine sediment, but carprofen had no adverse effects on renal function [144]. Some ketorolac- and ketoprofen-treated dogs had transient azotemia. In other studies, administration of carprofen to anesthetized healthy dogs had no adverse effects on renal function [149–153].

Meloxicam did not produce adverse renal effects in healthy dogs after short-term administration, with and without the cardiac inotropic and vasodilating agent, pimobendan [154]. In healthy dogs anesthetized and given acepromazine to produce hypotension, preanesthetic administration of meloxicam did not produce any alteration of kidney function, although generalization of the results from this model to other anesthetic protocols is difficult [155]. Healthy dogs administered meloxicam prior to anesthesia and an electrical nociceptive stimulus did not have decreased renal function associated with treatment [153].

Renal effects following deracoxib administration to dogs were reported by the manufacturer [156]. At high doses, there is a dose-dependent effect on renal tubules. It was well tolerated in most healthy dogs at up to 10 mg/kg for 6 months, but there is a potential for a dose-dependent renal tubular degeneration/regeneration at doses of 6 mg/kg or higher (clinically approved dose for long-term treatment is 1–2 mg/kg per day). Long-term administration of carprofen, etodolac, flunixin, ketoprofen, or meloxicam to dogs did not induce any evidence of kidney injury as measured by urinalysis and serum biochemistry [157].

The common theme in many of the studies cited above was that dogs were healthy, generally young, and NSAIDs were dosed once daily within the recommended range. Deviations from this study design, use of higher doses, longer duration of treatment, or administration to clinical patients with comorbidities could produce different results.

NSAID effects on kidneys in cats

Because it is often older cats that are treated with NSAIDs for degenerative joint disease (DJD), veterinarians and pet owners are concerned about the effects these drugs may have on kidney function. The effects of both short- and long-term use have attracted attention. One of the reasons for concern is a so-called "black box warning" issued by the FDA in 2010, which stated that "repeated use of meloxicam in cats has been associated with acute renal failure and death. Do not administer additional injectable or oral meloxicam to cats." This prompted several studies because overt and subclinical chronic kidney disease (CKD) is common in the population of cats most often treated with NSAIDs long term. Follow-up studies have helped to mitigate this concern. In cats with reduced renal function, but euvolemic, NSAIDs did not alter kidney function [158]. In their study, neither meloxicam nor acetylsalicylic acid had a measurable effect on urinary clearance of exogenously administered creatinine, serum creatinine concentration, or the protein-to-creatinine ratio. They concluded that kidney function of euvolemic cats with normal or reduced renal function is not dependent on COX function and, therefore, not likely impacted by NSAID administration.

Meloxicam is licensed for chronic use in cats in several countries (not in the US) and has been the drug recommended for long-term administration, by consensus, from a group of feline medicine experts [10]. Three important studies have concluded that chronic administration of meloxicam to cats can be both safe and effective. Oral meloxicam was safe and palatable for long-term treatment of DJD in cats when given with food at a dose of 0.01–0.03 mg/kg/day [159]. A follow-up study [160] with aged cats with CKD concluded that long-term therapy with meloxicam (0.02 mg/kg daily) can be administered safely. These cats tolerated meloxicam with daily administration despite their kidney disease. In an additional follow-up study, the same investigators [161] concluded that long-term management with oral meloxicam in cats did not reduce the lifespan of cats with pre-existent stable CKD and many cats had a better outcome associated with meloxicam treatment. A more recent study [162] showed that meloxicam did not adversely affect renal function in cats with CKD after 6 months of treatment at a dose of 0.02 mg/kg per day. However, the cats had a higher incidence of gastrointestinal effects and proteinuria compared to placebo-treated cats. These authors recommended monitoring urine protein in cats treated long-term with meloxicam to identify cats that may be at risk of developing worsening azotemia and hypertension.

These studies have resolved some, but not all, concerns about the use of meloxicam when administered to aged cats and to cats with CKD. It should be noted that the doses prescribed in these studies are lower than the approved label dose [61,62] and lower than the dose recommended in the review of NSAIDs in cats [10].

Studies have also been completed on another NSAID approved for cats, robenacoxib [51]. In safety studies using healthy cats, the data show that robenacoxib was well tolerated even when treatment was for longer, and at higher doses, than approved [163]. In a controlled study comparing robenacoxib and placebo in cats with kidney disease [164], 194 cats with osteoarthritis were given robenacoxib (1.0–2.4 mg/kg) or placebo once daily for 28 days. Forty of the cats had CKD. At the conclusion of the study, there were no differences between groups in frequencies of reported adverse events, body weight change, or results of serum or urine chemistry or hematology variables. Therefore, in this group of cats, robenacoxib at this dose had no measurable adverse effects on the kidneys.

The common concern for the effects of NSAIDs on the kidneys in cats prompted several feline pain management experts to publish a commentary to alleviate these concerns [143]. The title of the paper, "long-term use of non-steroidal anti-inflammatory drugs in cats with CKD: from controversy to optimism," shows the emphasis the authors intended to have regarding these concerns. Despite these studies and commentaries, the debate on the effects of meloxicam on feline kidneys continues. While some groups maintain that it can be used safely, others have discouraged its use [165].

Effects of NSAIDs on the liver

Because of their lipophilic chemistry, ability to diffuse into cells, and requirement for hepatic metabolism, any NSAID has the potential for causing liver injury. The liver is exposed to high concentrations of the parent drug and metabolites. Injury caused by NSAID administration can be idiosyncratic (unpredictable and non-dose related) or intrinsic (predictable and dose related) [166,167]. Toxicity resulting from high doses of acetaminophen and aspirin is intrinsic; reactions to other drugs tend to be idiosyncratic and unpredictable.

Prescribing NSAIDs for animals with hepatic disease has been questioned because of the role of the liver in metabolizing these drugs, but there is no evidence that prior hepatic disease predisposes a patient to NSAID-induced liver injury when properly dosed. Drug enzyme systems are remarkably preserved in hepatic disease, and pre-existing hepatic disease is not necessarily a contraindication for administration of an NSAID. Patients with liver disease may be more prone to gastrointestinal ulceration, and there is concern that administration of NSAIDs could increase the risk of this complication.

Carprofen has received the most attention related to drug-induced liver injury in small animal medicine, but the potential exists with all NSAIDs. Carprofen was approved by the FDA in October 1996 for relief of pain and inflammation in dogs [168]. Before this approval, it was registered for the treatment of dogs in Europe and was evaluated in clinical trials [169]. In studies in dogs with arthritis, it was effective and had a low incidence of adverse effects [169]. In longer term studies, in which carprofen was administered from 2 weeks to 5 years, the incidence of adverse reactions was only 1.3% [168]. Vomiting, diarrhea, anorexia, and lethargy were the most common adverse reactions documented. Attention was focused on the hepatic toxicity of carprofen because of a published report documenting liver injury in a series of dogs presented to a referral hospital [170]. In the report cited, 21 dogs were described in which carprofen was associated with acute, idiosyncratic hepatotoxicosis. Affected dogs had diminished appetites, vomited, and were icteric with elevations in hepatic enzymes and bilirubin. Dogs received the recommended dose and developed signs an average of 19 days after therapy was initiated. No predisposing conditions were identified, and most dogs recovered without further consequences following cessation of drug administration and supportive medical care. Many of the dogs in that report were Labrador Retrievers, but there is no additional evidence to show that this breed has an increased risk of carprofen hepatotoxicity [171]. Among other drugs, firocoxib caused fatty liver changes in young dogs when administered at high doses (manufacturer's data) [44]. Signs of hepatic injury are among the most common adverse events reported for carprofen to the FDA's Center for Veterinary Medicine adverse events reporting site (www.fda.gov).

Despite common recommendation by veterinarians, there is no evidence that dietary supplements such as silymarin (milk thistle, silybin, Marin®), S-adenosyl-methionine (SAMe, Denosyl®), or combinations of both (Denamarin®, NutraMax® Laboratories) have any benefit in preventing liver injury from NSAIDs. Idiosyncratic reactions are rare (1 in 1000 to 1 in 10,000 patients). Nevertheless, any unexplained increase in hepatic enzymes or bilirubin 7–90 days after initiating NSAID administration should be investigated. Fortunately, liver injury is generally reversible with supportive care and avoiding additional exposure to inciting causes.

Injury to cartilage

With chronic use, some NSAIDs have been shown to accelerate articular cartilage lesions in arthritic joints. However, this problem was primarily demonstrated experimentally when NSAIDs were administered at high doses in canine arthritis models. The significance in clinical patients when typical doses are administered is uncertain. Most of the currently used drugs have not been shown to accelerate the degradation of articular cartilage *in vivo* [172]. Similar studies have also been conducted in horses, with the conclusion in one review [12] that phenylbutazone does not have a deleterious effect on equine cartilage, but there is also no proof of benefits on inflammation-associated cartilage catabolism.

Blood coagulation effects: platelet inhibition and thrombotic abnormalities

NSAIDs can inhibit COX-1 and reduce thromboxane (TXA_2) synthesis in platelets, which inhibits platelet function. This can potentially lead to increased spontaneous bleeding (e.g., epistaxis), or increased bleeding associated with some surgical procedures. Aspirin, at low doses, is the most specific COX-1 inhibitor because the acetyl group (aspirin = acetylsalicylic acid) inhibits the COX in platelets irreversibly. Non-acetylated NSAIDs inhibit platelets only when their concentrations in blood are maintained at inhibitory levels. Therefore, the effects from non-aspirin NSAIDs are brief and rarely lead to clinical complications. However, the risk can be increased by co-administration of anticoagulants such as heparin during acute care treatment, or oral direct anticoagulants (apixaban and rivaroxaban) administered for long-term treatment.

Risks in people compared to animals

In the human literature, there has been a concern that COX-2-specific inhibitors may increase the risk of cardiovascular events, particularly myocardial infarction, thrombosis, stroke, and sudden death [173–175]. Similar problems have not been identified in animals. Cardiovascular safety is a concern in people using COX-2-selective drugs because these drugs preserve COX-1, which may promote platelet aggregation and vasoconstriction [173,174]. This is the reason that specific COX-2 inhibitors (rofecoxib and celecoxib) have been withdrawn or are rarely used in people [175]. It is likely that the high COX-2 selectivity of these drugs led to this increased risk [176–178].

Drug selection

There are many NSAID choices available to veterinarians (Box 24.1). It is not possible to define which NSAID drug is most efficacious and safest in an individual animal. Each medication has advantages and disadvantages. There are different dosage forms including injectable, oral solutions, oral transmucosal, conventional tablets, chewable tablets, equine pastes, and transdermal formulations. Initial dosing for healthy patients is well established (Table 24.2). Choice of product will depend on the clinical situation, owner preference, prior observed efficacy, and compliance. There are veterinary generic formulations of many of the popular drugs, and there are some human-labeled drugs that are used extra-label (e.g., aspirin, naproxen, meloxicam, and piroxicam).

COX-2 inhibition as selection criterion

After the discovery of the two isoenzymes, COX-1 and COX-2, there was a focus in drug development on highly selective COX-2 inhibitors. Drugs that emerged from this work were celecoxib, valdecoxib (discontinued), and rofecoxib (discontinued) [180]. At one time, these coxibs were among the top-selling prescription drugs of any category in human medicine. In veterinary medicine, with a few exceptions, there is little evidence that drugs with higher COX-1:COX-2 ratios produce fewer gastrointestinal or renal adverse effects than drugs with low ratios.

Deracoxib was the first veterinary drug in this group followed by firocoxib and robenacoxib. Mavacoxib and cimicoxib have been licensed for use in dogs in Europe. Although these drugs have a higher COX-1:COX-2 inhibitory ratio than older NSAIDs, clinical superiority has not been demonstrated in large patient populations. In fact, one of the veterinary drugs with selective

Table 24.2 Reported or regulatory agency approved dosages for NSAIDs in animals. The doses were derived from the approved label[a], published references listed in the text, and a veterinary drug handbook.

Drug	Cats	Dogs	Horses	Cattle
Aspirin	10 mg/kg q48 h, PO	10–20 mg/kg q8–12 h, PO	25–50 mg/kg q8 h, PO	100 mg/kg q12 h, PO
Carprofen	1–4 mg/kg given once by injection	4.4 mg/kg q24 h, or 2.2 mg/kg q12 h, PO	0.7 mg/kg q24 h, PO or IV	1.4 mg/kg, once, SC or IV
Deracoxib	1 mg/kg once, PO	3–4 mg/kg q24 h, PO for up to 7 days, then 1–2 mg/kg q24 h, PO	No dose established	No dose established
Etodolac	No dose established	10–15 mg/kg q24 h, PO	23 mg/kg q24 h, PO	No dose established
Firocoxib	1.5 mg/kg once, PO	5 mg/kg q24 h, PO	0.1 mg/kg q24 h, PO for up to 14 days, or 0.09 mg/kg q24 h, IV for up to 5 days	Not recommended
Flunixin	1 mg/kg once, IV, SC, or IM	1 mg/kg once, PO, IV, or IM	1 mg/kg q24 h, IM or IV for up to 5 days, or 1 mg/kg q24 h, PO	1–2 mg/kg q24 h, IV for up to 3 days
Grapiprant	Not established; 2 mg/kg used experimentally	2 mg/kg q24 h, PO (fasted produces better absorption)	Not established; likely requires higher than the 2 mg/kg canine dose	Not established
Meloxicam	0.1 mg/kg initial dose, PO, SC, or IV, then 0.05 mg/kg q24 h, then reduce dose to every other day, or 0.02 mg/kg q24 h, PO	0.2 mg/kg initial dose, PO, SC, or IV, then 0.1 mg/kg q24 h, PO	0.6 mg/kg q24 h, PO or IV	0.5 mg/kg q24 h, IM, IV, or SC
Naproxen	Not recommended	5 mg/kg initial dose, then 2 mg/kg q48 h, PO	10 mg/kg q12 h, PO	Not recommended
Phenylbutazone	6–8 mg/kg q12 h, PO	15–22 mg/kg q12 h, PO	4.4–8.8 mg/kg q24 h, PO (limit highest dose to 2–4 days); 2.2–4.4 mg/kg q24 h, IV for 2–4 days	17–25 mg/kg initial dose, then 2.5–5 mg/kg q24 h or 10–14 mg/kg q48 h, PO
Piroxicam	0.3 mg/kg q24 h, PO, or 1 mg per cat, q24 h, PO	0.3 mg/kg q24 or q48 h, PO	No dose established	Not recommended
Robenacoxib	1–2.4 mg/kg q24 h, PO	1–2 mg/kg q24 h, PO	No dose established	Not recommended
Mavacoxib	Not recommended	2 mg/kg once, PO, repeat in 14 days, then repeat q30 days for up to 6.5 months	Not recommended	Not recommended
Dipyrone (Metamizole)	25 mg/kg q8–12 h, IV, IM, or PO	25–35 mg/kg q8 h, IV, IM, or PO	30 mg/kg q12 h, IV for up to 3 days	20–50 mg/kg IM or IV or 40–50 mg/kg PO in some countries; regulatory concerns in some countries may prohibit its use
Acetaminophen (Paracetamol)	Do not use	25–35 mg/kg q6–8 h, PO	20–30 mg/kg q12 h, PO	50 mg/kg initial dose, then 30 mg/kg q6 h, PO

[a] Label dosing information including species, indicated uses, and precautionary warnings varies by regulatory jurisdiction. Appropriateness of use within the local regulatory environment should be verified by the prescribing veterinarian.
PO, oral; IV, intravenous; IM, intramuscular; SC, subcutaneous.
Source: Compiled from multiple sources including Papich [179], Elsevier.

COX-2 inhibitory action, deracoxib, was safe during an initial review [14], but gastrointestinal perforation and bleeding were associated with deracoxib use in dogs in a later report [109]. Studies that compare the efficacy of one NSAID versus another in any species are rare. In one canine efficacy study, firocoxib was compared to etodolac and carprofen and was shown in some measurements to have better improvement in lameness scores. Studies that have assessed safety among drugs have been scarce and of low statistical power. The results that are available, along with FOI summaries, indicate that approved NSAIDs have a similar incidence of vomiting and anorexia in dogs. Firocoxib may be an exception because it was associated with a lower incidence of vomiting and diarrhea compared to carprofen and etodolac and less melena compared to etodolac [44]. The studies with robenacoxib in cats have shown good safety and efficacy [51]. It was superior to meloxicam in a clinical study in cats [181] but was non-inferior to older NSAIDs such as ketoprofen in terms of safety and efficacy [58]. In studies performed in horses, or in intestinal tissues obtained from horses, there is some evidence that the COX-2 inhibitor firocoxib may lead to better restoration of intestinal integrity after an insult (e.g., equine colic) compared to the non-selective agent flunixin [126].

Selection of NSAIDs for dogs

For acute pain (e.g., postoperative pain), there is good evidence of efficacy from oral and injectable formulations, which has been published in various reports and reviews. Drugs discussed previously and listed in Tables 24.1 and 24.2 have been used in these instances. These drugs have been used in the short term to decrease fever and decrease pain from surgery or trauma. Some of these agents are available in an injectable form (meloxicam, robenacoxib, and carprofen), which allows for convenient in-hospital use. Proof of efficacy is provided in the approved labeling for this indication. Preoperative injections of carprofen in dogs were shown to be beneficial for decreasing postoperative pain after ovariohysterectomy [182]. Meloxicam has been reported to be effective in dogs for perioperative use and was shown to be superior to butorphanol in some pain assessments [183,184].

Oral NSAIDs may be used for acute treatment of myositis, arthritis, and postoperative pain, or they may be administered chronically for relief of osteoarthritis-related pain. Drugs that have been administered in the US to small animals are listed in Box 24.1, and some veterinarians have also used human-label drugs, but if this is considered, consult a reliable reference because the pharmacokinetics and dosages are different than in people. The approved traditional NSAID veterinary drugs used most often in dogs are carprofen, meloxicam, firocoxib, and deracoxib. Other drugs once available have been removed by the sponsor (tepoxalin, etodolac, and robenacoxib tablets). In countries outside the US, other NSAIDs approved for dogs include ketoprofen, mavacoxib, cimicoxib, and tolfenamic acid. Because all drugs on this list have undergone a review by the regulatory agencies in the country in which they are approved, there is substantial evidence of efficacy for this indication; however, there is no evidence in the approval that one agent is superior to another. The availability of grapiprant has increased the choices for treating chronic osteoarthritis in dogs. It was effective for the treatment of osteoarthritis in dogs [67], but results have varied for treatment of short-term postsurgical or experimental joint pain [68–70].

For long-term use, there are no controlled studies that indicate which drug is the safest and most effective. Because there are various choices of NSAIDs for treating dogs with osteoarthritis, selection can be frustrating for veterinarians. Like people, there may be greater differences among individuals in their response than there are differences among the drugs. Among the drugs available (Box 24.1), there may be variations among animals with respect to tolerance of adverse effects and clinical response. When drugs are compared to one another, it is difficult, using subjective measurements, to demonstrate differences between these drugs for reducing pain in animals. Clinical trials used for regulatory approval rarely compare one NSAID to another, and usually, the comparison is made to a control (placebo) treatment.

Selection of NSAIDs for cats

Excellent in-depth reviews are available for guidance on the use of NSAIDs in cats. Readers are encouraged to consult publications by other experts [7,9–11,185]. Treatment of DJD and other sources of long-term pain in cats has not been addressed adequately in the past, and these papers help raise awareness of these conditions.

Veterinarians have been reluctant to prescribe NSAIDs to cats because of a fear of adverse effects. The adverse effects of salicylates (aspirin) in cats are well documented. Cats are susceptible because of slow clearance and dose-dependent elimination. Affected cats may have hyperthermia, respiratory alkalosis, metabolic acidosis, methemoglobinemia, hemorrhagic gastritis, and kidney and liver injury. Cats also are prone to acetaminophen toxicosis because of their deficiency in the drug-metabolizing enzyme UDP-glucuronosyltransferase [186]. Despite the apparent sensitivity of cats to some adverse effects of NSAIDs, several NSAIDs have been used safely and approved by regulatory authorities for cats.

In the US, meloxicam injectable solution is approved by the FDA only for a single dose in cats at 0.3 mg/kg for postoperative pain. Meloxicam oral suspension is not approved for cats by the FDA [61], but the canine oral formulation is used extra-label. However, the oral suspension is licensed for cats in Europe, Australia, and New Zealand, even for long-term use. It is not approved for chronic treatment in the US but extra-label drug use in non-food animals is legal and, by consensus, was recommended by a group of feline medicine experts for repeated administration [10]. After the International Society of Feline Medicine and American Association of Feline Practitioners consensus guidelines were published [10], robenacoxib became available for cats in the US and Europe. Robenacoxib has favorable pharmacokinetic and safety properties that would make this an acceptable choice for repeated dosing [51].

Concerns regarding meloxicam are primarily associated with a high dose. According to a summary on the FDA-approved label [61], when cats were administered high doses (five times the recommended dose) of meloxicam, vomiting and other gastrointestinal problems were reported in some cats. With repeated doses (9 days) of 0.3 mg/kg per day to cats, inflamed gastrointestinal mucosa and ulceration were observed in three out of four cats. This high dose should not be used for more than a single administration. The consensus among experts is that meloxicam can, however, be safely administered to cats more than once [7,10,11]. As discussed under the section on renal adverse effects, meloxicam has been administered safely and long term at a dose of 0.01–0.03 mg/kg [159] and in aged cats with kidney disease at a dose of 0.02 mg/kg daily [160,161]. Some regimens recommend meloxicam in cats at 0.1 mg/kg initially, followed by decreasing doses to maintain effectiveness. One such regimen recommends that if a favorable response is seen in the first few days, increase the dose interval to once every 48–72 h, and then lower the dose to 0.05 mg/kg or less (0.025 mg/kg) if efficacy can be maintained. In Europe and other countries, the approved dose for cats is 0.05 mg/kg per day for chronic use with safety data from the sponsor to support this claim.

The recommended dose of robenacoxib has been optimized through PK-PD and safety studies [50,51,55–58,163]. The FDA-approved dose in the US is 1 mg/kg orally per day for a maximum of 3 days, while in the European Union the approved cat dose is 1–2.4 mg/kg body weight per day for up to 6 days. Availability of drug formulations differs between countries. In the US, there is a 6 mg unscored tablet for use in cats only; tablets were discontinued for use in the US for dogs. In Europe and other countries, it is also available as 5, 10, 20, and 40 mg tablets for dogs, and a 20 mg/mL injectable solution.

Carprofen (injectable solution) is approved for single-dose administration to cats in Europe. Repeated dosing of carprofen in cats has been discouraged because of reports of gastroduodenal toxicosis and high individual variation in half-life when administered at canine dose rates. There is one report of firocoxib administration in cats [187]. Firocoxib was effective for attenuating experimentally induced fever in cats at doses of 0.75–3 mg/kg (single dose).

Selection of NSAIDs for horses

The clinical pharmacology and use of NSAIDs in horses was thoroughly reviewed [12]. The short summary provided below cannot compare to the extensive amount of information provided in that review, and readers are encouraged to download that reference for a more extensive summary [12].

The administration of NSAIDs to horses traditionally has broken down into two choices. For acute pain, surgical pain, and colic pain, injections of flunixin meglumine are administered. For repeated oral doses for musculoskeletal pain and inflammation, phenylbutazone is most often administered. Phenylbutazone has been used more often than any other NSAID, and many experts still believe that it is the most cost-effective treatment, especially for oral treatment of musculoskeletal inflammation and pain. Flunixin meglumine is the most utilized injectable NSAID for acute soft tissue injury, endotoxemia, and abdominal pain [188]. Other NSAIDs have emerged on the market and are approved for horses, at least in some countries, or used extra-label. These alternatives also should be considered, depending on clinician preference [12,124,126,189]. These include injectable ketoprofen, the equine oral paste or injectable formulation of firocoxib, and meloxicam, which is approved in some countries. For example, meloxicam is approved in Europe to relieve pain associated with colic, and for acute and chronic pain associated with musculoskeletal disorders.

Occasionally meclofenamic acid is still used. In some countries (not the US), carprofen is licensed for use in horses at an IV dose of 0.7 mg/kg, which can be repeated once after 24 h. Dipyrone has been used for many years in horses, but only recently has an approved formulation been available (Zimeta®). This is approved for IV administration to treat pyrexia, but it is also used to treat colic pain and other forms of acute pain.

Flunixin has a long history in the treatment of acute pain and inflammation associated with colic in horses. The rationale for this treatment has focused on the inhibition of prostanoids that are responsible for hemodynamic changes during endotoxemia [127,128]. However, the non-selective NSAIDs may increase the risk of intestinal injury in horses, or delay restitution and healing [34,124–127,190]. These studies indicate that selective NSAIDs such as firocoxib may have a safety advantage [126].

Grapiprant, the unique NSAID approved for dogs, has been studied in horses [74]. Pharmacokinetic data are available, but no efficacy studies have been conducted. In pharmacokinetic studies, plasma concentrations did not reach the level reported to be effective in dogs. It is likely that at the canine dose, it will not reach therapeutic efficacy.

Acetaminophen was discussed in detail earlier in this chapter. Although some pharmacokinetic properties are favorable, and there is evidence of efficacy in models of pain, the effectiveness and doses for clinical indications or long-term use in naturally occurring pain have yet to be established.

NSAID selection for food animals

The administration of NSAIDs in food animals is regulated more closely than other animals because of the concern for residues that may end up in the food supply. Therefore, in most countries, the regulatory authorities limit the use to approved drugs and indications. Extra-label use requires justification and a reliable scientific estimate of the withdrawal time for milk and meat [191,192]. In the US, flunixin meglumine is FDA approved for the control of pyrexia in beef cattle with bovine respiratory disease and in dairy cattle with mastitis. It is also approved for the control of pain associated with foot rot in steers. There is also a unique transdermal formulation of flunixin (pour on) approved for control of pyrexia associated with bovine respiratory disease and acute bovine mastitis, and the control of pain associated with foot rot in cattle.

Ketoprofen is approved in cattle for the control of pyrexia associated with bovine respiratory disease (3 mg/kg subcutaneously). It is also approved in Europe for analgesic and antipyretic activity in pigs with respiratory infections and for mastitis–metritis–agalactia syndrome in the sow (3 mg/kg single-dose IM).

Meloxicam is approved in Europe, but not the US for use in cattle and pigs. Meloxicam is approved for use in cattle for fever and inflammation associated with respiratory infections and cattle with diarrhea (with fluid therapy). It is also approved in Europe to relieve postoperative pain following dehorning in calves and as supportive therapy in the treatment of acute mastitis. Meloxicam is approved in Europe for pigs for musculoskeletal indications, postoperative pain associated with minor soft tissue surgery such as castration, and for supportive therapy in sows after farrowing.

Other NSAIDs are considered off-label, and withdrawal times should be determined from a reliable source such as the Food Animal Residue Avoidance Databank (FARAD) [191]. Veterinarians should consult regulations in each country because some NSAIDs are approved for food animals in some countries, but not others. Unfortunately, there are no NSAIDs approved in the US for the most common sources of pain in cattle – dehorning and castration [192]. NSAIDs used off-label in food animals include aspirin, phenylbutazone (prohibited from use in dairy cattle), dipyrone (prohibited by the FDA), carprofen, and meloxicam (approved for use in Europe in cattle and pigs) [192–198]. Doses used in food animals are provided in other resources [189,192] and in Table 24.2.

References

1 Lees P. Analgesic, anti-inflammatory, antipyretic drugs. In: Riviere JE, Papich MG, eds. *Veterinary Pharmacology and Therapeutics*, 10th edn. Hoboken, NJ: John Wiley & Sons, 2018.

2 KuKanich B, Bidgood T, Knesl O. Clinical pharmacology of non-steroidal antiinflammatory drugs in dogs. *Vet Anaesth Analg* 2012; **39**(1): 69–90.

3 Monteiro-Steagall BP, Steagall PVM, Lascelles BDX. Systematic review of non-steroidal anti-inflammatory drug-induced adverse effects in dogs. *J Vet Intern Med* 2012; **27**(5): 1011–1019.

4 Lees P, Giraudel J, Landoni MF, *et al.* PK-PD integration and PK-PD modelling of non-steroidal anti-inflammatory drugs: principles and applications in veterinary pharmacology. *J Vet Pharmacol Ther* 2004; **27**(6): 491–502.

5 Lees P, Landoni MF, Giraudel J, *et al.* Pharmacodynamics and pharmacokinetics of non-steroidal anti-inflammatory drugs in species of veterinary interest. *J Vet Pharmacol Ther* 2004; **27**(6): 479–490.

6 Lascelles BDX, McFarland JM, Swann H. Guidelines for safe and effective use of NSAIDs in dogs. *Vet Ther* 2005; **6**(3): 237–250.

7 Gruen ME, Lascelles BDX, Colleran E, *et al.* 2022 AAHA pain management guidelines for dogs and cats. *J Am Anim Hosp Assoc* 2022; **58**(2): 55–76.

8 Monteiro BP, Lascelles BDX, Murrell J, *et al.* 2022 WSAVA guidelines for the recognition, assessment and treatment of pain. *J Small Anim Pract* 2023; **64**(4): 177–254.

9 Lascelles BDX, Court MH, Hardie EM, *et al.* Non-steroidal anti-inflammatory drugs in cats: a review. *Vet Anaesth Analg* 2007; **34**(4): 228–250.

10 Sparkes AH, Heiene R, Lascelles BDX, *et al.* ISFM and AAFP consensus guidelines: long-term use of NSAIDs in cats. *J Feline Med Surg* 2010; **12**(7): 521–538.

11 Steagall PV, Robertson S, Simon B, *et al.* 2022 ISFM consensus guidelines on the management of acute pain in cats. *J Feline Med Surg* 2022; **24**(1): 4–30.

12 Mercer MA, Davis JL, McKenzie HC. The clinical pharmacology and therapeutic evaluation of non-steroidal anti-inflammatory drugs in adult horses. *Animals (Basel)* 2023; **13**(10): 1597.

13 Coetzee JF. A review of analgesic compounds used in food animals in the United States. *Vet Clin North Am Food Anim Pract* 2013; **29**(1): 11–28.

14 Bergh MS, Budsberg SC. The Coxib NSAIDs: potential clinical and pharmacologic importance in veterinary medicine. *J Vet Intern Med* 2005; **19**(5): 633–643.

15 Papich MG. An update on non-steroidal anti-inflammatory drugs (NSAIDs) in small animals. *Vet Clin North Am Small Anim Pract* 2008; **38**(6): 1243–1266.

16 Vane JR, Botting RM. New insights into the mode of action of anti-inflammatory drugs. *Inflamm Res* 1995; **44**(1): 1–10.

17 Smith WL, Meade EA, DeWitt DL. Pharmacology of prostaglandin endoperoxide synthase isozymes-1 and -2. *Ann NY Acad Sci* 1994; **714**: 136–142.

18 Laneuville O, Breuer DK, DeWitt DL, *et al.* Differential inhibition of human prostaglandin endoperoxide synthases-1 and -2 by non-steroidal anti-inflammatory drugs. *J Pharm Exp Ther* 1994; **271**(2): 927–934.

19 Chandrasekharan NV, Dai H, Roos KL, *et al.* COX-3, a cyclooxygenase-1 variant inhibited by acetaminophen and other analgesic/antipyretic drugs: cloning, structure, and expression. *Proc Natl Acad Sci USA* 2002; **99**(21): 13926–13931.

20 Davies NM, Good RL, Roupe KA, *et al.* Cyclooxygenase-3: axiom, dogma, anomaly, enigma or splice error? - not as easy as 1, 2, 3. *J Pharm Pharm Sci* 2004; **7**(2): 217–226.

21 Wooten JG, Blikslager AT, Ryan KA, *et al.* Cyclooxygenase expression and prostanoid production in pyloric and duodenal mucosae in dogs after administration of non-steroidal anti-inflammatory drugs. *Am J Vet Res* 2008; **69**(4): 457–464.

22 Punke JP, Speas AL, Reynolds LR, *et al.* Effects of firocoxib, meloxicam, and tepoxalin on prostanoid and leukotriene production by duodenal mucosa and other tissues of osteoarthritic dogs. *Am J Vet Res* 2008; **69**(9): 1203–1209.

23 Konturek SJ, Konturek PC, Brzozowski T. Prostaglandins and ulcer healing. *J Physiol Pharmacol* 2005; **56**(Suppl 5): 5–31.

24 Brater DC. Effects of non-steroidal anti-inflammatory drugs on renal function: focus on cyclooxygenase-2 selective inhibition. *Am J Med* 1999; **107**(6): 65–70.

25 Lomas AL, Grauer GF. The renal effects of NSAIDs in dogs. *JAAHA* 2015; **51**(3):197–203.

26 Bertolini A, Ottani A, Sandrini M. Dual acting anti-inflammatory drugs: a reappraisal. *Pharmacol Res* 2001; **44**(6): 437–450.
27 Messenger KM, Wofford JA, Papich MG. Carprofen pharmacokinetics in plasma and in control and inflamed canine tissue fluid using in vivo ultrafiltration. *J Vet Pharmacol Ther* 2016; **39**(1):32–39.
28 Ricketts AP, Lundy KM, Seibel SB. Evaluation of selective inhibition of canine cyclooxygenase 1 and 2 by carprofen and other non-steroidal anti-inflammatory drugs. *Am J Vet Res* 1998; **59**(11): 1441–1446.
29 McKellar QA, Pearson T, Bogan JA, *et al.* Pharmacokinetics, tolerance and serum thromboxane inhibition of carprofen in the dog. *J Small Anim Pract* 1990; **31**(9): 443–448.
30 McKellar QA, Delatour P, Lees P. Stereospecific pharmacodynamics and pharmacokinetics of carprofen in the dog. *J Vet Pharmacol Ther* 1994; **17**(6): 447–454.
31 Bryant CE, Farnfield BA, Janicke HJ. Evaluation of the ability of carprofen and flunixin meglumine to inhibit activation of nuclear factor kappa B. *Am J Vet Res* 2003; **64**(2): 211–215.
32 Lees P, McKellar Q, May SA, *et al.* Pharmacodynamics and pharmacokinetics of carprofen in the horse. *Equine Vet J* 1994; **26**(3): 203–208.
33 Lees P, Aliabadi FS, Landoni MF. Pharmacodynamics and enantioselective pharmacokinetics of racemic carprofen in the horse. *J Vet Pharmacol Ther* 2002; **25**(6): 433–448.
34 Little D, Brown SA, Campbell NB, *et al.* Effects of the cyclooxygenase inhibitor meloxicam on recovery of ischemia-injured equine jejunum. *Am J Vet Res* 2007; **68**(6): 614–624.
35 Pairet M, van Ryn J. Experimental models used to investigate the differential inhibition of cyclooxygenase-1 and cyclooxygenase-2 by Non-steroidal anti-inflammatory drugs. *Inflamm Res* 1998; **47**(Suppl 2): S93–S101.
36 Warner TD, Giuliano F, Vojnovic I, *et al.* Non-steroid drug selectivities for cyclo-oxygenase-1 rather than cyclo-oxygenase-2 are associated with human gastrointestinal toxicity: a full in vitro analysis. *Proc Natl Acad Sci USA* 1999; **96**(13): 7563–7568.
37 Fox SM. Non-steroidal anti-inflammatory drugs. In: Carroll GL, ed. *Small Animal Anesthesia and Analgesia*. Ames, IA: Blackwell Publishing, 2008: 143–157.
38 Gierse JK, Staten NR, Casperson GF, *et al.* Cloning, expression, and selective inhibition of canine cyclooxygenase-1 and cyclooxygenase-2. *Vet Ther* 2002; **3**(3): 270–280.
39 McCann ME, Andersen DR, Zhang D, *et al.* In vitro effects and in vivo efficacy of a novel cyclo-oxygenase-2 inhibitor in dogs with experimentally induced synovitis. *Am J Vet Res* 2004; **65**(4): 503–512.
40 Glaser KB. Cyclooxygenase selectivity and NSAIDs: cyclooxygenase-2 selectivity of etodolac (LODINE). *InflammoPharmacology* 1995; **3**: 335–345.
41 Kay-Mugford P, Benn SJ, LaMarre J, *et al.* In vitro effects of non-steroidal anti-inflammatory drugs on cyclooxygenase activity in dogs. *Am J Vet Res* 2000; **61**(7): 802–810.
42 Wilson JE, Chandrasekharan NV, Westover KD, *et al.* Determination of expression of cyclooxygenase-1 and -2 isozymes in canine tissues and their differential sensitivity to non-steroidal anti-inflammatory drugs. *Am J Vet Res* 2004; **65**(6): 810–818.
43 Patrignani P, Panara MR, Greco A, *et al.* Biochemical and pharmacological characterization of the cyclooxygenase activity of human blood prostaglandin endoperoxide synthases. *J Pharmacol Exp Ther* 1994; **271**(3): 1705–1712.
44 US Food and Drug Administration. Freedom of Information Summary: Previcox Chewable Tablets (NADA 141–230). *Approval Date*: July 21, 2004. https://animaldrugsatfda.fda.gov/adafda/app/search/public/document/downloadFoi/768 (accessed September 2014).
45 Cox SR, Lesman SP, Boucher JF, *et al.* The pharmacokinetics of mavacoxib, a long-acting COX-2 inhibitor, in young adult laboratory dogs. *J Vet Pharmacol Ther* 2010; **33**(5): 461–470.
46 Cox SR, Liao S, Payne-Johnson M, *et al.* Population pharmacokinetics of mavacoxib in osteoarthritic dogs. *J Vet Pharmacol Ther* 2011; **34**(1): 1–11.
47 Gabrielsson J, Weiner D. *Pharmacokinetic and Pharmacodynamic Data Analysis: Concepts and Applications*, 5th edn. Stockholm, Sweden: Swedish Pharmaceutical Society, 2016: **87**. (Table 2.7).
48 Toutain PL, Reymond N, Laroute V, *et al.* Pharmacokinetics of meloxicam in plasma and urine of horses. *Am J Vet Res* 2004; **65**(11): 1542–1547.
49 Toutain PL, Cester CC. Pharmacokinetic-pharmacodynamic relationships and dose response to meloxicam in horses with induced arthritis in the right carpal joint. *Am J Vet Res* 2004; **65**(11): 1533–1541.
50 Pelligand L, King JN, Toutain PL, *et al.* Pharmacokinetic/pharmacodynamic modelling of robenacoxib in a feline tissue cage model of inflammation. *J Vet Pharmacol Ther* 2012; **35**(1): 19–32.
51 Lees P, Toutain PL, Elliott J, *et al.* Pharmacology, safety, efficacy and clinical uses of the COX-2 inhibitor robenacoxib. *J Vet Pharmacol Ther* 2022; **45**(4): 325–351.
52 Jung M, Lees P, Seewald W, King JN. Analytical determination and pharmacokinetics of robenacoxib in the dog. *J Vet Pharmacol Ther* 2009; **32**(1): 41–48.
53 Maitho TE, Lees P, Taylor JB. Absorption and pharmacokinetics of phenylbutazone in Welsh Mountain ponies. *J Vet Pharmacol Ther* 1986; **9**(1): 26–39.
54 King JN, Jung M, Maurer MP, *et al.* Effects of route of administration and feeding schedule on pharmacokinetics of robenacoxib in cats. *Am J Vet Res* 2013; **74**(3): 465–472.
55 Giraudel JM, Diquelou A, Laroute V, *et al.* Pharmacokinetic/pharmacodynamic modelling of NSAIDs in a model of reversible inflammation in the cat. *Br J Pharmacol* 2005; **146**(5): 642–653.
56 Giraudel JM, Diquelou A, Lees P, *et al.* Development and validation of a new model of inflammation in the cat and selection of surrogate endpoints for testing anti-inflammatory drugs. *J Vet Pharmacol Ther* 2005; **28**(3): 275–285.
57 Giraudel JM, King JN, Jeunesse EC, *et al.* Use of a pharmacokinetic/pharmacodynamics approach in the cat to determine a dosage regimen for the COX-2 selective drug robenacoxib. *J Vet Pharmacol Ther* 2009; **32**(1): 18–30.
58 Giraudel JM, Gruet P, Alexander DG, *et al.* Evaluation of orally administered robenacoxib versus ketoprofen for treatment of acute pain and inflammation associated with musculoskeletal disorders in cats. *Am J Vet Res* 2010; **71**(7): 710–719.
59 King JN, Rudaz C, Borer L, *et al.* In vitro and ex vivo inhibition of canine cyclooxygenase isoforms by robenacoxib: a comparative study. *Res Vet Sci* 2010; **88**(3): 497–506.
60 Hinz B, Brune K. Can drug removals involving cyclooxygenase-2 inhibitors be avoided? A plea for human pharmacology. *Trends Pharmacol Sci* 2008; **29**(8): 391–397.
61 US Food and Drug Administration. Freedom of Information Summary: Metacam Oral Suspension (NADA 141–213); and https://docs.boehringer-ingelheim.com/MSDS/Metacam_Injectable_Cat_PI
62 European Agency for the Evaluation of Medicinal Products. Meloxicam Summary Report. June 1997. EMEA/MRL/236/97.
63 Giraudel JM, Toutain PL, King JN, *et al.* Differential inhibition of cyclooxygenase isoenzymes in the cat by the NSAID robenacoxib. *J Vet Pharmacol Ther* 2009; **32**(1): 31–40.
64 Schmid VB, Spreng DE, Seewald W, *et al.* Analgesic and anti-inflammatory actions of robenacoxib in acute joint inflammation in the dogs. *J Vet Pharmacol Ther* 2009; **33**(20): 118–131.
65 Nagahisa A, Okumura T. Pharmacology of grapiprant, a novel EP4 antagonist: receptor binding, efficacy in a rodent postoperative pain model, and a dose estimation for controlling pain in dogs. *J Vet Pharmacol Ther* 2017; **40**(3): 285–292.
66 Sartini I, Giorgi M. Grapiprant: a snapshot of the current knowledge. *J Vet Pharmacol Ther* 2021; **44**(5): 679–688.
67 Rausch-Derra L, Huebner M, Wofford J, *et al.* A prospective, randomized, masked, placebo-controlled multisite clinical study of grapiprant, an EP 4 prostaglandin receptor antagonist (PRA), in dogs with osteoarthritis. *J Vet Intern Med* 2016; **30**(3): 756–763.
68 de Salazar Alcalá AG, Gioda L, Dehman A, *et al.* Assessment of the efficacy of firocoxib (Previcox®) and grapiprant (Galliprant®) in an induced model of acute arthritis in dogs. *BMC Vet Res* 2019; **15**(1): 309.
69 Budsberg SC, Kleine SA, Norton MM, *et al.* Comparison of two inhibitors of E-type prostanoid receptor four and carprofen in dogs with experimentally induced acute synovitis. *Am J Vet Res* 2019: **80**(11): 1001–1006.
70 Southern BL, Long SM, Barnes DN, *et al.* Preliminary evaluation of the effects of grapiprant compared with carprofen on acute pain and inflammation following ovariohysterectomy in dogs. *Am J Vet Res* 2022; **83**(7): ajvr.21.10.0162.
71 Rausch-Dera LC, Huebner M, Rhodes L. Evaluation of the safety of long-term, daily oral administration of grapiprant, a novel drug for treatment of osteoarthritic pain and inflammation, in healthy dogs. *Am J Vet Res* 2015; **76**(10): 853–859.
72 Lebkowska-Wieruszewska B, De Vito V, Owen H, *et al.* Pharmacokinetics of grapiprant, a selective EP 4 prostaglandin PGE 2 receptor antagonist, after 2 mg/kg oral and I.V. administrations in cats. *J Vet Pharmacol Ther* 2017; **40**(6): e11–e15.
73 Rausch-Derra LC, Rhodes L. Safety and toxicokinetic profiles associated with daily oral administration of grapiprant, a selective antagonist of the prostaglandin E2 EP4 receptor, to cats. *Am J Vet Res* 2016; **77**(7): 688–692.
74 Knych, H K, Seminoff K, McKemie DS. Detection of grapiprant following oral administration to exercised Thoroughbred horses. *Drug Test Analysis* 2018; **10**: 1237–1243.
75 Savides MC, Oehme FW, Nash SL, *et al.* The toxicity and biotransformation of single doses of acetaminophen in dogs and cats. *Toxicol Appl Pharmacol* 1984; **74**(1): 26–34.
76 Mburu DN, Mbugua LA, Skoglund LA, *et al.* Effects of paracetamol (acetaminophen) and acetylsalicylic acid on the post-operative course after experimental orthopaedic surgery in dogs. *J Vet Pharmacol Ther* 1988; **11**(2): 163–170.
77 Mburu DN. Evaluation of the anti-inflammatory effects of a low-dose of acetaminophen following surgery in dogs. *J Vet Pharmacol Ther* 1991; **14**(1): 109–111.
78 Hernández-Avalos I, Valverde A, Ibancovichi-Camarillo JA, *et al.* Clinical evaluation of postoperative analgesia, cardiorespiratory parameters and changes in liver and renal function tests of paracetamol compared to meloxicam and carprofen in dogs undergoing ovariohysterectomy. *PLoS ONE* 2020; **15**(2): e0223697.

79 Budsberg SC, Kleine SA, Norton MM, *et al.* Comparison of the effects on lameness of orally administered acetaminophen-codeine and carprofen in dogs with experimentally induced synovitis. *Am J Vet Res* 2020; **81**(8): 627–634.
80 Moore N, Salvo F, Duong M, *et al.* Does paracetamol still have a future in osteoarthritis? *The Lancet* 2016; **387**(10033): 2065–2066.
81 Toussaint K, Yang XC, Zielinski MA, *et al.* What do we (not) know about how paracetamol (acetaminophen) works? *J Clin Pharm Ther* 2010; **35**(6): 617–638.
82 Ohashi N, Kohno T. Analgesic effect of acetaminophen: a review of known and novel mechanisms of action. *Front Pharmacol* 2020; **11**: 580289.
83 Aronoff DM, Oates JA, Boutaud O. New insights into the mechanism of action of acetaminophen: its clinical pharmacologic characteristics reflect its inhibition of the two prostaglandin H2 synthases. *Clin Pharmacol Ther* 2005; **79**(1): 9–19.
84 Hinz B, Cheremina O, Brune K. Acetaminophen (paracetamol) is a selective cyclooxygenase-2 inhibitor in man. *FASEB J* 2008; **22**(2): 383–390.
85 Hinz B, Brune K. Can drug removals involving cyclooxygenase-2 inhibitors be avoided? A plea for human pharmacology. *Trends Pharmacol Sci* 2008; **29**(8): 391–397.
86 Kis B, Snipes JA, Busija DW. Acetaminophen and the cyclooxygenase-3 puzzle: sorting out facts, fictions, and uncertainties. *J Pharmacol Exp Ther* 2005; **315**(1): 1–7.
87 Pickering G, Esteve V, Loriot MA, *et al.* Acetaminophen reinforces descending inhibitory pain pathways. *Clin Pharmacol Ther* 2008; **84**(1): 47–51.
88 Sartini I, Łebkowska-Wieruszewska B, Lisowski A, *et al.* Pharmacokinetics of acetaminophen after intravenous and oral administration in fasted and fed Labrador Retriever dogs. *J Vet Pharmacol Ther* 2021; **44**(1): 28–35.
89 Madsen M, Enomoto H, Messenger K, *et al.* Effects of housing environment on oral absorption of acetaminophen in healthy Beagles. *Am J Vet Res* 2022; **83**(1):80–85.
90 Tueshaus T, McKemie DS, Kanarr K, *et al.* Pharmacokinetics and effects of codeine in combination with acetaminophen on thermal nociception in horses. *J Vet Pharmacol Ther* 2023; **46**(5): 311–325.
91 Mercer MA, McKenzie HC, Byron CR, *et al.* Pharmacokinetics and clinical efficacy of acetaminophen (paracetamol) in adult horses with mechanically induced lameness. *Equine Vet J* 2023; **55**(3): 524–533.
92 Mercer MA, McKenzie HC, Davis JL, *et al.* Pharmacokinetics and safety of repeated oral dosing of acetaminophen in adult horses. *Equine Vet J* 2020; **52**(1): 120–125.
93 Mercer MA, Davis JL, McKenzie HC, *et al.* Pharmacokinetics and efficacy of orally administered acetaminophen (paracetamol) in adult horses with experimentally induced endotoxemia. *J Vet Intern Med* 2023; **37**(2): 718–727.
94 Mercer MA, Davis JL, McKenzie HC, *et al.* Pharmacokinetics, pharmacodynamic efficacy, and safety of acetaminophen in adult horses with naturally occurring chronic lameness. *In Proc Am Assoc Equine Pract* 2021; **67**: 348–349.
95 Cascorbi I. The uncertainties of metamizole use. *Clin Pharmacol Ther* 2021; **109**(6): 1373–1375.
96 Pierre SC, Schmidt R, Brenneis C, *et al.* Inhibition of cyclooxygenases by dipyrone. *Br J Pharmacol* 2007; **151**(4): 494–503.
97 Giorgi MA, Łebkowska-Wieruszewska B, Lisowski A, *et al.* Pharmacokinetic profiles of the active metamizole metabolites after four different routes of administration in healthy dogs. *J Vet Pharmacol Ther* 2018; **41**(3): 428–436.
98 Zanuzzo FS, Teixeira-Neto FJ, Teixeira LR, *et al.* Analgesic and antihyperalgesic effects of dipyrone, meloxicam or a dipyrone–meloxicam combination in bitches undergoing ovariohysterectomy. *Vet J* 2015; **205**(1): 33–37.
99 Imagawa VH, Fantoni DT, Tatarunas AC, *et al.* The use of different doses of metamizol for post-operative analgesia in dogs. *Vet Anaesth Analg* 2011; **38**(4): 385–393.
100 Pereira MA, Campos KD, Gonçalves LA, *et al.* Cyclooxygenases 1 and 2 inhibition and analgesic efficacy of dipyrone at different doses or meloxicam in cats after ovariohysterectomy. *Vet Anaesth Analg* 2021; **48**(1): 7–16.
101 Teixeira LG, Martins LR, Schimites PI, *et al.* Evaluation of postoperative pain and toxicological aspects of the use of dipyrone and tramadol in cats. *J Feline Med Surg* 2020; **22**(6): 467–475.
102 Lebkowska-Wieruszewska B, Kim TW, Chea B, *et al.* Pharmacokinetic profiles of the two major active metabolites of metamizole (dipyrone) in cats following three different routes of administration. *J Vet Pharmacol Ther* 2018; **41**(2): 334–349.
103 Whittle BJ. Mechanisms underlying intestinal injury induced by anti-inflammatory COX inhibitors. *Eur J Pharmacol* 2004; **500**(1–3): 427–439.
104 Wolfe MM, Lichtenstein DR, Singh G. Gastrointestinal toxicity of non-steroidal antiinflammatory drugs. *N Engl J Med* 1999; **340**(24): 1888–1899.
105 Fortun PJ, Hawkey CJ. Non-steroidal antiinflammatory drugs and the small intestine. *Curr Opin Gastroenterol* 2005; **21**(2): 169–175.
106 Treinen-Moslen M, Kanz MF. Intestinal tract injury by drugs: importance of metabolite delivery by yellow bile road. *Pharmacol Ther* 2006; **112**(3): 649–667.
107 Hunt JR, Dean RS, Davis GN, *et al.* An analysis of the relative frequencies of reported adverse events associated with NSAID administration in dogs and cats in the United Kingdom. *Vet J* 2015; **206**(2): 183–190.
108 Bhalla N, Emberson J, Merhi A, *et al.* Vascular and upper gastrointestinal effects of non-steroidal anti-inflammatory drugs: meta-analyses of individual participant data from randomized trials. *Lancet* 2013; **382**(9894): 769–779.
109 Lascelles BDX, Blikslager AT, Fox SM, *et al.* Gastrointestinal tract perforation in dogs treated with a selective cyclooxygenase-2 inhibitor: 29 cases (2002–2003). *J Am Vet Med Assoc* 2005; **227**(7): 1112–1117.
110 Enberg TB, Braun LD, Kuzma AB. Gastrointestinal perforation in five dogs associated with the administration of meloxicam. *J Vet Emerge Crit Care* 2006; **16**(1): 34–43.
111 US Food and Drug Administration. Freedom of Information Summary: EtoGesic Tablets (NADA 141–108). Approval Date: July 22, 1998. www.fda.gov/ohrms/dockets/98fr/NADA141-108-FOIS082703.pdf.pdf (accessed September 2014).
112 Doig PA, Purbrook KA, Hare JE, *et al.* Clinical efficacy and tolerance of meloxicam in dogs with chronic osteoarthritis. *Can Vet J* 2000; **41**(4): 296–300.
113 Jones CJ, Steppe HK, Harmon BG, *et al.* In vivo effects of meloxicam and aspirin on blood, gastric mucosal, and synovial fluid prostanoid synthesis in dogs. *Am J Vet Res* 2002; **63**(11): 1527–1531.
114 Forsyth SF, Guilford WG, Haslett SJ, *et al.* Endoscopy of the gastroduodenal mucosa after carprofen, meloxicam and ketoprofen administration in dogs. *J Small Anim Pract* 1998; **39**(9): 421–424.
115 Lee YS, Kim H, Wu TX, *et al.* Genetically mediated interindividual variation in analgesic responses to cyclooxygenase inhibitory drugs. *Clin Pharmacol Ther* 2006; **79**(5): 407–418.
116 Satoh H, Amigas K, Ebara S, *et al.* Cyclooxygenase (COX)-1 and COX-2 both play an important role in the protection of the duodenal mucosa in cats. *J Pharmacol Exp Ther* 2013; **344**(1): 189–195.
117 Reimer ME, Johnston SA, Leib MS, *et al.* The gastrointestinal effects of buffered aspirin, carprofen, and etodolac in healthy dogs. *J Vet Intern Med* 1999; **13**(5): 472–477.
118 Nadeau JA, Andrews FM. Equine gastric ulcer syndrome: the continuing conundrum. *Equine Vet J* 2009; **41**(7): 611–615.
119 Tobin T, Chay S, Kamerling S, *et al.* Phenylbutazone in the horse: a review. *J Vet Pharmacol Ther* 1986; **9**(1): 1–25.
120 Whitfield-Cargile CM, Coleman MC, Cohen ND, *et al.* Effects of phenylbutazone alone or in combination with a nutritional therapeutic on gastric ulcers, intestinal permeability, and fecal microbiota in horses. *J Vet Intern Med* 2021; **35**(2): 1121–1130.
121 Richardson LM, Whitfield-Cargile CM, Cohen ND, *et al.* Effect of selective versus nonselective cyclooxygenase inhibitors on gastric ulceration scores and intestinal inflammation in horses. *Vet Surg* 2018; **47**(6): 784–791.
122 Pedersen SK, Cribb AE, Read EK, *et al.* Phenylbutazone induces equine glandular gastric disease without decreasing prostaglandin E2 concentrations. *J Vet Pharmacol Ther* 2018; **41**(2): 239–245.
123 Davis JL. Non-steroidal anti-inflammatory drug associated right dorsal colitis in the horse. *Equine Vet Educ* 2017; **29**(2): 104–113.
124 Marshall JF, Blikslager AT. The effect of non-steroidal anti-inflammatory drugs on the equine intestine. *Equine Vet J* 2011; **43**(s39): 140–144.
125 Tomlinson J, Blikslager A. Role of non-steroidal anti-inflammatory drugs in gastrointestinal tract injury and repair. *J Am Vet Med Assoc* 2003; **222**(7): 946–951.
126 Ziegler AL, Blikslager AT. Sparing the gut: COX-2 inhibitors herald a new era for treatment of horses with surgical colic. *Equine Vet Educ* 2020; **32**(11): 611–616.
127 Tomlinson JE, Blikslager AT. Effects of cyclooxygenase inhibitors flunixin and deracoxib on permeability of ischaemic-injured equine jejunum. *Equine Vet J* 2005; **37**(1): 75–80.
128 Moore JN. Non-steroidal anti-inflammatory drug therapy for endotoxemia: we're doing the right thing, aren't we? *Compendium Cont Education* 1989; **11**: 741–744.
129 McConnico RS, Morgan TW, Williams CC, *et al.* Pathophysiologic effects of phenylbutazone on the right dorsal colon in horses. *Am J Vet Res* 2008; **69**(11): 1496–1505.
130 Brzozowski T, Konturek PC, Konturek SJ, *et al.* Role of prostaglandins in gastroprotection and gastric adaptation. *J Physiol Pharmacol* 2005; **56**(Suppl 5): 33–55.
131 Hurley JW, Crandal LA. The effects of salicylates upon the stomach of dogs. *Gasteroenterology* 1964; **46**: 36–43.
132 Phillips BM. Aspirin-induced gastrointestinal microbleeding in dogs. *Toxicol Appl Pharmacol* 1973; **24**: 182–189.
133 Konturek JW, Dembinski A, Stoll R, *et al.* Mucosal adaptation to aspirin induced gastric damage in humans. Studies on blood flow, gastric mucosal growth, and neutrophil activation. *Gut* 1994; **35**(9): 1197–1204.
134 Taylor LA, Crawford LM. Aspirin-induced gastrointestinal lesions in dogs. *J Am Vet Med Assoc* 1968; **152**(6): 617–619.
135 Souza MH, de Lima OM , Jr Zamuner SR, *et al.* Gastritis increases resistance to aspirin-induced mucosal injury via COX-2-mediated lipoxin synthesis. *Am J Physiol Gastrointest Liver Physiol* 2003; **285**(1): G54–G61.

136 Wallace JL, Fiorucci S. A magic bullet for mucosal protection and aspirin is the trigger! *Trends Pharmacol Sci* 2003; **24**(7): 323–236.

137 Wallace JL, Zamuner SR, McKnight W, *et al.* Aspirin, but not NO-releasing aspirin (NCX-4016), interacts with selective COX-2 inhibitors to aggravate gastric damage and inflammation. *Am J Physiol Gastrointest Liver Physiol* 2004; **286**(1): G76–G81.

138 Fiorucci S, de Lima OM , Jr Mencarelli A, *et al.* Cyclooxygenase-2-derived lipoxin A4 increases gastric resistance to aspirin-induced damage. *Gastroenterology* 2002; **123**(5): 1598–1606.

139 Sennello KA, Leib MS. Effects of deracoxib or buffered aspirin on the gastric mucosa of healthy dogs. *J Vet Intern Med* 2006; **20**(60): 1291–1296.

140 Mathews KA, Doherty T, Dyson DH, *et al.* Nephrotoxicity in dogs associated with methoxyflurane anesthesia and flunixin meglumine analgesia. *Can Vet J* 1990; **31**(11): 766–771.

141 Mathews KA. Non-steroidal anti-inflammatory analgesics in pain management in dogs and cats. *Can Vet J* 1996; **37**(9): 539–545.

142 Gunson DE, Soma LR. Renal papillary necrosis in horses after phenylbutazone and water deprivation. *Vet Pathol* 1983; **20**(5): 603–610.

143 Monteiro B, Steagall PV, Lascelles BD, *et al.* Long-term use of non-steroidal anti-inflammatory drugs in cats with chronic kidney disease: from controversy to optimism. *J Small Anim Pract* 2019; **60**(8): 459–462.

144 Lobetti RG, Joubert KE. Effect of administration of non-steroidal anti-inflammatory drugs before surgery on renal function in clinically normal dogs. *Am J Vet Res* 2000; **61**(12): 1501–1506.

145 Gambaro G, Perazella MA. Adverse renal effects of anti-inflammatory agents: evaluation of selective and nonselective cyclooxygenase inhibitors. *J Intern Med* 2003; **253**(6): 643–652.

146 Rossat J, Maillard M, Nussberger JU, *et al.* Renal effects of selective cyclooxygenase-2 inhibition in normotensive salt-depleted subjects. *Clin Pharmacol Ther* 1999; **66**(1): 76–84.

147 Narita T, Sato R, Motoishi K, *et al.* The interaction between orally administered non-steroidal anti-inflammatory drugs and prednisolone in healthy dogs. *J Vet Med Sci* 2007; **69**(4): 353–363.

148 de Broe ME, Elseviers MM. Analgesic nephropathy. *N Engl J Med* 1998; **338**(7): 446–452.

149 Frendin JH, Boström IM, Kampa N, *et al.* Effects of carprofen on renal function during medetomidine-propofol-isoflurane anesthesia in dogs. *Am J Vet Res* 2006; **67**(12): 1967–1973.

150 Ko JCH, Miyabiyashi T, Mandsager RE, *et al.* Renal effects of carprofen administered to healthy dogs anesthetized with propofol and isoflurane. *Am J Vet Med Assoc* 2000; **217**(30): 346–349.

151 Bergmann HML, Nolte IJA, Kramer S. Effects of preoperative administration of carprofen on renal function and hemostasis in dogs undergoing surgery for fracture repair. *Am J Vet Res* 2005; **66**(8): 1356–1363.

152 Boström IM, Nyman GC, Lord PF, *et al.* Effects of carprofen on renal function and results of serum biochemical and hematologic analyses in anesthetized dogs that had low blood pressure during anesthesia. *Am J Vet Res* 2002; **63**(5): 712–721.

153 Crandell DE, Mathews KA, Dyson DH. Effect of meloxicam and carprofen on renal function when administered to healthy dogs prior to anesthesia and painful stimulation. *Am J Vet Res* 2004; **65**(10): 1384–1390.

154 Fusellier M, Desfontis JC, LeRoux A, *et al.* Effect of short-term treatment with meloxicam and pimobendan on the renal function in healthy beagle dogs. *J Vet Pharmacol Ther* 2008; **31**(20): 150–155.

155 Boström IM, Nyman G, Hoppe A, *et al.* Effects of meloxicam on renal function in dogs with hypotension during anaesthesia. *Vet Anaesth Analg* 2006; **33**(1): 62–69.

156 US Food and Drug Administration. Freedom of Information Summary: Deramaxx Chewable Tablets (NADA 141-203). Approval Date: August 21, 2002. www.fda.gov/downloads/AnimalVeterinary/Products/ApprovedAnimalDrug Products/ FOIADrugSummaries/ucm117640.pdf.

157 Luna SP, Basílio AC, Steagall PV, *et al.* Evaluation of adverse effects of long-term oral administration of carprofen, etodolac, flunixin meglumine, ketoprofen, and meloxicam in dogs. *Am J Vet Res* 2007; **68**(3): 258–264.

158 Surdyk KK, Brown CA, Brown SA. Evaluation of glomerular filtration rate in cats with reduced renal mass and administered meloxicam and acetylsalicylic acid. *Am J Vet Res* 2013; **74**(4): 648–651.

159 Gunew MN, Menrath VH, Marshall RD. Long-term safety, efficacy and palatability of oral meloxicam at 0.01–0.03 mg/kg for treatment of osteoarthritic pain in cats. *J Feline Med Surg* 2008; **10**(3): 235–241.

160 Gowan RA, Lingard AE, Johnston L, *et al.* Retrospective case–control study of the effects of long-term dosing with meloxicam on renal function in aged cats with degenerative joint disease. *J Feline Med Surg* 2011; **13**(10): 752–761.

161 Gowan RA, Baral RM, Lingard AE, *et al.* A retrospective analysis of the effects of meloxicam on the longevity of aged cats with and without overt chronic kidney disease. *J Feline Med Surg* 2012; **14**(12): 876–881.

162 KuKanich K, George C, Roush JK, *et al.* Effects of low-dose meloxicam in cats with chronic kidney disease. *J Feline Med Surg* 2021; **23**(2):138–148.

163 King JN, Hotz R, Reagan EL, *et al.* Safety of oral robenacoxib in the cat. *J Vet Pharmacol Ther* 2012; **35**(3): 290–300.

164 King JN, King S, Budsberg SC, *et al.* Clinical safety of robenacoxib in feline osteoarthritis: results of a randomized, blinded, placebo-controlled clinical trial. *J Feline Med Surg* 2016; **18**(8): 632–642.

165 Wun MK, Leister E, King T, *et al.* Acute kidney injury in 18 cats after subcutaneous meloxicam and an update on non-steroidal anti-inflammatory drug usage in feline patients in Australia. *Aust Vet J* 2023; **101**(3): 90–98.

166 Bjorkman D. Non-steroidal anti-inflammatory drug-associated toxicity of the liver, lower gastrointestinal tract, and esophagus. *Am J Med* 1998; **105**(Suppl 5A): 17S–21S.

167 Tolman KG. Hepatotoxicity of non-narcotic analgesics. *Am J Med* 1998; **105**(Suppl 1B): 13S–17S.

168 US Food and Drug Administration. Freedom of Information Summary: Rimadyl Tablets (NADA 141-053). Approval Date: October 25, 1996.

169 Vasseur PB, Johnson AL, Budsberg SC, *et al.* Randomized, controlled trial of the efficacy of carprofen, a non-steroidal antiinflammatory drug, in the treatment of osteoarthritis in dogs. *J Am Vet Med Assoc* 1995; **206**(6): 807–811.

170 MacPhail CM, Lappin MR, Meyer DJ, *et al.* Hepatocellular toxicosis associated with administration of carprofen in 21 dogs. *J Am Vet Med Assoc* 1998; **212**(120): 1895–1901.

171 Hickford FH, Barr SC, Erb HN. Effect of carprofen on hemostatic variables in dogs. *Am J Vet Res* 2001; **62**(10): 1642–1646.

172 Budsberg SC, Stoker AM, Johnston SA, *et al.* In vitro effects of meloxicam on metabolism in articular chondrocytes from dogs with naturally occurring osteoarthritis. *Am J Vet Res* 2013; **74**(9): 1198–1205.

173 Patrono C. Cardiovascular effects of cyclooxygenase-2 inhibitors: a mechanistic and clinical perspective. *Br J Clin Pharmacol* 2016; **82**(4): 957–964.

174 Mukherjee D, Nissen SE, Topol EJ. Risk of cardiovascular events associated with selective COX-2 inhibitors. *JAMA* 2001; **286**(8): 954–959.

175 Eisenberg RS. Learning the value of drugs – is rofecoxib a regulatory success story? *N Engl J Med* 2005; **352**(13): 1285–1287.

176 Fitzgerald GA. Coxibs and cardiovascular disease. *N Engl J Med* 2004; **351**(17): 1709–1711.

177 Topol EJ. Failing the public health – rofecoxib, Merck and the FDA. *N Engl J Med* 2004; **351**(17): 1707–1709.

178 Drazen JM. COX-2 inhibitors — a lesson in unexpected problems. *N England J Med* 2005; **352**(17): 1131–1132.

179 Papich MG. *Papich Handbook of Veterinary Drugs*, 5th edn. St. Louis, MO: Elsevier, 2021.

180 Fitzgerald GA, Patrono C. The coxibs, selective inhibitors of cyclooxygenase-2. *N Engl J Med* 2001; **345**(6): 433–442.

181 Kamata M, King JN, Seewald W, *et al.* Comparison of injectable robenacoxib versus meloxicam for peri-operative use in cats: results of a randomised clinical trial. *Vet J* 2012; **193**(1): 114–118.

182 Lascelles BDX, Cripps PJ, Jones A, *et al.* Efficacy and kinetics of carprofen, administered preoperatively or postoperatively, for the prevention of pain in dogs undergoing ovariohysterectomy. *Vet Surg* 1998; **27**(6): 568–582.

183 Mathews KA, Pettifer G, Foster R, *et al.* Safety and efficacy of preoperative administration of meloxicam, compared with that of ketoprofen and butorphanol in dogs undergoing abdominal surgery. *Am J Vet Res* 2001; **62**(6): 882–888.

184 Budsberg SC, Cross AR, Quandt JE, *et al.* Evaluation of intravenous administration of meloxicam for perioperative pain management following stifle joint surgery in dogs. *Am J Vet Res* 2002; **63**(11): 1557–1563.

185 Bennett D, Johnston P. Osteoarthritis in the cat. How should it be managed and treated? *J Feline Med Surg* 2012; **14**(1): 76–84.

186 Hjelle JJ, Grauer GF. Acetaminophen-induced toxicosis in dogs and cats. *J Am Vet Med Assoc* 1986; **188**(7): 742–746.

187 McCann ME, Rickes EL, Hora DF, *et al.* In vitro effects and in vivo efficacy of a novel cyclooxygenase-2 inhibitor in cats with lipopolysaccharide-induced pyrexia. *Am J Vet Res* 2005; **66**(7): 1278–1284.

188 Morresey PR. Therapeutic intervention strategies in endotoxemia. *Compend Contin Educ Vet* 2001; **23**: 925–931.

189 Valverde A, Gunkel CI. Pain management in horses and farm animals. *J Vet Emerg Crit Care* 2005; **15**(4): 295–307.

190 Cook VL, Meyer CT, Campbell NB, *et al.* Effect of firocoxib or flunixin meglumine on recovery of ischemic-injured equine jejunum. *Am J Vet Res* 2009; **70**(8): 992–1000.

191 Smith GW, Davis JL, Tell LA, *et al.* FARAD Digest: extralabel use of non-steroidal anti-inflammatory drugs in cattle. *J Am Vet Med Assoc* 2008; **232**(5): 697–701.

192 Wagner BK, Nixon E, Robles I, *et al.* Non-steroidal anti-inflammatory drugs: pharmacokinetics and mitigation of procedural-pain in cattle. *Animals* 2021; **11**(2): 282.
193 Coetzee JF, Mosher RA, KuKanich B, *et al.* Pharmacokinetics and effect of intravenous meloxicam in weaned Holstein calves following scoop dehorning without local anesthesia. *BMC Vet Res* 2012; **8**(1): 1–15.
194 Hirsch AC, Philipp H, Kleemann R. Investigation on the efficacy of meloxicam in sows with mastitis–metritis–agalactia syndrome. *J Vet Pharmacol Ther* 2003; **26**(5): 355–360.
195 Delatour P, Foot R, Foster AP, *et al.* Pharmacodynamics and chiral pharmacokinetics of carprofen in calves. *Br Vet J* 1996; **152**(2): 183–198.
196 Lohuis JACM, Werven TV, Brand A, *et al.* Pharmacodynamics and pharmacokinetics of carprofen, a non-steroidal anti-inflammatory drug, in healthy cows and cows with Escherichia coli endotoxin-induced mastitis. *J Vet Pharmacol Ther* 1991; **14**(3): 219–229.
197 Malreddy PR, Coetzee JF, KuKanich B, *et al.* Pharmacokinetics and milk secretion of gabapentin and meloxicam co-administered orally in Holstein-Friesian cows. *J Vet Pharmacol Ther* 2013; **36**(1): 14–20.
198 Mosher RA, Coetzee JF, Cull CA, *et al.* Pharmacokinetics of oral meloxicam in ruminant and preruminant calves. *J Vet Pharmacol Ther* 2012; **35**(4): 373–381.

25 Anesthetic and Analgesic Adjunctive Drugs

Daniel S.J. Pang
Faculty of Veterinary Medicine, University of Calgary, Calgary, Alberta, Canada and
Faculty of Veterinary Medicine, Université de Montréal, Saint-Hyacinthe, Québec, Canada

Chapter contents

Introduction, 420
Non-analgesic adjuncts, 420
Dantrolene, 420
Diphenhydramine, 421
Doxapram, 421
Famotidine, omeprazole, and pantoprazole, 423
Guaifenesin (GG, glyceryl guaiacolate ether), 424
Maropitant, 425
Methocarbamol, 427
Metoclopramide, 427
Ondansetron and dolasetron, 428
Procainamide, 428
Sodium nitroprusside, 429
Trazodone, 429
Vasopressin (arginine vasopressin, antidiuretic hormone) and desmopressin, 430
Analgesic adjuncts, 431
Amantadine and memantine, 431
Amitriptyline and nortriptyline, 432
Cannabinoids, 433
Gabapentin and pregabalin, 434
Tapentadol, 436
Tramadol, 436
References, 438

Introduction

Adjunctive drugs can be broadly described as drugs that fall outside common clinical use but may provide a benefit beyond that of more commonly used drugs or are less readily characterized because they play a supportive role in the provision of anesthesia and analgesia. Some of the drugs described in this chapter may enter the mainstream as evidence supporting their use grows, while others may remain unconventional, restricted to second- or third-line therapy, or fall out of use as alternatives are identified or emerging evidence fails to support their use. This chapter is divided into non-analgesic and analgesic adjuncts.

Non-analgesic adjuncts

Dantrolene

Dantrolene is a peripherally acting muscle relaxant, producing skeletal muscle relaxation through ryanodine receptor antagonism and inhibition of the dihydropyridine receptor calcium channel [1–3]. There are three isoforms of ryanodine receptors with RyR1 believed to be predominant in skeletal muscle. Receptors are located in organelle membranes (i.e., mitochondrial, endoplasmic and sarcoplasmic reticular, and nuclear). The primary effect of dantrolene is to reduce calcium release from the sarcoplasmic reticulum into the cytoplasm via the RyR1 receptor (a calcium channel), thereby dissociating excitation–contraction coupling. Its muscle-relaxing properties are limited to skeletal muscle though cardiac depression has been reported in dogs when administered at high doses (greater than 5 mg/kg) or in combination with verapamil [4]. At therapeutic intravenous (IV) doses (1–5 mg/kg) in dogs and cats, minute ventilation during general anesthesia is reduced through depression of both respiratory rate and tidal volume [5,6]. In humans, adverse effects are described as minor and include phlebitis, transient muscle weakness, and gastrointestinal upset [7].

Dantrolene is primarily indicated for the treatment and prevention of the pharmacogenetic disorder malignant hyperthermia (MH) [8–14], and rhabdomyolysis [15–19], with a potential role in cytoprotection and as an antiarrhythmic [2,3,20].

Shortly after MH was first reported in humans [21,22] and pigs [23,24], the successful use of dantrolene for the prevention and treatment of MH was published with the experiments performed in pigs [9]. It has since been used to treat MH in dogs [10] and horses [11].

Dantrolene is used in the prevention and treatment of exertional rhabdomyolysis in horses [16,18,25], though use in rhabdomyolysis in a dog [15] and tetanus in cats [19] has also been reported.

In horses given dantrolene before general anesthesia, there is a risk of hyperkalemia [26]. A study of six adult horses given oral dantrolene (6 mg/kg) or water 1 h before induction of general

Veterinary Anesthesia and Analgesia: The Sixth Edition of Lumb and Jones. Edited by Leigh Lamont, Kurt Grimm, Sheilah Robertson, Lydia Love and Carrie Schroeder.
© 2024 John Wiley & Sons, Inc. Published 2024 by John Wiley & Sons, Inc.
Companion website: www.wiley.com/go/lamont/anesthesia

anesthesia (crossover study design) found hyperkalemia (serum potassium > 5.5 mEq/L) occurred in four horses, with two of these horses having serum potassium concentrations > 7 mEq/L [26]. Three horses developed bradyarrhythmias associated with hyperkalemia. Dantrolene administration was also associated with reduced cardiac output (approximately 25–30%), heart rate, and arterial blood pressure (approximately 20%). No difference in recovery time was observed.

Dantrolene undergoes hepatic metabolism, primarily hydroxylation, in the dog and horse. Metabolites and up to 1% of unchanged dantrolene are excreted in urine and bile [27–29].

Dosages in horses are as follows: 1.9 mg/kg IV loading dose followed by oral dosing at 2.5 mg/kg every 60 min [28], or 2–4 mg/kg PO [11,16,18,26,29]. Notably, there is considerable interindividual variation in plasma concentrations following oral administration [16,26].

Dosages in dogs and cats are as follows: 1–3 mg/kg IV (low end of dose range for muscle relaxation and high end for the treatment of MH); 5–6 mg/kg PO once daily as prophylaxis. As seen with horses, oral dosing in dogs is associated with wide variability in plasma concentrations of dantrolene [30].

Dosages in pigs are as follows: 1–3 mg/kg IV for the treatment of MH; 5 mg/kg PO for prophylaxis.

Dantrolene is available as a powder for reconstitution (with sterile water). The two commercial formulations available are reconstituted to 0.33 mg/mL (Dantrium®) and 50 mg/mL (Ryanodex®). Solutions of reconstituted dantrolene are light sensitive and stable for 6 h [3]. Dantrolene is also available as 100 mg capsules.

Diphenhydramine

Diphenhydramine has a long history of perioperative use, particularly in dogs and cats undergoing mast cell tumor resection or exhibiting suspected allergic and anaphylactic reactions. It is an antihistamine, acting as a reversible competitive antagonist at the H_1 receptor [31,32]. Histamine receptors, of which there are at least four (H_1, H_2, H_3, and H_4), are widely distributed in the body, with H_1 present in the brain, airway smooth muscle, skin, gastrointestinal and genitourinary tracts, adrenal medulla, immune system, heart, and vascular endothelium (reviewed by Peters and Kovacic) [32]. Agonist activity at the H_1 receptor leads to phospholipase C activation and increased intracellular calcium, which, in turn, promotes airway smooth muscle contraction and catecholamine release from the adrenal medulla. In the vascular endothelium, H_1 receptor activation leads to nitric oxide formation and vasodilation. Additionally, increased intracellular calcium triggers a host of secondary signaling pathways, leading to vasodilation and increased cellular permeability.

Centrally, diphenhydramine's effect on histamine receptors in the brain is to cause drowsiness in people [31]. While this effect is often proposed in animals, there is little supporting evidence [33–35]. In a randomized, blinded, placebo-controlled clinical trial in dogs, diphenhydramine doses of 2–8 mg/kg intramuscular (IM) were not associated with sedation (observed for 30 min after administration), with sedation scores no different than the saline control group [33]. At the highest dose (8 mg/kg), there was a small increase in sedation score compared to baseline, but this was not statistically significant when compared with other groups. As an older drug, it is less selective than newer agents. It may be that higher doses, in the region of 10 mg/kg PO, are required to cause sedation in dogs [33]. In addition to its effects on the H_1 receptor, it also has antimuscarinic and antidopaminergic properties, which are likely to contribute to the adverse effects associated with high doses in dogs [31,36]. At doses of 30–45 mg/kg PO in dogs, diphenhydramine resulted in mydriasis, muscle tremors, increased muscle tone, head swaying, and hyperreactivity [36]. It is primarily used in humans for the management of motion sickness, as well as postoperative and opioid-induced nausea and vomiting [37]. In cats, a dose of 3 mg/kg PO resulted in behavioral changes within 30 min, reaching a peak effect at 1–2 h and lasting for over 4 h [38]. These effects included altered locomotion, increased muscle tone, tremors, hypersalivation, and vomiting. Effects on sleep were varied but included increased wakefulness and disrupted sleep patterns.

The benefits of diphenhydramine administration before mast cell tumor excision and in suspected anaphylaxis are unclear. Based on an earlier pharmacokinetic study showing plasma levels of diphenhydramine exceeding the therapeutic range in humans, Sanchez *et al.*, in a randomized, blinded, placebo-controlled trial, found no impact of diphenhydramine (1 mg/kg IV) on plasma histamine concentrations in dogs (n = 8) undergoing mast cell tumor resection (three dogs had grade 1 tumors, two had grade 2, two had grade 3, and one had grade 4) [39]. Intraoperatively, mean and diastolic arterial blood pressures were approximately 10–15 mmHg lower in the diphenhydramine group compared to control, with a small increase in cardiac index [39]. An *in vitro* study of a canine mast cell line found that diphenhydramine did not prevent histamine release [40]. Current treatment guidelines for anaphylaxis emphasize epinephrine for first-line therapy, with antihistamines described as having a "limited role" as a second- or third-line therapy, useful in managing cutaneous symptoms, if present [41,42]. In cutaneous allergic reactions in dogs, there is little evidence supporting the use of diphenhydramine [35].

The pharmacokinetics of diphenhydramine have been described in rabbits, camels, horses, sheep, and dogs [34,43–46]. In conscious dogs administered 1 mg/kg IV or 2 mg/kg IM, terminal half-life was reported to be approximately 4 and 7 h, respectively, with 88% bioavailability from IM injection [34]. No adverse effects were reported at these doses and with these routes of injection (the IV dose was given as a bolus over < 5 s) and resultant plasma levels were in the therapeutic range reported in humans. Oral diphenhydramine bioavailability in dogs is low (3–7%) [47].

Doses in dogs and cats are 1–4 mg/kg (every 8 h, PO, IM, or IV) and 0.5–1 mg/kg (every 12 h, PO or IM), respectively. In dogs, IM injection is preferred over IV use, with a described risk of hypotension/cardiovascular instability associated with the latter route [34]. The drug is supplied as a 50 mg/mL injectable formulation.

Doxapram

The analeptic (central nervous system [CNS] stimulant) agent doxapram has a long history of use in veterinary medicine and has been applied in a wide variety of situations including arousal from sedation/anesthesia [48–50], cardiopulmonary resuscitation (CPR) [51], stimulation of respiration in neonates and following drug-induced respiratory depression [52–60], and assessment of laryngeal function [61–63].

The mechanism of action leading to respiratory stimulation is likely a combination of central and peripheral effects [64–66]. Electrophysiological studies in cats and dogs showed increased activity of the respiratory nuclei of the medulla when given therapeutic doses of doxapram [64]. As the dose was increased, cortical stimulation occurred followed by convulsions. A safety margin of 20-60:1 was cited before onset of central stimulation and convulsions. Experimental evidence suggests that stimulation of respiration is dose dependent, with activation of peripheral aortic and carotid receptors occurring at doses (0.05–0.25 mg/kg IV) below those typically used clinically [65]. As the dose is increased (0.5–5.0 mg/kg IV), stimulation of respiratory and non-respiratory brainstem neurons occurs [65]. There is limited evidence for interspecies variability in the doxapram dose effective for respiratory stimulation versus CNS arousal. Low doses of doxapram are successful in eliciting respiratory stimulation in cats before cardiovascular or CNS stimulation occurs [64–66], but higher doses may be necessary in other species. It is unclear to what extent this dose dependency occurs in dogs and horses, with evidence of CNS arousal occurring at doses effective for respiratory stimulation [52,67–69].

The molecular mechanisms underlying peripheral and central control of respiration remain an active area of research. Recent evidence suggests involvement of two-pore domain potassium channels, and these channels may also be involved in the mechanism of inhalational anesthesia [70–72]. See [73] for a review.

Doxapram has the ability to significantly increase minute ventilation through an increase in both respiratory rate and tidal volume, leading to the term "pharmacologic ventilator" [74]. However, its effects are relatively short-lived, reflecting a rapid decline in plasma levels following an IV bolus [75]. Doxapram undergoes hepatic metabolism in dogs with renal excretion of metabolites. A similar pharmacokinetic profile is observed in horses with a rapid decline in plasma levels following IV bolus administration, extensive hepatic metabolism, and renal excretion of metabolites [76].

Doxapram also results in modest increases in arterial blood pressure and heart rate in humans [74]. While cardiovascular changes are short-lived in healthy animals (i.e., several minutes), one report of its use in dogs (1.5 mg/kg IV) rendered hypovolemic from controlled hemorrhage showed sustained increases in cardiac output and arterial blood pressure for up to 1 h [69]. Doxapram does not induce cardiac arrhythmias in dogs anesthetized with halothane or cycloproprane in the presence of epinephrine and hypercapnia and does not cause meaningful changes in hematology or serum biochemistry [77–78].

In healthy adult horses and those with experimentally induced respiratory disease, a dose of 0.3 mg/kg IV resulted in an approximately 50% increase in respiratory rate and tidal volume [79]. The duration of action was not described. During halothane anesthesia, preceded with acepromazine and thiopental in ponies, the addition of doxapram (0.05 mg/kg/min IV) resulted in a return of arterial carbon dioxide tension ($PaCO_2$) and pH to near normal levels, with an increase in respiratory rate (tidal volume was not measured) [67]. An increase in mean arterial blood pressure of approximately 20% without an accompanying increase in heart rate was observed during doxapram infusion. Interestingly, the infusion of doxapram was associated with a reduction in plane of anesthesia, necessitating an increase in halothane vaporizer setting.

In cats anesthetized with a preparation of alfaxalone–alfadolone (Saffan®), administration of doxapram (7.5 mg/kg IV) resulted in a 181% increase in minute ventilation, which lasted for several minutes [53]. A similar pattern was seen in cats anesthetized with thiopental [53]. At this dose, heart rates increased for several minutes during both thiopental and Saffan® anesthesia to approximately 15–20% above the pre-doxapram period. Recovery was faster in the Saffan® group with the addition of doxapram, while no change was observed in the thiopental group.

The use of doxapram in patients with a history of seizures is controversial [73]. While it is clear that cortical activity increases in a dose-dependent fashion, it is unclear if this constitutes proconvulsant activity. Care should be exercised when administering doxapram in patients with a history of seizures. As always, the use of appropriate dosing (i.e., to effect) is critical.

Two areas of active doxapram usage are in foal and calf neonatal medicine and assessment of laryngeal function in dogs. Retrospective data from a cohort of foals with hypoxic-ischemic encephalopathy (neonatal maladjustment syndrome) revealed doxapram (0.02–0.05 mg/kg/min IV) to be more effective than caffeine (loading dose of 7.5–12 mg/kg followed by 2.5–5 mg/kg/day PO via nasogastric tube) at reducing $PaCO_2$ for at least 12 h [55]. However, foals remained acidemic with no significant increase in pH. The reduction in $PaCO_2$ was achieved with an increase in tidal volume, without an increase in respiratory rate. No effects on heart rate were observed, and there was no difference in mortality rates. These data agreed with an earlier retrospective study in healthy foals showing no advantage of caffeine over saline in correcting respiratory acidosis created with isoflurane anesthesia [54]. Furthermore, a doxapram dosing regimen of 0.5 mg/kg followed by 0.03 mg/kg/min IV was as effective as 0.5 mg/kg followed by 0.08 mg/kg/min. Giguère *et al.* also reported an improvement in arterial oxygen tension (PaO_2) following doxapram administration, compared with saline control or caffeine [54]. The effects of doxapram in healthy foals differed from those observed in healthy adult horses, with a small but significant increase in heart rate observed in healthy foals regardless of doxapram dose. Doxapram also resulted in a modest increase in mean arterial blood pressure of approximately 10 mmHg. The mechanism of increased ventilation also differed; minute ventilation was increased in healthy foals as a result of increased respiratory rate and not tidal volume.

In calves, a comparison of doxapram (2 mg/kg IV) and theophylline (7 mg/kg IV) showed a marked increase in respiratory rate with doxapram but not theophylline [56]. Respiratory rate doubled 10 min after doxapram administration followed by a steady decline over the next 2 h (end of the recording period). The effect on $PaCO_2$ (maximal decrease of approximate 20 mmHg) and PaO_2 (maximal increase of approximate 15 mmHg) peaked 30 s following administration, followed by a steady return toward baseline over the recording period. Small increases in heart rate (120–155 beats/min) and systemic systolic arterial blood pressure (105–112 mmHg) were also observed without a significant change in cardiac output. A greater change (20 mmHg increase) was observed in systolic pulmonary arterial blood pressures. The authors concluded that the transient respiratory stimulation following doxapram administration could be beneficial in newborn calves when positive pressure ventilation was not possible. Similar results were observed in neonatal calves (2–15 h old) given doxapram at approximately 1 mg/kg IV, which resulted in a doubling of minute ventilation, an approximately 20% increase in PaO_2, and a 25% decrease in $PaCO_2$ [57]. Interestingly, a systematic review of doxapram use in human preterm infants did not identify a clear advantage associated with doxapram use over saline [80], and there is evidence that doxapram may cause cortical damage due to a reduction in cerebral blood flow [81–83].

Laryngeal paralysis in dogs manifests as a paradoxical movement of the arytenoid cartilages in affected dogs, with inward collapse of the arytenoid cartilages as subatmospheric thoracic pressure is generated during inspiration. While there are numerous studies evaluating the effect of doxapram on arytenoid cartilage motion in dogs, there appears only one in which both healthy and diseased (laryngeal paralysis) dogs were included [61]. In that study, following premedication with acepromazine (0.022 mg/kg IM in diseased dogs and 0.2 mg/kg IM in healthy dogs) and butorphanol (0.44 mg/kg IM), animals were preoxygenated for 5 min and general anesthesia induced with isoflurane delivered by mask. Doxapram was administered at 1.1 mg/kg IV following induction of general anesthesia. At baseline, the normalized glottal gap area was significantly larger in dogs with laryngeal paralysis during both inspiration and expiration. Following doxapram administration, the normalized glottal gap area at inspiration was significantly reduced in dogs with laryngeal paralysis compared to normal dogs, and the area during expiration was significantly greater in dogs with laryngeal paralysis. The dramatic changes observed (i.e., marked arytenoid adduction during inspiration) allowed for diagnosis but also led the authors to warn of the need to potentially intubate the airway to provide oxygen. Studies in healthy dogs consistently report increased laryngeal motion following doxapram administration (0.5–2.5 mg/kg IV) [63].

In horses, laryngeal function has been evaluated by comparing the following techniques: animals standing at rest with a twitch, at rest without twitch, manual occlusion of nostrils, post-exercise (lunging at canter), swallowing, doxapram (40 mg/kg IV), and xylazine (0.5 mg/kg IV) [62]. Subjectively, doxapram resulted in an increased respiratory rate in approximately half of the horses examined (total $n = 7$), but the most successful technique for stimulating deep breaths was manual nostril occlusion.

Using doxapram during CPR is no longer recommended, though this practice may persist. An internet survey of 600 veterinarians in small animal practice, with or without board certification in critical care and emergency medicine or anesthesia, showed that while doxapram was as frequently available to both specialists and practitioners (74% and 81%, respectively), a significantly higher percentage of general practitioners had used it during CPR (29% and 70%, respectively) [51]. This contrasts starkly with the current evidence-based CPR guidelines in which doxapram is not mentioned [84].

The use of doxapram at 0.1–0.2 mg/kg IV has also been suggested to facilitate recovery from general anesthesia in horses, when appropriate, by increasing the level of arousal and stimulating respiration, thereby speeding reduction in alveolar concentrations of inhalational agents [85].

Other species in which doxapram use has been recorded are cattle (1 mg/kg IV was effective in speeding recovery from xylazine), camels (0.05–0.13 mg/kg IV was effective at speeding recovery from xylazine in Bactrian camels), llamas (2.2 mg/kg IV was not effective in reversing xylazine), and southern elephant seals (appeared to cause CNS stimulation at 5 mg/kg when used to aid recovery from a range of drug combinations; therefore, authors recommended 2 mg/kg) [86–89].

Famotidine, omeprazole, and pantoprazole

Acid secretion in the stomach is initiated at the level of parietal cells by gastrin, histamine type-2 (H_2), and muscarinic (M_3) receptors. Receptor activation results in increased proton pump activity on the luminal side of the cell via calcium- or cAMP-dependent pathways. Several H_2 receptor antagonists (famotidine, ranitidine, and cimetidine) have been used clinically. Famotidine and ranitidine are 20–50 and 4–10 times more potent than cimetidine, respectively. Perioperative use is usually to offset risk of gastrointestinal ulceration, with common indications including stress- or non-steroidal anti-inflammatory drug (NSAID)-related abomasal and gastric ulcers in calves, foals, and horses, and following regurgitation during anesthesia in dogs.

In a crossover study of five healthy horses, a comparison of famotidine and ranitidine found a high degree of individual variation in measured gastric fluid pH following administration of either drug at a range of dosages [90]. Each horse received famotidine (0.5, 1, and 2 mg/kg) and raniditine (4.4 and 6.6 mg/kg) via nasogastric tube. For famotidine, gastric fluid pH increased above 6 in three of five horses receiving 0.5 mg/kg, five of five horses receiving 1 mg/kg, and three of five horses receiving 2 mg/kg. For ranitidine, gastric fluid pH increased above 6 in four of five horses receiving 4.4 mg/kg and five of five horses receiving 6.6 mg/kg. Ranitidine demonstrated a tendency to result in a longer elevation of gastric fluid pH (166 ± 106 min versus 98 ± 110 min; mean ± SD). The drug response varied considerably between horses, leading the authors to suggest a dose of 6.6 mg/kg ranitidine. Similar studies in 2–6-day-old foals and milk-fed calves resulted in recommended dosages of ranitidine of 6.6 mg/kg PO three times daily and 50 mg/kg PO three times daily, respectively [91–92]. However, more recent evidence highlights the risk of extrapolating the need for H_2 antagonists in critically ill foals without measurement of gastric pH [93]. This study found that almost 50% of hospitalized foals had a baseline gastric pH, which was alkaline. Data supporting the use of famotidine in calves and foals are not available.

Omeprazole and pantoprazole are proton pump inhibitors, which act on the proton pump located at the luminal surface of gastric parietal cells. Inhibition of acid secretion by proton pump inhibitors is cumulative in humans, requiring 2–4 days to achieve maximal inhibition [94]. This delay results from a combination of (1) increasing inhibition of parietal cells as dormant cells are activated following initial inhibition of active cells, (2) increased intestinal absorption of the drug as acid secretion is decreased in response to the drug's effects, and potentially (3) the impact of cytochrome P450 inhibition to decrease the drug's own metabolism. Proton pump inhibitors are metabolized by the cytochrome P450 system (CYP1A1/2 and CYP2D15 in dogs), and the pharmacokinetics of esomeprazole (the *S*-enantiomer of omeprazole) have been reported in dogs [95].

The delay to achieve maximal effect can be minimized with initial IV administration or use of enteric-coated formulations (though breaking or crushing coated tablets may reduce this benefit). Interestingly, the efficacy of proton pump inhibitors is increased with acid secretion (as occurs with feeding) and reduced when given in conjunction with H_2 receptor antagonists [96]. Human clinical evidence suggests that omeprazole is more effective at raising gastric pH above 3 (a level correlated with healing gastric and duodenal ulcers in humans) compared to H_2 receptor antagonists [97]. The dose in dogs and cats is 1–2.5 mg/kg PO once or twice daily [94,98,99], while the dose in horses and foals is 1–4 mg/kg PO once daily, with the low end of dose range for ulcer prevention and the higher end for treatment [100–102].

In 2-day-old calves, the pharmacokinetics of IV pantoprazole (1 mg/kg) have been studied and the terminal half-life reported to be 2.8 h, which is longer than that reported in foals (1.5 h), adult alpacas (0.5 h), and adult goats (0.7 h) [103–106]. In foals, pantoprazole (1.5 mg/kg IV) was effective at increasing gastric pH for up to 24 h following a single dose [104]. In alpacas, pantoprazole (2 mg/kg SC or 1 mg/kg IV, daily for 3 days) was effective at increasing third compartment pH above baseline within 4 or 12 h of initial administration, respectively [105].

The perioperative use of famotidine in dogs and cats is commonly performed in cases with suspected gastrointestinal ulceration or in patients at risk of ulceration. Recommended doses of famotidine in dogs and cats vary widely due to limited clinical data. In dogs, 0.1–0.5 mg/kg twice daily or 1 mg/kg once daily (PO, IV, SC, IM) has been advocated. In cats, 0.2–0.25 mg/kg once or twice daily

(IM, SC, PO, IV) has been suggested. Slow IV administration in cats is recommended based on anecdotal evidence that fast injection (i.e., less than 5 min) is associated with hemolysis from the benzyl alcohol component of the injectable formulation. However, a retrospective study where hospital policy was to administer famotidine over 5 min IV did not identify an effect on packed cell volume (PCV) [107]. The same study showed no change in PCV when cats received famotidine SC. There are limited clinical data demonstrating efficacy of famotidine in dogs, and omeprazole may be superior at raising gastric pH for a useful period of time [98,108]. A recent study in dogs with exercise-induced gastritis and clinically relevant gastric ulcers showed famotidine (approximately 1 mg/kg PO once daily) to be superior to no treatment in preventing gastric ulcers but inferior to omeprazole (approximately 0.85 mg/kg PO once daily) [108]. In healthy adult dogs, famotidine (0.5 mg/kg IV twice daily) resulted in a significant elevation of gastric pH above saline control and ranitidine, but did not raise pH as high, or for as long, as omeprazole (1 mg/kg PO once daily). Increasing the dosing frequency of famotidine to three times daily did not result in any improvement [98].

The preoperative use of omeprazole or esomeprazole shows variable results depending on dose and route of administration [95,109–111]. In one study, the administration of esomeprazole (two 1 mg/kg IV doses 12 h apart before induction of general anesthesia) resulted in a less acidic reflux but did not reduce the incidence of reflux [109]. In contrast, another study reporting the use of preoperative omeprazole (single 1 mg/kg PO dose at least 4 h before induction of general anesthesia) showed a reduction in the number of gastroesophageal reflux and regurgitation episodes [110]. A direct comparison between findings is difficult due to differences in study design. Zacuto *et al.* also had another treatment group, esomeprazole (1 mg/kg IV) with cisapride (1 mg/kg IV), which resulted in less acidic reflux but also a significant reduction in the number of reflux events compared to the control and omeprazole groups [109]. Esomeprazole (1 mg/kg, IV, SC, and enteric-coated formulation PO) was effective at increasing gastric pH in conscious dogs [95]. The duration that pH was ≥ 3 was longest with SC and PO administration, with an SC dose maintaining pH ≥ 3 for 80% of the 24-h observation period (in contrast to approximately 60% and 40% for the first and second 12-h periods after IV administration, respectively). Slightly greater efficacy (not statistically significant) and less variability were observed with once daily administration PO for 5 days. The pharmacokinetic profile of SC and PO administration is favorable in dogs, with bioavailability of approximately 100% and 70%, respectively [95]. Peak plasma concentrations were achieved between 1.8 and 0.8 h after PO administration on the first and fifth day, respectively. However, the terminal half-life is approximately 1 h regardless of route of administration (PO, SC, IV), indicating that once daily dosing is insufficient, with twice daily dosing recommended in dogs and cats [94,95]. Similar pharmacodynamic data were reported in dogs given omeprazole (approximately 0.5–1 mg/kg of an enteric-coated formulation PO, twice daily, for 5 days) in a randomized, blinded, placebo-controlled crossover study, with gastric pH maintained ≥ 3 for 90% of the 4-day observation period (days 2–5 of PO administration) [111]. Recently, a long-acting omeprazole formulation was evaluated in dogs [112]. Following a single injection (4 mg/kg IM), gastric pH ≥ 3 was maintained for over 60% of a 7-day observation period (peak effect on days 1–4). A study of the same formulation in horses (3.4–4.4 mg/kg IM) found it to be effective for up to 7 days after injection in four of seven horses studied [113].

There is currently no clear evidence supporting the use of one proton pump inhibitor over another in dogs or cats, but available evidence indicates that proton pump inhibitors are better than H_2 receptor antagonists at increasing gastric pH [94,98,99,108]. It is important to recognize that, while the incidence of gastroesophageal reflux is relatively high in anesthetized patients (up to approximately 50%) [114,115], the incidence of complications such as esophageal stricture formation is extremely low [116].

There is a theoretical concern with chronic proton pump inhibitor therapy resulting in a change in gastric fauna and bacterial overgrowth, potentially increasing the risk of pneumonia in patients predisposed to regurgitation, such as those with megaesophagus. Another potential concern is the effect of omeprazole to inhibit the cytochrome P450 system, specifically CYP2C19, responsible for diazepam metabolism [117,118]. There is currently no evidence that this is of clinical significance in veterinary medicine, and the large therapeutic margin of diazepam may reduce the risk of adverse events.

Famotidine is available as 10 mg tablets (other strengths may be available), an 8 mg/mL suspension, and a 10 mg/mL solution for injection.

Omeprazole is available as 20 and 40 mg capsules and is licensed as an oral paste in horses (370 mg/g of paste). Esomeprazole is available as 20 mg capsules and as injectable formulations (21.3 and 42.5 mg/mL). Pantoprazole is available as tablets (20 and 40 mg) and an injectable formulation (4 mg/mL).

Guaifenesin (GG, glyceryl guaiacolate ether)

Guaifenesin, originally derived from the *Guaiacum* genus of trees, is a centrally acting skeletal muscle relaxant with sedative properties primarily co-administered IV with injectable anesthetic agents for the induction and maintenance of general anesthesia in horses and ruminants. Historically, it was used for this indication in humans along with a role in the management of tetanus. It has been in use in veterinary anesthesia since the 1960s [119,120]. In humans, it is currently used exclusively as an expectorant [121]. The mechanism(s) of action of guaifenesin are largely unknown, but evidence from the 1950s suggests sites of action in both the brain (brainstem and subcortical regions) and spinal cord (polysynaptic reflex inhibition) via interneuron depression, resulting in sedation and muscle relaxation [120,122]. There is extremely limited evidence to suggest it has any analgesic properties and none are typically attributed [120]. It has a wide therapeutic margin, with doses resulting in cardiopulmonary adverse effects such as hypotension, respiratory depression, and apneustic breathing pattern, being approximately 70–80% greater than that required to induce recumbency in horses (75–150 mg/kg) [119–123]. When given to induce recumbency in ponies and horses (dose ranges of 109–134 mg/kg), plasma levels of guaifenesin ranged from 238,000 to 313,000 ng/mL [124,125].

Cardiovascular effects are mild when guaifenesin is administered on its own at recommended doses, with no change in heart rate, cardiac output, central venous pressure, or respiratory rate, and an approximately 20% decrease in mean arterial blood pressure [124,126]. Similarly, respiratory effects are minimal, and the physiologic changes associated with recumbency appear to have a greater effect than any respiratory depression from guaifenesin [127]. Minute ventilation is maintained as a result of increased respiratory rate offsetting a decrease in tidal volume, indicating a sparing effect on the respiratory muscles [124]. Schatzmann *et al.* found minimal changes in PaO_2 when horses were administered guaifenesin (100 mg/kg IV) but remained standing [127].

Overdose in horses results in a period of transient muscle spasm and mydriasis as the dose approaches 180 mg/kg IV, followed by loss of palpebral reflex, with death following respiratory or cardiac arrest at approximately 460 mg/kg [120]. Guaifenesin undergoes hepatic metabolism with glucuronidation followed by renal excretion. A sex difference in elimination has been identified in ponies with more rapid elimination in females [125]. The dose of guaifenesin required to achieve recumbency also shows a sex difference in ponies, with stallions requiring a higher dose than mares (130 versus 108 mg/kg IV) and a longer half-life (84 versus 60 min) [124]. Plasma half-life was approximately 75–80 min at doses of 88 and 134 mg/kg IV in adult horses, with no sex difference between geldings and mares, though geldings required a higher dose to achieve recumbency (163 versus 111 mg/kg IV) [124].

Guaifenesin is commonly prepared as a 5–15% solution with 0.9% saline or 5% dextrose solution, though it can also be solubilized in sterile water. There is a concentration-dependent risk of hemolysis which appears unrelated to the speed of administration [119,127,128]. Hemolysis has been documented in horses when the concentration exceeds a 15% solution, and in cattle when it exceeds 5% [119,127,129]. Intravascular thrombus formation is also dose related, and concentrations of greater than 7% are associated with increased risk of thrombosis [127,130,131]. This effect is related to solution concentration rather than speed of administration, with reported histologic changes including endothelial loss with formation of a fibrin clot [130]. With a 10% solution the thrombus is not occlusive [130].

Guaifenesin is prone to precipitate out of solution when stored below room temperature (22 °C), but this is reversible with gentle heating such as immersion in a warm water bath [120] or gradual warming in a microwave. Perivascular injection has been associated with tissue necrosis [120], and administration via an IV catheter is recommended. Urticaria attributed to guaifenesin has also been reported [132]. In the reported case, the horse also received xylazine, ketamine, butorphanol, bupivacaine, and isoflurane, but the timing of the appearance of urticaria and failure of recurrence during two subsequent anesthetic episodes without guaifenesin implicates a role for guaifenesin. Plasma histamine levels were slightly elevated (5.2 ± 7.1 ng/mL) compared with baseline (3.2 ± 2.4 ng/mL) when guaifenesin was given IV in combination with xylazine and ketamine to adult horses (n = 14) [133].

The inclusion of guaifenesin (with xylazine and ketamine) as part of a partial intravenous anesthesia (PIVA) protocol administered to mares with dystocia was associated with 25 times greater odds of death compared with α_2-adrenergic receptor agonist and ketamine PIVA (9 times greater odds), and α_2-adrenergic receptor agonist PIVA [134]. The authors suggested that the inclusion of guaifenesin contributed to greater ataxia and sedation in recovery.

In a study of the effect of numerous perianesthetic drugs (α_2-adrenergic receptor agonists, *S*-ketamine, lidocaine, rocuronium, atipamezole, acepromazine, butorphanol, benzodiazepines, and guaifenesin) on the lithium sensor used in lithium dilution cardiac output measurement, guaifenesin had minimal effect on sensor performance (< 10% bias) [135].

Maropitant

Maropitant is a neurokinin-1 (NK_1) receptor antagonist licensed as an antiemetic in dogs and cats. It is highly protein-bound and undergoes extensive hepatic metabolism by CYP3A, CYP2D15 (dogs), and CYP1A (cats) enzymes [136] [137]. Oral bioavailability is approximately 20% in dogs and 50% in cats [138].

Neurokinin receptor antagonism by maropitant reduces binding of the neuropeptide neurotransmitter substance P. Substance P is intimately involved in the brainstem nuclei (area postrema, nucleus tractus solitarius, and vagal dorsal motor nucleus) facilitating emesis [139].

The most frequently encountered and reported adverse effect of maropitant is pain on injection [140]. The commercial preparation is formulated with β-cyclodextrin to increase solubility and the binding relationship is temperature dependent. Metacresol is included as a preservative. Until recently, free, unbound maropitant was suspected to cause pain on injection and refrigerating the solution was investigated as a means of reducing this reaction. An injectate temperature of 4 °C was associated with a mild response ("twitching of the skin, licking of the fur, or digging at the injection site") in one out of 17 dogs; the remaining 16 dogs did not react to injection. In contrast, injections at 25 °C were associated with a painful response in nine out of 17 dogs, four of which were classified as moderate–severe ("short-term vocalization, jumping, wincing, prolonged yelping or aggression") [140]. This pattern of responses was reflected in concurrent visual analog scale (VAS) scores, with a significant increase in VAS score associated with the 25 °C injectate temperature compared to the 4 °C injectate temperature (or saline injectate, at both 4 °C and 25 °C) [140]. It appears that there is a role for the preservative, metacresol, in contributing to pain on injection [141]. A generic formulation of maropitant, using benzyl alcohol as a preservative, was found to cause less reaction on SC injection in dogs (total n = 32 dogs, crossover study) when compared with the formulation using metacresol [141]. Pain scores (as assessed with a VAS and a simple descriptive scale) were significantly lower with the benzyl alcohol formulation with no difference between injectate temperatures (4 °C and 25 °C), and VAS scores were approximately one-quarter to one-third those recorded for the metacresol formulation. In cats, the manufacturer reports a moderate response (retreating and vocalizing) to SC injection in 22.6% of cats (n = 133 total) receiving 1 mg/kg maropitant compared to 1.6% of cats (n = 62 total) receiving a placebo injection [137]. A significant response (retreating, hissing, scratching, and vocalizing) to SC injection was reported in 11.3% of cats (n = 133 total) given 1 mg/kg SC maropitant and in 1.6% of cats (n = 62 total) receiving placebo. The injectate temperature was not reported. Assessing the response to maropitant injection (1 mg/kg SC) in cats by blinded observers using a VAS found a VAS score ≥ 7/10 cm was awarded in 27.3% of cats (35/128 observations), in contrast with 4% (6/136 observations) in the saline injection group [142].

As an antiemetic, maropitant has been shown to be effective in cats and dogs in a variety of situations, including motion sickness, chemotherapy, and non-specific gastritis [138,143–149]. Its efficacy has compared favorably to metoclopramide, chlorpromazine, and ondansetron with a range of emetogens and clinical conditions [143,145,150].

Within anesthesia and analgesia, maropitant is primarily used for its antiemetic properties, with much of the work focused on reducing vomiting following opioid premedication (hydromorphone, morphine) [142,151–156]. The potential for maropitant to provide analgesia has also been studied [157–159].

The mechanism of maropitant as a potential analgesic is mediated via NK_1 receptors. These receptors have been identified at the following sites: sensory afferent nerves [160], spinal cord [161], brain, and viscera [162]. There is evidence of higher receptor concentrations of substance P in visceral versus somatic afferent fibers [163]. A minimum alveolar concentration (MAC)-sparing effect ranging from 16–30% has been shown in two nociceptive models: tail clamp (dogs) and ovary and ovarian ligament stimulation (dogs and cats) [157–159]. The range in MAC-sparing effect may reflect the different study models or doses used in each study, or both. A loading dose of 5 mg/kg IV followed by 150 μg/kg/h resulted in a MAC reduction of 16% after a tail clamp stimulus during sevoflurane anesthesia compared to control [157]. Administration of maropitant via the epidural route did not reduce MAC in the same model, and the authors suggested that inappropriate dose, failure to cross dural membranes, or a restricted site of action may have contributed [157]. In contrast, in a canine ovary and ovarian ligament stimulation model, a lower IV dose of maropitant (1 mg/kg IV followed by 30 μg/kg/h) resulted in a 24% decrease in the MAC of sevoflurane (maropitant plasma concentration of 112 ng/mL) [158]. Increasing the maropitant dose to 5 mg/kg IV followed by infusion at 150 μg/kg/h resulted in a small (non-significant) further reduction in MAC of 30% [158]. A similar study in cats (same nociceptive model and anesthetic agent) but with a single IV bolus of maropitant (1 mg/kg) resulted in a MAC reduction of 15% [159]. Increasing the dose of maropitant (5 mg/kg) did not lead to a further decrease in MAC [159]. When maropitant (1 mg/kg SC) is given in conjunction with a multimodal analgesic protocol (including methadone and meloxicam), in a randomized, blinded study, to cats undergoing ovariohysterectomy, the impact on reducing isoflurane requirement is less marked (approximately 0.25% isoflurane difference) [164]. In a randomized, blinded, controlled study, providing maropitant by continuous rate infusion (CRI) (30 or 100 μg/kg/h, after a 1 mg/kg IV loading dose) to cats undergoing ovariohysterectomy also receiving morphine (0.3 mg/kg IM) and acepromazine (0.05 mg/kg IM), maropitant was associated with lower postoperative pain scores compared with the control group [165]. However, there was no advantage to maropitant over other treatments (lidocaine CRI, ketamine CRI, lidocaine–ketamine CRI ± maropitant). A canine MAC_{BAR} study (n = 6 dogs) reported reductions in sevoflurane requirements of approximately 15% when maropitant (1 mg/kg SC) or maropitant combined with carprofen (4 mg/kg SC) was administered 60 min before an electrical stimulus [166].

Maropitant's antiemetic effect has been documented in dogs and cats receiving hydromorphone [151,152], morphine [142,153–156], or xylazine [138]. In cats, 1 mg/kg of maropitant administered 2 h before xylazine (0.44 mg/ kg IM) significantly reduced emesis by 76%, 90%, and 100% for the SC, PO, and IV routes of administration, respectively [138]. Additionally, administration of 1 mg/kg maropitant orally 24 h before xylazine administration resulted in a 66% reduction in emetic events [138]. Over a similar timeframe, female cats given maropitant (1 mg/kg SC) 20 h before premedication with morphine (0.1 mg/kg IM) and dexmedetomidine (0.02 mg/kg IM) vomited less (1/32 cats) than those given saline (20/34) [142].

When 1 mg/kg of maropitant was administered SC 1 h before hydromorphone (0.1 mg/kg IM) in healthy dogs (n = 9), emesis, retching, and nausea did not occur [151]. This compared to incidences of emesis, retching, and nausea of 66%, 11%, and 22%, respectively, in the saline control group (n = 9). Compared to the use of acepromazine as a strategy for reducing emesis following hydromorphone administration, maropitant is more effective [167,168]. When given IV to dogs 45–60 min before premedication with IM hydromorphone (0.1 mg/kg) and acepromazine (0.03 mg/kg), maropitant (1 mg/kg) prevented retching and vomiting (0/13 dogs). This contrasted with the saline control group, in which 6/13 dogs retched or vomited [152]. The same study did not find any difference in the incidence of gastroesophageal reflux between treatment groups (induction of anesthesia with propofol, maintenance with isoflurane, anesthesia time approximately 2.5 h). The time between administration of maropitant and the agent likely to cause emesis is important [154,168,169]. When maropitant (1 mg/kg SC) was given simultaneously with or 15, 30, 45, or 60 min before hydromorphone (0.1 mg/kg IM), retching or vomiting occurred in the simultaneous and 15-min treatment groups (60% and 20%, respectively) but not in the 30-, 45- or 60-min groups (n = 10 dogs per treatment group) [169]. When maropitant (1 mg/kg SC) was given concurrently with morphine (0.5 mg/kg IM) and acepromazine (0.05 mg/kg IM), the incidence of retching and vomiting (70% and 50%, respectively) was similar to the saline control group (n = 20 dogs per treatment group) [154]. By contrast, giving maropitant 30 min before morphine–acepromazine reduced the incidence of retching and vomiting (25% and 15%, respectively). Oral administration of maropitant (2–4 mg/kg) given 2 h before hydromorphone (0.1 mg/kg IM) in dogs appears similarly effective to SC administration in preventing vomiting [169]. Giving maropitant orally (1–3 mg/kg) up to 19 h before an emetogen (cisplatin) was effective in significantly reducing incidence of vomiting [144]. In cats, oral maropitant (2.5–3 mg/kg) given approximately 2 or 18 h before premedication with morphine (0.1 mg/kg IM) and dexmedetomidine (0.02 mg/kg IM) was effective at reducing the incidence of retching and vomiting (30–40% in the control group versus 4–13% in the maropitant group) [170,171].

The antiemetic efficacy of maropitant in the face of a wide range of emetogens likely reflects its central site of action at the common pathway governing emesis.

The impact of maropitant on nausea has been less clear than with retching/vomiting, reflecting differences in classifying nausea, blinding to treatment groups, choice of emetogen, and timing of administration [142,143,153–156,164,169–174]. Overall, maropitant is less effective in preventing nausea than retching/vomiting, with most studies showing no difference compared with saline control [142,143,153–155,164,170–174]. Compared to metoclopramide and ondansetron, in a low-dose cisplatin canine model for nausea, ondansetron outperformed both maropitant and metoclopramide [143]. Metoclopramide (0.5 mg/kg IV) did not reduce signs of nausea compared to saline control and maropitant (1 mg/kg IV) showed a minimal improvement, whereas ondansetron (0.5 mg/kg IV) attenuated signs associated with nausea. The authors suggested that 5-HT_3 serotonergic receptors (for which ondansetron is an antagonist) play a more important role in mediating nausea than NK_1 receptors. In that study, the antiemetics were infused over 15 min beginning 45 min after cisplatin administration. The same study found arginine vasopressin and cortisol served as biomarkers for nausea. Similarly, no advantage of maropitant (1 mg/kg SC) over metoclopramide (0.5 mg/kg SC) for preventing nausea was found in dogs premedicated with morphine (0.5 mg/kg SC) 45 min after maropitant or metoclopramide [155].

Limited evidence suggests a potential improvement in return to feeding and food consumption associated with maropitant [156,175]. A study from the manufacturer found that dogs undergoing ovariohysterectomy or castration surgery returned to feeding faster and consumed significantly more food when treated with maropitant (1 mg/kg SC, 45 min before morphine 0.5 mg/kg SC) versus saline [156]. These data should be interpreted with caution as perioperative analgesia was limited to a single dose of morphine and the presence of postoperative pain not assessed. In a comparison of preanesthetic treatment with maropitant (1 mg/kg SC) or morphine (0.5 mg/kg SC) in dogs undergoing ovariohysterectomy surgery, a higher proportion of dogs in the maropitant group (64.7% [11/17] versus 15.3% [2/13] in the morphine group) ate within 3 h of extubation [175]. Relatively high numbers of dogs in each treatment group received postoperative rescue analgesia with IV morphine (13/17 in the preanesthetic maropitant group and 10/13 in the preanesthetic morphine group). Further work is needed to corroborate these findings but improvements in return to normal function fit with the concept of enhanced recovery after surgery [176–178].

As the popularity of maropitant has grown, there is evidence that it is inappropriately prescribed in dogs for indications for which it has no efficacy [179].

The current label dose of the injectable maropitant formulation (10 mg/mL) in dogs is 1 mg/kg SC or 1 mg/kg IV (in dogs over 4 months old, over 1–2 min). In cats (over 4 months old), maropitant is labeled for IV use at 1 mg/kg over 1–2 min. Maropitant administered IV during general anesthesia (1 mg/kg over 2 min) in dogs premedicated with acepromazine (0.005 mg/kg IM)–butorphanol (0.2 mg/kg IM) or dexmedetomidine (0.005 mg/kg IM)–butorphanol (0.2 mg/kg IM), followed by induction of anesthesia with propofol and maintenance with isoflurane, has the potential to decrease arterial blood pressure [180]. The reduction in arterial blood pressure was greater in the acepromazine–butorphanol group, with a short period of mean arterial blood pressure below 60 mmHg during the period of injection. Minimal changes were observed in the dexmedetomidine–butorphanol group. Statistically significant decreases in arterial blood pressure (of approximately 10–15 mmHg) were observed in awake dogs, with a compensatory increase in heart rate. The mechanism of action underlying these blood pressure changes is unknown.

Pharmacokinetic data for maropitant are available for cats, dogs, chickens, horses, and rabbits [137,181–185].

Methocarbamol

Methocarbamol is a centrally acting muscle relaxant that selectively inhibits spinal and supraspinal polysynaptic reflexes through its action on interneurons, without direct effects on skeletal muscle [186,187]. It is commonly used in human medicine for back pain with a muscular component [188]. Use in veterinary medicine has historically been associated with tetanus [189–191], metaldehyde, 4-aminopyridine and pyrethrin/permethrin toxicity [192–198], and exertional rhabdomyolysis [199–200]. More recently, it has been successfully used for the management of acute muscle strain in combination with rest, physical therapy, and NSAIDs [201]. Higher doses may result in sedation, and this should be accounted for when used in combination with sedative and anesthetic agents.

Pharmacokinetics have been studied in dogs [202] and horses [199,200,203–205]. Therapeutic serum concentrations are achieved rapidly by an oral route of administration in dogs and horses [202,203]. Extensive hepatic metabolism (dealkylation and hydroxylation followed by conjugation) is followed by primarily urinary excretion of metabolites [202]. Guaifenesin is a metabolite of methocarbamol produced in low concentrations in horses [199,200].

The recommended dose of methocarbamol in cats and dogs is 40–60 mg/kg (PO, IV) three times daily for one day followed by 20–40 mg/kg (PO, IV) three times daily until symptoms resolve [201]. Higher doses may result in toxicity and potential effects of co-administration of drugs with CNS depressant effects should be considered [189,191,206]. One case series reported doses of 55–100 mg/kg IV every 30–60 min in dogs with tetanus, though its efficacy was questioned when compared to other muscle relaxants/sedatives employed [191]. Per rectum administration (55–200 mg/kg, up to 330 mg/kg/day per rectum every 6–8 h) has been reported when an IV formulation was not available [206]. Its use is associated with few adverse effects, with a human study finding the incidence of adverse events similar to that of placebo [188]. Administration of methocarbamol at therapeutic doses does not result in cardiopulmonary changes. Overdose may result in sedation and excessive muscle weakness with any effects being short-lived.

Methocarbamol is available as 500 mg and 750 mg tablets, and as a 100 mg/mL solution for injection.

Metoclopramide

Metoclopramide is primarily indicated as an antiemetic in small animals. It is less effective than maropitant as an antiemetic and its prevention of nausea varies between studies [143,150,155,207]. It has also been investigated for use in promoting gastric emptying and reduction of gastroesophageal reflux [208–210]. Metoclopramide is believed to increase gastroesophageal (lower esophageal) sphincter tone [211,212] and promote peristalsis of the duodenum along with an improvement in antropyloroduodenal coordination. Together, these effects promote gastric emptying in healthy dogs and cats [210,213]. Supporting evidence for its use in promoting gastric emptying in clinical cases is limited [208]. Following a dose of 0.3 mg/kg in dogs 1 week after gastropexy for correction of gastric dilatation-volvulus, metoclopramide did not promote gastric emptying [208]. Using manometry in conscious Beagles, a comparison of oral cisapride (0.5 mg/kg), metoclopramide (0.5 mg/kg), and placebo (gelatin capsule) found that only cisapride induced a significant increase in gastroesophageal sphincter pressure, with increased pressures at 4 and 7 h after administration [214]. Pressures recorded following metoclopramide did not differ from placebo.

In a comparison of two doses of metoclopramide (loading dose of 1 mg/kg then 1 mg/kg/h IV, or 0.4 mg/kg then 0.3 mg/kg/h IV) in dogs undergoing orthopedic surgery, the low and high doses of metoclopramide resulted in a reduction of the risk of gastroesophageal reflux by 34% and 54%, respectively [209]. Given the low risk of clinical sequelae following gastroesophageal reflux, the case for preemptive therapy is unclear. In dogs with laryngeal paralysis, a population susceptible to aspiration pneumonia, administration of metoclopramide (1 mg/kg IV loading dose followed by 1 mg/kg/h CRI) had no impact on the incidence of aspiration pneumonia (2/28 dogs in the control group, 4/33 dogs in the metoclopramide group, relative risk 0.59, 95% CI 0.12–3.0) [215]. The anesthetic protocol was standardized (no premedication, anesthetic induction with propofol, maintenance with isoflurane or sevoflurane, and buprenorphine 0.02 mg/kg IV given after orotracheal intubation).

Metoclopramide has multiple sites of action, including serotonin receptor antagonism in the CNS and dopamine (D_2) receptor antagonism in the CNS and gastrointestinal tract [139]. Its dopamine antagonist activity can result in extrapyramidal signs (muscle spasms, restlessness), even at recommended doses, as has been reported in humans, cattle, and a dog [216–218]. Metabolism is primarily hepatic with a high first-pass effect [219]. The recommended doses in dogs and cats are 0.25–0.5 mg/kg IV, IM, or PO every 8–12 h (higher doses may be required in refractory cases). For CRI, a loading dose of 0.4 mg/kg IV followed by 0.3–1 mg/kg/h is recommended.

The administration of metoclopramide in horses and ponies has shown limited efficacy [220]. Doses of 0.06–0.25 mg/kg caused restlessness, sedation, and occasionally colic. Lack of supporting evidence for beneficial large intestinal effects does not indicate its use in colic [221].

Use in cattle is limited as the dose effective at increasing reticular motility (0.3 mg/kg IM) in healthy animals is associated with extrapyramidal signs (restlessness then depression) [216]. The effects of the reported effective dose were short-lived, lasting approximately 20 min. Similarly, in calves, metoclopramide (0.1 mg/kg IM) was no better than saline at increasing abomasal motility or emptying rate [222].

Available formulations include 5 and 10 mg tablets, a 1 mg/mL oral solution, and a 5 mg/mL injectable solution.

Ondansetron and dolasetron

Ondansetron and dolasetron are serotonin (5-HT_3) receptor antagonists often administered as antiemetics before chemotherapy [223]. Ondansetron has been shown to be highly effective in cisplatin-induced nausea and emesis in dogs and doxorubicin-induced emesis in ferrets [143,224]. Cisplatin induces emesis through peripheral activity on the gastric mucosa to activate 5-HT_3 receptors in vagal and sympathetic afferents to the emetic center of the brainstem [225,226], and ondansetron and dolasetron block this pathway at the level of the emetic center. This mechanism of action differs from the centrally mediated antiemetic effects of maropitant (see above). Evidence suggests that these drugs can be successful in treating nausea and vomiting associated with renal and hepatic disease as well as gastroenteritis in dogs and cats [227–229]. Ondansetron has also been used successfully in treating a Chihuahua with obstructive sleep apnea, a condition in which serotonin plays a role in respiration and airway patency [230].

In comparisons between maropitant and ondansetron, the results are mixed, probably reflecting differences in cause of vomiting (peripherally versus centrally acting emetogens). Ondansetron (0.5 mg/kg PO or IV) has been shown to be less effective than maropitant in preventing emesis resulting from apomorphine administration, premedication with hydromorphone (0.1 mg/kg IM)–acepromazine (0.02 mg/kg IM)–glycopyrrolate (0.01 mg/kg IM), and following tranexamic acid administration in dogs, but more effective in a cisplatin model of nausea in dogs, and similarly effective in the management of emesis associated with parvoviral enteritis [143,150,174,228,231].

Evidence from clinical human literature does not suggest a difference in efficacy between dolasetron and ondansetron [232]. A similar comparison has not been studied in a clinical veterinary setting.

While adverse effects have not been reported in dogs and cats, in 2010, the United States Food and Drug Administration released a drug safety communication contraindicating the use of injectable dolasetron for the prevention of nausea and vomiting associated with chemotherapy in humans [233]. This resulted from evidence of electrocardiographic QT prolongation and torsade de pointes associated with IV administration. The warning did not extend to oral therapy.

Pharmacokinetics of ondansetron and dolasetron have been reported in dogs and cats [234–237]. In the dog, dolasetron undergoes hepatic metabolism, producing the active metabolite reduced dolasetron. This metabolite and the unchanged drug are both excreted in urine and feces [238]. Ondansetron metabolism is mediated by CYP3A4 in the liver with excretion of metabolites in urine and feces [239]. The pharmacokinetics of ondansetron are altered in cats with hepatic disease, with reduced clearance and increased plasma concentration [237]. Ondansetron dose in cats and dogs is 0.5–1 mg/kg twice daily (IV or PO) or 30 min before chemotherapy. A lower dose may be effective in reducing emesis associated with other emetogens. For example, 0.22 mg/kg IV reduced the incidence of emesis when co-administered with dexmedetomidine in cats [240]. The dose of dolasetron in dogs and cats is 0.6–1 mg/kg IV or PO, once daily.

Available formulations of ondansetron include 4 and 8 mg tablets, a 4 mg/5 mL oral solution, and a 2 mg/mL injectable solution. Dolasetron is available as 50 and 100 mg tablets and a 20 mg/mL solution.

Procainamide

Procainamide is a Class 1a (Singh-Vaughan Williams and Keefe classifications) antiarrhythmic agent with efficacy for the treatment of supraventricular and ventricular tachyarrhythmias. It is a derivative of the local anesthetic procaine (ester linkage replaced with amide). Through sodium channel blockade, it reduces the rate of rise of phase 0 of the cardiac action potential, raises the threshold potential, and prolongs the refractory period. It also has some anticholinergic effects. It is often used as a second-line therapy for ventricular tachycardia (VT) resistant to lidocaine.

A comparison between procainamide and lidocaine for the management of postoperative ventricular arrhythmias (i.e., ventricular premature contractions (VPCs), VT, R-on-T phenomenon, and multiform VPCs) in a mixed population of medium-to-large breed dogs showed these drugs to be equally effective in restoring sinus rhythm [241]. Procainamide was administered as a loading dose of 10 mg/kg IV over 5 min then an infusion of 20 μg/kg/min IV (lidocaine loading dose of 2 mg/kg IV, followed by 60 μg/kg/min IV). No adverse effects were associated with procainamide administration.

Efficacy in the treatment of atrial fibrillation is mainly from experimental models of induced arrhythmia studies in dogs, with one recent case report [242,243]. The clinical case report describes the successful use of procainamide (14.3 mg/kg IV over 15 min) to treat atrial fibrillation associated with pericardiocentesis and unresponsive to a single dose of lidocaine (1.2 mg/kg IV). Procainamide administration resulted in cardioversion to a sinus rhythm [242]. In Boxers with familial ventricular arrhythmias (including arrhythmogenic right ventricular cardiomyopathy), two studies have reported the efficacy of antiarrhythmic agents in terms of median survival time [244] and response of ventricular arrhythmias [245]. Caro-Vadillo *et al.* did not find a significant effect on median survival time (age and the presence of syncope were better predictors) between the following treatments: sotalol, mexiletine–atenolol, or procainamide (20–26 mg/kg PO every 8 h) [244]. Meurs *et al.*, in a comparison between procainamide (20–26 mg/kg PO every 8 h), atenolol, sotalol, or mexiletine–atenolol, found that only sotalol or mexiletine–atenolol were effective at reducing the number and severity of VPCs and heart rate [245]. However, none of the treatments resulted in an improvement in the incidence of syncope, though it is possible that the study was underpowered for this outcome.

There is limited evidence of its use in horses, with one report of failed therapy for ventricular extrasystoles and VT at a total dose of 20 mg/kg over two administrations given at a 2-h interval [246]. In a case report of a horse with atrial fibrillation, procainamide (20 mg/kg IV) was included as part of a successful treatment regimen (with sotalol and rest) following semisuccessful electrical cardioversion that converted the cardiac rhythm from atrial fibrillation to atrial tachycardia with variable AV conduction [247]. The pharmacokinetics of procainamide have been reported in horses where, unlike dogs [248], the active metabolite NAPA (*N*-acetylprocainamide) is produced which has class III antiarrhythmic activity (i.e., it prolongs the cardiac action potential) [249]. Recently, the pharmacokinetics of a sustained-release formulation of procainamide have been reported in dogs [250].

An effective dose in dogs is 10 mg/kg IV over 10 min followed by an infusion of 20 μg/kg/min [241]. Single or repeated bolus injection of 1–2 mg/kg IV may be effective in dogs for the management of short-duration ventricular ectopic activity associated with surgical manipulation or catecholamine release. The recommended dose in cats is a loading dose of 1–2 mg/kg slowly IV followed by an infusion of 10–20 μg/kg/min.

Toxicity manifests as a widening of the QRS complex, additional arrhythmias, and hypotension [245].

It is available as 250, 375, and 500 mg tablets and a 100 mg/mL solution for injection.

Sodium nitroprusside

Sodium nitroprusside (SNP) elicits arterial and venous dilation by liberating the potent endogenous vasodilator nitric oxide (NO). Cyanide ions are also produced as a by-product. For an in-depth review of NO physiology, the reader is referred to [251]. Following administration of SNP, its vascular effects are mediated locally in the vascular endothelium and underlying smooth muscle. NO production (from reaction with oxyhemoglobin, also generating methemoglobin) activates soluble guanylyl cyclase, increasing levels of cyclic guanosine monophosphate (cGMP) in the vascular musculature. cGMP inhibits entry of calcium into smooth muscle cells and increases uptake of intracellular calcium by smooth endoplasmic reticulum, resulting in vasodilation.

When delivered by IV infusion, SNP has a rapid onset and offset, allowing titration to effect. A dose range of 1–5 μg/kg/min has been reported to successfully reduce arterial blood pressure in a dog with phenylpropanolamine overdose and SNP has been used to induce hypotension in experimental studies in horses (0.1–1.5 μg/kg/min) and pigs (0.5–5 μg/kg/min) [252–255]. Close monitoring of systemic arterial blood pressure and heart rate and rhythm is essential due to the risk of inadvertent hypotension or reflex tachycardia.

Use of SNP during CPR ("sodium nitroprusside enhanced CPR") has been shown to provide neuroprotection in experimental models of cardiac arrest, though it is not currently known if this will translate to clinical use [256].

The rapid offset of SNP results from the short half-life of NO, which is rapidly oxidized to nitrite [257]. Cyanide ions, produced with NO from SNP, are metabolized by the liver to thiocyanate, which is then excreted by the kidneys [258]. In cases of overdose or hepatic or renal insufficiency, there is a risk of cyanide and thiocyanate toxicity. Toxicity manifests as tachycardia, hyperventilation, metabolic acidosis (as cyanide binds cytochrome oxidase, thereby inhibiting aerobic metabolism), and seizures. Toxicity can be treated with thiosulfate (6 mg/kg/h IV in dogs) [259–261]. Solutions of SNP are light sensitive, turning from a light orange/straw-colored solution when fresh (reconstituted with 5% dextrose) to dark brown/blue upon exposure to light. The solution should be discarded if this occurs.

Nitroprusside is available in 10 and 25 mg/mL solutions for injection following dilution.

Trazodone

Trazodone is a serotonin antagonist and reuptake inhibitor, with dose-dependent antagonist activity at 5-HT_{2A} and 5-HT_{2C} receptors and an inhibitory effect on serotonin reuptake [262]. As such, it may contribute to serotonin syndrome, when given concurrently with selective serotonin reuptake inhibitors, tricyclic antidepressants, or monoamine oxidase inhibitors [263,264]. It also has antagonist effects at histamine (H_{1A}) receptors and α_1- and α_2-adrenergic receptors [262]. Trazodone has become increasingly popular over recent years, prescribed for fear management and anxiolysis on a regular basis and perioperatively [263,265]. It is prescribed in humans for sleep disorders arising from a variety of causes. Despite widespread use, there is limited peer-reviewed veterinary literature available.

In an experimental cat study (n = 6), trazodone reduced activity (assessed via accelerometry) to 43–86% of pre-dosing values, with doses of 50, 75, and 100 mg/cat (corresponding to 10.6–16.7 mg/kg, 16–25 mg/kg, and 21–33 mg/kg PO, respectively) [266]. The highest dose (100 mg/cat) was most effective in reducing activity, with a peak effect at 2.5 h after dosing, but considerable interindividual variability in baseline and post-trazodone activity was reported. However, behavioral responses to a comprehensive physical examination (including abdominal palpation, otoscopic and ophthalmic examination, and mock venipuncture and cystocentesis with needle penetration of skin) performed 90 min after dosing were unchanged compared to placebo. Similarly, a stress score did not identify differences between placebo and the 100 mg/kg treatment. Heart and respiratory rates were unaffected by trazodone compared with placebo.

In a double-blinded, placebo-controlled, randomized crossover study (n = 10 cats) evaluating the effect of trazodone on transport and handling, trazodone (50 mg/cat, approximately 11 mg/kg PO) reduced signs of stress during transport and improved ease of handling [267]. Reduced stress (from "very tense" to "weakly relaxed") and improved tractability (from "restraint needed to examine safely" to "easy/relatively easy to examine") were identified. Sleepiness was identified as an adverse effect. Trazodone was given approximately 1–1.5 h before transport to the clinic and 1.5–2 h before physical examination.

As with cats, data from dogs is from a small number of studies, with variability in reported responses to trazodone. A randomized, placebo-controlled, double-blinded study did not identify differences in behaviors between treatments [268]. Dogs (n = 29) received either placebo or trazodone (2.8–10.8 mg/kg PO, every 12 h) with trazodone dose adjusted according to owner's wishes during a 4-week period following elective orthopedic surgery, during which activity restriction and confinement were prescribed. Behavioral assessments included greeting behavior, calmness, behavior on leash, and tolerance of confinement. The authors suggested several reasons for trial failure, including selection bias toward calmer dogs, caregiver placebo effect (owners performed behavioral assessments), placebo-by-proxy effect (owner beliefs altered interaction with their dog leading to a change in dog behavior), and lack of sensitivity in the behavioral assessment instrument. By contrast, a recent double-blinded, placebo-controlled crossover study in dogs (n = 20) found that trazodone (9–12 mg/kg PO) given 90 min before transport to a veterinary clinic was associated with reduced stress scores in the clinic, with most owners (18/20) correctly identifying when trazodone had been given [269]. Two earlier studies in dogs showed efficacy with trazodone, though both had limitations in study design, limiting data interpretation. A study of 36 dogs admitted for elective orthopedic surgery all received trazodone postoperatively for 4 weeks, with a subset of owners requesting a dose increase after week 2 (to 7 mg/kg PO every 8 h) [270]. Owners assessed behaviors (greeting behavior, calmness, behavior on leash, and tolerance of confinement). Compared to preoperative behavioral assessments, trazodone was associated with reduced intensity of greeting and overall calmness, but not response to owner commands or tendency to pull on leash walks. Trazodone was assessed as improving tolerance of postoperative confinement. Most owners reported an onset of drug effects within 45 min of dosing (16–90 min for 90% of owners) and a median duration of action of > 4 h (upper limit of observation period). A study of hospitalized dogs (most dogs were admitted to the surgery service) evaluated a convenience sample of 59 dogs prescribed trazodone (4.7 ± 1 mg/kg PO) by the supervising veterinarian, with a comparison group of dogs not prescribed trazodone (n = 58) [271]. Stress-related behavior scores were higher in the trazodone treatment group at baseline compared with the untreated group, but there was a significant reduction in these scores when assessed approximately 110 min following trazodone administration. One dog showed signs of aggression 60 min after trazodone administration.

In horses, 6 mg/kg PO induced mild sedation (based on a simple descriptive scale) in 7/8 horses, which lasted between 0.5 and 8 h after trazodone administration, with 4/8 horses remaining sedated at 12 h and no signs of sedation apparent at 24 h [272]. Higher doses (7.5 and 10 mg/kg PO) caused sedation within 20–30 min of administration that was generally mild (3/6 horses were heavily sedated at the higher dose) and lasted a few hours [273]. In the latter study, arrhythmias diagnosed by thoracic auscultation, without an ECG, were noted in 2/6 horses that received 10 mg/kg PO.

In goats, intended as a model for wild ruminants, a dose of 10 mg/kg PO resulted in a five- to sixfold increase in time spent sleeping and lying down, with reduced activity lasting approximately 4 h [274]. Eating and ruminating were unaffected.

Two studies have evaluated the effect of trazodone on the propofol requirement for induction of general anesthesia in dogs [275,276]. A retrospective study of dogs (n = 15) undergoing radiotherapy treatment showed a significant reduction in propofol dose (approximately 25%) when trazodone was given approximately 2 h before anesthesia (4.8 [2.9–7.3] mg/kg PO) [275]. Dogs were premedicated with alfentanil and atropine and served as their own controls. A prospective, randomized, unblinded study did not find an effect of trazodone (5–7 mg/kg PO 2 h before anesthesia) on the propofol dose requirement (dose administered over 20–30 seconds) compared with acepromazine (0.01–0.03 mg/kg IM 30 min before anesthesia) [276]. All dogs (n = 15 per treatment) were also given morphine (1 mg/kg IM 30 min before anesthesia). A MAC-sparing effect has been identified in dogs, with a 17% reduction in isoflurane MAC following trazodone (8 mg/kg PO) [277].

Trazodone is metabolized to an active metabolite, meta-chlorophenylpiperazine, which has agonist activity at the 5-HT_{2C} receptor, though its significance in animal species is unknown [273,278]. The primary route of elimination is renal (approximately 75%) with the remainder undergoing fecal elimination.

Pharmacokinetics have been described in dogs (PO, IV, per rectum), horses, pigeons, and goats [272,274,278–281]. Time to peak effect appears to vary markedly between individual dogs, with peak plasma concentrations achieved 445 ± 271 min after 8 mg/kg PO (n = 6 dogs), though onset of signs may be apparent within 45 min [270,280]. Pharmacokinetics have not been described in cats, but variability in behavioral responses may also reflect interindividual pharmacokinetic differences [266].

Adverse effects appear uncommon in dogs following PO dosing, with one report of hepatotoxicity in a dog attributed to trazodone (4 mg/kg PO once or twice daily) and reports of aggression following IV (3/6 dogs) and PO (1/59 dogs) administration [271,280,282]. Trazodone at doses between 1 and 30 mg/kg IV results in transient, dose-dependent reductions in heart rate and arterial blood pressure [283]. In cats (n = 12) given trazodone (approximately 11 mg/kg PO) 90–120 min before echocardiography, sedation was observed but there were minimal changes in cardiac measurements [284]. In horses, 4/8 horses exhibited sweating following oral trazodone (6 mg/kg), while IV dosing was associated with aggression, ataxia, tremors, and circling (2/2 horses, 2 mg/kg) and ataxia, tremors, circling, and sweating (1.5 mg/kg) [272,278].

Reported doses in dogs range from 3 to 12 mg/kg PO every 8–12 h [268,269,271,280] and those in cats range from 8 to 30 mg/kg PO [266,267,284]. Available formulations include 50, 100, 150, and 300 mg tablets.

Vasopressin (arginine vasopressin, antidiuretic hormone) and desmopressin

The primary perioperative indication for vasopressin is in CPR and refractory hypotension [84,285–288]. It is a potent vasoconstrictor, acting on V_{1a} receptors located in vascular smooth muscle, though it also displays activity at V_{1b} (anterior pituitary) and V_2 (renal collecting duct) receptors, and inhibits nitric oxide production [289,290]. Its analog, desmopressin (DDAVP), is used in the treatment of central diabetes insipidus [291–293] and management of coagulopathy [294–296].

Vasopressin is an alternative vasopressor to epinephrine for use during CPR, though there is no clear evidence supporting its role as a replacement for epinephrine. Recent veterinary CPR guidelines suggest its use (0.8 U/kg IV) on alternating rounds of CPR instead of epinephrine, though there is no evidence that it confers a benefit over epinephrine in humans [84,297]. Due to the lack of β_1-adrenergic receptor activity, it may reduce the risk of myocardial ischemia compared with epinephrine, though it will still cause coronary vasoconstriction. An additional potential advantage over epinephrine is that V_1 receptors, unlike α_1-adrenergic receptors, remain responsive in an acidic environment [298]. Reports of clinical use in the veterinary literature are mixed [285,287], with vasopressin showing no benefit over epinephrine in a randomized comparison using a standardized CPR technique [287] but associated with an improved rate of return to spontaneous circulation in a hospital-wide study [285]. A meta-analysis demonstrated a potential improvement in return of spontaneous circulation associated with its use, though contributing studies were predominantly in porcine models of ventricular fibrillation [288].

Vasopressin can be administered via the endotracheal route, if necessary, with one animal study suggesting that the same dose as that recommended for IV use is effective [299].

What has become clear from the Reassessment Campaign on Veterinary Resuscitation (RECOVER) initiative [300] is that there is wide variability in study design and reporting of animal models of CPR, making it difficult to draw firm conclusions from currently available experimental evidence. Anecdotal reports suggest the use of vasopressin in cases of refractory hypotension, though the available veterinary literature is sparse and human studies are contradictory [286,290,301–304]. This is likely a reflection of the heterogeneity of clinical and experimental studies [303]. Infusion rates of 0.5–5 mU/kg/min and 0.1–2.5 mU/kg/min have been suggested in dogs and foals, respectively [286,290,301]. Users should be aware of the potential for detrimental hypoperfusion of vascular beds resulting from the resultant vasoconstriction [305].

Desmopressn acetate (DDAVP), a synthetic analog of vasopressin with reduced vascular effects, is used for perioperative management of patients with von Willebrand disease [295,306,307] and management of central diabetes insipidus [291–293,308].

von Willebrand disease, the most common canine hereditary defect of hemostasis, is classified according to one of three subtypes, with type 1 being the least severe and most common, especially in Doberman Pinschers [309]. Management consists of both non-transfusion and transfusion therapy, based on disease severity and clinical presentation. Non-transfusion therapy includes appropriate patient management (i.e., good surgical technique, minimizing use of drugs with antiplatelet activity, careful handling) and DDAVP. Administration of 1 μg/kg SC or IV 30 min before surgery may support hemostasis, but the response is more variable in dogs than humans [295,306]. Administering DDAVP intranasally or into the conjunctival sac is commonly performed, but there is limited supporting evidence of its efficacy via this route in von Willebrand disease.

Other reported uses for DDAVP include support of hemostasis following administration of aspirin before surgery [310,311], as a prophylactic measure to manage postoperative diabetes insipidus following hypophysectomy [296], and administration to canine blood donors to increase von Willebrand factor production before blood collection for cryoprecipitate [312].

Injectable vasopressin is available as a 20 U/mL solution. DDAVP is available as a 4 μg/mL injectable solution, 0.1 and 0.2 mg tablets, 100 μg/mL spray, and a 0.01% solution for intranasal administration.

Analgesic adjuncts

Amantadine and memantine

The dopamine agonist and *N*-methyl-D-aspartate (NMDA) receptor antagonist amantadine was originally used as an antiviral agent [313,314] but has entered clinical use in human medicine for diseases and presentations as varied as Parkinson's disease [315], traumatic brain injury (TBI), and pain. Its continued use in the management of Parkinson's disease arose serendipitously from a patient with Parkinson's disease noticing an improvement in motor function wtaking amantadine for influenza [316]. Recent meta-analysis and systematic reviews have indicated a potential role for amantadine in TBI though further studies are required to confirm promising earlier findings [317,318]. Human studies have demonstrated improved arousal when amantadine was administered between 3 days and 4 weeks following TBI, and purported mechanisms are through CNS stimulation mediated by amantadine's dopaminergic activity and reduced neurotoxicity through its NMDA receptor antagonism [319,320]. Its use in animals is currently limited to an experimental model of TBI in rats where learning and hippocampal neuron survival were improved with amantadine administration 1 h following TBI [321].

Memantine, a derivative of amantadine, has similar pharmacological properties [322]. It has been used in dogs for compulsive disorders, though there is currently limited evidence of its use in pain management [265].

Amantadine has been used for analgesia, acting via NMDA receptor antagonism [323]. Its role as an analgesic appears to be limited to chronic pain, particularly where central sensitization may play a role, such as in chronic arthritis and limb amputation, though its efficacy appears variable [324–327]. In dogs with pelvic limb lameness and pain that was not alleviated by NSAID use, activity increased following 3 weeks of therapy combining meloxicam (0.1 mg/kg PO once daily) and amantadine (3–5 mg/kg PO once daily) [324]. Doses of 2–10 mg/kg PO 2–3 times daily have also been suggested. At these higher/more frequent doses, there is a possibility of CNS excitation. Pharmacokinetic data (from a single dose study) are supportive of 5 mg/kg PO twice daily dosing in dogs (a dose of 10 mg/kg PO twice daily was predicted to result in plasma levels associated with adverse effects in humans), though more work is needed to confirm this prediction [328,329]. Amantadine (14 mg/kg PO once daily with meloxicam 0.1 mg/kg PO) has also been reported as successful in managing chronic pain following bilateral pelvic fractures that was not responsive to meloxicam and gabapentin [330].

In cats, amantadine at a dose of 3–5 mg/kg PO once or twice daily has been suggested in cases of chronic arthritis [323,328,331]. A blinded, placebo-controlled, randomized crossover study of 13 cats with osteoarthritis found that amantadine (5 mg/kg PO once daily) was associated with reduced activity (as assessed via accelerometry) but improved owner-assessed outcomes (client-specific outcome measures) [331]. Amantadine was also associated with a higher proportion of owners reporting an improved quality of life for their cat. Over the course of the 3-week treatment period, the only adverse effect was vomiting, which occurred with a similar frequency in the amantadine and placebo groups. The study did not include a wash-out period between treatments, justified based upon the short half-life in cats [331,332]. In a thermal threshold testing model in healthy cats given oxymorphone to induce antinociception, amantadine did not result in any further antinociception; however, it may be that an acute nociception model in otherwise healthy cats may not be appropriate for assessing amantadine [333,334].

Amantadine (3 mg/kg PO twice daily) was associated with marked improvements in activity and interaction in a rhinoceros with suspected chronic osteoarthritis and neuropathic pain of the thoracic limbs that showed limited response to, or adverse effects associated with, phenylbutazone, pentosan polysulfate, and gabapentin [335].

Pharmacokinetic data are available for dogs, cats, and parrots [329,332,336]. In Greyhounds, the short half-life (approximately 5 h) indicates that twice daily oral dosing (5 mg/kg) may be preferable to once daily [329]. No adverse effects were reported. In cats, amantadine has high oral bioavailability and a half-life similar to that reported in dogs (approximately 5.5 h) following a dose of 5 mg/kg PO [332]. As for dogs, this suggests that twice daily dosing may be needed to maintain appropriate plasma concentrations. In orange-winged Amazon parrots (*Amazona amazonica*), a 5 mg/kg PO dose of amantadine, once daily, produced plasma concentrations considered therapeutic in dogs without causing adverse effects [336]. There is currently no species-specific pharmacodynamic data to support this dose. Based on renal elimination of minimally/partially metabolized drug in other species, the authors suggested that birds with renal disease may be at increased risk of developing toxicity [336]. Amantadine undergoes primarily renal excretion in dogs [337], and there are limited dose-response data from rats [338].

More work is required to clarify the potential role of amantadine and memantine in chronic pain, with a recent meta-analysis identifying a lack of strong evidence for its use in people with a range of neuropathic pain etiologies [327].

As a result of its dopaminergic properties, CNS stimulation is a predicted side effect from overdose, and caution should be exercised in patients receiving other dopamine agonists (e.g., the monoamine oxidase inhibitor selegiline), or agents inhibiting the reuptake of serotonin (e.g., the tricyclic antidepressants such as amitriptyline, and the selective serotonin reuptake inhibitors such as fluoxetine). Such combinations risk the occurrence of serotonin syndrome, a potentially fatal syndrome characterized by signs of

CNS stimulation, muscular tremors, and autonomic stimulation including tachycardia, tachypnea, and hypertension [339–342]. The risk is likely increased in the presence of hepatic insufficiency as monoamine oxidase inhibitors and selective serotonin reuptake inhibitors are metabolized by the CYP450 pathway. Specific to anesthesia, there is evidence from human medicine that the phenylpiperidine opioids (meperidine, fentanyl, and fentanyl's congeners, tramadol and methadone) all increase the CNS concentration of serotonin to varying degrees and in some instances have contributed to serotonin syndrome, although the risk to veterinary patients remains unknown [343,344].

A less studied use of amantadine and memantine involves their use as local anesthetics. Local anesthesia appears to be mediated through sodium channel-blocking properties in addition to NMDA receptor antagonism [338,345]. It remains to be seen if there are significant advantages over traditional local anesthetics such as lidocaine and bupivacaine.

It is possible that amantadine availability for animal use may become restricted in some jurisdictions [346].

Amantadine is available as 100 mg tablets and capsules and as a 10 mg/mL syrup. Memantine is available as 5 and 10 mg tablets and as a 2 mg/mL oral formulation.

Amitriptyline and nortriptyline

The tricyclic antidepressant amitriptyline is indicated for behavioral disorders (e.g., obsessive-compulsive disorder) [347], idiopathic feline lower urinary tract disease (IFLUTD) [348,349], and more recently, neuropathic pain states [350–352]. Tricyclic antidepressants are selective serotonin reuptake inhibitors, increasing synaptic levels of serotonin and norepinephrine. This appears to be the primary mechanism mediating their useful behavioral modification effects. However, other less well-understood mechanisms of action may also contribute to their clinical potential as analgesics [350]. These include sodium channel blockade [353], NMDA receptor antagonism [354], and antihistamine activity [355], but not opioid receptor activity [356].

Amitriptyline (1–2 mg/kg/day) is commonly prescribed for management of IFLUTD, though which mechanism(s) of action result in improved clinical signs is unclear: serotonin reuptake inhibition, antihistamine, and anticholinergic activity may be involved [348,349,357].

Use of amitriptyline in treating neuropathic pain remains largely anecdotal [207,350–352]. One case series of three dogs with neuropathic pain reported a positive response to amitriptyline (1.1–1.3 mg/kg PO twice daily) in two of the dogs [350]. Of these, one dog had signs consistent with mechanical allodynia and dysesthesia over the facial dermatome innervated by the infraorbital branch of the right trigeminal nerve. Following no apparent response to gabapentin (12.5 mg/kg PO twice daily), there was an improvement associated with amitriptyline (1.3 mg/kg PO twice daily), with clinical signs resolving over 6 weeks. Owner-initiated discontinuation of treatment was associated with a rapid return of clinical signs (in 3 days), leading to reinstitution and maintenance use of amitriptyline therapy. A second successful use of amitriptyline (1.1 mg/kg PO twice daily) was for management of intermittent lumbar pain with diffuse mechanical allodynia. Clinical signs improved within a week of initiating treatment and were resolved within one month. Again, discontinuing therapy was associated with a return of pain (in 2 days), resulting in long-term amitriptyline therapy. In the third case, in which there was mechanical allodynia secondary to ulnar and median nerve lesions, amitriptyline (1.4 mg/kg PO twice daily) did not improve clinical signs; however, there was improvement with gabapentin (14.3 mg/kg PO twice daily). Sedation, a common adverse effect of amitriptyline, was reported by the owners. In each of these three cases, initial trials with NSAIDs, steroids, and opioids for pain management were unsuccessful. It is also interesting that when one therapy fails, the addition of or switch to another may prove successful. This illustrates the potential complexity and challenge of treating these cases. A study of 13 dogs diagnosed with osteosarcoma receiving a combination of therapies (cimicoxib 2 mg/kg PO once daily; amitriptyline 1–1.5 mg/kg PO once daily; gabapentin 10 mg/kg PO every 8 h) and a battery of nociceptive tests (including investigator and owner behavioral assessments, quantitative sensory testing, activity level and quality of life assessment) failed to identify a clear benefit from the prescribed analgesics [358]. This highlights the difficulty in studying complex, dynamic, naturally occurring pain states, which is further complicated by use of poorly established effective analgesic therapies. Attributing analgesia to a single drug is often complicated in reported case series when animals are given multiple drugs concurrently [207,352].

A feline case of suspected neuropathic pain was thought to have developed following an initial femoral fracture repair, iatrogenic sciatic nerve trauma, and subsequent amputation [351]. Approximately 1 month after amputation, the cat was observed frequently shaking the stump though there were no signs associated with pain when the stump was palpated. This was believed to be a case of phantom limb pain. Initial treatment consisted of an IV infusion of morphine, ketamine, and lidocaine for 37 h, followed by oral transmucosal buprenorphine (approximately 0.03 mg/kg twice daily) and oral amitriptyline (approximately 2 mg/kg twice daily). The cat was ambulating normally at discharge. At follow-up 10 months later, no further shaking of the amputation stump was reported. There is increasing evidence of neuropathic pain in cases of Chiari-like malformation and syringomyelia [359], and it may also be implicated in some cases of head shaking in horses [360].

Hepatic metabolism of amitriptyline results in production of the active metabolite nortriptyline in dogs and humans [361]. Both amitriptyline and nortriptyline are also excreted unchanged in urine, and caution should, therefore, be exercised in animals with renal insufficiency. Nortriptyline is used clinically as a treatment for neuropathic pain in humans [362], though its use in animals has not been reported.

The recommended route of administration is oral [363]; transdermal application is not effective at raising plasma drug levels and intrathecal administration resulted in marked spinal cord pathology [354]. The pharmacokinetics of amitriptyline have been described in dogs and horses [329,364,365]. Further work is required to further understand the pharmacokinetics in horses as there is evidence of oral transmucosal absorption [364]. In a study of six horses, amitriptyline (1 mg/kg PO) administration was associated with significant reductions in heart rate (remaining within normal limits) and intestinal motility (for 2 h post-administration), with no respiratory changes observed [364]. One horse developed transient second-degree AV block at 30 min post-administration, which lasted for 2 h. Another horse developed ventricular premature contractions (1 per min) at 30 min post-administration (duration not reported). In dogs, amitriptyline pharmacokinetics may be altered depending on whether dogs are fed or fasted at the time of oral administration, with possible important differences in bioavailability, though limited sample sizes prevent firm conclusions from being drawn [329,365,366]. Fed Greyhounds given 4 mg/kg PO had low bioavailability (6%) and peak plasma levels below those considered therapeutic in humans [329]. In contrast, at a similar dose in fasted mixed-breed dogs, plasma levels were within the therapeutic range for humans [366]. Breed differences may also play a role in pharmacokinetic differences. Two fasted dogs vomited following oral amitriptyline administration, though it was unclear if this was drug related [329]. When given at 4 mg/kg IV to Greyhounds, the following adverse effects were observed: sedation, ataxia, transient tachycardia, polyphagia, and vomiting [329].

Adverse effects on the heart include tachycardia mediated via inhibition of cardiac sodium channels and an anticholinergic effect and potential fatal ventricular tachyarrhythmias from overdose (greater than approximately 15 mg/kg IV) in dogs and cats [367–369]. Ventricular tachyarrhythmias are preceded by prolongation of the QRS complex. No ECG abnormalities were detected in dogs receiving appropriate doses of amitriptyline (0.74–2.5 mg/kg PO every 12 h) for behavioral disorders [370]. Other signs of toxicity in conscious dogs include hypersalivation and vomiting. Common adverse effects at therapeutic doses are weight gain and sedation [357]. While there is a theoretical risk of triggering serotonin syndrome with the concurrent use of tricyclic antidepressants and monoamine oxidase inhibitors, this risk (at least in humans) is believed to be low with amitriptyline [344]. Treatment of amitriptyline toxicity includes alkalinization (with sodium bicarbonate) and lipid emulsion therapy [369].

Available formulations of amitriptyline include 10, 25, 50, 75, 100, and 150 mg tablets. Available formulations of nortriptyline include 10, 25, 50, and 75 mg tablets and a 10 mg/5 mL oral solution.

Cannabinoids

Use of the cannabis plant, *Cannabis spp*., has spanned thousands of years, for both its psychoactive and medicinal properties. There has been a renewed interest more recently as it has become legalized (under varying conditions, according to jurisdiction) and more readily accessible [371,372]. This is reflected in a rapid growth in the published human and veterinary literature, with several veterinary reviews available [373,374].

The active molecules of interest that derive from *Cannabis* are delta-9-tetrahydrocannabinol (THC) and cannabidiol (CBD). A somewhat simplified view is that THC exerts psychoactive effects and CBD exerts therapeutic effects. These cannabinoids act via cannabinoid receptors, primarily CB_1 and CB_2, which exist as part of an endogenous cannabinoid system with the following endogenous ligands (endocannabinoids): anandamide (*N*-arachidonoyl), 2-arachidonoyl glycerol, and 2-arachidonoyl ether. In addition to endocannabinoids, cannabimimetics (endogenous fatty acids) modulate the endogenous cannabinoid system [375,376]. CB_1 and CB_2 receptors are widely distributed in the body, including the central and peripheral nervous systems, the immune system, intestines, and skin, among others [374]. Receptor and ligand expression is likely to vary in different disease states and may present a route for therapeutic modulation of disease response [374]. To date, most clinical veterinary studies have focused on osteoarthritis, epilepsy, behavioral disorders, and atopic dermatitis, with varying quality of evidence [373,377]. Compounding the limited number of high-quality trials is variation in the cannabinoid or cannabimimetic molecules studied, methods of administration, and poorly established doses [374].

In osteoarthritis, there are a small number of higher quality clinical trials reported in a mix of dog breeds [207,378–380]. In a double-blinded, placebo-controlled, randomized, crossover trial of dogs with osteoarthritis (n = 16 dogs), CBD in oil (with measurable levels of THC but no evidence of psychoactive effects during the study) at a dose of 2 mg/kg twice daily PO for 4 weeks resulted in a significant reduction in pain scores (Canine Brief Pain Inventory and veterinary assessment) and increase in activity levels, but no improvement in lameness score or weight-bearing [378]. In this study, dogs also received a variety of other drugs including NSAIDs and nutritional joint supplements, with no change to treatment regimens during the study. Reported adverse effects included an increase in alkaline phosphatase (ALP) (mean of 323 versus 160 U/L in 9/16 dogs). A double-blinded, placebo-controlled, parallel group, randomized study in dogs with osteoarthritis compared three treatments (0.5 mg/kg CBD PO, 1.2 mg/kg CBD PO, and 0.5 mg/kg liposomal CBD PO, once daily; n = 5 dogs per treatment group) against placebo (n = 5 dogs), with each group treated for 4 weeks [379]. Pain was evaluated with the Helsinki Chronic Pain Index and veterinary assessments. No adverse effects were reported based on the evaluation of hematocrit and serum chemistry. There was a dose-dependent reduction in pain and increase in mobility in the 1.2 mg/kg CBD and 0.5 mg/kg/day liposomal CBD treatment groups. A double-blinded, placebo-controlled, crossover trial of dogs with osteoarthritis (n = 23), given a CBD-rich hemp oil (2.5 mg/kg twice daily PO, which also contained 0.3% THC) for 6 weeks (with no washout period, based on predicted half-life < 4 h), did not identify any improvement in the recorded outcome measures (activity, Canine Brief Pain Inventory, Liverpool Osteoarthritis in Dogs questionnaire, and gait analysis) [380]. In this study, approximately 50% of the dogs were also receiving an NSAID. Adverse effects included vomiting (2/23 dogs) and elevated ALP, aspartate aminotransferase (AST), or alanine transaminase (ALT) (14/23 dogs). It has been suggested that dosing follows an escalation schedule, with treatment for at least 14 days before a dose increase, if necessary [374]. Brioschi *et al.* compared CBD (2 mg/kg twice daily via oral transmucosal route for 12 weeks) combined with multimodal analgesia (gabapentin, amitriptyline, prednisone, or firocoxib) against multimodal analgesia alone in dogs with osteoarthritis in a randomized, parallel group study design (n = 9 receiving CBD protocol, n = 21 receiving multimodal analgesia protocol) [207]. Pain was assessed with the Canine Brief Pain Inventory, with scale items significantly lower in dogs during CBD treatment. No adverse effects in CBC or serum biochemistry parameters were noted, with observed somnolence and ataxia attributed to concurrent gabapentin, and some ptyalism associated with CBD administration. In all these studies, some of the reported improvements reflect statistical significance but fairly small changes in assessment scale scores. This may reflect multiple factors, including heterogeneity of osteoarthritis in the studied population, assessment scale sensitivity, interindividual variability in response to treatment, and small sample sizes, all of which underline the need for additional well-designed studies.

Similarly, high-quality evidence is also currently limited in studies of cannabinoids for the treatment of epilepsy, behavioral disorders, and atopic dermatitis [381–383].

The pharmacokinetics for some cannabinoids have been published for dogs, pigs, horses, and guinea pigs [378,384–393]. However, variations in formulation can affect absorption and bioavailability and, in dogs, cannabinoid absorption varies according to fasting state, so care should be taken when selecting a formulation and dose [387]. Oral bioavailability of CBD in dogs is low (approximately 19%), with extensive first pass metabolism and primarily fecal elimination [393–395]. Active metabolites are formed following hepatic metabolism in humans, though more work is required to understand their presence and effects in animal species [374,392,393,396]. Following oral administration of CBD in dogs, peak plasma levels are achieved between 1.5 to 5 h, with results varying between studies and with dose [378,384,387,391,392].

Importantly, there can be wide variability between cannabinoid product labels and actual content [397].

With the expansion of access to cannabinoids, there is increasing information available on toxicity and its management [394,398]. Toxicity manifests as a combination of clinical signs involving the neurologic, cardiovascular, and gastrointestinal systems, with common signs in dogs including ataxia, dullness/disorientation, mydriasis, urinary incontinence, hyperesthesia, tremors/shaking/twitching, bradycardia, and vomiting [394,398,399]. Prognosis following intoxication is generally good, with a reported LD_{50} exceeding 3000 mg/kg PO for THC [400]. The LD_{50} for CBD has not been described, though available reports suggest mortality is low following exposure [394,399]. A safety and tolerability study of CBD (doses up to 30.5 mg/kg PO), THC (doses up to 41.5 mg/kg PO), and CBD-THC combination (doses up to 13:8.4 mg/kg PO) in cats reported lethargy, hypothermia, ataxia, and protrusion of the nictitating membrane as the most common adverse effects, primarily associated with THC and CBD–THC [401]. A similar study in dogs suggests better tolerability of cannabinoids in this species compared to cats [396]. Cardiovascular changes (pale mucous membranes, bradycardia, and tachycardia) and tachypnea were similarly reported for each treatment.

Gabapentin and pregabalin

Gabapentin and pregabalin are structural analogs of γ-aminobutyric acid (GABA). Historically, gabapentin has been prescribed as an anticonvulsant in humans and veterinary species, but is being used increasingly for neuropathic, chronic, and perioperative pain. Previous systematic reviews and meta-analyses identified some promising results for a role in chronic and neuropathic pain, but a more recent meta-analysis shows that the evidence supporting their use for chronic postoperative pain remains unclear [402–406]. For acute postoperative pain in humans, current evidence indicates that any statistically significant reductions in pain scores are not clinically significant [407]. There is a growing body of veterinary literature describing its use in dogs [350,358,408–412], cats [413–417], horses [418–421], and cattle [422–424], though questions remain regarding its efficacy and appropriate dosing regimens.

The mechanism of action of gabapentin and pregabalin is not fully understood. They do not appear to interact with GABA, NMDA, or dopamine receptors, with most evidence indicating inhibition of voltage-gated calcium channels, with an intracellular site of action that requires active uptake [425–427]. Inhibition leads to a reduction of calcium influx, in turn reducing the release of a range of excitatory and inhibitory neurotransmitters, altering channel trafficking, and stimulating movement of channels away from neuronal cell membranes [426].

Pharmacokinetic data, primarily for gabapentin, are available for dogs [411,428], cats [414,429], horses [418,419,430], cattle [422–424], pigs [431], and horses [432]. In dogs, a short terminal half-life suggests the need for frequent dosing; this is supported by limited clinical evidence indicating that the therapeutic dose is in the range of 10–20 mg/kg PO two to three times daily [408,410]. Approximately 30% of the drug undergoes hepatic metabolism (to *N*-methyl-gabapentin), followed by renal elimination [428]. In humans, pregabalin shows favorable pharmacokinetics over gabapentin, with greater binding affinity for the voltage-gated calcium channel, linear pharmacokinetics, and non-saturable absorption from the gastrointestinal tract [433]. It remains to be seen to what extent these differences are present in animal species [429,432].

Since the previous edition of this textbook was published, several randomized, double-blinded clinical trials have been published and the following discussion will focus on these [434–436]. The most common population for these studies has been Chiari-like malformation and syringomyelia in Cavalier King Charles Spaniels, which is associated with neuropathic pain secondary to caudal cerebellar herniation and development of syringes in the spinal cord [434–436]. A randomized, placebo-controlled, double-blinded clinical trial in Cavalier King Charles Spaniels with Chiari-like malformation and syringomyelia (n = 8 dogs) found significant reductions in owner-rated pain scores using a numerical rating scale (including spontaneous vocalizations, phantom scratching, and exercise impairment) and improvement in quantitative sensory testing (reduced mechanical hyperalgesia, cold hyperalgesia, and allodynia) in dogs receiving pregabalin [434]. The mean difference in pain scale scores was 1 (scale range 0 to 10). Dogs were given pregabalin (5 mg/kg PO twice daily) or placebo for 14 days and all dogs also received an NSAID throughout the study period. Two dogs showed signs of sedation. Another study of Cavalier King Charles Spaniels with Chiari-like malformation and syringomyelia, using a randomized, placebo-controlled, double-blinded crossover design, reported reduced scratching and pain intensity (both owner and investigator assessed) and fewer scratching events (84% reduction) associated with pregabalin treatment (n = 12 dogs) [435]. All owners stated a preference for the period in which their dogs received pregabalin. Dogs received 150 mg pregabalin PO twice daily (13–19 mg/kg) for 21 days with a 2-day dose escalation, 2-day dose tapering, and 2-day washout period between treatments. The main adverse events reported were increased appetite (did not result in significant increase in body mass) and transient ataxia. A third randomized, blinded, crossover study in Cavalier King Charles Spaniels with Chiari-like malformation and syringomyelia (n = 33) found a significant improvement in quality of life associated with gabapentin (approximately 11.5 mg/kg PO three times daily) combined with carprofen (approximately 2.2 mg/kg PO once daily), in comparison with baseline scores or carprofen therapy alone [436]. Quality of life was owner-assessed using a visual analog scale (VAS) and showed a 10-mm reduction on the scale. A similar result was found with administration of the carbonic anhydrase inhibitor, topiramate (approximately 11 mg/kg PO three times daily). Blinding to treatment was incomplete as capsules containing gabapentin were labeled as such, limiting control of a placebo effect. Reported adverse effects were mild and self-limiting and included sedation, polyphagia, vomiting, diarrhea, and inappetence in four dogs. One dog in the gabapentin-carprofen group died, but the cause of death could not be determined (no necropsy performed).

Pharmacokinetic data for the use of pregabalin for analgesia in dogs suggest that plasma concentrations associated with analgesia in humans are achieved with a single dose of 4 mg/kg PO [437].

A randomized, blinded, placebo-controlled study of pregabalin (4 mg/kg PO three times daily) in 46 dogs (predominantly Dachshunds) initiated immediately before surgery for intervertebral disc herniation and continued for 5 days postoperatively found a significant reduction in pain scale scores (using a composite measure pain scale; mean reduction of 2.5 units on a 0–20 scale) and an increase in mechanical nociceptive thresholds [438]. Rescue analgesia requirements were low and similar in both treatment groups, and all dogs also had a fentanyl patch in place during the assessment period. Serum concentrations of pregabalin (sampled shortly before the next dose was administered) were highly variable, showing an approximately 30-fold difference between individuals.

A randomized, blinded, placebo-controlled clinical trial evaluating gabapentin in 29 dogs undergoing thoracic limb amputation did not identify an advantage of gabapentin over placebo (gelatin capsule) for postoperative pain [410]. Dogs received varying combinations of other analgesics (methadone, fentanyl, and NSAIDs), which may have made it difficult to identify a small treatment effect (the authors suggested the trial was underpowered) and the gabapentin dose (10 mg/kg total daily dose) may have been insufficient. A randomized, blinded, placebo-controlled clinical trial in a population of dogs undergoing hemilaminectomy surgery (n = 63 dogs total) included gabapentin (10 mg/kg PO twice daily) as an adjunctive analgesic (alongside levomethadone and a fentanyl patch) [408]. Compared to placebo, there was a non-significant reduction in pain scores. These mixed outcomes of gabapentin/pregabalin therapy may also reflect its mechanism of action in relation to the disease state, as voltage-gated calcium channels are upregulated following nerve injury and there is a delay for this to occur [439,440]. This could explain the lack of support for a role in acute postoperative pain in humans [407]. Further clinical studies are needed to better understand when gabapentin therapy is warranted.

In contrast to cats, gabapentin (20 mg/kg PO, 2 h before general anesthesia) has an isoflurane MAC-sparing effect (20% ± 14% reduction) in dogs, with no impact on cardiovascular variables [441]. Gabapentin (25–30 mg/kg PO) reduces fear behaviors in dogs with storm phobia when given approximately 90 min before exposure, with ataxia reported as an adverse effect [442].

Pharmacokinetic data for gabapentin in cats shows a high oral bioavailability (approximately 90%) and terminal half-life of around 3–4 h, with a suggested a dosing regimen of 8 mg/kg PO every 8 h, or 3 mg/kg PO every 6 h, in order to achieve plasma concentrations associated with analgesia in humans [414,443,444]. However, an increase in thermal threshold did not occur when gabapentin was administered orally at 5, 10, or 30 mg/kg in healthy cats [413]. These doses resulted in plasma drug concentrations in excess of those associated with analgesia in humans, leaving the authors to question the utility of gabapentin in healthy cats and the adequacy of the pain model. Sedation was not associated with gabapentin in this study at any dose, though it is a common adverse effect in dogs. The same investigators were not able to show a MAC-sparing effect of gabapentin on isoflurane despite achieving plasma drug concentrations almost double those reported to be effective in humans, though this does not rule out an analgesic effect [415]. In the presence of chronic kidney disease, plasma levels of gabapentin (10 mg/kg PO) were elevated to twice the concentration observed with the same dose in healthy cats and positively correlated with serum creatinine and serum symmetric dimethylarginine concentrations, indicating that dose reduction is necessary in cats with chronic kidney disease [444]. A randomized, blinded, placebo-controlled study in cats undergoing ovariohysterectomy (n = 15–19 cats per treatment group) did not identify a benefit of gabapentin (approximately 17 mg/kg PO twice daily) over meloxicam [417]. Rescue analgesia was required in all treatment groups as follows: gabapentin (25% of cats), meloxicam (13% of cats), and placebo (50% of cats). Two doses of gabapentin were given preoperatively, and a single dose of meloxicam (0.2 mg/kg SC) was given shortly before surgery. All cats also received buprenorphine perioperatively. Despite a lack of clear supporting evidence, it appears to be a popular choice for chronic musculoskeletal pain in cats [443]. The successful use of gabapentin (10 mg/kg PO every 8 h) was reported following polytrauma in two cases of road traffic accidents [416]. In each case, clinical signs were consistent with mechanical allodynia. Gabapentin was initiated when mechanical allodynia was observed 24–48 h following the surgical procedure and, in both cases, clinical signs resolved within 24 h, allowing a reduction of all administered analgesics. Importantly, a multimodal analgesic approach was used in both cases with cats also receiving opioids, NSAIDs, and locoregional analgesia. Chronic use of gabapentin in three cats (polytrauma or osteoarthritis) for between approximately 100–350 days (6.5 mg/kg PO twice daily) has been reported, without apparent adverse effects [445]. Pharmacokinetic data for pregabalin in cats indicate a longer terminal half-life compared to gabapentin which, along with linear pharmacokinetics, may make pregabalin preferable to gabapentin in this species [429,446]. Pregabalin (2 mg/kg PO twice daily) was associated with superficial dermatitis lesions in a cat with squamous cell carcinoma and clinical signs of neuropathic pain [447]. Lesions resolved with cessation of treatment and recurred when pregabalin was re-started (in response to recurrence of clinical neuropathic pain signs).

There has been increasing interest in gabapentin (13–30 mg/kg PO 1 to 1.5 h before transport) and pregabalin (5–10 mg/kg PO 1.5 h before transport) for anxiety and fear reduction in cats with both drugs appearing to be effective and associated with minimal, self-limiting adverse effects (sedation, ataxia, hypersalivation, and vomiting) [448–450]. Pregabalin is approved in Europe and the United States as a single oral dose (5 mg/kg 1.5 h before travel) to reduce anxiety before travel and veterinary visits [450].

In a study of gabapentin, reporting pharmacokinetic and behavioral data in horses, following 20 mg/kg PO or IV, no significant changes in heart rate or mean arterial blood pressure were recorded [419]. Sedation, scored as mild to moderate, occurred in all horses for 1 h following IV gabapentin. The frequency of drinking and standing at rest increased and decreased, respectively, over the 11-h observation period. Oral dosing of gabapentin had a lower bioavailability in horses (16%) compared to dogs (80%), which is likely to influence dosing requirements. No metabolites were detected in equine plasma, indicating that metabolism may be similar to that reported in humans, with the majority of drug excreted unchanged in urine. These pharmacokinetic data were in broad agreement with those previously reported in this species [418]. Oral dosing of gabapentin, up to 120 mg/kg PO twice daily, was not associated with sedation or ataxia, and vital signs and serum biochemistry values remained within the reference ranges [432]. By contrast, pregabalin appears to have considerably higher oral (nasogastric tube) bioavailability (> 90%) in horses, with a terminal half-life of 8 h [430].

There are few clinical reports of gabapentin use in horses [420,421,451]. In one randomized, blinded, crossover study (n = 14 horses) of chronic thoracic limb lameness (navicular syndrome, osteoarthritis, or collateral cartridge ossification), no advantage of including gabapentin (20 mg/kg in grain twice daily) in addition to an NSAID was identified [451]. Horses were evaluated with a subjective lameness score and various force plate measurements.

Gabapentin (2–3.3 mg/kg PO every 8 to 12 h) was included as part of a multimodal analgesic plan (with opioids, NSAIDs, locoregional analgesia, α_2-adrenergic receptor agonists, and ketamine at various times) in a horse following initial debridement of subsolar seromas, followed by infection and ongoing chronic laminitis and tendonitis [420]. Though difficult to specify the contribution of gabapentin, pain scores improved with initiation of gabapentin (along with concurrent perineural administration of bupivacaine) and no adverse effects were noted. In another reported case involving a pregnant mare following colic surgery, continuing signs of pain (circling and pawing with the affected hoof) were associated with femoral neuropathy and pelvic limb paresis [421]. Following a lack of response to xylazine, butorphanol, flunixin, and a lidocaine CRI, with adverse effects (marked sedation) during a detomidine CRI, gabapentin was begun (2.5 mg/kg PO every 8 h for 24 h, then every 12 h). Two h after giving gabapentin, during which time detomidine CRI (3 µg/ kg/h IV) and acepromazine (0.03 mg/kg IV every 6 h) were continued, the mare was less agitated and clinical signs improved over the following 36 h.

Pharmacokinetic and some pharmacodynamic data are available in adult cows [424] and calves [422,423]. A comparison of gabapentin (15 mg/kg PO once 1 h before dehorning) with flunixin, meloxicam, and meloxicam with gabapentin did not result in significant differences between groups or compared with placebo in plasma cortisol concentrations or eye temperature [423]. The results for mechanical nociceptive threshold were equivocal. Weight gain was the only parameter to show a difference between analgesic treatments and placebo. Average daily weight gain was greater in calves treated with meloxicam and gabapentin than placebo, gabapentin alone, or meloxicam alone. A combination of gabapentin (15 mg/kg PO) and meloxicam (0.5 mg/kg PO) resulted in plasma levels of gabapentin greater than 2 µg/mL (which is the threshold associated with analgesia in humans) for 15 h [422]. Compared with horses and dogs where maximal plasma concentrations were achieved within 2 h, peak concentrations in calves were not reached until 7 h post-administration. In adult Holstein-Friesian cows, the time to achieve maximal plasma concentrations of gabapentin (10–20 mg/kg PO co-administered with meloxicam 1 mg/kg PO) was also slow, taking over 8 h [424]. Both gabapentin and meloxicam concentrations in milk took 3 days to drop below the level of detection.

In dogs, approximately 30–35% of an administered dose of gabapentin undergoes hepatic metabolism while unchanged drug is excreted by the kidneys [428]. The metabolism of gabapentin has not been reported in the cat.

Gabapentin is available as tablets and capsules (100, 300, 400, 600, and 800 mg) and as a 50 mg/mL oral formulation. Pregabalin is available as capsules (25, 50, 75, 100, 150, 200, 225, and 300 mg) and as an oral solution (20 mg/mL).

Tapentadol

The analgesic agent tapentadol was designed with the aims of combining µ-opioid receptor agonism and norepinephrine reuptake inhibition without dependency on generating active metabolites, as is the case with tramadol [452,453]. Tapentadol has a higher affinity (approximately 50-fold) for the µ-opioid receptor compared to tramadol, but lower affinity compared to the M_1 metabolite of tramadol. Compared to tramadol, it has similar potency for inhibition of norepinephrine reuptake, and lesser potency (approximately fivefold) at inhibiting serotonin reuptake inhibition [452]. These activities, without a reliance on metabolism to an active metabolite, make tapentadol an attractive analgesic option though evidence of its use in veterinary species is limited. The pharmacokinetics have been described in dogs and cats [454–456]. In dogs, it has a low oral bioavailability (approximately 4%) and, as in humans, is expected to undergo extensive hepatic metabolism (glucuronidation) to generate inactive metabolites, of which tapentadol-*O*-glucuronide appears most important in dogs [455,456]. Oral dosing at 10, 20, and 30 mg/kg showed rapid absorption, with a terminal half-life of 3.5–4 h [456]. In a canine pharmacokinetic study, dose-related adverse effects (salivation, sedation, and panting) were described more frequently after IV administration [454]. The dose ranges were 1.4–3.9 mg/kg IV and 5.7–15.8 mg/kg PO. This contrasts with an oral pharmacokinetic study in which no adverse effects (no change in heart or respiratory rates and no sedation) were reported at doses of 10, 20, and 30 mg/kg PO [456]. In cats, bioavailability appears high after IM (94%) and SC (90%) injection with a terminal half-life of 2–3 h. Adverse effects (salivation, agitation, and panting lasting around 15–20 min) were reported at a dose of 5 mg/kg but were more common following IV rather than IM or SC administration [455].

Effective doses in dogs and cats are not well established [457,458]. In an acute pain model (thermal withdrawal latency; tail flick) in healthy Beagles, tapentadol (6.8 mg/kg IV) induced a significant increase in withdrawal latency that was similar to morphine (1.0 mg/kg IV) and lasted around 40 min with peak effect at 10 min [457]. In the same study, tramadol (6.8–10 mg/kg IV) had no effect on thermal thresholds. Tapentadol was associated with sedation, ataxia, hypersalivation, and diarrhea. An unblinded clinical study of 18 dogs with cranial cruciate rupture assessed 4 h after tapentadol (30 mg/kg PO) showed an improvement in subjective lameness assessment, with no change in gait analysis variables [459]. No sedation was reported. In a randomized, blinded, crossover, experimental study in healthy cats (n = 6), two different doses of tapentadol (approximately 6 and 11 mg/kg PO) increased thermal thresholds from baseline for 1- and 2-h post-administration, respectively; however, thermal thresholds were not significantly different from placebo. The 2-h duration of effect observed with the higher tapentadol dose was comparable to that observed in the buprenorphine (0.02 mg/kg IM) group [458]. Most cats hypersalivated following tapentadol administration, and this effect lasted up to 20 min.

Tapentadol is classified as a controlled substance in most jurisdictions. Oral formulations include 50, 75, and 100 mg tablets and a 20 mg/mL solution.

Tramadol

Tramadol is a racemic mixture and has been described as an "atypical" opioid due to the potential provision of analgesia via opioid and non-opioid (serotonin and norepinephrine reuptake inhibition) mechanisms [460]. Interestingly, both enantiomers of the parent compound and the M_1 metabolite (*O*-desmethyltramadol) contribute to analgesia. Norepinephrine reuptake inhibition results from activity of the (– or levo)-enantiomer of tramadol, serotonin (5-HT) reuptake inhibition results from activity of the (+ or dextro)-enantiomer of tramadol, and µ-opioid receptor agonism results from activity of the (+)-enantiomer of the M_1 metabolite and the (+)-enantiomer of tramadol [460–462]. It is, therefore, clear that the potential for interindividual as well as inter- and intraspecies variation in analgesic potency may occur as a result of variations in metabolism.

The pharmacokinetics of tramadol have been described in the dog [463–469], cat [468,470,471], horse [472–475], alpaca [476], llama [477], goat [478], piglet [479], and rhesus macaque [480].

In humans, metabolism of tramadol to the active M_1 metabolite is mediated by CYP2D6. In the dog, there appears to be limited production of the M_1 metabolite, indicating that analgesia is largely dependent on activity of the parent compound, concentrations of which display considerable interindividual variability (> 10-fold variation in plasma concentrations) [461,463–466,481]. A canine hepatic microsomal study has identified CYP2D15 as contributing to M_1 formation and CYP2B11/CYP3A12 as contributing to the predominant inactive

M_2 metabolite (*N*-desmethyltramadol) [469]. While the therapeutic plasma concentration of M_1 is unknown in the dog, measured levels are typically substantially below those associated with analgesia in humans. This may explain the variability in efficacy observed clinically, with a similar pattern observed in a subsection of humans who are "poor metabolizers" (i.e., those lacking the CYP2D6 isozyme) and consequently experience substantially lower analgesia from tramadol [482]. There is also evidence of genetic polymorphism in thoroughbred horses, which may explain the variation in plasma metabolite concentrations in this species [483]. As tramadol is excreted largely unchanged in urine, hepatic dysfunction would not be expected to result in complications with therapeutic dosing.

In cats, metabolism of tramadol is significant, resulting in M_1 metabolite concentrations associated with analgesia in humans [468,471,484]. Clearance was lower than reported in dogs, indicating that less frequent dosing may be effective. Excretion of parent drug and metabolites is suspected to be renal.

Tramadol may prove an effective analgesic in llamas as significant concentrations of the M_1 metabolite were detected following IV and IM administration, but clearance was similar to that reported in horses, which could make frequent dosing necessary [477]. In alpacas, a study of six adult animals discovered wide interindividual variation in oral absorption (ranging from 6% to 20%) and rapid clearance, with variable detection of the M_1 metabolite [476]. At doses of 3.4–4 mg/kg IV, adverse effects such as head tremor, ataxia, and star gazing were observed. A lower rate of infusion (i.e., the same dose but administered over 10 min) or oral dosing was not associated with side effects. Further work is needed to identify an effective dose in alpacas.

Lumbosacral epidural administration of tramadol (3 mg/kg) provided less effective and shorter acting analgesia than lidocaine (4 mg/kg) in adult goats undergoing castration with a rubber tension band [485].

Since the previous edition of this book, a systematic review and meta-analysis has been published on the use of tramadol for postoperative analgesia in dogs [486]. In reviewing 26 randomized clinical trials, including 848 dogs, the authors found that the certainty of evidence (a reflection of quality of evidence) supporting the use of tramadol for postoperative analgesia, specifically rescue analgesia requirement, was low or very low based on a four-point scale (high, moderate, low, and very low). Studies published up to 2020 were included in this analysis and grading reflects the poor quality of reporting, risk of bias, and imprecision, all of which are recognized and ongoing problems in the veterinary literature [487–491]. Disappointingly, none of the included studies performed a power calculation to estimate sample size and most (25/26) were designed as superiority trials, to identify a benefit of tramadol use. Together, this makes interpretation of existing data challenging, though evidence that tramadol does not make an important contribution to either postoperative analgesia or experimental nociceptive models continues to grow [457,481,492–494]. While there is probably some benefit to providing tramadol versus no analgesia (relative risk [RR]: 0.47; 95% CI: 0.26–0.85), its efficacy in reducing the highest pain score observed is questionable (standardized mean difference: −1.09; 95% CI: -2.34–0.16) [486]. When compared with different opioids (methadone, morphine, butorphanol, buprenorphine, codeine, and nalbuphine), there was no clear benefit associated with tramadol, with a possible exception for nalbuphine (tramadol may perform better; low certainty of evidence). There is some evidence that tramadol is less effective than NSAIDs, though the 95% CI for the RR is wide (RR: 2.27; 95% CI: 0.68–7.60). Unfortunately, weaknesses in study design, limitations of using different pain assessment scales, and inconsistencies in their application all contribute to difficulties in interpreting these data. The ongoing popularity of tramadol for chronic osteoarthritis pain management raises major concerns regarding the efficacy of analgesia provided [492,495]. A 26–36% sevoflurane MAC-reduction effect has been reported in dogs [496].

In horses, several pharmacokinetic studies of tramadol have been performed [471–473,475,483,497]. In contrast to humans, and similar to dogs, production of the unconjugated M_1 metabolite in horses is low, below the threshold associated with analgesia in humans [474]. However, in contrast to dogs, this does not represent a limitation of metabolism but rather very efficient glucuronidation (glucuronide-conjugated M_1 metabolite is rapidly produced following IV and PO dosing) [473,474]. The role of the glucuronide-conjugated M_1 metabolite in analgesia in horses is unclear. Similar to other species, large interindividual variability in M_1 metabolite production is also present in horses, with some of this variability perhaps explained by genetic polymorphism in CYP2D50 [473,474,483,497]. In addition to low concentrations of the M_1 metabolite, rapid clearance and short terminal half-life (approximately 2–3 h) may limit the tramadol's use in this species [473,474,483,497]. Repeated oral dosing (5 and 10 mg/kg every 12 h) resulted in accumulation of plasma tramadol (and extended terminal half-life) but not of its M_1 metabolite, though plasma concentrations continued to reflect widespread interindividual variability [497]. One horse, with a high plasma concentration, developed signs of colic though a clear causal relationship could not be established. Tramadol pharmacokinetics in foals (6–43 days old, administered 3 mg/kg IV) differed from that of adult horses, with a larger volume of distribution and faster clearance, though glucuronidation capability was reduced and different adverse effects were observed [475]. Between 13 and 43 days of age, transient inactivity and sedation were observed.

Dose-dependent adverse behavioral effects (muscle tremors, agitation, and circling) are observed following IV (1.5–3 mg/kg) but not oral administration (3–10 mg/kg) in horses [473,474,497]. Doses of tramadol greater than 3.1 mg/kg IV in horses were associated with significant (approximately 100%) increases in respiratory rate, 50% reductions in borborygmus, and trembling [498]. At lower doses (0.3 mg/kg IV), signs associated with CNS stimulation (i.e., head nodding) were observed.

Clinical data are increasingly available for both chronic and acute pain conditions. In four horses with chronic laminitis given oral tramadol (5 or 10 mg/kg twice daily), the higher dose resulted in a modest improvement in comfort (using a proxy measure of offloading frequency) [499]. Extradural administration (0.5–1 mg/kg) shows promise and may be a useful alternative route, providing analgesia and limiting CNS stimulation [500,501]. The extradural administration of tramadol has also been reported in cattle and lambs [502,503]. In horses, a dose of 2 mg/kg IV did not result in significant reductions in skin twitch latency or hoof withdrawal reflex during exposure to thermal stimulation [498]. While higher doses may have resulted in analgesia, the 2 mg/kg dose was selected as adverse effects were observed with higher doses.

Sedation was observed with tramadol doses greater than 2 mg/kg IV and at 4 mg/kg IM in dogs [466,504,505]. In cats, 1 mg/kg SC had variable behavioral effects with six of eight cats exhibiting signs of euphoria and two cats appearing dysphoric [506]. Reliance on renal excretion of parent drug and the active M_1 metabolite implies that renal dysfunction might result in increased adverse effects [507], though none have been reported in veterinary species.

In cats, the limited evidence available shows some promise for an analgesic effect of tramadol, which may reflect the increased production of the M_1 metabolite in this species [413,471]. Further research is needed to confirm these initial findings and establish effective doses. Oral administration at 8.6–11.6 mg/kg was effective at reducing the MAC of sevoflurane by approximately 40% [508]. Doses between 2 and 4 mg/kg PO have been associated with an increased thermal threshold in cats, and a dose of 4 mg/kg PO every 6 h has been proposed for providing analgesia [413]. An oral dose of 6 mg/kg provided similar levels of analgesia as 4 mg/kg IM for ovariohysterectomy surgery, though the author recognized a limitation of small sample size [509]. A comparison of meperidine (pethidine) and tramadol (2 and 4 mg/kg IM) found similar levels of analgesia, with an increased requirement for rescue analgesia in the meperidine group [510]. A 2 mg/kg IM dose of tramadol appeared to provide similar levels of analgesia as both morphine and control comparison groups (all cats also received medetomidine and ketamine) though the group sample size was estimated based on cardiovascular changes rather than pain assessment [511]. In cats exposed to mechanical stimulation, extradural administration of tramadol (1 mg/kg) was more effective than saline control but shorter lasting than extradural morphine [512]. A 2 mg/kg SC dose was no more effective than placebo following ovariohysterectomy when assessed with an interactive VAS and composite pain score, though there was a lower requirement for rescue analgesia compared with placebo [513]. A comparison of oral tramadol (3 mg/kg every 12 h) combined with a meloxicam spray to placebo with meloxicam spray in cats with osteoarthritis did not identify any advantage of including tramadol [514]. Similarly, 1 mg/kg SC did not substantially increase either pressure or thermal threshold responses in cats [506]. An important barrier to the use of tramadol in cats is the very low palatability of oral suspensions, which can trigger considerable hypersalivation. Formulating oral doses as capsules circumvents this problem [509,515]. A proprietary transdermal formulation of tramadol (200 mg/mL tramadol), administered at approximately 3 mg/kg either did not result in detectable plasma tramadol concentrations or concentrations greater than 100 times lower than an oral dose of 1 mg/kg [516]. Furthermore, the proprietary metered-dose applicators delivered an amount that exceeded the intended dose by up to 39%. In a randomized, placebo-controlled, blinded comparison of different doses of tramadol, in cats with osteoarthritis (0, 1, 2, and 4 mg/kg PO), activity and owner-assessed outcomes improved at the 2 mg/kg dose [515]. The frequency of adverse events was dose dependent, with mydriasis, euphoria, agitation, sedation, decreased appetite, and diarrhea observed most frequently. A case report of accidental tramadol overdose (80 mg/kg PO instead of 4 mg/kg PO) resulted in agitation, hypersalivation, head jerking, and hypertension after the first dose, followed by obtunded mentation, lateral recumbency, hypertension, tachycardia, abdominal distension, and pain after a further dose [264]. These signs were attributed to serotonin toxicity resulting from tramadol's effects as a serotonin reuptake inhibitor. The cat responded to supportive therapy (fluids, analgesia), an enema to relieve abdominal distension, and cyproheptadine (a serotonin receptor antagonist, 2 mg/kg PO once daily), with resolution of clinical signs over several days.

Tramadol is classified as a controlled substance in most jurisdictions. Available oral formulations include 50 and 100 mg tablets and a 5 mg/mL oral solution. Injectable formulations are approved in some countries.

References

1 Rosenberg H, Pollock N, Schiemann A, *et al.* Malignant hyperthermia: a review. *Orphanet J Rare Dis* 2015; **10**: 93.

2 Boys JA, Toledo AH, Anaya-Prado R, *et al.* Effects of dantrolene on ischemia-reperfusion injury in animal models: a review of outcomes in heart, brain, liver, and kidney. *J Investig Med* 2010; **58**: 875–882.

3 Inan S, Wei H. The cytoprotective effects of dantrolene: a ryanodine receptor antagonist. *Anesth Analg* 2010; **111**: 1400–1410.

4 Lynch C, Durbin CGJ, Fisher NA, *et al.* Effects of dantrolene and verapamil on atrioventricular conduction and cardiovascular performance in dogs. *Anesth Analg* 1986; **65**: 252–258.

5 Oliven A, Deal ECJ, Kelsen SG. Effect of dantrolene on ventilation and respiratory muscle activity in anaesthetized dogs. *Br J Anaesth* 1990; **64**: 207–213.

6 Bowman WC, Houston J, Khan HH, *et al.* Effects of dantrolene sodium on respiratory and other muscles and on respiratory parameters in the anaesthetised cat. *Eur J Pharmacol* 1979; **55**: 293–303.

7 Brandom BW, Larach MG, Chen MS, *et al.* Complications associated with the administration of dantrolene 1987 to 2006: a report from the North American Malignant Hyperthermia Registry of the Malignant Hyperthermia Association of the United States. *Anesth Analg* 2011; **112**: 1115–1123.

8 Bagshaw RJ, Cox RH, Rosenberg H. Dantrolene treatment of malignant hyperthermia. *J Am Vet Med Assoc* 1981; **178**: 1129.

9 Harrison GG. Control of the malignant hyperpyrexic syndrome in MHS swine by dantrolene sodium. *Br J Anaesth* 1975; **47**: 62–65.

10 Kirmayer AH, Klide AM, Purvance JE. Malignant hyperthermia in a dog: case report and review of the syndrome. *J Am Vet Med Assoc* 1984; **185**: 978–982.

11 Klein L, Ailes N, Fackelman GE, *et al.* Postanesthetic equine myopathy suggestive of malignant hyperthermia. *A case report. Vet Surg* 1989; **18**: 479–482.

12 Nelson TE. Malignant hyperthermia in dogs. *J Am Vet Med Assoc* 1991; **198**: 989–994.

13 Rand JS, O'Brien PJ. Exercise-induced malignant hyperthermia in an English springer spaniel. *J Am Vet Med Assoc* 1987; **190**: 1013–1014.

14 Waldron-Mease E, Klein LV, Rosenberg H, *et al.* Malignant hyperthermia in a halothane-anesthetized horse. *J Am Vet Med Assoc* 1981; **179**: 896–898.

15 Wells RJ, Sedacca CD, Aman AM, *et al.* Successful management of a dog that had severe rhabdomyolysis with myocardial and respiratory failure. *J Am Vet Med Assoc* 2009; **234**: 1049–1054.

16 McKenzie EC, Valberg SJ, Godden SM, *et al.* Effect of oral administration of dantrolene sodium on serum creatine kinase activity after exercise in horses with recurrent exertional rhabdomyolysis. *Am J Vet Res* 2004; **65**: 74–79.

17 McKenzie EC, Garrett RL, Payton ME, *et al.* Effect of feed restriction on plasma dantrolene concentrations in horses. *Equine Vet J Suppl* 2010; **38**: 613–617.

18 Edwards JG, Newtont JR, Ramzan PH, *et al.* The efficacy of dantrolene sodium in controlling exertional rhabdomyolysis in the Thoroughbred racehorse. *Equine Vet J* 2003; **35**: 707–711.

19 Takano K. Effect of dantrolene sodium upon the activity of the hind leg muscle of the cat with local tetanus. *Naunyn Schmiedebergs Arch Pharmacol* 1976; **293**: 195–196.

20 Zamiri N, Massé S, Ramadeen A, *et al.* Dantrolene improves survival after ventricular fibrillation by mitigating impaired calcium handling in animal models. *Circulation* 2014; **129**: 875–885.

21 Denborough MA, Lovell RRH. Anaesthetic deaths in a family. *Lancet* 1960; **276**: 45.

22 Denborough MA, Forster JFA, Lovell RRH, *et al.* Anesthetic deaths in a family. *Br J Anaesth* 1962; **34**: 395–396.

23 Jones EW, Nelson TE, Anderson IL, *et al.* Malignant hyperthermia of swine. *Anesthesiology* 1972; **36**: 42–51.

24 Hall LW, Woolf N, Bradley JW, *et al.* Unusual reaction to suxamethonium chloride. *Br Med J* 1966; **2**: 1305.

25 Aldrich K, Velez-Irizarry D, Fenger C, *et al.* Pathways of calcium regulation, electron transport, and mitochondrial protein translation are molecular signatures of susceptibility to recurrent exertional rhabdomyolysis in Thoroughbred racehorses. *PLoS ONE* 2021; **16**: e0244556.

26 McKenzie EC, Di Concetto S, Payton ME, *et al.* Effect of dantrolene premedication on various cardiovascular and biochemical variables and the recovery in healthy isoflurane-anesthetized horses. *Am J Vet Res* 2015; **76**: 293–301.

27 Wuis EW, Janssen MG, Vree TB, *et al.* Determination of a dantrolene metabolite, 5-(p-nitrophenyl)-2-furoic acid, in plasma and urine by high-performance liquid chromatography. *J Chromatogr* 1990; **526**: 575–580.

28 Court MH, Engelking LR, Dodman NH, *et al.* Pharmacokinetics of dantrolene sodium in horses. *J Vet Pharmacol Ther* 1987; **10**: 218–226.

29 DiMaio Knych HK, Arthur RM, Taylor A, *et al.* Pharmacokinetics and metabolism of dantrolene in horses. *J Vet Pharmacol Ther* 2011; **34**: 238–246.

30 Haraschak JL, Langston VC, Wang R, *et al.* Pharmacokinetic evaluation of oral dantrolene in the dog. *J Vet Pharmacol Ther* 2014; **37**: 286–294.

31 Zabirowicz ES, Gan TJ. Pharmacology of postoperative nausea and vomiting. In: Hemmings HC, Egan TD, eds. *Pharmacology and Physiology for Anesthesia*. Philadelphia, PA: Elsevier, 2019: 671–692.
32 Peters LJ, Kovacic JP. Histamine: metabolism, physiology, and pathophysiology with applications in veterinary medicine. *J Vet Emerg Crit Care (San Antonio)* 2009; **19**: 311–328.
33 Hofmeister EH, Egger CM. Evaluation of diphenhydramine as a sedative for dogs. *J Am Vet Med Assoc* 2005; **226**: 1092–1094.
34 Sanchez A, Valverde A, Sinclair M, *et al.* The pharmacokinetics of DPH after the administration of a single intravenous or intramuscular dose in healthy dogs. *J Vet Pharmacol Ther* 2016; **39**: 452–459.
35 Banovic F, Denley T, Blubaugh A, *et al.* Effect of diphenhydramine and cetirizine on immediate and late-phase cutaneous allergic reactions in healthy dogs: a randomized, double-blinded crossover study. *Vet Dermatol* 2020; **31**: e256–e258.
36 Barnett A, Iorio LC, Kreutner W, *et al.* Evaluation of the CNS properties of SCH 29851, a potential non-sedating antihistamine. *Agents Actions* 1984; **14**: 590–597.
37 Kranke P, Morin AM, Roewer N, *et al.* Dimenhydrinate for prophylaxis of postoperative nausea and vomiting: a meta-analysis of randomized controlled trials. *Acta Anaesthesiol Scand* 2002; **46**: 238–244.
38 Marzanatti M, Monopoli A, Trampus M, *et al.* Effects of nonsedating histamine H1-antagonists on EEG activity and behavior in the cat. *Pharmacol Biochem Behav* 1989; **32**: 861–866.
39 Sanchez A, Valverde A, Sinclair M, *et al.* Antihistaminic and cardiorespiratory effects of diphenhydramine hydrochloride in anesthetized dogs undergoing excision of mast cell tumors. *J Am Vet Med Assoc* 2017; **251**: 804–813.
40 Gamperl S, Stefanzl G, Willmann M, *et al.* In vitro effects of histamine receptor 1 antagonists on proliferation and histamine release in canine neoplastic mast cells. *Vet Med Sci* 2021; **7**: 57–68.
41 Cardona V, Ansotegui IJ, Ebisawa M, *et al.* World allergy organization anaphylaxis guidance 2020. *World Allergy Organ J* 2020; **13**: 100472.
42 Pang DSJ, Prebble M. Suspected anaphylaxis from intravenous cefazolin during general anaesthesia in a dog. *Vet Rec Case Rep* 2016; **4**: e000352.
43 Simons KJ, Chen X, Fraser TG, *et al.* Effect of cimetidine on the pharmacokinetics and pharmacodynamics of chlorpheniramine and diphenhydramine in rabbits. *Pharm Res* 1996; **13**: 301–304.
44 Wasfi IA, Abdel Hadi AA, Elghazali M, *et al.* Comparative pharmacokinetics of diphenhydramine in camels and horses after intravenous administration. *Vet Res Commun* 2003; **27**: 463–473.
45 Au-Yeung SC, Riggs KW, Gruber N, *et al.* The use of microdialysis for the study of drug kinetics: central nervous system pharmacokinetics of diphenhydramine in fetal, newborn, and adult sheep. *Drug Metab Dispos* 2007; **35**: 1285–1291.
46 Kumar S, Riggs KW, Rurak DW. Role of the liver and gut in systemic diphenhydramine clearance in adult nonpregnant sheep. *Drug Metab Dispos* 1999; **27**: 297–302.
47 Koyanagi T, Yamaura Y, Yano K, *et al.* Age-related pharmacokinetic changes of acetaminophen, antipyrine, diazepam, diphenhydramine, and ofloxacin in male cynomolgus monkeys and beagle dogs. *Xenobiotica* 2014; **44**: 893–901.
48 Hatch RC, Jernigan AD, Wilson RC, *et al.* Prompt arousal from fentanyl-droperidol-pentobarbital anesthesia in dogs: a preliminary study. *Can J Vet Res* 1986; **50**: 251–258.
49 Short CE. Doxapram for reversing xylazine sedation [letter]. *J Am Vet Med Assoc* 1984; **184**: 237, 258.
50 Zapata M, Hofmeister EH. Refinement of the dose of doxapram to counteract the sedative effects of acepromazine in dogs. *J Small Anim Pract* 2013; **54**: 405–408.
51 Boller M, Kellett-Gregory L, Shofer FS, *et al.* The clinical practice of CPCR in small animals: an internet-based survey. *J Vet Emerg Crit Care (San Antonio)* 2010; **20**: 558–570.
52 Roy RC, Stullken EH. Electroencephalographic evidence of arousal in dogs from halothane after doxapram, physostigmine, or naloxone. *Anesthesiology* 1981; **55**: 392–397.
53 Curtis R, Evans JM. The effect of doxapram hydrochloride on cats anaesthetized with either Saffan or thiopentone sodium. *J Small Anim Pract* 1981; **22**: 77–83.
54 Giguère S, Sanchez LC, Shih A, *et al.* Comparison of the effects of caffeine and doxapram on respiratory and cardiovascular function in foals with induced respiratory acidosis. *Am J Vet Res* 2007; **68**: 1407–1416.
55 Giguère S, Slade JK, Sanchez LC. Retrospective comparison of caffeine and doxapram for the treatment of hypercapnia in foals with hypoxic-ischemic encephalopathy. *J Vet Intern Med* 2008; **22**: 401–405.
56 Bleul U, Bircher B, Jud RS, *et al.* Respiratory and cardiovascular effects of doxapram and theophylline for the treatment of asphyxia in neonatal calves. *Theriogenology* 2010; **73**: 612–619.
57 Bleul U, Bylang T. Effects of doxapram, prethcamide and lobeline on spirometric, blood gas and acid-base variables in healthy new-born calves. *Vet J* 2012; **194**: 240–246.
58 Short CE, Cloyd GD, Ward JW. An evaluation of doxapram hydrochloride to control respiration in dogs during and after inhalation anesthesia. *Vet Med Small Anim Clin* 1970; **65**: 787–790.
59 Short CE, Cloyd GD. The use of doxapram hydrochloride with inhalation anesthetics in horses. *II. Vet Med Small Anim Clin* 1970; **65**: 260–261.
60 Short CE, Cloyd GD, Ward JW. The use of doxapram hydrochloride with intravenous anesthetics in horses. *I. Vet Med Small Anim Clin* 1970; **65**: 157–160.
61 Tobias KM, Jackson AM, Harvey RC. Effects of doxapram HCl on laryngeal function of normal dogs and dogs with naturally occurring laryngeal paralysis. *Vet Anaesth Analg* 2004; **31**: 258–263.
62 Archer RM, Lindsay WA, Duncan ID. A comparison of techniques to enhance the evaluation of equine laryngeal function. *Equine Vet J* 1991; **23**: 104–107.
63 Ranninger E, Kantyka M, Bektas RN. The Influence of anaesthetic drugs on the laryngeal motion in dogs: a systematic review. *Animals (Basel)* 2020; **10**: E530.
64 Funderburk WH, Oliver KL, Ward JW. Electrophysiologic analysis of the site of action of doxapram hydrochloride. *J Pharmacol Exp Ther* 1966; **151**: 360–368.
65 Hirsh K, Wang SC. Selective respiratory stimulating action of doxapram compared to pentylenetetrazaol. *J Pharmacol Exp Ther* 1974; **189**: 1–11.
66 Kato H, Buckley JP. Possible sites of action of the respiratory stimulant effect of doxapram hydrochloride. *J Pharmacol Exp Ther* 1964; **144**: 260–264.
67 Taylor PM. Doxapram infusion during halothane anaesthesia in ponies. *Equine Vet J* 1990; **22**: 329–332.
68 Soma LR, Kenny R. Respiratory, cardiovascular, metabolic and electroencephalographic effects of doxapram hydrochloride in the dog. *Am J Vet Res* 1967; **28**: 191–198.
69 Kim SI, Winnie AP, Collins VJ, *et al.* Hemodynamic responses to doxapram in normovolemic and hypovolemic dogs. *Anesth Analg* 1971; **50**: 705–710.
70 Pang DS, Robledo CJ, Carr DR, *et al.* An unexpected role for TASK-3 potassium channels in network oscillations with implications for sleep mechanisms and anesthetic action. *Proc Natl Acad Sci USA* 2009; **106**: 17546–17551.
71 Cotten JF. TASK-1 (KCNK3) and TASK-3 (KCNK9) tandem pore potassium channel antagonists stimulate breathing in isoflurane-anesthetized rats. *Anesth Analg* 2013; **116**: 810–816.
72 Trapp S, Aller MI, Wisden W, *et al.* A role for TASK-1 (KCNK3) channels in the chemosensory control of breathing. *J Neurosci* 2008; **28**: 8844–8850.
73 Yost CS. A new look at the respiratory stimulant doxapram. *CNS Drug Rev* 2006; **12**: 236–249.
74 Winnie AP, Collins VJ. The search for a pharmacologic ventilator. *Acta Anaesthesiol Scand Suppl* 1966; **23**: 63–71.
75 Bruce RB, Pitts JE, Pinchbeck F, *et al.* Excretion, distribution, and metabolism of doxapram hydrochloride. *J Med Chem* 1965; **8**: 157–164.
76 Sams RA, Detra RL, Muir WW. Pharmacokinetics and metabolism of intravenous doxapram in horses. *Equine Vet J Suppl* 1992; **11**: 45–51.
77 Huffington P, Craythorne NW. Effect of doxapram on heart rhythm during anesthesia in dog and man. *Anesth Analg* 1966; **45**: 558–563.
78 Sabiza S, Naddaf H, Jalali SM, *et al.* The effects of doxapram on haematology, serum biochemical parameters and erythrocyte oxidant/ antioxidant status in dogs anaesthetized with propofol. *Vet Med Sci* 2021; **7**: 586–592.
79 Aguilera-Tejero E, Pascoe JR, Smith BL, *et al.* The effect of doxapram-induced hyperventilation on respiratory mechanics in horses. *Res Vet Sci* 1997; **62**: 143–146.
80 Henderson-Smart DJ, Steer PA. Doxapram treatment for apnea in preterm infants. *Cochrane Database Syst Rev* 2001; **4**: CD000074.
81 Uehara H, Yoshioka H, Nagai H, *et al.* Doxapram accentuates white matter injury in neonatal rats following bilateral carotid artery occlusion. *Neurosci Lett* 2000; **281**: 191–194.
82 Roll C, Horsch S. Effect of doxapram on cerebral blood flow velocity in preterm infants. *Neuropediatrics* 2004; **35**: 126–129.
83 Dani C, Bertini G, Pezzati M, *et al.* Brain hemodynamic effects of doxapram in preterm infants. *Biol Neonate* 2006; **89**: 69–74.
84 Fletcher DJ, Boller M, Brainard BM, *et al.* RECOVER evidence and knowledge gap analysis on veterinary CPR. Part 7: clinical guidelines. *J Vet Emerg Crit Care (San Antonio)* 2012; **22**(Suppl 1): S102–S131.
85 Hubbell JAE, Muir WW. Considerations for induction, maintenance and recovery. In: Hubbell JAE, Muir WW, eds. *Equine Anesthesia: Monitoring and Emergency Therapy*, 2nd edn. St. Louis, MO: Saunders Elsevier, 2009: 381–396.
86 Zahner JM, Hatch RC, Wilson RC, *et al.* Antagonism of xylazine sedation in steers by doxapram and 4-aminopyridine. *Am J Vet Res* 1984; **45**: 2546–2551.
87 Riebold TW, Kaneps AJ, Schmotzer WB. Reversal of xylazine-induced sedation in llamas, using doxapram or 4-aminopyridine and yohimbine. *J Am Vet Med Assoc* 1986; **189**: 1059–1061.
88 Said AH. Some aspects of anaesthesia in the camel. *Vet Rec* 1964; **76**: 550.
89 Woods R, McLean S, Nicol S, *et al.* Antagonism of some cyclohexamine-based drug combinations used for chemical restraint of southern elephant seals (*Mirounga leonina*). *Aust Vet J* 1995; **72**: 165–171.

90 Murray MJ, Grodinsky C. The effects of famotidine, ranitidine and magnesium hydroxide/aluminium hydroxide on gastric fluid pH in adult horses. *Equine Vet J Suppl* 1992; **11**: 52–55.

91 Ahmed AF, Constable PD, Misk NA. Effect of orally administered cimetidine and ranitidine on abomasal luminal pH in clinically normal milk-fed calves. *Am J Vet Res* 2001; **62**: 1531–1538.

92 Sanchez LC, Lester GD, Merritt AM. Effect of ranitidine on intragastric pH in clinically normal neonatal foals. *J Am Vet Med Assoc* 1998; **212**: 1407–1412.

93 Sanchez LC, Lester GD, Merritt AM. Intragastric pH in critically ill neonatal foals and the effect of ranitidine. *J Am Vet Med Assoc* 2001; **218**: 907–911.

94 Marks SL, Kook PH, Papich MG, *et al.* ACVIM consensus statement: support for rational administration of gastrointestinal protectants to dogs and cats. *J Vet Intern Med* 2018; **32**: 1823–1840.

95 Hwang JH, Jeong JW, Song GH, *et al.* Pharmacokinetics and acid suppressant efficacy of esomeprazole after intravenous, oral, and subcutaneous administration to healthy Beagle dogs. *J Vet Intern Med* 2017; **31**: 743–750.

96 De Graef J, Woussen-Colle MC. Influence of the stimulation state of the parietal cells on the inhibitory effect of omeprazole on gastric acid secretion in dogs. *Gastroenterology* 1986; **91**: 333–337.

97 Huang JQ, Hunt RH. Pharmacological and pharmacodynamic essentials of H(2)-receptor antagonists and proton pump inhibitors for the practising physician. *Best Pract Res Clin Gastroenterol* 2001; **15**: 355–370.

98 Bersenas AM, Mathews KA, Allen DG, *et al.* Effects of ranitidine, famotidine, pantoprazole, and omeprazole on intragastric pH in dogs. *Am J Vet Res* 2005; **66**: 425–431.

99 Tolbert K, Bissett S, King A, *et al.* Efficacy of oral famotidine and 2 omeprazole formulations for the control of intragastric pH in dogs. *J Vet Intern Med* 2011; **25**: 47–54.

100 Andrews FM, Doherty TJ, Blackford JT, *et al.* Effects of orally administered enteric-coated omeprazole on gastric acid secretion in horses. *Am J Vet Res* 1999; **60**: 929–931.

101 Murray MJ. Suppression of gastric acidity in horses. *J Am Vet Med Assoc* 1997; **211**: 37–40.

102 Sanchez LC, Murray MJ, Merritt AM. Effect of omeprazole paste on intragastric pH in clinically normal neonatal foals. *Am J Vet Res* 2004; **65**: 1039–1041.

103 Olivarez JD, Kreuder AJ, Tatarniuk DM, *et al.* Pharmacokinetics and tissue levels of pantoprazole in neonatal calves after intravenous administration. *Front Vet Sci* 2020; **7**: 580735.

104 Ryan CA, Sanchez LC, Giguère S, *et al.* Pharmacokinetics and pharmacodynamics of pantoprazole in clinically normal neonatal foals. *Equine Vet J* 2005; **37**: 336–341.

105 Smith GW, Davis JL, Smith SM, *et al.* Efficacy and pharmacokinetics of pantoprazole in alpacas. *J Vet Intern Med* 2010; **24**: 949–955.

106 Smith JS, Mochel JP, Soto-Gonzalez WM, *et al.* Pharmacokinetics of pantoprazole and pantoprazole sulfone in goats after intravenous administration: a preliminary report. *Front Vet Sci* 2021; **8**: 744813.

107 de Brito Galvao JF, Trepanier LA. Risk of hemolytic anemia with intravenous administration of famotidine to hospitalized cats. *J Vet Intern Med* 2008; **22**: 325–329.

108 Williamson KK, Willard MD, Payton ME, *et al.* Efficacy of omeprazole versus high-dose famotidine for prevention of exercise-induced gastritis in racing Alaskan sled dogs. *J Vet Intern Med* 2010; **24**: 285–288.

109 Zacuto AC, Marks SL, Osborn J, *et al.* The influence of esomeprazole and cisapride on gastroesophageal reflux during anesthesia in dogs. *J Vet Intern Med* 2012; **26**: 518–525.

110 Panti A, Bennett RC, Corletto F, *et al.* The effect of omeprazole on oesophageal pH in dogs during anaesthesia. *J Small Anim Pract* 2009; **50**: 540–544.

111 Gaier A, Price J, Grubb L, *et al.* A prospective, randomized, masked, placebo-controlled crossover study for the effect of 10 mg omeprazole capsules on gastric pH in healthy dogs. *J Vet Intern Med* 2021; **35**: 887–891.

112 Odunayo A, Galyon G, Price J, *et al.* Evaluation of a long-acting injectable formulation of omeprazole in healthy dogs. *J Vet Intern Med* 2022; **36**: 1416–1421.

113 Sykes BW, Kathawala K, Song Y, *et al.* Preliminary investigations into a novel, long-acting, injectable, intramuscular formulation of omeprazole in the horse. *Equine Vet J* 2017; **49**: 795–801.

114 Adamama-Moraitou KK, Rallis TS, Prassinos NN, *et al.* Benign esophageal stricture in the dog and cat: a retrospective study of 20 cases. *Can J Vet Res* 2002; **66**: 55–59.

115 Wilson DV, Walshaw R. Postanesthetic esophageal dysfunction in 13 dogs. *J Am Anim Hosp Assoc* 2004; **40**: 455–460.

116 Pearson H, Darke PG, Gibbs C, *et al.* Reflux oesophagitis and stricture formation after anaesthesia: a review of seven cases in dogs and cats. *J Small Anim Pract* 1978; **19**: 507–519.

117 Andersson T, Cederberg C, Edvardsson G, *et al.* Effect of omeprazole treatment on diazepam plasma levels in slow versus normal rapid metabolizers of omeprazole. *Clin Pharmacol Ther* 1990; **47**: 79–85.

118 Hassan-Alin M, Andersson T, Niazi M, *et al.* A pharmacokinetic study comparing single and repeated oral doses of 20 mg and 40 mg omeprazole and its two optical isomers, S-omeprazole (esomeprazole) and R-omeprazole, in healthy subjects. *Eur J Clin Pharmacol* 2005; **60**: 779–784.

119 Funk KA. Glyceryl guaiacolate: a centrally acting muscle relaxant. *Equine Vet J* 1970; **2**: 173–178.

120 Funk KA. Glyceryl guaiacolate: some effects and indications in horses. *Equine Vet J* 1973; **5**: 15–19.

121 Seagrave J, Albrecht H, Park YS, *et al.* Effect of guaifenesin on mucin production, rheology, and mucociliary transport in differentiated human airway epithelial cells. *Exp Lung Res* 2011; **37**: 606–614.

122 Posner LP, Burns P. Injectable anesthetic agents. In: Riviere JE, Papich MG, eds. *Veterinary Pharmacology and Therapeutics*, 9th edn. Ames, IA: Wiley-Blackwell, 2009: 265–289.

123 Muir WW. Intravenous anesthetic drugs. In: Hubbell JAE, Muir WW, eds. *Equine Anesthesia: Monitoring and Emergency Therapy*, 2nd edn. St. Louis, MO: Saunders Elsevier, 2009: 243–259.

124 Hubbell JA, Muir WW, Sams RA. Guaifenesin: cardiopulmonary effects and plasma concentrations in horses. *Am J Vet Res* 1980; **41**: 1751–1755.

125 Davis LE, Wolff WA. Pharmacokinetics and metabolism of glyceryl guaiacolate in ponies. *Am J Vet Res* 1970; **31**: 469–473.

126 Tavernor WD. The influence of guaiacol glycerol ether on cardiovascular and respiratory function in the horse. *Res Vet Sci* 1970; **11**: 91–93.

127 Schatzmann U, Tschudi P, Held JP, *et al.* An investigation of the action and haemolytic effect of glyceryl guaiacolate in the horse. *Equine Vet J* 1978; **10**: 224–228.

128 Mostert JW, Metz J. Observations on the haemolytic activity of guaiacol glycerol ether. *Br J Anaesth* 1963; **35**: 461–464.

129 Wall R, Muir WW. Hemolytic potential of guaifenesin in cattle. *Cornell Vet* 1990; **80**: 209–216.

130 Herschl MA, Trim CM, Mahaffey EA. Effects of 5% and 10% guaifenesin infusion on equine vascular endothelium. *Vet Surg* 1992; **21**: 494–497.

131 Dickson LR, Badcoe LM, Burbidge H, *et al.* Jugular thrombophlebitis resulting from an anaesthetic induction technique in the horse. *Equine Vet J* 1990; **22**: 177–179.

132 Matthews NS, Light GS, Sanders EA, *et al.* Urticarial response during anesthesia in a horse. *Equine Vet J* 1993; **25**: 555–556.

133 Duke-Novakovski T, Jimenez CP, Fujiyama M, *et al.* Plasma histamine concentrations in horses administered sodium penicillin, guaifenesin-xylazine-ketamine and isoflurane with morphine or butorphanol. *Vet Anaesth Analg* 2021; **48**: 17–25.

134 Rioja E, Cernicchiaro N, Costa MC, *et al.* Perioperative risk factors for mortality and length of hospitalization in mares with dystocia undergoing general anesthesia: a retrospective study. *Can Vet J* 2012; **53**: 502–510.

135 Ambrisko TD, Kabes R, Moens Y. Influence of drugs on the response characteristics of the LiDCO sensor: an in vitro study. *Br J Anaesth* 2013; **110**: 305–310.

136 Benchaoui HA, Cox SR, Schneider RP, *et al.* The pharmacokinetics of maropitant, a novel neurokinin type-1 receptor antagonist, in dogs. *J Vet Pharmacol Ther* 2007; **30**: 336–344.

137 Zoetis. Cerenia (Maropitant Citrate) Package Insert. www.zoetisus.com/content/_assets/docs/Petcare/Cerenia/Cerenia-Tablets-and-Injectable-Solution-Combined-Marketing-Package-Insert.pdf (accessed September 2022).

138 Hickman MA, Cox SR, Mahabir S, *et al.* Safety, pharmacokinetics and use of the novel NK-1 receptor antagonist maropitant (Cerenia) for the prevention of emesis and motion sickness in cats. *J Vet Pharmacol Ther* 2008; **31**: 220–229.

139 Diemunsch P, Grelot L. Potential of substance P antagonists as antiemetics. *Drugs* 2000; **60**: 533–546.

140 Narishetty ST, Galvan B, Coscarelli E, *et al.* Effect of refrigeration of the antiemetic Cerenia (maropitant) on pain on injection. *Vet Ther* 2009; **10**: 93–102.

141 Deckers N, Ruigrok CA, Verhoeve HP, *et al.* Comparison of pain response after subcutaneous injection of two maropitant formulations to beagle dogs. *Vet Rec Open* 2018; **5**: e000262.

142 Martín-Flores M, Sakai DM, Learn MM, *et al.* Effects of maropitant in cats receiving dexmedetomidine and morphine. *J Am Vet Med Assoc* 2016; **248**: 1257–1261.

143 Kenward H, Elliott J, Lee T, *et al.* Anti-nausea effects and pharmacokinetics of ondansetron, maropitant and metoclopramide in a low-dose cisplatin model of nausea and vomiting in the dog: a blinded crossover study. *BMC Vet Res* 2017; **13**: 244.

144 de la Puente-Redondo VA, Tilt N, Rowan TG, *et al.* Efficacy of maropitant for treatment and prevention of emesis caused by intravenous infusion of cisplatin in dogs. *Am J Vet Res* 2007; **68**: 48–56.

145 de la Puente-Redondo VA, Siedek EM, Benchaoui HA, *et al.* The anti-emetic efficacy of maropitant (Cerenia) in the treatment of ongoing emesis caused by a wide range of underlying clinical aetiologies in canine patients in Europe. *J Small Anim Pract* 2007; **48**: 93–98.

146 Vail DM, Rodabaugh HS, Conder GA, *et al.* Efficacy of injectable maropitant (Cerenia) in a randomized clinical trial for prevention and treatment of cisplatin-induced emesis in dogs presented as veterinary patients. *Vet Comp Oncol* 2007; **5**: 38–46.
147 Rau SE, Barber LG, Burgess KE. Efficacy of maropitant in the prevention of delayed vomiting associated with administration of doxorubicin to dogs. *J Vet Intern Med* 2010; **24**: 1452–1457.
148 Ramsey DS, Kincaid K, Watkins JA, *et al.* Safety and efficacy of injectable and oral maropitant, a selective neurokinin 1 receptor antagonist, in a randomized clinical trial for treatment of vomiting in dogs. *J Vet Pharmacol Ther* 2008; **31**: 538–543.
149 Conder GA, Sedlacek HS, Boucher JF, *et al.* Efficacy and safety of maropitant, a selective neurokinin 1 receptor antagonist, in two randomized clinical trials for prevention of vomiting due to motion sickness in dogs. *J Vet Pharmacol Ther* 2008; **31**: 528–532.
150 Sedlacek HS, Ramsey DS, Boucher JF, *et al.* Comparative efficacy of maropitant and selected drugs in preventing emesis induced by centrally or peripherally acting emetogens in dogs. *J Vet Pharmacol Ther* 2008; **31**: 533–537.
151 Hay Kraus BL. Efficacy of maropitant in preventing vomiting in dogs premedicated with hydromorphone. *Vet Anaesth Analg* 2013; **40**: 28–34.
152 Johnson RA. Maropitant prevented vomiting but not gastroesophageal reflux in anesthetized dogs premedicated with acepromazine-hydromorphone. *Vet Anaesth Analg* 2014; **41**: 406–410.
153 Koh RB, Isaza N, Xie H, *et al.* Effects of maropitant, acepromazine, and electroacupuncture on vomiting associated with administration of morphine in dogs. *J Am Vet Med Assoc* 2014; **244**: 820–829.
154 Lorenzutti AM, Martín-Flores M, Litterio NJ, *et al.* Evaluation of the antiemetic efficacy of maropitant in dogs medicated with morphine and acepromazine. *Vet Anaesth Analg* 2016; **43**: 195–198.
155 Lorenzutti AM, Martín-Flores M, Litterio NJ, *et al.* A comparison between maropitant and metoclopramide for the prevention of morphine-induced nausea and vomiting in dogs. *Can Vet J* 2017; **58**: 35–38.
156 Ramsey D, Fleck T, Berg T, *et al.* Cerenia prevents perioperative nausea and vomiting and improves recovery in dogs undergoing routine surgery. *Intern J Appl Res Vet Med* 2014; **12**: 228–237.
157 Alvillar BM, Boscan P, Mama KR, *et al.* Effect of epidural and intravenous use of the neurokinin-1 (NK-1) receptor antagonist maropitant on the sevoflurane minimum alveolar concentration (MAC) in dogs. *Vet Anaesth Analg* 2012; 39: 201–205.
158 Boscan P, Monnet E, Mama K, *et al.* Effect of maropitant, a neurokinin 1 receptor antagonist, on anesthetic requirements during noxious visceral stimulation of the ovary in dogs. *Am J Vet Res* 2011; **72**: 1576–1579.
159 Niyom S, Boscan P, Twedt DC, *et al.* Effect of maropitant, a neurokinin-1 receptor antagonist, on the minimum alveolar concentration of sevoflurane during stimulation of the ovarian ligament in cats. *Vet Anaesth Analg* 2013; **40**: 425–431.
160 Inoue M, Kobayashi M, Kozaki S, *et al.* Nociceptin/orphanin FQ-induced nociceptive responses through substance P release from peripheral nerve endings in mice. *Proc Natl Acad Sci USA* 1998; **95**: 10949–10953.
161 Morris R, Cheunsuang O, Stewart A, *et al.* Spinal dorsal horn neurone targets for nociceptive primary afferents: do single neurone morphological characteristics suggest how nociceptive information is processed at the spinal level. *Brain Res Brain Res Rev* 2004; **46**: 173–190.
162 Mantyh PW, Gates T, Mantyh CR, *et al.* Autoradiographic localization and characterization of tachykinin receptor binding sites in the rat brain and peripheral tissues. *J Neurosci* 1989; **9**: 258–279.
163 Perry MJ, Lawson SN. Differences in expression of oligosaccharides, neuropeptides, carbonic anhydrase and neurofilament in rat primary afferent neurons retrogradely labelled via skin, muscle or visceral nerves. *Neuroscience* 1998; **85**: 293–310.
164 Swallow A, Rioja E, Elmer T, *et al.* The effect of maropitant on intraoperative isoflurane requirements and postoperative nausea and vomiting in dogs: a randomized clinical trial. *Vet Anaesth Analg* 2017; **44**: 785–793.
165 Corrêa JMX, Niella RV, Oliveira JNS, *et al.* Antinociceptive and analgesic effect of continuous intravenous infusion of maropitant, lidocaine and ketamine alone or in combination in cats undergoing ovariohysterectomy. *Acta Vet Scand* 2021; **63**: 49.
166 Fukui S, Ooyama N, Tamura J, *et al.* Interaction between maropitant and carprofen on sparing of the minimum alveolar concentration for blunting adrenergic response (MAC-BAR) of sevoflurane in dogs. *J Vet Med Sci* 2017; **79**: 502–508.
167 Valverde A, Cantwell S, Hernandez J, *et al.* Effects of acepromazine on the incidence of vomiting associated with opioid administration in dogs. *Vet Anaesth Analg* 2004; **31**: 40–45.
168 Claude AK, Dedeaux A, Chiavaccini L, *et al.* Effects of maropitant citrate or acepromazine on the incidence of adverse events associated with hydromorphone premedication in dogs. *J Vet Intern Med* 2014; **28**: 1414–1417.
169 Hay Kraus BL. Effect of dosing interval on efficacy of maropitant for prevention of hydromorphone-induced vomiting and signs of nausea in dogs. *J Am Vet Med Assoc* 2014; **245**: 1015–1020.
170 Martín-Flores M, Sakai DM, Mastrocco A, *et al.* Evaluation of oral maropitant as an antiemetic in cats receiving morphine and dexmedetomidine. *J Feline Med Surg* 2016; **18**: 921–924.
171 Martín-Flores M, Mastrocco A, Lorenzutti AM, *et al.* Maropitant administered orally 2–2.5 h prior to morphine and dexmedetomidine reduces the incidence of emesis in cats. *J Feline Med Surg* 2017; **19**: 876–879.
172 Hay Kraus BL. Efficacy of orally administered maropitant citrate in preventing vomiting associated with hydromorphone administration in dogs. *J Am Vet Med Assoc* 2014; **244**: 1164–1169.
173 Kanda T, Toda C, Morimoto H, *et al.* Antiemetic effect of oral maropitant treatment before the administration of brimonidine ophthalmic solution in healthy cats. *J Feline Med Surg* 2020; **22**: 557–563.
174 Kantyka ME, Meira C, Bettschart-Wolfensberger R, *et al.* Prospective, controlled, blinded, randomized crossover trial evaluating the effect of maropitant versus ondansetron on inhibiting tranexamic acid-evoked emesis. *J Vet Emerg Crit Care (San Antonio)* 2020; **30**: 436–441.
175 Marquez M, Boscan P, Weir H, *et al.* Comparison of NK-1 receptor antagonist (maropitant) to morphine as a pre-anaesthetic agent for canine ovariohysterectomy. *PLoS ONE* 2015; **10**: e0140734.
176 Armstrong T, Wagner MC, Cheema J, *et al.* Assessing analgesia equivalence and appetite following alfaxalone- or ketamine-based injectable anesthesia for feline castration as an example of enhanced recovery after surgery. *J Feline Med Surg* 2018; **20**: 73–82.
177 Hasiuk MM, Brown D, Cooney C, *et al.* Application of fast-track surgery principles to evaluate effects of atipamezole on recovery and analgesia following ovariohysterectomy in cats anesthetized with dexmedetomidine-ketamine-hydromorphone. *J Am Vet Med Assoc* 2015; **246**: 645–653.
178 Moser KL, Hasiuk MM, Armstrong T, *et al.* A randomized clinical trial comparing butorphanol and buprenorphine within a multimodal analgesic protocol in cats undergoing orchiectomy. *J Feline Med Surg* 2020; **22**: 760–767.
179 McCormack R, Olley L, Glanemann B, *et al.* Prospective observational study of the use of omeprazole and maropitant citrate in veterinary specialist care. *Sci Rep* 2020; **10**: 15727.
180 Chi TT, Hay Kraus BL. The effect of intravenous maropitant on blood pressure in healthy awake and anesthetized dogs. *PLoS ONE* 2020; **15**: e0229736.
181 Berryhill EH, Knych H, Edman JM, *et al.* Pharmacokinetics of single doses of maropitant citrate in adult horses. *J Vet Pharmacol Ther* 2019; **42**: 487–491.
182 Berryhill EH, Knych H, Chigerwe M, *et al.* Pharmacokinetics of maropitant citrate after oral administration of multiple doses in adult horses. *J Vet Pharmacol Ther* 2020; **43**: 282–287.
183 Lesman SP, Boucher JF, Grover GS, *et al.* The pharmacokinetics of maropitant citrate dosed orally to dogs at 2 mg/kg and 8 mg/kg once daily for 14 days consecutive days. *J Vet Pharmacol Ther* 2013; **36**: 462–470.
184 Mones AB, Petritz OA, Knych HK, *et al.* Pharmacokinetics of maropitant citrate in Rhode Island Red chickens (*Gallus gallus domesticus*) following subcutaneous administration. *J Vet Pharmacol Ther* 2022; **45**: 495–500.
185 Ozawa SM, Hawkins MG, Drazenovich TL, *et al.* Pharmacokinetics of maropitant citrate in New Zealand White rabbits (*Oryctolagus cuniculus*). *Am J Vet Res* 2019; **80**: 963–968.
186 Roszkowski AP. A pharmacological comparison of therapeutically useful centrally acting skeletal muscle relaxants. *J Pharmacol Exp Ther* 1960; **129**: 75–81.
187 Witkin LB, Spitaletta P, Galdi F, *et al.* Some neuropharmacologic effects of four mephenesin-like agents in mice. *Toxicol Appl Pharmacol* 1960; **2**: 264–269.
188 Valtonen EJ. A double-blind trial of methocarbamol versus placebo in painful muscle spasm. *Curr Med Res Opin* 1975; **3**: 382–385.
189 Simmonds EE, Alwood AJ, Costello MF. Magnesium sulfate as an adjunct therapy in the management of severe generalized tetanus in a dog. *J Vet Emerg Crit Care (San Antonio)* 2011; **21**:542–546.
190 Burkitt JM, Sturges BK, Jandrey KE, *et al.* Risk factors associated with outcome in dogs with tetanus: 38 cases (1987–2005). *J Am Vet Med Assoc* 2007; **230**: 76–83.
191 Bandt C, Rozanski EA, Steinberg T, *et al.* Retrospective study of tetanus in 20 dogs: 1988–2004. *J Am Anim Hosp Assoc* 2007; **43**: 143–148.
192 Boland LA, Angles JM. Feline permethrin toxicity: retrospective study of 42 cases. *J Feline Med Surg* 2010; **12**: 61–71.
193 Bates NS, Sutton NM, Campbell A. Suspected metaldehyde slug bait poisoning in dogs: a retrospective analysis of cases reported to the Veterinary Poisons Information Service. *Vet Rec* 2012; **171**: 324.
194 Richardson JA. Permethrin spot-on toxicosis in cats. *J Vet Emerg Crit Care* 2000; **10**: 103–106.
195 McLean MK, Khan S. A review of 29 incidents involving 4-aminopyridine in non-target species reported to the ASPCA Animal Poison Control Center. *J Med Toxicol* 2013; **9**: 418–421.
196 Peacock RE, Hosgood G, Swindells KL, *et al.* A randomized, controlled clinical trial of intravenous lipid emulsion as an adjunctive treatment for permethrin toxicosis in cats. *J Vet Emerg Crit Care (San Antonio)* 2015; **25**: 597–605.

197 Kuo K, Odunayo A. Adjunctive therapy with intravenous lipid emulsion and methocarbamol for permethrin toxicity in 2 cats. *J Vet Emerg Crit Care (San Antonio)* 2013; **23**: 436–441.
198 Draper WE, Bolfer L, Cottam E, *et al.* Methocarbamol CRI for symptomatic treatment of pyrethroid intoxication: a report of three cases. *J Am Anim Hosp Assoc* 2013; **49**: 325–328.
199 Muir WW, Sams RA, Ashcraft S. Pharmacologic and pharmacokinetic properties of methocarbamol in the horse. *Am J Vet Res* 1984; **45**: 2256–2260.
200 Muir WW, Sams RA, Ashcraft S. The pharmacology and pharmacokinetics of high-dose methocarbamol in horses. *Equine Vet J Suppl* 1992: 41–44.
201 Nielsen C, Pluhar GE. Diagnosis and treatment of hind limb muscle strain injuries in 22 dogs. *Vet Comp Orthop Traumatol* 2005; **18**: 247–253.
202 Bruce RB, Turnbull LB, Newman JH. Metabolism of methocarbamol in the rat, dog, and human. *J Pharm Sci* 1971; **60**: 104–106.
203 Cunningham FE, Fisher JH, Bevelle C, *et al.* The pharmacokinetics of methocarbamol in the Thoroughbred race horse. *J Vet Pharmacol Ther* 1992; **15**: 96–100.
204 Rumpler MJ, Colahan P, Sams RA. The pharmacokinetics of methocarbamol and guaifenesin after single intravenous and multiple-dose oral administration of methocarbamol in the horse. *J Vet Pharmacol Ther* 2014; **37**: 25–34.
205 Knych HK, Stanley SD, Seminoff KN, *et al.* Pharmacokinetics of methocarbamol and phenylbutazone in exercised Thoroughbred horses. *J Vet Pharmacol Ther* 2016; **39**: 469–477.
206 Dymond NL, Swift IM. Permethrin toxicity in cats: a retrospective study of 20 cases. *Aust Vet J* 2008; **86**: 219–223.
207 Brioschi FA, Di Cesare F, Gioeni D, *et al.* Oral transmucosal cannabidiol oil formulation as part of a multimodal analgesic regimen: effects on pain relief and quality of life improvement in dogs affected by spontaneous osteoarthritis. *Animals (Basel)* 2020; **10**: E1505.
208 Hall JA, Solie TN, Seim HB, *et al.* Effect of metoclopramide on fed-state gastric myoelectric and motor activity in dogs. *Am J Vet Res* 1996; **57**: 1616–1622.
209 Wilson DV, Evans AT, Mauer WA. Influence of metoclopramide on gastroesophageal reflux in anesthetized dogs. *Am J Vet Res* 2006; **67**: 26–31.
210 Husnik R, Gaschen FP, Fletcher JM, *et al.* Ultrasonographic assessment of the effect of metoclopramide, erythromycin, and exenatide on solid-phase gastric emptying in healthy cats. *J Vet Intern Med* 2020; **34**: 1440–1446.
211 Strombeck DR, Harrold D. Effect of gastrin, histamine, serotonin, and adrenergic amines on gastroesophageal sphincter pressure in the dog. *Am J Vet Res* 1985; **46**: 1684–1690.
212 Punto L, Mokka RE, Kairaluoma MI, *et al.* Effect of metoclopramide on the lower oesophageal sphincter. An experimental study in dogs. *Med Biol* 1977; **55**: 66–68.
213 Orihata M, Sarna SK. Contractile mechanisms of action of gastroprokinetic agents: cisapride, metoclopramide, and domperidone. *Am J Physiol* 1994; **266**: G665–G676.
214 Kempf J, Lewis F, Reusch CE, *et al.* High-resolution manometric evaluation of the effects of cisapride and metoclopramide hydrochloride administered orally on lower esophageal sphincter pressure in awake dogs. *Am J Vet Res* 2014; **75**: 361–366.
215 Milovancev M, Townsend K, Spina J, *et al.* Effect of metoclopramide on the incidence of early postoperative aspiration pneumonia in dogs with acquired idiopathic laryngeal paralysis. *Vet Surg* 2016; **45**: 577–581.
216 El-Khodery SA, Sato M. Ultrasonographic assessment of the reticular motility in cows after administration of different doses of metoclopramide and neostigmine. *Vet Res Commun* 2008; **32**: 473–480.
217 Watcha MF, White PF. Postoperative nausea and vomiting. Its etiology, treatment, and prevention. *Anesthesiology* 1992; **77**: 162–184.
218 Piana F, Minghella E. Extrapyramidal signs following a single intravenous dose of metoclopramide in an English Bulldog [letter]. *Vet Anaesth Analg* 2021; **48**: 977–978.
219 Bakke OM, Segura J. The absorption and elimination of metoclopramide in three animal species. *J Pharm Pharmacol* 1976; **28**: 32–39.
220 Kohn CW, Muir WW. Selected aspects of the clinical pharmacology of visceral analgesics and gut motility modifying drugs in the horse. *J Vet Intern Med* 1988; **2**: 85–91.
221 Sojka JE, Adams SB, Lamar CH, *et al.* Effect of butorphanol, pentazocine, meperidine, or metoclopramide on intestinal motility in female ponies. *Am J Vet Res* 1988; **49**: 527–529.
222 Wittek T, Constable PD. Assessment of the effects of erythromycin, neostigmine, and metoclopramide on abomasal motility and emptying rate in calves. *Am J Vet Res* 2005; **66**: 545–552.
223 Butler A, Hill JM, Ireland SJ, *et al.* Pharmacological properties of GR38032F, a novel antagonist at 5-HT3 receptors. *Br J Pharmacol* 1988; **94**: 397–412.
224 Sagrada A, Turconi M, Bonali P, *et al.* Antiemetic activity of the new 5-HT3 antagonist DAU 6215 in animal models of cancer chemotherapy and radiation. *Cancer Chemother Pharmacol* 1991; **28**: 470–474.
225 Fukui H, Yamamoto M, Sato S. Vagal afferent fibers and peripheral 5-HT3 receptors mediate cisplatin-induced emesis in dogs. *Jpn J Pharmacol* 1992; **59**: 221–226.
226 Miller AD, Nonaka S. Mechanisms of vomiting induced by serotonin-3 receptor agonists in the cat: effect of vagotomy, splanchnicectomy or area postrema lesion. *J Pharmacol Exp Ther* 1992; **260**: 509–517.
227 Ogilvie GK. Dolasetron: a new option for nausea and vomiting. *J Am Anim Hosp Assoc* 2000; **36**: 481–483.
228 Yalcin E, Keser GO. Comparative efficacy of metoclopramide, ondansetron and maropitant in preventing parvoviral enteritis-induced emesis in dogs. *J Vet Pharmacol Ther* 2017; **40**: 599–603.
229 Sullivan LA, Lenberg JP, Boscan P, *et al.* Assessing the efficacy of maropitant versus ondansetron in the treatment of dogs with parvoviral enteritis. *J Am Anim Hosp Assoc* 2018; **54**: 338–343.
230 Kopke MA, Wightman P, Ruaux CG. Obstructive sleep apnea in a Chihuahua successfully managed with ondansetron. *Clin Case Rep* 2019; **7**: 872–876.
231 Burke JE, Hess RS, Silverstein DC. Effectiveness of orally administered maropitant and ondansetron in preventing preoperative emesis and nausea in healthy dogs premedicated with a combination of hydromorphone, acepromazine, and glycopyrrolate. *J Am Vet Med Assoc* 2021; **260**: S40–S45.
232 Zarate E, Watcha MF, White PF, *et al.* A comparison of the costs and efficacy of ondansetron versus dolasetron for antiemetic prophylaxis. *Anesth Analg* 2000; **90**: 1352–1358.
233 United States Food and Drug Administration (FDA) Drug Safety Communication: Abnormal Heart Rhythms Associated with Use of Anzemet (Dolasetron Mesylate). 2010. www.fda.gov/drugs/drug-safety-and-availability/fda-drug-safety-communication-abnormal-heart-rhythms-associated-use-anzemet-dolasetron-mesylate (accessed September 2022).
234 Herndon AK, Quimby JM, Sieberg LG, *et al.* Preliminary pharmacokinetics of intravenous and subcutaneous dolasetron and pharmacodynamics of subcutaneous dolasetron in healthy cats. *J Feline Med Surg* 2018; **20**: 721–727.
235 Quimby JM, Lake RC, Hansen RJ, *et al.* Oral, subcutaneous, and intravenous pharmacokinetics of ondansetron in healthy cats. *J Vet Pharmacol Ther* 2014; **37**: 348–353.
236 Baek IH, Lee BY, Kang J, *et al.* Pharmacokinetic modeling and Monte Carlo simulation of ondansetron following oral administration in dogs. *J Vet Pharmacol Ther* 2015; **38**: 199–202.
237 Fitzpatrick RL, Wittenburg LA, Hansen RJ, *et al.* Limited sampling pharmacokinetics of subcutaneous ondansetron in healthy geriatric cats, cats with chronic kidney disease, and cats with liver disease. *J Vet Pharmacol Ther* 2016; **39**: 350–355.
238 Dow J, Francesco GF, Berg C. Comparison of the pharmacokinetics of dolasetron and its major active metabolite, reduced dolasetron, in dog. *J Pharm Sci* 1996; **85**: 685–689.
239 Somers GI, Harris AJ, Bayliss MK, *et al.* The metabolism of the 5HT3 antagonists ondansetron, alosetron and GR87442 I: a comparison of in vitro and in vivo metabolism and in vitro enzyme kinetics in rat, dog and human hepatocytes, microsomes and recombinant human enzymes. *Xenobiotica* 2007; **37**: 832–854.
240 Santos LC, Ludders JW, Erb HN, *et al.* A randomized, blinded, controlled trial of the antiemetic effect of ondansetron on dexmedetomidine-induced emesis in cats. *Vet Anaesth Analg* 2011; **38**: 320–327.
241 Chandler JC, Monnet E, Staatz AJ. Comparison of acute hemodynamic effects of lidocaine and procainamide for postoperative ventricular arrhythmias in dogs. *J Am Anim Hosp Assoc* 2006; **42**: 262–268.
242 Fries R, Saunders AB. Use of procainamide for conversion of acute onset AF following pericardiocentesis in a dog. *J Am Anim Hosp Assoc* 2012; **48**: 429–433.
243 Chou CC, Zhou S, Miyauchi Y, *et al.* Effects of procainamide on electrical activity in thoracic veins and atria in canine model of sustained atrial fibrillation. *Am J Physiol Heart Circ Physiol* 2004; **286**: H1936–H1945.
244 Caro-Vadillo A, Garcia-Guasch L, Carreton E, *et al.* Arrhythmogenic right ventricular cardiomyopathy in boxer dogs: a retrospective study of survival. *Vet Rec* 2013; **172**: 268.
245 Meurs KM, Spier AW, Wright NA, *et al.* Comparison of the effects of four antiarrhythmic treatments for familial ventricular arrhythmias in Boxers. *J Am Vet Med Assoc* 2002; **221**: 522–527.
246 Wijnberg ID, Ververs FF. Phenytoin sodium as a treatment for ventricular dysrhythmia in horses. *J Vet Intern Med* 2004; **18**: 350–353.
247 Barrell EA, Fiorenza LR, Perkins GA, *et al.* ECG of the Month. Persistent atrial tachycardia after cardioversion in a horse. *J Am Vet Med Assoc* 2015; **247**: 751–753.
248 Papich MG, Davis LE, Davis CA. Procainamide in the dog: antiarrhythmic plasma concentrations after intravenous administration. *J Vet Pharmacol Ther* 1986; **9**: 359–369.
249 Ellis EJ, Ravis WR, Malloy M, *et al.* The pharmacokinetics and pharmacodynamics of procainamide in horses after intravenous administration. *J Vet Pharmacol Ther* 1994; **17**: 265–270.

250 Thomason JD, Boothe D, KuKanich B, *et al.* Pharmacokinetic evaluation of a sustained-release compounded procainamide preparation after 24-h (acute) administration in normal dogs. *J Vet Cardiol* 2019; **24**: 58–63.

251 Forstermann U, Sessa WC. Nitric oxide synthases: regulation and function. *Eur Heart J* 2012; **33**: 829–837, 837a.

252 Ginn JA, Bentley E, Stepien RL. Systemic hypertension and hypertensive retinopathy following PPA overdose in a dog. *J Am Anim Hosp Assoc* 2013; **49**: 46–53.

253 Raisis AL, Mosing M, Hosgood GL, *et al.* The use of electrical impedance tomography (EIT) to evaluate pulse rate in anaesthetised horses. *Vet J* 2021; **273**: 105694.

254 Kurita T, Kawashima S, Morita K, *et al.* Assessment of cerebral and renal autoregulation using near-infrared spectroscopy under normal, hypovolaemic and post-fluid resuscitation conditions in a swine model: an observational study. *Eur J Anaesthesiol* 2019; **36**: 531–540.

255 Wilson KA, Raisis AL, Drynan EA, *et al.* Agreement between invasive blood pressure measured centrally and peripherally in anaesthetized horses. *Vet Anaesth Analg* 2018; **45**: 467–476.

256 Moore JC, Bartos JA, Matsuura TR, *et al.* The future is now: neuroprotection during cardiopulmonary resuscitation. *Curr Opin Crit Care* 2017; **23**: 215–222.

257 Kelm M. Nitric oxide metabolism and breakdown. *Biochim Biophys Acta* 1999; **1411**: 273–289.

258 Thomas C, Svehla L, Moffett BS. Sodium-nitroprusside-induced cyanide toxicity in pediatric patients. *Expert Opin Drug Saf* 2009; **8**: 599–602.

259 Michenfelder JD. Cyanide release from sodium nitroprusside in the dog. *Anesthesiology* 1977; **46**: 196–201.

260 Michenfelder JD, Tinker JH. Cyanide toxicity and thiosulfate protection during chronic administration of sodium nitroprusside in the dog: correlation with a human case. *Anesthesiology* 1977; **47**: 441–448.

261 Ivankovich AD, Braverman B, Shulman M, *et al.* Prevention of nitroprusside toxicity with thiosulfate in dogs. *Anesth Analg* 1982; **61**: 120–126.

262 Stahl SM. Mechanism of action of trazodone: a multifunctional drug. *CNS Spectr* 2009; **14**: 536–546.

263 Erickson A, Harbin K, MacPherson J, *et al.* A review of pre-appointment medications to reduce fear and anxiety in dogs and cats at veterinary visits. *Can Vet J* 2021; **62**: 952–960.

264 Indrawirawan Y, McAlees T. Tramadol toxicity in a cat: case report and literature review of serotonin syndrome. *J Feline Med Surg* 2014; **16**: 572–578.

265 Sinn L. Advances in behavioral psychopharmacology. *Vet Clin North Am Small Anim Pract* 2018; **48**: 457–471.

266 Orlando JM, Case BC, Thomson AE, *et al.* Use of oral trazodone for sedation in cats: a pilot study. *J Feline Med Surg* 2016; **18**: 476–482.

267 Stevens BJ, Frantz EM, Orlando JM, *et al.* Efficacy of a single dose of trazodone hydrochloride given to cats prior to veterinary visits to reduce signs of transport- and examination-related anxiety. *J Am Vet Med Assoc* 2016; **249**: 202–207.

268 Gruen ME, Roe SC, Griffith EH, *et al.* The use of trazodone to facilitate calm behavior after elective orthopedic surgery in dogs: results and lessons learned from a clinical trial. *J Vet Behav* 2017; **22**: 41–45.

269 Kim SA, Borchardt MR, Lee K, *et al.* Effects of trazodone on behavioral and physiological signs of stress in dogs during veterinary visits: a randomized double-blind placebo-controlled crossover clinical trial. *J Am Vet Med Assoc* 2022; **260**: 876–883.

270 Gruen ME, Roe SC, Griffith E, *et al.* Use of trazodone to facilitate postsurgical confinement in dogs. *J Am Vet Med Assoc* 2014; **245**: 296–301.

271 Gilbert-Gregory SE, Stull JW, Rice MR, *et al.* Effects of trazodone on behavioral signs of stress in hospitalized dogs. *J Am Vet Med Assoc* 2016; **249**: 1281–1291.

272 Moss AL, Hritz RL, Hector RC, *et al.* Investigation of the effects of orally administered trazodone on intraocular pressure, pupil diameter, physical examination variables, and sedation level in healthy equids. *Am J Vet Res* 2021; **82**: 138–143.

273 Davis JL, Schirmer J, Medlin E. Pharmacokinetics, pharmacodynamics and clinical use of trazodone and its active metabolite m-chlorophenylpiperazine in the horse. *J Vet Pharmacol Ther* 2018; **41**: 393–401.

274 Desmarchelier MR, Beaudry F, Ferrell ST, *et al.* Determination of the pharmacokinetics of a single oral dose of trazodone and its effect on the activity level of domestic pigeons (*Columba livia*). *Am J Vet Res* 2019; **80**: 102–109.

275 Walters K, Gittel C, Brearley JC. The effect of preanaesthetic oral trazodone hydrochloride on the induction dose of propofol: a preliminary retrospective study. *Vet Anaesth Analg* 2022: S1467–S2987(22)00073.

276 Murphy LA, Barletta M, Graham LF, *et al.* Effects of acepromazine and trazodone on anesthetic induction dose of propofol and cardiovascular variables in dogs undergoing general anesthesia for orthopedic surgery. *J Am Vet Med Assoc* 2017; **250**: 408–416.

277 Hoffman EA, Aarnes TK, Ricco Pereira CH, *et al.* Effect of oral trazodone on the minimum alveolar concentration of isoflurane in dogs. *Vet Anaesth Analg* 2018; **45**: 754–759.

278 Knych HK, Mama KR, Steffey EP, *et al.* Pharmacokinetics and selected pharmacodynamics of trazodone following intravenous and oral administration to horses undergoing fitness training. *Am J Vet Res* 2017; **78**: 1182–1192.

279 Prud'homme Y, Ferrell ST, Beaudry F, *et al.* Pharmacokinetics and clinical effects of a single oral dose of trazodone in the domestic goat (*Capra hircus*) as a model for wild ruminants. *J Zoo Wildl Med* 2021; **51**: 896–904.

280 Jay AR, Krotscheck U, Parsley E, *et al.* Pharmacokinetics, bioavailability, and hemodynamic effects of trazodone after intravenous and oral administration of a single dose to dogs. *Am J Vet Res* 2013; **74**: 1450–1456.

281 O'Donnell EM, Press SA, Karriker MJ, *et al.* Pharmacokinetics and efficacy of trazodone following rectal administration of a single dose to healthy dogs. *Am J Vet Res* 2020; **81**: 739–746.

282 Arnold A, Davis A, Wismer T, *et al.* Suspected hepatotoxicity secondary to trazodone therapy in a dog. *J Vet Emerg Crit Care (San Antonio)* 2021; **31**: 112–116.

283 Gomoll AW, Byrne JE. Trazodone and imipramine: comparative effects on canine cardiac conduction. *Eur J Pharmacol* 1979; **57**: 335–342.

284 Fries RC, Kadotani S, Vitt JP, *et al.* Effects of oral trazodone on echocardiographic and hemodynamic variables in healthy cats. *J Feline Med Surg* 2019; **21**: 1080–1085.

285 Hofmeister EH, Brainard BM, Egger CM, *et al.* Prognostic indicators for dogs and cats with cardiopulmonary arrest treated by cardiopulmonary cerebral resuscitation at a university teaching hospital. *J Am Vet Med Assoc* 2009; **235**: 50–57.

286 Dickey EJ, McKenzie H, Johnson A, *et al.* Use of pressor therapy in 34 hypotensive critically ill neonatal foals. *Aust Vet J* 2010; **88**: 472–477.

287 Buckley GJ, Rozanski EA, Rush JE. Randomized, blinded comparison of epinephrine and vasopressin for treatment of naturally occurring cardiopulmonary arrest in dogs. *J Vet Intern Med* 2011; **25**: 1334–1340.

288 Biondi-Zoccai GG, Abbate A, Parisi Q, *et al.* Is vasopressin superior to adrenaline or placebo in the management of cardiac arrest? *A meta-analysis. Resuscitation* 2003; **59**: 221–224.

289 Koshimizu TA, Nakamura K, Egashira N, *et al.* Vasopressin V1a and V1b receptors: from molecules to physiological systems. *Physiol Rev* 2012; **92**: 1813–1864.

290 Silverstein DC, Beer KA. Controversies regarding choice of vasopressor therapy for management of septic shock in animals. *J Vet Emerg Crit Care (San Antonio)* 2015; **25**: 48–54.

291 Schott HC. Water homeostasis and diabetes insipidus in horses. *Vet Clin North Am Equine Pract* 2011; **27**: 175–195.

292 Kranenburg LC, Thelen MH, Westermann CM, *et al.* Use of desmopressin eye drops in the treatment of equine congenital central diabetes insipidus. *Vet Rec* 2010; **167**: 790–791.

293 Simpson CJ, Mansfield CS, Milne ME, *et al.* Central diabetes insipidus in a cat with central nervous system B cell lymphoma. *J Feline Med Surg* 2011; **13**: 787–792.

294 Mansell PD, Parry BW. Changes in factor VIII: coagulant activity and von Willebrand factor antigen concentration after subcutaneous injection of desmopressin in dogs with mild hemophilia A. *J Vet Intern Med* 1991; **5**: 191–194.

295 Callan MB, Giger U. Effect of desmopressin acetate administration on primary hemostasis in Doberman Pinschers with type-1 von Willebrand disease as assessed by a point-of-care instrument. *Am J Vet Res* 2002; **63**: 1700–1706.

296 Hara Y, Masuda H, Taoda T, *et al.* Prophylactic efficacy of desmopressin acetate for diabetes insipidus after hypophysectomy in the dog. *J Vet Med Sci* 2003; **65**: 17–22.

297 Panchal AR, Bartos JA, Cabañas JG, *et al.* Part 3: adult basic and advanced life support: 2020 American Heart Association Guidelines for cardiopulmonary resuscitation and emergency cardiovascular care. *Circulation* 2020; **142**: S366–S468.

298 Fox AW, May RE, Mitch WE. Comparison of peptide and nonpeptide receptor-mediated responses in rat tail artery. *J Cardiovasc Pharmacol* 1992; **20**: 282–289.

299 Wenzel V, Lindner KH, Prengel AW, *et al.* Endobronchial vasopressin improves survival during cardiopulmonary resuscitation in pigs. *Anesthesiology* 1997; **86**: 1375–1381.

300 Reassessment Campaign on Veterinary Resuscitation (RECOVER). 2012. Available at: https://onlinelibrary.wiley.com/toc/14764431/2012/22/s1

301 Morales D, Madigan J, Cullinane S, *et al.* Reversal by vasopressin of intractable hypotension in the late phase of hemorrhagic shock. *Circulation* 1999; **100**: 226–229.

302 Cohn SM. Potential benefit of vasopressin in resuscitation of hemorrhagic shock. *J Trauma* 2007; **62**: S56–S57.

303 Russell JA. Bench-to-bedside review: vasopressin in the management of septic shock. *Crit Care* 2011; **15**: 226.

304 Murphy KM, Rishniw M, Silverstein DC. Use of vasopressors for treatment of vasodilatory hypotension in dogs and cats by Diplomates of the American College of Veterinary Emergency and Critical Care. *J Vet Emerg Crit Care (San Antonio)* 2022; **32**: 714–722.

305 Valverde A, Giguère S, Sanchez LC, *et al.* Effects of dobutamine, norepinephrine, and vasopressin on cardiovascular function in anesthetized neonatal foals with induced hypotension. *Am J Vet Res* 2006; **67**: 1730–1737.

306 Kraus KH, Turrentine MA, Jergens AE, *et al.* Effect of desmopressin acetate on bleeding times and plasma von Willebrand factor in Doberman pinscher dogs with von Willebrand's disease. *Vet Surg* 1989; **18**: 103–109.
307 Bebar KN, Sinnott V, Brooks MB. Recurrent hemorrhage caused by type 3 von Willebrand disease in a domestic long-haired cat. *J Vet Emerg Crit Care (San Antonio)* 2014; **24**: 326–331.
308 Fenn J, Kenny PJ, Scudder CJ, *et al.* Efficacy of hypophysectomy for the treatment of hypersomatotropism-induced diabetes mellitus in 68 cats. *J Vet Intern Med* 2021; **35**: 823–833.
309 Brooks MB, Catafalmo JL. Platelet disorders and von Willebrand disease. In: Ettinger SJ, Feldman EC, eds. *Textbook of Veterinary Internal Medicine*, 6th edn. St. Louis, MO: Elsevier Saunders, 2005: 1918–1929.
310 Di Mauro FM, Holowaychuk MK. Intravenous administration of desmopressin acetate to reverse acetylsalicylic acid-induced coagulopathy in three dogs. *J Vet Emerg Crit Care (San Antonio)* 2013; **23**: 455–458.
311 Sakai M, Watari T, Miura T, *et al.* Effects of DDAVP administrated subcutaneously in dogs with aspirin-induced platelet dysfunction and hemostatic impairment due to chronic liver diseases. *J Vet Med Sci* 2003; **65**: 83–86.
312 Jagodich TA, Holowaychuk MK. Transfusion practice in dogs and cats: an Internet-based survey. *J Vet Emerg Crit Care (San Antonio)* 2016; **26**: 360–372.
313 Grunert RR, McGahen JW, Davies WL. The in vivo antiviral activity of 1-adamantanamine (amantadine). I. Prophylactic and therapeutic activity against influenza viruses. *Virology* 1965; **26**: 262–269.
314 Lee SM, Yen HL. Targeting the host or the virus: current and novel concepts for antiviral approaches against influenza virus infection. *Antiviral Res* 2012; **96**: 391–404.
315 Hubsher G, Haider M, Okun MS. Amantadine: the journey from fighting flu to treating Parkinson disease. *Neurology* 2012; **78**: 1096–1099.
316 Schwab RS, England AC, Poskanzer DC, *et al.* Amantadine in the treatment of Parkinson's disease. *JAMA* 1969; **208**: 1168–1170.
317 Wheaton P, Mathias JL, Vink R. Impact of early pharmacological treatment on cognitive and behavioral outcome after traumatic brain injury in adults: a meta-analysis. *J Clin Psychopharmacol* 2009; **29**: 468–477.
318 Frenette AJ, Kanji S, Rees L, *et al.* Efficacy and safety of dopamine agonists in traumatic brain injury: a systematic review of randomized controlled trials. *J Neurotrauma* 2012; **29**: 1–18.
319 Saniova B, Drobny M, Kneslova L, *et al.* The outcome of patients with severe head injuries treated with amantadine sulphate. *J Neural Transm* 2004; **111**: 511–514.
320 Giacino JT, Whyte J, Bagiella E, *et al.* Placebo-controlled trial of amantadine for severe traumatic brain injury. *N Engl J Med* 2012; **366**: 819–826.
321 Wang T, Huang XJ, Van KC, *et al.* Amantadine improves cognitive outcome and increases neuronal survival after fluid percussion traumatic brain injury in rats. *J Neurotrauma* 2014; **31**: 370–377.
322 Ma HM, Zafonte RD. Amantadine and memantine: a comprehensive review for acquired brain injury. *Brain Inj* 2020; **34**: 299–315.
323 Robertson SA. Managing pain in feline patients. *Vet Clin North Am Small Anim Pract* 2008; **38**: 1267–1290, vi.
324 Lascelles BD, Gaynor JS, Smith ES, *et al.* Amantadine in a multimodal analgesic regimen for alleviation of refractory osteoarthritis pain in dogs. *J Vet Intern Med* 2008; **22**: 53–59.
325 Suzuki M. Role of N-methyl-D-aspartate receptor antagonists in postoperative pain management. *Curr Opin Anaesthesiol* 2009; **22**: 618–622.
326 Eisenberg E, Pud D. Can patients with chronic neuropathic pain be cured by acute administration of the NMDA receptor antagonist amantadine? *Pain* 1998; **74**: 337–339.
327 Collins S, Sigtermans MJ, Dahan A, *et al.* NMDA receptor antagonists for the treatment of neuropathic pain. *Pain Med* 2010; **11**: 1726–1742.
328 Pozzi A, Muir WW, Traverso F. Prevention of central sensitization and pain by N-methyl-D-aspartate receptor antagonists. *J Am Vet Med Assoc* 2006; **228**: 53–60.
329 Norkus C, Rankin D, Warner M, *et al.* Pharmacokinetics of oral amantadine in greyhound dogs. *J Vet Pharmacol Ther* 2015; **38**: 305–308.
330 Madden M, Gurney M, Bright S. Amantadine, an N-Methyl-D-Aspartate antagonist, for treatment of chronic neuropathic pain in a dog. *Vet Anaesth Analg* 2014; **41**: 440–441.
331 Shipley H, Flynn K, Tucker L, *et al.* Owner evaluation of quality of life and mobility in osteoarthritic cats treated with amantadine or placebo. *J Feline Med Surg* 2021; **23**: 568–574.
332 Siao KT, Pypendop BH, Stanley SD, *et al.* Pharmacokinetics of amantadine in cats. *J Vet Pharmacol Ther* 2011; **34**: 599–604.
333 Siao KT, Pypendop BH, Escobar A, *et al.* Effect of amantadine on oxymorphone-induced thermal antinociception in cats. *J Vet Pharmacol Ther* 2012; **35**: 169–174.
334 KuKanich B. Outpatient oral analgesics in dogs and cats beyond nonsteroidal anti-inflammatory drugs: an evidence-based approach. *Vet Clin North Am Small Anim Pract* 2013; **43**: 1109–1125.
335 Gardner BR, Rourke NL. Multimodal analgesia in a Southern White Rhinoceros (*Ceratotherium simum*) with pentosan polysulfate, gabapentin, amantadine and phenylbutazone to manage chronic pain. *Aust Vet J* 2021; **99**: 86–88.
336 Berg KJ, Sanchez-Migallon Guzman D, Knych HK, *et al.* Pharmacokinetics of amantadine after oral administration of single and multiple doses to orange-winged Amazon parrots (*Amazona amazonica*). *Am J Vet Res* 2020; **81**: 651–655.
337 Bleidner WE, Harmon JB, Hewes WE, *et al.* Absorption, distribution and excretion of amantadine hydrochloride. *J Pharmacol Exp Ther* 1965; **150**: 484–490.
338 Chen YW, Chu CC, Chen YC, *et al.* The local anesthetic effect of memantine on infiltrative cutaneous analgesia in the rat. *Anesth Analg* 2011; **113**: 191–195.
339 Crowell-Davis SL, Poggiagliolmi S. Understanding behavior: serotonin syndrome. *Compend Contin Educ Vet* 2008; **30**: 490–493.
340 Mohammad-Zadeh LF, Moses L, Gwaltney-Brant SM. Serotonin: a review. *J Vet Pharmacol Ther* 2008; **31**: 187–199.
341 Pugh CM, Sweeney JT, Bloch CP, *et al.* Selective serotonin reuptake inhibitor (SSRI) toxicosis in cats: 33 cases (2004–2010). *J Vet Emerg Crit Care (San Antonio)* 2013; **23**: 565–570.
342 Thomas DE, Lee JA, Hovda LR. Retrospective evaluation of toxicosis from selective serotonin reuptake inhibitor antidepressants: 313 dogs (2005–2010). *J Vet Emerg Crit Care (San Antonio)* 2012; **22**: 674–681.
343 Kitson R, Carr B. Tramadol and severe serotonin syndrome. *Anaesthesia* 2005; **60**: 934–935.
344 Gillman PK. Monoamine oxidase inhibitors, opioid analgesics and serotonin toxicity. *Br J Anaesth* 2005; **95**: 434–441.
345 Chen YW, Shieh JP, Chen YC, *et al.* Cutaneous analgesia after subcutaneous injection of memantine and amantadine and their systemic toxicity in rats. *Eur J Pharmacol* 2012; **693**: 25–30.
346 Gray A. Veterinary use of amantadine under threat. *Vet Rec* 2022; **191**: 11.
347 Overall KL, Dunham AE. Clinical features and outcome in dogs and cats with obsessive-compulsive disorder: 126 cases (1989–2000). *J Am Vet Med Assoc* 2002; **221**: 1445–1452.
348 Kraijer M, Fink-Gremmels J, Nickel RF. The short-term clinical efficacy of amitriptyline in the management of idiopathic feline lower urinary tract disease: a controlled clinical study. *J Feline Med Surg* 2003; **5**: 191–196.
349 Kruger JM, Conway TS, Kaneene JB, *et al.* Randomized controlled trial of the efficacy of short-term amitriptyline administration for treatment of acute, nonobstructive, idiopathic lower urinary tract disease in cats. *J Am Vet Med Assoc* 2003; **222**: 749–758.
350 Cashmore RG, Harcourt-Brown TR, Freeman PM, *et al.* Clinical diagnosis and treatment of suspected neuropathic pain in three dogs. *Aust Vet J* 2009; **87**: 45–50.
351 O'Hagan BJ. Neuropathic pain in a cat post-amputation. *Aust Vet J* 2006; **84**: 83–86.
352 Amengual Batle P, Rusbridge C, Nuttall T, *et al.* Feline hyperaesthesia syndrome with self-trauma to the tail: retrospective study of seven cases and proposal for an integrated multidisciplinary diagnostic approach. *J Feline Med Surg* 2019; **21**: 178–185.
353 Wang GK, Russell C, Wang SY. State-dependent block of voltage-gated Na+ channels by amitriptyline via the local anesthetic receptor and its implication for neuropathic pain. *Pain* 2004; **110**: 166–174.
354 Yaksh TL, Tozier N, Horais KA, *et al.* Toxicology profile of N-methyl-D-aspartate antagonists delivered by intrathecal infusion in the canine model. *Anesthesiology* 2008; **108**: 938–949.
355 Irman-Florjanc T, Stanovnik L. Tricyclic antidepressants change plasma histamine kinetics after its secretion induced by compound 48/80 in the rat. *Inflamm Res* 1998; **47**(Suppl 1): S26–S27.
356 Bohren Y, Karavelic D, Tessier LH, *et al.* Mu-opioid receptors are not necessary for nortriptyline treatment of neuropathic allodynia. *Eur J Pain* 2010; **14**: 700–704.
357 Chew DJ, Buffington CA, Kendall MS, *et al.* Amitriptyline treatment for severe recurrent idiopathic cystitis in cats. *J Am Vet Med Assoc* 1998; **213**: 1282–1286.
358 Monteiro BP, de Lorimier LP, Moreau M, *et al.* Pain characterization and response to palliative care in dogs with naturally-occurring appendicular osteosarcoma: an open label clinical trial. *PLoS ONE* 2018; **13**: e0207200.
359 Rusbridge C, Jeffery ND. Pathophysiology and treatment of neuropathic pain associated with syringomyelia. *Vet J* 2008; **175**: 164–172.
360 Newton SA, Knottenbelt DC, Eldridge PR. Headshaking in horses: possible aetiopathogenesis suggested by the results of diagnostic tests and several treatment regimes used in 20 cases. *Equine Vet J* 2000; **32**: 208–216.
361 Hucker HB, Balletto AJ, Demetriades J, *et al.* Urinary metabolites of amitriptyline in the dog. *Drug Metab Dispos* 1977; **5**: 132–142.
362 Dworkin RH, O'Connor AB, Backonja M, *et al.* Pharmacologic management of neuropathic pain: evidence-based recommendations. *Pain* 2007; **132**: 237–251.
363 Mealey KL, Peck KE, Bennett BS, *et al.* Systemic absorption of amitriptyline and buspirone after oral and transdermal administration to healthy cats. *J Vet Intern Med* 2004; **18**: 43–46.

364 Recchi L, Alvariza S, Benech A, *et al.* Pharmacokinetic study of oral amitriptyline in horses. *J Vet Pharmacol Ther* 2020; **43**: 381–384.
365 Norkus C, Rankin D, KuKanich B. Evaluation of the pharmacokinetics of oral amitriptyline and its active metabolite nortriptyline in fed and fasted Greyhound dogs. *J Vet Pharmacol Ther* 2015; **38**: 619–622.
366 Kukes VG, Kondratenko SN, Savelyeva MI, *et al.* Experimental and clinical pharmacokinetics of amitriptyline: comparative analysis. *Bull Exp Biol Med* 2009; **147**: 434–437.
367 Nattel S, Keable H, Sasyniuk BI. Experimental amitriptyline intoxication: electrophysiologic manifestations and management. *J Cardiovasc Pharmacol* 1984; **6**: 83–89.
368 Kwok YH, Mitchelson F. Comparison of the antimuscarinic activity of mianserin and amitriptyline in the cat superior cervical ganglion. *Naunyn Schmiedebergs Arch Pharmacol* 1981; **316**: 161–164.
369 Tsujikawa S, Matsuura T, Hori K, *et al.* Superior efficacy of lipid emulsion infusion over serum alkalinization in reversing amitriptyline-induced cardiotoxicity in guinea pig. *Anesth Analg* 2018; **126**: 1159–1169.
370 Reich MR, Ohad DG, Overall KL, *et al.* Electrocardiographic assessment of antianxiety medication in dogs and correlation with serum drug concentration. *J Am Vet Med Assoc* 2000; **216**: 1571–1575.
371 Kogan L, Schoenfeld-Tacher R, Hellyer P, *et al.* US veterinarians' knowledge, experience, and perception regarding the use of cannabidiol for canine medical conditions. *Front Vet Sci* 2018; **5**: 338.
372 Kogan LR, Hellyer PW, Silcox S, *et al.* Canadian dog owners' use and perceptions of cannabis products. *Can Vet J* 2019; **60**: 749–755.
373 Lima TM, Santiago NR, Alves ECR, *et al.* Use of cannabis in the treatment of animals: a systematic review of randomized clinical trials. *Anim Health Res Rev* 2022; **23**: 25–38.
374 R C Coelho MP, de O P Leme F, A Moreira F, *et al.* Current review of hemp-based medicines in dogs. *J Vet Pharmacol Ther* 2021; **44**: 870–882.
375 Abramo F, Campora L, Albanese F, *et al.* Increased levels of palmitoylethanolamide and other bioactive lipid mediators and enhanced local mast cell proliferation in canine atopic dermatitis. *BMC Vet Res* 2014; **10**: 21.
376 Valastro C, Campanile D, Marinaro M, *et al.* Characterization of endocannabinoids and related acylethanolamides in the synovial fluid of dogs with osteoarthritis: a pilot study. *BMC Vet Res* 2017; **13**: 309.
377 Morrow L, Belshaw Z. Does the addition of cannabidiol alongside current drug treatments reduce pain in dogs with osteoarthritis? *Vet Rec* 2020; **186**: 493–494.
378 Gamble LJ, Boesch JM, Frye CW, *et al.* Pharmacokinetics, safety, and clinical efficacy of cannabidiol treatment in osteoarthritic dogs. *Front Vet Sci* 2018; **5**: 165.
379 Verrico CD, Wesson S, Konduri V, *et al.* A randomized, double-blind, placebo-controlled study of daily cannabidiol for the treatment of canine osteoarthritis pain. *Pain* 2020; **161**: 2191–2202.
380 Mejia S, Duerr FM, Griffenhagen G, *et al.* Evaluation of the effect of cannabidiol on naturally occurring osteoarthritis-associated pain: a pilot study in dogs. *J Am Anim Hosp Assoc* 2021; **57**: 81–90.
381 Loewinger M, Wakshlag JJ, Bowden D, *et al.* The effect of a mixed cannabidiol and cannabidiolic acid based oil on client-owned dogs with atopic dermatitis. *Vet Dermatol* 2022; **33**: 329–e77.
382 McGrath S, Bartner LR, Rao S, *et al.* Randomized blinded controlled clinical trial to assess the effect of oral cannabidiol administration in addition to conventional antiepileptic treatment on seizure frequency in dogs with intractable idiopathic epilepsy. *J Am Vet Med Assoc* 2019; **254**: 1301–1308.
383 Corsetti S, Borruso S, Malandrucco L, *et al. Cannabis sativa* L. may reduce aggressive behaviour towards humans in shelter dogs. *Sci Rep* 2021; **11**: 2773.
384 Vaughn DM, Paulionis LJ, Kulpa JE. Randomized, placebo-controlled, 28-day safety and pharmacokinetics evaluation of repeated oral cannabidiol administration in healthy dogs. *Am J Vet Res* 2021; **82**: 405–416.
385 Schaefer N, Wojtyniak JG, Kettner M, *et al.* Pharmacokinetics of (synthetic) cannabinoids in pigs and their relevance for clinical and forensic toxicology. *Toxicol Lett* 2016; **253**: 7–16.
386 Williams MR, Holbrook TC, Maxwell L, *et al.* Pharmacokinetic evaluation of a cannabidiol supplement in horses. *J Equine Vet Sci* 2022; **110**: 103842.
387 Deabold KA, Schwark WS, Wolf L, *et al.* Single-dose pharmacokinetics and preliminary safety assessment with use of CBD-rich hemp nutraceutical in healthy dogs and cats. *Animals (Basel)* 2019; **9**: E832.
388 Ryan D, McKemie DS, Kass PH, *et al.* Pharmacokinetics and effects on arachidonic acid metabolism of low doses of cannabidiol following oral administration to horses. *Drug Test Anal* 2021; **13**: 1305–1317.
389 Polidoro D, Temmerman R, Devreese M, *et al.* Pharmacokinetics of cannabidiol following intranasal, intrarectal, and oral administration in healthy dogs. *Front Vet Sci* 2022; **9**: 899940.
390 Spittler AP, Helbling JE, McGrath S, *et al.* Plasma and joint tissue pharmacokinetics of two doses of oral cannabidiol oil in guinea pigs (*Cavia porcellus*). *J Vet Pharmacol Ther* 2021; **44**: 967–974.
391 Bartner LR, McGrath S, Rao S, *et al.* Pharmacokinetics of cannabidiol administered by 3 delivery methods at 2 different dosages to healthy dogs. *Can J Vet Res* 2018; **82**: 178–183.
392 Chicoine A, Illing K, Vuong S, *et al.* Pharmacokinetic and safety evaluation of various oral doses of a novel 1:20 THC:CBD cannabis herbal extract in dogs. *Front Vet Sci* 2020; **7**: 583404.
393 Samara E, Bialer M, Mechoulam R. Pharmacokinetics of cannabidiol in dogs. *Drug Metab Dispos* 1988; **16**: 469–472.
394 Brutlag A, Hommerding H. Toxicology of marijuana, synthetic cannabinoids, and cannabidiol in dogs and cats. *Vet Clin North Am Small Anim Pract* 2018; **48**: 1087–1102.
395 De Briyne N, Holmes D, Sandler I, *et al.* Cannabis, cannabidiol oils and tetrahydrocannabinol-what do veterinarians need to know. *Animals (Basel)* 2021; **11**: 892.
396 Vaughn D, Kulpa J, Paulionis L. Preliminary investigation of the safety of escalating cannabinoid doses in healthy dogs. *Front Vet Sci* 2020; **7**: 51.
397 Wakshlag JJ, Schwark WS, Deabold KA, *et al.* Pharmacokinetics of cannabidiol, cannabidiolic acid, Δ9-tetrahydrocannabinol, tetrahydrocannabinolic acid and related metabolites in canine serum after dosing with three oral forms of hemp extract. *Front Vet Sci* 2020; **7**: 505.
398 Meola SD, Tearney CC, Haas SA, *et al.* Evaluation of trends in marijuana toxicosis in dogs living in a state with legalized medical marijuana: 125 dogs (2005–2010). *J Vet Emerg Crit Care (San Antonio)* 2012; **22**: 690–696.
399 Amissah RQ, Vogt NA, Chen C, *et al.* Prevalence and characteristics of cannabis-induced toxicoses in pets: results from a survey of veterinarians in North America. *PLoS ONE* 2022; **17**: e0261909.
400 Thompson GR, Rosenkrantz H, Schaeppi UH, *et al.* Comparison of acute oral toxicity of cannabinoids in rats, dogs and monkeys. *Toxicol Appl Pharmacol* 1973; **25**: 363–372.
401 Kulpa JE, Paulionis LJ, Eglit GM, *et al.* Safety and tolerability of escalating cannabinoid doses in healthy cats. *J Feline Med Surg* 2021; **23**: 1162–1175.
402 Abbass K. Efficacy of gabapentin for treatment of adults with phantom limb pain. *Ann Pharmacother* 2012; **46**: 1707–1711.
403 Chaparro LE, Smith SA, Moore RA, *et al.* Pharmacotherapy for the prevention of chronic pain after surgery in adults. *Cochrane Database Syst Rev* 2013; **7**: CD008307.
404 Snedecor SJ, Sudharshan L, Cappelleri JC, *et al.* Systematic review and comparison of pharmacologic therapies for neuropathic pain associated with spinal cord injury. *J Pain Res* 2013; **6**: 539–547.
405 Zakkar M, Frazer S, Hunt I. Is there a role for gabapentin in preventing or treating pain following thoracic surgery? *Interact Cardiovasc Thorac Surg* 2013; **17**: 716–719.
406 Carley ME, Chaparro LE, Choinière M, *et al.* Pharmacotherapy for the prevention of chronic pain after surgery in adults: an updated systematic review and meta-analysis [editorial]. *Anesthesiology* 2021; **135**: 304–325.
407 Verret M, Lauzier F, Zarychanski R, *et al.* Perioperative use of gabapentinoids for the management of postoperative acute pain: a systematic review and meta-analysis. *Anesthesiology* 2020; **133**: 265–279.
408 Aghighi SA, Tipold A, Piechotta M, *et al.* Assessment of the effects of adjunctive gabapentin on postoperative pain after intervertebral disc surgery in dogs. *Vet Anaesth Analg* 2012; **39**: 636–646.
409 Plessas IN, Rusbridge C, Driver CJ, *et al.* Long-term outcome of Cavalier King Charles spaniel dogs with clinical signs associated with Chiari-like malformation and syringomyelia. *Vet Rec* 2012; **171**: 501.
410 Wagner AE, Mich PM, Uhrig SR, *et al.* Clinical evaluation of perioperative administration of gabapentin as an adjunct for postoperative analgesia in dogs undergoing amputation of a forelimb. *J Am Vet Med Assoc* 2010; **236**: 751–756.
411 Kukanich B, Cohen RL. Pharmacokinetics of oral gabapentin in greyhound dogs. *Vet J* 2011; **187**: 133–135.
412 Ruel HLM, Watanabe R, Evangelista MC, *et al.* Pain burden, sensory profile and inflammatory cytokines of dogs with naturally-occurring neuropathic pain treated with gabapentin alone or with meloxicam. *PLoS ONE* 2020; **15**: e0237121.
413 Pypendop BH, Siao KT, Ilkiw JE. Thermal antinociceptive effect of orally administered gabapentin in healthy cats. *Am J Vet Res* 2010; **71**: 1027–1032.
414 Siao KT, Pypendop BH, Ilkiw JE. Pharmacokinetics of gabapentin in cats. *Am J Vet Res* 2010; **71**: 817–821.
415 Reid P, Pypendop BH, Ilkiw JE. The effects of intravenous gabapentin administration on the minimum alveolar concentration of isoflurane in cats. *Anesth Analg* 2010; **111**: 633–637.
416 Vettorato E, Corletto F. Gabapentin as part of multi-modal analgesia in two cats suffering multiple injuries. *Vet Anaesth Analg* 2011; **38**: 518–520.
417 Steagall PV, Benito J, Monteiro BP, *et al.* Analgesic effects of gabapentin and buprenorphine in cats undergoing ovariohysterectomy using two pain-scoring systems: a randomized clinical trial. *J Feline Med Surg* 2018; **20**: 741–748.

418 Dirikolu L, Dafalla A, Ely KJ, *et al.* Pharmacokinetics of gabapentin in horses. *J Vet Pharmacol Ther* 2008; **31**: 175–177.
419 Terry RL, McDonnell SM, Van Eps AW, *et al.* Pharmacokinetic profile and behavioral effects of gabapentin in the horse. *J Vet Pharmacol Ther* 2010; **33**: 485–494.
420 Dutton DW, Lasnhnits KJ, Wegner K. Managing severe hoof pain in a horse using multimodal analgesia and a modified composite pain score. *Equine vet Educ* 2009; **21**: 37–43.
421 Davis JL, Posner LP, Elce Y. Gabapentin for the treatment of neuropathic pain in a pregnant horse. *J Am Vet Med Assoc* 2007; **231**: 755–758.
422 Coetzee JF, Mosher RA, Kohake LE, *et al.* Pharmacokinetics of oral gabapentin alone or co-administered with meloxicam in ruminant beef calves. *Vet J* 2011; **190**: 98–102.
423 Glynn HD, Coetzee JF, Edwards-Callaway LN, *et al.* The pharmacokinetics and effects of meloxicam, gabapentin, and flunixin in postweaning dairy calves following dehorning with local anesthesia. *J Vet Pharmacol Ther* 2013; **36**: 550–561.
424 Malreddy PR, Coetzee JF, Kukanich B, *et al.* Pharmacokinetics and milk secretion of gabapentin and meloxicam co-administered orally in Holstein-Friesian cows. *J Vet Pharmacol Ther* 2013; **36**: 14–20.
425 Chincholkar M. Analgesic mechanisms of gabapentinoids and effects in experimental pain models: a narrative review. *Br J Anaesth* 2018; **120**: 1315–1334.
426 Taylor CP. Mechanisms of analgesia by gabapentin and pregabalin--calcium channel alpha2-delta [Cavalpha2-delta] ligands. *Pain* 2009; **142**: 13–16.
427 Field MJ, Cox PJ, Stott E, *et al.* Identification of the alpha2-delta-1 subunit of voltage-dependent calcium channels as a molecular target for pain mediating the analgesic actions of pregabalin. *Proc Natl Acad Sci USA* 2006; **103**: 17537–17542.
428 Radulovic LL, Türck D, von Hodenberg A, *et al.* Disposition of gabapentin (neurontin) in mice, rats, dogs, and monkeys. *Drug Metab Dispos* 1995; **23**: 441–448.
429 Lamminen T, Doedée A, Hyttilä-Hopponen M, *et al.* Pharmacokinetics of single and repeated oral doses of pregabalin oral solution formulation in cats. *J Vet Pharmacol Ther* 2022; **45**: 385–391.
430 Mullen KR, Schwark W, Divers TJ. Pharmacokinetics of single-dose intragastric and intravenous pregabalin administration in clinically normal horses. *Am J Vet Res* 2013; **74**: 1043–1048.
431 Hampton CE, Queiroz-Williams P, Oubre MJ, *et al.* Pharmacokinetics of oral and compounded intravenous gabapentin in Duroc swine (*Sus Scrofa*). *J Vet Pharmacol Ther* 2021; **44**: 776–782.
432 Gold JR, Grubb TL, Cox S, *et al.* Pharmacokinetics and pharmacodynamics of repeat dosing of gabapentin in adult horses. *J Vet Intern Med* 2022; **36**: 792–797.
433 Bockbrader HN, Wesche D, Miller R, *et al.* A comparison of the pharmacokinetics and pharmacodynamics of pregabalin and gabapentin. *Clin Pharmacokinet* 2010; **49**: 661–669.
434 Sanchis-Mora S, Chang YM, Abeyesinghe SM, *et al.* Pregabalin for the treatment of syringomyelia-associated neuropathic pain in dogs: a randomised, placebo-controlled, double-masked clinical trial. *Vet J* 2019; **250**: 55–62.
435 Thoefner MS, Skovgaard LT, McEvoy FJ, *et al.* Pregabalin alleviates clinical signs of syringomyelia-related central neuropathic pain in Cavalier King Charles Spaniel dogs: a randomized controlled trial. *Vet Anaesth Analg* 2020; **47**: 238–248.
436 Plessas IN, Volk HA, Rusbridge C, *et al.* Comparison of gabapentin versus topiramate on clinically affected dogs with Chiari-like malformation and syringomyelia. *Vet Rec* 2015; **177**: 288.
437 Salazar V, Dewey CW, Schwark W, *et al.* Pharmacokinetics of single-dose oral pregabalin administration in normal dogs. *Vet Anaesth Analg* 2009; **36**: 574–580.
438 Schmierer PA, Tünsmeyer J, Tipold A, *et al.* Randomized controlled trial of pregabalin for analgesia after surgical treatment of intervertebral disc disease in dogs. *Vet Surg* 2020; **49**: 905–913.
439 Brennan FH, Noble BT, Wang Y, *et al.* Acute post-injury blockade of α2δ-1 calcium channel subunits prevents pathological autonomic plasticity after spinal cord injury. *Cell Rep* 2021; **34**: 108667.
440 Boroujerdi A, Zeng J, Sharp K, *et al.* Calcium channel alpha-2-delta-1 protein upregulation in dorsal spinal cord mediates spinal cord injury-induced neuropathic pain states. *Pain* 2011; **152**: 649–655.
441 Johnson BA, Aarnes TK, Wanstrath AW, *et al.* Effect of oral administration of gabapentin on the minimum alveolar concentration of isoflurane in dogs. *Am J Vet Res* 2019; **80**: 1007–1009.
442 Bleuer-Elsner S, Medam T, Masson S. Effects of a single oral dose of gabapentin on storm phobia in dogs: a double-blind, placebo-controlled crossover trial. *Vet Rec* 2021; **189**: e453.
443 Adrian D, Papich MG, Baynes R, *et al.* The pharmacokinetics of gabapentin in cats. *J Vet Intern Med* 2018; **32**: 1996–2002.
444 Quimby JM, Lorbach SK, Saffire A, *et al.* Serum concentrations of gabapentin in cats with chronic kidney disease. *J Feline Med Surg* 2022; **24**: 1260–1266.
445 Lorenz ND, Comerford EJ, Iff I. Long-term use of gabapentin for musculoskeletal disease and trauma in three cats. *J Feline Med Surg* 2013; **15**: 507–512.
446 Esteban MA, Dewey CW, Schwark WS, *et al.* Pharmacokinetics of single-dose oral pregabalin administration in normal cats. *Front Vet Sci* 2018; **5**: 136.
447 Clark L, Doyle RS, Shroeder S. Skin lesions following pregabalin administration in a cat. *Vet Anaesth Analg* 2017; **44**: 383–385.
448 van Haaften KA, Forsythe LRE, Stelow EA, *et al.* Effects of a single preappointment dose of gabapentin on signs of stress in cats during transportation and veterinary examination. *J Am Vet Med Assoc* 2017; **251**: 1175–1181.
449 Gurney M, Gower L. Randomised clinical trial evaluating the effect of a single preappointment dose of gabapentin on signs of stress in hyperthyroid cats. *J Feline Med Surg* 2022; **24**: e85–e89.
450 Lamminen T, Korpivaara M, Suokko M, *et al.* Efficacy of a single dose of pregabalin on signs of anxiety in cats during transportation-a pilot study. *Front Vet Sci* 2021; **8**: 711816.
451 Young JM, Schoonover MJ, Kembel SL, *et al.* Efficacy of orally administered gabapentin in horses with chronic thoracic limb lameness. *Vet Anaesth Analg* 2020; **47**: 259–266.
452 Raffa RB, Buschmann H, Christoph T, *et al.* Mechanistic and functional differentiation of tapentadol and tramadol. *Expert Opin Pharmacother* 2012; **13**: 1437–1449.
453 Tzschentke TM, Christoph T, Kögel B, *et al.* (-)-(1R,2R)-3-(3-dimethylamino-1-ethyl-2-methyl-propyl)-phenol hydrochloride (tapentadol HCl): a novel mu-opioid receptor agonist/norepinephrine reuptake inhibitor with broad-spectrum analgesic properties. *J Pharmacol Exp Ther* 2007; **323**: 265–276.
454 Giorgi M, Meizler A, Mills PC. Pharmacokinetics of the novel atypical opioid tapentadol following oral and intravenous administration in dogs. *Vet J* 2012; **194**: 309–313.
455 Lee HK, Lebkowska-Wieruszewska B, Kim TW, *et al.* Pharmacokinetics of the novel atypical opioid tapentadol after intravenous, intramuscular and subcutaneous administration in cats. *Vet J* 2013; **198**: 620–624.
456 Howard J, Aarnes TK, Dyce J, *et al.* Pharmacokinetics and pharmacodynamics after oral administration of tapentadol hydrochloride in dogs. *Am J Vet Res* 2018; **79**: 367–375.
457 Kögel B, Terlinden R, Schneider J. Characterisation of tramadol, morphine and tapentadol in an acute pain model in Beagle dogs. *Vet Anaesth Analg* 2014; **41**: 297–304.
458 Doodnaught GM, Evangelista MC, Steagall PVM. Thermal antinociception following oral administration of tapentadol in conscious cats. *Vet Anaesth Analg* 2017; **44**: 364–369.
459 Kieves NR, Howard J, Lerche P, *et al.* Effectiveness of tapentadol hydrochloride for treatment of orthopedic pain in dogs: a pilot study. *Can Vet J* 2020; **61**: 289–293.
460 Raffa RB, Friderichs E, Reimann W, *et al.* Opioid and nonopioid components independently contribute to the mechanism of action of tramadol, an 'atypical' opioid analgesic. *J Pharmacol Exp Ther* 1992; **260**: 275–285.
461 Raffa RB, Friderichs E, Reimann W, *et al.* Complementary and synergistic antinociceptive interaction between the enantiomers of tramadol. *J Pharmacol Exp Ther* 1993; **267**: 331–340.
462 Frink MC, Hennies HH, Englberger W, *et al.* Influence of tramadol on neurotransmitter systems of the rat brain. *Arzneimittelforschung* 1996; **46**: 1029–1036.
463 KuKanich B, Papich MG. Pharmacokinetics of tramadol and the metabolite O-desmethyltramadol in dogs. *J Vet Pharmacol Ther* 2004; **27**: 239–246.
464 Kukanich B, Papich MG. Pharmacokinetics and antinociceptive effects of oral tramadol hydrochloride administration in Greyhounds. *Am J Vet Res* 2011; **72**: 256–262.
465 Giorgi M, Del Carlo S, Saccomanni G, *et al.* Pharmacokinetics of tramadol and its major metabolites following rectal and intravenous administration in dogs. *N Z Vet J* 2009; **57**: 146–152.
466 McMillan CJ, Livingston A, Clark CR, *et al.* Pharmacokinetics of intravenous tramadol in dogs. *Can J Vet Res* 2008; **72**: 325–331.
467 Vettorato E, Zonca A, Isola M, *et al.* Pharmacokinetics and efficacy of intravenous and extradural tramadol in dogs. *Vet J* 2010; **183**: 310–315.
468 Perez Jimenez TE, Mealey KL, Grubb TL, *et al.* Tramadol metabolism to O-desmethyl tramadol (M1) and N-desmethyl tramadol (M2) by dog liver microsomes: species comparison and identification of responsible canine cytochrome P-450s (CYPs). *Drug Metab Dispos* 2016; **44**: 1963–1972.
469 Perez Jimenez TE, Mealey KL, Schnider D, *et al.* Identification of canine cytochrome P-450s (CYPs) metabolizing the tramadol (+)-M1 and (+)-M2 metabolites to the tramadol (+)-M5 metabolite in dog liver microsomes. *J Vet Pharmacol Ther* 2018; **41**: 815–824.
470 Pypendop BH, Ilkiw JE. Pharmacokinetics of tramadol, and its metabolite O-desmethyl-tramadol, in cats. *J Vet Pharmacol Ther* 2008; **31**: 52–59.
471 Cagnardi P, Villa R, Zonca A, *et al.* Pharmacokinetics, intraoperative effect and postoperative analgesia of tramadol in cats. *Res Vet Sci* 2011; **90**: 503–509.
472 Stewart AJ, Boothe DM, Cruz-Espindola C, *et al.* Pharmacokinetics of tramadol and metabolites O-desmethyltramadol and N-desmethyltramadol in adult horses. *Am J Vet Res* 2011; **72**: 967–974.

473 Knych HK, Corado CR, McKemie DS, *et al.* Pharmacokinetics and pharmacodynamics of tramadol in horses following oral administration. *J Vet Pharmacol Ther* 2013; **36**: 389–398.
474 Knych HK, Corado CR, McKemie DS, *et al.* Pharmacokinetics and selected pharmacodynamic effects of tramadol following intravenous administration to the horse. *Equine Vet J* 2013; **45**: 490–496.
475 Knych HK, Steffey EP, White AM, *et al.* Effects of age on the pharmacokinetics of tramadol and its active metabolite, O-desmethyltramadol following intravenous administration to foals. *Equine Vet J* 2016; **48**: 65–71.
476 Edmondson MA, Duran SH, Boothe DM, *et al.* Pharmacokinetics of tramadol and its major metabolites in alpacas following intravenous and oral administration. *J Vet Pharmacol Ther* 2012; **35**: 389–396.
477 Cox S, Martin-Jimenez T, van Amstel S, *et al.* Pharmacokinetics of intravenous and intramuscular tramadol in llamas. *J Vet Pharmacol Ther* 2011; **34**: 259–264.
478 de Sousa AB, Santos AC, Schramm SG, *et al.* Pharmacokinetics of tramadol and O-desmethyltramadol in goats after intravenous and oral administration. *J Vet Pharmacol Ther* 2008; **31**: 45–51.
479 Vullo C, Kim TW, Meligrana M, *et al.* Pharmacokinetics of tramadol and its major metabolite after intramuscular administration in piglets. *J Vet Pharmacol Ther* 2014; **37**: 603–606.
480 Kelly KR, Pypendop BH, Christe KL. Pharmacokinetics of tramadol following intravenous and oral administration in male rhesus macaques (*Macaca mulatta*). *J Vet Pharmacol Ther* 2015; **38**: 375–382.
481 Schütter AF, Tünsmeyer J, Kästner SBR. Influence of tramadol on acute thermal and mechanical cutaneous nociception in dogs. *Vet Anaesth Analg* 2017; **44**: 309–316.
482 Poulsen L, Arendt-Nielsen L, Brosen K, *et al.* The hypoalgesic effect of tramadol in relation to CYP2D6. *Clin Pharmacol Ther* 1996; **60**: 636–644.
483 Corado CR, McKemie DS, Young A, *et al.* Evidence for polymorphism in the cytochrome P450 2D50 gene in horses. *J Vet Pharmacol Ther* 2016; **39**: 245–254.
484 Pypendop BH, Siao KT, Ilkiw JE. Effects of tramadol hydrochloride on the thermal threshold in cats. *Am J Vet Res* 2009; **70**: 1465–1470.
485 Ajadi RA, Owanikin AO, Martins MM, *et al.* Effect of epidural tramadol and lignocaine on physiological and behavioural changes in goats subjected to castration with a high tension band. *N Z Vet J* 2012; **60**: 344–348.
486 Donati PA, Tarragona L, Franco JVA, *et al.* Efficacy of tramadol for postoperative pain management in dogs: systematic review and meta-analysis. *Vet Anaesth Analg* 2021; **48**: 283–296.
487 Rufiange M, Rousseau-Blass F, Pang DSJ. Incomplete reporting of experimental studies and items associated with risk of bias in veterinary research. *Vet Rec Open* 2019; **6**: e000322.
488 Munro BA, Bergen P, Pang DS. Randomization, blinding, data handling and sample size estimation in papers published in Veterinary Anaesthesia and Analgesia in 2009 and 2019. *Vet Anaesth Analg* 2022; **49**: 18–25.
489 Bennett RC. Reporting guidelines: has their use improved the quality of reporting in Veterinary Anaesthesia and Analgesia [editorial]. *Vet Anaesth Analg* 2022; **49**: 4–6.
490 Sargeant JM, Elgie R, Valcour J, *et al.* Methodological quality and completeness of reporting in clinical trials conducted in livestock species. *Prev Vet Med* 2009; **91**: 107–115.
491 Sargeant JM, Thompson A, Valcour J, *et al.* Quality of reporting of clinical trials of dogs and cats and associations with treatment effects. *J Vet Intern Med* 2010; **24**: 44–50.
492 Budsberg SC, Torres BT, Kleine SA, *et al.* Lack of effectiveness of tramadol hydrochloride for the treatment of pain and joint dysfunction in dogs with chronic osteoarthritis. *J Am Vet Med Assoc* 2018; **252**: 427–432.
493 Meunier NV, Panti A, Mazeri S, *et al.* Randomised trial of perioperative tramadol for canine sterilisation pain management. *Vet Rec* 2019; **185**: 406.
494 Piras LA, Mancusi D, Olimpo M, *et al.* Post-operative analgesia following TPLO surgery: a comparison between cimicoxib and tramadol. *Res Vet Sci* 2021; **136**: 351–359.
495 O'Neill DG, Brodbelt DC, Hodge R, *et al.* Epidemiology and clinical management of elbow joint disease in dogs under primary veterinary care in the UK. *Canine Med Genet* 2020; **7**: 1.
496 Seddighi MR, Egger CM, Rohrbach BW, *et al.* Effects of tramadol on the minimum alveolar concentration of sevoflurane in dogs. *Vet Anaesth Analg* 2009; **36**: 334–340.
497 Guedes AG, Knych HK, Soares JH, *et al.* Pharmacokinetics and physiological effects of repeated oral administrations of tramadol in horses. *J Vet Pharmacol Ther* 2014; **37**: 269–278.
498 Dhanjal JK, Wilson DV, Robinson E, *et al.* Intravenous tramadol: effects, nociceptive properties, and pharmacokinetics in horses. *Vet Anaesth Analg* 2009; **36**: 581–590.
499 Guedes A, Knych H, Hood D. Plasma concentrations, analgesic and physiological assessments in horses with chronic laminitis treated with two doses of oral tramadol. *Equine Vet J* 2016; **48**: 528–531.
500 Natalini CC, Robinson EP. Evaluation of the analgesic effects of epidurally administered morphine, alfentanil, butorphanol, tramadol, and U50488H in horses. *Am J Vet Res* 2000; **61**: 1579–1586.
501 DeRossi R, Modolo TJ, Maciel FB, *et al.* Efficacy of epidural lidocaine combined with tramadol or neostigmine on perineal analgesia in the horse. *Equine Vet J* 2013; **45**: 497–502.
502 Bigham AS, Habibian S, Ghasemian F, *et al.* Caudal epidural injection of lidocaine, tramadol, and lidocaine-tramadol for epidural anesthesia in cattle. *J Vet Pharmacol Ther* 2010; **33**: 439–443.
503 Habibian S, Bigham AS, Aali E. Comparison of lidocaine, tramadol, and lidocaine-tramadol for epidural analgesia in lambs. *Res Vet Sci* 2011; **91**: 434–438.
504 Monteiro ER, Junior AR, Assis HM, *et al.* Comparative study on the sedative effects of morphine, methadone, butorphanol or tramadol, in combination with acepromazine, in dogs. *Vet Anaesth Analg* 2009; **36**: 25–33.
505 Ronagh A, Sabiza S, Naddaf H, *et al.* Comparison of sedative and some cardiopulmonary effects of intramuscular medetomidine or medetomidine-tramadol in dogs. *Vet Anaesth Analg* 2020; **47**: 381–384.
506 Steagall PV, Taylor PM, Brondani JT, *et al.* Antinociceptive effects of tramadol and acepromazine in cats. *J Feline Med Surg* 2008; **10**: 24–31.
507 Barnung SK, Treschow M, Borgbjerg FM. Respiratory depression following oral tramadol in a patient with impaired renal function. *Pain* 1997; **71**: 111–112.
508 Ko JC, Abbo LA, Weil AB, *et al.* Effect of orally administered tramadol alone or with an intravenously administered opioid on minimum alveolar concentration of sevoflurane in cats. *J Am Vet Med Assoc* 2008; **232**: 1834–1840.
509 Bauquier SH. Randomised clinical trial comparing the perioperative analgesic efficacy of oral tramadol and intramuscular tramadol in cats. *J Feline Med Surg* 2022; **24**: 683–690.
510 Evangelista MC, Silva RA, Cardozo LB, *et al.* Comparison of preoperative tramadol and pethidine on postoperative pain in cats undergoing ovariohysterectomy. *BMC Vet Res* 2014; **10**: 252.
511 Zeiler GE, Dzikiti BT, Fosgate GT, *et al.* Anaesthetic, analgesic and cardiorespiratory effects of intramuscular medetomidine-ketamine combination alone or with morphine or tramadol for orchiectomy in cats. *Vet Anaesth Analg* 2014; **41**: 411–420.
512 Castro DS, Silva MF, Shih AC, *et al.* Comparison between the analgesic effects of morphine and tramadol delivered epidurally in cats receiving a standardized noxious stimulation. *J Feline Med Surg* 2009; **11**: 948–953.
513 Brondani JT, Luna SP, Marcello GC, *et al.* Perioperative administration of vedaprofen, tramadol or their combination does not interfere with platelet aggregation, bleeding time and biochemical variables in cats. *J Feline Med Surg* 2009; **11**: 503–509.
514 Monteiro BP, Klinck MP, Moreau M, *et al.* Analgesic efficacy of an oral transmucosal spray formulation of meloxicam alone or in combination with tramadol in cats with naturally occurring osteoarthritis. *Vet Anaesth Analg* 2016; **43**: 643–651.
515 Guedes AGP, Meadows JM, Pypendop BH, *et al.* Evaluation of tramadol for treatment of osteoarthritis in geriatric cats. *J Am Vet Med Assoc* 2018; **252**: 565–571.
516 Aldrich LA, Roush JK, KuKanich B. Plasma concentrations of tramadol after transdermal application of a single metered dose of a compounded tramadol gel to cats. *Am J Vet Res* 2021; **82**: 840–845.

26 Neuromuscular Blockade

Manuel Martin-Flores
Department of Clinical Sciences, College of Veterinary Medicine, Cornell University, Ithaca, New York, USA

Chapter contents

History of neuromuscular blocking agents, 448
Neuromuscular blocking agents in veterinary anesthesia, 448
Anatomy and physiology of the neuromuscular junction, 449
Neuromuscular blockade, 450
Pharmacology and nomenclature, 450
Nondepolarizing neuromuscular blocking agents, 450
Depolarizing neuromuscular blocking agents, 452
Novel nondepolarizing agents, 453
Monitoring neuromuscular transmission, 453
Muscle selection for monitoring neuromuscular transmission, 455
Factors affecting duration and recovery from neuromuscular blockade, 456
Reversal of neuromuscular blockade, 456
Acetylcholinesterase inhibitors, 456
Selective relaxant binding agents, 457
Reversal of succinylcholine, 457
Clinical strategies to minimize the risk of residual neuromuscular blockade, 458
References, 458

History of neuromuscular blocking agents

Long before its introduction to medical practice, curare was extracted primarily from plants, such as *Chondrodendron* species, by native South American aboriginal populations for use in quivers, arrows, or spears to hunt animals. Curare's site of action, the neuromuscular junction (NMJ), was described by Claude Bernard as early as 1844 through his well-known experiments using frog nerve–muscle preparations, demonstrating that direct muscle stimulation could be achieved while evoked contractions were abolished when motor nerves were stimulated in the presence of curare. This discovery was preceded by observations by Benjamin Brodie in 1812 who described that animals injected with curare could be kept alive if their lungs were ventilated. Later, in 1934, Henry Dale described the role of acetylcholine (ACh) in neuromuscular transmission. A multitude of studies that followed those original observations described the anatomy and function of the NMJ and the neurotransmitters involved. The NMJ and the events that result in neuromuscular transmission are now well understood and an immense amount of information has been made available since those initial reports.

Curare was first introduced to medical practice as a potential treatment for convulsive seizures and spasticity and as part of shock therapy. It was then recognized that the effects of curare could be useful in providing muscle relaxation during general anesthesia. The first report of the agent being used for this purpose occurred in 1942 by Dr. Harold Randall Griffith and his resident, Dr. Enid Johnson, during an appendectomy [1]. The synthesis of the alkaloid agent tubocurarine followed and its use during anesthesia began to gain traction. Further studies by Drs. John Halton and Cecil Gray with tubocurarine in 1946 laid the foundation for development of what became known as the "Liverpool anesthetic technique" – the first example of the concept of balanced anesthesia. The technique became popular and the practice of using deep planes of anesthesia to avoid movement was largely abandoned [2–4]. Within the next 10 years, the use of neuromuscular blockade for anesthesia in people had spread throughout the world.

Neuromuscular blocking agents in veterinary anesthesia

Possibly owing to more limited access to mechanical ventilators, or because most intubations and surgeries can be performed in veterinary species without the need for muscle paralysis, the uptake on incorporating neuromuscular blocking agents (NMBAs) into veterinary anesthesia has been much slower and more limited than in human anesthesiology. The depolarizing agent succinylcholine was first used for canine anesthesia in 1952 [5] and in 1954, Hall and Weaver described the use of the nondepolarizing agent gallamine coupled with positive-pressure ventilation as part of balanced anesthesia in the dog and cat [6]. Since those initial reports, a significant body of evidence relating to the effects, clinical use, monitoring, and antagonism of neuromuscular blockade in veterinary anesthesia has now accumulated. While our understanding of these agents has grown exponentially, NMBAs remain part of only a small proportion of all cases in veterinary anesthesia [7].

Veterinary Anesthesia and Analgesia: The Sixth Edition of Lumb and Jones. Edited by Leigh Lamont, Kurt Grimm, Sheilah Robertson, Lydia Love and Carrie Schroeder.
© 2024 John Wiley & Sons, Inc. Published 2024 by John Wiley & Sons, Inc.
Companion website: www.wiley.com/go/lamont/anesthesia

Anatomy and physiology of the neuromuscular junction

NMBAs exert their actions by interrupting transmission through the NMJ. The NMJ is composed of a presynaptic motor neuron and a postsynaptic skeletal muscle cell separated by the synaptic cleft (Fig. 26.1). The presynaptic cell originates in the spine and travels uninterrupted to the target muscle. It loses its myelin sheath when it approaches the synapse and branches to contact several muscle cells, composing what is known as a "motor unit." This presynaptic cell synthetizes and stores ACh in vesicles; both a reserve and a readily available population of ACh vesicles are found within this cell. Depolarization of the motor neuron results in an influx of Ca^{2+} via voltage-gated channels that triggers the mobilization of vesicles and the release of a large amount of ACh into the cleft. When two molecules of ACh interact with both α subunits of a nicotinic acetylcholine receptor (nAChR) located in the folds of the postsynaptic cell, a conformational change occurs within the receptor, allowing an influx of Na^+ into the skeletal muscle cell. Depolarization of the endplate terminal triggers the activation of voltage-gated Na^+ channels that propagate the action potential along the cell, signaling the process for muscular contraction [8,9]. The interaction between ACh and the nAChR is very brief, with its effects terminating almost immediately. Free ACh is promptly hydrolyzed by the acetylcholinesterase enzyme into choline and acetic acid [10]. The sudden and drastic reduction in the concentration of ACh in the cleft favors the movement of ACh away from the nAChR.

The amount of ACh released by the nerve is affected by the concentration of extracellular Ca^{2+}. The absence of Ca^{2+} would result in the absence of ACh release and muscular contractions, while doubling the concentration of Ca^{2+} would result in a 16-fold increase in the amount of released ACh. Under normal circumstances, only a fraction of the available vesicles of ACh are released; however, this fraction is more than sufficient for effective neuromuscular transmission. Moreover, only a small number of available nAChR need to be activated to cause maximal depolarization of the muscle cell. These redundancies in the process of neuromuscular transmission provide the NMJ with a substantial margin of safety and an immense reserve [11].

Pentameric nAChRs are found postsynaptically in the shoulders of the primary clefts, and presynaptically in the motor nerve. The postsynaptic receptor contains two α_1 subunits, which are the binding sites of ACh (and NMBAs). The fetal and mature forms of this receptor vary by only one subunit: a γ subunit in the fetal subtype, and the ε subunit in the mature form. β_1 and δ subunits complete the receptor. The fetal subtype, and a third subtype composed of α_7 subunits, are found during development, and are replaced by the mature form soon after birth; the adult form remains for life. The fetal and α_7 subtypes can also proliferate in abnormal situations that result in decreased muscle activity, such as poor innervation, prolonged immobilization, or increased muscle catabolism (e.g., inflammation). Opening time of the sodium channel and sensitivity to specific ligands are altered in these receptors. This explains in part why increased sensitivity to succinylcholine and decreased potency of nondepolarizing agents are observed in neonates or during abnormal states when other subtypes of the nAChR proliferate. Upregulation of receptors may also be involved in the differences observed during neuromuscular pathologies [12,13].

Presynaptic nAChR are also found in the NMJ. Through positive and negative feedback loops, presynaptic receptors control the mobilization and release of ACh. A negative feedback loop stops further release of the transmitter when the concentrations of ACh

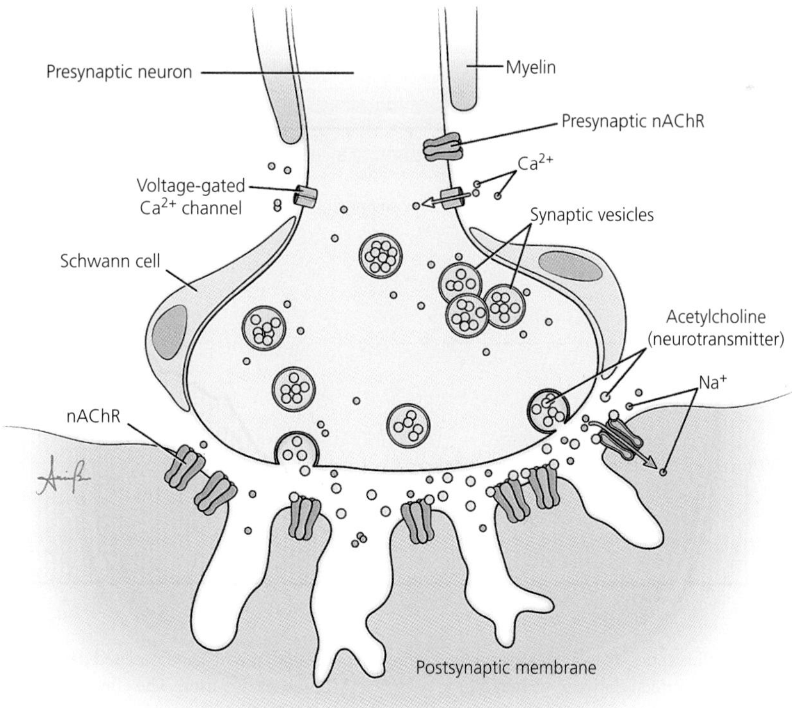

Figure 26.1 Representation of the neuromuscular junction and its main components. See text for details.

in the cleft are sufficiently high. In a complementary mechanism, a positive feedback loop signals the mobilization of reserve ACh toward the active zone, increasing the population of readily available ACh in preparation for the next stimulus. The latter mechanism may play a key role in the development of fade during repeated nerve stimulation when nondepolarizing NMBAs are used (discussed in the section on monitoring neuromuscular transmission). The depolarizing agent succinylcholine does not inhibit this receptor, explaining why no fade is observed when that agent is used [14].

Neuromuscular blockade

Neuromuscular transmission can be interrupted, producing paralysis, and thereby providing one of the main components of anesthesia (relaxation/immobility) without the need for excessively profound depression of the central nervous system. NMBAs do this through one of two main mechanisms: depolarization of the postsynaptic cell (depolarizing NMBA) or competitive antagonism of the nAChR (nondepolarizing NMBA).

Pharmacology and nomenclature

The effects of NMBAs are measured by quantitating the reduction in the evoked force of contraction (or a surrogate). Potency is determined by constructing a dose-response curve, which is composed of the responses to several submaximal doses (Fig. 26.2A). From that relationship, the effective doses that produce 50% and 95% depression of force of contraction (ED_{50} and ED_{95}, respectively) can be identified. The ED_{95} can be used to compare agents given at equipotent doses, or to compare the characteristics of multiples of the ED_{95}. The onset time is the interval between administration and a predetermined effect, typically 95% depression. Duration of action (sometimes called "duration of clinical or surgical block") is the time between injection and the return of 25% (sometimes 10%) of force of contraction. The recovery index is the time between 25% and 75% recovery of the evoked force of contraction and describes the slope (or speed) of recovery. Complete recovery of neuromuscular transmission requires more time and is reached when no residual weakness can be measured (Fig. 26.2B).

Nondepolarizing neuromuscular blocking agents

Nondepolarizing NMBAs exert their action through competitive antagonism of the nAChR receptors. The binding of a nondepolarizing NMBA with at least one α_1 subunit of the nicotinic receptor prevents the conformational change produced by ACh. Therefore, Na^+ influx, depolarization, and contraction do not occur. In general, nondepolarizing NMBAs are large, water-soluble molecules, with relatively low volumes of distribution (typically 0.2–0.4 L/kg) that do not cross the placenta or the blood–brain barrier. No sensory

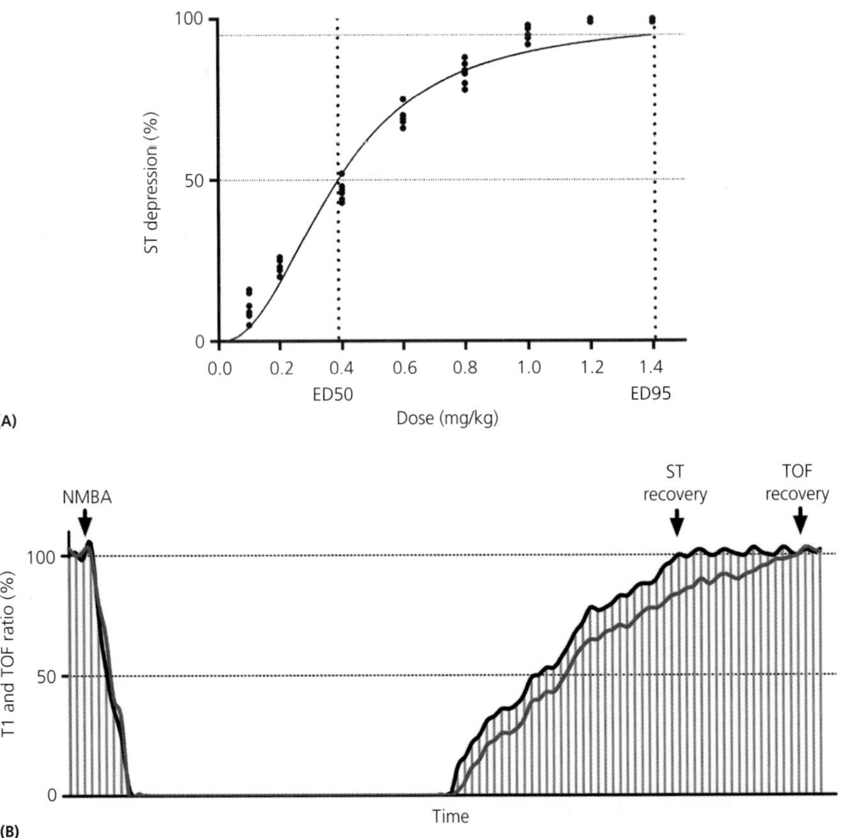

Figure 26.2 **A.** A dose-response curve illustrating responses to varying submaximal doses of an NMBA (simulated data). The depression in the magnitude (or height) of the single twitch (ST) is measured relative to its magnitude prior to NMBA administration. The effective dose producing 50% (ED_{50}) and 95% (ED_{95}) twitch depression can be calculated. Source: Dr. Daniel M. Sakai, with permission. **B.** An example of the time-course of neuromuscular block after administration of a nondepolarizing NMBA (simulated data). Time is shown on the x-axis and the magnitude of evoked responses for the first response (T1; black bars and line) to train-of-four (TOF) stimulation, and the TOF ratio (T4:T1; red line) are shown on the y-axis. Onset time is the period between NMBA administration and maximal effect. Notice that the magnitude of T1 returns earlier than the TOF ratio, making it a less sensitive indicator of partial block.

depression results from their use, therefore, other components of anesthesia, such as hypnosis and analgesia, need to be provided by different means. Onset time for neuromuscular blockade after injection of nondepolarizing agents is relatively slow, requiring 2–5 min to reach full effect. Both the onset and offset are progressive phenomena and respond to the concentration of drug at the site of action, the NMJ. Peak effect occurs with some delay (typically 1 min) after peak plasma concentration is reached, as the drug is transferred into the NMJ. Similar to other anesthetic agents, onset time is affected by cardiac output, muscle blood flow, and distance from the heart to each muscle. Therefore, onset time will vary between muscles. Moreover, the sensitivity of different muscles to the effects of an NMBA varies, with the diaphragm being characteristically resistant. That is, both the speed of action and the magnitude of the effect may differ between muscle groups after a dose is administered. In general, less potent agents have shorter onset times than more potent drugs. Owing to the margin of safety inherent to the NMJ, a large proportion of receptors need to be occupied before transmission is interrupted and contraction is abolished. Blockade occurs faster when larger numbers of molecules are administered, which is the case for less potent NMBAs. For each agent, increasing the dosage of the agent will accelerate onset and prolong duration.

The margin of safety associated with neuromuscular transmission has distinct clinical consequences. It is estimated that before any effect from an NMBA can be appreciated, approximately 70% of the nAChRs must be antagonized [15]. Therefore, a small dose that only interacts with a smaller proportion of receptors may not have a measurable impact on neuromuscular transmission and force of contraction. This observation is the basis for the *priming technique*, which was once popular when slower agents were commonplace. With this technique, a small and mostly clinically inconsequential dose of an NMBA is given during preoxygenation. After a few minutes, induction is performed followed by a larger dose of the NMBA. The intent is that the priming dose has already occupied a number of receptors without depressing the force of contraction. The second dose will produce a faster onset as it will act on "active" receptors. Onset time with a priming method produces faster paralysis than if the complete dose was administered at once. A second consequence of the margin of safety is that the neuromuscular effects from an initial dose will begin to dissipate while a large number of nAChRs are still occupied by the drug. A second dose, administered to prolong the duration of neuromuscular block, will therefore produce a larger and longer-lasting effect than the initial dose. This explains why anesthesiologists typically re-dose an NMBA with aliquots that are only a fraction (commonly 1/3 to 1/2) of the initial dose.

During offset, force of contraction is gradually restored until full neuromuscular transmission has recovered. Recovery occurs as the NMBA leaves the NMJ, a process closely related to a decay in plasma concentrations. Plasma concentrations will decrease because of redistribution, biotransformation, and excretion or, in particular cases, when binding agents are administered and the NMBA molecules are altered.

Nondepolarizing NMBAs are classified into two main chemical families: (1) benzylisoquinoliniums (e.g., atracurium, cisatracurium, and tubocurarine), and (2) aminosteroids (e.g., vecuronium, rocuronium, and pancuronium) (Table 26.1). In general, benzylisoquinolinium compounds are intermediate-acting NMBAs, with an expected duration of neuromuscular block of approximately 20–40 min. Agents of this family undergo extrahepatic paths of metabolism and most compounds are capable of releasing histamine upon injection. Aminosteroid compounds, on the other hand, do not generally cause histamine release and have fewer cardiovascular effects, although some agents may have a vagolytic effect leading to increased heart rate. Agents of this family undergo biotransformation

Table 26.1 Selected neuromuscular blocking agents (NMBAs) used in veterinary medicine.

Drug	Onset (min)[a]	Duration (min)[a]	Elimination	Intravenous dose (mg/kg)	Intravenous infusion (mg/kg/h)
Nondepolarizing agents					
Benzylisoquinoliniums					
Atracurium	3–5	20–40	Ester hydrolysis, Hoffmann elimination	Canine 0.1–0.2 Feline 0.1–0.25 Equine 0.07–0.15	Canine 0.18–0.36 Equine 0.17
Cisatracurium	3–5	30–40	Hoffmann elimination	Canine 0.075–0.3 Feline 0.05–0.3	
Aminosteroids					
Vecuronium	3–5	30–40	Hepatic metabolism biliary and renal excretion	Canine 0.05–0.1 Feline 0.025–0.1 Equine 0.1	
Rocuronium	1–2	20–30	Hepatic uptake and biliary excretion	Canine 0.1–0.6 Feline 0.1–0.6 Equine 0.3–0.6	Canine 0.2
Pancuronium	5	30–60	Hepatic metabolism and renal elimination of active metabolites	Canine 0.07–0.1 Feline 0.06–0.1 Equine 0.12	
Fumarate diesters					
Gantacurium	1–2	5	Ester hydrolysis, cysteine adduction	Canine 0.06 Feline 0.06	
Depolarizing agent					
Succinylcholine	1–2	6–20	Hydrolysis by plasma cholinesterase	Canine 0.3–0.4 Feline 0.1–0.2 Equine 0.12–0.15	

[a] Values listed for the nondepolarizing agents are based on canine studies.
Source: Compiled from Lee *et al.* [17]; Wright *et al.* [18]; Martin-Flores *et al.* [19]; Cottrell *et al.* [20]; Martin-Flores *et al.* [21].

and elimination via the liver or kidneys and, hence, clearance is altered when organ function is decreased. Modern agents in this family are largely considered intermediate-acting drugs with pancuronium (typically classified as long-acting) being an exception.

Atracurium is a benzylisoquinolinium compound comprising a mixture of 10 isomers of varying potency that undergoes enzymatic degradation by nonspecific esterases, which accounts for approximately two-thirds of its biotransformation [16]. These enzymes are distinct from acetylcholinesterase and plasma cholinesterase (also known as "pseudocholinesterase"). Hence, abnormal plasma cholinesterase concentrations do not affect degradation of atracurium. In addition, nonenzymatic degradation occurs spontaneously in the presence of normal pH and temperature via a process named "Hoffman elimination." Decreases in temperature and pH will delay nonenzymatic degradation, although it is unlikely that changes in pH observed under most clinical situations will have a noticeable impact. Moreover, changes in pH may also affect enzymatic hydrolysis in the opposite direction. Therefore, small changes in pH are unlikely to result in clinically relevant changes in duration of action of atracurium. For storage, atracurium is provided in a low-pH solution and should be kept refrigerated.

Degradation of atracurium by either pathway results in the production of laudanosine [22]. This byproduct has no neuromuscular blocking effects but can be a central nervous system stimulant. High concentrations of laudanosine can increase the minimum alveolar concentration of volatile anesthetics by as much as 30% [23]. Laudanosine elimination occurs mostly through bile (~70%) and urine (~30%) and, unlike its precursor atracurium, is dependent on hepatic function [24]. Therefore, hepatic disease is unlikely to substantially affect the duration of atracurium but can result in accumulation of laudanosine. As an example, laudanosine, but not atracurium, has been shown to accumulate during the anhepatic phase of liver transplant in pigs [25].

Like most benzylisoquinolinium relaxants, including tubocurarine, atracurium can release histamine upon administration, which may cause tachycardia and arterial hypotension. However, this is typically observed after several multiples of the ED_{95} are used [26].

Cisatracurium is one of the isomers that compose atracurium. It was developed in an attempt to decrease the risk of histamine release and improve atracurium's margin of safety. In humans, eight times the ED_{95} needs to be administered before clinical consequences of histamine release are observed; therefore, histamine release does not occur under normal clinical situations.

Like atracurium, cisatracurium is degraded via Hoffman elimination. Nonspecific enzymatic hydrolysis occurs at substantially lower rates than for atracurium [27]. As in the case for atracurium, laudanosine is a byproduct of metabolism; however, smaller quantities are formed as cisatracurium is more potent than atracurium so smaller doses are used to produce equivalent effects [28]. Like atracurium, duration of action is considered intermediate; however, since cisatracurium is more potent than atracurium and fewer molecules need to be administered, onset is slower.

Other examples in the benzylisoquinolinium family include the historically relevant agent tubocurarine (also known as "(+)-tubocurarine" or "*d*-tubocurarine") and mivacurium. Tubocurarine was considered a long-lasting agent that could release histamine at doses below the ED_{95}, hence, cardiovascular effects were common with its use. Mivacurium was introduced to clinical practice as an agent of short duration, owing to its rapid hydrolysis by plasma cholinesterase (pseudocholinesterase), a degradation path shared with succinylcholine [29]. Consequently, abnormally low levels of this enzyme increase the duration of action of this agent [30]. While mivacurium's effects are short-acting in people, differences in enzymatic activity in dogs result in long-lasting neuromuscular block in this species [31]. Like other agents of this family, mivacurium causes a dose-dependent release of histamine.

Of the aminosteroid NMBAs, pancuronium is longer-lasting, with a duration approximating or exceeding an hour [17]. Owing to its vagolytic effect, administration of pancuronium can result in increases in heart rate and arterial blood pressure [32,33].

Vecuronium results from demethylation of pancuronium and, unlike the parent compound, is not vagolytic and is largely devoid of any cardiovascular effects. An active (3-hydroxy) metabolite of vecuronium is produced during spontaneous deacetylation, which conserves 60–80% of the neuromuscular blocking potency. Vecuronium and its active metabolites are biotransformed by the liver and kidneys. Therefore, prolonged administration in the presence of decreased organ function is likely to result in accumulation [18].

Like vecuronium, rocuronium is an intermediate-acting NMBA, but with a lower potency and faster onset. At equipotent doses, rocuronium has a faster onset than vecuronium, mivacurium, and cisatracurium [34]. Metabolism of rocuronium is limited, and most of the drug is excreted unchanged through urine and bile. Like vecuronium, no hemodynamic alterations are observed at clinically useful doses (up to four times the ED_{95}) [35].

Depolarizing neuromuscular blocking agents

Succinylcholine is the only member of this family that is available for clinical use. The mechanism of action of succinylcholine is almost diametrically opposite to that of the nondepolarizing agents: succinylcholine binds to the nAChR and acts as an agonist. While the detailed mechanism of action is not fully understood, some key steps are known. Like ACh, succinylcholine binds the nAChR and depolarization of the membrane occurs. This opens voltage-gated Na^+ channels on the skeletal muscle cell resulting in muscle contraction. Closure and inactivation of the Na^+ channels only occurs when the membrane potential is reset. Normally, with ACh acting as the agonist at the nAChR, this is a very rapid process as ACh is hydrolyzed by the acetylcholinesterase enzyme in the synaptic cleft. Succinylcholine, however, is not metabolized by this enzyme and the drug remains at the NMJ for far longer. The Na^+ channels remain inactivated, transmission is blocked, and the muscle becomes flaccid. This depolarization-induced block (also called "Phase I block") is often preceded by an initial disorganized contraction of muscles (called "fasciculations") before relaxation follows [36]. Fasciculations typically last for a very short period, although sustained contraction (several minutes) has been observed in the masseter and adductor pollicis muscles in humans [37].

Recovery from depolarization or Phase I block induced by succinylcholine occurs as the drug redistributes out of the NMJ, a process that is facilitated by the decrease in the plasma concentration as the agent is hydrolyzed by the enzyme plasma cholinesterase (also known as "pseudocholinesterase") [36]. The enzyme is synthetized in the liver and, consequently, liver diseases may lead to lower levels of this enzyme and an increased duration of action of succinylcholine [38]. Abnormal plasma cholinesterase is present in individuals with a genetic mutation that affects the synthesis of the enzyme. In those cases, the duration of action of succinylcholine can be increased from an expected 10 min to 4 h [39]. A transfusion with whole blood or fresh frozen plasma might be required to terminate the effects of succinylcholine under those conditions.

The activity of plasma cholinesterase can be assessed in suspect individuals by measuring the dibucaine number. Dibucaine is a local anesthetic that inhibits the activity of the plasma cholinesterase enzyme. The activity of the abnormal form of the enzyme is resistant to this inhibition. The dibucaine number indicates the percentage of enzyme activity that is inhibited when exposed to dibucaine and shows whether normal or atypical plasma cholinesterase is present.

Under normal conditions in humans, succinylcholine produces a very fast onset and a short duration of action. There is species variation to these characteristics. A similar time-course is seen in cats; however, a longer duration (20–30 min) is commonly seen in dogs, likely due to lower enzymatic activity [19,40]. When the NMJ is exposed to increasing doses of the drug, usually through repeated boluses or continuous infusions, succinylcholine-induced block begins to assume the characteristics of a nondepolarizing (i.e., competitive) block and this phenomenon has been variably referred to as "Phase II," "desensitization," or "dual" block [36].

Unlike the nondepolarizing drugs, succinylcholine has several important effects on other organs. Interactions with muscarinic receptors can produce bradycardia, but interactions with sympathetic ganglia can increase circulating levels of catecholamines and result in tachycardia and hypertension. While no direct effect on the central nervous system occurs, increased intracranial and intraocular pressure have been reported [20,41–43]. Histamine release is possible following administration of this agent, and hence, swings in blood pressure should be expected. Hyperkalemia is also induced by administration of succinylcholine and may be fatal in individuals with muscle trauma or motor neuron defects [44,45].

Despite these drawbacks, succinylcholine remains in clinical use for humans, primarily (if not exclusively) due to its rapid onset. When a rapid sequence induction is necessary, succinylcholine produces acceptable intubating conditions faster than any other NMBA.

Novel nondepolarizing agents

Fumarate (olefinic isoquinolinium diester) compounds constitute a new family of nondepolarizing agents that are being developed. Several agents have been investigated, which provide either fast onset and ultra-short duration, or intermediate duration that can be shortened by a novel mechanism of reversal. While all agents have a potential for histamine release, this does not occur at clinically useful doses [46]. Gantacurium offers a fast onset and very short duration. In cats, gantacurium had an onset time of 1–1.5 min and a duration of 4–7 min to complete recovery [21]. This short duration is the consequence of different paths of metabolism: a slow pH-sensitive ester hydrolysis and a faster unique mechanism involving adduction of cysteine to the NMBA molecule. The adduction of cysteine occurs at the central fumarate bond, replacing chlorine. The resultant molecule has negligible neuromuscular blocking properties. This method of inactivation can be further accelerated by the administration of exogenous cysteine (L-cysteine) [47,48]. Analogues of gantacurium (CW 002 and CW 011) have also been synthesized to undergo slower cysteine adduction, yielding an intermediate duration of action. Predictably, their effects can be substantially shortened by the administration of L-cysteine [49]. Moreover, a newer agent (CW 1759-50) that is rapid-acting with a short duration like gantacurium, but with an improved cardiovascular profile, is also being studied [50]. These agents may soon be available for clinical use, and everything indicates they may result in better control of neuromuscular transmission blockade and recovery.

Monitoring neuromuscular transmission

Monitoring neuromuscular transmission is useful for titrating infusions of NMBAs, or for deciding when a dose should be repeated. It is necessary for assessing whether reversal is needed or even possible, and it is essential for avoiding inadvertent residual neuromuscular block. Neuromuscular function is monitored by stimulating a motor nerve and assessing the response evoked by that stimulus. The evoked responses can be assessed subjectively by observation or can be objectively measured. Measurements of isometric force of contraction (mechanomyography [MMG]) are widely considered the gold standard. The methodology is cumbersome as it requires that a limb be attached under tension to a force transducer. Commonly, either the distal end of the extremity or, in a more invasive fashion, a tendon, is secured to the transducer. A less invasive method of near-isometric force has been described, by suturing a tendon to the transducer [51,52]. Both methods of MMG are impractical for use in the operating room.

As alternatives, acceleromyography (AMG) and electromyography (EMG) can be utilized. Unlike MMG, AMG measures the acceleration of a freely moving limb and, therefore, avoids the need for setups that prevent movement. AMG is user-friendly, relatively inexpensive, and can be easily used in a clinical setting. Several handheld devices, as well as modules included in multiparameter monitors, are currently available. The method is reliable and a good surrogate for MMG; however, measurements are not interchangeable [52]. AMG has gained widespread acceptance as both a clinical and research tool [53] and, by helping to identify residual block, it can attenuate the consequences of this complication [54–56].

EMG measures the compound action potential at the muscle. Since it is cellular activation and not movement that is quantified, EMG is not affected by the position of the limb, or whether movement is opposed or not during stimulation. EMG correlates well with MMG and is more user-friendly as a clinical tool [57]. Both handheld devices and multiparameter monitors are available.

Prior to the development of these monitors, evoked responses were typically assessed visually in clinical settings. Subjective assessment is limited in that partial neuromuscular blockade cannot be appreciated unless the level of block is of considerable magnitude. Therefore, the method is not sufficiently sensitive to detect mild or shallow levels of residual block at extubation, which could result in severe complications.

Neuromuscular monitoring requires the electrical stimulation of a motor nerve. In veterinary medicine, the ulnar and fibular nerves are typically used for this purpose [58]. Facial nerves have also been used, but results obtained at the limbs do not always agree with those obtained at the face [58]. Stimulation of the nerve should be performed, if possible, away from the muscle that is being stimulated. For example, when stimulating the fibular nerve, it is preferable to place the electrodes lateral to the stifle, and not directly over the belly of the cranial tibial muscle (Fig. 26.3). Placing the electrodes directly over the muscle could result in direct muscle stimulation. Since NMBAs interrupt neuromuscular transmission, it is the transmission between nerve and muscle that should be tested. As shown originally by Claude Bernard almost two centuries ago, direct muscle stimulation may trigger a contraction even when neuromuscular transmission is blocked. To further minimize the risk of direct muscle stimulations, short square-wave pulses of 0.1–0.3 ms duration are typically used during stimulation; longer pulses are more likely to directly recruit muscle cells in the proximity to the electrodes. Square-wave pulses are preferred as they produce effective stimulation at lower currents than other

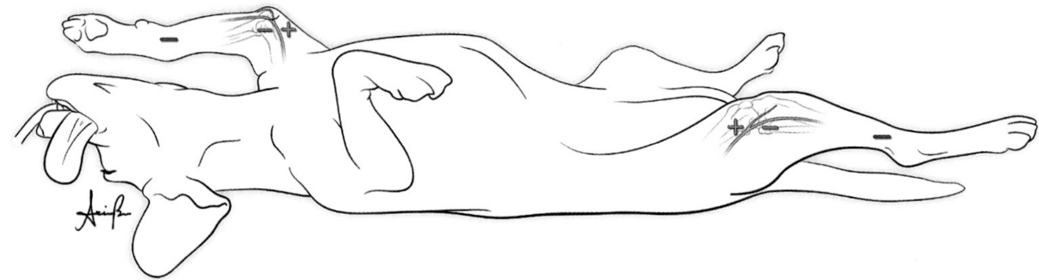

Figure 26.3 Electrode placement on the forelimb (ulnar nerve) or hindlimb (fibular nerve) of a dog for neuromuscular monitoring. In order to stimulate the nerve rather than directly stimulate the muscle belly, electrodes should not be placed directly over the muscle that is being stimulated.

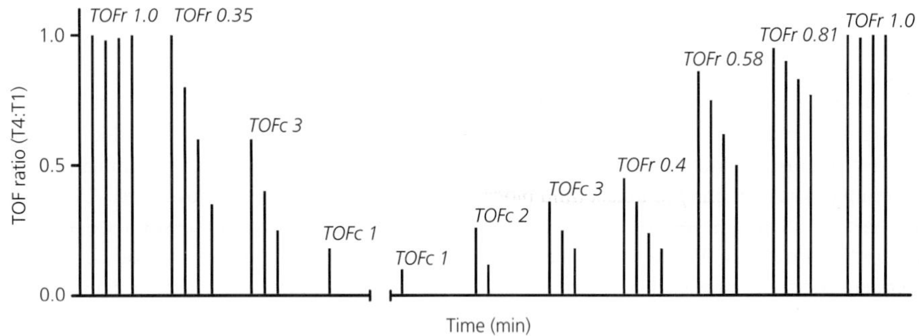

Figure 26.4 Representation of the train-of-four count (TOFc) and TOF ratio (TOFr) during onset and offset of nondepolarizing block. A fade can be observed between the first (T1) and fourth (T4) evoked responses in the presence of partial block. The number of responses to TOF disappear (from T4 to T1) during onset (first segment) and reappear (from T1 to T4) during recovery (second and third segments).

waveforms [59]. Supramaximal current is commonly used so that all fibers innervated can be recruited. Supramaximal current can be found for each individual by creating a dose-response curve, where the current is gradually increased until a plateau in the evoked response is measured. A current slightly higher than maximal is used thereafter. However, supramaximal current stimulation can be uncomfortable in lightly anesthetized animals. Submaximal currents, as discussed below with train-of-four, are better tolerated and can be safely used under certain conditions.

There are several patterns of stimulation that can be used. The simplest method is the "single twitch"' (ST), whereby a single pulse is delivered (typically every 10 s; 0.1 Hz), and the muscular twitch that it evokes is measured. Regardless of the method of quantification used (MMG, AMG, or EMG), it is the relative reduction in twitch magnitude that is plotted, not an absolute value. Hence, a precise baseline must be obtained, so that all subsequent values can be compared. For this reason, the ST is not used in the clinical setting; methods that do not require a baseline value are advantageous, as they allow the anesthesiologist to administer NMBAs during surgery and monitor the adequacy of neuromuscular transmission just prior to emergence. In addition, ST depression is an insensitive indicator of residual block. That is, when the magnitude of ST returns to normal, substantial weakness can still be identified by other means (Fig. 26.2B).

The use of ST is typically reserved for potency studies. Briefly, the percentage twitch depression (relative to pre-NMBA values) is plotted against a number of submaximal doses of the NMBA, and a dose-response curve is created (Fig. 26.2A). ST depression occurs from blockade of the postsynaptic nAChR, hence it is observed with the administration of depolarizing or nondepolarizing agents.

The "train-of-four" (TOF) was introduced to practice in the early 1970s after a series of now-classical studies by Ali, Utting, and Gray [60–64]. The TOF is composed of four stimuli administered every 0.5 s (2 Hz). Each train is repeated at least 10 s apart. Studies have shown that it is safe to use submaximal currents when monitoring the TOF as long as the current is sufficient to generate all four evoked responses [65,66]. Lower currents are less likely to be painful and are better tolerated by patients lightly anesthetized. There are several advantages to the use of TOF over ST, the main one being its sensitivity to detect partial blockade.

Prior to administration of an NMBA, all four responses to TOF stimulation are of equal magnitude. During the onset of neuromuscular blockade, all four twitches of the TOF decrease progressively until the "TOF count" (TOFc) equals zero (i.e., no responses to TOF) and blockade is complete. During block onset, twitch magnitude decreases and reaches zero in order of last to first twitch. In other words, T4 disappears first (TOFc = 3), followed by T3 (TOFc = 2), T2 (TOFc = 1), and finally T1 (TOFc = 0). During recovery from block, the reverse occurs, and twitches reappear from first to last. That is, T1 reappears and is then followed by T2, T3, and finally T4. The progressive increase in twitch magnitude during recovery also occurs in order, so that T4 recovery lags behind T1. This delay results in a visible (and measurable) fade. Once T1 recovers to its baseline magnitude, T4 will continue to increase until its pre-NMBA value is reached (Fig. 26.4). The decrease in the magnitude of T1 during TOF is analogous to the decrease seen when using ST. Therefore, T1 depression during TOF can also be used for potency studies and is attributed to postsynaptic block of nAChRs. Fade during repeated stimulation, however, is generally thought to be a consequence of presynaptic receptor blockade resulting in delayed

ACh mobilization. Because fade occurs with nondepolarizing drugs but is not observed during depolarizing or Phase I block induced by succinylcholine, this phenomenon is considered to be a feature of nondepolarizing blockade.

Fade is quantified by dividing the magnitude of T4 by that of T1 (T4:T1), which is known as the "TOF ratio" (TOFr). Measurement of the TOFr is useful for assessing neuromuscular function without a reference to baseline values; each TOF acts as its own reference. Therefore, a TOFr ≥ 1.0 (or 100%) is seen in the absence of neuromuscular blockade, and a TOFr < 1.0 is indicative of impaired neuromuscular transmission. As shown in Fig. 26.4, recovery of the TOFr lags behind the recovery of the magnitude of T1 (or ST), and hence, is a more sensitive indicator of partial block.

If neuromuscular impairment is substantial, that is, if the TOFr is < 0.5, fade can be easily observed. However, moderate to mild neuromuscular block (TOFr of 0.5–0.9) is not easily detected by visual inspection. It has been shown in humans, horses, and dogs, that our ability to identify modest changes in acceleration of the different components of the TOF is quite limited [55,56,67]. In dogs, the probability to detect impairment by observation of the TOF when the ratio is 0.7 was only 50% [56]. This inability to detect mild block is not dependent on the experience of the observers. Hence, visual assessment of the TOF cannot detect residual block reliably. The ability to accurately interpret TOFc and TOFr makes it possible to administer NMBAs during anesthesia without obtaining a baseline recording and improves safety by ensuring adequate neuromuscular function prior to extubation.

"Double burst stimulation" (DBS) uses the same general principles as TOF; repeated stimulation that can identify partial impairment without the need for baseline measurements. Unlike TOF, however, DBS is composed of two short tetanic stimulations (bursts) separated by a 750-ms interval [68]. Each burst is typically composed of three stimuli administered at 50 Hz, although some minor variations have been studied. The response to DBS is observed as two big twitches and, therefore, visual detection of any fade might be improved compared with TOF. However, similar limitations to visual assessment of TOF were observed when DBS was evaluated in dogs [56]. Hence, DBS seems to offer only minor advantages over TOF, and is likely to cause more discomfort.

The "post-tetanic count" (PTC) differs from the previous patterns in that it can help discern depths of neuromuscular block when no responses to TOF are present, that is, at quite profound levels of muscle paralysis. PTC is based on a physiological phenomenon known as "post-tetanic facilitation." Simply put, a tetanic stimulus increases intracellular Ca^{2+} in the presynaptic cell, leading to increased mobilization and release of ACh into the cleft for a short period of time (~90–120 s). This increased amount of ACh can transiently reverse the effects of competitive NMBAs. To measure the PTC, modern monitors deliver a sequence of impulses as follows: 15 s of ST at 1 Hz, 5 s of tetanic stimulation at 50 Hz, and 15 s of ST at 1 Hz (or a slight variation of this sequence). The number of ST responses that can be detected after tetanic facilitation is inversely related to the magnitude of block (i.e., the time of the return of T1) (Fig. 26.5) [69–71]. This pattern of stimulation is only reserved for profound depths of paralysis, and it should be noted that without tetanic facilitation, no responses would be detected during ST or TOF stimulation.

Muscle selection for monitoring neuromuscular transmission

Neuromuscular function is measured at a nerve-muscle unit, but results need to be extrapolated to the entire individual. This is complicated by the differences in potency and duration of NMBAs between muscles. For example, in most species, the diaphragm is among the most resistant muscles. After injection of an NMBA, the magnitude of block is less and recovery occurs faster at the diaphragm than at a limb, where monitoring is usually carried out. Return of spontaneous ventilation during offset of block does not necessarily indicate recovery from neuromuscular blockade in the patient; rather, it only indicates recovery of muscles responsible for ventilation. The well-known "curare cleft" in the capnograph is an indication of early recovery of the diaphragm in an otherwise relaxed individual. The relationship between the return of spontaneous ventilation and neuromuscular block measured at the limb was studied in dogs. It was shown that when tidal volume, peak inspiratory flow, and minute ventilation returned to pre-relaxation levels, substantial neuromuscular impairment was measured at the limbs (TOFr ≤ 0.2) [72]. In humans, neuromuscular function is typically measured at the adductor pollicis muscle, following stimulation of the ulnar nerve. This muscle recovers late relative to other important ones. For example, by the time neuromuscular function is restored at the adductor pollicis muscle, function has already

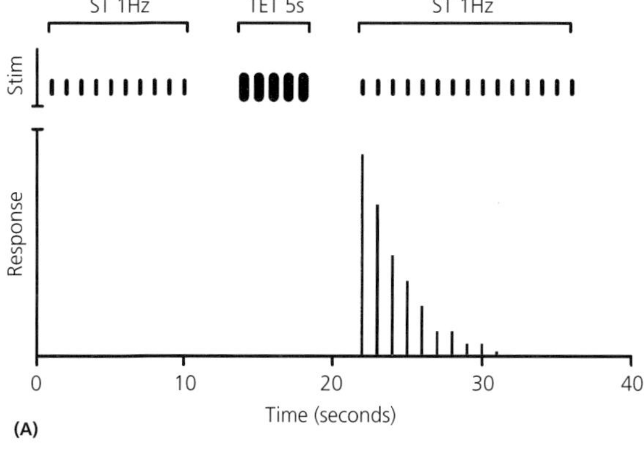

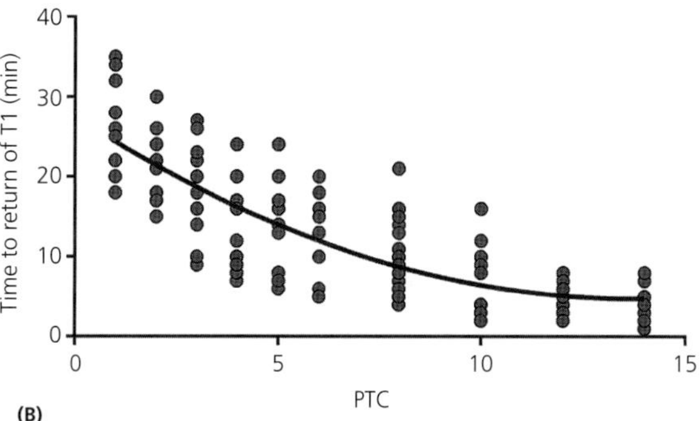

Figure 26.5 **A.** Representation of the post-tetanic count (PTC). The upper panel illustrates the pattern of stimuli. A period of single twitch (ST) stimulation at 1 Hz (1/s) is shown, followed by a tetanic (TET) stimulation (5 s at 5 Hz). After a 3-s pause, ST at 1 Hz resumes. The number of responses observed (bottom panel) after the TET stimulation constitutes the PTC and is inversely associated with the time required for recovery. **B.** Association between PTC and return of the first twitch of the train-of-four (T1) (simulated data). Note that no response to TOF or ST is visible without post-tetanic facilitation.

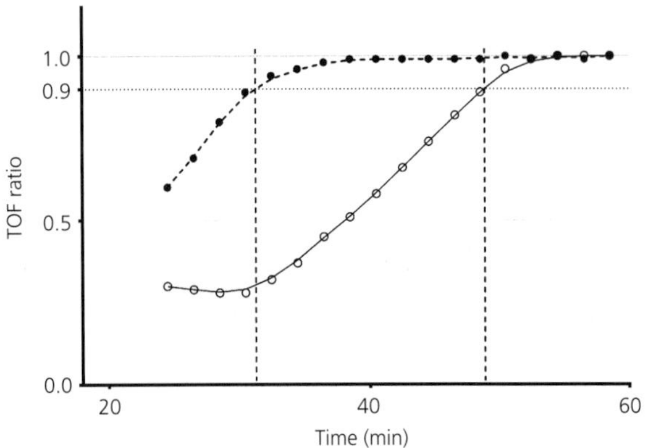

Figure 26.6 Recovery of the train-of-four (TOF) ratio in a dog measured simultaneously with electromyography (EMG) at the larynx (open circles) and a pelvic limb (black circles). Recovery at the larynx occurred more slowly than at the pelvic limb. Source: Adapted and redrawn based on Sakai *et al.* [74].

been restored at the larynx [73]. In dogs, a different relation was observed, and recovery of the larynx occurred later than at the pelvic limb [74,75] (Fig. 26.6). The implication is that complete recovery of function measured from stimulation of the fibular nerve in small animals may not necessarily ensure that laryngeal function will be normal. Therefore, it might be prudent to delay extubation a few minutes if neuromuscular function has just returned at the limbs.

Factors affecting duration and recovery from neuromuscular blockade

As previously mentioned, changes in temperature, enzyme activity, and, to a lesser extent, pH may affect the duration of certain agents, such as the benzylisoquinolinium compounds and succinylcholine. For the aminosteroidal relaxants, on the other hand, hepatic and renal function play a more important role.

NMBAs can interact with other drugs that may affect their potency or duration. Volatile anesthetics potentiate the effects of NMBAs, and smaller doses are needed when inhalational anesthetics are administered [76,77]. Some antibiotics, such as polymyxin and aminoglycosides, also potentiate the effects of NMBAs by affecting neurotransmitter release or action [78]. This effect appears to be more important when aminosteroidal relaxants are used, but it appears to be modest when benzylisoquinolinium agents are used. For example, in dogs and horses, gentamicin potentiates atracurium-induced block, but only minimally [79,80].

Changes in electrolyte concentrations will also affect neuromuscular function. As mentioned earlier, hypocalcemia will decrease the release of ACh, and therefore facilitate the effects of NMBAs. Magnesium can compete with Ca^{2+} and decrease the release of ACh. The effects of NMBAs can be greatly enhanced if magnesium is administered, and reversal may be difficult [81].

Recovery from neuromuscular blockade, even in the absence of any of the factors described above, is a variable phenomenon. For example, the time for spontaneous recovery after a single dose of atracurium or cisatracurium in healthy horses and dogs may vary by as much as 100% between individuals [55,82]. Recovery from neuromuscular blockade may also be affected by the context of administration. When vecuronium was administered to healthy dogs at different doses, the recovery period (defined in that study as the time between the return of T1 and a TOFr > 0.9) increased with higher doses. This is the case even when the recovery period was measured from the same baseline level of relaxation (and presumably similar plasma NMBA concentration) to the return of T1 [83]. As a result of this variability and the potential impact of several external factors, relying on an expected duration of time to consider an animal recovered from neuromuscular blockade carries a high risk for residual block after extubation. The potential negative clinical consequences of all factors affecting the duration or potency of blockade are greatly minimized if quantitative monitoring of neuromuscular blockade is used.

Table 26.2 Selected drugs for reversal of neuromuscular blockade in veterinary medicine.

Drug	Intravenous dose (mg/kg)
Acetylcholinesterase inhibitors	
Neostigmine	Canine 0.02–0.07 Feline 0.02–0.05 Equine 0.04
Edrophonium	Canine 0.1–0.5 Equine 0.5–1
Selective relaxant binding agent	
Sugammadex	Canine 8 Equine 4

Source: Compiled from Mosing *et al.* [58]; Mosing *et al.* [91]. Note that data on the dosage of sugammadex in companion animals is limited.

Reversal of neuromuscular blockade

Acetylcholinesterase inhibitors

Recovery from nondepolarizing neuromuscular block can be enhanced with an acetylcholinesterase inhibitor agent, such as neostigmine or edrophonium. These agents do not directly antagonize neuromuscular block; rather, they inhibit the activity of the acetylcholinesterase enzyme at the NMJ. As a result, ACh that is released into the cleft is allowed to accumulate. It is ACh that will compete for the nAChR with the nondepolarizing NMBA. This indirect mechanism for reversal is of clinical importance: accumulation of ACh will depend on its release, and some time will elapse before a sufficiently high concentration is reached. There is a limit to how much ACh can be released and accumulate within the cleft; this final concentration is insufficient to effectively compete with high concentrations of the NMBA. Profound neuromuscular block, which occurs with high concentrations of NMBA at the NMJ, cannot be reversed with these agents. The competition between NMBA and ACh is also biased in favor of the relaxant as binding of NMBA to only one α_1 subunit is required to block neuromuscular transmission, whereas two molecules of ACh are required for activation of the receptors. Hence, acetylcholinesterase inhibitors can enhance or accelerate recovery from block, but do not directly antagonize the nondepolarizing NMBAs. This process is relatively slow, and 5 to 15 min might be necessary after injection before function is fully restored. It should also be remembered that once the cholinesterase enzyme is fully inhibited, further doses of the reversal agents will have no more beneficial effects.

The two agents available, neostigmine and edrophonium, are similar in their effects but differ in their molecular mechanism of action (Table 26.2). The acetylcholinesterase enzyme has two active sites: an esteratic site, and an anionic site [84,85]. Neostigmine interacts with the enzyme to produce a carbamyl-ester complex at the esteratic site and competes with ACh as a substrate for the enzyme. The carbamylated enzyme is unable to hydrolyze ACh. The half-life of this bond ranges between 7 and 30 min [86]. Edrophonium does not possess a carbamyl group but forms an electrostatic bond with the anionic site of the acetylcholinesterase. The electrostatic bond is less stable than the chemical bond, and can be reversed by ACh, making edrophonium a weaker acetylcholinesterase inhibitor. As the half-life of the edrophonium–acetylcholinesterase enzyme complex is very short, edrophonium might be less effective as a reversal agent [86,87].

Similar to the NMBAs, the volumes of distribution for both reversal agents are relatively small, ranging between 0.7 and 1.0 L/kg, with an elimination half-time of approximately 1–2 h [67,88]. Hepatic biotransformation produces active metabolites that do not contribute to the reversal of blockade [89]. Both agents are primarily excreted by the kidneys. Hypothermia can delay reversal with neostigmine, likely due to reduced blood flow and a slower onset of action [90].

A wide range of doses of neostigmine have been used in dogs (0.0125–0.2 mg/kg); however, doses in the range of 0.02–0.07 mg/kg are used most commonly. Predictably, larger doses produce not only faster but less variable results in terms of speed of reversal [92]. The depth of neuromuscular block at the time of reversal also affects speed of recovery, as deeper levels of blockade are associated with higher concentrations of the NMBA at the NMJ. As mentioned earlier, complete block cannot be antagonized, and recovery times are no shorter if reversal agents are administered in the absence of any responses to TOF stimulation. It was historically suggested that "some degree of spontaneous recovery" should be present prior to administration of a reversal agent. Prior to the availability of peripheral nerve stimulators (PNS), this meant that either spontaneous ventilation or other movements should be observed before reversal in order to avoid administration during complete neuromuscular block. Now that PNS are widely available, reversal should be avoided while the TOFc is zero. Allowing further spontaneous recovery of neuromuscular transmission results in shorter and more predictable reversal times. In dogs, the time to reach a TOFr > 0.9 with administration of neostigmine (0.04 mg/kg) was reduced from 7 to 4 min if neostigmine was administered when the TOFc was 4 versus 2. Variability in the speed of recovery was also reduced [93]. When reversal with neostigmine is performed early during recovery from block, or when low doses of neostigmine are used, 10–15 min might be necessary before the TOFr is 0.9 at a limb [91,92].

The onset of action of edrophonium is shorter than that of neostigmine. In humans, time to peak antagonism after edrophonium was 2 min, compared with 11 min for neostigmine, when reversing tubocurarine [94]. Similar results were observed when reversing pancuronium [95]. There are some drawbacks to edrophonium. Being a "weaker" enzyme inhibitor, results are unpredictable when the drug is used if $\leq$ 2 responses to TOF are present during recovery from pancuronium [96]. When comparing neostigmine and edrophonium administered during profound levels of neuromuscular blockade (T1 < 5%), recovery was faster and more predictable with neostigmine [87]. Edrophonium is commonly used at doses ranging between 0.5 and 1.0 mg/kg in veterinary medicine.

Administration of acetylcholinesterase inhibitors results in increased circulating levels of Ach, which can produce potentially fatal bradyarrhythmias. Gastrointestinal activation may also be observed, which has been suggested as a cause of discomfort following gastrointestinal surgery in people. To avoid bradycardia, these agents are almost always administered with, or preceded by, antimuscarinic agents such as atropine or glycopyrrolate. The slower onset of glycopyrrolate compared with atropine might be better suited as a compliment to neostigmine. When atropine is used, an initial increase in heart rate might be observed owing to its fast onset. The combination of glycopyrrolate with edrophonium is poorly matched in terms of onset and if both agents are administered together bradycardia may ensue. An alternative is to administer the anticholinergic agent a minute prior to reversal. Both atropine and glycopyrrolate have been used successfully in veterinary anesthesia at doses of 0.02 and 0.01 mg/kg, respectively [93,97,98].

Selective relaxant binding agents

Sugammadex is the first selective relaxant binding agent (SRBA) marketed for clinical use. It is a modified γ-cyclodextrin that binds to rocuronium by encapsulating it in its lipophilic pocket [99]. The sugammadex–rocuronium complex constitutes an irreversible bond and is devoid of neuromuscular blocking effects. The complex is then excreted unchanged by the kidneys. As sugammadex binds to rocuronium, the plasma concentration of free rocuronium is drastically reduced, and the resulting concentration gradient favors its movement out of the NMJ. As long as sugammadex levels persist in plasma to "capture" rocuronium, this redistribution process will continue. As a result, both the plasma concentration of free rocuronium and the concentration at the NMJ fall promptly and neuromuscular transmission is restored [100,101]. Unlike reversal of neuromuscular blockade with acetylcholinesterase inhibitors, profound blockade can be reversed with sugammadex as long as sufficient molecules are administered to bind with rocuronium. Due to their structural similarities, vecuronium can also be reversed with sugammadex (Table 26.2). In dogs, sugammadex completely restored neuromuscular function in < 2 min when administered during complete rocuronium or vecuronium block [91]. Similar results (4 min to complete recovery) were shown in ponies after rocuronium-induced block [58].

The calabadions (calabadion 1 and calabadion 2) are first- and second-generation derivatives that are members of the cucurbituril family of drugs (commonly written as cucurbit[*n*]uril where *n* is the number of glycoluril units). These agents were developed as "molecular containers" to encapsulate both aminosteroidal and benzylisoquinolinium compounds and appear to quickly and completely reverse rocuronium- and cisatracurium-induced block. Unlike sugammadex, the calabadions are less-specific encapsulation agents and there is a risk of unintended encapsulation of other molecules with their administration [102,103].

Another agent that is undergoing investigation is L-cysteine for reversal of a novel class of NMBAs, the fumarates (e.g., gantacurium). Unlike sugammadex and the calabadions that work by encapsulating agents and carry an intrinsic risk of unintended encapsulation of other compounds, cysteine works by inactivating the NMBA. This process is not reversible, thus conferring safety against potential recurarization [47,49,104].

Reversal of succinylcholine

The depolarizing agent succinylcholine acts as an agonist at the nAChR and as such, depolarizing (Phase I) block cannot be reversed by competition with ACh. Thus, administration of an acetylcholinesterase inhibitor during Phase I block will not only fail to promote recovery but may also delay its onset. Neostigmine, but not edrophonium, also inhibits plasma cholinesterase, which is responsible for the degradation of succinylcholine. Hence, neostigmine may also contribute to delayed recovery from succinylcholine by this mechanism if administered during Phase I block [105]. Conversely, succinylcholine-induced Phase II block has many of the same features as competitive, nondepolarizing block and may be reversed by acetylcholinesterase inhibitors.

Clinical strategies to minimize the risk of residual neuromuscular blockade

Residual neuromuscular blockade, also called "postoperative residual curarization" (PORC), is a common and important complication with the use of NMBAs [106,107]. If unrecognized, even subtle degrees of weakness can have serious complications. Studies in volunteers show that laryngeal function is affected when the TOFr is between 0.6 and 0.9, leading to aspiration of solids; this is (mostly) prevented once the TOFr is > 0.9 [108,109]. In addition to muscular weakness, residual block (TOFr ~0.7) can depress carotid body chemoreceptors [110]. This occurs from interactions of the NMBA with neuronal nAChRs [111]. As a result, the expected ventilatory response to hypoxia is blunted [112–114]. Moreover, impairment of the chemoreflex response to hypoxia may persist even after reversal of block [115]. Large clinical studies also show that upper airway obstruction occurs more frequently when mild degrees of PORC are present [116] and these complications are observed soon after endotracheal extubation. In veterinary anesthesia, the early recovery period represents a particularly risky time, as oxygen support, airway instrumentation (even if noninvasive), and vital sign monitoring are often discontinued. Moreover, the effects of PORC may be exacerbated by hypothermia, residual effects of anesthetic drugs, and postoperative sedatives and analgesics, which are often administered during or soon after emergence from anesthesia. Hence, avoidance of PORC is of paramount importance, and efforts to ensure complete recovery of neuromuscular function are critical.

Different strategies can be used in combination to reduce the incidence and risks of PORC. Short- or intermediate-acting NMBAs are preferred over long-lasting agents [117]. If an extended duration of paralysis is needed during anesthesia, repeated small doses may be safer than an initial large dose of an NMBA, as the slope of recovery is flatter when large doses are used [83]. Constant rate infusions of NMBAs might appear convenient but carry an inherent risk of overdosing. If the infusion keeps the TOFc at zero, it is difficult to assess whether excessive drug delivery is leading to accumulation unless PTC is used. Repeated small doses at the reappearance of T1 during TOF reduce this risk and provide sufficient relaxation for most procedures. If an infusion is used, titration aiming to achieve a TOFc of 1 might be prudent to avoid inadvertently inducing excessive depth of blockade. Given the differences in recovery times for muscle groups, it is also recommended to document recovery of neuromuscular function at the limb for several minutes before the trachea is extubated.

Neuromuscular monitoring should be mandatory when these agents are used. Ideally, quantitative monitoring should be used as this has been shown to reduce the incidence of PORC and can detect partial recovery at the end of the procedure [54,118]. When this is the case, a TOFr ≥ 1.0 should be recorded prior to emergence from anesthesia. If a quantitative monitor is not available, a traditional PNS should be used. At least two twitches, and preferably four, should be detected before reversal with an acetylcholinesterase inhibitor is performed. As mentioned previously, mild PORC cannot be observed with qualitative PNS monitoring and the practice

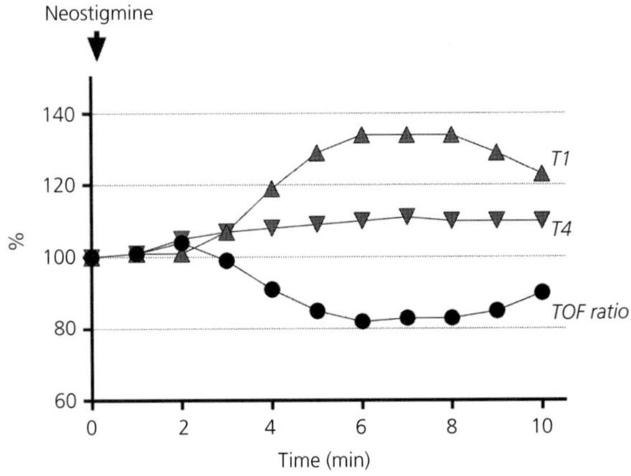

Figure 26.7 Force of contraction measured via mechanomyography (MMG) of the first (T1) and fourth (T4) evoked responses to train-of-four (TOF) stimulation, and TOF ratio (T4/T1) in an anesthetized dog. Neostigmine (0.04 mg/kg) and atropine (0.02 mg/kg) were administered IV when the TOF ratio had spontaneously recovered to 90% after vecuronium-induced neuromuscular block. A transient decrease in the TOF ratio is observed after neostigmine administration accompanied by an increase in the magnitude of T1 and a stable/slightly increased magnitude of T4. Source: Adapted and redrawn based on Romano *et al.* [122].

of relying on the passage of time to determine if NMBA effects have waned is risky. If complete recovery of function cannot be documented, reversing most patients might be the safest course of action, though the practice of "reverse all" (or most) will undoubtedly result in some animals receiving reversal agents unnecessarily. It has been suggested that administration of acetylcholinesterase inhibitors when residual paralysis is minimal (or absent) can result in paradoxical weakness, and that this may be the result of an excess of ACh at the NMJ [119–121]. Administration of neostigmine when the TOFr has recovered to ≥ 0.9 does produce a transient decrease in the TOFr. However, that reduction in the ratio is driven by an increase in the height of T1 relative to that of T4, and none of the evoked responses exhibit a reduction in magnitude (Fig. 26.7) [119,121,122]. It is unclear whether this represents weakness since the force of contraction of any individual response is not reduced. This phenomenon, however, can be avoided by using low doses of neostigmine (0.01–0.03 mg/kg) or by using edrophonium as the reversal agent [122,123].

References

1 Gillies D, Wynands JE. Harold Randall Griffith. The pioneer of the use of muscle relaxants in anaesthesia. *Br J Anaesth* 1986; **58**: 943–945.
2 Gray TC, Halton J. A milestone in Aanaesthesia?: (d-tubocurarine chloride). *Proc R Soc Med* 1946; **39**: 400–410.
3 Gray TC, Halton J. Curarine with balanced anaesthesia. *Br Med J* 1946; **2**: 293–295.
4 Gray TC, Halton J. Technique for the use of d-tubocurarine chloride with balanced anaesthesia. *Br Med J* 1946; **2**: 293–295.
5 Hall L. A report on the clinical use of bis (beta-dimethylaminoethyl)-succinate bisethiodide ("Brevedil, E" M and B2210) during anaesthesia in the dog. *Vet Rec* 1952; **64**: 491–493.
6 Hall L, Weaver B. Some notes on balanced anaesthesia for the dog and cat. *Vet Rec* 1954; **66**: 289–293.
7 Martin-Flores M, Sakai DM, Campoy L, *et al.* Survey of how different groups of veterinarians manage the use of neuromuscular blocking agents in anesthetized dogs. *Vet Anaesth Analg* 2018; **45**: 443–451.
8 Rahamimoff R, Lev-Tov A, Meiri H, *et al.* Regulation of acetylcholine liberation from presynaptic nerve terminals. *Monogr Neural Sci* 1980; **7**: 3–18.

9 Auerbach A. Activation of endplate nicotinic acetylcholine receptors by agonists. *Biochem Pharmacol* 2015; **97**: 601–618.
10 Booij LH. Neuromuscular transmission and its pharmacological blockade. Part 1: neuromuscular transmission and general aspects of its blockade. *Pharm World Sci* 1997; **19**: 1–12.
11 Rich MM. The control of neuromuscular transmission in health and disease. *Neuroscientist* 2006; **12**: 134–142.
12 Jeevendra Martyn JA, Fukushima Y, Chon JY, *et al.* Muscle relaxants in burns, trauma, and critical illness. *Int Anesthesiol Clin* 2006; **44**: 123–143.
13 Martyn JA, Richtsfeld M. Succinylcholine-induced hyperkalemia in acquired pathologic states: etiologic factors and molecular mechanisms. *Anesthesiology* 2006; **104**: 158–169.
14 Jonsson M, Gurley D, Dabrowski M, *et al.* Distinct pharmacologic properties of neuromuscular blocking agents on human neuronal nicotinic acetylcholine receptors: a possible explanation for the train-of-four fade. *Anesthesiology* 2006; **105**: 521–533.
15 Waud BE, Waud DR. The relation between the response to "train-of-four" stimulation and receptor occlusion during competitive neuromuscular block. *Anesthesiology* 1972; **37**: 413–416.
16 Fisher DM, Canfell PC, Fahey MR, *et al.* Elimination of atracurium in humans: contribution of Hofmann elimination and ester hydrolysis versus organ-based elimination. *Anesthesiology* 1986; **65**: 6–12.
17 Lee DD, Meyer RE, Sullivan TC, *et al.* Respiratory depressant and skeletal muscle relaxant effects of low-dose pancuronium bromide in spontaneously breathing, isoflurane-anesthetized dogs. *Vet Surg* 1998; **27**: 473–479.
18 Wright PM, Hart P, Lau M, *et al.* Cumulative characteristics of atracurium and vecuronium. A simultaneous clinical and pharmacokinetic study. *Anesthesiology* 1994; **81**: 59–68; discussion 27A.
19 Martin-Flores M, Pare MD, Campoy L, *et al.* The kalaemic and neuromuscular effects of succinylcholine in centronuclear myopathy: a pilot investigation in a canine model. *Eur J Anaesthesiol* 2015; **32**: 666–671.
20 Cottrell JE, Hartung J, Giffin JP, *et al.* Intracranial and hemodynamic changes after succinylcholine administration in cats. *Anesth Analg* 1983; **62**: 1006–1009.
21 Martin-Flores M, Cheetham J, Campoy L, *et al.* Effect of gantacurium on evoked laryngospasm and duration of apnea in anesthetized healthy cats. *Am J Vet Res* 2015; **76**: 216–223.
22 Agoston S, Vandenbrom RH, Wierda JM. Clinical pharmacokinetics of neuromuscular blocking drugs. *Clin Pharmacokinet* 1992; **22**: 94–115.
23 Shi WZ, Fahey MR, Fisher DM, *et al.* Laudanosine (a metabolite of atracurium) increases the minimum alveolar concentration of halothane in rabbits. *Anesthesiology* 1985; **63**: 584–588.
24 Ward S, Weatherley BC. Pharmacokinetics of atracurium and its metabolites. *Br J Anaesth* 1986; **58**(Suppl 1): 6S–10S.
25 Pittet JF, Tassonyi E, Schopfer C, *et al.* Plasma concentrations of laudanosine, but not of atracurium, are increased during the anhepatic phase of orthotopic liver transplantation in pigs. *Anesthesiology* 1990; **72**: 145–152.
26 Hughes R, Chapple DJ. The pharmacology of atracurium: a new competitive neuromuscular blocking agent. *Br J Anaesth* 1981; **53**: 31–44.
27 Welch RM, Brown A, Ravitch J, *et al.* The in vitro degradation of cisatracurium, the R, cis-R'-isomer of atracurium, in human and rat plasma. *Clin Pharmacol Ther* 1995; **58**: 132–142.
28 Fodale V, Santamaria LB. Laudanosine, an atracurium and cisatracurium metabolite. *Eur J Anaesthesiol* 2002; **19**: 466–473.
29 Savarese JJ, Ali HH, Basta SJ, *et al.* The clinical neuromuscular pharmacology of mivacurium chloride (BW B1090U). A short-acting nondepolarizing ester neuromuscular blocking drug. *Anesthesiology* 1988; **68**: 723–732.
30 Cerf C, Mesguish M, Gabriel I, *et al.* Screening patients with prolonged neuromuscular blockade after succinylcholine and mivacurium. *Anesth Analg* 2002; **94**: 461–466, table of contents.
31 Smith LJ, Moon PF, Lukasik VM, *et al.* Duration of action and hemodynamic properties of mivacurium chloride in dogs anesthetized with halothane. *Am J Vet Res* 1999; **60**: 1047–1050.
32 Booij LH, Edwards RP, Sohn YJ, *et al.* Cardiovascular and neuromuscular effects of Org NC 45, pancuronium, metocurine, and d-tubocurarine in dogs. *Anesth Analg* 1980; **59**: 26–30.
33 Fitzal S, Gilly H, Ilias W. Comparative investigations on the cardiovascular effects of Org NC 45 and pancuronium in dogs. *Br J Anaesth* 1983; **55**: 641–646.
34 Kopman AF, Klewicka MM, Kopman DJ, *et al.* Molar potency is predictive of the speed of onset of neuromuscular block for agents of intermediate, short, and ultrashort duration. *Anesthesiology* 1999; **90**: 425–431.
35 Levy JH, Davis GK, Duggan J, *et al.* Determination of the hemodynamics and histamine release of rocuronium (Org 9426) when administered in increased doses under N2O/O2-sufentanil anesthesia. *Anesth Analg* 1994; **78**: 318–321.
36 Appiah-Ankam J, Hunter J. Pharmacology of neuromuscular blocking drugs. *Contin Educ Anaesth Crit Care Pain* 2004; **4**: 2–7.
37 Smith CE, Saddler JM, Bevan JC, *et al.* Pretreatment with non-depolarizing neuromuscular blocking agents and suxamethonium-induced increases in resting jaw tension in children. *Br J Anaesth* 1990; **64**: 577–581.
38 Birch JH, Foldes FF, Rendell-Baker L. Causes and prevention of prolonged apnea with succinylcholine. *Curr Res Anesth Analg* 1956; **35**: 609–633.
39 Soliday FK, Conley YP, Henker R. Pseudocholinesterase deficiency: a comprehensive review of genetic, acquired, and drug influences. *AANA J* 2010; **78**: 313–320.
40 Cullen LK, Jones RS. The nature of suxamethonium neuromuscular block in the dog assessed by train-of-four stimulation. *Res Vet Sci* 1980; **29**: 281–288.
41 Minton MD, Grosslight K, Stirt JA, *et al.* Increases in intracranial pressure from succinylcholine: prevention by prior nondepolarizing blockade. *Anesthesiology* 1986; **65**: 165–169.
42 Chiu CL, Jaais F, Wang CY. Effect of rocuronium compared with succinylcholine on intraocular pressure during rapid sequence induction of anaesthesia. *Br J Anaesth* 1999; **82**: 757–760.
43 Lanier WL, Milde JH, Michenfelder JD. Cerebral stimulation following succinylcholine in dogs. *Anesthesiology* 1986; **64**: 551–559.
44 Cairoli VJ, Ivankovich AD, Vucicevic D, *et al.* Succinylcholine-induced hyperkalemia in the rat following radiation injury to muscle. *Anesth Analg* 1982; **61**: 83–86.
45 Stone WA, Beach TP, Hamelberg W. Succinylcholine-induced hyperkalemia in dogs with transected sciatic nerves or spinal cords. *Anesthesiology* 1970; **32**: 515–520.
46 Heerdt PM, Kang R, The A, *et al.* Cardiopulmonary effects of the novel neuromuscular blocking drug GW280430A (AV430A) in dogs. *Anesthesiology* 2004; **100**: 846–851.
47 Lien CA, Savard P, Belmont M, *et al.* Fumarates: unique nondepolarizing neuromuscular blocking agents that are antagonized by cysteine. *J Crit Care* 2009; **24**: 50–57.
48 Lien CA. Development and potential clinical impairment of ultra-short-acting neuromuscular blocking agents. *Br J Anaesth* 2011; **107**(Suppl 1): i60–i71.
49 Savarese JJ, McGilvra JD, Sunaga H, *et al.* Rapid chemical antagonism of neuromuscular blockade by L-cysteine adduction to and inactivation of the olefinic (double-bonded) isoquinolinium diester compounds gantacurium (AV430A), CW 002, and CW 011. *Anesthesiology* 2010; **113**: 58–73.
50 Savarese JJ, Sunaga H, McGilvra JD, *et al.* Preclinical pharmacology in the rhesus monkey of CW 1759-50, a new ultra-short acting nondepolarizing neuromuscular blocking agent, degraded and antagonized by L-cysteine. *Anesthesiology* 2018; **129**: 970–988.
51 Diaz LL, Zhang J, Heerdt PM. Comparative pharmacodynamics of pancuronium, cisatracurium, and CW002 in rabbits. *J Am Assoc Lab Anim Sci* 2014; **53**: 283–289.
52 Sakai DM, Romano M, Tseng CT, *et al.* Bias, limits of agreement, and percent errors between acceleromyography and mechanomyography in anesthetized dogs. *Vet J* 2018; **233**: 3–7.
53 Claudius C, Viby-Mogensen J. Acceleromyography for use in scientific and clinical practice: a systematic review of the evidence. *Anesthesiology* 2008; **108**: 1117–1140.
54 Murphy GS, Szokol JW, Avram MJ, *et al.* Intraoperative acceleromyography monitoring reduces symptoms of muscle weakness and improves quality of recovery in the early postoperative period. *Anesthesiology* 2011; **115**: 946–954.
55 Martin-Flores M, Campoy L, Ludders JW, *et al.* Comparison between acceleromyography and visual assessment of train-of-four for monitoring neuromuscular blockade in horses undergoing surgery. *Vet Anaesth Analg* 2008; **35**: 220–227.
56 Martin-Flores M, Sakai DM, Tseng CT, *et al.* Can we see fade? A survey of anesthesia providers and our ability to detect partial neuromuscular block in dogs. *Vet Anaesth Analg* 2019; **46**: 182–187.
57 Sakai DM, Martin-Flores M, Tomak EA, *et al.* Differences between acceleromyography and electromyography during neuromuscular function monitoring in anesthetized Beagle dogs. *Vet Anaesth Analg* 2015; **42**: 233–241.
58 Mosing M, Auer U, Bardell D, *et al.* Reversal of profound rocuronium block monitored in three muscle groups with sugammadex in ponies. *Br J Anaesth* 2010; **105**: 480–486.
59 Mundl WJ. A constant-current stimulator. *Physiol Behav* 1980; **24**: 991–993.
60 Ali HH, Utting JE, Nightingale DA, *et al.* Quantitative assessment of residual curarization in humans. *Br J Anaesth* 1970; **42**: 802–803.
61 Ali HH, Utting JE, Gray C. Stimulus frequency in the detection of neuromuscular block in humans. *Br J Anaesth* 1970; **42**: 967–978.
62 Ali HH, Utting JE, Gray TC. Quantitative assessment of residual antidepolarizing block. *I. Br J Anaesth* 1971; **43**: 473–477.
63 Ali HH, Utting JE, Gray TC. Quantitative assessment of residual antidepolarizing block. *II. Br J Anaesth* 1971; **43**: 478–485.
64 Ali HH, Wilson RS, Savarese JJ, *et al.* The effect of tubocurarine on indirectly elicited train-of-four muscle response and respiratory measurements in humans. *Br J Anaesth* 1975; **47**: 570–574.
65 Brull SJ, Ehrenwerth J, Silverman DG. Stimulation with submaximal current for train-of-four monitoring. *Anesthesiology* 1990; **72**: 629–632.

66 Silverman DG, Connelly NR, O'Connor TZ, *et al.* Accelographic train-of-four at near-threshold currents. *Anesthesiology* 1992; **76**: 34–38.
67 Ansermino JM, Sanderson PM, Bevan JC, *et al.* Acceleromyography improves detection of residual neuromuscular blockade in children. *Can J Anaesth* 1996; **43**: 589–594.
68 Engbaek J, Ostergaard D, Viby-Mogensen J. Double burst stimulation (DBS): a new pattern of nerve stimulation to identify residual neuromuscular block. *Br J Anaesth* 1989; **62**: 274–278.
69 Viby-Mogensen J, Howardy-Hansen P, Chraemmer-Jørgensen B, *et al.* Posttetanic count (PTC): a new method of evaluating an intense nondepolarizing neuromuscular blockade. *Anesthesiology* 1981; **55**: 458–461.
70 Vincent RD, Jr., Brockwell RC, Moreno MC, *et al.* Posttetanic count revisited: are measurements more reliable using the TOF-Watch accelerographic peripheral nerve stimulator? *J Clin Monit Comput* 2004; **18**: 33–37.
71 Sarrafzadeh-Rezaei F, Eddie Clutton R. The post-tetanic count during vecuronium-induced neuromuscular blockade in halothane-anaesthetized dogs. *Vet Anaesth Analg* 2009; **36**: 246–254.
72 Martin-Flores M, Sakai DM, Campoy L, *et al.* Recovery from neuromuscular block in dogs: restoration of spontaneous ventilation does not exclude residual blockade. *Vet Anaesth Analg* 2014; **41**: 269–277.
73 Hemmerling TM, Schmidt J, Hanusa C, *et al.* Simultaneous determination of neuromuscular block at the larynx, diaphragm, adductor pollicis, orbicularis oculi and corrugator muscles. *Br J Anaesth* 2000; **85**: 856–860.
74 Sakai DM, Martin-Flores M, Romano M, *et al.* Recovery from rocuronium-induced neuromuscular block was longer in the larynx than in the pelvic limb of anesthetized dogs. *Vet Anaesth Analg* 2017; **44**: 246–253.
75 Tseng CT, Sakai DM, Libin M, *et al.* Partial neuromuscular block impairs arytenoid abduction during hypercarbic challenge in anesthetized dogs. *Vet Anaesth Analg* 2017; **44**: 1049–1056.
76 Nagahama S, Nishimura R, Mochizuki M, *et al.* The effects of propofol, isoflurane and sevoflurane on vecuronium infusion rates for surgical muscle relaxation in dogs. *Vet Anaesth Analg* 2006; **33**: 169–174.
77 Kastrup MR, Marsico FF, Ascoli FO, *et al.* Neuromuscular blocking properties of atracurium during sevoflurane or propofol anaesthesia in dogs. *Vet Anaesth Analg* 2005; **32**: 222–227.
78 Sokoll MD, Gergis SD. Antibiotics and neuromuscular function. *Anesthesiology* 1981; **55**: 148–159.
79 Martinez EA, Mealey KL, Wooldridge AA, *et al.* Pharmacokinetics, effects on renal function, and potentiation of atracurium-induced neuromuscular blockade after administration of a high dose of gentamicin in isoflurane-anesthetized dogs. *Am J Vet Res* 1996; **57**: 1623–1626.
80 Hildebrand SV, Hill T. Interaction of gentamycin and atracurium in anaesthetised horses. *Equine Vet J* 1994; **26**: 209–211.
81 Martin-Flores M, Boesch J, Campoy L, *et al.* Failure to reverse prolonged vecuronium-induced neuromuscular blockade with edrophonium in an anesthetized dog. *J Am Anim Hosp Assoc* 2011; **47**: 294–298.
82 Chen IY, Liang YY, Chen KS, *et al.* Comparison of the neuromuscular blocking effects of cisatracurium during isoflurane or propofol anesthesia in dogs. *Vet Anaesth Analg* 2020; **47**: 454–462.
83 Lorenzutti AM, Zarazaga MP, Sakai DM, *et al.* Context-sensitive recovery of neuromuscular function from vecuronium in dogs: effects of dose and dosing protocol. *Vet J* 2019; **248**: 14–17.
84 Naguib M, Flood P, McArdle JJ, *et al.* Advances in neurobiology of the neuromuscular junction: implications for the anesthesiologist. *Anesthesiology* 2002; **96**: 202–231.
85 Wilson IB, Bergmann F. Studies on cholinesterase. VII. The active surface of acetylcholine esterase derived from effects of pH on inhibitors. *J Biol Chem* 1950; **185**: 479–489.
86 Wilson IB. The interaction of tensilon and neostigmine with acetylcholinesterase. *Arch Int Pharmacodyn Ther* 1955; **104**: 204–213.
87 Rupp SM, McChristian JW, Miller RD, *et al.* Neostigmine and edrophonium antagonism of varying intensity neuromuscular blockade induced by atracurium, pancuronium, or vecuronium. *Anesthesiology* 1986; **64**: 711–717.
88 Cronnelly R, Morris RB. Antagonism of neuromuscular blockade. *Br J Anaesth* 1982; **54**: 183–194.
89 Hennis PJ, Cronnelly R, Sharma M, *et al.* Metabolites of neostigmine and pyridostigmine do not contribute to antagonism of neuromuscular blockade in the dog. *Anesthesiology* 1984; **61**: 534–539.
90 Heier T, Clough D, Wright PM, *et al.* The influence of mild hypothermia on the pharmacokinetics and time course of action of neostigmine in anesthetized volunteers. *Anesthesiology* 2002; **97**: 90–95.
91 Mosing M, Auer U, West E, *et al.* Reversal of profound rocuronium or vecuronium-induced neuromuscular block with sugammadex in isoflurane-anaesthetised dogs. *Vet J* 2012; **192**: 467–471.
92 Martin-Flores M, Lorenzutti AM, Litterio NJ, *et al.* Speed of reversal of vecuronium neuromuscular block with different doses of neostigmine in anesthetized dogs. *Vet Anaesth Analg* 2017; **44**: 28–34.
93 Lorenzutti AM, Martin-Flores M, Baldivieso JM, *et al.* Evaluation of neostigmine antagonism at different levels of vecuronium-induced neuromuscular blockade in isoflurane anesthetized dogs. *Can Vet J* 2014; **55**: 156–160.
94 Cronnelly R, Morris RB, Miller RD. Edrophonium: duration of action and atropine requirement in humans during halothane anesthesia. *Anesthesiology* 1982; **57**: 261–266.
95 Ferguson A, Egerszegi P, Bevan DR. Neostigmine, pyridostigmine, and edrophonium as antagonists of pancuronium. *Anesthesiology* 1980; **53**: 390–394.
96 Kopman AF. Edrophonium antagonism of pancuronium-induced neuromuscular blockade in man: a reappraisal. *Anesthesiology* 1979; **51**: 139–142.
97 Martin-Flores M, Pare MD, Campoy L, *et al.* Neuromuscular blocking effects of cisatracurium and its antagonism with neostigmine in a canine model of autosomal-recessive centronuclear myopathy. *Br J Anaesth* 2015; **115**: 927–931.
98 Adams WA, Mark Senior J, Jones RS, *et al.* cis-atracurium in dogs with and without porto-systemic shunts. *Vet Anaesth Analg* 2006; **33**: 17–23.
99 Adam JM, Bennett DJ, Bom A, *et al.* Cyclodextrin-derived host molecules as reversal agents for the neuromuscular blocker rocuronium bromide: synthesis and structure-activity relationships. *J Med Chem* 2002; **45**: 1806–1816.
100 Bom A, Bradley M, Cameron K, *et al.* A novel concept of reversing neuromuscular block: chemical encapsulation of rocuronium bromide by a cyclodextrin-based synthetic host. *Angew Chem Int Ed Engl* 2002; **41**: 266–270.
101 Bom A, Clark JK, Palin R. New approaches to reversal of neuromuscular block. *Curr Opin Drug Discov Devel* 2002; **5**: 793–800.
102 Hoffmann U, Grosse-Sundrup M, Eikermann-Haerter K, *et al.* Calabadion: a new agent to reverse the effects of benzylisoquinoline and steroidal neuromuscular-blocking agents. *Anesthesiology* 2013; **119**: 317–325.
103 Ma D, Zhang B, Hoffmann U, *et al.* Acyclic cucurbit[n]uril-type molecular containers bind neuromuscular blocking agents in vitro and reverse neuromuscular block in vivo. *Angew Chem Int Ed Engl* 2012; **51**: 11358–11362.
104 Sunaga H, Malhotra JK, Yoon E, *et al.* Cysteine reversal of the novel neuromuscular blocking drug CW002 in dogs: pharmacodynamics, acute cardiovascular effects, and preliminary toxicology. *Anesthesiology* 2010; **112**: 900–909.
105 Sunew KY, Hicks RG. Effects of neostigmine and pyridostigmine on duration of succinylcholine action and pseudocholinesterase activity. *Anesthesiology* 1978; **49**: 188–191.
106 Murphy GS, Szokol JW, Marymont JH, *et al.* Residual paralysis at the time of tracheal extubation. *Anesth Analg* 2005; **100**: 1840–1845.
107 Murphy GS. Residual neuromuscular blockade: incidence, assessment, and relevance in the postoperative period. *Minerva anestesiologica* 2006; **72**: 97–109.
108 Eriksson LI, Sundman E, Olsson R, *et al.* Functional assessment of the pharynx at rest and during swallowing in partially paralyzed humans: simultaneous videomanometry and mechanomyography of awake human volunteers. *Anesthesiology* 1997; **87**: 1035–1043.
109 Sundman E, Witt H, Olsson R, *et al.* The incidence and mechanisms of pharyngeal and upper esophageal dysfunction in partially paralyzed humans: pharyngeal videoradiography and simultaneous manometry after atracurium. *Anesthesiology* 2000; **92**: 977–984.
110 Wyon N, Joensen H, Yamamoto Y, *et al.* Carotid body chemoreceptor function is impaired by vecuronium during hypoxia. *Anesthesiology* 1998; **89**: 1471–1479.
111 Jonsson M, Wyon N, Lindahl SG, *et al.* Neuromuscular blocking agents block carotid body neuronal nicotinic acetylcholine receptors. *Eur J Pharmacol* 2004; **497**: 173–180.
112 Eriksson LI, Sato M, Severinghaus JW. Effect of a vecuronium-induced partial neuromuscular block on hypoxic ventilatory response. *Anesthesiology* 1993; **78**: 693–699.
113 Eriksson LI. Reduced hypoxic chemosensitivity in partially paralysed man. A new property of muscle relaxants? *Acta Anaesthesiol Scand* 1996; **40**: 520–523.
114 Christensson E, Ebberyd A, Hårdemark Cedborg A, *et al.* Hypoxic ventilatory response after rocuronium-induced partial neuromuscular blockade in men with obstructive sleep apnoea. *Anaesthesia* 2020; **75**: 338–347.
115 Broens SJL, Boon M, Martini CH, *et al.* Reversal of partial neuromuscular block and the ventilatory response to hypoxia: a randomized controlled trial in healthy volunteers. *Anesthesiology* 2019; **131**: 467–476.
116 Murphy GS, Szokol JW, Marymont JH, *et al.* Residual neuromuscular blockade and critical respiratory events in the postanesthesia care unit. *Anesth Analg* 2008; **107**: 130–137.
117 Berg H, Roed J, Viby-Mogensen J, *et al.* Residual neuromuscular block is a risk factor for postoperative pulmonary complications. A prospective, randomised, and blinded study of postoperative pulmonary complications after atracurium, vecuronium and pancuronium. *Acta Anaesthesiol Scand* 1997; **41**: 1095–1103.
118 Murphy GS, Szokol JW, Marymont JH, *et al.* Intraoperative acceleromyographic monitoring reduces the risk of residual neuromuscular blockade and adverse

respiratory events in the postanesthesia care unit. *Anesthesiology* 2008; **109**: 389–398.

119 Caldwell JE. Reversal of residual neuromuscular block with neostigmine at one to four hours after a single intubating dose of vecuronium. *Anesth Analg* 1995; **80**: 1168–1174.

120 Herbstreit F, Zigrahn D, Ochterbeck C, *et al.* Neostigmine/glycopyrrolate administered after recovery from neuromuscular block increases upper airway collapsibility by decreasing genioglossus muscle activity in response to negative pharyngeal pressure. *Anesthesiology* 2010; **113**: 1280–1288.

121 Goldhill DR, Wainwright AP, Stuart CS, *et al.* Neostigmine after spontaneous recovery from neuromuscular blockade. Effect on depth of blockade monitored with train-of-four and tetanic stimuli. *Anaesthesia* 1989; **44**: 293–299.

122 Romano M, Martin-Flores M, Sakai DM, *et al.* Effects of neostigmine or edrophonium on force of contraction when administered at a train-of-four ratio of 0.9 in anesthetized dogs. *Vet Anaesth Analg* 2017; **44**: 1313–1320.

123 Fuchs-Buder T, Baumann C, De Guis J, *et al.* Low-dose neostigmine to antagonise shallow atracurium neuromuscular block during inhalational anaesthesia: a randomised controlled trial. *Eur J Anaesthesiol* 2013; **30**: 594–598.

27 Injectable Anesthetics

Stephanie M. Hamilton
Department of Companion Animals, Atlantic Veterinary College, University of Prince Edward Island, Charlottetown, Prince Edward Island, Canada

Chapter contents

Introduction, 462
Barbiturates, 463
  Chemical structure, 463
  Mechanism of action, 463
  Pharmacokinetics, 463
  Pharmacodynamics, 464
  Species-specific effects, 465
  Clinical use, 465
Propofol, 466
  Chemical structure, 466
  Mechanism of action, 466
  Pharmacokinetics, 466
  Pharmacodynamics, 467
  Species-specific effects, 467
  Clinical use, 468
  Fospropofol and other propofol prodrugs, 468
Dissociatives, 469
  Chemical structure, 469
  Mechanism of action, 469
  Pharmacokinetics, 469
  Pharmacodynamics, 470
  Species-specific effects, 471
  Clinical use, 472
Ketamine–propofol (ketofol), 472
Etomidate, 474
  Chemical structure, 474
  Mechanism of action, 474
  Pharmacokinetics, 474
  Pharmacodynamics, 474
  Species-specific effects, 476
  Clinical use, 476
  Etomidate analogs, 477
Alfaxalone, 477
  Chemical structure, 477
  Mechanism of action, 477
  Pharmacokinetics, 478
  Pharmacodynamics, 478
  Species-specific effects, 479
  Clinical use, 481
Other drugs, 481
  Metomidate, 481
  Chloral hydrate, 481
  Magnesium sulfate, 481
  Chloralose, 481
References, 482

Introduction

The drugs described below produce reliable sedation and anesthesia in veterinary patients. Most commonly, these agents are administered intravenously (IV) to induce an unconscious state suitable for intubation and transition to an inhaled anesthetic. However, when administered by either constant rate infusion, intermittent bolus, or intramuscularly (IM), injectable anesthetics can also be used to maintain anesthesia for short periods of time.

Ideally, all injectable anesthetics would be water soluble, have a long shelf-life, and be stable when exposed to heat and light. Only a small volume of drug would be needed to induce anesthesia, and these agents would have a large safety margin. Their duration of action would be short, with no cumulative effects, and they would be readily metabolized into non-toxic metabolites and/or excreted from the body. Their half-lives would be well characterized, as would their maximum residual limits so that withdrawal times could be established for animals destined for human consumption. Analgesia adequate for the procedure and some degree of muscle relaxation would also be produced by ideal injectable anesthetics. Most importantly perhaps, the ideal injectable anesthetic would not create unpredictable life-threatening changes in cardiovascular and respiratory function.

An injectable anesthetic that possesses all of these characteristics has not yet been produced. When selecting an injectable anesthetic, the practitioner should consider the pharmacokinetics and pharmacodynamics of the anesthetic, in addition to the patient's physical status, in order to select the most appropriate agent and dose for that individual patient.

Veterinary Anesthesia and Analgesia: The Sixth Edition of Lumb and Jones. Edited by Leigh Lamont, Kurt Grimm, Sheilah Robertson, Lydia Love and Carrie Schroeder.
© 2024 John Wiley & Sons, Inc. Published 2024 by John Wiley & Sons, Inc.
Companion website: www.wiley.com/go/lamont/anesthesia

Barbiturates

Barbiturates have been used in veterinary medicine for decades as both injectable anesthetics and anticonvulsants. For many years, thiopental was among the most commonly used injectable drugs for induction of anesthesia. However, over the past decade, its lack of availability in the United States and other countries has meant that veterinarians have increasingly turned to other non-barbiturate injectable anesthetic drugs.

Chemical structure

All of the drugs in this category are derivatives of barbituric acid, a combination of urea and malonic acid (Fig. 27.1). While barbituric acid does not have sedative or hypnotic properties, side chains added at position 5 in the pyrimidine nucleus impart hypnotic activity. The length of the side chain at position 5 influences the potency and the duration of action of these drugs, with longer side chains increasing potency. If a sulfur atom replaces the oxygen atom at position 2, an active barbiturate with a faster onset of action and a shorter duration is produced. In general, any modification of the barbiturate that increases the lipophilicity of the molecule will increase its potency while shortening the onset time and duration of action. Many barbiturates (thiopental, thiamylal, and methohexital) have asymmetric carbon atoms in one of the side chains attached to the barbiturate ring at position 5, which results in stereoisomers. Despite differences in potency of the stereoisomers (i.e., *S*(−)-enantiomers are nearly twice as potent as *R*(+)-enantiomers), barbiturates are supplied as racemic mixtures.

Commonly, barbiturates are classified by their duration of action (long, intermediate, short, and ultra-short) or their chemical structure. Thiobarbiturates (thiopental and thiamylal) are those with a sulfur atom at position 2, while oxybarbiturates (pentobarbital, phenobarbital, and methohexital) have an oxygen atom at position 2.

Historically, the ultra-short-acting thiobarbiturate, thiopental, was commonly used for anesthetic induction in veterinary medicine. In jurisdictions where it is still available, it is supplied as a yellow crystalline powder buffered with sodium bicarbonate, which is usually reconstituted with sterile water or saline to produce 2.5%, 5%, or 10% solutions. The resulting solution is alkaline (pH 10–11) and can cause tissue necrosis if injected perivascularly. The reconstituted solution is stable at room temperature for up to 1 week [1]. As the solution ages, crystals precipitate resulting in a progressive loss of potency; therefore, higher doses may be needed to induce anesthesia.

Thiamylal is an ultra-short-acting thiobarbiturate that differs from thiopental in that the ethyl radical in thiopental has been replaced with an allyl radical. While thiamylal was commonly used in veterinary medicine for some time, it is no longer commercially available.

Methohexital is an ultra-short-acting oxybarbiturate that possesses a methyl group at the N-1 position. This results in a drug that is twice as potent as thiopental, but also has an increased incidence of excitatory side effects. Methohexital sodium is supplied as a powder and is reconstituted with sterile water or saline to produce a 2.5% solution that is stable for up to 6 weeks if refrigerated [2].

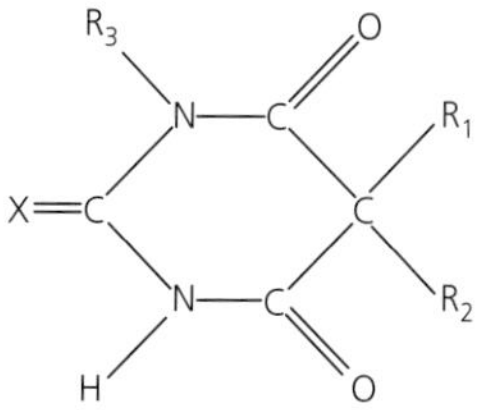

Pentobarbital is classified as a short-acting oxybarbiturate that is identical to methohexital but lacks a methyl group at the N-1 position. These substitutions result in a drug that has a longer duration of action (typically 1–2 h) and a lower margin of safety (anesthetic dose is 50–70% lethal dose). Pentobarbital has largely been replaced as a general anesthetic in most domestic species. It is still used as an injectable anesthetic in laboratory rodents, particularly in non-recovery procedures, and remains the primary ingredient in most commercially available veterinary euthanasia solutions. Pentobarbital is available in solutions of varying concentrations that, stored at room temperature, are stable for years.

Figure 27.1 General chemical structure of barbiturates.

Mechanism of action

Barbiturates produce central nervous system (CNS) depression by activating the ionotropic subtype of the γ-aminobutyric acid (GABA) receptor known as "$GABA_A$" [3]. Activation of the $GABA_A$ receptor increases transmembrane chloride conduction, resulting in hyperpolarization of the postsynaptic cell membrane. It appears that the barbiturates reduce the rate of dissociation of GABA from its receptor, which increases the duration of chloride channel opening. At increasing drug concentrations, barbiturates can mimic the action of GABA and activate the chloride channels directly [3,4]. Ultimately, inhibition of the postsynaptic neuron results in CNS depression and loss of consciousness.

Pharmacokinetics

Distribution of the barbiturates within the body is determined by factors such as time, protein binding, degree of ionization, and lipid solubility. Lipid solubility increases with the substitution of a sulfur molecule at carbon position 2 in the barbiturate ring. As previously stated, an increase in lipid solubility increases potency and shortens onset and duration of action. Protein binding correlates with lipid solubility, with barbiturates that are highly lipophilic (thiopental) also being highly bound to protein. Decreased protein binding due to displacement from binding sites by other drugs (aspirin and phenylbutazone) or hypoproteinemia can lead to increased drug effects.

The acid dissociation constant (pK_a) and pH of the environment can be used to predict the proportion of ionization of the barbiturates for any given condition. The pK_a is the pH at which the barbiturate exists 50% in the ionized and 50% in the non-ionized form. For a barbiturate to penetrate the lipid layer of a cell, it needs to be in the non-ionized form. Therefore, as blood becomes more acidic, more non-ionized drug exists. This leads to an increase in the barbiturate's CNS penetration and clinical effectiveness. The reverse is also true: with more alkaline blood, the ionized form is favored, and the anesthetic effect may be reduced.

Metabolism of the barbiturates occurs in the liver and is followed by excretion by the kidneys. Biotransformation (oxidation, *N*-dealkylation, desulfuration, and destruction of the barbituric acid ring structure) in the liver occurs primarily in the endoplasmic reticulum of hepatocytes and can result in hepatic enzyme induction (cytochrome P450 system) [5]. The reserve capacity of the liver is quite large; therefore, significant hepatic dysfunction must be present before there is a prolongation of the duration of action of barbiturates [6].

Thiopental

After IV administration of thiopental, the drug mixes within the blood and is delivered to body tissues in accordance with the rate of perfusion, the tissue affinity for the drug, and the relative concentration of thiopental in the blood and tissues. Well-perfused, small-volume tissues, such as the brain, equilibrate rapidly with the thiopental concentrations in the blood, inducing anesthesia. The concentration of thiopental in the blood and brain falls rapidly as the drug redistributes to less perfused muscular tissues, allowing the animal to regain consciousness. Dogs receiving 15 mg/kg of thiopental IV remained unresponsive to noxious stimuli (toe pinch) for 12 ± 6 min. Recovery to sternal recumbency took 52 ± 29 min and standing took place 77 ± 32 min after administration [7]. The principal factor limiting anesthetic duration after a single dose of thiopental is redistribution from the brain to other tissues [5]. Therefore, when thiopental is administered in large doses, as repeated doses, or as a constant rate infusion, recovery from anesthesia may be prolonged as lean tissues (e.g., muscle) approach equilibrium with the concentration of thiopental in the blood. This equilibrium progressively decreases the capacity of the tissues to remove the drug from the blood [8,9]. Additionally, obesity increases the mean disposition residence time of thiopental, and this is associated with a prolongation of terminal half-life, although the increased adipose mass will serve to remove more drugs from the blood and speed clinical recovery from a single bolus [10].

Pharmacokinetic parameters of thiopental have been described in dogs, horses, sheep, and rabbits [11,12]. The initial volume of distribution was 38.1 ± 18.4 mL/kg in dogs, 44.5 ± 9.1 mL/kg in sheep, and 38.6 ± 10.0 mL/kg in rabbits [12]. Horses and ponies had large volumes of distribution: 783 ± 128 mL/kg and 1127 ± 86 mL/kg, respectively [11]. The elimination half-life ($t_{1/2}$) was shown to be shortest in the rabbit (43.1 ± 3.4 min) and longest in the sheep (251.9 ± 107.8 min) [12]. The $t_{1/2}$ in the dog was 182.4 ± 57.9 min [12], and 147 ± 21 min in the horse [11,12].

Methohexital

A single dose of IV methohexital produces unconsciousness of short duration (8 ± 3 min in dogs). Recovery times compared to thiopental are faster with time to sternal recumbency and standing at 19 and 32 min, respectively [7]. Pharmacokinetic parameters in dogs receiving an IV dose of 10 mg/kg revealed both a rapid disposition phase (distribution half-life = 0.87 min) and a rapid elimination phase ($t_{1/2}$ = 24.1 min). The volume of distribution was 1602 ± 643 mL/kg while the total plasma clearance was 37.5 ± 8.07 mL/kg/min [7]. Administration of methohexital induces cardiopulmonary changes similar to thiopental. A recent study evaluating the effect of methohexital on laryngeal function dogs described adverse events after methohexital administration, including tachycardia, seizure-like activity, vomiting, and regurgitation [13].

Thiamylal

Mixed-breed dogs receiving 15 mg/kg of thiamylal IV remained unresponsive to toe pinch for 17 ± 9 min, returned to sternal recumbency in 55 ± 31 min, and were standing after 93 ± 46 min. Cardiopulmonary values in these dogs were similar to dogs receiving thiopental. Pharmacokinetics reveal a rapid disposition phase (distribution half-life = 38.9 min) and an extended elimination phase ($t_{1/2}$ = 666 min). The volume of distribution was 3352 ± 1887 mL/kg while the total plasma clearance was 3.21 ± 1.27 mL/kg/min [7]. A recent study using thiamylal to induce and maintain anesthesia in calves for approximately 2 h reported mean recovery times of over 5 h [14].

Pentobarbital

A single IV dose of 20 mg/kg of pentobarbital in mixed-breed dogs produces anesthesia of 64 ± 31 min. These dogs then needed 238 ± 52 min to return to sternal recumbency and 432 ± 22 min to stand [15]. Pentobarbital undergoes extensive hepatic metabolism and is totally dependent on the liver for biotransformation and elimination. Sheep and goats, however, are rapid metabolizers of the drug and require supplemental doses if anesthesia is to be maintained beyond 20–30 min.

Pharmacodynamics

Central nervous system

As noted previously, administration of barbiturates results in CNS depression and anesthesia. Following barbiturate administration, the electroencephalogram (EEG) is depressed in a dose-dependent fashion. With the administration of thiopental, the awake α pattern progresses to δ and θ waves until there is burst suppression and a flat EEG [16]. The barbiturates appear to possess cerebroprotectant properties. Cerebral metabolism of oxygen ($CMRO_2$) is reduced by up to 55% in a dose-dependent fashion [17]. Cerebral blood flow and intracranial pressure (ICP) are also decreased in parallel with the reduction in $CMRO_2$ [17]. Cerebral perfusion pressure, however, is usually not adversely affected because ICP decreases more than mean arterial pressure. Several studies have been performed evaluating thiopental as a cerebroprotectant and have shown that it may be of some clinical value. In dogs pretreated with thiopental and subjected to isolated brainstem ischemia, auditory evoked potentials were increased compared to those dogs that were not pretreated with thiopental [18]. Additionally, it was demonstrated that the mitigating effect of immediate post-arrest hypothermia in dogs with postischemic encephalopathy might be enhanced by thiopental [19]. These properties make thiopental an appropriate choice for patients with intracranial disease or a history of seizures. Methohexital has been associated with CNS excitation and epileptiform seizures, making it a poor choice for patients with seizures. Intraocular pressure is reduced slightly by thiopental administration [20].

Cardiovascular system

Administration of lower doses of thiopental results in a decrease in stroke volume and myocardial contractility [21]. A mild decrease in arterial blood pressure can be seen, but it is usually offset by a compensatory increase in heart rate. Venodilation after thiopental administration can lead to sequestration of red blood cells in the spleen, an increase in splenic size, and a decrease in packed cell volume. Vasodilation of cutaneous and skeletal blood vessels may also predispose the patient to hypothermia. Ventricular arrhythmias, particularly ventricular bigeminy, have also been demonstrated [22]. The incidence of these arrhythmias may be reduced with adequate ventilation and oxygenation prior to thiopental administration. Thiopental sensitizes the myocardium to epinephrine-induced arrhythmias in many species studied [23].

Respiratory system

Barbiturate administration for the induction of anesthesia causes dose-dependent depression of ventilatory centers, decreasing the brain's responsiveness to hypoxemia and hypercarbia [24]. There is a decrease in respiratory rate and minute ventilation [25]. Transient periods of apnea are commonly reported after large, rapidly administered doses of thiopental. Thiopental has also been shown to cause bronchoconstriction in the dog [26]. However, laryngeal reflexes may be less affected by thiopental administration compared to other induction agents; therefore, it may be a good choice for evaluation of laryngeal function [27]. Thiopental has also been shown to reduce mucociliary clearance in the dog [28].

Hepatic, renal, and gastrointestinal systems

Healthy patients have little change in hepatic or gastrointestinal function after induction of anesthesia with thiopental and only modest decreases in hepatic blood flow may be seen. Barbiturates stimulate an increase in microsomal enzymes, but only after 2 to 7 days of sustained drug administration [29].

While gastrointestinal effects such as diarrhea or intestinal stasis have not been reported with barbiturate administration, thiopental has been shown to decrease the tone of the lower esophageal sphincter in cats [30].

Renal blood flow may be decreased slightly by thiopental administration, most likely due to decreases in systemic blood pressure and cardiac output. A 15 mg/kg dose of thiopental in the dog resulted in a mean glomerular filtration rate of 2.04 ± 0.36 mL/min/kg, which did not differ significantly from other induction agents [31].

Fetal/neonatal effects

IV barbiturates easily cross the placenta and establish a dynamic equilibrium between maternal and fetal circulation. However, it should be remembered that the placental circulation passes through the liver before reaching the fetal CNS, thereby reducing overall drug exposure for most highly metabolized drugs. In a study performed on dogs, thiopental more profoundly depressed neurological reflexes in puppies born by cesarean section compared to propofol or epidural anesthesia [32]. Additionally, uterine blood flow transiently decreased in pregnant ewes induced with thiopental [33].

Analgesic effects

It should be noted that barbiturates do not produce antinociception (and analgesia only during unconsciousness); therefore, additional analgesics should be administered to patients undergoing painful procedures. In fact, at subanesthetic doses, the barbiturates may actually be hyperalgesic. However, this effect is controversial and is likely not clinically significant [34].

Species-specific effects

Canine

Documented breed-associated differences in anesthetic pharmacokinetics and pharmacodynamics are uncommon. However, among canine breeds, Greyhounds are relatively deficient in the hepatic microsomal enzymes that are needed to metabolize the thiobarbiturates. This deficiency, along with lean bodies and low-fat stores, potentially results in prolonged recoveries from thiopental anesthesia when larger doses are administered [29]. Barbiturate anesthetics are often not recommended for sighthound breeds (e.g., Greyhound, Irish Wolfhound, and Afghan Hound) but use of anesthetic-sparing premedications and minimal thiobarbiturate doses has allowed safe anesthetic induction in these breeds with minimal delay in recovery.

Equine

The pharmacokinetics of a single dose of thiopental at 11 mg/kg has been studied [11]. In that study, a three-compartment open model best described the disposition kinetics of thiopental. In plasma, thiopental has a very rapid initial distribution phase (distribution half-life = 1.4 ± 1.2 min and 1.3 ± 0.7 min in horses and ponies, respectively). While horses had a somewhat shorter $t_{1/2}$ (147 ± 21 min) than ponies (222 ± 44 min), no obvious difference in clearance of the drug between horses (3.5 ± 0.5 mL/kg/min) and ponies (3.6 ± 0.8 mL/kg/min) was noted [11].

Thiopental should not be administered to horses without prior sedation with an a_2-adrenergic receptor agonist, as significant excitement and incoordination may result. Additionally, anesthesia induction with guaifenesin and thiopental in horses that have just undergone maximal exercise is not recommended [35].

Ruminant

The pharmacokinetics of thiopental in sheep has also been described using a three-compartment open model [36]. The volume of distribution was 1005 ± 196 mL/kg, total body clearance was 3.5 ± 0.8 mL/kg/min, and $t_{1/2}$ was 196 ± 64 min in that study. Time of awakening was 36.6 ± 6.36 min [36]. The authors suggest that the relatively short duration of action of thiopental should be attributed mainly to elimination of the drug by hepatic metabolism and uptake by body fat [36]. This theory differs from the widely held belief that redistribution of thiopental terminates its anesthetic action. Toutain *et al.* propose that this is perhaps due to differences in regional blood flow between sheep and monogastric species, although this remains unestablished [36].

Swine

Barbiturates are effective anesthetic agents in swine limited only by the difficulty of attaining IV access in these species [37,38], although care should be used when administering thiopental to hypovolemic pigs as the anesthetic requirement for thiopental is reduced by approximately 35% in these animals [39]. Barbiturates do not trigger malignant hyperthermia in swine.

Clinical use

The induction doses of thiopental used in veterinary species are listed in Table 27.1. It should be noted that the dose required to induce anesthesia and facilitate endotracheal intubation is altered by premedications and the patient's physical status. Patients that are premedicated with other CNS depressants, or those that are hypovolemic, hypoproteinemic, acidotic, and/or uremic, will require less thiopental to induce anesthesia. Thiopental should be administered IV, preferably through a catheter, and the dose should be titrated to effect. Induction of anesthesia is rapid, occurring in approximately 20–30 s after administration. Because periods of apnea are often reported after induction of anesthesia with thiopental, equipment to facilitate intubation with a cuffed endotracheal tube, and to assist ventilation should be immediately available. The duration of action

Table 27.1 Barbiturate dosages in various species.

	Thiopental mg/kg IV	Pentobarbital mg/kg IV
Dog	8–22	2–30
Cat	8–22	2–15
Horse	4–15	
Cow	4–22	
Sheep	8–15	20–30
Llama	6–15	
Pig	5–12	

IV, intravenous.

of thiopental is quite short with the distribution/redistribution phase lasting 14.9 ± 3.3 min in dogs [6].

Perivascular administration of thiopental is associated with tissue necrosis, especially at higher concentrations (e.g., 5%). If inadvertent perivascular injection occurs, dilution of the drug should be attempted. This is best accomplished by injection of saline through the needle or catheter that still remains in place. At the same time, lidocaine can be injected to produce vasodilation and local anesthesia.

In order to reduce the incidence of ventricular arrhythmias, IV lidocaine has been investigated as a co-induction agent with thiobarbiturates. Thiopental administered IV to dogs at a dose of 11 mg/kg and lidocaine at a dose of 8.8 mg/kg produced a smooth induction with no arrhythmias and less cardiovascular depression as compared to thiopental alone [40]. This technique may not be suitable for all species since the IV administration of a relatively large dose of lidocaine may cause toxicity. Mixtures of thiopental and propofol (1:1) have also been used in the dog [41]. The dose of each drug required for induction was reduced and induction quality was similar to that of thiopental or propofol alone. Recovery times and quality of recovery were similar to those of propofol and superior to those of thiopental alone [41]. It should be noted that the mixture should inhibit bacterial growth and is bactericidal after 48 h against *Staphylococcus aureus, Escherichia coli, Pseudomonas aeruginosa,* and *Candida albicans* [42]. Mixtures of thiopental and propofol at a ratio of less than 1:1 do not maintain bactericidal properties [42]. Proper evaluation of drug stability in these mixtures is lacking, but they appear to maintain relatively normal potency.

Propofol

Propofol is chemically distinct from all other IV drugs used to induce or maintain anesthesia. Awakening from anesthesia has been found to be more rapid and complete with propofol than with other induction agents. It is this rapid return to consciousness with minimal residual effects that has made propofol such a popular anesthetic induction agent in both human and veterinary anesthesia. Its first use was reported in 1977 [43].

Chemical structure

Propofol is a substituted isopropylphenol (2,6-diisopropylphenol) that can be used to produce sedation, as well as to induce and maintain anesthesia (Fig. 27.2A). It is formulated as proprietary variations of an oil-in-water emulsion containing 1% propofol, 10% soybean oil, 2.25% glycerol, and 1.2% purified egg phosphatide. Propofol is relatively insoluble in aqueous solutions but is highly lipid soluble. It is a slightly viscous, milky white substance with a pH of 6.5–8.5. This formulation of propofol is stable at room temperature and is not light-sensitive. Most formulations do not contain preservatives and therefore will support bacterial or fungal growth; therefore, strict aseptic technique should be used when using multidose vials of propofol [44]. According to most labels, opened vials should be used or discarded before 6 h. When using propofol as a constant rate infusion, it would be prudent to discard IV tubing and administration sets every 12 h or if gross bacterial contamination occurs.

A lipid-free microemulsion formulation of propofol has been developed to increase vial shelf-life when broached, reduce infection risk by the addition of antimicrobial agents, reduce inherent emulsion instability, and reduce pain on injection [45,46]. It has a shelf-life of 28 days once the vial is opened. Additionally, a propofol formulation for the veterinary market containing benzyl alcohol has also been developed for use in dogs which has an increased shelf-life of 28 days once the vial is opened [47].

Mechanism of action

Like barbiturates, propofol appears to exert its anesthetic effects through an interaction with $GABA_A$ receptors [48]. Propofol also inhibits the *N*-methyl-D-aspartate (NMDA) receptor through modulation of channel gating which may also contribute to its CNS effects [49].

Pharmacokinetics

Propofol pharmacokinetics can be described by a two-compartment open model, with a rapid distribution phase followed by a slower clearance phase [51]. Following IV injection of propofol, it rapidly moves into the CNS resulting in induction of anesthesia. It is then rapidly redistributed from the brain to other tissues in the body, terminating its anesthetic action. In most species (cats are an exception), propofol undergoes rapid and extensive hepatic metabolism resulting in the production of inactive water-soluble sulfide and glucuronide metabolites. These are then excreted by the kidneys [52]. Clearance of propofol from the plasma exceeds hepatic blood flow, which emphasizes the importance of tissue uptake and suggests that extrahepatic metabolism or extrarenal excretion may occur [53]. In humans, there is no evidence of impaired elimination of propofol in patients with cirrhosis of the liver and extrahepatic metabolism has been confirmed in the anhepatic phase of liver transplant

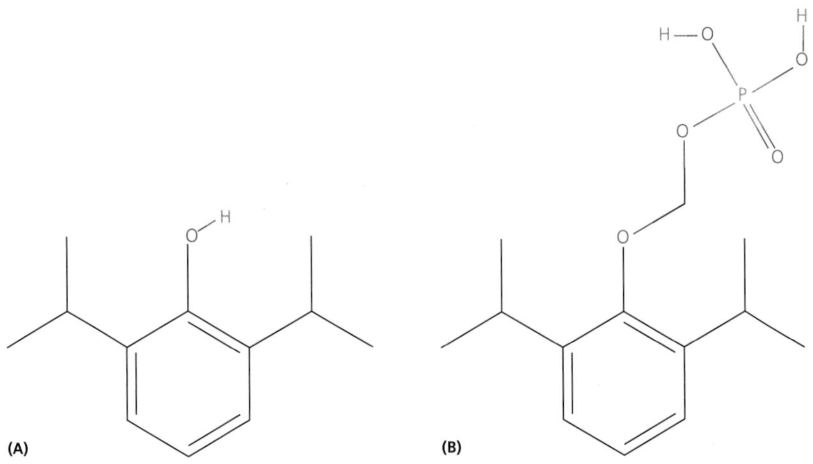

(A)

(B)

Figure 27.2 Chemical structure of **A.** propofol and **B.** fospropofol. Source: National Center for Biotechnology Information [50].

patients [53,54]. In cats, extrahepatic metabolism of propofol has been demonstrated in pulmonary tissue [55]. In cats with hepatic lipidosis, anesthetic induction with propofol for placement of a feeding tube did not increase morbidity or mortality despite the anticipated alteration of drug action [56].

The pharmacokinetics of propofol have been thoroughly studied in the dog [51,57,58]. Propofol's lipophilic nature results in a large apparent volume of distribution (17.9 L/kg) as well as steady-state volume of distribution (9.7 mL/kg) [51]. Due to the rapid redistribution of the drug into other tissues as well as rapid and extensive metabolism, the initial distribution half-life is short as is the rate of disappearance from plasma. Greyhounds appear to have a smaller apparent volume of distribution and steady-state volume of distribution, which suggests recovery from propofol anesthesia in Greyhounds will be slower [58]. Dogs greater than 8.5 years of age also have been shown to have a slower clearance rate compared to younger dogs [57]. The rapid distribution and clearance of propofol make it a suitable choice for maintenance of anesthesia by constant rate infusion of the drug in many species. In most species (except cats), propofol does not accumulate after repeated doses and/or prolonged infusion of the drug, so recovery from anesthesia remains rapid and of good quality [59,60].

Pharmacodynamics

Central nervous system

IV injection of propofol results in rapid CNS depression and induction of anesthesia. Much like the barbiturates, propofol reduces ICP and $CMRO_2$ [61]. Cerebral perfusion pressure is reduced slightly in patients with normal ICP, but in patients with elevated ICP, the drop in cerebral perfusion pressure is significant and may not be beneficial [62]. Brain responsiveness to carbon dioxide and cerebral metabolic autoregulation is maintained during propofol administration [61]; however, this response may be modified by concurrent administration of other drugs such as opioids. Propofol produces cortical EEG changes similar to barbiturates, including the incidence of burst suppression with the administration of high doses [61]. Propofol possesses anticonvulsant effects and can be used in the treatment of seizures [63,64].

Cardiovascular system

The most prominent cardiovascular effect of propofol administration is a decrease in arterial blood pressure. Decreases in systemic vascular resistance and cardiac output are also seen [65,66]. The magnitude of myocardial depression and vasodilation appear to be dependent on dose (and plasma concentration) [65]. These cardiovascular effects may be more profound in patients that are hypovolemic [67], geriatric, or have compromised left ventricular function [68]. Unlike thiopental, however, administration of propofol does not usually result in a compensatory increase in heart rate. Propofol does appear to sensitize the myocardium to epinephrine-induced arrhythmias but does not appear to be arrhythmogenic [69].

Respiratory system

Much like thiopental, propofol causes dose-dependent depression of ventilation and postinduction apnea (PIA), with transient cyanosis occurring regularly [70]. The incidence of apnea appears to be related to dose and rate of administration, with rapid injection rates making apnea more likely to occur [70]. The ventilatory response to hypoxemia [71] and carbon dioxide [72] is reduced by propofol [73], and the administration of opioids may enhance propofol's effect on ventilation [74]. Respiratory effects are also seen when propofol is administered as a constant rate infusion, with propofol decreasing tidal volume and respiratory rate [72].

Hepatic, renal, and gastrointestinal systems

Propofol does not adversely affect hepatic blood flow [75] or glomerular filtration rate in dogs [31]. In humans, propofol has been shown to be a very effective antiemetic. In fact, subanesthetic doses of propofol may be used postanesthesia to treat nausea and vomiting [76]; however, this effect has not been demonstrated in domestic animals.

Muscle

Like thiopental, propofol produces excellent muscle relaxation. Occasionally, however, myoclonic movements have been reported in both humans and dogs [77,78]. These movements resolve spontaneously.

Fetal/neonatal effects

Propofol readily crosses the placenta, but it is rapidly cleared from the neonatal circulation [79]. It is considered an acceptable choice for dogs undergoing cesarean section, as effects on healthy puppies are minimal [80].

Analgesic effects

Propofol produces neither antinociception nor hyperalgesia [34]. Animals undergoing painful procedures should therefore receive appropriate analgesics as part of the anesthetic plan.

Species-specific effects

Canine

Propofol can be administered IV for sedation and induction of anesthesia. It is also well suited to be used as a constant rate infusion for the maintenance of anesthesia. Propofol is often recommended for use in Greyhounds. The dose required for induction of anesthesia in Greyhounds is the same as mixed-breed dogs, but the recovery time is longer in Greyhounds [52].

As mentioned previously, the lipid-based emulsion formulation of propofol is capable of supporting microbial growth. In a retrospective study of clean wounds in dogs and cats, animals receiving propofol were 3.8 times more likely to develop wound infections compared to animals that did not receive propofol [81]. Causal mechanisms have not been established and the numerous confounding factors of wound infection rates would caution against overemphasizing the results of this study. However, strict aseptic technique should be followed when using propofol as an anesthetic and prompt disposal of unused drug should reduce the potential for drug contamination and any impact that would have on infection rates.

The lipid-free microemulsion formulation of propofol has been evaluated in the dog [82] and appears to be pharmacokinetically and pharmacodynamically similar to the lipid formulation. However, it has been reported that IV injection of the microemulsion formulation resulted in severe pain and complications in dogs [83].

Feline

Repeated daily administration of propofol can induce oxidative injuries to feline red blood cells [84]. Heinz body formation, facial edema, generalized malaise, anorexia, and diarrhea were all reported in one study in which cats received propofol on consecutive days. Heinz body formation was significantly increased by the third day of propofol administration and recovery times were significantly increased after the second consecutive day [84]. However, in another study, repeated propofol anesthesia was evaluated and no relevant hematologic changes were reported [85].

The formulation of propofol containing benzyl alcohol (Propoflo™28) has been evaluated in cats [47]. While there has been concern regarding this formulation due to potential adverse effects of benzyl alcohol on feline blood and nervous systems, it has been shown that administration to healthy cats of normal to high clinical doses of the formulation did not cause organ toxicity [47]. The lipid-free microemulsion formulation has also been evaluated in cats [46,86] and, when compared to the lipid-emulsion formulation, produces comparable pharmacokinetic, pharmacodynamic, and physiologic responses [46].

Equine

The clinical effects of propofol in the horse are similar to those seen in other species. IV administration of propofol following sedation produces rapid induction of anesthesia, a short duration of action, and a rapid, smooth recovery [87,88]. However, propofol can produce unpredictable behavioral responses and excitation at the time of induction, thereby limiting its use as a routine induction agent in adult horses [89]. These adverse effects at the time of induction appear to be prevented; however, by the IV administration of guaifenesin for 3 min prior to administration of propofol [90].

Propofol, either solely or in combination with other drugs, has been used effectively as a constant rate infusion in horses to maintain anesthesia [91–93]. While adverse events at induction were noted with propofol administration, horses appeared calm and coordinated in recovery [89]. This prompted the investigation of propofol, in combination with xylazine, as a potential modulator of recovery [94,95]. In these reports, it was noted that a combination of xylazine and propofol might be of some benefit as the quality of recovery was significantly improved [94,95].

The lipid-free microemulsion formulation of propofol has also been evaluated in the horse [96,97]. A 3-h continuous rate infusion produced similar cardiopulmonary and biochemical results to those reported when the lipid formulation was used [97]. However, in a different study of the pharmacokinetics, investigators urged caution when using propofol to maintain anesthesia due to variable kinetics, poor analgesia, and myoclonic activity [96].

Ruminant

Propofol has been satisfactorily used as an induction agent in sheep [98], goats [99], cows [100], and camelids [101]. Reported characteristics of propofol anesthesia in these species are similar to those reported in other veterinary species. Induction is rapid and smooth, duration of action is short, and recovery is of good quality. Cardiopulmonary effects are similar to those reported in other species.

The pharmacokinetics of propofol have been described in the goat. The mean $t_{1/2}$ was short (15.5 min), the volume of distribution at steady state was large (2.56 L/kg), and the clearance rate was rapid (275 mL/kg/min) [99]. These values differ from those obtained in sheep where the mean $t_{1/2}$ was 56.6 ± 13.1 min, volume of distribution was 1.037 ± 0.48 L/kg, and clearance was 85.4 ± 28.0 mL/kg/min [102].

Swine

Propofol does not induce malignant hyperthermia in susceptible swine [103]. As with other species, respiratory depression and apnea have been reported with propofol administration [104].

Clinical use

Propofol doses commonly used in veterinary patients are given in Table 27.2. It should be noted that the dose required to achieve endotracheal intubation is altered by premedications and the physical status of the patient. Patients that are debilitated and/or have received CNS depressants will often require less propofol for induction.

Propofol should be administered IV, preferably through a catheter, and the dose should be titrated to effect. Once administered, induction of anesthesia with propofol occurs within 20–30 s, although in states of low cardiac output, the lag period may be prolonged. The quality of induction with propofol is good with a smooth transition to unconsciousness. To reduce the incidence of PIA, it is often recommended that the titrated dose of propofol should be administered slowly (over 60–90 s); however, apnea may still occur. Transient apnea is seldom a problem (except when establishment of a patent airway is difficult or impossible such as with some oropharyngeal conditions) as long as the anesthetist is prepared to intubate with an endotracheal tube and assist or control ventilation until spontaneous respiration begins. Duration of unconsciousness ranges from 2–8 min and the quality of recovery is good.

While perivascular injection of propofol will not produce anesthesia, it is not associated with tissue necrosis. Pain on IV injection has been reported and appears to be associated with injection of propofol into smaller vessels, not necessarily perivascular injection. To decrease the incidence of injection pain, clinicians may choose to inject propofol into larger vessels, administer a small dose of lidocaine IV prior to propofol injection, or dilute the dose by administering propofol into a running IV fluid line.

Fospropofol and other propofol prodrugs

As stated previously, propofol is relatively insoluble in aqueous solutions and is therefore formulated as an oil-in-water emulsion. Disadvantages of this type of formulation have been discussed previously (e.g., pain at the injection site and potential bacterial contamination). Other drawbacks of the emulsion formulation include propofol infusion syndrome and hypertriglyceridemia with prolonged infusion. Research has therefore focused on finding alternative formulations or related drugs to address these issues. Fospropofol is a water-soluble prodrug of propofol licensed by the United States Food and Drug Administration [107]. It is chemically described as a 2,6-diisopropylphenoxymethyl phosphate disodium salt (Fig. 27.2B). Following administration, it is metabolized by alkaline phosphatase producing propofol, phosphate, and formaldehyde. The formaldehyde

Table 27.2 Propofol dosages in various species.

	Induction dose (mg/kg) IV	Constant rate infusion (mg/kg/min)
Dog	3[a]–10	0.2–0.6
Cat	5–10	0.2–1.0
Horse	2–3[a], 6–8	0.2–0.4
Foal	2	0.33
Donkey	2	0.21
Pig	2–3	0.1–0.2
Llama	2	0.4
Ferret	2–4	
Rabbit	2–10	0.6–0.9[b]
Sheep	2–6	0.3–0.4
Goat	3–6	0.3

[a] Premedicated
[b] Martin-Cancho *et al.* [105]; Terada *et al.* [106].
IV, intravenous.

is rapidly metabolized by aldehyde dehydrogenase in the liver and erythrocytes into formate. Systemic formaldehyde levels do not increase beyond those occurring from food and environmental intake or metabolism [107]. The available formulation of fospropofol is an aqueous, colorless, and clear solution supplied in a single dose vial at a concentration of 35 mg/mL. The pharmacokinetics are complex and reliable data on the kinetics are lacking as most publications on the subject have been retracted due to potential analytical errors [108]. In dogs, a single IV dose of 6 mg/kg of fospropofol resulted in a significantly slower onset (124 ± 15 s) and longer duration (1448 ± 155 s) of unconsciousness than propofol. This is unsurprising as the prodrug requires enzymatic conversion to the active drug [45]. In rabbits receiving infusions of fospropofol, the minimum infusion rate (MIR) was 2.0 mg/kg/min compared to 0.9 mg/kg/min for propofol and recovery time increased as the duration of infusion increased [109]. Rabbits receiving infusions of fospropofol for 6 or 8 h needed significantly more time (52 ± 6 and 84 ± 10 min, respectively) to recover than those receiving propofol (36 ± 7 and 48 ± 5 min, respectively) [109].

Additional water-soluble prodrugs of propofol have shown promise and are under investigation. HX0507 was found to have anesthetic effects similar to propofol and, in dogs, was found to cause similar dose-dependent hypotension but less dose-dependent respiratory depression [110]. Also, in development is HX0969w, a water-soluble ester prodrug of propofol that is similar to fospropofol, but releases γ-hydroxybutyrate instead of formaldehyde [111]. With modifications to the HX0969w molecule, studies in rats show greater water solubility, faster onset, and similar anesthetic effects as fospropofol [112].

While these new formulations are promising, they must offer significant advantages over the standard propofol emulsion to justify their incorporation into clinical practice.

Dissociatives

The dissociatives are phencyclidine derivatives that produce a so-called state of “dissociative anesthesia” characterized by dissociation of the thalamocortical and limbic systems causing a change in awareness [113]. Ketamine hydrochloride and tiletamine hydrochloride are the dissociative anesthetics most commonly used in veterinary medicine.

Chemical structure

Ketamine is 2-(o-chlorophenol)-2-(methylamino)-cyclohexanone hydrochloride (Fig. 27.3A). Two optical isomers of ketamine exist due to an asymmetric carbon. Most formulations contain the racemic mixture, but a purified *S*-ketamine formulation is available in some countries. The *S*(+)-enantiomer produces more intense analgesia, is metabolized more rapidly, and has a lower incidence of emergence reactions than the *R*(−)-enantiomer [114]. Racemic ketamine is available as a 10% aqueous solution. It has a pH of 3.5–5.5 and is preserved by benzethonium chloride.

Tietamine is 2-(ethylamino)-2-(2-thienyl)-cyclohexanone hydrochloride (Fig. 27.3B). It is only available in combination with the benzodiazepine, zolazepam, and is marketed under the names Telazol® and Zoletil®. Tiletamine–zolazepam combinations are available as a white powder that is reconstituted with 5 mL of diluent. The final concentrations of tiletamine and zolazepam depend on the product being used.

Mechanism of action

The dissociative anesthetics act on NMDA, opioid, monoaminergic, and muscarinic receptors. Additionally, they interact with voltage-gated calcium channels [116,117]. Interestingly, the dissociatives do not appear to interact with GABA receptors as the other injectable anesthetics do.

Ketamine and tiletamine are non-competitive antagonists at the NMDA receptor. They bind to the phencyclidine-binding site, which prevents glutamate, an excitatory neurotransmitter, from binding. Prevention of glutamate binding results in depression of the thalamocortical, limbic, and reticular activating systems.

Dissociatives have also been reported to have action at μ-, δ-, and κ-opioid receptors [118]. Activity at the opioid receptors imparts analgesic properties unlike other injectable anesthetics, although the clinical significance of this action at clinically relevant doses is debatable. Additionally, the dissociatives' interaction at monoaminergic receptors may also contribute to antinociception [117]. Because dissociative anesthesia is associated with anticholinergic symptoms (emergence delirium, bronchodilation, and sympathomimetic actions), it is thought that these drugs have antagonist activity at the muscarinic receptors [117]. However, many of these effects may also be related to the sympathetic nervous system-stimulating effects of ketamine and tiletamine.

Pharmacokinetics

The dissociatives are similar to other injectable anesthetics in that they have a rapid onset of action (especially when given IV), short duration, and are highly lipophilic. Unlike other injectable anesthetics, the dissociatives are effective when administered IM. Peak plasma concentrations occur within 1 min of IV administration and 10 min following IM injection. The high lipid solubility of the dissociatives ensures that the blood–brain barrier is crossed quickly, which establishes effective brain concentrations of the drugs [119].

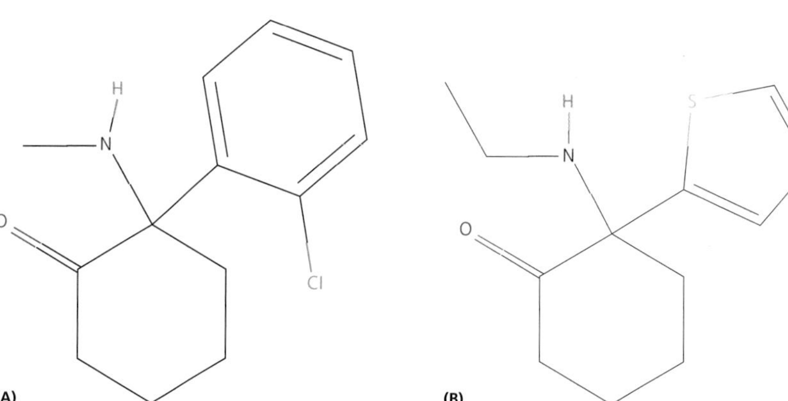

Figure 27.3 Chemical structure of **A.** ketamine and **B.** tiletamine. Source: National Center for Biotechnology Information [115].

In most species, metabolism of the dissociatives occurs in the liver. Ketamine is demethylated by hepatic microsomal enzymes producing the active metabolite norketamine. Eventually, norketamine is hydroxylated and then conjugated to form water-soluble and inactive glucuronide metabolites that are excreted by the kidney [120]. This process differs in the cat, where ketamine is biotransformed to norketamine, which is excreted unchanged in the urine [121]. Dissociatives should be used with care in animals with significant hepatic and/or renal dysfunction as prolonged anesthetic times may result.

Tiletamine also undergoes hepatic metabolism and renal excretion. Since tiletamine is only supplied with zolazepam, the action of the benzodiazepine should also be discussed. In cats, the duration of action of zolazepam is longer than that of tiletamine. This means that the CNS effects of the benzodiazepine (sedation) are present longer than those of tiletamine. In the dog, the reverse is true; the duration of action of tiletamine is longer than zolazepam. This means that the effects of the dissociative are observed, including muscle rigidity, sympathetic stimulation, and emergence delirium. Pigs appear to have a slow, calm recovery from tiletamine–zolazepam combinations, while in horses an agitated recovery may be seen if additional sedation is not provided. If significant plasma levels of tiletamine are present, reversal of the benzodiazepine with flumazenil may result in an anxious recovery.

Pharmacodynamics

Central nervous system

Dissociative anesthesia resembles a cataleptic state in which the patient does not appear to be asleep but does not respond to external stimuli. As mentioned previously, antagonism of the NMDA receptor leads to a dissociation of the limbic and thalamocortical systems [122]. Unlike other injectable anesthetics, the dissociatives increase cerebral blood flow and $CMRO_2$ [123]. Cerebral vasodilation and an increase in blood pressure results in an increase in ICP [122]. It appears that this increase in ICP can be attenuated if ventilation is controlled and animals remain eucapnic [124]. Administration of thiopental or a benzodiazepine has also been shown to reduce ketamine-induced increases in ICP [119]. Clinicians should still exercise caution, however, when using dissociatives in patients that have or are suspected of having increased ICP.

Eleptiform EEG patterns are seen after ketamine administration [125], resulting in the recommendation that dissociatives should be avoided in patients with seizure disorders. However, it has been shown that ketamine does not alter the seizure threshold in epileptic patients [126]. Additionally, there is evidence that ketamine possesses anticonvulsant as well as neuroprotective activity [127].

Abnormal behavior that may progress to emergence delirium may occur during recovery from dissociative anesthesia. Misrepresentation of visual and auditory stimuli may be responsible for this reaction [120]. A patient experiencing an emergence reaction may be ataxic, hyperreflexic, sensitive to touch, have increased motor activity, and may have a violent recovery. These reactions are usually temporary and usually resolve within a few hours. Administration of CNS depressants such as benzodiazepines, acepromazine, or α_2-adrenergic receptor agonists may decrease the incidence and/or the severity of these reactions [120].

Cardiovascular system

Ketamine has a direct negative cardiac inotropic effect [128], but it is usually overcome by central sympathetic stimulation. IV administration of ketamine increases systemic and pulmonary arterial pressures, heart rate, cardiac output, myocardial oxygen requirements, and cardiac work [129]. It is likely that these changes are the result of direct stimulation of the CNS leading to increased sympathetic nervous system outflow [130]. Ketamine also inhibits norepinephrine reuptake into postganglionic sympathetic nerve endings leading to an increased concentration of plasma catecholamines [131]. Critically ill patients may respond to induction of anesthesia with ketamine with a decrease in systemic blood pressure and cardiac output. The catecholamine stores and the sympathetic nervous system's compensatory mechanism may be exhausted, unveiling ketamine's negative inotropic effects [132]. While healthy animals are usually tolerant of increased cardiac work, myocardial oxygen requirements, and heart rate, ketamine should be used with caution in those animals that have severe cardiovascular disease (e.g., uncontrolled hypertension, cardiomyopathy, or heart failure), and/or are already tachycardic or dysrhythmic. Stimulation of the cardiovascular system in these patients may not be desirable.

Respiratory system

Unlike other injectable anesthetics, ketamine does not cause significant respiratory depression. Ventilatory responses to hypoxia and carbon dioxide are maintained in animals receiving ketamine as the sole anesthetic agent [133]. When ketamine is administered with other CNS depressants, significant respiratory depression can occur. Ketamine administration has been associated with an "apneustic" respiratory pattern, characterized by a prolonged inspiratory duration and relatively short expiratory time [134]. Despite this altered respiratory pattern, carbon dioxide levels and minute ventilation usually remain within normal limits.

Ketamine is a bronchial smooth muscle relaxant and causes bronchodilation and a decrease in airway resistance [135]. This makes it an attractive choice when anesthetizing animals with asthma or obstructive airway diseases such as chronic obstructive pulmonary disease. Pharyngeal and laryngeal reflexes remain intact when ketamine is used as the sole anesthetic agent [136]. It should be noted, however, that these reflexes are often uncoordinated and not protective. An endotracheal tube should always be placed to prevent aspiration. Maintaining a secure airway is especially important because ketamine increases salivation and respiratory tract secretions [119]. These can be reduced with the administration of an anticholinergic.

Hepatic, renal, and gastrointestinal systems

Laboratory tests that indicate hepatic or renal function are not altered by the administration of dissociatives. Gastrointestinal motility is unchanged after the administration of ketamine in the dog [137].

Analgesic effects

As previously discussed, the action of the dissociatives at NMDA and opioid receptors imparts analgesic properties. In fact, it has been demonstrated that subanesthetic doses of ketamine produce profound analgesia, especially in situations of somatic pain [116]. Additionally, blockade of the excitatory neurotransmitter glutamate at the NMDA receptor by the dissociatives is thought to play a role in preventing or minimizing central sensitization or wind-up pain. Therefore, preemptive administration of ketamine prior to painful stimuli may play a role in attenuating central sensitization [138,139].

Muscle

Unlike the previously discussed injectable anesthetic agents, the dissociatives produce little muscle relaxation. In fact, the dissociatives may cause muscle rigidity and often spontaneous movement of the limbs, trunk, and/or head. Substantial increases in intraocular pressure (IOP) are seen after ketamine administration which may be a result of increased tone of the extraocular muscles [140]. Muscle relaxation can be improved with the co-administration of benzodiazepines or α_2-adrenergic receptor agonists.

Fetal/neonatal effects

Ketamine crosses the placenta and enters fetal circulation. In a study evaluating neurologic reflexes in puppies born via cesarean section, anesthetic induction of the dam with ketamine and midazolam resulted in the most depression of neurologic reflexes when compared with other injectable induction drugs [32].

Species-specific effects

Canine

The dissociatives can be administered either IV or IM to produce a range of effects from sedation to anesthesia. Induction of anesthesia with ketamine alone can lead to muscle rigidity, spontaneous movement, and undesirable recoveries. Therefore, it is usually administered with a co-induction agent such as a benzodiazepine. Because tiletamine is supplied as a combination with zolazepam, there is no need for additional benzodiazepine for IV administration.

IM ketamine or tiletamine–zolazepam combinations are frequently combined with an α_2-adrenergic receptor agonist and an opioid to produce excellent immobilization with muscle relaxation and analgesia. Table 27.3 shows dosages of ketamine alone or in combination with other anesthetics commonly used in the dog. Table 27.4 shows common doses and usage of Telazol® in dogs.

Feline

The dissociatives have been used to produce a range of effects from sedation to anesthesia in cats. These drugs can be administered IV or IM. Ketamine is also absorbed through the oral mucosa. In particularly fractious cats, ketamine can be sprayed into the mouth to effectively induce sedation and facilitate the induction of anesthesia [141]. Copious salivation usually results due to the bitter taste and/or low pH of ketamine.

α_2-Adrenergic receptor agonists, benzodiazepines, and/or acepromazine are commonly administered in combination with IM ketamine. The combination of dexmedetomidine, ketamine, and an opioid produces excellent chemical restraint/anesthesia, muscle relaxation, and analgesia [142].

Tiletamine–zolazepam combinations (500 mg) have been reconstituted with xylazine (100 mg) and ketamine (400 mg) to form a potent chemical restraint/anesthesia cocktail that can be administered IM [143,144]. Care must be exercised when administering the drug combination as the overall volume is very small and accurate measurement is important. Additionally, careful patient monitoring to prevent profound hypothermia is required since prolonged recovery may result due to a reduction in metabolic rate. Flumazenil and/or an α_2-adrenergic receptor antagonist has been used to speed recovery from this combination. Table 27.5 shows common combinations and dosages of Telazol® in cats.

The use of tiletamine–zolazepam combinations in large felids, especially tigers, is not recommended. Adverse reactions, including delayed recovery, hindlimb paresis, hyperreflexia, seizures, and death have been reported [145].

Table 27.3 Commonly used ketamine dosages alone or in combination in dogs.

Agent	Dose (mg/kg)	Route	Duration (min)	Effect
Ketamine alone	10	IV	7–23	Short duration, anesthesia inadequate for surgery
Acepromazine Ketamine	0.2 10	IV	31–47	Clinical anesthesia, less muscle rigidity
Acepromazine Ketamine	0.22 11–18	IM		Restraint, spastic movements, prolonged recovery
Xylazine Ketamine	0.55–1.1 IM 22 IV to effect	IM/IV	28–36	Surgical anesthesia, muscle relaxation, analgesia for abdominal surgery
Atropine Xylazine Ketamine	0.04 1.1 11	IV	17–35	Increased risk with dogs with cardiopulmonary compromise
Atropine Xylazine Ketamine	0.04 1.1 22	IM	17–35	Increased risk with dogs with cardiopulmonary compromise
Medetomidine Ketamine	0.04 5	IM	25–35	Longer muscle relaxation and recovery than xylazine/ketamine
Diazepam Ketamine	0.28 5.5	IV		Suitable induction for sighthounds
Midazolam Ketamine	0.5 10	IV	10–16	Increased heart rate, mild respiratory depression, good muscle relaxation

IM, intramuscular; IV, intravenous.

Table 27.4 Commonly used tiletamine–zolazepam (Telazol®) dosages alone or in combination in dogs.

Agent	Dose (mg/kg)	Route	Duration (min)	Effect
Telazol®	9.9	IM	10–30	Rough recovery
Telazol®	6.6	IV	7–27	
Telazol® Xylazine Butorphanol	8.8 1.1 0.22	IM	100	Clinical anesthesia, good muscle relaxation, good analgesia
Butorphanol Telazol®	0.7 9.3–11.9	IM		Unsatisfactory sedation in vicious dogs
Acepromazine Telazol®	0.6–3.0 17.5–21.1	IM		Adequate sedation in vicious dogs

IM, intramuscular; IV, intravenous.

Table 27.5 Commonly used tiletamine–zolazepam (Telazol®) dosages alone or in combination in cats.

Agent	Dose (mg/kg)	Route	Duration (min)	Effect
Telazol® alone	6–40 (average 12.8)	IM	40–70	Salivation, apneustic breathing
Telazol® alone	12.8	IV	35–70	Salivation, apneustic breathing
Acepromazine Telazol®	0.1 3.4 ± 1.09	IM		Adequate anesthesia for castration
Telazol® Ketamine Xylazine	3.3 2.64 0.66	IM	34–52	Smooth induction and recovery, excellent muscle relaxation, good analgesia

IM, intramuscular; IV, intravenous.

Equine

The dissociatives, particularly ketamine, are used extensively in equine anesthesia. IV administration of the dissociatives rapidly and smoothly induces anesthesia provided that adequate sedation has been achieved prior to their administration. If the dissociatives are administered before adequate sedation has been provided, excitement will occur. Some muscle rigidity and involuntary movement may still occur when ketamine is used; therefore, it is frequently combined with a co-induction agent such as a benzodiazepine, α_2-adrenergic receptor agonist, or guaifenesin.

Anesthesia can be maintained by administering additional IV doses of ketamine. These doses may be administered as intermittent boluses or as a constant rate infusion. When used as a constant rate infusion, ketamine is frequently combined with sedatives and analgesic agents (e.g., α_2-adrenergic receptor agonists, guaifenesin, and opioids) in a combination commonly referred to as "triple drip." Commonly used doses for ketamine in combination with other anesthetic agents can be found in Table 27.6.

Tiletamine–zolazepam combinations can be administered IV to induce anesthesia in the horse after adequate sedation has been achieved. It should be noted, however, that recovery from tiletamine–zolazepam anesthesia is sometimes associated with excitement and incoordination if additional sedatives such as α_2-adrenergic receptor agonists are not administered, or anesthesia is not prolonged with inhalants [151]. Table 27.7 shows dosages for tiletamine in horses.

Ruminant

The dissociatives can be used in ruminants to induce anesthesia. Sedation and muscle relaxation are usually improved by the administration of an α_2-adrenergic receptor agonist or benzodiazepine prior to the administration of ketamine. Anesthesia can be maintained with a constant rate infusion of ketamine or by a combination of ketamine, guaifenesin, and xylazine.

Subanesthetic doses of ketamine (in combination with xylazine) have been administered to calves to produce sedation prior to castration [152]. This so-called "ketamine stun" technique may be an efficacious and cost-effective alternative or adjunct to local anesthesia for castration [152]. See Table 27.7 for dosages of the dissociatives in ruminants.

Swine

The dissociatives have been used extensively in swine for chemical restraint and anesthesia. Ketamine does not induce malignant hyperthermia in susceptible pigs, although its use in these animals has been controversial [153]. Similar to other species, ketamine as a sole anesthetic agent produces poor muscle relaxation so it is commonly combined with azaperone, benzodiazepines, and/or α_2-adrenergic receptor agonists for sedation and anesthesia. Tiletamine–zolazepam combinations are commonly reconstituted with 250 mg of xylazine and 250 mg of ketamine and used as an injectable anesthetic in swine [154]. See Table 27.7 for dosages of dissociative anesthetics in swine.

Clinical use

The tables mentioned previously list the commonly used doses of ketamine and tiletamine–zolazepam combinations, respectively. Both IV and IM routes of administration are listed. The total dose required to induce anesthesia will be affected by premedications, the patient's physical status, and route of administration. Clinicians should evaluate patients carefully to determine if the dosage needs to be altered.

Depending on the dose administered, IM injection of dissociatives produces effects ranging from rapid and reliable chemical immobilization to general anesthesia. Onset of action occurs within 10 min of IM injection. Duration of anesthesia is dependent on the dose administered but is usually longer following IM injection due to the higher overall dose. Reversal of the sedative/tranquilizer used in combination with the dissociative should not occur until the effects of the dissociative have waned. Early reversal of sedatives may lead to emergence delirium and a rough recovery.

IV administration of ketamine plus a benzodiazepine or tiletamine–zolazepam combinations results in anesthetic induction in approximately 45–90 s. The quality of induction is good, but clinicians should remember that ocular, laryngeal, and pharyngeal reflexes may remain intact. The eyes stay open, but the patient is anesthetized. Anesthetic duration of a single induction dose of ketamine–diazepam or tiletamine–zolazepam combinations is approximately 20 min. Recovery from IV dissociative administration is usually of good quality especially if other drugs (e.g., α_2-adrenergic receptor agonists) are co-administered or anesthesia is prolonged with inhalants.

Ketamine–propofol (ketofol)

A combination of ketamine and propofol, commonly referred to as "ketofol," has been studied in various clinical settings as an alternative anesthetic induction agent. It has been used extensively in humans for sedation and anesthesia in emergency procedures as it is thought to provide adequate sedation and analgesia with more stable hemodynamic and respiratory parameters compared to other injectable induction agents.

Mixtures of ketamine and propofol at 50:50 and 30:70 ratios are physically compatible and chemically stable in capped polypropylene syringes exposed to light and stored at room temperature for 3 h. Additionally, mixtures of propofol and ketamine in 5:1 and 6.7:1 ratios remained homogenous and physically stable for 6 h in a polypropylene syringe [155]. This ensures that ketamine and propofol delivered from the same syringe can be used in constant rate infusions and that the concentrations of the drugs delivered to patients are those calculated [156].

The combination of ketamine and propofol has been studied in domestic species. Five minutes after the induction of anesthesia in dogs premedicated with acepromazine and oxymorphone, ketofol (1:1 mixture, 2 mg/kg IV of each drug) increased heart rate, cardiac output, and calculated oxygen delivery. Mean arterial blood pressure and stroke volume remained unchanged while systemic vascular resistance was decreased. Respiratory depression (increased arterial partial pressure of carbon dioxide and hypoxemia) was reported, although the incidence of apnea was not different in dogs receiving propofol, ketofol, or ketamine and diazepam. Regardless of the agent used for induction of anesthesia, close monitoring of respiratory function is recommended [157]. In another study in dogs, a 1:1 mixture of ketamine and propofol reduced the dose of propofol required for the induction of anesthesia by 25% (4.0 ± 1.0 mg/kg versus 5.3 ± 1.1 mg/kg). Kennedy and Smith demonstrated that ketofol, when delivered as a constant rate infusion for 60 min, reduced the dose of propofol needed to maintain anesthesia by 50% (0.3 ± 0.1 mg/kg/min versus 0.6 mg/kg/min) [158]. Additionally, the cardiopulmonary effects of ketofol were similar to those reported by Riccó and Henao-Guerrero [157]. Martinez-Taboada and Leece [159] concluded that the quality of induction and tracheal intubation after ketofol was consistently good, and less variable compared to induction with propofol alone. Anesthesia

Table 27.6 Commonly used ketamine combination dosages in horses.

Agent	Dose (mg/kg)	Route	Duration (min)	Effect
Xylazine Ketamine	1.1 2.2	IV	12–35	Smooth induction and recovery, inadequate muscle relaxation
Xylazine Butorphanol Ketamine	1.1 0.1–0.2 2.2	IV	18–56 depending on breed	Behavioral changes, muscle relaxation, good analgesia
Xylazine Ketamine Methadone	1.1 2.2 0.1	IV		Satisfactory anesthesia
Methadone Acepromazine Xylazine Ketamine	0.1 0.15 1.1 2.2	IV		Inadequate anesthesia
Acepromazine Methadone Ketamine	0.04 0.04 2.0–2.5	IV	3–18	Muscle tremors
Guaifenesin Xylazine Ketamine	50 0.5 1.0	IV	120	Low blood pressure and hypoventilation
Guaifenesin Ketamine	50 1.5–2.2			Less cardiovascular depression than guaifenesin–barbiturate
Xylazine Diazepam Ketamine	1.1 0.1 2.0	IV		Supplement with 200–750 mg ketamine, maintain with inhalant, good muscle relaxation
Xylazine Temazepam Ketamine	1.1 0.044 2.2	IV		Longer recumbency
Romifidine Ketamine	0.1 2.0–2.2	IV	10–25	Initial limb rigidity, mild tremor
Romifidine Midazolam Ketamine	0.08 0.06 2.2	IV	25–40	May require additional dose of midazolam and ketamine, smooth recovery
Methotrimeprazine Midazolam Guaifenesin Ketamine	0.5 0.1 100 1.6	IV		Induction of anesthesia, smooth recovery
Detomidine Ketamine	0.02 2.2	IV	10–43	Required more time than xylazine–ketamine to assume recumbency, occasional poor recovery, longer hypertension
Guaifenesin Detomidine Ketamine	50 0.04 4	IV	140	Surgical anesthesia but may require additional ketamine during surgery, good recovery
Detomidine Butorphanol Ketamine	0.02 0.04 2.2	IV	18–67	Smooth induction, smooth recovery, muscle relaxation
Propofol Ketamine	1.0 1.0	IV		Doses are for induction of anesthesia after premedication with medetomidine and midazolam, good-quality induction, and recovery [146]
Xylazine Ketamine Propofol	0.016 0.03 0.1	IV		Doses are mg/kg/*min* for TIVA after premedication with xylazine and induction with ketamine, supplemental oxygen is recommended [147]
Propofol Ketamine	0.5 3.0	IV		Doses are for induction of anesthesia after premedication with xylazine [148]
Ketamine Medetomidine Propofol	1 0.00125 7.8–10.2 following a 0.5 loading dose	IV	160–190 (duration of TIVA)	Doses are mg/kg/*h* for TIVA, after premedication with medetomidine and induction with midazolam–ketamine, satisfactory anesthesia with minimal cardiovascular depression [149]
Propofol Ketamine	0.3–0.5 2.5–3.1	IV		Doses are for induction of anesthesia after premedication with xylazine, satisfactory inductions, and recoveries without clinically relevant adverse effects [150]

IM, intramuscular; IV, intravenous; TIVA, total intravenous anesthesia.

with ketofol was sufficient for castration in dogs premedicated with medetomidine [160].

The combination of ketamine and propofol is effective for the induction and maintenance of anesthesia in cats [161,162]. In cats undergoing ovariectomy, induction (2 mg/kg IV of each drug) and maintenance (10 mg/kg/h IV of each drug) of anesthesia with a 1:1 mixture of ketamine and propofol, resulted in smooth inductions and recoveries with extubation occurring quickly after cessation of the constant rate infusion (7.1 ± 2.5 min) [161]. The pharmacokinetics of ketofol in these cats was also described. Despite the rapid recovery

Table 27.7 Ketamine and tiletamine–zolazepam (Telazol®) dosages in various species.

Species	Dose of ketamine (mg/kg)	Dose of tiletamine–zolazepam (mg/kg)
Dog	5–10 IV	1 IV 3–6 IM
Cat	5–10 IV 5–15 IM	4–7 IM
Horse	2–2.2 IV (after adequate sedation)	1–3 IV (after adequate sedation)
Cattle	2–4 IV	2–4 IV
Pig	10 IM	6 IM

IM, intramuscular; IV, intravenous.

after ketofol infusion, propofol was quantifiable in most animals until 24 h after the infusion while ketamine was quantifiable for 8 h [162] albeit in concentrations less than what is considered effective.

Ketofol has also been used effectively in rabbits with doses of 5 mg/kg of each drug IV resulting in the loss of righting reflex in 11 ± 5 s with a duration of 374 ± 26 s. Hemodynamic function was well maintained, but hypoxemia was observed at this dose therefore oxygen supplementation is recommended [163].

A 3:1 mixture of propofol and ketamine has been studied in sheep and compared to propofol alone [102]. The combination of ketamine and propofol produced satisfactory anesthesia for superficial surgery and animals recovered quickly with the mean times to extubation, sternal recumbency, and standing being 5.3 ± 0.9, 11.2 ± 1.7, and 15.1 ± 2.2 min, respectively [102].

Simultaneous infusions of ketamine and propofol have been used to maintain anesthesia in ponies undergoing castration [164]. The combination provided satisfactory anesthesia and rapid, smooth recoveries with no evidence of excitement. The mean times to extubation, sternal recumbency, and standing were 1.9 ± 0.2, 8.4 ± 3.2, and 14.9 ± 10.1 min, respectively. Cardiopulmonary parameters were well maintained [164]. The pharmacokinetics of the simultaneous infusions were also described. The mean $t_{1/2}$ of propofol was 69.0 ± 8.0 min while ketamine was 89.8 ± 26.7 min. The mean residence times for propofol and ketamine were 87.1 ± 4.1 and 110.7 ± 8.2 min, respectively. The mean residence time for norketamine, the main metabolite of ketamine, was 144 ± 16 min [165].

Etomidate

Synthesized in 1964 and introduced into human medical practice in 1972, etomidate has been used as an induction and maintenance agent due to its minimal cardiopulmonary and cerebral protective effects [166,167]. Recent interest in etomidate derivatives such as methoxycarbonyl-etomidate (MOC-etomidate or MOC-ET) has resulted in an improved understanding of etomidate pharmacology and adverse effects.

Chemical structure

Etomidate is an imidazole derivative, ethyl 1-(1-phenylethyl)-1H-imidazole-5 carboxylate sulfate, which exists in two isomers, with only the *R*(+)-enantiomer producing hypnosis (Fig. 27.4). Etomidate is unstable in neutral solutions and is insoluble in water. It is supplied as a 0.2% solution in 35% propylene glycol with a pH of 6.9. Commercially available etomidate preparations have a high osmolality, which may result in some of its adverse effects, including the potential for erythrocyte damage.

Mechanism of action

Similar to other injectable anesthetics, etomidate has agonist activity at the GABA receptor [3]. Etomidate enhances the action of the inhibitory neurotransmitter GABA, which increases chloride conduction into the cell resulting in hyperpolarization of the postsynaptic neuron. The hyperpolarization of the postsynaptic neuron results in CNS depression and hypnosis.

Pharmacokinetics

The pharmacokinetics of etomidate have been described in cats and people as a three-compartment open model [168,169]. Etomidate is redistributed rapidly in the cat (0.05 h) and its $t_{1/2}$ is 2.89 h [169]. The volume of distribution at steady state is large (4.88 ± 2.25 L/kg in cats) and total clearance occurs at 2.47 ± 0.78 L/kg/h [169]. Etomidate penetrates the brain quickly, resulting in a rapid induction of anesthesia. Recovery from a single IV injection of etomidate is rapid due to redistribution of the drug from the brain to inactive tissue sites. Approximately, 75% of etomidate is bound to albumin, therefore conditions where albumin concentrations are decreased result in increases in the pharmacologically active drug [170]. The therapeutic index (LD_{50}/ ED_{50}) of etomidate in rats is quite large (26.0) as compared to thiopental (4.6) [171].

Etomidate undergoes hydrolysis of its ethyl ester sidechain that forms a water-soluble, pharmacologically inactive metabolite that is excreted in the urine, bile, and feces. Hepatic enzymes and plasma esterases carry out the hydrolysis. The hydrolysis of the drug is nearly complete as less than 3% of etomidate is excreted unchanged in the urine [172,173].

Pharmacodynamics

Central nervous system

The primary CNS effect of etomidate is hypnosis that is accomplished through GABA agonist activity. In cats, etomidate decreases the spontaneous firing of cortical neurons as well as the firing rate of neurons in the thalamus and reticular formation. This depression of neuronal activity likely contributes to anesthetic-induced unconsciousness [175].

Etomidate causes vasoconstriction of the cerebral vasculature and reduces cerebral blood flow and $CMRO_2$ [176,177]. Because mean arterial blood pressure is unchanged after etomidate administration, cerebral perfusion pressure is maintained [177]. As a result, previously elevated ICP is reduced after etomidate administration much like it is after thiopental administration [178,179]. In a canine model for cerebral hypoperfusion, cerebral oxygen extraction fraction did not change during hypotension when etomidate was administered. Therefore, it was concluded that etomidate may preserve the cerebral metabolic state [180]. Reducing the cerebral metabolic rate of oxygen consumption while lowering the rate of rise of ICP and producing immobilization may reduce the effects of a hypoxic insult to the brain of animals [181]. Etomidate produces changes in the EEG similar to barbiturates [179], but it has also been associated with grand mal seizures [182]. For this reason, some anesthetists argue against etomidate's use in patients with a history of seizures.

Cardiovascular system

IV administration of etomidate in healthy animals is characterized by cardiovascular stability. A single induction dose of etomidate results in minimal to no changes in heart rate, stroke volume, cardiac output, mean arterial blood pressure, central venous pressure, or cardiac index [183,184]. In a canine-isolated papillary muscle

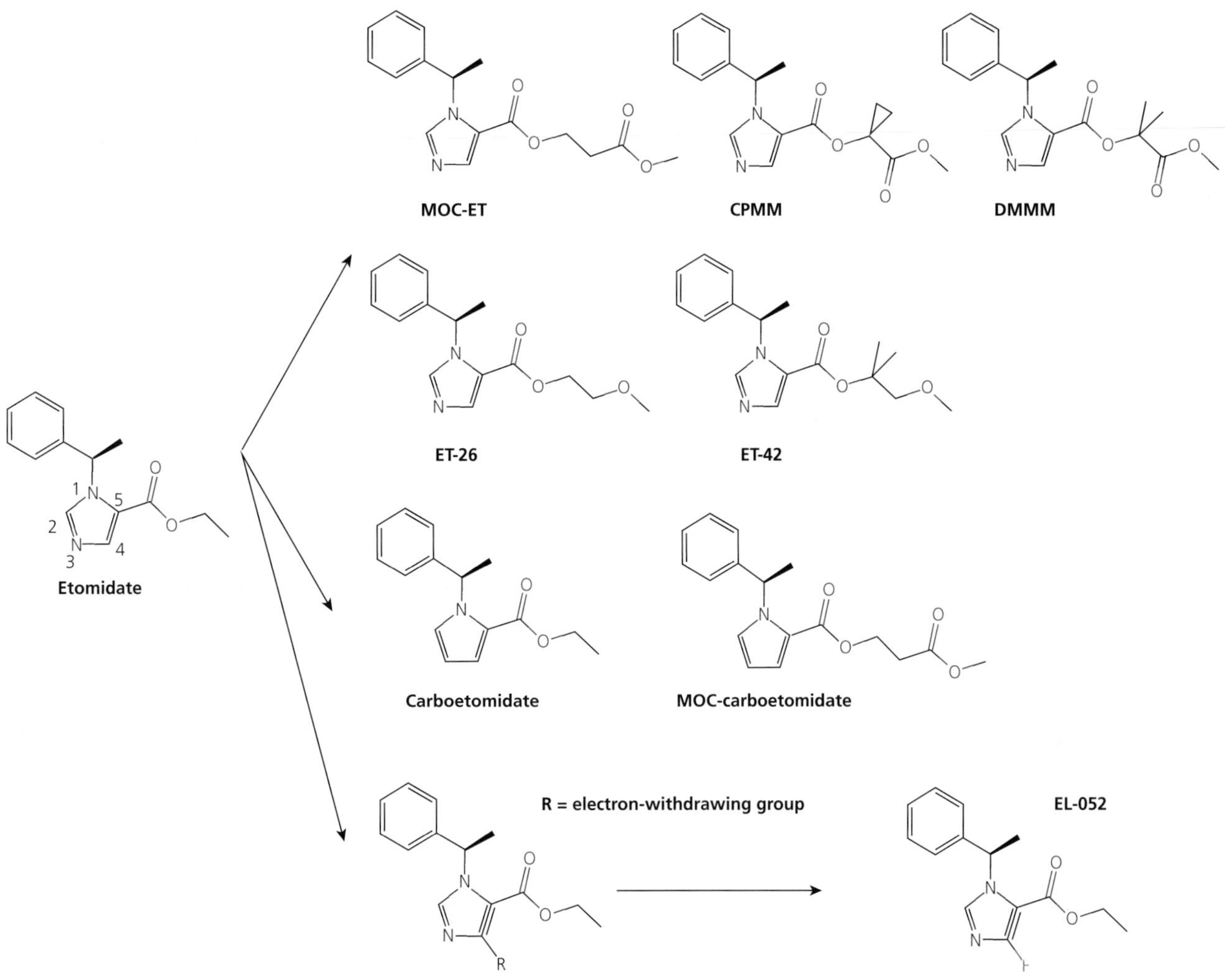

Figure 27.4 Chemical structure of etomidate and its analogs. MOC-ET, methoxycarbonyl-etomidate; CPMM, cyclopropyl-methoxycarbonyl-metomidate (renamed ABP-700); DMMM, dimethyl-methoxycarbonyl-metomidate; ET-26, methoxyethyl-etomidate; ET-42, methoxy-2-methylpropan-etomidate; MOC-carboetomidate, methoxycarbonyl-carboetomidate. Source: Jiang *et al.* [174].

preparation, etomidate produced less myocardial depression than an equally potent dose of thiopental [185]. Baroreceptor function and sympathetic nervous system responses appear to remain intact after etomidate administration, further contributing to hemodynamic stability [186]. When administered to hypovolemic dogs, etomidate produced minimal changes in cardiopulmonary variables [187]. In dogs with dilated cardiomyopathy, however, arterial blood pressure remains stable during etomidate anesthesia due to increases in arterial resistance and aortic impedance along with decreases in aortic compliance [188]. This indicates that arterial pressure is maintained due to an increase in left ventricular afterload, which adversely affects left ventricular systolic and diastolic performance in patients with impaired left ventricular function [188]. It should be emphasized that etomidate is usually only suitable for induction of anesthesia and that the greatest cardiovascular effects the patient is likely to experience will be due to the drugs used to maintain anesthesia (usually inhalant anesthetics), which may negate or alter any potential benefits from using etomidate.

Respiratory system

Etomidate has minimal effects on the respiratory system. PIA has been reported after rapid IV administration [189]. In most patients, any reduction in tidal volume that is seen after etomidate administration is usually offset by an increase in respiratory rate [166].

Hepatic, renal, and gastrointestinal systems

Etomidate does not decrease renal blood flow or glomerular filtration rate [31]. Hepatic and renal function tests are not affected by etomidate administration [168].

Endocrine system

Adrenocortical suppression has been documented after etomidate administration. Etomidate reduces adrenal steroidogenesis at several metabolic sites, including inhibition of the conversion of cholesterol to cortisol by the 11β-hydroxylase enzyme and suppression of the cholesterol-side chain cleavage enzyme [190–192]. This suppression of the adrenocortical system persists for up to 6 h in the dog [193] and 5 h in the cat [194]. This has been a proposed mechanism for the increased mortality in human patients observed in some studies following etomidate anesthesia. Care should be exercised when anesthetizing patients with existing adrenocortical disease (e.g., hypoadrenocorticism), highly stressed patients, or when etomidate is being used as a constant rate infusion to maintain anesthesia. Significant decreases in aldosterone and cortisol were noted in dogs receiving a 3-h constant rate infusion of etomidate. These decreases were dependent on both the dose and the duration of infusion [195]. Infusion of etomidate for long durations is not recommended.

Analgesic effects

Etomidate does not produce antinociception; therefore, patients undergoing painful procedures should have appropriate analgesics administered during the perioperative period.

Muscle

Myoclonus, dystonia, and tremor can occur with etomidate administration [196]. It is thought that this is the result of disinhibition of subcortical structures that normally suppress extrapyramidal motor activity [197]. Myoclonic activity can be decreased with adequate premedication and/or the IV administration of a benzodiazepine immediately prior to etomidate administration [196].

Pain on injection

IV administration of etomidate frequently results in pain. It is thought that this is due to the propylene glycol vehicle or the hyperosmolar nature of the commercial product. The incidence of pain can be lessened by administration of etomidate into a large vein, through a running IV line, or IV administration of an opioid immediately prior to etomidate administration [196].

Other considerations

The current formulation of etomidate in propylene glycol results in a solution with an osmolality of 4640 mOsm/L. This is hyperosmotic when compared to plasma (approximately 300 mOsm/L) and has been associated with intravascular hemolysis. In dogs, clinically significant hemolysis has been reported following prolonged administration of etomidate [198].

Species-specific effects

Canine

Despite side effects of administration such as vomiting, myoclonus, excitement, and hemolysis, etomidate still should be considered as an IV induction agent in patients with cardiovascular instability, increased ICP, and/or cirrhosis [199].

Feline

The pharmacokinetics of etomidate have been described in the cat and are detailed above. When used as an induction agent in normal cats, etomidate has been demonstrated to be an acceptable induction agent producing minimal cardiopulmonary effects [200]. Additionally, when investigated as an IV induction agent for cats with decreased cardiovascular reserve, etomidate administered at a dose of 1–2 mg/kg titrated to effect was determined to be effective. Excessive salivation was noted in all cats, however [200]. It should be noted, however, that due to the fragility of feline red blood cells, cats may be more likely to have intravascular hemolysis when etomidate is administered.

Equine

Etomidate is not used clinically in horses.

Ruminant

Etomidate has been studied in pregnant ewes. Fresno *et al.* studied the cardiovascular and acid–base effects of etomidate in the pregnant ewe and fetus [201]. It was determined that an IV bolus of 1 mg/kg of etomidate did not depress cardiovascular function in the ewe or fetus. When etomidate was administered as a constant rate infusion for 1 h, the maternal heart rate and blood pressure increased during the second half of the infusion and in the initial stages of recovery. Acid–base alterations led to transient but slight respiratory depression of the mother and fetus, which may have been due to a combination of etomidate and positioning of the animal [201]. Placental transfer of etomidate was also examined in pregnant ewes. It was determined that etomidate crosses the placenta rapidly and reaches the fetus in high amounts. However, cumulative effects of etomidate in the fetus were not demonstrated because fetal elimination occurred just as quickly as it did in the dam [202].

The inhibitory effects of etomidate on basal and ACTH-stimulated cortisol synthesis by isolated bovine adrenocortical cells have also been investigated. In concentrations likely to be achieved during anesthesia, etomidate blocks cortisol output by these isolated bovine cells [191].

Swine

Etomidate has been used as an IV induction agent in swine [203]. As in other species, etomidate provides cardiovascular stability, decreases cerebral blood flow, and renal blood flow remains essentially unchanged [204]. Additionally, etomidate does not trigger malignant hyperthermia in susceptible pigs [205].

Clinical use

Doses of etomidate commonly used in domestic species are given in Table 27.8. Clinicians should note that the dose needed to achieve endotracheal intubation is affected by the patient's physical status and prior administration of other CNS depressants (e.g., sedatives, tranquilizers, and opioids). Etomidate may be a reasonable anesthetic induction agent for those patients with some types of myocardial disease, cardiovascular instability, and/or intracranial lesions [199].

Induction of anesthesia with etomidate is rapid and endotracheal intubation is usually possible within 30 s of administration. As noted previously, pain on IV injection has been described. The incidence of injection pain may be reduced by IV administration of an opioid analgesic prior to etomidate injection, administration of etomidate through an IV catheter placed in a large vein, and/or administration of etomidate via a running IV line. Myoclonus following IV etomidate administration has also been described. Adequate premedication with sedatives such as benzodiazepines may reduce the incidence of myoclonic activity.

The duration of anesthesia after IV administration of etomidate is dose-dependent but awakening from a single dose of etomidate is more rapid than after barbiturate administration [166]. Anesthesia can be maintained by administering etomidate as a constant rate infusion as there is little evidence of cumulative drug effect. However, this practice is not recommended due to the previously discussed adrenocortical suppression and erythrocyte damage.

Table 27.8 Etomidate dosages in various species.

Species	Dose (mg/kg) IV
Dog	0.5–4.0
Cat	0.5–4.0
Pig	2–4

IV, intravenous.

Etomidate analogs

Efforts to produce an etomidate analog that maintains the desirable qualities of etomidate (rapid onset and recovery, excellent hemodynamic stability, and high therapeutic index) while minimizing the inhibition of adrenal steroid synthesis are ongoing. These analogs target modifications to the imidazole ring or the ester side chain of etomidate (Fig. 27.4). Carboetomidate replaces the imidazole ring with a pyrrole ring. The resulting drug does not suppress adrenocortical functioning; however, its sedation potency is seven times less than etomidate [206]. This reduction in potency causes a relatively slow onset of hypnosis compared to etomidate.

Methoxyethyl-etomidate (ET-26) leaves the imidazole ring of etomidate intact and instead modifies the ester side chain. Studies of ET-26 in rats and dogs reveal a sedative-hypnotic effect with maintenance of myocardial performance [207] and milder adrenal gland suppression [208]. Phase I clinical trials of ET-26 are imminent.

Methoxycarbonyl-etomidate (MOC-ET) was the first etomidate analog designed. While MOC-ET retained the rapid onset of hypnosis and hemodynamic stability of etomidate, its rapid metabolism resulted in a short duration of action [209]. This led to the adaptation of MOC-ET to cyclopropyl-methoxycarbonyl metomidate (CPMM). CPMM has been studied in rats [208] and dogs [210,211] showing hypnotic activity and a duration of action between that of MOC-ET and etomidate. Recovery from CPMM in these species was swift and adrenocortical suppression was significantly shorter than with etomidate. IV infusion of CPMM in dogs was associated with involuntary muscle movements and the incidence of these movements was higher during CPMM infusions than when etomidate was used [211]. CPMM was renamed ABP-700 and has undergone promising clinical trials in heathy human subjects. Adrenal gland function was preserved, few patients experienced pain on injection, and the incidence of postoperative nausea and vomiting was only moderate [212–214]. The development of ABP-700 is ongoing.

Alfaxalone

Alfaxalone has been used in veterinary medicine since its anesthetic properties were described in 1971 [215]. Because alfaxalone is poorly water soluble, it was originally combined with a weak anesthetic, alfadolone, and formulated in a 20% polyoxyethylated castor oil vehicle. Althesin® was formulated for human use while Saffan® was marketed for veterinary use. This combination of two neurosteroids was used to induce and/or maintain anesthesia in a variety of species, including cats, horses, pigs, and sheep [216]. However, the castor oil vehicle, Cremophor EL®, was associated with hyperemia in cats [217] and histamine release with resultant anaphylactic reactions in dogs [215]. A solution containing alfaxalone in a noncremophor (cyclodextrin) vehicle (Alfaxan-CD®) has been approved for dogs and cats. The cyclodextrin molecule is derived from starch and has a hydrophobic core in which the alfaxalone binds. This allows the mixture of alfaxalone and cyclodextrin to be dissolved in water. This formulation is not associated with histamine release [218], although one case of anaphylaxis associated with IV administration of alfaxalone in a dog has been reported [219].

Chemical structure

Alfaxalone (3α-hydroxy-5α-pregnane-11,20-dione) is a neuroactive steroid molecule capable of inducing anesthesia (Fig. 27.5). It is supplied as a 1% solution in 2-hydroxypropyl-β-cyclodextrin. The solution does not contain an antimicrobial preservative and

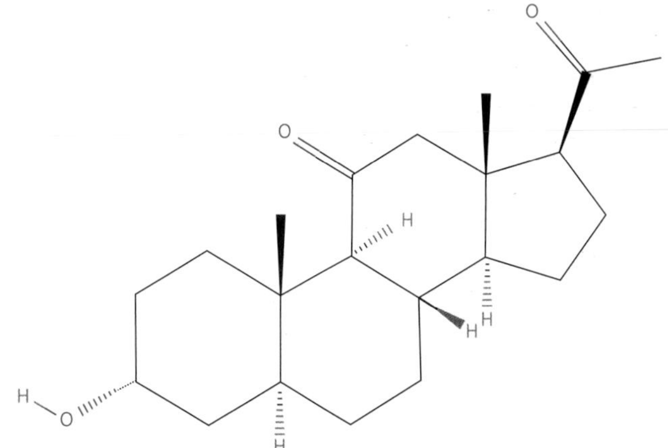

Figure 27.5 Chemical structure of alfaxalone. Source: National Center for Biotechnology Information [226].

supports the growth of *S. aureus* and *E. coli* (although less readily than propofol). The labeled shelf-life of this original, preservative-free formulation of alfaxalone varies between countries. In the United Kingdom, the vial is labeled as single use, while in the United States, it should be discarded 6 h after first puncture. In Australia, a vial stored at 4 °C can be used for 7 days. The microbial integrity of preservative-free alfaxalone has been evaluated [220]. In this study, no microbial contamination was found in alfaxalone stored at 4 °C for 7 days and handled with a protected port (closed system transfer device or nonclosed dispensing pin) [220]. A multidose formulation of alfaxalone containing the preservatives ethanol, benzethonium chloride, and chlorocresol extends the shelf-life of alfaxalone to 28 days [221]. The use and safety of these preservatives have been reviewed by Rowe *et al.* [222], and the formulation has been demonstrated to be pharmaceutically bioequivalent [223]. An experimental 4% solution of alfaxalone has been formulated and studied in remote delivery situations [224,225].

Mechanism of action

As with many of the other injectable anesthetic agents, alfaxalone produces CNS depression by activity at $GABA_A$ receptors [227], although there is evidence that the exact neurosteroid binding sites are separate from those of propofol and etomidate [228]. Typical $GABA_A$ receptors consist of 2α, 2β, and 1γ subunit with these subunits existing in numerous isoforms (e.g., α(1–6), β(1–3), and γ(1–3)). Recent evidence demonstrates that alfaxalone contacts α1β3γ2L $GABA_A$ receptors. In further describing the $GABA_A$ receptor structure, each subunit contains an *N*-terminal extracellular domain and a transmembrane domain with four α helices (M1 to M4). Each subunit interface is designated by the subunit and the helices forming the interface (e.g., α^+-β^-, where + corresponds to the M3 face and – is the M1 face). Within the receptor, alfaxalone binds to the transmembrane β^+-α^- inter subunit sites that are intracellular and adjacent to the sites for propofol and etomidate [228]. Binding of alfaxalone to the $GABA_A$ receptor causes movement of chloride into the cell resulting in hyperpolarization of the postsynaptic membrane. This, in turn, inhibits the pathways responsible for arousal and awareness. When present in lower concentrations, alfaxalone will modulate ion currents through the $GABA_A$ receptor. At higher concentrations, however, alfaxalone acts as a GABA agonist, similar to barbiturates [227].

Pharmacokinetics

The pharmacokinetics of IV alfaxalone have been determined in several species, including dogs, cats, horses, and rabbits. In dogs, the pharmacokinetics have been described using a non-compartmental model and a dose-dependent effect on the elimination half-life has been demonstrated [218]. After an IV dose of 2 mg/kg, the $t_{1/2}$ is 24 ± 1.9 min. A dose of 10 mg/kg IV increased the $t_{1/2}$ to 37.4 ± 1.6 min. There is also a dose-dependent effect on plasma clearance. Alfaxalone is cleared at 59.4 ± 12.9 mL/kg/min and 52.9 ± 12.8 mL/kg/min after 2 or 10 mg/kg IV, respectively [218]. The volume of distribution after a single dose of 2 mg/kg IV is 2.4 L/kg. The duration of anesthesia, $t_{1/2}$, and plasma clearance for alfaxalone in nonpremedicated Greyhounds are similar to those reported in Beagles [229]. Data has also been collected on dogs receiving 3 mg/kg IV alfaxalone followed by a constant rate infusion of 0.15 mg/kg/min for 90 or 180 min. The volume of distribution at steady state was 935.74 ± 170.25 and 1119.15 ± 190.65 mL/kg, the $t_{1/2}$ was 12 ± 2 and 13 ± 3 min, and clearance from the central compartment was 26.02 ± 4.41 and 27.74 ± 5.65 for the 90- and 180-min infusions, respectively [230].

In cats receiving a single 5 mg/kg IV dose, the volume of distribution was 1.8 L/kg, the mean terminal plasma $t_{1/2}$ was approximately 45 min, while mean plasma clearance was 25.1 ± 7.6 mL/kg/min [231]. The mean (standard deviation) bioavailability of an IM injection of 5 mg/kg alfaxalone in cats was 94.7 (19.8)%, and the mean $t_{1/2}$ and mean residence time following IM administration were 1.28 (0.21) and 2.09 (0.36) h, respectively [232].

In the horse, the volume of distribution after a 1 mg/kg IV dose was 1.6 ± 0.4 L/kg. The $t_{1/2}$ of a 1 mg/kg IV dose was 33.4 min, and the plasma clearance was 37.1 ± 11.1 mL/min/kg [233]. The median (range) values for volume of distribution, $t_{1/2}$, and clearance were 0.9 (0.9–1.2) L/kg, 59.8 (47.5–68.0) min, and 14.7 (12.1–16.0) mL/min/kg, respectively in horses receiving 2 mg/kg IV [234]. In foals premedicated with butorphanol, 3 mg/kg of alfaxalone IV had a mean plasma $t_{1/2}$ of 22.8 ± 5.2 min, and an observed plasma clearance and volume of distribution of 19.9 ± 5.9 mL/min/kg and 0.6 ± 0.2 L, respectively [235]. Alfaxalone as an IV constant rate infusion to maintain anesthesia in Standardbred horses has also been examined [236]. The infusion was administered for 180 min, and the median (range) IV infusion rate delivered was 3.1 (2.4–4.3) mg/kg/h. The volume of distribution was 1.60 ± 0.5 L/kg, the mean plasma $t_{1/2}$ was 41 min, and the plasma clearance was 25 ± 6.3 mL/min/kg [236].

Rabbits receiving alfaxalone at 5 mg/kg IV demonstrated a volume of distribution of 3.39 ± 0.64 L/kg, a $t_{1/2}$ of 1.59 h, and a clearance of 1.55 ± 0.27 L/kg/h [237].

There is evidence that alfaxalone is rapidly metabolized by the liver [238]. In the rat, it appears alfaxalone undergoes both cytochrome P450-dependent (Phase I) and conjugation-dependent (Phase II) hepatic metabolism [238]. Cats and dogs seem to form the same five Phase I metabolites of alfaxalone [239]. While cats produce alfaxalone sulfate and alfaxalone glucuronide in Phase II, dogs are observed to produce alfaxalone glucuronide [239]. While the exact mechanism of clearance is not known, it is likely that these metabolites are then primarily excreted in the urine [240].

Pharmacodynamics

Central nervous system

Alfaxalone administration produces unconsciousness and a dose-dependent reduction in EEG activity [235]. Cerebral blood flow, ICP, and cerebral metabolic oxygen demands are all decreased [241]. The duration of anesthesia and unresponsiveness to noxious stimuli increases with increasing dosages of alfaxalone in cats and dogs. In dogs anesthetized with halothane, alfaxalone administration resulted in EEG changes, including a shift in the dominant frequency band to δ from β, occasional burst suppression, and decreases in median and spectral edge frequency [242]. In dogs receiving 3.5 mg/kg followed by 0.15 mg/kg/min of alfaxalone IV, cerebral blood flow was significantly reduced as compared to dogs receiving propofol or isoflurane. However, alfaxalone maintained higher hypocapnic cerebrovascular reactivity to carbon dioxide [243].

Cardiovascular system

IV administration of alfaxalone produces dose-dependent cardiovascular depression in dogs and cats. Arterial blood pressure, cardiac output, and heart rate decreased in cats that were administered 15 and 50 mg/kg of IV alfaxalone. In those animals that received the 50 mg/kg dose, the decrease in systolic blood pressure was marked, and did not return to a clinically acceptable value for approximately 15–30 min [244]. In dogs that received 6 and 20 mg/kg of IV alfaxalone, heart rate increased while arterial blood pressure and mean pulmonary arterial pressure decreased in a dose-dependent fashion [245]. It should be noted, however, that when alfaxalone is administered to dogs and cats at clinically relevant doses (5 mg/kg in cats and 2 mg/kg in dogs), cardiovascular parameters remain quite stable [231]. Studies utilizing clinical doses of alfaxalone in horses [234–236,246], sheep [247–249], and swine [250,251] have also demonstrated clinically acceptable cardiovascular parameters.

Respiratory system

In dogs and cats, the administration of alfaxalone produces dose-dependent respiratory depression, with apnea being the most common side effect [244,245]. In dogs, the duration of apnea was related to the dose of alfaxalone administered [245]. Dose-dependent decreases in respiratory rate, minute volume, and arterial partial pressure of oxygen (PaO_2) were noted in both dogs and cats [244,245]. The arterial partial pressure of carbon dioxide ($PaCO_2$) increased in cats receiving 50 mg/kg and in dogs receiving 6 and 20 mg/kg [244,245]. Neither apnea nor increased $PaCO_2$ occurred in dogs that received 2 mg/kg of alfaxalone [245]. The rate of administration may affect the incidence of PIA. Premedicated dogs receiving alfaxalone at a rate of 0.5 mg/kg/min were less likely to experience PIA as compared to those receiving alfaxalone at a rate of 2 mg/kg/min [252]. However, a slower infusion rate did not have the same effect on the incidence of PIA in cats[253]. Decreased respiratory rate, hypoxemia, and increased $PaCO_2$ have been reported in other species receiving alfaxalone. While these effects are manageable, it is recommended that mechanisms to provide oxygen and assist ventilation are available when using alfaxalone.

Hepatic, renal, and gastrointestinal systems

To the author's knowledge, no controlled studies examining the effect of alfaxalone alone on hepatic or renal blood flow have been published. Studies involving alfaxalone–alfadolone have demonstrated that renal function in rats is only transiently altered, if changed at all [254,255], while a study in dogs showed that renal blood flow remained unchanged [256]. Administration of alfaxalone–alfadolone in Greyhounds decreased hepatic blood flow and hepatic oxygen supply [257]. As discussed previously, alfaxalone undergoes cytochrome P450 hepatic metabolism. Induction of the cytochrome P450 enzyme system leads to an increase in the rate of alfaxalone degradation, which may decrease the duration of anesthesia [238].

In patients with renal portal systems, such as reptiles, the site of alfaxalone injection may alter the effectiveness of alfaxalone. When injections are performed in the caudal portions of these animals, the injected drug may undergo first-pass extraction by the renal portal system and rapid metabolism by the liver. This reduces efficacy and plasma half-life of the injected drug. In studies performed on rattlesnakes and ball pythons, alfaxalone injections in the cranial third of the snakes produced more profound sedation with longer durations as compared to caudal injections [258–260].

Other effects

Alfaxalone is a steroid compound derived from progesterone; therefore, it is possible that sex-specific metabolism could produce pharmacokinetic differences between male and female animals. Previous publications have dismissed this possibility [218], however, this phenomenon has been demonstrated in several studies involving laboratory species. IV administration of alfaxalone to Sprague–Dawley rats demonstrated significant differences between sexes in plasma clearance, half-life, and mean residence time with reduced clearance and longer half-life and mean residence times in female rats [261]. These sex differences appear consistent regardless of route of administration as intraperitoneal alfaxalone produced longer sedation and anesthesia in female Sprague–Dawley rats [262,263], and IM alfaxalone with ketamine in female naked mole rats produced deeper sedation with more rapid onset and longer duration compared to males [264]. Similar results were found in mice receiving intraperitoneal xylazine and alfaxalone. Male C57BL/6J mice required 80–120 mg/kg of alfaxalone to produce surgical anesthesia compared to 40–80 mg/kg in females [265]. While sex differences have not been documented in clinical practice, population pharmacokinetics, and further investigation should be considered.

Species-specific effects

Canine

In a multicenter clinical trial involving 231 dogs, alfaxalone was found to be a safe and efficacious agent for the induction and maintenance of anesthesia [266]. In this study, the average induction dose for alfaxalone was 2.2 mg/kg in nonpremedicated dogs and 1.6 mg/kg in dogs that received premedications [266]. This reduction in the dose of alfaxalone needed for induction has been demonstrated in other studies [267,268].

As described previously, cardiovascular and respiratory parameters remain quite stable in dogs that are administered alfaxalone at clinically relevant doses, with PIA being the most commonly reported side effect [245]. When compared to etomidate, induction of anesthesia with alfaxalone resulted in tachycardia and an increase in cardiac index. Additionally, arterial blood pressure and systemic vascular resistance index were decreased, although both remained at clinically acceptable values [183]. When used in a clinical study involving dogs of poor anesthetic risk, alfaxalone did not produce significant changes in systolic blood pressure and was determined to be a clinically acceptable induction agent [269].

Alfaxalone has also been used as a constant rate infusion to maintain anesthesia in dogs and has been shown to be an effective anesthetic producing clinically acceptable hemodynamic values [270]. Constant rate infusions of alfaxalone produce effective anesthesia for surgical procedures [271,272]. Doses of 0.07 mg/kg/min adjusted to maintain adequate anesthetic depth [271] and 0.11 ± 0.01 mg/kg/min [272] produced satisfactory anesthesia in dogs undergoing ovariohysterectomy. In both studies, significant respiratory depression was observed; therefore, ventilatory monitoring is recommended [271,272].

Alfaxalone has also been evaluated in dogs less than 12 weeks of age and has been determined to be a suitable induction agent [273]. Additionally, alfaxalone has been used to induce anesthesia in dogs prior to cesarean section [274]. Seventy-four bitches were included in the study, 26 of which received alfaxalone to induce anesthesia. Puppy vigor scores were higher in those dogs receiving alfaxalone when compared to those receiving propofol, but survival rates 24 h after birth were similar between groups (97% for alfaxalone and 98% for propofol) [274]. In another retrospective study, neonatal mortality was unaffected by the use of IV alfaxalone to induce anesthesia [275]. In giant-breed dogs undergoing elective cesarean sections, alfaxalone was associated with higher Apgar scores [276]. However, when total intravenous anesthesia (TIVA) with alfaxalone (0.2 mg/kg/min) was used in dogs undergoing elective cesarean sections, puppy vigor was reduced at 5 and 60 min when compared to those dogs maintained with isoflurane [277].

Other studies of alfaxalone in dogs show that IV or IM administration of alfaxalone will briefly increase IOP [278] and reduce tear production [279–281]. Unlike some formulations of propofol, IV injection of alfaxalone does not cause pain on injection [83].

Recovery from alfaxalone anesthesia is longer compared to propofol and has been associated with adverse events such as paddling, rigidity, myoclonus, and vocalization [266,282]. However, these events lasted less than 2 min and did not result in injury or require treatment [282].

Alfaxalone is effective when administered IM in the dog with rapid absorption and onset of action. Cruz-Benedetti *et al.* [283] described moderate to deep sedation lasting approximately 35 min after 4 mg/kg IM. The pharmacokinetic data showed a volume of distribution of 1.94 ± 0.63 L/kg, a mean plasma $t_{1/2}$ of 29 ± 8 min, and a plasma clearance rate of 47.7 ± 14.1mL/min/kg. Of the 12 dogs included in the study, 10 of them exhibited paddling, trembling, nystagmus, and hypersensitivity to sounds [283]. Combinations of alfaxalone with other sedatives and opioids have been studied [281,284–288]. In most cases, the addition of a sedative and/or opioid improved the quality of sedation or anesthesia while maintaining acceptable cardiopulmonary function. It should be noted that with a high bioavailability, and especially in combination with other CNS depressants, IM alfaxalone can produce anesthesia with a loss of laryngeal reflexes [284]. Endotracheal tubes and mechanisms to provide oxygen and support ventilation should be available when administering these drugs.

Feline

Alfaxalone has been used for sedation as well as induction and maintenance of anesthesia in the cat. When used IV at clinically relevant doses to induce anesthesia, alfaxalone produces dose-dependent anesthesia and unresponsiveness to noxious stimuli [244]. As noted previously, cardiopulmonary parameters remain relatively stable, with hypoventilation and hypoxia being the most frequent side effects associated with administration of high doses of alfaxalone [244]. When compared to propofol, IV administration of alfaxalone resulted in similar and clinically acceptable inductions, cardiorespiratory variables, and recoveries [289,290]. In cats, 3–12 months of age, IV administration of alfaxalone produced a smooth induction of anesthesia with a rapid recovery [291]. Alfaxalone has also been demonstrated to be a suitable induction and maintenance agent in cats less than 12 weeks of age [292].

Intermittent IV bolus doses of alfaxalone to not appear to accumulate in the plasma nor do they increase recovery times, so alfaxalone can be used as a constant rate infusion to maintain anesthesia [231]. In cats premedicated with morphine and dexmedetomidine undergoing neutering procedures, alfaxalone induction and constant rate infusion (1.7 mg/kg and 0.18 mg/kg/min, respectively) were effective for surgical anesthesia [293].

Similar to the dog, minor adverse events have been noted during recovery in animals that have received alfaxalone. When compared to propofol, cats receiving alfaxalone were more likely to have episodes of paddling and trembling during recovery [294]. However, most recoveries were assessed as smooth overall and were similar to those cats receiving propofol [294].

As in the dog, alfaxalone is effective when administered by other routes. Subcutaneous (SC) administration of alfaxalone and butorphanol in hyperthyroid cats resulted in adequate sedation for oral administration of iodine-131 [295]. IM alfaxalone in combination with dexmedetomidine and hydromorphone resulted in prolonged recoveries with excitement, ataxia, and hyper-reactivity in all cats and therefore this route of administration for alfaxalone was not recommended [296]. However, subsequent studies involving IM administration have demonstrated effective sedation and anesthesia of good quality. Echocardiographic variables in cats receiving alfaxalone and dexmedetomidine IM showed minimal changes after blood donation [297]. IM combinations of alfaxalone, α_2-adrenergic receptor agonists, and opioids have produced anesthesia sufficient for minor procedures as well as surgery [296,298–300]. Recovery scores in cats receiving these IM alfaxalone combinations were not different from cats receiving IM dexmedetomidine and butorphanol [301], and were scored as excellent in cats administered alfaxalone, dexmedetomidine, and butorphanol [302].

Equine

Alfaxalone has been used to induce and maintain anesthesia in horses [303–305]. When administered to horses following xylazine and guaifenesin, 1 mg/kg of IV alfaxalone satisfactorily induced anesthesia, although tremors/shaking were reported [304]. When compared with ketamine, 1 mg/kg of alfaxalone with 0.02 mg/kg diazepam IV, produced shorter induction times (18 ± 4 s) with similar anesthesia times [305]. Recovery scores, however, were significantly worse in horses receiving alfaxalone [305]. Alfaxalone has also been administered as a constant rate infusion to maintain general anesthesia in horses undergoing field castration. In this study, alfaxalone at a dose of 2 mg/kg/h and medetomidine at a dose of 5 μg/kg/h were determined to be suitable for short-term field anesthesia in the horse [303]. Alfaxalone, along with remifentanil and dexmedetomidine, was sufficient for abdominal surgery in a foal, but recovery was prolonged [306].

The use of alfaxalone for the induction and maintenance of anesthesia has also been investigated in donkeys. IV alfaxalone induced anesthesia rapidly and was appropriate for surgical procedures. However, time to standing was longer and recovery scores were lower when compared to ketamine [307–309].

Ruminant

Alfaxalone has been shown to produce acceptable anesthesia while maintaining cardiovascular and respiratory function in sheep [247,249]. It has been demonstrated that a constant rate infusion of alfaxalone in desflurane anesthetized sheep reduced inhalant requirements while cardiorespiratory parameters remained similar to sheep anesthetized with desflurane alone [247]. In another study, a 2 mg/kg IV dose of alfaxalone produced minimal changes in cardiopulmonary and acid–base variables [249]. Alfaxalone has also been shown to have no effect on IOP in sheep; however, a marked miosis was observed [310].

IV alfaxalone for induction prior to isoflurane anesthesia is effective in goats. Goats receiving a dose of 2 mg/kg IV became unconscious quickly and smoothly and recovery scores were good to excellent [311]. The minimum infusion rate (MIR) of alfaxalone to prevent purposeful movement in goats is 0.16 mg/kg/h [312]. Fentanyl and midazolam lower the MIR in a dose-dependent manner [313,314]. Lidocaine, administered at doses of 3, 6, and 12 mg/kg/h, will also reduce MIR by 10, 30, and 30%, respectively [315].

Swine

Alfaxalone has been used to induce sedation and anesthesia in pigs. Alfaxalone alone or in combination with diazepam has been injected IM in pigs. This rapidly produced recumbency, deep sedation, and minimal side effects. It was noted that this combination may be useful for premedication in pigs, but that the volume of injectate would limit its use to small pigs [316]. IM dexmedetomidine and alfaxalone produced a deeper and better quality of sedation compared to dexmedetomidine and ketamine in Landrace × Large White pigs [317]. Intratesticular alfaxalone with lidocaine administered to piglets was sufficient for castration [318]. Intranasal alfaxalone at a dose of 1 or 2 mg/kg in Yucatan swine did increase sedation scores but did not facilitate handling or the performance of any clinical procedures [319].

Induction of anesthesia with IV alfaxalone has also been described in swine. In pigs premedicated with IM azaperone, IV alfaxalone resulted in satisfactory conditions for intubation with minimal side effects [320]. Maintenance of anesthesia in pigs with alfaxalone has also been described. TIVA with alfaxalone, ketamine, and dexmedetomidine was effective and resulted in higher respiratory rates and lower end-tidal carbon dioxide values as compared to pigs receiving propofol, ketamine, and dexmedetomidine [321]. IM alfaxalone in combination with butorphanol and medetomidine followed by IV alfaxalone for the maintenance of anesthesia was satisfactory and produced minimal cardiovascular side effects [251].

Other species

SC, IM, and IV administration of alfaxalone has been studied in several avian species with varying results. When used as the sole agent, alfaxalone produced varying levels of sedation and poor recoveries in peafowl [322], lovebirds [323], Quaker parrots [324], Mallard ducks [325], and budgerigars [326]. As with other species, the addition of other CNS depressants and or opioids may improve both the depth and quality of sedation in birds.

IM administration of alfaxalone has produced sedation, loss of righting reflex, and facilitated endotracheal intubation in rabbits [149,327–329]. Rousseau-Blass *et al.* [330] demonstrated that early oxygen supplementation after IM alfaxalone, dexmedetomidine, and midazolam resolved hypoxemia, but resulted in a decreased respiratory rate and increased $PaCO_2$. IM and SC administration have also been studied in guinea pigs [331–334], hedgehogs [335,336], and ferrets [337].

Sedation and anesthesia by immersion in alfaxalone have been demonstrated in goldfish and fire-bellied toads. Surgical anesthesia with a smooth induction and recovery with minimal side effects was produced by immersing goldfish in water containing 6 mg/L of alfaxalone [338]. Immersion in alfaxalone at a concentration of

Table 27.9 Alfaxalone dosages in various species.

Species	Intravenous induction of anesthesia (mg/kg)	Constant rate infusion (mg/kg/min)	Sedation dose (mg/kg)
Dog	0.5–2.2	0.07–0.12	
Cat	0.5–5.0	0.18	3.0 SC
Horse	1–3	0.033[a]	
Foal	3		
Sheep	1.2–2.6		
Pig	0.6–1.1		5.0 IM

[a] Administered with 5 μg/kg/h medetomidine
IM, intramuscular; SC, subcutaneous.

200 mg/L produced anesthesia in 10/11 toads and did not cause skin irritation or changes in pigmentation [339]. Adding dexmedetomidine to the alfaxalone did not potentiate the level of unconsciousness in fire-bellied toads and proved unsuitable for invasive procedures [340] while morphine provided superior antinociception compared to butorphanol [341].

Clinical use

Table 27.9 lists commonly used doses for alfaxalone. As with all injectable induction agents, the dose should be tailored according to concurrent drug administration and physical status.

As discussed previously, alfaxalone can be effective when administered IV or IM. However, due to volume of injection, the IM route of administration should be limited to small patients. A new formulation (40 mg/mL), RD0387, has been produced and studied [225,342].

While recovering from alfaxalone anesthesia, it is recommended that animals be left in a quiet, dark area where they are not handled or disturbed except for necessary monitoring. Paddling of the limbs, muscle twitching, hyper-reactivity, and ataxia have been reported in animals that are recovering from alfaxalone anesthesia. These reactions may be attenuated by the use of sedative agents.

Other drugs

The following injectable anesthetic agents are no longer routinely used in clinical practice but do have historical significance in the study of veterinary anesthesia or are occasionally of interest to laboratory investigators.

Metomidate

Metomidate is the first compound of the imidazole class of anesthetics that was designed as a non-barbiturate IV hypnotic drug. It is freely soluble in water, but aqueous solutions are unstable and should be used within 24 h. It was introduced initially as a hypnotic for pigs, horses [343], and a variety of avian species. When given by IV injection, metomidate produces loss of consciousness quickly. It has a short duration of action of less than 25 min; however, animals will sleep for several hours. Recovery in horses may be extremely violent [344].

Metomidate anesthesia is characterized by cardiovascular stability. Mild hypotension results initially, along with a decrease in heart rate and a slight decrease in cardiac output. Minute ventilation also remains stable with a slightly decreased respiratory rate but increased tidal volume. Metomidate produces profound muscle relaxation, but little analgesia, so it must be combined with analgesics for surgical procedures [344]. Further development of the imidazole compounds created the superior substance, etomidate, which has gained use in human and veterinary medicine.

Chloral hydrate

Chloral hydrate, 1,1,1-trichloro-2,2-dihydroxyethane, is a hypnotic that was first introduced in 1869. It is a crystalline substance that has a distinct odor and volatizes slowly at room temperature. It is readily soluble in water and aqueous solutions remain generally stable. Chloral hydrate is metabolized after administration to trichloroethanol, which is responsible for most of the observed effects.

Although the mechanism of action is unknown, it is likely that chloral hydrate interacts with the GABA receptor in a similar fashion as the other injectable anesthetics. When administered, chloral hydrate produces dose-dependent sedation. The dose required to produce anesthesia approaches the minimum lethal dose, so its margin of safety is quite narrow. The effects of an IV injection are slow to occur, which makes it difficult to assess the degree of sedation or depression. Even after slow administration, sedation continues to deepen for a few minutes after the injection is stopped, likely due to the lag time required for metabolism to trichloroethanol.

Myocardial contractility is reduced, resulting in hypotension. The respiratory system is mildly affected by chloral hydrate administration but at doses needed to produce anesthesia, respiratory depression can be severe. Ventricular fibrillation and sudden death in the recovery period have been reported. To mitigate the risk of death, the addition of either magnesium sulfate, pentobarbital, or both has been used.

Historically, chloral hydrate has been used for sedation in horses and cattle and was administered either IV or orally (PO). Chloral hydrate is irritating to the stomach and mucous membranes; its irritating nature means that perivascular injection results in necrosis and sloughing of the vessel wall and the surrounding tissues. If IV injection is continued until a surgical plane of anesthesia is reached, recovery will be prolonged.

Magnesium sulfate

Magnesium sulfate is probably better thought of as a muscle relaxant and CNS depressant rather than an injectable anesthetic. When combined with chloral hydrate, it hastens the onset of anesthesia, increases its depth, and reduces the toxicity associated with chloral hydrate. The recommended mixture is two parts chloral hydrate to one part magnesium sulfate.

Dilute solutions of magnesium sulfate have been used to induce anesthesia in small animal patients. However, magnesium sulfate administration results in global depression of the CNS, and respiratory arrest occurs frequently. Magnesium sulfate has been used for euthanasia, but it should only be administered after the animal is rendered unconscious with another anesthetic agent.

Chloralose

Chloralose is a solution prepared by heating glucose and chloral hydrate. Its use as an anesthetic is limited to laboratory animals being used in non-survival surgical experiments.

Anesthesia produced with chloralose is similar to chloral hydrate but the effects last 8–10 h. Compared to chloral hydrate, blood pressure is elevated, as is the heart rate and the respiratory rate [344]. Chloralose is transformed to chloraldehyde and glucose and the safety margin is relatively large. Recovery from chloralose anesthesia is slow and marked by paddling and muscle fasciculations. Consequently, there is little indication for its use in veterinary medicine.

References

1 Haws JL, Herman N, Clark Y, *et al.* The chemical stability and sterility of sodium thiopental after preparation. *Anesth Analg* 1998; **86**(1): 208–213.

2 Beeman CS, Dembo J, Bogardus A. Stability of reconstituted methohexital sodium. *J Oral Maxillofac Surg* 1994; **52**(4): 393–396.

3 Olsen RW, Li GD. GABA(A) receptors as molecular targets of general anesthetics: identification of binding sites provides clues to allosteric modulation. *Can J Anaesth* 2011; **58**(2): 206–215.

4 Tanelian DL, Kosek P, Mody I, *et al.* The role of the GABAA receptor/chloride channel complex in anesthesia. *Anesthesiology* 1993; **78**(4): 757–776.

5 Saidman LJ. Uptake, distribution, and elimination of barbiturates. In: Eger EI, ed. *Anesthetic Uptake and Action*, 2nd edn. Baltimore, MD: Williams & Wilkins, 1974: 264–285.

6 Brandon RA, Baggot JD. The pharmacokinetics of thiopentone. *J Vet Pharmacol Ther* 1981; **4**(2): 79–85.

7 Sams RA, Muir WW, Detra RL, *et al.* Comparative pharmacokinetics and anesthetic effects of methohexital, pentobarbital, thiamylal, and thiopental in Greyhound dogs and non-Greyhound, mixed-breed dogs. *Am J Vet Res* 1985; **46**(8): 1677–1683.

8 Russo H, Bressolle F. Pharmacodynamics and pharmacokinetics of thiopental. *Clin Pharmacokinet* 1998; **35**(2): 95–134.

9 Price HL. A dynamic concept of the distribution of thiopental in the human body. *Anesthesiology* 1960; **21**: 40–45.

10 Weiss M. How does obesity affect residence time dispersion and the shape of drug disposition curves? Thiopental as an example. *J Pharmacokinet Pharmacodyn* 2008; **35**(3): 325–336.

11 Abass BT, Weaver BM, Staddon GE, *et al.* Pharmacokinetics of thiopentone in the horse. *J Vet Pharmacol Ther* 1994; **17**(5): 331–338.

12 Ilkiw JE, Benthuysen JA, Ebling WF, *et al.* A comparative study of the pharmacokinetics of thiopental in the rabbit, sheep and dog. *J Vet Pharmacol Ther* 1991; **14**(2): 134–140.

13 Brown MB, Dugat DR, Lyon SD, *et al.* Comparison of methohexital and propofol as induction agents for evaluation of laryngeal function in healthy dogs. *Vet Surg* 2019; **48**(1): 70–78.

14 Kim A, Sasaki N, Lee I, *et al.* Analgesic and cardiopulmonary effects of premedication with tramadol in calves anesthetized with the infusion of guaifenesin and thiamylal. *J Vet Med Sci* 2021; **83**(12): 1988–1993.

15 Robinson EP, Sams RA, Muir WW. Barbiturate anesthesia in greyhound and mixed-breed dogs: comparative cardiopulmonary effects, anesthetic effects, and recovery rates. *Am J Vet Res* 1986; **47**(10): 2105–2112.

16 Kiersey DK, Bickford RG, Faulconer A, Jr. Electro-encephalographic patterns produced by thiopental sodium during surgical operations; description and classification. *Br J Anaesth* 1951; **23**(3): 141–152.

17 Albrecht RF, Miletich DJ, Rosenberg R, *et al.* Cerebral blood flow and metabolic changes from induction to onset of anesthesia with halothane or pentobarbital. *Anesthesiology* 1977; **47**(3): 252–256.

18 Guo J, White JA, Batjer HH. The protective effects of thiopental on brain stem ischemia. *Neurosurgery* 1995; **37**(3): 490–495.

19 Ebmeyer U, Safar P, Radovsky A, *et al.* Thiopental combination treatments for cerebral resuscitation after prolonged cardiac arrest in dogs. *Exploratory outcome study. Resuscitation* 2000; **45**(2): 119–131.

20 Hofmeister EH, Williams CO, Braun C, *et al.* Propofol versus thiopental: effects on peri-induction intraocular pressures in normal dogs. *Vet Anaesth Analg* 2008; **35**(4): 275–281.

21 Turner DM, Ilkiw JE. Cardiovascular and respiratory effects of three rapidly acting barbiturates in dogs. *Am J Vet Res* 1990; **51**(4): 598–604.

22 Muir WW. Thiobarbiturate-induced dysrhythmias: the role of heart rate and autonomic imbalance. *Am J Vet Res* 1977; **38**(9): 1377–1381.

23 Hayashi Y, Sumikawa K, Yamatodani A, *et al.* Myocardial sensitization by thiopental to arrhythmogenic action of epinephrine in dogs. *Anesthesiology* 1989; **71**(6): 929–935.

24 Hirshman CA, McCullough RE, Cohen PJ, *et al.* Hypoxic ventilatory drive in dogs during thiopental, ketamine, or pentobarbital anesthesia. *Anesthesiology* 1975; **43**(6): 628–634.

25 Quandt JE, Robinson EP, Rivers WJ, *et al.* Cardiorespiratory and anesthetic effects of propofol and thiopental in dogs. *Am J Vet Res* 1998; **59**(9): 1137–1143.

26 Hirota K, Ohtomo N, Hashimoto Y, *et al.* Effects of thiopental on airway calibre in dogs: direct visualization method using a superfine fibreoptic bronchoscope. *Br J Anaesth* 1998; **81**(2): 203–207.

27 Jackson AM, Tobias K, Long C, *et al.* Effects of various anesthetic agents on laryngeal motion during laryngoscopy in normal dogs. *Vet Surg* 2004; **33**(2): 102–106.

28 Forbes AR, Gamsu G. Depression of lung mucociliary clearance by thiopental and halothane. *Anesth Analg* 1979; **58**(5): 387–389.

29 Sams RA, Muir WW. Effects of phenobarbital on thiopental pharmacokinetics in greyhounds. *Am J Vet Res* 1988; **49**(2): 245–249.

30 Hashim MA, Waterman AE. Effects of thiopentone, propofol, alphaxalone-alphadolone, ketamine and xylazine-ketamine on lower oesophageal sphincter pressure and barrier pressure in cats. *Vet Rec* 1991; **129**(7): 137–139.

31 Chang J, Kim S, Jung J, *et al.* Evaluation of the effects of thiopental, propofol, and etomidate on glomerular filtration rate measured by the use of dynamic computed tomography in dogs. *Am J Vet Res* 2011; **72**(1): 146–151.

32 Luna SP, Cassu RN, Castro GB, *et al.* Effects of four anaesthetic protocols on the neurological and cardiorespiratory variables of puppies born by caesarean section. *Vet Rec* 2004; **154**(13): 387–389.

33 Alon E, Ball RH, Gillie MH, *et al.* Effects of propofol and thiopental on maternal and fetal cardiovascular and acid-base variables in the pregnant ewe. *Anesthesiology* 1993; **78**(3): 562–576.

34 Wilder-Smith OH, Kolletzki M, Wilder-Smith CH. Sedation with intravenous infusions of propofol or thiopentone. *Effects on pain perception. Anaesthesia* 1995; **50**(3): 218–222.

35 Hubbell JA, Hinchcliff KW, Schmall LM, *et al.* Anesthetic, cardiorespiratory, and metabolic effects of four intravenous anesthetic regimens induced in horses immediately after maximal exercise. *Am J Vet Res* 2000; **61**(12): 1545–1552.

36 Toutain PL, Brandon RA, Alvinerie M, *et al.* Thiopentone pharmacokinetics and electrocorticogram pattern in sheep. *J Vet Pharmacol Ther* 1983; **6**(3): 201–209.

37 Søfteland E, Framstad T, Thorsen T, *et al.* Evaluation of thiopentone-midazolam-fentanyl anaesthesia in pigs. *Lab Anim* 1995; **29**(3): 269–275.

38 Dyess DL, Tacchi E, Powell RQ, *et al.* Development of a protocol to provide prolonged general anesthesia to pregnant sows. *J Invest Surg* 1994; **7**(3): 235–242.

39 Weiskopf RB, Bogetz MS. Haemorrhage decreases the anaesthetic requirement for ketamine and thiopentone in the pig. *Br J Anaesth* 1985; **57**(10): 1022–1025.

40 Rawlings CA, Kolata RJ. Cardiopulmonary effects of thiopental/lidocaine combination during anesthetic induction in the dog. *Am J Vet Res* 1983; **44**(1): 144–149.

41 Ko JC, Golder FJ, Mandsager RE, *et al.* Anesthetic and cardiorespiratory effects of a 1:1 mixture of propofol and thiopental sodium in dogs. *J Am Vet Med Assoc* 1999; **215**(9): 1292–1296.

42 Joubert KE, Picard J, Sethusa M. Inhibition of bacterial growth by different mixtures of propofol and thiopentone. *J S Afr Vet Assoc* 2005; **76**(2): 85–89.

43 Kay B, Rolly G. I.C.I. 35868, a new intravenous induction agent. *Acta Anaesthesiol Belg* 1977; **28**(4): 303–316.

44 Wachowski I, Jolly DT, Hrazdil J, *et al.* The growth of microorganisms in propofol and mixtures of propofol and lidocaine. *Anesth Analg* 1999; **88**(1): 209–212.

45 McIntosh MP, Rajewski RA. Comparative canine pharmacokinetics–pharmacodynamics of fospropofol disodium injection, propofol emulsion, and cyclodextrin-enabled propofol solution following bolus parenteral administration. *J Pharm Sci* 2012; **101**(9): 3547–3552.

46 Cleale RM, Muir WW, Waselau AC, *et al.* Pharmacokinetic and pharmacodynamic evaluation of propofol administered to cats in a novel, aqueous, nano-droplet formulation or as an oil-in-water macroemulsion. *J Vet Pharmacol Ther* 2009; **32**(5): 436–445.

47 Taylor PM, Chengelis CP, Miller WR, *et al.* Evaluation of propofol containing 2% benzyl alcohol preservative in cats. *J Feline Med Surg* 2012; **14**(8): 516–526.

48 Ying SW, Goldstein PA. Propofol suppresses synaptic responsiveness of somatosensory relay neurons to excitatory input by potentiating GABA(A) receptor chloride channels. *Mol Pain* 2005; **1**: 2.

49 Orser BA, Bertlik M, Wang LY, *et al.* Inhibition by propofol (2,6 di-isopropylphenol) of the N-methyl-D-aspartate subtype of glutamate receptor in cultured hippocampal neurones. *Br J Pharmacol* 1995; **116**(2): 1761–1768.

50 National Center for Biotechnology Information. PubChem Compound Summary for CID 4943, Propofol; https://pubchem.ncbi.nlm.nih.gov/compound/Propofol and CID 3038498, Fospropofol; https://pubchem.ncbi.nlm.nih.gov/compound/Fospropofol (accessed June 2022).

51 Zoran DL, Riedesel DH, Dyer DC. Pharmacokinetics of propofol in mixed-breed dogs and greyhounds. *Am J Vet Res* 1993; **54**(5): 755–760.

52 Hay-Kraus BL, Greenblatt DJ, Venkatakrishnan K, *et al.* Evidence for propofol hydroxylation by cytochrome P4502B11 in canine liver microsomes: breed and gender differences. *Xenobiotica* 2000; **30**(6): 575–588.

53 Veroli P, O'Kelly B, Bertrand F, *et al.* Extrahepatic metabolism of propofol in man during the anhepatic phase of orthotopic liver transplantation. *Br J Anaesth* 1992; **68**(2): 183–186.

54 Servin F, Cockshott ID, Farinotti R, *et al.* Pharmacokinetics of propofol infusions in patients with cirrhosis. *Br J Anaesth* 1990; **65**(2): 177–183.

55 Matot I, Neely CF, Katz RY, *et al.* Pulmonary uptake of propofol in cats. Effect of fentanyl and halothane. *Anesthesiology* 1993; **78**(6): 1157–1165.

56 Posner LP, Asakawa M, Erb HN. Use of propofol for anesthesia in cats with primary hepatic lipidosis: 44 cases (1995–2004). *J Am Vet Med Assoc* 2008; **232**(12): 1841–1843.

57 Reid J, Nolan AM. Pharmacokinetics of propofol as an induction agent in geriatric dogs. *Res Vet Sci* 1996; **61**(2): 169–171.

58 Court MH, Hay-Kraus BL, Hill DW, *et al.* Propofol hydroxylation by dog liver microsomes: assay development and dog breed differences. *Drug Metab Dispos* 1999; **27**(11): 1293–1299.

59 Adam HK, Glen JB, Hoyle PA. Pharmacokinetics in laboratory animals of ICI 35 868, a new i.v. anaesthetic agent. *Br J Anaesth* 1980; **52**(8): 743–746.

60 Mandsager RE, Clarke CR, Shawley RV, *et al.* Effects of chloramphenicol on infusion pharmacokinetics of propofol in greyhounds. *Am J Vet Res* 1995; **56**(1): 95–99.

61 Artru AA, Shapira Y, Bowdle TA. Electroencephalogram, cerebral metabolic, and vascular responses to propofol anesthesia in dogs. *J Neurosurg Anesthesiol* 1992; **4**(2): 99–109.

62 Herregods L, Verbeke J, Rolly G, *et al.* Effect of propofol on elevated intracranial pressure. *Preliminary results. Anaesthesia* 1988; **43**(Suppl): 107–109.

63 Cheng MA, Tempelhoff R, Silbergeld DL, *et al.* Large-dose propofol alone in adult epileptic patients: electrocorticographic results. *Anesth Analg* 1996; **83**(1): 169–174.

64 Steffen F, Grasmueck S. Propofol for treatment of refractory seizures in dogs and a cat with intracranial disorders. *J Small Anim Pract* 2000; **41**(11): 496–499.

65 Goodchild CS, Serrao JM. Cardiovascular effects of propofol in the anaesthetized dog. *Br J Anaesth* 1989; **63**(1): 87–92.

66 Brüssel T, Theissen JL, Vigfusson G, *et al.* Hemodynamic and cardiodynamic effects of propofol and etomidate: negative inotropic properties of propofol. *Anesth Analg* 1989; **69**(1): 35–40.

67 Ilkiw JE, Pascoe PJ, Haskins SC, *et al.* Cardiovascular and respiratory effects of propofol administration in hypovolemic dogs. *Am J Vet Res* 1992; **53**(12): 2323–2327.

68 Pagel PS, Hettrick DA, Kersten JR, *et al.* Cardiovascular effects of propofol in dogs with dilated cardiomyopathy. *Anesthesiology* 1998; **88**(1): 180–189.

69 Kamibayashi T, Hayashi Y, Sumikawa K, *et al.* Enhancement by propofol of epinephrine-induced arrhythmias in dogs. *Anesthesiology* 1991; **75**(6): 1035–1040.

70 Muir WW III, Gadawski JE. Respiratory depression and apnea induced by propofol in dogs. *Am J Vet Res* 1998; **59**(2): 157–161.

71 Blouin RT, Seifert HA, Babenco HD, *et al.* Propofol depresses the hypoxic ventilatory response during conscious sedation and isohypercapnia. *Anesthesiology* 1993; **79**(6): 1177–1182.

72 Goodman NW, Black AM, Carter JA. Some ventilatory effects of propofol as sole anaesthetic agent. *Br J Anaesth* 1987; **59**(12): 1497–1503.

73 Ponte J, Sadler CL. Effect of thiopentone, etomidate and propofol on carotid body chemoreceptor activity in the rabbit and the cat. *Br J Anaesth* 1989; **62**(1): 41–45.

74 Taylor MB, Grounds RM, Mulrooney PD, *et al.* Ventilatory effects of propofol during induction of anaesthesia. Comparison with thiopentone. *Anaesthesia* 1986; **41**(8): 816–820.

75 Haberer JP, Audibert G, Saunier CG, *et al.* Effect of propofol and thiopentone on regional blood flow in brain and peripheral tissues during normoxia and hypoxia in the dog. *Clin Physiol* 1993; **13**(2): 197–207.

76 Apfel CC, Korttila K, Abdalla M, *et al.* A factorial trial of six interventions for the prevention of postoperative nausea and vomiting. *N Engl J Med* 2004; **350**(24): 2441–2451.

77 Smedile LE, Duke T, Taylor SM. Excitatory movements in a dog following propofol anesthesia. *J Am Anim Hosp Assoc* 1996; **32**(4): 365–368.

78 Nimmaanrat S. Myoclonic movements following induction of anesthesia with propofol: a case report. *J Med Assoc Thai* 2005; **88**(12): 1955–1957.

79 Andaluz A, Tusell J, Trasserres O, *et al.* Transplacental transfer of propofol in pregnant ewes. *Vet J* 2003; **166**(2): 198–204.

80 Doebeli A, Michel E, Bettschart R, *et al.* Apgar score after induction of anesthesia for canine cesarean section with alfaxalone versus propofol. *Theriogenology* 2013; **80**(8): 850–854.

81 Heldmann E, Brown DC, Shofer F. The association of propofol usage with postoperative wound infection rate in clean wounds: a retrospective study. *Vet Surg* 1999; **28**(4): 256–259.

82 Lee SH, Ghim JL, Song MH, *et al.* Pharmacokinetics and pharmacodynamics of a new reformulated microemulsion and the long-chain triglyceride emulsion of propofol in beagle dogs. *Br J Pharmacol* 2009; **158**(8): 1982–1995.

83 Michou JN, Leece EA, Brearley JC. Comparison of pain on injection during induction of anaesthesia with alfaxalone and two formulations of propofol in dogs. *Vet Anaesth Analg* 2012; **39**(3): 275–281.

84 Andress JL, Day TK, Day D. The effects of consecutive day propofol anesthesia on feline red blood cells. *Vet Surg* 1995; **24**(3): 277–282.

85 Bley CR, Roos M, Price J, *et al.* Clinical assessment of repeated propofol-associated anesthesia in cats. *J Am Vet Med Assoc* 2007; **231**(9): 1347–1353.

86 Wiese AJ, Lerche P, Cleale RM, *et al.* Investigation of escalating and large bolus doses of a novel, nano-droplet, aqueous 1% propofol formulation in cats. *Vet Anaesth Analg* 2010; **37**(3): 250–257.

87 Nolan AM, Hall LW. Total intravenous anaesthesia in the horse with propofol. *Equine Vet J* 1985; **17**(5): 394–398.

88 Mama KR, Steffey EP, Pascoe PJ. Evaluation of propofol as a general anesthetic for horses. *Vet Surg* 1995; **24**(2): 188–194.

89 Mama KR, Steffey EP, Pascoe PJ. Evaluation of propofol for general anesthesia in premedicated horses. *Am J Vet Res* 1996; **57**(4): 512–516.

90 Brosnan RJ, Steffey EP, Escobar A, *et al.* Anesthetic induction with guaifenesin and propofol in adult horses. *Am J Vet Res* 2011; **72**(12): 1569–1575.

91 Oku K, Ohta M, Katoh T, *et al.* Cardiovascular effects of continuous propofol infusion in horses. *J Vet Med Sci* 2006; **68**(8): 773–778.

92 Umar MA, Yamashita K, Kushiro T, *et al.* Evaluation of total intravenous anesthesia with propofol or ketamine–medetomidine–propofol combination in horses. *J Am Vet Med Assoc* 2006; **228**(8): 1221–1227.

93 Ishizuka T, Itami T, Tamura J, *et al.* Anesthetic and cardiorespiratory effects of propofol, medetomidine, lidocaine and butorphanol total intravenous anesthesia in horses. *J Vet Med Sci* 2013; **75**(2): 165–172.

94 Wagner AE, Mama KR, Steffey EP, *et al.* Evaluation of infusions of xylazine with ketamine or propofol to modulate recovery following sevoflurane anesthesia in horses. *Am J Vet Res* 2012; **73**(3): 346–352.

95 Steffey EP, Mama KR, Brosnan RJ, *et al.* Effect of administration of propofol and xylazine hydrochloride on recovery of horses after four hours of anesthesia with desflurane. *Am J Vet Res* 2009; **70**(8): 956–963.

96 Boscan P, Rezende ML, Grimsrud K, *et al.* Pharmacokinetic profile in relation to anaesthesia characteristics after a 5% micellar microemulsion of propofol in the horse. *Br J Anaesth* 2010; **104**(3): 330–337.

97 Rezende ML, Boscan P, Stanley SD, *et al.* Evaluation of cardiovascular, respiratory and biochemical effects, and anesthetic induction and recovery behavior in horses anesthetized with a 5% micellar microemulsion propofol formulation. *Vet Anaesth Analg* 2010; **37**(5): 440–450.

98 Lin HC, Purohit RC, Powe TA. Anesthesia in sheep with propofol or with xylazine-ketamine followed by halothane. *Vet Surg* 1997; **26**(3): 247–252.

99 Reid J, Nolan AM, Welsh E. Propofol as an induction agent in the goat: a pharmacokinetic study. *J Vet Pharmacol Ther* 1993; **16**(4): 488–493.

100 Cagnardi P, Zonca A, Gallo M, *et al.* Pharmacokinetics of propofol in calves undergoing abdominal surgery. *Vet Res Commun* 2009; **33**(Suppl 1): 177–179.

101 Duke T, Egger CM, Ferguson JG, *et al.* Cardiopulmonary effects of propofol infusion in llamas. *Am J Vet Res* 1997; **58**(2): 153–156.

102 Correia D, Nolan AM, Reid J. Pharmacokinetics of propofol infusions, either alone or with ketamine, in sheep premedicated with acepromazine and papaveretum. *Res Vet Sci* 1996; **60**(3): 213–217.

103 Foster PS, Hopkinson KC, Denborough MA. Propofol anaesthesia in malignant hyperpyrexia susceptible swine. *Clin Exp Pharmacol Physiol* 1992; **19**(3): 183–186.

104 Kaiser GM, Breuckmann F, Aker S, *et al.* Anesthesia for cardiovascular interventions and magnetic resonance imaging in pigs. *J Am Assoc Lab Anim Sci* 2007; **46**(2): 30–33.

105 Martin-Cancho MF, Lima JR, Luis L, *et al.* Relationship of bispectral index values, haemodynamic changes and recovery times during sevoflurane or propofol anaesthesia in rabbits. *Lab Anim-UK* 2006; **40**(1): 28–42.

106 Terada Y, Ishiyama T, Asano N, *et al.* Optimal doses of sevoflurane and propofol in rabbits. *BMC Res Notes* 2014; **7**(1): 820.

107 Fechner J, Ihmsen H, Jeleazcov C, *et al.* Fospropofol disodium, a water-soluble prodrug of the intravenous anesthetic propofol (2,6-diisopropylphenol). *Expert Opin Invest Drugs* 2009; **18**(10): 1565–1571.

108 Feng AY, Kaye AD, Kaye RJ, *et al.* Novel propofol derivatives and implications for anesthesia practice. *J Anaesthesiol Clin Pharmacol* 2017; **33**(1): 9–15.

109 Li R, Zhang W, Liu J, *et al.* Minimum infusion rates and recovery times from different durations of continuous infusion of fospropofol, a prodrug of propofol, in rabbits: a comparison with propofol emulsion. *Vet Anaesth Analg* 2012; **39**(4): 373–384.

110 Feng AY, Kaye AD, Kaye RJ, *et al.* Novel propofol derivatives and implications for anesthesia practice. *J Anaesthesiol Clin Pharmacol* 2017; **33**(1): 9–15.

111 Zhou Y, Yang J, Liu J, *et al.* Efficacy comparison of the novel water-soluble propofol prodrug HX0969w and fospropofol in mice and rats. *Br J Anaesth* 2013; **111**(5): 825–832.

112 Lang BC, Yang J, Wang Y, *et al.* An improved design of water-soluble propofol prodrugs characterized by rapid onset of action. *Anesth Analg* 2014; **118**(4): 745–754.

113 Reich DL, Silvay G. Ketamine: an update on the first twenty-five years of clinical experience. *Can J Anaesth* 1989; **36**(2): 186–197.

114 White PF, Ham J, Way WL, *et al.* Pharmacology of ketamine isomers in surgical patients. *Anesthesiology* 1980; **52**(3): 231–239.

115 National Center for Biotechnology Information. PubChem Compound Summary for CID 3821, Ketamine; https://pubchem.ncbi.nlm.nih.gov/compound/Ketamine and CID 26533, Tiletamine; https://pubchem.ncbi.nlm.nih.gov/compound/Tiletamine (accessed June 2022).

116 Annetta MG, Iemma D, Garisto C, *et al.* Ketamine: new indications for an old drug. *Curr Drug Targets* 2005; **6**(7): 789–794.

117 Hirota K, Lambert DG. Ketamine: its mechanism(s) of action and unusual clinical uses. *Br J Anaesth* 1996; **77**(4): 441–444.
118 Hustveit O, Maurset A, Oye I. Interaction of the chiral forms of ketamine with opioid, phencyclidine, sigma and muscarinic receptors. *Pharmacol Toxicol* 1995; 77(6): 355–359.
119 Stoelting RK. Nonbarbiturate induction drugs. In: Stoelting RK, ed. *Pharmacology and Physiology in Anesthetic Practice*. 3rd edn. Philadelphia: Lippincott, Williams & Wilkins, 1999: 140–157.
120 White PF, Way WL, Trevor AJ. Ketamine – its pharmacology and therapeutic uses. *Anesthesiology* 1982; **56**(2): 119–136.
121 Hanna RM, Borchard RE, Schmidt SL. Pharmacokinetics of ketamine HCl and metabolite I in the cat: a comparison of i.v., i.m., and rectal administration. *J Vet Pharmacol Ther* 1988; **11**(1): 84–93.
122 Takeshita H, Okuda Y, Sari A. The effects of ketamine on cerebral circulation and metabolism in man. *Anesthesiology* 1972; **36**(1): 69–75.
123 Dawson B, Michenfelder JD, Theye RA. Effects of ketamine on canine cerebral blood flow and metabolism: modification by prior administration of thiopental. *Anesth Analg* 1971; **50**(3): 443–447.
124 Pfenninger E, Dick W, Ahnefeld FW. The influence of ketamine on both normal and raised intracranial pressure of artificially ventilated animals. *Eur J Anaesthesiol* 1985; **2**(3): 297–307.
125 Kayama Y. Ketamine and e.e.g. seizure waves: interaction with anti-epileptic drugs. *Br J Anaesth* 1982; **54**(8): 879–883.
126 Celesia GG, Chen RC, Bamforth BJ. Effects of ketamine in epilepsy. *Neurology* 1975; **25**(2): 169–172.
127 Reder BS, Trapp LD, Troutman KC. Ketamine suppression of chemically induced convulsions in the two-day-old white leghorn cockerel. *Anesth Analg* 1980; **59**(6): 406–409.
128 Diaz FA, Bianco JA, Bello A, *et al.* Effects of ketamine on canine cardiovascular function. *Br J Anaesth* 1976; **48**(10): 941–946.
129 Haskins SC, Farver TB, Patz JD. Ketamine in dogs. *Am J Vet Res* 1985; **46**(9): 1855–1860.
130 Wong DH, Jenkins LC. An experimental study of the mechanism of action of ketamine on the central nervous system. *Can Anaesth Soc J* 1974; **21**(1): 57–67.
131 Baraka A, Harrison T, Kachachi T. Catecholamine levels after ketamine anesthesia in man. *Anesth Analg* 1973; **52**(2): 198–200.
132 Waxman K, Shoemaker WC, Lippmann M. Cardiovascular effects of anesthetic induction with ketamine. *Anesth Analg* 1980; **59**(5): 355–358.
133 Soliman MG, Brindle GF, Kuster G. Response to hypercapnia under ketamine anaesthesia. *Can Anaesth Soc J* 1975; **22**(4): 486–494.
134 Jaspar N, Mazzarelli M, Tessier C, *et al.* Effect of ketamine on control of breathing in cats. *J Appl Physiol Respir Environ Exerc Physiol* 1983; **55**(3): 851–859.
135 Hirshman CA, Downes H, Farbood A, *et al.* Ketamine block of bronchospasm in experimental canine asthma. *Br J Anaesth* 1979; **51**(8): 713–718.
136 Taylor PA, Towey RM. Ketamine anaesthesia. *Br Med J* 1971; **3**(5771): 432–a.
137 Fass J, Bares R, Hermsdorf V, *et al.* Effects of intravenous ketamine on gastrointestinal motility in the dog. *Intensive Care Med* 1995; **21**(7): 584–589.
138 Aida S, Yamakura T, Baba H, *et al.* Preemptive analgesia by intravenous low-dose ketamine and epidural morphine in gastrectomy: a randomized double-blind study. *Anesthesiology* 2000; **92**(6): 1624–1630.
139 Hamilton SM, Johnston SA, Broadstone RV. Evaluation of analgesia provided by the administration of epidural ketamine in dogs with a chemically induced synovitis. *Vet Anaesth Analg* 2005; **32**(1): 30–39.
140 Kovalcuka L, Birgele E, Bandere D, *et al.* The effects of ketamine hydrochloride and diazepam on the intraocular pressure and pupil diameter of the dog's eye. *Vet Ophthalmol* 2013; **16**(1): 29–34.
141 Wetzel RW, Ramsay EC. Comparison of four regimens for intraoral administration of medication to induce sedation in cats prior to euthanasia. *J Am Vet Med Assoc* 1998; **213**(2): 243–245.
142 Harrison KA, Robertson SA, Levy JK, *et al.* Evaluation of medetomidine, ketamine and buprenorphine for neutering feral cats. *J Feline Med Surg* 2011; **13**(12): 896–902.
143 Cistola AM, Golder FJ, Centonze LA, *et al.* Anesthetic and physiologic effects of tiletamine, zolazepam, ketamine, and xylazine combination (TKX) in feral cats undergoing surgical sterilization. *J Feline Med Surg* 2004; **6**(5): 297–303.
144 Cruz ML, Luna SP, de Castro GB, *et al.* A preliminary trial comparison of several anesthetic techniques in cats. *Can Vet J* 2000; **41**(6): 481–485.
145 Gunkel C, Lafortune M. Felids. In: West G, Heard D, Caulkett N, eds. *Zoo Animal and Wildlife Immobilization and Anesthesia*. Ames, IA: Blackwell Publishing, 2007: 443–458.
146 Tokushige H, Araki M, Kusano K, *et al.* A retrospective comparison of induction with thiopental/guaifenesin and propofol/ketamine in Thoroughbred racehorses anesthetized with sevoflurane and medetomidine during arthroscopic surgery. *J Equine Sci* 2019; **30**(2): 25–31.
147 Sage AM, Keating SC, Lascola KM, *et al.* Cardiopulmonary effects and recovery characteristics of horses anesthetized with xylazine-ketamine with midazolam or propofol. *Vet Anaesth Analg* 2018; **45**(6): 772–781.
148 Jarrett MA, Bailey KM, Messenger KM, *et al.* Recovery of horses from general anesthesia after induction with propofol and ketamine versus midazolam and ketamine. *J Am Vet Med Assoc* 2018; **253**(1): 101–107.
149 Umar MA, Yamashita K, Kushiro T, *et al.* Evaluation of total intravenous anesthesia with propofol or ketamine–medetomidine–propofol combination in horses. *J Am Vet Med Assoc* 2006; **228**(8): 1221–1227.
150 Posner LP, Kasten JI, Kata C. Propofol with ketamine following sedation with xylazine for routine induction of general anaesthesia in horses. *Vet Rec* 2013; **173**(22): 550.
151 Muir WW III, Lerche P, Robertson JT, *et al.* Comparison of four drug combinations for total intravenous anesthesia of horses undergoing surgical removal of an abdominal testis. *J Am Vet Med Assoc* 2000; **217**(6): 869–873.
152 Coetzee JF, Gehring R, Tarus-Sang J, *et al.* Effect of sub-anesthetic xylazine and ketamine ('ketamine stun') administered to calves immediately prior to castration. *Vet Anaesth Analg* 2010; **37**(6): 566–578.
153 Dershwitz M, Sréter FA, Ryan JF. Ketamine does not trigger malignant hyperthermia in susceptible swine. *Anesth Analg* 1989; **69**(4): 501–503.
154 Ko JC, Williams BL, Smith VL, *et al.* Comparison of Telazol, Telazol–ketamine, Telazol–xylazine, and Telazol–ketamine–xylazine as chemical restraint and anesthetic induction combination in swine. *Lab Anim Sci* 1993; **43**(5): 476–480.
155 Donnelly RF, Willman E, Andolfatto G. Stability of ketamine–propofol mixtures for procedural sedation and analgesia in the emergency department. *Can J Hosp Pharm* 2008; **61**(6).
156 Izgi M, Basaran B, Muderrisoglu A, *et al.* Evaluation of the stability and stratification of propofol and ketamine mixtures for pediatric anesthesia. *Paediatr Anaesth* 2018; **28**(3): 275–280.
157 Riccó CH, Henao-Guerrero N. Cardiovascular effects of orotracheal intubation following anesthetic induction with propofol, ketamine–propofol, or ketamine–diazepam in premedicated dogs. *J Am Vet Med Assoc* 2014: **244**.
158 Kennedy MJ, Smith LJ. A comparison of cardiopulmonary function, recovery quality, and total dosages required for induction and total intravenous anesthesia with propofol versus a propofol-ketamine combination in healthy Beagle dogs. *Vet Anaesth Analg* 2015; **42**(4): 350–359.
159 Martinez-Taboada F, Leece EA. Comparison of propofol with ketofol, a propofol-ketamine admixture, for induction of anaesthesia in healthy dogs. *Vet Anaesth Analg* 2014; **41**(6): 575–582.
160 Wamaitha MN, Mogoa EM, Mande JD. Evaluation of anesthesia produced by ketofol in acepromazine- or medetomidine-sedated dogs. *J Adv Vet Anim Res* 2019; **6**(2): 215–221.
161 Ravasio G, Gallo M, Beccaglia M, *et al.* Evaluation of a ketamine–propofol drug combination with or without dexmedetomidine for intravenous anesthesia in cats undergoing ovariectomy. *J Am Vet Med Assoc* 2012; **241**(10): 1307–1313.
162 Zonca A, Ravasio G, Gallo M, *et al.* Pharmacokinetics of ketamine and propofol combination administered as ketofol via continuous infusion in cats. *J Vet Pharmacol Ther* 2012; **35**(6): 580–587.
163 Santos M, Viñuela A, Vela AA, *et al.* Single-syringe ketamine–propofol for induction of anaesthesia in rabbits. *Vet Anaesth Analg* 2016; **43**(5): 561–565.
164 Flaherty D, Reid J, Welsh E, *et al.* A pharmacodynamic study of propofol or propofol and ketamine infusions in ponies undergoing surgery. *Res Vet Sci* 1997; **62**(2): 179–184.
165 Nolan A, Reid J, Welsh E, *et al.* Simultaneous infusions of propofol and ketamine in ponies premedicated with detomidine: a pharmacokinetic study. *Res Vet Sci* 1996; **60**(3): 262–266.
166 Nagel ML, Muir WW, Nguyen K. Comparison of the cardiopulmonary effects of etomidate and thiamylal in dogs. *Am J Vet Res* 1979; **40**(2): 193–196.
167 Tulleken CA, van Dieren A, Jonkman J, *et al.* Clinical and experimental experience with etomidate as a brain protective agent. *J Cereb Blood Flow Metab* 1982; **2**(Suppl 1): 92.
168 Van Hamme MJ, Ghoneim MM, Ambre JJ. Pharmacokinetics of etomidate, a new intravenous anesthetic. *Anesthesiology* 1978; **49**(4): 274–277.
169 Wertz EM, Benson GJ, Thurmon JC, *et al.* Pharmacokinetics of etomidate in cats. *Am J Vet Res* 1990; **51**(2): 281–285.
170 Meuldermans WE, Heykants JJ. The plasma protein binding and distribution of etomidate in dog, rat and human blood. *Arch Int Pharmacodyn Ther* 1976; **221**(1): 150–162.
171 Janssen PA, Niemegeers CJ, Marsboom RP. Etomidate, a potent non-barbiturate hypnotic. Intravenous etomidate in mice, rats, guinea-pigs, rabbits and dogs. *Arch Int Pharmacodyn Ther* 1975; **214**(1): 92.
172 Gooding JM, Corssen G. Etomidate: an ultrashort-acting nonbarbiturate agent for anesthesia induction. *Anesth Analg* 1976; **55**(2): 286–289.
173 Heykants JJ, Meuldermans WE, Michiels LJ, *et al.* Distribution, metabolism and excretion of etomidate, a short-acting hypnotic drug, in the rat. Comparative study of (R)-(+)-(--)-Etomidate. *Arch Int Pharmacodyn Ther* 1975; **216**(1): 113–129.

174 Jiang JH, Xu XQ, Jiang WG, *et al.* Discovery of the EL-0052 as a potential anesthetic drug. *Comput Struct Biotechnol J* 2021; **19**: 710–718.

175 Andrada J, Livingston P, Lee BJ, *et al.* Propofol and etomidate depress cortical, thalamic, and reticular formation neurons during anesthetic-induced unconsciousness. *Anesth Analg* 2012; **114**(3): 661–669.

176 Milde LN, Milde JH, Michenfelder JD. Cerebral functional, metabolic, and hemodynamic effects of etomidate in dogs. *Anesthesiology* 1985; **63**(4): 371–377.

177 Cold GE, Eskesen V, Eriksen H, *et al.* CBF and CMRO2 during continuous etomidate infusion supplemented with N2O and fentanyl in patients with supratentorial cerebral tumour. *A dose-response study. Acta Anaesthesiol Scand* 1985; **29**(5): 490–494.

178 Dearden NM, McDowall DG. Comparison of etomidate and althesin in the reduction of increased intracranial pressure after head injury. *Br J Anaesth* 1985; **57**(4): 361–368.

179 Ghoneim MM, Yamada T. Etomidate: a clinical and electroencephalographic comparison with thiopental. *Anesth Analg* 1977; **56**(4): 479–485.

180 Frizzell RT, Meyer YJ, Borchers DJ, *et al.* The effects of etomidate on cerebral metabolism and blood flow in a canine model for hypoperfusion. *J Neurosurg* 1991; **74**(2): 263–269.

181 Wauquier A. Profile of etomidate. A hypnotic, anticonvulsant and brain protective compound. *Anaesthesia* 1983; **38**(Suppl): 26–33.

182 Ebrahim ZY, DeBoer GE, Luders H, *et al.* Effect of etomidate on the electroencephalogram of patients with epilepsy. *Anesth Analg* 1986; **65**(10): 1004–1006.

183 Rodríguez JM, Muñoz-Rascón P, Navarrete-Calvo R, *et al.* Comparison of the cardiopulmonary parameters after induction of anaesthesia with alphaxalone or etomidate in dogs. *Vet Anaesth Analg* 2012; **39**(4): 357–365.

184 Sams L, Braun C, Allman D, *et al.* A comparison of the effects of propofol and etomidate on the induction of anesthesia and on cardiopulmonary parameters in dogs. *Vet Anaesth Analg* 2008; **35**(6): 488–494.

185 Kissin I, Motomura S, Aultman DF, *et al.* Inotropic and anesthetic potencies of etomidate and thiopental in dogs. *Anesth Analg* 1983; **62**(11): 961–965.

186 Priano LL, Bernards C, Marrone B. Effect of anesthetic induction agents on cardiovascular neuroregulation in dogs. *Anesth Analg* 1989; **68**(3): 344–349.

187 Pascoe PJ, Ilkiw JE, Haskins SC, *et al.* Cardiopulmonary effects of etomidate in hypovolemic dogs. *Am J Vet Res* 1992; **53**(11): 2178–2182.

188 Pagel PS, Hettrick DA, Kersten JR, *et al.* Etomidate adversely alters determinants of left ventricular afterload in dogs with dilated cardiomyopathy. *Anesth Analg* 1998; **86**(5): 932–938.

189 Choi SD, Spaulding BC, Gross JB, *et al.* Comparison of the ventilatory effects of etomidate and methohexital. *Anesthesiology* 1985; **62**(4): 442–447.

190 Fraser R, Watt I, Gray CE, *et al.* The effect of etomidate on adrenocortical function in dogs before and during hemorrhagic shock. *Endocrinology* 1984; **115**(6): 2266–2270.

191 Kenyon CJ, McNeil LM, Fraser R. Comparison of the effects of etomidate, thiopentone and propofol on cortisol synthesis. *Br J Anaesth* 1985; **57**(5): 509–511.

192 Wagner RL, White PF, Kan PB, *et al.* Inhibition of adrenal steroidogenesis by the anesthetic etomidate. *N Engl J Med* 1984; **310**(22): 1415–1421.

193 Dodam JR, Kruse-Elliott KT, Aucoin DP, *et al.* Duration of etomidate-induced adrenocortical suppression during surgery in dogs. *Am J Vet Res* 1990; **51**(5): 786–788.

194 Moon PF. Cortisol suppression in cats after induction of anesthesia with etomidate, compared with ketamine–diazepam combination. *Am J Vet Res* 1997; **58**(8): 868–871.

195 Qin B, Hu H, Cao B, *et al.* Effects of continuous infusion of etomidate at various dose rates on adrenal function in dogs. *BMC Anesthesiology* 2016; **16**(1): 2.

196 Muir WW III, Mason DE. Side effects of etomidate in dogs. *J Am Vet Med Assoc* 1989; **194**(10): 1430–1434.

197 Reddy RV, Moorthy SS, Dierdorf SF, *et al.* Excitatory effects and electroencephalographic correlation of etomidate, thiopental, methohexital, and propofol. *Anesth Analg* 1993; **77**(5): 1008–1011.

198 Moon PF. Acute toxicosis in two dogs associated with etomidate-propylene glycol infusion. *Lab Anim Sci* 1994; **44**(6): 590–594.

199 Robertson S. Advantages of etomidate use as an anesthetic agent. *Vet Clin North Am Small Anim Pract* 1992; **22**(2): 277–280.

200 Akkerdaas LC, Sap R, Hellebreker LJ. An alternative premedication and induction regime for cats with a decreased cardio-vascular reserve. *Vet Q* 1998; **20**(Suppl 1): S108.

201 Fresno L, Andaluz A, Moll X, *et al.* The effects on maternal and fetal cardiovascular and acid-base variables after the administration of etomidate in the pregnant ewe. *Vet J* 2008; **177**(1): 94–103.

202 Fresno L, Andaluz A, Moll X, *et al.* Placental transfer of etomidate in pregnant ewes after an intravenous bolus dose and continuous infusion. *Vet J* 2008; **175**(3): 395–402.

203 Clutton RE, Blissitt KJ, Bradley AA, *et al.* Comparison of three injectable anaesthetic techniques in pigs. *Vet Rec* 1997; **141**(6): 140–146.

204 Prakash O, Dhasmana KM, Verdouw PD, *et al.* Cardiovascular effects of etomidate with emphasis on regional myocardial blood flow and performance. *Br J Anaesth* 1981; **53**(6): 591–599.

205 Suresh MS, Nelson TE. Malignant hyperthermia: is etomidate safe? *Anesth Analg* 1985; **64**(4): 420–424.

206 Cotten JF, Forman SA, Laha JK, *et al.* Carboetomidate: a pyrrole analog of etomidate designed not to suppress adrenocortical function. *Anesthesiology* 2010; **112**(3): 637–644.

207 Liu X, Song H, Yang J, *et al.* The etomidate analog ET-26 HCl retains superior myocardial performance: comparisons with etomidate in vivo and in vitro. *PLoS ONE* 2018; **13**(1): e0190994. doi: 10.1371/journal.pone.0190994

208 Wang B, Yang J, Chen J, *et al.* An etomidate analogue with less adrenocortical suppression, stable hemodynamics, and improved behavioral recovery in rats. *Anesth Analg* 2017; **125**(2): 442–450.

209 Cotten JF, Husain SS, Forman SA, *et al.* Methoxycarbonyl-etomidate: a novel rapidly metabolized and ultra-short-acting etomidate analogue that does not produce prolonged adrenocortical suppression. *Anesthesiology* 2009; **111**(2): 240–249.

210 Yang J, Kang Y, Wang B, *et al.* Metabolite-inactive etomidate analogues alleviating suppression on adrenal function in Beagle dogs. *Eur J Pharm Sci* 2017; **99**: 343–349.

211 Campagna JA, Pojasek K, Grayzel D, *et al.* Advancing novel anesthetics: pharmacodynamic and pharmacokinetic studies of cyclopropyl-methoxycarbonyl metomidate in dogs. *Anesthesiology* 2014; **121**(6): 1203–1216.

212 Struys MMRF, Valk BI, Eleveld DJ, *et al.* A Phase 1, single-center, double-blind, placebo-controlled study in healthy subjects to assess the safety, tolerability, clinical effects, and pharmacokinetics–pharmacodynamics of intravenous cyclopropyl-methoxycarbonylmetomidate (ABP-700) after a single ascending bolus dose. *Anesthesiology* 2017; **127**(1): 20–35.

213 Valk BI, Absalom AR, Meyer P, *et al.* Safety and clinical effect of i.v. infusion of cyclopropyl-methoxycarbonyl etomidate (ABP-700), a soft analogue of etomidate, in healthy subjects. *Br J Anaesth* 2018; **120**(6): 1401–1411.

214 Valk BI, Struys MMRF. Etomidate and its analogs: a review of pharmacokinetics and pharmacodynamics. *Clin Pharmacokinet* 2021; **60**(10): 1253–1269.

215 Child KJ, Currie JP, Dis B, *et al.* The pharmacological properties in animals of CT1341--a new steroid anaesthetic agent. *Br J Anaesth* 1971; **43**(1): 2–13.

216 Hall LW. Althesin in the larger animal. *Postgrad Med J* 1972; **48**(Suppl 2): 55–58.

217 Dodman NH. Complications of saffan anaesthesia in cats. *Vet Rec* 1980; **107**(21): 481–483.

218 Ferré PJ, Pasloske K, Whittem T, *et al.* Plasma pharmacokinetics of alfaxalone in dogs after an intravenous bolus of Alfaxan-CD RTU. *Vet Anaesth Analg* 2006; **33**(4): 229–236.

219 Haworth M, McEwen M, Dixon B, *et al.* Anaphylaxis associated with intravenous administration of alphaxalone in a dog. *Aust Vet J* 2019; **97**(6): 197–201.

220 Whitehead MC, Vanetten CL, Jacob ME, *et al.* Microbial integrity of preservative-free alfaxalone in a multiple-use system for two storage conditions and three handling techniques. *Am J Vet Res* 2018; **79**(7): 704–710.

221 Jurox. Alfaxan Multidose IDX (Alfaxalone) [package insert]. Available at: www.fda.gov/media/135542/download?attachment (accessed June 2022).

222 Rowe RC, Sheskey PJ, Quinn ME. Monographs. In: Rowe RC, Sheskey PJ, Quinn ME, eds. *Handbook of Pharmaceutical Excipients*, 6th edn. London, UK: Pharmaceutical Press, 2009: 17–171.

223 Pasloske K, Ranasinghe MG, Sauer S, *et al.* The bioequivalence of a single intravenous administration of the anesthetic alfaxalone in cyclodextrin versus alfaxalone in cyclodextrin plus preservatives in cats. *J Vet Pharmacol Ther* 2018; **41**(3): 437–446.

224 Hector RC, Mama KR, Fisher MC, *et al.* Evaluation of two medetomidine-azaperone-alfaxalone combinations in captive Rocky Mountain Elk (*Cervus Elaphus Nelsoni*). *J Zoo Wildl Med* 2021; **51**(4): 825–833.

225 Patterson M, Caulkett N, Neuhaus P, *et al.* The utility of a novel formulation of alfaxalone in a remote delivery system. *Vet Anaesth Analg* 2021; **48**(4): 537–540.

226 National Center for Biotechnology Information. PubChem Compound Summary for CID 104845, Alfaxalone. https://pubchem.ncbi.nlm.nih.gov/compound/Alfaxalone (accessed June 2022).

227 Cottrell GA, Lambert JJ, Peters JA. Modulation of GABAA receptor activity by alphaxalone. *Br J Pharmacol* 1987; **90**(3): 491–500.

228 Ziemba AM, Szabo A, Pierce DW, *et al.* Alphaxalone binds in inner transmembrane β+-α- interfaces of α1β3γ2 γ-Aminobutyric acid type A receptors. *Anesthesiology* 2018; **128**(2): 338–351.

229 Pasloske K, Sauer B, Perkins N, *et al.* Plasma pharmacokinetics of alfaxalone in both premedicated and unpremedicated Greyhound dogs after single, intravenous administration of Alfaxan at a clinical dose. *J Vet Pharmacol Ther* 2009; **32**(5): 510–513.

230 Dehuisser V, Bosmans T, Devreese M, *et al.* Alfaxalone total intravenous anaesthesia in dogs: pharmacokinetics, cardiovascular data and recovery characteristics. *Vet Anaesth Analg* 2019; **46**(5): 605–612.

231 Whittem T, Pasloske KS, Heit MC, *et al.* The pharmacokinetics and pharmacodynamics of alfaxalone in cats after single and multiple intravenous administration

of Alfaxan at clinical and supraclinical doses. *J Vet Pharmacol Ther* 2008; **31**(6): 571–579.

232 Rodrigo-Mocholí D, Escudero E, Belda E, *et al.* Pharmacokinetics and effects of alfaxalone after intravenous and intramuscular administration to cats. *N Z Vet J* 2018; **66**(4): 172–177.

233 Goodwin WA, Keates HL, Pasloske K, *et al.* The pharmacokinetics and pharmacodynamics of the injectable anaesthetic alfaxalone in the horse. *Vet Anaesth Analg* 2011; **38**(5): 431–438.

234 Wakuno A, Aoki M, Kushiro A, *et al.* Clinical pharmacokinetics and pharmacodynamics of intravenous alfaxalone in young Thoroughbred horses premedicated with medetomidine and midazolam. *Vet Rec* 2019; **184**(13): 411.

235 Goodwin W, Keates H, Pasloske K, *et al.* Plasma pharmacokinetics and pharmacodynamics of alfaxalone in neonatal foals after an intravenous bolus of alfaxalone following premedication with butorphanol tartrate. *Vet Anaesth Analg* 2012; **39**(5): 503–510.

236 Goodwin WA, Pasloske K, Keates HL, *et al.* Alfaxalone for total intravenous anaesthesia in horses. *Vet Anaesth Analg* 2019; **46**(2): 188–199.

237 Marín P, Belda E, Laredo FG, *et al.* Pharmacokinetics and sedative effects of alfaxalone with or without dexmedetomidine in rabbits. *Res Vet Sci* 2020; **129**: 6–12.

238 Sear JW, McGivan JD. Metabolism of alphaxalone in the rat: evidence for the limitation of the anaesthetic effect by the rate of degradation through the hepatic mixed function oxygenase system. *Br J Anaesth* 1981; **53**(4): 417–424.

239 Warne LN, Beths T, Whittem T, *et al.* A review of the pharmacology and clinical application of alfaxalone in cats. *Vet J* 2015; **203**(2): 141–148.

240 Sear JW. Steroid anesthetics: old compounds, new drugs. *J Clin Anesth* 1996; **8**(3 Suppl): 91S–98S.

241 Rasmussen NJ, Rosendal T, Overgaard J. Althesin in neurosurgical patients: effects on cerebral hemodynamics and metabolism. *Acta Anaesthesiol Scand* 1978; **22**(3): 257–269.

242 Ambrisko TD, Johnson CB, Chambers P. Effect of alfaxalone infusion on the electroencephalogram of dogs anaesthetized with halothane. *Vet Anaesth Analg* 2011; **38**(6): 529–535.

243 Bini G, Bailey K, Voyvodic J, *et al.* Effects of propofol, alfaxalone and isoflurane on cerebral blood flow and cerebrovascular reactivity to CO2 in dogs. *Vet Anaesth Analg* 2020; **47**(6): 855.e2.

244 Muir W, Lerche P, Wiese A, *et al.* The cardiorespiratory and anesthetic effects of clinical and supraclinical doses of alfaxalone in cats. *Vet Anaesth Analg* 2009; **36**(1): 42–54.

245 Muir W, Lerche P, Wiese A, *et al.* Cardiorespiratory and anesthetic effects of clinical and supraclinical doses of alfaxalone in dogs. *Vet Anaesth Analg* 2008; **35**(6): 451–462.

246 Ohmura H, Okano A, Mukai K, *et al.* Cardiorespiratory and anesthetic effects of combined alfaxalone, butorphanol, and medetomidine in Thoroughbred horses. *J Equine Sci* 2016; **27**(1): 7–11.

247 Granados MM, Domínguez JM, Fernández-Sarmiento A, *et al.* Anaesthetic and cardiorespiratory effects of a constant-rate infusion of alfaxalone in desflurane-anaesthetised sheep. *Vet Rec* 2012; **171**(5): 125.

248 Moll X, Santos L, García F, *et al.* The effects on cardio-respiratory and acid-base variables of a constant rate infusion of alfaxalone-HPCD in sheep. *Vet J* 2013; **196**(2): 209–212.

249 Andaluz A, Felez-Ocaña N, Santos L, *et al.* The effects on cardio-respiratory and acid-basevariablesoftheanaestheticalfaxaloneina2-hydroxypropyl-β-cyclodextrin (HPCD) formulation in sheep. *Vet J* 2012; **191**(3): 389–392.

250 Duval JD, Pang JM, Boysen SR, *et al.* Cardiopulmonary effects of a partial intravenous anesthesia technique for laboratory swine. *J Am Assoc Lab Anim Sci* 2018; **57**(4): 376–381.

251 Bigby SE, Carter JE, Bauquier S, *et al.* The use of alfaxalone for premedication, induction and maintenance of anaesthesia in pigs: a pilot study. *Vet Anaesth Analg* 2017; **44**(4): 905–909.

252 Bigby SE, Beths T, Bauquier S, *et al.* Effect of rate of administration of propofol or alfaxalone on induction dose requirements and occurrence of apnea in dogs. *Vet Anaesth Analg* 2017; **44**(6): 1267–1275.

253 Bauquier SH, Warne LN, Carter JE, *et al.* Influence of two administration rates of alfaxalone at induction on its relative potency in cats: a pilot study. *J Feline Med Surg* 2017; **19**(2): 231–234.

254 Petersen JS, Shalmi M, Christensen S, *et al.* Comparison of the renal effects of six sedating agents in rats. *Physiol Behav* 1996; **60**(3): 759–765.

255 Chen CF, Chapman BJ, Munday KA. The effect of althesin, ketamine or pentothal on renal function in saline loaded rats. *Clin Exp Pharmacol Physiol* 1985; **12**(2): 99–105.

256 Patschke D, Passian J, Tarnow J, *et al.* Effect of althesin on renal perfusion in anaesthetized dogs. *Can Anaesth Soc J* 1975; **22**(2): 138–143.

257 Thomson IA, Fitch W, Hughes RL, *et al.* Effects of certain i.v. anaesthetics on liver blood flow and hepatic oxygen consumption in the Greyhound. *Br J Anaesth* 1986; **58**(1): 69–80.

258 Webb JK, Keller KA, Chinnadurai SK, *et al.* Optimizing the pharmacodynamics and evaluating cardiogenic effects of the injectable anesthetic alfaxalone in prairie rattlesnakes (*Crotalus Viridis*). *J Zoo Wildl Med* 2021; **52**(4): 1105–1112.

259 Yaw TJ, Mans C, Johnson SM, *et al.* Effect of injection site on alfaxalone-induced sedation in ball pythons (*Python regius*). *J Small Anim Pract* 2018; **59**(12): 747–751.

260 James LE, Williams CJ, Bertelsen MF, *et al.* Anaesthetic induction with alfaxalone in the ball python (*Python regius*): dose response and effect of injection site. *Vet Anaesth Analg* 2018; **45**(3): 329–337.

261 White KL, Paine S, Harris J. A clinical evaluation of the pharmacokinetics and pharmacodynamics of intravenous alfaxalone in cyclodextrin in male and female rats following a loading dose and constant rate infusion. *Vet Anaesth Analg* 2017; **44**(4): 865–875.

262 West SE, Lee JC, Johns TN, *et al.* Intraperitoneal alfaxalone and alfaxalone-dexmedetomidine anesthesia in Sprague–Dawley rats (*Rattus norvegicus*). *J Am Assoc Lab Anim Sci* 2020; **59**(5): 531–538.

263 Arenillas M, Gomez de Segura IA. Anaesthetic effects of alfaxalone administered intraperitoneally alone or combined with dexmedetomidine and fentanyl in the rat. *Lab Anim* 2018; **52**(6): 588–598.

264 Ambar N, Eshar D, Shrader TC, *et al.* Anesthetic effects of intramuscular alfaxalone-ketamine in naked mole rats (*Heterocephalus glaber*). *J Am Assoc Lab Anim Sci* 2020; **59**(5): 539–545.

265 Erickson RL, Blevins CE, Souza Dyer C, *et al.* Alfaxalone-xylazine anesthesia in laboratory mice (*Mus musculus*). *J Am Assoc Lab Anim Sci* 2019; **58**(1): 30–39.

266 Pasloske K, Gazzard B, Perkins N. *A Multi Centre Clinical Trial Evaluating the Efficacy and Safety of Alfaxan-CD RTU Administered to Dogs for Induction and Maintenance of Anesthesia.* Birmingham, UK: BSAVA Congress, April 7–10, 2005.

267 Pinelas R, Alibhai HI, Mathis A, *et al.* Effects of different doses of dexmedetomidine on anaesthetic induction with alfaxalone--a clinical trial. *Vet Anaesth Analg* 2014; **41**(4): 378–385.

268 Maddern K, Adams VJ, Hill NA, *et al.* Alfaxalone induction dose following administration of medetomidine and butorphanol in the dog. *Vet Anaesth Analg* 2010; **37**(1): 7–13.

269 Psatha E, Alibhai HI, Jimenez-Lozano A, *et al.* Clinical efficacy and cardiorespiratory effects of alfaxalone, or diazepam/fentanyl for induction of anaesthesia in dogs that are a poor anaesthetic risk. *Vet Anaesth Analg* 2011; **38**(1): 24–36.

270 Ambros B, Duke-Novakovski T, Pasloske KS. Comparison of the anesthetic efficacy and cardiopulmonary effects of continuous rate infusions of alfaxalone-2-hydroxypropyl-beta-cyclodextrin and propofol in dogs. *Am J Vet Res* 2008; **69**(11): 1391–1398.

271 Herbert GL, Bowlt KL, Ford-Fennah V, *et al.* Alfaxalone for total intravenous anaesthesia in dogs undergoing ovariohysterectomy: a comparison of premedication with acepromazine or dexmedetomidine. *Vet Anaesth Analg* 2013; **40**(2): 124–133.

272 Suarez MA, Dzikiti BT, Stegmann FG, *et al.* Comparison of alfaxalone and propofol administered as total intravenous anaesthesia for ovariohysterectomy in dogs. *Vet Anaesth Analg* 2012; **39**(3): 236–244.

273 O'Hagan B, Pasloske K, McKinnon C, *et al.* Clinical evaluation of alfaxalone as an anaesthetic induction agent in dogs less than 12 weeks of age. *Aust Vet J* 2012; **90**(9): 346–350.

274 Metcalfe S, Hulands-Nave A, Bell M, *et al.* Multicentre, randomised clinical trial evaluating the efficacy and safety of alfaxalone administered to bitches for induction of anaesthesia prior to caesarean section. *Aust Vet J* 2014; **92**(9): 333–338.

275 Schmidt K, Feng C, Wu T, *et al.* Influence of maternal, anesthetic, and surgical factors on neonatal survival after emergency cesarean section in 78 dogs: a retrospective study (2002 to 2020). *Can Vet J* 2021; **62**(9): 961–968.

276 Melandri M, Alonge S, Peric T, *et al.* Effects of alfaxalone or propofol on giant-breed dog neonates' viability during elective caesarean sections. *Animals (Basel)* 2019; **9**(11): 962. doi: 10.3390/ani9110962

277 Conde Ruiz C, Del Carro AP, Rosset E, *et al.* Alfaxalone for total intravenous anaesthesia in bitches undergoing elective caesarean section and its effects on puppies: a randomized clinical trial. *Vet Anaesth Analg* 2016; **43**(3): 281–290.

278 Hasiuk MM, Forde N, Cooke A, *et al.* A comparison of alfaxalone and propofol on intraocular pressure in healthy dogs. *Vet Ophthalmol* 2014; **17**(6): 411–416.

279 Costa D, Leiva M, Moll X, *et al.* Alfaxalone versus propofol in dogs: a randomised trial to assess effects on peri-induction tear production, intraocular pressure and globe position. *Vet Rec* 2015; **176**(3): 73.

280 Bauer BS, Ambros B. The effects of intravenous alfaxalone with and without premedication on intraocular pressure in healthy dogs. *Can J Vet Res* 2016; **80**(2): 156–161.

281 Mayordomo-Febrer A, Rubio M, Martínez-Gassent M, *et al.* Effects of morphine-alfaxalone-midazolam premedication, alfaxalone induction and sevoflurane maintenance on intraocular pressure and tear production in dogs. *Vet Rec* 2017; **180**(19): 474.

282 Maney JK, Shepard MK, Braun C, *et al.* A comparison of cardiopulmonary and anesthetic effects of an induction dose of alfaxalone or propofol in dogs. *Vet Anaesth Analg* 2013; **40**(3): 237–244.

283 Cruz-Benedetti IC, Bublot I, Ribas T, *et al.* Pharmacokinetics of intramuscular alfaxalone and its echocardiographic, cardiopulmonary and sedative effects in healthy dogs. *PLoS ONE* 2018; **13**(9): e0204553. doi: 10.1371/journal.pone.0204553

284 Kato K, Itami T, Nomoto K, *et al.* The anesthetic effects of intramuscular alfaxalone in dogs premedicated with low-dose medetomidine and/or butorphanol. *J Vet Med Sci* 2021; **83**(1): 53–61.

285 Arenillas M, Aguado D, Canfrán S, *et al.* Sedative effects of two doses of alfaxalone in combination with methadone and a low dose of dexmedetomidine in healthy Beagles. *Vet Anaesth Analg* 2020; **47**(4): 463–471.

286 Murdock MA, Riccó Pereira CH, Aarnes TK, *et al.* Sedative and cardiorespiratory effects of intramuscular administration of alfaxalone and butorphanol combined with acepromazine, midazolam, or dexmedetomidine in dogs. *Am J Vet Res* 2020; **81**(1): 65–76.

287 Micieli F, Chiavaccini L, Paré MD, *et al.* Comparison of the sedative effects of alfaxalone and methadone with or without midazolam in dogs. *Can Vet J* 2019; **60**(10): 1060–1064.

288 Lee J, Suh S, Choi R, *et al.* Cardiorespiratory and anesthetic effects produced by the combination of butorphanol, medetomidine and alfaxalone administered intramuscularly in Beagle dogs. *J Vet Med Sci* 2016; **77**(12): 1677–1680.

289 Taboada FM, Murison PJ. Induction of anaesthesia with alfaxalone or propofol before isoflurane maintenance in cats. *Vet Rec* 2010; **167**(3): 85–89.

290 Tamura J, Oyama N, Fukui S, *et al.* Comparison of the anesthetic effects between 5 mg/kg of alfaxalone and 10 mg/kg of propofol administered intravenously in cats. *J Vet Med Sci* 2021; **83**(1): 73–77.

291 Zaki S, Ticehurst K, Miyaki Y. Clinical evaluation of Alfaxan-CD(R) as an intravenous anaesthetic in young cats. *Aust Vet J* 2009; **87**(3): 82–87.

292 O'Hagan BJ, Pasloske K, McKinnon C, *et al.* Clinical evaluation of alfaxalone as an anaesthetic induction agent in cats less than 12 weeks of age. *Aust Vet J* 2012; **90**(10): 395–401.

293 Beths T, Touzot-Jourde G, Musk G, *et al.* Clinical evaluation of alfaxalone to induce and maintain anaesthesia in cats undergoing neutering procedures. *J Feline Med Surg* 2014; **16**(8): 609–615.

294 Mathis A, Pinelas R, Brodbelt DC, *et al.* Comparison of quality of recovery from anaesthesia in cats induced with propofol or alfaxalone. *Vet Anaesth Analg* 2012; **39**(3): 282–290.

295 Ramoo S, Bradbury LA, Anderson GA, *et al.* Sedation of hyperthyroid cats with subcutaneous administration of a combination of alfaxalone and butorphanol. *Aust Vet J* 2013; **91**(4): 131–136.

296 Grubb TL, Greene SA, Perez TE. Cardiovascular and respiratory effects, and quality of anesthesia produced by alfaxalone administered intramuscularly to cats sedated with dexmedetomidine and hydromorphone. *J Feline Med Surg* 2013; **15**(10): 858–865.

297 Reader RC, Yang VK, Babyak JM, *et al.* The effects of two intramuscular sedation protocols on echocardiographic variables in cats following sedation and blood donation. *J Vet Emerg Crit Care* 2021; **31**(2): 256–262.

298 Wheeler EP, Abelson AL, Lindsey JC, *et al.* Sedative effects of alfaxalone and hydromorphone with or without midazolam in cats: a pilot study. *J Feline Med Surg* 2021; **23**(12): 1109–1116.

299 Khenissi L, Nikolayenkova-Topie O, Broussaud S, *et al.* Comparison of intramuscular alfaxalone and ketamine combined with dexmedetomidine and butorphanol for castration in cats. *J Feline Med Surg* 2017; **19**(8): 791–797.

300 Fernandez-Parra R, Adami C, Dresco T, *et al.* Dexmedetomidine-methadone-ketamine versus dexmedetomidine-methadone-alfaxalone for cats undergoing ovariectomy. *Vet Anaesth Analg* 2017; **44**(6): 1332–1340.

301 Reader RC, Barton BA, Abelson AL. Comparison of two intramuscular sedation protocols on sedation, recovery and ease of venipuncture for cats undergoing blood donation. *J Feline Med Surg* 2019; **21**(2): 95–102.

302 Cremer J, Riccó CH. Cardiovascular, respiratory and sedative effects of intramuscular alfaxalone, butorphanol and dexmedetomidine compared with ketamine, butorphanol and dexmedetomidine in healthy cats. *J Feline Med Surg* 2018; **20**(10): 973–979.

303 Goodwin WA, Keates HL, Pearson M, *et al.* Alfaxalone and medetomidine intravenous infusion to maintain anaesthesia in colts undergoing field castration. *Equine Vet J* 2013; **45**(3): 315–319.

304 Keates HL, van Eps AW, Pearson MR. Alfaxalone compared with ketamine for induction of anaesthesia in horses following xylazine and guaifenesin. *Vet Anaesth Analg* 2012; **39**(6): 591–598.

305 Klöppel H, Leece EA. Comparison of ketamine and alfaxalone for induction and maintenance of anaesthesia in ponies undergoing castration. *Vet Anaesth Analg* 2011; **38**(1): 37–43.

306 Jones T, Bracamonte JL, Ambros B, *et al.* Total intravenous anesthesia with alfaxalone, dexmedetomidine and remifentanil in healthy foals undergoing abdominal surgery. *Vet Anaesth Analg* 2019; **46**(3): 315–324.

307 Loomes K. Alfaxalone total intravenous anaesthesia in a donkey foal. *Vet Anaesth Analg* 2020; **47**(5): 733–734.

308 Maney JK, Dzikiti BT. Evaluation of xylazine-alfaxalone anesthesia for field castration in donkey foals. *Vet Anaesth Analg* 2020; **47**(4): 547–551.

309 Maney JK, Durham HE Jr., Goucher KP, *et al.* Induction of anesthesia and recovery in donkeys sedated with xylazine: a comparison of midazolam-alfaxalone and midazolam-ketamine. *Vet Anaesth Analg* 2018; **45**(4): 539–544.

310 Torres MD, Andaluz A, García F, *et al.* Effects of an intravenous bolus of alfaxalone versus propofol on intraocular pressure in sheep. *Vet Rec* 2012; **170**(9): 226.

311 Oakleaf MH, Mama KR, Mangin LM, *et al.* Comparison of intravenous anesthetic induction doses and physiologic effects of ketamine or alfaxalone in goats undergoing surgery with isoflurane anesthesia. *Am J Vet Res* 2019; **80**(9): 819–824.

312 Ndawana PS, Dzikiti BT, Zeiler G, *et al.* Determination of the minimum infusion rate (MIR) of alfaxalone required to prevent purposeful movement of the extremities in response to a standardised noxious stimulus in goats. *Vet Anaesth Analg* 2015; **42**(1): 65–71.

313 Dzikiti TB, Ndawana PS, Zeiler G, *et al.* Determination of the minimum infusion rate of alfaxalone during its co-administration with midazolam in goats. *Vet Rec Open* 2015; **2**(1): e000065.

314 Dzikiti BT, Ndawana PS, Zeiler G, *et al.* Determination of the minimum infusion rate of alfaxalone during its co-administration with fentanyl at three different doses by constant rate infusion intravenously in goats. *Vet Anaesth Analg* 2016; **43**(3): 316–325.

315 Dzikiti BT, Ndawana PS, Dzikiti LN, *et al.* The minimum infusion rate of alfaxalone during its co-administration with lidocaine at three different doses by constant rate infusion in goats. *Vet Anaesth Analg* 2018; **45**(3): 285–294.

316 Santos González M, Bertrán de Lis BT, Tendillo Cortijo FJ. Effects of intramuscular alfaxalone alone or in combination with diazepam in swine. *Vet Anaesth Analg* 2013; **40**(4): 399–402.

317 Santos M, Bertrán de Lis BT, Tendillo FJ. Effects of intramuscular dexmedetomidine in combination with ketamine or alfaxalone in swine. *Vet Anaesth Analg* 2016; **43**(1): 81–85.

318 Hancock TM, Caulkett NA, Pajor EA, *et al.* An investigation of the effects of intratesticular alfaxalone and lidocaine during castration in piglets. *Vet Anaesth Analg* 2018; **45**(6): 858–864.

319 Hampton CE, Takawira C, Ross JM, *et al.* Sedation characteristics of intranasal alfaxalone in adult Yucatan Swine. *J Am Assoc Lab Anim Sci* 2021; **60**(2): 184–187.

320 Keates H. Induction of anaesthesia in pigs using a new alphaxalone formulation. *Vet Rec* 2003; **153**(20): 627–628.

321 Lervik A, Toverud SF, Krontveit R, *et al.* A comparison of respiratory function in pigs anaesthetised by propofol or alfaxalone in combination with dexmedetomidine and ketamine. *Acta Vet Scand* 2020; **62**(1): 14.

322 Hasse K, Crawford A, Gustafson D, *et al.* Plasma concentration and pharmacodynamics of intramuscular administration of alfaxalone in Indian peafowl (*Pavo Cristatus*). *J Zoo Wildl Med* 2022; **53**(1): 108–115.

323 Greunz EM, Limón D, Bertelsen MF. Alfaxalone Sedation in black-cheeked lovebirds (*Agapornis nigrigenis*) for non-invasive procedures. *J Avian Med Surg* 2021; **35**(2): 161–166.

324 Whitehead MC, Hoppes SM, Musser JMB, *et al.* The use of alfaxalone in Quaker parrots (*Myiopsitta monachus*). *J Avian Med Surg* 2019; **33**(4): 340–348.

325 Kruse TN, Messenger KM, Bowman AS, *et al.* Pharmacokinetics and pharmacodynamics of alfaxalone after a single intramuscular or intravascular injection in mallard ducks (*Anas platyrhynchos*). *J Vet Pharmacol Ther* 2019; **42**(6): 713–721.

326 Balko JA, Lindemann DM, Allender MC, *et al.* Evaluation of the anesthetic and cardiorespiratory effects of intramuscular alfaxalone administration and isoflurane in budgerigars (*Melopsittacus undulatus*) and comparison with manual restraint. *J Am Vet Med Assoc* 2019; **254**(12): 1427–1435.

327 Bradley MP, Doerning CM, Nowland MH, *et al.* Intramuscular administration of alfaxalone alone and in combination for sedation and anesthesia of rabbits (*Oryctolagus cuniculus*). *J Am Assoc Lab Anim Sci* 2019; **58**(2): 216–222.

328 Huynh M, Poumeyrol S, Pignon C, *et al.* Intramuscular administration of alfaxalone for sedation in rabbits. *Vet Rec* 2015; **176**(10): 255.

329 Reabel SN, Queiroz-Williams P, Cremer J, *et al.* Assessment of intramuscular administration of three doses of alfaxalone combined with hydromorphone and dexmedetomidine for endoscopic-guided orotracheal intubation in domestic rabbits (*Oryctolagus cuniculus*). *J Am Vet Med Assoc* 2021; **259**(10): 1148–1153.

330 Rousseau-Blass F, Pang DS. Hypoventilation following oxygen administration associated with alfaxalone-dexmedetomidine-midazolam anesthesia in New Zealand White rabbits. *Vet Anaesth Analg* 2020; **47**(5): 637–646.

331 Doerning CM, Bradley MP, Lester PA, *et al.* Effects of subcutaneous alfaxalone alone and in combination with dexmedetomidine and buprenorphine in guinea pigs (*Cavia porcellus*). *Vet Anaesth Analg* 2018; **45**(5): 658–666.

332 d'Ovidio D, Marino F, Noviello E, *et al.* Sedative effects of intramuscular alfaxalone in pet guinea pigs (*Cavia porcellus*). *Vet Anaesth Analg* 2018; **45**(2): 183–189.

333 Sixtus RP, Pacharinsak C, Gray CL, *et al.* Differential effects of four intramuscular sedatives on cardiorespiratory stability in juvenile guinea pigs (*Cavia porcellus*). *PLoS ONE* 2021; **16**(11): e0259559.

334 Álvarez ER, Solé LV, de Carellán Mateo AG. Comparison of subcutaneous sedation with alfaxalone or alfaxalone-midazolam in pet guinea pigs (*Cavia porcellus*) of three different age groups. *J Am Vet Med Assoc* 2022: 1–7.

335 Hawkins SJ, Doss GA, Mans C. Evaluation of subcutaneous administration of alfaxalone–midazolam and ketamine–midazolam as sedation protocols in African pygmy hedgehogs (*Atelerix albiventris*). *J Am Vet Med Assoc* 2020; **257**(8): 820–825.

336 Bellini L, Pagani G, Mollo A, *et al.* Evaluation of alfaxalone and dexmedetomidine for intramuscular restraint in European hedgehogs (*Erinaceus europaeus*). *Vet Rec* 2019; **185**(5): 145.

337 Milloway MC, Posner LP, Balko JA. Sedative and cardiorespiratory effects of intramuscular alfaxalone and butorphanol at two dosages in ferrets (*Mustela Putorius Furo*). *J Zoo Wildl Med* 2021; **51**(4): 841–847.

338 Leonardi F, Costa GL, Interlandi CD, *et al.* Immersion anaesthesia in goldfish (*Carassius auratus*) with three concentrations of alfaxalone. *Vet Anaesth Analg* 2019; **46**(1): 79–83.

339 Adami C, Spadavecchia C, Angeli G, *et al.* Alfaxalone anesthesia by immersion in oriental fire-bellied toads (*Bombina orientalis*). *Vet Anaesth Analg* 2015; **42**(5): 547–551.

340 Adami C, d'Ovidio D, Casoni D. Alfaxalone versus alfaxalone-dexmedetomidine anaesthesia by immersion in oriental fire-bellied toads (*Bombina orientalis*). *Vet Anaesth Analg* 2016; **43**(3): 326–332.

341 Adami C, d'Ovidio D, Casoni D. Alfaxalone-butorphanol versus alfaxalone-morphine combination for immersion anaesthesia in oriental fire-bellied toads (*Bombina orientalis*). *Lab Anim* 2016; **50**(3): 204–211.

342 Williams M, Caulkett N, Neuhaus P, *et al.* Comparison of the efficacy and safety of medetomidine-ketamine versus medetomidine-azaperone-alfaxalone combination in free-ranging rocky mountain bighorn sheep (*Ovis Canadensis*). *J Zoo Wildl Med* 2018; **49**(3): 662–670.

343 Hillidge CJ, Lees P, Serrano L. Investigations of azaperone-metomidate anaesthesia in the horse. *Vet Rec* 1973; **93**(11): 307–311.

344 Hall LW, Clarke KW. General pharmacology of the intravenous anaesthetics. In: Hall LW, Clarke KW, eds. *Veterinary Anesthesia*. Chichester, UK: Baillière Tindall, 1983: 74–93.

28 Inhalation Anesthetics

Eugene P. Steffey[1], Robert J. Brosnan[2] and Khursheed R. Mama[3]

[1] Emeritus Professor, Department of Surgical and Radiological Sciences, School of Veterinary Medicine, University of California–Davis, Davis, California, USA

[2] Department of Surgical and Radiological Sciences, School of Veterinary Medicine, University of California–Davis, Davis, California, USA

[3] Department of Clinical Sciences, College of Veterinary Medicine and Biomedical Sciences, Colorado State University, Fort Collins, Colorado, USA

Chapter contents

Introduction, 489
Physicochemical characteristics, 490
Chemical characteristics, 490
Physical characteristics, 491
Pharmacokinetics: uptake and elimination of inhalation anesthetics, 497
Anesthetic uptake: factors that determine the P_A of anesthetic, 497
Anesthetic elimination, 500
Anesthetic dose: the minimum alveolar concentration (MAC), 502
Pharmacodynamics: actions and toxicity of the volatile inhalation anesthetics on body systems, 504
Central nervous system, 505
Respiratory system, 508
Cardiovascular system, 509
Effects on the kidneys, 511
Effects on the liver, 512
Effects on skeletal muscle: malignant hyperthermia, 512
The gaseous anesthetic: nitrous oxide, 512
Dose, 512
Pharmacokinetics, 513
Pharmacodynamics, 513
Transfer of N_2O to closed gas spaces, 513
Diffusion hypoxia, 513
Interaction with respiratory gas monitoring, 514
Waste inhalation anesthetics, 514
Occupational exposure: trace concentrations of inhalation anesthetics, 514
Environmental implications of inhalation anesthetics, 515
References, 515

Introduction

Inhalation anesthetics are used widely for the anesthetic management of animals. They are unique among anesthetic drugs because they are administered, and in large part removed from the body, via the lungs. Their popularity arises in part because their pharmacokinetic characteristics favor predictable and rapid adjustment of anesthetic depth. In addition, a special apparatus is usually used to deliver the inhaled agents. This apparatus includes a source of oxygen (O_2) and a patient breathing circuit, which in turn usually includes an endotracheal tube or face mask, a means of eliminating carbon dioxide (CO_2), and a compliant gas reservoir. These components help minimize patient morbidity or mortality because they facilitate lung ventilation and improve arterial oxygenation. In addition, inhalation anesthetics in gas samples can be readily measured continuously. Measurement of inhalation anesthetic concentration enhances the precision and safety of anesthetic management beyond the extent commonly possible with injectable anesthetic agents.

Over the nearly 150 years that inhalation anesthesia has been used in clinical practice, less than 20 agents have actually been introduced and approved for general use with patients (Fig. 28.1) [1]. Less than 10 of these have a history of widespread clinical use in veterinary medicine, and only four are of current veterinary importance in North America. It is this group of anesthetics that is the focus of this chapter. Isoflurane remains the most widely used veterinary inhalation anesthetic in North America, with sevoflurane a close second. Other inhalation anesthetics include desflurane and the gaseous agent nitrous oxide (N_2O), which are used much less frequently. Halothane, once the most popular volatile anesthetic throughout the world, is no longer commercially distributed in North America. However, it remains available elsewhere (at least on a limited basis), and, considering the agent's widespread international distribution, we will continue to include information here on some actions of clinical importance to veterinary anesthesia.

Two additional volatile agents continue to receive brief attention for different reasons. Methoxyflurane, an agent popular during the period of about 1960 to 1990, has not been commercially available in North America for many years. However, because of some of its physicochemical characteristics, its inclusion here has value, especially to students of our clinical discipline and pharmacologists, and permits easy comparison to agents of more current interest. It remains commercially available in some global regions especially, for example, in the southern hemisphere. Enflurane, introduced for use in human patients in 1972 and still commercially available, has

Veterinary Anesthesia and Analgesia: The Sixth Edition of Lumb and Jones. Edited by Leigh Lamont, Kurt Grimm, Sheilah Robertson, Lydia Love and Carrie Schroeder.
© 2024 John Wiley & Sons, Inc. Published 2024 by John Wiley & Sons, Inc.
Companion website: www.wiley.com/go/lamont/anesthesia

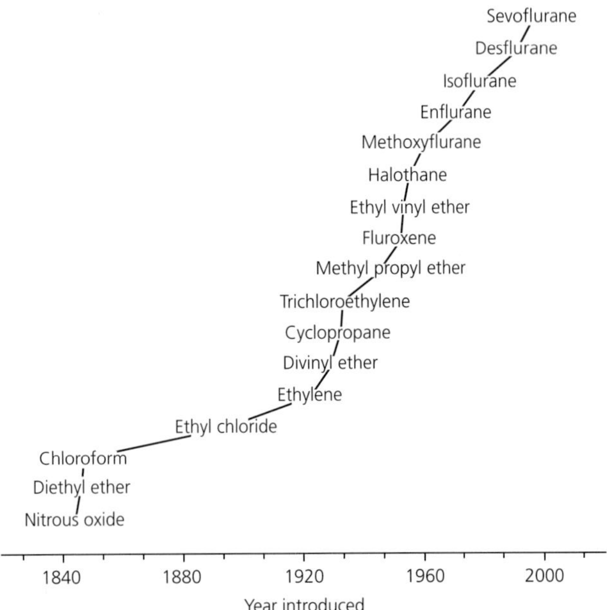

Figure 28.1 Inhalation anesthetics introduced for widespread clinical use. Source: Adapted from Eger [1].

```
Enflurane                    Cl  F      F
(Ethrane®)                   |   |      |
                         H - C - C - O - C - H
                             |   |      |
                             F   F      F

Desflurane                   F   H      F
(Suprane®, 1653)             |   |      |
                         F - C - C - O - C - H
                             |   |      |
                             F   F      F

Halothane                    Br  F
(Fluothane®)                 |   |
                         H - C - C - F
                             |   |
                             Cl  F

Isoflurane                   F   Cl     F
(Forane®, Aerrane®)          |   |      |
                         F - C - C - O - C - H
                             |   |      |
                             F   H      F

Nitrous oxide                  N
                              /
                            O ||
                              \
                               N

Sevoflurane                          F
(Ultane®, Sevoflo®)                  |
                             H   F - C - F
                             |       |
                         F - C - O - C - H
                             |       |
                             H   F - C - F
                                     |
                                     F
```

Figure 28.2 Chemical structure of inhalation anesthetics in current use for animals. Trade names are given in parentheses.

little or no use in veterinary practice in North America. Information on this volatile anesthetic was included in previous editions of this text. However, because enflurane is only in very limited and focused veterinary use elsewhere, we have deleted most information about this agent in the present chapter and refer interested readers to the fourth edition of this text for some coverage. Although of investigational and very limited human patient interest, a review of xenon is again not included in this animal patient-focused chapter.

In this edition, information on agents of largely historical interest again has not been included. Readers interested in aspects of these formerly used agents are referred to the earlier editions of this and other textbooks [2–6]. Examples of such agents are diethyl ether and chloroform. A more complete listing is noted in Fig. 28.1.

Physicochemical characteristics

The chemical structure of inhalation anesthetics and their physical properties determine their actions and safety of administration. An in-depth analysis of the impact of agent chemical structure and physical properties is beyond the scope of this chapter. However, brief discussion of aspects of Fig. 28.2 and Table 28.1 is appropriate because the physicochemical characteristics summarized determine and/or influence practical considerations of their clinical use. For example, they determine the form in which the agents are supplied by the manufacturer (e.g., as a gas or liquid) and account for the resistance of the anesthetic molecule to degradation by physical factors (e.g., heat and light) and substances it contacts during use (e.g., metal components of the anesthetic delivery apparatus and the CO_2 absorbents such as soda lime). The equipment necessary to safely deliver the agent to the patient (e.g., vaporizer and breathing circuit) is influenced by some of these properties, as are the agent's uptake, distribution within, and elimination (including potential for metabolic breakdown) from the patient. In summary, a knowledge and understanding of fundamental properties permits intelligent use of contemporary anesthetics.

Chemical characteristics

Most contemporary inhalation anesthetics are organic compounds, except N_2O (Fig. 28.2) (xenon is another notable inorganic anesthetic). Agents of current interest are further classified as either aliphatic (i.e., straight or branch chained) hydrocarbons or ethers (i.e., two organic radicals attached to an atom of oxygen; the general structure is ROR). In the continued search for a less reactive, more potent, nonflammable inhalation anesthetic, focus on halogenation (i.e., addition of fluorine, chlorine, or bromine) of these compounds has predominated. Chlorine and bromine especially convert many compounds of low anesthetic potency into more potent drugs. Historically, interest in fluorinated derivatives was delayed until the 1940s because of difficulties in synthesis, and thus quantities available for study were limited. Methods of synthesis, although difficult, improved considerably and facilitated new agent discovery (see Fig. 28.2). It is interesting that organic fluorinated compounds are a group of extreme contrasts – some are toxic, others are not; some are inert, others are highly reactive. In some anesthetics, fluorine is substituted for chlorine or bromine to improve stability, but at the expense of reduced anesthetic potency and solubility.

Halothane (see Fig. 28.2) is a halogenated, aliphatic saturated hydrocarbon (ethane). Predictions that a halogenated structure would confer non-flammability and molecular stability encouraged the development of halothane in the early 1950s. However, soon

Table 28.1 Some physical and chemical properties of inhalation anesthetics used clinically in animals.

Property	Desflurane	Enflurane	Halothane	Isoflurane	Methoxyflurane[a]	Nitrous oxide	Sevoflurane
Molecular weight (g)	168	185	197	185	165	44	200
Liquid specific gravity (20 °C) (g/mL)	1.47	1.52	1.86	1.49	1.42	1.42	1.52
Boiling point (°C)	23.5	57	50	49	105	-89	59
Vapor pressure (mmHg) at:							
20 °C	700[b]	172	243	240	23	–	160
24 °C	804	207	288	286	28	–	183
mL vapor/mL liquid at 20 °C	209.7	197.5	227	194.7	206.9	–	182.7
Preservative	None	None	Yes	None	Not available	None	Yes
Stability in:							
Soda lime	No	No	No	No	No	Yes	No
Ultraviolet light	Yes	Yes	No	Yes	No	Yes	??

[a]Methoxyflurane is no longer commercially available in the United States.
[b]Value from [7].

after clinical introduction, it was observed that the concurrent presence of halothane and catecholamines increased the incidence of cardiac arrhythmias, especially in human patients. An ether linkage in the molecule reduces the incidence of cardiac arrhythmias. Consequently, this chemical structure is a predominant characteristic of all agents, which have been developed or entered clinical use since the introduction of halothane (see Fig. 28.2).

Despite many favorable characteristics and improvements over earlier anesthetics (see Fig. 28.1) that included improved chemical stability, halothane is susceptible to decomposition. Accordingly, it is stored in dark bottles and a very small amount of a preservative, thymol, is added to slow decomposition. Thymol is much less volatile than halothane and over time concentrates within the devices used to control delivery of the volatile anesthetic (i.e., vaporizers) and causes them to malfunction. To achieve greater molecular stability, fluorine is substituted for chlorine or bromine in the anesthetic molecule. This chemical manipulation added shelf-life to the substance and negated the need for additives such as thymol. Unfortunately, the fluorine ion is also toxic to some tissues (e.g., kidneys), which is of clinical concern if the parent compound (e.g., historically, most notably methoxyflurane) is not resistant to metabolism (see Fig. 28.2).

Physical characteristics

Life is supported via a constant interchange of respiratory gases (O_2 and CO_2) between cells and the external environment and blood transport. Inhalation anesthetics similarly gain entrance and exit the body via the respiratory system and their movement from a container to sites of action in the central nervous system (CNS) involves similar considerations as respiratory gases. Early in the process of controlled transfer, the agent is diluted to an appropriate amount (partial pressure or concentration) and directed to the respiratory system in a gas mixture that contains enough O_2 to support life. The chain of events that ensues is influenced by many physical and chemical characteristics that can be quantitatively described (Tables 28.1–28.4). The practical clinical applications of these quantitative descriptions are reviewed here. Limited space does not permit in-depth review of all underlying principles, and readers interested in further background information are referred elsewhere [8,9].

The physical characteristics of importance to our understanding of the action of inhalation anesthetics can be conveniently divided into two general categories: those that determine the means by which the agents are administered and those that help determine their kinetics in the body. This information is applied in the clinical manipulation of anesthetic induction and recovery and in facilitating changes in anesthetic-induced CNS depression in a timely fashion.

Properties determining methods of administration

A variety of physical/chemical properties determine the means by which inhalation anesthetics are administered. These include characteristics such as boiling point, liquid density (specific gravity), and vapor pressure.

General principles: a brief review

Molecules are in a constant state of motion and exhibit a force of mutual attraction. The degree of attraction is evident by the state in which the substance exists (i.e., solid, liquid, or gas). Molecular motion increases as energy (e.g., in the form of heat) is added to the molecular aggregate and decreases as energy is removed. With increased motion, there is a reduction in the intermolecular forces; if conditions are extreme enough, a change in physical state may ensue. All substances exist naturally in a particular state but can be made to exist (at least in theory) in any or all phases by altering conditions. Water, as an example, exists as ice (mutual molecular attraction is great), liquid water, or water vapor (attraction considerably reduced) depending upon conditions.

Gas versus vapor

Inhalation anesthetics are either gases or vapors. In relation to inhalation anesthetics, the term "gas" refers to an agent, such as N_2O, that exists in its gaseous form at room temperature and sea level pressure. The term "vapor" indicates the gaseous state of a substance that at ambient temperature and pressure is a liquid. With the exception of N_2O, all the contemporary anesthetics fall into this category. Desflurane (see Table 28.1) is one volatile liquid that comes close to the transition stage and offers some unique (among the inhalation anesthetics) considerations to be discussed later in this chapter [7].

Whether inhalation agents are supplied as a gas or volatile liquid under ambient conditions, the same physical principles apply to each agent when it is in the gaseous state. Molecules move about in haphazard fashion at high speeds and collide with each other or the walls of the containing vessel. The force per unit area of the bombardment is measurable and referred to as "pressure." In the case of gases, if the space or volume in which the gas is enclosed is increased, the number of bombardments decreases (i.e., a smaller number of molecular collisions per unit time) and then the pressure decreases. The behavior of gases is predictably described by various gas laws. Relationships such as those described by Boyle's law (volume versus pressure), Charles's law (volume versus temperature), Gay-Lussac's law (temperature versus pressure), Dalton's law of

Table 28.2 Partition coefficients (solvent/gas) of some inhalation anesthetics at 37 °C.

Solvent	Desflurane	Enflurane	Halothane	Isoflurane	Methoxyflurane	Nitrous oxide	Sevoflurane
Water	–	0.78	0.82	0.62	4.50	0.47	0.60
Blood	0.42	2.00	2.54	1.46	15.00	0.47	0.68
Olive oil	18.70	96.00	224.00	91.00	970.00	1.40	47.00
Brain	1.30	2.70	1.90	1.60	20.00	0.50	1.70
Liver	1.30	3.70	2.10	1.80	29.00	0.38	1.80
Kidney	1.00	1.90	1.00	1.20	11.00	0.40	1.20
Muscle	2.00	2.20	3.40	2.90	16.00	0.54	3.10
Fat	27.00	83.00	51.00	45.00	902.00	1.08	48.00

Source: Tissue samples are derived from human sources. Data are from sources referenced in the 4th edition of this text.

Table 28.3 Blood/gas partition coefficients for desflurane, halothane, isoflurane, methoxyflurane, and sevoflurane in species of common clinical and/or research interest in veterinary medicine, including for comparison similarly derived values for humans.

Species	Desflurane	Halothane	Isoflurane	Methoxyflurane	Sevoflurane	Nitrous oxide
Cat	0.58	–	1.40	26.4	0.59	–
Cow	0.44	2.40 [10]	1.22	11.3	0.52	–
Dog	0.63	3.51 [10]	1.40	26.1	0.66	0.43 [11]
Goat	0.52	–	1.37	13.0	0.56	–
Horse	0.54	1.77 [10]	1.13	13.0	0.65	–
Pig	0.50	–	1.07	11.1	0.52	–
Rat	0.61	6.56 [12]	1.41	17.7	0.74	–
Rabbit	0.72	4.36 [13]	1.37	25.0	0.70	–
Sheep	0.50	–	1.24	13.2	0.56	–
Human	0.50	2.54 [12]	1.32	14.3	0.64	0.41 [11]

Note, some values reported in the present and the 5th editions of this text differ from earlier editions. Present and 5th edition values are taken primarily from the 2012 reported work of Soares *et al.* [14], except where indicated. Values are reported for 37 °C. A dash indicates the value was not found.

Table 28.4 Rubber or plastic/gas partition coefficients at room temperature.

Solvent	Desflurane	Enflurane	Halothane	Isoflurane	Methoxyflurane	Nitrous oxide	Sevoflurane	Reference
Rubber	–	74	120	62	630	1.2	–	[1]
	19	–	190	49	–	–	29	[15]
Poly(vinyl chloride)	–	120	190	110	–	–	–	[1]
	35	–	233	114	–	–	69	[15]
Poly(ethylene)	–	~2	26	~2	118	–	–	[1]
	16	–	128	58	–	–	31	[15]

These data are summarized from multiple sources as reported in Eger [1], with some differences in methods of determination. The data from Targ *et al.* [15] indicate more recently derived data which, unlike earlier data, were recorded following complete equilibration with these materials. Where there is overlap, the ranking of partition coefficients is consistent with halothane > isoflurane > sevoflurane > desflurane. Combining both groupings yields methoxyflurane > halothane > enflurane > isoflurane > sevoflurane > desflurane > N_2O.

partial pressure (the total pressure of a mixture of gases is equal to the sum of the partial pressures of all the gaseous substances present), and others are important to our overall understanding of aspects of respiratory and anesthetic gases and vapors. However, in-depth descriptions of these principles are beyond the scope of this chapter and readers are referred elsewhere for this information [9].

Methods of description

Quantities of inhalation anesthetic agent are usually characterized by one of three methods: pressure (e.g., in mmHg), concentration (in vol %), or mass (in mg or g). The form most familiar to clinicians is that of concentration (e.g., X% of agent A in relation to the whole gas mixture). Agent analysis monitoring equipment samples inspired and expired gases and provides readings for inhalation anesthetics. Precision vaporizers used to control delivery of inhalation anesthetics are calibrated in percentage of agent, and effective doses are almost always reported in percentages.

Pressure is also an important way of describing inhalation anesthetics and is further discussed under the heading of anesthetic potency. A mixture of gases in a closed container will exert pressure on the walls of the container. The individual pressure of each gas in a mixture of gases is referred to as its "partial pressure." As noted earlier, this expression of the behavior of a mixture of gases is known as Dalton's law, and its use in understanding inhalation anesthesia is inescapable. Use of the concept of partial pressure is important in understanding inhalation anesthetic action in a multiphase biologic system because, unlike concentration, the partial pressure of an agent is the same in different compartments that are in equilibrium with each other. That is, in contradistinction to concentration or volume percent, an expression of the relative ratio of gas molecules in a mixture, partial pressure is an expression of the absolute value.

Molecular weight and agent density are used in many calculations to convert from liquid to vapor volumes and mass. Briefly (and in simplified fashion), Avogadro's principle is that equal volume of all gases under the same conditions of temperature and pressure contain the same number of molecules (6.022×10^{23} [Avogadro's number] per gram molecular weight). Furthermore, under standard

Box 28.1 Example calculations to determine the volume of isoflurane vapor at 20 °C from 1 mL of isoflurane liquid.

Isoflurane specific gravity = 1.49 g/mL, therefore:
1 mL liquid isoflurane = 1 mL × 1.49 g/mL = 1.49 g

Since molecular weight of isoflurane = 185 g (from Table 28.1), then:
1.49 g ÷ 185 g = 0.0081 mol of liquid

Since 1 mol of gas = 22.4 L, then:
0.0081 mol × 22,400 mL/mol = 181.4 mL of isoflurane vapor at 0 °C and 1 atmosphere

But vapor is at 20 °C (293 K) not 0 °C (273 K), therefore:
181.4 mL × 293/273 = 194.7 mL vapor/mL liquid isoflurane at 20 °C and 1 atmosphere pressure (i.e., sea level)

For substantial variation in ambient pressure, the final figure noted above would have to be further "corrected" by a factor of (760/ambient barometric pressure)

conditions, the number of gas molecules in a gram molecular weight of a substance occupies 22.4 L. In order to compare properties of different substances of similar state, it is necessary to do so under comparable conditions; with respect to gases and liquids, this usually means with reference to pressure and temperature. Unless otherwise indicated, physical scientists have arbitrarily selected *standard conditions* as 0 °C (273 K in absolute scale) and 760 mmHg pressure (1 atmosphere at sea level). If conditions differ, appropriate temperature and/or pressure corrections must be applied to resultant data.

The weight of a given volume of liquid, gas, or vapor may be expressed in terms of its density or specific gravity. The density is an absolute value of mass (usually grams) per unit volume (for liquids, volume = 1 mL; for gases, 1 L at standard conditions). The specific gravity is a relative value; that is, the ratio of the weight of a unit volume of one substance to a similar volume of water, in the case of liquids, or air, in the case of gases (or vapors), under similar conditions. The value of both air and water is one. At least for clinical purposes, the value for density and specific gravity for an inhalation anesthetic is the same. Thus, for example, we can determine the volume of isoflurane gas (vapor) at 20 °C from 1 mL of isoflurane liquid according to the scheme given in Box 28.1. This type of calculation has practical applications. For example, to determine the savings in isoflurane liquid afforded by reducing the fresh gas (e.g., O_2) inflow rate, a series of calculations as presented in Box 28.2 can be made.

Box 28.2 Problem: Determine the savings in isoflurane liquid afforded by reducing the fresh gas (e.g., O_2) inflow rate from 6 Lpm (liters per minute) to 4 Lpm, given that the average delivered (vaporizer setting) concentration for 2 h is 3%.

Total isoflurane vapor delivered over 2 h (120 min) estimated at:

3%/100 × 6 Lpm = 0.18 Lpm × 120 min = 21.6 L/120 min = 21,600 mL/120 min

versus

3%/100 × 4 Lpm = 0.12 Lpm × 120 min = 14.4 L/120 min = 14,400 mL/120 min

Total vapor volume saved:

21,600 mL/120 min – 14,400 mL/120 min = 7200 mL vapor/120 min saved

Total liquid isoflurane volume saved/2 h (120 min):

7200 mL vapor ÷ 194.7 mL vapor/mL liquid = 36.98 mL of isoflurane liquid

(194.7 mL vapor/mL liquid can be calculated as in Box 28.1 or taken from Table 28.1)

The economic value of reducing isoflurane consumption can then be determined by calculating the product of the liquid volume saved and the purchase cost/mL of isoflurane liquid.

Vapor pressure Molecules of liquids are in constant random motion. Some of those in the surface layer gain sufficient velocity to overcome the attractive forces of neighboring molecules and in escaping from the surface, enter the vapor phase. The change in state from a liquid to a gas phase is known as "vaporization" or "evaporation." This process is dynamic and in a closed container that is kept at a constant temperature, eventually reaches an equilibrium whereby there is no further net loss of molecules to the gas phase (i.e., the numbers of molecules leaving and returning to the liquid phase are equal). The gas phase at this point is saturated.

Molecules of a vapor exert a force per unit area or pressure in exactly the same manner as molecules of a gas. The pressure (units of measure are mmHg) that the vapor molecules exert when the liquid and vapor phases are in equilibrium is known as the "vapor pressure." Thus, the vapor pressure of an anesthetic is a measure of its ability to evaporate; that is, it is a measure of the tendency for molecules in the liquid state to enter the gaseous (vapor) phase. The vapor pressure of a volatile anesthetic must be at least sufficient to provide enough molecules of anesthetic in the vapor state to produce anesthesia at ambient conditions. The *saturated vapor pressure* represents a maximum concentration of molecules in the vapor state that exists for a given liquid at each temperature. Herein lies a practical difference between substances classified as a gas or vapor; a gas can be administered over a range of concentrations from 0% to 100%, whereas the vapor has a ceiling that is dictated by its vapor pressure. The *saturated vapor concentration* can be easily determined by relating the vapor pressure to the ambient pressure. For example, in the case of isoflurane (see Table 28.1), a maximal concentration of 32% isoflurane is possible under usual conditions and 20 °C (i.e., [240/760] × 100 = 32%, where 760 mmHg is the barometric pressure at sea level). With other variables considered constant, the greater the vapor pressure, the greater the concentration of the drug deliverable to the patient. Therefore, again from Table 28.1, isoflurane, for example, is more volatile than methoxyflurane under similar conditions. The barometric pressure also influences the final concentration of an agent. For example, in locations such as Denver, Colorado, where the altitude is about 5000 feet above sea level and the barometric pressure is only about 635 mmHg, the saturated vapor concentration of isoflurane at 20 °C is now (240/635) × 100 = 37.8%.

It is important to recognize that the saturated vapor pressure at 1 atmosphere is unique for each volatile anesthetic agent and depends only on its temperature. In this case, the effect of barometric pressure can be neglected over ranges normally encountered in the practice of anesthesia. Thus, for a given agent, the graph of the saturated vapor pressure versus temperature is a curve as shown in Fig. 28.3. From this graph, it can be seen that if the temperature of the liquid is increased, more molecules escape the liquid phase and enter the gaseous phase. The greater number of molecules in the vapor phase results in a greater vapor pressure and vapor concentration. Conversely, if the liquid is cooled, the reverse occurs and vapor concentration decreases. Liquid cooling may occur not only as a result of ambient conditions but also as a natural consequence

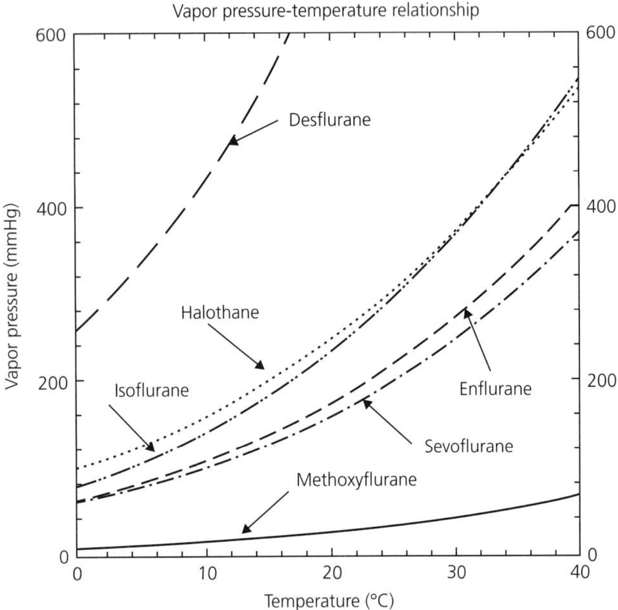

Figure 28.3 Vapor pressure as a function of temperature for six volatile anesthetics. Curves are generated from Antoine equations.

of the vaporization process. For example, during vaporization the "fastest" molecules at the surface escape first. With depletion of these "high-energy" molecules, the average kinetic energy of those left behind is reduced and there is a tendency for the temperature of the remaining liquid to fall if this process is not compensated for externally. As the temperature decreases, the vapor pressure, and thus the vapor concentration, also decreases.

Boiling point The *boiling point* of a liquid is defined as the temperature at which the vapor pressure of the liquid is equal to the atmospheric pressure. Customarily, the boiling temperature is stated at the standard atmospheric pressure of 760 mmHg. The boiling point decreases with increasing altitude because the vapor pressure does not change but the barometric pressure decreases. The boiling point of N_2O is −89 °C (see Table 28.1) at 1 atmosphere pressure at sea level. It is thus a gas under operating room conditions. Because of this, it is distributed for clinical purposes in steel tanks compressed to the liquid state at about 750 psi (pounds per square inch; 750 psi/14.9 psi [1 atmosphere] = 50 atmospheres pressure). As the N_2O gas is drawn from the tank, liquid N_2O is vaporized, and the over-riding gas pressure remains constant until no further liquid remains in the tank. At that point, only N_2O gas remains, and the gas pressure decreases from this point as remaining gas is vented from the tank. Consequently, the weight of the N_2O minus the weight of the tank rather than the gas pressure within the tank is a more accurate guide to the remaining amount of N_2O in the tank [16].

Desflurane also possesses an interesting consideration because its boiling point (see Table 28.1) is near room temperature. This characteristic accounted for an interesting engineering challenge in developing an administration device (i.e., a vaporizer) for routine use in the relatively constant environment of the operating room and limits further consideration of its use in all but a narrow range of circumstances commonly encountered in veterinary medical applications. For example, because of its low boiling point, even evaporative cooling has a large influence on vapor pressure and thus the vapor concentration of gas mixtures delivered to the patient.

Calculation of anesthetic concentration delivered by a vaporizer

The saturated vapor pressure of most volatile anesthetics is of such magnitude that the maximal concentration of anesthetic attainable at usual operating room conditions is above the range of concentrations that are commonly necessary for safe clinical anesthetic management. Therefore, some control of the delivered concentration is necessary and usually provided by a device known as a "vaporizer." The purpose of the vaporizer is to dilute the vapor generated from the liquid anesthetic with O_2 (or O_2 plus N_2O, or O_2 plus air mixtures) to produce a more satisfactory inspired anesthetic concentration. This anesthetic dilution is usually accomplished as indicated in the model shown in Fig. 28.4 by diverting the gas entering the vaporizer into two streams: one that enters the vaporizing chamber (anesthetic chamber volume: V_{anes}) and the other that bypasses the vaporizing chamber (dilution volume or $V_{dilution}$). If the vaporizer is efficient, the carrier gas passing through the vaporizing chamber becomes completely saturated to an anesthetic concentration (%) reflected by (anesthetic agent vapor pressure/atmospheric pressure) × 100, at the vaporizer chamber temperature. The resultant anesthetic concentration then is decreased (diluted) downstream by the second gas stream to a "working" concentration. In modern, precision, agent-specific vaporizers, no mental effort is required – just set the dial, as the manufacturers have precalibrated the vaporizer for accurate delivery of the dialed concentration (within some variability, say 10% of delivered concentration, allowance). Nevertheless, it is helpful to our overall understanding to know the principles underlying this convenience and how to apply these principles in the use of older, non-compensated measured flow vaporizers.

To calculate the anesthetic concentration from the vaporizer, one must know the vapor pressure of the agent (at the temperature of use), the atmospheric pressure, the fresh gas flow entering the vaporizing chamber, and the diluent gas flow. Then:

$$\%\ \text{Anesthetic} = \frac{\text{flow of anesthetic from the vaporizing chamber}}{\text{total gas flow}}$$

More detail for interested readers is given in Fig. 28.4.

Properties influencing drug kinetics: solubility

Anesthetic gases and vapors dissolve in liquids and solids. The solubility of an anesthetic is a major characteristic of the agent and has important clinical ramifications. For example, anesthetic solubility in blood and body tissues is a primary factor in the rate of uptake and its distribution within the body. It is therefore a primary determinant of the speed of anesthetic induction and recovery. Solubility in lipid bears a strong relationship to anesthetic potency, and its tendency to dissolve in anesthetic delivery components such as rubber goods influences equipment selection and other aspects of anesthetic management.

Solubility of gases

As previously mentioned, molecules of a gas that overlie a liquid surface are in random motion and some penetrate the liquid surface. After entering the liquid, they intermingle with the molecules of the liquid (i.e., the gas dissolves in the liquid). There is a net movement of the gas into the liquid until equilibrium is established between the dissolved gas in the liquid and the undissolved portion above the liquid. At this time, there is no further net gain of gas molecules by the liquid, and the number of gas molecules entering the liquid equals the number leaving. The gas molecules within the liquid exert the same pressure or tension that they exert in the

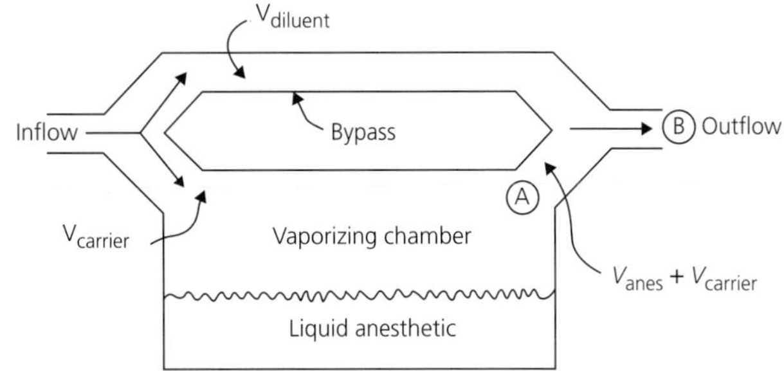

Steps:

1 The saturated *concentration* of anesthetic in the anesthetic vaporizing chamber and leaving it (ideally at Ⓐ above) is calculated knowing the saturated vapor pressure (P_{VP}) (from Table 28.1) and barometric pressure (P_B).
For example:

$$\text{Halothane \%} = \frac{243}{760} \times 100 = 32\% \tag{28.1}$$

2 The *volume* of anesthetic leaving the vaporizing chamber is the original volume of the carrier gas (O_2) entering the anesthetic vaporizing chamber ($V_{carrier}$) and the volume of anesthetic (V_{halo}) added to it.

$$\text{Halothane \%} = \frac{V_{halo}}{V_{carrier} + V_{halo}} \times 100 \tag{28.2}$$

Halothane % is known from eqn. 28.1 above and $V_{carrier}$ is known from control of a flowmeter (e.g., a measured flow vaporizer) or via the design characteristics of a commercial, agent-specific vaporizer that automatically "splits" the fresh gas flow from a single flow meter. In the first case, two gas flow controls are necessary, one for $V_{carrier}$ and one for an automatic fresh gas flow alteration. The equation is then solved for V_{halo} (expressed in mL of halothane vapor).
For example, if $V_{carrier}$ = 100 mL O_2, then:

$$32\% = \frac{V_{halo}}{100 + V_{halo}} \times 100$$

$$3200 + 32V_{halo} = 100V_{halo}$$

$$3200 = 68V_{halo}$$

$$V_{halo} = 47.1 \text{ mL halothane vapor}$$

3 V_{halo} is then contained in a total gas volume at Ⓑ of:

$$V_{total\ gas} = V_{halo} + V_{carrier} + V_{diluent} \tag{28.3}$$

Where $V_{diluent}$ is set by the anesthetist using a second gas control (i.e., flow meter; units here of mL/minute) or by the vaporizer design and dial setting.
Then, in our example for a $V_{diluent}$ of 1000 mL (in 1 minute):

$$V_{total} = 47.1 + 100 + 1000$$
$$= 1147 \text{ mL (rounded off)}$$

4 So the final halothane vapor concentration is determined by:

$$\text{Halothane \%} = \frac{V_{halo}}{V_{total}} \times 100$$

Again, in our example:

$$\text{Halothane \%} = \frac{47.1}{1147} = 4.1\%$$

Alternatively, with some basic algebraic work with the equations given above, the same numbers can be applied to the resultant formula given below to arrive at the anesthetic concentration. The condensed formula is:

$$\text{Anesthetic concentration (\%)} = \frac{V_{carrier} \cdot P_{VP} \cdot 100}{V_{diluent}(P_B - P_{VP}) + (V_{carrier} \cdot P_B)}$$

Figure 28.4 An anesthetic vaporizer model to assist in illustrating the principles associated with the calculation of the vapor concentration of an inhalation anesthetic emerging from a vaporizer. Conditions associated with halothane delivery in San Francisco (i.e., at sea level; barometric pressure = 760 mm Hg) at 20 °C are used as an example of general principles.

gas phase. If the pressure (i.e., the number of gas molecules overlying the liquid) is increased, more molecules pass into the liquid and the pressure within the liquid is increased. This net inward movement of gas molecules continues until a new equilibrium is established between the pressure of the gas in the liquid and that overlying the liquid. Alternatively, if the pressure of gas overlying the liquid is somehow decreased below that in the liquid, gas molecules escape from the liquid. This net outward movement of gas molecules from the liquid phase continues until equilibrium between the two phases is re-established.

The amount, that is, the total number of molecules of a given gas dissolving in a solvent, depends on the chemical nature of the gas itself, the partial pressure of the gas, the nature of the solvent, and the temperature. This relationship is described by Henry's law:

$$V = S \times P$$

where V is the volume of gas, P is the partial pressure of the gas, and S is the solubility coefficient for the gas in the solvent at a given temperature. Henry's law applies to gases that do not combine chemically with the solvent to form compounds.

Before leaving this basic information, a brief focus on a number of variations may be helpful. First, it is important to recognize that if the atmosphere that overlies the solvent is made up of a mixture of gases, then each gas dissolves in the solvent in proportion to the partial pressure of the individual gases. The total pressure exerted by the molecules of all gases within the solvent equals the total gas pressure lying above the solvent.

Within the body, there is a partition of anesthetic gases between blood and body tissues in accordance with Henry's law. This process can perhaps be better understood by visualizing a system composed of three compartments (e.g., gas, water, and oil) contained in a closed container (Fig. 28.5). In such a system the gas overlies the oil, which in turn overlies the water. Because there is a passive gradient from the gas phase to the oil, gas molecules move into the oil compartment. This movement in turn develops a gradient for the gas molecules in oil relative to water. If gas is continually added above the oil, there will be a continual net movement of the gas

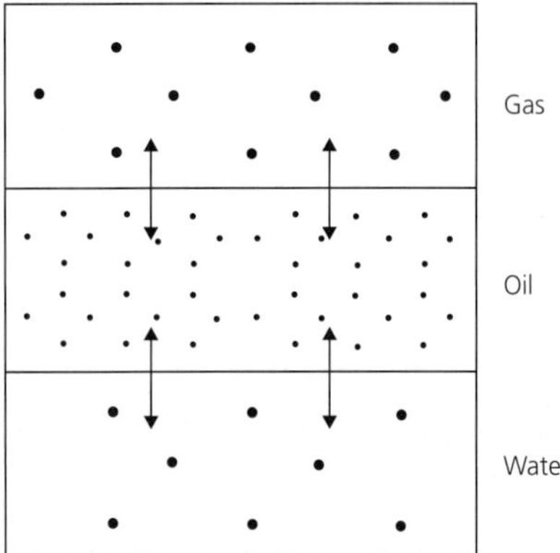

Figure 28.5 Diagrammatic representation of an anesthetic gas distributing itself among three compartments (gas, oil, and water). At equilibrium, the number of anesthetic molecules in the three compartments differs but the pressure exerted by the anesthetic molecules is the same in each compartment.

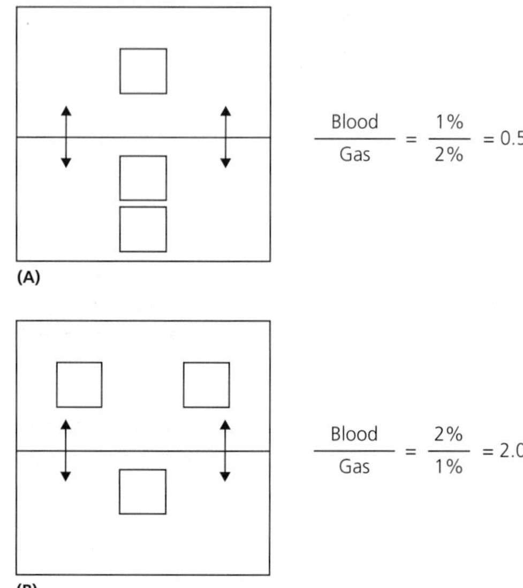

Figure 28.6 Illustration of two hypothetical gases (A. and B.) with varying blood/gas partition coefficients. See text for explanation. Source: Adapted from Eger [17].

molecules from the gas phase into both the oil and, in turn, the water. At a given temperature, when no more gas dissolves in the solvent, the solvent is said to be *fully saturated.* At this point, the pressure of the gas molecules within the three compartments will be equal but the amount (i.e., the number of molecules or volume of gas) partitioned between the two liquids will vary with the nature of the liquid and gas. Finally, it is important to understand that the amount of gas that goes into solution depends upon the temperature of the solvent. Less gas dissolves in a solvent as temperature increases, and more gas is taken up as solvent temperature decreases. For example, as water is heated, air bubbles appear inside the container as a result of the decreasing solubility of the air in water. Conversely, as blood is cooled from a normal body temperature (e.g., hypothermia), gases become more soluble in blood.

The extent to which a gas will dissolve in a given solvent is usually expressed in terms of its solubility coefficient (see Table 28.2). With inhalation anesthetics, solubility is most commonly measured and expressed as a partition coefficient (PC). Other measurements of solubility include the Bunsen and Ostwald solubility coefficients [9,17].

The PC is the concentration ratio of an anesthetic in the solvent and gas phases (e.g., blood and gas; Fig. 28.6) or between two tissue solvents (e.g., brain and blood; see Table 28.2). It thus describes the capacity of a given solvent to dissolve the anesthetic gas. That is, how the anesthetic will *partition* itself between the gas and the liquid solvent phases after equilibrium has been reached. Remember, anesthetic gas movement occurs because of a partial pressure difference in the gas and liquid solvent phases, so when there is no longer any anesthetic partial pressure difference, there is no longer any net movement of anesthetic and equilibrium has been achieved. Solvent/gas PCs are summarized in Table 28.2. Values noted in this table are for human tissues because they are most widely available in the anesthesia literature. Comparative data for blood solubility of desflurane, isoflurane, and sevoflurane in a variety of species of clinical interest in veterinary medicine are listed in Table 28.3. Regardless of the species, it is important to emphasize that many factors can alter anesthetic agent solubility [17–20]. Perhaps the most notable after the nature of the solvent is that of temperature.

Of all the PCs that have been described or are of interest, two are of particular importance in the practical understanding of anesthetic action. They are the blood/gas and the oil/gas solubility coefficients.

Blood/gas partition coefficient Blood/gas solubility coefficients (see Tables 28.2 and 28.3) provide a means for predicting the speed of anesthetic induction, recovery, and change of anesthetic depth. Assume, for example, that anesthetic A has a blood/gas PC value of 15. This means that the concentration of the anesthetic in blood will be 15 times greater at equilibrium than that in alveolar gas. Expressed differently, the same volume of blood, say 1 mL, will hold 15 times more anesthetic A than 1 mL of alveolar gas despite an equal partial pressure. Alternatively, consider anesthetic B with a PC of 1.4. This PC indicates that at equilibrium, the amount of anesthetic B is only 1.4 times greater in blood than it is in alveolar air. Comparing the PC of anesthetic A with that of anesthetic B indicates that anesthetic A is much more soluble in blood than B (nearly 11 times more soluble: 15/1.4). From this, and assuming other conditions are equal, anesthetic A will require a longer time of administration to attain a partial pressure in the body for a particular endpoint (say, anesthetic induction) than will anesthetic B. Also, since there is more anesthetic A contained in blood and other body tissues under similar conditions, elimination (and therefore anesthetic recovery) will be prolonged when compared to anesthetic B.

Oil/gas partition coefficient The oil/gas PC is another solubility characteristic of clinical importance (see Table 28.2). This PC describes the ratio of the concentration of an anesthetic in oil (olive oil is the standard) and gas phases at equilibrium. The oil/gas PC correlates directly with anesthetic potency (see Anesthetic dose: the minimum alveolar concentration (MAC) and Mechanism of action sections later in this chapter) and describes the capacity of lipids for anesthetic.

Other partition coefficients Solubility characteristics for various tissues (see Tables 28.2 and 28.3) and other media, such as rubber and plastic (see Table 28.4), are also important. For example, the solubility of a tissue determines in part the quantity of anesthetic removed from the blood to which it is exposed. The higher the tissue solubility, the longer it will take to saturate the tissue with anesthetic agent. Thus, other things considered equal, anesthetics that are very soluble in tissues will require a longer period for induction and recovery. If the amount of rubber goods in the apparatus used to deliver the anesthetic to the patient is substantial and the anesthetic agent solubility in rubber is large (as, for example, was common with equipment in use prior to the 21st century), the amount of uptake of anesthetic agent by the rubber may also be of clinical significance.

Pharmacokinetics: uptake and elimination of inhalation anesthetics

The aim in administering an inhalation anesthetic to a patient is to achieve an adequate partial pressure or tension of anesthetic (P_{anes}) in the central nervous system (CNS, e.g., brain; for purposes of this discussion considerations of anesthetic delivery to spinal cord sites of action are considered similar to those of the brain) to cause a desired level of CNS depression commensurate with the definition of general anesthesia. Anesthetic depth varies directly with P_{anes} in brain and spinal cord tissue. The rate of change of anesthetic depth is of obvious clinical importance and is directly dependent upon the rate of change in anesthetic tensions in the various media in which it is contained before reaching the brain. Thus, knowledge of the factors that govern these relationships is of fundamental importance to skillful control of general inhalation anesthesia.

Inhalation anesthetics are unique among the classes of drugs that are used to produce general anesthesia because they are administered via the lungs. The pharmacokinetics of the inhaled anesthetics describe the rate of their uptake by blood from the lungs, distribution in the body, and eventual elimination by the lungs and other routes. Readers seeking more in-depth coverage are directed to reviews by Eger [17,21,22] and Mapleson [23].

Inhalation anesthetics, similar to the gases of respiration (i.e., O_2 and CO_2), move down a series of partial pressure gradients from regions of higher tension to those of lower tension until equilibrium (i.e., equal pressure throughout the apparatus and body tissues) is established. Thus, on induction, the P_{anes} at its source in the vaporizer is high, as is dictated by the vapor pressure, and progressively decreases as anesthetic travels from vaporizer to patient breathing circuit, from circuit to lungs, from lungs to arterial blood, and finally, from arterial blood to body tissues (e.g., the brain; Fig. 28.7). Of these, the alveolar partial pressure of anesthetic, P_AAnes, is pivotal. The brain has a rich blood supply and the anesthetic in arterial blood, P_aAnes, rapidly equilibrates with brain tissue, P_{brain}Anes. Usually, gas exchange at the alveolar level is sufficiently efficient that the P_aAnes is close to P_AAnes. Thus, the P_{brain}Anes closely follows P_AAnes, and by controlling the P_AAnes there is a reliable indirect way for controlling P_{brain}Anes and anesthetic depth.

At this point, it may also be helpful to recall that although the partial pressure of anesthetic is of primary importance, we frequently define the clinical dose of an inhaled anesthetic in terms of concentration (*C*, i.e., vol %). As previously noted, this is because it is common practice for the clinician to regulate and/or measure respiratory and anesthetic gases in volume percent. In addition, in the gaseous phase, the relationship between the P_{anes} and the C_{anes} is a simple one:

$$P_{anes} = \text{fractional anesthetic concentration} \times \text{total ambient pressure}$$

The fractional anesthetic concentration is of course $C_{anes}/100$. However, as reviewed in the preceding section, in blood or tissues, the actual *quantity* of anesthetic depends on both the P_{anes} and the anesthetic solubility (as measured by the PC) within the solvent (e.g., blood or oil). Consequently, at equilibrium, the *partial pressure* of the gas in the alveoli and among tissue compartments will be equal, although *concentrations* will vary within these tissues.

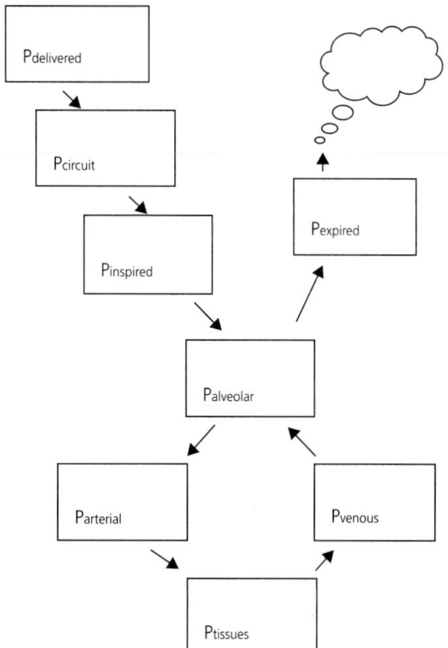

Figure 28.7 The flow pattern of inhalation anesthetic agents during anesthetic induction and recovery. Inhalation anesthesia may be viewed as the development of a series of partial pressure (tension) gradients. During induction, there is a high anesthetic tension in the vaporizer that decreases progressively as the flow of anesthetic gas moves from its source to the brain. Some of these gradients are easily manipulated by the anesthetist; others are not or are difficult to achieve.

Anesthetic uptake: factors that determine the P_A of anesthetic

The P_A of anesthetic is a balance between anesthetic input (i.e., delivery to the alveoli) and loss (uptake by blood and body tissues) from the lungs. A rapid rise in the P_A of anesthetic is associated with a rapid anesthetic induction or change in anesthetic depth. Factors that contribute to a rapid change in the P_A of anesthetic are summarized in Box 28.3.

Delivery to the alveoli

Delivery of anesthetic to the alveoli and therefore the rate of rise of the alveolar concentration or fraction (F_A) toward the inspired concentration or fraction (F_I) depends on the inspired anesthetic concentration itself and the magnitude of alveolar ventilation. Increasing either one of these or both increases the rate of rise of the P_A of anesthetic; that is, with other things considered equal, there is an increase in speed of anesthetic induction or change in anesthetic level.

Inspired concentration

The inspired concentration has a number of variables controlling it. First of all, the upper limit of inspired concentration is dictated

Box 28.3 Factors related to a rapid change in alveolar anesthetic tension (P_A).

Increased alveolar delivery
- Increased inspired anesthetic concentration
  - Increased vaporization of agent
  - Increased vaporizer dial setting
  - Increased fresh gas inflow
  - Decreased gas volume of patient breathing circuit
- Increased alveolar ventilation
  - Increased minute ventilation
  - Decreased deadspace ventilation

Decreased removal from the alveoli
- Decreased blood solubility of anesthetic
- Decreased cardiac output
- Decreased alveolar–venous anesthetic gradient

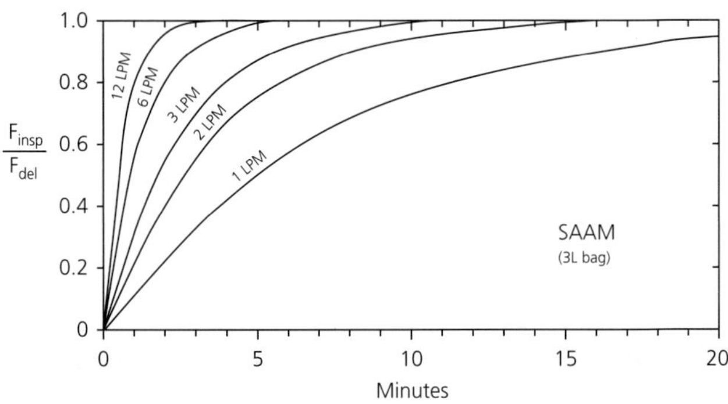

Figure 28.8 A comparison of the rate of increase of inspired halothane concentration toward a constant delivered concentration F_{insp}/F_{del} in a 7 L small animal anesthetic breathing circuit (SAAM) at fresh gas flow rates of 1, 3, 6, and 12 Lpm. Source: Eger [24].

by the agent vapor pressure, which in turn is dependent on temperature. This may be especially important in veterinary medicine considering the breadth of applications involving inhaled anesthesia and methods of vaporizing volatile anesthetics under widely diverse conditions (some environmental conditions are quite hostile).

Characteristics of the patient breathing system can also be a major factor in generating a suitable inspired concentration under usual operating room conditions. Characteristics of special importance include the volume of the system, the amount of rubber or plastic components of the system, the position of the vaporizer relative to the breathing circuit (i.e., within or outside the circuit), and the fresh gas inflow to the patient breathing circuit. The patient breathing circuit contains a gas volume that must be replaced with gas containing the desired anesthetic concentration. Thus, the volume of the breathing circuit serves as a buffer to delay the rise of anesthetic concentration. In the management of small animals (i.e., less than 10 kg), a nonrebreathing patient circuit and/or a relatively high fresh gas inflow into the patient breathing circuit is usually used, so there should *not* be a clinically important difference between the delivered (e.g., vaporizer dial setting) and the inspired concentration. That is, when the vaporizer dial setting is adjusted to the desired concentration setting, the fresh gas plus anesthetic flowing from the vaporizer almost immediately contains the dialed anesthetic vapor concentration. In addition, the total gas flow is high relative to the volume of the delivery circuit, so the anesthetic concentration in the inspired breath is rapidly increased. However, with larger animals (i.e., greater than 10 kg), a rebreathing (circle) patient circuit with a CO_2 absorber is most commonly used for inhalation anesthesia. The volume of this breathing circuit may be very large compared to fresh gas inflow. This volume markedly delays the rate of rise of inspired anesthetic concentration because the residual gas volume must be "washed out" and replaced by anesthetic containing fresh gas in order for the inspired concentration to increase to that delivered from the vaporizer (Fig. 28.8). In addition, rebreathing of exhaled gas (minus CO_2) occurs to varying degrees with these circuits. The inspired gas is composed of exhaled and fresh gases. Because the expired gas contains less anesthetic than the fresh gas, the inspired anesthetic gas concentration will be less than that of the fresh gas leaving the vaporizer.

In veterinary applications, the delaying influence of the circle circuit is most notable with anesthetic management of very large animals such as horses [24] and cattle and/or when using a closed-circuit fresh gas flow rate (i.e., where O_2 is the fresh gas and its inflow [plus anesthetic] to the circuit just meets the metabolic needs of the patient). With closed-circuit delivery, the fresh gas inflow is very low relative to the circuit volume [8,17,24].

Table 28.5 Vaporizer positioning within or outside a circle patient rebreathing circuit influences inspired anesthetic concentration.

Factor	Vaporizer positioning	
	Out of circuit	In circuit
Increase ventilation	Decrease	Increase
Increase fresh gas (O_2) inflow to circuit	Increase	Decrease

The high solubility of some anesthetics (e.g., methoxyflurane; see Table 28.4) in rubber and plastic delays development of an appropriate inspired anesthetic concentration. The loss of anesthetic to these equipment "sinks" increases the apparent volume of the anesthetic circuitry and may, in some cases, be clinically important (e.g., the use of rubber hoses and a large rubber rebreathing bag on circuits designed for anesthetic management of horses). With the newest inhalation anesthetics and more modern anesthetic delivery equipment, this issue is of minor or no clinical importance.

Positioning the vaporizer in relation to the patient breathing circuit will influence inspired anesthetic concentration [23,25]. For example, with the vaporizer positioned within a circle rebreathing circuit, a decrease in inspired concentration will follow an increase in fresh gas inflow to the circuit, whereas an increase in inspired concentration will result if the vaporizer is positioned outside the circuit (Table 28.5). With the loss of methoxyflurane to clinical practice, nearly all, if not all, vaporizers in use in North America are agent-specific, precision vaporizers. This style of vaporizer is always placed upstream and outside the patient's breathing circuit.

Alveolar ventilation

An increase in alveolar ventilation increases the rate of delivery of inhalation anesthetic to the alveolus (Fig. 28.9). If unopposed by blood and tissue uptake of anesthetic, alveolar ventilation would rapidly increase the alveolar concentration of anesthetic so that within minutes, the alveolar concentration would equal the inspired concentration. However, in reality, the input created by alveolar ventilation is countered by absorption of anesthetic into blood. Predictably, hypoventilation decreases the rate at which the alveolar

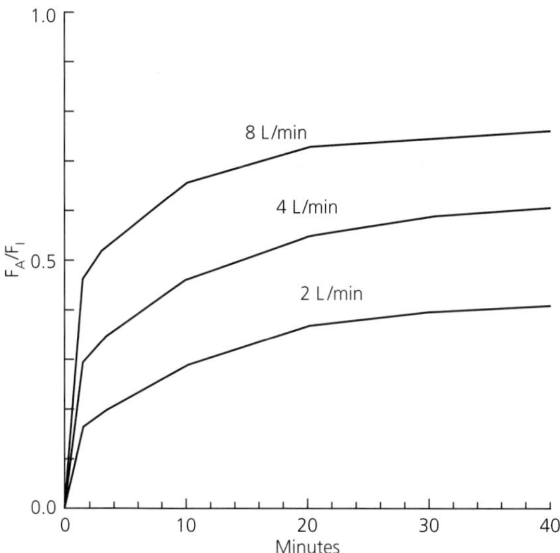

Figure 28.9 The effect of ventilation on the rise of the alveolar (F_A) concentration of halothane toward the inspired (F_I) concentration. As noted, the F_A:F_I ratio increases more rapidly as ventilation is increased from 2 to 8 L/min. Source: Eger [17], with permission of Wolters Kluwer Health, Inc.

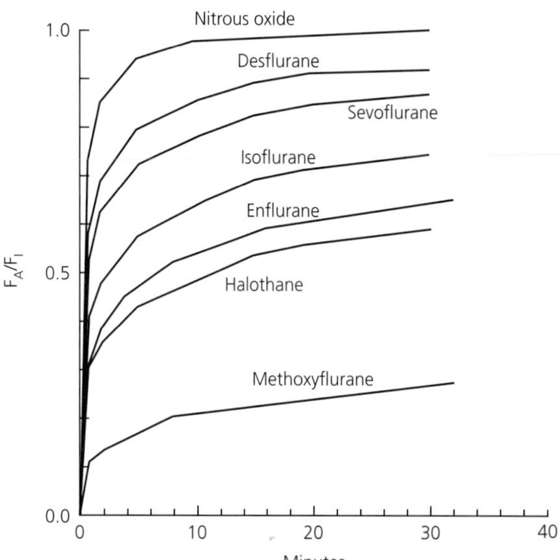

Figure 28.10 The rise in the alveolar (F_A) anesthetic concentration toward the inspired (F_I) concentration. Note the rise is most rapid with the least soluble anesthetic, N_2O, and slowest with the most soluble anesthetic, methoxyflurane. All data are from studies of humans. Source: The curves are redrawn from Eger [1]; Eger [27].

concentration increases over time compared to the inspired concentration (i.e., anesthetic induction is slowed). Alveolar ventilation is altered by changes in anesthetic depth (increased depth usually means decreased ventilation), mechanical ventilation (usually increased ventilation), and deadspace ventilation (i.e., for constant minute ventilation, a decrease in deadspace ventilation results in an increase in alveolar ventilation).

Alveolar ventilation and thus the alveolar anesthetic concentration can also be influenced by administering a potent inhalation anesthetic such as halothane in conjunction with N_2O. Very early in the administration of N_2O (during the period of large volume uptake; the first 5–10 min of delivery), the rate of rise of the alveolar concentration of the concurrently administered inhalation anesthetic is increased. This is commonly referred to as the "second gas effect," and this phenomenon can be applied clinically to speed anesthetic induction [17,21,26].

Removal from alveoli: uptake by blood

As noted by Eger [17], anesthetic uptake is the product of three factors: solubility (S, the blood/gas solubility; see Table 28.3), cardiac output (CO), and the difference in the anesthetic partial pressure between the alveolus and venous blood returning to the lungs ($P_A - P_{\bar{V}}/P_{bar}$), expressed in mmHg; that is:

$$\text{Uptake} = S \times \text{CO}\left(P_A - P_{\bar{V}} / P_{bar}\right)$$

where P_{bar} = barometric pressure in mmHg. Note that if any of these three factors equals zero, there is no further uptake of anesthetic by blood.

Solubility

As previously discussed, the solubility of an inhalation anesthetic in blood and tissues is characterized by its partition coefficient (PC; see Tables 28.2 and 28.3). Remember that a PC describes how an inhalation anesthetic distributes itself between two phases or two solvents (e.g., the quantity of agent in blood and alveoli [gas] or blood and muscle, respectively) once equilibrium is established (i.e., when the anesthetic partial pressure is equal). Based on blood/gas PCs, inhalation anesthetics range from highly soluble (methoxyflurane) to poorly soluble (N_2O, desflurane, and sevoflurane). Agents such as halothane and isoflurane are intermediate.

Compared to an anesthetic with high blood solubility (PC), an agent with low blood solubility is associated with a more rapid equilibration because a smaller amount of anesthetic must be dissolved in the blood before equilibrium is reached with the gas phase. In the case of the agent with a high blood/gas PC, the blood acts like a large "sink" into which the anesthetic is poured and accordingly, blood is "reluctant" to give up the agent to other tissues (such as the brain). The blood serves as a conduit for drug delivery to the brain and as such can be visualized as a pharmacologically inactive reservoir that is interposed between the lungs and the agent's site of desired pharmacologic activity (i.e., brain). Therefore, an anesthetic agent with a low blood/gas PC is usually more desirable than a highly soluble agent, because it is associated with (1) a more rapid anesthetic induction (i.e., more rapid rate of rise in alveolar concentration during induction; Fig. 28.10); (2) more precise control of anesthetic depth (i.e., alveolar concentration during the anesthetic maintenance); and (3) a more rapid elimination of anesthetic and recovery (i.e., a rapid decrease in alveolar concentration during recovery).

Cardiac output

The amount of blood flowing through the lungs and on to body tissues also influences anesthetic uptake from the lungs. The greater the CO, the more blood passes through the lungs carrying away anesthetic from the alveoli. Thus, a large CO, like increased anesthetic agent blood solubility, delays the alveolar rise of P_{anes} (Fig. 28.11). Patient excitement is an example in which a relatively

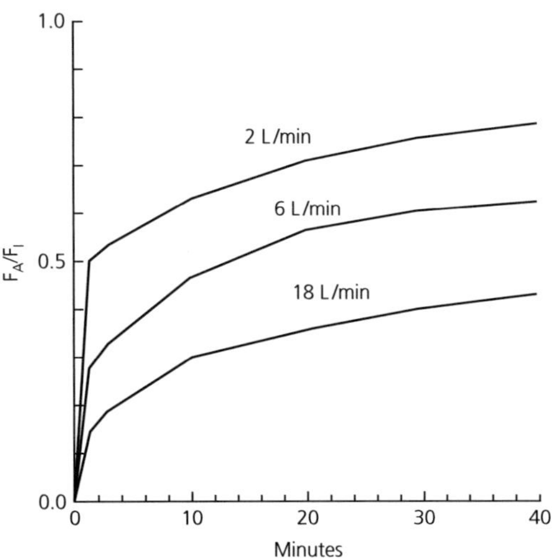

Figure 28.11 The effect of cardiac output on the rise of the alveolar (F_A) concentration of halothane toward the inspired (F_I) concentration. As noted, the F_A:F_I ratio increases more rapidly as cardiac output is decreased from 18 to 2 L/min. Source: Eger [17], with permission of Wolters Kluwer Health, Inc.

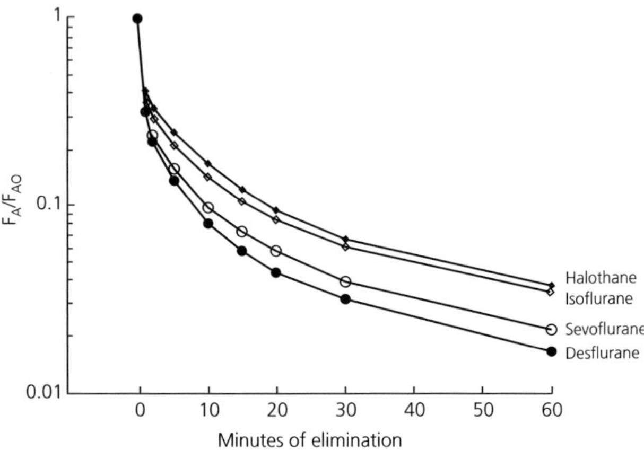

Figure 28.12 The fall in alveolar (F_A) concentration relative to the alveolar concentration at the end of anesthesia (F_{AO}). Note that the newest, most insoluble, volatile anesthetic, desflurane, is eliminated in humans more rapidly than the other contemporary potent anesthetics. Not shown is information for methoxyflurane. If present, the curve for methoxyflurane would appear above that for halothane. Source: Reproduced with permission from Eger [27].

large CO is anticipated. Conversely, a reduced CO should be anticipated with a patient with poor myocardial function or severe bradycardia. Such a situation would be associated with an increase in the rate of rise of the P_A of the anesthetic and this, along with other factors, makes the anesthetic induction more rapid and risky.

Alveolar to venous anesthetic partial pressure difference

The magnitude of difference in anesthetic partial pressure between the alveoli and mixed venous blood returning to the lungs is related to the amount of uptake of anesthetic by tissues. It is not surprising that the largest gradient occurs during induction. Once the tissues no longer absorb anesthetic (i.e., equilibrium is reached), there is no longer any uptake of anesthetic from the lungs because $P_{\bar{v}} = P_A$ (i.e., the mixed venous blood returning to the lungs contains as much anesthetic as when it left the lungs). The changes in gradient between the initiation of induction and equilibration result in part from the relative distribution of CO. In this regard, it is important to recognize that roughly 70–80% of the CO is normally directed to only a small volume of body tissues in a lean individual [28,29]. Tissues such as the brain, heart, hepatoportal system, and kidneys represent only about 10% of the body mass but normally receive about 75% of the total blood flow each minute. As a result, these highly perfused tissues equilibrate rapidly with arterial anesthetic partial pressure when compared to other body tissues (actual timing is influenced by agent solubility). Since the venous anesthetic pressure or tension equals that in the tissue within 10 or 15 min, about 75% of the blood returning to the lungs is the same as the alveolar tension. This presumes there has been no change in arterial anesthetic partial pressure during this time and thus uptake is reduced. Skin and muscle comprise the major bulk of the body (about 50% in humans) but at rest receive only about 15–20% of the CO, so saturation of these tissues takes hours to accomplish. Fat is a variable component of body bulk and receives only a small proportion of blood flow. Consequently, anesthetic saturation of this tissue is very slow because all anesthetics are considerably more soluble in fat than other tissue groups (see Table 28.2).

Other factors can influence the magnitude of the alveolar to arterial anesthetic partial pressure gradient. For example, abnormalities of ventilation/perfusion result in an alveolar–arterial gradient proportional to the degree of abnormality [17,30,31]. Others include loss of anesthetic via the skin [32–34] and into closed gas spaces [17,21,26], and metabolism [17,21].

Overview

The rate at which the alveolar anesthetic concentration increases relative to the inspired concentration (i.e., the rate of change in anesthetic level) is often summarized as a plot of the ratio of F_A:F_I versus time. The position of individual curves representing different anesthetics on a plot is related to the solubility characteristics of the anesthetics (see Fig. 28.10). The shape of the graph of F_A:F_I versus time is similar for all anesthetics (see Fig. 28.10). There is a rapid rise initially that results from the effect of alveolar ventilation bringing anesthetic into the lung. There is then a decrease in the rate of rise of the curve as uptake by the blood occurs. With time, the highly perfused tissues of the body equilibrate with incoming blood so that eventually about three-quarters of the total blood flow returning to the heart has the same anesthetic partial pressure as it had when it left the lungs. Thus, further uptake from the lung is decreased and the rate of approach of the F_A to F_I over time is further decreased.

Anesthetic elimination

Recovery from inhalation anesthesia results from the elimination of anesthetic from the CNS. This requires a decrease in alveolar anesthetic partial pressure (concentration), which in turn fosters a decrease in arterial and then CNS anesthetic partial pressure (see Box. 28.3). Prominent factors accounting for recovery are the same as those for anesthetic induction. The percent clearance of an inhaled anesthetic can be expressed as:

$$\%\ \text{Clearance} = 100 \times \frac{V_A}{(\text{agent blood/gas PC} \times \text{CO}) + V_A} \qquad [35]$$

Therefore, factors such as alveolar ventilation (V_A), CO, and especially agent solubility greatly influence recovery from inhalation anesthesia. Indeed, the graphic curves representing the washout of anesthetic from alveoli versus time (Fig. 28.12) are essentially inverses of the

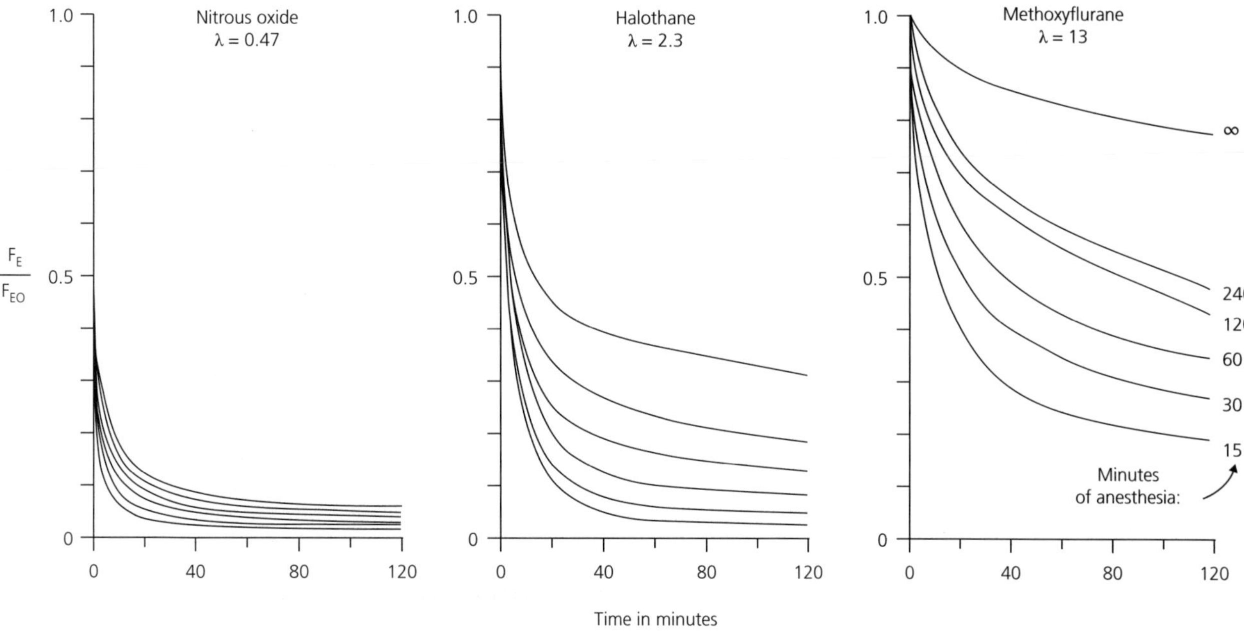

Figure 28.13 The decrease in the alveolar (F_E) anesthetic concentration from the concentration at the time of breathing circuit disconnect (i.e., the beginning of recovery from anesthesia; F_{EO}) is influenced by both the solubility (λ) of anesthetic and the duration of anesthesia. Source: Stoelting and Eger [36], with permission of Wolters Kluwer Health, Inc.

wash-in curves. That is, the wash-out of the less soluble anesthetics is high at first (i.e., rapid wash-out by ventilation of the lung functional residual capacity), then rapidly declines to a lower output level that continues to decrease but at a slower rate. The wash-out of more soluble agents is also high at first, but the magnitude of decrease in alveolar anesthetic concentration is less and decreases more gradually with time (see Fig. 28.12).

An important factor during the wash-out period is the duration of anesthesia. This effect and a comparison of this effect between three agents spanning a range of blood solubilities are summarized in Fig. 28.13 [36]. Times to recovery from anesthesia in, for example, rats correlate with values for blood solubility of anesthetics (Fig. 28.14) [37]. If a patient rebreathing anesthetic circuit (e.g., circle system) is in use and the patient is not disconnected from the circuit at the end of anesthesia, the circuit itself may also reduce the rate of recovery, just as the circuit was shown to decrease the rate of rise of anesthetic during induction. This influence of rebreathing circuits can be reduced by directing high flow rates of anesthetic-free O_2 into the anesthetic circuit (i.e., applying principles of a non-rebreathing circuit).

Other factors that are important to varying degrees for inhalation anesthetic elimination from the body include percutaneous loss, intertissue diffusion of agents, and metabolism. While some transcutaneous movement of inhalation agent occurs, the amount under consideration is small [32–35,38]. Intertissue diffusion is of theoretical interest, but its clinical importance is limited [35,39,40]. In this regard, the impact of obesity on recovery from anesthesia may be important to consider clinically [35]. Metabolism may also play a small role with some inhalation anesthetics (e.g., methoxyflurane and perhaps even halothane), especially when associated with prolonged anesthesia [39,41–43].

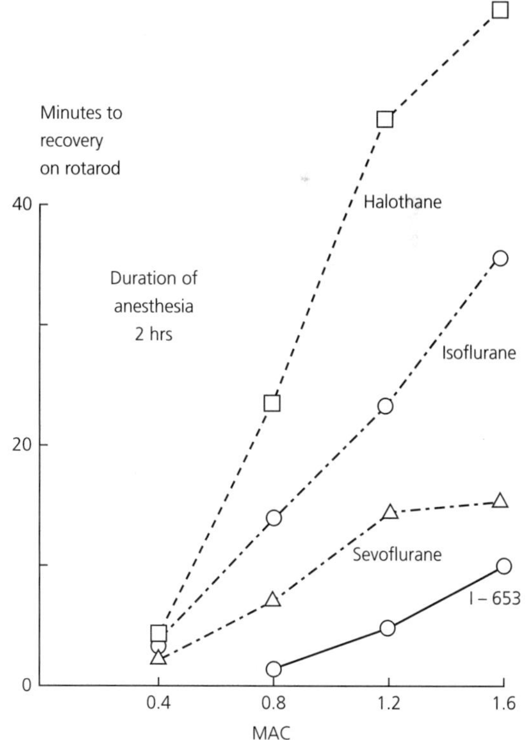

Figure 28.14 Increasing the delivered concentration of inhalation anesthetic increased the time to recovery of the motor coordination necessary to remain atop a 6 cm rod rotating at 8 rpm. The duration of anesthesia was constant for all trials. Source: Eger and Johnson [37], with permission of Wolters Kluwer Health, Inc.

A special consideration associated with recovery following use of N_2O deserves comment. *Diffusion hypoxia* is a possibility at the end of N_2O administration when the patient breathes air immediately rather than O_2 for at least a brief transition period (i.e., 5–10 min) [44–46]. In this case, a large volume of N_2O returns to the lungs from the blood. This early rapid inflow of N_2O to the lung displaces other gases within the lung. If at this time the patient is breathing air (only about 21% O_2) rather than 100% O_2, N_2O dilutes alveolar O_2, further reducing O_2 partial pressure from levels found in ambient air. This may cause life-threatening reductions in arterial oxygenation. Since the major effect is in the first few minutes after discontinuing N_2O, the condition can be prevented by administering high-inspired fractions of O_2 at the conclusion of N_2O administration rather than allowing the patient to immediately breathe ambient air.

Biotransformation

Most inhalation anesthetics are not chemically inert [47]. They undergo varying degrees of metabolism, primarily in the liver but also to lesser degrees in the lung, kidney, and intestinal tract [41,48–51]. The importance of this is two-fold. First, in a very limited way, metabolism may facilitate anesthetic recovery. Second, and more important, is the potential for acute and chronic toxicities by intermediate or end metabolites of inhalation agents, especially involving the kidneys, liver, and reproductive organs [41,51].

The magnitude of metabolism of inhalation anesthetic agents varies greatly and is determined by a variety of factors, including the chemical structure, hepatic enzyme activity (cytochrome P450 enzymes located in the endoplasmic reticulum of the hepatocyte), the blood concentration of the anesthetic [52], disease states, and genetic factors (i.e., some species and individuals are more active metabolizers of these drugs than others, e.g., humans versus rats).

An indication of the extent of biotransformation of contemporary inhalation anesthetics is given in Table 28.6. The degradation of sevoflurane occurs *in vivo* to about the same extent as isoflurane, perhaps a bit more depending on circumstances, and as indicated by transient postanesthetic increases in blood and urinary fluoride levels in rats [53–57], dogs [56], horses [58–60], swine [61], and humans [62]. The peak serum fluoride concentrations observed in humans during and following sevoflurane anesthesia are low, and nephrotoxicity is not expected [62,63]. Desflurane resists degradation *in vivo* [61,64,65]. The increase in serum inorganic fluoride is much smaller than that found with isoflurane [61,64,65].

For further information on the biotransformation of inhalation anesthetics in general and specific details regarding individual anesthetic agents, readers are referred to reviews by Baden and Rice [41], Mazze and Fujinaga [51], and Njoku *et al.* [66].

Table 28.6 Biotransformation of inhalation anesthetics in humans.

Anesthetic	% of Anesthetic metabolized	Reference
Methoxyflurane	50–75	[43,50]
Halothane	20–46	[43,49,67]
Sevoflurane	2–5	[62,68]
Enflurane	2–8	[43,69]
Isoflurane	0.2	[70]
Desflurane	0.02	[65]
Nitrous oxide	0.004	[71,72]

Anesthetic dose: the minimum alveolar concentration (MAC)

In 1963, Merkel and Eger described what became the standard index of anesthetic potency for inhalation anesthetics, *MAC* [73]. MAC is defined as the minimum alveolar concentration of an anesthetic at 1 atmosphere that produces immobility in 50% of subjects exposed to a supramaximal noxious stimulus. Thus, MAC corresponds to the effective $dose_{50}$ or ED_{50}; half of the subjects are anesthetized, and half have not yet reached that "level." The dose that corresponds to the ED_{95} (95% of the individuals are anesthetized), at least in humans, is 20–40% greater than MAC [74]. Anesthetic potency of an inhaled anesthetic is inversely related to MAC (i.e., potency = 1/MAC). From information presented earlier, it also follows that MAC is inversely related to the oil/gas PC. Thus, a very potent anesthetic such as methoxyflurane, which has a high oil/ gas PC has a low MAC, whereas an agent with a low oil/gas PC has a high MAC.

A number of characteristics of MAC deserve emphasis [17]. First, the "A" in MAC represents *alveolar* concentration, not inspired or delivered (as, for example, from a vaporizer). This is important because the alveolar concentration is easily monitored with contemporary technology. Also, as we reviewed earlier, after sufficient time for equilibration (minutes), alveolar partial pressure will closely approximate arterial and brain (CNS) anesthetic partial pressures.

Second, MAC is defined in terms of volumes percent of 1 atmosphere and therefore represents an anesthetic partial pressure (P) at the anesthetic site of action (i.e., remember $P_x = (C/100)\ P_{bar}$, where P_x stands for the partial pressure of the anesthetic in the gas mixture, C is the anesthetic concentration in vol % and P_{bar} is the barometric or total pressure of the gas mixture). Thus, although the concentration at MAC for a given agent may vary depending on ambient pressure conditions (e.g., sea level versus high altitude), the anesthetic partial pressure always remains the same. For example, MAC for isoflurane in healthy cats is reported as 1.63 volumes %. The study reporting this value was conducted at near sea level conditions at Davis, California (i.e., P_{bar} of 760 mmHg). Based on discussion above, MAC of 1.63% represents an alveolar isoflurane partial pressure (P_{iso}) of 11.6 mmHg. In comparison, for the same dog at Mexico City (elevation 2240 m above sea level; P_{bar} = 584 mmHg), the alveolar P_{iso} at MAC is expected to be the same as determined at Davis, California (i.e., 11.6 mmHg); however, MAC (i.e., the alveolar concentration) would be about 2.17%.

Finally, it is important to note that MAC is determined in healthy animals under laboratory conditions in the *absence* of other drugs and circumstances common to clinical use that may modify the requirements for anesthesia. General techniques for determining MAC in animals are given elsewhere [17,75–79]. In determining MAC in humans, the initial surgical skin incision has been the standard noxious stimulus used [17]. For the determination of MAC in smaller animals (mice to dogs and pigs) [17,80,81], the standard stimulus has been application of a forceps or other surgical clamp to the base of the tail or the base of the dewclaw of the limb (e.g., pigs [78]), while electrical stimulus applied beneath the oral mucus membranes is most commonly used in larger species such as horses [76].

The MAC values for contemporary inhalation anesthetics for a variety of mammals commonly encountered in veterinary medicine are summarized in Table 28.7A, while the ED_{50} values for non-mammalian species are given in Table 28.7B. Values for humans are also given for comparison. For values of agents of historical interest such as methoxyflurane, enflurane, or diethyl ether, readers are referred to the review in an earlier edition of this book or elsewhere [17,81].

Since its original introduction, the MAC concept has been extended to other stimulus endpoints in an effort to better define and understand the anesthetic state. For example, Stoelting *et al.* [82] determined the value for MAC of an anesthetic at which humans opened their eyes on verbal command during emergence from anesthesia; this has been termed "MAC-awake." The verbal stimulus is of course less intense than the surgical incision in humans and thus the response occurs at a lower concentration of anesthetic than movement following incision. The end-tidal concentration preventing movement in response to tracheal intubation (MAC for intubation) is more stimulating to humans than surgical incision and was described by Yakaitis *et al.* [83,84]. Roizen *et al.* [85] reported an even greater alveolar concentration necessary to prevent adrenergic response (rise in endogenous catecholamines) to skin incision (also in human patients) compared to the concentration necessary to just prevent movement; this is known as "MAC–BAR." Similarly, Boscan *et al.* showed that ovarian/ovarian ligament traction increased sevoflurane MAC compared to tail clamp in dogs [86]. Thus, a group of response curves is possible and dependent upon the strength of the stimulus applied.

In a single species the variability in MAC (response to a noxious stimulus) is generally small and is not substantially influenced by gender, duration of anesthesia, variation of $PaCO_2$ (from 10 to 90 mmHg), metabolic alkalosis or acidosis, variation in PaO_2 (from 40 to 500 mmHg), moderate anemia, or moderate hypotension (see Table 28.7A) [17,81,87]. Even between species, the variability in MAC for a given agent is usually not large. However, there is at least one notable exception (see Table 28.7A). In humans, the MAC for N_2O is 104%, making it the least potent of the inhalation anesthetics currently used in this species. Its potency in other species is less than half that in humans (i.e., around 200%). Because the N_2O MAC is above 100%, it cannot be used by itself at 1 atmosphere pressure in any species and still provide adequate amounts of O_2. Consequently, and assuming that MAC values for combinations of inhaled anesthetics are additive, N_2O is usually administered with another more potent agent to thereby reduce the concentration of the second agent necessary for anesthesia (see Fig. 28.15). However, because of the potency difference between animals and humans, the amount of reduction differs in an important way. For example, administration of 60% N_2O with halothane reduces the amount of halothane needed to produce MAC by about 55% in healthy humans (see Fig. 28.15) but reduces it only by about 20–30% in dogs. As noted in Fig. 28.15, the response of other animals most closely resembles the dog. Some factors that are known to influence MAC are given in Table 28.8.

Equipotent doses (i.e., equivalent concentrations of different anesthetics at MAC) are useful for comparing effects of inhalation anesthetics on vital organs. In this regard, anesthetic dose is commonly defined in terms of multiples of MAC (i.e., 1.5- or 2.0-times MAC, or simply 1.5 MAC or 2.0 MAC). From the preceding discussion, therefore, the ED_{50} equals MAC or 1.0 MAC and represents a light level of anesthesia (clearly inadequate in 50% of otherwise unmedicated, healthy animals). The ED_{95} is 1.2 to 1.4 MAC, and 2.0 MAC represents a deep level of anesthesia, in some cases even an anesthetic overdose. The authors will use the concept of MAC multiples later to compare drug effects and contrast pharmacodynamics of multiple doses of a specific drug.

In concluding this introduction to MAC, a few additional comments are warranted with further details available in recent publications and below in the section on CNS actions. Inhalation anesthetics act in the CNS to cause immobility, analgesia, and unconsciousness. Immobility is now known to reflect the activity of inhalation anesthetics on the spinal cord [88–90], but equi-MAC may not translate to equivalent potency in the brain, at least when evaluated with regards to analgesic and hypnotic potency [91]. Regardless, and despite the fact that ". . .MAC has withstood the test of time. . .," a recent editorial [92] (from which this quote was taken) in response to a publication in the same issue of the journal *Anesthesiology* [93] notes, ". . . in an era of precision medicine, we should use more precise terminology. It is time to call a MAC (minimum alveolar concentration) a MAC (***median*** alveolar concentration)."

Table 28.7A MAC values (%) for a variety of mammals at sea level or near sea level conditions.

Species	Desflurane	Halothane	Isoflurane	Sevoflurane	Nitrous oxide
Cat	9.79 [94] 10.27 [95]	0.99 [96,97] 1.14 [98] 1.19 [99]	1.28 [100] 1.50 [97] 1.61 [99] 1.63 [101] 1.90 [95] 2.21 [102]	2.58 [103] 3.07 [97] 3.41 [95]	255 [98]
Cow		0.76 [104] (calf)	1.14 [105]		223 [104] (calf)
Dog	7.2 [106] 7.68–8.19 [107] 10.3 [108]	0.86 [109] 0.87 [98,110,111] 0.89 [112,113] 0.92 [114] 0.93 [115]	1.28 [101] 1.30 [116] 1.31 [117] 1.39 [101] 1.39–1.50 [118]	2.10 [119] 2.36 [113]	188 [110] 222 [98]
Ferret		1.01 [120]	1.52 [120] 1.74 [121]		267 [120]
Goat		1.29 [122] 1.3 [123]	1.2 [89] 1.23 [124] 1.29 [122] 1.31 [125] 1.43 [126] 1.5 [123]	2.33 [122]	
Horse	7.02 [127] 8.06 [128]	0.88 [76] 0.95 [129] 1.02 [130] 1.05 [131]	1.31 [76] 1.43 [132] 1.44 [133] 1.64 [134]	2.31 [135] 2.84 [60]	205 [136]
Monkey		0.89 [98] 1.15 [137]	1.28 [137] 1.46 [116]		200 [98]

(Continued)

Table 28.7A *(Continued)*

Species	Desflurane	Halothane	Isoflurane	Sevoflurane	Nitrous oxide
Mouse	6.6–9.1[a] [138]	0.95 [139] 1.00 [140] 1.19–1.37[a] [138]	1.31–1.77[a] [138] 1.35 [139] 1.41 [140]	2.7 [141]	150 [142] 275 [140]
Pig	10.00 [78]	0.90 [143] 0.91 [144] 1.25 [145]	1.45 [146] 1.48 [143] 1.51 [116] 1.55 [147] 1.75 [148] 2.04 [78]	1.97 [149] 2.12 [143] 2.53 [150] 2.66 [151]	162 [147] 195 [148] 277 [145]
Rabbit	8.90 [106]	0.80 [152] 0.82 [153] 1.05 [154] 1.39 [155] 1.42 [156] 1.44 [157] 1.56 [158]	2.05 [155] 2.07 [156] 2.12 [157]	3.70 [159]	
Rat	5.72 [160] 6.48 [161] 6.85 [162] 7.10 [163]	0.81 [164] 0.95 [165] 1.02 [166] 1.03 [139] 1.10 [167] 1.11 [168] 1.13 [169,170] 1.17 [171] 1.23 [162]	1.17 [164] 1.28 [172] 1.30 [173] 1.38 [168] 1.46 [139] 1.46 [162] 1.58 [121,165]	2.99 [166] 2.40 [167] 2.50 [53]	136 [174] 155 [175] 204 [176] 221 [177] 235 [177]
Sheep		0.97 [178]	1.58 [178]		
Human (30–60 years)	6.00 [179]	0.73 [180] 0.74 [181,182] 0.77 [183]	1.15 [184]	1.58 [185] 1.71 [186] 1.83 [187] 1.84 [188] 1.85 [189] 1.9 [190] 2.05 [159]	104 [191]

[a] Absolute value related to strain.
Note, some variability within and across species is likely associated with the technique of measurement of alveolar anesthetic concentration [79].

Table 28.7B ED_{50} values for a variety of non-mammals at sea level or near sea level conditions.

	Desflurane	Halothane	Isoflurane	Sevoflurane	Nitrous oxide
Birds:					
Chicken		0.85 [77]	1.15 [192]		
Cockatoo			1.44 [193]		
Crane			1.34 [194]		
Duck		1.04 [195]	1.30 [195]		
Guinea fowl			1.45 [196]	2.9 [197]	220 [196]
Hawk			2.05 [198]		
Parrot, Amazon			1.47 [193]		
Parrot, African Gray			1.91 [193]		
Parrot, thick-billed			1.07 [199]		
Pigeon			1.51 [196] 1.45 [200]		154 [196]
Other:					
Goldfish		0.76 [201]			
Toad		0.67 [202]			82.2 [202]

Pharmacodynamics: actions and toxicity of the volatile inhalation anesthetics on body systems

All contemporary inhalation anesthetic agents in one way or another influence vital organ function. Some actions are inevitable and accompany the use of all agents, whereas other actions are a special or prominent feature of one or a number of the agents. In addition, dose–response relationships of inhalation anesthetics are not necessarily parallel. Differences in action, and especially undesirable action, of specific anesthetic agents, form the basis for selecting one agent over another for a particular patient and/or procedure. Undesirable actions also provide primary impetus for development of new agents and/or anesthetic techniques.

Data from healthy animals exposed to equipotent alveolar concentrations of these drugs under controlled circumstances provide foundational information for this review. In other cases, results of studies of human volunteers form the basis of our understanding of some drug actions because actions in animals of common clinical focus in veterinary medicine have not been described. Because animals are commonly allowed to breathe spontaneously during clinical management of general anesthesia (versus controlled mechanical ventilation), investigational results obtained from spontaneously breathing test animals are often considered baseline by veterinarians. However, in the broader anesthesiology and pharmacology literature, results of studies from human volunteers or animals administered precise amounts of inhalation anesthetics during controlled ventilation (and normocapnia) most commonly form the basis of comparison of pharmacodynamic differences. It is important to stress that many variables other than mode of ventilation commonly accompany anesthetic management of animals in both clinical and laboratory settings. These variables influence drug pharmacokinetics and pharmacodynamics and may cause individuals to respond differently from test subjects that were studied under standardized conditions. Such confounding variables include species, duration of anesthesia, noxious (painful) stimulation, co-existing disease, concurrent medications, variation in body temperature, and extremes of age, as examples.

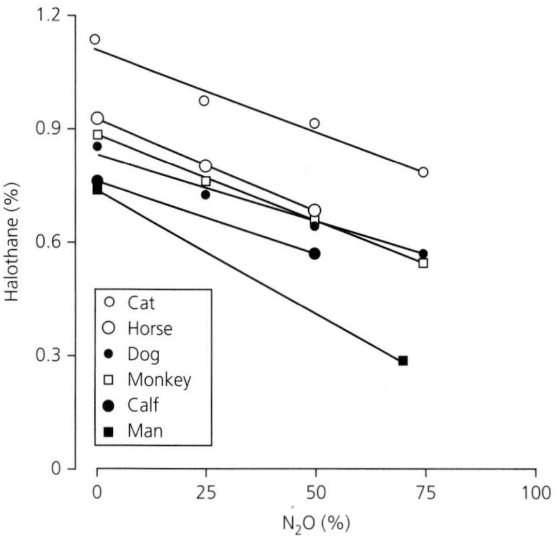

Figure 28.15 When N_2O is combined with halothane the alveolar concentration of halothane at MAC is decreased. However, the halothane sparing imposed by N_2O is less in animals compared to humans. Source: Reproduced with permission from Steffey and Eger [203].

Central nervous system

Inhalation anesthetics affect the CNS in many ways. Mostly these agents are selected because they induce a reversible, dose-related state of CNS (somatic, motor), but also hemodynamic and endocrine unresponsiveness to noxious stimulation, that is, a state of general anesthesia. Interestingly, although clinical anesthesia was introduced more than 150 years ago, the mechanisms and sites by which general anesthetics (including inhalation anesthetics) cause unresponsiveness to surgical or other forms of noxious stimulation remain unknown [221]. Inhalation anesthetics influence electrical activity of the brain, cerebral metabolism, cerebral perfusion, intracranial pressure, and analgesia – issues of critical importance to the anesthetic management of animals. Our systematic review will start with a focus on mechanisms of action of inhalation anesthetics within the CNS.

Mechanism of action

Molecular mechanisms of action

Background Ever since the first public demonstration of diethyl ether in 1846, the molecular determinants of inhaled anesthetic action have remained elusive [221]. As a class, inhaled anesthetics

Table 28.8 Some factors that influence the value of MAC (anesthetic requirement).

No change	Increase	Decrease
Arterial blood pressure > 50 mmHg [204]	Drugs causing CNS stimulation:	Drugs causing CNS depression[a]:
Atropine, glycopyrrolate, scopolamine [96]	Amphetamine	Other inhaled anesthetic; N_2O [26]
Duration of anesthesia	Ephedrine	Injectable anesthetics:
Gender	Morphine (horse) [131]	Ketamine [206]
Hyperkalemia, hypokalemia	Laudanosine [158]	Lidocaine [102,115]
Metabolic acid-base change	Physostigmine [205]	Thiopental [207]
PaO_2 > 40 mmHg	Hyperthermia (to 42 °C)	Preanesthetic medications:
$PaCO_2$ 15–95 mmHg		Acepromazine [208–210]
		Diazepam [211–213]
		Detomidine [133]
		Fentanyl [214]
		Medetomidine [215,216]
		Meperidine [217]
		Midazolam [218]
		Morphine [219]
		Xylazine [134]
		Other:
		Adenosine
		Central anticholinergic [205]
		5-HT antagonist [220]
		Arterial blood pressure < 50 mmHg
		Hyponatremia
		Hypothermia
		Increasing adult age
		PaO_2 < 40 mmHg
		$PaCO_2$ > 95 mmHg
		Pregnancy

[a] The list of example drugs is intended to be representative, not exhaustive. The list is summarized from previous reviews [17,75,81] except where indicated by reference numbers.

exhibit unusual actions that set them apart from most other pharmacologic agents. Most drugs rely on a unique molecular size, shape, volume, charge, polarity, functional group, or other structural motif in order to bind with a specific target molecule and induce a functional change, as set forth by Fisher's Schloss und Schlüssel (lock and key) description of specific enzyme–substrate or protein–drug interactions [222]. Yet inhaled anesthetics share no chemical or structural commonalities; they range in composition from single atoms (xenon) and diatomic elements (nitrogen) to inorganic molecules (N_2O) and hydrocarbons of varying lengths containing any number of halogens and organic functional groups, including alkanes (chloroform, halothane), alkenes (trichloroethylene), alcohols (ethanol), ethers (isoflurane, sevoflurane, and desflurane), and combinations thereof (ethyl vinyl ether, fluroxene). Even endogenous by-products of metabolism such as CO_2 [223], ammonia [224], and ketones [225] exert anesthetic effects. Such chemical diversity among drug "keys" is incongruent with classical notions of drug–ligand interactions.

Inhaled anesthetic efficacy is not limited to humans and domestic mammals. These drugs can reversibly immobilize all vertebrate and invertebrate animals in which they have been studied, including worms, fish, amphibians, reptiles, and birds. In fact, efficacy is not limited to the animal kingdom, as inhaled anesthetics can even prevent movement in protozoa [226] and plants (those with touch-sensitive contractile leaves) [227]. It is unknown why these pharmacologic effects should be conserved across such diverse phyla, especially since most anesthetics are not found in nature and there is no obvious selective pressure underlying anesthetic sensitivity. It suggests, perhaps, that the molecular mechanism underlying inhaled anesthetic action involves interactions with cellular components that are essential to all life. Indeed, given that we are surrounded by potential anesthetics – from the nitrogen [228] in the air we breathe to the volatile essential oils [229] in the food we eat – there may have been evolutionary pressure to minimize sensitivity of target sites at the concentrations these "natural anesthetics" are present within the environment.

Molecular sites: lipid and aqueous theories Meyer [230] and Overton [231] noted that narcotic potency correlated with anesthetic solubility in oil from which they concluded that the cell lipid membrane served as the site of anesthetic action. However, non-specific lipid theories do not adequately explain effect differences between anesthetic stereoisomers [232] or the existence of the anesthetic cut-off effect and non-immobilizers, compounds that lack an immobilizing effect at concentrations predicted by the Meyer–Overton hypothesis to produce general anesthesia [233]. More recently, Cantor [234,235] hypothesized that anesthetics may alter molecular composition and forces within a bilayer plane and cause a change in the lateral pressure profile exerted upon proteins within the lipid membrane, a theory that was supported by several computer simulation models [236–239]. However, using an experimental assay to detect changes in lipid bilayer properties, neither isoflurane, halothane, nor cyclopropane was found to produce detectable membrane effects at clinically relevant concentrations [240].

Miller [241] and Pauling [242] each proposed an aqueous site of action whereby the ordering of water into gas hydrates or clathrates alters electrical conductance across the cell membrane to produce unconsciousness. However, anesthetic MAC correlates better with lipid solubility than with hydrate dissociation pressure [243,244]. In addition, enthalpy for anesthetic hydrate formation is much greater than calculated for *in vivo* hypothermia MAC studies [109], and the extreme transience of anesthetic clathrate formation with reduced water concentration at anesthetic binding sites [245] makes a bulk aqueous phase site of action unlikely.

Molecular sites: protein Inhaled anesthetics bind proteins and can modulate their function even in the absence of a lipid environment [246]. Presynaptically, volatile anesthetics inhibit calcium channel function in the terminal bouton of the neuron and bind soluble N-ethylmaleimide-sensitive attachment proteins (SNAP) and SNAP receptor (SNARE) and associated proteins to decrease neurotransmitter release [247–255]. The magnitude of these effects is much greater at excitatory glutamatergic synapses than at inhibitory GABA-ergic synapses, resulting in reduced excitatory neurotransmission relative to inhibitory neurotransmission [256,257]. Inhaled anesthetics also act postsynaptically to potentiate inhibitory cell targets such as γ-aminobutyric acid type A ($GABA_A$) receptors, glycine receptors, and two-pore domain potassium channels; these same agents inhibit excitatory cell targets such as *N*-methyl-d-aspartate (NMDA) receptors, α-amino-3-hydroxy-5-methyl-4-isoxazole-propionic acid (AMPA) receptors, neuronal nicotinic acetylcholine receptors, and voltage-gated sodium channels [221,232,258–264].

Inability to identify a single target critical to anesthetic action may in fact suggest that immobility is the product of multiple cell receptor and ion channel target modulations [265] acting in a combination of in-parallel and in-series cell pathways and neuronal circuits to decrease cell excitability [266]. Such a model, in which the anesthetic MAC greatly exceeds the dissociation constant between the anesthetic and its relevant protein targets, also predicts steep dose responses (large Hill coefficients) and additive combinatorial effects that are hallmarks of most inhaled anesthetic actions both *in vivo* [267] and *in vitro* [268]. Multiple relevant sites of action would also explain why loss of anesthetic efficacy at one cellular target consequently produces greater anesthetic modulation of other putative cellular targets at MAC [269,270].

How can a single inhaled anesthetic modulate so many different protein targets? At MAC, aqueous phase drug concentrations are around 300 μM or more, depending on the agent, which implies low-affinity drug binding of protein targets [271,272]. Indeed, any hydrocarbon – not just conventional inhaled anesthetics – appears able to modulate anesthetic-sensitive ion channels and receptors when present at sufficiently high concentrations, limited only by the molar water solubility of the drug itself. However, according to the Molar Water Solubility Hypothesis, if a hydrocarbon's saturated aqueous phase concentration is less than a critical cut-off value specific for a given receptor, then the drug fails to modulate that receptor's function [273–275]. This suggests that anesthetic binding may occur at allosterically active amphipathic pockets in the protein that are normally occupied by water with a high dissociation constant (k_d). When an anesthetic agent is present at sufficiently high concentrations relative to the water k_d, the drug displaces the water molecule from this site and induces a change in protein structure and function. Although this implies that access to this amphipathic site is not dependent on drug structure, the type and strength of the subsequent protein–drug molecular interaction – and hence the direction (positive or negative) and magnitude (efficacy) of receptor modulation – certainly would be.

Anatomic sites of action

Inhaled anesthetics cause immobility, amnesia, and unconsciousness, but these distinct endpoints are achieved via actions at different CNS sites [88–90]. In an experimental goat model in which the cerebral circulation was isolated from the rest of the body, selective brain isoflurane administration more than doubled the anesthetic requirement for immobility compared to whole-body isoflurane administration. This demonstrated that the spinal cord, and not the brain, is principally responsible for preventing movement during surgery with inhaled anesthetics [89]. Within the spinal cord, immobility is most likely produced by depression of locomotor neuronal networks located in the ventral horn [276].

In contrast, amnestic effects of inhaled anesthetics are produced by actions within the brain, most probably within the amygdala and hippocampus [277]. Lesions created within the amygdala of rats can block amnestic actions of sevoflurane [278]. Patch clamp recordings *in vitro* of murine amygdala slice preparations also show decreased synaptic transmission at 1 MAC of isoflurane due to inhibition of glutamatergic currents and potentiation of $GABA_A$ receptor currents [279]. Moreover, infusion of a selective 5-HT_7 receptor agonist bilaterally into the basolateral amygdala in rats can actually reverse memory impairment caused by sevoflurane [280]. On electroencephalography, hippocampal-dependent θ-rhythm frequency slows in proportion to the amnestic effects observed with subanesthetic concentrations of isoflurane in rats [281]. Furthermore, mutant mice lacking the gene encoding either the α_4 or β_3 subunits of $GABA_A$ receptors are resistant to isoflurane depression of hippocampus-dependent learning and memory [282,283], and antagonism of α_5 subunit-containing $GABA_A$ receptors restores hippocampal-dependent memory during sevoflurane administration [284].

Consciousness in humans is commonly assessed by testing for voluntary responses to verbal commands. In animals, behavioral tests of consciousness include presence of a righting reflex, movement in response to non-noxious stimuli, and spontaneous interaction with the environment. Cholinergic stimulation of the prefrontal cortex, but not the parietal cortex, causes wakefulness and spontaneous movement in rats breathing 1.9–2.4% sevoflurane. Stimulation of the central medial thalamus via infusions of antibodies against the voltage gated K^+ channel $K_v1.2$ restores ambulation and exploring behavior in rats breathing 0.5 MAC sevoflurane or desflurane [285]. Activation of dopaminergic neurons within the ventral tegmental area of the midbrain in rats or mice using electrical or optogenetic stimulation restores the righting reflex during isoflurane or sevoflurane anesthesia [286,287]. Finally, electrical or glutamatergic stimulation of neurons in the parabrachial nucleus of the pons can also cause return of righting in mice anesthetized with isoflurane or sevoflurane [288,289]. Collectively, these findings suggest that volatile anesthetics produce unconsciousness through actions at multiple discrete sites within the pons, midbrain, thalamus, and possibly cerebral cortex.

At concentrations above MAC, it is presumed that inhaled anesthetics sufficiently depress cortical function to prevent animals from experiencing motivational-affective dimensions of pain [290]. Additionally, concentrations of modern volatile agents (halothane, enflurane, isoflurane, sevoflurane, and desflurane) between 0.8 and 1.0 MAC decrease, but do not ablate, wind-up, and central sensitization and so may help prevent heightened postoperative pain sensitivity; however, higher concentrations of contemporary drugs offer no further benefit in this regard [291,292]. Volatile anesthetic concentrations between 0.4 and 0.8 MAC decrease withdrawal responses to noxious stimuli, but lower concentrations can actually cause hyperalgesia with a peak effect at 0.1 MAC [293,294] due to potent nicotinic cholinergic receptor inhibition [295]. In contrast, the gaseous anesthetics xenon and N_2O produce analgesia via glutamatergic receptor inhibition [296] and, in the case of N_2O, through additional modulation of noradrenergic-opioid receptor pathways [297]. Anatomically, analgesic actions occur both supraspinally and within the dorsal horn of the spinal cord and are likely responsible for greater blunting of autonomic responses associated with these gases compared to the modern volatile agents [298].

Electroencephalographic effects

The electroencephalogram (EEG) is used to help identify pathologic brain disorders and predict outcome of brain insults. Studies have shown that general anesthesia alters EEG parameters; however, all anesthetics do not produce exactly the same changes in EEG pattern as dose (anesthetic depth) increases; therefore, the generic correlation of the raw EEG with anesthetic dose is not precise. Indeed, despite some weak correlations and its usefulness as an indication of changing anesthetic depth, no parameter has had sensitivity and specificity sufficient to justify use of the EEG alone as a reliable index of anesthetic depth [299]. With technological advances in recent years, research has focused on use of processed EEG parameters (e.g., the bispectral index) as improved descriptions of anesthetic states. Additional information on this topic is available in Chapter 10.

In general, as the depth of anesthesia increases from awake states, the electric activity of the cerebral cortex becomes desynchronized. Using isoflurane as an example of the general EEG response to volatile anesthetics [1], there is initially an increased frequency of the EEG activity (alveolar concentrations less than 0.4 MAC). With further increases in anesthetic concentration, a decrease in frequency and increased amplitude of the EEG waves occur. The wave amplitude increases to a peak (about 1.0 MAC) and then, with further dose increase, it progressively declines (burst suppression occurs at about 1.5 MAC, that is, bursts of slow high-voltage activity separated by electrical silence) and eventually becomes flat line. With isoflurane, an isoelectric pattern occurs at about 2.0 MAC, while at the other extreme, it is not seen with halothane until > 3.5 MAC. Electrical silence does not occur with enflurane. The two newest volatile anesthetics, sevoflurane and desflurane, cause dose-related changes similar to those of isoflurane [300–302]. Systematic studies of EEG activity in humans [303] and dogs [304] showed that enflurane was associated with spontaneous or noise-initiated intensified seizures. In addition, enflurane induces seizure activity that is associated with substantial increases in cerebral blood flow and cerebral metabolic use of O_2. The EEG responses of desflurane, sevoflurane, and isoflurane are similar [300–302] and all three can suppress drug-induced convulsive behavior [305–309]. However, there are reports of seizure activity in animals [119,310] and human patients [311,312] during sevoflurane anesthesia.

Cerebral metabolism

All volatile anesthetics decrease cerebral metabolic rate (cerebral oxygen consumption [$CMRO_2$]). The magnitude of decrease is least with halothane but similar with isoflurane, sevoflurane, and desflurane [119,300,305,313,314].

Cerebral blood flow and cerebral perfusion pressure

Anesthetic goals for patients having, or at risk for, intracranial hypertension should include reduction of intracranial pressure (ICP), maintenance of cerebral perfusion pressure (CPP), and matching cerebral blood flow (CBF) to a reduced $CMRO_2$.

According to the Monro–Kellie doctrine [315,316], three volumes are contained within the calvarium: brain parenchyma, cerebrospinal fluid, and blood; an increase in volume of one component will increase ICP unless compensated by a decrease in one or both of the other intracranial component volumes. Most inhaled agents cause cerebral vasodilation, thereby increasing brain blood volume and ICP. This effect is greatest with halothane, less with enflurane, isoflurane, and desflurane, and least with sevoflurane [317,318]. The gas anesthetics currently in use have divergent effects; N_2O causes more cerebral vasodilation than equipotent doses of volatile anesthetics [319], whereas xenon has little effect on ICP and cerebral vascular tone [320].

CPP is defined as the difference between mean arterial blood pressure (MAP) and ICP; it represents the driving pressure for blood flow to the brain. The potent volatile agents depress cardiovascular function and decrease MAP, and thus decrease CPP [321]. Nonetheless, CBF typically increases due to dose-dependent cerebral vasodilation that reduces vascular resistance [322], despite dose-dependent reductions in EEG activity and $CMRO_2$. Through possible actions on nitric oxide synthase [323–326], cyclooxygenase, [323], adenylate cyclase [327], and ATP-sensitive K^+ channels [328], vasodilation caused by potent volatile anesthetics leads to a loss of cerebrovascular autoregulation, reflected by an uncoupling of cerebral perfusion from cerebral oxygen demand. Increased CBF from N_2O is accompanied by an actual increase in metabolic rate of the cerebral cortex if administered alone [329], but not when co-administered with a potent volatile agent such as isoflurane [330,331]. Xenon minimally affects $CMRO_2$ [332] and preserves normal cerebrovascular autoregulation [333].

In addition to specific agent effects, anesthetic modulation of cerebral hemodynamics depends upon agent dose, anesthetic time, animal species studied, and hyper- or hypoventilation. At 0.5 MAC, cerebrovascular autoregulation during anesthesia with potent inhaled agents is slowed or obtunded; however, at concentrations greater than MAC, cerebrovascular autoregulation is significantly and progressively diminished as CBF becomes simply a function of CPP [334,335]. Blood flow also increases throughout most of the brain as a function of anesthetic duration, presumably due to time-dependent increases in nitric oxide synthase inhibition [336]. Carbon dioxide tension further affects autoregulation. Although halothane tends to increase CBF regardless of ventilation status [337], cerebrovascular autoregulation may be better preserved at a given MAC-multiple of a haloether anesthetic when hyperventilation is maintained concurrently [338]. The converse also appears true: autoregulation is lost and CBF is increased at lower inhaled anesthetic doses when animals are allowed to hypoventilate [339], although this interaction between CO_2 and agent is greater with isoflurane than for sevoflurane [340].

Intracranial pressure

Although most anesthetic effects on cerebral hemodynamics are similar among humans and small animal research models, the same does not hold true for horses, and perhaps other very large animal species. Intracranial pressure (ICP) in awake horses remains constant irrespective of head position [341], but cerebral vasodilation during inhalant anesthesia causes large increases in ICP – sometimes similar in magnitude to values seen with severe head trauma in human patients – that is exacerbated by dorsal recumbency, head-down positioning, hypercapnia during spontaneous ventilation, and anesthetic time during controlled ventilation [342–345]. Surprisingly, over a wide range of perfusion pressures, isoflurane-anesthetized horses maintain regional CBF relatively constant, albeit at a low flow that may still place animals at risk for tissue hypoxia [346]. Blood flow to the thoracolumbar spinal cord is particularly low, and further reduction may predispose to postanesthetic myelomalacia in horses [347].

Respiratory system

Inhalation anesthetics depress respiratory system function. The volatile agents in particular decrease ventilation in a drug- and species-specific manner. Depending on conditions, including species of interest, some of the most commonly considered measures of breathing effectiveness, that is, breathing rate and depth (tidal volume), may not be revealing or may even be misleading. In general, spontaneous ventilation progressively decreases as inhalation anesthetic dose is increased because at low doses tidal volume decreases more than frequency increases. As anesthetic dose is further increased, respiratory frequency also decreases. In otherwise unmedicated animals (including humans) anesthetized with volatile agents, respiratory arrest occurs at 1.5–3.0 MAC (Table 28.9). The overall decrease in minute ventilation and the likely variable increase in deadspace ventilation (resulting in an increase in the deadspace to tidal volume ratio, V_D/V_T, from a normal of about 0.3 to 0.5 or more) result in a reduction in alveolar ventilation. Decreases in alveolar ventilation are out of proportion to decreases in CO_2 production (O_2 utilization is decreased by general anesthesia), such that $PaCO_2$ increases (Fig. 28.16). In addition, the normal stimulation of ventilation caused by increased $PaCO_2$ (or decreased PaO_2) is depressed by the inhalation anesthetics, presumably via the action of these agents directly on the medullary and peripheral (aortic and carotid body) chemoreceptors [348–351].

Bronchospasm is associated with some conditions that contribute to increased airway resistance. A variety of early studies indicated that among anesthetics available at the time, halothane was the most effective bronchodilator [352,353]. That effect is believed to result, at least partially, from decreased cholinergic neurotransmission [354,355]. Therefore, it was often recommended for patients at risk of bronchospasm. The work of Hirschman *et al.* suggests that isoflurane and perhaps enflurane were as effective in decreasing experimentally produced airway resistance and therefore were good alternatives to halothane [356,357]. Recent work with isoflurane, sevoflurane, and desflurane indicates that relaxation of constricted bronchial muscles by these agents at least equals or exceeds that caused by halothane [355,358,359].

Avoiding airway irritation during administration of inhalation anesthetics is important, especially during induction of anesthesia because it may cause breath holding, coughing, and laryngospasm (particularly in some species such as primates, both human and nonhuman) that in turn result in arterial oxyhemoglobin desaturation. At least in humans, none of the potent inhalation anesthetics seem to have irritant properties at subanesthetic concentrations. However, patient objection and airway irritation are evident with desflurane (and to a lesser degree with isoflurane [360]) at concentrations of 7% or greater [361,362] and as a result, desflurane is not commonly used for anesthetic induction of human patients.

Arterial carbon dioxide tension

The $PaCO_2$ is the most frequently used measure of respiratory system response to general anesthetics. All contemporary inhalation anesthetics depress alveolar ventilation and increase $PaCO_2$ in dose-related fashion. Fig. 28.16 summarizes the effects of inhalation anesthetics in humans, the species for which data are most complete [349,363–367].

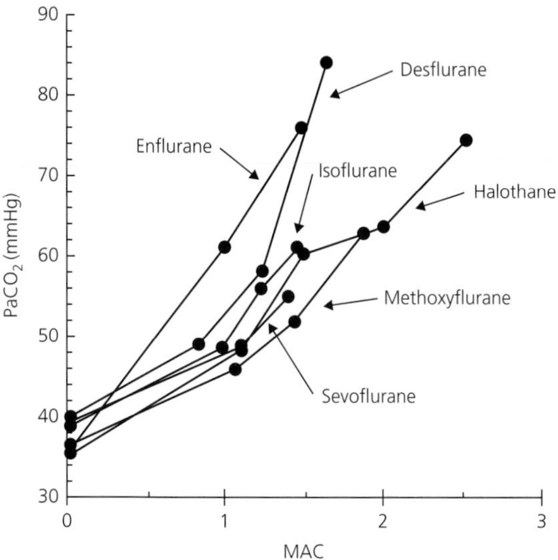

Figure 28.16 Respiratory response to an increase in the alveolar concentration (expressed as a multiple of MAC) of inhalation anesthetics in humans. Source: Data are taken from multiple sources Fourcade *et al.* [349]; Lockhart *et al.* [363]; Munson *et al.* [364]; Larson *et al.* [365]; Doi and Ikeda [366]; Calverley *et al.* [367].

Table 28.9 Apneic Index (AI) in various species.

Species	Desflurane		Halothane		Isoflurane	
	MAC	AI	MAC	AI	MAC	AI
Cat	NA	NA	NA	NA	1.63	2.4 [101]
Dog	7.2	2.4 [361]	0.87	2.9 [111]	1.28	2.5 [101]
Horse	NA	NA	0.88	2.6 [76]	1.31	2.3 [76]
Pig	9.8	1.6 [361,368]	NA	NA	NA	NA
Rat	NA	NA	1.11	2.3 [369]	1.38	3.1 [170]
Human	7.25	1.8 [363]	0.77	2.3 [363]	1.15	1.7 [363]

Minimum alveolar concentration (MAC) is given in vol % and the AI is a ratio of the end-tidal anesthetic concentration at apnea and MAC. Similar data are not currently available for sevoflurane. NA, not available.

Because appropriate data in the species of interest to veterinary anesthetists are incomplete, rank order of the magnitude of hypoventilation caused by the four contemporary volatile anesthetics at a common alveolar dose cannot be expressed with authority. Indeed, species variability is an important confounder (see below).

Factors influencing respiratory effects

Mode of ventilation

Ventilation is often assisted or controlled during inhalation anesthesia to compensate for the anesthetic-induced respiratory depression. Controlled mechanical ventilation is used to predictably maintain a normal or some other specific $PaCO_2$, during anesthesia. Assisted ventilation (i.e., the anesthetist augments tidal volume, but the animal determines its own breathing frequency) is used to attempt to improve the efficiency of oxygenating arterial blood and reduce the work of breathing but is usually not effective in substantially lowering $PaCO_2$ compared to circumstances associated with spontaneous ventilation (i.e., the animal controls both the rate and depth of breathing) [370,371].

Duration of anesthesia

Respiratory function, including $PaCO_2$, is little changed for as long as up to 10 h of constant, low-dose halothane (or methoxyflurane) dogs [372,373]. This is also supported by studies of humans [374] anesthetized with constant low-dose halothane. However, in horses anesthetized for 5 h with a constant dose of 1.2 MAC isoflurane, a substantial temporal increase in $PaCO_2$ was noted [375]. A similar but more modest trend was noted in horses when halothane was used for anesthesia [376,377]. At least in some species, if the alveolar dose of halothane is increased above about 1–1.3 MAC and maintained constant at a heightened level, the magnitude of change in hypoventilation also worsens with time [373]. Conversely, there is evidence for recovery from the ventilatory depressant effects of volatile anesthetics in humans [367].

Surgery and other noxious stimulation

Noxious stimulation may result in sufficient central nervous stimulation to lessen the ventilatory depression of inhalation anesthetics [378–381]. This effect is diminished with increasing anesthetic depth.

Concurrent drugs

In humans, the substitution of N_2O for an equivalent amount of a concurrently administered volatile agent such as isoflurane results in a lower $PaCO_2$ than that seen with the volatile agent alone [26]. However, in dogs and monkeys anesthetized with halothane, ventilation was at least as, and sometimes more, depressed when N_2O was substituted for a portion of the halothane [382,383]. The addition of opioid drugs such as morphine may increase the respiratory depression produced by an inhalation anesthetic [116,131,132,380].

Cardiovascular system

All volatile inhalation anesthetics cause dose-dependent and drug-specific changes in cardiovascular performance. The magnitude and sometimes direction of change may be influenced by other variables that often accompany general anesthesia (Box 28.4). The mechanisms of cardiovascular effects are diverse but often include direct myocardial depression and a decrease in sympathoadrenal activity.

Cardiac output

All of the volatile anesthetics can decrease cardiac output (CO). The magnitude of change is dose-related and dependent upon agent. In general, among the contemporary agents in use with animals, halothane is most depressing to CO [1,384–386]. Desflurane in many ways is similar in cardiovascular action to isoflurane while sevoflurane has characteristics resembling both halothane and isoflurane. All of the newer volatile anesthetics tend to preserve CO at clinically useful concentrations, facilitated by reductions in systemic vascular resistance [128,361,387–394]. However, the direct effect of volatile agents on CO (if vascular resistance is maintained) is often a

Box 28.4 Factors that influence cardiovascular effects of inhalation anesthetics.

Anesthetic dose
Duration of anesthesia
Concurrent drug therapy
Intravenous fluid therapy
Magnitude of $PaCO_2$
Mechanical ventilation
Noxious stimulation

decrease in stroke volume as a result of dose-related depression in myocardial contractility [1,128,361,391,395–397].

The effect of inhalation anesthetics on heart rate (HR) is variable and depends on agent and species. For example, in humans, HR is not substantially altered with halothane anesthesia but is usually increased by isoflurane, desflurane, and sevoflurane [393,398,399]. Compared to conditions in awake, calm dogs, HR is increased with all four of the anesthetics listed [390,394]. There is evidence to suggest that differences between agents in the degree of increase in HR in dogs are explained by differences in their vagolytic activity [392]. In the dog, the HR usually remains constant over a range of clinically useful alveolar concentrations in the absence of other modifying factors (e.g., noxious stimulation) [384,385,390,394,400,401].

Cardiac rhythm and catecholamines

Inhalation anesthetics may increase the automaticity of the myocardium and the likelihood of propagated impulses from ectopic sites, especially from within the ventricle [402]. While spontaneous dysrhythmias were most notable with earlier inhalation anesthetics (e.g., halothane), it appears that none of the three most recently introduced ether-derivative agents predispose the heart to extrasystoles. However, adrenergic agonist-associated dysrhythmias may be exaggerated by the presence of inhalant anesthetics [403]. The association of cardiac dysrhythmias with adrenergic drugs and anesthetic agents has received extensive study.

Halothane markedly reduces the amount of epinephrine necessary to cause ventricular premature contractions [404]. There is some evidence that deeper levels of halothane decrease this incidence [405–407], but this is not a consistent finding [408]. Enflurane and methoxyflurane are less likely to sensitize the heart to arrhythmogenic effects of epinephrine, and isoflurane, desflurane, and sevoflurane are least arrhythmogenic [1,407,409–414]. The potential for dysrhythmias follows administration of most catecholamine-type drugs, although the magnitude of such potential varies with the drug co-administered [414–419] and other associated conditions [420].

Regional blood flow

A fundamental principle of circulatory function is that blood flow is sufficient to deliver adequate amounts of O_2 and nutrients to tissues and to remove metabolic waste. However, tissues have very different requirements for blood flow per unit volume of tissue and these tissue-specific blood flow requirements change with conditions (e.g., basal versus exercise or "flight or fight"). In general, blood flow to each tissue is usually maintained at a level only slightly more than that required for metabolic activity by the tissue. Unfortunately, inhalation anesthetics not only reduce total blood flow (i.e., CO) but also impact the distribution of blood flow to tissues. In most patients, the changes are qualitatively similar for all the contemporary agents, but in others, agents have clear differences. Dose of anesthetic and species differences add further impact to their ultimate effect. Detailed information on the many permutations of anesthetic effects on regional blood flow is not available for all species and is beyond the scope of this chapter. However, references are included here as an introduction to this much broader topic [388,421–424].

Arterial blood pressure

Volatile anesthetics cause a dose-dependent decrease in arterial blood pressure (Fig. 28.17) [60,101,112,128,384,388,394,424–427]. In general, the dose-related decrease in arterial blood pressure is similar regardless of the species studied [76,112,384,386,389, 425–428]. The dose-related decrease in blood pressure with all four of the contemporary agents is usually related to a decrease in stroke volume but in some cases (agent and/or species), a decrease in peripheral vascular resistance may play an important role. This common scenario in animals differs from results generally reported from studies with humans anesthetized with isoflurane, sevoflurane, and desflurane, where pressure decreases primarily from a decrease in systemic vascular resistance [22,429]. Indices of anesthetic influence on cardiovascular collapse are given in Table 28.10 [176,369,384].

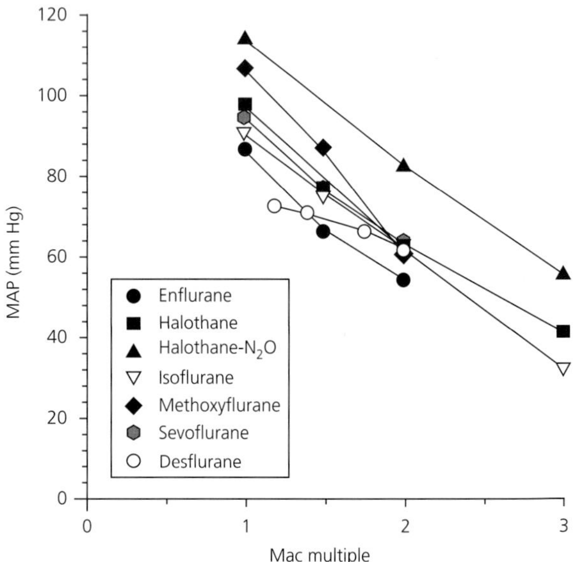

Figure 28.17 Inhalation anesthetics cause a dose (expressed as multiples of MAC)-dependent decrease in mean arterial blood pressure (MAP) in dogs whose ventilation is mechanically controlled to produce eucapnia. Source: Data are from multiple sources Steffey *et al.* [112]; Klide [385]; Merin *et al.* [388]; Mutoh *et al.* [394]; Steffey *et al.* [425].

Table 28.10 Anesthetic-induced cardiovascular depression as expressed by cardiovascular anesthetic indices.

Species	Desflurane	Halothane	Isoflurane
Dog[a]	2.84		2.69
Pig[b]	2.45		3.02
Rat[c]		3.0	5.7

[a]The anesthetic concentration causing death in ventilated dogs related to MAC [361].
[b]Mean fatal dose related to MAC [368].
[c]Heart concentration of anesthetic at cardiovascular failure related to heart concentration of anesthetic at establishment of anesthesia [176,369].

Factors influencing circulatory effects

A variety of circumstances associated with the anesthetic management of veterinary patients may add to or oppose the primary effects of the anesthetic. The most profound modifications of drug action are usually on cardiovascular function. They may include mechanical ventilation and alterations in $PaCO_2$, noxious (surgical) stimulation, duration of anesthesia, and co-existing drugs.

Mode of ventilation and $PaCO_2$

There may be considerable difference in the cardiovascular effects of inhalation anesthetics in animals breathing spontaneously compared to when their breathing is mechanically controlled (e.g., intermittent positive-pressure ventilation or IPPV) to produce and maintain a normal $PaCO_2$. In general, cardiovascular function is usually depressed during IPPV relative to spontaneous ventilation. This results from either the direct mechanical actions (i.e., intermittent elevation of intrathoracic pressure and resultant decrease in venous return to the heart) or lessening of the indirect pharmacologic action of $PaCO_2$ [430], or both. Carbon dioxide has pharmacologic actions important to these considerations. For example, an increased $PaCO_2$ has direct depressant actions on the heart and smooth muscle of the peripheral blood vessels (i.e., vessel dilation) but indirect (via sympathetic nervous system) stimulation of circulatory function. In generally healthy, sympathetically intact animals, the stimulatory actions of hypercapnia usually predominate, so increased CO and arterial blood pressure usually accompany an increase in $PaCO_2$, becoming lower when $PaCO_2$ is normalized [60,370,386,426,428,431–436].

Noxious stimulation

Noxious stimulation during anesthesia modifies the circulatory effect of inhalation anesthetics via stimulation of the sympathetic nervous system. An increase in arterial blood pressure and HR (CO) commonly accompanies noxious stimulation [85,380,381,437,438]. The response is anesthetic dose related. For example, Roizen *et al.* [85] and Yasuda *et al.* [437] showed that deeper levels of halothane and enflurane decreased or prevented surgically induced increases in serum norepinephrine levels in human patients. Anesthetic doses that block the response are in the range of 1.5–2.0 MAC [85,437]. Similar responses have been reported for animals as well [439–444].

Duration of anesthesia

Some cardiovascular effects of inhalation anesthetics may change with duration of anesthesia. For example, in humans, halothane anesthesia lasting 5–6 h is associated with an increase in values of some measures of cardiovascular function such as CO and HR [432,445]. Similarly, varying degrees of time-related changes have been reported with enflurane [367], desflurane [399,446,447], and others [398,446–450]. Temporal changes in cardiovascular function have also been reported in a variety of animals with halothane [373,376,451,452], isoflurane [375,451,453], and sevoflurane [453]. Dose of anesthetic [373,389,454] and body posture during anesthesia [377,455] apparently also play a temporal role in some species.

The causes of these changes remain unclear. *In vitro*, depression of the cat papillary muscle exposed to a constant concentration of halothane does not vary over a 3-h period [456]. This observation suggests that temporal effects associated with inhalation anesthetics are not the result of improved intrinsic cardiac function. Studies of human volunteers have shown that temporal responses to halothane can be prevented if the subjects are given propranolol before anesthesia, suggesting the mechanism is related to increasing sympathetic nervous system activity [457].

Usually, the temporal changes associated with inhalation anesthetics are of only minor or no concern to the clinician. However, such changes must be considered in interpreting results of laboratory studies in which these agents are used for anesthetic management.

Concurrent drugs

Drugs administered immediately before or in conjunction with inhalation anesthetics (preanesthetic medication, injectable anesthetic induction drugs, vasoactive and cardiotonic drugs, etc.) may influence cardiovascular function by altering the anesthetic requirement (i.e., MAC and thereby increased or decreased anesthetic level) or by their own direct action on cardiovascular performance or sympathetic nervous system function.

For example, N_2O is used on occasion to substitute for a portion of a potent inhalation anesthetic. Because of its own anesthetic potency (albeit low; remember the MAC for N_2O in animals is in the range of 2 atmospheres; see Table 28.7A), its use may facilitate delivery of a reduced amount of the potent volatile agent, and thereby contribute to some cardiovascular sparing. Nitrous oxide may depress the myocardium directly, but these effects are usually counterbalanced by its sympathomimetic effect, resulting in a net improvement in cardiovascular function compared to conditions without N_2O. In animal patients, the magnitude of N_2O effect is limited and species-dependent [136,203,382,383,425,458,459].

Injectable drugs such as acepromazine, α_2-adrenergic receptor agonists, alfaxalone, dissociatives (e.g., ketamine), opioids, propofol, and others are frequently administered to animals as part of their anesthetic management. They confound the primary effects of the inhalation anesthetics and may accentuate cardiovascular depression. On the other hand, sympathomimetic drugs such as ephedrine [460], dopamine, and dobutamine [461,462], and norepinephrine, and phenylephrine are frequently given to counteract unwanted cardiovascular depression of the anesthetic.

Effects on the kidneys

It is generally regarded that clinically used volatile inhalation anesthetics produce similar mild, reversible, dose-related decreases in renal blood flow, and glomerular filtration rate and that such changes largely reflect an anesthetic-induced decrease in CO [429]. However, some studies show little or no change in these kidney-related parameters [53,422,463,464].

As a consequence of the anesthetic-induced decrease in glomerular filtration, healthy anesthetized animals commonly produce a smaller volume of concentrated urine compared to when awake. An increase in serum urea nitrogen, creatinine, and inorganic phosphate may accompany prolonged anesthesia [465–468]. The reduction in renal function is highly influenced by the animal's state of hydration and hemodynamics during anesthesia [469]. Intravenous fluid therapy and prevention of a marked reduction in renal blood flow will lessen or counteract the tendency for reduced renal function. In most cases, especially in healthy animals, effects of inhalation anesthesia on renal function are rapidly reversed after anesthesia.

Among the inhalation anesthetics, methoxyflurane was the most nephrotoxic. Although it is no longer available in North America for use in human or animal patients, it is of pathophysiologic interest and therefore will be briefly reviewed. In humans and some strains of rats, methoxyflurane caused renal failure that was characterized not by oliguria but by a large urine volume (polyuria) unresponsive to vasopressin [41]. This was caused by the biotransformation of methoxyflurane and the large release of free fluoride ion (both in peak levels and in the prolonged exposure due to high adipose accumulation of methoxyflurane during anesthesia) that in turn caused direct damage to the renal tubules. Although renal injury in animals is rare, it has been reported in dogs when methoxyflurane was used in combination with tetracycline antibiotics [470] and flunixin [470].

With the possible exception of enflurane and sevoflurane, the breakdown of other inhalation anesthetics does not pose a risk of fluoride-induced nephrotoxicity. Biotransformation of enflurane and sevoflurane by humans following moderate duration of anesthesia causes serum inorganic fluoride concentrations to increase even beyond the 50 μmol/L level, which is normally considered the nephrotoxic threshold in humans [41,429,471,472]. However, clinical, histological, or biochemical evidence of injury related to increases in fluoride has only rarely been reported in human patients. The over-riding consensus is that sevoflurane has little potential for nephrotoxicity as a result of defluorination [41,429].

Two factors may explain the general lack of injury despite the body's ability to degrade sevoflurane. In 1977, Mazze *et al.* proposed that the area under the serum fluoride concentration versus time curve may be a more important determinant of nephrotoxicity than peak serum fluoride concentration [473]. Because sevoflurane is poorly soluble and is rapidly eliminated via the lungs, the duration of its availability for biotransformation is notably limited. Subsequently, Kharasch *et al.* proposed another consideration [474]. Sevoflurane is primarily metabolized by the liver while hepatic and renal sites are important for methoxyflurane breakdown. The relative lack of intrarenal anesthetic defluorination may markedly reduce its nephrotoxic potential [475]. Studies have confirmed the increase in serum fluoride in horses anesthetized with sevoflurane [58–60]. In these reports, the magnitude and time course of fluoride increase were similar to those reported for humans. As with humans, there has been no evidence of untoward renal effects associated with the increase in fluoride in horses.

Early reports of sevoflurane noted its degradation by CO_2 absorbents such as soda lime and Baralyme [54,62]. A nephrotoxic breakdown product, Compound A, is produced [54]. Compound A can cause renal injury and death in rats [476] and the concentration threshold for nephrotoxicity in rats [477–479] is within the range of concentrations that may be found associated with the anesthetic management of human patients [480]. However, reports of nephrotoxicity in humans are rare [475] and point to alternative mechanisms of toxicity such as species-dependent metabolic degradation of Compound A to directly nephrotoxic compounds. Not surprisingly, Compound A is formed in the breathing circuits used for animals (except non-rebreathing circuits which do not use CO_2 absorbent) [481]. The ultimate importance of *in vitro* sevoflurane degradation to the well-being of veterinary patients such as dogs, cats, and horses [59] remains to be established. Regardless, because of concerns associated with anesthetic management of human patients, most commercially available absorbents now used in North America no longer contain KOH or NaOH.

Effects on the liver

Depression of hepatic function and hepatocellular damage may be caused by the action of volatile anesthetics. Effects may be mild and transient or permanent, and injury may be by direct or indirect action. Studies by Reilly *et al.* [482] suggested that halothane (but likely also other potent inhalation anesthetics) substantially inhibits drug-metabolizing capacity in the liver. A reduction in intrinsic hepatic clearance of drugs, along with anesthetic-induced alteration of other pharmacokinetically important variables (e.g., reduced hepatic blood flow), delays drug removal, and may increase plasma drug concentration during anesthesia. Examples of such circumstances have been reported [206,217,482–484]. Prolonged or increased (relative to conditions in the unanesthetized animal) plasma concentrations of some drugs have important toxic implications, especially in physiologically compromised patients.

All of the potent inhalation anesthetics are capable of causing hepatocellular injury by reducing liver blood flow and oxygen delivery. However, available data suggest that of the four contemporary volatile anesthetics, isoflurane is most likely to better maintain liver O_2 delivery and thus is the agent least likely to produce hepatocyte injury. Sevoflurane and desflurane are similar to isoflurane, whereas halothane produces the most striking adverse changes [41,388,421,422,424,485–490]. Results of studies indicate that confounding factors, including N_2O [491], concurrent hypoxia [489,492–494], prior induction of hepatic drug-metabolizing enzymes [495,496], mode of ventilation [497], and positive end-expired pressure [498] may worsen conditions and increase the likelihood of hepatocellular damage.

It now appears that halothane produces two types of hepatotoxicity in susceptible individuals. One is a mild, self-limiting postanesthetic form of hepatocellular damage and associated increase in serum concentrations of liver enzymes. Signs of hepatotoxicity occur shortly after anesthetic exposure. The other is a rare, severe, often fatal hepatotoxicity with delayed onset. The fulminant hepatopathy appears limited to human patients (i.e., "halothane hepatitis") and is thought to be an immune-mediated toxicity [499,500]. The mechanism of halothane hepatitis may also be genetically associated [501]. The increased incidence of hepatic injury associated with halothane is the principal factor leading to the decrease in use of halothane for human patients nearly three decades ago.

Effects on skeletal muscle: malignant hyperthermia

Malignant hyperthermia (MH) is a potentially life-threatening pharmacogenetic myopathy that is most commonly reported in susceptible human patients [502,503] and swine [504]. However, reports of its occurrence in other species exist [505–511]. Its clinicopathological, histopathological, and genetic basis has recently been further described for the horse [512–514]. All of the four contemporary volatile anesthetics can initiate MH, but halothane is the most potent triggering agent (relative to other inhalation anesthetics) [503]. The syndrome is characterized by a rapid rise in cellular metabolic activity that, if not treated quickly, causes death. Monitoring of temperature, CO_2 production, and other signs of metabolic imbalance (e.g., arterial blood gases and pH) is warranted in susceptible/suspected patients. Patients that are known to be susceptible to MH can usually be anesthetized safely. Avoidance of triggering agents and prophylactic dantrolene given before anesthesia is effective in blocking the onset of MH [503].

The gaseous anesthetic: nitrous oxide

Nitrous oxide (N_2O) was introduced into clinical practice more than 150 years ago. Since then, its use has formed the basis for more general anesthetic techniques for human patients than any other single inhalation agent [26]. Its widespread use resulted from many desirable properties, including low blood solubility (see Table 28.2), limited cardiovascular and respiratory system depression, and minimal toxicity [26]. The origin of its clinical use in the anesthetic management of animal patients in the early 1960s arose from its clinical use with human patients rather than from objective species-specific supporting evidence.

Dose

Nitrous oxide is not the ideal anesthetic for humans or animals. As discussed earlier in this chapter, N_2O is not a potent anesthetic (see Table 28.7A) and will not anesthetize a fit, healthy individual when given alone. To maximize the benefits of N_2O, it is usually used in high-inspired concentrations. However, as the concentration of N_2O is increased, there is a change in the proportion and partial pressure of the various other constituents of the inspired breath, notably O_2. Consequently, to avoid hypoxemia, 75% of the inspired breath is the highest fraction that can be safely administered under conditions at sea level. Use of N_2O at locations above sea level requires a lower N_2O concentration to ensure an adequate P_IO_2.

Nitrous oxide has less value in the anesthetic management of animals than in that of humans because the anesthetic potency of N_2O in most animals studied is only about half (or less) that found for humans (e.g., MAC for the dog is about 200% versus about 100% for humans; see Table 28.7A) [17,203]. Thus, the value of N_2O in veterinary clinical practice is as an anesthetic adjuvant, that is, accompanying other inhaled or injectable drugs. Since the effects of N_2O on vital organ function (including cardiovascular and respiratory) in the absence of hypoxemia are small (but *not* necessarily inconsequential) in most veterinary patients, benefit is most commonly afforded by allowing a certain reduction in the amount of the primary, more potent, inhaled or injectable anesthetic agents.

Pharmacokinetics

Nitrous oxide's low blood solubility (see Table 28.2) is responsible for its rapid onset of action. Although it does not have the potency to produce anesthesia by itself, it may be used to speed induction of inhalation anesthesia as a result of its own (albeit limited) CNS effects and, as mentioned earlier, also by augmenting the uptake of a concurrently administered, more potent volatile anesthetic such as halothane, the "second gas effect" [17,26,515,516]. When a high concentration of N_2O is given concurrently in a mixture with an inhalation agent (e.g., N_2O plus halothane), the alveolar concentration of the simultaneously administered anesthetic (halothane) increases more rapidly than when the "second" gas had been administered without N_2O. The second gas effect is the result of an increased inspiratory volume secondary to the large volume of N_2O taken up [515] and a concentrating effect on the second gas in a smaller volume (and thus increased gradient for transfer to blood) as a result of the uptake of the large volume of N_2O [17,516]. Results of a more recent study with desflurane confirm previous findings for the second gas effect [517].

Pharmacodynamics

As noted previously, N_2O's effects on cardiovascular and respiratory function (other than reducing the inspired O_2 concentration) are small compared to other inhalation anesthetics. It does depress myocardial function directly, but its sympathetic stimulation properties counteract some of the direct depression (its own as well as that from accompanying volatile anesthetics) [203,518]. As a result of its sympathetic nervous system activation, it may contribute to a desirable increased arterial blood pressure [136,519] or an undesirable increased incidence of cardiac arrhythmias [520,521]. There is evidence to suggest that its use contributes to myocardial ischemia in some circumstances [522–525]. Overall, a conservative outlook regarding N_2O use relative to respiration and circulation is that significant concern is warranted only in patients with initially compromised function [526,527]. As with any agent, its advantages and disadvantages should be considered on an individual patient basis.

N_2O has little or no effect on liver and kidney function [528–530]. Although there is evidence of N_2O-induced interference with production of red and white blood cells by bone marrow, the risk of adverse outcomes to a subject exposed under most clinical veterinary circumstances is little or none [529,531]. However, prolonged exposure to N_2O causes megaloblastic hematopoiesis and polyneuropathy. Seriously ill patients may have increased sensitivity to these toxicities. Problems result from N_2O-induced inactivation of the vitamin B_{12}-dependent enzyme methionine synthase, an enzyme that controls inter-relations between vitamin B_{12} and folic acid metabolism [532]. Although an occasional patient may develop signs suggestive of vitamin B_{12} and folic acid deficiency after an anesthetic technique that includes N_2O, this is a rare event in human and animal patients [529,533]. Prolonged occupational or abusive exposure to N_2O may be equally harmful and should be considered in management plans of veterinary practices [41,529,534,535]. In this regard, it is important to recognize that while use of commercially available charcoal adsorbers used to scavenge patient breathing circuit effluent gases effectively capture volatile anesthetics, they are ineffective in removing N_2O, most of which is rapidly eliminated in the exhaled breath. The extent of biotransformation (to molecular N_2) is very small and mainly by intestinal flora (see Table 28.6) [41,71,72].

Transfer of N_2O to closed gas spaces

Gas spaces exist or may exist in the body under a variety of conditions. For example, gas is normally found in the stomach and intestines. The gut is a dynamic reservoir; the gas it contains is freely movable into and out of it according to the laws of diffusion. The gas in the gut originates from air swallowing, normal production from bacterial processes, chemical reactions, and diffusion from the blood. There is marked variability in both composition and volume of stomach and bowel gas (e.g., herbivore versus carnivore). There are other natural air cavities, such as the air sinuses and the middle ear, and then there are circumstances in which air may be electively or inadvertently introduced as part of diagnostic or therapeutic actions (e.g., pneumoencephalogram, pneumocystogram, endoscopy, vascular air emboli, and others).

Potential problems associated with gas spaces arise when an animal breathing air is given a gas mixture containing a high partial pressure of N_2O [17,26]. Nitrogen (N_2) is the major component of air (80%) and of most gas spaces within the body (methane, CO_2, and hydrogen are also found in variable quantities in the gut). When N_2O is introduced into the inspired breath, a re-equilibration of gases in the gas space begins with N_2O quickly entering and N_2 slowly leaving. That is, because of its greater blood solubility the volume of N_2O that can be transported to a closed gas space is many times the volume of N_2 that can be carried away [17]. For example, the blood/gas PC for N_2O is 0.47 (see Table 28.2), whereas that for N_2 is about 0.015 [536]. Thus, N_2O is more than 30 times more soluble in blood than N_2 (0.47/0.015). The result of the net transfer of gas to the gas space can be manifested as an increase in volume (e.g., with the gut [537,538], pneumothorax [538], or blood embolus [539,540]), an increase in pressure (e.g., middle ear [541,542], or pneumoencephalogram [543]), or both (as the distending limits of the compliant container are reached). Usually, air is used to inflate the cuff of an endotracheal tube. This cuff is another relatively compliant, enclosed air space. Nitrous oxide will similarly expand this gas space and may increase the pressure exerted on the tracheal wall [544–546].

Diffusion hypoxia

A further consideration for the differential movement of N_2O and N_2 occurs at the end of anesthesia when N_2O is discontinued. Because of the large volume of N_2O stored in the body during anesthesia and the unequal change of N_2O for N_2, a deficiency in blood oxygenation may occur at the end of anesthesia if air is abruptly substituted for N_2O. As discussed earlier in this chapter, this condition is referred to as "diffusion hypoxia" [44,45]. The rapid outpouring of N_2O from the blood into the lung results in a transient but marked decrease in alveolar PO_2 with a resultant decrease in PaO_2.

Interaction with respiratory gas monitoring

Routine monitoring of expired CO_2 is of well-established importance in the operating room of veterinary hospitals. Nitrous oxide interferes with the accurate detection of CO_2 with some, especially older vintage monitoring devices. This interaction must be considered in decisions regarding the purchasing of equipment and overall anesthetic management plan. A more complete summary of the advantages and disadvantages of N_2O use is available elsewhere [26]. Brief summaries of practical considerations for N_2O use in veterinary practice are also available [547,548].

Waste inhalation anesthetics

Occupational exposure: trace concentrations of inhalation anesthetics

Operating room personnel are often exposed to low concentrations of inhalation anesthetics. Contamination of ambient air occurs via vaporizer filling, known and unknown leaks in the patient breathing circuit, and careless spillage of liquid agents. Another source of anesthetic gas exposure is disconnection of a patient from an anesthetic machine at the end of a procedure without first flushing the system with anesthetic-free gas and allowing the patient to expire into the machine for several minutes. Measurable amounts of anesthetic gases and vapors are present in operating room air under a variety of conditions [549–556]. As shown by various studies, personnel inhale and retain these agents for some time [557,558]. The slow rate of elimination of some vapors (especially the more blood-soluble agents such as halothane) allows accumulation of retained trace anesthetic quantities from one day to the next.

Concern is raised because epidemiologic studies of humans and laboratory studies of animals have suggested that chronic exposure to trace levels of anesthetics *may* constitute a health hazard. The possibility that chronic exposure to low levels of anesthetic agents constitutes a hazard to health science personnel has attracted and maintained worldwide interest since the early 1970s. Of particular concern are reports that inhaled anesthetics possess mutagenic, carcinogenic, or teratogenic potential. Depending on the point in life at which exposure occurs, there is concern that these underlying mechanisms in turn may result in an increased incidence of fetal death, spontaneous abortion, birth defects, or cancer in exposed workers [559–561]. However, to date, no genotoxic effect of long-term or short-term exposure to inhaled anesthetics has been demonstrated in humans and ". . .the conclusion from both animal and human studies is that there is no carcinogenic risk either from exposure to the currently used inhaled anesthetics" [41].

Although the data to date, especially regarding effects on human reproduction, remain equivocal, a firm cause-and-effect relationship between chronic exposure to trace levels of anesthetics and human health problems does not exist. Although the risk of long-term exposure to trace concentrations of anesthetics for those in operating room conditions appears minimal, current evidence is suggestive enough to cause concern and to encourage practices to reduce the contamination by anesthetics of operating room personnel. Indeed, within the United States, there are three federal agencies concerned with possible hazards associated with exposure to waste anesthetic gases: the National Institute for Occupational Safety and Health (NIOSH), an agency of the Department of Health, Education, and Welfare, the Occupational Safety and Health Administration (OSHA), an agency of the Department of Labor, and the Food and Drug Administration (FDA). Levels of exposure have been recommended and published by NIOSH as 2.0 parts per million (ppm) for volatile agents and 25 ppm for N_2O [559]. In this regard, inexpensive methods to reduce and control anesthetic exposure by operating room personnel are available and should be used (Box 28.5). Indeed, the spillage of inhalation anesthetic agents into the operating room environment has been reduced significantly since the 1970s by the widespread introduction of anesthetic delivery equipment scavenging systems. However, with the exception of anesthetic adsorbent systems, most systems in use deposit the waste gases directly and unchanged into the atmosphere.

Frequent monitoring of actual levels of anesthetic gas/vapor is of obvious value and is encouraged in specialized circumstances and/or environments of high use. Likely the greatest impact results from educating personnel about the potential problem of waste anesthetic gases and methods for controlling exposure levels [559–562]. For further information on this subject, readers are directed to a more complete report of current knowledge and conclusions from available data that have been developed by the American Society of Anesthesiologists (ASA) Task Force on Trace Anesthetic Gases of the ASA Committee on Occupational Health of Operating Room Personnel [563]. Commentary and recommendations on control of waste anesthetic gases in the veterinary medical workplace have also been articulated by the American College of Veterinary Anesthesia and Analgesia (www.acvaa.org/veterinarians/guidelines; *Control of Waste Anesthetic Gas*) [564].

While exposure of personnel during anesthetic delivery equipment preparation and clean-up, inhalation anesthetic induction procedures, and when working with anesthetic equipment that is not leak-free is most notable, the postanesthetic recovery period is not without concern. In human hospitals, postanesthetic care personnel interacting with patients recovering from anesthesia are also exposed to gases eliminated from those patients. Studies of human postanesthetic care circumstances have reported quantities of volatile anesthetic concentrations that in some cases approach NIOSH recommended maximum exposure limits [565,566]. Similar circumstances are undoubtedly also present in veterinary medicine, particularly those veterinary hospitals (small and large animal patients) with large daily inhalation anesthesia requirements. For example, horses recovering from inhalation anesthesia in a relatively small room with limited fresh air changes per unit time can likely raise the concentration of exhaled inhalation anesthetic

Box 28.5 Methods to reduce occupational exposure to inhalation anesthetics in the operating room.

1. Educate personnel.
2. Use waste gas *scavenger* to collect gas from the adjustable pressure relief (pop-off) valve of the patient breathing circuit and ventilator.
3. Conduct *regular inspections* and *maintenance* to detect and repair leaks in anesthetic machines and patient breathing circuits, piped gas supplies (N_2O), etc.
4. *Alter work practices* (e.g., minimize leaks around face mask, turn off vaporizer/fresh gas flow when patient breathing circuit not attached to patient).
5. Adequately ventilate operating rooms and recovery rooms/areas.
6. Monitor room trace anesthetic gas levels.

considerably and in such cases likewise approach or perhaps exceed OSHA recommended maximum amounts. Additional helpful information on this subject may be found at the ASA website (www.asahq.org; *Operating Room Design Manual May 2022*).

Environmental implications of inhalation anesthetics

Research and commentary regarding the impact (or lack of impact) of contemporary general anesthetic gases and vapors on the global environment have been ongoing in the medical literature since early concerns were publicly voiced about stratospheric ozone destruction by man-made halogenated organic compounds [567,568] and biomedical contributions to the global atmosphere of exponentially increasing concentrations of N_2O, and other "greenhouse gases" [569].

Before proceeding to focus on anesthetic gases, a brief review of selected aspects of atmospheric science seems appropriate. Earth is surrounded by an atmosphere that gradually changes its composition (via molecular diffusion) with altitude. The inner two layers of our atmosphere important to life are the innermost (closest to earth) troposphere (upper limit at about 5–10 miles above the earth's surface) and the outer of these two layers, the stratosphere (reaching up to 30 miles above earth). Circumstances associated with the uppermost layers of our environment, the mesosphere, thermosphere, and exosphere, are not important to the present discussion. Life on earth depends on solar energy. Of the sunlight that ultimately reaches the earth's surface, some is reflected upward again as infrared radiation. Emission of infrared radiation into space is an important mechanism by which the earth's temperature is regulated, that is, the heat caused by infrared radiation is absorbed by "greenhouse gases" such as water vapor, carbon dioxide, ozone, methane, and others, which in turn slows the energy's escape from the troposphere and thus regulates climatic conditions by trapping the heat. Therefore, the greenhouse effect is an essential environmental prerequisite for life on earth as without it, conditions on earth would be far too cold to sustain the ecosystem as we know it. Additions (quantitative and qualitative) to greenhouse gases distort and accelerate the natural process and result in more such gases in the atmosphere than are necessary to regulate and maintain an ideal temperature on earth; global warming is a consequence. The other layer associated with this discussion, the stratospheric ozone layer, shields the earth's surface from the sun's harmful ultraviolet (UV) radiation.

The major atmospheric effects that result from emission of inhalation anesthetics are their contributions to ozone depletion in the stratosphere and to greenhouse warming in the troposphere. The stratospheric ozone layer is known to be damaged by the rapid, widespread global usage, and subsequent atmospheric presence, of volatile, synthetic, long-lived organochlorine- and bromine-containing compounds (chlorofluorocarbons [CFCs]). Indeed, knowledge of ozone depletion by CFCs was one of the major environmental issues of the 20th century and is sure to continue in a major way well into the 21st century. The CFCs causing most of the original worldwide concern regarding destruction of the ozone layer were those used as refrigerants, aerosol propellants, cleaning solutions, and foaming agents [570,571].

As halogenated compounds, all of the contemporary volatile anesthetics are in theory potentially destructive to the ozone layer [572–574]. In effect, however, only chlorine-containing halothane and, much less so, isoflurane, are of concern in this regard (substances that contain only fluorine do not harm the ozone layer). In addition, the relative contribution of these two volatile agents has been estimated to be at most only 0.01% of the annual global release of CFCs [572], and thus their resulting impact on ozone depletion is comparatively small [574,575]. Historically, CFCs have been considered the dominant ozone-depleting substances but N_2O shares many similarities with the CFCs and N_2O emission has been highlighted as ". . . the single most important ozone-depleting emission and is expected to remain the largest throughout the 21st century . . ." [576]. The inhalation anesthetics, including N_2O, are not regulated by the 1987 Montreal Protocol on Substances that Deplete the Ozone Layer (the Montreal Protocol to the Vienna Convention for the Protection of the Ozone Layer is an international agreement designed to protect the ozone layer, ratified by 197 states) [577]. Although the magnitude of stratospheric impact of halothane and isoflurane is controversial, there is increasing concern that as a result of the effectiveness of the Montreal Protocol and associated efforts to decrease CFCs globally, the influence of the volatile anesthetics on ozone depletion is becoming proportionally more important [574].

As noted previously, both N_2O and the volatile agents affect global warming. The impact of the volatile agents is small relative to the much larger players such as CO_2 and methane, so present debate relates more to their potential status [574,575,578–581]. For example, in their recently published assessment of the impact on global climate of general anesthetic gases, Sulbaek Andersen *et al.* [575] estimated that "the inhaled anesthetics released during the approximately 200 million anesthetic procedures performed globally each year, globally have a climate impact that is approximately 0.01% . . . of that of the CO_2 released from global fossil fuel combustion." Regardless, the majority of impacts of inhalation anesthetics are due to desflurane, which has the highest heat trapping effect of the inhalation anesthetics [578,579,582,583], and N_2O which is released to the atmosphere in the greatest quantity [570,572,573,575,578,583]. In an attempt to provide contemporary comparative relevance, Ryan and Nielsen [578] note that, on an hourly basis and given the US average of 398 g of CO_2 emissions/mile of auto driving, ". . . using desflurane equates with driving 235–470 miles per hour of anesthetic use, whereas sevoflurane and isoflurane equate with driving 18 and 20–40 miles per hour of anesthetic use, respectively."

In conclusion, while the contributions of N_2O and volatile anesthetics are relatively low compared to other produced substances, they are intrinsically potent greenhouse gases and as such have the potential to cause harm. Accordingly, factors to reduce waste and minimize the impact of these agents on both environmental and occupational health should be considered. Recent reviews focusing on these subjects are available for further in-depth information applicable to inhalation anesthetic use in clinical veterinary medical practice (ASA website, www.asahq.org; *Greening the Operating Room and Perioperative Arena: Environmental Sustainability for Anesthesia Practice*) [584–587].

References

1 Eger EI II. *Isoflurane (Forane): A Compendium and Reference*, 2nd edn. Madison, WI: Anaquest, 1985.

2 Soma LR. *Textbook of Veterinary Anesthesia*. Baltimore, MD: Williams & Wilkins, 1971.

3 Hall LW. *Wright's Veterinary Anaesthesia and Analgesia*, 7th edn. London, UK: Baillière Tindall, 1971.

4 Lumb WV, Jones EW. *Veterinary Anesthesia*. Philadelphia, PA: Lea & Febiger, 1973.

5 Short CE. Inhalant anesthetics. In: Short CE, ed. *Principles & Practice of Veterinary Anesthesia*. Baltimore, MD: Williams & Wilkins, 1987: 70–90.

6 Steffey EP, Mama KR. Inhalation anesthetics. In: Tranquilli WJ, Thurmon JC, Grimm KA, eds. *Lumb and Jones' Veterinary Anesthesia and Analgesia*, 4th edn. Ames, IA: Blackwell Publishing, 2007: 355–393.

7 Susay SR, Smith MA, Lockwood GG. The saturated vapor pressure of desflurane at various temperatures. *Anesth Analg* 1996; **83**: 864–866.
8 Lowe HJ, Ernst EA. *The Quantitative Practice of Anesthesia: Use of Closed Circuit*. Baltimore, MD: Williams & Wilkins, 1981.
9 Hill DW. *Physics Applied to Anaesthesia*, 4th edn. London, UK: Butterworth, 1980.
10 Webb AI, Weaver BMQ. Solubility of halothane in equine tissues at 37°C. *Br J Anaesth* 1981; **53**: 479–486.
11 Kety SS, Harmel MH, Broomell HT, *et al.* The solubility of nitrous oxide in blood and brain. *J Biol Chem* 1948; **173**: 487–496.
12 Wahrenbrock EA, Eger EI II, Laravuso RB, *et al.* Anesthetic uptake – of mice and men (and whales). *Anesthesiology* 1974; **40**: 19–23.
13 Coburn CM, Eger EI II. The partial pressure of isoflurane or halothane does not affect their solubility in rabbit blood or brain or human brain: inhaled anesthetics obey Henry's law. *Anesth Analg* 1986; **65**(9): 960–963.
14 Soares JHN, Brosnan RJ, Fukushima FB, *et al.* Solubility of haloether anesthetics in human and animal blood. *Anesthesiology* 2012; **117**(1): 48–55.
15 Targ AG, Yasuda N, Eger EI II. Solubility of I-653, sevoflurane, isoflurane, and halothane in plastics and rubber composing a conventional anesthetic circuit. *Anesth Analg* 1989; **69**: 218–225.
16 Haskins S, Sansome AL. A time-table for exhaustion of nitrous oxide cylinders using cylinder pressure. *Vet Anesth* 1979; **6**: 6–8.
17 Eger EI II. *Anesthetic Uptake and Action*. Baltimore, MD: Williams & Wilkins, 1974.
18 Mapleson WW, Allott PR, Steward A. The variability of partition coefficients for halothane in the rabbit. *Br J Anaesth* 1972; **44**: 650.
19 Eger RR, Eger EI II. Effect of temperature and age on the solubility of enflurane, halothane, isoflurane, and methoxyflurane in human blood. *Anesth Analg* 1985; **64**: 640–642.
20 Lerman J, Schmitt-Bantel BI, Gregory GA, *et al.* Effect of age on the solubility of volatile anesthetics in human tissues. *Anesthesiology* 1986; **65**(3): 307–312.
21 Eger EI II. Uptake and distribution. In: Miller RD, ed. *Anesthesia*, 5th edn. Philadelphia, PA: Churchill Livingstone, 2000: 74–95.
22 Eger EI II, Eisenkraft JB, Weiskopf RB. *The Pharmacology of Inhaled Anesthetics*, 2nd edn. San Francisco, CA: Dannemiller Memorial Educational Foundation, 2003.
23 Mapleson WW. Pharmacokinetics of inhalational anaesthetics. In: Nunn JF, Utting JE, Brown BR Jr., eds. *General Anaesthesia*, 5th edn. London, UK: Butterworths, 1989: 44–59.
24 Steffey EP, Howland D Jr. Rate of change of halothane concentration in a large animal circle anesthetic system. *Am J Vet Res* 1977; **38**(12): 1993–1996.
25 Mapleson WW. The concentration of anaesthetics in closed circuits, with special reference to halothane. *I. Theoretical studies. Br J Anaesth* 1960; **32**: 298–309.
26 Eger EI II. *Nitrous Oxide/N2O*. New York: Elsevier, 1985.
27 Eger EI II. Desflurane animal and human pharmacology: aspects of kinetics, safety, and MAC. *Anesth Analg* 1992; **75**: S3–S9.
28 Webb AI. The effect of species differences in the uptake and distribution of inhalant anesthetic agents. In: Grandy J, Hildebrand S, McDonell W, *et al.*, eds. *Proceedings of the Second International Congress of Veterinary Anesthesia*. Santa Barbara, CA: Veterinary Practice Publishing Co., 1985: 27–32.
29 Staddon GE, Weaver BMQ, Webb AI. Distribution of cardiac output in anaesthetized horses. *Res Vet Sci* 1979; **27**: 38–45.
30 Eger EI II, Severinghaus JW. Effect of uneven pulmonary distribution of blood and gas on induction with inhalation anesthetics. *Anesthesiology* 1964; **25**: 620–626.
31 Stoelting RK. The effect of right to left shunt on the rate of increase of arterial anesthetic concentration. *Anesthesiology* 1972; **36**: 352–356.
32 Stoelting RK, Eger EI II. Percutaneous loss of nitrous oxide, cyclopropane, ether and halothane in man. *Anesthesiology* 1969; **30**(3): 278–283.
33 Fassoulaki A, Lockhart SH, Freire BA, *et al.* Percutaneous loss of desflurane, isoflurane, and halothane in humans. *Anesthesiology* 1991; **74**: 479–483.
34 Lockhart SH, Yasuda N, Peterson N, *et al.* Comparison of percutaneous losses of sevoflurane and isoflurane in humans. *Anesth Analg* 1991; **72**: 212–215.
35 Eger EI II, Saidman LJ. Illustrations of inhaled anesthetic uptake, including intertissue diffusion to and from fat. *Anesth Analg* 2005; **100**: 1020–1033.
36 Stoelting RK, Eger EI II. The effects of ventilation and anesthetic solubility on recovery from anesthesia: an in vivo and analog analysis before and after equilibration. *Anesthesiology* 1969; **30**(3): 290–296.
37 Eger EI II, Johnson BH. Rates of awakening from anesthesia with I-653, halothane, isoflurane, and sevoflurane – a test of the effect of anesthetic concentration and duration in rats. *Anesth Analg* 1987; **66**: 977–983.
38 Cullen BF, Eger EI II. Diffusion of nitrous oxide, cyclopropane, and halothane through human skin and amniotic membrane. *Anesthesiology* 1972; **36**: 168–173.
39 Carpenter RL, Eger EI II, Johnson BH, *et al.* Does the duration of anesthetic administration affect the pharmacokinetics or metabolism of inhaled anesthetics in humans? *Anesth Analg* 1987; **66**: 1–8.
40 Laster MJ, Taheri S, Eger EI, *et al.* Visceral losses of desflurane, isoflurane, and halothane in swine. *Anesth Analg* 1991; **73**: 209–212.
41 Baden JM, Rice SA. Metabolism and toxicity of inhaled anesthetics. In: Miller RD, ed. *Anesthesia*, 5th edn. New York: Churchill Livingstone, 2000: 147–173.
42 Cahalan MK, Johnson BH, Eger EI II. Relationship of concentrations of halothane and enflurane to their metabolism and elimination in man. *Anesthesiology* 1981; **54**: 3–8.
43 Carpenter RL, Eger EI II, Johnson BH, *et al.* The extent of metabolism of inhaled anesthetics in humans. *Anesthesiology* 1986; **65**: 201–206.
44 Fink BR. Diffusion anoxia. *Anesthesiology* 1955; **16**: 511–519.
45 Rackow H, Salanitre E, Frumin MH. Dilution of alveolar gases during nitrous oxide excretion in man. *J Appl Physiol* 1961; **16**(4): 723–728.
46 Sheffer L, Steffenson JL, Birch AA. Nitrous oxide-induced diffusion hypoxia in patients breathing spontaneously. *Anesthesiology* 1972; **37**: 436–439.
47 Van Dyke RA, Chenoweth MB, van Poznak A. Metabolism of volatile anesthetics. I. Conversion in vivo of several anesthetics to 14-CO_2 and chloride. *Biochem Pharmacol* 1964; **13**: 1239–1247.
48 Stier A, Alter H, Hessler O, *et al.* Urinary excretion of bromide in halothane anesthesia. *Anesth Analg* 1964; **43**: 723–728.
49 Rehder K, Forbes J, Alter H, *et al.* Halothane biotransformation in man: a quantitative study. *Anesthesiology* 1967; **28**: 711–715.
50 Holaday DA, Rudofsky S, Treuhaft PS. The metabolic degradation of methoxyflurane in man. *Anesthesiology* 1970; **33**(6): 579–593.
51 Mazze RI, Fujinaga M. Biotransformation of inhalational anaesthetics. In: Nunn JF, Utting JE, Brown BR, eds. *General Anaesthesia*, 5th edn. London, UK: Butterworths, 1989: 73–85.
52 Sawyer DC, Eger EI II, Bahlman SH, *et al.* Concentration dependence of hepatic halothane metabolism. *Anesthesiology* 1971; **34**: 230–235.
53 Cook TL, Beppu WJ, Hitt BA, *et al.* Renal effects and metabolism of sevoflurane in Fischer 344 rats: an in-vivo and in-vitro comparison with methoxyflurane. *Anesthesiology* 1975; **43**: 70–77.
54 Wallin RF, Regan BM, Napoli MD, *et al.* Sevoflurane: a new inhalational anesthetic agent. *Anesth Analg* 1975; **54**: 758–766.
55 Cook TL, Beppu WJ, Hitt BA, *et al.* A comparison of renal effects and metabolism of sevoflurane and methoxyflurane in enzyme-induced rats. *Anesth Analg* 1975; **54**: 829–835.
56 Martis L, Lynch S, Napoli MD, *et al.* Biotransformation of sevoflurane in dogs and rats. *Anesth Analg* 1981; **60**: 186–191.
57 Rice SA, Dooley JR, Mazze RI. Metabolism by rat hepatic microsomes of fluorinated ether anesthetics following ethanol consumption. *Anesthesiology* 1983; **58**: 237–241.
58 Aida H, Mizuno Y, Hobo S, *et al.* Cardiovascular and pulmonary effects of sevoflurane anesthesia in horses. *Vet Surg* 1996; **25**: 164–170.
59 Driessen B, Zarucco L, Steffey EP, *et al.* Serum fluoride concentrations, biochemical and histopathological changes associated with prolonged sevoflurane anaesthesia in horses. *J Vet Med A Physiol Pathol Clin Med* 2002; **49**: 337–347.
60 Steffey EP, Mama KR, Galey F, *et al.* Effects of sevoflurane dose and mode of ventilation on cardiopulmonary function and blood biochemical variables in horses. *Am J Vet Res* 2005; **66**(4): 606–614.
61 Koblin DD, Weiskopf RB, Holmes MA, *et al.* Metabolism of I-653 and isoflurane in swine. *Anesth Analg* 1989; **68**: 147–149.
62 Holaday DA, Smith FR. Clinical characteristics and biotransformation of sevoflurane in healthy human volunteers. *Anesthesiology* 1981; **54**: 100–106.
63 Frink EJ Jr, Malan TP Jr., Brown EA, *et al.* Plasma inorganic fluoride levels with sevoflurane anesthesia in morbidly obese and nonobese patients. *Anesth Analg* 1993; **76**: 1333–1337.
64 Koblin DD, Eger EI II, Johnson BH, *et al.* I-653 resists degradation in rats. *Anesth Analg* 1988; **67**: 534–539.
65 Sutton TS, Koblin DD, Gruenke LD, *et al.* Fluoride metabolites after prolonged exposure of volunteers and patients to desflurane. *Anesth Analg* 1991; **73**: 180–185.
66 Njoku D, Laster MJ, Gong DH, *et al.* Biotransformation of halothane, enflurane, isoflurane, and desflurane to trifluoroacetylated liver proteins: association between protein acylation and hepatic injury. *Anesth Analg* 1997; **84**(1): 173–178.
67 Cascorbi HF, Blake DA, Helrich M. Differences in the biotransformation of halothane in man. *Anesthesiology* 1970; **32**: 119–123.
68 Shiraishi Y, Ikeda K. Uptake and biotransformation of sevoflurane in humans: a comparative study of sevoflurane with halothane, enflurane and isoflurane. *J Clin Anesth* 1990; **2**(6): 377–380.
69 Chase RE, Holaday DA, Fiserova-Bergerova V, *et al.* The biotransformation of ethrane in man. *Anesthesiology* 1971; **35**(3): 262–267.
70 Holaday DA, Fiserova-Bergerova V, Latto IP, *et al.* Resistance of isoflurane to biotransformation in man. *Anesthesiology* 1975; **43**: 325–332.
71 Hong K, Trudell JR, O'Neil JR, *et al.* Biotransformation of nitrous oxide. *Anesthesiology* 1980; **53**: 354–355.
72 Hong K, Trudell JR, O'Neil JR, *et al.* Metabolism of nitrous oxide by human and rat intestinal contents. *Anesthesiology* 1980; **52**: 16–19.

73 Merkel G, Eger EI II. A comparative study of halothane and halopropane anesthesia: including method for determining equipotency. *Anesthesiology* 1963; **24**(3): 346–357.
74 deJong RH, Eger EI II. MAC expanded: AD50 and AD95 values of common inhalation anesthetics in man. *Anesthesiology* 1975; **42**: 408–419.
75 Stanski DR. Monitoring depth of anesthesia. In: Miller RD, ed. *Anesthesia*, 5th edn. Philadelphia, PA: Churchill Livingstone, 2000: 1087–1116.
76 Steffey EP, Howland D Jr., Giri S, *et al.* Enflurane, halothane and isoflurane potency in horses. *Am J Vet Res* 1977; **38**: 1037–1039.
77 Ludders JW, Mitchell GS, Schaefer SI. Minimum anesthetic dose and cardiopulmonary response for halothane in chickens. *Am J Vet Res* 1988; **49**: 929–933.
78 Eger EI II, Johnson BH, Weiskopf RB, *et al.* Minimum alveolar concentration of I-653 and isoflurane in pigs: definition of a supramaximal stimulus. *Anesth Analg* 1988; **67**: 1174–1177.
79 Steffey EP. Methodology for determining minimum alveolar concentration: a critical appraisal. *Vet Anes Anal* 2017; **44**: 2–6.
80 Eger EI II, Saidman LJ, Brandstater B. Minimal alveolar anesthetic concentration: a standard of anesthetic potency. *Anesthesiology* 1965; **26**: 756–763.
81 Quasha AL, Eger EI II, Tinker JH. Determination and applications of MAC. *Anesthesiology* 1980; **53**(4): 315–334.
82 Stoelting RK, Longnecker DE, Eger EI II. Minimum alveolar concentrations in man on awakening from methoxyflurane, halothane, ether and fluroxene anesthesia: MAC awake. *Anesthesiology* 1970; **33**: 5–9.
83 Yakaitis RW, Blitt CD, Angiulo JP. End-tidal halothane concentration for endotracheal intubation. *Anesthesiology* 1977; **47**: 386–388.
84 Yakaitis RW, Blitt CD, Angiulo JP. End-tidal enflurane concentration for endotracheal intubation. *Anesthesiology* 1979; **50**: 59–61.
85 Roizen MF, Horrigan RW, Frazer BM. Anesthetic doses blocking adrenergic (stress) and cardiovascular responses to incision – MAC BAR. *Anesthesiology* 1981; **54**: 390–398.
86 Boscan P, Monnet E, Mama K, *et al.* A dog model to study ovary, ovarian ligament and visceral pain. *Vet Anaesth Analg* 2011; **38**(3): 260–266.
87 Drummond JC, Patel PM. Cerebral physiology and the effects of anesthetics and techniques. In: Miller RD, ed. *Anesthesia*, 5th edn. Philadelphia, PA: Churchill Livingstone, 2000: 695–733.
88 Rampil IJ, Mason P, Singh H. Anesthetic potency (MAC) is independent of forebrain structures in the rat. *Anesthesiology* 1993; **78**: 707–712.
89 Antognini JF, Schwartz K. Exaggerated anesthetic requirements in the preferentially anesthetized brain. *Anesthesiology* 1993; **79**: 1244–1249.
90 Rampil IJ. Anesthetic potency is not altered after hypothermic spinal cord transection in rats. *Anesthesiology* 1994; **80**: 606–610.
91 Ryu K H, Song K, Lim T-Y, *et al.* Does Equi-minimum alveolar concentration value ensure equivalent analgesic or hypnotic potency? A comparison between desflurane and sevoflurane. *Anesthesiology* **128**: 1092–1098.
92 Kharasch ED. Anesthetic MAC: origin, utility, and nomenclature revisited. *Anesthesiology* 2022; **136**: 885–887.
93 Hendrickx JFA, De Wolf AM. End-tidal anesthetic concentration: monitoring interpretation, and clinical application. *Anesthesiology* 2022; **136**: 985–996.
94 McMurphy RM, Hodgson DS. The minimum alveolar concentration of desflurane in cats. *Vet Surg* 1995; **24**: 453–455.
95 Barter LS, Ilkiw JE, Steffey EP, *et al.* Animal dependence of inhaled anaeshtetic requirements in cats. *Br J Anaesth* 2004; **92**(2): 275–277.
96 Webb AI, McMurphy RM. Effect of anticholinergic preanesthetic medicaments on the requirements of halothane for anesthesia in the cat. *Am J Vet Res* 1987; **48**: 1733–1736.
97 Ide T, Sakurai Y, Aono M, *et al.* Minimum alveolar anesthetic concentrations for airway occlusion in cats: a new concept of minimum alveolar anesthetic concentration airway occlusion response. *Anesth Analg* 1998; **86**(1): 191–197.
98 Steffey EP, Gillespie JR, Berry JD, *et al.* Anesthetic potency (MAC) of nitrous oxide in the dog, cat and stumptail monkey. *J Appl Physiol* 1974; **36**: 530–532.
99 Drummond JC, Todd MM, Shapiro HM. Minimal alveolar concentrations for halothane, enflurane, and isoflurane in the cat. *J Am Vet Med Assoc* 1983; **182**: 1099–1101.
100 Ilkiw JE, Pascoe PJ, Fisher LD. Effect of alfentanil on the mimimum alveolar concentration of isoflurane in cats. *Am J Vet Res* 1997; **58**(11): 1274–1279.
101 Steffey EP, Howland D Jr. Isoflurane potency in the dog and cat. *Am J Vet Res* 1977; **38**: 1833–1836.
102 Pypendop BH, Ilkiw JE. The effects of intravenous lidocaine administration on the minimum alveolar concentration of isoflurane in cats. *Anesth Analg* 2005; **100**(1): 97–101.
103 Doi M, Yunoki H, Ikeda K. The minimum alveolar concentration of sevoflurane in cats. *J Anesth* 1988; **2**: 113–114.
104 Steffey EP, Howland D Jr. Halothane anesthesia in calves. *Am J Vet Res* 1979; **40**: 372–376.
105 Cantalapierdra AG, Villanueva B, Pereira JL. Anaesthetic potency of isoflurane in cattle: determination of the minimum alveolar concentration. *Vet Anaesth Analg* 2000; **27**(1): 22–26.
106 Doorley MB, Waters SJ, Terrell RC, Robinson JL. MAC of I-653 in Beagle dogs and New Zealand white rabbits. *Anesthesiology* 1988; **69**: 89–92.
107 Wang BG, Tang J, White PF, *et al.* The effect of GP683, an adenosine kinase inhibitor, on the desflurane anesthetic requirement in dogs. *Anesth Analg* 1997; **85**: 675–680.
108 Hammond RA, Alibhai HIK, Walsh KP, *et al.* Desflurane in the dog; minimum alveolar concentration (MAC) alone and in combination with nitrous oxide. *J Vet Anaesth* 1994; **21**: 21–23.
109 Eger EI II, Saidman LJ, Brandstater B. Temperature dependence of halothane and cylcopropane anesthesia in dogs: correlation with some theories of anesthetic action. *Anesthesiology* 1965; **26**(6): 764–770.
110 Eger EI II, Brandstater B, Saidman LJ, *et al.* Equipotent alveolar concentrations of methoxyflurane, halothane, diethyl ether, fluroxene, cyclopropane, xenon, and nitrous oxide in the dog. *Anesthesiology* 1965; **26**(6): 771–777.
111 Regan MJ, Eger EI II. Effect of hypothermia in dogs on anesthetizing and apneic doses of inhalation agents. Determination of the anesthetic index (apnea/MAC). *Anesthesiology* 1967; **28**(4): 689–700.
112 Steffey EP, Farver TB, Woliner MJ. Circulatory and respiratory effects of methoxyflurane in dogs: comparison of halothane. *Am J Vet Res* 1984; **45**: 2574–2579.
113 Kazama T, Ikeda K. Comparison of MAC and the rate of rise of alveolar concentration of sevoflurane with halothane and isoflurane in the dog. *Anesthesiology* 1988; **68**: 435–438.
114 Steffey EP, Eger EI II. Hyperthermia and halothane MAC in the dog. *Anesthesiology* 1974; **41**(4): 392–396.
115 Himez RS Jr., DiFazio CA, Burmey RC. Effects of lidocaine on the anesthetic requirements of nitrous oxide and halothane. *Anesthesiology* 1977; **47**: 437–440.
116 Steffey EP, Baggot JD, Eisele JH, *et al.* Morphine–isoflurane interaction in dogs, swine and rhesus monkeys. *J Vet Pharmacol Ther* 1994; **17**: 202–210.
117 Schwieger IM, Szlam F, Hug CC. Absence of agonistic or antagonistic effect of flumazenil (Ro 15-1788) in dogs anesthetized with enflurane, isoflurane, or fentanyl- enflurane. *Anesthesiology* 1989; **70**(3): 477–481.
118 Schwartz AE, Maneksha FR, Kanchuger MS, *et al.* Flumazenil decreases the minimum alveolar concentration of isoflurane in dogs. *Anesthesiology* 1989; **70**(5): 764–767.
119 Scheller MS, Nakakimura K, Fleischer JE, Zornow MH. Cerebral effects of sevoflurane in the dog: comparison with isoflurane and enflurane. *Br J Anaesth* 1990; **65**: 388–392.
120 Murat I, Housmans PR. Minimum alveolar concentrations of halothane, enflurane, and isoflurane in ferrets. *Anesthesiology* 1988; **68**(5): 783–787.
121 Imai A, Steffey EP, Farver TB, *et al.* Assessment of isoflurane-induced anesthesia in ferrets and rats. *Am J Vet Res* 1999; **60**(12): 1577–1583.
122 Hikasa Y, Okuyama K, Kakuta T, *et al.* Anesthetic potency and cardiopulmonary effects of sevoflurane in goats: comparison with isoflurane and halothane. *Can J Vet Res* 1998; **62**: 299–306.
123 Antognini JF, Eisele PH. Anesthetic potency and cardiopulmonary effects of enflurane, halothane, and isoflurane in goats. *Lab Anim Sci* 1993; **43**: 607–610.
124 Doherty TJ, Rohrbach BW, Geiser DR. Effect of acepromazine and butorphanol on isoflurane minimum alveolar concentration in goats. *J Vet Pharmacol Ther* 2002; **25**: 65–67.
125 Doherty TJ, Rohrbach BW, Ross L, Schultz H. The effect of tiletamine and zolazepam on isoflurane minimum alveolar concentration in goats. *J Vet Pharmacol Ther* 2002; **25**(3): 233–235.
126 Doherty TJ, Will WA, Rohrbach BW, Geiser DR. Effect of morphine and flunixin meglumine on isoflurane minimum alveolar concentration in goats. *Vet Anaesth Analg* 2004; **31**(2): 97–101.
127 Tendillo FJ, Mascias A, Santos M, *et al.* Anesthetic potency of desflurane in the horse: determination of the minimum alveolar concentration. *Vet Surg* 1997; **26**(4): 354–357.
128 Steffey EP, Woliner MJ, Puschner B, Galey F. Effects of desflurane and mode of ventilation on cardiovascular and respiratory functions and clinicopathologic variables in horses. *Am J Vet Res* 2005; **66**(4): 669–677.
129 Steffey EP, Willits N, Woliner M. Hemodynamic and respiratory responses to variable arterial partial pressure of oxygen in halothane-anesthetized horses during spontaneous and controlled ventilation. *Am J Vet Res* 1992; **53**: 1850–1858.
130 Pascoe PJ, Steffey EP, Black WD, *et al.* Evaluation of the effect of alfentanil on the minimum alveolar concentration on halothane in horses. *Am J Vet Res* 1993; **54**: 1327–1332.
131 Bennett RC, Steffey EP, Kollias-Baker C, *et al.* Influence of morphine sulfate on the halothane sparing effect of xylazine hydrochloride in horses. *Am J Vet Res* 2004; **65**(4): 519–526.
132 Steffey EP, Eisele JH, Baggot JD. Interactions of morphine and isoflurane in horses. *Am J Vet Res* 2003; **64**(2): 166–175.

133 Steffey EP, Pascoe PJ. Detomidine reduces isoflurane anesthetic requirement (MAC) in horses. *Vet Anaesth Analg* 2002; **29**(4): 223–227.
134 Steffey EP, Pascoe PJ, Woliner MJ, *et al.* Effects of xylazine hydrochloride during isoflurane-induced anesthesia in horses. *Am J Vet Res* 2000; **61**(10): 1225–1231.
135 Aida H, Mizuno Y, Hobo S, *et al.* Determination of the minimum alveolar concentration (MAC) and physical response to sevoflurane inhalation in horses. *J Vet Med Sci* 1994; **56**: 1161–1165.
136 Steffey EP, Howland D Jr. Potency of halothane-N_2O in the horse. *Am J Vet Res* 1978; **39**: 1141–1146.
137 Tinker JH, Sharbough FW, Michenfelder TD. Anterior shift of the dominant EEG rhythm during anesthesia in the Java monkey. *Anesthesiology* 1977; **46**: 252–259.
138 Sonner JM, Gong D, Eger EI II. Naturally occurring variability in anesthetic potency among inbred mouse strains. *Anesth Analg* 2000; **91**: 720–726.
139 Mazze RI, Rice SA, Baden JM. Halothane, isoflurane, and enflurane MAC in pregnant and nonpregnant female and male mice and rats. *Anesthesiology* 1985; **62**: 339–342.
140 Deady JR, Koblin DD, Eger EI II, *et al.* Anesthetic potencies and the unitary theory of narcosis. *Anesth Analg* 1981; **60**: 380–384.
141 Dahan A, Sarton E, Teppema L, *et al.* Anesthetic potency and influence of morphine and sevoflurane on respiration in mu-opioid receptor knockout mice. *Anesthesiology* 2001; **94**: 824–832.
142 Miller KW, Paton WDM, Smith EB, *et al.* Physiochemical approaches to the mode of action of general anesthetics. *Anesthesiology* 1972; **36**: 339–351.
143 Lerman J, Oyston JP, Gallagher TM, *et al.* The minimum alveolar concentration (MAC) and hemodynamic effects of halothane, isoflurane, and sevoflurane in newborn swine. *Anesthesiology* 1990; **73**: 717–721.
144 Tranquilli WJ, Thurmon JC, Benson GJ, *et al.* Halothane potency in pigs (Sus. scrofa). *Am J Vet Res* 1983; **44**: 1106–1107.
145 Weiskopf R, Bogetz MS. Minimum alveolar concentrations (MAC) of halothane and nitrous oxide in swine. *Anesth Analg* 1984; **63**: 529–532.
146 Lundeen G, Manohar M, Parks C. Systemic distribution of blood flow in swine while awake and during 1.0 and 1.5 MAC isoflurane anesthesia with or without 50% nitrous oxide. *Anesth Analg* 1983; **62**: 499–512.
147 Eisele PH, Talken L, Eisele JH Jr. Potency of isoflurane and nitrous oxide in conventional swine. *Lab Anim Sci* 1985; **35**: 76–78.
148 Tranquilli WJ, Thurmon JC, Benson GJ. Anesthetic potency of nitrous oxide in young swine (Sus scrofa). *Am J Vet Res* 1985; **46**: 58–61.
149 Gallagher TM, Burrows FA, Miyasaka K, *et al.* Sevoflurane in newborn swine: anesthetic requirements (MAC) and circulatory responses. *Anesthesiology* 1987; **67**: A503.
150 Hecker KE, Baumert JH, Horn N, *et al.* Minimum anesthetic concentration of sevoflurane with different xenon concentrations in swine. *Anesth Analg* 2003; **97**(5): 1364–1369.
151 Manohar M, Parks CM. Porcine systemic and regional organ blood flow during 1.0 and 1.5 minimum alveolar concentrations of sevoflurane anesthesia without and with 50% nitrous oxide. *J Pharmacol Exp Ther* 1984; **231**(3): 640–648.
152 Wear R, Robinson S, Gregory GA. Effect of halothane on baroresponse of adult and baby rabbits. *Anesthesiology* 1982; **56**: 188–191.
153 Davis NL, Nunnally RL, Malinin TI. Determination of the minimum alveolar concentration (MAC) of halothane in the white New Zealand rabbit. *Br J Anaesth* 1975; **47**: 341–345.
154 Sobair ATH, Cottrell DF, Camburn MA. Focal heat stimulation for the determination of the minimum alveolar concentration of halothane in the rabbit. *Vet Res Commun* 1997; **21**: 149–159.
155 Drummond JC. MAC for halothane, enflurane, and isoflurane in the New Zealand white rabbit: and a test for the validity of MAC determinations. *Anesthesiology* 1985; **62**(3): 336–339.
156 Imai A, Steffey EP, Ilkiw JE, *et al.* Comparison of clinical signs and hemodynamic variables used to monitor rabbits during halothane- and isoflurane-induced anesthesia. *Am J Vet Res* 1999; **60**(10): 1189–1195.
157 McLain GE, Sipes IG, Brown B, Thompson MF. The noncompetitive N-methyl-D-aspartate receptor antagonist, MK-810 profoundly reduces volatile anesthetic requirements. *Neuropharmacology* 1989; **28**: 677–681.
158 Shi WZ, Fahey MR, Fisher DM, *et al.* Increase in minimum alveolar concentration (MAC) of halothane by laudanosine in rabbits. *Anesth Analg* 1985; **64**: 282.
159 Scheller MS, Saidman LJ, Partridge BL. MAC of sevoflurane in humans and the New Zealand white rabbit. *Can J Anaesth* 1988; **35**: 153–157.
160 Eger EI II, Johnson BH. MAC of I-653 in rats, including a test of the effect of body temperature and anesthetic duration. *Anesth Analg* 1987; **66**: 974–977.
161 Yost CS, Hampson AJ, Leonoudakis D, *et al.* Oleamide potentiates benzodiazepine-sensitive g-aminobutyric acid receptor activity but does not alter minimum alveolar anesthetic concentration. *Anesth Analg* 1998; **86**: 1294–1300.
162 Laster MJ, Liu J, Eger EI II, *et al.* Electrical stimulation as a substitute for the tail clamp in the determination of minimum alveolar concentration. *Anesth Analg* 1993; **76**: 1310–1312.
163 Taheri S, Halsey MJ, Liu J, *et al.* What solvent best represents the site of action of inhaled anesthetics in humans, rats, and dogs? *Anesth Analg* 1991; **72**: 627–634.
164 Vitez TS, White PF, Eger EI II. Effects of hypothermia on halothane MAC and isoflurane MAC in the rat. *Anesthesiology* 1974; **41**: 80–81.
165 Cole DJ, Kalichman MW, Shapiro HM, *et al.* The nonlinear potency of sub-MAC concentrations of nitrous oxide in decreasing the anesthetic requirement of enflurane, halothane, and isoflurane in rats. *Anesthesiology* 1990; **73**: 93–99.
166 Steffey MA, Brosnan RJ, Steffey EP. Assessment of halothane and sevoflurane anesthesia in spontaneously breathing rats. *Am J Vet Res* 2003; **64**(4): 470–474.
167 Crawford MW, Lerman J, Saldivia V, *et al.* Hemodynamic and organ blood flow responses to halothane and sevoflurane anesthesia during spontaneous ventilation. *Anesth Analg* 1992; **75**: 1000–1006.
168 White PF, Johnston RR, Eger EI II. Determination of anesthetic requirement in rats. *Anesthesiology* 1974; **40**: 52–57.
169 Strout CD, Nahrwold MC. Halothane requirement during pregnancy and lactation in rats. *Anesthesiology* 1981; **55**: 322–323.
170 Roizen MF, White PF, Eger EI II, *et al.* Effects of ablation of serotonin or norepinephrine brain-stem areas on halothane and cyclopropane MACs in rats. *Anesthesiology* 1978; **49**: 252–255.
171 Waizer PR, Baez S, Orkin LR. A method for determining minimum alveolar concentration of anesthetic in the rat. *Anesthesiology* 1973; **39**: 394–397.
172 Russell GB, Graybeal JM. Differences in anesthetic potency between Sprague–Dawley and Long–Evans rats for isoflurane but not nitrous oxide. *Pharmacology* 1995; **50**: 162–167.
173 Rampil IJ, Laster M. No correlation between quantitative electroencephalographic measures and movement response to noxious stimuli during isoflurane anesthesia in rats. *Anesthesiology* 1992; **77**(5): 920–925.
174 DiFazio CA, Brown RE, Ball CG, *et al.* Additive effects of anesthetics and theories of anesthesia. *Anesthesiology* 1972; **36**: 57–63.
175 Russell GB, Graybeal JM. Direct measurement of nitrous oxide MAC and neurologic monitoring in rats during anesthesia under hyperbaric conditions. *Anesth Analg* 1992; **75**: 995–999.
176 Wolfson B, Hebrick WD, Lake CL, *et al.* Anesthetic indices – further data. *Anesthesiology* 1978; **48**: 187–190.
177 Gonsowski CT, Eger EI II. Nitrous oxide minimum alveolar anesthetic concentration in rats is greater than previously reported. *Anesth Analg* 1994; **79**: 710–712.
178 Palahniuk RJ, Shnider SM, Eger EI II. Pregnancy decreases the requirement for inhaled anesthetic agents. *Anesthesiology* 1974; **41**: 82–83.
179 Rampil IJ, Lockhart SH, Zwass MS, *et al.* Clinical characteristics of desflurane in surgical patients – minimum alveolar concentration. *Anesthesiology* 1991; **74**: 429–433.
180 Miller RD, Wahrenbrock EA, Schroeder CF, *et al.* Ethylene–halothane anesthesia: addition or synergism? *Anesthesiology* 1969; **31**: 301–304.
181 Saidman LJ, Eger EI II. Effect of nitrous oxide and of narcotic premedication on the alveolar concentration of halothane required for anesthesia. *Anesthesiology* 1964; **25**: 302–306.
182 Gibbons RT, Steffey EP, Eger EI II. The effect of spontaneous versus controlled ventilation on the rate of rise of alveolar halothane concentration in dogs. *Anesth Analg* 1977; **56**: 32–34.
183 Saidman LJ, Eger EI II, Munson ES, *et al.* Minimum alveolar concentrations of methoxyflurane, halothane, ether and cyclopropane in man: correlation with theories of anesthesia. *Anesthesiology* 1967; **28**: 994–1002.
184 Stevens WC, Dolan WM, Gibbons RD, *et al.* Minimum alveolar concentrations (MAC) of isoflurane with and without nitrous oxide in patients of various ages. *Anesthesiology* 1975; **42**: 197–200.
185 Kimura T, Watanabe S, Asakura N, *et al.* Determination of end-tidal sevoflurane concentration for tracheal intubation and minimum alveolar anesthetic concentration in adults. *Anesth Analg* 1994; **79**: 378–381.
186 Katoh T, Ikeda K. The minimum alveolar concentration (MAC) of sevoflurane in humans. *Anesthesiology* 1987; **66**: 301–304.
187 Katoh T, Ikeda K. The effect of clonidine on sevoflurane requirements for anaesthesia and hypnosis. *Anaesthesia* 2005; **52**: 364–381.
188 Katoh T, Ikeda K. The effects of fentanyl on sevoflurane requirements for loss of consciousness and skin incision. *Anesthesiology* 1998; **88**: 18–24.
189 Katoh T, Kobayashi S, Suzuki A, *et al.* The effect of fentanyl on sevoflurane requirements for somatic and sympathetic responses to surgical incision. *Anesthesiology* 1999; **90**(2): 398–405.
190 Suzuki A, Katoh T, Ikeda K. The effect of adenosine triphosphate on sevoflurane requirements for minimum alveolar anesthetic concentration and minimum alveolar anesthetic concentration awake. *Anesth Analg* 1998; **86**(1): 179–183.
191 Hornbein TF, Eger EI II, Winter PM, *et al.* The minimum alveolar concentration on nitrous oxide in man. *Anesth Analg* 1982; **61**: 553–556.
192 Martin-Jurado O, Vogt R, Knutter APN, *et al.* Effect of inhalation of isoflurane at end-tidal concentrations greater than, equal to, and less than the minimum

anesthetic concentration on bispectral index in chickens. *Am J Vet Res* 2008; **69**(10): 1254–1261.
193 Curro TG, Brunson DB, Paul-Murphy J. Determination of the ED50 of isoflurane and evaluation of the isoflurane-sparing effect of butorphanol in cockatoos (Cacatua spp.). *Vet Surg* 1994; **23**: 429–433.
194 Ludders JW, Rode J, Mitchell GS. Isoflurane anesthesia in sandhill cranes (Grus canadensis): minimal anesthetic concentration and cardiopulmonary dose–response during spontaneous and controlled breathing. *Anesth Analg* 1989; **68**: 511–516.
195 Ludders JW, Mitchell GS, Rode J. Minimal anesthetic concentration and cardiopulmonary dose response of isoflurane in ducks. *Vet Surg* 1990; **19**: 304–307.
196 Fitzgerald G, Blais D. Effect of nitrous oxide on the minimal anesthetic dose of isoflurane in pigeons and red-tailed hawks. In: *Proceedings of the 4th International Congress of Veterinary Anaesthesia*, Utrecht, Netherlands, 1991: 27.
197 Escobar A, Valadao CAA, Brosnan RJ, *et al.* Effects of butorphanol on the minimum anesthetic concentration for sevoflurane in guineafowl (Numida meleagris). *Am J Vet Res* 2012; **73**(2): 183–188.
198 Pavez JC, Hawkins MG, Pascoe PJ, *et al.* Effect of fentanyl target-controlled infusions on isoflurane minimum anaesthetic concentration and cardiovascular function in red-tailed hawks (Buteo jamaicensis). *Vet Anaesth Analg* 2011; **38**(4): 344–351.
199 Mercado JA, Larsen RS, Wack RF, *et al.* Minimum anesthetic concentration of isoflurane in captive thick-billed parrots (Rhynchopsitta pachyrhyncha). *Am J Vet Res* 2008; **69**(2): 189–194.
200 Smith J, Mason DE, Muir WW III. The influence of midazolam on the minimum anesthetic concentration of isoflurane in racing pigeons. *Vet Surg* 1993; **22**(6): 546–547.
201 Cherkin A, Catchpool JF. Temperature dependence of anesthesia in goldfish. *Science* 1964; **144**: 1460–1462.
202 Shim CY, Andersen NB. The effects of oxygen on minimal anesthetic requirements in the toad. *Anesthesiology* 1971; **34**: 333–337.
203 Steffey EP, Eger EI II. Nitrous oxide in veterinary practice and animal research. In: Eger EI II, ed. *Nitrous Oxide/N2O*. New York, NY: Elsevier, 1984: 305–312.
204 Wouters P, Doursout MF, Merin RG, *et al.* Influence of hypertension on MAC of halothane in rats. *Anesthesiology* 1990; **72**: 843–845.
205 Zucker J. Central cholinergic depression reduces MAC for isoflurane in rats. *Anesth Analg* 1991; **72**: 790–795.
206 White PF, Johnston RR, Pudwill CR. Interaction of ketamine and halothane in rats. *Anesthesiology* 1975; **42**: 179–186.
207 Stone DJ, Moscicki JC, DiFazio CA. Thiopental reduces halothane MAC in rats. *Anesth Analg* 1992; **74**: 542–546.
208 Doherty TJ, Geiser DR, Rohrbach BW. Effect of acepromazine and butorphanol on halothane minimum alveolar concentration in ponies. *Equine Vet J* 1997; **29**(5): 374–376.
209 Heard DJ, Webb AI, Daniels RT. Effect of acepromazine on the anesthetic requirement of halothane in the dog. *Am J Vet Res* 1986; **47**: 2113–2116.
210 Webb AI, Obrien JM. The effect of acepromazine maleate on the anesthetic potency of halothane and isoflurane. *J Am Anim Hosp Assoc* 1988; **24**(6): 609–615.
211 Matthews NS, Dollar NS, Shawley RV. Halothane-sparing effect of benzodiazepines in ponies. *Cornell Vet* 1990; **80**: 259–265.
212 Hellyer PW, Mama KR, Shafford HL, *et al.* Effects of diazepam and flumazenil on minimum alveolar concentrations for dogs anestetized with isoflurane or a combination of isoflurane and fentanyl. *Am J Vet Res* 2001; **62**(4): 555–560.
213 Perisho JA, Buechel DR, Miller RD. The effect of diazepam on minimum alveolar anesthetic requirement (MAC) in man. *Can Anaesth Soc J* 1971; **18**: 536.
214 Murphy MR, Hug CC Jr. The anesthetic potency of fentanyl in terms of its reduction of enflurane MAC. *Anesthesiology* 1982; **57**: 485–488.
215 Ewing KK, Mohammed HO, Scarlett JM, *et al.* Reduction of isoflurane anesthetic requirement by medetomidine and its restoration by atipamezole in dogs. *Am J Vet Res* 1993; **54**: 294–299.
216 Gross ME, Clifford CA, Hardy DA. Excitement in an elephant after intravenous administration of atropine. *J Am Vet Med Assoc* 1994; **205**(10): 1437–1438.
217 Steffey EP, Martucci R, Howland D, *et al.* Meperidine–halothane interaction in dogs. *Can Anaesth Soc J* 1977; **24**(4): 459–467.
218 Melvin MA, Johnson BH, Quasha AL, *et al.* Induction of anesthesia with midazolam decreases halothane MAC in humans. *Anesthesiology* 1982; **57**(3): 238–241.
219 Lambert-Zechovsky N, Bingen E, Bourillon A, *et al.* Effects of antibiotics on the microbial intestinal ecosystem. *Dev Pharmacol Ther* 1984; **7**(1): 150–157.
220 Doherty TJ, McDonell WN, Dyson DH, *et al.* The effect of a 5-hydroxytryptamine antagonist (R51703) on halothane MAC in the dog. *J Vet Pharmacol Ther* 1995; **18**: 153–155.
221 Sonner JM, Antognini JF, Dutton RC, *et al.* Inhaled anesthetics and immobility: mechanisms, mysteries, and minimum alveolar anesthetic concentration. *Anesth Analg* 2003; **97**(3): 718–740.
222 Fischer E. Einfluss der configuration auf die wirkung der enzyme. *Der Dtsch Chem Ges* 1894; **27**: 2985–2993.
223 Brosnan RJ, Eger EI II, Laster MJ, *et al.* Anesthetic properties of carbon dioxide in the rat. *Anesth Analg* 2007; **105**(1): 103–106.
224 Brosnan RJ, Yang L, Milutinovic PS, *et al.* Ammonia has anesthetic properties. *Anesth Analg* 2007; **104**(6): 1430–1433.
225 Won A, Oh I, Liao M, *et al.* The minimum alveolar anesthetic concentration of 2-, 3-, and 4- alcohols and ketones in rats: relevance to anesthetic mechanisms. *Anesth Analg* 2006; **102**(5): 1419–1426.
226 Nunn JF, Sturrock JE, Willis EJ, *et al.* The effect of inhalational anaesthetics on the swimming velocity of Tetrahymena pyriformis. *J Cell Sci* 1974; **15**: 537–554.
227 Livingston JS. On the anaesthetic effects of chloroform, ether, and amylene on sensitive plants. *Trans Bot Soc Edinburgh* 1860; **6**: 323–325.
228 Winter PM, Burce DL, Bach MJ, *et al.* The anesthetic effect of air at atmospheric pressure. *Anesthesiology* 1975; **42**: 658–661.
229 Brosnan RJ, Ramos K, Aguiar AJA, *et al.* Anesthetic pharmacology of the mint extracts L-carvone and methyl salicylate. *Pharmacology* 2022; **107**: 167–178.
230 Meyer H. Zur theorie der alkoholnarkose. *Naunyn-Schmiedeberg Arch Pharmacol* 1899; **42**: 109–118.
231 Overton CE. *Studies of Narcosis*. London, UK: Chapman and Hall, 1991.
232 Brosnan R, Gong D, Cotten J, *et al.* Chirality in anesthesia II: stereoselective modulation of ion channel function by secondary alcohol enantiomers. *Anesth Analg* 2006; **103**(1): 86–91.
233 Koblin DD, Chortkoff BS, Laster MJ, *et al.* Polyhalogenated and perfluorinated compounds that disobey the Meyer–Overton hypothesis. *Anesth Analg* 1994; **79**: 1043–1048.
234 Cantor RS. Breaking the Meyer–Overton rule: predicted effects of varying stiffness and interfacial activity on the intrinsic potency of anesthetics. *Biophys J* 2001; **80**(5): 2284–2297.
235 Cantor RS. Breaking the Meyer–Overton rule: predicted effects of varying stiffness and interfacial activity on the intrinsic potency of anesthetics. *Biophys J* 2001; **80**: 2284–2297.
236 Fabian B, Sega M, Voloshin VP, *et al.* Lateral pressure profile and free volume properties in phospholipid membranes containing anesthetics. *J Phys Chem B* 2017; **121**: 2814–2824.
237 Booker RD, Sum AK. Biophysical changes induced by xenon on phospholipid bilayers. *Biochem Biophys Acta* 2013; **1828**: 1347–1356.
238 Reigada R. Atomistic study of lipid membranes containing chloroform: looking for a lipid-mediated mechanism of anesthesia. *PLoS ONE* 2013; **8**: e52631.
239 Darvas M, Hoang PN, Picaud S, *et al.* Anestheti molecules embedded in a alipid membrane: a computer simulation study. *Phys Chem Chem Phys* 2012; **14**: 12956–12969.
240 Herold KF, Sanford RL, Lee W, *et al.* Clinical concentrations of chemically diverse general anesthetics minimally affect lipid bilayer properties. *Proc Natl Acad Sci USA* 2017; **114**: 3109–3114.
241 Miller SL. A theory of gaseous anesthetics. *Proc Natl Acad Sci USA* 1961; **47**: 1515–1524.
242 Pauling L. A molecular theory of general anesthesia. *Science* 1961; **134**: 15–21.
243 Miller KW, Paton WD, Smith EB. Site of action of general anaesthetics. *Nature* 1965; **206**: 574–577.
244 Eger EI II, Lundgren C, Miller SL, *et al.* Anesthetic potencies of sulfur hexafluoride, carbon tetrafluoride, chloroform and ethrane in dogs: correlation with the hydrate and lipid theories of anesthetic action. *Anesthesiology* 1969; **30**(2): 129–135.
245 Willenbring D, Xu Y, Tang P. The role of structured water in mediating general anesthetic action on alpha4beta2 nAChR. *Phys Chem Chem Phys* 2010; **12**: 10263–10269.
246 Franks NP, Lieb WR. Do general anaesthetics act by competitive binding to specific receptors? *Nature* 1984; **310**: 599–602.
247 Xie Z, McMillan K, Pike CM, *et al.* Interaction of anesthetics with neurotransmitter release machinery proteins. *J Neurophysiol* 2013; **109**: 758–767.
248 Nagele P, Mendel JB, Placzek WJ, *et al.* Volatile anesthetics bind rat synaptic snare proteins. *Anesthesiology* 2005; **103**: 768–778.
249 Miao N, Frazer MJ, Lynch C III. Volatile anesthetics depress Ca2+ transients and glutamate release in isolated cerebral synaptosomes. *Anesthesiology* 1995; **83**: 593–603.
250 Wang HY, Eguchi K, Yamashita T, *et al.* Frequency-dependent block of excitatory neurotransmission by isoflurane via dual presynaptic mechanisms. *J Neurosci* 2020; **40**: 4103–4115.
251 Hemmings HC Jr., Yan W, Westphalen RI, *et al.* The general anesthetic isoflurane depresses synaptic vesicle exocytosis. *Mol Pharmacol* 2005; **67**: 1591–1599.
252 Torturo CL, Zhoụ ZY, Ryan TA, *et al.* Isoflurane inhibits dopaminergic synaptic vesicle exocytosis coupled to CaV2.2 in rat midbrain neurons. *eNeuro* 2019: 6.
253 Wu XS, Sun JY, Evers AS, *et al.* Isoflurane inhibits transmitter release and the presynaptic action potential. *Anesthesiology* 2004; **100**: 663–670.

254 Herring BE, Xie Z, Marks J, *et al.* Isoflurane inhibits the neurotransmitter release machinery. *J Neurophysiol* 2009; **102**: 1265–1273.

255 Baumgart JP, Zhou ZY, Hara M, *et al.* Isoflurane inhibits synaptic vesicle exocytosis through reduced Ca2+ influx, not Ca2+-exocytosis coupling. *Proc Natl Acad Sci USA* 2015; **112**: 11959–11964.

256 Wesphalen RI, Hemmings HC Jr. Volatile anesthetic effects on glutamate versus GABA release from isolated rat cortical nerve terminals: basal release. *J Pharmacol Exp Ther* 2006; **316**: 208–215.

257 Westphalen RI, Hemmings HC Jr. Volatile anesthetic effects on glutamate versus GABA release from isolated rat cortical nerve terminals: 4-aminopyridine-evoked release. *J Pharmacol Exp Ther* 2006; **316**: 216–223.

258 Yamakura T, Harris RA. Effects of gaseous anesthetics nitrous oxide and xenon on ligand-gated ion channels. *Comparison with isoflurane and ethanol. Anesthesiology* 2000; **93**: 1095–1101.

259 Ogata J, Shiraishi M, Namba T, *et al.* Effects of anesthetics on mutant N-methyl-D-asparate receptors expressed in Xenopus oocytes. *J Pharmacol Exp Ther* 2006; **318**; 434–443.

260 Krasowski MD, Harrison NL. The actions of ether, alcohol and alkane general anaesthetics on BABAA and glycine receptors and the effects of TM2 and TM3 mutations. *Br J Pharmacol* 2000; **129**: 731–743.

261 Violet JM, Downie DL, Nakisa RC, *et al.* Differential sensitivities of mammalian neuronal and muscle nicotinic acetylcholine receptors to general anesthetics. *Anesthesiology* 1997; **86**: 866–874.

262 Lin LH, Chen LL, Zirrolli JA, *et al.* General anesthetics potentiate gamma-aminobutyric acid actions on gamma-aminobutyric acid A receptors expressed by Xenopus oocytes: lack of involvement of intracellular calcium. *J Pharmacol Exp Ther* 1992; **263**: 569–578.

263 Downie DL, Hall AC, Lieb WR, *et al.* Effects of inhalational general anaesthetics on native glycine receptors in rat medullary neurons and recombinant glycine receptors in Xenopus oocytes. *Br J Pharmacol* 1996; **118**: 493–502.

264 Liu C, Au JD, Zou HL, *et al.* Potent activation of the human tandem pore domain K channel TRESK with clinical concentrations of volatile anesthetics. *Anesth Analg* 2004; **99**: 1715–1722.

265 Eckenhoff RG, Johansson JS. On the relevance of 'clinically relevant concentrations' of inhaled anesthetics in in vitro experiments. *Anesthesiology* 1999; **91**: 856–860.

266 Shafer SL, Hendrickx JFA, Flood P, *et al.* Additivity versus synergy: a theoretical analysis of implications for anesthetic mechanisms. *Anesth Analg* 2008; **107**(2): 507–524.

267 Eger EI II, Tang M, Liao M, *et al.* Inhaled anesthetics do not combine to produce synergistic effects regarding minimum alveolar anesthetic concentration in rats. *Anesth Analg* 2008; **107**(2): 479–485.

268 Brosnan RJ. Does anesthetic additivity imply a similar molecular mechanism of anesthetic action at N-methyl-D-aspartate receptors? *Anesth Analg* 2011; **112**: 568–573.

269 Brosnan RJ. GABA-A receptor antagonism increases NMDA receptor inhibition by isoflurane at a minimum alveolar concentration. *Vet Anaesth Analg* 2011; **38**(3): 231–239.

270 Brosnan RJ. Increased NMDA receptor inhibition at an increased sevoflurane MAC. *BMC Anesthesiol* 2012; **12**: 9.

271 Franks NP, Lieb WR. Selective actions of volatile general anaesthetics at molecular and cellular levels. *Br J Anaesth* 1993; **71**: 65–76.

272 Franks NP, Lieb WR. Temperature dependence of the potency of volatile general anesthetics implications for in vitro experiments. *Anesthesiology* 1996; **84**: 716–720.

273 Brosnan RJ, Pham TL. Hydrocarbon molar water solubility predicts NMDA vs GABAA receptor modulation. *BMC Pharmacol Toxicol* 2014; **15**: 62.

274 Brosnan RJ, Pham TL. GABAA receptor modulation by phenyl ring compounds is associated with a water solubility cut-off value. *Pharmacology* 2016; **98**: 13–19.

275 Brosnan RJ, Pham TL. Anesthetic-sensitive ion channel modulation is associated with a molar water solubility cut-off. *BMC Pharmacol Toxicol* 2018; **19**: 57.

276 Jinks SL, Atherley RJ, Dominguez CL, *et al.* Isoflurane disrupts central pattern generator activity and coordination in the lamprey isolated spinal cord. *Anesthesiology* 2005; **103**: 567–575.

277 Eger EI II, Xing Y, Pearce R, *et al.* Isoflurane antagonizes the capacity of flurothyl or 1,2-dichlorohexafluorocyclobutane to impair fear conditioning to context and tone. *Anesth Analg* 2003; **96**: 1010–1018.

278 Alkire MT, Nathan SV. Does the amygdala mediate anesthetic-induced amnesia? Basolateral amygdala lesions block sevoflurane-induced amnesia. *Anesthesiology* 2005; **102**: 754–760.

279 Ranft A, Kurz J, Deuringer M, *et al.* Isoflurane modulates glutamatergic and GABAergic neurotransmission in the amygdala. *Eur J Neurosci* 2004; **20**: 1276–1280.

280 Zhang F, Feng X, Zeng Q, *et al.* Sevoflurane induced amnesia inhibits hippocampal Arc expression partially through 5-hydroxytryptamine-7 receptors in the bilateral basolateral amygdala in rats. *Neurosci Lett* 2014; **562**: 13–18.

281 Perauansky M, Rau V, Ford T, *et al.* Slowing of the hippocampal theta rhythm correlates with anesthetic-induced amnesia. *Anesthesiology* 2010; **113**: 1299–1309.

282 Rau V, Iyer SV, Oh I, *et al.* Gamma-aminobutyric acid type A receptor alpha 4 subunit knowckout mice are resistant to the amnesic effect of isoflurane. *Anesth Analg* 2009; **109**: 1816–1822.

283 Rau V, Oh I, Liao M, *et al.* Gamma-aminobutyric acid type A receptor beta3 subunit forebrain-specific knowckout mice are resistant to the amnestic effect of isoflurane. *Anesth Analg* 2011; **113**: 500–504.

284 Zurek AA, Bridgwater EM, Orser BA. Inhibition of alpha5 gamma-aminobutyric acid type A receptors restore recognition memory after general anesthesia. *Anesth Analg* 2012; **114**: 845–855.

285 Alkire MT, Asher CD, Franciscus AM, Hahn EL. Thalamic microinfusion of antibody to a voltage-gated potassium channel restores consciousness during anesthesia. *Anesthesiology* 2009; **110**: 766–773.

286 Solt K, Van Dort CJ, Chemali JJ, *et al.* Electrical stimulation of the ventral tegmental area induces reanimation from general anesthesia. *Anesthesiology* 2014; **121**: 311–319.

287 Boyden ES, Brown EN, Solt K. Optogenetic activation of dopamine neurons in the ventral tegmental area induces reanimation from general anesthesia. *Proc Natl Acad Sci USA* 2016; **113**: 12826–12831.

288 Muindi F, Kenny JD, Taylor NE, *et al.* Electrical stimulation of the parabrachial nucleus induces reanimation from isoflurane general anesthesia. *Behav Brain Res* 2016; **306**: 20–25.

289 Wang TX, Xiong B, Xu W, *et al.* Activation of parabrachial nucleus glutamatergic neurons accelerates reanimation from sevoflurane anesthesia in mice. *Anesthesiology* 2019; **130**: 106–118.

290 Melzack R, Casey KL. Sensory, motivational and control determinants of pain; a new conceptual model. In: Kenshalo D, ed. *The Skin Senses*. Tallahassee, FL: Thomas, 1967: 423–443.

291 O'Connor TC, Abram SE. Inhibition of nociception-induced spinal sensitization by anesthetic agents. *Anesthesiology* 1995; **82**: 259–266.

292 Mitsuyo T, Dutton RC, Antognini JF, *et al.* The differential effects of halothane and isoflurane on windup of dorsal horn neurons selected in unanesthetized decerebrated rats. *Anesth Analg* 2006; **103**(3): 753–760.

293 Zhang Y, Eger EI, Dutton RC, *et al.* Inhaled anesthetics have hyperalgesic effects at 0.1 minimum alveolar anesthetic concentration. *Anesth Analg* 2000; **91**: 462–466.

294 Sonner J, Li J, Eger EI. Desflurane and nitrous oxide, but not nonimmobilizers, affect nociceptive responses. *Anesth Analg* 1998; **86**(3): 629–634.

295 Flood P, Sonner JM, Gong D, *et al.* Isoflurane hyperalgesia is modulated by nicotinic inhibition. *Anesthesiology* 2002; **97**: 192–198.

296 Yamakura T, Harris RA. Effects of gaseous anesthetics nitrous oxide and xenon on ligand-gated ion channels. *Comparison with isoflurane and ethanol. Anesthesiology* 2000; **93**: 1095–1101.

297 Zhang C, Davies MF, Guo TZ, *et al.* The analgesic action of nitrous oxide is dependent on the release of norepinephrine in the dorsal horn of the spinal cord. *Anesthesiology* 1999; **91**: 1401–1407.

298 Nakata Y, Goto T, Ishiguro Y, *et al.* Anesthetic doses of sevoflurane to block cardiovascular responses to incision when administered with xenon or nitrous oxide. *Anesthesiology* 1999; **91**: 369–373.

299 Dwyer RC, Rampil IJ, Eger EI II, Bennett HL. The electroencephalogram does not predict depth of isoflurane anesthesia. *Anesthesiology* 1994; **81**: 403–409.

300 Scheller MS, Tateishi A, Drummond JC, *et al.* The effects of sevoflurane on cerebral blood flow, cerebral metabolic rate for oxygen, intracranial pressure, and the electroencephalogram are similar to those of isoflurane in the rabbit. *Anesthesiology* 1988; **68**: 548–552.

301 Rampil IJ, Weiskopf RB, Brown JG, *et al.* I-653 and isoflurane produce similar dose-related changes in the electroencephalogram of pigs. *Anesthesiology* 1988; **69**: 298–302.

302 Rampil IJ, Lockhart SH, Eger EI II, *et al.* The electroencephalographic effects of desflurane in humans. *Anesthesiology* 1991; **74**: 434–439.

303 Neigh JL, Garman JK, Harp JR. The electroencephalographic pattern during anesthesia with Ethrane: effects of depth of anesthesia, $PaCO_2$ and nitrous oxide. *Anesthesiology* 1971; **35**: 482–487.

304 Joas TA, Stevens WC, Eger EI II. Electroencephalographic seizure activity in dogs during anaesthesia: studies with Ethrane, fluroxene, halothane, chloroform, divinyl ether, diethyl ether, methoxyflurane, cyclopropane and forane. *Br J Anaesth* 1971; **43**: 739–745.

305 Todd MM, Drummond JC. A comparison of the cerebrovascular and metabolic effects of halothane and isoflurane in the cat. *Anesthesiology* 1984; **60**: 276–282.

306 Karasawa F. The effects of sevoflurane on lidocaine-induced convulsions. *J Anesth* 1991; **5**(1): 60–67.

307 Fukuda H, Hirabayashi Y, Shimizu R, *et al.* Sevoflurane is equivalent to isoflurane for attenuating bupivacaine-induced arrhythmias and seizures in rats. *Anesth Analg* 1996; **83**: 570–573.

308 Murao K, Shingu K, Tsushima K, *et al.* The anticonvulsant effects of volatile anesthetics on penicillin-induced status epilepticus in cats. *Anesth Analg* 2000; **90**(1): 142–147.

309 Murao K, Shingu I, Tsushima K, *et al.* The anticonvulsant effects of volatile anesthetics on lidocaine-induced seizures in cats. *Anesth Analg* 2000; **90**(1): 148–155.

310 Osawa M, Shingu K, Murakawa M, *et al.* Effect of sevoflurane on central nervous system electrical activity in cats. *Anesth Analg* 1994; **79**: 52–57.

311 Woodforth IJ, Hicks RG, Crawford MR, *et al.* Electroencephalographic evidence of seizure activity under deep sevoflurane anesthesia in a nonepileptic patient. *Anesthesiology* 1997; **87**: 1579–1582.

312 Komatsu H, Tale S, Endo S, *et al.* Electrical seizures during sevoflurane anesthesia in two pediatric patients with epilepsy. *Anesthesiology* 1994; **81**: 1535–1537.

313 Cucchiara RF, Theye RA, Michenfelder JD. The effects of isoflurane on canine cerebral metabolism and blood flow. *Anesthesiology* 1974; **40**: 571–574.

314 Lutz LJ, Milde JH, Milde LN. The cerebral functional, metabolic, and hemodynamic effects of desflurane in dogs. *Anesthesiology* 1990; **73**: 125–131.

315 Munro A. *Observations on the Structure and Functions of the Nervous System.* Edinburgh: William Creech, 1783.

316 Kellie G. Account of the appearances observed in the dissection of two of three individuals presumed to have perished in the storm of the 3rd, and whose bodies were discovered in the vicinity of Leith on the morning of the 4th, November 1821: with some reflections on the pathology of the brain. *Trans Medico- Chirurgical Soc Edinb* 1824; **1**: 84–169.

317 Artru AA. Relationship between cerebral blood volume and CSF pressure during anesthesia with halothane or enflurane in dogs. *Anesthesiology* 1983; **58**(6): 533–539.

318 Holmstrom A, Akeson J. Desflurane increases intracranial pressure more and sevoflurane less than isoflurane in pigs subjected to intracranial hypertension. *J Neurosurg Anesthesiol* 2004; **16**: 136–143.

319 Lam AM, Mayberg TS, Eng CC, *et al.* Nitrous oxide-isoflurane anesthesia causes more cerebral vasodilation than an equipotent dose of isoflurane in humans. *Anesth Analg* 1994; **78**: 462–468.

320 Fukuda T, Nakayama H, Yanagi K, *et al.* The effects of 30% and 60% xenon inhalation on pial vessel diameter and intracranial pressure in rabbits. *Anesth Analg* 2001; **92**: 1245–1250.

321 Fraga M, Rama-Macerias P, Rodino S, *et al.* The effects of isoflurane and desflurane on intracranial pressure, cerebral perfusion pressure, and cerebral arteriovenous oxygen content difference in normocapnic patients with supratentorial brain tumors. *Anesthesiology* 2003; **98**: 1085–1090.

322 Matta BF, Heath KJ, Tipping K, *et al.* Direct cerebral vasodilatory effects of sevoflurane and isoflurane. *Anesthesiology* 1999; **91**: 677–680.

323 Moore LE, Kirsch J, Helfaer MA, *et al.* Nitric oxide and prostanoids contribute to isoflurane-induced cerebral hyperemia in pigs. *Anesthesiology* 1994; **80**: 1328–1337.

324 Iadecola C. Does nitric oxide mediate the increases in cerebral blood flow elicited by hypercapnia? *Proc Natl Acad Sci USA* 1992; **89**: 3913–3916.

325 Sjakste N, Baumane L, Meirena D, *et al.* Drastic increase in nitric oxide content in rat brain under halothane anesthesia revealed by EPR method. *Biochem Pharmacol* 1999; **58**: 1955–1959.

326 Todd MM, Wu B, Warner DS, *et al.* The dose-related effects of nitric oxide synthase inhibition on cerebral blood flow during isoflurane and pentobarbital anesthesia. *Anesthesiology* 1994; **80**: 1128–1136.

327 Kant GJ, Muller TW, Lenox RH, *et al.* In vivo effects of pentobarbital and halothane anesthesia on levels of adenosine 3′, 5′-monophosphate and guanosine 3′, 5′-monophosphate in rat brain regions and pituitary. *Biochem Pharmacol* 1980; **29**: 1891–1896.

328 Iida H, Ohata H, Iida M, *et al.* Isoflurane and sevoflurane induced vasodilation of cerebral vessels via ATP-sensitive K+ channel activation. *Anesthesiology* 1998; **89**: 954–960.

329 Pelligrino DA, Miletich DJ, Hoffman WE, *et al.* Nitrous oxide markedly increases cerebral cortical metabolic rate and blood flow in the goat. *Anesthesiology* 1984; **60**: 405–412.

330 Reasoner DK, Warner DS, Todd MM, *et al.* Effects of nitrous oxide on cerebral metabolic rate in rats anaesthetized with isoflurane. *Br J Anaesth* 1990; **65**: 210–215.

331 Drummond JC, Scheller MS, Todd MM. The effect of nitrous oxide on cortical cerebral blood flow during anesthesia with halothane and isoflurane, with and without morphine in the rabbit. *Anesth Analg* 1987; **66**: 1083–1089.

332 Frietsch T, Bogdanski R, Blobner M, *et al.* Effects of xenon on cerebral blood flow and cerebral glucose utilization in rats. *Anesthesiology* 2001; **94**: 290–297.

333 Fink H, Blobner M, Bogdanski R, *et al.* Effects of xenon on cerebral blood flow and autoregulation: an experimental study in pigs. *Br J Anaesth* 2000; **84**: 221–225.

334 Strebel S, Lam AM, Matta B, *et al.* Dynamic and static cerebral autoregulation during isoflurane, desflurane, and propofol anesthesia. *Anesthesiology* 1995; **83**: 66–76.

335 Hoffman WE, Edelman G, Kochs E, *et al.* Cerebral autoregulation in awake versus isoflurane-anesthetized rats. *Anesth Analg* 1991; **73**: 753–757.

336 McPherson RW, Kirsch J, Tobin J, *et al.* Cerebral blood flow in primates is increased by isoflurane over time and is decreased by nitric oxide synthase inhibition. *Anesthesiology* 1994; **80**: 1320–1327.

337 Alexander SC, Wollman H, Cohen PJ, *et al.* Cerebrovascular response to P_aCO_2 during halothane anesthesia in man. *J Appl Physiol* 1964; **19**: 561–565.

338 Scheller MS, Todd MM, Drummond JC. Isoflurane, halothane, and regional cerebral blood flow at various levels of $PaCO_2$ in rabbits. *Anesthesiology* 1986; **64**(5): 598–605.

339 McPherson RW, Brian JE, Traysman RJ. Cerebrovascular responsiveness to carbon dioxide in dogs with 1.4% and 2.8% isoflurane. *Anesthesiology* 1989; **70**(5):843–851.

340 Nishiyama T, Matsukawa T, Yokoyama T, *et al.* Cerebrovascular carbon dioxide reactivity during general anesthesia: a comparison between sevoflurane and isoflurane. *Anesth Analg* 1999; **89**: 1437–1441.

341 Brosnan RJ, LeCouteur RA, Steffey EP, *et al.* Direct measurement of intracranial pressure in adult horses. *Am J Vet Res* 2002; **63**(9): 1252–1256.

342 Brosnan RJ, Steffey EP, LeCouteur RA, *et al.* Effects of body position on intracranial and cerebral perfusion pressures in isoflurane-anesthetized horses. *J Appl Physiol* 2002; **92**: 2542–2546.

343 Brosnan RJ, Steffey EP, LeCouteur RA, *et al.* Effects of ventilation and isoflurane end-tidal concentration on intracranial and cerebral perfusion pressures in horses. *Am J Vet Res* 2003; **64**(1): 21–25.

344 Brosnan RJ, Steffey EP, LeCouteur RA, *et al.* Effects of duration of isoflurane anesthesia and mode of ventilation on intracranial and cerebral perfusion pressures in horses. *Am J Vet Res* 2003; **64**(11): 1444–1448.

345 Brosnan RJ, Esteller-Vico A, Steffey EP, *et al.* Effects of head-down positioning on regional central nervous system perfusion in isoflurane-anesthetized horses. *Am J Vet Res* 2008; **69**(6): 737–743.

346 Brosnan RJ, Steffey EP, LeCouteur RA, *et al.* Effects of isoflurane anesthesia on cerebrovascular autoregulation in horses. *Am J Vet Res* 2011; **72**(1): 18–24.

347 Trim CM. Postanesthetic hemorrhagic myelopathy or myelomalacia? *Vet Clin North Am Equine Pract* 1997; **13**: 73–77.

348 Knill RL, Kieraszewicz HT, Dodgson BG, *et al.* Chemical regulation of ventilation during isoflurane sedation and anaesthesia in humans. *Br J Anaesth* 1983; **49**: 957–963.

349 Fourcade HE, Stevens WC, Larson CP Jr., *et al.* The ventilatory effects of forane, a new inhaled anesthetic. *Anesthesiology* 1971; **35**: 26–31.

350 Hirshman CA, McCullough KE, Cohen PJ, *et al.* Depression of hypoxic ventilatory response by halothane, enflurane and isoflurane in dogs. *Br J Anaesth* 1977; **49**: 947–962.

351 Knill RL, Manninen PH, Clement JL. Ventilation and chemoreflexes during enflurane sedation and anaesthesia in man. *Can Anaesth Soc J* 1979; **26**: 353–360.

352 Coon RL, Kampinc JP. Hypocapnic bronchoconstriction and inhalation anesthetics. *Anesthesiology* 1975; **43**: 635–641.

353 Klide AM, Aviado DM. Mechanism for the reduction in pulmonary resistance induced by halothane. *J Pharmacol Exp Ther* 1967; **158**: 28–35.

354 Tobias JD, Hirshman CA. Attenuation of histamine-induced airway constriction by albuterol during halothane anesthesia. *Anesthesiology* 1990; **72**: 105–110.

355 Habre W, Petak F, Sly PD, *et al.* Protective effects of volatile agents against methacholine- induced bronchoconstriction in rats. *Anesthesiology* 2001; **94**: 348–353.

356 Hirshman CA, Bergman NA. Halothane and enflurane protect against bronchospasm in an asthma dog model. *Anesth Analg* 1978; **57**: 629–633.

357 Hirshman CA, Edelstein H, Peetz S, *et al.* Mechanism of action of inhalational anesthesia on airways. *Anesthesiology* 1982; **56**: 107–111.

358 Mazzeo AJ, Cheng EY, Bosnjak ZJ, *et al.* Differential effects of desflurane and halothane on peripheral airway smooth muscle. *Br J Anaesth* 1996; **76**: 841–846.

359 Wiklund CU, Lim S, Lindsten U, *et al.* Relaxation by sevoflurane, desflurane and halothane in the isolated guinea-pig trachea via inhibition of cholinergic neurotransmission. *Br J Anaesth* 1999; **83**(3): 422–429.

360 Doi M, Ikeda K. Airway irritation produced by volatile anaesthetics during brief inhalation: comparison of halothane, enflurane, isoflurane and sevoflurane. *Can J Anaesth* 1993; **40**: 122–126.

361 Eger EI II. *Desflurane (Suprane): A Compendium and Reference.* Rutherford, NJ: Healthpress Publishing Group, 1993.

362 Terriet MF, Desouza GJA, Jacobs JS, *et al.* Which is most pungent: isoflurane, sevoflurane or desflurane? *Br J Anaesth* 2000; **85**: 305–307.

363 Lockhart SH, Rampil IJ, Yasuda N, *et al.* Depression of ventilation by desflurane in humans. *Anesthesiology* 1991; **74**: 484–488.

364 Munson ES, Larson CP Jr., Babad AA, *et al.* The effects of halothane, fluroxene and cyclopropane on ventilation: a comparative study in man. *Anesthesiology* 1966; **27**(6): 716–728.

365 Larson CP Jr., Eger EI II, Muallem M, *et al.* The effects of diethyl ether and methoxyflurane on ventilation: II. *A comparative study in man. Anesthesiology* 1969; **30**(2): 174–184.

366 Doi M, Ikeda K. Respiratory effects of sevoflurane. *Anesth Analg* 1987; **66**: 241–244.
367 Calverley RK, Smith NT, Jones CW, *et al.* Ventilatory and cardiovascular effects of enflurane anesthesia during spontaneous ventilation in man. *Anesth Analg* 1978; **51**: 610–618.
368 Weiskopf RB, Holmes MA, Rampil IJ, *et al.* Cardiovascular safety and actions of high concentrations of I-653 and isoflurane in swine. *Anesthesiology* 1989; **70**: 793–799.
369 Wolfson B, Kielar CM, Lake C, *et al.* Anesthetic Index – a new approach. *Anesthesiology* 1973; **38**: 583–586.
370 Hodgson DS, Steffey EP, Grandy JL, *et al.* Effects of spontaneous, assisted, and controlled ventilation in halothane-anesthetized geldings. *Am J Vet Res* 1986; **47**: 992–996.
371 Steffey EP, Wheat JD, Meagher DM, *et al.* Body position and mode of ventilation influences arterial pH, oxygen and carbon dioxide tensions in halothane–anesthetized horses. *Am J Vet Res* 1977; **38**: 379–382.
372 Brandstater B, Eger EI II, Edelist G. Constant-depth halothane anesthesia in respiratory studies. *J Appl Physiol* 1965; **20**(2): 171–174.
373 Steffey EP, Farver TB, Woliner MJ. Cardiopulmonary function during 7 h of constant- dose halothane and methoxyflurane. *J Appl Physiol* 1987; **63**: 1351–1359.
374 Fourcade HE, Larson CP Jr., Hickey RF, *et al.* Effects of time on ventilation during halothane and cyclopropane anesthesia. *Anesthesiology* 1972; **36**: 83–88.
375 Steffey EP, Hodgson DS, Dunlop CI, *et al.* Cardiopulmonary function during 5 hours of constant-dose isoflurane in laterally recumbent, spontaneously breathing horses. *J Vet Pharmacol Ther* 1987; **10**: 290–297.
376 Steffey EP, Kelly AB, Woliner MJ. Time-related responses of spontaneously breathing laterally recumbent horses to prolonged anesthesia with halothane. *Am J Vet Res* 1987; **48**: 952–957.
377 Steffey EP, Kelly AB, Hodgson DS, *et al.* Effect of body posture on cardiopulmonary function in horses during five hours of constant-dose halothane anesthesia. *Am J Vet Res* 1990; **51**: 11–16.
378 France CJ, Plumer HM, Eger EI II, *et al.* Ventilatory effects of isoflurane (Forane) or halothane when combined with morphine, nitrous oxide and surgery. *Br J Anaesth* 1974; **46**: 117–120.
379 Eger EI II, Dolan WM, Stevens WC, *et al.* Surgical stimulation antagonizes the respiratory depression produced by Forane. *Anesthesiology* 1972; **36**: 544–549.
380 Steffey EP, Eisele JH, Baggot JD, *et al.* Influence of inhaled anesthetics on the pharmacokinetics and pharmacodynamics of morphine. *Anesth Analg* 1993; **77**: 346–351.
381 Steffey EP, Pascoe PJ. Xylazine blunts the cardiovascular but not the respiratory response induced by noxious stimulation in isoflurane anesthetized horses (abstract). *Proceedings of the 7th International Congress of Veterinary Anaesthesia,* 2000.
382 Steffey EP, Gillespie RJ, Berry JD, *et al.* Circulatory effects of halothane and halothane–nitrous oxide anesthesia in the dog: spontaneous ventilation. *Am J Vet Res* 1975; **36**(2): 197–200.
383 Steffey EP, Gillespie JR, Berry JD, *et al.* Cardiovascular effects with the addition of N_2O to halothane in stump-tailed macaques during spontaneous and controlled ventilation. *J Am Vet Med Assoc* 1974; **165**: 834–837.
384 Steffey EP, Howland D Jr. Potency of enflurane in dogs: comparison with halothane and isoflurane. *Am J Vet Res* 1978; **39**: 673–677.
385 Klide AM. Cardiovascular effects of enflurane and isoflurane in the dog. *Am J Vet Res* 1976; **37**: 127–131.
386 Steffey EP, Howland D Jr. Comparison of circulatory and respiratory effects of isoflurane and halothane anesthesia in horses. *Am J Vet Res* 1980; **41**: 821–825.
387 Eger EI II. New inhaled anesthetics. *Anesthesiology* 1994; **80**: 906–922.
388 Merin RG, Bernard JM, Doursout MF, *et al.* Comparison of the effects of isoflurane and desflurane on cardiovascular dynamics and regional blood flow in the chronically instrumented dog. *Anesthesiology* 1991; **74**(3): 568–574.
389 Weiskopf RB, Holmes MA, Eger EI II, *et al.* Cardiovascular effects of I-653 in swine. *Anesthesiology* 1988; **69**: 303–309.
390 Pagel PS, Kampine JP, Schmeling WT, *et al.* Comparison of the systemic and coronary hemodynamic actions of desflurane, isoflurane, halothane, and enflurane in the chronically instrumented dog. *Anesthesiology* 1991; **74**: 539–551.
391 Warltier DC, Pagel PS. Cardiovascular and respiratory actions of desflurane: is desflurane different from isoflurane? *Anesth Analg* 1992; **75**: S17–S31.
392 Picker O, Scheeren TWL, Arndt JO. Inhalation anaesthetics increase heart rate by decreasing cardiac vagal activity in dogs. *Br J Anaesth* 1988; **87**(5): 748–754.
393 Malan TP, DiNardo JA, Isner J, *et al.* Cardiovascular effects of sevoflurane compared with those of isoflurane in volunteers. *Anesthesiology* 1995; **83**: 918–928.
394 Mutoh T, Nishimura R, Kim HY, *et al.* Cardiopulmonary effects of sevoflurane, compared with halothane, enflurane, and isoflurane, in dogs. *Am J Vet Res* 1997; **58**(8): 885–890.
395 Pagel PS, Kampine JP, Schmeling WT, *et al.* Influence of volatile anesthetics on myocardial contractility in vivo – desflurane versus isoflurane. *Anesthesiology* 1991; **74**: 900–907.
396 Pagel PS, Kampine JP, Schmeling WT, *et al.* Evaluation of myocardial contractility in the chronically instrumented dog with intact autonomic nervous system function: effects of desflurane and isoflurane. *Acta Anaesthesiol Scand* 1993; **37**(2): 203–210.
397 Boban M, Stowe DF, Buljubasic N, *et al.* Direct comparative effects of isoflurane and desflurane in isolated guinea pig hearts. *Anesthesiology* 1992; **76**: 775–780.
398 Stevens WC, Cromwell TH, Halsey MJ, *et al.* The cardiovascular effects of a new inhalation anesthetic, Forane, in human volunteers at constant arterial carbon dioxide tension. *Anesthesiology* 1971; **35**: 8–16.
399 Weiskopf RB, Cahalan MK, Eger EI II, *et al.* Cardiovascular actions of desflurane in normocarbic volunteers. *Anesth Analg* 1991; **73**: 143–156.
400 Bernard JM, Wouters PF, Doursout MF, *et al.* Effects of sevoflurane and isoflurane on cardiac and coronary dynamics in chronically instrumented dogs. *Anesthesiology* 1990; **72**: 659–662.
401 Clarke KW, Alibhai HIK, Lee YHL, *et al.* Cardiopulmonary effects of desflurane in the dog during spontaneous and artificial ventilation. *Res Vet Sci* 1996; **61**: 82–86.
402 Price HL. The significance of catecholamine release during anesthesia. *Br J Anaesth* 1966; **38**: 705–711.
403 Katz RL, Epstein RA. The interaction of anesthetic agents and adrenergic drugs to produce cardiac arrhythmias. *Anesthesiology* 1968; **29**: 763–784.
404 Raventos J. The action of fluothane: a new volatile anaesthetic. *Br J Pharmacol* 1956; **11**: 394–409.
405 Muir BJ, Hall LW, Littlewort MCG. Cardiac irregularities in cats under halothane anaesthesia. *Br J Anaesth* 1959; **31**: 488–489.
406 Ueda I, Hirakawa M, Arakawa K, Kamaya H. Do anesthetics fluidize membranes? *Anesthesiology* 1986; **64**: 67–72.
407 Joas TA, Stevens WC. Comparison of the arrhythmic doses of epinephrine during Forane, halothane, and fluroxene anesthesia in dogs. *Anesthesiology* 1971; **35**(1): 48–53.
408 Muir WW III, Hubbell JAE, Flaherty S. Increasing halothane concentration abolishes anesthesia-associated arrhythmias in cats and dogs. *J Am Vet Med Assoc* 1988; **192**: 1730–1735.
409 Moore MA, Weiskopf RB, Eger EI II, *et al.* Arrhythmogenic doses of epinephrine are similar during desflurane or isoflurane anesthesia in humans. *Anesthesiology* 1993; **79**(5): 943–947.
410 Munson ES, Tucker WK. Doses of epinephrine causing arrhythmia during enflurane, methoxyflurane and halothane anesthesia in dogs. *Can Anaesth Soc J* 1975; **22**: 495–501.
411 Navarro R, Weiskopf RB, Moore MA, *et al.* Humans anesthetized with sevoflurane or isoflurane have similar arrhythmic response to epinephrine. *Anesthesiology* 1994; **80**: 545–549.
412 Weiskopf RB, Eger EI II, Holmes MA, *et al.* Epinephrine-induced premature ventricular contractions and changes in arterial blood pressure and heart rate during I-653, isoflurane, and halothane anesthesia in swine. *Anesthesiology* 1989; **70**: 293–298.
413 Johnston RR, Eger EI II, Wilson C. A comparative interaction of epinephrine with enflurane, isoflurane and halothane in man. *Anesth Analg* 1976; **55**: 709–712.
414 Hikasa Y, Okabe C, Takase K, *et al.* Ventricular arrhythmogenic dose of adrenaline during sevoflurane, isoflurane, and halothane anaesthesia either with or without ketamine or thiopentone in cats. *Res Vet Sci* 1996; **60**: 134–137.
415 Tucker WK, Rackstein AD, Munson ES. Comparison of arrhythmic doses of adrenaline, metaraminol, ephedrine, and phenylephrine, during isoflurane and halothane anesthesia in dogs. *Br J Anaesth* 1974; **46**: 392–396.
416 Maze M, Smith CM. Identification of receptor mechanisms mediating epinephrine- induced arrhythmias during halothane anesthesia in the dog. *Anesthesiology* 1983; **59**: 322–326.
417 Light GS, Hellyer PW, Swanson CR. Parasympathetic influence on the arrhythmogenicity of graded dobutamine infusions in halothane-anesthetized horses. *Am J Vet Res* 1992; **53**(7): 1154–1160.
418 Lemke KA, Tranquilli WJ, Thurmon JC, *et al.* Alterations in the arrhythmogenic dose of epinephrine after xylazine or medetomidine administration in halothane-anesthetized dogs. *Am J Vet Res* 1993; **54**: 2132–2138.
419 Lemke KA, Tranquilli WJ, Thurmon JC, *et al.* Alterations in the arrhythmogenic dose of epinephrine after xylazine or medetomidine administration in isoflurane-anesthetized dogs. *Am J Vet Res* 1993; **54**: 2139–2144.
420 Robertson BJ, Clement JL, Knill RL. Enhancement of the arrhythmogenic effect of hypercarbia by surgical stimulation during halothane anaesthesia in man. *Can Anaesth Soc J* 1981; **28**: 342.
421 Gelman S, Fowler KC, Smith LR. Liver circulation and function during isoflurane and halothane anesthesia. *Anesthesiology* 1984; **61**(6): 726–731.
422 Bernard JM, Doursout MF, Wouters P, *et al.* Effects of enflurane and isoflurane on hepatic and renal circulations in chronically instrumented dogs. *Anesthesiology* 1991; **74**(2): 298–302.

423 Bernard JM, Doursout MF, Wouters P, *et al.* Effects of sevoflurane and isoflurane on hepatic circulation in the chronically instrumented dog. *Anesthesiology* 1992; **77**(3): 541–545.

424 Frink EJ Jr., Morgan SE, Coetzee A, *et al.* The effects of sevoflurane, halothane, enflurane, and isoflurane on hepatic blood flow and oxygenation in chronically instrumented Greyhound dogs. *Anesthesiology* 1992; **76**: 85–90.

425 Steffey EP, Gillespie JR, Berry JD, *et al.* Circulatory effects of halothane and halothane–nitrous oxide anesthesia in the dog: controlled ventilation. *Am J Vet Res* 1974; **35**: 1289–1293.

426 Steffey EP, Howland D Jr. Cardiovascular effects of halothane in the horse. *Am J Vet Res* 1978; **39**: 611–615.

427 Pypendop BH, Ilkiw JE. Hemodynamic effects of sevoflurane in cats. *Am J Vet Res* 2004; **65**(1): 20–25.

428 Steffey EP, Gillespie JR, Berry JD, *et al.* Cardiovascular effect of halothane in the stump-tailed macaque during spontaneous and controlled ventilation. *Am J Vet Res* 1974; **35**: 1315–1319.

429 Stoelting RK. *Inhaled Anesthetics. Pharmacology and Physiology in Anesthetic Practice*, 3rd edn. Philadelphia, PA: Lippincott-Raven, 1999: 36–76.

430 Cullen DJ, Eger EI II. Cardiovascular effects of carbon dioxide in man. *Anesthesiology* 1974; **41**: 345–349.

431 Grandy JL, Hodgson DS, Dunlop CI, *et al.* Cardiopulmonary effects of halothane anesthesia in cats. *Am J Vet Res* 1989; **50**: 1729–1732.

432 Bahlman SH, Eger EI II, Halsey MJ, *et al.* The cardiovascular effects of halothane in man during spontaneous ventilation. *Anesthesiology* 1972; **36**: 494–502.

433 Cromwell TH, Stevens WC, Eger EI II, *et al.* The cardiovascular effects of compound 469 (Forane) during spontaneous ventilation and CO_2 challenge in man. *Anesthesiology* 1971; **35**(1): 17–25.

434 Cullen LK, Steffey EP, Bailey CS, *et al.* Effect of high $PaCO_2$ and time on cerebrospinal fluid and intraocular pressure in halothane-anesthetized horses. *Am J Vet Res* 1990; **51**: 300–304.

435 Smith NT, Eger EI II, Stoelting RK, *et al.* The cardiovascular and sympathomimetic response to the addition of nitrous oxide to halothane in man. *Anesthesiology* 1970; **32**(5): 410–421.

436 Yamashita K, Tsubakishita S, Futaoka S, *et al.* Cardiovascular effects of medetomidine, detomidine and xylazine in horses. *J Vet Med Sci* 2000; **62**(10): 1025–1032.

437 Yasuda N, Weiskopf RB, Cahalan MK, *et al.* Does desflurane modify circulatory responses to stimulation in humans? *Anesth Analg* 1991; **73**: 175–179.

438 Zbinden AM, Petersenfelix S, Thomson DA. Anesthetic depth defined using multiple noxious stimuli during isoflurane/oxygen anesthesia. II. Hemodynamic responses. *Anesthesiology* 1994; **80**(2): 261–267.

439 Antognini JF, Berg K. Cardiovascular responses to noxious stimuli during isoflurane anesthesia are minimally affected by anesthetic action in the brain. *Anesth Analg* 1995; **81**: 843–848.

440 March PA, Muir WW III. Minimum alveolar concentration measures of central nervous system activation in cats anesthetized with isoflurane. *Am J Vet Res* 2003; **64**(12): 1528–1533.

441 Love L, Egger C, Rohrbach B, *et al.* The effect of ketamine on the MACBAR of sevoflurane in dogs. *Vet Anaesth Analg* 2011; **38**(4): 292–300.

442 Yamashita K, Frukawa E, Itami T, *et al.* Minimum alveolar concentratin for blunting adrenergic responses (MAC-BAR) of sevoflurane in dogs. *J Vet Med Sci* 2012; **74**(4): 507–511.

443 Hofmeister EH, Brainard BM, Sams LM, *et al.* Evaluation of induction characteristics and hypnotic potency of isoflurane and sevoflurane in healthy dogs. *Am J Vet Res* 2008; **69**(4): 451–456.

444 Schmeling WT, Ganjoo P, Staunton M, *et al.* Pretreatment with dexmedetomidine: altered indices of anesthetic depth for halothane in the neuraxis of cats. *Anesth Analg* 1999; **88**: 625–632.

445 Eger EI II, Smith NT, Stoelting RK, *et al.* Cardiovascular effects of halothane in man. *Anesthesiology* 1970; **32**(5): 396–409.

446 Eger EI II, Bowland T, Ionescu P, *et al.* Recovery and kinetic characteristics of desflurane and sevoflurane in volunteers after 8-h exposure, including kinetics of degradation products. *Anesthesiology* 1997; **87**(3): 517–526.

447 Tayefeh F, Larson MD, Sessler DI, *et al.* Time-dependent changes in heart rate and pupil size during desflurane or sevoflurane anesthesia. *Anesth Analg* 1997; **85**(12): 1362–1366.

448 Cullen BF, Eger EI II, Smith NT, *et al.* Cardiovascular effects of fluroxene in man. *Anesthesiology* 1970; **32**(3): 218–230.

449 Libonati M, Cooperman LH, Price HL. Time-dependent circulatory effects of methoxyflurane in man. *Anesthesiology* 1971; **34**: 439–444.

450 Gregory GA, Eger EI II, Smith NT. The cardiovascular effects of diethyl ether in man. *Anesthesiology* 1971; **34**(1): 19–24.

451 Dunlop CI, Steffey EP, Miller MF, *et al.* Temporal effects of halothane and isoflurane in laterally recumbent ventilated male horses. *Am J Vet Res* 1987; **48**: 1250–1255.

452 Steffey EP, Dunlop CI, Cullen LK, *et al.* Circulatory and respiratory responses of spontaneously breathing, laterally recumbent horses to 12 hours of halothane anesthesia. *Am J Vet Res* 1993; **54**: 929–936.

453 Yamanaka T, Oku K, Koyama H, *et al.* Time-related changes of the cardiovascular system during maintenance anesthesia with sevoflurane and isoflurane in horses. *J Vet Med Sci* 2001; **63**(5): 527–532.

454 Whitehair KJ, Steffey EP, Willits NH, *et al.* Recovery of horses from inhalation anesthesia. *Am J Vet Res* 1993; **54**: 1693–1702.

455 Steffey EP, Woliner MJ, Dunlop C. Effects of 5 hours of constant 1.2 MAC halothane in sternally recumbent, spontaneously breathing horses. *Equine Vet J* 1990; **22**: 433–436.

456 Shimosato S, Yasuda I. Cardiac performance during prolonged halothane anaesthesia in the cat. *Br J Anaesth* 1978; **50**: 215–219.

457 Price HL, Skovsted P, Pauca AL, *et al.* Evidence for beta-receptor activation produced by halothane in normal man. *Anesthesiology* 1970; **32**(5): 389–395.

458 Bahlman SH, Eger EI II, Smith NT, *et al.* The cardiovascular effects of nitrous oxide–halothane anesthesia in man. *Anesthesiology* 1971; **35**(3): 274–285.

459 Eisele JH Jr. Cardiovascular effects of nitrous oxide. In: Eger EI II, ed. *Nitrous Oxide/N2O*. New York: Elsevier, 1985: 125–156.

460 Grandy JL, Hodgson DS, Dunlop CI, *et al.* Cardiopulmonary effects of ephedrine in halothane-anesthetized horses. *J Vet Pharmacol Ther* 1989; **12**: 389–396.

461 Dyson DH, Pascoe PJ. Influence of preinduction methoxamine, lactated ringer solution, or hypertonic saline solution infusion or postinduction dobutamine infusion on anesthetic-induced hypotension in horses. *Am J Vet Res* 1990; **51**(1): 17–21.

462 Swanson CR, Muir WW III, Bednarski RM, *et al.* Hemodynamic responses in halothane-anesthetized horses given infusions of dopamine or dobutamine. *Am J Vet Res* 1985; **46**: 365–371.

463 Priano LL, Marrone B. Effect of halothane on renal hemodynamics during normovolemia and acute hemorrhagic hypovolemia. *Anesthesiology* 1985; **63**(4): 357–364.

464 Gelman S, Fowler KC, Smith LR. Regional blood flow during isoflurane and halothane anesthesia. *Anesth Analg* 1984; **63**(6): 557–566.

465 Steffey EP, Zinkl J, Howland D Jr. Minimal changes in blood cell counts and biochemical values associated with prolonged isoflurane anesthesia of horses. *Am J Vet Res* 1979; **40**(11): 1646–1648.

466 Steffey EP, Farver T, Zinkl J, *et al.* Alterations in horse blood cell count and biochemical values after halothane anesthesia. *Am J Vet Res* 1980; **41**(6): 934–939.

467 Stover SM, Steffey EP, Dybdal NO, *et al.* Hematologic and biochemical values associated with multiple halothane anesthesias and minor surgical trauma of horses. *Am J Vet Res* 1988; **49**: 236–241.

468 Steffey EP, Giri SN, Dunlop CI, *et al.* Biochemical and haematological changes following prolonged halothane anaesthesia in horses. *Res Vet Sci* 1993; **55**: 338–345.

469 Nunez E, Steffey EP, Ocampo L, *et al.* Effects of alpha-2 adrenergic receptor agonists on urine production in horses deprived of food and water. *Am J Vet Res* 2004; **65**(10): 1342–1346.

470 Pedersoli WM. Blood serum inorganic ionic fluoride tetracycline and methoxyflurane anesthesia in dogs. *J Am Anim Hosp Assoc* 1977; **13**: 242–246.

471 Mazze RI, Trudell JR, Cousins MJ. Methoxyflurane metabolism and renal dysfunction: clinical correlation in man. *Anesthesiology* 1971; **35**: 247–252.

472 Leiman BC, Katz J, Stanley TH, *et al.* Removal of tracheal secretions in anesthetized dogs: balloon catheters versus suction. *Anesth Analg* 1987; **66**: 529–533.

473 Mazze RI, Calverley RK, Smith NT. Inorganic fluoride nephrotoxicity: prolonged enflurane and halothane anesthesia in volunteers. *Anesthesiology* 1977; **46**: 265–271.

474 Kharasch ED, Hankins DC, Thummel KE. Human kidney methoxyflurane and sevoflurane metabolism – intrarenal fluoride production as a possible mechanism of methoxyflurane nephrotoxicity. *Anesthesiology* 1995; **82**(3): 689–699.

475 Ikeda S, Makino H. A round trip: the Japanese contribution to the development of sevoflurane. *Anesthe Analg* 2022; **134**: 432–439.

476 Morio M, Fujii K, Satoh N, *et al.* Reaction of sevoflurane and its degradation products with soda lime. *Anesthesiology* 1992; **77**: 1155–1164.

477 Gonsowski CT, Laster MJ, Eger EI II, *et al.* Toxicity of compound A in rats: effect of a 3-hour administration. *Anesthesiology* 1994; **80**: 556–565.

478 Gonsowski CT, Laster MJ, Eger EI II, *et al.* Toxicity of compound A in rats: effect of increasing duration of administration. *Anesthesiology* 1994; **80**: 566–573.

479 Kandel L, Laster MJ, Eger EI II, *et al.* Nephrotoxicity in rats undergoing a 1 hour exposure to compound A. *Anesth Analg* 1995; **81**: 559–563.

480 Frink EJ Jr., Malan TP Jr., Isner RJ, *et al.* Renal concentrating function with prolonged sevoflurane or enflurane anesthesia in volunteers. *Anesthesiology* 1994; **80**: 1019–1025.

481 Muir WW III, Gadawski JE. Cardiorespiratory effects of low-flow and closed circuit inhalation anesthesia, using sevoflurane delivered with an in-circuit vaporizer and concentrations of compound A. *Am J Vet Res* 1998; **59**(5): 603–608.

482 Reilly CS, Wood AJJ, Koshakji RP, *et al.* The effect of halothane on drug disposition: contribution of changes in intrinsic drug metabolizing capacity and hepatic blood flow. *Anesthesiology* 1985; **63**: 70–76.

483 Pearson GR, Bogan JA, Sanford J. An increase in the half-life of pentobarbitone with the administration of halothane in sheep. *Br J Anaesth* 1973; **45**: 586–591.

484 Smith CM, Steffey EP, Baggot JD, *et al.* Effects of halothane anesthesia on the clearance of gentamicin sulfate in horses. *Am J Vet Res* 1988; **49**(1): 19–22.

485 Subcommittee of the National Halothane Study of the Committee on Anesthesia NAoS-NRC. Summary of the National Halothane Study: possible association between halothane anesthesia and postoperative hepatic necrosis. *JAMA* 1966; **197**: 121–134.

486 Inman WHW, Mushin WW. Jaundice after repeated exposure to halothane: an analysis of reports to the Committee on Safety of Medicines. *BMJ J* 1974; **1**: 5–10.

487 Holmes MA, Weiskopf RB, Eger EI II, *et al.* Hepatocellular integrity in swine after prolonged desflurane (I-653) and isoflurane anesthesia: evaluation of plasma alanine aminotransferase activity. *Anesth Analg* 1990; **71**: 249–253.

488 Eger EI II, Johnson BH, Ferrell LD. Comparison of the toxicity of I-653 and isoflurane in rats: a test of the effect of repeated anesthesia and use of dry soda lime. *Anesth Analg* 1987; **66**: 1230–1233.

489 Strum DP, Eger EI II, Johnson BH, *et al.* Toxicity of sevoflurane in rats. *Anesth Analg* 1987; **66**: 769–773.

490 Eger EI II, Johnson BH, Strum DP, *et al.* Studies of the toxicity of I-653, halothane, and isoflurane in enzyme-induced, hypoxic rats. *Anesth Analg* 1987; **66**: 1227–1230.

491 Ross JAS, Monk SJ, Duffy SW. Effect of nitrous oxide on halothane-induced hepatotoxicity in hypoxic, enzyme-induced rats. *Br J Anaesth* 1984; **56**(5): 527–533.

492 Shingu K, Eger EI II, Johnson BH. Hypoxia per se can produce hepatic damage without death in rats. *Anesth Analg* 1982; **61**: 820–823.

493 Shingu K, Eger EI II, Johnson BH. Hypoxia may be more important than reductive metabolism in halothane-induced hepatic injury. *Anesth Analg* 1982; **61**: 824–827.

494 Whitehair KJ, Steffey EP, Woliner MJ, *et al.* Effects of inhalation anesthetic agents on response of horses to 3 hours of hypoxemia. *Am J Vet Res* 1996; **57**: 351–360.

495 Reynolds ES, Moslen MT. Liver injury following halothane anesthesia in phenobarbital- pretreated rats. *Biochem Pharmacol* 1974; **23**: 189–195.

496 Reynolds ES, Moslen MT. Halothane hepatotoxicity: enhancement by polychlorinated biphenyl pretreatment. *Anesthesiology* 1977; **47**(1): 19–27.

497 Cooperman LH, Warden JC, Price HL. Splanchnic circulation during nitrous oxide anesthesia and hypocarbia in normal man. *Anesthesiology* 1968; **29**: 254–258.

498 Johnson EE, Hedley-Whyte J. Continuous positive-pressure ventilation and choledochoduodenal flow resistance. *J Appl Physiol* 1975; **39**: 937–942.

499 Davis M, Eddleston ALWF, Neuberger JM, *et al.* Halothane hepatitis. *N Engl J Med* 1980; **303**(19): 1123–1124.

500 Kitteringham NR, Kenna JG, Park BK. Detection of autoantibodies directed against human hepatic endoplasmic reticulum in sera from patients with halothane- associated hepatitis. *Br J Clin Pharmacol* 1995; **40**(4): 379–386.

501 Farrell G, Prendergast D, Murray M. Halothane hepatitis: detection of a constitutional susceptibility factor. *N Engl J Med* 1985; **313**: 1310–1315.

502 Denborough MA, Forster JFP, Lovell RRH. Anaesthetic deaths in a family. *Br J Anaesth* 1962; **34**: 395–396.

503 Gronert GA, Antognini JF, Pessah IN. Malignant hyperthermia. In: Miller RD, ed. *Anesthesia*, 5th edn. Philadelphia, PA: Churchill Livingstone, 2000: 1033–1052.

504 Hall LW, Woolf N, Bradley JWP, *et al.* Unusual reaction to suxamethonium chloride. *BMJ* 1966; **2**: 1305.

505 Kirmayer AH, Klide AM, Purvance JE. Malignant hyperthermia in a dog: case report and review of the syndrome. *J Am Vet Med Assoc* 1984; **185**: 978–983.

506 Deuster PA, Bockman EL, Muldoon SM. In vitro responses of cat skeletal muscle to halothane and caffeine. *J Appl Physiol* 1985; **58**: 521–528.

507 Bagshaw RJ, Cox RH, Knight DH, *et al.* Malignant hyperthermia in a greyhound. *J Am Vet Med Assoc* 1978; **172**: 61.

508 Rosenberg H, Waldron-Mease E. Malignant hyperpyrexia in horses: anesthetic sensitivity proven by muscle biopsy (abstract). In: *Annual Meeting of the American Society of Anesthesiologists*, 1977: 333–334.

509 Hildebrand SV, Howitt GA. Succinylcholine infusion associated with hyperthermia in ponies anesthetized with halothane. *Am J Vet Res* 1983; **44**: 2280–2284.

510 Short C, Paddleford RR. Malignant hyperthermia in the dog – letter. *Anesthesiology* 1973; **39**: 462–463.

511 deJong RH, Heavner JE, Amory DW. Malignant hyperpyrexia in the cat. *Anesthesiology* 1974; **41**: 608–609.

512 Aleman M, Brosnan RJ, Williams DC, *et al.* Malignant hyperthermia in a horse anesthetized with halothane. *J Vet Intern Med* 2005; **19**: 363–367.

513 Aleman M, Riehl J, Aldridge BM, *et al.* Association of a mutation in the ryanodine receptor 1 gene with equine malignant hyperthermia. *Muscle Nerve* 2004; **30**(3): 356–365.

514 Aleman M, Aldridge BM, Riehl J, *et al.* Equine malignant hyperthermia. *Proc Am Assoc Equine Pract* 2004; **50**: 51–54.

515 Epstein RM, Rackow H, Salanitre E, *et al.* Influence of the concentration effect on the uptake of anesthetic mixtures: the second gas effect. *Anesthesiology* 1964; **25**: 364–371.

516 Stoelting RK, Eger EI II. An additional explanation for the second gas effect: a concentrating effort. *Anesthesiology* 1969; **30**(3): 273–277.

517 Taheri S, Eger EI. A demonstration of the concentration and second gas effects in humans anesthetized with nitrous oxide and desflurane. *Anesth Analg* 1999; **89**: 774–780.

518 Fukunaga AF, Epstein RM. Sympathetic excitation during nitrous oxide–halothane anesthesia in the cat. *Anesthesiology* 1973; **39**: 23–36.

519 Pypendop BH, Ilkiw JE, Imai A, *et al.* Hemodynamic effects of nitrous oxide in isoflurane-anesthetized cats. *Am J Vet Res* 2003; **64**(3): 273–278.

520 Liu WS, Wong KC, Port JD, *et al.* Epinephrine-induced arrhythmia during halothane anesthesia with the addition of nitrous oxide, nitrogen or helium in dogs. *Anesth Analg* 1982; **61**: 414–417.

521 Lampe GH, Donegan JH, Rupp SM, *et al.* Nitrous oxide and epinephrine-induced arrhythmias. *Anesth Analg* 1990; **71**: 602–605.

522 Philbin DM, Foex P, Drummond G, *et al.* Postsystolic shortening of canine left ventricle supplied by a stenotic coronary artery when nitrous oxide is added in the presence of narcotics. *Anesthesiology* 1985; **62**: 166–174.

523 Leone BJ, Philbin DM, Lehot JJ, *et al.* Gradual or abrupt nitrous oxide administration in a canine model of critical coronary stenosis induces regional myocardial dysfunction that is worsened by halothane. *Anesth Analg* 1988; **67**: 814–822.

524 Nathan HJ. Nitrous oxide worsens myocardial ischemia in isoflurane-anesthetized dogs. *Anesthesiology* 1988; **68**: 407–416.

525 Diedericks J, Leone BJ, Foex P, *et al.* Nitrous oxide causes myocardial ischemia when added to propofol in the compromised canine myocardium. *Anesth Analg* 1993; **76**: 1322–1326.

526 Saidman LJ, Hamilton WK. We should continue to use nitrous oxide. In: Eger EI II, ed. *Nitrous Oxide/N2O*. New York: Elsevier, 1985: 345–353.

527 Eger EI II, Lampe GH, Wauk LZ, *et al.* Clinical pharmacology of nitrous oxide: an argument for its continued use. *Anesth Analg* 1990; **71**: 575–585.

528 Lampe GH, Wauk LZ, Whitendale P, *et al.* Nitrous oxide does not impair hepatic function in young or old surgical patients. *Anesth Analg* 1990; **71**: 606–609.

529 Brodsky JB. Toxicity of nitrous oxide. In: Eger EI II, ed. *Nitrous Oxide/N2O*. New York: Elsevier, 1985: 259–279.

530 Lampe GH, Wauk LZ, Donegan JH, *et al.* Effect on outcome of prolonged exposure of patients to nitrous oxide. *Anesth Analg* 1990; **71**: 586–590.

531 Waldman FM, Koblin DD, Lampe GH, *et al.* Hematologic effects of nitrous oxide in surgical patients. *Anesth Analg* 1990; **71**: 618–624.

532 Nunn JF, Chanarin I. Nitrous oxide inactivates methionine synthetase. In: Eger EI II, ed. *Nitrous Oxide/N2O*. New York: Elsevier, 1985: 211–233.

533 Koblin DD, Tomerson BW, Waldman FM, *et al.* Effect of nitrous oxide on folate and vitamin B12 metabolism in patients. *Anesth Analg* 1990; **71**: 610–617.

534 Layzer RB, Fishman RA, Schafer JA. Neuropathy following abuse of nitrous oxide. *Neurology* 1978; **28**: 504–506.

535 Layzer RB. Myeloneuropathy after prolonged exposure to nitrous oxide. *Lancet* 1978; **2**: 1227–1230.

536 Weathersby PK, Homer LD. Solubility of inert gases in biological fluids and tissues: a review. *Undersea Biomed Res* 1980; **7**: 277–296.

537 Steffey EP, Johnson BH, Eger EI II, *et al.* Nitrous oxide increases the accumulation rate and decreases the uptake of bowel gases. *Anesth Analg* 1979; **58**: 405–408.

538 Eger EI II, Saidman LJ. Hazards of nitrous oxide anesthesia in bowel obstruction and pneumothorax. *Anesthesiology* 1965; **26**(1): 61–66.

539 Steffey EP, Gauger GE, Eger EI II. Cardiovascular effects of venous air embolism during air and oxygen breathing. *Anesth Analg* 1974; **53**: 599–604.

540 Munson ES, Merrick HC. Effect of nitrous oxide on venous air embolism. *Anesthesiology* 1966; **27**: 783–787.

541 Davis I, Moore JRM, Lahiri SK. Nitrous oxide and the middle ear. *Anaesthesia* 1979; **34**: 147–151.

542 Perreault L, Normandin N, Plamondon L, *et al.* Middle ear pressure variations during nitrous oxide and oxygen anaesthesia. *Can Anaesth Soc J* 1982; **29**(5): 428–434.

543 Saidman LJ, Eger EI II. Change in cerebrospinal fluid pressure during pneumoencephalography under nitrous oxide anesthesia. *Anesthesiology* 1965; **26**(1): 67–72.

544 Stanley TH, Kawamura R, Graves C. Effects of N_2O on volume and pressure of endotracheal tube cuffs. *Anesthesiology* 1974; **41**: 256–262.

545 Stanley TH. Effects of anesthetic gases on endotracheal tube cuff gas volumes. *Anesth Analg* 1974; **53**(3): 480–482.

546 Stanley TH. Nitrous oxide and pressures and volumes of high- and low-pressure endotracheal tube cuffs in intubated patients. *Anesthesiology* 1975; **42**: 637–640.

547 Bednarski RM. Advantages and guidelines for using nitrous oxide. *Vet Clin North Am Small Anim Pract* 1992; **22**: 313–314.
548 Klide AM, Haskins SC. Precautions when using nitrous oxide. *Vet Clin North Am Small Anim Pract* 1992; **22**: 314–316.
549 Linde HW, Bruce DL. Occupational exposure of anesthetists to halothane, nitrous oxide and radiation. *Anesthesiology* 1969; **30**: 363–368.
550 Whitcher CE, Cohen EN, Trudell JR. Chronic exposure to anesthetic gases in the operating room. *Anesthesiology* 1971; **35**: 348–353.
551 Ward GS, Byland RR. Concentrations of methoxyflurane and nitrous oxide in veterinary operating rooms. *Am J Vet Res* 1982; **43**: 360–362.
552 Ward GS, Byland RR. Concentrations of halothane in veterinary operating and treatment rooms. *J Am Vet Med Assoc* 1982; **180**: 174–177.
553 Milligan JE, Sablan JL, Short CE. A survey of waste anesthetic gas concentrations in U.S. Airforce veterinary surgeries. *J Am Vet Med Assoc* 1980; **177**: 1021–1022.
554 Dreesen DW, Jones GL, Brown J, *et al.* Monitoring for trace anesthetic gases in a veterinary teaching hospital. *J Am Vet Med Assoc* 1981; **179**: 797–799.
555 Manley SV, McDonell WF. Recommendations for reduction of anesthetic gas pollution. *J Am Vet Med Assoc* 1980; **176**: 519–524.
556 Manley SV, Taloff P, Aberg N, *et al.* Occupational exposure to waste anesthetic gases in veterinary practice. *California Vet* 1982; **36**: 14–19.
557 Pfaffli P, Nikki P, Ahlman K. Halothane and nitrous oxide in end-tidal air and venous blood of surgical personnel. *Ann Clin Res* 1972; **4**: 273–277.
558 Corbett TH. Retention of anesthetic agents following occupational exposure. *Anesth Analg* 1973; **52**: 614–618.
559 Ad Hoc Committee on Effects of Trace Anesthetic Agents on Health of Operating Room Personnel. *Waste Anesthetic Gases in Operating Room Air: A Suggested Program to Reduce Personnel Exposure.* Park Ridge, IL: American Society of Anesthesiologists, 1983.
560 Cohen EN, Bellville JW, Brown BW. Anesthesia, pregnancy, and miscarriage: a study of operating room nurses and anesthetists. *Anesthesiology* 1971; **35**: 343–347.
561 Cohen EN, Brown BW Jr., Bruce DL, *et al.* A survey of anesthetic health hazards among dentists. *J Am Dental Assoc* 1975; **90**: 1291–1296.
562 Lecky JH. Anesthetic pollution in the operating room: a notice to operating room personnel. *Anesthesiology* 1980; **52**: 157–159.
563 Berry A, McGregor DG, Baden JM, *et al. Waste Anesthetic Gases: Information for Management in Anesthetizing Areas and The Postanesthetic Care Unit (PACU).* Park Ridge, IL: American Society of Anesthesiologists, 2005.
564 American College of Veterinary Anesthesiologists Ad Hoc Committee on Waste Anesthetic Gas Pollution and Its Control. Commentary and recommendations on control of waste anesthetic gases in the workplace. *J Am Vet Med Assoc* 1996; **209**: 75–77.
565 Sessler DI, Badgwell JM. Exposure of postoperative nurses to exhaled anesthetic gases. *Anesth Analg* 1998; **87**: 1083–1088.
566 Summer G, Lirk P, Hoerauf K, *et al.* Sevoflurane in exhaled air of operating room personnel. *Anesth Analg* 2003; **97**(4): 1070–1073.
567 Cicerone RJ, Stolarski RS, Walters S. Stratospheric ozone destruction by man-made chlorofluoromethanes. *Science* 1974; **185**(4157): 1165–1167.
568 Fox JWC, Fox EJ, Villanueva R. Stratospheric ozone destruction and halogenated anaesthetics. *Lancet* 1975; **1**: 864.
569 Sherman SJ, Cullen BF. Nitrous oxide and the greenhouse effect. *Anesthesiology* 1988; **68**(5): 816–817.
570 Rowland FS. Chlorofluorocarbons and the depletion of stratospheric ozone. *Am Sci* 1989; **77**: 36–45.
571 Rowland FS. Stratospheric ozone depletion. *Phil Trans R Soc London B Biol Sci* 2006; **361**(1469): 769–790.
572 Logan M, Farmer JG. Anaesthesia and the ozone layer. *Br J Anaesth* 1989; **63**(6): 645–647.
573 Ishizawa Y. General anesthetic gases and the global environment. *Anesth Analg* 2011; **112**(1): 213–217.
574 Langbein T, Sonntag H, Trapp D, *et al.* Volatile anaesthetics and the atmosphere: atmospheric lifetimes and atmospheric effects of halothane, enflurane, isoflurane, desflurane and sevoflurane. *Br J Anaesth* 1999; **82**(1): 66–73.
575 Sulbaek Andersen MP, Nielsen OJ, Wallington TJ, *et al.* Assessing the impact on global climate from general anesthetic gases. *Anesth Analg* 2012; **114**(5): 1081–1085.
576 Ravishankara AR, Daniel JS, Portmann RW. Nitrous oxide (N_2O): the dominant ozone-depleting substance emitted in the 21st century. *Science* 2009; **326**: 123–125.
577 United Nations. Montreal Protocol on Substances that Deplete the Ozone Layer. www.unep.org/ozonaction/who-we-are/about-montreal-protocol (accessed September 2022).
578 Ryan SM, Nielsen CJ. Global warming potential of inhaled anesthetics: application to clinical use. *Anesth Analg* 2010; **111**(1): 92–98.
579 Sulbaek Andersen MP, Sander SP, Nielsen O, *et al.* Inhalation anaesthetics and climate change. *Br J Anaesth* 2010; **105**(6): 760–766.
580 Ryan S. Sustainable anesthesia. *Anesth Analg* 2012; **114**(5): 921–923.
581 Mychaskiw G II, Eger EI II. A different perspective on anesthetics and climate change. *Anesth Analg* 2013; **116**(3): 734–735.
582 Sulbaek Andersen MP, Nielsen OJ, Karpichev B, *et al.* Atmospheric chemistry of isoflurane, desflurane, and sevoflurane: kinetics and mechanisms of reactions with chlorine atoms and OH radicals and global warming potentials. *J Phys Chem* 2012; **116**: 5806–5820.
583 Sherman J, Le C, Lamers V, Eckelman M. Life cycle greenhouse gas emissions of anesthetic drugs. *Anesth Analg* 2012; **114**(5): 1086–1089.
584 Varughese S, Ahmed R. Environmental and occupational considerations of anesthesia: a narrative review and update. *Anesth Analg* 2021; **133**: 826–835.
585 Chol BJJ, Chen CL. The triple bottom line and stabilization wedges: a framework for perioperative sustainability. *Anesth Analg* 2022; **134**: 475–485.
586 White SM, Shelton CL, Gelb AW, *et al.* Principles of environmentally-sustainable anaesthesia: a global consensus statement from the World Federation of Societies of Anaesthesiologists. *Anaesthesia* 2022; **77**: 201–212.
587 Devlin-Hegedus JA, McGain F, Harris RD, *et al.* Action guidance for addressing pollution from inhalational anaesthetics. *Anaesthesia* 2022; **77**: 1023–1029.

29 Local Anesthetics

Eva Rioja Garcia
Optivet Referrals, Havant, Hampshire, UK

Chapter contents

Introduction, 526
Pharmacology, 526
Molecular mechanism of action, 526
Mechanism of blockade of neural tissue, 528
Chemical structure, 530
Physicochemical properties, 530
Clinical pharmacology, 531
Pharmacokinetics, 531
Mixtures of local anesthetics, 537
Tachyphylaxis, 538
Specific drugs and clinical uses, 538
Aminoesters, 538
Aminoamides, 539
Special formulations, 540
Adverse effects, 541
Systemic toxicity, 541
Local toxicity, 544
Methemoglobinemia, 544
Toxicosis (oral ingestion), 545
Allergic reactions, 545
References, 545

Introduction

Local anesthetics reversibly block the generation and propagation of electrical impulses in nerves, thereby causing sensory and motor blockade. Their use dates from the late 1880s when cocaine was first used for ophthalmologic procedures by Carl Köller and Sigmund Freud. However, cocaine was found to be highly toxic and addictive and, since then, new agents with better pharmacologic profiles and less potential for systemic toxicity have been developed. Today, local anesthetics are the mainstay analgesic drugs used for local and regional anesthetic techniques in the perioperative period. These techniques cause complete desensitization of a localized area of the body, allowing a reduction in general anesthetic requirements and promoting greater cardiorespiratory stability. Sustained analgesia when a long-acting local anesthetic is used is also beneficial in the recovery period. Apart from these advantages, there is new evidence in veterinary anesthesia that locoregional techniques, when used as part of a balanced anesthetic protocol, may reduce the risk of perianesthetic mortality [1]. There is also moderate-quality evidence in humans that regional anesthesia may reduce the risk of developing persistent postoperative pain for up to 18 months in some type of surgeries [2]. In recent years, the surge in interest in locoregional anesthesia in veterinary medicine has meant the introduction of numerous new techniques and increased the use of local anesthetics worldwide.

In addition to locoregional applications related to nerve impulse blockade, the local anesthetic lidocaine may also be administered systemically for a variety of indications, including management of ventricular arrhythmias, improvement of intestinal motility following ischemia-reperfusion-injury, reduction in general anesthetic requirements, and systemic analgesia.

Pharmacology

Molecular mechanism of action

Local anesthetics are considered primarily ion channel blockers, acting mainly on voltage-gated Na^+ channels. However, they also block voltage-dependent K^+ and Ca^{2+} channels, though with lower affinity [3–7]. Some studies also suggest that local anesthetics act on intracellular sites involved in the signal transduction of G-protein-coupled receptors [8]. This range of molecular targets may explain some of the adverse and toxic effects that this group of drugs produces on various organ systems.

Ten different genes encode voltage-gated Na^+ channels and they are differentially expressed throughout the major excitable tissues.

Veterinary Anesthesia and Analgesia: The Sixth Edition of Lumb and Jones. Edited by Leigh Lamont, Kurt Grimm, Sheilah Robertson, Lydia Love and Carrie Schroeder.
© 2024 John Wiley & Sons, Inc. Published 2024 by John Wiley & Sons, Inc.
Companion website: www.wiley.com/go/lamont/anesthesia

For example, sensory neurons express mainly $Na_V1.7$ and $Na_V1.8$ Na^+ channels, whereas cardiac cells, breast, and colon cancer metastatic cells express $Na_V1.5$ [9]. While all of the current clinically available local anesthetics are nonselective, it is possible that in the future there will be subtype-selective Na^+ channel blockers [9].

The most important mechanism of action leading to local anesthesia involves the blockade of inward Na^+ currents through voltage-gated Na^+ channels, thereby impeding membrane depolarization and nerve excitation and conduction [10]. The Na^+ channel is a multimolecular complex with a large α-subunit composed of almost 2000 amino acids that traverses the cell membrane several times. This subunit forms the channel's pore and gating apparatus [10]. Some smaller auxiliary β-subunits influence the activation–inactivation states of the channel [11]. The α-subunit consists of four domains (I to IV) each containing six helical segments (S1 to S6) that wrap around and form a bell-shaped central channel. Segments S5 and S6, and the P loop between them, form the channel or pore. The S4 segments in each domain have positively charged arginine or lysine molecules and form the voltage-sensing module. The inactivation gate is formed by a short intracellular loop between domains III and IV (Fig. 29.1) [9,12]. The binding site for local anesthetic, antiarrhythmic and anticonvulsant drugs, is formed by amino acid residues in the S6 segments of domains I, II, and IV, which contribute to a single drug-binding site within the pore [12]. Because this binding site is localized within the pore, it is only accessible when the Na^+ channel is open [13].

The channel is a gated conduit for Na^+ ions and exists in three different gating states: resting (closed), open, and inactivated (Fig. 29.2), depending on the membrane potential and timing. At resting membrane potential (−70 mV), the S4 segments are in the "down" position, making the channel non-conductive. During depolarization, the channel opens by outward spiral rotation of the S4 segments allowing rapid influx of Na^+ ions down the electrical and chemical gradients. This conformational change exposes the receptor site of the inactivation gate, located between domains III and IV, which leads to channel inactivation after only a few milliseconds. Only by repolarization of the cell membrane does the channel recover to the resting state from the inactivated state [11,14].

There is evidence that local anesthetics may interact with the lipid membrane, altering its fluidity, causing membrane expansion, and thus reducing Na^+ conductance [15]; however, this does not completely explain the mechanism of action of modern clinically used local anesthetics.

The "modulated-receptor hypothesis" proposes that local anesthetics have high binding affinity for the Na^+ channel in its open and inactivated states, but low affinity for the resting state [10,16]. Lipid-soluble drug forms are thought to enter and leave the receptor via a hydrophobic region of the membrane, while charged less lipid-soluble forms pass via a hydrophilic region (the inner channel pore) [16]. The hydrophilic pathway is open only when the gates of the channel are open, which causes cumulative binding of

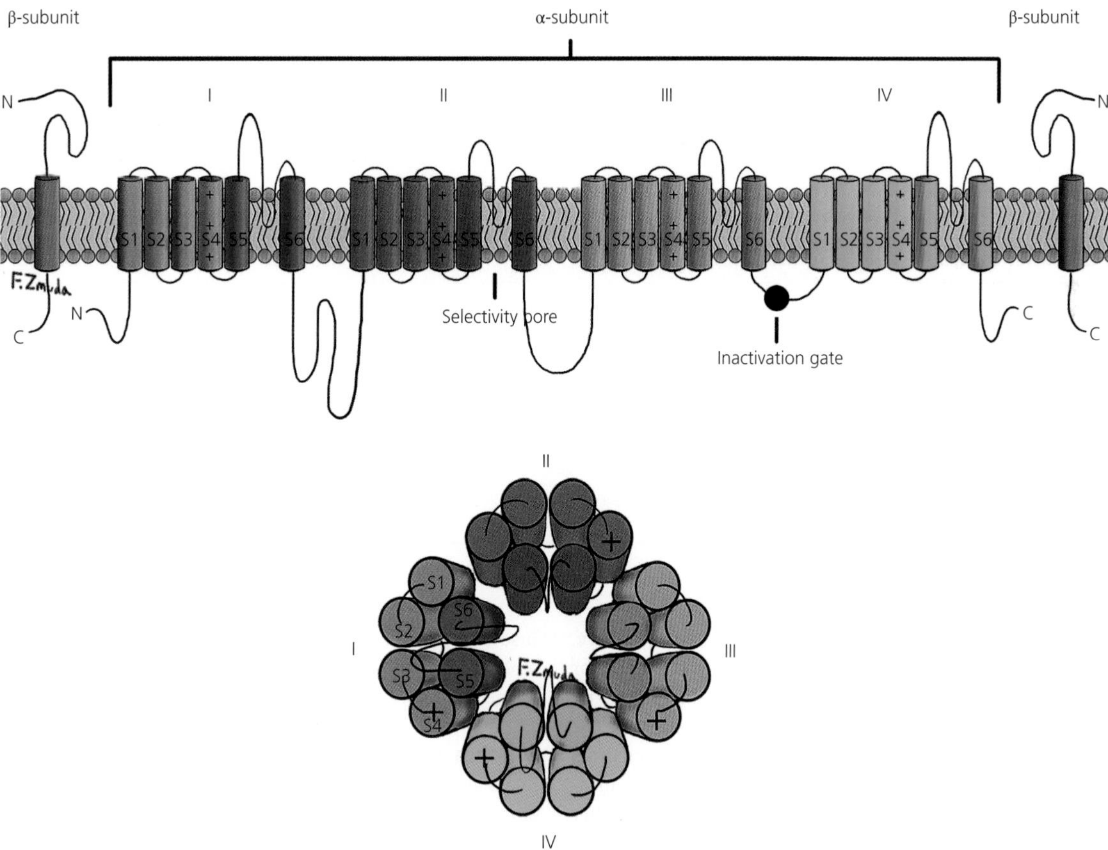

Figure 29.1 Structure of the voltage-gated Na^+ channel. I through IV represent distinct domains of the α-subunit. S1 through S6 represent helical segments within each domain that wrap around and form a bell-shaped central channel. Segments S5 and S6, and the P loop between them, form the channel or pore. The S4 segments in each domain have positively charged arginine or lysine molecules and form the voltage-sensing module. The inactivation gate is formed by a short intracellular loop between domains III and IV. Source: Taylor and McLeod [9], with permission of Elsevier.

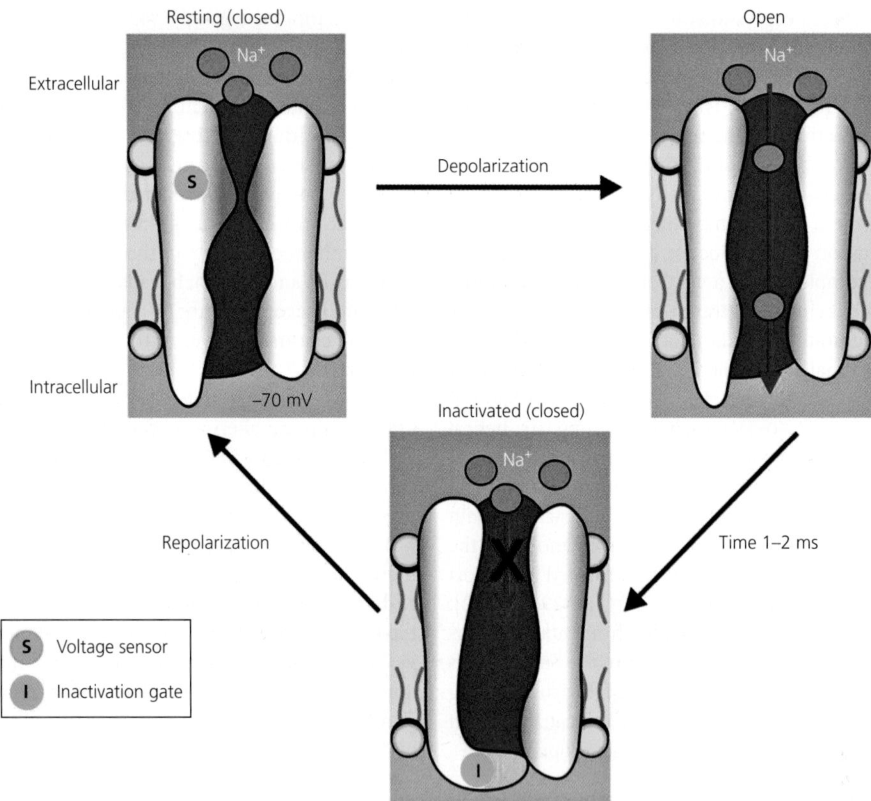

Figure 29.2 The Na⁺ channel has two gates: an activation ("voltage sensor") and an inactivation gate. At resting membrane potential, the channel exists in its resting (closed) state. Depolarization of the membrane causes outward rotation of the voltage-sensing module causing opening of the channel, allowing Na⁺ ions to flow intracellularly. Within 1–2 ms, the inactivation gate closes automatically (inactivated channel), allowing repolarization to occur. Repolarization leads to conformational changes with closure of the activation gate and opening of the inactivation gate within 2–5 ms (i.e., the refractory period). Following repolarization, the channel is in a resting state again.

Table 29.1 Classification of nerve fibers by Erlanger and Gasser and order of blockade.

Classification	Diameter (μm)	Myelin	Conduction (m/s)	Location	Function	Order of blockade
Aα	12–20	+	70–120	Afferent/efferent for muscles and joints	Afferent proprioception; efferent motor	5
Aβ	5–12	+	30–70	Efferent to muscle; afferent sensory nerve	Motor and sensory (touch and pressure)	4
Aγ	3–6	+	15–30	Efferent to muscle spindles	Muscle tone	3
Aδ	2–5	+	12–30	Afferent sensory nerve	Pain (fast), touch, temperature (cold)	2
B	< 3	+	3–15	Preganglionic sympathetic	Autonomic	1
C	0.4–1.2	–	0.5–2	Postganglionic sympathetic; afferent sensory nerve	Autonomic, pain (slow), temperature, some mechanoreceptors and reflex responses	2

Source: Adapted from Khurana *et al.* [28].

local anesthetics to the Na⁺ channel when the channels are active. The "guarded-receptor hypothesis" proposes that the receptor for local anesthetics is located inside the channel and that the drug binds to this receptor with constant affinity [17]. Access to the receptor is regulated by the channel gates and therefore the channel needs to be open for the receptor to be accessible to the local anesthetic. Increasing the frequency of stimulation increases the number of Na⁺ channels in the open and inactive states, which increases the binding of local anesthetics.

Both of these hypotheses explain the property of tertiary amine local anesthetics whereby the depth of the block increases with repetitive membrane depolarization, which has been termed "use-dependent block" or "phasic block" [18,19]. On the other hand, blockade obtained on unstimulated nerves is constant, which is termed "tonic block" [18,19].

Mechanism of blockade of neural tissue

Local anesthetics show a differential pattern of sensory and motor blockade that can be observed clinically when applied to peripheral nerves and the central neuraxis [20,21]. Vasodilation occurs first, followed by loss of sensation of temperature, sharp pain, light touch, and finally loss of motor activity (Table 29.1) [22]. This property is called "differential block" and was first described by Gasser and Erlanger in 1929 when they observed that, within myelinated A fibers, cocaine reduced compound action potentials from slower and smaller fibers more rapidly than from faster and larger fibers [23]. However, this differential block *in vivo* cannot be simply explained by the size of the fiber, but rather is influenced by numerous factors, including type of fiber (size and myelination), frequency of stimulation, length of nerve exposed to the local anesthetic, and choice and concentration of local anesthetic drug.

Initially, it was hypothesized that the differential block produced by local anesthetics when applied to peripheral nerves was due to a greater susceptibility of small, unmyelinated C fibers compared to larger, myelinated A fibers. However, *in vitro* [24] and *in vivo* studies [18,25] have shown that A-fiber susceptibility to phasic and tonic block is actually greater than that of C fibers, with the order of blockade from fastest to slowest being $A\gamma > A\delta = A\alpha > A\beta > C$. This would suggest that motor and proprioceptive deficits should occur prior to loss of nociception, but this is opposite to what is clinically observed.

Anatomic features such as myelination may also account for some differences in susceptibility, since myelin can effectively pool anesthetic molecules close to the axon membrane [26]. Experimental studies have found that unmyelinated fibers are less sensitive to lidocaine than myelinated fibers [27]. This is contrary to clinical observations of differential block, which is manifested by the loss of small fiber-mediated sensation (e.g., temperature) two or more dermatomes beyond the sensory limit for large fiber-mediated sensations.

Exposure length of the nerve to the local anesthetic may in part explain differential block *in vivo*, as smaller fibers need a shorter length exposed than larger fibers for block to occur [29]. This has been called the "critical length" to completely block conduction which, in myelinated fibers, corresponds to three or more nodes of Ranvier [30]. Therefore, larger fibers with greater internodal distances are less susceptible to local anesthetic blockade.

The somatotopic fascicular organization of peripheral nerve fibers may also influence the order of blockade. Early investigations of the brachial plexus in humans observed that nerve fibers in the mantle or peripheral bundles innervate primarily motor fibers of the proximal limb, whereas fibers localized more internally within the nerve innervate the distal limb, with sensory fibers being localized in the center bundles [31,32]. This could partially explain why in certain nerve trunks such as the brachial plexus, onset of anesthesia proceeds from proximal to distal as the local anesthetic penetrates the nerve down a concentration gradient. This is especially true when high concentrations of local anesthetics are used [32]. The recovery from the block may not follow the same pattern due to the intrinsic vascularization of nerves, which may contribute to the observed recovery of distal portions of the limb occurring before more proximal areas [32].

However, this somatotopic distribution of nerve fibers within nerves may not be consistent in different nerves or across species. What seems to be clear is that there is a high degree of somatic organization within mammalian nerves: each fascicle contains motor or sensory fibers innervating very specific areas of skin or specific muscles (Fig. 29.3) [33]. This distribution of fibers may also explain the partial blockade that is sometimes observed clinically.

Another important mechanism of local anesthetic blockade is the phenomenon of decremental conduction, which describes the diminished ability of successive nodes of Ranvier to propagate the impulse in the presence of a local anesthetic [35]. This principle explains why the propagation of an impulse can be stopped even if none of the nodes has been rendered completely inexcitable [30], as

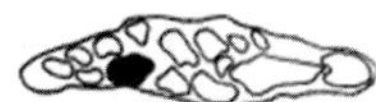

Carpal tunnel

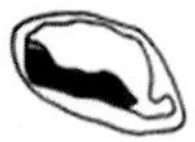

Distal forearm

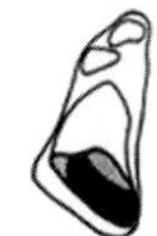

Proximal forearm

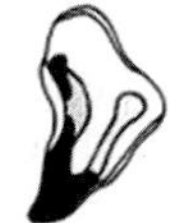

Distal arm

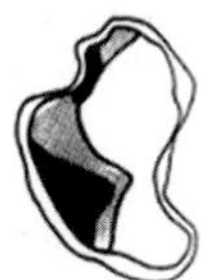

Proximal arm

Figure 29.3 Camera lucida drawings of the median nerve from a *Macaca mulatta* monkey in which the nerve fibers of an individual digital nerve (in this case, the radial digital nerve of the thumb) were exposed to horseradish peroxidase. Sections from the nerve from the carpal tunnel to proximal arm show that these nerve fibers mainly remain closely packed together (black, dense labeling), but there is some scattering of a few of the nerve fibers (stippled areas, sparse labeling). Source: Brushart [34].

occurs, for example, with low concentrations of local anesthetics. Concentrations of local anesthetic that block 74–84% of the sodium conductance at successive nodes cause a progressive decrease in amplitude of the impulse, until it eventually decays below the threshold [30]. Higher concentrations that block more than 84% of the sodium conductance at three consecutive nodes will prevent impulse propagation completely [30]. This explains why blocks of greater extent and duration result from injection of small-volume/high-concentration solutions versus large-volume/low-concentration solutions, despite the same total drug dose [36].

Some authors suggest that a large portion of the sensory information transmitted by peripheral nerves is carried via coding of electrical signals in after-potentials and after-oscillations [37]. Sub-blocking concentrations of local anesthetics can suppress these intrinsic oscillatory after-effects of impulse discharge without significantly affecting action potential conduction [38]. Thus, another possible mechanism of blockade of nerve function, especially at low concentrations of local anesthetics, is by disruption of coding of electrical information [19].

When local anesthetics are administered in the central neuraxis (epidurally or intrathecally) or systemically, they may possess other mechanisms of analgesic action at the level of the spinal cord in addition to those previously discussed. Local anesthetics inhibit other ion channels such as K^+ or Ca^{2+} channels at the level of the dorsal horn of the spinal cord. This may affect central neuroprocessing of sensory information, thereby contributing to their antinociceptive effects [39–41]. In addition to ion channels, nociceptive transmission is mediated by several neurotransmitters in the dorsal horn, such as the tachykinins (e.g., substance P). Local anesthetics have been shown to inhibit substance P binding and evoked increases in intracellular Ca^{2+} [42]. Additionally, local anesthetics also inhibit glutamatergic transmission in spinal dorsal horn neurons, reducing *N*-methyl-D-aspartate (NMDA)- and neurokinin-mediated postsynaptic depolarizations [43,44].

Chemical structure

Clinically useful local anesthetic drugs are composed of a lipophilic, benzene ring with different substitutions (aromatic ring), and a hydrophilic amine group (tertiary or quaternary amine), which are linked through an intermediate chain, either an ester or an amide. Depending on the type of link, local anesthetics are classified as (1) aminoesters which are hydrolyzed by plasma cholinesterase (also known as "butyrylcholinesterase" or "pseudocholinesterase"), or (2) aminoamides which are metabolized by the liver.

Physicochemical properties

The physicochemical properties influencing local anesthetic activity include molecular weight, pK_a, lipid solubility, and degree of protein binding (Table 29.2) [45,46].

The molecular weight of clinically used local anesthetics is very similar, ranging between 220 and 288 Da. The diffusion coefficient is thus not significantly affected and molecular weight does not seem to be an important factor determining differences in activity of local anesthetics [45]. However, changes in molecular weight due to alkyl substitutions may influence other properties such as lipid solubility and pK_a.

All clinically useful local anesthetics are weak bases, and as such they exist in equilibrium between the neutral, non-ionized, lipid-soluble form (B) and the ionized (charged), water-soluble form (BH^+). They are formulated as acidic solutions of hydrochloride salts (pH 4–7), which are more highly ionized and water soluble.

The receptor for local anesthetics appears to be located within the pore of the Na^+ channel close to the cytoplasm [13] and only the ionized, charged form of the local anesthetic can interact with this receptor [47]. Local anesthetics can cross the cell membrane in two different ways: (1) the ionized form can pass through the open sodium channel, and (2) the non-ionized, lipophilic form can penetrate through the lipid membrane. The latter seems to be the main method for local anesthetics to access the cell (Fig. 29.4).

The pK_a of a drug is the pH at which the two forms exist in equal concentrations and is alkaline (pH > 7.4) for all clinically used local anesthetics.

$$pK_a = pH - \log\left([B]/[BH^+]\right)$$

The higher the pK_a, the greater the degree of ionization or proportion of local anesthetic in the ionized, charged hydrophilic form at physiologic pH, and the slower the onset of action. On the other hand, a local anesthetic with a low pK_a will have a greater proportion of the non-ionized, lipid-soluble form at physiologic pH and a more rapid onset of action.

Lipid solubility is the main determinant of intrinsic local anesthetic potency, and it will determine the clinically relevant concentrations needed to produce effective conduction blockade [48–50]. Increasing lipid solubility facilitates the penetration through lipid membranes, potentially hastening onset of action; however, highly lipid-soluble agents will also become sequestered within the myelin and other lipid compartments. Thus, the net effect of increasing lipid solubility is delayed onset of action of local anesthetics [51]. On the other hand, sequestration of local anesthetic in myelin and other lipid compartments creates a depot for slow release of the

Table 29.2 Physicochemical properties and relative potencies of clinically used local anesthetics.

Local anesthetic	pK_a [a]	% Ionized (at pH 7.4)	Lipid solubility[b]	% Protein binding	Relative anesthetic potency[c]	Relative potency for CNS toxicity[d]	CV:CNS ratio[e]
Ester-linked							
Low potency, short duration							
Procaine	8.89	97	100	6	1	0.3	3.7
Chloroprocaine	9.06	95	810	7	1	0.3	3.7
High potency, long duration							
Tetracaine	8.38	93	5822	94	8	2	ND
Amide-linked							
Intermediate potency and duration							
Lidocaine	7.77	76	366	64	2	1	7.1
Mepivacaine	7.72	61	130	77	2	1.4	7.1
Prilocaine	8.02	76	129	55	2	1.2	3.1
Intermediate potency, long duration							
Ropivacaine	8.16	83	775	94	6	2.9	2
High potency, long duration							
Bupivacaine	8.1	83	3420	95	8	4	2
Levobupivacaine	8.1	83	3420	> 97	8	2.9	2
Etidocaine	7.87	66	7317	94	6	2	4.4

[a] Measured with spectrophotometric method at 36 °C, except prilocaine and ropivacaine measured at 25 °C.
[b] Partition coefficients expressed as relative concentrations (mol/L) in octanol and buffer at 36 °C, except prilocaine and ropivacaine measured at 25 °C.
[c] Potency relative to procaine.
[d] Potency relative to lidocaine.
[e] Cardiovascular (CV) to central nervous system (CNS) toxicity ratio. CV denotes the disappearance of pulse and CNS denotes the onset of seizures.
Source: Data obtained from Liu [46]; Strichartz *et al.* [48]. ND, no data.

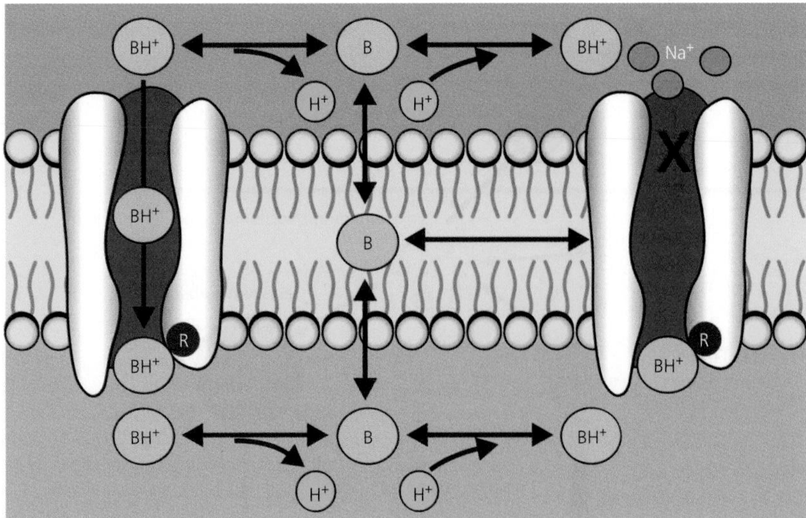

Figure 29.4 The cell membrane lipid bilayer with the Na^+ channel. Local anesthetics exist as a neutral base (B) and an ionized form (BH^+) in equilibrium. The neutral form is lipid soluble and easily crosses the cell membrane. The ionized form is more water soluble and can cross through the open channel. The neutral form can cause membrane expansion and closure of the Na^+ channel. The ionized form interacts with its receptor on the intracellular side of the Na^+ channel.

drug, increasing the duration of the effect [51]. It has also been postulated that more lipophilic drugs such as bupivacaine may be less likely to travel by bulk flow than less lipophilic drugs such as mepivacaine, and therefore, more hydrophilic local anesthetics may have greater ability to spread further [52].

The degree of protein binding also influences activity of local anesthetics, as only the unbound, free fraction is pharmacologically active. Higher protein binding is associated with increased duration of action. This cannot be explained by slower dissociation kinetics from the Na^+ channel, as this dissociation occurs within seconds regardless of the degree of protein binding [53]. Increased duration of action of highly protein-bound local anesthetics is probably associated with other membrane or extracellular proteins [54].

Lidocaine, procaine, and tetracaine are achiral molecules, while levobupivacaine and ropivacaine are pure *S*(−)-enantiomers [45,55]. The rest of the clinically available local anesthetics are racemic mixtures of the *R*(+)- and *S*(−)-enantiomers in a 50:50 mixture. Although both enantiomers have the same physicochemical properties, they have different affinities for the ion channels of Na^+, K^+, and Ca^{2+}, with the *R*(+)-enantiomer having greater *in vitro* potency and thus greater therapeutic efficacy but also greater potential for systemic toxicity [56,57]. There is less potential for nervous and cardiac toxicity with the *S*(−)-enantiomer compared with the *R*(+)-enantiomer or the racemic mixture [58].

Studies *in vitro* have characterized the relative potencies of local anesthetic agents, which depend not only on their physicochemical properties (i.e., lipid solubility) but also on the individual nerve fibers and frequency of stimulation [59]. However, *in vivo* potencies do not necessarily correlate with *in vitro* studies [60], because of the complex interaction of factors, including site of administration, dose, and volume of local anesthetics, and other environmental factors.

Local anesthetics with an amide group, high pK_a, and lower lipid solubility show greater differential blockade, with more potent blockade of C fibers than of fast-conducting A fibers [51,61]. This is believed to be due to the slower diffusion across permeability barriers present in A fibers. The relative order of differential rate of blockade is chloroprocaine > ropivacaine > bupivacaine, levobupivacaine > lidocaine, mepivacaine > etidocaine [62,63]. This is especially true at low concentrations and the differential rate of blockade tends to disappear as local anesthetic concentrations increase.

Clinical pharmacology

Pharmacokinetics

Absorption

Disposition of local anesthetics within the body after local administration is governed by several competing factors, including bulk flow, diffusion and binding to neural and non-neural structures, and vascular uptake (Fig. 29.5). The rate and extent of systemic absorption of the local anesthetic are important as toxic plasma concentrations may be achieved. Therefore, local anesthetics with lower systemic absorption will have a greater margin of safety. Systemic absorption depends on several factors, including the site of injection (i.e., vascularity), the intrinsic lipid solubility and vasoactivity of the agent, the dose administered, the presence of additives such as vasoconstrictors, other formulation factors that modify local drug residence and release, the influence of the nerve block in the region (i.e., vasodilation), and the (patho)physiologic state of the patient [45].

In general, areas with greater vascularity will have more extensive and rapid systemic drug absorption than areas with more fat, regardless of the agent used [19]. Areas with greater vascularity will have a greater peak plasma concentration (C_{max}) and a shorter time-to-peak plasma concentration (T_{max}). In an experimental study in pigs, lidocaine rate of absorption following subcutaneous administration was highest in the pectoral region, followed by the face and neck, with the slowest being the abdomen [64]. With regard to specific blocks, the degree of systemic absorption is as follows, in decreasing order: intercostal > epidural > brachial plexus > sciatic/femoral [65]. Following administration of lidocaine in an inverted L nerve block in cows, the serum C_{max} was 572 ng/mL, which occurred at T_{max} 0.52 h, while lidocaine via a caudal epidural block was

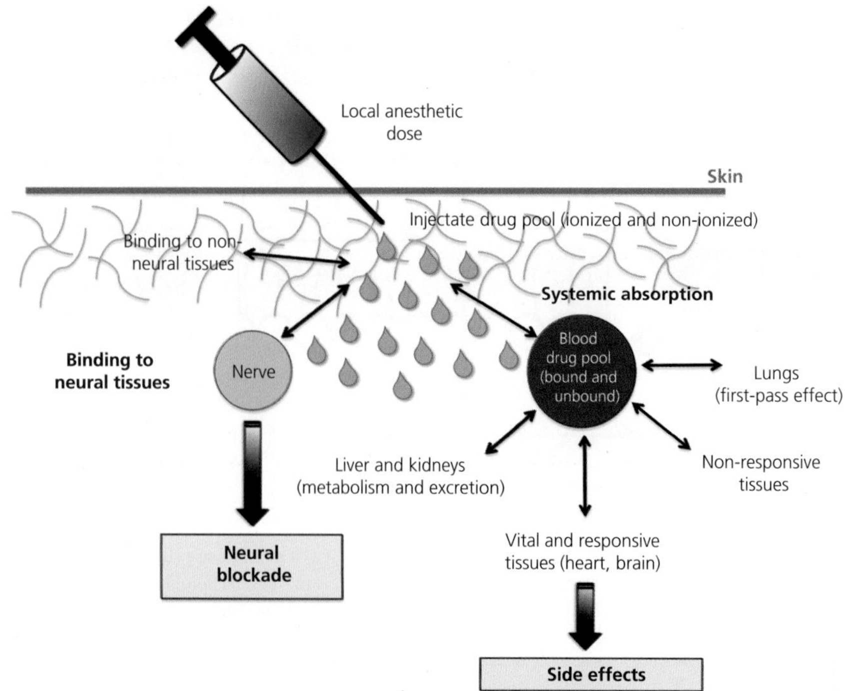

Figure 29.5 Disposition of local anesthetics within the body following peripheral administration.

undetectable in serum [66]. Systemic absorption of local anesthetic drugs is much lower after spinal (intrathecal) than after epidural administration [67,68]. Normally, the greatest risk of systemic toxicity coincides with T_{max} in arterial blood, which will vary from 5 to 45 min after injection, depending on the site of the block, speed of injection, and drug injected [45]. However, T_{max} is independent of the dose injected [69]. Faster speed of injection is associated with greater C_{max}, and therefore with increased risk of systemic toxicity [70].

Physicochemical properties of local anesthetics will also influence systemic absorption. In general, drugs with greater lipid solubility and protein binding will result in lower systemic absorption and C_{max} [45]. Therefore, shorter-acting amide drugs such as lidocaine and mepivacaine will be absorbed into the systemic circulation more readily than longer-acting bupivacaine, ropivacaine, and levobupivacaine, probably because of binding of the latter to neural and non-neural lipid-rich tissues [19]. Another factor influencing the rate of absorption is the intrinsic vasoactivity of the local anesthetic. Most clinically used local anesthetics cause vasodilation when applied locally, with the exceptions of ropivacaine and levobupivacaine [71,72]. The vasoconstrictive activity of ropivacaine and levobupivacaine results in slower absorption and therefore longer T_{max} values [73,74].

The addition of a vasoconstrictor, such as epinephrine, will counteract the inherent vasodilating effects on the local vasculature induced by most agents, delaying their systemic absorption. Hyaluronidase is another additive occasionally added to local anesthetics to improve their anesthetic effect by causing depolymerization of interstitial hyaluronic acid and thus increasing the permeability of the tissues; however, hyaluronidase also enhances systemic absorption and the risk of systemic toxicity (see the section on Additives later in this chapter).

There are some formulations, such as local anesthetic-loaded liposomes, polylactide microspheres, or cyclodextrin inclusion complexes, among others, which are designed to cause a slow release of the drug, providing a local depot of local anesthetic which significantly decreases systemic absorption and prolongs the duration of effect [69,75,76]. When liposome-encapsulated lidocaine was administered epidurally to dogs, the C_{max} was lower while the T_{max} and the duration of effect (170 versus 61 min) were significantly longer compared to regular lidocaine [75]. In sheep, intercostal administration of bupivacaine–dexamethasone microspheres prolonged the duration of the block up to 13 days, with plasma concentrations remaining 10 times below the convulsive concentration [77]. Liposome-encapsulated lidocaine has also been administered topically to cats at a dose of 15 mg/kg, which proved to be safe, with C_{max} well below the toxic plasma levels for that species [78]. Administration of different slow-release lidocaine formulations for sciatic nerve block in postoperative pain models in rats produced analgesia from 3 days up to 1 week and inhibited the development of hyperalgesia [79,80]. A number of newer formulations of local anesthetics have been approved for use in animals that greatly reduce systemic absorption, thereby limiting the extent of their effect to the surgical area, prolonging the analgesic effect, and reducing C_{max} and the possibility of systemic toxicity. These are discussed later in this chapter in the Special formulations section.

Distribution

After absorption into the bloodstream, aminoester local anesthetics are rapidly hydrolyzed by plasma cholinesterases, and their distribution into body tissues is limited. Aminoamide local anesthetics are widely distributed into different body organs and tissues. The degree of tissue distribution and binding is normally represented by the pharmacokinetic parameter known as the "apparent volume of distribution at steady state" (V_{dss}), which is usually paralleled by the degree of protein binding [45]. Only the free, active fraction of the drug, and not the protein-bound fraction, governs tissue concentration and degree of entry into the central nervous system (CNS) [81].

Amide-type local anesthetics bind primarily to α_1-acid glycoprotein (AAG) in the plasma and to a lesser extent to albumin [82,83]. In dogs, increasing concentrations of AAG caused an increase in total serum concentration but a decrease in the free fraction, V_{dss}, and elimination half-life of lidocaine [81,84]. Because AAG is an acute-phase protein, its circulating levels will be increased during trauma, surgery, cancer, or any inflammatory state. Therefore, although the total concentration of local anesthetic in plasma will be greater, reflecting the increase in AAG, the unbound (active) drug fraction will remain similar [45,85].

Amide-type local anesthetics in venous blood undergo first-pass pulmonary uptake, which effectively decreases the plasma concentration of the drug temporarily [86,87]. Consequently, the lungs are able to attenuate the toxic effects after accidental intravenous injections of local anesthetics. In animals with right-to-left cardiac shunts, the pulmonary first-pass effect is absent and there is an increased risk of toxicity. The pulmonary uptake of a local anesthetic is mostly dependent on its physicochemical properties, mainly lipid solubility and pK_a. More lipid-soluble agents undergo greater pulmonary uptake and those with lower pK_a values will have a greater fraction of the non-ionized base form, which is the form that accumulates in the lung [88]. Decreasing blood pH (i.e., acidemia) decreases the degree of pulmonary uptake of local anesthetics, which may contribute to increased plasma concentrations and promote toxicity [86,88]. The rank order of pulmonary uptake in rat lung slices was found to be bupivacaine > etidocaine > lidocaine [88]. Others have also found greater uptake of prilocaine compared to bupivacaine and mepivacaine in isolated perfused rat lungs, with little evidence of pulmonary metabolism [89]. The mean pulmonary uptake of lidocaine after IV administration in dogs has been calculated to be 63.6% [87]. There is evidence of a pulmonary contribution to lidocaine metabolism using rat pulmonary microsomes *in vitro* [90]. After an intravenous bolus injection in rabbits, the pulmonary uptake of levobupivacaine was greater than that of ropivacaine (31% versus 23%) [91].

Local anesthetic agents also distribute rapidly and extensively into milk and muscle at concentrations proportional to those in the bloodstream. Drugs that diffuse most readily into milk are those that are relatively lipophilic, non-ionized, not strongly protein-bound, and with low molecular weights [92]. Following an inverted L nerve block with 100 mL of 2% lidocaine in adult Holstein cows, the lidocaine C_{max} in milk was 300 ng/mL compared with serum C_{max} of 572 ng/mL; T_{max} in milk was 1.75 h compared with serum T_{max} of 0.52 h [66]. The last measurable time of lidocaine detection in milk after inverted L block was 32.5 h with a mean concentration of 46 ng/mL [66]. On the other hand, following caudal epidural administration of 0.22 mg/kg of lidocaine, there was no detectable lidocaine concentration present in any serum or milk sample [66]. The current Food Animal Residue Avoidance Database (FARAD) withdrawal intervals reflect these differences, with a 4-day meat withdrawal and 72 h milk withdrawal following infiltrative lidocaine administration, but only a 1-day meat withdrawal and 24-h milk withdrawal following epidural lidocaine administration. The European Medicines Agency (EMA), on the other hand, establishes a 28-day withdrawal period for meat and 15-day milk withdrawal after lidocaine administration by any route.

Local anesthetic drugs also cross the placenta and appear in the fetus following administration to the pregnant animal. Ester-linked local anesthetic agents are rapidly metabolized and placental transfer is limited [45]. Amide-linked local anesthetic agents can become "trapped" in their ionized forms on the more acidotic fetal side of the placenta, and therefore their net transfer across the placenta is increased [93]. In pregnant ewes, as fetal blood pH decreased from 7.35 to 7.10, the fetal–maternal ratio (F:M) for lidocaine increased from 0.76 to 1.21 [93]. Apart from the pH, the degree of local anesthetic binding to both maternal and fetal plasma proteins is also an important determinant of placental transfer of local anesthetics, as only the unbound, free drug crosses the placenta [94]. Since fetal AAG content and binding are less than maternal [95], the F:M of highly protein-bound local anesthetics such as bupivacaine (F:M = 0.36) is lower than less protein-bound drugs such as lidocaine (F:M = 1) [94,96]. The placental transfer of levobupivacaine and ropivacaine is similar to bupivacaine in pregnant ewes [97].

An important consideration when choosing a local anesthetic agent in the pregnant animal is the ability of the neonate to metabolize and excrete the drug after birth. Studies in sheep show that back-transfer of bupivacaine, but not of lidocaine, from the fetus to the mother occurs [94,96]. Lidocaine and its metabolites monoethylglycinexylidide (MEGX) and glycinexylidide (GX) were detected in fetal urine within 1–2 h following intravenous infusion of lidocaine to pregnant ewes [94]. These studies suggest that lidocaine might be a better option in pregnant animals since the fetus/neonate will be able to readily eliminate the drug. They also suggest that if high plasma concentrations of local anesthetic in maternal blood are likely (i.e., large volumes used for local blockade or inadvertent intravenous administration), it would be beneficial to delay delivery in the case of bupivacaine, but there would be no benefit in doing so in the case of lidocaine [94].

Metabolism

Ester-linked local anesthetics are cleared mainly in the blood by plasma cholinesterase (also known variably as butyrylcholinesterase, non-specific cholinesterase, or pseudocholinesterase), where they undergo ester hydrolysis. Esterases present in the liver, red blood cells, and synovial fluid also contribute to the clearance of these drugs [98–100]. Among the ester agents, chloroprocaine is cleared most rapidly due to its faster hydrolysis rate. *In vitro* half-lives tend to be very short for the ester-linked drugs, ranging from 11 s for chloroprocaine in human plasma [101] to 9 s and 12 s for procaine in equine whole blood and plasma, respectively [98], and up to several minutes for tetracaine [45]. *In vivo* terminal half-lives are typically longer, probably reflecting slow uptake from the site of administration and/or wide distribution within the body [45,102]. The terminal half-life of procaine in horses after intravenous administration is 50 min with an apparent volume of distribution of 6.7 L/kg [102]. The hydrolysis products of procaine, chloroprocaine, and tetracaine appear to be pharmacologically inactive. Procaine and benzocaine are hydrolyzed to *para*-aminobenzoic acid (PABA) which may, however, cause rare allergic reactions [45].

Cocaine undergoes ester hydrolysis in plasma and liver, but also *N*-demethylation in the liver to norcocaine, which subsequently undergoes further hydrolysis [100]. Cocaine is rarely used in veterinary medicine, but illegal use in horses or dogs before races to increase performance and delay the time to exhaustion is possible [103]. Procaine also possesses CNS stimulatory effects and its use is banned in racehorses [102].

Amide-linked local anesthetics are almost exclusively metabolized in the liver by microsomal enzymes (CYP450). Phase I reactions involve hydroxylation, *N*-dealkylation, and *N*-demethylation, followed by Phase II reactions where the metabolites are conjugated with amino acids or glucuronide into less active and inactive metabolites. Clearance values differ among species, but typically the rank order of clearance is prilocaine > etidocaine > lidocaine > mepivacaine > ropivacaine > bupivacaine [45]. In humans, prilocaine is cleared most rapidly, with blood clearance values that exceed liver blood flow, indicating extrahepatic metabolism in this species [45]. Hydrolysis of prilocaine produces *ortho*-toluidine (*o*-toluidine), a metabolite that oxidizes hemoglobin to methemoglobin (MHb) [104].

Lidocaine undergoes hydroxylation and *N*-demethylation in the liver. Its two main metabolites are monoethylglycinexylidide (MEGX) and glycinexylidide (GX) in dogs [105], rabbits [106], rats [107], cats [108], horses [109,110], goats [111], and chickens [112], but these metabolites have not been detected in cows [113]. Of these metabolites, MEGX in particular has significant activity (approximately, 70% that of lidocaine) and could potentially contribute to its toxicity during prolonged intravenous infusions [45,110]. Another metabolite of lidocaine, 2,6-xylidine, is of interest in food-producing animals as it has been shown to have genotoxic and carcinogenic potential following ingestion in humans. Other amides such as mepivacaine, bupivacaine, and ropivacaine undergo mainly *N*-dealkylation and hydroxylation. These agents produce the less toxic metabolite pipecoloxylidide (PPX) [114]. The *N*-dealkylated metabolite of bupivacaine, *N*-desbutylbupivacaine, is about half as cardiotoxic as bupivacaine, but less toxic to the CNS in rat studies [115]. Some amide metabolites are further conjugated to glucuronide before they are eliminated in the urine or bile [116].

Excretion

Local anesthetics are poorly water soluble, which limits renal excretion of the unchanged drug. The hydrolysis metabolites of ester-linked local anesthetics are mainly excreted in urine [117]. Similarly, the metabolites of amide-linked local anesthetics are eliminated in urine or bile. A small portion of amide-type local anesthetics is excreted unchanged in urine (4–7% for lidocaine, 6% for bupivacaine, and 16% for mepivacaine in humans; 1.7–2.9% for lidocaine in horses) [118–120].

Factors affecting pharmacokinetics and activity

Patient factors, such as age, may influence the pharmacokinetics of local anesthetics. Absorption of lidocaine from laryngeal spray was higher in dogs less than 20 days of age compared to 2–3-month-old puppies [121]. The volume of distribution and the elimination half-life of lidocaine were greater in neonatal lambs compared with adult sheep [122]. In a pharmacokinetic study of lidocaine in puppies, the elimination rate constant from the central compartment (k_{10}) was lower, and the elimination half-life was longer in 3–16-day old compared with 6-month-old puppies [123]. When comparing neonatal lambs with adult sheep, hepatic clearance of lidocaine was similar but renal clearance of unchanged drug was greater in the neonate, probably due to decreased protein binding, lower urine pH, and decreased tubular reabsorption because of higher urine flow rates [122]. Plasma hydrolysis of ester-linked local anesthetics is also affected by age, as observed in human neonates and infants where plasma cholinesterase activity was half that of adults [124]. In geriatric animals, hepatic clearance of local anesthetics may be decreased, and half-life increased [125,126].

Increased nerve sensitivity to local anesthetics seems to be present during pregnancy with faster onset of conduction blockade [127]. Acute progesterone treatment had no effect on bupivacaine-induced conduction blockade in the isolated rabbit vagus nerve; therefore, this effect is unlikely to be a direct effect of progesterone on the cell membrane but may involve hormonal effects on protein synthesis [128]. Pregnant ewes were found to clear lidocaine more rapidly, but bupivacaine and ropivacaine more slowly than non-pregnant ewes [129,130]. This difference may be explained by lidocaine's clearance being more dependent on hepatic blood flow, which is increased during pregnancy, whereas clearance of bupivacaine and ropivacaine is more dependent on hepatic enzymatic activity, which may be inhibited during pregnancy [45].

Hepatic disease can decrease the rate of metabolism of amide-linked local anesthetics. Plasma cholinesterase activity is also reduced in the presence of liver disease and during pregnancy, which will decrease the rate of hydrolysis of ester-linked local anesthetics [131,132]. In general, standard doses may be administered to animals with hepatic disease for single-dose neural blockade but repeated doses, dosing intervals, and continuous rate infusions need to be adjusted to avoid accumulation and toxicity [45]. A decrease in hepatic blood flow, as can occur during general anesthesia, cardiac disease, or any condition decreasing cardiac output, will decrease hepatic clearance of local anesthetics, especially those more dependent on hepatic blood flow such as lidocaine [45,133]. The V_{dss} and clearance (*Cl*) of intravenous lidocaine were significantly decreased in anesthetized compared to awake horses (0.4 versus 0.79 L/kg and 15 versus 29 mL/kg/min, respectively) [134], and in anesthetized compared to awake cats (1.4 versus 1.9 L/kg and 21 versus 26 mL/kg/min, respectively) [108]. Hepatic clearance of other amide-linked local anesthetics such as mepivacaine or bupivacaine is more dependent on activity of hepatic enzymes and the effect of reduced hepatic blood flow is less pronounced.

Renal failure decreases plasma cholinesterase activity by 40% in humans [135]. Aminoamides are excreted mainly as water-soluble metabolites, which may accumulate in animals with renal failure and contribute to CNS toxicity if they are active (e.g., MEGX and GX) [133].

Fasting has been shown to decrease hepatic clearance of lidocaine in horses [120]. Gastrointestinal disease (e.g., equine colic) may also affect clearance of aminoamide local anesthetics that depend mainly on hepatic blood flow, such as lidocaine, especially if cardiac output is significantly reduced. However, pharmacokinetic parameters of intravenous lidocaine in horses undergoing abdominal surgery for colic are similar to those of healthy, awake horses, with V_{dss} and *Cl* values of 0.7 L/kg and 25 mL/kg/min [136]. It was hypothesized that the cardiac output of the horses included in that study might have been increased, rather than decreased [136].

Interestingly, diabetes mellitus increases hepatic clearance of lidocaine, although the excretion of the metabolite MEGX is impaired [137,138].

Concomitant administration of local anesthetics with other drugs may affect their distribution and elimination kinetics. Drugs that decrease plasma or red cell esterase activity, such as neostigmine or acetazolamide, will prolong half-life of ester-linked local anesthetics [139,140]. When CYP1A2 and CYP3A4 inhibitors, such as erythromycin, are co-administered with aminoamide local anesthetics, their hepatic clearance may decrease [141]. β-Adrenergic receptor blocking drugs reduce liver perfusion and inhibit the activity of hepatic microsomal metabolizing enzymes responsible for the metabolism of aminoamide local anesthetics; hence, greater plasma concentration and decreased elimination will occur when these drugs are co-administered [142].

Co-administration of different classes of local anesthetics may also affect their pharmacokinetic parameters. The rate of hydrolysis of chloroprocaine is reduced by concomitant administration of bupivacaine or etidocaine, but not when it is co-administered with lidocaine or mepivacaine [139,143].

Temperature may also affect the pharmacokinetics and pharmacodynamics of local anesthetics. Lidocaine's ability to block nerve impulses, both *in vitro* and *in vivo*, is potentiated by cooling [144,145]. Conversely, lidocaine uptake by mammalian sciatic nerve is reduced by cooling, with a 45% decrease when the temperature falls from 37 °C to 20 °C [146]. Some clinical studies in humans have observed an increase in the speed of onset of various types of blocks when the temperature of the local anesthetic solution was increased to 37 °C [147–150], although this effect has not been consistent [151,152]. Cooling of the local anesthetic solution increases the pK_a and the relative amount of ionized active form, while warming the solution decreases the pK_a and increases the amount of non-ionized lipid-soluble form [146]. These pK_a changes may explain the increased potency of local anesthetics with cooling and the hastening of onset of action with warming.

Baricity is one of the most important physical properties of local anesthetics during subarachnoid or intrathecal administration as it will affect the distribution and spread of the solution, and therefore impact the characteristics of the block [153]. Baricity of a local anesthetic solution is the calculated ratio of the density of the solution to the density of the cerebrospinal fluid (CSF), both measured at the same temperature, which is normally 37 °C. Density is the weight in grams of 1 mL of the solution, and it is inversely related to its temperature [154]. An isobaric solution has a baricity ratio of 1. If the ratio is > 1, the solution is hyperbaric, and if it is < 1, it is hypobaric. At room temperature, most commercially available local anesthetic solutions are isobaric with respect to the CSF, but when they are warmed to body temperature, they become hypobaric [154]. The densities of commercial 2% lidocaine and 0.5% and 0.75% bupivacaine are lower than that of human CSF at 37 °C, which makes them relatively hypobaric [155]. Dilution of these solutions with water makes them increasingly hypobaric [155]. When local anesthetics are mixed with dextrose or hypertonic saline, the resulting solution is hyperbaric [154,156]. Neurotoxicity has been observed with hyperbaric bupivacaine when high concentrations and doses are administered intrathecally in dogs (≥ 10 mg of 1% or 2% bupivacaine in 10% glucose solution), but not with low concentrations and doses (5 mg of 0.5% bupivacaine in 10% glucose solution) [157]. High concentrations and doses of hypobaric bupivacaine (20 mg of 2% bupivacaine in water) were not associated with neurotoxicity when administered intrathecally to dogs [157].

Hypobaric solutions, when injected into the subarachnoid space, will migrate to non-dependent areas, because their density is lower than that of the CSF, while hyperbaric solutions will migrate to dependent areas. This migration allows preferential blockade to occur on the surgical side, with unilateral spinal anesthesia being possible when low doses of local anesthetics are used [158]. Isobaric solutions will migrate to both sides of the spinal cord, causing bilateral spinal block. In humans, it is reported that unilateral spinal block results in a four-fold reduction of the incidence of clinically relevant hypotension with more stable cardiovascular parameters as compared with conventional bilateral spinal block [159]. Because only small amounts of local anesthetic solution are injected, the extent of spinal block is reduced, and the resolution of sensory and motor blockade is faster [159].

Mixtures of local anesthetic agents with additives such as solvents or vasoconstrictors, or with other drugs such as opioids, may alter the density and baricity of the solution. When 0.125–0.5% bupivacaine solutions are mixed with fentanyl (0.005%), sufentanil (0.005%), or morphine (0.1%), the resultant solutions are hypobaric [160]. The mixture of 2% lidocaine and epinephrine (1:200,000) results in a hyperbaric solution [160].

There is some variation in the density of the CSF among individuals [161]. Density of the CSF may also be influenced by physiologic status (e.g., density is decreased during pregnancy in humans) [162]. Therefore, there may be some interindividual variation in clinical response to intrathecal solutions, especially with those that are marginally hypo- or hyperbaric [153].

Additives

Epinephrine (adrenaline)

Epinephrine has been used as an adjunct to local anesthetics for more than a century. The rationale behind its use is that it causes vasoconstriction and therefore decreases the systemic absorption of the local anesthetic agent, which decreases the dose of local anesthetic required and prolongs its duration of effect [163,164]. Decreased systemic absorption also reduces the local anesthetic C_{max}, which decreases the probability of systemic toxicity. Several studies have demonstrated decreased C_{max} of local anesthetics when administered with epinephrine both in peripheral and neuraxial blocks [164–167]. In general, the greatest effects are observed with shorter-acting rather than with longer-acting agents.

In addition to this pharmacokinetic interaction, epinephrine seems to have analgesic effects on its own when administered epidurally or intrathecally by stimulating α_2-adrenergic receptors, thereby inhibiting presynaptic neurotransmitter release from C and Aδ fibers in the substantia gelatinosa of the spinal cord dorsal horn [168–170]. It has also been shown that α_2-adrenergic receptors can modify certain K^+ channels in the axons of peripheral nerves, potentiating the impulse-blocking actions of local anesthetics [171,172]. A later study in rats also showed that local infiltration of epinephrine causes cutaneous anesthesia mediated by activation of local α_1-adrenergic receptors [173]. Therefore, it seems that pharmacokinetic and pharmacodynamic interactions between epinephrine and local anesthetics are responsible for the increased duration and intensity of the block when administered in combination.

A potential concern when epinephrine is co-administered with local anesthetics is a decrease in peripheral nerve or spinal cord blood flow, which could cause nerve or spinal cord ischemia. However, research studies with radiolabeled microspheres in dogs and cats show that epinephrine injected intrathecally causes regional dural vasoconstriction but does not reduce spinal cord or cerebral blood flow [174,175]. This is supported by many years of clinical experience using epinephrine-containing solutions for neuraxial anesthesia and the absence of observed detrimental effects on spinal cord function [172,176]. *In vitro* studies in rats showed that sciatic nerve blood flow is reduced by injection of lidocaine without epinephrine, but that the reduction is more pronounced when epinephrine (5 μg/mL) is added [177]. However, a more recent *in vivo* rat study using radiolabeled microspheres showed that lidocaine with or without epinephrine (10 μg/mL) does not reduce sciatic nerve or surrounding skeletal muscle blood flow [178]. The authors of this study concluded that mechanisms other than local vasoconstriction might contribute to the prolongation of lidocaine peripheral nerve blockade by epinephrine.

Systemic absorption of epinephrine administered in combination with local anesthetics can also cause cardiovascular effects characterized by an increase in heart rate, stroke volume, and cardiac output, and a decrease in peripheral vascular resistance [179]. A study in humans also showed an improvement in left ventricular diastolic function with epinephrine added to local anesthetics, in contrast with norepinephrine, which impaired it [179]. Excessive plasma concentrations of epinephrine could precipitate tachycardia and arrhythmias.

The recommended concentrations of epinephrine for addition to local anesthetic solutions for clinical use range between 1:400,000 (1 mg/400 mL or 2.5 μg/mL) and 1:200,000 (1 mg/200 mL or 5 μg/mL] [172]. A 1:200,000 concentration can be obtained by adding 0.1 mL of a 1:1000 epinephrine solution (0.1 mg) into 20 mL of local anesthetic solution. Concentrations in excess of 5 μg/mL do not provide any additional decrease in C_{max} and should therefore be avoided in light of the potential for systemic side effects [45]. Market preparations of local anesthetics that contain epinephrine have lower pH values than plain or freshly prepared solutions. The lower pH of these epinephrine-containing preparations could potentially decrease the amount of non-ionized form, thereby slowing the onset of action.

Phenylephrine and methoxamine

Other vasoconstrictors such as phenylephrine or methoxamine may be added to prolong the duration of the effect of local anesthetics by decreasing their systemic absorption [180]. Some degree of pharmacodynamic interaction may also exist as the infiltration of these α_1-adrenergic receptor agonists caused cutaneous anesthesia in rats [173]. But in contrast with epinephrine, these other agents lack α_2-adrenergic receptor effects and, therefore, potential interactions with local anesthetics mediated by these receptors are not possible. Moreover, phenylephrine, but not epinephrine, caused a significant decrease in sciatic nerve and skeletal muscle blood flow when administered in combination with lidocaine [178], which could potentially cause complications due to nerve ischemia.

Vasoconstrictors should be avoided for blockade of areas with erratic blood supply or without good collateral perfusion (e.g., intravenous regional anesthesia, teat blocks, or large areas of skin) because of the possibility of vasoconstriction-induced tissue ischemia and necrosis.

Phentolamine

Phentolamine, a non-selective α-adrenergic receptor antagonist, has been shown to reverse prolonged local anesthetic-induced block when administered in combination with vasoconstrictors [181]. A commercial preparation of phentolamine mesylate (OraVerse®) has been approved for the reversal of soft tissue anesthesia and the associated functional deficits resulting from local dental anesthesia in humans.

Hyaluronidase

Hyaluronidase, an enzyme that depolymerizes hyaluronic acid, the main cement of the interstitium, may be added to local anesthetics to improve tissue penetration and thereby shorten onset and increase spread of the block [182]. The addition of hyaluronidase raises the pH of the anesthetic solution to a slightly more physiologic level, which may contribute to the shortening of onset by increasing the amount of non-ionized drug. However, local anesthetic C_{max} and the risk of systemic toxicity may also increase. Human studies show diverse results with respect to improved efficacy. Some human studies show better quality of peribulbar or retrobulbar block and shorter onset of action when hyaluronidase is added at concentrations as low as 3.5 IU/mL to mixtures of 0.5% or 0.75% bupivacaine and 2% lidocaine [183–185], while others show no benefit when hyaluronidase is added at concentrations as high as 150 IU/mL to a mixture of 0.75% bupivacaine and 2% lidocaine for peribulbar block [186,187]. Hyaluronidase added to bupivacaine with epinephrine (1:200,000) for brachial plexus block did not increase the speed of onset of anesthesia or reduce the incidence of inadequate nerve block in humans [188]. When used in infiltration anesthesia, hyaluronidase added at 15 IU/mL to 1% lidocaine increased the area of desensitized skin, but pain on injection also increased compared with plain 1% lidocaine in humans [189]. The addition of hyaluronidase seems particularly advantageous in ophthalmic blocks in humans, as it has been shown to limit the acute intraocular pressure increase secondary to periocular injection and seems to have a protective effect against local anesthetic-induced myotoxicity resulting in postoperative strabismus [190]. In dogs, the addition of 400 IU of hyaluronidase to 1.06 mg/kg of 0.5% levobupivacaine for lumbosacral epidural block decreased the onset from 15 to 5 min, but it also decreased the duration of block, while dermatomal spread was unchanged [191]. Another study in dogs looking at the effects of hyaluronidase added to ropivacaine or bupivacaine for femoral–ischiatic blocks showed highly variable onset and offset times and no difference compared to the addition of saline [192]. The addition of hyaluronidase to lidocaine for infiltration block does not delay wound healing [193].

Sodium bicarbonate

The pH of commercially available local anesthetic solutions is normally acidic to enhance stability and solubility and extend shelf-life [194,195]. Alkalinization of the solution by addition of sodium bicarbonate causes an increase in the amount of local anesthetic in the non-ionized form, which is the lipid-soluble fraction able to cross the axonal membrane, thereby shortening the onset of the block. The intensity and duration of the block may also increase due to an increase in the transmembrane pH gradient, causing ion trapping of the ionized active form inside the nerve. The efficacy of alkalinization depends on the local anesthetic solution, the site of the block, and the concurrent addition of epinephrine.

Buffering of 1% lidocaine, 1% mepivacaine, or 0.5% bupivacaine with sodium bicarbonate for intradermal administration does not affect the onset, extent, and duration of skin anesthesia in humans [196,197]. Addition of bicarbonate to lidocaine for median nerve block in humans increased the rate of motor block without changing the onset or extent of sensory block [198]. Similarly, alkalinization of 1% lidocaine or 0.25% bupivacaine to a pH of 7.4 did not prolong infraorbital nerve block duration in rats [199]. Studies using buffered local anesthetics during epidural anesthesia show conflicting results. Some studies show shorter onset of epidural block when 1.5–2% lidocaine, 2% mepivacaine, or 0.5% bupivacaine solutions are alkalinized with bicarbonate [200–202], while others show no shortening of onset with buffered 2% lidocaine or 0.5% bupivacaine [203–205]. The alkalinization of 0.75% ropivacaine solution does not decrease sensory or motor block onset but increases the duration of the epidural block [206]. In femoral and sciatic nerve blocks, the effects of alkalinization on the onset of sensory analgesia and motor block were more evident with 2% mepivacaine, but for brachial plexus axillary block, the greatest effect was observed with 2% lidocaine [202]. Nonetheless, in studies where hastening of block onset occurred with alkalinization, the decrease was less than 5 min when compared with commercial preparations. In addition, it seems that the effect of alkalinization is mainly observed when epinephrine is also added to the solution [207]. Thus, the value of alkalinization of local anesthetics appears debatable as a clinically useful tool to improve anesthesia [19].

Alkalinization has a greater effect when the local anesthetic is administered into an acidic environment, as with intravesicular instillation where the urine is normally acidic. Intravesicular instillation of 5% lidocaine buffered with an equal volume of 8.4% sodium bicarbonate to a pH of 8.0 provided local anesthesia of the bladder submucosa as indicated by the rapid decrease in pain scores in human patients with interstitial cystitis [208]. However, intravesicular administration of alkalinized lidocaine for up to three consecutive days had no apparent beneficial effect on decreasing recurrence rate and severity of clinical signs in cats with obstructive idiopathic lower urinary tract disease [209].

Buffered local anesthetics also have a greater effect when topically administered to the cornea. The corneal permeability of topically applied lidocaine increased when the pH of the solution was buffered from 5.2 to 7.2, with greater concentrations of lidocaine found in the aqueous humor [210,211].

Buffering of the local anesthetic solution with bicarbonate decreases pain on injection when administered subcutaneously and also decreases pain when an epidural catheter is inserted [194,195,212]. Reduction of pain on injection seems to be enhanced by additional warming of the solution to body temperature [212].

The most common dose of sodium bicarbonate used is 0.1 mEq per mL of local anesthetic solution. The addition of bicarbonate may cause precipitation of the solution, especially with bupivacaine and etidocaine when the pH rises above 7.0 [213]. Mepivacaine may also precipitate at a pH above neutral within 20 min [214]. Therefore, it is recommended to use the mixed solution immediately after the addition of sodium bicarbonate.

Carbon dioxide

Carbonation of local anesthetics by adding carbon dioxide (CO_2) is sometimes used to decrease onset and improve quality of the block. The addition of CO_2 to a solution of lidocaine decreased the amount of lidocaine needed to achieve conduction block *in vitro* [215]. This potentiation of local anesthetic block is possibly due to a decreased intracellular pH, causing ion trapping. Carbonated lidocaine administered epidurally shortened the onset and improved the block in humans [216,217]; however, it did not offer any advantage over the hydrochloride salt for caudal epidural anesthesia in horses [218].

α_2-Adrenergic receptor agonists

The addition of α_2-adrenergic receptor agonist drugs to local anesthetics during regional blocks is being increasingly used in veterinary medicine. Clonidine has been extensively used in humans to prolong the duration of intrathecal, epidural, and peripheral nerve blocks. Meta-analyses and systematic reviews clearly show an analgesic benefit from the addition of clonidine to local anesthetics [219]. In large animals, epidural or intrathecal xylazine has been used in combination with lidocaine since the early 1990s to prolong the analgesic effect [220]. In dogs, a study showed that xylazine administered epidurally in combination with lidocaine produced the longest analgesic effect compared with clonidine, detomidine, romifidine, and dexmedetomidine, which may be attributed to xylazine's local anesthetic-like properties and its lower lipophilicity compared with the other α_2-adrenergic receptor agonists [221]. Medetomidine administered either perineurally or systemically (0.01 mg/kg) in combination with mepivacaine for radial nerve block in dogs prolonged the duration of sensory and motor blockade, with residual sensory blockade persisting beyond the observable sedative effects [222].

Dexmedetomidine is now the most widely used α_2-adrenergic receptor agonist regional anesthesia adjuvant in humans and animals. Studies in rats showed that administration of dexmedetomidine in combination with bupivacaine or ropivacaine enhances sensory and motor blockade in sciatic nerve block without inducing neurotoxicity [223,224]. In fact, addition of dexmedetomidine to ropivacaine for sciatic nerve block in rats not only prolonged the duration of sensory and motor block, but also markedly reduced ropivacaine-induced neurotoxicity dose-dependently [225]. Evidence in humans supports block prolongation from 1–8 h when dexmedetomidine is added depending on the type of block and local anesthetic used, but it also increases the incidence of bradycardia and sedation intraoperatively [226].

Several studies involving the addition of dexmedetomidine to hindlimb nerve blocks in dogs, both experimental and clinical, report contradictory results. Some studies showed that dexmedetomidine, at doses ranging between 0.15 and 2 μg/kg, combined with ropivacaine for sciatic and saphenous or femoral nerve blocks prolonged the duration of sensory but not motor blockade [227,228]. Another study showed that sciatic and femoral nerve blocks using bupivacaine plus dexmedetomidine (0.1 μg/kg) had a similar degree and duration of analgesia (up to 24 h) compared with epidural bupivacaine plus buprenorphine [229]. However, a two-center study using 0.5 μg/kg dexmedetomidine in combination with ropivacaine for sciatic and femoral nerve block did not reduce the use of postoperative methadone compared with ropivacaine alone [230].

Epidural administration of dexmedetomidine and bupivacaine in dogs undergoing pelvic limb surgery provided a similar degree of analgesia compared with bupivacaine plus morphine; however, the increased duration of motor blockade was a clinical concern [231].

In cats, dexmedetomidine has also been used in combination with local anesthetics. A clinical study showed that dexmedetomidine combined with bupivacaine intraperitoneally during ovariohysterectomy produced a similar duration and degree of analgesia than bupivacaine combined with epinephrine [232]. An experimental study in cats using dexmedetomidine combined with bupivacaine for sciatic and femoral nerve blocks could not demonstrate a benefit in terms of degree and duration of analgesia compared with bupivacaine alone, although the results may have been influenced by the administration of atipamezole [233].

The increased duration of analgesia caused by adding α_2-adrenergic receptor agonists to local anesthetics is postulated to be due to hyperpolarization of C fibers through blockade of the so-called "hyperpolarization-activated cation current" [234,235]. α-Adrenergic receptors do not seem to be implicated as administration of α-adrenergic receptor antagonists neither reverses the conduction block nor decreases the duration of the block [234–236].

Mixtures of local anesthetics

Local anesthetic mixtures of aminoamide agents consisting of an intermediate-acting agent, such as lidocaine or mepivacaine, combined with a long-acting agent, such as bupivacaine, are used in the belief that the combination will provide a shorter block onset and a similar duration than the long-acting agent administered alone. However, these mixtures produce unpredictable and variable clinical results. Clinical studies in humans using a 50:50 mixture of lidocaine or mepivacaine with bupivacaine or ropivacaine for peripheral nerve blocks show a shorter onset of effect, but also a shorter duration of action, compared with the administration of bupivacaine or ropivacaine alone [237–239]. The epidural or intrathecal combination of lidocaine and bupivacaine in cows [240], cats [241], and humans [242–245] produced similar sensory block onset than either agent alone, and the duration was intermediate between the two agents or similar to bupivacaine.

When chloroprocaine, a short-onset, short-duration-of-action aminoester local anesthetic, is administered prior to bupivacaine, the duration of bupivacaine-induced blockade is decreased. This may be due to an inhibitory effect caused by chloroprocaine metabolites on the Na^+ channel receptor site for bupivacaine [246]. Mixing commercial preparations of chloroprocaine and bupivacaine resulted in a pH of 3.6 and nerve blockade with characteristics of a chloroprocaine block [247]. When the pH of the mixture was increased to 5.56, the nerve block resembled that of bupivacaine. Therefore, mixing commercially available solutions of local anesthetics results in unpredictable blockade that will depend on a number of factors, including the pH of the final mixture [247]. Furthermore, local anesthetic toxicity of combinations of drugs is additive [248].

Tachyphylaxis

Tachyphylaxis to local anesthetics is defined as a decrease in duration, segmental spread, or intensity of a regional block despite repeated constant dosages [249]. In 1969, Bromage described that repeated injection of a constant dose of epidural lidocaine led to a reduction in both the number of dermatomes blocked and the duration of the block [250]. The incidence of this phenomenon in veterinary medicine is unknown, and probably is largely unrecognized. Tachyphylaxis appears neither to be linked to structural or pharmacologic properties of the local anesthetics, nor the technique or mode of administration, as it can occur with both ester- and amide-linked local anesthetics and with either neuraxial or peripheral nerve blocks [250–253]. Bromage found that tachyphylaxis to local anesthetics is promoted by longer interanalgesic intervals between injections [250]. If local anesthetic injections were repeated at intervals short enough to prevent return of pain or at intervals with pain of less than 10 min duration, tachyphylaxis did not occur and augmentation of the analgesic effect was noted. Conversely, if the patient experienced pain between local anesthetic administrations for more than 10 min, tachyphylaxis occurred more rapidly.

The mechanisms underlying tachyphylaxis may involve both pharmacokinetic and pharmacodynamic aspects. Suggested pharmacokinetic mechanisms include local edema, increased epidural protein concentration, changes in local anesthetic distribution in the epidural space, a decrease in perineural pH (limiting the diffusion of local anesthetic from the epidural space to binding sites at the Na^+ channel), an increase in epidural blood flow, or an increase in local metabolism (favoring clearance of local anesthetics from the epidural space) [249]. Other pharmacodynamic mechanisms have also been suggested, such as antagonistic effects of nucleotides or increased Na^+ concentration, increased afferent input from nociceptors, or receptor downregulation of Na^+ channels [249]. A human study with repeated injections of epidural lidocaine showed lack of changes in the distribution or rate of elimination of lidocaine from the epidural space [253] and another study in rats failed to show an effect of tissue pH on the development of tachyphylaxis to bupivacaine [251].

Tachyphylaxis to local anesthetics does not result from reduced drug effectiveness at the nerve itself [254], but it seems to be mainly mediated by a spinal site of action [255]. Tachyphylaxis and central hyperalgesia seem to be related, as evidenced by studies in rats, where tachyphylaxis occurred only under conditions where they concurrently developed hyperalgesia in the tested paw [256]. If only non-noxious motor tests were used to test the duration of the block, tachyphylaxis did not occur. Moreover, it has been shown that drugs that prevent hyperalgesia at spinal sites, such as NMDA receptor antagonists [256] and nitric oxide synthase inhibitors [257], prevent the development of tachyphylaxis. Therefore, it seems that a spinal nitric oxide pathway is involved in the development of tachyphylaxis to local anesthetics [243]. Additionally, descending pathways do not seem necessary for the development of tachyphylaxis since it occurs even after spinal cord transection at the tenth thoracic level in rats [255].

Local anesthetic switching has also been proposed when tachyphylaxis to a local anesthetic agent develops. This approach has been successful in humans with cancer-related pain in whom intrathecal morphine and bupivacaine were not effective and substitution of bupivacaine with lidocaine improved analgesia [258].

Specific drugs and clinical uses

Aminoesters

Proparacaine (proxymetacaine)

This aminoester is used as a topical anesthetic for the cornea and is commercialized as a 0.5% preparation. It is reported to produce quick desensitization of the cornea (within 1 min) and a duration of maximal corneal anesthesia of 25 min in dogs [259] but only 5 min in cats [260]. Reduced corneal sensitivity lasts up to 55 min in dogs and 25 min in cats after 2 drops of the commercial preparation. One of the reported side effects of topical local anesthetics in the eye is that they reduce tear production due to reduced corneal sensation. Also, if used repeatedly, topical local anesthetics may slow corneal healing [261].

Oxybuprocaine

This ester of *para*-aminobenzoic acid is also used for topical anesthesia of the cornea and is commercialized as a 0.4% ophthalmic solution. It is reported to cause rapid desensitization of the cornea (within 1 min) and to have a duration of up to 45 min in dogs [262].

Procaine

This agent has a quick onset and short duration of effect (30–60 min) because of its rapid hydrolysis in blood [19]. Epinephrine may be added to prolong its duration of effect. Its potential for systemic toxicity is minimal, but it occasionally causes allergic reactions due to a hydrolysis metabolite (PABA).

Procaine is used in veterinary medicine for infiltration and nerve blocks at concentrations of 1–2% [263]. It is rarely used for topical anesthesia, as it is not very effective via this route [263]. In humans, it is sometimes administered intrathecally for short procedures [264].

Intravenous procaine is a CNS stimulant in horses [102]. Because of this property, and its analgesic effect when used for peripheral nerve blocks, it has been illegally used in racehorses [263]. Procaine is sometimes added to drug formulations (i.e., procaine penicillin) to prolong the duration of effect.

Benzocaine

This agent is also a fast-acting and short-lasting local anesthetic, available exclusively for topical anesthesia. It causes methemoglobinemia in several animal species and therefore it is no longer used in clinical practice. Benzocaine is also an anesthetic for fish when added to water [265].

Chloroprocaine

This agent is similar to procaine, with a fast onset and short duration of action (30–60 min). It is available in concentrations of 1% to 3%. It is not widely used in veterinary medicine, but in humans, its use has re-emerged for short-duration epidural and intrathecal anesthesia because it is associated with a lower incidence of transient neurologic symptoms compared with lidocaine [266]. It may also be used for local infiltration blocks when a short duration of effect is required.

Tetracaine

Tetracaine is also called amethocaine. It is rarely used in veterinary medicine. In humans, it is most commonly used for intrathecal anesthesia because it has a fast onset (3–5 min) and its effect lasts 2–3 h [267]. It is rarely used for other forms of regional anesthesia due to its extremely slow onset and potential for systemic toxicity [267]. It is an excellent topical anesthetic and because of this property, it is included in topical anesthetic solutions such as ophthalmological preparations (0.5% and 1.0% aqueous solutions, or a 0.5% viscous formulation). A study in horses showed that the viscous formulation resulted in the greatest decrease in corneal sensitivity and the longest duration of action (30 min) compared with aqueous solutions of proparacaine or tetracaine (20 min) [268]. The absorption of tetracaine from mucous membranes is very rapid and several fatalities have been reported after its use for endoscopic procedures in humans [269]. Human studies have shown that tetracaine topical preparations, including a lidocaine–tetracaine patch (Synera®, Rapydan®), provide faster and better dermal anesthesia than the eutectic mixture of lidocaine and prilocaine (EMLA® cream) [270,271].

Aminoamides

Lidocaine

Lidocaine remains the most versatile and most widely used local anesthetic in veterinary medicine because of its fast onset, moderate duration of effect, and moderate toxicity. It is available as 0.5%, 1%, 1.5%, and 2% solutions. Lidocaine is used for infiltration anesthesia, peripheral nerve blocks, epidural and intrathecal blocks, and intravenous regional anesthesia. The duration of plain lidocaine is approximately 1 h, which can be prolonged up to 3–4 h with the addition of epinephrine [19]. It is also commonly used topically for laryngeal desensitization before tracheal intubation (2%, 4%, or 10% spray solution). For dermal anesthesia, it is available in different formulations such as the eutectic mixture with prilocaine (2.5% EMLA® cream), as patches of lidocaine alone (5% Lidoderm®), mixed with tetracaine (Synera®, Rapydan®), or mixed with bupivacaine (Tri-Solfen®) (see Special formulations section later in this chapter).

Lidocaine has numerous non-anesthetic uses when administered intravenously. It is a Class Ib antiarrhythmic drug. It also reduces the requirements for inhalational anesthetics when administered intravenously in different species, including dogs [272–274], cats [275], goats [111], horses [276,277], and calves [278]. It is also an analgesic drug for different types of pain when administered systemically, as shown in human patients [279,280] and experimental studies in laboratory animals [281,282]. Administration of intravenous lidocaine (2 mg/kg bolus followed by 0.05 mg/kg/min) produced thermal antinociception in horses [283]. However, it did not affect the thermal threshold in cats (plasma concentrations up to 4.3 μg/mL) [284], or the electrical threshold in dogs (2 mg/kg IV bolus followed by an infusion of up to 0.1 mg/kg/min) [285].

The mechanism by which systemically administered lidocaine produces analgesia is uncertain but is thought to include action at Na^+, Ca^{2+}, and K^+ channels and the NMDA receptor [39–41,43,44]. Lidocaine also possesses anti-inflammatory effects, which may be important in producing analgesia because inflammatory mediators augment neuronal excitability [286]. In addition, some studies show that lidocaine administered as an intravenous infusion perioperatively may improve gastrointestinal motility, reducing reflux, jejunal distension, and peritoneal fluid accumulation, and preventing the development of postoperative ileus in horses with colic of varying etiologies [287–289]. This beneficial effect on motility may be especially true in cases with small intestinal lesions and ischemia-reperfusion injury, and it may be enhanced if lidocaine is administered early during the intraoperative period [290]. However, a single-center study showed no effect on the prevalence of postoperative reflux, total reflux volume, and duration of reflux, or postoperative survival in horses undergoing surgical management of small intestinal disease [291]. In healthy horses, lidocaine administration as an intravenous infusion has no effect on gastrointestinal transit time [292] or may prolong it [293].

The disposition of lidocaine after intravenous administration has been described for sheep [122], dogs [105,123,294], cats [108], horses [134], cows [113], and chickens [112] (Table 29.3).

Mepivacaine

This agent has a pharmacologic profile very similar to lidocaine, with a slightly longer duration of effect (up to 2 h), probably because of slightly less intrinsic vasodilatory properties. It is available at concentrations from 0.5% to 2%. Its use in clinical practice is similar to lidocaine, except that it is not routinely used for intravenous regional anesthesia or for obstetric procedures due to its very slow metabolism in the fetus and newborn [267]. Unlike lidocaine, mepivacaine is not an effective topical anesthetic [267]. It is the preferred agent for diagnostic peripheral nerve blocks in horses because of its lower neurotoxicity compared with other local anesthetics [295].

Bupivacaine

This is a highly lipophilic agent, about four times as potent as lidocaine, and with slow onset of action (20–30 min) and a long duration of effect (3–10 h) [267]. It is used in concentrations, ranging from 0.125% to 0.75%. Its clinical uses include infiltrative, peripheral nerve, epidural, and intrathecal blocks. Bupivacaine is not used for topical anesthesia, and it is not recommended for intravenous regional anesthesia because of its high cardiotoxicity potential. It possesses intrinsic differential blocking properties, especially at low concentrations, and therefore is indicated when sensory blockade accompanied by minimal motor dysfunction is desired.

Table 29.3 Pharmacokinetic parameters (mean ± SD) of intravenous lidocaine in domestic species.

	$t_{1/2}$ (minutes)	V_{dss} (L/kg)	*Cl* (mL/kg/min)
Dog [294]	68.1 ± 10.9	1.38 ± 0.08	27.5 ± 6
Cat [108]	100 ± 28	1.39 ± 0.37	26 ± 2.7
Horse [134]	79 ± 41	0.79 ± 0.16	29 ± 7.6
Cattle [113]	63.6 ± 42	3.3 ± 1.6	42.2 ± 20.5
Sheep [122]	30.9	NA	41.2

$t_{1/2}$, terminal half-life; V_{dss}, apparent volume of distribution in steady state; *Cl*, total body clearance.

Levobupivacaine

This is the S(−)-enantiomer ("levorotatory" isomer) of bupivacaine, with slightly less cardiotoxic potential than the racemic mixture. Its physicochemical properties and clinical uses are the same as bupivacaine.

Ropivacaine

This agent is structurally related to mepivacaine and bupivacaine, but it is marketed as the pure S(−)-enantiomer to reduce the cardiotoxicity associated with the R(+)-enantiomer. It is slightly less potent than bupivacaine and is available in concentrations of up to 1%. Its clinical uses are the same as bupivacaine, with similar onset of effect, a marginally shorter sensory blockade (up to 6 h), and a slightly lower degree of motor blockade at equipotent doses [251]. It has a biphasic effect on peripheral vasculature, causing vasoconstriction at concentrations below 0.5% and vasodilation at concentrations over 1% [296].

Special formulations

In addition to standard local anesthetic preparations, there are several special formulations that improve topical absorption and/or prolong their effects (Table 29.4). These formulations include encapsulation in liposomes, association with biopolymers, complexation in cyclodextrins, incorporation into transdermal non-liposomal carriers, and other carrier systems. These carriers present in different physical states, including solids (patches), semisolids (gel, cream, and ointment), and liquids (emulsion and dispersion).

Lidocaine dermal patches and eutectic creams

Lidocaine patches are made of a nonwoven polyester felt backing with adhesive material, and commercially available products contain 5% lidocaine (50 mg of lidocaine per gram of adhesive, with a total of 700 mg lidocaine per patch measuring 10 × 14 cm). They consist of a single-layer matrix that allows lidocaine to diffuse across the different layers of the skin via passive diffusion down a concentration gradient. The patch itself is an occlusive delivery system that prevents water loss from the skin, increasing the hydration of the stratum corneum, and therefore enhancing the absorption of the drug through the skin [297]. The pharmacokinetics of lidocaine patches have been described in different species, with a low systemic absorption observed in cats [298], dogs [299,300], and horses [301,302] when they were applied to intact, clipped, and surgically prepared skin. When they were applied on a surgical incision in dogs, the area under the curve lidocaine plasma concentration was significantly higher than when applied on intact skin [303], although these levels were well below the reported concentrations measured when lidocaine is administered intravenously at clinically recommended doses [273].

Table 29.4 Clinically relevant local anesthetic commercial preparations, indications, and doses.

Local anesthetic	Commercial preparations	Indications	Doses
Procaine	Novocaine Procasel Adrenacaine Dalocain Isocain (with epinephrine)	Infiltration Nerve blocks	Maximum dose: 2–4 mg/kg
Lidocaine	Topical: EMLA cream (with prilocaine) Xylocaine Intubeaze Lidoderm patches Tri-Solfen (with bupivacaine) Injectable: Lidocaine HCl Lignocaine Xylocaine (some with epinephrine)	Topical (dermal, mucous membranes, wounds) Infiltration Nerve blocks Interpleural Epidural Intrathecal[a] Intravenous (IV)	Maximum dose: 6–10 mg/kg (Ca) 3–5 mg/kg (Fe) 6 mg/kg (Eq, Bo, Ov, Cp, Sw) IV infusion dose: 1–2 mg/kg bolus, 30–50 μg/kg/min awake (Ca) 1–2 mg/kg bolus, 50–200 μg/kg/min under general anesthesia (Ca) 1.3 mg/kg bolus, 25–50 μg/kg/min (Eq, Bo)
Mepivacaine	Carbocaine Intra-Epicaine Vetacaine	Infiltration Nerve blocks Interpleural Epidural Intrathecal[a] Intra-articular	Maximum dose: 5–6 mg/kg (Ca, Eq, Bo, Ov, Cp, Sw) 2–3 mg/kg (Fe) Intra-articular dose: 1–2 mg/kg
Bupivacaine	Topical: Tri-Solfen (with lidocaine) Injectable: Marcaine Nocita	Topical (wounds) Infiltration Nerve blocks Interpleural Epidural Intrathecal[a]	Maximum dose: 2 mg/kg (Ca, Eq, Bo, Ov, Cp, Sw) 1–1.5 mg/kg (Fe)
Levobupivacaine	Chirocaine	Infiltration Nerve blocks Interpleural Epidural Intrathecal[a]	Maximum dose: 3 mg/kg (Ca, Eq, Bo, Ov, Cp, Sw) 1.5 mg/kg (Fe)
Ropivacaine	Naropin	Infiltration Nerve blocks Interpleural Epidural Intrathecal[a]	Maximum dose: 3 mg/kg (Ca, Eq, Bo, Ov, Cp, Sw) 1.5 mg/kg (Fe)

[a] Intrathecal dose is one-tenth of epidural dose.
Ca, Canine; Fe, Feline; Eq, Equine; Bo, Bovine; Ov, Ovine; Cp, Caprine; Sw, Swine.

The efficacy of lidocaine patches to provide analgesia in clinical conditions has been evaluated in dogs undergoing ovariohysterectomy and hemilaminectomy surgery, with no improvement of postoperative pain scores when they are used in combination with other analgesic therapies [304,305]. A study in horses showed a reduction in the visual analog scale scores to pinprick when a 5% lidocaine cream was used, but not when lidocaine patches were applied proximal to the carpus [302]. Another later study in horses showed that lidocaine patches applied over the withers and saddle area increased local thermal and mechanical nociceptive thresholds under experimental conditions [306]. This study also tested eutectic cream mixtures of lidocaine with prilocaine and lidocaine with tetracaine and found a greater intensity and longer duration of local thermal and mechanical antinociception compared to the lidocaine patches in horses [306].

Lidocaine–bupivacaine gel (Tri-Solfen®)

A commercially available topical anesthetic in a gel base (Tri-Solfen®) consisting of 5% lidocaine hydrochloride and 0.5% bupivacaine hydrochloride, mixed with epinephrine 1:2000 for hemostasis, and 0.5% cetrimide as an antiseptic, has been registered in Australia and New Zealand since 2006 to provide pain relief in lambs and calves. It has also been approved in 2022 in the United Kingdom for the alleviation of pain in pigs. When applied directly over the disbudding wound, this preparation was reported to be effective to mitigate postoperative pain in calves [307,308], causing no toxic effects or negative impact on wound healing at doses up to five times the recommended dose, and with evidence of lower levels of bacterial colonization [309]. It has also been shown to reduce pain in lambs following mulesing, castration, and tail docking [310,311], in dairy cows during treatment of hoof lesions [312], and in piglets following castration [313].

Liposome-encapsulated bupivacaine (Nocita®)

Liposome-encapsulated bupivacaine (Nocita®) is a sterile, nonpyrogenic, preservative-free, aqueous suspension of multivesicular lipid-based particles containing bupivacaine at a concentration of 13.3 mg/mL. The liposomes are microscopic structures made of nonconcentric lipid bilayers resembling a honeycomb-like matrix designed to allow a gradual release of bupivacaine from the vesicles for 72 h, as the lipid bilayers break down. Liposome-encapsulated bupivacaine was approved by the United States Food and Drug Administration (FDA) in 2016 in dogs for single-dose infiltration into the surgical site for cranial cruciate ligament surgery at a dose of 5.3 mg/kg. In 2018, it also obtained FDA approval for peripheral nerve blocks for onychectomy in cats at a dose of 5.3 mg/kg per paw (10.6 mg/kg total dose). If a greater volume is needed, it may be mixed with 0.9% saline or another isotonic solution (e.g., Lactated Ringer's solution) in a 1:1 ratio [314]. Mixing the product with sterile water or another hypotonic solution is not recommended as this may disrupt the liposomes.

Several studies have shown that locally infiltrated liposome-encapsulated bupivacaine is more effective than placebo (significantly lower pain scores) in dogs undergoing stifle surgery [315], and at least as effective as local infiltration with 0.5% bupivacaine hydrochloride (similar postoperative pain scores) in dogs undergoing tibial plateau leveling osteotomy [316] and in cats undergoing ovariohysterectomy [317]. Dogs administered liposome-encapsulated bupivacaine, however, were less likely to require rescue analgesia and received lower amounts of opioids than dogs administered 0.5% bupivacaine hydrochloride [316].

There are also some pre-clinical studies in horses using liposome-encapsulated bupivacaine for perineural analgesia in experimentally induced lameness. Compared with bupivacaine hydrochloride at milligram-equivalent doses, liposome-encapsulated bupivacaine ameliorated forelimb lameness in most horses (5/6), and with a similar duration of effect (median 4.5 h) [318]. However, in another study using a different experimental model of lameness, horses treated with bupivacaine hydrochloride had reduced mechanical nociceptive thresholds and improved objective lameness parameters for only 1 h post-block compared with a duration of up to 24 h in horses treated with liposome-encapsulated bupivacaine [319].

Dual-acting bupivacaine–meloxicam extended-release polymer

A novel formulation of bupivacaine hydrochloride combined with a low dose of meloxicam (HTX-011) using extended-release polymer technology was approved for use in humans in 2021 by the FDA, and in several other countries, including the European Union and United Kingdom (Zynrelef™). It is instilled locally around the incision site after surgery to produce postoperative analgesia up to 72 h. Pre-clinical studies in pigs showed the ability of meloxicam to reduce local tissue inflammation, thereby lessening the drop in tissue pH in the incision after surgery compared with control, which was associated with potentiated and prolonged analgesic activity of bupivacaine [320].

Adverse effects

Systemic toxicity

Local anesthetic drugs may cause CNS and cardiac toxicity at high plasma concentrations. Plasma concentrations are determined by the rate of drug absorption into the systemic circulation, but the most common reason for excessive plasma concentrations is the inadvertent direct intravascular injection of the local anesthetic solution while performing peripheral or neuraxial blocks. Local anesthetics vary considerably in their potency at causing systemic toxic reactions, and generally, this potency follows the same rank order as their potency at producing nerve blockade [321]. More lipid-soluble drugs (i.e., bupivacaine) are more potent at causing systemic toxicity than less lipid-soluble agents (i.e., lidocaine or mepivacaine), and the $S(-)$-enantiomers (i.e., levobupivacaine or ropivacaine) are less toxic than the $R(+)$-enantiomers, or than the racemic mixture of both [322–325].

The dose of a local anesthetic causing systemic toxicity will depend on the route and speed of administration (rapid intravenous administration will be more likely to cause high plasma levels), the species involved, and patient factors (such as acid–base balance, serum potassium levels, and whether the animal is under anesthesia).

The clinical incidence of systemic toxicity in domestic animals is unknown. The incidence of systemic toxicity associated with regional anesthetic blocks in humans is estimated to be around 1 in 10,000, with peripheral blocks having the highest incidence (7.5 in 10,000) [326,327].

Central nervous system toxicity

CNS toxic signs follow a progression as the plasma concentration of local anesthetic increases (Fig. 29.6). At low doses, all local anesthetics are effective anticonvulsants, and they also have sedative effects [328]. In conscious, unsedated humans, the initial signs of local anesthetic CNS toxicity include tongue numbness,

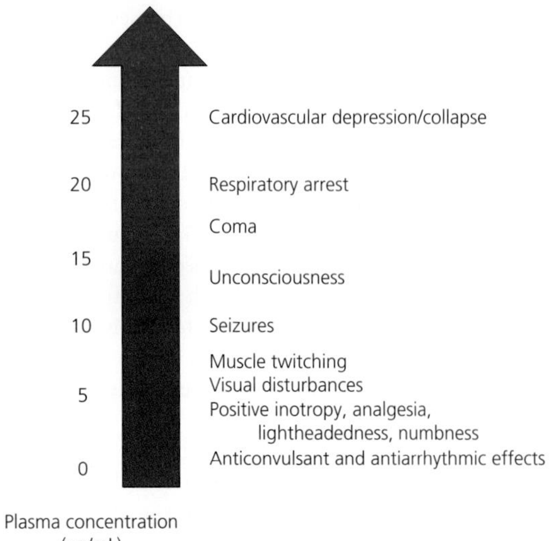

Figure 29.6 Progressive signs of lidocaine systemic toxicity with increasing plasma concentrations. Note that concentrations are approximate and depend on various factors (see text for details).

light-headedness, dizziness, drowsiness, paresthesia of sight and sound, and acute anxiety, or even fear of death [329]. In horses, this has been described as alteration in visual function, rapid eye blinking, anxiety, mild sedation, and ataxia [287,288,330]. As the plasma level rises, local anesthetics inhibit inhibitory cortical neurons in the temporal lobe or the amygdala, allowing facilitatory neurons to function in an unopposed fashion, resulting in increased excitatory activity, which first leads to muscle twitching followed by grand mal seizures [321,328]. As the plasma concentration increases further, local anesthetics can inhibit both inhibitory and facilitatory pathways, resulting in CNS depression, unconsciousness, and coma [321,328].

Not all local anesthetics produce signs of aura, such as drowsiness or excitement, before the onset of seizures. With highly lipophilic, highly protein-bound agents such as bupivacaine, the excitement phase can be brief and mild, and the first signs may be bradycardia, cyanosis, and unconsciousness [331].

CNS toxicity is generally assumed to precede cardiovascular toxicity. This derives from studies in conscious sheep where the doses and plasma drug concentrations associated with cardiovascular collapse (defined as the disappearance of pulsatile blood pressure) and CNS toxicity (signified by the onset of seizures) were calculated as the CV:CNS ratio. Values for the CV:CNS ratio for various local anesthetics in conscious sheep are much greater than 1, supporting this notion [323,332].

In humans, the frequency of seizures and accompanying cardiovascular changes associated with various regional block techniques have been reviewed. There is a significant difference between the rate of seizure development with caudal > brachial plexus > epidural blocks, with no adverse cardiovascular or pulmonary effects occurring during seizures [333].

In conscious dogs, the mean cumulative dose required for convulsive activity was 4 mg/kg for tetracaine, 5 mg/kg for bupivacaine, 8 mg/kg for etidocaine, and 22 mg/kg for lidocaine in one study [13]. In another study, administration of intravenous infusions of lidocaine (8 mg/kg/min), bupivacaine (2 mg/kg/min), or ropivacaine (2 mg/kg/min) caused generalized seizures at an average dose of 21 mg/kg of lidocaine, 4 mg/kg of bupivacaine, and 5 mg/kg of ropivacaine in conscious dogs [334]. The first seizure activity observed with lidocaine toxicity in dogs was tonic extension at an infused dose of 12 mg/kg, followed by running activity after 23 mg/kg, and with tonic-clonic seizures occurring at an infused dose of 33 mg/kg [335]. The plasma concentration of lidocaine causing muscle tremors was 2.7 μg/mL after administration of a total dose of 11.1 mg/kg IV to conscious dogs [336]. The onset of seizures occurred when lidocaine plasma concentrations reached 8.2 μg/mL in another study involving awake dogs [337].

In conscious horses, the mean toxic plasma concentration of lidocaine causing muscle fasciculations was determined to be 3.24 μg/mL (range 1.85–4.53 μg/mL), and it did not change regardless of speed of administration [330]. Such plasma concentrations may be achieved during prolonged lidocaine IV infusions of greater than 12 h in postcolic surgery horses [338,339].

In lightly anesthetized and ventilated cats, seizures occurred after administration of 12 mg/kg of lidocaine and 5 mg/kg of bupivacaine given at intravenous infusion rates of 16 mg/kg/min and 4 mg/kg/min, respectively [340]. The onset of seizures occurred with lidocaine plasma concentrations of 19.6 μg/mL [341]. The CV:CNS toxicity ratio for drug dosage was 4.0 with lidocaine and 4.8 with bupivacaine in cats [340].

In conscious sheep, the doses of infused lidocaine, bupivacaine, and ropivacaine necessary to produce convulsions were 6.8 mg/kg, 1.6 mg/kg, and 3.5 mg/kg, respectively [342]. Therefore, the ratio of the mean convulsant doses (lidocaine/bupivacaine/ropivacaine) was approximately 5:1:2 [342].

There is an inverse relationship between the seizure threshold dose of local anesthetics and the arterial CO_2 tension [343]. This may be due to an increase in cerebral blood flow during hypercapnia causing increased delivery of drug to the brain and/or a decrease in plasma protein binding of local anesthetics causing an increase in free drug [344]. Hypoxemia also increases the CNS and cardiovascular toxicity of local anesthetics [345].

Cardiovascular toxicity

At low concentrations, most local anesthetics have an antiarrhythmic effect, but at higher concentrations, they produce cardiac toxicity. Local anesthetics block cardiac Na^+ channels and decrease the maximum rate of rise of Phase 0 of the action potential, leading to a pronounced and evolving inhibition of cardiac conduction [346]. Electrocardiographic changes include prolonged PR and QRS intervals and a prolonged refractory period [346–348]. The cardiovascular effects of local anesthetics are complex and non-linear, including direct effects on cardiac conduction, cardiac contractility, and vascular smooth muscle, as well as indirect effects mediated by the CNS [321].

All local anesthetics cause myocardial depression with small intravenous doses that cause no overt CNS toxicity [325,349]. At subconvulsant doses, heart rate may increase slightly and the QRS complex may widen, but there are no major effects on blood pressure and cardiac output [325,349]. These effects are mild and rapidly reversed, with no qualitative differences among local anesthetics [325]. At the onset of convulsions, there is a profound sympathetic response associated with all local anesthetics, which reverses the induced myocardial depression causing tachycardia and increased blood pressure and cardiac output [324,325,342]. Convulsant doses of all longer-acting local anesthetics cause marked arrhythmias, typically ventricular tachycardia, that may progress to ventricular fibrillation or cardiovascular collapse [324,350]. Supraconvulsant doses of lidocaine cause profound hypotension, bradycardia, decreases in myocardial contractility, respiratory arrest, and ultimately asystole [324,342].

It has been postulated that the CNS toxic effects may be involved in the production of serious cardiotoxicity because of the onset of respiratory failure accompanied by hypoxia, bradycardia, hypercapnia, and acidosis [328].

While all local anesthetics cause direct negative inotropic effects, the shorter-acting local anesthetics such as lidocaine and mepivacaine are less arrhythmogenic than the longer-acting ones, such as bupivacaine or ropivacaine [324,350]. These differences are caused by differences in the kinetics of binding and unbinding from various ion channels [351,352]. While both shorter- and longer-acting agents have similar rates of binding to cardiac Na^+ channels, the longer-acting agents have slower unbinding rates, hence predisposing to cardiac arrhythmias [321]. The *R*(+)-enantiomers of the more lipophilic local anesthetics have slower unbinding rates than the *S*(−)-enantiomers, thereby making them even more arrhythmogenic [351,352].

No ventricular arrhythmias were observed with cardiotoxic doses of lidocaine in conscious dogs [324]. Ventricular tachycardia with no hemodynamic impairment was observed in only one of eight conscious sheep with lidocaine and one of seven with mepivacaine [350]. In contrast, ventricular arrhythmias occurred in one of six conscious dogs with cardiotoxic doses of ropivacaine and five of six with bupivacaine [324]. Polymorphic ventricular tachycardia accompanied by decreased cardiac output occurred in 7 of 10 conscious sheep receiving bupivacaine, 4 of 11 with levobupivacaine, and 5 of 12 with ropivacaine [350]. Even though the newer local anesthetics ropivacaine and levobupivacaine appear to be less cardiotoxic than bupivacaine (judging by the larger doses tolerated before the onset of serious arrhythmias), they must not be regarded as totally safe [353].

General anesthesia has a substantial impact on toxicity, mortality, and pharmacokinetics of various local anesthetics and distorts pharmacokinetic–pharmacodynamic relationships. In a study in halothane-anesthetized sheep, the pre-existing myocardial depression from halothane was markedly exacerbated by infusions of lidocaine, mepivacaine, prilocaine, bupivacaine, levobupivacaine, or ropivacaine [350]. The cardiovascular toxic effects of each local anesthetic were also prolonged in anesthetized sheep compared with conscious sheep, and concurrently, the blood drug concentrations were markedly increased under general anesthesia. However, no serious arrhythmias occurred in any anesthetized sheep. Despite the exaggerated cardiovascular effects of the local anesthetics when the sheep were anesthetized, none of them died, whereas approximately 15% died from fatal cardiac arrhythmias when conscious [350].

As the K^+ gradient across cardiac myocyte membranes is the most important factor in establishing the membrane potential, hyperkalemia can markedly increase local anesthetic toxicity. Under conditions of hyperkalemia (5.4 mEq/L) in dogs, the cardiotoxic doses of both lidocaine and bupivacaine were halved compared to conditions of normokalemia, while the seizure-inducing doses did not change for either agent [354]. Conversely, hypokalemia decreases local anesthetic cardiotoxicity [354].

Box 29.1 Guidelines for treatment of local anesthetic systemic toxicity.

Central nervous system toxicity
1. Intubate trachea, administer O_2, and ventilate
2. Treat seizures with a benzodiazepine

Cardiac arrest
1. Start basic cardiopulmonary resuscitation
2. Administer epinephrine at low doses (≤ 1 μg/kg IV)
3. AVOID lidocaine, vasopressin, calcium channel blockers, and β-blockers
4. Administer a 20% lipid emulsion IV:
   - Initial bolus 1.5–4 mL/kg over 1 min
   - Continue with CRI at 0.25 mL/kg/min for 30–60 min
   - If non-responsive administer additional boluses of 1.5 mL/kg (up to a maximum of 7 mL/kg)
   - CRI may be continued at 0.5 mL/kg/h until clinical signs improve (24 h maximum)

CRI, constant rate infusion.
Source: Adapted from Neal *et al.* [355]; Fernandez *et al.* [365].

Treatment of systemic toxicity

When signs of systemic toxicity are noted, the administration of local anesthetic should be discontinued. Treatment of systemic toxicity is primarily supportive (Box 29.1). Oxygenation and ventilation are the main goals. It may be necessary to intubate the trachea and mechanically ventilate the animal to avoid or reverse hypoxemia, hypercapnia, and acidosis, all of which promote toxicity. If grand mal seizures are present, an anticonvulsant drug may be administered. If cardiovascular depression is also present, barbiturates or propofol are not recommended and treatment with a benzodiazepine is preferable.

Cardiovascular toxicity induced by lidocaine or mepivacaine is usually mild and reversible with the use of positive inotropic drugs and fluid support [19]. Cardiac arrhythmias produced by longer-acting local anesthetics such as bupivacaine (i.e., ventricular tachycardia or fibrillation) are usually malignant and refractory to routine treatment. In these cases, cardiopulmonary resuscitation should be immediately instituted, and defibrillation initiated if necessary. In humans, the guidelines of the American Society of Regional Anesthesia and Pain Medicine recommend using low doses of epinephrine (< 1 μg/kg) and avoiding vasopressin [355]. Calcium channel blockers should not be administered as their cardiodepressant effects are exaggerated [356]. Amiodarone rather than lidocaine is indicated to treat ventricular arrhythmias in this setting [356]. In cases of refractory cardiac arrest, it is recommended to use an intravenous lipid emulsion (i.e., Intralipid® 20%), which has been shown to reverse refractory arrhythmias caused by highly lipophilic local anesthetics in different experimental models [357,358] and in human clinical reports [359–361].

In a rodent model of bupivacaine-induced asystole in animals pretreated with an intravenous lipid solution, the median lethal dose (LD_{50}) of bupivacaine increased by 48% [357]. In a dog model of bupivacaine-induced cardiotoxicity (10 mg/kg IV), cardiopulmonary resuscitation was instituted for 10 min and then dogs received similar volumes of either intravenous saline fluid or a 20% lipid solution (4 mL/kg over 2 min, followed by 0.5 mL/kg/min over 10 min) [358]. Notably, all dogs in the saline control group failed to regain spontaneous circulation and died, while all dogs treated with the lipid solution survived, achieving near baseline blood pressure and heart rate values within 30 min of its administration [358]. Later studies in rats have demonstrated the potential adverse effects of epinephrine administered at high doses during lipid emulsion rescue with a higher incidence of ventricular arrhythmias, hyperlactatemia, hypoxia, acidosis, and pulmonary edema [362,363]. Another study in rats also demonstrated worse outcomes when vasopressin was administered alone or in combination with epinephrine compared with a lipid emulsion [364].

The exact mechanism of action of lipid emulsions is unknown and is likely multifactorial, but it is thought to be related to improved myocardial performance and a "lipid sink" effect, which postulates that the lipophilic local anesthetic is sequestered into a lipid compartment within the bloodstream [365].

Propofol should not be administered as a substitute for intravenous lipid emulsions as its lipid content is too low (10%) and the large doses required would induce profound cardiovascular depression.

Local toxicity

Neurotoxicity

Exposure of the peripheral or central nervous systems to local anesthetics can cause direct damage, although this complication is rare. Mechanisms of local anesthetic neurotoxicity remain speculative, but some studies suggest injury to Schwann cells, which is time and concentration dependent [366], inhibition of fast axonal transport, disruption of the blood–nerve barrier, decreased neural blood flow with associated ischemia [367], and disruption of cell membrane integrity due to a detergent property of local anesthetics [368].

All local anesthetics are potentially neurotoxic and neurotoxicity parallels anesthetic potency. The *in vitro* rank order of potency for cytotoxicity is procaine ≤ mepivacaine < lidocaine < chloroprocaine < ropivacaine < bupivacaine, based on the LD_{50} for neuronal cells [295]. Neurotoxicity is also related to the concentration of local anesthetic. Clinically relevant concentrations of local anesthetics are considered safe for peripheral nerves [369]. The spinal cord and nerve roots, on the other hand, are more prone to injury [19]. Intrathecal administration of 8% lidocaine, 2% bupivacaine, and 1% tetracaine, but not of 2% chloroprocaine and 2% ropivacaine, caused histopathologic changes in the spinal cord and neurologic deficits in rabbits [370]. The cytotoxic effect of lidocaine and bupivacaine is concentration dependent, with higher concentrations causing death of all cells in culture. In contrast, mepivacaine, ropivacaine, procaine, and chloroprocaine did not kill all cells even at very high concentrations [295].

The effects of local anesthetics on spinal cord blood flow appear to be benign, and do not seem responsible for spinal cord neurotoxicity. Intrathecal administration of lidocaine, mepivacaine, bupivacaine, and tetracaine causes vasodilation and increases spinal cord blood flow, whereas ropivacaine causes vasoconstriction and decreases spinal cord blood flow, with both effects being concentration dependent [72].

The incidence of long-term neurologic injury in human patients undergoing spinal anesthesia is 0–0.02% [327]. Therefore, it seems to be a relatively safe technique in clinical practice if properly performed using clinically appropriate local anesthetic concentrations.

Myotoxicity

Local anesthetics can cause toxicity to skeletal muscle. Experimentally, all local anesthetics have the potential for myotoxicity at clinically relevant concentrations. Myotoxicity is concentration dependent, as observed in a study in rabbits where extraocular muscle injection with 0.75% bupivacaine caused acute myonecrosis and degeneration, compared with only scattered and significantly fewer areas of mild muscle fiber degeneration with 0.38% bupivacaine, and no muscle degeneration observed when the injection was with 0.19% bupivacaine [371]. Bupivacaine seems to be more myotoxic than other local anesthetics as judged by the larger extent of muscle lesions observed [372]. The mechanism of local anesthetic-induced muscle toxicity is likely to be related to dysregulation of intracellular calcium concentration and/or alterations in mitochondrial bioenergetics [373].

In most cases, local anesthetic-induced myonecrosis appears to be regenerative and clinically imperceptible. However, bupivacaine and ropivacaine produced irreversible skeletal muscle damage characterized by calcific myonecrosis observed 4 weeks after peripheral nerve blockade in a study in pigs [372].

Clinically relevant myopathy and myonecrosis have been described in humans after receiving continuous peripheral blocks, infiltration of wound margins, trigger point injections, and peri- and retrobulbar blocks [374].

Chondrotoxicity

Local anesthetics are sometimes injected intra-articularly in clinical practice. Local anesthetic chondrotoxicity has been demonstrated both *in vivo* and *in vitro* in both animal and human cartilage [375–378]. Clinically, chondrolysis has been associated with the use of intra-articular local anesthetic pain pumps in humans [379,380].

The chondrotoxicity exhibited by local anesthetics is time and concentration dependent. *In vitro* bovine chondrocyte viability decreased after just 15 min of exposure to 1% lidocaine, and longer exposures to 1% and 2% lidocaine further reduced chondrocyte viability [376]. Chondrocyte viability was reduced to a larger extent when exposed to 2% lidocaine compared to 1% lidocaine [376]. This study also showed that the intact articular surface is not protective against local anesthetic chondrotoxicity [376].

In vitro exposure of equine chondrocytes to 0.5% bupivacaine, 2% lidocaine, or 2% mepivacaine for 30 or 60 min revealed that bupivacaine is the most chondrotoxic of the three local anesthetics and that mepivacaine is the least toxic [377]. Ropivacaine is also significantly less toxic than bupivacaine and lidocaine in both intact human articular cartilage and chondrocyte culture [381,382]. The marked chondrotoxicity exhibited by bupivacaine and lidocaine is mainly due to necrosis rather than apoptosis [377].

In conclusion, evidence suggests that there is a greater risk for chondrolysis with longer exposure to a higher concentration of local anesthetics, such as with a pain pump, than with a single injection, and that mepivacaine seems to be the least toxic and consequently the preferred drug for intra-articular administration.

Methemoglobinemia

Methemoglobin (MHb) formation may be induced by certain local anesthetics in several animal species and humans. MHb is produced by oxidative damage to the hemoglobin molecule. Specifically, the iron of the heme group is oxidized to the ferric (Fe^{3+}) form. In this state, it cannot bind oxygen (O_2), and therefore blood oxygen-carrying capacity is decreased. The physiologic range of MHb in the blood is 0–2% [383]. Concentrations of MHb of 10–20% are tolerated well, but higher levels are often associated with clinical signs, and levels above 70% may cause death [383]. Oxidative denaturation of hemoglobin can cause Heinz body formation (precipitated hemoglobin or globin subunits), which is irreversible, decreases the lifespan of red blood cells, and causes hemolysis.

The local anesthetics more often associated with MHb formation are the aminoester benzocaine, and the aminoamide prilocaine. Administration of a 2 s spray of benzocaine (estimated dose 56 mg) to the mucous membranes of the nasopharynx of dogs, cats, ferrets, monkeys, rabbits, and miniature pigs induced MHb formation ranging from 3.5–38% 15–60 min after administration in more than 95% of the animals tested [384]. In sheep, intranasal administration of topical benzocaine for 2 s caused MHb in half of the animals tested, ranging from 16–26%, and a 10 s spray caused MHb levels of up to 50.5% [385,386]. Dermal administration of benzocaine has also been implicated in clinical cases of methemoglobinemia in dogs and cats [387–388]. An *N*-hydroxy metabolite of benzocaine (i.e., *o*-toluidine) is the likely active MHb-forming substance [385]. Prilocaine has been implicated in cases of methemoglobinemia in mothers and fetuses following epidural administration for labor [389] and following topical administration for dental procedures in humans [383]. Topical lidocaine did not induce MHb formation in sheep or monkeys, but it may be associated with MHb formation in cats and humans [385,390].

When MHb levels are 30% or higher, clinical signs of tissue hypoxia occur including cyanosis, dyspnea, nausea, vomiting, and tachycardia [383,387]. Lethargy, stupor, and shock occur when MHb levels approach 55% [383,388]. Animals with chronic methemoglobinemia may only present with Heinz body anemia and lethargy [388]. Chocolate brown-colored blood together with clinical signs that are not responsive to O_2 therapy are suggestive of methemoglobinemia. Definitive diagnosis is made by measuring the MHb concentration with co-oximetry or spectrophotometry. Blood smears will reveal the presence of Heinz bodies in the red blood cells.

Traditional first-line therapy of methemoglobinemia consists of slow intravenous administration of 1% methylene blue solution (4 mg/kg in dogs, 1–2 mg/kg in cats) [391–393]. The action of methylene blue depends on the availability of reduced nicotinamide adenine dinucleotide phosphate (NADPH) within red blood cells [383]. This dose can be repeated in dogs, but caution should be exercised in cats as repeated injections of methylene blue can markedly aggravate subsequent hemolysis without further lowering MHb content [394]. Glucose should also be administered because it is the major source of reduced nicotinamide adenine dinucleotide (NADH) in red blood cells, which is necessary to form NADPH, which is in turn needed for methylene blue to be effective [383]. In severe cases, a blood transfusion may be required.

Toxicosis (oral ingestion)

Topical preparations containing lidocaine, benzocaine, and tetracaine are found in many prescription and non-prescription products, such as ointments, teething gels, suppositories, and aerosols. These topical local anesthetic preparations can be hazardous if ingested or inappropriately applied to animals. Between 1995 and 1999, the American Society for the Prevention of Cruelty to Animals (ASPCA) Animal Poison Control Center (APCC) consulted on more than 70 cases of local anesthetic toxicosis in a variety of animal species [395]. Benzocaine toxicosis cases reported to the ASPCA APCC involved either ingestion of topical preparations or application of a laryngeal spray before endotracheal intubation. Clinical signs in cats and ferrets with benzocaine toxicosis included varying degrees of vomiting, depression, cyanosis, dyspnea, and tachypnea [395]. Other signs observed with local anesthetic toxicosis in different species include prolonged sedation, vasodilation (leading to hypotension), cardiac arrhythmias, respiratory depression, tremors and seizures, and death [395].

Allergic reactions

Ester-type local anesthetics (e.g., procaine) are associated with a higher incidence of allergic reactions due to a *para*-aminobenzoic acid (PABA) metabolite. Amide-type agents do not undergo such metabolism and rarely cause allergic reactions. However, preservative compounds (i.e., methylparaben and sodium metabisulfite) used in preparations of amide-type local anesthetics are metabolized to PABA and may cause allergies [396,397]. Therefore, it is recommended that animals known to be allergic to ester-type local anesthetics be treated with a preservative-free amide-type agent [396].

True allergic reactions to amide-type local anesthetics are rare in humans but have been documented [398]. The incidence in veterinary species appears to be extremely rare. Anaphylactic reactions are characterized by bronchospasm, upper airway edema, vasodilation, increased capillary permeability, and cutaneous wheal and flare. Rapid intervention with airway maintenance, O_2 therapy, epinephrine administration, and volume expansion is essential to avoid a fatal outcome.

References

1 Redondo JI, Bilbao I, Costa C, *et al.* Mortalidad anestésica en perros en España. Proyecto COMPLRED 2016–2021. *Proceedings of the Southern European Veterinary Conference 2021. Online virtual conference.* October 19–22, 2021.

2 Weinstein EJ, Levene JL, Cohen MS, *et al.* Local anaesthetics and regional anaesthesia versus conventional analgesia for preventing persistent postoperative pain in adults and children. *Cochrane Database Syst Rev* 2018; **6**(6): CD007105.

3 Komai H, McDowell TS. Local anesthetic inhibition of voltage-activated potassium currents in rat dorsal root ganglion neurons. *Anesthesiology* 2001; **94**: 1089–1095.

4 Olschewski A, Hempelmann G, Vogel W, *et al.* Blockade of Na + and K + currents by local anesthetics in the dorsal horn neurons of the spinal cord. *Anesthesiology* 1998; **88**: 172–179.

5 Xiong ZL, Strichartz GR. Inhibition by local anesthetics of Ca^{2+} channels in rat anterior pituitary cells. *Eur J Pharmacol* 1998; **363**: 81–90.

6 Sugiyama K, Muteki T. Local anesthetics depress the calcium current of rat sensory neurons in culture. *Anesthesiology* 1994; **80**: 1369–1378.

7 Scholz A. Mechanisms of (local) anaesthetics on voltage-gated sodium and other ion channels. *Br J Anaesth* 2002; **89**: 52–61.

8 Hollmann MW, Wieczorek KS, Berger A, *et al.* Local anesthetic inhibition of G protein-coupled receptor signaling by interference with Galpha(q) protein function. *Mol Pharmacol* 2001; **59**: 294–301.

9 Taylor A, McLeod G. Basic pharmacology of local anaesthetics. *BJA Educ* 2020; **20**(2): 34–41.

10 Fozzard HA, Lee PJ, Lipkind GM. Mechanism of local anesthetic drug action on voltage-gated sodium channels. *Curr Pharm Des* 2005; **11**(21): 2671–2686.

11 Catterall WA. From ionic currents to molecular mechanisms: the structure and function of voltage-gated sodium channels. *Neuron* 2000; **26**(1): 13–25.

12 Catterall WA, Swanson TM. Structural basis for pharmacology of voltage-gated sodium and calcium channels. *Mol Pharmacol* 2015; **88**(1): 141–150.

13 Narahashi T, Frazier DT. Site of action and active form of local anesthetics. *Neurosci Res* 1971; **4**: 65–99.

14 Wann KT. Neuronal sodium and potassium channels: structure and function. *Br J Anaesth* 1993; **71**(1): 2–14.

15 Yun I, Cho ES, Jang HO, *et al.* Amphiphilic effects of local anesthetics on rotational mobility in neuronal and model membranes. *Biochim Biophys Acta* 2002; **1564**(1): 123–132.

16 Hille B. Local anesthetics: hydrophilic and hydrophobic pathways for the drug-receptor reaction. *J Gen Physiol* 1977; **69**(4): 497–515.

17 Starmer CF, Grant AO, Strauss HC. Mechanisms of use-dependent block of sodium channels in excitable membranes by local anesthetics. *Biophys J* 1984; **46**(1): 15–27.

18 Huang JH, Thalhammer JG, Raymond SA, *et al.* Susceptibility to lidocaine of impulses in different somatosensory afferent fibers of rat sciatic nerve. *J Pharmacol Exp Ther* 1997; **292**: 802–811.

19 Lin Y, Liu SS. Local anesthetics. In: Barash PG, Cullen BF, Stoelting RK, *et al.*, eds. *Clinical Anesthesia*, 8th edn. Philadelphia, PA: Wolters Kluwer, 2017: 564–584.

20 Stevens RA, Bray JG, Artuso JD, *et al.* Differential epidural block. *Reg Anesth* 1992; **17**: 22–25.

21 Sakura S, Sumi M, Yamada Y, *et al.* Quantitative and selective assessment of sensory block during lumbar epidural anaesthesia with 1% or 2% lidocaine. *Br J Anaesth* 1998; **81**: 718–722.

22 Nathan PW. Observations on sensory and sympathetic function during intrathecal analgesia. *J Neurol Neurosurg Psychiatry* 1976; **39**: 114–121.

23 Gasser HS, Erlanger J. Role of fibre size in the establishment of nerve block by pressure or cocaine. *Am J Physiol* 1929; **88**: 581–591.

24 Gissen AJ, Covino BG, Gregus J. Differential sensitivities of mammalian nerve fibers to local anesthetic agents. *Anesthesiology* 1980; **53**: 467–474.

25 Gokin AP, Philip B, Strichartz GR. Preferential block of small myelinated sensory and motor fibers by lidocaine: in vivo electrophysiology in the rat sciatic nerve. *Anesthesiology* 2001; **95**: 1441–1454.

26 Strichartz G, Pastijn E, Sugimoto K. Neural physiology and local anesthetic action. In: Cousins MJ, Carr DB, Horlocker TT, Bridenbaugh PO, eds. *Cousins & Bridenbaugh's Neural Blockade in Clinical Anesthesia and Pain Medicine*, 4th edn. Philadelphia, PA: Lippincott Williams & Wilkins, 2009: 26–47.

27 Jaffe RA, Rowe MA. Differential nerve block. Direct measurements on individual myelinated and unmyelinated dorsal root axons. *Anesthesiology* 1996; **84**: 1455–1464.

28 Khurana I, Khurana A, Kowlgi NG. The nerve. In: *Textbook of Medical Physiology*, 3rd edn, E-book. India: Elsevier Health Sciences, 2020: 51–72.

29 Raymond SA, Steffensen SC, Gugino LD, *et al.* The role of length of nerve exposed to local anesthetics in impulse blocking action. *Anesth Analg* 1989; **68**: 563–570.

30 Fink BR. Mechanisms of differential axial blockade in epidural and subarachnoid anesthesia. *Anesthesiology* 1989; **70**: 851–858.

31 de Jong RH, Wagman IH. Physiological mechanisms of peripheral nerve block by local anesthetics. *Anesthesiology* 1963; **24**: 684–727.

32 Winnie AP, Tay CH, Patel KP, *et al.* Pharmacokinetics of local anesthetics during plexus blocks. *Anesth Analg* 1977; **56**(6): 852–861.

33 Stewart JD. Peripheral nerve fascicles: anatomy and clinical relevance. *Muscle Nerve* 2003; **28**(5): 525–541.

34 Brushart TM. Central course of digital axons within the median nerve of *Macaca mulatta*. *J Comp Neurol* 1991; **311**(2): 197–209.

35 Condouris GA, Goebel RH, Brady T. Computer simulation of local anesthetic effects using a mathematical model of myelinated nerve. *J Pharmacol Exp Ther* 1976; **196**: 737–745.

36 Nakamura T, Popitz-Bergez F, Birknes J, *et al.* The critical role of concentration for lidocaine block of peripheral nerve in vivo. Studies of function and drug uptake in the rat. *Anesthesiology* 2003; **99**: 1187–1197.

37 Waikar SS, Thalhammer JG, Raymond SA, *et al.* Mechanoreceptive afferents exhibit functionally-specific activity dependent changes in conduction velocity. *Brain Res* 1996; **721**: 91–100.

38 Raymond SA. Subblocking concentrations of local anesthetics: effects on impulse generation and conduction in single myelinated sciatic nerve axons in frog. *Anesth Analg* 1992; **75**: 906–921.

39 Olschewski A, Wolff M, Bräu ME, *et al.* Enhancement of delayed-rectifier potassium conductance by low concentrations of local anaesthetics in spinal sensory neurones. *Br J Pharmacol* 2002; **136**: 540–549.

40 Olschewski A, Schnoebel-Ehehalt R, Li Y, *et al.* Mexiletine and lidocaine suppress the excitability of dorsal horn neurons. *Anesth Analg* 2009; **109**: 258–264.

41 Ku WH, Schneider SP. Multiple T-type Ca^{2+} current subtypes in electrophysiologically characterized hamster dorsal horn neurons: possible role in spinal sensory integration. *J Neurophysiol* 2011; **106**: 2486–2498.

42 Li YM, Wingrove DE, Too HP, *et al.* Local anesthetics inhibit substance P binding and evoked increases in intracellular Ca^{2+}. *Anesthesiology* 1995; **82**: 166–173.

43 Nagy I, Woolf CJ. Lignocaine selectively reduces C fibre-evoked neuronal activity in rat spinal cord in vitro by decreasing N-methyl-D-aspartate and neurokinin receptor-mediated post-synaptic depolarizations: implications for the development of novel centrally acting analgesics. *Pain* 1996; **64**: 59–70.

44 Furutani K, Ikoma M, Ishii H, *et al.* Bupivacaine inhibits glutamatergic transmission in spinal dorsal horn neurons. *Anesthesiology* 2010; **112**: 138–143.

45 Mather LE, Tucker GT. Properties, absorption and disposition of local anesthetic agents. In: Cousins MJ, Carr DB, Horlocker TT, Bridenbaugh PO, eds. *Cousins & Bridenbaugh's Neural Blockade in Clinical Anesthesia and Pain Medicine*, 4th edn. Philadelphia, PA: Lippincott Williams & Wilkins, 2009: 48–95.

46 Liu SS. Local anesthetics and analgesia. In: Ashburn MA, Rice LJ, eds. *The Management of Pain*. New York: Churchill Livingstone, 1997: 141–170.

47 Butterworth JF, Strichartz GR. Molecular mechanisms of local anesthetics: a review. *Anesthesiology* 1990; **72**: 711–734.

48 Strichartz GR, Sanchez V, Arthur R, *et al.* Fundamental properties of local anesthetics II. Measured Octanol: Buffer partition coefficients and pKa, values of clinically used drugs. *Anesth Analg* 1990; **71**: 158–170.

49 Bräu ME, Vogel W, Hempelmann G. Fundamental properties of local anesthetics: half-maximal blocking concentrations for tonic block of Na^+ and K^+ channels in peripheral nerve. *Anesth Analg* 1998; **87**: 885–889.

50 Covino BG, Wildsmith JAW. Clinical pharmacology of local anesthetic agents. In: Cousins MJ, Bridenbaugh PO, eds. *Neural Blockade in Clinical Anesthesia and Management of Pain*, 3rd edn. Philadelphia, PA: Lippincott-Raven, 1998: 97–128.

51 Gissen AJ, Covino BG, Gregus J. Differential sensitivity of fast and slow fibers in mammalian nerve II. Margin of safety for nerve transmission. *Anesth Analg* 1982; **61**: 561–569.

52 Burm AG, Vermeulen NP, van Kleef JW, *et al.* Pharmacokinetics of lignocaine and bupivacaine in surgical patients following epidural administration. Simultaneous investigation of absorption and disposition kinetics using stable isotopes. *Clin Pharmacokinet* 1987; **13**(3): 191–203.

53 Ulbricht W. Kinetics of drug action and equilibrium results at the node of Ranvier. *Physiol Rev* 1981; **61**: 785–828.

54 Salinas FV, Liu SL, Scholz AM. Ion channel ligands, sodium channel blockers, local anesthetics. In: Evers AS, Maze M, eds. *Anesthetic Pharmacology, Physiologic Principles and Clinical Practice*. Philadelphia, PA: Churchill Livingstone, 2004: 507–537.

55 Leone S, di Cianni S, Casati A, *et al.* Pharmacology, toxicology and clinical use of new long acting local anesthetics, ropivacaine and levobupivacaine. *Acta Biomed* 2008; **79**: 92–105.

56 Aberg G. Toxicological and local anesthetic effects of optically active isomers of two local anesthetic compounds. *Acta Pharmacol Toxicol Scand* 1972; **31**: 273–286.

57 Lee-Son MB, Wang GK, Concus A, *et al.* Stereoselective inhibition of neuronal sodium channels by local anesthetics. *Anesthesiology* 1992; **77**: 324–335.

58 Huang YF, Pryor ME, Veering BT, *et al.* Cardiovascular and central nervous system effects of intravenous levobupivacaine and bupivacaine in sheep. *Anesth Analg* 1998; **86**: 797–804.

59 Wildsmith JA, Brown DT, Paul D, *et al.* Structure–activity relationships in differential nerve block at high and low frequency stimulation. *Br J Anaesth* 1989; **63**: 444–452.

60 Pateromichelakis S, Prokopiou AA. Local anaesthesia efficacy: discrepancy between in vitro and in vivo studies. *Acta Anaesthesiol Scand* 1988; **32**: 672–675.

61 Wildsmith JA, Gissen AJ, Takman B, *et al.* Differential nerve blockade: esters v. amides and the influence of pKa. *Br J Anaesth* 1987; **59**: 379–384.

62 Ford DJ, Raj PP, Singh P, *et al.* Differential peripheral nerve block by local anesthetics in the cat. *Anesthesiology* 1984; **60**: 28–33.

63 Markham A, Faulds D. Ropivacaine. A review of its pharmacology and therapeutic use in regional anaesthesia. *Drugs* 1996; **52**: 429–449.

64 Mottura AA, Procickieviez O. The fate of lidocaine infiltrate during abdominoplasty and a comparative study of absorption of local anesthetic in 3 different regions: experimental studies in a porcine model. *Aesthet Surg J* 2001; **21**: 418–422.

65 Tucker GT, Moore DC, Bridenbaugh PO, *et al.* Systemic absorption of mepivacaine in commonly used regional block procedures. *Anesthesiology* 1972; **37**: 277–387.

66 Sellers G, Lin HC, Riddell MG, *et al.* Pharmacokinetics of lidocaine in serum and milk of mature Holstein cows. *J Vet Pharmacol Ther* 2009; **32**: 446–450.

67 Sum DC, Chung PC. Plasma lidocaine level during spinal or epidural anesthesia in geriatric patients. *Ma Zui Xue Za Zhi* 1993; **31**: 59–63.

68 Clement R, Malinovsky JM, Le Corre P, *et al.* Cerebrospinal fluid bioavailability and pharmacokinetics of bupivacaine and lidocaine after intrathecal and epidural administrations in rabbits using microdialysis. *J Pharmacol Exp Ther* 1999; **289**: 1015–1021.

69 Estebe JP, Le Corre P, du Plessis L, *et al.* The pharmacokinetics and pharmacodynamics of bupivacaine-loaded microspheres on a brachial plexus block model in sheep. *Anesth Analg* 2001; **93**: 447–455.

70 Jiang X, Wen X, Gao B, *et al.* The plasma concentrations of lidocaine after slow versus rapid administration of an initial dose of epidural anesthesia. *Anesth Analg* 1997; **84**: 570–573.

71 Johns RA, DiFazio CA, Longnecker DE. Lidocaine constricts or dilates rat arterioles in a dose-dependent manner. *Anesthesiology* 1985; **62**: 141–144.

72 Iida H, Ohata H, Iida M, *et al.* The differential effects of stereoisomers of ropivacaine and bupivacaine on cerebral pial arterioles in dogs. *Anesth Analg* 2001; **93**: 1552–1556.

73 Ala-Kokko TI, Partanen A, Karinen J, *et al.* Pharmacokinetics of 0.2% ropivacaine and 0.2% bupivacaine following caudal blocks in children. *Acta Anaesthesiol Scand* 2000; **44**: 1099–1102.

74 Karmakar MK, Aun CS, Wong EL, *et al.* Ropivacaine undergoes slower systemic absorption from the caudal epidural space in children than bupivacaine. *Anesth Analg* 2002; **94**: 259–265.

75 Mashimo T, Uchida I, Pak M, *et al.* Prolongation of canine epidural anesthesia by liposome encapsulation of lidocaine. *Anesth Analg* 1992; **74**: 827–834.

76 Tofoli GR, Cereda CM, de Araujo DR. Pharmacokinetic and local toxicity studies of liposome-encapsulated and plain mepivacaine solutions in rats. *Drug Deliv* 2010; **17**: 68–76.

77 Dräger C, Benziger D, Gao F, *et al.* Prolonged intercostal nerve blockade in sheep using controlled-release of bupivacaine and dexamethasone from polymer microspheres. *Anesthesiology* 1998; **89**: 969–979.

78 Fransson BA, Peck KE, Smith JK, *et al.* Transdermal absorption of a liposome-encapsulated formulation of lidocaine following topical administration in cats. *Am J Vet Res* 2002; **63**: 1309–1312.

79 Tobe M, Obata H, Suto T, *et al.* Long-term effect of sciatic nerve block with slow-release lidocaine in a rat model of postoperative pain. *Anesthesiology* 2010; **112**: 1473–1481.

80 Wang CF, Pancaro C, Gerner P, Strichartz G. Prolonged suppression of postincisional pain by a slow-release formulation of lidocaine. *Anesthesiology* 2011; **114**: 135–149.

81 Marathe PH, Shen DD, Artru AA, *et al.* Effect of serum protein binding on the entry of lidocaine into brain and cerebrospinal fluid in dogs. *Anesthesiology* 1991; **75**: 804–812.

82 Shand DG. Alpha 1-acid glycoprotein and plasma lidocaine binding. *Clin Pharmacokinet* 1984; **9**: 27–31.

83 Tucker G. Pharmacokinetics of local anaesthetics. *Br J Anaesth* 1986; **58**: 717–731.

84 De Rick AF, Belpaire FM, Dello C, Bogaert MG. Influence of enhanced alpha-1-acid glycoprotein concentration on protein binding, pharmacokinetics and antiarrhythmic effect of lidocaine in the dog. *J Pharmacol Exp Ther* 1987; **241**: 289–293.

85 Belpaire FM, de Rick A, Dello C, *et al.* Alpha 1-acid glycoprotein and serum binding of drugs in healthy and diseased dogs. *J Vet Pharmacol Ther* 1987; **10**: 43–48.

86 Palazzo MG, Kalso EA, Argiras E, *et al.* First pass lung uptake of bupivacaine: effect of acidosis in an intact rabbit lung model. *Br J Anaesth* 1991; **67**: 759–763.

87 Krejcie TC, Avram MJ, Gentry WB, *et al.* A recirculatory model of the pulmonary uptake and pharmacokinetics of lidocaine based on analysis of arterial and mixed venous data from dogs. *J Pharmacokinet Biopharm* 1997; **25**: 169–190.

88 Post C, Andersson RG, Ryrfeldt A, *et al.* Physico-chemical modification of lidocaine uptake in rat lung tissue. *Acta Pharmacol Toxicol (Copenh)* 1979; **44**: 103–109.

89 Geng WP, Ebke M, Foth H. Prilocaine elimination by isolated perfused rat lung and liver. *Naunyn Schmiedebergs Arch Pharmacol* 1995; **351**: 93–98.

90 Aoki M, Okudaira K, Haga M, *et al.* Contribution of rat pulmonary metabolism to the elimination of lidocaine, midazolam, and nifedipine. *Drug Metab Dispos* 2010; **38**: 1183–1188.

91 Ohmura S, Sugano A, Kawada M, *et al.* Pulmonary uptake of ropivacaine and levobupivacaine in rabbits. *Anesth Analg* 2003; **97**: 893–897.

92 Puente NW, Josephy PD. Analysis of the lidocaine metabolite 2, 6-dimethylaniline in bovine and human milk. *J Anal Toxicol* 2001; **25**(8): 711–715.

93 Biehl D, Shnider SM, Levinson G, *et al.* Placental transfer of lidocaine: effects of fetal acidosis. *Anesthesiology* 1978; **48**: 409–412.

94 Kennedy RL, Bell JU, Miller RP, *et al.* Uptake and distribution of lidocaine in fetal lambs. *Anesthesiology* 1990; **72**: 483–489.

95 Hamshaw-Thomas A, Reynolds F. Placental transfer of bupivacaine, pethidine and lignocaine in the rabbit. Effect of umbilical flow rate and protein content. *Br J Obstet Gynaecol* 1985; **92**: 706–713.

96 Kennedy RL, Miller RP, Bell JU, *et al.* Uptake and distribution of bupivacaine in fetal lambs. *Anesthesiology* 1986; **65**: 247–253.

97 Santos AC, Karpel B, Noble G. The placental transfer and fetal effects of levobupivacaine, racemic bupivacaine, and ropivacaine. *Anesthesiology* 1999; **90**: 1698–1703.

98 Tobin T, Blake JW, Sturma L, *et al.* Pharmacology of procaine in the horse: procaine esterase properties of equine plasma and synovial fluid. *Am J Vet Res* 1976; **37**: 1165–1170.

99 Calvo R, Carlos R, Erill S. Effects of disease and acetazolamide on procaine hydrolysis by red blood cell enzymes. *Clin Pharmacol Ther* 1980; **27**: 179–183.

100 Matsubara K, Kagawa M, Fukui Y. In vivo and in vitro studies on cocaine metabolism: ecgonine methyl ester as a major metabolite of cocaine. *Forensic Sci Int* 1984; **26**: 169–180.

101 Kuhnert BR, Kuhnert PM, Philipson EH, *et al.* The half-life of 2-chloroprocaine. *Anesth Analg* 1986; **65**: 273–278.

102 Tobin T, Blake JW. A review of the pharmacology, pharmacokinetics and behavioral effects of procaine in Thoroughbred horses. *Br J Sports Med* 1976; **10**: 109–116.

103 McKeever KH, Hinchcliff KW, Gerken DF, *et al.* Effects of cocaine on incremental treadmill exercise in horses. *J Appl Physiol* 1993; **75**: 2727–2733.

104 Hjelm M, Ragnarsson B, Wistrand P. Biochemical effects of aromatic compounds. 3. Ferrihaemoglobinaemia and the presence of p-hydroxy-o-toluidine in human blood after the administration of prilocaine. *Biochem Pharmacol* 1972; **21**: 2825–2834.

105 Wilcke JR, Davis LE, Neff-Davis CA, *et al.* Pharmacokinetics of lidocaine and its active metabolites in dogs. *J Vet Pharmacol Ther* 1983; **6**: 49–57.

106 Kammerer RC, Schmitz DA. Lidocaine metabolism by rabbit-liver homogenate and detection of a new metabolite. *Xenobiotica* 1986; **16**: 681–690.

107 Oda Y, Imaoka S, Nakahira Y, *et al.* Metabolism of lidocaine by purified rat liver microsomal cytochrome P-450 isozymes. *Biochem Pharmacol* 1989; **38**: 4439–4444.

108 Thomasy SM, Pypendop BH, Ilkiw JE, *et al.* Pharmacokinetics of lidocaine and its active metabolite, monoethylglycinexylidide, after intravenous administration of lidocaine to awake and isoflurane-anesthetized cats. *Am J Vet Res* 2005; **66**: 1162–1166.

109 Valverde A, Gunkelt C, Doherty TJ, *et al.* Effect of a constant rate infusion of lidocaine on the quality of recovery from sevoflurane or isoflurane general anaesthesia in horses. *Equine Vet J* 2005; **37**: 559–564.

110 Dickey EJ, McKenzie HC III, Brown KA, *et al.* Serum concentrations of lidocaine and its metabolites after prolonged infusion in healthy horses. *Equine Vet J* 2008; **40**: 348–352.

111 Doherty T, Redua MA, Queiroz-Castro P, *et al.* Effect of intravenous lidocaine and ketamine on the minimum alveolar concentration of isoflurane in goats. *Vet Anaesth Analg* 2007; **34**: 125–131.

112 Da Cunha AF, Messenger KM, Stout RW, *et al.* Pharmacokinetics of lidocaine and its active metabolite monoethylglycinexylidide after a single intravenous administration in chickens (*Gallus domesticus*) anesthetized with isoflurane. *J Vet Pharmacol Ther* 2012; **35**: 604–607.

113 Cox S, Wilson J, Doherty T. Pharmacokinetics of lidocaine after intravenous administration to cows. *J Vet Pharmacol Ther* 2012; **35**: 305–308.

114 Webb AI, Pablo LS. Local anesthetics. In: Riviere JE, Papich MG, eds. *Veterinary Pharmacology and Therapeutics*, 9th edn. Ames, IA: Wiley-Blackwell, 2009: 381–400.

115 Rosenberg PH, Heavner JE. Acute cardiovascular and central nervous system toxicity of bupivacaine and desbutylbupivacaine in the rat. *Acta Anaesthesiol Scand* 1992; **36**: 138–141.

116 Harkins JD, Karpiesiuk W, Tobin T, *et al.* Identification of hydroxyropivacaine glucuronide in equine urine by ESI+/MS/MS. *Can J Vet Res* 2000; **64**: 178–183.

117 O'Brien JE, Abbey V, Hinsvark O, *et al.* Metabolism and measurement of chloroprocaine, an ester-type local anesthetic. *J Pharm Sci* 1979; **68**: 75–78.

118 Reynolds F. Metabolism and excretion of bupivacaine in man: a comparison with mepivacaine. *Br J Anaesth* 1971; **43**: 33–37.

119 Rowland M, Thomson PD, Guichard A, Melmon KL. Disposition kinetics of lidocaine in normal subjects. *Ann N Y Acad Sci* 1971; **179**: 383–398.

120 Engelking LR, Blyden GT, Lofstedt J, *et al.* Pharmacokinetics of antipyrine, acetaminophen and lidocaine in fed and fasted horses. *J Vet Pharmacol Ther* 1987; **10**: 73–82.

121 Hastings CL, Brown TC, Eyres RL, *et al.* The influence of age on plasma lignocaine levels following tracheal spray in young dogs. *Anaesth Intensive Care* 1985; **13**: 392–394.

122 Morishima HO, Finster M, Pedersen H, *et al.* Pharmacokinetics of lidocaine in fetal and neonatal lambs and adult sheep. *Anesthesiology* 1979; **50**: 431–436.

123 Hastings CL, Brown TC, Eyres RL, *et al.* The influence of age on lignocaine pharmacokinetics in young puppies. *Anaesth Intensive Care* 1986; **14**: 135–139.

124 Zsigmond EK, Downs JR. Plasma cholinesterase activity in newborns and infants. *Can Anaesth Soc J* 1971; **18**: 278–285.

125 Abernethy DR, Greenblatt DJ. Impairment of lidocaine clearance in elderly male subjects. *J Cardiovasc Pharmacol* 1983; **5**: 1093–1096.

126 Veering BT, Burm AG, van Kleef JW, *et al.* Epidural anesthesia with bupivacaine: effects of age on neural blockade and pharmacokinetics. *Anesth Analg* 1987; **66**: 589–593.

127 Datta S, Lambert DH, Gregus J, *et al.* Differential sensitivities of mammalian nerve fibers during pregnancy. *Anesth Analg* 1983; **62**: 1070–1072.

128 Bader AM, Datta S, Moller RA, *et al.* Acute progesterone treatment has no effect on bupivacaine-induced conduction blockade in the isolated rabbit vagus nerve. *Anesth Analg* 1990; **71**: 545–548.

129 Santos AC, Pedersen H, Morishima HO, *et al.* Pharmacokinetics of lidocaine in nonpregnant and pregnant ewes. *Anesth Analg* 1988; **67**: 1154–1158.

130 Santos AC, Arthur GR, Lehning EJ, *et al.* Comparative pharmacokinetics of ropivacaine and bupivacaine in nonpregnant and pregnant ewes. *Anesth Analg* 1997; **85**: 87–93.

131 Gentz HD, Schlicht I, Wiederholt W. Pseudocholinesterase in patients with and without liver diseases. *Med Klin* 1978; **73**: 1422–1426.

132 Venkataraman BV, Iyer GY, Narayanan R, *et al.* Erythrocyte and plasma cholinesterase activity in normal pregnancy. *Indian J Physiol Pharmacol* 1990; **34**: 26–28.

133 Waller ES. Pharmacokinetic principles of lidocaine dosing in relation to disease state. *J Clin Pharmacol* 1981; **21**: 181–194.

134 Feary DJ, Mama KR, Wagner AE, *et al.* Influence of general anesthesia on pharmacokinetics of intravenous lidocaine infusion in horses. *Am J Vet Res* 2005; **66**: 574–580.

135 Calvo R, Carlos R, Erill S. Procaine hydrolysis defect in uraemia does not appear to be due to carbamylation of plasma esterases. *Eur J Clin Pharmacol* 1983; **24**(4): 533–535.

136 Feary DJ, Mama KR, Thomasy SM, *et al.* Influence of gastrointestinal tract disease on pharmacokinetics of lidocaine after intravenous infusion in anesthetized horses. *Am J Vet Res* 2006; **67**: 317–322.

137 Peeyush M, Ravishankar M, Adithan C, *et al.* Altered pharmacokinetics of lignocaine after epidural injection in type II diabetics. *Eur J Clin Pharmacol* 1992; **43**: 269–271.

138 Gawrońska-Szklarz B, Musiał DH, Pawlik A, *et al.* Effect of experimental diabetes on pharmacokinetic parameters of lidocaine and MEGX in rats. *Pol J Pharmacol* 2003; **55**: 619–624.

139 Raj PP, Ohlweiler D, Hitt BA, *et al.* Kinetics of local anesthetic esters and the effects of adjuvant drugs on 2-chloroprocaine hydrolysis. *Anesthesiology* 1980; **53**: 307–314.

140 Calvo R, Carlos R, Erill S. Effects of disease and acetazolamide on procaine hydrolysis by red blood cell enzymes. *Clin Pharmacol Ther* 1980; **27**: 179–183.

141 Olkkola KT, Isohanni MH, Hamunen K, *et al.* The effect of erythromycin and fluvoxamine on the pharmacokinetics of intravenous lidocaine. *Anesth Analg* 2005; **100**: 1352–1356.

142 Tesseromatis C, Kotsiou A, Tsagataki M, *et al.* In vitro binding of lidocaine to liver tissue under the influence of propranolol: another mechanism of interaction? *Eur J Drug Metab Pharmacokinet* 2007; **32**: 213–217.

143 Lalka D, Vicuna N, Burrow SR, *et al.* Bupivacaine and other amide local anesthetics inhibit the hydrolysis of chloroprocaine by human serum. *Anesth Analg* 1978; **57**: 534–539.

144 Rosenberg PH, Heavner JE. Temperature-dependent nerve-blocking action of lidocaine and halothane. *Acta Anaesthesiol Scand* 1980; **24**: 314–320.

145 Butterworth JF, Walker FO, Neal JM. Cooling potentiates lidocaine inhibition of median nerve sensory fibers. *Anesth Analg* 1990; **70**: 507–511.

146 Sanchez V, Arthur GR, Strichartz GR. Fundamental properties of local anesthetics. I. The dependence of lidocaine's ionization and octanol: buffer partitioning on solvent and temperature. *Anesth Analg* 1987; **66**: 159–165.

147 Heath PJ, Brownlie GS, Herrick MJ. Latency of brachial plexus block. The effect on onset time of warming local anaesthetic solutions. *Anaesthesia* 1990; **45**: 297–301.

148 Han SS, Lee SC, Ro YJ, *et al.* Warming the epidural injectate improves first sacral segment block: a randomised double-blind study. *Anaesth Intensive Care* 2010; **38**: 690–694.

149 Liu FC, Liou JT, Day YJ, *et al.* Effect of warm lidocaine on the sensory onset of epidural anesthesia: a randomized trial. *Chang Gung Med J* 2009; **32**: 643–649.

150 Lee R, Kim YM, Choi EM, *et al.* Effect of warmed ropivacaine solution on onset and duration of axillary block. *Korean J Anesthesiol* 2012; **62**: 52–56.

151 Chilvers CR. Warm local anaesthetic – effect on latency of onset of axillary brachial plexus block. *Anaesth Intensive Care* 1993; **21**: 795–798.

152 Kristoffersen E, Sloth E, Husted JC, *et al.* Spinal anaesthesia with plain 0.5% bupivacaine at 19 degrees C and 37 degrees C. *Br J Anaesth* 1990; **65**: 504–507.

153 Greene NM. Distribution of local anesthetic solutions within the subarachnoid space. *Anesth Analg* 1985; **64**: 715–730.

154 Imbelloni LE, Moreira AD, Gaspar FC, *et al.* Assessment of the densities of local anesthetics and their combination with adjuvants: an experimental study. *Rev Bras Anestesiol* 2009; **59**: 154–165.

155 Horlocker TT, Wedel DJ. Density, specific gravity, and baricity of spinal anesthetic solutions at body temperature. *Anesth Analg* 1993; **76**: 1015–1018.

156 McLeod GA. Density of spinal anaesthetic solutions of bupivacaine, levobupivacaine, and ropivacaine with and without dextrose. *Br J Anaesth* 2004; **92**: 547–551.

157 Ganem EM, Vianna PT, Marques M, *et al.* Neurotoxicity of subarachnoid hyperbaric bupivacaine in dogs. *Reg Anesth* 1996; **21**: 234–238.

158 Kaya M, Oguz S, Aslan K, *et al.* A low-dose bupivacaine: a comparison of hyperbaric and hypobaric solutions for unilateral spinal anesthesia. *Reg Anesth Pain Med* 2004; **29**: 17–22.

159 Casati A, Fanelli G. Unilateral spinal anesthesia. *State of the art. Minerva Anestesiol* 2001; **67**: 855–862.

160 Richardson MG, Wissler RN. Densities of dextrose-free intrathecal local anesthetics, opioids, and combinations measured at 37 degrees C. *Anesth Analg* 1997; **84**: 95–99.

161 Lui AC, Polis TZ, Cicutti NJ. Densities of cerebrospinal fluid and spinal anaesthetic solutions in surgical patients at body temperature. *Can J Anaesth* 1998; **45**: 297–303.

162 Richardson MG, Wissler RN. Density of lumbar cerebrospinal fluid in pregnant and nonpregnant humans. *Anesthesiology* 1996; **85**: 326–330.

163 Bernards CM, Kopacz DJ. Effect of epinephrine on lidocaine clearance in vivo: a microdialysis study in humans. *Anesthesiology* 1999; **91**: 962–968.

164 Kuchembuck NL, Colahan PT, Zientek KD, *et al.* Plasma concentration and local anesthetic activity of procaine hydrochloride following subcutaneous administration to horses. *Am J Vet Res* 2007; **68**: 495–500.

165 Burm AG, van Kleef JW, Gladines MP, *et al.* Epidural anesthesia with lidocaine and bupivacaine: effects of epinephrine on the plasma concentration profiles. *Anesth Analg* 1986; **65**: 1281–1284.

166 Karmakar MK, Ho AM, Law BK, *et al.* Arterial and venous pharmacokinetics of ropivacaine with and without epinephrine after thoracic paravertebral block. *Anesthesiology* 2005; **103**: 704–711.

167 Ratajczak-Enselme M, Estebe JP, Rose FX, *et al.* Effect of epinephrine on epidural, intrathecal, and plasma pharmacokinetics of ropivacaine and bupivacaine in sheep. *Br J Anaesth* 2007; **99**: 881–890.

168 Reddy SV, Maderdrut JL, Yaksh TL. Spinal cord pharmacology of adrenergic agonist- mediated antinociception. *J Pharmacol Exp Ther* 1980; **213**: 525–533.

169 Collins JG, Kitahata LM, Matsumoto M, *et al.* Spinally administered epinephrine suppresses noxiously evoked activity of WDR neurons in the dorsal horn of the spinal cord. *Anesthesiology* 1984; **60**: 269–725.

170 Sonohata M, Furue H, Katafuchi T, *et al.* Actions of noradrenaline on substantia gelatinosa neurones in the rat spinal cord revealed by in vivo patch recording. *J Physiol* 2004; **555**: 515–526.

171 Sinnott CJ, Cogswell III LP, Johnson A, *et al.* On the mechanism by which epinephrine potentiates lidocaine's peripheral nerve block. *Anesthesiology* 2003; **98**: 181–188.

172 Niemi G. Advantages and disadvantages of adrenaline in regional anaesthesia. *Best Pract Res Clin Anaesth* 2005; **19**: 229–245.

173 Shieh JP, Chu CC, Wang JJ, *et al.* Epinephrine, phenylephrine, and methoxamine induce infiltrative anesthesia via alpha1-adrenoceptors in rats. *Acta Pharmacol Sin* 2009; **30**: 1227–1236.

174 Kozody R, Palahniuk RJ, Wade JG, *et al.* The effect of subarachnoid epinephrine and phenylephrine on spinal cord blood flow. *Can Anaesth Soc J* 1984; **31**: 503–508.

175 Porter SS, Albin MS, Watson WA, *et al.* Spinal cord and cerebral blood flow responses to subarachnoid injection of local anesthetics with and without epinephrine. *Acta Anaesthesiol Scand* 1985; **29**: 330–338.

176 Neal JM. Effects of epinephrine in local anesthetics on the central and peripheral nervous systems: neurotoxicity and neural blood flow. *Reg Anesth Pain Med* 2003; **28**: 124–134.

177 Myers RR, Heckman HM. Effects of local anesthesia on nerve blood flow: studies using lidocaine with and without epinephrine. *Anesthesiology* 1989; **71**: 757–762.

178 Palmer GM, Cairns BE, Berkes SL, *et al.* The effects of lidocaine and adrenergic agonists on rat sciatic nerve and skeletal muscle blood flow in vivo. *Anesth Analg* 2002; **95**: 1080–1086.

179 Niwa H, Hirota Y, Sibutani T, *et al.* The effects of epinephrine and norepinephrine administered during local anesthesia on left ventricular diastolic function. *Anesth Prog* 1991; **38**: 221–226.

180 Henslee TM, Hodson SB, Lamy CJ, *et al.* Vasoconstrictive agents commonly used in combination with local anesthetics: a literature review. *J Foot Surg* 1987; **26**: 504–510.

181 Yagiela JA. What's new with phentolamine mesylate: a reversal agent for local anaesthesia? *SAAD Dig* 2011; **27**: 3–7.

182 Kirby CK, Eckenhoff JE, Looby JP. The use of hyaluronidase with local anesthetic agents in nerve block and infiltration anesthesia. *Surgery* 1949; **25**: 101–104.

183 Dempsey GA, Barrett PJ, Kirby IJ. Hyaluronidase and peribulbar block. *Br J Anaesth* 1997; **78**: 671–674.

184 Nicoll JM, Treuren B, Acharya PA, *et al.* Retrobulbar anesthesia: the role of hyaluronidase. *Anesth Analg* 1986; **65**: 1324–1328.

185 Kallio H, Paloheimo M, Maunuksela EL. Hyaluronidase as an adjuvant in bupivacaine- lidocaine mixture for retrobulbar/peribulbar block. *Anesth Analg* 2000; **91**: 934–937.

186 Crawford M, Kerr WJ. The effect of hyaluronidase on peribulbar block. *Anaesthesia* 1994; **49**: 907–908.

187 Brydon CW, Basler M, Kerr WJ. An evaluation of two concentrations of hyaluronidase for supplementation of peribulbar anaesthesia. *Anaesthesia* 1995; **50**: 998–1000.

188 Keeler JF, Simpson KH, Ellis FR, *et al.* Effect of addition of hyaluronidase to bupivacaine during axillary brachial plexus block. *Br J Anaesth* 1992; **68**: 68–71.

189 Nevarre DR, Tzarnas CD. The effects of hyaluronidase on the efficacy and on the pain of administration of 1% lidocaine. *Plast Reconstr Surg* 1998; **101**: 365–369.

190 Etesse B, Beaudroit L, Deleuze M, *et al.* Hyaluronidase: here we go again. *Ann Fr Anesth Reanim* 2009; **28**: 658–665.

191 DeRossi R, de Barros AL, Silva-Neto AB, *et al.* Hyaluronidase shortens levobupivacaine lumbosacral epidural anaesthesia in dogs. *J Small Anim Pract* 2011; **52**: 195–199.

192 Gray TR, Dzikiti BT, Zeiler GE. Effects of hyaluronidase on ropivacaine or bupivacaine regional anaesthesia of the canine pelvic limb. *Vet Anaesth Analg* 2019; **46**(2): 214–225.

193 Wohlrab J, Finke R, Franke WG, *et al.* Clinical trial for safety evaluation of hyaluronidase as diffusion enhancing adjuvant for infiltration analgesia of skin with lidocaine. *Dermatol Surg* 2012; **38**: 91–96.

194 Morris R, McKay W, Mushlin P. Comparison of pain associated with intradermal and subcutaneous infiltration with various local anesthetic solutions. *Anesth Analg* 1987; **66**: 1180–1182.

195 McKay W, Morris R, Mushlin P. Sodium bicarbonate attenuates pain on skin infiltration with lidocaine, with or without epinephrine. *Anesth Analg* 1987; **66**: 572–574.

196 Christoph RA, Buchanan L, Begalla K, *et al.* Pain reduction in local anesthetic administration through pH buffering. *Ann Emerg Med* 1988; **17**: 117–120.

197 Jones JS, Plzak C, Wynn BN, *et al.* Effect of temperature and pH adjustment of bupivacaine for intradermal anesthesia. *Am J Emerg Med* 1998; **16**: 117–120.

198 Ririe DG, Walker FO, James RL, *et al.* Effect of alkalinization of lidocaine on median nerve block. *Br J Anaesth* 2000; **84**: 163–168.

199 Buckley FP, Duval Neto G, Fink BR. Acid and alkaline solutions of local anesthetics: duration of nerve block and tissue pH. *Anesth Analg* 1985; **64**: 477–482.
200 Capogna G, Celleno D, Varrassi G, *et al.* Epidural mepivacaine for cesarean section: effects of a pH-adjusted solution. *J Clin Anesth* 1991; **3**: 211–214.
201 Benzon HT, Toleikis JR, Dixit P, *et al.* Onset, intensity of blockade and somatosensory evoked potential changes of the lumbosacral dermatomes after epidural anesthesia with alkalinized lidocaine. *Anesth Analg* 1993; **76**: 328–332.
202 Capogna G, Celleno D, Laudano D, *et al.* Alkalinization of local anesthetics. Which block, which local anesthetic? *Reg Anesth* 1995; **20**: 369–377.
203 Stevens RA, Chester WL, Grueter JA, *et al.* The effect of pH adjustment of 0.5% bupivacaine on the latency of epidural anesthesia. *Reg Anesth* 1989; **14**: 236–239.
204 Verborgh C, Claeys MA, Camu F. Onset of epidural blockade after plain or alkalinized 0.5% bupivacaine. *Anesth Analg* 1991; **73**: 401–404.
205 Gaggero G, Meyer O, van Gessel E, *et al.* Alkalinization of lidocaine 2% does not influence the quality of epidural anaesthesia for elective caesarean section. *Can J Anaesth* 1995; **42**: 1080–1084.
206 Ramos G, Pereira E, Simonetti MP. Does alkalinization of 0.75% ropivacaine promote a lumbar peridural block of higher quality? *Reg Anesth Pain Med* 2001; **26**: 357–362.
207 Sinnott CJ, Garfield JM, Thalhammer JG, *et al.* Addition of sodium bicarbonate to lidocaine decreases the duration of peripheral nerve block in the rat. *Anesthesiology* 2000; **93**: 1045–1052.
208 Henry R, Patterson L, Avery N, *et al.* Absorption of alkalized intravesical lidocaine in normal and inflamed bladders: a simple method for improving bladder anesthesia. *J Urol* 2001; **165**: 1900–1903.
209 Zezza L, Reusch CE, Gerber B. Intravesical application of lidocaine and sodium bicarbonate in the treatment of obstructive idiopathic lower urinary tract disease in cats. *J Vet Intern Med* 2012; **26**: 526–531.
210 Zehetmayer M, Rainer G, Turnheim K, *et al.* Topical anesthesia with pH-adjusted versus standard lidocaine 4% for clear corneal cataract surgery. *J Cataract Refract Surg* 1997; **23**: 1390–1393.
211 Fuchsjäger-Mayrl G, Zehetmayer M, Plass H, *et al.* Alkalinization increases penetration of lidocaine across the human cornea. *J Cataract Refract Surg* 2002; **28**: 692–696.
212 Nakayama M, Munemura Y, Kanaya N, *et al.* Efficacy of alkalinized lidocaine for reducing pain on intravenous and epidural catheterization. *J Anesth* 2001; **15**: 201–203.
213 Mader TJ, Playe SJ, Garb JL. Reducing the pain of local anesthetic infiltration: warming and buffering have a synergistic effect. *Ann Emerg Med* 1994; **23**: 550–554.
214 Peterfreund RA, Datta S, Ostheimer GW. pH adjustment of local anesthetic solutions with sodium bicarbonate: laboratory evaluation of alkalinization and precipitation. *Reg Anesth* 1989; **14**: 265–270.
215 Bokesch PM, Raymond SA, Strichartz GR. Dependence of lidocaine potency on pH and PCO_2. *Anesth Analg* 1987; **66**: 9–17.
216 Bromage PR, Burfoot MF, Crowell DE, *et al.* Quality of epidural blockade. 3. Carbonated local anaesthetic solutions. *Br J Anaesth* 1967; **39**: 197–209.
217 Gosteli P, van Gessel E, Gamulin Z. Effects of pH adjustment and carbonation of lidocaine during epidural anesthesia for foot or ankle surgery. *Anesth Analg* 1995; **81**: 104–109.
218 Schelling CG, Klein LV. Comparison of carbonated lidocaine and lidocaine hydrochloride for caudal epidural anesthesia in horses. *Am J Vet Res* 1985; **46**: 1375–1377.
219 Brummett CM, Williams BA. Additives to local anesthetics for peripheral nerve blockade. *Int Anesthesiol Clin* 2011; **49**: 104–116.
220 Grubb TL, Riebold TW, Huber MJ. Comparison of lidocaine, xylazine, and xylazine/ lidocaine for caudal epidural analgesia in horses. *J Am Vet Med Assoc* 1992; **201**: 1187–1190.
221 Pohl VH, Carregaro AB, Lopes C, *et al.* Epidural anesthesia and postoperatory analgesia with alpha-2 adrenergic agonists and lidocaine for ovariohysterectomy in bitches. *Can J Vet Res* 2012; **76**(3): 215–220.
222 Lamont LA, Lemke KA. The effects of medetomidine on radial nerve blockade with mepivacaine in dogs. *Vet Anaesth Analg* 2008; **35**: 62–68.
223 Brummett CM, Norat MA, Palmisano JM, *et al.* Perineural administration of dexmedetomidine in combination with bupivacaine enhances sensory and motor blockade in sciatic nerve block without inducing neurotoxicity in rat. *Anesthesiology* 2008; **109**: 502–511.
224 Brummett CM, Padda AK, Amodeo FS, *et al.* Perineural dexmedetomidine added to ropivacaine causes a dose-dependent increase in the duration of thermal antinociception in sciatic nerve block in rat. *Anesthesiology* 2009; **111**: 1111–1119.
225 Xue X, Fan J, Ma X, *et al.* Effects of local dexmedetomidine administration on the neurotoxicity of ropivacaine for sciatic nerve block in rats. *Mol Med Rep* 2020; **22**(5): 4360–4366.
226 Kirksey MA, Haskins SC, Cheng J, *et al.* Local anesthetic peripheral nerve block adjuvants for prolongation of analgesia: a systematic qualitative review. *PLoS ONE* 2015; **10**(9): e0137312.
227 Trein TA, Floriano BP, Wagatsuma JT, *et al.* Effects of dexmedetomidine combined with ropivacaine on sciatic and femoral nerve blockade in dogs. *Vet Anaesth Analg* 2017; **44**(1): 144–153.
228 Marolf V, Ida KK, Siluk D, *et al.* Effects of perineural administration of ropivacaine combined with perineural or intravenous administration of dexmedetomidine for sciatic and saphenous nerve blocks in dogs. *Am J Vet Res* 2021; **82**(6): 449–458.
229 Bartel AK, Campoy L, Martin-Flores M, *et al.* Comparison of bupivacaine and dexmedetomidine femoral and sciatic nerve blocks with bupivacaine and buprenorphine epidural injection for stifle arthroplasty in dogs. *Vet Anaesth Analg* 2016; **43**(4): 435–443.
230 Marolf V, Selz J, Picavet P, *et al.* Effects of perineural dexmedetomidine combined with ropivacaine on postoperative methadone requirements in dogs after tibial plateau levelling osteotomy: a two-centre study. *Vet Anaesth Analg* 2022; **49**(3): 313–322.
231 O O, Smith LJ. A comparison of epidural analgesia provided by bupivacaine alone, bupivacaine + morphine, or bupivacaine + dexmedetomidine for pelvic orthopedic surgery in dogs. *Vet Anaesth Analg* 2013; **40**(5): 527–536.
232 Benito J, Monteiro B, Beaudry F, *et al.* Efficacy and pharmacokinetics of bupivacaine with epinephrine or dexmedetomidine after intraperitoneal administration in cats undergoing ovariohysterectomy. *Can J Vet Res* 2018; **82**(2): 124–130.
233 Evangelista MC, Doodnaught GM, Fantoni DT, *et al.* Sciatic and femoral nerve blockade using bupivacaine alone, or in combination with dexmedetomidine or buprenorphine in cats. *Vet Rec* 2017; **180**(24): 592.
234 Kroin JS, Buvanendran A, Beck DR, *et al.* Clonidine prolongation of lidocaine analgesia after sciatic nerve block in rats is mediated via the hyperpolarization-activated cation current, not by alpha-adrenoreceptors. *Anesthesiology* 2004; **101**: 488–494.
235 Brummett CM, Hong EK, Janda AM, *et al.* Perineural dexmedetomidine added to ropivacaine for sciatic nerve block in rats prolongs the duration of analgesia by blocking the hyperpolarization-activated cation current. *Anesthesiology* 2011; **115**: 836–843.
236 Leem JW, Choi Y, Han SM, *et al.* Conduction block by clonidine is not mediated by alpha-2-adrenergic receptors in rat sciatic nerve fibers. *Reg Anesth Pain Med* 2000; **25**: 620–625.
237 Ribotsky BM, Berkowitz KD, Montague JR. Local anesthetics. Is there an advantage to mixing solutions? *J Am Podiatr Med Assoc* 1996; **86**: 487–491.
238 Cuvillon P, Nouvellon E, Ripart J, *et al.* A comparison of the pharmacodynamics and pharmacokinetics of bupivacaine, ropivacaine (with epinephrine) and their equal volume mixtures with lidocaine used for femoral and sciatic nerve blocks: a double-blind randomized study. *Anesth Analg* 2009; **108**: 641–649.
239 Gadsden J, Hadzic A, Gandhi K, *et al.* The effect of mixing 1.5% mepivacaine and 0.5% bupivacaine on duration of analgesia and latency of block onset in ultrasound- guided interscalene block. *Anesth Analg* 2011; **112**: 471–476.
240 Vesal N, Ahmadi M, Foroud M, *et al.* Caudal epidural anti-nociception using lidocaine, bupivacaine or their combination in cows undergoing reproductive procedures. *Vet Anaesth Analg* 2013; **40**(3): 328–332.
241 Lawal FM, Adetunji A. A comparison of epidural anaesthesia with lignocaine, bupivacaine and a lignocaine-bupivacaine mixture in cats. *J S Afr Vet Assoc* 2009; **80**: 243–246.
242 Seow LT, Lips FJ, Cousins MJ, *et al.* Lidocaine and bupivacaine mixtures for epidural blockade. *Anesthesiology* 1982; **56**: 177–183.
243 Kaukinen S, Kaukinen L, Eerola R. Epidural anaesthesia with mixtures of bupivacaine-lidocaine and etidocaine-lidocaine. *Ann Chir Gynaecol* 1980; **69**: 281–286.
244 Magee DA, Sweet PT, Holland AJ. Epidural anaesthesia with mixtures of bupivicaine and lidocaine. *Can Anaesth Soc J* 1983; **30**: 174–178.
245 Jacobsen J, Husum B, von Staffeldt H, *et al.* The addition of lidocaine to bupivacaine does not shorten the duration of spinal anesthesia: a randomized, double-blinded study of patients undergoing knee arthroscopy. *Anesth Analg* 2011; **113**: 1272–1275.
246 Corke BC, Carlson CG, Dettbarn WD. The influence of 2-chloroprocaine on the subsequent analgesic potency of bupivacaine. *Anesthesiology* 1984; **60**: 25–27.
247 Galindo A, Witcher T. Mixtures of local anesthetics: bupivacaine-chloroprocaine. *Anesth Analg* 1980; **59**: 683–685.
248 Mets B, Janicki PK, James MF, *et al.* Lidocaine and bupivacaine cardiorespiratory toxicity is additive: a study in rats. *Anesth Analg* 1992; **75**: 611–614.
249 Kottenberg-Assenmacher E, Peters J. Mechanisms of tachyphylaxis in regional anesthesia of long duration. *Anasthesiol Intensivmed Notfallmed Schmerzther* 1999; **34**: 733–742.
250 Bromage PR, Pettigrew RT, Crowell DE. Tachyphylaxis in epidural analgesia: I. Augmentation and decay of local anesthesia. *J Clin Pharmacol J New Drugs* 1969; **9**: 30–38.
251 Baker CE, Berry RL, Elston RC. Effect of pH of bupivacaine on duration of repeated sciatic nerve blocks in the albino rat. Local Anesthetics for Neuralgia Study Group. *Anesth Analg* 1991; **72**: 773–778.

252 Wang C, Liu H, Wilder RT, *et al.* Effects of repeated injection of local anesthetic on sciatic nerve blocks response. *J Huazhong Univ Sci Technolog Med Sci* 2004; **24**: 497–499.

253 Mogensen T, Simonsen L, Scott NB, *et al.* Tachyphylaxis associated with repeated epidural injections of lidocaine is not related to changes in distribution or the rate of elimination from the epidural space. *Anesth Analg* 1989; **69**: 180–184.

254 Lipfert P, Holthusen H, Arndt JO. Tachyphylaxis to local anesthetics does not result from reduced drug effectiveness at the nerve itself. *Anesthesiology* 1989; **70**: 71–75.

255 Wang C, Sholas MG, Berde CB, *et al.* Evidence that spinal segmental nitric oxide mediates tachyphylaxis to peripheral local anesthetic nerve block. *Acta Anaesthesiol Scand* 2001; **45**: 945–953.

256 Lee KC, Wilder RT, Smith RL, *et al.* Thermal hyperalgesia accelerates and MK-801 prevents the development of tachyphylaxis to rat sciatic nerve blockade. *Anesthesiology* 1994; **81**: 1284–1293.

257 Wilder RT, Sholas MG, Berde CB. NG-nitro-L-arginine methyl ester (L-NAME) prevents tachyphylaxis to local anesthetics in a dose-dependent manner. *Anesth Analg* 1996; **83**: 1251–1255.

258 Mercadante S, Villari P, Ferrera P, *et al.* Local anesthetic switching for intrathecal tachyphylaxis in cancer patients with pain. *Anesth Analg* 2003; **97**: 187–189.

259 Herring IP, Bobofchak MA, Landry MP, *et al.* Duration of effect and effect of multiple doses of topical ophthalmic 0.5% proparacaine hydrochloride in clinically normal dogs. *Am J Vet Res* 2005; **66**(1): 77–80.

260 Binder DR, Herring IP. Duration of corneal anesthesia following topical administration of 0.5% proparacaine hydrochloride solution in clinically normal cats. *Am J Vet Res* 2006; **67**(10): 1780–1782.

261 Peyman GA, Rahimy MH, Fernandes ML. Effects of morphine on corneal sensitivity and epithelial wound healing: implications for topical ophthalmic analgesia. *Br J Ophthalmol* 1994; **78**(2): 138–141.

262 Douet JY, Michel J, Regnier A. Degree and duration of corneal anesthesia after topical application of 0.4% oxybuprocaine hydrochloride ophthalmic solution in ophthalmically normal dogs. *Am J Vet Res* 2013; **74**(10): 1321–1326.

263 Mama KR, Steffey EP. Local anesthetics. In: Adams HR, ed. *Veterinary Pharmacology and Therapeutics*, 8th edn. Ames, IA: Blackwell, 2001: 343–359.

264 Axelrod EH, Alexander GD, Brown M, *et al.* Procaine spinal anesthesia: a pilot study of the incidence of transient neurologic symptoms. *J Clin Anesth* 1998; **10**: 404–409.

265 Heo GJ, Shin G. Efficacy of benzocaine as an anaesthetic for Crucian carp (Carassius carassius). *Vet Anaesth Analg* 2010; **37**: 132–135.

266 Forster JG, Rosenberg PH. Revival of old local anesthetics for spinal anesthesia in ambulatory surgery. *Curr Opin Anaesthesiol* 2011; **24**: 633–637.

267 Butterworth JF. Clinical pharmacology of local anesthetics. In: Cousins MJ, Carr DB, Horlocker TT, Bridenbaugh PO, eds. *Cousins & Bridenbaugh's Neural Blockade in Clinical Anesthesia and Pain Medicine*, 4th edn. Philadelphia, PA: Lippincott Williams & Wilkins, 2009: 96–113.

268 Sharrow-Reabe KL, Townsend WM. Effects of action of proparacaine and tetracaine topical ophthalmic formulations on corneal sensitivity in horses. *J Am Vet Med Assoc* 2012; **241**(12): 1645–1649.

269 Patel D, Chopra S, Berman MD. Serious systemic toxicity resulting from use of tetracaine for pharyngeal anesthesia in upper endoscopic procedures. *Dig Dis Sci* 1989; **34**: 882–884.

270 Lander JA, Weltman BJ, So SS. EMLA and amethocaine for reduction of children's pain associated with needle insertion. *Cochrane Database Syst Rev* 2006; **19**(3): CD004236.

271 Sawyer J, Febbraro S, Masud S, *et al.* Heated lidocaine/tetracaine patch (Synera, Rapydan) compared with lidocaine/prilocaine cream (EMLA) for topical anaesthesia before vascular access. *Br J Anaesth* 2009; **102**: 210–215.

272 Muir WW, Wiese AJ, March PA. Effects of morphine, lidocaine, ketamine, and morphine-lidocaine-ketamine drug combination on minimum alveolar concentration in dogs anesthetized with isoflurane. *Am J Vet Res* 2003; **64**: 1155–1160.

273 Valverde A, Doherty TJ, Hernandez J, *et al.* Effect of lidocaine on the minimum alveolar concentration of isoflurane in dogs. *Vet Anaesth Analg* 2004; **31**: 264–271.

274 Wilson J, Doherty TJ, Egger CM, *et al.* Effects of intravenous lidocaine, ketamine, and the combination on the minimum alveolar concentration of sevoflurane in dogs. *Vet Anaesth Analg* 2008; **35**: 289–296.

275 Pypendop BH, Ilkiw JE. The effects of intravenous lidocaine administration on the minimum alveolar concentration of isoflurane in cats. *Anesth Analg* 2005; **100**: 97–101.

276 Dzikiti TB, Hellebrekers LJ, van Dijk P. Effects of intravenous lidocaine on isoflurane concentration, physiological parameters, metabolic parameters and stress-related hormones in horses undergoing surgery. *J Vet Med A Physiol Pathol Clin Med* 2003; **50**: 190–195.

277 Rezende ML, Wagner AE, Mama KR, *et al.* Effects of intravenous administration of lidocaine on the minimum alveolar concentration of sevoflurane in horses. *Am J Vet Res* 2011; **72**: 446–451.

278 Vesal N, Spadavecchia C, Steiner A, *et al.* Evaluation of the isoflurane-sparing effects of lidocaine infusion during umbilical surgery in calves. *Vet Anaesth Analg* 2011; **38**: 451–460.

279 Yardeni IZ, Beilin B, Mayburd E, *et al.* The effect of perioperative intravenous lidocaine on postoperative pain and immune function. *Anesth Analg* 2009; **109**: 1464–1469.

280 Swenson BR, Gottschalk A, Wells LT, *et al.* Intravenous lidocaine is as effective as epidural bupivacaine in reducing ileus duration, hospital stay, and pain after open colon resection: a randomized clinical trial. *Reg Anesth Pain Med* 2010; **35**: 370–376.

281 Ness TJ. Intravenous lidocaine inhibits visceral nociceptive reflexes and spinal neurons in the rat. *Anesthesiology* 2000; **92**: 1685–1691.

282 Smith LJ, Shih A, Miletic G, *et al.* Continual systemic infusion of lidocaine provides analgesia in an animal model of neuropathic pain. *Pain* 2002; **97**: 267–273.

283 Robertson SA, Sanchez LC, Merritt AM, *et al.* Effect of systemic lidocaine on visceral and somatic nociception in conscious horses. *Equine Vet J* 2005; **37**: 122–127.

284 Pypendop BH, Ilkiw JE, Robertson SA. Effects of intravenous administration of lidocaine on the thermal threshold in cats. *Am J Vet Res* 2006; **67**: 16–20.

285 MacDougall LM, Hethey JA, Livingston A, *et al.* Antinociceptive, cardiopulmonary, and sedative effects of five intravenous infusion rates of lidocaine in conscious dogs. *Vet Anaesth Analg* 2009; **36**: 512–522.

286 Doherty TJ, Seddighi MR. Local anesthetics as pain therapy in horses. *Vet Clin North Am Equine Pract* 2010; **26**: 533–549.

287 Brianceau P, Chevalier H, Karas A, *et al.* Intravenous lidocaine and small-intestinal size, abdominal fluid, and outcome after colic surgery in horses. *J Vet Intern Med* 2002; **16**: 736–741.

288 Malone E, Ensink J, Turner T, *et al.* Intravenous continuous infusion of lidocaine for treatment of equine ileus. *Vet Surg* 2006; **35**: 60–66.

289 Torfs S, Delesalle C, Dewulf J, *et al.* Risk factors for equine postoperative ileus and effectiveness of prophylactic lidocaine. *J Vet Intern Med* 2009; **23**: 606–611.

290 Guschlbauer M, Feige K, Geburek F, *et al.* Effects of in vivo lidocaine administration at the time of ischemia and reperfusion on in vitro contractility of equine jejunal smooth muscle. *Am J Vet Res* 2011; **72**: 1449–1455.

291 Salem SE, Proudman CJ, Archer DC. Has intravenous lidocaine improved the outcome in horses following surgical management of small intestinal lesions in a UK hospital population? *BMC Vet Res* 2016; **12**(1): 157.

292 Elfenbein JR, Robertson SA, MacKay RJ, *et al.* Systemic and anti-nociceptive effects of prolonged lidocaine, ketamine, and butorphanol infusions alone and in combination in healthy horses. *BMC Vet Res* 2014; **10**(Suppl 1): S6.

293 Rusiecki KE, Nieto JE, Puchalski SM, *et al.* Evaluation of continuous infusion of lidocaine on gastrointestinal tract function in normal horses. *Vet Surg* 2008; **37**: 564–570.

294 Ngo LY, Tam YK, Tawfik S, *et al.* Effects of intravenous infusion of lidocaine on its pharmacokinetics in conscious instrumented dogs. *J Pharm Sci* 1997; **86**: 944–952.

295 Perez-Castro R, Patel S, Garavito-Aguilar ZV, *et al.* Cytotoxicity of local anesthetics in human neuronal cells. *Anesth Analg* 2009; **108**: 997–1007.

296 Cederholm I, Evers H, Lofstrom JB. Skin blood flow after intradermal injection of ropivacaine in various concentrations with and without epinephrine evaluated by laser Doppler flowmetry. *Reg Anesth* 1992; **17**: 322–328.

297 Riviere JE, Papich MG. Potential and problems of developing transdermal patches for veterinary applications. *Adv Drug Deliv Rev* 2001; **50**(3): 175–203.

298 Ko JC, Maxwell LK, Abbo LA, *et al.* Pharmacokinetics of lidocaine following the application of 5% lidocaine patches to cats. *J Vet Pharmacol Ther* 2008; **31**(4): 359–367.

299 Weiland L, Croubels S, Baert K, *et al.* Pharmacokinetics of a lidocaine patch 5% in dogs. *J Vet Med A Physiol Pathol Clin Med* 2006; **53**(1): 34–39.

300 Ko J, Weil A, Maxwell L, *et al.* Plasma concentrations of lidocaine in dogs following lidocaine patch application. *J Am Anim Hosp Assoc* 2007; **43**(5): 280–283.

301 Bidwell LA, Wilson DV, Caron JP. Lack of systemic absorption of lidocaine from 5% patches placed on horses. *Vet Anaesth Analg* 2007; **34**(6): 443–446.

302 Andreoni V, Giorgi M. Evaluation of plasma detectable concentrations of two lidocaine transdermal formulations and their analgesic effect in the horse. *J Equine Vet Sci* 2009; **29**(9): 681–686.

303 Joudrey SD, Robinson DA, Kearney MT, *et al.* Plasma concentrations of lidocaine in dogs following lidocaine patch application over an incision compared to intact skin. *J Vet Pharmacol Ther* 2015; **38**(6): 575–580.

304 Merema DK, Schoenrock EK, Le Boedec K, *et al.* Effects of a transdermal lidocaine patch on indicators of postoperative pain in dogs undergoing midline ovariohysterectomy. *J Am Vet Med Assoc* 2017; **250**(10): 1140–1147.

305 Re Bravo V, Aprea F, Bhalla RJ, *et al.* Effect of 5% transdermal lidocaine patches on postoperative analgesia in dogs undergoing hemilaminectomy. *J Small Anim Pract* 2019; **60**(3): 161–166.

306 Söbbeler FJ, Kästner SB. Effects of transdermal lidocaine or lidocaine with prilocaine or tetracaine on mechanical superficial sensation and nociceptive thermal thresholds in horses. *Vet Anaesth Analg* 2018; **45**(2): 227–233.
307 Espinoza C, Lomax S, Windsor P. The effect of a topical anesthetic on the sensitivity of calf dehorning wounds. *J Dairy Sci* 2013; **96**(5): 2894–2902.
308 Cuttance EL, Mason WA, Yang DA, *et al.* Effects of a topically applied anaesthetic on the behaviour, pain sensitivity and weight gain of dairy calves following thermocautery disbudding with a local anaesthetic. *N Z Vet J* 2019; **67**(6): 295–305.
309 Sheil M, Chambers M, Polkinghorne A, *et al.* Topical application of lidocaine and bupivacaine to disbudding wounds in dairy calves: safety, toxicology and wound healing. *Animals (Basel)* 2021; **11**(3): 869.
310 Lomax S, Sheil M, Windsor PA. Impact of topical anaesthesia on pain alleviation and wound healing in lambs after mulesing. *Aust Vet J* 2008; **86**(5): 159–168.
311 Lomax S, Dickson H, Sheil M, *et al.* Topical anaesthesia alleviates short-term pain of castration and tail docking in lambs. *Aust Vet J* 2010; **88**(3): 67–74.
312 Ferrador AM. *Use of Tri-Solfen to Control Pain during Treatment of Hoof Lesions in Dairy Cows.* Dissertation Universidade de Lisboa, Faculdade de Medicina Veterinária, 2018.
313 Sheil M, De Benedictis GM, Scollo A, *et al.* Efficacy of intra-operative topical wound anaesthesia to mitigate piglet castration pain – a large, multi-centred field trial. *Animals (Basel)* 2021; **11**(10): 2763.
314 NOCITA® (Bupivacaine Liposome Injectable Suspension) (2018b) Package Insert. Leawood, KS. Aratana Therapeutics. https://assets-eu-01.kc-usercontent.com/43db687c-fb47-015f-c990-00802940e2bc/9e1f56d5-5b93-4691-9fe2-ea6514b2d793/2019_NocitaPckg_Insert_10mL-NO%20BARCODE.pdf (accessed June 2022)
315 Lascelles BD, Rausch-Derra LC, Wofford JA, *et al.* Pilot, randomized, placebo-controlled clinical field study to evaluate the effectiveness of bupivacaine liposome injectable suspension for the provision of post-surgical analgesia in dogs undergoing stifle surgery. *BMC Vet Res* 2016; **12**(1): 168.
316 Reader RC, McCarthy RJ, Schultz KL, *et al.* Comparison of liposomal bupivacaine and 0.5% bupivacaine hydrochloride for control of postoperative pain in dogs undergoing tibial plateau leveling osteotomy. *J Am Vet Med Assoc* 2020; **256**(9): 1011–1019.
317 Gordon-Evans WJ, Suh HY, Guedes AG. Controlled, non-inferiority trial of bupivacaine liposome injectable suspension. *J Feline Med Surg* 2020; **22**(10): 916–921.
318 Le KM, Caston SS, Hossetter JM, *et al.* Comparison of analgesic and tissue effects of subcutaneous perineural injection of liposomal bupivacaine and bupivacaine hydrochloride in horses with forelimb lameness induced via circumferential clamp. *Am J Vet Res* 2020; **81**(7): 551–556.
319 Moorman VJ, Pezzanite LM, Griffenhagen GM. Liposomal bupivacaine provides longer duration analgesia than bupivacaine hydrochloride in an adjustable sole-pressure model of equine lameness. *Am J Vet Res* 2022; **83**(4): 298–304.
320 Ottoboni T, Quart B, Pawasauskas J, *et al.* Mechanism of action of HTX-011: a novel, extended-release, dual-acting local anesthetic formulation for postoperative pain. *Reg Anesth Pain Med* 2020; **45**: 117–123.
321 Mather LE. The acute toxicity of local anesthetics. *Expert Opin Drug Metab Toxicol* 2010; **6**: 1313–1332.
322 Aberg G. Toxicological and local anesthetic effects of optically active isomers of two local anesthetic compounds. *Acta Pharmacol Toxicol Scand* 1972; **31**: 273–286.
323 Santos AC, DeArmas PE. Systemic toxicity of levobupivacaine, bupivacaine, and ropivacaine during continuous intravenous infusion to nonpregnant and pregnant ewes. *Anesthesiology* 2001; **95**: 1256–1264.
324 Feldman HS, Arthur GR, Covino BG. Comparative systemic toxicity of convulsant and supraconvulsant doses of intravenous ropivacaine, bupivacaine, and lidocaine in the conscious dog. *Anesth Analg* 1989; **69**: 794–801.
325 Rutten AJ, Nancarrow C, Mather LE, *et al.* Hemodynamic and central nervous system effects of intravenous bolus doses of lidocaine, bupivacaine, and ropivacaine in sheep. *Anesth Analg* 1989; **69**: 291–299.
326 Faccenda KA, Finucane BT. Complications of regional anaesthesia: incidence and prevention. *Drug Saf* 2001; **24**: 413–442.
327 Auroy Y, Benhamou D, Bargues L, *et al.* Major complications of regional anesthesia in France: the SOS Regional Anesthesia Hotline Service. *Anesthesiology* 2002; **97**: 1274–1280.
328 Cox B, Durieux ME, Marcus MAE. Toxicity of local anaesthetics. *Best Pract Res Clin Anaesth* 2003; **17**: 111–136.
329 Marsch S, Schaefer H, Castelli I. Unusual psychological manifestation of systemic local anaesthetic toxicity. *Anesthesiology* 1998; **88**: 532–533.
330 Meyer GA, Lin HC, Hanson RR, *et al.* Effects of intravenous lidocaine overdose on cardiac electrical activity and blood pressure in the horse. *Equine Vet J* 2001; **33**: 434–437.
331 Rosenberg P, Kalso E, Tuominen M, *et al.* Acute bupivacaine toxicity as a result of venous leakage under the tourniquet cuff during a bier block. *Anesthesiology* 1983; **58**: 95–98.
332 Morishima HO, Pedersen H, Finster M, *et al.* Bupivacaine toxicity in pregnant and nonpregnant ewes. *Anesthesiology* 1985; **63**: 134–139.
333 Brown DL, Ransom DM, Hall JA, *et al.* Regional anesthesia and local anesthetic-induced systemic toxicity: seizure frequency and accompanying cardiovascular changes. *Anesth Analg* 1995; **81**: 321–328.
334 Liu PL, Feldman HS, Giasi R, *et al.* Comparative CNS toxicity of lidocaine, etidocaine, bupivacaine, and tetracaine in awake dogs following rapid intravenous administration. *Anesth Analg* 1983; **62**: 375–379.
335 Hofman WF, Jerram DC, Gangarosa LP. Cardiorespiratory and behavioral reactions to the lidocaine-induced convulsions in the dog. *Res Commun Chem Pathol Pharmacol* 1977; **16**: 581–591.
336 Lemo N, Vnuk D, Radisic B, *et al.* Determination of the toxic dose of lidocaine in dogs and its corresponding serum concentration. *Vet Rec* 2007; **160**: 374–375.
337 Wilcke JR, Davis LE, Neff-Davis CA. Determination of lidocaine concentrations producing therapeutic and toxic effects in dogs. *J Vet Pharmacol Ther* 1983; **6**: 105–111.
338 Milligan M, Kukanich B, Beard W, *et al.* The disposition of lidocaine during a 12-hour intravenous infusion to postoperative horses. *J Vet Pharmacol Ther* 2006; **29**: 495–499.
339 Navas de Solis C, McKenzie HC. Serum concentrations of lidocaine and its metabolites MEGX and GX during and after prolonged intravenous infusion of lidocaine in horses after colic surgery. *J Equine Vet Sci* 2007; **27**: 398–404.
340 Chadwick HS. Toxicity and resuscitation in lidocaine- or bupivacaine-infused cats. *Anesthesiology* 1985; **63**: 385–390.
341 de Jong RH, Ronfeld RA, DeRosa RA. Cardiovascular effects of convulsant and supraconvulsant doses of amide local anesthetics. *Anesth Analg* 1982; **61**(1): 3–9.
342 Nancarrow C, Rutten AJ, Runciman WB, *et al.* Myocardial and cerebral drug concentrations and the mechanisms of death after fatal intravenous doses of lidocaine, bupivacaine, and ropivacaine in the sheep. *Anesth Analg* 1989; **69**: 276–283.
343 Heavner JE, Badgwell JM, Dryden CF Jr., *et al.* Bupivacaine toxicity in lightly anesthetized pigs with respiratory imbalances plus or minus halothane. *Reg Anesth* 1995; **20**: 20–26.
344 Burney RG, DiFazio CA, Foster JA. Effects of pH on protein binding of lidocaine. *Anesth Analg* 1978; **57**: 478–480.
345 Heavner JE, Dryden CF Jr., Sanghani V, *et al.* Severe hypoxia enhances central nervous system and cardiovascular toxicity of bupivacaine in lightly anesthetized pigs. *Anesthesiology* 1992; **77**: 142–147.
346 Beecroft C, Davies G. Systemic toxic effects of local anaesthetics. *Anaesth Intensive Care Med* 2010; **11**: 98–100.
347 Mazoit JX, Boico O, Samii K. Myocardial uptake of bupivacaine: II. Pharmacokinetics and pharmacodynamics of bupivacaine enantiomers in the isolated perfused rabbit heart. *Anesth Analg* 1993; **77**: 477–482.
348 Chang DH, Ladd LA, Wilson KA, *et al.* Tolerability of large-dose intravenous levobupivacaine in sheep. *Anesth Analg* 2000; **91**: 671–679.
349 Huang YF, Upton RN, Runciman WB. I.V. bolus administration of subconvulsive doses of lignocaine to conscious sheep: myocardial pharmacokinetics. *Br J Anaesth* 1993; **70**: 326–332.
350 Copeland SE, Ladd LA, Gu SQ, *et al.* The effects of general anesthesia on the central nervous and cardiovascular system toxicity of local anesthetics. *Anesth Analg* 2008; **106**: 1429–1439.
351 Valenzuela C, Snyders DJ, Bennett PB, *et al.* Stereoselective block of cardiac sodium channels by bupivacaine in guinea pig ventricular myocytes. *Circulation* 1995; **92**: 3014–3024.
352 Valenzuela C, Delpon E, Tamkun MM, *et al.* Stereoselective block of a human cardiac potassium channel (Kv1.5) by bupivacaine enantiomers. *Biophys J* 1995; **69**: 418–427.
353 Mather L, Chang D. Cardiotoxicity with modern local anaesthetics: is there a safe choice? *Drugs* 2001; **61**: 333–342.
354 Avery P, Redon D, Schaenzer G, *et al.* The influence of serum potassium on the cerebral and cardiac toxicity of bupivacaine and lidocaine. *Anesthesiology* 1984; **61**: 134–138.
355 Neal JM, Mulroy MF, Weinberg GL. American Society of Regional Anesthesia and Pain Medicine checklist for managing local anesthetic systemic toxicity: 2012 version. *Reg Anesth Pain Med* 2012; **37**: 16–18.
356 Weinberg GL. Current concepts in resuscitation of patients with local anesthetic cardiac toxicity. *Reg Anesth Pain Med* 2002; **27**: 568–575.
357 Weinberg GL, VadeBoncouer T, Ramaraju GA, *et al.* Pretreatment or resuscitation with a lipid infusion shifts the dose-response to bupivacaine-induced asystole in rats. *Anesthesiology* 1998; **88**: 1071–1075.
358 Weinberg G, Ripper R, Feinstein DL, *et al.* Lipid emulsion infusion rescues dogs from bupivacaine-induced cardiac toxicity. *Reg Anesth Pain Med* 2003; **28**: 198–202.
359 Rosenblatt MA, Abel M, Fischer GW, *et al.* Successful use of a 20% lipid emulsion to resuscitate a patient after a presumed bupivacaine-related cardiac arrest. *Anesthesiology* 2006; **105**: 217–218.

360 Warren JA, Thoma RB, Georgescu A, *et al.* Intravenous lipid infusion in the successful resuscitation of local anesthetic-induced cardiovascular collapse after supraclavicular brachial plexus block. *Anesth Analg* 2008; **106**: 1578–1580.
361 Sonsino DH, Fischler M. Immediate intravenous lipid infusion in the successful resuscitation of ropivacaine-induced cardiac arrest after infraclavicular brachial plexus block. *Reg Anesth Pain Med* 2009; **34**: 276–277.
362 Weinberg GL, di Gregorio G, Ripper R, *et al.* Resuscitation with lipid versus epinephrine in a rat model of bupivacaine overdose. *Anesthesiology* 2008; **108**: 907–913.
363 Hiller DB, Gregorio GD, Ripper R, *et al.* Epinephrine impairs lipid resuscitation from bupivacaine overdose: a threshold effect. *Anesthesiology* 2009; **111**: 498–505.
364 Gregorio G, Schwartz D, Ripper R, *et al.* Lipid emulsion is superior to vasopressin in a rodent model of resuscitation from toxin-induced cardiac arrest. *Crit Care Med* 2009; **37**: 993–999.
365 Fernandez AL, Lee JA, Rahilly L, *et al.* The use of intravenous lipid emulsion as an antidote in veterinary toxicology. *J Vet Emerg Crit Care* 2011; **21**: 309–320.
366 Yang S, Abrahams MS, Hurn PD, *et al.* Local anesthetic Schwann cell toxicity is time and concentration dependent. *Reg Anesth Pain Med* 2011; **36**: 444–451.
367 Kalichman MW. Physiologic mechanisms by which local anesthetics may cause injury to nerve and spinal cord. *Reg Anesth* 1993; **18**: 448–452.
368 Kitagawa N, Oda M, Totoki T. Possible mechanism of irreversible nerve injury caused by local anesthetics: detergent properties of local anesthetics and membrane disruption. *Anesthesiology* 2004; **100**: 962–967.
369 Selander D. Neurotoxicity of local anesthetics: animal data. *Reg Anesth* 1993; **18**: 461–468.
370 Yamashita A, Matsumoto M, Matsumoto S, *et al.* A comparison of the neurotoxic effects on the spinal cord of tetracaine, lidocaine, bupivacaine, and ropivacaine administered intrathecally in rabbits. *Anesth Analg* 2003; **97**: 512–519.
371 Zhang C, Phamonvaechavan P, Rajan A, *et al.* Concentration-dependent bupivacaine myotoxicity in rabbit extraocular muscle. *J AAPOS* 2010; **14**: 323–327.
372 Zink W, Bohl JR, Hacke N, *et al.* The long term myotoxic effects of bupivacaine and ropivacaine after continuous peripheral nerve blocks. *Anesth Analg* 2005; **101**: 548–554.
373 Nouette-Gaulain K, Sirvent P, Canal-Raffin M, *et al.* Effects of intermittent femoral nerve injections of bupivacaine, levobupivacaine, and ropivacaine on mitochondrial energy metabolism and intracellular calcium homeostasis in rat psoas muscle. *Anesthesiology* 2007; **106**: 1026–1034.
374 Zink W, Graf BM. Local anesthetic myotoxicity. *Reg Anesth Pain Med* 2004; **29**: 333–340.
375 Gomoll AH, Kang RW, Williams JM, *et al.* Chondrolysis after continuous intraarticular bupivacaine infusion: an experimental model investigating chondrotoxicity in the rabbit shoulder. *Arthroscopy* 2006; **22**: 813–819.
376 Karpie JC, Chu CR. Lidocaine exhibits dose- and time-dependent cytotoxic effects on bovine articular chondrocytes in vitro. *Am J Sports Med* 2007; **35**: 1621–1627.
377 Park J, Sutradhar BC, Hong G, *et al.* Comparison of the cytotoxic effects of bupivacaine, lidocaine, and mepivacaine in equine articular chondrocytes. *Vet Anaesth Analg* 2011; **38**: 127–133.
378 Dragoo JL, Braun HJ, Kim HJ, *et al.* The in vitro chondrotoxicity of single-dose local anesthetics. *Am J Sports Med* 2012; **40**: 794–799.
379 Hansen BP, Beck CL, Beck EP, *et al.* Postarthroscopic glenohumeral chondrolysis. *Am J Sports Med* 2007; **35**: 1628–1634.
380 Rapley JH, Beavis RC, Barber FA. Glenohumeral chondrolysis after shoulder arthroscopy associated with continuous bupivacaine infusion. *Arthroscopy* 2009; **25**: 1367–1373.
381 Piper SL, Kim HT. Comparison of ropivacaine and bupivacaine toxicity in human articular chondrocytes. *J Bone Joint Surg Am* 2008; **90**: 986–991.
382 Grishko V, Xu M, Wilson G, *et al.* Apoptosis and mitochondrial dysfunction in human chondrocytes following exposure to lidocaine, bupivacaine, and ropivacaine. *J Bone Joint Surg Am* 2010; **92**: 609–618.
383 Rehman HU. Methemoglobinemia. *West J Med* 2001; **175**: 193–196.
384 Davis JA, Greenfield RE, Brewer TG. Benzocaine-induced methemoglobinemia attributed to topical application of the anesthetic in several laboratory animal species. *Am J Vet Res* 1993; **54**: 1322–1326.
385 Guertler AT, Lagutchik MS, Martin DG. Topical anesthetic-induced methemoglobinemia in sheep: a comparison of benzocaine and lidocaine. *Fundam Appl Toxicol* 1992; **18**: 294–298.
386 Lagutchik MS, Mundie TG, Martin DG. Methemoglobinemia induced by a benzocaine- based topically administered anesthetic in eight sheep. *J Am Vet Med Assoc* 1992; **201**: 1407–1410.
387 Wilkie DA, Kirby R. Methemoglobinemia associated with dermal application of benzocaine cream in a cat. *J Am Vet Med Assoc* 1988; **192**: 85–86.
388 Harvey JW, Sameck JH, Burgard FJ. Benzocaine-induced methemoglobinemia in dogs. *J Am Vet Med Assoc* 1979; **175**: 1171–1175.
389 Poppers PJ, Mastri AR. Maternal and foetal methaemoglobinaemia caused by prilocaine. *Acta Anaesthesiol Scand Suppl* 1969; **37**: 258–263.
390 Martin DG, Watson CE, Gold MB, *et al.* Topical anesthetic-induced methemoglobinemia and sulfhemoglobinemia in macaques: a comparison of benzocaine and lidocaine. *J Appl Toxicol* 1995; **15**: 153–158.
391 Jaffey JA, Harmon MR, Villani NA, *et al.* Long-term treatment with methylene blue in a dog with hereditary methemoglobinemia caused by cytochrome b5 reductase deficiency. *J Vet Intern Med* 2017; **31**: 1860–1865.
392 Vasiliadou E, Karakitsou V, Kazakos G, *et al.* Hereditary methemoglobinemia in a cyanotic cat presented for ovariohysterectomy. *Can Vet J* 2019; **60**(5): 502–506.
393 Fidanzio F, Corsini A, Spindler KP, *et al.* Suspected drinking water poisoning in a domestic kitten with methemoglobinemia. *Vet Sci* 2021; **8**(11): 243.
394 Harvey JW, Keitt AS. Studies of the efficacy and potential hazards of methylene blue therapy in aniline-induced methaemoglobinaemia. *Br J Haematol* 1983; **54**: 29–41.
395 Welch SL. Local anesthetic toxicosis. *Vet Med* 2000; **95**: 670–673.
396 Eggleston ST, Lush LW. Understanding allergic reactions to local anesthetics. *Ann Pharmacother* 1996; **30**: 851–857.
397 Dooms-Goossens A, de Alam AG, Degreef H, *et al.* Local anesthetic intolerance due to metabisulfite. *Contact Derm* 1989; **20**: 124–126.
398 Bina B, Hersh EV, Hilario M, *et al.* True allergy to amide local anesthetics: a review and case presentation. *Anesth Prog* 2018; **65**(2): 119–123.

SECTION 4

Body Fluids and Fluid Therapy

30 Acid–Base Physiology

Peter D. Constable[1] and William W. Muir[2]
[1] College of Veterinary Medicine, University of Illinois at Urbana–Champaign, Urbana, Illinois, USA
[2] Gillespie College of Veterinary Medicine (LMU-CVM) at Lincoln Memorial University, Harrogate, Tennessee, USA

Chapter contents

Introduction, 555
Acids and bases, 556
pH, 556
pK_a and the Henderson–Hasselbalch equation, 557
Temperature effects on acid–base balance, 557
Mechanisms to minimize changes in blood pH, 558
Chemical buffers, 558
Respiratory system, 559
Renal system, 559
Approaches to evaluating acid–base balance, 559
Traditional (bicarbonate-centric) approach, 559
Base excess (buffer-centric) approach, 563
Physicochemical approach (simplified strong ion approach), 564
Anion gap and cNa^+–cCl^- difference, 565
Strong ion gap, 567
Clinical acid–base disturbances, 568
Disorders of PCO_2, 568
Disorders in strong ion difference, 569
Disorders in A_{TOT}, 571
Free-water abnormalities (combined disorders in SID and A_{TOT}), 571
Evaluations of acid–base balance, 571
References, 572

Introduction

A fundamental principle of physiology is homeostasis: the maintenance of constant conditions through dynamic equilibrium of the body's internal environment. An important component of homeostasis is the regulation of "acid–base balance," a term introduced by Henderson in 1908 [1]. Current understanding of acid–base physiology is evolving but similar to many scientific fields, the timeline for the historical development of analytical methods has greatly impacted the clinical interpretation of acid–base disorders. What once was a purely descriptive science has become far more quantitative and mechanistically based, contributing significantly to a more comprehensive understanding of the multiple factors responsible for acid–base regulation in health and disease.

Central to all schemes of acid–base balance is the understanding that metabolism of food (carbohydrates, fats, and proteins) results in the predictable production of work, heat, and waste products such as carbon dioxide (CO_2) and hydrogen ions. Indeed, normal metabolic processes are responsible for the production of thousands of millimoles of carbon dioxide (CO_2; volatile acid) and potentially hundreds of milliequivalents of nonvolatile hydrogen ions (fixed acid) daily. Individual differences in the amount of CO_2 and hydrogen ions (H^+) produced are influenced by diet, basal metabolic rate, activity, and body temperature. Animals consuming high-protein diets produce CO_2 and excess quantities of H^+ precursors, whereas animals consuming diets high in plant material produce CO_2 and excess quantities of bicarbonate ion (HCO_3^-) precursors. The CO_2 that is produced is combined with water, catalyzed by carbonic anhydrase, to form carbonic acid (H_2CO_3). The formation of carbonic acid from CO_2 and water (H_2O) (eqn 30.1) and the subsequent generation of H^+ and HCO_3^- (eqn 30.2) provide a focal point for almost all discussions of acid–base balance.

Starting in 1917, plasma hydrogen ion activity (aH^+) and CO_2 content, as well as plasma bicarbonate concentration ($cHCO_3^-$) were the only relevant acid–base quantities that could be conveniently and accurately measured in the laboratory. Henderson's studies emphasized that large quantities of CO_2 are produced by metabolizing cells and that CO_2 is in equilibrium with H^+ and HCO_3^-, such that:

$$CO_2 + H_2O \rightleftarrows H_2CO_3 \tag{30.1}$$

$$H_2CO_3 \rightleftarrows H^+ + HCO_3^- \tag{30.2}$$

Combining eqns 30.1 and 30.2 yields:

$$CO_2 + H_2O \rightleftarrows H_2CO_3 \rightleftarrows H^+ + HCO_3^- \tag{30.3}$$

It is important to emphasize that carbonic anhydrase catalyzes the interconversion of CO_2 and H_2CO_3 and that current-day technologies have advanced the science of acid–base homeostasis far beyond that available in 1917 and Henderson's introduction of the

Veterinary Anesthesia and Analgesia: The Sixth Edition of Lumb and Jones. Edited by Leigh Lamont, Kurt Grimm, Sheilah Robertson, Lydia Love and Carrie Schroeder.
© 2024 John Wiley & Sons, Inc. Published 2024 by John Wiley & Sons, Inc.
Companion website: www.wiley.com/go/lamont/anesthesia

term "acid–base balance." Regardless, the central importance of H^+ regulation to cell function and animal health cannot be overemphasized and led Hastings to state: "Tiny though it is, I suppose no constituent of living matter has so much power to influence biological behavior" [2].

Acid–base homeostasis involves the integrated normal activity of the lungs, kidney, liver, and gastrointestinal tract (Fig. 30.1). The lung removes CO_2; the kidneys remove H^+ as fixed acids (i.e., acid produced from sources other than CO_2 and not excreted by the lungs), ammonium, and non-metabolizable (fixed) strong cations such as Na^+ and K^+ and strong anions such as Cl^- and sulfate; the liver metabolizes protein; and the gastrointestinal tract regulates the absorption of water, nutrients, and minerals, and eliminates wastes. This chapter reviews the basic principles that determine acid–base balance and their integration into both descriptive and quantitative approaches to acid–base abnormalities in animals. Other more specific texts should be consulted for a more comprehensive review of the subject [3–8].

Acids and bases

pH

Most formal definitions of acids or bases when applied to biologic solutions utilize the Brønsted–Lowry concept, which classifies acids as proton donors and bases as proton acceptors. A more appropriate working definition, however, may be that acids are substances that increase H^+ ion activity (aH^+), the preferred chemical term for protons in aqueous solutions [9]. Hydrogen ion activity is preferred to the term H^+ ion concentration ($[H^+]$) for a number of reasons. First, a proton unaccompanied by an electron shell is much smaller than elements such as Na^+ or Cl^- or any molecule. The proton is therefore more appropriately viewed as a highly reactive electromotive force or free energy source in solution rather than a concentration. Second, the strength of an acid and resultant acidity of a solution are determined, in part, by its activity coefficient, a factor influenced by temperature and ionic strength that determines the degree of dissociation. The glass electrode that is used to determine pH provides a measure of the hydrogen ion activity referenced to that of standard buffers, and theoretically $[H^+]$ can be calculated by multiplying aH^+ by the activity coefficient. However, the activity coefficient for the proton in water cannot be accurately estimated and is < 1 in vertebrate fluids because the ionic strength approximates 0.15 *M* and the fluids are not infinitely dilute (ionic strength ≈ 0 *M*, the value where the activity concentration = 1). In other words, use of the term $[H^+]$ is based on an incorrect assumption that the activity coefficient is 1. Third, the concept of pH is historically based as a symbol for the "power of hydrogen" and defined as the negative value of the log to the base 10 of hydrogen ion activity, $-\log_{10}(aH^+)$. The logarithmic expression was developed to simplify the notation necessary to describe the large amounts of H^+ produced and the changes of aH^+ observed in nature and chemical experiments. This means of expression, although cumbersome mathematically, defines the nonlinear relationship between pH and aH^+ (Fig. 30.2):

$$\text{pH} = -\log_{10}\left(aH^+\right) = \log_{10}\left(1/aH^+\right) \quad (30.4)$$

Fourth, the variability in pH is much less than that of aH^+, and the distribution of aH^+ is usually skewed in vertebrate fluids. Consequently, pH is more accurately expressed as mean ± SD than aH^+. Finally, because the proton is so reactive in water, it exists fleetingly in many forms, with the hydronium ion (H_3O^+) being the predominant form. As such, use of the term "hydrogen ion concentration," which suggests a constant state over time, is misleading and inaccurate when applied to protons in water.

Because a base is defined as a H^+ (proton) acceptor, each acid dissociates into H^+ and a potential H^+ acceptor, or conjugate base. For example, H_2CO_3 in aqueous solution dissociates into H^+ and its conjugate base HCO_3^- (eqn 30.2). Substances that are strong acids

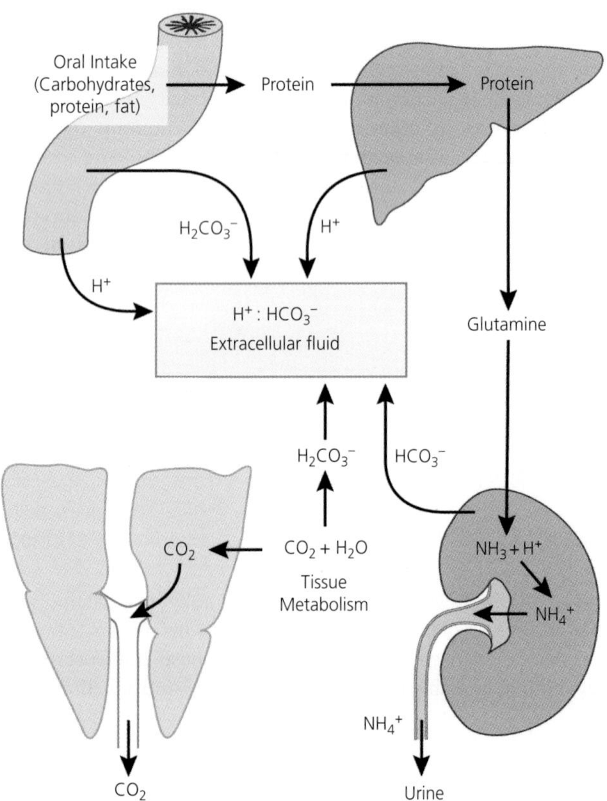

Figure 30.1 The lung, kidney, liver, and gastrointestinal tract aid in acid–base homeostasis.

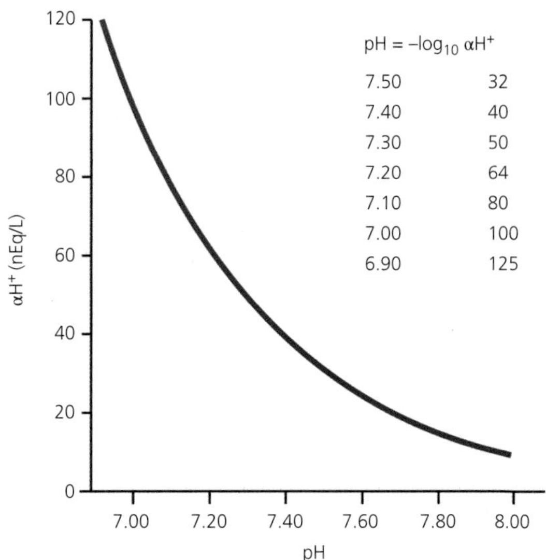

Figure 30.2 Relationship between aH^+ and pH. The relationship is curvilinear.

have weak conjugate bases and vice versa. Interestingly, water, the most abundant solvent in the body, can function as both an acid (H_3O^+; proton donor) or a base (H_2O; proton acceptor) depending on local conditions ($H_3O^+ \leftrightarrow H^+ + H_2O$). At normal pH (7.40), temperature (37–38 °C), and ionic strength (0.15 *M*), water is the most abundant base in the body.

Physiologically and clinically, the formation of acids and therefore H^+ production are emphasized in acid–base regulation because the end-products of ingestion, absorption, and metabolism, as well as that of many pathophysiologic processes, are protons or CO_2.

Regardless of conversion issues and the relatively narrow range (20–150 nEq/L) over which changes in aH^+ occur in biologic fluids, the concept of pH has persisted and is routinely reported on all pH and blood gas analyzers.

pK_a and the Henderson–Hasselbalch equation

The development of methods to measure pH in blood by Hasselbalch (1912) and CO_2 content and $cHCO_3^-$ in plasma or serum by Van Slyke (1917) led to the widespread adoption of the Henderson–Hasselbalch equation and subsequent characterization of acid–base disturbances as being either respiratory or non-respiratory (metabolic) in origin. The presence of many chemical equilibriums in blood (e.g., phosphates and sulfates) and the law of mass action produce many potential equilibrium equations that could be used to explain acid–base balance. The reasons why the carbonic acid equilibrium equation (eqn 30.3) was chosen to describe acid–base balance were (1) historical (methods were available to determine CO_2 content); (2) HCO_3^- is quantitatively the most important buffer in extracellular fluid; and (3) the carbonic acid equation includes a volatile substance (CO_2). The respiratory system in air-breathing vertebrates is an open system in that CO_2 can leave the system (body) rapidly by an increase in minute ventilation. As a consequence, the buffering ability of HCO_3^- in an open system is much greater than that in a closed system, such as a test tube that is capped. This is best appreciated by expressing eqn 30.3 in the reverse direction, such that:

$$H^+ + HCO_3^- \rightleftarrows H_2CO_3 \rightleftarrows CO_2 + H_2O \qquad (30.5)$$

Continuous removal of CO_2 by ventilation in an open system drives the reaction to the right and therefore greatly assists the rapid removal of excess protons from the body.

The law of mass action states that the rate (velocity) of a reaction is dependent on the concentration of the reactants, the dissociation constant (*K*) for the reaction, as well as the temperature and ionic strength of the solution. For mammalian fluids such as blood, plasma, and serum, changes in temperature and ionic strength are relatively small, and consequently, their effects can be ignored for clinical purposes. It is important to note that this is not the case for ectothermic ("cold-blooded" animals).

The rate of dissociation (r) for an uncharged monoprotic acid (HA) can be characterized as:

$$HA \rightarrow H^+ + A^- \qquad (30.6)$$

using the concentration of HA (*c*HA) and dissociation constant K_1,

$$r_1 = K_1 \times cHA \qquad (30.7)$$

Similarly:

$$H^+ + A^- \rightarrow HA \qquad (30.8)$$

and using the hydrogen ion activity and the concentration of A^- (cA^-):

$$r_2 = K_2 \times aH^+ \times cA^- \qquad (30.9)$$

which at equilibrium results in $r_1 = r_2$, or the following mass action equation:

$$K_2/K_1 = K_a = aH^+ \times cA^-/cHA \qquad (30.10)$$

where K_a is the dissociation constant for the uncharged monoprotic acid HA. Applying this general approach to carbonic acid, an uncharged diprotic acid (H_2CO_3) using the dissociation reaction described in eqn 30.3, Henderson derived:

$$aH^+ = K_a \times PCO_2/cHCO_3^- \qquad (30.11)$$

Henderson used the concentration of dissolved molecular CO_2 instead of H_2CO_3 because H_2CO_3 could not be measured. Hasselbalch then introduced PCO_2 into Henderson's equation and applied Sørensen's logarithmic format, producing the Henderson–Hasselbalch equation for carbonic acid, arguably the most famous equation in biology:

$$pH = pK_a + \log_{10}\left(cHCO_3^-/S \times PCO_2\right) \qquad (30.12)$$

where pH is $-\log_{10}(aH^+)$, pK_a is $= -\log_{10}(K_a)$, and *S* (0.0307 {mmol/L}/mmHg) is the solubility of CO_2 in the solution. In blood, plasma, and serum, pK_a is termed the apparent dissociation constant (pK_1') for carbonic acid, with a value at 37 °C of 6.095 when blood is analyzed and 6.105 when plasma or serum is analyzed.

The Henderson–Hasselbalch equation has been rewritten for clinical explanatory purposes as follows:

$$\begin{aligned} pH &= pK_a + \log_{10}\left([\text{base}]/[\text{acid}]\right) \\ &= pK_a + \log_{10}\left([\text{kidney function}]/[\text{lung function}]\right) \qquad (30.13) \end{aligned}$$

This equation is an oversimplification of acid–base regulation because it ignores the role of non-bicarbonate buffers such as hemoglobin, albumin, globulins, and phosphate, ignores the role of the liver in amino-acid metabolism and bicarbonate formation, and implies that the time required for renal adaptation to an acute acid–base disturbance (typically hours to days) is similar to the time required for respiratory adaptation to an acute acid–base disturbance (typically minutes). It is therefore time to retire eqn 30.13.

Temperature effects on acid–base balance

Increases or decreases in body temperature are frequently encountered in animals during anesthesia and surgery. Increases in body temperature may be caused by systemic disease, stress, increases in skeletal muscle activity (inadequate relaxation), and/or infectious and genetic disorders (malignant hyperthermia). Hypothermia is a common consequence of anesthesia and surgery and is much more profound in small animals (< 8 to 10 kg) because of their larger body surface area to body mass ratio. Decreases in body temperature are potentiated by cleaning solutions (water or alcohol), cold exposure (stainless steel tables), illness (shock), drugs that cause vasodilation (phenothiazine drugs, inhalant anesthesia), and muscle relaxants (neuromuscular blocking drugs). Changes in body temperature affect the pH of all body fluids. Decreases in body temperature increase pH and vice versa such that blood pH increases by 0.015–0.020 units for every 1 °C decrease in body temperature [10]. Changes in pH with body temperature are expected because of known temperature-induced changes on dissociation constants (pK_a) and the solubility of CO_2 in blood. For example, as body temperature decreases, the pK_a and blood solubility of CO_2 increase, producing an increase in pH and decrease in PCO_2 (Table 30.1). These temperature-dependent changes in both intracellular and extracellular pH are believed to be important in maintaining a constant relative alkalinity to that of water. This ensures constant net protein charge and structure, thereby preserving protein activity and function [11,12]. The most important dissociable group responsible for the maintenance of a constant net protein charge is the imidazole ring of histidine, in that the fractional dissociation of imidazole–histidine remains constant as temperature changes and varies with pH during isothermal conditions. This regulation of imidazole–histidine dissociation to maintain acid–base balance is termed *alpha-stat* regulation in contrast to the *pH-stat* regulation concept wherein pH values are maintained constant (Table 30.2) [12,13,14].

Both the alpha-stat and pH-stat concepts of acid–base balance have been used to interpret pH and blood gases in humans with body temperatures higher or lower than normal [14]. Proponents of the pH-stat hypothesis argue that it is important to maintain a constant pH of 7.40 and PCO_2 of 40 mmHg at any temperature, whereas proponents of the alpha-stat strategy attempt to keep a constant relative alkalinity. Proponents of the pH-stat strategy realize that if the pH and PCO_2 were kept constant at pH of 7.40 and PCO_2 of 40 mmHg during hypothermia, the animal would be acidemic, but they argue that pH-stat-oriented therapy reduces morbidity [15]. Proponents of alpha-stat-oriented therapy argue similarly and point out that blood flow to vital organs, particularly cerebral blood flow, becomes pressure-dependent (loss of autoregulation) with pH-stat management. From a practical standpoint, pH and PCO_2 do not need to be corrected for temperature unless absolute values at the animal's current temperature are required. Determining the pH and blood gases (PO_2, PCO_2) from a blood sample taken from a hypothermic animal (the temperature at which most blood gas machines are calibrated is 37 °C) enables interpretation of acid–base abnormalities for appropriate therapeutic decisions. This last statement is made with the knowledge that the pH and blood gas values obtained are correct only at 37 °C and do not represent the actual values at the animal's current body temperature (unless it is 37 °C). The clinical utility of using an alpha-stat approach is that only one reference range is needed (that obtained at 37 °C), whereas a pH-stat approach requires a reference range for every potential temperature (Table 30.2).

Table 30.1 Effect of temperature on blood PCO_2 and pH. All blood pH and gas analyzers measure blood at 37 °C (shaded) and reference ranges for blood pH and gas tensions should be obtained at a temperature of 37 °C.

Temperature (°C)	PCO_2	pH
20	19	7.65
25	24	7.58
30	30	7.50
35	37	7.43
36	38	7.41
37	40	7.40
38	42	7.39
39	44	7.37
40	45	7.36

Table 30.2 Comparison of pH-stat and alpha-stat regulation of acid–base balance.

Concept	Purpose	Total CO_2	α-Imidazole and buffering	Enzyme structure and function
pH-stat	Constant pH	Increases	Altered net protein charge, buffering decreased	Altered and activity decreased
Alpha-stat	Constant relative alkalinity	Constant	Constant net protein charge, buffering constant	Normal and activity maximal

Mechanisms to minimize changes in blood pH

Maintenance of pH within a narrow range of values is vital to normal tissue enzyme activity and cell viability. The body uses three principal mechanisms to minimize or buffer changes in blood pH. Chemical buffers act within seconds (extracellular buffers) or up to 4 h (intracellular buffers) of a pH shift and constitute the first line of defense against changes in pH. The respiratory system, via central and peripheral chemoreceptors, responds within seconds to minutes to resist changes in pH by regulating the partial pressure of CO_2 (physiologic buffering). For example, an increase in proton formation will drive the reaction in eqn 30.5 to the right and increase PCO_2 that can be eliminated from the animal by increased minute ventilation. Finally, protons produced by non-respiratory mechanisms (non-respiratory acidosis) are excreted by the kidney in the urine over a period of hours or days (Fig. 30.3).

Chemical buffers

Chemical buffers are substances that minimize changes in the pH of a solution when an acid or base is added. A buffer solution consists of a weak acid and its conjugate base and is most effective when the pH is within 1.0 to 1.5 pH units of its dissociation constant (pK_a) [16] (Table 30.3). Alterations in blood, interstitial, and intracellular fluid pH are immediately buffered (modified) by chemical buffer systems, as described by the mass action equation (eqn 30.10).

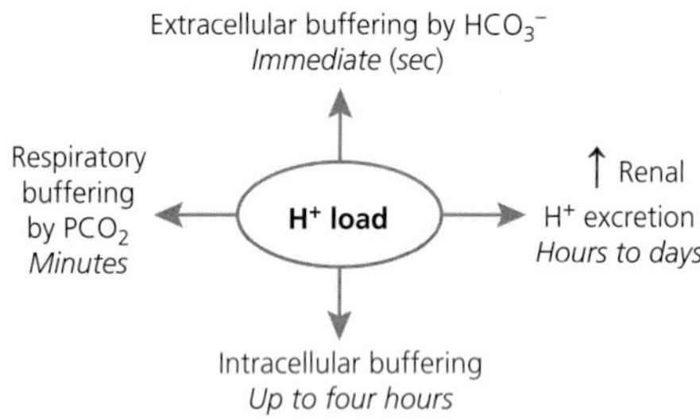

Figure 30.3 Body buffering mechanisms.

Table 30.3 pK_a values of important chemical buffers[a].

Compound	pK_a
Lactic acid	3.9
3-Hydroxybutyric acid	4.7
Creatinine	5.0
Organic phosphates	6.0–7.5
Carbonic acid (H_2CO_3)	6.1
Imidazole group of histidine (protein)	6.4–6.7
Oxygenated hemoglobin	6.7
Inorganic phosphates	6.8
α-Amino (amino terminal)	7.4–7.9
Deoxygenated hemoglobin (protein)	7.9
Ammonium (NH_4^+)	9.2
Bicarbonate (HCO_3^-)	9.8

[a] pK_a values are approximate and represent a mix of values obtained at room temperature or 37 °C. Compounds with pK_a values in the range of 6.4 to 8.4 are most useful as buffers in biological systems. The pK_a values for the imidazole group of histidine and for the α-amino (amino terminal) groups are for those side groups in proteins. The pK_a range for organic phosphates refers to such intracellular compounds as ATP, ADP, and 2,3-DPG.

For the weak acid HA, as pH decreases (aH$^+$ increases), cA$^-$ decreases, and cHA increases by equal amounts, keeping the total amount of A_{TOT} (A_{TOT} = cHA + cA$^-$) the same.

The principal chemical buffers are the bicarbonate (HCO_3^-/H_2CO_3), protein (Prot/H-Prot$^+$), and phosphate (HPO_4^{2-}/$H_2PO_4^-$) systems. In rapidly growing animals, bone can readily contribute calcium carbonate and calcium phosphate to the extracellular fluid, thereby increasing the buffering capacity. Functionally, anytime there is a decreased pH in the body, the buffer (HCO_3^-, Prot, HPO_4^{2-}) at physiologic pH accepts the excess proton, converting the buffer to its conjugate acid (H_2CO_3, H-Prot$^+$, $H_2PO_4^-$) [17]. Because the body can have only one pH in a well-mixed fluid compartment, the ratio of the acid to salt forms of the various buffer pairs in solution can always be predicted by the relevant mass action equation (isohydric principle), providing their concentration and dissociation constant (pK_a) are known [18]. In other words, with knowledge of the behavior of one buffer pair, one can predict the behavior of all the other buffer pairs in solution. As pointed out above, the HCO_3^-/H_2CO_3 buffer pair is most frequently used to determine acid–base status in clinical practice because it is the most prominent chemical buffer in the extracellular fluid and in the presence of carbonic anhydrase, carbonic acid forms CO_2, which is eliminated by alveolar ventilation. Thus, during normal conditions, the body can be considered an "open" system.

Approximately, 60% of the body's chemical buffering capacity occurs by intracellular phosphates and proteins. Inorganic and organic (ATP, ADP, and 2,3-DPG) phosphates possess pK_a values that range from 6.0 to 7.5, making them ideal chemical buffers over a wide range of potential intracellular pH values. The most important intracellular protein-dissociable group is the imidazole ring of the amino-acid histidine (pK_a 6.4–6.7). The α-amino groups of proteins (pK_a 7.4–7.9) play a secondary but important role in intracellular buffering.

Hemoglobin contributes approximately 80% of the non-bicarbonate buffering capacity of whole blood and with other intracellular proteins is responsible for three-fourths of the chemical buffering power of the body. Plasma proteins, particularly albumin, typically contain 16 histidine and 1 α-amino groups, with some species differences, and collectively are responsible for approximately 20% of the non-bicarbonate buffering capacity of whole blood.

Inorganic phosphate (pK_a 6.8) and creatinine (pK_a 5.0) are the major buffers in carnivore and omnivore urine because renal tubular pH (typically 5.5–6.5) is within 1.0 to 1.5 units of their pK_a [19].

Respiratory system

The respiratory system provides a route by which pH can be regulated by varying the partial pressure of carbon dioxide (PCO_2) in blood (Fig. 30.1). Chemoreceptors throughout the body, but particularly those located in the carotid body and medulla oblongata, monitor changes in pH and PCO_2 and adjust breathing (tidal volume and frequency) to maintain a normal pH. The association of protons with $cHCO_3^-$ and the subsequent formation of CO_2 and H_2O is an example of very rapid chemical buffering (closed system), whereas subsequent elimination of CO_2 by the lung via increased ventilation (open physiologic system) requires a longer response time (usually minutes). Changes in blood PCO_2 also have important consequences for hemoglobin's affinity for oxygen and its buffering capacity. Increases in PCO_2 decrease blood pH and decrease hemoglobin affinity for oxygen (Bohr effect: shifting the oxygen–hemoglobin curve to the right). This decrease in the oxygen affinity of hemoglobin is advantageous in tissues, allowing hemoglobin to release more oxygen for metabolism. Non-oxygenated hemoglobin in turn can transport more CO_2 in the form of hemoglobin carbamino compounds to the lungs (Haldane effect).

Renal system

The synthesis of new HCO_3^- and excretion of excess H$^+$ emphasizes the role of the kidneys in both chemical and physiologic buffering (Fig. 30.1). Although relatively slow (hours to days), compared with the lungs (minutes) and chemical buffering (seconds), the kidney serves as the principal means by which acids produced by metabolic processes (not owing to CO_2 production) are ultimately eliminated (Fig. 30.3). Protons produced by metabolic processes are excreted in the urine in combination with weak anions (titratable acidity), primarily phosphate and to a lesser extent creatinine, and in a much smaller amount as free protons [19,20].

The term "titratable acidity" may be considered synonymous with urinary phosphate concentration but actually represents the buffering effect of all weak acids in urine, including creatinine and urate. Although titratable acidity is frequently emphasized when the renal role in acid–base balance is discussed, the much more important mechanism for acid excretion during severe metabolic acidosis is urinary ammonium excretion (Fig. 30.4); however, it can take up to five days for the maximal rate of urinary ammonium excretion to be obtained [21]. Ammonium (NH_4^+) is produced in the proximal tubule primarily from glutamine metabolism to α-ketoglutarate and NH_3, a process that simultaneously generates HCO_3^- that is returned to the plasma.

Approaches to evaluating acid–base balance

Three conceptual frameworks for describing acid–base balance are currently used to describe acid–base balance (Fig. 30.5) [22,23]. In chronologic order of development, the three approaches are the traditional approach, which is bicarbonate-centric in that it utilizes the Henderson–Hasselbalch equation; the base excess approach, which is buffer-centric in that it is based on the buffering ability of hemoglobin and plasma proteins in the Van Slyke equation; and the physicochemical approach, which is based on three fundamental laws of chemistry, the law of mass action, the conservation of mass, and the requirement for electroneutrality.

Traditional (bicarbonate-centric) approach

Traditional descriptions of acid–base balance and acid–base abnormalities are based on the Brønsted–Lowry definition (proton donor) of an acid and base and the Henderson–Hasselbalch equation to determine pH. The terms "acidemia" and "alkalemia" are used to describe whether the blood pH is acid or alkaline, respectively. The terms "acidosis" and "alkalosis" are used to describe the abnormal or pathologic (-osis) state due to the accumulation or decrease of protons in the body. Importantly, the terms "acidosis" and "alkalosis" must always be preceded by the descriptor respiratory or non-respiratory (metabolic). The Henderson–Hasselbalch equation characterizes all acid–base disturbances as being either respiratory or non-respiratory because of the body's production and elimination of volatile (dissolved CO_2, H_2CO_3) and non-volatile or fixed (e.g., lactic, ketoacid, and uremic) acids, respectively.

Clinically, the terms "respiratory" and "non-respiratory" (*metabolic)* have been used to imply the respective roles of the lung and kidney in acid–base regulation. The term "non-respiratory" frequently replaces metabolic in many discussions of acid–base imbalance because it incorporates all mechanisms responsible for

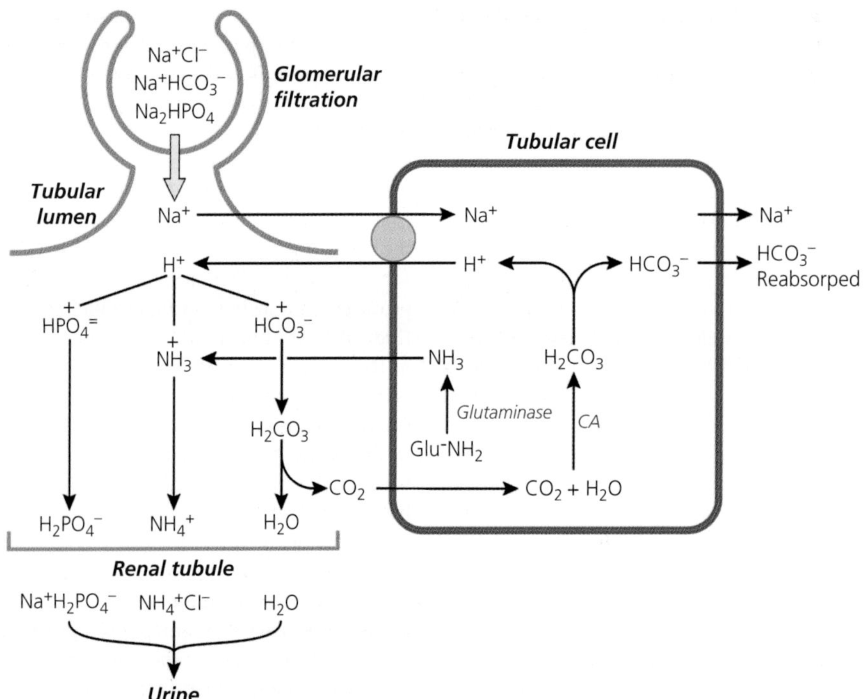

Figure 30.4 Reabsorption and regeneration of sodium bicarbonate ion (HCO_3^-) in the renal tubules. Bicarbonate reabsorption in the proximal tubule coincides with H^+ secretion. Bicarbonate regeneration in the renal tubules coincides with titration of phosphate by H^+ and ammonium formation.

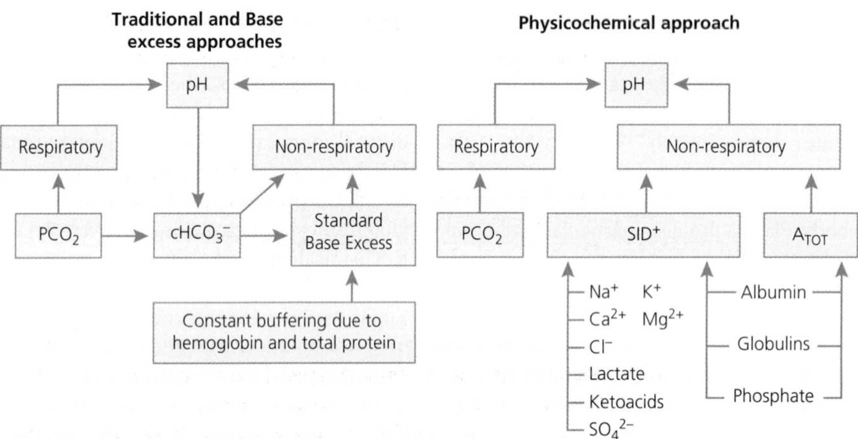

Figure 30.5 Summary of three approaches to describe an acid–base imbalance. All three approaches use the partial pressure of carbon dioxide (PCO_2, mmHg) to evaluate the respiratory component of acid–base balance. The left panel summarizes the traditional (bicarbonate-centric) and base excess (buffer-centric) approaches to evaluate the non-respiratory component of acid–base balance. The traditional approach uses plasma bicarbonate concentration ($cHCO_3^-$); however, plasma $cHCO_3^-$ does not provide an independent measure of an acid–base change because it is directly calculated from PCO_2 and pH and is therefore dependent on their values. The base excess approach uses Standard Base Excess (SBE) by assigning a fixed buffer value to extracellular fluid; however, SBE does not provide an independent measure of an acid–base change because it is calculated from PCO_2 and pH and assumes a constant buffer value for blood and extracellular fluid. The right panel summarizes the physicochemical approach to evaluating the non-respiratory component of acid–base balance. This approach uses strong ion difference (SID, mmol/L difference in charge between strong cations and anions in plasma) and the total weak acid concentration (A_{TOT}, mmol of dissociable groups/L). Source: Adapted from Constable [24].

acid–base imbalance other than the production of CO_2 and carbonic acid (H_2CO_3). Therefore, only four primary acid–base abnormalities are possible when using the traditional approach to acid–base evaluation: respiratory acidosis, non-respiratory acidosis, respiratory alkalosis, and non-respiratory alkalosis (Table 30.4; Fig. 30.6).

The traditional approach posits that primary acid–base abnormalities arise from altered PCO_2 or $cHCO_3^-$ (Fig. 30.5). A fundamental flaw with using the traditional approach and the Henderson–Hasselbalch equation is that blood $cHCO_3^-$ cannot be an independent predictor of blood pH because $cHCO_3^-$ is calculated from blood pH and PCO_2!

Table 30.4 Traditional characteristics of primary acid–base disturbances as assessed using the Henderson–Hasselbalch equation.

Disorder[a]	pH	aH^+	Primary disturbance	Compensatory response
Respiratory acidosis	↓	↑	↑ PCO_2	↑ $cHCO_3^-$
Respiratory alkalosis	↑	↓	↓ PCO_2	↓ $cHCO_3^-$
Non-respiratory acidosis	↓	↑	↓ $cHCO_3^-$	↓ PCO_2
Non-respiratory alkalosis	↑	↓	↑ $cHCO_3^-$	↑ PCO_2

[a] In this table, the descriptor non-respiratory is used in preference to the descriptor metabolic. aH^+, proton activity; $cHCO_3^-$, bicarbonate concentration in plasma or serum.

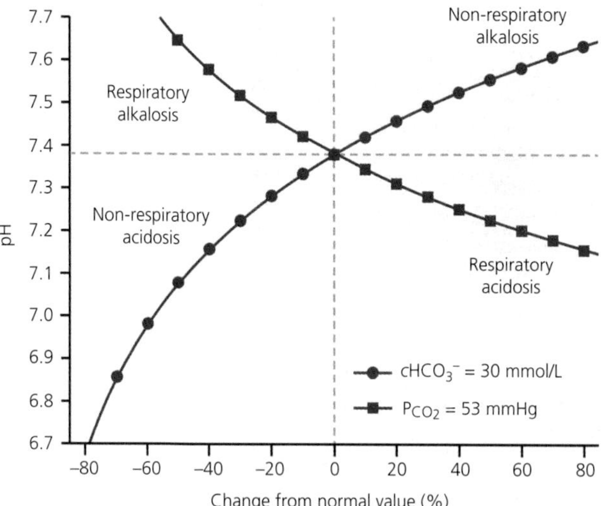

Figure 30.6 Spiderplot characterizing the curvilinear relationship between plasma pH and blood PCO_2 to evaluate the respiratory component of an acid–base disturbance in neonatal calves, and the curvilinear relationship between blood pH and plasma bicarbonate concentration ($cHCO_3^-$) to evaluate the non-respiratory component. The spider plot was obtained by systematically varying one input variable, while holding the other input variable at their normal value for calf plasma. The dashed lines indicate that pH = 7.38 when PCO_2 and $cHCO_3^-$ are at their reference mean values. The four quadrants reflect the four primary acid–base disturbances identified in Table 30.4. Source: Adapted from Constable [23].

In the traditional approach, simple acid–base abnormalities occur only when either PCO_2 or $cHCO_3^-$ are responsible for the acid–base disturbance. Mixed acid–base abnormalities are caused by disturbances in both PCO_2 or $cHCO_3^-$. Mixed acid–base abnormalities may be additive (respiratory and non-respiratory acidosis) or offsetting (respiratory alkalosis and non-respiratory acidosis) with regard to their ability to influence pH (Table 30.5) [25]. Offsetting mixed acid–base abnormalities occur when two primary acid–base abnormalities produce opposite effects on plasma pH. Animals with offsetting mixed acid–base abnormalities have both acidosis and alkalosis but do not necessarily demonstrate acidemia or alkalemia because the offsetting change might be partially (i.e., returns pH toward normal) or fully compensatory in which case blood pH will be normal. Observations that should lead to suspicions of a mixed acid–base disturbance when evaluating blood gas and pH values include [25]:

- the presence of a normal pH with abnormal PCO_2 or $cHCO_3^-$
- a pH change in a direction opposite to that predicted for the known primary disorder
- PCO_2 and $cHCO_3^-$ changing in opposite directions.

Table 30.5 Classification of mixed acid–base disorders according to the traditional bicarbonate-centric (Henderson–Hasselbalch) approach.

Classification	Effect on the pH
Mixed respiratory disorders	
Acute and chronic respiratory acidosis	Additive
Acute and chronic respiratory alkalosis	Additive
Mixed respiratory and non-respiratory disorders	
Respiratory acidosis and non-respiratory acidosis	Additive
Respiratory acidosis and non-respiratory alkalosis	Offsetting
Respiratory alkalosis and non-respiratory acidosis	Offsetting
Respiratory alkalosis and non-respiratory alkalosis	Additive
Mixed non-respiratory disorders	
Non-respiratory acidosis and non-respiratory alkalosis	Offsetting
Normal plus high anion gap non-respiratory acidosis	Additive
Mixed high anion gap non-respiratory acidosis	Additive
Mixed normal anion gap non-respiratory acidosis	Additive
Triple disorders	
Non-respiratory acidosis, non-respiratory alkalosis, and respiratory acidosis	Final pH is function of relative dominance of acidifying and alkalinizing processes
Non-respiratory acidosis, non-respiratory alkalosis, and respiratory alkalosis	Final pH is function of relative dominance of acidifying and alkalinizing processes

Mixed acid–base disorders can be classified based on the origin of the primary disturbances as mixed respiratory disturbances, mixed non-respiratory and respiratory disturbances, mixed non-respiratory disturbances, and triple disorders. They also can be classified based on their effect on an animal's pH in additive combinations, offsetting combinations, and occasionally triple disorders (Table 30.5). In additive combinations, both primary disorders tend to change pH in the same direction (e.g., respiratory acidosis and non-respiratory acidosis), whereas in offsetting combinations, the primary disorders tend to change the pH in opposite directions (e.g., respiratory alkalosis and non-respiratory acidosis). The final pH reflects the dominant of the two offsetting disorders in offsetting combinations.

Secondary or compensatory (adaptive) acid–base changes frequently occur in response to most primary acid–base abnormalities and aid in buffering or minimizing changes in plasma pH. Respiratory acid–base abnormalities, for example, are generally compensated for by controlled, oppositely directed changes in non-respiratory function (Table 30.6). In simple acid–base abnormalities such as primary respiratory acidosis caused by hypoventilation, the kidney compensates by producing non-respiratory alkalosis (Table 30.4).

Respiratory compensation for primary non-respiratory acidosis is accomplished by increasing alveolar ventilation and CO_2 excretion by the lungs. Non-respiratory acidosis is characterized by a decrease in blood $cHCO_3^-$ and pH, and a decrease in PCO_2 (respiratory alkalosis), caused by secondary hyperventilation. Non-respiratory alkalosis is characterized by an increase in blood $cHCO_3^-$ and pH, and an increase in PCO_2, owing to compensatory hypoventilation (respiratory acidosis) (Table 30.4).

In primary respiratory acid–base disorders, the compensation occurs in two phases. The first phase consists of titration of protons

Table 30.6 Compensatory responses in primary acid–base disorders as evaluated using the traditional (bicarbonate-centric) approach. Equations should be regarded as rough "rules of thumb," and species-to-species variation in equation values should be expected.

Disorder	Primary change	Expected range of compensation
Non-respiratory acidosis	↓ $cHCO_3^-$	$\Delta PCO_2 = 1 - 1.13 \times (\Delta cHCO_3^-)$ $PCO_2 = cHCO_3^- + 15$ PCO2 = 0.7 × cHCO3⁻ ± 3 (dogs)
Non-respiratory alkalosis	↑ $cHCO_3^-$	PCO_2 increases variably PCO_2 increases 0.6 mmHg for each new 1 mmol/L increase in $cHCO_3^-$ $PCO_2 = 0.7 \times cHCO_3^- \pm 3$ (dogs)
Respiratory acidosis, Acute	↑ PCO_2	$cHCO_3^-$ increases 1 mmol/L and pH decreases 0.05 units for every 10 mmHg increase in PCO_2 $cHCO_3^- = 0.15 \times PCO_2 \pm 2$ (dogs)
Respiratory acidosis, Chronic	↑ PCO_2	$cHCO_3^-$ increases 3.5 mmol/L and pH decreases 0.07 units for every 10 mmHg increase in PCO_2 $cHCO_3^- = 0.35 \times PCO_2 \pm 2$ (dogs)
Respiratory alkalosis, Acute	↓ PCO_2	$cHCO_3^-$ falls 2 mmol/L and pH increases 0.1 units for each 10 mmHg fall in PCO_2 $cHCO_3^- = 0.25 \times PCO_2 \pm 2$ (dogs)
Respiratory alkalosis, Chronic	↓ PCO_2	$cHCO_3^-$ falls 5 mmol/L and pH increases 0.15 units for each 10 mmHg fall in PCO_2 $cHCO_3^- = 0.55 \times PCO_2 \pm 2$ (dogs)

$cHCO_3^-$, bicarbonate concentration.

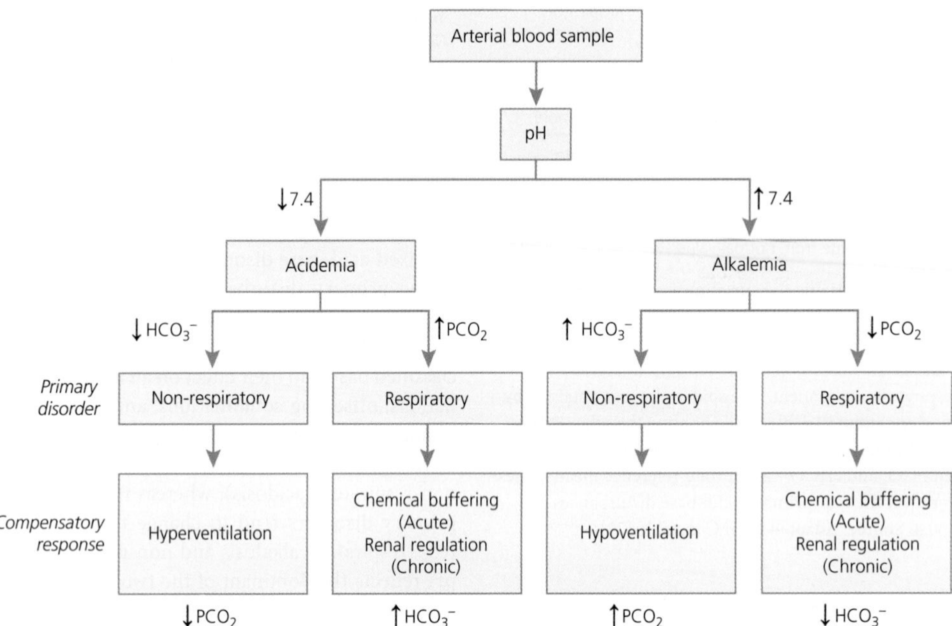

Figure 30.7 Analysis of simple acid–base disorders according to the traditional approach. An arterial blood sample is preferred for analysis when clinical abnormalities of the respiratory system are identified, or the presence of a cardiovascular anatomic shunt is suspected.

by non-bicarbonate buffers, and the second phase reflects renal compensation of the acid–base disorder, by increasing or decreasing HCO_3^- and Cl^- excretion in the urine (Fig. 30.7). Primary respiratory acidosis is characterized by increased PCO_2 due to alveolar hypoventilation, leading directly to decreased pH and an associated increase in blood $cHCO_3^-$. Renal compensation occurs by titration of non-bicarbonate buffers, an increase in net acid and Cl^- excretion by the kidneys, and increased HCO_3^- reabsorption and production by the kidneys. Primary respiratory alkalosis is characterized by decreased PCO_2 due to alveolar hyperventilation, leading directly to increased pH and a compensatory decrease in blood $cHCO_3^-$. The initial compensation in respiratory alkalosis is caused by release of H^+ from non-bicarbonate buffers within cells. The second phase is mediated by a compensatory decrease in net acid excretion by the kidneys.

When analyzing secondary changes in a given acid-base disorder, it is important to remember the following three points:

- With the exception of chronic respiratory alkalosis, compensation does not return the pH to normal. The pH almost always trends toward the primary condition.
- Overcompensation does not occur.
- Sufficient time must elapse for compensation to reach a steady state, at which time the expected compensation can be estimated (see Table 30.6).

The question that often arises when analyzing simple acid–base abnormalities that demonstrate both respiratory acidosis and non-respiratory alkalosis is, "Which is the primary problem and is there a secondary and/or compensatory event?" The answer is not always obvious, although simple primary acid–base abnormalities generally change pH in the direction of the primary disorder.

For example, an animal with respiratory acidosis and compensatory non-respiratory alkalosis would have a pH that tended to be acidemic (below the reference range; e.g., a pH of 7.31). Mixed respiratory and non-respiratory acid–base abnormalities are much more difficult to decipher, and like simple acid–base abnormalities must be carefully evaluated in the context of an animal's disease, and other available diagnostic information.

Because non-respiratory acidosis is so frequently associated with disease processes in animals, two indices of acid–base balance have been developed to enable quantitative evaluation of the non-respiratory component of an acid–base abnormality: standard bicarbonate and base excess. Standard bicarbonate was the first index to be developed, and it represents the concentration of bicarbonate in plasma after the whole-blood sample has been equilibrated to a PCO_2 of 40 mmHg at 37 °C. This index purportedly quantifies the non-respiratory component of an acid–base abnormality; however, standard bicarbonate is no longer used because it is increased in acute respiratory acidosis and initially required two additional measurements using a tonometer. Methods to estimate standard bicarbonate using a nomogram or calculate standard bicarbonate from other acid–base values have been developed. These methods have the advantage that tonometry is not required; however, nomograms are cumbersome and slow to use, and the equation is based on the calculated value for base excess. Consequently, base excess has become widely used to evaluate the non-respiratory component of an acid–base abnormality.

Base excess (buffer-centric) approach

Buffering and buffer values are foundational concepts when acid–base balance is interpreted using the base excess approach, and consequently, the approach is best described as buffer-centric or buffer-centered. The base excess of blood (BE_b) quantitates the mmols of strong acid (such as HCl) or strong base (such as NaOH) required to titrate 1 L of blood to pH 7.40 at 37 °C while the PCO_2 is held constant at 40 mmHg. BE_b from healthy humans is defined as 0 mmol/L with a reference range of −2.3 to +2.3 mmol/L. A positive BE_b value indicates base excess (non-respiratory alkalosis), whereas a negative BE_b value indicates a base deficit (non-respiratory acidosis) [4].

Values for BE_b were initially read from a graphical calculating device called a "nomogram," which is a two-dimensional diagram that provides an approximate graphical computation of a relationship between two or more entities. Since 1977, BE_b has been calculated using the Van Slyke equation [26], and the nomogram is no longer used to provide the value for BE_b. The Van Slyke equation takes the following general form for human arterial (oxygenated) blood when temperature = 37 °C, pH = 7.40, and PCO_2 = 40 mmHg, with Z providing an adjustment for the effect of changes in hematocrit assuming a fixed value for the mean hemoglobin concentration in erythrocytes [27], such that:

$$BE_b = \{\Delta cHCO_3^- + \beta \times (pH - 7.40)\} \times (1 - Z) \quad (30.14)$$

In eqn 30.14, $\Delta cHCO_3^-$ is the difference between the actual $cHCO_3^-$ and the reference value at blood pH = 7.40 and PCO_2 = 40 mmHg, β is the overall buffer value for blood (an index of buffering ability that is determined primarily by the blood hemoglobin concentration) and pH is the measured pH.

Valid initial criticisms of the base excess approach were that BE_b did not reflect the *in vivo* changes observed during CO_2 titration in humans and dogs [28,29] because the calculated value for BE_b was obtained from *in vitro* studies. This criticism was empirically addressed by assuming a substantial amount of *in vivo* acid–base buffering was occurring in the extracellular fluid volume. Assuming an approximate ratio of 1 part blood volume to 2 parts interstitial fluid volume in adult mammals, a hemoglobin concentration of 5 g/dL (one-third the typical value for human blood of 15 g/dL) has been generally accepted to provide a clinically useful model for the *in vivo* buffer response to an acid–base disturbance (Fig. 30.5). The value for Standard Base Excess (SBE) in mmol/L, also called "extracellular base excess" (BE_{ecf}), is calculated using a hemoglobin concentration of 5 g/dL in eqn 30.14, providing the following equation [30]:

$$SBE = BE_{ecf} = (cHCO_3^- - 24.8) + 16.2 \times (pH - 7.40) \quad (30.15)$$

Equation 30.15 uses reference values for $cHCO_3^-$ of 24.8 mmol/L and pH of 7.40, based on a reference value for PCO_2 of 40 mmHg and *S* of 0.0307 {mmol/L}/mmHg [30]. Equation 30.15 also assumes that the value for Z in eqn 30.14 = 0.

All modern automated blood gas analyzers report BE_b and SBE values calculated from the buffering characteristics of human blood. The difference between BE_b and SBE is small, and only one of the two base excess values should be used clinically and reported in clinical studies, with the preference being SBE because it more closely reflects the *in vivo* response to an acid–base disturbance. The buffering characteristics of dog blood and bovine blood are different from that of human blood, whereas the buffering characteristics of equine blood appear to be similar to that of human blood. Cattle [31], dog [32], and pig [33,34] base excess nomograms have been developed that differ from that of human blood; however, these nomograms are rarely used because commercial blood gas analyzers are programmed specifically for human blood. The routine use of human values for BE_b and SBE equations is suspected to create minimal error for clinical use in domestic animals, although the error may be more important in research studies [22,23,32].

Bicarbonate distribution space

Clinically, a negative value for SBE represents a base deficit (non-respiratory acidosis) that is most accurately corrected by intravenous administration of sodium bicarbonate. The amount of sodium bicarbonate required (the value for SBE in mmol/L) has traditionally been multiplied by the apparent distribution space of bicarbonate in L (equivalent to 0.3 × body weight (kg) in adult mammals [35] and 0.4 × body weight (kg) in neonatal mammals), reflecting the extracellular fluid volume in healthy animals, such that:

$$\text{Base}\left(Na^+HCO_3^-\right)\text{needed} = SBE \times (0.3 \times \text{body weight in kg}) \quad (30.16)$$

A positive value for SBE represents a base excess (non-respiratory alkalosis) that is usually best corrected by intravenous administration of isotonic saline (0.9 % NaCl), such that:

$$\text{Acid}\left(Na^+Cl^-\right)\text{needed} = SBE \times (0.3 \times \text{body weight in kg}) \quad (30.17)$$

It should be noted that equations 30.16 and 30.17 use the 100-year-old acid–base terms of Van Slyke *et al.* that predates the current Brønsted–Lowry definition of acid (proton donor) and base (proton acceptor), in that a base is a non-metabolizable cation such as sodium and an acid is a non-metabolizable anion such as chloride.

It should also be noted that the distribution space for intravenously administered bicarbonate, called the "apparent bicarbonate space" (ABS; units of L per kg body weight) in eqn 30.16 and 30.17, uses a 1960 estimate derived from rapid intravenous administration of 5% sodium bicarbonate solution over 10 min in nine adult humans with blood pH and standard bicarbonate concentrations within the reference range [35]. This study suggested that the typical extracellular fluid volume was 30% of body weight [35]. Studies in humans, dogs, and calves have subsequently demonstrated that the ABS is not a fixed value (such as the typical extracellular fluid volume) but is dependent on the initial plasma $cHCO_3^-$.

A recent study [36] in critically ill neonatal calves with marked acidemia (median pH, 7.00; range, 6.58 to 7.26) and varying degrees of non-respiratory (metabolic) acidosis demonstrated that the ABS was nonlinearly related to jugular venous $cHCO_3^-$ and negatively related to jugular venous PCO_2 (Fig. 30.8). The negative linear relationship between ABS and PCO_2 was consistent with eqn 30.5, in that administered intravenously administered bicarbonate buffers excess protons, resulting in excretion of CO_2.

The two equations can be simplified for clinical application in neonatal animals, such that:

$$\text{ABS} = 0.4 + 1/c\text{HCO}_3^- \quad (30.18)$$

$$\text{ABS} = 0.85 - 0.008 \times \text{PCO}_2 \quad (30.19)$$

For neonates, we, therefore, suggest the amount (mmol) of bicarbonate needed to correct the non-respiratory acid–base abnormality be calculated from SBE and $cHCO_3^-$ in mmol/L as follows:

$$\text{mmol HCO}_3^- \text{ needed} = \text{SBE} \times \left(0.4 + 1/c\text{HCO}_3^-\right) \times \left(\text{body weight in kg}\right) \quad (30.20)$$

It remains to be determined whether these new equations also apply to adult animals where the typical extracellular fluid volume in L is 0.3 × body weight in kg [35] instead of 0.4 × body weight in kg [36]. Until such studies are completed, we suggest the following equation should be used in adult animals:

$$\text{mmol HCO}_3^- \text{ needed} = \text{SBE} \times \left(0.3 + 1/c\text{HCO}_3^-\right) \times \left(\text{body weight in kg}\right) \quad (30.21)$$

Physicochemical approach (simplified strong ion approach)

A physicochemical description of acid–base balance was first introduced by Henderson in 1928 [3], formalized by Singer and Hastings in 1948 [37], expanded to include plasma buffers by Stewart in 1981 [5,38], and simplified by Constable in 1997 [16,39]. The physicochemical approach is based on a fundamental assumption that quantitatively important chemical reactions in plasma are those of simple ions in solution. This assumption can be made because the quantitatively important cations (Na^+, K^+, Ca^{2+}, and Mg^{2+}) and anions (Cl^-, HCO_3^-, Protein$^-$, L-lactate$^-$, and sulfate^{2-}) in plasma bind each other in a salt-type manner at physiologic pH [16,38,40].

Strong ions are electrically charged substances that are completely dissociated in plasma at body pH and therefore exert no buffering effect. The most important strong cations in plasma are Na^+, K^+, Ca^{2+}, and Mg^{2+}, and the most important strong anions in plasma are Cl^-, lactate, β-hydroxybutyrate, acetoacetate, and sulfate [16]. The sum of the strong cation charge in plasma exceeds that of the strong anion charge, and Stewart termed this difference the "strong ion difference" (SID), which can be regarded as a collective unit of positive charge with a net cation charge of +1 per mmol [5,38]. An increase in SID correlates with non-respiratory alkalosis, whereas a decrease in SID correlates with non-respiratory acidosis.

The physicochemical approach is based on three fundamental laws of chemistry [5,16,38]:

- Electroneutrality must be maintained, in that the sum of all positively charged ions in solution must equal the sum of all negatively charged ions
- The mass action law. Bicarbonate and a lumped group of non-bicarbonate buffers are only partially dissociated at physiologic pH, being described by an apparent dissociation constant for carbonic acid in plasma (K_1'), and a lumped dissociation constant (K_a) for non-bicarbonate buffers with the anionic dissociated form (A^-) having a concentration cA^-, and the undissociated form (HA) having a concentration cHA
- Conservation of mass for a lumped group of non-bicarbonate buffers with total concentration of A_{TOT}, such that $A_{TOT} = cHA + cA^-$

Stewart developed a polynomial equation in 1981 based on the three fundamental laws that indicated pH was dependent on eight variables [5]. Constable demonstrated in 1997 that two of Stewart's

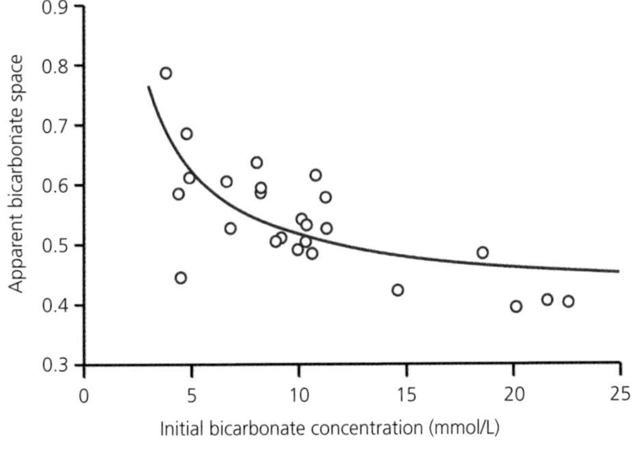

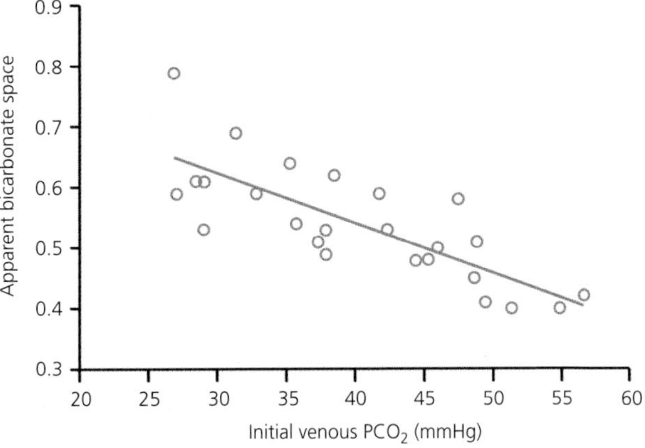

Figure 30.8 Relationship between the calculated apparent bicarbonate space (L/kg body weight) and the initial jugular venous bicarbonate concentration (left panel) and jugular venous carbon dioxide tension (PCO_2) in 25 neonatal calves with diarrhea, acidemia, and non-respiratory acidosis. Calves received a hypertonic sodium bicarbonate and glucose solution that was administered over a period of 1 h. Values for apparent bicarbonate space were determined at the end of the infusion. Lines represent the results of nonlinear regression analysis. Source: Figures Adapted from Trefz *et al.* [36].

eight variables were redundant, resulting in development of the simplified strong ion equation [16] that contained six variables, such that:

$$\mathrm{pH} = \log_{10}\left(2\times \mathrm{SID}\Big/\left[\begin{array}{l} K_1'\times S\times \mathrm{PCO_2} + K_a \times \mathrm{A_{TOT}} - K_a\times \mathrm{SID} \\ +\sqrt{\left\{\begin{array}{l}\left(K_1'\times S\times \mathrm{PCO_2} + K_a\times \mathrm{SID} + K_a\times \mathrm{A_{TOT}}\right)^2 \\ -4K_a^{\,2}\times \mathrm{SID}\times \mathrm{A_{TOT}}\end{array}\right\}}\end{array}\right]\right) \tag{30.22}$$

Equation 30.22 was termed the "Constable equation" in 2008 [41]; the equation indicates that plasma pH is dependent on three independent variables, the plasma carbon dioxide tension (PCO_2), the difference in charge at physiologic pH assigned to strong cations and strong anions in plasma (SID), and A_{TOT} (Fig. 30.5) as well as three constants, K_a, S (the solubility of CO_2 in plasma) and K_1'.

An algebraically simpler, but equivalent equation to eqn 30.22 where $pK_a = -\log_{10}(K_a)$ and $pK_1' = -\log_{10}(K_1')$ is the following expression [16]:

$$\mathrm{pH} = pK_1' + \log_{10}\left(\left\{\mathrm{SID} - \mathrm{A_{TOT}}\Big/\left(1+10^{(pKa-\mathrm{pH})}\right)\right\}\Big/S\times \mathrm{PCO_2}\right) \tag{30.23}$$

It is important to note that in solutions that do not contain a non-bicarbonate buffer, eqn 30.23 simplifies to the Henderson–Hasselbalch equation because A_{TOT} = 0 mmol/L and SID = $cHCO_3^-$ [16]. Equation 30.22 similarly simplifies to the Henderson–Hasselbalch equation in solutions where A_{TOT} = 0 mmol/L.

Although the Constable equation provides a mechanistic physicochemical description of acid–base balance, application of the equation to vertebrate plasma requires accurate estimates for A_{TOT}, K_a, and SID to be physiologically and clinically useful [16,22,23]. Stewart assigned different values for A_{TOT} and K_a and did not provide a method for their experimental determination. Constable developed a method applying nonlinear regression to paired pH-PCO_2 data values obtained by CO_2 tonometry of plasma to experimentally determine values for A_{TOT} and K_a and permit calculation of more accurate estimates for SID [16]. Mean SID and A_{TOT} values for selected animals have been experimentally determined (Table 30.7), with the K_a value approximating that of the imidazole dissociable group in histidine.

Blood PCO_2 provides an independent measure of the respiratory component of plasma pH. SID and A_{TOT} provide independent measures of the non-respiratory component of plasma pH. Therefore, when using the strong ion approach for acid–base analysis, there are two respiratory acid–base disorders and four primary non-respiratory (metabolic) acid–base disorders (Fig. 30.5). Non-respiratory acidosis is further defined by being either decreased SID or increased A_{TOT}, whereas non-respiratory alkalosis is characterized by either increased SID or decreased A_{TOT} relative to reference mean values (Fig. 30.9; Table 30.8).

Table 30.7 Comparative experimentally determined mean values for pH, PCO_2, SID, and A_{TOT} of venous blood at 37 °C in selected domestic animals.

Animal	pH	PCO_2 (mmHg)	SID (mmol/L)	A_{TOT} (mmol/L)	Reference
Horse	7.43	44	40	14.0	[16]
Horse	7.42	47	43	14.9	[42]
Human	7.37	45	37	17.2	[43]
Cat	7.35	30	30	24.3	[44]
Cattle	7.43	43	44	22.9	[45]
Calf	7.38	53	42	18.5	[46]
Dog	7.40	37	27	17.4	[47]
Pigeon	7.43	41	34	7.8	[48]

These mechanisms include alterations in the concentrations of strong (fully dissociated) ions as assessed by the anion gap and SID and the concentration of non-bicarbonate plasma buffers (primarily serum proteins; A_{TOT}) (Fig. 30.5). Note that non-respiratory (metabolic) acid–base disturbances can be brought about by changes in the concentration of strong ions or weak ions. These ions can be routinely measured (e.g., Cl^-) or not (e.g., lactate and ketoacids). Those that are not routinely measured are referred to as "unmeasured ions."

In summary, the physicochemical approach posits that acid–base disorders are caused by changes in three independent factors (PCO_2, SID, and A_{TOT}) that can change independently to each other, with the change directly and predictably resulting in changes in pH. It should be noted, however, that changes in temperature can affect all the independent variables, a consideration that has special importance during surgery and anesthesia, especially in ectothermic animals [6,13].

Anion gap and cNa^+–cCl^- difference

The anion gap (AG), like SID, is calculated on the basis of the principle of electroneutrality and is used clinically to estimate the concentration of unmeasured anions in plasma or serum (Fig. 30.10). The AG is a useful tool to assess mixed acid–base disorders [49–51] particularly when using the traditional or base excess approach. Chemically, there is no AG because electroneutrality must be maintained at all times and the "AG" is the difference between the concentration of unmeasured anions (cUA^-) and unmeasured cations (cUC^+). The AG is calculated using four quantitatively important cations and anions that are routinely measured and change appreciably in their concentrations in a variety of clinical conditions. The two cations measured are the plasma or serum

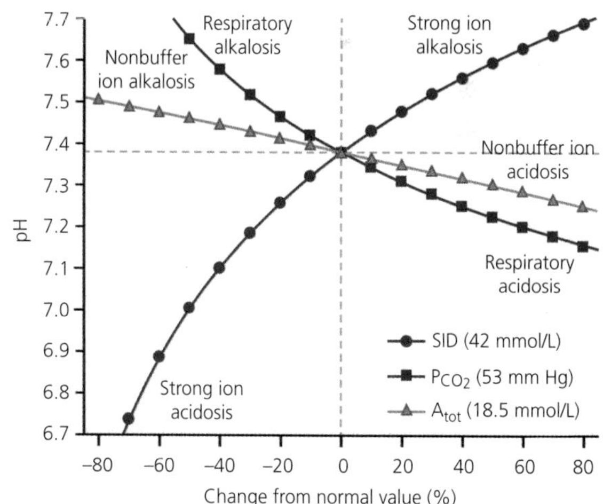

Figure 30.9 Spiderplot characterizing the curvilinear relationship between plasma pH and blood PCO_2 to evaluate the respiratory component of an acid–base disturbance, the curvilinear relationship between blood pH and plasma strong ion difference (SID) to evaluate the SID component, and the linear relationship between blood pH and A_{TOT} to evaluate the buffer ion component. The spider plot was obtained by systematically varying one input variable, while holding the other input variables at their normal values for calf plasma. The dashed lines indicate that pH = 7.38 when PCO_2, SID, and A_{TOT} are at their reference mean values. The four quadrants identify the six primary acid–base disturbances identified by the physicochemical approach. Source: Adapted from Constable [23].

Table 30.8 Causes of non-respiratory (metabolic) acid–base abnormalities classified according to the physicochemical approach.

SID acidosis (↓ SID)	SID alkalosis (↑ SID)
Hyperchloremic acidosis (↑ Cl^-_{corr})	**Hypochloremic alkalosis (↓ Cl^-_{corr})**
Loss of Na^+ relative to Cl^-	Gain of Na^+ relative to Cl^-
Diarrhea	Isotonic or hypertonic $NaHCO_3$ administration
Gain of Cl^- relative to Na^+	Loss of Cl^- relative to Na^+
Fluid therapy (0.9% NaCl, 7.2% NaCl, KCl-supplemented fluids)	Vomiting of stomach contents
Retention of Cl^- relative to Na^+	Thiazide or loop diuretics
Renal failure	**Concentration alkalosis (↑ Na^+)**
Hypoadrenocorticism	Pure water loss
Organic acidosis (↑ unmeasured strong anions)	Water deprivation
Uremic, keto- or lactic acidosis	Diabetes insipidus
Toxicities	Hypotonic fluid loss
Ethylene glycol	Vomiting
Salicylate	Non-oliguric renal failure
Dilution acidosis (↓ Na^+)	Postobstructive diuresis
With hypervolemia	
Severe liver disease	
Congestive heart failure	
Nephrotic syndrome	
With normovolemia	
Psychogenic polydipsia	
Hypotonic fluid infusion	
With hypovolemia	
Vomiting	
Diarrhea	
Hypoadrenocorticism	
Third space loss	
Diuretic administration	
A_{TOT} acidosis (↑ A_{TOT})	**A_{TOT} alkalosis (↓ A_{TOT})**
Hyperalbuminemia	**Hypoalbuminemia**
Water deprivation	Decreased production
Hyperphosphatemia	Chronic liver disease
Translocation	Acute phase response to inflammation
Tumor cell lysis	Malnutrition/starvation
Tissue trauma/rhabdomyolysis	Extracorporeal loss
Increased intake	Protein-losing nephropathy
Phosphate-containing enemas	Protein-losing enteropathy
Intravenous phosphate	Sequestration
Decreased loss	Inflammatory effusions
Renal failure	Vasculitis
Urethral obstruction	
Uroabdomen	

Source: Modified from Constable [39].

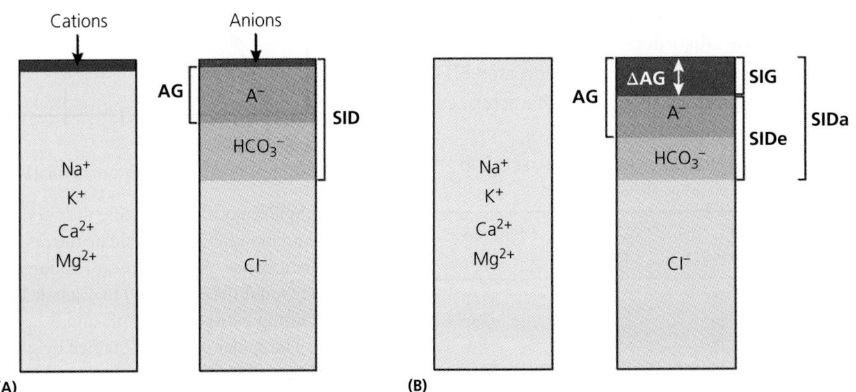

Figure 30.10 **A.** Cation and anion equivalency diagrams can be used to illustrate the relationship among the anion gap (AG), strong ion difference (SID), and strong ion gap (SIG). **B.** Cation and anion equivalency diagrams can also be used to illustrate the difference between an abnormal and baseline AG (ΔAG). The ΔAG is quantitatively similar to the strong ion gap (SIG) or difference between the SID apparent (SIDa) and SID effective (SIDe): SIG = SIDa–SIDe.

concentrations of sodium (cNa^+) and potassium (cK^+). The two anions measured are the plasma or serum concentrations of chloride (cCl^-) and bicarbonate ($cHCO_3^-$). The law of electroneutrality requires the following:

$$cNa^+ + cK^+ + cUC^+ = cCl^- + cHCO_3^- + cUA^- \quad (30.24)$$

or, when applied clinically:

$$AG = cUC^+ - cUA^- = \left(cNa^+ + cK^+\right) - \left(cCl^- + cHCO_3^-\right) \quad (30.25)$$

Based on eqn 30.24, every time there is a decrease in $cHCO_3^-$, either cCl^- or cUA^- must be increased to maintain electroneutrality. When titrated HCO_3^- is replaced by Cl^- in non-respiratory acidosis, the difference (cUA^- - cUC^+; and consequently, the AG) will remain the same (called "hyperchloremic" or "normal AG acidosis"). When titrated HCO_3^- is replaced by UA^-, the difference (cUA^- - cUC^+; i.e., the AG) will increase while cCl^- remains the same (called "normochloremic" or "high AG acidosis") [52,53]. Negatively charged proteins, phosphates, sulfates, and organic acids (e.g., L-lactate, β-hydroxybutyrate, acetoacetate, and uremic anions) constitute the UA^- [51,54,55].

An increase in AG clinically implies an accumulation of organic acids in the body [50], and assuming no laboratory error, a large increase in AG is always due to a large increase in the concentration of unmeasured strong anions in plasma. However, a mild increase in AG also occurs by an increase in the net negative charge on serum proteins due to hyperproteinemia [52]. Hypoalbuminemia is the most common cause of a decrease in AG, and each decrease in albumin concentration of 1 g/dL produces a decrease of approximately 2.5–3.0 mmol/L in the AG. A patient with concurrent lactic acidosis and hypoalbuminemia may therefore have a normal AG. Thus, AG alone can be clinically misleading in elucidating some complex mixed acid–base disorders. It should be noted that the AG can increase because of excessive exposure of serum to air, resulting in a decrease in $cHCO_3^-$ and increase in AG of 6.5 ± 2.3 mmol/L after 2 h [56].

Similar to AG, the cNa^+–cCl^- difference (average value in health animals approximates 36 mmol/L) is potentially useful for initial assessment of those non-respiratory acid–base disturbances not associated with an increase in unmeasured anions (Table 30.9) [57,58]. If cNa^+ is normal, hypochloremia increases its value and is an indication of metabolic alkalosis, whereas hyperchloremia decreases the cNa^+–cCl^- difference and is an indication of hyperchloremic acidosis [8]. In addition, the chloride to sodium (cCl^-:cNa^+) ratio (normal range 0.75–0.79) serves as a simple method to quantify the role of hyperchloremia in acid–base disturbances. An increased cCl^-:cNa^+ ratio (> 0.79) has an acidifying effect, and a decreased ratio (< 0.75) has an alkalinizing effect. Animals with metabolic acidosis and an increased cCl^-:cNa^+ generally have hyperchloremia as the cause of acidosis. A normal cCl^-:cNa^+ and metabolic acidosis indicate a mixed acidosis. The cNa^+–cCl^- and cCl^-:cNa^+ can be used in conjunction with the AG to identify disorders in hydration and acid–base balance (Box 30.1).

Strong ion gap

The strong ion gap (SIG) represents the concentration of unmeasured strong ions in plasma. The SIG, similar to AG, is based on the requirement for electroneutrality, but differs from the AG in that it has a value approximating 0 mmol/L in healthy subjects (Fig. 30.10). A positive value for SIG is very rare and usually indicates the presence of laboratory error. A negative value for SIG quantifies the concentration of unmeasured strong anions in plasma. Confusion

Box 30.1 Relative changes in cNa^+_0 and cCl^-_0 as an index of disorders in hydration or acid–base balance or both.

a Proportionate change in cNa^+_0 and cCl^-_0 are always due to the disturbances of hydration alone.
- Dehydration
  - cNa^+_0 ↑ and cCl_0 ↑
- Overhydration
  - cNa^+_0 ↓ and cCl_0 ↓

b Changes in cCl^-_0 without any change in cNa^+_0 are always due to disturbances of acid-base alone.
- Respiratory acidosis or non-respiratory alkalosis
  - cNa^+_0 and cCl^-_0 ↓
- Respiratory alkalosis or hyperchloremic acidosis
  - cNa^+_0 and cCl_0 ↑

c Disproportionate changes in cNa^+_0 and cCl^-_0 are due to disturbances in both hydration and acid–base balance.
- Dehydration plus respiratory acidosis or non-respiratory alkalosis
  - cNa^+_0 ↑ and cCl^-_0
- Dehydration plus respiratory alkalosis or non-respiratory acidosis
  - cNa^+_0 ↑ and cCl^-_0 ↑↑
- Overhydration plus respiratory alkalosis or hyperchloremic acidosis
  - cNa^-_0 ↓ and cCl^-_0
- Overhydration plus respiratory acidosis or non-respiratory alkalosis
  - cNa^+_0 ↓ and cCl^- ↓↓

Source: Adapted from Emmett and Seldin [57].

Table 30.9 Primary non-respiratory acid–base disorders and respiratory compensation.

Non-respiratory disorder	cNa^+–cCl^-	AG	TCO_2	Respiratory compensation	Biochemical profile
Alkalosis					
Hypoalbuminemia	N	N,↓	↑	No	↓ cAlbumin
Hypochloremia	↑	N	↑	No	↓ $cCl^-_{corrected}$
Concentration	↑	N	↑	Yes	↑ cNa^+
Acidosis					
Hyperalbuminemia	N	N,↑	↓	No	↑ cAlbumin
Hyperphosphatemia	N	N,↑	↓	No	↑ cInorganic phosphate
Hyperchloremia	↓	N	↓	Yes	↑ $cCl^-_{corrected}$
Dilution	↓	N	↓	Yes	↓ cNa^+
Organic	N	↓	↓	Yes	Specific assays required

cNa^+ – cCl^-, difference between sodium and chloride concentration; AG, anion gap; TCO_2, total CO_2; ↑, increase; N, normal; and ↓, decrease. See the text for limitations in using cNa^+–cCl^- difference and AG; $cCl^-_{corrected}$, see eqn 30.30. Source: Adapted from de Morais and Muir [58].

exists in the way SIG is calculated in that there are two SIGs; the first equation was developed by Kellum *et al.* in 1995 [59] that is a direct extension of the AG concept, and the second equation was developed by Constable *et al.* in 1998 [54] that is a direct extension of the physicochemical approach to acid–base balance.

Kellum *et al.* defined the SIG as the difference between the apparent strong ion difference (SIDa) and the effective strong ion difference (SIDe). The value for SIDa is the difference between measured strong cation charge and strong anion charge in plasma. Equations for SIDa vary, depending on the availability, cost, and clinical value of measuring quantitatively important strong cations and strong anions, but a commonly used equation is:

$$\text{SIDa} = \left(c\text{Na}^+ + c\text{K}^+ + c\text{Ca}^{2+} + c\text{Mg}^{2+}\right) - \left(c\text{Cl}^- + c\text{L-lactate}^-\right) \quad (30.26)$$

where $c\text{Ca}^{2+}$ + $c\text{Mg}^{2+}$ represent the charge assigned to these divalent ions in mEq/L. The value for SIDe is calculated from the three quantitatively important buffer anions in human plasma (bicarbonate, albumin, and phosphate), with bicarbonate (in mmol/L) being calculated using the Henderson–Hasselbalch equation and albumin (in g/L) and phosphate (in mmol/L) being calculated using linear pH equations developed by Figge *et al.* [60] for human plasma, such that:

$$\begin{aligned}\text{SIDe} = {} & c\text{HCO}_3^- + c\text{Albumin}^- \times (0.123 \times \text{pH} - 0.631) \\ & + c\text{Phosphate}^- \times (0.309 \times \text{pH} - 0.469)\end{aligned} \quad (30.27)$$

The SIG is then calculated as the difference between SIDa and SIDe, such that:

$$\text{SIG} = \text{SIDa} - \text{SIDe} \quad (30.28)$$

Constable *et al.* developed a different SIG equation by algebraic rearrangement of the simplified strong ion equation in terms of other factors [54], such that:

$$\text{SIG} = \text{A}_{\text{TOT}} / \left(1 + 10^{\text{p}K_a - \text{pH}}\right) - \text{AG} \quad (30.29)$$

Equation 30.29 provides a simpler method for calculating SIG than that provided by eqns 30.26 and 30.27 and is theoretically more accurate for species other than humans, in that species-specific values for A_{TOT} and p*K*a are used (Table 30.7).

Very few studies have formally compared the predictive ability of the two methods for calculating SIG; however, the predictive ability of eqn 30.29 in critically ill cattle with abomasal volvulus was greater than that of eqn 30.28 [54], and the predictive ability of both methods for calculating SIG was greater than that for AG [54].

An alternative method for quantifying unmeasured strong anions in plasma, called the "Fencl method," was introduced in 1993 [61]. The Fencl method attempts to take into account the effect that changes in sodium, chloride, and plasma protein concentrations exert on plasma pH. Although the method has been applied to a variety of domestic animals [45,62–65], Fencl's method has been formally evaluated in the pig where it was found to be "a biased and imprecise predictor of unmeasured strong ion concentration" [62], and in cattle where it had reduced explanatory power relative to SIG calculated using eqn 30.29 [45]. In summary, Fencl's method is considered "too imprecise for use in species other than humans" [54]. Accordingly, Fencl's method is currently not recommended for evaluating acid–base imbalances in domestic animals.

Clinical acid–base disturbances

Acid–base disturbances occur when an abnormality in one of the principal independent determinants of pH (e.g., PCO_2, SID, or A_{TOT}) occurs (Figs. 30.5, 30.9; Table 30.8). So-called "simple" acid–base disturbances include both the primary process and the compensatory response. That is, if a sustained primary disturbance occurs in PCO_2, a compensatory change of regulated magnitude normally occurs in the SID and vice versa. If the primary disturbance results from a change in A_{TOT}, however, ventilatory compensation does not occur but renal excretion of chloride is altered. Therapeutic success or failure depends on interventions that adjust the independent variables [16,66,67].

Disorders of PCO_2

Primary respiratory disturbances result from increases in PCO_2 (respiratory acidosis) or decreases in PCO_2 (respiratory alkalosis). CO_2 tension can be changed by alveolar ventilation, which has a profound effect on pH, and combined evaluation of pH and PCO_2 can be used to make descriptive decisions regarding the primary process for the observed acid–base abnormality (Table 30.10). Because PaCO_2 is inversely related to alveolar ventilation, measurement of PaCO_2 provides direct information about the adequacy of alveolar ventilation. Respiratory acidosis is therefore caused by and synonymous with hypoventilation, whereas respiratory alkalosis is caused by and synonymous with hyperventilation.

Principal disorders associated with respiratory acidosis are airway obstruction, respiratory center depression (e.g., drugs or neurologic disorders), cardiopulmonary arrest (PaCO_2 may be below normal during cardiopulmonary resuscitation), neuromuscular diseases, diaphragmatic hernia, chest wall trauma, and inadequate mechanical ventilation. Therapy for respiratory acidosis should be directed toward elimination of the underlying cause of alveolar hypoventilation. Ventilatory assistance should be provided when necessary. It is clinically important to note that respiratory acidosis is not an indication for bicarbonate therapy. Administration of sodium bicarbonate to conscious animals will increase pH and decrease ventilatory drive, thus worsening hypoxemia and hypercapnia in animals with primary respiratory acidosis. Treatment for hypercapnia in animals with chronic pulmonary disease should be directed toward the underlying disease.

Principal causes of respiratory alkalosis are hypoxia, low cardiac output, severe anemia, pulmonary disease (stimulation of peripheral reflexes, e.g., pneumonia), hyperventilation mediated by the central nervous system (e.g., drugs, central nervous system inflammation or tumor, liver disease, fear, or pain), and overzealous mechanical ventilation. Hypocapnia itself is not a major threat to the well-being of animals with respiratory alkalosis. The arterial pH in chronic primary respiratory alkalosis is usually normal or slightly alkalemic owing to efficient renal compensation in this setting.

Table 30.10 Primary processes associated with changes in PaCO_2 and pH.

PaCO_2	pH	Primary process
Normal	Normal	None
Normal	High	Non-respiratory alkalosis, respiratory alkalosis
Normal	Low	Non-respiratory acidosis, respiratory acidosis
High	Normal	Respiratory acidosis, non-respiratory alkalosis
High	High	Non-respiratory alkalosis
High	Low	Respiratory acidosis
Low	Normal	Chronic respiratory alkalosis
Low	High	Respiratory alkalosis
Low	Low	Non-respiratory acidosis

Therapy for the underlying disease responsible for hypocapnia should be the primary focus in animals with respiratory alkalosis. Notably, PCO_2 is a primary determinant of cerebral blood flow. Overventilation and low PCO_2 reduces cerebral blood flow and predisposes to cerebral ischemia [68,69].

Disorders in strong ion difference

Changes in strong ion difference (SID) are usually recognized in the traditional approach to acid–base balance by changes in $cHCO_3^-$ or BE [22,23,59]. A decrease in SID causes a strong ion acidosis, whereas an increase in SID causes a strong ion alkalosis (Fig. 30.9; Table 30.8). There are three common mechanisms by which SID can change (Table 30.11): (1) changing plasma cCl^-; (2) increasing the concentration of unidentified strong anions (cXA^-) in plasma; and (3) changing the free-water content of plasma [61,67].

The selection of intravenous fluids during anesthesia should always consider effects on the SID and A_{TOT}, although conventional rates of fluid administration (10 mL/kg/h) for up to 3 h do not affect acid–base balance [70,71]. Intravenous infusion of larger volumes at faster rates (> 30 mL/kg/h) of either a crystalloid or synthetic colloid (e.g., hydroxyethyl starch) drives the SID and A_{TOT} of the extracellular fluid toward the SID and A_{TOT} of the fluid being administered. The acid–base changes induced by the crystalloid depend upon the fluid's effect on SID and A_{TOT}. A reduction in SID has an acidifying effect and an increase in SID has an alkalinizing effect. Since crystalloids do not contain A_{TOT} they dilute the extracellular fluid A_{TOT} causing an alkalinizing effect. If the fluid's SID is greater than the plasma SID this will also cause an alkalinizing effect. The extent of the changes in SID and A_{TOT} depends upon the amount and rate of crystalloid administered. NaCl 0.9% has a SID of 0 mEq/L and always reduces plasma SID, producing an acidifying effect [72,73]. The ideal SID of a "balanced" crystalloid solution should be approximately 25 mmol/L in order to counteract the A_{TOT} dilutional alkalosis produced by the fluid being administered: commercial crystalloids do not contain A_{TOT} [70,73,74]. The addition of metabolizable strong anions like L-lactate and acetate do contribute to the fluid SID on administration but they are usually rapidly metabolized on infusion and should therefore not be included as strong anions when calculating solution SID. In contrast, the addition of slowly metabolizable strong anions such as D-lactate and gluconate should be included in the estimation of solution SID [23,74–76]. Notably, the SID of 0.9% NaCl (normal saline) is 0 mmol/L, and infusions of large volumes of this fluid can produce hyperchloremic non-respiratory acidosis [70,74] (Fig 30.11). This is also true for Ringer's solution, 5% dextrose, and 7.2% hypertonic saline solutions [74].

Figure 30.11 tells a clear and compelling story, 0.9% NaCl and similar solutions with SID = 0 mmol/L decrease plasma pH in a dose-dependent manner when rapidly infused intravenously. Based on normal values for human plasma, the intravenous administration of a crystalloid solution with an effective SID less than 25 mEq/L is always acidifying, whereas the administration of a crystalloid solution with an effective SID greater than 25 mEq/L is always alkalinizing (Fig. 30.11). This prediction has been experimentally verified by an *in vitro* study [77]. Currently, available formulations of Lactated Ringer's (L-lactate concentration, 28 mmol/L) and Acetated Ringer's (acetate concentration, 27 mmol/L; gluconate, 23 mmol/L) are very mildly alkalinizing when infused into humans and domestic animals. Historic formulations of Lactated Ringer's solution contained approximately equimolar amounts of L-lactate (14 mmol/L) and D-lactate (14 mmol/L) and consequently were mildly acidifying when infused rapidly.

Table 30.11 Causes for changes in plasma strong ion difference (SID).

Chloride abnormalities	
Decrease in cCl^- corrected	→ Hypochloremic alkalosis
Increase in cCl^- corrected	→ Hyperchloremic acidosis
Unmeasured strong anion abnormalities	
Increase in cXA^-	→ Organic acidosis
Free-water abnormalities	
Increase in cNa^+ due to decreased plasma-free water	→ "Concentration" alkalosis
Decrease in cNa^+ due to increased plasma-free water	→ "Dilution" acidosis

cXA^-, unidentified strong anions.

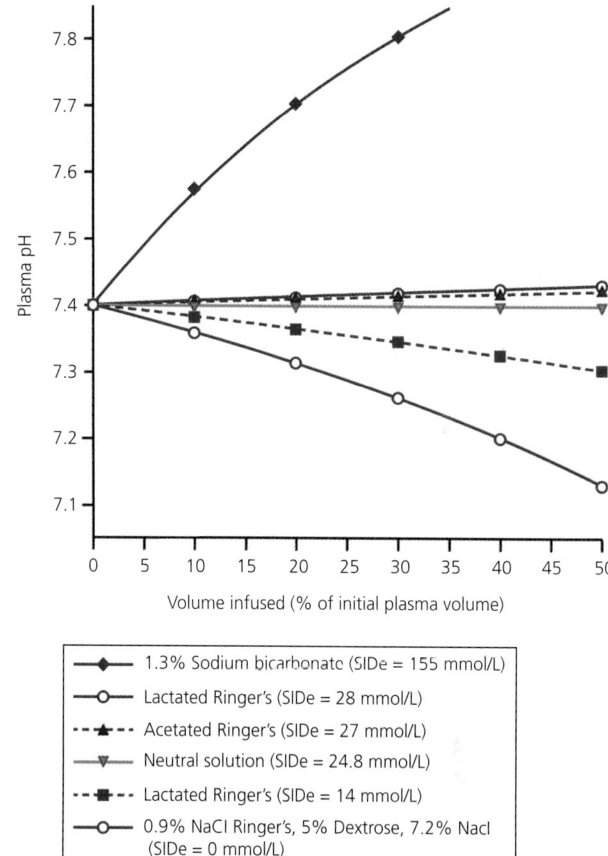

Figure 30.11 Graphic representation of the theoretic effect of rapid intravenous administration of six crystalloid solutions on plasma pH in humans. SIDe is the effective difference between the solution charge of strong cations and strong anions, such as L-lactate and acetate, that are rapidly metabolized in plasma. The figure assumes that Lactated Ringer's solution formulation that contains L-lactate (28 mmol/L) that is rapidly metabolized, or the historic formulation that contained L-lactate (14 mmol/L) that is rapidly metabolized and D-lactate (14 mmol/L) that is very slowly metabolized. Acetated Ringer's solution contains acetate (27 mmol/L) that is rapidly metabolized and gluconate (23 mmol/L) that is slowly metabolized. Source: Adapted from Constable [74].

Isonatremic chloride abnormalities

If there is no change in the water content of plasma, plasma cNa^+ will be normal. Other strong cations (e.g., K^+) are regulated for purposes other than acid–base balance, and their concentration never changes sufficiently to affect SID substantially [52,53]. Consequently, SID changes only as a result of changes in strong anions when water content is normal. If cNa^+ remains constant, changes in cCl^- can substantially increase or decrease SID [78]. Evaluation of cCl^- must be considered in conjunction with the cNa^+ because cCl^- can change for reasons other than a change in water balance (see Box 30.1) [52]. The animal's cCl^- is therefore "corrected" for changes in cNa^+, applying a formula developed for use in people and adapted for use in small and large animals:

$$cCl^-_{corrected} = cCl^- \times cNa^+_{normal}/cNa^+ \quad (30.30)$$

where cCl^- and cNa^+ are the animal's plasma Cl^- and Na^+ concentrations. The ideal cNa^+ is the normal cNa^+ for the species being evaluated. Suggested normal values for cNa^+ in dogs are 144 to 152 mmol/L [47,79], whereas for cats they range from 148 to 160 mmol/L [44,79]. In large animals, normal cNa^+ is approximately 138 mmol/L in horses [42] and 142 mmol/L in cattle. Normal cCl^- is approximately 111–121 mmol/L for dogs [47,79], 110–126 mmol/L for cats [44,79], 101 mmol/L for horses [16,42], and 102 mmol/L for cattle. These values may vary for different laboratories and different analyzers. An increase or decrease in $cCl^-_{corrected}$ indicates that cCl^- is responsible at least in part for the changes in SID. An increase in $cCl^-_{corrected}$ (i.e., an increase in cCl^- relative to cNa^+) results in a hyperchloremic non-respiratory acidosis, whereas a decrease in $cCl^-_{corrected}$ (i.e., a decrease in cCl^- relative to cNa^+) results in hypochloremic non-respiratory alkalosis. A $cCl^-_{corrected}$ to normal in the presence of abnormal observed cCl^- indicates that SID changes are caused by dilution acidosis or concentration alkalosis.

The principal causes of hyperchloremic acidosis and hypochloremic alkalosis are listed in Box 30.2. Treatment of hyperchloremic acidosis should be directed at correction of the underlying disease. Administration of $NaHCO_3$, when pH values are < 7.20 will tend to correct hyperchloremic acidosis because 1.3% sodium bicarbonate has an SID greater than plasma (Fig. 30.11).

Chloride-responsive hypochloremic alkalosis can be caused by excessive loss of Cl^- relative to Na^+ or by administration of substances containing more Na^+ than Cl^- compared with ECF (e.g., $NaHCO_3$). The former can occur following the administration of diuretics that cause Cl^- loss (e.g., furosemide) or when the lost fluid has a low or negative SID, (e.g., acute vomiting). Chloride administration is essential for the treatment of chloride-responsive hypochloremic alkalosis. Renal Cl^- conservation is ordinarily enhanced in hypochloremic states and renal Cl^- reabsorption does not return to normal until plasma cCl^- is restored to normal or near normal [22]. In situations where expansion of extracellular volume is desired, intravenous infusion of 0.9% NaCl is the treatment of choice. This solution has an SID of 0 and will decrease plasma SID [70,74]. If hypokalemia is present, KCl should be added to the fluid. If volume expansion is not necessary, Cl^- can be administered using salts without Na^+ (e.g., ammonium chloride, potassium chloride, calcium chloride, and magnesium chloride). These salts should correct the alkalosis because Cl^- is given together with cations that are regulated within narrow limits for purposes unrelated to acid–base balance [22,23]. Chloride-resistant hypochloremic alkalosis can occur in animals through hyperadrenocorticism and primary hyperaldosteronism. Increased mineralocorticoid activity causes sodium retention and urinary chloride loss in these diseases and both will increase SID. Administration of chloride will not correct the metabolic alkalosis because of chloruresis. Fortunately, metabolic alkalosis in these animals is usually very mild.

Box 30.2 Principal causes of chloride abnormalities.

Hypochloremic alkalosis[a] (↓cCl^- corrected)

- Excessive loss of chloride relative to sodium
  - Vomiting of stomach contents
  - Gastric reflux in horses with ileus
  - Abomasum volvulus (ruminants)
  - Vagal indigestion with internal vomiting (ruminants)
  - Therapy with thiazides or loop diuretics
  - Hyperadrenocorticism
- Excessive gain of sodium relative to chloride
  - Sodium bicarbonate therapy

Hyperchloremic acidosis[b] (↑cCl^- corrected)

- Excessive loss of sodium relative to chloride
  - Diarrhea
- Excessive gain of chloride relative to sodium
  - Fluid therapy (e.g., 0.9% NaCl and KCl supplemental fluids)
  - Salt poisoning
  - Total parenteral nutrition
  - Ammonium chloride or potassium chloride therapy
- Chloride retention
  - Renal failure
  - Renal tubular acidosis
- Hypoadrenocorticism
- Diabetes mellitus
- Drug induced (e.g., acetazolamide and spironolactone)

[a] Chronic respiratory acidosis will cause a compensatory decrease in corrected Cl^-.
[b] Chronic respiratory alkalosis will cause a compensatory increase in corrected Cl^-.
Source: Adapted from de Morais and Muir [58].

Isonatremic organic acid abnormalities

Accumulation of metabolically produced organic strong anions (e.g., L-lactate, D-lactate, acetoacetate, and β-hydroxybutyrate) or addition of exogenous organic strong anions (e.g., salicylate, glycolate from ethylene glycol poisoning, and formate from methanol poisoning) can cause non-respiratory acidosis because these strong anions decrease SID [22,23]. Addition of some inorganic strong anions (e.g., SO_4^{2-} during renal failure) will resemble organic acidosis because SID decreases without changing electrolytes. The most frequently encountered causes of organic acidosis are listed in Table 30.12.

Treatment of organic acidosis should be directed toward the primary disorder and stabilization of the animal. Sodium bicarbonate should be used cautiously because metabolism of accumulated organic anions will normalize SID and increase HCO_3^-. The initial goal in animals with severe organic acidosis is to raise systemic pH to an acceptable value of > 7.20 and treat the primary disease.

Table 30.12 Principal disorders of the unidentified strong ions.

Disorder	Strong anions
Uremic acidosis	SO_4^{2-} and other anions of renal failure
Diabetic ketoacidosis, ketosis, pregnancy toxemia	β-hydroxybutyrate, acetoacetate
L-Lactic acidosis	L-Lactate
D-Lactic acidosis	D-Lactate
Salicylate intoxication	Salicylate
Ethylene glycol toxicity	Glycolate
Methanol toxicity	Formate

[XA^-], unidentified strong anions.
Source: Adapted from de Morais and Muir [58].

Disorders in A_{TOT}

Albumin, globulins, and inorganic phosphate are non-bicarbonate (nonvolatile) weak acids and collectively are the major contributors to A_{TOT} (see Fig. 30.5) [8,22,23]. Consequently, changes in their concentrations will change pH. Hypoalbuminemia will decrease A_{TOT} and cause a non-respiratory alkalosis (Fig. 30.9; Tables 30.8, 30.9). Although rare except for water deprivation, an increase in albumin concentration can cause non-respiratory acidosis, owing to an increase in A_{TOT}. Phosphate also contributes to A_{TOT} and is normally present in plasma at a low concentration. Severe hyperphosphatemia will increase A_{TOT}, resulting in non-respiratory acidosis. Treatment for hyperalbuminemic acidosis, hyperphosphatemic acidosis, and hypoalbuminemic alkalosis should be directed at the underlying cause. The administration of sodium bicarbonate shifts phosphorus into cells and expands the extracellular fluid volume and can be used as adjuvant therapy in patients with hyperphosphatemic acidosis [80].

Free-water abnormalities (combined disorders in SID and A_{TOT})

Changing the water content of body fluid compartments will dilute or concentrate both strong cations and strong anions as well as all non-bicarbonate buffers [22,23,74]. Consequently, SID and A_{TOT} will change by the same proportion with changes in free water. Although increases or decreases in SID and A_{TOT} have opposite effects on pH, the effect of SID on pH predominates; for example, an increase in plasma-free water decreases SID (acidifying effect) and A_{TOT} (alkalinizing effect), with the overall effect being mild acidification because there are similar percent changes in SID and A_{TOT}. For comparison, a decrease in plasma-free water increases SID (alkalinizing effect) and A_{TOT} (acidifying effect), with the overall effect being mild alkalinization because there are similar percent changes in SID and A_{TOT}. Changes in plasma-free water can be identified by evaluating the cNa^+. An increase in SID caused by water loss increases in cNa^+ and results in concentration alkalosis, whereas a decrease in SID caused by decreases in cNa^+ results in dilutional acidosis. Principal causes of free-water abnormalities are listed in Box 30.3. Therapy for dilution acidosis and concentration alkalosis should be directed at the underlying cause responsible for changing cNa^+. If necessary, cNa^+ and plasma osmolality should be corrected [78].

Box 30.3 Principal causes of free-water abnormalities.

Concentration alkalosis (↑cNa^+)

- Pure-water deficit
  - Primary hypodipsia
  - Diabetes Insipidus
  - Fever
  - Inadequate access to water
  - High environmental temperature
- Hypotonic fluid loss
  - Vomiting
  - Peritonitis
  - Pancreatitis
  - Non-oliguric renal failure
  - Post-obstructive diuresis
- Sodium gain
  - Salt poisoning
  - Hypertonic fluid administration (e.g., hypertonic saline and sodium bicarbonate)
  - Hyperaldosteronism
  - Hyperadrenocorticism

Dilution acidosis (↓cNa^+)

- Severe liver disease
- Nephrotic syndrome
- Advanced renal failure
- Congestive heart failure
- Psychogenic polydipsia
- Excessive sweating in horses
- Hypotonic fluid administration (e.g., 0.45% NaCl solution)
- Vomiting
- Diarrhea
- Uroabdomen
- Hypoadrenocorticism
- Diuretic administration

Source: Adapted from de Morais and Muir [58].

Evaluations of acid–base balance

A systematic stepwise approach should be followed in animals with suspected acid–base disorders. Thorough assessment of acid–base status requires blood gas and pH analysis and serum biochemical analysis, with blood samples being obtained from a major vein or any artery.

If the primary clinical interest is acid–base assessment, then a jugular venous blood sample should be anerobically obtained in a 1 to 3 mL polypropylene syringe that has been previously coated internally with sodium heparin (by drawing sodium heparin into the syringe barrel and then expelling all heparin from the barrel before blood collection). Air bubbles are removed from the blood in the syringe after blood collection by tapping on the syringe held vertically with the hub uppermost. This causes small bubbles to float to the syringe hub, from where they coalesce and are eliminated by expelling a small volume of blood. The syringe is capped to prevent loss of CO_2 and addition of O_2 to the blood sample, and the syringe is placed on ice (4 °C) until analysis. This minimizes any time-related changes in pH, PCO_2, and SBE that occur when blood is held at room temperature after collection [81–83]. If the primary interest is evaluation of the respiratory system, an arterial blood sample should be obtained in the same manner, but the sample should be kept at body temperature until analyzed, which should be completed as soon as possible. This is because keeping blood in polypropylene syringes in iced water (0 °C) facilitates oxygen diffusion through the syringe barrel, resulting in a post-collection increase in PO_2 [81–83]. Blood samples for gas and pH analysis should not be collected into partially evacuated (vacutainer) tubes as this sampling method does not provide an anaerobic sample [81].

If serum total protein, albumin, and phosphate concentrations are approximately normal, then acid–base status should be evaluated using blood pH, PCO_2, and SBE or $cHCO_3^-$. There are four primary acid–base abnormalities: respiratory acidosis, respiratory alkalosis, non-respiratory acidosis, and non-respiratory alkalosis (Fig. 30.6). This is the base excess or traditional (Henderson-Hasselbalch) approach (Fig. 30.5). The possibility of a mixed respiratory and non-respiratory acid–base disorder should be assessed by calculating the expected compensation (see Table 30.6). The presence of unidentified anions should be investigated by calculating the AG using eqn 30.25.

If serum total protein, albumin, or phosphate concentrations are markedly abnormal, then acid–base status should be evaluated using blood pH, PCO_2, measured SID_4 ($cNa^+ + cK^+ - cCl^- - c$L-lactate$^-$), and A_{TOT} (calculated from the plasma concentration of total protein or albumin). There are six primary acid–base abnormalities: respiratory acidosis, respiratory alkalosis, strong ion acidosis, strong ion alkalosis, non-bicarbonate buffer ion acidosis, and non-bicarbonate buffer ion alkalosis (Fig. 30.9). This is the physicochemical (simplified strong ion) approach (Fig. 30.5). The presence of unidentified strong ions should be investigated by calculating the SIG using eqn 30.29 and species-specific values for A_{TOT} and pK_a (Table 30.7). General anesthesia produces dose-dependent respiratory and cardiovascular depression, thereby predisposing animals to the development of respiratory and non-respiratory acidosis that can exaggerate or complicate a pre-existing acid–base imbalance. The application of physicochemical methods for the analysis, diagnosis, and treatment of acid–base disorders compels clinicians to consider a more comprehensive set of potential causes for acid–base disturbances and by doing so, focuses diagnostic approaches and refines therapeutic decisions.

References

1 Henderson LJ. The theory of neutrality regulation in the animal organism. *Am J Physiol* 1908; **21**:427–448.
2 Hastings AB. Acid-base measurements in vitro. *Ann N Y Acad Sci* 1966; **133**: 15–24.
3 Henderson LJ. *Blood. A Study in General Physiology*. New Haven: Yale University Press, 1928: 1–397.
4 Siggaard-Andersen O. *The Acid-Base Status of the Blood*, 4th ed. Munksgaard, Copenhagen: Munksgaard, 1974: 1–229.
5 Stewart PA. *How to Understand Acid-base: A Quantitative Acid-base Primer for Biology and Medicine*. New York, NY: Elsevier, 1981.
6 Truchot JP. *Comparative Aspects of Extracellular Acid-Base Balance*. New York, NY: Springer-Verlag, 1987: 1–248.
7 Jones NL. *Blood Gases and Acid-base Physiology*. New York: Thieme, 1987.
8 Kellum JA, Elbers PWG, eds. *Stewart's Textbook of Acid-base*. Raleigh, NC: Lulu Enterprises (www.Lulu.com), 2009.
9 Davis RP. Logland: a Gibbsian view of acid-base balance. *Am J Med* 1967; **42**: 159–162.
10 Rosenthal TB. The effect of temperature on the pH of blood and plasma in vitro. *J Biol Chem* 1948; **173**: 25–30.
11 Reeves RB. An imidazole alphastat hypothesis for vertebrate acid-base regulation: tissue carbon dioxide content and body temperature in bullfrogs. *Resp Physiol* 1972; **14**: 219–236.
12 Cameron JN. Acid-base homeostasis: past and present perspectives. *Physiol Zoology* 1989; **62**: 845–865.
13 Nattie EE. The alpha-stat hypothesis in respiratory control and acid-base balance. *J Appl Physiol* 1990; **69**: 1201–1207.
14 Settergren G. pH-stat, alpha-stat versus temperature correction. *J Cardiothorac Anesth* 1989; **3**: 526–527.
15 Murkin JM, Martzke JS, Buchan AM, *et al.* A randomized study of the influence of perfusion technique and pH management strategy in 316 patients undergoing coronary artery bypass surgery. I. Mortality and cardiovascular morbidity. *J Thorac Cardiovasc Surg* 1995; **110**: 340–348.
16 Constable PD. A simplified strong ion model for acid-base equilibria: application to horse plasma. *J Appl Physiol* 1997; **83**: 297–311.
17 Burton RF. The roles of buffers in body fluids: mathematical analysis. *Resp Physiol* 1973; **18**: 34–42.
18 Watson PD. Modeling the effects of proteins on pH in plasma. *J Appl Physiol* 1999; **86**: 1421–1427.
19 Constable PD, Gelfert CC, Fürll M, *et al.* Application of strong ion difference theory to urine and the relationship between urine pH and net acid excretion in cattle. *Am J Vet Res* 2009; **70**: 915–925.
20 Constable PD, Megahed AA, Hiew MW. Measurement of urine pH and net acid excretion and their association with urine calcium excretion in periparturient dairy cows. *J Dairy Sci* 2019; **102**: 11370–11383.
21 Sartorius OW, Roemmelt JC, Pitts RF, *et al.* The renal regulation of acid-base balance in man. IV. The nature of the renal compensations in ammonium chloride acidosis. *J Clin Invest* 1949; **28**: 423–439.
22 Constable PD. Clinical assessment of acid-base status: comparison of the Henderson–Hasselbalch and strong ion approaches. *Vet Clin Path* 2000; **29**: 115–128.
23 Constable PD. Acid-base assessment: when and how to apply the Henderson–Hasselbalch equation and strong ion difference theory. *Vet Clin North Am Food Anim Pract* 2014; **30**: 295–316.
24 Constable PD. Clinical assessment of acid–base status: strong ion difference theory. *Vet Clin North Am Food Anim Pract* 1999; **15**: 447–471.
25 Adams LG, Polzin DJ. Mixed acid-base disorders. *Vet Clin North Am Small Anim Pract* 1989; **19**: 307–326.
26 Siggaard-Andersen O. The van Slyke equation. *Scand J Clin Lab Invest Supplementum* 1977; **146**: 15–20.
27 Lang W, Zander R. The accuracy of calculated base excess in blood. *Clin Chem Lab Med* 2002; **40**: 404–410.
28 Schwartz WB, Relman AS. A critique of the parameters used in the evaluation of acid-base disorders: whole-blood buffer base and standard bicarbonate compared with blood pH and plasma bicarbonate concentration. *New Engl J Med* 1963; **268**:1382–1388.
29 Brown Jr EB, Clancy RL. In vivo and in vitro CO_2 blood buffer curves. *J Appl Physiol* 1965; **20**: 885–889.
30 Clinical Laboratory Standards Institute (CLSI). *Blood Gas and pH Analysis and Related Measurements; Approved Guideline - 2nd edn. CLSI Document C46-A2.* Wayne, PA: Clinical and Laboratory Standards Institute, 2009.
31 Phillips GD. The assessment of blood acid-base parameters in ruminants. *Brit Vet J* 1970; **126**: 325–332.
32 Emuakpor DS, Maas AH, Ruigrok TJ, *et al.* Acid-base curve nomogram for dog blood. *Pflügers Archiv* 1976; **363**: 141–147.
33 Weiskopf RB, Townsley MI, Riordan KK, *et al.* Acid-base curve and alignment nomograms for swine blood. *J Appl Physiol* 1983; **54**: 978–983.
34 Hannon JP. Construction of acid-base alignment nomograms to estimate buffer base and base-excess concentrations in arterial blood from immature pigs. *Am J Vet Res* 1984; **45**: 1918–1923.
35 Mellemgaard K, Astrup P. The quantitative determination of surplus amounts of acid or base in the human body. *Scand J Clin Lab Invest* 1960; **12**: 187–199.
36 Trefz FM, Lorenz I, Constable PD. Dependence of the apparent bicarbonate space on initial plasma bicarbonate concentration and carbon dioxide tension in neonatal calves with diarrhea, acidemia, and metabolic acidosis. *J Vet Intern Med* 2021; **35**: 644–654.
37 Singer RB, Hastings AB. An improved clinical method for the estimation of disturbances of the acid-base balance of human blood. *Medicine* 1948; **27**: 223–242.
38 Stewart PA. Modern quantitative acid-base chemistry. *Can J Physiol Pharmacol* 1983; **61**: 1444–1461.
39 Constable PD. Comparative animal physiology and adaptation. In: Kellum JA, Elbers PWG, eds. *Stewart's Textbook of Acid-Base Physiology*. Raleigh, NC: Lulu Enterprises (www.Lulu.com), 2009: 305–320.
40 Van Leeuwen AM. Net cation equivalency ('base binding power') of the plasma proteins. *Acta Medica Scandinavica* 1964; **176**(Suppl 422).
41 Kurtz I, Kraut J, Ornekian V, *et al.* Acid-base analysis: a critique of the Stewart and bicarbonate-centered approaches. *Am J Renal Physiol* 2008; **294**: F1009–F1031.
42 Stämpfli HR, Misiaszek S, Lumsden JH, *et al.* Weak acid-concentration Atot and dissociation constant Ka of plasma proteins in racehorses. *Eq Vet J* 1999; **31**: 438–442.
43 Staempfli HR, Constable PD. Experimental determination of net protein charge and Atot and Ka on nonvolatile buffers in human plasma. *J Appl Physiol* 2003; **95**: 620–630.
44 McCullough SM, Constable PD. Calculation of the total plasma concentration of nonvolatile weak acids and the effective dissociation constant of nonvolatile buffers in the plasma for use in the strong ion approach to acid-base balance in cats. *Am J Vet Res* 2003; **64**: 1047–1051.
45 Constable PD. Calculation of variables describing plasma nonvolatile weak acids for use in the strong ion approach to acid-base balance in cattle. *Am J Vet Res* 2002; **63**: 482–490.
46 Constable PD, Stämpfli HR, Navetat H, *et al.* Use of a quantitative strong ion approach to determine the mechanism for acid-base abnormalities in sick calves with or without diarrhea. *J Vet Intern Med* 2005; **19**: 581–589.
47 Constable PD, Stämpfli HR. Experimental determination of net protein charge and Atot and Ka of nonvolatile buffers in canine plasma. *J Vet Intern Med* 2005; **19**: 507–514.
48 Stämpfli H, Taylor M, McNicoll C, *et al.* Experimental determination of net protein charge, Atot, and Ka of nonvolatile buffers in bird plasma. *J Appl Physiol* 2006; **100**: 1831–1836.
49 Oh MS, Carroll HJ. Current concepts. The anion gap. *New Engl J Med* 1977; **297**: 814–817.
50 Gabow PA. Disorders associated with high altered gap. *Kidney Int* 1985; **27**: 472–483.
51 Constable PD, Streeter RN, Koenig GJ, *et al.* Determinants and utility of the anion gap in predicting hyperlactatemia in cattle. *J Vet Intern Med* 1997; **11**: 71–79.
52 Constable PD. Hyperchloremic acidosis: the classic example of strong ion acidosis. *Anesth Analg* 2003; **96**: 919–922.
53 Handy JM, Soni N. Physiological effects of hyperchloraemia and acidosis. *Br J Anaesth* 2008; **101**: 141–150.
54 Constable PD, Hinchcliff KW, Muir WW III. Comparison of anion gap and strong ion gap as predictors of unmeasured strong ion concentration in plasma and serum from horses. *Am J Vet Res* 1998; **59**: 881–887.

55 Trefz FM, Constable PD, Lorenz I. Quantitative physicochemical analysis of acid-base balance and clinical utility of anion gap and strong ion gap in 806 neonatal calves with diarrhea. *J Vet Intern Med* 2015; **29**: 678–687.

56 Nanji A, Blank D. Spurious increases in the anion gap due to exposure of serum to air. *N Engl J Med* 1982; **307**: 190–191.

57 Emmett M, Seldin DW. Evaluation of acid-base disorders from plasma composition. In: Seldin DW, Giebisch G, eds. *The Regulation of Acid-base Balance*. New York, NY: Raven, 1989: 259–268.

58 de Morais HAS, Muir WW. Strong ions and acid-base disorders. In: Bonagura JD, Kirk RW, eds. *Kirk's Current Veterinary Therapy*, 12th edn. Philadelphia, PA: WB Saunders, 1995: 121–127.

59 Kellum JA, Kramer DJ, Pinsky MR. Strong ion gap: a methodology for exploring unexplained anions. *J Crit Care* 1995; **10**: 51–55.

60 Figge J, Mydosh T, Fencl V. Serum proteins and acid-base equilibria: a follow-up. *J Lab Clin Med* 1992; **120**: 713–719.

61 Fencl V, Leith DE. Stewart's quantitative acid-base chemistry: applications in biology and medicine. *Resp Physiol* 1993; **91**: 1–16.

62 Frischmeyer KJ, Moon PF. Evaluation of quantitative acid-base balance and determination of unidentified anions in swine. *Am J Vet Res* 1994; **55**: 1153–1157.

63 Whitehair KJ, Haskins SC, Whitehair JG, *et al.* Clinical applications of quantitative acid-base chemistry. *J Vet Intern Med* 1995; **9**: 1–11.

64 Hopper K, Epstein SE, Kass PH, *et al.* Evaluation of acid-base disorders in dogs and cats presenting to an emergency room. Part 2: comparison of anion gap, strong ion gap, and semiquantitative analysis. *J Vet Emerg Crit Care* 2014; **24**: 502–508.

65 Zeiler GE, Fuller A, Kamerman P, *et al.* Describing acid-base balance using three different methods of analysis in a feline acute haemorrhage-resuscitation model. *Vet Anaesth Analg* 2022; **49**: 65–75.

66 Corey HE. Stewart and beyond: new models of acid-base balance. *Kidney Int* 2003; **64**: 777–787.

67 Wooten EW. Science review: quantitative acid-base physiology using the Stewart model. *Crit Care* 2004; **8**: 448–452.

68 Raichle ME, Plum F. Hyperventilation and cerebral blood flow. *Stroke* 1972; **3**: 566–575.

69 Yoon S, Zuccarello M, Rapoport RM. PCO_2 and pH regulation of cerebral blood flow. *Front Physiol* 2012; **3**: 365.

70 Morgan JT. The meaning of acid-base abnormalities in the intensive care unit: Part III: effects of fluid administration. *Crit Care* 2005; **9**: 204–211.

71 Valverde A, Hatcher ME, Stämpfli HR. Effects of fluid therapy on total protein and its influence on calculated unmeasured anions in the anesthetized dog. *J Vet Emerg Crit Care* 2008; **18**: 480–487.

72 Langer T, Ferrari M, Zazzeron L, *et al.* Effects of intravenous solutions on acid-base equilibrium: from crystalloids to colloids and blood components. *Anaesthesiol Intensive Ther* 2014; **46**: 350–360.

73 Muir W. Effect of intravenously administered crystalloid solutions on acid-base balance in domestic animals. *J Vet Intern Med* 2017; **31**:1371–1381.

74 Constable PD. In response: letters to the editor. *Anesth Analg* 2004; **98**: 271–272.

75 Müller KR, Gentile A, Klee W, *et al.* Importance of the effective strong ion difference of an intravenous solution in the treatment of diarrheic calves with naturally-acquired acidemia and strong ion (metabolic) acidosis. *J Vet Intern Med* 2012; **26**: 674–683.

76 Weinberg L, Collins N, Van Mourik K, *et al.* Plasma-Lyte 148: a clinical review. *World J Crit Care Med* 2016; **5**:235–250.

77 Morgan TJ, Venkatesh B, Hall J. Crystalloid strong ion difference determines metabolic acid-base change during in vitro hemodilution. *Crit Care Med* 2002; **30**: 157–160.

78 Lloyd P. Strong ion calculator – a practical bedside application of modern quantitative acid-base physiology. *Crit Care Resus* 2004; **6**: 285–294.

79 Hopper K, Epstein SE, Kass PH, *et al.* Evaluation of acid-base disorders in dogs and cats presenting to an emergency room. Part 1: comparison of three methods of acid-base analysis. *J Vet Emerg Crit Care* 2014; **24**: 493–501.

80 Barsotti G, Lazzeri M, Cristofano C, *et al.* The role of metabolic acidosis in causing uremic hyperphosphatemia. *Miner Electrolyte Metab* 1986; **12**: 103–106.

81 Noël PG, Couëtil L, Constable PD. Effects of collecting blood into plastic heparinised Vacutainer® tubes and storage conditions on blood gas analysis values in horses. *Eq Vet J* 2010; **42**: 91–97.

82 Kennedy SA, Constable PD, Sen I, *et al.* Effects of syringe type and storage conditions on results of equine blood gas and acid-base analysis. *Am J Vet Res* 2012; **73**: 979–987.

83 Tinkler SH, Couëtil LL, Kennedy SA, *et al.* Effect of the size of evacuated blood collection tubes on total carbon dioxide concentration in equine plasma. *J Am Vet Med Assoc* 2012; **241**: 922–926.

31 Treatment of Coagulation and Platelet Disorders

Benjamin M. Brainard
Department of Small Animal Medicine and Surgery, College of Veterinary Medicine, University of Georgia, Athens, Georgia, USA

Chapter contents

Introduction, 574
The cell-based model of hemostasis, 574
Coagulation and platelet function testing, 575
  Platelet function testing (primary hemostasis), 575
  Coagulation testing (secondary hemostasis), 575
Anticoagulant therapy, 575
  Antiplatelet drugs, 575
  Coagulation inhibitors, 576
Fibrinolytic drugs, 577
Procoagulant therapies, 577
Drugs that support coagulation, 578
References, 578

Introduction

Interest in the process of both normal and disordered hemostasis in the veterinary patient has experienced resurgence in recent years. This is due in part to the availability of newer tests and techniques that can better illustrate the process and products of coagulation. At the same time, new understanding of the formation of clots *in vivo* has made it clear that traditional testing provides only a limited view into the actual mechanisms and pathophysiology of clot formation and platelet function.

The cell-based model of hemostasis

The cell-based model of hemostasis provides a framework for understanding the complex interactions between cellular components, soluble factors, and the vascular endothelium in the formation of a clot. In some cases, this model explains why certain conditions (e.g., factor deficiencies) have a particular hemostatic phenotype. Coagulation as described by this model consists of three phases: initiation, amplification, and propagation [1].

The vast majority of coagulation *in vivo* occurs as a result of tissue factor (TF, factor III) initiation of the extrinsic coagulation cascade (as opposed to contact activation via the intrinsic coagulation cascade [also termed the "contact-activation pathway"], which may occur on the surfaces of foreign materials like intravenous catheters) [2]. TF is exposed following intimal injury of a blood vessel and may also be present on the surface of circulating monocytes and microparticles, especially in the setting of systemic inflammation. Microparticles are small membrane blebs released from activated endothelial cells, platelets, or leukocytes. The other important player in the initiation of coagulation is the platelet. Following activation, the platelet undergoes a shape change, and anionic phospholipids such as phosphatidyl serine are exposed on the outer platelet membrane. These phospholipids provide a surface for the assembly of coagulation factors into complexes that promote clot amplification [3]. In the initiation step, exposed TF comes into contact with activated factor VII (fVIIa) and activated factor X (fXa), forming a TF-fVIIa-fXa complex [1]. A small amount of thrombin (factor IIa) is generated by this complex.

The small amount of thrombin released in the initiation step promotes the amplification stage, where additional platelets and coagulation factors V, VIII, and XI are activated [2]. Thrombin is generated in the propagation phase from complexes of these factors assembled on cell membranes. The tenase complex, composed of factors IXa, VIIIa, and calcium, activates coagulation factor X. The presence of factor Xa then allows formation of the prothrombinase complex, which is composed of factors Xa, Va, and calcium. The prothrombinase complex is an extremely efficient complex that promotes the formation of thrombin (factor IIa) from prothrombin, which then catalyzes the formation of fibrin from fibrinogen [4].

Endogenous coagulation inhibitors are present at each stage of the coagulation process to prevent excessive thrombin formation. Tissue factor pathway inhibitor (TFPI) is a potent inhibitor of the TF-fVIIa-Xa complex [1]. Antithrombin acts to inhibit factors Xa and IIa. The protein C/protein S system supports the inhibition of factors Va and VIIIa. Patients with urinary losses of antithrombin and humans with congenital low concentrations of protein C are thought to have an increased risk for the development of thromboembolism. Dogs with sepsis have decreased activities of protein C

Veterinary Anesthesia and Analgesia: The Sixth Edition of Lumb and Jones. Edited by Leigh Lamont, Kurt Grimm, Sheilah Robertson, Lydia Love and Carrie Schroeder.
© 2024 John Wiley & Sons, Inc. Published 2024 by John Wiley & Sons, Inc.
Companion website: www.wiley.com/go/lamont/anesthesia

and antithrombin [5]. Dogs with sepsis have also been reported to have increased thrombin-activatable fibrinolysis inhibitor (TAFI) activity [6]. TAFI is activated in the presence of thrombin and acts to decrease the speed of fibrinolysis or clot breakdown.

Coagulation and platelet function testing

The complex *in vivo* physiology of clot formation is very difficult to mimic *in vitro*. Most laboratory tests of coagulation function are focused on individual aspects of the coagulation process.

Platelet function testing (primary hemostasis)

Platelet function may be assessed using tools such as optical or impedance aggregometry, which document the response of platelets (in platelet-rich plasma or whole blood, respectively) to discrete agonists such as adenosine diphosphate (ADP), collagen, or arachidonic acid [7]. Most aggregometry testing is performed under low shear settings, which do not necessarily reflect the *in vivo* physiology of the high-shear condition of flowing blood. The PFA-100 (Siemens-Dade Behring) is a whole blood test that aspirates blood through a small aperture using a vacuum [8]. The aperture is coated with a combination of either epinephrine and collagen or ADP and collagen. As platelets pass through the aperture, they are activated by the agonists and form a plug, stopping the flow of blood. The time it takes for this to occur is termed the "closure time" and is measured in seconds. In dogs with von Willebrand disease (vWD, which impairs the ability of platelets to tether and adhere to sites of vascular injury) and in animals treated with drugs that decrease platelet activity, the closure time is prolonged [9]. This is a rapid, benchtop test that can be used to assess an animal's risk of bleeding due to platelet function abnormalities. Low hematocrits and platelet counts less than 90×10^9 platelets/L may cause prolonged closure times unrelated to platelet function.

Buccal mucosal bleeding time (BMBT) is another test that can diagnose platelet function abnormalities. It is simple and can be done rapidly as part of a presurgical screen. To perform this test, the buccal mucosa is exposed and a standard incision (5 mm long and 1 mm deep) is made using a SimPlate® device [10]. Once the incision is made, the area is observed for the formation of a gel-like platelet plug. The *bleeding time* is defined as the time until bleeding has ceased and is between 3–5 min in normal animals. Because cats have a small buccal surface, the oral mucosal bleeding time (OMBT) is performed instead, by making the incision in the gums above the upper canine tooth [11]. Cats generally need to be sedated or anesthetized for this test. As with the PFA, the BMBT will be prolonged if patients have thrombocytopenia ($< 75 \times 10^9$ platelets/L).

Coagulation testing (secondary hemostasis)

Assessment of coagulation factor activity is generally performed using citrated plasma but may also be assessed in whole blood systems. Most tests monitor for the formation of a fibrin clot by exposing citrated plasma to calcium in combination with an activating substance and report the time until clot formation (which may be sensed optically or mechanically) as the clotting time [12]. The prothrombin time (PT) is initiated using a mixture of TF and phospholipid and primarily assesses the extrinsic and common pathway of coagulation (i.e., factors VII, X, V, II). Activated partial thromboplastin time (aPTT) is initiated with a strong contact activator such as kaolin and reflects activity in the intrinsic and common pathways (i.e., factors XII, XI, IX, VIII, X, V, II). The thrombin time is dependent on the blood fibrinogen concentration and assesses only the formation of fibrin in the common pathway following the addition of thrombin. Modifications of both PT and aPTT have been developed to use citrated whole blood for coagulation testing as well [13]. The activated clotting time (ACT) adds whole blood to diatomaceous earth (a strong contact activator) and measures the time until it forms into a clot. The reference intervals for coagulation times of normal animals vary depending on methodology and technique.

Viscoelastic coagulation testing using techniques such as thromboelastography (TEG), rotational thromboelastometry (ROTEM), or Sonoclot use citrated whole blood to evaluate both primary and secondary hemostasis, in addition to fibrinolysis [14]. Viscoelastic testing displays the change in viscosity as blood gels into a clot and can identify both hypocoagulable and hypercoagulable states. Transfusion algorithms based on intraoperative viscoelastic monitoring have resulted in more targeted transfusion strategies and decreased waste of blood products in human medicine [15]. Viscoelastic techniques have been described in dogs, cats, and horses [16–18].

Anticoagulant therapy

In human medicine, arterial thromboses are thought to result from activation or hyperactivity of platelets, while venous thrombosis or thromboembolism is more associated with blood stasis and activation of coagulation factors [19]. While these two pathophysiologic consequences dictate different treatment approaches, the reality in veterinary medicine balances the need for patient safety and ease of administration. For this reason, most anticoagulants used in veterinary medicine are antiplatelet agents that can be administered orally. Injectable anticoagulants that target the coagulation cascade are also used, especially in hospitalized patients, and newer oral anticoagulants may provide a safer approach to providing tailored long-term anticoagulation in veterinary patients.

Antiplatelet drugs

Platelet activation results in a series of events that allow the platelet to adhere to sites of vascular damage (tethered by molecules such as von Willebrand Factor and collagen) and also cause the release of substances that support coagulation and activate adjacent platelets. Molecules released from activated platelets include ADP, thromboxane, serotonin, and calcium. Because there are specific receptors for many of these agonists, antiplatelet agents have been designed to affect the binding or release of these agonists.

Aspirin (acetylsalicylic acid, ASA) decreases platelet responsiveness and has been evaluated in most domestic species. Aspirin exerts an antiplatelet effect by irreversible inhibition of platelet cyclo-oxygenase (COX), which produces thromboxane A_2 (TXA_2) from arachidonic acid in response to platelet activation [20,21]. TXA_2 is a potent vasoconstrictor and platelet activator, although platelet responses vary between species and individuals. In dogs, aspirin at various doses has been recommended to decrease platelet activity in patients with immune-mediated hemolytic anemia (IMHA) and other diseases that are associated with hypercoagulable states (e.g., protein-losing nephropathy) [5]. In many of these cases, a low dose of aspirin (0.5–1.0 mg/kg PO q 12 h) has been recommended, although the efficacy of these lower doses on platelet aggregation is unclear [22]. Interestingly, certain breeds or families of dogs may not be as responsive to aspirin-mediated platelet inhibition [23]. The same may be true in humans, and a syndrome of "aspirin resistance" has been described [24]. In cats, aspirin has been recommended for thromboprophylaxis in animals with hypertrophic cardiomyopathy, although efficacy for inhibition of platelet aggregation or for prevention of intracardiac thrombus formation has not been definitively demonstrated [21,25]. Aspirin has been used to treat horses with jugular venous thrombosis. Other veterinary-labeled non-steroidal anti-inflammatory drugs may cause transient impairment of platelet function in dogs, which is unlikely to cause clinically significant perioperative bleeding unless used in patients with other comorbidities that decrease platelet function (e.g., vWD).

Clopidogrel (Plavix®, Sanofi Synthelabo, New York) is an irreversible antagonist of the platelet $P2Y_{12}$ receptor, one of two ADP receptors on the platelet surface. In dogs, cats, and horses, clopidogrel effectively decreases platelet aggregation in response to ADP [11,26,27]. Clopidogrel is a prodrug, requiring hepatic biotransformation to an active compound. Co-administration of drugs that affect the hepatic P450 enzyme system may alter the pharmacokinetics of clopidogrel; however, recent studies do not indicate a clinically relevant interaction with proton pump inhibitors in dogs [28]. As with aspirin, there are human patients who do not demonstrate decreased platelet aggregation following clopidogrel therapy. The mechanism may be altered hepatic processing or variations of platelet receptor affinity, and this phenomenon likely occurs in veterinary species as well [29,30].

Because both aspirin and clopidogrel result in irreversible inhibition of platelet function, it is necessary for patients to release new platelets to regain platelet function. In animals with normal bone marrow function, a new platelet population is generally present 5–7 days after cessation of antiplatelet medications, although clinical response to platelet agonists may return prior to this point. Aspirin and clopidogrel are frequently prescribed for veterinary patients diagnosed with hypercoagulable conditions because they are generally well tolerated, easily administered at home, and not associated with adverse events such as hemorrhage when used individually. When clopidogrel and aspirin were used together in human patients, the antithrombotic effects were more pronounced, but there was also an increased incidence of gastrointestinal bleeding [31].

Coagulation inhibitors

Warfarin is an oral vitamin K epoxide reductase antagonist that prevents the hepatic recycling of vitamin K, resulting in decreased coagulation factor production. It impairs the production of vitamin K-dependent coagulation factors (i.e., II, VII, IX, and X) [32]. Warfarin is difficult to titrate. Clinical use requires initial weekly measurements of PT, a tightly regulated diet, and a strict dosing schedule to minimize the chances for hemorrhage. Warfarin therapy has been used as a component of medical management in dogs with venous thrombi [33] and was also utilized in a small number of cats with hypertrophic cardiomyopathy. However, in those cats, its use was associated with a shorter survival time [25]. The effects of warfarin can be antagonized using either oral vitamin K (phytonadione) therapy or by transfusions of fresh frozen or stored plasma [34]. Despite the fact that warfarin is administered orally, it is not frequently used in veterinary medicine due to the potential severity of complications and difficulty in ensuring owner compliance.

Other oral anticoagulant medications such as rivaroxaban (Xarelto®, Bayer Healthcare) and apixaban (Eliquis®, Pfizer/Bristol-Myers Squibb) have recently been introduced for human patients [35,36]. These drugs are inhibitors of activated coagulation factor X (Xa) and have shown equivalent or superior effect to warfarin in a number of human studies. In cats and dogs, rivaroxaban displays dose-dependent anticoagulant activity [35,36]. Apixaban also appears to have dose-dependent pharmacodynamic activity in dogs, cats, and horses [37–39]. In horses, apixaban has very low oral bioavailability, which can be overcome with increased doses [40]. There is not an easily available reversal agent to treat overdose of the anti-Xa medications, short of transfusions of fresh frozen plasma. Studies in veterinary medicine that will provide clearer information on dosing guidelines and safety of the anti-Xa drugs are ongoing. Plasma drug concentrations for rivaroxaban and apixaban can be measured directly or estimated using specifically calibrated anti-Xa activity assays [41]. Higher plasma drug concentrations (potentially above the therapeutic target range) will result in prolongations of traditional coagulation tests (e.g., PT or aPTT).

Heparins are another class of drugs commonly used for anticoagulation in veterinary species. The use of both unfractionated heparin (UFH) and low-molecular-weight heparins (LMWH) has been described in many animal species. They have been used to treat many conditions associated with potential or actual thrombosis [42,43]. All heparins are injectable drugs and may be given by either the intravenous or subcutaneous route. Heparins enhance the inhibitory effect of antithrombin on activated coagulation factors X and II. LMWH is a smaller molecule and primarily inhibits factor Xa activity. Heparins are indicated for anticoagulation in patients with gross thrombosis, or for those in danger of thrombotic complications, especially in the perioperative period [44].

UFH has been used in the treatment of dogs with IMHA, pulmonary thromboembolism, and other prothrombotic conditions [44]. There is no evidence to support preincubation of fresh frozen plasma with UFH in the context of disseminated intravascular coagulation (DIC), and this practice may actually decrease the amount of available antithrombin in the plasma [45]. In addition, UFH is frequently used for anticoagulation during cardiopulmonary bypass and hemodialysis procedures. Postoperative UFH and LMWH administration has been described in dogs following adrenal gland resection [46] and may be used during other vascular procedures. In horses, UFH may result in anemia caused by agglutination of red blood cells. This adverse event is rapidly reversed following the cessation of UFH therapy [47].

In people, LMWH has a more favorable pharmacokinetic profile (once-daily dosing) and a decreased risk of hemorrhage compared to UFH. It may be safer in the perioperative period for this reason, although this has not been specifically studied in veterinary patients. Of the LMWHs available, dalteparin (Fragmin®, Pfizer) and enoxaparin (Lovenox®, Sanofi) have been most studied in veterinary medicine. Direct comparisons between these and UFH have been performed in cats [43] and dogs [48] with more focused studies available in horses [49] and other species. Although the pharmacokinetics in humans are amenable to once-daily dosing, the pharmacodynamic studies available for veterinary species suggest that multiple doses may be required to maintain anti-factor Xa activity in the presumed therapeutic range. The utility of LMWH versus UFH for thromboprophylaxis in veterinary medicine is not clear. The use of a newer synthetic LMWH, fondaparinux, has been described in cats [50].

Human guidelines for dosing of heparin are based on anti Xa activity (aXa), and targets vary for prophylactic or therapeutic dosing. Target therapeutic aXa levels for UFH (measured at 4 h after administration of a dose) are 0.35–0.7 U/mL, while prophylactic levels are approximately 10% of these [51,52]. LMWH targets for therapeutic aXa levels are 0.5–1.0 U/mL and 0.1–0.3 U/mL for

Table 31.1 Doses of anticoagulant and antiplatelet drugs used in veterinary medicine.

Drug	Species	Dose	Comments
Aspirin	Dog	5 mg/kg PO q24 h [20]	Analgesic dose higher
	Cat	81 mg/cat PO q48–72 h [25]	Questionable efficacy at either dose
		5 mg/kg PO q48 h [21]	No decrease in platelet function
	Horse	5 mg/kg PO q24 h [26]	
		10 mg/kg [54]	Effective; single dose
Clopidogrel	Dog	1–3 mg/kg PO q24 h [27,44]	
	Cat	18.75 mg/cat PO q24 h [11]	
	Horse	2 mg/kg PO q24 h [26]	
Warfarin	Dog	0.22 mg/kg PO q12–24 h [55]	Adjust using PT or INR
	Cat	0.06–0.09 mg/kg PO q24 h [56]	Monitor PT
Unfractionated heparin	Dog	150–300 U/kg SC q8 h [16,42,44]	Adjust to target aPTT or anti-Xa levels
		20–50 U/kg/h IV	Loading dose of 100 U/kg IV may be given prior to IV constant rate infusion in dogs [44]
	Cat	150–300 U/kg SC q6–8 h [43,44]	May result in anemia
	Horse	40–150 U/kg SC q12 h [57]	
Low-molecular-weight heparin	Dog	Dalteparin 150 U/kg SC q8 h [58,59]	
		Dalteparin 100–175 U/kg SC q8 h [44]	
		Enoxaparin 0.8 mg/kg SC q6 h [44,60]	
	Cat	Dalteparin 75–200 IU/kg SC q6–8 h [43,44,61]	
		Enoxaparin 0.75–1 mg/kg SC q6–12 h [43,44,62]	
	Horse	Dalteparin 50 U/kg SC q12 h [63,71]	
		Enoxaparin 40–80 U/kg SC q24 h [64]	
Rivaroxaban	Dog	0.5–2 mg/kg PO q 24 h [44,65]	When used in combination with clopidogrel a lower dose (i.e., 0.5–1 mg/kg) should be targeted
	Cat	2.5 mg/cat PO q 24 h [35]	
		0.5–1 mg/kg PO q24 h [44]	

aPTT, activated partial thromboplastin time; INR, international normalized ratio; PO, per os; PT, prothrombin time; SC, subcutaneous.

prophylaxis. In dogs, due to limited availability of rapid aXa testing, UFH is usually dose adjusted by measuring serial aPTT until the aPTT is extended to 1.5–2 times the normal value [53]. These guidelines will vary depending on the type of machine used to measure aPTT, and using some methodologies, a prolongation closer to 1.2–1.5 times normal aPTT may be indicated [16]. Guidance for dosing regimens for most anticoagulant medications in small animal species has been reviewed in Table 31.1 [44].

Fibrinolytic drugs

In animals that have developed venous or arterial thrombi, blood flow and oxygen delivery may be restored through the use of fibrinolytic drugs that encourage the dissolution of clots *in vivo*. The primary drugs that have been used for clot dissolution are tissue plasminogen activator (tPA) and streptokinase. Streptokinase is no longer available in many countries. tPA is a potent activator of plasmin, which breaks down fibrin into fibrinopeptides A and B. If the fibrin has been cross-linked by activated factor XIII, dissolution by plasmin also results in the generation of d-dimers [66]. Systemic administration of tPA can be associated with hemorrhage, and rapid reperfusion of thrombosed areas following tPA administration may lead to reperfusion injury [67]. Local administration of tPA using catheter-guided delivery may mitigate some side effects of systemic administration. When used for clot dissolution in cats with aortic thromboembolism, approximately 50% of cats experienced rapid reperfusion of thrombosed limbs [68]. This percentage is similar to that reported for cats receiving supportive care (treatment of congestive heart failure, analgesia) without specific fibrinolytic therapy, and most cats experienced side effects including azotemia, neurologic signs, and sudden death [68]. tPA usage in dogs has been infrequently reported in clinical settings, although it has been used experimentally [69].

Procoagulant therapies

There are very few procoagulant therapies available to the veterinarian. The majority are topical products including hemostatic gels and solubilized liquid thrombin, which are applied directly to the source of hemorrhage. In patients with hemorrhage due to clotting factor deficiency, products such as fresh frozen plasma or stored plasma may be appropriate to restore clotting function. In patients with anticoagulant rodenticide toxicosis or some forms of hepatic disease (especially in cats), the administration of vitamin K (phytonadione) at 1–5 mg/kg/day either PO or SC may allow the body to support production of necessary factors. Cryoprecipitate contains high concentrations of von Willebrand Factor, factor V, and fibrinogen and is useful for acute treatment of hemorrhage due to vWD. Both frozen and lyophilized platelet concentrates are available for dogs and can be used to address hemorrhage due to thrombocytopenia [70].

A drug that is available to human medicine and that has been used in dogs to a small degree is recombinant activated factor VII (fVIIa; Novoseven®, Novo Nordisk, Denmark). Its mechanism is explained as follows: although physiologic levels of fVIIa only result in small amounts of thrombin, the larger dose used with rfVIIa results in sufficient thrombin formation to allow coagulation to proceed. Activated factor VII is indicated for the cessation of bleeding in patients with hemophilia or other coagulation factor deficiencies and has been used to correct hemostatic testing abnormalities in fVII-deficient Beagles [71]. fVIIa has also been used to stop bleeding in human patients with severe trauma and coagulopathy [72]. In this context, it effectively stops or slows bleeding without a concomitant increase in the incidence of thrombosis. While this represents a possible indication for use of fVIIa in veterinary patients, the effectiveness of therapy and immunogenicity of the compound itself have not been extensively studied.

If an iatrogenic coagulopathy has developed secondary to the use of heparin molecules, protamine may be used to reverse the effects of heparin. Protamine forms 1:1 complexes with heparins (UFH more so than LMWH). When administered in excess, it may cause anticoagulation. Dosing recommendations are 1–1.5 mg of protamine per 100 units of heparin administered [73]. Because heparin is rapidly metabolized, if 30 min have elapsed following heparin administration, the protamine dose is halved and then subsequently halved 30 min later [73]. Protamine may cause histamine release and hypotension or bradycardia if administered rapidly IV and has sometimes been reported to cause fatal anaphylactic reactions in humans, which may be related to prior exposure to protamine-containing insulin products (e.g., protamine-zinc insulin) [74]. Although these reactions have not been reported in veterinary medicine, protamine should be administered slowly, especially in patients who may have prior sensitization.

Drugs that support coagulation

Other drugs may be used to augment coagulation by strengthening the fibrin clot. The lysine analogues aminocaproic acid and tranexamic acid are classified as antifibrinolytic agents because of their ability to limit clot breakdown in normal and pathologic circumstances. Both of these drugs work by occupying the lysine binding site on plasmin. This prevents its association with fibrin and consequently stabilizes the clot (plasmin binds to lysine residues on fibrin to initiate fibrinolysis). Antifibrinolytic agents are not indicated for treatment of DIC but may be useful in the treatment of perioperative bleeding, especially in patients with otherwise normal coagulation competency. They may also be used topically to treat mucosal bleeding.

Antifibrinolytics are used in equine nasal surgery, where extensive hemorrhage can occur [75]. Other authors have considered their use in dogs with hemoperitoneum or other conditions where the maintenance of clot integrity is critical [76]. Pharmacokinetic and pharmacodynamic analyses of single doses of both antifibrinolytic agents have been published for dogs, but the safety and efficacy in cats has not been evaluated [77,78]. The perioperative use of aminocaproic acid has been described in Greyhounds due to the tendency of this breed to develop postoperative hemorrhage 48–72 h following surgery [79]. The authors hypothesized, based on the onset of hemorrhage, that the bleeding occurred due to the breakdown of formed clots, and that Greyhounds may be hyperfibrinolytic in some circumstances.

References

1 McMichael M. New models of hemostasis. *Top Companion Anim Med* 2012; **27**: 40–45.

2 Smith SA. The cell-based model of coagulation. *J Vet Emerg Crit Care* 2009; **19**: 3–10.

3 Mann KG, Krishnaswamy S, Lawson JH. Surface-dependent hemostasis. *Semin Hematol* 1992; **29**: 213–226.

4 Kalafatis M. Coagulation factor V: a plethora of anticoagulant molecules. *Curr Opin Hematol* 2005; **12**: 141–148.

5 De Laforcade AM. Diseases associated with thrombosis. *Top Companion Anim Med* 2012; **27**: 59–64.

6 Jessen LR, Wiinberg B, Kjelgaard-Hansen M, *et al.* Thrombin-activatable fibrinolysis inhibitor activity in healthy and diseased dogs. *Vet Clin Pathol* 2010; **39**: 296–301.

7 Born G, Patrono C. Antiplatelet drugs. *Br J Pharmacol* 2006; **147**(Suppl 1): S241–S251.

8 Jandrey KE. Assessment of platelet function. *J Vet Emerg Crit Care* 2012; **22**: 81–98.

9 Callan MB, Giger U. Assessment of a point-of-care instrument for identification of primary hemostatic disorders in dogs. *Am J Vet Res* 2001; **62**: 652–658.

10 Brooks M, Catalfamo J. Buccal mucosa bleeding time is prolonged in canine models of primary hemostatic disorders. *Thromb Haemost* 1993; **70**: 777–780.

11 Hogan DF, Andrews DA, Green HW, *et al.* Antiplatelet effects and pharmacodynamics of clopidogrel in cats. *J Am Vet Med Assoc* 2004; **225**: 1406–1411.

12 Babski DM, Brainard BM, Krimer PM, *et al.* Sonoclot evaluation of whole blood coagulation in healthy adult dogs. *J Vet Emerg Crit Care* 2012; **22**: 646–652.

13 Dixon-Jimenez AC, Brainard BM, Cathcart CJ, *et al.* Evaluation of a point-of-care coagulation analyzer (Abaxis VSPro) for identification of coagulopathies in dogs. *J Vet Emerg Crit Care* 2013; **23**: 402–407.

14 Ganter MT, Hofer CK. Coagulation monitoring: current techniques and clinical use of viscoelastic point-of-care coagulation devices. *Anesth Analg* 2008; **106**: 1366–1375.

15 Whiting P, Al M, Westwood M, *et al.* Viscoelastic point-of-care testing to assist with the diagnosis, management and monitoring of haemostasis: a systematic review and cost-effectiveness analysis. *Health Technol Assess* 2015; **19**: 1–228, v–vi.

16 Babski DM, Brainard BM, Ralph AG, *et al.* Sonoclot(R) evaluation of single- and multiple-dose subcutaneous unfractionated heparin therapy in healthy adult dogs. *J Vet Intern Med* 2012; **26**: 631–638.

17 Epstein KL, Brainard BM, Lopes MA, *et al.* Thrombelastography in 26 healthy horses with and without activation by recombinant human tissue factor. *J Vet Emerg Crit Care* 2009; **19**: 96–101.

18 Banerjee A, Blois SL, Wood RD. Comparing citrated native, kaolin-activated, and tissue factor-activated samples and determining intraindividual variability for feline thromboelastography. *J Vet Diagn Invest* 2011; **23**: 1109–1113.

19 Mackman N. Triggers, targets and treatments for thrombosis. *Nature* 2008; **451**: 914–918.

20 Brainard BM, Meredith CP, Callan MB, *et al.* Changes in platelet function, hemostasis, and prostaglandin expression after treatment with nonsteroidal antiinflammatory drugs with various cyclooxygenase selectivities in dogs. *Am J Vet Res* 2007; **68**: 251–257.

21 Cathcart CJ, Brainard BM, Reynolds LR, *et al.* Lack of inhibitory effect of acetylsalicylic acid and meloxicam on whole blood platelet aggregation in cats. *J Vet Emerg Crit Care* 2012; **22**: 99–106.

22 McLewee N, Archer T, Wills R, *et al.* Effects of aspirin dose escalation on platelet function and urinary thromboxane and prostacyclin levels in normal dogs. *J Vet Pharmacol Ther* 2018; **41**: 60–67.

23 Johnson GJ, Leis LA, King RA. Thromboxane responsiveness of dog platelets is inherited as an autosomal recessive trait. *Thromb Haemost* 1991; **65**: 578–580.

24 Berent R, Sinzinger H. "Aspirin – resistance"? A few critical considerations on definition, terminology, diagnosis, clinical value, natural course of atherosclerotic disease, and therapeutic consequences. *Vasa* 2011; **40**: 429–438.

25 Smith SA, Tobias AH, Jacob KA, *et al.* Arterial thromboembolism in cats: acute crisis in 127 cases (1992–2001) and long-term management with low-dose aspirin in 24 cases. *J Vet Intern Med* 2003; **17**: 73–83.

26 Brainard BM, Epstein KL, LoBato D, *et al.* Effects of clopidogrel and aspirin on platelet aggregation, thromboxane production, and serotonin secretion in horses. *J Vet Intern Med* 2011; **25**: 116–122.

27 Brainard BM, Kleine SA, Papich MG, *et al.* Pharmacodynamic and pharmacokinetic evaluation of clopidogrel and the carboxylic acid metabolite SR 26334 in healthy dogs. *Am J Vet Res* 2010; **71**: 822–830.

28 Thames BE, Lovvorn J, Papich MG, *et al.* The effects of clopidogrel and omeprazole on platelet function in normal dogs. *J Vet Pharmacol Ther* 2017; **40**(2): 130–139.

29 Vadasz D, Sztriha LK, Sas K, *et al.* Aspirin and clopidogrel resistance: possible mechanisms and clinical relevance. Part I: concept of resistance. *Ideggyogy Sz* 2012; **65**: 377–385.

30 Ueda Y, Li RHL, Nguyen N, *et al.* A genetic polymorphism in P2RY1 impacts response to clopidogrel in cats with hypertrophic cardiomyopathy. *Sci Rep* 2021; **11**(1): 12522.

31 Palacio S, Hart RG, Pearce LA, *et al.* Effect of addition of clopidogrel to aspirin on mortality: systematic review of randomized trials. *Stroke* 2012; **43**: 2157–2162.

32 Waddell LS, Poppenga RH, Drobatz KJ. Anticoagulant rodenticide screening in dogs: 123 cases (1996–2003). *J Am Vet Med Assoc* 2013; **242**: 516–521.

33 Winter RL, Sedacca CD, Adams A, *et al.* Aortic thrombosis in dogs: presentation, therapy, and outcome in 26 cases. *J Vet Cardiol* 2012; **14**: 333–342.

34 Logan JC, Callan MB, Drew K, *et al.* Clinical indications for use of fresh frozen plasma in dogs: 74 dogs (October through December 1999). *J Am Vet Med Assoc* 2001; **218**: 1449–1455.

35 Dixon-Jimenez AC, Brainard BM, Brooks MB, *et al.* Pharmacokinetic and pharmacodynamic evaluation of oral rivaroxaban in healthy adult cats. *J Vet Emerg Crit Care* 2016; **26**: 619–629.

36 Bae J, Kim H, Kim W, *et al.* Therapeutic monitoring of rivaroxaban in dogs using thromboelastography and prothrombin time. *J Vet Intern Med* 2019; **33**: 1322–1330.

37 Myers JA, Wittenburg LA, Olver CS, *et al.* Pharmacokinetics and pharmacodynamics of the factor Xa inhibitor apixaban after oral and intravenous administration to cats. *Am J Vet Res* 2015; **76**: 732–738.

38 He K, Luettgen JM, Zhang D, *et al.* Preclinical pharmacokinetics and pharmacodynamics of apixaban, a potent and selective factor Xa inhibitor. *Eur J Drug Metab Pharmacokinet* 2011; **36**: 129–139.

39 Mischke R, Teuber M, Tiede A. Measurements of endogenous thrombin potential using the CAT method in cats: reference values and influence of the direct factor Xa inhibitor apixaban. *Res Vet Sci* 2019; **127**: 113–121.

40 Wallace GE, McKaba VF, Reinhart JM, *et al.* Pharmacokinetics and pharmacodynamics of intravenous and oral apixaban in horses. *J Vet Pharmacol Ther* 2021; **44**: 724–732.

41 Douxfils J, Adcock DM, Bates SM, *et al.* 2021 update of the International Council for Standardization in Haematology Recommendations for Laboratory Measurement of Direct Oral Anticoagulants. *Thromb Haemost* 2021; **121**: 1008–1020.

42 Pittman JR, Koenig A, Brainard BM. The effect of unfractionated heparin on thrombelastographic analysis in healthy dogs. *J Vet Emerg Crit Care* 2010; **20**: 216–223.

43 Alwood AJ, Downend AB, Brooks MB, *et al.* Anticoagulant effects of low-molecular weight heparins in healthy cats. *J Vet Intern Med* 2007; **21**: 378–387.

44 Blais MC, Bianco D, Goggs R, *et al.* Consensus on the Rational Use of Antithrombotics in Veterinary Critical Care (CURATIVE): Domain 3-Defining antithrombotic protocols. *J Vet Emerg Crit Care* 2019; **29**: 60–74.

45 Rozanski EA, Hughes D, Giger U. The effect of heparin and fresh frozen plasma on antithombin III activity, prothrombin time and activated partial thromboplastin time in critically ill dogs. *J Vet Emerg Crit Care* 2001; **11**: 15–21.

46 Kyles AE, Feldman EC, de Cock HE, *et al.* Surgical management of adrenal gland tumors with and without associated tumor thrombi in dogs: 40 cases (1994–2001). *J Am Vet Med Assoc* 2003; **223**: 654–662.

47 Moore JN, Mahaffey EA, Zboran M. Heparin-induced agglutination of erythrocytes in horses. *Am J Vet Res* 1987; **48**: 68–71.

48 Morris TA, Marsh JJ, Konopka R, *et al.* Anti-thrombotic efficacies of enoxaparin, dalteparin, and unfractionated heparin in venous thrombo-embolism. *Thromb Res* 2000; **100**: 185–194.

49 Schwarzwald CC, Feige K, Wunderli-Allenspach H, *et al.* Comparison of pharmacokinetic variables for two low-molecular-weight heparins after subcutaneous administration of a single dose to horses. *Am J Vet Res* 2002; **63**: 868–873.

50 Fiakpui NN, Hogan DF, Whittem T, *et al.* Dose determination of fondaparinux in healthy cats. *Am J Vet Res* 2012; **73**: 556–561.

51 Monagle P, Chalmers E, Chan A, *et al.* Antithrombotic therapy in neonates and children: American College of Chest Physicians Evidence-Based Clinical Practice Guidelines, 8th edn. *Chest* 2008; **133**: 887S–968S.

52 Hirsh J, Bauer KA, Donati MB, *et al.* Parenteral anticoagulants: American College of Chest Physicians Evidence-Based Clinical Practice Guidelines, 8th edn. *Chest* 2008; **133**: 141S–159S.

53 Breuhl EL, Moore G, Brooks MB, *et al.* A prospective study of unfractionated heparin therapy in dogs with primary immune-mediated hemolytic anemia. *J Am Anim Hosp Assoc* 2009; **45**: 125–133.

54 Segura D, Monreal L, Espada Y, *et al.* Assessment of a platelet function analyser in horses: reference range and influence of a platelet aggregation inhibitor. *Vet J* 2005; **170**: 108–112.

55 Neff-Davis CA, Davis LE, Gillette EL. Warfarin in the dog: pharmacokinetics as related to clinical response. *J Vet Pharmacol Ther* 1981; **4**: 135–140.

56 Smith SA, Kraft SL, Lewis DC, *et al.* Pharmacodynamics of warfarin in cats. *J Vet Pharmacol Ther* 2000; **23**: 339–344.

57 Feige K, Schwarzwald CC, Bombeli T. Comparison of unfractioned and low molecular weight heparin for prophylaxis of coagulopathies in 52 horses with colic: a randomised double-blind clinical trial. *Equine Vet J* 2003; **35**: 506–513.

58 Mischke R, Grebe S, Jacobs C, *et al.* Amidolytic heparin activity and values for several hemostatic variables after repeated subcutaneous administration of high doses of a low molecular weight heparin in healthy dogs. *Am J Vet Res* 2001; **62**: 595–598.

59 Mischke R, Grebe S. The correlation between plasma anti-factor Xa activity and haemostatic tests in healthy dogs, following the administration of a low molecular weight heparin. *Res Vet Sci* 2000; **69**: 241–247.

60 Lunsford KV, Mackin AJ, Langston VC, *et al.* Pharmacokinetics of subcutaneous low molecular weight heparin (enoxaparin) in dogs. *J Am Anim Hosp Assoc* 2009; **45**: 261–267.

61 Mischke R, Schmitt J, Wolken S, *et al.* Pharmacokinetics of the low molecular weight heparin dalteparin in cats. *Vet J* 2012; **192**: 299–303.

62 Van de Wiele CM, Hogan DF, Green HW, *et al.* Antithrombotic effect of enoxaparin in clinically healthy cats: a venous stasis model. *J Vet Intern Med* 2010; **24**: 185–191.

63 Whelchel DD, Tennent-Brown BS, Giguere S, Epstein KL. Pharmacodynamics of multi-dose low molecular weight heparin in healthy horses. *Vet Surg* 2013; **42**(4): 448–454.

64 Schwarzwald CC, Feige K, Wunderli-Allenspach H, *et al.* Comparison of pharmacokinetic variables for two low-molecular-weight heparins after subcutaneous administration of a single dose to horses. *Am J Vet Res* 2002; **63**: 868–873.

65 Yang VK, Cunningham SM, Rush JE, de Laforcade A. The use of rivaroxaban for the treatment of thrombotic complications in four dogs. *J Vet Emerg Crit Care* 2016; **26**: 729–736.

66 Griffin A, Callan MB, Shofer FS, *et al.* Evaluation of a canine D-dimer point-of-care test kit for use in samples obtained from dogs with disseminated intravascular coagulation, thromboembolic disease, and hemorrhage. *Am J Vet Res* 2003; **64**: 1562–1569.

67 Welch KM, Rozanski EA, Freeman LM, *et al.* Prospective evaluation of tissue plasminogen activator in 11 cats with arterial thromboembolism. *J Feline Med Surg* 2010; **12**: 122–128.

68 Guillaumin J, Gibson RM, Goy-Thollot I, Bonagura JD. Thrombolysis with Tissue Plasminogen Activator (TPA) in feline acute aortic thromboembolism: a retrospective study of 16 cases. *J Feline Med Surg* 2019; **21**: 340–346.

69 Hong TT, Huang J, Lucchesi BR. Effect of thrombolysis on myocardial injury: recombinant tissue plasminogen activator vs. alfimeprase. *Am J Physiol Heart Circ Physiol* 2006; **290**: H959–H967.

70 Goggs R, Brainard BM, LeVine DN, *et al.* Lyophilized platelets versus cryopreserved platelets for management of bleeding in thrombocytopenic dogs: a multicenter randomized clinical trial. *J Vet Intern Med* 2020; **34**: 2384–2397.

71 Callan MB, Aljamali MN, Margaritis P, *et al.* A novel missense mutation responsible for factor VII deficiency in research Beagle colonies. *J Thromb Haemost* 2006; **4**: 2616–2622.

72 Sorensen B, Fries D. Emerging treatment strategies for trauma-induced coagulopathy. *Br J Surg* 2012; **99**(Suppl 1): 40–50.

73 Plumb DC. *Veterinary Drug Handbook*, 5th edn. Ames, IA: Blackwell, 2005.

74 Weiler JM, Freiman P, Sharath MD, *et al.* Serious adverse reactions to protamine sulfate: are alternatives needed? *J Allergy Clin Immunol* 1985; **75**: 297–303.

75 Ross J, Dallap BL, Dolente BA, *et al.* Pharmacokinetics and pharmacodynamics of epsilon-aminocaproic acid in horses. *Am J Vet Res* 2007; **68**: 1016–1021.

76 Kelmer E, Marer K, Bruchim Y, *et al.* Retrospective evaluation of the safety and efficacy of tranexamic acid (Hexakapron) for the treatment of bleeding disorders in dogs. *Isr J Vet Med* 2013; **68**: 94–100.

77 Brown JC, Brainard BM, Fletcher DJ, *et al.* Effect of aminocaproic acid on clot strength and clot lysis of canine blood determined by use of an in vitro model of hyperfibrinolysis. *Am J Vet Res* 2016; **77**: 1258–1265.

78 Osekavage KE, Brainard BM, Lane SL, *et al.* Pharmacokinetics of tranexamic acid in healthy dogs and assessment of its antifibrinolytic properties in canine blood. *Am J Vet Res* 2018; **79**: 1057–1063.

79 Marin LM, Iazbik MC, Zaldivar-Lopez S, *et al.* Retrospective evaluation of the effectiveness of epsilon aminocaproic acid for the prevention of postamputation bleeding in retired racing Greyhounds with appendicular bone tumors: 46 cases (2003–2008). *J Vet Emerg Crit Care* 2012; **22**: 332–340.

32 Clinical Pharmacology and Administration of Fluid, Electrolyte, and Blood Component Solutions

Amandeep S. Chohan[1] and Elizabeth B. Davidow[2]

[1] Department of Surgical and Radiological Sciences, School of Veterinary Medicine, University of California–Davis, Davis, California, USA
[2] Timberline Veterinary Emergency and Specialty, Seattle, Washington, USA

Chapter contents

Physiology of body fluids, 580
- Total body water, 580
- Solute composition of various body fluid compartments, 581
- Movement of water between intracellular and extracellular fluid compartments, 581
- Fluid shifts between intravascular (plasma) and interstitial fluid compartments, 581
- Endothelial glycocalyx model of transvascular fluid exchange and modification of Starling's equation, 582

Different types of fluids used in clinical practice, 582
- Crystalloids, 582

Perioperative fluid therapy, 588
- Liberal versus restrictive approach, 588
- Monitoring fluid balance, 589
- Individualized goal-directed fluid therapy, 589
- Improving the utility of dynamic indices of preload responsiveness, 591
- Microvasculature and fluid therapy, 591

Electrolytes, 592
- Sodium, 592
- Calcium, 593
- Potassium, 593

Transfusion therapy, 595
- Blood component therapy, 595
- Transfusion compatibility testing, 599
- Transfusion considerations for massive blood loss, 600
- Blood administration, 600
- Adverse effects of transfusion, 600

Alternatives to allogenic blood transfusions, 602
- Autologous transfusion, 602
- Blood substitutes, 603

Strategies to minimize perioperative blood loss, 603

References, 603

Physiology of body fluids

The body is principally composed of water, a triatomic molecule composed of two hydrogen molecules bound by covalent bonds to one oxygen molecule (H–O–H). Water behaves like a charged molecule: a dipole created by negatively charged oxygen and positively charged hydrogen. This polarity is responsible for imparting many of water's chemical and physical properties such as high surface tension, high specific heat, high heat of vaporization, low vapor pressure, and a high boiling point. Because of water's ionizing nature, substances dissolved in water segregate into individual components. Water also exists in an ionized form, composed of a negatively charged hydroxyl ion (OH^-) and a positively charged protonated ion (H_3O^+). The aqueous milieu created by water provides the framework where all the metabolic and enzymatic processes take place.

Total body water

Water is the single most abundant compound in the body, making up the majority of body weight. On average, water constitutes approximately 60% of adult mammalian body weight. Age, body composition, and sex can influence total body water (TBW). Neonatal animals have greater TBW compared to adults (80% versus 60%), and an age-related decrease has been described in companion animals during the first six months of life [1]. Adipose tissue has less water content compared to lean body tissues like muscle, so estimation of TBW needs to consider body condition since obesity can lead to overestimation.

To understand distribution of body water, the body fluids can be thought of as existing in two major compartments: intracellular fluid (ICF) and extracellular fluid (ECF). ECF can be further divided into two compartments: interstitial fluid (ISF) that surrounds the cells, and intravascular fluid (IVF) that is contained within the vessels. The largest volume of water in the body is contained within the cells, making ICF the largest contributor to body weight. Of TBW, about two-thirds (i.e., 40% of body weight) is ICF. The remaining one-third of TBW (i.e., 20% of body weight) is ECF where it is distributed between ISF and IVF in a ratio of 3:1. About three-quarters of ECF (i.e., 15% of body weight) is ISF that bathes the cells and one-quarter of ECF (i.e., 5% of body weight) is IVF (i.e., plasma volume).

Veterinary Anesthesia and Analgesia: The Sixth Edition of Lumb and Jones. Edited by Leigh Lamont, Kurt Grimm, Sheilah Robertson, Lydia Love and Carrie Schroeder.
© 2024 John Wiley & Sons, Inc. Published 2024 by John Wiley & Sons, Inc.
Companion website: www.wiley.com/go/lamont/anesthesia

Solute composition of various body fluid compartments

In addition to water, body fluid compartments also contain varying concentrations of different solutes (Table 32.1). This heterogeneity is because the membranes separating fluid compartments have different permeability characteristics for various solutes. The ICF and ECF are separated by cell membranes, while capillary endothelium separates ISF and IVF. Endothelium is freely permeable to water and various ionic solutes, and the concentration of these is similar in ISF and IVF. On the other hand, the cell membrane is freely permeable to water, but by utilizing various carrier proteins, active transport and passive diffusion mechanisms maintain a specific intracellular milieu, resulting in very different solute concentrations in ICF compared to ECF (Table 32.1). The Gibbs–Donnan equilibrium results in slightly different concentrations of cations and anions in the ISF and IVF (i.e., plasma), but clinically this difference is negligible and the plasma concentration of various ions is considered to be a reflection of ECF solute concentrations. The major cation in ECF is Na^+, with Cl^- and HCO_3^- being the most abundant anions. In contrast, the major cations in ICF are K^+ and Mg^{2+}, and the most common anions are organic phosphates and proteins.

Movement of water between intracellular and extracellular fluid compartments

Movement of water between ICF and ECF is governed by the osmotic gradient created by the differing concentrations of solutes between these two fluid compartments. The concentrations of solutes within a solution determine osmolality, which is dependent only on the number of particles in solution and not on their chemical formula, valence, molecular weight (MW), or size. Osmotic pressure due to solutes is expressed as milliosmoles per kilogram of water (mOsm/kg). In biologic fluids, the difference between *osmolarity* (solute osmotic concentration per unit volume of solution) and *osmolality* (solute osmotic concentration per unit mass of solvent) is not significant, and the milliosmolar concentration of a solution can be expressed as milliosmolarity or milliosmolality of solution.

Osmolality (i.e., the number of osmotically active particles) in part determines the volume of water in ECF and ICF. Solutes that cannot cross the cell membrane contribute to effective osmolality (or tonicity) and are called "effective osmoles." On the other hand, solutes that can freely diffuse across the cell membrane (like urea) are called "ineffective osmoles" and do not contribute to fluid shifts across cell membranes since they are in equilibrium on both sides of the semipermeable membrane. Osmosis is the movement of water across the semipermeable membrane from an area of lower (low solute concentration) to higher (high solute concentration) osmotic pressure.

Table 32.1 Solute composition of various body compartments.

Ions	Extracellular fluid (mEq/L)		Intracellular fluid (mEq/L)
	Interstitial fluid	Intravascular fluid (plasma)	
Na^+	145	142	12
K^+	4	5	140
Ca^{2+}	2	2	4
Mg^{2+}	2	2	34
Cl^-	112	104	4
HCO_3^-	27	24	12
HPO_4^{2-}, $H_2PO_4^-$	2	2	40
$Protein^-$	1	14	50

In both the plasma and ISF, osmolality is mainly the result of ions such as Na^+, K^+, Cl^-, HCO_3^-, glucose, and urea. Large molecules like albumin, though an important component of colloid osmotic pressure (COP), contribute little to osmolality. Being the most abundant cation in ECF, Na^+ and its associated anions are responsible for the majority of ECF osmolality. The ECF osmolality (essentially the plasma osmolality) can be estimated by using the following formula:

$$\text{Plasma osmolality (mOsm/kg)} = 2([Na^+]+[K^+]) + \frac{[\text{Glucose}]}{18} + \frac{[\text{BUN}]}{2.8}$$

where Na^+ and K^+ are expressed in mEq/L, and glucose and blood urea nitrogen (BUN) are expressed in mg/dL. Glucose is an effective osmole by not being freely permeable through cell membranes, but urea is not an effective osmole because it is freely permeable across cell membranes. The concentration of all effective and ineffective osmoles is referred to as "plasma osmolality," but the concentration of only effective osmoles refers to "effective osmolality" or "tonicity." When the concentrations of various solutes on either side of the cell membrane are not disturbed (e.g., equilibrium), the fluid is in osmotic equilibrium (same osmolality), and there is no gradient for the movement of water between the two fluid compartments. If there is extracellular loss of free water, the concentration of solutes increases in the ECF, leading to generation of higher osmolality (i.e., osmotic pressure) compared to ICF, resulting in osmotic pull causing net movement (osmosis) of water through the cell membrane into the ECF until a new osmotic equilibrium is achieved. Hence, water is lost from the ICF to replace an ECF free water deficit.

Osmolality can be either measured or calculated (as described earlier). Osmolality is measured clinically by freezing point depression of a serum sample. Normal serum osmolality is around 300 mOsm/kg. Clinically, the measured osmolality may not be equal to the calculated value, and the difference between the two (osmolal gap) can be used to predict the presence of unmeasured solutes (such as ethylene glycol and acetone).

Fluid shifts between intravascular (plasma) and interstitial fluid compartments

Fluid shifts between IVF (plasma) and ISF compartments occur at the level of capillaries. The fundamental principles that govern movement were described by Starling in 1896 [2]. Fluid movement across the capillary wall is determined by the imbalance between the osmotic absorption pressure created by plasma proteins (COP) and the capillary hydrostatic pressure. The capillary endothelial barrier slowly leaks plasma proteins into ISF. Staverman's osmotic reflection coefficient, σ, can be used to quantify the degree of leakiness of capillary membrane to any particular solute. It ranges from 1 (i.e., 100% reflection or not permeable) to 0 (i.e., no reflection or completely permeable). For a membrane separating solutions of a single solute at two different concentrations, the principle of irreversible thermodynamics states that

$$\frac{J_v}{A} = L_p[\Delta P - \sigma \Delta \pi]$$

where J_v is the volume filtration rate per unit membrane area A, L_p represents the hydraulic permeability, ΔP the difference in hydrostatic pressures, and $\Delta \pi$ is the difference in osmotic pressures across the membrane.

IVF and ISF each contain many solutes (species "n"). Therefore, to describe the movement of fluid across the capillary wall, the above equation can be written as:

$$\frac{J_v}{A} = L_p\left[\Delta P - \sum_{i=1}^{n} \sigma n \Delta \pi n\right]$$

where $\sum_{i=1}^{n} \sigma n \Delta \pi n$ represents the sum of the difference in osmotic pressure exerted across the capillary wall by all the solutes in IVF and ISF. In the above equation, ΔP describes the difference between local capillary blood pressure (P_c) and ISF hydrostatic pressure (P_i). In most microvascular beds, the capillary wall is freely permeable to water and other ionic solutes like Na^+, K^+, and glucose because of their very small σ of ≤ 0.1. In other words, they are ineffective osmoles in this scenario and do not contribute to water distribution between ISF and IVF. Only the macromolecular solutes (like proteins) with high σ, and which are present in significantly different concentrations across the capillary wall, will contribute to generation of osmotic gradients ($\sigma\Delta\pi$). If π_p is the osmotic pressure generated by plasma proteins (COP) in IVF and π_i is the osmotic pressure generated by macromolecules in ISF, then the above equation can be written as the conventional expression for Starling's equation as follows:

$$\frac{J_v}{A} = L_p\left[(P_c - P_i) - \sigma(\pi_p - \pi_i)\right]$$

Under normal circumstances, P_c is much greater than P_i, producing a hydrostatic pressure gradient at the arterial end that favors movement of fluid out of the capillary into the interstitium. Capillary blood pressure is decreased from the arteriolar to venous end of the capillary, while the π_p stays almost the same, resulting in an oncotic pressure gradient that favors the movement of fluid from the interstitium into the capillaries at the venous end [3]. Altogether there is a net filtration pressure that is responsible for the movement of water out of the capillaries into the interstitium. Some of the filtered fluid is normally returned back to the circulation via the lymphatic system.

Endothelial glycocalyx model of transvascular fluid exchange and modification of Starling's equation

As the understanding of microcapillary structure has evolved, it has been proposed that the filtration properties of the capillary wall actually reside in an endothelial surface layer (ESL) that is composed of a matrix of membrane bound complex sugars called the endothelial glycocalyx (EG). The matrix covers the intercellular clefts and the endothelial cells on the luminal side of the capillaries [4,5]. Traditional Starling's forces describe that the fluid filtered at the arteriolar end of the capillary is absorbed back into the circulation at the venous end under the influence of the dominant osmotic pressure gradient generated by the difference, $\pi_p - \pi_i$. Recently, it has been shown that the effect of π_i on fluid exchange at the capillary level is much less than predicted by Starling's original equation. It is now established that many capillaries filter fluid into the ISF throughout their length, and absorption at the venous end of the capillaries does not take place. Plasma protein oncotic pressure (COP) opposes this filtration but does not change the direction of net filtration (i.e., filtration is always occurring toward the ISF). Most of the filtered fluid returns to the circulation via lymphatics. The EG layer separates plasma from a subglycocalyx space that contains a very small amount of protein. This subglycocalyx COP (π_g) should replace π_i in the Starling's equation to determine the transcapillary flow (J_v):

$$\frac{J_v}{A} = L_p\left[(P_c - P_i) - \sigma(\pi_p - \pi_g)\right]$$

Low protein concentration in the subglycocalyx space results in a low value of π_g causing a higher value for ($\pi_p - \pi_g$), that is, a bigger opposing force against the transcapillary flow (J_v) that occurs under the influence of differences in hydrostatic pressures around the capillary membrane ($P_c - P_i$). The fact that the low value of π_g results in low J_v, coupled with the important contribution of lymph flow in various tissues in returning fluid back into circulation, are critical features on which the glycocalyx model of transvascular fluid exchange is based.

An index of vascular permeability is transcapillary escape rate of albumin (TCERA). In humans, it is about 5% of the plasma albumin per hour. This rate could double during surgery or increase 20% or more in septic patients. Evidence points to a compromised EG in those patients. Loss of plasma albumin causes reduction in π_p leading to an increase in J_v. Increasing the π_p (COP) in septic patients with synthetic or natural colloids will decrease J_v and prolong vascular expansion compared to crystalloids, though the use of artificial colloids is controversial in septic patients (see discussion below).

Different types of fluids used in clinical practice

Crystalloids

Crystalloid solutions are prepared by dissolving crystalline compounds in water. Most of the clinically used crystalloids are either polyionic sodium-based or dextrose solutions in water. Crystalloids are classified mostly based on their tonicity relative to plasma.

Isotonic crystalloids

Isotonic crystalloids have similar tonicity/osmolality compared to the plasma. This means that administration of isotonic fluids will not cause any change in the solute concentration of the ECF. There will not be any alteration in the net osmotic forces that might trigger the water movement between ICF and ECF. Hence, the isotonic crystalloid fluid will stay within the ECF, and no alteration in ICF volume will take place unless previous free water loss occurred from the ICF compartment. After intravenous administration, isotonic crystalloids stay within the ECF and redistribute into the IVF and ISF. This redistribution occurs according to the normal fluid distribution in the body so that within 30–60 min post infusion, only about one-quarter of the administered amount remains intravascular and the rest moves out to the ISF [6,7]. The most commonly used isotonic fluids and their constituents can be found in Table 32.2.

Isotonic fluids contain mixtures of various electrolytes found in plasma with or without additives, which affect the acid–base status of the patient. Some crystalloids contain dextrose. Except for physiological (or "normal") saline (0.9% NaCl), most of the commonly used crystalloids contain a precursor for bicarbonate production such as lactate or acetate and gluconate ions (Lactated Ringer's solution [LRS], or Normosol® and Plasma-Lyte®, respectively). Lactate ions undergo either oxidation or gluconeogenesis primarily in the liver, although kidneys and muscle tissues also participate to

Table 32.2 Characteristics of various isotonic crystalloids compared to plasma.

Fluid (isotonic, replacement)	Electrolytes (mEq/L)					Buffers (mEq/L)			Osmolarity (mOsm/L)	pH
	Na^+	Cl^-	K^+	Ca^{2+}	Mg^{2+}	Lactate	Acetate	Gluconate		
0.9% NaCl	154	154	0	0	0	0	0	0	308	5.0
Lactated Ringer's solution	130	109	4	3	0	28	0	0	272	6.5
Plasma-Lyte®-148	140	98	5	0	3	0	27	23	294	5.5
Normosol®-R	140	98	5	0	3	0	27	23	294	6.4
Plasma-Lyte®-A	140	98	5	0	3	0	27	23	294	
Plasma	142	104	5	5	3		HCO_3^- = 24		300	7.4

some extent. During glycogenesis, lactate is converted to glucose via pyruvate, and this process utilizes H^+. So lactate also has a bicarbonate-sparing effect. Acetate is metabolized mostly in muscle, and gluconate can be metabolized by most tissues. Because these crystalloids increase bicarbonate level in the plasma, they have been called "alkalinizing fluids." 0.9% sodium chloride, on the other hand, is an "acidifying solution" due to plasma bicarbonate dilution (dilutional acidosis) and high Cl^- content that can decrease the strong ion difference and cause hyperchloremic metabolic acidosis [8–10]. The composition of some crystalloids more closely matches plasma (e.g., LRS, Plasma-Lyte®-148, Normosol®-R) compared to others (e.g., 0.9% NaCl), and they are considered balanced isotonic crystalloids in comparison to unbalanced crystalloids. Another way of looking at crystalloids is from the standpoint of their clinical use. Most of the isotonic crystalloids, because of their similar osmolality and solute composition to plasma, do not cause osmotic water shift from blood cells to plasma and can be used for emergency volume resuscitation and are, therefore, called "replacement fluids."

To understand the clinical use of various crystalloids, it is imperative to understand which body compartment is deficient in fluid (intravascular/perfusion versus intracellular/hydration) [11]. When isotonic crystalloids are used for replenishment of IVF and electrolyte deficits, about 75% of the fluid redistributes to ISF. Therefore, relatively large volumes are usually administered to replenish intravascular deficits. In dogs, Silverstein *et al.* demonstrated the potential of isotonic fluids to increase the blood volume [12]. Immediately following the infusion of fluid, the blood volume increased by 76%, more than 3–4.5 times the increase following hypertonic fluid and colloids. However, at 30 min post infusion, the increase was only 35%. The initial increase in blood volume was attributed to the greater volume of isotonic crystalloids administered. More importantly, the authors also calculated the efficacy ratio (ER; increase in blood volume compared to the volume of fluid infused), and isotonic fluid had an ER of only 0.4 at 30 min post infusion. Typically, three to four times the deficit volume of crystalloid fluids is recommended to replenish the intravascular space.

Shock, hemorrhage, and severe volume deficit due to diarrhea, vomiting, excessive diuresis, or third spacing constitute common scenarios when these fluids are administered. Crystalloids are also administered during most elective surgery procedures in healthy patients. It is often recommended that patients with shock should receive up to one blood volume (e.g., 80–90 mL/kg in dogs) in an hour, starting with one-quarter to one-third of the shock dose given incrementally with constant monitoring for desired endpoints to guide fluid therapy further (i.e., goal-directed fluid therapy). A typical fluid rate used for patients under general anesthesia is 5–10 mL/kg/h [13,14], although recent trends have been to reduce these rates further in patients without risk factors for perioperative fluid loss.

Slight variability in composition and concentration of various solutes (electrolytes and buffers) in different isotonic crystalloids (see Table 32.2) may make administration of one solution preferable in certain clinical situations. Patients with hypochloremic metabolic alkalosis and hypercalcemia may benefit from the use of 0.9% saline [15,16]. Alkalinizing fluids are not used very commonly in adult dehydrated cattle because metabolic acidosis is not a common occurrence except in cases of grain overload, hepatic lipidosis, chronic ketosis, or kidney disease [17,18]. Patients that are acidotic may benefit from the use of alkalinizing fluids. LRS can contain either a racemic mixture of both L-lactate (i.e., *S*(+)-lactate) and D-lactate (i.e., *R*(−)-lactate), or just L-lactate. Fluids containing acetate might have a more profound alkalinizing effect, as dogs cannot metabolize D-lactate as readily [15].

Various isotonic crystalloids have different Na^+ ion concentrations, giving them a range of osmolalities (see Table 32.2). In severe electrolyte disturbances, it is recommended to use a fluid with a Na^+ concentration closest to that of the patient for resuscitation to avoid rapid changes in Na^+ ion concentration (Na^+ concentration should not change more than 0.5–1 mEq/L/h). While resuscitating patients with head trauma or cerebral edema, replacement crystalloid solutions with the highest Na^+ concentration (i.e., 0.9% NaCl) will be least likely to reduce plasma osmolality that might favor the movement of water into brain cells. With a Na^+ content of 130 mEq/L, LRS is relatively hypotonic compared to plasma and has been associated with increased intracranial pressure in some models of traumatic brain injury [19,20].

ISF accumulation/edema can occur after excessive fluid administration, especially in patients suffering from oliguric renal failure, cardiac insufficiency, head trauma, pulmonary contusions, or decreased COP. In clinical scenarios characterized by active intracavitary (abdominal or thoracic) or intracranial bleeding, aggressive fluid administration to achieve normotensive resuscitation endpoints before surgical control of bleeding is achieved could increase hydrostatic pressure and might lead to disruption of blood clots and worsening of bleeding. "Hypotensive" fluid resuscitation is often advocated in these patients, aiming to achieve the lower limit of clinically acceptable mean arterial pressure (60 mmHg, corresponding to a minimally adequate perfusion pressure of various vital organ systems). Others suggest delayed fluid resuscitation until hemostasis is achieved; however, the risk of anesthetizing hemodynamically unstable patients should be weighed against the perceived risk of volume resuscitation. The veterinarian should also be cognizant of the possibility of excessive hemodilution of clotting factors, platelets, plasma protein, and red blood cells (RBCs) when large volumes of fluid are administered [6,7,21]. This may be even more relevant in patients undergoing surgical procedures associated with more blood loss or patients that already have pre-existing coagulopathies, hypoproteinemia, or anemia.

Due to the presence of Ca^{2+} ions in LRS, it is recommended that blood products not be administered in the same fluid line since Ca^{2+} may antagonize common anticoagulants, leading to microemboli. Studies have concluded that rapid transfusion rates for whole blood (WB) or packed red blood cells (PRBCs) can be safely used with LRS [22] and that LRS can be safely used to dilute citrate phosphate dextrose preserved PRBCs in emergency settings [23]. Because of the liver's major contribution to lactate metabolism, there has been some concern about the use of LRS in patients with hepatic insufficiency. However, studies have failed to show any increase in blood lactate levels after LRS administration [24,25]. Hyperlactatemia is common in cancer patients due to use of anaerobic glycolysis by neoplastic cells, but a study in dogs suffering from lymphoma showed only a transient increase in lactate levels that became normal after 2 h of infusion of LRS [26]. Large quantities of rapidly administered acetate solutions can cause vasodilation due to release of adenosine from muscles that could cause hypotension, especially in hypovolemic patients [27–29].

Hypertonic crystalloids

Hypertonic solutions have an increased tonicity/osmolality compared to plasma. Administration of hypertonic fluids will increase osmotic pressure in the IVF and set up a gradient for the movement of water from ISF as well as ICF (with lesser osmotic pressure; lower solute concentration). The most commonly used hypertonic fluids in clinical practice are hypertonic saline solutions (HSSs; Table 32.3). The reflection coefficient of Na^+ for cell membranes is maintained close to 1 by the Na^+-K^+ ATPase pump, whereas the reflection coefficient of the endothelial membrane is only 0.1. This means that most of the movement of water after HSS administration is from the ICF rather than ISF [30]. Hence, fluid is pulled out of the cells (cellular dehydration) and interstitium into the intravascular space. Analysis of transcapillary driving pressures (governed by Starling's forces) supports an immediate plasma volume expansion under the effect of HSS that rapidly reverses the transcapillary pressure gradient from a small filtration force under normal physiologic conditions to a large absorptive force (osmotic pressure gradient). Due to a very low reflection coefficient of capillary endothelium for Na^+, the generated osmotic pressure is transmitted across the capillary endothelium to the cell membrane and is responsible for pulling the water out of cells. As HSS itself does little to address TBW deficits, it is imperative that hypertonic therapy be followed by administration of appropriate follow-up fluids (isotonic crystalloids, colloids, or blood products). In cattle, it was recommended, after using hypertonic fluids, to administer fluids ororuminally if the animal does not consume more than 5 gallons of fluid orally [17,31]. HSSs are unbalanced crystalloids and are available in various concentrations having very high osmolality compared to plasma (see Table 32.3). Clinically, 7.5% HSS is most commonly used. Although mannitol is also another hyperosmotic agent, its osmotic effects are typically delayed by 15–30 min [32] and effects are not as profound as 7.5% NaCl because its osmolarity is only half (1250 mOsm/L for 25% mannitol) as much. The discussion here will focus on HSS only.

Table 32.3 Characteristics of various hypertonic saline solutions compared to plasma.

Composition	Hypertonic saline solutions					Normal saline	Plasma
	3%	5%	7.2%	7.5%	23%	0.9%	
Na^+ (mEq/L)	513	856	1232	1283	4004	154	142
Cl^- (mEq/L)	513	856	1232	1283	4004	154	104
Osmolarity (mOsm/L)	1026	1712	1464	2566	8008	308	300

In hypovolemic animals (hemorrhagic shock models), plasma volume expansion at the end of an HSS bolus/infusion given over 1–10 min at a dose of 4–8 mL/kg varied from 10 to 21 mL/kg with higher doses causing more volume expansion. However, HSS quickly equilibrated within ECF so that after 1–3 h, there was minimal plasma volume expansion [33–36]. In normovolemic dogs, Silverstein *et al.* showed that the ER (defined as the relative increase in blood volume in relation to the volume infused) was maximum with HSS immediately post infusion (2.7 ± 0.5; approximately three times that of other fluid types) and was still higher at 30 min post infusion compared to isotonic crystalloids and synthetic colloids [12]. In order to prolong the duration of effect, HSS was combined with a colloid (6% dextran 70 [HSD]) that not only increased the extent of immediate plasma volume expansion but the plasma volume expansion persisted 3 h later [34,35]. Other available colloids like hydroxyethyl starch (HES) can also be combined with HSS. This hypertonic–hyperoncotic combination constitutes "small-volume fluid resuscitation" [17]. Usually, it is constituted by diluting 23.4% HSS with the colloid in the ratio of 1:2.5, or the two can be used separately (2–6 mL/kg of 7% HSS plus 4–10 mL/kg of colloid) [17,31].

Cardiovascular effects of HSS administration are characterized by an increase in preload, heart rate, and myocardial contractility and a decrease in systemic vascular resistance (SVR), leading to an increase in cardiac output (CO) [37–39]. Beneficial immunomodulatory effects have been described characterized by decreased interaction of neutrophils with endothelial cells, reduced neutrophilic activation, and improved activity of lymphocytes and natural killer T cells [40–42]. HSSs have also been shown to reduce cytotoxic edema and improve splanchnic and muscle capillary perfusion in animal injury models of soft tissue contusions, hemorrhagic shock, and superior mesenteric artery occlusion [43–47].

Most of the clinical and experimental literature on HSS/HSD suggests its application in the management of hemorrhagic hypovolemic shock [33–36,48,49]. Another area where HSS has been shown to be beneficial is in the management of intracranial hypertension. Although brain trauma management foundation guidelines [50] still recommend mannitol as the primary hyperosmolar therapy (Level II evidence), new evidence has been emerging that shows hypertonic saline to be a better choice [51–56]. Benefits of hypertonic resuscitation have also been documented in the canine model of gastric dilation-volvulus-induced obstructive shock [57], canine model of bile-induced pancreatitis [58], and murine models of acute pancreatitis [59,60]

Large animal practice has found HSS/HSD to be particularly helpful where the patient's large blood volume makes volume expansion challenging. Oral rehydration therapy has been suggested as acceptable if the calf or cattle is $< 8\%$ dehydrated, but a combination of HSS intravenous therapy plus oral rehydration was shown to be successful if dehydration was $\geq 8\%$ [17,31]. Use of hypertonic–hyperoncotic resuscitation has been described in horses with endotoxemia [61,62], in calves with endotoxemia [63] or diarrhea [64–66], and in adult endotoxemic cattle [67].

Use of HSS in patients with uncontrolled hemorrhage can lead to increased bleeding and worsened outcome compared to isotonic resuscitation. However, studies demonstrate that if the hemorrhage is controlled, then HSS can improve hemodynamic variables and final outcomes [68–70]. It has been shown that if a bolus of hypertonic–hyperoncotic fluid (4 mL/kg) is administered slowly (over about 12 min) compared to 1 min, blood loss was significantly reduced and survival improved [69,71].

Pre-existing dehydration has been suggested as a contraindication to administration of HSS because a dehydrated intracellular environment could decrease the efficacy of intravascular hypertonic fluid resuscitation. Studies performed in dehydrated hemorrhagic swine [72] and sheep [73,74] models with preinfusion plasma osmolalities of 325–340 mOsm/L showed that administration of 4 mL/kg of 7.5% NaCl achieved hemodynamic stability and an increase in plasma volume similar to euvolemic animals. When a rapid onset of action is desired, HSS can in fact be considered as an adjunct with isotonic resuscitation to correct hypovolemia in dehydrated patients. A recent study in endurance horses showed that horses resuscitated with 2 L of HSS followed by 5 L of isotonic saline achieved normal packed cell volume (PCV) and total protein (TP) compared to horses that received 7 L of 0.9% sodium chloride alone that demonstrated residual hemoconcentration [75]. Keeping in mind the diuresis that occurs after HSS administration and mobilization of ICF to the intravascular space with the potential to be filtered, the possibility of subsequent dehydration must be considered in veterinary patients, especially when appropriate follow-up fluid administration is delayed or impossible (e.g., some field conditions).

HSS has been associated with cardiac arrhythmias, bradycardia, hypotension, and volume overload. Such effects are noted mostly when high doses of higher concentration HSS are administered at a very fast rate [76]. The recommended administration regimen of 7.5% NaCl at a dose of 4–6 mL/kg given at a rate no faster than 1 mL/kg/min is not usually associated with complications. Use of recommended doses rarely causes any consistent blood chemistry abnormalities, but the potential for hypernatremia, hyperchloremic metabolic acidosis, hyperosmolar renal failure, and hypokalemia should be considered especially if pre-existing electrolyte abnormalities or repeated dosing with HSS are considered [8–10,21]. Ajito *et al.* [77] administered doses of 2.5, 5, and 15 mL/kg of 7.2% NaCl at a rate of 1.6 mL/kg/min to anesthetized Beagle dogs. Administering 5 mL/kg caused only transient elevations in Na^+ (153 at 3 min; 165 at 5 min; baseline 142) that returned to below 160 mEq/L at the end of infusion, whereas a dose of 15 mL/kg led to consistent hypernatremia (161–174 mEq/L) from 10 to 90 min after initiation of infusion. A study conducted in dogs showed that the maximum tolerated dose of 7.5% NaCl was 20 mL/kg, although that dose caused transient neurological signs like pacing and lethargy, which resolved within 24 h [78].

Hypotonic crystalloids

Hypotonic crystalloid solutions have lower tonicity/osmolality than plasma (Table 32.4). Dextrose in water is a source of free water because the dextrose is metabolized leaving water that is free of osmotic particles. Dextrose administration decreases ECF solute concentration compared to ICF, creating an osmotic pressure gradient for movement of water from the ECF to ICF (cellular swelling). Less than 10% of infused hypotonic fluid remains in the IVF space after 30–60 min. Due to their large volume of distribution and potential for cellular swelling, hypotonic fluids are not indicated for intravenous volume replenishment. They are used mostly to provide maintenance needs of patients in which water intake is absent because they are anorexic (no feed intake), unable to drink, and/or fluid losses are not beyond normal physiologic losses (unlike vomiting, diarrhea, etc.) [79].

Maintenance fluid requirements can be calculated in several ways [80,81]. The simple empirical formula of 40 mL/kg/day (in large dogs) or 60 mL/kg/day (small dogs and cats) can be used. Since water requirements are tied to metabolism, daily maintenance energy expenditure (and water requirement) may be calculated as 140 kcal × body weight $(kg)^{0.75}$ [80]. Another formula used to calculate maintenance water requirement is [30 × body weight (kg)] + 70, but if the patient weight is less than 2 kg or more than 50 kg, then it is proposed to use the caloric requirement to calculate the maintenance fluid requirements [80,81]. One milliliter of water is required for every kcal of energy consumed. The ongoing physiologic fluid losses may consist of insensible (feces, saliva, skin, and respiratory tract) and/or sensible (urinary) losses. These losses are typically hypotonic in nature with low Na^+ and high K^+ compared to that of ECF [81]. Hypotonic fluids are manufactured to match this composition (Table 32.4). However, in patients with normal renal function, isotonic replacement fluids with some added K^+ can also be used for maintenance purposes because kidneys can excrete excess electrolytes. This is a frequently used method in many veterinary clinics due to a combination of economic pressures to maintain low inventory as well as lack of familiarity with maintenance/hypotonic crystalloids. Other major indications for hypotonic crystalloids involve free water supplementation (e.g., hypernatremia and diabetes insipidus), dextrose supplementation during hypoglycemia, and perioperative fluid therapy for patients at risk of volume overload (i.e., congestive heart failure).

It is important to administer these fluids at a slow rate so that sudden and excessive dilution of plasma solutes is avoided as the reduced ECF osmolality could cause cellular swelling (cerebral edema). It is advisable to monitor electrolyte concentrations in patients receiving hypotonic fluids.

Colloids

Colloids are composed of macromolecular particles suspended in a crystalloid fluid solution. In the absence of increased microvascular permeability, their movement is limited across the endothelium, and they are less able to accumulate in the interstitium. This results

Table 32.4 Characteristics of commonly available hypotonic crystalloids compared to plasma.

Fluid	Electrolytes (mEq/L)					Buffers (mEq/L)			Osmolarity (mOsm/L)	pH	Glucose (g/L)
	Na^+	Cl^-	K^+	Ca^{2+}	Mg^{2+}	Lactate	Acetate	Gluconate			
0.45% NaCl	77	77	0	0	0	0	0	0	154	5.0	0
0.45% NaCl with 2.5% dextrose	77	77	0	0	0	0	0	0	280	4.5	25
Plasma-Lyte®-M with 5% dextrose	40	40	16	5	3	12	12	0	376	5.5	50
Normosol®-M with 5% dextrose	40	40	13	0	3	0	16	0	364	5.5	50
Dextrose 5%	0	0	0	0	0	0	0	0	252	4.0	50
Plasma	142	104	5	5	3		HCO_3^- = 24		300	7.4	

in a longer dwell time within the IVF compartment compared to crystalloids, and they can pull fluid into the IVF compartment based on their oncotic properties. Colloidal oncotic pressure is the osmotic pressure generated by the colloids in solution and is determined by the number of particles rather than their size. In clinical practice, colloids are mostly used in patients requiring oncotic support (hypoproteinemia) to prevent ISF accumulation or in hypovolemic patients as a resuscitative fluid [82–87]. Colloidal preparations can be classified as consisting of blood component products (discussed later in this chapter) or synthetic compounds (discussed below).

Synthetic colloids

Synthetic colloids contain compounds composed of three major groups: the hydroxyethylstarch derivatives, dextrans, and gelatins. Most of the following discussion revolves around HES solutions due to their common use in clinical practice, but some basics about dextrans and gelatins are also presented.

Hydroxyethyl starches

HESs are the synthetic colloid preparations most commonly used in both human and veterinary medicine. Chemically, HES preparations are modified polymers of amylopectin, a polysaccharide very similar to glycogen. The polymers are suspended in saline or a balanced electrolyte crystalloid solution. Different preparations of HES with variable structural characteristics (Table 32.5) have different physicochemical properties governed by three main variables: mean molecular weight (MW), molar substitution (MS), and C2:C6 ratio. It is important to understand these differences in order to appreciate the clinical variability with respect to the pharmacokinetics, pharmacodynamics, and adverse effect profile of various HES preparations [88–90]. HESs are typically identified by three numbers (e.g., 6% HES 130/0.4). The first number dictates the concentration of the solution, the second represents the manufactured mean MW in kilodaltons (kDa), and the third indicates the MS.

The concentration of HES influences the initial volume expansion. 6% solutions are iso-oncotic, and 10% solutions are hyperoncotic with considerably more volume expansion. MW is the weight-averaged (M_w) or number-averaged (M_n) size of the polymers. Since the polymers actually are of varying length (ranging from a few thousand to few million daltons), this parameter is only an average. HESs are arbitrarily classified by the manufactured mean MW into high-MW (> 400 kDa), medium-MW (200–400 kDa), and low-MW (< 200 kDa) preparations. As M_w takes into account the individual weights of different particles, it is influenced by the presence of large molecules in the system and will give a larger value compared to the M_n that represents the total weight of all the molecules divided by the number of molecules. The ratio M_w:M_n provides an index of the polydispersity (that is, the variation in particle size). It is important to understand that the given MW applies to the colloidal preparation *in vitro* because soon after these fluids are administered to a patient, the low-MW fraction is excreted by the kidneys and larger molecules are progressively hydrolyzed by serum α-amylase, resulting in a narrow distribution of MWs with an *in vivo* mean MW that is lower than the mean MW of the infused preparation. The decrease in COP after initial excretion of the low-MW fraction is partly compensated for by the availability of a greater number of small MW molecules created by metabolism (cleavage) of larger molecules.

Molar substitution (MS) describes the degree of substitution of glucose molecules with hydroxyethyl groups. This substitution increases the polymer solubility and inhibits the metabolism of the polymer by amylase. The degree of MS can be calculated in two ways. One method, termed the "degree of substitution" (DS), is calculated by the number of substituted glucose residues divided by the total number of glucose residues. With the second method, MS is calculated as the average number of hydroxyethyl residues per glucose unit. More than one substitution can occur at each glucose residue, so the MS could be higher than the DS. The value of 0.4 in the 6% HES 130/0.4 indicates that there are four hydroxyethyl residues on average per 10 glucose subunits. Based on DS, HESs have been referred to as "hetastarch" (≥ 0.7), "hexastarch" (0.6), "pentastarch" (0.5), and "tetrastarch" (0.4). The greater the MS, the harder it is to metabolize the HES.

The C2:C6 ratio describes the pattern of hydroxyethylation and also impacts the pharmacokinetics of HES preparations. Hydroxyethyl groups at position C2 of the glucose molecule inhibit the access of α-amylase to the substrate more efficiently than the C6 position. HES products with high MW, larger C2:C6 ratio, and greater MS are metabolized slowly and have prolonged persistence in plasma. Based on these physicochemical properties, HES preparations can be classified in a more clinically relevant way as slowly degradable (e.g., hetastarch) or rapidly degradable (e.g., Voluven® or Vetstarch®) preparations (see Table 32.5).

Pharmacokinetics and pharmacodynamics of various HES preparations are complex in part due to their polydisperse nature [91]. After intravenous administration, particles having MWs below the renal threshold (45–60 kDa) are quickly filtered into the urine. Additionally, small amounts diffuse into the interstitium of tissues, eventually redistribute, and are subsequently eliminated. A transient proportion is stored in tissues and degraded by the reticuloendothelial system. Larger molecules are retained in the plasma for a

Table 32.5 Characteristics of hydroxyethyl starch (HES) preparations commonly used in veterinary anesthesia.

Type of HES	HES product	Physicochemical properties					Carrier	COP (mmHg)	Osmolarity (mOsm/L)	Plasma volume expansion (%)
		Concentration	Weight (kDa)		MS	C2:C6				
			Molecular	Number average						
Rapidly degradable	Tetrastarch (Voluven®, Vetstarch®)	6%	130	70–80	0.4	9:1	Saline	High 30s	308	130
Slowly degradable	Hetastarch (Hextend®)	6%	670		0.75	4–5:1	Balanced	Low 30s	307	100
	Hetastarch (Hespan®)	6%	450	69	0.7	4:1	Saline	Low 30s	309	100

MS, molar substitution; COP, colloidal osmotic pressure.

variable period of time subject to their metabolism by α-amylase. Metabolism is, in turn, influenced by the physicochemical properties of the particular HES preparations as described earlier [88–90]. The resulting smaller fractions after metabolism are further excreted in urine. Studies in animals and humans have demonstrated significantly more accumulation of slowly degradable HES preparations compared to rapidly degradable preparations, especially after repeated administration [91]. Clearance of tetrastarches has been shown to be about 23 times faster than hetastarch and five times greater than pentastarch. The pharmacokinetics of HES have been described in dogs and horses [92–94]. Species-specific differences in plasma amylase activity have also been documented and contribute to the variable half-life of HES in different species. Relative to humans, amylase activity has been shown to be greater in dog plasma [92] and less in equine plasma [93].

The pharmacodynamics of synthetic colloid fluids are related to the volume and duration of intravascular volume expansion and may be influenced by many factors including dose, speed of administration, specific colloid preparation, microvascular permeability, species of animal, and preinfusion intravascular volume status [88–91,95]. Iso-oncotic (6%) preparations of HES have been associated with similar increase in intravascular volume compared to the volume administered, while the hyperoncotic preparations (10%) can expand volume up to 145% by pulling fluid from the interstitial space [88,89]. The initial increase in plasma volume is the result of COP of the colloidal preparation administered and is mostly attributed to the large number of small MW particles. As these smaller molecules are removed from the circulation during the first few hours, a significant decrease in COP occurs, translating clinically into reduced effect on plasma volume expansion over time. Due to the presence of the remaining large MW particles in the plasma, the concentration of the colloidal preparation (mass per unit volume) may still be quite high, but the COP will be low.

Slowly degradable preparations have a longer plasma half-life, but this does not translate into an increased duration of volume expansion. In spite of minimal plasma accumulation of tetrastarch, studies in orthopedic [96,97] and cardiac [98] surgeries have demonstrated its duration of effect (at similar concentration) to be comparable to pentastarch [99] and hetastarch [96,100]. It is important to understand that though the clearance and residual plasma concentration of HES are affected by their physicochemical properties (mainly MS and C2:C6 ratio [101]), the COP depends upon the number of osmotically active particles and not on the concentration of HES [88–90,95]. In a given volume of HES solution, there will be more particles of lower MW product compared to an HES preparation with higher MW translating into a greater COP at similar plasma concentrations.

The effect of hetastarch on COP has been described in healthy ponies and horses, hypoproteinemic dogs and horses, hypovolemic, and hypotensive dogs under anesthesia, and dogs undergoing orthopedic surgery [82,83,102–107]. Effects of various HES preparations on COP do not seem to last beyond 24 h. It is important to remember that variables like health status [104,105], pre-existing volume status [82,91,95], concurrent fluid therapy [106,108], dose [107], type of preparation [83,93,102], and anesthesia [109] all have the potential to influence plasma COP, meaning that results of different studies must be evaluated carefully. A study in horses reported that COP was higher in the group receiving tetrastarch (130/0.4) compared to hetastarch (600/0.75) but returned to baseline at 24 h [83]. Due to its ability to provide colloidal oncotic support and prolonged intravascular retention, HES has proven to be better at providing intravascular support and improvement in hemodynamic indices compared to crystalloids [82–87].

Adverse events have been associated with HES use in clinical patients. It is important to point out that results from *in vitro* studies cannot be directly extrapolated to clinical scenarios (*in vivo*) as the side-effect profile is heavily impacted by the *in vivo* pharmacokinetic behavior of various HES products and slowly degradable preparations (hetastarch and pentastarch) carry more risk compared to rapidly degradable preparations (tetrastarches) [88–90].

All types of fluids have the potential to cause dilutional coagulopathy, but the HES solutions also impact hemostasis directly by altering both primary and secondary hemostasis [88]. HES decreases the expression of platelet surface GP IIb-IIIa complex and also physically coats the surface of platelets, causing decreased interaction of agonists like soluble fibrinogen and von Willebrand factor (vWF) with this receptor, thus preventing platelet aggregation. HES also decreases factor VIII/vWF complex concentration, possibly due to accelerated elimination of this complex after binding to HES. These adverse effects have clinically translated into increased blood loss perioperatively. Use of rapidly degradable HES preparations (HES 130/0.4) caused lower blood loss in various types of surgeries in humans compared to slowly degradable HES preparations (HES 200/0.5, HES 450/0.7, and HES 600/0.75) [96,110,111]. Desmopressin has been suggested as a treatment option for mild coagulopathy associated with HES administration [112]. Studies in dogs [103,106,113–118] and horses [62,83,102,107,119] have also reported dose-related effects [107,116,117,119,120] of hetastarch and tetrastarch on platelet function and factor VIII/vWF complex [115–117,119–121] *in vitro* and *in vivo* but have failed to document increases in clinical bleeding [103,106,113]. Several of these studies documented less impact on hemostasis when tetrastarches were used [83,107,116,121]. Human studies [122,123] have shown that HES preparations formulated in a balanced carrier solution containing Ca^{2+} ions cause less impairment of hemostasis compared to 0.9% sodium-chloride-based formulations. Similar *in vitro* comparisons in dogs [115] and horses [119] did not show improved platelet function as assessed by estimation of platelet closure times. Concerns about hyperchloremic metabolic acidosis with 0.9% sodium chloride formulations have also been expressed [88].

A multicenter blinded trial in severely septic human patients revealed that HES 130/0.42 was associated with more mortality and need for renal replacement therapy compared to the Ringer's acetate group [124]. A meta-analysis in humans revealed an increased risk of acute kidney injury (AKI) in critically ill patients receiving HES preparations [125]. In dogs and cats, retrospective studies have shown conflicting impacts of HES on renal function [126–130]. One study revealed the use of 10% HES 200/0.5 and its increasing dose as a risk factor for AKI [126]. Other studies did not show any risk of AKI with 6% HES 130/0.4, but one study documented an association between the length of administration of 6% HES 130/0.4 and grade of AKI within 10 days of HES administration [127]. A case report documented exacerbation of renal dysfunction in a dog with pre-existing azotemia that received a 10 mL/kg dose of 6% HES 130/0.4 in an effort to increase its osmotic pressure [131]. A subgroup analysis in two studies specifically performed in septic small animal patients did not reveal any association between HES and AKI [129–130]. Due to different doses and types of HES products, no standardization of AKI definition, and small sample size, it is difficult to draw any firm conclusions. Experimental studies did not reveal any association between 6% HES 130/0.4 and biomarkers of AKI within 3 or 72 h post-HES bolus (20 mL/kg) administration [132,133]. Furthermore, a randomized clinical trial in dogs undergoing shock resuscitation with 6% HES 130/0.4 or Hartmann's solution did not reveal any difference in urinary biomarkers of AKI [134].

Reports indicating a low incidence of anaphylactoid reactions, increases in α-amylase level, and tissue accumulation of slowly degradable preparations causing pruritus in humans have been published [88,90]. In cats, hetastarch has been associated with vomiting if administered too rapidly.

Most of the dosage recommendations in veterinary patients are extrapolated from manufacturer's and human literature rather than veterinary-specific studies, but it seems appropriate to not exceed a dose of 20 mL/kg/day for various types of HES formulations although doses of up to 50 mL/kg/day have been suggested in the past for tetrastarches due to their relatively less negative impact on hemostasis [83,107,116,121]. Increased blood loss was reported in dogs when a > 30 mL/kg dose of hetastarch was used [135,136]. A few studies in horses have suggested a hetastarch dose of 10 mL/kg/day is well tolerated [62,93].

Dextrans

Dextrans are linear polysaccharide molecules and include a low (10% dextran 40) and high (6% dextran 70) MW preparation in 0.9% saline. Smaller molecules are removed by glomerular filtration with bigger molecules staying in circulation longer and eventually being metabolized by dextranase enzyme systems in the kidney, liver, and spleen to produce carbon dioxide and water. Due to the importance of glomerular filtration in excretion of dextrans, half-life can be increased in patients with renal insufficiency. Dextrans are hyperoncotic compared to plasma and cause plasma volume expansion that can be more than the volume infused (dextran 40 > dextran 70).

Dextrans have been used to improve microcirculatory blood flow (especially dextran 40) and as thromboprophylaxis to prevent deep vein thrombosis in humans. Complications associated with their use include anaphylactic reactions, renal function impairment (especially with dextran 40), and impaired hemostasis (inhibited platelet aggregation, dose-dependent hyperfibrinolysis, decreased levels of vWF, and factor VIII:C activity) [136–141]. They can also coat the surface of RBCs, interfering with cross-matching procedures. A maximum dose of 10–20 mL/kg/day in dogs and 5–10 mL/kg/day in cats has been suggested to minimize adverse effects.

Gelatins

Gelatins are large MW polydisperse proteins formed by hydrolysis of bovine collagen. Three modified newer generation gelatin preparations are succinylated or modified fluid gelatins, urea-cross-linked gelatins, and oxy-cross-linked gelatins (oxypolygelatins). Gelatin preparations have similar average MWs (30–35 kDa) and are supplied in concentrations of 3.5–5.5% [142]. The small size of gelatin molecules makes them susceptible to glomerular filtration, which is the main route of elimination. The half-life of oxypolygelatin has been suggested at 2–4 h in dogs [138]. The distribution of total dose administered by 24 h is 71% in urine, 16% extravascular, and 13% remains in the plasma [142]. Rapid renal excretion means less plasma retention, and though similar side effects on coagulation compared to other synthetic colloids are reported, their magnitude is less [138,143,144]. Urea-cross-linked gelatins have been associated with anaphylactoid reactions due to histamine release that were blocked by prophylactic use of histamine blockers [145]. Although there are no standard guidelines for gelatin dosages in veterinary species, a dose of 5 mL/kg for oxypolygelatin in dogs has been recommended [138].

Clinical implications of synthetic colloid use in veterinary medicine

Most of the studies in veterinary medicine have looked at the effect of HES, dextrans, and gelatins in healthy animals and have documented dose-related deterioration in both primary and secondary hemostasis but failed to show exacerbation of clinical bleeding. A meta-analysis in humans documented increased blood loss with HES compared to crystalloid therapy in perioperative settings [146], and recent human guidelines published for trauma patients recommended avoiding use of HES due to the adverse impact on hemostasis [147]. As effects of synthetic colloids on hemostasis are directly linked to their plasma concentration, it is reasonable to assume that if they are used in dosages higher than the maximum recommended, are used repeatedly, are used when there is decreased clearance (e.g., renal impairment), or are used in patients with pre-existing bleeding diatheses, the potential to increase clinical bleeding does exist.

Renal filtration is the major route of HES excretion, and urine osmolality and specific gravity are increased in dogs administered HES 600/0.75 [148]. Hyperviscosity of the urine after glomerular filtration of colloid molecules theoretically causing tubular obstruction due to stasis of urine flow seems the most likely mechanism of renal impairment [90,140,141]. A case report and a retrospective study in critically ill dogs revealed a positive association between the histopathological evidence of osmotic nephrosis and the severity of renal tubular vacuolization with administration of 6% HES 130/0.4 and cumulative dose of 6% HES 600/0.75, respectively [131,149]. Based on the present evidence [126–134,149], the use of HES in dogs and cats poses a limited risk for AKI when HESs are administered at a relatively low dose and for shorter periods of time. The possibility of renal dysfunction may exist, especially in critically ill patients with pre-existing renal compromise, warranting renal function monitoring (urine output, creatinine, BUN, etc.) and use of minimal amounts of synthetic colloids in such scenarios. Also, hyperoncotic preparations seem to potentiate this issue so it might be advisable to use iso-oncotic preparations of synthetic colloids when possible [90,140,141].

Perioperative fluid therapy

Liberal versus restrictive approach

The objective of perioperative fluid therapy is to maintain circulatory volume so that end-organ perfusion and oxygen delivery are not compromised. The traditional approach to achieving this goal entails administration of replacement crystalloids at a dose rate that could vary between 5 and 20 mL/kg/h [13,14]. This high rate of fluid administration was expected to offset the transient intraoperative hypovolemia due to fluid deprivation during preoperative fasting, vasodilation associated with anesthetic drugs, third spacing of intravascular fluids, insensible fluid losses, and intraoperative fluid or blood loss [150,151]. With emerging evidence, most of these physiologic theories are being reexamined. Present perioperative patient management does not advocate prolonged fasting times [152], with patients usually having access to water up until the time of surgery. Additionally, blood volume has been shown to stay normal even after prolonged fasting [153]. The concept of third spacing of fluids during surgery [154] and fluid loading of normovolemic patients to prevent intraoperative hypotension [155] has also been questioned.

Stress associated with surgery and anesthesia leads to neuroendocrine responses mediated by stimulation of the hypothalamic–pituitary–adrenal axis, activation of the renin–angiotensin–aldosterone system, and atrial natriuretic peptide and vasopressin release. All of these compensatory mechanisms can alter fluid dynamics independent of renal function [156]. In dogs, antidiuretic hormone concentration increased [157] and urine production decreased after morphine premedication [158], but did not change during anesthesia and surgery when patients received conventional fluid therapy [159] or increased crystalloid fluid administration [7].

Anesthesia- and surgery-related physiological effects cease or decrease at the end of surgery, possibly resulting in a patient who has been given a relatively large quantity of fluids. Postoperatively, such patients end up gaining body weight [159,160]. This positive fluid balance and weight gain mostly occurs in the ECF and has been shown to be associated with a host of abnormalities including increased lung water, decreased pulmonary function, increased infection rate, reduced gut motility, decreased PCV, decreased TP, and a decrease in body temperature eventually translating into increased morbidity and mortality [160–163]. The Confidential Enquiry into Perioperative Small Animal Fatalities (CEPSAF) revealed that cats receiving fluids (likely not goal-directed dosing) were four times more likely to die, and the authors speculated that excessive fluid administration causing fluid overload could be a cause [164]. Restrictive intraoperative fluid administration could improve postoperative pulmonary function and hypoxemia [165–167].

What constitutes restrictive or liberal fluid therapy is still a question of debate because different randomized controlled trials in humans have used different fluid regimens [168]. Evidence from human anesthesia suggests that low-risk patients undergoing low-to-moderate-risk surgery benefit from liberal intraoperative fluid therapy (20–40 mL/kg total dose) resulting in reduced postoperative complications like dizziness, pain, nausea, vomiting, drowsiness, and reduced hospital length of stay [167,169,170]. Restrictive fluid therapy in humans was shown to be beneficial in high-risk patients undergoing major abdominal surgeries [171,172] and was not associated with renal function compromise [166], but findings from a recently published large prospective randomized controlled trial on perioperative fluid therapy in humans were somewhat contradictory. The Restrictive versus Liberal Fluid Therapy in Major Abdominal Surgery (RELIEF) trial conducted in 2983 patients undergoing major abdominal surgery revealed a significantly higher incidence of acute renal injury (8.6% versus 5.0%), need for renal replacement therapy (0.9% versus 0.3%), and surgical site infection (16.5% versus 13.6%) when a restrictive fluid therapy regimen to achieve zero net fluid balance was used intraoperatively and for 24 h postoperatively [173]. Overall, median fluid volume received intraoperatively and in the first 24 h postoperatively in the RELIEF trial was ~6 mL/kg/h and ~1 mL/kg/h in the restricted group and ~11 mL/kg/h and ~1.5 mL/kg/h in the liberal group, respectively.

No impact on systolic blood pressure was noticed in dogs receiving fluid rates between 0 and 15 mL/kg/h [174], and increasing fluid rates from 0 to 30 mL/kg/h did not cause any change in urine production or oxygen delivery under anesthesia [7]. Though not based on any specific clinical evidence nor accepted universally, the AAHA/AAFP fluid therapy guidelines in dogs and cats [175] have suggested initially starting fluid administration at 3 mL/kg/h in cats and 5 mL/kg/h in dogs. In short procedures, minimal fluid volume will be administered with these suggested rates, so it is important to closely assess the patient's hydration and volume status as well as total fluid volume delivered.

Monitoring fluid balance

As measurement of ICF and ISF is not easily accomplished, estimation of IVF volume status is typically undertaken in clinical practice. There is no single variable that can assess the intravascular volume status, which creates some difficulties for application of goal-directed fluid therapy. Furthermore, it is important to do serial evaluations of a patient to optimize volume status. Clinical examination (mucous membrane color, capillary refill time, pulse rate and quality, temperature of extremities, mentation, skin turgor, moistness of mucous membranes, peripheral edema, thoracic auscultation for crackles, papilledema, respiration rate, pulse oximetry, blood pressure, urine output, and serial body weights), invasive hemodynamic monitoring to obtain objective data (direct blood pressure monitoring, CO monitoring, cardiac filling pressures including central venous pressure [CVP] and pulmonary artery occlusion pressure, pulse pressure variation [PPV] and stroke volume variation [SVV], and transesophageal echocardiography), and laboratory data (arterial and venous blood gases, electrolyte status, and renal function evaluation) all should be used in conjunction to estimate the volume status. Information on various macrovascular (CVP, arterial blood pressure, and urine output) and microvascular (lactate concentration and clearance, base excess, and mixed or central venous oxygen saturation) perfusion parameters help dictate the state of critical oxygen delivery to the tissues [176,177]. Early goal-directed therapy to normalize some of these endpoints has been shown to improve outcomes [178].

Therapy with synthetic colloids should ideally be monitored using colloid osmometry to measure COP rather than relying on the refractometric analysis because the relationship between COP and refractive index may be different for plasma proteins versus synthetic colloid [179]. There is a poor correlation between the changes in COP and TP as measured by a refractometer after administration of a high-MW HES formulation (hetastarch) and dextran 70. Both of these synthetic colloids push the refractometric reading toward 4.5 g/dL [180]. Recently published studies in dogs showed that low-MW 6% HES 130/0.4 formulation (VetStarch®) and 4% succinylated gelatin can also interfere with refractometric measurement of total plasma protein, pushing its reading toward 4.3 g/dL, and this interference could last up to 3 h [181,182]. Refractometric total solids (TS) readings could decrease after colloid administration due to dilutional effects, and this could be falsely interpreted as a need for additional colloidal support, leading to fluid overload [95].

Individualized goal-directed fluid therapy

The eventual goal of fluid administration is to improve venous return resulting in an improvement in stroke volume (SV). Venous return depends on the gradient between mean circulatory filling pressure (MCFP) and right atrial pressure and the resistance to blood flow in venous circulation. Physiologically, about 70% of the blood volume is *unstressed* (volume of blood in the vasculature at zero transmural pressure) and the remainder is *stressed* (volume of blood that must be removed from the vasculature to drop transmural pressure to zero from existing values) [183]. The stressed volume is a major determinant of venous return and is responsible for generating blood flow by increasing transmural pressure across blood vessels resulting in increased MCFP [184,185]. An unpredictable distribution of administered fluids between stressed and unstressed volumes may in part be responsible for fluid unresponsiveness in certain patients as only about 50% of critically ill human patients respond to fluid challenge with a significant increase in

SV [186,187]. It is important to recognize patients that are not fluid responsive (non-responders) to avoid ineffective or deleterious fluid overloading [188]. Although no standard fluid therapy guidelines have been devised as yet, an individualized fluid therapy approach called "individualized goal-directed therapy" based on objective feedback from a patient's fluid responsiveness has been shown to improve outcomes [189–192].

At the core of fluid responsiveness is the Frank–Starling curve [193,194]. In the case of responders, the heart is operating on the ascending part of this curve and they respond with a 10–15% increase in their SV or CO when a fluid bolus is administered to augment the preload [195,196]. The Marik–Philips curve illustrates the relationship between preload and extravascular lung water (EVLW) [197]. Non-responders operate on the flat part of the Frank–Starling curve resulting in minimal improvement in SV, but, at the same time, the administered fluid results in an increase in EVLW and tissue edema. These curves are influenced by changes in patient physiology imposed by various diseases that necessitate an individualized approach to fluid therapy. Although considered simultaneously, it is important to appreciate the distinction between volume status and fluid responsiveness since a patient that is fluid responsive may not be hypovolemic and vice versa due to changes in vascular permeability, capillary leakage, changes in cardiac function, vascular tone, and complex local and systemic implications of EG damage. Assessment of fluid responsiveness can minimize unnecessary fluid administration, especially in patients predisposed to fluid overload, and may aid in ascertaining the need for inotropic and/or vasopressor therapy.

Both static and dynamic indices of preload responsiveness have been described. A parameter is considered static if it is measured at a single time point, whereas a dynamic parameter is measured in real time in response to a change in preload. Based on the Frank–Starling curve, an increase in SV may be expected with fluid administration if the preload is low. This is why the markers of cardiac preload were proposed to predict fluid responsiveness. However, studies have shown that CVP, pulmonary capillary occlusion pressure, and end-diastolic dimensions of the ventricle are unreliable and generally late indicators of fluid overload, alterations in blood volume, and fluid responsiveness [194,198]. CVP is a poor indicator of right atrial pressure, cardiac filling pressure, and preload changes because the pressure and volume relationship of the ventricle is not linear and CVP is affected by lung, cardiac, and intrathoracic pressures [199,200]. In dogs, it was also shown that CVP performs poorly compared to dynamic indices to evaluate fluid responsiveness [201,202]. The filling pressures may still be helpful to evaluate volume status of the patient such that a low value may justify fluid administration and a high value should prompt stopping or reducing the fluid administration. Originally, pulmonary artery catheterization (PAC) was used to guide optimal oxygen delivery in high-risk surgical patients but, due to morbidity and mortality increases associated with the use of the PAC itself, and failure to show any clear benefit, it fell out of favor [203–205].

The position of cardiac performance on the Frank–Starling curve is best understood by performing functional hemodynamic testing or the use of heart–lung interactions in mechanically ventilated patients by evaluating respiratory variation in various dynamic indices of preload responsiveness [195,196,206–210]. Functional hemodynamic testing involves administration of an intravenous fluid bolus or performance of a passive leg raise maneuver to shift volume into the central circulation and augment preload [195,196,211,212]. It is desirable to use as small a fluid bolus as possible to assess fluid responsiveness to further minimize the potential for fluid overload. A meta-analysis in humans revealed that a mini-fluid challenge can successfully predict fluid responsiveness [213]. A mini-fluid bolus approach has been reported in dogs using 3–5 mL/kg LRS or Hartmann's solution administered over 1–5 min [213–217], but the use of 10–20 mL/kg LRS bolus over 5–15 min was reported most often [202,218–222]. Colloids have also been used for fluid challenges in humans [223], and this has been reported in one dog study that used 10 mL/kg of 6% HES 130/0.4 as a fluid bolus that was administered over 13 min [201]. Various veterinary studies have reported a fluid responsiveness rate anywhere from 38% to 100% in healthy and normovolemic dogs under anesthesia [214,201,217,219,221, 222], in dogs undergoing anesthesia for orthopedic or oncologic surgery [220,218], or dogs undergoing abdominal surgery [202]. The variation in fluid responsiveness could be the result of different patient populations, size of the fluid bolus, rate of bolus administration, and modality used to evaluate the change in CO or SV [223,224].

A change in arterial blood pressure is commonly used in veterinary clinical settings as a surrogate for changes in SV or CO, but it is important to appreciate the limitations of this assumption as alterations in SVR may have significant impacts on arterial blood pressure in hypotensive and/or hypovolemic patients [224,225]. Studies in spontaneously breathing anesthetized dogs have demonstrated the inability of mean arterial pressure to discriminate between fluid responders and non-responders in spite of an increase in CO or SV [201,202,216,220–222]. Various modalities to measure CO have been utilized in anesthetized dogs to evaluate fluid responsiveness including transpulmonary thermodilution [219,221,222], transesophageal echocardiography [218,220], transthoracic echocardiography [201,214–216], uncalibrated pulse contour analysis (PCA) [217], and esophageal Doppler [202]. Many minimally invasive and non-invasive flow monitoring modalities provide real-time, continuous, and beat-by-beat SV information that is particularly useful when response to a fluid challenge needs to be evaluated. These modalities hold the potential for clinical utility in veterinary medicine, but they should be thoroughly evaluated for their agreement and trending ability with a reference method to measure SV and CO [226,227]. An uncalibrated PCA method does not require any calibration with a reference method, but its performance may suffer during hemodynamic instability and when significant changes in SVR occur [228]. The pressure recording analytical method (PRAM) (incorporated into Most Care Up®) is an uncalibrated PCA method that showed good precision and trending ability with bolus pulmonary artery thermodilution (PATD) CO measurement in dogs under stable circulatory conditions [229] and has been recently used to measure a response to a small volume fluid bolus in dogs [217]. However, in dynamic circulatory conditions created by a hemorrhagic shock dog model [230], and use of various sympathomimetics [231], PRAM revealed a high bias, low precision, and low concordance when compared with bolus PATD CO measurement. Another uncalibrated PCA device (FloTrac/Vigileo®) was found unsuitable to monitor CO in dogs when it was compared with indicator dilution techniques [232,233]. Other non-invasive methods to measure CO, like electrical velocimetry [234] and pulse wave transit time [235], have also been evaluated in dogs.

Different variables related to aortic blood flow have been evaluated in dogs using Doppler technology that could yield information about CO and have been studied in the context of fluid responsiveness [214,215,221,236]. In anesthetized dogs, a > 14.7% change in the velocity time integral (VTI) after a fluid challenge as measured by transthoracic echocardiography tracked closely to the change in SV (> 15%) measured by transpulmonary thermodilution, suggesting that change in the aortic VTI may serve as a surrogate marker for change in SV to predict fluid responsiveness [221]. Another study in conscious dogs with a variety of clinical conditions revealed that an aortic flow VTI of ≤ 10.3 cm showed a sensitivity of 84.6% and a specificity of 100% to predict fluid responsiveness [215]. Although CO obtained from an esophageal Doppler monitor did not show good agreement with bolus PATD CO [237], an abstract in dogs reported a correlation coefficient of 0.9 between the bolus PATD SV and stroke distance (SD) (i.e., the VTI obtained from the descending aorta by the esophageal Doppler) in a hemorrhagic dog model, suggesting that changes in SD may serve as a surrogate marker of changes in SV induced by fluid challenge [236]. Furthermore, the SD variation increased with hemorrhage and decreased when the blood was retransfused. The same abstract showed an increase in descending aortic peak velocity index with hemorrhage and a decrease when the blood was retransfused. Two more studies in dogs revealed significantly higher aortic peak velocity in responders compared to non-responders with one study showing an area under the receiver operating characteristic curve of 0.95 for prediction of fluid responsiveness, suggesting that changes in aortic blood flow peak velocity could provide information about fluid responsiveness [214,215].

Heart–lung interactions are a dynamic index of volume responsiveness that do not require fluid administration and rely on respiratory variation in preload caused by cyclic alterations in pleural and transpulmonary pressure during mechanical ventilation [202,206–210,238,239]. Reduction in venous return during inspiration with positive-pressure ventilation is the major determinant of the variation in these dynamic indices. According to the Frank–Starling principle, diastolic filling of the ventricles determines the myocardial stretch and hence SV as related to myocardial contractility. In hypovolemic states, the variation in dynamic indices is high, and the left ventricular contractility depends on the preload to a greater extent. In other words, the ventricle operates on the ascending limb of the Frank–Starling curve. As the volume expands, the left ventricular function shifts in the rightward direction on the Frank–Starling curve and causes an observed decrease in dynamic indices variation.

Preload changes result in stroke volume variation (SVV) during inspiration and expiration. In addition, it has been shown that pulse pressure variation (PPV) and systolic pressure variation (SPV) can be used as surrogate markers of SVV and could be easily employed in clinical settings where arterial catheters are placed and patients are ventilated mechanically [202,207–210]. The plethysmographic variability index (PVI) is a non-invasive dynamic index of preload responsiveness that evaluates changes in perfusion index as obtained by a pulse oximeter (Masimo™ Radical-7®) [202]. Various canine studies have suggested that SVV > 11–14.7% [217,239], PPV > 7–16% [201,202,217,219,220,240], SPV > 4.1–7.4 mmHg [217,220], PVI > 11–14% [201,202,217,241], and caudal vena cava distensibility index of 24% [214] predict fluid responsiveness with good sensitivity and specificity. A few human and canine studies have suggested PPV to be a better index of fluid responsiveness compared to SPV and PVI [202,208,217].

An abbreviated echocardiogram ("cardiac point-of-care ultrasound") is also being used increasingly due to its rapid, non-invasive, and real-time ability to evaluate patient volume status [242]. Estimation of volume status mostly focuses on the subjective assessment of atrial and ventricular lumen size, ventricular wall thickness, and cardiac contractility, all of which require minimal training to learn [243,244]. Studies performed in dogs and cats revealed these changes to be proportional to the severity of hypovolemia [245].

Improving the utility of dynamic indices of preload responsiveness

The difference in cutoff values, sensitivity, and specificity of various dynamic indices among different studies is a reflection of a lack of standardization of the volume and rate of fluid administration and ventilatory parameters, including tidal volume, peak inspiratory pressure, and positive end-expiratory pressure, and is also affected by patient–ventilator asynchrony, changes in respiratory system compliance, changes in vascular tone, arrhythmias, right heart failure, and intra-abdominal hypertension [223,246–251]. The proportion of responders to fluid bolus has not been shown to be influenced by the type of fluid [223]. In clinical veterinary settings, tidal volumes are often altered, patients may buck the ventilator, many patients undergo minimally invasive laparoscopic procedures coupled with increased intra-abdominal pressure, and critically ill patients may have cardiac arrhythmias or be exposed to vasoactive drugs to support arterial blood pressure. In order to improve the utility of published thresholds for dynamic indices, it is important to understand the context of the published study and the clinical scenario in which the dynamic index will be employed.

One should refrain from interpretation of these tests in isolation since they are not 100% sensitive and specific. Every patient has an individual set of Frank–Starling and Marik–Philips curves that are influenced by various physiological and pathological factors. Understanding of the individual's physiology should allow clinicians to estimate the impact of fluid administration in patients but obviously without absolute certainty. Also, it is important to understand that fluid responsiveness does not equate to fluid requirement unless there is clear cut evidence of benefit to a patient's hemodynamic status as well as a lack of associated risks and various confounding factors [252–255]. Administration of fluids to the point of lack of fluid responsiveness could lead to fluid overload and hemodilution that could be detrimental to the patient [255].

Microvasculature and fluid therapy

Arterioles, capillaries, and venules are the structural components of the microcirculation and are the conduit of oxygen and nutrient delivery to the tissues. As described above, the endothelial glycocalyx (EG) is a protective layer of carbohydrate scaffold that coats the luminal surface of endothelium and plays a vital role in cell signaling and transvascular permeability [4,5,256]. The EG is composed of proteoglycans, glycosaminoglycans, and glycoproteins. Together with the mobile or soluble protein components, including albumin and antithrombin, it constitutes the ESL. The ESL regulates vascular permeability and controls local inflammation. Its system-wide degradation has been associated with severity of illness, increased vascular permeability, and exacerbated systemic inflammation via soluble heparan sulfate and low-MW hyaluronan that are shed into the circulation after EG damage [257–258]. Though clinicians rely heavily on the measurement of macrocirculatory perfusion parameters like CO and arterial blood pressure, it has been demonstrated that despite their normalization, heterogeneity in capillary blood flow could still persist [259,260]. There is evidence that ESL degradation can alter microcirculation resulting in reduced capillary blood flow [261].

EG biomarkers are components of the ESL that are released into circulation after degradation and data supports an association between the concentration of biomarkers like hyaluronan, syndecan, and heparan sulfate and the volume of fluid administered (that is, excessive fluid therapy itself degrades the ESL). Inflammation and shock can result in ESL degradation even before any fluid therapy is administered via proinflammatory cytokines like tumor necrosis factor-α, matrix metalloproteinases released by activated leukocytes, ischemia and reperfusion, reactive oxygen species, and bacterial components like lipopolysaccharides. Hemodilution caused by crystalloids leads to a reduction in ESL thickness and an increase in vascular permeability. In addition, bolus fluid therapy results in degradation of the EG and increased vascular permeability due to release of atrial and brain natriuretic peptides (ANP and BNP) from the atria and ventricles during myocardial stretch [262,263]. Fluid loading in human surgical patients resulted in a parallel increase in ANP and EG biomarkers syndecan-1 and hyaluronan in serum [264]. A rapid volume expansion with a balanced isotonic crystalloid in a canine hemorrhagic model, however, did not show an increase in ANP but did reveal an increase in hyaluronan concentration and enhanced inflammatory response indicated by increased plasma concentrations of interleukin-6 and interleukin-10 [265].

Although the clinical relevance of ESL degradation with fluid therapy is not yet clear, it may promote microcirculatory dysfunction, inflammation, and coagulation. It is therefore advisable to avoid excessive hemodilution and hypervolemia. Careful fluid titration should be considered in septic patients suffering from vasodilation and microcirculatory dysfunction due to lack of hemodynamic coherence between the macro- and microcirculations [259,266,267]. At the same time, caution is advised in restricting fluid volume in non-septic patients as a recent randomized controlled trial revealed a higher rate of AKI and surgical site infection in patients receiving restrictive fluid therapy [173]. There is also some evidence that rapid fluid administration may result in more heterogeneity in microcirculatory blood flow and higher inflammatory cytokines due to amplified EG degradation; slower fluid administration may help achieve similar endpoints without deleterious effects on the EG [268,269].

The question about the type of fluid (crystalloids or colloids) to be used for volume expansion has long been debated. The relatively higher efficacy of colloids to restore intravascular volume has been shown in patients without systemic disease [270]. However, more recent clinical studies in systemically ill people have failed to support these findings and suggested a colloid-to-crystalloid volume expansion ratio of 1:1 to 1:1.5 [271]. Damage to the EG caused by systemic illness results in fluid extravasation of both colloids and crystalloids resulting in loss of the volume efficacy effect of colloids [272,273]. In addition, the duration of the volume expansion by colloids is reduced under systemic inflammatory conditions due to increased vascular permeability. Although there is some evidence that colloids may be associated with less ESL degradation [274–276], altering the fluid choice to optimize microcirculation based on its potential beneficial or detrimental impact on ESL is premature. In the absence of any clear-cut benefit on mortality, the human literature does not advocate the use of one over another type of fluid [277].

Electrolytes

Sodium

Sodium is the most abundant cation in the ECF (see Table 32.1). Embedded in the cell membrane, Na^+-K^+ ATPase maintains a relatively low intracellular concentration of Na^+. The concentration of Na^+ in the serum is a reflection of the amount of Na^+ relative to total ECF and does not provide any indication about the content of total body sodium. Disorders of sodium are mostly the result of changes in the amount of body water so changes in Na^+ concentration should be viewed as changes in free water content of the body. In response to changes in intravascular volume, antidiuretic hormone (ADH), signals from baroreceptors and osmoreceptors, thirst mechanisms, the renin–angiotensin–aldosterone (RAAS), and ANP all act accordingly to promote homeostasis of volume and tonicity of body fluids via regulation of Na^+ and water balance [278].

Hypernatremia could result from hypotonic dehydration (resulting in hypovolemic hypernatremia), a deficit of free water (resulting in normovolemic hypernatremia), or ingestion or iatrogenic administration of high sodium-containing fluids (resulting in hypervolemia) [279]. Hypernatremia results in cellular dehydration (especially of brain cells) as water moves from the ICF to the ECF. Shrinking of brain tissue can cause tearing of blood vessels, resulting in subarachnoid and intracerebral hemorrhage [278].

The pathophysiological consequences of hypernatremia are determined mainly by the rapidity of onset of hypernatremia rather than the absolute value. Under chronic circumstances (> 2–3 days), brain cells increase intracellular osmolality by accumulation of osmotically active solutes called "idiogenic osmoles" [280,281]. Lien *et al.* [281] found that hypernatremia in rats increased concentrations of myoinositol, bataine, glycerophosphorylcholine, phosphocreatine, glutamine, glutamate, and taurine in the brain. Idiogenic osmoles help maintain intracellular volume and prevent efflux of fluid. Hence, in chronic hypernatremia, rapid correction of the sodium level could decrease extracellular osmolality and favor the movement of water into brain cells, causing cerebral edema. If hypernatremia is of relatively acute onset (< 24 h), rapid correction is better tolerated because idiogenic osmoles are not yet present.

Intracranial hemorrhage and neuronal dehydration associated with hypernatremia could result in muscle weakness, lethargy, ataxia, seizure, coma, and death [279]. Treatment should involve correction of the underlying problem and fluid administration to replenish free water content. In hypovolemic hypernatremic patients, intravascular volume deficits should be corrected using a fluid that is isotonic to the patient followed by correction of the free water deficit with fluids like 5% dextrose or 2.5% dextrose in 0.45% saline [282]. The formula given below is used to calculate the free water deficit (FWD):

$$\text{FWD} = [(\text{Serum Na}^+/140) - 1] \times \text{Body weight (kg)} \times 0.6$$

It is recommended that in cases of chronic hypernatremia, free water deficits should be corrected slowly over 48–72 h so that Na^+ concentration does not decrease at a rate that exceeds 0.5 mEq/L/h to avoid cerebral edema.

Hyponatremia can result from gain of free water or loss of sodium. Variable pathophysiology could result in hyponatremia that may be characterized by normal osmolality (e.g., pseudohyponatremia), hyperosmolality (e.g., extreme hyperglycemia), or hypo-osmolality (seen most commonly clinically). Hyponatremia with hypo-osmolality could be further divided into hyponatremia with hypovolemia (e.g., gastrointestinal losses, third space loss, Addison's disease, etc.), hypervolemia (e.g., congestive heart failure, cirrhosis, nephrotic syndrome, etc.), or euvolemia (e.g., myxedema coma, administration of hypotonic fluids, syndrome of inappropriate secretion of ADH [SIADH], etc.) [278,283]. In people and dogs, SIADH is characterized by secretion of ADH in the absence of hyperosmolality or hypovolemia and may cause hyponatremia [284,285]. In perioperative settings, SIADH has been associated with the use of various anesthetic drugs including opioids [284,286]. Sympathetic stimulation due to pain associated with surgical procedures can also cause ADH release in the absence of volume contraction. All these factors can lead to renal retention of water and development of hyponatremia in surgical patients [278]. Transurethral resection of prostate (TURP) syndrome is an established cause of hyponatremia in human anesthetic patients due to intravascular absorption of irrigation fluids causing hypotonic hyponatremia [287]. However, a case series describing a small number of dogs undergoing this procedure did not show hyponatremia [288].

Pathophysiological consequences of hyponatremia depend on its rate of development. A decrease in serum sodium concentration can generate an osmotic gradient across the blood–brain barrier that would cause movement of water into brain cells causing cerebral edema. Clinical signs typically do not develop unless the concentration drops below 125 mEq/L and include ataxia, vomiting, depression, seizures, and coma [289]. During chronic hyponatremia, the recommended Na^+ correction rate is not more than 0.5 mEq/L/h. If correction is faster, higher plasma osmolality can cause efflux of water from brain cells (cellular dehydration), producing the clinical syndrome of osmotic demyelination or central pontine myelinolysis [290,291]. Treatment of hyponatremia will partly depend upon the volume status of the patient. An approach using 3% saline has been described for correction of hyponatremia [284].

Calcium

Calcium is a divalent cation involved in many biologic processes, of which its effects on cardiac smooth muscle, vascular smooth muscle, and blood coagulation are particularly important to the anesthesiologist [292]. In addition, calcium is involved in skeletal muscle contraction, neuronal conduction, synaptic transmission, and hormone secretion and acts as a major intracellular messenger required for many cellular functions. Approximately 99% of the total body calcium is stored as hydroxyapatite in the skeletal tissue, and the rest is divided between the ICF and ECF compartments. Calcium exists in three biologic forms: (1) in plasma as ionized or free calcium (iCa^{2+}); (2) complexed or chelated to phosphate, sulfate, bicarbonate, citrate, and lactate; and (3) protein-bound calcium [293]. The biologically active form is the iCa^{2+}. The serum level of calcium is controlled by parathyroid hormone (PTH), calcitonin, and calcitriol (1,25-dihydroxycholecalciferol). These hormones act at the level of bone, kidneys, and gastrointestinal tract to regulate calcium homeostasis [292].

Hypocalcemia is common in critically ill small animal patients, in horses suffering from colic, and sick cattle and has been shown to carry a poor prognosis [18,31,61,294,295]. Inhalant anesthesia decreases total and ionized calcium concentrations in horses [296,297]. Hypocalcemia could occur due to impaired PTH release (primary and secondary hypoparathyroidism, post-thyroidectomy, post-parathyroidectomy), impaired calcitriol synthesis (acute or chronic renal failure, malabsorptive syndromes, liver insufficiency, etc.), and chelation of serum calcium (sodium phosphate enemas, bicarbonate therapy, blood products containing citrate, ethylene glycol toxicity, saponification of fat in pancreatitis or steatitis, etc.) [292,295,298]. Hypoalbuminemia/hypoproteinemia could decrease total calcium concentration though formulas traditionally used to correct total calcium concentration for changes in albumin concentration have been shown to be erroneous, and it is advisable to always measure iCa^{2+} concentration [299].

The severity of clinical signs depends upon the magnitude and the rapidity of onset of hypocalcemia. Pathophysiological consequences are due to a decrease in threshold membrane potential (TMP) resulting in increased membrane excitability as neural membranes become more permeable to sodium. Hyperkalemia and hypomagnesemia potentiate the cardiac and neuromuscular effects of hypocalcemia [283]. Clinical signs are attributable to neuromuscular irritability and include tetany, seizures, restlessness or excitation, facial rubbing, muscle tremors, tachycardia, hyperthermia, hypotension, and cardiopulmonary arrest [283]. The electrocardiogram may reveal a prolonged QT interval. Symptomatic acute hypocalcemia should be treated with calcium gluconate (10% solution at a dose of 0.5–1.5 mL/kg), administered intravenously slowly over 15–20 min with continuous heart rate and rhythm monitoring.

Hypercalcemia could result from increased resorption of calcium from bones (hyperparathyroidism, hypercalcemia of malignancy, etc.), increased absorption from the gastrointestinal tract (hypervitaminosis D, granulomatous diseases, antipsoriasis creams, vitamin D rodenticides, etc.), or decreased renal excretion (acute or chronic renal failure) [283]. Hydrogen ions can compete with iCa^{2+} for binding sites on albumin, hence acidemia can increase ionized calcium concentration [300]. Hypercalcemia can result in neuromuscular, cardiovascular, gastrointestinal, renal, and skeletal muscle abnormalities [283,292]. Clinical signs may be characterized by nausea, anorexia, constipation, abdominal pain, polyuria, polydipsia, and soft tissue mineralization [283]. Electrocardiographic changes are characterized by QT interval shortening, prolonged PR interval, and a widened QRS complex.

Treatment of hypercalcemia should involve correction of dehydration, promotion of calciuresis, inhibition of bone resorption, and treatment of the underlying disease process [283,292]. Calcium-free fluids, especially 0.9% NaCl, are preferred as they competitively inhibit renal tubular calcium reabsorption [283]. Once the patient is properly hydrated, use of a loop diuretic (furosemide) can be considered to promote calciuresis with regular monitoring of serum electrolytes. Additionally, glucocorticoids, bisphosphonates (pamidronate, etidronate disodium, etc.), and calcitonin could be used to treat some tumor-associated hypercalcemias and decrease bone resorption [283,292]. Effects of various drugs used during anesthesia, including CNS and cardiovascular effects, can be influenced by changes in calcium concentration, including inhalant anesthetics, local anesthetics, and non-depolarizing muscle relaxants [292].

Potassium

Potassium is the most abundant intracellular cation (see Table 32.1). About 95% of total body potassium is present intracellularly with only 5% in the ECF. Clearly, the routine measurement of plasma potassium concentration gives little indication of total body potassium content. Plasma potassium concentration is a reflection of intake (nutrition), gastrointestinal loss, renal function, and transcellular potassium shifts [301]. The major causes of hyperkalemia involve increased intake (mostly iatrogenic overadministration of potassium-containing fluids), decreased renal excretion (urethral obstruction, ruptured bladder, anuric or oliguric renal failure, hypoadrenocorticism, drugs, etc.), translocation from ICF to ECF (acute mineral acidosis, insulin deficiency, tumor lysis syndrome, drugs, reperfusion injury, hyperkalemic periodic paralysis, etc.), and pseudohyperkalemia (hemolysis especially in Japanese dog breeds, thrombocytosis, and samples collected in Na^+/K^+ EDTA) [301,302]. In addition, hyperkalemia has also been documented in two Greyhounds [303], a Rottweiler [304], and large felids during general anesthesia [305,306].

The normally high gradient between ICF and ECF potassium is maintained by the Na^+-K^+ ATPase pump. In the resting state, permeability of the cell membrane is approximately 100 times higher for K^+ than Na^+ ions and the resting membrane potential (RMP) is largely determined by the intracellular to extracellular K^+ gradient as described by the Nernst and Goldman-Hodgkin-Katz equations [307]. Most of the effects seen due to alterations in ECF [K^+] are the result of alterations in the RMP, which may have a profound impact on electrophysiologic function particularly noticeable in excitable cell membranes like cardiac tissue [308].

Hyperkalemia results in a decreased concentration gradient of K^+ across the cell membrane, resulting initially in an increased or less negative RMP, causing cell membrane excitability to increase due to a reduced gradient between RMP and threshold membrane potential (TMP). If the RMP reaches TMP, then depolarization occurs. This results in opening of voltage-gated fast Na^+ channels causing an influx of Na^+ ions. The number of voltage-gated fast Na^+ channels that open during generation of the action potential (phase 0) is influenced by the RMP. If the RMP is less negative than normal at the start of depolarization, some voltage-gated fast Na^+ channels remain in the inactivated (closed) state, decreasing the rate of rise of phase 0 of the action potential (V_{max}) due to reduced magnitude of inward Na^+ current [309–311]. As ECF [K^+] continues to rise, depression of myocardial conduction results as the proportion of voltage-gated fast Na^+ channels participating in generation of inward Na^+ current to cause depolarization are reduced. The decrease in V_{max} results in slowing of impulse conduction through the myocardium and prolongation of membrane depolarization resulting in prolonged duration of P wave, PR interval, and QRS complex on the electrocardiogram. Atrial and ventricular myocytes are more sensitive to the effects of hyperkalemia compared to the sinoatrial node, atrioventricular node, and internodal fibers due to their dependence on voltage-gated fast Na^+ channels, whereas depolarization in nodal tissues is dependent upon slow Ca^{2+} channels [312]. During phases 2 and 3 of the cardiac action potential, the inward rectifying potassium current (I_{Kr}) is responsible for K^+ efflux and is sensitive to the ECF [K^+] [313]. As the levels rise, the K^+ conductance through these currents is increased, resulting in more K^+ leaving the myocytes per unit time. It leads to an increase in the slope of phases 2 and 3 causing shortening of the repolarization time. This has been speculated to result in early electrocardiographic changes associated with hyperkalemia, characterized by tenting of T waves, shortening of the QT interval, and ST segment depression [314,315].

Clinical signs include muscle weakness and cardiac toxicity that is especially apparent at concentrations > 7.5 mEq/L. Concurrent hypocalcemia, hyponatremia, acidemia, and hypovolemia can exacerbate the cardiac deterioration at lower concentrations [283,301,308]. Changes in the electrocardiogram due to hyperkalemia have been described [308], and the mechanism for these changes has been discussed earlier. As the concentration of potassium in ECF increases from mild to severe, changes in the electrocardiogram are characterized by increasing amplitude and narrowing of the T wave (tenting), shortening of the QT interval, prolongation of the PR interval, widening of the QRS complex, decreasing amplitude and widening of the P wave, disappearance of the P wave, atrial standstill, extreme bradycardia, sinoventricular rhythm and eventually sine wave appearance of the QRS complex, followed by ventricular fibrillation or ventricular asystole. These ECG changes are inconsistent and influenced by other variables including acid–base balance, rate of K^+ increase, and concurrent electrolyte anomalies [308,316]. It should also be noted that various tachyarrhythmias are possible with mild increases in plasma potassium concentrations.

Treatment involves use of calcium salts for cardiac protection, initiation of movement of potassium from ECF to ICF, and removal of potassium from the body via diuresis with fluids or relief of urinary obstruction if present [301]. Peritoneal dialysis or hemodialysis are viable options for refractory hyperkalemia [283]. Although the use of potassium-free fluids in patients with hyperkalemia has been suggested, in cats with urethral obstruction, there was no difference in the rate of reduction of potassium with either Normosol®-R or 0.9% sodium chloride [317]. Intravenous administration of calcium raises the TMP so that the gradient between the RMP and TMP is re-established, resulting in restoration of membrane excitability. Calcium therapy starts to work within minutes and the response typically lasts anywhere between 30 and 60 min [301]. A slow bolus administration (10–20 min) of 10% calcium gluconate at a dose of 50–150 mg/kg (0.5–1.5 mL/kg) with continuous monitoring of the ECG should be considered as fast administration could cause bradycardia. Approximately one-third of the dose should be administered if calcium chloride is used [283].

Calcium administration does not do anything to lower the potassium concentration. To move the potassium intracellularly and decrease the serum potassium concentration, intravenous dextrose can be administered with or without insulin, though dextrose alone is slow to resolve hyperkalemia and may not be fully effective. Insulin facilitates the movement of glucose into the cells and potassium moves in the same direction (intracellularly), though an independent mechanism resulting in Na^+-K^+ ATPase pump activation (especially in the muscles) has been suggested [318]. Regular crystalline insulin should be used at a dose of 0.25–0.5 U/kg of body weight. Dextrose (dilute 50%) at a dose of 2 g (4 mL) per unit of insulin administered should be given simultaneously. Onset of treatment effect is about 30 min and it could last for about an hour [188]. The potential for iatrogenic hypoglycemia exists with insulin-dextrose therapy and once initial stabilization is achieved, dextrose supplementation may be required until euglycemia is reached. Intravenous administration of sodium bicarbonate results in alkalosis that in turn causes hydrogen ions to move from ICF to ECF and potassium moves into the ICF in exchange. The recommended dose is 1–2 mEq/kg, but concerns about paradoxical cerebrospinal acidosis, hyperosmolality, and the patient's ability to ventilate should be considered beforehand. Also, bicarbonate therapy will cause hypocalcemia that may be counterproductive if calcium salts have been used for their cardioprotective effects [283]. Therapy takes effect in about 15 min and could last for an hour. Use of a β_2-adrenergic receptor agonist has been described to treat hyperkalemia by stimulating the Na^+-K^+ ATPase pump that occurs independent of insulin [319].

Hypokalemia is the result of dilution (from potassium-depleted fluids), decreased dietary intake, increased urinary excretion (chronic renal failure, postobstructive diuresis, diuretics, mineralocorticoid excess, etc.), increased gastrointestinal loss (vomiting, diarrhea), and intracellular shift (alkalosis, glucose/insulin-containing fluids, β-adrenergic receptor agonists, etc.) [283,301,320]. Refractory hypokalemia could occur in the presence of hypomagnesemia [281]. Clinical signs of hypokalemia are characterized by neuromuscular function disturbances due to hyperpolarization, especially when the concentration is below 2.5 mEq/L, and include cervical ventroflexion, respiratory paralysis, anorexia, vomiting, decreased gastrointestinal motility, and lethargy [283,321]. Electrocardiographic abnormalities could include ST segment depression, decreased amplitude or inversion of T wave, increased P wave amplitude, and prolonged PR and QRS intervals, but life-threatening arrhythmias are uncommon [283]. Treatment involves parenteral supplementation with potassium chloride or potassium phosphate as additives to the crystalloids. It is important to remember that potassium supplementation rate should generally not exceed 0.5–1 mEq/kg/h because of cardiotoxic effects of potassium on cardiac conduction [283]. If potassium-supplemented fluids are used during anesthesia, it is important to have another catheter placed with a second fluid bag attached without additional potassium in case there is a need for fluid bolus administration. In addition, careful mixing of fluid bags with added potassium should be accomplished to avoid accidental potassium bolus.

Transfusion therapy

While crystalloids and synthetic colloids can provide cardiovascular support by improving hemodynamic variables, in situations of significant blood loss or coagulopathy, blood products become necessary. However, blood products are costly, have a more limited shelf-life, need specific storage conditions, and are highly immunogenic due to the presence of biologic products like proteins and cells (transfusions can be considered a liquid transplant). Thus, it is important to adequately determine when a transfusion is necessary, which components are needed, and how to best deliver the blood safely. There are limited publications in the veterinary literature specifically about use of transfusions in the perioperative period and during anesthesia. However, an understanding of available blood components and their usage, indications for autologous transfusions, and new information about transfusions in situations of massive blood loss can help guide practice.

Blood component therapy

Red blood cell products

Red blood cell (RBC) products are indicated in anemic patients to improve their oxygen-carrying capacity. Oxygen delivery (DO_2) is the product of cardiac output (CO) and arterial oxygen content (CaO_2):

$$DO_2 = CO \times CaO_2$$

where $CaO_2 = (PaO_2 \times 0.003) + (SaO_2 \times Hb \times 1.34)$. In this equation, PaO_2 is partial pressure of oxygen in arterial blood, SaO_2 is saturation of hemoglobin with oxygen in arterial blood, and 1.34 is the number of milliliters of oxygen each 1 g of hemoglobin (Hb) can carry.

The transfusion trigger is the concentration of hemoglobin below which the DO_2 decreases to an extent that anaerobic metabolism starts. Although there is still a deficiency of literature defining a transfusion trigger in human surgical patients with substantial blood loss, in stable anemic patients RBC administration is recommended when the hemoglobin concentration falls below 6 g/dL (corresponding to a PCV of approximately 18% in most species as Hb occupies 1/3 of the RBC) [322]. In small animals, it has been suggested that a PCV of 15–18% may be a reasonable transfusion trigger [323]. In euvolemic cattle, a hemoglobin level of 5 g/dL (i.e., a PCV of ~15%) is recommended, and in cattle undergoing surgery, having pulmonary disease or in late pregnancy, a transfusion trigger value of 7 g/dL (i.e., a PCV of ~21%) has been suggested [324]. A PCV of 20% has been suggested as the transfusion trigger in horses [325].

However, the use of only the hemoglobin level or PCV as a transfusion trigger should be avoided, and any decision to transfuse should be based on an individual patient's intravascular volume status, presence of ongoing bleeding, signs of organ ischemia, duration (acute versus chronic), extent of anemia, and cardiopulmonary physiologic parameters [322]. In acute settings, animals lack the compensatory changes that occur during chronic anemia such as (1) a right-shifted oxyhemoglobin dissociation curve due to increased synthesis of 2,3-diphosphoglycerate (2,3-DPG) (facilitating oxygen release to tissues); (2) diversion of blood flow away from skeletal, skin, and splanchnic circulation toward coronary and cerebral circulations secondary to alterations in sympathetic tone; and (3) recruitment of capillaries to facilitate tissue oxygen extraction [326]. Conversely, in the face of chronic anemia, some compensatory adaptations to chronic anemia may be diminished by the cardiovascular side effects of anesthesia.

Intraoperative blood loss can be monitored by visual assessment of the surgical field, estimating the amount of blood on the drapes and floor, and collecting and weighing gauze and lap sponges. The amount of blood on gauze and lap sponges can be estimated by subtracting the weight of dry gauze and lap sponges from the weight of blood-soaked ones (assuming 1 g weight = 1 mL of blood). If no lavage fluid is used, the volume of blood collected in the suction bottle can be measured directly. If the bottle contains a mixture of blood and fluid, the following formula can be used to estimate blood loss [327]:

$$\text{Blood loss (mL)} = \frac{\text{PCV of suctioned fluid} \times \text{Volume in canister (mL)}}{\text{Preoperative patient PCV}}$$

It is also helpful to look at blood loss as a percentage of the total blood volume to estimate severity, as animals under anesthesia are often not as able to compensate for significant blood loss as an awake patient can. Profound hemodynamic changes occur in anesthetized animals when approximately 15–20% of their blood volume is acutely lost and its impact on oxygen delivery may be more profound because of depressed cardiovascular reflexes under anesthesia [82,328].

Traditional transfusion triggers are based on PCV, and allowable blood loss will be greater in patients with a high PCV at the start of anesthesia. However, intraoperative changes in PCV and TS can be difficult to interpret in the face of intraoperative fluid therapy and the timing of measurement after blood loss. When whole blood (WB) is lost acutely, the ratio of RBCs to plasma stays the same. The PCV only begins to decline after intraoperative fluid administration or after IVF shifts, and other compensatory mechanisms result in plasma volume expansion and hemodilution [324]. Often a drop in TS will be the first sign of acute blood loss as splenic contraction may maintain the hematocrit initially. Alternatively, a decrease in PCV and TS due to fluid administration in a surgery without significant hemorrhage may represent hemodilution, and a better estimate of actual blood loss may be obtained by rechecking the values after fluid redistribution has occurred (often several hours later).

Monitoring for indices of inadequate perfusion and oxygenation should not only involve standard intraoperative monitoring like blood pressure, heart rate, electrocardiography, and pulse oximetry but should also include lactate, base excess, mixed venous saturation/central venous saturation, and/or echocardiography when applicable [176,177,322,325]. It has been shown that blood loss under anesthesia may decrease CO without the expected changes in heart rate and blood pressure due to blunting of the baroreceptor response [328].

Thus, these standard cardiovascular parameters monitored in veterinary anesthesia may not identify the severity of blood loss. Careful monitoring of physical blood loss as described above in conjunction with perfusion parameters like lactate and base excess may yield a better perspective on compromised oxygen delivery and need for improved oxygen-carrying capacity.

Various reasons for transfusion of WB or PRBCs in veterinary patients include anemia due to blood loss, hemolysis, and erythropoietic failure [329–335]. Once the decision has been made to provide RBCs, there are several products that can be chosen.

Fresh whole blood

Fresh whole blood (FWB) is commonly used in clinical veterinary medicine due to its ready availability from in-house donors. It has all the components of blood including RBC, plasma proteins, platelets, and labile and stable coagulation factors. If held at room temperature, it should be used within 4–6 h of collection due to the potential for bacterial growth [323]. Its use should be restricted to patients with massive blood loss or those that are missing multiple components. FWB can be transfused at varying rates depending on the rate of blood loss and size of the volume deficit. The dose can be estimated as each 2 mL/kg will raise the PCV by 1% [336,337], or more precisely calculated using the following formula where blood volume is estimated to be 88 mL/kg in a dog, 80 mL/kg in a horse, and 66 mL/kg in a cat [323,325]:

$$\text{FWB (mL)} = \frac{[\text{PCV}_{\text{required}} - \text{PCV}_{\text{recipient}}]}{\text{PCV}_{\text{donor}}} \times \text{Body weight (kg)} \times \text{Blood volume (mL/kg)}$$

If not used within 6 h, FWB can be stored in a refrigerator at 1–6 °C for 28 days if CPDA-1 is used as a preservative, or 30 days if acid citrate dextrose (ACD) is used.

Stored whole blood

Stored refrigerated WB retains its ability to form a strong clot through the first 14 days of storage. Although canine refrigerated platelets lose activity over time, the ability to aggregate into a strong clot is not lost until after day 14 [338]. After day 14, stored WB is best used for supplementing oxygen-carrying capacity in a hypoproteinemic patient or a patient with lost circulatory blood volume. The dose can be calculated as for FWB.

Packed red blood cells

PRBCs are prepared by separating the RBCs from plasma using a hard spin in a refrigerated centrifuge. Units of PRBCs contain RBCs, a small amount of plasma, white blood cells (WBCs), platelets, and a small amount of anticoagulant. A unit of PRBC obtained from a unit of WB contains approximately the same oxygen-carrying capacity as a unit of WB but in a smaller volume. Transfusion with PRBCs is indicated in patients that need improvement in their oxygen-carrying capacity but are otherwise normovolemic and have no clotting abnormalities. In severe thrombocytopenia, risk of bleeding is also affected by degree of anemia, and RBCs can reduce the risk of bleeding in such patients by scavenging nitric oxide, leading to an increase in platelet activity. The higher hematocrit following PRBC administration can push the platelets toward the endothelial wall to improve contact and increase production of thromboxane by platelets at the injury site and help reduce shear stress [339,340]. If initial collection of PRBC is done in CPDA-1, the product can be stored at 4 °C for approximately 20 days. If nutrient additive solutions are added, the storage time can be extended (35 days with Nutricel® or Optisol® and 37 days with Adsol®) [323]. The hematocrit of PRBC products can vary considerably, but for dogs, if the PCV of PRBC is approximately 60%, then the volume required to raise the recipient PCV can be calculated as below [341]:

$$\text{PRBC (mL)} = 1.5\ \text{mL} \times \text{Desired\%increase in PCV} \times \text{Body weight (kg)}$$

If the PCV is higher, the formula listed above for WB can be used.

Plasma products

Plasma products are indicated perioperatively to treat significant coagulopathy. These may be used prophylactically in patients with known coagulopathies or perioperatively if active bleeding occurs. The type of product used depends on the coagulopathy being treated.

Fresh frozen plasma

Fresh frozen plasma (FFP) is plasma separated by a hard spin from WB that is frozen within 8 h of collection. In addition to plasma proteins and clotting factors, FFP is rich in labile clotting factors V and VIII and vWF. Units of FFP can be stored up to 1 year in a freezer maintained at −20 to −30 °C and can be used prophylactically prior to surgery in patients with known significant inherited or acquired coagulopathies. They can also be used perioperatively if active bleeding due to coagulopathy occurs and prothrombin time (PT) is greater than 1.5 times normal, activated partial thromboplastin time (APTT) is greater than 2 times normal, or international normalized ratio (INR) is greater than 2 [322]. Units of FFP can be thawed at room temperature or in a warm water bath maintained at 37 °C. They should be placed in a sealed plastic bag before placement in a water bath to prevent contamination of the ports. The recommended dosage for treatment of vitamin K antagonist rodenticide toxicity is 10–20 mL/kg [342] and 15–30 mL/kg is required to treat coagulopathy associated with hemophilia A or von Willebrand disease (vWD) [343].

Frozen plasma

If FFP is stored for more than 1 year it is called "frozen plasma" (FP). If, at initial separation from WB, it is not frozen within 24 h or if the FFP is thawed and refrozen, then too it is called "frozen plasma." It differs from FFP in the lack of labile clotting factors V and VIII and vWF. Units of FP can be kept frozen at −20 °C for 5 years from the date of collection. Though the labile clotting factors and anticoagulant proteins are not active, FP can be used for treatment of vitamin K-dependent (factors II, VII, IX, and X) coagulopathies like rodenticide toxicity [323,344]. Also, it can potentially be used as a source of albumin to provide COP support [323].

Cryoprecipitate (cryo)

Cryoprecipitate (cryo) can be prepared from FFP within 12 months of collection. It is formed by slow thawing at 0–6 °C. A white precipitate forms and both the plasma and precipitated fractions are separated by centrifugation and refrozen. The precipitated fraction is called "cryoprecipitate" and serves as a concentrated source of labile factors V and VIII, vWF, and fibrinogen. It should be used within 12 months from the date of initial blood draw. Cryoprecipitate is the treatment of choice for prophylaxis or active bleeding in dogs with hemophilia A or vWD [343,345,346]. Recommended dosing for cryoprecipitate is 1 unit per 10 kg of body weight. A lyophilized commercial canine cryoprecipitate product is available that can be stored for 18 months in the refrigerator prior to rehydration (Canine Cryoprecipitate, Lyophilized, Animal Blood Resources International, Stockbridge, MI).

The supernatant produced in the process of procuring cryoprecipitate is called "cryo-poor plasma" (CPP). This blood product lacks labile clotting factors but still contains the non-labile factors II, VII, IX, and X, so it can be used for the treatment of coagulopathies associated with rodenticide toxicity [347].

Albumin products

Albumin constitutes 50–60% of the total plasma protein and provides 75–80% of COP in healthy animals. It also has other important physiologic functions including transport of various substrates and drugs, buffer capacity, scavenging of free radicals, mediation of coagulation, and wound healing [348]. Many critically ill patients suffer from hypoalbuminemia that could result in ISF accumulation including pulmonary edema, impaired wound healing, improper transport of various anesthetic drugs, hypercoagulability, and systemic organ dysfunction [349,350]. Hypoalbuminemia has been associated with a poor prognosis in both human and veterinary patients. In critically ill patients, the relationship between albumin and COP is not as predictable as expected and edema formation results from complex pathophysiological processes involving changes in capillary permeability, lymphatic function, plasma COP, albumin kinetics, and extracellular matrix structure. The most common form of species-specific albumin supplementation for COP support has been in the form of plasma transfusions. However, a large volume of plasma will be required to supply a relatively small amount of albumin; it is estimated that 22.5 mL/kg of plasma will be required to raise the albumin level by 0.5 g/dL [323]. Consequently, a large amount of fluid will accompany the plasma transfusion that potentially could lead to transfusion-associated circulatory overload (TACO). Two concentrated forms of albumin, human serum albumin (HSA) and canine serum albumin (CSA), have been used as sources of albumin in veterinary species. The use of bovine serum albumin in dogs has also been described [351].

Human serum albumin

Use of HSA has been reported mostly in small animal patients though its use in horses has also been described [352–357]. Use of 25% hyperoncotic and 5% iso-oncotic preparations have been reported in retrospective studies in critically ill small animal patients [352–355] and prospectively in healthy animals [358–360].

The prospective studies in healthy dogs [358–360] were undertaken to study any potential adverse effects with the use of HSA. In these studies, a few dogs developed immediate hypersensitivity reactions (anaphylactoid reactions) characterized by vomiting, facial edema, tachypnea, collapse, and hypotension. In addition, some dogs developed delayed hypersensitivity reactions 5–13 days after the initial transfusion characterized by facial edema, limb edema, pruritus, shifting limb lameness, vomiting, lethargy, inappetence, ecchymoses, lymphadenopathy, diarrhea, and cutaneous lesions indicative of vasculitis. Two of the dogs in one study suffered fatal consequences [358]. The delayed hypersensitivity was shown to be characterized by antigen–antibody complex deposition in various tissues, a characteristic of type III hypersensitivity [356,358,360]. Also, HSA transfusion led to a prolonged immunoglobulin E (IgE) immune response in healthy dogs as shown by positive intradermal testing [360].

Initial retrospective studies conducted in critically ill small animal patients receiving HSA showed fewer adverse reactions. In a study conducted by Mathews and Barry [352], out of 64 dogs and two cats, facial edema was reported in only two dogs while transfusing HSA, but no information was available about delayed reactions. Another study conducted in 73 critically ill dogs showed no fulminant anaphylaxis but minor complications in 27% of animals characterized by tachypnea, tachycardia, increased body temperature, peripheral edema, and ventricular arrhythmias [353]. Delayed reactions were seen in three dogs 5–14 days after administration characterized by edema, urticaria, lameness, pyrexia, vomiting, cutaneous lesions, and generalized pain. A recent study in 418 dogs and 170 cats using 5% HSA showed diarrhea, hyperthermia, or tremors in 43.5% of dogs and 36.5% of cats but there were no severe hypersensitivity reactions [350]. However, a more recent report identified delayed type III hypersensitivity reaction with acute kidney failure and death in two dogs given HSA for septic peritonitis [355]. Given the severe sequelae, HSA should only be considered in severely compromised small animal patients where all other options have been exhausted.

Canine serum albumin

Fortunately, CSA is now available (Lyophilized canine albumin, Animal Blood Resources International, Dixon, CA). The product is derived from canine source donor plasma using a heat shock process. It is available as a lyophilized preparation in 5 g vials that can be reconstituted with sodium chloride solution. It can be used as a hyperosmotic 16% solution (166 mg/mL) or an iso-osmotic 5% (50 mg/mL) preparation. The 16% solution can be used in hypotensive patients with low albumin concentrations with a goal of achieving acute volume expansion and maintenance of intravascular volume.

The use of CSA in postoperative management of dogs after source control surgery for septic peritonitis has been reported [361]. Fourteen dogs were divided into two groups with one group receiving CSA and the other group receiving clinician-directed therapy (CDT). They used 800 mg/kg of 5% CSA for 6 h in the CSA group. Doppler blood pressure, albumin concentration, and COP were significantly higher at 2 h post infusion, and the albumin concentration was significantly higher at 24 h post infusion in the CSA group compared to the CDT group. No difference was noticed in COP at the 24 h time point. Both groups received similar amounts of crystalloids and synthetic colloids during their hospitalization. The authors speculated that HES (COP 32.7 mmHg) administration during subsequent hospitalization masked the effect of 5% CSA (COP 22 mmHg) on COP. Only one dog showed an increase in respiration rate during the transfusion that resolved with slowing of the administration rate. Two safety studies of two different CSA products have been conducted in healthy purpose-bred Beagle dogs which were given a dose of 1 g/kg repeatedly for several weeks [362,363]. Two dogs had minor reactions. One dog, during the second weekly infusion, developed pallor and prolonged capillary refill time that resolved on slowing the infusion and another vomited once during its second infusion and had no other signs. The investigators concluded that healthy dogs tolerated the repeated infusion well without any evidence of physical or biochemical abnormality.

In spite of the favorable experimental data and physiologic benefits from the use of albumin, literature in human medicine has not been able to demonstrate significant benefits with its use for initial resuscitation over sodium chloride solution in terms of improvement in morbidity and mortality [364,365]. However, albumin is recommended as the colloid of choice in patients with sepsis and septic shock. It also appears useful in conjunction with furosemide in treatment of acute lung injury and in support of patients with cirrhosis and severe ascites [366].

Platelet products

Platelet transfusions in human patients are done for prophylactic as well as therapeutic purposes. A prospective study in humans revealed that out of 7401 platelet transfusions performed in 503 patients, about 74% were prophylactic in nature, 18% were therapeutic, and 8% were administered prior to surgery or invasive procedures in patients with coagulopathy or at high risk of bleeding [367]. In the perioperative setting, prophylactic platelet transfusion should be considered if the platelet count is $< 50 \times 10^9$/L [322]. The need for therapy, including any prophylactic treatment in patients with platelet counts in the range of $50–100 \times 10^9$/L, should be based on potential for platelet dysfunction, anticipated or ongoing hemorrhage, and the risk of bleeding in a confined space (e.g., brain) [322]. Platelet transfusion may be indicated in patients with normal platelet counts if there is suspected or known platelet dysfunction (e.g., antiplatelet drug exposure or congenital thrombopathies).

Aside from invasive procedures associated with high risk of bleeding, in humans, platelets are recommended for prophylaxis only if the count is $< 10 \times 10^9$/L [368,369]. In actively bleeding patients, therapeutic platelet transfusion is warranted if the count is $< 20 \times 10^9$/L [368,369].

In veterinary medicine, the indications for platelet transfusions are similar but specific platelet products are used less commonly due to issues with storage and expense. WB is the most readily available veterinary blood product that serves as a source of platelets and should be used within 8 h of collection. While the platelets in FWB last longer in circulation, canine platelets in stored WB maintain activity for up to 14 days [338]. WB should ideally be used in patients that are anemic and also have thrombocytopenia or thrombocytopathia. A dose of 10 mL/kg is expected to raise the platelet count by 10,000/μL [370,371]. In non-anemic patients, this volume of transfused RBCs may lead to polycythemia and volume overload. Advantages of using FWB are that no platelets are lost during processing and there is less activation of platelets than if they were obtained by centrifugation [371].

Platelet-rich plasma

Platelet-rich plasma (PRP) is produced from FWB using a "soft spin" centrifugation technique. The supernatant plasma contains the platelets and is separated from the PRBCs [370]. The recommended dose of PRP is 1 unit per 10 kg of body weight. Use of WB to produce PRP has also been described in cattle and horses [372].

Platelet concentrate

Platelet concentrate (PC) can be prepared from PRP by "hard spin" centrifugation. The supernatant (platelet-poor plasma) is expressed into a satellite bag attached to the PRP bag, leaving about 35–70 mL of concentrated platelets. A canine study revealed a mean platelet yield of 8×10^{10} per unit of PC and that about 25% of platelets are lost during the process of making PC from FWB [373]. The use of automated blood cell separators for canine plateletpheresis has been described that gave a mean platelet yield of 3.3×10^{11} platelets in a mean collected volume of 246 mL [374]. The recommended dose of PC is 1 unit per 10 kg of body weight and a maximum rise in platelet count of 40,000/μL is expected [370]. Fresh platelet products, including both PRP and PC, are stored at 20–24 °C with gentle continuous or intermittent agitation for 5 days when prepared using a closed collection system [370]. Despite evidence of a short life span *in vivo*, cold-stored (refrigerated) platelets retain hemostatic capability and use is increasing in human trauma medicine [375].

Frozen platelet concentrate

Frozen PC can be made by stabilizing apheresed platelets with 6% dimethyl sulfoxide (DMSO) or 2% DMSO and ThromoboSol® (a mixture of amiloride, adenosine, and sodium nitroprusside, second messenger effectors that inhibit platelet function) [376]. Valeri *et al.* showed that canine platelets preserved with 6% DMSO and kept at −80 °C for 1 year had a 70% recovery rate with a half-life of 2 days versus 3.5 days for fresh platelets [377]. Moreover, the platelets were effective in stopping clinical bleeding in thrombocytopenic dogs [378]. Another canine study revealed 49% platelet recovery when preserved with 6% DMSO compared to 44% with 2% DMSO and ThromboSol®. The half-life was approximately 2 days compared to 3.8 days for fresh platelets [376]. Because the platelets retain the ability to be activated with a reasonable half-life, they hold promise for the management of life-threatening bleeding in severely thrombocytopenic or thrombocytopathic dogs. Cryopreserved platelets with 6% DMSO are available in the veterinary market (Leukoreduced Frozen Canine Platelet Concentrate, Animal Blood Resources International, Dixon, CA). The recommended dose is 1 unit/10 kg body weight given over 4 h. Studies evaluating this commercial product indicated a decreased recovery rate of platelets at 59% and increased activation of platelets as indicated by flow cytometry and aggregometry [379,380].

Lyophilized platelets

Lyophilized platelets (LYO) are stabilized using an aldehyde cross-linking of membrane proteins and lipids and then lyophilized. Units of LYO can be stored in a refrigerator for up to 2 years and can be reconstituted with 0.9% sodium chloride immediately before administration [381]. Experimental data show that LYO act like normal platelets (as demonstrated by binding to collagen, damaged endothelium, vWF, and the cell membrane receptors), are activated normally, and bind fibrinogen [382,383]. In an experimental canine model of thrombocytopenia and platelet dysfunction induced by cardiac bypass, an infusion of LYO led to improvement in venous bleeding times that peaked at 20–30 min after infusion compared to the control group [384]. An initial prospective multicenter trial compared the use of LYO and PC in 37 dogs with thrombocytopenia and evidence of active bleeding [385]. Twenty-two dogs received LYO and 15 received PC. The incidence of transfusion reactions was low in both groups and there was no difference in hospitalization time and mortality between groups. A commercial canine LYO product using trehalose-stabilized platelets was available (StablePlateRX, Bodevet, Rockville, MD) but is currently off the market. A prospective multicenter trial compared the use of this LYO with cryopreserved platelets for control of bleeding in thrombocytopenic dogs. Eighty-eight dogs were enrolled with 50 receiving LYO and 38 receiving CPP. At 1 h post-administration, both the bleeding score and hematocrit had improved more in the LYO group; and LYO were non-inferior compared to CPP for bleeding score and hematocrit at 24 h, change in platelet count, need for additional RBC units, and survival to discharge [386]. There is also potential for LYO to be used as a hemostatic agent even if the platelet count and function are normal. In a swine model of liver injury, administration of LYO led to 80% survival compared to 20% in the placebo group [387]. One of the pigs in the LYO group had evidence of thrombi in other locations on necropsy indicating the risk of thromboembolic potential.

Transfusion compatibility testing

Once the decision has been made to transfuse, compatibility testing should be undertaken if the transfusion is not an emergency. If excessive bleeding is a risk, typing and cross-matching should be considered prior to surgical procedures.

Blood typing

Blood groups are based on the expression of RBC surface antigens and are important in transfusion compatibility. The number and type of significant blood groups varies among different domestic animal species.

Dogs

In dogs, recognized blood types include dog erythrocytic antigen (DEA) 1, 3, 4, 5, and 7 [323,388,389]. The DEA 1 system is the most antigenic. Due to the absence of naturally occurring alloantibodies, the first transfusion from a DEA 1-positive donor to a DEA 1-negative recipient should not cause an immune reaction to the erythrocytes. However, the second such transfusion will often lead to a severe hemolytic reaction if enough time has elapsed to allow an immune response to develop [390]. It has been shown that naturally occurring alloantibodies are present in some dogs for DEA 3, DEA 5, and DEA 7 [323,391–393]. These alloantibodies can result in transfusion reactions that are usually mild or delayed and a significantly shorter half-life of transfused RBCs may be noticed [394]. At present, a dog is considered a universal donor if it is DEA 4 positive and negative for all the other DEA antigens. Dal, a more recently discovered antigen, exists at a high frequency in dogs but is missing in some Dalmatians and also in some other breeds [395,396]. *In vitro* antibodies against Dal induce a strong agglutination reaction and could cause a severe transfusion reaction. Kai is another recently discovered antigen [396]. Based on population prevalence, it has been speculated that DEA 1 compatibility testing could decrease the risk of acute transfusion reaction by 24% and, by decreasing exposure to other DEA systems, the risk of acute and delayed transfusion reactions could be reduced by an additional 8% [323]. In-house blood typing kits are available for DEA 1 and are recommended for dogs prior to transfusion when at all possible. The Association of Veterinary Hematology and Transfusion Medicine (AVHTM) Transfusion Reaction Small Animal Consensus Statement (TRACS) strongly recommends using DEA 1-negative blood for DEA 1-negative dogs and DEA 1-positive blood for DEA 1-positive dogs. DEA 1-negative can be given to a DEA 1-positive blood in an emergency or if DEA 1-positive blood is not available [397].

Cats

Cat blood group types include A, B, and AB. An additional feline blood group antigen, Mik, has also been identified [398]. Distribution of these blood types varies geographically with the highest prevalence of type B reported in Australia (36% of the population) [399]. The incidence of type B has been reported at 6% in the United States [400]. Blood group B is more prevalent among some pure-bred cats, including Birman (18%), Devon Rex (41%), Cornish Rex (31%), British Shorthair (36%), and Scottish Fold (19%) [401]. Type AB has been reported to occur in less than 1% of the general cat population, although the prevalence may actually be higher, as new typing methodologies appear better at identifying these cats [402]. Blood type A cats may have low titers of natural alloantibodies that can cause shortened RBC survival if type B blood is given. On the other hand, type B cats have naturally occurring alloantibodies against type A in high titers and that can cause a fatal reaction even if 1 mL of type A blood is transfused [403,404]. Type AB cats have neither alloantibody but should receive either AB or A type RBC products because of the strong anti-A alloantibodies present in type B blood products. Most cats have the Mik antigen, but in cats without Mik, naturally occurring alloantibodies can lead to a hemolytic transfusion reaction even without having received a previous transfusion [398]. In simple terms, the likelihood of a severe transfusion reaction is much higher in cats compared to dogs if an unmatched transfusion is performed. In-house typing kits are readily available for cats and it is strongly recommended that all cats are typed prior to transfusion and given type-specific blood [397,405].

In cases where transfusion is necessary and either no feline blood is available, or the cat is type B and no type B blood is available, canine blood can be used. This xenotransfusion can be lifesaving in emergencies, but the RBCs are very short lived in circulation, with hemolysis usually occurring within 48 h. Xenotransfusion can only be performed once as a second canine transfusion will result in a severe life-threatening acute hemolytic reaction [406].

Horses

In horses, there are eight blood groups with more than 30 red cell antigens recognized [325]. Approximately 90% of horses do not have naturally occurring alloantibodies but the most common are to Aa and Ca. Full blood typing for horses is available through only a few diagnostic laboratories [407], but a stall side test is now available for Ca (Quick Test BT, Equine, Alvedia, Limonest, France). Chances of adverse reactions increase if either the donor or recipient is a mare that has been bred previously. Thus, it is recommended to use blood from male horses or mares that have never been pregnant as preferred donors. It is also preferable to consider donors that are negative for factors Aa and Qa to prevent sensitization of brood mares against the alloantigens most frequently involved in neonatal isoerythrolysis [325].

Ruminants

In cattle, the likelihood of reaction during first transfusion is low due to a lack of naturally occurring alloantibodies or low titers in the serum. However, cows with J-negative antigen on the RBCs may have J antibodies that can cause a reaction on a first transfusion if J-positive donor cells are used [408]. Although this reaction seems to be of minor clinical significance, the ideal donor cow should have J-negative RBCs.

Other ruminants also appear to have low circulating naturally occurring antibodies. Goats have six blood group systems, sheep have eight, and camelids have at least six group factors [409].

Pigs

Pigs have 16 recognized blood groups. The A-O group is most important and is very similar to the human ABO group but without a B antigen. While hemolytic reactions do not seem to occur with a first transfusion, incompatible A-O transfusions may cause pulmonary hypertension and other adverse events. These reactions seem to be related to anti-A antibodies in plasma so use of PRBCs is safer. Cross-matching should always be performed prior to additional transfusions [410].

Cross-matching

Cross-matching determines the serological compatibility between recipient and donor blood and is based on an agglutination reaction. It detects naturally occurring alloantibodies or alloantibodies produced as a result of previous exposure to incompatible blood products. The major cross-match evaluates the compatibility between donor RBCs and recipient plasma/serum. The minor cross-match assesses compatibility between the recipient's RBCs and donor plasma/serum. In dogs, cross-matching is strongly recommended if transfusion history is unknown, if hemolytic reaction is noticed during the first transfusion, or in any dog who has been previously transfused more than 4 days prior, independent of initial typing and cross-matching results [390,391,397]. Cross-matching should be considered prior to a first transfusion in dogs due to the presence of naturally occurring antibodies to other antigens and possible influence on RBC life span [323]. In cats, both typing and cross-matching are recommended before an initial transfusion because of identification of the Mik antigen with naturally occurring alloantibodies and the potential for a severe transfusion reaction [397,403–405]. In horses, cross-matching is recommended if a second transfusion is needed more than 4–7 days after a first transfusion or if any reaction is noted during the first transfusion [325]. Cattle serum carries minimal agglutinating antibodies and cross-match is usually of little benefit in predicting a transfusion reaction unless a hemolytic test using complement is performed [324]. Standard cross-matching procedures [323] can be found in many texts. A gel cross-match kit is now available for dogs and cats that simplifies the procedure (RapidVet®-H, DMS Laboratories Inc., Flemington, NJ). A gel cross-match kit is also available for horses [411].

Transfusion considerations for massive blood loss

Massive transfusion (MT) involves administration of WB or blood components in an amount that is more than the patient's blood volume in 24 h or more than half of the blood volume in 3 h [412]. Human studies have shown that increasing the ratios of plasma and platelets relative to PRBCs early in the resuscitation phase leads to improvement in outcome [413–415]. Due to these new developments, MT protocols (also known as "substantial bleeding protocols" [SBP] or "trauma exsanguination protocol" [TEP]) have been developed [416]. The PROMMTT (Prospective, observational, multicenter, major trauma transfusion) study showed that in the initial 6 h, mortality was decreased in patients who received higher plasma:RBC and platelet:RBC ratios [417]. A meta-analysis of the impact of MT protocols with increased ratios of plasma and platelets showed that these protocols significantly reduced the overall mortality for trauma patients [418].

There are limited veterinary studies of MT. One veterinary canine study with MT had a high mortality rate of 74% with 100% mortality in dogs with elevated clotting times [412]. Another study in three cats that received MT revealed 67% survival [332]. A dog with aortic laceration that received MT and five units of PRBCs, three units of FFP, and 1.2 L of autotransfused blood survived [419].

Blood administration

Due to the higher viscosity of PRBCs, administration can be facilitated by diluting the cells with warm 0.9% sodium chloride and using the largest possible catheter for venous access. Various RBC products can be warmed by wrapping in a sealed plastic bag and putting in a water bath maintained at 37 °C. Medications and calcium containing fluids should not be given in the same line while administering blood products [323]. Intravenous administration is preferred but blood may be given by the intraosseous route in neonates and animals with difficult vascular access. In healthy dogs, more than 90% of delivered RBCs can be seen in the peripheral circulation after intraosseous administration [420]. The initial rate of administration is usually 0.5 mL/kg over the first 15 min to monitor for any adverse effects of transfusion [336]. The rate can be increased to 10–20 mL/kg/h if no adverse effects are detected. In patients with heart disease, the rate should be less and in cats, rates of 4 mL/kg/h, 10 mL/kg/h, and 60 mL/kg/h have been described in cardiovascular anomalies, normovolemia, and hypovolemic shock, respectively [329,397]. Ideally, blood transfusion is finished within 4 h due to the potential risk of bacterial overgrowth in blood maintained at room temperature. In settings of substantial bleeding or trauma, blood can be given as rapidly as possible. This is facilitated by using short length and larger gauge catheters.

RBCs and all plasma products should be administered with a filter to avoid administration of microthrombi. An in-line 170–260 μm filter is most appropriate for canine blood products. An 18-μm microaggregate filter can be used in cats. Different types of pumps are available to allow administration of a specified volume over a specific time, but this delivery technique can potentially influence the half-life of transfused RBCs [397]. A study in dogs showed significantly shorter RBC life span when a syringe pump and microaggregate filter were used compared to gravity flow and an in-line filter [421]. Studies have also shown increased hemolysis of canine PRBC when administered with peristaltic and rotary pumps. In dogs, administration with an in-line filter and gravity flow or a specifically evaluated piston pump (Hospira Plum A+® infusion pump, Hospira Inc, Lake Forest, IL) is recommended [397]. In cats, use of a syringe pump and a microaggregate filter (18 μm) resulted in acceptable RBC survival [397,422].

Adverse effects of transfusion

Transfusion reactions are categorized as immune-mediated or non-immunologic as well as acute or delayed [323]. Immunologic reactions are often against RBCs, plasma proteins, WBCs, or platelet antigens. Non-immunologic reactions can be related to administration, contamination, additives, and storage. The incidence of transfusion reaction varies from 0% to 38% in the veterinary literature, depending on species, blood product, and reaction definitions [324,333,409,423].

Clinical signs of reactions can include fever, tachycardia, dyspnea, vomiting, tremors, face rubbing, hives, hemolysis, and, in horses, signs of colic [324,333,409,423]. Regardless of the species, transfusion reaction signs typical for conscious animals may be masked or absent in anesthetized patients [424]. American Society of Anesthesiologists practice guidelines recommend that patients should be monitored carefully for urticaria, hypotension, tachycardia, increased peak airway pressure, hyperthermia, hemoglobinuria, decreased urine output, and evidence of increased microvascular bleeding [322]. If any of these are seen, transfusion should be stopped, and appropriate diagnostic testing should be ordered.

Premedication with antihistamines or antipyretic medications has shown no utility in either human or veterinary medicine and is not recommended [423,424].

Febrile non-hemolytic transfusion reactions (FNHTRs) are the most common adverse events with veterinary transfusions, defined as a temperature of more than 39 °C and increase of more than 1 °C from the pretransfusion temperature during or within 4 h of transfusion where external warming and other reactions have been ruled out [423]. These reactions are mostly associated with leukocyte-derived cytokines and/or circulating antileukocyte antibodies in the recipient against donor leukocytes. In people, the use of leukoreduction filters while collecting blood components appears to decrease the incidence of these reactions [397]. If a fever is noted, the transfusion should be paused while vital signs are checked. The unit should also be double checked for identification, expiration date, and any visual evidence of particulate matter or discoloration that could indicate a storage problem or bacterial contamination. A sample should be drawn from both the patient and the unit to check for hemolysis. If fever is the only clinical sign seen, the unit is correct and not discolored, and the patient's sample is not hemolyzed, the transfusion may be restarted at a slower rate [425].

Fever can also be an early sign of a transfusion transmitted infection, an *acute hemolytic transfusion reaction* (AHTR), or *transfusion-related acute lung injury* (TRALI), so if the patient is unstable, the unit is hemolyzed or discolored, or the patient's sample is hemolyzed, the transfusion should not be restarted and further investigation is warranted [425].

AHTRs can either be immunologic or related to storage or administration issues. Immunologic AHTRs are characterized by intravascular hemolysis and are antigen–antibody, type II hypersensitivity reactions primarily mediated by immunoglobulin G (IgG). They occur due to sensitized alloantibody-mediated incompatibilities (such as a DEA 1-negative dog sensitized after receiving DEA 1-positive blood) or due to the presence of natural alloantibodies (like naturally occurring anti-A antibodies in a type B cat) [390,403]. The antigen–antibody interaction causes activation of complement and cytokines and can result in hyperbilirubinemia, hyperbilirubinuria, hemolysis, hemoglobinuria, an inadequate increase in PCV, hypotension, fever, and/or tachycardia seen during or within 24 h of transfusion [423]. The incidence of AHTR can be greatly decreased by blood typing and cross-matching prior to transfusion. Non-immunologic AHTR can be minimized by proper blood storage and checking blood units for hemolysis prior to administration [425].

Non-immune-mediated hemolysis can happen because of overheating, freezing of the blood bag or mixing with hypotonic fluids. Signs of hemoglobinemia and/or hemoglobinuria can be noticed during transfusion without other associated signs of an AHTR. However, severe clinical signs were documented in four dogs after transfusion with blood that was hemolyzed due to improper storage [426]. It is recommended to check RBC units for hemolysis prior to administration. Consistent with human guidelines, units with greater than 1% hemolysis should not be used [397].

TRALI is defined as respiratory distress with bilateral pulmonary edema on imaging and hypoxemia (PaO_2/F_IO_2 < 300 mmHg or SpO_2 < 90% on room air) that occurs within 6 h of transfusion, without evidence of left atrial hypertension or an alternate risk factor for acute respiratory distress syndrome (ARDS) [427]. In humans, the TRALI incidence has been reported to be between 0.08% and 15% [428]. A study in small animals reported the incidence of veterinary acute lung injury after transfusion to be 3.7% [429]. In humans, it has been reported with all types of blood products, but FFP has been implicated most frequently [428].

Bioactive mediators of TRALI can include antibodies and, additionally, products that accumulate during storage [430]. Antileukocyte antibodies from the donor plasma can interact with recipient leukocyte antigens leading to neutrophil and complement activation that can produce endothelial damage and capillary leakage. In other cases, the clinical condition of the patient causes endothelial activation and sequestration of neutrophils. Then, when transfusion of biologically active mediators such as lipids and cytokines occurs, these sequestered neutrophils release oxidases and proteases that cause endothelial cell damage and capillary leakage, resulting in TRALI. The clinical picture of TRALI includes tachypnea, tachycardia, and hypoxemia with or without fever with no evidence of circulatory overload. Differentials include TACO, AHTRs, anaphylactoid reactions, or an underlying respiratory disease not related to the transfusion [425]. Radiographs and echocardiography are recommended to rule out cardiac disease and other differentials [425]. Treatment is mainly supportive and may include only oxygen supplementation in minor cases or mechanical ventilation in severe cases. Usually, TRALI is self-limiting and human patients recover within 96 h [428].

In human medicine, development of TRALI has been particularly associated with plasma transfusion from parturient female donors, and use of plasma from male and non-parturient female donors decreases the incidence of TRALI significantly [431]. RBC alloantibodies are not increased in dogs with repeated pregnancies, but WBC alloantibodies have not been studied [432].

Some blood products have significant colloidal potential and administration to normovolemic animals or animals with compromised cardiac or pulmonary function predisposes them to hypervolemia, known as TACO. Clinical signs include dyspnea, cyanosis, pulmonary edema, increased CVP, and pulmonary venous distension on thoracic radiographs. Echocardiography and measurement of NTproBNP are used for diagnosis in humans and should be considered in veterinary patients [425]. Treatment involves discontinuing the transfusion, oxygen supplementation, and diuretics.

Allergic reactions are the result of an IgE antibody-mediated type I hypersensitivity reaction and are caused by soluble substances in the donor plasma that bind to preformed IgE antibodies on mast cells in the recipient, causing release of histamine. These reactions can range from mild hives to severe anaphylaxis causing hypotension and shock. Vomiting might also be a sign of an allergic transfusion reaction in dogs [425]. If the only signs are hives or a single episode of vomiting, and no other signs are observed, the transfusion can be temporarily interrupted and an antihistamine administered [425]. If anaphylaxis is suspected, immediate treatment with epinephrine is warranted and the transfusion should be discontinued [425].

Bacterial contamination of blood components is rare but can lead to sepsis [433]. Bacteria can originate from inadequately screened donors or from the venipuncture site. In a case series of 14 cats, contamination of blood products was linked to *Serratia marcescens* contamination of a jar containing alcohol-soaked cotton balls and a bag of saline solution used during venipuncture [434]. Signs of sepsis in six cats in this report included vomiting, diarrhea, collapse, and acute death. If vomiting occurs, a full set of vital signs should be obtained. If sepsis is suspected, the transfusion should be stopped immediately and a Gram stain and blood culture should be obtained directly from the unit and the patient [425].

Metabolic and hemostatic complications similar to humans have been described in dogs after MTs that included hypocalcemia, hypomagnesemia, thrombocytopenia, elevations in clotting times (PT and APTT), and hypothermia [396]. Thrombocytopenia and dilutional coagulopathy occur from dilution of clotting factors and platelets with factor-depleted stored blood, resulting in prolongation of coagulation times. Elevation in clotting times was a poor prognostic indicator in the above study in dogs with MT. Hypocalcemia and hypomagnesemia likely arise from binding of anticoagulant citrate to ionized calcium and magnesium. Following transfusion, citrate is usually metabolized quite fast by the liver but, under circumstances of rapid administration, could cause hypocalcemia. In addition, citrate metabolism may be slowed in patients with poor liver function, hypothermia, or decreased perfusion to the liver. Symptomatic hypocalcemia (muscle tremors, arrhythmias, hypotension, etc.) should be treated using calcium gluconate (50–150 mg/kg of 10% solution) or calcium chloride (5–10 mg/kg of 10% solution). Stored blood usually is at a temperature of 4 °C and, if administered without warming, could potentially cause arrhythmias and decreased CO initially in addition to hypothermia, although these adverse effects also depend on the rate of administration [435].

During storage, RBCs undergo a series of biologic and biochemical changes collectively referred to as "storage lesions." There is progressive depletion of ATP and 2,3-DPG, decreased deformability of RBCs, decrease in the pH of stored units due to glycolysis, and increased potassium content of the unit due to RBC lysis. In humans, transfusion-associated hyperkalemia can occur but RBCs from most dog breeds (except some like Akitas and Shiba Inus) are low in intracellular potassium so hyperkalemia from stored RBC products is less of a problem in most dogs [436]. Hyperkalemia has been reported in 20% (2/10) of dogs with MT and also in one dog that was given 28-day-old PRBCs [412,436].

In cats, the half-life of transfused RBCs is approximately 35–38 days for compatible transfusions and decreases to only 1–2 h if a type B cat receives type A blood, and approximately 2 days when type B blood is given to a type A cat [323]. The half-life of allogenic transfused RBCs in cattle has been shown to be 2–4 days with a rapid loss of 10–15% of cells occurring in the first 24 h [324]. Previous studies using radioactive RBC labeling techniques have reported that transfused RBCs survive less than a week in the horse and sometimes less than 2 days, but a recent study using biotin-labeled RBCs reported an average life span of 20 days in allogenic RBC transfusions [437].

Alternatives to allogenic blood transfusions

Because of the potential complications associated with the use of allogenic blood products and to help conserve blood products, alternative strategies have been examined to reduce the need for blood products in the perioperative settings.

Autologous transfusion

Autologous transfusion involves administering blood to a patient that was previously collected from that patient. By using one's own blood, the risks associated with the transmission of infectious diseases or transfusion reactions are minimized. Three forms of autologous transfusion strategies have been explored.

Preoperative autologous blood donation

Preoperative autologous blood donation (PABD) provides a supply of safe blood for patients scheduled to undergo an elective surgical procedure that could potentially be associated with significant blood loss. Patients donate their own blood in advance and it is stored for their own use. Data from human meta-analyses on PABD revealed a 63% reduction in allogenic blood transfusions but an increased overall transfusion of RBCs by 30% (both allogenic and autologous) in patients that undertook the donation. A decline in the patient's hemoglobin by an average of 1.23 g/dL from before PABD to immediately prior to surgery was reported [438–440]. Use of PABD has been described especially in total joint replacement surgeries in humans [441]. In veterinary medicine, PABD has been described in horses that were scheduled for sinus surgeries and in cats that underwent craniotomies [442,443]. In cats, the median time from donation until surgery was 12 days. The predonation median PCV was 30% (approximately 10 g/dL hemoglobin) and the PCV before surgery was 26% (approximately 8.7 g/dL hemoglobin), a decrease (1.3 g/dL) similar to that reported in humans [438,443]. Preoperatively, mild anemia was noticed in 3/15 cats. Eleven of 15 cats that received an autologous transfusion perioperatively did not require an allogenic transfusion. Some inherent limitations to this technique would include the need for advanced planning, cost, need for sedation in veterinary patients, risk of bacterial contamination, and the fact that some patients may experience perioperative anemia thereby increasing the likelihood that transfusion is needed. In addition, waste of unneeded PABD units of blood products has been reported to vary from 18% to above 50% in humans [444,445]. Waste may be decreased by using the PABD unit for other animals, but this would require infectious disease screening, blood typing, and cross-matching, all of which add to the expense.

Acute normovolemic hemodilution

Acute normovolemic hemodilution (ANH) involves removal of a patient's WB before anticipated surgical blood loss. It is performed shortly before or after induction of anesthesia. The circulating blood volume is restored by using crystalloids or colloids in a ratio of 3:1 or 1:1, respectively [446]. The blood is collected in standard blood collection bags and stored in the operating room at room temperature. Collected blood is administered within 6–8 h so that there is little deterioration of platelets and clotting factors. The main benefit of ANH is reduction in RBC losses when WB with lower PCV is lost after ANH is completed. A decrease in blood viscosity caused by hemodilution decreases peripheral resistance and CO can be increased. Although arterial oxygen content (CaO_2) is decreased, DO_2 is maintained by the increase in CO. When performing ANH, a target PCV of 25% is usual but should be dictated by the anticipated blood loss, pre-existing volume status, type of surgical procedure, PCV before ANH, presence of any other comorbidities, and institutional policies. In order to calculate the amount of blood that could be collected to achieve a desired PCV, the following formula may be used:

$$\text{Collected blood (mL)} = \frac{[\text{EBV} \times (H_o - H_f)]}{H_{av}}$$

where EBV is effective circulating blood volume calculated as body weight (kg) times the volume of blood (mL/kg), H_o is the original PCV of the patient before ANH, H_f is the targeted PCV, and H_{av} is the average of H_o and H_f. In humans, ANH has been successfully utilized during surgical procedures for radical prostatectomy, hip and knee arthroplasty, and vascular surgeries. A relative drop of 31% in the frequency of allogenic transfusion has been reported [438,446–449]. There are also rare case reports of ANH in veterinary medicine [450].

Cell salvage

Autologous transfusion using cell salvage methodology is a technique by which blood lost intra- or postoperatively is collected, washed, and administered to the patient [451]. Relatively simple methods of blood salvage involve using sterile vacuum suction tips or a syringe and tubing system for blood aspiration connected to an attached reservoir for collection [452]. If the blood has been in contact with serosal surfaces for more than an hour, defibrination occurs that precludes the need for an anticoagulant but when blood is collected from a site of fresh and rapid hemorrhage, anticoagulant will be required. The blood collected via these methods should be transfused within 4–6 h of collection compared to ANH which can be kept for up to 8 h.

Use of a semiautomated autotransfusion cell separator system (Electa Autotransfusion Cell Separator, Dideco, Mirandola, Italy) was described in a case series of dogs with hemoabdomen [451]. Blood is directly suctioned from the surgical field into a reservoir where automatic mixing with the anticoagulant takes place. It is then moved to a centrifugation bowl system, a process called "priming," followed by "washing" to remove plasma, activated clotting factors, anticoagulants, complement, and systemic medications. After completion of the washing phase, the "emptying" phase moves the blood to a reinfusion bag. The authors speculated that by using the above technique, they were able to reduce the transfusion requirement. Meta-analysis in humans has shown that cell salvage techniques lead to 38% relative and 21% absolute reduction in the risk of exposure to allogenic RBC transfusion [453].

An in-line leukoreduction filter is used during transfusion of salvaged cells to reduce the nucleated cell count and bacterial load delivered to the patient. In humans, salvaged cell solutions used for administration are equal or superior to blood bank units with regard to cell morphology, pH, red cell osmotic resistance, and levels of 2,3-DPG [454,455]. The contraindication often given to using these techniques is in patients with neoplasia, to avoid iatrogenic hematogenous spread. However, this risk is reduced as the process of cell salvage and use of leukoreduction filters remove tumor cells. Studies in humans have failed to document an increase in any adverse outcomes when cell salvage techniques were employed in perioperative oncologic settings [455–458]. Septicemia does not appear to be a major complication of cell salvaging [456,459]. If less sophisticated methods of autotransfusion are used and enteric contamination is suspected or hemoabdomen is from a suspected splenic hemangiosarcoma, autotransfusion should be avoided. Hemolysis, hypocalcemia, and coagulopathy are complications of autotransfusion and have been seen in dogs [435]. To avoid hemolysis as a result of collection technique, it is recommended to keep the needle or suction tip below the surface of the blood to avoid air interface damage and to keep the maximum vacuum settings between 100 and 300 mmHg [460]. Ionized calcium should be checked after autotransfusion and treatment should be considered if there are clinical signs of hypocalcemia or if the ionized calcium is < 0.9 mmol/L [425].

Blood substitutes

Use of oxygen-carrying solutions as an alternative to blood transfusion has been researched for decades. Early versions of hemoglobin-based oxygen carriers (HBOC) were associated with nephrotoxic effects and a short intravascular half-life [461]. These were improved by ultrapurification to remove RBC stromal elements and polymerization of hemoglobin units with glutaraldehyde [462,463]. Oxyglobin® was a clinically approved ultrapurified glutaraldehyde-polymerized bovine-derived hemoglobin solution for use in dogs with anemia [463,464]. It contained 13 g/dL hemoglobin concentration in a modified Ringer's solution with a pH of 7.8 and an osmolality of 300 mOsm/kg. It could be stored at room temperature for 3 years from the date of manufacture and there was no need for a cross-match [465–467]. While it was approved for use only in dogs, it was used off label in other species including cats [468–470] and ponies [471]. However, cell-free hemoglobin can lead to high blood pressure and can damage the kidneys. Oxyglobin® is now produced by Hemoglobin Oxygen Therapeutics (Soulderton, PA) but is no longer commercially available. The human product, Hemopure (Hemoglobin Oxygen Therapeutics) is only readily available in South Africa. However, several HBOC products can be obtained for people under compassionate use rules. Research in this area is ongoing [472].

Strategies to minimize perioperative blood loss

Selective and non-selective inhibitors of cyclooxygenase enzymes including carprofen, meloxicam, deracoxib, and aspirin can impair hemostasis by inhibiting platelet function to variable extents [473–475]. In addition, antiplatelet drugs such as clopidogrel also inhibit platelet function with effects in cats lasting for approximately 7 days after stopping drug administration [476]. The CURATIVE guidelines on rational use of antithrombotic agents in dogs and cats recommend discontinuing antithrombotic drugs prior to surgery and antiplatelet drugs 5–7 days prior in animals at low to moderate risk of thrombosis. In animals at high risk of thrombosis, these medications should not be discontinued but close attention should be paid to hemostasis [477]. Desmopressin can improve hemostasis during invasive procedures such as biopsy and surgery. Use of desmopressin acetate (DDAVP) has been shown to improve primary hemostasis in dogs with aspirin-induced platelet dysfunction, von Willebrand's disease, and chronic liver disease [478,479].

Antifibrinolytic drugs prevent the breakdown of clots. In humans, their use has been associated with significant reductions in blood loss during and after surgery [480,481]. Aprotinin reduced the probability of RBC transfusion requirement by a relative 34% and appeared more effective than lysine analogs ε-aminocaproic acid and tranexamic acid. In the veterinary literature, two studies [482,483] documented the use of ε-aminocaproic acid in retired running Greyhounds undergoing amputation and gonadectomy and its use was associated with significantly lower postoperative blood loss. American Society of Anesthesiologists practice guidelines recommend considering antifibrinolytic therapy as prophylaxis in patients undergoing cardiopulmonary bypass, having liver surgery, or in other surgical cases at high risk for excessive bleeding [322].

Maintenance of near-normothermia is important in the perioperative period because hypothermia can increase surgical blood loss [484]. In elective hip arthroplasty procedures, a drop in core body temperature of 1.6 °C resulted in a 500 mL increase in blood loss and a significant increase in need for allogenic blood transfusion [485,486]. Hypothermia can influence both platelet function and clotting factor activity adversely [487,488].

References

1 MacIntire DK. Pediatric fluid therapy. *Vet Clin North Am Small Anim Pract* 2008; **38**: 621–627.

2 Starling EH. On the absorption of fluids from the connective tissue spaces. *J Physiol* 1896; **19**: 312–326.

3 Landis EM, Pappenheimer JR. Exchange of substances through capillary walls. In: Hamilton WF, Dow P, eds. *Handbook of Physiology, Section 2: Circulation II*. Washington, DC: American Physiological Society, 1963: 961–1034.

4 Woodcock TE, Woodcock TM. Revised Starling equation and the glycocalyx model of transvascular fluid exchange: an improved paradigm for prescribing intravenous fluid therapy. *Br J Anaesth* 2012; **108**: 384–394.

5 Levick JR, Michel CC. Microvascular fluid exchange and revised Starling principle. *Cardiovascular Res* 2010; **87**: 198–210.

6 Valverde A, Gianotti G, Rioja-Garcia E, *et al.* Effects of high volume, rapid fluid therapy on cardiovascular function and hematological values during isoflurane-induced hypotension in healthy dogs. *Can J Vet Res* 2012; **76**: 99–108.

7 Muir WW, Kitjawornrat A, Ueyama Y, *et al.* Effects of intravenous administration of lactated Ringer's solution on hematologic, serum biochemical, rheological, hemodynamic, and renal measurements in healthy isoflurane-anesthetized dogs. *J Am Vet Med Assoc* 2011; **239**: 630–637.

8 Kolsen-Peterson JA, Nielsen JO, Tonnesen E. Acid base and electrolyte changes after hypertonic saline (7.5%) infusion: a randomized controlled clinical trial. *Scand J Clin Lab Invest* 2005; **65**: 13–22.

9 Hopper K, Epstein SE. Incidence, nature, and etiology of metabolic acidosis in dogs and cats. *J Vet Intern Med* 2012; **26**: 1107–1114.

10 Handy JM, Soni N. Physiological effects and hyperchloremia and acidosis. *Br J Anaesth* 2008; **101**: 141–150.

11 Tonozzi CC, Rudloff E, Kirby R. Perfusion versus hydration: impact on the fluid therapy plan. *Compend Contin Edu Vet* 2009: E1–E14.

12 Silverstein DC, Aldrich J, Haskins SC, *et al.* Assessment of changes in blood volume in response to resuscitative fluid administration in dogs. *J Vet Emerg Crit Care* 2005; **15**: 185–192.

13 Kudnig ST, Mama K. Guidelines for perioperative fluid therapy. *Compend Contin Edu Pract Vet* 2003; **25**: 102–111.

14 Bednarski R, Grimm K, Harvey R, *et al.* AAHA anesthesia guidelines for dogs and cats. *J Am Anim Hosp Assoc* 2011; **47**: 377–385.

15 Schenck PA, Chew DJ, Nagode LA, *et al.* Disorders of calcium: hypercalcemia and hypocalcemia. In: Dibartola SP, ed. *Fluid, Electrolyte, and Acid-Base Disorders in Small Animal Practice*, 4th edn. St. Louis, MO: Elsevier, 2012: 120–194.

16 Schaer M. Therapeutic approach to electrolyte emergencies. *Vet Clin North Am Small Anim Pract* 2008; **38**: 513–533.

17 Smith GW. Supportive therapy of the toxic cow. *Vet Clin North Am Food Anim Pract* 2005; **21**: 595–614.

18 Roussel AJ, Cohen ND, Holland PS, *et al.* Alterations in acid-base and serum electrolyte concentrations in cattle: 632 cases (1984–1994). *J Am Vet Med Assoc* 1998; **212**: 1769–1775.

19 Pinto FC, Capone-Neto A, Prist R, *et al.* Volume replacement with lactated Ringer's or 3% hypertonic saline solution during combined experimental hemorrhagic shock and traumatic brain injury. *J Trauma* 2006; **60**: 758–764.

20 Ramming S, Shackford SR, Zhuang J, *et al.* The relationship of fluid balance and sodium administration to cerebral edema formation and intracranial pressure in a porcine model of brain injury. *J Trauma* 1994; **37**: 705–713.

21 Schmall LM, Muir WW, Robertson JT. Haematological, serum electrolyte and blood gas effects of small volume hypertonic saline in experimentally induced hemorrhagic shock. *Equine Vet J* 1990; **22**: 278–283.

22 Lorenzo M, Davis JW, Negin S, *et al.* Can Ringer's lactate be used safely with blood transfusions? *Am J Surg* 1998; **175**: 308–310.

23 Cull DL, Lally KP, Murphy KD. Compatibility of packed erythrocytes and Ringer's lactate solution. *Surg Gynecol Obstet* 1991; **173**: 9–12.

24 Goldstein SM, MacLean LD. Ringers lactate infusion with severe hepatic damage: effect on arterial lactate level. *Can J Surg* 1972; **15**: 318–321.

25 Didwania A, Miller J, Kassel D, *et al.* Effect of intravenous lactated Ringer' solution infusion on the circulating lactate concentration: Part 3. Results of a prospective, randomized, double-blind, placebo-controlled trial. *Crit Care Med* 1997; **25**: 1851–1854.

26 Vall DM, Ogilvie GK, Fettman MJ, *et al.* Exacerbation of hyperlactatemia by infusion of lactated Ringer's solution in dogs with lymphoma. *J Vet Intern Med* 1990; **4**: 228–232.

27 Steffen RP, McKenzie JE, Bockman EL, *et al.* Changes in dog gracilis muscle adenosine during exercise and acetate infusion. *Am J Physiol* 1983; **244**: H387–H395.

28 Saragoca MA, Bessa AM, Mulinari RA, *et al.* Sodium acetate, an arterial vasodilator: haemodynamic characterization in normal dogs. *Proc Eur Dial Transplant Assoc* 1985; **21**: 221–224.

29 Keshaviah PR. The role of acetate in the etiology of symptomatic hypotension. *Artif Organs* 1982; **6**: 378–387.

30 Strandvik GF. Hypertonic saline in critical care: a review of literature and guidelines for use in hypotensive states and raised intracranial pressure. *Anaesthesia* 2009; **64**: 990–1003.

31 Constable P. Fluid and electrolyte therapy in ruminants. *Vet Clin North Am Food Anim Pract* 2003; **19**: 557–597.

32 Barry KG, Berman AR. Mannitol infusion. Part III. The acute effect of the intravenous infusion of mannitol on blood and plasma volume. *N Engl J Med* 1961; **264**: 1085–1088.

33 Velasco IT, Pontieri V, Rocha e Silva M, *et al.* Hyperosmotic NaCl and severe hemorrhagic shock. *Am J Physiol* 1980; **239**: H664–H673.

34 Smith GJ, Kramer GC, Perron P, *et al.* A comparison of several hypertonic solutions for resuscitation of bled sheep. *J Surg Res* 1985; **39**: 517–528.

35 Velasco IT, Rocha e Silva M, Oliveira MA, *et al.* Hypertonic and hyperoncotic resuscitation from severe hemorrhagic shock in dogs: a comparative study. *Crit Care Med* 1989; **17**: 261–264.

36 Schertel ER, Valentine AK, Rademakers AM, *et al.* Influence of 7% NaCl on the mechanical properties of the systemic circulation in hypovolemic dogs. *Circ Shock* 1990; **31**: 203–214.

37 Wildenthal K, Mierzwiak DS, Mitchell JH. Acute effects of increased serum smolality on left ventricular performance. *Am J Physiol* 1969; **216**: 898–904.

38 Kien ND, Kramer GC. Cardiac performance following hypertonic saline. *Braz J Med Biol Res* 1989; **22**: 245–248.

39 Gazitua MC, Scott JB, Swindall B. Resistance responses to local changes in plasma osmolality in three vascular beds. *Am J Physiol* 1971; **220**: 384–391.

40 Pascual JL, Khwaja KA, Chaudhury P, *et al.* Hypertonic saline and microcirculation. *J Trauma* 2003; **54**: S133–S140.

41 Ciesla DJ, Moore EE, Silliman CC, *et al.* Hypertonic saline attenuation of polymorphonuclear cytotoxicity: timing is everything. *J Trauma* 2000; **48**: 388–395.

42 Hirsh M, Dyugovaskaya L, Bashenko Y, *et al.* Reduced rate of bacterial translocation and improved variables of natural killer cell and T-cell activity in rats surviving controlled hemorrhagic shock and treated with hypertonic saline. *Crit Care Med* 2002; **30**: 861–867.

43 Rocha e Silva M, Poli de Figueiredo LF. Small volume hypertonic resuscitation of circulatory shock. *Clinics* 2005; **60**: 159–172.

44 Vajda K, Szabo A, Boros M. Heterogeneous microcirculation in the rat small intestine during hemorrhagic shock: quantification of the effects of hypertonic-hyperoncotic resuscitation. *Eur Surg Res* 2004; **36**: 338–344.

45 Zhao L, Wang B, You G, *et al.* Effects of different resuscitation fluids on the rheologic behavior of red blood cells, blood viscosity and plasma viscosity in experimental hemorrhagic shock. *Resuscitation* 2009; **80**: 253–258.

46 Jonas J, Heimann A, Strecker U, *et al.* Hypertonic/hyperoncotic resuscitation after intestinal superior mesenteric artery occlusion: early effects on circulation and intestinal reperfusion. *Shock* 2000; **14**: 24–29.

47 Mittlmeier T, Vollmar B, Menger MD, *et al.* Small volume hypertonic hydroxyethyl starch reduces acute microvascular dysfunction after closed soft tissue trauma. *J Bone Joint Surg* 2003; **85B**: 126–132.

48 Schmall LM, Muir WW, Robertson JT. Haematological, serum electrolyte and blood gas effects of small volume hypertonic saline in experimentally induced hemorrhagic shock. *Equine Vet J* 1990; **22**: 278–283.

49 Wade CE, Grady JJ, Kramer GC. Efficacy of hypertonic saline dextran fluid resuscitation for patients with hypotension from penetrating trauma. *J Trauma* 2003; **54**: S144–S148.

50 Bratton SL, Chestnut RM, Ghajar J, *et al.* Brain trauma foundation guidelines for the management of severe traumatic brain injury. *II Hyperosmolar therapy. J Neurotrauma* 2007; **24**(S1): S14–S21.

51 Zornow MH, Todd MM, Moore SS. The acute cerebral effects of changes in plasma osmolality and oncotic pressure. *Anesthesiology* 1987; **67**: 936–941.

52 Qureshi AI, Silson DA, Traystman RJ. Treatment of elevated intracranial pressure in experimental intracerebral hemorrhage: comparison between mannitol and hypertonic saline. *Neurosurgery* 1999; **44**: 1055–1063.

53 Kamel H, Navi BB, Nakagawa K, *et al.* Hypertonic saline versus mannitol for the treatment of elevated intracarial pressure: a meta-analysis of randomized clinical trials. *Crit Care Med* 2011; **39**: 554–559.

54 Mortazavi MM, Romeo AK, Deep A, *et al.* Hypertonic saline for treating intracranial pressure: literature review with meta-analysis. *J Neurosurg* 2012; **116**: 210–221.

55 Shackford SR, Schmoker JD, Zhuang J. The effect of hypertonic resuscitation on pial arteriolar tone after brain injury and shock. *J Trauma* 1994; **37**: 899–908.

56 Doyle JA, Davis DP, Hoyt DB. The use of hypertonic saline in the treatment of traumatic brain injury. *J Trauma* 2001; **50**: 367–383.

57 Schertel ER, Allen DA, Muir WW, *et al.* Evaluation of a hypertonic saline-dextran solution for treatment of dogs with shock induced by gastric-dilation-volvulus. *J Am Vet Med Assoc* 1997; **210**: 226–230.

58 Horton JW, Dunn CW, Burnweit CA, *et al.* Hypertonic saline-dextran resuscitation of acute canine bile-induced pancreatitis. *Am J Surg* 1989; **158**: 48–56.

59 Machado MC, Coelho AM, Pontieri V, *et al.* Local and systemic effects of hypertonic solution (NaCl 7.5%) in experimentally acute pancreatitis. *Pancreas* 2006; **32**: 80–86.

60 Shields CJ, Sookhai S, Ryan L, *et al.* Hypertonic saline attenuates end organ damage in experimental model of acute pancreatitis. *Br J Surg* 2000; **87**: 1336–1340.

61 Pantaleon LG, Furr MO, McKenzie HC, *et al.* Cardiovascular and pulmonary effects of hetastarch plus hypertonic saline solutions during experimental endotoxemia in anesthetized horses. *J Vet Intern Med* 2006; **20**: 1422–1428.

62 Pantaleon LG, Furr MO, McKenzie HC, *et al.* Effects of small- and large-volume resuscitation on coagulation and electrolytes during experimental endotoxemia in anesthetized horses. *J Vet Intern Med* 2007; **21**: 1374–1379.

63 Constable PD, Schmall LM, Muir WW, *et al.* Hemodynamic responses of endotoxemic calves to treatment with small-volume hypertonic saline solution. *Am J Vet Res* 1991; **52**: 990–998.

64 Constable PD, Gohar HM, Morin DE, *et al.* Use of hypertonic saline-dextran solution to resuscitate hypovolemic calves with diarrhea. *Am J Vet Res* 1996; **57**: 97–104.

65 Koch A, Kaske M. Clinical efficacy of intravenous hypertonic saline solution or hypertonic bicarbonate solution in the treatment of inappetent calves with neonatal diarrhea. *J Vet Intern Med* 2008; **22**: 202–211.

66 Senturk S. Effects of a hypertonic saline solution and dextran 70 combination in the treatment of diarrheic dehydrated calves. *J Vet Med A Physiol Pathol Clin Med* 2003; **50**: 57–61.

67 Tyler JW, Welles EG, Erskine RJ, *et al.* Clinical and clinicopathologic changes in cows with endotoxin-induced mastitis treated with small volumes of isotonic or hypertonic sodium chloride administered intravenously. *Am J Vet Res* 1994; **55**: 278–287.

68 Gross D, Landau EH, Klin B, *et al.* Treatment of uncontrolled hemorrhagic shock with hypertonic saline solution. *Surg Gynecol Obstet* 1990; **170**: 106–112.

69 Bruttig SP, O'Benar J, Wade CE, *et al.* Benefit of slow infusion of hypertonic saline/dextran in swine with uncontrolled aortotomy hemorrhage. *Shock* 2005; **24**: 92–96.

70 Landau EG, Gross D, Assalia A, *et al.* Treatment of uncontrolled hemorrhagic shock with hypertonic saline and external counter pressure. *Ann Emerg Med* 1989; **18**: 1039–1043.

71 Stern SA, Kowalenko T, Younger J, *et al.* Comparison of the effects of bolus vs. slow infusion of 7.5% NaCl/6% dextran-70 in a model of near-lethal uncontrolled hemorrhage. *Shock* 2000; **14**: 616–622.

72 McKirnan MD, Williams RL, Limjoco U, *et al.* Hypertonic saline/dextran vs. lactated Ringer's treatment for hemorrhage in dehydrated swine. *Circ Shock* 1994; **44**: 238–246.

73 Ho HS, Sondeen JL, Dubick MA, *et al.* The renal effects of 7.5% NaCl-6% dextran-70 versus lactated Ringer's resuscitation of hemorrhage in dehydrated sheep. *Shock* 1996; **5**: 289–297.

74 Sondeen JL, Gunther RA, Dubick MA. Comparison of 7.5% NaCl/6% dextran-70 resuscitation of hemorrhage between euhydrated and dehydrated sheep. *Shock* 1995; **3**: 63–68.

75 Fielding CL, Magdesian KG. A comparison of hypertonic (7.2%) and isotonic (0.9%) saline for fluid resuscitation in horses: a randomized, double-blinded, clinical trial. *J Vet Intern Med* 2011; **25**: 1138–1143.

76 Kramer GC. Hypertonic resuscitation: physiologic mechanisms and recommendations for trauma care. *J Trauma* 2003; **54**: S89–S99.

77 Ajito T, Suzuki K, Iwabuchi S. Effect of intravenous infusion of 7.2% hypertonic saline solution on serum electrolytes and osmotic pressure in healthy Beagles. *J Vet Med Sci* 1999; **61**: 637–641.

78 Dubick MA, Zaucha GM, Korte DW Jr., *et al.* Acute and subacute toxicity of 7.5% hypertonic saline-6% dextran-70 (HSD) in dogs. 2. Biochemical and behavioral responses. *J Appl Toxicol* 1993; **13**: 49–55.

79 Mensack S. Fluid therapy: options and rational administration. *Vet Clin North Am Small Anim Pract* 2008; **38**: 575–586.

80 Wellman ML, DiBartola SP, Kohn CW. Applied physiology of body fluids in dogs and cats. In: Dibartola SP, ed. *Fluid, Electrolyte, and Acid-Base Disorders in Small Animal Practice*, 4th edn. St. Louis, MO: Elsevier, 2012: 2–25.

81 Silverstein DC. Daily intravenous fluid therapy. In: Silverstein D, Hopper K, eds. *Small Animal Critical Care Medicine*. St. Louis, MO: Saunders, 2009: 271–275.

82 Muir WW, Wiese AJ. Comparison of lactated Ringer's solution and physiologically balanced 6% hetastarch plasma expander for the treatment of hypotension induced via blood withdrawal in isoflurane anesthetized dogs. *Am J Vet Res* 2004; **65**: 1189–1194.

83 Epstein KL, Bergren A, Giguere S, *et al.* Cardiovascular, colloid osmotic pressure, and hemostatic effects of 2 formulations of hydroxyethyl starch in healthy horses. *J Vet Intern Med* 2014; **28**: 223–233.

84 Aarnes TK, Bednarski RM, Lerche P, *et al.* Effect of intravenous administration of lactated Ringer's solution or hetastarch for the treatment of isoflurane induced hypotension in dogs. *Am J Vet Res* 2009; **70**: 1345–1353.

85 Hallowell GD, Corley KT. Preoperative administration of hydroxyethyl starch or hypertonic saline to horses with colic. *J Vet Intern Med* 2006; **20**: 980–986.

86 Hiltebrand LB, Kimberger O, Arnberger M, *et al.* Crystalloids versus colloids for goal-directed fluid therapy in major surgery. *Crit Care* 2009; **13**: R40–R53.

87 Mcllory DR, Kharasch ED. Acute intravascular volume expansion with rapidly administered crystalloid or colloid in the setting of moderate hypovolemia. *Anesth Analg* 2003; **96**: 1572–1577.

88 Westphal M, James MFM, Kozek-Langenecker S, *et al.* Hydroxyethyl starches, different products-different effects. *Anesthesiology* 2009; **111**: 187–202.

89 Kozek-Langenecker S. Effects of hydroxyethyl starch solutions on hemostasis. *Anesthesiology* 2005; **103**: 654–660.

90 Boldt J. Modern rapidly degradable hydroxyethyl starches: current concepts. *Anesth Analg* 2009; **108**: 1574–1582.

91 Jungheinrich C, Neff TA. Pharmacokinetics of hydroxyethyl starch. *Clin Pharmacokinet* 2005; **44**: 681–699.

92 Yacobi A, Gibson TP, McEntegrat CM, *et al.* Pharmacokinetics of high molecular weight hydroxyethyl starch in dogs. *Res Commun Chem Pathol Pharmacol* 1982; **36**: 199–204.

93 Meiseter D, Hermann M, Mathis GA. Kinetics of hydroxyethyl starch in horses. *Schweiz Arch Tierheilkd* 1992; **134**: 329–339.

94 Thompson WL, Fukushima T, Rutherford RB, *et al.* Intravascular persistence, tissue storage, and excretion of hydroxyethyl starch. *Surg Gynecol Obstet* 1970; **131**: 965–972.

95 Hughes D. Fluid therapy with artificial colloids: complications and controversies. *Vet Anaesth Analg* 2001; **28**: 111–118.

96 Gandhi SD, Weiskopf RB, Jungheinrich C, *et al.* Volume replacement therapy during major orthopaedic surgery using Voluven (hydroxyethyl starch 130/0.4) or hetastarch. *Anesthesiology* 2007; **106**: 1120–1127.

97 Langeron O, Doelberg M, Ang ET, *et al.* Voluven®, a lower substituted novel hydroxyethyl starch (HES 130/0.4) causes fewer effects on coagulation in major orthopaedic surgery than HES 200/0.5. *Anesth Analg* 2001; **92**: 855–862.

98 Gallandat Huet RC, Siemons AW, Baus D, *et al.* A novel hydroxyethyl starch (Voluven®) for effective perioperative plasma volume substitution in cardiac surgery. *Can J Anaesth* 2000; **47**: 1207–1215.

99 Ickx BE, Bepperling F, Melot C, *et al.* Plasma substitution effects of a new hydroxyethyl starch HES 130/0.4 compared with HES 200/0.5 during and after extended acute normovolaemic hemodilution. *Br J Anaesth* 2003; **91**: 196–202.

100 James MF, Latoo MY, Mythen MG, *et al.* Plasma volume changes associated with two hydroxyethyl starch colloids following acute hypovolaemia in volunteers. *Anaesthesia* 2004; **59**: 738–742.

101 Madjdpour C, Dettori N, Frascarol P, *et al.* Molecular weight of hydroxyethyl-starch: is there an effect on blood coagulation and pharmacokinetics? *Br J Anaesth* 2005; **94**: 569–576.

102 Jones PA, Tomasic M, Gentry PA. Oncotic, hemodilutional, and hemostatic effects of isotonic saline and hydroxyethyl starch solutions in clinically normal ponies. *Am J Vet Res* 1997; **58**: 541–548.

103 Smiley LE, Garvey MS. The use of hetastarch as adjunct therapy in 26 dogs with hypoalbuminemia: a phase two clinical trial. *J Vet Intern Med* 1994; **8**: 195–202.

104 Moore LE, Garvey MS. The effect of hetastarch on serum colloid oncotic pressure in hypoalbuminemic dogs. *J Vet Intern Med* 1996; **10**: 300–303.

105 Jones PA, Bain FT, Byars TD, *et al.* Effect of hydroxyethyl starch infusion on colloid oncotic pressure in hypoproteinemic horses. *J Am Vet Med Assoc* 2001; **218**: 1130–1135.

106 Chohan AS, Greene SA, Grubb TL, *et al.* Effects of 6% hetastarch (600/0/75) or lactated Ringer's solution on hemostatic variables and clinical bleeding in healthy dogs anesthetized for orthopedic surgery. *Vet Anaesth Analg* 2011; **38**: 94–105.

107 Viljoen A, Page PC, Fosgate GT, *et al.* Coagulation, oncotic and haemodilutional effects of a third-generation hydroxyethyl starch (130/0.4) solution in horses. *Equine Vet J* 2014; **46**: 739–744.

108 Wendt-Hornickle EL, Snyder LBC, Tang R, *et al.* The effects of lactated Ringer's solution (LRS) or LRS and 6% hetastarch on colloid osmotic pressure, total protein and osmolality in healthy horses under general anesthesia. *Vet Anaesth Analg* 2011; **38**: 336–343.

109 Wright BD, Hopkins A. Change in colloid osmotic pressure as a function of anesthesia and surgery in the presence and absence of isotonic fluid administration in dogs. *Vet Anaesth Analg* 2008; **35**: 282–288.

110 Kozek-Langenecker SA, Jungheinrich C, Sauermann W, *et al.* The effects of hydroxyethyl starch 130/0.4 (6%) on blood loss and use of blood products in major surgery: a pooled analysis of randomized clinical trials. *Anesth Analg* 2008; **107**: 382–390.

111 Gandhi S, Warltier D, Weiskopf R, *et al.* Volume substitution with HES 130/0.4 Voluven) versus HES 450/0.7 (hetastarch) during major orthopedic surgery. *Crit Care* 2005; **9**(Suppl 1): P206.

112 Conroy JM, Fishman RL, Reeves ST, *et al.* The effects of desmopressin and 6% hydroxyethyl starch on factor VIII:C. *Anesth Analg* 1996; **83**: 804–807.

113 Zoran DL, Jergens AE, Riedesel DH, *et al.* Evaluation of hemostatic analytes after use of hypertonic saline solution combined with colloids for resuscitation of dogs with hypovolemia. *Am J Vet Res* 1992; **53**: 1791–1796.

114 Smart L, Jandrey KE, Wierenga JR, *et al.* The effect of hetastarch (670/0.75) in vivo on platelet closure time in the dog. *J Vet Emerg Crit Care* 2009; **19**: 444– 449.

115 Wierenga JR, Jandrey KE, Haskins SC, *et al.* In vitro comparison of the effects of two forms of hydroxyethyl starch solutions on platelet function in dogs. *Am J Vet Res* 2007; **68**: 605–609.

116 McBride D, Hosgood GL, Mansfield CS, *et al.* The effect of hydroxyethyl starch 130/0.4 and 200/0.5 on canine platelet function in vitro. *Am J Vet Res* 2013; **74**: 1133–1137.

117 McBride D, Hosgood G, Smart L, *et al.* Platelet closure time in dogs with hemorrhagic shock treated with hydroxyethyl starch 130/0.4 or 0.9% NaCl. In: *Proceedings of the 18th International Veterinary Emergency and Critical Care Society Meeting*, 2012: 701.

118 Gauthier V, Bersenas A, Holowaychuk M, *et al.* Effect of synthetic colloid administration of coagulation in dogs with systemic inflammation. In: *Proceedings of the 18th International Veterinary Emergency and Critical Care Society Meeting*, 2012: 697.
119 Blong AE, Epstein KL, Brainard BM. In vitro effects of hydroxyethyl starch solutions on coagulation and platelet function in horses. *Am J Vet Res* 2013; **74**: 713–720.
120 Classen J, Adamik KN, Weber K, *et al.* In vitro effect of hydroxyethyl starch 130/0/42 on canine platelet function. *Am J Vet Res* 2012; **73**: 1908–1912.
121 Bacek LM, Martin LG, Spangler EA, *et al.* Determination of the in vitro effects of two forms of hydroxyethyl starch solutions on thromboelastography and coagulation parameters in healthy dogs. In: *Proceedings of the 17th International Veterinary Emergency and Critical Care Society Meeting*, 2011: 732.
122 Boldt J, Haish G, Suttner S, *et al.* Effects of a new modified, balanced hydroxyethyl starch preparations (Hextend) on measures of coagulation. *Br J Anaesth* 2002; **89**: 722–728.
123 Deusch E, Thaler U, Kozek-Langenecker SA. The effects of high molecular weight hydroxyethyl starch solutions on platelet function. *Anesth Analg* 2004; **99**: 665–668.
124 Perner A, Hasse N, Guttormsen AB, *et al.* Hydroxyethyl starch 130/0.42 versus Ringer's acetate in severe sepsis. *N Engl J Med* 2012; **73**: 124–134.
125 Zarychanski R, Abou-Setta AM, Turgeon AF, *et al.* Association of hydroxyethyl starch administration with mortality and acute kidney injury in critically ill patients requiring volume resuscitation: a systematic review and meta-analysis. *JAMA* 2013; **309**: 678–688.
126 Hayes G, Benedicenti L, Mathews K. Retrospective cohort study on the incidence of acute kidney injury and death following hydroxyethyl starch (HES 10% 250/0.5/5:1) administration in dogs (2007–2010). *J Vet Emerg Crit Care* 2015; **26**: 35–40.
127 Sigrist NE, Kalin N, Dreyfus A. Changes in serum creatinine concentration and acute kidney injury (AKI) grade in dogs treated with hydroxyethyl starch 130/0.4 from 2013 to 2015. *J Vet Intern Med* **2017**; 31: 434–441.
128 Sigrist NE, Kalin N, Dreyfus A. Effects of hydroxyethyl starch 130/0.4 on serum creatinine concentration and development of acute kidney injury in nonazotemic cats. *J Vet Intern Med* 2017; **31**: 1749–1756.
129 Yozova ID, Howard J, Adamik KN. Retrospective evaluation of the effects of administration of tetrastarch (hydroxyethyl starch 130/0.4) on plasma creatinine concentration in dogs (2010–2013): 201 dogs. *J Vet Emerg Crit Care* 2016; **26**: 568–577.
130 Yozova ID, Howard J, Adamik KN. Effect of tetrastarch (hydroxyethyl starch 130/0.4) on plasma creatinine concentration in cats: a retrospective analysis (2010–2015). *J Feline Med Surg* 2017; **19**: 1073–1079.
131 Bae J, Soliman M, Kim H, *et al.* Rapid exacerbation of renal function after administration of hydroxyethyl starch in a dog. *J Vet Med Sci* 2017; **79**: 1591–1595.
132 Boyd CJ, Claus MA, Raisis AL, *et al.* Evaluation of biomarkers of kidney injury following 4% succinylated gelatin and 6% hydroxyethyl starch 130/0.4 administration in a canine hemorrhagic shock model. *J Vet Emerg Crit Care* 2019; **29**: 132–142.
133 Diniz MS, Teixeira-Neto FJ, Celeita-Rodríguez N, *et al.* Effects of 6% tetrastarch and lactated Ringer's solution on extravascular lung water and markers of acute renal injury in hemorrhaged, isoflurane-anesthetized healthy dogs. *J Vet Intern Med* 2018; **32**: 712–721.
134 Boyd C, Claus M, Sharp C, *et al.* Biomarkers of acute kidney injury in dogs after 6% hydroxyethyl starch 130/0.4 or hartmann's solution: a randomized blinded clinical trial. *J Vet Emerg Crit Care* 2019; **29**: 306–314.
135 Garzon AA, Cheng C, Lerner B, *et al.* Hydroxyethyl starch (HES) and bleeding: an experimental investigation of its effect on hemostasis. *J Trauma* 1967; **7**: 757–766.
136 Thompson WL, Gadsen RH. Prolonged bleeding time and hypofibrinogenemia in dogs after infusion of hydroxyethyl starch and dextran. *Transfusion* 1965; **5**: 440–446.
137 Concannon KT, Haskins SC, Feldman BF. Hemostatic defects associated with two infusion rates of dextran 70 in dogs. *Am J Vet Res* 1992; **53**: 1369–1375.
138 Glowaski MM, Massat-Moon PF, Erb HN, *et al.* Effects of oxypolygelatin and dextran 70 on hemostatic variables in dogs. *Vet Anaesth Analg* 2003; 3**0**: 202–210.
139 Heath MF, Evans RJ, Hayes LJ. Dextran-70 inhibits equine platelet aggregation induced by PAF but not by other agonists. *Equine Vet J* 1998; **30**: 408–411.
140 Mailloux L, Swartz CD, Dappizzi R, *et al.* Acute renal failure after administration of low-molecular weight dextran. *N Engl J Med* 1967; **277**: 1113–1118.
141 Zwaveling JH, Meulenbelt J, van Xanten NH, *et al.* Renal failure associated with the use of dextran-40. *Neth J Med* 1989; **35**: 321–326.
142 Mitra S, Khandelwal P. Are all colloids same? How to select the right colloid? *Ind J Anaesth* 2009; **53**: 592–607.
143 de Jonge E, Levi M, Berends F, *et al.* Impaired haemostasis by intravenous administration of a gelatin-based plasma expander in human subjects. *Thromb Haemost* 1998; **79**: 286–290.
144 Mortelmans YJ, Vermaut G, Verbruggen AM, *et al.* Effects of 6% hydroxyethyl starch and 3% modified fluid gelatin on intravascular volume and coagulation during intraoperative hemodilution. *Anesth Analg* 1995; **81**: 1235–1242.
145 Lorenz W, Duda D, Dick W, *et al.* Incidence and clinical importance of perioperative histamine release: randomized study of volume loading and antihistamines after induction of anesthesia. *Lancet* 1994; **343**: 933–940.
146 Rasmussen KC, Secher NH, Pedersen T. Effect of perioperative crystalloid or colloid fluid therapy on hemorrhage, coagulation competence, and outcome: a systematic review and stratified meta-analysis. *Medicine* 2016; **95**: e4498.
147 Spahn DR, Bouillon B, Cerny V, *et al.* The European guideline on management of major bleeding and coagulopathy following trauma. *Crit Care* 2019; **23**: 98.
148 Smart L, Hopper K, Aldrich J, *et al.* The effect of hetastarch (670/0.75) on urine specific gravity and osmolality in the dog. *J Vet Intern Med* 2009; **23**: 388–391.
149 Schmid SM, Cianciolo RE, Drobatz KJ, *et al.* Postmortem evaluation of renal tubular vacuolization in critically ill dogs. *J Vet Emerg Crit Care* 2019; **29**: 279–287.
150 Shires T, Williams J, Broen F. Acute changes in extracellular fluids associated with major surgical procedures. *Ann Surg* 1961; **154**: 803–810.
151 Virtue RW, LeVine DS, Aikawa JW. Fluid shifts during the surgical period: RISA and S35 determinations following glucose, saline or lactate infusions. *Ann Surg* 1965; **163**: 523–528.
152 Savvas I, Rallis T, Raptopoulos D. The effect of pre-anesthetic fasting time and type of food on gastric content volume and acidity in dogs. *Vet Anaesth Analg* 2009; **36**: 539–546.
153 Jacob M, Chappel D, Conzen P, *et al.* Blood volume is normal after pre-operative overnight fasting. *Acta Anesthesiol Scand* 2008; **52**: 522–529.
154 Brandstrup B, Svensen C, Engquist A. Hemorrhage and operation cause a contraction of the extracellular space needing replacement - evidence and implications? *A systematic review. Surgery* 2006; **139**: 419–432.
155 Jackson R, Reid JA, Thorburn J. Volume preloading is not essential to prevent spinal- induced hypotension at Caesarean section. *Br J Anaesth* 1995; **75**: 262–265.
156 Iijima T. Complexity of blood volume control system and its implications in perioperative fluid management. *J Anesth* 2009; **23**: 534–542.
157 Hauptman JG, Richter MA, Wood SL, *et al.* Effects of anesthesia, surgery, and intravenous administration of fluids on antidiuretic hormone concentration in healthy dogs. *Am J Vet Res* 2000; **61**: 1273–1276.
158 Robertson SA, Hauptman JG, Nachreiner RF, *et al.* Effects of acetylpromazine or morphine on urine production in halothane-anesthetized dogs. *Am J Vet Res* 2001; **62**: 1922–1927.
159 Boscan P, Pypendop BH, Siao KT, *et al.* Fluid balance, glomerular filtration rate, and urine output in dogs anesthetized for an orthopedic surgical procedure. *Am J Vet Res* 2010; **71**: 497–596.
160 Rahbari NN, Zimmermann JB, Schmidt T, *et al.* Meta-analysis of standard, restrictive and supplemental fluid administration in colorectal surgery. *Br J Surg* 2009; **96**: 331–341.
161 Chappell D, Jacob M, Hoffmann-Kiefer K, *et al.* A rational approach to perioperative fluid management. *Anesthesiology* 2008; **109**: 723–740.
162 Holte K, Sharrock NE, Kehlet H. Pathophysiology and clinical implications of perioperative fluid excess. *Br J Anaesth* 2002; **89**: 622–632.
163 Cotton BA, Guy JS, Morris JA, *et al.* The cellular, metabolic, and systemic consequences of aggressive fluid resuscitation strategies. *Shock* 2006; **26**: 115–121.
164 Brodbelt DC, Pfeiffer DU, Young LE, *et al.* Risk factors for anaesthetic-related death in cats: results from the Confidential Enquiry into Perioperative Small Animal Fatalities (CEPSAF). *Br J Anaesth* 2007; **99**: 617–623.
165 Holte K, Foss NB, Anderson J, *et al.* Liberal or restrictive fluid administration in fast-track colonic surgery: a randomized double-blinded study. *Br J Anaesth* 2007; **99**: 500–508.
166 Brandstrup B, Tonnesen H, Beier-Holgersen R, *et al.* Effect of intravenous fluid restrictions on postoperative complications: comparison of two perioperative fluid regimens: a randomized assessor-blinded multicenter trial. *Ann Surg* 2003; **238**: 641–648.
167 Yogendran S, Asokumar B, Cheng DC, *et al.* A prospective randomized double blinded study of the effect of intravenous fluid therapy on adverse outcome on outpatient surgery. *Anesth Analg* 1995; **80**: 682–686.
168 Bundgaard-Nielson M, Secher NH, Kehlet H. 'Liberal' vs. 'Restrictive' perioperative fluid therapy - a critical assessment of the evidence. *Acta Anaesthesiol Scand* 2009; **53**: 843–851.
169 Lambert KG, Wakim JH, Lambert NE. Preoperative fluid bolus and reduction of postoperative nausea and vomiting in patients undergoing laparoscopic gynecologic surgery. *AANA J* 2009; **77**: 110–114.
170 Holte K, Klarskov B, Christensen DS, *et al.* Liberal versus restrictive fluid administration to improved recovery after laproscopic cholecystectomy: a randomized, double blinded study. *Ann Surg* 2004; **240**: 892–899.
171 Nisanevich V, Felsenstein I, Almogy G, *et al.* Effect of intraoperative fluid management on outcome after intraabdominal surgery. *Anesthesiology* 2005; **103**: 25–32.
172 Joshi GP. Intraoperative fluid restriction improves outcome after major elective gastrointestinal surgery. *Anesth Analg* 2005; **101**: 601–605.

173 Myles PS, Bellomo R, Corcoran T, *et al.* Australian and New Zealand College of Anaesthetists Clinical Trials Network, the Australian and New Zealand Intensive Care Society Clinical Trials Group. Restrictive versus Liberal fluid therapy for major abdominal surgery. *N Engl J Med* 2018; **378**: 2263–2274.

174 Gaynor JS, Wertz EM, Kesel LM, *et al.* Effect of intravenous administration of fluids on packed cell volume, blood pressure, total protein and blood glucose concentration in healthy halothane anesthetized dogs. *J Am Vet Med Assoc* 1996; **208**: 2013–2015.

175 Davis H, Jensen T, Johnson A, *et al.* 2013 AAHA/AAFP fluid therapy guidelines for dogs and cats. *J Am Anim Hosp Assoc* 2013; **49**: 149–159.

176 Butler AL. Goal-directed therapy in small animal critical care. *Vet Clin North Am Sm Anim Pract* 2011; **41**: 817–838.

177 Hayes GM, Mathews K, Boston S, *et al.* Low central venous oxygen saturation is associated with increased mortality in critically ill dogs. *J Small Anim Pract* 2011; **52**: 433–440.

178 Rivers E, Nguyen B, Havstad S, *et al.* Early goal-directed therapy in the treatment of severe sepsis and septic shock. *N Engl J Med* 2001; **345**: 1368–1377.

179 Concannon KT. Colloid osmotic pressure and the clinical use of colloidal solutions. *J Vet Emerg Crit Care* 2002; **3**: 49–62.

180 Bumpus SE, Haskins SC, Kass PH. Effect of synthetic colloids on refractometric readings of total solids. *J Vet Emerg Crit Care* 1998; **8**: 21–26.

181 Yam E, Hosgood G, Rossi G, *et al.* Synthetic colloid fluids, (6% hydroxyethyl starch 130/0.4 and 4% succinylated gelatin), interfere with measurement of total plasma protein in vitro. *Vet Clin Pathol* 2018; **47**: 575–587.

182 Yam E, Boyd CJ, Hosgood G, *et al.* (2019) Hydroxyethyl starch 130/0.4 and succinylated gelatin (4%) interferes with refractometry in dogs with hemorrhagic shock. *Vet Anaesth Analg* 2019; **46**: 579–586.

183 Rothe CF. Reflex control of veins and vascular capacitance. *Physiol Rev* 1983; **63**: 1281–1342.

184 Gelman S. Venous function and central venous pressure: a physiologic story. *Anesthesiology* 2008; **108**: 735–748.

185 Magder S. Volume and its relationship to cardiac output and venous return. *Crit Care* 2016; **20**: 271.

186 Michard F, Teboul JL. Predicting fluid responsiveness in ICU patients: a critical analysis of the evidence. *Chest* 2002; **121**: 2000–2008.

187 Messina A, Longhini F, Coppo C, *et al.* Use of the fluid challenge in critically ill adult patients: a systematic review. *Anesth Analg* 2017; **125**: 1532–1543.

188 Renner J, Scholz J, Bein B. Monitoring fluid therapy. *Best Pract Res Clin Anesthesiol* 2009; **23**: 159–171.

189 Kehlet H, Bundgaard-Nielson M. Goal-directed perioperative fluid therapy. *Anesthesiology* 2009; **110**: 453–455.

190 Bednarczyk JM, Fridfinnson JA, Kumar A, *et al.* Incorporating dynamic assessment of fluid responsiveness into goal directed therapy: a systematic review and meta-analysis. *Crit Care Med* 2017; **45**: 1538–1545.

191 Som A, Maitra S, Bhattacharjee S, *et al.* Goal directed fluid therapy decreases postoperative morbidity but not mor- tality in major non-cardiac surgery: a meta-analysis and trial sequential analysis of randomized controlled trials. *J Anesth* 2017; **31**: 66–81.

192 Jessen MK, Vallentin MF, Holmberg MJ, *et al.* Goal directed hemodynamic therapy during general anesthesia for noncardiac surgery: a systematic view and meta-analysis. *B J Anaesth* 2022; **128**: 416–433.

193 Cherpanath TG, Geerts BF, Lagrand WK, *et al.* Basic concepts of fluid responsiveness. *Neth Heart J* 2013; **21**: 530–536.

194 Guerin L, Monnet X, Teboul JL. Monitoring volume and fluid responsiveness: from static to dynamic indicators. *Best Pract Res Clin Anesth* 2013; **17**: 177–185.

195 Cecconi M, Parsons AK, Rhodes A. What is a fluid challenge? *Curr Opin Crit Care* 2011; **17**: 290–295.

196 Carsetti A, Cecconi M, Rhodes A. Fluid bolus therapy: monitoring and predicting fluid responsiveness. *Curr Opin Crit Care* 2015; **21**: 388–394.

197 Marik PE, Lemson J. Fluid responsiveness: an evolution of our understanding. *Br J Anaesth* 2014; **112**: 620–622.

198 Osman D, Ridel C, Ray P, *et al.* Cardiac filling pressures are not appropriate to predict hemodynamic response to volume challenge. *Crit Care Med* 2007; **35**: 64–68.

199 Marik PE, Baram M, Vahid B. Does central venous pressure predict fluid responsiveness? A systematic review of the literature and the tale of seven mares. *Chest* 2008; **134**: 172–178.

200 Marik PE, Cavallazzi R. Does the central venous pressure predict fluid responsiveness? An updated meta-analysis and a plea for some common sense. *Crit Care Med* 2013; **41**: 1774–1781.

201 Sano H, Seo J, Wightman P, *et al.* Evaluation of pulse pressure variation and pleth variability index to predict fluid responsiveness in mechanically ventilated isoflurane-anesthetized dogs. *J Vet Emerg Crit Care* 2018; **28**: 301–309.

202 Drozdzynska MJ, Chang YM, Stanzani G, *et al.* Evaluation of the dynamic predictors of fluid responsiveness in dogs receiving goal-directed fluid therapy. *Vet Anaesth Analg* 2018; **45**: 22–30.

203 Vincent JL. The pulmonary artery catheter. *J Clin Monit Comput* 2012; **26**: 341–345.

204 Marik PE. Obituary: pulmonary artery catheter 1970 to 2013. *Ann Intensive Care* 2013; **28**: 38.

205 Harvey S, Harrison DA, Singer M, *et al.* Assessment of clinical effectiveness of pulmonary artery catheters in management of patients in intensive care (PACMan): a randomized controlled trial. *Lancet* 2005; **366**: 472–477.

206 Araos J, Kenny JS, Rousseau-Blass F, *et al.* Dynamic prediction of fluid responsiveness during positive pressure ventilation: a review of the physiology underlying heart-lung interactions and a critical interpretation. *Vet Anaesth Analg* 2020; **47**: 3–14.

207 Michard F. Changes in arterial pressure during mechanical ventilation. *Anesthesiology* 2005; **103**: 419–428.

208 Marik PE, Cavallazi R, Vasu T, *et al.* Dynamic changes in arterial waveform derived variables and fluid responsiveness in mechanically ventilated patients: a systematic review of literature. *Crit Care Med* 2009; **37**: 2642–2647.

209 Thiele R, Durieux ME. Arterial waveform analysis for the anesthesiologist: past, present, and future concepts. *Anesth Analg* 2011; **113**: 766–776.

210 Michard F, Teboul JL. Using heart-lung interactions to assess fluid responsiveness during mechanical ventilation. *Crit Care* 2000; **4**: 282–289.

211 Monnet X, Teboul JL. Passive leg raising: five rules, not a drop of fluid! *Crit Care* 2015; **19**: 18.

212 Paranjape VV, Shih AC, Garcia-Pereira FL. Use of a modified passive leg-raising maneuver to predict fluid responsiveness during experimental induction and correction of hypovolemia in healthy isoflurane-anesthetized pigs. *Am J Vet Res* 2019; **80**: 24–32.

213 Messina A, Dell'Anna A, Baggiani M, *et al.* Functional hemodynamic tests: a systematic review and a metanalysis on the reliability of the end-expiratory occlusion test and of the mini-fluid challenge in predicting fluid responsiveness. *Crit Care* 2019; **23**: 264.

214 Bucci M, Rabozzi R, Guglielmini C, *et al.* Respiratory variation in aortic blood peak velocity and caudal vena cava diameter can predict fluid responsiveness in anaesthetised and mechanically ventilated dogs. *Vet J* 2017; **227**: 30–35.

215 Oricco S, Rabozzi R, Meneghini C, *et al.* Usefulness of focused cardiac ultrasonography for predicting fluid responsiveness in conscious, spontaneously breathing dogs. *Am J Vet Res* 2019; **80**: 369–377.

216 Rabozzi R, Oricco S, Meneghini C, *et al.* Evaluation of the caudal vena cava diameter to abdominal aortic diameter ratio and the caudal vena cava respiratory collapsibility for predicting fluid responsiveness in a heterogeneous population of hospitalized conscious dogs. *J Vet Med Sci* 2020; **82**: 337–344.

217 Skouropoulou D, Lacitignola L, Di Bella C, *et al.* Intraoperative assessment of fluid responsiveness in normotensive dogs under isoflurane anaesthesia. *Vet Sci* 2021; **8**: 26.

218 Fantoni DT, Ida KK, Gimenes AM, *et al.* Pulse pressure variation as a guide for volume expansion in dogs undergoing orthopedic surgery. *Vet Anaesth Analg* 2017; **44**: 710–718.

219 Celeita-Rodríguez N, Teixeira-Neto FJ, Garofalo NA, *et al.* Comparison of the diagnostic accuracy of dynamic and static preload indexes to predict fluid responsiveness in mechanically ventilated, isoflurane anesthetized dogs. *Vet Anaesth Analg* 2019; **6**: 276–288.

220 Gonçalves LA, Otsuki DA, Pereira MA, *et al.* Comparison of pulse pressure variation versus echocardiography-derived stroke volume variation for prediction of fluid responsiveness in mechanically ventilated anesthetized dogs. *Vet Anaesth Analg* 2020; **47**: 28–37.

221 de Oliveira GCV, Teixeira-Neto FJ, Dalmagro TL, *et al.* Use of aortic flow indexes derived from transthoracic echocardiography to evaluate response to a fluid challenge in anesthetized dogs. *Vet Anaesth Analg* 2021; **48**: 187–197.

222 Dalmagro TL, Teixeira-Neto FJ, Celeita-Rodríguez N, *et al.* Comparison between pulse pressure variation and systolic pressure variation measured from a peripheral artery for accurately predicting fluid responsiveness in mechanically ventilated dogs. *Vet Anaesth Analg* 2021; **48**: 501–508.

223 Toscani L, Aya HD, Antonakaki D, *et al.* What is the impact of fluid challenge technique on diagnosis of fluid responsiveness? A systematic review and meta-analysis. *Critical Care* 2017; **21**: 207–219.

224 Cecconi M, Hofer C, Teboul JL, *et al.* Fluid challenges in intensive care: the FENICE study: a global inception cohort study. *Intensive Care Med* 2015; **41**: 1529–1537.

225 Pierrakos C, Velissaris D, Scolletta S, *et al.* Can changes in arterial pressure be used to detect changes in cardiac index during fluid challenge in patients with septic shock? *Intensive Care Med* 2012; **38**: 422–428.

226 Critchley LA, Critchley JA. A meta-analysis of studies using bias and precision statistics to compare cardiac output measurement techniques. *J Clin Monit Comput* 1999; **15**: 85–91.

227 Critchley LA, Critchley LA, Yang XX, *et al.* Assessment of trending ability of cardiac output monitors by polar plot methodology. *J Cardiothorac Vasc Anesth* 2011; **25**: 536–546.

228 Grensemann J. Cardiac output monitoring bypulse contour analysis, the technical basis of less-invasive techniques. *Front Med* 2018; **5**: 64.

229 Briganti A, Evangelista F, Centonze P, *et al.* A preliminary study evaluating cardiac output measurement using Pressure Recording Analytical Method (PRAM) in anaesthetized dogs. *BMC Vet Res* 2018; **14**: 72.

230 Chohan AS, Pascoe PJ. Experimental evaluation of a pressure related analytical method (PRAM), a pulse contour analysis method, to calculate cardiac output during progressive hypovolemia and volume restoration in Beagle dogs. *Vet Anaesth Analg* 2021; **48**: 984.e3.

231 Chohan AS, Pascoe PJ. Experimental evaluation of a Pressure Recording Analytical Method (PRAM), a pulse contour análisis method, for monitoring cardiac output in dogs. *Vet Anaesth Analg* 2023; **50**: e107–e108.

232 Valverde A, Gianotti G, Rioja E, *et al.* Comparison of cardiac output determined by arterial pulse pressure waveform analysis method (FloTrac/Vigileo) versus lithium dilution method in anesthetized dogs. *J Vet Emerg Crit Care* 2011; **21**: 328–334.

233 Bektas RN, Kutter AP, Hartnack S, *et al.* Evaluation of a minimally invasive non-calibrated pulse contour cardiac output monitor (FloTrac/Vigileo) in anaesthetized dogs. *Vet Anaesth Analg* 2012; **39**: 464–471.

234 Sasaki K, Mutoh T, Kawashima R, *et al.* Electrical velocimetry for non-invasive cardiac output and stroke volume variation measurements in dogs undergoing cardiovascular surgery. *Vet Anaesth Analg* 2017; **44**: 7–16.

235 Sano H, Chambers JP. Ability of pulse wave transit time to detect changes in stroke volume and to estimate cardiac output compared to thermodilution technique in isoflurane-anaesthetised dogs. *Vet Anaesth Analg* 2017; **44**: 1057–1067.

236 Chohan AS, Pascoe PJ. Evaluation of transesophageal Doppler in Beagle dogs as an aid to provide goal directed fluid therapy. *Vet Anaesth Analg* 2019; **46**: 831.e4.

237 Canfrán S, Cediel R, Sández I, *et al.* Evaluation of an oesophageal Doppler device for monitoring cardiac output in anaesthetised healthy normotensive dogs. *J Small Anim Pract* 2015; **56**: 450–455.

238 Monnet X, Marik PE, Teboul JL. Prediction of fluid responsiveness:an update. *Ann Intensive Care* 2016; **6**: 111.

239 Mesquida J, Kim HK, Pinsky MR. Effect of tidal volume, intrathoracic pressure, and cardiac contractility on variations in pulse pressure, stroke volume, and intrathoracic blood volume. *Intensive Care Med* 2011; **37**: 1672–1679.

240 Endo Y, Tamura J, Ishizuka T, *et al.* Stroke Volume Variation (SVV) and Pulse Pressure Variation (PPV) as indicators of fluid responsiveness in sevoflurane anesthetized mechanically ventilated euvolemic dogs. *J Vet Med Sci* 2017; **79**: 1437–1445.

241 Endo Y, Kawase K, Miyasho T, *et al.* Plethysmography variability index for prediction of fluid responsiveness during graded haemorrhage and transfusion in sevoflurane anaesthetized mechanically ventilated dogs. *Vet Anaesth Analg* 2017; **44**: 1303–1312.

242 Mackenzie DC, Noble VE. Assessing volume status and fluid responsiveness in the emergency department. *Clin Exp Emerg Med* 2014; **1**: 67–77.

243 Durkan, SD, Rush J, Rozanski E. Echocardiographic findings in dogs with hypovolemia [Abstract]. *J Vet Emerg Crit Care* 2005; **15**: S1–S13.

244 Campbell FE, Kittleson MD. The effect of hydration status on the echocardiographic measurements of normal cats. *J Vet Intern Med* 2007; **21**: 1008–1015.

245 Fine DM, Durham HE Jr., Rossi NF, *et al.* Echocardiographic assessment of hemodynamic changes produced by two methods of inducing fluid deficit in dogs. *J Vet Intern Med* 2010; **24**: 348–353.

246 Teboul JL, Monnet X. Pulse pressure variation and ARDS. *Minerva Anesthesiol* 2013; **79**: 398–407.

247 Diaz F, Erranz B, Donoso A, *et al.* Influence of tidal volume on pulse pressure variation and stroke volume variation during experimental intra-abdominal hypertension. *BMC Anesthesiol* 2015; **15**: 127.

248 Nouira S, Elatrous S, Dimassi S, *et al.* Effects of norepinephrine on static and dynamic preload indicators in experimental hemorrhagic shock. *Crit Care Med* 2005; **33**: 2339–2343.

249 Diniz MS, Teixeira-Neto FJ, Candido TD, *et al.* Effects of dexmedetomidine on pulse pressure variation changes induced by hemorrhage followed by volume replacement in isoflurane-anesthetized dogs. *J Vet Emerg Crit Care* 2014; **24**: 681–692.

250 Hadian M, Severyn DA, Pinsky MR. The effects of vasoactive drugs on pulse pressure and stroke volume variation in postoperative ventilated patients. *J Crit Care* 2011; **26**: 328.e1–8.

251 Mair S, Tschirwahn J, Gotz S, *et al.* Applicability of stroke volume variation in patients of a general intensive care unit a longitudinal observational study. *J Clin Monit Comput* 2017; **31**: 1177–1187.

252 Magder S. Fluid status and fluid responsiveness. *Curr Opin Crit Care* 2010; **16**: 289–296.

253 Navarro LH, Bloomstone JA, Auler JO Jr., *et al.* Perioperative fluid therapy: a statement from the International Fluid Optimization Group. *Perioper Med (London)* 2015; **4**: 3.

254 Pinsky MR. Cardiopulmonary interactions: physiologic basis and clinical applications. *Ann Am Thorac Soc* 2018; **15**: S45–S48.

255 Takala J. Volume responsive, but does the patient need volume? *Intensive Care Med* 2016; **42**: 1461–1463.

256 Reines BP, Ninham BW. Structure and function of the endothelial surface layer: unraveling the nanoarchitecture of biological surfaces. *Q Rev Biophys* 2019; **52**: e13.

257 Akbarshahi H, Axelsson JB, Said K, *et al.* TLR4 dependent heparan sulphate-induced pancreatic inflammatory response is IRF3-mediated. *J Transl Med* 2011; **9**: 219.

258 Scheibner KA, Lutz MA, Boodoo S, *et al.* Hyaluronan fragments act as an endogenous danger signal by engaging TLR2. *J Immunol* 2006; **177**: 1272–1281.

259 De Backer D, Donadello K, Sakr Y, *et al.* Microcirculatory alterations in patients with severe sepsis: impact of time of assessment and relationship with outcome. *Crit Care Med* 2013; **41**: 791–799.

260 Tachon G, Harrois A, Tanaka S, *et al.* Microcirculatory alterations in traumatic hemorrhagic shock. *Crit Care Med* 2014; **42**: 1433–1441.

261 Cabrales P, Vazquez BY, Tsai AG, *et al.* Microvascular and capillary perfusion following glycocalyx degradation. *J Appl Physiol* 2007; **102**: 2251–2259.

262 Chen W, Gassner B, Borner S, *et al.* Atrial natriuretic peptide enhances microvascular albumin permeability by the caveolae-mediated transcellular pathway. *Cardiovasc Res* 2012; **93**: 141–151.

263 Chappell D, Bruegger D, Potzel J, *et al.* Hypervolemia increases release of atrial natriuretic peptide and shedding of the endothelial glycocalyx. *Crit Care* 2014; **18**: 538.

264 Belavi´c M, Sotošek TokmadŽi´c V, Fiši´c E, *et al.* The effect of various doses of infusion solutions on the endothelial glycocalyx layer in laparoscopic cholecystectomy patients. *Minerva Anestesiol* 2018; **84**: 1032–1043.

265 Smart L, Boyd CJ, Claus MA, *et al.* Large-volume crystalloid fluid is associated with increased hyaluronan shedding and inflammation in a canine hemorrhagic shock model. *Inflammation* 2018; **41**: 1515–1523.

266 Marik PE, Byrne L, van Haren F. Fluid resuscitation in sepsis: the great 30 mL per kg hoax. *J Thor Dis* 2020; **12**(Suppl. 1): S37–S47.

267 Macdonald SPJ, Keijzers G, Taylor DM, *et al.* Restricted fluid resuscitation in suspected sepsis associated hypotension (REFRESH): a pilot randomised controlled trial. *Intensive Care Med* 2018; **44**: 2070–2078.

268 Turek Z, Cerny V, Parizkova R, *et al.* Prolonged hypervolemic hemodilution decreases functional capillary density of ileal mucosa in pigs revealed by sidestream dark-field imaging. *J Zhejiang Univ Sci B* 2011; **2**: 867–874.

269 Yu TC, Yang FL, Hsu BG, *et al.* Deleterious effects of aggressive rapid crystalloid resuscitation on treatment of hyperinflammatory response and lung injury induced by hemorrhage in aging rats. *J Surg Res* 2014; **187**: 587–595.

270 Jacob M, Chappell D, Hofmann-Kiefer K, *et al.* The intravascular volume effect of Ringer's lactate is below 20%: a prospective study in humans. *Crit Care* 2012; **16**: R86.

271 Zazzeron L, Gattinoni L, Caironi P. Role of albumin, starches and gelatins versus crystalloids in volume resuscitation of critically ill patients. *Curr Opin Crit Care* 2016; **22**: 428–436.

272 Chelazzi C, Villa G, Mancinelli P, *et al.* Glycocalyx and sepsis-induced alterations in vascular permeability. *Crit Care* 2015; **19**: 26.

273 Fleck A, Hawker F, Wallace PI, *et al.* Increased vascular permeability: a major cause of hypoalbuminaemia in disease and injury. *Lancet* 1985; **325**: 781–784.

274 Müller RB, Ostrowski SR, Haase N, *et al.* Markers of endothelial damage and coagulation impairment in patients with severe sepsis resuscitated with hydroxyethyl starch 130/0.42 vs Ringer acetate. *J Crit Care* 2016; **32**: 16–20.

275 Torres LN, Sondeen JL, Dubick MA, *et al.* Systemic and microvascular effects of resuscitation with blood products after severe hemorrhage in rats. *J Trauma Acute Care Surg* 2014; **77**: 716–723.

276 Kozar RA, Peng Z, Zhang R, *et al.* Plasma restoration of endothelial glycocalyx in a rodent model of hemorrhagic shock. *Anesth Analg* 2011; **112**: 1289–1295.

277 Lewis SR, Pritchard MW, Evans DJ, *et al.* Colloids versus crystalloids for fluid resuscitation in critically ill people. *Cochrane Database Syst Rev* 2018; **8**: CD000567.

278 Dibartola SP. Disorders of sodium and water: hypernatremia and hyponatremia. In: Dibartola SP, ed. *Fluid, Electrolyte and Acid-Base Disorders in Small Animal Practice*, 4th edn. St. Louis, MO: Elsevier, 2012: 45–79.

279 Androgue HJ, Madias NE. Hypernatremia. *N Engl J Med* 2000; **342**: 1493–1499.

280 Pollock AS, Arieff AI. Abnormalities of cell volume regulation and their functional consequences. *Am J Physiol* 1980; **239**: F195–F205.
281 Willard M. Therapeutic approach to chronic electrolyte disorders. *Vet Clin North Am Small Anim Pract* 2008; **38**: 535–541.
282 Lien YH, Shapiro JI, Chan L. Effects of hypernatremia on organic brain osmoles. *J Clin Invest* 1990; **85**: 1427–1435.
283 Schaer M. Therapeutic approach to electrolyte emergencies. *Vet Clin North Am Small Anim Pract* 2008; **38**: 513–533.
284 Ellison DH, Berl T. The syndrome of inappropriate antidiuresis. *N Engl J Med* 2007; **356**: 2064–2072.
285 Houston DM, Allen DG, Kruth SA, *et al.* Syndrome of inappropriate antidiuretic hormone secretion in a dog. *Can Vet J* 1989; **30**: 423.
286 Kokko H, Hall PD, Afrin LB. Fentanyl associated syndrome of inappropriate antidiuretic hormone secretion. *Pharmacotherapy* 2002; **22**: 1188–1192.
287 Demirel I, Ozer AB, Bayar MK, *et al.* TRUP syndrome and severe hyponatremia under general anesthesia. *BMJ Case Rep* 2012; **BCR-2012**: 006899.
288 Liptak JM, Brutsher SP, Monnet E, *et al.* Transurethral resection in the management of urethral and prostatic neoplasia in 6 dogs. *Vet Surg* 2004; **33**: 505–516.
289 Toll J, Barr SC, Hickford FH. Acute water intoxication in a dog. *J Vet Emerg Crit Care* 1999; **9**: 19–22.
290 O'Brien DP, Kroll RA, Johnson GC, *et al.* Myelinolysis after correction of hyponatremia in two dogs. *J Vet Intern Med* 1994; **8**: 40–48.
291 Churcher RK, Wason ADJ, Eaton A. Suspected myelinolysis following rapid correction of hyponatremia in a dog. *J Am Anim Hosp Assoc* 1999; **35**: 492–497.
292 Aguilera IM, Vaughan RS. Calcium and the anesthetist. *Anaesthesia* 2000; **55**: 779–790.
293 Schenck PA, Chew DJ. Calcium: total or ionized? *Vet Clin North Am Sm Anim Pract* 2008; **38**: 497–502.
294 Holowaychuk MK, Martin LG. Review of hypocalcemia in septic patients. *J Vet Emerg Crit Care* 2007; **17**: 348–358.
295 Borer KE, Corley KTT. Electrolyte disorders in horses with colic. Part 2: calcium, sodium, chloride and phosphate. *Equine Vet Educ* 2006; **18**: 320–325.
296 Grubb TL, Benson GJ, Foreman JH, *et al.* Hemodynamic effects of ionized calcium in horses anesthetized with halothane or isoflurane. *Am J Vet Res* 1999; **60**: 1430–1435.
297 Gasthuys F, de Moor A, Parmentier D, *et al.* Cardiovascular effects of low dose calcium chloride infusions during halothane anesthesia in dorsally recumbent ventilated ponies. *J Am Vet Med Assoc* 1991; **38**: 728–736.
298 Dhupa N, Proulx J. Hypocalcemia and hypomagnesemia. *Vet Clin North Am Sm Anim Pract* 1998; **28**: 587–608.
299 Sharp CR, Kerl ME, Mann FA. A comparison of total calcium, corrected calcium, and ionized calcium concentrations as indicators of calcium homeostasis among hypoalbuminemic dogs requiring intensive care. *J Vet Emerg Crit Care* 2009; **19**: 571–578.
300 Brennan SF, O'Donovan J, Mooney CT. Changes in canine ionized calcium under three storage conditions. *J Small Anim Pract* 2006; **47**: 383–386.
301 Dibartola SP, de Morais HA. Disorders of potassium: hypokalemia and hyperkalemia. In: Dibartola SP, ed. *Fluid, Electrolyte and Acid-Base Disorders in Small Animal Practice*, 4th edn. St. Louis, MO: Elsevier, 2012: 92–119.
302 Kablack KA, Embertson RM, Bernard WV, *et al.* Uroperitoneum in the hospitalized equine neonates: retrospective study of 31 cases. *Equine Vet J* 2000; **32**: 505–508.
303 Jones SJ, Mama KR, Brock NK, *et al.* Hyperkalemia during general anesthesia in two Greyhounds. *J Am Vet Med Assoc* 2019; **254**: 1329–1334.
304 Tong CW, Balakrishnan A, Wynn RM. Recurrent hyperkalemia during general anesthesia in a dog. *Front Vet Sci* 2020; **7**: 210.
305 Reilly S, Seddighi MR, Steeil JC, *et al.* Selected clinical, biochemical, and electrolyte alterations in anesthetized captive Tigers (*Panthera Tigris*) and lions (*Panthera Leo*). *J Zoo Wildl Med* 2014; **45**: 328–334.
306 McEntire MS, Ramsay EC, Price J, *et al.* The effects of procedure duration and atipamezole administration on hyperkalemia in Tigers (*Panthera Tigris*) and lions (*Panthera Leo*) anesthetized with alpha-2 agonists. *J Zoo Wildl Med* 2020; **51**: 490–496.
307 Guyton AC, Hall JE. *Textbook of Medical Physiology*, 14th edn. Philadelphia, PA: Elsevier, 2021: 63–77.
308 Tag TL, Day TK. Electrocardiographic assessment of hyperkalemia in dogs and cats. *J Vet Emerg Crit Care* 2008; **18**: 61–67.
309 Dananberg J. Electrolyte abnormalities affecting the heart. In: Schwartz GR, ed. *Principles and Practice of Emergency Medicine*, 4th edn. Baltimore, MD: Williams & Wilkins, 1999: 425–427.
310 Quick G, Bastani B. Prolonged asystolic hyperkalemic cardiac arrest with no neurologic sequelae. *Ann Emerg Med* 1994; **24**: 305–311.
311 Parham WA, Mehdirad AA, Biermann KM, *et al.* Hyperkalemia revisited. *Tex Heart Inst J* 2006; **33**: 40–47.
312 Norman BC, Côté E, Barrett KA. Wide-complex tachycardia associated with severe hyperkalemia in three cats. *J Feline Med Surg* 2006; **8**: 372–378.
313 Roden DM, Lazzara R, Rosen M, *et al.* Multiple mechanisms in the long-QT syndrome. Current knowledge, gaps, and future directions. The SADS Foundation Task Force on LQTS. *Circulation* 1996; **94**: 1996–2012.
314 Dittrich KL, Walls RM. Hyperkalemia: ECG manifestations and clinical considerations. *J Emerg Med* 1986; **4**: 449–455.
315 Ettinger PO, Regan TJ, Oldewurtel HA. Hyperkalemia, cardiac conduction, and the electrocardiogram: a review. *Am Heart J* 1974; **88**: 360–371.
316 Parks J. Electrocardiographic abnormalities from serum electrolyte imbalance due to feline urethral obstruction. *J Am Anim Hosp Assoc* 1975; **11**: 102–109.
317 Drobatz KJ, Cole SG. The influence of crystalloid type on acid-base and electrolyte status of cats with urethral obstruction. *J Vet Emerg Crit Care* 2008; **18**: 355–361.
318 Ho K. A critically swift response: insulin-stimulated potassium and glucose transport in skeletal muscle. *Clin J Am Soc Nephrol* 2011; **6**: 1513–1516.
319 Carvalhanna V, Burry L, Lapinsky SE. Management of severe hyperkalemia without hemodialysis: case report and literature review. *J Crit Care* 2006; **21**: 316–321.
320 Borer KE, Corley KTT. Electrolyte disorders in horses with colic. Part 1: potassium and magnesium. *Equine Vet J* 2006; **18**: 266–271.
321 Haldane S, Graves TK, Bateman S, *et al.* Profound hypokalemia causing respiratory failure in a cat with hyperaldosteronism. *J Vet Emerg Crit Care* 2007; **17**: 202–207.
322 American Society of Anesthesiologists. Practice guidelines for perioperative blood management; An updated report by the American Society of Anesthesiologists task force on perioperative blood management. *Anesthesiology* 2015; **122**: 241–275.
323 Davidow B. Transfusion medicine in small animals. *Vet Clin North Am Small Anim Pract* 2013; **43**: 735–756.
324 Divers TJ. Blood component transfusion. *Vet Clin North Am Food Anim Pract* 2005; **21**: 615–622.
325 Mudge MC. Acute hemorrhage and blood transfusions in horses. *Vet Clin North Am Equine Pract* 2014; **30**: 427–436.
326 Herbert P, van der Linden P, Biro G, *et al.* Physiologic aspects of anemia. *Crit Care Med* 2004; **20**: 187–212.
327 Jutkowitz LA. Blood transfusion in the perioperative period. *Clin Tech Small Anim Pract* 2004; **2**: 75–82.
328 Teixeira-Neto FJ, Luna S, Cruz MA, *et al.* A study of the effect of hemorrhage on the cardiorespiratory actions of halothane, isoflurane and sevoflurane in the dog. *Vet Anaesth Analg* 2007; **34**: 107–116.
329 Weingart C, Giger U, Kohn B. Whole blood transfusion in 91 cats: a clinical evaluation. *J Fel Med Surg* 2004; **6**: 139–148.
330 Klaser DA, Reine NJ, Hohenhaus AE. Red blood cell transfusion in cats: 126 cases (1999). *J Am Vet Med Assoc* 2005; **226**: 920–923.
331 Castellanos I, Couto CG, Gray TL. Clinical use of blood products in cats: a retrospective study (1997–2000). *J Vet Intern Med* 2004; **18**: 529–532.
332 Roux FA, Deschamps JY, Blais MC, *et al.* Multiple red cell transfusion in 27 cats (2003–2006). *J Fel Med Surg* 2008; **10**: 213–218.
333 Hurcombe SD, Mudge MC, Hinchcliff KW. Clinical and clinicopathologic variables in adult horses receiving blood transfusion. *J Am Vet Med Assoc* 2007; **231**: 267–274.
334 Kerl ME, Hohenhaus AE. Packed red blood cell transfusions in dogs: 131 case (1989). *J Am Vet Med Assoc* 1993; **202**: 1495–1499.
335 Callan MB, Oakley DA, Shofer ES, *et al.* Canine red blood cell transfusion practice. *J Am Anim Hosp Assoc* 1996; **32**: 303–311.
336 Kuo KW, McMichael M. Small animal transfusion medicine. *Vet Clin North Am Small Anim Pract* 2020; **50**: 1203–1214.
337 Reed N, Espadas I, Lalor SM, *et al.* Assessment of five formulae to predict post-transfusion packed cell volume in cats. *J Fel Med Surg* 2014; **16**: 651–656.
338 Edwards TH, Darlington DN, Pusateri AE, *et al.* Hemostatic capacity of canine chilled whole blood over time. *J Vet Crit Care* 2021; **31**: 239–246.
339 Valeri CR, Khuri S, Ragno G. Nonsurgical bleeding diathesis in anemic thrombocytopenic patients: role of temperature, red blood cells, platelets, and plasma-clotting proteins. *Transfusion* 2007; **47**: 206S–248S.
340 Valeri CR, Cassidy G, Pivacek LE, *et al.* Anemia-induced increase in the bleeding time: implications for treatment of nonsurgical blood loss. *Transfusion* 2001; **41**: 977–983.
341 Sort JL, Diehl S, Seshadri R, *et al.* Accuracy of formulas used to predict posttransfusion packed cell volume rise in anemic dogs. *J Vet Emerg Crit Care* 2012; **22**: 428–434.
342 Brooks MB, Wardrop KJ. Stability of hemostatic proteins in canine fresh frozen plasma units. *Vet Clin Pathol* 2001; **30**: 91–95.
343 Stokol T, Parry B. Efficacy of fresh-frozen plasma and cryoprecipitate in dogs with von Willebrand's disease or hemophilia A. *J Vet Intern Med* 1998; **12**: 84–92.
344 Urban R, Couto CG, Iazbik MC. Evaluation of hemostatic activity of canine frozen plasma for transfusion by thromboelastography. *J Vet Intern Med* 2013; **27**: 964–969.

345 Stokol T, Parry BW. Stability of canine factor VIII and von Willebrand factor antigen concentration in the frozen state. *Res Vet Sci* 1995; **59**: 156–159.

346 Ching YNLH, Meyers KM, Brassard JA, *et al.* Effect of cryoprecipitate and plasma on plasma von Willebrand factor multimers and bleeding time in Doberman Pinschers with type-I von Willebrand's disease. *Am J Vet Res* 1994; **55**: 102–110.

347 Cheung H, Jandrey KE, Burges J, *et al.* An in vitro study of canine cryopoor plasma to correct vitamin K-dependent coagulopathy in dogs. *J Vet Emerg Crit Care* 2021; **31**: 231–238.

348 Throop JL, Kerl ME, Cohn LA. Albumin in health and disease: protein metabolism and function. *Comp Cont Educ Vet* 2004; **26**: 932–939.

349 Mazzaferro EM, Rudloff E, Kirby R. The role of albumin replacement in the critically ill veterinary patient. *J Vet Emerg Crit Care* 2002; **12**: 113–124.

350 Vigano F, Perissinotto L, Bosco V. Administration of 5% human serum albumin in critically ill small animal patients with hypoalbuminemia: 418 dogs and 170 cats (1994–2008). *J Vet Emerg Crit Care* 2010; **20**: 237–243.

351 Mosley CAE, Matthews KA. The use of concentrated serum albumin in canines. *Vet Anesth Analg* 2005; **32**: 14–15.

352 Mathews K, Barry M. The use of 25% human serum albumin: outcome and efficacy in raising serum albumin and systemic blood pressure in critically ill dogs and cats. *J Vet Emerg Crit Care* 2005; **15**: 110–118.

353 Trow A, Rozanski E, de Laforcade A, *et al.* Evaluation of the use of human albumin in critically ill dogs: 73 cases (2003–2006). *J Am Vet Med Assoc* 2008; **233**: 607–612.

354 Vigano F, Perissinotto L, Bosco V. Administration of 5% human serum albumin in critically ill small animal patients with hypoalbuminemia: 418 dogs and 170 cats (1994–2008). *J Vet Emerg Crit Care* 2010; **20**: 237–243.

355 Mazzaferro EM, Balakrishnan A, Hackner SG, *et al.* Delayed type III hypersensitivity reaction with acute kidney injury in two dogs following administration of concentration human albumin during treatment for hypoalbuminemia secondary to septic peritonitis. *J Vet Emerg Crit Care* 2020; **30**: 574–580.

356 Powell C, Thompson L, Murtaugh RJ. Type III hypersensitivity reaction with immune complex deposition in 2 critically ill dogs administered human serum albumin. *J Vet Emerg Crit Care* 2013; **23**: 598–604.

357 DeWitt SF, Paradis MR. Use of human albumin as a colloidal therapy in the hypoproteinemic equine [Abstract]. *J Vet Intern Med* 2004; **14**: S8.

358 Francis AH, Martin L, Haldorson GJ, *et al.* Adverse reactions suggestive of type III hypersensitivity in six healthy dogs given human albumin. *J Am Vet Med Assoc* 2007; **320**: 873–879.

359 Cohn LA, Kerl ME, Lenox CE, *et al.* Response of healthy dogs to infusion of human serum albumin. *Am J Vet Res* 2007; **68**: 657–663.

360 Martin LG, Luther TY, Alperin DC, *et al.* Serum antibodies against human albumin in critically ill and healthy dogs. *J Am Vet Med Assoc* 2008; **232**: 1004–1009.

361 Craft EM, Powell LL. The use of canine-specific albumin in dogs with septic peritonitis. *J Vet Emerg Crit Care* 2012; **22**: 631–639.

362 Enders B, Musulin S, Holowaychuk M, *et al.* Repeated infusion of lyophilized canine albumin safely and effectively increases serum albumin and colloid osmotic pressure in healthy dogs [Abstract]. *J Vet Emerg Crit Care* 2018; **28**(S1): S5.

363 Smith CL, Ramsey NB, Parr AM, *et al.* Evaluation of a novel canine albumin solution in normal Beagles [Abstract]. *J Vet Emerg Crit Care* 2009; **19**(Suppl): A3.

364 Finfer S, Bellomo R, Boyce N, *et al.* A comparison of albumin and saline for fluid resuscitation in the intensive care unit. *N Engl J Med* 2004; **350**: 2247–2256.

365 Roberts I, Blackhall K, Alderson P, *et al.* Human albumin solution for resuscitation and volume expansion in critically ill patients. *Cochrane Database Syst Rev* 2011; **11**: CD001208.

366 Melia D, Post B. Human albumin solutions in intensive care: A review. *J Intensive Care Soc* 2021; **22**: 248–254.

367 Greeno E, McCullough J, Weisdorf D. Platelet utilization and the transfusion trigger: a prospective analysis. *Transfusion* 2007; **47**: 201–205.

368 Petrides M, Stack G, Cooling L, *et al. Practical Guide to Transfusion Medicine.* Bethesda, MD: AABB Press, 2007.

369 Callow CR, Swindell R, Randall W, *et al.* The frequency of bleeding complications in patients with haematological malignancy following the introduction of a stringent prophylactic platelet transfusion policy. *Br J Haematol* 2002; **118**: 677–682.

370 Abrams-Ogg AC. Triggers for prophylactic use of platelet transfusions and optimal platelet dosing in thrombocytopenic dogs and cats. *Vet Clin North Am Small Anim Pract* 2003; **33**: 1401–1418.

371 Callan MB, Appleman EH, Sachais BS. Canine platelet transfusions. *J Vet Emerg Crit Care* 2009; **19**: 401–415.

372 Clemmons RM, Bliss EL, Dorsey-Lee MR, *et al.* Platelet function, size and yield in whole blood and in platelet-rich plasma prepared using different centrifugation force and time in domestic and food-producing animals. *Thromb Haemost* 1983; **50**: 838–843.

373 Abrams-Ogg ACG, Kruth SA, Carter RF, *et al.* Preparation and transfusion of canine platelet concentrates. *Am J Vet Res* 1993; **54**: 635–642.

374 Callan MB, Appleman EH, Shofer FS, *et al.* Clinical and clinicopathologic effects of plateletpheresis on healthy donor dogs. *Transfusion* 2008; **48**: 2214–2221.

375 Mack JP, Miles J, Stolla. Cold-stored platelets: review of studies in humans. *Transfus Med Rev* 2020; **34**: 221–226.

376 Appleman EH, Sachais BS, Patel R, *et al.* Cryopreservation of canine platelets. *J Vet Intern Med* 2009; **23**: 138–145.

377 Valeri CR, Feingold H, Marchionni LD. A simple method for freezing human platelets using 6 per cent dimethyl-sulfoxide and storage at -80 degrees C. *Blood* 1974; **43**: 131–136.

378 Valeri CR, Feingold H, Melaragno AJ, *et al.* Cryopreservation of dog platelets with dimethyl sulfoxide: therapeutic effectiveness of cryopreserved platelets in the treatment of thrombocytopenic dogs, and the effect of platelet storage at -80 degrees C. *Cryobiology* 1986; **23**: 387–394.

379 Guillaumin J, Jandrey KE, Norris JW, *et al.* Assessment of a dimethyl-sulfoxide-stabilized frozen canine platelet concentrate. *Am J Vet Res* 2008; **69**: 1580–1586.

380 Guillaumin J, Jandrey KE, Norris JW, *et al.* Analysis of a commercial dimethyl-sulfoxide-stabilized frozen canine platelet concentrate by turbidimetric aggregometry. *J Vet Emerg Crit Care* 2010; **20**: 571–577.

381 Bode AP, Fischer TH. Lyophilized platelets: fifty years in the making. *Artif Cells Blood Substit Immobil Biotechnol* 2007; **35**: 125–133.

382 Read MS, Reddick RL, Bode AP, *et al.* Preservation of hemostatic and structural properties of rehydrated lyophilized platelets: potential for long-term storage of dried platelets for transfusion. *Proc Natl Acad Sci USA* 1995; **92**: 397–401.

383 Fischer TH, Merricks EP, Bode AP, *et al.* Thrombus formation with rehydrated, lyophilized platelets. *Hematology* 2002; **7**: 359–369.

384 Bode AP, Lust RM, Read MS, *et al.* Correction of the bleeding time with lyophilized platelet infusions in dogs on cardiopulmonary bypass. *Clin Appl Thromb Hemost* 2008; **14**: 38–54.

385 Davidow EB, Brainard B, Martin LG, *et al.* Use of fresh platelet concentrate or lyophilized platelets in thrombocytopenic dogs with clinical signs of hemorrhage: a preliminary trial in 37 dogs. *J Vet Emerg Crit Care* 2012; **22**: 116–125.

386 Goggs R, Brainard BM, LeVine D, *et al.* Lyophilized platelets versus cryopreserved platelets for management of bleeding in thrombocytopenic dogs: a multicenter randomized clinical trial. *J Vet Intern Med* 2020; **34**: 2384–2397.

387 Hawksworth JS, Elster EA, Fryer D, *et al.* Evaluation of lyophilized platelets as an infusible hemostatic agent in experimental non-compressible hemorrhage in swine. *J Thromb Haemost* 2009; **7**: 1663–1671.

388 Symons M, Bell K. Canine blood groups: description of 20 specificities. *Anim Genet* 1992; **23**: 509–515.

389 Symons M, Bell K. Expansion of the canine A blood group system. *Anim Genet* 1991; **22**: 227–235.

390 Giger U, Gelens CJ, Callan MB, *et al.* An acute hemolytic transfusion reaction caused by dog erythrocyte antigen 1.1 incompatibility in a previously sensitized dog. *J Am Vet Med Assoc* 1995; **206**: 1358–1362.

391 Kessler RJ, Reese J, Chang D, *et al.* Dog erythrocyte antigens 1.1, 1.2, 3, 4, 7, and Dal blood typing and cross-matching by gel column technique. *Vet Clin Pathol* 2010; **39**: 306–316.

392 Callan MB, Jones LT, Giger U. Hemolytic transfusion reactions in a dog with an alloantibody to a common antigen. *J Vet Intern Med* 1995; **9**: 277–279.

393 Spada E, Proverbio D, Vinals Florez LM, *et al.* Prevalence of naturally occurring antibodies against dog erythrocyte antigen 7 in a population of dog erythrocyte antigen 7-negative dogs from Spain and Italy. *Am J Vet Res* 2016; **77**: 877–881.

394 Swisher SN, Young LE, Trabold N. In vitro and in vivo studies of the behavior of canine erythrocyte-isoantibody systems. *Ann N Y Acad Sci* 1962; **97**: 15–25.

395 Blais MC, Berman L, Oakley DA, *et al.* Canine Dal blood type: a red cell antigen lacking in some Dalmatians. *J Vet Intern Med* 2007; **21**: 281–286.

396 Ebelt AK, Fuchs S, Weber C, *et al.* Survey of blood groups DEA1, DEA4, DEA5, Dal, and Kai 1/Kai 2 in different canine breeds from a diagnostic laboratory in Germany. *Front Vet Sci* 2020; **7**: 85.

397 Davidow EB, Blois SL, Goy-Thollot I, *et al.* Association of Veterinary Hematology and Transfusion Medicine (AVHTM) Transfusion Reaction Small Animal Consensus Statement (TRACS) Part 2: Prevention and monitoring. *J Vet Emerg Crit Care* 2021; **31**: 167–188.

398 Weinstein NM, Blais MC, Harris K, *et al.* A newly recognized blood group in domestic shorthair cats: the Mik red cell antigen. *J Vet Intern Med* 2007; **21**: 287–292.

399 Malik R, Griffin DL, White JD, *et al.* The prevalence of feline A/B blood types in the Sydney region. *Aust Vet J* 2005; **83**: 38–44.

400 Giger U, Kilrain CG, Filippich LJ, *et al.* Frequencies of feline blood groups in the United States. *J Am Vet Med Assoc* 1989; **195**: 1230–1232.

401 Giger U, Bucheler J, Patterson DF. Frequency and inheritance of A and B blood types in feline breeds of the United States. *J Hered* 1991; **82**: 15–20.

402 Proverbio D, Spada E, Baggiani L, *et al.* Comparison of gel column agglutination with monoclonal antibodies and card agglutination methods for assessing the

feline AB group system and a frequency study of feline blood types in northern Italy. *Vet Clin Pathol* 2011; **40**: 32–39.
403 Giger U, Bucheler J. Transfusion of type-A and type-B blood to cats. *J Am Vet Med Assoc* 1991; **198**: 411–418.
404 Giger U, Akol KG. Acute hemolytic transfusion reaction in an Abyssinian cat with blood type B. *J Vet Intern Med* 1990; **4**: 315–316.
405 Martinez-Sogues L, Blois SL, Mazanilla EG, *et al.* Exploration of risk factors for non-survival and for transfusion-associated complications in cats receiving red blood cell transfusions: 450 cases (2009–2017). *J Sm Anim Pract* 2020; **61**: 177–184.
406 Le Gal A, Thomas EK, Humm KR. Xenotransfusion of canine blood to cats: a review of 49 cases and their outcome. *J Small Anim Pract* 2020; **61**: 156–162.
407 Proverbio D, Perego R, Baggiani L, *et al.* Prevalence of Ca blood type and alloantibodies in a population of horses from Italy. *Animals (Basel)* 2020; **10**: 1179.
408 Stormont CJ. Blood groups in animals. *Adv Vet Sci Comp Med* 1991; **36**: 9–55.
409 Luethy D, Stefanovski D, Salber R, *et al.* Prediction of packed cell volume after whole blood transfusion in small ruminants and South American camelids: 80 cases (2006–2016). *J Vet Intern Med* 2017; **31**: 1900.
410 Smith DM, Newhouse M, Naziruddin B, *et al.* Blood groups and transfusions in pigs. *Xenotransplantation* 2006; **13**: 186–194.
411 Luethy D, Owens SD, Stefanovski D, *et al.* Comparison of tube, gel, and immunochromatic strip methods for evaluation of blood transfusion compatibility in horses. *J Vet Intern Med* 2016; **30**: 1864–1871.
412 Jutkowitz LA, Rozanski EA, Moreau JA, *et al.* Massive transfusion in dogs: 15 cases (1997–2001). *J Am Vet Med Assoc* 2002; **220**: 1664–1669.
413 Holcomb JB, Wade CE, Michalek JE, *et al.* Increased plasma and platelet to red blood cell ratios improves outcome in 466 massively transfused civilian trauma patients. *Ann Surg* 2008; **248**: 447–458.
414 Zink KA, Sambasivan CN, Holcomb JB, *et al.* A high ratio of plasma and platelets to packed red blood cells in the first 6 hours of massive transfusion improves outcomes in a large multicenter study. *Am J Surg* 2009; **197**: 565–570.
415 Shaz BH, Dente CJ, Nicholas J, *et al.* Increased number of coagulation products in relationship to red blood cell products transfused improves mortality in trauma patients. *Transfusion* 2010; **50**: 493–500.
416 Nunez TC, Young PP, Holcomb JB, *et al.* Creation, implementation, and maturation of a massive transfusion protocol for the exsanguinating trauma patient. *J Trauma* 2010; **68**: 1498–1505.
417 Holcomb JB, del Junco DJ, Fox EE, *et al.* The prospective observational multicenter major trauma transfusion (PROMMTT) study: comparative effectiveness of a time-varying treatment with competing risk. *J Am Med Assoc* 2013; **148**: 127–136.
418 Consunji R, Elseed A, El-Menyar A, *et al.* The effect of massive transfusion protocol implementation on the survival of trauma patients; a systematic review and meta-analysis. *Blood Transfus* 2020; **18**: 434–445.
419 Buckley GJ, Aktay SA, Rozanski EA. Massive transfusion and surgical management of iatrogenic aortic laceration associated with cystocentesis in a dog. *J Am Vet Med Assoc* 2009; **235**: 288–291.
420 Clark CH, Woodley CH. The absorption of red blood cells after parenteral injection at various sites. *Am J Vet Res* 1959; **10**: 1062–1066.
421 McDevitt RI, Ruaux CG, Baltzer WI. Influence of transfusion technique on survival of autologous red blood cells in the dog. *J Vet Emerg Crit Care* 2011; **21**: 209–216.
422 Heikes B, Ruaux CG. Syringe and aggregate filter administration does not effect survival of transfused autologous feline red blood cells. *J Vet Emerg Crit Care* 2014; **24**: 162–167.
423 Davidow EB, Blois SL, Goy-Thollot I, *et al.* Association of Veterinary Hematology and Transfusion Medicine (AVHTM) Transfusion Reaction Small Animal Consensus Statement (TRACS) Part 1: Definitions and clinical signs. *J Vet Emerg Crit Care* 2021; **31**: 141–166.
424 Bruce JA, Kriese-Anderson L, Bruce AM, *et al.* Effect of premedication and other factors on the occurrence of acute transfusion reactions in dogs. *J Vet Emerg Crit Care* 2015; **25**: 620–630.
425 Odunayo A, Nash KJ, Davidow EB, *et al.* Association of Veterinary Hematology and Transfusion Medicine (AVHTM) Transfusion Reaction Small Animal Consensus Statement (TRACS) Part 3: Diagnosis and treatment. *J Vet Emerg Crit Care* 2021; **31**: 189–203.
426 Patterson J, Rousseau A, Kessler RJ, *et al.* In vitro lysis and acute transfusion reactions with hemolysis caused by inappropriate storage of canine red blood cell products. *J Vet Intern Med* 2011; **25**: 927–933.
427 Vlaar APJ, Toy P, Fung M, *et al.* A consensus redefinition of transfusion-related acute lung injury. *Transfusion* 2019; **59**: 2465–2476.
428 Vlaar APJ, Juffermans NP. Transfusion related acute lung injury - clinical review. *Lancet* 2013; **382**: 984–994.
429 Thomovsky E, Bach J. Incidence of acute lung injury in dogs receiving transfusion. *J Am Vet Med Assoc* 2014; **244**: 170–174.
430 Looney MR. Current concepts in TRALI pathogenesis. *ISBT Sci Ser* 2016; **11**(S1): 206–210.
431 Palfi M, Berg S, Ernerudh J, *et al.* A randomized controlled trial of transfusion-related acute lung injury: is plasma from multiparous blood donors dangerous? *Transfusion* 2001; **41**: 317–322.
432 Blais MC, Rozanski EA, Hale AS, *et al.* Lack of evidence of pregnancy-induced alloantibodies in dogs. *J Vet Intern Med* 2009; **23**: 462–465.
433 Hillyer CD, Josephson CD, Blajchman MA, *et al.* Bacterial contamination of blood components: risks, strategies, and regulation: joint ASH and AABB educational session in transfusion medicine. *Hematology Am Soc Hematol Edu Program* 2003: 575–589.
434 Hohenhaus AE, Drustin LM, Garvey MS. *Serratia marcescens* contamination of feline whole blood in a hospital blood bank. *J Am Vet Med Assoc* 1997; **210**: 794–798.
435 Maxwell MJ, Wilson MJA. Complications of blood transfusion. *Contin Educ Anaesth Crit Care Pain* 2006; **6**: 225–229.
436 Nickel JR, Shih A. Anesthesia case of the month. *J Am Vet Med Assoc* 2011; **239**: 1429–1431.
437 Mudge MC, Walker NJ, Borjesson DL, *et al.* Post-transfusion survival of biotin-labeled allogenic RBCs in adult horses. *Vet Clin Pathol* 2012; **41**: 56–62.
438 Forgie MA, Wells PS, Laupacis A, *et al.* Preoperative autologous donation decreased allogeneic transfusion by relative 63 percent, but increases exposure to all red blood cell transfusion by 30 percent: results of a meta-analysis. International Study of Perioperative Transfusion (ISPOT) Investigators. *Arch Int Med* 1998; **158**: 610–616.
439 Henry DA, Carless PA, Moxey AJ, *et al.* Pre-operative autologous donation for minimizing perioperative allogeneic blood transfusion. *Cochrane Database Syst Rev* 2002; **2**: CD003602.
440 Carless P, Moxey A, O'Connell D, *et al.* Autologous transfusion techniques: a systematic review of their efficacy. *Transfusion Med* 2004; **14**: 123–144.
441 Sinclair KC, Clarke HD, Noble BN. Blood management in total knee arthroplasty: a comparison of techniques. *Orthopedics* 2009; **32**: 19.
442 Mudge MC, Macdonald MH, Owens SD, *et al.* Comparison of 4 blood storage methods in a protocol for equine pre-operative autologous donation. *Vet Surg* 2004; **33**: 475–486.
443 Fusco JV, Hohenhaus AE, Aiken SW, *et al.* Autologous blood collection and transfusion in cats undergoing partial craniectomy. *J Am Vet Med Assoc* 2000; **216**: 1584–1588.
444 Mijovic A, Britten C, Regan F, *et al.* Preoperative autologous blood donation for bone marrow harvests: are we wasting donors' time and blood? *Transfus Med* 2006; **16**: 57–62.
445 Bess RS, Lenke LG, Bridwell KH, *et al.* Wasting of preoperatively donated autologous blood in the surgical treatment of adolescent idiopathic scoliosis. *Spine* 2006; **31**: 2375–2380.
446 Monk TG, Goodnough LT, Pulley DD, *et al.* Acute normovolemic hemodilution can replace preoperative autologous blood donation as a standard of care for autologous blood procurement in radical prostatectomy. *Anesth Analg* 1997; **85**: 953–958.
447 Monk TG, Goodnough LT, Brecher ME, *et al.* A prospective randomized comparison of three blood conservation strategies for radical prostatectomy. *Anesthesiology* 1999; **91**: 24–33.
448 Oishi CS, d'Lima DD, Morris BA, *et al.* Hemodilution with other blood reinfusion techniques in total hip arthroplasty. *Clin Orthop* 1997; **339**: 132–139.
449 Schmied H, Schiferer A, Sessler DI, *et al.* The effects of red-cell scavenging, hemodilution, and active warming on allogeneic blood requirements in patients undergoing hip or knee arthroplasty. *Anesth Analg* 1998; **86**: 387–391.
450 Joubert KE. Acute normovoaemic haemodilution - 2 case studies. *J S Afr Vet Assoc* 2008; **79**: 46–49.
451 Hirst C, Admantos S. Autologous blood transfusion following red blood cell salvage for the management of blood loss in 3 dogs with hemoperitoneum. *J Vet Emerg Crit Care* 2012; **22**: 355–360.
452 Higgs VA, Rudloff E, Kirby R, *et al.* Autologous blood transfusion in dogs with thoracic or abdominal hemorrhage: 25 cases (2007–2012). *J Vet Emerg Crit Care* 2015; **25**: 731–738.
453 Carless PA, Henry DA, O'Connell D, *et al.* Cell salvage for minimizing perioperative allogenic blood transfusion. *Cochrane Database Syst Rev* 2010; **4**: CD001888.
454 Serrick CJ, Scholz M, Melo A, *et al.* Quality of red blood cells using autotransfusion devices: a comparative analysis. *J Extra Corpor Technol* 2003; **35**: 28–34.
455 Kirkpatrick UJ, Adams RA, Lardi A, *et al.* Rheological properties and function of blood cells in stored bank blood and salvaged blood. *Br J Haematol* 1998; **101**: 364–368.
456 Esper SA, Waters JH. Intra-operative cell salvage: a fresh look at the indications and contraindications. *Blood Transfus* 2011; **9**: 139–147.
457 Catling S, Williams S, Freites O, *et al.* Use of a leucocyte filter to remove tumour cells from intra-operative cell salvage blood. *Anaesthesia* 2008; **63**: 1332–1338.

458 Waters JH, Donnenberg AD. Blood salvage and cancer surgery: should we do it? *Transfusion* 2009; **49**: 2016–2018.

459 Waters JH, Tuohy MJ, Hobson DF, *et al.* Bacterial reduction by cell salvage washing and leukocyte depletion filtration. *Anesthesiology* 2003; **99**: 652–655.

460 Gregoretti S. Suction-induced hemolysis at various vacuum pressures: implications for intraoperative blood salvage. *Transfusion* 1996; **36**: 57–60.

461 Bull BS, Bull MH. The salvaged blood syndrome: a sequel to mechanochemical activation of platelets and leukocytes? *Blood Cells* 1990; **16**: 5–20.

462 Reid TJ. Hb-based oxygen carriers: are we there yet? *Transfusion* 2003; **43**: 280–287.

463 Haney CR, Buehler PW, Gulati A. Purification and chemical modifications of hemoglobin in developing hemoglobin based oxygen carriers. *Adv Drug Deliv Rev* 2000; **40**: 153–169.

464 Muir WW, Wellman LM. Hemoglobin solutions and tissue oxygenation. *J Vet Intern Med* 2003; **17**: 127–135.

465 Rentko VT, Wohl J, Murtaugh R, *et al.* A clinical trial of hemoglobin-based oxygen-carrying (HBOC) fluid in the treatment of anemia in dogs. *J Vet Intern Med* 1996; **10**: 177.

466 Rentko VT, Pearce LB, Moon-Massat PF, *et al.* Pharmacokinetics of a hemoglobin based O2 carrier in dogs [Abstract]. *J Vet Intern Med* 2003; **17**: 407.

467 Driessen B, Jahr JS, Lurie F, *et al.* Arterial oxygenation and oxygen delivery after hemoglobin-based oxygen carrier infusion in canine hypovolemic shock: a dose-response study. *Crit Care Med* 2003; **31**: 1771–1779.

468 Gibson GR, Callan MB, Hoffmann V, *et al.* Use of hemoglobin based oxygen carrying solutions in cats: 72 cases (1998–2000). *J Am Vet Med Assoc* 2002; **221**: 96–102.

469 Weingart C, Kohn B. Clinical use of a hemoglobin-based oxygen carrying solution (Oxyglobin) in 48 cats (2002–2006). *J Feline Med Surg* 2008; **10**: 431–438.

470 Wehausen CE, Kirby R, Rudloff E. Evaluation of the effects of bovine hemoglobin glutamer-200 on systolic arterial blood pressure in hypotensive cats: 44 cases (1997–2008). *J Am Vet Med Assoc* 2011; **238**: 909–914.

471 Belgrave RL, Hines MT, Keegan RD, *et al.* Effects of polymerized ultrapurified bovine hemoglobin blood substitute administrated to ponies with normovolemic anemia. *J Vet Intern Med* 2002; **16**: 396–403.

472 Jahr JS, Guinn NR, Lowery DR, *et al.* Blood substitutes and oxygen therapeutics: a review. *Anesth Analg* 2021; **132**: 119–129.

473 Brainard BM, Meredith CP, Callan MB, *et al.* Changes in platelet function, hemostasis, and prostaglandin expression after treatment with nonsteroidal anti-inflammatory drugs with various cyclooxygenase selectivities in dogs. *Am J Vet Res* 2007; **68**: 251–257.

474 Blois SI, Allen DG, Wood D, *et al.* Effects of aspirin, carprofen, deracoxib, and meloxicam on platelet function and systemic prostaglandin concentrations in healthy dogs. *Am J Vet Res* 2010; **71**: 349–358.

475 Mullins KB, Thomason JM, Lunsford KV, *et al.* Effects of carprofen, meloxicam and deracoxib on platelet function in dogs. *Vet Anaesth Analg* 2012; **39**: 206–217.

476 Hogan DF, Andrews DA, Green HW, *et al.* Antiplatelet effects and pharmacodynamics of clopidogrel in cats. *J Am Vet Med Assoc* 2004; **225**: 1406–1411.

477 Brainard BM, Buriko Y, Good J, *et al.* Consensus on the Rational Use of Antithrombotics in Veterinary Critical Care (CURATIVE): Domain 5 - Discontinuation of anticoagulant therapy in small animals. *J Vet Emerg Crit Care* 2019; **29**: 88–97.

478 Callan MB, Giger U. Effect of desmopressin acetate administration on primary hemostasis in Doberman Pinschers with type-1 von Willebrand disease as assessed by a point-of-care instrument. *Am J Vet Res* 2002; **63**: 1700–1706.

479 Sakai M, Watari T, Miura T, *et al.* Effects of DDAVP administration subcutaneously in dogs with aspirin induced platelet dysfunction and hemostatic impairment due to chronic liver disease. *J Vet Med Sci* 2003; **65**: 83–86.

480 Henry DA, Carless PA, Moxey AJ, *et al.* Anti-fibrinolytic use for minimizing perioperative allogenic blood transfusion. *Cochrane Database Syst Rev* 2011; **16**: CD001886.

481 Berenholtz SM, Pham JC, Garrett-Mayer E, *et al.* Effect of epsilon aminocaproic acid on red-cell transfusion requirements in major spinal surgery. *Spine* 2009; **34**: 2096–2103.

482 Marin LM, Iazbik MC, Zaldivar-Lopez S, *et al.* Retrospective evaluation of epsilon aminocaproic acid for the prevention of postamputation bleeding in retired racing Greyhounds with appendicular bone tumors: 46 cases (2003–2008). *J Vet Emerg Crit Care* 2012; **22**: 332–340.

483 Marin LM, Iazbik MC, Zaldivar-Lopez S, *et al.* Epsilon aminocaproic acid for the prevention of delayed postoperative bleeding in retired racing Greyhounds undergoing gonadectomy. *Vet Surg* 2012; **41**: 594–603.

484 Rajagopalan S, Mascha E, Na Jie, *et al.* The effects of mild perioperative hypothermia on blood loss and transfusion requirement. *Anesthesiology* 2008; **108**: 71–77.

485 Schmied H, Kurz A, Sessler DI, *et al.* Mild intraoperative hypothermia increases blood loss and allogeneic transfusion requirements during total hip arthroplasty. *Lancet* 1996; **347**: 289–292.

486 Schmied H, Schiferer A, Sessler DI, *et al.* The effects of red-cell scavenging, hemodilution, and active warming on allogeneic blood requirement in patients undergoing hip or knee arthroplasty. *Anesth Analg* 1998; **86**: 387–391.

487 Felfernig M, Blaicher A, Kettner SC, *et al.* Effects of temperature on partial thromboplastin time in heparinized plasma in vitro. *Eur J Anaesthesiology* 2001; **18**: 467–470.

488 Shimokawa M, Kitaguchi K, Kawaguchi M, *et al.* The influence of induced hypothermia for hemostatic function on temperature-adjusted measurements in rabbits. *Anesth Analg* 2003; **96**: 1209–1213.

SECTION 5

Physiology and Anesthetic Management

33 Cardiovascular Physiology

William W. Muir
Gillespie College of Veterinary Medicine (LMU-CVM) at Lincoln Memorial University, Harrogate, Tennessee, USA

Chapter contents

Introduction, 615
Comparative cardiovascular morphology and shunting, 617
The mammalian cardiovascular system, 619
- Anatomy, 619
- Metabolism, 620
- Electrophysiology and electrocardiogram, 620

Excitation–contraction coupling, 626
The actin-activated myosin chemomechanical ATPase cycle, 629
Myocardial contraction and relaxation, 629
The vascular system, 631
- Large arteries and veins, 633
- Small arteries, 633
- Resistance vessels, 633
- Capillaries, 634
- Transcapillary fluid exchange, 635
- Veins, venules, and venous capacitance, 638

Smooth muscle metabolism, 638
Smooth muscle contraction and relaxation, 638
Blood, 640
Lymphatic system, 641
Hemodynamics and cardiac function, 642
- Blood flow, 642
- Blood pressure, 644
- Resistance, 646
- Preload and afterload, 647

The cardiac cycle and pressure–volume loop, 647
Assessment of cardiac function, 650
Oxygen delivery and oxygen consumption, 653
Neurohumoral and local control mechanisms, 654
- Neurohormonal mechanisms, 656
- Local mechanisms, 658

Special circulations, 658
- Coronary circulation, 658
- Cerebral circulation, 659
- Pulmonary circulation, 659
- Splanchnic circulation, 660
- Renal circulation, 660

References, 660

Introduction

The cardiovascular system is a closed tubular arrangement that consists of the heart, blood vessels, and blood. The purpose of the cardiovascular system is to circulate blood and other essential materials, especially oxygen, remove waste products, and maintain homeostatic control of the body's temperature, pH, and cellular environment. The purpose of the heart is to pump blood in quantities sufficient to meet the body's oxygen demands. The purpose of the vasculature is to distribute blood to tissues, maintain adequate parenchymal perfusion, and facilitate the cellular exchange of nutrients for waste products. Blood transports oxygen, carbon dioxide, nutrients, waste, and hormones; regulates pH, temperature, and fluid balance; and protects the body from blood loss and foreign invaders via clotting mechanisms and the immune response, respectively. Schematically, the cardiovascular system of mammals is a circuit comprised of two circulations (i.e., systemic and pulmonary) in series (Fig. 33.1).

Oxygen is essential for maintaining normal cellular metabolic function in all tissues. Relatively brief periods (2–3 min) of cerebral or cardiac anoxia, for example, can produce devastating consequences that threaten life even if blood flow is restored. Oxygenated blood returning from the lungs enters the left atrium and then the left ventricle and is pumped into the aorta and coronary circulation. The aorta, in conjunction with an elaborate array of large arteries, distributes blood throughout the systemic circulation to the tissue beds of each body organ (e.g., brain, heart, kidney, skeletal muscle, etc.). Large arteries transition to smaller arteries and eventually into arterioles (i.e., resistance vessels) that distribute and regulate blood flow and oxygen delivery to capillary beds (i.e., exchange vessels) based upon their oxygen demand. Capillaries provide a surface area that is over three orders of magnitude larger than the aorta and are the primary sites for tissue oxygen, carbon dioxide, and nutrient exchange. Capillary beds coalesce to form venules that return deoxygenated blood, carbon dioxide, and metabolic waste products to small and large veins that transition into the venae cavae. The venae cavae return deoxygenated blood to the right atrium and subsequently the right ventricle and pulmonary artery. Pulmonary capillaries exchange carbon dioxide for oxygen

Veterinary Anesthesia and Analgesia: The Sixth Edition of Lumb and Jones. Edited by Leigh Lamont, Kurt Grimm, Sheilah Robertson, Lydia Love and Carrie Schroeder.
© 2024 John Wiley & Sons, Inc. Published 2024 by John Wiley & Sons, Inc.
Companion website: www.wiley.com/go/lamont/anesthesia

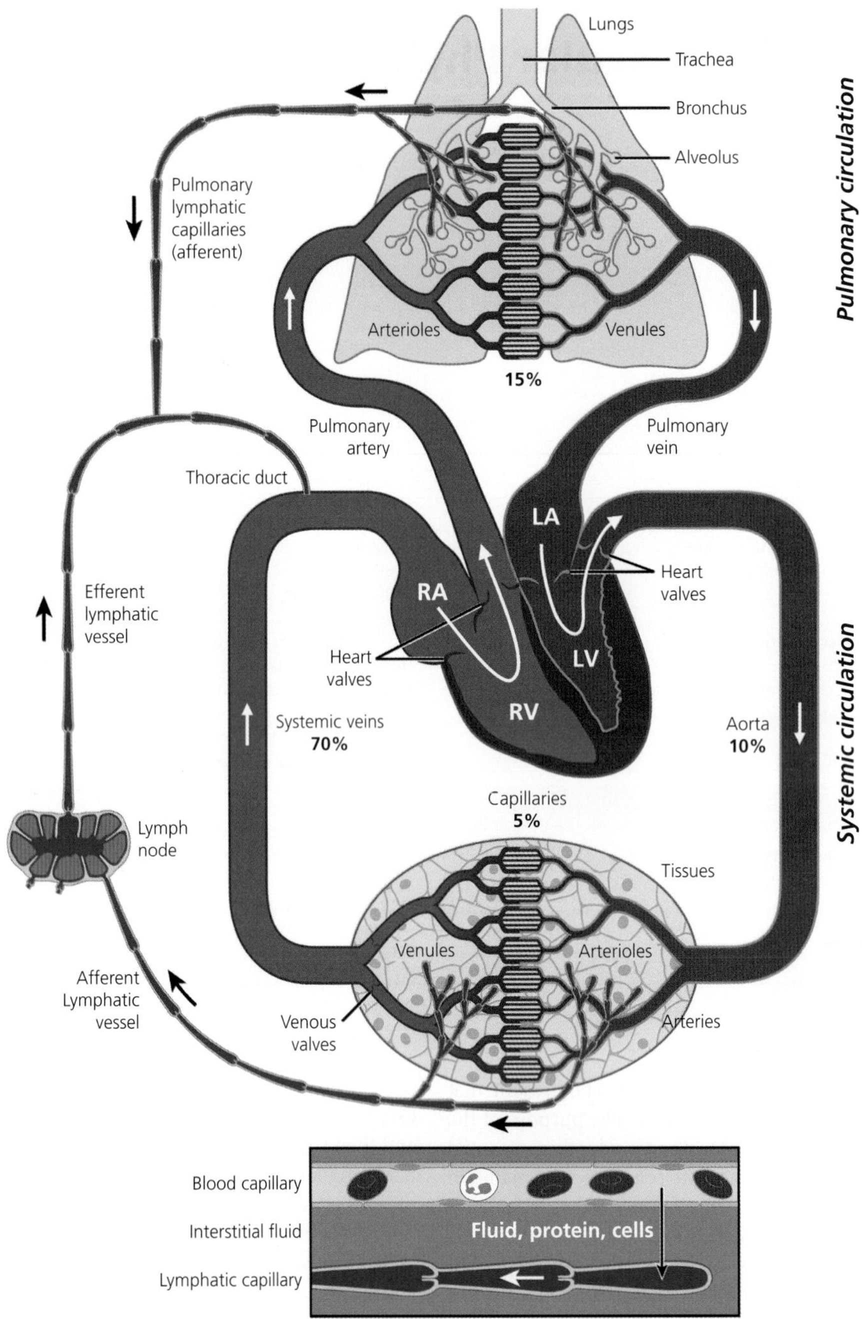

Figure 33.1 The mammalian circulatory systems consist of the heart, two circulations, pulmonary and systemic, and the lymphatic system. Blood returning to the right atrium (RA) from the systemic veins (70% blood volume) enters the right ventricle (RV) and is pumped into the pulmonary artery and oxygenated in the capillaries of the lung (15% blood volume). Oxygenated blood returns to the left atrium (LA) enters the left ventricle (LV), is pumped into the aorta and arterial conduits (10% blood volume), and distributed to capillaries (5% blood volume). Deoxygenated blood (blue); oxygenated blood (red); lymph (green). The lymphatic system regulates tissue fluid homeostasis by transporting interstitial fluid (i.e., lymph) to the venous system via the thoracic duct.

and return oxygenated blood to the left atrium thus completing the circuit. The body's circulatory system also includes a network of lymph vessels, nodes, and organs (e.g., thymus and tonsils) in parallel with the vascular system that actively maintain interstitial fluid homeostasis by regulating filtered plasma (i.e., lymph) accumulation, preventing infection (i.e., immune response), and removing or destroying bacteria and toxins (Fig. 33.1).

The circulation of fluid (i.e., blood and lymph) throughout the body depends on a normally functioning heart, blood vessels, blood volume, and lymphatic system. Since blood flow is responsible for the uptake, delivery, and elimination of all drugs including anesthetic drugs, a functional appreciation of cardiovascular anatomy and circulatory dynamics are required for safe anesthetic practice. This chapter reviews the anatomy and physiology of the cardiovascular and lymphatic systems of mammals and summarizes the general effects of anesthesia and anesthetic drugs on their function.

Comparative cardiovascular morphology and shunting

All vertebrate animals have a heart and circulatory systems (i.e., pulmonary, systemic, and lymphatic) although this can vary substantially among genera. The heart exhibits intrinsic electrical and mechanical properties that ensure the delivery of blood to closed (i.e., blood is contained within blood vessels) systemic and pulmonary circulations (Table 33.1). The lymphatic circulatory system is an open network of tissues, vessels, and organs that moves filtered interstitial fluid (i.e., lymph) back into the bloodstream. The American Veterinary Medical Association lists fish, ferrets, rabbits, hamsters, birds, gerbils, rodents, frogs, turtles, snakes, and lizards among others as exotic species. Several of these species have unique circulatory systems and not all have a four-chambered heart (Fig. 33.2) [1,2]. Current opinions regarding circulatory system architectures, "open" or "closed" configurations, and different species' unique circulatory characteristics are beyond the scope of this chapter; however, the opinion that the heart and circulation of amphibians and reptiles (i.e., three chambers with cardiac and vascular shunts) are functionally inefficient intermediate steps to the four-chambered heart of birds and mammals is considered obsolete [1–3]. It is more likely that cardiac and vascular shunts represent an adaptive phenotypic trait providing various genera with the ability to regulate blood flow depending upon cellular respiration and environmental requirements.

Table 33.1 Intrinsic properties of the heart.

Term	Description
Chronotropy*	Heart rate
Bathmotropy	Excitability
Dromotropy	Conduction
Inotropy	Force
Lusitropy	Relaxation
Clinotropy	Velocity

* tropy = change.

The fish heart consists of four parts that includes two primary chambers, an entrance, and an exit, and its cardiovascular system is considered to consist of a single-cycle (i.e., one "circulation") closed-loop circulatory system (Fig. 33.2). Amphibians have a three-chambered heart (i.e., two atria and one ventricle) and are considered to have a "double" circulatory system (arterial and venous). The ventricle is incompletely separated by a partial septum into two pumps that results in less mixing of oxygenated and deoxygenated blood. Blood returning to the heart is pumped into two circulations: one carries blood to the lungs and skin for oxygenation, and the other delivers oxygenated blood to the rest of the body (Fig. 33.2).

The systemic circulation of reptiles, like other vertebrates, consists of arterial, venous, and lymphatic vessels. The hearts of many reptiles including turtles, snakes, and lizards consist of two atria and a single ventricle that delivers blood to two circulatory routes; however, blood is only oxygenated in the lungs. The single ventricle has an incomplete muscular ridge that acts to divide the ventricle

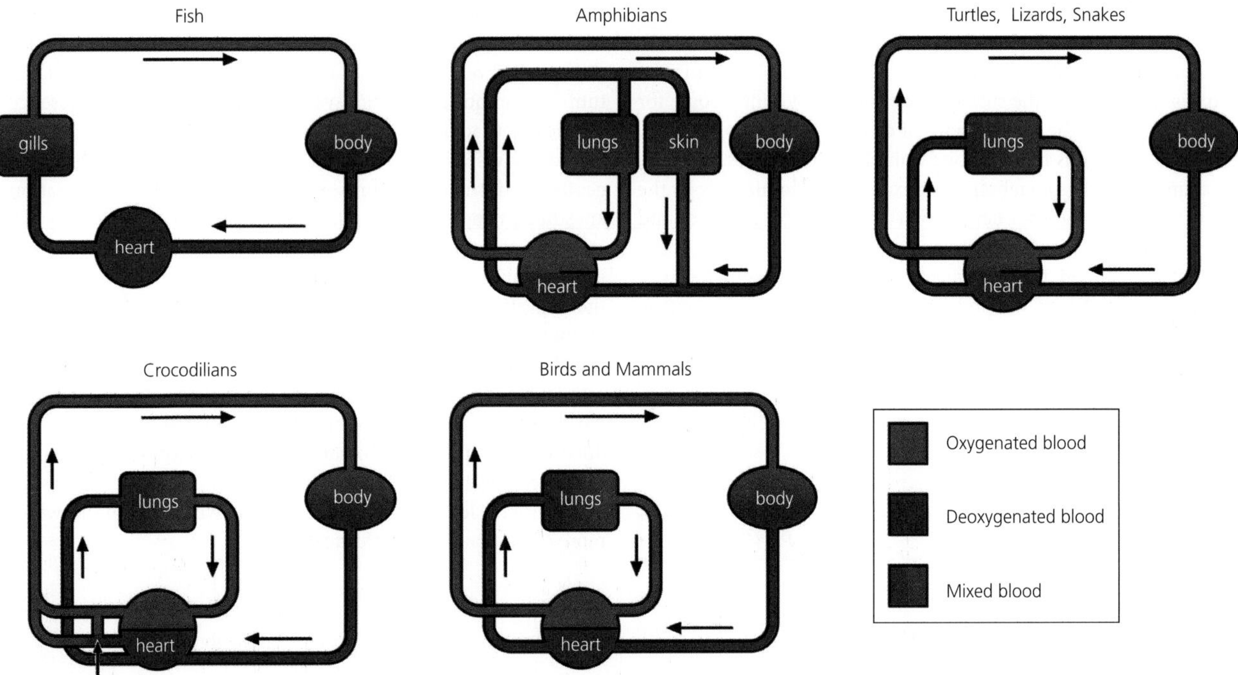

Figure 33.2 The circulatory systems of vertebrates. Birds and mammals have a closed vascular system and complete ventricular septum. The hearts of turtles, lizards, and snakes consist of two atrial chambers and two ventricular chambers separated by an incomplete ventricular septum. The heart of crocodilians is completely divided into four chambers but retains a dual aortic arch system. The foramen of Panizza located near the RV and LV outflow tracts allows blood to bypass the lungs when submerged. Note that the ventricular septum is absent or incomplete in fish, amphibians, turtles, lizards, and snakes. Source: Adapted from Hicks [2].

into two major chambers minimizing the mixing of oxygenated and deoxygenated blood (Fig. 33.2) [2,4]. The pulmonary artery and right and left aortic arches originate from specific anatomical sites (i.e., cavum pulmonale and cavum venosum) [5]. The sinus venosus is occasionally considered to be an additional chamber classifying the non-crocodilian heart as an atypical "four-chambered" organ [5]. The pulmonary artery is equipped with a muscular sphincter that when contracted diverts blood flow through the incomplete ventricular septum into the left ventricle and out the aorta producing a right-to-left (R-L) shunt estimated to equal 60–70% of the venous return. Both pulmonary and systemic arterial vascular resistance and the degree of contraction of the muscular ridge control the magnitude and direction of cardiac shunting in reptiles [2]. For example, deoxygenated blood mixes with oxygenated blood during diastole but not during systole when the contraction process causes the ventricle to function as a dual chamber pressure pump. Factors that control the direction and magnitude of R-L shunting during diving and breath-holding include the size of the shunt orifice, the pressure gradient between the chambers or vessels that produce the shunt, and the "downstream" resistance to flow (Table 33.2) [2]. Both diving and breath-holding also increase peripheral vascular resistance resulting in bradycardia, a normal response in reptiles, leading to the redirection of blood flow to the brain and the heart. Reptiles switch from aerobic to anaerobic glycolysis during extended breath-holding resulting in restricted pulmonary blood flow and R-L shunting of blood to ensure that blood flow continues to the systemic circulation [4]. The resumption of normal breathing reverses these events, decreasing pulmonary resistance, increasing heart rate, and reducing R-L shunting. These physiologic changes can be pharmacologically induced by dissociative anesthetics (e.g., ketamine and tiletamine), α_2-adrenergic receptor agonists (e.g., medetomidine and dexmedetomidine), or propofol and should be anticipated [4].

Snakes possess a vertebral venous plexus comprised of a network of spinal veins located within and around the vertebral column. The plexus is supported by the surrounding bones providing a route for venous return and the maintenance of cerebral blood supply [5]. A renal portal system is found in birds, amphibians, reptiles, and fish, suggesting that drugs metabolized or excreted predominantly by the liver will undergo a greater hepatic first-pass effect (e.g., opioids and most anesthetics) [6]. Venous blood returning from the tail and hindlimbs is filtered through the kidneys and through the liver. Valves located between the abdominal and femoral veins regulate blood flow through the kidneys especially during times of water conservation. Parenteral drug administration of potentially nephrotoxic drugs into the tail or caudal extremities is generally not recommended because of the potential for nephrotoxicity [7]. The administration of non-nephrotoxic drugs into the caudal extremities does not pose a risk [6]. Reptiles have a lymphatic system but lack lymph nodes. The lymph vessels have muscular dilations referred to as "lymph hearts" that propel lymph into the venous system [5].

The circulatory anatomy of crocodilians is unique among reptiles and more like birds and mammals (i.e., four separate heart chambers and a complete ventricular septum), thus preventing intracardiac R-L shunting. However, crocodilians retain the dual aortic arch system found in many reptiles [2]. The left aortic arch originates from the right ventricle next to the pulmonary artery, and the right aortic arch originates from the left ventricle. Importantly, the left and right aortic arches of crocodilians communicate via the foramen of Panizza located close to the heart (Fig. 33.2). This anatomic arrangement permits systemic venous blood to bypass the pulmonary circulation. The consequences of R-L and left-to-right (L-R) shunts can have important consequences for anesthesia (Box 33.1). An R-L shunt bypasses the lungs diverting deoxygenated blood back into the systemic circulation, whereas an L-R shunt recirculates pulmonary venous (oxygenated) blood back into the pulmonary circulation. Physiologic L-R shunting in reptiles is not thought to contribute to pulmonary circulation overload due to the ability of blood to be shunted either L-R or R-L, although it can contribute to pulmonary overcirculation in mammals. Autonomic tone, neurohumoral substances, and the activity of pulmonary stretch and chemoreceptors control pulmonary and systemic vascular resistances in reptiles and the direction and magnitude of cardiac shunting. Ventilatory status, particularly in diving animals, thermoregulation, feeding, and digestion may also influence cardiac shunting. For example, most reptiles breathe intermittently with long periods of apnea. Parasympathetic tone increases during apnea resulting in bradycardia and increased pulmonary vascular resistance promoting the development of R-L shunting [2].

The heart of birds and mammals is comprised of four chambers: two thin-walled atria separated by an interatrial septum, and two thick-walled ventricles separated by a complete interventricular septum. The unique respiratory system of birds includes the presence of air sacs that facilitate gas exchange throughout the inspiratory and expiratory respiratory cycle. Intrapulmonary or intracardiac (congenital malformation) shunts can affect the onset and elimination of anesthetic drug effects in birds and mammals, particularly when inhalant anesthetics are administered (Box 33.1). The speed of inhalant anesthetic induction is determined by how fast the anesthetic partial pressure is reached in the brain, which is determined by the rate of anesthetic inflow into the lungs, the rate of anesthetic transfer to the blood, and the rate of anesthetic transfer from the arterial blood to the brain. Inhalant anesthetics with a low blood-gas partition coefficient (low solubility) are generally expected to produce a more rapid induction and recovery in normal mammals. For example, anesthetic induction and washout in healthy pigs is more rapid with the less soluble desflurane than with sevoflurane, which is more rapid than with isoflurane [8].

Table 33.2 Physiologic effects of cardiac shunting in mammals.

Physiologic effect	Direction of shunt
Decreased arterial oxygen content	R-L
Decreased carbon dioxide removal	R-L
Decreased lung plasma filtration	R-L
Erythrocytosis	R-L
Increased heart rate	R-L
Increased arterial oxygen content	L-R
Increased carbon dioxide removal	L-R
Reduced ventilation–perfusion mismatch	L-R
Pulmonary overperfusion	L-R
Renin–angiotensin system activation	L-R

R-L, right-to-left shunt; L-R, left-to-right shunt.

Box 33.1 Effect of intracardiac shunts on anesthetic induction.

L-R shunt
IV anesthetic: little effect on induction
Inhalant anesthetic: little effect on induction

R-L shunt
IV anesthetic: rapid induction; blood bypasses lungs and goes to brain
Inhalant anesthetic: slower induction with less soluble inhalants

An L-R cardiac shunt has minimal or no effect on the onset or elimination of injectable or inhalant anesthetics in mammals (Box 33.1). The rate of inhalant anesthetic induction is unchanged even though recirculation of blood through the lungs promotes a more rapid rate of rise in alveolar partial pressure. The speed of induction increases following the administration of an intravenous anesthetic to animals that have an R-L shunt due to its immediate transfer to the brain. An R-L shunt slows the rate of inhalant anesthetic induction and elimination, and this effect is more pronounced with less soluble anesthetics (e.g., isoflurane, sevoflurane, and desflurane) compared to a more soluble anesthetic (e.g., halothane). This effect is dependent upon the size of the shunt and the dilutional effect of shunted blood, which contains no volatile anesthetic. One study demonstrated that the rate of rise of the end-tidal concentration of the comparatively soluble anesthetic halothane was not significantly affected by an R-L intracardiac shunt in children [9].

The mammalian cardiovascular system

Anatomy

The boundaries of the cardiac chambers in mammals are easily defined by the great veins (i.e., cranial and caudal venae cavae) that return blood to the right atrium, the smaller pulmonary veins that return oxygenated blood from the lung to the left atrium, the coronary sulcus (i.e., groove) that demarcates the atria from the ventricles, and the anterior (i.e., ventral) and posterior (i.e., dorsal) interventricular sulci that contain branches of the left circumflex coronary artery that separate the right and left ventricles (Fig. 33.3). All four chambers of the heart are easily visualized (Fig. 33.3A). The ventral interventricular branch of the left main coronary artery, occasionally referred to as the "left anterior descending coronary artery" in humans, provides blood supply to the ventricular septum and left ventricular free wall. The dorsal interventricular artery, generally an extension of the left circumflex coronary artery (the other major branch of the left main coronary artery), provides blood supply to most of the left ventricle. The right coronary artery provides blood supply to the right ventricular free wall and occasionally a large portion of the left ventricle (Fig. 33.3B). Anatomical differences in the anatomy of the coronary circulation among species account for dissimilarities in the source and distribution of myocardial blood flow. The left interventricular (i.e., anterior descending) coronary artery and its diagonal branches supply a larger mass of myocardium than the circumflex in humans, swine, rats, and nonhuman primates. The circumflex artery supplies the largest mass of cardiac muscle in dogs, cats, horses, and cattle although there is considerable species variation. Dogs have an extensive collateral coronary circulation (i.e., a network of tiny blood vessels that are not open under normal conditions but open during reduced blood flow), while pigs, monkeys, and humans do not. Cardiac veins empty into the great cardiac vein, which empties into the right atrium via the coronary sinus and accounts for over 90% of the venous return from the heart. Small capillary-like vessels (Thebesian veins) are present throughout the endocardium and drain directly into the cardiac chambers accounting for approximately 4% of the heart's venous return.

Blood returning from the systemic circulation (i.e., venous return) and pulmonary veins empties into the right and left atrium, respectively. The ventricles are the major pumping chambers of the heart and are separated from the atria by a fibrous skeleton of dense connective tissue (i.e., fibrous trigone) that anchors the atrioventricular (AV) (i.e., tricuspid and mitral) and semilunar (i.e., pulmonic and aortic) heart valves. The tricuspid valve is located between the right atrium and right ventricle and the mitral valve between the left atrium and left ventricle. The pulmonic valve is located between the right ventricle and pulmonary artery and the aortic valve between the left ventricle and aorta. Once the process of cardiac contraction is initiated, almost simultaneous contraction of

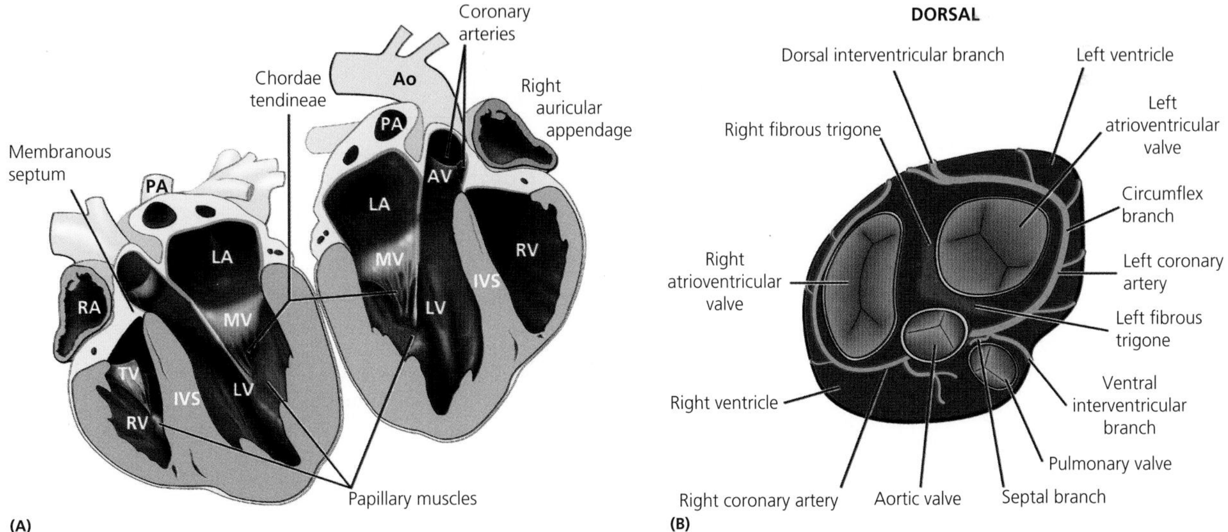

Figure 33.3 **A.** The mammalian heart is comprised of two thin-walled (i.e., right, and left atria) and two thick-walled chambers (i.e., right and left ventricles) and contains a highly reactive and diffuse vascular network (i.e., coronary circulation). The thin-walled right atrium (RA) and left atrium (LA) are separated from each other by a membranous septum. The interventricular muscular septum (IVS) lies between the right and left ventricles. The tricuspid valve (TV) and mitral valve (MV) lie between the RA and RV and the LA and LV, respectively. The pulmonary and aortic (AV) valves separate the RV and LV from the pulmonary artery (PA) and aorta (Ao), respectively. **B.** A fibrous trigone located at the center of the heart provides the scaffolding for the heart valves, atria, and ventricles. The right and left coronary arteries emerge from the base of the aorta and supply blood to all the chambers of the heart including the heart valves.

the atria is followed by nearly synchronous and simultaneous contraction of the ventricles. Cardiac contraction produces pressure changes that are responsible for AV and semilunar valve opening and closing and the production of audible heart sounds. Fibrous bands (i.e., chordae tendineae) originating from papillary muscles located on the inner wall of the ventricular chambers are attached to the free edges of the AV valve leaflets and limit valve prolapse into the atria during ventricular contraction thereby preventing the regurgitation of blood into the atrium (Fig. 33.3A). Alterations in heart chamber geometry (e.g., stretch, dilation, or hypertrophy) produced by changes in blood volume, ventricular deformation (pericardial tamponade), incompetent heart valves, or disease (e.g., tumors and scarring) can have profound effects on ventricular pressures, blood flow, and myocardial function.

Metabolism

The maintenance of normal cardiac electrical and mechanical activity is dependent upon the energy (i.e., adenosine triphosphate [ATP]) derived from multiple metabolic pathways. Mitochondria generate more than 95% of the ATP used by the heart, in addition to regulating intracellular calcium concentrations, cell signaling, and coordinated cell death. A detailed description of these pathways is beyond the scope of this chapter and is more appropriately described in reviews and texts specifically dedicated to this subject [10,11]. The heart produces ATP when mitochondrial oxidative phosphorylation is fueled by electrons generated by dehydrogenation of carbon fuels (i.e., fats and carbohydrates) and the oxidation (i.e., electron transfer) of nicotinamide adenine dinucleotide (NADH) and flavin adenine dinucleotide ($FADH_2$). NADH and $FADH_2$ are primarily produced by fatty acid oxidation, the citric acid cycle, and to a minor extent, by the pyruvate dehydrogenase reaction and glycolysis (Fig. 33.4). Oxidative phosphorylation is responsible for approximately 60–90% of the ATP formation in the heart during normal non-ischemic conditions with the remainder derived from the citric acid cycle. The citric acid cycle is dependent upon acetyl-CoA formed by the decarboxylation of pyruvate and the oxidation of fatty acids (Fig. 33.4) [10]. Approximately 60–70% of ATP hydrolysis is consumed by cardiac contraction, while the remaining 30–40% is used to maintain the ion pumps and sarcoplasmic reticulum Ca^{2+} ATPase. The rate of oxidative phosphorylation is directly linked to the rate of ATP hydrolysis so that ATP concentrations remain constant during intense exercise or changes in neurohumoral activity (e.g., variations in catecholamine concentrations) [11].

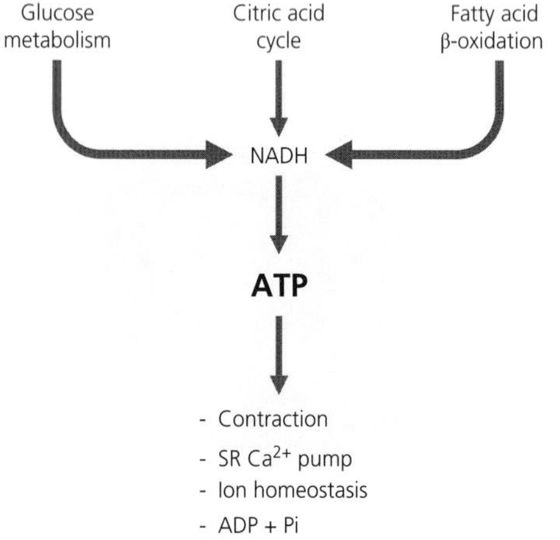

Figure 33.4 ATP is primarily produced (60–90%) by mitochondrial oxidative phosphorylation of free fatty acids but can also be generated by glycolysis (10–40%). Dehydrogenation reactions produced by the fatty acid β-oxidation pathway, citric acid cycle, and glycolysis generate reducing equivalents (i.e., NADH) that deliver electrons to the electron transport chain resulting in ATP formation. Adenosine triphosphate (ATP) and its metabolite (adenosine diphosphate) provide energy for myocardial contraction, membrane pump activity, and ion homeostasis, NADH, reduced nicotinamide adenine dinucleotide.

Electrophysiology and electrocardiogram

A highly integrated series of electrical, metabolic, and mechanical events are required to produce normal cardiac contractile function (i.e., excitation–contraction coupling). Notably, myocardial contraction is preceded by, and will not occur without, electrical activation although normal or near-normal electrical activity is possible without myocardial contraction (e.g., electrical–mechanical uncoupling, electrical–mechanical dissociation, and pulseless electrical activity [PEA]). PEA is the presence of organized cardiac electrical activity, other than ventricular fibrillation or ventricular tachycardia, that should produce a pulse, but does not. The cardiac cell membrane (sarcolemma) is a highly specialized lipid bilayer that contains protein-associated channels, pumps, enzymes, and exchangers in an architecturally organized, yet fluid (i.e., reorganizable and movable) medium [12]. The molecular composition and fluidity (i.e., freely movable membrane protein and lipid constituents) of cardiac membranes determine their ion transport/exchange and membrane-associated electrical properties, as well as the ability to generate and propagate electrical impulses [12,13]. The unequal distribution (i.e., concentrations) of various ions (i.e., sodium, potassium, chloride, and calcium) across the sarcolemma and its permeability to these ions are responsible for the development of the resting membrane potential. Resting membrane potential can be estimated by the Nernst equation or more accurately determined by the Goldman–Hodgkin–Katz constant-field equation [12] as shown below.

Nernst equation for potassium ions:

$$E = \frac{RT}{zF} \ln \frac{[K^+]_o}{[K^+]_i}$$

$$E_K = 2.303 \frac{RT}{zF} \log_{10} \frac{[K^+]_o}{[K^+]_i}$$

$$E_K = -61 \log_{10} \frac{[150\ \text{mEq/L}]_i}{[4\ \text{mEq/L}]_o} = -96\ \text{mV}$$

where E is electromotive force; 2.303 is the conversion of ln to $\log_{10}$; C_i and C_o are ion concentrations inside (i) and outside (o) the cell membrane; R is the gas constant; T is absolute temperature in Kelvin; z is valence of the ion (in this case, 1); F is the Faraday constant; and mV is millivolts at 37 °C.

Goldman–Hodgkin–Katz equation:

$$E_m = -\frac{RT}{F} \ln \frac{P_{Na}[Na^+]_i + P_K[K^+]_i + P_{Cl}[Cl^-]_o}{P_{Na}[Na^+]_o + P_K[K^+]_o + P_{Cl}[Cl^-]_i}$$

where E_m is the resting membrane potential and P_{Na} (0.04), P_K (1.0), and P_{Cl} (0.45) are the relative permeabilities of the membrane at rest, and other terms are defined above.

Transmembrane changes in the electric potential (i.e., action potential) generated by cardiac cells are the result of transmembrane ion fluxes (active properties) that generate currents through voltage- and ligand-gated membrane channels (Fig. 33.5; Table 33.3) [12,14,15]. The term "gated" refers to the opening (activation) or closing (deactivation or inactivation) of ion channels. Ion channels are characterized by their ionic selectivity, conductance, gating characteristics, and density. The channel gating mechanisms control ion passage and are composed of both activation and inactivation gates, which are voltage- and frequently time-dependent (e.g., sodium channels). The functional configuration of the gates determines channel state: activated or open, inactivated or closed, and resting (i.e., capable of being activated) [13]. The directional movement (inward or outward) of the various ions ultimately depends on channel state and the electrochemical driving force (i.e., equilibrium potential minus membrane potential) for each ion. The electrochemical driving force, as illustrated by the Nernst equation, is composed of an electric force and the transmembrane ion concentration gradient. It should be noted that most local anesthetics (e.g., lidocaine, bupivacaine, etc.) demonstrate use- (i.e., frequency-) dependent block [16,17]. Use-dependent block is the phenomenon exhibited by cardiac cells when, in the presence of a drug, increases in stimulation rate (i.e., chronotropy) produce a more pronounced drug effect because more drug molecules are able to enter the channel and cause more inactivation than during slower rates of stimulation [16].

Excitability (i.e., bathmotropy), or the ability of the cardiac cell membrane to be activated, generate, and propagate an electric potential (action potential), is a fundamental intrinsic property of cardiac cells [12,13]. The cardiac action potential (AP) morphology and duration vary considerably from that of nerves and skeletal muscle (Fig. 33.6A) [15]. The cardiac muscle AP arises from a more negative membrane potential (−90 versus −70 mV), may be of similar magnitude, but is much longer in duration (150–300 versus 1 ms) than APs recorded from nerve or skeletal muscle (Fig. 33.6A). Cardiac AP magnitude and duration also vary depending on the type of cardiac cell that generates them (Fig. 33.6B). Five characteristic phases of the cardiac AP are discernible in most cardiac cells: phase 0, or the phase of rapid depolarization, is caused by the rapid and relatively large influx of sodium ions (i.e., fast inward current) into the cell; phase 1, the early repolarization phase, is caused by the transient outward movement of potassium ions; phase 2, the plateau phase, is attributed to the continued, but decreased, entry of sodium ions and a large, but slower, influx of calcium ions (i.e., slow inward current) into the cell; phase 3 is the phase of membrane repolarization during which the membrane potential returns to its resting value primarily due to potassium efflux (i.e., outward current) from the cell; and phase 4 is a resting phase in atrial and ventricular muscle cells during which membrane pumps (i.e., Na^+–K^+ ATPase, Ca^{2+} pumps), and exchange mechanisms maintain the negative membrane potential and keep intracellular ion concentrations more or less constant prior to initiation of the next AP. For example, the Na^+–Ca^{2+} exchanger (NCX) or antiporter membrane protein removes calcium from cells helping to restore normal transmembrane electrolyte concentrations (Fig. 33.5; Table 33.3) but is reversible, moving Ca^{2+} out or into the cell depending on the prevailing electrochemical driving forces for Ca^{2+} and Na^+. Notably, a great deal of interest has been focused upon repolarization currents (I_K) due to their importance in determining membrane resting potential, AP duration, and their involvement in repolarization abnormalities (i.e., inhomogeneities or dispersion of the QT interval) including long QT syndrome [18,19]. Long QT syndrome is

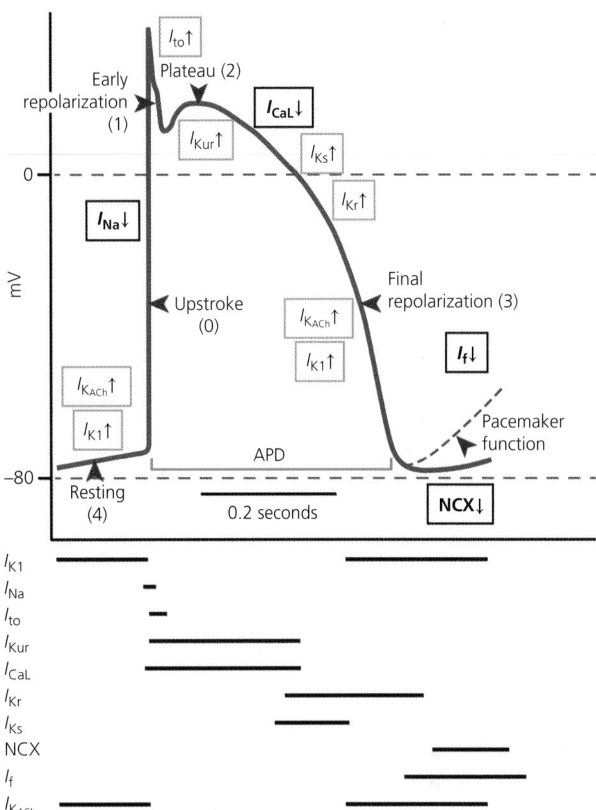

Figure 33.5 The normal action potential has five phases: Resting (4), Upstroke or depolarization (0), Early repolarization (1), Plateau (2), and Late or final repolarization (3). Gradual depolarization occurs at the end of phase 3 during phase 4 (blue dotted line) in automatic tissues (e.g., sinus node; Purkinje fibers). The inward currents, I_{Na}, I_{Ca}, I_f, and the sodium-calcium exchanger (NCX) are shown in bold black lined boxes. NCX is electrogenic and can generate an inward or outward current depending upon the membrane potential. Outward currents, I_{KACh}, I_{K1}, I_{to}, I_{Kur}, I_{Kr}, and I_{Ks} are shown in light gray lined boxes. The action potential duration (APD) in ventricular muscle cells is usually > 100 milliseconds. Source: Grant [15], Nature Publishing Group.

Table 33.3 Cardiac action potential (AP) currents.

Current	Abbreviation	Effect	AP phase
Sodium	I_{Na}	Rapid depolarization	Phase 0
Transient outward	I_{to}	Transient repolarization	Phase 1
Delayed rectifier	I_{Kur}	Rapid repolarization	Phase 1
L-type calcium	I_{CaL}	Plateau depolarizations	Phase 2
Delayed rectifier	I_{Ks}	Slow repolarization	Phase 3
Delayed rectifier	I_{Kr}	Rapid repolarization	Phase 3
Inward rectifier	I_{K1}	Resting membrane potential	Phases 3, 4
Muscarinic potassium	I_{KAch}	Inwardly rectifying SA node pacemaker	Phase 4
Pacemaker	I_f	Hyperpolarization-activated inward pacemaker current	Phase 4
Other Currents			
T-type calcium	I_{CaT}	Transient depolarization	Phase 2
ADP activated potassium	I_{KATP}	Inward rectification	Phases 1, 2
Na^+–Ca^{2+} exchanger	NCX	Electrogenic exchange; reversible	All phases

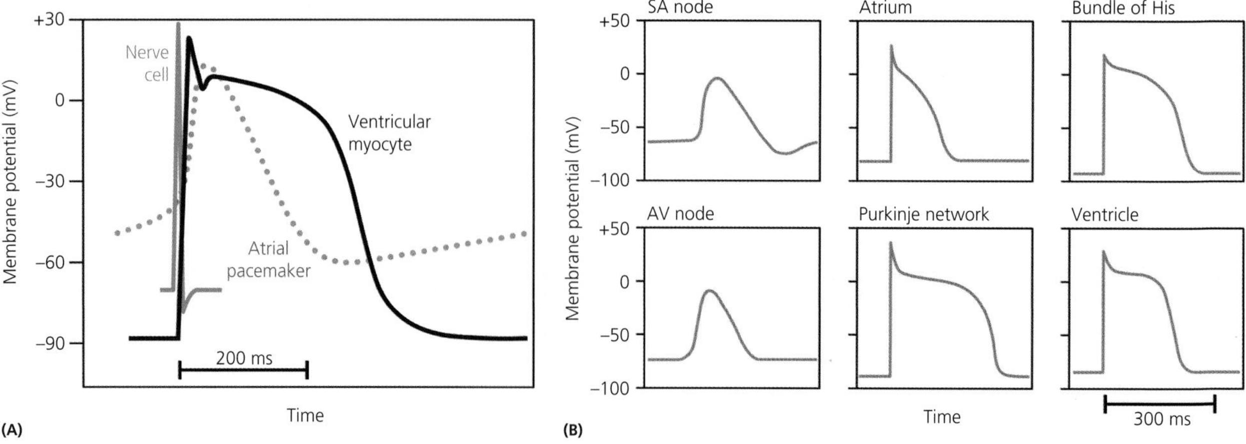

Figure 33.6 **A.** Nerve cell action potentials (light blue) are much shorter in duration (e.g., sodium based 1–2 ms) than cardiac muscle cell action potentials (black). Automatic cells determine heart rate (e.g., atrial pacemaker: orange). **B.** Action potential magnitudes and durations from various cardiac tissues.

Table 33.4 Intrinsic rate, action potential duration, and conduction velocity in cardiac tissues of larger mammals[a].

Cardiac tissue	Intrinsic rate	APD (ms)	Conduction velocity (m/second)
Sinoatrial node	50–80	80–120	0.01–0.05
Atrial muscle[b]	–	120–200	1.0
Atrioventricular node	20–40	80–120	0.01–0.05
Bundle of His	20–40	120–200	1.5
Purkinje fibers	5–20	300–450	2–4
Ventricular muscle[b]	–	150–250	1.0

APD, action potential duration.
[a] APD decreases and conduction velocity increases as intrinsic rate increases.
[b] Atrial and ventricular muscle is not normally automatic.

an uncommon hereditary or drug-induced condition (e.g., select antiarrhythmics, antidepressants, antipsychotics, antimicrobials, and opioids), in which AP duration becomes longer and may become highly variable among ventricular myocytes leading to electrical instability and the risk of reentrant induced torsades de pointes and ventricular fibrillation [20–22].

The speed of conduction of the cardiac electrical impulse (i.e., dromotropy) is determined by the magnitude and rate of sodium influx into the cardiac muscle cells and is directly related to the rate of voltage change (dV/dt) during phase 0 (Fig. 33.5; Table 33.4) [23]. A large dV/dt indicates more rapid depolarization of the cell membrane and more rapid conduction of the cardiac impulse through cardiac tissue [12]. The change (d) in transmembrane potential (V) is determined by the transmembrane ionic current (I_{ion}) and the membrane capacitance (C_m; 1 μF/cm^2) provided by the charge separation across the lipid bilayer:

$$dV/dt = 1/C_m \times I_{ion}$$

Ion movement occurs due to the activity of voltage-gated ion channels, pumps, and exchangers [13]. A negative I_{ion} indicates the inward flow of positive ions into the cell and produces a positive dV/dt, which depolarizes (i.e., makes the inside of the cells more positive) the membrane potential. A positive I_{ion} indicates an outward flow of positive ions, which repolarizes the membrane potential by generating a negative dV/dt. The generation of the cardiac AP results from the time-, voltage-, and concentration-dependent evolution of I_{ion} and represents the contribution of multiple ion-selective mechanisms for ion movement across the cardiac cell membrane (Fig. 33.5) [23]. Current flows from a depolarized cell to its neighboring less depolarized cells via intercellular resistive pathways known as "gap junctions." Gap junctions are hydrophilic intercellular protein channels (i.e., connexons) composed of six connexin proteins that allow ions and electrical impulses to pass between cells through regulated hydrophilic channels [23]. Voltage-gated ionic channels and gap junctions are depressed (i.e., resistance is increased) by anesthetic drugs through direct interaction with their protein subunits, thereby interfering with cardiac excitability, transmission, and propagation of electrical impulses [24–26].

Calcium enters cardiac cells through L-type calcium channels during phase 2 of the AP triggering intracellular calcium release from the sarcoplasmic reticulum, which is important for normal cellular contraction. Since calcium enters the cell more slowly than sodium (i.e., slow inward calcium current) and from a less negative membrane potential, cardiac cells with a reduced resting membrane potential (e.g., the sinoatrial [SA] and atrioventricular [AV] nodes) demonstrate a considerably smaller phase 0 dV/dt and slower conduction velocity compared to those with a more negative resting membrane potential (e.g., atrial and ventricular muscle and Purkinje cells) [11–13]. Potassium efflux from cardiac cells is controlled by a variety of mechanisms, including the concentration difference of potassium across the membrane and changes in membrane permeability to potassium as the membrane potential changes (Table 33.3). The channels responsible for repolarization (phase 3) are major determinants of cardiac AP duration and cardiac cell refractoriness (Fig. 33.7). The duration of the cardiac AP and refractoriness have important clinical implications relative to the amount of calcium that enters the cell during depolarization (i.e., longer AP duration permits more calcium entry) and the potential for arrhythmia development, respectively [12,27]. Arrhythmias develop if there are large differences (i.e., inhomogeneities) in myocyte AP duration (e.g., > 20–40 ms) among groups of adjacent cardiac cells because of the potential for electrical impulses to re-enter cells that have rapidly repolarized and regained excitability and conduction capabilities (i.e., reentry). Cardiac cells with particularly long AP durations are thought to predispose to dispersion of refractoriness and afterdepolarizations (i.e., afterpotentials) that leads to electrical instability and cardiac arrhythmias [27–29].

Phase 4, diastolic depolarization, endows the heart with the unique property of automaticity (i.e., self-excitation). SA automaticity

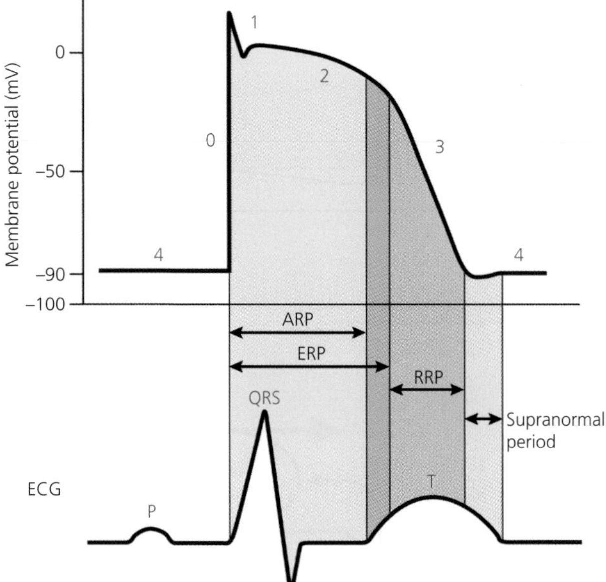

Figure 33.7 Absolute (ARP), effective (ERP), and relative (RRP) refractory periods. During the ARP the cell is incapable of generating an electrical response (i.e., action potential). ERP: An electrical response can be generated during the ERP but is not conducted. RRP: A greater than normal stimulus can generate a conducted response. The functional refractory period (FRP; not shown) is the shortest interval between two consecutively conducted responses. Supranormal period: the period following the RRP during which a smaller than normal stimulus can generate a conducted action potential.

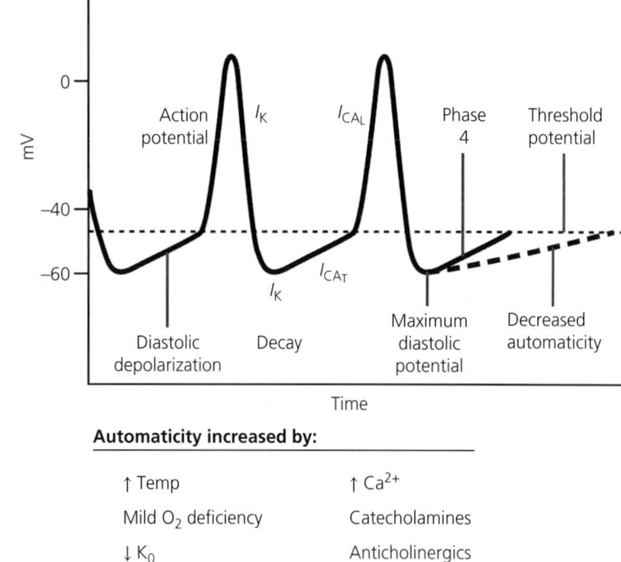

Figure 33.8 The transmembrane potential of the sinoatrial node (i.e., normal pacemaker) is characterized by a maximum diastolic potential ≅ 60 mV that depolarizes toward threshold (i.e., phase 4 diastolic depolarization), a slow phase 0 caused by I_{Ca}, and a relatively rapid repolarization due to I_K. The rate of phase 4 diastolic depolarization (i.e., automaticity) can be increased by increases in temperature, calcium, mild oxygen deficiency, catecholamines, decreases in extracellular potassium concentration, and anticholinergic drugs (e.g., atropine). Increases in extracellular potassium concentration and I_f inhibitors (e.g., ivabradine) decrease diastolic depolarization.

is produced by depolarizing membrane currents and is influenced by local factors, including temperature, pH, and blood gases (PO_2 and PCO_2), extracellular potassium concentration, catecholamines, and various hormones (Fig. 33.8). Cells in the SA and AV nodes and specialized atrial and ventricular muscle cells (i.e., Purkinje) cells are automatic (Table 33.4) [30]. The resting membrane potential of these cells depolarizes toward a threshold potential, which when reached triggers the development of an AP. The ionic processes responsible for phase 4 diastolic depolarization vary among the various specialized tissues of the heart primarily because of differences in their resting membrane potential and cell type (e.g., SA node, AV node, and Purkinje cell), but all are dependent upon the funny current (I_f), a mixed sodium–potassium current that activates upon hyperpolarization [31]. The funny current, first described in SA node myocytes as an inward current activated during hyperpolarization, determines the end of an AP, the steepness of phase 4 depolarization, and the frequency of AP firing [31]. Cells in the SA and AV nodes have comparatively less negative maximum diastolic potentials (-65 mV) compared to cardiac muscle and Purkinje cells (≥ -90 mV) and depend upon I_f, the entry of calcium ions (i.e., inward calcium current), and a progressive decrease in membrane permeability to potassium efflux for their automaticity [12,13,31,32]. Automatic cells in atrial specialized pathways and the ventricular Purkinje network have a more negative maximum diastolic potential (≥ -90 mV) and depend more upon I_f [32]. The principal mechanisms responsible for altering automaticity are changes in the threshold potential, the rate of phase 4 depolarization, and the maximum diastolic potential following repolarization. The cardiac tissue with the most rapid rate of phase 4 depolarization (normally the SA node) is termed the "pacemaker" and determines the heart rate (HR). The cardiac pacemaker normally activates (i.e., overdrives) and, therefore, resets the automaticity of slower or subsidiary pacemakers, thereby preventing other potential pacemakers from controlling HR (i.e., overdrive suppression; Fig. 33.9A) [32]. Overdrive suppression of subsidiary pacemakers is caused by activation of the sodium–potassium (Na^+–K^+) pump, leading to membrane hyperpolarization and a longer time required to reach threshold (Fig. 33.9B) [13]. Subsidiary pacemakers are depressed by fast HRs because the Na^+–K^+ pump is more active at faster rates, resulting in a more negative maximum diastolic potential. Clinically, the administration of anticholinergic drugs (e.g., atropine and glycopyrrolate) can produce increases in sinus rate that eliminate (i.e., overdrive suppress) infrequent or slower automatic ventricular arrhythmias. Alternatively, ivabradine, a drug that selectively and specifically inhibits the cardiac pacemaker current I_f, slows HR [33].

The average of the voltage vectors produced by all the APs produced by activation of each cardiac cell is responsible for the body surface electrocardiogram (ECG; a graphical representation of the electrical depolarization and repolarization of the heart) (Fig. 33.10). Initiation of an electric impulse in the SA node is followed by rapid transmission of a wave of depolarization throughout the atria, giving rise to the P wave. Repolarization of the atria gives rise to the T_a wave, which is small and difficult to identify in smaller animals (e.g., rats, rabbits, dogs, cats, etc.) but becomes obvious in larger animals (e.g., horses and cattle) because the total atrial tissue mass is substantial enough to generate an electromotive force that can be detected electrocardiographically from the body surface. Similarly, depolarization of the SA and AV nodes does not normally generate a large enough electromotive force to be recorded at the body surface. Once the wave of depolarization

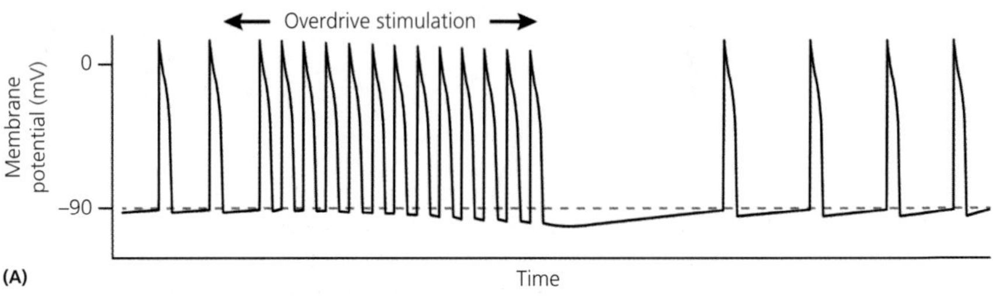

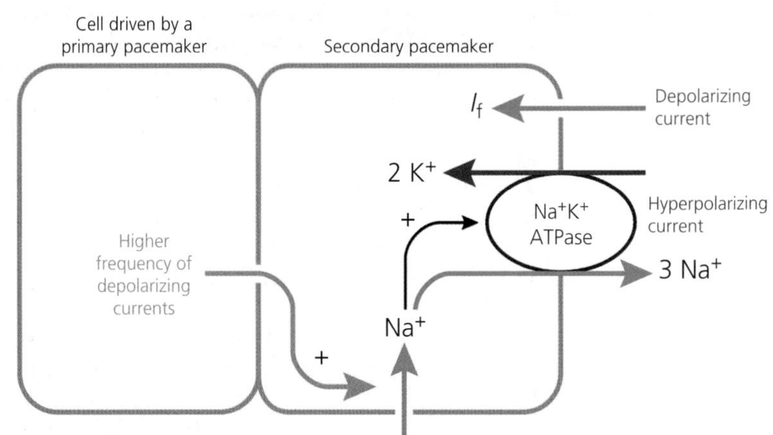

Figure 33.9 **A.** Overdrive suppression occurs when a higher frequency of activation suppresses automaticity. Usually interpreted to mean that increase SA node firing suppresses other pacemaker sites. **B.** Overdrive suppression is mediated by enhanced Na^+–K^+ ATPase pump activity. Increased frequency of depolarizations increases intracellular Na^+ stimulating the electrogenic (i.e., moves more Na^+ outward than K^+ inward) Na^+–K^+ ATPase pump thereby generating an outward (hyperpolarizing) current across the cell membrane and a more negative membrane potential, counteracting the depolarizing I_f current, thus slowing the rate of phase 4 diastolic depolarization and suppressing spontaneous impulse initiation.

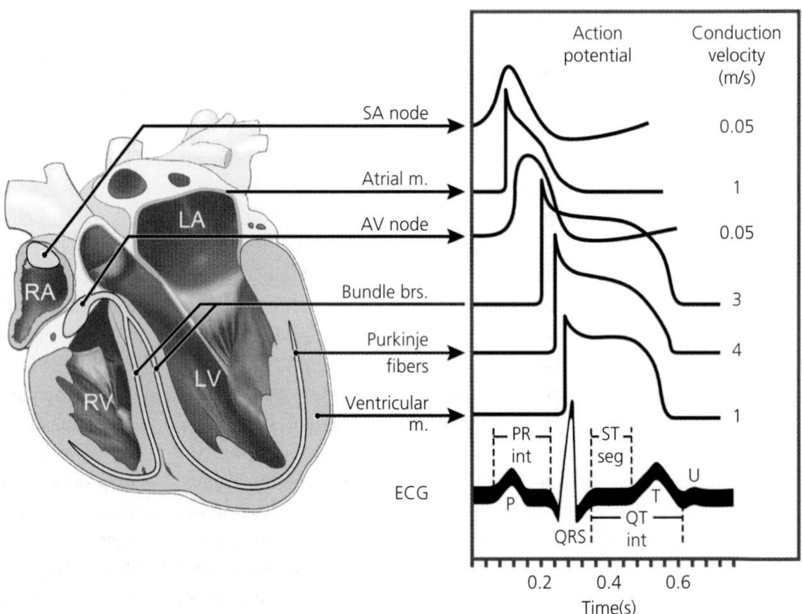

Figure 33.10 The electrocardiogram (ECG) is the average of the voltage vectors produced by the electrical activation (i.e., action potentials) of the heart during a cardiac cycle. SA, sinoatrial node; AV, atrioventricular node; brs, branches; int, interval; LA, left atrium; LV, left ventricle; m, muscle; RA, right atrium; RV, right ventricle; seg, segment.

reaches the AV node, conduction is slowed because of its less negative resting membrane potential (i.e., −40 to −60 mV) and reduced slope (dV/dt) of phase 0 (Fig. 33.6B). This is especially evident when the AV node is stimulated at higher rates due to a phenomenon called "decremental conduction," which is characterized by poor propagation of the electrical impulse due to progressive decreases in membrane potential and AP dV/dt. Increased parasympathetic tone also produces marked slowing of AV nodal conduction, leading to first-degree, second-degree, and, occasionally, third-degree AV block. Many drugs used for anesthesia, including opioids, α_2-adrenergic receptor agonists, and occasionally acepromazine, can increase parasympathetic tone, causing sinus slowing and bradyarrhythmias. The use of anticholinergic drugs (e.g., atropine and glycopyrrolate) is generally effective therapy in these situations but not when AV block is caused by inflammation or structural disease (e.g., fibrosis and calcification). Caution is indicated when atropine or glycopyrrolate are co-administered with α_2-adrenergic receptor agonists due to their potential to produce or exacerbate ventricular arrhythmias. α_2-Adrenergic receptor agonist–anticholinergic drug combinations that produce cardiac arrhythmias are likely due to increases in the rate–pressure product and myocardial oxygen consumption, or myocardial ischemia in conjunction with functional impairment of autonomic tone (i.e., dysautonomia) [34,35].

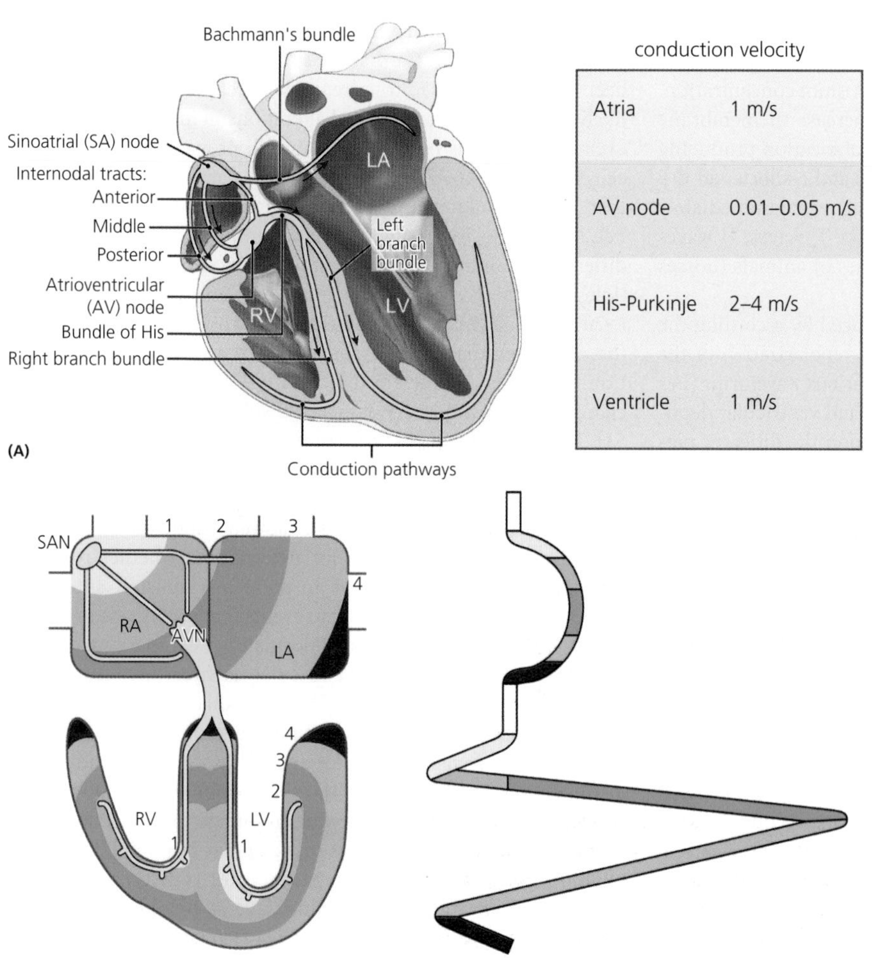

Figure 33.11 A. The specialized conducting pathways of the heart include the sinoatrial node, the atrial internodal pathways, the atrioventricular node and His bundle, and the right and left bundle branches. Bachmann's bundle facilitates electrical signal transmission to the left atrium. The conduction velocity of the electrical signal varies in different cardiac tissues. **B.** The sequence of electrical conduction in the atrial and ventricles (1–4) from initiation (yellow) to termination (dark blue) in relation to the development of the ECG.

The conduction of the electrical impulse through the AV node provides time for the atria to contract (i.e., atrial priming or kick) prior to activation and contraction of the ventricles. The delay in ventricular depolarization is responsible for the PR or PQ interval of the ECG (Fig. 33.10). This delay is functionally important, particularly at faster HRs, because it enables atrial contraction to contribute to ventricular filling. It is worth remembering that cells of the AV node depend upon both sodium and calcium ions for the generation and conduction of their AP. Thus, cells of the AV node are extremely sensitive to drugs that block transmembrane calcium flux, including excessive doses of anesthetic drugs and calcium channel antagonists (e.g., verapamil and diltiazem). Excessive doses of injectable or inhalant anesthetic drugs can produce post-repolarization refractoriness, a phenomenon wherein cardiac cells remain refractory to electric activation after complete repolarization. This phenomenon is likely to produce AV block as HR increases. In addition, increases in parasympathetic tone in the presence of drugs or diseases (e.g., inflammation and ischemia) that interfere with conduction of the electric impulse through the AV node can lead to ECG sinus bradycardia and first-degree (prolonged PR interval), second-degree (blocked P wave), or third-degree (dissociation of P from the QRS complex) AV block.

Once the electrical impulse has traversed the AV node, it is rapidly transmitted via specialized pathways to ventricular muscle cells. Bundles of Purkinje cells (the right and left bundle branches) transmit the electrical impulse to the ventricular septum and the right and left ventricular wall papillary muscles, respectively, via the moderator band in the right ventricle and the left anterior and posterior divisions of the left bundle branch, in the left ventricle (Fig. 33.11A). Purkinje fibers conduct the electric impulse at relatively rapid speeds (3–4 m/s) throughout the ventricles. Purkinje cells and midmyocardial (M) cells located at the terminal ends of the Purkinje bundle branches and in the middle of the ventricular walls, respectively, have the longest AP durations and, therefore, serve as physiological "gates" preventing reentry or recycling of electric impulses into the ventricular myocardium [36,37]. The comparatively long duration of Purkinje and M cell APs is also considered to be one cause for the development of U waves in the ECG (Fig. 33.10). It is important to remember that the electrical transmission of the cardiac AP ultimately depends on spatial variation in myocardial cell refractoriness and the maintenance of uniform (isotropic) cell-to-cell resistive and capacitive (passive force) membrane properties that are largely determined by low-resistance gap or nexus junctions between cells [38,39].

The interval beginning immediately after the terminal S wave of the QRS complex (J point) and the ventricular repolarization T wave is referred to as the "ST segment." Elevation or depression of the ST segment (±0.2 mV or greater) from the isoelectric line is indicative of myocardial hypoxia or ischemia caused by low cardiac output (CO), hypotension, anemia, pericarditis, or cardiac contusion, and suggests the potential for arrhythmias to develop. The ST segment is followed by, and may slur into, the T wave [40].

The configuration and magnitude of the T wave vary considerably among species and are particularly influenced by changes in HR, blood temperature, and the extracellular potassium concentration. Hyperkalemia, for example, produces an increase in membrane conductance to potassium and shortens repolarization producing large magnitude, spiked, or pointed T waves and a shortened QT interval. U waves, when present, can be distinguished immediately following the T wave (Fig. 33.10) [36,41]. Like T_a waves, U waves are more frequently observed in larger species of animals (horses and cattle).

As described previously, the ECG is produced by recording the electrically synchronized depolarization and repolarization of the atria and ventricles. The morphology of the various waveforms (i.e., P, QRS, and T waves) that characterize atrial and ventricular depolarization and repolarization is dependent upon the different patterns of depolarization, electrode placement, the size of the cardiac chambers (e.g., hypertrophy increases the electromotive force generated), the orthogonal direction of the dominant electromotive force, resistance to electrical signal transmission (i.e., fat, fluid, and air), and a host of electrode, equipment, and environmental factors (e.g., electrical noise). P wave morphology will vary depending on where within the crescent-shaped SA node electrical activation originates and spreads into the right atrium. The electrical signal is then transmitted via intra-atrial and interatrial specialized pathways that depolarize the right and left atrial (e.g., Bachmann's bundle) muscle fibers, respectively (Fig. 33.11A). The right atrium is normally activated before the left atrium since the electrical signal normally originates in the SA node. This sequence of activation (i.e., right atrium then left atrium) may be hard to appreciate in smaller animals (e.g., rats, rabbits, cats, and small dogs) since their atrial muscle mass is relatively small and the electrical activation process is completed in a shorter time compared to larger animals (e.g., pigs, horses, goats, and cattle). The larger atrial muscle mass in large animals or in larger smaller species (e.g., dogs) with an enlarged left atrium can often be identified by a bifid P wave. Once the atrial electrical signal traverses the AV node, it activates the rapidly conducting Purkinje fiber network. Bundles of Purkinje fibers form the right and left bundle branches, which distribute the wave of depolarization to the respective papillary muscles and ventricular muscle cells of the right and left ventricles generating the QRS wave that represents ventricular depolarization (Figs. 33.10 and 33.11B). Purkinje fibers penetrate a short distance from the subendocardium in smaller animal species (Category I: rats, rabbits, cats, and dogs) while larger animal species have evolved a more diffuse Purkinje fiber distribution that extends close to the subepicardium (Category II: sheep, goats, cattle, pigs, and horses). This difference in Purkinje fiber anatomical distribution ensures the synchrony of ventricular activation and contraction. Fiber-to-fiber spread of the ventricular myocardial electrical signal occurs from the endpoints of the Purkinje fibers in the subendocardium of Category I (i.e., smaller) species (Fig. 33.12A) or wherever Purkinje fibers terminate in Category II (i.e., larger) species (Fig. 33.12B). Orthogonal (i.e., X, Y, Z; ECG leads: I, aVf, V10) ECG lead placement illustrates differences in the dominant ventricular electrical activation forces, spatial orientation, and pattern of ventricular depolarization generated by animals in Category I (e.g., cats, dogs, and humans) and Category II (Category IIA: sheep, goats, and cattle; Category IIB: pigs and horses) (Fig. 33.13).

Several inhalant (e.g., halothane, isoflurane, and enflurane) and injectable (e.g., thiopental, propofol, and opioids) anesthetic drugs are known to sensitize the myocardium to catecholamines or facilitate torsadogenicity resulting in the development of cardiac arrhythmias [42–45]. Cardiac sensitization to anesthetic drugs has been linked to cardiac α_1-adrenerigc receptor stimulation and is likely produced by drug-related alterations in intracellular calcium cycling, alterations in electrical impulse propagation, and muscle cell excitability [46,47]. Anesthetic drugs, particularly volatile anesthetics, are also known to interact with multiple cardiac ion channels. Halothane, isoflurane, and sevoflurane depress ion channels at different minimum alveolar anesthetic concentration (MAC) multiples: sodium (> 2 MAC), calcium (~30% at > 2 MAC), potassium (~20% at > 1 MAC), and chloride (> 2 MAC) [48]. Inhibition of these channels may alter AP shape (i.e., triangulation) and conduction velocity and these are the two most common proarrhythmic changes in the cardiac AP associated with volatile anesthetics [48–51]. Triangulation allows more time for Na^+–Ca^{2+} exchange, reactivation of the sodium current, reduced synchronization of APs, and facilitation of re-excitation predisposing to the development of early afterdepolarizations [50,51]. Slowed conduction and tissue refractoriness are key factors for determining whether reentrant arrhythmias occur. In addition to these mechanisms, autonomic nervous system imbalances lead to events that predispose to cardiac repolarization and conduction abnormalities, coronary vasospasm, and unifocal or multifocal ventricular tachycardias. Autonomic imbalance may be responsible for the cardiac arrhythmias attributed to the concurrent administration of anticholinergic (e.g., atropine) and α_2-adrenerigc receptor agonist (e.g., medetomidine and dexmedetomidine) drugs [34]. γ-Aminobutyric acid type A ($GABA_A$) anesthetics (i.e., propofol, etomidate, and alfaxalone) acting on various $GABA_A$ subunits (α, β, γ) may also inhibit postganglionic vagal input (i.e., reduce M_2 receptor activity) to the heart provoking sinus tachycardia while several opioids, particularly methadone, are known to lengthen the QT interval predisposing to ventricular arrhythmias [52,53].

In summary, the active (i.e., ion movement) and passive (resistive and capacitive) properties of cardiac cell membranes determine the heart's excitability (i.e., bathmotropy), automaticity (i.e., chronotropy), conduction (i.e., dromotropy), rhythmicity, and refractoriness. Injectable and inhalant anesthetic drugs produce alterations in cardiac ion channels and transmembrane ion flux that may impair mechanical contraction or induce cardiac arrhythmias [42,46,47,54,55].

Excitation–contraction coupling

Excitation–contraction coupling refers to the process whereby electrical activation of myocardial cells is transformed into muscle contraction [56–59]. The process begins with depolarization of the cardiac cell membrane and ends with sarcomere and subsequently muscle fiber shortening. The normal extracellular [Ca^{2+}] is 10^{-3} M compared with an intracellular [Ca^{2+}] of 10^{-7} M. The electrical activation of the sarcolemma and its extensions (i.e., transverse [T] tubules) into the cell interior initiates an influx of calcium ions through L-type calcium channels that trigger the release (i.e., calcium-induced calcium release [CICR]) of calcium from ryanodine-sensitive Ca^{2+} release channels in the sarcoplasmic reticulum [59]. CICR raises the intracellular calcium concentration from 10^{-7} to 10^{-5} M resulting in myosin–actin cycling and sarcomere contraction (Fig. 33.14). While most calcium ions enter the cardiac cell through voltage-dependent L-type calcium channels (i.e., dihydropyridine channel or DHP channel), some calcium ions enter via the Na^+–Ca^{2+} exchanger (NCX) mechanism [37]. Voltage-dependent calcium channels are of two types (Table 33.3): a fast but transient (i.e., T-type) channel that is

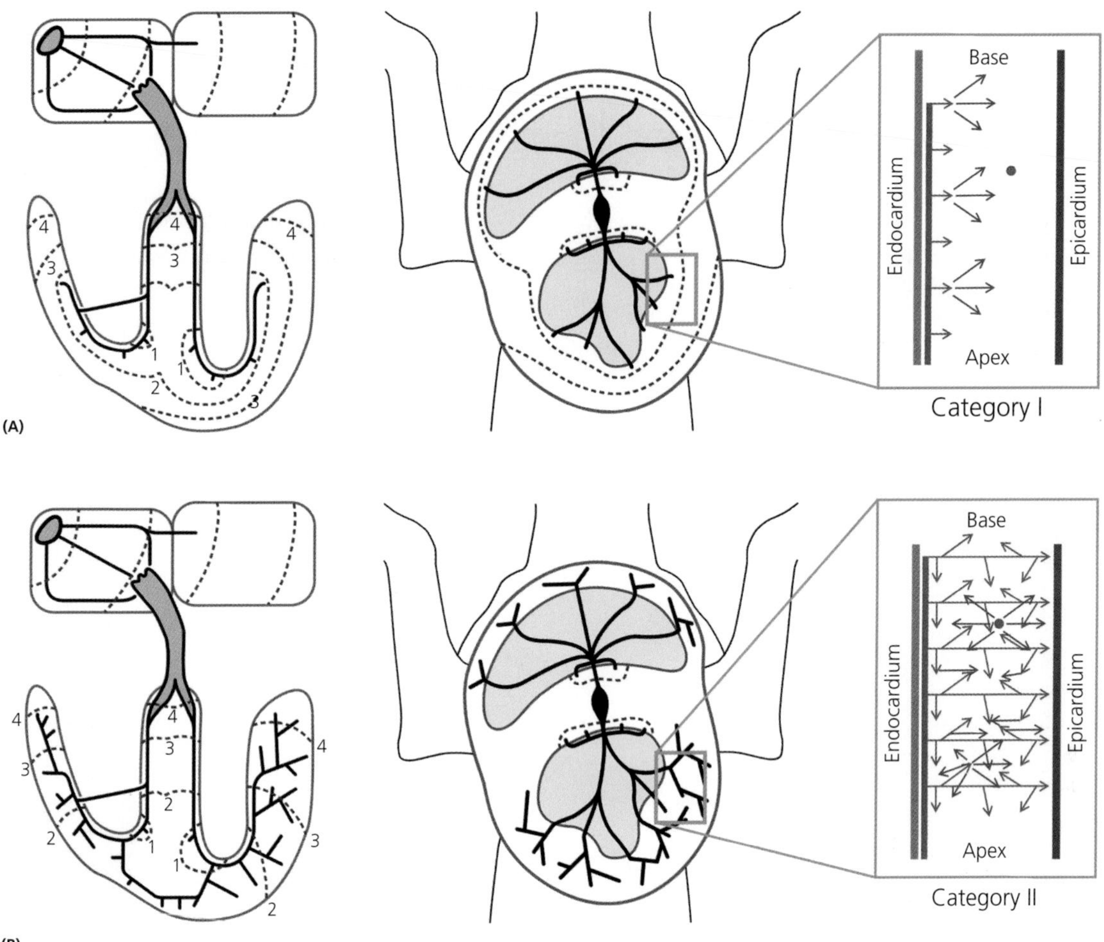

Figure 33.12 **A.** Depolarization reaches every point in the myocardium by traveling rapidly in specialized pathways and slowly from muscle fiber to muscle fiber. Hearts from larger animals (e.g., horses, cattle) or hearts from species with large ancestors (e.g., sheep and goats) require more complete penetration of Purkinje fibers to achieve adequate synchronization of contraction. **B.** Conduction velocity along His–Purkinje fibers (red arrows) is ~2–4 m/s for all animals. Conduction patterns within the ventricular myocardium from the endpoint of the Purkinje fiber network (red dot) are responsible for different patterns of ventricular activation and body surface ECG patterns: Category 1 (e.g., guinea pig, rabbits, dog, cat, and humans); Category IIA (e.g., goat and cow); Category IIB (e.g., horse, pig, dolphins). Source: Dr. Robert Hamlin, with permission.

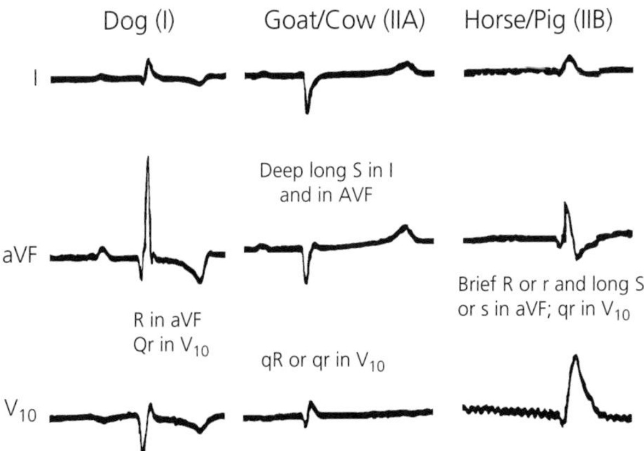

Figure 33.13 QRS patterns in orthogonal (i.e., X, Y. Z: I, aVf, V10) ECG leads in Category I (e.g., cat, dog, and human) and Category II (e.g., Category IIA: sheep, goat, and cattle; Category IIB: pigs and horses) animals. Source: Dr. Robert Hamlin, with permission.

activated earlier and at more negative potentials than L-type channels and is believed to play a role in activation of pacemaker cells; and a slow, long-lasting (i.e., L-type) channel that is opened by cellular depolarization and is responsible for excitation–contraction coupling. T-type channels are insensitive to sodium channel blockers (e.g., lidocaine or tetrodotoxin) and calcium antagonists [57]. L-type channels are sensitive to specific types of calcium antagonists (e.g., verapamil, diltiazem, and nifedipine-like compounds) [57,58]. The L-type channels are more prevalent in atrial and ventricular muscle cells than are T-type channels, open at less negative potentials, and account for the latter phases of calcium channel opening [56]. Both channels are physiologically linked via specialized bridging or spanning (i.e., "foot") proteins that connect them to the ryanodine-sensitive Ca^{2+} release channels in the sarcoplasmic reticulum. The foot structures are part of a high-molecular-weight protein complex termed the "ryanodine receptor" (RyR) because of its affinity for the insecticide ryanodine [60]. Multiple RyR isoforms exist and cardiac RyRs are of the RyR2 type [60]. Any drug that prolongs channel opening triggered by

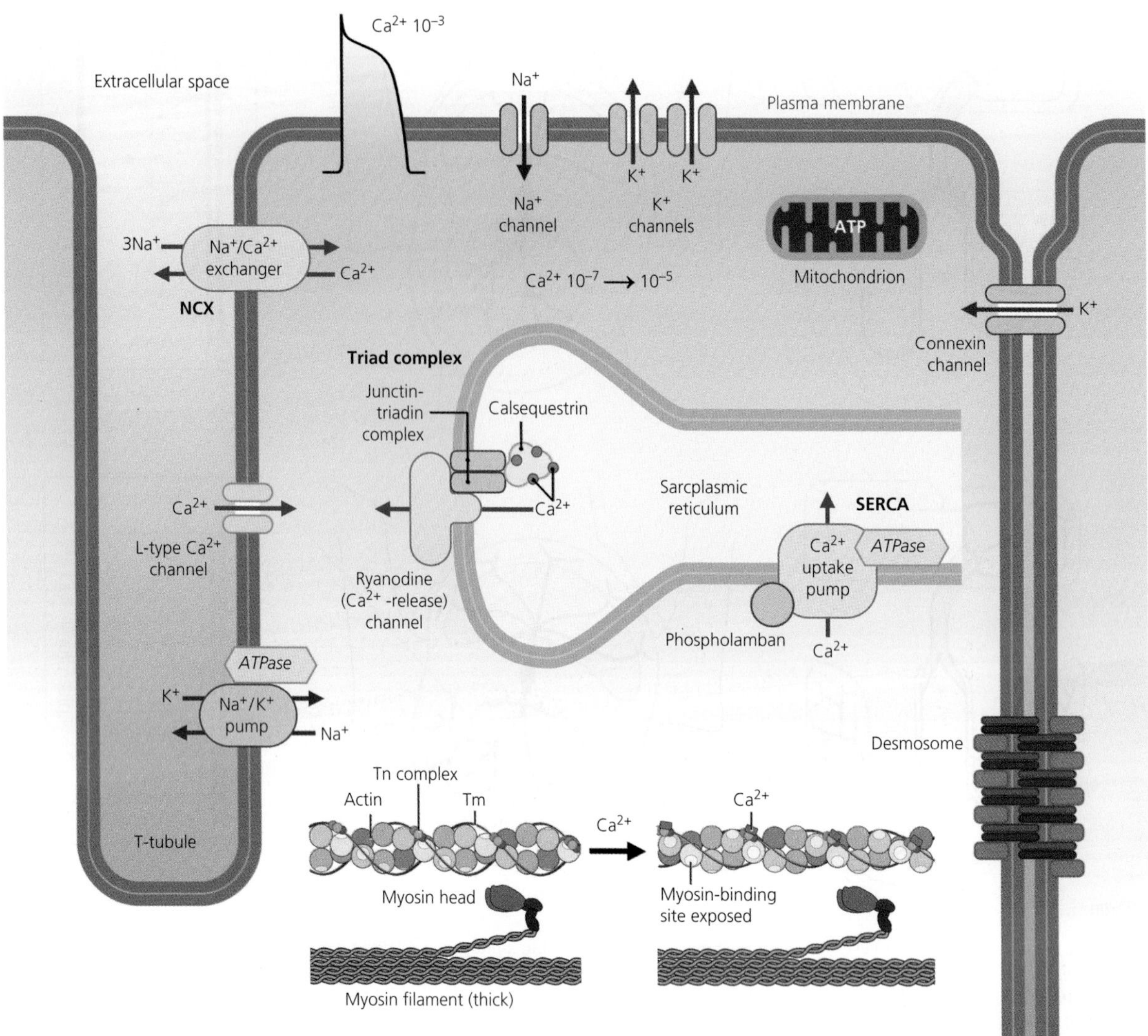

Figure 33.14 Cardiac muscle cell excitation–contraction coupling. Cardiac muscle cells (cardiomyocytes) are surrounded by a surface membrane with tubular invaginations (T-tubules). The T-tubular network assists action potential propagation into the cytoplasm of cardiac muscle cells. Calcium enters the cardiac cell during phase 2 of the action potential via L-type calcium channels (i.e., dihydropyridine receptors). The junctin, triadin, calsequestrin, and ryanodine receptor form a quaternary complex (i.e., foot protein) that triggers normal intracellular Ca^{2+} release from the sarcoplasmic reticulum (SR) by a process termed "calcium-induced calcium release" (CICR). Increases in intracellular calcium (10^{-7} to 10^{-5} *M*) activates the regulatory protein troponin (Tn) complex (i.e., Tn-C on the thin (i.e., actin) filament allowing binding of thick filament myosin heads to attach to exposed binding sites on the thin filament (inset) resulting in filament sliding, sarcomere shortening and muscle contraction. Calcium is transported back into the sarcoplasmic reticulum (SR) by the SR-Ca^{2+} ATPase pump (SERCA) and out of the cell by the sodium-calcium exchanger (NCX), located in the surface membrane. Phospholamban modulates Ca^{2+} pump reuptake of calcium into the SR. Metabolism of adenosine triphosphate (ATP) and formation of adenosine diphosphate and inorganic phosphate, and reuptake of calcium by the SR cause sarcomere relaxation. Small quantities of cytosolic Ca^{2+} stimulate mitochondrion resynthesis of ATP.

cytoplasmic Ca^{2+} will also promote RyR activation and increase cytoplasmic [Ca^{2+}]. For example, mutations in the skeletal muscle isoform of the ryanodine receptor Ca^{2+}-release channel (RyR1) are responsible for susceptibility to malignant hyperthermia and can be triggered by inhalant anesthetics (e.g., halothane, isoflurane, sevoflurane, and succinylcholine) [61,62]. Membrane-bound inositol 1,4,5-trisphosphate receptors (IP_3R) provide a second pathway for internal Ca^{2+} release [63]. Their subcellular localization in atrial, ventricular, and Purkinje fibers is about 50-fold less than RyR2s in ventricular myocytes. They are believed to modulate transcription, amplify RyR2 Ca^{2+} signals, and provide independent cellular activation through diverse pathways that generate IP_3. The activation of IP_3Rs by select agonists (e.g., angiotensin II, endothelin, and norepinephrine) is believed to be important in development of cardiac arrhythmias, hypertrophy and heart failure [63]. Notably, inhalant (i.e., halothane, isoflurane, sevoflurane, and desflurane) and injectable (i.e., propofol, etomidate, and midazolam) anesthetics produce dose-dependent inhibition of the cardiac L-type calcium current by interacting with and inhibiting DHP and RyR calcium channels thereby reducing CICR and the force of cardiac contraction [64–67].

The actin-activated myosin chemomechanical ATPase cycle

Cardiac muscle cells (myocytes) are composed of repeating core contractile units called "sarcomeres" (Fig. 33.15A). Sarcomeres contain the contractile proteins actin (i.e., thin) and myosin (i.e., thick) filaments, which are the smallest functional units of striated cardiac muscle cells. The thin actin filaments have plus and minus ends and are attached at their plus end to structural proteins (i.e., Z bands) that separate each sarcomere (Fig. 33.15B) [68]. Each actin filament contains two helical strands of actin intertwined with tropomyosin, which has periodic troponin complexes. Increases in intracellular calcium-ion concentration initiated during phase 2 of the cardiac AP and amplified by CICR serve as the catalyst for actin–myosin interaction and sarcomere shortening. More specifically, calcium ions bind to the regulatory protein troponin C (Tn-C; C for calcium) and remove the inhibitory function of troponin I (Tn-I; I for inhibitor) on the chemical interaction between actin and myosin thick filaments, allowing actin–myosin crossbridges to form (Fig. 33.15C). Myosin heavy chain (MHC) is the actin-activated molecular motor of muscle thick filaments that forms crossbridges with actin pulling the thin actin filament over the thicker myosin filament toward the center of the sarcomere, thereby shortening the sarcomere [68,69]. Two functionally distinct isoforms of myosin, alpha (α) and beta (β), are present in mammalian hearts both containing ATPase and actin-binding domains. The isoforms are structurally similar and are key determinants of sarcomere force generation and shortening velocity [70]. The α isoform is more highly expressed in the atria and ventricles of smaller mammals (i.e., mice and rats), whereas the β isoform predominates in the ventricles of larger mammals (i.e., pig, dogs, and humans) [71]. β-Myosin has lower ATPase activity and produces slower actin sliding velocities than α-myosin but is able to generate greater force [72].

Cardiac MHCs are comprised of two domains: heavy meromyosin (HMM) and light meromyosin (LMM). HMM is subdivided into subfragments (S1 and S2) (Fig. 33.15D). The S1 subfragment is comprised of two actin-activated ATPase globular heads (the motor domain) followed by a converter domain and a lever arm. The essential light chain (ELC) and regulatory light chain (RLC) comprise the lever arm. Both the ELC and RLC in conjunction with myosin-binding protein C (MyBPC) modulate sarcomere activity, intermolecular interactions between the two myosin S1 heads, and the conversion of chemical energy (ATP) into heat (i.e., Fenn effect) and mechanical work (Fig. 33.15C) [73–75]. The force produced by myosin motors is fueled by ATP hydrolysis resulting in the sequential release of inorganic phosphate (P_i) and ADP, strong actin–myosin binding, and the swing of the lever arm. The swing of the lever arm pulls the actin (i.e., power stroke) causing the sarcomere to shorten. The lever arm merges with the coiled-coil tail of HMM (i.e., S2 subfragment) and connects to LMM molecules that are packed with the tails of other LMM molecules forming the backbone of the thick filament (Fig. 33.15C) [68,76].

Pairs of myosin S1 heads encircle the thick filament in a helical or quasi-helical fashion and exist in one of three transitional states: active, disordered relaxed (DRX; approximately 50–60%), and super-relaxed (SRX; approximately 40–50%) [77,78]. The SRX state is "off" or "hibernating." SRX myosin S1 heads are folded back ("parked" or "docked") along the thick filament. Parked S1 heads have markedly reduced ATPase activity, cannot bind to actin, and provide a method for regulating cardiac contractility in response to changes in loading conditions (i.e., preload and afterload) [79,80]. Activation of cardiac muscle only involves free heads in the DRX state. Myosin S1 heads in the DRX state display a flexible or free ("swaying") position (Fig. 33.15C). Their partnered blocked myosin S1 head is docked onto its S2 tail and cannot bind to actin. Intermolecular interactions between myosin S1 heads and their S2 tails, ELC, RLC, and MyBPC favor the DRX or SRX states and are collectively referred to as the "interacting-heads motif" (IHM) [68]. The regulatory protein MyBPC modulates force generation by maintaining the SRX ("off") state [79,81–83]. Phosphorylation of the RLC releases one (i.e., free head) or both of the two myosin S1 heads, and increases myosin S1 step size, the velocity of sarcomeric shortening, isometric force, and power generation [68]. These interactions modulate the kinetics of actin–myosin crossbridge formation, myosin ATPase activity, and calcium utilization thereby acting as molecular regulators of muscle force and velocity generation [84]. Notably, stress sensed by the myosin thick filament destabilizes the SRX state releasing myosin S1 heads from their docked state and transitioning them from an "off" to an active state (i.e., positive cooperativity) [68,78,85]. Cycling of the myosin S1 heads (i.e., velocity of lever-arm swinging; number that synchronously swing and form strong attachments) produces the force, velocity, and power needed for contraction [86,87].

Important steps in the actin-activated myosin chemomechanical ATPase cycle (i.e., "swinging lever-arm" model) include (Fig. 33.16): (1) ATP hydrolysis to ADP and P_i and adoption of a bent or "cocked" (pre-power stroke) position by the myosin S1 head; (2) weak binding of the myosin S1 head containing ADP and P_i to actin; (3) transition of the myosin S1 head from a weak to strong binding state upon P_i release and lever-arm swinging pulling the actin filament toward the center of the sarcomere ("swinging lever-arm" model); (4) adoption of a post-power stroke position associated with ADP release; and (5) binding of ATP to the myosin S1 head weakening its interaction with actin.

The rate of P_i release is the rate limiting step that determines the duration that myosin S1 heads are strongly bound to actin. The velocity of actin filament sliding until the myosin S1 heads detach is determined by ADP release (i.e., detachment rate [k_{det}]) [84,87,88]. Cyclic asynchronous ATP-driven actin–myosin mechanosensing and biased Brownian motion driven by increased ionic strength are responsible for the lever-arm swing, myosin displacement, sarcomere shortening, and force development [89,90]. Maximum velocity of contraction (V_{max}) is derived from the unitary displacement divided by the myosin head detachment rate. Thus, the load-dependent attachment rate, overall cycle rate, amount of time that myosin is attached to actin, and the total number of myosin S1 heads in the active state (i.e., duty ratio) determine the developed force (F), sliding velocity (V_{max}), and amount of ATP consumed [90–93].

Myocardial contraction and relaxation

Increases in intracellular calcium facilitate increased myosin ATPase activity. Therefore, intracellular calcium concentration serves as the principal factor for determining the rate at which crossbridges attach and detach. The rate of crossbridge detachment and the number of interacting crossbridges (e.g., baseline: 20–30% of total crossbridges) is the basis for the force–velocity relationship that determines cardiac contractility [84,87,94,95].

The concept of optimal sarcomere length serves as the explanation for the Frank–Starling law of the heart and predicts an increase in contractile force when sarcomeres are stretched (e.g., increased

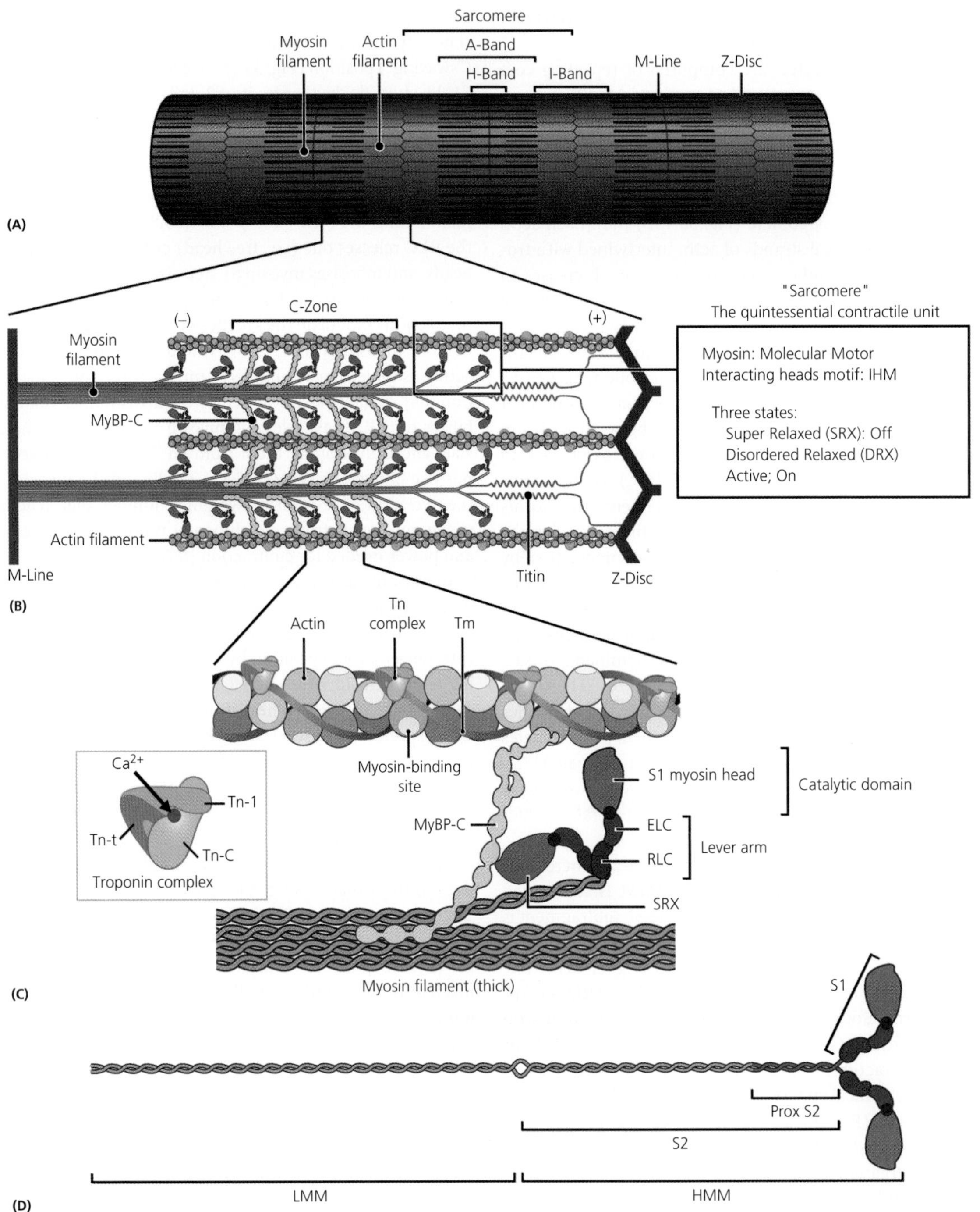

Figure 33.15 **A.** Cardiac muscle cells contain sarcomeres, mitochondria, and a sarcoplasmic reticulum that occupy ~60%, 35%, and 5% of the cell volume, respectively. Sarcomeres contain an overlapping array of thin (actin) and thick (myosin) protein filaments that produces a striated or banded (i.e., A, H, I) appearance. Sarcomeres are separated by Z-discs (i.e., bands). **B.** The left half of a sarcomere illustrates the polarized (-/+) thin actin filament connected to the Z-disc and the myosin thick filament connected to the center of the sarcomere (M-line). The mechanosensing protein titin regulates myosin length and connects myosin to the M-line and Z-Disc. Myosin-binding protein C (MyBPC) modulates the force of contraction. **C.** Actin–myosin crossbridges are formed when myosin heads bind to myosin-binding sites on the actin filament. Myosin access to actin-binding sites is regulated by the troponin (Tn) complex comprised of three regulatory proteins: troponin I, troponin T, troponin C. An increase in intracellular calcium concentration increases calcium binding to Tn-C repositioning tropomyosin (Tm) and exposing myosin-binding sites on actin filaments to myosin heads. Myosin heads exist in free, disorganized (DRX), and folded-back, super relaxed (SRX), or docked (i.e., parked) states, collectively referred to as the "interacting-heads motif" (IHM). Myosin head binding is regulated by interactions among the MyBPC, the converter domain (dark dot), essential light chain (ELC) and the regulatory light chain (RLC). **D.** The myosin filament is composed of heavy meromyosin (HMM) that includes subfragment 1 (myosin S1 head [S1], essential light chain [ELC], regulatory light chain [RLC]) and subfragment 2 (S2) that transitions to a coiled-coil tail and then into light meromyosin (LMM). S2 tails combine with other light meromyosin (LMM) tails to form the thick myosin filament.

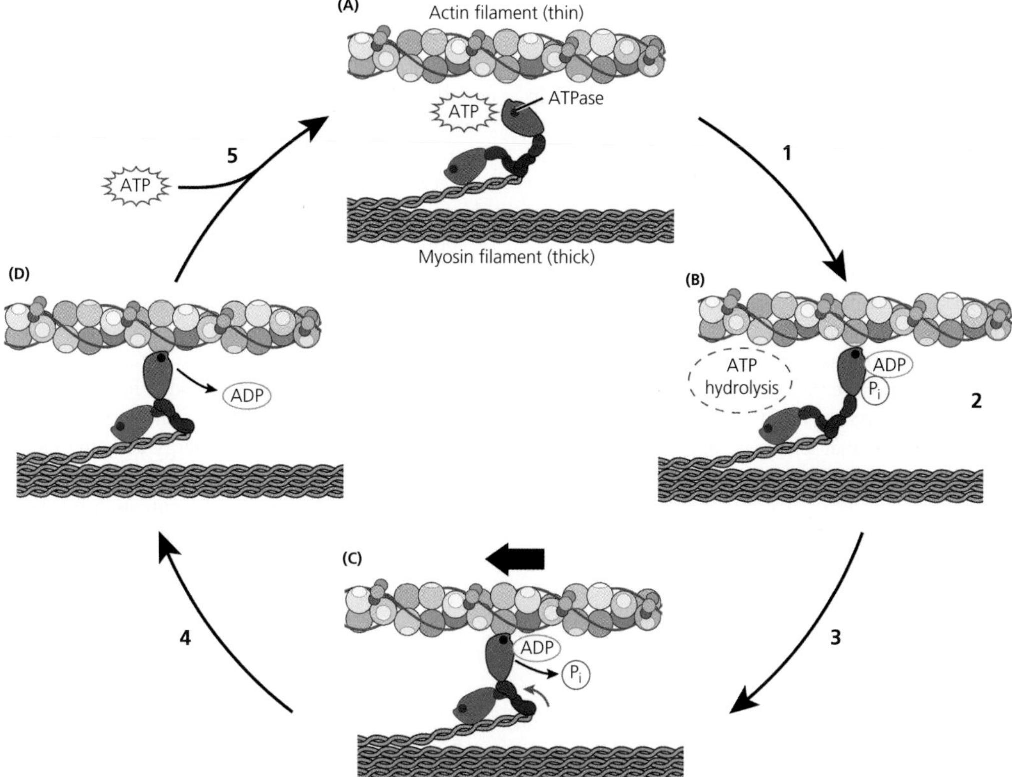

Figure 33.16 The actin-activated myosin chemomechanical ATPase cycle (i.e., ATP binding, hydrolysis, Pi release, ADP release). **A.** ATP binds to the ATPase containing the myosin S1 globular head ("molecular motor") weakening its interaction with actin thereby freeing the myosin S1 head so that the lever arm can cock into a pre-power stroke DRX position. **B.** One myosin S1 head is in the folded back SRX (docked on the coiled-coil S2 tail) state and the other is in the post-stroke DRX state (1). ATP hydrolysis transitions the myosin S1 head from a weak to strong binding state with actin (2). **C.** Pi release is associated with a leftward shift (leftward arrow) of the lever arm and movement of the actin filament to the left (3). The swing of the lever arm is responsible for force production (power stroke). **D.** ADP dissociates, forming the rigor state (4). Binding of ATP to myosin S1 head dissociates it from actin forming the post-rigor state (5).

ventricular volume) to their optimal length (i.e., approximately 2.2 μm) [94–96]. It is unlikely, however, that this explanation provides an adequate explanation of the Frank–Starling effect since sarcomeres rarely change length even during dilated forms of heart failure [37]. The more probable reason for Starling's law of the heart is that sarcomere loading increases troponin C affinity for calcium and RLC phosphorylation leading to increased activation of the myofilament and sarcomere shortening without increases in sarcomere length or additional increases in intracellular calcium [96,97].

Decreased interaction between actin and myosin filaments is directly related to a decrease in $[Ca^{2+}]_i$ and signals the beginning of the actin–myosin uncoupling process and myocardial relaxation [98]. Three principal mechanisms are responsible for reducing intracellular calcium-ion concentration and the subsequent decrease in cardiac contractile force. Depolarization-triggered increases in intracellular calcium increase the activity of the calcium regulatory protein calmodulin. Calmodulin serves as an intracellular calcium sensor and, when activated (i.e., calmodulin-calcium complex), stimulates the active extrusion of calcium by pumps in the sarcolemma. Phosphorylation of the phospholamban-modulated calcium pump increases calcium uptake by the sarcoplasmic reticulum and enhances the activity of the Na^+–Ca^{2+} exchanger (NCX) (Fig. 33.14) [99]. Calcium transported by the sarcoendoplasmic reticulum calcium transport ATPase (SERCA) lowers the cytosolic calcium concentration and removes calcium from Tn-C [100]. The reduced intracellular calcium induces a conformational change in the troponin complex allowing Tn-I inhibition of the actin-binding site. Upon completion of the chemomechanical cycle, a new ATP binds to the myosin S1 head displacing ADP and restoring the initial sarcomere length, and the entire cycle is ready to be repeated (Fig. 33.16).

Most intravenous anesthetic drugs (e.g., barbiturates, ketamine, and propofol), and in particular the inhalation anesthetics, produce dose-dependent decreases in cardiac contractility by decreasing calcium influx through L-type channels, decreasing calcium release from the sarcoplasmic reticulum, and decreasing Tn-C sensitivity to calcium [101–110]. Anesthetic drugs also interfere with the reuptake of calcium by the sarcoplasmic reticulum ultimately leading to depletion of intracellular calcium [98,106,107,111,112]. Notably, the effects of both injectable and inhalant anesthetics on the chemomechanical mechanisms responsible for myocardial contraction and relaxation require reexamination using updated contemporary experimental technologies.

The vascular system

The function of the vascular system (arteries, capillaries, and veins) is to transport blood, nutrients, and oxygen to tissues, remove waste products (e.g., carbon dioxide), protect tissues, and stop bleeding. Blood vessels larger than 100–150 μm comprise the macrocirculation, while those that are smaller than 100 μm constitute the microcirculation [113]. The largest blood vessels are not embedded in organs and function as conduits for the delivery of blood to and from the heart, lungs, and peripheral tissues. Small vessels (i.e., < 100 μm) are embedded in organs and are actively involved in regulating blood flow or exchange processes. The pulmonary artery and aorta deliver blood to the pulmonary and systemic circulations, respectively. The pulmonary circulation receives its blood supply from the right ventricle via the pulmonary artery while the nutrient supply of the lung parenchyma is provided by the bronchial arteries. The systemic circulation receives its blood supply from the left ventricle via the aorta. The left ventricle, aorta, and other large arteries comprise the high-pressure portion of the systemic circulation while the right ventricle, pulmonary artery, left atrium, and all the veins are considered low pressure (i.e., < 20–30 mmHg). Vessels of the systemic circulation undergo repeated division into smaller and smaller parallel vascular beds that terminate in arterioles (i.e., the smallest arteries at 10–30 μm) that subdivide and transition into capillaries (5–10 μm).

Blood vessels can be functionally categorized as primarily elastic, compliant conduits (e.g., large arteries: aorta), muscular arteries (e.g., distributive arteries: femoral artery), sphincter or resistance vessels (e.g., arterioles), exchange vessels (e.g., capillaries), capacitance vessels (e.g., venules and veins), large conduit veins, and shunt vessels (e.g., arteriovenous anastomoses) [114]. All vessels have an endothelial surface and all but capillaries contain varying proportions of elastic fibers, smooth muscle, and fibrous tissue (Fig. 33.17). The tunica media is composed mostly of smooth muscle and elastic connective tissue, and the outer layer, the tunica externa (i.e., tunica adventitia), contains fibrous collagen fibers. The proportion of elastic connective tissue to smooth muscle determines the vessel's principal function (i.e., conduit, resistive, or capacitive). Larger arteries possess a high proportion of elastic tissue in comparison to smooth muscle and fibrous tissues found in veins (Fig. 33.17). These structural differences allow the aorta to stretch during ventricular contraction and the ejection of blood. The potential (stored) energy imparted to the elastic fibers of the stretched proximal aorta is returned as kinetic (motion) energy assisting blood flow (i.e., the Windkessel effect) [115]. Thus, the highly elastic architecture of the aorta aids in converting pulsatile (non-uniform) flow to continuous blood flow (Fig. 33.18). The Windkessel effect is believed to be responsible for up to 50% of peripheral blood flow in most animals during normal resting HRs.

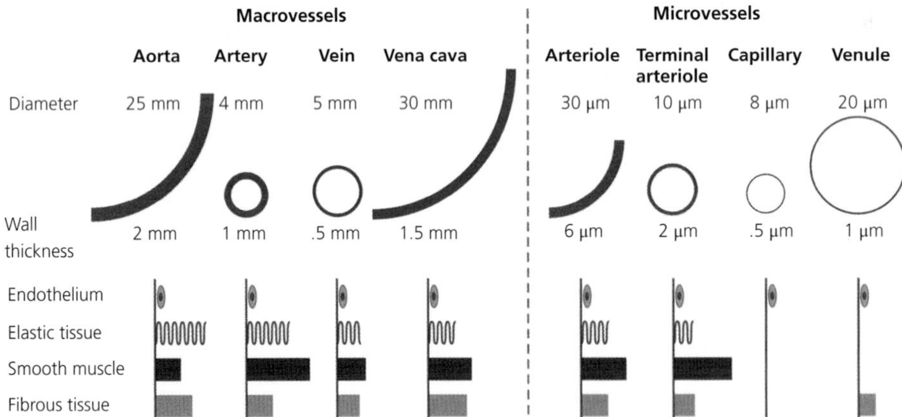

Figure 33.17 Blood vessel types, diameter, and wall thickness. Note the differences in vessel diameter, elastic tissue, and smooth muscle between arteries and veins.

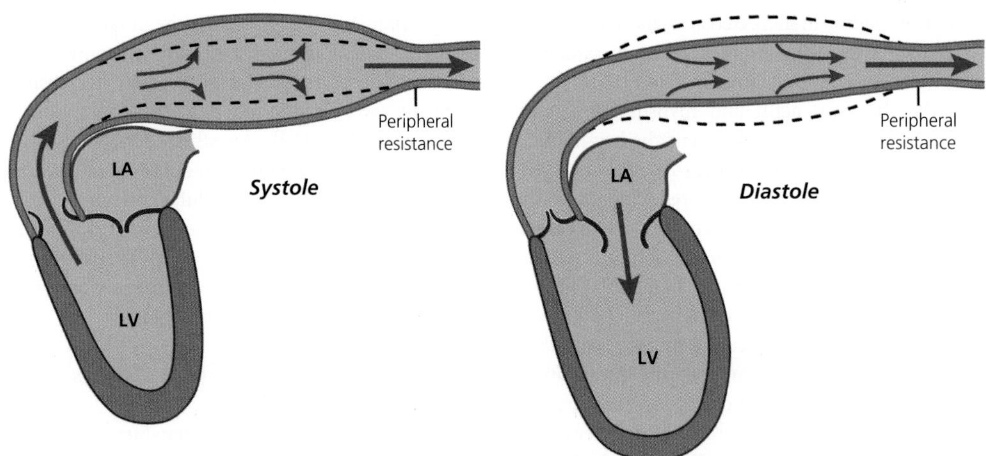

Figure 33.18 Aortic distensibility (i.e., compliance) and elasticity (i.e., ability to resume its normal shape after being stretched) are often conflated with stiffness. Aortic elasticity is responsible for the Windkessel effect wherein the aorta is distended during systole and recoils during diastole. Large distensible elastic arteries briefly store blood (i.e., hydraulic accumulator) during systole and distribute blood during diastole.

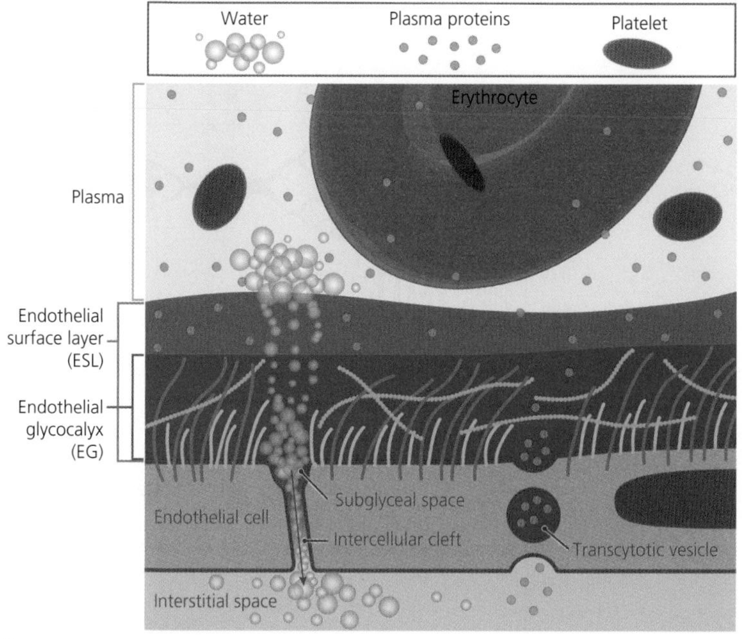

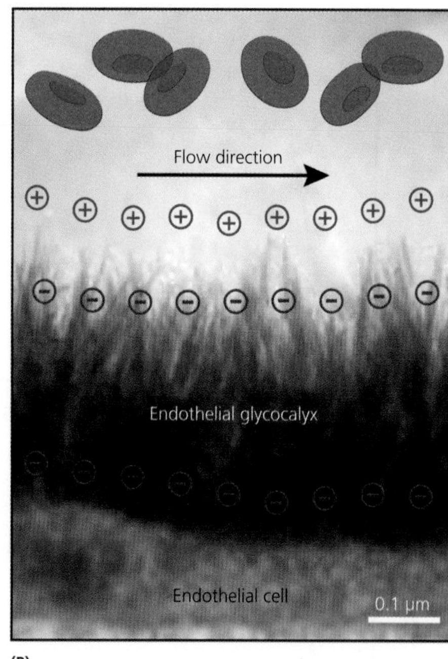

Figure 33.19 **A.** The endothelial surface layer (ESL) is a multilayered structure that covers the endothelial surface of most blood vessels. It is composed of water, a dense inner layer of sulfated proteoglycans (e.g., syndecans, glypicans) and a less dense outer layer of covalently bound glycosaminoglycans (GAGs: heparan sulfate, chondroitin sulfate, and hyaluronan), glycoproteins, and plasma proteins. Transcytosis of albumin via caveolae is an important means for its transport across the endothelium. **B.** The electroviscous effects of the glycocalyx attenuate blood cell–vessel wall interactions and influences the permeability of larger negatively charged molecules (e.g., albumin).

The luminal surface of all blood vessels is lined by endothelial cells (i.e., tunica intima; Fig. 33.17) that are covered with a multilayered endothelial surface layer (Fig. 33.19A). The glycocalyx is a thin layer of negatively charged (anionic) material composed of syndecans, glypicans, glycoproteins, and polysaccharides that extends from the surface of vascular endothelial cells and binds plasma proteins and soluble glycosaminoglycans (Fig. 33.19A) [116,117]. Endothelial cells are dynamic and have both metabolic and synthetic functions exerting autocrine, paracrine, and endocrine actions that modulate smooth muscle contraction and relaxation, platelet and leukocyte adherence, thrombosis, and thrombolysis. Endothelial cells generate and maintain the glycocalyx [117,118], a voluminous water-phobic (negatively charged) intravascular compartment that plays an important role in maintaining vascular wall homeostasis, red and white blood cell movement, and vessel wall permeability in capillaries (Fig. 33.19B) [117–120]. Pathologic loss of the glycocalyx initiates breakdown of the vascular barrier and has been linked to ischemia, systemic inflammatory response, sepsis, and volume overload [117,121–123].

Large arteries and veins

Large elastic arteries serve as conduits through which blood is transported to the periphery (Fig. 33.17). The elasticity of large arteries opposes the stretching effect that the blood pressure produces following ventricular contraction. For example, the initial stretching of the aorta produced by ventricular ejection is opposed by the elastic tissue in the vessel walls, which returns the aorta and large arteries to their original dimension once the pressure imposed by ventricular ejection subsides (i.e., the Windkessel effect) [115]. The degree to which the larger arteries can be stretched depends on the ratio of elastic to collagen fibers and fibrous tissue. Systemic veins are more than 30 times more distensible (i.e., compliant) than systemic arteries (Fig. 33.20A) and the lumped systemic circulation (i.e., arteries, capillaries, and veins) is more compliant than the lumped pulmonary circulation (Fig. 33.20B) [124].

Small arteries

Peripheral muscular arteries contain greater percentages of smooth muscle compared to elastic tissue, thereby providing greater control over vessel diameter, vascular resistance, and the regulation of blood flow (Fig. 33.17). The amount of smooth muscle determines the vessel's resting tone (i.e., myogenic basal tone), the ability to respond to an increase in blood pressure, and the amount of stress relaxation (i.e., vasoconstriction followed by delayed relaxation; Bayliss effect), and reverse stress relaxation (i.e., vessel contraction due to fall in blood volume) [125,126]. Stress relaxation is characterized by a rapid initial increase in resting tone caused by an increase in pressure that declines gradually during the next several minutes. The blood pressure decreases because of smooth muscle myofilament rearrangement. Reverse stress relaxation is the reverse of this process [125].

The most distal branches of peripheral feed arteries terminate in "resistance vessels" that control the distribution of blood flow. These vessels contain a predominance of smooth muscle, are densely innervated by the sympathetic nervous system, and include arterioles, metarterioles, and arteriovenous anastomoses.

Resistance vessels

Resistance vessels include the muscular arterioles, metarterioles (i.e., short vessels that link arterioles and capillaries), and arteriovenous anastomoses (Fig. 33.17). The small arteries and arterioles represent the primary vessels involved in the distribution of blood

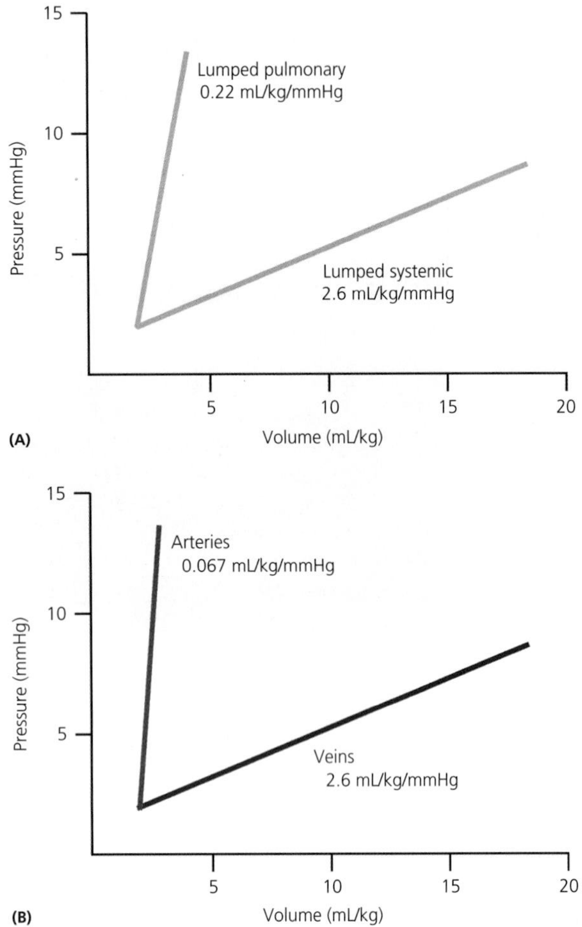

Figure 33.20 **A.** Lumped (i.e., arteries, capillaries, veins) pulmonary and systemic compliance (i.e., V/P). Lumped pulmonary compliance is less than lumped systemic compliance. A small increase in pulmonary blood volume causes a much larger increase in pulmonary pressure. **B.** Systemic arteries are much less compliant than systemic veins. Source: Adapted from Green [124].

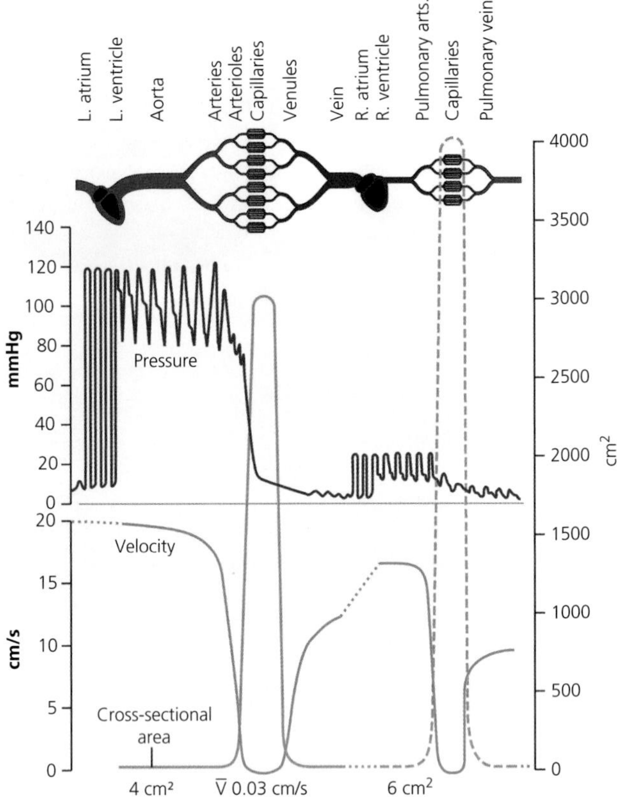

Figure 33.21 Blood pressure (mmHg), flow velocity (cm/s), and vascular cross-sectional area (cm^2) in the systemic vasculature. As blood approaches the capillaries, blood pressure and blood flow velocity decrease and cross-sectional area increase.

flow and regulation of arterial blood pressure. Notably, approximately 50–60% of the pressure drop between the aorta and capillaries occurs across terminal arterioles and metarterioles (Fig. 33.21). Functionally, precapillary resistance vessels (i.e., sphincter vessels) help to regulate the number of open capillaries and, therefore, the size of the capillary bed that is available for exchange processes. The relatively thick-walled muscular arterioles and sphincter vessels are regulated by a variety of neural, humoral, and local metabolic factors and are the principal determinants of the total amount of blood flow distributed to all tissues of the body (Table 33.5). Arteriovenous anastomoses bypass the capillary by connecting arterioles to small veins. These vessels reduce or totally interrupt blood flow to capillaries and are densely populated by both α_1- and α_2-adrenergic receptors [127]. Arteriovenous anastomoses possess smooth muscle cells throughout their entire length and are found in the greatest numbers in the skin and extremities (ears, feet, and hooves) of most species [127,128]. When open, they shunt arterial blood to venous plexuses in the limbs and play an important role in temperature regulation. Their identification in the intestine, kidney, liver, and skeletal muscles suggests their importance as a separate blood flow regulatory mechanism for controlling nutrient blood flow in these tissues. α_2-Adrenergic receptor agonists have been demonstrated to cause redistribution of CO away from less vital organs [129].

Table 33.5 Factors producing vasodilation or vasoconstriction.

Vasoconstriction	Vasodilation
Systemic	
Increased noradrenergic discharge	Activation of cholinergic dilators in skeletal muscle
Circulating catecholamines	Bradykinin
Angiotensin II	Histamine
Arginine vasopressin	Kallikrein
Serotonin (5-HT_B receptors)	Endothelin B
Endothelin A	Substance P (axon reflex)
Neuropeptide Y	PGI_2, PGE_2
Thromboxane A_2	
PgA_2, $PGF_2\alpha$	
Reactive oxygen species (superoxide, hydroxyl radical)	
Local	
Decreased temperature	Increased temperature
Increased PO_2	Decreased PO_2
	Increased H^+, K^+, lactic acid, H_2S
	Increased NO
	Adenosine

Capillaries

The microcirculation includes the smallest blood vessels in the body and consists of the terminal arterioles, the capillary network (4–8 μm) and venules ($\lesssim$ 10–100 μm) (Fig. 33.17).

The microcirculation is embedded within organs and responsible for the exchange of oxygen (O_2), carbon dioxide (CO_2), nutrients, metabolites, and fluid between blood and tissue. Exchange occurs by three processes: passive diffusion, filtration, and pinocytosis (e.g., fluid endocytosis). A single layer of endothelial cells, normally covered by the glycocalyx, separates the intravascular volume from the interstitial fluid volume (Fig. 33.19A) [117]. The glycocalyx, part liquid and part solid, becomes denser closer to the endothelial cell surface and serves as the major barrier to transcapillary flow of macromolecules larger than 15 nm [130]. The dense inner region is composed of a network of membrane-bound and membrane-attached proteoglycans, glycosaminoglycans, glycoproteins, and adherent plasma proteins extending out from the endothelial surface (Fig. 33.19A) [115]. The capillary wall, therefore, is a three-layered structure consisting of the glycocalyx on the luminal surface, the basement membrane on the abluminal surface, and endothelial cells in between. The intravascular volume consists of the glycocalyx, plasma volume, and red cell volume. The glycocalyx is normally the dynamic and active interface between plasma and the endothelial cell surface acting as a semipermeable molecular sieve with respect to anionic macromolecules such as albumin and other plasma proteins, whose size and structure determine their ability to penetrate the layer (Fig. 33.19B) [117–121]. The normal glycocalyx is impermeable to red blood cells (RBCs) and molecules larger than 70 kDa and semipermeable to albumin (molecular weight ~69 kDa; diameter ~7 nm; reflection coefficient 0.79–0.9) [129]. Increasing evidence, however, suggests that albumin transport from blood plasma to the interstitial fluid may occur via plasmalemmal vesicles (i.e., transcytosis) thereby serving as large pore (i.e., 20–70 nm) equivalents (Fig. 33.19A). For example, hydrostatic pressure-dependent activation of albumin transcytosis in the lung microvasculature increases interstitial colloid osmotic pressure (COP) enhancing fluid flux across the endothelium, reducing intravascular pressure. Functionally, amphiphilic (i.e., having both hydrophilic and hydrophobic parts) molecules like albumin help to sustain and regulate the vascular and glycocalyx permeability [130,131].

There are three types of capillaries: continuous non-fenestrated, fenestrated, and discontinuous or sinusoidal (Fig. 33.22A) [132]. Their distribution, porosity, and numbers vary in different tissue beds depending on tissue metabolism (O_2 requirements) and the importance of fluid exchange. Continuous non-fenestrated capillaries with tight junctions are present in all tissues of the body except epithelia and cartilage. They have a functional pore size of approximately 5 nm that permits the diffusion of water, small solutes, and lipid-soluble materials into the interstitial fluid. The term "pore" is not a simple opening but refers to any path through (e.g., transcytosis) or between (e.g., intercellular cleft) endothelial cells that allows fluid to pass.

Specialized continuous non-fenestrated capillaries are found throughout most of the central nervous system (CNS), enteric nervous system, retina, and in the thymus (Fig. 33.22B). The endothelial cells are bound together by tight junctions with an effective pore size of < 1 nm [132]. Endothelial cells in the brain and spinal cord are tightly opposed by zonula occludens (i.e., tight junctions) with few interendothelial breaks and are responsible for the blood–brain barrier. The blood–brain barrier is only permeable to the smallest non-lipid-soluble molecules. Breaks within the interendothelial cell junctions produced by trauma or inflammation are the primary path for increased porosity and transvascular fluid filtration. Aquaporins (i.e., water channels) are present within continuous, but not fenestrated, vascular endothelial cells [133]. Aquaporins selectively facilitate the rapid transport of fluid across epithelial and endothelial cells but are also found in other tissues such as muscle and nerve cells. Aquaporins mediate osmotic water transport across plasma membranes and function as membrane channels for water alone or for water plus small molecules [132]. Anesthetic drugs (e.g., propofol, isoflurane, and sevoflurane) are known to influence aquaporin expression and water homeostasis, but additional research is required to determine the clinical relevance of these findings [134,135].

Fenestrated (i.e., windowed) capillaries with diaphragmed fenestrae and small gaps between adjacent endothelial cells are present in skin, connective tissue, kidney, intestinal mucosa, endocrine and exocrine glands, and the choroid plexus (Fig. 33.22B). The basement membrane of these capillaries is continuous. Their upper pore size is in the range of 6–12 nm [132]. Fenestrated capillaries with open fenestrae (i.e., "windows,") span the endothelial lining (Fig. 33.22B). Windows permit the rapid exchange of water and solutes. Open fenestrated capillaries are present in the kidney cortex and medulla, the gastrointestinal mucosa, and the lymph nodes.

Sinusoidal capillaries (sinusoids) resemble fenestrated capillaries but are discontinuous and are characterized by gaps between adjacent endothelial cells. The basement membrane and glycocalyx are absent, and interstitial fluid is part of the plasma volume in sinusoidal tissues (spleen, liver, bone marrow, and endocrine organs; Fig. 33.22B). Plasma proteins (e.g., albumin) secreted by liver cells pass easily through the sinusoids into the bloodstream through pores as large as 200–280 nm [132]. Phagocytic cells monitor the passing blood in sinusoidal tissues, engulfing damaged RBCs, pathogens, and cellular debris.

Transcapillary fluid exchange

Capillary fluid exchange is governed by two primary processes: diffusion and filtration. Diffusion is the movement of a specific molecule from an area of high concentration to a low concentration. Fick's law of diffusion describes solute exchange (J_s) as

$$J_s = DA/M_T C_D$$

where D is the diffusion coefficient, A is the capillary surface area, M_T is the membrane thickness, and C_D is the transmembrane concentration gradient or difference. The diffusion coefficient is determined by the diffusion medium and the qualities characteristic of the diffusion particle such as the molecular weight, molecular shape, ionic charge, and lipid solubility. Filtration is the movement of fluid and molecules from an area of high pressure to one of low pressure. Fluid exchange (i.e., fluid flux [J_v]) by filtration is determined by four primary factors (P_c, P_i, π_c, and π_i) according to a dynamic equilibrium originally hypothesized by Starling but formulated by others (i.e., Starling principle of capillary fluid exchange), wherein

$$J_v = K_f\left(P_c - P_i\right) - \sigma\left(\pi_c - \pi_i\right)$$

where, in the classical Starling equation, J_v is fluid flux across the capillary (positive for filtration, and negative for reabsorption), P_c and P_i are capillary and interstitial hydrostatic pressures, π_c and π_i are the plasma and interstitial colloid osmotic pressures, K_f is the capillary filtration coefficient, and σ is the osmotic reflection coefficient for all plasma proteins [136–139]. The filtration coefficient (K_f) indicates the resistance of the capillary wall to fluid flow and is determined by the surface area, the number and radius of capillary pores, the capillary wall thickness, and the viscosity of the fluid being filtered. The osmotic reflection coefficient (σ) is an indicator

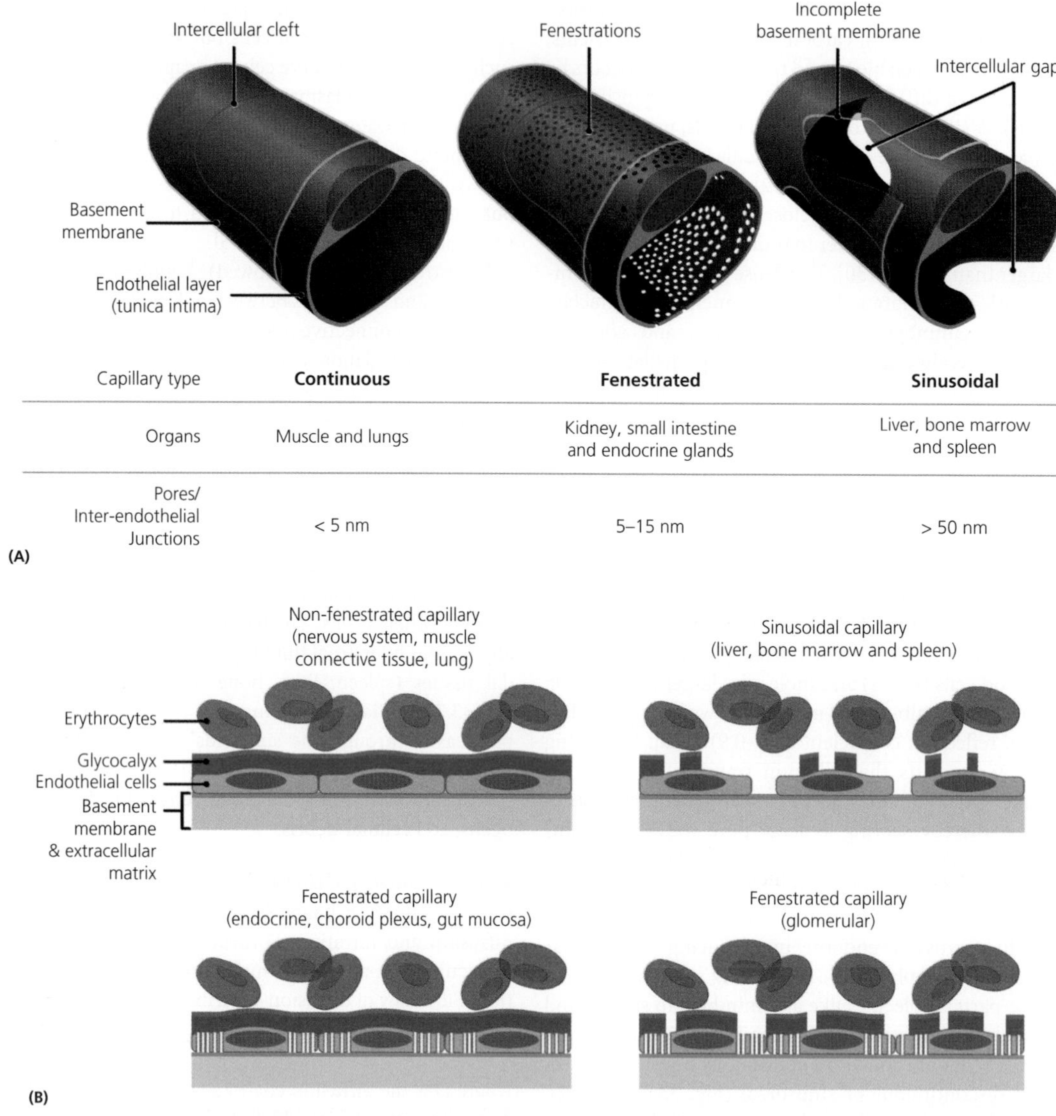

Figure 33.22 **A.** Types of capillaries: sinusoidal, fenestrated, and continuous or non-fenestrated. **B.** Capillaries and associated glycocalyx and basement membrane. Fenestrated capillaries exist in most tissues. Non-sinusoidal non-fenestrated capillaries have a continuous basement membrane. Interendothelial cell breaks between cell junctions are the primary pathway for transvascular fluid flux.

of transvascular protein transport (i.e., a reflection coefficient of 0 implies that the substance is freely permeable and 1 implies that the substance does not pass through the membrane). The initial osmotic reflection coefficient for albumin and most colloid solutions (i.e., > 70 kDa) is close to 1 in normal animals since most capillary membranes are impermeable to large colloids. Providing that all factors can be accurately measured or approximated, net fluid flux across the capillary wall can be estimated by the Starling equation [139]. Historically, Starling's principle of capillary fluid flux suggested fluid filtration at the arterial end of the capillary and fluid reabsorption at the venous end of the capillary. Lymph vessels were assumed to carry excess interstitial fluid back to the venous circulation. It is now understood, however, that non-fenestrated capillaries normally filter fluid throughout their entire length, fluid flux to the interstitial space is under a dominant hydrostatic pressure gradient (capillary pressure P_c minus P_i), and that the effect of π_c on transvascular fluid exchange is much less than predicted [119]. The low protein concentration within the subglycocalyx intercellular spaces accounts for low J_v and lymph flow in most tissues during normal physiologic conditions. Absorption through capillaries and venules does not occur except in abnormal physiologic conditions or disease states. During normal conditions, π_c opposes but does not reverse filtration, and most of the filtered plasma returns to the circulation as lymph [120]. The glycocalyx covers the endothelial intercellular clefts in fenestrated capillaries, separating plasma from an almost protein-free subglycocalyx space (Fig. 33.19). The subglycocalyx COP (π_g) replaces π_i as a determinant of transcapillary fluid flux (J_v). The fluid at the abluminal side of the glycocalyx is separated from the pericapillary interstitial fluid by the tortuous path through the intercellular clefts. Plasma proteins, including albumin, can escape to the interstitial space through the intercellular clefts or via transcytosis (i.e., large pores) and are responsible for the increased J_v observed during endothelial inflammatory states. Importantly, J_v can be modified by many factors including drugs

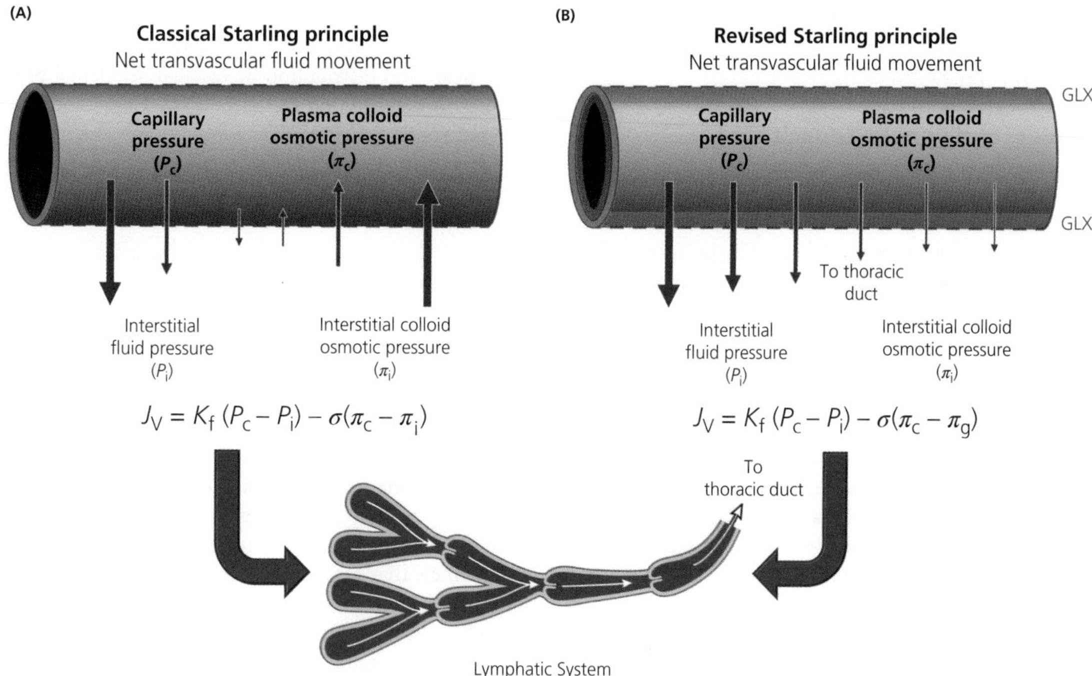

Figure 33.23 Classical and revised Starling principle of transcapillary fluid flux. **A.** Classical: Transcapillary fluid flux is determined by four classic Starling forces (P_c, P_i, π_c, and π_i). Blue arrows indicate net force imbalance and the direction and magnitude of fluid filtration and absorption. **B.** Revised: Starling equation forces predicted by the glycocalyx-cleft model (P_c, P_i, π_c, and π_g). Fluid filtration reabsorption is primarily due to capillary hydrostatic pressure (P_c). Blue arrows indicate fluid filtration from the capillary throughout its length. These diagrams assume the filtration coefficient and the osmotic reflection coefficient are minimally affected.

and intravenous fluid replacement regimens that produce fluid overload. A more accurate depiction of transcapillary fluid flux is represented by the revised Starling equation (Fig. 33.23):

$$J_v = K_f\left(P_c - P_i\right) - \sigma\left(\pi_p - \pi_g\right)$$

where π_g is the COP of the ultrafiltrate on the underside of the glycocalyx. π_g is normally very low, for two reasons; σ is high, or the outward flow of the ultrafiltrate prevents protein diffusion between the subglycocalyx fluid and the pericapillary interstitial fluid.

The filtration of fluid across the microvascular endothelial barrier constitutes the primary mechanism for removal of excess fluid from the bloodstream, the formation of lymph, and increases in interstitial fluid volume particularly during excess IV fluid administration [140]. Increases in P_c (e.g., volume overload, venous obstruction, and heart failure) and increases K_f (e.g., histamine, cytokines, and kinins) or decreases in π_p (e.g., hypoproteinemia) can lead to fluid accumulation in the interstitial space, resulting in edema particularly when the lymphatic circulation is impaired (Box 33.2). Interstitial edema increases the diffusion distance for oxygen and other nutrients and collapses capillaries in swollen tissue (capillary no-reflow), especially in encapsulated organs (e.g., brain and kidney) compromising cellular metabolism and impairing nutritive tissue perfusion. Edema formation and capillary no-reflow (i.e., capillary occlusion by swollen endothelial or muscle cells) also act to limit the diffusional removal of potentially toxic by-products of cellular metabolism. Edema is facilitated by an increase in P_c but also by degradation of the glycocalyx [141]. Decreases in P_c (hypotension and hypovolemia) and increases in π_p (hyperproteinemia and dehydration) favor fluid retention or fluid reabsorption into the vascular compartment (autotransfusion) and reduce the potential for fluid to accumulate in interstitial space [142]. Anesthesia, anesthetic drugs, the volume (mL/kg) and rate (mL/kg/min) of fluid administration, the type of fluid administered, and the anesthetic protocol can produce important effects on the Starling forces and the glycocalyx that lead to interstitial fluid accumulation [121,143]. For example, many anesthetic drugs and anesthetic techniques decrease P_c, causing a transient fluid reabsorption from the interstitial space and hemodilution. If the anesthetic drug or technique produces mild precapillary vasodilation, however, P_c may increase, promoting transcapillary fluid flux and interstitial fluid accumulation (e.g., edema). Several anticancer drugs (e.g., doxorubicin), anesthetic drugs, (e.g., morphine and meperidine), and drug diluents (e.g., cremophor EL) produce histamine release, thereby

Box 33.2 Causes of increased interstitial fluid volume (i.e., edema).

Increased hydrostatic pressure
- Arterial dilatation
- Venular constriction
- Increased systemic or pulmonary venous pressures

Decreased capillary osmotic pressure gradient
- Decreased plasma protein (i.e., albumin)
- Accumulation of interstitial osmotic substances (i.e., colloids)

Increased capillary permeability (i.e., endotheliopathy)
- Inflammation (i.e., cytokines)
- Substance P
- Histamine
- Kinins

Obstructed lymph flow
- Lymph vessel obstruction
- Lymphangitis

Fluid overload

increasing K_f and tissue fluid accumulation [144–146]. Fluid overload degrades the glycocalyx promoting interstitial fluid accumulation (Table 33.5) [147].

Veins, venules, and venous capacitance

Veins are composed of an endothelial lining, elastic tissue, smooth muscle, and fibrous tissue while venules have an endothelium surrounded by fibrous tissue (Fig. 33.17). Like capillaries, the walls of the smallest venules are very porous and serve as major sites for fluid exchange. Fluid and macromolecular exchange occur most prominently at venular cell junctions where phagocytic white blood cells migrate from the blood into surrounding infected or diseased tissues. Some venules act as postcapillary sphincters. Venules then merge into small veins which are about two times as numerous as arterioles and arteries and are the most compliant vessels in the body (i.e., capacitance vessels) [148]. Sympathetic tone (i.e., venoconstriction) has an important function in regulating capillary hydrostatic pressure. Small and larger veins contain increasing amounts of fibrous tissue in addition to smooth muscle and elastic tissue, although their walls are much thinner than comparably sized arteries. Larger veins (i.e., > 2 mm) contain valves that act in conjunction with external compression (i.e., contracting muscles) and pressure differences in the abdominal and thoracic cavities to facilitate the return flow of blood to the right atrium [149]. The systemic venous system is 30 times more compliant (i.e., distensible) than the systemic arterial system and a major blood reservoir containing 60–70% of the blood volume during resting conditions (Figs. 33.1 and 33.20; Table 33.6). Splanchnic and cutaneous veins, unlike skeletal muscle veins, have a high density of α_1- and α_2-adrenergic receptors, which, when activated, help to mobilize blood into the circulation when needed (see section on splanchnic circulation) [148,150,151].

Adjustments in venous capacitance are important in blood volume distribution and maintaining an effective or "stressed" circulating blood volume. Stressed volume (V_s) is the intravascular blood volume required to produce a measurable increase in transmural blood pressure and is a primary determinant of venous return. Unstressed volume (V_{us}) is the intravascular volume of blood required to fill the circulatory system to capacity without increasing the vascular transmural pressure [152]. V_{us} provides a recruitable reservoir of blood that can be mobilized (e.g., during exercise, trauma, and hemorrhage) to preserve V_s. Only V_s is hemodynamically active [152]. The mean circulatory filling pressure (MCFP) is the pressure within the circulatory system when the heart is stopped and blood pressure throughout the systemic circulatory system stabilizes [152]. Some physiologists believe that MCFP and right atrial pressure are the main determinants of venous return and, therefore, CO (e.g., venous return curves), thereby neglecting the importance of the heart and distribution of vascular segmental pressures and volumes in determining CO [152–154]. Contemporary evidence, however, suggests that cardiac contraction is the driving force for venous return and CO and that venous return curves are misleading mythical abstractions that should be removed from educational materials [154–157].

Table 33.6 Distribution of blood volume and average number of vessels.

Segment	% of Intravascular volume	Average number of individual vessels
Aorta	2.0	1
Large arteries	4.0	40
Main arterial branches	3.4	600
Terminal branches	1.7	1800
Small arteries	2.7	40 × 10^6
Arterioles	1.0	400 × 10^6
Capillaries, postcapillary venules	3.9	7.600 × 10^6
Venules	25.6	1200 × 10^6
Small veins	18.6	80 × 10^6
Main venous branches	18.5	600
Large veins	15.2	40
Vena cava	3.4	2

Smooth muscle metabolism

Vascular smooth muscle metabolism of carbohydrates and fatty acids is characterized by a substantial production of lactic acid even under fully oxygenated conditions [158,159]. While the role of aerobic production of lactate in the energetics of smooth muscle has not been completely defined, it likely serves as a mechanism affording optimal coordination and modulation of glucose supply and linking oxidative energy production to energy demand. The vascular smooth muscle membrane contains microdomains and ion channels that regulate cellular metabolism and cellular function. These include but are not limited to a host of G-protein-coupled receptors (GPCRs), second messengers (e.g., adenylate cyclase and phospholipase C), kinases (e.g., rho kinase, protein kinase C, and protein kinase A), and ion channels (e.g., L-type calcium channels and K_{ATP} channels) in close proximity that regulate vascular smooth muscle function [158,159].

Smooth muscle contraction and relaxation

Smooth muscle is involuntary in non-striated muscle and fundamentally different from skeletal and cardiac muscle in terms of structure, function, regulation of contraction, and excitation–contraction coupling. Vascular smooth muscle is divided into two subgroups: single-unit (unitary) and multiunit smooth muscle. Unitary vascular smooth muscle predominates at precapillary sphincter sites and is characterized by spontaneous activity initiated by pacemaker areas that are activated by stretch. Unitary vascular smooth muscle operates to maintain a constant local blood flow despite changing perfusion pressures [158]. Multiunit smooth muscle fibers are present in larger arteries and veins, are under CNS control, do not usually respond to stretch, and override unitary smooth muscle in order to regulate the distribution of body blood flow [160,161]. Smooth muscle cell contraction is regulated by receptor and mechanical (stretch) activation of the contractile proteins, actin and myosin. A change in membrane potential initiated by APs can also trigger contraction. All three mechanisms (i.e., stretch, receptor, and AP) lead to increases in cytosolic Ca^{2+} ($[Ca^{2+}]_i$) [159]. Increases in cytosolic Ca^{2+} via Ca^{2+} channels (i.e., receptor-operated Ca^{2+} channels) increase Ca^{2+} release from intracellular stores in the sarcoplasmic reticulum. Contractile activity in smooth muscle is determined primarily by the phosphorylation of the myosin light chain (MLC). Intracellular Ca^{2+} combines with the protein calmodulin and the Ca^{2+}-calmodulin complex activates MLC kinase (MLCK), phosphorylating MLC, which results in the interaction of myosin with actin and contraction (Fig. 33.24). Energy released from ATP results in the cycling of myosin–actin crossbridges and contraction. Low levels of phosphorylation of the MLC maintain basal levels of vascular smooth muscle tone [162]. Sensitization of the contractile proteins to Ca^{2+} is signaled by the RhoA/Rho kinase pathway inhibiting dephosphorylation of tyrosine light chain, thereby maintaining sustained force generation.

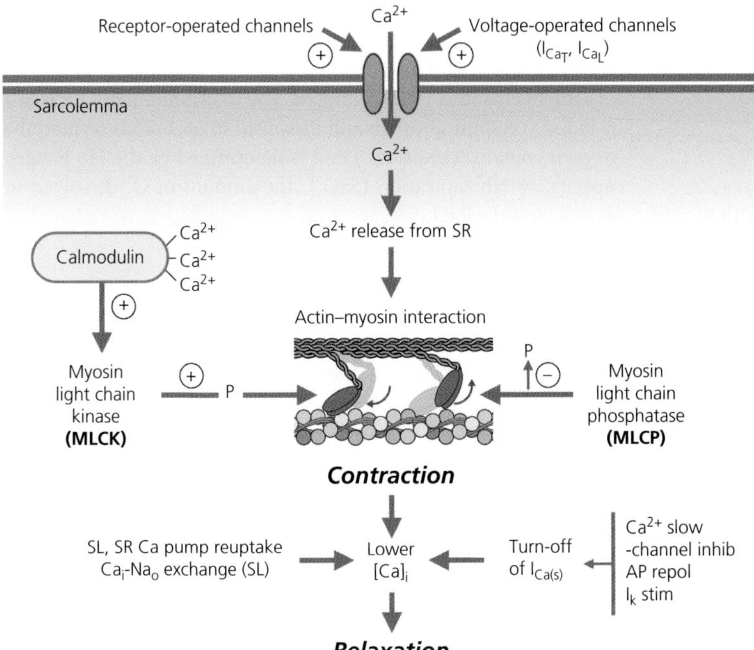

Figure 33.24 Vascular smooth muscle excitation–contraction coupling. Calcium entry into smooth muscle cells through L-type channels located in the caveolae of the cell membrane is initiated by depolarization, hormones, or neurotransmitters. Intracellular calcium stimulates the release of calcium from the sarcoplasmic reticulum (SR) by way of ryanodine receptors and IP_3. Some agonists act on smooth muscle membrane receptors (not shown) to stimulate phosphatidylinositol turnover and the production of inositol triphosphate (IP_3) and diacylglycerol (DAG). IP_3 releases calcium from the SR and DAG activates protein kinase C, which stimulates the activity of the voltage-dependent slow calcium channels. Increases in intracellular calcium also interact with calmodulin to form a calcium–calmodulin complex that stimulates myosin light chain kinase (MLCK), which together with intracellular calcium facilitates actin–myosin interaction. Contraction terminates when myosin light chain phosphatase (MLCP) dephosphorylates the myosin light chain and intracellular calcium is reduced by sarcolemmal (SL) intracellular calcium–extracellular sodium exchange, SR reuptake, and when the slow calcium channels turn off.

Plasmalemmal calcium (Ca^{2+}) channels are the principal routes whereby Ca^{2+} enters vascular smooth muscle cells [162]. Various types of Ca^{2+} channels have been identified including voltage-operated Ca^{2+} channels (VOCCs), receptor-operated Ca^{2+} channels (ROCCs), and store-operated Ca^{2+} channels (SOCCs). ROCCs are further subdivided into ligand-gated Ca^{2+} channels and second messenger-operated Ca^{2+} channels [162]. ROCCs can be blocked by calcium antagonists (e.g., verapamil, diltiazem, or nifedipine) [160]. All play a role in increasing intracellular Ca^{2+} concentration, but VOCCs are believed to be crucial in the physiologic regulation of vascular smooth muscle tone. Cytosolic $[Ca^{2+}]$ is reduced by plasma membrane Ca^{2+} ATPase (PMCA), sarcoplasmic reticulum Ca^{2+} ATPase (SERCA), the Na^+–Ca^{2+} exchanger (NCX), and cytosolic Ca^{2+}-binding proteins (e.g., calmodulin). Both PMCA-mediated Ca^{2+} extrusion and SERCA-mediated Ca^{2+} uptake play a major role in decreasing vascular smooth muscle $[Ca^{2+}]_i$. Various agonist (e.g., norepinephrine, epinephrine, angiotensin II, endothelin, etc.) induce smooth muscle contraction by binding to GPCRs that stimulate phospholipase C, which activates the membrane lipid phosphatidylinositol 4,5-bisphosphate (PIP_2) to catalyze the formation of two second messengers: inositol trisphosphate (IP_3) and diacylglycerol (DAG). Activation of IP_3 receptor channels is believed to play a primary physiologic role in intracellular Ca^{2+} mobilization. The binding of IP_3 to receptors on the sarcoplasmic reticulum results in the release of Ca^{2+} into the cytosol (Fig. 33.24). Notably, this calcium-induced calcium release (CICR) mechanism is considered essential for maintaining cellular Ca^{2+} homeostasis in vascular smooth muscle cells [161,162].

In addition to the Ca^{2+}-dependent activation of MLCK, MLC phosphorylation is also regulated by MLC phosphatase (MLCP) that removes high-energy phosphate from MLC, thereby initiating smooth muscle relaxation (Fig. 33.24) [162]. Smooth muscle relaxation occurs as a result of removal of the contractile stimulus, decreases in $[Ca^{2+}]_i$, and an increase in MLCP activity, or by a substance that directly inhibits the contractile mechanism. A decrease in the $[Ca^{2+}]_i$ by Ca^{2+} uptake into the sarcoplasmic reticulum is dependent on ATP hydrolysis. Sarcoplasmic Ca^{2+} binding proteins (e.g., calmodulin) also contribute to decreased intracellular Ca^{2+} concentrations. The plasma membrane also contains NCXs and Ca^{2+}–Mg^{2+} ATPases, providing an additional mechanism for reducing the concentration of activator Ca^{2+} inside the cell [160,162].

Most volatile and intravenous anesthetics, including ketamine, inhibit vascular smooth muscle contractile activity at clinically relevant concentrations [163–165]. Vasoconstriction caused by many common endogenous and exogenous receptor agonists including epinephrine, norepinephrine, dopamine, dobutamine, and phenylephrine is blunted by anesthetic drugs [165]. Receptor-operated activation, VOCCs, SERCA, and myofilament Ca^{2+} sensitivity are inhibited by all currently available volatile and injectable anesthetics [160,161]. Isoflurane, sevoflurane, propofol, and benzodiazepines inhibit smooth muscle contraction by blocking calcium channels, especially the VOCCs, and by raising intracellular cyclic adenosine monophosphate (cAMP) and cyclic guanosine monophosphate (cGMP). Volatile anesthetic-induced suppression of smooth muscle contraction is also attributable to mechanisms independent of $[Ca^{2+}]_i$, which involve the depression of Ca^{2+} sensitization mediated by protein kinase C [165]. ATP-sensitive potassium (K_{ATP}) channels present in vascular smooth muscle cells play an important role in the vascular responses to a variety of pharmacological and endogenous vasodilators [166]. The K_{ATP} channels are inhibited by intracellular ATP and by sulphonylurea agents. Pharmacological vasodilators are used to lower arterial blood pressure (e.g., cromakalim and pinacidil) and many anesthetics, including isoflurane, sevoflurane, and propofol, directly activate K_{ATP} channels resulting in K^+ exit from the cell and membrane hyperpolarization [163–167]. The associated membrane hyperpolarization closes voltage-dependent Ca^{2+} channels, which leads to a reduction in intracellular Ca^{2+} and vasodilation [166]. Isoflurane activates K_{ATP} channels via protein kinase A activation [167]. By contrast, hypotension after systemic propofol administration is mainly caused by its direct relaxation effect on vascular smooth muscle [163]. Notably, K_{ATP} channels are also activated by pathophysiological conditions, such as hypoxia, ischemia, acidosis, and septic shock [166].

Blood

Blood is a non-Newtonian (i.e., viscosity changes when flow rate changes) viscous fluid (i.e., 3.5–5.5 cP) composed of approximately 60% plasma and 40% blood cells and is responsible for carrying oxygen and nutrients to tissues and transporting the by-products of cellular metabolism (e.g., CO_2, drugs metabolites) to the organs of elimination. This suspension of red and white blood cells and platelets in plasma is responsible for maintaining a normal internal environment, defending against infections and toxins (immunity), and preventing or limiting hemorrhage (hemostasis) [168,169]. Blood volume averages 5.5–8.5% of body weight in many animal species, but this varies with fitness level (Table 33.7).

RBCs (i.e., erythrocytes) contain the iron-rich protein hemoglobin (Hb). Hemoglobin exists as a tetramer (i.e., molecular weight, 64 kDa) consisting of two α and two β polypeptide chains. Each polypeptide chain contains heme and a central iron molecule that can bind oxygen [168]. Heme must be in the reduced or ferrous state (Fe^{2+}) to bind oxygen. Hemoglobin's affinity for oxygen is determined by the partial pressure of carbon dioxide (PCO_2), pH, body temperature, the RBC concentration of 2,3-diphosphoglycerate (2,3-DPG) and the chemical structure of Hb (Fig. 33.25A) [171]. RBC 2,3-DPG concentration controls Hb oxygen release to tissues [171]. A decrease in pH or increase in RBC PCO_2, 2,3-DPG, or temperature decreases Hb's affinity for oxygen and vice versa thereby helping to maintain a physiologically relevant P_{50} (i.e., PO_2 where Hb is 50% saturated with oxygen). Mammalian P_{50} values normally range between 23 to 28 mmHg and are used as a comparative indicator of Hb affinity for oxygen (Fig. 33.25A) [172].

Oxygen delivery (DO_2) to tissues is an essential function of blood and is primarily dependent upon the blood hemoglobin (Hb) concentration since oxygen is relatively insoluble in plasma (i.e., 0.003 mL O_2 per 100 mL of plasma per mmHg). Therefore, 100 mL of plasma carries approximately 0.3 mL (i.e., vol %) O_2 when the partial pressure of O_2 (PaO_2) is 100 mmHg (e.g., 0.003 mL × 100 mmHg). Hemoglobin's oxygen-binding capacity (i.e., the amount of oxygen that chemically combines with Hb) is 1.34–1.39 mL/g Hb when 100% saturated. Oxygen-binding capacity does not include oxygen dissolved in plasma. This indicates that the amount of O_2 carried by blood with a Hct of 45% (i.e., Hb = 1/3 Hct; 1/3 × 45 = 15 g/dL Hb) is approximately 20 mL/100 mL (i.e., 15 g/dL × 1.34 mL = 20.1 mL/dL) if each gram of hemoglobin carries 1.34 mL of O_2 and is 100% saturated. The total amount of O_2 carried by blood (i.e., bound to Hb and dissolved in plasma) is termed the "oxygen content" (i.e., CaO_2) and is determined by the Hb oxygen capacity, % Hb saturation (SaO_2), the amount of O_2 dissolved in plasma, and the PaO_2:

$$CaO_2 = \left[\left(1.34 \times Hb\right) \times SaO_2\right] + \left(0.003 \times PaO_2\right)$$

The CaO_2 is 20.4 mL/dL when blood PaO_2 is 100 mmHg and [Hb] is 15 g/dL (i.e., CaO_2 = ([1.34 mL × 15 g/dL) × 1] + (0.003 × 100) = 20.4 mL) emphasizing the importance of hemoglobin as an oxygen

Table 33.7 Average blood volume in select animal species.

Animal	Blood volume (mL/kg)
Dog	80 > 90 in racing Greyhounds
Cat	55
Horse	75
Cow	60
Sheep	60
Goat	70
Pig	65
Rabbit	60
Rat	65
Poultry	65
Monkey	65
Human	75

Source: Adapted from Burke [170].

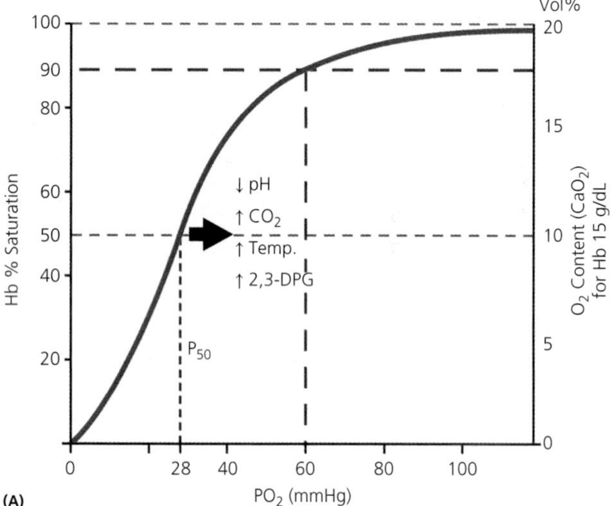

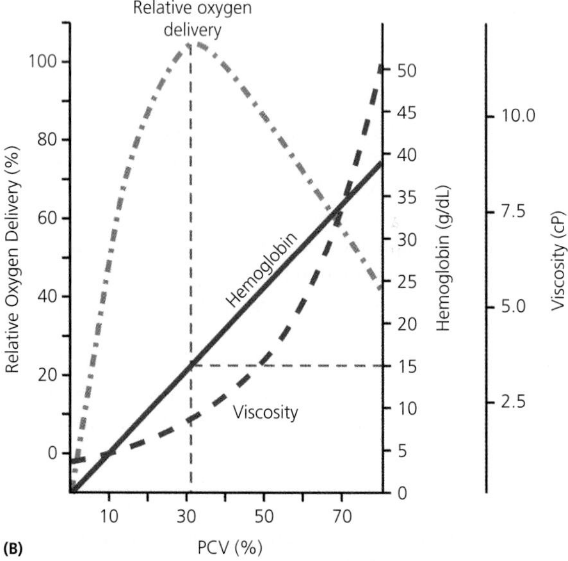

Figure 33.25 The oxyhemoglobin-dissociation relationship. **A.** Hemoglobin (Hb) saturation with oxygen (O_2) versus the partial pressure of oxygen (PO_2). The relationship is right shifted (Hb has less affinity for O_2) when pH is decreased (i.e., acidosis) and carbon dioxide [CO_2]), body temperature, and 2,3-diphosphoglycerate (2,3-DPG) are increased. **B.** Oxygen delivery is dependent upon blood Hb concentration and viscosity. Viscosity increases as Hb concentration increases. Oxygen delivery (DO_2) is maximal at a PCV of approximately 30%.

carrier. Tissue oxygen delivery DO_2 is determined by systemic blood flow (Q) or CO multiplied by CaO_2:

$$DO_2 = Q \times CaO_2$$

DO_2 is significantly influenced by [Hb] and blood viscosity during normal resting conditions (Fig. 33.25B).

Methemoglobin is a stable oxidized form of Hb that is spontaneously produced when the iron contained within the Hb molecule is oxidized to the ferric state (Fe^{3+}). This form of Hb cannot bind oxygen and is usually below 3% of the total Hb concentration. Hemoglobin is maintained in the ferrous state (Fe^{2+}) inside RBCs by reduced NADH–methemoglobin reductase. Carboxyhemoglobin (e.g., carbon monoxide poisoning), sulfhemoglobin, and cyanmethemoglobin are other forms of Hb that interfere with Hb's ability to carry oxygen. The binding of oxygen to hemoglobin has important vasoregulatory effects by promoting Hb binding of nitric oxide (NO) and the formation of *S*-nitrosohemoglobin (SNO) [173–176]. Current evidence suggests that deoxygenation of hemoglobin is accompanied by an allosteric transition of SNO (i.e., transitions from R [relaxed]-oxygenated to T [tense]-deoxygenated state) that releases NO [177]. The release of NO relaxes vessels and increases blood flow [177,178]. Thus, by sensing the physiological oxygen gradient in tissues, Hb exploits conformational changes in SNO to bring about changes in local blood flow and oxygen delivery (Fig. 33.26).

Tissue oxygen deprivation induced by inadequate PaO_2, low blood flow, low [Hb], or exposure to substances that limit Hb's O_2 carrying capabilities (e.g., carbon monoxide) activates genes that initiate angiogenesis, glucose metabolism, and increase the production of hypoxia-inducible factor (HIF) as well as activates fibroblasts in the renal cortex to increase erythropoietin synthesis and the differentiation of proerythroblasts to RBCs [179,180].

Cell-free Hb (e.g., arising from hemolysis) is maintained in the ferrous (Fe^{2+}) state and reacts with NO to inhibit NO signaling [178,181]. Cell-free heme and iron also promote oxidative and inflammatory injury via activation of macrophages and monocytes [182,183]. Homeostatic protective pathways that normally limit these NO and oxidation reactions include haptoglobin- and hemopexin-mediated sequestration of hemoglobin monomers, dimers, and heme [182,183]. Hemoxygenase and biliverdin reductase signaling detoxify heme and iron and provide catalytic antioxidant, antiproliferative, and anti-inflammatory effects. There is little to no information regarding the effects of anesthetic drugs on Hb oxygen affinity and what little literature does exist suggests that inhalational anesthetic drugs do not change the oxygen dissociation curve or jeopardize tissue oxygenation [184]. Notably, several local anesthetics (e.g., prilocaine and benzocaine) and drug diluent excipients (e.g., benzyl alcohol) are known to predispose to methemoglobinemia, especially in cats [185,186]. In addition, sevoflurane has been demonstrated to inhibit the accumulation and expression of HIF following ischemia reperfusion injury [187].

Lymphatic system

The lymphatic system is part of the circulatory and immune systems and consists of a dense and diffuse network of lymph channels (i.e., lymph capillaries), lymph vessels, nodes, ducts, organs (e.g., bone marrow and thymus), and tissues (e.g., tonsils and spleen) [188]. Lymphatic capillaries exist in all vascularized organs and tissues except retina, bone, and brain [189,190]. The interstitial space is the primary source of lymph [191]. Like peripheral tissue beds, a

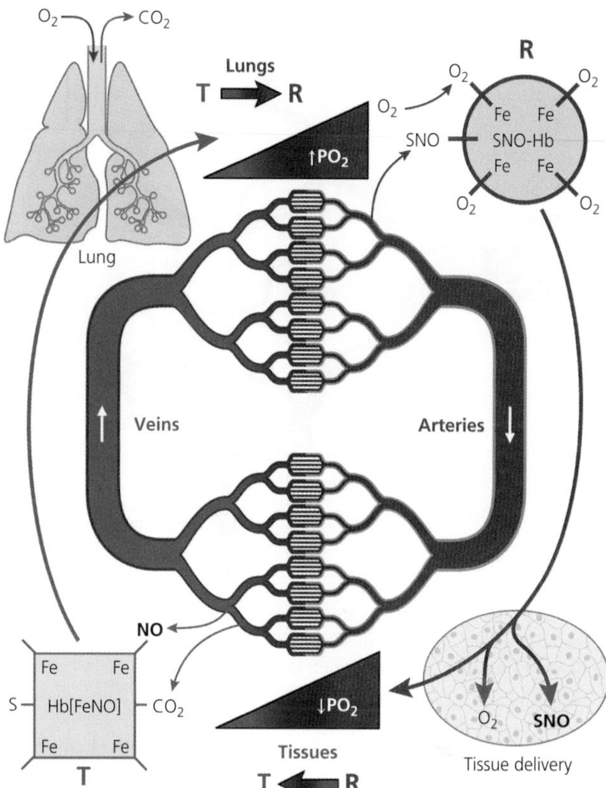

Figure 33.26 Red blood cell Hb alternates between R (relaxed or oxygenated) and T (tense and deoxygenated) states depending on PO_2 and PCO_2. Blood oxygenation in the lung produces the R state and promotes *S*-nitrosylated Hb (SNO-Hb) formation. Endothelial nitric oxide (NO) synthase is responsible for the production of the NO group in SNO-Hb. RBCs offload O_2 as Hb senses falling PO_2 in tissues, triggering the release of NO thereby increasing blood flow to tissues. Source: Adapted from McMahon *et al.* [177].

glymphatic system of perivascular channels, formed by astroglia cells, provides efficient elimination of fluid, soluble proteins, and metabolic wastes from the CNS [192].

Systemic lymph (i.e., filtered plasma) is formed as an ultrafiltrate of the capillary microcirculation supplemented by proteins of cellular origin (i.e., 25% extracellular, 32% from cytoplasm, 21% from nucleus, and 11% from plasma membrane). Lymph contains large numbers of lymphocytes that are essential for the development of the adaptive immune response [193,194]. Lymph vessels contain smooth muscle within their walls and function to provide the one-way transport of interstitial fluid, proteins, lipids, and waste products back to the circulation blood via the thoracic duct and other lymph vessel-venous anastomoses (Figs. 33.1 and 33.27). Interstitial fluid balance is critically modulated by interstitial fluid pressure and lymphatic vessel smooth muscle contractions. Lymph nodes filter the interstitial fluid containing phagocytic cells (e.g., macrophages and monocytes) and proteolytic enzymes that break down bacteria, viruses, and waste products [188,190]. Lymphatic drainage is mainly driven by NO-dependent rhythmic contractions of lymph vessel smooth muscle and local skeletal muscle contractions (i.e., lymphatic pump) [188]. Lymphatic capillaries (lacteals) collect interstitial fluid (lymph) and chylomicrons (triglycerides, phospholipids, cholesterol, and proteins) that is eventually returned to the cranial vena cava and right atrium after passing through a series of

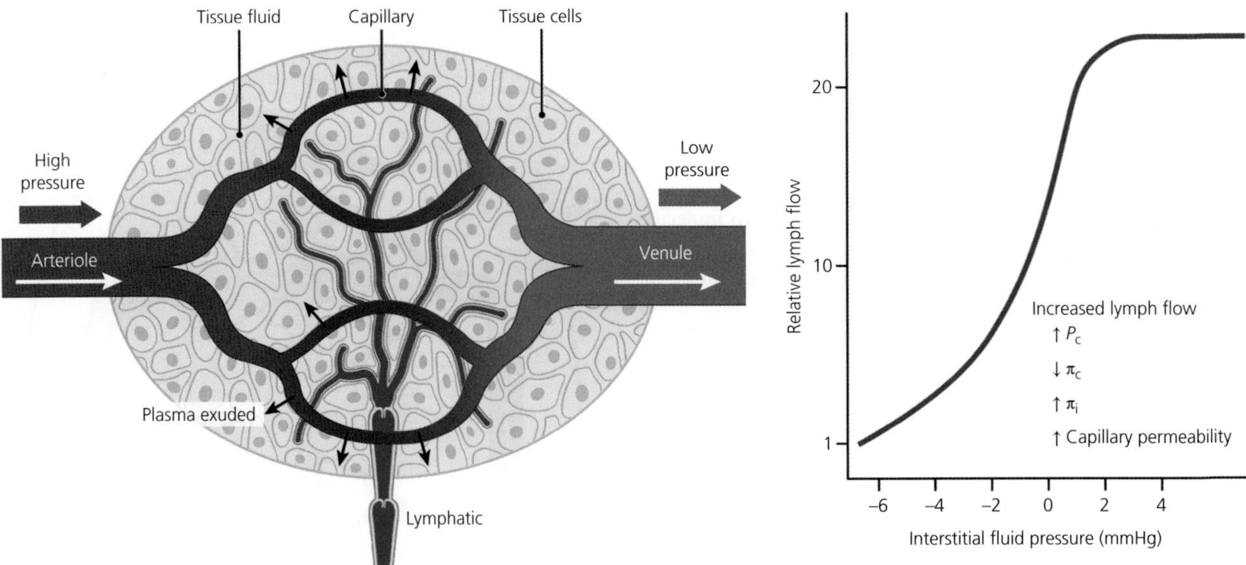

Figure 33.27 Lymphatic capillaries (green) collect and transfer interstitial tissue fluid (i.e., lymph) to larger afferent collecting vessels that drain into lymph nodes. Black arrows indicate outward transvascular fluid flux. Increases in capillary hydrostatic pressure (P_c), interstitial oncotic pressure (π_i), and capillary permeability increase lymph flow. Decreases in capillary oncotic pressure (π_c) increase lymph flow. Source: Adapted from Shang *et al.* [189].

lymph vessels and lymph nodes (Fig. 33.1) [189]. Lymphatic capillaries do not have a basement membrane but are lined with a single layer of partly overlapping lymphatic endothelial cells (LECs) [189,190]. The LECs are anchored to the extracellular matrices and function as primary valves that unidirectionally control lymph fluid drainage when interstitial pressure increases (Fig. 33.27). LECs modulate the inflammatory response by secreting chemokines for recruitment of immune (e.g., dendritic) cells into the lymphatic system. Toll-like receptors (TLRs) are highly expressed in LECs and contribute to lipopolysaccharide-induced lymphangiogenesis by chemotactic recruitment of macrophages [195,196]. TLRs also act as the first line of host defense against microbial infection and are pivotal in the development of both innate and adaptive immune responses [197].

Hemodynamics and cardiac function

Hemodynamics is the study of blood flow and the circulation of blood [198]. Direct (i.e., invasive; invading the circulatory system) and indirect (i.e., non-invasive; not entering the body) methods for assessing hemodynamic events include a host of both singular (e.g., pressure and blood flow velocity) and derived (e.g., resistance and ejection fraction) parameters that may include simultaneous measures of temporally related electrical (e.g., ECG), mechanical (e.g., transit times), and acoustic (e.g., heart sounds) events [199]. Blood pressure and blood flow velocity decrease as the total vascular cross-sectional area increases ensuring adequate exchange of nutrients and gases (Fig. 33.21). Hemodynamic measures should be accurate (i.e., closeness of the measurement to the true value) and precise (i.e., closeness of repeated measurements to each other) and are used to identify normal and abnormal physiology, confirm optimal tissue perfusion, and develop therapeutic plans. Uninterrupted recordings of dynamic (i.e., continuously changing) cardiovascular events provide the most clinically relevant information.

The primary function of the heart is to pump blood. Succinct definitions of terms used to describe cardiac function should be employed (Box 33.3). Many terms, however, are often controversial and occasionally ambiguous. The reasons for this include the use of different abbreviations to describe the same item (e.g., stroke volume abbreviated as SV or V_s), the conflation of diverse terms (e.g., cardiac function versus performance), and the application of terms developed from *in vitro* experiments to *in vivo* events (e.g., afterload) [200]. For example, there are more than 20 different definitions for the commonly used terms "preload" and "afterload" [200]. Furthermore, three terms (i.e., "performance," "inotropy," and "contractility") commonly employed to describe cardiac function are often conflated but have different meanings. Cardiac performance is determined by measuring changes in blood flow (i.e., cardiac output) and inotropy is determined by measuring changes in myocardial force [201,202]. Both are load (i.e., preload, afterload, and heart rate) dependent [201–203]. Conversely, cardiac contractility is load-independent (Box 33.3) [204–206].

Blood flow

Blood flow (Q) is determined by the driving pressure (i.e., $P_1 - P_2$) and the resistance to flow (R) as derived by the hydraulic equivalent of Ohm's law ($I = E/R$) where I is current flow, E is electromotive force (i.e., voltage), and R is resistance.

$$Q = \left(P_1 - P_2\right)/R$$

Resistance to blood flow (e.g., systemic vascular resistance [SVR]) is determined by blood vessel geometry (i.e., vessel radius, length, and morphology), compliance, blood volume, and the characteristics of the fluid medium (i.e., rheological properties), key among which is blood viscosity (η). The steady, non-pulsatile, laminar flow of Newtonian fluids (i.e., homogenous fluids, such as water or saline, where viscosity does not change with flow velocity or tube geometry) is described by the Hagen–Poiseuille equation:

$$\left(P_1 - P_2\right) = Q \times 8L\eta/\pi r^4$$

Box 33.3 Definitions for popular hemodynamic terms.

Afterload: operationally defined in terms of the external factors that oppose or prevent muscle fiber shortening. *In vitro* afterload is the weight (load) the muscle fiber or sarcomere must lift or shorten against. *In vivo* indices of afterload include total peripheral resistance, peak systolic pressure, ventricular wall tension during ejection, and arterial (aortic input) impedance (i.e., the hindrance to blood flow into a great artery imposed by its stiffness; the combination of both resistance and reactance).

Capacitance: the relationship between volume and distending pressure in a vessel, vascular bed, or circulation. Vascular capacitance curves are constructed from the relationship between blood volume and mean circulatory filling pressure.

Cardiac performance: the heart's ability to pump blood (i.e., cardiac output) that is determined by heart rate and stroke volume. Cardiac performance is load- (i.e., preload, afterload, heart rate) dependent regardless of changes in force development or the velocity of muscle shortening (see Preload, Afterload). Both stroke volume and cardiac output are inversely related to afterload when preload is held constant.

Compliance: the ratio of the change in volume (ΔV) to a change in pressure (ΔP) in a vessel; the ability of a blood vessel or chamber to distend.

Contractility: the actin-activated, intrinsic, kinetically controlled, chemomechanical processes responsible for the development of force and velocity. Contractility is load-independent.

Force-frequency relationship (Bowditch, treppe, staircase effect, chronotropic-inotropy): operationally defined as an increase in the force of cardiac contraction in response to an increase in heart rate.

Heart rate: operationally defined as the number of times the heart beats in 1 min. Heart rate or frequency-dependent increases in sarcomere force and velocity occur in all mammals.

Heterometric autoregulation (Cyon–Frank–Starling mechanism): operationally defined as a change (increase/decrease) in the force of contraction in response to a directionally similar change in muscle fiber or sarcomere length (i.e., length-dependent).

Homeometric autoregulation (von Anrep effect *in vivo*; slow force response *in vitro*): operationally defined as a progressive increase in force leading to a decrease in left ventricular end-diastolic pressure that occurs after an initial increase in afterload or attributed to angiotensin II release and an increase in the calcium transient through activation of the Na^+-Ca^{2+} exchanger.

Inotropy: the ability of a muscle to develop force. Inotropy is load- (i.e., preload, afterload, heart rate) dependent.

Mean circulatory filling pressure: the average pressure in the circulatory system when the heart is acutely stopped, blood is redistributed, and all pressures are the same throughout the system.

Preload: operationally defined as the initial muscle fiber or sarcomere length (i.e., *in vitro*) just prior to muscle contraction. *In vivo*, preload is often described in terms of the end-diastolic volume, end-diastolic pressure, or end-diastolic wall stress.

Stressed volume: the volume of blood in the venous system, in addition to the unstressed volume, that increases the transmural pressure above zero. The sum of stressed (~30% of total) and unstressed (~70% of total) volumes is the total blood volume in the venous system during normal resting conditions.

Unstressed volume: the volume of blood in the venous system required to fill the vasculature to a transmural pressure of 0 mmHg.

Ventricular elastance ("stiffness"): operationally defined as a change in pressure for a given change in volume (d*P*/d*V* mmHg/mL). Greater ventricular elastance increases the tendency for the wall to recoil toward its original volume on removal of the distending force; the lower the elastance, the higher the compliance.

Ventricular–vascular coupling: represents the interaction between the ventricle and the elastance of the corresponding great artery (e.g., aorta, pulmonary artery) expressed as a dimensionless ratio between the end-systolic elastance of the ventricle (E_{es}) and the aorta or pulmonary trunk (E_a) at a time when muscle fibers have maximally contracted, and the ventricle has ejected its stroke volume.

Source: Adapted from Norton [200].

Therefore

$$Q = (P_1 - P_2)\pi r^4 / 8L\eta$$

where $P_1 - P_2$ is the driving pressure, L is the length of the tube, η is the viscosity of the fluid, r^4 is the radius to the fourth power, and $8/\pi$ is a constant of proportionality. The maintenance of laminar flow (i.e., smooth regular paths) is a fundamental assumption of the Hagen–Poiseuille equation [207]. This equation is frequently used to determine blood flow but must be kept in perspective since blood is not a homogenous fluid (i.e., it is non-Newtonian), viscosity is not constant but varies with flow rate, blood vessels are not rigid but distensible and progressively decrease in radius, and blood flow is only intermittently laminar, may contain vortices (i.e., regions in which flow revolves around an axis line), and may be turbulent. Vascular resistance and autoregulatory processes regulate the distribution of blood flow throughout the body [208,209]. Pulsatile blood flow is generally considered to be laminar in large straight vessels and takes the form of a parabola but can become turbulent where blood vessels curve or branch, or when constrictions are encountered (Fig. 33.28). Turbulence is predicted by a dimensionless number, Reynolds number (*Re*):

$$Re = \rho D v / \eta$$

where ρ is the fluid density, D is the vessel diameter, and v is the mean blood flow velocity (Fig. 33.28) [210]. Blood viscosity (η) is inversely proportional to *Re*. *Re* values greater than 2000 suggest the development of turbulent blood flow that produces periodic wave fluctuations and vibrations of surrounding tissue structures leading to murmurs and, with time, weakening of the supporting elements of the vessel wall resulting in vascular dilation (i.e., aneurysm). Anemia and chronic or acute hemodilution (e.g., fluid therapy) reduce hematocrit and blood viscosity, increasing *Re* and the potential for a "functional" or "innocent" cardiac murmur. Flow restrictions caused by congenital diseases (e.g., aortic or pulmonic stenosis) produce an increase in blood flow velocity as predicted by the continuity equation (i.e., total blood flow through different areas of a continuous intact vascular system must be equal;

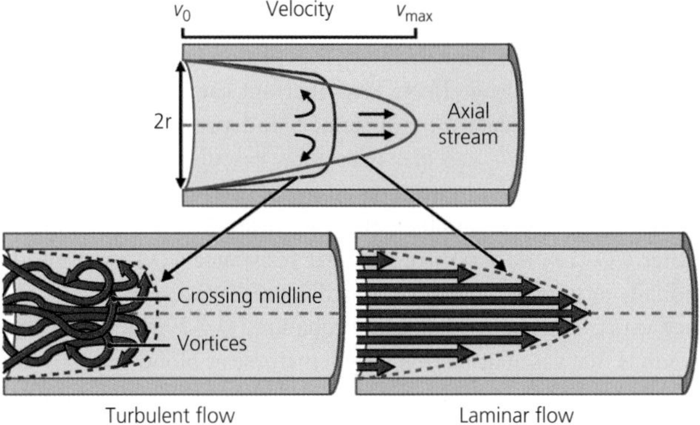

Figure 33.28 Velocity profile for laminar (i.e., blood moves in ordered, parallel layers; straight red arrows) and turbulent (i.e., chaotic; curved and circular red arrows) blood flow. Velocity is highest in the center of the blood vessel during laminar flow. Turbulence occurs at a critical flow rate as determined by the Reynolds (*Re*) number. An increased perfusion pressure is required during turbulent blood flow to maintain tissue perfusion. v, mean velocity; D, vessel diameter; ρ, blood density; η, blood viscosity.

therefore, blood flow through a narrowed orifice must increase). Blood flow immediately downstream from narrowed or partially obstructed vessels often contains vortices and becomes turbulent. Cardiac (e.g., aortic, pulmonic stenosis) and vascular diseases (e.g., thrombophlebitis) that narrow blood vessels increase blood flow velocity across the area of constriction producing turbulence and murmurs. The heart must produce a greater pressure to pump turbulent blood flow resulting in increased work and myocardial oxygen consumption (i.e., MVO_2). Blood flow velocity and the pressure gradient across a constricted orifice can be quantified using Doppler echocardiography and the Bernoulli equation:

$$\Delta P = 4v^2$$

where ΔP is the pressure change and v is blood flow velocity with the assumption that velocity distal to the obstruction is significantly greater than the velocity proximal to the obstruction and is, therefore, ignored [211].

Blood flow distribution is determined by tissue metabolism and oxygen requirements (Table 33.8). Tissues with higher oxygen demand, therefore, receive a greater percentage of the CO. Anesthetic drugs are delivered to the various tissues based upon the distribution of CO. Approximately 75% of the CO is distributed to "vessel-rich" group tissues (heart, brain, liver, kidney, and adrenal glands) compared to muscle group (muscle and skin) or "vessel-poor" group (fat, bone, and cartilage) tissues during resting conditions (Fig. 33.29) [212]. Blood flow distribution changes during stressful conditions (e.g., fear and pain exercise) and influences the onset, magnitude, and duration of drug-related effects. Regulatory control of blood flow and compensatory responses are integrated through the combined effects of central and peripheral nervous system activity, the influence of circulating (humoral) vasoactive substances, and local tissue mediators. These regulatory processes maintain blood flow at an appropriate level while distributing blood to meet the needs of tissue beds that have the greatest oxygen demand.

Table 33.8 Distribution of blood flow (i.e., cardiac output) during resting conditions.

Organ	% of Total
Heart	5
Brain	15
Kidneys	20
Splanchnic organs	25
Skeletal muscle	20
Skin	5
Other	10

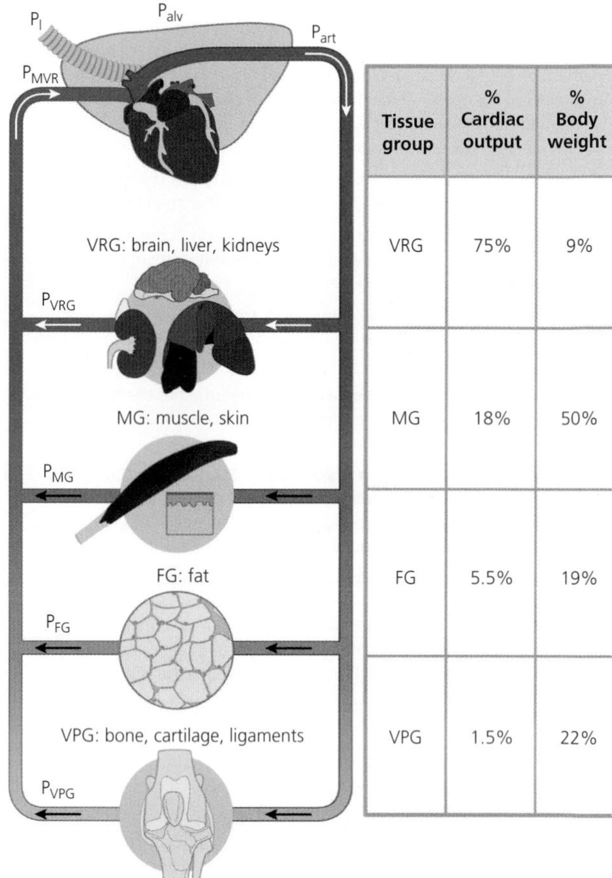

Figure 33.29 Regulation of cardiac output to various tissue groups based upon tissue type (i.e., vessel-rich group, muscle group, fat group, and vessel-poor group), percent of cardiac output, and percent body weight. Vessel-rich group tissues receive the greatest percentage of cardiac output based upon tissue weight and rapidly equilibrate with anesthetic drugs.

Blood pressure

Blood pressure is the force that moves blood and is exerted against vascular walls. Measurement of arterial blood pressure is one of the fastest and most informative methods for assessing cardiovascular function and, when done correctly, provides an indication of hemodynamic trends, drug effects, and aberrant cardiovascular events. The factors that determine arterial blood pressure include HR, stroke volume (SV), vascular resistance, vascular compliance, and blood volume. The volume of blood in the vascular system and vascular tone are key variables affecting arterial blood pressure. If either CO (i.e., flow [Q]) or vascular resistance (R) increase individually or together, pressure (P) will increase (i.e., $P = Q \times R$), and vice versa. The Hagen–Poiseuille equation ($Q = P/R$; $R = 8L\eta / r^4\pi$) predicts that vascular resistance will increase as blood viscosity and vessel length increase and vessel radius decreases [206]. Clinically, a mean arterial blood pressure greater than 60 mmHg is required to provide adequate blood flow to most organs realizing that both systolic (P_s) and diastolic (P_d) arterial pressures provide additional information. Mean arterial blood pressure can be estimated as:

$$P_m = P_d + 1/3\left(P_s - P_d\right) \text{ or } P_m = \left(2/3 \times P_d\right) + \left(1/3 \times P_s\right)$$

where P_m, P_s, and P_d are mean (m), systolic (s), and diastolic (d) blood pressures, respectively (Fig. 33.30A) [213]. P_s increases, and P_m and P_d decrease in more distal conduit arteries (Fig. 33.30B). The difference between P_s and P_d is known as the "arterial pulse pressure" (PP = $P_s - P_d$). The P_s, P_d, and P_m can be measured, calculated, or estimated using invasive (direct) vascular catheterization or non-invasive (indirect) Doppler or oscillometric techniques.

Intravascular pressure exerts tension on the vessel wall as described by the law of Laplace:

$$T = \Pr/2h \text{ or } P = 2hT/r$$

where T is wall tension, P is developed pressure, r is the internal radius, and h is the chamber or vessel wall thickness [214]. Tension is a key determinant of tissue myocardial oxygen consumption

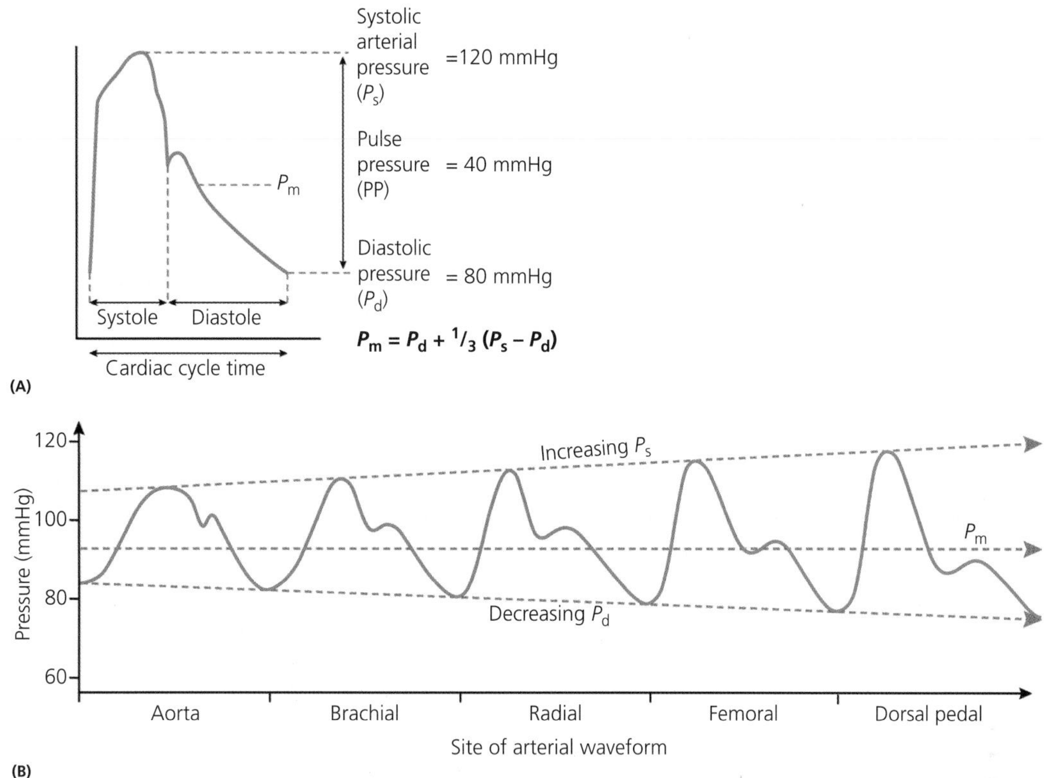

Figure 33.30 **A.** Arterial blood pressure. The mean arterial pressure (P_m) represents the area under the arterial pressure curve divided by the duration of the cardiac cycle. P_m is estimated by adding one-third of the difference between the systolic arterial pressure (P_s) and diastolic arterial pressure (P_d) to P_d. P_s minus P_d is the pulse pressure (PP). PP is normally about 40 mmHg. **B.** P_s increases and P_m and P_d decreases as arteries decrease in diameter.

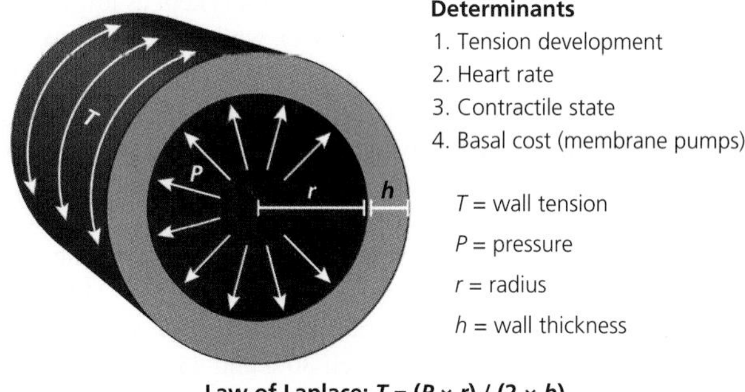

Figure 33.31 Determinants of myocardial oxygen consumption (MVO_2). Myocardial oxygen consumption is estimated by the law of Laplace: ventricular wall tension is proportional to ventricular radius and intraventricular pressure divided by two times the wall thickness. Ventricular wall tension and heart rate are the two principal determinants of MVO_2.

(MVO_2) and factors that increase tension development by cardiac muscle cells, the rate of tension development, or the number of tension generating cycles (e.g., increased HR) will increase MVO_2 (Fig. 33.31) [215].

The arterial pulse pressure ($PP = P_s - P_d$), pulse pressure waveform, and pulse pressure variation provide valuable information regarding changes in vascular compliance, vessel tone, vascular volume, and fluid responsiveness [214–217]. Increases or decreases in pulse pressure are suggestive of cardiovascular disease. For example, increases in PP (i.e., > 60 mmHg) suggest aortic regurgitation or vasodilation (e.g., sepsis), while decreases in PP (i.e., < 20 mmHg) suggest severe cardiogenic shock, cardiac tamponade, massive pulmonary embolism, or tension pneumothorax.

Pressure values and pressure waveform morphology change as the pressure wave travels peripherally, with systolic pressure increasing and mean and diastolic pressures decreasing (Fig. 33.30B). Pulse pressure is proportional to the volume of blood ejected from the ventricle (i.e., SV) during normal physiologic conditions but may vary during disease. Drugs (e.g., acepromazine) or diseases (e.g., hyperdynamic septic shock) that produce arterial dilation increase vascular compliance, causing a rapid rise, short duration, a rapid fall in the arterial waveform, and an increased pulse pressure [217]. Situations that produce vasoconstriction decrease vascular compliance and produce a longer-duration pulse waveform and a slower fall in the systolic to diastolic blood pressure value, thereby decreasing pulse pressure. The diastolic component of the arterial pressure waveform can contain secondary and sometimes tertiary pressure waveforms, particularly if the measuring site is in a peripheral artery at a distance from the heart [218]. Secondary and tertiary pulse-wave fluctuations may be indicative of normal or elevated vascular tone in response to sympathetic nervous system activity or the vascular effects of vasoactive drugs (e.g., dexmedetomidine or catecholamines).

Traditionally, arterial and central venous pressures values and waveform morphology have been used to assess cardiovascular status during anesthesia [218–220]. Emphasis is placed upon maximum and minimum acceptable values, waveform contour, pulse pressure variation, and expected changes associated with anesthetic drugs or vasoactive therapies (e.g., vasopressors and fluid administration). Caution is advised when assessing central venous pressure, however, due to its dependence on multiple variables including blood volume, HR, venous return, right ventricular function, and pulmonary arterial pressure [219].

Resistance

Factors opposing blood flow (i.e., afterload) are described and quantitated in terms of resistance, hindrance, and impedance. These terms are frequently conflated but are not the same and should not be used interchangeably. The Hagen–Poiseuille equation is the popular method employed for reporting vascular resistance (R):

$$R = 8L\eta/\pi r^4$$

R is usually derived by dividing the change in pressure by flow (i.e., $R = (P_1 - P_2)/Q$) and although convenient is arguably the least accurate since, as stated previously, blood is not a Newtonian fluid, vessels are not rigid tubes, and blood flow is not laminar in all parts of the arterial tree. The rheological term that characterizes blood flow conditions (i.e., blood flow velocity) is "shear rate," which is a function of blood flow velocity and vascular geometry. Blood viscosity is shear rate (i.e., blood flow velocity) dependent. Viscosity decreases as shear rate increases according to this equation:

$$\eta = \text{shear stress}\left(\text{dynes/cm}^2\right)/\text{shear rate}\left(\text{s}^{-1}\right)$$

where η is viscosity and shear stress is the force applied during pulsatile blood flow between theoretic parallel layers of blood in the blood vessel [221,222]. Shear rate gradually increases and blood viscosity decreases as large arteries become smaller and is greatest in the capillaries regardless of low blood flow rates [223,224]. This phenomenon (decreased blood viscosity in smaller vessels) is known as the "Fåhræus–Lindqvist effect" and is attributed to the centralization (i.e., central streaming) of RBCs, reduced RBC numbers (Fåhræus effect) at the vessel wall ("plasma skimming"), and RBC deformability. Rephrasing, as the diameter of the vessel decreases, the concentration of RBCs decreases (Fåhræus effect) and blood viscosity also decreases (Fåhræus–Lindqvist effect) [225]. Viscosity in capillaries is low because RBCs pass through capillaries single file in the center of the capillary. Blood viscosity is, therefore, dependent upon the RBC concentration (hematocrit), RBC deformability and aggregability, plasma viscosity, temperature, and blood flow conditions [226,227]. Notably, blood viscosity is rarely measured or calculated in most studies reporting vascular resistance although it can be responsible for significant effects in smaller blood vessels, during hemodilution, and in low blood flow states. Maintaining normal blood viscosity sustains microcirculatory blood flow and supports coherence between macrovascular and microvascular perfusion (i.e., hemodynamic coherence) [228–231].

Vascular hindrance (R_h) varies with blood viscosity (η) and vessel geometry (i.e., radius, length) and the number of blood vessels arranged in parallel over which the resistance measurement is being made [232]. Vascular hindrance (R_h) is

$$R_h = R/\eta$$

An increase in viscosity is known to produce compensatory vasodilation [233,234].

Impedance (Z) is defined as the ratio between the frequency components of the local blood pressure and blood flow waveforms [235]. Impedance includes both the resistance (R) and reactance (i.e., changes in vessel compliance or stiffness) of the vessel wall to pulsatile changes in intravascular pressure

$$Z_L = R_p + R$$

where Z_L represents longitudinal impedance, which is the sum of the pulsatile (R_p) and steady non-pulsatile components of longitudinal arterial resistance (R) [235,236]. Under normal (non-stressed) conditions, the steady resistive non-pulsatile component (R) represents approximately 85–90% of the total impedance to blood flow while the pulsatile component (R_p) comprises the remaining 10–15%. This fact (R = 85–90% of Z_L) is the principal reason why investigators and clinicians are usually satisfied with the determination of vascular resistance from blood flow and driving pressure (i.e., Hagen–Poiseuille equation: $R = P/Q$). The components of Z change substantially, however, during heart failure or pharmacological manipulation [237]. Aortic input impedance (Zi) is the ratio of pressure and flow at the aortic root and is dependent upon aortic elastance or compliance [235,236]. Impedance to blood flow, therefore, is viewed as having a resistive (steady-state [R]) component due primarily to the arterioles and a reactive (pulsatile [R_p]) component due to vessel wall properties (i.e., compliance, elastance, and pulse-wave reflection). Low systolic arterial pressure enables more complete ventricular ejection, maintains low myocardial oxygen demands, and provides little stimulus for producing hypertrophy. High diastolic pressure ensures adequate coronary blood flow and myocardial perfusion because most of myocardial blood flow occurs during ventricular relaxation. Increases in systolic and diastolic pressures increase myocardial work, oxygen consumption, and energy requirements and decrease myocardial perfusion [215]. Ideally, the best match between the heart's pumping activity and the vascular response to the ejection of blood (ventricular–vascular coupling) is obtained when myocardial work is kept as low as possible (i.e., relatively low systolic pressure), while adequate myocardial and peripheral tissue perfusion (i.e., higher diastolic pressure) is maintained [238]. Anesthesia and fluid therapy generally decrease hematocrit and plasma protein concentrations leading to decreases in blood viscosity, which, when combined with a decrease in impedance (i.e., vasodilation and vessel smooth muscle relaxation), favorably affect ventricular–vascular coupling, providing that hypotension (e.g., $P_m < 60$ mmHg) does not occur [239–242].

The optimum hematocrit for transporting oxygen varies among species and generally ranges between 30% and 45% [243]. Splenic contraction (e.g., dogs and horses) provides additional RBCs (i.e., increases hematocrit) and oxygen-carrying capacity during times of stress or exercise [244]. Excessively elevated hematocrits (e.g., polycythemia; > 65%) and hyperproteinemia (e.g., dehydration) dramatically increase blood viscosity and myocardial work due to an increase in RBC aggregability and rouleaux formation resulting in an increase in R_p (i.e., Z) and a decrease in oxygen delivery to tissues. Hemodilution (e.g., isovolumic hemodilution) can be beneficial in reducing blood viscosity and is used during anesthesia to improve oxygen delivery to tissues [245,246]. Blood flow is more dependent upon plasma viscosity in smaller vessels (< 100 μm) and capillaries [246]. The viscous properties of plasma and its effects on wall shear stress, nitric oxide production, and functional capillary density, therefore, are particularly significant for maintaining microcirculatory flow [247,248]. Hematocrit values less than 30%, however, jeopardize blood oxygen content, microcirculatory blood flow, and tissue oxygenation. Anesthesia and fluid therapy generally produce favorable effects on hematocrit, RBC deformability, and plasma protein concentration, leading to alterations in blood viscosity, which decrease impedance and improve ventricular–vascular coupling [241,242].

Preload and afterload

Preload is the stretch (i.e., increased muscle length) or load imposed on a muscle fiber or the myocardial wall at the end of diastole just before contraction begins (Box 33.3) [249]. End-diastolic muscle length (i.e., *in vitro*), end-diastolic volume (EDV), end-diastolic pressure (EDP), and ventricular wall stress have all been used as measures of preload. Sarcomere length provides the most meaningful measure of preload but is impossible to measure *in vivo*. The EDV is directly related to the degree of stretch imposed on myocardial sarcomeres and, therefore, provides the most accurate *in vivo* preload determinant. Preload is usually explained in terms of the Frank–Starling relationship where the force generated by ventricular contraction occurs in direct relation to the end-diastolic fiber length (i.e., heterometric autoregulation) [250]. Increases in cardiac muscle resting tension likely increase sensitivity to calcium, resulting in an increase in contractile force [251]. The Frank–Starling relationship serves as an important compensatory mechanism for maintaining SV when afterload or contractility is acutely changed (Fig. 33.32) [252]. Notably, preload is affected by afterload [253]. Increases in afterload decrease the volume of blood pumped by the heart with each beat (i.e., SV), which results in increased end-systolic volume (ESV) that augments EDV (i.e., preload).

Afterload is the force opposing ventricular ejection (Box 33.3) [249]. Although conceptually straightforward use of the term "afterload" suffers from multiple definitions and incomplete understanding of what the term represents. Afterload in isolated muscle tissues (i.e., *in vitro*) is the external force that inhibits the muscle (i.e., sarcomere) from shortening [200]. In contrast, afterload in intact animals changes continuously throughout ventricular ejection and is more accurately described by the hindrance or impedance to blood flow during ventricular ejection. An acute increase in arterial blood pressure increases ventricular EDV and decreases SV. The increased ventricular EDV increases ventricular wall stretch and contractile force via the Frank–Starling mechanism (i.e., heterometric autoregulation). This, however, is followed by a progressive decrease in the EDV to near-normal values and a sustained increase in SV (i.e., homeometric autoregulation; von Anrep effect; Box 33.3). Multiple mechanisms are responsible for this response including release of angiotensin II and endothelin, activation of the mineralocorticoid receptor and myocardial Na^+–H^+ exchanger, increase in intracellular Na^+ concentration, and augmentation of the Ca^{2+} transient amplitude through the Na^+–Ca^{2+} exchanger (NCX). The net effect of all of these mechanisms is an increased SV at a lower diastolic volume [254]. The major reason for interest in afterload is because of its inverse relationship with SV in failing hearts and its direct correlation with myocardial oxygen consumption (i.e., MVO_2) as a result of an increase in ventricular wall tension (Fig. 33.31) [215]. The effects of anesthetic drugs on afterload and homeometric autoregulation require further investigation.

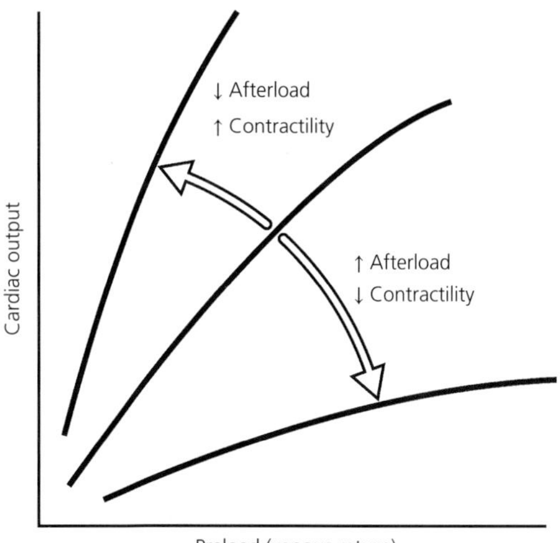

Figure 33.32 Frank–Starling curves. Increases in afterload and decreases in contractility shift the cardiac output–preload relationship down and to the right. Increases in contractility and decreases in afterload shift the cardiac output–preload relationship up and to the left.

The cardiac cycle and pressure–volume loop

Detailed illustrations of the cardiac cycle (i.e., Wiggers diagram) are used to explain the time-related relationships among the various electrical, mechanical (e.g., pressure, volume, and flow), and acoustic (Table 33.9) components of cardiac contraction and relaxation (Fig. 33.33A) [255]. The diagram provides a pictorial representation of all the major events that occur during one cardiac cycle. Similarly, the ventricular pressure–volume (PV) loop provides a real-time image of changes in ventricular pressure plotted against ventricular volume (Fig. 33.33B) [256,257]. Changes in the PV loop are used to illustrate and quantitate changes in cardiac function: preload, afterload, contractility, and ventricular–vascular coupling [256–258]. Various components of the cardiac cycle and PV loop for both the right and left ventricles are qualitatively similar, although quantitatively different.

The P wave of the surface ECG is a reasonable starting point to begin a description of the cardiac cycle since electric activity precedes mechanical activity (Fig. 33.33A). Electrical impulses originating in the SA node are rapidly transmitted from the right to the left atrium by atrial specialized fibers (i.e., Bachmann's bundle) causing generation of the P wave and almost simultaneous contraction of the right and left atria. Bifid P waves representing electrical activation of the right and then left atria are frequently observed in ECGs obtained from larger animals (e.g., horses and cattle) due to the increased size and volume of the atria, and the time required to traverse the increased muscle mass. Atrial contraction increases intra-atrial pressure, producing the "a" wave of the atrial pressure curve. Both right and left atria function as reservoirs and conduits for blood transfer and, upon contraction (i.e., atrial kick), prime the ventricles contributing approximately 10–30% of the ventricular blood volume at resting HRs and becoming more important at faster HRs. The reflected pressure wave from the atrial kick and structural vibrations in the AV valves prior to ventricular contraction are responsible for the fourth heart sound (S_4, atrial gallop) that generally remains inaudible in small animals (e.g., dogs and cats) but is frequently auscultated in larger animals (e.g., horses and cattle) or in animals with dilated and stiffened ventricles (Table 33.9). Ventricular contraction is signaled by the R wave and begins after a variable delay (i.e., PR interval), during which the electrical impulse traverses the AV node. Once the ventricle is electrically activated, ventricular contraction raises intracavitary pressure to a value greater than in the atrium closing the AV (i.e., tricuspid and mitral) valves. The AV valves bulge into their respective atria due to the

Table 33.9 Normal heart sounds and auscultation locations.

Sequence	Nomenclature	Associated events
First heart sound	S_1	Mitral and tricuspid valves close
Second heart sound	S_2	Aortic and pulmonary valves close
Third heart sound	S_3	Ventricular filling*
Fourth heart sound	S_4	Atrial filling*

S_1 mitral (radiates dorsally); S_2 aortic (radiates cranially);
*Auscultable with enlarged heart chambers and in healthy large animals (e.g., > 250 kg)

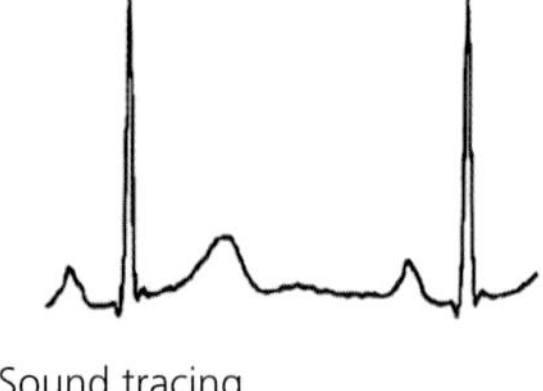

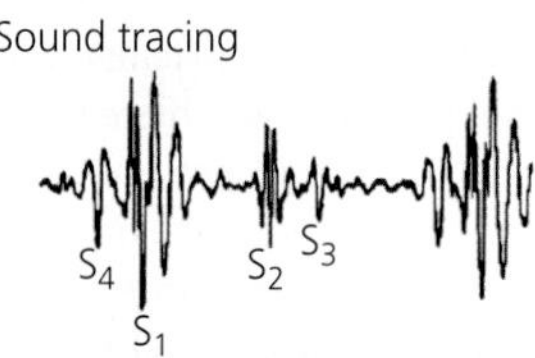

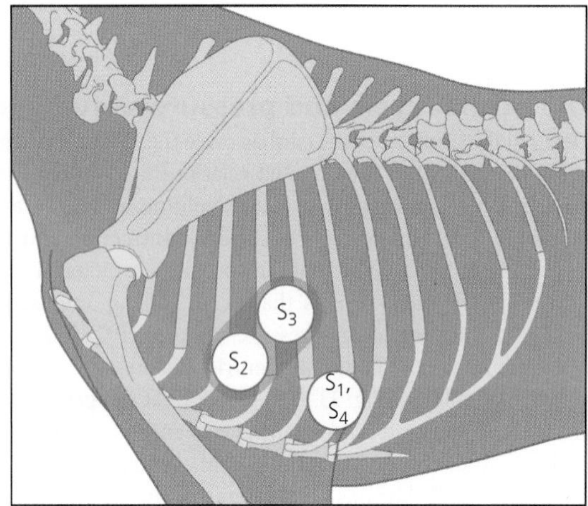

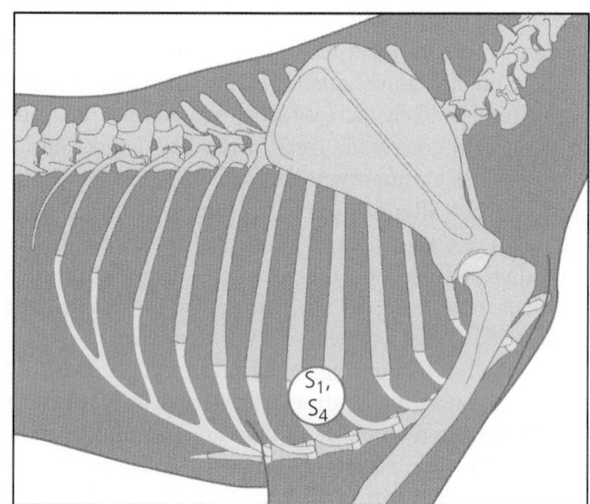

increased pressures in their respective ventricles, thereby decreasing atrial volume and giving rise to the "c" wave of the atrial pressure curve. The AV valves are prevented from completely prolapsing into the atrial chambers by cord-like fibrous structures (i.e., chordae tendineae) that connect ventricular papillary muscles to the edges of the tricuspid and the mitral valves. The sudden development of tension in the contracting ventricular myocardium and tensing of the chordae tendineae coincident with AV valve closure are responsible for the first heart sound (S_1; Table 33.9). The rapid increase in ventricular pressure while both the AV and semilunar (i.e., aortic and pulmonic) valves are closed produces isovolumic contraction (Fig. 33.33A,B). Once ventricular pressure exceeds that in the aorta or pulmonary artery, the semilunar valves open and ventricular ejection begins (Fig. 33.33A). The initial portion of the ejection phase of the cardiac cycle coincides with an abrupt decrease in ventricular volume, a large increase in aortic flow velocity, and a decrease in the venous pressure curve since the AV valves are drawn toward the apex of the heart thereby increasing the volume of the atria (i.e., the "x descent" following the "c" wave of the atrial pressure curve; Fig. 33.33A). Ventricular pressure exceeds aortic pressure during the first one-third of ventricular ejection (i.e., the rapid ejection period), reaches equilibrium with aortic pressure, and thereafter declines more rapidly than aortic pressure because of the onset of ventricular relaxation. Once the ventricular pressure decreases to values below the arterial pressure, the semilunar valves close. Closure of the semilunar valves is associated with the development of an incisura (i.e., dicrotic notch) in the arterial pressure waveform, the second heart sound (S_2), and the end of ventricular systole. The second heart sound is composed of both aortic (A_2) and pulmonic (P_2) components and is frequently split (10–15 ms) during slow HRs and in larger species (e.g., horses and cattle) [259]. The volume of blood ejected by the ventricle (i.e., SV) is the difference between ventricular EDV and ESV

$$SV = EDV - ESV$$

The period between closure of the semilunar valves and opening of the AV valves and the beginning of ventricular filling is termed "isovolumic relaxation" (Fig. 33.33A,B). Isovolumic relaxation is characterized by a rapid decrease in ventricular pressure and no change in ventricular volume. Once ventricular pressure falls below atrial pressure, the AV valves open, initiating a phase of rapid ventricular filling and producing the third heart sound (S_3; ventricular gallop; Table 33.9). The third heart sound is believed to be caused by vibrations in the ventricular walls once they reach their elastic limit during ventricular filling. The third sound is frequently heard in larger species (horses and cattle) or in dogs and cats with dilated ventricular chambers due to cardiac disease [260]. Ventricular filling proceeds more gradually after the initial rapid filling phase, whereas ventricular pressure and volume increase nonlinearly during late diastole (Fig. 33.33B). The slope of the PV curve (dP/dV) during ventricular filling is an index of ventricular elasticity, and its inverse (dV/dP) is used to assess ventricular compliance [257]. The ventricular filling phase continues as blood returns to the atria from the systemic and pulmonary circulations until the cardiac cycle is reinitiated by the next SA nodal electrical impulse.

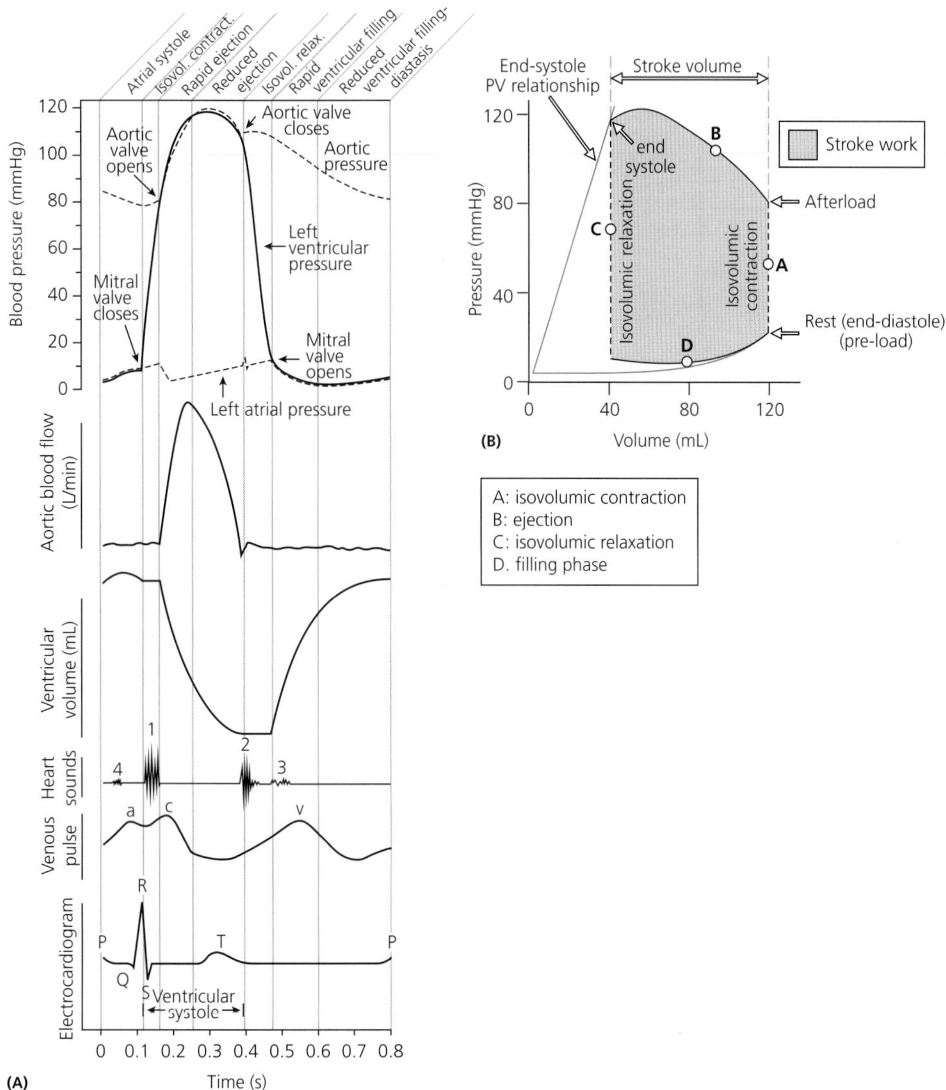

Figure 33.33 **A.** The cardiac cycle (i.e., Wiggers diagram) illustrates the temporal relationship between mechanical, acoustical, and electrical events during systole and diastole. **B.** The pressure–volume (PV) loop is a time-independent illustration of ventricular contraction used to derive load-independent indices of cardiac function (i.e., contractility) via the end-systolic PV relationship.

A PV loop represents the simultaneous changes in pressure and volume that take place during a single cardiac contraction and is represented as an irregular rectangle, inscribed in a counterclockwise fashion, in which intraventricular pressure is plotted on the *y*-axis against ventricular volume on the *x*-axis [257,261]. Analysis of the PV loop begins at point (B) and occurs at end-diastole (i.e., at the onset of systole as demarcated by closure of the AV valves and the first heart sound; Fig. 33.34A). The coordinates of this point are EDV and EDP. The ratio of EDV to EDP is a measure of static ventricular compliance, and the ratio of EDP to EDV is a measure of static ventricular stiffness. The relative slope of the ventricular filling line from A to B (Fig. 33.34A) is an estimate of dynamic ventricular compliance ($C_{dynamic}$) and the steepness of the slope is a measure of dynamic stiffness.

Ventricular pressure increases rapidly from B to C once the AV valves close, but there is no change in volume (i.e., isovolumetric contraction) until the semilunar valve opens at C (Fig. 33.34A) and blood begins to be ejected into the aorta. Ventricular pressure changes minimally during the ventricular ejection from C to D (i.e., isotonic contraction; Fig. 33.34A) but ventricular volume decreases. The change in ventricular volume represented by the horizontal distance between BC and DA (Fig. 33.34A) is the SV, and the ratio (SV/EDV) is the ejection fraction (EF).

$$EF = SV/EDV$$

The EF is the percentage of the EDV the ventricle pumps into the aorta during each contraction and ranges from 50–60% in healthy animals. The EF is considered a "gold standard" for assessing the general health of the cardiovascular system [262,263].

Closure of the semilunar valves (i.e., point D) indicates the end of systole. The ratio of end-systolic pressure (ESP) to ESV (ESP/ESV) is a measure of end-systolic elastance or stiffness of the ventricle contracting from any given EDV. The slope of the end-systolic pressure–volume relationship (ESPVR) obtained from ventricular contractions during decreases in ventricular volume is a load-independent measure of myocardial contractility [261]. This slope

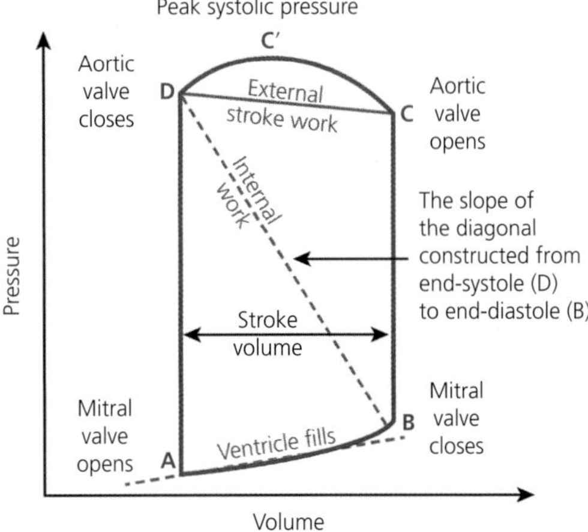

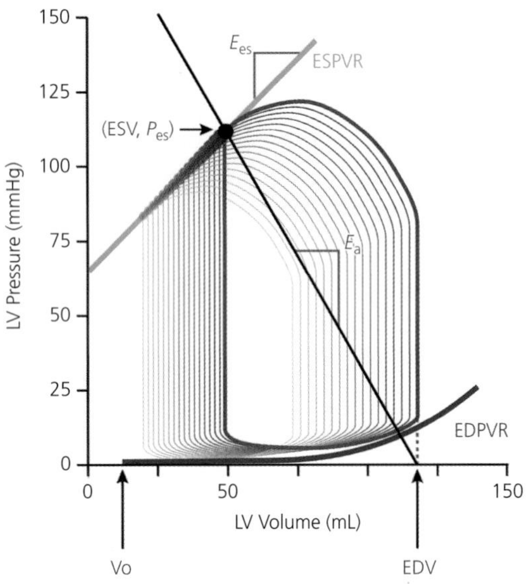

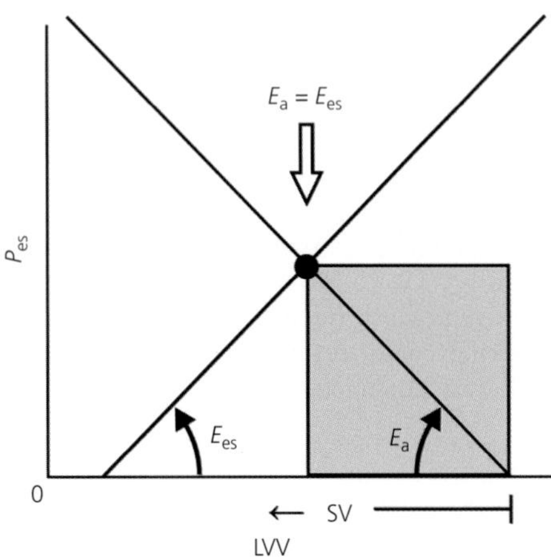

Figure 33.34 Ventricular PV loops provide a quantitative approach for determining cardiac contractility independent of preload, afterload, and heart rate. The E_a/E_{es} ratio is a measure of ventricular–arterial coupling. The E_a/E_{es} ranges from 0.6–1.2 in normal hearts. P_{es}, end-systolic pressure; SV, stroke volume; ESV, end-systolic volume; LVV, left ventricular volume; EDPVR, end-diastolic pressure–volume relationship; ESPVR, end-systolic pressure–volume relationship; E_{es}, end-systolic elastance (i.e., slope is an index of contractility; E_a, effective arterial elastance (i.e., index of afterload).

(E_{es}) is believed to be the most useful and accurate load-independent estimate of cardiac contractility currently available (Fig. 33.34B). The ventricular pressure falls quickly once the semilunar valves close (i.e., D to A; isovolumetric relaxation; Fig. 33.34A) and the ventricles begin to fill once the AV valves open.

Arterial elastance (E_a), a measure of the opposition to ventricular ejection (i.e., afterload), is the slope of a line that starts at the EDV and goes through the end-systolic PV point (Fig. 33.34B). E_a can also be calculated (i.e., $E_a = P_{es}/SV$) [261]. The E_a/E_{es} ratio is a measure of ventricular–arterial coupling and is normally close to 1.0 implying that the ventricular and arterial systems are optimally coupled (Fig. 33.34C) [264,265]. Ventricular–arterial uncoupling occurs when the E_a/E_{es} ratio is > 1.0.

The total area within the PV loop represents the total work performed by the ventricle against the opposition to ejection (i.e., afterload) imposed by arterial pressure and the stiffness (i.e., elastance) of the arterial wall. Total work is comprised of both internal work (i.e., cycling of heavy meromyosin heads and stretching the series elastic elements) and external work (i.e., moving a volume of blood against a resistance). Total work is a measure of myocardial oxygen consumption (MVO_2) and, along with oxygen delivery (DO_2), is used to estimate energetic balance (MVO_2/DO_2) and oxygen extraction ratio ($O_2ER = MVO_2/DO_2$) [215].

Thus, ventricular PV loops allow calculation of: (1) intracardiac ventricular pressures, (2) ventricular compliance, (3) myocardial contractility, (4) SV, and (5) myocardial oxygen consumption. In addition, the ratio of pulsatile aortic pressure to SV is an estimate of arterial stiffness and, like E_a/E_{es}, can be used to monitor changes in ventricular–vascular coupling [266].

The cardiac cycle and PV loop illustrate the hemodynamic events that occur during cardiac contraction and relaxation (Figs. 33.33 and 33.34). Clinically, M-mode echocardiography and two-dimensional color-flow Doppler echocardiography provide a dynamic representation of cardiac function (Fig. 33.35) [267]. For example, CO can be quantitatively estimated non-invasively (e.g., via echocardiography) as the product of HR and SV:

$$CO = HR \times SV$$

$$SV = LVOT\ area \times LVOT\ VTI$$

where LVOT area is the left ventricular outflow tract area and LVOT VTI is the velocity time integral.

Assessment of cardiac function

Assessment of cardiac contractile function (i.e., systolic function) encompasses multiple physical and image-based methods for determining performance (i.e., CO), inotropy (i.e., force), and contractility (i.e., force and velocity) (Box 33.4) [268–270]. Measurements of CO and inotropy are load-dependent and, therefore, must account for changes in either preload or afterload to explain hemodynamic and cardiovascular functional changes. Cardiac contractility is load-independent and, therefore, requires methods of measurement that are not sensitive to changes in preload, afterload, or HR [69,206]. Contractility is generally described by shifts of the force–velocity–length relationship, shifts in the ventricular function curve (e.g., shifts in the Frank–Starling relationship) when preload and afterload are held constant, or by changes in E_{es} (Fig. 33.36) [89,257,261,265]. Available indices used to evaluate cardiac contractile function generally fall into one of four broad categories: (1) isovolumic contraction phase indices, (2) ejection phase

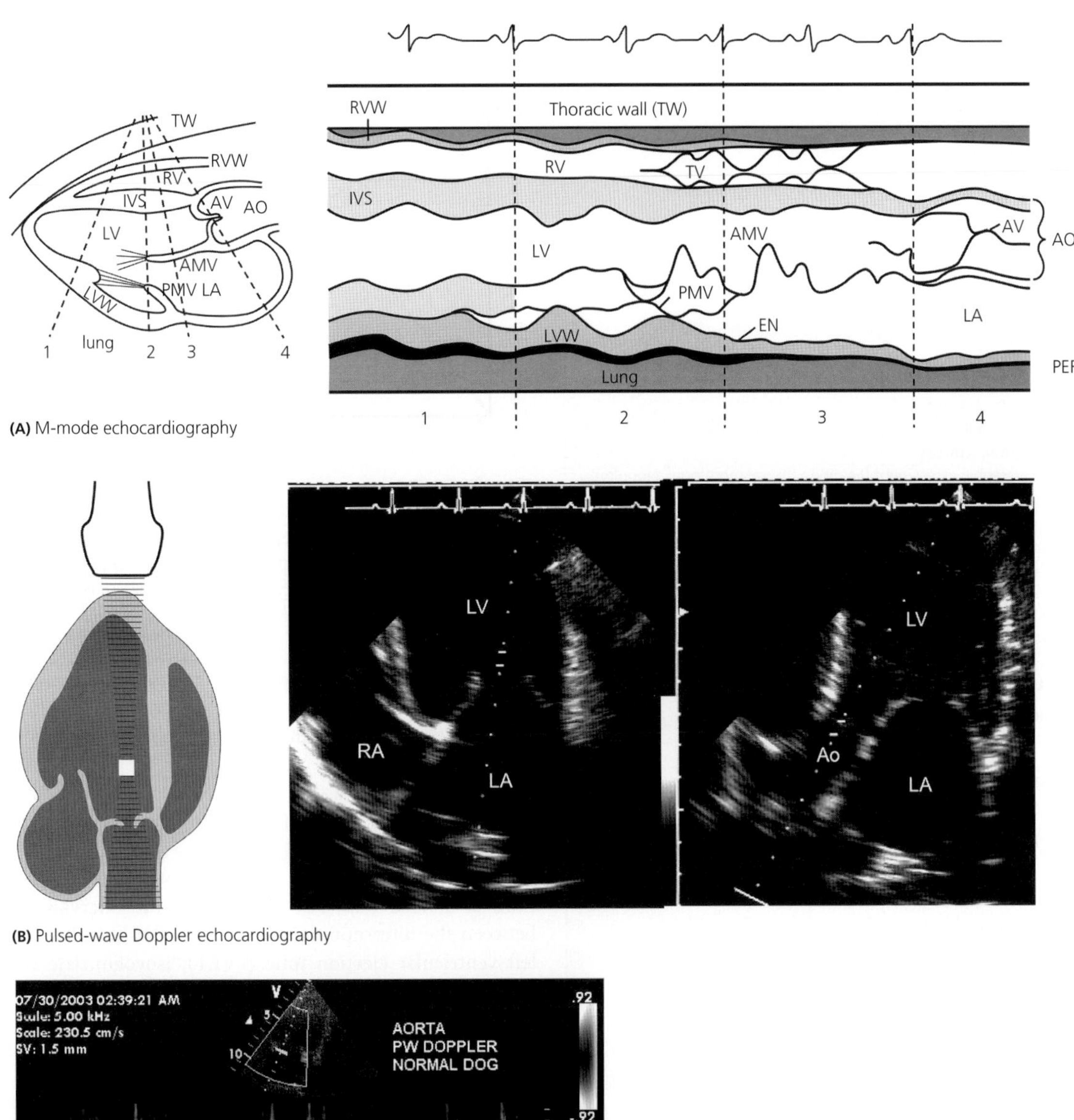

Figure 33.35 Non-invasive methods of assessing cardiac function. **A.** M-mode and pulsed-wave Doppler echocardiography produce dynamic real-time relationships in cardiac function in animals; **B.** Pulsed-wave Doppler echocardiography illustrating cardiac chambers; **C.** Left ventricular aortic outflow tract (LVOT) illustrating blood flow velocity. RVW, right ventricular wall; RV, right ventricle chamber; TV, tricuspid valve; IVS, interventricular septum; LV, left ventricular chamber; AMV, anterior mitral valve; PMV, posterior mitral valve; AV, aortic valve; AO, aorta; EN, endocardium; LVW, left ventricular wall.

indices, (3) PV relationship indices, and (4) stress–strain relationship indices.

The $dLVP/dt_{max}$ and $dLVP/dt_{max}$ divided by left ventricular end-diastolic volume (LVEDV), termed "preload-adjusted (i.e., PA) left ventricular dP/dt_{max}" or "$PALVdP/dt_{max}$," are sensitive indicators of changes in contractility during properly controlled experimental conditions or when $dLVP/dt_{max}$ is normalized to EDV ($PALVdP)/dt_{max}$) [271–274]. An even more robust expression of contractility can be obtained from the ventricular PV loop by determining the slope of the straight line formed when graphing stroke work (mean

Box 33.4 Examples of hemodynamic indices of systolic and diastolic function

Systolic function

1 **Isovolumic indices**
 a Echocardiographic assessment (M-mode, two-dimensional, Doppler)
 b dP/dt_{max}, dP/dt_{40}, and $dP/dt/V_{ed}$
 c V_{max}
 d Power; rate of change of power
2 **Ejection phase indices**
 a Echocardiographic assessment (M-mode, two-dimensional, Doppler)
 b Cardiac output
 c Ejection fraction, (EDV – ESV)/EDV
 d Stroke work
 e Maximum velocity of circumferential shortening
 f Left ventricular ejection time
 g Pre-ejection period
3 **Pressure–volume indices**
 a Echocardiographic assessment (M-mode, two-dimensional, Doppler)
 b E_{es} and E_{max}
 c End-systolic pressure–volume ratios
 d T_{max} (time to E_{max})
4 **Stress–strain indices**
 a Elastic stiffness (stress/strain)
 b End-systolic stress–volume ratio
 c Echocardiographic derived 2D strain

Diastolic function

1 **Isovolumic relaxation indices** (pressure derived)
 a Echocardiographic assessment (M-mode, two-dimensional, Doppler)
 b dP/dt_{min}
 c Time constant of left ventricular pressure fall (τ)
 d Relaxation time
 e $-dT/dt$ (tension fall)
2 **Diastolic filling indices**
 a dP/dV
 b Peak filling rate (dV/dt_{max})
 c Chamber stiffness (dP/dV versus P)
3 **End-diastolic indices**
 a End-diastolic pressure
 b End-diastolic P/V ratio
4 **Interval-derived indices**
 a Echocardiographic assessment (M-mode, two-dimensional, Doppler)
 b Time to $-dP/dt_{min}$; time to 50% $-dP/dt_{min}$
 c Diastolic filling time
 d Isovolumic relaxation period
 e Time from minimal left ventricular dimension to mitral valve opening
5 **Stress–strain indices**
 a Echocardiographic LV global diastolic strain rate (DSr avg)

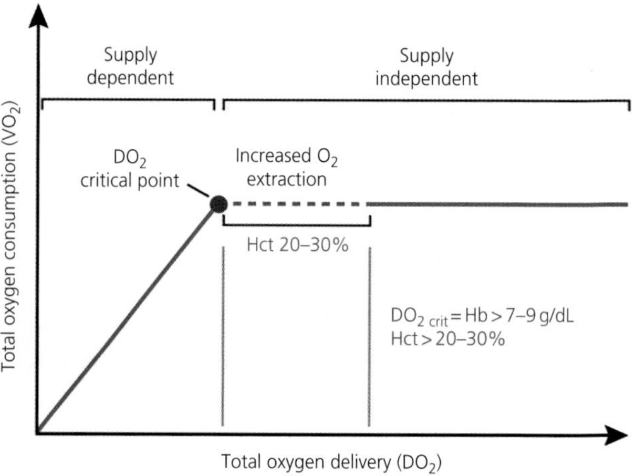

Figure 33.36 Oxygen consumption (VO_2) is not normally limited by oxygen delivery ($DO_2 = CO \times CaO_2$) and oxygen extraction ($OE = CaO_2 - C\bar{v}O_2$) (i.e., supply independent). Decreases in cardiac output (blood flow) to critically low values (e.g., hemorrhagic shock, heart failure) produce situations where VO_2 can become DO_2 dependent (i.e., supply dependent). CaO_2, arterial oxygen content; $C\bar{v}O_2$, venous oxygen content.

pressure during ejection × SV) against decreasing EDV as EDV is reduced by partial venous inflow occlusion (preload recruitable stroke work [PRSW]) [261]. Measures of contractility extracted from families of PV loops (e.g., E_{es}, V_0) generated in response to IV doses of known positive or negative inotropes (e.g., dobutamine, isoflurane) and vasoactive compounds (e.g., phenylephrine, isoflurane) indicate that E_{es} and the volume-axis intercept, V_0, provide a relatively good measure of the left ventricular contractility index because it is less sensitive to afterload compared to other indices [242]. It is important to note, however, that the methodological techniques used to manipulate preload or afterload are important. Changes in preload induced by administering IV fluids or removal of blood, occlusion of the caudal vena cava, or by changing afterload via physical constriction of the aorta produce a different result than changing preload or afterload pharmacologically (e.g., methoxamine, phenylephrine to increase afterload; nitroprusside, isoflurane to decrease preload). Differences arise due to the additional vasoactive, inotropic, clinotropic, lusitropic, chronotropic, and dromotropic properties that these drugs produce [202,263]. The PV loop produces more information about contraction and relaxation of the ventricle than any other method of expressing either systolic or diastolic function. It allows direct measurement of EDV (preload), ESV, SV, and EDP and permits calculation of EDP/EDV (elastance), PRSW, E_{es}, E_a, E_a/E_{es}, and the slope of the PV curve during ventricular filling. If the loops were interrupted (*z*-axis modulation) at a fixed rate (i.e., every 2 ms) the intervals (durations) between the interruptions could be used to calculate $dLVP/dt_{max}$, left ventricular ejection time (LVET), isovolumetric contraction time (IVCT), and IVCT/LVET [273]. The IVCT/LVET relates inversely to EF, can be obtained non-invasively, and is considered to be the "gold standard" of ventricular systolic function in clinical cardiology [274].

Less invasive assessment of E_{es} has been approximated by myocardial stress, magnetic resonance elastography, or from a single PV loop for which volume is estimated non-invasively by echocardiography and pressure is estimated indirectly from peak systemic systolic arterial pressure using sphygmomanometry [275]. Despite arithmetic "corrections," estimates of volume (by echocardiography) and pressure (e.g., sphygmomanometer) are at best estimates. "True" ESV obtained by echocardiography is limited by geometrical considerations, precision, and reproducibility, while "true" ESP differs from peak pressure in non-central arteries with peripheral arterial peak pressure variably and significantly higher than that realized by the ventricle at end-systole [276]. Regardless, evaluation of contractility estimated from a single PV loop obtained by non-invasive measurements has produced accurate predictions of patient outcomes [276,277]. In addition, segmental strain curves obtained non-invasively by trans-diaphragmatic two-dimensional echocardiographic images and speckle tracking analysis have been demonstrated to produce a load-independent measure of the cardiac contractile state [278]. The PV relationship has been used to assess the effects of most anesthetic drugs on cardiac function [279–281].

Lusitropy (i.e., rate of myocardial relaxation) refers to the ability of the myocardium to relax following excitation–contraction coupling and is fundamentally important to an understanding of cardiac performance [112,282]. The most popular and clinically relevant definition of *diastole* states that relaxation begins with the closure of the aortic valve, which is indicated by the second heart sound (S_2, Fig. 33.33A). Diastole is thereafter divided into four phases: (1) isovolumic relaxation, (2) early rapid ventricular filling, (3) slow (i.e., reduced) ventricular filling (diastasis), and (4) atrial systole (during sinus rhythm). Mechanical factors, loading factors, inotropic activity, HR, and synchronicity (patterns of relaxation) are the major determinants of lusitropy [112,283–285]. Factors and interventions that alter relaxation are of special interest because of their importance in determining ventricular compliance or stiffness. A partial list of methods used to quantitatively describe relaxation includes pressure, volume-derived, and interval indices (Box 33.4). Indices of isovolumetric relaxation (i.e., the rate of ventricular pressure decline; $-dP/dt$) and the time constant for relaxation (τ) are useful for measuring the active phase of relaxation and reflect the dissociation of actin–myosin linkages because of reuptake of cytoplasmic calcium by the sarcoplasmic reticulum. Both indices are influenced by myocardial systolic function, ventricular loading conditions (preload and afterload), and HR and are, therefore, considered to be load-dependent.

Drugs used as preanesthetic medication or for intravenous or inhalation anesthesia often produce profound effects on the cardiovascular system and indices of cardiac function (Table 33.10). While the arterial effects of anesthetic dugs are well-recognized, consideration should also be given to effects on venous physiology, unstressed vascular volume (V_{us}), and venous return. The venous vascular effects of anesthetics on the effective or stressed circulating blood volume (V_s) are much more complex than originally surmised and can be responsible for precipitous and dramatic decreases in venous return and cardiac function [286,287].

Oxygen delivery and oxygen consumption

The importance of adequate oxygen delivery (DO_2) cannot be overemphasized because reduced oxygen consumption (VO_2) and the development of increasing oxygen debt are directly linked to increased morbidity and mortality [288–291]. Once DO_2 falls below the minimum threshold for tissue metabolic requirements an oxygen supply–demand imbalance occurs (Fig. 33.36). Inadequate DO_2 increases oxygen debt and promotes anaerobic metabolism [289]. The severity of oxygen debt and anaerobic metabolism can be quantitated by their metabolic correlates, lactic acid and negative base excess (i.e., base deficit) [291]. Lactate accumulation and base deficit are used clinically, to quantitate the onset and severity of oxygen debt, the probability of death (LD_{50}), and the therapeutic reversal of oxygen debt [292].

Tissue oxygen consumption (VO_2) is determined by cellular metabolic rate. The VO_2 can be determined by the Fick, or oxygen consumption, equation [293]:

$$VO_2 = CO\left(CaO_2 - C\bar{v}O_2\right)$$

where CaO_2 is arterial oxygen content and $C\bar{v}O_2$ is mixed venous oxygen content. The Fick equation is rearranged to derive oxygen delivery ($DO_2 = CO \times CaO_2$), oxygen extraction ($OE = CaO_2 - C\bar{v}O_2$), and the oxygen extraction ratio ($OER = CaO_2 \times C\bar{v}O_2/CaO_2$), noting that all of the equations contain the term "CaO_2" and are, therefore, mathematically coupled [293]. Arterial blood oxygen content (CaO_2) is approximately 20–21 mL of O_2/dL of blood when Hb concentration is 15 g/dL; each gram of hemoglobin carries 1.34 mL O_2/g Hb; the SaO_2 is 100%; and the PaO_2 is 100 mmHg (room air):

$$CaO_2 = \left[\left(Hb \times 1.34\right) \times SaO_2\right] + \left(0.003 \times PaO_2\right)$$

The venous blood oxygen content ($C\bar{v}O_2$) is generally 14–15 mL/dL during resting states yielding an OER of 0.2 to 0.3 (20–30%).

Table 33.10 Effects of clinically relevant doses of commonly administered anesthetic drugs.[a]

Drug	HR	ABP	CO	Cardiac contractile force	MCFP	Vasomotor tone	Baroreceptor reflex activity	Sympathetic nervous system activity	Splanchnic venous capacitance	Venous return
Inhalant anesthetic	↑↓±	↓↓	↓↓	↓	↓↓	↓↓	↓↓	↓↓	↑↑	↓↓
Injectable hypnotic										
Propofol	±↓	↓↓	↓	↓	↓	↓	↓	↓	↑↑	↓↓
Etomidate	±	↓	↓	↓	±↓	±↓	±↓	±↓	↑	±↓
Barbiturate	±↑	±	↓	↓	±↓	↓	↓	↓	↑	↓
Alfaxalone	±↓	↓	↓	±↓	±↓	±↓	↓	↓	↑	↓
Dissociative										
Ketamine	↑	↑	↑±	↑±	–	–	–	–↑	–	–
Tiletamine	↑	↑	↑±	↑±	–	–	–	–↑	–	–
Opioid										
Morphine	↓	–↓	–↓	–↓	–	–	–↓	–↓	–	–↓
Hydromorphone	↓	–↓	–↓	–↓	–	–	–↓	–↓	–	–↓
Fentanyl	↓	–↓	–↓	–↓	–	–	–↓	–↓	–	–↓
α_2-Adrenergic receptor agonist	↓↓	↑→↓	↓↓	–↓	↑→↓	↑→↓	–↓	–	↓→↑	↑→↓
Benzodiazepine										
Diazepam Midazolam	–	–	–↓	–	–↓	–↓	–	–↓	–↓	–↓
Phenothiazine										
Acepromazine	±↓	↓	–↓	–↓	↓	↓	↓	↓	↑	↓
Local anesthetic										
Lidocaine	±↑	↓	–↓	–↓	↓	↓	–	↓	↑	↓

HR, heart rate; ABP, arterial blood pressure; CO, cardiac output; MCFP, mean circulatory filling pressure.
[a]Clinically relevant dosages are generally equal to or less than those recommended by the manufacturer. Idealized effects expected from normal healthy dogs.
↑, increase; ↓, decrease; ±, increase or decrease; –, little or no change; ↑→↓, increase followed by decease; ↓→↑, decrease followed by increase.

Decreased Hb concentration (e.g., parasitism, hemorrhage, and hemodilution) causes OE to increase to maintain the requisite oxygen delivery required by metabolizing tissues. The critical Hb concentration, DO_{2Crit}, and OER_{Crit} are approximately 4 g/dL, 5–7 mL/kg/min, and 0.6 (60%), respectively, in normal healthy dogs (Fig. 33.36) [294,295]. Higher concentrations of most anesthetics, including ketamine, are known to decrease tolerance to anemia and OER in a dose-dependent manner purportedly due to anesthetic-induced blunting of CO and alterations in blood flow distribution among organ systems [296,297]. It is important to recognize that most experimental studies detailing anesthetic drug effects in animals and humans frequently include additional derived or calculated variables (e.g., CO, SVR, stroke work, and MVO_2) that provide additional information regarding drug-related effects. Mathematic coupling occurs when one variable either directly or indirectly contains the whole or components of a second variable [298,299]. This can lead to erroneous results and invalid conclusions in studies involving these derived and/or calculated variables.

Neurohumoral and local control mechanisms

Blood flow is regulated by the integration of supraregional (i.e., CNS), regional, and local factors (Box 33.5). These regulatory elements coordinate immediate and long-term adjustments in total vascular resistance, vascular capacitance, blood volume, blood pressure, and CO. CNS regulation depends on three components: afferent input, central integration and processing, and efferent output [300]. Continuous adjustments in cardiovascular system function and reflex responses help to modulate and buffer changes in blood volume, pressure, and flow in order to sustain oxygen and nutrient delivery to tissues (Fig. 33.37; Box 33.6). The autonomic nervous system exerts a major influence on the regulation of cardiovascular function [301]. Peripheral receptors, including baroreceptors, mechanoreceptors, and chemoreceptors, sense and respond to changes in blood flow, blood pressure, blood volume, and blood-gas tensions. These sensory signals are integrated in "control centers" located in the hypothalamus, pons, and medulla from which a host of neurohumoral responses are elicited. The autonomic nervous system regulates the release of neurotransmitters (e.g., norepinephrine and acetylcholine) that activate adrenergic and cholinergic receptors that modify cardiac performance and vascular tone (Table 33.11). Minute-to-minute changes in blood flow are also regulated by local control mechanisms, which integrate with nervous system activity [302]. Many of the cardiac and vasoactive effects produced by neurotransmitters and circulating substances are mediated by the activation of G-protein-coupled receptors (GPCRs) [303]. GPCRs are transmembrane heterotrimeric G-proteins composed of α, β and γ subunits and are located in the membranes of cardiomyocytes, fibroblasts, endothelial cells, and vascular smooth muscle cells. They convert extracellular signals into intracellular responses and are activated by neurotransmitters, neuropeptides, hormones, glycoproteins, and a variety

Box 33.5 Neurohumoral factors that regulate blood flow, pressure, and volume.

Immediate (short term)

1 Autonomic nervous system (sympathetic and parasympathetic)
Regulate heart rate and vessel tone and capacity
2 Vascular baroreceptor or pressoreceptor reflexes (stretch receptors)
Regulate heart rate and vessel tone and capacity
3 Cardiac stretch receptors
Regulate heart rate and vessel tone and capacity
4 Chemoreceptor reflexes (sense changes in oxygen and carbon dioxide [hydrogen ions])
Regulate heart rate and vessel tone
5 Blood borne (humoral) responses (epinephrine and norepinephrine)
Regulate heart rate, vessel tone, and cardiac contractility
6 Local factors: arteriolar oxygen partial pressure; local metabolites (carbon dioxide, hydrogen ions, and lactate); myogenic autoregulation
Regulate vessel tone to changes in blood pressure in order to maintain tissue blood flow

Intermediate

1 Transcapillary fluid shifts and the lymphatic system
Regulate fluid filtration and reabsorption
2 Hormonal responses (renin–angiotensin–aldosterone system)
Regulate vessel tone and salt and water retention

Long term

1 Oral fluid consumption
Regulate body water and electrolytes
2 Renal control system (vasopressin [ADH], aldosterone, and atrial natriuretic peptide)
Regulate total body water and renal fluid output
3 Hormonal response (i.e., kidney cell erythropoietin release) to low oxygen
Regulate red blood cell production

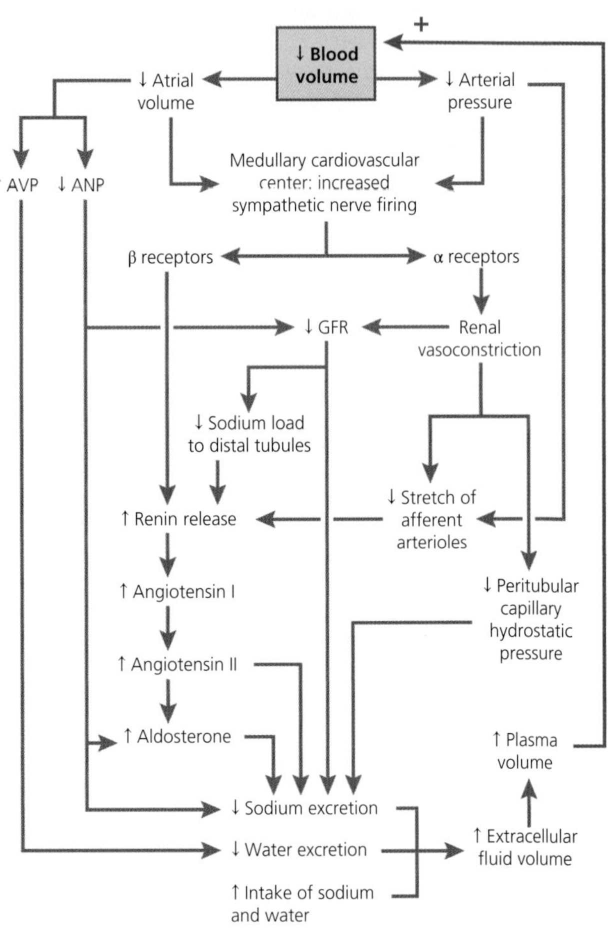

Figure 33.37 Neurohumoral response to a decrease in blood volume. AVP, arginine vasopressin; ANP, atrial natriuretic peptide; GFR, glomerular filtration rate.

Box 33.6 Cardiovascular and pulmonary reflexes and effects.

Abdominocardiac reflex: Mechanical stimulation of the abdominal viscera causes changes in heart rate, usually slowing; rarely causes extrasystoles.

Anrep effect: Increases in aortic pressure results in a positive inotropic effect, augmented resistance to outflow in the heart.

Atrial stretch-receptor reflex: Atrial distension causes the release of atrial natriuretic peptide (ANP) from the atria, resulting in diuretic activity, vasodilation, inhibition, and aldosterone secretion. ANP is an endogenous antagonist of angiotensin II. Sinus and supraventricular tachycardias are common stimuli for this response.

Bainbridge reflex: An increase in heart rate initiated by stretch-sensitive mechanoreceptors in the great veins and right and left atria. The reflex is primarily attributed to an increase in venous return and withdrawal of vagal tone. A **reverse Bainbridge reflex** is used to explain a decrease in heart rate during an acute decrease in venous return.

Baroreceptor reflex (i.e., high-pressure baroreceptor [mechanoreceptor] reflex): Stretch-sensitive mechanoreceptors in the carotid sinus and aortic arch decreases heart rate in response to increases in arterial blood pressure. A decrease in arterial pressure produces hyperventilation, and an increase in arterial blood pressure causes respiratory depression and ultimately apnea.

Bayliss effect: A mechanism by which vessels keep organ blood supply constant. Increased blood pressure induces reactive vasoconstriction thereby limiting increases in blood flow and vice versa.

Bezold–Jarisch reflex: Afferent and efferent pathways in the vagus nerve stimulation of cardiac, primarily ventricular, chemoreceptors or stretch receptors (mechanoreceptors), induce sinus bradycardia, hypotension, and peripheral vasodilation. Stretch of ventricular mechanoreceptors is responsible for syncope when standing.

Branham's sign: Slowing of the heart rate following compression or excision of an arteriovenous fistula (e.g., patent ductus arteriosus ligation).

Chemoreceptor reflex: Systemic hypoxia or hypercarbia cause bradycardia, coronary vasodilation, and systemic vasoconstriction.

Cough reflex: Stimulation of the larynx, trachea, or main bronchi or chemical stimulation throughout the respiratory tree result in cough or endotracheal tube precipitates bradycardia.

Craniocardiac reflex: Stimulation of cranial nerves (olfactory, ophthalmic, and trigeminal), resulting in bradycardia and hypotension (depressor effects).

Cushing reflex: Increases in intracranial pressure result in Cushing's triad (i.e., increasing systolic blood pressure and widened pulse pressure, bradycardia, and irregular respiration) theorized to be caused by increased sympathetic and parasympathetic (i.e., vagal tone) activation form increases in cerebral and peripheral blood pressures, respectively.

Diving reflex (i.e., oxygen-conserving reflex): Stimulation of the trigeminal nerve (i.e., cranial nerve five) by cold temperature, pressure of immersion) causes activation of the vagus nerve and sympathetic chain causing bradycardia, systemic vasoconstriction, and cerebral vasodilation.

Hering–Breuer reflex: Effects of the vagus in the control of respiration – lung inflation arrests inspiration, and lung deflation initiates inspiration

Low-pressure baroreceptor reflex: Low-pressure baroreceptors in the large systemic veins, pulmonary vessels, and walls of the right atrium and ventricles sense changes in wall tension and are involved with the regulation of blood volume. Increases in blood volume increases atrial natriuretic peptide (ANP) and antidiuretic hormone secretion, inhibits constriction of renal arterioles and increases heart rate (see: Bainbridge reflex).

Oculocardiac reflex (Aschner's reflex): Pressure on the eyeball causes bradycardia, vasoconstriction, and cerebral vasodilation

Pulmonary chemoreflex: Stimulation of C-fiber endings (juxtapulmonary capillary receptors [J receptors]) by tissue damage. Fluid accumulation of cytokines produces sinus bradycardia, hypotension, shallow breathing and apnea, bronchoconstriction, and mucous secretion (e.g., isoflurane administration).

Respiratory sinus arrhythmia: Cyclical changes in heart rate coincident with normal respiration. Heart increases during inspiration and decreases during expiration.

Vagovagal reflex: Afferent and efferent pathways in the vagus nerve. Stimulation or irritation of the larynx or trachea by a laryngoscope or endotracheal tube precipitates bradycardia.

Vasovagal reflex (Barcroft–Edholm reflex): Initiated by a decrease in venous return to the heart (e.g., hypovolemia, orthostasis, compression of the inferior vena cava, micturition, increased intrathoracic pressure, and regional analgesia), causing sinus bradycardia and vasodilation. The term has come to include neurocardiogenic syncope, carotid sinus syndrome, and micturition syncope in human patients.

Venorespiratory reflex: Increases in right atrial pressure stimulate increases in respiration.

Table 33.11 Cardiovascular effects of autonomic nervous system activity.

Cardiovascular tissue	Sympathetic		Parasympathetic	
	Primary receptor type	Effect	Primary receptor type	Effect
SA node	β_1	↑ HR	M_2	↓ HR
Atria	β_1	↑ Excitability ↑ Conduction	M_2	↓ Excitability ↓ Conduction
AV node	β_1	↑ Conduction	M_2	↓ Conduction
Ventricle	β_1	↑ Contractility ↑ Excitability ↑ Conduction ↑ Lusitropy	$M_{1\text{-}5}$	Little to no effect
Coronary arteries	β_2	Vasodilation	M_3, M_5 (Endo-NO)	Vasodilation
	α_1, α_2	Vasoconstriction	M_1, M_3 (SM)	Vasoconstriction
Arteries	β_2 α_1, α_2	Vasodilation Vasoconstriction	M_3	Vasodilation
Arterioles	α_1, α_2	Vasoconstriction	M_3	Vasodilation
Large and small veins	β_2 α_1, α_2	Vasodilation Vasoconstriction	M_3	Vasodilation

Muscarinic M_3 receptor subtype mediates cholinergic endothelium-dependent vasodilation and endothelium-independent vasoconstriction. Endo-NO, endothelial nitric oxide; SM, smooth muscle.

of anesthetic drugs including opiates and α_2-adrenergic receptor agonists [303,304]. There are four main classes of G-proteins (i.e., $G\alpha_{stimulatory}$ [$G\alpha_s$], $G\alpha_{inhibitory}$ [$G\alpha_i$], $G\alpha_q$, and $G\alpha_{12/13}$) allowing for diverse signaling transduction functions. Once activated, GPCRs modify the function of a variety of intracellular signaling molecules, enzymes, and ion channels leading to changes in cAMP concentrations and the degree of phosphorylation of proteins that either stimulate or inhibit the activity of effector proteins. The Gαs and Gαi stimulate or depress, respectively, the effector enzyme adenylate cyclase thereby increasing or decreasing the second messenger cAMP, protein kinase A, and phosphorylation of intracellular proteins that regulate cellular responses (Fig. 33.38).

Most anesthetic drugs blunt the neurohormonal and sensory (input), neural integration (processing), and effector (output) mechanisms that control cardiovascular function [305–308]. Inhalation anesthetics in particular blunt compensatory responses to blood loss, trauma, fluid administration and resuscitative drugs (e.g., catecholamines and/or vasopressors) and, when administered in excessive amounts, can totally abolish homeostatic control mechanisms [308–312]. Normally, a decrease in arterial blood pressure in conscious animals (e.g., blood loss, bradycardia, and poor cardiac performance) is sensed by central and peripheral high-pressure

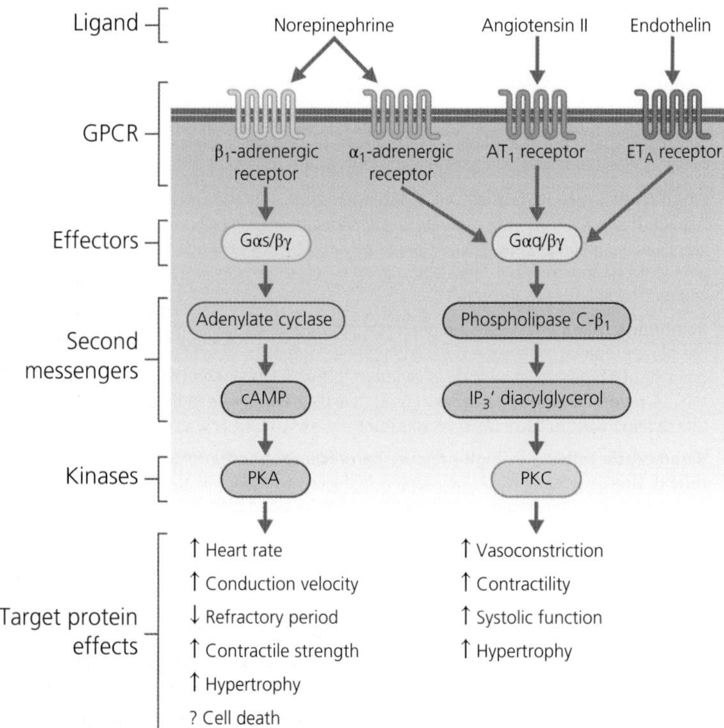

Figure 33.38 Activation of various G-protein-coupled receptors (GPCRs) regulate cardiovascular function through modulation of multiple target proteins. β_1-Adrenerigc receptors function through $G\alpha s/\beta\gamma$, adenylate cyclase, and protein kinase A (PKA). α_1-Adrenergic, angiotensin II type 1 (AT_1), and Endothelin-1 (ET_A) receptors signal through $G\alpha q/\beta\gamma$, phospholipase C-β_1 and protein kinase C (PKC). Norepinephrine also activates α_2-adrenergic receptors that regulate vascular tone. The effects of anesthetic drugs on these neurohumoral signaling systems are unclear and require continued investigation.

vascular receptors (i.e., baroreceptors), which are the most important short-term determinants of arterial blood pressure. Output from these receptors triggers readjustments in CNS autonomic output, which compensates for small changes in arterial blood pressure. Local myogenic autoregulation also helps to protect the brain, heart, liver, mesentery, and skeletal muscle from small changes in blood pressure. If arterial blood pressure is reduced to a point that tissue blood flow is negatively affected, baroreceptor-triggered responses produce increases in HR, cardiac contractility, and vascular tone. Epinephrine and norepinephrine are released from the adrenal gland during severe decreases in mean blood pressure (< 40–60 mmHg) exacerbating these effects. In addition, blood flow is redistributed to the lungs, heart, and brain (i.e., central circulation) and away from the skin, skeletal muscle, kidney, and splanchnic viscera (i.e., from the unstressed vascular volume [V_{us}] to the effective or stressed vascular volume [V_s]) [313]. Similarly, peripheral chemoreceptors sense changes in blood gases (i.e., PO_2, PCO_2) and the acute onset of hypoxemia or hypercarbia (i.e., respiratory acidosis) activates autonomic responses that induce tachycardia and peripheral vasoconstriction.

Neurohormonal mechanisms

Neurohormonal factors, including osmoreceptors in the hypothalamus, antidiuretic hormone released by neurons in the supraoptic and paraventricular nuclei, aldosterone secreted by the adrenal cortex, renin and erythropoietin produced by the kidney, and atrial natriuretic peptide released by stretch-sensitive atrial muscle cells, are all integrally involved in maintaining plasma volume, the production of RBCs, and preserving blood volume (Fig. 33.37) [314,315].

Arterial baroreceptors are stretch receptors (mechanoreceptors) located in the carotid sinus and aortic arch which respond to decreases in arterial blood pressure and the rate of change of blood pressure by incremental increases in the rate of electrical impulses (i.e., baroreceptor reflex). Impulses from the carotid sinus baroreceptors are carried by the carotid sinus and glossopharyngeal nerve (cranial nerve IX), while impulses from the aortic arch are carried by the vagus nerve (cranial nerve X) to the nucleus tractus solitarius in the brain. The signals are processed and initiate an effector response that adjusts parasympathetic and sympathetic outflow returning arterial blood pressure to its normal range. For example, parasympathetic nervous system activity increases and sympathetic nervous system activity decreases when arterial pressure increases above the normal set point. The increased parasympathetic activity to the SA node decreases HR. Simultaneously, decreased sympathetic activity reduces HR and myocardial contractility and results in vasodilation in arterioles and small veins. Baroreceptor activity is minimal at mean arterial blood pressures below 60 mmHg but progressively increases as mean arterial pressure rises above 60 mmHg, reaching a maximum at approximately 180 mmHg. Most baroreceptors have a set point of approximately 100 mmHg. Decreases in arterial blood pressure (P_m < 60 mmHg) decrease the firing rate of the carotid sinus nerve which decreases parasympathetic activity to the heart and increases sympathetic activity to the heart and blood vessels, thereby increasing HR and blood flow, and redistributing blood volume from V_{us} to V_s. Anesthetic drugs interfere with the baroreceptor reflex [316]. Inhalation anesthetics depress normal baroreflex responsiveness and diminish sympathetic output from the CNS [308,309]. The degree of baroreceptor depression depends upon the rate of drug administration and the depth of anesthesia produced.

Low-pressure cardiac mechanoreceptors located in the atria, ventricles, and pulmonary veins help to minimize changes in systemic blood pressure in response to changes in blood volume [314]. These cardiac stretch receptors respond to comparatively small changes in pressure or stretch. The atria contain two types of low-pressure receptors located at the venoatrial junctions. An increase in atrial volume activates both types of atrial mechanoreceptors, sending impulses to the medulla via vagal afferents. Depending on the prevailing HR, arterial blood pressure, and venous return, HR may increase or decrease [317]. Increases in venous return and atrial distension usually cause a withdrawal of vagal tone and enhancement of sympathetic outflow increasing HR (i.e., Bainbridge reflex) and vice versa (i.e., reverse Bainbridge reflex; Box 33.6). Atrial distension also decreases sympathetic output to renal afferent arterioles resulting in vasodilation and decreases in vasopressin (antidiuretic hormone) release, thereby reducing fluid reabsorption in the renal tubular collecting ducts and increasing urine flow. The rapid loss of free water into the urine helps return circulating blood volume to normal values. In addition to these neural responses, atrial natriuretic peptide (ANP) and brain natriuretic peptide (BNP) are released into the bloodstream (Fig. 33.37) [318]. ANP is produced in atrial cardiomyocytes in response to atrial distension and increases sodium excretion by the kidney with an accompanying increase in water loss. BNP has a similar effect to ANP and is produced by ventricular muscle cells in response to increases in myocardial stretch [319].

Ventricular mechanoreceptors located in the ventricular endocardium discharge in parallel with changes in ventricular pressure and produce effects that help to regulate systemic blood pressure and myocardial work. Ventricular distension, however, also stimulates powerful depressor reflexes that decrease HR and peripheral vascular resistance, resulting in bradycardia and hypotension (i.e., Bezold–Jarisch reflex) [320–322]. Impulses initiated by either ventricular distention or the injection of select chemicals (e.g., capsaicin or serotonin) into the coronary arteries can produce the Bezold–Jarisch reflex, which is also called the "coronary chemoreflex" (Box 33.6) [322].

The carotid artery and aortic arch contain specialized sensory chemoreceptors termed the "carotid and aortic bodies" [323]. The carotid and aortic bodies are innervated by the glossopharyngeal (i.e., cranial nerve IX) and vagus (i.e., cranial nerve X) nerves and receive the highest blood flow per gram of tissue weight of any organ within the body. They are sensitive to changes in arterial oxygen tension below 60 mmHg, increases in carbon dioxide tension greater than 45 mmHg, and pH less than 7.30 [323]. They are depressed by hypothermia. Increases in afferent activity from the chemoreceptors increase minute ventilation, restoring arterial blood pH, carbon dioxide, and/or oxygen to normal.

The kidney is the major site for activation of the renin–angiotensin–aldosterone system (RAAS) [324,325]. The RAAS produces peptides that demonstrate autocrine (i.e., on the cells where they are being produced), paracrine (i.e., on neighboring cells), or endocrine (i.e., on a distant organ or tissue via systemic circulation) effects. Renin is produced by the juxtaglomerular cells of the kidney and is secreted into the circulation during hypotension or hypovolemia [324]. This enzyme cleaves angiotensinogen, produced by the liver, to angiotensin I, thereby initiating an enzymatic cascade that generates peptides that regulate blood pressure, cell growth, apoptosis, and electrolyte balance. Angiotensin I is hydrolyzed by angiotensin-converting enzyme (ACE1) producing the octapeptide, angiotensin II. Angiotensin II acts on angiotensin II type 1 and type 2 receptors (i.e., AT1R and AT2R) promoting vasoconstriction, inflammation, salt and water reabsorption, and oxidative stress via AT1R activation [325]. Angiotensin-converting enzyme 2 (ACE2) is expressed in various organ systems including the cardiovascular system, kidneys, lungs, and brain, and exerts important actions to maintain cardiovascular homeostasis. ACE2 activation is the dominant mechanism for counter-regulating the effects of angiotensin II by metabolizing it into the beneficial peptide Angiotensin-(1–7). Angiotensin-(1–7) binds to Mas 1 receptors (i.e., ACE2/Ang-(1–7)/MasR axis) present on cardiomyocytes, cardiac fibroblasts, and endothelial cells limiting the oxidative and inflammatory effects of angiotensin II and producing cardioprotective effects (Fig. 33.39) [326]. The impact of anesthesia and anesthetic drugs on the RAAS and homeostasis requires further investigation [327].

The hypothalamus is directly involved in the hormonal control of cardiovascular responses. Arginine vasopressin (antidiuretic hormone) is produced in the hypothalamus and is transported through nerve cell axons to the posterior pituitary [328,329]. Under normal circumstances, the pituitary releases vasopressin in response to increases in plasma solute (Box 33.5). Vasopressin acts on the collecting ducts of the kidney, where it stimulates water conservation, thereby returning plasma osmolality (and volume) to normal. Vasopressin is a vasoconstrictor, especially in mesenteric vessels; therefore, the presence of circulating vasopressin is influential in

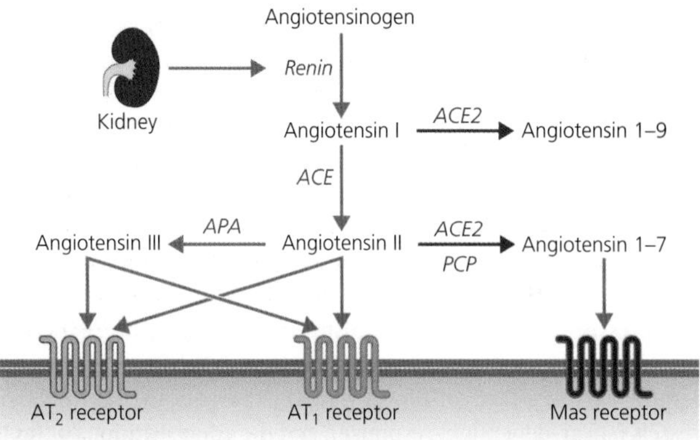

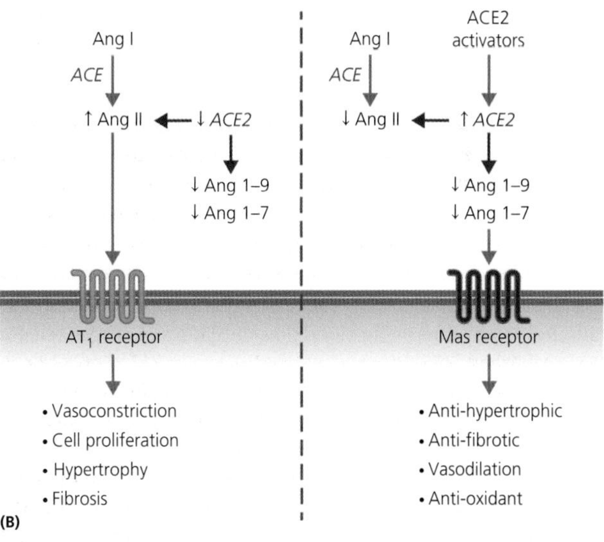

Figure 33.39 Enzymatic cascade of the renin–angiotensin system (RAAS), receptor systems, and the biological effects mediated by angiotensin II (Ang II) and angiotensin-(1–7) (Ang 1–7). **A.** Angiotensinogen is cleaved by renin to Ang I. Ang I is cleaved by angiotensin-converting enzyme (ACE) to Ang II, which is cleaved by ACE2 to Ang 1–7. Ang II acts on angiotensin II type 1 and type 2 receptors: AT_1R, AT_2R. **B.** Ang 1–7 acts on Mas receptors (MasR) and counterbalances AT_1R effects. Decreased ACE2 shifts the balance to the AT_1R resulting in disease. Increased ACE2 (e.g., ACE2 activators) shifts the balance to the Ang 1–7/MasR leading to mitigating disease. APA, aminopeptidase A; PCP, prolyl carboxypeptidase.

Table 33.12 Mechanisms responsible for blood flow control of special circulations[a].

Circulation	Mechanism	Vasoactive metabolites	Mechanical effects
Coronary	Local vasoactive metabolites most important	Hypoxia, adenosine, K^+, H_2O_2, and redox signaling	Reduced blood flow during systole
Cerebral	Local vasoactive metabolites most important	High PCO_2 and H^+	Increased ICP decreases blood flow
Pulmonary	Local vasoactive metabolites most important	Low P_AO_2, endothelin-1 (ET-1), thromboxane, prostacyclin (PGI), nitric oxide (NO)	Lung inflation decreases blood flow
Splanchnic	Local vasoactive metabolites most important	Low PO_2, high PCO_2 and H^+, adenosine, serotonin, histamine, bradykinin, prostaglandins	Abdominal distention decreases blood flow; fluid overload
Renal	Myogenic tone and tubuloglomerular feedback most important	ATP, adenosine, nitric oxide, PGE_2	Fluid overload causes renal impairment and decreased urine output

[a] Sympathetic tone is the most important regulator of skin and skeletal muscle blood flow during resting conditions. ICP, intracranial pressure.

the redistribution of systemic blood flow [330]. Vasopressin release by the pituitary can also occur in the absence of changes in plasma osmolality. Examples of non-osmotic stimuli that cause the release of vasopressin are pain, stress, hypoxia, heart failure, and vascular volume depletion. Some anesthetic drugs are associated with increased circulating levels of arginine vasopressin, including opioids (morphine and meperidine) and barbiturates [328].

Local mechanisms

Autoregulation is the ability of blood vessels to adjust blood flow in accordance with metabolic needs despite changes in tissue perfusion pressure [331–333]. Mechanisms that contribute to changes in vascular tone include responses to intraluminal pressure (myogenic response), the effects of blood flow on the endothelial lining of vessels (shear-dependent response), and the concentrations of metabolic factors on vessels (metabolic response). The myogenic mechanism is a type of autoregulation that responds almost immediately to changes in arterial blood pressure by increasing smooth muscle contraction in response to increases in arterial pressure and vice versa. The vasoconstriction or dilation helps to maintain a constant tissue blood flow. Similarly, increases in blood flow velocity increase wall shear stress and the release of nitric oxide from the vascular endothelium producing vasodilation and vice versa [334]. The metabolic response occurs after longer periods (30 s) of low tissue blood flow. Increases in tissue oxygen demand or decreases in oxygen tension release vasodilatory substances (e.g., CO_2, H^+, K^+) and vasodilatory prostaglandins (e.g., PGI_2) that relax vascular smooth muscle, thereby improving blood flow until normal oxygen tension is reestablished [335].

In summary, vascular tone and tissue perfusion are modulated by host neurogenic, neurohumoral, and local factors that determine tissue blood flow [336–339]. Collectively, these factors determine the number of perfused (RBC-containing) capillaries, known as the "functional capillary density." Whether a given capillary remains open or closed depends on the contractile state of the terminal arterioles located near the entrance to the capillary bed.

Special circulations

Special circulations include those organs that control or modulate their own blood flow using methods that override those described by Poiseuille's law (see section on hemodynamics and cardiac function) [340]. Active hyperemia is the concept that organ blood flow is proportional to metabolic activity and the production of vasodilator metabolites (CO_2, H^+, K^+, lactate, and adenosine). Reactive hyperemia occurs in response to a prior period of decreased blood flow (i.e., ischemia). The coronary, cerebral, pulmonary, and splanchnic circulations are primarily dependent on local metabolic activity for regulation of blood flow while renal blood flow is primarily determined by myogenic tone and tubuloglomerular feedback (Table 33.12). Skin and skeletal muscle blood flow are primarily determined by changes in sympathetic tone. Skin arterioles have a high density of α_1-adrenergic receptors that when activated cause vasoconstriction. It is noteworthy that anesthetic drugs and anesthesia blunt all normal compensatory responses and autoregulatory mechanisms that mobilize and redistribute blood to tissues that are in highest demand. These effects are due to their direct vasodilatory effects and depression of sympathoadrenal activation [160,161,341].

Coronary circulation

The heart has the highest oxygen consumption per tissue mass of all organs in the resting body and receives most of its blood flow during diastole (Fig. 33.40). Myocardial arterial oxygen extraction is 70–80%, compared with 25% for most other organs. The heart receives approximately 5% of the CO and possesses a rich capillary network, three to four times denser than skeletal muscle, to achieve this high extraction [342–346]. Species differences in coronary artery anatomy and its regulation are responsible for different patterns of myocardial perfusion and the heart's response to ischemia [347–349].

Flow across the resting myocardium is usually dependent upon the pressure gradient between the aortic root ("coronary driving pressure") and the right atrium although coronary perfusion pressure in the left ventricle is more accurately determined as the difference between the aortic diastolic pressure and left ventricular end-diastolic pressure. Under normal conditions the driving pressure is fully maintained along epicardial conduit vessels with little pressure loss in the distal epicardial arteries. Intracoronary arterial pressure declines in the microvasculature (< 100 μm) reaching a value of 20–30 mmHg across the capillaries [346]. The majority of coronary blood flow occurs during diastole and decreases by 50% or more during isovolumic contraction in intramyocardial vessels compared to epicardial arteries (Fig. 33.40) [346]. Blood flow resumes during isovolumic relaxation. The primary determinants of resistance to blood flow in the myocardium include extravascular compression of intramural coronary vessels (30–40% of total resistances), the contractile state of the myocardium, and HR [343]. In addition, systolic ventricular torsion also increases coronary

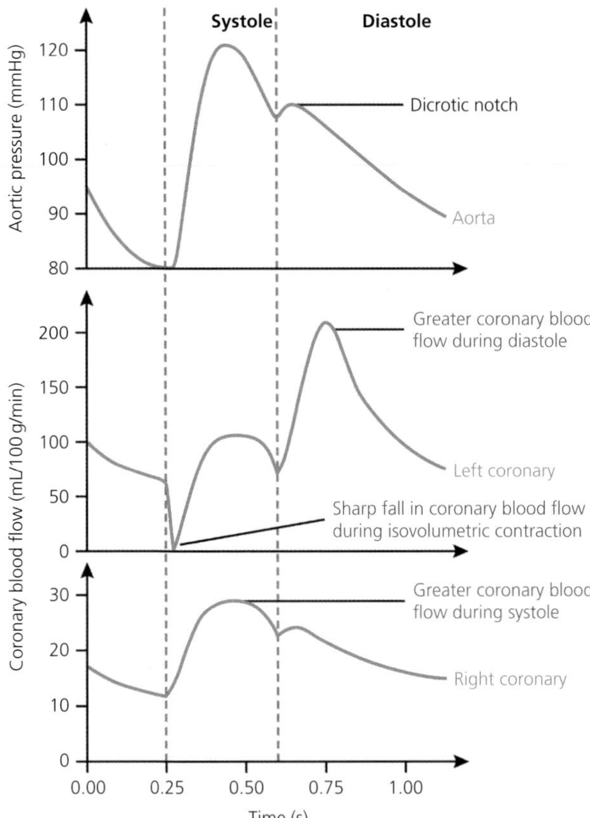

Figure 33.40 Coronary artery blood flow during systole and diastole. Left coronary artery blood flow is greatest during diastole. The right ventricle develops less force so right coronary artery blood flow is greatest during systole. Source: Chambers *et al.* [350], Cambridge University Press.

resistance to a point that systolic flow within the myocardium may be zero or negative during systole.

Coronary blood flow is mainly determined by local metabolic activity, oxygen demand, and HR (Table 33.12) [351]. Autoregulatory myogenic and metabolic mechanisms coordinate the interaction between intracoronary driving pressure and microvascular resistance to maintain adequate flow across capillaries for substrate delivery and metabolite removal. The vascular endothelium is the final common pathway controlling vasomotor tone (coronary autoregulation) and, like all other vessels, nitric oxide production plays a major role [352–353]. Local regulatory mechanisms maintain blood flow within the physiologic range but fail during hypotension when flows become strongly dependent on the driving pressure. Coronary arteries receive their innervation through bilateral vagal (parasympathetic) fibers from the cardiac plexus at the base of the aorta and sympathetic nerves from the stellate ganglion [354]. Factors that lower arterial blood pressure (hypovolemia), increase ventricular diastolic pressure (heart failure), or decrease diastolic time (tachycardia) lower the subendocardial to subepicardial flow ratio predisposing to subendocardial ischemia, ST segment changes, and cardiac arrhythmias. Increases in HR impinge on diastolic time more than systolic time thereby decreasing perfusion time. Anesthesia and anesthetics drugs decrease myocardial perfusion by increasing HR, lowering arterial blood pressure, and impairing ventricular function.

Cerebral circulation

The brain has little capacity for anaerobic metabolism or storing energy and is therefore dependent upon an uninterrupted blood flow. Cerebral autoregulation maintains stable cerebral blood flow during changes in arterial blood pressure (i.e., cerebral perfusion pressure [CPP]) ranging from 50–150 mmHg [355]. Cerebral blood flow (CBF) is dependent on CPP and inversely proportional to cerebrovascular resistance (CVR):

$$\text{CBF} = \text{CPP}/\text{CVR} = (\text{MAP} - \text{ICP})/\text{CVR}$$

where MAP is the mean arterial pressure and ICP is the intracranial pressure. If intracranial pressure is stable, CPP is replaceable by MAP. Both myogenic and local metabolic factors determine CBF, with local metabolic factors being the most important. For example, increases in the arterial partial pressure of carbon dioxide ($PaCO_2$) of 1 mmHg decrease CVR and increase CBF by approximately 3–4%, and vice versa (Table 33.5) [356–358]. Severe hypocapnia can, therefore, markedly increase CVR and decrease CBF, predisposing to brain ischemia. Myogenic tone decreases in response to decreased pressure and vice versa. If CPP increases or decreases, the myogenic reflex results in vasoconstriction or vasodilation, respectively [355]. Cerebral vasoreactivity is also modulated by astrocytes and microglia that secrete neurotransmitters with vasoactive properties [356]. Such neurotransmitters include acetylcholine and nitric oxide that are potent vasodilators, and serotonin and neuropeptide Y that cause vasoconstriction [356]. Endothelial mechanisms also include the cellular secretion of the vasodilator nitric oxide as well as the vasoconstrictors thromboxane A_2 and endothelin-1. Inhalation and dissociative (e.g., ketamine and tiletamine) anesthetics have been demonstrated to increase CBF, while most hypnotics and sedatives (e.g., propofol, alfaxalone, etomidate, and dexmedetomidine) reduce CBF [359].

Pulmonary circulation

The lung is unique among all organs in that it receives the entire CO, contains approximately 10–15% of the total blood volume, and serves as an important blood reservoir stabilizing left ventricular SV and CO (Fig. 33.1) [360,361]. The primary purpose of the pulmonary circulation is gas exchange [362]. The right ventricle and pulmonary circulation buffer dynamic changes in blood volume and flow resulting from respiration, positional changes, and changes in left ventricular CO [360]. This low-pressure system has limited ability to control the regional distribution of blood flow resulting in the potential for the pulmonary capillaries to collapse [363]. Mild increases in pulmonary arterial blood pressure normally distend and recruit pulmonary capillaries, decreasing pulmonary vascular resistance. Pulmonary blood flow is determined by the difference between inflow and outflow pressures unless the surrounding pressure (i.e., alveolar pressure) is greater than the outflow pressure [363]. Pulmonary blood flow, therefore, is often described in terms of a "Starling resistor" where the pressure surrounding a collapsible tube influences the fluid flow through it. Low vascular pressure also predisposes the lung to the so-called "waterfall effect" wherein pulmonary venous pressure may be below alveolar pressure and therefore only intermittently permits blood flow. Pulmonary blood flow is particularly influenced by gravity in larger animals (e.g., adult horses and cattle) resulting in the regional redistribution of pulmonary blood flow during anesthesia [362,363]. Excessive and prolonged inspiratory pressure during anesthesia and mechanical ventilation can markedly reduce or stop pulmonary blood flow leading to marked reductions CO and arterial blood pressure [364].

The bronchial circulation (i.e., bronchial arteries) supplies oxygenated arterial blood to the lung parenchyma. Although physical factors have an important role in determining both pulmonary and bronchial blood flow, local vasoactive metabolites and low alveolar oxygen tension (P_AO_2) determine pulmonary parenchymal blood flow (Table 33.12). Low P_AO_2 produces vasoconstriction of intrapulmonary arteries [365]. Alveolar hypoxia activates mitochondrial sensors increasing the production of reactive oxygen species that depolarize pulmonary artery smooth muscle cells leading to the activation of voltage-gated calcium channels, increases in cytosolic calcium, and vasoconstriction [365]. The primary site of action is in small extra-alveolar vessels. During hypoxic conditions the pulmonary vessels constrict increasing pulmonary arterial pressure [366,367]. This response distends and recruits under-perfused pulmonary vessels effectively shunting blood to better ventilated alveoli and resulting in an improved ventilation–perfusion ratio. Hypoxic pulmonary vasoconstriction (HPV) functions as a negative feedback mechanism for matching ventilation and perfusion and is minimally inhibited by recommended doses of anesthetic drugs, including propofol [368,369].

Splanchnic circulation

The splanchnic circulation includes multiple organs, contains approximately 20% of total blood volume, and receives approximately 25% of the CO (Table 33.8) [370,371]. Splanchnic vessels, particularly veins, are highly compliant and serve as one of the body's largest blood volume reservoirs. Local metabolites regulate tissue perfusion during normal resting conditions (Table 33.12). Splanchnic veins and the spleen, however, also contain a high population of α_1- and α_2-adrenergic receptors that are highly sensitive to adrenergic stimulation [148,150,151,372–374]. For example, the volume of blood that can be mobilized from the spleen, liver, and intestine of hemorrhaged dogs ranges from 6% to 30% of their total blood depending upon the severity of hemorrhage [375]. If arterial blood pressure decreases substantially, sympathoadrenal stimulation causes splanchnic arterial constriction, increasing the pressure in capacitance vessels and expelling splanchnic blood into the systemic circulation [152]. Active mobilization of splanchnic blood volume is almost entirely the result of β_2- and α_1-adrenergic receptor activation [373]. Both β_2- and α_1-adrenergic receptors act in concert to maximally shift blood from the splanchnic vasculature into the systemic circulation by decreasing splanchnic vascular capacitance and intrahepatic vascular resistance [375–377]. These processes deliver blood to the systemic circulation and can effectively compensate for up to 50–60% of lost blood volume. Inhalant and injectable anesthetic drugs including benzodiazepines (e.g., midazolam) blunt the ability of the splanchnic circulation to mobilize blood [378–380]. This effect may be more important than the arterial vasodilatory or negative cardiac inotropic effects of anesthetic drugs when considering the potential causes for arterial hypotension and/or low CO during anesthesia.

Renal circulation

Myogenic tone and tubuloglomerular feedback are the two most important mechanisms that regulate renal blood flow during resting conditions (Table 33.12) [381,382]. Increases in arterial blood pressure stretch smooth muscle cells in the walls of afferent arterioles perfusing the glomerulus causing them to contract, thereby increasing vascular resistance and minimizing a change in glomerular blood flow. Decreases in arterial blood pressure cause the smooth muscle cells to relax, decreasing vascular resistance and maintaining blood flow.

The juxtaglomerular apparatus is a specialized structure formed by the glomerular afferent arteriole and the distal convoluted tubule. Renin is the key regulator of the renin–angiotensin–aldosterone system and is critically involved in salt, volume, and blood pressure homeostasis. Renin is mainly produced and released into the circulation by juxtaglomerular epithelioid cells (i.e., macula densa) located in the walls of the distal nephron and constricts renal afferent arterioles as they enter the glomerular capillary network [382]. Elevated sodium concentration in the distal tubule triggers the macula densa to release ATP and adenosine that stimulates the juxtaglomerular cells of the afferent arteriole to contract, thereby decreasing glomerular blood flow and filtration rate, and vice versa. The vasodilator, nitric oxide, modulates this response [383]. Changes in sympathetic tone also modulate renal blood flow during resting conditions. Increases in sympathetic tone reduce renal blood flow, filtrate formation, and urine output while decreases in sympathetic tone result in vasodilation, increased blood flow, and increased urine output.

References

1 Reiber CL, McGaw IJ. A review of the 'open' and 'closed' circulatory systems: new terminology for complex invertebrate circulatory systems in light of current findings. *Int J Zool* 2009: 1–8.

2 Hicks JW. The physiological and evolutionary significance of cardiovascular shunting patterns in reptiles. *News Physiol Sci* 2002; **17**: 241–245.

3 Moore JE Jr., Bertram CD. Lymphatic system flows. *Annu Rev Fluid Mech* 2018; **50**: 459–482.

4 Kik MJL, Mitchell MA. Reptile cardiology: a review of anatomy and physiology, diagnostic approaches, and clinical disease. *Semin Avian Exot Pet Med* 2005; **14**: 52–60.

5 Girling SJ, Hynes B. Cardiovascular and haemopoietic systems. In: Girling SJ, Raiti P, eds. *BSAVA Manual of Reptiles*, 2nd edn. Quedgeley, Gloucester, UK: BSAVA, 2004: 243–260.

6 Holz PH. Anatomy and physiology of the reptile renal portal system. *Vet Clin Exotic Am Pract* 2020; **23**(1): 103–114.

7 Holz PH, Burger JP, Pasloske K, *et al.* Effect of injection site on carbenicillin pharmacokinetics in the carpet python, *Morelia spilota. J Herp Med Surg* 2002; **12**(4): 12–16.

8 Yasuda N, Targ AG, Eger EI, *et al.* Pharmacokinetics of desflurane, sevoflurane, isoflurane, and halothane in pigs. *Anesth Analg* 1990; **71**(4): 340–348.

9 Huntington JH, Malviya S, Voepel-Lewis T, *et al.* The effect of a right-to-left intracardiac shunt on the rate of rise of arterial and end-tidal halothane in children. *Anesth Analg* 1999; **88**(4): 759–762.

10 Stanley WC, Recchia FA, Lopaschuk GD. Myocardial substrate metabolism in the normal and failing heart. *Physiol Rev* 2005; **85**(3): 1093–1129.

11 Opie LH. Fuels. Aerobic and anaerobic metabolism. In: Opie LH, ed. *Heart Physiology: From Cell to Circulation*, 4th edn. Philadelphia, PA; Lippincott Williams & Wilkins, 2004: 306–354.

12 Opie LH. Channels, pumps, and exchangers. In: Opie LH, ed. *Heart Physiology: From Cell to Circulation*, 4th edn. Philadelphia, PA: Lippincott Williams & Wilkins, 2004: 73–118.

13 Kléber AG, Rudy Y. Basic mechanisms of cardiac impulse propagation and associated arrhythmias. *Physiol Rev* 2004; **84**(2): 431–488.

14 Nattel S, Carlsson L. Innovative approaches to anti-arrhythmic drug therapy. *Nat Rev Drug Discov* 2006; **5**(12): 1034–1049.

15 Grant AO. Cardiac ion channels. *Circ Arrhythm Electrophysiol* 2009; **2**(2): 185–194.

16 Starmer CF, Grant AO, Strauss HC. Mechanisms of use-dependent block of sodium channels in excitable membranes by local anesthetics. *Biophys J* 1984; **46**(1): 15–27.

17 Scholz A. Mechanisms of (local) anaesthetics on voltage-gated sodium and other ion channels. *Br J Anaesth* 2002; **89**(1): 52–61.

18 Hauneke R, Fassl J, Rossiant R, *et al.* Effects of volatile anesthetics on cardiac ion channels. *Anaesthesiol* 2004; **48**: 547–561.

19 Booker PD, Whyte SD, Ladusans EJ. Long QT syndrome and anaesthesia. *Br J Anaesth* 2003; **90**(3): 349–366.

20 Behzadi M, Joukar S, Beik A. Opioids and cardiac arrhythmia: a literature review. *Med Princ Pract* 2018; **27**(5): 401–414.

21 Krantz MJ, Mehler PS. Synthetic opioids and QT prolongation. *Arch Intern Med* 2003; **163**(13): 1615.

22 Ehret GB, Desmeules JA, Broers B. Methadone-associated long QT syndrome: improving pharmacotherapy for dependence on illegal opioids and lessons learned for pharmacology. *Expert Opin Drug Saf* 2007; **6**(3): 289–303.

23 Carmeliet E. Conduction in cardiac tissue. *Historical reflections. Physiol Rep* 2019; **7**(1): e13860.

24 Burt JM, Spray DC. Volatile anesthetics block intercellular communication between neonatal rat myocardial cells. *Circ Res* 1989; **65**: 829–836.

25 Turner LA, Polic S, Hoffmann RG, *et al.* Actions of volatile anesthetics on ischemic and nonischemic Purkinje fibers in the canine heart: regional action potential characteristics. *Anesth Analg* 1993; **76**(4): 726–733.

26 Weigt HU, Kwok WM, Rehmert GC, *et al.* Voltage-dependent effects of volatile anesthetics on cardiac sodium current. *Anesth Analg* 1997; **84**(2): 285–293.

27 The 'Sicilian Gambit'. A new approach to the classification of antiarrhythmic drugs based on their actions on arrhythmogenic mechanisms. The Task Force of the Working Group on Arrhythmias of the European Society of Cardiology. *Eur Heart J* 1991; **12**(10): 1112–1131.

28 Dhein S, Seidel T, Salameh A, *et al.* Remodeling of cardiac passive electrical properties and susceptibility to ventricular and atrial arrhythmias. *Front Physiol* 2014; **5**: 424.

29 Osadchii OE. Role of abnormal repolarization in the mechanism of cardiac arrhythmia. *Acta Physiol (Oxf)* 2017; **220**(Suppl 712): 1–71.

30 Vetulli HM, Elizari MV, Naccarelli GV, *et al.* Cardiac automaticity: basic concepts and clinical observations. *J Interv Card Electrophysiol* 2018; **52**(3): 263–270.

31 DiFrancesco D. The role of the funny current in pacemaker activity. *Circ Res* 2010; **106**(3): 434–446.

32 Noble D, Noble SJ. A model of sino-atrial node electrical activity based on a modification of the DiFrancesco-Noble (1984) equations. *Proc R Soc Lond B Biol Sci* 1984; **222**(1228): 295–304.

33 Petite SE, Bishop BM, Mauro VF. Role of the funny current inhibitor ivabradine in cardiac pharmacotherapy: a systematic review. *Am J Ther* 2018; **25**(2): e247–e266.

34 Robertson D, Goldberg MR, Tung CS, *et al.* Use of alpha 2 adrenoreceptor agonists and antagonists in the functional assessment of the sympathetic nervous system. *J Clin Invest* 1986; **78**(2): 576–581.

35 Congdon JM, Marquez M, Niyom S, *et al.* Evaluation of the sedative and cardiovascular effects of intramuscular administration of dexmedetomidine with and without concurrent atropine administration in dogs. *J Am Vet Med Assoc* 2011; **239**(1): 81–89.

36 Antzelevitch C, Shimizu W, Yan GX, *et al.* The M cell: its contribution to the ECG and to normal and abnormal electrical function of the heart. *J Cardiovasc Electrophysiol* 1999; **10**(8): 1124–1152.

37 Lukas A. Electrophysiology of myocardial cells in the epicardial, midmyocardial, and endocardial layers of the ventricle. *J Cardiovasc Pharmacol Ther* 1997; **2**(1): 61–72.

38 Spach MS, Dolber PC. Discontinuous anisotropic propagation. In: Rosen MR, Janse MJ, Wit AL, eds. *Cardiac Electrophysiology: A Textbook*. Mount Kisco, NY: Futura, 1990: 517–534.

39 Spach MS, Dolber PC, Heidlage JF. Influence of the passive anisotropic properties on directional differences in propagation following modification of the sodium conductance in human atrial muscle. A model of reentry based on anisotropic discontinuous propagation. *Circ Res* 1988; **62**(4): 811–832.

40 Kléber AG. ST-segment elevation in the electrocardiogram: a sign of myocardial ischemia. *Cardiovasc Res* 2000; **45**(1): 111–118.

41 di Bernardo D, Murray A. Origin on the electrocardiogram of U-waves and abnormal U-wave inversion. *Cardiovasc Res* 2002; **53**(1): 202–208.

42 Staikou C, Stamelos M, Stavroulakis E. Impact of anaesthetic drugs and adjuvants on ECG markers of torsadogenicity. *Br J Anaesth* 2014; **112**(2): 217–230.

43 Hayashi Y, Kamibayashi T, Sumikawa K, *et al.* Adrenoceptor mechanism involved in thiopental-epinephrine-induced arrhythmias in dogs. *Am J Physiol* 1993; **265**(4 Pt 2): H1380–H1385.

44 Kamibayashi T, Hayashi Y, Sumikawa K, *et al.* Enhancement by propofol of epinephrine-induced arrhythmias in dogs. *Anesthesiology* 1991; **75**(6): 1035–1040.

45 Bednarski RM, Majors LJ. Ketamine and the arrhythmogenic dose of epinephrine in cats anesthetized with halothane and isoflurane. *Am J Vet Res* 1986; **47**(10): 2122–2125.

46 Cárceles MD, Laorden ML, Hernandez J, *et al.* Halothane, isoflurane and enflurane potentiate the effect of noradrenaline on ventricular automaticity in the rat heart: evidence of the involvement of both alpha- and beta-adrenoceptors. *J Pharm Pharmacol* 1990; **42**(3): 186–190.

47 Kulier AH, Turner LA, Vodanovic S, *et al.* Multiple agents potentiate alpha1-adrenoceptor-induced conduction depression in canine cardiac purkinje fibers. *Anesthesiology* 2000; **92**(6): 1713–1721.

48 Himmel HM. Mechanisms involved in cardiac sensitization by volatile anesthetics: general applicability to halogenated hydrocarbons? *Crit Rev Toxicol* 2008; **38**: 773–803.

49 Batchvarov VN, Behr ER. QRS-ST-T triangulation with repolarization shortening as a precursor of sustained ventricular tachycardia during acute myocardial ischemia. *J Arrhythm* 2015; **31**(2): 118–120.

50 Hondeghem LM. Relative contributions of TRIaD and QT to proarrhythmia. *J Cardiovasc Electrophysiol* 2007; **18**(6): 655–657.

51 Roden DM. Predicting drug-induced QT prolongation and torsades de pointes. *J Physiol* 2016; **594**(9): 2459–2468.

52 Bentzen BH, Grunnet M. Central and peripheral GABA(A) receptor regulation of the heart rate depends on the conscious state of the animal. *Adv Pharmacol Sci* 2011; **2011**: 578273.

53 Etaee F, Tobin M, Vuppala S, *et al.* Effects of opioid receptor agonist and antagonist medications on electrocardiogram changes and presentation of cardiac arrhythmia: review article. *J Interv Card Electrophysiol* 2022; **63**(2): 471–500.

54 Bujubasic N, Marijic J, Berczi V, *et al.* Differential effects of etomidate, propofol and midazolam on calcium and potassium channel currents in canine myocardial cells. *Anesthesiology* 1996; **85**: 1092–1099.

55 Hatakeyama N, Ito Y, Momose Y. Effects of sevoflurane, isoflurane, and halothane on mechanical and electrophysiologic properties of canine myocardium. *Anesth Analg* 1993; **76**(6): 1327–1332.

56 Bers DM. Cardiac excitation–contraction coupling. *Nature* 2002; **415**(6868): 198–205.

57 Opie LH. Excitation–contraction coupling and calcium. In: Opie LH, ed. *Heart Physiology: From Cell to Circulation*, 4th edn. Philadelphia, PA: Lippincott Williams & Wilkins, 2004: 159–185.

58 Greenstein JL, Winslow RL. Integrative systems models of cardiac excitation–contraction coupling. *Circ Res* 2011; **108**(1): 70–84.

59 Eisner DA. Caldwell JL, Kistamás K, *et al.* Calcium and excitation–contraction coupling in the heart. *Circ Res* 2017; **121**: 181–195.

60 Laver DR. Ca2+ stores regulate ryanodine receptor Ca2+ release channels via luminal and cytosolic Ca2+ sites. *Clin Exp Pharmacol Physiol* 2007; **34**(9): 889–896.

61 Diaz-Sylvester PL, Porta M, Copello JA. Halothane modulation of skeletal muscle ryanodine receptors: dependence on Ca2+, Mg2+, and ATP. *Am J Physiol Cell Physiol* 2008; **294**(4): C1103–C1112.

62 Cieniewicz A, Trzebicki J, Mayzner-Zawadzka E, *et al.* Malignant hyperthermia – what do we know in 2019? *Anaesthesiol Intensive Ther* 2019; **51**: 69–177.

63 Hund TJ, Ziman AP, Lederer WJ, *et al.* The cardiac IP3 receptor: uncovering the role of 'the other' calcium-release channel. *J Mol Cell Cardiol* 2008; **45**(2): 159–161.

64 Bosnjak ZJ. Cardiac effects of anesthetics. In: Blanck TJJ, Wheeler DM, eds. *Mechanisms of Anesthetic Action in Skeletal, Cardiac and Smooth Muscles*. New York, NY: Plenum Press, 1991: 91–98.

65 Bosnjak ZJ, Supan FD, Rusch NJ. The effects of halothane, enflurane, and isoflurane on calcium current in isolated canine ventricular cells. *Anesthesiology* 1991; **74**(2): 340–345.

66 Zhou W, Fontenot JH, Liu S, *et al.* Modulation of cardiac calcium channels by propofol. *Anesthesiology* 1997; **86**: 670–675.

67 Hobai IA. Anesthetics, the ryanodine receptors, and the heart. *Anesthesiology* 2017; **126**: 373–375.

68 Trivedi DV, Nag S, Spudich A, *et al.* The myosin family of mechanoenzymes: from mechanisms to therapeutic approaches. *Annu Rev Biochem* 2020; **89**: 667–693.

69 Kawas RF, Anderson RL, Ingle SRB, *et al.* A small-molecule modulator of cardiac myosin acts on multiple stages of the myosin chemomechanical cycle. *J Biol Chem* 2017; **292**(40): 16571–16577.

70 Batters C, Veigel C, Homsher E, *et al.* To understand muscle you must take it apart. *Front Physiol* 2014; **5**: 90.

71 Nikitina LV, Kopylova GV, Shchepkin DV, *et al.* Investigations of molecular mechanisms of actin–myosin interactions in cardiac muscle. *Biochem (Mosc)* 2015; **80**(13): 1748–1763.

72 Reiser PJ, Portman MA, Ning XH, *et al.* Human cardiac myosin heavy chain isoforms in fetal and failing adult atria and ventricles. *Am J Physiol Heart Circ Physiol* 2001; **280**(4): H1814–H1820.

73 Gibbs CL. Cardiac energetics and the Fenn effect. *Basic Res Cardiol* 1987; **82**(Suppl 2): 61–68.

74 Nagayama T, Takimoto E, Sadayappan S, *et al.* Control of in vivo left ventricular [correction] contraction/relaxation kinetics by myosin-binding protein C: protein kinase A phosphorylation dependent and independent regulation. *Circulation* 2007; **116**(21): 2399–2408.

75 Heling LWHJ, Geeves MA, Kad NM. MyBP-C: one protein to govern them all. *J Muscle Res Cell Motil* 2020; **41**(1): 91–101.

76 Rüegg C, Veigel C, Molloy JE, *et al.* Molecular motors: force and movement generated by single myosin II molecules. *News Physiol Sci* 2002; **17**: 213–218.

77 Squire JM. Muscle myosin filaments: cores, crowns and couplings. *Biophys Rev* 2009; **1**(3): 149.

78 Anderson RL, Trivedi DV, Sarkar SS, *et al.* Deciphering the super relaxed state of human β-cardiac myosin and the mode of action of mavacamten from myosin molecules to muscle fibers. *Proc Natl Acad Sci USA* 2018; **115**(35): E8143–E8152.

79 McNamara JW, Li A, Dos Remedios CG, *et al.* The role of super-relaxed myosin in skeletal and cardiac muscle. *Biophys Rev* 2015; **7**(1): 5–14.

80 Alamo L, Ware JS, Pinto A, *et al.* Effects of myosin variants on interacting-heads motif explain distinct hypertrophic and dilated cardiomyopathy phenotypes. *Elife* 2017; **6**: e24634.

81 Sweeney HL, Holzbaur ELF. Motor proteins. *Cold Spring Harb Perspect Biol* 2018; **10**(5): a021931.

82 Kampourakis T, Ponnam S, Sun YB, *et al.* Structural and functional effects of myosin-binding protein-C phosphorylation in heart muscle are not mimicked by serine-to-aspartate substitutions. *J Biol Chem* 2018; **293**(37): 14270–14275.

83 McNamara JW, Singh RR, Sadayappan S. Cardiac myosin binding protein-C phosphorylation regulates the super-relaxed state of myosin. *Proc Natl Acad Sci USA* 2019; **116**(24): 11731–11736.

84 Janssen PML. Myocardial relaxation in human heart failure: why sarcomere kinetics should be center-stage. *Arch Biochem Biophys* 2019; **661**: 145–148.

85 Tang W, Yengo CM. Inter-filament co-operativity is crucial for regulating muscle contraction. *J Physiol* 2018; **596**(1): 17–18.

86 Landesberg A, Livshitz L, Ter Keurs HE. The effect of sarcomere shortening velocity on force generation, analysis, and verification of models for crossbridge dynamics. *Ann Biomed Eng* 2000; **28**(8): 968–978.

87 Liu C, Kawana M, Song D, *et al.* Controlling load-dependent kinetics of β-cardiac myosin at the single-molecule level. *Nat Struct Mol Biol* 2018; **25**(6): 505–514.

88 Houdusse A, Sweeney HL. How myosin generates force on actin filaments. *Trends Biochem Sci* 2016; **41**(12): 989–997.

89 Sequeira V, van der Velden J. Historical perspective on heart function: the Frank–Starling Law. *Biophys Rev* 2015; 7(4): 421–447.

90 Piazzesi G, Caremani M, Linari M, *et al.* Thick filament mechano-sensing in skeletal and cardiac muscles: a common mechanism able to adapt the energetic cost of the contraction to the task. *Front Physiol* 2018; **9**: 736.

91 Sweeney HL, Houdusse A, Robert-Paganin J. Myosin structures. *Adv Exp Med Biol* 2020; **1239**: 7–19.

92 Katz AM. Structure, biochemistry, and biophysics; the contractile proteins. In: Katz AM, ed. *Physiology of the Heart*, 5th edn. Philadelphia, PA: Lippincott Williams & Wilkins, 2011: 88–106.

93 Fujita K, Ohmachi M, Ikezaki K, *et al.* Direct visualization of human myosin II force generation using DNA origami-based thick filaments. *Commun Biol* 2019; **2**: 437.

94 Opie LH. Myocardidal contraction and relaxation. In: Opie LH, ed. *Heart Physiology: From Cell to Circulation*, 4th edn. Philadelphia, PA: Lippincott Williams & Wilkins, 2004: 221–246.

95 Muir WW, Hamlin RL. Myocardial contractility: historical and contemporary considerations. *Front Physiol* 2020; **11**: 222.

96 Toepfer CN, West TG, Ferenczi MA. Revisiting Frank–Starling: regulatory light chain phosphorylation alters the rate of force redevelopment (ktr) in a length-dependent fashion. *J Physiol* 2016; **594**(18): 5237–5254.

97 Sevrieva IR, Brandmeier B, Ponnam S, *et al.* Cardiac myosin regulatory light chain kinase modulates cardiac contractility by phosphorylating both myosin regulatory light chain and troponin I. *J Biol Chem* 2020; **295**(14): 4398–4410.

98 Eisner DA, Caldwell JL, Trafford AW, *et al.* The control of diastolic calcium in the heart: basic mechanisms and functional implications. *Circ Res* 2020; **126**(3): 395–412.

99 Scranton K, John S, Escobar A, *et al.* Modulation of the cardiac Na^+-Ca^{2+} exchanger by cytoplasmic protons: molecular mechanisms and physiological implications. *Cell Calcium* 2020; **87**: 102140.

100 Stammers AN, Susser SE, Hamm NC, *et al.* The regulation of sarco(endo)plasmic reticulum calcium-ATPases (SERCA). *Can J Physiol Pharmacol* 2015; **93**(10): 843–854.

101 Gelissen HP, Epema AH, Henning RH, *et al.* Inotropic effects of propofol, thiopental, midazolam, etomidate, and ketamine on isolated human atrial muscle. *Anesthesiology* 1996; **84**(2): 397–403.

102 Blanck TJ, Chiancone E, Salviati G, *et al.* Halothane does not alter Ca2+ affinity of troponin C. *Anesthesiology* 1992; **76**(1): 100–105.

103 Meng T, Bu W, Ren X, *et al.* Molecular mechanism of anesthetic-induced depression of myocardial contraction. *FASEB J* 2016; **30**(8): 2915–2925.

104 Haworth RA, Goknur AB. Inhibition of sodium/calcium exchange and calcium channels of heart cells by volatile anesthetics. *Anesthesiology* 1995; **82**(5): 1255–1265.

105 Kongsayreepong S, Cook DJ, Housmans PR. Mechanism of the direct, negative inotropic effect of ketamine in isolated ferret and frog ventricular myocardium. *Anesthesiology* 1993; **79**(2): 313–322.

106 Pagel PS, Kampine JP, Schmeling WT, *et al.* Reversal of volatile anesthetic-induced depression of myocardial contractility by extracellular calcium also enhances left ventricular diastolic function. *Anesthesiology* 1993; **78**(1): 141–154.

107 Rusy BF, Komai H. Anesthetic depression of myocardial contractility: a review of possible mechanisms. *Anesthesiology* 1987; **67**(5): 745–766.

108 Lynch C III, Frazer MJ. Depressant effects of volatile anesthetics upon rat and amphibian ventricular myocardium: insights into anesthetic mechanisms of action. *Anesthesiology* 1989; **70**(3): 511–522.

109 Schmidt U, Schwinger RH, Böhm S, *et al.* Evidence for an interaction of halothane with the L-type Ca2+ channel in human myocardium. *Anesthesiology* 1993; **79**(2): 332–339.

110 Wilde DW, Davidson BA, Smith MD, *et al.* Effects of isoflurane and enflurane on intracellular Ca2+ mobilization in isolated cardiac myocytes. *Anesthesiology* 1993; **79**(1): 73–82.

111 Humphrey LS, Stinson DC, Humphrey MJ, *et al.* Volatile anesthetic effects on left ventricular relaxation in swine. *Anesthesiology* 1990; **73**(4): 731–738.

112 Constable P, Muir W III, Sisson D. Clinical assessment of left ventricular relaxation. *J Vet Intern Med* 1999; **13**(1): 5–13.

113 Guven G, Hilty MP, Ince C. Microcirculation: physiology, pathophysiology, and clinical application. *Blood Purif* 2020; **49**(1–2): 143–150.

114 Shepard JT, Vanhoutte P. Components of the cardiovascular system: how structure is geared to function. In: Shepard JT, Vanhoutte P, eds. *The Human Cardiovascular System: Facts and Concepts*. New York, NY: Raven, 1979: 5–8.

115 Westerhof N, Lankhaar JW, Westerhof BE. The arterial Windkessel. *Med Biol Eng Comput* 2009; **47**(2): 131–141.

116 Reines BP, Ninham BW. Structure and function of the endothelial surface layer: unraveling the nanoarchitecture of biological surfaces. *Q Rev Biophys* 2019; **52**: e13.

117 Gaudette S, Hughes D, Boller M. The endothelial glycocalyx: structure and function in health and critical illness. *J Vet Emerg Crit Care (San Antonio)* 2020; **30**(2): 117–134.

118 Jedlicka J, Becker BF, Chappell D. Endothelial glycocalyx. *Crit Care Clin* 2020; **36**(2): 217–232.

119 Levick JR, Michel CC. Microvascular fluid exchange and the revised Starling principle. *Cardiovasc Res* 2010; **87**(2): 198–210.

120 Woodcock TE, Woodcock TM. Revised Starling equation and the glycocalyx model of transvascular fluid exchange: an improved paradigm for prescribing intravenous fluid therapy. *Br J Anaest* 2012; **108**(3): 384–394.

121 Chappell D, Westphal M, Jacob M. The impact of the glycocalyx on microcirculatory oxygen distribution in critical illness. *Curr Opin Anaesthesiol* 2009; **22**(2): 155–162.

122 Rodrigues SF, Granger DN. Role of blood cells in ischaemia-reperfusion induced endothelial barrier failure. *Cardiovasc Res* 2010; **87**(2): 291–299.

123 Kundra P, Goswami S. Endothelial glycocalyx: role in body fluid homeostasis and fluid management. *Indian J Anaesth* 2019; **63**(1): 6–14.

124 Green JR. Circulatory mechanics. In: *Fundamental Cardiovascular and Pulmonary Physiology*, 2nd edn. Philadelphia, PA: Lea and Febiger, 1987: 59–80.

125 Waghmare LS, Srivastava TK. Conceptualizing physiology of arterial blood pressure regulation through the logic model. *Adv Physiol Educ* 2016; **40**(4): 477–479.

126 Voets T, Nilius B. TRPCs, GPCRs and the Bayliss effect. *EMBO J* 2009; **28**(1): 4–5.

127 Roosterman D, Goerge T, Schneider SW, *et al.* Neuronal control of skin function: the skin as a neuroimmunoendocrine organ. *Physiol Rev* 2006; **86**(4): 1309–1379.

128 Molyneux GS, Haller CJ, Mogg K, *et al.* The structure, innervation and location of arteriovenous anastomoses in the equine foot. *Equine Vet J* 1994; **26**(4): 305–312.

129 Lawrence CJ, Prinzen FW, de Lange S. The effect of dexmedetomidine on nutrient organ blood flow. *Anesth Analg* 1996; **83**(6): 1160–1165.

130 Woodcock TE, Michel CC. Advances in the Starling principle and microvascular fluid exchange; consequences and implications for fluid therapy. *Front Vet Sci* 2021; **8**: 623671.

131 Dull RO, Chignalia AZ. The glycocalyx and pressure-dependent transcellular albumin transport. *Cardiovasc Eng Technol* 2020; **11**(6): 655–662.

132 Sarin H. Physiologic upper limits of pore size of different blood capillary types and another perspective on the dual pore theory of microvascular permeability. *J Angiogenes Res* 2010; **2**: 14.

133 Verkman AS. Aquaporins in clinical medicine. *Annu Rev Med* 2012; **63**: 303–316.

134 Yang WC, Zhou LJ, Zhang R, *et al.* Effects of propofol and sevoflurane on aquaporin-4 and aquaporin-9 expression in patients performed gliomas resection. *Brain Res* 2015; **1622**: 1–6.

135 Demirgan S, Akyol O, Temel Z, *et al.* Isoflurane exposure in infant rats acutely increases aquaporin 4 and does not cause neurocognitive impairment. *Bosn J Basic Med Sci* 2019; **19**(3): 257–264.

136 Starling EH. On the absorption of fluids from the connective tissue spaces. *J Physiol* 1896; **19**: 312–326.

137 Landis EM. Microinjection studies of capillary permeability. II. The relation between capillary pressure and the rate of which fluid passes through the walls of single capillaries. *Am J Physiol* 1927; **82**(2): 217–238.
138 Pappenheimer JR, Soto-Rivera A. Effective osmotic pressure of the plasma proteins and other quantities associated with the capillary circulation in the hindlimbs of cats and dogs. *Am J Physiol* 1948; **152**(3): 471–491.
139 Taylor AE. Capillary fluid filtration. Starling forces and lymph flow. *Circ Res* 1981; **49**(3): 557–575.
140 Reed RK, Rubin K. Transcapillary exchange: role and importance of the interstitial fluid pressure and the extracellular matrix. *Cardiovasc Res* 2010; **87**(2): 211–217.
141 Woodcock TA. Plasma volume, tissue oedema, and the steady-state Starling principle. *BJA Educ* 2017; **17**(2): 74–78.
142 Dull RO, Hahn RG. Transcapillary refill: the physiology underlying fluid reabsorption. *J Trauma Acute Care Surg* 2021; **90**(2): e31–e39.
143 Becker BF, Chappell D, Bruegger D, *et al.* Therapeutic strategies targeting the endothelial glycocalyx: acute deficits, but great potential. *Cardiovasc Res* 2010; **87**(2): 300–310.
144 Eschalier A, Lavarenne J, Burtin C, *et al.* Study of histamine release induced by acute administration of antitumor agents in dogs. *Cancer Chemother Pharmacol* 1988; **21**(3): 246–250.
145 Robinson EP, Faggella AM, Henry DP, *et al.* Comparison of histamine release induced by morphine and oxymorphone administration in dogs. *Am J Vet Res* 1988; **49**: 1699–1701.
146 Lorenz W, Schmal A, Schult H, *et al.* Histamine release and hypotensive reactions in dogs by solubilizing agents and fatty acids: analysis of various components in cremophor El and development of a compound with reduced toxicity. *Agents Actions* 1982; **12**(1–2): 64–80.
147 Jacobs R, Jonckheer J, Malbrain M. Fluid overload FADEs away! Time for fluid stewardship. *J Crit Care* 2018; **48**: 458–461.
148 Hainsworth R. Vascular capacitance: its control and importance. *Rev Physiol Biochem Pharmacol* 1986; **105**: 101–173.
149 Caggiati A, Phillips M, Lametschwandtner A, *et al.* Valves in small veins and venules. *Eur J Vasc Endovasc Surg* 2006; **32**(4): 447–452.
150 Elsner D, Stewart DJ, Sommer O, *et al.* Postsynaptic alpha 1- and alpha 2-adrenergic receptors in adrenergic control of capacitance vessel tone in vivo. *Hypertension* 1986; **8**(11): 1003–1014.
151 Noble BJ, Drinkhill MJ, Myers DS, *et al.* Reflex control of splanchnic blood volume in anaesthetized dogs. *J Physiol* 1998; **513**(Pt 1): 263–272.
152 Gelman S. Venous function and central venous pressure: a physiologic story. *Anesthesiology* 2008; **108**(4): 735–748.
153 Guyton AC, Lindsey AW, Abernathy B, *et al.* Venous return at various right atrial pressures and the normal venous return curve. *Am J Physiol* 1957; **189**: 609–615.
154 Beard DA, Feigl EO. Understanding Guyton's venous return curves. *Am J Physiol Heart Circ Physiol* 2011; **301**(3): H629–H633.
155 Levy MN. The cardiac and vascular factors that determine systemic blood flow. *Circ Res* 1979; **44**: 739–747.
156 Brengelmann GL. A critical analysis of the view that right atrial pressure determines venous return. *J Appl Physiol* 2003; **94**: 849–859.
157 Reddi BA, Carpenter RH. Venous return: cardiomythology? *Clin Med (Lond)* 2007; **7**(1): 35–36.
158 Webb RC. Smooth muscle contraction and relaxation. *Adv Physiol Educ* 2003; **27**(1–4): 201–206.
159 Clifford PS. Local control of blood flow. *Adv Physiol Educ* 2011; **35**(1): 5–15.
160 Akata T. Cellular and molecular mechanisms regulating vascular tone. Part 1: basic mechanisms controlling cytosolic Ca2+ concentration and the Ca2+-dependent regulation of vascular tone. *J Anesth* 2007; **21**(2): 220–231.
161 Akata T. Cellular and molecular mechanisms regulating vascular tone. Part 2: regulatory mechanisms modulating Ca2+ mobilization and/or myofilament Ca2+ sensitivity in vascular smooth muscle cells. *J Anesth* 2007; **21**(2): 232–242.
162 Goulopoulou S, Webb RC. Symphony of vascular contraction: how smooth muscle cells lose harmony to signal increased vascular resistance in hypertension. *Hypertension* 2014; **63**(3): e33–e39.
163 Chang KS, Davis RF. Propofol produces endothelium-independent vasodilation and may act as a Ca2+ channel blocker. *Anesth Analg* 1993; **76**(1): 24–32.
164 Akata T, Izumi K, Nakashima M. Mechanisms of direct inhibitory action of ketamine on vascular smooth muscle in mesenteric resistance arteries. *Anesthesiology* 2001; **95**: 452–462.
165 Akata T. General anesthetics and vascular smooth muscle: direct actions of general anesthetics on cellular mechanisms regulating vascular tone. *Anesthesiology* 2007; **106**(2): 365–391.
166 Tykocki NR, Boerman EM, Jackson WF. Smooth muscle ion channels and regulation of vascular tone in resistance arteries and arterioles. *Compr Physiol* 2017; **7**(2): 485–581.
167 Tanaka K, Kawano T, Nakamura A, *et al.* Isoflurane activates sarcolemmal adenosine triphosphate-sensitive potassium channels in vascular smooth muscle cells: a role for protein kinase A. *Anesthesiology* 2007; **106**(5): 984–991.
168 Burton AC. Composition of blood. In: Burton AC, ed. *Physiology and Biophysics of the Circulation*, 2nd edn. Chicago, IL: Year Book, 1972: 15–21.
169 Davies KJ. Adaptive homeostasis. *Mol Aspects Med* 2016; **49**: 1–7.
170 Burke JD. Blood volume in mammals. *Physiological Zoology*, 1954; **27**: 1–21.
171 Ahmed MH, Ghatge MS, Safo MK. Hemoglobin: structure, function and allostery. *Subcell Biochem* 2020; **94**: 345–382.
172 Cambier C, Wierinckx M, Clerbaux T, *et al.* Haemoglobin oxygen affinity and regulating factors of the blood oxygen transport in canine and feline blood. *Res Vet Sci* 2004; **77**(1): 83–88.
173 Lima B, Forrester MT, Hess DT, *et al.* S-nitrosylation in cardiovascular signaling. *Circ Res* 2010; **106**(4): 633–646.
174 Doctor A, Stamler JS. Nitric oxide transport in blood: a third gas in the respiratory cycle. *Compr Physiol* 2011; **1**(1): 541–568.
175 Chen K, Pittman RN, Popel AS. Nitric oxide in the vasculature: where does it come from and where does it go? *A quantitative perspective. Antioxid Redox Signal* 2008; **10**(7): 1185–1198.
176 Schechter AN, Gladwin MT. Hemoglobin and the paracrine and endocrine functions of nitric oxide. *N Engl J Med* 2003; **348**(15): 1483–1485.
177 McMahon TJ, Moon RE, Luschinger BP, *et al.* Nitric oxide in the human respiratory cycle. *Nat Med* 2002; **8**(7): 711–717.
178 Sonveaux P, Lobysheva II, Renon O, *et al.* Transport and peripheral bioactivities of nitrogen oxides carried by red blood cell hemoglobin: role in oxygen delivery. *Physiology* 2007; **22**: 97–112.
179 MacIntyre NR. Tissue hypoxia: implications for the respiratory clinician. *Respir Care* 2014; **59**(10): 1590–1596.
180 Corrado C, Fontana S. Hypoxia and HIF signaling: one axis with divergent effects. *Int J Mol Sci* 2020; **21**(16): 5611.
181 Rifkind JM, Nagababu E, Ramasamy S. The quaternary hemoglobin conformation regulates the formation of the nitrite-induced bioactive intermediate and the dissociation of nitric oxide from this intermediate. *Nitric Oxide* 2011; **24**(2): 102–109.
182 Silva G, Jeney V, Chora A, *et al.* Oxidized hemoglobin is an endogenous proinflammatory agonist that targets vascular endothelial cells. *J Biol Chem* 2009; **284**(43): 29582–29595.
183 Alayash AI, Patel RP, Cashon RE. Redox reactions of hemoglobin and myoglobin: biological and toxicological implications. *Antioxid Redox Signal* 2001; **3**(2): 313–327.
184 Lanza V, Mercadante S, Pignataro A. Effects of halothane, enflurane, and nitrous oxide on oxyhemoglobin affinity. *Anesthesiology* 1988; **68**(4): 591–594.
185 Wilkie DA, Kirby R. Methemoglobinemia associated with dermal application of benzocaine cream in a cat. *J Am Vet Med Assoc* 1988; **192**(1): 85–86.
186 Guay J. Methemoglobinemia related to local anesthetics: a summary of 242 episodes. *Anesth Analg* 2009; **108**(3): 837–845.
187 Yu F, Tong LJ, Cai DS. Sevoflurane inhibits neuronal apoptosis and expressions of HIF-1 and HSP70 in brain tissues of rats with cerebral ischemia/reperfusion injury. *Eur Rev Med Pharmacol Sci* 2020; **24**(9): 5082–5090.
188 Choi I, Lee S, Hong YK. The new era of the lymphatic system: no longer secondary to the blood vascular system. *Cold Spring Harb Perspect Med* 2012; **2**(4): a006445.
189 Shang T, Liang J, Kapron CM, *et al.* Pathophysiology of aged lymphatic vessels. *Aging (Albany NY)* 2019; **11**(16): 6602–6613.
190 Kesler CT, Liao S, Munn LL, *et al.* Lymphatic vessels in health and disease. *Wiley Interdiscip Rev Syst Biol Med* 2013; **5**(1): 111–124.
191 Stewart RH. A modern view of the interstitial space in health and disease. *Front Vet Sci* 2020; **7**: 609583.
192 Jessen NA, Munk AS, Lundgaard I, *et al.* the glymphatic system: a beginner's guide. *Neurochem Res* 2015; **40**(12): 2583–2599.
193 Chaplin DD. Overview of the immune response. *J Allergy Clin Immunol* 2010; **125**(2 Suppl 2): S3–S23.
194 Hansen KC, D'Alessandro A, Clement CC, *et al.* Lymph formation, composition and circulation: a proteomics perspective. *Int Immunol* 2015; **27**(5): 219–227.
195 Kang S, Lee SP, Kim KE, *et al.* Toll-like receptor 4 in lymphatic endothelial cells contributes to LPS-induced lymphangiogenesis by chemotactic recruitment of macrophages. *Blood* 2009; **113**(11): 2605–2613.
196 Hemmi H, Akira S. TLR signaling and the function of dendritic cells. *Chem Immunol Allergy* 2005; **86**: 120–135.
197 Akira S, Takeda K, Kaisho T. Toll-like receptors: critical proteins linking innate and acquired immunity. *Nat Immunol* 2001; **2**(8): 675–680.
198 Secomb TW. Hemodynamics. *Compr Physiol* 2016; **6**(2): 975–1003.
199 Scheeren TWL, Ramsay MAE. New developments in hemodynamic monitoring. *J Cardiothorac Vasc Anesth* 2019; **33**(Suppl 1): S67–S72.
200 Norton JM. Toward consistent definitions for preload and afterload. *Adv Physiol Educ* 2001; **25**(1): 53–61.
201 Ross J. Cardiac function and myocardial contractility: a perspective. *J Am Coll Cardiol* 1983; **1**: 52–62.
202 Sonnenblick EH. Instantaneous force-velocity-length determinants in the contraction of heart muscle. *Circ Res* 1965; **16**: 441–451.

203 Ross J, Franklin D, Sasayama S. Preload, afterload, and the role of afterload mismatch in the descending limb of cardiac function. *Eur J Cardiol* 1976; **4**(Suppl): 77–86.

204 Brutsaert DL, Sonnenblick EH. Cardiac muscle mechanics in the evaluation of myocardial contractility and pump function: problems, concepts, and directions. *Prog Cardiovasc Dis* 1973; **16**(3): 337–361.

205 Kass DA, Maughan WL, Guo ZM, *et al.* Comparative influence of load versus inotropic states on indexes of ventricular contractility: experimental and theoretical analysis based on pressure–volume relationships. *Circulation* 1987; **76**(6): 1422–1436.

206 Monge García MI, Jian Z, Settels JJ, *et al.* Determinants of left ventricular ejection fraction and a novel method to improve its assessment of myocardial contractility. *Ann Intensive Care* 2019; **9**(1): 48.

207 Sutera SP, Skalak R. The history of Poiseuille's law. *Ann Rev Fluid Mech* 1993; **25**: 1–19.

208 Guyton AC. Regulation of cardiac output. *N Engl J Med* 1967; **277**(15): 805–812.

209 Guyton AC. Regulation of cardiac output. *Anesthesiology* 1968; **29**(2): 314–326.

210 He S, Seddighi M. Transition of transient channel flow after a change in Reynolds number. *J Fluid Mech* 2015; **764**: 395–427.

211 Yoganathan AP, Cape EG, Sung HW, *et al.* Review of hydrodynamic principles for the cardiologist: applications to the study of blood flow and jets by imaging techniques. *J Am Coll Cardiol* 1988; **12**(5): 1344–1353.

212 Eger EI. Tissue groups arranged by solubility and perfusion characteristics. In: *Anesthetic Uptake and Action*. Baltimore, MD: Williams & Wilkins, 1974: 88–94.

213 Westerhof BE, van Gemert MJC, van den Wijngaard JP. Pressure and flow relations in the systemic arterial tree throughout development from newborn to adult. *Front Pediatr* 2020; **8**: 251.

214 Basford JR. The Law of Laplace and its relevance to contemporary medicine and rehabilitation. *Arch Phys Med Rehabil* 2002; **83**(8): 1165–1170.

215 Guensch DP, Fischer K, Jung C, *et al.* Relationship between myocardial oxygenation and blood pressure: experimental validation using oxygenation-sensitive cardiovascular magnetic resonance. *PLoS ONE* 2019; **14**(1): e0210098.

216 Thiele RH, Durieux ME. Arterial waveform analysis for the anesthesiologist: past, present, and future concepts. *Anesth Analg* 2011; **113**(4): 766–776.

217 Boysen SR, Gommeren K. Assessment of volume status and fluid responsiveness in small animals. *Front Vet Sci* 2021; **8**: 630643.

218 Barbeito A, Mark JB. Arterial and central venous pressure monitoring. *Anesthesiol Clin* 2006; **24**(4): 717–735.

219 Marik PE, Baram M, Vahid B. Does central venous pressure predict fluid responsiveness? A systematic review of the literature and the tale of seven mares. *Chest* 2008; **34**(1): 172–178.

220 Marik PE. Noninvasive cardiac output monitors: a state-of-the-art review. *J Cardiothorac Vasc Anesth* 2013; **27**(1): 121–134.

221 Eckmann DM, Bowers S, Stecker M, *et al.* Hematocrit, volume expander, temperature, and shear rate effects on blood viscosity. *Anesth Analg* 2000; **91**(3): 539–545.

222 Reinhart WH. Molecular biology and self-regulatory mechanisms of blood viscosity: a review. *Biorheology* 2001; **38**(2–3): 203–212.

223 Ercan M, Koksal C. The relationship between shear rate and vessel diameter. *Anesth Analg* 2003; **96**(1): 307; author reply 307–308.

224 Pries AR, Secomb TW, Gaehtgens P, *et al.* Blood flow in microvascular networks. *Experiments and simulation. Circ Res* 1990; **67**(4): 826–834.

225 Ascolese M, Farina A, Fasano A. The Fåhræus–Lindqvist effect in small blood vessels: how does it help the heart? *J Biol Phys* 2019; **45**(4): 379–394.

226 Lasala PA, Chien S, Michelsen CB. Hemorrheology: what is the ideal hematocrit? In: Askanasi J, Starker RM, Weissman C, eds. *Fluid and Electrolyte Management in Critical Care*. Boston, MA: Butterworth, 1986: 203–213.

227 Goto Y, Sakakura S, Hatta M, *et al.* Hemorrheological effects of colloidal plasma substitutes infusion. *A comparative study. Acta Anaesthesiol Scand* 1985; **29**(2): 217–223.

228 Cabrales P, Intaglietta M, Tsai AG. Increase plasma viscosity sustains microcirculation after resuscitation from hemorrhagic shock and continuous bleeding. *Shock* 2005; **23**(6): 549–555.

229 Martini J, Carpentier B, Chávez Negrete A, *et al.* Beneficial effects due to increasing blood and plasma viscosity. *Clin Hemorheol Microcirc* 2006; **35**(1–2): 51–57.

230 Negrete A, Tsai AG, Forconi S, *et al.* Cardiovascular benefits in moderate increases of blood and plasma viscosity surpass those associated with lowering viscosity: experimental and clinical evidence. *Clin Hemorheol Microcirc* 2010; **44**(2): 75–85.

231 Arnemann PH, Hessler M, Kampmeier T, *et al.* Resuscitation with hydroxyethyl starch maintains hemodynamic coherence in ovine hemorrhagic shock. *Anesthesiology* 2020; **132**(1): 131–139.

232 Olson RM. In vivo blood viscosity and hindrance. *Am J Physiol* 1964; **206**: 955–961.

233 Whittaker SR, Winton FR. The apparent viscosity of blood flowing in the isolated hindlimb of the dog, and its variation with corpuscular concentration. *J Physiol* 1933; **78**(4): 339–369.

234 Chen RY, Carlin RD, Simchon S, *et al.* Effects of dextran-induced hyperviscosity on regional blood flow and hemodynamics in dogs. *Am J Physiol* 1989; **256**(3 Pt 2): H898–H905.

235 O'Rourke MF, Pauca A, Jiang XJ. Pulse wave analysis. *Br J Clin Pharmacol* 2001; **51**(6): 507–522.

236 O'Rourke MF. Vascular impedance in studies of arterial and cardiac function. *Physiol Rev* 1982; **62**(2): 570–623.

237 Zelis R, Flaim SF, Liedtke AJ, *et al.* Cardiocirculatory dynamics in the normal and failing heart. *Annu Rev Physiol* 1981; **43**: 455–476.

238 Little WC, Cheng CP. Left ventricular–arterial coupling in conscious dogs. *Am J Physiol* 1991; **261**(1 Pt 2): H70–H76.

239 Kouraklis G, Karayannacos P, Sechas M, *et al.* The influence of hemodilution on left ventricular function. *Int Angiol* 1990; **9**(1): 38–42.

240 Wood NB. Aspects of fluid dynamics applied to the larger arteries. *J Theor Biol* 1999; **199**(2): 137–161.

241 Deryck YL, Brimioulle S, Maggiorini M, *et al.* Systemic vascular effects of isoflurane versus propofol anesthesia in dogs. *Anesth Analg* 1996; **83**(5): 958–964.

242 Hettrick DA, Pagel PS, Warltier DC. Isoflurane and halothane produce similar alterations in aortic distensibility and characteristic aortic impedance. *Anesth Analg* 1996; **83**(6): 1166–1172.

243 Crowell JW, Smith EE. Determinant of the optimal hematocrit. *J Appl Physiol* 1967; **22**(3): 501–504.

244 Hsia CC, Johnson RL Jr., Dane DM, *et al.* The canine spleen in oxygen transport: gas exchange and hemodynamic responses to splenectomy. *J Appl Physiol (1985)* 2007; **103**(5): 1496–1505.

245 Chapler CK, Cain SM. The physiologic reserve in oxygen carrying capacity: studies in experimental hemodilution. *Can J Physiol Pharmacol* 1986; **64**(1): 7–12.

246 Leone BJ, Spahn DR. Anemia, hemodilution, and oxygen delivery. *Anesth Analg* 1992; **75**(5): 651–653.

247 Cabrales P, Tsai AG, Intaglietta M. Microvascular pressure and functional capillary density in extreme hemodilution with low- and high-viscosity dextran and a low-viscosity Hb-based O2 carrier. *Am J Physiol Heart Circ Physiol* 2004; **287**(1): H363–H373.

248 Tsai AG, Acero C, Nance PR, *et al.* Elevated plasma viscosity in extreme hemodilution increases perivascular nitric oxide concentration and microvascular perfusion. *Am J Physiol Heart Circ Physiol* 2005; **288**(4): H1730–H1739.

249 Rothe C. Toward consistent definitions for preload and afterload--revisited. *Adv Physiol Educ* 2003; **27**(1–4): 44–45; author reply 89–90.

250 Suga H, Igarashi Y, Yamada O, *et al.* Mechanical efficiency of the left ventricle as a function of preload, afterload, and contractility. *Heart Vessels* 1985; **1**(1): 3–8.

251 Cazorla O, Lacampagne A. Regional variation in myofilament length-dependent activation. *Pflugers Arch* 2011; **462**(1): 15–28.

252 Katz AM. Ernest Henry Starling, his predecessors, and the 'Law of the Heart'. *Circulation* 2002; **106**: 2986–2992.

253 Schotola H, Sossalla ST, Renner A, *et al.* The contractile adaption to preload depends on the amount of afterload. *ESC Heart Fail* 2017; **4**(4): 468–478.

254 Cingolani HE, Pérez NG, Cingolani OH, *et al.* The Anrep effect: 100 years later. *Am J Physiol Heart Circ Physiol* 2013; **304**(2): H175–H182.

255 Mitchell JR, Wang JJ. Expanding application of the Wiggers diagram to teach cardiovascular physiology. *Adv Physiol Educ* 2014; **38**(2): 170–175.

256 Sagawa K. The end-systolic pressure–volume relation of the ventricle: definition, modifications and clinical use. *Circulation* 1981; **63**(6): 1223–1227.

257 Burkhoff D, Mirsky I, Suga H. Assessment of systolic and diastolic ventricular properties via pressure–volume analysis: a guide for clinical, translational, and basic researchers. *Am J Physiol Heart Circ Physiol* 2005; **289**(2): H501–H512.

258 Kass DA, Kelly RP. Ventriculo-arterial coupling: concepts, assumptions, and applications. *Ann Biomed Eng* 1992; **20**(1): 41–62.

259 Welker FH, Muir WW. An investigation of the second heart sound in the normal horse. *Equine Vet J* 1990; **22**(6): 403–407.

260 Ettinger SJ, Suter PF. Heart sounds and phonocardiography. In: Canine Cardiology. *Philadelphia*, PA: WB Saunders, 1970: 12–39.

261 Bastos MB, Burkhoff D, Maly J, *et al.* Invasive left ventricle pressure–volume analysis: overview and practical clinical implications. *Eur Heart J* 2020; **41**(12): 1286–1297.

262 Monge García MI, Jian Z, Settels JJ, *et al.* Determinants of left ventricular ejection fraction and a novel method to improve its assessment of myocardial contractility. *Ann Intensive Care* 2019; **9**(1): 48.

263 McDonald M, Virani S, Chan M, *et al.* CCS/CHFS heart failure guidelines update: defining a new pharmacologic standard of care for heart failure with reduced ejection fraction. *Can J Cardiol* 2021; **37**(4): 531–546.

264 Antonini-Canterin F, Poli S, Vriz O, *et al.* The ventricular–arterial coupling: from basic pathophysiology to clinical application in the echocardiography laboratory. *J Cardiovasc Echogr* 2013; **23**(4): 91–95.

265 De Tombe PP, Jones S, Burkhoff D, *et al.* Ventricular stroke work and efficiency both remain nearly optimal despite altered vascular loading. *Am J Physiol* 1993; **264**(6 Pt 2): H1817–H1824.

266 Pavlopoulos H, Nihoyannopoulos P. Pulse pressure/stroke volume: a surrogate index of arterial stiffness and the relation to segmental relaxation and longitudinal systolic deformation in hypertensive disease. *Eur J Echocardiogr* 2009; **10**(4): 519–526.
267 Anavekar NS, Oh JK. Doppler echocardiography: a contemporary review. *J Cardiol* 2009; **54**(3): 347–358.
268 Geerts BF, Aarts LP, Jansen JR. Methods in pharmacology: measurement of cardiac output. *Br J Clin Pharmacol* 2011; **71**(3): 316–330.
269 Spinale FG. Assessment of cardiac function--basic principles and approaches. *Compr Physiol* 2015; **5**(4): 1911–1946.
270 Bombardini T. Myocardial contractility in the echo lab: molecular, cellular and pathophysiological basis. *Cardiovasc Ultrasound* 2005; **3**: 27.
271 Sarazan DR, Parish ST. An evaluation of the utility of LVdP/dt_{40}, QA interval, LVdP/dt_{min} and Tau as indicators of drug-induced changes in contractility and lusitropy in dogs. *J Pharmacol Toxicol Methods* 2017; **85**: 1–21.
272 Sarazan RD, Kroehle JP, Main BW. Left ventricular pressure, contractility and dP/dt(max) in nonclinical drug safety assessment studies. *J Pharmacol Toxicol Methods* 2012; **66**(2): 71–78.
273 Blaudszun G, Licker MJ, Morel DR. Preload-adjusted left ventricular dP/dtmax: a sensitive, continuous, load-independent contractility index. *Exp Physiol* 2013; **98**(10): 1446–1456.
274 Biering-Sørensen T, Mogelvang R, Schnohr P, *et al.* Cardiac time intervals measured by tissue Doppler imaging M-mode: association with hypertension, left ventricular geometry, and future ischemic cardiovascular diseases. *J Am Heart Assoc* 2016; **5**(1): e002687.
275 Smiseth OA, Torp H, Opdahl A, *et al.* Myocardial strain imaging: how useful is it in clinical decision making? *Eur Heart J* 2016; **37**(15): 1196–1207.
276 Senzaki H, Chen CH, Kass DA. Single-beat estimation of end-systolic pressure–volume relation in humans. A new method with the potential for noninvasive application. *Circulation* 1996; **94**(10): 2497–2506.
277 Brinke EA, Klautz RJ, Verwey HF, *et al.* Single-beat estimation of the left ventricular end-systolic pressure–volume relationship in patients with heart failure. *Acta Physiol (Oxf)* 2010; **198**(1): 37–46.
278 Mirea O, Vallecilla C, Claus P, *et al.* Experimental validation of the prestretch-strain relationship as a non-invasive index of left ventricular myocardial contractility. *PLoS ONE* 2020; **15**(2): e0228027.
279 Swanson CR, Muir WW III. Simultaneous evaluation of left ventricular end-systolic pressure–volume ratio and time constant of isovolumic pressure decline in dogs exposed to equivalent MAC halothane and isoflurane. *Anesthesiology* 1988; **68**(5): 764–770.
280 Pagel PS, Kampine JP, Schmeling WT, *et al.* Comparison of the systemic and coronary hemodynamic actions of desflurane, isoflurane, halothane, and enflurane in the chronically instrumented dog. *Anesthesiology* 1991; **74**(3): 539–551.
281 Pagel PS, Schmeling WT, Kampine JP, *et al.* Alteration of canine left ventricular diastolic function by intravenous anesthetics in vivo. Ketamine and propofol. *Anesthesiology* 1992; **76**(3): 419–425.
282 Brutsaert DL, Rademakers FE, Sys SU, *et al.* Analysis of relaxation in the evaluation of ventricular function of the heart. *Prog Cardiovasc Dis* 1985; **28**(2): 143–163.
283 Ogunyankin KO. Assessment of left ventricular diastolic function: the power, possibilities, and pitfalls of echocardiographic imaging techniques. *Can J Cardiol* 2011; **27**(3): 311–318.
284 Zhao W, Choi JH, Hong GR, *et al.* Left ventricular relaxation. *Heart Fail Clin* 2008; **4**(1): 37–46.
285 Nagueh SF. Non-invasive assessment of left ventricular filling pressure. *Eur J Heart Fail* 2018; **20**(1): 38–48.
286 Pagel PS, Grossman W, Haering JM, *et al.* Left ventricular diastolic function in the normal and diseased heart. Perspectives for the anesthesiologist (1). *Anesthesiology* 1993; **79**(4): 836–854.
287 Noel-Morgan J, Muir WW. Anesthesia-associated relative hypovolemia: mechanisms, monitoring, and treatment considerations. *Front Vet Sci* 2018; **5**: 53.
288 Schumacker PT, Cain SM. The concept of a critical oxygen delivery. *Intensive Care Med* 1987; **13**(4): 223–239.
289 Dunham CM, Siegel JH, Weireter L, *et al.* Oxygen debt and metabolic acidemia as quantitative predictors of mortality and the severity of the ischemic insult in hemorrhagic shock. *Crit Care Med* 1991; **19**(2): 231–243.
290 Shoemaker WC, Appel PL, Kram HB. Role of oxygen debt in the development of organ failure sepsis, and death in high-risk surgical patients. *Chest* 1992; **102**(1): 208–215.
291 Rixen D, Siegel JH. Bench-to-bedside review: oxygen debt and its metabolic correlates as quantifiers of the severity of hemorrhagic and post-traumatic shock. *Crit Care* 2005; **9**(5): 441–453.
292 Siegel JH, Fabian M, Smith JA, *et al.* Oxygen debt criteria quantify the effectiveness of early partial resuscitation after hypovolemic hemorrhagic shock. *J Trauma* 2003; **54**(5): 862–880.
293 Schumacker PT, Long GR, Wood LD. Tissue oxygen extraction during hypovolemia: role of hemoglobin P50. *J Appl Physiol (1985)* 1987; **62**(5): 1801–1807.
294 Van der Linden P, Schmartz D, De Groote F, *et al.* Critical haemoglobin concentration in anaesthetized dogs: comparison of two plasma substitutes. *Br J Anaesth* 1998; **81**(4): 556–562.
295 Cain SM. Oxygen delivery and uptake in dogs during anemic and hypoxic hypoxia. *J Appl Physiol Respir Environ Exerc Physiol* 1977; **42**(2): 228–234.
296 Van der Linden P, Gilbart E, Engelman E, *et al.* Effects of anesthetic agents on systemic critical O2 delivery. *J Appl Physiol (1985)* 1991; **71**(1): 83–93.
297 Van der Linden P, De Hert S, Mathieu N, *et al.* Tolerance to acute isovolemic hemodilution. Effect of anesthetic depth. *Anesthesiology* 2003; **99**(1): 97–104.
298 Archie JP Jr. Mathematic coupling of data: a common source of error. *Ann Surg* 1981; **193**(3): 296–303.
299 Walsh TS, Lee A. Mathematical coupling in medical research: lessons from studies of oxygen kinetics. *Br J Anaesth* 1998; **81**(2): 118–120.
300 Dampney RA. Central neural control of the cardiovascular system: current perspectives. *Adv Physiol Educ* 2016; **40**(3): 283–296.
301 McCorry LK. Physiology of the autonomic nervous system. *Am J Pharm Educ* 2007; **71**(4): 78.
302 Segal SS. Regulation of blood flow in the microcirculation. *Microcirculation* 2005; **12**(1): 33–45.
303 Hollmann MW, Strumper D, Herroeder S, *et al.* Receptors, G proteins, and their interactions. *Anesthesiology* 2005; **103**(5): 1066–1078.
304 Wang J, Gareri C, Rockman HA. G-protein-coupled receptors in heart disease. *Circ Res* 2018; **123**(6): 716–735.
305 Arimura H, Bosnjak ZJ, Hoka S, *et al.* Modifications by halothane of responses to acute hypoxia in systemic vascular capacitance, resistance, and sympathetic nerve activity in dogs. *Anesth Analg* 1991; **73**(3): 319–326.
306 McCallum JB, Stekiel TA, Bosnjak ZJ, *et al.* Does isoflurane alter mesenteric venous capacitance in the intact rabbit? *Anesth Analg* 1993; **76**(5): 1095–1105.
307 Nakamura K, Terasako K, Toda H, *et al.* Mechanisms of inhibition of endothelium-dependent relaxation by halothane, isoflurane, and sevoflurane. *Can J Anaesth* 1994; **41**(4): 340–346.
308 Vatner SF. Effects of anesthesia on cardiovascular control mechanisms. *Environ Health Perspect* 1978; **26**: 193–206.
309 Zimpfer M, Sit SP, Vatner SF. Effects of anesthesia on the canine carotid chemoreceptor reflex. *Circ Res* 1981; **48**(3): 400–406.
310 Mayer N, Zimpfer M, Raberger G, *et al.* Fentanyl inhibits the canine carotid chemoreceptor reflex. *Anesth Analg* 1989; **69**(6): 756–762.
311 Uggeri MJ, Proctor GJ, Johns RA. Halothane, enflurane, and isoflurane attenuate both receptor- and non-receptor-mediated EDRF production in rat thoracic aorta. *Anesthesiology* 1992; **76**(6): 1012–1017.
312 Ickx BE, Rigolet M, Van der Linden PJ. Cardiovascular and metabolic response to acute normovolemic anemia. Effects of anesthesia. *Anesthesiology* 2000; **93**(4): 1011–1016.
313 Skillman JJ, Eltringham WK, Goldensen RH, *et al.* Transcapillary refilling after hemorrhage in the splenectomized dog. *J Surg Res* 1968; **8**(2): 57–67.
314 Isbister JP. Physiology and pathophysiology of blood volume regulation. *Transfus Sci* 1997; **18**(3): 409–423.
315 Wadei HM, Textor SC. The role of the kidney in regulating arterial blood pressure. *Nat Rev Nephrol* 2012; **8**(10): 602–609.
316 Daniel M, Weiskopf RB, Noorani M, *et al.* Fentanyl augments the blockade of the sympathetic response to incision (MAC-BAR) produced by desflurane and isoflurane: desflurane and isoflurane MAC-BAR without and with fentanyl. *Anesthesiology* 1998; **88**(1): 43–49.
317 Crystal GJ, Salem MR. The Bainbridge and the 'reverse' Bainbridge reflexes: history, physiology, and clinical relevance. *Anesth Analg* 2012; **114**(3): 520–532.
318 Zhang YH, Youm JB, Earm YE. Stretch-activated non-selective cation channel: a causal link between mechanical stretch and atrial natriuretic peptide secretion. *Prog Biophys Mol Biol* 2008; **8**(1): 1–9.
319 Goetze JP, Bruneau BG, Ramos HR, *et al.* Cardiac natriuretic peptides. *Nat Rev Cardiol* 2020; **17**(11): 698–717.
320 Aviado DM, Guevara Aviado D. The Bezold–Jarisch reflex. A historical perspective of cardiopulmonary reflexes. *Ann N Y Acad Sci* 2001; **940**: 48–58.
321 Kinsella SM, Tuckey JP. Perioperative bradycardia and asystole: relationship to vasovagal syncope and the Bezold–Jarisch reflex. *Br J Anaesth* 2001; **86**(6): 859–868.
322 Campagna JA, Carter C. Clinical relevance of the Bezold–Jarisch reflex. *Anesthesiology* 2003; **98**(5): 1250–1260.
323 Lindsey BG, Nuding SC, Segers LS, *et al.* Carotid bodies and the integrated cardiorespiratory response to hypoxia. *Physiology (Bethesda)* 2018; **33**(4): 281–297.
324 Persson PB. Renin: origin, secretion and synthesis. *J Physiol* 2003; **552**(Pt 3): 667–671.
325 Bader M, Ganten D. Update on tissue renin–angiotensin systems. *J Mol Med (Berl)* 2008; **86**(6): 615–621.

326 Patel VB, Zhong JC, Grant MB, *et al.* Role of the ACE2/angiotensin 1–7 axis of the renin–angiotensin system in heart failure. *Circ Res* 2016; **118**(8): 1313–1326.

327 Mirenda JV, Grissom TE. Anesthetic implications of the renin–angiotensin system and angiotensin-converting enzyme inhibitors. *Anesth Analg* 1991; **72**(5): 667–683.

328 Philbin DM, Coggins CH. The effects of anesthesia on antidiuretic hormone. *Contemp Anesth Pract* 1980; **3**: 29–38.

329 Maybauer MO, Maybauer DM, Enkhbaatar P, *et al.* Physiology of the vasopressin receptors. *Best Pract Res Clin Anaesthesiol* 2008; **22**(2): 253–263.

330 Bankir L, Bichet DG, Morgenthaler NG. Vasopressin: physiology, assessment and osmosensation. *J Intern Med* 2017; **282**(4): 284–297.

331 Armstead WM. Cerebral blood flow autoregulation and dysautoregulation. *Anesthesiol Clin* 2016; **34**(3): 465–477.

332 Olsson RA. Local factors regulating cardiac and skeletal muscle blood flow. *Annu Rev Physiol* 1981; **43**: 385–395.

333 Carlson BE, Arciero JC, Secomb TW. Theoretical model of blood flow autoregulation: roles of myogenic, shear-dependent, and metabolic responses. *Am J Physiol Heart Circ Physiol* 2008; **295**(4): H1572–H1579.

334 Cengel A, Sahinarslan A. Nitric oxide and cardiovascular system. *Anadolu Kardiyol Derg* 2006; **6**(4): 364–368.

335 Davis MJ, Hill MA. Signaling mechanisms underlying the vascular myogenic response. *Physiol Rev* 1999; **79**(2): 387–423.

336 Popel AS, Johnson PC. Microcirculation and hemorheology. *Annu Rev Fluid Mech* 2005; **37**: 43–69.

337 Sriram K, Salazar Vázquez BY, Tsai AG, *et al.* Autoregulation and mechanotransduction control the arteriolar response to small changes in hematocrit. *Am J Physiol Heart Circ Physiol* 2012; **303**(9): H1096–H1106.

338 Yetik-Anacak G, Catravas JD. Nitric oxide and the endothelium: history and impact on cardiovascular disease. *Vascul Pharmacol* 2006; **45**(5): 268–276.

339 Watts SW. Endothelin receptors: what's new and what do we need to know? *Am J Physiol Regul Integr Comp Physiol* 2010; **298**(2): R254–R260.

340 Sawdon M. Characteristics of special circulations. *Anesth Int Care Med* 2013; **14**(2): 68–71.

341 Barile L, Fominskiy E, Di Tomasso N, *et al.* Acute normovolemic hemodilution reduces allogenic red blood cell transfusion in cardiac surgery: a systematic review and meta-analysis of randomized trials. *Anesth Analg* 2017; **124**(3): 743–752.

342 Ramanathan T, Skinner H. Coronary blood flow. *Contin Educ Anaesth Crit Care Pain* 2005; **5**: 61–64.

343 Feigl EO. Coronary autoregulation. *J Hypertens Suppl* 1989; **7**(4): S55–S58.

344 Rowe GG. Responses of the coronary circulation to physiologic changes and pharmacologic agents. *Anesthesiology* 1974; **41**(2): 182–196.

345 Schelbert HR. Anatomy and physiology of coronary blood flow. *J Nucl Cardiol* 2010; **17**(4): 545–554.

346 Christensen GC, Campeti FD. Anatomic and functional studies of the coronary circulation in the dog and pig. *Am J Vet Res* 1959; **20**: 18–23.

347 Sethna DH, Moffitt EA. An appreciation of the coronary circulation. *Anesth Analg* 1986; **65**: 294–305.

348 Esperança Pina JA, Correia M, O'Neill JG. Morphological study on the thebesian veins of the right cavities of the heart in the dog. *Acta Anat (Basel)* 1975; **92**: 310–320.

349 Goodwill AG, Dick GM, Kiel AM, *et al.* Regulation of coronary blood flow. *Compr Physiol* 2017; **7**(2): 321–382.

350 Chambers D, Huang C, Matthews G. Cardiac anatomy and function. In: Chambers D, Huang C, Matthews G, eds. *Basic Physiology for Anaesthetists*. Cambridge, UK: Cambridge University Press: 2015: 111–116.

351 Tune JD, Richmond KN, Gorman MW, *et al.* Role of nitric oxide and adenosine in control of coronary blood flow in exercising dogs. *Circ* 2000; **101**: 2942–2948.

352 Denn MJ, Stone HL. Autonomic innervation of dog coronary arteries. *J Appl Physiol* 1976; **41**: 30–35.

353 Greyson CR. The right ventricle and pulmonary circulation: basic concepts. *Rev Esp Cardiol* 2010; **63**: 81–95.

354 Silverman A, Petersen NH. Physiology, cerebral autoregulation. In: *Stat Pearls [Internet]*. Treasure Island, FL: StatPearls Publishing, 2021.

355 Hamel E. Perivascular nerves and the regulation of cerebrovascular tone. *J Appl Physiol (1985)* 2006 Mar; **100**(3): 1059–1064.

356 Yoshihara M, Bandoh K, Marmarou A. Cerebrovascular carbon dioxide reactivity assessed by intracranial pressure dynamics in severely head injured patients. *J Neurosurg* 1995; **82**(3): 386–393.

357 Nadeem M, Murray D, Boylan G, *et al.* Blood carbon dioxide levels and adverse outcome in neonatal hypoxic-ischemic encephalopathy. *Am J Perinatol* 2010; **27**(5): 361–365.

358 Slupe AM, Kirsch JR. Effects of anesthesia on cerebral blood flow, metabolism, and neuroprotection. *J Cereb Blood Flow Metab* 2018; **38**(12): 2192–2208.

359 West JB. Comparative physiology of the pulmonary circulation. *Compr Physiol* 2011; **1**(3): 1525–1539.

360 Suresh K, Shimoda LA. Lung circulation. *Compr Physiol* 2016; **6**(2): 897–943.

361 Gillespie JR, Tyler WS, Eberly VE. Pulmonary ventilation and resistance in emphysematous and control horses. *J Appl Physiol* 1966; **21**(2): 416–422.

362 West JB. Blood flow to the lung and gas exchange. *Anesthesiology* 1974; **41**(2): 124–138.

363 Robinson NE. Some functional consequences of species differences in lung anatomy. *Adv Vet Sci Comp Med* 1982; **26**: 1–33.

364 Michard F. Changes in arterial pressure during mechanical ventilation. *Anesthesiology* 2005; **103**(2): 419–428.

365 Dunham-Snary KJ, Wu D, Sykes EA, *et al.* Hypoxic pulmonary vasoconstriction: from molecular mechanisms to medicine. *Chest* 2017; **151**(1): 181–192.

366 Lumb AB, Slinger P. Hypoxic pulmonary vasoconstriction: physiology and anesthetic implications. *Anesthesiology* 2015; **122**(4): 932–946.

367 MacEachern KE, Smith GL, Nolan AM. Characteristics of the in vitro hypoxic pulmonary vasoconstrictor response in isolated equine and bovine pulmonary arterial rings. *Vet Anaesth Analg* 2004; **31**(4): 239–249.

368 Van Keer L, Van Aken H, Vandermeersch E, *et al.* Propofol does not inhibit hypoxic pulmonary vasoconstriction in humans. *J Clin Anesth* 1989; **1**(4): 284–288.

369 Benumof JL. Isoflurane anesthesia and arterial oxygenation during one-lung ventilation. *Anesthesiology* 1986; **64**(4): 419–422.

370 Harper D, Chandler B. Splanchnic circulation. *BJA Educ* 2016; **16**(2): 66–71.

371 Gelman S, Mushlin PS. Catecholamine-induced changes in the splanchnic circulation affecting systemic hemodynamics. *Anesthesiology* 2004; **100**(2): 434–439.

372 Hainsworth R, Karim F. Responses of abdominal vascular capacitance in the anaesthetized dog to changes in carotid sinus pressure. *J Physiol* 1976; **262**(3): 659–677.

373 Shigemi K, Brunner MJ, Shoukas AA. Alpha- and beta-adrenergic mechanisms in the control of vascular capacitance by the carotid sinus baroreflex system. *Am J Physiol* 1994; **267**(1 Pt 2): H201–H210.

374 Rothe CF. Reflex control of veins and vascular capacitance. *Physiol Rev* 1983; **63**(4): 1281–1342.

375 Carneiro JJ, Donald DE. Blood reservoir function of dog spleen, liver, and intestine. *Am J Physiol* 1977; **232**(1): H67–H72.

376 Mellander S, Johansson B. Control of resistance, exchange, and capacitance functions in the peripheral circulation. *Pharmacol Rev* 1968; **20**(3): 117–196.

377 Mellander S. On the control of capillary fluid transfer by precapillary and postcapillary vascular adjustments. A brief review with special emphasis on myogenic mechanisms. *Microvasc Res* 1978; **15**(3): 319–330.

378 Gelman S, Reves JG, Harris D. Circulatory responses to midazolam anesthesia: emphasis on canine splanchnic circulation. *Anesth Analg* 1983; **62**(2): 135–139.

379 Hoka S, Yamaura K, Takenaka T, *et al.* Propofol-induced increase in vascular capacitance is due to inhibition of sympathetic vasoconstrictive activity. *Anesthesiology* 1998; **89**(6): 1495–1500.

380 Yamazaki M, Stekiel TA, Bosnjak ZJ, *et al.* Effects of volatile anesthetic agents on in situ vascular smooth muscle transmembrane potential in resistance- and capacitance-regulating blood vessels. *Anesthesiology* 1998; **88**(4): 1085–1095.

381 Burke M, Pabbidi MR, Farley J, *et al.* Molecular mechanisms of renal blood flow autoregulation. *Curr Vasc Pharmacol* 2014; **12**(6): 845–858.

382 Zehra T, Cupples WA, Braam B. Tubuloglomerular feedback synchronization in nephrovascular networks. *J Am Soc Nephrol* 2021; **32**(6): 1293–1304.

383 Tojo A, Onozato ML, Fujita T. Role of macula densa neuronal nitric oxide synthase in renal diseases. *Med Mol Morphol* 2006; **39**(1): 2–7.

34 Anesthesia for Cardiopulmonary Bypass

Khursheed R. Mama
Department of Clinical Sciences, College of Veterinary Medicine and Biomedical Sciences, Colorado State University, Fort Collins, Colorado, USA

Chapter contents

Introduction, 667
The circuitry and patient cannulation, 667
  The external circuit, 667
  Patient cannulation, 668
Systemic responses – pathobiology, 669
Drugs and interventions used during cardiopulmonary bypass, 669
  Antibiotics, 669
  Steroids, 669
  Antifibrinolytics, 669
  Anticoagulation and reversal, 669
  Hypothermia, 669
Preanesthetic preparation, 670
  Patient evaluation, 670
  Anesthesia setup, 670
  Medications, 670
The sequence of events and terminology, 671
References, 673

Introduction

The term "cardiopulmonary bypass" is broadly applied to the procedure by which blood is diverted away from the heart and lungs while also providing oxygenated blood to other organs to sustain viability. There is a long history of the use of animals, predominantly pigs and sheep, for cardiovascular surgical training and research. Additionally, over the past three decades, animals, most notably dogs (albeit there are occasional reports of cats [1]), have been anesthetized with varying frequency in the clinical arena to facilitate surgical procedures involving the heart (and lungs) [2–15]. Although perioperative morbidity is common (e.g., dysrhythmias, bleeding, phrenic nerve damage, hypoventilation, and hypoxemia), acute survival (off pump to recovery) percentages from the aforementioned reports are generally high, even 100%. Longer-term survival, however, is variable, with wide-ranging complications including hemorrhage, thromboembolism, pleural effusion, heart failure, and sudden death being reported.

The focus of this chapter is to introduce the reader to cardiopulmonary bypass as used to facilitate cardiac surgery in canine patients. Challenges associated with this as a clinical tool have been reviewed [16]. Although anesthesia management is reviewed here, much of the chapter is devoted to introducing the basics of circuitry and instrumentation used to facilitate cardiopulmonary bypass and the considerations (e.g., cardiac protection and management of coagulation) that arise as a result. As the reader is no doubt aware, many cardiac procedures may be performed on the beating heart, sometimes with the added utilization of inflow occlusion and hypothermia. This chapter is limited to a discussion of the management of clinical canine patients where cardiopulmonary bypass is necessary to facilitate cardiac surgery.

The circuitry and patient cannulation

The external circuit

The circuit external to the patient consists of a reservoir for blood and fluids used to prime the pump, a membrane (versus bubble) [17] oxygenator of appropriate size (pediatric size is commonly used for small- to medium-sized dogs), ventilating system, pumps (roller or centrifugal) [18,19] of varying number (three to five) to facilitate circulation of blood, a heat exchanger, and circulating heating/cooling water bath to permit initial cooling and subsequent warming of the patient (Fig. 34.1). Tubing appropriate to the patient's size (so that excessive hemodilution resulting from excessive prime volume, exposure to circuit components, and subsequent red blood cell trauma can be minimized) connects these parts and is attached to lines from/to the patient. As the lung is no longer functional during this process, an oxygen flowmeter (or oxygen and air flowmeters along with an oxygen blender to vary the oxygen fraction) and vaporizer are connected to the circuit to facilitate the delivery of inhaled anesthetic as needed. Maintenance of anesthesia with parenterally administered injectable drugs has also been described [14]. Newer bypass circuits have an independent pump and tubing mechanism for the delivery of cardioplegic solutions, arterial and/or venous in-line monitors (to record temperature, hematocrit,

Veterinary Anesthesia and Analgesia: The Sixth Edition of Lumb and Jones. Edited by Leigh Lamont, Kurt Grimm, Sheilah Robertson, Lydia Love and Carrie Schroeder.
© 2024 John Wiley & Sons, Inc. Published 2024 by John Wiley & Sons, Inc.
Companion website: www.wiley.com/go/lamont/anesthesia

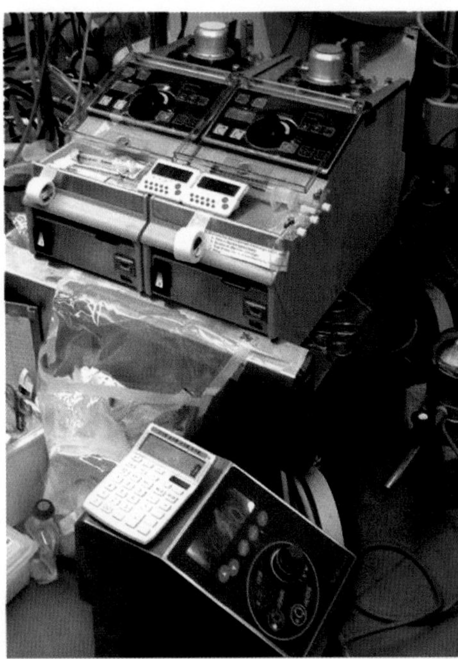

Figure 34.1 Standard and pediatric cardiopulmonary bypass pumps.

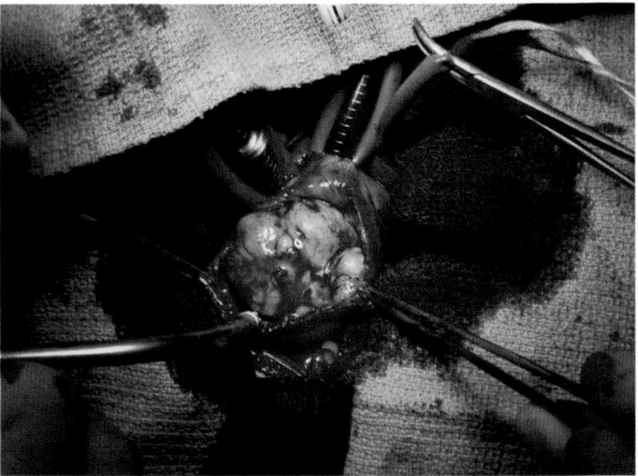

Figure 34.2 Bicaval cannulation for removal of a right atrial mass (in the center of the picture). The caudal vena cava is in the 11 o'clock position and cranial vena cava in the 1 o'clock position. Tape ties are pulled up around each cava, to prevent blood leakage into the right atrium. The cardiotomy sucker in the 7 o'clock position is in place to drain any coronary sinus flow.

saturation, etc.), and safety devices (e.g., bubble detector and flow sensors). A more complete description and diagram of bypass circuitry available for human cardiopulmonary bypass are available in other medical texts [20].

Although the personnel responsible for the anesthetic management of the patient should have a general understanding of the external circuitry used, the author's experience has been that an individual with specialized training in perfusion should be responsible for ensuring functionality of the external circuitry and bypass equipment. The anesthesia personnel will, however, need to be in constant communication and provide the perfusionist with patient-specific information, such as the hematocrit and calculated blood volume. This information will be used to determine the pump prime volume with a target hematocrit of 25–30% to optimize capillary flow and oxygen-carrying capacity during bypass when hypothermia causes an increase in blood viscosity [21]. The perfusionist may request crystalloid fluids, synthetic colloids, blood, plasma or packed red cells (usually in smaller patients), and additives such as mannitol, sodium bicarbonate, and heparin to add to the pump prime. Steroids are added to the pump prime in some circumstances but with decreasing frequency. The perfusion team may also request a vaporizer and inhalant anesthetic consistent with what the anesthesia team is using for the patient. Additional details regarding types and sizes of oxygenators, calculation of pump prime volume, components of prime solution, types and sizes of tubing, etc. may be found elsewhere [21–23].

Patient cannulation

Patient cannulation is performed by the surgical team. A lateral thoracotomy is the preferred approach in the dog if the cardiac procedure to be performed allows for this; a median sternotomy approach is a feasible alternative. Commonly, arterial (oxygenated) blood is actively returned (using a pump) to the patient via a cannula placed in the femoral or carotid artery. It is important that the anesthesia team is aware of which site will be used and, specifically for the femoral vessels, which limb will be utilized, so they do not place the arterial catheter to monitor systemic arterial blood pressure in the same limb. The arterial cannula is either placed first or at the same time as the thoracotomy is performed if there are two surgeons. Early placement facilitates a quicker connection to the bypass circuitry if the patient's status deteriorates during placement of the venous cannula(e).

Bicaval or atrial venous cannulation is performed by the surgical team depending on the procedure to be performed. For procedures involving the right heart, bicaval cannulation is preferred to minimize blood in the surgical field and minimize compromise to venous drainage if the heart is retracted during the procedure (Fig. 34.2). The venous line connected to the cannula passively drains the majority of blood returned to the heart into the reservoir of the bypass circuit. Blood returning from the thebesian veins, coronary sinus, and systemic collaterals can usually be drained by appropriate (depending on the nature of the surgery) placement of these cannulas to reduce the risk of right ventricular distention. As this is a gravity-dependent process, the height of the patient above the reservoir is an important consideration. Suction may be cautiously applied to venous drainage if needed. An additional left ventricular vent line may be placed to minimize left ventricular distention and warming resulting from drainage of systemic, pericardial, and bronchopulmonary collaterals and thebesian veins [20]. A surgical suction cannula is also available and may be connected with a line to the reservoir.

Placement of the aforementioned cannulas facilitates extracorporeal circulation and a bloodless surgical field but does not offer a mechanism for myocardial protection. An additional cannula is, therefore, placed for administration of cardioplegia. This cannula may be placed such that flow of cardioplegic solution is anterograde via an aortic root cannula located on the cardiac side of the aortic cross clamp, or retrograde via a balloon catheter in the coronary sinus. Cardioplegic solutions are administered to stop cardiac activity once the aortic cross clamp is placed to reduce energy requirements, protect myocardial cells, and scavenge free radicals. Cardioplegic solutions may be blood-based (sanguineous) or crystalloid-based, with additives for cardiac protection (e.g., mannitol or lidocaine) and high levels of potassium to stop electrical activity.

Sanguineous solutions are thought to provide better oxygen delivery and scavenging of free radicals, especially for longer procedures [20,23]. Additional myocardial protection is achieved using systemic and/or local hypothermia (using iced saline slush around the heart if appropriate and with adequate protection of the phrenic nerve).

Systemic responses – pathobiology

Although cardiopulmonary bypass offers ideal conditions for surgical intervention, the processes involved also generate real or potential negative effects on a multitude of organ systems. These have been reviewed extensively and many continue to form the basis of ongoing study [24–27]. Briefly, contact of blood components with the cardiopulmonary bypass circuitry (tubing, pump, and oxygenator) rapidly results in significant activation of the inflammatory cascade not dissimilar to that occurring in sepsis. Surgical processes also contribute and together these result in platelet, white blood cell, complement, and cytokine activation. The consequences of this inflammatory response can be far reaching, influencing coagulation, which, in turn, can increase microemboli and bleeding and result in organ dysfunction. This is, therefore, an area of significant investigation both into how anesthetic drugs or/and modifications in circuit components (e.g., heparin-bonded circuits) might favorably modulate these responses to benefit the patient. A few of the common medications and strategies that aim to maximize patient outcome in light of these changes are presented in the next section.

Drugs and interventions used during cardiopulmonary bypass

Antibiotics

Owing to the invasive nature of the surgical procedure and inflammatory changes resulting from bypass, a broad-spectrum antibiotic is administered prior to and at fixed intervals during surgery.

Steroids

Historically, because of the many cellular and humoral changes that occur during cardiopulmonary bypass, steroid use has been advocated. Although steroid administration is associated with an increase in blood glucose, which, in turn, is associated with a poor neurologic outcome, considerations such as improved hemodynamic stability, lower rates of postoperative atrial fibrillation, and reduced myocardial injury and inflammation have generally outweighed concerns [28–30]. More recently, while use may still be advocated in children even though evidence of benefit is limited [31], steroid use is considered equivocal in adults with some studies suggesting increased risk of myocardial infarction and lack of benefit to outcome. A meta-analysis suggests that dose may have a significant impact on results following steroid use with low doses being considered potentially beneficial and high doses potentially detrimental [32]. Steroids are no longer routinely administered to dogs prior to cardiopulmonary bypass at the author's institution.

Antifibrinolytics

Both lysine analogs (e.g., ε-aminocaproic acid and tranexamic acid) that inhibit proteases through antagonism of free plasmin, and nonspecific protease (or plasmin) and kalikrein inhibitors (e.g., aprotinin) have been used preoperatively with to the aim of reducing the need for post-bypass transfusion in human patients [33–35]. The lysine analogs act as antifibrinolytics and help prevent dissolution of the clot, while aprotinin has both antifibrinolytic and anti-inflammatory actions. While aprotinin was used in both human and canine patients and was effective at reducing transfusion requirements perioperatively, there was suggestion of increased risk of renal, neurologic, and cardiovascular complications and anaphylaxis, which led to its (temporary) withdrawal. Both tranexamic and aminocaproic acid continue to be used in human patients although dosing guidelines (dosage and timing of administration) vary. Seizures are more commonly reported with tranexamic acid as compared to aminocaproic acid but both are effective at decreasing the need for transfusions in people [36]. Our current practice is to use ε-aminocaproic acid prior to and during cardiopulmonary bypass and until chest wall closure. Following assessment of coagulation parameters and clinical signs, additional drug may be administered during the postoperative period.

Anticoagulation and reversal

Heparin is approved and routinely utilized in human patients for anticoagulation during cardiopulmonary bypass despite the large individual variability in its actions. An initial dose of 300–400 IU/kg of unfractionated heparin has been recommended for human patients and has also been used in clinical canine patients. In the author's experience, the activated clotting time (ACT) following administration of this dose to dogs is typically greater than 1000 s when blood is sampled approximately 10 min after administration; an ACT greater than 400–480 s (in hypothermic patients) is considered by most to be adequate to initiate bypass. Repeated (often partial) dosing is considered necessary if ACT values approach this, while the patient is still connected to the bypass circuit. With the availability of heparin-coated circuits, both initial and repeat dosing may need to be adjusted.

Low-molecular-weight heparin (e.g., dalteparin and enoxaparin) and other anticoagulants that result in direct Factor IIa (thrombin) inhibition (e.g., argatroban and dabigratran), in addition to antiplatelet medications (e.g., clopidogrel) and factor Xa inhibitors (e.g., apixaban and rivaroxaban), are increasingly available for use in the management of (anti)coagulation in humans. Some of these have been studied and used in dogs and cats, but specific studies of their use during cardiopulmonary bypass are lacking [37–40]; however, they are often used for weeks to months postoperatively to prevent clot formation.

The effects of heparin are reversed with protamine sulfate at the conclusion of cardiopulmonary bypass. As discussed later, slow administration is advised as protamine is reported to cause significant hypotension in dogs when administered rapidly [41].

Hypothermia

This is a strategy commonly used during cardiopulmonary bypass to reduce metabolic rate and oxygen consumption. Hypothermia preserves high-energy phosphate stores and reduces excitatory neurotransmitter release, calcium-mediated enzyme induction, and cell destruction [42,43]. The reduction in oxygen demand allows for lower pump flow rates, which, in turn, reduces cell trauma and embolic events and provides better surgical visualization. However, it is not without negative aspects. These include, but are not limited to, changes in drug disposition, coagulation, acid–base and electrolyte values, and increases in blood glucose, viscosity, and cardiac arrhythmogenicity. Extreme hypothermia can also affect the ability to successfully defibrillate the patient.

Of significant importance to the anesthesia team is how pH and blood gas values are managed with body temperature changes. Recall that the solubility of carbon dioxide (and oxygen) in blood increases with hypothermia, while its content remains constant. Hence, the pCO_2 value decreases and pH increases. The influence of temperature on pH results from a change in carbon dioxide solubility (as stated above) and another mechanism that is independent of solubility. The latter mechanism by which pH is influenced is related to the fact that water, a weak solution of acid and base, is a primary solvent in body systems, and its dissociation is directly influenced by temperature. As body temperature decreases, the tendency of water to dissociate to its ionized components (H^+ and OH^-) decreases. Changes in blood pH parallel temperature-related changes for water but are tempered by the buffering capability of the amino acid histidine (and its five-membered imidazole ring). Hence, blood pH remains higher than the pH of neutrality for water at a given temperature [21,43,44].

Alpha-stat management of acid–base balance allows pH and carbon dioxide tensions to follow thermodynamic dissociation changes but keeps the total carbon dioxide constant. The term "alpha" refers to the ratio of unprotonated to protonated histidine. Relevant to the clinician, pH and blood gas values are not corrected for body temperature, but interpreted and managed as they would be at 37 °C. Conversely, pH-stat management consists of holding temperature-corrected values at normal (at 37 °C) as the patient is cooled. In adult human patients, for various reasons including better maintenance of cerebral autoregulation and prevention of stroke, alpha-stat management is most common, and this has also been the management strategy with which the author is familiar for dogs [21,22]. In young children, where the risk for microemboli to cause stroke is negligible, it has been suggested that pH-stat management may improve outcomes by increasing cerebral perfusion. A prospective study in children less than 9 months of age at the time of surgery, however, did not show any difference in neurologic development at either a 2- or 4-year follow-up. Interestingly, a trend to lower postoperative morbidity was observed [45].

Preanesthetic preparation

Patient evaluation

In addition to an accurate body weight and routine physical assessment and laboratory evaluation (including complete blood count, serum chemistry profile, and urinalysis), the patient should have a coagulation profile (prothrombin time [PT], partial thromboplastin time [PTT], thromboelastography, and fibrinogen) and ACT (once anesthetized) assessed, and a blood type and cross-match performed. A complete cardiac evaluation and medication history should also be available. This information forms the basis of discussion among team members of any special considerations for the individual patient. For example, it may be in the patient's best interest to have certain medications (e.g., enalapril) discontinued in advance of anesthesia and surgery, while others (e.g., pimobendan) may be administered. It is increasingly common in our practice to administer oral antiemetics (e.g., maropitant) 8–12 h before anesthesia; gabapentin or trazodone is also considered in active dogs where there are concerns that preoperative sedation with an opioid and benzodiazepine will not be adequate. While there are reports in people suggesting QT prolongation and cardiac excitability following trazodone [46], we have not observed this in our patient population. If pulmonary hypertension is observed, sildenafil may be given PO prior to anesthesia. If a patient presents with abdominal or pleural effusion, drainage of the same may be considered.

Anesthesia setup

A small animal anesthesia machine and ventilator should be checked for functionality and absence of leaks. Standard catheterization (arterial, venous, and central venous multilumen or Swan-Ganz catheters, if desired) and intubation equipment in appropriate sizes should be available. As the patient will be anticoagulated, atraumatic catheter placement is followed by wrapping the catheter sites. A physiologic monitor with the capability to monitor heart rate and rhythm, direct arterial blood pressures, central venous/pulmonary arterial pressures, end-tidal carbon dioxide, oxygen saturation, and both rectal and esophageal temperature should be available. A tool to monitor the neuromuscular junction (e.g., peripheral nerve stimulator and accelerometer), coagulation status (ACT block or PT/INR [prothrombin time/international normalized ratio]), and urinary catheter and collection system should also be readied. It is the author's preference also to have a Doppler non-invasive blood pressure monitor, respirometer, and positive end-expiratory pressure (PEEP) valve available. Multiple syringe pumps, intravenous (IV) fluids, colloids, blood product and medication/administration supplies, blood gas syringes, pressure bags, etc., are also best kept in an easily accessed location.

Additional supplies that should be available include a pacing unit and leads, defibrillator with both external and internal paddles, and tracheostomy supplies (in the event of need for postanesthesia ventilation). An epidural catheter may be considered (generally after coagulation status is normalized) to assist in postoperative pain management.

Medications

In addition to drugs used for anesthesia (Table 34.1), numerous other medications (Tables 34.2 and 34.3) should be available and, in some cases, drawn up. These include anticholinergics, inotropes, vasopressors, antiarrhythmics, furosemide, electrolytes, sodium bicarbonate, heparin, an antifibrinolytic, a neuromuscular blocking agent, and protamine. Insulin may be necessary for treatment of hyperglycemia. Although it is our practice to use an opioid, benzodiazepine, inhaled anesthetic, and neuromuscular blocking agent or balanced anesthesia plan, other anesthesia techniques have been described [13,14].

Table 34.1 Suggested anesthesia drugs for dogs undergoing cardiopulmonary bypass.

Drug	Dose (mg/kg or as noted)
Premedication	
Hydromorphone or	0.1, SC, IM
Methadone	0.7 SC, IM
Midazolam	0.1 SC, IM
Atropine or	0.02, SC, IM
Glycopyrrolate	0.01, SC, IM
Anesthesia induction	
Fentanyl	0.01, IV
Midazolam	0.2, IV
Etomidate or	0.5, IV
Alfaxalone	0.5, IV
Anesthesia maintenance (balanced technique)	
Fentanyl	0.35–0.7 μg/kg/min, IV CRI
Midazolam	0.35–0.7 μg/kg/min, IV CRI
Isoflurane or sevoflurane	Dosed to effect
Cisatracurium or atracurium	0.1–0.25, IV
Local anesthetic nerve blocks for postoperative analgesia	Per individual preference and drug

Table 34.2 Anticholinergics, inotropes, vasopressors, and antiarrhythmic medications for dogs anesthetized for cardiopulmonary bypass.

Drug	Bolus dose (mg/kg, IV)	Infusion dose (μg/kg/min, IV)
Atropine	0.02–0.04	NA
Lidocaine	1–3	80–100
Amiodarone	2 (over 10 min)	10–12
Esmolol	0.1	70–100
Diltiazem	0.24 (slowly)	6
Dobutamine	NA	5–10
Dopamine	NA	2–10
Milrinone	0.05	0.5
Epinephrine	0.005–0.05	0.05–0.2
Phenylephrine	0.002–0.005	1–3
Norepinephrine	NA	0.1–0.2

Table 34.3 Adjunct drug doses for dogs undergoing anesthesia for cardiopulmonary bypass.

Drug	Dose (IV)
Heparin	300–400 IU/kg
Cefoxitin or cefazolin	22 mg/kg every 90 min
ε-Aminocaproic acid	50–100 mg/kg loading dose over 30 min; 10–15 mg/kg/h, IV CRI
Furosemide	0.5–2.0 mg/kg
Protamine	3 mg/kg or 1.3 mg/mg heparin over 30 min

The sequence of events and terminology

Much of what is described here is experientially based from work in two institutions. The author recognizes that other approaches are viable and better suited to other environments.

Following a quick assessment on the morning of surgery and confirmation of the medication and fasting status, the dog is premedicated. Premedication is administered subcutaneously or intramuscularly and generally consists of a non-histamine-releasing opioid such as hydromorphone or methadone. Midazolam and an anticholinergic may be concurrently administered. After approximately 30 min, during which time the anesthesia equipment has been checked for function and drug infusions verified, the dog is brought to the anesthesia induction area and instrumented with an ECG, Doppler, and cephalic IV catheter. Oxygen, IV fluids, and anesthesia drug infusions (which in our practice consist of fentanyl and midazolam) are started. As many dogs are being treated for heart failure, IV fluid administration is conservatively maintained in the range 1–2 mL/kg/h. Anesthesia is induced with IV fentanyl and midazolam along with a low dose of a hypnotic agent (e.g., etomidate, alfaxalone, or propofol) if needed. Following endotracheal intubation and connection to the anesthesia machine, additional equipment, including a pulse oximeter, capnograph, and esophageal temperature probe, are placed. Additional catheters to facilitate arterial and central venous blood pressure measurements and blood sampling for pH, blood gas, glucose, acid–base status, electrolytes, packed cell volume (PCV) and total protein (TP), and ACT and PT are placed. Support at this stage may consist of an inotrope to maintain blood pressure and an antiarrhythmic if arrhythmias are observed and of consequence to the patient. The patient is ventilated to maintain a normal arterial carbon dioxide tension, which is verified with a blood gas sample taken after the arterial catheter is in place. If other abnormalities are noted in pH, blood gas, acid–base, electrolyte, or glucose values, attempts are made to correct these. External heat is typically not provided in these patients at this stage since patient cooling will occur with initiation of bypass.

While the surgical site is being clipped, prophylactic antibiotics are administered and repeated at 90-min intervals during anesthesia. A loading dose (followed by an infusion) of ε-aminocaproic acid is also started at this time.

Following movement of the dog into the operating room and appropriate positioning, a rectal temperature probe is placed. If neuromuscular blocking agents are to be used, a peripheral nerve stimulator with accelerometer is placed. The central venous line is connected for monitoring central venous pressure. A baseline ACT or PT is taken prior to administration of heparin and commonly another blood sample is taken for measurement of pH, blood gases, electrolytes, glucose, lactate, PCV, and TP. The patency of the urine collection system bag is verified, and the bag emptied if necessary.

The surgeons begin working on placement of the femoral (or carotid) cannula and may simultaneously or subsequently begin the thoracotomy. This is usually a good time to have internal defibrillator paddles set up on the surgical table. Heparin is given and the ACT or PT is rechecked within 10 min following administration. If a neuromuscular blocking agent is to be used, it may be administered at this time. Fentanyl and midazolam infusions are continued, and the inhalant and inotropes are adjusted as necessary to normalize blood pressure while maintaining an appropriate anesthetic plane. As surgeons manipulate the heart to place the cannulas, hypotension resulting from changes in cardiac filling and arrhythmias may be seen and are treated as necessary to minimize influence on blood pressure and/or chance of premature fibrillation. PEEP at 2.5–5.0 cmH_2O is applied after the chest is open in an effort to maintain oxygenation if it does not impair visualization by the surgeon [47,48]. Alternatively, it may be applied once the pericardial sling is in place.

Occasionally, a dog may lose blood or fibrillate during cannula placement. Treatment is appropriate to the cause and in some cases might include a rapid transition to extracorporeal circulation. If the process goes uneventfully, then the planned transition to partial bypass is initiated by unclamping the venous lines (connected to the venous cannulas) and starting the arterial pump. It should be kept in mind that flow is no longer pulsatile, so monitors will tend to record only a mean value once the heart stops ejecting. It is common for blood pressure to decrease significantly during this transition to extracorporeal circulation. This is thought to be due in part to abrupt changes in volume, hematocrit, colloid oncotic pressure, and viscosity. The perfusionist will adjust the pump flow to vary the mean arterial pressure with the traditional goal in adult humans being to maintain pressure between 40 and 70 mmHg [20]; recently, higher pressures have been suggested in human patients due to the beneficial impact on neurological outcome. The perfusionist may request a vasoconstrictor such as phenylephrine to assist in maintenance of blood pressure if the pump flow rate is deemed to be adequate for the size of the patient.

This is also the time when the perfusionist starts to take over the administration of the inhaled anesthetic, and mechanical ventilation may be reduced or stopped as the heart stops ejecting blood. PEEP is maintained as it has been shown in dogs to benefit oxygenation at least transiently without negative impact on cardiac output [47–49]. Injectable anesthetic infusions are frequently decreased as the patient is cooled. This is done despite demonstrated decreases in concentrations resulting from hemodilution and pump sequestration for drugs such as fentanyl due to the decrease in metabolic rate with hypothermia (which, in turn, decreases anesthetic requirements) and changes in protein binding (which increase the free drug fraction) [50,51]. If atracurium or cisatracurium is used for neuromuscular blockade, significant increases in dosing interval will be noted with hypothermia. Antifibrinolytic medications, when used, are usually continued at least until conclusion of bypass, but increasingly until the chest wall is closed. Blood for pH, blood gases, acid–base, blood glucose and electrolyte values, ACT/PT, and PCV/TP may be obtained from the perfusionist, who is also able to administer medications (e.g., antibiotics, neuromuscular blocking agents) as necessary; IV lines may continue to be used, but it should be noted that vascular flow patterns are altered and this may have an additional influence on drug kinetics. Peripheral vasoconstriction resulting from hypothermia is also common.

As the patient cools, the cardiac rhythm, if not already altered from primary disease and manipulation, will often change and ventricular fibrillation may be noted. Although one can attempt to defibrillate electrically at this time, success is limited in profoundly hypothermic patients. Hence, it is best to place the patient on total bypass as soon as feasible. To do this, the surgeon places the aortic cross clamp and administers cardioplegic solution as previously described to stop electrical activity. Once the aortic cross clamp has been placed, the ventilator is turned off if this was not done previously. The perfusionist now assumes full responsibility for patient management while the surgical team works on the heart. The anesthesia team serves a supportive role during this period.

As the cardiac procedure is reaching its end, the anesthesia, surgical, and perfusion teams must be in communication to transition the patient off bypass successfully. It is worthwhile to check blood values just prior to coming off the pump. It should be kept in mind that potassium values may be abnormally high due to the administration of cardioplegic solution, but no intervention is necessary as this effect will resolve once cardiac circulation resumes. Infusions of antiarrhythmic, inotropic, and vasoactive drugs are usually started at this time in an effort to load them prior to coming off bypass; bolus doses may be used as needed. Although epinephrine or a combination of dobutamine and dopamine has been successfully used, the author's preference has been to transition the dog off bypass with dobutamine and phenylephrine. It has further been our experience that dogs do not typically require antihypertensive medications such as nitroprusside. However, these should be available as their necessity has been described by others. The perfusionist will also start to warm the patient at this time in anticipation of transitioning off bypass.

Ventricular fibrillation may be noted during this period or after removal of the aortic cross clamp. If defibrillation is unsuccessful after a few attempts, it may be wise to let the heart rest and warm, while the dog is still on partial bypass. Although there is no absolute guideline, clinical experience suggests that if defibrillation attempts are unsuccessful during weaning from the pump, warming the patient to between 33 and 35 °C usually results in success. On rare occasions, the dog may need to be paced temporarily. The patient may also spontaneously resume a normal electrical rhythm and gradually begin to eject blood with cardiovascular support as warming continues. The surgeon will ask the anesthesia team to help de-air the heart by using the ventilator to give a large breath or series of breaths and move blood into the heart. Transesophageal echocardiography may also be used to verify the absence of air in the left heart prior to cardiac closure. Ventilation is resumed once the heart begins to eject blood as noted by return of pulsatile flow on the arterial line. The perfusionist will gradually decrease the pump's contribution to circulation as the heart resumes functioning.

Once the heart is pumping adequately, cannulas can be removed and protamine administration started. Doses between 2 and 6 mg/kg or 1.3 mg/mg heparin have been described. Selection of dose should be made after consideration of duration of heparin administration, ACT/PT values, and body temperature. Significant hypotension may be seen with protamine administration in dogs, which is thought to be primarily associated with histamine release, but increased central nitric oxide release has also been implicated [41,52]. With slow administration, anaphylactoid reactions are still possible and in part are thought to be due to excessive complement activation resulting from the formation of heparin-protamine complexes. In some patients, anaphylactoid reactions may be mediated via immunoglobulin E antibodies. The responses can be immediate or delayed. Protamine has also been reported to affect platelet number and function, enhance fibrinolysis, and decrease clot strength, which, in turn, can contribute to bleeding [53–55]. Given that there may be other causes of hypotension (e.g., surgical bleeding) during this period, communication between the surgical and anesthesia teams is critical to determine the cause and extent. pH, blood gases, blood glucose, acid–base status and electrolytes, PCV/TP, and ACT are checked as needed during this period and abnormal values are addressed. Urine output is also assessed at this time, keeping in mind that it is not unusual to see discoloration related to hemolysis following bypass. It is fairly common, despite the use of high potassium-containing cardioplegic solutions, to see potassium values decrease during this phase. Calcium values also tend to be low and supplementation may help correct protamine-induced hypotension. Although magnesium may be used in a patient where difficulty is encountered during defibrillation attempts, treatment of hypomagnesemia is usually deferred until the patient is in the critical care unit owing to the potential for hypotension with administration. Fresh whole blood can be administered concurrently with or after protamine to provide platelets and coagulation factors.

The closure of the chest wall is managed as for any thoracotomy; a chest drain is placed. If blood gases are suggestive of hypoxemia relative to the F_IO_2, furosemide may be administered. The team may also elect to maintain these patients on a ventilator for the immediate postoperative phase either via the orotracheal tube or, if less sedation is desirable, a tracheotomy. Typically, anesthesia infusions are reduced during body wall closure. Intercostal or intrapleural local anesthetic blocks may be performed. The supportive infusions and IV fluids (crystalloid, colloid, and blood products) are titrated as necessary. If available, a cell salvage device can be a useful tool to conserve blood. At the conclusion of surgery, the critical care team verifies and rewraps all catheters, the chest tube, etc., and the patient is then transitioned to them for postoperative care. In addition to evaluation of blood gases, electrolytes, blood glucose and lactate, coagulation parameters may be rechecked at this time.

Given the complexity of the process and relatively infrequent nature with which cardiopulmonary bypass is currently performed in veterinary medicine, it is imperative that lines of communication between the anesthesia, perfusion, surgery, and critical care teams are maintained to maximize the possibility of a successful outcome.

References

1 Brourman JD, Schertel ER, Holt DW, *et al.* Cardiopulmonary bypass in the cat. *Vet Surg* 2002; **31**: 412–417.

2 Klement P, Feindel CM, Scully HE, *et al.* Mitral valve replacement in dogs. Surgical technique and post operative management. *Vet Surg* 1987; **16**: 231–237.

3 Kombtebedde J, Ilkiw JE, Follette DM, *et al.* Resection of subvalvular aortic stenosis. Surgical and perioperative management in seven dogs. *Vet Surg* 1993; **22**: 419–430.

4 Monnet E, Orton EC, Gaynor JS, *et al.* Open resection of subvalvular aortic stenosis in dogs. *J Am Vet Med Assoc* 1996; **209**: 1255–1261.

5 Monnet E, Orton E, Gaynor J, *et al.* Diagnosis and surgical repair of partial atrioventricular septal defects in two dogs. *J Am Vet Med Assoc* 1997; **211**: 567–572.

6 Orton EC, Herndon GD, Boon JA, *et al.* Influence of open surgical correction on intermediate-term outcome in dogs with subvalvular aortic stenosis: 44 cases (1991–1998). *J Am Vet Med Assoc* 2000; **216**: 364–367.

7 Lew LJ, Fowler JD, Egger CM, *et al.* Deep hypothermic low flow cardiopulmonary bypass in small dogs. *Vet Surg* 1997; **26**: 281–289.

8 Orton EC, Mama K, Hellyer P, *et al.* Open surgical repair of tetralogy of Fallot in two dogs. *J Am Vet Med Assoc* 2001; **219**: 1089–1093.

9 Martin JM, Orton EC, Boon JA, *et al.* Surgical correction of double-chambered right ventricle in dogs. *J Am Vet Med Assoc* 2002; **6**: 770–774.

10 Griffiths LG, Orton EC, Boon JA. Evaluation of techniques and outcomes of mitral valve repair in dogs. *J Am Vet Med Assoc* 2004; **224**: 1941–1945.

11 Orton EC, Hackett TB, Mama K, *et al.* Technique and outcome of mitral valve replacement in dogs. *J Am Vet Med Assoc* 2005; **226**: 1508–1511.

12 Tanaka R, Shimizu M, Hoshi K, *et al.* Efficacy of open patch-grafting under cardiopulmonary bypass for pulmonic stenosis in small dogs. *Aust Vet J* 2009; **87**: 88–92.

13 Kanemoto I, Taguchi, D, Yokoyama S, *et al.* Open heart surgery with deep hypothermia and cardiopulmonary bypass in small and toy dogs. *Vet Surg* 2010; **39**: 674–679.

14 Uechi M, Mizukoshi T, Mizuno T, *et al.* Mitral valve repair under cardiopulmonary bypass in small-breed dogs: 48 cases (2006–2009). *J Am Vet Med Assoc* 2012; **240**: 1194–2012.

15 Rodriguez AL, Mama KR, Wagner AE, *et al.* Retrospective evaluation of plasma biochemical values in dogs anesthetized for cardiopulmonary bypass and influence on anesthetic mortality. In: *Proceedings of the 9th World Congress of Veterinary Anesthesia 2006*, Santos, Brazil, 2006; 131.

16 Pelosi A, Anderson LK, Paugh J, *et al.* Challenges of cardiopulmonary bypass – a review of the veterinary literature. *Vet Surg* 2013; **42**: 119–136.

17 Iwahashi H, Yuri K, Nose Y. Development of the oxygenator: past, present and future. *J Artif Organs* 2004; **7**: 111–120.

18 Nishinaka T, Nishida H, Endo M, *et al.* Less blood damage in the impeller centrifu gal pump. A comparative study with the roller pump in open heart surgery. *Artif Organs* 1996; **20**: 707–710.

19 Linneweber J, Chow TW, Kawamura M, *et al.* In vitro comparison of blood pump induced platelet microaggregates between a centrifugal and roller pump during cardiopulmonary bypass. *Int J Artif Organs* 2002; **25**: 549–555.

20 Nyhan D and Johns RA. Anesthesia for cardiac surgery procedures. In: Miller RD, ed. *Miller's Anesthesia*, 6th edn. Philadelphia, PA: Elsevier Churchill Livingstone, 2005: 1941–2004.

21 Nussmeier NA, Hauser MC, Sarwar MF, *et al.* Anesthesia for cardiac surgical procedures. In: Miller RD, Eriksson LI, Fleisher LA, *et al.*, eds. *Miller's Anesthesia*, 7th edn. Philadelphia, PA: Elsevier Churchill Livingstone, 2010: 1889–1975.

22 Greeley WJ, Berkowitz DH, Nathan AT. Anesthesia for pediatric cardiac surgery. In: Miller RD, Eriksson LI, Fleisher LA, *et al.*, eds. *Miller's Anesthesia*, 7th edn. Philadelphia, PA: Churchill Livingstone Elsevier, 2010: 2599–2652.

23 Orton EC. Inflow occlusion and cardiopulmonary bypass. *Small Animal Thoracic Surgery*. Baltimore, MD: Williams & Wilkins, 1995: 185–201.

24 Gravlee GP, Davis RE, Utley JR, eds. *Cardiopulmonary Bypass: Principles and Practice*. Baltimore, MD: Williams & Wilkins, 1993.

25 Knudsen F, Andersen LW. Immunological aspects of cardiopulmonary bypass. *J Cardiothorac Anesth* 1990; **4**: 245–258.

26 Hirai S. Systemic inflammatory response syndrome after cardiac surgery under cardiopulmonary bypass. *Ann Thorac Cardiovasc Surg* 2003; **9**: 365–370.

27 Hammon JW Jr, Edmunds HL Jr. Extracorporeal circulation: organ damage. In: Cohn LH, Edmunds LH Jr, eds. *Cardiac Surgery in the Adult*. New York, NY: McGraw Hill, 2003: 361–368.

28 Aarts LP, Boonstra PW, Rakhorst G, *et al.* Prophylactic use of dexamethasone in cardiopulmonary bypass. *Chest* 2004; **126**: 854S.

29 Engleman RM, Rousou JA, Flack JE, *et al.* Influence of steroids on complement and cytokine generation after cardiopulmonary bypass. *Ann Thorac Surg* 1994; **60**: 801–804.

30 Tilman VS, Savvas G, Gotz JKW, *et al.* Effects of dexamethasone on intravascular and extravascular fluid balance in patients undergoing coronary bypass surgery with cardiopulmonary bypass. *Anesthesiology* 2002; **96**: 827–834.

31 Gibbison B, Villalobos Lizardi JC, Aviles Martinez KI, *et al.* Prophylactic corticosteroids for paediatric heart surgery with cardiopulmonary bypass. *Cochrane Database Syst Rev* 2020; **10**: CD013101.

32 Chai T, Zhuang X, Tian M, *et al.* Meta-analysis: shouldn't prophylactic corticosteroids be administered during cardiac surgery with cardiopulmonary bypass? *Front Surg* 2022; **9**: 832205.

33 Troianos CA, Sypula RW, Lucas DM, *et al.* The effect of prophylactic epsilon-aminocaproic acid on bleeding, transfusions, platelet function and fibrinolysis during coronary artery bypass grafting. *Anesthesiology* 1999; **91**: 430–435.

34 American Society of Anesthesiologists. Practice guidelines for perioperative blood transfusion and adjuvant therapies: an updated report by the American Society of Anesthesiologists Task Force on Perioperative Blood Transfusion and Adjuvant Therapies. *Anesthesiology* 2006; **105**: 198–208.

35 Kovesi T, Royston D. Pharmacological approaches to reducing allogenic blood exposure. *Vox Sang* 2003; **84**: 2–10.

36 Aggarwal NK, Subramanian A. Antifibrinolytics and cardiac surgery: the past, the present and the future. *Ann Card Anaesth* 2020; **23**: 193–199.

37 Gagnon AL, Scansen BA, Olver C, *et al.* Phase I clinical trial of an antithrombotic drug protocol combining apixaban and clopidogrel in dogs. *J Vet Cardiol* 2021; **36**: 105–114.

38 Bae J, Kim H, Kim W, *et al.* Therapeutic monitoring of rivaroxaban in dogs using thromboelastography and prothrombin time. *J Vet Intern Med* 2019; **33**: 1322–1330.

39 Brainard BM, Kleine SA, Papich MG, *et al.* Pharmacodynamic and pharmacokinetic evaluation of clopidogrel and the carboxylic acid metabolite SR 26334 in healthy dogs. *Am J Vet Res* 2010; **71**: 822–830.

40 Mischke R, Schmitt J, Wolken S, *et al.* Pharmacokinetics of low molecular weight heparin dalteparin in cats. *Vet J* 2012; **192**: 299–303.

41 Stoelting RK, Henry DP, Verburg KM, *et al.* Haemodynamic changes and circulating histamine concentrations following protamine administration to patients and dogs. *Can Anaesth Soc J* 1984; **5**: 534–540.

42 Little DM. *Hypothermia. Anesthesiology* 1959; **20**: 842–877.

43 Davies LK. Hypothermia: physiology and clinical use. In: Gravlee GP, Davis RE, Utley JR, eds. *Cardiopulmonary Bypass: Principles and Practice*. Baltimore, MD: Williams & Wilkins, 1993: 140–154.

44 Alston TA. Blood gases and pH during hypothermia: the "-stats." *Int Anesthesiol Clin* 2004; **42**: 73–80.

45 Bellinger DC, Wypij D, du Plessis AJ, *et al.* Developmental and neurologic effects of alpha-stat versus pH-stat strategies for deep hypothermic cardiopulmonary bypass in infants. *J Thorac Cardiovasc Surg* 2001; **121**: 374–383.

46 Laiwala RC, Srinivasan S. Mind the heart – evaluating the arrhythmogenic potential of trazodone. *Am J Geriatr Psychiatry* 2017; **25**: S108–S109.

47 Rustomjee T, Wagner A, Orton EC. Effect of 5 cm of water positive end-expiratory pressure on arterial oxygen tension in dogs during and after thoracotomy. *Vet Surg* 1994; **4**: 307–310.

48 Kudnig ST, Monnet E, Riquelme M, *et al.* Effect of positive end-expiratory pressure on oxygen delivery during 1-lung ventilation for thoracoscopy in normal dogs. *Vet Surg* 2006; **35**: 534–542.

49 Riquelme M, Monnet E, Kudnig ST, *et al.* Cardiopulmonary effects of positive end-expiratory pressure during one-lung ventilation in anesthetized dogs with a closed thoracic cavity. *Am J Vet Res* 2005; **66**: 978–983.

50 Mets B. The pharmacokinetics of anesthetic drugs and adjuvants during cardiopulmonary bypass. *Acta Anaesthesiol Scand* 2000; **44**: 261–273.

51 Hall RI. Cardiopulmonary bypass and the systemic inflammatory response: effects on drug action. *J Cardiothorac Vasc Anesth* 2002; **18**: 83–98.

52 Hamada Y, Kameyama Y, Narita H, *et al.* Protamine after heparin produces hypotension resulting from decreased sympathetic outflow secondary to increased nitric oxide in the central nervous system. *Anesth Analg* 2005; **100**: 33–37.

53 Lindblad B, Wajefuield TW, Whitehouse WM, *et al.* The effect of protamine sulfate on platelet function. *Scand J Thorac Cardiovasc Surg* 1988; **22**: 55–59.

54 Nielsen VG. Protamine enhances fibrinolysis by decreasing clot strength: role of tissue factor-initiated thrombin generation. *Ann Thorac Surg* 2006; **81**: 1720–1727.

55 Bailey CJ, Koenigshof AM. The effects of protamine sulfate on clot formation time and clot strength thromboelastography variables for canine blood samples. *Am J Vet Res* 2014; **75**: 338–343.

35 Cardiac Pacemakers and Anesthesia

Barret J. Bulmer
Tufts Veterinary Emergency Treatment and Specialties, Walpole, Massachusetts, USA

Chapter contents

Introduction, 674
Artificial pacemakers, 674
Pacemaker modalities, 675
Anesthetic management, 676
Patient evaluation, 676
Temporary pacemaker implantation, 677
Permanent pacemaker implantation, 677
Considerations for anesthesia, 677
Complications, 678
Pacemaker patients undergoing non-cardiac procedures, 678
References, 678

Introduction

Cardiac anesthesia and surgery can generally be described as high risk, high reward. Pacemaker implantation exemplifies this since no other group of patients has such a high risk of sudden asystole and death, but yet can have a dramatic improvement in quality of life with successful implantation. The anesthetist can have a significant impact on the management of perioperative risk through understanding the surgical procedure and the needs of the cardiologist, selecting drugs and techniques that minimize the effects on heart rhythm and function, and having an emergency plan should severe bradycardia or asystole occur. Since pacemaker implantation can extend the lifespan of many animals, it is becoming more common to perform non-cardiac elective and emergency procedures on animals with pacemakers.

Since the first report of pacemaker implantation in a dog with complete heart block [1], artificial pacemakers have become a mainstay for dogs, and less commonly cats, for bradyarrhythmia management. Because of the increasing number of pacemaker implantations, there are two common scenarios that will be encountered by the anesthetist: (1) anesthesia for pacemaker implantation or pacemaker system modification in a patient with a bradyarrhythmia or (2) anesthesia of a patient with a previously implanted and functional artificial pacing system undergoing an unrelated medical or surgical procedure [2]. While anesthesia delivery to these patients can be challenging, by better understanding implantation procedures, the function of pacemakers, and interactions of anesthetic and hemodynamic supportive drugs, overall anesthetic risk can be reduced.

Artificial pacemakers

Permanent transvenous artificial pacemakers are comprised of one or more pacing leads and a pulse generator (Fig. 35.1). The pacing lead wire delivers the electrical impulses to the heart and serves as the sensing electrode to detect native electrical activity. The lead consists of three parts: (1) the conductor (a coil of wire that conducts the electrical current), (2) lead insulation, and (3) a lead connector. Attachment of a transvenous pacemaker lead to the endocardial surface is most often accomplished using either passive (e.g., tined) or active fixation (e.g., fixed or retractable helical screw) leads (Fig. 35.2). Many leads incorporate a steroid eluting reservoir in an attempt to reduce scar tissue formation, which, if it were to occur, could contribute to unacceptably high pacing thresholds.

The pacemaker lead is the weakest link of the implantable artificial pacemaker system. It serves a passive function to deliver current developed from the pulse generator to the heart and to relay signals from the heart to the pulse generator. At a stimulus rate of 70 beats/min, the heart contracts 36.8 million times per year. Respiration, along with motion induced by ventricular and atrial contraction and closure of the tricuspid valve, exposes transvenous leads to profound mechanical stresses of flexion, torsion, and elongation that must be combated. Despite ever-improving lead technology, failure related to conductor fracture, insulation breakage, or lead dislodgement and failure at the header remain recognized complications (Fig. 35.3) [3].

The pulse generator contains the battery and computer circuitry controlling the timing of electrical impulses sent to the heart,

Veterinary Anesthesia and Analgesia: The Sixth Edition of Lumb and Jones. Edited by Leigh Lamont, Kurt Grimm, Sheilah Robertson, Lydia Love and Carrie Schroeder.
© 2024 John Wiley & Sons, Inc. Published 2024 by John Wiley & Sons, Inc.
Companion website: www.wiley.com/go/lamont/anesthesia

the sensing threshold of the pacing lead, and the response to sensed electrical activity. Pulse generator technology has progressed with the incorporation of advanced circuitry and microprocessors providing telemetrically programmable pacing parameters and a wealth of diagnostic data to help monitor and manage arrhythmias [4]. These advancements have allowed the development of more sophisticated and physiologic pacing modalities.

Pacemaker modalities

Pacemakers implanted in dogs most often employ a single lead that paces the apex of the ventricle (e.g., right ventricle for a single transvenous lead) irrespective of atrial activity. More advanced pacing systems may employ a single-lead physiologic pacemaker (e.g., coordinates native atrial depolarization with ventricular stimulation) [5], a dual-lead system to pace the atria and ventricles, or a three-lead system to pace the atria along with simultaneous activation of the right and left ventricles [6]. Programmed pacemaker modalities are most often described using a five-letter code (Table 35.1). The NBG coding system is a joint project between the **N**orth American Society of Pacing and Electrophysiology (NASPE) and the **B**ritish Pacing and Electrophysiology **G**roup (BPEG). Although some newer pulse generators defy description by the NBG code, most pacemakers implanted in veterinary patients employ only the first three or four letters. However, with a potential increase in implantation of cardiac defibrillators in dogs [7,8], veterinary medicine may have need of the complete five-letter NBG code.

The first position in the code indicates the chamber paced, the second indicates the chamber sensed, the third indicates the response to spontaneous depolarizations, and the fourth commonly describes rate modulation. Hence a VVIR pacemaker paces and

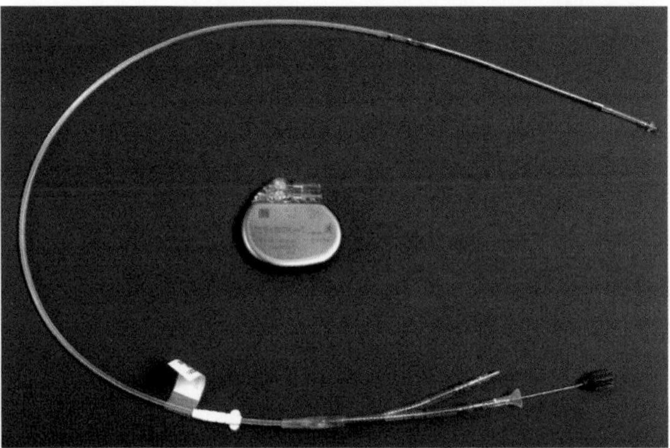

Figure 35.1 A dual-chamber pulse generator (both atrial and ventricular ports are present) along with a transvenous pacemaker lead. This particular lead has two floating atrial electrodes which enables atrioventricular (AV) sequential pacing in dogs with AV block using only a single pacemaker lead.

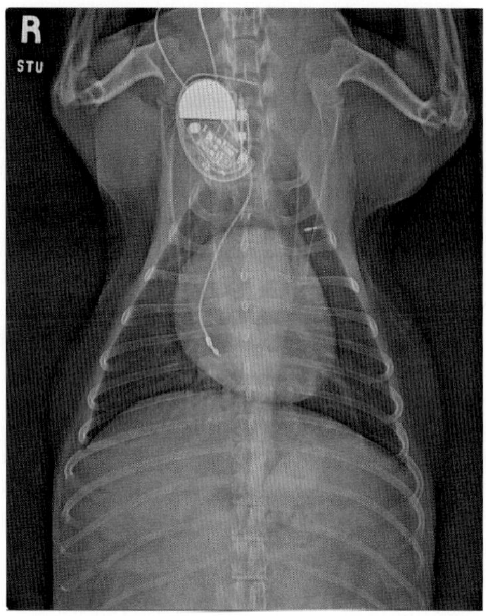

Figure 35.3 Radiograph from a dog that had loss of pacemaker capture on a recheck examination. Failure to pace was related to fracture of the pacing lead at its junction with the header.

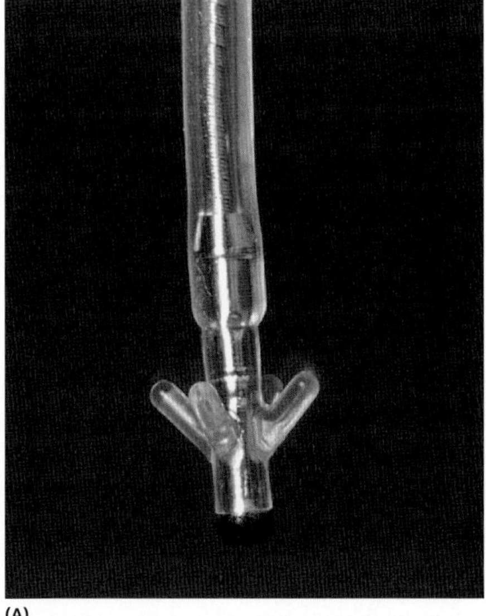

(A)

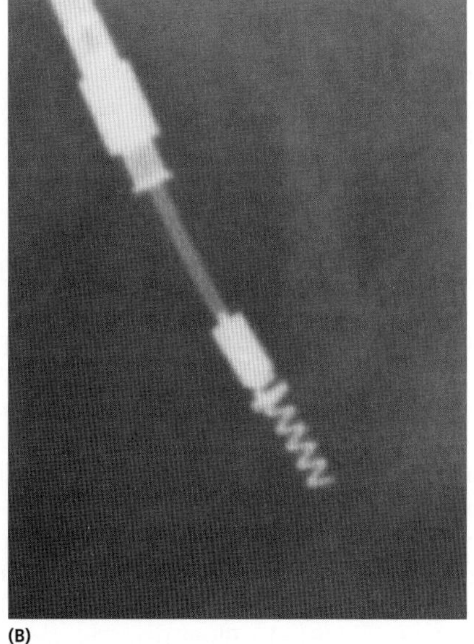

(B)

Figure 35.2 **A.** Tined (passive) pacemaker leads employ small plastic "fins" to entangle within the trabeculae carneae to enhance short-term lead security. **B.** Active fixation leads have either a fixed or a retractable helical screw to penetrate and adhere to the myocardium.

Table 35.1 The five-letter NBG coding system description of pacemaker modalities.

I Chamber paced	II Chamber sensed	III Response to a sensed impulse	IV Programmable functions/rate modulation	V Anti-tachycardia function
V = ventricle A = atrium D = dual (V and A) O = none	V = ventricle A = atrium D = dual (V and A) O = none	I = inhibited T = triggered D = dual (I and T) O = none	P = programmable M = multiprogrammable C = communicating R = rate modulation O = none	P = pacing S = shock D = dual (P and S) O = none

NBG, joint project between the North American Society of Pacing and Electrophysiology (NASPE) and the British Pacing and Electrophysiology Group (BPEG).

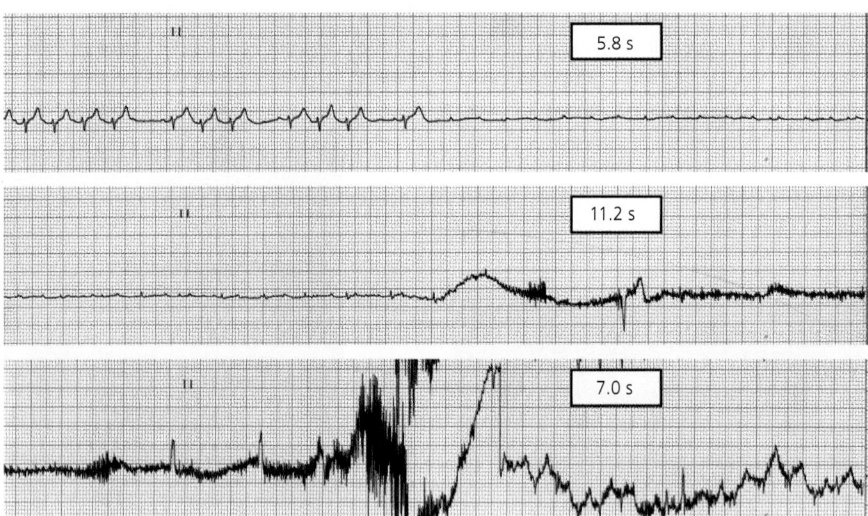

Figure 35.4 Continuous lead II ECG (25 mm/s) from a cat that presented for acute onset "seizure-like" activity. The episodes were triggered by intermittent, sustained atrioventricular (AV) block with lack of a stable ventricular escape focus. In this particular ECG, an absence of AV conduction or stable ventricular escape focus persisted for approximately 24 s. The artifact in the ECG was produced by movement accompanying the syncopal episode. Emergency pacemaker implantation was performed and the cat survived without recurrence of episodes for more than 2 years.

senses only the ventricle. In response to a sensed impulse, a VVIR pacemaker is inhibited until there is another period of quiescence in the sensed chamber. If no impulse is detected in a VVIR pacemaker at the end of a programmable lower rate interval, a ventricular stimulus will be delivered. The fourth position, most commonly an R, represents rate modulation wherein an activity sensor (e.g., accelerometer, respiratory rate, and QT interval) is able to increase the programmed heart rate during activity. A VDD pacemaker paces only the ventricle, but it senses both the atrium and ventricle. Delivery of a stimulating electrical impulse to the ventricle is triggered by a sensed atrial impulse and it is inhibited by a sensed ventricular impulse. A DDD pacemaker is able to sense and pace both the atrium and the ventricle. Biventricular (BiV) pacing implies simultaneous pacing of the right ventricular apex and left ventricular free wall.

Most pacemakers are programmed to discharge only on demand (synchronous pacing). However, on rare occasions pacemakers may be programmed (often temporarily) to an asynchronous pacing mode (e.g., VOO). In this modality, the ventricle is paced at a fixed rate independent of the underlying rhythm. Depending on the pulse generator, placement of a strong magnetic field over the generator may change the programming from synchronous to asynchronous. If the installed unit is an implantable cardioverter defibrillator, placement of a magnet over the generator usually turns off defibrillation. Asynchronous pacing can increase the likelihood that a pacemaker impulse may fall on the T-wave of a spontaneous beat, causing an R on T event, which may lead to ventricular fibrillation. The avoidance of asynchronous pacing will reduce this risk.

Anesthetic management

The most common indications for pacemaker implantation in dogs and cats are high-grade second- and third-degree atrioventricular (AV) block, sick sinus syndrome (SSS), and persistent atrial standstill. In humans, pacemaker implantation for these indications is usually performed on an outpatient basis with local anesthetic techniques, limiting the need for an anesthesiologist's involvement. However, to facilitate cooperation by veterinary patients, most artificial pacing systems are placed during general anesthesia [9,10]. Currently, there is no evidence that anesthetics alter the stimulation threshold of pacemakers [11]; therefore, the primary considerations when formulating an anesthetic plan are focused on (1) the utility of placing a temporary pacing system and (2) selection of anesthetic drug and techniques that do not adversely affect the animal's underlying cardiac status during the implantation procedures.

Patient evaluation

Patients may have considerable variability in their ventricular rate and underlying rhythm. Atropine response tests are often performed during initial patient workup and provide guidance as to whether anticholinergics will be beneficial. Cats with third-degree AV block have ventricular escape rates that far exceed those seen in most dogs [12]. The median heart rate reported in 21 cats with third-degree AV block was 120 beats/min (range 80–140) [12]. In the author's experience, cats with intermittent high-grade AV block (as opposed to sustained third-degree AV block) are the most unstable, often exhibiting ventricular asystole presumably related to overdrive suppression of ventricular escape foci (Fig. 35.4). The intermittent nature of AV block can also make diagnosis more challenging as the presence of sinus rhythm on examination does not exclude an intermittent arrhythmogenic cause for "seizure-like" activity [13].

Additional testing, such as blood chemistries and complete blood counts, is also useful in helping identify primary or secondary changes such as renal insufficiency or electrolyte abnormalities. It should be emphasized that blood collection via jugular venipuncture should not be performed in these patients. Hematoma formation can delay or prevent successful transvenous lead placement, especially when transvenous temporary pacing is employed wherein both jugular veins are commonly used. Patients with a previously implanted transvenous pacing lead should never be injected or bled from that jugular vein since accidental damage to the pacing lead could result. A thorough evaluation of the patient's cardiac status is important as canine valvular disease, feline myocardial disease, or volume overload related to long-standing bradycardia may influence anesthetic candidacy along with short- and long-term outcome post-pacemaker implantation.

Temporary pacemaker implantation

Despite the increasing frequency of pacemaker implantation, anesthetic and procedural times remain long enough that animals with symptomatic bradyarrhythmias may become unstable with irreversible asystole. A report from an experienced veterinary cardiology center reported mean procedural times of 94.9 and 133.5 min and mean anesthesia times of 137.9 and 179.1 min for implantation of single- and dual-chamber pacing systems, respectively [14]. Therefore, placement of a temporary pacing system in the event that a ventricular escape focus becomes unstable, or a prolonged period of sinus arrest occurs, would seem prudent.

Either a transvenous or transthoracic [15] method is most often used to achieve temporary cardiac pacing. Transesophageal placement of a pacing lead or electrophysiologic catheter may capture the atria but would be less suitable for temporary pacing in dogs with AV block [16,17]. Prior to beginning the procedure, intravenous antibiotics are administered to reduce the risk of lead contamination, vegetative endocarditis, and phlebitis. Temporary transvenous pacing requires placement of a catheter introducer into the jugular (or lateral saphenous) vein under mild sedation or local anesthesia. If local anesthetics (e.g., lidocaine or bupivacaine) are used in animals with an escape rhythm, the smallest dose possible is recommended owing to the potential inhibition of myocardial sodium channels and inadvertent suppression of the escape rhythm. Fluoroscopic guidance can be used to maneuver a temporary pacing lead, via the catheter introducer, through the right atrium, across the tricuspid valve, and into the right ventricle. After appropriate positioning, the temporary pacing lead is connected to an external temporary pulse generator and artificial pacing can commence. This permits control of heart rate during induction and prevents anesthetic drug-induced alterations. Transvenous pacing, in comparison with transthoracic pacing, has the advantage of myocardial stimulation without pain or thoracic skeletal muscle stimulation [15]. The disadvantages include the technical skill needed for placement of the catheter introducer and lead (especially if the patient is only lightly sedated), risk for vascular/cardiac perforation or infection, risk for lead dislodgement/loss of ventricular capture with lack of resumption of the ventricular escape focus leading to asystole, and the need for an external cardiac pulse generator and sterile temporary pacing lead.

Transthoracic temporary cardiac pacing generally employs an external cardiovertor defibrillator with pacing capabilities and a pair of disposable transthoracic patch electrodes. The left and right precordia are shaved, conductive paste is placed on the surface of the electrodes, and the adhesive patches are placed on the left and right side of the chest directly over the precordial impulse [15]. Often the electrodes are secured with elastic non-adhesive bandaging material to maintain skin contact during muscle contraction and patient movement. In most cases, anesthesia with rapid-acting injectable anesthetics is subsequently induced and testing for ventricular capture is performed. The disadvantages of transthoracic temporary pacing are the requirement for higher current output in comparison with transvenous pacing, the need for general anesthesia because of the pain induced by a required higher current output, thoracic skeletal muscle stimulation during cardiac pacing that may make permanent pacemaker placement more challenging, the potential risk in very large dogs of incomplete ventricular capture, and the need for a defibrillator with pacing capabilities. To avoid skeletal muscle stimulation when using transthoracic pacing, the cardiologist may test for ventricular capture and then turn off temporary pacing unless hemodynamically significant bradyasystole develops. Alternatively, neuromuscular junction-blocking drugs may be administered, requiring the availability of controlled ventilation methods. Neuromuscular junction-blocking drugs may not abolish all muscle activity since the pacing current may be high enough to cause direct muscle depolarization.

Temporary pacing systems should not be used without concurrent careful patient monitoring. If the temporary transvenous pacing lead were to dislodge from the endocardial surface or if the transthoracic electrodes failed to capture the ventricle, the ECG monitor will often still record the pacing spike in the absence of myocardial stimulation. Detection of a QRS complex following the pacing spike and monitoring of the arterial pulse allow confirmation of cardiac contraction. Temporary pacemakers should be viewed as a backup should asystole occur and not be relied upon to replace careful patient monitoring.

Permanent pacemaker implantation

Permanent pacemaker system implantation is usually performed under general anesthesia. Protocols may vary, but the over-riding goal is to maintain the intrinsic heart rate until the pacemaker can be activated. After the pacemaker has become active, protocol choice is of minimal importance. The most common transvenous technique involves identification, isolation, and incision of the jugular vein. The pacemaker lead, often with the help of a stylet and fluoroscopic guidance, is advanced through the cranial vena cava and right atrium, across the tricuspid valve, and into the apex of the right ventricle. A pulse generator pocket is often formed in the neck or dorsally between the scapulae and, if necessary, the lead is tunneled under the skin to connect to the pulse generator. Following connection/activation of permanent pacing, threshold testing to ensure good ventricular capture is often performed, the lead and generator are secured in place, and the incision(s) are closed. Alternative techniques are available for placement of epicardial pacemaker leads [18,19] in cases of pacemaker revision or for the initial implantation in very small dogs, cats, and puppies.

Considerations for anesthesia

The use of anticholinergic drugs should be carefully considered based on the type of underlying rhythm, the expected response (as many animals with high-grade AV block have no meaningful increase in heart rate), and the cardiologist's preferences. The use of atropine or glycopyrrolate may increase the sinus rate in animals with responsive AV block or SSS. If responsive, these animals may develop tachyarrhythmias where the heart rate exceeds the upper limit of the pulse generator. Although this is not a problem for the patient, it may make it difficult to determine if the lead placement is suitable, and if the pulse generator settings are adequate to take over pacing when the effects of the anticholinergic eventually wane. Anticholinergics can also cause an initial transient increase in vagal tone, which may cause a temporary worsening of the underlying rhythm before any beneficial response is seen.

Anesthetic drug selection often incorporates classes that are thought to have minimal, or manageable, effects on conduction and heart rate. Dissociative anesthetics such as ketamine typically cause an increased heart rate through increased sympathetic nervous system activity. However, in animals with maximally stimulated sympathetic nervous systems, significant myocardial depression may occur [20]. Benzodiazepine premedication may provide some reduction in anesthetic dose requirements, but excitation may be induced in some animals.

Hypnotic drugs such as propofol, alfaxalone, and barbiturates have been used with varying success. Propofol infusion is a technique that allows titration of depth of anesthesia without excessive depression of conduction. With all intravenous drug administration, it should be remembered that animals with extremely low heart rates usually have low cardiac output and prolonged drug distribution (onset of effect), and doses result in higher initial plasma concentrations. Slower, careful administration is required when dosing to effect.

Opioid drugs have been used for sedation and analgesia prior to pacemaker implantation. They are reversible with specific antagonists and generally have minimal effects on myocardial contractility. However, most opioids, especially at higher doses, can enhance vagal tone and promote AV blockade. Anticholinergics will often minimize these effects.

Inhalant anesthetics allow the rapid titration of anesthetic depth. Many pacemakers have been placed during inhalant anesthesia, but effects on Ca^{2+} currents and other ion fluxes, along with effects on conduction, have cautioned some to avoid inhalant administration until temporary or permanent pacing is established.

Following anesthesia, sedation is often desirable to facilitate a smooth recovery and minimize risk of lead dislodgement. α_2-Adrenergic receptor agonists are not recommended for pacemaker placement, but acepromazine, benzodiazepines, and sedating opioids have all been used successfully.

Complications

Severe bradyarrhythmia or hypotension during pacemaker implantation requires rapid treatment. The use of β_1-adrenergic receptor agonists such as isoproterenol, dobutamine, dopamine, or epinephrine may improve dromotropy and stimulate escape rates. However, the routine use of positive dromotropes may also potentiate mechanically triggered ventricular early depolarizations, which may lead to ventricular tachycardia or fibrillation. Drugs and equipment should be readied for administration, but withheld until clearly needed.

Ventricular arrhythmias during lead placement typically indicate that the lead has traversed the tricuspid valve. Treatment of ventricular early depolarizations with antiarrhythmic drugs such as lidocaine is often reserved for those patients with severe arrhythmias, and who are not relying on a ventricular escape rhythm for sustaining life.

Pacemaker patients undergoing non-cardiac procedures

Often the anesthetist is called upon to anesthetize patients with pacemakers for other emergent and elective procedures. Consultation with a cardiologist is advisable to assess the adequacy of the programmed parameters and battery life, the expected response to atrial, ventricular, or ectopic complexes, the severity of myocardial or valvular dysfunction, and recommendations for perioperative antibiotic prophylaxis. If possible, anesthesia should be performed in the same facility where the pacemaker programmer is located so that changes in pacing rate, threshold, or sensing algorithm can be made, if necessary. A contemporary ECG recording with the planned surgical procedure is recommended prior to induction of anesthesia.

Patients with rate-responsive, ventricular demand pacemakers (e.g., VVIR) often have a programmed lower rate limit at or below 80 beats/min. This may not be adequate to maintain arterial blood pressure in the face of inhalant anesthetic-induced vasodilation (e.g., isoflurane). It is often advantageous to increase the minimum rate to a level appropriate for anesthesia (e.g., 120 beats/min). If the surgery also has a high likelihood of producing significant chest wall movement, it may be necessary to turn off rate responsiveness to avoid inappropriate pacemaker-derived tachycardia.

In most instances, artificial pacemakers are incompatible with magnetic resonance imaging. Similarly, high-frequency signals accompanying electrocautery may produce numerous complications with implanted pacemakers, including induction of arrhythmias, increased pacing rate in rate-responsive pacemakers, asynchronous pacing, inhibition of pacing, or electrical resetting. Therefore, monopolar electrocautery should ideally be avoided in pacemaker patients unless the pulse generator documentation specifically allows it. Some precautions that may be useful if electrocautery cannot be avoided include pacemaker reprogramming, using short, intermittent bursts at the lowest energy level, avoiding contact between the electrocautery probe and the pacemaker, placement of the return electrode as far from the pulse generator as possible, ensuring that the current pathway does not intersect the pulse generator, and the use of bipolar electrocautery.

Antimicrobial prophylaxis is important in pacemaker patients undergoing procedures associated with bacteremia (e.g., dental cleaning). Various protocols exist, but the goal is to reduce the risk associated with bacterial seeding of the transvenous lead and subsequent phlebitis and endocarditis, which may require surgical removal of the pacing lead.

References

1 Buchanan JW, Dear MG, Pyle RL, *et al.* Medical and pacemaker therapy of complete heart block and congestive heart failure in a dog. *J Am Vet Med Assoc* 1968; **152**(8): 1099–1109.

2 De Carellán Mateo AG, Casamián-Sorrosal D. The perioperative management of small animals with previously implanted pacemakers undergoing anesthesia. *Vet Anaesth Analg* 2022; **49**(1): 7–17.

3 Borek PP, Wilkoff BL. Pacemaker and ICD leads: strategies for long-term management. *J Interv Card Electrophysiol* 2008; **23**(1): 59–72.

4 Ohm OJ, Danilovic D. Improvements in pacemaker energy consumption and functional capability: four decades of progress. *Pacing Clin Electrophysiol* 1997; **20**(1 Pt 1): 2–9.

5 Bulmer BJ, Sisson DD, Oyama MA, *et al.* Physiologic VDD versus nonphysiologic VVI pacing in canine 3rd-degree atrioventricular block. *J Vet Intern Med* 2006; **20**(2): 257–271.

6 Estrada AH, Maisenbacher HW III, Prosek R, *et al.* Evaluation of pacing site in dogs with naturally occurring complete heart block. *J Vet Cardiol* 2009; **11**(2): 79–88.

7 Nelson OL, Lahmers S, Schneider T, *et al.* The use of an implantable cardioverter defibrillator in a Boxer dog to control clinical signs of arrhythmogenic right ventricular cardiomyopathy. *J Vet Intern Med* 2006; **20**(5): 1232–1237.
8 Pariaut R, Saelinger C, Vila J, *et al.* Evaluation of shock waveform configuration on the defibrillation capacity of implantable cardioverter defibrillators in dogs. *J Vet Cardiol* 2012; **14**(3): 389–398.
9 Musselman EE, Rouse GP, Parker AJ. Permanent pacemaker implantation with transvenous electrode placement in a dog with complete atrioventricular heart block, congestive heart failure and Stokes–Adams syndrome. *J Small Anim Pract* 1976; **17**(3): 149–162.
10 Sisson D, Thomas WP, Woodfield J, *et al.* Permanent transvenous pacemaker implantation in forty dogs. *J Vet Intern Med* 1991; **5**(6): 322–331.
11 Veve I, Melo LF. Anesthesia for pacemaker insertion. *Semin Cardiothorac Vasc Anesth* 2000; **4**(3): 138–143.
12 Kellum HB, Stepien RL. Third-degree atrioventricular block in 21 cats (1997–2004). *J Vet Intern Med* 2006; **20**(1): 97–103.
13 Penning VA, Connolly DJ, Gajanayake I, *et al.* Seizure-like episodes in 3 cats with intermittent high-grade atrioventricular dysfunction. *J Vet Intern Med* 2009; **23**(1): 200–205.
14 Genovese DW, Estrada AH, Maisenbacher HW, *et al.* Procedure times, complication rates, and survival times associated with single-chamber versus dual-chamber pacemaker implantation in dogs with clinical signs of bradyarrhythmia: 54 cases (2004–2009). *J Am Vet Med Assoc* 2013; **242**(2): 230–236.
15 DeFrancesco TC, Hansen BD, Atkins CE, *et al.* Noninvasive transthoracic temporary cardiac pacing in dogs. *J Vet Intern Med* 2003; **17**(5): 663–667.
16 Sanders RA, Green HW III, Hogan DF, *et al.* Efficacy of transesophageal and transgastric cardiac pacing in the dog. *J Vet Cardiol* 2010; **12**(1): 49–52.
17 Chapel EH, Sanders RA. Efficacy of two commercially available cardiac pacing catheters for transesophageal atrial pacing in dogs. *J Vet Cardiol* 2012; **14**(3): 409–414.
18 Fox PR, Matthiesen DT, Purse D, *et al.* Ventral abdominal, transdiaphragmatic approach for implantation of cardiac pacemakers in the dog. *J Am Vet Med Assoc* 1986; **189**(10): 1303–1308.
19 Nelson DA, Miller MW, Gordon SG, *et al.* Minimally invasive transxiphoid approach to the cardiac apex and caudoventral intrathoracic space. *Vet Surg* 2012; **41**(8): 915–917.
20 Chamberlain JH, Seed RG, Undre N. Myocardial depression by ketamine. Haemodynamic and metabolic observations in animals. *Anaesthesia* 1981; **36**(4): 366–370.

36 Pathophysiology and Anesthetic Management of Patients with Cardiovascular Disease

Sandra Z. Perkowski[1] **and Mark A. Oyama**[2]

[1] BluePearl Specialty and Emergency Pet Hospital, Malvern, Pennsylvania, USA

[2] Department of Clinical Sciences and Advanced Medicine, School of Veterinary Medicine, University of Pennsylvania, Philadelphia, Pennsylvania, USA

Chapter contents

Introduction, 680
Preanesthetic evaluation, 680
Electrocardiography, 680
Thoracic radiography, 681
Echocardiography, 681
Blood-based cardiac markers, 682
Cooperation between the cardiologist and anesthesiologist, 682
Anesthesia for specific conditions, 683
Conditions associated with volume overload, 683
Right-to-left shunting congenital defects, 687
Conditions associated with pressure overload, 688
Diastolic dysfunction-associated diseases, 689
Diseases associated with arrhythmias, 691
Hypotension, 692
Shock, 693
References, 694

Introduction

In animals with suspected cardiac disease, care must be taken both prior to and during anesthesia to assess the heart's ability to (1) provide adequate cardiac output and tissue perfusion, (2) maintain low venous pressures and prevent congestion, and (3) avoid arrhythmias. The preanesthetic database should include the medical history and physical examination, with particular attention to cardiac and pulmonary auscultation, inspection of the jugular veins, and palpation of peripheral arterial pulses. Commonly considered diagnostics include electrocardiography (ECG), thoracic radiography, echocardiography, and noninvasive blood pressure measurement. The use of cardiac-specific blood-based markers such as N-terminal pro-B-type natriuretic peptide (NTproBNP) and cardiac troponin I (cTnI) as part of the preanesthetic work-up in animals with suspected cardiac disease may be included. The decision regarding if and how to anesthetize patients with cardiac disease relies on the appropriate selection and interpretation of these and other diagnostic tests.

Preanesthetic evaluation

Electrocardiography

ECG is the gold standard for the evaluation of cardiac arrhythmias. However, in the absence of arrhythmias, the sensitivity of ECG to detect underlying cardiac dysfunction and disease is relatively poor. The ECG should be evaluated for heart rate, mean electrical axis (when applicable), rhythm, and criteria for cardiac chamber enlargement. The reader is referred to several excellent reviews of ECG interpretation for further information [1–3]. ECG findings that most commonly impact anesthesia include abnormalities of rate (either bradycardia or tachycardia) or criteria for chamber enlargement. In cats, abnormalities of mean electrical axis are occasionally detected with underlying structural disease, such as cardiomyopathy.

Clinically important bradycardias include second- or third-degree atrioventricular nodal (AV) block, sinus arrest or block, sinus bradycardia, and, less commonly, atrial standstill. The presence of AV block, sinus arrest/block, and sinus bradycardia is often challenged by administration of vagolytic agents such as atropine or glycopyrrolate. Complete resolution of the bradycardia following challenge usually indicates that the bradycardia is due to physiologic high resting vagal tone, and bradycardia occurring while under anesthesia can often be effectively treated with repeated administration of atropine or glycopyrrolate. Incomplete resolution or absence of response to vagolytic challenge often indicates injury or disease of the cardiac conduction system and additional diagnostics, such as thoracic radiography, echocardiography, serial ECG, or 24-h ambulatory ECG (Holter) monitoring should be pursued prior to anesthesia. Depending on the response to vagolytic challenge, some dogs with partial responses can be safely anesthetized with proper selection of anesthetic agents, monitoring, and/or availability of temporary artificial cardiac pacing. Most instances of sinus block/arrest or sinus bradycardia that are part of a pronounced respiratory sinus arrhythmia are vagally mediated and present little risk for anesthesia. In contrast, most cases of high-grade second-degree AV block, third-degree AV block, and atrial standstill indicate the presence of either primary cardiac disease or severe electrolyte or acid-base disturbances and are associated with a significant increase in anesthetic risk. Various forms of bradycardia can also be present in

Veterinary Anesthesia and Analgesia: The Sixth Edition of Lumb and Jones. Edited by Leigh Lamont, Kurt Grimm, Sheilah Robertson, Lydia Love and Carrie Schroeder.
© 2024 John Wiley & Sons, Inc. Published 2024 by John Wiley & Sons, Inc.
Companion website: www.wiley.com/go/lamont/anesthesia

patients with sick sinus syndrome (SSS) wherein intermittent periods of bradycardia and tachycardia both occur.

Clinically important tachycardias include supraventricular tachycardia (SVT), ventricular tachycardia (VT), and atrial fibrillation (AF) or flutter. Sinus tachycardia due to pain, hyperthyroidism, congestive heart failure, and drugs/toxins (e.g., theophylline, terbutaline, and theobromine) can also be present. The impact of tachyarrhythmias on anesthesia depends on the rate, frequency, and duration of such arrhythmias. Very rapid, frequent, and sustained tachyarrhythmias decrease diastolic filling time and cardiac output (CO) while increasing myocardial oxygen demand. Tachyarrhythmias such as sustained SVT, VT, and AF are often associated with clinically significant primary cardiac disease, such as degenerative mitral valve disease in the dog or various forms of cardiomyopathy in both the dog and cat. Ventricular arrhythmias are also common in dogs with extra-cardiac disease, especially diseases of the abdomen such as splenic or hepatic neoplasia or gastric dilation-volvulus. Thus, further diagnostics such as thoracic radiography, echocardiography, Holter monitoring, abdominal ultrasound, and serum chemistry are usually pursued in animals with tachyarrhythmias. In cases wherein arrhythmias appear to be due solely to extra-cardiac causes such that echocardiography reveals normal cardiac structure and function, anesthesia often can be achieved with minimal additional risk.

Thoracic radiography

Thoracic radiography is an extremely useful tool in assessing patients with cardiac disease. Cardiac disease results in activation of neurohormonal responses that serve to increase cardiac preload via renal retention of fluid and sodium. The resultant volume overload produces eccentric cardiac hypertrophy, the severity of which reflects the degree of injury and neurohormonal activity. Thus, radiographic heart size is an excellent surrogate marker of disease severity and risk for congestive heart failure (CHF). Evaluation of radiographic heart size is confounded by variables such as radiographic technique, patient body weight, chest conformation, and breed. Standardized measurement techniques such as the vertebral heart size (VHS) are useful to minimize variability and increase diagnostic value. The VHS system has been extensively reviewed elsewhere [4–6]. Briefly, the long and short axes of the heart are measured from the right or left lateral projection and these measurements are indexed to the number of vertebral bodies starting from the cranial aspect of the fourth thoracic vertebra (Fig. 36.1). The sum of the vertebral length and width of the heart represents the VHS. The range of VHS in healthy dogs and cats is 8.5–10.5 and 6.9–8.1 vertebra, respectively. Although these ranges are generally regarded as applicable across a wide range of breeds and ages, some reports indicate slightly different ranges, although only two of the studies had at least 100 subjects (Table 36.1). As a preanesthetic test, VHS is useful in determining the severity of canine degenerative mitral valve disease in geriatric patients with the typical left-sided systolic murmur. In the authors' experience, regardless of the intensity of the murmur, dogs with VHS < 11.0–11.5 are at low risk for spontaneous development of CHF, whereas those with VHS > 11.5–12.0 are at higher risk. Coupled with inspection of the pulmonary veins and pulmonary parenchymal pattern, VHS helps assess the risk of induced CHF secondary to IV fluid administration (at 5–10 mL/kg/h) while under anesthesia.

In species and diseases other than canine degenerative mitral valve disease, the authors regard VHS as a useful means to assess the risk of induced or spontaneous CHF in dogs with dilated cardiomyopathy and cats with hypertrophic or restrictive cardiomyopathy. In instances of suspected canine or feline cardiomyopathy, detailed echocardiographic evaluation of systolic and diastolic function can supplement radiographic findings.

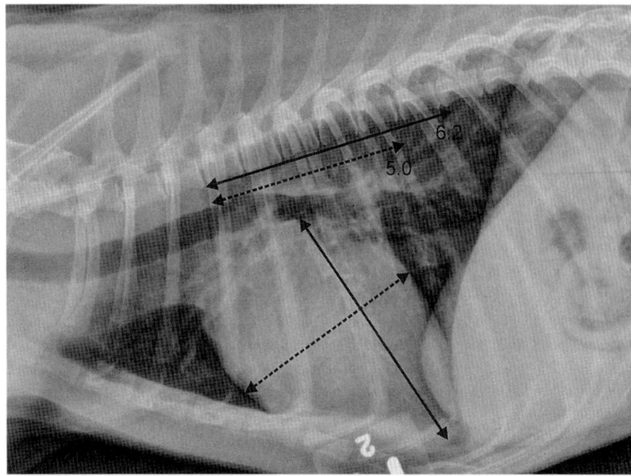

Figure 36.1 Right lateral thoracic radiograph from a 13-year-old female spayed Toy Poodle demonstrating the vertebral heart size (VHS) measurement technique. The length of the cardiac silhouette is measured from a point ventral to the carina of the trachea to the apex of the heart and the width of the silhouette is measured along the widest portion of the heart perpendicular to the long axis. The ventral border of the caudal vena cava is often used as the starting point for the width measurement. The length and width measurements are compared with the number of vertebral bodies starting from the cranial aspect of the fourth vertebral body. In this instance, the length of the silhouette is 6.2 vertebra and the width is 5.0 vertebra, yielding an overall VHS of 11.2.

Table 36.1 Reported mean (SD) radiographic vertebral heart size from various studies in dogs and cats.

Species/Breed	*n*	Mean (SD)	Comments
Canine/Beagle [7]	19	10.3 (0.4)	
Canine/Greyhound [8]	42	10.5 (0.1)	
Canine/Whippet [9]	44	11.0 (0.5)	Right lateral recumbency
		11.3 (0.5)	Left lateral recumbency
Canine/Rottweiler [9]	38	9.8 (0.1)	
Canine/Cavalier King Charles Spaniel [6]	10	10.8 (0.49)	
Canine/mixed [10]	63	9.8 (0.6)	Right lateral recumbency
		9.5 (0.8)	Left lateral recumbency
Canine/puppies [11]	11	10.0 (0.5)	3 months
		9.8 (0.4)	6 months
		9.9 (0.6)	12 months
	6	10.3 (0.6)	36 months
Canine/Boxer [12]	20	11.6 (0.8)	
Canine/Labrador Retriever [12]	25	10.8 (0.6)	
Canine/German Shepherd [12]	20	9.7 (0.7)	
Canine/Doberman [12]	20	10.0 (0.6)	
Canine/Cavalier King Charles Spaniel [12]	20	10.6 (0.5)	
Canine/Yorkshire Terrier [12]	22	9.7 (0.5)	
Canine/mixed [4]	100	9.7 (0.5)	
Feline/mixed [13]	50	7.3 (0.49)	Right lateral recumbency
		7.3 (0.55)	Left lateral recumbency
Feline/mixed [5]	100	7.5 (0.3)	

Echocardiography

Echocardiography represents the gold standard for the clinical evaluation of cardiac structure and function. It is less useful than thoracic radiography in trying to determine the presence or likelihood of CHF manifested as pulmonary edema. Echo provides data regarding ventricular and atrial chamber dimensions, thickness of the ventricular walls and interventricular septum, pattern of blood flow through the heart and proximal portions of the great vessels, myocardial contractility, and morphology of valve structure (Table 36.2). Echo should be performed by individuals not only proficient in image acquisition but also with an adequate familiarity with the pathophysiology of the most common cardiac diseases since interpretation of the echocardiographic-derived data is necessary to assess the impact of changes on anesthetic risk. Measurements from individual animals are interpreted using reference ranges from healthy animals indexed to body weight. The most accurate reference ranges utilize indices indexed to the body weight raised to the power of approximately 1/3, providing a single range of values applicable across all body weights (Table 36.3) [14].

Diseases that result in volume overload (e.g., eccentric hypertrophy) such as canine mitral valve disease, dilated cardiomyopathy (DCM), and patent ductus arteriosus (PDA), result in increased diastolic chamber dimensions, whereas diseases that result in concentric hypertrophy such as feline hypertrophic cardiomyopathy (HCM), systemic hypertension, and congenital subaortic stenosis (SAS), result in increased diastolic and systolic ventricular wall thickness. Diseases that produce decreased contractility, such as DCM, result in increased systolic chamber dimensions. Interpretation of the echocardiogram relies on both subjective and objective evaluation. Because of many breed peculiarities with respect to chest conformation and imaging planes, objective data should always be compared against the subjective evaluation of the sonographer. In fact, subjective estimation of cardiac function by experienced echocardiographers possesses a better correlation with angiographic evaluation than many of the routine objective calculations [15]. Thus, objective measurements should align closely with the trained echocardiographer's subjective assessment of cardiac morphology and function, and discrepancies between the two often indicate measurement errors due to suboptimal imaging planes.

Echocardiographic studies are typically obtained by imaging through the thorax, but images can also be obtained with the use of an intraesophageal probe or transesophageal echocardiography (TEE). TEE, by virtue of its closer proximity to the heart, renders highly detailed views of the heart and great vessels and is often used in patients whose chest conformation or body weight precludes high-quality transthoracic imaging. The high resolution and visual acuity of TEE images facilitate cardiac catheterization procedures, such as device occlusion of PDA or balloon valvuloplasty of valvular pulmonic stenosis (PS). The TEE probe consists of a flexible and steerable shaft (similar to an endoscope) with a phased array ultrasound transducer at its tip. Biplane TEE utilizes two transducers positioned at right-angles from each other whereas multiplane TEE utilizes a single transducer that can be rotated within the scope's housing to permit imaging along any plane from 0° to 180°. In veterinary patients, TEE examination is performed under general anesthesia or heavy sedation, and the TEE probe is inserted through a mouth gag into the patient's oropharynx and esophagus. The probe is positioned over the heart base and multiple imaging planes of the heart can be obtained by switching between the two transducers (biplane) or by rotating the transducer within the probe housing (multiplane) (Fig. 36.2). Excellent reviews of biplane TEE imaging technique and planes in the dog and cat are available [16,17].

Table 36.2 Common echocardiographic measurements and calculations.

Measurement	Commonly used abbreviation(s)
Left ventricle at end-diastole	
Left ventricular end-diastolic dimension; values that are indexed or normalized to the animal's body weight commonly utilize an "i" or "n" (i.e., iLVEDD or LVIDdN)	LVEDD, LVIDd, LVd
Thickness of the left ventricular posterior wall	LVPWd
Thickness of the interventricular septum	IVSd
Left ventricle at end-systole	
Left ventricular end-systolic dimension; values that are indexed or normalized to the animal's body weight commonly utilize an "i" or "n" (i.e., iLVESD or LVIDsN)	LVESD, LVIDs, LVs
Thickness of the left ventricular posterior wall	LVPWs
Thickness of the interventricular septum	IVSs
Diameter of the aortic root	AoD
Diameter of the left atrium	LAD
Ratio of the aortic to left atrium diameter	LA:Ao, LAD:AoD
Fractional shortening [(LVEDD – LVEDSD)/LVEDD] × 100%	FS%

Table 36.3 Upper and lower bounds of the 95th percentile confidence interval (CI) for indexed echocardiographic formula constants in healthy dogs. The constants multiplied by the body weight (BW in kg) raised to an exponential power provide a single reference range across all body weights for the indicated measurements.

Measurement	95% CI boundary	Formula (BW in kg)
iLVIDd	1.35–1.73	iLVIDd = LVIDd/$BW^{0.294}$
iLVIDs	0.79–1.14	iLVIDs = LVIDs/$BW^{0.315}$
iIVSd	0.33–0.52	iIVSd = IVSd/$BW^{0.241}$
iIVSs	0.48–0.71	iIVSs = IVSs/$BW^{0.240}$
iLVPWd	0.33–0.53	iLVPWd = LVPWd/$BW^{0.232}$
iLVPWs	0.53–0.78	iLVPWs = LVPWs/$BW^{0.222}$
iLAD	0.64–0.90	iLAD = LAD/$BW^{0.345}$
iAoD	0.68–0.89	iAoD = AoD/$BW^{0.341}$

Source: Adapted from Cornell *et al.* [14].

Blood-based cardiac markers

The heart is an active endocrine organ. In the case of the sympathomimetic and renin–angiotensin–aldosterone systems, the heart is an end-organ target of neurohormonal activity, whereas in the case of atrial and B-type natriuretic peptide (ANP, BNP), the heart is a source of neurohormonal production. Measurement of ANP, BNP, and NTproBNP (a precursor of BNP) can help differentiate cardiac versus respiratory etiology of respiratory signs, detect occult cardiomyopathy, and provide prognostic information [18–21]. In the setting of anesthesia, the natriuretic peptides, in addition to markers of cardiac tissue injury, such as cTnI, are probably most useful in helping to ascertain the risk of occult cardiomyopathy in cats during the preanesthetic work-up. In selected populations of cats that are at high risk for cardiomyopathy, such as adult cats with a heart murmur, gallop, or arrhythmia, NTproBNP assay detects clinically significant occult cardiomyopathy with moderate sensitivity and specificity [19,20]. Elevated values warrant additional diagnostics such as echocardiography to achieve a definitive diagnosis and help formulate anesthetic recommendations. Natriuretic or troponin assay as part of the preanesthetic work-up prior to routine elective surgery (e.g., spay or neuter) is not currently recommended as the low prevalence of cardiomyopathy in these populations will result in many false positive results.

Cooperation between the cardiologist and anesthesiologist

Animals with pre-existing cardiac disease often undergo evaluation by a cardiology specialist prior to anesthesia. Depending on findings, cardiologists might make recommendations regarding

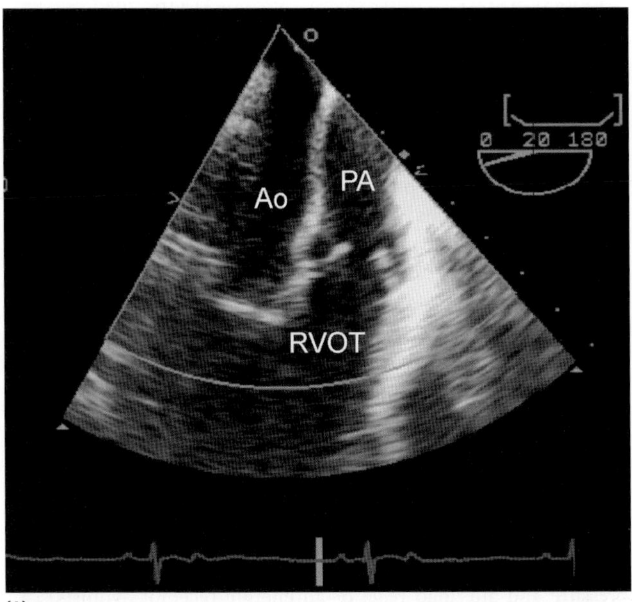

(A)

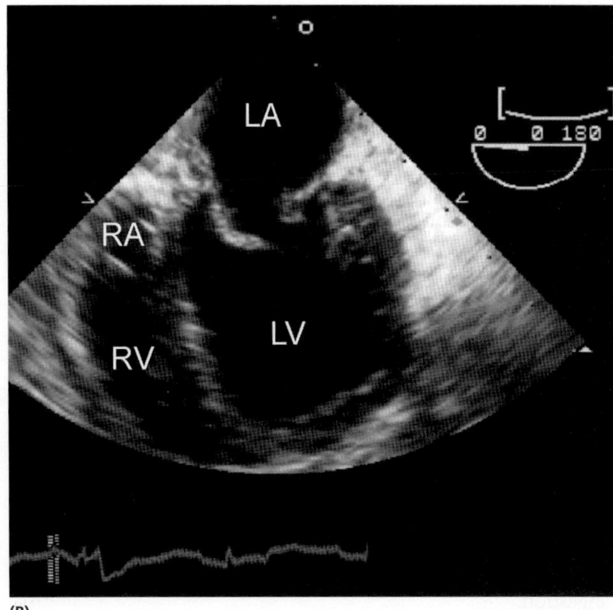

(B)

Figure 36.2 Transesophageal echocardiography (TEE) in dogs. **A.** Dog with congenital pulmonic stenosis showing the incomplete opening and abnormal thickness of the pulmonic valve leaflets from the cranial transverse probe position (RVOT, right ventricular outflow tract; Ao, aorta; PA, pulmonary artery). **B.** Dog with congenital mitral stenosis showing incomplete opening of the mitral valve leaflets and from the middle transverse position (LA, left atrium; LV, left ventricle; RV, right ventricle; RA, right atrium).

chronic medications and recheck exams following anesthesia and resolution of the animal's primary problem. In the authors' opinion, cardiologists should refrain from routinely including specific anesthesia recommendations as part of their consult barring specific requests from the anesthesiologist. The goal of the preanesthetic cardiology consult is to provide the anesthesiologist with information regarding diagnosis and severity of cardiac disease so that the anesthesiologist can make appropriate plans. Good communication and division of duties between the cardiologist and anesthesiologist are essential for proper patient care.

Anesthesia for specific conditions

When anesthetizing any animal with cardiovascular disease, maintaining CO and tissue perfusion is a primary goal. How that goal is best achieved will differ depending on the underlying cardiac condition.

CO is the product of stroke volume and heart rate and decreases in either of these can lead to a low output state. Conversely, fast heart rates, either atrial (e.g., AF) or ventricular in origin, can also lead to a low output state, since diastolic filling times are decreased and/or the atrial contribution (atrial "kick") to ventricular filling is decreased. To determine accurately the reasons for a decrease in stroke volume, it is important to ascertain whether it is due to a change in preload, afterload (increased systemic vascular resistance [SVR]), and/or contractility of the left ventricle. All of these variables are interdependent. For example, chronic excess preload can cause ventricular over-distension and systolic dysfunction. Myocardial contractility and stroke volume also may be affected by indirect causes such as pericardial effusion, inflammatory cytokines, and anesthetic agents.

Valvular heart lesions and/or septal defects lead to changes in the loading conditions of the heart and the approach to the patient changes accordingly. For example, the left ventricle is volume overloaded in mitral regurgitation and pressure overloaded in subaortic stenosis. Compensatory mechanisms differ between conditions and can include chamber enlargement, myocardial hypertrophy, changes in vascular tone, and alterations in sympathetic activity. Changes in myocardial compliance and chronic myocardial dysfunction may follow. Anesthetic management requires an understanding of the alterations in loading conditions so that compensatory mechanisms may be preserved, and problems may be anticipated and avoided before they occur.

Conditions associated with volume overload

Mitral valve insufficiency/regurgitation

Mitral valve regurgitation (MR) can be caused by primary incompetence of the valve leaflets (e.g., myxomatous mitral valve degeneration [MMVD], bacterial endocarditis, congenital malformation) or secondarily to dilation of the annular ring in diseases that cause eccentric hypertrophy secondary to systolic dysfunction (e.g., DCM). MMVD is the most common cause of MR, having a prevalence of approximately 30% in small-breed dogs over the age of 10 years. Regardless of the initial cause, the presence of MR induces further eccentric hypertrophy and annular dilation in a vicious cycle wherein "MR begets further MR."

MR results in volume overload of the left ventricle and left atrium. With incompetence of the mitral valve, the outflow of the left ventricle is divided between the relatively high-pressure/low-compliance outflow tract through the aorta and arterial tree, and the low-pressure/high-compliance outflow route across the incompetent mitral valve into the left atrium. This mismatch in afterload conditions can result in MR volumes representing a high percentage of total stroke volume. This regurgitant fraction can be as high as 50–70% of total stroke volume, highlighting the often-severe degree of volume overload within the left ventricle and atrium. Thoracic radiography is particularly useful in dogs with MMVD such that the radiographic heart size is proportional to the severity of MR. In many cases of uncomplicated MMVD, radiographic inspection of the cardiac silhouette, pulmonary vessels, and pulmonary parenchyma provides sufficient information regarding severity of disease and risk for CHF and helps guide the need for chronic medical therapy.

Although the volume work of the left ventricle is increased, left ventricular systolic wall tension is minimally increased, as the presence of MR allows a large percentage of the work to be done at low pressure. Thus, in most small-breed dogs (body weight < 15 kg) with MR, systolic contractility often appears normal or even hypercontractile when assessed by echocardiography. In larger breed dogs, systolic dysfunction secondary to MR is much more common, for reasons that are poorly understood. Thus, preanesthetic echocardiography to detect systolic dysfunction is often of greater value in large- than small-breed dogs.

The time course for the development of MR influences the severity of symptoms. If the MR develops slowly over time, the left atrium compensates with gradual dilation, and some dogs with severe amounts of MR can be asymptomatic. However, if the MR occurs acutely, as in the case of bacterial endocarditis or acute ruptured primary chordae tendinae, the sudden volume overload can lead to a rapid increase in left atrial pressures and severe pulmonary congestion.

Chronic medical therapy for MR involves reduction in preload (diuretics such as furosemide and spironolactone), reduction in arterial afterload (vasodilators such as angiotensin-converting enzyme inhibitors [ACEIs], and pimobendan), and maintenance of adequate systolic contractility (positive inotropes such as pimobendan). Initiation of medical therapy prior to elective anesthesia should be considered for newly diagnosed cases of MR.

Anesthetic considerations

The primary goal of anesthesia in the patient with MR is to maintain forward aortic flow while minimizing regurgitant flow and development of pulmonary edema (Box 36.1). The volume of regurgitant flow across the mitral valve is related to the size of the regurgitant orifice (which is related to ventricular size), the time available for retrograde flow, and the pressure gradient across the dysfunctional valve [22]. Patients with chronic, compensated MR will be sensitive to changes in ventricular loading conditions and preload should generally be maintained during anesthesia [23]. Overzealous fluid administration should be avoided; however, to avoid ventricular distension and resultant changes in regurgitant flow. Maintenance fluid rates of 2–4 mL/kg/h are generally recommended. Preload reduction may be helpful in some cases. Heart rates should be maintained at a normal or slightly above normal rate to help maintain smaller left ventricular volumes and minimize MR secondary to annular dilation. Bradycardia also increases the duration of systolic contraction and the time available for regurgitant flow.

Most patients with MR benefit greatly from afterload reduction. By reducing afterload, the left ventricular systolic pressures required for ejection from the ventricle to the aorta and arterial vasculature decrease, optimizing forward flow. This, in turn, decreases the pressure gradient from the left ventricle to the left atrium during systole and decreases regurgitant flow. Adequate depth of anesthesia and anesthetic agents that promote arteriolar dilation and maintenance of heart rate are generally recommended. In contrast, administration of drugs that cause increases in systemic blood pressure and afterload (e.g., α_2-adrenergic receptor agonists) can impair forward flow, increase regurgitant flow, and cause rapid deterioration of patients with MR. In early compensated MR, LV contractility may be preserved, but patients with significant MR may benefit from inotropic support with a drug such as dobutamine (5–15 μg/kg/min) (Table 36.4).

Premedication may be required in some cases to decrease the anxiety of the animal and stress during patient handling, minimizing catecholamine release, tachycardia, and increased myocardial work. Ideally, patients should receive supplemental oxygen after receiving sedative medication, but the stress of restraint for oxygen administration should be considered. If preoperative sedation is necessary, opioid receptor agonists are generally the drug class of choice since they usually cause minimal cardiovascular depression at clinically useful doses, with left ventricular contractility, CO, and systemic blood pressure being well maintained. In healthy animals, opioids cause behavioral changes ranging from sedation to excitement; however, in depressed or critically ill patients, opioids usually cause sedation. Opioids may cause dose-dependent bradycardia by stimulation of the vagal nerve [24]. Heart rate should be monitored and an anticholinergic drug such as glycopyrrolate or atropine administered if beneficial. Some animals with MR may also have pulmonary hypertension (PHT) and right heart failure. Increased carbon dioxide secondary to opioid-induced hypoventilation can increase pulmonary pressures and may be of concern in those animals with PHT.

Box 36.1 Hemodynamic goals in patients with mitral valve regurgitation.

Preload: usually increased; some reduction may help decrease regurgitant flow
Afterload: decreases help minimize regurgitant flow
Contractility: unrecognized myocardial depression is possible
Rate: modest increases help maintain smaller left ventricular volume

Table 36.4 Inotropic and vasopressor drugs, adrenergic receptor binding, and standard dose range for dogs and cats.

Drug	α_1	α_2	β_1	β_2	Dose	Comments
Epinephrine	5+	3+	4+	2+	0.01–1 μg/kg/min 0.02–0.2 mg/kg bolus	Primarily β effects at lower doses; increasing α effects at higher doses For cardiac arrest
Norepinephrine	5+	5+	3+	0/1+	0.01–0.1 μg/kg/min	β_2 effect not evident clinically
Dobutamine	0/1+	0	4+	2+	5–15 μg/kg/min	Positive inotropic effects, β_2 effect decreases afterload
Phenylephrine	5+	2+	0	0	0.2–2 μg/kg/min	
Dopamine	1–5+	2+	3+	2+		Actions are dependent on dose:
					1–3 μg/kg/min	Acts primarily on dopamine-1 receptors in renal and splanchnic vasculature to produce vasodilation
					5–10 μg/kg/min > 10 μg/kg/min	Primarily β effects Primarily α effects
Ephedrine	2+	1+	3+	1+	0.05–0.5 mg/kg	Primary action by an indirect effect; direct and indirect effects (norepinephrine release)

A combination of an opioid receptor agonist (e.g., fentanyl, methadone, or hydromorphone) or agonist/antagonist (e.g., butorphanol and buprenorphine) and a benzodiazepine tranquilizer (diazepam or midazolam) may be used to sedate patients for chest radiographs or echocardiography. This combination provides sedation with minimal cardiovascular depression [25–27]. The use of fentanyl may be more likely to cause clinically significant bradycardia. Reversal may be accomplished by using an opioid receptor antagonist such as naloxone and/or a benzodiazepine antagonist such as flumazenil. Phenothiazine tranquilizers such as acepromazine in low doses may be beneficial in some patients with MR because they calm the patient, decrease afterload, and decrease the incidence of arrhythmias. Acepromazine should only be used after careful consideration; however, since α_1-adrenergic receptor antagonism may cause hypotension, not only by decreasing SVR, but also by causing venodilation and decreased preload. In conscious dogs, intravenous acepromazine (0.01–0.05 mg/kg) decreased mean arterial pressure (MAP) and stroke index, but did not significantly change SVR, heart rate, or cardiac index [28].

In general, a carefully titrated anesthetic induction is preferred in the cardiac patient with continuous monitoring of cardiovascular parameters. Although no one best technique exists, a high-dose opioid technique including an opioid and a benzodiazepine tranquilizer with or without low-dose propofol, etomidate, and/or alfaxalone is often advocated for induction to maintain systolic function in patients with severe myocardial dysfunction. Premedicaton with maropitant 30–60 min prior to induction is helpful in preventing emesis if hydromorphone or etomidate are being used [29]. MR patients with minimal systolic dysfunction may be anesthetized with other protocols using propofol or alfaxalone, (remembering to avoid excessive increases in SVR).

The primary advantages of opioids are lack of myocardial depression and maintenance of hemodynamic stability. Most opioid receptor agonists, with the exception of meperidine, lack negative inotropic effects with clinically used doses. Hydromorphone, methadone, fentanyl, or synthetic fentanyl derivatives such as remifentanil [30–34] are usually preferred. μ-Opioid receptor agonists such as fentanyl and its analogs, although relatively free of direct cardiovascular effects, can cause a significant vagally mediated bradycardia that would result in decreased CO. The extent of the bradycardia is dependent on the dose and rate of drug administration, and the use of any opioid in high doses can produce excessive bradycardia. Some anesthesiologists prefer to administer anticholinergics such as glycopyrrolate prior to high-dose opioids used during induction to avoid extreme swings in heart rate. Vagally mediated bradycardia induced by fentanyl (e.g., at 5 μg/kg IV) can sometimes be useful in ameliorating the sympathomimetic effects of other induction agents such as alfaxalone and help prevent significant changes in heart rate during induction. Other adjunctive drugs are commonly used, including benzodiazepine tranquilizers such as midazolam or diazepam.

A low dose of propofol given as a slow infusion is often used as an induction agent in patients with MR or other cardiac disease. Propofol acts as a vasodilator and can decrease afterload while maintaining heart rate. Rapid administration of large doses of propofol should generally be avoided owing to potentially profound cardiovascular effects, including vasodilation, decreased cardiac contractility, and hypotension [35–41]. In patients with poor systolic function, propofol induction requirements can be reduced by concurrent administration of other drugs in a balanced induction protocol, including an opioid, a benzodiazepine, and/or etomidate. Co-administration of propofol and etomidate decreases the required doses of each individual drug. While one study found that midazolam co-induction decreased the induction dose of propofol and improved the quality of induction, it did not improve cardiopulmonary variables in critically ill dogs [40]. Etomidate is a useful anesthetic induction agent in any animal with cardiac disease associated with poor systolic function [42–45]. Left ventricular pressures, mean aortic pressure, and coronary blood flow do not change significantly in healthy dogs receiving up to 2.5 mg/kg for induction. Etomidate is not arrhythmogenic and may also be useful in animals with cardiac conduction abnormalities. The addition of midazolam decreases the etomidate induction dose required with no change in cardiopulmonary function [45]. An opioid is also used as part of this induction protocol. Alfaxalone has a rather large therapeutic index and can also be used to induce animals with heart disease, although dose-dependent adverse effects such as tachycardia can be seen after larger doses are given rapidly [46–51]. The administration of fentanyl prior to alfaxalone can decrease induction requirements and ameliorate changes in heart rate.

Maintenance of anesthesia can be achieved with an opioid (e.g., fentanyl or remifentanil), propofol infusion, and/or alfaxalone infusion (or some combination of these) with or without an inhalant agent. Etomidate infusions are not recommended owing to the potential for hemolysis associated with the high osmolality of the commercially available formulations and also concerns related to prolonged adrenocortical suppression [52–54]. A single bolus injection of 2 mg/kg etomidate reduces the adrenocortical response to anesthesia and surgery for 2–6 h, and longer infusions have been associated with prolonged adrenocortical suppression and higher mortality rates in critically ill multiple-trauma patients [55].

The hemodynamic changes associated with dexmedetomidine administration include bradycardia and increased SVR and are generally to be avoided. When given as a constant rate infusion without a loading bolus, plasma concentrations are lower and may reduce cardiovascular side effects, although increased blood pressure and decreased heart rate still occur [56]. Use of vatinoxan (MK-467), a peripheral α_2-adrenergic receptor antagonist, in combination with medetomidine may reduce the increase in SVR and may expand the potential utility of α_2-adrenergic receptor agonists in patients with myocardial disease. However, further research to establish the safety of this combination in patients with heart disease is needed.

Most of the commonly used inhalant agents (e.g., isoflurane, sevoflurane, and desflurane) tend to preserve myocardial contractility at light anesthetic planes. The advantages of inhalant anesthetics for maintenance of anesthesia include their dose-dependent cardiovascular effects, the ability to rapidly adjust the depth of anesthesia, and their suppression of sympathetic responses associated with surgical stress. Disadvantages include myocardial depression, systemic hypotension (due to decreased contractility or vasodilation), and lack of postoperative analgesia. Mild decreases in SVR coupled with adequate systolic function may reduce regurgitant fraction and are goals of anesthetizing patients with MR. Decreased preload and decreased systolic function associated with deep planes of inhalant anesthesia are not recommended; therefore, multimodal "balanced" anesthetic techniques are often advocated.

Patients on medication for heart disease are generally continued on their medications (especially diuretics, calcium channel blockers, antiarrhythmics, and inotropic drugs) until the time of anesthesia. Pimobendan acts as both a positive inotrope (by increasing calcium binding to the myofibrils) and as a vasodilator (by acting as a phosphodiesterase 3 inhibitor) and is usually given on the day of anesthesia. However, hypotension may be more pronounced under anesthesia in patients receiving ACEIs such as enalapril and some anesthesiologists prefer to delay giving enalapril until after recovery. It is always prudent to have inotropic and venoconstrictor agents immediately available for the management of intraoperative hypotension since fluid administration is often contraindicated.

Dilated cardiomyopathy

Dilated cardiomyopathy (DCM) is defined as idiopathic systolic dysfunction and is accompanied by eccentric dilation and volume overload as the heart's generation of normal forward stroke volume decreases. The resulting left ventricular dilation involves the mitral valve annulus creating secondary MR, which further contributes to volume overload. DCM is common in large-breed dogs, and in particular the Doberman Pinscher, Irish Wolfhound, and Great Dane. DCM is relatively uncommon in cats following the recognition of taurine deficiency and subsequent reformulation of commercial diets. Taurine deficiency is occasionally seen in dogs, in particular, the Cocker Spaniel. Some dogs receiving grain-free diets are also noted to have moderate-to-severely decreased contractility.

DCM predisposes to CHF in addition to ventricular arrhythmias. In most cases, heart failure is left-sided (pulmonary edema) but can occasionally be right-sided (ascites, pleural effusion). Frequent ventricular arrhythmias can cause activity intolerance, syncope, and sudden cardiac death. A combination of echocardiography, thoracic radiography, and ECG is typically used to diagnose and stage the severity of DCM. Holter monitoring is commonly performed to screen at-risk dogs for ventricular premature beats, which is an early sign of disease. Chronic therapy is targeted toward reduction of preload (diuretics such as furosemide and spironolactone), reduction of afterload (ACEIs and pimobendan), and increased contractility (positive inotropes such as pimobendan and digoxin). Suppression of ventricular arrhythmias is performed acutely using lidocaine or procainamide continuous rate infusion (CRI), and chronically using sotalol or amiodarone. β-Adrenergic receptor antagonists (β-blockers) are occasionally used as an adjunctive ventricular antiarrhythmic but, owing to their negative inotropic effects, caution should be exercised in animals with severe systolic dysfunction or active CHF.

Many cases of DCM are further complicated by the development of AF. AF is particularly common in Great Danes, Mastiffs, Irish Wolfhounds, and other giant breed dogs with DCM. The rapid ventricular rate associated with AF increases myocardial oxygen demand and reduces CO as diastolic filling time decreases. Hence, therapy of AF involves reduction of AV conduction and slowing of ventricular heart rate. The most common agents used include digoxin, calcium channel blockers (e.g., diltiazem), and β-blockers.

Many dogs with early DCM are asymptomatic. Older, large-breed dogs that have occasional ventricular early depolarizations (VPCs) before or during anesthesia, which do not resolve following anesthesia, may benefit from examination by a cardiologist. Some cases of occult DCM are only diagnosed after unexplained VPCs are noticed during and after anesthesia, prompting consultation with a cardiologist.

Anesthetic considerations

Anesthetic considerations for DCM patients are similar to those of animals with MR, with the added concerns of decreased systolic function (which may be severe), CHF, and increased incidence of cardiac arrhythmias. Additionally, dogs with cardiomyopathy often have a significant downregulation of β-adrenergic receptors in the heart, although receptor affinity does not change [57], making these animals more resistant to treatment with a positive inotrope. Dogs with significant systolic dysfunction probably benefit from inotropic drug support (e.g., dobutamine or dopamine) during anesthesia.

Ventricular arrhythmias can be seen during anesthesia in animals with DCM. Antiarrhythmic drugs such as lidocaine and procainamide should be available but are often reserved for cases where the frequency of abnormal beats creates significant blood pressure or CO decreases. Although often unnecessary, esmolol, a short-acting β-blocker, may be given as an infusion as indicated (0.5 mg/kg loading bolus followed by an infusion of 0.01–0.2 mg/kg/min to reduce the frequency of ventricular premature contractions associated with sympathetic stimulation). The dose rate may be adjusted as needed to minimize any negative inotropic and bradycardic effects associated with β-receptor blockade. In addition to blood pressure monitoring (direct or indirect), monitoring of end-tidal CO_2 can be helpful under anesthesia, as a secondary means of monitoring CO.

In dogs with concurrent DCM and AF, electrocardioversion may be considered (if the patient is a candidate) at the beginning of anesthesia. The increased ventricular filling following resynchronization of the atria and ventricles can improve CO. Alternatively, drugs that slow the sinus rate and conduction through the AV node, such as fentanyl, can be used during anesthesia. Anticholinergic agents are to be avoided in dogs with AF but may be useful for dogs with DCM without AF that are bradycardic under anesthesia. Fentanyl at a dose of 5–40 μg/kg/h can be an effective anesthetic in sick dogs when used as a primary agent in combination with oxygen and ventilation in those animals that do not tolerate inhalant anesthetics. Remifentanil has an elimination half-life shorter than that of fentanyl, with rapid recovery times regardless of the duration of infusion, although either opioid is suitable for an infusion technique. Infusion of remifentanil at 0.25–0.5 μg/kg/min with propofol at 0.2 mg/kg/min produces little change in mean arterial blood pressures in healthy dogs, although the heart rate decreases with increasing doses of remifentanil [34].

Left-to-right shunting congenital defects – ventricular septal defect and patent ductus arteriosus

Both ventricular septal defect (VSD) and patent ductus arteriosus (PDA) permit left-to-right shunting, which produces volume overload of the pulmonary circulation and left heart. As the physiologic response to the increased pulmonary circulation progresses, pulmonary and right ventricular pressures may increase, resulting in minimal or reverse flow (right-to-left shunt). Anesthesia without consideration of drug selection and patient management on SVR (and blood pressure) and pulmonary and right ventricular pressure may result in reverse shunt flow and rapid deterioration of the patient's condition. Careful echocardiographic evaluation prior to anesthesia and careful perianesthetic monitoring of patients can facilitate anesthetic management of patients with cardiovascular shunts.

Many VSDs in dogs and cats are relatively small and the volume of the shunt is not sufficient to cause CHF. In contrast, the majority of animals with PDA will suffer from left-sided heart failure within the first year of life if the defect is not corrected. PDA is common in dogs and less so in cats, whereas VSD is more common in cats than in dogs. Both PDA and VSD generate characteristic murmurs that often permit a presumptive diagnosis based on the physical examination findings alone. In both diseases, a combination of echocardiography and thoracic radiography facilitates a definitive diagnosis and permits assessment of shunt volume and risk for heart failure. In general, the extent of left ventricular eccentric hypertrophy and degree of left atrial dilation reflect the magnitude of the shunt.

The extent of shunting depends not only on the cross-sectional area of the lesion, but also on the relative pressures and compliance of the right and left portions of the circulation. Low pressure and compliance of the pulmonary circulation and right ventricle relative to the systemic circulation and left ventricle promote left-to-right shunting. Interventions that either increase right-sided pressure or decrease left-sided pressure decrease the shunt severity, at least to the point where flow reverses through the shunt when hypoxemia and polycythemia can develop. Hence systemic arterial vasodilators can be used to reduce the shunt volume, as can surgical interventions such as pulmonary artery banding, which increase pressure within the right ventricle.

Anesthetic considerations

In animals with VSD or PDA, the degree and magnitude of shunt flow are dependent upon relative outflow resistances, which are determined by the size of the defect or ductus and the difference between systemic and pulmonary resistance. With simple left-to-right shunting, pulmonary blood flow is increased, and the right ventricle and pulmonary vasculature can be pressure or volume overloaded; some degree of pulmonary hypertension (PHT) may be present. Further increases in pulmonary blood flow are avoided by preventing increases in SVR. In addition, manipulations that decrease pulmonary vascular resistance (PVR) (hypocapnia, alkalemia, spontaneous ventilation, and deep anesthesia) can also increase the magnitude of left-to-right shunt flow.

In many cases, heart failure is not yet present, and the animal is relatively young and active and may become excited with restraint. Almost any anesthetic agent that does not significantly alter SVR may be used safely for premedication, induction, or maintenance. Drugs that significantly increase SVR, including the α_2-adrenergic receptor agonists (e.g., dexmedetomidine) are generally avoided. Repair of PDA may be accomplished by surgical ligation or transvascular occlusion, with the rate of survival being similar between the two techniques [58], although arrhythmias and hypotension are commonly reported [59].

If not corrected within the first year, a significant percentage of dogs with PDA will develop CHF. For those cases in which some degree of CHF is present, considerations are similar to those for patients with volume overload (see earlier). An opioid-based induction technique with benzodiazepine tranquilizer and etomidate, alfaxalone, or propofol followed by inhalant anesthesia or propofol infusion, or a combination of fentanyl/remifentanil and propofol infusion can all be used [33,58,59]. Propofol can result in clinically significant changes in cardiac shunt direction and arterial desaturation; however, due to a decrease in SVR [60]. This decrease is usually dependent on the dose and rapidity with which the propofol is given.

Diastolic pressures are often low in these patients owing to the shunting of blood from the systemic circulation to the lower resistance pulmonary circulation. A characteristic change in the arterial waveform may be seen with ligation of the PDA, including a decrease in the pulse pressure, increase in mean and diastolic pressures, and reappearance of a dicrotic (reflected) wave (Fig. 36.3). Hypotension may be pronounced in some patients due to the low diastolic pressures and is generally treated with the use of an inotrope such as dobutamine (see Table 36.4), which helps maintain myocardial function and heart rate while avoiding increases in SVR. However, significant decreases in SVR must also be avoided, especially in those patients with significant PHT in which shunt flows may reverse in the face of inhalant anesthetic-associated arteriolar dilation. These patients will benefit from the administration of a vasoconstrictor (e.g., dopamine or phenylephrine; see Table 36.4) to maintain baseline SVR. A sudden decrease in arterial oxygen saturation due to venous admixture as monitored with a pulse oximeter or arterial blood gas may be an early indicator of shunt reversal.

If surgery is to be performed on a relatively young animal for repair of a congenital heart defect, the progressive maturation of the autonomic nervous system and cardiovascular responses must be taken into account. In puppies, the adrenergic vasoconstrictor response is not fully developed until after 8 weeks of age [61]. Similarly, although chronotropic responsiveness is apparent at 1 week, the inotropic response to sympathetic stimulation does not fully develop until after 8 weeks of age [62]. Neonatal patients typically have a higher heart rate and lower arterial blood pressure and SVR than adults. In addition, the cardiovascular response to sympathomimetic agents may be less pronounced in the neonatal or pediatric patient than the adult animals of similar species [63–65].

Right-to-left shunting congenital defects

Tetralogy of Fallot and reverse patent ductus arteriosus

Tetralogy of Fallot (TF) and reverse patent ductus arteriosus (rPDA) are uncommon congenital heart defects in dogs and are rare in cats. The pathophysiology of both TF and rPDA involves right-to-left shunting and systemic hypoxemia. In the case of rPDA, concurrent

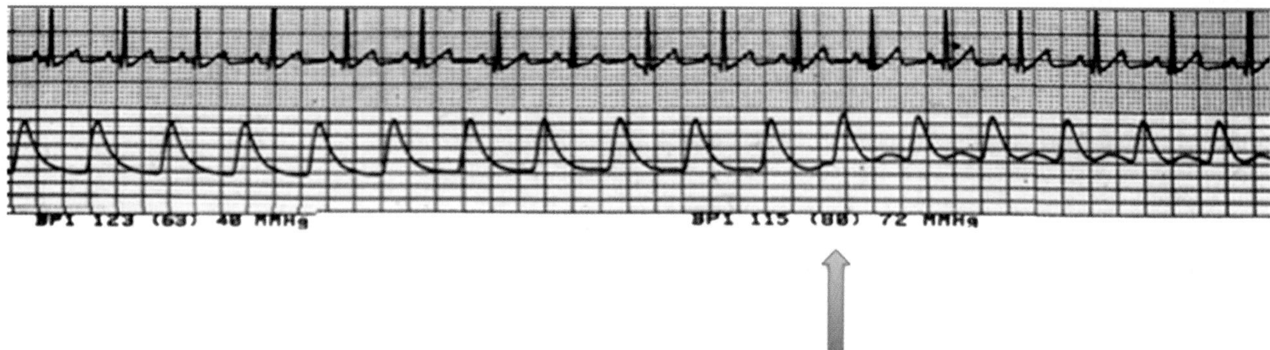

Figure 36.3 Output from a patient monitor during occlusion of a patent ductus arteriosus (PDA) showing the electrocardiogram and arterial pressure waveform. Notice the rapid increase in diastolic arterial blood pressure and the appearance of a dicrotic (reflected) wave during diastole immediately following occlusion (blue arrow). These changes are characteristic of decreased flow through the PDA and can be used to help identify the vessel during surgery.

pulmonary hypertension (PHT) is present. TF is caused by defects in the fetal conotruncal formation resulting in a dextro- or rightward-positioned aortic root, VSD, PS/pulmonic hypoplasia, and secondary right ventricular concentric hypertrophy. The presence of the pulmonic lesion creates pressure overload of the right ventricle sufficient to cause right ventricular to left ventricular shunting through the VSD. The dextropositioned aorta further contributes to admixture of unoxygenated blood into the systemic circulation. rPDA is characterized by a large cylindrical ductus arteriosus and the development of progressive PHT over the animal's first 6–8 months of life. The PHT increases pulmonary artery pressures sufficiently to "reverse" the flow through the ductus arteriosus and shunt blood from the pulmonary circulation to the systemic circulation. Animals with TF or rPDA often display poor growth, activity intolerance, weakness, fainting, and cyanosis. Echocardiography and radiography help provide a definitive diagnosis and assessment of disease severity. ECG abnormalities commonly include right axis shift, interventricular conduction abnormalities, ST segment changes, and occasionally ventricular arrhythmias. The degree of hypoxemia can be assessed through pulse oximetry or arterial blood gas analysis. Chronic hypoxemia stimulates red blood cell production and polycythemia is an important component of the pathophysiology of right-to-left defects. Clinical signs in animals with TF or rPDA are usually due to hypoxemia and polycythemia, and CHF is very rare in both conditions. A packed cell volume (PCV) as high as 70–75% is not uncommon, and activity intolerance, organ dysfunction, and clotting abnormalities commonly occur at these extreme values. Periodic phlebotomy is used to maintain PCV at or below 65%.

The balance between the right- and left-sided pressures affects the extent of shunting, and interventions that lower SVR such as arterial vasodilators can potentiate signs. Signs of weakness or cyanosis are common during attempted exercise as systemic arterial vasodilation to the animal's skeletal muscle occurs. Affected animals are sometimes prescribed non-selective β-blockers such as propranolol to try and limit the amount of β_2-adrenergic receptor-mediated vasodilation during activity.

Anesthetic considerations

Goals of anesthesia for the patient with TF or other reverse shunt disorders are to maintain SVR and arterial pressures while minimizing changes in PVR and pulmonary pressures. As right-to-left shunting increases so does arterial oxygen desaturation. Patients with significant PHT can be sensitive to changes in preload. Hypotension secondary to hypovolemia or vasodilation should be avoided and treated immediately if it occurs.

Premedication with an intramuscular opioid may be useful as struggling and sympathetic stimulation with restraint can increase right-to-left flow. These drugs should, however, be used judiciously as hypoventilation can lead to hypercarbia and respiratory acidosis, which can increase PVR and reverse shunting. Hypoxemia and hypotension can occur quickly in these patients. Preoxygenation prior to induction of anesthesia is extremely important, not only to address the underlying chronic hypoxemia that occurs in these animals, but also as a means of decreasing PVR. Other manipulations that can help decrease PVR include lowering the hematocrit to < 60% prior to anesthesia and hyperventilation with the maintenance of relative hypocarbia and respiratory alkalosis during anesthesia. Care must be taken with controlled ventilation, as increases in intrathoracic pressure with mechanical ventilation or the use of positive end-expiratory pressure can increase PVR and the magnitude of right-to-left shunt flow.

Patients with TF often have a dynamic component to the stenotic lesion and increases in heart rate may exacerbate the pulmonary outflow obstruction and reverse shunting [23]. An opioid-based induction technique is often used with or without etomidate, although significant decreases in heart rates should be avoided, especially if fentanyl or remifentanil is used. All catheters and injection ports should be cleared of bubbles to avoid systemic air embolization.

SVR must be maintained in these patients, as excessive hypotension will increase the right-to-left flow. Phenylephrine, an α-adrenergic receptor agonist that causes arterial and venous vasoconstriction, can be useful in reversing right-to-left shunting during anesthesia, although other pressor agents such as norepinephrine or dopamine may also be used.

Conditions associated with pressure overload

Subaortic stenosis and pulmonic stenosis

Subaortic stenosis (SAS) and pulmonic stenosis (PS) are common congenital valvular defects in the dog. SAS and PS lead to a chronic systolic pressure increase in the left or right ventricle, respectively, with a resultant increase in wall tension and a compensatory increase in ventricular wall thickness or concentric hypertrophy. The increase in ventricular muscle mass and the increase in myocardial work required to generate increased systolic pressures result in an increased demand for coronary blood flow and myocardial oxygen delivery. In theory, the resulting risk for ischemia is greatest during periods of tachycardia and leads to myocardial necrosis, replacement fibrosis, and development of ventricular arrhythmias. In young dogs with severe SAS, the risk for syncope or sudden arrhythmic death is high, whereas the risk of left-sided CHF is typically recognized in much older dogs. Right ventricular concentric hypertrophy, even in cases of severe PS, appears to be better tolerated than cases of left ventricular hypertrophy. Sudden death in dogs with severe PS is relatively uncommon, although clinical signs such as activity intolerance or syncope occur. In the authors' experience, CHF, in the form of ascites, is more common in dogs with PS.

Chronic medical management of severe SAS or PS often involves β-blockers to reduce heart rate and myocardial oxygen demand. Echocardiography is an extremely useful modality to assess the severity of the SAS or PS lesion and the extent of concentric hypertrophy. ECG, 24-h ambulatory ECG (Holter) monitoring, and cardiac troponin assay are useful to evaluate cardiac rhythm and to detect ST segment elevation or depression, which is suggestive of myocardial ischemia. In both SAS and PS, arterial vasodilators should be used with caution as a decrease in arterial blood pressure increases the pressure gradient across the stenotic valve and can lead to increased myocardial work, severe hypotension, and decreased coronary perfusion pressure.

Anesthetic considerations

Patients with SAS or PS often have poor ventricular compliance; thus, it is critically important to maintain adequate preload in these animals. Maintaining an adequate venous return by insuring a full intravascular volume to fill the non-compliant ventricular chamber will help optimize diastolic filling and CO, although volume overload should be avoided. In addition, these patients are dependent on maintenance of a normal sinus rhythm and atrial "kick" to optimize ventricular filling. Tachycardia must be avoided to limit myocardial oxygen deficit (Box 36.2). The stenosis may also have a dynamic component, becoming more pronounced at rapid heart rates.

Box 36.2 Hemodynamic goals in patients with pulmonic or subaortic stenosis.

Preload: optimize intravascular volume to maintain filling of non-compliant ventricle
Afterload: already elevated, but relatively fixed
Contractility: usually not impaired in most patients
Rate: avoid bradycardia (decreased CO), avoid tachycardia (myocardial oxygen deficit)

Afterload is elevated, but relatively fixed due to the stenosis at the level of the valve. Vasodilation and reductions in vascular tone generally do little to relieve the fixed afterload from a stenotic valve, but rather decrease preload and reduce coronary perfusion pressure.

When managing the patient with SAS or PS, it is important to minimize hypotension and treat aggressively if it develops. Volume is the first treatment for hypotension in these patients, followed by the use of a vasoconstrictor such as phenylephrine or norepinephrine (see Table 36.4). Contractility is generally maintained, although inotropes may be helpful in patients with severe SAS or PS with ventricular dysfunction. Dopamine may be preferred to dobutamine since the former will maintain or increase SVR and may be more effective at treating inhalant anesthetic-associated hypotension [66,67], whereas dobutamine maintains or decreases SVR such that the MAP changes little despite an increase in cardiac contractility [68–70]. Norepinephrine may increase MAP by increasing CO, rather than by causing significant increases in SVR, in dogs anesthetized with isoflurane [71]. In some patients with SAS or PS, the obstruction also has a dynamic component, which may be accentuated by reductions in ventricular size, as occurs with increases in heart rate or contractility or decreases in preload or afterload. In patients with PS, increases in PVR may be minimized by maintaining a high F_IO_2 and low $PaCO_2$.

Premedication of patients with SAS or PS may decrease the anxiety of the animal and stress during patient handling and help prevent unnecessary increases in heart rate. Care must be taken, however, to ensure adequate venous return (preload) and optimal diastolic filling. Ideally, patients should receive supplemental oxygen after receiving any medication. If preoperative sedation is necessary, opioids are generally the drugs of choice since they cause minimal cardiovascular depression, although hypoventilation may be of concern in patients with PS. Antiarrhythmic therapy should be instituted to maintain a normal sinus rhythm as needed [72].

Dogs with SAS are at increased risk for bacterial endocarditis of the aortic and mitral valves. Perioperative antibiotics should be considered for surgical conditions that result in bacteremia.

Diastolic dysfunction-associated diseases

Hypertrophic cardiomyopathy and restrictive cardiomyopathy

Hypertrophic cardiomyopathy (HCM) and restrictive cardiomyopathy (RCM) are common cardiomyopathies in cats but are rare in dogs. Both HCM and RCM are characterized by diastolic dysfunction as opposed to DCM, which is primarily a disease of systolic function. The pathophysiology of HCM involves idiopathic concentric hypertrophy of the left ventricle, increased myocardial oxygen demand, myocardial ischemia, and development of left ventricular outflow tract (LVOT) obstruction due to systolic anterior motion (SAM) of the mitral valve leaflets. The pathophysiology of RCM involves idiopathic fibrosis of the left ventricle muscle with resultant diastolic dysfunction in the absence of appreciable concentric hypertrophy. Thus, while the gross appearance of the left ventricle is different between HCM and RCM, the underlying pathophysiology involving diastolic performance is similar.

Diastolic dysfunction results in the inability of the ventricle to properly relax during diastole. The non-compliant left ventricle requires increased pressure to fill properly and the resultant increase in left atrial pressure and volume overload predisposes to CHF. In cats, left-sided CHF can manifest as either pulmonary edema, pleural effusion, or both. Both ventricular arrhythmias due to suspected ischemia and systemic thromboembolism are common in cats with HCM or RCM. It is prudent to evaluate any cat for cardiomyopathy that has unexplained ventricular premature contractions during the perianesthetic period.

The presence of SAM in cases of HCM is multifactorial and incompletely understood. Likely mechanisms for the development of SAM include abnormal mitral leaflet morphology, interventricular septal hypertrophy, misalignment of the papillary muscle and chordae tendinae apparatus due to concentric hypertrophy, and increased flow rates through the narrowed LVOT, which "pulls" the mitral leaflets into the outflow tract. HCM with LVOT obstruction due to SAM is often termed "hypertrophic obstructive cardiomyopathy" (HOCM), and HOCM makes up as much as 50% of all HCM cases. The presence of the LVOT obstruction is akin to animals with SAS. The resulting left ventricular pressure overload further stimulates concentric hypertrophy and increases myocardial oxygen demand. Therapy for HOCM involves reductions in ventricular contractility, heart rate, and outflow tract pressure gradient, which reduce the degree of SAM. Commonly used agents include β-blockers such as atenolol or calcium channel blockers such as diltiazem. Systemic hypertension secondary to chronic kidney disease and hyperthyroidism are common comorbidities in geriatric cats with HCM or HOCM. Overly aggressive arterial vasodilators should be avoided as a reduction in SVR will increase the pressure gradient across the LVOT, potentiate SAM, and increase myocardial oxygen demand. Chronic therapy of HCM, HOCM, and RCM includes preload reduction using diuretics, heart rate control using β-blockers or calcium channel blockers, and antithrombosis using aspirin or clopidogrel. ACEIs are also often prescribed but used with caution due to their arterial vasodilatory potential.

Anesthetic considerations

Anesthesia in cats with HCM is directed at optimizing diastolic filling, both by maintaining relatively low heart rates and by avoiding drugs that may increase cardiac contractility (Box 36.3). Optimizing preload and ventricular filling can be useful. Afterload reduction may worsen the obstruction and marked decreases in arterial pressures are poorly tolerated. Decreases in aortic pressure will contribute to inadequate coronary perfusion and potential myocardial ischemia. In contrast, increasing afterload may decrease SAM and outflow tract obstruction. One study found complete resolution of dynamic outflow obstruction in cats with HCM or SAM receiving medetomidine [73]. Medetomidine, an α_2-adrenergic receptor agonist, causes vasoconstriction and increased SVR, which are both potentially desirable effects in HCM with LVOT obstruction. However, systolic function should be carefully evaluated prior to administration of α_2-adrenergic receptor agonists, and ultimately drugs that can be titrated carefully (e.g., phenylephrine) may be better choices during the anesthetic period [74].

Positive inotropic activity can potentially increase dynamic outflow tract obstruction in addition to myocardial oxygen consumption.

Box 36.3 Hemodynamic goals in patients with hypertrophic cardiomyopathy.

Preload: optimize intravascular volume to maintain filling of non-compliant ventricle
Afterload: maintain or augment, manage hypotension with vasoconstrictor titrated to effect
Contractility: reduction may be helpful
Rate: avoid tachycardia, modest reductions in rate preferred

Ketamine or tiletamine can cause catecholamine release, tachycardia, and increased myocardial contractility and oxygen consumption [75–77]. These agents may also predispose to arrhythmias. Therefore, other anesthetic agents are often preferred. Intramuscular administration of alfaxalone and methadone in healthy cats with or without a low dose of ketamine, provided sedation with no clinically significant effect on echocardiographic variables [78]. Similarly, intramuscular alfaxalone alone or combined with butorphanol had no significant effect on echocardiographic variables, while providing enough sedation for diagnostic procedures [79]. Intravenous bolus administration of alfaxalone can cause dose-dependent cardiopulmonary depression [80]. When given as an intravenous infusion, cardiac index did not change in spontaneously ventilated cats [81]. Low doses of an opioid such as fentanyl or methadone may be given as part of the induction technique. Induction with etomidate, which has a minimal effect on cardiovascular contractility, and a benzodiazepine tranquilizer such as midazolam or diazepam, is often used when venous access is available. Decreased SVR due to decreased sympathetic nervous system activity, which accompanies loss of consciousness, should be anticipated with any anesthetic protocol and appropriate contingency measures considered before induction.

Hypotension occurs with relative frequency in healthy cats anesthetized with inhalation anesthetics. Pressure support for cats with HCM under anesthesia usually involves the use of vasopressors such as phenylephrine, an α_1-adrenergic receptor agonist with little or no β-activity. Phenylephrine increases SVR with little direct effect on the myocardium. In cats with HCM without LVOT anesthetized with isoflurane, both phenylephrine and dopamine increased systemic and arterial blood pressure, although only dopamine increased cardiac index [74]. Plasma levels of cTnI, measured as a marker of cardiac injury, increased in response to hypotension but were not different between the two groups. Phenylephrine or norepinephrine may still be preferred in those cases with LVOT.

Pericardial effusion

The pericardium encloses the heart within the sheet of fibroelastic tissue and the space between the epicardial surface of the heart and the parietal pericardium normally contains a small volume of fluid, the purpose of which is to lubricate the heart and provide a friction-free environment. Pericardial effusion is the abnormal accumulation of large volumes of fluid within the pericardial space, which exerts external compressive forces on the heart. The term "cardiac tamponade" is used to describe situations in which the volume of pericardial effusion is sufficient to decrease cardiac filling markedly, leading to poor CO and shock. In the case of pericardial effusion, the diastolic dysfunction that occurs is not due to an intrinsic abnormality of the myocardium but rather an external compression and restriction of diastolic filling of the heart. Common causes of pericardial effusion include cardiac neoplasia and idiopathic pericarditis in dogs, and CHF and feline infectious peritonitis in cats. Less common is infectious pericarditis or uremic pericarditis.

Common clinical findings in animals with cardiac tamponade include muffled heart sounds, dyspnea, weakness, collapse, pallor, hypotension, tachycardia, and right heart failure (typically ascites or chylothorax). ECG and thoracic radiography can reveal low amplitude QRS complexes and electrical alternans, and a globoid cardiac silhouette, respectively. Echocardiography is particularly useful in confirming the presence of pericardial effusion and detecting heart base masses. Hemangiosarcoma of the right atrium/auricle or chemodectoma associated with the aortic root are two common tumors associated with pericardial effusion.

Therapy involves pericardiocentesis, which provides immediate relief and improvement in CO. Animals with pericardial effusion are very sensitive to changes in preload and diuresis should not be routinely performed unless the animal is volume overloaded, as this can worsen tamponade, further reduce CO, and aggravate clinical signs. In cases with severe ascites, abdominocentesis can be performed to improve respiration and comfort. Chronic pericardial effusion often necessitates surgical pericardiectomy; however, the decision whether to pursue this course is influenced by the etiology of the effusion.

Anesthetic considerations

In the presence of tamponade, intrapericardial pressures determine venous return, and the ventricle can become small and underloaded despite a compensatory increase in right and left ventricular filling pressures to maintain cardiac filling. Stroke volume becomes limited and CO becomes dependent on compensatory mechanisms, including peripheral vasoconstriction to maintain venous return, tachycardia, and increased contractility.

The goal of anesthesia is to select agents that will preserve these compensatory mechanisms and maintain forward flow. Intravenous fluids should be administered prior to induction of anesthesia to optimize preload and maintain cardiac-filling pressures. Small (2–5 mL/kg) boluses of crystalloid or colloids at induction given to optimize preload can offset anesthetic-associated venodilation while avoiding the worsening of pericardial effusion that can occur with longer-term fluid therapy. Drugs that cause myocardial depression, bradycardia, or vasodilation should be avoided. Ketamine, because of its sympathomimetic effects, may be helpful in preserving heart rate and blood pressure [75–77]. However, larger doses can induce hypotension in those animals that are already under maximum sympathetic stress or in critically ill patients [82,83]. Alfaxalone may similarly be helpful in preserving heart rate and blood pressure. An opioid technique can be used, although anticholinergics may be required to preserve heart rate. Regardless of anesthetic technique, it is often beneficial to use a multimodal approach with careful monitoring and titration of drug effect.

Any manipulation that may decrease venous return should be avoided. Controlled positive-pressure ventilation with large tidal volumes may significantly decrease preload and CO. Since thoracotomy for pericardiectomy is usually the surgical treatment for pericardial effusion, positive-pressure ventilation using smaller volumes (lower peak inspiratory pressure) with a higher respiratory rate should be used. Pericardiocentesis may be indicated prior to induction of anesthesia in some animals with severe hemodynamic compromise in order to optimize cardiac filling and stroke volume.

Diseases associated with arrhythmias

Arrhythmogenic diseases resulting in tachycardia

Common tachycardias and associated cardiac diseases include ventricular tachycardia (VT) (seen in Boxer arrhythmogenic right ventricular cardiomyopathy [ARVC], feline cardiomyopathy, DCM, and SAS), atrial fibrillation (AF) (seen in MMVD and DCM), supraventricular tachycardia (SVT) (seen in DCM and MMVD), and accessory pathway-mediated SVT in Labrador Retrievers. Common to all pathological tachycardias is the increase in myocardial oxygen demand and progressive decrease in diastolic filling time. The exact heart rate at which a tachycardia goes from beneficial to detrimental is dependent on many factors, including the origin of the tachycardia (i.e., sinus versus ectopic), species, breed (primarily related to body size), underlying systolic and diastolic function of the heart, and presence of eccentric or concentric hypertrophy. In general, ectopic heart rates > 250 beats/min in cats and small-breed dogs and > 200 beats/min in large-breed dogs are regarded as sufficiently tachycardic to warrant intervention. Clinical findings associated with tachycardia include signs of diminished CO, such as weakness, syncope, pallor, disorientation, hypothermia, or cold extremities. Arterial blood pressure may be normal during tachycardia and reduced CO, but it is due to compensatory arteriolar constriction. Anesthesia with subsequent arteriolar dilation may result in profound hypotension even though the heart rate does not decrease significantly. Tachycardias, especially VT, can predispose to ventricular fibrillation and sudden death.

Treatment is centered on addressing any underlying cardiac disease or heart failure, and administration of specific antiarrhythmic agents. Commonly used agents for acute treatment of ventricular arrhythmias during anesthesia include lidocaine, procainamide, and short-acting parenteral β-blockers such as esmolol. Acute therapy for AF or SVT includes parenteral esmolol or calcium channel blockers such as diltiazem. Chronic therapy of ventricular arrhythmias often uses sotalol or mexiletine or less commonly amiodarone, and chronic therapy of AF or supraventricular arrhythmias uses oral digoxin, diltiazem and/or β-blockers, and occasionally sotalol. Owing to the potential for side effects, lidocaine and procainamide are uncommonly used in cats. Electrocardioversion of tachyarrhythmias may be appropriate for some patients and is often performed just after induction of anesthesia.

Arrhythmogenic diseases resulting in bradycardia

Common bradycardias include second- and third-degree (complete) AV nodal block, sick sinus syndrome (SSS), and atrial standstill. Bradycardia is relatively uncommon in cats but does occur. All cases of bradycardia detected with auscultation during the preanesthetic physical examination should be further evaluated with an ECG and other diagnostics as indicated. SSS is commonly seen in Miniature Schnauzers, whereas AV nodal block is often detected in larger breed dogs, such as the Labrador Retriever. Bradycardia can be detected in association with underlying structural heart disease, but often occurs in isolation, and is thought to represent primary disease of the cardiac conduction system. Idiopathic degeneration of the sinus node, AV node, and other conduction tissue is often assumed. In some cases, acute inflammatory injury to the heart (i.e., myocarditis) is suspected. Bradycardia secondary to electrolyte abnormalities such as severe hyperkalemia can occur in cases of renal disease, uncontrolled hyperadrenocorticism, soft tissue injury, and other conditions.

The exact heart rate at which bradycardia becomes clinically significant depends on the underlying cardiac function, species, and breed. Periods of asystole lasting > 5–8 s are usually sufficient to cause weakness or syncope. Chronic bradycardia with heart rates < 50 beats/min is often associated with activity intolerance, lethargy, weakness, or syncope in dogs. It should be remembered that resting heart rates during sleep can be relatively low compared to values during normal activity. However, the rate during sleep may be a better indicator of the patient's acceptable heart rate during anesthesia. Any time arterial blood pressure becomes heart rate dependent during anesthesia, intervention to increase the heart rate should be considered because it represents a point where stroke volume cannot increase further to maintain CO. In rare instances, CHF due to excessively slow rates occurs. In the authors' experience, chronic symptomatic bradycardia in the cat is rare as most cats maintain escape rates at or near 100 beats/min, which is sufficient to maintain an acceptable quality of life.

Therapy of bradycardia includes correction of underlying electrolyte abnormalities and support of heart rate through parenteral or oral parasympatholytic (e.g., atropine, glycopyrrolate, and probanthine bromide) or sympathomimetic (e.g., isoproterenol, terbutaline, and theophylline) agents. Standard diagnostics performed in animals with bradycardia include bloodwork, ECG, echocardiography, and radiography. Commonly, the influence of native vagal tone on the bradycardia is determined by ECG examination before and after administration of atropine, with the presumption that early or mild conduction system disease (such as asymptomatic intermittent second-degree AV block) can be differentiated from high resting vagal tone by an abnormal response to atropine. Rarely do cases of symptomatic AV block or SSS demonstrate a normal response to atropine, indicating the presence of structural disease of the conduction system.

In cases that are poorly responsive to medical therapy, artificial pacing can be performed. Permanent transvenous or epicardial pacemaker implantation is considered in animals with bradycardia sufficient to cause clinical signs. Temporary transvenous or transthoracic artificial pacing can also be performed in instances where temporary worsening of relatively benign bradycardia could occur, for instance, during anesthesia (see below).

Anesthetic considerations

The goal of anesthesia in the patient with a known cardiac rhythm disturbance is to avoid further deterioration of the rhythm. Arrhythmias should be evaluated prior to anesthesia in terms of both their electrical stability (or lack thereof) and their hemodynamic consequences. Any electrolyte abnormalities should be corrected prior to induction. Stress during restraint of the animal should be minimized if at all possible. Very low doses of acepromazine in combination with an opioid may be helpful as a premedication in some animals with ventricular arrhythmias. In the case of tachycardias that are ventricular in origin, drugs such as propofol, alfaxalone, or etomidate, which have little to no effect on cardiac conduction, may be preferred for induction. An opioid and/or benzodiazepine may also be used as part of the induction technique. A single dose of lidocaine can be given prior to induction to determine the efficacy of this agent in suppressing the ventricular arrhythmia and is occasionally continued as a CRI throughout the procedure, depending on the severity of the arrhythmia. However, VPCs must be differentiated from other ventricular complexes such as escape beats or VT secondary to hyperkalemia, as lidocaine administration in those cases may cause immediate asystole. Alternatively, procainamide may be given intravenously and has a longer duration of action than lidocaine. Drugs such as ketamine that can cause catecholamine release and increased heart rate are usually avoided.

SVT can be difficult to differentiate from VT. In those patients with known SVT, vagomimetic drugs such as fentanyl or a fentanyl analog such as remifentanil may be useful, as these drugs can cause a pronounced decrease in sinus rate mediated through the vagus nerve [84–86]. In these patients, drugs that increase AV nodal conduction (e.g., anticholinergics) are generally avoided. In the case of severe SVT, esmolol may be loaded intravenously and given as a CRI, although the β-receptor blockade can also lead to negative inotropic effects.

For the patient with SSS or heart block, the goal of anesthesia is to prevent the worsening of the bradycardia (e.g., asystole) with drug administration. A relatively high dose of atropine or glycopyrrolate is often given prior to anesthesia to avoid the consequences of a sudden increase in vagal tone. Ketamine–benzodiazepine, alfaxalone, propofol, and etomidate may all be used for induction. Drugs known to cause bradyarrhythmias, such as α_2-adrenergic receptor agonists, should be avoided. A temporary transvenous pacemaker is ideally placed prior to induction of anesthesia or transthoracic artificial pacing pads may be used as needed. During artificial pacing, blood pressure should be carefully monitored as paced beats result in atypical sequences of ventricular depolarization, and coupled with the loss of synchronized atrial activity, CO can be markedly reduced despite successful electrical capture of the heart. In the authors' experience, transthoracic pacing often results in inadequate CO if relied upon for anything other than brief periods of time. Heart rates can decrease dramatically upon induction with the relative decrease in sympathetic tone. Dobutamine, dopamine, or isoproterenol infusions [87] should be prepared prior to anesthetic induction if a temporary pacemaker has not been placed.

Hypotension

Systemic blood pressure is dependent on CO and SVR and must be maintained above the minimum level required to maintain cerebral, coronary, and renal perfusion. Mean arterial blood pressures (MAPs) less than 65–70 mmHg are generally considered inadequate for maintaining optimal blood flow to tissues. In patients that are hypovolemic and hemodynamically unstable, neural and neurohormonal mechanisms can increase SVR and minimize apparent changes in blood pressure, while decreasing blood flow and oxygen delivery to the tissues. Patients that are compensating by increasing SVR can have a precipitous decrease in blood pressure following induction of anesthesia.

CO is determined by stroke volume and heart rate, although stroke volume can also be affected by changes in vascular resistance. Decreases in stroke volume may be seen secondary to decreased venous return (decreased preload), often caused by underlying fluid deficits or peripheral vasodilation (decreased SVR), leading to a relative fluid deficit. In addition, stroke volume may be decreased due to decreased myocardial contractility, increased SVR (increased afterload), and/or cardiac arrhythmias. Induction of anesthesia and the subsequent decreases in sympathetic stimulation can lead to decreases in heart rate, preload, and cardiac contractility, all of which will affect CO. Similarly, administration of vagomimetic opioids (e.g., fentanyl and remifentanil) can reduce heart rate and affect blood pressure, although they are frequently recommended for use as adjunct anesthetics in patients with cardiovascular compromise to reduce inhalant anesthetic requirements.

Duration of hypotension is important in determining ultimate clinical outcome in both cardiac and non-cardiac patients [88], so early recognition is key. Methods for recognition of hypotension can include monitoring changes in heart rate and rhythm, measuring decreases in MAP below 60–65 mmHg, and/or assessing changes in tissue perfusion (e.g., decreases in central venous oxygen saturation and increases in serum lactate). Tachycardia is generally considered a major compensatory response to fluid/blood loss and hypovolemia, although increases in heart rate may also be seen due to inadequate anesthesia, hypercarbia, hypoxemia, or drug administration (e.g., anticholinergics). In addition, the use of vagomimetic drugs such as fentanyl may mask the early compensatory increase in heart rate in response to changes in preload.

Arterial blood pressure may be measured using non-invasive measuring techniques, including Doppler ultrasonographic flow probes and oscillometric measuring devices, or invasively using a direct arterial line and blood pressure transducer. Central venous pressure (CVP) is often used as an indicator of volume status in a given patient. However, a review of the literature found a very poor relationship between CVP and blood volume and the inability of CVP change to predict the hemodynamic response to a fluid challenge [89]. Changes in parameters related to tissue oxygenation such as lactate, blood pH, base deficit, and central venous oxygen saturation are being used with increasing frequency to assess the adequacy of fluid resuscitation and inotropic and/or pressor support. Other dynamic variables used to assess fluid responsiveness, such as pulse pressure variation and systolic pressure variation, may be useful in patients undergoing mechanical ventilation [90].

In any animal, the underlying cause of hypotension should be identified and corrected as rapidly as possible. Hypotension is common during anesthesia due to inadequate preoperative fluid replacement, failure to keep up with intraoperative fluid and/or blood loss, and dose-dependent effects of anesthetics on CO and SVR. Rapid administration of high volumes of crystalloid fluid (e.g., Plasma-Lyte® and Lactated Ringer's solution) has a minimal effect in improving arterial blood pressure during isoflurane-induced hypotension in normovolemic dogs unless the anesthetic plane is also lightened [91,92]. Although CO and stroke volume improve, arterial blood pressure does not change significantly due to decreases in SVR. Colloid administration using relatively large volumes of hetastarch (hydroxyethyl starch [HES]) or dextran 70 [91,93] may increase both cardiac index and blood pressure in anesthetized animals. However, long-term administration of synthetic colloids has been associated with acute kidney injury and increased mortality in human patients with sepsis. The use of other colloids such as fresh frozen plasma and packed red blood cells can also be considered. The underlying disease process, evaluation of ongoing losses and changes in volume status, and close monitoring of changes in PCV, total solids, and determinants of tissue oxygenation should all be used in determining the rate and type of fluids administered to the patient.

Higher fluid rates are usually needed in emergent patients with pre-existing deficits or ongoing blood losses. Low diastolic pressures (< 40 mmHg), large position-associated changes in blood pressure, or difficulty in tolerating positive-pressure ventilation may all alert the clinician to the presence of inadequate volume. In some cases, maintenance of anesthesia may need to be changed from an inhalant to an injectable technique, which causes less myocardial depression and vasodilation than most inhalant techniques.

Pharmacological support

Pharmacological support may be required if hypotension is severe and does not respond to fluid therapy or changes in anesthetic depth.

In addition, patients with cardiovascular disease may not tolerate fluid administration. Drugs are selected for cardiovascular support based on the patient's condition and underlying hemodynamic disturbance, the physiologic response desired, the pharmacology of the available drugs, and clinician experience and opinion. The principal effects include changes in heart rate (chronotropism), contractility (inotropism), myocardial conduction velocity (dromotropism), rhythm, and peripheral vasodilation or vasoconstriction, which influences preload and afterload.

For many years, the choice of agent was made depending primarily on its effects on myocardial function and vascular resistance as determinants of blood pressure. More recently, attention has also been focused on changes in venous capacitance and preload, as well as the distribution of blood flow to the various organs. For example, norepinephrine (0.1–1 μg/kg/min) acts on both α- and β-adrenergic receptors, although it acts primarily as a vasoconstrictor due to its predominant effects at α-adrenergic receptors. Norepinephrine increases arterial vascular tone (afterload), but also increases venoconstriction (preload), which can improve venous return and CO. In healthy dogs anesthetized with isoflurane, norepinephrine increased MAP, CO, and oxygen delivery in a dose-dependent manner, while SVR did not significantly change [71]. In contrast, dobutamine (5–15 μg/kg/min) acts primarily at β-adrenergic receptors, improving cardiac contractility if systolic function is decreased. In addition, β_2-adrenergic receptor-mediated vasodilation may decrease afterload and improve forward flow and tissue perfusion, despite no change in measured blood pressure. Changes in blood lactate, pH, base deficit, and central venous oxygen saturation are often used clinically to help determine what changes in flow are occurring at the tissue level. Drugs used to treat hypotension are discussed in more detail in other chapters.

Shock

The therapeutic priority in patients with circulatory shock is oxygen delivery to the tissues. Sequelae to decreased CO, decreased SVR, and/or decreased blood oxygen content include tissue hypoxia, systemic inflammation, and organ dysfunction. In order to achieve this goal, fluid resuscitation, including blood transfusion, and the use of vasopressors (see Table 36.4) may be required, although the optimal strategy, including choice of fluid for resuscitation and hemodynamic goals, is still controversial in both the human and the veterinary literature.

Selection of target indices for monitoring the hemodynamic response to therapy has changed over the last several years. Blood pressure is relatively easy to measure and is often used as a primary measurement for evaluating the severity of circulatory shock and the adequacy of resuscitation. Blood pressure is also a major criterion used in separating septic syndrome from septic shock [94]. Blood pressure monitoring has serious limitations; however, it assumes that changes in blood pressure values are directly related to altered blood flow (i.e., SVR is unchanged). In the early stages of hemorrhage, neurohormonal mechanisms may maintain blood pressure near normal (at the expense of perfusion to selected tissues) by increasing SVR.

Shoemaker *et al.* first introduced the concept of goal-directed resuscitation in the 1980s, after noting that survivors of high-risk surgical procedures had a higher cardiac index and oxygen delivery in concert with an increased oxygen demand compared with non-survivors [95,96]. Changes in MAP lagged changes in cardiac index, and by the time hypovolemia and low flow to the tissues were of sufficient magnitude to produce severe hypotension, the deteriorating circulatory condition was well advanced [97].

Early goal-directed therapy, involving manipulation of cardiac preload, afterload, and contractility to balance oxygen delivery with oxygen demand, has been used in human patients with systemic inflammatory response syndrome as a means to slow progression to severe sepsis and septic shock [98]. The systemic inflammatory response syndrome is a continuum, with circulatory abnormalities, including intravascular volume depletion, peripheral vasodilation, myocardial depression, and increased tissue metabolic needs causing an imbalance between systemic oxygen delivery and oxygen demand. Changes in vital signs, CVP, and urinary output have proven to be poor indicators of effective hemodynamic resuscitation and fail to detect tissue hypoxia. More recently, researchers have chosen alternative targets to monitor successful therapy, including normalized values for mixed venous oxygen saturation (as a substitute for cardiac index as a target of hemodynamic therapy), arterial lactate concentration, base deficit, and pH. The Early Goal-Directed Therapy (EGDT) trial by Rivers *et al.* [98] found that, during the first 6 h of therapy, there was no significant difference in mean heart rate or CVP between the EGDT group and standard therapy group. MAP was maintained at ≥ 65 mmHg in both groups with the use of vasopressors and CVP was maintained at ≥ 8 mmHg with the use of crystalloid fluid boluses. However, patients in the early goal-directed groups first received red blood cells to maintain a hematocrit of ≥ 30% if the central venous oxygen saturation (venous blood gas from jugular central line) fell below 70%, and then received dobutamine to improve cardiac contractility if central venous oxygen saturation remained below 70%. Choice of the alternative target indices in the early stages of treatment improved survival rates by 16% in human patients with severe sepsis and served as the basis for recommendations made following the Surviving Sepsis Campaign in 2004 and 2008 [99,100]. Recommendations also included either dopamine or norepinephrine as a first-line vasopressor, although vasopressin or phenylephrine may also be used. A resuscitation protocol using blood pressure, central venous oxygen saturation, CVP, lactate, base deficit, and hematocrit has been evaluated in dogs with sepsis secondary to pyometra, with central venous oxygen saturation and base deficit being the best predictors of non-survival [101].

In terms of the type and amount of fluid used for resuscitation, no definitive proof can be found in the literature that supports the superiority of one type of fluid over another for fluid resuscitation in acute trauma or septic patients [102–104]. Crystalloids are the primary first line of fluid resuscitation with balanced electrolyte solutions such as Lactated Ringer's solution and Plasma-Lyte® preferred over 0.9% NaCl. High chloride solutions such as 0.9% NaCl may cause renal vasoconstriction and contribute to acute kidney injury in people [105]. In experimental models of sepsis, high chloride solutions may increase circulating inflammatory molecules, such as tumor necrosis factor-α, IL-10, and IL-6, and impair microcirculatory function compared to more balanced solutions [106]. An important advantage that colloids have over crystalloids is that they can induce a more rapid and persistent plasma expansion due to the larger increase in colloid oncotic pressure. In addition, resuscitation with large volumes of crystalloids has been associated with tissue edema and hyperchloremic metabolic acidosis. However, crystalloids are less expensive and research findings have shown no survival benefit when colloids are administered.

A review of critically ill human patients [107] with trauma or burns or after surgery found no evidence that resuscitation with colloids reduced the risk of death compared with resuscitation with crystalloids. Rather, impaired coagulation, an increase in clinical bleeding, and acute kidney injury are frequently reported with some types of HES used in humans [108,109]. In addition, recent reports in the human literature, including the Efficacy of Volume Substitution and Insulin Therapy in Severe Sepsis (VISEP) study [110], found that patients receiving HES for resuscitation had lower survival rates and more pronounced kidney dysfunction than patients resuscitated with crystalloids. Perner *et al.* [111] showed an increased risk of death (at day 90) in patients with severe sepsis who received fluid resuscitation with 6% HES in Ringer's acetate compared with patients resuscitated with Ringer's acetate alone (6S trial). Renal dysfunction was also more pronounced in the HES group. How these findings relate to fluid resuscitation in the septic or bleeding patient in the acute perioperative period is unknown, but HES has been removed from the human market in Europe and is under review in the United States. It is not known if these results can be extrapolated to veterinary medicine, due to species-specific differences in HES metabolism. In addition, products may differ. For example, Vetstarch® is composed of a relatively homogeneous group of molecules, while Hespan®, is composed of a more heterogeneous group of molecules. The larger molecules tend to be retained in the intravascular space for a more prolonged period and may have a more significant impact on coagulopathy and other side effects. A consensus on the use of synthetic colloids in veterinary medicine has not been reached. Several retrospective studies in dogs have resulted in conflicting results [112,113]. In non-azotemic cats, retrospective studies have found no association between HES administration and kidney injury [114].

Other colloids may be used for resuscitation. Whole blood, red blood cells, and fresh frozen plasma may all be used to expand intravascular volume and provide colloidal support. In addition, administration of whole blood or red blood cells can restore oxygen-carrying capacity in patients that are bleeding or anemic for other reasons. Risks associated with red blood cell administration include transfusion reactions, and many patients are blood-typed or cross-matched prior to transfusion. Human serum albumin (HSA, 25%) has also been used in canine patients with markedly varied success. In human patients, the SAFE study found no difference in the overall mortality rates of ICU patients treated with albumin and saline [115]. However, in a subgroup of patients with brain injury, relative risk was higher in patients assigned to the albumin-treated group than the saline-treated group. Conversely, in a subset of patients with sepsis, relative risk was decreased in patients receiving albumin. One of the first retrospective reports of HSA administration in critically ill canine and feline patients [116] found that administration of an average of 5 mL/kg increased albumin levels and systemic blood pressure. However, two of the 64 dogs developed facial edema and five animals died during or immediately after transfusion. In healthy dogs receiving HSA, three of nine dogs developed facial edema and urticaria within days of receiving the transfusion and two dogs developed severe hypertension [117]. One of the nine dogs developed a severe anaphylactoid reaction within 10 min of receiving the infusion. Two out of two dogs receiving a second infusion had a similar severe anaphylactoid reaction. Martin *et al.* [118] found that administration of HSA resulted in antibody formation in both healthy and critically ill patients, with the onset time being shorter in healthy dogs. Interestingly, two of the 57 control dogs also had anti-HSA antibodies, despite never having received an infusion. Canine albumin is now commercially available in the United States and a number of other countries. Allergic reactions occur with some regularity but tend to be less severe than those seen with HSA. In dogs with septic peritonitis, albumin levels remained increased 24 h after receiving 5% canine albumin [119].

References

1 Tilley LP, Burtnick NL. *ECG for the Small Animal Practitioner*. Jackson, WY: Teton NewMedia, 1999.

2 Fuentes VL, Johnson LR, Dennis D, eds. *Canine and Feline Cardiorespiratory Medicine*, 2nd edn. Quedgeley, Gloucester, UK: British Small Animal Veterinary Association, 2013.

3 Tilley LP, Smith FW, Oyama MA, Sleeper MM, eds. *Manual of Canine and Feline Cardiology*, 4th edn. St. Louis, MO: Saunders Elsevier, 2013.

4 Buchanan JW, Bucheler J. Vertebral scale system to measure canine heart size in radiographs. *J Am Vet Med Assoc* 1995; **206**: 194–199.

5 Litster AL, Buchanan JW. Vertebral scale system to measure heart size in radiographs of cats. *J Am Vet Med Assoc* 2000; **216**: 210–214.

6 Hansson K, Haggstrom J, Kvart C, *et al.* Interobserver variability of vertebral heart size measurements in dogs with normal and enlarged hearts. *Vet Radiol Ultrasound* 2005; **46**: 122–130.

7 Kraetschmer S, Ludwig K, Meneses F, *et al.* Vertebral heart scale in the Beagle dog. *J Small Anim Pract* 2008; **49**: 240–243.

8 Marin LM, Brown J, McBrien C, *et al.* Vertebral heart size in retired racing Greyhounds. *Vet Radiol Ultrasound* 2007; **48**: 332–334.

9 Bavegems V, Van Caelenberg A, Duchateau L, *et al.* Vertebral heart size ranges specific for whippets. *Vet Radiol Ultrasound* 2005; **46**: 400–403.

10 Greco A, Meomartino L, Raiano V, *et al.* Effect of left vs. right recumbency on the vertebral heart score in normal dogs. *Vet Radiol Ultrasound* 2008; **49**: 454–455.

11 Sleeper MM, Buchanan JW. Vertebral scale system to measure heart size in growing puppies. *J Am Vet Med Assoc* 2001; **219**: 57–59.

12 Lamb CR, Wikeley H, Boswood A, *et al.* Use of breed-specific ranges for the vertebral heart scale as an aid to the radiographic diagnosis of cardiac disease in dogs. *Vet Rec* 2001; **148**: 707–711.

13 Ghadiri A, Avizeh R, Rasekh A, *et al.* Radiographic measurement of vertebral heart size in healthy stray cats. *J Feline Med Surg* 2008; **10**: 61–65.

14 Cornell CC, Kittleson MD, Della TP, *et al.* Allometric scaling of M-mode cardiac measurements in normal adult dogs. *J Vet Intern Med* 2004; **18**: 311–321.

15 Mueller X, Stauffer JC, Jaussi A, *et al.* Subjective visual echocardiographic estimate of left ventricular ejection fraction as an alternative to conventional echocardiographic methods: comparison with contrast angiography. *Clin Cardiol* 1991; **14**: 898–902.

16 Loyer C, Thomas WP. Biplane transesophageal echocardiography in the dog: technique, anatomy, and imaging planes. *Vet Radiol Ultrasound* 1995; **36**: 212–226.

17 Kienle RD, Thomas WP, Rishniw M. Biplane transesophageal echocardiography in the normal cat. *Vet Radiol Ultrasound* 1997; **38**: 288–298.

18 Fox PR, Oyama MA, Reynolds C, *et al.* Utility of plasma N-terminal pro-brain natriuretic peptide (NT-proBNP) to distinguish between congestive heart failure and non-cardiac causes of acute dyspnea in cats. *J Vet Cardiol* 2009; **11**(Suppl 1): S51–S61.

19 Fox PR, Rush JE, Reynolds CA, *et al.* Multicenter evaluation of plasma N-terminal probrain natriuretic peptide (NT-pro BNP) as a biochemical screening test for asymptomatic (occult) cardiomyopathy in cats. *J Vet Intern Med* 2011; **25**: 1010–1016.

20 Wess G, Daisenberger P, Mahling M, *et al.* Utility of measuring plasma N-terminal pro-brain natriuretic peptide in detecting hypertrophic cardiomyopathy and differentiating grades of severity in cats. *Vet Clin Pathol* 2011; **40**: 237–244.

21 Hezzell MJ, Boswood A, Chang YM, *et al.* The combined prognostic potential of serum high-sensitivity cardiac troponin I and N-terminal pro-B-type natriuretic peptide concentrations in dogs with degenerative mitral valve disease. *J Vet Intern Med* 2012; **26**: 302–311.

22 Yoran C, Yellin EL, Becker RM, *et al.* Dynamic aspects of acute mitral regurgitation: effects of ventricular volume, pressure and contractility on the effective regurgitant orifice area. *Circulation* 1979; **60**: 170–176.

23 Nussmeier NA, Hauser MC, Sarwar MF, *et al.* Anesthesia for cardiac surgical procedures. In: Miller RD, Eriksson LI, Fleisher LA, *et al.*, eds. *Miller's Anesthesia*, 7th edn. Philadelphia, PA: Churchill Livingstone Elsevier, 2010: 2599–2652.

24 Reitan JA, Stengart KB, Wynmore MC, *et al.* Central vagal control of fentanyl induced bradycardia during halothane anesthesia. *Anaesth Analg* 1978; **57**: 31–36.

25 Smith LJ, Yi JK, Bjorling DE, *et al.* Effects of hydromorphone or oxymorphone, with or without acepromazine, on preanesthetic sedation, physiologic values, and histamine release in dogs. *J Am Vet Med Assoc* 2001; **218**: 1101–1105.

26 Flacke JW, Davis LJ, Flacke WE, *et al.* Effects of fentanyl and diazepam in dogs deprived of autonomic tone. *Anesth Analg* 1985; **64**: 1053–1059.

27 Machado CG, Dyson DH, Mathews KA. Evaluation of induction by use of a combination of oxymorphone and diazepam or hydromorphone and diazepam and maintenance of anesthesia by use of isoflurane in dogs with experimentally induced hypovolemia. *Am J Vet Res* 2005; **66**: 1227–1237.

28 Rangel JPP, Monteiro ER, Bitti FS, *et al.* Hemodynamic, respiratory and sedative effects of progressively increasing doses of acepromazine in conscious dogs. *Vet Anaesth Analg* 2020; **47**: 447–453.
29 Hay Kraus BL. Effect of dosing interval on efficacy of maropitant for prevention of hydromorphone-induced vomiting and signs of nausea in dogs. *J Am Vet Med Assoc* 2014; **245**:1015–1020.
30 Grimm KA, Tranquilli WJ, Gross DR, *et al.* Cardiopulmonary effects of fentanyl in conscious dogs and dogs sedated with a continuous rate infusion of medetomidine. *Am J Vet Res* 2005; **66**: 1222–1226.
31 Michelsen LG, Salmenpera M, Hug CC, *et al.* Anesthetic potency of remifentanil in dogs. *Anesthesiology* 1996; **84**: 865–872.
32 Marques MG, Cancelli CHB, Fernandes CMS, *et al.* Effect of a constant rate infusion of remifentanil hydrochloride on left ventricular systolic and diastolic function in propofol-anesthetized dogs. *Am J Vet Res* 2018; **79**: 1261–1267.
33 Gimenes AM, de Araujo Aguiar AJ, Perri SHV, *et al.* Effect of intravenous propofol and remifentanil on heart rate, blood pressure and nociceptive response in acepromazine premedicated dogs. *Vet Anaesth Analg* 2011; **38**: 54–62.
34 Musk GC, Flaherty DA. Target-controlled infusion of propofol combined with variable rate infusion of remifentanil for anaesthesia of a dog with patent ductus arteriosus. *Vet Anaesth Analg* 2007; **34**: 359–364.
35 De Hert SG, Vermeyen KM, Adriaensen HF. Influence of thiopental, etomidate, and propofol on regional myocardial function in the normal and acute ischemic heart segment in dogs. *Anesth Analg* 1990; **70**: 600–607.
36 Coetzee A, Fourie P, Coetzee J, *et al.* Effect of various propofol plasma concentrations on regional myocardial contractility and left ventricular afterload. *Anesth Analg* 1989; **69**: 473–483.
37 Ismail EF, Kim S, Ramez Salem M, *et al.* Direct effects of propofol on myocardial contractility in in situ canine hearts. *Anesthesiology* 1992; **77**: 964–972.
38 Nakaigawa Y, Akazawa S, Shimizu R, *et al.* Effects of graded infusion rates of propofol on cardiovascular haemodynamics, coronary circulation and myocardial metabolism in dogs. *Br J Anaesth* 1995; **75**: 616–621.
39 Ilkiw JE, Pascoe PJ, Haskins SC, *et al.* Cardiovascular and respiratory effects of propofol administration in hypovolemic dogs. *Am J Vet Res* 1992; **53**: 2323–2327.
40 Aguilera R, Sinclair M, Valverde A, *et al.* Dose and cardiopulmonary effects of propofol alone or with midazolam for induction of anesthesia in critically ill dogs. *Vet Anaesth Analg* 2020; **47**:472–480.
41 Pagel PS, Schmeling WT, Kampine JP, *et al.* Alteration of canine left ventricular diastolic function by intravenous anesthetics in vivo: ketamine and propofol. *Anesthesiology* 1992; **76**: 419–425.
42 Nagel ML, Muir WW, Nguyen K. Comparison of the cardiopulmonary effects of etomidate and thiamylal in dogs. *Am J Vet Res* 1979; **40**: 193–196.
43 P Pascoe P, Ilkiw J, Haskins S, *et al.* Cardiopulmonary effects of etomidate in hypovolemic dogs. *Am J Vet Res* 1992; **53**: 2178–2182.
44 Gooding JM, Weng JT, Smith RA, *et al.* Cardiovascular and pulmonary responses following etomidate induction of anesthesia in patients with demonstrated cardiac disease. *Anesth Analg* 1979; **58**: 40–41.
45 Keating SCJ, Sage AM, Ambrisko T, *et al.* The effect of midazolam or lidocaine administration prior to etomidate induction of anesthesia on heart rate, arterial pressure, intraocular pressure and serum cortisol concentration in healthy dogs. *Vet Anaesth Analg* 2020; **47**: 160–167.
46 Muir W, Lerche P, Wiese A, *et al.* The cardiorespiratory and anesthetic effects of clinical and supraclinical doses of alfaxalone in dogs. *Vet Anaesth Analg* 2008; **35**: 451–462.
47 Dehuisser V, Bosmans T, Devreese M, *et al.* Alfaxalone total intravenous anaesthesia in dogs: pharmacokinetics, cardiovascular data and recovery characteristics. *Vet Anaesth Analg* 2019: **46**: 605–612.
48 Hampton EC, Riebold TW, LeBlanc NL, *et al.* Effects of intravenous administration of tiletamine-zolazepam, alfaxalone, ketamine, diazepam, and propofol for induction of anesthesia in healthy dogs before and during anesthesia maintained with isoflurane. *Am J Vet Res* 2019; **80**: 33–44.
49 Bennett KJ, Seddighi R, Moorhead KA, *et al.* Effect of fentanyl on the induction dose and minimum infusion rate of alfaxalone preventing movement in dogs. *Vet Anaesth Analg* 2019; **46**: 173–181.
50 Psatha E, Alibhai HI, Jimenez-Lozano A, *et al.* Clinical efficacy and cardiorespiratory effects of alfaxalone, or diazepam/fentanyl for induction of anaesthesia in dogs that are a poor anaesthetic risk. *Vet Anesth Analg* 2011; **38**: 24–36.
51 Rodríguez JM, Munoz-Rascón P, Navarrete-Calvo R, *et al.* Comparison of the cardiopulmonary parameters after induction of anaesthesia with alphaxalone or etomidate in dogs. *Vet Anaesth Analg* 2012; **39**: 357–365.
52 Moon PF. Acute toxicosis in two dogs associated with etomidate–propylene glycol infusion. *Lab Anim Sci* 1994; **44**: 590–594.
53 Dodam JR, Kruse-Elliott KT, Aucoin DP, *et al.* Duration of etomidate induced adrenocortical suppression during surgery in dogs. *Am J Vet Res* 1990; **51**: 786–788.
54 Wagner RL, White PF, Kan PB, *et al.* Inhibition of adrenal steroidogenesis by the anesthetic etomidate. *N Engl J Med* 1984; **310**: 1415–1421.
55 Ledingham IM, Watt I. Influence of sedation on mortality in critically ill multiple trauma patients. *Lancet* 1983; **1**(8336): 1270.
56 Nagashima JK, Goncalves LA, Pereira MAA, *et al.* Microcirculation assessment of dexmedetomidine constant rate infusion during anesthesia of dogs with sepsis from pyometra: a randomized clinical study. *Vet Anaesth Analg* 2022; **49**: 536–545.
57 Badino P, Odore R, Re G. Are so many adrenergic receptor subtypes really present in domestic animal tissues? *A pharmacological perspective. Vet J* 2005; **170**: 163–174.
58 Ranganathan B, LeBlanc N, Scollan KF, *et al.* Comparison of major complication and survival rates begween surgical ligation and use of a canine ductal occlude device for treatment of dogs with left-to-right shunting patent ductus arteriosus. *J Am Vet Med Assoc* 2018; **253**: 1046–1052.
59 Parisi C, Phillips V, Ferreira J, *et al.* Anaesthetic management and complications of transvascular patent ductus arteriosus occlusion in dogs. *Vet Anaesth Analg* 2020; **47**: 581–587.
60 Williams GD, Jones TK, Hanson KA, *et al.* The hemodynamic effects of propofol in children with congenital heart disease. *Anesth Analg* 1999; **89**: 1411–1416.
61 Boatman DL, Shaffer RA, Dixon RL, *et al.* Function of vascular smooth muscle and its sympathetic innervation in the newborn dog. *J Clin Invest* 1965; **44**: 241–246.
62 Boatman DL, Brody MJ. Cardiac responses to adrenergic stimulation in the newborn dog. *Arch Int Pharmacodyn Ther* 1967; **170**: 1–11.
63 Driscoll DJ, Gillette PC, Lewis RM, *et al.* Comparative hemodynamic effects of isoproterenol, dopamine, and dobutamine in the newborn dog. *Pediatr Res* 1979; **13**: 1006–1009.
64 Park IS, Michael LH, Driscoll DJ. Comparative response of the developing canine myocardium to inotropic agents. *Am J Physiol* 1982; **242**: H13–H18.
65 Manders WT, Pagani M, Vatner SF. Depressed responsiveness to vasoconstrictor and dilator agents and baroreflex sensitivity in conscious, newborn lambs. *Circulation* 1979; **60**: 945–955.
66 Rosati M, Dyson DH, Sinclair MD, *et al.* Response of hypotensive dogs to dopamine hydrochloride and dobutamine hydrochloride during deep isoflurane anesthesia. *Am J Vet Res* 2007; **68**: 483–494.
67 Pascoe PJ, Ilkiw JE, Pypendop BH. Effects of increasing infusion rates of dopamine, dobutamine, epinephrine and phenylephrine in healthy anesthetized cats. *Am J Vet Res* 2006; **67**: 1491–1499.
68 Abdul-Rasool IH, Chamberlain JH, Swan PC, *et al.* Cardiorespiratory and metabolic effects of dopamine and dobutamine infusions in dogs. *Crit Care Med* 1987; **15**: 1044–1050.
69 Vatner SF, McRitchie RJ, Braunwald E. Effects of dobutamine on left ventricular performance, coronary dynamics and distribution of cardiac output in conscious dogs. *J Clin Invest* 1974; **53**: 1265–1273.
70 Orchard CH, Chakrabarti MK, Sykes MK. Cardiorespiratory responses to an i.v. infusion of dobutamine in the intact anaesthetized dog. *Br J Anaesth* 1982; **54**: 673–679.
71 Kojima K, Ishizuka T, Sasaki N, *et al.* Cardiovascular effects of dose escalating of norepinephrine in healthy dogs anesthetized with norepinephrine. *Vet Anaesth Analg* 2021; **48**: 654–662.
72 De Moraes AN, Dyson DH, O'Grady MR, *et al.* Plasma concentrations and cardiovascular influence of lidocaine infusions during isoflurane anesthesia in healthy dogs and dogs with subaortic stenosis. *Vet Surg* 1998; **27**: 486–497.
73 Lamont LA, Bulmer BJ, Sisson DD, *et al.* Doppler echocardiographic effects of medetomidine on dynamic left ventricular outflow tract obstruction in cats. *J Am Vet Med Assoc* 2002; **221**: 1276–1281.
74 Wiese AJ, Barter LS, Ilkiw JE, *et al.* Cardiovascular and respiratory effects of incremental doses of dopamine and phenylephrine in the management of isoflurane-induced hypotension in cats with hypertrophic cardiomyopathy. *Am J Vet Res* 2012; **73**: 908–916.
75 White PF, Way WL, Trevor AJ. Ketamine – its pharmacology and therapeutic uses. *Anesthesiology* 1982; **56**: 119–136.
76 Haskins SC, Farver TB, Patz JD. Ketamine in dogs. *Am J Vet Res* 1985; **46**: 1855–1860.
77 Pascoe PJ, Ilkiw JE, Craig C, *et al.* The effects of ketamine on the minimum alveolar concentration of isoflurane in cats. *Vet Anaesth Analg* 2007; **34**: 31–39.
78 Lazzarini E, Martinellui E, Brioschi A, *et al.* Intramuscular alfaxalone and methadone with or without ketamine in healthy cats:effects on sedations and echocardiographic measurements. *Vet Anaesth Analg* 2020; **47**: 621–630.
79 Ribas T, Bublot I, Junot S, *et al.* Effects of intramuscular sedation with alfaxalone and butorphanol on echocardiographic measurements in healthy cats. *J Feline Med Surg* 2015; **17**: 530–536.
80 Muir W, Lerche P, Wiese A, *et al.* The cardiorespiratory and anesthetic effects of clinical and supraclinical doses of alfaxalone in cats. *Vet Anaesth Analg* 2009; **36**: 42–54.
81 Pypendop BH, Barter LS, Pascoe PJ, *et al.* Hemodynamic effect of subclinical, clinical and supraclinical plasma alfaxalone concentrations in cats. *Vet Anaesth Analg* 2019; **46**: 597–604.

82 Lippman M, Appel PL, Mok MS, *et al.* Sequential cardiorespiratory patterns of anesthetic induction with ketamine in critically ill patients. *Crit Care Med* 1983; **11**: 730–734.

83 Jacobson JD, Hartsfield SM. Cardiovascular effects of intravenous bolus administration and infusion of ketamine–midazolam in isoflurane-anesthetized dogs. *Am J Vet Res* 1993; **54**: 1715–1720.

84 Joshi GP, Warner DS, Twersky RS, *et al.* A comparison of remifentanil and fentanyl adverse effect profile in a multicenter phase IV study. *J Clin Anesth* 2002; **14**: 494–499.

85 Nosier RK, Ficke DJ, Kundu A, *et al.* Sympathetic and vascular consequences from remifentanil in humans. *Anesth Analg* 2003; **96**: 1645–1650.

86 Allweiler S, Broadbelt DC, Borer K, *et al.* The isoflurane-sparing and clinical effects of a constant rate infusion of remifentanil in dogs. *Vet Anaesth Analg* 2007; **34**: 388–393.

87 Overgaard CB, Dzavik V. Inotropes and vasopressors. Review of physiology and clinical use in cardiovascular disease. *Circulation* 2008; **118**: 1047–1056.

88 Walsh M, Devereaux PJ, Garg AX, *et al.* Relationship between intraoperative mean arterial pressure and clinical outcomes after noncardiac surgery: towards an empirical definition of hypotension. *Anesthesiology* 2013; **119**: 507–515.

89 Marik PE, Baram M, Vahid B. Does central venous pressure predict fluid responsiveness? A systematic review of the literature and the tale of seven mares. *Chest* 2008; **134**: 172–178.

90 Fantoni ET, Ida KK, Gimenes AM, *et al.* Pulse pressure variation as a guide for volume expansion in dogs undergoing orthopedic surgery. *Vet Anaesth Analg* 2017; **44**: 710–718.

91 Aarnes TK, Bednarski RM, Lerche P, *et al.* Effect of intravenous administration of Lactated Ringer's solution or Hetastarch for the treatment of isoflurane-induced hypotension in dogs. *Am J Vet Res* 2009; **70**: 1345–1353.

92 Valverde A, Gianotti G, Rioja-Garcia E, *et al.* Effects of high-volume, rapid-fluid therapy on cardiovascular function and hematological values during isoflurane-induced hypotension in healthy dogs. *Can J Vet Res* 2012; **76**: 99–108.

93 Sinclair MD, Dyson DH. The impact of acepromazine on the efficacy of crystalloid, dextran or ephedrine treatment in hypotensive dogs under isoflurane anesthesia. *Vet Anaesth Analg* 2012; **39**: 563–573.

94 Bone RC, Balk RA, Cerra FB, *et al.* Definitions for sepsis and organ failure and guidelines for the use of innovative therapies in sepsis. The ACCP/SCCM Consensus Conference Committee, American College of Chest Physicians/Society of Critical Care Medicine. *Crit Care Med* 1992; **20**: 864–874.

95 Shoemaker WC, Appel PL, Kram HB. Hemodynamic and oxygen transport responses in survivors and nonsurvivors of high-risk surgery. *Crit Care Med* 1983; **21**: 977–990.

96 Shoemaker WC, Appel P, Bland R. Use of physiologic monitoring to predict outcome and to assist in clinical decision in critically ill postoperative patients. *Am J Surg* 1983; **146**: 43–50.

97 Wo CC, Shoemaker WE, Appel PL, *et al.* Unreliability of blood pressure and heart rate to evaluate cardiac output in emergency resuscitation and critical illness. *Crit Care Med* 1993; **21**: 218–223.

98 Rivers E, Nguyen B, Havstad S, *et al.* Early goal-directed therapy in the treatment of severe sepsis and septic shock. *N Engl J Med* 2001; **345**: 1368–1377.

99 Dellinger RP, Carlet JM, Masur H, *et al.* Surviving Sepsis Campaign: guidelines for management of severe sepsis and septic shock. *Crit Care Med* 2004; **32**: 858–873.

100 Dellinger RP, Levy MM, Carlet JM, *et al.* Surviving Sepsis Campaign: international guidelines for management of severe sepsis and septic shock. *Crit Care Med* 2008; **36**: 296–327.

101 Conti-Patara A, de Araujo Caldeira J, de Mattos-Junior E, *et al.* Changes in tissue perfusion parameters in dogs with severe sepsis/septic shock in response to goal – directed hemodnamic optimization at admission to ICU and the relation to outcome. *J Vet Emerg Crit Care* 2012; **22**: 409–418.

102 Bouglé A, Harrois A, Duranteau J. Resuscitative strategies in traumatic hemorrhagic shock. *Ann Intensive Care* 2013; **3**: 1.

103 The National Heart, Lung, and Blood Institute Acute Respiratory Distress Syndrome (ARDS) Clinical Trials Network. Comparison of two fluid-management strategies in acute lung injury. *N Engl J Med* 2006; **354**: 2564–2575.

104 Mapstone J, Roberts I, Evans P. Fluid resuscitation strategies: a systematic review of animal trials. *J Trauma* 2003; **55**: 571–589.

105 Chowdhury AH, Cox EF, Francis ST, *et al.* A randomized, controlled, double-blind crossover study on the effects of 2-L infusions of 0.9% saline and Plasma-Lyte 148 on renal blood flow velocity and renal cortical tissue perfusion in healthy volunteers. *Ann Surg* 2012; **256**: 18–24.

106 Santacruz CA, De Backer D, Taccone FS, *et al.* Effects of different crystalloid solutions on hemodynamics, peripheral perfusion, and the microcirculation in experimental abdominal sepsis. *Anesthesiology* 2016; **125**: 744–754.

107 Perel P, Roberts I. Colloids versus crystalloids for fluid resuscitation in critically ill patients. *Cochrane Database Syst Rev* 2011; (3): CD000567; update: Perel P, Roberts I, Ker K. *Cochrane Database Syst Rev* 2013; (2): CD000567.

108 Groeneveld AB, Navickis RJ, Wilkes MM. Update on the comparative safety of colloids: a systematic review of clinical studies. *Ann Surg* 2011; **253**: 470–483.

109 Choi SJ, Ahn HJ, Chung SS, *et al.* Hemostatic and electrolyte effects of hydroxyethyl starches in patients undergoing posterior lumbar interbody fusion using pedicle screws and cages. *Spine* 2010; **35**: 829–834.

110 Brunkhorst FM, Engel C, Bloos F, *et al.* Intensive insulin therapy and pentastarch resuscitation in severe sepsis. *N Engl J Med* 2008; **358**: 125–139.

111 Perner A, Haase N, Guttormsen AB, *et al.* Hydroxyethyl starch 130/0/42 versus Ringer's acetate in severe sepsis. *N Engl J Med* 2012; **367**: 124–134.

112 Sigrist NE, Kalin N, Dreyfus A. Changes in serum creatinine concentration and acute kidney injury (AKI) grade in dogs treated with hydroxyethyl starch 130/0.4 from 2013 to 2015. *J Vet Intern Med* **2017**; 31: 434–441.

113 Hayes G, Benedicenti L, Mathew K. Retrospective cohort study on the incidence of acute kidney injury and death following hydroxyethyl starch (HES 10% 250/0/5/5:1) administration in dogs (2007–2010). *J Vet Emerg Crit Care* 2016; **26**: 35–40.

114 Sigrist NE, Kalin N, Dreyfus A. Effects of hydroxyethyl starch 130/0.4 on serum creatinine concentration and development of acute kidney injury in nonazotemic cats. *J Vet Intern Med* 2017; **31**: 1749–1756.

115 Finfer S, Bellomo R, Boyce N, *et al.* A comparison of albumin and saline for fluid resuscitation in the intensive care unit. *N Engl J Med* 2004; **350**: 2247–2256.

116 Mathews KA, Barry M. The use of 25% human serum albumin: outcome and efficacy in raising serum albumin and systemic blood pressure in critically ill dogs and cats. *J Vet Emerg Crit Care* 2005; **15**: 110–118.

117 Cohn LA, Kerl ME, Lenox CE, *et al.* Response of healthy dogs to infusions of human serum albumin. *Am J Vet Res* 2007; **68**: 657–663.

118 Martin LG, Luther TY, Alperin DC, *et al.* Serum antibodies against human albumin in critically ill and healthy dogs. *J Am Vet Med Assoc* 2008; **232**: 1004–1009.

119 Craft EM, Powell LL. The use of canine-specific albumin in dogs with septic peritonitis. *J Vet Emerg Crit Care* 2012; **22**: 631–639.

37 Respiratory Physiology and Pathophysiology

Carolyn L. Kerr[1] **and Francisco J. Teixeira-Neto**[2]
[1] Department of Clinical Studies, Ontario Veterinary College, University of Guelph, Guelph, Ontario, Canada
[2] Faculdade de Medicina Veterinária e Zootecnia, Universidade Estadual Paulista (UNESP), Botucatu, Brazil

Chapter contents

Introduction, 697
Key concepts and lung volumes, 697
Respiratory function in conscious and anesthetized animals, 700
Neural control of ventilation, 700
Pulmonary ventilation, 702
Pulmonary perfusion, 713
Ventilation–perfusion relationships, 718
Effects of anesthesia on ventilation, pulmonary perfusion, and ventilation–perfusion relationships, 721
Oxygen transport, 737
Carbon dioxide transport, 740
References, 743

Introduction

Maintenance of adequate respiratory function is a principal requirement for safe anesthesia. The respiratory system is responsible for eliminating carbon dioxide (CO_2) via adjustments in alveolar ventilation per minute ($\dot{V}_A$), and for transferring oxygen from the alveoli to mixed venous blood (pulmonary artery blood) at the pulmonary capillary level. In conscious resting, mammals breathing air (fraction of inspired oxygen [F_IO_2] of 0.21) at sea level, CO_2 partial pressure in arterial blood ($PaCO_2$), and oxygen partial pressure in arterial blood (PaO_2) usually range from 35 to 45 mmHg and from 90 to 110 mmHg, respectively, with some variation among species (Table 37.1). These gas partial pressures reflect adequate CO_2 elimination and oxygen uptake to meet tissue metabolic requirements in normal patients at rest.

During general anesthesia, there is a tendency for PaO_2 to be lower and $PaCO_2$ to be elevated above that observed in the same species while conscious and breathing the same F_IO_2 [1–5]. Depending on the species and health of the individual patient, sedation alone may also result in deterioration of normal gas exchange [6–8]. Alteration in the efficacy of the gas exchange associated with sedation and/or general anesthesia results from changes in $\dot{V}_A$, pulmonary perfusion ($\dot{Q}$), or alveolar ventilation–perfusion ratios ($\dot{V}_A/\dot{Q}$) within the lung. Numerous factors, including species, influence the degree and nature of lung dysfunction in the perioperative period. However, within a species, the degree of change in lung function associated with anesthesia is significantly greater in individuals with underlying respiratory disease.

Strategies employed to manage the changes in respiratory function associated with sedation and general anesthesia include increasing the F_IO_2 delivered to a patient, establishing an artificial airway, and supporting ventilation through mechanical means. In certain instances, pharmaceutical interventions are warranted to address either underlying conditions or counter the side-effects of diagnostic or therapeutic interventions. Further details regarding current strategies used to support veterinary patients' respiratory function during anesthesia are provided in Chapter 38. While many strategies used in veterinary anesthesia are also employed in humans, veterinary species differ in terms of lung structure, body size, and the circumstances in which they are anesthetized. As such, it is important to consider the evidence surrounding the risks and benefits of the various interventions in the veterinary context as the goals and means to achieve them may be different than in humans. While perioperative morbidity and mortality are clearly linked to respiratory dysfunction, with appropriate interventions, the risks can be minimized, and outcomes optimized.

This chapter aims to provide a review of respiratory physiology with emphasis on pathophysiological changes in respiratory function associated with sedation and general anesthesia. Several excellent reviews of basic respiratory physiology exist, and the reader is encouraged to consult these works for further detail [9,10].

Key concepts and lung volumes

The primary function of the respiratory system is to eliminate CO_2 produced by cell metabolism to the atmosphere and to transfer oxygen from the atmosphere to deoxygenated blood. Other functions include regulation of acid–base balance, via adjustment of CO_2 partial pressure (PCO_2) in blood; defense against pollutants and microorganisms that may be inhaled; and metabolism of vasoactive peptides by enzymes in lung cells (e.g., bradykinin and angiotensin).

Respiration is the total process whereby oxygen is supplied to and used by cells and CO_2 is eliminated by means of partial pressure

Veterinary Anesthesia and Analgesia: The Sixth Edition of Lumb and Jones. Edited by Leigh Lamont, Kurt Grimm, Sheilah Robertson, Lydia Love and Carrie Schroeder.
© 2024 John Wiley & Sons, Inc. Published 2024 by John Wiley & Sons, Inc.
Companion website: www.wiley.com/go/lamont/anesthesia

Table 37.1 Arterial blood gas and acid–base values for various species.

Species	Body weight (kg)	n	Conditions	pHa	$PaCO_2$ (mmHg)	PaO_2 (mmHg)	HCO_3^-(mEq/L)	Reference
Rat	0.207	10	Awake, chronic catheter	7.44	32.7		21.5	[11]
	0.305	8	Awake, prone, chronic catheter	7.467	39.8		28.7	[12]
Rabbit	3.1	NS	Awake, catheter	7.388	32.8	86	21	[13]
	3.5	20	Awake, catheter	7.47	28.5	89.2	20.2	[14]
Cat	2.5–5.1	8	Unsedated, chronic catheter, prone	7.41	28.0	108	18	[15]
	3–8	10	Unsedated, not restrained, chronic catheter	7.426	32.5	108	22.1	[16]
Dog	18.8	8	Unsedated, chronic trach/catheter, standing	7.383	39.0	103.8	22.1	[17]
	12.2	22	Chronic catheters, lateral recumbency	7.40	35	102	21	[18]
Sheep	33	NS	Awake, catheter	7.44	40.9	96	27.6	[13]
	24.5	11	Unsedated, prone, carotid loop	7.48	33	92		[19]
Goat	18	6	Unsedated, standing	7.46	36.5	101		[20]
	47.6	6	Unsedated, standing, catheter	7.45	35.3	94.5	24.1	[21]
	46.6	6	Unsedated, standing	7.45	41.1	87.1	27.6	[22]
Calf	31–57	4	Standing, unsedated, aortic catheter	7.39	40	81	24	[23]
	48–66	20	Unanesthetized, catheter	7.37	42.8	93.6	23.6	[24]
Cow	517	7	Awake, unsedated, standing	7.40	39.6	83.1	24.4	[25]
	641	7	Awake, unsedated, standing	7.435	38.7	95.1	25.5	[a]
Horse	402	6	Awake, unsedated, standing	7.39	41.1	80.7	24.5	[25]
Pony	147	19	Standing, aortic catheter	7.40	40	88.7	24.4	[26]

n, sample size; NS, not specified; trach, tracheostomy.
[a] Warren R and McDonell WN; unpublished observations.

gradients. It is dependent on the integrated action of the respiratory and cardiovascular systems. *Ventilation* is the movement of gas in and out of the lungs. The ventilatory requirement for homeostasis varies with metabolic rate, and therefore varies with the animal species, age, body mass, level of activity, body temperature, and depth of anesthesia.

The volume of gas within the respiratory system is subdivided into four different volumes. Occasionally, it is desirable to consider two or more of the volumes together. Such combinations are termed "pulmonary capacities" (Fig. 37.1):

1 *Tidal volume* (V_T) is the volume of air that moves in and out of the respiratory system (conducting airways and alveoli) in one breath.
2 *Inspiratory reserve volume* (IRV) is the volume of air that can be inspired over and above the normal V_T.
3 *Expiratory reserve volume* (ERV) is the amount of air that can be expired by forceful expiration after a normal expiration.
4 *Residual volume* (RV) is the air remaining in the lungs after a maximal expiration.
5 *Inspiratory capacity* (IC) is the V_T plus the inspiratory reserve volume. This is the amount of air that can be inhaled starting after a normal expiration and distending the lungs to the maximum amount.
6 *Functional residual capacity* (FRC) is the expiratory reserve volume plus the residual volume. This is the amount of air remaining in the lungs after a normal expiration. From a mechanical viewpoint, at FRC, the inward "pull" of the lungs due to their elasticity equals the outward "pull" of the chest wall.
7 *Vital capacity* (VC) is the inspiratory reserve volume plus the V_T plus the expiratory reserve volume. This is the maximum amount of air that can be expelled from the lungs after first filling them to their maximum capacity.
8 *Total lung capacity* (TLC) is the inspiratory reserve volume plus the V_T plus the expiratory reserve volume plus the residual volume, or the maximum volume to which the lungs can be expanded with the greatest possible inspiratory effort (or by full inflation to 30 cmH_2O airway pressure when a patient is anesthetized).

Most of these volumes cannot be measured in conscious animals (Fig. 37.1), because to do so requires cooperation of the test subject. The TLC, FRC, and RV reported in mammalian species are summarized in Table 37.2. The TLC is generally estimated by inflation of the lung to pressures above 30 cmH_2O in anesthetized animals. Values for TLC are reasonably similar among the domestic species when compared on a body-weight basis, but the total volume varies from less than 2 mL in mice to over 45 L in horses and cows. The volume of gas remaining in the lungs at the end of a normal expiration (that is, the FRC) varies considerably among species and can rapidly change within an individual patient. Increased abdominal volume from any source (e.g., near-term gravid uterus, bowel distension, obesity, or large abdominal tumor) will tend to move the diaphragm forward and lessen the FRC. Conversely, overnight fasting increased the FRC of ponies by about 16% [27]. Changes in body position, specifically, changing from standing to lateral or dorsal recumbency can significantly alter FRC in humans and in some veterinary species [27–29]. Few actual measurements have been made of this phenomenon in relation to animals in health and disease, but the consequences for ventilation and arterial oxygenation in patients with severe lung disease or during anesthesia are consistent with a decrease in FRC.

Minute ventilation ($\dot{V}_E$), calculated as V_T times breathing frequency (*f*), is the volume of air that moves in and out of the respiratory system (conducting airways and alveoli) over 1 min. It is only the fraction of $\dot{V}_E$ that effectively ventilates the alveoli over 1 min ($\dot{V}_A$) that determines gas exchange.

Under normal conditions, $\dot{V}_E$ is matched with CO_2 production per minute ($\dot{V}CO_2$) to maintain $PaCO_2$ within physiological ranges (Table 37.1). Factors that influence CO_2 production and $\dot{V}_E$ include species, age, body mass, level of activity, body temperature, and depth of anesthesia. Although basal metabolic rate and CO_2 production per unit body mass are significantly higher in small mammals (mice and rats) than in large animal species (horses and cows), normal $PaCO_2$ values are not substantially different. This is explained by the fact that $\dot{V}_E$ (and $\dot{V}_A$) is significantly higher in mice and rats [32] than in horses and cows when indexed to body mass [25,36–38]. The $\dot{V}_E$ recorded in several animal species is presented in Table 37.3.

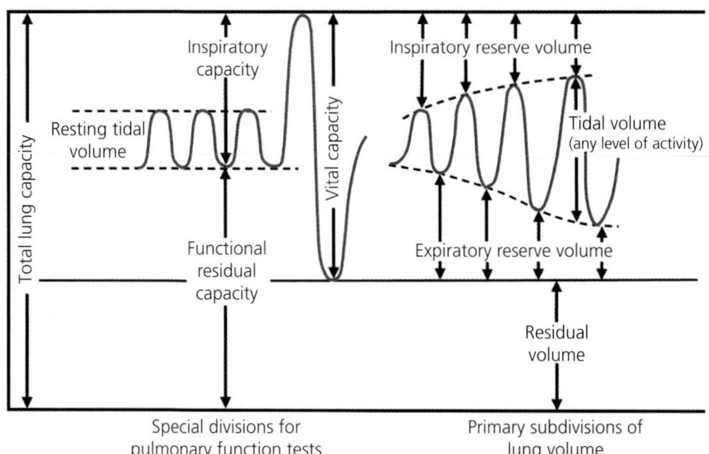

Figure 37.1 Lung volumes and capacities. Only V_T (obtained using a tightly fitting face mask attached to a pneumotachograph or by placing the animal in a whole-body barometric plethysmography chamber) and FRC (obtained by an open-circuit nitrogen washout technique) can be measured in conscious animals since the other measurements require cooperation of the subject being studied or general anesthesia. Source: Adapted from Gallivan *et al.* [30]; Liu *et al.* [31].

Table 37.2 Lung volumes for various mammalian species.

Species	Body weight (kg)	*n*	Conditions	TLC		FRC (mL/kg)	RV (mL/kg)	Reference
				mL	mL/kg			
Mouse	0.020	NS	Anesthetized	1.57	78.5	25.0	19.5	[32]
Rat	0.31	NS	Anesthetized, prone	12.2	39.4	6.8	4.2	[32]
Rabbit	3.14	NS	Anesthetized, supine	111	35.4	11.6	6.4	[32]
Cat	3.7	4	Anesthetized			17.8		[33]
Dog	18.6	6	Awake, prone	2090	112.4	53.6	16.7	[34]
	9.2	140	Unsedated, 1-year old			44.8		[35]
Sheep	24.5	4	Unsedated, prone, nasal endotracheal tube			45.3		[19]
Goat	46.4	6	Unsedated, standing, face mask			49.6		[22]
Cow	517	7	Awake, standing			39.4		[30]
	537	5	Anesthetized, prone	45,377	84.5	31.9	16.1	[30]
Horse	485		Anesthetized, prone	44,800	92.4	36.3	19.0	[28]
	402	6	Awake, standing			51.3		[30]
	394	4	Anesthetized, prone, lung inflated to 35 cmH_2O, starved 18 h	45,468	115.4	37.9		[30]
	450–822	6	Conscious, standing			35.6		[27]
Pony	164–288	8	Conscious, standing			39.9		[27]

n, sample size; NS, not specified; TLC, total lung capacity; FRC, functional residual capacity; RV, residual volume.

Table 37.3 Breathing frequency (*f*), tidal volume (V_T), and minute ventilation ($\dot{V}_E$) for various species.

Species	Mean body weight (kg)	*n*	Conditions	*f* (breaths/min)	V_T		$\dot{V}_E$		Reference
					mL	mL/kg	mL/min	mL/kg/min	
Mouse	0.02	NS	Awake, prone	163.4	0.15	7.78	24.5	1239	[32]
	0.032	NS	Anesthetized	109	0.18	5.63	21.0	720	[32]
Rat	0.113	NS	Awake, prone	85.5	0.87	7.67	72.9	646	[32]
	0.305	NS	Awake, pleth	103	2.08	6.83	213	701	[32]
Cat	3.8	4	Unanesthetized, pleth	22	30	7.9	664	174	[39]
	3.7	NS	Anesthetized	30	34	9.2	960	310	[32]
Dog	18.6	6	Awake, prone, chronic trach, intubated	13	309	16.6	3818	205	[34]
	18.8	8	Awake, standing, chronic trach, intubated	16.5	314	16.9	4963	264	[17]
Sheep	32–37	4	Awake, standing, mask	38	289	8.3	10,400	297	[40]
Goat	36.3	3	Awake, standing, mask	13.6	470	12.9	6313	174	[20]
Pig	46.4	6	Awake, standing, mask	26	483	10.4	11,900	256	[22]
	47.6	6	Awake, standing, mask	17.6	602	12.6	10,540	221	[21]
	12.9	4	Awake, standing	13.1	209	15.9	2731	208	[41]
Cow	517 Holstein	7	Awake, standing, mask	23.7	3676	7.1	85,977	166	[25]
	405 Jersey	11	Awake, standing, mask	28.6	3360	8.3	94,870	234	[38]
Calf	43–73 Hereford	8	4–6 weeks old, standing, sling	26.7	403	15.1	10,290	385	[42]
Horse	402	6	Awake, standing, mask	11.8	4253	10.6	49,466	123	[25]
	483	6	Awake, standing, mask	15.5	4860	10.1	74,600	154	[37]
	486	15	Awake, standing, mask (some sedated) (mask V_D not removed)	10	7300	15.0	79,000	163	[36]
Pony	147	19	Awake, standing, mask	19.0	1370	9.3	26,380	180	[26]

n, sample size; NS, not specified; pleth, whole-body plethysmograph; trach, tracheostomy.

Respiratory function in conscious and anesthetized animals

When considering respiratory function and dysfunction in the clinical setting, it is useful to evaluate the respiratory system in terms of its major components: neural control, structures involved in achieving ventilation (upper airway and the bellows mechanism, including the thoracic wall and diaphragm), and lung parenchyma where the matching of ventilation and perfusion results in gas exchange (Fig. 37.2). Alterations of arterial blood gas values occur due to changes in (1) the neural control of ventilation by sedative, opioid, or anesthetic depression and/or central nervous system (CNS) disease; (2) upper airway or lower airway patency by muscle relaxation or spasm; or (3) the bellows mechanism of the thorax through decreased inspiratory muscle tone (diaphragm and intercostal muscles) by anesthetic drugs, neuromuscular paralysis, space-occupying lesions of the thorax, or a change in the diaphragm shape, location, or function; and (4) the parenchyma, such as an abnormal alveolar–capillary membrane or less than optimal matching between $\dot{V}_A$ and $\dot{Q}$.

Neural control of ventilation

The movement of air in and out of the lungs in a rhythmic ventilatory pattern is determined by a complex network of neurons located in the brainstem (*medulla oblongata* and *pons*), which receive neural input from central and peripheral chemoreceptors, the cerebral cortex, and from pulmonary receptors (Fig. 37.3) [44]. Respiratory neurons include those located in the pontine respiratory group (lateral parabrachial and Kölliker–Fuse areas) and several medullary areas, most notably the retrotrapezoid nucleus, the Bötzinger and preBötzinger complexes, the rostral (nucleus ambiguous) and caudal ventral respiratory groups (nucleus parambigualis and nucleus retroambigualis), and a dorsal respiratory group of neurons located in the nucleus tractus solitarius [44]. Current understanding of respiratory processing and control mechanisms are described in detail elsewhere [43–45]. Normal respiratory rhythmicity originates from neuronal activity in a subset of respiratory neurons, referred to as the "central pattern generator," which initiates inspiration by increasing efferent nerve signals to the external intercostal muscles and diaphragm. The intercostal nerves, which originate from the ventral branch of spinal thoracic nerves, provide motor innervation to the intercostal muscles; while the phrenic nerve, which originates from branches of cervical nerves (between the fourth and seventh cervical vertebrae), is responsible for the contraction of the diaphragm. Inspiration, which is an active process that involves contraction of external intercostal muscles and diaphragm, is terminated through inhibition of the inspiratory neurons by the pontine respiratory group, also known as the "pneumotaxic center," and by afferent nerve impulses originating from pulmonary stretch receptors. In most species, expiration occurs passively, without any muscular effort (*equidae* being a notable exception). In some circumstances, such as during exercise, expiratory neurons in the medulla can become activated, resulting in contraction of the expiratory muscles (abdominal and internal intercostal muscles) [43,46]. Respiratory control mechanisms monitor the chemical composition of blood (pH, $PaCO_2$, and PaO_2), the effort exerted by

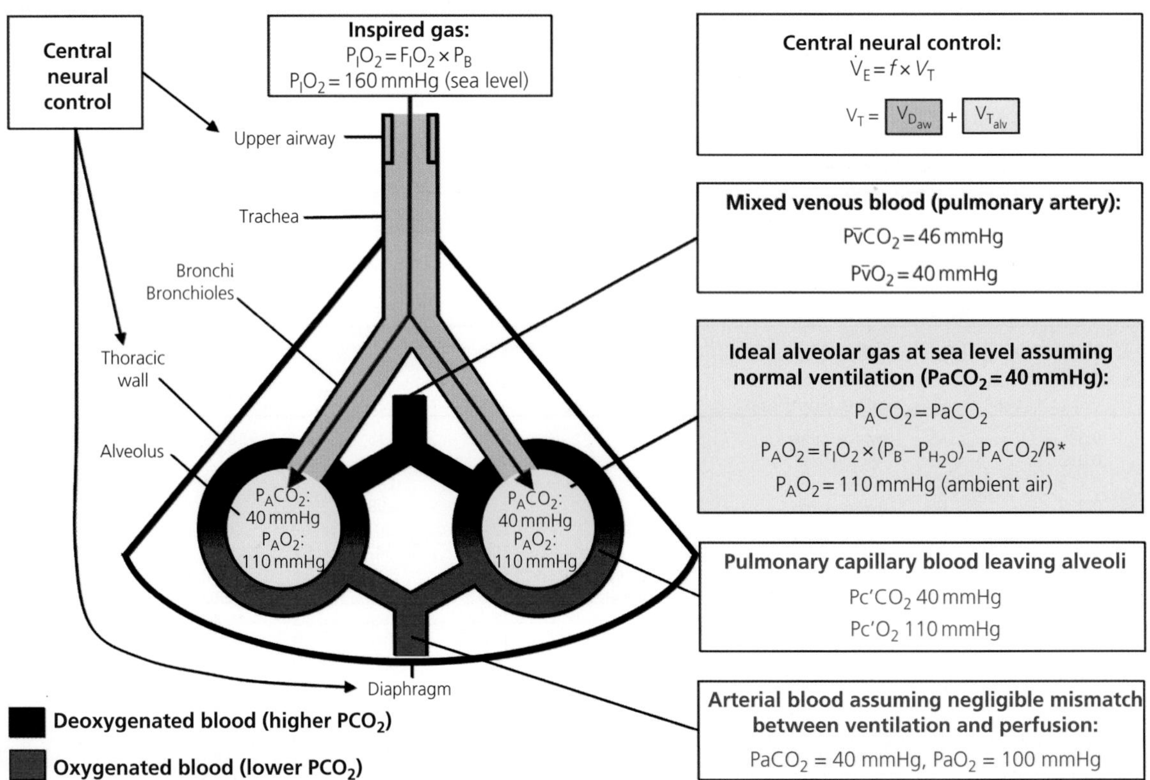

Figure 37.2 Diagrammatic representation of the neural control, bellows mechanism (diaphragm and thoracic wall), and matching of pulmonary artery (mixed venous) blood and alveolar gas in the lung under ideal conditions. Minute volume ($\dot{V}_E$), respiratory frequency (*f*), tidal volume (V_T), airway deadspace ($V_{D_{aw}}$) (colored blue), alveolar tidal volume ($V_{T_{alv}}$) (colored yellow), and representative inspired (P_I), alveolar (P_A), mixed venous ($P\bar{v}$), end-capillary (Pc′), and arterial (Pa) partial pressures of oxygen and carbon dioxide are also illustrated (see the text for a detailed explanation). *Respiratory quotient (R) represents the relative ratio of carbon dioxide production to oxygen consumption (assumed to be 0.9 in conscious healthy dogs). Source: Adapted from Walters *et al.* [43].

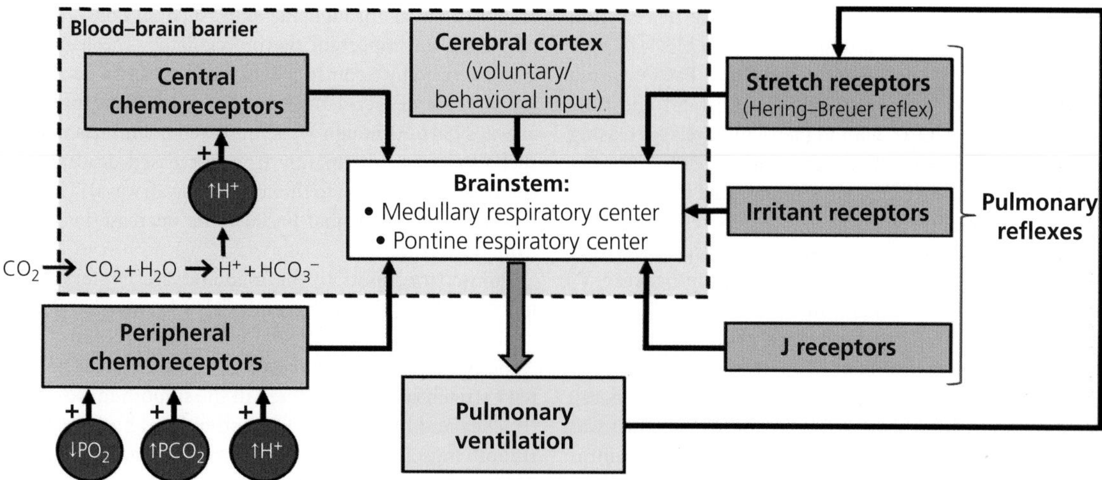

Figure 37.3 Diagrammatic representation of the neural control of ventilation. The medullary respiratory center receives multiple inputs and coordinates activity of respiratory muscles and adjusts pulmonary ventilation (see text for detailed explanation). Source: Adapted from Lyons and Kevin [46].

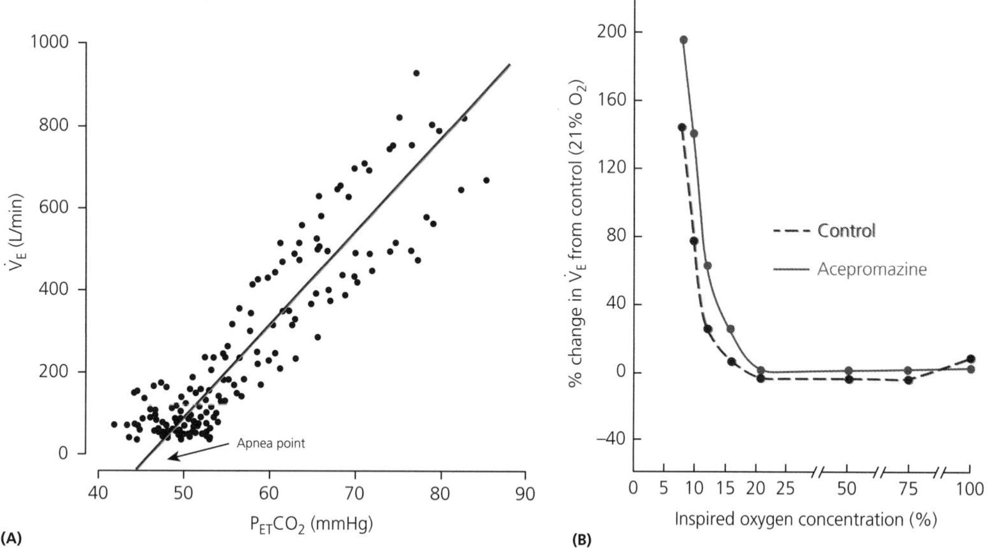

Figure 37.4 **A.** Effects of hypercapnia on $\dot{V}_E$ in conscious horses. End-tidal CO_2 partial pressure ($P_{ET}CO_2$) was used as an indicator of hypercapnia induced by CO_2 rebreathing. **B.** Effects of changes in inspired oxygen concentration on percent changes in $\dot{V}_E$ from baseline (inspired oxygen = 21%) recorded in conscious horses (control), and in horses that received a tranquilizer (acepromazine). Source: Adapted from Gauvreau *et al.* [48]; Muir and Hamlin [50].

respiratory muscles, and the presence of foreign material within the airway, providing input to the brainstem to alter the bronchomotor tone, duration of inspiration, airflow velocity on inspiration and expiration, and respiratory frequency.

Central and *peripheral chemoreceptors* provide the major afferent input to the respiratory neurons in the medulla and pons as illustrated in Fig. 37.3 [44–46]. The central chemoreceptors, located primarily on the ventral surface of the medulla, as well as in other locations within the CNS, are responsible for maintaining a tonic ventilatory drive at normal baseline $PaCO_2$ levels and for increasing $\dot{V}_E$ in response to increasing $PaCO_2$ levels [47]. The effect of $PaCO_2$ on central chemoreceptor activity occurs indirectly via changes in cerebrospinal fluid (CSF) hydrogen ion concentration (pH) as CO_2 readily crosses the blood–brain barrier and reacts with water to form carbonic acid (H_2CO_3), which in turn dissociates into H^+ and bicarbonate (HCO_3^-) (Fig. 37.3). The CSF exhibits poor buffering capacity and any change in PCO_2 within the CNS is quickly reflected as a change in pH [44,46]. The correlation between $\dot{V}_E$ and progressively increasing CO_2 levels in conscious horses is shown in Fig. 37.4A. Anesthetic drugs alter the relationship between $\dot{V}_E$ and $PaCO_2$ by decreasing central chemoreceptor sensitivity to increasing CO_2 levels and by inhibiting neuronal activity within the respiratory center of the brainstem.

Peripheral chemoreceptors are primarily responsible for the ventilatory response to decreases in PaO_2 (Fig. 37.3) [44]. These receptors respond faster than central chemoreceptors and are located within the highly vascular carotid and aortic bodies, although the role of the chemoreceptors in the aortic bodies in mature animals is believed to play a less significant role [44]. As PaO_2 levels fall, peripheral chemoreceptors increase input to the respiratory center in the brainstem to increase $\dot{V}_E$, a response referred to as the "hypoxic ventilatory drive." Peripheral chemoreceptor also play an important role in the maintenance of normal $PaCO_2$ and arterial pH and are responsible for 30–50% of the tonic drive to ventilate. In sheep, goats, calves, pigs, and ponies, carotid body denervation causes hypoventilation, hypoxemia, and hypercapnia [23,41].

In general, there is tight physiologic control over $PaCO_2$ with a quasi-linear relationship between $\dot{V}_E$ and $PaCO_2$ (and end-tidal CO_2 partial pressure [$P_{ET}CO_2$]), with higher CO_2 levels increasing $\dot{V}_E$ as illustrated in Fig. 37.4A [48]. Species differences in response to progressive increases in $PaCO_2$ or $P_{ET}CO_2$ induced by increasing inspired CO_2 exist, with horses being slightly less responsive and burrowing or diving animals being much less responsive than humans [48–50]. Unlike the quasi-linear relationship between $\dot{V}_E$ and increasing CO_2 levels, the change in $\dot{V}_E$ evoked by changes in PaO_2 is curvilinear. While $\dot{V}_E$ remains relatively constant with PaO_2 values above 70 mmHg, an exponential increase in $\dot{V}_E$ occurs as PaO_2 falls below 60–70 mmHg in mature animals [44,46,49]. As illustrated in Fig. 37.4B, when the F_IO_2 in conscious horses was decreased from approximately 1 (100% inspired oxygen concentration) to 0.16 (16% inspired oxygen concentration), there was no substantial change in $\dot{V}_E$; however, as F_IO_2 was decreased below 0.16, an inspired oxygen concentration that would result in PaO_2 < 60 mmHg, $\dot{V}_E$ increased exponentially [50].

Metabolic acid–base disturbances trigger a compensatory response in ventilation through peripheral chemoreceptors. A decrease in plasma pH originating from non-respiratory causes stimulates peripheral chemoreceptors and increases $\dot{V}_E$. The decrease in $PaCO_2$ secondary to the increase in ventilatory drive reduces the impact of metabolic acidosis on blood/extracellular pH. The compensatory decrease in $PaCO_2$ in animals with metabolic acidosis is self-limiting because of a decrease in central chemoreceptor activity associated with the alkalinization of CSF pH, which limits further reductions in $PaCO_2$. Therefore, respiratory compensation of metabolic acidosis may only partially offset the impact of the metabolic acid–base disturbance on pH [46,51]. The decreased $\dot{V}_E$ and compensatory increase in $PaCO_2$ during metabolic alkalosis is also limited because rising PCO_2 levels within the CNS increase the ventilatory drive [51].

The respiratory compensation of metabolic acid–base disturbances can be estimated in dogs. To date, there is limited data to allow calculation of the expected respiratory compensation of metabolic acid–base disturbances in cats, but it appears that the feline species have a limited ability to reduce the impact of metabolic acidosis on pH through an increase in pulmonary ventilation [51]. In dogs with primary metabolic acidosis, for each mEq/L of decrease in plasma HCO_3^- from normal values (e.g., 20 mEq/L), a compensatory decrease in $PaCO_2$ of 0.7 mmHg is expected to occur [51,52]. Changes in $PaCO_2$ of the same magnitude but in an opposite direction occur during metabolic alkalosis. Calculating the expected respiratory compensation to metabolic acid–base derangements is useful to differentiate simple from mixed acid–base disturbances and the reader is referred to the specialized literature for further details [51,52]. From an anesthesiologist's perspective, it is important to understand that anesthetic drugs may decrease central and peripheral chemoreceptor activity, increasing $PaCO_2$ and inhibiting the respiratory compensation to metabolic acidosis.

The cerebral cortex also provides input to the medullary respiratory center, mediating behavioral/voluntary changes in pulmonary ventilation (Fig. 37.3). Behavioral changes such as fear, anxiety, excitement, and pain are thought to be particularly important in small animal species and will often increase ventilatory drive and cause hypocapnia (low $PaCO_2$)/primary respiratory alkalosis because of increased $\dot{V}_E$ and $\dot{V}_A$ [53]. Heat stress/hyperthermia may also increase the ventilatory drive, particularly in animals with limited ability to sweat through the skin, such as dogs. In these species, panting is an important thermoregulatory mechanism. Panting is characterized by a controlled increase in *f* and a decrease in V_T with the purpose of increasing evaporative heat loss through the upper airways [54]. Although $\dot{V}_E$ is increased in animals that are panting, such change results mainly from increased deadspace ventilation (increased ventilation to the conducting airways). Therefore, $PaCO_2$ may be close to normal because the decrease in V_T prevents $\dot{V}_A$ from increasing.

Pulmonary inputs to the medullary respiratory center include the *pulmonary stretch receptors* (also known as "slowly adapting stretch receptors"), *J receptors*, and *irritant receptors* (also known as "rapidly adapting stretch receptors") (Fig. 37.3) [44,46]. The pulmonary stretch receptors, located in the smooth muscle of the airways (trachea and bronchi) [55], are stimulated by distension of airway smooth muscle (enlargement of airway cross-sectional area) as lung volume increases during inspiration [56]. As there is an increase in the frequency of depolarization from these receptors caused by the conditions described above, a negative feedback mechanism (the Hering–Breuer reflex) determines termination of inspiration and prevents lung over-inflation [44,46]. Although the role of pulmonary stretch receptors in controlling inspiration in adult humans is now believed to be minor, in several veterinary species including dogs, cats, and rabbits, it appears to play a significant role in the regulation of V_T [44,57]. The J receptors are nerve endings located in the pulmonary interstitium and the conducting airways. Stimulation of J receptors by inflammation results in rapid, shallow breathing, mucus production, and bronchoconstriction [44]. Irritant receptors are nerve endings located in the epithelial cells of the conducting airways that are activated by noxious stimuli such as gases/chemicals and suspended particles [44]. Activation of these receptors will alter the ventilatory rhythmic pattern and may lead to rapid/shallow breathing. Sniffing and sneezing are caused by the presence of irritants in the nasal cavity, whereas stimulation of laryngeal and pharyngeal irritant receptors may cause cough, mucus secretion, or, in severe situations, laryngospasm, bronchospasm, and apnea.

Pulmonary ventilation

Physics of respiratory gases and the alveolar gas equation

Respiratory gases (oxygen, CO_2, and nitrogen) can be measured as percent of total volume represented by each gas in the mixture (%) or according to their partial pressure in millimeters of mercury (mmHg) or kilopascals (1 kPa = 7.5 mmHg). Gases dissolve in fluids and diffuse across membranes (e.g., alveolar–capillary membrane) according to their partial pressures [58]. Dalton's law states that the total partial pressure of a gas mixture equals the sum of the partial pressure of each gas. The partial pressure of each gas is calculated by multiplying the percent volume of each gas in the mixture by the barometric pressure (P_B), that is, the pressure exerted by the atmosphere, and is expressed in mmHg or kPa (Fig. 37.5). Because the degree of collision among gas molecules is influenced by the gravitational forces exerted by the earth, the partial pressure of a single gas or gas mixture will vary according to the altitude in relation to sea level [58]. While the partial pressure of a gas or gas mixture decreases in proportion to the decrease in barometric pressure at higher altitudes, the percent volume of gas in the mixture remains constant with changes in altitude and barometric pressure. As such, F_IO_2 is the same at sea level or the top of Mount Everest (21%), the highest peak on earth (8848 meters above sea level). However, because P_B at Mount Everest is about one-third of that at

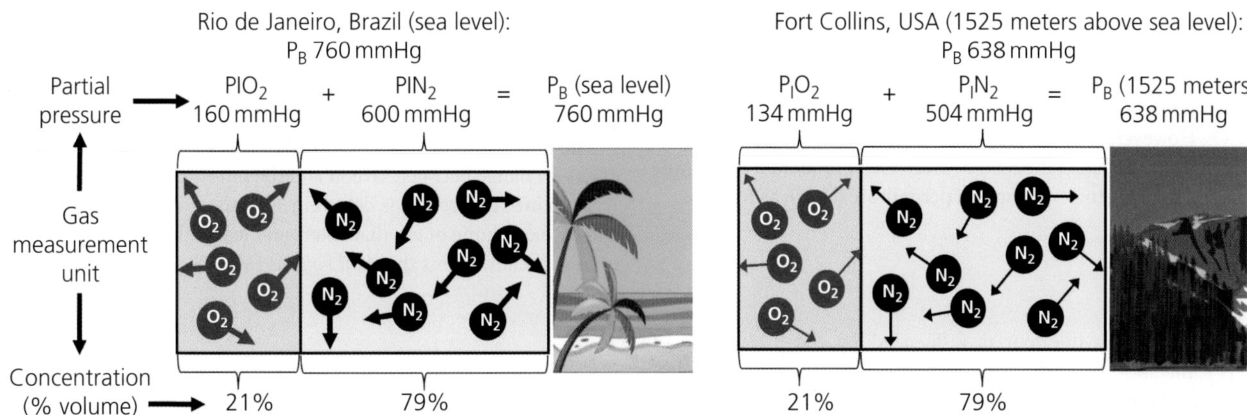

Figure 37.5 Diagrammatic representation of the influence of variations in altitude on ambient air assuming negligible air humidity (i.e., water vapor partial pressure = zero) (see text for explanation). P_IO_2, inspired partial pressure of oxygen; P_IN_2, inspired partial pressure of nitrogen; P_B, barometric pressure.

Table 37.4 Composition of respiratory gases expressed as percent volume (%) and as partial pressure (mmHg) at sea level for air and 100% oxygen.

Gas	Inspired gas (breathing air): P_{H_2O} = 9 mmHg[a]		Alveolar gas (breathing air): P_{H_2O} = 47 mmHg[b]	
	Percent volume	Partial pressure	Percent volume	Partial pressure
Nitrogen	79%	593 mmHg	79%	563 mmHg
Oxygen	20.95%	157 mmHg	15.3%	109 mmHg
Carbon dioxide	0.04%	0.3 mmHg	5.7%	41 mmHg
Total sum[c]	100%	751 mmHg	100%	713 mmHg
Gas	**Inspired gas (breathing 100% oxygen): P_{H_2O} = 0 mmHg**		**Alveolar gas (breathing 100% oxygen): P_{H_2O} = 47 mmHg[b]**	
	Percent volume	**Partial pressure**	**Percent volume**	**Partial pressure**
Nitrogen	3%	23 mmHg	3%	21 mmHg
Oxygen	97%	737 mmHg	91.3%	651 mmHg
Carbon dioxide	–	–	5.7%	41 mmHg
Total sum[c]	100%	760 mmHg	100%	713 mmHg

[a] Water vapor partial pressure assuming 51% relative humidity at 20 °C ambient temperature.
[b] Water vapor partial pressure assuming alveolar gas fully saturated with water and warmed (37 °C) after passing through the conducting airways.
[c] Total sum of partial pressures will equal atmospheric pressure at sea level (760 mmHg) if water vapor pressure is added.
Source: Data taken from Hlastala [58].

sea level (253 mmHg and 760 mmHg, respectively), oxygen partial pressure in inspired gas (P_IO_2) at this altitude will be markedly low (53 mmHg, calculated as $F_IO_2 \times P_B$), leading to a degree of hypoxemia that is incompatible with life. While extremely high altitudes (above 5500 meters or 18,000 feet) generally cannot sustain developed forms of life due to the low P_IO_2, another more realistic example of the impact of altitude on inspired gases is illustrated in Fig. 37.5. Compared to Rio de Janeiro (Brazil), located at sea level, the P_IO_2 in Fort Collins (United States), located 1525 meters above sea level, is reduced from 160 mmHg to 134 mmHg due to altitude. Oxygen partial pressure in alveolar gas (P_AO_2), calculated on the basis of the *alveolar gas equation*, will be approximately 105 mmHg and 85 mmHg at sea level and an altitude of 1525 meters, respectively. Assuming that the *alveolar to arterial oxygen gradient* ($P(A\text{-}a)O_2$) is normally between 5 and 15 mmHg, normal PaO_2 levels in Rio de Janeiro and Fort Collins are estimated to be approximately 95–100 mmHg and 75–80 mmHg, respectively.

The water vapor partial pressure (P_{H_2O}) decreases the P_B and should be subtracted from the altitude-based barometric pressure if ambient air humidity is elevated. In the presence of water vapor, the sum of the partial pressures of a gas mixture should be equal to P_B minus P_{H_2O} (Table 37.4). For simplicity, it is typically assumed that water vapor partial pressure is zero in ambient air and the sum of partial pressure of gases equals the barometric pressure at a given altitude (Table. 37.4). While water vapor partial pressure in inspired gas is probably zero in a patient receiving 100% medical oxygen without humidification, this simplification may stray from reality if relative air humidity and ambient temperature are elevated. If the relative air humidity is 51%, water vapor pressure of ambient air is 9 mmHg at 20 °C [58].

The composition of alveolar gas differs from inspired dry air because, in addition to oxygen and nitrogen, it contains saturated water vapor and CO_2 that diffused out of pulmonary capillary blood, according to the *alveolar gas equation* (Fig. 37.2, Table 37.4):

$$P_AO_2 = F_IO_2 \times \left(P_B - P_{H_2O}\right) - \frac{P_ACO_2}{R}$$

Where P_AO_2 is oxygen partial pressure in alveolar gas, F_IO_2 is the fraction of inspired oxygen, P_B is the barometric pressure, P_{H_2O} is the water vapor pressure, P_ACO_2 is the alveolar CO_2 partial pressure, and R is the respiratory quotient. As inspired gases are warmed and humidified after passing through the conducting airways, water vapor partial pressure increases to 47 mmHg at 37 °C (Fig. 37.2, Table 37.4). Carbon dioxide is highly diffusible across the alveolar–capillary membrane; therefore, P_ACO_2 is assumed to be equal to $PaCO_2$. However, to account for the metabolic rate, P_ACO_2 should be divided by the R, that is, the ratio between CO_2 production per minute ($\dot{V}CO_2$) and oxygen consumption per minute ($\dot{V}O_2$), as follows:

$$R = \frac{\dot{V}CO_2}{\dot{V}O_2}$$

The respiratory quotient is influenced by the diet/source of energy metabolism and varies with the percentage of carbohydrates, proteins, and fats being oxidized. Oxidative metabolism of carbohydrates, proteins, and fats results in R values of 1, 0.8, and 0.7, respectively [58]. The reason for this difference is that when oxygen fuels carbohydrate metabolism, one molecule of CO_2 is formed for each molecule of oxygen consumed; during oxidative metabolism of fats, a large share of the oxygen combines with hydrogen atoms from the fats to form water instead of CO_2. In humans consuming a Western diet, R has been determined to be 0.8 while studies in healthy conscious dogs report an R-value of 0.9 [43]. The respiratory quotient can be altered by species, breed, nutritional state, hormonal circadian rhythm, and level of activity. Because of changes in the energy metabolism, R values ranging from 0.7 to 0.8 have been reported in critically ill dogs [59].

Kinetics of carbon dioxide elimination

The ideal gas exchange between pulmonary capillary blood and the alveoli is illustrated in Fig. 37.2. As the CO_2 in mixed venous blood (CO_2 partial pressure in mixed venous blood [$P\bar{v}CO_2$]) reaches the pulmonary capillaries, it equilibrates with P_ACO_2. The rate of CO_2 removal from the alveoli to ambient air, and consequently the P_ACO_2 and the CO_2 partial pressure in end-pulmonary capillary blood ($Pc'CO_2$), is determined by the volume of air flowing in and out of alveoli over 1 min, that is, $\dot{V}_A$ [9]. The $PaCO_2$, which averages CO_2 of the end-capillary blood from all alveoli, indicates the adequacy of $\dot{V}_A$. It is important to understand the variables that influence CO_2 removal to manage $\dot{V}_A$ and $PaCO_2$ in the perianesthetic setting.

The flow of gas in and out of the lungs is an essential component of gas exchange between alveoli and the pulmonary capillary blood. As explained before, $\dot{V}_E$, is determined by the *breathing frequency* (*f*) and by the volume of gas that enters and leaves the mouth or nostrils in each breath, that is the *tidal volume* (V_T) (Fig. 37.2, Table 37.3).

$$\dot{V}_E = f \times V_T$$

Gas exchange takes place only at the level of the alveolar–capillary barrier, more specifically in alveoli that are ventilated and perfused. Areas of the respiratory tract that receive ventilation but that do not participate in gas exchange, are referred to as "deadspace." Because the upper airways and tracheobronchial tree do not participate in gas exchange, the relative volume necessary to fill these structures during tidal breathing is termed "airway deadspace" ($V_{D_{aw}}$). The conducting airways are not the only component of the respiratory system responsible for deadspace ventilation, however, ventilated but not perfused alveoli also contribute to deadspace. The volume of these alveolar units is referred to as "alveolar deadspace" ($V_{D_{alv}}$). "Physiologic deadspace" ($V_{D_{phys}}$) is the total deadspace volume, which includes $V_{D_{aw}}$ and $V_{D_{alv}}$ (Fig. 37.6A):

$$V_{D_{phys}} = V_{D_{aw}} + V_{D_{alv}}$$

Although $\dot{V}_E$ is commonly measured to evaluate pulmonary ventilation, the important factor in pulmonary gas exchange is the rate at which *alveolar air* is exchanged with atmospheric air. Alveolar ventilation per minute ($\dot{V}_A$) is described by:

$$\dot{V}_A = \left(V_T - V_{D_{phys}}\right) \times f \text{ or } \dot{V}_A = \dot{V}_E - \dot{V}_{D_{phys}}$$

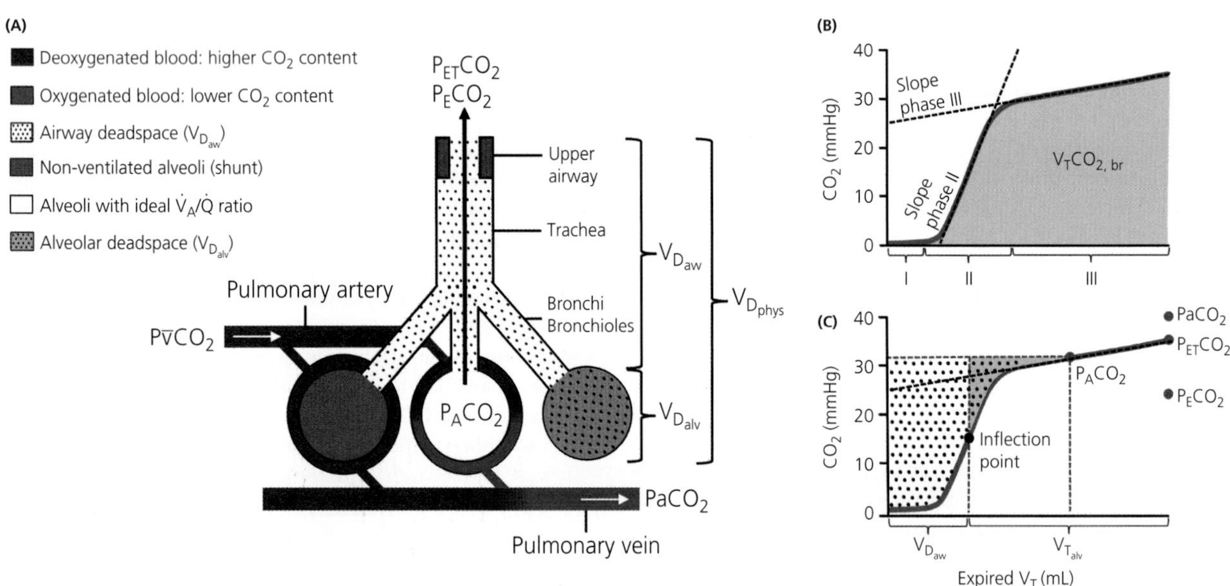

Figure 37.6 **A.** Diagrammatic representation of ventilation-to-perfusion relationships in relation to deadspace ventilation and the kinetics of carbon dioxide elimination. **B.** and **C.** Graphic representation of expired carbon dioxide partial pressure changes in relation to expired V_T (volumetric capnography) (see the text for detailed explanation).

The formula above accounts for the volume of gas that enters and leaves the physiologic deadspace per minute ($\dot{V}_{D_{phys}}$). With the use of volumetric capnography (further discussed below in this section), $\dot{V}_A$ can be measured. Alternatively, the *alveolar ventilation equation* can be used to quantitate $\dot{V}_A$. In this equation, $\dot{V}CO_2$ is CO_2 production per minute, P_ACO_2 is the CO_2 partial pressure in the alveolus, which is assumed to be equal to $PaCO_2$, and *K* is a constant:

$$\dot{V}_A = K \times \frac{\dot{V}CO_2}{PaCO_2}$$

From this equation, it is evident that $\dot{V}_A$ is inversely correlated with $PaCO_2$. If $\dot{V}_A$ is reduced by 50%, and $\dot{V}CO_2$ is unchanged (stable metabolism), $PaCO_2$ will double and vice versa. Pulmonary ventilation ($\dot{V}_E$ and $\dot{V}_A$) in the resting state should match the CO_2 production at the basal metabolic rate, which may vary among animal species and breeds [60]. Because energy expenditure and basal metabolic rate are significantly higher at birth and progressively decrease as aging occurs [60], $\dot{V}_E$ and $\dot{V}_A$ are significantly higher in neonatal and pediatric patients than in adult animals. The clinical implication of higher $\dot{V}_E$ and $\dot{V}_A$ in younger patients is that respiratory depression caused by anesthetic agents can rapidly lead to severe hypercapnia and hypoxemia in these individuals.

Based on the second formula above ($\dot{V}_A = \dot{V}_E - \dot{V}_{D_{phys}}$), isolating $\dot{V}_E$ on one side of the equation shows that $\dot{V}_E$ is the sum of $\dot{V}_{D_{phys}}$ and $\dot{V}_A$. However, during a single breath, gas exchange will depend on the fraction of V_T that goes beyond the $V_{D_{phys}}$, and effectively ventilates alveoli that are perfused. While both fractions of a V_T are useful to consider as independent variables, over time, there is some mixing between the gas in the $V_{D_{aw}}$ and the alveolar gas due to diffusion of gases, a phenomenon facilitated by the movement created by the beating heart [61]. This "mixing" action probably explains why $PaCO_2$ levels are usually not all that elevated in smaller dogs or cats showing a very shallow tachypneic breathing pattern wherein V_T must be near $V_{D_{aw}}$. It probably also explains why insufflation of 15 L/min oxygen deep into the trachea in an apneic horse will maintain PaO_2 values in the 50–60 mmHg range (Dr. Wayne McDonell, personal observation).

Experimentally, $V_{D_{phys}}$ has been evaluated in animals using several techniques that are influenced to varying degrees by pulmonary ventilation and perfusion abnormalities ($\dot{V}_A/\dot{Q}$ mismatch and shunt). As clinicians and researchers, it is important to consider the methodology and the factors influencing the measurement as it may alter the interpretation of the results [62–64]. Initial studies in humans measured $V_{D_{aw}}$ using the single-breath nitrogen washout test (Fowler's technique), which involves plotting the partial pressure of nitrogen in expired gas of a single breath after a maximal voluntary inspiration of 100% oxygen [9,65]. However, the Fowler technique is technically challenging to perform in conscious animals due to the need for voluntary maximum inspiration.

Physiologic deadspace to tidal volume ratio ($V_{D_{phys}}/V_T$), which is the proportion of V_T that does not contribute to gas exchange, has been determined through application of the Bohr equation:

$$\frac{V_{D_{phys}}}{V_T} = \frac{P_ACO_2 - P_{\bar{E}}CO_2}{P_ACO_2}$$

In this equation, P_ACO_2 represents mean alveolar CO_2 partial pressure and $P_{\bar{E}}CO_2$ is the average CO_2 partial pressure in mixed expired gas collected during a single breath. Effectively, the greater the amount of gas from alveolar units that are ventilated and non-perfused ($V_{D_{alv}}$) that is added to the exhaled breath, the greater the reduction of $P_{\bar{E}}CO_2$ below P_ACO_2, thereby indicating a greater proportion of deadspace ventilation in relation to V_T. However, before the advent of volumetric capnography, measurement of P_ACO_2 required complex methodology applicable only to the research setting (for example, multiple inert gas elimination technique) [25,66]. Therefore, $PaCO_2$ has been substituted for P_ACO_2 in the calculation (Bohr–Enghoff equation) as follows:

$$\frac{V_{D_{phys}}}{V_T} = \frac{PaCO_2 - P_{\bar{E}}CO_2}{PaCO_2}$$

The presence of perfused non-ventilated alveoli (shunt) or alveoli with low ventilation-to-perfusion ($\dot{V}_A/\dot{Q}$) ratio does not increase true $V_{D_{alv}}$; however, the calculated $V_{D_{phys}}/V_T$ ratio using the Enghoff modification of the Bohr equation is impacted by ventilation-to-perfusion inequalities caused by shunt and areas of low $\dot{V}_A/\dot{Q}$ ratio as these abnormalities will add CO_2-rich mixed venous blood to arterial blood, increasing $PaCO_2$, and resulting in greater overestimation of $V_{D_{phys}}/V_T$ by the Bohr–Enghoff equation. Specifically, any calculation that replaces P_ACO_2 with $PaCO_2$ will artificially increase the deadspace determination in the presence of poorly ventilated (low $\dot{V}_A/\dot{Q}$ ratio) and non-ventilated alveoli (shunt) due to rising $PaCO_2$ levels, assuming constant V_T [62–64]. In patients with lower-than-expected PaO_2 values in relation to the F_IO_2, the impact of shunt and low $\dot{V}_A/\dot{Q}$ regions on gas exchange should be considered when applying these calculations to patient ventilatory management.

In addition to the Bohr–Enghoff $V_{D_{phys}}/V_T$, the *alveolar deadspace fraction* ($V_{D_{alv}}/V_T$), that is the fraction of V_T that ventilates non-perfused alveoli, has been proposed to be estimated by replacing $P_{\bar{E}}CO_2$ with $P_{ET}CO_2$ [67]:

$$\frac{V_{D_{alv}}}{V_T} = \frac{PaCO_2 - P_{ET}CO_2}{PaCO_2}$$

Calculation of $V_{D_{alv}}/V_T$ as described above will result in a significantly smaller deadspace value as it reflects only a fraction of total (physiologic) deadspace [62–64]. Under normal circumstances, $P_{ET}CO_2$ is up to 5 mmHg lower than $PaCO_2$ because of dilution of alveolar gas, which contains CO_2, with gas from deadspace which does not contain CO_2. As a simplification of the formula above, $V_{D_{alv}}$ is considered to be increased if the arterial to end-tidal CO_2 gradient ($P(a\text{-}ET)CO_2$) is abnormally high. In this case, because P_ACO_2 is replaced by $PaCO_2$, $V_{D_{alv}}/V_T$ and $P(a\text{-}ET)CO_2$ will also increase in the presence of $\dot{V}_A/\dot{Q}$ mismatch caused by shunted flow and a low $\dot{V}_A/\dot{Q}$ ratio leading to oxygenation impairment, in a similar way as the Bohr–Enghoff $V_{D_{phys}}/V_T$ [68]. Therefore, in the presence of the above-described conditions, an increase in $V_{D_{alv}}/V_T$ and $P(a\text{-}ET)CO_2$ reflects an increase in the scatter of $\dot{V}_A/\dot{Q}$ mismatch in the lung rather than only an increase in $V_{D_{alv}}$.

In the research setting, $V_{D_{phys}}/V_T$ can be determined by collecting arterial blood gas samples to measure $PaCO_2$ as an equivalent to P_ACO_2 as well as collecting exhaled gases in a mixing chamber, or Douglas bag, to measure CO_2 in mixed expired gas ($P_{\bar{E}}CO_2$) in large animals (horses and cows) and dogs [25,69]. More recently, with the introduction of volumetric capnography for monitoring patients during mechanical ventilation, $V_{D_{phys}}/V_T$ can be more practically and reliably measured in intubated small animals [70]. Volumetric capnography is the graphic representation of expired CO_2 versus expired V_T measured using a capnograph and a pneumotachometer (device that measures flow over time) placed at the end of an endotracheal tube.

The diagram in Fig. 37.6A shows the composition of deadspace and its relationship with alveoli presenting different ventilation-to-perfusion ratios. If alveoli present an ideal ventilation-to-perfusion ratio ($\dot{V}_A/\dot{Q} = 1$), an equilibrium is established between deoxygenated (mixed venous) blood with higher CO_2 content entering the pulmonary capillary and alveolar CO_2 (P_ACO_2). The mixed expired CO_2 in each tidal breath reflects the average CO_2 from alveoli that are effectively ventilated and perfused over a range of $\dot{V}_A/\dot{Q}$ ratios, which contribute to CO_2 elimination, and alveoli that are ventilated but not perfused ($V_{D_{alv}}$), which do not contribute to CO_2 elimination. An increase in $V_{D_{alv}}$, lowers CO_2 in mixed expired gas (P_ECO_2) and increases the gradient between P_ACO_2 (or $PaCO_2$ according to the Bohr–Enghoff equation) and P_ECO_2 [62–64].

The kinetics of CO_2 elimination assessed by the volumetric capnography curve has three distinct phases (Fig. 37.6B). Phase I represents exhaled gas from the upper airways, which does not contain CO_2. Phase II represents expired gas from the lower portions of the airways mixed with CO_2-rich alveolar gas, which causes a rapid rise in CO_2. Phase III is the expired volume that represents pure alveolar gas as the CO_2 curve flattens and plateaus. The slope of phase III reflects the emptying of alveoli with different time constants. In patients with small airway disease/bronchoconstriction, or with lung disease, resistance to gas flow may differ substantially among alveolar units [71]. During expiration, alveoli where the conducting airways offer low resistance to gas flow empty first ("fast" alveoli), whereas poorly ventilated alveolar units due to increased resistance to gas flow take longer to empty. Because alveoli with different time constants differ in the speed they are emptied during expiration, the slope of phase III increases [71]. The area under the CO_2 curve represents the total amount of CO_2 exhaled during a single breath ($V_TCO_{2,br}$). The CO_2 eliminated per minute, which is assumed to be equivalent to CO_2 production per minute ($\dot{V}CO_2$), is calculated by multiplying the respiratory rate (*f*) by the $V_TCO_{2,br}$.

The airway–alveolar interface, identified as the inflection point of phase II, is the limit between exhaled gas from lower conducting airways (bronchioles) and CO_2-rich alveolar gas (Fig. 37.6C). The expired volume below and above the inflection point represents the airway deadspace ($V_{D_{aw}}$) and the alveolar tidal volume ($V_{T_{alv}}$), respectively. The CO_2 level at the midpoint of phase III slope, starting at the inflection point and ending at the end-tidal partial pressure of CO_2 ($P_{ET}CO_2$), represents the average CO_2 of all alveolar units (P_ACO_2) [64,66,72]. Studies measuring P_ACO_2 by the multiple inert gas elimination technique have validated P_ACO_2 measured by volumetric capnography [66,72].

The area above the volumetric capnography curve, which reflects deadspace ventilation, shows that $V_{D_{phys}}$ ($V_{D_{aw}} + V_{D_{alv}}$) calculations based on the Bohr equation (Fig. 37.7A) are overestimated when $PaCO_2$ is used to replace P_ACO_2 in the Enghoff modification of the original formula (Bohr–Enghoff equation) (Fig. 37.7B).

In heathy individuals, $V_{D_{phys}}$ is representative of $V_{D_{aw}}$ as $V_{D_{alv}}$ is negligible. In normal conscious humans at rest, $V_{D_{phys}}$ is approximately 2 mL/kg (150 mL) and V_T is 6–7 mL/kg of ideal body weight (assuming a V_T of 450–500 mL in a 75 kg adult human), resulting in a $V_{D_{phys}}/V_T$ ratio of approximately 30% [65]. Veterinary species in general have significantly larger deadspace volumes (indexed to body weight) than humans. Under normal conditions, $V_{D_{aw}}$ remains relatively constant, however, V_T can change for a variety of reasons (e.g., thermoregulation, excitement, and acid–base disturbances) and therefore alter the relative amount of deadspace per V_T. As such, it is important to consider the deadspace volume as well as V_T indexed to ideal body weight, particularly as it relates to both anesthetic equipment and mechanical ventilation settings. In an experimental setting, unsedated normal tracheostomized dogs breathing quietly through a standard endotracheal tube had a $V_{D_{phys}}$ of 5.9 mL/kg [17]. In conscious healthy horses and cows breathing through a face mask, the Bohr–Enghoff $V_{D_{phys}}$ (calculated using a correction factor for the added deadspace represented by the face-mask) was about 5.2 and 3.7 mL/kg [25]. Recent observations in anesthetized dogs receiving mechanical ventilation have confirmed that $V_{D_{aw}}$ estimated by volumetric capnography is substantially larger in the canine species (6.5–7.6 mL/kg) than the $V_{D_{aw}}$ calculated using the single-breath nitrogen washout test (Fowler's method) in humans (2 mL/kg) [65,69,70]. Although some of the measured

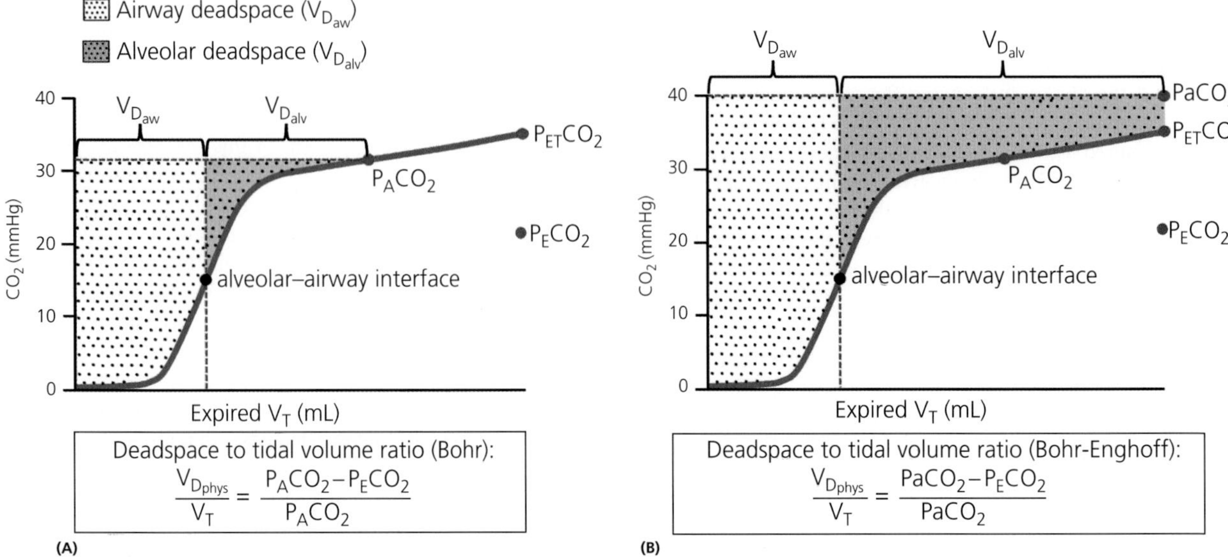

Figure 37.7 Graphic representation of expired carbon dioxide partial pressure changes in relation to expired V_T (volumetric capnography) showing the area used to calculate deadspace volumes according to the **A.** Bohr and **B.** Bohr–Enghoff equations.

differences in deadspace between humans and animals can be attributed to the use of the Bohr–Enghoff equation, which overestimates the $V_{D_{phys}}/V_T$ ratio, the use of this method likely did not have a major influence because measurements were obtained under conditions where alveolar deadspace, shunt, and $\dot{V}_A/\dot{Q}$ mismatch were minimal (standing horses and cows, healthy conscious and anesthetized dogs) [73]. Because of differences in $V_{D_{phys}}$ between animal species and humans, V_T settings during mechanical ventilation cannot be directly extrapolated from humans to animals, as discussed further in Chapter 38.

The relationship between $\dot{V}_E$, $\dot{V}_A$, and $\dot{V}_{D_{phys}}$ is critical to understanding the kinetics of CO_2 in both health and disease. Clinically, an increase in total deadspace volume ($V_{D_{phys}}$) can be due to a change in $V_{D_{aw}}$ (either physiologic due to bronchodilation or iatrogenic with artificial airways/apparatus deadspace) and/or $V_{D_{alv}}$. An increase in *f* with a reduction in V_T, and therefore the creation of a higher $V_{D_{phys}}/V_T$ ratio, is extremely common in conscious animals for a variety of reasons, including thermoregulation. In healthy animals, $\dot{V}_A$ and as a result, $PaCO_2$ are maintained within physiological limits through central and peripheral chemoreceptor stimulation as previously discussed. In disease states, increases in $V_{D_{alv}}$ commonly occur with low pulmonary perfusion pressures secondary to a low cardiac output (CO), pulmonary thromboembolism, severe airway disease, and acute respiratory distress syndrome (ARDS) [74–77]. An increase in $V_{D_{alv}}$ does not necessarily impair arterial oxygenation (PaO_2) if the capillary flow that bypasses ventilated alveoli is perfusing well-ventilated lung areas. $PaCO_2$ levels can also be maintained within normal levels when there is an increase in $V_{D_{alv}}$ by increasing *f* or V_T to maintain $\dot{V}_A$. Arterial blood gases (PaO_2 and $PaCO_2$) may therefore be maintained within normal ranges in awake spontaneously breathing animals with increases in $V_{D_{alv}}$. In patients with underlying disease and patients under general anesthesia, a compensatory increase in $\dot{V}_A$ in the face of increased $V_{D_{alv}}$ may not occur. In these instances, $PaCO_2$ will rise due to a reduction in $\dot{V}_A$. In addition to impacting $PaCO_2$ values, decreases in $\dot{V}_A$ associated with an increase in $\dot{V}_{D_{phys}}$ may also have an impact on a patient's oxygenation by lowering the P_AO_2 if inspired gases are not enriched with oxygen (Table 37.5).

Effects of altered alveolar ventilation

While changes in deadspace may not necessarily impact the ability to achieve adequate gas exchange, when $\dot{V}_A$ is altered significant changes in P_ACO_2 and P_AO_2 can occur (Fig. 37.2, Table 37.5). As previously discussed, $\dot{V}_A$ is inversely correlated with $PaCO_2$ as described by the alveolar ventilation equation ($\dot{V}_A = K \times \dot{V}CO_2/PaCO_2$). Hyperventilation occurs when $\dot{V}_A$ is excessive relative to metabolic rate; as a result, $PaCO_2$ is reduced. An increase in *f*, referred to as "tachypnea," may not result in hyperventilation if a decrease in V_T prevents $\dot{V}_E$ and $\dot{V}_A$ from increasing. Hypoventilation is present when $PaCO_2$ rises because $\dot{V}_A$ is low relative to $\dot{V}CO_2$. The effects of hypoventilation on P_AO_2 and PaO_2 in a healthy dog breathing ambient air or 100% oxygen are illustrated in Table 37.5. In an individual breathing ambient air at sea level with normal $\dot{V}_A$ (e.g., $PaCO_2$ = 36 mmHg), P_AO_2 is predicted to be approximately 110 mmHg by the alveolar gas equation. If there is a decrease in $\dot{V}_A$ (e.g., $PaCO_2$ increases from 36 mmHg to 72 mmHg), P_AO_2 decreases from 110 mmHg to approximately 70 mmHg because of rising CO_2 levels within the alveoli. Considering that the alveolar to arterial oxygen gradient ($P(A\text{-}a)O_2$) is 5–15 mmHg for a healthy individual breathing ambient air, PaO_2 can be predicted to be decreased from 95–105 during normal ventilation to 55–65 mmHg during hypoventilation. If air is replaced by 100% oxygen in inspired gas ($F_IO_2 = 0.97$), P_AO_2 will be markedly increased (612 mm Hg) despite severe hypoventilation. Although $P(A\text{-}a)O_2$ may increase over time due to absorption atelectasis caused by elevated F_IO_2, PaO_2 can be estimated to be approximately 500 mmHg in the presence of severe hypoventilation with an F_IO_2 close to 1.0.

Pulmonary mechanics

Fluctuating pressure gradients between the airway opening and the alveoli cause air to flow in and out of the lungs. The factors that contribute to these pressure gradients and the measurement of their magnitude are referred to as "pulmonary mechanics." During spontaneous breathing, a negative pressure gradient between the airway opening (mouth, nostrils, or the interface between the breathing circuit and the endotracheal tube) and the alveoli/pleural cavity is responsible for the inflow of gas to the lungs. In anesthetized patients, a mechanical ventilator is commonly used to create a positive pressure gradient between the airway opening (endotracheal tube) and the alveoli to generate flow of gases into the lungs during inspiration. Factors that influence the development of a pressure gradient between the airway opening and the alveoli include the elasticity of the lungs, thoracic cage, and diaphragm (chest wall), in addition to the resistance to flow between these two regions. These properties determine the normal distribution of airflow within the lung and the energy expended to achieve optimal ventilation (work of breathing). Both anesthesia and disease can alter the elastic properties and resistance of the respiratory system, impacting the ability to achieve adequate alveolar ventilation. While pulmonary physical characteristics are generally measured on the whole lung in the clinical setting, regional differences in physical properties are also important in determining normal distribution of ventilation.

Pressures measured in the respiratory system are illustrated in Fig. 37.8. By convention transpulmonary pressure (P_L) is the difference in pressure across the entire respiratory system, from the

Table 37.5 The effects of hypoventilation on gas exchange in a dog breathing ambient air or 100% oxygen.

Normal ventilation, ambient air ($PaCO_2$ = 36 mmHg and F_IO_2 = 0.21)	Hypoventilation, ambient air ($PaCO_2$ = 72 mmHg and F_IO_2 = 0.21)	Hypoventilation, 100% oxygen ($PaCO_2$ = 72 mmHg and F_IO_2 = 0.97)
P_AO_2 = (760–47) × 0.21 – 40[a] P_AO_2 = 110 mmHg PaO_2 = 95 to 105 mmHg[b]	P_AO_2 = (760–47) × 0.21–80[a] P_AO_2 = 70 mmHg PaO_2 = 55 to 65 mmHg[b]	P_AO_2 = (760–47) × 0.97–80[a] P_AO_2 = 612 mmHg PaO_2 = 450 to 520 mmHg[c]

[a] $P_AO_2 = (P_B - P_{H_2O}) \times F_IO_2 - (P_ACO_2/R)$ where P_AO_2 is the oxygen partial pressure in alveolar gas, P_B is the local barometric pressure (760 mmHg at sea level), P_{H_2O} is the water vapor pressure after humidification of inspiratory gases (47 mmHg), F_IO_2 is the inspired oxygen fraction (0.21 for ambient air and 0.97 mmHg for 100% oxygen), and the second term is calculated by considering P_ACO_2 as equal to $PaCO_2$ and dividing it by the respiratory quotient (0.9 in healthy dogs) [43].
[b] PaO_2 levels assuming a normal alveolar to arterial oxygen gradient for ambient air ($P(A\text{-}a)O_2$ = 5 to 15 mmHg).
[c] PaO_2 levels considering that the use of 100% in inspired gas increases $P(A\text{-}a)O_2$ due to absorption atelectasis.

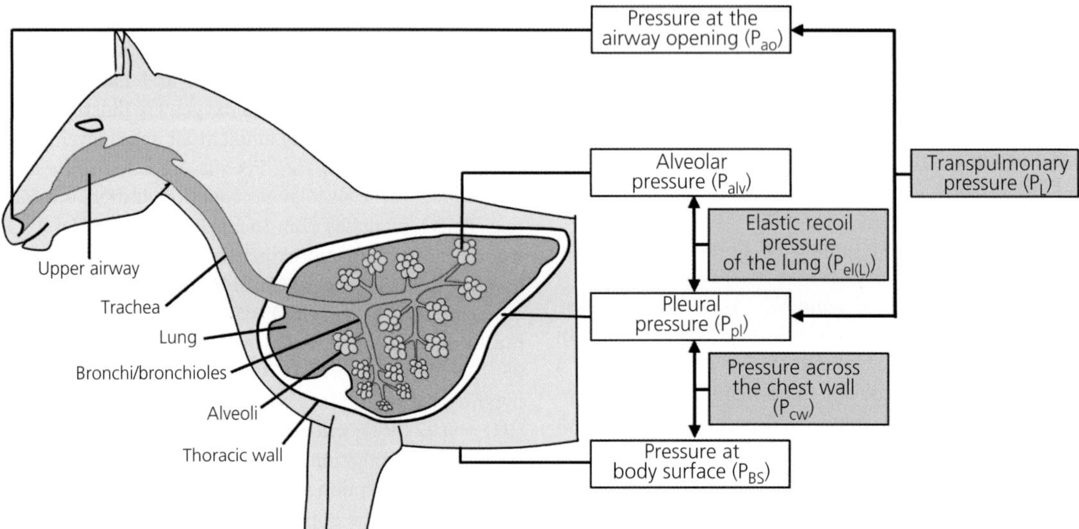

Figure 37.8 Diagrammatic representation of pressures (white boxes) and of pressure gradients (gray boxes) measured across the respiratory system (see text for explanation). Source: Adapted from Loring *et al.* [78].

pressure at the airway opening (P_{ao}) to the pleural pressure (P_{pl}); however, intensive care specialists and anesthesiologists often define P_L as the difference between alveolar and pleural pressures ($P_{alv}-P_{pl}$), creating some confusion in the literature [10,78]. The pressure gradient from atmospheric pressure (taken as P_{ao}) to the pleural space (P_{pl}) is responsible for the movement of air to and from the lungs during spontaneous breathing. The P_{ao} is always 0 cmH_2O at 1 atmosphere throughout the respiratory cycle in non-instrumented, conscious, and spontaneously breathing animals. With initiation of inspiration, as active muscular effort enlarges the pleural cavity through expansion of the thoracic wall and contraction of the diaphragm, P_{pl} becomes more negative and causes P_{alv} to become slightly sub-atmospheric (negative). The slightly negative pressure gradient between P_{ao} (0 cmH_2O) and P_{alv} (e.g., −1 cmH_2O) drives airflow from the mouth/nostrils to the alveoli, and lung volume increases. In contrast to inspiration, expiration is normally passive and depends on the elastic recoil of the lungs, diaphragm, and intercostal muscles, which causes P_{pl} to become less negative and returns the lungs to a resting position, that is, to FRC. The horse is a notable exception in that abdominal muscle contraction plays a part in normal expiratory activity, producing a biphasic mode of exhalation. As the P_{pl} becomes less negative, P_{alv} may slightly increase above atmospheric pressure. Reversal of the pressure gradient during expiration ($P_{alv} > P_{ao}$) causes air to flow from the alveoli to the airway opening/atmosphere [49,79].

The pressure difference between the airway opening and the pleural space, P_L (Fig. 37.8), can be measured using a differential pressure transducer connected to the airway opening to measure P_{ao} (face mask or endotracheal tube) and to an esophageal balloon placed in the thoracic esophagus to provide a surrogate measure of P_{pl}. The change in lung volume (or V_T) can be measured using a spirometer, a body plethysmograph, or a pneumotachometer [10].

The pressure gradient between the alveoli and the pleural cavity ($P_{alv}-P_{pl}$) is traditionally defined as *elastic recoil pressure of the lung* ($P_{el(L)}$) (Fig. 37.8 and 37.9) [78]. In spontaneously breathing subjects, $P_{el(L)}$ measured at the end of inspiration provides an estimate of the lung's ability to deflate/return to its resting position (FRC). In anesthetized individuals receiving positive-pressure ventilation, $P_{alv}-P_{pl}$ provides an assessment of the positive pressure applied to the lung tissue per se, excluding the effects of the chest wall and abdomen [80].

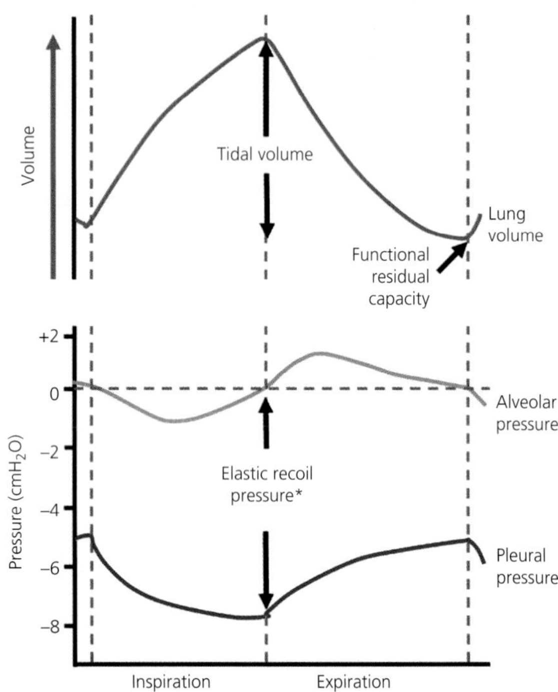

Figure 37.9 Changes in lung volume, alveolar, and pleural pressures during spontaneous breathing. Note that difference between alveolar and pleural pressure at the end of inspiration (*elastic recoil pressure of the lung*) may also be referred to as "transpulmonary pressure" in some literature. Source: Ewart [79], Elsevier.

In spontaneously breathing animals, the relationship between change in pleural pressure (ΔP_{pl}) and the resultant change in lung volume (ΔV) is known as "respiratory system compliance" (C_{RS}) or "total compliance" [9,61].

$$C_{RS} = \frac{\Delta V\ (L)}{\Delta P_{pl}\ (cmH_2O)}$$

As shown by the formula above, C_{RS} describes the ability of the lungs to distend in response to a change in pleural pressure. Compliance provides a measure of how stiff the lung is and is inversely correlated with elastance, that is, the force causing the lungs to recoil to FRC. C_{RS} is also known as "total compliance" because both the lungs and chest wall (thoracic wall and diaphragm) provide an elastic resistance to lung expansion on inspiration. However, in spontaneously breathing animals, the contribution of the latter to the total respiratory system compliance is not captured when intrapleural pressures are measured due to the effort exerted by the inspiratory muscles. When the chest wall and diaphragm are partially or completely relaxed (and do not contribute any effort to breathing), however, as often occurs during general anesthesia, they become an important contributor to the elastic resistance to inspiration and total compliance (C_{RS}). During general anesthesia, the relationship of C_{RS} to the individual compliance of the lungs (C_L) and chest wall (C_{CW}) is additive, because the lungs and chest wall are arranged concentrically and can be expressed as:

$$\frac{1}{C_{RS}} = \frac{1}{C_L} + \frac{1}{C_{CW}}$$

During positive-pressure ventilation, the pressure gradient that drives gas into the lungs is no longer negative and is determined by the difference between airway pressure measured at end-inspiration and end-expiration (ΔP_{aw}). Therefore, in anesthetized patients receiving mechanical ventilatory support, C_{RS} is measured as the ratio between change in lung volume ΔV (that is the V_T delivered by the ventilator) and the change in airway pressure (ΔP_{aw}) during a mechanical breath:

$$C_{RS} = \frac{\Delta V\ (L)}{\Delta P_{aw}\ (cmH_2O)}$$

Prior to the advent of spirometry, in anesthetized patients receiving positive-pressure ventilation, airway pressures at end-inspiration and end-expiration were used for pressure determinations, and ventilator settings (volume displaced by the bellows) were used for volume calculations. As further described in Chapter 38, with the use of modern anesthesia ventilators incorporating built-in flow sensors (built-in spirometry) or with the use of stand-alone multiparameter monitors incorporating flow sensors that are placed between the endotracheal tube and the breathing circuit (near patient spirometry), more accurate determination of changes in volume and pressure can be obtained during mechanical ventilation [81,82]. The difference in how C_{RS} is measured in spontaneously breathing versus animals receiving positive-pressure ventilation is an important concept for the veterinary clinician as the contribution of the different components (lung and/or chest wall) to total compliance needs to be considered when interpreting values and when implementing ventilatory support strategies.

Compliance is further characterized as either dynamic, static, or quasistatic. In spontaneously breathing animals, *dynamic compliance* describes changes in lung volume per unit change in pleural pressure in the presence of airflow. If the patient is receiving mechanical ventilation in a volume-controlled mode without an inspiratory pause (period of zero flow at the end of inspiration), then dynamic compliance is measured as the change in lung volume per unit change in airway pressure (peak inspiratory pressure minus end-expiratory pressure) (Fig. 37.10A). Dynamic C_{RS} is altered by changes in the *elastic properties of the respiratory system* and by changes in *airway resistance* (R_{aw}). *Static* and *quasistatic* C_{RS} describes changes in lung volume per unit change in pressure during a brief pause at end-inspiration (zero airflow). Because patient cooperation is required, static compliance measurements are often performed in anesthetized animals receiving mechanical ventilatory support with an inspiratory pause (Fig. 37.10B) [30,83–85]. The pause at end-inspiration, before passive expiration begins, must be long enough to allow airflow to equilibrate between alveoli with faster and slower filling rates, the latter reflective of areas with heightened resistance to airflow that may be increased during

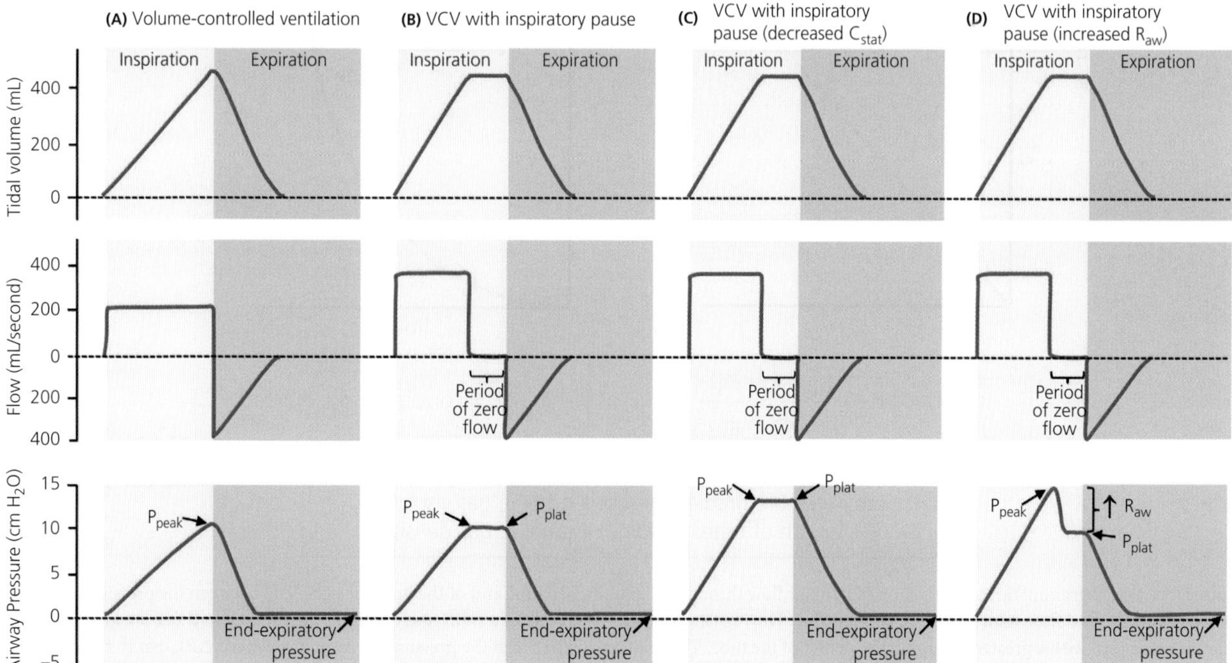

Figure 37.10 Diagrammatic representation of changes in lung volume (tidal volume), flow, and airway pressure measured at the distal end of an endotracheal tube in a normal anesthetized individual during: **A.** Volume-controlled ventilation (VCV) without an inspiratory pause. **B.** VCV with an inspiratory pause (period of zero flow at end-inspiration). **C.** During constant volume ventilation, an increase in the gradient between plateau pressure (P_{plat}) and end-expiratory pressure occurs with a decrease in static or quasistatic C_{RS}. **D.** An increase in the gradient between peak inspiratory pressure (P_{peak}) and P_{plat} occurs with an increase in R_{aw}.

pathological conditions (e.g., bronchitis/pneumonia in small animals and small airway disease in horses) [84,85]. If the duration of the inspiratory pause is between 0.5 and 2 s, frictional resistance imposed by the airways may impact measurements in humans; therefore compliance measurements are better defined as quasistatic [84,85]. Once gas flow distribution has been completed, that is, the resistive properties of the respiratory system are overcome, the ratio between V_T and the change in airway pressure (plateau minus end-expiratory pressure) reflects solely the elastic properties of the respiratory system (static or quasistatic C_{RS}) (Fig. 37.10C). Lungs develop low static compliance (become stiffer) with a reduction in lung volume, such as occurs with regional atelectasis, pulmonary edema, or fibrosis. In the case of dynamic compliance, increases in R_{aw} can contribute to decreases in compliance measurements. For example, asthma (heaves, recurrent airway obstruction) in horses and asthma (bronchopulmonary disease) in cats decreases dynamic lung compliance via increased R_{aw} [86,87].

As previously mentioned in this section, for gas to flow into the lungs, a pressure gradient must be developed to overcome, in addition to the elastic resistance, the nonelastic resistance of the respiratory system. The relationship between the pressure gradient and gas flow illustrated in Fig. 37.11A is analogous to a fundamental principle of physics, referred to as Ohm's law, wherein voltage (equivalent to pressure gradient along a tube) is proportional to current (equivalent to gas flow) multiplied by resistance [88].

$$\text{Voltage} = \text{Current} \times \text{Resistance}$$

Or in terms of gas flow:

$$\Delta P = \text{Flow rate} \times \text{Resistance}$$

Rearranging Ohm's law to determine resistance:

$$\text{Resistance} = \frac{\Delta P}{\text{Flow Rate}}$$

According to the Hagen–Poiseuille equation, *laminar* gas flow through an *unbranched* straight tube is proportional to the pressure gradient across the tube and the fourth power of the radius of the tube, and inversely proportional to the viscosity of the gas and length of the tube:

$$\text{Flow rate} = \frac{\Delta P \times \pi \times (\text{radius})^4}{8 \times \text{viscosity} \times \text{length of tube}}$$

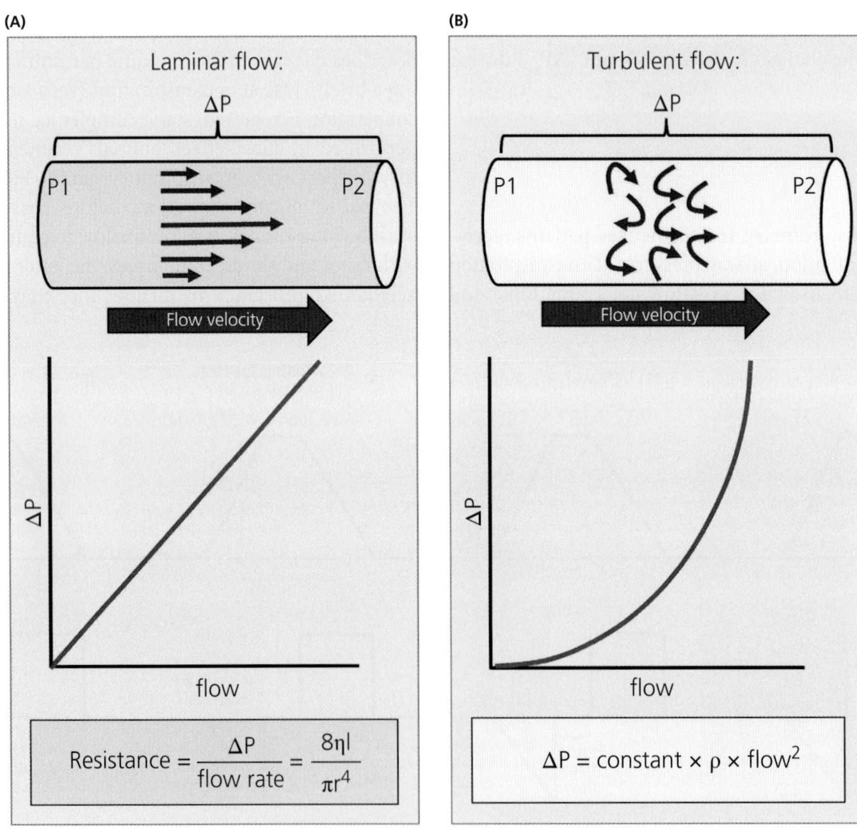

Figure 37.11 **A.** Diagrammatic representation of laminar flow through an unbranched tube and of the linear relationship between the pressure gradient across a tube (ΔP) and flow velocity during laminar flow. During laminar flow, molecules of a fluid (gas or liquid) are moving in a smooth and streamlined pattern with a greater velocity at the center of the tube. The relationship between the pressure gradient developed (ΔP), that is, the drop in pressure as gas flows down an unbranched tube, and the flow rate follows a linear pattern [89,90]. Because the pressure gradient equals resistance to gas flow, *resistance* (R) can be calculated as R = ΔP/flow rate. **B.** Diagrammatic representation of turbulent flow through an unbranched tube and of the nonlinear relationship between ΔP and flow velocity during turbulent flow (see text for explanation). Source: Adapted from Mitchell and Cheesman [89].

By combining Ohm's law and the Hagen–Poiseuille equation (substituting Hagen–Poiseuille's determinants of flow into Ohm's law), the resistance to laminar gas flow can be established:

$$\text{Resistance} = \frac{8 \times \text{viscosity} \times \text{length of tube}}{\pi \times (\text{radius})^4}$$

Resistance to laminar flow therefore increases with an increase in the tube length or a reduction in tube radius. The significance of this equation for the anesthetist is the impact of the diameter of a patient's airway on the resistance to gas flow. An increase in resistance can result from a variety of conditions such as bronchospasm, congenital or acquired anatomic abnormalities in the airway, and/or the presence of mucus, exudates, foreign bodies, or tumors within the airway lumen [89,90]. If a narrow endotracheal tube is used in a patient with an already increased airway resistance due to respiratory disease (e.g., tracheal collapse or brachycephalic airway syndrome), there may be a dramatic increase in resistance to airflow during anesthesia with spontaneous ventilation. For example, if the diameter of the upper airway is reduced by 50% due to pathology or secondary to the placement of a small endotracheal tube, the R_{aw} goes up 16-fold. Of note, with laminar flow, viscosity is the only gas property to influence resistance.

While the above relationship between gas flow, pressure gradient, and resistance is valid during laminar flow, when flow rate exceeds a critical velocity, it becomes turbulent as gas molecules swirl and turn in a chaotic pattern rather than in an orderly manner. In this circumstance, the relationship between the pressure gradient as gas flows through a straight tube (ΔP) and the flow rate is no longer linear. Fig. 37.11B shows the physics of *turbulent* flow. In this case, ΔP will depend on gas density and the squared flow as follows [89,90]:

$$\Delta P = \text{constant} \times \text{gas density} \times \text{flow}^2$$

With turbulent flow, the change in pressure is inversely proportional to the fifth power of the radius of the tube (Fanning equation); therefore, airway radius has an even greater impact on air flow than with laminar flow [91]. In a *straight unbranched tube*, the transition from laminar flow to turbulent flow can be estimated by the Reynold number (Re), a nondimensional number that is derived from gas velocity, tube diameter, gas density, and gas viscosity.

$$\text{Re} = \frac{\text{linear gas velocity} \times \text{tube diameter} \times \text{gas density}}{\text{gas viscosity}}$$

As the Reynolds number increases above 2000, air flow becomes progressively more turbulent. While airway resistance and its determinants are generally explained in terms of *laminar* flow, the structure of airways results in a mix of laminar and turbulent flow in the major airways. In addition to the variables included in calculating the Reynolds number, branching and/or irregularities in the tube predispose to turbulent flow. In general, resistance to gas flow is significantly greater with turbulent flow relative to laminar flow and turbulent flow is dependent on gas density and not viscosity. Because flow may become turbulent during pathological conditions that include narrowing/partial obstruction of the airways, incorporating helium, a gas with less density relative to oxygen or air, as a carrier gas with oxygen (mixture of 70% helium and 30% oxygen) may reduce resistance to gas flow [92,93]. As gas flow is usually laminar in the distal airways (and therefore not influenced by gas density), helium, which has a viscosity similar to air, may be less useful in animals with mild-to-moderate bronchoconstriction of the distal airways but it may have a positive impact in the presence of severe bronchospasm affecting the whole bronchial tree, as gas flow is likely turbulent under these circumstances [89]. In anesthetized horses, an alveolar recruitment maneuver with a mixture of 70% helium and 30% oxygen increased dynamic C_{RS} and improved pulmonary oxygen exchange (decreased $P(\text{A-a})O_2$) when compared to 100% oxygen [93]. However, dynamic C_{RS} is altered by the resistive and elastic properties of the respiratory system, and it remains to be demonstrated that the use of helium as a carrier gas would improve pulmonary mechanics by reducing resistance to gas flow in horses [93].

During spontaneous ventilation, the relationship between the pressure gradient across the respiratory system during inspiration, that is, the pressure at the airway opening (P_{ao}) minus the pleural pressure (P_{pl}) and the rate of inspiratory airflow (usually expressed in liters per second, L/s) is known as R_{aw} (expressed in $cmH_2O/L/s$) [61,79].

$$R_{aw} = \frac{(P_{ao} - P_{pl})}{\text{Flow rate}}$$

Airway resistance can be calculated during mechanical ventilation if using a volume-controlled mode with an inspiratory pause during anesthesia (Fig. 37.10D). Considering that plateau pressure (P_{plat}) recorded at the end of an inspiratory pause is the pressure that reflects the elastic properties of the respiratory system, while peak inspiratory pressure (P_{peak}) is the pressure that is necessary to overcome both the frictional resistance imposed by the airways (resistance) and the elastic properties of the respiratory system, R_{aw} is calculated as the gradient between P_{peak} and P_{plat}, divided by the flow rate [84,85]:

$$R_{aw} = \frac{(P_{peak} - P_{plat})}{\text{Flow rate}}$$

In conscious animals, measurement of R_{aw} can be obtained by simultaneous determination of instantaneous airflow with a pneumotachometer connected to the airway opening (mouth or nostrils) via a facemask and of the gradient between P_{ao} and P_{pl} (estimated by an esophageal balloon catheter), using a differential pressure transducer. The upper airways including the nasal cavity, pharynx, and larynx are major determinants of resistance to airflow within the respiratory system, generally contributing over 50% of the total R_{aw} [79]. Due to the extensive branching of the airways and dramatic increase in total airway area toward the periphery of the lung, despite the narrow radius, airflow velocity in bronchioles is very low and follows a laminar pattern. Therefore, the relative contribution of the small airways and bronchioles to total R_{aw} is low (< 10%) unless marked lower airway disease/bronchospasm is present [79]. As with lung compliance, resistance to airflow changes with lung volume. As lung volume decreases, R_{aw} increases, with dramatic increases occurring at lung volumes below FRC.

Presence of turbulent flow and increased R_{aw} directly impact the *work of breathing*, which is the energy spent by respiratory muscles (measured in joules) for air to flow in and out of the lungs. Work of breathing is measured as the product of pressure changes across the respiratory system (P_{ao} – P_{pl} in spontaneously breathing animals) and the volume of gas moved (V_T) [89,90]. Because inspiration is an active process that involves contraction of the diaphragm and chest wall muscles, most of the work done occurs during inspiration [89,90]. Respiratory work is further divided into elastic work (required to overcome the recoil of the lung) and resistive work (required to overcome the frictional opposition or resistance to airflow) [89,90]. As is discussed in Chapter 38, turbulent flow and increased R_{aw} are likely to be present in dogs with brachycephalic airway syndrome or collapsed trachea and horses with severe bronchospasm secondary small airway disease (heaves). The consequent increase in the respiratory work may lead to fatigue of inspiratory muscles, therefore, mechanical ventilatory support may be required in these patients.

Distribution of ventilation

The distribution of inspired gases during inspiration is not completely homogenous throughout the lung, with gravity playing a major role in regional pulmonary ventilation. Specifically, due to the weight of the lung in the thorax, P_{pl} is more negative (sub-atmospheric) in the uppermost part of the thorax relative to the lowermost portion and the negative pressure gradient between the alveoli and the pleural cavity ($P_{alv} - P_{pl}$) is greater in dorsal lung compared to ventral lung areas. Therefore, the average alveolar size is larger in the uppermost areas and smaller in the lowermost areas of the lung at end-expiration (Fig. 37.12A) [94,95]. Since larger alveoli have lower compliance (they are less distensible), they expand less on inspiration, and air preferentially enters the more compliant lowermost alveoli (Fig. 37.12B), producing a vertical gradient of ventilation distribution in standing animals breathing quietly [96–98]. This tendency for preferential ventral ventilation in the lung may also be associated with regional chest wall and diaphragmatic movement. During anesthesia, the distribution of ventilation becomes more uneven and may even reverse so that the uppermost lung of a laterally recumbent horse is receiving most of the ventilation.

Local resistance to air flow and compliance are the two major determinants of regional distribution of ventilation [79] (Fig. 37.13). Alveoli within regions with normal resistance and compliance completely fill during slow and fast tidal breathing, while alveoli that are poorly complaint due to inflammation/fluid accumulation in the interstitium (e.g., in pneumonia) only partially fill during inspiration. If there is increased resistance to airflow due to narrowing of the small airways caused by mucus, bronchoconstriction, or foreign material, these alveolar units take longer to fill and empty during tidal breathing and are referred to as "slow" alveoli. Slow alveoli also tend to be under-distended during inspiration (less ventilated than perfused), especially at faster respiratory frequencies [79]. Slow alveoli contrast with alveoli that completely fill regardless of the breathing pattern ("fast alveoli"). Uneven distribution of ventilation, leading to areas of low $\dot{V}_A/\dot{Q}$ and gas exchange impairment (lower-than-expected PaO_2 values) occur in lung disease due to areas with poor compliance or increased resistance to airflow.

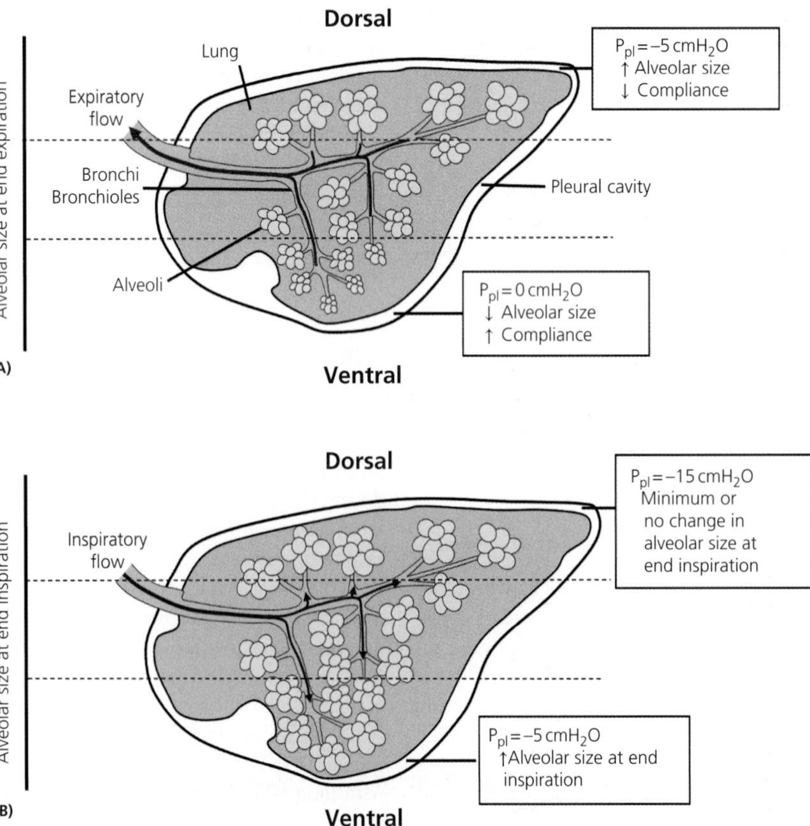

Figure 37.12 Relative alveolar size at end-expiration and end-inspiration and distribution of ventilation in standing horse. **A.** End-expiration: In the uppermost lung regions alveoli are close to their maximum size (i.e., are less compliant) because P_{pl} is more sub-atmospheric (negative) in dorsal regions. In the lowermost lung regions, P_{pl} is less negative, alveoli are more compliant because P_{pl} is less sub-atmospheric. **B.** End-inspiration: As P_{pl} become more negative causing the lungs to expand, ventilation (inspiratory flow) is directed preferentially to smaller/more compliant alveoli located in lowermost and intermediate lung regions.

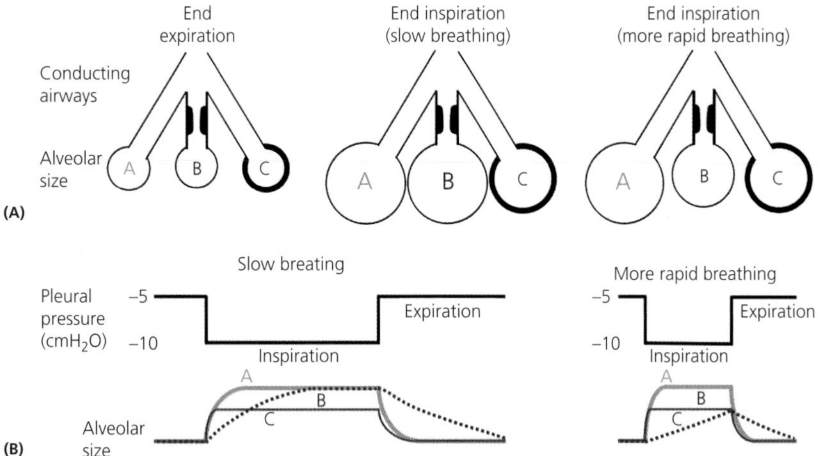

Figure 37.13 **A.** Relative alveolar size at end-expiration and end-inspiration during slow breathing versus more rapid breathing in alveoli with varying resistance and compliance. Alveoli labeled A represent normal resistance and compliance; alveoli labeled B represent high resistance and normal compliance; and alveoli labeled C represent normal resistance and low compliance. **B.** Graphical representation of changes in pleural pressure and alveolar size during slow breathing and more rapid breathing in alveoli with varying resistance and compliance (A, B, and C). See text for explanation. Source: Adapted from Robinson [49].

Pulmonary perfusion

The pulmonary circulation is a low-pressure system composed of highly compliant arterial vessels that offer low resistance to blood flow. Because pulmonary arterial tree vessels are relatively thin-walled and compliant, the pulmonary circulation can accommodate large increases in blood flow without an appreciable increase in mean pulmonary arterial pressure (MPAP) under physiological conditions. One notable exception is horses, where MPAP increases from 25–30 mmHg at rest to values above 80 mmHg during galloping because the pulmonary vasculature cannot dilate to accommodate the large increase in pulmonary blood flow/CO that occurs during high-intensity exercise [99]. The pulmonary hypertension caused by the increase in pulmonary blood flow is considered a major factor that contributes to exercise-induced pulmonary hemorrhage in equine species [100]. The extensive branching of the pulmonary arterial tree increases the vascular surface area available for gas exchange. Although this is followed by a progressive reduction in the diameter of arterial vessels, when the multiple arterial branches are arranged in parallel, the total cross-sectional area of the pulmonary arterial tree is greatly increased; hence, vascular resistance is lower in the pulmonary than in the systemic circulation even though it accepts the same volume of blood per unit of time. Interestingly, there are differences among species, with horses having higher pulmonary artery pressures at rest than humans and dogs [101,102]. Typically, MPAP values in resting conscious horses are in the range of 25–30 mmHg while in dogs MPAP values are approximately 15 mmHg [101–103]. Higher pulmonary artery pressure values observed in large animal species are necessary to overcome the large vertical hydrostatic pressure gradient and provide perfusion to the uppermost areas of the lungs.

In the absence of intracardiac shunting, the pulmonary blood flow generated by the right ventricle equals the aortic blood flow generated by the left ventricle. The total blood flow to the lungs ($\dot{Q}_T$), is determined by the gradient between arterial MPAP and left atrial pressure (LAP) and by pulmonary vascular resistance (PVR), as follows:

$$\dot{Q}_T = \frac{(MPAP - LAP)}{PVR}$$

While LAP is difficult to measure unless under experimental conditions, invasive hemodynamic monitoring with a pulmonary artery catheter allows continuous measurement of MPAP and intermittent measurement of pulmonary artery occlusion pressure (PAOP), a surrogate of LAP. As illustrated in Fig. 37.14A,B, PAOP is measured by gently inflating a balloon at the distal end of the catheter until it is "wedged" into a distal branch of the pulmonary artery. This creates a static column of blood between the catheter tip and the left atrium, and the pressure measured at the catheter tip after occlusion of blood flow will be equivalent to the pulmonary vein and LAP if there is no obstruction of blood flow between the pulmonary artery and the left ventricle [104]. PAOP is considered a close estimate of left ventricular end-diastolic pressure (LVEDP), although there are situations where this proximity may not hold true [104].

In addition to CO determinations by the thermodilution technique (that is equivalent to $\dot{Q}_T$) (Fig. 37.14C), a pulmonary artery catheter allows measurement of pulmonary perfusion pressure (Fig. 37.14D), that is, the gradient between MPAP and PAOP, while PVR is calculated as follows:

$$PVR = \frac{(MPAP - PAOP)}{\dot{Q}_T}$$

Distribution of pulmonary perfusion

For many years, it was believed that gravity was a primary determinant of the distribution of pulmonary blood flow. Specifically, a vertical perfusion gradient was thought to direct more blood flow to lower lung regions compared to upper lung regions in both conscious and anesthetized animals [96,105]. Current evidence suggests that distribution of pulmonary blood flow is governed by other factors, such as the branching pattern of the pulmonary arterial tree and regional differences in PVR, with little gravitational dependence in quadrupeds [106–108]. While some of the conflicting results can be attributed to inaccurate methods of determining blood flow distribution, a heterogeneous pattern of lung perfusion has been documented in conscious standing horses, with a larger proportion of the blood flow being directed toward the uppermost (caudo-dorsal) lung regions, against gravitational forces [106]. In standing humans, gravity bears some influence on the

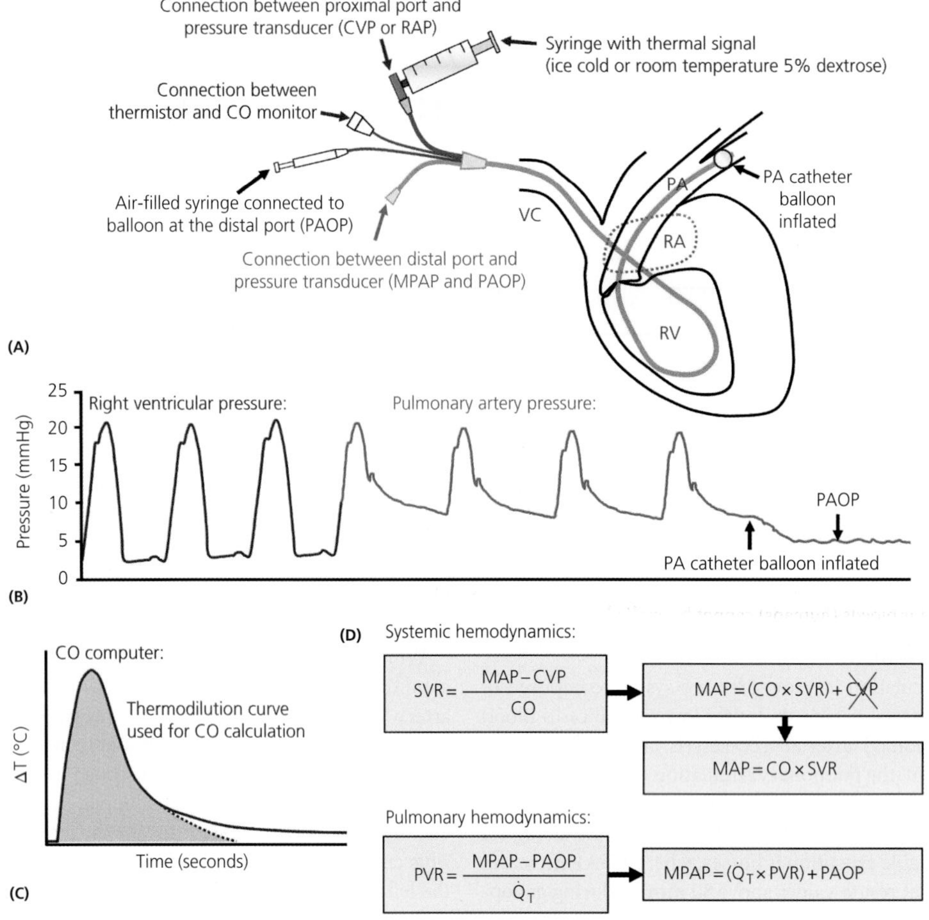

Figure 37.14 Hemodynamic monitoring with a pulmonary artery (PA) catheter. **A.** Correct anatomical positioning of a PA catheter. As the PA catheter is advanced through the vena cava (VC) and right atrium (RA) and reaches the right ventricle (RV), the balloon located at its tip is inflated and the catheter is advanced until the balloon is wedged into a branch of the PA. **B.** Pressure waveforms observed during PA catheterization which can be used to guide positioning of the PA catheter (alternatively, the procedure can be performed under fluoroscopic guidance). **C.** Measurement of cardiac output (CO) by a PA catheter is based on the area under the thermodilution curve. A fast response thermistor located at the tip of the PA catheter detects changes in blood temperature (ΔT) induced by injection of a room temperature or ice-cold 5% dextrose bolus into the proximal port of the PA catheter which is also used to monitor central venous pressure (CVP) or right atrial pressure (RAP). **D.** Because CVP (or RAP) is often near 0 mmHg its contribution is minor and the major determinants of mean arterial pressure (MAP) are CO and systemic vascular resistance (SVR). In the pulmonary circulation, increases in mean pulmonary arterial pressure (MPAP) are not only a result of increases in pulmonary vascular resistance (PVR) and pulmonary blood flow ($\dot{Q}_T$) (which is equivalent to CO), but increases in pulmonary artery occlusion pressure (PAOP) (a surrogate measure of pulmonary vein pressure/left atrial pressure [LAP]) may also contribute.

distribution of pulmonary blood flow as demonstrated in experiments with varying gravitational forces; however, it likely plays less of a role in supine positions [61,109].

The historical gravitational effects on distribution of lung perfusion have been commonly divided, and functionally described, as a three- or four-zone system in humans according to J. B. West, as illustrated in Fig. 37.15 [96,110]. While the relevance of linking the zones to specific regions of the lung may not be as applicable in quadrupeds in the awake or anesthetized state, the relationship of pulmonary artery, pulmonary vein, and alveolar pressures is still relevant and warrants consideration. Specifically, perfusion of pulmonary capillaries is not only determined by the gradient between arterial and venous pressure, such as in the systemic circulation, but also by alveolar pressure. Zone I represents alveoli that are not perfused, as alveolar pressure (P_{alv}) is greater than pulmonary artery (P_{PA}) and pulmonary vein (P_{PV}) pressures. In zone II, P_{PA} is greater than P_{alv}, and the difference between the two is the driving pressure for blood flow through the pulmonary capillaries. In zone III, P_{PA} and P_{PV} both exceed P_{alv}, and the capillary vessels are fully distended, with perfusion being determined by the pressure difference between P_{PA} and P_{PV}. In zone IV, the flow per unit of lung is reduced in comparison to zone III. This occurs because, as lung interstitial pressure (P_{int}) increases above venous pressure (P_{PV}), capillary perfusion pressure becomes governed by the gradient between P_{PA} and P_{int} [111]. In zone IV blood flow may cease altogether if P_{int} increases above P_{PA}, such as in the development of interstitial pulmonary edema. While the exact mechanism for the reduced flow in the most dependent lung regions is unknown, an increase in vascular resistance of the extra-alveolar pulmonary vessels, hypoxic pulmonary vasoconstriction (HPV), or the anatomical structure of the vasculature are potential mechanisms [9,10]. Prior to the research cited above, it was thought that when the body position was altered, and an animal became recumbent, pulmonary blood

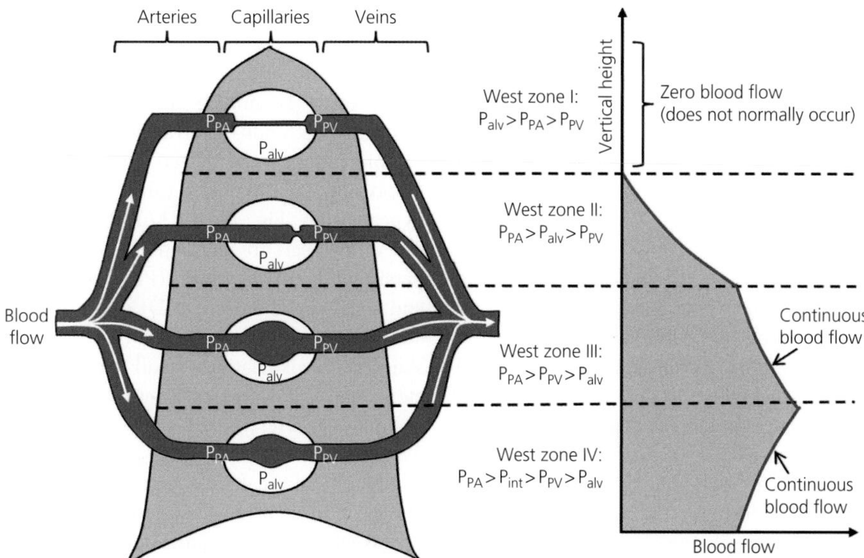

Figure 37.15 Diagrammatic illustration of gravitational blood flow distribution within the lung. Although the vertical gradient of blood flow distribution originally developed for bipeds (humans) cannot be applied to quadrupeds, the pattern of blood flow governed by the relationship between alveolar pressure (P_{alv}), pulmonary artery pressure (P_{PA}), pulmonary vein pressure (P_{PV}), and interstitial pressure (P_{int}) should be considered when analyzing the heterogeneity of lung perfusion (see text for further explanation). Source: Adapted from Chambers *et al.* [110].

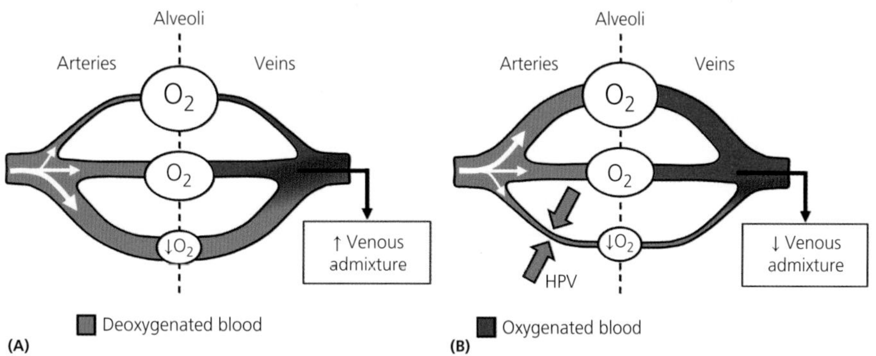

Figure 37.16 **A.** During ventilation-to-perfusion mismatch in the absence of hypoxic pulmonary vasoconstriction (HPV), a relatively large proportion of mixed venous blood (white arrows) flows past non-ventilated alveoli or alveoli with low oxygen partial pressure (↓ O_2). Arterial oxygen levels decrease because deoxygenated blood is mixed with oxygenated end-capillary blood (increased venous admixture). **B.** HPV (blue arrows) triggered by alveoli with low oxygen partial pressures (↓ O_2) diverts mixed venous blood toward better-ventilated lung areas (white arrows), improving the matching between ventilation and perfusion and decreasing venous admixture. Source: Adapted from Sommer *et al.* [115].

flow would realign along gravitational lines consistent with the new body position [96,105].

Hypoxic pulmonary vasoconstriction

Unlike smooth muscle in systemic arteries, which dilates in response to hypoxia, pulmonary arterial smooth muscle contracts when exposed to low oxygen partial pressures, a response referred to as "hypoxic pulmonary vasoconstriction" (HPV). The contractile response of pulmonary artery smooth muscle cells to hypoxia has been shown to be an inherent characteristic, with endothelial cells now regarded as modulators of the response [112–114]. Activation of a mitochondrial sensor in the smooth muscle cell in response to hypoxia results in closure of potassium channels, opening of calcium channels, and subsequent activation of the contractile apparatus within the smooth muscle cells [113]. This local response diverts mixed venous blood from poorly ventilated lung areas to better-ventilated alveoli, thus helping to minimize the increase in venous admixture and oxygenation impairment caused by low $\dot{V}_A/\dot{Q}$ and shunt (Fig. 37.16) [112,115]. HPV develops when the alveolar oxygen partial pressure falls to less than 100 mmHg in the normal lung, and the response is maximal when the oxygen tension is approximately 30 mmHg [112]. There is an apparent difference in the strength of the HPV response to whole lung hypoxia in various species [116], based on exposure of animals to high altitude and excised lung studies [117–119]. Cattle and swine have a strong reflex, whereas ponies, cats, and rabbits have an intermediate response, and sheep and dogs show less response. It appears, however, that under normal conditions even species with a weak hypoxic pulmonary reflex are capable of considerable blood flow diversion in response to regional areas of low alveolar oxygen partial pressure [116,118]. Interestingly, the response varies with time and repeat exposure to low oxygen conditions [112]. While HPV plays a major role in diverting blood flow from the pulmonary circulation to the placenta during fetal life, the anesthesiologist should be aware that HPV may assume an important role in maintaining oxygenation in mature animals with lung pathology. Anesthetic drugs have the potential to inhibit HPV to various degrees and aggravate $\dot{V}_A/\dot{Q}$ mismatch caused by pre-existing lung disease (discussed later).

Pulmonary hypertension

Understanding the factors that cause an abnormal increase in pulmonary artery pressure is important because anesthesia of animals with conditions leading to pulmonary hypertension may be required. Although a pulmonary artery catheter (Fig. 37.14) is the gold standard method for evaluating pulmonary hypertension, diagnosis of pulmonary hypertension in dogs is based on the measurement of tricuspid regurgitation velocity using Doppler echocardiography and on echocardiographic signs of pulmonary hypertension [120]. Fig. 37.17 illustrates the pathophysiological changes that may result in pulmonary hypertension in animals.

Pulmonary hypertension has been classified according to its origin as precapillary, postcapillary, or mixed (pre- and postcapillary). Precapillary pulmonary hypertension, also known as "pulmonary arterial hypertension," is caused by abnormalities on the arterial side of the pulmonary circulation and occurs when MPAP is abnormally increased because of an increase in PVR secondary to lung disease associated with arterial vasoconstriction, and/or pulmonary thromboembolism. Precapillary pulmonary hypertension also occurs in severe forms of heartworm disease in dogs (dirofilariasis) [120,121]. Lung disease leading to alveolar hypoxia (low alveolar PO_2) also has the potential to cause pulmonary hypertension (defined in humans as MPAP > 25 mmHg) because of a vasoconstrictive response (increased PVR) in alveoli exposed to low PO_2, that is, HPV. In dogs, pulmonary hypertension is associated with a diverse spectrum of respiratory diseases, most commonly obstructive disorders, and estimates of systolic pulmonary artery pressures > 47 mmHg using Doppler echocardiography were associated with non-survival [122].

Congenital cardiac defects leading to increased total pulmonary blood flow ($\dot{Q}_T$) may also cause pulmonary arterial (precapillary) hypertension (Fig. 37.17) [120,121]. Because pressures on the left side of the heart are higher than on the right side of the circulation, persistent ductus arteriosus (PDA), ventricular septal defect (VSD), and atrial septal defect (ASD) often result in arterial blood being added to mixed venous blood (left-to-right shunt) in dogs. If the shunted flow is relatively small (e.g., PDA with small ductal diameter, small VSD), the resulting increase in blood flow through the pulmonary artery may not result in significant pulmonary hypertension because the pulmonary vasculature is highly compliant and can accommodate the increase blood volume. However, in their most severe forms, these congenital defects may be associated with significant pulmonary arterial hypertension ultimately resulting in shunt reversal.

PDA is one of the most common congenital cardiac defects in dogs, accounting for up to 30% of congenital defects in this species. Direction of blood flow through the PDA is determined by the pressure gradient between the aorta and the pulmonary artery. Usually, when PDA is detected in young dogs, there is a continuous left-to-right shunt because pressures and vascular resistance are higher in the aorta than in the pulmonary artery. Blood flow though the duct is dependent on ductal diameter. In case of a very large PDA causing excessive increases in $\dot{Q}_T$, hypertrophy of smooth muscle from small pulmonary arteries/increased PVR occurs to protect pulmonary capillaries from volume overload. Precapillary pulmonary hypertension secondary to increased PVR can precipitate reversal

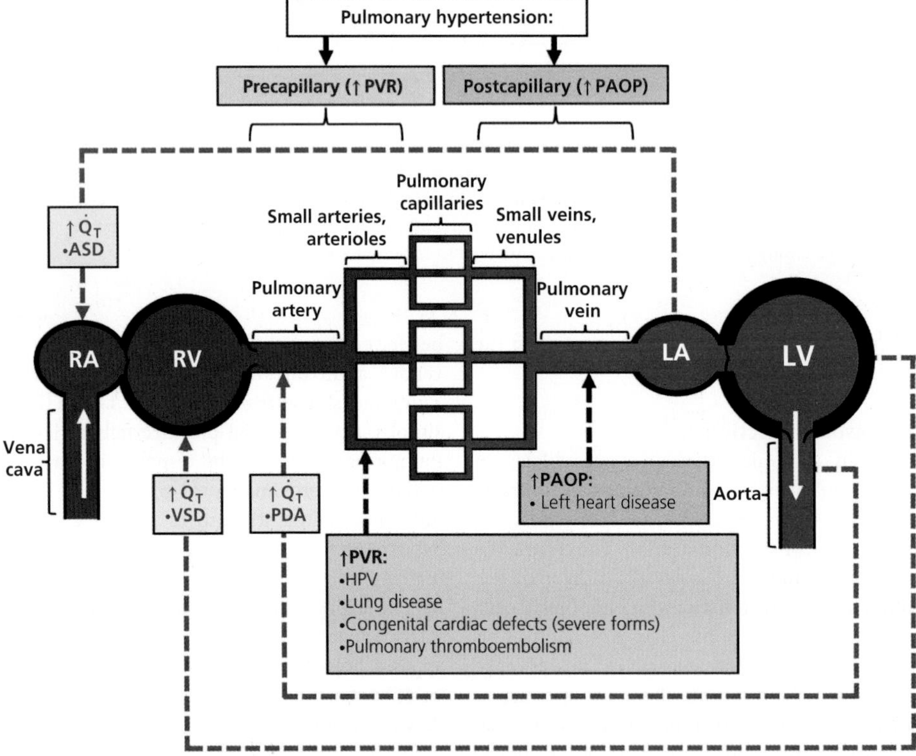

Figure 37.17 Pathophysiological changes that result in pulmonary hypertension in animals at rest (see text for explanation).

of shunt and cause cyanosis, while volume overload of the left atrium and left ventricle results in left-sided heart failure. Cyanosis due to right-to-left shunt is relatively uncommon in young dogs with PDA and may be more often observed in animals that live into adulthood [123–125]. Contrasting with PDA in dogs, where the incidence of pulmonary hypertension estimated by Doppler echocardiography is relatively low, ranging from 3% in 5-month-old dogs (median age) to 22% in animals older than 5 years [124], pulmonary hypertension is more frequently associated with PDA in cats with up to 46% of animals presenting with this complication [126]. Right-to-left shunting associated with severe pulmonary hypertension may also occur more frequently in cats than in dogs [125,126]. Anesthesia is unlikely to be performed in animals with PDA and right-to-left shunting because ductal closure may be contraindicated under these circumstances. Although there might be a concern that decreases in SVR/hypotension induced by general anesthesia could reverse the shunt from left-to-right to right-to-left because aortic pressures could fall below pulmonary artery pressures, precipitating cyanosis, there are no complications related to shunt reversal (hypoxemia/cyanosis) reported in dogs anesthetized with isoflurane for transvascular PDA occlusion [127]. However, the absence of studies reporting shunt reversal in dogs undergoing anesthesia for PDA correction must be interpreted with care. If anesthesia is performed in animals with severe pulmonary hypertension where pulmonary artery pressures approach aortic pressures, drug-induced hypotension could in theory reverse the shunt and precipitate cyanosis/hypoxemia.

Pulmonary hypertension of postcapillary origin (also known as "pulmonary venous hypertension") (Fig. 37.17), is characterized by elevated pressures on the venous side of the pulmonary circulation (PAOP > 15 mmHg in humans). Postcapillary pulmonary hypertension caused by left-sided congestive heart failure is the result of passive backward transmission of elevated left ventricular filling pressures (LVEDP and LAP) increasing pressures in the pulmonary veins, capillaries, and arteries. Chronic left-sided congestive heart failure secondary to myxomatous mitral valve disease or dilated cardiomyopathy is a common cause of postcapillary pulmonary hypertension in dogs with at least 40–70% of cases affected [128,129]. At this time, the incidence of postcapillary pulmonary hypertension secondary to left-sided congestive heart failure is smaller in cats (17%) than in dogs (> 70%) [130].

Pulmonary edema

Pulmonary edema is defined as an increase in pulmonary extravascular water. In its more severe form, alveoli are flooded with transudate (hydrostatic pulmonary edema) or exudate fluid (increased permeability pulmonary edema) [131,132]. Movement of fluid across capillary membranes was first described by Starling and has since been refined and described by the following equation [131,132]:

$$J_v = K\left[\left(P_{cap} - P_{int}\right) - \sigma\left(\pi_{cap} - \pi_{int}\right)\right]$$

Where J_v is the flow rate of transudated fluid across the endothelium which, in equilibrium, will be equal to the lymphatic drainage; K is the filtration coefficient or leakiness of fluid from the endothelium to the interstitium (also known as "hydraulic conductance"); P_{cap} is the hydrostatic pressure in the pulmonary capillary; P_{int} is the hydrostatic pressure in the interstitial space; σ (sigma) is the protein reflection coefficient, which is an expression of the permeability of the endothelium to albumin; π_{cap} is the oncotic pressure in the pulmonary capillaries (mainly determined by albumin); and π_{int} is the oncotic pressure in the interstitium [131–133]. In the normal lung P_{int} is slightly negative compared to P_{cap}, which results in the movement of fluid from the microvasculature to the interstitium. However, interstitial edema does not occur under normal circumstances because this is matched by lymphatic system's ability to remove the filtrate from the interstitium. If there are no changes in the normal endothelial structure, intravascular oncotic pressure (π_{cap}) is higher than in the interstitium (π_{int}), which also helps to retain fluid within the intravascular space [131–133].

It has been traditionally accepted that the fluid balance in the lungs and other tissues obeys the classical Starling equation described above. However, with the evolving knowledge of the role of the endothelial glycocalyx in fluid dynamics across the capillaries, this classical view has been reassessed as it may not fully reflect the transvascular movement of fluid at the capillary level [133,134]. The glycocalyx, which is a layer of proteoglycans and glycoproteins lining the luminal aspect of capillaries, serves as a barrier to the efflux of plasma proteins (albumin) and therefore helps to maintain the Starling forces that prevent pulmonary edema. In the revised Starling equation, the oncotic pressure gradient is between the intravascular space and the protein-free space beneath the glycocalyx. In this construct, pulmonary edema develops as P_{cap} and J_v increase and/or lymphatic drainage decreases [133,134]. Damage to the endothelial glycocalyx by shear stress induced by fluid resuscitation, or by inflammatory mechanisms associated with sepsis may increase the risk of pulmonary edema caused by excess fluid administration in hypovolemic and septic animals [135,136].

There are three basic mechanisms responsible for pulmonary edema: (1) increased hydrostatic forces within the microvasculature, (2) increased microvascular permeability, and (3) low plasma oncotic pressure (hypoalbuminemia). The third mechanism does not appear to play an important role in causing lung edema per se. However, hypoalbuminemia may contribute to pulmonary edema when it occurs concomitantly with the other two mechanisms. *Hydrostatic pulmonary edema* occurs when increased P_{cap} causes fluid accumulation within the interstitium and leakage of fluid floods alveoli with transudate fluid [131,132]. Hydrostatic pulmonary edema occurs in animals presenting in advanced stages of left-sided congestive heart failure (e.g., degenerative mitral valve disease and dilated cardiomyopathy in dogs, hypertrophic cardiomyopathy in cats) or animals receiving excessive amounts of intravenous fluids [128,137,138]. Left-sided heart disease leading to severe diastolic dysfunction may precipitate hydrostatic pulmonary edema as excessive LAP and LVEDP will increase pressures in vessels located proximally in the pulmonary circulation (pulmonary vein, and pulmonary capillary pressures) [128]. Doppler echocardiography is an important tool to evaluate the degree of diastolic dysfunction and risk of pulmonary edema in the latter patients [128,139]. A restrictive fluid therapy strategy should be adopted during anesthesia if a restrictive pattern of diastolic function (suggested by elevated LVEDP) is identified by Doppler echocardiography in small animals [128,137,139,140].

Although less common, pulmonary edema can occur secondary to upper airway obstruction, a condition referred to as "negative-pressure pulmonary edema" or "postobstructive pulmonary edema." The etiology is likely multifactorial; however, excessively negative intrathoracic/alveolar pressures, generated by contraction of inspiratory muscles against an obstructed upper airway, lead to an increase in venous return to the right side of the heart and an increase in hydrostatic pressures in the pulmonary vasculature. In combination with greater negative alveolar pressures under these circumstances, transvascular fluid filtration is increased, precipitating interstitial and alveolar edema [141,142]. In one retrospective study of noncardiogenic pulmonary edema diagnosed in 23 dogs and 3 cats, lung edema resulting from airway obstruction was recorded in 8 animals [143]. Hemorrhagic/negative-pressure pulmonary edema is a rare but potentially fatal complication reported in horses with acute upper airway obstruction during recovery from anesthesia [142,144]. The hemorrhagic nature of pulmonary edema (presence of pink frothy fluid in the airways) in this species is likely a result of injury to pulmonary capillaries and alveolar membranes caused by the extremely negative intrathoracic/airway pressure [142,144].

Increased permeability pulmonary edema occurs when damage to the microvascular endothelial surface layer and alveolar epithelium leads to leakage of protein-rich fluid from the microvasculature to the interstitial compartment and alveoli [131,132]. In humans, increased permeability pulmonary edema is a characteristic of acute respiratory distress syndrome (ARDS). Direct causes of acute lung injury (ALI) leading to ARDS in humans include pneumonia, aspiration of gastric contents, inadequate ventilator settings leading to alveolar overdistension, inhalation injury, pulmonary contusion, pulmonary vasculitis, and drowning. Humans may also develop ARDS secondary to indirect injury to the lungs, which may occur due to sepsis not involving the lungs, major trauma, pancreatitis, severe burns, non-cardiogenic shock, drug overdose, and multiple transfusions [145]. Based on the criteria for the diagnosis of veterinary ARDS in small animals and foals published in 2007 [146], the most frequent cause of lung injury leading to increased permeability pulmonary edema and signs of ARDS was aspiration pneumonia in dogs and systemic inflammatory response syndrome without sepsis in cats [147]. Current evidence shows that acute necrotizing pancreatitis may be an important cause of indirect lung injury in dogs, as this disease has been associated with recruitment of pulmonary intravascular macrophages (PIMs) and histological evidence of lung inflammation [148,149]. While anesthesia of animals with increased permeability pulmonary edema and/or ARDS is rarely necessary, when required, a protective ventilatory support strategy is highly recommended to avoid further lung injury and is discussed further in Chapter 38.

Ventilation–perfusion relationships

Ventilation–perfusion relationships and gas exchange

To achieve optimal gas exchange with the least amount of energy expenditure, ventilation and perfusion would not necessarily be uniform throughout the lung but rather would be matched in order to achieve optimal oxygenation and CO_2 removal. In fact, when an arterial blood gas sample is analyzed for efficacy of gas exchange, it must be borne in mind that PaO_2 and $PaCO_2$ values reflect the blood flow from millions of alveoli with varying $\dot{V}_A/\dot{Q}$ ratios. A mismatch between ventilation and perfusion, more specifically increased areas of low $\dot{V}_A/\dot{Q}$ ratio and shunt (perfusion of non-ventilated regions), has a major impact on oxygen uptake by the lung. Since CO_2 is more diffusible across the alveolar–capillary barrier than oxygen, the presence of low $\dot{V}_A/\dot{Q}$ regions leads to decreased PaO_2 levels before $PaCO_2$ is increased [9,96,150,151].

A diagrammatic representation of $\dot{V}_A/\dot{Q}$ relationships is detailed in Fig. 37.18A. Ideal matching between ventilation and perfusion occurs when the $\dot{V}_A/\dot{Q}$ ratio is 1. In the conscious resting animal with normal lung function, gas exchange is optimal because the relative distribution of $\dot{V}_A/\dot{Q}$ ratios is centralized toward the prevalence of alveoli with a $\dot{V}_A/\dot{Q}$ ratio close to 1 (Fig. 37.18B) As alveolar units become less ventilated (areas of low $\dot{V}_A/\dot{Q}$ ratio), there is a progressive increase in the amount of mixed venous blood added to end-capillary blood, known as "venous admixture." One extreme is to have perfused alveoli or areas of the lung with no ventilation such that blood passing through such a region is not oxygenated. This is referred to as "intrapulmonary shunt" and has a $\dot{V}_A/\dot{Q}$ ratio equal to zero [150]. The major consequence of adding mixed venous blood ($P\bar{v}O_2$ = 40 mmHg) to pulmonary end-capillary blood is a decrease in PaO_2 and arterial oxygen content (CaO_2). Oxygenation impairment secondary to areas of low $\dot{V}_A/\dot{Q}$ ratio and shunt may be observed in animals with pulmonary disease (pneumonia, neoplasia, and lung edema) or during general anesthesia. Although arterial oxygenation can be impaired, CO_2 elimination may not be compromised during the early stages of pulmonary disease. In fact, severe hypoxemia (PaO_2 < 60 mmHg) caused by areas of low $\dot{V}_A/\dot{Q}$ and shunt may be associated with normal or below normal $PaCO_2$ (respiratory alkalosis) due to stimulation of peripheral chemoreceptors located in the carotid body by low PaO_2 (hypoxic drive), which mediates an increase in $\dot{V}_A$ through increases in *f* and V_T [53,150]. This is possible because CO_2 is 20 times more diffusible across the alveolar–capillary membrane than oxygen and there is an inverse relationship between $\dot{V}_A$ and $PaCO_2$. In animals that have a reduced central respiratory drive (due to disease or secondary to drugs including opioids and general anesthetics), low $\dot{V}_A/\dot{Q}$ and shunt may contribute to rising $PaCO_2$ levels. Because areas of low $\dot{V}_A/\dot{Q}$ are partially ventilated, hypoxemia caused by low $\dot{V}_A/\dot{Q}$ can be counteracted by increasing alveolar oxygen partial pressure (P_AO_2) via oxygen supplementation (i.e., increasing F_IO_2). If a patient that is ventilated fails to respond to an increase in F_IO_2, shunt should be suspected as the major cause of oxygenation impairment.

As capillary blood flow decreases in relation to the ideal in ventilated alveoli (areas of high $\dot{V}_A/\dot{Q}$ ratio), there is an increase in the fraction of total ventilation that does not contribute to gas exchange, that is *wasted ventilation* [150]. *Alveolar deadspace* ($V_{D_{alv}}$) is an extreme instance of a high $\dot{V}_A/\dot{Q}$ ratio, where alveoli are ventilated but are not perfused. As explained above, $V_{D_{alv}}$ adds to the *airway deadspace* ($V_{D_{aw}}$) to form the *physiologic deadspace* ($V_{D_{phys}}$). An increase in $V_{D_{alv}}$ per se does not impact gas exchange if there is a compensatory increase in $\dot{V}_A$ [150]. However, if the ventilatory response is obliterated or reduced by anesthetic drugs, $PaCO_2$ will increase.

Based on radioisotope studies evaluating distribution of blood flow in pulmonary capillaries across the lung tissue, the vertical gradient of perfusion and ventilation is minimal in standing dogs with a horizontal lung [107,152]. Matching of vertical perfusion and ventilation gradients in conscious horses is such that there is little difference in $\dot{V}_A/\dot{Q}$ in different lung regions [97,106]. Studies using a multiple inert gas elimination technique in horses suggest that the scatter of $\dot{V}_A/\dot{Q}$ ratios in conscious horses is very similar to that seen in people [153]. No regions of low $\dot{V}_A/\dot{Q}$ were identified, but a minor shunt component (less than 3% of CO) was observed. A high $\dot{V}_A/\dot{Q}$ area was identified (constituting 3–17% of the total), and the extent of this area was correlated with lower pulmonary artery pressures [153] (Fig. 37.19).

Measurement of ventilation-to-perfusion mismatch in clinical practice

Matching between ventilation and perfusion is measured in the research setting by the multiple inert gas elimination technique. However, this method is not applicable to the clinical setting. When the P_B, F_IO_2, $PaCO_2$, and R are known, the P_AO_2 can be calculated as

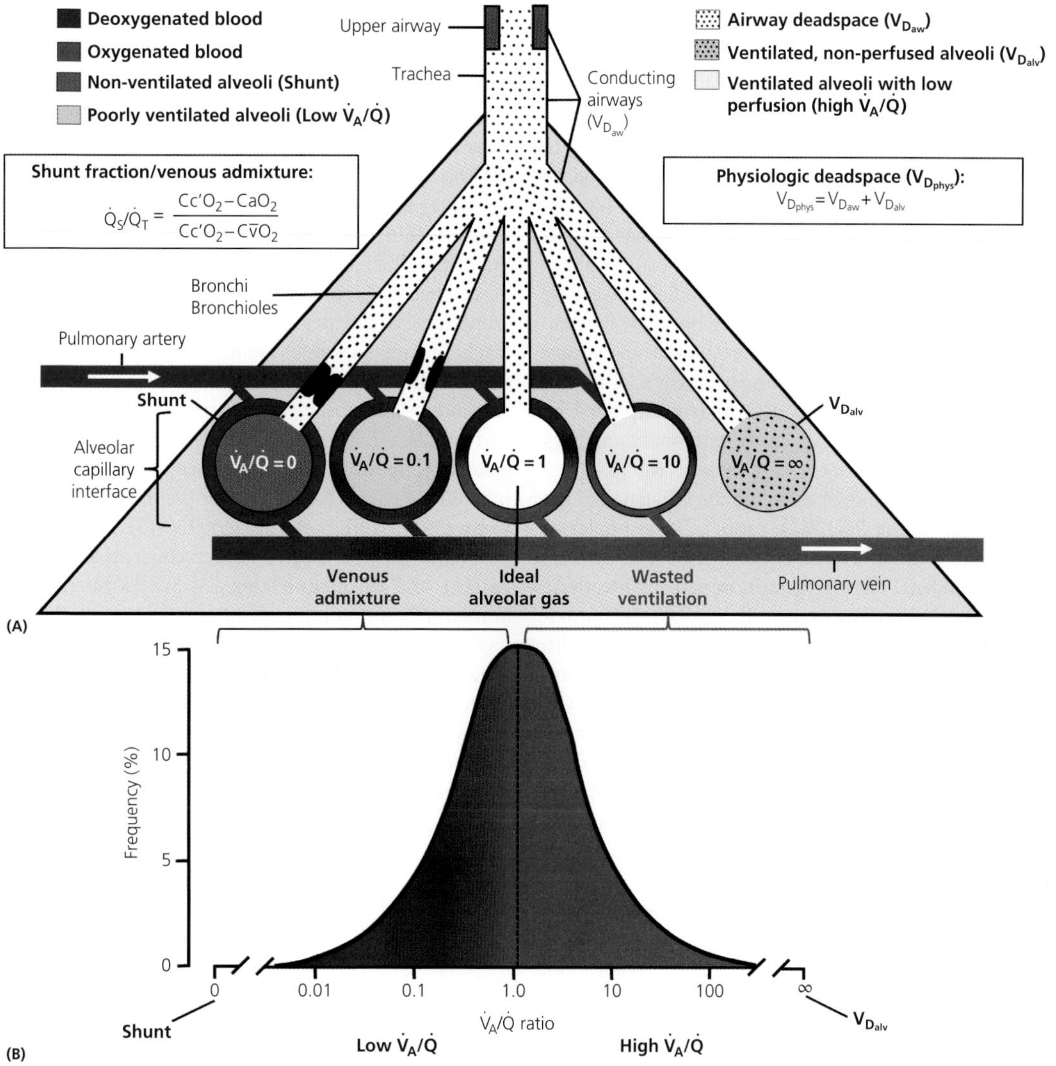

Deoxygenated blood
Oxygenated blood
Non-ventilated alveoli (Shunt)
Poorly ventilated alveoli (Low $\dot{V}_A/\dot{Q}$)
Upper airway
Trachea
Conducting airways ($V_{D_{aw}}$)
Airway deadspace ($V_{D_{aw}}$)
Ventilated, non-perfused alveoli ($V_{D_{alv}}$)
Ventilated alveoli with low perfusion (high $\dot{V}_A/\dot{Q}$)

Shunt fraction/venous admixture:

$$\dot{Q}_S/\dot{Q}_T = \frac{Cc'O_2 - CaO_2}{Cc'O_2 - C\bar{v}O_2}$$

Physiologic deadspace ($V_{D_{phys}}$):

$$V_{D_{phys}} = V_{D_{aw}} + V_{D_{alv}}$$

Bronchi
Bronchioles
Pulmonary artery
Shunt
Alveolar capillary interface
$\dot{V}_A/\dot{Q} = 0$
$\dot{V}_A/\dot{Q} = 0.1$
$\dot{V}_A/\dot{Q} = 1$
$\dot{V}_A/\dot{Q} = 10$
$\dot{V}_A/\dot{Q} = \infty$
$V_{D_{alv}}$
Venous admixture
Ideal alveolar gas
Wasted ventilation
Pulmonary vein
(A)

Frequency (%)
15
10
5
0
0
0.01
0.1
1.0
10
100
∞
$\dot{V}_A/\dot{Q}$ ratio
Shunt
Low $\dot{V}_A/\dot{Q}$
High $\dot{V}_A/\dot{Q}$
$V_{D_{alv}}$
(B)

Figure 37.18 **A.** Diagrammatic representation of ventilation-to-perfusion ($\dot{V}_A/\dot{Q}$) ratios. Deoxygenated mixed venous blood (blue) from the pulmonary artery is distributed to the alveoli with different $\dot{V}_A/\dot{Q}$ ratios. Optimal gas exchange/transfer of oxygen from alveoli to pulmonary capillary blood occurs as the $\dot{V}_A/\dot{Q}$ ratio approaches 1. As the $\dot{V}_A/\dot{Q}$ ratio decreases ($\dot{V}_A/\dot{Q} = 0.1$), there is an increase in poorly oxygenated (mixed venous) blood added to oxygenated blood (increased venous admixture). Intrapulmonary shunt ($\dot{V}_A/\dot{Q}$ ratio = 0) occurs when alveoli or areas of lung are perfused but do not receive ventilation. As the $\dot{V}_A/\dot{Q}$ ratio increases above 1 ($\dot{V}_A/\dot{Q} = 10$), there is wasted ventilation because a greater proportion of $\dot{V}_A$ is ineffective and does not participate in gas exchange. The alveolar deadspace represents completely wasted ventilation because ventilated alveoli are not perfused, representing a $\dot{V}_A/\dot{Q}$ ratio equal to infinity (∞). **B.** The percent distribution of alveolar units in a normal lung. Gas exchange is optimized when alveoli with a $\dot{V}_A/\dot{Q}$ ratio close to 1 prevail and alveoli with low or high $\dot{V}_A/\dot{Q}$ ratios represent much lower percentages of lung parenchyma. Source: Adapted from Petersson and Glenny [150].

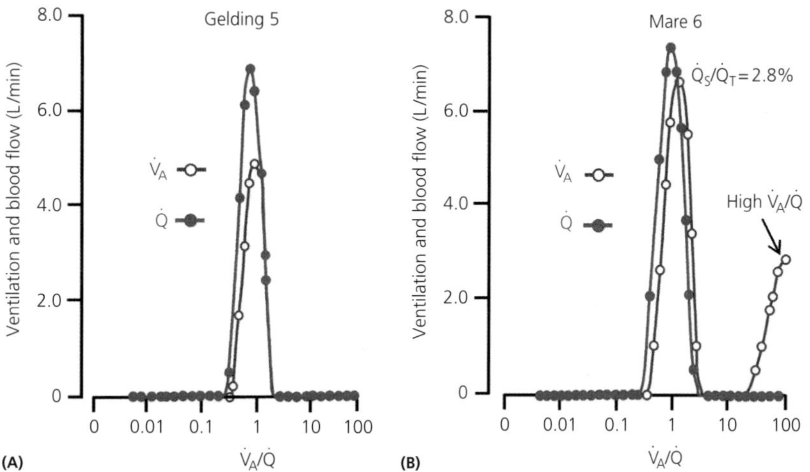

Figure 37.19 Ventilation-to-perfusion ($\dot{V}_A/\dot{Q}$) ratios measured by inert gas elimination in two conscious standing horses. **A.** The first horse presented with a unimodal $\dot{V}_A/\dot{Q}$ ratio centered on 1. **B.** The second horse presented with a bimodal distribution with a $\dot{V}_A/\dot{Q}$ ratio centered on 1 and an additional high $\dot{V}_A/\dot{Q}$ ratio. There was also minor shunting ($\dot{Q}_S/\dot{Q}_T$) corresponding to 2.8% of total blood flow. Animals were clinically healthy and a shunt fraction ranging from 1.1 to 2.8% was recorded in 5/8 horses. Areas with high $\dot{V}_A/\dot{Q}$ ratio identified in 5/8 horses were explained by poor perfusion of upper lung regions due to lower pulmonary artery pressures. Source: Reproduced with permission from Hedenstierna *et al.* [153], John Wiley & Sons.

previously described (Fig. 37.2, Table 37.4). The difference between this value and the PaO_2 (that is, the *alveolar to arterial oxygen gradient*, $P(A\text{-}a)O_2$) provides a measure of the relative efficiency of gas exchange. The $P(A\text{-}a)O_2$ increases with hypoxemia caused by $\dot{V}_A/\dot{Q}$ mismatch (areas of low $\dot{V}_A/\dot{Q}$), shunt, and diffusion impairment, but not in the case of hypoxemia caused by hypoventilation (increased $PaCO_2$) or low P_IO_2 [9,150,151]. The $P(A\text{-}a)O_2$ ranges from 5–15 mmHg in an animal breathing ambient air and is usually less than 150 mmHg in a healthy patient breathing 100% oxygen. Healthy individuals breathing high F_IO_2 levels (≥ 0.8) show an increase in $P(A\text{-}a)O_2$ over time because of absorption atelectasis. Collapse of poorly ventilated alveolar units ($\dot{V}_A/\dot{Q} < 0.15$) is precipitated by high F_IO_2 because the transfer of oxygen to pulmonary capillary blood exceeds the inspired gas flow entering these alveoli [154].

A more clinically practical way of assessing the efficiency of gas exchange is by measuring the PaO_2/F_IO_2 ratio, as it is simpler to calculate and provides a rough assessment of $P(A\text{-}a)O_2$ under certain conditions. The normal PaO_2/F_IO_2 ratio in patients breathing ambient air ($F_IO_2 = 0.21$) and 100% oxygen ($F_IO_2 > 0.90$) is approximately 500. In patients breathing air, low PaO_2/F_IO_2 ratio with normal or below normal $PaCO_2$ levels suggests the presence of oxygenation impairment caused by low $\dot{V}_A/\dot{Q}$ and/or shunt. However, particularly in individuals breathing ambient air, this index may not differentiate hypoxemia caused by alveolar hypoventilation from hypoxemia secondary to low $\dot{V}_A/\dot{Q}$ and shunt. The PaO_2/F_IO_2 is also insensitive to detect hypoxemia caused by low P_IO_2 at high altitudes (discussed previously). A more detailed description of the assessment of hypoxemia is provided in Chapter 38.

If the patient has a pulmonary artery catheter and a second catheter placed in an artery of the systemic circulation for measuring blood gases and hemoglobin concentration in mixed venous blood and in arterial blood, respectively, *shunt fraction* ($\dot{Q}_S/\dot{Q}_T$) can be measured as follows (Fig. 37.18):

$$\frac{Q_S}{Q_T} = \frac{Cc'O_2 - CaO_2}{Cc'O_2 - C\overline{v}O_2}$$

Where $Cc'O_2$ is the oxygen content in end-capillary blood, estimated based on the assumption that oxygen partial pressure in end-capillary blood ($Pc'O_2$) equals that of ideal alveolar gas (P_AO_2) according to the *alveolar gas equation* (Fig. 37.2); while CaO_2 and $C\overline{v}O_2$ are the arterial and mixed venous oxygen content, respectively.

Shunt fraction is the percentage of total blood flow generated by the right ventricle (i.e., $\dot{Q}_T$) that reaches the left ventricle without exposure to ventilated areas of the lung. Shunted flow is divided into intrapulmonary and anatomic shunt. *Intrapulmonary shunt* occurs when mixed venous (pulmonary arterial) blood perfuses non-ventilated areas of the lung ($\dot{V}_A/\dot{Q} = 0$). *Anatomic shunt* is blood flow that bypasses lung parenchyma (that is, the portion of the lung where there is gas exchange), moving directly from the right side of the heart to the left side of the heart. Anatomic shunt can be either physiologic or pathologic, as in some congenital cardiac diseases (e.g., PDA with right-to-left shunt, as explained previously). *Physiologic anatomic shunt* corresponds to the outflow from bronchial and Thebesian veins (a network of vessels that irrigate the myocardium in mammals) that drains directly into the left heart [150,151,155,156]. The presence of a small physiologic anatomic shunt (2 to 5% of $\dot{Q}_T$) explains why, in conscious individuals breathing ambient air, PaO_2 is slightly lower than P_AO_2 [150,151,156]. As explained before, intrapulmonary shunt ($\dot{V}_A/\dot{Q} = 0$) plays a major role in causing oxygenation impairment in patients with severe lung disease and in some animal species during general anesthesia. *Pathologic anatomic shunt* is a major cause of increased shunt fraction in animals with congenital heart diseases leading to severe hypoxemia/cyanosis.

The terms "venous admixture" and "shunt fraction" do not mean the same thing, although they are often used interchangeably in the literature, which causes some confusion. While shunt fraction is the percentage of $\dot{Q}_T$ going past non-ventilated areas of the lung, venous admixture is the degree of admixture of mixed venous blood (including mixed venous blood from areas of low $\dot{V}_A/\dot{Q}$ and shunted flow) with pulmonary end-capillary blood that would be required to produce the observed difference between the arterial and the end-capillary oxygen partial pressure. True *shunt fraction* can be calculated by the formula described above only in patients breathing 100% oxygen ($F_IO_2 > 0.9$), as the impact of low $\dot{V}_A/\dot{Q}$ units on venous admixture is eliminated [150,151]. However, if the patient is breathing lower inspired oxygen concentrations (e.g., $F_IO_2 = 0.21$ to 0.6), the calculation above is better referred to as "venous admixture" as it will represent not only shunted flow but also the blood flow going past low $\dot{V}_A/\dot{Q}$ units.

Finally, if one knows the inspired oxygen concentration and the PaO_2 and assumes that arterial–venous oxygen extraction is normal, an *isoshunt diagram* can be used to provide a convenient and reasonably accurate estimate of the magnitude of pulmonary shunt flow (Fig. 37.20) [157]. Fig. 37.20 also illustrates the poor response,

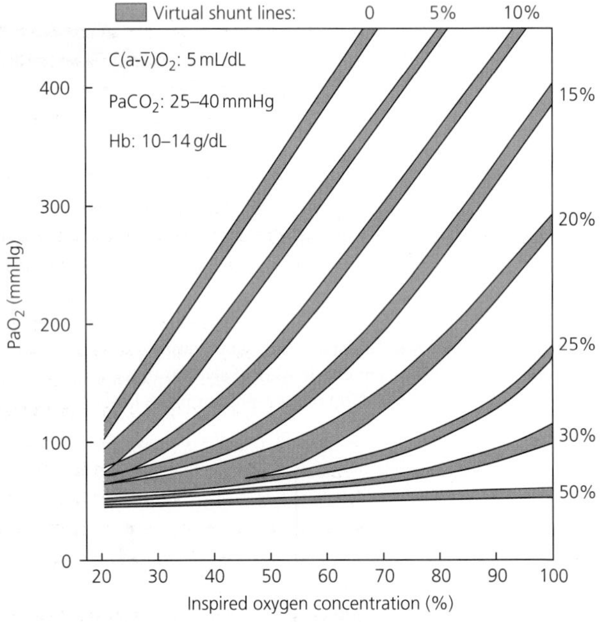

Figure 37.20 An isoshunt diagram depicting the relationship between inspired oxygen concentration, PaO_2, and various degrees of venous admixture or pulmonary shunt. Shunt flow is expressed as a percentage of cardiac output, ranging from 0 to 50%. The arteriovenous (a-$\overline{v}$) oxygen content difference is assumed to be 5 mL per 100 mL of blood, reflecting a normal cardiac output. The shunt bands have been drawn to include the range of hemoglobin (Hb) and arterial carbon dioxide partial pressure ($PaCO_2$) levels shown. Note that at the higher levels of shunt flow (30–50%), there is little improvement in arterial oxygen levels even when the inspired oxygen concentration is 100%. Also note that if the inspired oxygen concentration and PaO_2 are known, it is possible to obtain a quick estimate of the degree of venous admixture or shunt flow. Source: Adapted from Benatar *et al.* [157].

in terms of improving PaO_2, that will occur with increased inspired-oxygen concentrations when shunt flows exceed 30%.

Effects of anesthesia on ventilation, pulmonary perfusion, and ventilation–perfusion relationships

Influence of anesthetic drugs on neural control of ventilation

Injectable and inhalant anesthetic agents and some sedative/analgesic drugs used during the perioperative period decrease the ventilatory response to increases in $PaCO_2$ and decreases in PaO_2 in a dose-dependent manner. This occurs secondary to suppression of neuronal activity in the medulla and pons, decreased central and peripheral chemoreceptor activity, as well as inhibition of mechanoreceptors throughout the respiratory system [44].

The typical hypoventilation and the resulting hypercapnia observed in spontaneously breathing anesthetized animals is not harmful per se if extracellular/blood pH is not markedly decreased (< 7.20) and hypoxemia is prevented by increasing F_IO_2. However, if general anesthesia is induced in animals with uncorrected metabolic acidosis, suppression of chemoreceptor activity leading to increased $PaCO_2$ above physiologic ranges (> 45 mmHg) has the potential to precipitate a mixed acid–base disturbance (metabolic acidosis and respiratory acidosis) that may result in severe acidemia (pH < 7.10–7.20) [52]. The effects of the latter on homeostasis during general anesthesia may be translated into poor cardiovascular function and hypotension refractory to catecholamines [158]. In addition to metabolic disease, in patients with pre-existing impaired gas exchange prior to sedation/anesthesia, appropriate selection of drugs and the management of the clinical consequences associated with the effects on the neural control of ventilation will improve outcomes.

To determine drug effects on the neural control of ventilation *in vivo*, the change in $\dot{V}_E$ in response to alterations in environmental conditions (hypoxia, hyperoxia, hypercapnia, and hypocapnia) can be measured in experimental settings. In conscious normal mammals, the CO_2 response curve, which is the graphic representation of the change in $\dot{V}_E$ in response to increases in $PaCO_2$ or $P_{ET}CO_2$ is relatively linear (Fig. 37.4A). The effects of drugs on the neural control of ventilation are determined by measuring changes in respiratory pattern (most notably frequency) and the degree of respiratory depression as assessed by $PaCO_2$, in addition to the ventilatory response to increased CO_2 and decreased PaO_2 with different drug doses or combinations.

Inhalant and injectable anesthetic drugs

The anesthetic index, calculated by dividing the end-tidal anesthetic concentration that induces apnea (cessation of breathing for 60 s) by the minimum alveolar concentration (MAC), provides an assessment of the central respiratory depressant effects of inhalant anesthetics [159,160]. Inhalant anesthetics in current use cause progressive increases in $PaCO_2$ as the anesthetic dose is increased from 1 MAC to 1.5 and 2 MAC multiples [4]. Although the degree of hypercapnia observed with equipotent concentrations of sevoflurane and isoflurane, ranging from 1 to 2 MAC is similar [4], the anesthetic index was reported to be larger for sevoflurane (3.45 MAC) than for isoflurane (2.65 MAC) in dogs, suggesting that sevoflurane causes less respiratory depression at higher equipotent anesthetic concentrations than does isoflurane [161].

As noted above, CO_2 is a major determinant of ventilatory drive in normal mammals under typical environmental conditions. All inhalant general anesthetic agents in current use produce a dose-dependent decrease in the ventilatory response to CO_2. Therefore, for any given $PaCO_2$, the $\dot{V}_E$ is lower than in a conscious animal and the CO_2 response curve is shifted downward and to the right as illustrated in Fig. 37.21A [162]. The reduced sensory input and central sensitivity to CO_2 produce a marked fall in $\dot{V}_E$, usually through a dose-related decrease in V_T, with a variable effect on breathing frequency depending on the inhalant anesthetic. As a result of these changes, $PaCO_2$ levels increase as the anesthetic dose is increased when animals breathe spontaneously [2,4,163,164]. The degree of hypercapnia at equipotent doses of inhalant anesthetic agents varies with the species and the degree of surgical stimulation [4,160,163–165]. Afferent sensory input from surgical stimulation will stimulate the respiratory center in the brainstem and increase

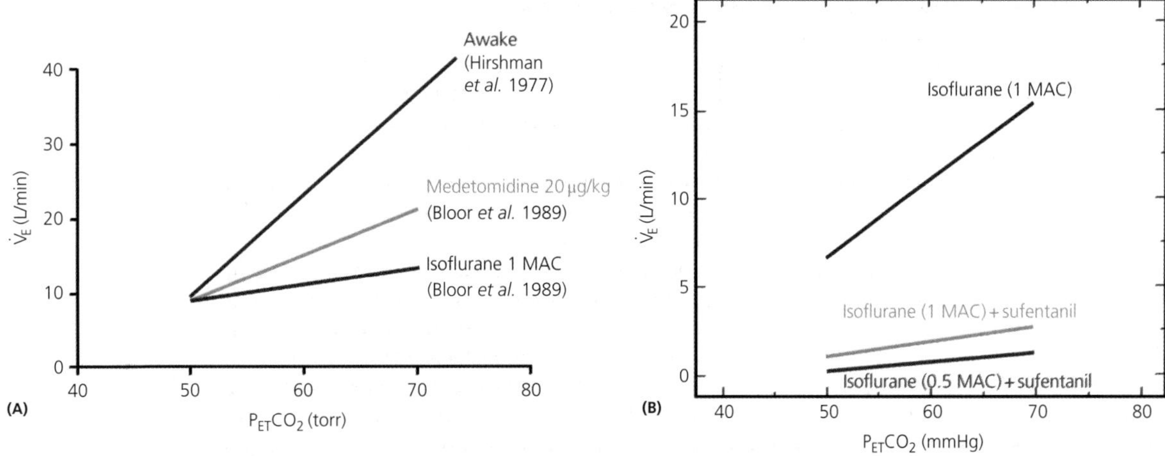

Figure 37.21 **A.** Increases in minute ventilation in response to increasing end-tidal CO_2 partial pressure ($P_{ET}CO_2$) induced by CO_2 rebreathing (CO_2 response curves). Data were recorded in dogs that were conscious (awake), dogs anesthetized with 1 minimum alveolar concentration (MAC) of isoflurane, and dogs that received intravenous medetomidine (20 µg/kg over 30 min, with data recorded 15 min after medetomidine administration and discontinuation of isoflurane). **B.** Carbon dioxide response curves recorded in dogs anesthetized with isoflurane alone (1 MAC) or anesthetized with isoflurane (1 and 0.5 MAC) plus an intravenous infusion of sufentanil. A decrease in the slope of the CO_2 response curves denotes drug-induced decreases in central chemoreceptor sensitivity to CO_2. Source: Adapted from Bloor *et al.* [162]; Abdul-Rasool and Ward [173].

the ventilatory drive. Therefore, the respiratory depression induced by general anesthetics is usually less in the presence of surgical stimulation. Noxious stimulation however will not alter ventilatory drive during general anesthesia if afferent sensory input is blocked by local/regional anesthesia techniques. Of the inhalant anesthetics, halothane produces the least increase in $PaCO_2$ during spontaneous respiration, whereas, at equipotent doses, isoflurane, sevoflurane, and desflurane produce somewhat higher and similar $PaCO_2$ levels in most species [4,163,166–168]. In ruminants, the degree of hypercapnia is greater with equipotent inhalant anesthetic doses than for horses, and horses show more respiratory depression than monkeys, cats, and dogs [4,160,163,165,169,170]. Clinically, swine, ferrets, rabbits, and rats also seem to be more prone to hypercapnia, whereas deep-diving seals may become totally apneic during light levels of anesthesia or with opioid-only sedation [167,171,172].

The *apneic threshold* can be defined as the $PaCO_2$ level at which spontaneous ventilatory effort ceases due to loss of central respiratory drive (e.g., low $PaCO_2$ or high CSF pH [relative to the set-point]). A $PaCO_2$ reduction of 5–9 mmHg from normal resting values through voluntary hyperventilation in conscious humans, or by artificial ventilation of deeply sedated or anesthetized animals, produces apnea. The distance between the resting normal $PaCO_2$ level and the apneic threshold is relatively constant (i.e., 4–6 mmHg less than the normal resting level) irrespective of the anesthetic depth [174,175]. Because inhalant and injectable anesthetics reset the apneic threshold to a higher level, $PaCO_2$ must be higher than the normal range for the animal species for spontaneous breathing efforts to occur during general anesthesia [176]. It is a common practice to provide mechanical ventilation in anesthetized animals simply by adjusting the number of mandatory breaths (*f*) and the V_T (or inspiratory pressure) delivered by the ventilator (i.e., $\dot{V}_E$) to maintain $PaCO_2$ levels within normal ranges (35–45 mmHg), without having to resort to neuromuscular blocking agents to abolish spontaneous respiratory efforts. This technique may not be effective, however, if $\dot{V}_E$ delivered by the mechanical ventilator is less than necessary to maintain eucapnia. On the other hand, if the ventilator is adjusted to deliver a relatively large $\dot{V}_E$, the resultant decrease in $PaCO_2$ (hypocapnia) can lead to a more prolonged period of apnea after discontinuation of mechanical ventilation at the end of anesthesia. One practical way of reducing the period of apnea following mechanical ventilation is to decrease $\dot{V}_E$ by lowering the ventilator respiratory rate to allow $PaCO_2$ to increase above the apneic threshold toward the end of anesthesia. In anesthetized horses, adjusting controlled mechanical ventilation to allow higher $P_{ET}CO_2$ values (60 mmHg) results in a more rapid return of spontaneous ventilation at the end of anesthesia when compared to animals where mechanical ventilation was adjusted to achieve a $P_{ET}CO_2$ of 40 mmHg [177]. When weaning a patient from ventilatory support, if the animal is apneic for more than 30 s to 1 min, the anesthesiologist can intermittently provide manually assisted breaths while allowing $PaCO_2$ to rise to a level where the apneic threshold is again exceeded, and spontaneous ventilation resumes. Depending on the residual analgesic or anesthetic drug levels, the latter typically occurs at elevated $PaCO_2$ levels.

Among the contemporary injectable anesthetic agents, propofol is known for inducing respiratory depression and transient apnea in a similar fashion as thiopental in small animals [178]. The injectable anesthetic alfaxalone, may also cause respiratory depression/apnea after rapid intravenous administration. In dogs sedated with dexmedetomidine–methadone, incidence of post-induction apnea did not differ between induction of anesthesia with propofol and alfaxalone [179]. However, when both agents were administered at a faster rate to induce anesthesia (2 mg/kg/min and 4 mg/kg/min for alfaxalone and propofol, respectively) 100% of animals developed apnea lasting for at least 30 s; while a slower rate of administration (0.5 mg/kg/min and 1.0 mg/kg/min for alfaxalone and propofol, respectively), reduced the incidence of apnea to 25% for both anesthetic agents [179]. In dogs, current evidence therefore favors the slow titration of injectable anesthetics to achieve the desired depth of anesthesia to minimize post-induction respiratory depression/apnea [179,180]. Use of propofol as part of a total intravenous anesthesia technique often results in significant respiratory depression/apnea that requires mechanical ventilatory support in animals [181,182]. There is some evidence that total intravenous anesthesia with alfaxalone might be favored when mechanical ventilation is not available in cats because of less respiratory depression relative to that observed with propofol [182]. However, evidence in dogs undergoing elective surgery points out that maintenance of anesthesia with propofol (mean infusion rate 0.37 ± 0.09 mg/kg/min) or alfaxalone (mean infusion rate 0.11 ± 0.01 mg/kg/min) results in a similar degree of hypoventilation [183].

Although ketamine may be associated with less respiratory depression than other injectable anesthetics, when dissociative anesthetics are used in combination with other drugs during clinical anesthesia, they may also contribute to apnea or reduced $\dot{V}_E$. For example, post-induction apnea was more common in dogs after administration of propofol–ketamine (2 mg/kg each) than after propofol (4 mg/kg) alone [184]. Similarly, induction of anesthesia with propofol–ketamine in dogs for laryngeal examination resulted in lower hemoglobin saturation (87%) than propofol alone (94%), an observation attributed to a reduced central ventilatory drive and associated hypoventilation [185]. In cats, pulmonary ventilation may be decreased when supratherapeutic doses of ketamine are used, but the slope of the CO_2 response curve is not altered in comparison to the conscious state [186]. In horses, short-term anesthesia with α_2-adrenergic receptor agonists and ketamine alone or in combination benzodiazepines and/or guaifenesin induces some degree of respiratory depression (increased $PaCO_2$), although less than that observed with inhalant anesthetics [187–189]. During anesthesia produced with tiletamine–zolazepam or halothane in horses, $PaCO_2$ levels will increase by 5–10 mmHg if the inspired oxygen concentration is increased from 21–30% to 90–100% [190,191]. The latter is attributed to a reduction in chemoreceptor activity associated with higher PaO_2 levels [44]. Other studies have shown a trend toward greater respiratory depression (i.e., higher $PaCO_2$ levels) in spontaneously breathing, isoflurane-anesthetized horses inhaling an inspired oxygen concentration approaching 100% compared to 50% oxygen [192]. Greater respiratory depression associated with high F_IO_2 has been reported in other species under general anesthesia, including the rabbit [193]. Although there is a decrease in respiratory drive observed in spontaneously breathing animals during anesthesia with increased F_IO_2 levels, oxygen supplementation is still recommended to minimize the risk of hypoxemia, particularly in the equine [187,188,190,192,194,195].

As described previously, in conscious individuals $\dot{V}_E$ steeply increases when PaO_2 falls below 60 mmHg, with the slope of the curve approaching infinity as PaO_2 falls to 30–40 mmHg [196] (Fig. 37.4B). Compared to the conscious state, most general anesthetics suppress peripheral chemoreceptor activity and inhibit the hypoxic ventilatory drive in a dose-related fashion (Fig. 37.22) [197–202]. Early studies demonstrated that isoflurane causes less suppression of the hypoxic ventilatory drive compared to halothane

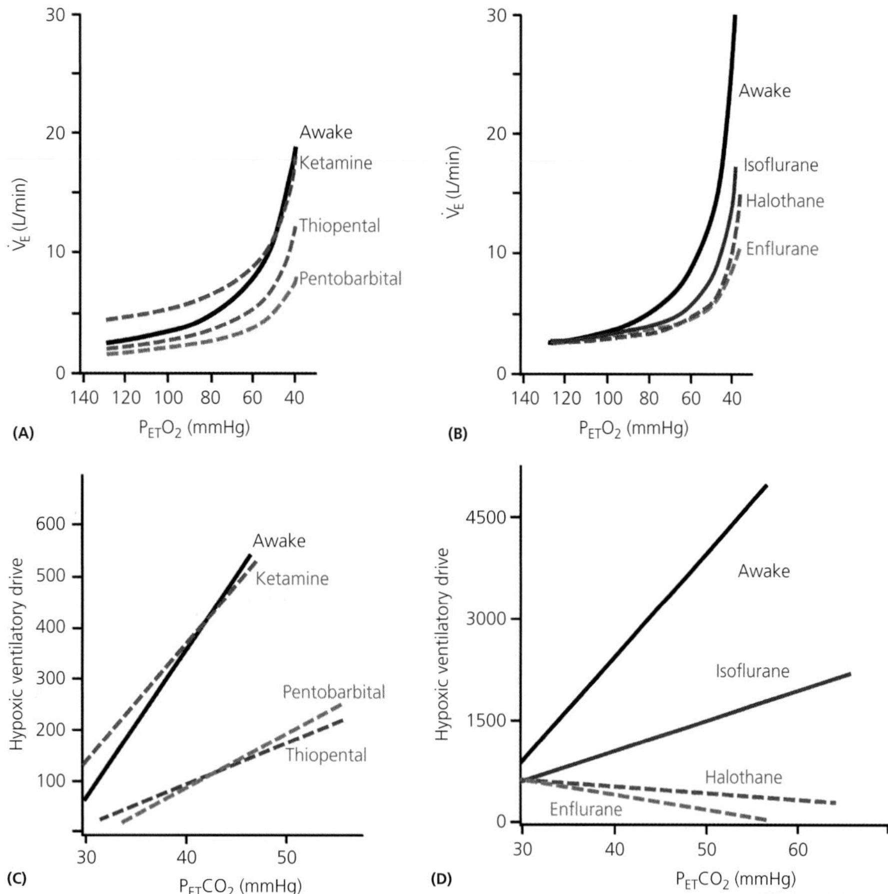

Figure 37.22 **A.** and **B.** Relationship between progressive decreases in expired oxygen partial pressure ($P_{ET}O_2$) and minute ventilation ($\dot{V}_E$) in dogs anesthetized with injectable and inhalant anesthetics ($n = 6$). A rightward shift of the curve in comparison to the awake state denotes suppression of the hypoxic ventilatory drive. **C.** and **D.** Effects of carbon dioxide levels (end-tidal carbon dioxide, $P_{ET}CO_2$) on the hypoxic ventilatory drive with injectable and inhalant anesthetics in dogs ($n = 6$). A decrease in the slope of the linear regression line denotes suppression of the hypoxic ventilatory drive during conditions of hypercapnia (increased $P_{ET}CO_2$). Source: Adapted from Hirshman *et al.* [197]; Hirshman *et al.* [198].

and enflurane (Fig. 37.22) [198]; and sevoflurane appears to cause less suppression of the hypoxic ventilatory drive than isoflurane [202]. While barbiturates (thiopental and pentobarbital) are known for inhibiting the hypoxic ventilatory drive, intravenous ketamine (10 mg/kg, followed by 0.5 mg/kg/min) was shown to preserve the ventilatory response to low PaO_2 levels in dogs under experimental conditions (Fig. 37.22) [197]. In human subjects, propofol inhibits the hypoxic ventilatory response even when administered at subanesthetic doses to produce sedation without loss of consciousness [201].

Anesthetic drugs that suppress the hypoxic ventilatory drive should be used cautiously for induction of anesthesia in animal species where endotracheal intubation is associated with a greater degree of difficulty, such as lagomorphs (rabbits) and rodents, or if the equipment necessary to perform endotracheal intubation and artificially ventilate the lungs is not readily available. If prolonged apnea occurs during induction of anesthesia, failure to establish a patent airway for oxygen supplementation and positive-pressure ventilation will quickly precipitate an episode of severe hypoxemia/tissue hypoxia, and an anesthetic fatality. For anesthesiologists who are less experienced with endotracheal intubation in rabbits, a species-specific supraglottic airway device (laryngeal mask) may facilitate more rapid establishment of a patent airway for oxygen supplementation and artificial ventilation of the lungs if necessary [203,204].

Sedatives and hypnotics

Mild to moderate sedation with α_2-adrenergic receptor agonists alone usually does not result in clinically relevant changes in arterial blood gases in most species. However, when relatively high doses of α_2-adrenergic receptor agonists are combined with opioids or ketamine to produce deeper levels of sedation/chemical restraint, some degree of gas exchange impairment (increased $PaCO_2$ and decreased PaO_2) can be observed in small animal species breathing room air (Fig. 37.23A,B) [205–208]. In ruminants, the degree of impaired gas exchange associated with α_2-adrenergic receptor agonists alone, administered at doses sufficient to induce recumbency, can be marked [7,209]. When arterial blood gas changes associated with α_2-adrenergic receptor agonist combinations are observed, they cannot be explained only by a centrally mediated decrease in $\dot{V}_E$ and $\dot{V}_A$, as the increase in $PaCO_2$ per se does not justify the decrease in arterial oxygenation observed after administration of these drug combinations. While the decrease in $\dot{V}_E$ and increase in $PaCO_2$ induced by injectable/inhalant anesthetics appears to be related to the CNS depressant effects of these drugs, $\dot{V}_A/\dot{Q}$ mismatch likely contributes to the decrease in PaO_2 in animals receiving

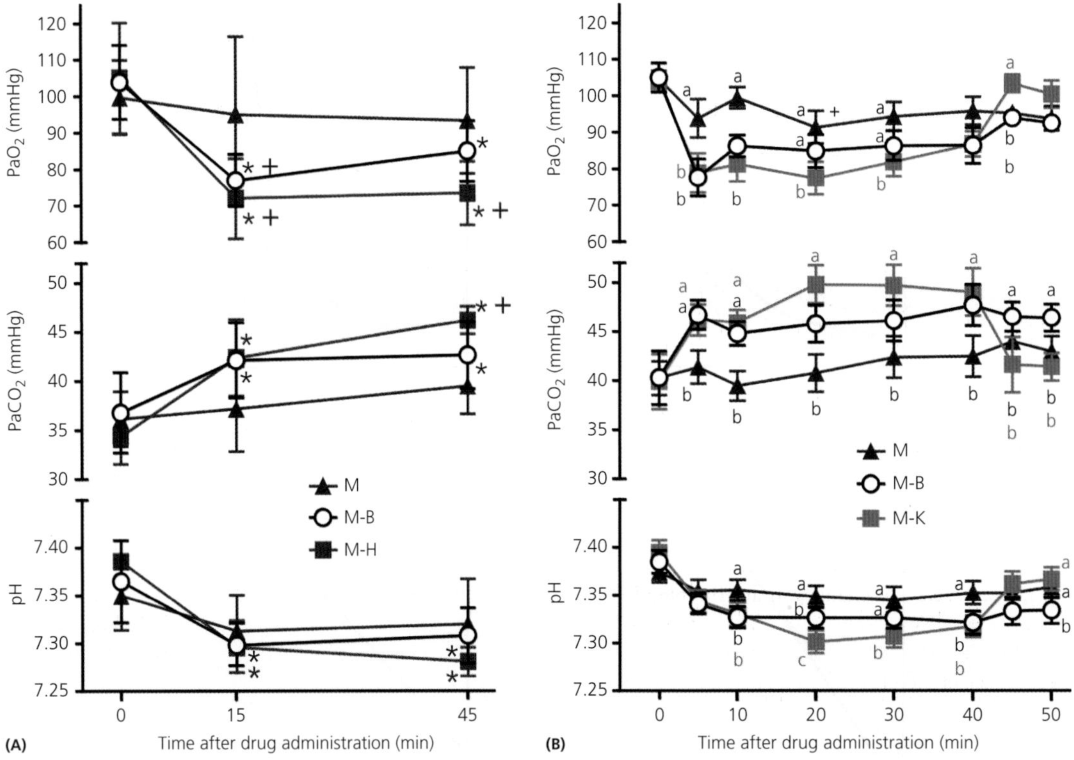

Figure 37.23 **A.** Arterial blood gas changes observed in six healthy mixed breed dogs (mean ± standard deviation) after intravenous administration of 20 μg/kg of medetomidine (M) alone or combined with 0.2 mg/kg of butorphanol (M-B) or 0.1 mg/kg of hydromorphone (M-H) in a randomized crossover design. *Significant difference from baseline (time 0). +Significant difference from medetomidine alone. **B.** Arterial blood gas changes observed in six healthy dogs (mean ± standard deviation) after intramuscular administration of 30 μg/kg of medetomidine (M) alone or combined with 0.2 mg/kg of butorphanol (M-B) or 3 mg/kg of ketamine (M-K) in a randomized crossover design.[a,b,c] For a given time point, treatment group means followed by different letters are significantly different from each other (a>b>c). Source: Adapted from Ko *et al.* [205]; Kuo and Keegan [206].

injectable/inhalant anesthetics and α_2-adrenergic receptor agonist drug combinations.

Experimental data in dogs suggests that high doses of medetomidine administered intravenously (20 μg/kg) inhibit the ventilatory response to increased CO_2 levels in comparison to the awake state, but such effect is less than that observed during isoflurane anesthesia (Fig. 37.21A) [162,198]. Dexmedetomidine-induced sedation has also been shown to impair the ventilatory response to hypoxemia and hypercapnia in humans [210]. In dogs that were receiving a fentanyl infusion (5 μg/kg/min) during recovery from isoflurane anesthesia, intravenous dexmedetomidine administration (2.5 μg/kg) resulted in significant respiratory depression ($PaCO_2$ > 45 mmHg) when compared to placebo or acepromazine (0.05 mg/kg) [207]. Therefore, caution should be exerted when α_2-adrenergic receptor agonists are used to provide sedation during recovery from general anesthesia because of the potential for respiratory depression particularly when oxygenation will not be monitored or the ability to provide oxygen supplementation is not available. Relatively low doses of α_2-adrenergic receptor agonists are commonly administered after discontinuation of inhalant anesthesia in horses with the goal of improving the quality of recovery [211,212]. However, administration of α_2-adrenergic receptor agonists and other anesthetic adjuvants to horses in the recovery room should be delayed until strong spontaneous breathing efforts are present, if measures to support ventilatory support are not available, as apnea may be precipitated if these drugs are administered to animals that are in a deep plane of anesthesia.

Phenothiazines (acepromazine) and butyrophenones (droperidol) may increase the hypoxic ventilatory drive, possibly by blocking the effects of endogenous dopamine on peripheral chemoreceptors [50,213,214]. Interestingly, in humans and cats, intravenous dopamine (3–5 μg/kg/min) inhibits the ventilatory response to low PaO_2 due to depression of peripheral chemoreceptor (carotid body) output [215,216]. In human patients with heart failure breathing ambient air, intravenous dopamine has also been shown to decrease $\dot{V}_E$ despite decreased oxygen saturation and increased $P_{ET}CO_2$, although the clinical significance of this in the management of clinical veterinary patients is unknown [217].

Opioids

Opioids are known for inducing respiratory depression. In knockout mice lacking μ-opioid receptors, morphine and other pure μ-opioid receptor agonists do not induce respiratory depression, demonstrating that the adverse ventilatory effects induced by these drugs are largely mediated by stimulation of μ-opioid receptors [218,219]. Experimental evidence obtained in conscious human subjects provides ample evidence that pure μ-opioid receptor agonists suppress the ventilatory response to hypercapnia [220]. Contrasting with pure μ-opioid receptor agonists, drugs that act as μ-opioid receptor antagonists and κ-opioid receptor agonists (butorphanol and nalbuphine) have a limited (ceiling) effect on the ventilatory response to increasing CO_2 levels [221,222] and can reverse the respiratory depression induced by pure μ-opioid receptor agonists [223–225]. In humans not experiencing pain, opioid-induced respiratory depression (decreased $\dot{V}_E$) is further aggravated by use of high F_IO_2 [226]. However, the clinical significance of respiratory depression caused by hyperoxia associated with high F_IO_2 in animals receiving opioids is presently unclear.

Opioids may induce panting in some species, most notably dogs [227–229]. In conscious dogs, panting is more frequently observed after administration of pure μ-opioid receptor agonists (oxymorphone) than after μ-opioid receptor antagonists/κ-opioid receptor agonists (butorphanol) [230]. This reaction is thought to be mediated by the hypothalamic thermoregulatory center that resets as if the body temperature was increased (though it is not). Because panting is an important thermoregulatory mechanism in canine species, opioid administration to conscious dogs may decrease body temperature [54]. Interestingly, an increase in body temperature leading to clinically relevant hyperthermia is observed after opioid administration in cats, which is attributed to drug-induced changes in the thermoregulatory center [231]. Although panting is commonly observed after opioid administration in canine species, relatively high doses of methadone (0.5–1 mg/kg) or morphine (1.0 mg/kg) administered intravenously do not cause clinically relevant changes in arterial blood gases in healthy conscious dogs [232]. Administration of hydromorphone (0.2 mg/kg) subcutaneously, or liposome-encapsulated hydromorphone (2.0 mg/kg, subcutaneously), increased $PaCO_2$ and decreased PaO_2 from baseline values in dogs [233]. However, blood gas changes were mild in the latter study, and in most cases, $PaCO_2$ values were not increased above the high normal range (45 mmHg), and PaO_2 values were not decreased below the low normal range (80 mmHg) [233]. Butorphanol does not induce significant changes in arterial blood gases when administered to conscious dogs at a dose of 0.3 mg/kg intravenously [234], or even when larger doses (up to 0.8 mg/kg) are administered in spontaneously ventilating dogs anesthetized with halothane [235]. However, in human subjects anesthetized with 50% nitrous oxide in oxygen, butorphanol was shown to inhibit the increase in $\dot{V}_E$ in response to increasing CO_2 levels [236]. While administration of opioid analgesics to conscious non-painful horses may result in excitatory behavior, arterial blood gases are unaltered [237–239]. In isoflurane-anesthetized horses, morphine administered intravenously at doses, ranging from 0.15 to 0.25 mg/kg does not induce respiratory depression, while supratherapeutic doses (2.0 mg/kg) cause significant respiratory depression/hypercapnia [240,241].

Pure μ-opioid receptor agonists (methadone, 0.25–0.75 mg/kg; morphine, 0.25–1.0 mg/kg) combined with intramuscular acepromazine (0.05 mg/kg) induce sedative effects with minimal evidence of respiratory depression based on arterial blood gases in healthy dogs [242,243]. Intravenous or intramuscular administration of acepromazine (0.05 mg/kg) combined with butorphanol (0.4 mg/kg) or nalbuphine (0.5 mg/kg) in cats induces mild sedation without evidence of respiratory acidosis based on venous blood gases [244]. In animals, the respiratory depressant effects of opioids are evident when these drugs are administered intravenously during general anesthesia [240,245–247]. Respiratory depression/apnea associated with intraoperative opioid administration often requires mechanical ventilatory support in anesthetized animals [245,247,248]. Constant rate infusion of short-acting pure μ-opioid receptor agonists (e.g., sufentanil) in isoflurane-anesthetized dogs causes the CO_2 response curve to become nearly flat, suggesting that these drugs produce marked inhibition of central chemoreceptor activity during general anesthesia (Fig. 37.21B) [173]. Studies in cats under light anesthesia with α-chloralose and urethane have shown that morphine (0.15 mg/kg) depresses ventilation at hyperoxia but does not alter the ventilatory response (increase in $\dot{V}_E$) to hypoxia [249].

Administration of μ-opioid receptor agonists as premedication may also impair ventilation during recovery from anesthesia. Clinical evidence in healthy dogs undergoing surgery (ovariohysterectomy and castration) indicates that premedication with hydromorphone 0.2 mg/kg, intramuscularly may result in higher $PaCO_2$ in comparison to the use of butorphanol 0.4 mg/kg, intramuscularly [250]. When μ-opioid receptor agonists are used as premedication, the degree of respiratory depression is usually mild and well tolerated by healthy animals undergoing elective surgeries [250]. However, caution should be exerted when these drugs are administered to sick animals or patients with respiratory disease, as they may have a greater impact on ventilation and lead to clinically relevant hypercapnia and hypoxemia. During recovery from general anesthesia in dogs, persistent respiratory depression caused by opioids resulting in low hemoglobin saturation (e.g., pulse oximetry < 94%) can occur while the patient is breathing ambient air and is often accompanied by excessive residual sedation and delayed extubation (lack of return of swallowing reflex). These signs can be reversed by slow intravenous titration of a μ-opioid receptor antagonist (naloxone 1–5 μg/kg) or a μ-opioid receptor antagonist/κ-opioid receptor agonist (butorphanol 0.05–0.1 mg/kg). In dogs, intravenous naloxone at 1 μg/kg increments every 2 min can be administered until the breathing frequency and amplitude of spontaneous respiratory efforts are increased to the point of normalizing pulse oximetry saturation (≥ 95%), and there is an improvement in the levels of consciousness/return of the swallowing reflex allowing orotracheal tube removal. Because respiratory depression and analgesia are clinical effects associated with μ-opioid receptor stimulation, slow titration until achieving the desired effect is important to avoid reversal of the analgesic effects. The elimination half-life of intravenous naloxone is relatively short in dogs (37 min) [251]. Therefore, clinicians should be aware of possible recurrence of respiratory depression and the need for additional opioid reversal over time [252]. In the case of opioid intoxication, much higher doses of naloxone (40 μg/kg) are necessary to reverse the adverse effects/respiratory depression induced by the opioid and there may be the need for repeated administration of high doses in case of an inadequate response. Pharmacokinetic studies in dogs suggest that the intranasal route (4 mg via a commercially available fixed-dose naloxone atomizer; mean dose of 0.17 mg/kg) may represent an effective alternative to intravenous naloxone administration in emergency situations of opioid intoxication [251].

Effects of sedation and anesthesia on pulmonary ventilation and mechanics

In addition to reducing central respiratory drive as discussed above, sedation and anesthesia can alter pulmonary ventilation by changing the volume of the lung, absolute or relative amount of deadspace (physiological and apparatus deadspace) in relation to V_T, and the mechanical properties of the respiratory system. While the changes associated with anesthesia can be considered individually, it is important to recognize that alterations in individual components of the respiratory system are not independent. For example, changes in lung volume influence the mechanical properties of the respiratory system, and vice versa.

Ventilation and lung volumes

A reduction in lung volume, specifically the lung volume at end-expiration (FRC), is one of the major physiologic changes associated with general anesthesia and recumbency [61,253–256]. While not extensively studied in all species, a reduction in FRC observed with general anesthesia has been demonstrated in several species, including humans, horses, and dogs [27–29,256,257]. In recumbent humans, FRC is reduced by about 20% with the induction of general anesthesia [256,257]. While a reduced FRC does not necessarily result in atelectasis, it is a commonly recognized sequela to the reduction of lung volume associated with recumbency and relaxation/paralysis of respiratory muscles induced by anesthesia. Atelectasis has been reported to occur in up to 90% of adult human patients with normal cardiopulmonary function undergoing general anesthesia, with up to 20–25% of the lung becoming atelectatic or poorly ventilated as assessed by computed tomography [254,258].

One study in beagle dogs showed no change in FRC associated with thiopental anesthesia; however, sedation and both sternal and lateral recumbency have been shown to reduce FRC in deep-chested dogs [29,259]. While measurement of FRC has rarely been performed in dogs, with advances in thoracic imaging, specifically computed tomography, changes in lung volume and the development of atelectasis during anesthesia have been evaluated more extensively. In dogs sedated and maintained in sternal recumbency, minimal atelectasis is evident on computed tomography images; however, mild attenuation of aeration/atelectasis occurs in lateral or dorsally recumbent dogs during sedation and/or general anesthesia breathing spontaneously or receiving mechanical ventilation [260–263]. In horses and cows, the decrease in FRC with the onset of recumbency and general anesthesia may be marked, as much as 50–70%. This has been directly measured by helium dilution [27,264] and open-circuit nitrogen washout [28] and is consistent with imaging studies showing reduced lung aeration [265,266]. The reduction in FRC seems to be primarily related to the positional change from an upright posture to recumbency and, in horses, is greater in lateral or dorsal recumbency compared to sternal positioning [28]. Laterally recumbent horses and cows have a smaller FRC compared to the conscious state and radiographic images indicate that the dependent lung is poorly aerated [265,266]. Studies using nuclear scintigraphy and computed tomography have clearly demonstrated that there is markedly less ventilation of the dependent lung of horses in lateral and dorsal recumbency during anesthesia [267,268]. In horses, the reduction in lower lung volume is accompanied by atelectasis and may be influenced by the degree of obesity or body conformation, a finding consistent with studies in humans [269,270].

The acute reduction in FRC and development of atelectasis associated with anesthesia has been primarily attributed to three factors: (1) alterations in chest wall (thoracic wall and diaphragm) function and configuration with a resultant increase in P_{pl} (globally with regional differences), (2) low distal airway/alveolar pressures (P_{alv}), and (3) loss of functional surfactant. The former two mechanisms are believed to be the major mechanisms contributing to the development of atelectasis in healthy humans and in some animal species under anesthesia while surfactant dysfunction is recognized to contribute to the development of atelectasis in patients with pre-existing lung injury and/or patients receiving long-term mechanical ventilatory support [257,271].

Alterations in chest wall function and configuration are responsible for most of the reduction in FRC associated with anesthesia, particularly in large animal species such as horses and cows. In conscious animals, the outward recoil of the chest wall results in a sub-atmospheric pressure within the pleural cavity (P_{pl}). The pressure difference between the inside (alveoli) and the outside of the lung (pleural cavity) ($P_{alv} - P_{pl}$), is responsible for maintaining the alveoli open throughout the respiratory cycle (inspiration and expiration). Induction of anesthesia results in relaxation of the chest wall (thoracic wall and diaphragm), which in turn increases P_{pl} (it becomes less negative) and decreases the outward pull on the lung. Cranial migration of the diaphragm, increased transfer of pressure from the abdominal cavity to the thorax, and the weight of the lung within the chest wall also contribute to an increased (less negative) P_{pl}, most notably in the dependent lung regions. When the pressure outside the lungs (P_{pl}) exceeds the pressure within the airways and alveoli (P_{alv}), *compression atelectasis* develops. Because of their long-sloping diaphragm (notably horses), anatomy of their gastrointestinal tract, and their body mass, large animal species are more prone to compression of the lungs and atelectasis in dependent zones when recumbent relative to small animal species. In horses and cows, with the onset of anesthesia and movement into lateral recumbency, there is radiographic evidence of a marked change in the two-dimensional lung silhouette and the position of the diaphragm [265,266]. In ponies anesthetized with halothane, the diaphragmatic outline moved forward in both sternal and lateral recumbency, although the forward shift was considerably greater in lateral recumbency [265]. When the ponies were positioned in dorsal recumbency, the diaphragmatic outline moved toward the dependent spine region. With minor variations, observations of 315–400 kg cattle were very similar [266]. The positional alteration of the diaphragmatic silhouette concurs with the reduction in FRC noted by Sorenson and Robinson when ponies were moved from sternal to lateral or dorsal recumbency [28]. In addition to changes in position of the diaphragm, the tonic activity of the lateral chest wall, especially that provided by the serratus ventralis muscle, may be decreased in anesthetized horses, and it is postulated that this phenomenon reduces the stabilization of the lateral chest wall and likely contributes to the loss of FRC in this species [272].

In addition to loss of lung volume secondary to compression, distal airway and alveolar pressures (P_{alv}) may also contribute to the loss of lung volume and atelectasis during anesthesia [271]. Reduction in airway radius or even obstruction of small airways secondary to compression (as described above), constriction, or the presence of intraluminal material (e.g., mucus) may reduce ventilation to distal lung units. Absorption of gases from the regions of lung that are poorly ventilated but still perfused may subsequently result in the development of *absorption atelectasis*. The development of the latter is influenced by the characteristics of the gases in the distal lung unit. In individuals breathing ambient air, alveolar gas contains approximately 79% of nitrogen (Table 37.4). Because nitrogen is insoluble in blood, it is not absorbed from the alveoli to capillary blood and may have a role in preventing alveolar units with low $\dot{V}_A/\dot{Q}$ ratio from collapsing (acting as a "nitrogen skeleton"). If alveolar nitrogen is largely replaced by oxygen by using high F_IO_2 (> 0.8), the flow of oxygen from alveoli to capillary blood in low $\dot{V}_A/\dot{Q}$ units exceeds flow of inspired gas (oxygen) entering these alveoli, causing these lung units to become progressively smaller until they collapse [154]. High F_IO_2 in the perianesthetic period has been demonstrated to lead to a greater degree of atelectasis in horses, dogs, cats, and humans, an observation consistent with absorption of gases in distal airways and alveoli [61,191,253,261,262,273].

There are several important consequences resulting from a decrease in lung volume at end-expiration. Most importantly, a reduced FRC predisposes a patient to $\dot{V}_A/\dot{Q}$ mismatching and intrapulmonary shunting of blood secondary to the development of atelectasis [256]. Due to compression of lung parenchyma during anesthesia, a portion of blood supplying the lung will flow by collapsed ($\dot{V}_A/\dot{Q} = 0$) and/or poorly ventilated alveoli ($\dot{V}_A/\dot{Q}$ ratio between 0.01 and 0.1) without achieving adequate oxygenation (assuming HPV does not divert blood to well-ventilated lung units), thereby contributing to a reduction in oxygen levels in the blood leaving the lung (i.e., increased venous admixture) [274], as discussed previously. Although oxygenation impairment/low PaO_2 is the major consequence of atelectatic lung areas, an increase in $\dot{Q}s/\dot{Q}_T$ through the lung also adds CO_2-rich mixed venous blood to oxygenated blood, further aggravating hypercapnia caused by a decrease in $\dot{V}_A$ during anesthesia. In addition to impacting gas exchange function of the lung, changes in lung volume also influence pulmonary mechanics, with pulmonary resistance increasing and compliance decreasing with a reduction in FRC/atelectasis.

To minimize the loss of lung volume and the development of atelectasis associated with anesthesia and recumbency, several strategies have been investigated including the use of negative-pressure ventilation, positive-pressure ventilation, and varying inspired gas composition. Early mechanical ventilators were designed to create a negative (sub-atmospheric) pressure around the thorax to enlarge the chest wall and pull gas into the lungs by creating a negative intrapleural pressure. This was achieved by encasing the whole body (except the head) inside a cylinder that intermittently generated a sub-atmospheric pressure. These early ventilators, also called "iron lungs," were widely used during the 1950s to provide mechanical ventilation in patients who suffered from paralysis of diaphragm caused by poliomyelitis. Due to the required equipment and limited access to the patient's thorax, ventilatory support using negative-pressure ventilation is not in common use today. Application of intermittent positive pressure to oxygen or air/oxygen mixtures supplying the lungs is now commonly used during veterinary medicine to maintain alveolar ventilation. Depending on the strategy, positive-pressure ventilation may establish a positive pressure gradient between the alveoli and pleural space such that loss of lung volume and atelectasis does not occur. However, the level of applied positive pressure and its resulting P_{alv} may not be enough to overcome the increased P_{pl} in the dependent lung zones, therefore the latter may remain closed throughout the respiratory cycle. Even if inspiratory pressures are set to a level that is high enough to open up atelectatic lung areas during inspiration, if there is no positive end-expiratory pressure (PEEP) or if the level of PEEP is inadequate to keep the alveoli open during expiration, the intermittent opening and closure of alveoli (tidal recruitment) will lead to ventilator-induced lung injury, specifically atelectrauma [275,276]. Reversal of atelectasis during anesthesia may require an alveolar recruitment maneuver, that is, the temporary application of high inspiratory airway pressures to open up atelectatic lung areas, followed by mechanical ventilation with an adequate PEEP level to prevent loss of lung volume and recurrence of atelectasis [93,262,277,278]. As high F_IO_2 levels have been shown to contribute to absorption atelectasis, the use of varying inspired F_IO_2 and/or supplementation of inspired gases with less soluble gases such as helium have been investigated [93,194,279,280]. Inspired gas concentrations, alveolar recruitment maneuvers, and PEEP adjustment during mechanical ventilation are discussed in greater detail in Chapter 38.

Ventilation and deadspace

As previously discussed, $\dot{V}_A$ and the maintenance of normal $PaCO_2$ levels can be influenced by alterations in deadspace and the $V_{D_{phys}}/V_T$ relationship. In anesthetized patients, deadspace can be altered through a change in either $V_{D_{phys}}$ (airway or alveolar) or mechanical (apparatus) deadspace. Airway deadspace can increase with positional changes such as extension of the head and neck, high airway pressures associated with positive-pressure ventilation, and bronchodilation [281,282].

While bypassing the upper airways through use of a tracheostomy or placement of an endotracheal tube (of appropriate length) decreases total deadspace (physiologic and apparatus deadspace), anesthetic equipment, including facemasks, excessively long endotracheal tubes that protrude outside the mouth/nostrils, and airway adaptors placed between the breathing circuit and the endotracheal tube for airway gas sampling/analysis or spirometry can dramatically increase apparatus and total deadspace, with possible clinical relevance, particularly in small patients [283]. While an increase in deadspace will not alter $\dot{V}_A$ if a compensatory change in V_T and/or f occurs, as one may expect to occur in a conscious healthy individual, an increase in deadspace due to anesthesia equipment, combined with an unchanged or decreased V_T associated with general anesthesia, can significantly increase $V_{D_{phys}}/V_T$, reduce $\dot{V}_A$, and contribute to hypercapnia.

As previously discussed, changes in expired nitrogen concentration over a single breath after the patient inhales 100% oxygen can be used to estimate deadspace values in an experimental setting (single-breath nitrogen washout), while volumetric capnography is the current clinical gold standard to determine $V_{D_{phys}}$, $V_{D_{alv}}$, $V_{D_{aw}}$, and effective alveolar ventilation per minute [$\dot{V}_A = (V_T - V_{D_{phys}}) \times f$]. In general, $V_{D_{phys}}$ does not change significantly in healthy human patients during general anesthesia with either spontaneous or artificial ventilation [257]. In healthy spontaneously breathing horses with normal cardiovascular function placed in dorsal recumbency, $V_{D_{phys}}/V_T$ ratio measured according to the Bohr equation by volumetric capnography was approximately 0.35–0.39 and remained relatively stable over 3 h of general anesthesia [68]. In anesthetized dogs receiving positive-pressure ventilation, $V_{D_{phys}}/V_T$ ratio calculated using the Bohr–Enghoff equation, was approximately 0.6, and remained stable throughout a 60-min period [69]. Use of high airway pressures (typically with high PEEP levels) during mechanical ventilation can, however, result in an increase in P_{alv} and $V_{D_{alv}}$ by impairing alveolar perfusion [284]. A decrease in pulmonary perfusion from a variety of causes including a reduced CO associated with anesthesia or an embolic event, can also lead to an increase in $V_{D_{alv}}$ [281]. In hemodynamically compromised small animal or large animal patients, an increase in $P(a\text{-}ET)CO_2$ may not reflect only impaired pulmonary perfusion if there is significant oxygenation impairment secondary to areas of low $\dot{V}_A/\dot{Q}$ and intrapulmonary shunting of blood.

Ventilation and lung mechanics

As previously described, the mechanical properties of the respiratory system, specifically regional compliance and resistance, determine the normal distribution of airflow within the lung and the energy expended to achieve optimal ventilation. Changes in the upper and lower airways, thoracic cage, and diaphragm associated with anesthesia produce marked changes in airway resistance and pulmonary compliance. While thoracic and lung tissues contribute to overall pulmonary resistance, the relative change over time in healthy subjects is believed to be minor relative to the airways. While changes in lung mechanical properties are significant with anesthesia, interpretation of measurements of both pulmonary resistance and compliance during anesthesia is difficult because changes in lung volume per se will alter these values [79,257].

The latter is particularly relevant when considering the etiology of such changes. Absolute values for pulmonary resistance and compliance are influenced by many factors including the method of measurement, airway device and diameter, patient size, and method of ventilation. Further discussion regarding the measurement of pulmonary mechanics during anesthesia is provided in Chapter 38.

At rest under normal circumstances (nasal breathing), the upper airways (nasal cavity, pharynx, and larynx) are responsible for more than 50% of the total R_{aw}. With sedation and anesthesia in horses, alar and pharyngeal muscles relax, reducing the diameter of the upper airways, further increasing the resistance to breathing and increasing the relative contribution of the upper airways to total R_{aw} [285–287]. In some patients, the consequences of an increase in upper airway resistance may be limited to an increase in the patient's effort to achieve alveolar ventilation. This is typically characterized by an increase in abdominal movement during inspiration with minimal or paradoxical (inward-moving) chest wall movement. The latter respiratory pattern is due to a greater impact of anesthetics on the function of intercostal muscles versus the diaphragm. Upper airway obstruction following sedation or induction of general anesthesia may also occur, particularly in patients with structurally abnormal upper airways, such as in brachycephalic dogs and cats, or patients with pathology of the upper airways. In the equine placed in dorsal recumbency for prolonged periods, congestion and tissue swelling of the nasopharyngeal structures are particularly common. For obligate nasal breathers (e.g., cats and horses), bypassing the nasopharynx by placing an orotracheal tube, nasotracheal tube (horses), or supraglottic airway device (cats) reduces upper airway resistance and the work of breathing, ensuring a patent airway during anesthesia [287]. Further discussion regarding the relative risk and benefits of different airway devices is provided in chapters dedicated to specific species management. In contrast to the upper airways, most currently used injectable and inhalant anesthetics result in a dose-dependent bronchodilation in addition to inhibiting airway vagal reflexes and bronchoconstriction [175,288–291]. One notable exception is desflurane, which may cause an increase in R_{aw} due to bronchoconstriction at higher doses (1.5–2.0 MAC) [290,292]. Airway resistance is, however, influenced by lung volume, with lower lung volumes resulting in an increase in resistance, particularly as lung volumes approach RV [293].

In general, in humans, an overall increase in R_{aw} (excluding the effect of upper airways) occurs with anesthesia. It is unknown if this is due to the reduction in lung volume or change in airflow rates, two variables that impact resistance measurements [61]. During an anesthetic period, however, R_{aw} generally remains stable in healthy human patients receiving ventilatory support [61]. There are few studies evaluating conscious versus anesthetized respiratory mechanics in veterinary species using consistent methodology that take into consideration the effect of lung volume and airflows, therefore it is difficult to make conclusions regarding the effects of anesthesia alone. In one study evaluating cows anesthetized for 3 h with halothane, R_{aw} tended to increase, however, the degree of change was only significant in fed cows [294]. The latter also was reported to become tympanic, therefore, it is possible that the change over time in R_{aw} was related to a loss of lung volume. In anesthetized mechanically ventilated healthy dogs placed in lateral or dorsal recumbency for orthopedic procedures, R_{aw} did not significantly increase over a 120-min period [295]. Resistance was also unchanged in healthy sedated recumbent foals receiving ventilatory support over a 24-h period [296].

Similar to the decrease in lung volumes with anesthesia, total respiratory system compliance (C_{RS}) is reduced during anesthesia. It is important to emphasize that decreased C_{RS} in anesthetized animals may be the result of decreases in lung (C_L) and chest wall (C_{CW}) compliance. Development of anesthesia-related atelectasis and severe lung disease will reduce C_{RS} because of poor C_L. Factors that are external to the lung, such as loss of respiratory muscle tone/muscle paralysis (diaphragm and intercostal muscles) induced by anesthetic drugs, obesity, increased intra-abdominal volume and pressure, and chest wall conformation (barrel-chested dogs) will result in a less compliant chest wall (decreased C_{CW}) and contribute to a reduced C_{RS} during anesthesia [297]. Although an independent assessment of C_L and C_{CW} would allow the anesthetist to identify the cause of decreased C_{RS} and to direct the clinical conduct to improve overall compliance, as described previously, in the clinical setting C_{RS} is often measured during anesthesia with positive-pressure ventilation. Specifically, total C_{RS} (either dynamic or static/quasistatic C_{RS}), is calculated as the ratio between the V_T (mL) and the driving pressure (cm H_2O) (inspiratory minus end-expiratory pressures) during mechanical ventilation. However, comparison of compliance measurements among veterinary species requires indexing values to ideal body weight (mL/cmH_2O/kg). Analysis of C_{RS} measurements indexed to body weight shows that adult horses present significantly lower C_{RS} (0.4 mL/cmH_2O/kg) than dogs (1.3 mL/cmH_2O/kg) during anesthesia and positive-pressure ventilation [93,297].

In healthy human patients, the decrease in C_{RS} with anesthesia is believed to be due to the reduction in lung volume [257]. The timeline of changes in lung volume with changes in compliance, are consistent with the latter etiology. In healthy dogs maintained under general anesthesia in a clinical setting, quasistatic C_{RS} has been shown to be relatively stable over time, but it is reduced in obese animals and animals with a barrel-shaped chest [295,297]. Although there is a paucity of data in the literature, adequate preoperative fasting appears to be important to minimize the decrease in C_{RS} and improve gas exchange during general anesthesia in ruminants. In one study, a progressive decrease in dynamic C_{RS} was recorded during a 90-min period of halothane anesthesia in nonfasted cows and in cows that were deprived of food for 48 h and water for 12 h prior to anesthesia [294]. However, dynamic C_{RS} was decreased to a greater extent in nonfasted than in fasted cows and these changes in pulmonary mechanics were associated with progressive worsening of gas exchange (higher $PaCO_2$ and lower PaO_2 values), probably because of a greater degree of atelectasis associated with the development of abdominal tympany in cows that were not fasted before anesthesia [294].

Effects of anesthesia on pulmonary perfusion and hypoxic pulmonary vasoconstriction

Pulmonary perfusion is driven by the gradient between MPAP and LAP. Inhalant anesthetics have a major impact on the perfusion of systemic organs due to dose-dependent decreases in mean arterial pressure (MAP) and/or CO. The effects of inhalant anesthetics on pulmonary circulation, however, are less obvious as increasing doses of inhalant anesthetics (from 1.0 to 1.5–2.0 MAC) did not cause significant changes in MPAP in spontaneously breathing dogs, despite reduction of MAP in a dose-related manner (Fig. 37.24A) [4]. In mechanically ventilated horses anesthetized with sevoflurane, MPAP was significantly decreased from values observed in conscious animals, although changes in MPAP were not observed between MAC multiples (Fig. 37.24B) [298]. Absence of changes in MPAP occurred despite dose-related decreases in MAP and CO (Fig. 37.24B) [298]. Ventilated but poorly perfused lung areas (high $\dot{V}_A/\dot{Q}$ ratio), apparently caused by low MPAP, appear to be relatively common finding

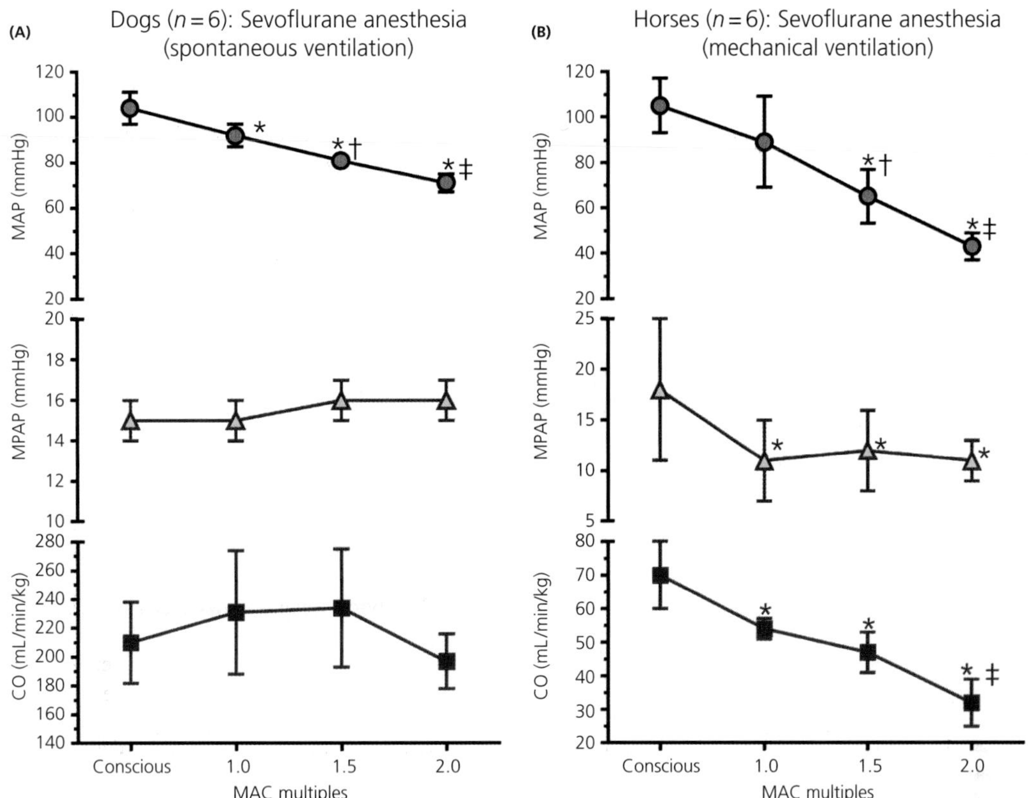

Figure 37.24 Effects of increasing doses of sevoflurane expressed as multiples of minimum alveolar concentration (MAC) on mean arterial pressure (MAP), mean pulmonary arterial pressure (MPAP), and cardiac output (CO) in **A.** spontaneously breathing dogs, and **B.** mechanically ventilated horses. * Significant difference from value recorded when animals were conscious; † Significant difference from value recorded at 1.0 MAC; ‡ Significant difference from value recorded at 1.5 MAC. Source: Adapted from Mutoh *et al.* [4]; Aida *et al.* [298].

in standing conscious horses [153,299]. Although general anesthesia decreases CO and MPAP compared to the conscious state in equine species, areas of high $\dot{V}_A/\dot{Q}$ ratio are paradoxically decreased from values recorded during the conscious state in dorsal recumbency anesthetized horses [299].

Major changes in CO during anesthesia will influence arterial and mixed venous blood oxygenation. In a patient with a relatively large intrapulmonary shunt (e.g., 50% of shunted flow leading to hypoxemia/low PaO_2), arterial oxygenation will be further impaired if CO is significantly decreased by anesthesia or hemorrhage. This effect is secondary to a decrease in mixed venous blood PO_2 and not to a direct effect of low CO on gas exchange within the lungs [300,301]. Because oxygen delivery is decreased by low CO, a compensatory increase in oxygen extraction by tissues reduces the PO_2/hemoglobin saturation in mixed venous blood. As the pulmonary artery blood with lower-than-normal PO_2 and hemoglobin saturation (e.g., 30 mmHg and 57%) reaches ventilated alveoli, it will not be fully oxygenated and the blood leaving these alveolar units will further aggravate the oxygenation impairment caused by the intrapulmonary shunt [300,301]. Based on this physiologic concept, the anesthesiologist should consider means to improve CO (e.g., inotropic and/or fluid administration) in patients where poor hemodynamic function is coinciding with hypoxemia caused by intrapulmonary shunting during anesthesia.

General anesthesia and mechanical ventilation may decrease perfusion in specific areas of the lung through decreases in $\dot{Q}_T$, which may contribute to an increase in $V_{D_{alv}}$ if perfusion is completely abolished in some lung areas. As previously discussed, ventilated lung areas where capillary blood flow is absent because P_{alv} is greater than arterial and venous pressures (West zone I) (Fig. 37.15) can be increased in anesthetized patients receiving mechanical ventilation, especially if high inspiratory pressures and/or high levels of PEEP are used. Due to relationship between $P_{ET}CO_2$ and $PaCO_2$ in mammalian species with normal lungs, monitoring $P_{ET}CO_2$ provides a quick and non-invasive tool to assess the adequacy of ventilation in patients under general anesthesia. Under normal circumstances, the $P_{ET}CO_2$ (which represents the CO_2 eliminated from alveoli that are ventilated and perfused) is up to 5 mmHg less than $PaCO_2$, as alveolar CO_2 is diluted with gas from the airways, which does not contain CO_2 [302]. However, in the event of decreased lung perfusion during anesthesia contributing to an abnormally high $V_{D_{alv}}$, the $P(a\text{-}ET)CO_2$ will often increase above 5 mmHg. As previously noted, the anesthesiologist should also be aware that the use of $P(a\text{-}ET)CO_2$ as an index that reflects solely pulmonary/alveolar deadspace is limited in the presence of significant low $\dot{V}_A/\dot{Q}$ areas and intrapulmonary shunting [62,68]. Mixed venous blood bypassing ventilated alveoli (shunted flow) and areas with low $\dot{V}_A/\dot{Q}$ ratios adds CO_2-rich blood to the arterial side leading to an increase in $PaCO_2$ and overestimation of pulmonary/alveolar deadspace based on the Enghoff method [62,68]. For practical purposes, the anesthesiologist may suspect that intrapulmonary shunting is increased, and therefore bears a greater influence on $P(a\text{-}ET)CO_2$ calculations, by evaluating PaO_2 values while the animal is breathing an inspired oxygen concentration close to 100%; if PaO_2 is near 500 mmHg, intrapulmonary shunting is likely to be minimal, and pulmonary/alveolar deadspace is likely the major determinant of the P(a-ET)CO_2 gradient.

In hemodynamically unstable patients, if P(a-ET)CO_2 is elevated or increases over time, there could be an increase in pulmonary/alveolar deadspace secondary to poor pulmonary perfusion, which should be investigated. Identification and resolution of the cause of abnormally high P(a-ET)CO_2 is paramount to avoid the development of further complications during anesthesia. For practical purposes, in anesthetized small animals presenting a clearly distinguishable phase III (alveolar plateau) in the capnogram, an increased discrepancy between $P_{ET}CO_2$ and $PaCO_2$ (P(a-ET)CO_2 > 5 mmHg) may provide a rough estimate that $V_{D_{alv}}/V_T$ is increased. In otherwise healthy anesthetized animals receiving constant volume mechanical ventilation, a temporal increase in P(a-ET)CO_2 may suggest poor pulmonary perfusion secondary to low CO caused by surgical factors such as intraoperative hemorrhage/shock [75,76]. Similar changes secondary to low CO caused by obstruction of venous return (vena cava) or aortic flow during surgical manipulation of the abdominal cavity may be observed in small animal anesthesia.

In anesthetized horses, P(a-ET)CO_2 gradients of 10 mmHg or higher are a common finding and this difference historically was thought to arise as consequence of increased pulmonary/alveolar deadspace in this species [67,303]. The degree of underestimation of $PaCO_2$ by $P_{ET}CO_2$ in dorsally recumbent horses is higher during emergency colic surgery than during elective arthroscopic surgery (Fig. 37.25A,B) [303]. High airway pressures (> 30 cmH_2O) are frequently necessary to provide mechanical ventilation in colic horses with poor chest wall compliance associated with a distended abdomen; the elevated P_{alv} generated by mechanical ventilation under these circumstances likely has a negative impact on lung perfusion because of compression of pulmonary capillaries. However, because of the significant increase in shunted flow observed during routine anesthesia in horses, P(a-ET)CO_2 and $V_{D_{alv}}/V_T$ calculations based on the Enghoff method may not only reflect an increase in pulmonary/alveolar deadspace but should be considered global indices of gas exchange efficiency (Fig. 37.25A,B) [68]. Therapeutic measures to improve CO/pulmonary perfusion (e.g., initiating or increasing dobutamine infusion rate) should be considered if P(a-ET)CO_2 is excessively increased. In the case of high airway pressures observed during anesthesia for colic surgery, the surgeon should expedite abdominal decompression to minimize the negative impact of distended bowel on chest wall compliance. An improvement in lung perfusion in these cases may also be associated with increases in PaO_2 due to better $\dot{V}_A/\dot{Q}$ matching.

Besides influencing gas exchange, pulmonary perfusion is an important factor to consider when evaluating the pharmacokinetics of injectable anesthetics/anesthetic adjuvants, as drugs are subject to *first-pass pulmonary uptake*, that is, the instantaneous extraction of a drug from the circulation by lung tissue [304]. *Pulmonary retention* is related to the percentage of the injected dose that remains in the lungs after the first-pass period [304]. While metabolism will not necessarily occur in the lungs, drugs that are substantially retained

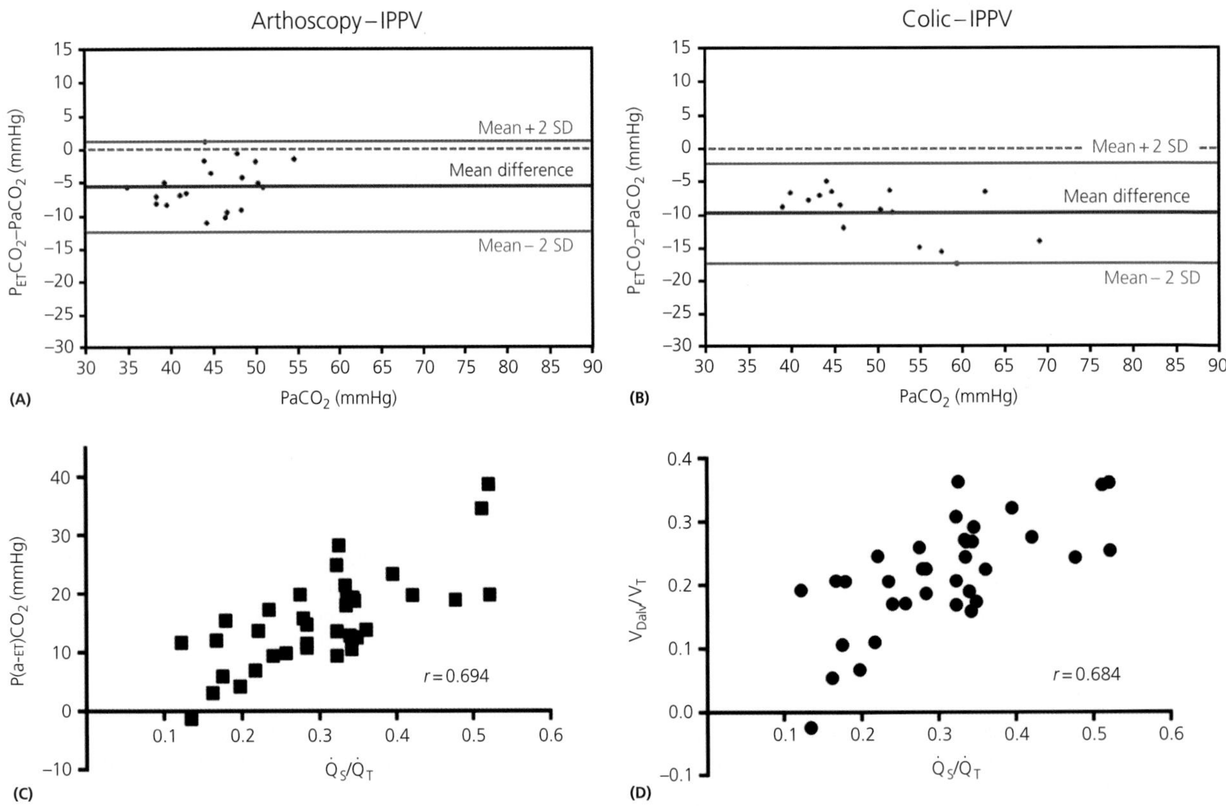

Figure 37.25 **A.** and **B.** Discrepancy between arterial ($PaCO_2$) and end-tidal CO_2 ($P_{ET}CO_2$) in dorsally recumbent horses anesthetized with isoflurane that received intermittent positive-pressure ventilation (IPPV) during arthroscopy and colic surgery. **C.** and **D.** Correlation between arterial to end-tidal CO_2 gradient (P(a-ET)CO_2) or alveolar deadspace fraction ($V_{D_{alv}}/V_T$) with shunt fraction ($\dot{Q}_S/\dot{Q}_T$) in dorsally recumbent spontaneously breathing horses anesthetized with isoflurane and a medetomidine constant rate infusion. SD, standard deviation; *r*, Pearson's correlation coefficient. Source: Adapted from Mosing *et al.* [68]; Koenig *et al.* [303].

in the lungs after the first-pass period are released back into the blood stream as incoming blood concentrations decrease. Propofol undergoes significant first-pass pulmonary retention in animals and man but there is no definitive evidence that this drug is metabolized in the lung. Although studies have suggested that the lungs take part in the metabolism/elimination of propofol in humans [305], this has been a matter of dispute [306,307]. In human surgical patients, propofol was shown to undergo extensive first-pass pulmonary retention (28.4%) but was released back into the circulation, as indicated by comparable propofol concentration versus time curves obtained from blood entering the lungs (mixed venous blood collected from a pulmonary artery catheter) and from blood exiting the lungs (arterial blood collected from a radial artery catheter) [306]. In sheep, 30% of a propofol dose was eliminated during first-pass through the lungs [308]. However, the study could not determine if elimination was attributed to true drug metabolism in the lung or to distribution into a deep lung compartment [308]. In pentobarbital anesthetized cats, first-pass pulmonary retention of propofol is relatively large (60%) and is significantly reduced when fentanyl is administered 30 s before propofol injection, but not when fentanyl is administered 3 or 10 min before propofol [309,310]. Propofol and its metabolites are mainly excreted in urine and an extremely small fraction of propofol is exhaled though the lungs. Because the concentration of propofol in expired gas correlates well with plasma concentrations, monitoring of expired propofol concentrations may have a clinical application in the future [311–313]. Other drugs used during anesthesia such as thiopental, ketamine, opioids, local anesthetics, benzodiazepines, and catecholamines (norepinephrine and dopamine) can be taken up by the lungs and more specific details on handling of these drugs by lung tissue in humans and animal species are available elsewhere [304].

Anesthesia and hypoxic pulmonary vasoconstriction

As discussed previously, HPV is a physiologic mechanism whereby a decrease in alveolar PO_2 causes constriction of adjacent arterioles. In the presence of gas exchange impairment/hypoxemia due to areas of low $\dot{V}_A/\dot{Q}$ ratio or shunt, HPV may improve arterial oxygenation by diverting pulmonary blood flow to better-aerated regions of the lung. Comparison of the effects of anesthetic drugs on PaO_2 and shunt fraction during one-lung ventilation has been used extensively to indirectly assess the effects of inhalant or intravenous anesthetics on HPV in humans, but this model fails to evaluate the effects of lung regions with low PaO_2 on the vascular tone of adjacent arterioles. On the other hand, *in vitro* studies using isolated lung preparations ventilated with low F_IO_2 may be able to demonstrate drug effects on HPV but may not be directly extrapolated to clinical situations.

Attenuation of HPV by some anesthetic drugs may in part explain the lower than expected PaO_2 values observed during general anesthesia. Early experimental studies in the 1970s using a perfused lung model in cats and dogs originally postulated that inhalant anesthetics could inhibit HPV, and that this could lead to an increase in the proportion of mixed venous blood flowing through areas of low $\dot{V}_A/\dot{Q}$ ratio or non-ventilated lung areas (shunt), thereby contributing to a decrease in PaO_2 during anesthesia [314]. This postulation was later confirmed using isolated rat lung preparations, which showed that HPV was inhibited by inhalant agents (halothane, methoxyflurane, and ether), but remained unaffected by injectable anesthetics (barbiturates and ketamine) [315]. Other *in vitro* studies supported the observation that all contemporary inhalant anesthetics (isoflurane, sevoflurane, and desflurane) would block HPV and that this effect could, at least in part, explain the absolute or relative hypoxemia observed in animals receiving inhalant anesthesia [316–318]. Although isoflurane was reported to inhibit HPV [316,319–321], some early studies failed to show a consistent effect of this inhalant on HPV/arterial oxygenation in anesthetized animals and humans due to methodological issues, including lack of comparison of the HPV response to that of non-anesthetized individuals, the confounding effect of other concurrently administered drugs (e.g., pentobarbital anesthesia), or the lack of comparison of the pressor response to alveolar hypoxia at a fixed pulmonary artery flow [322–325]. Because the pressor response of pulmonary arterial vessels to low alveolar PO_2 (i.e., HPV) is also flow dependent, the effects of drugs on HPV should be compared at a similar pulmonary artery flow [326,327].

The effects of inhalant anesthetics on HPV are controversial at best. Studies performed during one-lung ventilation in humans have suggested that sevoflurane and desflurane inhibit HPV in a similar fashion as isoflurane because of absence of differences in PaO_2 among these drugs [328–331]. However, sevoflurane and desflurane did not inhibit the pressor response to low alveolar PO_2 at a similar CO/pulmonary flow range in piglets [332]. In chronically instrumented dogs, the increase in pulmonary artery pressure in response to alveolar hypoxia (due to low F_IO_2) at a similar pulmonary artery flow indicates that isoflurane, but not sevoflurane or desflurane, inhibits HPV in comparison to the HPV observed in the conscious state (Fig. 37.26A,B) [327,333]. Based on the same methodology, ketamine did not alter HPV while propofol potentiated HPV in comparison to the HPV observed in conscious state in dogs (Fig. 37.26C,D) [334].

Although some experimental models provide evidence that the pressor response to low alveolar PO_2 is maintained by propofol, ketamine, desflurane, and sevoflurane [327,332–334], there is no evidence that any one anesthetic drug is associated with better arterial oxygenation during one-lung ventilation, with the exception of propofol [328–331,335,336]. In conscious animals presenting with lung disease associated with areas of low $\dot{V}_A/\dot{Q}$ ratio and shunt, HPV may represent an important mechanism that prevents further oxygenation impairment. Under these circumstances, the anesthesiologist could opt for drugs that are more likely to preserve the HPV response observed during the conscious state (i.e., propofol, ketamine, sevoflurane, and desflurane).

Effects of anesthesia on ventilation–perfusion relationships

All forms of general anesthesia are associated with some degree of deterioration in pulmonary gas exchange. A decrease in arterial oxygenation that cannot be explained by hypoventilation/hypercapnia is commonly observed in otherwise healthy animals undergoing general anesthesia. An increased $P(A\text{-}a)O_2$ resulting in lower-than-expected PaO_2 levels is usually attributed to a mismatch between ventilation and perfusion of the lungs ($\dot{V}_A/\dot{Q}$ mismatch); more specifically due to areas of low $\dot{V}_A/\dot{Q}$ ratio (between 0.01 and 0.1) or areas of the lungs that are perfused but not ventilated ($\dot{V}_A/\dot{Q}$ ratio = 0). Development of atelectasis of dependent lung regions resulting in shunted flow to the lungs ($\dot{V}_A/\dot{Q}$ ratio = 0) combined with the inhibition of HPV is the main cause of oxygenation impairment during general anesthesia. As previously discussed, factors such as body mass, obesity, type of recumbency, intrabdominal volume/pressure, and inspired oxygen concentration, may contribute to development of atelectasis and poor lung compliance

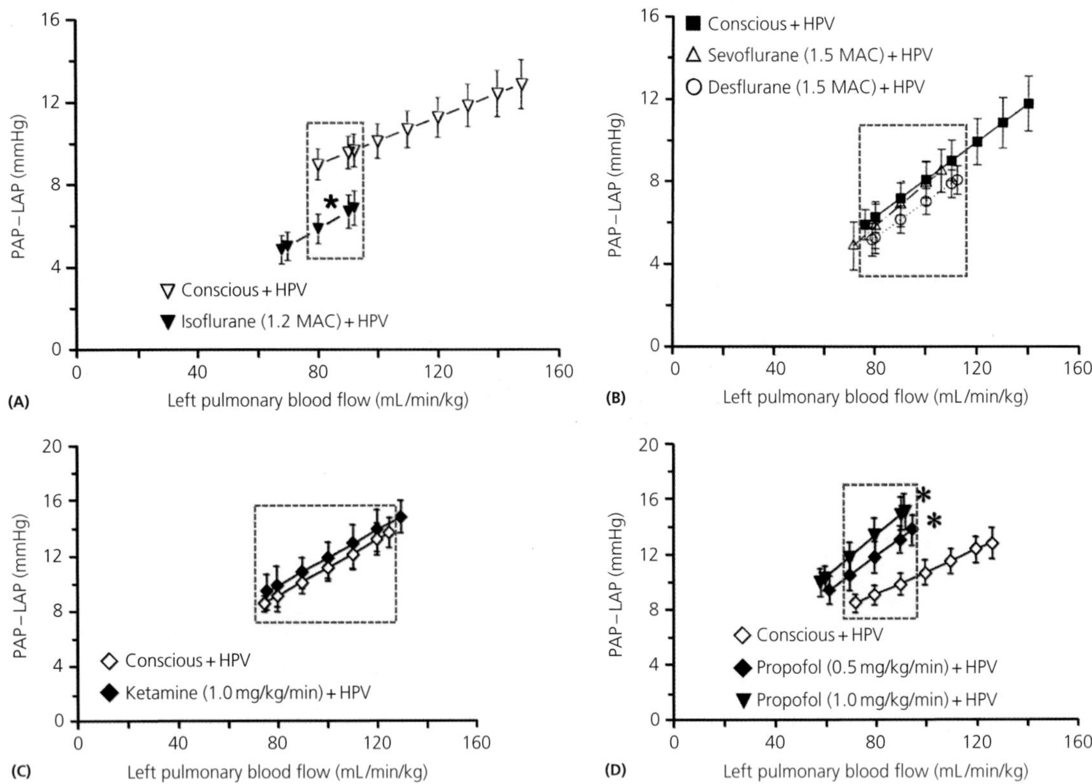

Figure 37.26 Relationships between pulmonary perfusion pressure (pulmonary artery pressure [PAP] minus left atrial pressure [LAP]) and changes in left pulmonary artery blood flow in conscious and anesthetized dogs where hypoxic pulmonary vasoconstriction (HPV) was induced by lowering the inspired oxygen fraction. When compared to the conscious state, a decrease in pressure at the same flow range denotes inhibition of HPV and vice versa (dashed red squares). **A.** Isoflurane (1.2 minimum alveolar concentration [MAC]) attenuates HPV compared to the conscious state. **B.** Sevoflurane and desflurane (1.5 MAC) do not alter HPV compared to the conscious state. **C.** Ketamine does not alter HPV compared to the conscious state. **D.** Propofol potentiates HPV compared to the conscious state. *Significant difference from HPV observed in conscious dogs. Source: Adapted from Lennon and Murray [327]; Lesitsky *et al.* [333]; Nakayama and Murray [334].

during anesthesia [27,28,261,268,337]. There are species differences in the development of $\dot{V}_A/\dot{Q}$ mismatch and shunt. Horses are particularly prone to develop a large shunt (> 15–20% of CO) due to the presence of large areas of alveolar collapse during anesthesia, with body positioning in dorsal recumbency resulting in larger areas of atelectasis and shunt when compared to lateral recumbency (Figs. 37.27 and 37.28) [268,299]. As previously noted, because of their body mass, large animal species are more prone to compression of the lungs leading to atelectasis than small animals. More specifically, in horses, compression of the lungs by gravitational forces acting on the chest wall, and by abdominal viscera pushing the diaphragm forward, are of greater magnitude than in dogs and cats, explaining why this species develops more atelectasis/shunted blood flow during anesthesia (Figs. 37.27 and 37.28).

In humans, atelectasis that develops after induction of anesthesia may extend into the postoperative period and cause some degree of oxygenation impairment after recovery and has been associated with a higher incidence of postoperative complications (e.g., pneumonia) [338,339]. Evidence of the negative impact of intraoperative atelectasis in the postanesthetic period in veterinary species is currently lacking.

The gold standard method for assessing the matching between ventilation and perfusion of the lung ($\dot{V}_A/\dot{Q}$) is the multiple inert gas elimination technique, which has advanced the understanding of the mechanism of gas exchange impairment during anesthesia in humans and animal species [299,301,340,341]. In normal conscious humans, a bimodal distribution of $\dot{V}_A/\dot{Q}$ ratios has been identified, with one mode centered around the ratio of 1 and another, smaller mode, within low $\dot{V}_A/\dot{Q}$ regions [341].

Fig. 37.29 shows changes in ventilation and perfusion matching evaluated by a multiple inert gas elimination technique in conscious and anesthetized horses [299]. The relative distribution of ventilation and perfusion in conscious standing animals with normal lungs is centered around 1, which is the ideal matching between ventilation and perfusion to achieve optimal gas exchange. A small area of high $\dot{V}_A/\dot{Q}$ ratio (between 10 and 100) and of shunted flow ($\dot{V}_A/\dot{Q} = 0$), which represents < 3% of total pulmonary blood flow ($\dot{Q}_S/\dot{Q}_T < 3\%$), may also be observed in healthy horses in a quadrupedal position (Fig. 37.29A) [153,299]. After induction of anesthesia in horses breathing spontaneously, there is a marked increase in shunt flow, which often exceeds 30% of total pulmonary blood flow ($\dot{Q}_S/\dot{Q}_T > 30\%$) when animals are positioned in dorsal recumbency. Such increases in shunt flow result in oxygenation impairment characterized by marked increases in $P(A\text{-}a)O_2$ (Fig. 37.29B). Use of conventional mechanical ventilation with zero end-expiratory pressure (ZEEP) or 10 cm H_2O of PEEP does not consistently decrease the shunt in dorsally recumbent horses and may contribute to further decreases in PaO_2 if inotropic support is not used to counteract the negative effects of positive-pressure ventilation on pulmonary blood flow (CO) (Fig. 37.29C,D).

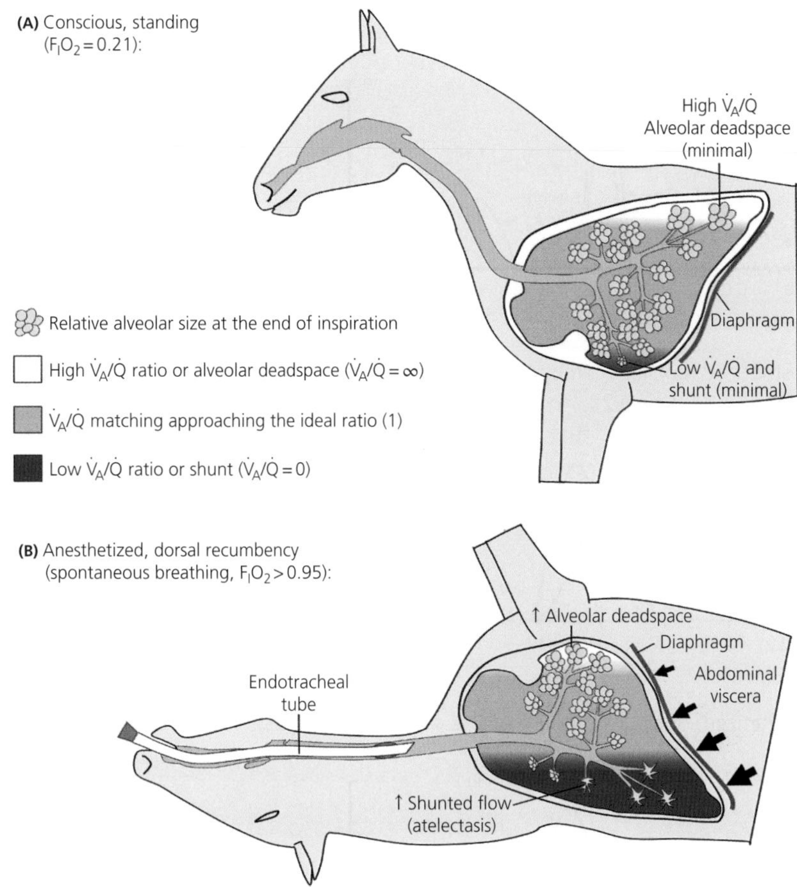

Figure 37.27 Effect of anesthesia and postural changes on $\dot{V}_A/\dot{Q}$ matching in horses. **A.** In conscious standing horses, most of the lung has $\dot{V}_A/\dot{Q}$ matching approaching the ideal ratio (1). **B.** During general anesthesia in spontaneously breathing horses positioned in dorsal recumbency, compression of the lung tissue by the weight of abdominal viscera and cephalad displacement of the diaphragm contributes to a marked increase in shunt because of atelectasis of dependent areas of both lungs. Alveolar deadspace may also be increased because of decreased pulmonary blood flow and MPAP induced by anesthesia in relation to the conscious state.

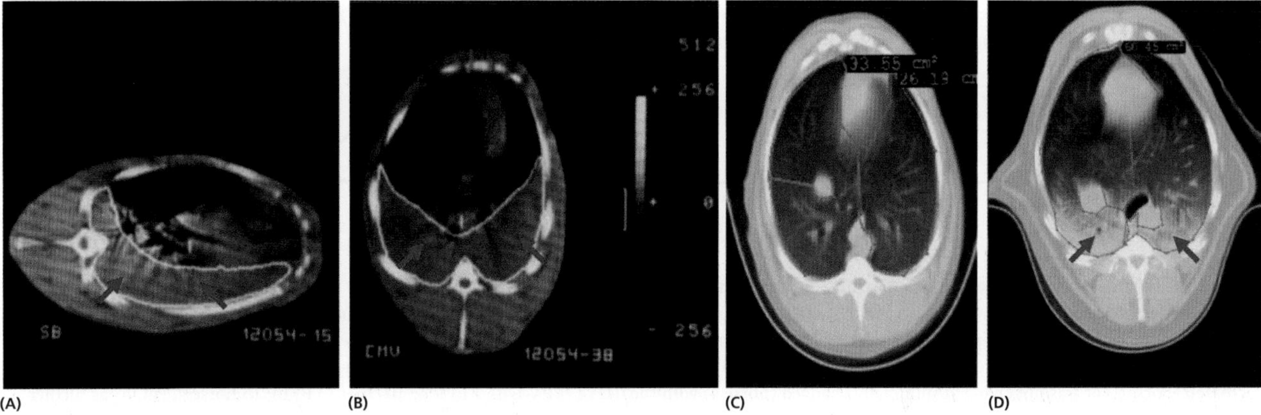

Figure 37.28 **A.** and **B.** Computed tomography images of the lungs of a spontaneously breathing pony anesthetized with an inspired oxygen concentration close to 100% in **A.** lateral and **B.** dorsal recumbency. The large dense areas of dependent lung regions encircled by white lines (arrows) were identified as atelectatic lung tissue by histology. **C.** and **D.** Computed tomography images of the lungs of a dog anesthetized in dorsal recumbency with an inspired oxygen concentration of **C.** 40% oxygen, or **D.** 100% oxygen receiving mechanical ventilation in a volume-controlled mode (V_T = 15 mL/kg, inspiration to expiration ratio = 1:2, and 25% inspiratory hold). Use of 40% oxygen eliminated the dense (atelectatic) lung areas observed with 100% oxygen (arrows). Note that the dense atelectatic areas observed in **D.** dorsally recumbent dogs inspiring 100% oxygen are less extensive than in **B.** dorsally recumbent horses inhaling a similar oxygen concentration. Source: Reproduced from Staffieri *et al.* [261], with permission of American Veterinary Medical Association; Nyman *et al.* [268], with permission of John Wiley & Sons, Inc.

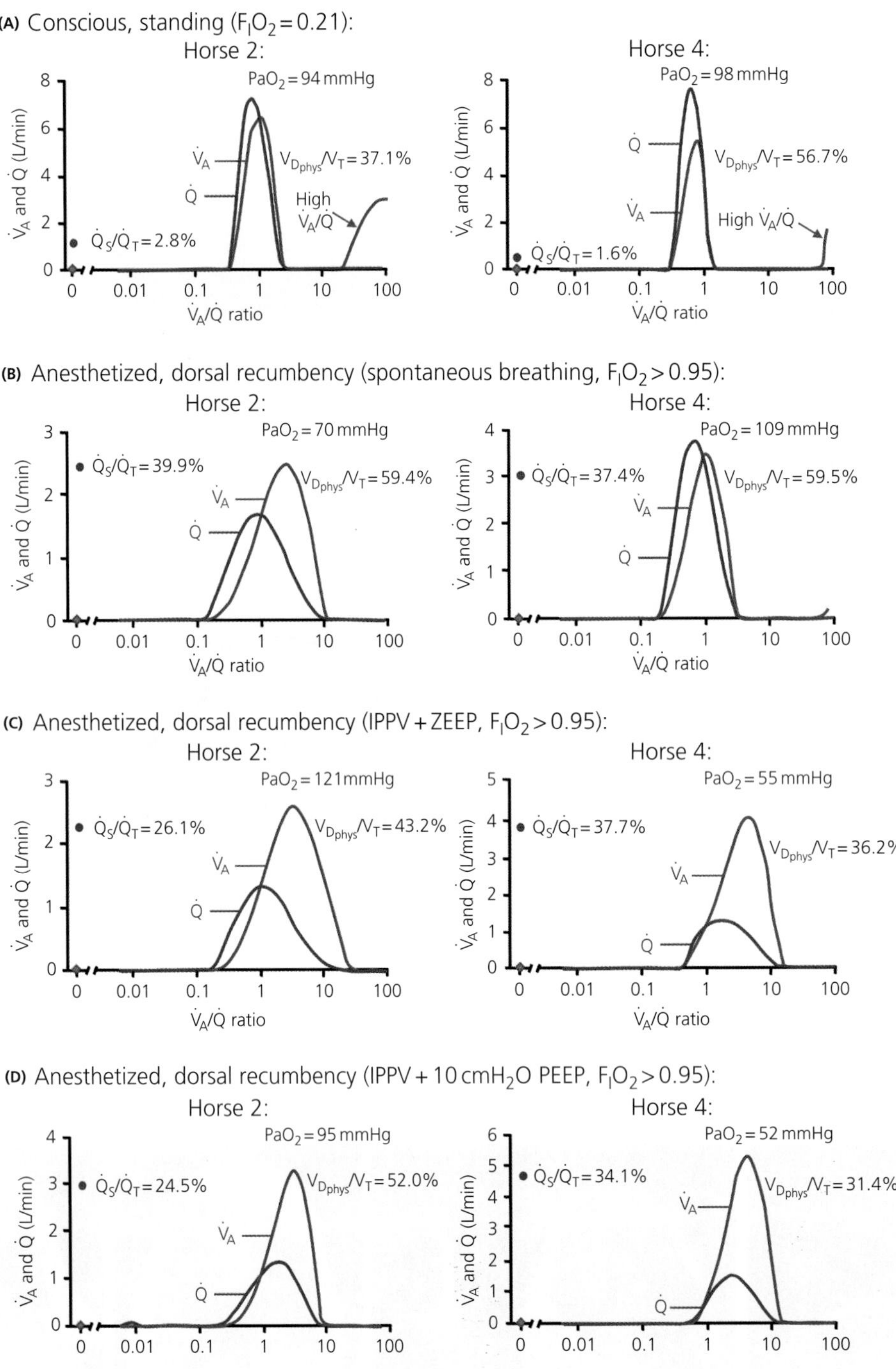

Figure 37.29 Examples of $\dot{V}_A/\dot{Q}$ matching as measured using the multiple inert gas elimination technique in two horses (horse 2 and horse 4) while conscious and anesthetized with halothane. **A.** Conscious, standing; **B.** Anesthetized, dorsal recumbency, spontaneous breathing; **C.** Anesthetized, dorsal recumbency, intermittent positive-pressure ventilation (IPPV) with zero end-expiratory pressure (ZEEP); **D.** Anesthetized, dorsal recumbency, IPPV with 10 cmH_2O positive end-expired pressure (PEEP). Notice that the large shunt that developed during anesthesia in dorsal recumbency was only slightly decreased (horse 2) or was not changed/minimally changed (horse 4) with the use of IPPV with ZEEP or 10 cmH_2O PEEP. In horse 4, PaO_2 was further decreased by IPPV in comparison to PaO_2 during spontaneous breathing because mechanical ventilation resulted in a major decrease in CO/pulmonary blood flow. Source: Adapted from Nyman and Hedenstierna [299].

An increase in $V_{D_{phys}}/V_T$ may also occur due to an increase in $V_{D_{alv}}$ ($\dot{V}_A/\dot{Q}$ ratio = ∞ [infinity]) associated with decreased pulmonary blood flow/CO and MPAP in anesthetized horses. In conscious animals, increased deadspace ventilation can be compensated for by an increase in $\dot{V}_A$ to maintain $PaCO_2$ levels within physiological ranges. During general anesthesia, increased $V_{D_{phys}}/V_T$ (caused by increases in $V_{D_{alv}}$) may aggravate hypercapnia in spontaneously breathing patients as the ventilatory response to increased CO_2 is suppressed.

As the predominant mechanism responsible for the increase in intrapulmonary shunt during anesthesia in humans with normal lungs is compression atelectasis, the use of lower F_IO_2 by mixing oxygen and air in inspired gas per se does not abolish atelectasis during anesthesia and surgery [342]. However, current guidelines for lung protective mechanical ventilation in anesthetized human patients include the recommendation to set the F_IO_2 after intubation to ≤ 0.4 with subsequent adjustments in F_IO_2 to the lowest value necessary to maintain oxygen saturation monitored by pulse oximetry ≥ 94% (strength of recommendation: weak) [343].

Current evidence indicates that lower F_IO_2 values (e.g., 0.4) may decrease intrapulmonary shunt in those animal species where compression atelectasis is less likely to play a major role in causing oxygenation impairment (e.g., dogs and cats) [261,273]. A study in horses anesthetized with halothane and positioned in lateral recumbency suggests that a low F_IO_2 (0.3) results in less respiratory depression/hypercapnia and less $\dot{V}_A/\dot{Q}$ mismatch (decreased P(A-a) O_2 secondary to a smaller shunt fraction) in comparison to a high F_IO_2 (> 0.85) [190]. However, as the duration of anesthesia was extended to 4 h with 30% inspired oxygen, PaO_2 decreased to levels characterized as clinically relevant hypoxemia (PaO_2 = 96 ± 13 mmHg at 30 min versus PaO_2 = 60 ± 4 mmHg at 240 min). Qualitatively similar findings were observed in spontaneously breathing horses anesthetized with isoflurane in dorsal recumbency, where a 50% inspired oxygen concentration decreased P(A-a) O_2 but increased the risk of hypoxemia (PaO_2 = 70 ± 18 mmHg after 90 min of anesthesia) in comparison to > 95% inspired oxygen (178 ± 114 mmHg after 90 min of anesthesia) (Fig. 37.30A) [192]. Although the use of 100% oxygen as the carrier gas may result in greater $\dot{V}_A/\dot{Q}$ mismatch from absorption atelectasis, anesthesia with

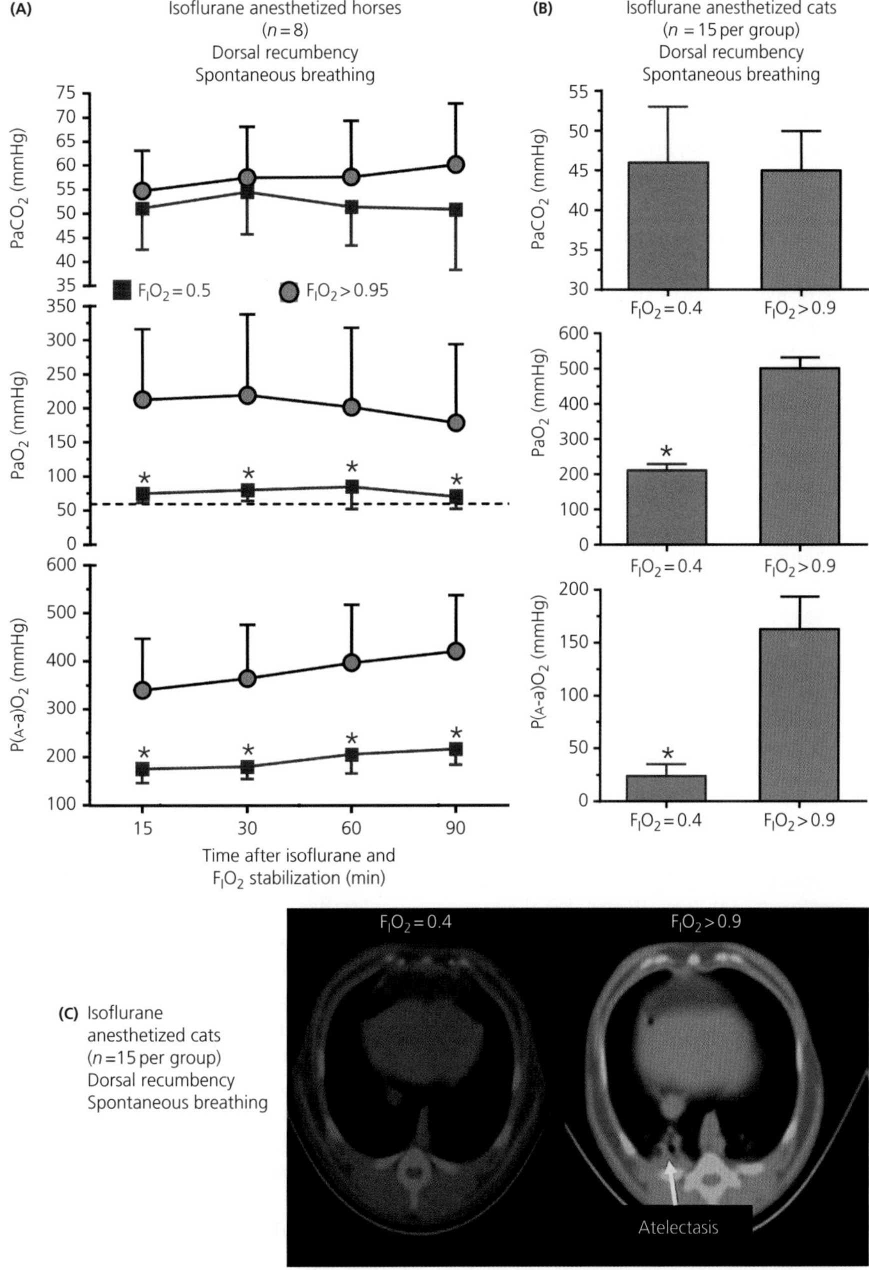

Figure 37.30 **A.** and **B.** Effects of a decrease in inspired oxygen concentration (F_IO_2) during isoflurane anesthesia in spontaneously breathing, dorsally recumbent horses and cats (see text for explanation). **C.** Computed tomography images of the lungs of an isoflurane-anesthetized spontaneously breathing cat in dorsal recumbency with F_IO_2 = 0.4 and > 0.9. *Significantly lower than high F_IO_2. Source: Adapted from Crumley *et al.* [192]; Staffieri *et al.* [273], with permission of Elsevier.

high F_IO_2 still is safer in spontaneously breathing horses because it may prevent hypoxemia under these circumstances. Experimental studies carried out during conventional mechanical ventilation in dorsally recumbent horses (V_T = 15 mL/kg and *f* adjusted to maintain eucapnia) have shown that inhaling a 50% oxygen concentration does not reduce the $\dot{Q}_S/\dot{Q}_T$ in comparison to a > 95% oxygen concentration (*n* = 5 per group) [194]. Contrasting with the high incidence of hypoxemia during anesthesia with lower F_IO_2 (0.3–0.5) in spontaneously breathing horses, use of 40% inspired oxygen in isoflurane-anesthetized cats not receiving mechanical ventilatory support resulted in greater optimization of oxygen transfer from alveoli to capillary blood ($P(A\text{-}a)O_2$ = 24 ± 11 mmHg with F_IO_2 = 0.4 versus $P(A\text{-}a)O_2$ = 163 ± 31 mmHg with F_IO_2 > 0.9) and was not associated with hypoxemia (Fig. 37.30B) [273]. Computed tomography images confirmed that decreases in F_IO_2 from > 0.9 to 0.4 decreased atelectatic areas of the lungs, likely because of decreased absorption atelectasis (Fig. 37.30C). In mechanically ventilated isoflurane-anesthetized dogs, computed tomography also showed that 40% inspired oxygen reduced poorly aerated and non-aerated lung areas in comparison to 100% oxygen, probably because of decreased absorption atelectasis [261] (Fig. 37.28B). Reduction of atelectasis with 40% oxygen in dogs resulted in lower $P(A\text{-}a)O_2$ than with 100% oxygen (36 ± 12 mmHg versus 177 ± 49 mmHg). Use of lower F_IO_2 may reduce lung collapse without increasing the risk of hypoxemia in small animal species (dogs and cats). However, at present, there is no evidence to support the potential benefits of preventing absorption atelectasis during the early recovery phase and postanesthetic period in normal veterinary patients.

In contrast to other species, intravenous injection of α_2-adrenergic receptor agonists has been reported to cause moderate (PaO_2 < 60 mmHg) to severe (PaO_2 < 40 mmHg) hypoxemia in sheep [209,344]. The severity of hypoxemia is highly variable among different breeds and among individual animals of the same breed [345]; however, it may be life-threatening in animals with pre-existing respiratory disease or in individual animals that have greater sensitivity to this adverse reaction. In addition to low PaO_2 levels, $PaCO_2$ may be normal or below normal values [209]; hypocapnia observed concurrently with hypoxemia is likely caused by an increase in $\dot{V}_E$ secondary to activation of peripheral chemoreceptors by low PaO_2 levels (hypoxic ventilatory drive).

Experimental evidence shows that hypoxemia caused by sedation with α_2-adrenergic receptor agonists in sheep is the result of an increase in shunted flow ($\dot{Q}_S/\dot{Q}_T$) secondary to an inflammatory response in the lungs/pulmonary edema [345,346]. Studies using a pulmonary artery catheter (Fig. 37.14), have shown that the oxygenation impairment caused by α_2-adrenergic receptor agonists in anesthetized sheep is associated with pulmonary hypertension (MPAP > 25 mmHg) and significant increases in PAOP, which often exceeds the threshold associated with pulmonary edema caused by increased hydrostatic pressure (PAOP > 15–18 mmHg) [345,346] (Fig. 37.31A). The marked increase in PAOP (> 15–18 mmHg), reported 2 min after intravenous dexmedetomidine (2 μg/kg) in sevoflurane-anesthetized sheep, suggests that early development of oxygenation impairment/pulmonary edema is secondary to increased hydrostatic pressure in the microcirculation, which leads to the movement of fluid from the intravascular compartment to the alveolar interstitium/alveolar lumen [345] (Fig. 37.31A).

Sheep are particularly susceptible to the adverse effects of α_2-adrenergic receptor agonists on the pulmonary circulation where significant increases in MPAP and PAOP are observed after relatively small cumulative doses of medetomidine (1.5 μg/kg, intravenously) [346]. Based on the pathophysiology of pulmonary hypertension discussed previously, cumulative doses of medetomidine (0.5 to 4.0 μg/kg/min) likely cause pre- and postcapillary pulmonary hypertension (increases in MPAP secondary to increases in PVR and PAOP, respectively) [346]. This response contrasts with a study evaluating progressively increasing doses of medetomidine (1 to 20 μg/kg intravenously) in conscious dogs, where only a high dose (20 μg/kg) significantly increased PAOP and MPAP [347] (Fig. 37.31B). However, even when medetomidine was administered at doses that may cause clinically relevant increases in pulmonary capillary hydrostatic pressure (PAOP > 15–18 mmHg), there was no evidence of pulmonary edema as PaO_2 was not significantly altered in healthy dogs (Fig. 37.31B). Collectively, these results suggest that elevated hydrostatic pressure is not the only factor that triggers the pulmonary edema/oxygenation impairment observed following α_2-adrenergic receptor agonist administration in sheep.

Damage of the capillary endothelium and type-1 alveolar cells, intra-alveolar hemorrhage/edema, and interstitial edema has been reported 60 min after intravenous xylazine (0.15 mg/kg) administration to sheep [348]. Besides the pulmonary edema of hydrostatic origin, it has been proposed that damage to lung parenchyma/pulmonary edema may also result from an inflammatory component that involves activation of pulmonary intravascular macrophages (PIMs) [348]. These are phagocytic cells that play an important role in removing particulate material from the circulation in some animal species (ruminants, pigs, and cats) [349]. It appears that PIMs are activated early during the course of pulmonary edema, as these cells present morphological changes 3 min after α_2-adrenergic receptor agonist injection in sheep [348].

Besides damage to lung parenchyma *in vitro*, studies have also shown that α_2-adrenergic receptor agonists induce airway smooth muscle contraction in sheep but not in other species such as cattle and horses [350–352]. Bronchoconstriction, combined with lung edema, may be responsible for the increase airway resistance (R_{aw}) observed following intravenous medetomidine administration in halothane-anesthetized sheep receiving mechanical ventilation [346]. Increased R_{aw}/bronchoconstriction might be caused by proinflammatory mediators (cytokines) secondary to lung damage or by direct stimulation of α_2-adrenergic receptors located in airway smooth muscle [351]. Besides increasing R_{aw}, α_2-adrenergic receptor agonists also decrease dynamic compliance of the respiratory system (C_{RS}), which can be attributed to a decrease in lung compliance due to pulmonary hemorrhage/edema, although dynamic C_{RS} may also decrease if resistance to gas flow (R_{aw}) is elevated, as explained previously.

α_2-Adrenergic receptor agonists that cannot cross the blood–brain barrier and are devoid of sedative/analgesic effects also induce hypoxemia and pulmonary inflammation/edema, providing evidence that these adverse effects are mediated by peripheral α_2-adrenergic receptor stimulation [344,346,348]. Intravenous administration of vatinoxan (0.75 mg/kg), a peripheral α_2-adrenergic receptor antagonist that does not cross the blood–brain barrier, can prevent hypoxemia caused by a high dose of xylazine in sheep (0.5 mg/kg, intravenously) without an apparent effect on sedation [353] (Fig. 37.32). Although these results suggest that vatinoxan may be a promising option to prevent the adverse pulmonary effects of α_2-adrenergic receptor agonists in this species, its use was associated with more severe histopathological changes in the lung which requires further investigation [353]. α_2-Adrenergic receptor

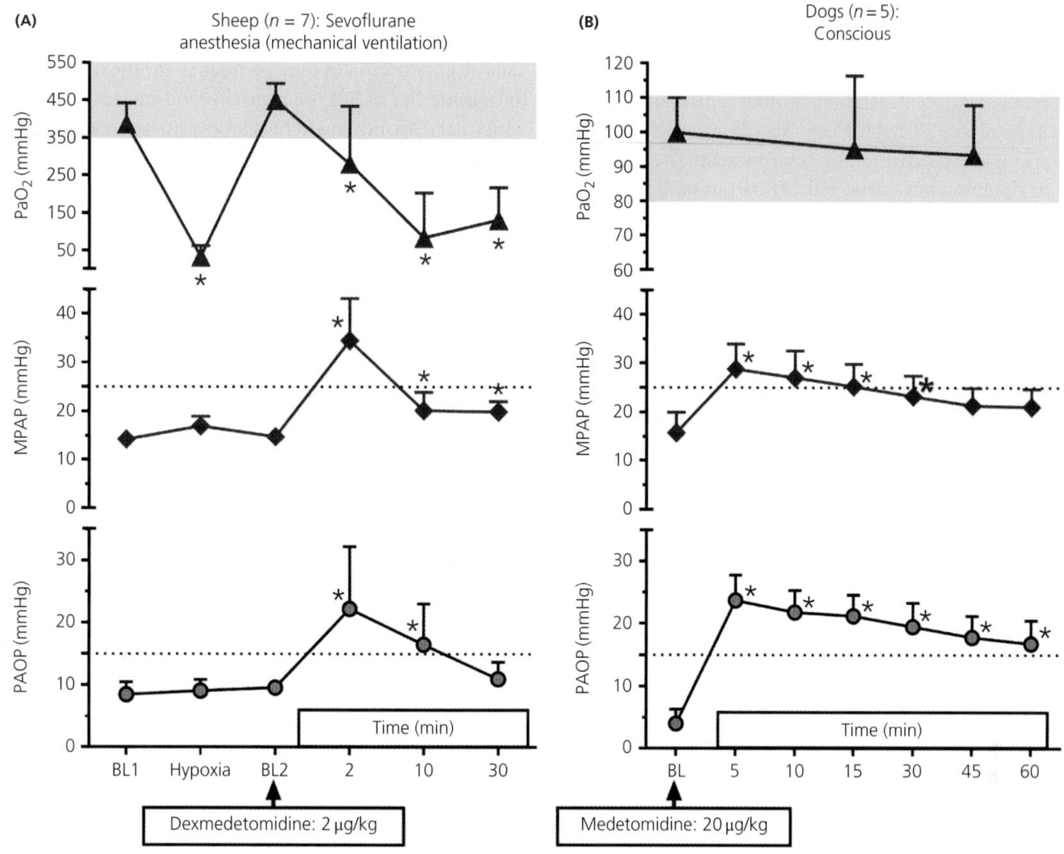

Figure 37.31 Hemodynamic changes in pulmonary circulation and PaO_2 observed before and after intravenous α_2-adrenergic receptor agonist administration (mean and standard deviation) in sheep and dogs. **A.** In sevoflurane-anesthetized sheep receiving mechanical ventilation with an F_IO_2 of 1.0 (BL1), a decrease in F_IO_2 to 0.1 (Hypoxia) caused a marked decrease in PaO_2 (< 40 mmHg) but did not increase MPAP likely due to inhibition of hypoxic pulmonary vasoconstriction by sevoflurane. After F_IO_2 was increased again to 1.0 (BL2), a small dose of dexmedetomidine (2 μg/kg, intravenously) transiently increased MPAP and PAOP to values characterizing pulmonary hypertension (MPAP > 25 mmHg) and excessive increases in pulmonary capillary pressure (PAOP > 15 mmHg) (indicated by dashed lines). These changes were paralleled by a longer-lasting oxygenation impairment, as shown by the lower-than-expected PaO_2 values (gray shaded area) persisting for 30 min after dexmedetomidine administration. **B.** In conscious dogs, a high dose of medetomidine (20 μg/kg intravenously) induced longer-lasting increases MPAP and PAOP, with values that characterize pulmonary hypertension and excessive increases in pulmonary capillary pressure (indicated by dashed lines), but these changes were not accompanied by a decrease in PaO_2 below normal ranges for animals breathing ambient air (gray shaded area). See text for further explanation. BL1, baseline recorded with F_IO_2 = 1.0; Hypoxia data recorded after reducing F_IO_2 to 0.1; BL2 baseline recorded after returning F_IO_2 to 1.0, before dexmedetomidine injection; BL, baseline recorded before medetomidine injection in animals breathing ambient air (F_IO_2 = 0.21); *Significantly different from baseline. Source: Adapted from Kästner *et al.* [345]; Pypendop and Verstegen [347].

agonists are potent sedatives and analgesics that are useful as premedication in sheep. To minimize their adverse effects on respiratory function in this species, intravenous administration should be avoided, and the lowest possible dose used to attain a satisfactory sedative effect; their use in sheep with pre-existing respiratory disease is contraindicated [354].

Oxygen transport

Arterial oxygen content

Oxygen is transported from the lungs to tissues largely in chemical combination with hemoglobin, with only a small fraction of total arterial oxygen content (CaO_2) dissolved in plasma (PaO_2). Mammalian hemoglobin consists of four-unit molecules. Each unit molecule contains a heme group, which is a protoporphyrin consisting of four pyrroles with a central ferrous ion (Fe^{2+}). Oxygen combines reversibly with the Fe^{2+} in proportion to the PO_2. At complete saturation, each gram of hemoglobin combines with approximately 1.36 mL of oxygen. This is the total carrying capacity of hemoglobin, or four oxygen molecules combined with each hemoglobin molecule [355,356]. The total oxygen content of arterial blood, in mL of oxygen per deciliter (100 mL) of blood, is calculated as follows:

$$CaO_2 = (SaO_2 \times Hb \times 1.36) + (PaO_2 \times 0.0031)$$

The first part of the equation corresponds to the amount of oxygen carried by hemoglobin in mL/dL, where SaO_2 is the hemoglobin saturation in arterial blood (expressed as fraction), Hb is the hemoglobin concentration (g/dL), and 1.36 is the maximum oxygen-carrying capacity of fully saturated hemoglobin. The second part of the equation corresponds to the amount of oxygen dissolved in blood (mL/dL), calculated as PaO_2 multiplied by the solubility coefficient of oxygen in 1 deciliter of blood (0.0031) [355,356].

The oxyhemoglobin dissociation curve and the Bohr effect

As most of the oxygen is carried by hemoglobin, it is important to understand the oxyhemoglobin dissociation curve, which describes the relationship between hemoglobin saturation and PO_2 (Fig. 37.33A). The ability of hemoglobin to combine with oxygen depends on the PO_2 in the surrounding environment. The sigmoidal shape of the oxyhemoglobin curve reflects its physiologic role in uploading oxygen in the lungs and offloading oxygen to the tissues.

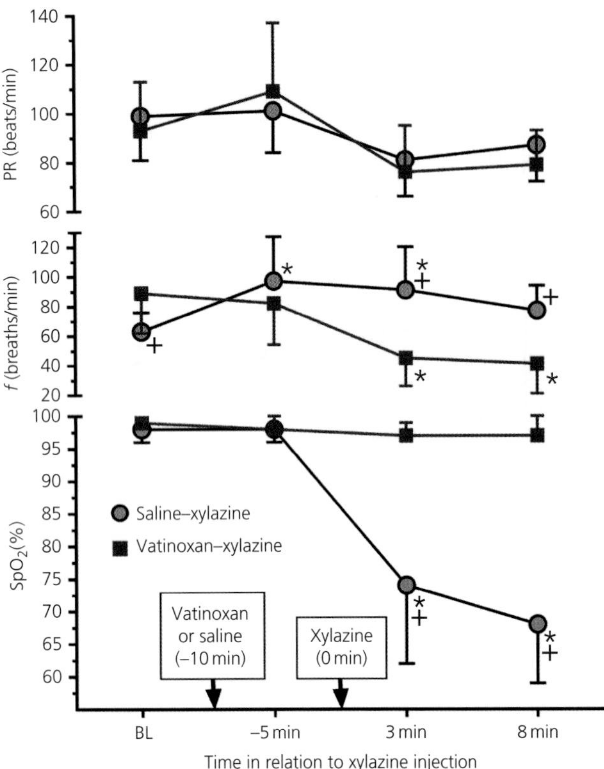

Figure 37.32 Effects of a peripheral α_2-adrenergic receptor antagonist, vatinoxan (0.75 mg/kg, intravenously, $n = 7$), or saline ($n = 7$) administered 10 min before sedation with intravenous xylazine (0.5 mg/kg) in sheep (mean and standard deviation). PR, pulse rate; *f*, breathing frequency; SpO_2, pulse oximetry hemoglobin saturation; BL, baseline. Source: Adapted from Adam *et al.* [353].

At the pulmonary capillary level, hemoglobin has a high affinity to oxygen, being almost fully saturated in a normal conscious animal. This affinity translates into a tendency for the oxyhemoglobin curve to become flat as PO_2 in arterial blood increases above 70 mmHg, which corresponds to a hemoglobin saturation above 94% [355,356]. At the systemic capillary level, transfer of oxygen from blood to tissues is facilitated by the decrease in hemoglobin's affinity for oxygen. This is reflected by the steeper slope of the oxyhemoglobin curve at PO_2 values less than 60 mmHg. At a PO_2 of 40 mmHg, which is the oxygen tension typically found in mixed venous blood draining systemic capillaries, the hemoglobin saturation falls to approximately 75% and the total oxygen content in mixed venous blood is approximately 24–25% less than in arterial blood [355,356].

The position of the oxyhemoglobin curve is dynamic and is modified according to changes in metabolic status. Physiological conditions that signal an increase in metabolic activity such as increased temperature, high PCO_2, and low pH decrease the affinity of hemoglobin for oxygen and cause a rightward shift of the oxyhemoglobin dissociation curve (Fig. 37.33B). Physiological changes that signal decreased metabolic activity (decreased temperature, low PCO_2, and increased pH) increase the affinity of hemoglobin for oxygen and cause a leftward shift of the oxyhemoglobin dissociation curve [355,356]. Certain enzyme systems aid the dissociation of oxygen from hemoglobin, the most completely studied being the enzyme system producing 2,3-diphosphoglycerate (2,3-DPG). This enzyme is a byproduct of glycolysis within the red blood cells that enhances the dissociation of oxygen from hemoglobin by competing with oxygen for the binding site. Anemia, chronic hypoxemia, and acclimation to high altitude reduce oxygen content in blood and stimulate glycolysis. Increased glycolysis and 2,3-DPG production during these clinical conditions facilitate unloading of oxygen at the tissue level. A lowered level of this enzyme, as occurs with stored blood used for transfusion, increases the affinity of hemoglobin for oxygen and shifts the dissociation curve to the left [355,356]. While changes in 2,3-DPG levels are a major factor influencing the loading and unloading of oxygen in humans, in some animal species, including cats and ruminants, hemoglobin affinity for oxygen is less affected by 2,3-DPG. In these species, chloride ions (Cl^-) play a greater role in modifying hemoglobin oxygen affinity [357–359]. As red blood cells reach the capillaries of the systemic circulation, rising CO_2 levels originating from tissue aerobic activity form HCO_3^- inside

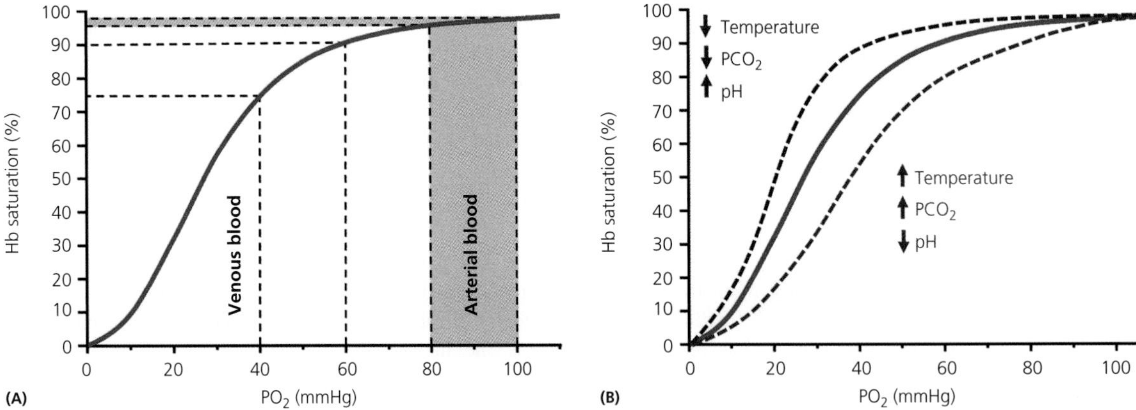

Figure 37.33 **A.** Oxyhemoglobin curve describing the relationship between hemoglobin (Hb) saturation and oxygen partial pressure (PO_2). **B.** Effect of changes in temperature, pH, and partial pressure of carbon dioxide (PCO_2) on the affinity of hemoglobin for oxygen (hemoglobin curve) (see text for explanation).

these cells. In a mechanism named "chloride shift" or "Hamburger effect" (see further details below), the HCO_3^- is driven out of red blood cells to plasma in exchange for Cl^-. The increase in Cl^- inside the red blood cells, in a similar fashion as 2,3-DPG, reduces affinity of hemoglobin for oxygen, facilitating the unloading of oxygen to tissues [357–359].

In 1904, the Danish physiologist Christian Bohr first showed that increased PCO_2 decreases the affinity of hemoglobin for oxygen [360]. The effects of changes in pH and PCO_2 on the affinity of hemoglobin for oxygen (*Bohr effect*) play an important role in facilitating the uploading of oxygen in the lungs and its subsequent transfer to tissues (Fig. 37.33B) [361]. As CO_2 is eliminated by alveolar ventilation, the decrease in PCO_2 and increase in pH at the pulmonary capillary level augments the affinity of hemoglobin for oxygen (leftward shift of the oxyhemoglobin curve), facilitating the uploading of oxygen to pulmonary capillary blood. In the systemic capillaries, as CO_2 produced by metabolic activity is transferred from tissues to capillary blood, the resultant increase in PCO_2 levels and decrease in pH reduces the affinity of hemoglobin for oxygen (rightward shift of the dissociation curve), facilitating the unloading of oxygen from hemoglobin to tissues [361].

The oxyhemoglobin dissociation curves are not superimposed in all mammals but have a similar sigmoidal shape among mammalian species (Fig. 37.34) [356,362]. The oxygen partial pressure at which hemoglobin saturation is 50% (P_{50}) provides a comparative measure of the affinity of hemoglobin for oxygen, and this value varies between species. Slightly higher P_{50} values are found in dogs and rabbits in comparison to horses, cattle, and elephants suggesting that small animals are better adapted to oxygen delivery at the tissue level than large animal species (Fig. 37.34A) [356,362]. Also, P_{50} is reduced in septic patients and carbon monoxide poisoning, whereas the reverse has been encountered in chronic anemia. Since tissues require a given volume of oxygen per unit time, the hemoglobin concentration of blood has a significant influence on oxygen content and delivery to the tissues.

South American camelids (e.g., llamas and alpacas), have genetically coded changes in hemoglobin that increase its affinity for oxygen and result in lower P_{50} values in comparison to other mammal species (Fig. 37.34B) [363–365]. The relatively low P_{50} in Andean camelids is an important adaptation for life in their natural environment, where altitudes above 4000 meters decrease P_IO_2 from 160 mmHg (sea level) to 95 mmHg or less. Because of their relatively low P_{50} (22.7 mmHg), denoting high affinity of hemoglobin for oxygen, llamas were reportedly able to maintain a high SaO_2 (> 92%) when PaO_2 values were already at hypoxemic levels (51–53 mmHg) due to the high altitude (P_IO_2 = 107 mmHg at 3420 meters where P_B is 511 mmHg) [363]. By comparison, in humans, SaO_2 is reduced to 86–87% at a PaO_2 of 51–53 mmHg. While increased hemoglobin affinity for oxygen is physiologically advantageous because CaO_2 is maintained despite hypoxemic conditions/low PaO_2, unloading of oxygen at the tissue level may be reduced. However, high-altitude camelids present a very effective mechanism of oxygen transfer to tissues [363,364].

Hypoxemia

"Hypoxemia" is a term that specifically refers to abnormally low PaO_2 or hemoglobin saturation in arterial blood. Hypoxemia can be caused by low P_IO_2, hypoventilation, and anything that causes venous admixture (including low $\dot{V}_A/\dot{Q}$ ratio, shunt, and diffusion impairment). As explained before, hypoxemia caused by hypoventilation, low $\dot{V}_A/\dot{Q}$ ratio, and shunt are of particular interest to the anesthesiologist. Another important factor that may contribute to hypoxemia in anesthetized animals, that is not related to gas exchange impairment across the alveolar–capillary membrane, is a decrease in mixed venous oxygen saturation secondary to low CO during anesthesia in the face of a large pre-existing shunt, as discussed previously [300,301]. *Diffusion limitation* across the alveolar–capillary membrane may play an important role in the development of hypoxemia in some circumstances. Diffusion of oxygen to capillary blood can be limited by interstitial edema or fibrotic thickening of the alveolar–capillary membrane (interstitial lung disease), or when there is an extremely short capillary transit time [151]. In humans with interstitial lung disease, diffusion limitation most commonly causes hypoxemia during exercise as under these circumstances the decrease in capillary transit time does not allow enough time for oxygen to equilibrate between the alveolar gas and end-capillary blood [150,366]. Mild hypoxemia (PaO_2 between 60 and 80 mmHg) observed during heavy exercise in horses is the

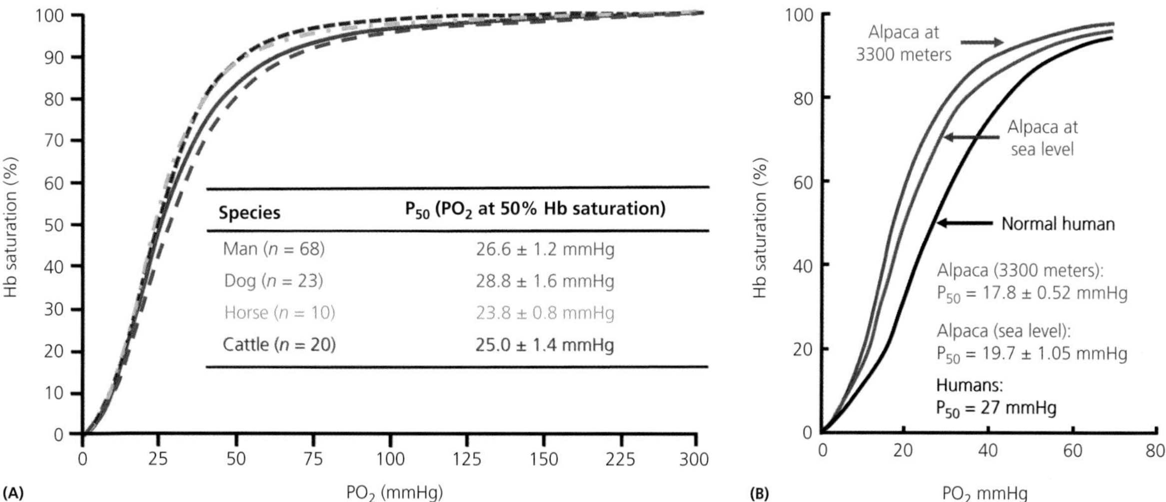

Figure 37.34 **A.** Oxyhemoglobin curves in man, dogs, horses, and cattle. The oxygen partial pressure at which hemoglobin is 50% saturated (P_{50}) is presented. **B.** Oxyhemoglobin curves in alpacas at high altitudes (3300 meters) and sea level in comparison to the human oxyhemoglobin curve (see text for explanation). Source: Adapted from Clerbaux *et al.* [362]; Sillau *et al.* [364].

Table 37.6 Classification of hypoxemia according to arterial oxygen partial pressure (PaO_2) and arterial hemoglobin saturation (SaO_2).

Classification	PaO_2	SaO_2	Percent decrease in CaO_2[a]
Normal	80 to 100 mmHg	95 to 98%	Reference value[b]
Mild hypoxemia	60 to < 80 mmHg	90 to < 95%	3 to 7%
Moderate hypoxemia	40 to < 60 mmHg	75 to < 90%	8 to 24%
Severe hypoxemia	20 to < 40 mmHg	32 to < 75%	25 to 68%

[a] CaO_2 calculated assuming a constant hemoglobin concentration (15 mL/dL).
[b] Reference CaO_2 value estimated as 20.2 mL/dL (PaO_2 100 mmHg, SaO_2 97.7%, and Hb concentration 15 g/dL).

result of diffusion limitation, which is precipitated by the shorter transit time of blood through the capillaries associated with the increase in CO during exercise [367].

Based on PaO_2 and SaO_2 values, hypoxemia can be classified as mild, moderate, or severe (Table 37.6). Classification of the severity of hypoxemia considers the magnitude of the change in PaO_2 on SaO_2 and the impact on oxygen content. For instance, if PaO_2 decreases from 100 (SaO_2 = 0.977) to 50 mmHg (SaO_2 = 0.85), hypoxemia is classified as moderate because CaO_2 decreases by only 13% (e.g., from 20.2 to 17.5 mL/dL) as 85% of hemoglobin is still saturated. However, if PaO_2 falls below 40 mmHg, critical hemoglobin desaturation is observed because of the steep slope of the oxyhemoglobin curve (Fig. 37.33). If PaO_2 falls to approximately 27 mmHg, hemoglobin saturation is only 50%. At this level of desaturation, hypoxemia is classified as severe since CaO_2 falls by nearly 50% of the normal value (from 20.2 to 10.3 mL/dL).

As explained before, an increase in F_IO_2 by 100% oxygen administration can markedly increase PaO_2 if intrapulmonary shunt is not the source of oxygenation impairment. However, this increased PaO_2 results in a relatively small increase in CaO_2 if hemoglobin saturation is already close to 100% while the animal is breathing ambient air. In a conscious individual breathing ambient air (F_IO_2 = 0.21) with a PaO_2 (100 mmHg), 1 deciliter (100 mL) of blood will hold 0.3 mL of oxygen dissolved in solution. If oxygen bound to hemoglobin is considered (hemoglobin saturation = 97.7% at a PaO_2 of 100 mmHg and hemoglobin concentration = 15 g/dL), total oxygen content increases to approximately 20.2 mL of oxygen per 100 mL of blood, or about 70 times as much as plasma. An increase in F_IO_2 from 0.21 to > 0.9 increases PaO_2 by fivefold (from 100 to 500 mmHg), but CaO_2 will increase only by 9% (from 20.2 to 22.0 mL/dL), as nearly all hemoglobin is already saturated when PaO_2 is 100 mmHg (97.7%). Although this increase in oxygen content is relatively small, it may be of clinical relevance in patients whose oxygen-carrying capacity is already compromised by severe anemia (e.g., hematocrit < 15% or hemoglobin < 5 g/dL). The PaO_2 level is also of some importance because oxygen transfers from blood to tissues by diffusion, and the process occurs at a rate proportional to the difference in oxygen tension between plasma and tissues. Preoxygenation of the lungs, preferentially via a sealed face mask attached to a breathing circuit filled with 100% oxygen, is recommended for added safety before induction of anesthesia in anemic animals, as the decrease in CaO_2 is more likely to achieve critical levels if mild-to-moderate hypoxemia occurs in patients with an already reduced oxygen-carrying capacity.

As hypoxemia becomes severe, cyanosis (blue-purple tinge) of mucous membranes can be observed because deoxygenated hemoglobin is dark red. However, cyanotic mucous membranes may not be perceived if the animal is anemic. Blood gas analyzers directly measure PO_2 in plasma through polarographic electrodes, while hemoglobin saturation is often calculated from PO_2 based on the human oxyhemoglobin dissociation curve. A more accurate measurement of hemoglobin saturation would require the use of species-specific algorithms, or the direct measurement of hemoglobin saturation via a blood gas analyzer equipped with a CO-oximeter. Pulse oximeters are non-invasive tools that measure hemoglobin saturation by absorption and transmission of two wavelengths of light (red and infrared light) through the tongue or other anatomic structures in animal species. Conventional pulse oximeters, however, are unable to detect other forms of hemoglobin that cannot bind to oxygen and will provide erratic hemoglobin saturation values in the presence of carboxyhemoglobin or methemoglobin [368,369]. Similarly, calculation of hemoglobin saturation from PO_2 using a blood gas analyzer not equipped with a CO-oximeter will lead to an erroneous estimation of hemoglobin saturation under these circumstances. If dyshemoglobinemias are suspected (e.g., methemoglobinemia or carboxyhemoglobinemia due to carbon monoxide poisoning), or if there is a discrepancy between PaO_2 measured by blood gas analysis and hemoglobin saturation measured by conventional pulse oximetry, an accurate measure of hemoglobin saturation can be obtained via CO-oximetry, which can measure concentrations of oxyhemoglobin, deoxyhemoglobin, and other forms of hemoglobin (including methemoglobin and carboxyhemoglobin), or via non-invasive multiple wavelength pulse CO-oximetry technology [370–372].

Carbon dioxide transport

Carbon dioxide is 20 times more soluble in water than oxygen. Its solubility coefficient is 0.0308 mmol/mmHg, which corresponds to 0.066 mL/mmHg/100 mL of blood. Therefore, the amount of CO_2 dissolved in 100 mL of venous and arterial blood is approximately 3 mL ($P\bar{v}CO_2$ = 46 mmHg) and 2.5 mL ($PaCO_2$ = 40 mmHg), respectively; the difference is eliminated by alveolar ventilation [373]. Because CO_2 has a much higher solubility and diffusing capability when compared to oxygen, its partial pressure in pulmonary capillary blood and the alveoli will be virtually the same [373]. This rapid equilibration ensures that CO_2 elimination by the lungs is not impaired in the face of a large intrapulmonary shunt if the ventilatory response in alveoli that are ventilated and perfused is preserved.

Arterial CO_2 levels are a function of CO_2 elimination and production, and under normal circumstances, $PaCO_2$ levels are maintained within narrow limits. During high-intensity exercise, the production of CO_2 is increased enormously, whereas during anesthesia, production likely decreases. Elimination of CO_2 depends on pulmonary blood flow ($\dot{Q}_T$) and alveolar ventilation ($\dot{V}_A$). Normally, CO_2 production ($\dot{V}CO_2$) parallels oxygen consumption ($\dot{V}O_2$) according to the respiratory quotient (R). As explained previously, the ratio between $\dot{V}CO_2$ and $\dot{V}O_2$ varies according to the diet and source of energy metabolism [58]. Although the value varies depending on the diet, R equals 0.8 at steady state in humans and may differ in animals. Due to the blood buffer systems, CO_2 transport to the lungs for excretion occurs with little change in blood pH.

Carbon dioxide content in blood and the Haldane effect

The total amount of CO_2 produced in tissues by aerobic metabolism is transported to the lungs in three ways: (1) *as gas dissolved in blood*; (2) as *HCO_3^-*; and (3) as *carbamino compounds* [356,373]. Carbon dioxide produced by the tissues diffuses down a concentration gradient to capillary blood in the systemic circulation in a process that is coupled with the transfer of oxygen from capillary

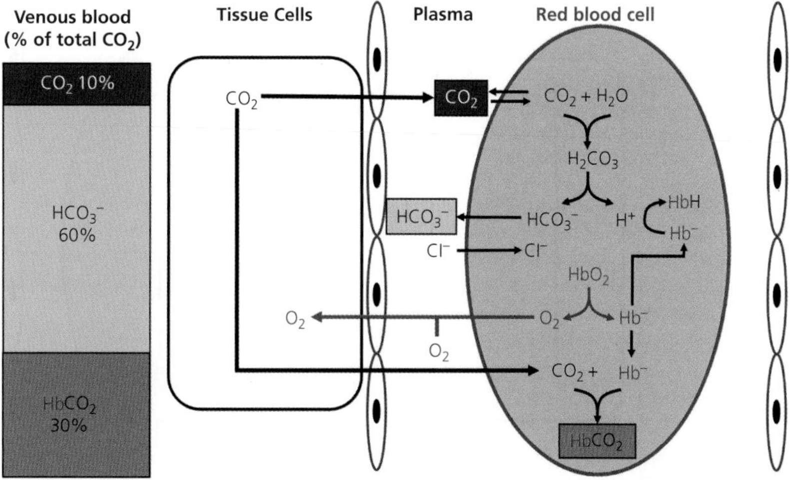

Figure 37.35 Carbon dioxide and oxygen transport at the tissue level. As oxygen is delivered to tissues there is an increase in CO_2 carrying capacity (CO_2 content) in venous blood attributable to deoxyhemoglobin (Hb^-). See text for explanation.

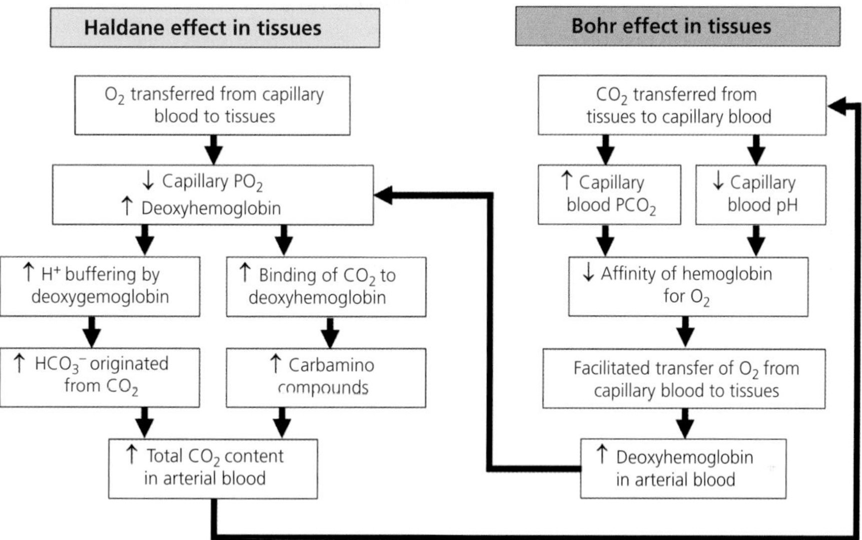

Figure 37.36 Interplay between the Haldane and Bohr effects in tissues.

blood to tissues. The transport of CO_2 and O_2 at the tissue level is summarized in Fig. 37.35. Typically, the PCO_2 of mixed venous blood draining tissues and organs of the systemic circulation is slightly higher than the PCO_2 of arterial blood ($P\bar{v}CO_2$ = 46 mmHg versus $PaCO_2$ = 40 mmHg). However, most CO_2 is transported in mixed venous blood as *plasma HCO_3^-* or combined with hemoglobin *as carbamino compounds*, with *CO_2 dissolved in blood* representing a smaller fraction of total CO_2 content. Because CO_2 is a nonpolar molecule, it readily diffuses across the lipid membrane of red blood cells, where carbonic anhydrase catalyzes the hydration of CO_2 to H_2CO_3 and its dissociated form (HCO_3^- and H^+). This reaction occurs within red blood cells but not in plasma of vertebrates, which does not contain carbonic anhydrase. A buildup of hydrogen within the cell would prevent further conversion of HCO_3^- from H_2CO_3. However, as oxyhemoglobin (HbO_2) releases oxygen to tissues, deoxyhemoglobin (Hb^-) buffers the hydrogen ion released by H_2CO_3, further shifting the reaction toward the generation of HCO_3^-, which increases the total CO_2 content in blood. The newly formed HCO_3^- anion is exported from the red blood cell to plasma in exchange for Cl^- in a mechanism named the "chloride shift" or "Hamburger effect." Approximately 60% of total CO_2 content in venous blood is transported as HCO_3^- [373]. As hemoglobin unloads oxygen to tissues, total CO_2 content increases because CO_2 reversibly binds to the amino groups ($-NH_2$) of deoxyhemoglobin to form *carbamino compounds* ($HbCO_2$), which is the second most important form of CO_2 transport and corresponds to 30% of total CO_2 content in mixed venous blood. Finally, the remaining 10% of the total CO_2 content is present in venous blood as CO_2 dissolved in solution [373]. The *Haldane effect* is the increase in CO_2 carrying capacity (total CO_2 content) that occurs with a decrease in PO_2. At the tissue level, the Haldane effect is explained by: (1) the buffering action of deoxygenated hemoglobin which combines with hydrogen ions released by H_2CO_3 and contributes to an increase in plasma HCO_3^- and (2) the reversible combination between deoxyhemoglobin and CO_2 forming carbamino compounds. The interplay between the Bohr (effect of changes in pH and PCO_2 on hemoglobin's affinity for oxygen) and Haldane effects at the tissue level is detailed in Fig. 37.36.

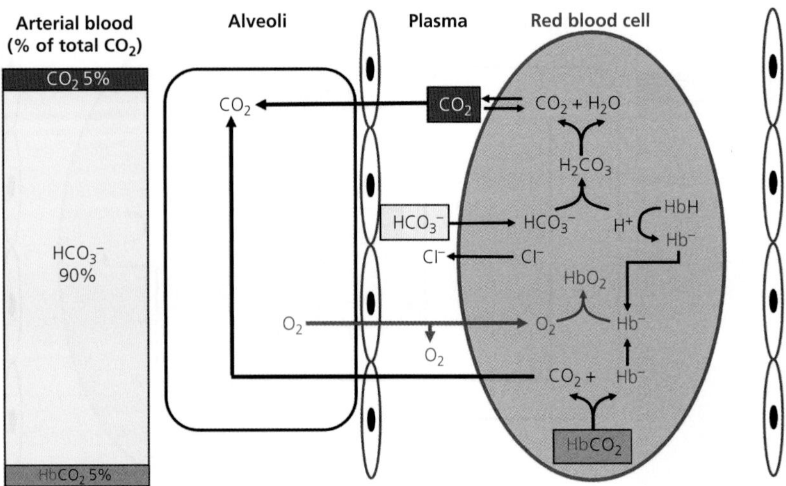

Figure 37.37 Carbon dioxide and oxygen transport at the alveoli (see text for explanation).

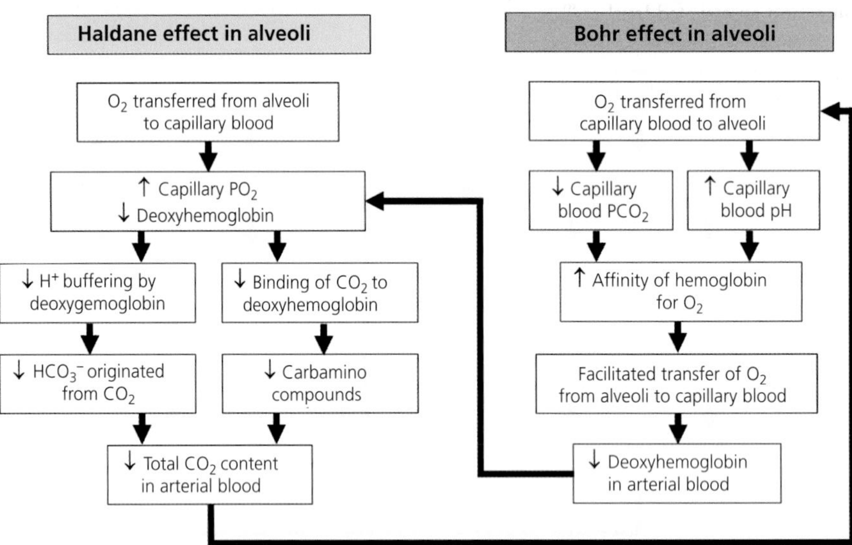

Figure 37.38 Interplay between the Haldane and Bohr effects in the alveoli.

Once mixed venous blood reaches the lung, the partial pressure of CO_2 decreases from 46 mmHg to approximately 40 mmHg in end-capillary blood. The difference corresponds to the amount of CO_2 eliminated by alveolar ventilation. However, CO_2 transported as gas dissolved in plasma is not the only source of CO_2 eliminated by alveolar ventilation. A large proportion of exhaled CO_2 originates from carbamino compounds ($HbCO_2$) and HCO_3^-. As illustrated in Fig. 37.37, as CO_2 is eliminated by alveolar ventilation, the relative contribution of CO_2 dissolved in plasma to total CO_2 content is reduced from 10% in venous blood to 5% in arterial blood, whereas the carbamino compounds have their relative contribution to total CO_2 reduced from 30% in venous blood to 5% in arterial blood; the remaining CO_2 (90%) is transported in arterial blood as HCO_3^-. As CO_2 is transferred from plasma to ventilated alveoli, the decrease in pulmonary capillary PCO_2 shifts the $H_2CO_3 \rightleftharpoons HCO_3^-$ reaction toward the formation of CO_2 and H_2O. Additionally, as oxygen is transferred from alveoli to capillary blood, an increase in HbO_2 reduces CO_2 carrying capacity by decreasing the amount of Hb^- available to form carbamino compounds. In summary, the Haldane effect in the lungs (decreased total CO_2 content at high PO_2 levels in pulmonary capillary blood) is explained by: (1) decreased amount of Hb^- which limits the buffering of hydrogen ions released by H_2CO_3 and shifts the equation toward the formation of H_2CO_3 with its subsequent dissociation into CO_2 and H_2O, and (2) decreased availability of Hb^- to combine with CO_2 and form carbamino compounds. The interplay between the Bohr and Haldane effects at the alveolar–capillary barrier is detailed in Fig. 37.38.

Hypercapnia and hypocapnia

Fig. 37.39, shows that CO_2 content changes significantly with changes in $PaCO_2$. As previously mentioned, hyperventilation occurs when $\dot{V}_A$ is excessive relative to the metabolic rate and as a result, $PaCO_2$ is reduced. Hypoventilation is present when $\dot{V}_A$ is low

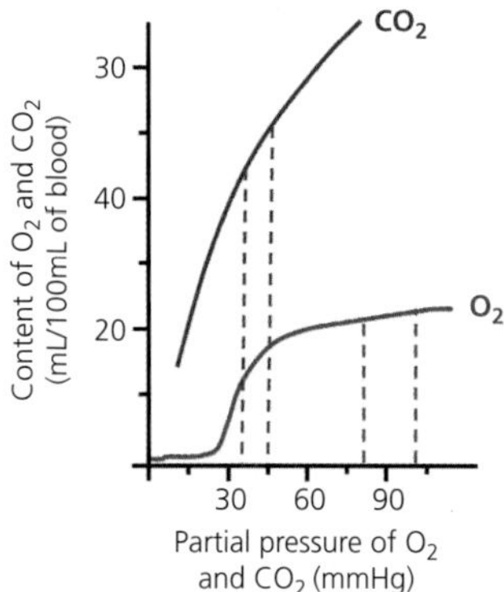

Figure 37.39 Correlation between partial pressures and content of CO_2 and O_2 in blood. Normal ranges of partial pressures of CO_2 (35–45 mmHg, blue dashed lines) and of O_2 (80–100 mmHg, red dashed lines) in arterial blood are shown (see text for explanation). Source: Adapted from Arthurs and Sudhakar [373].

relative to metabolic rate, and $PaCO_2$ rises. A lowered $PaCO_2$ level is referred to as "hypocapnia" and an elevated level as "hypercapnia," whereas normal $PaCO_2$ is termed "eucapnia." Most, but not all, of the common mammalian species, have a normal resting $PaCO_2$ level close to 40 mmHg (Table 37.2). Hypercapnia and hypocapnia produce respiratory acidosis and alkalosis, respectively, because CO_2 in the body is in dynamic equilibrium with H_2CO_3 and, ultimately, hydrogen ion concentration [H^+]:

$$CO_2 + H_2O \rightleftarrows H_2CO_3 \rightleftarrows H^+ + HCO_3^-$$

The normal pH is slightly more acidic in venous blood (7.34 to 7.43) than in arterial blood (7.35 to 7.45) because of higher PCO_2 in venous blood. *Acidemia* and *alkalemia* are defined as a plasma pH below or above, respectively, the normal range for the species in question. Concurrent metabolic acid–base disturbances and the presence or absence of renal compensation of the respiratory acid–base disturbance will determine the actual degree of pH change accompanying hypocapnia or hypercapnia.

During acute respiratory acidosis (e.g., general anesthesia in a spontaneously ventilating patient), there can be a small compensatory increase in plasma HCO_3^-. In dogs and cats with acute respiratory acidosis, HCO_3^- has been estimated to increase by 0.15 mmol/L for each mmHg increase in PCO_2 above normal (e.g., PCO_2 = 36 mmHg) [52,53]. Hemoglobin contributes to the increase in HCO_3^- during acute respiratory acidosis, as deoxygenated hemoglobin (Hb^-) will neutralize the hydrogen ions released from H_2CO_3, shifting the $H_2CO_3 \rightleftharpoons HCO_3^-$ equation toward the formation of HCO_3^-. If hypercapnia persists for several days, chronic respiratory acidosis is associated with a renal compensatory response. The kidneys eliminate the excess acid load via excretion of ammonium chloride ($NH_4^+Cl^-$) [53]. Increased excretion of Cl^- is paralleled by increased reabsorption of HCO_3^- by renal tubular cells, resulting in a state of hypochloremic metabolic alkalosis (decreased plasma Cl^- and increased plasma HCO_3^-), which may be able to minimize or neutralize the impact of chronic respiratory acidosis on pH. The compensatory renal response to chronic acidosis is estimated to increase plasma HCO_3^- by 0.35 mmol/L for each mmHg of increase in PCO_2 in dogs but current data does not allow the estimation of the renal compensation to chronic respiratory acidosis in cats [53].

References

1 Hall LW, Gillespie JR, Tyler WS. Alveolar-arterial oxygen tension differences in anaesthetized horses. *Br J Anaesth* 1968; **40**: 560–568.
2 Steffey EP, Wheat JD, Meagher DM, *et al.* Body position and mode of ventilation influences arterial pH, oxygen, and carbon dioxide tensions in halothane-anesthetized horses. *Am J Vet Res* 1977; **38**: 379–382.
3 Hall LW. Oxygenation of pulmonary vein blood in conscious and anaesthetised ponies. *Equine Vet J* 1979; **11**: 71–75.
4 Mutoh T, Nishimura R, Kim HY, *et al.* Cardiopulmonary effects of sevoflurane, compared with halothane, enflurane, and isoflurane, in dogs. *Am J Vet Res* 1997; **58**: 885–890.
5 Hodgson DS, Dunlop CI, Chapman PL, *et al.* Cardiopulmonary effects of anesthesia induced and maintained with isoflurane in cats. *Am J Vet Res* 1998; **59**: 182–185.
6 Enouri SS, Kerr CL, McDonell WN, *et al.* Effects of a peripheral alpha2 adrenergic-receptor antagonist on the hemodynamic changes induced by medetomidine administration in conscious dogs. *Am J Vet Res* 2008; **69**: 728–736.
7 Rioja E, Kerr CL, Enouri SS, *et al.* Sedative and cardiopulmonary effects of medetomidine hydrochloride and xylazine hydrochloride and their reversal with atipamezole hydrochloride in calves. *Am J Vet Res* 2008; **69**: 319–329.
8 Borges LP, Nishimura LT, Carvalho LL, *et al.* Behavioral and cardiopulmonary effects of dexmedetomidine alone and in combination with butorphanol, methadone, morphine or tramadol in conscious sheep. *Vet Anaesth Analg* 2016; **43**: 549–560.
9 West JB, Luks AM. *West's Respiratory Physiology. The Essentials, 11th edn.* Philadelphia, PA: Wolters Kluwer, 2021.
10 Lumb AB, Thomas C. *Nunn and Lumb's Applied Respiratory Physiology*, 9th edn. Edinburgh, UK: Elsevier, 2021.
11 Libermann IM, Capano A, Gonzalez F, *et al.* Blood acid–base status in normal albino rats. *Lab Anim Sci* 1973; **23**: 862–865.
12 Lai YL, Tsuya Y, Hildebrandt J. Ventilatory responses to acute CO2 exposure in the rat. *J Appl Physiol Respir Environ Exerc Physiol* 1978; **45**: 611–618.
13 Lahiri S. Blood oxygen affinity and alveolar ventilation in relation in body weight in mammals. *Am J Physiol* 1975; **229**: 529–536.
14 Neutze JM, Wyler F, Rudolph AM. Use of radioactive microspheres to assess distribution of cardiac output in rabbits. *Am J Physiol* 1968; **215**: 486–495.
15 Dyson DH, Allen DG, Ingwersen W, *et al.* Effects of saffan on cardiopulmonary function in healthy cats. *Can J Vet Res* 1987; **51**: 236–239.
16 Herbert DA, Mitchell RA. Blood gas tensions and acid–base balance in awake cats. *J Appl Physiol* 1971; **30**: 434–436.
17 McDonell WN. Ventilation and acid–base equilibrium with methoxyflurane anesthesia in dogs. MSc Thesis, University of Guelph, 1969.
18 Horwitz LD, Bishop VS, Stone HL, *et al.* Cardiovascular effects of low-oxygen atmospheres in conscious and anesthetized dogs. *J Appl Physiol* 1969; **27**: 370–373.
19 Wanner A, Reinhart ME. Respiratory mechanics in conscious sheep: response to methacholine. *J Appl Physiol Respir Environ Exerc Physiol* 1978; **44**: 479–482.
20 Bakima M, Gustin P, Lekeux P, *et al.* Mechanics of breathing in goats. *Res Vet Sci* 1988; **45**: 332–336.
21 Forster HV, Bisgard GE, Klein JP. Effect of peripheral chemoreceptor denervation on acclimatization of goats during hypoxia. *J Appl Physiol Respir Environ Exerc Physiol* 1981; **50**: 392–398.
22 Mesina JE Jr., Bisgard GE, Robinson GM. Pulmonary function changes in goats given 3-methylindole orally. *Am J Vet Res* 1984; **45**: 1526–1531.
23 Bisgard GE, Vogel JH. Hypoventilation and pulmonary hypertension in calves after carotid body excision. *J Appl Physiol* 1971; **31**: 431–437.
24 Donawick WJ, Baue AE. Blood gases, acid–base balance, and alveolar-arterial oxygen gradient in calves. *Am J Vet Res* 1968; **29**: 561–567.
25 Gallivan GJ, McDonell WN, Forrest JB. Comparative ventilation and gas exchange in the horse and the cow. *Res Vet Sci* 1989; **46**: 331–336.
26 Orr JA, Bisgard GE, Forster HV, *et al.* Cardiopulmonary measurements in nonanesthetized, resting normal ponies. *Am J Vet Res* 1975; **36**: 1667–1670.
27 McDonell W, Hall LW. Functional residual capacity in conscious and anaesthetized horses. *Br J Anaesth* 1974; **46**: 802–803.
28 Sorenson PR, Robinson NE. Postural effects on lung volumes and asynchronous ventilation in anesthetized horses. *J Appl Physiol Respir Environ Exerc Physiol* 1980; **48**: 97–103.
29 Rozanski EA, Bedenice D, Lofgren J, *et al.* The effect of body position, sedation, and thoracic bandaging on functional residual capacity in healthy deep-chested dogs. *Can J Vet Res* 2010; **74**: 34–39.
30 Gallivan GJ, McDonell WN, Forrest JB. Comparative pulmonary mechanics in the horse and the cow. *Res Vet Sci* 1989; **46**: 322–330.
31 Liu NC, Adams VJ, Kalmar L, *et al.* Whole-body barometric plethysmography characterizes upper airway obstruction in 3 brachycephalic breeds of dogs. *J Vet Intern Med* 2016; **30**: 853–865.

32 Lai YL. Comparative ventilation of the normal lung. In: Parent RA, ed. *Treatise of Pulmonary Toxicology Vol 1: Comparative Biology of the Normal Lung*. Boca Raton, FL: CRC Press, 1992: 219–224.

33 Crosfill ML, Widdicombe JG. Physical characteristics of the chest and lungs and the work of breathing in different mammalian species. *J Physiol* 1961; **158**: 1–14.

34 Gillespie DJ, Hyatt RE. Respiratory mechanics in the unanesthetized dog. *J Appl Physiol* 1974; **36**: 98–102.

35 Mauderly JL. Effect of age on pulmonary structure and function of immature and adult animals and man. *Fed Proc* 1979; **38**: 173–177.

36 Gillespie JR, Tyler WS, Eberly VE. Pulmonary ventilation and resistance in emphysematous and control horses. *J Appl Physiol* 1966; **21**: 416–422.

37 Willoughby RA, McDonell WN. Pulmonary function testing in horses. *Vet Clin North Am Large Anim Pract* 1979; **1**: 171–196.

38 Keith IM, Bisgard GE, Manohar M, *et al.* Respiratory effects of pregnancy and progesterone in Jersey cows. *Respir Physiol* 1982; **50**: 351–358.

39 Fordyce WE, Tenney SM. Role of the carotid bodies in ventilatory acclimation to chronic hypoxia by the awake cat. *Respir Physiol* 1984; **58**: 207–221.

40 Hales JR, Webster ME. Respiratory function during thermal tachypnoea in sheep. *J Physiol* 1967; **190**: 241–260.

41 Verbrugghe C, Laurent P, Bouverot P. Chemoreflex drive of ventilation in the awake miniature pig. *Respir Physiol* 1982; **47**: 379–391.

42 Bisgard GE, Ruiz AV, Grover RF, *et al.* Ventilatory control in the Hereford calf. *J Appl Physiol* 1973; **35**: 220–226.

43 Walters LM, Ogilvie GK, Salman MD, *et al.* Repeatability of energy expenditure measurements in clinically normal dogs by use of indirect calorimetry. *Am J Vet Res* 1993; **54**: 1881–1885.

44 Ewart SL. Control of ventilation. In: Klein BG, ed. *Cunningham's Textbook of Veterinary Physiology*, 6th edn. St. Louis, MO: Elsevier, 2020: 560–567.

45 Levitzky MG. Control of breathing. In: Levitzky MG, ed. *Pulmonary Physiology*, 9th edn. New York, NY: McGraw-Hill, 2018: 206–234.

46 Lyons C, Kevin LG. Respiration: control of ventilation. *Anaesth Intensive Care Med* 2021; **22**: 174–178.

47 Nattie E, Li A. Central chemoreceptors: locations and functions. *Compr Physiol* 2012; **2**: 221–254.

48 Gauvreau GM, Wilson BA, Schnurr DL, *et al.* Oxygen cost of ventilation in the resting horse. *Res Vet Sci* 1995; **59**: 168–171.

49 Robinson N. The respiratory system. In: Muir WW, Hubbell J, eds. *Equine Anesthesia: Monitoring and Emergency Therapy*, 2nd edn. St. Louis, MO: Saunders, 2009: 11–36.

50 Muir WW, Hamlin RL. Effects of acetylpromazine on ventilatory variables in the horse. *Am J Vet Res* 1975; **36**: 1439–1442.

51 DiBartola SP. Metabolic acid–base disorders. In: DiBartola SP, ed. *Fluid, Electrolyte, and Acid–Base Disorders*, 4th edn. St. Louis, MO: Elsevier Saunders, 2012: 253–286.

52 de Morais HA, Leiseweitz AL. Mixed acid–base disorders. In: DiBartola SP, ed. *Fluid, Electrolyte, and Acid–Base Disorders in Small Animal Practice*, 4th edn. St. Louis, MO: Elsevier Sanders, 2012: 302–315.

53 Johnson RA, de Morais HA. Respiratory acid–base disorders. In: DiBartola SP, ed. *Fluid, Electrolyte, and Acid–Base Disorders*, 4th edn. St. Louis, MO: Elsevier Saunders, 2012: 287–301.

54 Robertshaw D. Mechanisms for the control of respiratory evaporative heat loss in panting animals. *J Appl Physiol (1985)* **2006**; 101: 664–668.

55 Bartlett D Jr., Jeffery P, Sant'ambrogio G, *et al.* Location of stretch receptors in the trachea and bronchi of the dog. *J Physiol* 1976; **258**: 409–420.

56 Guz A, Trenchard DW. Pulmonary stretch receptor activity in man: a comparison with dog and cat. *J Physiol* 1971; **213**: 329–343.

57 Lumb AB, Horncastle E. Pulmonary physiology. In: Hemmings HC Jr., Egan TD, eds. *Pharmacology and Physiology for Anesthesia*, 2nd edn. Philadelphia, PA: Elsevier, 2019: 586–608.

58 Hlastala MP. Ventilation. In: Laurent GJ, Sharpiro SD, eds. *Encyclopedia of Respiratory Medicine*, 1st edn. Cambridge, MA: Academic Press, 2006: 428–434.

59 Walton RS, Wingfield WE, Ogilvie GK. Energy expenditure in 104 postoperative and traumatically injured dogs with indirect calorimetry. *J Vet Emerg Crit Care* 1996; **6**: 71–79.

60 Speakman JR, van Acker A, Harper EJ. Age-related changes in the metabolism and body composition of three dog breeds and their relationship to life expectancy. *Aging Cell* 2003; **2**: 265–275.

61 Kavanagh BP, Hedenstierna G. Respiratory physiology and pathophysiology. In: Gropper MA, Cohen NH, Eriksson LI, *et al.*, eds. *Miller's Anesthesia*, 9th edn. Philadelphia, PA: Elsevier, 2020: 354–383.

62 Tusman G, Sipmann FS, Böhm SH. Rationale of dead space measurement by volumetric capnography. *Anesth Analg* 2012; **114**: 866–874.

63 Bourgoin P, Baudin F, Brossier D, *et al.* Assessment of Bohr and Enghoff dead space equations in mechanically ventilated children. *Respir Care* 2017; **62**: 468–474.

64 Kremeier P, Böhm SH, Tusman G. Clinical use of volumetric capnography in mechanically ventilated patients. *J Clin Monit Comput* 2020; **34**: 7–16.

65 Levitzky MG. Alveolar ventilation. In: Levitzky MG, ed. *Pulmonary Physiology*, 9th edn. New York, NY: McGraw-Hill, 2018: 59–92.

66 Tusman G, Sipmann FS, Borges JB, *et al.* Validation of Bohr dead space measured by volumetric capnography. *Intensive Care Med* 2011; **37**: 870–874.

67 Moens Y. Arterial-alveolar carbon dioxide tension difference and alveolar dead space in halothane anaesthetised horses. *Equine Vet J* 1989; **21**: 282–284.

68 Mosing M, Böhm SH, Rasis A, *et al.* Physiologic factors influencing the arterial-to-end-tidal CO_2 difference and the alveolar dead space fraction in spontaneously breathing anesthetised horses. *Front Vet Sci* 2018; **5**: 58.

69 Mosing M, Staub L, Moens Y. Comparison of two different methods for physiologic dead space measurements in ventilated dogs in a clinical setting. *Vet Anaesth Analg* 2010; **37**: 393–400.

70 Bumbacher S, Schramel JP, Mosing M. Evaluation of three tidal volumes (10, 12 and 15 mL kg(-1)) in dogs for controlled mechanical ventilation assessed by volumetric capnography: a randomized clinical trial. *Vet Anaesth Analg* 2017; **44**: 775–784.

71 Mosing M, Iff I, Hirt R, *et al.* Evaluation of variables to describe the shape of volumetric capnography curves during bronchoconstriction in dogs. *Res Vet Sci* 2012; **93**: 386–392.

72 Fletcher R, Jonson B, Cumming G, *et al.* The concept of deadspace with special reference to the single breath test for carbon dioxide. *Br J Anaesth* 1981; **53**: 77–88.

73 Tang Y, Turner MJ, Baker AB. Effects of alveolar dead-space, shunt and V/Q distribution on respiratory dead-space measurements. *Br J Anaesth* 2005; **95**: 538–548.

74 Tornabene VW, Fortune JB, Wagner PD, *et al.* Gas exchange after pulmonary fat embolism in dogs. *J Thorac Cardiovasc Surg* 1979; **78**: 589–599.

75 Dubin A, Murias G, Estenssoro E, *et al.* End-tidal CO_2 pressure determinants during hemorrhagic shock. *Intensive Care Med* 2000; **26**: 1619–1623.

76 Teixeira-Neto FJ, Luna SP, Cruz ML, *et al.* A study of the effect of hemorrhage on the cardiorespiratory actions of halothane, isoflurane and sevoflurane in the dog. *Vet Anaesth Analg* 2007; **34**: 107–116.

77 Murias G, Blanch L, Lucangelo U. The physiology of ventilation. *Respir Care* 2014; **59**: 1795–1807.

78 Loring SH, Topulos GP, Hubmayr RD. Transpulmonary pressure: the importance of precise definitions and limiting assumptions. *Am J Respir Crit Care Med* 2016; **194**: 1452–1457.

79 Ewart SL. Overview of respiratory function: ventilation of the lungs. In: Klein BG, ed. *Cunningham's Textbook of Veterinary Physiology*, 6th edn. St. Louis, MO: Elsevier, 2020: 518–531.

80 Grieco DL, Chen L, Brochard L. Transpulmonary pressure: importance and limits. *Ann Transl Med* 2017; **5**: 285.

81 Moens YP, Gootjes P, Ionita JC, *et al.* In vitro validation of a Pitot-based flow meter for the measurement of respiratory volume and flow in large animal anaesthesia. *Vet Anaesth Analg* 2009; **36**: 209–219.

82 Morgenroth S, Thomas J, Cannizzaro V, *et al.* Accuracy of near-patient vs. inbuilt spirometry for monitoring tidal volumes in an in-vitro paediatric lung model. *Anaesthesia* 2018; **73**: 972–979.

83 Corcoran BM. Static respiratory compliance in normal dogs. *J Small Anim Pract* 1991; **32**: 438–442.

84 Barberis L, Manno E, Guérin C. Effect of end-inspiratory pause duration on plateau pressure in mechanically ventilated patients. *Intensive Care Med* 2003; **29**: 130–134.

85 Henderson WR, Sheel AW. Pulmonary mechanics during mechanical ventilation. *Respir Physiol Neurobiol* 2012; **180**: 162–172.

86 Dye JA, McKiernan BC, Rozanski EA, *et al.* Bronchopulmonary disease in the cat: historical, physical, radiographic, clinicopathologic, and pulmonary functional evaluation of 24 affected and 15 healthy cats. *J Vet Intern Med* 1996; **10**: 385–400.

87 Hoffman AM, Oura TJ, Riedelberger KJ, *et al.* Plethysmographic comparison of breathing pattern in heaves (recurrent airway obstruction) versus experimental bronchoconstriction or hyperpnea in horses. *J Vet Intern Med* 2007; **21**: 184–192.

88 Lumb AB, Thomas C. Respiratory system resistance. In: Lumb AB, Thomas C, eds. *Nunn and Lumb's Applied Respiratory Physiology*, 9th edn. Edinburgh, UK: Elsevier, 2021: 27–41.

89 Mitchell V, Cheesman K. Gas, tubes and flow. *Anaesth Intensive Care Med* 2007; **8**: 7–10.

90 Kaminsky DA. What does airway resistance tell us about lung function? *Respir Care* 2012; **57**: 85–96.

91 Lumb AB, Thomas C. Elastic forces and lung volumes. In: Lumb AB, Thomas C, eds. *Nunn and Lumb's Applied Respiratory Physiology*, 9th edn. Edinburgh, UK: Elsevier, 2021: 14–26.

92 Papamoschou D. Theoretical validation of the respiratory benefits of helium-oxygen mixtures. *Respir Physiol* 1995; **99**: 183–190.

93 Hopster K, Duffee LR, Hopster-Iversen CCS, *et al.* Efficacy of an alveolar recruitment maneuver for improving gas exchange and pulmonary mechanics in anesthetized horses ventilated with oxygen or a helium-oxygen mixture. *Am J Vet Res* 2018; **79**: 1021–1027.

94 Derksen FJ, Robinson NE. Esophageal and intrapleural pressures in the healthy conscious pony. *Am J Vet Res* 1980; **41**: 1756–1761.

95 Olson LE, Lai-Fook SJ. Pleural liquid pressure measured with rib capsules in anesthetized ponies. *J Appl Physiol (1985)* **1988**; 64: 102–107.
96 West JB. State of the art: ventilation–perfusion relationships. *Am Rev Respir Dis* 1977; **116**: 919–943.
97 Amis TC, Pascoe JR, Hornof W. Topographic distribution of pulmonary ventilation and perfusion in the horse. *Am J Vet Res* 1984; **45**: 1597–1601.
98 Schramel J, Nagel C, Auer U, *et al.* Distribution of ventilation in pregnant Shetland ponies measured by Electrical Impedance Tomography. *Respir Physiol Neurobiol* 2012; **180**: 258–262.
99 Pelletier N, Leith DE. Cardiac output but not high pulmonary artery pressure varies with FIO2 in exercising horses. *Respir Physiol* 1993; **91**: 83–97.
100 Manohar M, Hutchens E, Coney E. Pulmonary haemodynamics in the exercising horse and their relationship to exercise-induced pulmonary haemorrhage. *Br Vet J* 1993; **149**: 419–428.
101 Elkins RC, Milnor WR. Pulmonary vascular response to exercise in the dog. *Circ Res* 1971; **29**: 591–599.
102 Erickson BK, Erickson HH, Coffman JR. Pulmonary artery, aortic and oesophageal pressure changes during high intensity treadmill exercise in the horse: a possible relation to exercise-induced pulmonary haemorrhage. *Equine Vet J Suppl* 1990; **9**: 47–52.
103 Stpeanek J, Christen P. Pulmonary arterial pressure in conscious and anaesthetized dogs. *Bull Physiopathol Respir (Nancy)* 1975; **11**: 295–304.
104 Lampert BC. Right heart catheterization. In: Vasan RS, Sawyer DB, eds. *Encyclopedia of Cardiovscular Research and Medicine*. Oxford, UK: Elsevier, 2018: 298–306.
105 Porcelli RJ. Pulmonary hemodynamics. In: Parent RA, ed. *Treatise on Pulmonary Toxicology*, Vol **1**. Boca Raton, FL: CRC Press, 1992: 241–270.
106 Hlastala MP, Bernard SL, Erickson HH, *et al.* Pulmonary blood flow distribution in standing horses is not dominated by gravity. *J Appl Physiol (1985)* **1996**; 81: 1051–1061.
107 Glenny RW, Lamm WJ, Albert RK, *et al.* Gravity is a minor determinant of pulmonary blood flow distribution. *J Appl Physiol (1985)* **1991**; 71: 620–629.
108 Pelletier N, Robinson NE, Kaiser L, *et al.* Regional differences in endothelial function in horse lungs: possible role in blood flow distribution? *J Appl Physiol (1985)* **1998**; 85: 537–542.
109 Galvin I, Drummond GB, Nirmalan M. Distribution of blood flow and ventilation in the lung: gravity is not the only factor. *Br J Anaesth* 2007; **98**: 420–428.
110 Chambers D, Huang C, Matthews G. Ventilation–perfusion zones in the lung. In: Chambers D, Huang C, Matthews G, eds. *Basic Physiology for Anaesthetists*, 2nd edn. Cambridge, UK: Cambridge University Press, 2019: 71–73.
111 McLean SR, Lohser J. Physiology of the lateral decubitus position, open chest and one-lung ventilation. In: Slinger PS, ed. *Principles and Practice of Anesthesia for Thoracic Surgery*, 1st edn. New York, NY: Springer, 2011: 93–105.
112 Lumb AB, Slinger P. Hypoxic pulmonary vasoconstriction: physiology and anesthetic implications. *Anesthesiology* 2015; **122**: 932–946.
113 Dunham-Snary KJ, Wu D, Sykes EA, *et al.* Hypoxic pulmonary vasoconstriction: from molecular mechanisms to medicine. *Chest* 2017; **151**: 181–192.
114 Lumb AB, Thomas C. The pulmonary circulation. In: Lumb AB Thomas C, eds. *Nunn and Lumb's Applied Respiratory Physiology*, 9th edn. Edinburgh, UK: Elsevier, 2021: 73–87.
115 Sommer N, Strielkov I, Pak O, *et al.* Oxygen sensing and signal transduction in hypoxic pulmonary vasoconstriction. *Eur Respir J* 2016; **47**: 288–303.
116 Robinson NE. Some functional consequences of species differences in lung anatomy. *Adv Vet Sci Comp Med* 1982; **26**: 1–33.
117 Tucker A, McMurtry IF, Reeves JT, *et al.* Lung vascular smooth muscle as a determinant of pulmonary hypertension at high altitude. *Am J Physiol* 1975; **228**: 762–767.
118 Marshall BE, Marshall C, Benumof J, *et al.* Hypoxic pulmonary vasoconstriction in dogs: effects of lung segment size and oxygen tension. *J Appl Physiol Respir Environ Exerc Physiol* 1981; **51**: 1543–1551.
119 Elliott AR, Steffey EP, Jarvis KA, *et al.* Unilateral hypoxic pulmonary vasoconstriction in the dog, pony and miniature swine. *Respir Physiol* 1991; **85**: 355–369.
120 Reinero C, Visser LC, Kellihan HB, *et al.* ACVIM consensus statement guidelines for the diagnosis, classification, treatment, and monitoring of pulmonary hypertension in dogs. *J Vet Intern Med* 2020; **34**: 549–573.
121 Kellihan HB, Stepien RL. Pulmonary hypertension in dogs: diagnosis and therapy. *Vet Clin North Am Small Anim Pract* 2010; **40**: 623–641.
122 Jaffey JA, Wiggen K, Leach SB, *et al.* Pulmonary hypertension secondary to respiratory disease and/or hypoxia in dogs: clinical features, diagnostic testing and survival. *Vet J* 2019; **251**: 105347.
123 Pyle RL, Park RD, Alexander AF, *et al.* Patent ductus arteriosus with pulmonary hypertension in the dog. *J Am Vet Med Assoc* 1981; **178**: 565–571.
124 Boutet BG, Saunders AB, Gordon SG. Clinical characteristics of adult dogs more than 5 years of age at presentation for patent ductus arteriosus. *J Vet Intern Med* 2017; **31**: 685–690.
125 Greet V, Bode EF, Dukes-McEwan J, *et al.* Clinical features and outcome of dogs and cats with bidirectional and continuous right-to-left shunting patent ductus arteriosus. *J Vet Intern Med* 2021; **35**: 780–788.
126 Bascuñán A, Thieman Mankin KM, *et al.* Patent ductus arteriosus in cats (Felis catus): 50 cases (2000–2015). *J Vet Cardiol* 2017; **19**: 35–43.
127 Parisi C, Phillips V, Ferreira J, *et al.* Anaesthetic management and complications of transvascular patent ductus arteriosus occlusion in dogs. *Vet Anaesth Analg* 2020; **47**: 581–587.
128 Schober KE, Hart TM, Stern JA, *et al.* Detection of congestive heart failure in dogs by Doppler echocardiography. *J Vet Intern Med* 2010; **24**: 1358–1368.
129 Borgarelli M, Abbott J, Braz-Ruivo L, *et al.* Prevalence and prognostic importance of pulmonary hypertension in dogs with myxomatous mitral valve disease. *J Vet Intern Med* 2015; **29**: 569–574.
130 Vezzosi T, Schober KE. Doppler-derived echocardiographic evidence of pulmonary hypertension in cats with left-sided congestive heart failure. *J Vet Cardiol* 2019; **23**: 58–68.
131 Matthay MA, Quinn TE. Pulmonary edema. In: Laurent GJ, Shapiro SD, eds. *Encyclopedia of Respiratory Medicine*. Oxford, UK: Academic Press, 2006: 544–550.
132 Lumb AB, Thomas C. Pulmonary vascular disease. In: Lumb AB, Thomas C, eds. *Nunn and Lumb's Applied Respiratory Physiology*, 9th edn. Edinburgh, UK: Elsevier, 2021: 339–348.
133 Collins SR, Blank RS, Deatherage LS, *et al.* Special article: the endothelial glycocalyx: emerging concepts in pulmonary edema and acute lung injury. *Anesth Analg* 2013; **117**: 664–674.
134 Woodcock TE, Woodcock TM. Revised Starling equation and the glycocalyx model of transvascular fluid exchange: an improved paradigm for prescribing intravenous fluid therapy. *Br J Anaesth* 2012; **108**: 84–394.
135 Chappell D, Bruegger D, Potzel J, *et al.* Hypervolemia increases release of atrial natriuretic peptide and shedding of the endothelial glycocalyx. *Crit Care* 2014; **18**: 538.
136 Uchimido R, Schmidt EP, Shapiro NI. The glycocalyx: a novel diagnostic and therapeutic target in sepsis. *Crit Care* 2019; **23**: 16.
137 Schober KE, Bonagura J, Scansen BA, *et al.* Estimation of left ventricular filling pressure by use of Doppler echocardiography in healthy anesthetized dogs subjected to acute volume loading. *Am J Vet Res* 2008; **69**: 1034–1049.
138 Hansen B. *Fluid overload*. *Front Vet Sci* 2021; **8**: 668688.
139 Schober KE, Chetboul V. Echocardiographic evaluation of left ventricular diastolic function in cats: hemodynamic determinants and pattern recognition. *J Vet Cardiol* 2015; **17**(Suppl 1): S102–S133.
140 Teixeira-Neto FJ, Valverde A. Clinical application of the fluid challenge approach in goal-directed fluid therapy: what can we learn from human studies? *Front Vet Sci* 2021; **8**: 701377.
141 Bhattacharya M, Kallet RH, Ware LB, *et al.* Negative-pressure pulmonary edema. *Chest* 2016; **150**: 927–933.
142 Tute AS, Wilkins PA, Gleed RD, *et al.* Negative pressure pulmonary edema as a post-anesthetic complication associated with upper airway obstruction in a horse. *Vet Surg* 1996; **25**: 519–523.
143 Drobatz KJ, Saunders HM, Pugh CR, *et al.* Noncardiogenic pulmonary edema in dogs and cats: 26 cases (1987–1993). *J Am Vet Med Assoc* 1995; **206**: 1732–1736.
144 Kollias-Baker CA, Pipers FS, Heard D, *et al.* Pulmonary edema associated with transient airway obstruction in three horses. *J Am Vet Med Assoc* 1993; **202**: 1116–1118.
145 Ranieri VM, Rubenfeld GD, Thompson BT, *et al.* Acute respiratory distress syndrome: the Berlin Definition. *J Am Med Assoc* 2012; **307**: 2526–2533.
146 Wilkins PA, Otto CM, Baumgardner JE, *et al.* Acute lung injury and acute respiratory distress syndromes in veterinary medicine: consensus definitions: the Dorothy Russell Havemeyer Working Group on ALI and ARDS in Veterinary Medicine. *J Vet Emerg Crit Care* 2007; **17**: 333–339.
147 Boiron L, Hopper K, Borchers A. Risk factors, characteristics, and outcomes of acute respiratory distress syndrome in dogs and cats: 54 cases. *J Vet Emerg Crit Care (San Antonio)* 2019; **29**: 173–179.
148 Vrolyk V, Wobeser BK, Al-Dissi AN, *et al.* Lung inflammation associated with clinical acute necrotizing pancreatitis in dogs. *Vet Pathol* 2017; **54**: 129–140.
149 Vrolyk V, Singh B. Animal models to study the role of pulmonary intravascular macrophages in spontaneous and induced acute pancreatitis. *Cell Tissue Res* 2020; **380**: 207–222.
150 Petersson J, Glenny RW. Gas exchange and ventilation–perfusion relationships in the lung. *Eur Respir J* 2014; **44**: 1023–1041.
151 Levitzky MG. Ventilation–perfusion relationships. In: Levitsky MG, ed. *Pulmonary Physiology*, 9th edn. New York, NY: McGraw-Hill, 2018: 124–141.
152 Amis TC, Jones HA, Hughes JM. A conscious dog model for study of regional lung function. *J Appl Physiol Respir Environ Exerc Physiol* 1982; **53**: 1050–1054.
153 Hedenstierna G, Nyman G, Kvart C, *et al.* Ventilation–perfusion relationships in the standing horse: an inert gas elimination study. *Equine Vet J* 1987; **19**: 514–519.

154 Dantzker DR, Wagner PD, West JB. Proceedings: instability of poorly ventilated lung units during oxygen breathing. *J Physiol* 1974; **242**: 72.

155 Moir TW, Driscol TE, Eckstein RW. Thebisian drainage in the left heart of the dog. *Circ Res* 1964; **14**: 245–249.

156 Ravin MB, Epstein RM, Malm JR. Contribution of Thebesian veins to the physiologic shunt in anesthetized man. *J Appl Physiol* 1965; **20**: 1148–1152.

157 Benatar SR, Hewlett AM, Nunn JF. The use of iso-shunt lines for control of oxygen therapy. *Br J Anaesth* 1973; **45**: 711–718.

158 Kimmoun A, Ducrocq N, Sennoun N, *et al.* Efficient extra- and intracellular alkalinization improves cardiovascular functions in severe lactic acidosis induced by hemorrhagic shock. *Anesthesiology* 2014; **120**: 926–934.

159 Regan MJ, Eger EI II. Effect of hypothermia in dogs on anesthetizing and apneic doses of inhalation agents. Determination of the anesthetic index (Apnea/MAC). *Anesthesiology* 1967; **28**: 689–700.

160 Steffey EP, Howland D Jr. Isoflurane potency in the dog and cat. *Am J Vet Res* 1977; **38**: 1833–1836.

161 Galloway DS, Ko JC, Reaugh HF, *et al.* Anesthetic indices of sevoflurane and isoflurane in unpremedicated dogs. *J Am Vet Med Assoc* 2004; **225**: 700–704.

162 Bloor BC, Abdul-Rasool I, Temp J, *et al.* The effects of medetomidine, an alpha 2-adrenergic agonist, on ventilatory drive in the dog. *Acta Vet Scand Suppl* 1989; **85**: 65–70.

163 Steffey EP, Howland D Jr. Potency of enflurane in dogs: comparison with halothane and isoflurane. *Am J Vet Res* 1978; **39**: 573–577.

164 Hikasa Y, Okuyama K, Kakuta T, *et al.* Anesthetic potency and cardiopulmonary effects of sevoflurane in goats: comparison with isoflurane and halothane. *Can J Vet Res* 1998; **62**: 299–306.

165 Steffey EP, Gillespie JR, Berry JD, *et al.* Cardiovascular effects of halothane in the stump-tailed macaque during spontaneous and controlled ventilation. *Am J Vet Res* 1974; **35**: 1315–1319.

166 Steffey EP, Woliner MJ, Puschner B, *et al.* Effects of desflurane and mode of ventilation on cardiovascular and respiratory functions and clinicopathologic variables in horses. *Am J Vet Res* 2005; **66**: 669–677.

167 Steffey MA, Brosnan RJ, Steffey EP. Assessment of halothane and sevoflurane anesthesia in spontaneously breathing rats. *Am J Vet Res* 2003; **64**: 470–474.

168 Grosenbaugh DA, Muir WW. Cardiorespiratory effects of sevoflurane, isoflurane, and halothane anesthesia in horses. *Am J Vet Res* 1998; **59**: 101–106.

169 Steffey EP, Howland D Jr., Giri S, *et al.* Enflurane, halothane, and isoflurane potency in horses. *Am J Vet Res* 1977; **38**: 1037–1039.

170 Steffey EP, Howland D Jr. Halothane anesthesia in calves. *Am J Vet Res* 1979; **40**: 372–376.

171 McDonell W. Anesthesia of the harp seal. *J Wildl Dis* 1972; **8**: 287–295.

172 Flecknell PA, Roughan JV, Hedenqvist P. Induction of anaesthesia with sevoflurane and isoflurane in the rabbit. *Lab Anim* 1999; **33**: 41–46.

173 Abdul-Rasool IH, Ward DS. Ventilatory and cardiovascular responses to sufentanil infusion in dogs anesthetized with isoflurane. *Anesth Analg* 1989; **69**: 300–306.

174 Hornbein TF. Anesthetics and ventilatory control. In: Covino BG FH, Rehder K, Strichartz G, eds. *Effects of Anesthesia*. Bethesda, MD: American Physiologic Society, 1985: 75–90.

175 Evgenov OV, Liang Y, Jiang Y, *et al.* Pulmonary pharmacology and inhaled anesthetics. In: Gropper MA, Cohen NH, Eriksson LI, *et al.*, eds. *Miller's Anesthesia*, 9th edn. Philadelphia, PA: Elsevier, 2020: 540–571.

176 Boden AG, Harris MC, Parkes MJ. Apneic threshold for CO_2 in the anesthetized rat: fundamental properties under steady-state conditions. *J Appl Physiol (1985)* **1998**; 85: 898–907.

177 Thompson KR, Bardell D. The effect of two different intra-operative end-tidal carbon dioxide tensions on apnoeic duration in the recovery period in horses. *Vet Anaesth Analg* 2016; **43**: 163–170.

178 Quandt JE, Robinson EP, Rivers WJ, *et al.* Cardiorespiratory and anesthetic effects of propofol and thiopental in dogs. *Am J Vet Res* 1998; **59**: 1137–1143.

179 Bigby SE, Beths T, Bauquier S, *et al.* Effect of rate of administration of propofol or alfaxalone on induction dose requirements and occurrence of apnea in dogs. *Vet Anaesth Analg* 2017; **44**: 1267–1275.

180 Muir WW III, Gadawski JE. Respiratory depression and apnea induced by propofol in dogs. *Am J Vet Res* 1998; **59**: 157–161.

181 Liehmann L, Mosing M, Auer U. A comparison of cardiorespiratory variables during isoflurane-fentanyl and propofol-fentanyl anaesthesia for surgery in injured cats. *Vet Anaesth Analg* 2006; **33**: 158–168.

182 Campagna I, Schwarz A, Keller S, *et al.* Comparison of the effects of propofol or alfaxalone for anaesthesia induction and maintenance on respiration in cats. *Vet Anaesth Analg* 2015; **42**: 484–492.

183 Suarez MA, Dzikiti BT, Stegmann FG, *et al.* Comparison of alfaxalone and propofol administered as total intravenous anaesthesia for ovariohysterectomy in dogs. *Vet Anaesth Analg* 2012; **39**: 236–244.

184 Lerche P, Nolan AM, Reid J. Comparative study of propofol or propofol and ketamine for the induction of anaesthesia in dogs. *Vet Rec* 2000; **146**: 571–574.

185 McKeirnan KL, Gross ME, Rochat M, *et al.* Comparison of propofol and propofol/ketamine anesthesia for evaluation of laryngeal function in healthy dogs. *J Am Anim Hosp Assoc* 2014; **50**: 19–26.

186 Jaspar N, Mazzarelli M, Tessier C, *et al.* Effect of ketamine on control of breathing in cats. *J Appl Physiol Respir Environ Exerc Physiol* 1983; **55**: 851–859.

187 Brock N, Hildebrand SV. A comparison of xylazine-diazepam-ketamine and xylazine-guaifenesin-ketamine in equine anesthesia. *Vet Surg* 1990; **19**: 468–474.

188 Kerr CL, McDonell WN, Young SS. A comparison of romifidine and xylazine when used with diazepam/ketamine for short duration anesthesia in the horse. *Can Vet J* 1996; **37**: 601–609.

189 McMurphy RM, Young LE, Marlin DJ, *et al.* Comparison of the cardiopulmonary effects of anesthesia maintained by continuous infusion of romifidine, guaifenesin, and ketamine with anesthesia maintained by inhalation of halothane in horses. *Am J Vet Res* 2002; **63**: 1655–1661.

190 Cuvelliez SG, Eicker SW, McLauchlan C, *et al.* Cardiovascular and respiratory effects of inspired oxygen fraction in halothane-anesthetized horses. *Am J Vet Res* 1990; **51**: 1226–1231.

191 Marntell S, Nyman G, Hedenstierna G. High inspired oxygen concentrations increase intrapulmonary shunt in anaesthetized horses. *Vet Anaesth Analg* 2005; **32**: 338–347.

192 Crumley MN, McMurphy RM, Hodgson DS, *et al.* Effects of inspired oxygen concentration on ventilation, ventilatory rhythm, and gas exchange in isoflurane-anesthetized horses. *Am J Vet Res* 2013; **74**: 183–190.

193 Rousseau-Blass F, Pang DS. Hypoventilation following oxygen administration associated with alfaxalone-dexmedetomidine-midazolam anesthesia in New Zealand White rabbits. *Vet Anaesth Analg* 2020; **47**: 637–646.

194 Hubbell JA, Aarnes TK, Bednarski RM, *et al.* Effect of 50% and maximal inspired oxygen concentrations on respiratory variables in isoflurane-anesthetized horses. *BMC Vet Res* 2011; **7**: 23.

195 Kerr CL, McDonell WN, Young SS. Cardiopulmonary effects of romifidine/ketamine or xylazine/ketamine when used for short duration anesthesia in the horse. *Can J Vet Res* 2004; **68**: 274–282.

196 Weil JV, Byrne-Quinn E, Sodal IE, *et al.* Hypoxic ventilatory drive in normal man. *J Clin Invest* 1970; **49**: 1061–1072.

197 Hirshman CA, McCullough RE, Cohen PJ, *et al.* Hypoxic ventilatory drive in dogs during thiopental, ketamine, or pentobarbital anesthesia. *Anesthesiology* 1975; **43**: 628–634.

198 Hirshman CA, McCullough RE, Cohen PJ, *et al.* Depression of hypoxic ventilatory response by halothane, enflurane and isoflurane in dogs. *Br J Anaesth* 1977; **49**: 957–963.

199 Ponte J, Sadler CL. Effect of thiopentone, etomidate and propofol on carotid body chemoreceptor activity in the rabbit and the cat. *Br J Anaesth* 1989; **62**: 41–45.

200 Ponte J, Sadler CL. Effect of halothane, enflurane and isoflurane on carotid body chemoreceptor activity in the rabbit and the cat. *Br J Anaesth* 1989; **62**: 33–40.

201 Blouin RT, Seifert HA, Babenco HD, *et al.* Propofol depresses the hypoxic ventilatory response during conscious sedation and isohypercapnia. *Anesthesiology* 1993; **79**: 1177–1182.

202 Karanovic N, Pecotic R, Valic M, *et al.* The acute hypoxic ventilatory response under halothane, isoflurane, and sevoflurane anaesthesia in rats. *Anaesthesia* 2010; **65**: 227–234.

203 Engbers S, Larkin A, Rousset N, *et al.* Comparison of a supraglottic airway device (v-gel(®)) with blind orotracheal intubation in rabbits. *Front Vet Sci* 2017; **4**: 49.

204 Wenger S, Müllhaupt D, Ohlerth S, *et al.* Experimental evaluation of four airway devices in anaesthetized New Zealand White rabbits. *Vet Anaesth Analg* 2017; **44**: 529–537.

205 Ko JC, Fox SM, Mandsager RE. Sedative and cardiorespiratory effects of medetomidine, medetomidine-butorphanol, and medetomidine-ketamine in dogs. *J Am Vet Med Assoc* 2000; **216**: 1578–1583.

206 Kuo WC, Keegan RD. Comparative cardiovascular, analgesic, and sedative effects of medetomidine, medetomidine-hydromorphone, and medetomidine-butorphanol in dogs. *Am J Vet Res* 2004; **65**: 931–937.

207 Keating SC, Kerr CL, Valverde A, *et al.* Cardiopulmonary effects of intravenous fentanyl infusion in dogs during isoflurane anesthesia and with concurrent acepromazine or dexmedetomidine administration during anesthetic recovery. *Am J Vet Res* 2013; **74**: 672–682.

208 Enouri SS, Kerr CL, McDonell WN, *et al.* Cardiopulmonary effects of anesthetic induction with thiopental, propofol, or a combination of ketamine hydrochloride and diazepam in dogs sedated with a combination of medetomidine and hydromorphone. *Am J Vet Res* 2008; **69**: 586–595.

209 Celly CS, McDonell WN, Young SS, *et al.* The comparative hypoxaemic effect of four alpha 2 adrenoceptor agonists (xylazine, romifidine, detomidine and medetomidine) in sheep. *J Vet Pharmacol Ther* 1997; **20**: 464–471.

210 Lodenius Å, Ebberyd A, Hårdemark Cedborg A, *et al.* Sedation with dexmedetomidine or propofol impairs hypoxic control of breathing in healthy male volunteers: a non-blinded, randomized crossover study. *Anesthesiology* 2016; **125**: 700–715.

211 Santos M, Fuente M, Garcia-Iturralde R, *et al.* Effects of alpha-2 adrenoceptor agonists during recovery from isoflurane anaesthesia in horses. *Equine Vet J* 2003; **35**: 170–175.

212 Woodhouse KJ, Brosnan RJ, Nguyen KQ, *et al.* Effects of postanesthetic sedation with romifidine or xylazine on quality of recovery from isoflurane anesthesia in horses. *J Am Vet Med Assoc* 2013; **242**: 533–539.

213 Ward DS. Stimulation of hypoxic ventilatory drive by droperidol. *Anesth Analg* 1984; **63**: 106–110.

214 Murphy DJ, Renninger JP, Schramek D. Respiratory inductive plethysmography as a method for measuring ventilatory parameters in conscious, non-restrained dogs. *J Pharmacol Toxicol Methods* 2010; **62**: 47–53.

215 Ide T, Shirahata M, Chou CL, *et al.* Effects of a continuous infusion of dopamine on the ventilatory and carotid body responses to hypoxia in cats. *Clin Exp Pharmacol Physiol* 1995; **22**: 658–664.

216 Dahan A, Ward D, van den Elsen M, *et al.* Influence of reduced carotid body drive during sustained hypoxia on hypoxic depression of ventilation in humans. *J Appl Physiol (1985)* **1996**; 81: 565–572.

217 van de Borne P, Oren R, Somers VK. Dopamine depresses minute ventilation in patients with heart failure. *Circulation* 1998; **98**: 126–131.

218 Dahan A, Sarton E, Teppema L, *et al.* Anesthetic potency and influence of morphine and sevoflurane on respiration in mu-opioid receptor knockout mice. *Anesthesiology* 2001; **94**: 824–832.

219 Romberg R, Sarton E, Teppema L, *et al.* Comparison of morphine-6-glucuronide and morphine on respiratory depressant and antinociceptive responses in wild type and mu-opioid receptor deficient mice. *Br J Anaesth* 2003; **91**: 862–870.

220 Camporesi EM, Nielsen CH, Bromage PR, *et al.* Ventilatory CO_2 sensitivity after intravenous and epidural morphine in volunteers. *Anesth Analg* 1983; **62**: 633–640.

221 Romagnoli A, Keats AS. Ceiling effect for respiratory depression by nalbuphine. *Clin Pharmacol Ther* 1980; **27**: 478–485.

222 Talbert RL, Peters JI, Sorrells SC, *et al.* Respiratory effects of high-dose butorphanol. *Acute Care* 1988; **12**(Suppl 1): 47–56.

223 Freye E, Azevedo L, Hartung E. Reversal of fentanyl related respiratory depression with nalbuphine. Effects on the CO_2-response curve in man. *Acta Anaesthesiol Belg* 1985; **36**: 365–374.

224 Bowdle TA, Greichen SL, Bjurstrom RL, *et al.* Butorphanol improves CO_2 response and ventilation after fentanyl anesthesia. *Anesth Analg* 1987; **66**: 517–522.

225 McCrackin MA, Harvey RC, Sackman JE, *et al.* Butorphanol tartrate for partial reversal of oxymorphone-induced postoperative respiratory depression in the dog. *Vet Surg* 1994; **23**: 67–74.

226 Niesters M, Mahajan RP, Aarts L, *et al.* High-inspired oxygen concentration further impairs opioid-induced respiratory depression. *Br J Anaesth* 2013; **110**: 837–841.

227 Jacobson JD, McGrath CJ, Smith EP. Cardiorespiratory effects of four opioid-tranquilizer combinations in dogs. *Vet Surg* 1994; **23**: 299–306.

228 Cullen LK, Raffe MR, Randall DA, *et al.* Assessment of the respiratory actions of intramuscular morphine in conscious dogs. *Res Vet Sci* 1999; **67**: 141–148.

229 Smith LJ, Yu JK, Bjorling DE, *et al.* Effects of hydromorphone or oxymorphone, with or without acepromazine, on preanesthetic sedation, physiologic values, and histamine release in dogs. *J Am Vet Med Assoc* 2001; **218**: 1101–1105.

230 Dyson DH, Atilola M. A clinical comparison of oxymorphone-acepromazine and butorphanol-acepromazine sedation in dogs. *Vet Surg* 1992; **21**: 418–421.

231 Posner LP, Pavuk AA, Rokshar JL, *et al.* Effects of opioids and anesthetic drugs on body temperature in cats. *Vet Anaesth Analg* 2010; **37**: 35–43.

232 Maiante AA, Teixeira-Neto FJ, Beier SL, *et al.* Comparison of the cardio-respiratory effects of methadone and morphine in conscious dogs. *J Vet Pharmacol Ther* 2009; **32**: 317–328.

233 Wunsch LA, Schmidt BK, Krugner-Higby LA, *et al.* A comparison of the effects of hydromorphone HCl and a novel extended release hydromorphone on arterial blood gas values in conscious healthy dogs. *Res Vet Sci* 2010; **88**: 154–158.

234 Trim CM. Cardiopulmonary effects of butorphanol tartrate in dogs. *Am J Vet Res* 1983; **44**: 329–331.

235 Quandt JE, Raffe MR, Robinson EP. Butorphanol does not reduce the minimum alveolar concentration of halothane in dogs. *Vet Surg* 1994; **23**: 156–159.

236 Zucker JR, Neuenfeldt T, Freund PR. Respiratory effects of nalbuphine and butorphanol in anesthetized patients. *Anesth Analg* 1987; **66**: 879–881.

237 Robertson JT, Muir WW, Sams R. Cardiopulmonary effects of butorphanol tartrate in horses. *Am J Vet Res* 1981; **42**: 41–44.

238 Carregaro AB, Neto FJ, Beier SL, *et al.* Cardiopulmonary effects of buprenorphine in horses. *Am J Vet Res* 2006; **67**: 1675–1680.

239 Figueiredo JP, Muir WW, Sams R. Cardiorespiratory, gastrointestinal, and analgesic effects of morphine sulfate in conscious healthy horses. *Am J Vet Res* 2012; **73**: 799–808.

240 Steffey EP, Eisele JH, Baggot JD. Interactions of morphine and isoflurane in horses. *Am J Vet Res* 2003; **64**: 166–175.

241 Clark L, Clutton RE, Blissitt KJ, *et al.* Effects of peri-operative morphine administration during halothane anaesthesia in horses. *Vet Anaesth Analg* 2005; **32**: 10–15.

242 Bitti FS, Campagnol D, Rangel JP, *et al.* Effects of three methadone doses combined with acepromazine on sedation and some cardiopulmonary variables in dogs. *Vet Anaesth Analg* 2017; **44**: 237–245.

243 Monteiro ER, Rabello TA, Rangel JPP, *et al.* Effects of 3 morphine doses, in combination with acepromazine, on sedation and some physiological parameters in dogs. *Can J Vet Res* 2019; **83**: 235–240.

244 Costa GP, Monteiro ER, Marques ÉJ, *et al.* Sedative effects of acepromazine in combination with nalbuphine or butorphanol, intramuscularly or intravenously, in healthy cats: a randomized, blinded clinical trial. *J Feline Med Surg* 2021; **23**: 540–548.

245 Nolan AM, Reid J. The use of intraoperative fentanyl in spontaneously breathing dogs undergoing orthopaedic surgery. *J Vet Anaesth* 1991; **18**: 30–39.

246 Steffey EP, Baggot JD, Eisele JH, *et al.* Morphine-isoflurane interaction in dogs, swine and rhesus monkeys. *J Vet Pharmacol Ther* 1994; **17**: 202–210.

247 Garofalo NA, Teixeira-Neto FJ, Pereira CD, *et al.* Cardiorespiratory and neuroendocrine changes induced by methadone in conscious and in isoflurane anaesthetised dogs. *Vet J* 2012; **194**: 398–404.

248 Leibetseder EN, Mosing M, Jones RS. A comparison of extradural and intravenous methadone on intraoperative isoflurane and postoperative analgesia requirements in dogs. *Vet Anaesth Analg* 2006; **33**: 128–136.

249 Berkenbosch A, Teppema LJ, Olievier CN, *et al.* Influences of morphine on the ventilatory response to isocapnic hypoxia. *Anesthesiology* 1997; **86**: 1342–1349.

250 Campbell VL, Drobatz KJ, Perkowski SZ. Postoperative hypoxemia and hypercarbia in healthy dogs undergoing routine ovariohysterectomy or castration and receiving butorphanol or hydromorphone for analgesia. *J Am Vet Med Assoc* 2003; **222**: 330–336.

251 Wahler BM, Lerche P, Ricco Pereira CH, *et al.* Pharmacokinetics and pharmacodynamics of intranasal and intravenous naloxone hydrochloride administration in healthy dogs. *Am J Vet Res* 2019; **80**: 696–701.

252 Copland VS, Haskins SC, Patz J. Naloxone reversal of oxymorphone effects in dogs. *Am J Vet Res* 1989; **50**: 1854–1858.

253 Hedenstierna G. Gas exchange during anaesthesia. *Br J Anaesth* 1990; **64**: 507–514.

254 Reber A, Engberg G, Sporre B, *et al.* Volumetric analysis of aeration in the lungs during general anaesthesia. *Br J Anaesth* 1996; **76**: 760–766.

255 Rothen HU, Sporre B, Engberg G, *et al.* Airway closure, atelectasis and gas exchange during general anaesthesia. *Br J Anaesth* 1998; **81**: 681–686.

256 Wahba RW. Perioperative functional residual capacity. *Can J Anaesth* 1991; **38**: 384–400.

257 Lumb AB, Thomas C. Anaesthesia. In: Lumb AB, Thomas C, eds. *Nunn and Lumb's Applied Respiratory Physiology*, 9th edn. Edinburgh, UK: Elsevier, 2021: 244–267.

258 Hedenstierna G, Tokics L, Reinius H, *et al.* Higher age and obesity limit atelectasis formation during anaesthesia: an analysis of computed tomography data in 243 subjects. *Br J Anaesth* 2020; **124**: 336–344.

259 Lai YL, Rodarte JR, Hyatt RE. Respiratory mechanics in recumbent dogs anesthetized with thiopental sodium. *J Appl Physiol Respir Environ Exerc Physiol* 1979; **46**: 716–720.

260 Barletta M, Almondia D, Williams J, *et al.* Radiographic evaluation of positional atelectasis in sedated dogs breathing room air versus 100% oxygen. *Can Vet J* 2014; **55**: 985–991.

261 Staffieri F, Franchini D, Carella GL, *et al.* Computed tomographic analysis of the effects of two inspired oxygen concentrations on pulmonary aeration in anesthetized and mechanically ventilated dogs. *Am J Vet Res* 2007; **68**: 925–931.

262 De Monte V, Grasso S, De Marzo C, *et al.* Effects of reduction of inspired oxygen fraction or application of positive end-expiratory pressure after an alveolar recruitment maneuver on respiratory mechanics, gas exchange, and lung aeration in dogs during anesthesia and neuromuscular blockade. *Am J Vet Res* 2013; **74**: 25–33.

263 Ambrosio AM, Carvalho-Kamakura TPA, Ida KK, *et al.* Ventilation distribution assessed with electrical impedance tomography and the influence of tidal volume, recruitment and positive end-expiratory pressure in isoflurane-anesthetized dogs. *Vet Anaesth Analg* 2017; **44**: 254–263.

264 McDonell W. The effect of anesthesia on pulmonary gas exchange and arterial oxygenation in the horse. PhD Thesis, University of Cambridge, 1974.

265 McDonell WN, Hall LW, Jeffcott LB. Radiographic evidence of impaired pulmonary function in laterally recumbent anaesthetised horses. *Equine Vet J* 1979; **11**: 24–32.

266 Watney GC. Radiographic evidence of pulmonary dysfunction in anaesthetised cattle. *Res Vet Sci* 1986; **41**: 162–171.

267 Hornof WJ, Dunlop CI, Prestage R, *et al.* Effects of lateral recumbency on regional lung function in anesthetized horses. *Am J Vet Res* 1986; **47**: 277–282.

268 Nyman G, Funkquist B, Kvart C, *et al.* Atelectasis causes gas exchange impairment in the anaesthetised horse. *Equine Vet J* 1990; **22**: 317–324.

269 Moens Y, Lagerweij E, Gootjes P, *et al.* Distribution of inspired gas to each lung in the anaesthetised horse and influence of body shape. *Equine Vet J* 1995; **27**: 110–116.

270 Damia G, Mascheroni D, Croci M, *et al.* Perioperative changes in functional residual capacity in morbidly obese patients. *Br J Anaesth* 1988; **60**: 574–578.

271 Zeng C, Lagier D, Lee JW, *et al.* Perioperative pulmonary atelectasis: Part I. *Biology and mechanisms. Anesthesiology* 2022; **136**: 181–205.

272 Benson GJ, Manohar M, Kneller SK, *et al.* Radiographic characterization of diaphragmatic excursion in halothane-anesthetized ponies: spontaneous and controlled ventilation systems. *Am J Vet Res* 1982; **43**: 617–621.

273 Staffieri F, De Monte V, De Marzo C, *et al.* Effects of two fractions of inspired oxygen on lung aeration and gas exchange in cats under inhalant anaesthesia. *Vet Anaesth Analg* 2010; **37**: 483–490.

274 Hedenstierna G, Tokics L, Strandberg A, *et al.* Correlation of gas exchange impairment to development of atelectasis during anaesthesia and muscle paralysis. *Acta Anaesthesiol Scand* 1986; **30**: 183–191.

275 Pavone L, Albert S, DiRocco J, *et al.* Alveolar instability caused by mechanical ventilation initially damages the nondependent normal lung. *Crit Care* 2007; **11**: R104.

276 Pavone LA, Albert S, Carney D, *et al.* Injurious mechanical ventilation in the normal lung causes a progressive pathologic change in dynamic alveolar mechanics. *Crit Care* 2007; **11**: R64.

277 Hopster K, Kästner SB, Rohn K, *et al.* Intermittent positive pressure ventilation with constant positive end-expiratory pressure and alveolar recruitment manoeuvre during inhalation anaesthesia in horses undergoing surgery for colic, and its influence on the early recovery period. *Vet Anaesth Analg* 2011; **38**: 169–177.

278 Canfrán S, Gómez de Segura IA, Cediel R, *et al.* Effects of a stepwise lung recruitment manoeuvre and positive end-expiratory pressure on lung compliance and arterial blood oxygenation in healthy dogs. *Vet J* 2012; **194**: 89–93.

279 Varner KM, Hopster K, Driessen B. Comparison of various types of inert gas components on efficacy of an alveolar recruitment maneuver in dorsally recumbent anesthetized horses. *Am J Vet Res* 2019; **80**: 631–636.

280 Staffieri F, Bauquier SH, Moate PJ, *et al.* Pulmonary gas exchange in anaesthetised horses mechanically ventilated with oxygen or a helium/oxygen mixture. *Equine Vet J* 2009; **41**: 747–752.

281 Hedenstierna G, McCarthy G. The effect of anaesthesia and intermittent positive pressure ventilation with different frequencies on the anatomical and alveolar deadspace. *Br J Anaesth* 1975; **47**: 847–852.

282 Tusman G, Suarez-Sipmann F, Böhm SH, *et al.* Monitoring dead space during recruitment and PEEP titration in an experimental model. *Intensive Care Med* 2006; **32**: 1863–1871.

283 Casati A, Fanelli G, Torri G. Physiological dead space/tidal volume ratio during face mask, laryngeal mask, and cuffed oropharyngeal airway spontaneous ventilation. *J Clin Anesth* 1998; **10**: 652–655.

284 Maisch S, Reissmann H, Fuellekrug B, *et al.* Compliance and dead space fraction indicate an optimal level of positive end-expiratory pressure after recruitment in anesthetized patients. *Anesth Analg* 2008; **106**: 175–181.

285 Lavoie JP, Pascoe JR, Kurpershoek CJ. Effect of head and neck position on respiratory mechanics in horses sedated with xylazine. *Am J Vet Res* 1992; **53**: 1652–1657.

286 Broadstone RV, Gray PR, Robinson NE, *et al.* Effects of xylazine on airway function in ponies with recurrent airway obstruction. *Am J Vet Res* 1992; **53**: 1813–1817.

287 Tomasic M, Mann LS, Soma LR. Effects of sedation, anesthesia, and endotracheal intubation on respiratory mechanics in adult horses. *Am J Vet Res* 1997; **58**: 641–646.

288 Brown RH, Zerhouni EA, Hirshman CA. Comparison of low concentrations of halothane and isoflurane as bronchodilators. *Anesthesiology* 1993; **78**: 1097–1101.

289 Yamakage M. Effects of anaesthetic agents on airway smooth muscles. *Br J Anaesth* 2002; **88**: 624–627.

290 Dikmen Y, Eminoglu E, Salihoglu Z, *et al.* Pulmonary mechanics during isoflurane, sevoflurane and desflurane anaesthesia. *Anaesthesia* 2003; **58**: 745–748.

291 Myers CF, Fontao F, Jánosi TZ, *et al.* Sevoflurane and desflurane protect cholinergic-induced bronchoconstriction of hyperreactive airways in rabbits. *Can J Anaesth* 2011; **58**: 1007–1015.

292 Nyktari V, Papaioannou A, Volakakis N, *et al.* Respiratory resistance during anaesthesia with isoflurane, sevoflurane, and desflurane: a randomized clinical trial. *Br J Anaesth* 2011; **107**: 454–661.

293 Westbrook PR, Stubbs SE, Sessler AD, *et al.* Effects of anesthesia and muscle paralysis on respiratory mechanics in normal man. *J Appl Physiol* 1973; **34**: 81–86.

294 Blaze CA, LeBlanc PH, Robinson NE. Effect of withholding feed on ventilation and the incidence of regurgitation during halothane anesthesia of adult cattle. *Am J Vet Res* 1988; **49**: 2126–2129.

295 Bradbrook CA, Clark L, Dugdale AH, *et al.* Measurement of respiratory system compliance and respiratory system resistance in healthy dogs undergoing general anaesthesia for elective orthopaedic procedures. *Vet Anaesth Analg* 2013; **40**: 382–389.

296 Kerr CL, Keating SCJ, Arroyo LG, *et al.* Cardiopulmonary effects and recovery characteristics associated with 2 sedative protocols for assisted ventilation in healthy neonatal foals. *Can J Vet Res* 2021; **85**: 251–260.

297 Asorey I, Pellegrini L, Canfrán S, *et al.* Factors affecting respiratory system compliance in anaesthetised mechanically ventilated healthy dogs: a retrospective study. *J Small Anim Pract* 2020; **61**: 617–623.

298 Aida H, Mizuno Y, Hobo S, *et al.* Cardiovascular and pulmonary effects of sevoflurane anesthesia in horses. *Vet Surg* 1996; **25**: 164–170.

299 Nyman G, Hedenstierna G. Ventilation–perfusion relationships in the anaesthetised horse. *Equine Vet J* 1989; **21**: 274–281.

300 Takala J. Hypoxemia due to increased venous admixture: influence of cardiac output on oxygenation. *Intensive Care Med* 2007; **33**: 908–911.

301 Wagner PD. The multiple inert gas elimination technique (MIGET). *Intensive Care Med* 2008; **34**: 994–1001.

302 Bhavani-Shankar K, Moseley H, Kumar AY, *et al.* Capnometry and anaesthesia. *Can J Anaesth* 1992; **39**: 617–632.

303 Koenig J, McDonell W, Valverde A. Accuracy of pulse oximetry and capnography in healthy and compromised horses during spontaneous and controlled ventilation. *Can J Vet Res* 2003; **67**: 169–174.

304 Boer F. Drug handling by the lungs. *Br J Anaesth* 2003; **91**: 50–60.

305 Dawidowicz AL, Fornal E, Mardarowicz M, *et al.* The role of human lungs in the biotransformation of propofol. *Anesthesiology* 2000; **93**: 992–997.

306 He YL, Ueyama H, Tashiro C, *et al.* Pulmonary disposition of propofol in surgical patients. *Anesthesiology* 2000; **93**: 986–991.

307 Hiraoka H, Yamamoto K, Miyoshi S, *et al.* Kidneys contribute to the extrahepatic clearance of propofol in humans, but not lungs and brain. *Br J Clin Pharmacol* 2005; **60**: 176–182.

308 Kuipers JA, Boer F, Olieman W, *et al.* First-pass lung uptake and pulmonary clearance of propofol: assessment with a recirculatory indocyanine green pharmacokinetic model. *Anesthesiology* 1999; **91**: 1780–1787.

309 Matot I, Neely CF, Katz RY, *et al.* Fentanyl and propofol uptake by the lung: effect of time between injections. *Acta Anaesthesiol Scand* 1994; **38**: 711–715.

310 Matot I, Neely CF, Katz RY, *et al.* Pulmonary uptake of propofol in cats. *Effect of fentanyl and halothane. Anesthesiology* 1993; **78**: 1157–1165.

311 Grossherr M, Hengstenberg A, Meier T, *et al.* Discontinuous monitoring of propofol concentrations in expired alveolar gas and in arterial and venous plasma during artificial ventilation. *Anesthesiology* 2006; **104**: 786–790.

312 Takita A, Masui K, Kazama T. On-line monitoring of end-tidal propofol concentration in anesthetized patients. *Anesthesiology* 2007; **106**: 659–664.

313 Colin P, Eleveld DJ, van den Berg JP, *et al.* Propofol breath monitoring as a potential tool to improve the prediction of intraoperative plasma concentrations. *Clin Pharmacokinet* 2016; **55**: 849–859.

314 Sykes MK, Loh L, Seed RF, *et al.* The effect of inhalational anaesthetics on hypoxic pulmonary vasoconstriction and pulmonary vascular resistance in the perfused lungs of the dog and cat. *Br J Anaesth* 1972; **44**: 776–788.

315 Bjertnaes LJ. Hypoxia-induced vasoconstriction in isolated perfused lungs exposed to injectable or inhalation anesthetics. *Acta Anaesthesiol Scand* 1977; **21**: 133–147.

316 Marshall C, Lindgren L, Marshall BE. Effects of halothane, enflurane, and isoflurane on hypoxic pulmonary vasoconstriction in rat lungs in vitro. *Anesthesiology* 1984; **60**: 304–308.

317 Ishibe Y, Gui X, Uno H, *et al.* Effect of sevoflurane on hypoxic pulmonary vasoconstriction in the perfused rabbit lung. *Anesthesiology* 1993; **79**: 1348–1353.

318 Loer SA, Scheeren TW, Tarnow J. Desflurane inhibits hypoxic pulmonary vasoconstriction in isolated rabbit lungs. *Anesthesiology* 1995; **83**: 552–556.

319 Mathers J, Benumof JL, Wahrenbrock EA. General anesthetics and regional hypoxic pulmonary vasoconstriction. *Anesthesiology* 1977; **46**: 111–114.

320 Naeije R, Lambert M, Lejeune P, *et al.* Cardiovascular and blood gas responses to inhaled anaesthetics in normoxic and hypoxic dogs. *Acta Anaesthesiol Scand* 1986; **30**: 538–544.

321 Domino KB, Borowec L, Alexander CM, *et al.* Influence of isoflurane on hypoxic pulmonary vasoconstriction in dogs. *Anesthesiology* 1986; **64**: 423–429.

322 Ewalenko P, Stefanidis C, Holoye A, *et al.* Pulmonary vascular impedance vs. resistance in hypoxic and hyperoxic dogs: effects of propofol and isoflurane. *J Appl Physiol (1985)* **1993**; 74: 2188–2193.

323 Rogers SN, Benumof JL. Halothane and isoflurane do not decrease PaO2 during one-lung ventilation in intravenously anesthetized patients. *Anesth Analg* 1985; **64**: 946–954.

324 Benumof JL, Augustine SD, Gibbons JA. Halothane and isoflurane only slightly impair arterial oxygenation during one-lung ventilation in patients undergoing thoracotomy. *Anesthesiology* 1987; **67**: 910–915.

325 Naeije R, Lejeune P, Leeman M, *et al.* Effects of propofol on pulmonary and systemic arterial pressure-flow relationships in hyperoxic and hypoxic dogs. *Br J Anaesth* 1989; **62**: 532–539.

326 Shoukas AA, Brunner MJ, Frankle AE, *et al.* Carotid sinus baroreceptor reflex control and the role of autoregulation in the systemic and pulmonary arterial pressure-flow relationships of the dog. *Circ Res* 1984; **54**: 674–682.

327 Lennon PF, Murray PA. Attenuated hypoxic pulmonary vasoconstriction during isoflurane anesthesia is abolished by cyclooxygenase inhibition in chronically instrumented dogs. *Anesthesiology* 1996; **84**: 404–414.

328 Abe K, Mashimo T, Yoshiya I. Arterial oxygenation and shunt fraction during one-lung ventilation: a comparison of isoflurane and sevoflurane. *Anesth Analg* 1998; **86**: 1266–1270.

329 Pagel PS, Fu JL, Damask MC, *et al.* Desflurane and isoflurane produce similar alterations in systemic and pulmonary hemodynamics and arterial oxygenation in patients undergoing one-lung ventilation during thoracotomy. *Anesth Analg* 1998; **87**: 800–807.

330 Wang JY, Russell GN, Page RD, *et al.* Comparison of the effects of sevoflurane and isoflurane on arterial oxygenation during one lung ventilation. *Br J Anaesth* 1998; **81**: 850–853.

331 Wang JY, Russell GN, Page RD, *et al.* A comparison of the effects of desflurane and isoflurane on arterial oxygenation during one-lung ventilation. *Anaesthesia* 2000; **55**: 167–173.

332 Kerbaul F, Bellezza M, Guidon C, *et al.* Effects of sevoflurane on hypoxic pulmonary vasoconstriction in anaesthetized piglets. *Br J Anaesth* 2000; **85**: 440–445.

333 Lesitsky MA, Davis S, Murray PA. Preservation of hypoxic pulmonary vasoconstriction during sevoflurane and desflurane anesthesia compared to the conscious state in chronically instrumented dogs. *Anesthesiology* 1998; **89**: 1501–1508.

334 Nakayama M, Murray PA. Ketamine preserves and propofol potentiates hypoxic pulmonary vasoconstriction compared with the conscious state in chronically instrumented dogs. *Anesthesiology* 1999; **91**: 760–771.

335 Van Keer L, Van Aken H, Vandermeersch E, *et al.* Propofol does not inhibit hypoxic pulmonary vasoconstriction in humans. *J Clin Anesth* 1989; **1**: 284–288.

336 Abe K, Shimizu T, Takashina M, *et al.* The effects of propofol, isoflurane, and sevoflurane on oxygenation and shunt fraction during one-lung ventilation. *Anesth Analg* 1998; **87**: 1164–1169.

337 Hedenstierna G, Edmark L. Mechanisms of atelectasis in the perioperative period. *Best Pract Res Clin Anaesthesiol* 2010; **24**: 157–169.

338 Benoît Z, Wicky S, Fischer JF, *et al.* The effect of increased FIO(2) before tracheal extubation on postoperative atelectasis. *Anesth Analg* 2002; **95**: 1777–1781.

339 Lindberg P, Gunnarsson L, Tokics L, *et al.* Atelectasis and lung function in the postoperative period. *Acta Anaesthesiol Scand* 1992; **36**: 546–553.

340 Baumgardner JE, Hedenstierna G. Ventilation/perfusion distributions revisited. *Curr Opin Anaesthesiol* 2016; **29**: 2–7.

341 Bindslev L, Hedenstierna G, Santesson J, *et al.* Ventilation perfusion distribution during inhalation anaesthesia. Effects of spontaneous breathing, mechanical ventilation and positive end-expiratory pressure. *Acta Anaesthesiol Scand* 1981; **25**: 360–371.

342 Joyce CJ, Baker AB. What is the role of absorption atelectasis in the genesis of perioperative pulmonary collapse? *Anaesth Intensive Care* 1995; **23**: 691–696.

343 Young CC, Harris EM, Vacchiano C, *et al.* Lung-protective ventilation for the surgical patient: international expert panel-based consensus recommendations. *Br J Anaesth* 2019; **123**: 898–913.

344 Celly CS, McDonell WN, Black WD, *et al.* Cardiopulmonary effects of clonidine, diazepam and the peripheral alpha 2 adrenoceptor agonist ST-91 in conscious sheep. *J Vet Pharmacol Ther* 1997; **20**: 472–478.

345 Kästner SB, Ohlerth S, Pospischil A, *et al.* Dexmedetomidine-induced pulmonary alterations in sheep. *Res Vet Sci* 2007; **83**: 217–226.

346 Celly CS, McDonell WN, Black WD. Cardiopulmonary effects of the alpha2-adrenoceptor agonists medetomidine and ST-91 in anesthetized sheep. *J Pharmacol Exp Ther* 1999; **289**: 712–720.

347 Pypendop BH, Verstegen JP. Hemodynamic effects of medetomidine in the dog: a dose titration study. *Vet Surg* 1998; **27**: 612–622.

348 Celly CS, Atwal OS, McDonell WN, *et al.* Histopathologic alterations induced in the lungs of sheep by use of alpha2-adrenergic receptor agonists. *Am J Vet Res* 1999; **60**: 154–161.

349 Brain JD, Molina RM, DeCamp MM, *et al.* Pulmonary intravascular macrophages: their contribution to the mononuclear phagocyte system in 13 species. *Am J Physiol* 1999; **276**: L146–L154.

350 LeBlanc PH, Eberhart SW, Robinson NE. In vitro effects of alpha 2-adrenergic receptor stimulation on cholinergic contractions of equine distal airways. *Am J Vet Res* 1993; **54**: 788–792.

351 Papazoglou L, Raptopoulos D, Kounenis G. The effect of xylazine on the isolated sheep trachea. *J Vet Pharmacol Ther* 1995; **18**: 216–219.

352 Manning MM, Broadstone RV. Effects of alpha 2-adrenergic receptor agonist and antagonist drugs on cholinergic contraction in bovine tracheal smooth muscle in vitro. *Am J Vet Res* 1995; **56**: 930–935.

353 Adam M, Lindén J, Raekallio M, *et al.* Effects of vatinoxan on xylazine-induced pulmonary alterations in sheep. *J Vet Pharmacol Ther* 2022; **45**: 117–125.

354 Kästner SB. A2-agonists in sheep: a review. *Vet Anaesth Analg* 2006; **33**: 79–96.

355 Levitzky MG. Transport of oxygen and carbon dioxide in blood. In: Levitzky MG, ed. *Pulmonary Physiology*, 9th edn. New York, NY: McGraw-Hill, 2018: 157–178.

356 Ewart SL. Gas transport in the blood. In: Klein, BG, ed. *Cunningham's Textbook of Veterinary Physiology*, 6th edn. St. Louis, MO: Elsevier, 2020: 550–559.

357 Bunn HF. Regulation of hemoglobin function in mammals. *Amer Zool* 1980; **20**: 199–211.

358 Cambier C, Detry B, Beerens D, *et al.* Effects of hyperchloremia on blood oxygen binding in healthy calves. *J Appl Physiol (1985)* **1998**; 85: 1267–1272.

359 Prange HD, Shoemaker JL Jr., Westen EA, *et al.* Physiological consequences of oxygen-dependent chloride binding to hemoglobin. *J Appl Physiol (1985)* **2001**; 91: 33–38.

360 Bohr C, Hasselbalch K, Krogh A. Ueber einen in biologischer beziehung wichtigen einfluss, den die kohlensäurespannung des blutes auf dessen sauerstoffbindung übt. *Skand Arch Physiol* 1904; **16**: 402–412.

361 Jensen FB. Red blood cell pH, the Bohr effect, and other oxygenation-linked phenomena in blood O_2 and CO_2 transport. *Acta Physiol Scand* 2004; **182**: 215–227.

362 Clerbaux T, Gustin P, Detry B, *et al.* Comparative study of the oxyhaemoglobin dissociation curve of four mammals: man, dog, horse and cattle. *Comp Biochem Physiol Comp Physiol* 1993; **106**: 687–694.

363 Banchero N, Grover RF, Will JA. Oxygen transport in the llama (*Lama glama*). *Respir Physiol* 1971; **13**: 102–115.

364 Sillau AH, Cueva S, Valenzuela A, *et al.* O_2 transport in the alpaca (*Lama pacos*) at sea level and at 3,300 m. *Respir Physiol* 1976; **27**: 147–155.

365 Weber RE. High-altitude adaptations in vertebrate hemoglobins. *Respir Physiol Neurobiol* 2007; **158**: 132–142.

366 Levitzky MG. Mechanics of breathing. In: Levitzky MG, ed. *Pulmonary Physiology*, 9th edn. New York, NY: McGraw-Hill, 2018: 13–58.

367 Wagner PD, Gillespie JR, Landgren GL, *et al.* Mechanism of exercise-induced hypoxemia in horses. *J Appl Physiol (1985)* **1989**; 66: 1227–1233.

368 Barker SJ, Tremper KK, Hyatt J. Effects of methemoglobinemia on pulse oximetry and mixed venous oximetry. *Anesthesiology* 1989; **70**: 112–117.

369 Hampson NB. Pulse oximetry in severe carbon monoxide poisoning. *Chest* 1998; **114**: 1036–1041.

370 Feiner JR, Bickler PE. Improved accuracy of methemoglobin detection by pulse CO-oximetry during hypoxia. *Anesth Analg* 2010; **111**: 1160–1167.

371 Love L, Singer M. Anesthesia case of the month. *Methemoglobinemia. J Am Vet Med Assoc* 2013; **242**: 753–756.

372 Sández I, Márquez F, López A, *et al.* Detection of methaemoglobinaemia in a Pomeranian dog using pulse co-oximetry. *Vet Anaesth Analg* 2019; **46**: 708–710.

373 Arthurs GJ, Sudhakar M. Carbon dioxide transport. *Continuing Ed in Anaesth Crit Care Pain* 2005; **5**: 207–210.

38 Oxygen Therapy, Mechanical Ventilation, and Anesthetic Management of Patients with Respiratory Disease

Francisco J. Teixeira-Neto[1] and Carolyn L. Kerr[2]
[1] Faculdade de Medicina Veterinária e Zootecnia, Universidade Estadual Paulista (UNESP), Botucatu, Brazil
[2] Department of Clinical Studies, Ontario Veterinary College, University of Guelph, Guelph, Ontario, Canada

Chapter contents

Introduction, 750
Oxygen therapy, 751
Physiologic effects of oxygen therapy, 751
Strategies for oxygen supplementation, 752
Oxygen toxicity, 755
Mechanical ventilation during anesthesia, 755
Evolution of mechanical ventilators used in veterinary and human anesthesia, 756
Modes of mechanical ventilation utilized during anesthesia, 764
Monitoring pulmonary mechanics during mechanical ventilation, 770
Strategies for reducing atelectasis during mechanical ventilation, 773
Effects of mechanical ventilation on cardiovascular function, 777
Ventilator-induced lung injury, 778
Mechanical ventilation during anesthesia in humans and veterinary species, 780
Anesthesia for bronchoscopy, 782
Anesthesia for intrathoracic procedures, 783
Separation of the lungs and one-lung ventilation (OLV), 786
Anesthetic management of patients with respiratory disease, 788
Anesthesia and upper respiratory disease, 788
Anesthesia and lower airway disease, 802
Anesthesia and pleural space disease, 804
Anesthesia and pulmonary parenchymal disease, 806
Anesthesia and pulmonary hypertension, 809
References, 811

Introduction

Sedation and general anesthesia can produce profound changes in respiratory function, with the degree of change depending on drugs employed, species involved, depth of anesthesia, surgical procedure, and the health of the individual animal. Of greatest concern is significant reduction in gas exchange causing inadequate oxygen delivery to vital tissues and/or carbon dioxide (CO_2) removal from the body.

The aim of oxygen supplementation/therapy is to increase the alveolar oxygen partial pressure (P_AO_2) to a level that achieves a target arterial hemoglobin oxygen saturation (SaO_2), most commonly > 94%. This objective is achieved by increasing the inspired oxygen fraction (F_IO_2) in both intubated and non-intubated patients. Oxygen supplementation may be necessary before induction of general anesthesia, during anesthesia, and into the postanesthetic period.

To prevent a decrease in SaO_2/hypoxemia caused by the decreased minute ventilation ($\dot{V}_E$) induced by anesthetic drugs, it is common practice to increase the F_IO_2 in spontaneously breathing patients. However, in animal species where atelectasis plays a major role in causing oxygenation impairment during anesthesia (e.g., horses), use of a high F_IO_2 (> 0.8) may not abolish or prevent the development of hypoxemia [1,2].

The use of mechanical ventilators to provide positive-pressure ventilatory support has become a routine component of anesthesia management in both small and large animal referral hospitals. While mechanical ventilatory support has variable effects on PaO_2 in animals with respiratory disease or in the presence of significant atelectasis, it is an effective means of preventing the increase in arterial carbon dioxide partial pressure ($PaCO_2$) caused by anesthetic drugs. Supporting ventilation by an artificial means, in addition to counteracting the negative effects of anesthesia on gas exchange, will also decrease the work of breathing, which may be particularly beneficial in animals presenting with clinical conditions associated with fatigue of respiratory muscles [3]. Mechanical ventilation is an essential support measure for patients that are undergoing intrathoracic procedures including thoracoscopy, thoracotomy, and/or one-lung ventilation (OLV). It is important for the clinician to understand the physiologic effects of oxygen therapy and mechanical ventilation, in addition to their indications and contraindications, to maximize their benefits and minimize any potential negative effects associated with their use. In addition to standard perianesthetic patient preparation, use of balanced anesthetic techniques, monitoring, and supportive care, specific considerations for managing patients with underlying respiratory disease that require anesthesia for a variety of procedures are discussed below.

Veterinary Anesthesia and Analgesia: The Sixth Edition of Lumb and Jones. Edited by Leigh Lamont, Kurt Grimm, Sheilah Robertson, Lydia Love and Carrie Schroeder.
© 2024 John Wiley & Sons, Inc. Published 2024 by John Wiley & Sons, Inc.
Companion website: www.wiley.com/go/lamont/anesthesia

Oxygen therapy

Inspired oxygen supplementation is routinely performed in both the perianesthetic period and intensive care setting. Overall, oxygen therapy aims to prevent hypoxemia by maintaining arterial hemoglobin oxygen saturation above 94%. Hypoxemia refers to an abnormally low PaO_2 or SaO_2 compromising the oxygen content in arterial blood (CaO_2), which may lead to an inadequate oxygen supply to tissues. Animals may be considered hypoxemic when PaO_2 levels are < 80 mmHg and SaO_2 is < 95% [4]. Oxygen supplementation to maintain hemoglobin saturation above 90% (or PaO_2 > 60 mmHg) may be acceptable (assuming normal hemoglobin levels) as the CaO_2 will be close to values observed when hemoglobin is fully saturated. Depending on the species and health of the individual animal, oxygen supplementation may be required prior to, during, or following anesthesia to prevent hypoxemia.

Physiologic effects of oxygen therapy

Supplementation of inspired gases with oxygen, either alone or with ventilatory support, results in an increase in P_AO_2, as described by the *alveolar gas equation* (Chapter 37, Fig. 37.2, and Table 37.5). The impact of altering F_IO_2 on P_AO_2 with varying levels of alveolar ventilation is highlighted in Fig. 38.1. If alveolar ventilation is decreased by 50% of its normal resting value, P_AO_2 in an individual breathing ambient air at sea level is predicted to decrease from values close to 100 mmHg to < 50 mmHg (effect related to CO_2 build-up within the alveoli). However, if F_IO_2 is increased from 0.21 (ambient air) to values between 0.3 and 0.4 (or more), alveolar oxygen will be maintained above 100 mmHg despite severe hypoventilation.

When matching of alveolar ventilation and perfusion ($\dot{V}_A/\dot{Q}$) within the lung is close to ideal, minimal $\dot{V}_A/\dot{Q}$ mismatch (lung areas with low $\dot{V}_A/\dot{Q}$ ratio) or intrapulmonary shunt ($\dot{V}_A/\dot{Q}$ ratio = 0) are present, and the alveolar–capillary membrane is normal, an increase in P_AO_2 induced by enriching the inspired oxygen concentration will significantly raise PaO_2 as illustrated in Fig. 38.2. Although increasing F_IO_2 and P_AO_2 can be an effective means of preventing hypoxemia caused by hypoventilation, $\dot{V}_A/\dot{Q}$ mismatch, and diffusion impairment (thickening of the alveolar–capillary barrier), its effects on hypoxemia caused by intrapulmonary shunt are dependent on the percentage of mixed-venous blood that bypasses ventilated lung areas, specifically, the *shunt fraction* ($\dot{Q}_s/\dot{Q}_T$). As there is a progressive increase in $\dot{Q}_s/\dot{Q}_T$, the gradient between alveolar and arterial oxygen partial pressures (P(A-a)O_2) increases to the point where high percentages of shunted flow (≥ 30%) results in little or no improvement in PaO_2 in response to inspired oxygen concentrations approaching 100% [6]. Therefore, whenever progressive increases in F_IO_2 fail to improve arterial oxygenation, a major increase in shunt flow should be suspected and the possible causes investigated and treated.

Anesthetized healthy dogs and cats typically have relatively low levels of venous admixture (< 10%) originating from lung areas with a low $\dot{V}_A/\dot{Q}$ ratio and from intrapulmonary shunting ($\dot{V}_A/\dot{Q}$ = 0), therefore, oxygen supplementation results in PaO_2 values approaching theoretical P_AO_2 levels. Studies evaluating the respiratory effects of inhalant or injectable anesthetics in spontaneously breathing dogs and cats receiving oxygen (F_IO_2 > 0.9) have reported PaO_2 levels greater than 450 mmHg that remain constant over time periods typical of clinical anesthesia [7–13]. Although PaO_2 values ≥ 450 mmHg result in 100% SaO_2, these values are less than the predicted P_AO_2 (> 600 mmHg) probably because of normal physiologic shunt (bronchial veins and myocardial thebesian veins that bypass the lung) as well as shunted flow in some alveolar units due to atelectasis. Experimental research has shown that the use of F_IO_2

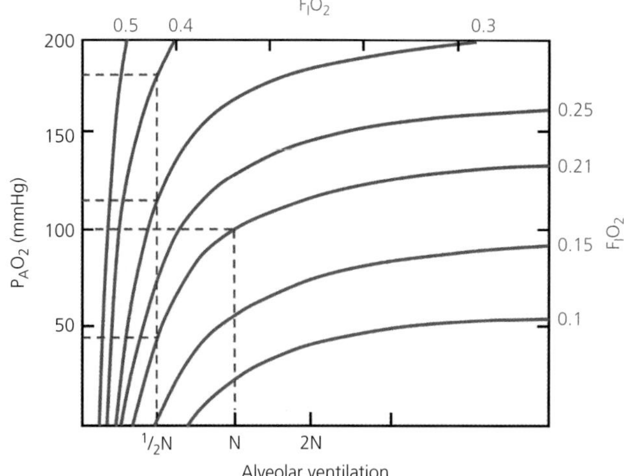

Figure 38.1 Effect of varying F_IO_2 levels with various degrees of alveolar hypoventilation and hyperventilation on alveolar oxygen partial pressure (P_AO_2) at sea level (barometric pressure of 760 mmHg). Alveolar ventilation is displayed on the x-axis with N representing normal alveolar ventilation and P_AO_2 is on the y-axis (see text for explanation). Source: Modified from Nunn [5], reproduced with permission of Elsevier.

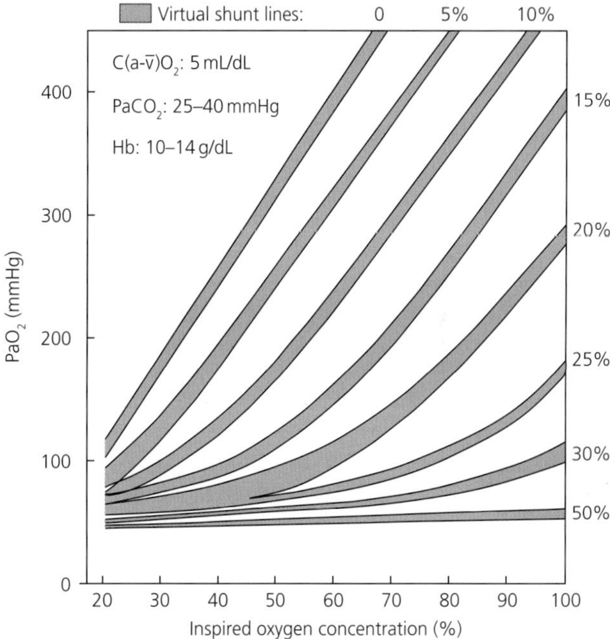

Figure 38.2 An isoshunt diagram depicting the relationship between inspired oxygen concentration, PaO_2, and various degrees of venous admixture or pulmonary shunt. Shunt flow is expressed as a percentage of cardiac output, ranging from 0 to 50%. The arteriovenous (a-$\bar{v}$) oxygen content difference is assumed to be 5 mL per 100 mL of blood, reflecting a normal cardiac output. The shunt bands have been drawn to include the range of hemoglobin (Hb) and $PaCO_2$ levels shown. Note that at the higher levels of shunt flow (30–50%), there is little improvement in arterial oxygen levels even when the inspired oxygen concentration is 100%. Also note that if the inspired oxygen concentration and PaO_2 are known, it is possible to obtain a quick estimate of the degree of venous admixture or shunt flow. Source: Redrawn from Benatar *et al.* [6], with permission.

of 0.4 during anesthesia in small animals reduced atelectasis in comparison to an $F_IO_2 > 0.9$ [14,15]. The impact of different F_IO_2s on the development of atelectasis over time in healthy dogs and cats has yet to be demonstrated.

During procedures performed under deep sedation or with short-duration intravenous anesthesia, a minimum F_IO_2 of 0.3 (which can be easily achieved by using flow-by oxygen or by supplementing oxygen through a face mask) is recommended to minimize the risk of hypoxemia due to hypoventilation and $\dot{V}_A/\dot{Q}$ mismatching. Evidence to support this recommendation includes reports of impaired oxygenation as reflected by PaO_2 values below 65 mmHg in dogs sedated with an α_2-adrenergic receptor agonist, either alone or in combination with an opioid, in addition to reports of cyanosis and low PaO_2 values during induction of anesthesia with injectable anesthetics when supplemental oxygen is not provided [16–19]. In some animals receiving oxygen supplementation, PaO_2 may not increase as predicted based on the delivered F_IO_2. Small animal patients with pulmonary parenchymal disease typically have clinically significant alveolar–capillary diffusion barriers, $\dot{V}_A/\dot{Q}$ mismatching, and increased shunt fraction. These patients may have lower-than-expected increases in PaO_2 associated with oxygen therapy [20–23].

Recumbency and general anesthesia of mature large animal patients commonly produce significant $\dot{V}_A/\dot{Q}$ mismatch and intrapulmonary shunting of blood due to anesthesia-related atelectasis [1,24]. Thus, despite normal lung parenchyma prior to anesthesia, these patients have a reduced and variable response to oxygen supplementation when recumbent. Horses breathing ambient air with an intravenous anesthetic regimen commonly have PaO_2 values in the range of 50–70 mmHg during recumbency [25,26]. During inhalational anesthesia with 100% oxygen as the carrier gas, laterally recumbent spontaneously breathing healthy horses have PaO_2 values that typically range from 300 to 350 mmHg; horses in dorsal recumbency often have lower levels, ranging from 200 to 300 mmHg [2]. Unlike the dog and cat, where PaO_2 levels usually remain stable over time during general anesthesia with an $F_IO_2 > 0.95$, PaO_2 values often decrease over time in the equine, particularly when they are positioned in dorsal recumbency [2,27–30]. While oxygen supplementation is generally administered to reduce the risk of hypoxemia, high F_IO_2 during general anesthesia (to either spontaneously breathing or mechanically ventilated patients) can contribute to atelectasis in numerous species, including dogs, cats, horses, and humans [14,15,31–34]. Absorption of oxygen, which is more soluble than nitrogen, into the bloodstream and out of the alveoli, is responsible for the atelectasis associated with high inspired F_IO_2. If the degree of atelectasis resulting from absorption is significant, it can contribute to an increase in the $P(\text{A-a})O_2$ gradient. In larger species such as the horse, the contribution of absorption of alveolar gases relative to the development of atelectasis because of compression of alveoli by abdominal contents may be minor, but its significance may vary with body position and the specific inspired oxygen level [24,27,35,36]. In humans, atelectasis attributed to high F_IO_2 values has been associated with an increased incidence of postoperative hypoxemia and respiratory complications [37]. The presence of atelectasis has been associated with progression of lung injury in human patients and in numerous experimental animal models of lung injury receiving ventilatory support (see below). In veterinary species, the clinical significance of anesthesia-associated atelectasis without hypoxemia on lung health in the patient with no pre-existing pulmonary disease is yet undetermined. Irrespective of the impact on the creation or progression of lung injury, the presence of atelectasis may affect the quality of thoracic imaging and may warrant consideration when evaluating and comparing images to those obtained while the animal is exposed to a lower F_IO_2 or following application of specific ventilator strategies aimed at maintaining lung volume [38]. In humans, administration of 100% oxygen via face mask prior to and during the induction of general anesthesia (i.e., preoxygenation) has been a relatively standard procedure to increase the time to hemoglobin desaturation once oxygen is withdrawn, as occurs during orotracheal intubation. However, this technique is now being called into question as it has been shown to result in a greater degree of atelectasis compared with inspiring lower oxygen fractions such as 60 or 80% [33]. Although preoxygenation is not always accomplished in healthy veterinary patients, it is recommended in cases where a prolonged time from induction of anesthesia to securing an airway is anticipated, or in animals with respiratory disease. Relative to the situation in human anesthesia, when oxygen is administered via a non-sealed face mask to veterinary species in the clinical setting, it is unlikely that F_IO_2 values will be greater than 0.8 unless an unusually tight-fitting face mask is utilized [39,40].

Spontaneously breathing anesthetized patients receiving oxygen supplementation may experience higher $PaCO_2$ levels than animals breathing either room air or an $F_IO_2 < 0.5$ [27,31,39,41]. Horses anesthetized with halothane receiving an F_IO_2 of 0.3 versus > 0.85 had significantly lower $PaCO_2$ levels [27]. Similar findings have been reported in horses under injectable anesthesia [31]. Dogs that were preoxygenated prior to induction of anesthesia also had a tendency toward an increased $PaCO_2$ compared with dogs breathing room air [39]. Maintenance of PaO_2 above levels that increase peripheral chemoreceptor input into the respiratory center in the brainstem (PaO_2 > 60–70 mmHg) is likely the main mechanism responsible for a greater degree of hypoventilation in animals receiving oxygen supplementation compared to animals breathing a lower F_IO_2 during anesthesia.

Strategies for oxygen supplementation

In intubated patients connected to an anesthetic machine equipped with oxygen and air flowmeters, the flow rate of gases entering the breathing circuit can be adjusted to achieve a variable F_IO_2 (e.g., 0.4). Most veterinary anesthesia machines, however, do not permit adjustment of F_IO_2 because they are equipped with only an oxygen flowmeter and therefore deliver an $F_IO_2 > 0.95$ in an animal with a sealed airway (for example, with an endotracheal tube or laryngeal mask in place). In non-intubated patients, there are numerous different strategies/techniques which are described below that are used to increase a patient's F_IO_2.

Low-flow oxygen systems

In conscious, sedated, or anesthetized non-intubated patients, F_IO_2 can be increased above 0.3 by administering oxygen at the level of the nares, nasopharynx, or trachea. Oxygen supplementation in non-intubated patients is commonly provided using low-flow systems that deliver a maximum oxygen flow rate of 15 L/min. These systems include (1) *flow-by oxygen* near the nostrils/mouth; (2) supply of *oxygen by face mask*; and (3) *supply of oxygen by nasal, nasopharyngeal, or nasotracheal catheter*. The efficacy of these systems in increasing F_IO_2 will be dependent on the amount of dilution of the inspired gases with room air. For example, in animals that present with tachypnea, the inspiratory flow may greatly exceed the flow rate provided by the external oxygen source. As a result, the F_IO_2 will be less than expected because ambient air will enter the lungs to a greater degree when compared to an animal that is breathing at a slower respiratory rate, a phenomenon referred to as "air entrainment" [42]. In animals receiving oxygen supplementation through a nasal catheter, dilution of inspired oxygen may also occur if the animal breathes through its mouth, as commonly occurs in dogs [42].

Flow-by oxygen supplementation, which consists of placing an oxygen source within approximately 2 cm of a patient's nostrils and mouth, is the easiest and simplest way of increasing F_IO_2 during emergency situations in small animals. Oxygen flow rates typically used in small animals with this technique range from 100–200 mL/kg/min and the resulting F_IO_2 has been reported to be 0.24 to 0.45 [42,43]. Unfortunately, the efficacy of this strategy is reduced in uncooperative patients as they typically move their heads away from the oxygen source.

Oxygen supplementation via a face mask attached to an anesthesia breathing circuit is an effective means of increasing F_IO_2 in dogs, cats, neonatal foals, and calves. In many animals, sedation may be required for the animal to accept placement of a face mask. If a tight-fitting face mask is attached to a small animal anesthesia breathing circuit delivering 100 mL/kg/min of oxygen, it may result in F_IO_2 levels > 0.8. In dogs, providing oxygen (100 mL/kg/min) through a tightly fitting face mask attached to a breathing circuit for 3 min prior to induction of anesthesia increased inspired oxygen concentration to 90%; while flow-by oxygen supplementation at the same rate resulted in an inspired concentration of 30% [40]. The time to desaturation (defined as a pulse oximetry hemoglobin saturation of 90%) after propofol-induced apnea was significantly longer in dogs receiving preoxygenation by a face mask (approximately 3 min [187 ± 67 s]) than in animals receiving flow-by oxygen (approximately 1 min [66 ± 17 s]) [40], consistent with a previous publication assessing preoxygenation with a facemask in healthy dogs [39]. Oxygen supplementation by face mask before inhalant anesthesia is a practical means of reducing the risk of hypoxemia caused by injectable induction agents in patients with respiratory disease. Although commonly used before induction of general anesthesia in small animals, face masks may not be suitable for delivering oxygen for prolonged periods due to lack of patient tolerance and the need for personnel to hold the mask to the animal.

Delivery of oxygen using a nasal catheter is suitable for long-term oxygen supplementation. Animals with respiratory disease may have a nasal oxygen system in place prior to anesthesia and/or require oxygen supplementation using this system following anesthesia. A short nasal catheter, consisting of two 1 cm long prongs designed for people, has been used to deliver oxygen with some success in dogs; however, they are easily dislodged and only fit a small subset of animals. Longer nasopharyngeal catheters, generally constructed of soft flexible material, ideally with multiple fenestrations, can be placed further into the nasal cavity and are less likely to be dislodged. They have been shown to be effective in delivering oxygen in a variety of species [44–48]. To avoid patient discomfort during catheter placement, a local anesthetic jelly is applied to the nostrils, followed by instillation of a local anesthetic solution into the nasal cavity with the animal's head extended upwards. Sedation may be required in uncooperative patients and additional care should be taken not to exceed the recommended maximum dose of local anesthetic to avoid toxic effects in cats or other small patients. Catheters can be placed unilaterally or bilaterally in the ventral nasal meatus and extended distally into the nasal cavity or nasopharynx. In most dogs, advancing the catheter to the level of the medial canthus of the eye places its tip within the nasal cavity, while advancing it further to the level of the vertical ramus of the mandible places the catheter within the nasopharynx. In conscious animals, delivering oxygen at a flow rate of 30–150 mL/kg/min through a nasal cannula can result in an F_IO_2 of 0.3 to 0.7 (depending on species) [44,45,48]. Higher flow rates, while improving PaO_2, can result in low patient tolerance and nasal mucosal damage [45,48]. In dogs, gastric tympany secondary to aerophagia has also been reported with high flow rates [49]. The effects of progressively increasing oxygen flow rates (from 50 to 200 mL/kg/min) through unilateral or bilateral nasal catheters in dogs and neonatal foals are illustrated in Fig. 38.3 [44,45]. As oxygen flow rates are increased, there are progressive increases in F_IO_2 and PaO_2, without significant changes in $PaCO_2$, from values obtained while animals are breathing room air [44,45]. Oxygen supplementation with bilateral catheters may result in slightly higher F_IO_2 and PaO_2 in comparison to a unilateral nasal catheter. Patient tolerance to higher oxygen flow rates has also been reported to improve when nasal catheters are placed bilaterally compared to unilaterally in dogs [44]. To minimize the risk of oxygen toxicity caused by prolonged exposure to high F_IO_2 levels and other adverse reactions (low patient tolerance, excessive drying/irritation of the nasal mucosa, and aerophagia/gastric distension), the oxygen flow rate should be adjusted to the minimum necessary to maintain an acceptable hemoglobin saturation/PaO_2 level (e.g., saturation > 90% or PaO_2 > 60 mmHg). If a nasal catheter fails to maintain arterial oxygenation with high oxygen flow rates (> 150–200 mL/kg/min), or if the work of breathing does not improve despite increased oxygen levels, escalation to other methods of oxygen supplementation (high-flow nasal oxygen therapy) or invasive mechanical ventilation should be considered.

In horses sedated with detomidine and butorphanol, a nasal catheter providing 15 L/min (approximately, 30 mL/kg/min) of oxygen for 3 min increased PaO_2 immediately after induction of anesthesia to 83 ± 20 mmHg (mean ± standard deviation) in comparison to PaO_2 measured at the same time point in horses not receiving oxygen supplementation (56 ± 12 mmHg) [50]. Although this procedure appears effective to ameliorate the decrease in PaO_2 immediately after induction of anesthesia with an injectable anesthetic, oxygenation relative to horses that were not administered nasal oxygen was not different after 30 min of anesthesia, and to date, there is no evidence to support routine preanesthetic nasal oxygen administration in healthy horses. Oxygen insufflation into the nasal cavity or trachea via a nasotracheal or orotracheal tube is commonly used in horses during recovery from general anesthesia. Delivery of 15 L/min oxygen through a nasotracheal catheter has been shown to result in PaO_2 values greater than 90 mmHg in laterally recumbent horses during anesthetic recovery [51].

Administration of oxygen using a percutaneous transtracheal system has been described in foals in respiratory distress, as well as in healthy standing horses, and therefore should be considered for use in equine patients with impaired oxygenation [47,52].

Commercially available oxygen cages and hoods constructed of clear acrylic or plexiglass are available for use in small animals. Some commercially available cage designs permit the control of oxygen levels, environmental temperature, and humidity within the cage and are very effective for long-term oxygen supplementation in small patients. Both systems are suitable for use prior to or following anesthesia but not during periods where access to the patient is required. Helmets designed for pediatric humans have been used to increase F_IO_2 and deliver continuous positive airway pressure (CPAP) in dogs recovering from anesthesia [53].

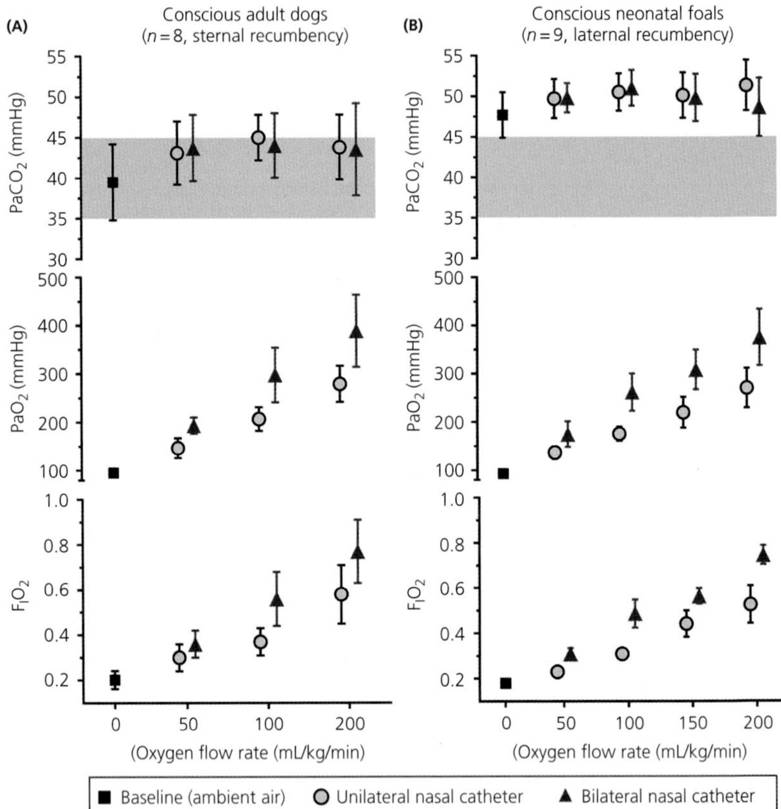

Figure 38.3 Effects of oxygen supplementation through unilateral or bilateral catheters advanced to the level of the nasopharynx on F_IO_2, PaO_2, and $PaCO_2$, (mean ± standard deviation) in conscious adult dogs **(A.)** and in neonatal foals **(B.)**. The F_IO_2 in both studies was measured by an intratracheal catheter connected to an airway gas analyzer. The gray shaded area shows the $PaCO_2$ range considered normal for most species (35 to 45 mmHg). See text for further explanation. Source: Data compiled from Dunphy *et al.* [44]; Wong *et al.* [45].

High-flow oxygen systems

In contrast to low-flow oxygen therapy systems discussed above, where the maximum oxygen flow rate is limited to 15 L/min, *high-flow nasal oxygen therapy* (HFNOT) systems can deliver up to 60 L/min of humidified and heated oxygen or oxygen-enriched air. The system includes an oxygen cylinder (or oxygen concentrator), an air mixer, a humidifier, heated tubing of varying sizes, and purpose-made nasal prongs [42,54]. While low-flow systems result in variable effects on F_IO_2 because of variations in $\dot{V}_E$ and peak inspiratory flow, HFNOT systems reliably achieve the target F_IO_2 level because the high flow delivered to the airway exceeds the patient's peak inspiratory flow [55]. In addition to a more reliable increase in F_IO_2 than traditional oxygen supplementation systems, HFNOT systems create a low level of CPAP, which may increase the functional residual capacity (FRC) and improve matching between ventilation and perfusion within the lungs, while still permitting the patient to breathe spontaneously [56–58]. The CPAP associated with HFNOT may also stent the airways opened, decreasing the work of breathing and mitigating the need for invasive mechanical ventilation in some patients [56]. The relative humidity of inspired gas provided by HFNOT systems is close to 100% at a temperature between 34 and 37 °C, thereby reducing the sensation of respiratory distress or mouth dryness in humans [59]. Because inspired gas flow is heated and humified, HFNOT may also result in better patient tolerance by not desiccating the nasal mucosa [59].

Based on human recommendations, the soft silicone binasal prongs used for HFNOT should occlude up to 50% of the nares in veterinary patients [56,60,61]. Preliminary canine studies have shown that the ability of HFNOT to achieve the target F_IO_2 and CPAP is dependent on the flow rate of oxygen or oxygen-enriched air delivered to the patient. Oxygen flow rates between 1 to 2 L/kg/min achieve F_IO_2 levels > 0.95 in dogs [56] (Fig. 38.4).

Despite the advantages of HFNOT over traditional oxygen supplementation systems, there are some conditions that may limit the clinical utility of HFNOT systems in veterinary patients, including patient intolerance, and the need to adapt the bilateral nasal prongs made for pediatric and adult humans to a variety of head sizes and conformations. In very small patients, it has been suggested to apply only one nasal prong as placement of bilateral pediatric nasal prongs may occlude more than 50% of the nares and impair expiratory flow [62]. Another disadvantage is the decrease in F_IO_2 below the target level in animals that are open-mouth breathing because the oxygen-rich gas delivered by the HFNOT system is diluted with ambient air entering through the mouth. Although it is possible that the HFNOT systems are less affected by panting/open-mouth breathing, this hypothesis has not yet been evaluated [42,54]. Although morbidity associated with HFNOT is considered minimal, aerophagia leading to gastric distension is a potential complication of this therapy in dogs and may require placement of an orogastric tube [56,62,63].

HFNOT has the potential for use during the perianesthetic period or when orotracheal intubation is not feasible in anesthetized/deeply sedated patients. Because of the flow-dependent increase in pharyngeal pressures/CPAP reported in dogs receiving 100% oxygen at flow rates ≥ 1 L/kg/min [56], the use of HFNOT may be particularly useful to reduce the inspiratory work of breathing and alleviate signs of upper airway obstruction of dogs with brachycephalic obstructive airway syndrome (BOAS). In one case series report, application of HFNOT to brachycephalic dogs with clinical signs of upper airway obstruction (dyspnea/inspiratory stridor)

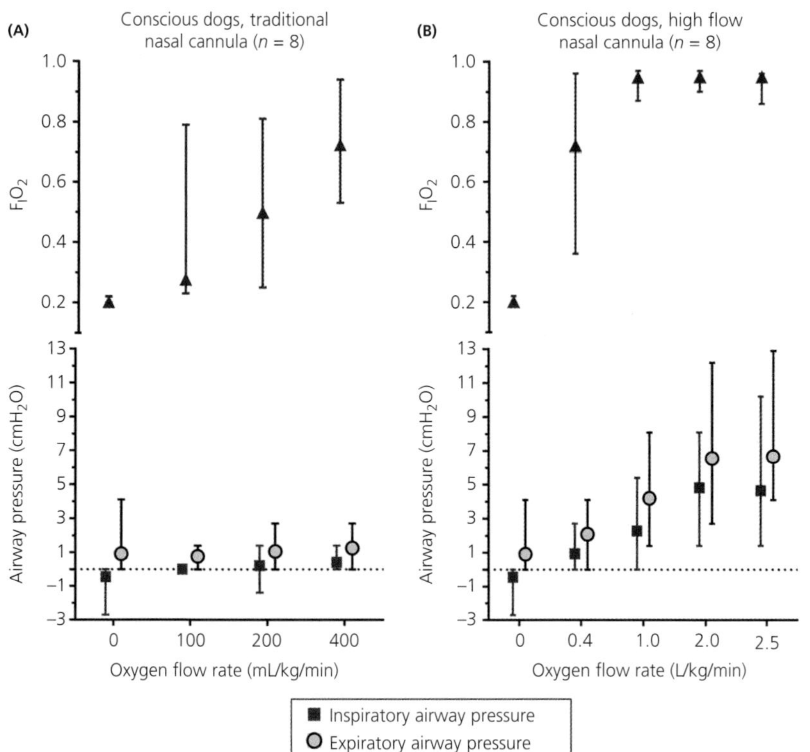

Figure 38.4 Effects of oxygen supplementation on airway pressure and F_IO_2 (mean and lower-upper range) measured at the level of the oropharynx in dogs using **A.** a traditional nasal cannula and **B.** a high-flow nasal cannula. Treatments were administered in randomized crossover design and included non-sedated patients (traditional nasal cannula) and sedated/non-sedated animals (high-flow nasal cannula). With the high-flow nasal oxygen therapy (HFNOT) system, the heated and humidified oxygen source was selected to deliver an F_IO_2 of 1.0. Notice that low-flow oxygen supplementation (traditional nasal cannula) does not provide continuous positive airway pressure (CPAP) and has variable effects on F_IO_2, while the HFNOT adjusted to deliver oxygen flow rates between 1 to 2 L/kg/min can produce low to moderate levels of continuous positive airway pressure (CPAP) levels and reliably results in F_IO_2 close to the target level (1.0). Increasing the oxygen flow rate above 2 L/kg/min did not induce additional changes in CPAP and F_IO_2 and increased patient intolerance. Source: Data compiled from Jagodich *et al.* [56].

during recovery from anesthesia improved the respiratory pattern (decreased inspiratory stridor) [62]. However, results were limited by the small number of animals ($n = 5$) and by the lack of another group not receiving HFNOT for comparison [54]. In another case series report, HFNOT set to deliver 1 L/kg/min of 100% oxygen (33 °C) was evaluated in non-intubated dogs anesthetized with propofol for bronchoscopy [64]. Of the four animals enrolled in this study, two animals showed transient hypoxemia (pulse oximetry saturation of 84% and 92% lasting < 1 min) during or after completion of bronchoalveolar lavage [64]. Delivery of high-flow nasal oxygen may not be enough to counteract hypoxemia secondary to bronchoalveolar lavage, but conclusions of this case series were also limited by the small number of animals and by the lack of a control treatment.

HFNOT systems have also been evaluated in animals with hypoxemic respiratory failure, where the most frequent pathology was pneumonia/aspiration pneumonia [65–68]. Collective analysis of these studies shows that HFNOT should be considered if traditional oxygen supplementation methods fail to improve patient's oxygenation or cannot mitigate the increased respiratory effort/work of breathing. Under these circumstances, HFNOT may be effective in improving PaO_2 and reducing signs of dyspnea, thereby avoiding escalation to invasive mechanical ventilation in some cases.

Oxygen toxicity

It has long been recognized that high inspired oxygen levels (over 70%) when administered for prolonged periods will produce pulmonary dysfunction and even death in previously healthy laboratory and domestic animals [69]. Studies in animals with experimentally induced lung injury have also demonstrated that lung injury is negatively impacted by high F_IO_2 [70–73]. The onset of pulmonary damage in healthy animals seems to require $F_IO_2 > 0.7$, producing PaO_2 values exceeding 450 mmHg and "prolonged exposure," generally longer than the period usually associated with clinical veterinary anesthesia. While high F_IO_2 may promote atelectasis, there is no evidence that the use of 100% oxygen as the carrier gas during anesthesia negatively impacts outcomes in clinical veterinary patients. In critically ill humans, current recommendations include avoiding supramaximal PaO_2 and maintaining PaO_2 and SaO_2 within a physiologic range [74–77]. Therefore, in the critical care setting, if spontaneously breathing patients receive oxygen supplementation, or if escalation to invasive mechanical ventilation is necessary, the general approach is to adjust the F_IO_2 to the point where PaO_2 levels are in the range of 60–80 mmHg with hemoglobin oxygen saturation levels between 90–94% [76]. With severe pulmonary parenchymal injury in humans, there is current discussion of targeting some degree of "permissive hypoxemia" [78–80]. To date, the impact of permissive hypoxemia on mortality has not been clearly demonstrated [80,81].

Mechanical ventilation during anesthesia

Mechanical ventilators can be described as flow generators, driving gas into the lungs by creating a pressure gradient between the airway opening (P_{ao}, pressure measured at the distal end of the endotracheal tube as airway pressure) and the alveoli (P_{alv}, alveolar pressure). Inspiration ceases after the peak airway pressure (P_{peak}) or volume set on the ventilator is achieved and, once the expiratory valve is opened, the elastic recoil of the lungs and chest wall results in passive expiration.

While intensive care unit (ICU) ventilators vent exhaled gases out into the environment, anesthesia ventilators are designed to allow rebreathing of expired gases. The primary goals of mechanical ventilation during anesthesia are to optimize gas exchange and reduce the work of breathing while minimizing the risk of iatrogenic lung injury. In addition to its beneficial effects on respiratory function, mechanical ventilation may facilitate the control of depth of inhalant anesthesia when compared to spontaneous breathing. In anesthetized, spontaneously breathing animals, changes in the respiratory pattern (respiratory rate [*f*] and tidal volume [V_T]) leading to variations in minute ventilation ($\dot{V}_E = f \times V_T$) will modify the rate at which the alveolar (end-tidal) anesthetic concentration approaches the inspired anesthetic concentration. As a practical example, if an animal hypoventilates significantly (decreased $\dot{V}_E$) immediately after induction of anesthesia, the decreased $\dot{V}_E$ will slow down the rate of rise in end-tidal anesthetic concentration, potentially delaying the time until an adequate depth of anesthesia is achieved. Alternatively, if the animal receives mechanical ventilation and the $\dot{V}_E$ is adjusted to prevent hypoventilation, the end-tidal anesthetic concentration will increase more rapidly.

Evolution of mechanical ventilators used in veterinary and human anesthesia

The first mention of mechanical ventilation in the form of positive-pressure ventilation dates back to the mid-1500s when the Dutch physician at the University of Padua (Italy) Andreas Vesalius observed that "... life may be restored to the animal, an opening must be attempted in the trunk of the trachea, into which a tube of reed or cane should be put; you will then blow into this, so that the lung may rise again and take air" [82]. Early mechanical ventilators were designed to establish a negative (sub-atmospheric) pressure around the thorax to enlarge the chest wall and pull gas into the lungs by creating a negative intrapleural/alveolar pressure. After the development of rudimentary models of negative-pressure ventilators between the second half of the 1800s and early 1900s, the first negative-pressure ventilator effectively used for life support in humans with respiratory muscle paralysis was developed from studies in curare-paralyzed cats by Philip Drinker and Louis Agassiz Shaw in the United States. These ventilators were named "iron lungs" and became widely used for life support in human patients suffering from respiratory muscle paralysis secondary to poliomyelitis during the 1950s [83].

Due to the required equipment and limited access to the patient's thorax, abdomen, and limbs, ventilatory support using negative-pressure ventilation cannot be applied to anesthesia machines designed for use in the operating room or the modern ICU setting. Instead, mechanical ventilation under these circumstances can be more effectively adopted by applying positive pressure to the airways. When William Thomas Green Morton performed the first official demonstration that surgery could be carried out without pain by administration of an inhalant anesthetic on October 16, 1846 (Ether Day), early inhalant anesthetic delivery systems were simple inhalers whose aim was to evaporate the anesthetic agent as a function of the patient's own breath. This rudimentary equipment evolved during the first decades of the 20th century to anesthesia machines that allowed precise administration of an anesthetic gas flow independent of the patient's breathing effort. Further developments included CO_2 absorption and the circle breathing system, which allowed rebreathing of inhalant anesthetics and oxygen. However, it was only in the 1950s that anesthesia ventilators were effectively integrated into inhalant anesthetic delivery systems [84,85] (Fig. 38.5).

The bellows-type ventilator

Conventional anesthesia ventilators used in veterinary practice operate solely in a volumetric mode where the user adjusts the inspiratory flow and/or inspiratory time to achieve the target volume displaced by the bellows or, alternatively, the target P_{peak} (Fig. 38.6A and B). As discussed further below, the volume displaced by the bellows may not accurately reflect the V_T delivered to the animal [86]. There are two types of ventilators according to the movement of the bellows during expiration: ascending and descending bellows. Early ventilators were designed with bellows that descended during expiration (Fig. 38.5E and F). Unfortunately, in case of a leak in the circuit and/or accidental disconnection of the breathing circuit, the operator may be unaware of ventilator failure because a descending bellows will continue to move upwards during inspiration and downwards during expiration as gravity will cause the bellows to fill with ambient air. In contrast, ascending bellows ventilators have the advantage of providing an early warning in case of disconnection or a large leak in the breathing circuit because the bellows will not move upwards during expiration. Providing that the fresh gas flow (FGF) delivered by the flowmeter is not elevated, small leaks within the breathing circuit can also be detected by an ascending bellows as it will not completely fill/reach the top of its housing during expiration. Because there is a requirement for a compressed gas source to drive the ascending bellows downwards during inspiration and generate the tidal breath, these devices are classified as pneumatic ventilators. While older models did not require electricity, several bellows-type ventilators used in veterinary medicine incorporate electronically controlled parameters (e.g., respiratory rate and inspiratory time or inspiration-to-expiration [I:E] ratio) and require both compressed gas and electricity to function (Fig. 38.6A and B). Ventilators designed for use in the magnetic resonance imaging environment require only compressed gas and do not have electronic components.

The interval at which each mechanical breath is initiated is set by the respiratory rate control knob. Because termination of each mechanical breath occurs after a predetermined time has elapsed, which corresponds to the inspiratory time, these devices are classified as time-cycled ventilators. In some electronically controlled bellows-type ventilators, the inspiratory time is indirectly defined by adjusting the respiratory rate and the I:E ratio (Fig. 38.6A), whereas for other ventilators, there is a control knob to adjust the inspiratory time, and the I:E ratio is indirectly defined as a function of the inspiratory time and breathing frequency (Fig. 38.6B).

Fig. 38.7 illustrates a circle breathing circuit attached to an ascending bellows-type ventilator. These ventilators are also known as "double circuit ventilators," meaning that the drive gas and the breathing gas circuit exist in two separate circuits. During inspiration (Fig. 38.7A), the driving gas (compressed air or oxygen) is routed into the bellows housing, which causes the bellows to move downwards. Airway pressure increases as the bellows is compressed, and the V_T is delivered to the patient. The degree of compression of the bellows/V_T delivered to the patient is set by adjusting the inspiratory flow knob until the volume displaced by the bellows (as shown by a volume scale located in the bellows housing) matches the target V_T. However, the volume displaced by the bellows may be an inaccurate estimate of the actual V_T delivered to the patient [86] as the inspired V_T is not solely determined by the volume displaced by the bellows. Inspired V_T will also be influenced by compliance and leaks within the breathing circuit and by the FGF. As an alternative to setting a predefined V_T based on the volume displaced by the bellows, the inspiratory flow may be adjusted until P_{peak} (assessed by the breathing circuit pressure gauge) increases to a certain level.

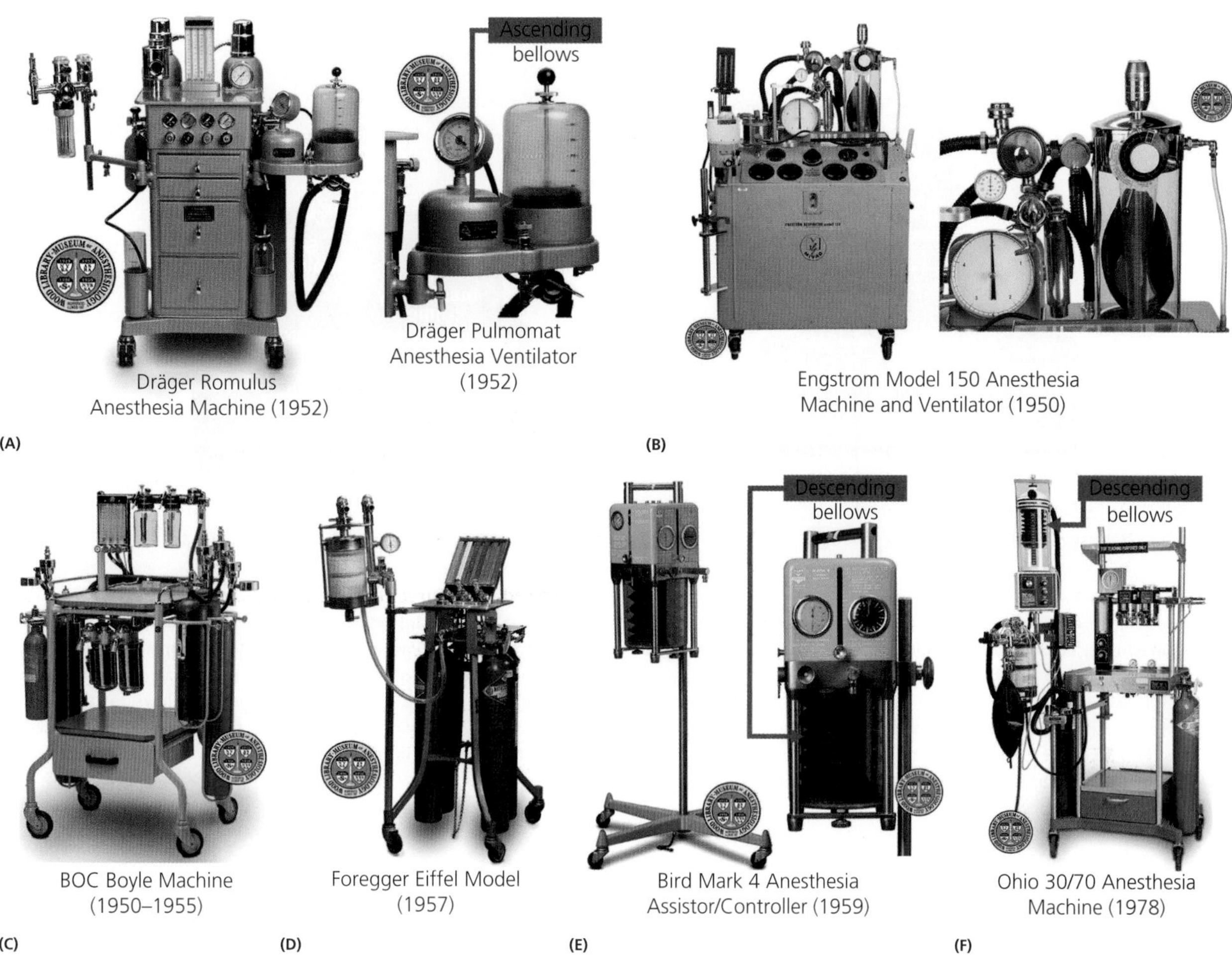

Figure 38.5 Early models of anesthesia ventilators incorporated into anesthetic delivery systems. **A.** and **B.** The Dräger Romulus (Germany) and the Engstrom Model 150 (Sweden) were integrated with ventilators that applied positive pressure to the airways to expand the lungs during inspiration. During expiration, negative pressure was applied to the airways to "remove residual air from the lungs," a concept that is no longer utilized. The ascending bellows design (classification based on the movement of the bellows during expiration) of the Dräger Pulmomat ventilator is still used by contemporary anesthesia ventilators. **C.** and **D.** The BOC Boyle Machine (United Kingdom) and the Foregger Eiffel Anesthesia Machines (USA) did not incorporate anesthesia ventilators and ventilation had to be performed by manually squeezing the reservoir bag. **E.** As mechanical ventilation became increasingly popular in human anesthesia in North America, the Bird Corporation developed a stand-alone anesthesia ventilator that could be integrated into pre-existing anesthesia machines by replacing the reservoir bag of the circle circuit with a descending bellows ventilator (Bird Mark 4). **F.** Ohio Medical Products began integrating anesthesia ventilators into their equipment in the 1960s. Source: Reproduced with permission from the Wood Library Museum of Anesthesiology.

Delivery of pressurized drive gas into the bellows housing is interrupted during expiration. As passive expiration occurs through the elastic recoil of the lungs and chest wall, the bellows fills with expired gas and fresh gas entering the circuit, while the *exhalation valve* opens to allow the drive gas to be vented out to the room or the exterior/anesthetic gas absorber through the scavenge outlet (Fig. 38.7B). When the bellows is full, excess FGF will cause pressure build-up within the breathing circuit. As pressure in the circuit reaches 2–4 cmH_2O, the ventilator pop-off valve (also known as the "spill valve") opens and excess breathing circuit gas is vented out through the scavenge outlet (Fig. 38.7C). Because of the weight of the passive bellows and of the pressure necessary to open the ventilator pop-off valve, ascending bellows ventilators typically result in an intrinsic positive end-expiratory pressure (PEEP) of 2–4 cmH_2O. In large animal anesthesia machines, the weight of the ascending bellows results in higher intrinsic pressures.

Influence of gas compression, breathing circuit compliance, and fresh gas flow on ventilator performance

During mechanical ventilation, part of the volume displaced by the bellows may get compressed within the breathing circuit before reaching the lungs. *Gas compression losses* cause the volume delivered to the lungs (inspired V_T) to be less than the volume displaced by the bellows. The volume of compressed gas within one ventilator model was found to increase linearly at a ratio of 3.8 mL for every 1 cmH_2O increase in airway pressure [88]. Also, part of the volume generated by the ventilator may not reach the patient because of the *compliance of the breathing circuit*. The latter is defined as the change in volume (distension of breathing circuit tubing) caused by an increase in pressure (mL/cmH_2O). Breathing circuit compliance losses causing a decrease in inspired V_T depend on the level of positive pressure achieved within the circuit, and on the diameter and length of the corrugated tubing. According to international standards, breathing circuit compliance losses should ideally be less than

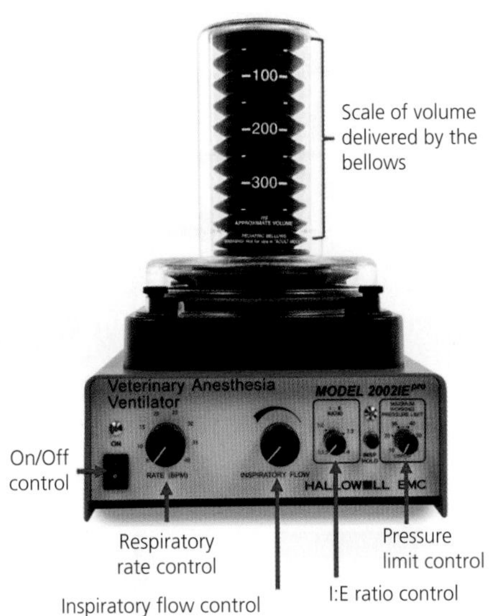

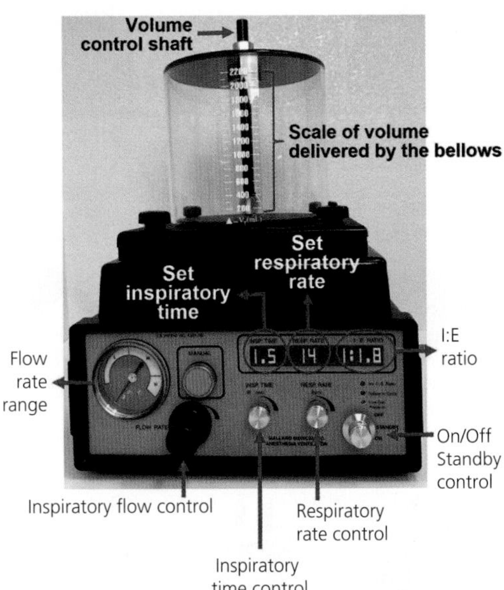

Figure 38.6 Examples of time-cycled, electronically controlled, ascending bellows ventilators designed for veterinary use that can be fitted into pre-existing anesthesia machines. These ventilators operate only in volume-control mode (mandatory breaths only), where the operator sets the breathing rate, I:E ratio (or inspiratory time), and the volume displaced by the bellows. Some ventilators incorporate a pressure limit control to prevent an excessive increase in peak airway pressure (P_{peak}). The inspiratory flow control knob adjusts the flow of compressed gas (e.g., oxygen) that drives the bellows downwards, regulating volume that enters the breathing circuit. During small animal anesthesia, the inspired V_T may differ substantially from the volume displaced by the bellows [86], therefore it may be preferable to perform pressure-limited ventilation by adjusting the inspiratory flow to achieve a target P_{peak} (based on the pressure gauge of the breathing circuit) instead of a target volume.

1 mL per cm H_2O of distending pressure for every 1 meter of tubing [89]. If that is the case and the anesthesia circuit for medium/large size dogs is 3 meters in total length for the inspiratory and expiratory limbs, mechanical ventilation to a P_{peak} of 10 cmH_2O will result in a delivered V_T of 30 mL less than the volume displaced by the bellows. Besides compliance and gas compression losses, which may vary according to tubing characteristics and total internal volume of the breathing circuit, leaks within the breathing circuit are an important source of discrepancy between the volume delivered by the bellows and inspired V_T. Therefore, to prevent accidents such as failure to properly ventilate an anesthetized animal, a thorough preanesthetic assessment of the ventilator, including a leak test of the breathing circuit, should be performed prior to use.

In a conventional anesthesia apparatus, the portion of FGF entering the breathing circuit during inspiration adds to the volume delivered by the bellows to the lungs and increases P_{peak}, an effect known as "fresh gas coupling" (Fig. 38.7A) [86,87,90,91]. Activation of the oxygen flush valve during inspiration, which delivers a high flow of 100% oxygen directly into the breathing circuit, will also generate excessively high P_{peak} values and increase inspired V_T if the apparatus does not incorporate an appropriately adjusted inspiratory pressure limiter (maximum airway pressure-control) (Fig. 38.6A). If FGF is relatively low (e.g., $\leq$ 50 mL/kg/min), the added volume to the V_T delivered by the bellows may not be clinically relevant; however, if FGF is high (relative to the size of the patient), it can substantially increase the V_T. As shown in Table 38.1, in an anesthetized dog weighing 20 kg, where the ventilator is set to deliver 15 mL/kg based on the bellows scale (300 mL), with a respiratory rate of 10 breaths/min and an I:E ratio of 1:2 (2 s of inspiratory time), if the FGF is set at 1 L/min (50 mL/kg/min), approximately 16.6 mL of fresh gas will enter the breathing circuit every second. Therefore, during the inspiratory phase of each mechanical breath (2 s), a total volume of 33.3 mL is added to the volume of gas delivered by the bellows. When this added FGF volume is balanced against losses from breathing circuit compliance and gas compression, one may expect that the inspired V_T will be close to 300 mL because the relatively small volume added by the FGF during inspiration (33.3 mL) will be close to breathing circuit compliance and gas compression losses (39 mL) (Table 38.1). If FGF is increased from 1 to 4 L/min, 66.6 mL of fresh gas will be entering the breathing circuit every second, which could potentially increase the inspired V_T from 294 mL (14.7 mL/kg) to 379 mL (19 mL/kg) (Table 38.1). While fresh gas coupling may have a smaller impact on the V_T delivered for medium-sized/large dogs, this effect may be particularly hazardous during anesthesia of animals weighing $\leq$ 5 kg. If the FGF is increased from 1 to 4 L/min in a 3.3 kg cat, the inspired V_T may increase by approximately 126%, from 48 mL (14.5 mL/kg) to 113 mL (34.2 mL/kg). Such supraphysiological V_T, in addition to being harmful to the lungs, will result in elevated P_{peak} and could result in greater cardiovascular depression due to decreased venous return and cardiac output. In contrast, the effects of FGF on the V_T in a large animal anesthesia ventilator are not clinically relevant. Assuming a V_T delivered by a large animal ventilator (based on the scale of the bellows housing) is 6 L for a 500 kg horse and the inspiratory time is set at 2 s, the additional volume generated by a 6 L/min FGF will represent less than 5% of the set V_T (6 L plus 200 mL of FGF) and will likely be minimized by breathing circuit compliance and gas compression losses.

As discussed below, modern anesthesia ventilators either *decouple* the FGF from the inspired V_T or *compensate* for the effect of FGF by adjusting the inspired volume generated by the ventilator to achieve the user-set V_T [87,90,91]. When using a ventilator that does not decouple or compensate for changes in FGF, the user must exert

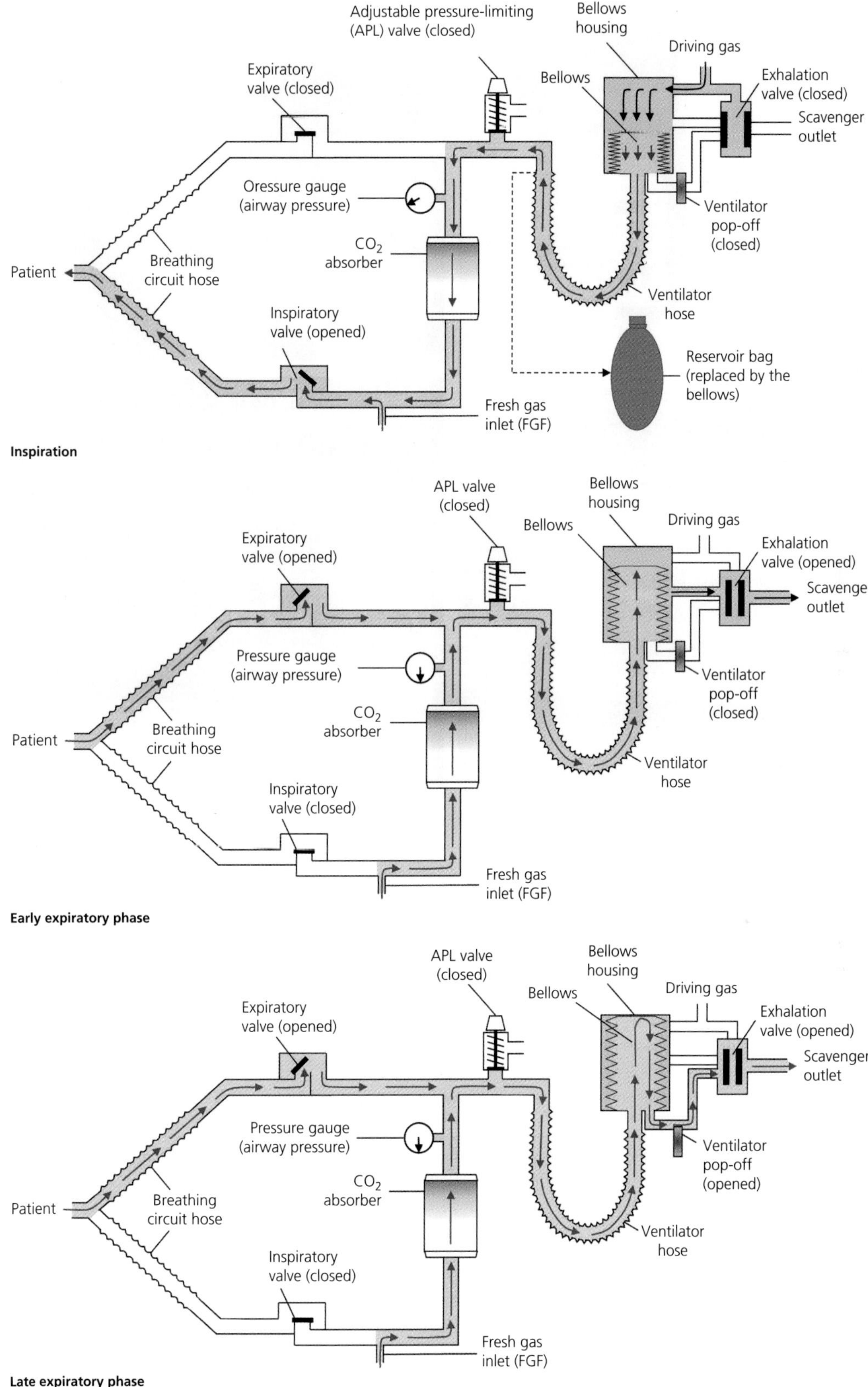

Figure 38.7 Dynamics of gas flow in a breathing circuit of a conventional anesthesia apparatus equipped with a bellows-type ventilator. See text for further details. Source: Adapted from Bokoch and Weston [87].

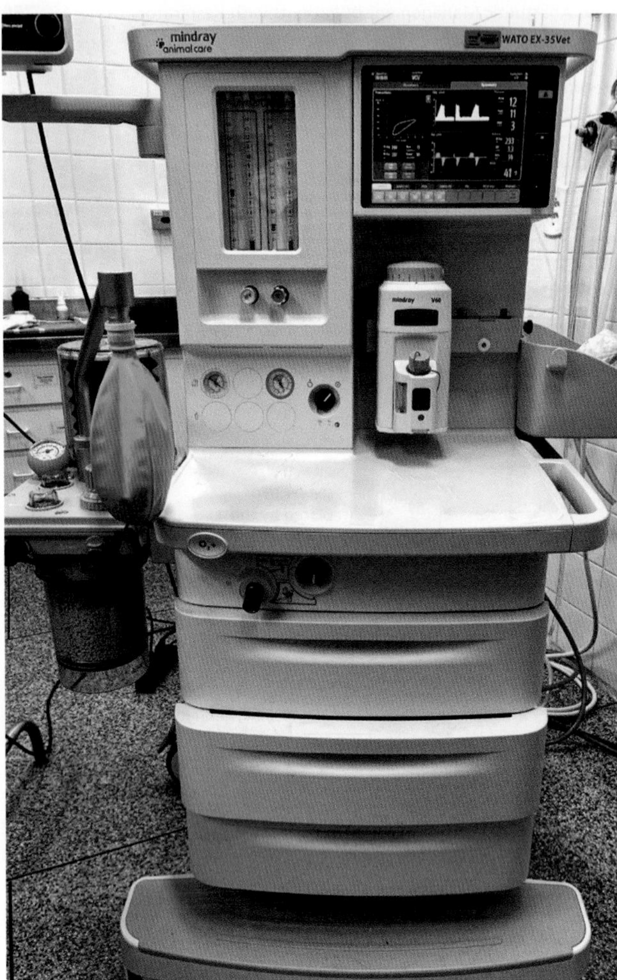

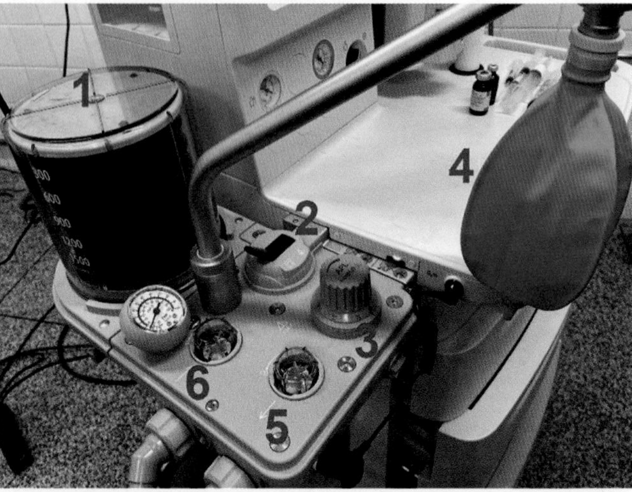

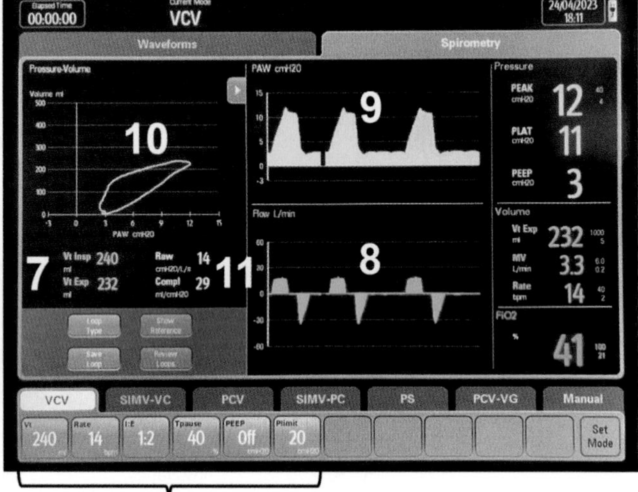

Figure 38.8 Modern anesthesia workstation (EX-35Vet, Mindray Animal Care) incorporating an ascending bellows ventilator (1). Interchange between spontaneous and mechanical ventilation is performed by a switch (2). The pop-off (adjustable pressure-limiting [APL]) valve) (3) and the reservoir bag (4) remain active only during spontaneous ventilation. During mechanical ventilation, flow sensors placed close to the inspiratory (5) and expiratory (6) valves of the breathing circuit provide accurate monitoring of inspired V_T and expired V_T (7) and allow display of the inspiratory and expiratory flow curves over time (8). A pressure transducer within the breathing circuit monitors airway pressures during inspiration and expiration and allows the graphical display of airway pressure changes over time (9). Continuous monitoring of airway pressure and volume changes throughout the respiratory cycle provides the graphical display of pressure–volume (P–V) loops (10). Airway resistance (R_{aw}) is calculated from the difference between plateau pressure (P_{plat}) and positive end-expiratory pressure (PEEP) divided by the peak expiratory flow, while compliance (Compl) is calculated as the ratio between tidal volume (V_T) and the driving pressure (P_{plat} – PEEP).

Table 38.1 Effects of fresh gas flow (FGF), breathing circuit compliance, and gas compression on the inspired tidal volume (V_T) in a 20 kg dog and in a 3.3 kg cat anesthetized with a bellows-type ventilator where the volume delivered by the bellows was adjusted to 15 mL/kg.

	Volume delivered by the bellows	FGF entering the breathing circuit	FGF/volume added during inspiration[a]	Breathing circuit compliance losses[b]	Gas compression losses[c]	Inspired V_T[d]	% difference between bellows and inspired V_T
20 kg dog	300 mL (15 mL/kg)	1 L/min (16.6 mL/s)	33.3 mL	9 mL (P_{peak} = 10 cmH_2O)	30 mL (P_{peak} = 10 cmH_2O)	294 mL (14.7 mL/kg)	−2%
		2 L/min (33.3 mL/s)	66.6 mL	10.8 mL (P_{peak} = 12 cmH_2O)	36 mL (P_{peak} = 12 cmH_2O)	320 mL (16 mL/kg)	+7%
		4 L/min (66.6 mL/s)	133.2 mL	12.6 mL (P_{peak} = 14 cmH_2O:	42 mL (P_{peak} = 14 cmH_2O:	379 mL (19.0 mL/kg)	+26%
3.3 kg cat	50 mL (15 mL/kg)	1 L/min (16.6 mL/s)	33.3 mL	8.1 mL (P_{peak} = 9 cmH_2O)	27 mL (P_{peak} = 9 cmH_2O)	48 mL (14.5 mL/kg)	−4%
		2 L/min (33.3 mL/s)	66.6 mL	10.8 mL (P_{peak} = 12 cmH_2O)	36 mL (P_{peak} = 12 cmH_2O)	70 mL (21.2 mL/kg)	+40%
		4 L/min (66.6 mL/s)	133.2 mL	16.2 mL (P_{peak} = 18 cmH_2O)	54 mL (P_{peak} = 18 cmH_2O	113 mL (34.2 mL/kg)	+126%

[a] Assuming a fixed inspiratory time (2 s): 10 breaths/min and I:E ratio = 1:2.

[b] Assuming a compliance loss of 0.3 mL per 1 cmH_2O of distending pressure for every 1 m of breathing circuit corrugated tubing (1.5 m inspiratory hose + 1.5 m expiratory hose = 3 m of tubing length).

[c] Assuming a gas compression loss of 3 mL for every 1 cm H_2O of distending pressure.

[d] Inspired V_T = Volume delivered by the bellows + (Volume added during inspiration by the FGF – [breathing circuit compliance losses + gas compression losses]).

FGF, fresh gas flow; V_T, tidal volume; P_{peak}, peak airway pressure.

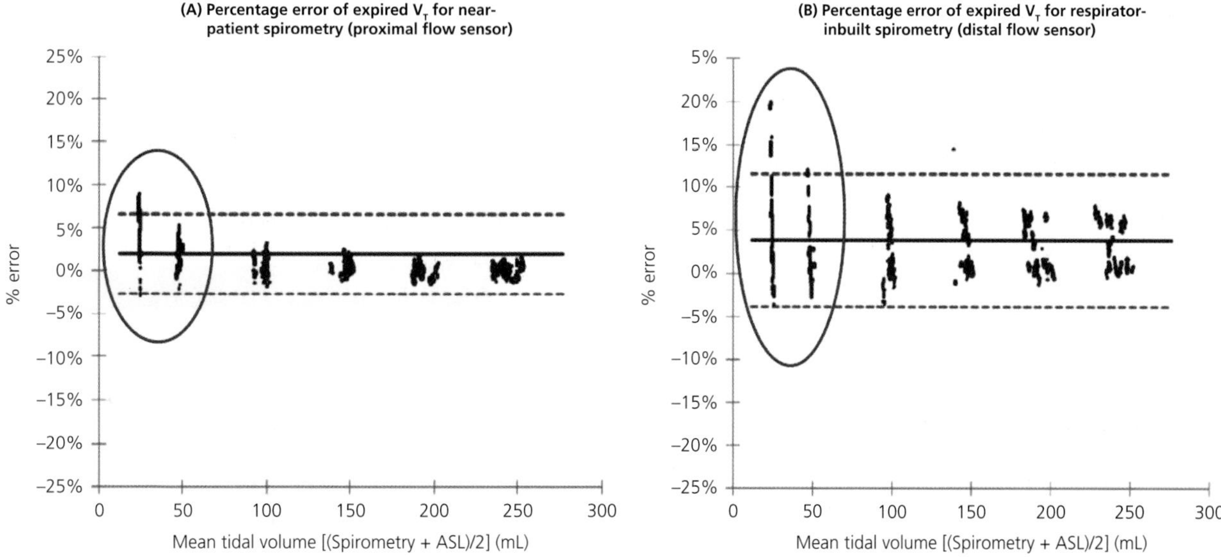

Figure 38.9 Bland–Altmann plots showing percentage error of expired V_T measured by proximal and distal flow sensors in relation to V_Ts generated by a pediatric lung model (ASL). **A.** Near-patient spirometer (pediatric D-Lyte, GE Healthcare) and **B.** Variable orifice inbuilt spirometer (Aisys CS², GE Healthcare). The mean bias (continuous line) and precision (dashed lines) show better agreement and precision of the near-patient spirometer with the V_Ts generated by the simulated lung model. Differences were most significant with V_Ts used in pediatric/neonatal humans or animals weighing ≤ 5 kg (V_T ≤ 50 mL, red ovals), suggesting that near-patient spirometry could be preferable under these circumstances. Source: Morgenroth *et al.* [98]; reproduced with permission.

caution when adjusting the FGF on the anesthetic machine. If FGF is increased, the circuit pressure should be monitored, and the inspiratory flow (tidal volume control) reduced to maintain P_{peak} at a target value to avoid lung overdistention. As accurate measurement of inspired and expired V_T (via spirometry) is not readily available in many veterinary anesthesia ventilators, the operator may adjust the inspiratory flow to achieve a target P_{peak} (e.g., 8–10 cmH_2O for medium-sized dogs). Further adjustments in P_{peak} and respiratory rate are performed with the aim of maintaining end-tidal carbon dioxide partial pressure ($P_{ET}CO_2$) within a predefined range (e.g., between 35 and 45 mmHg).

Modern anesthesia ventilators

Modern anesthesia ventilators incorporate many features that were previously available only in ICU ventilators. Some ventilators incorporate pressure transducers that permit the accurate measurement of breathing circuit pressure and can display airway pressure-time curves. Advanced anesthesia ventilators also incorporate flow sensors (spirometers) placed between the breathing circuit and the endotracheal tube (proximal or near-patient spirometry) or placed near the inspiratory and expiratory valves (distal or inbuilt spirometry) of the breathing circuit and display flow-time curves (Fig. 38.8). Numerical integration of the flow signal by the ventilator permits accurate monitoring of inspired and expired V_T on a breath-by-breath basis. In addition to these variables, incorporation of flow sensors and airway pressure transducers to anesthesia ventilators provides real-time monitoring of pressure–volume (P–V) loops, that is, the graphic display of changes in airway pressure (ΔP) plotted as a function of changes in lung volume (ΔV), and of changes in flow versus changes in lung volume (flow-volume loops) [92]. These parameters, combined with arterial blood gases and other non-invasive monitoring tools (capnography and pulse oximetry), provide the basis for adjusting ventilation parameters. For anesthesia ventilators that do not incorporate built-in flow sensors, a multiparameter monitor that uses a near-patient/proximal flow sensor (Pitot tube) originally designed for humans can be used to accurately monitor V_T in small animals [92,93]. This same flow sensor refashioned to fit between a large animal endotracheal tube and the Y-piece of a large animal anesthesia machine has been used to accurately monitor V_T during mechanical ventilation in horses and other large animals [94,95].

Monitoring V_T by means of proximal/near-patient flow sensors more accurately reflects the actual V_T delivered during mechanical ventilation in pediatric/neonatal humans than distal flow sensors placed near the expiratory valve [96,97]. For an ascending bellows human anesthesia ventilator (Aisys CS², GE Healthcare), V_T measurements provided by a proximal flow sensor also resulted in more accurate and precise estimates of V_T than a variable orifice flow sensor placed near the inspiratory and expiratory valves of the breathing circuit (Fig. 38.9) [98]. Although proximal flow sensors have some disadvantages (e.g., inaccuracy in the presence of excess humidity) in comparison to distal flow sensors, their performance may be superior for neonatal/pediatric humans and for animals weighing ≤ 5 kg [98]. This difference in performance may be explained by different sensor technologies and the fact that sensors placed near the endotracheal tube may achieve better signal-to-noise ratio; that is, the level of the desired signal (flow) is higher in comparison to the level of background noise/interference (which causes inaccuracy). The reader is referred to the specialized literature for additional details regarding advantages and disadvantages of different flow sensors used in anesthesia ventilators [92,99].

As previously described, there are two types of ventilators according to the movement of the bellows during expiration (ascending and descending bellows). Modern anesthesia ventilators usually incorporate the ascending bellows design, which allows visualization of leaks within the breathing circuit as the bellows does not completely fill during expiration. One disadvantage of bellows ventilators is the consumption of higher amounts of compressed gas (air or oxygen compressed within a cylinder) [87,90,91]. One veterinary anesthesia ventilator uses a turbine to generate the compressed gas (ambient air) necessary for driving the ventilator bellows (Veta 5, Mindray Animal Health). A potential problem associated with ventilators that use compressed gas to drive the ventilator bellows is excessive V_T delivery (and possibly barotrauma) if there is a communication due to a tear or leak between the bellows and the housing assembly because high-pressure driving gas can enter the patient circuit. Inhalant anesthetic concentrations within the breathing circuit may be abnormally low as breathing circuit contamination by drive gas will lead to a dilutional effect. If the bellows is driven by compressed air, breathing circuit contamination by the drive gas will lower the inspired oxygen concentration [87,90,91].

The major advantage of modern anesthesia ventilators is that changes in FGF do not alter their ability to deliver an accurate V_T. This is achieved by either the ventilator reducing the volume delivered to compensate for the FGF entering the circuit during inspiration (*fresh gas flow compensation*) or by preventing fresh gas from entering the breathing circuit during inspiration (*fresh gas decoupling*). Fresh gas flow compensation is used by bellows-type ventilators, whereas fresh gas decoupling has been used by piston-driven ventilators originally designed for human anesthesia [87,90,91]. Accuracy of inspired V_T can also be guaranteed by compensation for losses caused by compliance of the breathing circuit with some ventilators [87,90,91]. Advanced anesthesia workstations perform a mandatory self-test before the machine becomes fully operational. Among other safety checks, the pre-use self-test may quantify volume losses caused by compliance of the breathing circuit (mL/cmH_2O) and by small leaks (Fig. 38.10). These measurements are considered when the electronically adjusted V_T is delivered to the patient (breathing circuit compliance compensation). To guarantee optimal ventilator performance, the pre-use self-test should be repeated every time the hoses and other components of the breathing circuit are changed between anesthetic procedures and the flow sensors should be calibrated as per manufacturer recommendations.

Fig. 38.11 illustrates the dynamics of gas flow of an advanced anesthesia workstation equipped with an ascending bellows-type ventilator. During inspiration (Fig. 38.11A), pressurized gas enters the bellows housing, driving the bellows downwards to deliver the V_T. The bellows contains a mixture of exhaled gas and fresh gas, that will add to the fresh gas entering the circuit (fresh gas inlet). The V_T set by the user on the screen of the ventilator electronically controls the gas flow that enters the bellows housing and drives the bellows downward, using data integrated from inspiratory and expiratory flow sensors to deliver an accurate V_T. A stable V_T delivered by the ventilator is guaranteed by a feedback signal provided by the inspiratory flow sensor placed near the inspiratory valve. The inspired V_T is not altered by the FGF because the volume delivered by the bellows is constantly adjusted to compensate for the volume added by the FGF, and as mentioned, for breathing circuit compliance losses identified during the mandatory pre-use self-test. The expired V_T is measured by a flow sensor placed near the expiratory valve and data from inspiratory and expiratory flow sensors is used by some anesthesia ventilators to compensate for compliance losses (Fig. 38.11B). Because the inspired V_T does not account for small leaks around the endotracheal tube or supraglottic device, assessment of ventilation should be based on expired V_T. While the bellows moves toward the top of the housing during passive expiration, the pop-off valve (spill or pressure relief valve) of the ventilator remains closed and only the drive gas exits through the exhalation valve to the scavenge system. Once the bellows is filled, pressure built up within the system opens the ventilator pop-off valve and allows excess gas from the breathing circuit to exit to the scavenge system (not shown) [87,90,91].

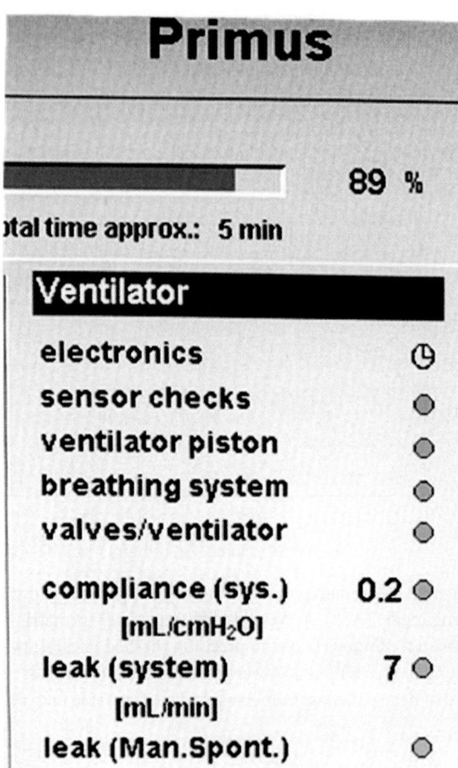

Figure 38.10 Screenshot of the mandatory self-test of the Dräger Primus Anesthesia Workstation with a pediatric circle system. After pressurizing the system to 30 cmH_2O (pop-off/APL valve set to 30 cm H_2O), breathing circuit compliance was 0.2 mL/cmH_2O and leak was 7 mL/min. The green light means that the parameter passed the self-test according to manufacturer standards. The volume delivered by the piston-driven ventilator, in addition to being decoupled from the fresh gas flow, will compensate for compliance losses to deliver an accurate V_T.

While the bellows-type ventilator is the most common type of ventilator used in veterinary medicine, newer ventilator technologies are available in modern anesthesia workstations originally designed for humans, including piston, volume reflective, and turbine ventilators. The reader is referred to the literature for more details on these newer anesthesia workstations [87]. One piston-driven ventilator has been specifically designed for use in large animals (Tafonius, Hallowell EMC) and is described in Chapter 6. An electrically driven piston ventilator (Fig. 38.12) functions as a single-circuit ventilator as there is not a second circuit with compressed gas to drive the piston. Instead, a stepped electric motor controls the movement of a piston within a cylinder to deliver the inspired V_T. This driving mechanism has the advantage of significantly reducing the use of compressed gas, but in the event of a power failure, it will depend on limited battery backup [90]. The inspired V_T is accurately delivered because of: (1) the low compliance of the piston chamber and the accuracy of the stepped electric motor; (2) the volume displaced by the piston is increased to compensate for breathing circuit compliance losses assessed during the pre-use self-test (compliance compensation) (Fig. 38.10); and (3) the FGF is decoupled during inspiration (decoupling valve closed) (Fig. 38.12A) [87,90,91]. During inspiration, the piston delivers a mixture of exhaled and fresh gas, and the FGF entering the circuit is diverted to the reservoir bag, which remains active during mechanical ventilation. In contrast

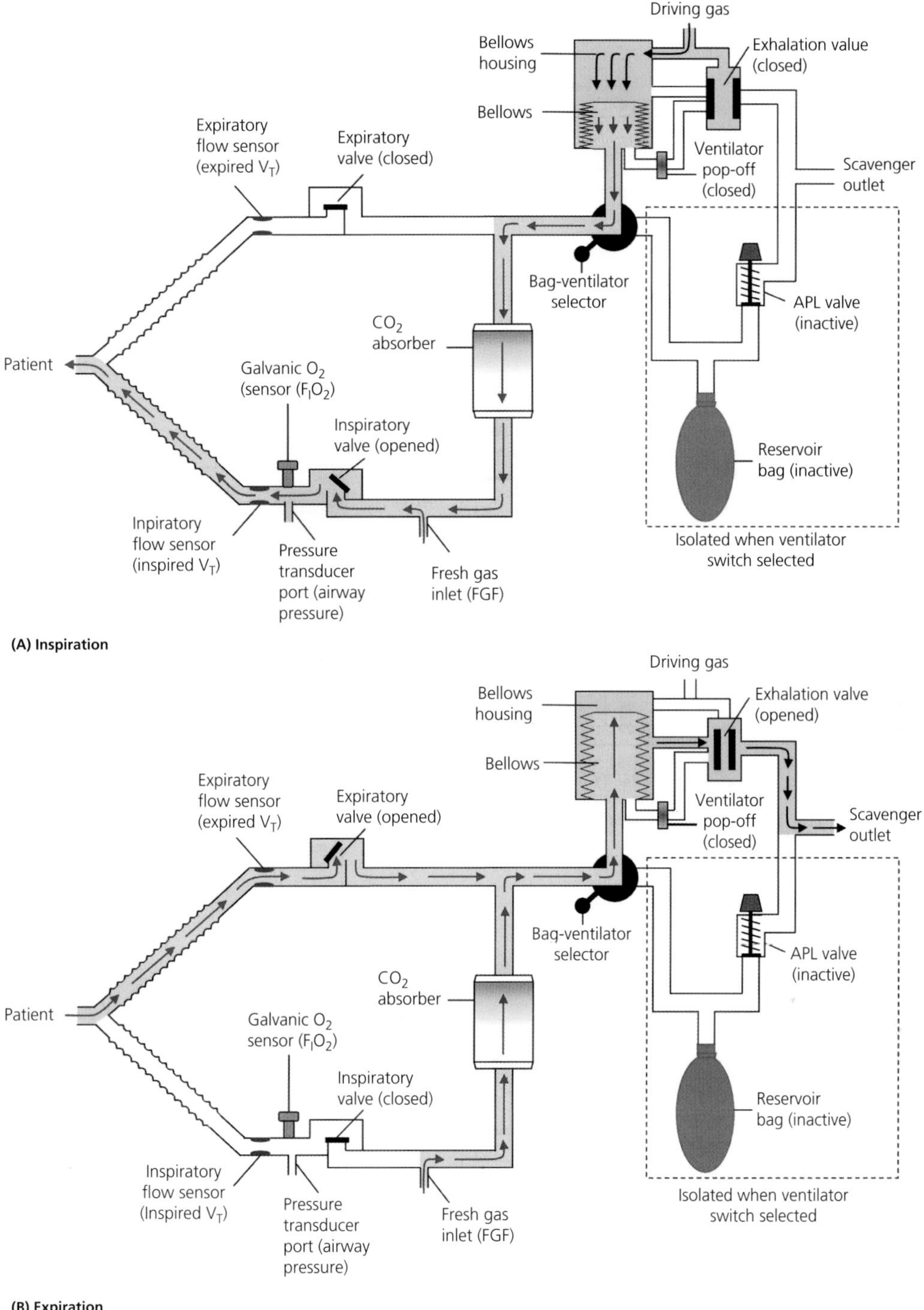

Figure 38.11 Dynamics of gas flow during **A.** inspiration, and **B.** expiration in a breathing circuit of an advanced anesthesia apparatus equipped with a bellows-type ventilator (Aysis anesthesia workstation, GE Healthcare). The bellows-type ventilator is positioned distal to the expiratory valve of the breathing circuit. Notice that the reservoir bag and the APL (pop-off) valve are isolated (inactive) during mechanical ventilation. After the bellows reaches the top of the housing during expiration, excess gas within the breathing circuit opens the ventilator pop-off valve once the pressure exceeds 2 cmH_2O and exits to the scavenge outlet (not shown). See text for further explanation. Source: Modified from Bokoch and Weston [87].

to a bellows ventilator, excess circuit gas is vented through the scavenge outlet during inspiration (Fig. 38.12A). Expired gases pass through the CO_2 absorber and initially fill the reservoir bag. As the decoupling valve opens, a mixture of expired and fresh gas from the reservoir bag and FGF entering the circuit fills the ventilator as the piston moves downwards to its original position (Fig. 38.12B).

Unlike the bellows-type ventilator where the movement of the bellows can be directly visualized through its transparent housing, the piston within the cylinder is usually concealed from view by the operator. With the ascending bellows ventilator, an accidental disconnection or a large leak within the breathing circuit can be rapidly detected as the bellows will not fill during expiration; while smaller

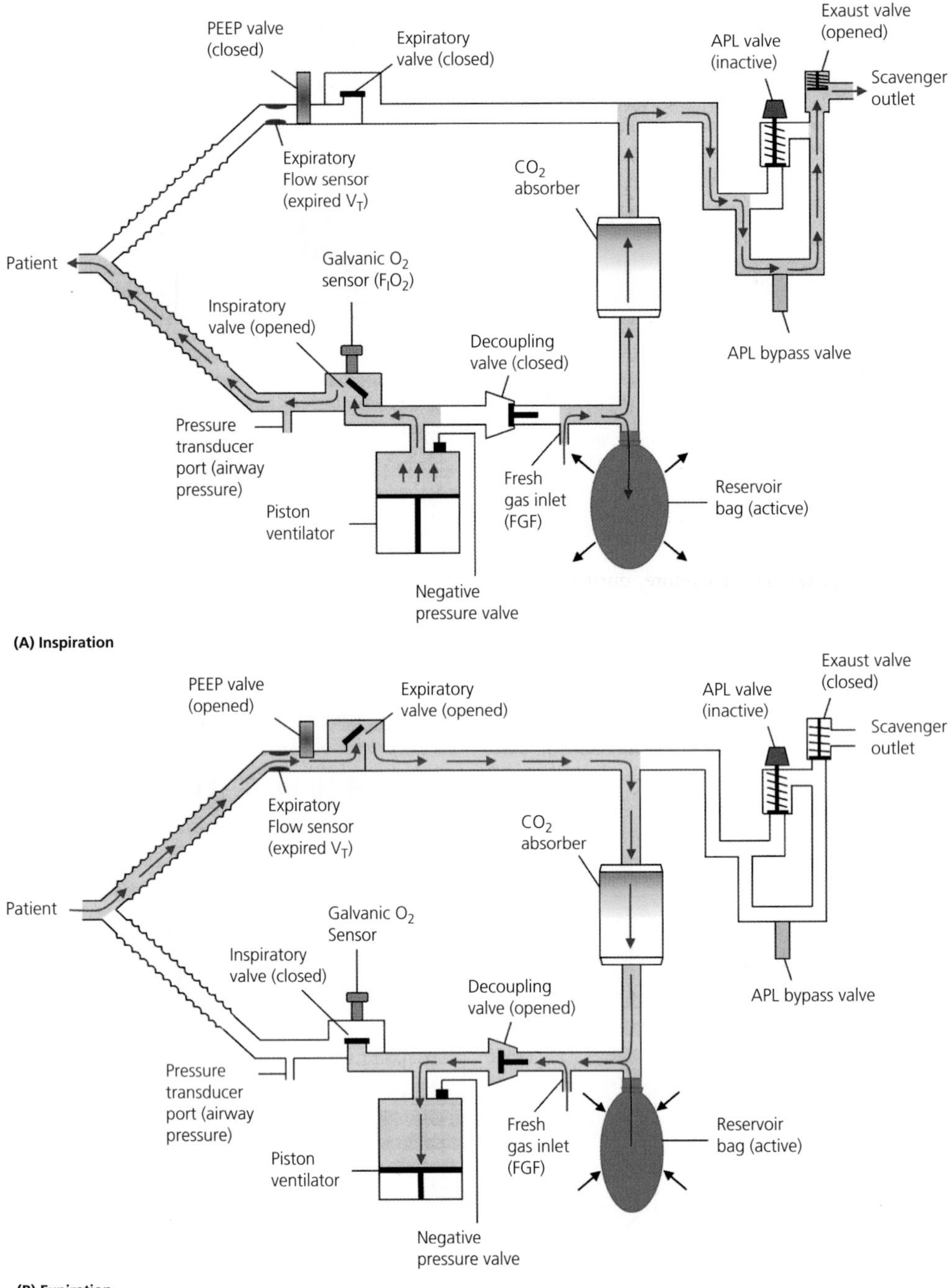

Figure 38.12 Dynamics of gas flow during **A.** inspiration, and **B.** expiration in a modern anesthesia apparatus equipped with a piston ventilator (Fabius GS anesthesia system, Dräger). A piston-type ventilator is located between the fresh gas inlet and the inspiratory valve. Notice that the rebreathing bag remains active during mechanical ventilation and excess gas exits the breathing circuit during inspiration. See text for further explanation. Source: Modified from Bokoch and Weston [87].

leaks will cause the bellows to incompletely fill. A leak in a piston-driven ventilator may be more difficult to detect. If a leak is present, during expiration the cylinder will fill with ambient air by activation of a negative-pressure valve, diluting inspired gases with air, decreasing F_IO_2, and reducing anesthetic gas concentration within the circuit (possibly leading to patient awareness). Collapse of the reservoir bag, which contains a mixture of expired and fresh gas during mechanical ventilation, provides the user with an alert of a large leak/disconnection in the breathing circuit of a piston ventilator.

Modes of mechanical ventilation utilized during anesthesia

Continuous mandatory ventilation

In continuous mandatory ventilation (CMV), also known as "controlled ventilation," the ventilator delivers all mechanical breaths at predefined intervals according to the respiratory rate set by the operator. Continuous mandatory modes of ventilation are typically time cycled, that is termination of the inspiratory phase occurs after a certain time has elapsed. As explained above, for some ventilators, the inspiratory time is directly adjusted by the operator, while for other machines inspiratory time is indirectly adjusted via changes in the I:E ratio and respiratory rate.

Volume-controlled ventilation (VCV)

When a standard VCV mode is chosen, the operator selects the V_T to be delivered (target variable), in addition to other variables (e.g., respiratory rate, I:E ratio or inspiratory time, and the PEEP level). In VCV mode, the V_T is the independent variable as it will remain constant, whereas P_{peak} is the dependent variable as it will change in case of modifications in respiratory system compliance (C_{RS}) and airway resistance (R_{aw}). The inspiratory flow, which is automatically adjusted by the ventilator to achieve the target V_T, will remain constant throughout inspiration (square wave flow-time curve). Because of the constant inspiratory flow pattern, airway pressure measured within the breathing circuit (that is equivalent to P_{ao}) increases in a quasilinear fashion until the end of inspiration (Fig. 38.13A). The peak increase in airway pressure (P_{peak}) recorded at the end of constant flow inspiration reflects the combined effects of airway resistance (R_{aw}) and compliance of the respiratory system (C_{RS}) on airway pressures [100–103]. Therefore, during conventional mechanical ventilation with a constant V_T, a temporal increase in P_{peak} suggests a decrease in C_{RS} or an increase in R_{aw}, and vice versa (Fig. 38.13B and C):

$$P_{peak}\left(cmH_2O\right)=\frac{R_{aw}}{C_{RS}}$$

In healthy lungs, it is assumed that the increase in airway pressure will rapidly equilibrate with P_{alv}, expanding alveoli across the lung tissue. However, in VCV mode without an inspiratory pause, the absence of a plateau pressure (P_{plat}) at the end of inspiration could favor an unequal distribution of inspiratory flow, leading to preferential volume delivery to alveoli with faster-filling rates (Fig. 38.14). Alternatively, VCV may allow maintenance of a P_{plat} during inspiration [100–103]. This goal can be achieved by adding an inspiratory pause (period of zero flow) after the target V_T is achieved, which is usually defined by the operator as percent of total inspiratory time. Maintenance of a P_{plat} may theoretically allow a more homogenous distribution of gas flow across the lung (Fig. 38.14).

A pause in inspiratory flow during VCV allows measurement of P_{peak} at the end of constant inspiratory flow (when the target V_T is delivered) and of P_{plat} at the end of the inspiratory pause (Fig. 38.15A).

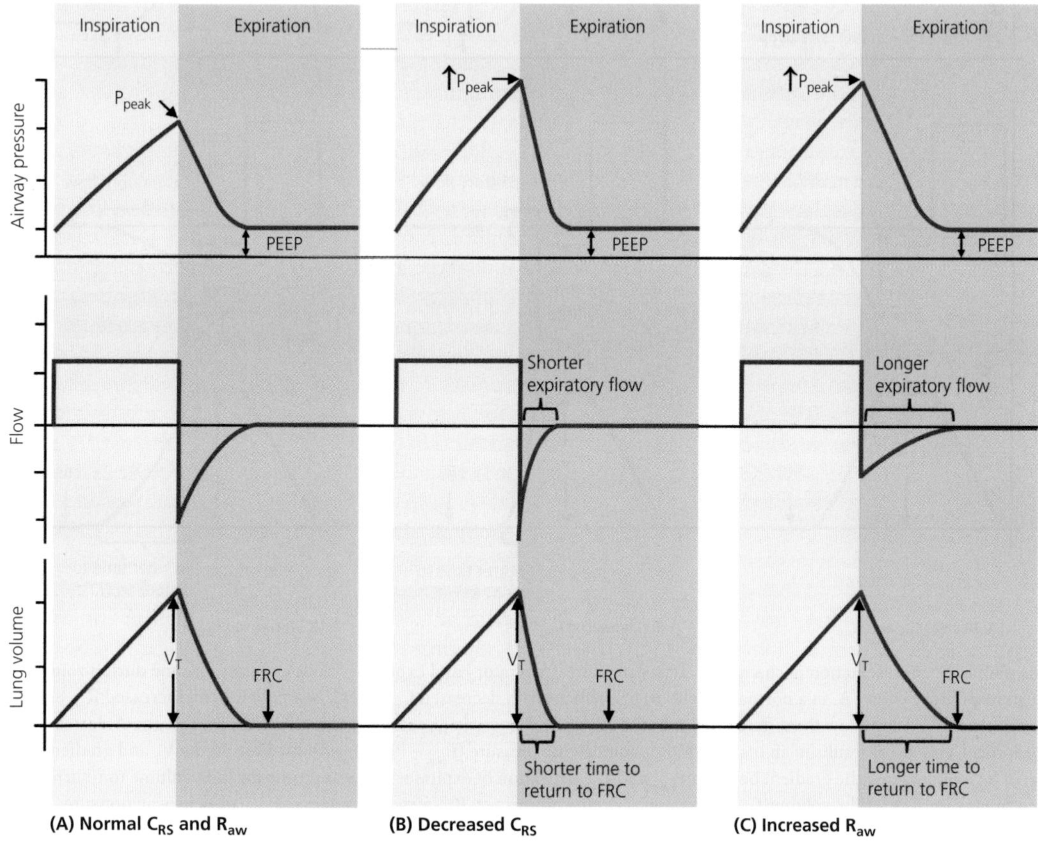

Figure 38.13 Diagrammatic representation of changes in airway pressure, inspiratory and expiratory flow, and lung volume during volume-controlled ventilation without an inspiratory pause: **A.** in a normal patient, **B.** in a patient with decreased C_{RS}, and **C.** in a patient with increased R_{aw}. A decrease in C_{RS} or an increase in R_{aw} will increase P_{peak} while V_T remains unaltered. During passive expiration, a decrease in C_{RS} (or an increase in its reciprocal elastance) accelerates lung emptying as the time until expiratory flow returns to zero and the time until lung volume returns to its resting position (FRC) is shortened. Otherwise, increased R_{aw} slows lung emptying and the flow-time curve takes longer to reach zero while lung volume takes longer to return to FRC. V_T, tidal volume; C_{RS}, respiratory system compliance; R_{aw}, airway resistance; P_{peak}, peak airway pressure; PEEP, positive end-expired pressure; FRC, functional residual capacity. Source: Partially modified from Kaczka *et al.* [104].

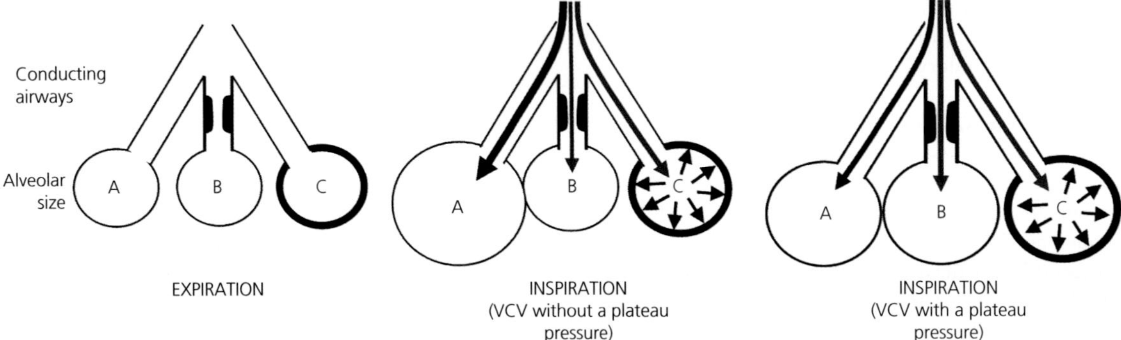

Figure 38.14 Diagrammatic representation of distribution of inspiratory gas flow during volume-controlled ventilation (VCV) in alveoli with different filling rates: (A) small airways with normal resistance to flow leading to alveoli with normal compliance ("fast" alveoli); (B) small airways with high resistance to flow ("slow" alveoli); and (C) alveoli with low compliance. In the case of constant inspiratory flow leading to a quasilinear increase in airway pressure (i.e., positive-pressure ventilation without a plateau pressure), gas flow is preferentially distributed to 'fast' alveoli, which may be overdistended. Maintenance of a plateau pressure during inspiration theoretically favors homogeneous gas distribution to alveoli with different filling rates.

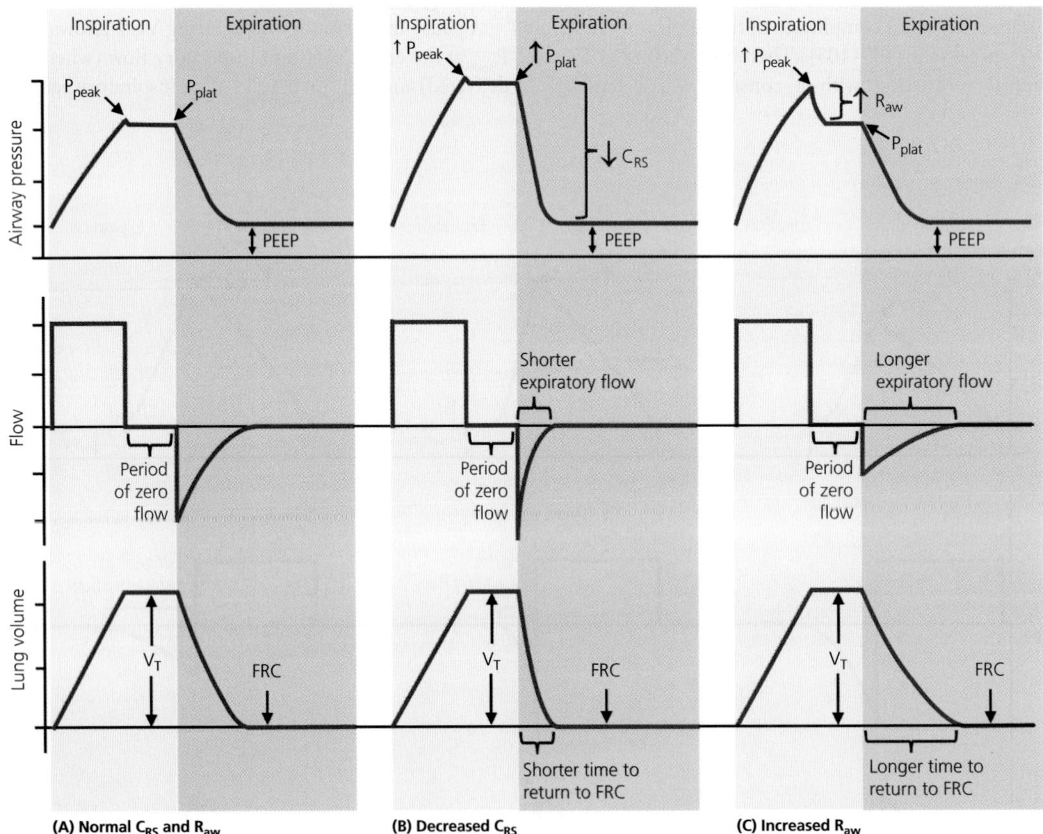

Figure 38.15 Diagrammatic representation of changes in airway pressure, inspiratory and expiratory flow, and lung volume during volume-controlled ventilation with an inspiratory pause: **A.** in a normal patient, **B.** in a patient with decreased C_{RS} and **C.** in a patient with increased R_{aw}. Setting an inspiratory pause during VCV may allow the differentiation of the effects of changes in C_{RS} and R_{aw} on pulmonary mechanics. A decrease in C_{RS} (or an increase in its reciprocal, elastance) results in an increase in P_{plat} and driving pressure (P_{plat} – PEEP), without altering the V_T and gradient between P_{peak} and P_{plat}. An increase in R_{aw} will increase the gradient between P_{peak} and P_{plat}. Duration of expiratory flow and time for lung volume to return to FRC follow the pattern explained in Fig. 38.13. V_T, tidal volume; C_{RS}, respiratory system compliance; R_{aw}, airway resistance; P_{peak}, peak airway pressure; P_{plat}, plateau pressure; PEEP, positive end-expired pressure; FRC, functional residual capacity. Source: Partially modified from Kaczka *et al.* [104].

The P_{plat} (and the driving pressure, calculated as the gradient between P_{plat} and the PEEP level) is influenced by V_T and by C_{RS}. Therefore, during mechanical ventilation with a constant V_T, an increase in P_{plat} or driving pressure over time is indicative of a decrease in C_{RS} (Fig. 38.15B):

$$P_{plat}\left(cmH_2O\right)=\frac{V_T}{C_{RS}}$$

As explained before, the P_{peak} recorded in VCV mode is the distending pressure of the lungs that is necessary to overcome the resistive and viscoelastic properties of the respiratory system (R_{aw} and C_{RS}, respectively). In humans, the P_{plat} recorded at the end of an inspiratory pause (period of zero flow) of at least 0.5 s, may reflect the distending pressure of the lungs that is necessary to overcome viscoelastic properties of the respiratory system (C_{RS}) per se, without the confounding effects of R_{aw} [100,103]. Analysis of the airway pressure-time curve and the gradient between P_{peak} and P_{plat} during VCV with an inspiratory pause of at least 0.5 s may allow the discrimination of the effects of C_{RS} and R_{aw} on airway pressures [100,103] (Fig. 38.15B and C).

Animals may have low C_{RS} because of obesity, increased intra-abdominal volume caused by pregnancy, distended abdominal viscera, pneumoperitoneum, shape of the chest wall (dogs with barrel-shaped chest conformation), atelectasis, and pleural/parenchymal lung disease. As explained before, during ventilation in volume-controlled mode, V_T will remain constant while airway pressure increases or decreases as a function of changes in C_{RS}. If V_T and respiratory frequency are adjusted appropriately, $\dot{V}_E$ and normal $PaCO_2$ levels can be maintained despite decreases in C_{RS} related to patient positioning or the surgical procedure (e.g., pneumoperitoneum) [101,105]. Since a decrease in C_{RS} will increase airway pressure during constant volume ventilation, modern anesthesia machines allow adjusting the maximum airway pressure in VCV mode, that is, inspiratory flow will be interrupted before preset V_T is achieved if the airway pressure limit set by the operator is exceeded.

Airway resistance may also increase because of anesthetic equipment (e.g., relatively narrow/kinked endotracheal tube, narrow tubing of the breathing circuit) or because of pathophysiological changes in the airways (e.g., brachycephalic syndrome in dogs, tracheal stenosis, and partial obstruction of the airways by thick/viscous secretions or foreign material). The use of an inspiratory pause during VCV may be advantageous because it may allow discrimination of changes in pulmonary mechanics caused by increased R_{aw} from those caused by decreased C_{RS} (Fig. 38.16).

Pressure-controlled ventilation (PCV)

The PCV mode is characterized by a decelerating flow-time curve during inspiration. Unlike the VCV mode, the operator selects the maximum inspiratory pressure (P_{max}) rather than the V_T to be delivered to the patient. During PCV, the P_{max} is the independent variable while V_T is the dependent variable. Specifically, the P_{max} set by the operator will remain constant while V_T will vary as a function of changes in C_{RS} and R_{aw}. Therefore, if C_{RS} decreases or R_{aw} increases, inspiratory airflow and V_T will decrease, and vice versa (Fig. 38.17) [104,106].

During inspiration, following a rapid rise in airway pressure, which coincides with the peak inspiratory flow, pressure increases in a more curvilinear fashion until the target airway pressure (P_{max}) is achieved. The decelerating flow may reach zero before the expiratory valve opens and passive expiration begins creating an inspiratory pause/P_{plat} (Fig. 38.17). Because the ventilator generates a decelerating inspiratory flow, PCV does not result in a peak rise in airway pressure (P_{peak}) that is observed at the end of a constant inspiratory flow (VCV mode). For some anesthesia ventilators the rise time (T_{slope}), that is the time elapsed for airway pressure to increase from PEEP to P_{max} in PCV mode, can be adjusted. An increase in T_{slope} in relation to the total inspiratory time will lower the peak increase in inspiratory flow and shorten the period of zero flow during inspiration, and vice versa (Fig. 38.18).

When using PCV, the anesthesiologist must be aware that changes in chest wall compliance associated with specific surgical conditions, such as laparoscopic surgery associated pneumoperitoneum, could decrease C_{RS} and lead to some degree of alveolar collapse/hypoventilation because V_T will fall [105]. Therefore, if there is a decrease in expired V_T monitored by the flow sensor during PCV, the operator may need to reset airway pressure to a higher value to maintain V_T and prevent hypercapnia.

Dual-controlled ventilation

VCV has the advantage of maintaining a constant V_T and $\dot{V}_E$; however, it may result in high airway pressures. Conversely, PCV does not guarantee that V_T and $\dot{V}_E$ are maintained but has the advantage of reducing alveolar stress by limiting the maximum airway pressure delivered to the lung [106]. To overcome the disadvantages of decreased V_T and $\dot{V}_E$ in face of decreased C_{RS} and increased R_{aw} during PCV, some anesthesia ventilators incorporate the option to perform a volume-targeted (or volume-guaranteed) PCV mode. This ventilation mode, also known as "dual-mode ventilation," combines the advantages of VCV and PCV (delivery of a fixed V_T and decelerating inspiratory flow resulting in lower airway pressures). In volume-targeted PCV, the user selects the V_T while the

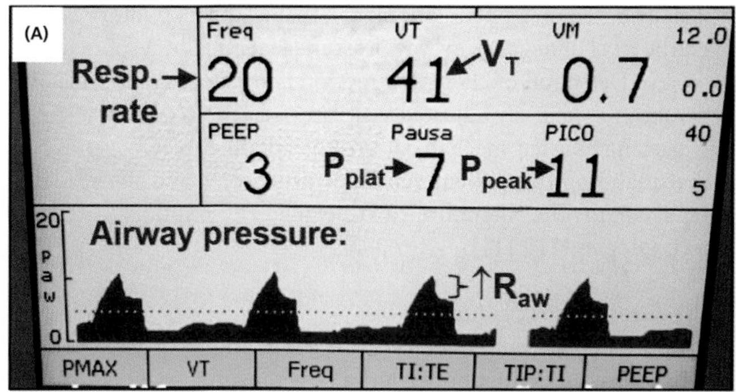

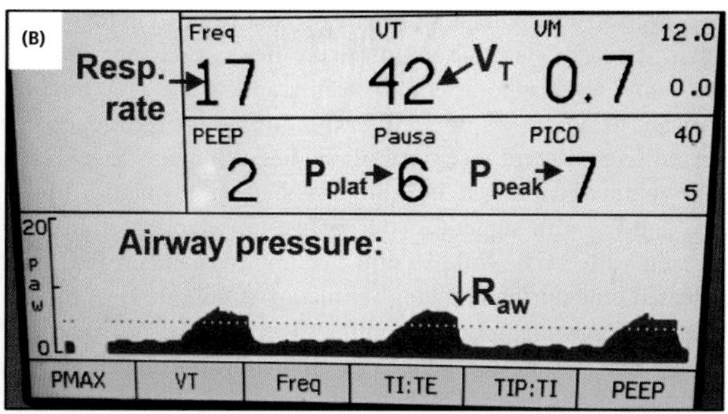

Figure 38.16 Screenshots of an anesthesia ventilator (Dräger Fabius Plus, Drägerwerk AG & Co.) used for a 3.8 kg cat anesthetized with isoflurane during volume-controlled ventilation. The ventilator was adjusted to obtain an expired V_T of approximately 40 mL (10–11 mL/kg) with an inspiratory pause of 40% of inspiratory time. The respiratory rate was set to maintain $P_{ET}CO_2$ close to 35–40 mmHg. **A.** After a 3 mm internal diameter endotracheal tube was placed, the airway pressure tracing is suggestive of increased R_{aw} and there is an increased gradient between P_{peak} and P_{plat}. **B.** Immediately after the 3 mm tube was replaced by a 4 mm inner diameter endotracheal tube, the gradient between P_{peak} and P_{plat} decreased, denoting a decrease in R_{aw}. $P_{ET}CO_2$, end-tidal carbon dioxide partial pressure; P_{peak}, peak airway pressure; P_{plat}, plateau pressure; R_{aw}, airway resistance; V_T, expired tidal volume. Source: Drägerwerk AG & Co.

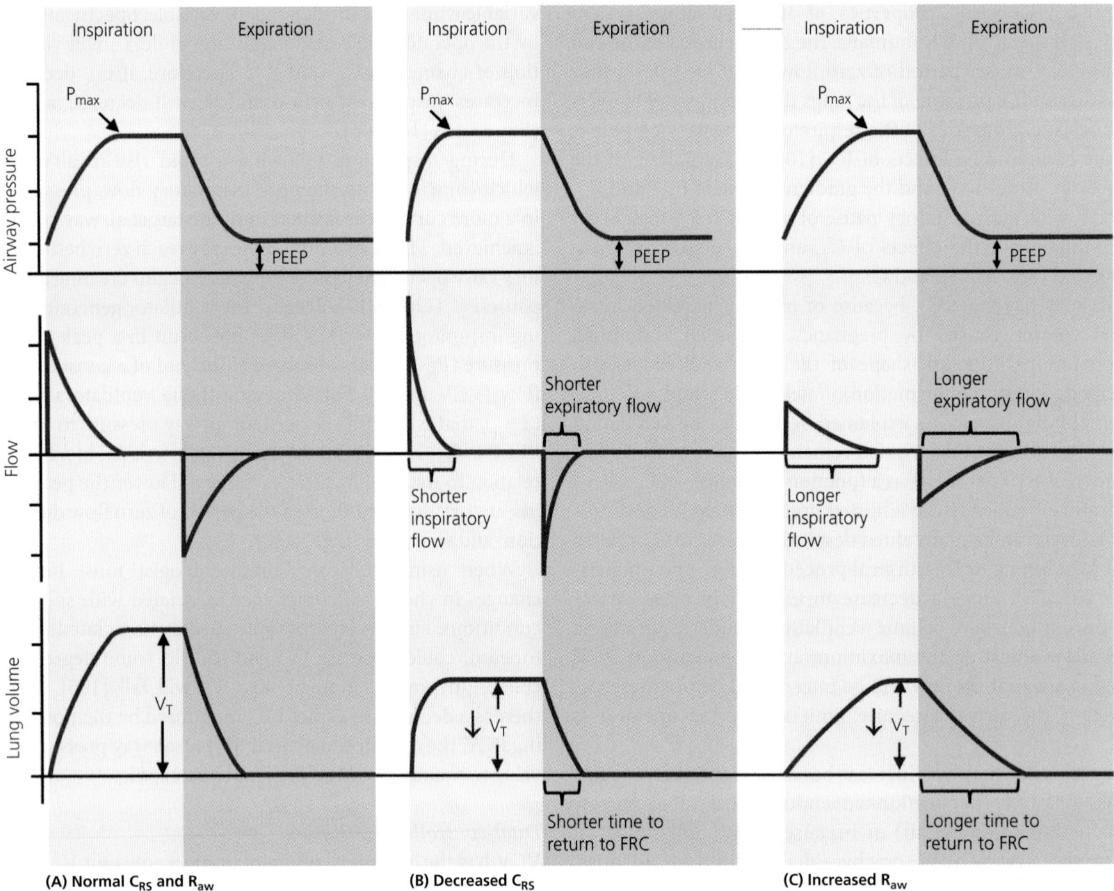

Figure 38.17 Diagrammatic representation of changes in airway pressure, inspiratory and expiratory flow, and lung volume during pressure-controlled ventilation: **A.** in a normal patient, **B.** in a patient with decreased C_{RS}, and **C.** in a patient with increased R_{aw}. Notice that as inspiratory flow decelerates, airway pressure increases in a more curvilinear fashion compared to volume-controlled ventilation and there is no P_{peak}. Because airway pressure set by the user is kept constant, inspiratory/expiratory flow and consequently V_T will change as a function of changes in C_{RS} and R_{aw}. In a more rigid lung (decreased C_{RS}), inspiratory/expiratory flow is decreased and more quickly returns to zero. The decrease in airflow results in decreased V_T. If R_{aw} is increased, inspiratory/expiratory flow also decreases, resulting in a decrease in V_T. V_T, tidal volume; C_{RS}, respiratory system compliance; R_{aw}, airway resistance; P_{max}, maximum inspiratory pressure; PEEP, positive end-expired pressure; FRC, functional residual capacity. Source: Partially modified from Kaczka *et al.* [104].

ventilator adjusts the lowest possible airway pressure to achieve the preset volume [101,107]. In healthy dogs undergoing abdominal surgery (ovariohysterectomy), PCV targeting a V_T of 10 mL/kg improved airway dynamics (lower P_{peak}) and resulted in higher C_{RS} but without a detectable improvement in gas exchange ($PaCO_2$, PaO_2, and alveolar-to-arterial oxygen gradient $P(A\text{-}a)O_2$ in comparison to VCV (V_T = 10 mL/kg) during the intraoperative period [108]. Recent meta-analysis studies in humans have shown that volume-guaranteed PCV improves airway dynamics (lower P_{peak} and P_{plat} with higher C_{RS}) during two-lung ventilation in comparison with VCV, while an effective improvement in PaO_2 was detected only during one-lung ventilation (OLV) [109]. Although these findings might apply to animals without lung disease, these results may not be reproduced in animals with lung disease. A summary of the differences between controlled ventilation modes (VCV, PCV, and volume-guaranteed PCV) is presented in Table 38.2.

Assisted and assisted-controlled ventilation modes

Assisted and assisted-controlled ventilation modes may be available in some anesthesia ventilators. In the *assisted mode*, the ventilator detects a trigger signal from the patient, that is, the commencement of a spontaneous breathing effort, to provide a synchronized mechanical breath. The trigger signal of anesthesia ventilators is usually based on a pneumatic signal, that is, the inspiratory flow or on the level of negative airway pressure generated by a spontaneous breath. Detection of chest wall motion and diaphragmatic electromyograms (neurally adjusted ventilatory assist) are other forms of triggering assisted mechanical breaths adopted in ICU ventilators that may improve patient-ventilator synchrony, and the reader is referred to the literature for detailed descriptions of these technologies [110,111].

Pressure support ventilation

Pressure support ventilation (PSV) is a modality of assisted ventilation where the ventilator delivers a target inspiratory pressure with a decelerating flow pattern when a spontaneous breathing effort is detected [101]. Delivery of an assisted breath is based on the level of negative airway pressure or the inspiratory flow generated by a spontaneous breathing effort. The operator can increase the sensitivity of the triggering mechanism either by decreasing the inspiratory flow or by adjusting the level of negative airway pressure to a

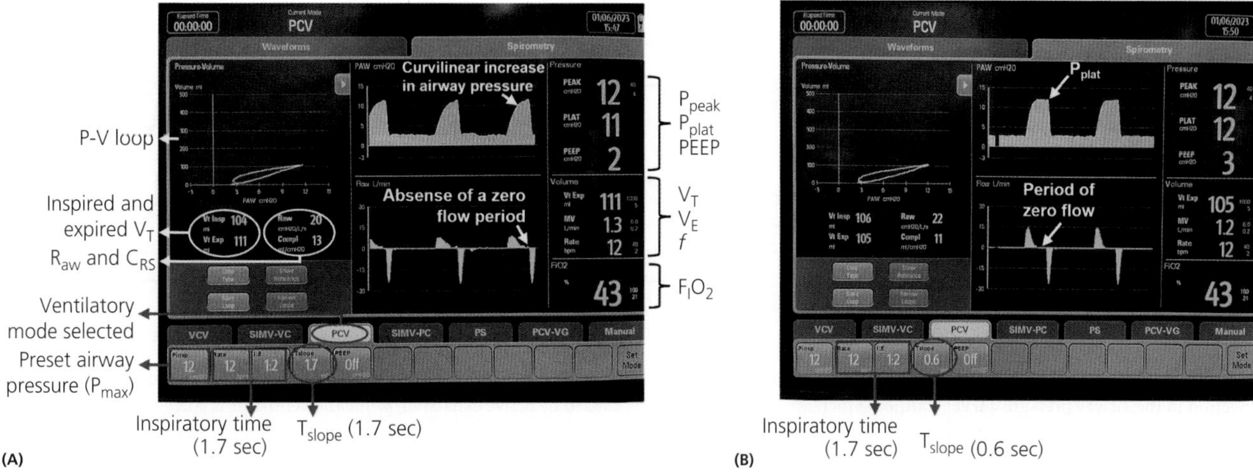

Figure 38.18 Airway pressure and flow curves recorded during pressure-controlled ventilation in a 10 kg dog (9 kg ideal body weight) anesthetized with isoflurane and a constant rate infusion of fentanyl. The P_{max} was adjusted to 12 cmH_2O aiming to deliver a V_T of approximately 12 mL/kg (108 mL based on ideal body weight) at a respiratory frequency of 12 breaths/min and an I:E ratio of 1:2, which resulted in an inspiratory time of 1.7 s. **A.** Notice that when the rise time (T_{slope}) was adjusted to match the inspiratory time (1.7 s), there was no period of zero flow and the pressure rose in a curvilinear fashion until reaching P_{max}. The measured P_{peak} (P_{max}) cannot be considered equivalent to the P_{peak} measured in VCV mode because it was measured at the end of the period of decelerating flow and not at the end of a period of constant inspiratory flow that is typical of VCV. The measured P_{plat} also cannot be considered reliable because there is no period of zero flow before passive expiration begins. **B.** Notice that when the T_{slope} is adjusted to 0.6 s (approximately, 35% of inspiratory time), a period of zero flow is created before passive expiration begins. This results in the formation of a plateau in the airway pressure curve, which allows correct measurement of P_{plat}. $P_{max,}$ maximum inspiratory pressure; V_T, tidal volume; P_{plat}, plateau pressure.

Table 38.2 Summary characteristics of volume-controlled ventilation (VCV), pressure-controlled ventilation (PCV), and dual-controlled (volume-guaranteed PCV) ventilation.

	Volume-controlled ventilation	Pressure-controlled ventilation	Dual-controlled ventilation
Breathing pattern	Only mandatory breaths	Only mandatory breaths	Only mandatory breaths
Termination of inspiratory flow	Time cycled	Time cycled	Time cycled
Inspiratory flow pattern	Constant (square wave) flow	Decelerating flow	Decelerating flow
Target variable	V_T	P_{max} [a]	V_T
Advantages	Allows maintenance of $\dot{V}_E$ and $PaCO_2$ regardless of changes in C_{RS} and R_{aw} If an inspiratory pause is added, quasistatic C_{RS} and R_{aw} (P_{peak} – P_{plat}) can be assessed	Lower airway pressures +/– better compliance than VCV	Combines the advantages of VCV and PCV
Disadvantages	Higher airway pressures (P_{peak}) than PCV	$\dot{V}_E$ and $PaCO_2$ influenced by changes in C_{RS} and R_{aw} Cannot assess R_{aw} by the gradient between P_{peak} and P_{plat} (typical P_{peak} in VCV not measured)	Cannot assess R_{aw} by the gradient between P_{peak} and P_{plat} (typical P_{peak} in VCV not measured)

[a] The target pressure set in PCV mode is better defined as P_{max} as true P_{peak} (as measured at the end of constant inspiratory flow in VCV mode) cannot be measured with the decelerating flow that is characteristic of PCV. VCV, volume-controlled ventilation; PCV, pressure-controlled ventilation; V_T, tidal volume; $\dot{V}_E$, minute ventilation; C_{RS}, respiratory system compliance; R_{aw}, airway resistance; P_{peak}, peak airway pressure; P_{plat}, plateau pressure.

less negative value, and vice versa. During PSV mode, delivery of mechanical breaths is dependent on the degree of central ventilatory drive. Therefore, depending on the suppression of central nervous system (CNS) sensitivity to CO_2 and the level of relaxation of respiratory muscles by anesthetic drugs, the number of patient-triggered mechanical breaths will vary and result in varying degrees of decreased $\dot{V}_E$/hypercapnia or may even result in apnea. Ventilators often offer PSV with safety backup ventilation to provide the patient with mandatory ventilation in case of complete suppression of the CNS ventilatory drive or excessive respiratory muscle relaxation/paralysis [101]. This mode of ventilation can be adopted for weaning the animal from the ventilator when there is enough ventilatory drive for the patient to initiate spontaneous breaths.

Another fundamental difference between controlled ventilation modes (VCV, PCV, and volume-guaranteed PCV) and PSV is the mechanism of termination of inspiratory flow (also known as "cycling mechanism") [112,113]. As explained before, termination of inspiratory flow, that is the transition between inspiration and expiration, in controlled ventilation modes occurs after a certain time has elapsed (inspiratory time), as defined by the operator. Cycling (that is passive exhalation) in PSV mode occurs after the

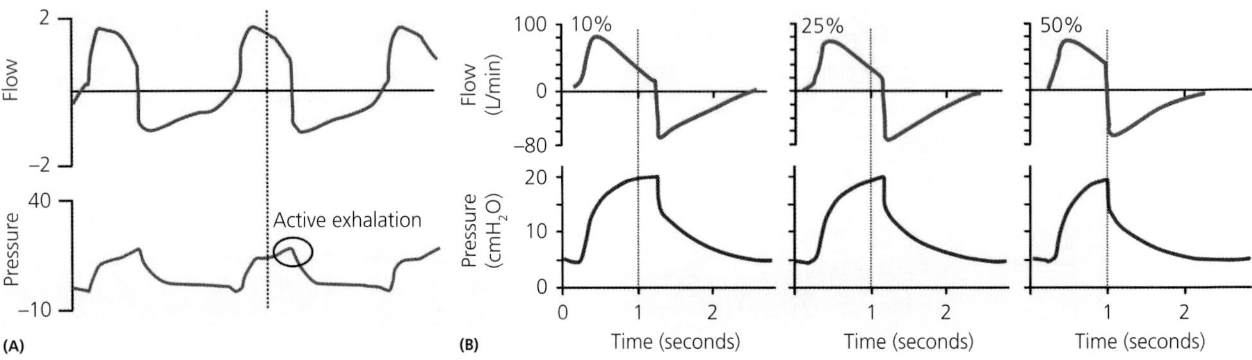

Figure 38.19 Changes in inspiratory and expiratory flow and airway pressure during pressure support ventilation (PSV). **A.** The oval shows an abnormal deflection in the airway pressure curve (additional increase in airway pressure) caused by active exhalation while the ventilator is still generating inspiratory flow. **B.** Lung model showing flow-cycling (end of inspiration) at 10%, 25%, and 50% of peak inspiratory flow. Notice that when the percent of peak flow is increased, there is a shortening of inspiratory flow, which may avoid patient-ventilator asynchrony caused by delayed cycling. Source: Hess [112]; Gentile [113], reproduced with permission.

inspiratory flow decelerates to a certain percentage of its peak. Typically, the end of inspiration can be set at 25% of peak inspiratory flow to avoid breath holding (period of zero flow during inspiration), which may be uncomfortable to a patient that is spontaneously breathing. Although patient-ventilator asynchrony is avoided during PSV as the patient initiates the mechanical breaths, asynchrony may still occur if the duration of inspiratory flow exceeds the time of an active exhalation effort, a phenomenon known as "delayed cycling." If the patient tries to exhale while positive airway pressure is still being applied to the airway, the major consequence of delayed cycling is the creation of PEEP, which may also impair the triggering of assisted breaths. Avoidance of patient-ventilator asynchrony caused by delayed cycling can be achieved by shortening the inspiratory flow by increasing the percent of peak inspiratory flow at which the ventilator cycles to exhalation (Fig. 38.19A and B). Adjusting the flow-cycling is of great relevance in ICU patients that are on PSV and the reader is referred to the literature for further details [112,113].

Spontaneous intermittent mandatory ventilation

Spontaneous intermittent mandatory ventilation (SIMV) is an *assisted-controlled* ventilation modality provided by some anesthesia ventilators. This ventilation mode allows mandatory mechanical breaths as selected by the operator (controlled ventilation) and patient-triggered mechanical breaths (assisted ventilation), with the mandatory breaths either in volume-control (SIMV-VCV) or pressure-control (SIMV-PCV) mode [101]. During the expiratory phase following a mandatory breath, there is a trigger window at late expiration (set by the operator as *percentage of expiratory time*) where the ventilator algorithm responds to a pneumatic signal (negative airway pressure or inspiratory flow generated by the patient) with assisted mechanical breaths either in volume-control (constant flow and volume targeted) or pressure-control (decelerating flow and pressure-targeted) mode. A pressure-targeted flow cycled breath (PSV mode) is delivered if the patient makes spontaneous breathing efforts at any time during expiration outside the triggering window. If the patient has an increased ventilatory drive and assisted mechanical breaths superimpose on the time interval programmed by the ventilator to deliver a mandatory breath, pre-programmed breaths are canceled, avoiding patient-ventilator asynchrony (Fig. 38.20).

Anesthesia ventilators with SIMV capabilities often present the flow and pressure curves originating from patient-triggered breaths with a distinctive color, or another graphic hallmark, to allow the operator to discriminate patient-triggered from mandatory breaths. The SIMV mode (either in pressure- or volume-control mode) can be selected for maintenance of general anesthesia; absence of patient-triggered breaths during anesthesia can be achieved by setting a proper $\dot{V}_E$ (based on f and V_T during SIMV-VCV or f and P_{max} during SIMV-PCV) to maintain eucapnia and by ensuring an adequate depth of anesthesia. Alternatively, spontaneous breathing efforts can be abolished by administering a neuromuscular blocking agent during anesthesia. The SIMV mode can be useful as an alternative to controlled modes of ventilation (VCV and PCV) in animals with spontaneous breathing efforts despite proper $\dot{V}_E$ and adequate depth of anesthesia (Fig 38.20). At the end of anesthesia, weaning the animal off the ventilator can be achieved by reducing the number of mandatory breaths to allow CO_2 to build-up and increase central ventilatory drive; once ventilatory drive is judged to be adequate, as observed by the number of patient-triggered breaths, the ventilation mode can be switched to assisted (PSV), before allowing the patient to resume spontaneous ventilation.

Monitoring pulmonary mechanics during mechanical ventilation

Pressure–volume (P–V) loops

Dynamic P–V loops, which graphically present changes in airway pressure (ΔP) on the x-axis and changes in lung volume (ΔV) on the y-axis during a mechanical breath, provide important information regarding R_{aw} and C_{RS}. A summary of changes in dynamic P–V loops that may occur during VCV and PCV are illustrated in Fig. 38.21. Analysis of dynamic P–V loops reveals that lung volume during inspiration is less than lung volume recorded at the same airway pressure during expiration. The difference in lung volume during inflation and deflation occurs because some of the energy spent to distend the lungs is lost during deflation. The dissipating energy during lung inflation/deflation (defined by the area within the P–V loop), named "hysteresis," is attributed to alveolar recruitment during inspiration and de-recruitment during expiration, alveolar surface tension/surfactant, gas absorption, and stress relaxation of lung tissue [114,115].

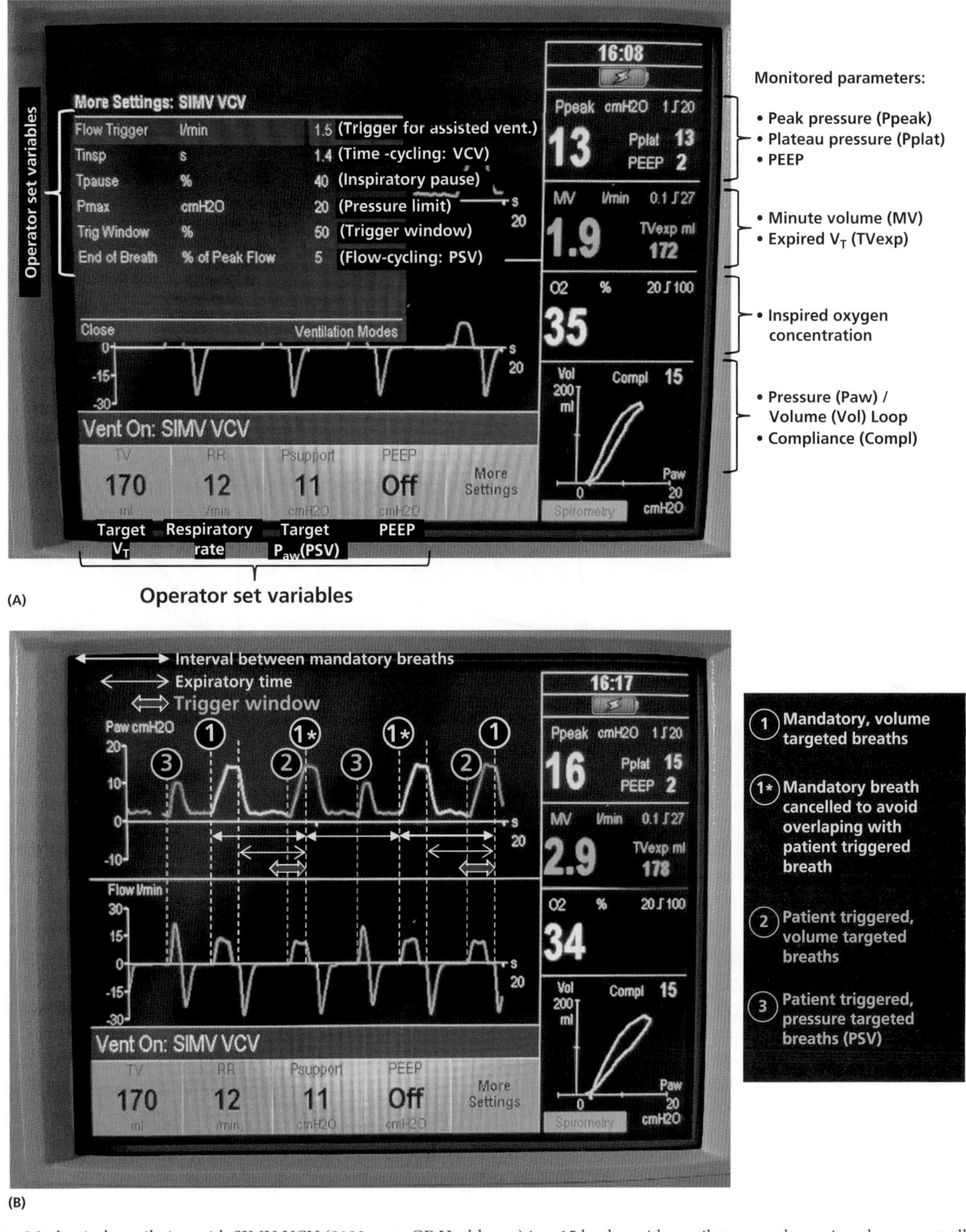

Figure 38.20 Mechanical ventilation with SIMV-VCV (9100c nxt, GE Healthcare) in a 15 kg dog with ventilator asynchrony in volume-controlled ventilation (VCV) mode, despite an adequate depth of anesthesia and a $P_{ET}CO_2$ between 32–34 mmHg (pulse oximetry = 98% with an F_IO_2 = 0.35). **A.** Ventilation mode was switched to SIMV-VCV (operator settings shown). **B.** The airway pressure and flow curves of mandatory volume-targeted breaths are displayed in yellow and green, respectively, while patient-triggered breaths are displayed in blue. Patient-triggered, volume-targeted breaths (blue), are delivered only during the trigger window after a mandatory breath (window set at 50% of expiratory time); spontaneous breathing efforts outside the trigger window initiate pressure-targeted breaths (PSV). Notice that if patient-triggered breaths coincide with the timing of mandatory breaths, the mandatory cycle is canceled to avoid asynchrony (overlapping between assisted and controlled breaths).

Standard veterinary anesthesia ventilators or older model human anesthesia workstations adapted for veterinary use usually can perform mechanical ventilation only in volume-controlled mode, without the option for adding an inspiratory pause. The user sets the inspiratory flow necessary to achieve a target V_T. Tidal volume monitoring may be restricted to the visual analysis of the volume displaced on the ventilator bellows during inspiration, which strays from the actual inspired V_T [86], while airway pressure is monitored by a pressure gauge incorporated into the breathing circuit. If the anesthesia apparatus does not incorporate flow sensors and pressure transducers, pulmonary mechanics can be monitored in small and large animal species by a near-patient

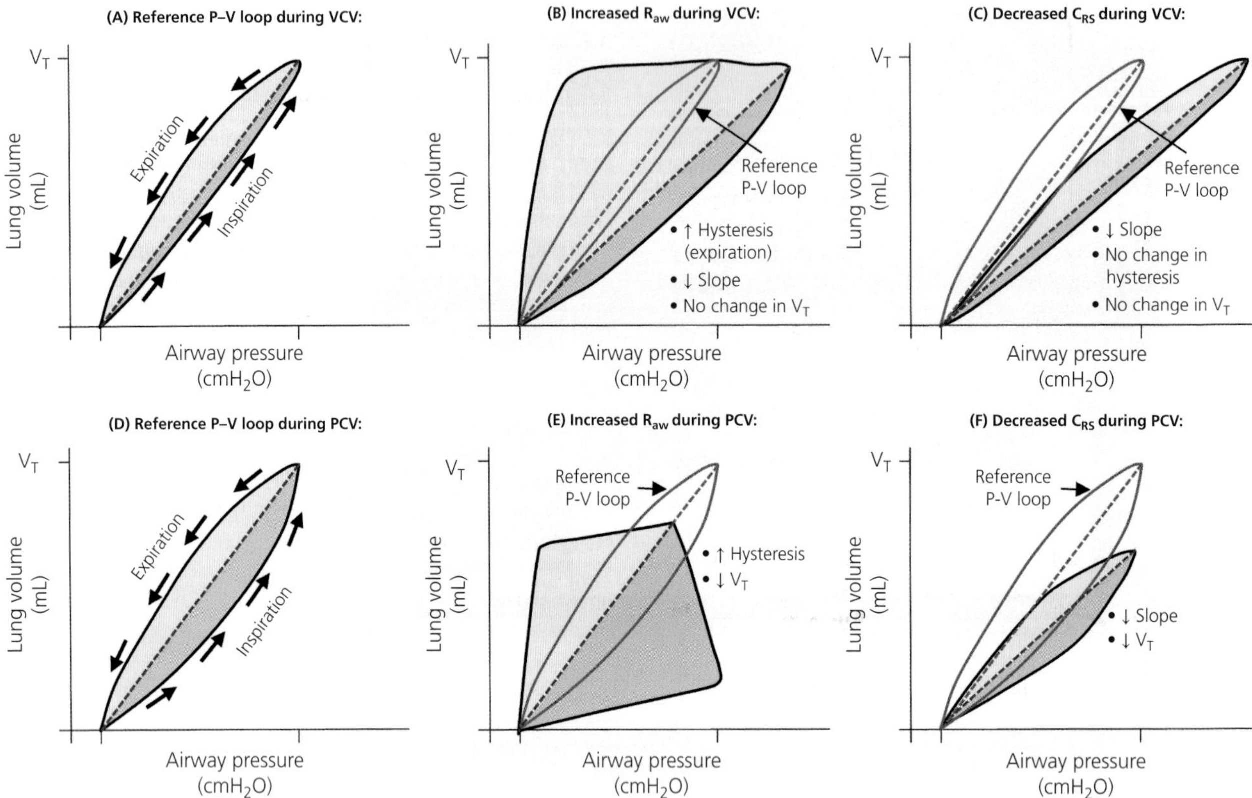

Figure 38.21 Diagrammatic representation of dynamic P–V loops recorded during volume-controlled ventilation (VCV) and pressure-controlled ventilation (PCV) in dogs. **A.** Reference pressure–volume (P–V) loop during VCV. The inspiratory limb is a near-straight line because airway pressure increases in a quasilinear fashion with lung volume during VCV. The slope is represented by the red dotted line. **B.** An increase in R_{aw} during VCV may increase the area of the expiratory limb (hysteresis) due to an increase in resistive expiratory work. The slope also decreases during VCV because P_{peak} increases to compensate for the increase in R_{aw}. **C.** A decrease in C_{RS} during VCV decreases the slope of the P–V loop while hysteresis may not be significantly altered. **D.** Reference loop during PCV. The inspiratory limb has a more rounded shape compared to VCV because of the decelerating inspiratory flow. **E.** An increase in R_{aw} during PCV increases hysteresis during inspiration and expiration (box-shaped P–V loop) while the slope may be unaltered. **F.** A decrease in C_{RS} decreases the slope of the P–V loop during PCV. V_T, tidal volume; C_{RS}, respiratory system compliance; R_{aw}, airway resistance; P_{peak}, peak airway pressure.

spirometer (Pitot tube-based flow sensor), originally designed for use during mechanical ventilation in humans [93–95]. The original flow sensor (adult and pediatric D-lite) can be used in small animals or other species with a maximum $V_T < 2$ L; whereas the sensor remodeled into a larger scale (H-lite) can be used during anesthesia in large animals (e.g., horses). The sensor, placed between the endotracheal tube and the Y-piece of the breathing circuit, provides real-time monitoring of inspired and expired V_T, inspired and expired minute volume, P_{peak}, P_{plat}, PEEP, C_{RS}, and P–V loops (Fig. 38.22).

Compliance of the respiratory system and airway resistance

Dynamic C_{RS} can be measured during VCV as the ratio between the change in lung volume (V_T) and the change in airway pressure (difference between P_{peak} and PEEP):

$$\text{Dynamic } C_{RS}\left(\text{mL/cmH}_2\text{O}\right)=\frac{V_T(\text{mL})}{P_{peak}-\text{PEEP}\left(\text{cmH}_2\text{O}\right)}$$

The P_{peak} generated by a constant inspiratory flow during VCV is the pressure necessary to overcome the resistive and viscoelastic properties of the respiratory system [100–102]. Therefore, decreased dynamic C_{RS} is not only attributed to factors that decrease lung (atelectasis and pulmonary edema) and chest wall (increased intra-abdominal pressure and obesity) compliance, but also to factors that increase R_{aw} (narrow/kinked endotracheal tube, viscous secretions in the airways, and bronchoconstriction) [100–102].

Static C_{RS}, measured as the ratio between V_T and the driving pressure (P_{plat} − PEEP) during conditions of zero flow, allows evaluation of the viscoelastic properties of the respiratory system per se, without the confounding effects of the frictional component of the work done (R_{aw}) [100–102].

$$\text{Static } C_{RS}\left(\text{mL/cmH}_2\text{O}\right)=\frac{V_T(\text{mL})}{P_{plat}-\text{PEEP}\left(\text{cmH}_2\text{O}\right)}$$

In humans, a P_{plat} created by the inspiratory hold (period of zero flow at end-inspiration) should last for at least 2–5 s to allow measurement of true P_{alv} after gas flow distribution between alveoli with faster and slower filling rates (Fig. 38.14) [100,103]. If the duration of the inspiratory pause is between 0.5 and 2 s, it may still mostly overcome the frictional resistance imposed by the airways, but such compliance measurements are better defined as quasistatic [100,103].

The algorithm used to calculate C_{RS} may significantly impact evaluation of pulmonary mechanics. During VCV without an

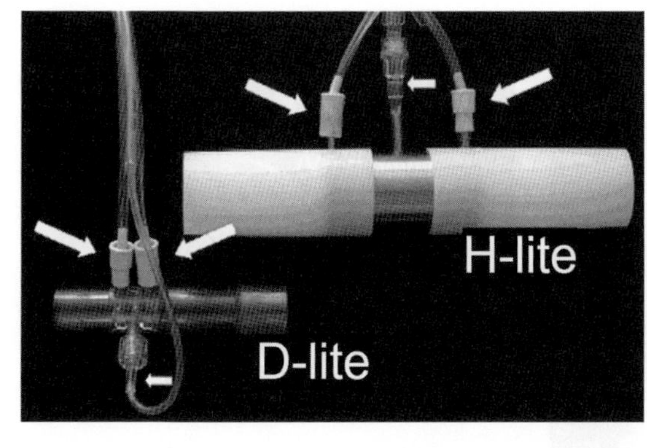

(A)

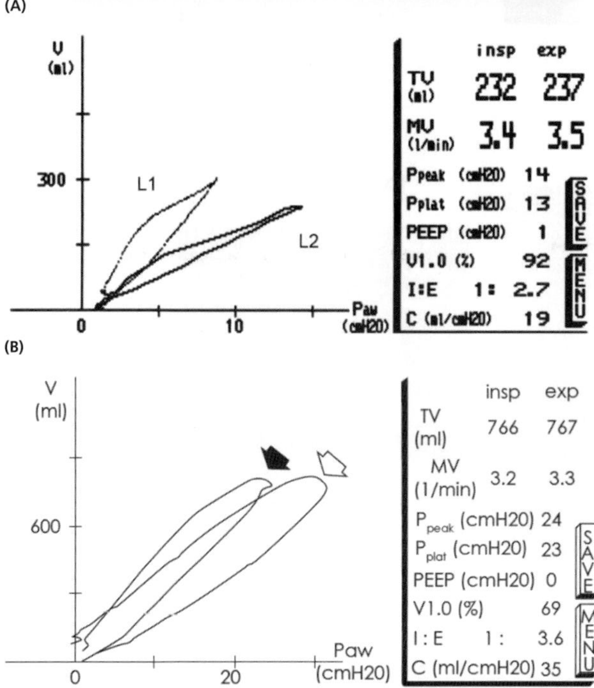

Figure 38.22 **A.** Pitot tube-based spirometer/flow sensor designed for human anesthesia that is compatible for use in small animals (D-lite, GE/Datex-Ohmeda) and the same sensor remodeled into a larger scale for use in large animals (H-lite). **B.** Pressure–volume (P–V) loops measured by the D-lite sensor in a 26 kg dog undergoing laparoscopic ovariectomy under pneumoperitoneum (intra-abdominal pressure of 15 mmHg). Compared to the P–V loop recorded before abdominal insufflation (L1), the decreased slope observed after induction of pneumoperitoneum (L2), suggests worsening (decreased) dynamic C_{RS}. **C.** Pressure–volume loops measured by the H-lite sensor in a 400 kg horse undergoing colic surgery in dorsal recumbency. Compared to the loop recorded before the abdominal cavity was opened (white arrow), the increased slope observed after abdominal decompression (black arrow) suggests an improvement (increase) in dynamic C_{RS}. For the H-Lite actual tidal volumes (TV) and dynamic compliance (C) are obtained by multiplying the displayed values by 5. Source: Reproduced from Calice *et al.* [93]; Moens et al. [94], with permission from Elsevier.

inspiratory pause, compliance measurements provided by the ventilator should be considered dynamic. If there is an inspiratory pause during VCV and the manufacturer's algorithm calculates C_{RS} from P_{plat}, compliance measurements can be considered quasistatic or static, depending on the duration of the inspiratory pause (Fig. 38.23). Close hemodynamic monitoring should be performed, especially if longer periods of inspiratory hold are performed (> 25% of inspiratory time). Maintaining alveolar distension for longer periods could have negative hemodynamic consequences attributed to longer-lasting decreases in vena caval blood flow and stroke volume (due to increased P_{pl} during mechanical ventilation) and to more prolonged increases in right ventricular (RV) afterload secondary to compression of pulmonary capillaries in West zones I and II during the inspiratory hold [116].

Compliance measurements usually are not indexed to body weight in adult humans. However, because of the large variation in body mass and size of the lungs among veterinary species, C_{RS} should be indexed to body weight (mL/cmH_2O/kg). In dorsally recumbent adult horses undergoing VCV with zero end-expiratory pressure (F_IO_2 > 90%), dynamic C_{RS} may be close to 0.4 mL/cmH_2O/kg, which is considerably less than C_{RS} in anesthetized dogs (F_IO_2 = 50%) during VCV and with 2–6 cmH_2O PEEP (1.3 mL/cmH_2O/kg) [117,118]. Poor C_{RS} typically found during mechanical ventilation in large animal species is caused by impaired lung and chest wall compliance. Compression atelectasis associated with relaxation and cranial displacement of the diaphragm is a major contributing factor to the decrease in lung compliance observed in horses [1,119,120]. Factors such as increased intra-abdominal pressure, pregnancy, and obesity may further aggravate compression atelectasis and lead to greater decreases in C_{RS}. Factors found to influence C_{RS} in mechanically ventilated dogs include body weight, body condition score, and shape of the chest wall [118,121]. Three types of chest wall conformation are recognized in dogs: barrel-chested (wide chest at the sternum), deep-chested (narrow chest at the sternum), and intermediate-chested (chest area at sternum between the deep and barrel-shaped chest). In dogs with a barrel-shaped thorax, C_{RS} may be reduced by approximately 20% in comparison to dogs with intermediate chest wall shape. Similar decreases in C_{RS} may be observed in dogs that are overweight (high body condition score) in comparison to dogs with normal body condition scores (Fig. 38.24) [118].

Strategies for reducing atelectasis during mechanical ventilation

Development of atelectasis during anesthesia is associated with oxygenation impairment and decreased lung compliance. Conventional mechanical ventilation, which often improves $\dot{V}_E$ and prevents hypercapnia, may fail to reopen atelectatic lung areas and increase PaO_2 levels. If poor lung compliance (decreased C_{RS}) and low PaO_2 values in relation to the F_IO_2 (PaO_2/F_IO_2 ratio < 300 mmHg) are observed, a temporary increase in airway pressures aiming to reopen atelectatic lung areas, that is, an alveolar recruitment maneuver (ARM), may be considered to increase C_{RS} and PaO_2 levels. In the *open-lung approach*, originally developed for clinical use in humans with acute respiratory distress syndrome (ARDS) during mechanical ventilation, collapsed alveoli are opened by temporary application of elevated inspiratory pressures and post-recruitment PEEP is applied to prevent recurrence of atelectasis [122]. In addition to an improvement in pulmonary mechanics and gas exchange, preventing cyclic alveolar collapse reduces the progression of lung injury associated with mechanical ventilation in ARDS patients because of improved homogeneity in alveolar distention throughout the lung parenchyma [123,124]. In addition to their use in humans with ARDS in the ICU setting, ARMs are an effective means to increase C_{RS} and PaO_2 levels in anesthetized humans not suffering from ARDS, or those undergoing cardiac and thoracic surgeries [125]. Systematic reviews in humans have recommended routine use of ARMs followed by PEEP after induction of

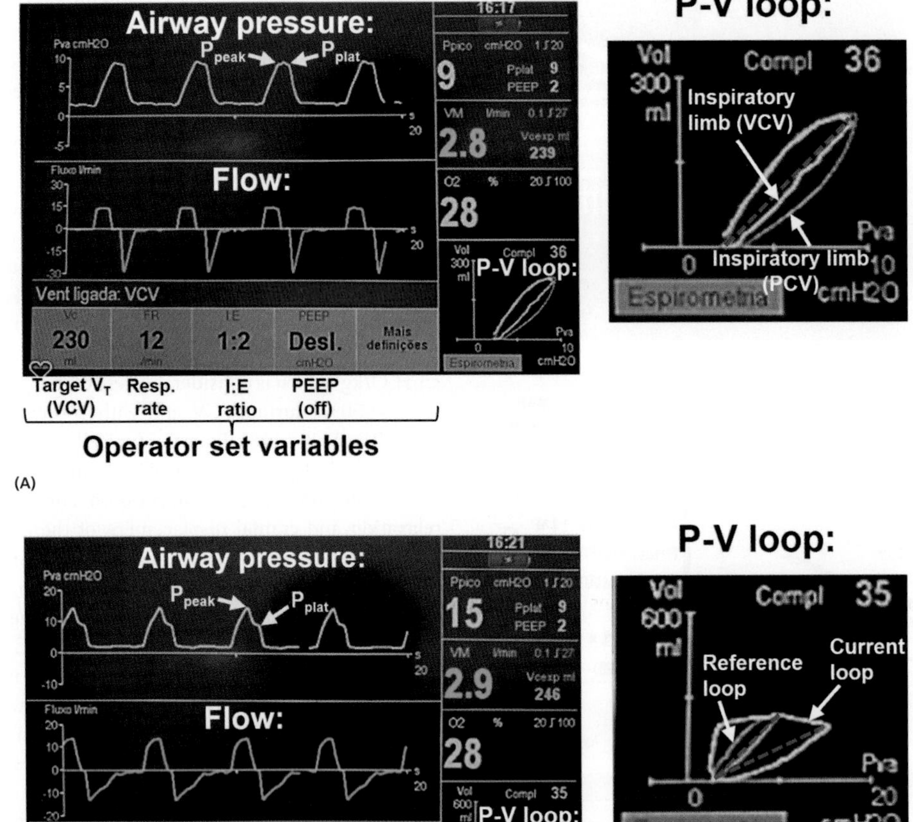

Figure 38.23 Airway pressure and flow curves and dynamic pressure–volume (P–V) loops recorded during volume controlled ventilation (VCV) (9100c nxt, GE Healthcare) in a 23 kg dog (ideal body weight) anesthetized with isoflurane. **A.** The ventilator was set to deliver a V_T (Vc) of 10 mL/kg (230 mL) at a respiratory frequency (FR) of 12 breaths/min and a 1:2 inspiration-to-expiration ratio (I:E). The end-inspiratory hold was set to 40%. Peak inspiratory pressure (P_{peak}), plateau pressure (P_{plat}), minute volume (VM = expired V_T × respiratory frequency), and respiratory system compliance [Compl = expired $V_T/(P_{plat}$ – PEEP)] are shown on the left-hand side of the screen. Compliance measurements are quasistatic because the duration of inspiratory pause was between 0.5–2 s (0.66 s). The inspiratory limb of the dynamic P–V loop shows a quasilinear increase in airway pressure during VCV (arrow). The P–V loop stored when the same animal was under pressure-controlled ventilation (PCV) shows that the inspiratory limb has a more rounded shape during PCV (arrow). The slope of the P–V loop is shown by the dashed red line. **B.** Screenshot recorded after the cuffed endotracheal tube was kinked in the same animal under VCV. The airway pressure tracing is suggestive of increased R_{aw} and there is an increased gradient between peak (15 cmH_2O) and plateau pressure (9 cmH_2O). The dynamic P–V loop shows increased expiratory resistance (area above the slope of the P–V loop – dashed red line). The slope is decreased because P_{peak} increased with increased R_{aw}. Quasistatic C_{RS} remained constant (35–36 mL/cmH_2O, or 1.5 mL/cmH_2O/kg) after partial obstruction of the endotracheal tube.

general anesthesia, and in the face of declining hemoglobin saturation [125].

Despite the potential benefits of ARMs followed by PEEP, some individuals may not respond favorably to an open-lung approach (Fig. 38.25) and the potential benefits should be weighed against the negative physiological impact of high alveolar pressures on hemodynamic function [126]. Elevated airway pressures (P_{alv}) during an ARM increase intrathoracic (P_{pl}) and transpulmonary pressures (gradient between alveolar [P_{alv}] and pleural pressure [P_{pl}]), reducing venous return through the vena cava [127,128]. In addition, distension of the alveolar wall by elevated P_{alv} leads to compression of pulmonary capillaries and increases pulmonary vascular resistance (PVR)/RV afterload, which may further contribute to the decrease in stroke volume/cardiac output caused by the ARM [127–129]. For these reasons, this technique cannot be applied to hemodynamically unstable or hypovolemic individuals and close hemodynamic monitoring is necessary during lung recruitment maneuvers. Furthermore, ARMs may need to be interrupted and the target increase in airway pressure may not be achieved if cardiovascular compromise develops (e.g., severe hypotension). Inotropic/vasopressor drugs and/or intravenous fluid boluses may be initiated in anticipation of the hemodynamic

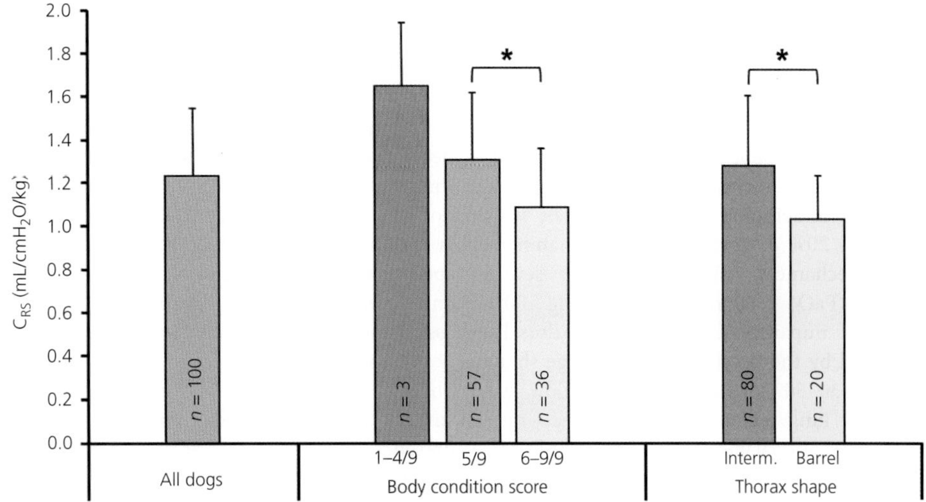

Figure 38.24 Influence of body condition score (underweight, 1–4; normal, 5; overweight, 6–9) and thorax shape (intermediate shaped [Interm.] and barrel-shaped [Barrel]) on C_{RS} during volume-controlled ventilation in anesthetized healthy dogs ($n = 100$). The V_T (8–12 mL/kg) was set according to actual body weight and an inspiratory pause of 20% was added after the preset V_T was achieved. Source: Reproduced from Asorey *et al.* [118], with permission. *Significant difference between groups ($p < 0.05$).

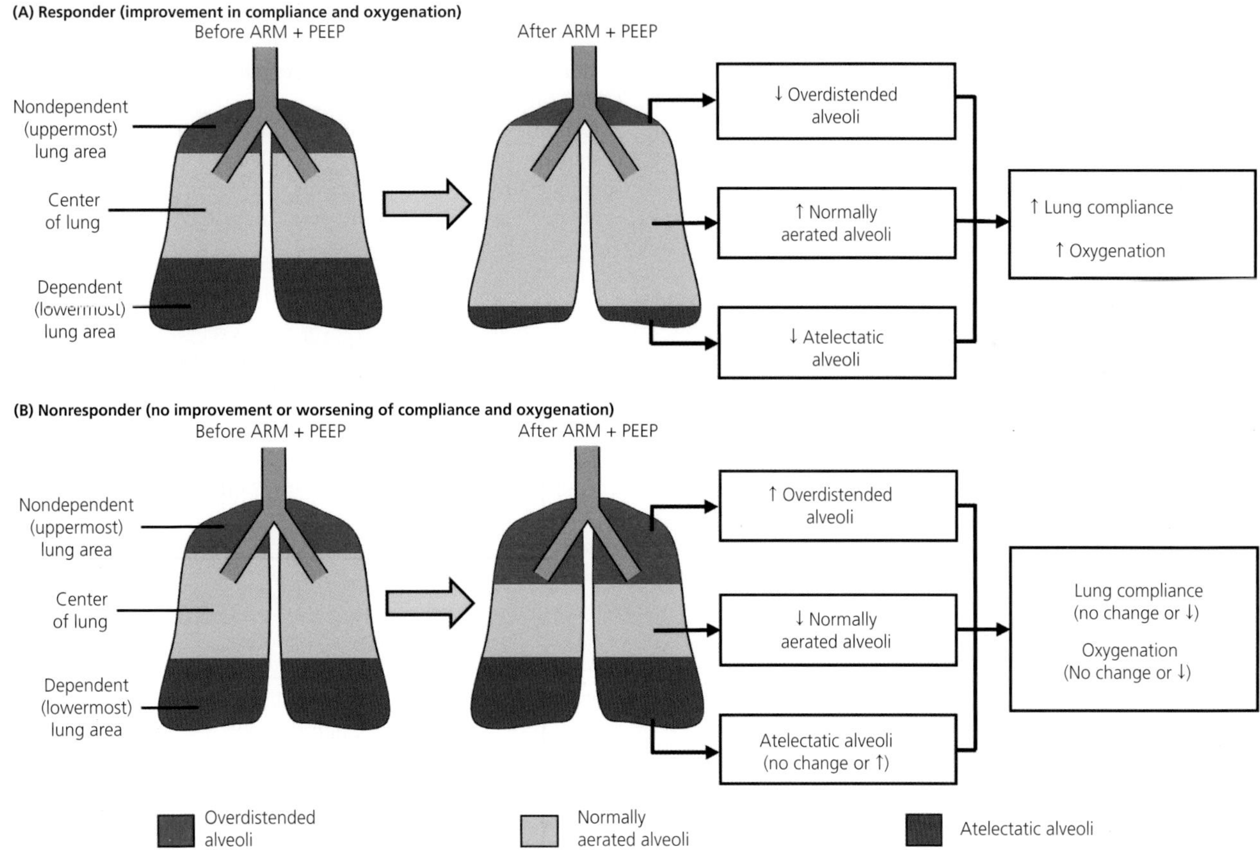

Figure 38.25 Effects of an alveolar recruitment maneuver followed by open-lung positive end-expiratory pressure (ARM + PEEP) on the distribution of lung aeration considering two possible phenotypes: **A.** responder to lung recruitment; **B.** nonresponder to lung recruitment. Source: Adapted from Pensier *et al.* [126].

compromise in animals that present arterial blood pressures that are approaching the lower acceptable range (60 and 90 mmHg for mean and systolic arterial pressure, respectively).

The degree of alveolar collapse leading to decreased C_{RS} and oxygenation impairment varies substantially among mammalian species and there is no evidence supporting the routine use of ARMs in veterinary anesthesia. Incidence of hypoxemia is high in dorsally recumbent horses undergoing elective surgeries, with reports showing that up to 20% of dorsally recumbent animals receiving conventional mechanical ventilation develop severe intraoperative hypoxemia (PaO_2 < 60%) while breathing 100% oxygen [2]. Oxygenation impairment observed in dorsally recumbent horses is caused by the development of a large shunt fraction, which may exceed 30–50% of pulmonary blood flow, due to atelectasis of dependent lung regions and these effects may persist despite the use of conventional mechanical ventilation [1,24]. Although recruitment maneuvers may be useful in this scenario, one must be aware of the cardiovascular depressant effects caused by the high airway pressures (60–80 cmH_2O) that may be necessary to improve PaO_2 in equine species [130], and of the possibility of such elevated pressures to cause alveolar overdistension/inflammation in horses [131]. In anesthetized horses subjected to an ARM reaching a P_{peak} of 60 cmH_2O, histological analysis of lung tissue revealed overdistended lung areas but there was no cytological (bronchoalveolar lavage) or histopathological evidence of lung injury [131]. However, compared to the groups of conscious horses and spontaneously breathing anesthetized horses, an increased expression of pro-inflammatory cytokines (interleukin 1-β and 6) matrix metalloproteinases (MMP 1 and 9) was observed in the lung tissue of groups that received conventional mechanical ventilation alone or combined with an ARM, suggesting that mechanical ventilation per se might be associated with early stages of lung injury [131]. Despite controversies regarding its clinical application, lung recruitment maneuvers should be considered to improve arterial oxygen levels in severely hypoxemic horses (PaO_2 < 60 mmHg) undergoing surgery in dorsal recumbency [130,132–134]. If a decision has been made to apply an ARM in horses with colic, this procedure should be performed after abdominal decompression/exposure of the large colon, which may allow some improvement in C_{RS} and PaO_2 levels. In contrast to the situation in horses, the degree of oxygenation impairment caused by atelectasis is significantly less during routine anesthesia in small animal species. Currently, the use of ARMs followed by PEEP in small animal anesthesia may be considered in selected clinical conditions associated with poor C_{RS} due to atelectasis and low PaO_2/F_IO_2 ratio (< 300 mmHg) or hypoxemia. These conditions may be caused by obesity, increased intra-abdominal pressure (e.g., laparoscopic surgery under pneumoperitoneum), diaphragmatic hernia, or presence of poorly aerated areas due to lung disease.

Recruitment maneuvers can be performed in several ways as illustrated in Fig. 38.26. The simplest way of performing lung recruitment in humans involves a temporary increase in airway pressure to 30–40 cmH_2O lasting up to 30–40 s, while monitoring the patient for adverse effects such as hemodynamic compromise [101,135] (Fig. 38.26A). A temporary increase in airway pressure to 40 cmH_2O for 20 s, followed by 5 cmH_2O PEEP has been successfully applied to increase arterial oxygenation and static C_{RS} in healthy dogs undergoing laparoscopy [136]. Much higher airway pressures (60–80 cmH_2O for 10–12 s), have been reported to recruit alveoli and promote an increase in PaO_2 levels in dorsally recumbent horses undergoing elective or emergency (colic) surgeries [130,134].

Continuous positive airway pressure (CPAP) is a tool originally designed for non-invasive ventilation in non-intubated, spontaneously breathing patients. However, if the anesthesia ventilator has the option for performing CPAP, this ventilation

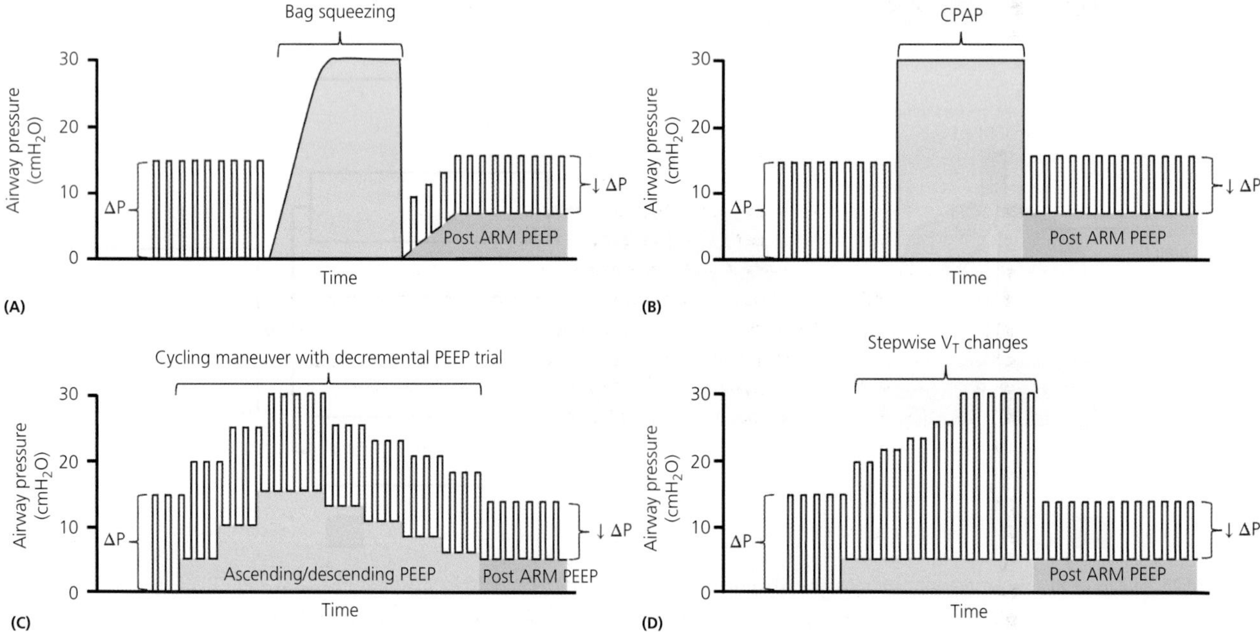

Figure 38.26 Diagrammatic representation of airway pressure–time curves of alveolar recruitment maneuvers (ARMs). **A.** Manual recruitment with bag squeezing. **B.** Recruitment with continuous CPAP. **C.** Cycling maneuver with decremental positive PEEP trial. **D.** Stepwise V_T changes. Effective alveolar recruitment should decrease the driving pressure (ΔP, gradient between inspiratory and end-expiratory pressure) and increase C_{RS}. CPAP, continuous positive airway pressure; PEEP, positive end-expired pressure; V_T, tidal volume; C_{RS}, respiratory system compliance. Source: Partially modified from Ball *et al.* [101].

mode may be selected in intubated patients to achieve an elevated airway pressure for a short period of time (e.g., 30 cmH_2O for 20 s), before returning to a standard mechanical ventilation protocol and post-recruitment PEEP, which aims to keep the alveoli opened [38,101,136] (Fig. 38.26B). However, most anesthesia machines do not have the option for CPAP. In this case, with the spontaneous mode selected, the rebreathing bag is manually squeezed with the pop-off (APL) valve closed/semi-closed to achieve the target airway pressure for the desired length of time. This technique may be used to improve oxygenation and expand the lungs in small animal species (dogs and cats) with diaphragmatic hernia. In this case, the increase in airway pressure should be applied after reduction of the visceral contents herniated into the thoracic cavity, while the surgeon is guiding the increase in airway pressure by visually assessing lung expansion within the thoracic cavity (see discussion below regarding re-expansion pulmonary edema). The maximum airway pressure can be limited to 30 cmH_2O or less, pending the severity of cardiovascular depression (e.g., hypotension) observed during the recruitment maneuver. Cats with a diaphragmatic hernia may be more sensitive to the negative cardiovascular effects of ARMs, therefore a reduced maximum airway pressure is initially recommended (≤ 20 cmH_2O).

Alveolar recruitment may also be performed using *cycling maneuvers*, which have three distinct phases: (1) hemodynamic conditioning; (2) recruitment; and (3) decremental PEEP trial (Fig. 38.26C and 38.27). During the hemodynamic conditioning phase, before the lung's opening pressure is achieved, inspiratory pressures and PEEP are progressively increased with ventilation in PCV mode while the driving pressure (gradient between P_{max} and PEEP) is held constant. Theoretically, pulmonary tissue stress is less than during CPAP maneuvers. Stepwise increases in airway pressure may reduce the possibility of overdistension of ventilated lung areas as it progressively spreads across the collapsed lung tissue, opening atelectatic alveoli in a more controlled manner than with CPAP maneuvers [101,135]. Stepwise increases in airway pressures also identify individuals with occult hypovolemia, who may not tolerate the higher airway pressures that are necessary to open collapsed lung areas [135]. If severe hypotension is identified during this phase, the procedure is interrupted, and intravenous fluid boluses and/or sympathomimetics are administered before the cycling maneuver is reinstituted. During the recruitment phase, while PEEP is maintained at the maximum target level (e.g., 15 cmH_2O for 30 s), the driving pressure can be temporarily increased by adjusting P_{max} to achieve inspiratory pressures that are necessary to open collapsed lung areas (e.g., 30 cmH_2O). The decremental PEEP trial is the last phase of a cycling maneuver and aims to determine the lowest PEEP level that will prevent de-recruitment or re-collapse of lung tissue. As PEEP is progressively reduced in 2 cmH_2O steps, it will reach the closing pressure, that is the pressure at which alveoli collapse [135]. Identification of the closing pressure can be performed by measuring the quasistatic C_{RS} at the end of each stepwise decrease in PEEP during VCV with an inspiratory pause. The post-recruitment PEEP level can be adjusted based on the PEEP that resulted in highest quasistatic C_{RS} during the decremental PEEP trial + 2 cmH_2O [135,137–139].

Effects of mechanical ventilation on cardiovascular function

In general, greater cardiovascular depression occurs in anesthetized animals receiving positive-pressure ventilation compared to anesthetized animals that are permitted to breathe spontaneously. Mechanical ventilation alters cardiovascular function directly through changes in intrapleural and alveolar pressures. Cardiovascular function is also indirectly modified by mechanical ventilation via changes in $PaCO_2$ levels. A decrease in $\dot{V}_E$ due to low respiratory frequency and/or low V_T set on the ventilator will cause varying degrees of hypercapnia. In conscious dogs and humans, hypercapnia increases endogenous catecholamine levels leading to a cardiovascular stimulant effect (increased heart rate, cardiac output, and arterial blood pressure, and decreased systemic vascular resistance [SVR]). Although general anesthetics can potentially blunt the sympathetic stimulation caused by high $PaCO_2$ levels, studies in anesthetized mechanically ventilated horses have shown that hypercapnia increases circulating plasma epinephrine and norepinephrine levels and results in cardiovascular stimulation [140,141]. In humans under general anesthesia, mild hypercapnia ($PaCO_2$ up to 60 mmHg) during mechanical ventilation increases subcutaneous tissue oxygen tension, which may contribute to oxidative killing of surgical pathogens by neutrophils and reduce the rate of surgical infection [142]. However, cardiovascular depression/poor responsiveness to exogenous catecholamines can occur in the face of severe acidemia (pH < 7.2).

In most patients, mechanical ventilation depresses cardiovascular function by decreasing venous return. The blood flow entering the heart through the vena cava (VR) is directly proportional to the gradient between the mean circulatory filling pressure (MCFP) of the venous circulation and right atrial pressure (RAP) divided by the resistance to blood flow in the venous circulation.

$$VR = \frac{MCFP - RAP}{\text{Venous resistance}}$$

The MCFP is determined by the stressed volume (V_s), which represents the blood volume that exerts pressure inside the veins and effectively contributes to VR; while the unstressed volume (V_{us}) is the blood that keeps small veins and venules minimally opened and does not contribute significantly to VR [143,144]. Changes in VR during spontaneous breathing and during mechanical ventilation are illustrated in Fig. 38.28. During spontaneous breathing, VR transiently increases because the gradient between MCFP and RAP increases as P_{pl} become more negative during inspiration. In contrast, mechanical ventilation decreases the gradient between MCFP and RAP as P_{pl} increases during inspiration. According to the Frank–Starling mechanism, as VR and preload are decreased, RV stroke volume decreases on the next heartbeat. Under normal circumstances, decreases in preload/stroke volume induced by mechanical breaths are relatively small. However, in hypovolemic animals, the inspiratory rise in P_{pl} caused by mechanical ventilation induces larger decreases in VR/preload, which may result in significant cardiovascular depression. An excessively large V_T delivered by the ventilator may also induce greater decreases in VR/preload, mimicking the effects of hypovolemia.

In addition to the effects on VR, distension of the alveolar wall caused by the rise in alveolar pressure (P_{alv}) increases RV afterload because of compression of pulmonary capillaries in West zones I and II. The increase in RV afterload opposes RV ejection and may contribute to the decrease in RV stroke volume (Fig. 38.29) [116,145].

On the left side of the circulation, increases in pleural (P_{pl}) and alveolar (P_{alv}) pressures induced by mechanical breaths cause intermittent increases and decreases in aortic blood flow and left ventricular (LV) stroke volume (Fig. 38.29). Aortic blood flow and LV stroke volume transiently decrease because of the inspiratory decrease in preload/RV stroke volume as discussed before; however, the maximum decrease in aortic

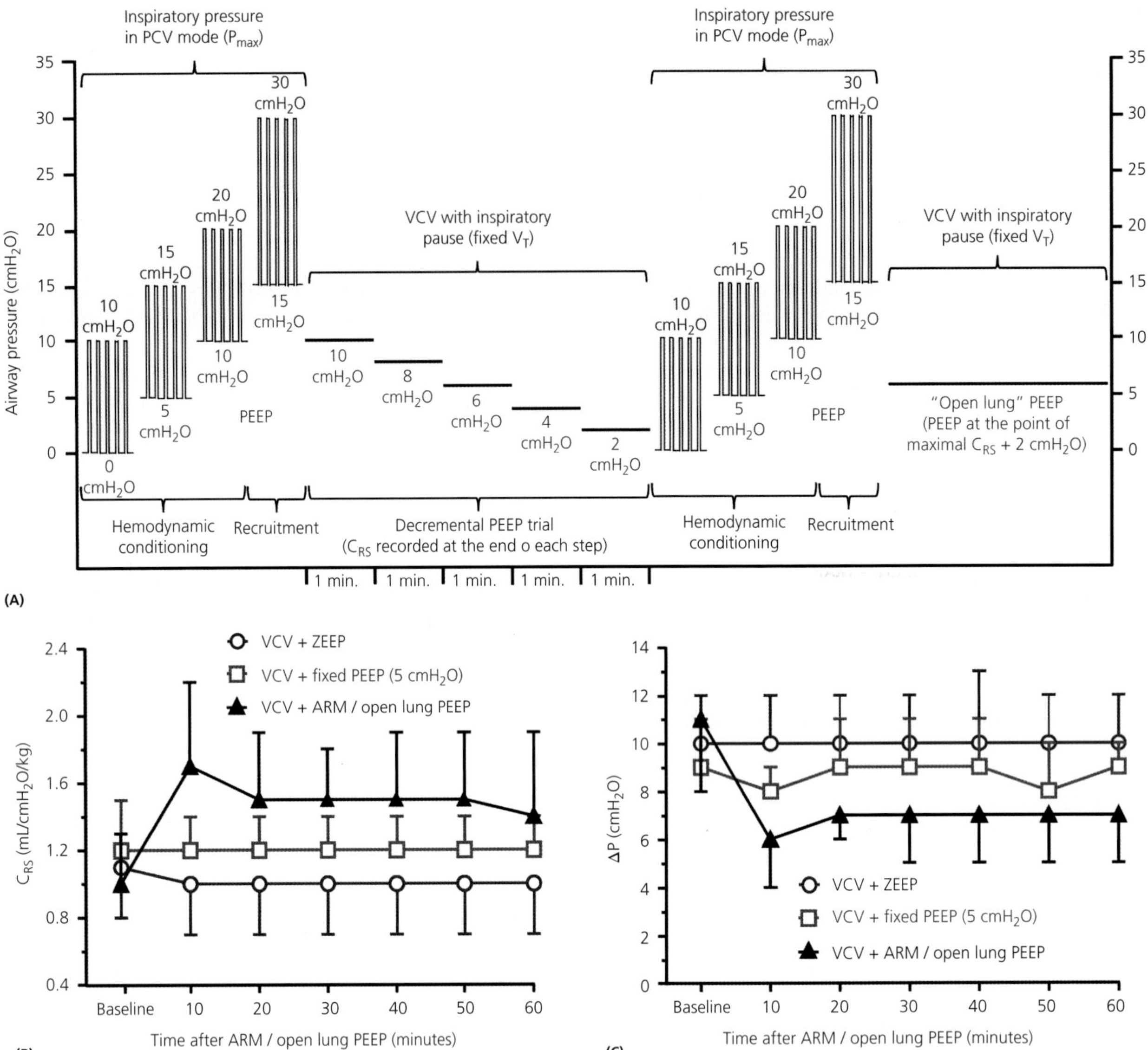

Figure 38.27 Example of a cycling maneuver followed by decremental PEEP trial in anesthetized dogs. **A.** Progressive increases in P_{max} and PEEP are performed in PCV mode (hemodynamic conditioning phase). Each step may last for a fixed number of breaths (e.g., 5 breaths). After a maximum PEEP level is achieved, the driving pressure (P_{max} – PEEP) is increased to achieve the lung's opening pressure (recruitment phase). After lung recruitment, progressive decreases in PEEP are performed with a fixed V_T in VCV mode with an inspiratory pause lasting ≥ 0.5 s (decremental PEEP trial phase). Quasistatic C_{RS}, measured after 1 minute at each stepwise decrease in PEEP, is used to identify the lowest PEEP associated with maximum C_{RS}. After a new recruitment was performed, anesthesia was maintained in VCV + PEEP associated with maximum C_{RS} + 2 cmH_2O (open-lung PEEP). **B.** and **C.** In healthy dogs anesthetized under VCV a cycling maneuver (ARM + open-lung PEEP) resulted in higher quasistatic C_{RS} and lower ΔP than animals anesthetized under VCV + PEEP (5 cmH_2O) and VCV + ZEEP. PEEP, positive end-expired pressure; P_{max}, maximum airway pressure; PCV, pressure-controlled ventilation; V_T, tidal volume; VCV, volume-controlled ventilation; C_{RS}, respiratory system compliance; ARM, alveolar recruitment maneuver; ZEEP, zero end-expired pressure; ΔP, driving pressure. Source: Data compiled from García-Sanz *et al.* [138].

flow/LV stroke volume caused by this mechanism will only be detected a few heartbeats later, during expiration, reflecting the time needed for blood to travel through the pulmonary circulation. On the other hand, an inspiratory increase in aortic flow/LV stroke volume occurs because of increased LV preload and decreased LV afterload caused by increased P_{alv} and by increased P_{pl}, respectively, as illustrated in Fig. 38.29. Because patients that are hypovolemic have larger variations in aortic flow/LV stroke volume induced by mechanical breaths, heart–lung interactions during mechanical ventilation provide the physiologic basis for assessment of fluid responsiveness, that is, the determination of whether a patient will respond or not to intravascular volume expansion with increases in stroke volume/cardiac output [116,145].

Ventilator-induced lung injury

Precise monitoring of V_T and airway pressure during positive-pressure ventilation is critical because inappropriate mechanical ventilator settings can cause lung damage. Currently, it is recognized that there are four basic mechanisms that contribute, either alone or in combination, to lung injury associated with mechanical ventilation: barotrauma, volutrauma, atelectrauma, and biotrauma. Barotrauma,

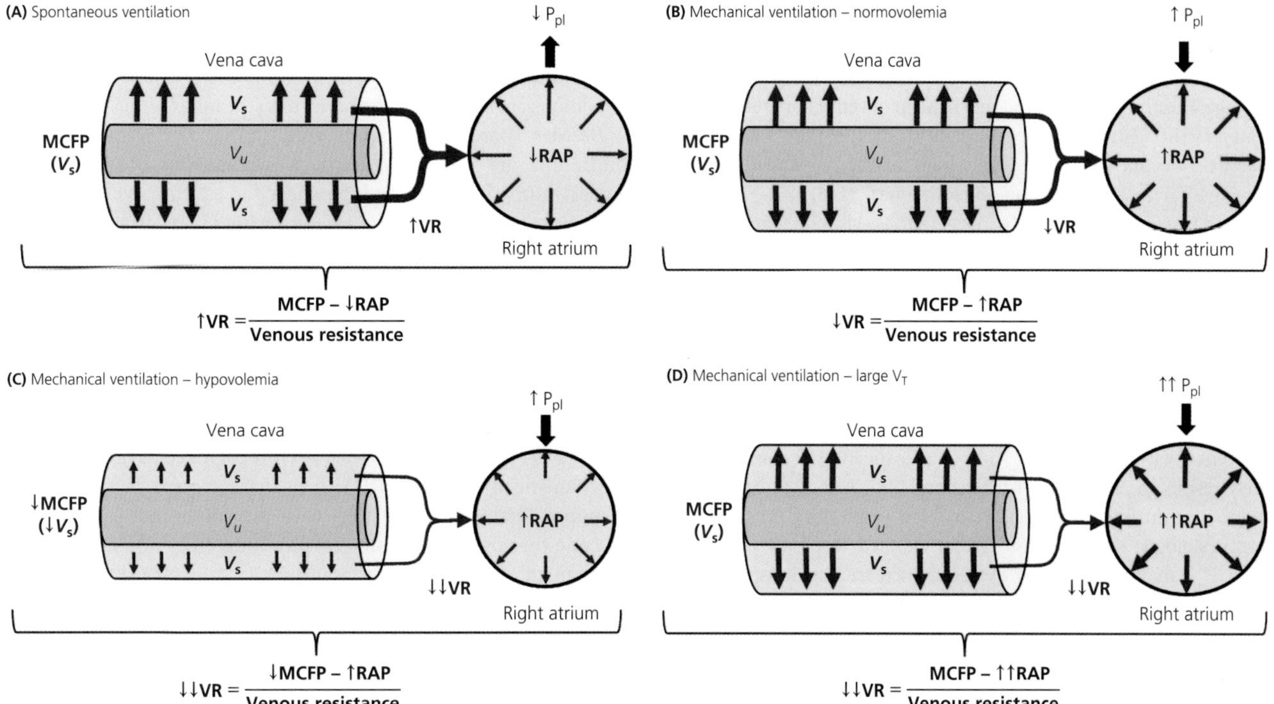

Figure 38.28 Diagrammatic representation of inspiratory changes in venous return (VR) during spontaneous and mechanical ventilation. **A.** During spontaneous ventilation, the decrease in P_{pl} during inspiration increases right atrial transmural pressure (the difference between pressure inside and outside an elastic organ) and transiently decreases RAP. Venous return increases because the gradient between MCFP and RAP is increased. **B.** During mechanical ventilation, the increase in P_{pl} during inspiration decreases right atrial transmural pressure and RAP is increased. Venous return decreases because the gradient between MCFP and RAP is reduced. **C.** Greater decreases in VR are induced by mechanical ventilation in hypovolemic patients because the decrease in MCFP (due to a decrease in V_s) further reduces the gradient between MCFP and RAP. **D.** Mechanical ventilation with a large V_T can mimic the effects of hypovolemia on VR and preload. A supraphysiological V_T results in larger increases in P_{pl}, and causes greater increases in RAP, which further reduces VR. V_s, stressed volume; V_{us}, unstressed volume; VR, venous return; MCFP, mean circulatory filling pressure; RAP, right atrial pressure; P_{pl}, pleural pressure.

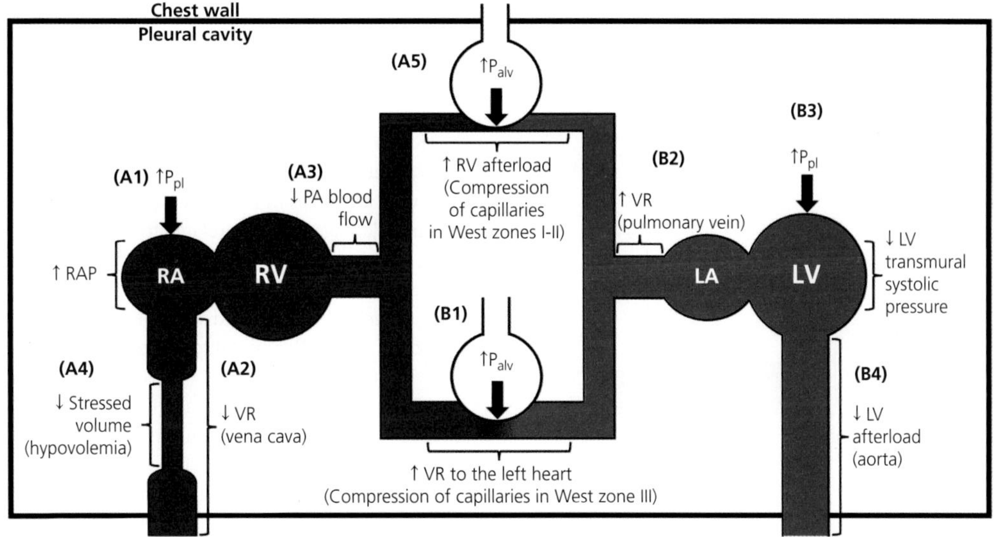

Figure 38.29 Heart–lung interactions during mechanical ventilation. Mechanisms that cause intermittent decreases and increases in aortic blood flow/LV stroke volume are described in sequences A1 to A5 and B1 to B4, respectively. The increase in P_{pl} induced by mechanical breaths increases RAP (A1), which leads to a decrease in VR and RV preload (A2). PA blood flow and RV stroke volume are decreased (A3). The impairment in VR induced by mechanical ventilation is magnified by hypovolemia, which decreases the stressed blood volume (A4). The increase in P_{alv} induced by mechanical breaths causes compression of capillaries not engorged with blood (West zones I and II) and increases RV afterload (A5), contributing to further decreases in PA blood flow/RV stroke volume (A3). The maximum decrease in aortic blood flow/LV stroke volume is detected during expiration because of the delay associated with transit of blood flow through the pulmonary circulation. Increased P_{alv} squeezes blood out of capillaries in West zone III (B1) and increases venous return to the left heart (B2). Increased P_{pl} during inspiration (B3) decreases LV systolic transmural pressure (the pressure difference between the inside and the outside of LV during systole), consequently decreasing LV afterload (B4). The increase in LV preload (B1 and B2), combined with the decrease in LV afterload (B3 and B4) increases LV stroke volume during inspiration. P_{pl}, pleural pressure; RAP, right atrial pressure; VR, venous return; RV, right ventricle; PA, pulmonary artery; P_{alv}, alveolar pressure; RA, right atrium; LA, left atrium; LV, left ventricle. Source: Adapted from Michard *et al.* [116].

initially defined as excessively high airway pressures/P_{alv} causing lung damage, was the first proposed mechanism of ventilator-induced lung injury (VILI). However, experimental studies in the 1980s showed that VILI occurs when excessively high airway pressures/P_{alv} causes excessive alveolar expansion (volutrauma) [146,147]. Therefore, elevated inspiratory pressure (equivalent to P_{alv}) is more likely to result in VILI if it results in excessive increases in lung volume. This fundamental concept was shown by experimental studies demonstrating that mechanical ventilation with high airway pressures (P_{peak} of 45 cmH_2O) did not result in evidence of lung damage/inflammation when lung expansion was limited by low chest wall compliance (Fig. 38.30) [146]. Barotrauma is currently defined as lung injury caused by high transpulmonary pressures, that is the pressure difference between inside (P_{alv}) and outside the lung (P_{pl}), which effectively results in alveolar overdistension [148]. Although barotrauma may occur during VCV because of high inspiratory pressures, the anesthesiologist should consider that elevated inspiratory pressures (high P_{alv}) may not result in excessive increases in transpulmonary pressure (alveolar overdistension) if P_{pl} is also increased because chest wall compliance is markedly reduced, as in morbidly obese animals or animals with marked increases in intra-abdominal pressure. As an example, standard mechanical ventilator settings (V_T of 12–15 mL/kg) in horses with colic and severe abdominal distension may, on some occasions, result in P_{peak} values that exceed 45 cmH_2O. Although no specific measurements of transpulmonary pressures have been performed in horses under these circumstances, the decrease in P_{peak} that is noticeable after the surgeon removes the distended bowel from the abdominal cavity suggests that the cause of vof the chest wall by abdominal viscera. Therefore, high inspiratory pressures under these conditions are less likely to be harmful to the lungs.

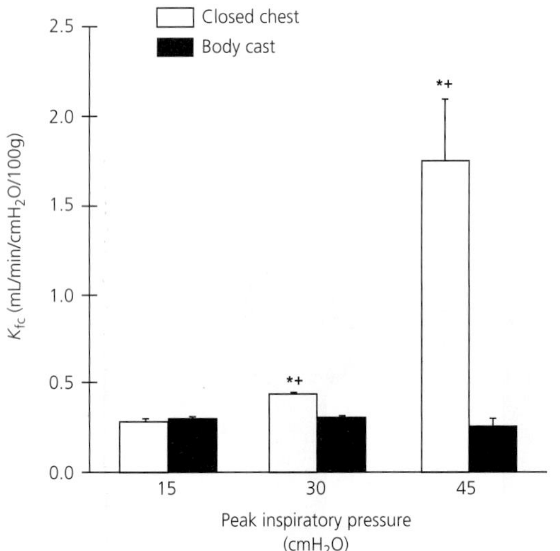

Figure 38.30 Effects of mechanical ventilation with peak inspiratory pressures of 15, 30, and 45 cmH_2O on capillary filtration coefficient (K_{fc}) in the lungs of rabbits with normal chest wall compliance (Closed chest, white bar) and in rabbits where lung expansion was restricted by a full body plaster cast surrounding the chest wall and abdomen. The body cast was molded while rabbits were breathing spontaneously (Body cast, black bars). The increase in K_{fc} was observed only when elevated airway pressures resulted in increased lung volume (Closed chest group), which likely resulted in high transpulmonary pressures ($P_{alv} - P_{pl}$). Source: Reproduced from Hernandez *et al.* [146], with permission.
* Significantly higher than 15 cmH_2O in Closed chest group.
† Significantly higher than Body cast group at the same peak inspiratory pressure.

Besides barotrauma and volutrauma, atelectrauma, and biotrauma are now recognized as mechanisms of VILI [148]. Atelectrauma is caused by high shear forces from cyclic opening and closure of atelectatic alveoli, which can trigger a local inflammatory response and injure the alveolar–capillary membrane [148]. The alveolar instability caused by the intermittent opening and closure of atelectatic lung areas, named "tidal recruitment," occurs when the level of inspiratory pressure is large enough to open atelectatic alveoli, but these alveoli subsequently collapse during expiration because the level of end-expiratory pressure is insufficient to keep them open throughout the ventilatory cycle [149–151]. Biotrauma has been recognized as an important mechanism of VILI in ARDS. It is characterized as a biological response, including activation of a pro-inflammatory cytokine cascade that promotes injury even in lung areas not subjected to mechanical stress and in extrapulmonary organs [148]. Although data are lacking in veterinary medicine, it has been recognized that a lung-protective ventilation strategy in humans with ARDS, aimed at minimizing mechanical stress to the lungs by use of low V_Ts, may attenuate the systemic inflammatory response and associated multiple organ failure, contributing to a decrease in mortality [123,152–154].

Mechanical ventilation during anesthesia in humans and veterinary species

Experimental animal models of ARDS show that application of PEEP with a relatively small V_T is less injurious to the lung than ventilation with a large V_T in the absence of PEEP [147]. In the medical field, the importance of VILI and its negative impact on clinical outcomes was first established in humans with ARDS [123,153–155]. Historically, routine anesthesia in humans was performed with relatively high V_T (10–15 mL/kg) without PEEP in most instances [156]. While the concept of lung-protective ventilation with low V_T ($\leq$ 6 mL/kg) and high PEEP (> 12 cmH_2O) has been a standard procedure for long-term ventilation in humans with ARDS in the ICU setting for more than 20 years [157], ventilation strategies for routine anesthesia in humans only started to change with advances in the understanding of mechanisms of VILI, where lung damage is closely related to the amplitude of cyclic stretch of lung parenchyma induced by mechanical ventilation [158]. In human patients without lung disease undergoing anesthesia for elective surgeries, mechanical ventilation with lower V_T (6 mL/kg) and 10 cmH_2O PEEP may reduce lung inflammation compared to a higher V_T (12 mL/kg) [159]. A reduction in V_T from values $\geq$ 10 mL/kg to < 8 mL/kg also improves the clinical outcome (lower incidence of postoperative pneumonia/respiratory failure and shorter duration of hospital stay) in human patients without ARDS in the operating room [160,161]. To prevent postoperative pulmonary complications, current guidelines for protective mechanical ventilation in human patients undergoing surgery recommend targeting a V_T of 6–8 mL/kg based on predicted (ideal) body weight and an initial PEEP level of 5 cmH_2O [162].

Ventilator settings in veterinary species cannot be directly extrapolated from recommendations in humans for several reasons including: (1) minute ventilation ($V_T \times f$) should be adjusted according to the CO_2 production (metabolic rate), which can vary among animals and man; (2) the V_T adjusted on the ventilator may vary among species because of differences in airway deadspace ($V_{D_{aw}}$) and physiological space ($V_{D_{phys}}$), which lead to differences in effective alveolar ventilation ($\dot{V}_A$); and (3) the maximum airway pressure and driving pressure (gradient between P_{plat} and PEEP) may differ among animals and man because of differences in C_{RS}, which is affected by body mass (large versus small animals), shape of chest wall, intra-abdominal volume/pressure, and degree of atelectasis, among other factors. Tidal volume adjustments however should be based on ideal (predicted) body weight as variable degrees of alveolar overdistension/higher driving pressures may occur if V_T calculation is based on actual body weight in obese animals [163]. In animals with poor body condition scores, calculation of V_T based on actual body weight instead of ideal body weight could result in alveolar sub-distension/atelectasis.

A critical point to consider is the size of mechanical breaths delivered to veterinary patients because the V_T must be large enough to overcome the airway deadspace ($V_{D_{aw}}$) and expand the alveoli ($V_{T_{alv}}$), according to the formula:

$$V_T = V_{D_{aw}} + V_{T_{alv}}$$

Typically, the $V_{D_{aw}}$ measured by the single nitrogen washout (Fowler's) technique in adult humans is 150 mL (2 mL/kg for an adult averaging 75 kg) [164]. Therefore, a V_T between 6–8 mL/kg (450–600 mL for 75 kg adult human) is large enough to overcome the deadspace represented by the conducting airways, effectively expanding the alveoli during inspiration without causing alveolar overdistension or cyclic alveolar opening and closure (tidal recruitment), especially when combined with a moderate PEEP level (5 cmH_2O or more). However, a V_T currently recommended for routine ventilation during anesthesia in humans (e.g., 6 mL/kg) may not be large enough to go past the $V_{D_{aw}}$ measured in dogs by volumetric capnography (6.5 to 7.6 mL/kg) and effectively expand the alveoli [165].

As explained in Chapter 37, CO_2 removal by the lungs and $PaCO_2$ levels depend on the fraction of V_T that goes beyond the physiological deadspace ($V_{D_{phys}}$), which is the sum of areas of the respiratory system that do not participate in gas exchange, including the conducting airways ($V_{D_{aw}}$) and alveoli that are ventilated but not perfused (alveolar deadspace [$V_{D_{alv}}$]):

$$V_{D_{phys}} = V_{D_{aw}} + V_{D_{alv}}$$

Therefore, the rate of CO_2 removal is better described by the effective alveolar ventilation per minute ($\dot{V}_A$) than by the minute ventilation ($\dot{V}_E$), because the former considers the $V_{D_{phys}}$:

$$\dot{V}_A = \left(V_T - V_{D_{phys}}\right) \times f$$

Fig. 38.31 shows deadspace calculations using volumetric capnography in a dog anesthetized with isoflurane receiving mechanical ventilation (VCV mode). As discussed in Chapter 37, the Enghoff modification of the Bohr equation for calculating the physiological deadspace to tidal volume ratio ($V_{D_{phys}}/V_T$) may overestimate true $V_{D_{phys}}$ in the presence of increased areas of low alveolar ventilation-to-perfusion ($\dot{V}_A/\dot{Q}$) ratio and shunt. The PaO_2/F_IO_2 ratio close to 500 mmHg (480 mmHg) in Fig. 38.31 demonstrates that venous admixture/shunt is minimal; therefore, the Bohr–Enghoff formula may provide a reasonable estimate of true $V_{D_{phys}}/V_T$. For this dog, $V_{D_{phys}}$ was 7 mL/kg (6.4 mL/kg of $V_{D_{aw}}$ and 0.6 mL/kg of $V_{D_{alv}}$) and mechanical ventilation with a standard V_T adopted in humans (6 mL/kg) would be inappropriate because it would only ventilate deadspace. Airway deadspace calculations based on the volumetric capnography curve (6.4 mL/kg) show a larger $V_{D_{aw}}$ than values considered physiological in humans (2 mL/kg). Other species may also

Temperature-corrected arterial blood gases (F_IO_2 = 0.43):

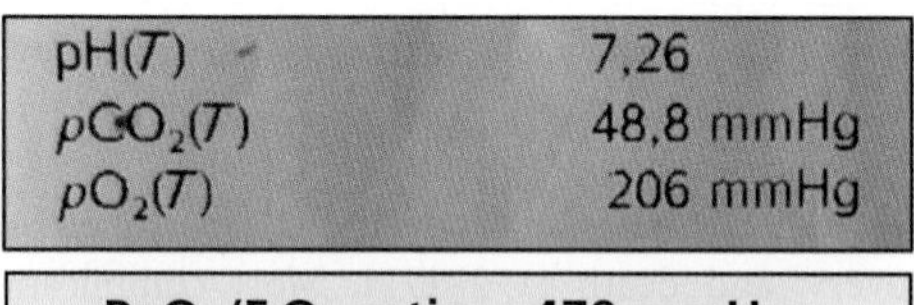

PaO_2/F_IO_2 ratio = 479 mmHg

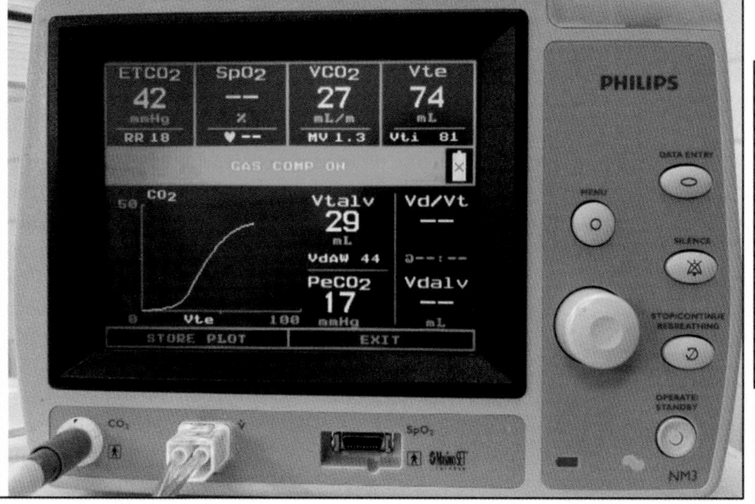

Deadspace calculations (Volumetric capnography curve):

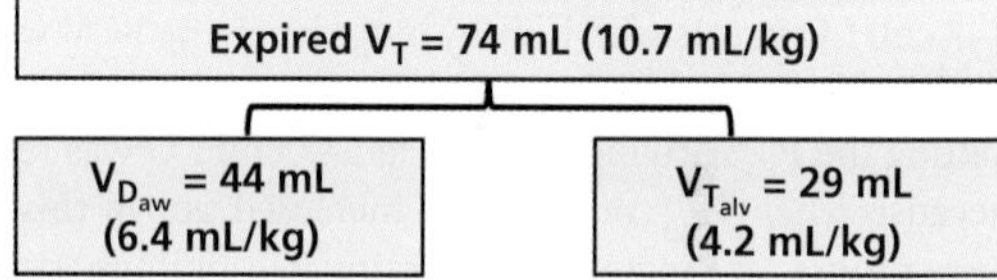

Deadspace calculations (Bohr-Enghoff):

$$V_{D_{phys}}/V_T = \frac{PaCO_2 - PeCO_2}{PaCO_2}$$

$$V_{D_{phys}}/V_T = \frac{48.8\ \text{mmHg} - 17\ \text{mmHg}}{48.8\ \text{mmHg}}$$

$$V_{D_{phys}}/V_T = 0.65$$

$$V_{D_{phys}} = V_{D_{phys}}/V_T \times \text{Expired } V_T$$

$$V_{D_{phys}} = 48\ \text{mL (7 mL/kg)}$$

$$V_{D_{alv}} = V_{D_{phys}} - V_{D_{aw}}$$

$$V_{D_{alv}} = 4\ \text{mL (0.6 mL/kg)}$$

Figure 38.31 Arterial blood gases and deadspace volume calculations using data from volumetric capnography (plotting of expired CO_2 and expired V_T) in a healthy dog (6.9 kg) anesthetized with isoflurane and receiving mechanical ventilation in VCV mode (target V_T 12 mL/kg [83 mL], I:E ratio 1:2, *f* 18 breaths/min, F_IO_2 0.43). See text for further explanation. V_T, tidal volume; VCV, volume-controlled ventilation; $V_{D_{phys}}/V_T$, physiologic deadspace to tidal volume ratio; $PeCO_2$, partial pressure of CO_2 in mixed expired gas; $V_{D_{aw}}$, airway deadspace; $V_{D_{phys}}$, physiological deadspace; $V_{D_{alv}}$, alveolar deadspace; $V_{T_{alv}}$, alveolar tidal volume.

present a larger $V_{D_{aw}}$ and $V_{D_{phys}}$, which could also impact extrapolation of V_T currently recommended for mechanical ventilation in humans. In conscious healthy horses and cows breathing through a face mask, the Bohr–Enghoff $V_{D_{phys}}$ (calculated using a correction factor for the added deadspace represented by the facemask) was about 5.2 and 3.7 mL/kg, respectively [166].

The use of low V_T (8 mL/kg) has been evaluated in anesthetized dogs; however, a real benefit in terms of improved clinical outcome (decreased postanesthetic respiratory complications) has not been identified [167,168]. In addition, one canine study showed that a V_T of 8 mL/kg results in less than ideal $\dot{V}_A$ leading to hypercapnia/respiratory acidosis despite the use of high breathing rates (> 30 breaths/min) [167]. In this same study, computerized tomography also provided evidence that the low V_T (8 mL/kg) resulted in a greater degree of atelectasis/poorly aerated lung areas in comparison to a V_T of 15 mL/kg plus 5 cmH_2O of PEEP [167]. As $V_{D_{aw}}$ tends to remain relatively constant, $V_{D_{phys}}$ can be further increased by an increase in $V_{D_{alv}}$ during clinical anesthesia. Under these circumstances, mechanical ventilation with V_T in the range that approaches the deadspace represented by the conducting airways (6–8 mL/kg) could result in even higher degrees of hypercapnia despite attempts to maintain $\dot{V}_A$ by increasing the number of mandatory breaths (*f*). While data are lacking for most species, current evidence still supports the use of V_Ts in the range of 10–15 mL/kg during routine anesthesia in most species as no real benefit has been shown with V_Ts recommended in humans to provide "protective lung ventilation." If anesthesia ventilators that incorporate flow sensors that allow accurate adjustment of V_T are not available, P_{peak} is often adjusted along with respiratory rate to maintain eucapnia based on capnography in small animal practice.

During PCV, the target airway pressure (P_{max}) will vary according to the species as they differ in their C_{RS}. Also, specific conditions such as decreased C_{RS} due to obesity, pneumoperitoneum, or thoracic shape (barrel-chested dogs) may require a higher P_{max} to provide effective alveolar ventilation. The P_{max} can be initially set at 5–7 cmH_2O in cats with healthy lungs receiving PCV with zero end-expiratory pressure (driving pressure between 5–7 cmH_2O) [169]. Setting the P_{max}/driving pressure at 5–7 cmH_2O was recommended because when P_{max} values were increased above this range there were progressive increases in overinflated pulmonary parenchyma upon computed tomography [169]. To date, there are no published studies evaluating the P_{max} during PCV in canine species; however, clinical experience has shown that in non-obese medium-sized dogs with healthy lungs, the P_{max} can be initially set at 8–10 cmH_2O; taking into consideration that there is an intrinsic PEEP of at least 2 cmH_2O in a bellows-type ventilator, this level of P_{max} will result in a driving pressure of 6–8 cmH_2O.

In humans, avoidance of 100% oxygen as carrier gas and maintenance of PEEP during mechanical ventilation are strategies used to reduce atelectasis and improve oxygen transfer from alveoli to arterial blood (decrease the $P(A\text{-}a)O_2$ and increase PaO_2/F_IO_2 ratio). As explained in Chapter 37, collapse of poorly ventilated alveolar units ($\dot{V}_A/\dot{Q} < 0.15$) is precipitated by high F_IO_2 (> 0.8) because the transfer of oxygen to pulmonary capillary blood exceeds the inspired gas flow entering these alveoli [170]. As the predominant mechanism responsible for the increase in intrapulmonary shunt during anesthesia in humans with normal lungs is compression atelectasis, the use of lower F_IO_2 by mixing oxygen and air in inspired gas per se does not abolish atelectasis during anesthesia and surgery [171]. However, current guidelines for lung-protective mechanical ventilation in anesthetized human patients include the recommendation to set the F_IO_2 after intubation to ≤ 0.4 with subsequent adjustments in F_IO_2 to the lowest value necessary to maintain oxygen saturation monitored by pulse oximetry ≥ 94% (strength of recommendation: weak) [162].

A reduction in the inspired oxygen concentration from 100% to 40% during VCV (V_T adjusted to 15 mL/kg) in dogs reduced atelectasis and poorly aerated lung areas, recognized as dense lung areas upon computed tomography, and improved oxygen transfer from alveoli to arterial blood (decreased $P(A\text{-}a)O_2$) despite lower PaO_2 values in comparison to animals receiving 100% oxygen [15]. During VCV in dogs (V_T adjusted to 12 mL/kg), a reduction in inspired oxygen from 100% to 40% while maintaining zero end-expiratory pressure or the use of 100% oxygen with PEEP (5 cmH_2O) after an ARM (CPAP of 40 cmH_2O applied for 20 s) resulted in higher PaO_2/F_IO_2 ratio, improved pulmonary mechanics (increased compliance), and increased lung aeration in comparison to 100% oxygen and zero end-expiratory pressure [38]. While the use of lower F_IO_2 may be a feasible alternative to improve lung function during mechanical ventilation in dogs with healthy lungs, reducing the F_IO_2 from values > 95% to 50% during conventional VCV did not reduce the large shunt fraction/venous admixture that develops in dorsally recumbent, isoflurane-anesthetized horses [35].

Anesthesia for bronchoscopy

While lower airway procedures in large animals can be performed using sedation and topical anesthesia, general anesthesia is required to permit bronchoscopy in companion animals. General considerations when performing anesthesia for bronchoscopy include the impact of the patient's underlying condition on respiratory function, potential for bronchospasm, overall impairment of gas exchange function of the lung during and following the intervention, reduction in airway lumen by the bronchoscope increasing R_{aw} and the work of breathing, and a potential lack of a sealed airway throughout the bronchoscopy procedure, which could lead to environmental pollution and impair efficacy of positive-pressure ventilation. Reported complications associated with bronchoscopy (with or without bronchoalveolar lavage) in companion animals include hypoxemia, hemodynamic changes (bradycardia, tachycardia, hypotension, and hypertension), pneumothorax, bronchospasm, prolonged anesthetic recovery, and death [172–177]. Most complications that occur during anesthesia are transient and improve over time with oxygen supplementation, ventilatory support, and/or specific interventions such as thoracocentesis; however, mortality during anesthesia in feline patients undergoing bronchoscopy may be higher compared to that observed with other interventions [172].

Management of anesthesia

Most canine and feline patients scheduled for bronchoscopy have clinically significant underlying respiratory disease that warrants a thorough history, preoperative physical examination, and diagnostic work up, including chest radiography. In general, sedation of small animal patients with opioid analgesics is routinely performed due to their mild sedative and antitussive properties [172]. Inclusion of anticholinergics in premedication protocols may not prevent bronchospasm; however, they can be included based on other indications [178]. Preoxygenation of patients prior to induction of anesthesia with injectable anesthetics and subsequent delivery of oxygen using an anesthetic breathing circuit is recommended. Methods used to secure the airway prior to bronchoscopy in cats include a sterilized standard endotracheal tube or a supraglottic airway device [172,179], while sterilized standard orotracheal tubes are generally used in dogs. Anesthesia may be initially maintained with either an inhalant anesthetic or an injectable anesthetic. As the patient's cardiopulmonary status can change rapidly during endoscopic airway procedures, it is recommended that monitoring devices such as an electrocardiogram (ECG), blood pressure monitor, pulse oximeter, and capnograph are in use prior to initiation of any airway procedure.

Several different strategies can be used to facilitate oxygen delivery during airway examination and sample collection. A bronchoscope swivel adapter placed between the patient's end of the breathing circuit and endotracheal tube permits use of an endoscope with an endotracheal tube or supraglottic device (Fig. 38.32). Use of a bronchoscope adapter avoids the need to disconnect an intubated patient from the breathing circuit during the exam, allowing more effective oxygen supplementation/high F_IO_2 levels to be provided throughout the procedure. Of concern for the anesthesiologist is the narrowing of the trachea (in non-intubated patients) or of the endotracheal tube by the bronchoscope, which will increase R_{aw} and the work of breathing. Therefore, intubation should be performed with an endotracheal tube with the largest internal diameter possible and if possible, mechanical ventilation should be considered to improve gas exchange and reduce the work of breathing, especially in patients that are already dyspneic and experiencing respiratory muscle fatigue due to increased work of breathing.

Providing oxygen (from the anesthesia machine or alternative oxygen source) via a catheter that is suitable for insertion into the trachea with or without an orotracheal tube in place is an alternative option. In patients that are too small to permit passage of a scope through an endotracheal tube and/or placement of a catheter beside the scope, it may be possible to deliver oxygen through one of the endoscope channels. With the latter technique, low oxygen flows should be used, and care taken to ensure adequate expiratory airflow to prevent gas trapping in the lungs and development of a pneumothorax. To minimize potential environmental contamination and personnel exposure to inhalant anesthetics, injectable agents such as propofol or alfaxalone, administered as an infusion or intermittent boluses are generally preferred to maintain anesthesia during bronchoscopy if it is not feasible to use a bronchoscope swivel adapter with a breathing circuit. During anesthetic recovery following bronchoscopy, continued supplementation of inspired gases with oxygen and monitoring of the patient's adequacy of oxygenation is highly recommended. Further recommendations regarding preanesthetic patient preparation and anesthetic management for patients with specific respiratory diseases are provided below.

Anesthesia for intrathoracic procedures

Indications for thoracic exploration in companion animals typically include spontaneous pneumothorax, lung lobe torsion, intrathoracic or thoracic mass lesions, traumatic lesions to the thorax, diaphragmatic hernia, congenital vascular anomalies such as persistent right aortic arch or persistent ductus arteriosus, pericardial disease, chylothorax, and pyothorax [180–185]. In addition, esophageal foreign bodies and/or esophageal perforations are relatively common in companion animals, and in some instances, they may require thoracic exploration for removal and repair, respectively [186]. Although less common, in the equine and bovine, pleuropneumonia, pericarditis, and traumatic injuries to the thorax, resulting in a pneumothorax and/or diaphragmatic hernia may be indications for thoracic exploration and surgical repair [187–190]. Diagnostic or therapeutic interventions related to intrathoracic structures may be performed using an intercostal thoracotomy, median sternotomy in small/medium-sized animals, or a thoracoscopic approach. In some instances, more than one surgical technique may be required to achieve the desired outcome, particularly when thoracoscopy is the initial technique employed, therefore, the anesthetist should be prepared for multiple surgical approaches [183,184,191,192].

In most species, intrathoracic procedures are performed under general anesthesia; however, in adult cows and horses, both thoracotomy and thoracoscopy have been performed in standing sedated animals using local anesthetic techniques [187,190,193]. Although an incomplete mediastinum is possible in large animal species, in mature horses and cattle, the mediastinum is commonly reported to be complete [190,193,194]. As such, despite lung collapse on the side of surgery, adequate gas exchange can be maintained due to the function of the contralateral lung when the surgery is performed with the horse or cow standing, assuming it does not have similar pathology. Like large animals, dogs and cats generally have a

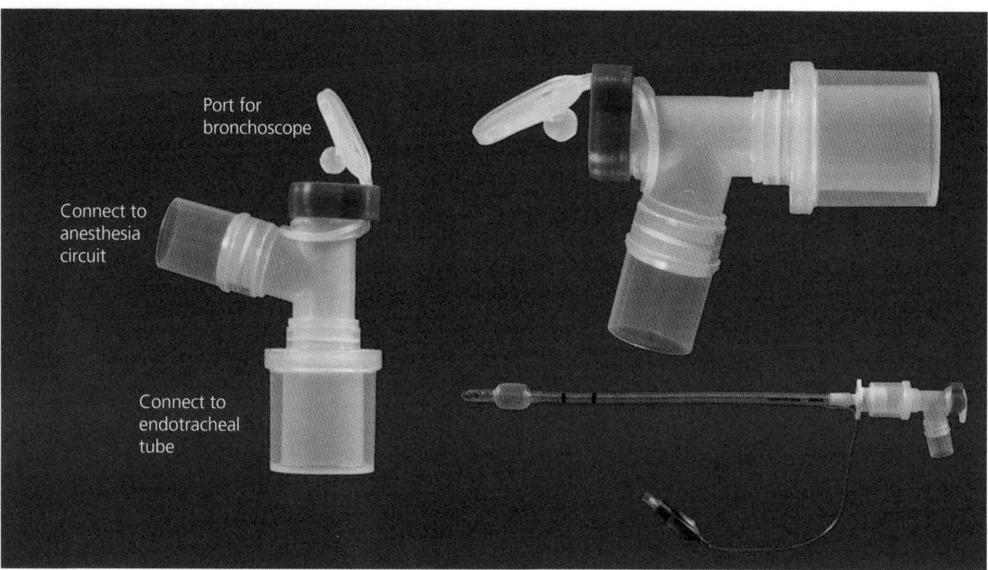

Figure 38.32 Bronchoscopy can be performed in intubated anesthetized patients receiving oxygen supplementation and mechanical ventilation using a bronchoscope swivel adapter. Source: www.dmsveterinary.com/product/mila-15mm-tracheal-tube-connector-double-swiveling.

complete mediastinum; however, when any veterinary patient is under general anesthesia, ventilatory support is generally required once the pleural space is entered even if the contralateral thoracic space and lung are normal. Traditional two-lung ventilation is generally used during intrathoracic procedures under general anesthesia; however, as will be discussed below, one-lung ventilation (OLV) is feasible in dogs and may provide optimal surgical conditions for some intrathoracic procedures. Thoracoscopy under general anesthesia with two-lung ventilation may be performed with or without intrathoracic CO_2 insufflation to facilitate visualization of intrathoracic structures [180,185,194,195]. In the cat during general anesthesia, CO_2 insufflation pressures greater than 3 mmHg result in significant cardiovascular side effects and are not recommended in this species [196–198]. In the horse and dog during general anesthesia, use of thoracic CO_2 insufflation is described, and the cardiopulmonary effects can be marked. Insufflation of the thoracic cavity should not be undertaken unless required and in-depth cardiopulmonary monitoring is recommended [187,199–202].

Complications and outcomes associated with thoracic interventions are dependent on the primary disease and concurrent conditions; however, in general, major intraoperative concerns include the potential reduction in pulmonary gas exchange both during and following the procedure, iatrogenic injury to intrathoracic structures, as well as a deterioration in cardiovascular performance associated with ventilatory support, reduced venous return, vasodilation, and/or hemorrhage [183,191]. Postoperatively, pneumothorax and pleural effusion are frequently reported, particularly if patients have clinical signs associated with pulmonary or pleural disease preoperatively [181,186,191]. Cellulitis and abscessation of the thoracotomy site have been reported in horses with pleuropneumonia following thoracic exploration [189]. Commonly encountered conditions involving the respiratory system that require either thoracoscopy or thoracotomy are discussed further below.

Management of anesthesia

Prior to anesthesia, the surgical approach should be reviewed with the surgical team to facilitate planning for patient positioning, management of ventilation, including the need for OLV or thoracic insufflation, as well as a postoperative patient management plan, including the optimal approach to analgesic management. Intrathoracic procedures are major surgeries with potential for considerable reduction in respiratory and cardiovascular function intraoperatively and a thorough preoperative assessment of the patient is strongly recommended. In addition, a complete blood count (CBC), serum biochemistry, and thoracic radiographs are highly recommended in all patients undergoing intrathoracic procedures with additional diagnostic imaging such as ultrasound and computed tomography as appropriate. In patients with pre-existing respiratory disease, preoperative arterial blood gas analysis can provide information regarding lung function if it is available. Patients with intrapulmonary masses should be evaluated for metastasis, and changes in hepatic or renal function, in addition to the effects of the mass on respiratory function. Cardiovascular assessment with an ECG, echocardiographic evaluation, and blood pressure measurement are appropriate for patients with pre-existing cardiac disease. For patients with a history of trauma, an ECG and arterial blood gas are also highly recommended preoperatively due to the potential presence of arrhythmias and gas exchange impairment.

Whenever possible, patients should be normovolemic with adequate hemoglobin concentrations prior to intrathoracic procedures as blood loss is a potential complication [184]. Preoperative fluid therapy may therefore include crystalloid, artificial colloid, and/or blood product administration. In cases where significant hemorrhage is anticipated, preoperative blood typing or crossmatching is warranted. Medications aimed at optimizing cardiopulmonary function should be maintained preoperatively. In patients with pre-existing pneumothorax or pleural effusion, air and/or fluid should be removed from the intrathoracic space immediately prior to anesthesia, to minimize the patient's work of breathing and improve gas exchange during anesthetic induction. In cases with rapidly accumulating intrathoracic air or fluid, measures to permit repeated chest evacuation, such as a chest tube should be in place prior to induction of anesthesia.

The specific anesthetic protocol used for thoracic procedures should be tailored to the individual patient. Systemic administration of non-steroidal anti-inflammatory agents (NSAIDs), sedatives, and opioid analgesics, with regional anesthesia (paravertebral or intercostal nerve block) or infiltration of local anesthetic at surgery sites, generally provides suitable conditions for thoracoscopy in the standing adult horse or cow [187,189,190,193,194,203]. Monitoring of the patient's PaO_2 is recommended and oxygen administration through nasal catheter(s) is indicated if hemoglobin saturation falls below 95% [190,203].

Recommendations for small animal patients undergoing general anesthesia include preoxygenation of the patient if there is any pre-existing impairment of pulmonary function, use of rapid induction strategies to secure a sealed airway quickly, use of mechanical ventilatory support during the thoracic procedure or earlier if indicated, providing hemodynamic support as required (inotrope/vasopressor infusions and antiarrhythmic medications), employing active warming strategies to maintain the patient's body temperature, and using multiple approaches to manage postoperative pain. In general, a balanced anesthetic technique using a combination of inhalant anesthetics and infusions of minimum alveolar concentration (MAC)-reducing agents such as opioids, lidocaine (except cats), and ketamine can be used to maintain a suitable plane of anesthesia while providing intraoperative analgesia and minimizing the cardiovascular depression induced by inhalant anesthetics. In cases where pulmonary tissue is being resected or there is a risk of air leak, inhalant agents are ideally avoided to prevent environmental contamination. Neuromuscular blocking agents are not routinely used in veterinary patients undergoing intrathoracic procedures as adequate muscle relaxation is typically achieved with the protocols discussed above.

Critical to the success of intrathoracic procedures performed during general anesthesia is the use of appropriate ventilatory support techniques. While ventilation can be supported manually for a short period of time, mechanical ventilation should be available for any intrathoracic intervention planned under general anesthesia. This will permit consistent ventilation using set volumes or pressures while freeing up the anesthetist to monitor and manage other aspects of anesthesia such as providing appropriate and timely hemodynamic support. In cases with significant pulmonary parenchymal disease or pleural effusion, the clinician should be prepared to provide ventilatory support immediately after anesthetic induction while in some patients, spontaneous ventilation may be feasible before thoracotomy or thoracoscopy. In patients undergoing a thoracotomy or thoracoscopy, once the thoracic cavity is open to the atmosphere and intrapleural pressure equilibrates with atmospheric pressure, the patient's breathing effort will not be able to create a negative intrapleural pressure and normal airflow into the ipsilateral lung. As previously noted, in most healthy dogs and cats, the mediastinum is complete; however, it may be disrupted in cases with thoracic disease and entry to the chest may impact both lungs. For some intrathoracic procedures in canine patients, controlling ventilation to the right and left lungs independently may be desirable, and techniques to achieve such conditions are discussed below. In most cases requiring separation of the lungs, ventilation is initiated using a standard orotracheal tube, and therefore whole lung ventilation is conducted until the patient is prepared and positioned for surgery. Placement of an endobronchial blocker or performing selective endobronchial intubation to initiate OLV is then performed to minimize lung movement and improve surgical visualization.

With traditional (non-PEEP) ventilatory support, opening of the pleural cavity via a thoracotomy or thoracoscopy typically results in a decrease in PaO_2 because of venous admixture associated with $\dot{V}_A/\dot{Q}$ mismatch and intrapulmonary shunting of blood [190,193,203–207]. The latter is attributed to a decrease in FRC (to below closing capacity) associated with the loss of the elastic recoil of the chest wall and its associated negative intrapleural pressure [204]. The significance of the fall in PaO_2 will be dependent on the patient's baseline oxygenation; however, in most companion animals without primary lung disease, hemoglobin oxygen saturation is generally well maintained during intrathoracic procedures. While the use of PEEP and conservative V_T settings (< 15 mL/kg) may not influence outcomes in patients with healthy lungs, in patients with lung injury, the use of ventilatory strategies that minimize lung collapse and maintain alveolar recruitment, as discussed above, should be employed to prevent further lung injury. In terms of lung mechanical properties, as FRC is reduced, the compliance of the lung will decrease; however, the overall impact on the patient may be variable depending on the contribution of the chest wall, as total respiratory compliance (C_{RS}) is the sum of both lung and chest wall compliance. For example, during thoracoscopy, C_{RS} may not change significantly, while it may increase in a patient undergoing a median sternotomy because the constraint imposed by the chest wall on total C_{RS} has been removed. In the latter circumstance, if the patient is receiving ventilatory support with a preset pressure target (PCV mode) and the P_{max} is not decreased once the thorax is open, $PaCO_2$ will generally fall due to excessive alveolar ventilation associated with an increase in V_T. Irrespective of the surgical approach, if the V_T delivered to the patient is maintained (VCV mode), changes in $PaCO_2$ will be minimal after the thorax is opened [205,208].

Recommended monitoring during intrathoracic procedures under general anesthesia includes pulse oximetry, capnography, ECG, direct arterial blood pressure, blood gas analysis, and body temperature. While end-tidal CO_2 monitoring may be a useful tool to adjust mechanical ventilation in healthy dogs, $P_{ET}CO_2$ may not reliably assess adequacy of ventilation in dogs undergoing thoracotomy [209,210]. Despite its limited ability to evaluate adequacy of ventilation, $P_{ET}CO_2$ monitoring and determination of $P(a\text{-}ET)CO_2$ by serial arterial blood gas analysis may provide important information related to changes in alveolar deadspace and lung perfusion in patients undergoing thoracic surgery.

Arterial blood gas analysis will provide an accurate measure of $PaCO_2$ as well as information regarding the patient's oxygenation and degree of intrapulmonary shunting of blood. In terms of lung mechanical properties, airway pressure should also be monitored and if available, spirometry will provide additional information regarding pulmonary mechanics to help guide ventilatory support as described above. In small animal patients, if it is not possible to monitor blood pressure invasively, a Doppler blood pressure monitor is recommended in addition to an oscillometric technique, as it can be used repeatedly over a short period of time, and it has an audible signal permitting the anesthesiologist to continuously evaluate the pulse rate, rhythm, and quality of peripheral perfusion. Arrhythmias are relatively common in patients undergoing thoracic procedures due to underlying cardiovascular disease, hemodynamic alterations associated with the intervention, or direct myocardial irritation, therefore the clinician should monitor the ECG continuously and have antiarrhythmics available.

Small animal patients with chronic pleural space disease (e.g., chronic diaphragmatic hernia or chylothorax) may have concurrent pulmonary parenchymal disease and/or lung lobe collapse, which will be further injured by rapid re-expansion during surgery. The pathophysiology of pulmonary re-expansion injury (i.e., re-expansion pulmonary edema) is complex but includes mechanical stress leading to increases in the pulmonary microvascular permeability secondary to the abrupt re-expansion of the lungs, and infiltration of immune cells [211,212]. In humans, re-expansion pulmonary edema is a rare but potentially fatal complication that may occur after rapid re-expansion of chronically collapsed/atelectatic lungs secondary to pneumothorax, hemothorax, and pleural effusion [211,212]. Although objective data are lacking in the veterinary literature, rapid re-expansion of the lungs during surgery in cats with chronic diaphragmatic hernia may carry high risk of fatality because of re-expansion pulmonary edema [213]. Therefore, in cases of diaphragmatic hernia where chronic alveolar collapse is suspected, extra caution should be exerted when applying progressively increasing inspiratory pressures and increased PEEP levels to reopen collapsed alveoli. Visual assessment of the reopening of collapsed lung (which changes from a dark color to a light pink) by the surgeons may help to guide the anesthesiologist when recruiting collapsed areas. Pulmonary edema has been observed in some individuals in the early postoperative period, which has led to various recommendations such as limited crystalloid volume administration, use of colloids, administration of diuretics, and administration of corticosteroids. Despite the lack of published evidence, gradual re-expansion of chronically collapsed lung might carry a lower risk of complications compared to rapid re-expansion of the lung intraoperatively. When considering alveolar recruitment maneuvers (ARMs) previously discussed in this chapter, a stepwise increase in airway pressures by using a cycling maneuver approach could be an option to minimize sudden re-expansion of the collapsed lung after the abdominal viscera are removed from the thorax.

Placement of at least one thoracic tube prior to chest closure is routine in patients at risk of intrapleural air or fluid accumulation following thoracoscopy or thoracotomy. At the end of the surgical intervention, the anesthesia-surgery team needs to communicate when the chest is closed to ensure removal of intrapleural air and closure of the chest tubes prior to recovery from anesthesia.

Recommended analgesic techniques used in patients undergoing a thoracotomy include regional anesthesia techniques (e.g., intercostal nerve block, serratus plane block, paravertebral nerve block, and placement of bupivacaine liposomal injectable suspension at wound closure), epidural analgesia with opioids, and systemic analgesia with opioids, ketamine, lidocaine, dexmedetomidine, and NSAIDs. In clinical patients, using more than one approach is highly recommended. Epidural morphine administration is an effective means of providing analgesia for thoracotomies in small animals [214,215]. As morphine is more soluble in water than in fat, epidural administration of this opioid at the level of the lumbosacral space results in relatively high concentrations in the cerebrospinal fluid, which favors its cranial spread within the medulla and the extension of its analgesic effects up to the level of thoracic dermatomes [216].

More recently, an ultrasound-guided erector spinae block adopted in humans for pain control in thoracic surgery has been evaluated in cadaveric studies performed in dogs (level of the ninth thoracic transverse process) [217,218]. A bilateral erector spinae block has been used in anesthetized dogs undergoing sternotomies [219], whereas another case series not including a control group reported that epidural morphine, combined with an ultrasound-guided erector spinae plane block with bupivacaine, provided adequate intra- and postoperative pain control for lateral thoracotomies in dogs [220]. A serratus block is another interfascial plane block that provides analgesia for thoracotomies in humans [221] that has been evaluated in cadaveric studies in dogs [222]. However, like the erector spinae block, published evidence of its effectiveness for controlling pain in thoracic surgery is based on a case series study with a small number of animals [223].

Intrapleural instillation and infiltration of local anesthetic around chest tube insertion sites have also been shown to be safe and improve postoperative analgesia in dogs [224–226]. When local anesthetic techniques are employed, bupivacaine or ropivacaine are generally preferred due to the longer duration of action relative to lidocaine. Due to potential toxicity, the total dose of bupivacaine should not exceed 2 mg/kg in dogs, whereas the dose of ropivacaine should not exceed 3 mg/kg in this species.

Separation of the lungs and one-lung ventilation (OLV)

Functional separation of the lungs can be performed during anesthesia for a variety of indications. In veterinary medicine, the most common indications are to facilitate thoracoscopic or minimally invasive thoracic surgery or to isolate one lung from another when contamination from one lung to the other is undesirable [227]. In the latter instance, patients are generally undergoing lung lobectomy to remove the affected lobe [192,228–231]. Controlling the distribution of ventilation in patients with a bronchopleural fistula, pulmonary bullae, disruption of the tracheobronchial tree, or other severe unilateral lung disease are less common indications for isolation of the lungs during ventilatory support [227,229]. Theoretically, the need for ventilation of both lungs versus selective ventilation of one lung influences what strategy is optimal for the intended procedure. To achieve independent ventilation of the right and left lungs, placement of a double-lumen endotracheal tube is necessary. When ventilation of one lung and collapse of the alternative lung will provide the necessary conditions, options include selective endobronchial intubation using a single-lumen endotracheal tube, placement of a double-lumen endotracheal tube, or use of a bronchial blocker (Fig. 38.33) [227,232,233].

With some bronchial blockers and double-lumen endotracheal tubes, it is also feasible to ventilate one lung and maintain static lung inflation using CPAP with varying F_IO_2 levels in the alternate lung [227,229]. In veterinary medicine, determination of the best strategy for an individual patient will be dependent on the size of the patient, available equipment (endoscopic equipment and specialized airway devices), surgical approach, and experience of the anesthesia and surgical team. Irrespective of the type of equipment used, fiberoptic bronchoscopy is recommended either during or immediately following placement to ensure the correct location of the double-lumen tube or blocker, although this may not be feasible in very small patients. When the latter is not feasible, video-assisted thoracoscopic verification of airway device placement has been used and fluoroscopic guidance of airway devices suitable for OLV has been described in an experimental setting [230,234]. A brief description of the technique and physiologic consequences of selective lung ventilation is provided below. Depending on the planned intervention, patients may be placed in lateral recumbency, with the ventilated lung in the dependent position, or dorsal recumbency.

As noted, placement of a double-lumen endotracheal tube creates functional separation of the right and left lung, permitting either independent ventilation of both lungs, ventilation of one lung, and either application of CPAP or zero airway pressure on the alternative lung. Several different double-lumen tube designs exist; however, due to anatomical differences in humans and veterinary species, patient size, and airway configuration, their use is generally limited to medium-sized dogs (10–25 kg) that can be managed with standard

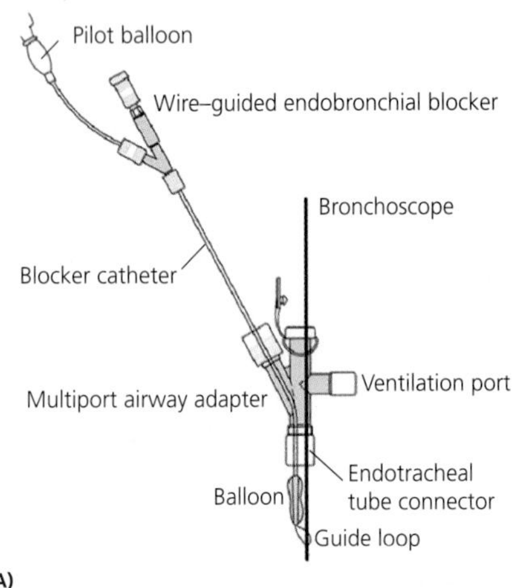

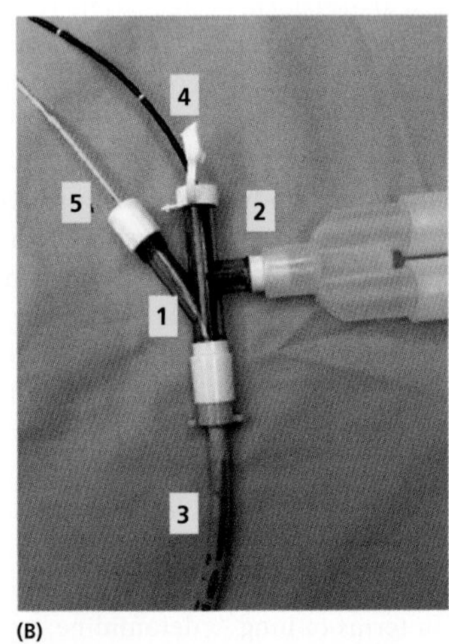

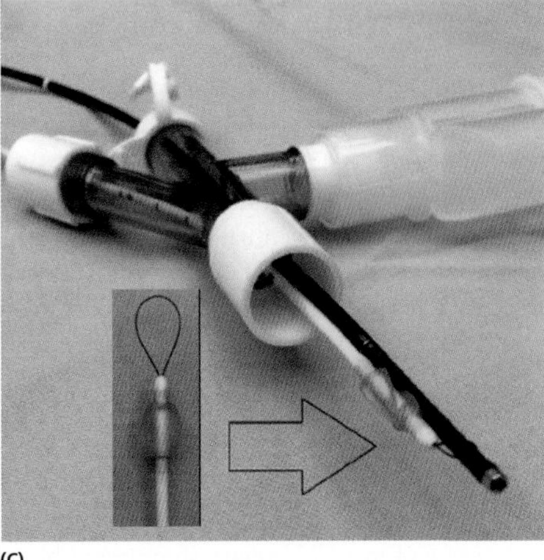

Figure 38.33 **A.** A wire-guided endobronchial blocker originally developed for one-lung ventilation in children can be used for one-lung ventilation using a standard endotracheal tube in small animals. **B.** A multiport airway adapter (1) connects the breathing circuit (2) to the endotracheal tube (3). The multiport adapter has two working channels used to insert a bronchoscope (4) and an endobronchial blocker (5). **C.** The endobronchial blocker has a wire loop to attach its tip to the bronchoscope and a balloon that is inflated to occlude the bronchus after it is properly positioned under guidance of the bronchoscope. Source: Fabila *et al.* [232], with permission from the Indian Journal of Anaesthesia; Wu *et al.* [233], Wolters Kluwer Health / CCBY 4.0.

orotracheal tubes with internal diameters of 6.5 to 10 mm. Double-lumen endotracheal tubes are supplied in varying configurations, lengths, and internal and external diameters, variables that must be considered on an individual patient basis. In general, left-sided double-lumen tubes, which have a longer tube that fits into the left mainstem bronchus and a shorter tube terminating above the carina, are commonly used due to the anatomy of the right mainstem bronchus and right apical lobe in humans as well as veterinary species. Specifically, the short distance from the tracheal carina to the right apical lobe, as well as anatomical variation between individual patients, make consistent blocking of the right lung more challenging and prone to failure in both humans and dogs [227,235].

Endobronchial blockers, which are also available in different sizes and configurations, are long catheters with inflatable cuffs at the distal tip designed to occlude an airway. The blocker can be placed before the endotracheal tube so that they both reside within the trachea independently, or it can be placed through an endotracheal tube under bronchoscopic guidance once the patient is intubated (Fig. 38.33). Verification of the position of the device is similar to that described for double-lumen endotracheal tubes. Once in place, the cuff on the blocker can be inflated, isolating the portion of the lung distal to the endobronchial blocker cuff from the trachea. Some blockers have a lumen within the catheter that permits application of either negative pressure or positive pressure to the isolated lung region. The former facilitates collapsing the lung and the latter permits delivery of continuous airway pressure to maintain lung volume without fluctuations in lung size. In cases where use of a double-lumen tube or bronchial blocker is not possible (unsuitable or unavailable), advancement of an endotracheal tube, of sufficient length, into a mainstem bronchus can create isolation of a lung lobe and OLV. This procedure has been described for use in large dogs due to the limitations in length of double-lumen endotracheal tubes and bronchial blockers [231].

The physiologic effect of separate lung ventilation strategies will vary depending on how each lung is managed. While physiologic effects of ventilation are anticipated to be equivalent to that observed with traditional ventilation when independent ventilation of both lungs is provided (e.g., with a double-lumen endotracheal tube and two separate ventilators), a decrease in PaO_2 is observed when ventilation is limited to one lung [208,236–239]. The latter is a result of continued perfusion of the non-ventilated lung (shunted blood flow). As explained in Chapter 37, hypoxic pulmonary vasoconstriction (HPV) can minimize the oxygenation impairment caused by the increase in shunted flow during OLV because mixed-venous blood is redirected from non-ventilated lung regions with low P_AO_2 to ventilated lung areas. Numerous factors have been shown to reduce HPV during OLV, including underlying lung disease, sepsis, hypocapnia, hypothermia, Trendelenburg position, and systemic vasodilators [235,240]. While inhalant anesthetic agents were historically considered to be inhibitors of HPV, when delivered at doses at or below 1 MAC they have been demonstrated to result in a similar degree of intrapulmonary shunting compared to injectable anesthetic regimens; therefore, they are no longer considered contraindicated for clinical use during OLV [235,239,240]. Factors that may potentiate HPV include hypercapnia, hyperthermia, metabolic acidosis, and hypertension [235]. The clinical implications of the latter variables in controlling HPV have not been studied in veterinary medicine to date.

In addition to the continued perfusion of the non-ventilated lung, alteration of $\dot{V}_A/\dot{Q}$ relationships in the ventilated lung can also contribute to a reduction in PaO_2 in patients undergoing OLV. The latter may be influenced by underlying disease, ventilatory strategy, patient hemodynamics, and positioning [235,240,241]. One of the best predictors of the ability of a patient to tolerate OLV, is their PaO_2 while receiving two-lung ventilation in the position required for surgery [235]. Patients with severe lung dysfunction may not have adequate capacity of the non-surgical lung to permit safe OLV. Ensuring adequate PaO_2 levels prior to initiation of OLV with arterial blood gas analysis is highly recommended. The ventilatory strategy used for the ventilated lung may also impact patient arterial oxygen levels. A recruitment maneuver at the start of OLV is recommended in humans to minimize atelectasis in the ventilated lung and has been used in clinical veterinary patients [229,235]. Decreased pulmonary perfusion due to hemodynamic causes (e.g., hypotension) may be associated with pre-existing $\dot{V}_A/\dot{Q}$ abnormalities in both lungs even before initiation of OLV, and this will further impair gas exchange and exacerbate hypoxemia after the lung is isolated. In terms of patient positioning, the incidence of hypoxemia is higher when human patients are in a supine position (equivalent to dorsal recumbency in quadrupeds) [235,240]. As the right lung is larger (about 55% of the total volume) than the left lung (45%), human patients that are positioned in right lateral recumbency for OLV of the right lung (left thoracotomy) present better arterial oxygen levels than individuals positioned in left lateral recumbency for OLV of the left lung (right thoracotomy). Similar discrepancy in lung sizes exists in animals, and it is anticipated that patients having OLV of the right lung while positioned in right lateral recumbency for left thoracotomy would be at less risk of hypoxemia compared to animals positioned left lateral recumbency (ventilation of the left lung) for right thoracotomy.

Investigations of the cardiopulmonary effects of closed-thorax OLV have been carried out in healthy experimental dogs anesthetized with isoflurane positioned in lateral recumbency, with and without PEEP of the dependent ventilated lung [236–238]. Consistent with reports in other species, including humans, a substantial decrease in PaO_2 is observed with initiation of OLV. These studies found that tissue oxygen delivery was not significantly different during OLV versus the control bilateral lung ventilation, despite the large increase in $P(A\text{-}a)O_2$ gradients, and the increase in venous admixture. The maintenance of tissue oxygen supply occurred because CO was maintained and because the use of 100% oxygen as the inhalational carrier gas resulted in PaO_2 levels during OLV that were high enough to produce nearly full hemoglobin oxygen saturation, despite the increase in $P(A\text{-}a)O_2$ gradient. Similar findings have been reported in normal dogs undergoing OLV with an open thoracic cavity [208]. Although it did not affect oxygen delivery in the healthy dogs studied, the use of PEEP in the ventilated lung did improve PaO_2 levels, consistent with reducing intrapulmonary shunting and the inclusion of PEEP was therefore recommended in clinical patients [238]. The delivery of CPAP to the non-ventilated lung has also been shown experimentally to maintain PaO_2 in dogs undergoing OLV while placed in right lateral recumbency [239].

In many of the experimental studies described to date, the V_T and respiratory rate were maintained at similar levels before and after initiation of OLV with VCV and $PaCO_2$ increased in all studies, although the values remained within acceptable limits, an effect likely due to the creation of increased deadspace ventilation with the relatively large V_Ts delivered to the one lung [208,236,237]. With PCV, as expected, conversion to OLV without changing ventilatory variables resulted in an increase in $PaCO_2$ [239].

In veterinary medicine, numerous case series and case reports of patients undergoing OLV for a variety of procedures, including lung lobectomy for pulmonary mass removal, thymoma removal, correction of persistent right aortic arch, and pericardial fenestration, have been published [182,183,228,229,231,242–244]. In clinical patients, balanced anesthetic protocols that include local anesthesia and injectable analgesics that permit inhalant anesthetics to be maintained below 1 MAC or injectable anesthetic regimens (propofol) are recommended. Ventilatory strategies that include PEEP levels of 3–5 cmH_2O and reduced V_Ts (< 10 mL/kg) when converting from two to OLV to prevent overinflation of the ventilated lung are suggested, although the specific V_T should ideally be adjusted to the individual patient based on gas exchange and pulmonary mechanics measurements as discussed.

In the event of hypoxemia during OLV: (1) the F_IO_2 to the ventilated lung should be maximized; (2) placement of the endobronchial blocker/double-lumen endotracheal tube/endotracheal tube should be verified; (3) patient hemodynamics should be supported to achieve normotension; and (4) lung recruitment of the ventilated lung with subsequent application of PEEP, if not in use, should be initiated. If PaO_2 levels do not increase to satisfactory levels (generally considered a PaO_2 above 60 mmHg), two-lung ventilation should be resumed. If a double-lumen endotracheal tube or bronchial blocker with lumen to the blocked lung is in place, CPAP can be delivered to reduce atelectasis in the non-ventilated lung [229,239].

Complications reported during OLV in veterinary patients include inability to achieve OLV or displacement of the airway devices and subsequent failure of OLV during surgery, in addition to inadequate PaO_2 [180,227]. In some instances, surgical access is inadequate despite OLV, and conversion to a thoracotomy is required. Inadvertent entrapment of an endobronchial blocker tip by a surgical stapler has also been reported [245].

Anesthetic management of patients with respiratory disease

Patients with respiratory disease may require anesthesia for procedures related or unrelated to their respiratory disease. Unfortunately, sedation and anesthesia of these patients are associated with an increased risk of anesthetic morbidity and mortality. To reduce such risks, when developing an anesthetic plan, it is important for clinicians to understand (1) the underlying pathophysiology of the condition and its consequences as they relate to anesthesia; (2) the presence and nature of any concurrent conditions; and (3) the proposed diagnostic and/or therapeutic intervention and its potential complications. Knowledge of the required positioning of the patient during interventions will also assist with anesthetic preparation and case management.

Patients presenting to a veterinary hospital in respiratory distress may need to be triaged and supported prior to obtaining a history and complete physical examination. In some instances, additional specific information in the history relative to the respiratory disorder is relevant to anesthesia as discussed below; otherwise, it is assumed that standard history and physical examination are appropriate. In general, proactive review and discussion of possible complications and challenges among veterinary team members will increase preparedness and improve patient outcomes. Respiratory diseases with substantial implications related to anesthesia will be discussed in detail below, and while all potential disorders are not covered, the principles and practices applied to these conditions are often transferrable to other situations. As previously noted, when specific aspects of anesthetic management are not discussed, it is assumed standard practices including balanced anesthetic protocols with appropriate supportive therapies and analgesic strategies are appropriate.

Anesthesia and upper respiratory disease

Anesthesia may be indicated in patients with upper airway disease or dysfunction for procedures that may or may not be associated with their airway. In animals with upper airway disease, resistance to airflow (R_{aw}) and the work of breathing are often increased. These changes can be exacerbated due to the relaxation of the upper airways induced by sedation and anesthesia. Of greatest concern is the potential for severe hypoventilation and/or airway obstruction; however, numerous other factors should be considered depending on the patient's underlying condition, as discussed below.

General approach to the management of animals with a difficult airway

Securing an airway to maintain its patency, minimize the risk of aspiration, and permit administration of oxygen, with or without an inhalant anesthetic, is a key component of anesthetic management. Differences in degree of difficulty in securing an airway exist among species; however, access to appropriate equipment and pre-anesthetic preparation result in successful airway management in most patients. Unfortunately, challenges in establishing an airway can occur in patients with normal airways due to laryngospasm or in patients with abnormalities secondary to a variety of factors including anatomic conformation (e.g., brachycephalic breeds), foreign bodies, structural abnormalities (e.g., temporomandibular joint disease), masses intrinsic or extrinsic to the airway, inflammation, and/or fluid accumulation. Successful management of the patient, including prevention of hypoxemia caused by induction of anesthesia with injectable agents and rapidly securing a patent airway, may be impacted by preoperative planning and emergency preparation.

The American Society of Anesthesiologists (ASA) has published guidelines for the management of the difficult airway [246]. While no definitive guidelines exist in veterinary medicine, the principles of preparing in advance of anesthetic induction, providing oxygen supplementation during attempts at establishing an airway, enlisting assistance, and attempting alternative strategies or awakening the patient can be applied to the veterinary situation. More detail on management of the difficult airway can be found in Chapter 5. Further recommendations for airway management of animals with pre-existing respiratory diseases are discussed below.

Canine brachycephalic obstructive airway syndrome

Characteristics and pathophysiology

Individuals identified as being affected with brachycephalic airway syndrome, or brachycephalic obstructive airway syndrome (BOAS), have a combination of primary and secondary abnormalities that result in a reduced airway diameter and partial to complete airway obstruction [247,248]. Not all brachycephalic dogs are affected by BOAS; however, a large percentage of dogs within certain breeds, most notably English and French Bulldogs, Pugs, and Boston Terriers, meet the criteria for classification as being affected by BOAS [249–251]. Common primary abnormalities in dogs affected with BOAS include stenotic nares, abnormal nasal turbinate morphology, elongated soft palate, redundant pharyngeal soft tissues, macroglossia, and hypoplastic trachea [250,251]. As anticipated based on the turbulent airflow characteristics of the upper airways and the relationship of luminal radius to resistance to airflow (Chapter 37), the reduction in upper airway diameter results in a dramatic increase in airway resistance (R_{aw}) and the work of breathing. To compensate for the upper airway obstruction, a greater transpulmonary pressure gradient ($P_{ao} - P_{pl}$) is required to generate adequate inspiratory flow. Unfortunately, greater negative intraluminal pressure can exacerbate collapse of the upper airway structures into the air passages and further increase R_{aw}. Secondary structural alteration to the airways as a result of the changes in intraluminal pressure and flow that are observed in BOAS patients include soft palate hyperplasia, pharyngeal hyperplasia, laryngeal collapse, tonsillar hyperplasia, and eversion, eversion of laryngeal saccules, and bronchial collapse [247,252–256].

Clinical signs reported in dogs with BOAS include increased respiratory noise, snoring, stridor, inspiratory dyspnea, exercise intolerance, heat intolerance, syncope, cyanosis, and collapse. Case presentation to the veterinary hospital may vary tremendously. In some instances, clinical signs may be evident during elective physical examination with owners unaware of any abnormalities, while in other instances, dogs may present on an urgent basis with life-threatening hypoxemia and/or hyperthermia. An increase in thoracic and abdominal muscular effort associated with inspiration is often present at rest during physical examination and it is exacerbated with exercise or when the animal is placed in a stressful environment. Longer inspiratory times, and shorter expiratory times are also characteristic of the condition [257]. Severely affected dogs may develop respiratory obstruction during sleep when pharyngeal muscles relax, resulting in altered sleep patterns [258]. The latter has drawn comparisons between this condition and obstructive sleep apnea in humans, with the English Bulldog being considered a naturally occurring animal model of the human condition [258].

The presence of lower airway or pulmonary parenchymal disease is highly variable in dogs with BOAS. Although large prospective studies have not been performed, higher $PaCO_2$ and lower PaO_2 values have been reported in French Bulldogs presenting for BOAS surgery in one investigation as well as in a group of brachycephalic dogs presenting to a referral hospital for a variety of procedures [259,260]. In both studies, $PaCO_2$ was elevated above normal values suggesting chronic habituation to hypoventilation while changes in PaO_2 were relatively mild and consistent with reduced alveolar ventilation. As mentioned, however, some dogs may present with cyanosis, indicative of severe reductions in PaO_2, which may be secondary to reduced alveolar ventilation, $\dot{V}_A/\dot{Q}$ mismatch, or intrapulmonary shunting associated with pulmonary parenchymal disease [261]. Aspiration pneumonia was reported as an underlying cause of hypoxemia in one retrospective study assessing brachycephalic dogs admitted to a referral hospital [261]. Post-obstructive pulmonary edema, also known as "negative-pressure pulmonary edema," as reported in other species, including humans and horses, has also been suggested to be a contributing factor in cases with acute severe hypoxemia [262]. Excessive negative airway pressures caused by severe upper airway obstruction increase venous return to the right side of the heart and increase pulmonary artery pressure. This effect, in combination with decreased left heart function, results in excessive increases in pulmonary capillary hydrostatic pressures leading to pulmonary edema as fluid moves out of pulmonary capillaries into the lung interstitial tissue and alveolar lumen [262]. Early experimental models of upper airway obstruction (nasal and laryngeal) in dogs reported impaired oxygenation over several weeks postoperatively and it was concluded that both hypoventilation and $\dot{V}_A/\dot{Q}$ disturbances contributed to the hypoxemia [263]. In the latter study, however, dogs were noted to have difficulty eating; therefore, aspiration pneumonia may have contributed to the hypoxemia observed.

In addition to abnormalities related to the respiratory system, gastrointestinal signs including gagging, ptyalism, regurgitation, and vomiting are reported in many BOAS patients, with the severity of signs correlating with the severity of respiratory compromise [264–266]. The nature of the gastrointestinal abnormalities may vary with breed, with French Bulldogs having a higher prevalence of gastrointestinal signs compared to English Bulldogs and Pugs [265–268]. Further investigation into the gastrointestinal dysfunction in this group of patients has shown the presence of gastritis, esophagitis, gastroesophageal reflux, atony of the lower esophageal sphincter, and sliding hiatal hernia [265,268,269]. Regurgitation and vomiting are of particular concern in the perioperative period as they are associated with aspiration pneumonia, esophagitis, esophageal stricture, and airway obstruction [270–272]. Reported incidence of regurgitation in patients hospitalized for surgical correction of BOAS ranged from 9.1% to 34.5% [264,267,273] with postoperative rates being higher than preoperative rates in one retrospective study [273]. Large negative intrathoracic pressure created during inspiration secondary to partial airway obstruction is believed to contribute to the increased incidence of gastrointestinal dysfunction in this group of dogs [269]. Underlying gastroesophageal junction abnormalities, hiatal hernia, and/or esophageal dysmotility likely also contribute to the presence of gastrointestinal disease [269,273–276]. Reduction in frequency of gastrointestinal events, such as regurgitation and vomiting reported by owners, and improvement in gastrointestinal lesions, as assessed by endoscopy, following surgical interventions to alleviate the upper airway obstruction have been reported, strengthening the relationship between respiratory dysfunction and gastrointestinal disease in dogs with BOAS [265–267,277].

Brachycephalic dogs have also been shown to have a higher resting vasovagal tone than dogs of other breeds, which may predispose them to bradycardia [278]. In a sample of brachycephalic dogs, arterial blood pressure assessed using an oscillometric technique was demonstrated to be higher than in control dogs [259]. Others have reported higher packed cell volume and indices compatible with hypercoagulability, potentially due to the low PaO_2 levels and chronic inflammation [259]. Ocular conformation in brachycephalic dogs, and particularly those with BOAS, predisposes them to corneal injury [249,279].

Surgical interventions have consistently been shown to reduce undesirable respiratory and gastrointestinal signs and improve the quality of life, as judged by owners and physical examination findings, in a large percentage of brachycephalic dogs [250,264, 267,280–283]. Techniques currently performed for BOAS include staphylectomy, alarplasty, turbinectomy, vestibuloplasty, laryngeal sacculectomy, and tonsillectomy [247]. Brachycephalic dogs have a higher reported incidence of complications, including death, in the perioperative period compared to non-brachycephalic breeds when anesthetized for a variety of procedures [273,277,284–287]. The reported perioperative morbidity and mortality associated with airway surgery in this patient population range from 6 to 51.1% and 0 to 6.6%, respectively [250,264,277,287–290]. English Bulldogs were reported to have a higher anesthetic complication rate, including death, when compared with other brachycephalic dogs in one retrospective study [290]. Reports on the impact of brachycephalic dog age on anesthetic outcomes associated with airway surgery have been variable. Young dogs were reported to have a higher incidence of regurgitation in one study, and a higher complication rate in another; however, it is recognized that dogs with more severe disease may present at a younger age [273,291]. Anesthetic risk in brachycephalic dogs that had undergone corrective airway surgery was reduced in one study; however, the risk relative to non-brachycephalic dogs was not assessed prospectively and it may remain higher in the brachycephalic population [287]. A preoperative risk score, based on preoperative data, to predict the risk of major complications or death for dogs presenting for surgical treatment of BOAS syndrome was created based on retrospective data from two centers and subsequently validated in a third center [292]. Risk of a negative outcome was successfully predicted based on a 10-point score (BRisk score), determined by assigning a score to the animal's breed (English or French Bulldog versus other brachycephalic breeds), surgical history, procedures planned, body condition score, level of compromise at admission, and rectal temperature upon admission [292]. Based on highly accessible data, the BRisk score, can help inform owners regarding the risk of a negative outcome as well as prepare staff and resources prior to corrective surgery [292].

Management of anesthesia

Overall, the specific concerns related to BOAS during the perianesthetic period include the potential development of respiratory distress, hypoxemia, and/or airway obstruction (partial or complete), and the predisposition to regurgitation and aspiration [262,293]. The surgical location also makes anesthetic monitoring of the patient's depth of anesthesia using jaw tone or eye reflexes more challenging as well as poses a greater risk of unobserved airway disconnection or gastric regurgitation. Maintaining hemodynamic stability and preventing corneal trauma, are also of concern and may prove more challenging than in non-BOAS patients. Having a clearly communicated perioperative plan developed with the entire veterinary team, that extends for at least 24 h postoperatively, is highly recommended [262,277,294].

Prior to anesthesia, it is important that a thorough history, including the owner's perception of their animal's condition is obtained. Unfortunately, owners are often unaware of their dog's abnormalities and risks associated with surgery and anesthesia [279]. Specific questions regarding the dog's respiratory noise, exercise tolerance, activity levels, and gastrointestinal signs should therefore be included rather than interpretive questions that rely on the owner's opinion regarding normal canine behavior (activity levels) and physical symptoms (e.g., respiratory noise and heat tolerance). Current medications including NSAIDs, corticosteroids, and gastrointestinal medications are particularly relevant as they will influence perioperative patient medical management.

Physical examination including auscultation of the laryngeal region and thorax should be performed, although referred upper airway sounds can make auscultation challenging in many dogs. Inspiratory stridor over the laryngeal region is an indicator of laryngeal dysfunction which may impact the ease of intubation as well as the planned surgical intervention [295]. Hyperthermia may be present in patients presenting in respiratory distress and should be considered during initial patient stabilization; however, acquisition of rectal temperature can be stressful, and it may be prudent to stabilize the animal prior to obtaining this measurement.

Several investigators have used scoring systems to characterize the severity of respiratory symptoms and facilitate prediction of outcomes and/or complications following surgical intervention [264,265,292]. The BRisk score provides risk of mortality or major complications during the period of hospitalization [292]. Inclusion of a 3-min trot test and evaluation of pulmonary mechanics using whole-body plethysmography can provide further information regarding the patient's airflow obstruction [295,296]. The latter is not routinely available for clinical use, but it has been used to objectively assess other measures of respiratory dysfunction in BOAS patients as well as the outcome associated with different surgical and medical treatments [291,295,297].

Although patients may be systemically healthy, routine presurgical diagnostic testing should include a CBC, serum biochemistry, and thoracic radiographs to screen for inflammatory lung disease and to provide baseline values in the event of complications postoperatively. Additional tests such as esophageal contrast studies, ultrasound, or fluoroscopy are recommended based on individual clinical signs. Patients showing a marked increase in respiratory effort and/or signs of impaired oxygenation should have further assessment of respiratory function performed. Arterial blood gas sampling and analysis is ideal; however, if this is not feasible, measurement of hemoglobin oxygen saturation with pulse oximetry is informative in some patients. While the latter tool is readily available, the limitations of pulse oximetry need to be considered when interpreting individual patient measurements [298]. In patients presenting with severe disease, an ECG and blood pressure measurement may also provide additional useful information preoperatively. Because of the high incidence of pulmonary hypertension in animals with clinical signs of BOAS, echocardiographic evaluation should be considered. For elective procedures, overweight dogs should have a nutritional consultation and weight loss plan implemented prior to surgery as obesity has been associated with severity of clinical signs in Bulldogs and Pugs with BOAS [296].

To date, no large prospective clinical study has been performed to assess the optimal perioperative medical management of gastrointestinal dysfunction in BOAS patients. Due to the high prevalence of gastric and esophageal disease in most dogs with BOAS, routine preoperative administration of a proton pump inhibitor is recommended [269,299–301]. While the treatment may not prevent gastroesophageal reflux and regurgitation in all dogs, it will increase the gastric pH and may prevent secondary esophageal lesions from developing. The duration of treatment may vary based on the individual patient's clinical signs as well as ease of treatment. Patients with a history of regurgitation have an increased incidence of perioperative regurgitation and may benefit from a longer preoperative course of therapy if feasible [268,273]. The prokinetic cisapride has shown positive effects in BOAS dogs and is currently recommended over metoclopramide, which has shown variable effects on gastroesophageal reflux and regurgitation; however, it may not be readily available. Many clinicians include metoclopramide despite a lack of strong evidence supporting its use at clinically recommended doses [251,300,302]. Maropitant, a neurokinin-1 (NK_1) receptor antagonist, is an effective antiemetic when administered prior to preanesthetic medication and is therefore recommended in patients with a history of vomiting [303–306]. Routine inclusion of histamine type-2 (H_2) antagonists/proton pump inhibitors and mucosal protectants, such as sucralfate, in the perioperative management of BOAS patients is more controversial; however, when used on a short-term basis, they have a low incidence of side effects and may offer beneficial effects in patients with severe gastrointestinal disease.

Once a procedure is scheduled, it is recommended that the brachycephalic patient be admitted on the day of surgery with minimal wait time before premedication to minimize the impacts of stress and anxiety. Prescribing oral behavioral modifying drugs to reduce pre-appointment fear may also be considered [307].

The impact of fasting time on the risk of regurgitation, gastroesophageal reflux, and/or vomiting in both normal and dogs affected with BOAS is not known at this time. At present, there is inadequate data to make recommendations for a universal fasting period prior to anesthesia [308,309]. Common recommendations include overnight fasting (minimum fasting period of 6 h) and free access to water until premedication.

Prior to administration of preanesthetic medication, the anesthesia workstation should be prepared. In addition to the standard equipment, orotracheal tubes in a range of sizes, facemasks, and monitors including a pulse oximeter should be readily available. Laryngoscopes with different blade sizes and/or styles, should be available to facilitate intubation. Despite the presence of an orotracheal tube, the work of breathing in brachycephalic dogs will likely be higher than in a non-brachycephalic dog of similar weight due to their relatively small airway radius and tendency for overweight body condition scores. As such, it is recommended that a suitable mechanical ventilator be available and prepared for use. Equipment that can be used to suction the oropharyngeal area should also be readily available in the induction and recovery areas.

In general, the choice of premedication agents will be dependent on the patient's temperament and co-existing medical conditions, planned diagnostic and/or surgical intervention, and clinician preference. When patients are scheduled for relatively non-invasive procedures such as airway surgery only, it is recommended that μ-opioid receptor agonists are not used due to their association with regurgitation and vomiting, particularly when administered alone via the intramuscular (IM) or subcutaneous (SC) route [306,310–313]. In mature quiet dogs, low doses of sedative agents alone may be sufficient, with opioid analgesic agents added if required once the patient is anesthetized with a secure airway. If opioid analgesics are included in the premedication, methadone or buprenorphine are currently recommended options as they are associated with a lower incidence of vomiting [313]. Panting is also associated with μ-opioid receptor agonists, which can worsen airway obstruction in patients with severe disease. Some authors have recommended the exclusion of α_2-adrenergic receptor agonists due to concerns related to airway obstruction associated with profound muscle relaxation. While high doses of α_2-adrenergic receptor agonists should be avoided, premedication with dexmedetomidine (2 μg/kg IM) in combination with methadone (0.3 mg/kg IM) has been shown to provide good sedation without an increase in complications in ASA I or II brachycephalic dogs prior to anesthetic induction when compared to acepromazine (0.02 mg/kg IM) and methadone (0.3 mg/kg IM) [314]. When α_2-adrenergic receptor agonists are not included in the premedication regimen, including anticholinergics such as glycopyrrolate in the animal's premedication offers the advantage of maintaining heart rate and reducing oropharyngeal secretions. While anticholinergics have not been demonstrated to increase the risk of aspiration pneumonia, atropine has been shown to reduce lower esophageal sphincter tone [270,315–318]. While the decision to include anticholinergics prophylactically in the premedication regimen remains controversial, their use to treat bradycardia once a secure and sealed airway is established is warranted.

Induction of anesthesia using a rapidly acting injectable anesthetic such as propofol or alfaxalone is ideal to ensure a rapid transition to a secure and sealed airway; however, this should be performed following preoxygenation for 3–5 min using a facemask. The latter has been shown to prolong the time to hemoglobin desaturation and will permit a brief airway examination prior to intubation should the patient become apneic [39,40]. If preoxygenation using a mask is not tolerated, preoxygenation using a flow-by technique can be used; however, the time to desaturation will be shorter compared to that obtained with a mask [40]. Irrespective of the technique used, the patient's eyes should be well lubricated prior to induction to minimize risk of corneal abrasion.

Prior to intubation, a rapid oropharyngeal exam should be performed. Further examination may be warranted in individual patients with signs of laryngeal dysfunction. Orotracheal intubation is generally performed using direct visualization facilitated by use of a laryngoscope while the patient is maintained in sternal recumbency with the head and neck elevated. The cuff on the orotracheal tube should be inflated to create a seal as soon as the orotracheal tube is in place and the seal should intermittently be verified throughout anesthesia. If standard placement of an endotracheal tube is not possible due to challenges associated with visualization, a stylet, such as a semi-rigid urinary catheter can be used as a guide for the endotracheal tube to facilitate intubation. Oxygen can be insufflated through the catheter while the endotracheal tube is placed. If it is not possible to place an orotracheal tube, the catheter can be used to provide oxygen while a tracheostomy is performed. As the catheter is rigid, care must be taken to not damage the airways and excessive flows should be avoided if severe airway narrowing is present. If available, a small-diameter endoscope can also be used as a stylet for the endotracheal tube. Because the trachea is often hypoplastic in dogs with BOAS, it may not be possible to insert an endotracheal tube of the same size that would be typically inserted in a non-brachycephalic dog of similar body mass. For example, while a 9.5 mm internal diameter endotracheal tube would easily fit in a 20 kg mongrel dog, an English Bulldog of similar weight may allow placement of an endotracheal tube with an internal diameter of only 6.5 mm (Fig. 38.34A). Inasmuch as the endotracheal tube will further reduce diameter of an already narrowed airway, resulting in greater increases in R_{aw} and the work of breathing, providing mechanical ventilatory support during anesthesia is strongly advised (Fig. 38.34B). Dog breeds that are typically diagnosed with BOAS (e.g., English and French Bulldogs, Pugs, and Boston Terriers) have a barrel-shaped chest and often are obese, factors that are known to decrease C_{RS} during anesthesia (Fig. 38.34B) [118]. In these dogs, due to their increased R_{aw} and decreased C_{RS}, VCV or PCV volume-guaranteed may be preferred over a standard PCV mode as previously discussed in the mechanical ventilation section.

Once a secure airway is in place and oxygen supplementation initiated, a variety of techniques and anesthetic agents can be used to maintain anesthesia, including inhalant anesthetics, infusions of injectable anesthetics, or a combination of both. The goal should be to use a protocol that results in a smooth, excitement-free recovery while minimizing residual sedation and upper airway relaxation. In terms of inhalant anesthetics, some clinicians might prefer sevoflurane over isoflurane because the former has a pharmacokinetic profile that favors faster recoveries from anesthesia. However, clinical data shows that the quality and duration of recovery are comparable between these inhalant anesthetics in canine species [319,320]. Use of infusions of injectable anesthetics may result in more prolonged anesthetic recoveries when compared to inhalant anesthetics and therefore may be less desirable unless inhalant anesthetics are contraindicated for other reasons. If constant rate infusions of opioids are indicated to provide intraoperative analgesia and reduce inhalant requirements, fentanyl and remifentanil are suitable agents [321,322]. While remifentanil is the ideal agent for prolonged infusions because it is devoid of cumulative effects [323], fentanyl is still an effective drug for intraoperative use in dogs with BOAS because, differently from humans, this opioid does not accumulate during prolonged infusions in dogs (i.e., its plasma sensitive half-life is unaltered by infusion duration in this species) [324]. If prolonged recoveries are attributed to residual effects of pure μ-opioid receptor agonists, partial reversal with a μ-opioid receptor antagonist (naloxone) or a μ-opioid antagonist/κ-opioid agonist (butorphanol) should be considered.

Care should be taken when positioning the patient. Even with optimal positioning such as sternal recumbency with head elevated, or lateral recumbency with the oropharyngeal area elevated, the oropharynx should be surveyed routinely for gastric contents. This is particularly important when the patient is moved repeatedly during anesthesia [325]. If reflux is noted, the oral cavity and esophagus should be cleared immediately, and the esophagus and mouth flushed with warm water followed by gentle suctioning prior to recovery. Intraoperatively, monitoring of oxygenation, ventilation, and thermoregulation should be performed on a regular basis in addition to hemodynamic monitoring tailored to the patient. Pulse oximetry and capnography can be monitored continuously; ideally, blood gas analysis is performed intermittently to verify accuracy and gain further insight into potential impairment of oxygenation in critical patients.

Irrespective of the surgical or diagnostic procedures being performed, addition of local anesthetic techniques should be considered to reduce the reliance on opioid analgesics in the postoperative period. Bilateral maxillary blocks may reduce the need for additional opioid and anesthetic drug use intraoperatively in patients undergoing BOAS-related airway procedures [326,327]. Unfortunately, inadvertent puncture of the maxillary artery resulting in retrobulbar hemorrhage/hematoma is a potential complication of this block [328]. Analgesic adjuncts such as intravenous lidocaine (50 μg/kg/min) and ketamine (10 μg/kg/min) infusions can also be added to opioid infusions to provide additional analgesia and improve intraoperative stability during longer procedures if necessary. Corticosteroids are often administered in patients undergoing airway surgery and may be administered prior to anesthesia or in the perioperative period; however, their use will preclude the administration of NSAIDs for postoperative analgesia because of increased risk of toxicity.

Although there is not extensive objective evidence to support their use, vasoconstrictors such as phenylephrine or oxymetazoline, applied topically in the upper airways, may reduce swelling prior to recovery. Depending on the surgical procedure, a system for delivering oxygen using nasal catheters or prongs may be placed prior to extubation, and oxygen delivered via this route. The routine preplacement of nasotracheal catheters has also been described [283,329]. Normothermia should be achieved prior to initiation of recovery to prevent shivering associated with low body temperature. Although hypothermia is often observed following prolonged anesthesia, hyperthermia should also be avoided during the recovery phase as panting secondary to elevated body temperature can worsen signs of upper airway obstruction in dogs with BOAS.

Recovery from anesthesia is a particularly critical phase in animals with BOAS as most complications related to surgery and anesthesia are observed during this period. Dogs with BOAS who have not had airway surgery are still at increased risk of postoperative complications. Adverse events frequently reported in brachycephalic dogs in the postoperative period include respiratory distress, hypoxemia, prolonged time to extubation, airway obstruction (partial or complete), regurgitation, vomiting, and aspiration [250,264,277,287–289]. The recovery period is particularly challenging in brachycephalic patients following airway surgery due to the associated soft tissue swelling. In some cases where severe airway swelling is present, it is appropriate to place a temporary tracheostomy tube prior to recovery. Potentially life-threatening events, primarily related to the patency of the airway, have been reported up to 24 h postoperatively; therefore, intensive monitoring is currently recommended for at least this period following airway surgery [277]. Having a clean set of orotracheal tubes, laryngoscope, facemask, tracheostomy tubes, and additional short-acting injectable anesthetic available prior to initiation of recovery will permit rapid reestablishment of general anesthesia and a patent airway if necessary. Recovering dogs with BOAS in sternal recumbency following airway suctioning, with their tongue pulled out of the oral cavity, and head and neck slightly elevated, may improve their ability to ventilate with the least amount of respiratory effort. Dogs with BOAS tolerate the presence of an orotracheal tube at greater levels of wakefulness when compared with normal dogs, probably because it provides an unobstructed airway and reduces the work of breathing. Most clinicians recommend discontinuing oxygen supplementation while the patient still has the orotracheal tube in place to verify that an F_IO_2 of 0.21 is tolerated, as judged by the maintenance of oxygen hemoglobin saturation (Fig. 38.34C and D). The orotracheal tube can be maintained in place until the dog shows resistance to the tube by pawing at the mouth or chewing the tube. Immediately following extubation, oxygen supplementation using a facemask or flow-by technique can be provided to increase the F_IO_2 which will help maintain oxygenation if mild hypoventilation or $\dot{V}_A/\dot{Q}$ mismatching are present. Ideally, oxygenation is assessed using arterial blood gas analysis in patients at risk of hypoxemia in recovery; however, if arterial blood gas analysis is not available or feasible during the immediate post-extubation period, pulse oximetry is a suitable alternative as it may still provide additional clinically relevant information during recovery relative to visual observation of mucus membrane color [298]. If an acute decrease in pulse oximetry hemoglobin saturation (SpO_2) to values below 95% and the displayed heart rate matches the pulse rate taken by other means (palpation or blood pressure tracing), a change in management is indicated. While SpO_2/F_IO_2 ratio is advocated for monitoring critically ill patients, an accurate F_IO_2 is generally not available during recovery with either facemask or flow-by oxygen delivery [330,331].

To reduce airway soft tissue swelling postoperatively, systemic corticosteroids such as dexamethasone can be administered unless there are specific contraindications [264,283]. Aerosolized epinephrine has also been shown to improve airflow in BOAS patients, with Pugs showing a greater response relative to Bulldogs [297]. During recovery from anesthesia, caution should be exerted to avoid confusing an animal displaying dysphoric/excitatory behavior associated with opioid administration from an animal that is agitated because of an obstructed airway. If the dog becomes dysphoric, low doses of dexmedetomidine (1–2 μg/kg diluted in saline and slowly titrated to effect) or acepromazine (0.01–0.02 mg/kg) administered intravenously and titrated to effect are effective at calming the patient; however, if the patient cannot achieve adequate airflow, interventions are required immediately. Depending on the facilities and clinician preference, dogs may be placed on non-invasive ventilatory support using HFNOT, CPAP, or following orotracheal intubation, traditional positive-pressure ventilation, for a variable period to wait for airway inflammation to subside [53,62,65,332,333]. Provision of CPAP in animals with

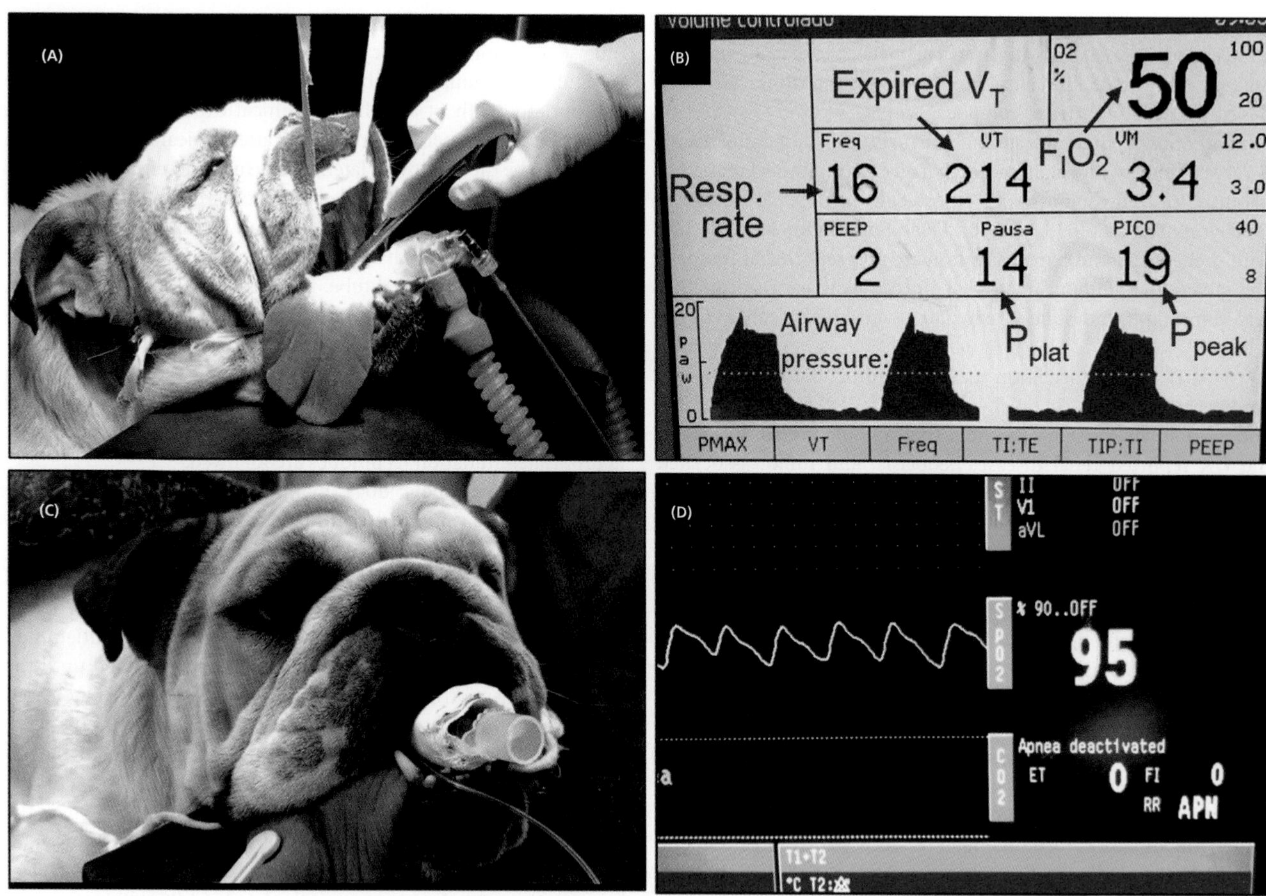

Figure 38.34 **A.** Surgical correction of BOAS in an English Bulldog (body weight 20 kg) that allowed intubation with a 6.5 internal diameter tube. **B.** Anesthesia was maintained with isoflurane and the animal received VCV (target V_T 10 mL/kg) with a 40% inspiratory pause. The large gradient between P_{peak} and P_{plat} (5 mmHg) denotes increased R_{aw}. The C_{RS} [$V_T/(P_{plat}$ – PEEP)] indexed to body weight is low (0.9 mL/cmH_2O/kg) compared to values reported in intermediate-chested dogs (1.3 mL/cmH_2O/kg). Source: Asorey *et al.* [118]. **C.** and **D.** Recovery in sternal recumbency with the endotracheal tube in place and a pulse oximeter in the tongue. Hemoglobin saturation is 95% while animal is breathing ambient air. Notice that the animal is awake (eyes opened) while still intubated and the endotracheal tube is protected by a mouth gag made of soft material to prevent the animal from tearing the tube. VCV, volume-controlled ventilation; V_T, tidal volume; P_{peak}, peak airway pressure; P_{plat}, plateau pressure; R_{aw}, airway resistance; C_{RS}, respiratory system compliance; PEEP, positive end-expired pressure.

inspiratory stridor after orotracheal tube removal may stent the airways open and reduce signs of dyspnea. Helmets, originally developed for non-invasive ventilatory support in humans with respiratory failure, are a potential alternative for providing CPAP and oxygen-enriched air in dogs with signs of upper airway obstruction after orotracheal tube removal. Helmets adjusted to deliver CPAP of 5 cmH_2O with ambient air (F_IO_2 = 0.21) were reported as an effective means of improving arterial oxygenation in healthy dogs recovering from general anesthesia [53]. Computed tomography assessment has shown that a CPAP of 5 cmH_2O provided by a helmet increases the internal diameter of the larynx in normal healthy dogs [334], suggesting that this level of CPAP might reduce inspiratory dyspnea and the work of breathing commonly observed after extubation in dogs with BOAS. HFNOT is another means of increasing F_IO_2 along with low levels of CPAP (up to 5 cmH_2O) that may improve signs of respiratory distress in dogs with BOAS recovering from anesthesia (Fig. 38.4) [56,62].

If means to provide prolonged non-invasive ventilatory support (CPAP) are not available or airway patency does not improve over time, placement of a nasotracheal catheter or tracheostomy tube are alternative option to invasive mechanical ventilation. Tracheostomy tubes, both temporary and permanent, are associated with high complication rates; however, they can provide a useful strategy for short- and long-term management in select cases [335,336].

Feline brachycephalic obstructive airway syndrome

Characteristics and pathophysiology

Brachycephaly is a characteristic of certain feline breeds but substantially less literature exists regarding its impact on the health and welfare of this species relative to the canine [337,338]. To date, there is little information regarding anesthetic morbidity and mortality in cats affected with BOAS. Dyson *et al.* reported a higher anesthetic complication rate in Himalayan cats, a breed characterized by brachycephaly [284]. Persian, Himalayan, British Shorthair, Bernese, Scottish Fold, and Exotic Shorthair cats are considered brachycephalic breeds; however, Persian and Exotic Shorthair are considered extreme brachycephalic breeds with associated severe symptoms related to their altered facial conformation [339]. The reported structural respiratory abnormalities in cats include stenotic nares and abnormal nasal turbinates [251,340,341]. Unlike brachycephalic dogs, an elongated soft palate appears to be very rare in cats [342]. Difficulty breathing, increased respiratory noise, sneezing, decreased airflow, nasal discharge, and reduced activity levels are reported clinical signs associated with brachycephaly in cats [251,340,343]. Surgery to reduce the nasal obstruction to airflow has been described with low rates of complication [344,345].

In addition to the respiratory abnormalities, ophthalmic disease is very common with epiphora, corneal ulceration, corneal sequestra, keratitis, and entropion being reported in a high percentage of brachycephalic cats [338,343,346]. Dental malalignment, difficulty with prehension, and hypersalivation are also reported at frequencies greater than in non-brachycephalic cats, whereas regurgitation and vomiting have not been associated with brachycephaly in the feline [347].

To date, little information exists regarding the prevalence of cardiovascular disease in brachycephalic cats. A report on disorders and mortality in Persian cats under first-opinion veterinary care in the UK reported renal disease, neoplasia, and tumor-associated disorders as the major causes of death; however, the significance of brachycephaly on their cat's overall wellbeing is underappreciated by owners [348].

Management of anesthesia

The major anesthetic concern for brachycephalic feline patients is related to the risk of airway obstruction in the perioperative period. Corneal trauma is also a significant risk due to their facial conformation [346].

Preoperative history, work up, and preparation should be tailored to the individual patient. Like brachycephalic dogs, obtaining a thorough and complete history with client education regarding underlying disease is recommended. Routine patient preanesthetic preparation, including fasting times, is suitable based on the current state of knowledge.

Prior to sedating a brachycephalic cat, the workstation should be set up to include a variety of endotracheal tubes and facemasks. To date, there are no comparative studies evaluating different anesthesia protocols in brachycephalic cats and the associated outcomes. The following recommendations therefore reflect current opinions based on experience and the reader is referred to the literature on general anesthetic management in feline patients [349]. The specific anesthetic protocol should be tailored to the individual patient based on their behavior, underlying disease(s), and proposed surgical intervention. After premedication, cats should be monitored continuously for respiratory obstruction. Preoxygenation will minimize the risk of hypoxemia during oropharyngeal examination and placement of the orotracheal tube. Anticholinergic agents decrease oropharyngeal secretions and may indirectly reduce the incidence of laryngospasm during induction of anesthesia; therefore, they should be considered as part of a preanesthetic protocol if the patient is not receiving an α_2-adrenergic receptor agonist and no other contraindications exist.

To minimize the risk of hypoxemia and laryngospasm during induction of anesthesia brachycephalic cats should be preoxygenated for at least 3 min with a face mask attached to a breathing circuit with the oxygen flowmeter adjusted to deliver a high flow rate (> 200 mL/kg/min). Intravenous agents such as propofol or alfaxalone are suitable anesthetic induction agents as they have the advantage of being rapid acting with a short duration of effect, which permits titration to a suitable anesthetic depth of anesthesia to permit intubation. Actual doses of intravenous anesthetics will depend on the level of sedation/CNS depression achieved after premedication and on the severity of systemic disease if present. Topical administration of 2% lidocaine (0.1 mL) to the arytenoid cartilages should be performed while visualizing the larynx with a laryngoscope and the face mask repositioned while the anesthesiologist waits for the latency period of topical lidocaine. Attempts at intubation should only be performed once the patient is at an appropriate depth of anesthesia. Clinical experience dictates that intubation can be performed 45–60 s after topical lidocaine, which appears to be the minimum latency to achieve desensitization of the arytenoids. In the event of a failed intubation (e.g., due to anatomical abnormalities), the anesthesiologist may attempt to pass a small semi-rigid stylet through the arytenoids and use it as a guide for inserting the endotracheal tube. If the cat develops laryngospasm, the depth of anesthesia should be evaluated, and additional anesthetic administered if required before subsequent attempts at intubation are repeated. Use of rocuronium (1 mg/kg) was reported to reverse severe laryngospasm and produce appropriate conditions for intubation in a cat [350], although this is rarely required if appropriate intubation techniques are followed.

As in brachycephalic dogs, maintenance of anesthesia can be achieved using a variety of techniques. General principles of reducing the need for intra- and postoperative opioid analgesics by incorporating local anesthetic techniques may offer the advantage of reducing respiratory depression during recovery. Careful swabbing/suctioning of the airway should be performed prior to initiation of recovery and intensive monitoring should be performed until the cat is showing control of the head and airflow is such that increased inspiratory effort is not causing patient distress. To prevent laryngospasm during recovery from anesthesia, extubation in the cat should not be delayed as is practiced in the dog. Positioning the cat in sternal or lateral recumbency with the tongue extended out of the oral cavity and the mouth open following extubation often provides optimal airflow until the animal has regained greater control of laryngeal muscles. In some cases, the head may need manual support to prevent closing of the mouth. Supplemental oxygen should be provided in the early post-extubation phase using a facemask or by placing the cat in an oxygen-enriched environment. In non-intubated, spontaneously breathing cats anesthetized with an injectable regimen (intramuscular dexmedetomidine, ketamine, and buprenorphine), non-invasive ventilatory support provided by a helmet adjusted to deliver a CPAP of 5 cmH_2O with an F_IO_2 of 0.21 improved arterial oxygen levels [351]. However, currently, there are no studies evaluating the benefits and feasibility of CPAP and oxygen supplementation provided by helmets in cats with BOAS recovering from general anesthesia. Patients that have undergone airway surgery may benefit from postoperative overnight hospitalization with observation due to possible airway swelling; however, there are no large-scale studies reporting details related to complications following upper airway surgery in cats.

Canine laryngeal paralysis

Characteristics and pathophysiology

The upper respiratory tract, including the larynx, provides most of the resistance to airflow at rest in the normal animal due to the rapid (relative to that in lower airways) and turbulent airflow as described in Chapter 37 [352]. Laryngeal dysfunction can dramatically increase the resistance to breathing by reducing airway radius and, when disease is bilateral, it can lead to complete airway obstruction. During inspiration, contraction of the paired *cricoarytenoideus dorsalis muscle* normally abducts the arytenoid cartilages and vocal folds, thereby widening the glottis. During swallowing, the arytenoid cartilages are adducted, and the vocal folds are brought together though contraction of several internal laryngeal muscles to prevent aspiration of material into the trachea.

The caudal laryngeal nerve, a terminal branch of the recurrent laryngeal nerve arising from the vagus nerve in the thorax, innervates all intrinsic muscles of the larynx except for the *cricothyroideus muscle*, which is innervated by the cranial laryngeal nerve, arising from the vagus nerve in the proximal cervical region.

Congenital and acquired laryngeal paralysis have been described in the canine [353,354]. A hereditary mode of transmission has been reported in numerous breeds [353–355]. Acquired laryngeal paralysis can result from damage to the neural control of the larynx (central or peripheral lesions involving the nerves innervating the larynx), disease affecting the laryngeal muscles, or neuromuscular junction disorders [354]. For dogs in which a specific etiology is not identified, the condition has historically been referred to as "idiopathic laryngeal paralysis." At present, Labrador Retrievers, Golden Retrievers, Newfoundlands, Irish Setters, and Brittany Spaniels are the most common breeds affected with acquired laryngeal paralysis of unknown cause [354]. More recently, it has been recognized that, for many dogs, the disease is progressive with generalized signs becoming evident as the dog ages. "Laryngeal paralysis" associated with "generalized polyneuropathy," "late-onset laryngeal paralysis," or "geriatric-onset laryngeal paralysis polyneuropathy syndrome" are terms that are currently used to identify the disease in dogs with progressive generalized disease [354,356].

Irrespective of the etiology, laryngeal paralysis is characterized by impaired abduction and adduction of the arytenoid cartilages and vocal folds, either unilaterally or bilaterally resulting in the vocal cords assuming a paramedian position. Clinical signs of laryngeal paralysis may include a change in phonation (bark), coughing, dysphagia, or gagging, increased inspiratory sounds, decreased exercise tolerance, respiratory distress, cyanosis, hyperthermia, and collapse [354]. Dogs are generally more severely affected in hot weather and during or immediately after exercise; however, the severity of symptoms associated with laryngeal paralysis can vary tremendously [354]. Hypoxemia can be marked in severely affected dogs with only minor changes in $PaCO_2$ levels. Hypoventilation (elevated $PaCO_2$) may be the underlying cause of impaired oxygenation and cyanosis in some cases; however, pneumonia secondary to aspiration or negative-pressure pulmonary edema caused by upper airway obstruction may also contribute to hypoxemia by increasing the diffusion barrier for oxygen at the alveolar–capillary level, $\dot{V}_A/\dot{Q}$ mismatching, and/or intrapulmonary shunting. As mentioned, several other conditions may be responsible for acquired laryngeal paralysis and dogs may have other clinically significant diseases related to their primary condition. For example, generalized polyneuropathy may be present and may be detected on neurological examination. Esophageal dysmotility is present in many cases with late-onset idiopathic laryngeal paralysis and may manifest as gastroesophageal reflux, regurgitation, and/or aspiration pneumonia [357].

Clinical diagnosis of laryngeal paralysis is made based on laryngeal examination performed under heavy sedation or light planes of general anesthesia. Examination may involve direct visual examination and/or video-endoscopy. A lack of abduction of arytenoid cartilages during inspiration, laxity of the vocal cords, and edema of the corniculate processes are supportive of the diagnosis [358]. Experimentally, insufflation of CO_2 to stimulate respiration with assessment of laryngeal function using video-endoscopy through a laryngeal mask airway has been demonstrated to be effective in dogs with surgically created laryngeal paralysis [359]. As will be discussed, anesthesia can influence the assessment of laryngeal paralysis by inhibiting abduction of arytenoid cartilages and leading to a false positive diagnosis.

Medical management including patient weight loss, anti-inflammatory medication, and exercise restriction is recommended for patients with unilateral laryngeal paralysis and/or mild clinical signs. When laryngeal paralysis is bilateral and/or symptoms impact a dog's quality of life, surgery is recommended. Results may vary with the underlying etiology of the disease, breed, and comorbidities [356,360]. Unilateral arytenoid lateralization is the technique most used currently as it has been shown to improve the quality of life in dogs with significant presurgical symptoms [251,354,356,360–363]. The most common postsurgical complication is aspiration pneumonia [361,362,364]. Rates of aspiration pneumonia of 18.6, 31.8, and 31.8% at 1, 3, and 4 years postoperatively were reported in a large retrospective study of 232 dogs having unilateral arytenoid lateralization [364]. In this study, factors predisposing to aspiration included esophageal disease and use of opioids postoperatively [364].

Management of anesthesia

The presence of underlying respiratory disease that could predispose the patient to hypoxemia, the potential for impaired airway patency, and the risk of regurgitation and aspiration are the major anesthetic concerns for patients with laryngeal paralysis in the perioperative period. As with patients with BOAS, the surgical location makes anesthetic monitoring of patient's depth of anesthesia using jaw tone or eye reflexes more challenging. Surgical location also poses a potentially greater risk of unobserved regurgitation and disconnection or obstruction of the anesthetic breathing circuit.

A thorough history including exercise tolerance, concurrent diseases, previous anesthetics, and current medications is required. A physical examination including in-depth examination of the respiratory and neurological systems is indicated. As discussed, many patients have an associated progressive generalized neurological disease. Megaesophagus, myasthenia gravis, hypothyroidism, or neoplasia should be considered as possible concurrent conditions [354]. CBC, serum biochemical profile, urinalysis, thyroid function screening, and thoracic radiographs are considered standard in mature patients. Further diagnostic procedures such as video fluoroscopy and measurement of serum antibodies against acetylcholine receptors to test for canine myasthenia gravis may be indicated based on examination and preliminary diagnostic test results.

Information to support a change in routine fasting times for patients undergoing general anesthesia to diagnose and/or treat laryngeal paralysis does not exist; therefore, a standard fasting period is recommended. Medical management prior to anesthesia to reduce the risk of aspiration pneumonia and/or gastrointestinal complications includes antiemetics such as maropitant, proton pump inhibitors, and prokinetics [300]. Maropitant administered 30 min to 1 h prior to preanesthetic medication has consistently been shown to reduce the incidence of vomiting following preanesthetic administration in healthy dogs [303,305,306]. The prokinetic cisapride has been demonstrated to increase lower esophageal pressure and reduce gastroesophageal reflux in normal dogs [302,365]. It was also shown to reduce the incidence of aspiration in clinical patients having unilateral arytenoid lateralization in one relatively small study using historical controls [366]. In the latter study, a total dose of 1 mg/kg of cisapride was administered by an intravenous infusion over approximately 90 min prior to surgery (increasing doses based on response to infusion). Of 50 dogs receiving cisapride, three had reported adverse clinical signs during the infusion; however, no further adverse effects were reported. Metoclopramide, another prokinetic, has had variable results on outcomes in dogs, with one study demonstrating a reduction in gastroesophageal reflux while others have shown no impact on gastroesophageal reflux or regurgitation and aspiration [364,367,368]. To date, evidence to support routine administration of metoclopramide in patients with the goal of reducing regurgitation and aspiration is lacking [300,354,368].

Preoxygenation is recommended prior to and during anesthetic induction to prevent hypoxemia during laryngeal examination. Numerous studies, as recently reviewed by Ranninger *et al.* [369], have been performed to determine the best anesthetic protocol to permit assessment of laryngeal function by direct visualization or video laryngoscopy. Direct comparison between studies is challenging due to differences in study design, study population, drug doses, and drug administration techniques; however, in general, premedication has been shown to be beneficial. This is potentially due to reduced doses of injectable anesthetics subsequently required to facilitate examination. The use of hydromorphone or morphine is not recommended in patients with laryngeal dysfunction because opioid-induced vomiting may increase the risk of aspiration. However, methadone, butorphanol, or buprenorphine are frequently used and have not been shown to have a deleterious effect on outcomes. Recently, dexmedetomidine alone or in combination with butorphanol or hydromorphone was shown to permit assessment of laryngeal function by video laryngoscopy in normal dogs [370]. Specifically, following an initial dose of dexmedetomidine (3 μg/kg IV), administered alone or in combination with an opioid (0.3 mg/kg of butorphanol or 0.1 mg/kg of hydromorphone), additional dexmedetomidine (2 μg/kg doses) was administered (up to a maximum of 15 μg/kg) to prevent jaw movement and permit evaluation of the laryngeal function before and after intravenous doxapram administration (1 mg/kg) [370]. Although no complications related to vomiting and aspiration pneumonia were reported after dexmedetomidine/hydromorphone in this study, it is still advisable to avoid this opioid in dogs with laryngeal dysfunction. Vomiting is commonly observed after dexmedetomidine in cats and emesis may also occur following this drug in canine species and this possibility should be considered by the anesthesiologist as it could lead to aspiration pneumonia in animals with laryngeal paralysis.

In terms of anesthetic induction agents, thiopental was shown to be superior to other injectable agents in early studies evaluating impact on laryngeal function; however, it is not readily available and propofol has consistently been shown to be a suitable alternative [371–373]. When alfaxalone has been compared to propofol, the results have been variable with some showing equivalency while others report a greater negative impact on laryngeal function relative to propofol [371,372,374–376]. Laryngeal function was shown to be superior after a period of anesthesia maintained with isoflurane following induction with propofol or alfaxalone relative to that observed immediately following induction of anesthesia with either intravenous agent, although maintenance of anesthesia with an injectable regimen was not evaluated [377]. While assessment could be delayed for a period after induction with injectables and orotracheal intubation, the impact of intubation prior to assessment of laryngeal function is unknown and the potential for environmental contamination with inhalant agents should be considered. Doxapram, a CNS stimulant, transiently increases respiratory rate and V_T in dogs and has been administered intravenously at 0.25 to 2.5 mg/kg to improve the assessment of laryngeal function in dogs [370,372,376,378,379] (Fig. 38.35). As laryngeal obstruction may worsen following administration of doxapram in dogs with laryngeal dysfunction, the team should be prepared to quickly intervene in this scenario [369,378]. Other reported side effects of doxapram include tachycardia, hypertension, arrhythmias, muscle rigidity, hyperthermia, and seizures; however, these would appear to be rare events as they have not been reported in canine clinical trials [369].

Following orotracheal intubation, anesthesia is generally maintained with an inhalant anesthetic and adjunctive agents such as systemically administered lidocaine and opioids when required to achieve adequate analgesia and to decrease inhalant anesthetic concentrations. As for patients undergoing BOAS-related surgery, butorphanol, buprenorphine, or methadone are commonly recommended analgesic agents with hydromorphone and morphine being considered unsuitable due to their association with vomiting and regurgitation. Use of NSAIDs should be based on the individual's history of corticosteroid use and gastrointestinal status. Prior to discontinuing anesthesia, the oropharyngeal region should be carefully examined and suctioned to remove any excess fluid. It is important that the patient is normothermic to prevent shivering or panting during recovery. Preplacement of a nasal oxygen catheter prior to recovery should be considered in patients with underlying lower airway or pulmonary parenchymal disease that may require

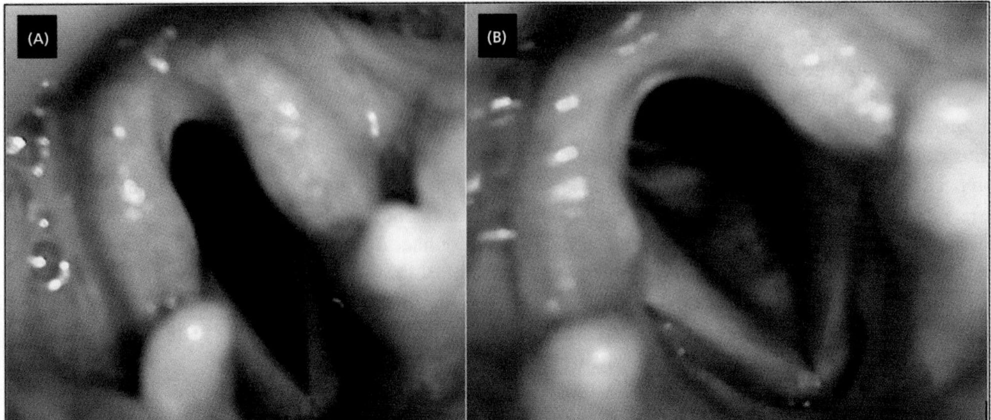

Figure 38.35 **A.** Abduction of the arytenoid cartilages prior to administration of doxapram in a dog sedated with dexmedetomidine. **B.** Maximal abduction of the arytenoid cartilages on inspiration of the same dog after intravenous doxapram administration (1 mg/kg). Source: DeGroot *et al.* [370], with permission from John Wiley & Sons, Inc.

oxygen supplementation. Patients are generally recovered in lateral recumbency with the laryngeal region elevated. Sedation may be required during recovery and low doses of acepromazine (0.02 mg/kg) or dexmedetomidine (1 μg/kg, titrated to effect) are generally effective if there are no specific contraindications. Intensive monitoring should continue for 12–24 h postoperatively to permit rapid interventions should regurgitation and aspiration occur.

Canine tracheal collapse

Characteristics and pathophysiology

Narrowing of the tracheal lumen can occur from numerous causes, including trauma, intraluminal tracheal masses, compressive extraluminal masses, tracheal hypoplasia, and tracheomalacia. The most common form of tracheal collapse is characterized by softened tracheal rings resulting in dorsoventral flattening of the trachea with collapse of the dorsal tracheal membrane, which may be weakened or redundant, into the tracheal lumen. The extrathoracic (cervical) or intrathoracic trachea or both may be affected as well as the bronchial walls [380]. Although less common, malformed tracheal rings, with cartilage that deviates dorsally into the trachea into what is described as a W shape, are also present in some dogs [381]. The underlying cause of tracheal collapse is unknown; however, it is likely multifactorial and may vary with the specific characteristics (malformation versus tracheomalacia). Based on breed prevalence, genetic factors likely play a role in combination with infectious and environmental contributions. Breeds most affected by tracheal collapse are toy or small breeds including Yorkshire Terriers, Pomeranians, Toy Poodles, Chihuahuas, Maltese, and Pugs [381].

Clinical signs may develop at any age; however, most studies report onset at 6–8 years of age [381]. Coughing, which is often described as "goose-honking," gagging, stridor, reduced exercise tolerance, and dyspnea are commonly reported clinical signs [381]. The severity of disease on presentation for veterinary examination can vary tremendously with some dogs appearing normal on physical examination. In these dogs, gentle tracheal palpation can generally elicit a cough. Other dogs may present on an emergency basis with severe dyspnea and cyanosis. The location of the tracheal collapse will impact the timing of the obstruction to airflow observed on physical examination. In dogs with dysfunction of the cervical portion of the trachea, the negative airway pressure generated during inspiration causes dynamic collapse of the airway. If the intrathoracic portion of the airway is affected, the dynamic collapse will be observed during forced exhalation, such as occurs during coughing. Dogs with cervical tracheal obstruction therefore present with an increase in inspiratory effort while dogs with thoracic tracheal disease exhibit abnormal signs during expiration. Many dogs are affected at multiple locations and therefore exhibit signs of dyspnea during inspiration and expiration [382]. Laryngeal paralysis has been documented as a complicating factor in up to 30% of cases with tracheal collapse [383]. Bronchomalacia, small airway disease, and pneumonia are also present in approximately 20% of dogs with tracheal collapse. Chronic inflammation and impaired mucociliary clearance likely contribute to the lower airway disease. Pulmonary function testing may be available to further characterize the respiratory obstruction but is not routinely available.

Other comorbidities reported in dogs with tracheal collapse include obesity, cardiomegaly, pulmonary hypertension, mitral valve disease, hepatomegaly, and endocrinopathies [381,384]. A causal association between tracheal collapse and the mentioned comorbidities has not been established and concurrent diagnosis likely reflects the age and breed predisposition for cardiovascular and endocrine disease in these dogs.

Diagnosis of tracheal collapse is based on physical examination, diagnostic imaging, and tracheobronchoscopy [381]. Fluoroscopic examination of patients while awake is preferred to radiographic examination due to the dynamic nature of the collapse. Computed tomography if available may also provide additional information regarding the severity and extent of airway dysfunction. During tracheobronchoscopy, a bronchoalveolar lavage may be performed to characterize the extent of lower airway disease.

Medical management of tracheal collapse, which is regarded as palliative not curative, involves multimodal therapy aimed at reducing inflammation and the predisposition for coughing. Antitussives, anti-inflammatories (steroidal drugs), anxiolytics, bronchodilators, and antibiotics are often prescribed based on the patient's severity of disease following diagnostic work up. In addition to medical management, interventions currently recommended in some patients include extraluminal tracheal prostheses or intraluminal stent placement. General anesthesia is typically required for both a thorough diagnostic work up and for therapeutic interventions. Patients with a confirmed or suspected diagnosis of tracheal collapse may also be anesthetized for non-airway-related reasons (e.g., dental or abdominal procedures).

Outcomes and mean survival times of dogs presenting with varying severity of disease and subsequent medical and/or interventional surgical management have been reported [382,384–387]. In general, the disease is progressive but dogs presenting with mild-to-moderate clinical signs show an improvement in clinical symptoms with medical management while dogs with severe clinical symptoms, as judged by respiratory noise, coughing, and dyspnea, have a superior outcome when managed with an intervention such extraluminal prosthesis or intratracheal stent placement. Perioperative mortality following extraluminal prosthesis is reported to occur in approximately 5% of cases [385,387]. The reported rate of major complications following extraluminal prosthesis or intratracheal stent placement is approximately 40%. Tracheal tears, laryngeal paralysis, and pneumonia are reported with extraluminal repair and stent fracture, while tissue ingrowth, progressive tracheal collapse, and stent dislodgement are reported following intraluminal stent placement [382,385,387].

Management of anesthesia

The potential for impaired airway patency leading to marked increases in R_{aw} and the work of breathing, stimulation of the cough reflex, and augmentation of hypoxemia due to underlying respiratory disease are the major anesthetic concerns for patients with tracheal collapse in the perioperative period. In patients undergoing intraluminal stenting, the need to share the airway during the stent placement and to prevent post-procedural coughing are aspects that require consideration. For patients with pre-existing laryngeal dysfunction and those patients developing postsurgical laryngeal paralysis, strategies to minimize risks discussed in the laryngeal paralysis section are applicable.

Physical examination, CBC, biochemistry profile, urinalysis, thoracic radiographs, as well as imaging performed to characterize the tracheal disease, should be performed prior to anesthesia. Auscultation of the upper airways should be included during the physical examination to screen for laryngeal disease. Further cardiovascular diagnostic tests such as ECG and cardiac ultrasound should be recommended based on the physical examination and thoracic radiographic results. Patients should be maintained on their medical management regimen up to the perioperative period to minimize coughing and inflammation of the airways. As noted above, general anesthesia to permit tracheobronchoscopy and/or airway sample collection (tracheal wash or bronchoalveolar lavage) may be performed prior to stent placement. During the exam, the degree and location of airway collapse can be assessed (Fig. 38.36). After careful planning and treatment of underlying conditions, animals may undergo a second anesthetic procedure for placement of an intraluminal stent or placement of external ring prostheses (Fig. 38.37) [388].

In addition to the standard workstation and monitoring equipment set up, endotracheal tubes with embedded radiopaque markings in various sizes and lengths should be available when intraluminal stent placement is planned. Equipment to permit oxygen insufflation during tracheobronchoscopy should be available as discussed above (Anesthesia for bronchoscopy).

To date, there are no studies comparing outcomes with different protocols in patients undergoing diagnostic or therapeutic procedures related to tracheal collapse. Due to their antitussive properties, opioid analgesics are routinely included with low doses of sedative agents in the premedication regimen. Butorphanol provides adequate analgesia for minimally invasive procedures (endoluminal stent placement); however, when more invasive procedures such as extraluminal prosthesis placement are planned, a μ-opioid receptor agonist such as methadone is recommended for perioperative analgesia. Adding an anticholinergic to the premedication is recommended if there are no contraindications as airway secretions, which can elicit coughing, will be reduced.

Preoxygenation and upper airway examination should be performed before intubation. As in patients with BOAS or laryngeal paralysis, the intravenous agents propofol or alfaxalone are suitable anesthetic induction agents. Lidocaine administered intravenously at 1–2 mg/kg intravenously prior to or during anesthetic induction with propofol or alfaxalone with subsequent intubation has variable impact on the frequency of coughing [389–392]. In dogs premedicated with methadone or acepromazine, lidocaine at 1.5–2 mg/kg was reported to reduce the incidence of cough while dogs that had dexmedetomidine included in the premedication prior to 2 mg/kg of lidocaine did not demonstrate a reduced incidence of coughing [389,390]. Importantly, the incidence of cough reported in dogs receiving lidocaine systemically at induction ranges from 7 to 52% [389–393]. Fentanyl administered at 7 μg/kg IV was shown to be superior to 2 mg/kg lidocaine IV at suppressing cough in dogs receiving alfaxalone for induction of anesthesia; however, 9% of dogs were reported to have coughed during intubation [393]. In methadone-premedicated dogs where endotracheal intubation was performed after achieving a moderate plane of anesthesia (propofol titrated to abolish the medial palpebral reflex), co-administration of lidocaine (2 mg/kg IV) resulted in a relatively low incidence of coughing (7%) [390]. Anesthetic induction with propofol alone (43% incidence of coughing) increased the likelihood of coughing during endotracheal intubation by 10 times in comparison to propofol and IV lidocaine [390]. Although no studies have been completed to date in dogs with tracheal collapse, for those dogs who have a history of coughing, recommendations include ensuring antitussives are continued prior to anesthesia, opioid analgesics are included in the premedication regimen, intubation is performed at a moderate depth of anesthesia (injectable titrated until loss of medial palpebral reflex), and lidocaine 1.5–2.0 mg/kg is administered as part of the induction protocol.

During airway examination and endoluminal stent placement, maintenance of anesthesia with injectable agents (propofol or alfaxalone), administered as boluses or as an intravenous infusion, will reduce the potential for environmental contamination as maintaining a sealed airway with no leaks is difficult with inhalant anesthetics. For patients with tracheal collapse that are undergoing extraluminal stent placement or procedures unrelated to the airway, maintenance of anesthesia with an inhalant anesthetic regimen is suitable with ventilatory support provided as required. Ideally, spontaneous breathing is maintained during anesthesia for endoluminal stent placement as there may be periods when positive-pressure ventilation is not feasible. In patients with cervical tracheal collapse undergoing endoluminal stent placement through the endotracheal tube, the endotracheal tube can be extended

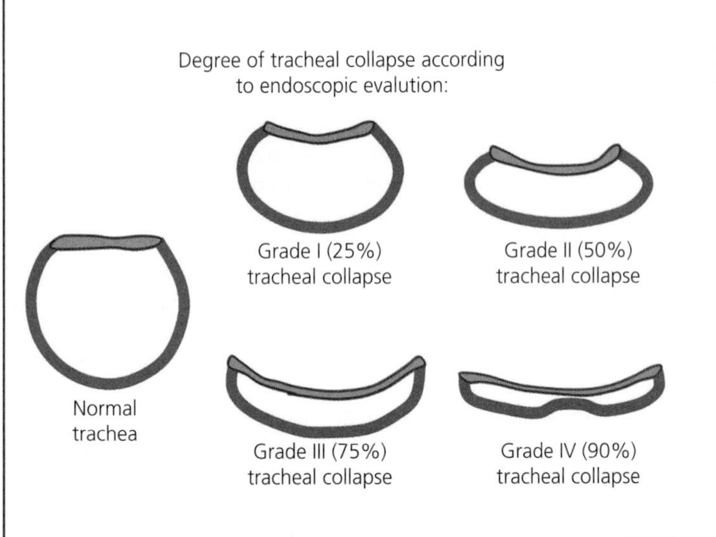

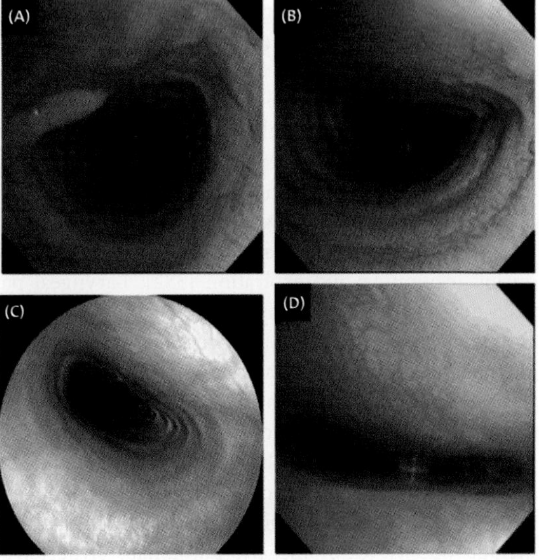

Figure 38.36 Classification of severity of tracheal collapse based on lumen reduction assessed by endoscopy/bronchoscopy. **A.** Grade I (25% loss of tracheal lumen). **B.** Grade II (50% loss of tracheal lumen). **C.** Grade III (75% loss of tracheal lumen). **D.** Grade IV (90% or nearly complete loss of tracheal lumen). Source: Reproduced from Tappin *et al.* [388], with permission from John Wiley & Sons, Inc.

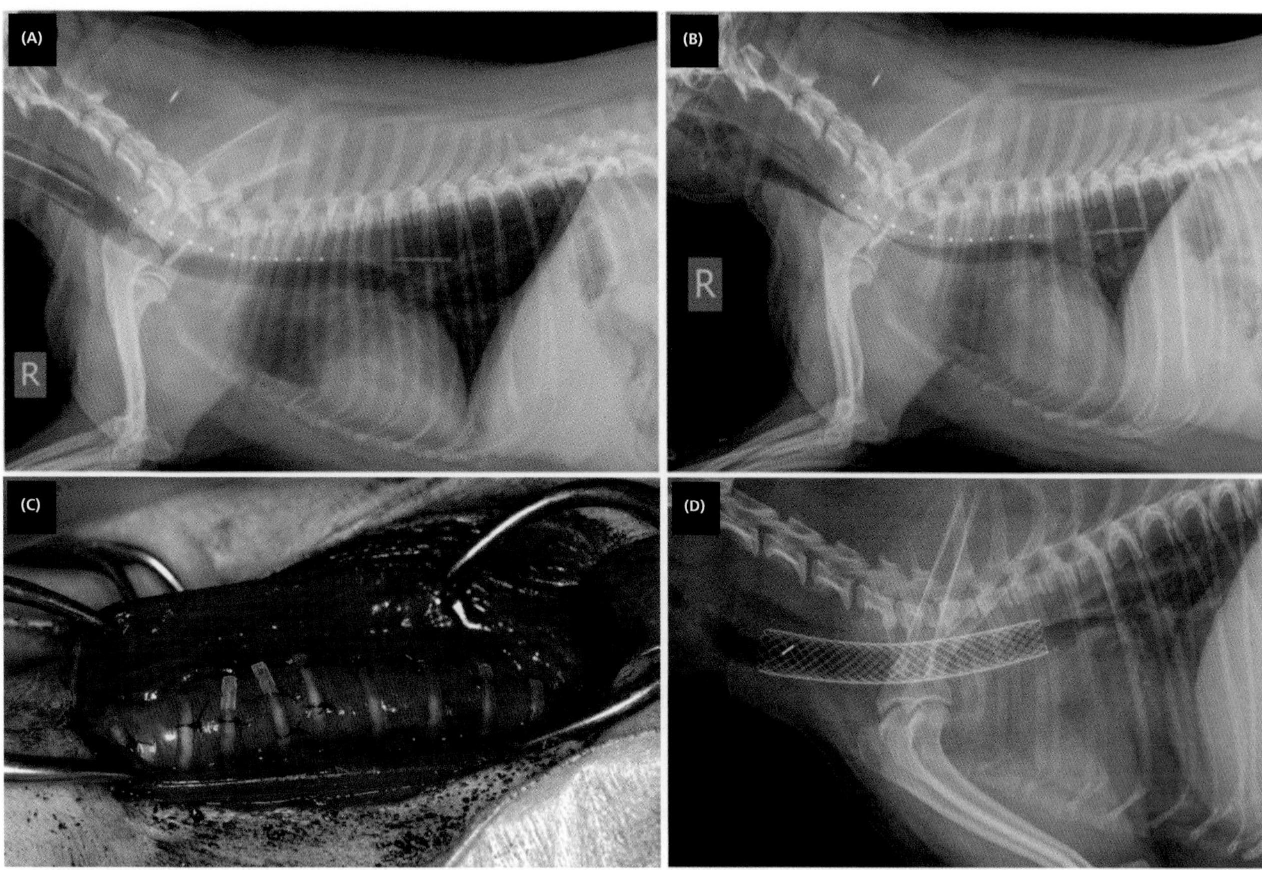

Figure 38.37 Radiographic assessment of tracheal collapse in an anesthetized animal (top images) and treatment options that involve general anesthesia in dogs (bottom images). **A.** The radiographic image seems normal when taken during a positive-pressure breath (20 cmH_2O) applied during inspiration, which can be achieved by squeezing the reservoir bag with the pop-off (APL) valve closed. **B.** In contrast, the radiographic image taken at the end of expiration shows tracheal collapse across the thoracic inlet. This animal would benefit from PEEP administration during anesthesia to minimize tracheal collapse throughout the ventilatory cycle, except during radiographic assessment of tracheal collapse. **C.** External ring prostheses placed to support a collapsing trachea. **D.** A tapered tracheal stent placed in an 11-year-old female Yorkshire terrier that also presented with bilateral bronchial collapse. Source: Reproduced from Tappin *et al.* [388], with permission from John Wiley & Sons, Inc.

beyond the collapsed region if feasible initially, with subsequent repositioning performed using fluoroscopy [394]. If the latter is not available, the endotracheal tube can be inserted to the level of the third rib as a guide. Alternatively, the procedure may be performed with the endotracheal tube placed just beyond the larynx [394]. Lubricant should be placed on the tube and gentle cuff inflation should be performed to minimize tracheal irritation which may predispose the patient to coughing during recovery. When tracheal procedures are being performed, the potential development of a pneumothorax should be considered if deterioration in ventilation or oxygenation develops.

Irrespective of the procedure undertaken, prior to anesthetic recovery, the airway should be examined and carefully suctioned to remove excess fluid or debris. Avoiding excitement and coughing in addition to ensuring analgesia is critical during recovery. Low doses of sedatives such as acepromazine (0.01 mg/kg) or dexmedetomidine (1 μg/kg) can facilitate a smooth recovery. Butorphanol is a suitable postoperative analgesic when minimally invasive procedures such as bronchoscopy or endoluminal tracheal stenting are occurring or when local anesthesia can be included in the protocol. Invasive procedures such as extraluminal stent placement require the use of opioid analgesics with greater analgesic efficacy such as methadone. Including NSAIDs in the perioperative analgesic regimen if no contraindications exist (for example, concurrent corticosteroids) is recommended. Oxygen supplementation may be required during anesthetic recovery. The technique used can be tailored to the individual patient needs and resources available. As patients are generally small, an oxygen-enriched environment created with an oxygen hood or cage is often suitable. Patients with tracheal collapse that are recovering from anesthesia but have not undergone airway stabilization techniques may require oxygen supplementation during recovery. In severe cases, nasotracheal catheterization and/or emergency stent placement may be indicated.

Equine guttural pouch disease

Guttural pouches are extensions of the Eustachian tubes which connect the pharynx to the middle ear. Of domesticated veterinary species, the equine is the only species with guttural pouches. In the adult horse, each pouch is approximately 500 mL in volume with medial and lateral compartments. The pouches communicate with the pharynx via a pharyngeal orifice located in the lateral and caudal aspect of the pharynx, rostral and ventral to the dorsal pharyngeal recess. The maxillary artery, internal and external carotid arteries, and cranial nerves VII, IX, X, XI, and XII as well as the mandibular nerve (branch of cranial nerve V), the sympathetic trunk, and cranial cervical ganglion are either located in or adjacent to the guttural pouches and can be affected by the primary disease or have the potential to be damaged during interventions involving the guttural pouches.

Equine guttural pouch tympany

Characteristics and pathophysiology Distention of the guttural pouch, referred to as "tympany," is generally reported in foals in the first few weeks of life [395–400]. Arabian and Paint horse foals are overrepresented in some regions; however, the condition has been reported in a variety of breeds, including Warmbloods, Thoroughbreds, Standardbreds, and Quarter horses [395–400]. Causes of the condition include alteration of the structure of the pharyngeal opening of the pouch such that it acts as a one-way valve to capture air and fluid within the pouch, upper airway inflammation, persistent coughing, or pharyngeal muscle dysfunction [401]. The condition is usually unilateral but can be bilateral and is more common in fillies than colts. A hereditary link has been established in some breeds [401].

On physical examination, there is usually marked tympanic distention noted in the parotid region that is nonpainful on palpation. Both sides can be affected even with unilateral disease as one pouch may encroach medially on the other side. Stridor can range from mild to severe depending on the degree of airway obstruction. Severe distention can result in dyspnea and dysphagia, with secondary aspiration pneumonia and empyema of the guttural pouches. Diagnosis is performed by radiographic and endoscopic examination of the pharynx and guttural pouches.

Initial patient management generally involves decompressing the pouches by placing a catheter into the pharyngeal opening, a procedure performed using endoscopy. Many patients can be managed medically with an indwelling catheter placed into the affected pouch; however, surgery may be required in some cases [401]. Traditional surgical techniques include creating a connection between the affected and non-affected pouches, altering the opening of the guttural pouch into the pharynx on the affected side, or creating a new opening into the pharynx with the foal under general anesthesia in dorsal or lateral recumbency. Alternatively, a minimally invasive approach using transendoscopic electrocautery or laser can be used. The latter may be performed with the foal under general anesthesia or sedation [395,396,399]. Overall, success following surgical interventions is high, although repeat surgeries are frequently required to achieve complete resolution of the condition [399,401].

Management of sedation and/or general anesthesia In addition to standard perioperative concerns related to sedation and general anesthesia, concerns for foals with guttural pouch tympany relate to underlying respiratory disease, and potential development of further compromise of upper airway airflow during the perioperative period. Intraoperative damage to vessels with subsequent hemorrhage or nerve injury is possible due to the location of major vessels and nerves in the surgical field [397,401].

A standard history, including determination of current medications and information regarding the degree of respiratory compromise and prior anesthetic events should be obtained. Preanesthetic diagnostic work up in foals presenting with tympany should include a thorough physical examination, CBC, biochemistry profile, and radiographs of the pharyngeal region and thorax. Endoscopy is generally performed as part of the diagnostic plan. In most cases, surgery is not undertaken in the first few weeks of life; however, if surgery is required in this period, serum IgG should be measured to ensure adequacy of passive transfer of antibodies. In foals with clinical signs related to pneumonia (fever, increased respiratory effort, and/or impaired gas exchange), medical management should be initiated, and if required, general anesthesia scheduled after resolution of pneumonia. Alternatively, surgery could be performed under sedation if feasible.

Preoperative medications routinely administered include NSAIDs such as flunixin meglumine in addition to antimicrobials. An intravenous catheter should be placed to facilitate sedative and analgesic administration. Sedation with xylazine and butorphanol has been reported to provide adequate conditions for surgery with laser in some foals [395,396]. In patients undergoing general anesthesia, surgery is ideally scheduled when the foal is not compromised due to underlying pulmonary disease as previously mentioned. Medical management, including decompression of the pouches using indwelling catheters, can be considered while the patient is stabilized. Immediately prior to general anesthesia, decompression of tympany is recommended if pharyngeal distention is creating upper airway obstruction. For cases undergoing general anesthesia, preoxygenation is recommended prior to induction of general anesthesia if the foal has any pulmonary parenchymal disease. This can be achieved using nasal catheters or a facemask connected to the anesthetic breathing circuit once the foal is sedated and manually restrained. Sedation can be accomplished with either a benzodiazepine (midazolam or diazepam) or an α_2-adrenergic receptor agonist based on the patient's age and hemodynamic status [402]. Injectable anesthetic induction techniques (ketamine or propofol titrated to effect) are recommended over inhalational agents alone as the latter has been associated with a higher morbidity in foals [403]. Maintenance of anesthesia can be achieved through a variety of techniques including injectable, inhalant, or a combination of techniques [398,399]. Opioids are typically used to provide intraoperative analgesia. Monitoring of cardiovascular and respiratory function throughout anesthesia is ideally performed with ECG, direct blood pressure monitoring, capnography, and pulse oximetry measured continuously, with intermittent arterial blood gas analysis. As the surgical site is located near the head, the intra-arterial catheter can be placed in the lateral metatarsal artery to facilitate monitoring of blood pressure and sampling for gas analysis. Monitoring of body temperature and use of warming devices to prevent hypothermia are also recommended along with standard fluid therapy protocols. Postoperative analgesia with an opioid analgesic in combination with an NSAID is standard while corticosteroid administration may be required in some cases to reduce soft tissue swelling [398–401]. Respiratory obstruction is generally minimal following surgery, however, an orotracheal tube can be maintained until the foal is standing to minimize the risk of inadequate airflow during recovery.

Equine guttural pouch mycosis

Characteristics and pathophysiology Mycotic infection located within the guttural pouches can affect horses at any age but the factors that predispose a horse to developing an infection are unknown. [401]. *Aspergillus* is the most common fungus associated with the condition. Lesions are typically located on the dorsal wall of the guttural pouch and in most cases the disease is unilateral. Clinical signs arise due to secondary mycotic erosion of tissues, including nerves and vessels within and adjacent to the pouches. Epistaxis is the most commonly reported clinical sign, however, cranial nerve damage resulting in dysphagia, which may present as coughing or nasal discharge with particulate food material and/or aspiration pneumonia is also reported either in isolation or with epistaxis. Other clinical signs resulting from cranial nerve injury include laryngeal hemiplegia, facial paralysis, and Horner's syndrome. Pain in the head and cranial cervical region may be present. Radiographs may reveal fluid in the guttural pouches. Definitive diagnosis is generally determined by endoscopy.

The infection can spontaneously resolve, however, the mortality associated with guttural pouch mycosis is high in horses with epistaxis due to hemorrhage. Medical management involves treating the fungal infection with oral and topical antifungal agents as well as daily flushing of the pouches. Supportive therapy such as intravenous balanced crystalloids and/or blood may be required in addition to nutritional support and systemic anti-inflammatories to reduce neuritis [401]. In horses with epistaxis, surgery may be undertaken to occlude affected arteries using balloon catheters, microcoils, or nitinol plugs with the goal of reducing the risk of mortality associated with hemorrhage [401,404]. Depending on the surgical technique used and individual circumstances, the procedures may be performed with the horse standing or under general anesthesia.

Management of sedation and/or anesthesia The major concerns related to sedation and/or general anesthesia of the horse with guttural pouch mycosis for arterial occlusion relate to the hemodynamic stability of the patient associated with hypovolemia, the potential for hemorrhage, and/or neurological abnormalities including ataxia, blindness, and collapse following arterial occlusion [404–408]. In horses with dysphagia, underlying aspiration pneumonia may be present and gas exchange impairment may be aggravated once the horse is recumbent. Ataxia, blindness, weakness, and laryngeal paralysis are all postoperative risks that could impair recovery from general anesthesia.

In addition to a standard history including current medications and prior surgeries, the number of episodes and the timing of any epistaxis events should be obtained. Diagnostic work up of patients presenting for sedation and general anesthesia should include a thorough physical examination, CBC, and serum biochemistry. Further work up such as thoracic radiography should be based on results of the physical examination. In hypovolemic patients, fluid therapy with crystalloids and blood products to reestablish blood volume and ensure normal oxygen-carrying capacity of the blood should be performed prior to surgery.

During sedation, restraining the head in an elevated position is important to prevent increases in pressures in affected arteries prior to ligation [409]. In general, sedation can be achieved by titrating α_2-adrenergic receptor agonists to effect with an opioid analgesic such as butorphanol or morphine included in the protocol. For standing procedures, additional α_2-adrenergic receptor agonists can be administered as required by intermittent boluses or via an infusion [405,410]. In general, infusions will reduce the total dose of sedative administered and the variation in level of sedation. An initial intravenous dose of detomidine (5–10 μg/kg) followed by an intravenous infusion (5–10 μg/kg/h) provides good quality sedation for standing surgery [411]. Opioid analgesics such as morphine (0.05 mg/kg) or butorphanol (0.05 mg/kg) can also be added to the protocol. While acepromazine is often administered to horses prior to standing surgery in combination with α_2-adrenergic receptor agonists, it should be avoided in any horse with hypovolemia due to its vasodilating effect. Local anesthesia can be delivered topically in the nostril to facilitate endoscopy as well as infiltrated subcutaneously at the surgery site [405]. Horses should be monitored throughout the procedure. The veterinary team should be available to rapidly induce anesthesia in the horse in the event of complications that could endanger the horse or personnel. Induction of general anesthesia may be required in an emergency when hemorrhage cannot be controlled with the horse standing.

For horses undergoing general anesthesia, standard anesthesia, and supportive drug protocols are appropriate. ECG, direct arterial blood pressure (lateral metatarsal site), capnography, and blood gas analysis with repeated packed cell volume/total protein measurements (if significant hemorrhage occurs intraoperatively) should be included as part of the monitoring protocol. The anesthetist should be prepared to adjust fluid therapy, including the need for a blood transfusion, based on intraoperative blood loss.

Equine laryngeal paralysis

Characteristics and pathophysiology

Several different pathological conditions may affect the equine laryngeal region; however, the most common condition resulting in surgical intervention is recurrent laryngeal neuropathy. The disease is characterized by progressive reduction in abduction and adduction of the arytenoid cartilages, most commonly on left side, though it can be bilateral. The severity of the laryngeal dysfunction is generally scored using the Havermeyer laryngeal 1–4 grading system with 4 being the most severely affected. Although the cause is unknown, progressive axonopathy, specifically loss of large, myelinated axons in the recurrent laryngeal nerves, is responsible for neurogenic atrophy of the musculature of the larynx [412]. Breeds commonly reported to be affected include Thoroughbreds, Warmbloods, and various draft breeds. Poor exercise performance and an increase in exercise-induced stridor are typical clinical signs [413–416]. Horses with recurrent laryngeal neuropathy generally do not have concurrent medical conditions but laryngeal paralysis secondary to guttural pouch mycosis, cervical trauma, neoplasia, or inflammatory processes have been rarely described [416,417].

Definitive diagnosis of recurrent laryngeal neuropathy or laryngeal dysfunction associated with other disease processes is accomplished with endoscopy in the non-sedated horse at rest and/or during exercise [416]. Both α_2-adrenergic receptor agonists and acepromazine influence the scoring of laryngeal dysfunction via endoscopy, therefore, physical restraint is recommended during the initial assessment of laryngeal function at rest [418]. Ultrasound has been added to the typical diagnostic work up of horses with laryngeal paralysis to assess the degree of laryngeal muscle atrophy and screen for concurrent laryngeal diseases [419].

In cases of recurrent laryngeal neuropathy, surgery may be undertaken when performance is impaired. Laryngoplasty, ventriculectomy, ventriculocordectomy, reinnervation of the caudal arytenoideus dorsalis muscle, and arytenoidectomy have all been described with unilateral laryngoplasty and ventriculocordectomy most commonly performed [420]. Traditionally, these procedures are conducted during general anesthesia with the horse in lateral recumbency. More recently, laryngoplasty and ventriculectomy have been performed with the horse standing under sedation to avoid the risks of general anesthesia, improve visibility, and anatomical orientation, and permit more accurate assessment of arytenoid abduction intraoperatively [413,421]. Overall, the prognosis for return to performance after laryngoplasty is good, although nonracing horses have a better prognosis. Postoperative complications are numerous and include dysphagia leading to coughing, chronic tracheitis and bronchitis, lung abscess formation, and pneumonia [416].

Management of sedation and anesthesia

Preanesthetic preparation should include a thorough physical examination with focus on the respiratory system. Standard preoperative diagnostic tests, such as a CBC or blood gas analysis with packed cell volume, total protein, and blood urea nitrogen or creatinine are appropriate unless co-existing disease is detected on physical examination. Preoperative fasting time of 8 to 12 h with water freely available is typically recommended. Non-steroidal anti-inflammatories are routinely administered pre- and postoperatively.

As noted, there are several advantages to performing laryngeal surgery with the horse standing, including the reduced risk of neuropathy and myopathy associated with recumbency and general anesthesia. Sedation protocols that include acepromazine (0.03 mg/kg IV) followed by an α_2-adrenergic receptor agonist administered as an infusion or intermittent boluses are typically employed. Opioid analgesics, such as butorphanol (0.05 mg/kg) or morphine (0.05 mg/kg), are added to improve the quality of sedation and provide intraoperative analgesia. Local anesthesia of the operative field can be achieved with either local infiltration of the site or by performing a unilateral cervical plexus (C2 and C3) block [413,422]. Placing ear plugs and a hood with a blinker on the surgery side is also recommended [413].

In cases in which general anesthesia is required, routine anesthetic protocols including standard monitoring and fluid therapy are suitable. Direct arterial pressure should be measured from the lateral metatarsal artery and the anesthetist should ensure they have ready access to an intravenous access port if using a jugular vein for fluid and drug administration. Intubation can occasionally be difficult in horses with unilateral laryngeal paralysis; therefore, the anesthetist should be prepared to use a smaller endotracheal tube to minimize trauma of the laryngeal structures during intubation in patients with severe clinical signs. The surgical team may also request the use of a small orotracheal tube if ventriculectomy is being performed to assist with access to the surgical site. Alternatively, intermittent extubation may be considered intraoperatively [416].

Anesthesia and lower airway disease

Patients may require sedation and/or general anesthesia for further diagnostic work up of their airway disease or for unrelated conditions. General considerations for patients undergoing bronchoscopy are discussed above. In general, patients with lower airway disease typically have an increase in lower airway resistance, which may be exacerbated by anesthesia because of a decrease in mucociliary clearance and accumulation of airway secretions. Feline and equine asthma are discussed below in more detail; however, the principles of anesthetic management also apply to canine patients with chronic bronchitis.

Feline asthma

Characteristics and pathophysiology

Feline asthma is an inflammatory lower airway disease currently estimated to affect 1–5% of cats [423]. Major characteristics of asthma in cats include airway inflammation, airway hyperresponsiveness, and airflow limitation. The etiology of the disease is believed to be due to a Type I hypersensitivity to inhaled allergens with genetic, epigenetic, and environmental factors involved in the pathophysiology [424,425]. Cats generally present for clinical signs, such as coughing, wheezing, or respiratory distress at 4–5 years of age; however, more subtle signs may be evident in younger cats [423]. Siamese cats may be overrepresented, but the disease has been reported in all breeds [426,427]. Fluctuations in clinical signs are relatively common and may correlate with exposure to allergens. As with presenting complaints, physical examination findings may vary considerably, with some cats being asymptomatic and others exhibiting tachypnea, wheezing, increased expiratory effort, and open-mouth breathing [428,429]. A cough can generally be elicited with gentle tracheal palpation. A CBC may show elevated total leukocyte and eosinophil counts and eosinophilic inflammation is present in bronchoalveolar lavage fluid [428,429]. Radiographic findings can also be highly variable with some cats having normal radiographic findings while others have bronchial, interstitial, bronchointerstitial, or alveolar patterns. Lobar collapse may be present in some cats which is attributed to airway obstruction with respiratory secretions [428]. Further diagnostic testing including thoracic ultrasound, thoracic computed tomography, and pulmonary function testing may help to characterize the degree of severity of the disease and airflow obstruction, although the availability of the latter is limited for clinical patients. Cats with chronic bronchitis, pulmonary parasitic disease, or heartworm-associated respiratory disease may be confounded with asthmatic cats, and the definitive diagnosis of asthma may not be known when the patient requires anesthesia, particularly when scheduled for bronchoscopy and bronchoalveolar lavage [423,428,429]. Therapy of cats with mild-moderate asthma includes environmental management, optimization of body weight, glucocorticoids, and bronchodilators as required. When cats present in respiratory distress, oxygen therapy, bronchodilators, glucocorticoids, and in some cases, sedation may be required [423].

As noted above, asthma is a relatively common airway disease in cats therefore anesthesia may be required for routine procedures that do not involve the airways. In addition, general anesthesia may also be required to permit procedures such as bronchoscopy and/or bronchoalveolar lavage to obtain a definitive diagnosis of asthma and rule out other diseases involving the airways. In humans, the risk of perioperative morbidity and mortality is higher in patients with asthma, particularly when their condition is unstable; however, this information is currently unknown for cats [430,431]. Bronchospasm is reported to occur in about 9% of human patients with asthma during the perioperative period [432]. Although not specific to asthma, in cats undergoing bronchoscopy and bronchoalveolar lavage while receiving jet ventilation (180 breaths/min delivered by a specialized jet ventilator) a 38% complication rate was reported, with 24% of the complications considered mild [173]. Three percent of cats in the latter investigation were reported to develop a pneumothorax during the procedure [173]. A similar incidence of pneumothorax development was described in a more recent retrospective study (2.5%) [172].

Management of anesthesia

General concerns for patients with asthma include the potential development of bronchospasm, increased R_{aw} leading to impaired expiration/gas trapping within the lungs, and/or hypoxemia during or after anesthesia [430,431]. Overall, perianesthetic goals should include minimizing airway secretions, avoidance of airway manipulation at light planes of anesthesia, and using strategies that minimize the risk of laryngospasm and hypoxemia.

Prior to anesthesia, the patient should have a thorough history with documentation of current medications, followed by a diagnostic work up including a physical examination with pulmonary and cardiac auscultation, CBC, serum biochemistry profile, and thoracic radiographs. The latter will help rule out other cardiopulmonary diseases and provide further information regarding the severity of lung involvement. As noted, clinical signs can fluctuate, and elective procedures should be performed when the patient is not exhibiting signs of significant respiratory dysfunction.

Preanesthetic administration of terbutaline systemically (0.01 mg/kg IM or SC) may be considered prior to performing bronchoscopy and/or bronchoalveolar lavage and in cats with asthma undergoing anesthesia for non-airway procedures [423]. Although this treatment is thought to reduce the incidence of bronchospasm in cats undergoing bronchoalveolar lavage, to date, no prospective study has evaluated its efficacy [172,173,423]. Similarly, to date, there are no studies evaluating the outcome of different anesthetic protocols in cats with naturally occurring asthma. General recommendations include premedicating cats with opioids such as butorphanol or methadone, and an anticholinergic. Due to their potential association with histamine release, morphine and meperidine are not recommended opioid analgesics in patients with reactive airways. Although anticholinergics may increase the viscosity of airway secretions, they are effective bronchodilators and may reduce the risk of laryngospasm secondary to oropharyngeal secretions. Additional sedation can be achieved if required by adding acepromazine, midazolam, or alfaxalone. Experimentally, dexmedetomidine reduced histamine-induced bronchoconstriction in healthy dogs and reduced indicators of airway inflammation in a murine model of asthma [433,434]. Although α_2-adrenergic receptor agonists may be suitable sedatives, their use in combination with anticholinergics, without concurrent peripheral α_2-adrenergic receptor antagonist administration is not recommended because of a severe hypertensive response [435]. When used in combination with opioid analgesics, α_2-adrenergic receptor agonists can reduce arterial hemoglobin oxygen saturation in healthy animals breathing room air and oxygen supplementation should be available [17,436].

Preoxygenation prior to anesthetic induction, if tolerated, will minimize the risk of hypoxemia during anesthetic induction. Ideally, monitoring of hemoglobin oxygen saturation (SpO_2 on a peripheral site such as the paw) is initiated prior to induction of anesthesia, along with ECG assessment of cardiac rhythm and rate. Induction of anesthesia with an injectable anesthetic will provide a smooth transition to general anesthesia and propofol is often used in asthmatic patients as it produces airway smooth muscle relaxation and reduces R_{aw} [432]. Ketamine has also been shown to result in relaxation of airway musculature and may be preferred in some hemodynamically unstable patients. Ketamine is typically combined with a benzodiazepine to improve musculoskeletal relaxation and facilitate intubation [437]. The effects of alfaxalone on airway smooth muscle have not been reported, however, based on its clinical effects, it is anticipated to have similar effects as propofol and ketamine. When endotracheal intubation is performed, lidocaine should be applied topically to the larynx 45–60 s before intubation is attempted to avoid laryngospasm and endotracheal tube placement should not be attempted if the patient is at a light plane of anesthesia [438]. In cats with asthma, an endotracheal tube with the largest internal diameter possible should be placed to minimize the impact of the tube on overall R_{aw} (Fig. 38.16). Use of a feline supraglottic airway device may also be a suitable means to protect the airway in select patients [172]. Isoflurane and sevoflurane both consistently produce bronchodilation and reduce R_{aw}; however, the latter may offer slightly greater effect and it is therefore the preferred inhalant agent in humans with asthma [432]. Desflurane is not recommended as it may cause airway irritation and increase R_{aw} at higher concentrations (2 MAC) [432].

Anesthesia can be maintained under spontaneous ventilation. Depending on the disease severity and the associated increase in R_{aw}, work of breathing, or deficits in arterial oxygenation, mechanical ventilatory support may be required. In such cases, the goal should be to provide a long expiratory phase to prevent gas trapping associated with lower airway obstruction. The latter can be accomplished by using a short inspiratory time (e.g., < 1.5 s) and a small I:E ratio (e.g., ≥ 1:3). Extubation is recommended when patients are still at a deep plane of anesthesia unless it is specifically contraindicated due to other concurrent conditions. If patients are receiving glucocorticoids, NSAIDs are contraindicated, and alternative strategies must be employed to ensure adequate analgesia postoperatively.

Signs of bronchospasm, which can occur at any time during the perianesthetic period, include an increase in respiratory effort during spontaneous ventilation. An increased R_{aw} and reduced dynamic C_{RS} ($V_T/[P_{peak} - PEEP]$) is indicated by an increase in P_{peak} if the cat is receiving VCV. If an advanced anesthesia ventilator is available, adding an inspiratory pause during VCV may facilitate identification of increased R_{aw} by analyzing the gradient between P_{peak} and P_{plat} (Fig. 38.16). Otherwise, it may be possible to qualitatively appreciate increased R_{aw} and decreased dynamic C_{RS} during manual compression of the reservoir bag, as higher P_{peak} (recorded by the manometer of the breathing circuit) is needed to achieve adequate chest excursion. Impaired gas exchange will be evident as cyanosis, a decrease in SpO_2 and PaO_2, and an increase in $P_{ET}CO_2$ or $PaCO_2$ [176,432]. A classic obstructive expiratory pattern on the capnograph may be observed: an obtuse α angle that can be described as a "shark fin." The plane of anesthesia should be assessed and deepened if the patient's hemodynamic status permits, and aerosolized albuterol administered via the endotracheal tube. Additional treatments include systemic terbutaline, corticosteroids, anticholinergics, or a low dose of epinephrine (0.005–0.01 mg/kg, SC or IV). Inspired gases should be supplemented with oxygen if the patient is breathing room air. The decision to induce general anesthesia to reestablish an airway in a conscious (i.e., post-extubation) patient will be determined by the severity of gas exchange impairment and the patient's work of breathing.

Equine asthma (non-infectious lower airway disease)

Characteristics and pathophysiology

Lower airway disease in the equine is common, with etiologic factors, including environmental and infectious factors [439]. Recently, the term "equine asthma" has been proposed to include horses with a spectrum of clinical signs ranging from mild inflammatory airway disease to those exhibiting signs of recurrent airway obstruction [440]. Horses with asthma may have a variety of clinical signs, including a cough, reduced performance, increased work of breathing and, when severe, impaired gas exchange. Physical examination findings may be very mild or may reveal nostril flaring while the animal is at rest, an increase in abdominal expiratory effort, nasal discharge, expiratory wheezes, and inspiratory crackles. Pulmonary function tests available in some referral centers can detect an increase in R_{aw}, increased maximal change in pleural pressure (ΔP_{pl}), and a reduced dynamic C_{RS} [439]. The severity of the disease is often episodic with clinical signs precipitated by exposure to specific antigens such as moldy hay or pasture allergens [441]. Bronchoalveolar lavage sampling typically reveals neutrophilic inflammation. Treatment includes environmental modification to reduce allergen exposure, corticosteroids, and bronchodilators. Therapeutics may be administered systemically or via inhalation [439].

Management of anesthesia

Patients with severe airway disease may have impaired gas exchange during episodes of airway inflammation and bronchospasm. An increased $P(A\text{-}a)O_2$ difference leading to lower-than-expected PaO_2 levels due to atelectasis is not uncommon in normal horses during general anesthesia; however, this may be exacerbated in horses with pre-existing $\dot{V}_A/\dot{Q}$ mismatching associated with severe asthma. In addition, increased R_{aw} in cases of severe asthma contributes to an increase in work of breathing which in turn may contribute to reduced ventilation during general anesthesia in spontaneously breathing horses.

Preanesthetic history should include the horse's degree of respiratory compromise during rest and exercise as well as medications being administered. If the patient is exhibiting clinical signs consistent with impaired gas exchange, arterial blood gas analysis prior to anesthesia in addition to routine preoperative physical examination and diagnostics is recommended. Pulmonary function testing if available can provide a method to trend an individual horse's response to therapy and characterize the severity of their disease. Horses with acute exacerbations of clinical signs should not undergo elective procedures until stabilized and in horses with continued gas exchange impairment (hypercapnia and hypoxemia), procedures should be performed with the horse standing using sedation and local/regional anesthesia rather than general anesthesia whenever possible. As dorsal recumbency is associated with the greatest risk of hypoxemia [2,24], if general anesthesia is required, lateral recumbency is the preferred position if feasible for the intended procedure.

Prior to anesthesia, patients should be maintained on medications and exposure to known allergens such as dusty hay or straw eliminated to minimize the risk of relapse in their condition. Fortunately, sedatives and general anesthetics routinely used in horses result in relaxation of airway smooth muscle. Xylazine was shown to reduce R_{aw} and increase dynamic C_{RS} in ponies exhibiting lower airway obstruction following a challenge with dusty hay [442]. Ketamine, isoflurane, and sevoflurane have also been shown to produce bronchodilation as discussed above. Monitoring of direct arterial blood pressure, arterial blood gas, ECG, capnography, and respiratory mechanics is ideal for prolonged procedures performed under general anesthesia. Ventilatory support with low rates (6–7 breaths per min) and long expiratory times (I:E ratio of 1:3 or 1:4) should be used to avoid gas trapping in the lungs leading to dynamic hyperinflation/intrinsic PEEP during expiration. Modern piston-driven large animal anesthesia ventilators allow an inspiratory pause to be set in VCV mode (Tafonius, Hallowell EMC). In horses with severe bronchospasm secondary to asthma, the use of an inspiratory pause could theoretically allow recognition of an increase in R_{aw} by an increase in the gradient between P_{peak} and P_{plat}. With either spontaneous or positive-pressure ventilation, setting a target $PaCO_2$ of 50–60 mmHg (permissive hypercapnia) can be adopted. In humans with severe obstructive airway disease, the development of gas trapping can occur due to inadequate/slow emptying of the lungs during expiration. Increased P_{peak} during VCV, decreased V_T and hypercapnia during PCV, and increased PEEP during the expiratory phase are all indicators of increased R_{aw} and gas trapping caused by severe small airway disease in humans [443].

Strategies used to address hypoxemia during anesthesia include employing lung recruitment maneuvers as discussed above, supporting hemodynamics, and administering aerosolized albuterol (salbutamol) via a metered dose inhaler into the endotracheal tube [130,134,444,445]. Adverse side effects of the latter treatment include sweating, ventricular tachycardia, and hypotension; therefore, hemodynamics should be monitored during treatment [444,446].

Anesthesia and pleural space disease

Pleural space disease is relatively common in veterinary species either in isolation or in combination with other conditions, including pulmonary parenchymal disease (contusions, neoplasia, pneumonia, and bullae), mediastinal masses, esophageal disease (perforation), infectious diseases such as feline infectious peritonitis, diaphragmatic hernia, coagulopathies, and/or cardiovascular disease. The presence of air or fluid in the thoracic cavity, or disruption of the normal chest wall or diaphragm anatomy (penetrating chest wound or a diaphragmatic hernia), can dramatically influence respiratory function. Patients may present on an urgent basis and require immediate intervention to address the underlying condition.

Pneumothorax and/or pleural effusion

In normal patients, the pleural space is under negative pressure relative to the atmosphere, which maintains lung volume at end expiration, facilitates venous return (Fig. 38.28A), and influences myocardial performance. Air can enter the chest through the thoracic wall, esophagus, or respiratory system creating a pneumothorax. Traumatic pneumothorax or pneumothorax resulting from an esophageal foreign body is generally detected during physical examination and diagnosed with ultrasound and radiographic imaging in patients presenting with a history of trauma or inappropriate consumption of foreign objects. Spontaneous pneumothorax can occur in association with inflammatory, infectious, or neoplastic disease of the lung. In the dog, primary spontaneous pneumothorax has also been reported with ruptured pulmonary bullae or blebs leading to an air leak between the lung and pleural space [191,447,448]. In large animals, spontaneous pneumothorax has been reported in patients with pleuropneumonia or bronchopneumonia, presumably secondary to air leaks from the lung parenchyma [449,450]. Irrespective of the cause of the pneumothorax, clinical signs are dependent on the volume of air within the thoracic space, with some patients exhibiting only minor changes in respiratory rate and effort, while others present in respiratory distress. Additional clinical signs consistent with pneumothorax include cyanosis, lack of lung sounds on auscultation of the dorsal lung fields, fever, tachycardia, depression, inappetence, exercise intolerance, and cough [447,449,450]. Diagnosis of pneumothorax is generally based on radiographic and ultrasonographic findings [191,449–451].

A small volume of fluid (0.1–0.3 mL/kg) resides in the intrapleural space; however, abnormal accumulation of fluid can result from many different conditions with the categorization of the fluid including transudates, modified transudates (e.g., chylous effusions), or exudates (e.g., hemorrhagic effusions). Congestive heart failure, neoplasia, and pleuropneumonia are a few of the more common causes of pleural effusion in veterinary species [451,452]. Cytologic evaluation with bacterial culture of pleural fluid acquired via thoracocentesis is required to confirm the nature of the effusion.

Major concerns for patients that require anesthesia with air or fluid accumulation in the chest include the nature of the underlying disease, the presence of concurrent disease, and the impact of the air or fluid within the pleural space on cardiopulmonary function. In many instances, when anesthesia is required, an intrathoracic intervention is planned; however, in some cases, such as a stable or resolving pneumothorax post-trauma, non-thoracic injuries may require general anesthesia to permit intervention.

Management of anesthesia

The patient's respiratory function, hemodynamic status, level of hydration, and cardiac performance should all be critically evaluated and appropriately managed prior to anesthesia. In many instances, patients with pleural space disease will have undergone an extensive diagnostic work up prior to anesthesia. Animals with a history of trauma should have an ECG performed prior to induction of anesthesia, if possible, to investigate potential arrhythmias [453]. Measurement of serum cardiac troponin I levels may also provide information regarding the probability of subsequent arrhythmias in dogs with blunt chest trauma [453].

In addition to oxygen supplementation and appropriate analgesic therapy, preoperative preparation should include removal of pleural fluid and/or air prior to induction of anesthesia. The specific anesthetic protocol used can be tailored to the individual patient. If pulmonary contusions are present, it is generally preferrable for the patient to maintain spontaneous ventilation during anesthesia, to avoid further injury to the lung. A means to evacuate pleural fluid or air is ideally established prior to and maintained during anesthesia, with easy access to the system by the anesthesia team members when the patient is not undergoing an intrathoracic procedure.

Development of pneumothorax during routine anesthesia in animals and humans is a rare event, but it may occur if emphysematous bullae or smaller blebs in the pulmonary parenchyma are ruptured by positive-pressure ventilation [454]. In animals with traumatic pneumothorax and/or pulmonary contusions, anesthesia for correction of other problems (e.g., fractures) should be postponed until there is an improvement in the clinical signs related to the respiratory system. To minimize further complications in animals with pre-existing pneumothorax, anesthesia should be maintained under spontaneous ventilation and animals should receive an inspired oxygen concentration close to 100%. When mechanical ventilation is required, adjusting the ventilator to deliver a relatively low V_T ($\leq$ 8 mL/kg) or adjusting the volume delivered by the ventilator to result in a relatively low P_{peak} ($\leq$ 8 cmH_2O in small animals) is advisable to minimize the risk of positive-pressure ventilation causing pneumothorax secondary to rupture of a previously injured area of the lung. Aggravation of a previously existing pneumothorax or the development of pneumothorax during anesthesia with VCV is noticed by progressive increases in P_{peak} as lung compliance rapidly worsens. A vicious cycle known as "tension pneumothorax" may quickly develop. Specifically, lung volume progressively decreases as positive-pressure ventilation causes more gas to become entrapped into the pleural cavity, and the animal will quickly become hypoxemic/cyanotic. If the anesthesiologist faces this scenario, mechanical ventilation should be interrupted, and thoracocentesis and/or rapid placement of a chest tube should be completed to prevent a cardiac arrest.

Prior to anesthetic recovery, a system to provide oxygen supplementation and thoracic drainage should be in place. In general, patients with pleural space disease should be monitored intensively for at least 24 h postoperatively.

Diaphragmatic hernia

In veterinary patients, defects or rents in the diaphragm are commonly acquired secondary to trauma, such as motor vehicle collisions, kicks, thoracic wounds, or falls [455–457]. Although less common, congenital defects in the diagram, such as congenital peritoneopericardial hernia, hiatal hernia, diaphragmatic diverticulum, and retrosternal diaphragmatic hernia, are also encountered [455,458,459]. Dyspnea and an abdominal breathing pattern secondary to severe lung collapse are common clinical signs in small animals presenting with acute traumatic rupture of the diaphragm. The severity of clinical signs is generally related to the degree of lung compression caused by the migration of the abdominal viscera into the thoracic cavity. Some animals present with a chronic diaphragmatic hernia and a history of anorexia, vomiting, or exercise intolerance [456,457]. In some instances, the defect is discovered incidentally on imaging studies or during abdominal exploration, or when clinical signs develop after a known traumatic event (sometimes years later). Clinical signs only develop when abdominal organs are displaced into the chest cavity resulting in impaired organ function, respiratory compromise, and/or pain. Diaphragmatic defects in large animals are usually identified when animals present for colic or abdominal pain due to intestinal incarceration [455,460].

Thoracic imaging generally establishes a diagnosis of a diaphragmatic defect in dogs and cats. In large animals, diagnosis is challenging, and it is often determined intraoperatively [455,460,461]. Results of thoracic auscultation, thoracic radiography, thoracic ultrasonography, and rectal examination in large animals may result in a diagnosis or suggest diaphragmatic incarceration of abdominal viscera in the thoracic cavity [455].

Surgical correction is generally performed through a standard midline laparotomy with removal of incarcerated viscera from the thorax back into the abdomen followed by closure of the diaphragmatic tear. Successful thoracoscopic repair of a diaphragmatic rent, however, has been reported in the equine [455]. In general, depending on concurrent injuries, survival rates for dogs and cats that undergo surgery for correction of traumatic diaphragmatic hernias are good, with reported survival to discharge of approximately 80–90% [456,457,462]. In the equine, overall prognosis for horses presenting with diaphragmatic defects is poor. In horses with operable lesions, the prognosis may be fair (approximately 70%) for survival [460,461].

Major anesthetic concerns for patients with diaphragmatic hernia include impaired respiratory function, in particular the ability to oxygenate throughout the perianesthetic period, re-expansion pulmonary edema, hemodynamic depression as a result of the presence of abdominal viscera within the thorax, induction of arrhythmias associated with surgical manipulations within the thoracic cavity, hemorrhage, viscera rupture, prolonged surgical time, and presence of pneumothorax and pleural effusion following closure of the defect [455,463].

Management of anesthesia

Hemodynamically unstable patients should be stabilized prior to anesthesia with appropriate fluid therapy and sympathomimetics if necessary. Patients with impaired oxygenation or an increased respiratory effort should receive oxygen supplementation prior to and during the induction of anesthesia. In small animal patients, preoxygenation with a facemask may be effective unless there is severe hypoxemia secondary to a large increase in intrapulmonary shunting of blood [39,40]. Consideration should be given to maintaining the patient in a head-up position throughout induction, surgical preparation, and the surgical approach to minimize compression atelectasis. In large animals, intranasal or intratracheal insufflation with oxygen can be used prior to induction of anesthesia [47,50,464]. Intensive monitoring of the patient's hemodynamic status is recommended throughout anesthesia, ideally with invasive blood pressure techniques and an ECG. Patients can be hemodynamically unstable during anesthesia and the use of balanced anesthetic techniques with local anesthesia and inotropic/vasopressor support is highly recommended to optimize cardiovascular and respiratory status. Mechanical ventilation with 100% oxygen should be instituted immediately after orotracheal intubation. If a VCV mode is chosen in small animals with abdominal viscera herniated into the thoracic cavity, adjusting the ventilator to deliver low V_Ts ($\leq$ 8 mL/kg) is initially recommended to minimize the risk of excessive distension of pulmonary parenchyma that remains functional/not collapsed. If a standard veterinary anesthesia ventilator that does not allow precise measurement of V_T is utilized, it is advisable to adjust the volume delivered by the ventilator according to the P_{peak} monitored by the manometer measuring pressure within the breathing circuit. Although there are no published studies evaluating the clinical outcome of different ventilation strategies in animals with diaphragmatic hernia, initially limiting the P_{peak} to 7–8 cmH_2O in cats or 10 cmH_2O in dogs should be considered to reduce the risk of alveolar overdistention. If a decelerating flow, pressure-targeted ventilation (PCV) mode is adopted as a protective lung strategy, maximum airway pressures can be adjusted as above.

In animals with acute lung collapse/atelectasis caused by the displacement of abdominal viscera into the thoracic cavity, moderate (hemoglobin saturation < 90%) to severe hypoxemia (hemoglobin saturation < 75%) may persist despite the use of high F_IO_2 (> 0.9) and mechanical ventilation. Besides poor arterial oxygenation, the presence of large areas of atelectasis (stiff lung) will also result in low C_{RS}. Following removal of the abdominal organs from the thoracic cavity (which may involve the stomach, liver, spleen, and segments of the small intestine) the lungs should be gradually expanded by slowly increasing maximum inspiratory pressure (directly or by small stepwise increases in V_T; Fig. 38.26D) combined with progressively increasing PEEP levels if possible. If an advanced anesthesia ventilator is available for use in small animals, a cycling maneuver as described in Figs. 38.26C and 38.27 can be performed [138,139]. A commercially available piston-driven large animal ventilator (Tafonius, Hallowell EMC) is also capable of performing ARMs through progressive increases and decreases in PEEP in large animals [117]. Clinical observations have indicated that cats with diaphragmatic hernia are more sensitive to the cardiovascular depression-associated cycling maneuvers; therefore, smaller stepwise increases in PEEP and maximum inspiratory pressures (P_{max}) are preferred (e.g., 3 cm H_2O instead of 5 cmH_2O) and the maximum increase in PEEP and P_{max} in this species can be initially limited to 10-12 cmH_2O and 20–25 cmH_2O, respectively. As explained above, slow progressive increases in airway pressure, which can be achieved by cycling maneuvers as previously described, are advisable to reopen collapsed alveoli as opposed to sudden exposure of lung parenchyma to high airway pressures (e.g., temporary administration of a CPAP of 30–40 cmH_2O; Fig. 38.26B), which could potentially lead to alveolar rupture, lung inflammation/edema, and hemorrhage in diseased lungs [101,125]. ARMs have been shown to improve pulmonary oxygen gas exchange and respiratory mechanics (increased C_{RS}) in healthy dogs and horses but their impact on outcomes has not been evaluated in animals with a diaphragmatic hernia [38,117,130,134,136,138,139,465]. If the anesthesia ventilator in use does not incorporate advanced methods of ventilation used in ARMs, the anesthesiologist can manually perform a recruitment maneuver by closing the pop-off (APL) valve and progressively increasing the airway pressures by manually squeezing the rebreathing bag (Fig. 38.26A). This procedure is ideally performed under the guidance of the surgeon observing the expansion of collapsed lung areas. Contraindications of ARMs include hemodynamic instability (e.g., hypotension), cor pulmonale (right-sided heart failure), lung emphysema, and bronchopleural fistula. If hypotension is present, animals should be properly stabilized with fluids and sympathomimetics, if necessary, before an ARM is initiated [466].

Following closure of the diaphragmatic rent, air should be removed from the thorax, a procedure generally performed using a catheter placed through the diaphragm. As oxygen supplementation and pleural fluid or air evacuation from the thorax may also be required following recovery from anesthesia, appropriate systems should be pre-placed prior to anesthetic recovery in small animals and if feasible in large animals.

Anesthesia and pulmonary parenchymal disease

While general considerations related to bronchoscopy and thoracic exploration are discussed above, further considerations related to anesthetic management of patients with intrapulmonary masses, lung lobe torsions, and pneumonia are provided below.

Intrapulmonary masses

Removal of primary lung tumors or metastatic lesions may be performed for diagnostic purposes and to prolong and/or improve a patient's quality of life. Patients with intrapulmonary masses may also require anesthesia for non-thoracic procedures. In either case, when the type of lung cancer is known, it is recommended that further information regarding the nature of the cancer is obtained from current veterinary oncology texts and/or consultation with veterinary oncologists.

Management of anesthesia

Anesthetic considerations for human patients with lung cancer are summarized as the "4 Ms" which include (1) Mass effects; (2) Metabolic effects; (3) Metastases; and (4) Medications [235], which may provide a useful mnemonic to consider when presented with veterinary patients with suspected lung cancer. In essence, a thorough physical examination and diagnostic work up of any patient with intrapulmonary disease scheduled for anesthesia should be performed to detect concurrent disease including acid-base/electrolyte abnormalities, anemia, and effects associated with the size and location of the lung mass as well as any metastases. In consultation with the surgical team, the surgical approach, potential surgical complications, and perioperative analgesic plan can be discussed and developed. Current medications should be reviewed to determine if there are contraindications to any analgesics routinely used such as NSAIDs. Specific considerations related to the intrathoracic procedure are discussed above.

Canine lung lobe torsion

Characteristics and pathophysiology

Torsion of a lung lobe along its long axis is a rare but life-threatening disease reported in both dogs and cats [467–470]. Underlying conditions that may predispose a patient to the condition include pleural effusion, pneumonia, and pneumothorax; however, it may also occur spontaneously in healthy animals. Most commonly, middle-aged, large-breed, and deep-chested dogs such as Afghan hounds are affected [467,471]. Pugs also appear to be predisposed to the condition and juvenile dogs less than one year have been reported with lung lobe torsions [472,473]. Presenting clinical signs are variable and include lethargy, anorexia, coughing, hemoptysis, dyspnea, vomiting, and exercise intolerance [467,469,473,474].

Pyrexia, tachypnea, or dyspnea with increased respiratory effort may be present on physical examination and auscultation may reveal muffled heart sounds, harsh lung sounds, crackles and wheezes, and decreased lung sounds over a portion of the lung field [467,470,472–474]. Complete blood cell count, biochemistry profile, and cytology of pleural fluid may be consistent with an ongoing inflammatory process and/or reveal underlying concurrent disease. Diagnostic imaging routinely performed includes radiography, ultrasonography, and computed tomography which may identify the affected lobe and presence of pleural effusion. Bronchoscopy may reveal an occluded bronchus. Diagnosis may be challenging with differential conditions including pneumonia, neoplasia, and pulmonary thromboembolism, and definitive diagnosis may occur during exploration of the thorax [475]. Surgical removal of the affected lung lobe via an intercostal thoracotomy following medical stabilization of the patient is required [475]. Survival for dogs undergoing lung lobectomy appears to have risen with discharge rates of up to 92% recently reported [467,474]. Cats may also have a high rate of survival to discharge rate although fewer reports are available [470].

Management of anesthesia

Oxygen supplementation should be provided to any patient with signs of impaired oxygenation and thoracocentesis should be performed to remove excess pleural fluid prior to anesthesia. Hematology, serum chemistry, and blood gas analysis results should be used to guide fluid and electrolyte therapy during patient stabilization prior to and during anesthesia. If a large amount of pleural fluid is present, it may be necessary to place a chest tube to achieve adequate thoracic drainage.

Oxygen supplementation should be continued into the preanesthetic period. The general principles for intrathoracic procedures discussed above should be followed with adjustments made based on the individual patient. Ventilatory support with 100% oxygen may be required immediately following induction of anesthesia, due to the presence of pleural effusion. As the total lung volume will be reduced due to loss of the affected lung lobe, V_Ts that are traditionally employed in small animal anesthesia (12–15 mL/kg based on ideal body weight) may result in variables degrees of hyperdistention of alveoli located in the remaining functional lung areas. Therefore, if a VCV mode with an inspiratory pause is adopted during anesthesia, it is suggested that the V_T should be adjusted to a normal driving pressure (gradient between P_{plat} and PEEP). Although there are no published studies specifically evaluating the normal driving pressure during mechanical ventilation in small animals, clinical experience has shown that most healthy non-obese dogs receiving VCV with a target V_T of 12–15 mL/kg require a driving pressure of approximately 7–10 cmH_2O; healthy cats require a lower driving pressure (5–7 cmH_2O). Adjusting the V_T according to a target driving pressure is suggested as a means of avoiding overdistention of aerated lung parenchyma in patients that have lost functional lung areas due to lung lobe torsion of a lung tumor. If standard veterinary equipment that does not allow accurate V_T adjustment is used, the volume delivered by the ventilator can be adjusted to deliver a target P_{peak} (limited to 7–8 cmH_2O in cats and to 10 cmH_2O in dogs) to minimize the risk of alveolar overdistension. Reported intraoperative complications include cardiopulmonary arrest, hypotension, and hemorrhage [472,474]. A thoracostomy tube should be placed prior to recovery to facilitate removal of pleural effusion in the postoperative period.

Pneumonia

In humans, postoperative respiratory dysfunction is extremely common, particularly following intrathoracic surgery [476–478]. In this population, pre-existing pulmonary disease, duration of anesthesia, advanced patient age, obesity, intrathoracic procedures, and presence of a nasogastric tube postoperatively have been identified as significant risk factors for postoperative respiratory complications [476,479]. A reduction in function of normal respiratory defenses such as the mucociliary clearance mechanism, presence of atelectasis, and stress- and drug-induced immunosuppression likely all contribute to the development of impaired respiratory function following general anesthesia and surgery [478,480]. Stress and general anesthesia have been shown to cause immunomodulation, most commonly immunosuppression, in animal models of infectious disease [481].

Although there are no large clinical trials reporting outcomes in veterinary patients with pre-existing pneumonia undergoing anesthesia to date, general anesthesia, and elective surgery are not recommended in these patients to minimize the risk of perioperative respiratory dysfunction and potential exacerbation of disease severity. Neonatal or pediatric equine and ruminant patients with pneumonia may present for non-elective exploratory laparotomy, patent urachal resection, or orthopedic procedures. Additional comorbidities in these patients may include persistence of fetal circulation and failure of passive transfer of colostral antibodies. Small animals with upper airway and/or gastrointestinal disease with pneumonia secondary to aspiration of foreign material may require anesthesia for endoscopy or abdominal procedures [271,354,482]. *Pulmonary aspiration* is defined as the inhalation of oropharyngeal or gastric contents into the larynx and lower respiratory tract [483]. The latter occurs due to suppression or dysfunction of cough and laryngeal reflexes (laryngospasm). Aspiration pneumonia associated with frequent regurgitation is a common finding in dogs and cats with megaesophagus. Although this condition is managed medically in most instances, animals may need to undergo anesthesia to place a feeding tube. Thoracotomy for surgical correction of a persistent fourth aortic arch is necessary if the megaesophagus is caused by this congenital vascular ring abnormality [484,485]. Animals with congenital or acquired cleft palate frequently have pneumonia and may require surgical correction of the defect. Drugs used in the perianesthetic period can reduce tone in the lower and upper esophageal sphincters, leading to regurgitation of stomach contents, thereby predisposing the patient to this catastrophic anesthetic complication. Epidemiologic data from a large multicenter study involving approximately 140,000 canine patients reported that the incidence of aspiration pneumonia following anesthesia and sedation in dogs (1 case for every 590 procedures) was much higher than the incidence reported in people (1 case for every 2000 to 7100 anesthetic procedures) [270,486]. Increased odds for aspiration pneumonia after anesthesia in dogs were observed in the presence of patient-related factors (megaesophagus or pre-existing respiratory or neurologic disease), anesthesia-related factors (regurgitation during anesthesia or the use of hydromorphone for induction), and surgical factors (laparotomy, upper airway surgery, neurosurgery, thoracotomy, and endoscopy) [270].

Management of anesthesia

In patients with pre-existing pneumonia, anesthesia should be delayed until clinical signs have resolved to minimize the risk of intra- and postoperative respiratory complications. In patients with pneumonia that require anesthesia on an urgent basis, it is important to evaluate their preoperative condition thoroughly to initiate appropriate therapy, and plan for postoperative supportive therapy, including oxygen supplementation. Physical examination with thorough auscultation and percussion as well as appropriate laboratory testing based on patient signalment is recommended. Assessment of a patient's fluid status is particularly important as dehydration may be present in severely affected patients and may influence prognosis [487]. Thoracic radiography and ultrasonography, pulse oximetry, and/or arterial blood gas analysis can provide further information about the severity and distribution of pulmonary disease and the degree of gas exchange impairment. As explained in Chapter 37, pneumonia may cause areas of low $\dot{V}_A/\dot{Q}$ ratio and varying degrees of intrapulmonary shunt resulting in lower-than-expected PaO_2 values, and even hypoxemia, or signs of ARDS in advanced cases. Inflammatory changes in the lung parenchyma may alter pulmonary mechanics due to poor lung/respiratory system compliance.

In some cases, local or neuraxial anesthesia may provide adequate conditions to permit diagnostic or therapeutic procedures to be performed and may reduce the risks associated with general anesthesia, including the progression of pneumonia. In patients requiring general anesthesia, the anesthetist should utilize a protocol that includes preoxygenation, rapid intubation, and oxygen supplementation with the ability to provide ventilatory support if required. When mechanical ventilation is utilized, a protective ventilatory strategy described above should be employed. In brief, low V_Ts with adequate PEEP to prevent alveolar collapse should be considered. In addition to routine hemodynamic monitoring, assessment of gas exchange and airway pressures should be included. Planning for postanesthetic respiratory support, such as oxygen supplementation and/or mechanical ventilation, should be considered for patients with gas exchange abnormalities. If hypoxemia is present, mechanical ventilation and ARMs may be attempted to increase the PaO_2/FiO_2 ratio and improve C_{RS}. Appropriate disinfection of anesthetic equipment should be performed after anesthetizing a patient with pneumonia to prevent disease transmission.

In animals at risk of aspiration that require general anesthesia, general preventive strategies to minimize the risk of aspiration include adhering to preoperative fasting periods, using premedication agents that minimize the risk of vomiting/regurgitation, using rapid anesthetic induction techniques, optimizing patient positioning during anesthesia, and maintaining a secure airway by ensuring a properly inflated endotracheal tube cuff from anesthetic induction through recovery. In adult animals, standard preoperative fasting periods should be followed based on species. Shorter fasting periods are currently recommended for neonatal, pediatric, and diabetic animals, while longer fasting periods are adopted for ruminants. Upon induction of anesthesia, it is crucial that the animal is maintained in sternal recumbency with the neck and head kept at an elevated position to minimize the risk of regurgitation. After rapid placement of an endotracheal tube, the cuff should be immediately inflated before the animal is moved to another position (e.g., lateral or dorsal recumbency) to reduce the likelihood of aspiration in case regurgitation occurs. To minimize the risk of aspiration after endotracheal intubation, the animal's head should be angled to facilitate draining of any regurgitant fluid accumulated in the oropharyngeal cavity throughout anesthesia. If regurgitation occurs, lavage and suction of the fluid within the oropharynx should be carefully performed. During anesthesia, the endotracheal tube cuff pressure should be high enough to seal the airway and prevent any regurgitant fluid from reaching the lower airways/lungs. It is recommended that cuff pressure should be maintained between 20–30 cm H_2O in humans, as pressures below this range may result in a defective seal, allowing gastric contents and bacterially colonized oral secretions to reach the lower airways and lungs; conversely, excessively high cuff pressures may compromise the microcirculation of the tracheal mucosa and lead to ischemic lesions [488,489]. Excessively high cuff pressures have been implicated as the causative factor of postanesthetic tracheal lesions in dogs, cats, and horses, which may range from tracheal mucosal inflammation/irritation to tracheal rupture/necrosis [490–494]. Although veterinary anesthesiologists may consider human recommendations (cuff pressure between 20–30 cmH_2O) as adequate for small animal patients, this pressure range applies only to low-pressure/high-volume cuffs found in endotracheal tubes designed for human use, where intracuff pressure approaches the pressure exerted by the cuff on the lateral tracheal wall. Veterinary endotracheal tubes available for medium-sized animals (e.g., swine and foals) and for large animals (e.g., adult horses and cattle) are equipped with high pressure/low volume cuffs, where the correlation between intracuff pressure and the lateral tracheal wall pressure is unknown [492,494]. In adult horses intubated with a 30 mm internal diameter endotracheal tube, a cuff pressure of 80–100 cmH_2O reduced the extent of tracheal mucosal damage compared to an intracuff pressure of 120 cmH_2O, while providing protection against aspiration of liquid into the lungs [492]. Although there are no recommendations for cuff pressure in large animals, placement of an endotracheal tube with a larger internal diameter that can be easily passed through the larynx should be encouraged because it will require a lower volume of air within the cuff to create a seal and minimize damage to the tracheal mucosa.

Routine measurement of cuff pressure using specific devices that allow cuff pressure adjustment is not common in veterinary anesthesia. Especially during prolonged procedures, there is a tendency for cuff pressure to decrease over time and such monitoring would allow readjusting intracuff pressures to adequate values. Instead of inflating the cuff to a target pressure (e.g., 20–30 cmH_2O), prevention of air leaks between the endotracheal tube and the tracheal lumen can be achieved by inflating the cuff using a *minimum occlusive volume*. This technique is performed while the pop-off (APL) valve is temporarily closed. The rebreathing bag is manually compressed to create a positive airway pressure of 20 cmH_2O and, if an audible air leak is perceived, the cuff is progressively inflated by adding relatively small volumes using a graduated syringe until leakage is no longer perceived. According to a recent study in dogs undergoing general anesthesia, adjustment of the minimum occlusive volume according to the technique described above resulted in cuff pressures within the target range of 20–30 cmH_2O in only 14% of animals, while cuff overinflation and underinflation were observed in 76% and 14% of patients, respectively [495].

When feasible, animals at risk of aspiration should be recovered in a sternal position with their head elevated above the shoulders. Removal of the endotracheal tube should be delayed until the swallowing reflex is present. To remove any foreign material that may have accumulated in the trachea proximal to the endotracheal tube cuff (and not removed by airway suctioning), it has traditionally been recommended that the endotracheal tube cuff remain inflated during extubation; however, evidence to support this strategy as being effective is limited.

Anesthesia and pulmonary hypertension

Detailed knowledge of pulmonary artery (PA) pressures at rest, during exercise, and in disease states in different species is variable. In dogs, pulmonary hypertension (PH) is defined as mean PA pressure > 25 mmHg at rest, and similar values are currently used to define PH in cats [496,497]. In large animals, a consensus on what constitutes PH is not yet available; however, in the equine, mean PA pressures > 35 mmHg at rest are considered consistent with PH [498]. The three basic hemodynamic mechanisms that may cause PH include: (1) increased PVR; (2) increased pulmonary blood flow; and (3) increased pulmonary vein pressure. As described in Chapter 37 (Fig. 37.17), PH caused by increased PVR and increased pulmonary blood flow is classified according to its anatomic location as precapillary PH, while postcapillary PH results from increased pulmonary vein pressure caused by left-sided congestive heart failure. On some occasions, PH can be of pre- and postcapillary origin. Current canine guidelines divide PH into six groups based on pathological etiology: Group 1: Pulmonary arterial hypertension (caused by contraction of small arteries); Group 2: PH caused by left heart disease; Group 3: PH caused by lung disease/hypoxia; Group 4: PH caused by intraluminal PA obstruction (pulmonary thromboembolism); 5: PH caused by parasitic disease; and 6: PH resulting from unclear/multifactorial mechanisms [497]. PH in Groups 1, 3, 4, 5, and 6 have different etiologies, although they share a common hemodynamic mechanism (increased PVR) and anatomic location (precapillary PH). The primary hemodynamic mechanism involved in group 2 PH is an increase in pulmonary vein pressures. Therefore group 2 PH is also classified according to its anatomic location as postcapillary PH, although an increase in PVR (precapillary PH) might also be involved [496].

In animals with precapillary PH, increased PVR has most often been attributed to respiratory disease, parasitic disease (canine dirofilariasis), thromboembolic disease, or multifactorial/unclear mechanisms [496]. Increased pulmonary blood flow/increased PVR may occur in some congenital cardiovascular defects leading to left-to-right shunting of blood within the circulation, including persistent ductus arteriosus, atrial/ventricular septal defects, and aortopulmonary window [496,498,499]. Increased PVR secondary to pulmonary disease and/or hypoxia has been recognized as a major causative factor of precapillary PH. Hypoxic pulmonary vasoconstriction (HPV) is a physiologic mechanism whereby a decrease in alveolar PO_2 causes constriction of adjacent arterioles. Although HPV aims to maintain arterial oxygenation and $\dot{V}_A/\dot{Q}$ matching by diverting pulmonary blood flow from poorly ventilated (low $\dot{V}_A/\dot{Q}$) or non-ventilated (shunted flow) alveoli to better-ventilated lung areas, in patients with chronic respiratory diseases, HPV can cause an overall increase in PVR and lead to PH with the subsequent development of right-sided heart failure [498,500,501]. Within the canine population, PH secondary to respiratory disease has been more often identified in small-breed dogs and the more common complaints include syncope (64%), cough (56%), and respiratory difficulty (32%) [502]. Obstructive large airway disorders (tracheal/mainstream bronchial collapse, bronchomalacia, and BOAS), bronchiectasis, bronchiolar disease, emphysema, pulmonary fibrosis, neoplasia, and other parenchymal lung diseases have been associated with PH in dogs [503]. Definitive diagnosis of the underlying respiratory disease in dogs presenting with PH may be challenging in some cases because of the need for more invasive procedures requiring general anesthesia, including tracheobronchoscopy, bronchoalveolar lavage fluid cytology, and histopathology (emphysema and pulmonary fibrosis).

The increase in pulmonary vein pressure observed in postcapillary PH is commonly attributed to left heart disease (e.g., myxomatous mitral valve disease [MMVD] and dilated cardiomyopathy in dogs) or, more rarely, to compression of a large pulmonary vein, such as could occur with the presence of an intrathoracic tumor [496,498]. The reported prevalence of PH in dogs with MMVD ranges from 14 to 53% [504–508]. In a retrospective study of 212 dogs with MMVD, graded as B2 or C according to the American College of Veterinary Internal Medicine, 39% of animals presented echocardiographic signs of PH [504]. PH was more commonly observed in animals with signs of congestive heart failure (grade C) and was associated with poorer prognosis for long-term survival when compared to animals with MMVD without PH [504]. Although PH has been largely overlooked in cats, one study showed that 17% of cats with left-sided heart disease (22 of 131 animals) also presented echocardiographic evidence of PH [509]. Cardiomyopathies (hypertrophic, end-stage hypertrophic, restrictive, unclassified, and dilated cardiomyopathy) accounted for most cases of PH in cats (n = 15), whereas a smaller proportion of animals presented with PH associated with congenital cardiac defects (n = 5), and the remaining two cats showed evidence of PH associated with other causes [510].

While definitive recognition of PH may require invasive hemodynamic monitoring using a PA (Swan–Ganz) catheter, echocardiography is used to diagnose PH in companion animals and can provide useful information regarding cardiac morphologic and functional changes in the equine [496,498,510]. Diagnosis of and classification of PH in dogs has been the focus of an American College of Veterinary Internal Medicine consensus statement and more recent articles have also called attention to PH in cats as a frequently overlooked complication of several disease states [496,497]. Echocardiographic signs of PH in dogs include an abnormally dilated PA and the presence of a pulmonic valve regurgitant jet detected using color Doppler studies. The increase in RV afterload caused by PH leads to eccentric dilation/hypertrophy of the right ventricle and tricuspid valve dysplasia/regurgitation. Increased RV afterload/pressure may cause flattening of the interventricular septum on short axis echocardiographic views. If tricuspid regurgitation secondary to PH is present, measurement of peak tricuspid regurgitation velocity (TRV) by placing the spectral Doppler over the regurgitant jet ultimately allows estimation of systolic pulmonary artery pressure (SPAP). Although SPAP derived from TRV has been traditionally used to grade the severity of PH in veterinary medicine, these measurements are subject to several flaws and recent guidelines have recommended using the peak TRV along with a number of different anatomic sites with echocardiographic signs of PH (PA, ventricles, and right atrium/vena cava) to classify the probability of PH [496].

Although data in the veterinary literature are lacking, 30-day mortality rates in human patients with PH undergoing elective, non-cardiac, and non-obstetric surgeries have been reported to range between 3 and 18%, increasing to 5–50% for emergency procedures [511]. The major cause of death during the perianesthetic period is related to RV failure. If anesthesia is to be performed in patients with PH, outcomes may be improved by a multidisciplinary approach aiming to provide proper preanesthetic risk assessment, treatment optimization, and advanced perioperative planning [511].

Precapillary pulmonary hypertension

Management of anesthesia

A thorough preoperative assessment including CBC, biochemistry profile, chest radiographs, ECG, and echocardiogram is recommended in patients with suspected PH. In some patients, assessment of coagulation status may also be indicated. In general, patients may be receiving and should continue therapy prior to anesthesia to support cardiovascular function and reduce PVR and PA pressures. Dogs with previously diagnosed PH may be on treatment with sildenafil, a phosphodiesterase type 5 enzyme inhibitor, which induces relaxation of smooth muscle cells located in PA vessels, decreasing PVR and PA pressures without significantly impacting systemic arterial pressures [502,512,513]. According to one case series study, sildenafil (target dose of 2–4 mg/kg a day) administered for 30 days in dogs with PH associated with respiratory disease ($n = 25$) significantly decreased the pressure gradient across the tricuspid valve in survivors (from 83.0 ± 17.4 mmHg to 55.4 ± 17.4 mmHg) [502]. Despite the elevated mortality rate associated with respiratory disease and PH (32% after 1 month of therapy, 50% after 6 months, and 85% after 5 years), and the lack of a placebo group not receiving sildenafil, quality-of-life scores assigned by the owners were improved after 30 days of sildenafil therapy [502]. Pimobendan has been combined with sildenafil in the treatment of dogs that develop right-sided heart failure secondary to PH of respiratory origin [514]. Pimobendan increases inotropism by sensitizing myocardial proteins to calcium and has vasodilating properties via its actions as a phosphodiesterase type 3 inhibitor. Although pimobendan was shown to increase survival time and reduce the reoccurrence of pulmonary edema in dogs with left-sided congestive heart failure caused by MMVD [515,516], one study showed that pimobendan combined with sildenafil in dogs with PH secondary to respiratory disease ($n = 16$) did not impact long-term survival when compared to dogs treated with sildenafil alone ($n = 12$) [514].

Because drugs used to treat PH and general anesthetics (e.g., isoflurane) can decrease SVR, the clinician should consider the use of vasopressors to treat intra-anesthetic hypotension. Evidence suggests that sildenafil, despite its pulmonary vasodilating properties, does not appear to impact peripheral vascular tone and systemic arterial pressure during anesthesia. In human patients with PH that were anesthetized for valvular heart surgery, sildenafil (50 mg, administered orally 10 min before induction of anesthesia) decreased systolic and mean PA pressures 30 min after its administration, without significantly altering mean arterial pressure or SVR in comparison to a placebo control group [512]. Pimobendan has systemic vasodilatory properties which could potentially contribute to hypotension during anesthesia. A recent randomized crossover study performed in six healthy Beagle dogs showed that one single dose of pimobendan (0.15 mg/kg), administered intramuscularly during isoflurane anesthesia, decreased SVR and diastolic blood pressure in comparison to placebo controls [517]. However, these results may not be extrapolated to the clinical scenario because animals with PH and right-sided heart failure are likely to be receiving chronic treatment with oral pimobendan by the time anesthesia is performed.

Table 38.3 summarizes the factors that can increase PVR and aggravate PH, including management strategies for the perianesthetic period.. In addition to providing adequate sedation and analgesia to avoid stress and pain, small animals should be preoxygenated by delivery of 100% oxygen through a face mask for at least 3 min to ensure significant increases in alveolar PO_2, to prevent hypoxemia caused by hypoventilation during induction of anesthesia. Elevated $PaCO_2$ levels/respiratory acidosis are known to potentiate HPV [500,518]. Although mechanical ventilation may prevent hypercapnia caused by anesthetic drugs, patients with PH may be less tolerant of the hemodynamic effects of positive-pressure ventilation. As discussed before (Fig. 38.29), positive-pressure breaths decrease venous return by increasing P_{pl} and increase RV afterload by distending alveoli and compressing pulmonary capillaries. Therefore, in patients with PH, positive-pressure ventilation has the potential to further increase RV afterload and PVR, which could precipitate cardiovascular collapse in a patient with right-sided heart failure secondary to PH. To minimize the potential negative impact of mechanical ventilation on RV function, human guidelines for anesthesia in patients with PH have recommended avoiding high P_{plat} and the use of low V_T (5–7 mL/kg) and low PEEP levels [511]. However, direct extrapolation of V_Ts adopted in humans to animal species might not be possible. As previously discussed, V_Ts in the order of ≤ 8 mL/kg are more likely to approach the airway deadspace volume of normal dogs and would likely result in hypercapnia (which could also be detrimental in PH) despite the use of high breathing rates. In the absence of veterinary evidence, the use of a low P_{plat} (or low P_{peak} if only a volumetric ventilator is available) is recommended in veterinary patients with PH. Plateau pressure or P_{peak} can be initially limited to 6–8 cmH_2O in small animal species with PH. However, it must be acknowledged that these adjustments may not prevent hypercapnia despite the use of high breathing rates. Provided the animal is hemodynamically stable, inspiratory pressures can be further increased to address hypercapnia based on $P_{ET}CO_2$ or, ideally, $PaCO_2$ values derived from blood gas analysis.

Central venous pressure (CVP) monitoring has limited ability to predict fluid responsiveness status. However, increased CVP (> 6–8 mmHg in dogs) is expected to occur with RV failure secondary to PH, and with circulating volume overload. For more invasive/prolonged procedures in patients with PH, insertion of a central venous catheter for monitoring CVP along with invasive blood pressure monitoring is advisable, as onset of hypotension/tachycardia coinciding with increased CVP often indicates RV failure and cardiovascular collapse [511]. Positive inotropes (e.g., dobutamine and dopamine) may be used to treat hypotension during anesthesia in animals with echocardiographic evidence of right-sided heart failure [511].

Since low SVR, in addition to low cardiac output, may contribute to hypotension during general anesthesia, and considering that certain drugs used in the treatment of PH associated with heart failure may also decrease SVR (e.g., pimobendan and angiotensin-converting enzyme [ACE] inhibitors), vasopressor agents should also be considered for treatment of hypotension. *In vitro* studies support the use of vasopressin to treat hypotension during the perioperative period because this agent does not elicit a contractile response in the PA but is a potent vasoconstrictor of systemic arteries [519,520]. However, if α_1-adrenergic receptor agonists such as norepinephrine are used to increase SVR and treat hypotension, their potential to increase PVR should be considered. Therefore, α_1-adrenergic receptor agonists such as norepinephrine should be carefully titrated to effect as higher doses may increase PVR (Table 38.3).

General recommendations of anesthetic management should be followed. Animals with PH secondary to respiratory disease could present with variable degrees of respiratory distress/hypoxemia. Therefore, mechanical ventilation with 100% oxygen during anesthesia, along with oxygen supplementation during the perianesthetic period is advisable. The clinician should also consider that more invasive diagnostic procedures (e.g., bronchoscopy and bronchoalveolar lavage) could aggravate or precipitate hypoxemia due to limitations in providing oxygen supplementation under these circumstances, particularly in very small patients. With proper preanesthetic planning and discussion of the risks involved, outcomes can be optimized.

Table 38.3 Summary of factors that can increase pulmonary vascular resistance (PVR) and their management during the anesthetic/perianesthetic period in patients with pre-existing pulmonary hypertension.

Factors that may increase PVR	Anesthetic/perianesthetic management for patients with pre-existing pulmonary hypertension
High sympathetic tone	Avoid stress (provide adequate sedation) and pain (provide analgesia)
Low alveolar (P_AO_2) and arterial (PaO_2) oxygen partial pressures	Provide oxygen supplementation during the perianesthetic period Use a high F_IO_2 during anesthesia
Hypercapnia/respiratory acidosis	Provide mechanical ventilation to maintain eucapnia if respiratory depression/hypercapnia is significant
High P_{plat} and elevated PEEP levels during mechanical ventilation	If mechanical ventilation is required, avoid the use of PEEP, and adjust ventilator to deliver a low P_{plat} (or low P_{peak} if using a volumetric ventilator) Note that hypercapnia may increase PVR during protective mechanical ventilation
Vasopressor agents used to treat hypotension	Avoid high doses of norepinephrine (> 0.5 μg/kg/min) which are more likely to increase PVR Consider vasopressin constant rate infusion to increase SVR and arterial pressure without altering PVR
α_2-Adrenergic receptor agonists, ketamine	Increased PVR and MPAP are observed with high doses of α_2-adrenergic receptor agonists, therefore avoid these drugs, or use low doses, if necessary Avoid high doses of ketamine
Low mixed-venous PO_2	Optimize tissue perfusion (inotropes, fluid therapy) to maintain mixed-venous (or central venous) PO_2 > 40 mmHg

PVR, pulmonary vascular resistance; SVR, systemic vascular resistance; PEEP, positive end-expired pressure; P_{plat}, plateau pressure; P_{peak}, peak pressure; MPAP, mean pulmonary arterial pressure.

Postcapillary pulmonary hypertension

Management of anesthesia

Canine patients with MMVD may require anesthesia for a variety of reasons. In these cases, it should be acknowledged that the presence of PH is a hallmark of severe left-sided congestive heart failure, where elevated LV filling pressures and retrograde blood flow through the degenerated mitral valve cause excessive increases in left atrial and pulmonary vein pressures, ultimately leading to increased hydrostatic pressure within the pulmonary capillaries and PH. Therefore, animals with PH secondary to MMVD may be more likely to develop hydrostatic pulmonary edema associated with fluid overload during anesthesia.

Besides conventional therapy with diuretics and ACE inhibitors, animals with MMVD grade B2 or above commonly receive pimobendan treatment. Randomized controlled studies performed in animals with MMVD have shown that pimobendan combined with conventional therapy, compared to animals receiving only conventional therapy, increases survival time by 1.9 to 2.5 times, and reduces the reoccurrence of pulmonary edema [515,516]. If echocardiographic evidence of PH is also present, pimobendan is frequently combined with sildenafil therapy with the aim of decreasing pulmonary arterial pressures.

While the drugs described above can ameliorate signs of heart disease and increase long-term survival, their potential impact on anesthesia should be considered. The use of ACE inhibitors aims to decrease LV afterload by causing arterial vasodilation. However, in healthy dogs, administration of the ACE inhibitor benazepril for one week, with the last dose administered 90 minutes before anesthesia, was reported to increase the intensity of intra-anesthetic hypotension and the number of interventions required to correct moderate-to-severe hypotensive crises in comparison to a placebo control treatment [521]. As previously discussed, one single dose of pimobendan during isoflurane anesthesia could also result in greater decreases in SVR and lower diastolic blood pressure compared to a placebo control [517]. Considering the potential of drugs used in the treatment of MMVD to aggravate hypotension during general anesthesia, the clinician should be prepared to rapidly intervene with vasopressor agents (e.g., norepinephrine) or drugs with mixed vasopressor/inotropic action (e.g., ephedrine and dopamine) if hypotension develops following induction of anesthesia. Unless there is clear evidence of circulating volume deficits, administration of fluid boluses with the aim of stabilizing arterial blood pressure should be avoided in animals with PH associated with heart disease.

In companion animals, preference is generally given to premedication with opioids alone, which may result in adequate sedation without significantly interfering with myocardial contractility, but combination of opioids with low doses of other drugs (e.g., acepromazine or dexmedetomidine) may be necessary to achieve a satisfactory level of sedation in some patients. Preoxygenation with 100% oxygen delivered though a face mask for at least 3 min immediately before induction of anesthesia with an injectable agent should be routinely performed. General guidelines for maintenance of anesthesia include an inhalant anesthetic, combined with locoregional anesthesia and/or infusions of drugs that provide intraoperative analgesia and reduce inhalant requirements. Monitoring should include ECG, arterial blood pressure, pulse oximetry, and capnography, and use of mechanical ventilation is advisable to optimize gas exchange and to prevent hypercapnia. Although data is lacking, in large animal patients with PH, locoregional anesthesia should be considered. If general anesthesia is required, similar principles discussed above should be considered.

References

1 Nyman G, Funkquist B, Kvart C, *et al.* Atelectasis causes gas exchange impairment in the anaesthetised horse. *Equine Vet J* 1990; **22**: 317–324.
2 Day TK, Gaynor JS, Muir WW III, *et al.* Blood gas values during intermittent positive pressure ventilation and spontaneous ventilation in 160 anesthetized horses positioned in lateral or dorsal recumbency. *Vet Surg* 1995; **24**: 266–276.
3 Barton L. Respiratory muscle fatigue. *Vet Clin North Am Small Anim Pract* 2002; **32**: 1059–1071.
4 Haskins SC. Hypoxemia. In: Silverstein DC, Hopper K, eds. *Small Animal Critical Care Medicine*, 2nd edn. St. Louis, MO: WB Saunders, 2015: 81–86.
5 Nunn JF. *Applied Respiratory Physiology*, 3rd edn. London, UK: Butterworth, 1987.
6 Benatar SR, Hewlett AM, Nunn JF. The use of iso-shunt lines for control of oxygen therapy. *Br J Anaesth* 1973; **45**: 711–718.
7 Steffey EP, Farver TB, Woliner MJ. Circulatory and respiratory effects of methoxyflurane in dogs: comparison of halothane. *Am J Vet Res* 1984; **45**: 2574–2579.
8 Steffey EP, Howland D Jr. Isoflurane potency in the dog and cat. *Am J Vet Res* 1977; **38**: 1833–1836.
9 Ambros B, Duke-Novakovski T, Pasloske KS. Comparison of the anesthetic efficacy and cardiopulmonary effects of continuous rate infusions of alfaxalone-2-hydroxypropyl-beta-cyclodextrin and propofol in dogs. *Am J Vet Res* 2008; **69**: 1391–1398.

10 Mutoh T, Nishimura R, Kim HY, *et al.* Cardiopulmonary effects of sevoflurane, compared with halothane, enflurane, and isoflurane, in dogs. *Am J Vet Res* 1997; **58**: 885–890.

11 Hikasa Y, Kawanabe H, Takase K, *et al.* Comparisons of sevoflurane, isoflurane, and halothane anesthesia in spontaneously breathing cats. *Vet Surg* 1996; **25**: 234–243.

12 Pypendop BH, Ilkiw JE. Hemodynamic effects of sevoflurane in cats. *Am J Vet Res* 2004; **65**: 20–25.

13 Ingwersen W, Allen DG, Dyson DH, *et al.* Cardiopulmonary effects of a ketamine hydrochloride/acepromazine combination in healthy cats. *Can J Vet Res* 1988; **52**: 1–4.

14 Staffieri F, De Monte V, De Marzo C, *et al.* Effects of two fractions of inspired oxygen on lung aeration and gas exchange in cats under inhalant anaesthesia. *Vet Anaesth Analg* 2010; **37**: 483–490.

15 Staffieri F, Franchini D, Carella GL, *et al.* Computed tomographic analysis of the effects of two inspired oxygen concentrations on pulmonary aeration in anesthetized and mechanically ventilated dogs. *Am J Vet Res* 2007; **68**: 925–931.

16 Haskins SC, Patz JD, Farver TB. Xylazine and xylazine-ketamine in dogs. *Am J Vet Res* 1986; **47**: 636–641.

17 Enouri SS, Kerr CL, McDonell WN, *et al.* Cardiopulmonary effects of anesthetic induction with thiopental, propofol, or a combination of ketamine hydrochloride and diazepam in dogs sedated with a combination of medetomidine and hydromorphone. *Am J Vet Res* 2008; **69**: 586–595.

18 Rolfe NG, Kerr CL, McDonell WN. Cardiopulmonary and sedative effects of the peripheral α2-adrenoceptor antagonist MK 0467 administered intravenously or intramuscularly concurrently with medetomidine in dogs. *Am J Vet Res* 2012; **73**: 587–594.

19 Smith JA, Gaynor JS, Bednarski RM, *et al.* Adverse effects of administration of propofol with various preanesthetic regimens in dogs. *J Am Vet Med Assoc* 1993; **202**: 1111–1115.

20 Hopper K, Haskins SC, Kass PH, *et al.* Indications, management, and outcome of long-term positive-pressure ventilation in dogs and cats: 148 cases (1990–2001). *J Am Vet Med Assoc* 2007; **230**: 64–75.

21 Campbell VL, King LG. Pulmonary function, ventilator management, and outcome of dogs with thoracic trauma and pulmonary contusions: 10 cases (1994–1998). *J Am Vet Med Assoc* 2000; **217**: 1505–1509.

22 Lee JA, Drobatz KJ, Koch MW, *et al.* Indications for and outcome of positive-pressure ventilation in cats: 53 cases (1993–2002). *J Am Vet Med Assoc* 2005; **226**: 924–931.

23 Palmer JE. Ventilatory support of the critically ill foal. *Vet Clin North Am Equine Pract* 2005; **21**: 457–486.

24 Nyman G, Hedenstierna G. Ventilation-perfusion relationships in the anaesthetised horse. *Equine Vet J* 1989; **21**: 274–281.

25 Kerr CL, McDonell WN, Young SS. A comparison of romifidine and xylazine when used with diazepam/ketamine for short duration anesthesia in the horse. *Can Vet J* 1996; **37**: 601–609.

26 Kerr CL, McDonell WN, Young SS. Cardiopulmonary effects of romifidine/ketamine or xylazine/ketamine when used for short duration anesthesia in the horse. *Can J Vet Res* 2004; **68**: 274–282.

27 Cuvelliez SG, Eicker SW, McLauchlan C, *et al.* Cardiovascular and respiratory effects of inspired oxygen fraction in halothane-anesthetized horses. *Am J Vet Res* 1990; **51**: 1226–1231.

28 Steffey EP, Wheat JD, Meagher DM, *et al.* Body position and mode of ventilation influences arterial pH, oxygen, and carbon dioxide tensions in halothane-anesthetized horses. *Am J Vet Res* 1977; **38**: 379–382.

29 Gleed RD, Dobson A. Improvement in arterial oxygen tension with change in posture in anaesthetised horses. *Res Vet Sci* 1988; **44**: 255–259.

30 Hall LW, Gillespie JR, Tyler WS. Alveolar-arterial oxygen tension differences in anaesthetized horses. *Br J Anaesth* 1968; **40**: 560–568.

31 Marntell S, Nyman G, Hedenstierna G. High inspired oxygen concentrations increase intrapulmonary shunt in anaesthetized horses. *Vet Anaesth Analg* 2005; **32**: 338–347.

32 Staffieri F, Bauquier SH, Moate PJ, *et al.* Pulmonary gas exchange in anaesthetised horses mechanically ventilated with oxygen or a helium/oxygen mixture. *Equine Vet J* 2009; **41**: 747–752.

33 Edmark L, Kostova-Aherdan K, Enlund M, *et al.* Optimal oxygen concentration during induction of general anesthesia. *Anesthesiology* 2003; **98**: 28–33.

34 Hedenstierna G, Edmark L. Mechanisms of atelectasis in the perioperative period. *Best Pract Res Clin Anaesthesiol* 2010; **24**: 157–169.

35 Hubbell JA, Aarnes TK, Bednarski RM, *et al.* Effect of 50% and maximal inspired oxygen concentrations on respiratory variables in isoflurane-anesthetized horses. *BMC Vet Res* 2011; **7**: 23.

36 Crumley MN, McMurphy RM, Hodgson DS, *et al.* Effects of inspired oxygen concentration on ventilation, ventilatory rhythm, and gas exchange in isoflurane-anesthetized horses. *Am J Vet Res* 2013; **74**: 183–190.

37 Duggan M, Kavanagh BP. Pulmonary atelectasis: a pathogenic perioperative entity. *Anesthesiology* 2005; **102**: 838–854.

38 De Monte V, Grasso S, De Marzo C, *et al.* Effects of reduction of inspired oxygen fraction or application of positive end-expiratory pressure after an alveolar recruitment maneuver on respiratory mechanics, gas exchange, and lung aeration in dogs during anesthesia and neuromuscular blockade. *Am J Vet Res* 2013; **74**: 25–33.

39 McNally EM, Robertson SA, Pablo LS. Comparison of time to desaturation between preoxygenated and nonpreoxygenated dogs following sedation with acepromazine maleate and morphine and induction of anesthesia with propofol. *Am J Vet Res* 2009; **70**: 1333–1338.

40 Ambros B, Carrozzo MV, Jones T. Desaturation times between dogs preoxygenated via face mask or flow-by technique before induction of anesthesia. *Vet Anaesth Analg* 2018; **45**: 452–458.

41 Rousseau-Blass F, Pang DS. Hypoventilation following oxygen administration associated with alfaxalone-dexmedetomidine-midazolam anesthesia in New Zealand White rabbits. *Vet Anaesth Analg* 2020; **47**: 637–646.

42 Ramesh M, Thomovsky E, Johnson P. Conventional versus high-flow oxygen therapy in dogs with lower airway injury. *Can J Vet Res* 2021; **85**: 241–250.

43 Manning AM. Oxygen therapy and toxicity. *Vet Clin North Am Small Anim Pract* 2002; **32**: 1005–1020.

44 Dunphy ED, Mann FA, Doham JR, *et al.* Comparison of unilateral versus bilateral nasal catheters for oxygen administration in dogs. *J Vet Emerg Crit Care* 2002; **12**: 245–251.

45 Wong DM, Alcott CJ, Wang C, *et al.* Physiologic effects of nasopharyngeal administration of supplemental oxygen at various flow rates in healthy neonatal foals. *Am J Vet Res* 2010; **71**: 1081–1088.

46 Gordon D, Clark-Price S, Keating S, *et al.* Evaluation of nasal oxygen administration at various flow rates and concentrations in conscious, standing adult horses. *J Equine Vet Sci* 2023; **123**: 104250.

47 Floriano D, Watkins AR, Hopster K. Intratracheal oxygen administration increases FIO2 and PaO2 compared with intranasal administration in healthy, standing horses. *Am J Vet Res* 2022; **83**: 450–454.

48 Mann FA, Wagner-Mann C, Allert JA, *et al.* Comparison of intranasal and intratracheal oxygen administration in healthy awake dogs. *Am J Vet Res* 1992; **53**: 856–860.

49 Fitzpatrick RK, Crowe DT. Nasal oxygen administration in dogs and cats: experimental and clinical investigations. *J Am Anim Hosp Assoc* 1986; **22**: 293–300.

50 van Oostrom H, Schaap MW, van Loon JP. Oxygen supplementation before induction of general anaesthesia in horses. *Equine Vet J* 2017; **49**: 130–132.

51 McMurphy RM, Cribb PH. Alleviation of postanesthetic hypoxemia in the horse. *Can Vet J* 1989; **30**: 37–41.

52 Hoffman AM, Viel L. A percutaneous transtracheal catheter system for improved oxygenation in foals with respiratory distress. *Equine Vet J* 1992; **24**: 239–241.

53 Staffieri F, Crovace A, De Monte V, *et al.* Noninvasive continuous positive airway pressure delivered using a pediatric helmet in dogs recovering from general anesthesia. *J Vet Emerg Crit Care (San Antonio)* 2014; **24**: 578–585.

54 Whitney J, Keir I. Clinical review of high-flow nasal oxygen therapy in human and veterinary patients. *Front Vet Sci* 2023; **10**: 1070881.

55 Wettstein RB, Shelledy DC, Peters JI. Delivered oxygen concentrations using low-flow and high-flow nasal cannulas. *Respir Care* 2005; **50**: 604–609.

56 Jagodich TA, Bersenas AME, Bateman SW, *et al.* Comparison of high flow nasal cannula oxygen administration to traditional nasal cannula oxygen therapy in healthy dogs. *J Vet Emerg Crit Care (San Antonio)* 2019; **29**: 246–255.

57 Corley A, Caruana LR, Barnett AG, *et al.* Oxygen delivery through high-flow nasal cannulae increase end-expiratory lung volume and reduce respiratory rate in post-cardiac surgical patients. *Br J Anaesth* 2011; **107**: 998–1004.

58 Riera J, Pérez P, Cortés J, *et al.* Effect of high-flow nasal cannula and body position on end-expiratory lung volume: a cohort study using electrical impedance tomography. *Respir Care* 2013; **58**: 589–596.

59 Milési C, Boubal M, Jacquot A, *et al.* High-flow nasal cannula: recommendations for daily practice in pediatrics. *Ann Intensive Care* 2014; **4**: 29.

60 Lenglet H, Sztrymf B, Leroy C, *et al.* Humidified high flow nasal oxygen during respiratory failure in the emergency department: feasibility and efficacy. *Respir Care* 2012; **57**: 1873–1878.

61 Ward JJ. High-flow oxygen administration by nasal cannula for adult and perinatal patients. *Respir Care* 2013; **58**: 98–122.

62 Jagodich TA, Bersenas AME, Bateman SW, *et al.* Preliminary evaluation of the use of high-flow nasal cannula oxygen therapy during recovery from general anesthesia in dogs with obstructive upper airway breathing. *J Vet Emerg Crit Care (San Antonio)* 2020; **30**: 487–492.

63 Daly JL, Guenther CL, Haggerty JM, Keir I. Evaluation of oxygen administration with a high-flow nasal cannula to clinically normal dogs. *Am J Vet Res* 2017; **78**: 624–630.

64 de Jaureguizar Tesas MR, Matson H, Tappin S, Thomas E. The use of High-Flow Nasal Oxygen Therapy in 4 dogs undergoing bronchoscopy. *Front Vet Sci* 2023; **10**: 1088103.

65 Jagodich TA, Bersenas AME, Bateman SW, *et al.* High-flow nasal cannula oxygen therapy in acute hypoxemic respiratory failure in 22 dogs requiring oxygen support escalation. *J Vet Emerg Crit Care (San Antonio)* 2020; **30**: 364–375.

66 Keir I, Daly J, Haggerty J, Guenther C. Retrospective evaluation of the effect of high flow oxygen therapy delivered by nasal cannula on PaO2 in dogs with moderate-to-severe hypoxemia. *J Vet Emerg Crit Care (San Antonio)* 2016; **26**: 598–602.

67 Pouzot-Nevoret C, Hocine L, Nègre J, *et al.* Prospective pilot study for evaluation of high-flow oxygen therapy in dyspnoeic dogs: the HOT-DOG study. *J Small Anim Pract* 2019; **60**: 656–662.

68 Frischer R, Daly J, Haggerty J, Guenther C. High-flow nasal cannula improves hypoxemia in dogs failing conventional oxygen therapy. *J Am Vet Med Assoc* 2022; **261**: 210–216.

69 Kallet RH, Matthay MA. Hyperoxic acute lung injury. *Respir Care* 2013; **58**: 123–141.

70 Knight PR, Kurek C, Davidson BA, *et al.* Acid aspiration increases sensitivity to increased ambient oxygen concentrations. *Am J Physiol Lung Cell Mol Physiol* 2000; **278**: L1240–L1247.

71 Thiel M, Chouker A, Ohta A, *et al.* Oxygenation inhibits the physiological tissue-protecting mechanism and thereby exacerbates acute inflammatory lung injury. *PLoS Biol* 2005; **3**: e174.

72 Aggarwal NR, D'Alessio FR, Tsushima K, *et al.* Moderate oxygen augments lipopolysaccharide-induced lung injury in mice. *Am J Physiol Lung Cell Mol Physiol* 2010; **298**: L371–L381.

73 Minkove S, Dhamapurkar R, Cui X, *et al.* Effect of low-to-moderate hyperoxia on lung injury in preclinical animal models: a systematic review and meta-analysis. *Intensive Care Med Exp* 2023; **11**: 22.

74 Barbateskovic M, Schjørring OL, Krauss SR, *et al.* Higher vs lower oxygenation strategies in acutely Ill adults: a systematic review with meta-analysis and trial sequential analysis. *Chest* 2021; **159**: 154–173.

75 Hochberg CH, Semler MW, Brower RG. Oxygen toxicity in critically ill adults. *Am J Respir Crit Care Med* 2021; **204**: 632–641.

76 Fichtner F, Moerer O, Weber-Carstens S, *et al.* Clinical guideline for treating acute respiratory insufficiency with invasive ventilation and extracorporeal membrane oxygenation: evidence-based recommendations for choosing modes and setting parameters of mechanical ventilation. *Respiration* 2019; **98**: 357–372.

77 Chu DK, Kim LH, Young PJ, *et al.* Mortality and morbidity in acutely ill adults treated with liberal versus conservative oxygen therapy (IOTA): a systematic review and meta-analysis. *Lancet* 2018; **391**: 1693–1705.

78 MacIntyre NR. Supporting oxygenation in acute respiratory failure. *Respir Care* 2013; **58**: 142–150.

79 Martin DS, Grocott MP. Oxygen therapy in critical illness: precise control of arterial oxygenation and permissive hypoxemia. *Crit Care Med* 2013; **41**: 423–432.

80 Nishimoto K, Umegaki T, Ohira S, *et al.* Impact of permissive hypoxia and hyperoxia avoidance on clinical outcomes in septic patients receiving mechanical ventilation: a retrospective single-center study. *Biomed Res Int* 2021; **2021**: 7332027.

81 Girardis M, Busani S, Damiani E, *et al.* Effect of conservative vs conventional oxygen therapy on mortality among patients in an intensive care unit: the Oxygen-ICU Randomized Clinical Trial. *JAMA* 2016; **316**: 1583–1589.

82 Slutsky AS. History of mechanical ventilation from vesalius to ventilator-induced lung injury. *Am J Respir Crit Care Med* 2015; **191**: 1106–1115.

83 Brawn NMT. Negative pressure noninvasive ventilation (NPNIV): history, rationale, and application. *Nocturnal Non-Invasive Ventilation* 2015 Oct **1**: 27–71.

84 Wilkinson D. Evolution of the anaesthetic machine. *Curr Anaesth Crit Care* 1991; **2**: 51–56.

85 Romero-Ávila P, Márquez-Espinós C, Cabrera Afonso JR. Historical development of the anesthetic machine: from Morton to the integration of the mechanical ventilator. *Braz J Anesthesiol* 2021; **71**: 148–161.

86 Topulos SP, Topulos GP, Abelson AL, *et al.* Predicting the effect of fresh gas flow on tidal volume in volume-controlled mechanically ventilated dogs. *Vet Anaesth Analg* 2023; **50**: 57–62.

87 Bokoch MP, Weston SD. Inhaled anesthetics: delivery systems. In: Gropper M, Eriksson L, Fleisher L, *et al.*, eds. *Miller's Anesthesia*, 9th ed. Philadelphia, PA: Elsevier, 2019: 572–637.

88 Forbat AF, Her C. Correction for gas compression in mechanical ventilators. *Anesth Analg* 1980; **59**: 488–493.

89 Standardization ISO. *Standards* 2023. www.iso.org/standards.html (accessed June 2023).

90 Areti YK, Garcia ER. Anesthesia ventilators. In: Vancanti C, Sikka P, Urman RD, *et al.*, eds. *Essential Clinical Anesthesia*. New York, NY: Cambridge University Press, 2011: 138–143.

91 Jain RK, Swaminathan S. Anaesthesia ventilators. *Indian J Anaesth* 2013; **57**: 525–532.

92 Eisenkraft JB. Monitoring pressure, volume, and flow in the anesthesia breathing system. In: Press CU, ed. *Monitoring in Anesthesia and Perioperative Care*. New York, NY: Cambridge University Press, 2011: 171–184.

93 Calice I, Moens Y. Modern spirometry supports anesthetic management in small animal clinical practice: a case series. *J Am Anim Hosp Assoc* 2016; **52**: 305–311.

94 Moens YP, Gootjes P, Ionita JC, *et al.* In vitro validation of a Pitot-based flow meter for the measurement of respiratory volume and flow in large animal anaesthesia. *Vet Anaesth Analg* 2009; **36**: 209–219.

95 Moens YPS. Clinical application of continuous spirometry with a pitot-based flow meter during equine anaesthesia. *Equine Vet Educ* 2010; **22**: 354–360.

96 Cannon ML, Cornell J, Tripp-Hamel DS, *et al.* Tidal volumes for ventilated infants should be determined with a pneumotachometer placed at the endotracheal tube. *Am J Respir Crit Care Med* 2000; **162**: 2109–2112.

97 Castle RA, Dunne CJ, Mok Q, *et al.* Accuracy of displayed values of tidal volume in the pediatric intensive care unit. *Crit Care Med* 2002; **30**: 2566–2574.

98 Morgenroth S, Thomas J, Cannizzaro V, *et al.* Accuracy of near-patient vs. inbuilt spirometry for monitoring tidal volumes in an in-vitro paediatric lung model. *Anaesthesia* 2018; **73**: 972–979.

99 Schena E, Massaroni C, Saccomandi P, *et al.* Flow measurement in mechanical ventilation: a review. *Med Eng Phys* 2015; **37**: 257–264.

100 Henderson WR, Sheel AW. Pulmonary mechanics during mechanical ventilation. *Respir Physiol Neurobiol* 2012; **180**: 162–172.

101 Ball L, Dameri M, Pelosi P. Modes of mechanical ventilation for the operating room. *Best Pract Res Clin Anaesthesiol* 2015; **29**: 285–299.

102 Bigatello L, Pesenti A. Respiratory physiology for the anesthesiologist. *Anesthesiology* 2019; **130**: 1064–1077.

103 Barberis L, Manno E, Guérin C. Effect of end-inspiratory pause duration on plateau pressure in mechanically ventilated patients. *Intensive Care Med* 2003; **29**: 130–134.

104 Kaczka DW, Chiitilian HV, Melo MFV. Respiratory monitoring. In: Gropper M, Eriksson L, Fleisher L, *et al.*, eds. *Miller's Anesthesia*, 9th edn. Philadelphia, PA: Elsevier, 2019: 1298–1339.

105 Aydın V, Kabukcu HK, Sahin N, *et al.* Comparison of pressure and volume-controlled ventilation in laparoscopic cholecystectomy operations. *Clin Respir J* 2016; **10**: 342–349.

106 Campbell RS, Davis BR. Pressure-controlled versus volume-controlled ventilation: does it matter? *Respir Care* 2002; **47**: 416–424.

107 Assad OM, El Sayed AA, Khalil MA. Comparison of volume-controlled ventilation and pressure-controlled ventilation volume guaranteed during laparoscopic surgery in Trendelenburg position. *J Clin Anesth* 2016; **34**: 55–61.

108 Fantoni DT, Ida KK, Lopes TF, *et al.* A comparison of the cardiopulmonary effects of pressure controlled ventilation and volume controlled ventilation in healthy anesthetized dogs. *J Vet Emerg Crit Care (San Antonio)* 2016; **26**: 524–530.

109 Schick V, Dusse F, Eckardt R, *et al.* Comparison of volume-guaranteed or -targeted, pressure-controlled ventilation with volume-controlled ventilation during elective surgery: a systematic review and meta-analysis. *J Clin Med* 2021; **10**: 1276.

110 Clement KC. Ventilator triggering. *J Pediatr Intensive Care* 2013; **2**: 11–18.

111 Pettenuzzo T, Aoyama H, Englesakis M, *et al.* Effect of neurally adjusted ventilatory assist on patient-ventilator interaction in mechanically ventilated adults: a systematic review and meta-analysis. *Crit Care Med* 2019; **47**: e602–e609.

112 Parthasarathy S, Jubran A, Tobin MJ. Cycling of inspiratory and expiratory muscle groups with the ventilator in airflow limitation. *Am J Respir Crit Care Med* 1998; **158**: 1471–1478.

113 Hess DR. Ventilator waveforms and the physiology of pressure support ventilation. *Respir Care* 2005; **50**: 166–186.

114 Escolar JD, Escolar A. Lung hysteresis: a morphological view. *Histol Histopathol* 2004; **19**: 159–166.

115 Harris RS. Pressure-volume curves of the respiratory system. *Respir Care* 2005; **50**: 78–98.

116 Michard F. Changes in arterial pressure during mechanical ventilation. *Anesthesiology* 2005; **103**: 419–428.

117 Hopster K, Duffee LR, Hopster-Iversen CCS, *et al.* Efficacy of an alveolar recruitment maneuver for improving gas exchange and pulmonary mechanics in anesthetized horses ventilated with oxygen or a helium-oxygen mixture. *Am J Vet Res* 2018; **79**: 1021–1027.

118 Asorey I, Pellegrini L, Canfrán S, *et al.* Factors affecting respiratory system compliance in anaesthetised mechanically ventilated healthy dogs: a retrospective study. *J Small Anim Pract* 2020; **61**: 617–623.

119 McDonell WN, Hall LW, Jeffcott LB. Radiographic evidence of impaired pulmonary function in laterally recumbent anaesthetised horses. *Equine Vet J* 1979; **11**: 24–32.

120 Sorenson PR, Robinson NE. Postural effects on lung volumes and asynchronous ventilation in anesthetized horses. *J Appl Physiol Respir Environ Exerc Physiol* 1980; **48**: 97–103.

121 Bradbrook CA, Clark L, Dugdale AH, *et al.* Measurement of respiratory system compliance and respiratory system resistance in healthy dogs undergoing general anaesthesia for elective orthopaedic procedures. *Vet Anaesth Analg* 2013; **40**: 382–389.

122 Lachmann B. Open up the lung and keep the lung open. *Intensive Care Med* 1992; **18**: 319–321.

123 Amato MB, Barbas CS, Medeiros DM, *et al.* Effect of a protective-ventilation strategy on mortality in the acute respiratory distress syndrome. *N Engl J Med* 1998; **338**: 347–354.

124 Satalin J, Andrews P, Gatto LA, *et al.* "Open the lung and keep it open": a homogeneously ventilated lung is a 'healthy lung'. *Ann Transl Med* 2016; **4**: 141.

125 Hartland BL, Newell TJ, Damico N. Alveolar recruitment maneuvers under general anesthesia: a systematic review of the literature. *Respir Care* 2015; **60**: 609–620.

126 Pensier J, de Jong A, Hajjej Z, *et al.* Effect of lung recruitment maneuver on oxygenation, physiological parameters and mortality in acute respiratory distress syndrome patients: a systematic review and meta-analysis. *Intensive Care Med* 2019; **45**: 1691–1702.

127 Nielsen J, Nilsson M, Fredén F, *et al.* Central hemodynamics during lung recruitment maneuvers at hypovolemia, normovolemia and hypervolemia. A study by echocardiography and continuous pulmonary artery flow measurements in lung-injured pigs. *Intensive Care Med* 2006; **32**: 585–594.

128 Nielsen J, Østergaard M, Kjaergaard J, *et al.* Lung recruitment maneuver depresses central hemodynamics in patients following cardiac surgery. *Intensive Care Med* 2005; **31**: 1189–1194.

129 Jardin F, Vieillard-Baron A. Right ventricular function and positive pressure ventilation in clinical practice: from hemodynamic subsets to respirator settings. *Intensive Care Med* 2003; **29**: 1426–1434.

130 Hopster K, Kästner SB, Rohn K, *et al.* Intermittent positive pressure ventilation with constant positive end-expiratory pressure and alveolar recruitment manoeuvre during inhalation anaesthesia in horses undergoing surgery for colic, and its influence on the early recovery period. *Vet Anaesth Analg* 2011; **38**: 169–177.

131 Hopster K, Jacobson B, Hopster-Iversen C, *et al.* Histopathological changes and mRNA expression in lungs of horses after inhalation anaesthesia with different ventilation strategies. *Res Vet Sci* 2016; **107**: 8–15.

132 Auckburally A, Nyman G. Review of hypoxaemia in anaesthetized horses: predisposing factors, consequences and management. *Vet Anaesth Analg* 2017; **44**: 397–408.

133 Mosing M, Senior JM. Maintenance of equine anaesthesia over the last 50 years: Controlled inhalation of volatile anaesthetics and pulmonary ventilation. *Equine Vet J* 2018; **50**: 282–291.

134 Hopster K, Rohn K, Ohnesorge B, *et al.* Controlled mechanical ventilation with constant positive end-expiratory pressure and alveolar recruitment manoeuvres during anaesthesia in laterally or dorsally recumbent horses. *Vet Anaesth Analg* 2017; **44**: 121–126.

135 Tusman G, Böhm SH. Prevention and reversal of lung collapse during the intraoperative period. *Best Pract Res Clin Anaesthesiol* 2010; **24**: 183–197.

136 Di Bella C, Lacitignola L, Grasso S, *et al.* An alveolar recruitment maneuver followed by positive end-expiratory pressure improves lung function in healthy dogs undergoing laparoscopy. *Vet Anaesth Analg* 2018; **45**: 618–629.

137 Suarez-Sipmann F, Böhm SH, Tusman G, *et al.* Use of dynamic compliance for open lung positive end-expiratory pressure titration in an experimental study. *Crit Care Med* 2007; **35**: 214–221.

138 García-Sanz V, Aguado D, Gómez de Segura IA, *et al.* Comparative effects of open-lung positive end-expiratory pressure (PEEP) and fixed PEEP on respiratory system compliance in the isoflurane anaesthetised healthy dog. *Res Vet Sci* 2019; **127**: 91–98.

139 García-Sanz V, Canfrán S, Gómez de Segura IA, *et al.* Effect of recumbency and body condition score on open-lung positive end-expiratory pressure and respiratory system compliance following a stepwise lung recruitment manoeuvre in healthy dogs during general anaesthesia. *Res Vet Sci* 2020; **132**: 177–185.

140 Wagner AE, Bednarski RM, Muir WW III. Hemodynamic effects of carbon dioxide during intermittent positive-pressure ventilation in horses. *Am J Vet Res* 1990; **51**: 1922–1929.

141 Khanna AK, McDonell WN, Dyson DH, *et al.* Cardiopulmonary effects of hypercapnia during controlled intermittent positive pressure ventilation in the horse. *Can J Vet Res* 1995; **59**: 213–221.

142 Akça O, Doufas AG, Morioka N, *et al.* Hypercapnia improves tissue oxygenation. *Anesthesiology* 2002; **97**: 801–806.

143 Gelman S. Venous function and central venous pressure: a physiologic story. *Anesthesiology* 2008; **108**: 735–748.

144 Teixeira-Neto FJ, Valverde A. Clinical application of the fluid challenge approach in goal-directed fluid therapy: what can we learn from human studies? *Front Vet Sci* 2021; **8**: 701377.

145 Mahmood SS, Pinsky MR. Heart-lung interactions during mechanical ventilation: the basics. *Ann Transl Med* 2018; **6**: 349.

146 Hernandez LA, Peevy KJ, Moise AA, *et al.* Chest wall restriction limits high airway pressure-induced lung injury in young rabbits. *J Appl Physiol (1985)* **1989**; 66: 2364–2368.

147 Dreyfuss D, Saumon G. Ventilator-induced lung injury: lessons from experimental studies. *Am J Respir Crit Care Med* 1998; **157**: 294–323.

148 Beitler JR, Malhotra A, Thompson BT. Ventilator-induced lung injury. *Clin Chest Med* 2016; **37**: 633–646.

149 Steinberg JM, Schiller HJ, Halter JM, *et al.* Alveolar instability causes early ventilator-induced lung injury independent of neutrophils. *Am J Respir Crit Care Med* 2004; **169**: 57–63.

150 Pavone L, Albert S, DiRocco J, *et al.* Alveolar instability caused by mechanical ventilation initially damages the nondependent normal lung. *Crit Care* 2007; **11**: R104.

151 Pavone LA, Albert S, Carney D, *et al.* Injurious mechanical ventilation in the normal lung causes a progressive pathologic change in dynamic alveolar mechanics. *Crit Care* 2007; **11**: R64.

152 Ranieri VM, Rubenfeld GD, Thompson BT, *et al.* Acute respiratory distress syndrome: the Berlin Definition. *JAMA* 2012; **307**: 2526–2533.

153 Parsons PE, Eisner MD, Thompson BT, *et al.* Lower tidal volume ventilation and plasma cytokine markers of inflammation in patients with acute lung injury. *Crit Care Med* 2005; **33**: 1–6.

154 Brower RG, Matthay MA, Morris A, *et al.* Ventilation with lower tidal volumes as compared with traditional tidal volumes for acute lung injury and the acute respiratory distress syndrome. *N Engl J Med* 2000; **342**: 1301–1308.

155 Ranieri VM, Suter PM, Tortorella C, *et al.* Effect of mechanical ventilation on inflammatory mediators in patients with acute respiratory distress syndrome: a randomized controlled trial. *JAMA* 1999; **282**: 54–61.

156 Wanderer JP, Ehrenfeld JM, Epstein RH, *et al.* Temporal trends and current practice patterns for intraoperative ventilation at U.S. academic medical centers: a retrospective study. *BMC Anesthesiol* 2015; **15**: 40.

157 Bein T, Grasso S, Moerer O, *et al.* The standard of care of patients with ARDS: ventilatory settings and rescue therapies for refractory hypoxemia. *Intensive Care Med* 2016; **42**: 699–711.

158 Tschumperlin DJ, Oswari J, Margulies AS. Deformation-induced injury of alveolar epithelial cells. Effect of frequency, duration, and amplitude. *Am J Respir Crit Care Med* 2000; **162**: 357–362.

159 Wolthuis EK, Choi G, Dessing MC, *et al.* Mechanical ventilation with lower tidal volumes and positive end-expiratory pressure prevents pulmonary inflammation in patients without pre-existing lung injury. *Anesthesiology* 2008; **108**: 46–54.

160 Serpa Neto A, Cardoso SO, Manetta JA, *et al.* Association between use of lung-protective ventilation with lower tidal volumes and clinical outcomes among patients without acute respiratory distress syndrome: a meta-analysis. *JAMA* 2012; **308**: 1651–1659.

161 Futier E, Constantin JM, Paugam-Burtz C, *et al.* A trial of intraoperative low-tidal-volume ventilation in abdominal surgery. *N Engl J Med* 2013; **369**: 428–437.

162 Young CC, Harris EM, Vacchiano C, *et al.* Lung-protective ventilation for the surgical patient: international expert panel-based consensus recommendations. *Br J Anaesth* 2019; **123**: 898–913.

163 Araos J, Lacitignola L, de Monte V, *et al.* Evaluation of lung aeration and respiratory system mechanics in obese dogs ventilated with tidal volumes based on ideal vs. *current body weight. Front Vet Sci* 2021; **8**: 704863.

164 Levitzky MG. Alveolar ventilation. In: *Pulmonary Physiology*, 9th edn. New York, NY: McGraw-Hill, 2018: 59–92.

165 Bumbacher S, Schramel JP, Mosing M. Evaluation of three tidal volumes (10, 12 and 15 mL kg(-1)) in dogs for controlled mechanical ventilation assessed by volumetric capnography: a randomized clinical trial. *Vet Anaesth Analg* 2017; **44**: 775–784.

166 Gallivan GJ, McDonell WN, Forrest JB. Comparative ventilation and gas exchange in the horse and the cow. *Res Vet Sci* 1989; **46**: 331–336.

167 De Monte V, Bufalari A, Grasso S, *et al.* Respiratory effects of low versus high tidal volume with or without positive end-expiratory pressure in anesthetized dogs with healthy lungs. *Am J Vet Res* 2018; **79**: 496–504.

168 Rodrigues RR, Ambrósio AM, Engbruch AM, *et al.* Intraoperative protective mechanical ventilation in dogs: a randomized clinical trial. *Front Vet Sci* 2022; **9**: 842613.

169 Martins ARC, Ambrósio AM, Fantoni DT, *et al.* Computed tomography assessment of tidal lung overinflation in domestic cats undergoing pressure-controlled mechanical ventilation during general anesthesia. *Front Vet Sci* 2022; **9**: 842528.

170 Dantzker DR, Wagner PD, West JB. Proceedings: instability of poorly ventilated lung units during oxygen breathing. *J Physiol* 1974; **242**: 72.

171 Joyce CJ, Baker AB. What is the role of absorption atelectasis in the genesis of perioperative pulmonary collapse? *Anaesth Intensive Care* 1995; **23**: 691–696.

172 Tucker PK, MacFarlane P. Incidence of perianaesthetic complications experienced during feline bronchoscopy: a retrospective study. *J Feline Med Surg* 2019; **21**: 959–966.

173 Johnson LR, Drazenovich TL. Flexible bronchoscopy and bronchoalveolar lavage in 68 cats (2001–2006). *J Vet Intern Med* 2007; **21**: 219–225.

174 Bianco Z, Bukoski A, Masseau I, *et al.* Risk factors and outcomes in dogs with respiratory disease undergoing diagnostic airway lavage. *Front Vet Sci* 2020; **7**: 165.

175 Cooper ES, Schober KE, Drost WT. Severe bronchoconstriction after bronchoalveolar lavage in a dog with eosinophilic airway disease. *J Am Vet Med Assoc* 2005; **227**: 1257–1262.
176 Perez TE, Tucker M, Grubb T, *et al.* Anesthesia case of the month inability to ventilate due to feline asthma exacerbated by general anesthesia and bronchoalveolar lavage. *J Am Vet Med Assoc* 2015; **247**: 605–609.
177 Hooi KS, Defarges AM, Sanchez AL, *et al.* Comparison of bronchoscopic and nonbronchoscopic bronchoalveolar lavage in healthy cats. *Am J Vet Res* 2018; **79**: 1209–1216.
178 Kirschvink N, Leemans J, Delvaux F, *et al.* Bronchodilators in bronchoscopy-induced airflow limitation in allergen-sensitized cats. *J Vet Intern Med* 2005; **19**: 161–167.
179 Dear JD, Johnson LR. Lower respiratory tract endoscopy in the cat: diagnostic approach to bronchial disease. *J Feline Med Surg* 2013; **15**: 1019–1027.
180 Scharf VF. Updates in thoracoscopy. *Vet Clin North Am Small Anim Pract* 2022; **52**: 531–548.
181 Matiasovic M, Halfacree ZJ, Moores A, *et al.* Surgical management of impalement injuries to the trunk of dogs: a multicentre retrospective study. *J Small Anim Pract* 2018; **59**: 139–146.
182 MacIver MA, Case JB, Monnet EL, *et al.* Video-assisted extirpation of cranial mediastinal masses in dogs: 18 cases (2009–2014). *J Am Vet Med Assoc* 2017; **250**: 1283–1290.
183 Nucci DJ, Hurst KC, Monnet E. Retrospective comparison of short-term outcomes following thoracoscopy versus thoracotomy for surgical correction of persistent right aortic arch in dogs. *J Am Vet Med Assoc* 2018; **253**: 444–451.
184 Radlinsky MG. Complications and need for conversion from thoracoscopy to thoracotomy in small animals. *Vet Clin North Am Small Anim Pract* 2009; **39**: 977–984.
185 Plesman R, Johnson M, Rurak S, *et al.* Thoracoscopic correction of a congenital persistent right aortic arch in a young cat. *Can Vet J* 2011; **52**: 1123–1128.
186 Carey Beer AJ, Hernon T, Halfacree Z, *et al.* Complications associated with and outcome of surgical intervention for treatment of esophageal foreign bodies in dogs. *J Am Vet Med Assoc* 2022; **260**: 622–627.
187 Vachon AM, Fischer AT. Thoracoscopy in the horse: diagnostic and therapeutic indications in 28 cases. *Equine Vet J* 1998; **30**: 467–475.
188 Malone ED, Farnsworth K, Lennox T, *et al.* Thoracoscopic-assisted diaphragmatic hernia repair using a thoracic rib resection. *Vet Surg* 2001; **30**: 175–178.
189 Hilton H, Aleman M, Madigan J, *et al.* Standing lateral thoracotomy in horses: indications, complications, and outcomes. *Vet Surg* 2010; **39**: 847–855.
190 Michaux H, Nichols S, Babkine M, *et al.* Description of thoracoscopy and associated short-term cardiovascular and pulmonary effects in healthy cattle. *Am J Vet Res* 2014; **75**: 468–476.
191 Dickson R, Scharf VF, Michael AE, *et al.* Surgical management and outcome of dogs with primary spontaneous pneumothorax: 110 cases (2009–2019). *J Am Vet Med Assoc* 2021; **258**: 1229–1235.
192 Bleakley S, Duncan CG, Monnet E. Thoracoscopic lung lobectomy for primary lung tumors in 13 dogs. *Vet Surg* 2015; **44**: 1029–1035.
193 Peroni JF, Robinson NE, Stick JA, *et al.* Pleuropulmonary and cardiovascular consequences of thoracoscopy performed in healthy standing horses. *Equine Vet J* 2000; **32**: 280–286.
194 Peroni JF, Horner NT, Robinson NE, *et al.* Equine thoracoscopy: normal anatomy and surgical technique. *Equine Vet J* 2001; **33**: 231–237.
195 Wormser C, Singhal S, Holt DE, *et al.* Thoracoscopic-assisted pulmonary surgery for partial and complete lung lobectomy in dogs and cats: 11 cases (2008–2013). *J Am Vet Med Assoc* 2014; **245**: 1036–1041.
196 Griffin MA, Sutton JS, Hunt GB, *et al.* Video-assisted thoracoscopic resection of a noninvasive thymoma in a cat with myasthenia gravis using low-pressure carbon dioxide insufflation. *Vet Surg* 2016; **45**: O28–O33.
197 Mayhew PD, Pascoe PJ, Giuffrida MA, *et al.* Cardiorespiratory effects of variable pressure thoracic insufflation in cats undergoing video-assisted thoracic surgery. *Vet Surg* 2019; **48**: O130–O137.
198 Mayhew PD, Pascoe PJ, Shilo-Benjamini Y, *et al.* Effect of one-lung ventilation with or without low-pressure carbon dioxide insufflation on cardiorespiratory variables in cats undergoing thoracoscopy. *Vet Surg* 2015; **44**: 15–22.
199 Faunt KK, Cohn LA, Jones BD, *et al.* Cardiopulmonary effects of bilateral hemithorax ventilation and diagnostic thoracoscopy in dogs. *Am J Vet Res* 1998; **59**: 1494–1498.
200 Daly CM, Swalec-Tobias K, Tobias AH, *et al.* Cardiopulmonary effects of intrathoracic insufflation in dogs. *J Am Anim Hosp Assoc* 2002; **38**: 515–520.
201 Polis I, Gasthuys F, Gielen I, *et al.* The effects of intrathoracic pressure during continuous two-lung ventilation for thoracoscopy on the cardiorespiratory parameters in sevoflurane anaesthetized dogs. *J Vet Med A Physiol Pathol Clin Med* 2002; **49**: 113–120.
202 Bohaychuk-Preuss KS, Carrozzo MV, Duke-Novakovski T. Cardiopulmonary effects of pleural insufflation with CO(2) during two-lung ventilation in dorsally recumbent anesthetized horses. *Vet Anaesth Analg* 2017; **44**: 483–491.
203 Röcken M, Mosel G, Barske K, *et al.* Thoracoscopic diaphragmatic hernia repair in a warmblood mare. *Vet Surg* 2013; **42**: 591–594.
204 Yoshida H, Takaori M. Pulmonary gas exchange and ventilation-perfusion relationships during hypocapnia and thoracotomy in anaesthetized dogs. *Can J Anaesth* 1991; **38**: 527–532.
205 Rustomjee T, Wagner A, Orton EC. Effect of 5 cm of water positive end-expiratory pressure on arterial oxygen tension in dogs during and after thoracotomy. *Vet Surg* 1994; **23**: 307–310.
206 Kudnig ST, Monnet E, Riquelme M, *et al.* Cardiopulmonary effects of thoracoscopy in anesthetized normal dogs. *Vet Anaesth Analg* 2004; **31**: 121–128.
207 Kudnig ST, Monnet E, Riquelme M, *et al.* Effect of positive end-expiratory pressure on oxygen delivery during 1-lung ventilation for thoracoscopy in normal dogs. *Vet Surg* 2006; **35**: 534–542.
208 Kudnig ST, Monnet E, Riquelme M, *et al.* Effect of one-lung ventilation on oxygen delivery in anesthetized dogs with an open thoracic cavity. *Am J Vet Res* 2003; **64**: 443–448.
209 Teixeira-Neto FJ, Carregaro AB, Mannarino R, *et al.* Comparison of a sidestream capnograph and a mainstream capnograph in mechanically ventilated dogs. *J Am Vet Med Assoc* 2002; **221**: 1582–1585.
210 Wagner AE, Gaynor JS, Dunlop CI, *et al.* Monitoring adequacy of ventilation by capnometry during thoracotomy in dogs. *J Am Vet Med Assoc* 1998; **212**: 377–379.
211 Mahfood S, Hix WR, Aaron BL, *et al.* Reexpansion pulmonary edema. *Ann Thorac Surg* 1988; **45**: 340–345.
212 Sohara Y. Reexpansion pulmonary edema. *Ann Thorac Cardiovasc Surg* 2008; **14**: 205–209.
213 Stampley AR, Waldron DR. Reexpansion pulmonary edema after surgery to repair a diaphragmatic hernia in a cat. *J Am Vet Med Assoc* 1993; **203**: 1699–1701.
214 Pascoe PJ, Dyson DH. Analgesia after lateral thoracotomy in dogs. Epidural morphine vs. intercostal bupivacaine. *Vet Surg* 1993; **22**: 141–147.
215 Carregaro AB, Freitas GC, Lopes C, *et al.* Evaluation of analgesic and physiologic effects of epidural morphine administered at a thoracic or lumbar level in dogs undergoing thoracotomy. *Vet Anaesth Analg* 2014; **41**: 205–211.
216 Steagall PVM, Simon BT, Teixeira-Neto FJ, *et al.* An update on drugs used for lumbosacral epidural anesthesia and analgesia in dogs. *Front Vet Sci* 2017; **4**: 68.
217 Pirsaharkhiz N, Comolli K, Fujiwara W, *et al.* Utility of erector spinae plane block in thoracic surgery. *J Cardiothorac Surg* 2020; **15**: 91.
218 Portela DA, Castro D, Romano M, *et al.* Ultrasound-guided erector spinae plane block in canine cadavers: relevant anatomy and injectate distribution. *Vet Anaesth Analg* 2020; **47**: 229–237.
219 Ferré BMI, Drozdzynska M, Vettorato E. Ultrasound-guided bilateral erector spinae plane block in dogs undergoing sternotomies anaesthetised with propofol-dexmedetomidine continuous infusion. *Vet Res Commun* 2022; **46**: 1331–1337.
220 Gómez Fernández L, Huuskonen V, Potter J. The combination of an ultrasound-guided erector spinae plane (ESP) block and epidural morphine as effective intra-operative adjuncts to opioid premedication in six dogs undergoing lateral thoracotomy. *Vet Rec Case Rep* 2021; **9**: e152.
221 Khalil AE, Abdallah NM, Bashandy GM, *et al.* Ultrasound-guided serratus anterior plane block versus thoracic epidural analgesia for thoracotomy pain. *J Cardiothorac Vasc Anesth* 2017; **31**: 152–158.
222 Freitag FA, Gaio TS, Dos Santos AA, *et al.* Ultrasound-guided superficial serratus plane block in dog cadavers: an anatomical evaluation and volume dispersion study. *Vet Anaesth Analg* 2020; **47**: 88–94.
223 Bosak VL, Piontkovsky RJ, Mazur Dos Santos A, *et al.* Ultrasound-guided superficial serratus plane block in multimodal analgesia for three dogs undergoing surgical correction of persistent ductus arteriosus. *Vet Anaesth Analg* 2022; **49**: 330–332.
224 Thompson SE, Johnson JM. Analgesia in dogs after intercostal thoracotomy. A comparison of morphine, selective intercostal nerve block, and interpleural regional analgesia with bupivacaine. *Vet Surg* 1991; **20**: 73–77.
225 Stobie D, Caywood DD, Rozanski EA, *et al.* Evaluation of pulmonary function and analgesia in dogs after intercostal thoracotomy and use of morphine administered intramuscularly or intrapleurally and bupivacaine administered intrapleurally. *Am J Vet Res* 1995; **56**: 1098–1109.
226 Bernard F, Kudnig ST, Monnet E. Hemodynamic effects of interpleural lidocaine and bupivacaine combination in anesthetized dogs with and without an open pericardium. *Vet Surg* 2006; **35**: 252–258.
227 Pascoe PJ, Mayhew PD. Anesthesia for thoracoscopy. In: Fransson BA, Mayhew PD, eds. *Small Animal Laparoscopy and Thoracoscopy*. Ames, IA: John Wiley and Sons, Inc., 2015: 255–273.
228 Lansdowne JL, Monnet E, Twedt DC, *et al.* Thoracoscopic lung lobectomy for treatment of lung tumors in dogs. *Vet Surg* 2005; **34**: 530–535.
229 Adami C, Axiak S, Rytz U, *et al.* Alternating one lung ventilation using a double lumen endobronchial tube and providing CPAP to the non-ventilated lung in a dog. *Vet Anaesth Analg* 2011; **38**: 70–76.

230 Mayhew PD, Culp WT, Pascoe PJ, *et al.* Evaluation of blind thoracoscopic-assisted placement of three double-lumen endobronchial tube designs for one-lung ventilation in dogs. *Vet Surg* 2012; **41**: 664–670.
231 Mayhew PD, Hunt GB, Steffey MA, *et al.* Evaluation of short-term outcome after lung lobectomy for resection of primary lung tumors via video-assisted thoracoscopic surgery or open thoracotomy in medium- to large-breed dogs. *J Am Vet Med Assoc* 2013; **243**: 681–688.
232 Fabila TS, Menghraj SJ. One lung ventilation strategies for infants and children undergoing video assisted thoracoscopic surgery. *Indian J Anaesth* 2013; **57**: 339–344.
233 Wu C, Liang X, Liu B. Selective pulmonary lobe isolation with Arndt pediatric endobronchial blocker for an infant: a case report. *Med (Baltimore)* 2019; **98**: e18262.
234 Mayhew PD, Chohan A, Hardy BT, *et al.* Cadaveric evaluation of fluoroscopy-assisted placement of one-lung ventilation devices for video-assisted thoracoscopic surgery in dogs. *Vet Surg* 2020; **49**: O93–O101.
235 Slinger P, Campos JH. Anesthesia for thoracic surgery. In: Gropper MACN, Eriksson LI, Fleisher LA, *et al.*, eds. *Miller's Anesthesia*, 9th ed. Philadelphia, PA: Elsevier, 2020: 1648–1716.
236 Cantwell SL, Duke T, Walsh PJ, *et al.* One-lung versus two-lung ventilation in the closed-chest anesthetized dog: a comparison of cardiopulmonary parameters. *Vet Surg* 2000; **29**: 365–373.
237 Riquelme M, Monnet E, Kudnig ST, *et al.* Cardiopulmonary changes induced during one-lung ventilation in anesthetized dogs with a closed thoracic cavity. *Am J Vet Res* 2005; **66**: 973–977.
238 Riquelme M, Monnet E, Kudnig ST, *et al.* Cardiopulmonary effects of positive end-expiratory pressure during one-lung ventilation in anesthetized dogs with a closed thoracic cavity. *Am J Vet Res* 2005; **66**: 978–983.
239 Floriano BP, Trein TA, Wagatsuma JT, *et al.* Pulmonary hemodynamics and alveolar oxygenation in healthy dogs anesthetized with propofol or isoflurane during one-lung ventilation in a closed-thoracic experimental model. *Am J Vet Res* 2017; **78**: 1117–1125.
240 Karzai W, Schwarzkopf K. Hypoxemia during one-lung ventilation: prediction, prevention, and treatment. *Anesthesiology* 2009; **110**: 1402–1411.
241 Campos JH, Feider A. Hypoxia during one-lung ventilation-a review and update. *J Cardiothorac Vasc Anesth* 2018; **32**: 2330–2338.
242 Case JB, Maxwell M, Aman A, *et al.* Outcome evaluation of a thoracoscopic pericardial window procedure or subtotal pericardectomy via thoracotomy for the treatment of pericardial effusion in dogs. *J Am Vet Med Assoc* 2013; **242**: 493–498.
243 Dupré GP, Corlouer JP, Bouvy B. Thoracoscopic pericardectomy performed without pulmonary exclusion in 9 dogs. *Vet Surg* 2001; **30**: 21–27.
244 Townsend S, Oblak ML, Singh A, *et al.* Thoracoscopy with concurrent esophagoscopy for persistent right aortic arch in 9 dogs. *Vet Surg* 2016; **45**: O111–O118.
245 Levionnois OL, Bergadano A, Schatzmann U. Accidental entrapment of an endobronchial blocker tip by a surgical stapler during selective ventilation for lung lobectomy in a dog. *Vet Surg* 2006; **35**: 82–85.
246 Apfelbaum JL, Hagberg CA, Connis RT, *et al.* 2022 American Society of Anesthesiologists practice guidelines for management of the difficult airway. *Anesthesiology* 2022; **136**: 31–81.
247 Dupré G, Heidenreich D. Brachycephalic syndrome. *Vet Clin North Am Small Anim Pract* 2016; **46**: 691–707.
248 Liu NC, Troconis EL, Kalmar L, *et al.* Conformational risk factors of Brachycephalic Obstructive Airway Syndrome (BOAS) in Pugs, French Bulldogs, and Bulldogs. *PLoS ONE* 2017; **12**: e0181928.
249 Ladlow J, Liu NC, Kalmar L, *et al.* Brachycephalic obstructive airway syndrome. *Vet Rec* 2018; **182**: 375–378.
250 Riecks TW, Birchard SJ, Stephens JA. Surgical correction of brachycephalic syndrome in dogs: 62 cases (1991–2004). *J Am Vet Med Assoc* 2007; **230**: 1324–1328.
251 Phillips H. Updates in upper respiratory surgery. *Vet Clin North Am Small Anim Pract* 2022; **52**: 339–368.
252 Heidenreich D, Gradner G, Kneissl S, *et al.* Nasopharyngeal dimensions from computed tomography of Pugs and French Bulldogs with brachycephalic airway syndrome. *Vet Surg* 2016; **45**: 83–90.
253 Meola SD. Brachycephalic airway syndrome. *Top Companion Anim Med* 2013; **28**: 91–96.
254 Auger M, Alexander K, Beauchamp G, *et al.* Use of CT to evaluate and compare intranasal features in brachycephalic and normocephalic dogs. *J Small Anim Pract* 2016; **57**: 529–536.
255 De Lorenzi D, Bertoncello D, Drigo M. Bronchial abnormalities found in a consecutive series of 40 brachycephalic dogs. *J Am Vet Med Assoc* 2009; **235**: 835–840.
256 Yoon H, Yu J, An G, *et al.* CT and radiographic evaluation of bronchial collapsibility at forced expiration in asymptomatic brachycephalic dogs. *Vet Radiol Ultrasound* 2020; **61**: 167–180.
257 Bernaerts F, Talavera J, Leemans J, *et al.* Description of original endoscopic findings and respiratory functional assessment using barometric whole-body plethysmography in dogs suffering from brachycephalic airway obstruction syndrome. *Vet J* 2010; **183**: 95–102.
258 Hendricks JC, Kline LR, Kovalski RJ, *et al.* The English Bulldog: a natural model of sleep-disordered breathing. *J Appl Physiol (1985)* **1987**; 63: 1344–1350.
259 Hoareau GL, Jourdan G, Mellema M, *et al.* Evaluation of arterial blood gases and arterial blood pressures in brachycephalic dogs. *J Vet Intern Med* 2012; **26**: 897–904.
260 Sławuta P, Nicpoń J, Domańska S. Influence of the wing-of-the-nostrils correction procedure on the change of the acid-base balance parameters and oxygen concentration in the arterial blood in French Bulldogs. *Pol J Vet Sci* 2011; **14**: 77–80.
261 Hoareau GL, Mellema MS, Silverstein DC. Indication, management, and outcome of brachycephalic dogs requiring mechanical ventilation. *J Vet Emerg Crit Care (San Antonio)* 2011; **21**: 226–235.
262 Downing F, Gibson S. Anaesthesia of brachycephalic dogs. *J Small Anim Pract* 2018; **59**: 725–733.
263 Ogura JH, Nelson JR, Suemitsu M, *et al.* Relationship between pulmonary resistance and changes in arterial blood gas tension in dogs with nasal obstruction, and partial laryngeal obstruction. *Ann Otol Rhinol Laryngol* 1973; **82**: 668–683.
264 Poncet CM, Dupré GP, Freiche VG, *et al.* Long-term results of upper respiratory syndrome surgery and gastrointestinal tract medical treatment in 51 brachycephalic dogs. *J Small Anim Pract* 2006; **47**: 137–142.
265 Poncet CM, Dupré GP, Freiche VG, *et al.* Prevalence of gastrointestinal tract lesions in 73 brachycephalic dogs with upper respiratory syndrome. *J Small Anim Pract* 2005; **46**: 273–279.
266 Kaye BM, Rutherford L, Perridge DJ, *et al.* Relationship between brachycephalic airway syndrome and gastrointestinal signs in three breeds of dog. *J Small Anim Pract* 2018; **59**: 670–673.
267 Haimel G, Dupré G. Brachycephalic airway syndrome: a comparative study between Pugs and French Bulldogs. *J Small Anim Pract* 2015; **56**: 714–719.
268 Vangrinsven E, Broux O, Massart L, *et al.* Diagnosis and treatment of gastro-oesophageal junction abnormalities in dogs with brachycephalic syndrome. *J Small Anim Pract* 2021; **62**: 200–208.
269 Freiche V, German AJ. Digestive diseases in brachycephalic dogs. *Vet Clin North Am Small Anim Pract* 2021; **51**: 61–78.
270 Ovbey DH, Wilson DV, Bednarski RM, *et al.* Prevalence and risk factors for canine post-anesthetic aspiration pneumonia (1999–2009): a multicenter study. *Vet Anaesth Analg* 2014; **41**: 127–136.
271 Darcy HP, Humm K, Ter Haar G. Retrospective analysis of incidence, clinical features, potential risk factors, and prognostic indicators for aspiration pneumonia in three brachycephalic dog breeds. *J Am Vet Med Assoc* 2018; **253**: 869–876.
272 Kogan DA, Johnson LR, Jandrey KE, *et al.* Clinical, clinicopathologic, and radiographic findings in dogs with aspiration pneumonia: 88 cases (2004–2006). *J Am Vet Med Assoc* 2008; **233**: 1742–1747.
273 Fenner JVH, Quinn RJ, Demetriou JL. Postoperative regurgitation in dogs after upper airway surgery to treat brachycephalic obstructive airway syndrome: 258 cases (2013–2017). *Vet Surg* 2020; **49**: 53–60.
274 Reeve EJ, Sutton D, Friend EJ, *et al.* Documenting the prevalence of hiatal hernia and oesophageal abnormalities in brachycephalic dogs using fluoroscopy. *J Small Anim Pract* 2017; **58**: 703–708.
275 Broux O, Clercx C, Etienne AL, *et al.* Effects of manipulations to detect sliding hiatal hernia in dogs with brachycephalic airway obstructive syndrome. *Vet Surg* 2018; **47**: 243–251.
276 Eivers C, Chicon Rueda R, Liuti T, *et al.* Retrospective analysis of esophageal imaging features in brachycephalic versus non-brachycephalic dogs based on videofluoroscopic swallowing studies. *J Vet Intern Med* 2019; **33**: 1740–1746.
277 Lindsay B, Cook D, Wetzel JM, *et al.* Brachycephalic airway syndrome: management of postoperative respiratory complications in 248 dogs. *Aust Vet J* 2020; **98**: 173–180.
278 Doxey S, Boswood A. Differences between breeds of dog in a measure of heart rate variability. *Vet Rec* 2004; **154**: 713–717.
279 Packer RM, Hendricks A, Tivers MS, *et al.* Impact of facial conformation on canine health: brachycephalic obstructive airway syndrome. *PLoS ONE* 2015; **10**: e0137496.
280 Torrez CV, Hunt GB. Results of surgical correction of abnormalities associated with brachycephalic airway obstruction syndrome in dogs in Australia. *J Small Anim Pract* 2006; **47**: 150–154.
281 Pohl S, Roedler FS, Oechtering GU. How does multilevel upper airway surgery influence the lives of dogs with severe brachycephaly? Results of a structured pre- and postoperative owner questionnaire. *Vet J* 2016; **210**: 39–45.
282 Seneviratne M, Kaye BM, Ter Haar G. Prognostic indicators of short-term outcome in dogs undergoing surgery for brachycephalic obstructive airway syndrome. *Vet Rec* 2020; **187**: 403.

283 Carabalona JPR, Le Boedec K, Poncet CM. Complications, prognostic factors, and long-term outcomes for dogs with brachycephalic obstructive airway syndrome that underwent H-pharyngoplasty and ala-vestibuloplasty: 423 cases (2011–2017). *J Am Vet Med Assoc* 2021; **260**: S65–S73.

284 Dyson DH, Maxie MG, Schnurr D. Morbidity and mortality associated with anesthetic management in small animal veterinary practice in Ontario. *J Am Anim Hosp Assoc* 1998; **34**: 325–335.

285 Gaynor JS, Dunlop CI, Wagner AE, *et al.* Complications and mortality associated with anesthesia in dogs and cats. *J Am Anim Hosp Assoc* 1999; **35**: 13–17.

286 Gruenheid M, Aarnes TK, McLoughlin MA, *et al.* Risk of anesthesia-related complications in brachycephalic dogs. *J Am Vet Med Assoc* 2018; **253**: 301–306.

287 Doyle CR, Aarnes TK, Ballash GA, *et al.* Anesthetic risk during subsequent anesthetic events in brachycephalic dogs that have undergone corrective airway surgery: 45 cases (2007–2019). *J Am Vet Med Assoc* 2020; **257**: 744–749.

288 Ree JJ, Milovancev M, MacIntyre LA, *et al.* Factors associated with major complications in the short-term postoperative period in dogs undergoing surgery for brachycephalic airway syndrome. *Can Vet J* 2016; **57**: 976–980.

289 Fasanella FJ, Shivley JM, Wardlaw JL, *et al.* Brachycephalic airway obstructive syndrome in dogs: 90 cases (1991–2008). *J Am Vet Med Assoc* 2010; **237**: 1048–1051.

290 Oda A, Wang WH, Hampton AK, *et al.* Perianesthetic mortality in English Bulldogs: a retrospective analysis in 2010 - 2017. *BMC Vet Res* 2022; **18**: 198.

291 Liu NC, Oechtering GU, Adams VJ, *et al.* Outcomes and prognostic factors of surgical treatments for brachycephalic obstructive airway syndrome in 3 breeds. *Vet Surg* 2017; **46**: 271–280.

292 Tarricone J, Hayes GM, Singh A, Davis G. Development and validation of a brachycephalic risk (BRisk) score to predict the risk of complications in dogs presenting for surgical treatment of brachycephalic obstructive airway syndrome. *Vet Surg* 2019; **48**: 1253–1261.

293 Grubb T. Anesthesia for patients with respiratory disease and/or airway compromise. *Top Companion Anim Med* 2010; **25**: 120–132.

294 Costa RS, Abelson AL, Lindsey JC, *et al.* Postoperative regurgitation and respiratory complications in brachycephalic dogs undergoing airway surgery before and after implementation of a standardized perianesthetic protocol. *J Am Vet Med Assoc* 2020; **256**: 899–905.

295 Riggs J, Liu NC, Sutton DR, *et al.* Validation of exercise testing and laryngeal auscultation for grading brachycephalic obstructive airway syndrome in Pugs, French Bulldogs, and English Bulldogs by using whole-body barometric plethysmography. *Vet Surg* 2019; **48**: 488–496.

296 Liu NC, Adams VJ, Kalmar L, *et al.* Whole-body barometric plethysmography characterizes upper airway obstruction in 3 brachycephalic breeds of dogs. *J Vet Intern Med* 2016; **30**: 853–865.

297 Franklin PH, Liu NC, Ladlow JF. Nebulization of epinephrine to reduce the severity of brachycephalic obstructive airway syndrome in dogs. *Vet Surg* 2021; **50**: 62–70.

298 Farrell KS, Hopper K, Cagle LA, *et al.* Evaluation of pulse oximetry as a surrogate for PaO(2) in awake dogs breathing room air and anesthetized dogs on mechanical ventilation. *J Vet Emerg Crit Care (San Antonio)* 2019; **29**: 622–629.

299 Panti A, Bennett RC, Corletto F, *et al.* The effect of omeprazole on oesophageal pH in dogs during anaesthesia. *J Small Anim Pract* 2009; **50**: 540–544.

300 Marks SL, Kook PH, Papich MG, *et al.* ACVIM consensus statement: support for rational administration of gastrointestinal protectants to dogs and cats. *J Vet Intern Med* 2018; **32**: 1823–1840.

301 Lotti F, Twedt D, Warrit K, *et al.* Effect of two different pre-anaesthetic omeprazole protocols on gastroesophageal reflux incidence and pH in dogs. *J Small Anim Pract* 2021; **62**: 677–682.

302 Kempf J, Lewis F, Reusch CE, *et al.* High-resolution manometric evaluation of the effects of cisapride and metoclopramide hydrochloride administered orally on lower esophageal sphincter pressure in awake dogs. *Am J Vet Res* 2014; **75**: 361–366.

303 Hay Kraus BL. Efficacy of maropitant in preventing vomiting in dogs premedicated with hydromorphone. *Vet Anaesth Analg* 2013; **40**: 28–34.

304 Hay Kraus BL. Efficacy of orally administered maropitant citrate in preventing vomiting associated with hydromorphone administration in dogs. *J Am Vet Med Assoc* 2014; **244**: 1164–1169.

305 Claude AK, Dedeaux A, Chiavaccini L, *et al.* Effects of maropitant citrate or acepromazine on the incidence of adverse events associated with hydromorphone premedication in dogs. *J Vet Intern Med* 2014; **28**: 1414–1417.

306 Johnson RA. Maropitant prevented vomiting but not gastroesophageal reflux in anesthetized dogs premedicated with acepromazine-hydromorphone. *Vet Anaesth Analg* 2014; **41**: 406–410.

307 Erickson A, Harbin K, MacPherson J, *et al.* A review of pre-appointment medications to reduce fear and anxiety in dogs and cats at veterinary visits. *Can Vet J* 2021; **62**: 952–960.

308 Viskjer S, Sjöström L. Effect of the duration of food withholding prior to anesthesia on gastroesophageal reflux and regurgitation in healthy dogs undergoing elective orthopedic surgery. *Am J Vet Res* 2017; **78**: 144–150.

309 Tsompanidou P, Robben JH, Savvas I, *et al.* The effect of the preoperative fasting regimen on the incidence of gastro-oesophageal reflux in 90 dogs. *Animals (Basel)* 2021; **12**: 64.

310 Valverde A, Cantwell S, Hernández J, *et al.* Effects of acepromazine on the incidence of vomiting associated with opioid administration in dogs. *Vet Anaesth Analg* 2004; **31**: 40–45.

311 Wilson DV, Evans AT, Miller R. Effects of preanesthetic administration of morphine on gastroesophageal reflux and regurgitation during anesthesia in dogs. *Am J Vet Res* 2005; **66**: 386–390.

312 Koh RB, Isaza N, Xie H, *et al.* Effects of maropitant, acepromazine, and electroacupuncture on vomiting associated with administration of morphine in dogs. *J Am Vet Med Assoc* 2014; **244**: 820–829.

313 Blancquaert JP, Lefebvre RA, Willems JL. Emetic and antiemetic effects of opioids in the dog. *Eur J Pharmacol* 1986; **128**: 143–150.

314 Petruccione I, Murison PJ, Flaherty D, *et al.* Comparison between dexmedetomidine and acepromazine in combination with methadone for premedication in brachycephalic dogs undergoing surgery for brachycephalic obstructive airway syndrome. *Vet Anaesth Analg* 2021; **48**: 305–313.

315 Strombeck DR, Harrold D. Effects of atropine, acepromazine, meperidine, and xylazine on gastroesophageal sphincter pressure in the dog. *Am J Vet Res* 1985; **46**: 963–965.

316 Galatos AD, Raptopoulos D. Gastro-oesophageal reflux during anaesthesia in the dog: the effect of preoperative fasting and premedication. *Vet Rec* 1995; **137**: 479–483.

317 Sanmiguel CP, Hagiike M, Mintchev MP, *et al.* Effect of electrical stimulation of the LES on LES pressure in a canine model. *Am J Physiol Gastrointest Liver Physiol* 2008; **295**: G389–G394.

318 van der Hoeven CW, Attia A, Deen L, *et al.* The influence of anaesthetic drugs on the lower oesophageal sphincter in propofol/nitrous oxide anaesthetized dogs. Pressure profilometry in an animal model. *Acta Anaesthesiol Scand* 1995; **39**: 822–826.

319 Johnson RA, Striler E, Sawyer DC, Brunson DB. Comparison of isoflurane with sevoflurane for anesthesia induction and recovery in adult dogs. *Am J Vet Res* 1998; **59**: 478–481.

320 Bennett RC, Fancy SP, Walsh CM, *et al.* Comparison of sevoflurane and isoflurane in dogs anaesthetised for clinical surgical or diagnostic procedures. *J Small Anim Pract* 2008; **49**: 392–397.

321 Monteiro ER, Teixeira-Neto FJ, Campagnol D, *et al.* Effects of remifentanil on the minimum alveolar concentration of isoflurane in dogs. *Am J Vet Res* 2010; **71**: 150–156.

322 Williamson AJ, Soares JHN, Pavlisko ND, *et al.* Isoflurane minimum alveolar concentration sparing effects of fentanyl in the dog. *Vet Anaesth Analg* 2017; **44**: 738–745.

323 Hoke JF, Cunningham F, James MK, *et al.* Comparative pharmacokinetics and pharmacodynamics of remifentanil, its principle metabolite (GR90291) and alfentanil in dogs. *J Pharmacol Exp Ther* 1997; **281**: 226–232.

324 Iizuka T, Nishimura R. Context-sensitive half-time of fentanyl in dogs. *J Vet Med Sci* 2015; **77**: 615–617.

325 Torrente C, Vigueras I, Manzanilla EG, *et al.* Prevalence of and risk factors for intraoperative gastroesophageal reflux and postanesthetic vomiting and diarrhea in dogs undergoing general anesthesia. *J Vet Emerg Crit Care (San Antonio)* 2017; **27**: 397–408.

326 De Gennaro C, Vettorato E, Corletto F. Evaluation of bilateral maxillary nerve block in dogs undergoing surgery for brachycephalic obstructive airway syndrome. *Can Vet J* 2022; **63**: 67–73.

327 Cremer J, Sum SO, Braun C, *et al.* Assessment of maxillary and infraorbital nerve blockade for rhinoscopy in sevoflurane anesthetized dogs. *Vet Anaesth Analg* 2013; **40**: 432–439.

328 Loughran CM, Raisis AL, Haitjema G, *et al.* Unilateral retrobulbar hematoma following maxillary nerve block in a dog. *J Vet Emerg Crit Care (San Antonio)* 2016; **26**: 815–818.

329 Senn D, Sigrist N, Forterre F, *et al.* Retrospective evaluation of postoperative nasotracheal tubes for oxygen supplementation in dogs following surgery for brachycephalic syndrome: 36 cases (2003–2007). *J Vet Emerg Crit Care (San Antonio)* 2011; **21**: 261–267.

330 Carver A, Bragg R, Sullivan L. Evaluation of PaO2 /FiO2 and SaO2 /FiO2 ratios in postoperative dogs recovering on room air or nasal oxygen insufflation. *J Vet Emerg Crit Care (San Antonio)* 2016; **26**: 437–445.

331 Calabro JM, Prittie JE, Palma DA. Preliminary evaluation of the utility of comparing SpO2 /FiO2 and PaO2 /FiO2 ratios in dogs. *J Vet Emerg Crit Care (San Antonio)* 2013; **23**: 280–285.

332 Stabile M, Lacitignola L, Piemontese MR, *et al.* Comparison of CPAP and oxygen therapy for treatment of postoperative hypoxaemia in dogs. *J Small Anim Pract* 2021; **62**: 351–358.

333 Ceccherini G, Lippi I, Citi S, *et al.* Continuous Positive Airway Pressure (CPAP) provision with a pediatric helmet for treatment of hypoxemic acute respiratory failure in dogs. *J Vet Emerg Crit Care (San Antonio)* 2020; **30**: 41–49.

334 Rondelli V, Guarracino A, Iacobellis P, *et al.* Evaluation of the effects of helmet continuous positive airway pressure on laryngeal size in dogs anesthetized with propofol and fentanyl using computed tomography. *J Vet Emerg Crit Care (San Antonio)* 2020; **30**: 543–549.

335 Stordalen MB, Silveira F, Fenner JVH, *et al.* Outcome of temporary tracheostomy tube-placement following surgery for brachycephalic obstructive airway syndrome in 42 dogs. *J Small Anim Pract* 2020; **61**: 292–299.

336 Gobbetti M, Romussi S, Buracco P, *et al.* Long-term outcome of permanent tracheostomy in 15 dogs with severe laryngeal collapse secondary to brachycephalic airway obstructive syndrome. *Vet Surg* 2018; **47**: 648–653.

337 Geiger M, Schoenebeck JJ, Schneider RA, *et al.* Exceptional changes in skeletal anatomy under domestication: the case of brachycephaly. *Integr Org Biol* 2021; **3**: obab023.

338 Farnworth MJ, Chen R, Packer RM, *et al.* Flat feline faces: is brachycephaly associated with respiratory abnormalities in the domestic cat (*Felis catus*)? *PLoS ONE* 2016; **11**: e0161777

339 Plitman L, Černá P, Farnworth MJ, *et al.* Motivation of owners to purchase pedigree cats, with specific focus on the acquisition of brachycephalic cats. *Animals (Basel)* 2019; **9**: 394.

340 Ginn JA, Kumar MS, McKiernan BC, *et al.* Nasopharyngeal turbinates in brachycephalic dogs and cats. *J Am Anim Hosp Assoc* 2008; **44**: 243–249.

341 Schlueter C, Budras KD, Ludewig E, *et al.* Brachycephalic feline noses: CT and anatomical study of the relationship between head conformation and the nasolacrimal drainage system. *J Feline Med Surg* 2009; **11**: 891–900.

342 Corgozinho KB, Pereira AN, Cunha SC, *et al.* Recurrent pulmonary edema secondary to elongated soft palate in a cat. *J Feline Med Surg* 2012; **14**: 417–419.

343 Anagrius KL, Dimopoulou M, Moe AN, *et al.* Facial conformation characteristics in Persian and Exotic Shorthair cats. *J Feline Med Surg* 2021; **23**: 1089–1097.

344 Trostel CT, Frankel DJ. Punch resection alaplasty technique in dogs and cats with stenotic nares: 14 cases. *J Am Anim Hosp Assoc* 2010; **46**: 5–11.

345 Berns CN, Schmiedt CW, Dickerson VM, *et al.* Single pedicle advancement flap for treatment of feline stenotic nares: technique and results in five cases. *J Feline Med Surg* 2020; **22**: 1238–1242.

346 Featherstone HJ, Sansom J. Feline corneal sequestra: a review of 64 cases (80 eyes) from 1993 to 2000. *Vet Ophthalmol* 2004; **7**: 213–227.

347 Sieslack J, Farke D, Failing K, *et al.* Correlation of brachycephaly grade with level of exophthalmos, reduced airway passages and degree of dental malalignment in Persian cats. *PLoS ONE* 2021; **16**: e0254420.

348 O'Neill DG, Romans C, Brodbelt DC, *et al.* Persian cats under first opinion veterinary care in the UK: demography, mortality and disorders. *Sci Rep* 2019; **9**: 12952.

349 Robertson SA, Gogolski SM, Pascoe P, *et al.* AAFP feline anesthesia guidelines. *J Feline Med Surg* 2018; **20**: 602–634.

350 Doodnaught GM, Pang DS. Intubation following high-dose rocuronium in a cat with protracted laryngospasm. *JFMS Open Rep* 2017; **3**: 2055116917733642.

351 Di Bella C, Araos J, Lacitignola L, *et al.* Effects of continuous positive airway pressure administered by a helmet in cats under general anaesthesia. *J Feline Med Surg* 2021; **23**: 337–343.

352 Ewart SL. Overview of respiratory function: ventilation of the lungs. In: Klein BG, ed. *Cunningham's Textbook of Veterinary Physiology*, 6th ed. St. Louis, MO: Elsevier, 2020: 518–531.

353 Millard RP, Tobias KM. Laryngeal paralysis in dogs. *Compend Contin Educ Vet* 2009; **31**: 212–219.

354 MacPhail CM. Laryngeal disease in dogs and cats: an update. *Vet Clin North Am Small Anim Pract* 2020; **50**: 295–310.

355 Letko A, Minor KM, Friedenberg SG, *et al.* A CNTNAP1 missense variant is associated with canine laryngeal paralysis and polyneuropathy. *Genes (Basel)* 2020; **11**: 1426.

356 Sample SJ, Stilin A, Binversie EE, *et al.* Late-onset laryngeal paralysis: owner perception of quality of life and cause of death. *Vet Med Sci* 2020; **6**: 306–313.

357 Tarvin KM, Twedt DC, Monnet E. Prospective controlled study of gastroesophageal reflux in dogs with naturally occurring laryngeal paralysis. *Vet Surg* 2016; **45**: 916–921.

358 Monnet E. Surgical treatment of laryngeal paralysis. *Vet Clin North Am Small Anim Pract* 2016; **46**: 709–717.

359 Sakai DM, Martin-Flores M, Jones AK, *et al.* Laryngeal mask airway and transient hypercapnic hyperpnea for video-endoscopic assessment of unilateral laryngeal paralysis in dogs. *Vet Surg* 2018; **47**: 543–548.

360 Bookbinder LC, Flanders J, Bookbinder PF, *et al.* Idiopathic canine laryngeal paralysis as one sign of a diffuse polyneuropathy: an observational study of 90 cases (2007–2013). *Vet Surg* 2016; **45**: 254–260.

361 Hammel SP, Hottinger HA, Novo RE. Postoperative results of unilateral arytenoid lateralization for treatment of idiopathic laryngeal paralysis in dogs: 39 cases (1996–2002). *J Am Vet Med Assoc* 2006; **228**: 1215–1220.

362 Snelling SR, Edwards GA. A retrospective study of unilateral arytenoid lateralisation in the treatment of laryngeal paralysis in 100 dogs (1992–2000). *Aust Vet J* 2003; **81**: 464–468.

363 Nelissen P, White RA. Arytenoid lateralization for management of combined laryngeal paralysis and laryngeal collapse in small dogs. *Vet Surg* 2012; **41**: 261–265.

364 Wilson D, Monnet E. Risk factors for the development of aspiration pneumonia after unilateral arytenoid lateralization in dogs with laryngeal paralysis: 232 cases (1987–2012). *J Am Vet Med Assoc* 2016; **248**: 188–194.

365 Zacuto AC, Marks SL, Osborn J, *et al.* The influence of esomeprazole and cisapride on gastroesophageal reflux during anesthesia in dogs. *J Vet Intern Med* 2012; **26**: 518–525.

366 Ogden J, Ovbey D, Saile K. Effects of preoperative cisapride on postoperative aspiration pneumonia in dogs with laryngeal paralysis. *J Small Anim Pract* 2019; **60**: 183–190.

367 Wilson DV, Evans AT, Mauer WA. Influence of metoclopramide on gastroesophageal reflux in anesthetized dogs. *Am J Vet Res* 2006; **67**: 26–31.

368 Milovancev M, Townsend K, Spina J, *et al.* Effect of metoclopramide on the incidence of early postoperative aspiration pneumonia in dogs with acquired idiopathic laryngeal paralysis. *Vet Surg* 2016; **45**: 577–581.

369 Ranninger E, Kantyka M, Bektas RN. The influence of anaesthetic drugs on the laryngeal motion in dogs: a systematic review. *Animals (Basel)* 2020; **10**: 530.

370 DeGroot WD, Tobias KM, Browning DC, *et al.* Examination of laryngeal function of healthy dogs by using sedation protocols with dexmedetomidine. *Vet Surg* 2020; **49**: 124–130.

371 Smalle TM, Hartman MJ, Bester L, *et al.* Effects of thiopentone, propofol and alfaxalone on laryngeal motion during oral laryngoscopy in healthy dogs. *Vet Anaesth Analg* 2017; **44**: 427–434.

372 Labuscagne S, Zeiler GE, Dzikiti BT. Effects of chemical and mechanical stimulation on laryngeal motion during alfaxalone, thiopentone or propofol anaesthesia in healthy dogs. *Vet Anaesth Analg* 2019; **46**: 435–442.

373 Brown MB, Dugat DR, Lyon SD, *et al.* Comparison of methohexital and propofol as induction agents for evaluation of laryngeal function in healthy dogs. *Vet Surg* 2019; **48**: 70–78.

374 Ambros B, Gaunt MC, Duke-Novakovski T, *et al.* Effects of alfaxalone, thiopental, or propofol and diazepam on laryngeal motion in healthy dogs. *Can Vet J* 2018; **59**: 791–795.

375 Norgate D, Ter Haar G, Kulendra N, *et al.* A comparison of the effect of propofol and alfaxalone on laryngeal motion in nonbrachycephalic and brachycephalic dogs. *Vet Anaesth Analg* 2018; **45**: 729–736.

376 Radkey DI, Hardie RJ, Smith LJ. Comparison of the effects of alfaxalone and propofol with acepromazine, butorphanol and/or doxapram on laryngeal motion and quality of examination in dogs. *Vet Anaesth Analg* 2018; **45**: 241–249.

377 Kapaldo N, McMurphy R, Hodgson D, *et al.* Laryngeal function in normal dogs administered isoflurane following partial clearance of alfaxalone or propofol. *Vet Anaesth Analg* 2021; **48**: 493–500.

378 Tobias KM, Jackson AM, Harvey RC. Effects of doxapram HCl on laryngeal function of normal dogs and dogs with naturally occurring laryngeal paralysis. *Vet Anaesth Analg* 2004; **31**: 258–263.

379 Miller CJ, McKiernan BC, Pace J, *et al.* The effects of doxapram hydrochloride (dopram-V) on laryngeal function in healthy dogs. *J Vet Intern Med* 2002; **16**: 524–528.

380 Johnson LR, Pollard RE. Tracheal collapse and bronchomalacia in dogs: 58 cases (7 /2001–1 /2008). *J Vet Intern Med* 2010; **24**: 298–305.

381 Della Maggiore A. An update on tracheal and airway collapse in dogs. *Vet Clin North Am Small Anim Pract* 2020; **50**: 419–430.

382 Weisse C, Berent A, Violette N, *et al.* Short-, intermediate-, and long-term results for endoluminal stent placement in dogs with tracheal collapse. *J Am Vet Med Assoc* 2019; **254**: 380–392.

383 Johnson L. Tracheal collapse. Diagnosis and medical and surgical treatment. *Vet Clin North Am Small Anim Pract* 2000; **30**: 1253–1266.

384 Congiusta M, Weisse C, Berent AC, *et al.* Comparison of short-, intermediate-, and long-term results between dogs with tracheal collapse that underwent multimodal medical management alone and those that underwent tracheal endoluminal stent placement. *J Am Vet Med Assoc* 2021; **258**: 279–289.

385 Chisnell HK, Pardo AD. Long-term outcome, complications and disease progression in 23 dogs after placement of tracheal ring prostheses for treatment of extrathoracic tracheal collapse. *Vet Surg* 2015; **44**: 103–113.

386 Jeung SY, Sohn SJ, An JH, *et al.* A retrospective study of theophylline-based therapy with tracheal collapse in small-breed dogs: 47 cases (2013–2017). *J Vet Sci* 2019; **20**: e57.

387 Tinga S, Thieman Mankin KM, Peycke L, *et al.* Comparison of outcome after use of extra-luminal rings and intra-luminal stents for treatment of tracheal collapse in dogs. *Vet Surg* 2015; **44**: 858–865.
388 Tappin SW. Canine tracheal collapse. *J Small Anim Pract* 2016; **57**: 9–17.
389 Cerasoli I, Nannarone S, Schauvliege S, *et al.* The effects of intravenous lidocaine before propofol induction in premedicated dogs. *J Small Anim Pract* 2016; **57**: 435–440.
390 Thompson KR, Rioja E. Effects of intravenous and topical laryngeal lidocaine on heart rate, mean arterial pressure and cough response to endotracheal intubation in dogs. *Vet Anaesth Analg* 2016; **43**: 371–378.
391 Panti A, Cafrita IC, Clark L. Effect of intravenous lidocaine on cough response to endotracheal intubation in propofol-anaesthetized dogs. *Vet Anaesth Analg* 2016; **43**: 405–411.
392 Jolliffe CT, Leece EA, Adams V, *et al.* Effect of intravenous lidocaine on heart rate, systolic arterial blood pressure and cough responses to endotracheal intubation in propofol-anaesthetized dogs. *Vet Anaesth Analg* 2007; **34**: 322–330.
393 Bravo VR, Palomba N, Corletto F, *et al.* Comparison between intravenous lidocaine and fentanyl on cough reflex and sympathetic response during endotracheal intubation in dogs. *Vet Anaesth Analg* 2020; **47**: 481–489.
394 Clarke DL. Interventional radiology management of tracheal and bronchial collapse. *Vet Clin North Am Small Anim Pract* 2018; **48**: 765–779.
395 Tate LP Jr., Blikslager AT, Little ED. Transendoscopic laser treatment of guttural pouch tympanites in eight foals. *Vet Surg* 1995; **24**: 367–372.
396 Blazyczek I, Hamann H, Deegen E, *et al.* Retrospective analysis of 50 cases of guttural pouch tympany in foals. *Vet Rec* 2004; **154**: 261–264.
397 Bell C. Pharyngeal neuromuscular dysfunction associated with bilateral guttural pouch tympany in a foal. *Can Vet J* 2007; **48**: 192–194.
398 Sparks HD, Stick JA, Brakenhoff JE, *et al.* Partial resection of the plica salpingopharyngeus for the treatment of three foals with bilateral tympany of the auditory tube diverticulum (guttural pouch). *J Am Vet Med Assoc* 2009; **235**: 731–733.
399 Krebs W, Schmotzer WB. Laser fenestrated salpingopharyngeal fistulas for treatment of bilateral guttural pouch tympany in a foal. *Equine Vet Educ* 2007; **19**: 419–423.
400 Schambourg MA, Marcoux M, Celeste C. Salpingoscopy for the treatment of recurrent guttural pouch tympany in a filly. *Equine Vet Educ* 2006; **18**: 231–237.
401 Freeman DE. Update on disorders and treatment of the guttural pouch. *Vet Clin North Am Equine Pract* 2015; **31**: 63–89.
402 Kerr CL, Bouré LP, Pearce SG, *et al.* Cardiopulmonary effects of diazepam-ketamine-isoflurane or xylazine-ketamine-isoflurane during abdominal surgery in foals. *Am J Vet Res* 2009; **70**: 574–580.
403 Johnston GM, Eastment JK, Wood J, *et al.* The confidential enquiry into perioperative equine fatalities (CEPEF): mortality results of Phases 1 and 2. *Vet Anaesth Analg* 2002; **29**: 159–170.
404 Lepage OM, Piccot-Crézollet C. Transarterial coil embolisation in 31 horses (1999–2002) with guttural pouch mycosis: a 2-year follow-up. *Equine Vet J* 2005; **37**: 430–434.
405 Genton M, Farfan M, Tesson C, *et al.* Balloon catheter occlusion of the maxillary, internal, and external carotid arteries in standing horses. *Vet Surg* 2021; **50**: 546–555.
406 Bonilla AG, Scansen BA, Hurcombe SD, *et al.* Potential for iatrogenic coil embolization of the caudal cerebellar artery during treatment of internal carotid artery bifurcation in two horses with guttural pouch mycosis. *J Am Vet Med Assoc* 2015; **247**: 1427–1432.
407 Dobesova O, Schwarz B, Velde K, *et al.* Guttural pouch mycosis in horses: a retrospective study of 28 cases. *Vet Rec* 2012; **171**: 561.
408 Greet V, Bode EF, Dukes-McEwan J, *et al.* Clinical features and outcome of dogs and cats with bidirectional and continuous right-to-left shunting patent ductus arteriosus. *J Vet Intern Med* 2021; **35**: 780–788.
409 Caffey SR, Lund CM, Farnsworth KD, *et al.* Effects of head position on internal and external carotid pressures in standing sedated horses. *Can J Vet Res* 2021; **85**: 127–130.
410 Cousty M, Tricaud C, De Beauregard T, *et al.* Ligation of the ipsilateral common carotid artery and topical treatment for the prevention of epistaxis from guttural pouch mycosis in horses. *Vet Rec* 2016; **178**: 44.
411 Cruz AM, Kerr CL, Bouré LP, *et al.* Cardiovascular effects of insufflation of the abdomen with carbon dioxide in standing horses sedated with detomidine. *Am J Vet Res* 2004; **65**: 357–362.
412 Hahn CN, Matiasek K, Dixon PM, *et al.* Histological and ultrastructural evidence that recurrent laryngeal neuropathy is a bilateral mononeuropathy limited to recurrent laryngeal nerves. *Equine Vet J* 2008; **40**: 666–672.
413 Rossignol F, Vitte A, Boening J, *et al.* Laryngoplasty in standing horses. *Vet Surg* 2015; **44**: 341–347.
414 Hawkins JF, Tulleners EP, Ross MW, *et al.* Laryngoplasty with or without ventriculectomy for treatment of left laryngeal hemiplegia in 230 racehorses. *Vet Surg* 1997; **26**: 484–491.
415 Kraus BM, Parente EJ, Tulleners EP. Laryngoplasty with ventriculectomy or ventriculocordectomy in 104 draft horses (1992–2000). *Vet Surg* 2003; **32**: 530–538.
416 Abdul-Rasool IH, Ward DS. Ventilatory and cardiovascular responses to sufentanil infusion in dogs anesthetized with isoflurane. *Anesth Analg* 1989; **69**: 300–306.
417 McCarrel TM, Woodie JB. Update on laryngeal disorders and treatment. *Vet Clin North Am Equine Pract* 2015; **31**: 13–26.
418 Lindegaard C, Husted L, Ullum H, *et al.* Sedation with detomidine and acepromazine influences the endoscopic evaluation of laryngeal function in horses. *Equine Vet J* 2007; **39**: 553–556.
419 Chalmers HJ, Yeager AE, Cheetham J, *et al.* Diagnostic sensitivity of subjective and quantitative laryngeal ultrasonography for recurrent laryngeal neuropathy in horses. *Vet Radiol Ultrasound* 2012; **53**: 660–666.
420 Ducharme NG, Rossingnol F. Larynx. In: Auer JA, Stick JA, Kummerle JM, *et al.*, eds. *Equine Surgery*, 5th edn. St. Louis, MO: Elsevier, 2019: 568–590.
421 Cramp PA, Prange T, Nickels FA. Standing equine surgery of the upper respiratory tract. *Vet Clin North Am Equine Pract* 2014; **30**: 111–141.
422 Campoy L, Morris TB, Ducharme NG, *et al.* Unilateral cervical plexus block for prosthetic laryngoplasty in the standing horse. *Equine Vet J* 2018; **50**: 727–732.
423 Trzil JE. Feline asthma: diagnostic and treatment update. *Vet Clin North Am Small Anim Pract* 2020; **50**: 375–391.
424 Reinero CR, DeClue AE, Rabinowitz P. Asthma in humans and cats: is there a common sensitivity to aeroallegens in shared environments? *Environ Res* 2009; **109**: 634–640.
425 van Eeden ME, Vientós-Plotts AI, Cohn LA, *et al.* Serum allergen-specific IgE reactivity: is there an association with clinical severity and airway eosinophilia in asthmatic cats? *J Feline Med Surg* 2020; **22**: 1129–1136.
426 Moise NS, Wiedenkeller D, Yeager AE, *et al.* Clinical, radiographic, and bronchial cytologic features of cats with bronchial disease: 65 cases (1980–1986). *J Am Vet Med Assoc* 1989; **194**: 1467–1473.
427 Adamama-Moraitou KK, Patsikas MN, Koutinas AF. Feline lower airway disease: a retrospective study of 22 naturally occurring cases from Greece. *J Feline Med Surg* 2004; **6**: 227–233.
428 Lee EA, Johnson LR, Johnson EG, *et al.* Clinical features and radiographic findings in cats with eosinophilic, neutrophilic, and mixed airway inflammation (2011–2018). *J Vet Intern Med* 2020; **34**: 1291–1299.
429 Grotheer M, Hirschberger J, Hartmann K, *et al.* Comparison of signalment, clinical, laboratory and radiographic parameters in cats with feline asthma and chronic bronchitis. *J Feline Med Surg* 2020; **22**: 649–655.
430 Bayable SD, Melesse DY, Lema GF, *et al.* Perioperative management of patients with asthma during elective surgery: a systematic review. *Ann Med Surg (Lond)* 2021; **70**: 102874.
431 Woods BD, Sladen RN. Perioperative considerations for the patient with asthma and bronchospasm. *Br J Anaesth* 2009; **103**: i57–i65.
432 Evgenov OVL, Jiang Y, Blair JL. Pulmonary pharmacology and inhaled anesthetics. In: Gropper M, Eriksson L, Fleisher L, *et al.*, eds. *Miller's Anesthesia*, 9th edn. Philadelphia, PA: Elsevier, 2020: 540–571.
433 Groeben H, Mitzner W, Brown RH. Effects of the alpha2-adrenoceptor agonist dexmedetomidine on bronchoconstriction in dogs. *Anesthesiology* 2004; **100**: 359–363.
434 Zhou Y, Du X, Wang Q, *et al.* Dexmedetomidine protects against Airway Inflammation and Airway Remodeling in a Murine Model of chronic asthma through TLR4/NF-κB signaling pathway. *Mediators Inflamm* 2023; **2023**: 3695469.
435 Siao KT, Pypendop BH, Honkavaara J, *et al.* Hemodynamic effects of dexmedetomidine, with and without MK-467, following intramuscular administration in cats anesthetized with isoflurane. *Vet Anaesth Analg* 2017; **44**: 1101–1115.
436 Selmi AL, Mendes GM, Lins BT, *et al.* Evaluation of the sedative and cardiorespiratory effects of dexmedetomidine, dexmedetomidine-butorphanol, and dexmedetomidine-ketamine in cats. *J Am Vet Med Assoc* 2003; **222**: 37–41.
437 DeYoung DW, Paddleford RR, Short CE. Dissociative anesthetics in the cat and dog. *J Am Vet Med Assoc* 1972; **161**: 1442–1445.
438 Jones TL, Boyer K, Chapman K, *et al.* Evaluation of the time to desensitization of the larynx of cats following topical lidocaine application. *J Feline Med Surg* 2021; **23**: 563–567.
439 Wilson ME, Robinson NE. Recurrent airway obstruction and inflammatory airway disease. In: Sprayberry KA, Robinson NE, eds. *Robinson's Current Therapy in Equine Medicine 7*. St. Louis, MO: Elsevier, 2015: 257–261.
440 Couetil L, Cardwell JM, Leguillette R, *et al.* Equine asthma: current understanding and future directions. *Front Vet Sci* 2020; **7**: 450.
441 Mazan MR. Update on noninfectious inflammatory diseases of the lower airway. *Vet Clin North Am Equine Pract* 2015; **31**: 159–185.
442 Broadstone RV, Gray PR, Robinson NE, *et al.* Effects of xylazine on airway function in ponies with recurrent airway obstruction. *Am J Vet Res* 1992; **53**: 1813–1817.
443 Hess DR, Kacmarek RM. Pressure and volume ventilation. In: Hess DR, Kacmarek RM, eds. *Essentials of Mechanical Ventilation*, 4th edn. New York, NY: McGraw-Hill Education, 2019: 61–72.

444 Robertson SA, Bailey JE. Aerosolized salbutamol (albuterol) improves PaO2 in hypoxaemic anaesthetized horses – a prospective clinical trial in 81 horses. *Vet Anaesth Analg* 2002; **29**: 212–218.
445 Dupont J, Gougnard A, Salciccia A, *et al.* Comparison of single-breath continuous positive airway pressure manoeuvre with inhaled salbutamol to improve oxygenation in horses anaesthetized for laparotomy. *Vet Anaesth Analg* 2022; **49**: 85–94.
446 Casoni D, Spadavecchia C, Adami C. Cardiovascular changes after administration of aerosolized salbutamol in horses: five cases. *Acta Vet Scand* 2014; **56**: 49.
447 Howes CL, Sumner JP, Ahlstrand K, *et al.* Long-term clinical outcomes following surgery for spontaneous pneumothorax caused by pulmonary blebs and bullae in dogs – a multicentre (AVSTS Research Cooperative) retrospective study. *J Small Anim Pract* 2020; **61**: 436–441.
448 Gilday C, Odunayo A, Hespel AM. Spontaneous pneumothorax: pathophysiology, clinical presentation and diagnosis. *Top Companion Anim Med* 2021; **45**: 100563.
449 Boy MG, Sweeney CR. Pneumothorax in horses: 40 cases (1980–1997). *J Am Vet Med Assoc* 2000; **216**: 1955–1959.
450 Slack JA, Thomas CB, Peek SF. Pneumothorax in dairy cattle: 30 cases (1990–2003). *J Am Vet Med Assoc* 2004; **225**: 732–735.
451 Cole L, Pivetta M, Humm K. Diagnostic accuracy of a lung ultrasound protocol (Vet BLUE) for detection of pleural fluid, pneumothorax and lung pathology in dogs and cats. *J Small Anim Pract* 2021; **62**: 178–186.
452 Ruiz MD, Vessières F, Ragetly GR, *et al.* Characterization of and factors associated with causes of pleural effusion in cats. *J Am Vet Med Assoc* 2018; **253**: 181–187.
453 Biddick AA, Bacek LM, Fan S, *et al.* Association between cardiac troponin I concentrations and electrocardiographic abnormalities in dogs with blunt trauma. *J Vet Emerg Crit Care (San Antonio)* 2020; **30**: 179–186.
454 Haynes D, Baumann MH. Pleural controversy: aetiology of pneumothorax. *Respirology* 2011; **16**: 604–610.
455 Abu-Seida A. Diagnostic and treatment challenges for diaphragmatic hernia in equids: a concise review of literature. *J Equine Vet Sci* 2021; **106**: 103746.
456 Schmiedt CW, Tobias KM, Stevenson MA. Traumatic diaphragmatic hernia in cats: 34 cases (1991–2001). *J Am Vet Med Assoc* 2003; **222**: 1237–1240.
457 Legallet C, Thieman Mankin K, Selmic LE. Prognostic indicators for perioperative survival after diaphragmatic herniorrhaphy in cats and dogs: 96 cases (2001–2013). *BMC Vet Res* 2017; **13**: 16.
458 Morgan KRS, Singh A, Giuffrida MA, *et al.* Outcome after surgical and conservative treatments of canine peritoneopericardial diaphragmatic hernia: a multi-institutional study of 128 dogs. *Vet Surg* 2020; **49**: 138–145.
459 Burns CG, Bergh MS, McLoughlin MA. Surgical and nonsurgical treatment of peritoneopericardial diaphragmatic hernia in dogs and cats: 58 cases (1999–2008). *J Am Vet Med Assoc* 2013; **242**: 643–650.
460 Romero AE, Rodgerson DH. Diaphragmatic herniation in the horse: 31 cases from 2001–2006. *Can Vet J* 2010; **51**: 1247–1250.
461 Hart SK, Brown JA. Diaphragmatic hernia in horses: 44 cases (1986–2006). *J Vet Emerg Crit Care (San Antonio)* 2009; **19**: 357–362.
462 Gibson TW, Brisson BA, Sears W. Perioperative survival rates after surgery for diaphragmatic hernia in dogs and cats: 92 cases (1990–2002). *J Am Vet Med Assoc* 2005; **227**: 105–109.
463 Clutton RE, Boyd C, Richards DL, *et al.* Anaesthetic problems caused by diaphragmatic hernia in the horse: a review of four cases. *Equine Vet J Suppl* 1992; **11**: 30–33.
464 Wilson DV, Schott HC II, Robinson NE, *et al.* Response to nasopharyngeal oxygen administration in horses with lung disease. *Equine Vet J* 2006; **38**: 219–223.
465 Canfrán S, Gómez de Segura IA, Cediel R, *et al.* Effects of a stepwise lung recruitment manoeuvre and positive end-expiratory pressure on lung compliance and arterial blood oxygenation in healthy dogs. *Vet J* 2012; **194**: 89–93.
466 Canfrán S, Gómez de Segura IA, Cediel R, *et al.* Effects of fluid load on cardiovascular function during stepwise lung recruitment manoeuvre in healthy dogs. *Vet J* 2013; **197**: 800–805.
467 Neath PJ, Brockman DJ, King LG. Lung lobe torsion in dogs: 22 cases (1981–1999). *J Am Vet Med Assoc* 2000; **217**: 1041–1044.
468 Schultz RM, Peters J, Zwingenberger A. Radiography, computed tomography and virtual bronchoscopy in four dogs and two cats with lung lobe torsion. *J Small Anim Pract* 2009; **50**: 360–363.
469 Hambrook LE, Kudnig ST. Lung lobe torsion in association with a chronic diaphragmatic hernia and haemorrhagic pleural effusion in a cat. *J Feline Med Surg* 2012; **14**: 219–223.
470 Benavides KL, Rozanski EA, Oura TJ. Lung lobe torsion in 35 dogs and 4 cats. *Can Vet J* 2019; **60**: 60–66.
471 Rossanese M, Wustefeld-Janssens B, Price C, *et al.* Long-term survival after treatment of idiopathic lung lobe torsion in 80 cases. *Vet Surg* 2020; **49**: 659–667.
472 Murphy KA, Brisson BA. Evaluation of lung lobe torsion in Pugs: 7 cases (1991–2004). *J Am Vet Med Assoc* 2006; **228**: 86–90.
473 Latimer CR, Lux CN, Sutton JS, *et al.* Lung lobe torsion in seven juvenile dogs. *J Am Vet Med Assoc* 2017; **251**: 1450–1456.
474 Park KM, Grimes JA, Wallace ML, *et al.* Lung lobe torsion in dogs: 52 cases (2005–2017). *Vet Surg* 2018; **47**: 1002–1008.
475 Fossum TW. Surgery of the lower respriatory system. In: Fossum TW, ed. *Small Animal Surgery*, 5th edn. Philadelphia, PA: Elsevier, 2019: 884–915.
476 Gallart L, Canet J. Postoperative pulmonary complications: understanding definitions and risk assessment. *Best Pract Res Clin Anaesthesiol* 2015; **29**: 315–330.
477 Kaufmann K, Heinrich S. Minimizing postoperative pulmonary complications in thoracic surgery patients. *Curr Opin Anaesthesiol* 2021; **34**: 13–19.
478 Kiefer J MM, Roizen MF, Fleisher LA. Anesthetic implications of concurrent diseases. In: Gropper MA, Eriksson LI, Fleisher LA, *et al.*, eds. *Miller's Anesthesia*, 9th edn. Philadelphia, PA: Elsevier, 2020: 999–1064.
479 Fisher BW, Majumdar SR, McAlister FA. Predicting pulmonary complications after nonthoracic surgery: a systematic review of blinded studies. *Am J Med* 2002; **112**: 219–225.
480 Ackerman RS, Luddy KA, Icard BE, *et al.* The effects of anesthetics and perioperative medications on immune function: a narrative review. *Anesth Analg* 2021; **133**: 676–689.
481 Layton R, Layton D, Beggs D, *et al.* The impact of stress and anesthesia on animal models of infectious disease. *Front Vet Sci* 2023; **10**: 1086003.
482 Sherman R, Karagiannis M. Aspiration pneumonia in the dog: a review. *Top Companion Anim Med* 2017; **32**: 1–7.
483 Marik PE. Aspiration pneumonitis and aspiration pneumonia. *N Engl J Med* 2001; **344**: 665–671.
484 Fingeroth JM, Fossum TW. Late-onset regurgitation associated with persistent right aortic arch in two dogs. *J Am Vet Med Assoc* 1987; **191**: 981–983.
485 Loughin CA, Marino DJ. Delayed primary surgical treatment in a dog with a persistent right aortic arch. *J Am Anim Hosp Assoc* 2008; **44**: 258–261.
486 Janda M, Scheeren TW, Nöldge-Schomburg GF. Management of pulmonary aspiration. *Best Pract Res Clin Anaesthesiol* 2006; **20**: 409–427.
487 Arroyo MG, Slovis NM, Moore GE, *et al.* Factors associated with survival in 97 horses with septic pleuropneumonia. *J Vet Intern Med* 2017; **31**: 894–900.
488 Akça O. Endotracheal tube cuff leak: can optimum management of cuff pressure prevent pneumonia? *Crit Care Med* 2007; **35**: 1624–1626.
489 Hamilton VA, Grap MJ. The role of the endotracheal tube cuff in microaspiration. *Heart Lung* 2012; **41**: 167–172.
490 Alderson B, Senior JM, Dugdale AH. Tracheal necrosis following tracheal intubation in a dog. *J Small Anim Pract* 2006; **47**: 754–756.
491 Mitchell SL, McCarthy R, Rudloff E, *et al.* Tracheal rupture associated with intubation in cats: 20 cases (1996–1998). *J Am Vet Med Assoc* 2000; **216**: 1592–1595.
492 Touzot-Jourde G, Stedman NL, Trim CM. The effects of two endotracheal tube cuff inflation pressures on liquid aspiration and tracheal wall damage in horses. *Vet Anaesth Analg* 2005; **32**: 23–29.
493 Wylie C, Foote A, Rasotto R, *et al.* Tracheal necrosis as a fatal complication of endotracheal intubation. *Equine Vet Edu* 2015; **27**: 170–175.
494 Ferreira TH, Allen M, De Gasperi D, *et al.* Impact of endotracheal tube size and cuff pressure on tracheal and laryngeal mucosa of adult horses. *Vet Anaesth Analg* 2021; **48**: 891–899.
495 Hung WC, Ko JC, Weil AB, *et al.* Evaluation of endotracheal tube cuff pressure and the use of three cuff inflation syringe devices in dogs. *Front Vet Sci* 2020; **7**: 39.
496 Reinero C, Visser LC, Kellihan HB, *et al.* ACVIM consensus statement guidelines for the diagnosis, classification, treatment, and monitoring of pulmonary hypertension in dogs. *J Vet Intern Med* 2020; **34**: 549–573.
497 Rolph KE, Cavanaugh SM. Feline pulmonary hypertension: are we overlooking an important comorbidity? *J Feline Med Surg* 2022; **24**: e636–e646.
498 Slack J. Pulmonary hypertension. In: Robinson NE, Sprayberry KA, eds. *Current Therapy in Equine Medicine* 6. St. Louis, MO: Saunders Elsevier, 2009: 216–220.
499 Jung S, Orvalho J, Griffiths LG. Aortopulmonary window characterized with two- and three-dimensional echocardiogram in a dog. *J Vet Cardiol* 2012; **14**: 371–375.
500 Tarry D, Powell M. Hypoxic pulmonary vasoconstriction. *Br J Anaesth Educ* 2017; **17**: 208–213.
501 Dixon PM. Pulmonary artery pressures in normal horses and in horses affected with chronic obstructive pulmonary disease. *Equine Vet J* 1978; **10**: 195–198.
502 Johnson LR, Stern JA. Clinical features and outcome in 25 dogs with respiratory-associated pulmonary hypertension treated with sildenafil. *J Vet Intern Med* 2020; **34**: 65–73.
503 Jaffey JA, Wiggen K, Leach SB, *et al.* Pulmonary hypertension secondary to respiratory disease and/or hypoxia in dogs: clinical features, diagnostic testing and survival. *Vet J* 2019; **251**: 105347.
504 Borgarelli M, Abbott J, Braz-Ruivo L, *et al.* Prevalence and prognostic importance of pulmonary hypertension in dogs with myxomatous mitral valve disease. *J Vet Intern Med* 2015; **29**: 569–574.
505 Borgarelli M, Zini E, D'Agnolo G, *et al.* Comparison of primary mitral valve disease in German Shepherd dogs and in small breeds. *J Vet Cardiol* 2004; **6**: 27–34.

506 Guglielmini C, Civitella C, Diana A, *et al.* Serum cardiac troponin I concentration in dogs with precapillary and postcapillary pulmonary hypertension. *J Vet Intern Med* 2010; **24**: 145–152.

507 Schober KE, Hart TM, Stern JA, *et al.* Detection of congestive heart failure in dogs by Doppler echocardiography. *J Vet Intern Med* 2010; **24**: 1358–1368.

508 Serres FJ, Chetboul V, Tissier R, *et al.* Doppler echocardiography-derived evidence of pulmonary arterial hypertension in dogs with degenerative mitral valve disease: 86 cases (2001–2005). *J Am Vet Med Assoc* 2006; **229**: 1772–1778.

509 Vezzosi T, Schober KE. Doppler-derived echocardiographic evidence of pulmonary hypertension in cats with left-sided congestive heart failure. *J Vet Cardiol* 2019; **23**: 58–68.

510 Kellihan HB, Stepien RL. Pulmonary hypertension in dogs: diagnosis and therapy. *Vet Clin North Am Small Anim Pract* 2010; **40**: 623–641.

511 Price LC, Martinez G, Brame A, *et al.* Perioperative management of patients with pulmonary hypertension undergoing non-cardiothoracic, non-obstetric surgery: a systematic review and expert consensus statement. *Br J Anaesth* 2021; **126**: 774–790.

512 Shim JK, Choi YS, Oh YJ, *et al.* Effect of oral sildenafil citrate on intraoperative hemodynamics in patients with pulmonary hypertension undergoing valvular heart surgery. *J Thorac Cardiovasc Surg* 2006; **132**: 1420–1425.

513 Bach JF, Rozanski EA, MacGregor J, *et al.* Retrospective evaluation of sildenafil citrate as a therapy for pulmonary hypertension in dogs. *J Vet Intern Med* 2006; **20**: 1132–1135.

514 Murphy LA, Russell N, Bianco D, *et al.* Retrospective evaluation of pimobendan and sildenafil therapy for severe pulmonary hypertension due to lung disease and hypoxia in 28 dogs (2007–2013). *Vet Med Sci* 2017; **3**: 99–106.

515 Häggström J, Boswood A, O'Grady M, *et al.* Effect of pimobendan or benazepril hydrochloride on survival times in dogs with congestive heart failure caused by naturally occurring myxomatous mitral valve disease: the QUEST study. *J Vet Intern Med* 2008; **22**: 1124–1135.

516 Mizuno M, Yamano S, Chimura S, *et al.* Efficacy of pimobendan on survival and reoccurrence of pulmonary edema in canine congestive heart failure. *J Vet Med Sci* 2017; **79**: 29–34.

517 Enokizono M, Mandour AS, Komeda S, *et al.* Hemodynamic effect of pimobendan following intramuscular and intravenous administration in healthy dogs: a pilot study. *Front Vet Sci* 2022; **9**: 969304.

518 Ketabchi F, Egemnazarov B, Schermuly RT, *et al.* Effects of hypercapnia with and without acidosis on hypoxic pulmonary vasoconstriction. *Am J Physiol Lung Cell Mol Physiol* 2009; **297**: L977–L983.

519 Price LC, Wort SJ, Finney SJ, *et al.* Pulmonary vascular and right ventricular dysfunction in adult critical care: current and emerging options for management: a systematic literature review. *Crit Care* 2010; **14**: R169.

520 Currigan DA, Hughes RJ, Wright CE, *et al.* Vasoconstrictor responses to vasopressor agents in human pulmonary and radial arteries: an in vitro study. *Anesthesiology* 2014; **121**: 930–936.

521 Coleman AE, Shepard MK, Schmiedt CW, *et al.* Effects of orally administered enalapril on blood pressure and hemodynamic response to vasopressors during isoflurane anesthesia in healthy dogs. *Vet Anaesth Analg* 2016; **43**: 482–494.

39 Physiology, Pathophysiology, and Anesthetic Management of Patients with Neurologic Disease

Tatiana H. Ferreira[1] and Starr Cameron[2]
[1]Department of Surgical Sciences, School of Veterinary Medicine, University of Wisconsin, Madison, Wisconsin, USA
[2]Department of Medical Sciences, School of Veterinary Medicine, University of Wisconsin, Madison, Wisconsin, USA

Chapter contents

Introduction, 822
Anatomy of the nervous system, 822
Central nervous system, 822
Peripheral nervous system, 825
Physiology of the central nervous system, 829
Brain physiology, 829
Spinal cord physiology, 832
Effects of vasoactive drugs, sedatives, and anesthetics, 832
Vasoactive drugs, 832
Sedatives and anesthetics, 832
Pathophysiology and anesthetic management of specific neurological conditions, 835
Central nervous system conditions, 835
Peripheral nervous system conditions, 839
References, 840

Introduction

Anesthetic management of patients with neurological disorders undergoing diagnostic and/or surgical procedures is common in veterinary medicine. Knowledge of normal anatomy and physiology as well as pathophysiology of the central, peripheral, somatic, and autonomic nervous systems allows the anesthetic provider to understand the impact of sedation and anesthesia on normal physiology as well as disease processes. Whether a patient is anesthetized for evaluation or management of neurologic conditions or suffers from comorbidities related to the nervous system, a solid foundational knowledge of the nervous system is important to ensure appropriate and optimal patient care while decreasing patient morbidity and mortality.

Anatomy of the nervous system

The nervous system is anatomically divided into the central nervous system, containing the brain and spinal cord, and the peripheral nervous system, containing the cranial and spinal nerves. Functionally, the nervous system can be divided into somatic and autonomic nervous system components, each with afferent and efferent fibers.

Central nervous system

The central nervous system (CNS) contains the brain and spinal cord and is made up of gray and white matter. Gray matter is composed of neuronal cell bodies and is located more superficially in the brain and more deeply (i.e., centrally) within the spinal cord. There are also some deeper regions of gray matter within the brain known as "nuclei." White matter is composed of nerve fibers (axons) and is located deeper within the brain and more superficially within the spinal cord. The meninges are composed of three layers of connective tissue within the CNS: the dura, arachnoid, and pia mater. The dura mater is the most superficial layer and, in the vertebral column, the space between the bone and the dura mater is the epidural space. Within the skull, the dura mater is fused to the periosteum and, therefore, is considered a potential space. Because there is no epidural space intracranially, the venous sinuses are located within the dura mater of the brain. The arachnoid is the middle layer of the meninges while the pia mater is the innermost layer. The pia mater is only one cell thick and is fused to the surface of the brain and the spinal cord. Within the vertebral canal, the subarachnoid space is located between the arachnoid and pia mater layers and contains cerebrospinal fluid (CSF). The meninges extend around the spinal nerve roots with some reaching the level of the intervertebral foramina.

When CSF collection is performed, a spinal needle is inserted into the subarachnoid space either at the level of the cerebellomedullary cistern cranially, or the lower lumbar region caudally. In dogs and cats, the L5–L6 vertebral space is recommended for obtaining CSF. In large-breed dogs, the L4–L5 vertebral space can often be used if obtaining CSF from the L5–L6 space is unsuccessful. Local anesthetic and analgesic agents may be administered either in the epidural or subarachnoid spaces; species-specific descriptions of these techniques may be found in the local anesthetic and analgesic techniques chapters in this text.

Brain

Anatomically, the brain can be divided into five regions: the telencephalon (cerebral cortex and basal ganglia), diencephalon (thalamus, hypothalamus, epithalamus, subthalamus, and metathalamus),

Veterinary Anesthesia and Analgesia: The Sixth Edition of Lumb and Jones. Edited by Leigh Lamont, Kurt Grimm, Sheilah Robertson, Lydia Love and Carrie Schroeder.
© 2024 John Wiley & Sons, Inc. Published 2024 by John Wiley & Sons, Inc.
Companion website: www.wiley.com/go/lamont/anesthesia

mesencephalon (midbrain), metencephalon (pons and cerebellum), and myelencephalon (medulla oblongata) (Fig. 39.1). Functionally and clinically, the telencephalon and diencephalon together make up the prosencephalon or forebrain. The midbrain, pons, and medulla form the brainstem. There are 12 pairs of cranial nerves; a list of the nerves and their innervation is provided in Table 39.1.

The cerebral cortex or telencephalon is where sensory information from the environment is consciously perceived and voluntary motor functions are initiated. The telencephalon is divided into right and left hemispheres. In mammals, except mice and rats, the cerebral cortex is composed of gyri and sulci and classified as gyrencephalic. The brains of fish, reptiles, birds, mice, and rats are smooth and lack these characteristic folds and are referred to as lissencephalic. The presence of gyri allows a significantly increased number of neurons without increasing the size of the cranium or skull. The gyri are divided into lobes including the frontal, parietal,

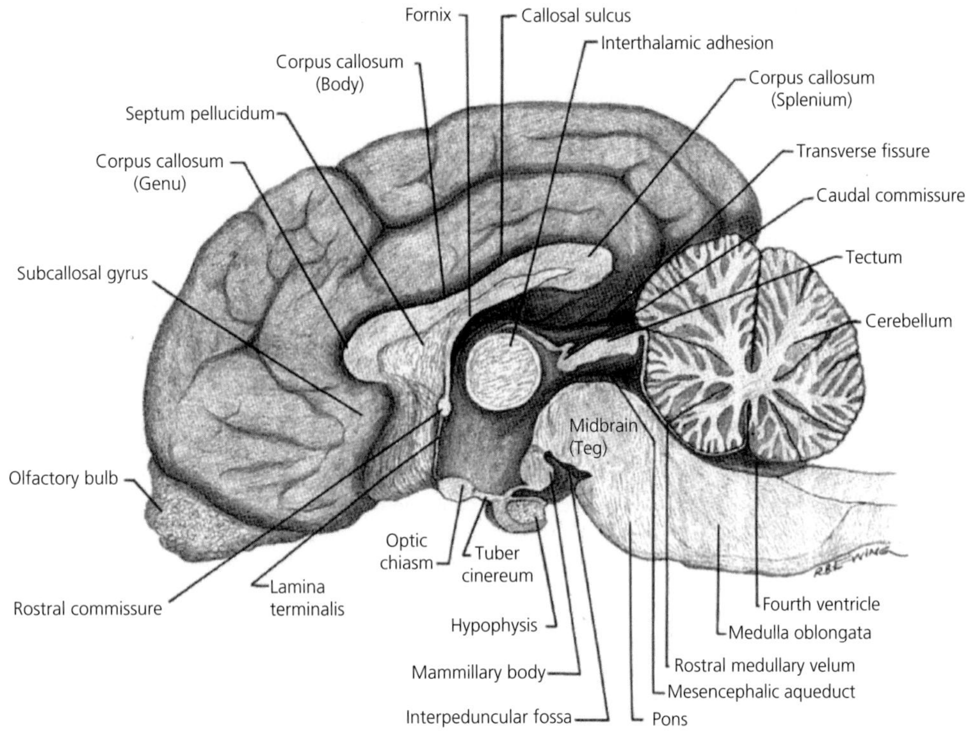

Figure 39.1 Sagittal section of the canine brain. Teg, tegmentum. Source: Jenkins [1], with permission.

Table 39.1 Cranial nerves and their innervation.

Cranial nerve number	Cranial nerve name	Classification	Function/innervation
I	Olfactory	Sensory	Olfaction
II	Optic	Sensory	Vision
III	Oculomotor	Motor	Somatic motor information to dorsal, medial, ventral rectus, ventral oblique, and levator palpebrae superioris muscles of the eye Parasympathetic innervation to pupil (constriction)
IV	Trochlear	Motor	Somatic motor innervation to dorsal oblique muscle of eye
V	Trigeminal	Mixed	Somatic motor innervation to muscles of mastication and tensor tympani muscle Sensory innervation to most of the face and muzzle
VI	Abducens	Motor	Somatic motor innervation to lateral rectus and retractor bulbi muscles of the eye
VII	Facial	Mixed	Somatic motor innervation to muscles of facial expression and stapedius muscles Sensory innervation of inner pinnae Sensory innervation to rostral two-thirds of tongue Parasympathetic innervation to salivary, lacrimal, palatine, and nasal glands
VIII	Vestibulocochlear	Sensory	Vestibular function and hearing
IX	Glossopharyngeal	Mixed	Somatic motor innervation to larynx and pharynx Sensory innervation of pharynx and caudal third of tongue Parasympathetic innervation of salivary glands (parotid and zygomatic)
X	Vagus	Mixed	Somatic motor innervation to larynx and pharynx Sensory innervation of pharynx Parasympathetic innervation to viscera
XI	Accessory	Motor	Somatic motor innervation to larynx
XII	Hypoglossal	Motor	Somatic motor innervation to the tongue

temporal, and occipital lobes. The olfactory bulb is the most rostral part of the telencephalon and is where the axons of the olfactory nerves terminate.

The diencephalon, specifically the thalamus, receives all sensory information (except olfaction) and projects to sensory areas of the telencephalon. Efferent, or motor, pathways also course from the cerebral cortex through the thalamus to the brainstem. The hypothalamus is important in maintaining homeostasis as it is the neurologic control center for the endocrine system and the autonomic nervous system. The axons of cranial nerve II (optic nerve) terminate within the diencephalon after coursing through the optic chiasm.

The mesencephalon, or midbrain, is the most rostral part of the brainstem. The midbrain contains sensory and motor tracts, as well as the rostral and caudal colliculi, which are associated with visual and auditory reflexes, respectively. The nuclei of cranial nerves III (oculomotor nerve) and IV (trochlear nerve) are located within the mesencephalon. The midbrain is connected to the cerebellum via the rostral cerebellar peduncles.

The metencephalon, or pons, also contains sensory and motor pathways and the nuclei associated with cranial nerve V (trigeminal nerve). The cerebellum is also part of the metencephalon and is located dorsal to the brainstem. The pons is connected to the cerebellum via the middle cerebellar peduncles. The cerebellum has two hemispheres and a centrally located vermis. It receives sensory information directly from afferent pathways, including the vestibular system, and motor information from the cerebral cortex. While the cerebellum does not initiate movement, it is responsible for integrating sensory and motor input to create smooth, controlled, and coordinated movements.

The myelencephalon, or medulla, contains sensory and motor tracts, as well as nuclei for the remaining pairs of cranial nerves VI through XII, including cranial nerve X (vagus nerve), which innervates organs within the thorax and abdomen. In addition, nerve centers for vital body functions, including regulation of blood pressure, heart rate, and respiration, are located within the medulla.

The blood–brain barrier (BBB) is a semipermeable membrane made up of microvascular endothelial cells that restrict free movement of particles from the blood into the brain parenchyma and CSF. The BBB allows carbon dioxide, oxygen, small lipid-soluble substances, and general anesthetics to cross from the blood into the brain. The BBB is made up of pericytes, tight junctions between capillary endothelial cells, a layer of astrocyte foot processes that surround the capillaries, and the basal lamina (or basement membrane). Several areas of the brain, including the hypothalamus, area postrema, and the pineal gland, are outside the BBB as these regions contain sensors for monitoring osmolarity, glucose levels, and pH, and are important for providing information for maintenance of homeostasis. While the BBB fulfills a protective function by preventing possible toxins and limiting pathogens from entering the CNS, it also limits therapeutic options by excluding many drugs from entering. Permeability of the BBB may increase in the face of inflammation or increased intracranial pressure.

The CSF is a clear, colorless fluid produced by the choroid plexus and the ependymal lining cells within the ventricles of the brain and is an ultrafiltrate of plasma. It is produced at a rate of 0.02 mL/min in cats and 0.05 mL/min in dogs [2,3]. Compared to plasma, CSF has a lower concentration of protein, glucose, calcium, and potassium and a higher concentration of sodium, chloride, and magnesium [4]. The CSF is present within the lateral, third, and fourth ventricles of the brain, and within the central canal and subarachnoid space of the spinal cord. The CSF flows from the lateral ventricles, located within the cerebral cortex, into the third ventricle, located between the thalamus and hypothalamus. From here, it flows into the fourth ventricle, located ventral to the cerebellum and dorsal to the medulla. These ventricles can be clearly seen on magnetic resonance imaging (MRI) (Fig. 39.2). Caudally, the fourth ventricle becomes continuous with the central canal of the spinal cord and bilateral apertures within the ventricle allow CSF to flow into the subarachnoid space. The CSF passes from the subarachnoid space through arachnoid villi, which act as one-way valves, to the dural sinuses where it is absorbed. The arachnoid villi are located within the venous sinuses, as well as the spinal veins.

The blood supply to the arterial circle, or the "Circle of Willis" as termed in human medicine, is the main arterial supply to the brain. There are several anatomical species differences that can have clinical implications. In dogs (and in humans), the arterial circle is formed by the joining of the basilar artery and the left and right internal carotid arteries. In the cow, the maxillary and vertebral arteries form this arterial supply. In the cat and sheep, the maxillary artery, via the rete mirabile, forms the arterial circle. The rete mirabile is a network of branches of the maxillary artery located in the

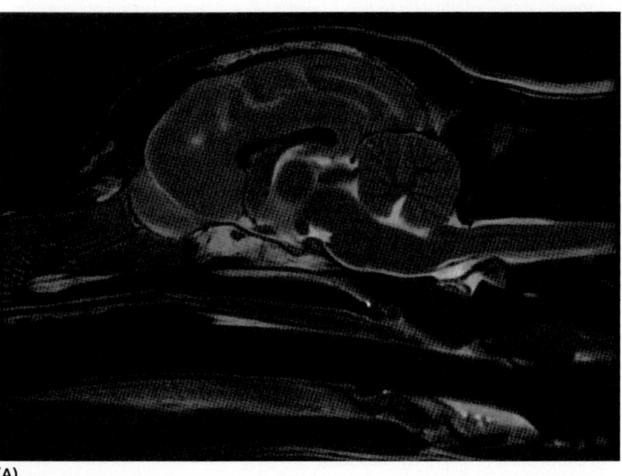
(A)

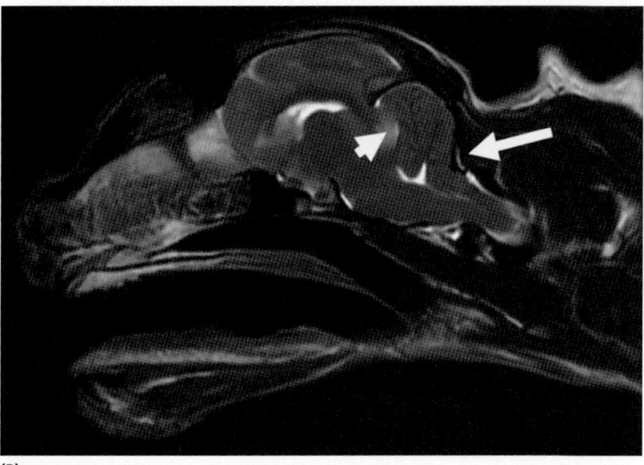
(B)

Figure 39.2 T2-weighted magnetic resonance imaging (MRI) sagittal views. **A.** Normal canine brain. **B.** Feline brain with signs of foramen magnum (arrow) and transtentorial (arrowhead) herniation secondary to a large intracranial tumor. Source: Images courtesy of Dr. Starr Cameron.

cavernous sinus on the ventral surface of the calvarium. The blood from the cavernous sinus drains from the nasal cavity. A countercurrent heat exchange mechanism between the rete mirabile (arterial) and cavernous sinus (venous) may play a role in thermoregulation of the brain. Because of this anatomic variation, using a spring-held mouth gag in cats may increase the risk of neurologic complications associated with anesthesia, including cortical blindness and hearing deficits [5–7]. One study identified changes in electroretinogram (ERG) and brainstem auditory evoked responses (BAER) in anesthetized cats when mouth gags were used compared to no changes when mouth gags were not used [8]. From the arterial circle, the rostral, middle, and caudal cerebral arteries supply the prosencephalon. The blood supply to the brainstem arises as branches from the basilar artery.

The venous system including the venous sinuses and veins of the CNS is valveless, meaning blood can flow in either direction. Associated vessels have thin walls without muscular layers and the veins drain into the larger venous sinuses. The cerebral cortex contains the dorsal and ventral cerebral veins as well as the great cerebral vein which drains the deeper cortex. The major veins of the brainstem include the dorsal and ventral cerebellar veins, pontine veins, and medullary veins. The dorsal sagittal sinus, straight sinus, and paired transverse sinuses are located dorsally. Paired rostral and caudal cavernous sinuses, as well as the sigmoid, basilar, and petrosal sinuses, are located ventrally within the calvarium. The venous sinuses are located within the meninges and drain into the internal jugular, maxillary, and vertebral veins and into the venous plexus.

Spinal cord

Rostrally, the spinal cord is continuous with the myelencephalon, or medulla, of the brainstem and is a complex network of ascending and descending tracts. It is located within the spinal, or vertebral, canal and is surrounded by the meninges, which are composed of the dura mater, arachnoid, and pia mater. The epidural space contains epidural fat, blood vessels, and lymphatics. The CSF passes through the central canal of the spinal cord and flows around the spinal cord within the subarachnoid space. The pia mater is one cell thick and lies directly on the spinal cord.

Anatomically, the spinal cord is divided longitudinally into four major regions: cervical, thoracic, lumbar, and sacral. The caudal (coccygeal) segments are associated with the tail and contain nerves. Each segment of the spinal cord has a pair (right and left) of spinal nerves that exit through the intervertebral foramen. The dorsal root carries sensory (afferent) information and the ventral root carries motor (efferent) information. Just inside the intervertebral foramina, the dorsal and ventral roots combine and exit as the associated spinal nerve for that segment of spinal cord. The number of vertebrae and spinal cord segments varies with species. Spinal nerve C1 exits through a foramen in C1 and the spinal nerves C2–C7 exit cranial to the associated vertebrae. Spinal nerve C8 exits between C7 and T1, and spinal nerves T1–L3 exit caudal to the associated vertebrae. The vertebrae and spinal cord segments are misaligned to varying degrees due to differential growth rates during development. For example, in the lumbar region of the dog, spinal cord segments L5, L6, and L7 all lie within the region of the L4 vertebra. In medium to large-breed dogs, the spinal cord terminates at approximately L6–L7, and in small-breed dogs and cats, the spinal cord terminates at approximately S1. In large animals, including horses, ruminants, and swine, the spinal cord terminates mid-sacrum. These anatomic differences are important to note when considering diagnostic and therapeutic procedures involving the subarachnoid and epidural spaces.

Clinically and functionally, the spinal cord is divided into four segments based on innervation: C1–C5, C6–T2, T3–L3, and L4–S3. The cervical (C6–T2 segments) and lumbosacral (L4–S3 segments) intumescences supply the lower motor neurons to the thoracic and pelvic limbs, respectively. Lesions within the cervical segments (C1–C5 and C6–T2) can cause tetraparesis, hemiparesis, tetraplegia, or hemiplegia. Cervical pain is also common with lesions in this region but may or may not be present. Lesions within the T3–L3 or L4–S3 segments may cause paraparesis or paraplegia and, depending on the etiology, lesions may cause back pain (Fig. 39.3).

Caudal to the lumbar intumescence, the spinal cord tapers into a region called the "conus medullaris," which consists of sacral and caudal segments. The filum terminale is a strand of glial and ependymal cells that extends from the end of the spinal cord. This region is covered by a dural sac, creating a space within the subarachnoid space filled with CSF. As the sacral and caudal spinal roots move caudally past the conus medullaris, each exits at an intervertebral foramen. These roots are collectively known as the "cauda equina."

The spinal cord has an H- or butterfly-shaped center of gray matter, which is divided into the dorsal, lateral, and ventral horns (Fig. 39.4). The dorsal horn contains sensory neurons. The lateral horn is located in the thoracolumbar (T1–L4, specifically) and sacral segments and contains motor neurons that innervate the viscera. The ventral horn contains cell bodies of somatic motor neurons, which are also called lower motor neurons. The white matter surrounds the gray matter of the spinal cord and is divided into three funiculi. The dorsal funiculus contains only sensory fiber tracts in several mammalian species including the dog, while the lateral and ventral funiculi carry both sensory and motor fiber tracts.

Cranially, the subclavian artery branches to become the vertebral artery, which enters the vertebral canal at the atlas (first cervical vertebra). Segmental spinal arteries enter the spinal cord via the intervertebral foramen where they divide into dorsal and ventral branches. The ventral branches connect via the longitudinal ventral spinal artery (which runs in the ventral median fissure of the spinal cord) and supply the ventral gray matter and ventral funiculus. The dorsal branch supplies the dorsal gray matter. Other branches of the segmental spinal arteries supply the lateral funiculus. Blood flow in the gray matter of the spinal cord is four times that of the white matter, and blood flow to the thoracolumbar region of the spinal cord has been shown to be 40% less compared to the cervical and lumbosacral regions [9]. There is less gray matter in the thoracolumbar region of the spinal cord, which accounts for the reduced blood flow.

The venous system of the CNS is valveless and vertebral veins communicate directly with the cranial venous sinus described above. Lying ventral to the spinal cord is the internal vertebral venous plexus, which extends the entire length of the spinal canal. This flat, thin-walled valveless network is paired and is a frequent source of hemorrhage during neurosurgery. The sinus diverges at the intervertebral foramen and then converges over the vertebral body. At the level of the intervertebral foramen, the sinus communicates with the intervertebral veins and exits the foramen with the spinal nerve roots where they drain into larger vessels, including the azygous vein and caudal vena cava.

Peripheral nervous system

The peripheral nervous system (PNS) is divided into afferent (sensory) and efferent (motor) components. Sensory neurons receive

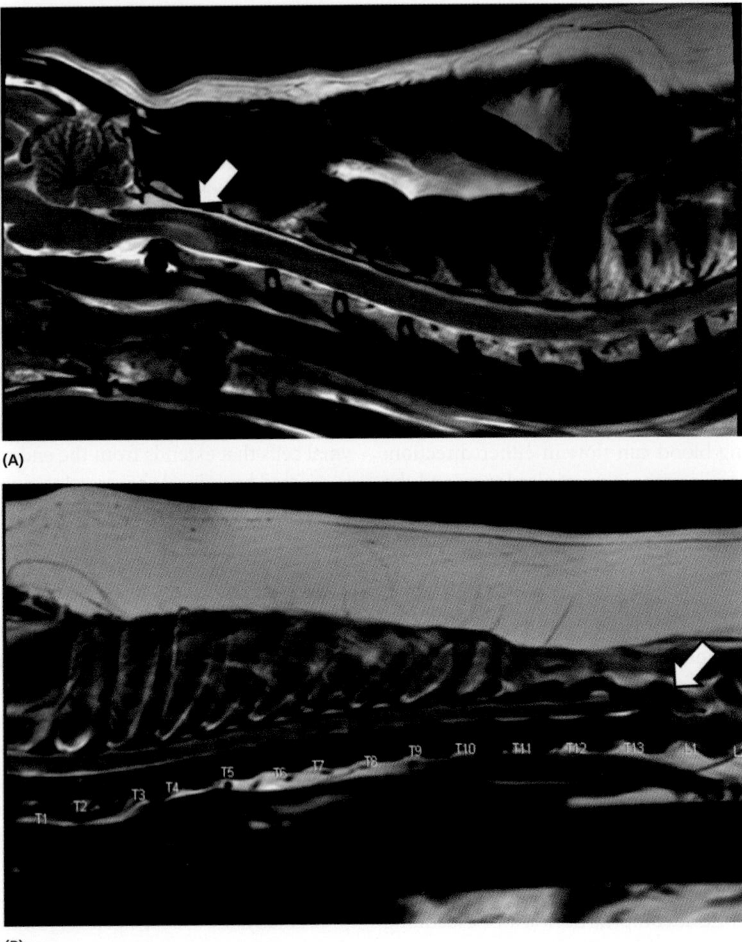

Figure 39.3 T2-weighted magnetic resonance image (MRI) sagittal views. **A.** Cervical spine in a cat with an intramedullary C1–C2 myelopathy (arrow) most consistent with feline ischemic myelopathy. **B.** Thoracic spine in a dog with an acute intervertebral disc extrusion at the T13–L1 disc space (arrow). Source: Images courtesy of Dr. Starr Cameron.

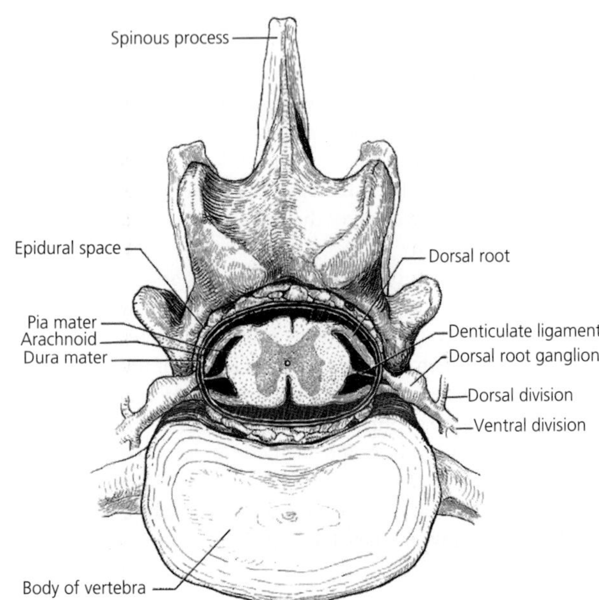

Figure 39.4 Transverse section of the spinal cord within the vertebral canal. Note the adipose tissue and blood vessels in the epidural space. Source: Jenkins [1], with permission.

information from peripheral receptors and transmit this information via action potentials to the CNS for integration and interpretation. Sensory neurons enter the intervertebral foramen as part of the spinal nerve and then enter the dorsal horn of the spinal cord via the dorsal nerve root. Efferent information leaves the ventral horn of the spinal cord via the ventral nerve root before becoming the spinal nerve and then motor neurons. There are two divisions of motor neurons within the PNS: somatic motor neurons, which innervate skeletal muscle, and autonomic motor neurons, which innervate cardiac muscle, smooth muscle, and some glands.

Myelin, produced by oligodendrocytes within the CNS and by Schwann cells within the PNS, insulates the axons of nerves and expedites transmission of electrical activity. The nodes of Ranvier, which are the spaces or gaps between myelin along the axon, allow saltatory conduction to take place which greatly expedites signal transmission. Therefore, nerves that are myelinated have considerably faster conduction velocities compared to unmyelinated nerves. In addition, large fiber nerves also have faster conduction velocities compared to small fiber nerves. The largest and fastest nerve fibers are called Type A and innervate somatic nerves. Type B fibers are also myelinated but are smaller than Type A and make up the preganglionic nerves of the autonomic nervous system. Type C are small unmyelinated nerve fibers with the slowest conduction velocity. Type C fibers transmit postganglionic information within the autonomic nervous system, as well as sensory information regarding temperature, pain, and touch.

Somatic nervous system

The somatic nervous system contains both afferent (sensory) and efferent (motor) nerves. Afferent fibers transmit environmental and peripheral sensory information regarding pain, temperature, and pressure, as well as sight and hearing. The cutaneous region innervated by one specific sensory spinal nerve is called a dermatome, and the presence or absence of sensation in dermatomes can be useful to isolate a particular sensory nerve that is affected by a lesion. Skeletal muscles contain specialized sensory receptors. Muscle spindles provide information on muscle length and are located within the extrafusal fibers of skeletal muscles. Golgi tendon organs provide information about muscle tension and are located within the tendons. All of these are examples of the information transmitted by the general somatic afferent system.

Neuromuscular junction transmission

Motor neurons are found in both cranial and spinal nerves and form synapses with skeletal, smooth, or cardiac muscle fibers at the neuromuscular junction. The motor endplate is the specific region where the nerve meets the muscle, with most muscle fibers having one neuromuscular junction per muscle fiber. The neurotransmitter acetylcholine (ACh) is released from the presynaptic neuron and crosses the synaptic cleft to bind to receptors on the postsynaptic muscle membrane. Depending on the strength of the stimulus and the amount of ACh released, this action potential may cause muscle contraction. Even without action potentials, ACh is constantly being released in small amounts which causes miniature endplate potentials.

In a resting state, there is an excess of sodium ions outside the muscle membrane and an excess of potassium ions inside the muscle membrane, creating a negatively charged environment inside the muscle. The electrical difference between the two sides of the membrane is 90 mV. Once a nerve is stimulated, an action potential travels down the axon and reaches the presynaptic terminal of the nerve where ACh is present in small synaptic vesicles. These vesicles fuse with the presynaptic membrane and ACh is released. ACh diffuses across the cleft and reaches the postsynaptic muscle membrane where it binds reversibly to nicotinic receptors. There are five subunits of the nicotinic receptor, and when two ACh molecules bind to the two α subunits, an allosteric change in conformation of the membrane proteins occurs. Sodium ions flow into the muscle membrane and potassium ions flow out of the muscle membrane, causing a change in the electrical charge, which is called depolarization. If the change in charge inside the muscle membrane is greater than 45 mV, then muscle contraction usually occurs. There is an overabundance of ACh released by an action potential into the neuromuscular junction, which acts as a safety margin to ensure adequate binding. Excess ACh is broken down by the enzyme acetylcholinesterase into acetic acid and choline and then recycled and returned to the presynaptic nerve. The impulses are transmitted through the T-tubules of the sarcolemma of the muscle membrane, causing a release of calcium from the sarcoplasmic reticulum and muscle contraction.

In addition to the presynaptic nerve and postsynaptic muscle receptors described above, there are other postsynaptic receptors located outside the neuromuscular junction on the muscle membrane and these are called extrajunctional (or extrasynaptic) receptors. These receptors, which normally play a very small role in neuromuscular transmission, proliferate after denervation or muscle injury and may cause an exaggerated response that can be detected after a depolarizing neuromuscular blocking agent (i.e., succinylcholine) has been administered.

Autonomic nervous system

The autonomic nervous system (ANS) is responsible for regulating the body's internal environment and helping to maintain homeostasis. Most of the functions of the ANS are under subconscious control and include maintaining heart rate and blood pressure, thermoregulation, controlling micturition, and managing gastrointestinal secretions, although the gastrointestinal tract does have additional nervous system components. The ANS consists of afferent pathways, CNS integration (brain and spinal cord), and two efferent pathways: the sympathetic (flight or fight) and parasympathetic (rest and digest) systems.

Within the diencephalon, the hypothalamus facilitates regulation of both the sympathetic and parasympathetic nervous systems, along with the cerebral cortex and brainstem. Both systems are always active, and activity can be increased or decreased to control organ function and response. Most organs have both sympathetic and parasympathetic innervation, creating reciprocal effects. For example, the heart has sympathetic innervation which increases heart rate and contractility, and parasympathetic innervation which has opposing effects. Sympathetic innervation of the gastrointestinal tract causes relaxation while parasympathetic innervation causes contraction. Unlike the somatic system which has one efferent neuron, efferent information from the ANS is conducted via two (preganglionic and postganglionic) neurons. The preganglionic neuron is within the CNS, and the postganglionic neuron is within the PNS.

The general visceral afferent fibers carry afferent (sensory) information to the CNS and that information is then used to control internal homeostasis and bodily functions via the efferent components of the ANS. Afferent information from cranial nerves VII, IX, and X travels along the solitary tract within the medulla and synapses within the solitary nucleus. Axons then travel to other regions of the brainstem (parasympathetic system) or spinal cord (sympathetic system) to control visceral functions or project to the thalamus for conscious perception of sensory information. Afferent information regarding taste travels via cranial nerves VII and IX. Blood pressure and tissue oxygenation levels are monitored by baroreceptors and chemoreceptors located in arteries and information is transmitted to cranial nerves IX and X. Additionally, sensory information from the olfactory and limbic regions is carried along the solitary tract to the solitary nucleus to allow the ANS to respond to smells and emotions, respectively.

ACh is the neurotransmitter for all preganglionic synapses within the sympathetic and parasympathetic systems, as well as for postganglionic synapse transmission in the parasympathetic system. In postganglionic sympathetic synapses, norepinephrine is the main neurotransmitter secreted; however, some sympathetic postganglionic synapses, such as those that supply sweat glands and blood vessels of skeletal muscles, secrete ACh. ACh receptors are either nicotinic or muscarinic. Nicotinic receptors are found in all preganglionic synapses of the ANS and at the somatic neuromuscular junction. Muscarinic receptors are located in effector cells at postganglionic synapses of the parasympathetic nervous system and in cholinergic postganglionic synapses of the sympathetic nervous system. A list of selected effects of sympathetic and parasympathetic nervous system transmission can be found in Table 39.2.

Table 39.2 Selected effects of sympathetic and parasympathetic nervous system transmission.

Organ	Sympathetic		Parasympathetic	
	Action	Receptor	Action	Receptor
Heart				
Rate	Increase	β_1	Decrease	M
Contractility	Increase	β_1	Decrease	M
Blood vessels				
Arteries	Vasoconstriction	α_1		
Veins	Vasoconstriction	α_2		
Skeletal muscle	Vasodilation	β_2		
Bronchioles	Bronchodilation	β_2	Bronchoconstriction	M
Salivary glands	Increase secretion	α_1	Increase secretion	
Gastrointestinal tract	Relaxation	α_2	Contraction	M
Kidney	Renin secretion	β_1		
Ureter	Contraction	α_1	Relaxation	M
Urinary bladder	Relaxation	β_2	Contraction	M
Internal urethral sphincter	Contraction	α_1	Relaxation	M
Uterus	Contraction	α_1	Variable	
Eye				
Iris dilator muscle	Contraction (mydriasis)	α_1		
Iris sphincter muscle			Contraction (miosis)	M
Ciliary muscle	Relaxation	β_2	Contraction	M
Adipose tissue	Lipolysis	β_1		
Sweat glands	Increase secretion	α_1		
Hair follicles	Contraction (piloerection)	α_1		

M, muscarinic.
Source: Adapted from Hall and Hall [4]; Glick [12].

Sympathetic nervous system

Often referred to as the "fight or flight system," the sympathetic nervous system is most active during times of stress. It discharges as a unit, and the effects are widespread and last longer than those of the parasympathetic system. ACh is the neurotransmitter between preganglionic and postganglionic neurons within the sympathetic system. Norepinephrine is the main neurotransmitter used between postganglionic neurons and the effector organ within the sympathetic nervous system. Norepinephrine acts as an agonist at α_1-, α_2-, β_1-, and β_2-adrenergic receptors. For sweat glands, the receptor is cholinergic, except in horses where the receptor is β_2-adrenergic [10].

Visceral sensory (afferent) information travels along sympathetic nerves to the dorsal horn of the spinal cord. There, interneurons receive information from visceral and somatic afferent nerves. The sympathetic system has short preganglionic and long postganglionic axons. The efferent preganglionic neurons of the sympathetic nervous system are located within the gray matter of the thoracolumbar spinal cord, specifically the T1–L5 spinal cord segments (Fig. 39.5). The axons leave via the ventral nerve root to join the spinal nerve of the associated spinal cord segment and then synapse in a ganglion at one of three locations. Some preganglionic neurons synapse in the sympathetic chain ganglion located along the lateral aspect of the vertebral column (paravertebral). These synapses can occur within ganglia at the same segmental level of the chain, or they may synapse rostrally or caudally which allows for multiple possible synapses. This more diffuse distribution accounts for the widespread effects of sympathetic innervation. The postganglionic neurons then travel to innervate blood vessels, sweat glands, and pilomotor muscles. Other preganglionic neurons travel through the sympathetic chain without synapsing. These neurons then synapse on prevertebral ganglia that supply visceral organs and glands within the thoracic or abdominal cavities. The prevertebral ganglia include the celiac, cranial, and caudal mesenteric ganglia.

Lastly, other preganglionic neurons of the sympathetic nervous system travel from the thoracolumbar region of the spinal cord via the splanchnic nerve to the adrenal medulla where they synapse on chromaffin cells. These neurons release ACh which acts at nicotinic receptors located on chromaffin cell membranes, stimulating these cells to release epinephrine (80% in dogs, 60% in cats) and norepinephrine (20% in dogs, 40% in cats) into circulation [11]. Epinephrine causes vasodilation within skeletal muscles and bronchodilation within the airways, while norepinephrine causes vasoconstriction, increased cardiac activity, and pupillary dilation.

Parasympathetic nervous system

The parasympathetic nervous system of the ANS also has preganglionic and postganglionic neurons. In contrast to the sympathetic preganglionic fibers, the efferent parasympathetic preganglionic axons are long and tend to synapse either within or very near the target organ, meaning that the postganglionic fibers are quite short. The parasympathetic nervous system efferent nuclei are located within the brainstem or sacral spinal cord segments, leading this portion of the ANS to be referred to as the craniosacral component. The preganglionic nuclei of the parasympathetic nervous system are located within the nuclei of cranial nerves III, VII, IX, and X, adjacent to the somatic nuclei of these cranial nerves (Fig. 39.5). The preganglionic parasympathetic nucleus (often called the "Edinger–Westphal nucleus") of the oculomotor nerve (cranial nerve III) is located within the midbrain. The postganglionic neuron stimulates the iris (pupillary) sphincter and ciliary muscles of the eye to cause pupillary constriction. Postganglionic fibers from the facial and glossopharyngeal nerves (cranial nerves VII and IX, respectively) innervate salivary glands. The parasympathetic nucleus of the vagus nerve (cranial nerve X) provides efferent control to the heart, lungs, gastrointestinal tract, liver, pancreas, and gallbladder.

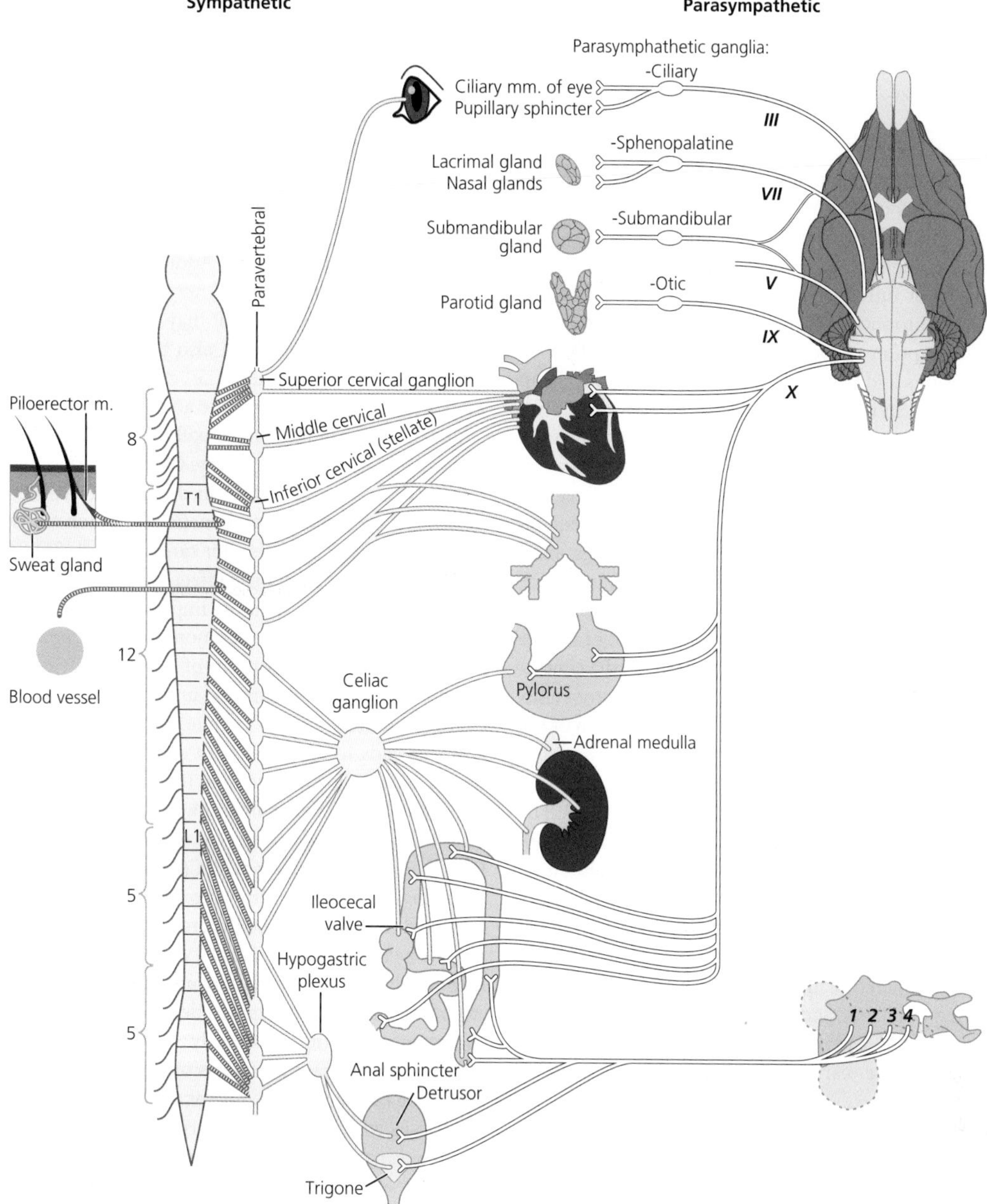

Figure 39.5 The sympathetic and parasympathetic nervous systems. Note the distribution of cranial nerves III, VII, V, IX, and X.

The sacral segments of the parasympathetic nervous system regulate bladder control, the internal urethral sphincter, smooth rectal muscles, and the reproductive organs. During micturition, postganglionic parasympathetic neurons cause detrusor muscle contraction and urethral relaxation for urine voiding.

Preganglionic neurons of the parasympathetic system release ACh which acts on nicotinic receptors of the postganglionic neurons. Postganglionic neurons also release ACh but the receptors at the effector organs are mostly muscarinic.

Physiology of the central nervous system

Brain physiology

Cerebral perfusion pressure and intracranial pressure

According to the Monro–Kellie doctrine, the brain is enclosed in the rigid structure of the skull and an equilibrium must exist between the volumes of brain parenchyma, interstitial and CSF fluid, and arterial/venous blood; therefore, an increase in one component or the addition of another (e.g., hematoma, skull fracture, and tumor) must cause a decrease in the remaining components [13,14]. Additionally, an increase in the volume of any constituent can result in an increase in intracranial pressure (ICP). Blood and CSF are the main volume buffering components; thus, initial compensatory mechanisms such as a decrease in cerebral blood volume (CBV), and/or a shift of CSF from the brain into the spinal canal, or even absorption of CSF will prevent major increases in ICP [15]. This stage is often characterized as the compensated state of increased ICP. While changes in cerebral venous volume occur rapidly, "spatial compensation" of CSF happens more slowly, so its ability to mitigate acute increases in ICP is limited [14,16]. Therefore, once these compensatory mechanisms are exhausted, marked elevations in ICP can occur leading to decreased cerebral perfusion pressure (CPP), defined as the difference between mean arterial blood pressure (MAP) and ICP (i.e., CPP = MAP − ICP), and increased risk of cerebral ischemia [14,15]. Significant increases in ICP can also result in compression of brain tissue against the tentorium, falx, and foramen magnum and potential brain herniation, which is characterized as the decompensated state of increased ICP [15,16].

Some causes of increased ICP include space-occupying lesions (i.e., intracranial hemorrhage, hematoma, tumor, abscess), cerebral edema (i.e., due to head injury, or hypoxic or ischemic encephalopathy), venodilation, and a decrease in venous drainage (i.e., head-down position, jugular vein obstruction/compression, and increased right heart or intrathoracic pressures) [14–17]. In addition, increased CSF production (i.e., choroid plexus tumor) or impeded CSF reabsorption or outflow (i.e., flow obstruction by space-occupying lesions and Chiari malformation) can result in an increase in CSF volume and ICP [14,15].

As a result of increased ICP, a physiologic response known as the "Cushing reflex" occurs, which has classically been reported as an increase in systolic blood pressure, bradycardia, and an irregular (Cheyne–Stokes) breathing pattern [18–21]; however, subsequent studies led to refinement of Cushing's original findings [22]. Initially, both blood pressure and heart rate may rise due to sympathetic activation [22–24] as MAP increases to maintain CPP. Over time, hypertension persists in the face of elevated ICP, but heart rate begins to decrease. The mechanism resulting in bradycardia continues to be debated with some suggesting it is a baroreceptor reflex while others propose it is a result of intracranial compression of the vagus nerve [24]. Finally, once the brainstem is compressed and the respiratory center is compromised by increased ICP, irregular breathing and even apnea (respiratory arrest) can ensue [24]. The Cushing reflex has also been recognized in cases of decreased CPP (< 15 mmHg) in humans [25]. As bradycardia is a late component of the physiologic response, focusing on this symptom may result in the patient being subjected to a prolonged period of intracranial hypertension prior to intervention, resulting in a higher incidence of complications [25]. Therefore, in the human literature, monitoring for systemic hypertension and tachycardia as potential early indicators of increased ICP and impaired brain perfusion has been recommended to facilitate earlier intervention and improved outcomes [25].

Regulation of cerebral blood flow

The brain is an organ with high metabolic demand. Despite this high demand for energy substrates (mainly oxygen and glucose) to maintain homeostasis, extreme fluctuations in cerebral blood flow (CBF) are not tolerated due to the non-compliant cranium and meninges. Thus, tight control and regulation of tissue pressure (i.e., ICP) is required because increases in CBV will lead to increases in ICP, and vice versa [26,27]. Several key factors contribute to regulation of CBF including the arterial partial pressure of carbon dioxide ($PaCO_2$), MAP, cerebral metabolic rate (CMR), and the ANS [27]. For simplicity, regulators of CBF may be classified as chemical, myogenic, and neurogenic factors [26].

Chemical regulation of cerebral blood flow

Chemical regulation involves changes in CMR, $PaCO_2$, and arterial partial pressure of oxygen (PaO_2). Increases in neuronal activity lead to increased CMR, which is directly related to the change in CBF, a phenomenon known as "flow-metabolism coupling" [26,28]. Flow-metabolism coupling is a complex physiologic process involving metabolic, glial, neuronal, and vascular factors [26,28]. Local by-products, including potassium ions, hydrogen ions, lactate, adenosine, and adenosine triphosphate modulate vascular tone and likely contribute to the mechanism of neurovascular coupling [27,29]. It is thought that neurotransmitters, especially glutamate (released with increased or excitatory neuronal activity), are the main factors augmenting activity-induced blood flow due to the release of nitric oxide leading to cerebral vasodilation [27,28,30]. Oxygen concentration modulates the contribution of different signaling pathways, and reduced oxygen concentration can lead to adenosine release, contributing to vasodilation. Additionally, astrocytes also mediate neurovascular coupling, and nerves innervating cerebral vessels release neurotransmitters that may also be involved in this process [26,27,30,31]. The CMR can also be influenced by the functional state of the nervous system (i.e., awake versus sleep), and can be extremely high during epileptic activity, for example.

A decrease in temperature will decrease CMR and CBF in animals [32–34]. More specifically, CMR decreases by 6% per degree Celsius drop in temperature in dogs [35]. Hypothermia has been shown to have a consistently beneficial effect on neurologic outcomes in small and large animals after cardiac arrest [36]. Hyperthermia is associated with the opposite effect on CMR and CBF [35]. As such, modest hypothermia or, more importantly, the avoidance of hyperthermia may be a consideration in anesthetizing patients with conditions in which elevations of CMR or CBF may be of concern.

The cerebrovasculature is uniquely and highly sensitive to changes in $PaCO_2$ [27,31]. An acute decrease in $PaCO_2$ in healthy animals leads to an increase in cerebral vascular resistance and a decrease in CBF; conversely, an increase in $PaCO_2$ has the opposite effect but is of a higher magnitude (Fig. 39.6) [31]. In monkeys, a linear relationship between both CBV and $PaCO_2$ and CBF and $PaCO_2$ was observed when $PaCO_2$ ranged between 15–76 mmHg [37]. In dogs, a potential maximal cerebral vasodilatory effect occurred at between 60–70 mmHg; however, cerebrovascular responsiveness to CO_2 seems to vary depending on species, experimental design, anesthetic drugs used, and CO_2 levels [38]. Additionally, while a sustained decrease in $PaCO_2$ due to prolonged hyperventilation (approximately 5–6 h) lowers CBF to some extent, it may return to baseline values over time because brain interstitial pH is one of the major regulators of CBF. Brain interstitial pH initially rises with an acute decrease in $PaCO_2$, but then falls during sustained hyperventilation as lactate accumulates and bicarbonate falls [39–41]. As such, anesthetic management of intracranial

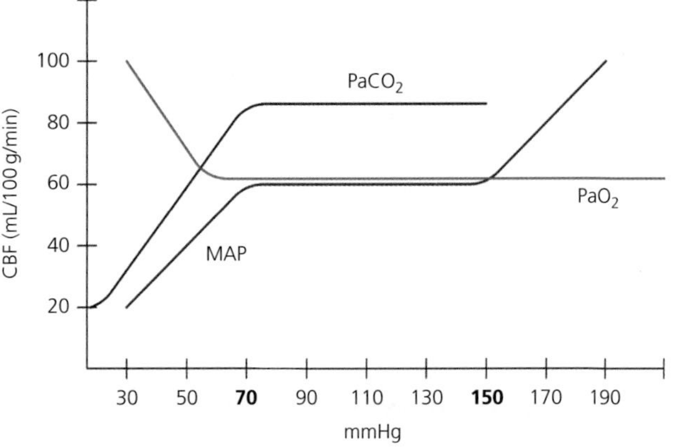

Figure 39.6 Representation of the effects of arterial partial pressure of oxygen (PaO_2), arterial partial pressure of carbon dioxide ($PaCO_2$), and mean arterial blood pressure (MAP) on cerebral blood flow (CBF).

hypertension with modest hyperventilation (discussed later) may only be employed as a relatively temporary strategy. Furthermore, because of the metabolic changes associated with a decrease in $PaCO_2$, patients subjected to sustained hyperventilation (hypocapnia) may be at risk of developing intracranial hypertension with restoration of normocapnia as this is accompanied by CSF acidosis, significant increases in CBF, and ultimately increased ICP. Sustained hypoventilation (hypercapnia), once corrected to normocapnia, may result in a significant decrease in CBF, and the patient may, theoretically, be at risk of ischemia [26]. The change in brain extracellular pH and CBF after acute changes in $PaCO_2$ happens because CO_2 diffuses across the BBB [27,31]. However, changes in pH due to metabolic acidosis (instead of respiratory acidosis) have little effect on CBF because hydrogen ions do not cross the BBB.

The cerebrovasculature is also sensitive to changes in PaO_2 but only in hypoxic conditions (PaO_2 < 60 mmHg) (Fig. 39.6), leading to cerebral vasodilation and a rapid increase in CBF (but not CMR) [31]. This sensitivity to PaO_2 is dependent on the $PaCO_2$ level. For instance, hypercapnia increases cerebrovascular sensitivity to hypoxia, and both have synergistic effects, but the vasodilatory effect of hypoxia predominates over the vasoconstrictive effect of hypocapnia [42]. Additionally, the changes in CBF due to oxygen seem to be related to oxygen content rather than oxygen tension (PaO_2) because decreases in oxygen content from anemia and hemodilution also result in an increase in CBF [43,44]. The mechanism involved in hypoxia-mediated cerebral vasodilation may involve neurogenic (neuraxial chemoreceptors) and local humoral factors [26,31].

The impact of hematocrit (i.e., blood viscosity) on CBF is controversial [45]. Anemia results in decreased cerebral vascular resistance and an increase in CBF, but as mentioned above, this response seems to be related to the decrease in oxygen content [43]. However, a study in rats demonstrated that increased viscosity decreased CBF, but only in conditions where CBF was already elevated (i.e., not in control animals) [46].

Myogenic regulation of cerebral blood flow

Myogenic regulation of CBF is related to the local vascular smooth muscle response to changes in intraluminal pressure in the cerebrovasculature. An increase in MAP leads to an increase in transmural vessel tension resulting in depolarization of vascular smooth muscle and a reduction in vascular diameter (i.e., constriction) [27]; conversely, vasodilation happens when MAP and transmural tension decrease [16]. Autoregulation of CBF is classically defined as the ability of the brain circulation to alter its resistance to maintain constant CBF within a range of MAP [47]. The lower and upper limits of CBF autoregulation likely occur at approximately 70 and 150 mmHg, respectively (Fig. 39.6). Above and below this MAP range, CBF becomes pressure-dependent and will vary linearly with CPP [26]. There is some controversy in the literature regarding the lower limit of CBF autoregulation and values ranging from 50–70 mmHg of MAP have been suggested [27,31,48]. The initial characterization of the lower limit of CBF autoregulation at approximately 50–60 mmHg seems to originate from Lassen's study in 1959 [47]. One complicating factor is that some authors use CPP instead of MAP on the x-axis [31], which would naturally bring the lower limit value down because CPP = MAP – ICP. There is also significant variation between species as well as the conditions (awake versus anesthetized) and drugs used during the studies assessing the limits of cerebral autoregulation [49]; there is certainly not enough evidence to form conclusions regarding all drugs and drug combinations used clinically across all species. Furthermore, significant interindividual variation has been reported [48,49], and it is not valid to assume that autoregulation of CBF will be preserved at a MAP as low as 50 mmHg in an individual, in a broader population, or every anesthetic situation. In addition, in the normal CNS, while there is a blood flow reserve that acts as a buffer and protects against significant reductions in blood flow (i.e., hypotension), this reserve may be compromised in some clinical situations [48]. As such, defining the lower threshold of MAP below which a clinical patient is at substantial risk of ischemic injury is not easy. The authors prefer to use 70 mmHg as the lower limit of CBF autoregulation for clinical case management (Fig. 39.6).

Newer evidence suggests this topic is much more complex than commonly presented. Cerebral autoregulation does not always maintain constant perfusion through the MAP range of 70–150 mmHg, but CBF is still directly affected by changes in perfusion pressure [31]. CBF is only kept constant (i.e., the "classic" description of autoregulation) with gradual changes in blood pressure, as in nocturnal MAP changes or changes due to treatment for hypertension. For rapid changes in blood pressure (i.e., over minutes or seconds – such as those happening during surgery), CBF is more unstable and can undergo large, rapid fluctuations [27]. Slow changes in blood pressure and their effect on CBF align better with the "static autoregulation" model, whereas the impact of faster changes on CBF is more consistent with the "dynamic autoregulation" model [27,31]. Therefore, despite normal autoregulatory mechanisms, CBF may still vary with changes in blood pressure. One common misconception is that chronic hypertension leads to impairment of autoregulation (i.e., that brain vessels may become dependent on higher MAP to maintain perfusion) but treatment to lower MAP is not associated with a decrease in CBF [27].

Additionally, the effects of arterial blood gases and blood pressure are interdependent in their regulation of CBF, and it is difficult to determine the impact of each individual parameter when they change simultaneously [31]. For instance, dogs with severe hypotension showed no change in CBF following changes in $PaCO_2$ because the vessels had already reached maximal dilation; therefore, blood pressure is a critical component of CBF [31,50].

Neurogenic regulation of cerebral blood flow

Neurogenic regulation of CBF contributes to cerebral autoregulation and can buffer surges in perfusion pressure. The cerebrovasculature is innervated by adrenergic fibers (with epinephrine, norepinephrine, dopamine, and neuropeptide Y as transmitters), cholinergic fibers (with ACh, and vasoactive intestinal peptide as transmitters), and sensory fibers (with calcitonin gene-related peptide, substance P, and pituitary adenylate cyclase-activating polypeptide as transmitters) as part of the sympathetic, parasympathetic, and trigeminal nervous systems, respectively [27,31]. The exact influence of cerebral vasomotor nerves is not well understood. Despite some controversies, the sympathetic nervous system generally prevents increases in CBF during resting conditions and contributes to autoregulation of CBF during rapid changes in blood pressure [27]. However, it is difficult to assess the effects of the sympathetic nervous system in isolation, as many other confounding variables are usually present. Cholinergic innervation in the brain can lead to vasodilation and further release of nitric oxide locally, but it does not seem to play a major role in autoregulation [27]. The influence of the sympathetic and parasympathetic nervous systems on CBF control seems to be species-specific [31], so caution is advised when extrapolating across species.

Luxury perfusion

Vasomotor paralysis, which is impaired ability of vessels to respond to $PaCO_2$ and perfusion pressure, or a loss of regional CBF autoregulation can happen in some pathological conditions leading to inadequate cerebral perfusion and hypoxia (i.e., ischemic stroke and tumor) [51–53]. Therefore, regional CBF within ischemic areas may become passively dependent on perfusion pressure, which can result in excessive blood flow relative to local metabolic demands in the face of normal or high perfusion pressure, a phenomenon called "luxury perfusion syndrome" [51,54–56]. Additionally, paradoxical flow responses can happen in some patients with these pathological conditions following an increase or decrease in $PaCO_2$ [51,57]. In the case of decreased cerebral vascular resistance (i.e., increased $PaCO_2$ or drugs that cause cerebral vasodilation), blood may be shunted away from areas of vasomotor paralysis to normal areas of the brain, a phenomenon called "intracerebral steal syndrome" [51]. On the other hand, an increase in cerebral vascular resistance (i.e., decreased $PaCO_2$) may lead to blood shunting into areas of vasomotor paralysis, a phenomenon called "inverse intracerebral steal" or "Robin Hood syndrome," which could be deleterious to normal areas of the brain [51,54].

Spinal cord physiology

The spinal cord extends rostrally from the brainstem and ends caudally within the lumbar or sacral spinal segments, depending on the species. Each segment of the spinal cord contains a pair (right and left) of spinal nerves that contain both afferent (sensory) and efferent (motor) information. Spinal cord blood flow (SCBF) is maintained via autoregulation when MAP is between 60–150 mmHg [58]. When MAP falls below 60 mmHg, SCBF is significantly reduced in dogs. Interestingly, SCBF seems to decrease with dobutamine infusions that increase MAP in healthy horses, which is concerning as low spinal cord perfusion could predispose the animal to myelopathy [59,60]. In healthy horses anesthetized with isoflurane, a significant decrease in SCBF was found with MAP levels of 100 mmHg, specifically in the thoracolumbar spinal cord region [60]. Hemodilution increases SCBF if the patient is normotensive; however, in cases of hypotension, there may be increased risk of ischemia due to limited ability to vasodilate [45]. In situations of acute blood loss representing approximately 20% of total blood volume, no changes in SCBF were detected; however, when tetracaine was administered in the subarachnoid space, a significant decrease in SCBF was detected [61].

The response of SCBF to oxygen and carbon dioxide levels is very similar to that of the brain. Hypoxia significantly increases SCBF with maximal flow reached at PaO_2 levels of 30–40 mmHg [62]. Additionally, hypocapnia decreases SCBF while hypercapnia increases SCBF, with $PaCO_2$ levels of 85 mmHg resulting in double the normocapnic SCBF [9,62].

Studies evaluating the relationship between CSF and SCBF revealed no significant change in blood flow with changes in the volume of CSF; however, elevations in CSF pressure significantly reduced SCBF [63].

Effects of vasoactive drugs, sedatives, and anesthetics

Vasoactive drugs

Most drugs used to decrease blood pressure (i.e., sodium nitroprusside and calcium channel blockers) lead to cerebral vasodilation but CBF may increase or be maintained [64–66]. The effects of catecholamine agonists and antagonists on cerebral physiology depend on baseline blood pressure, the magnitude of changes in blood pressure, autoregulation, and the status of the BBB [26]. In general, in cases where autoregulation is preserved but baseline blood pressure is outside autoregulatory limits, drug-induced increases in blood pressure will typically increase CBF. If baseline blood pressure is within the limits of autoregulation, drug-induced increases in blood pressure may not significantly change CBF because of activation of normal autoregulatory mechanisms [26]. There is also significant variation in drug effects on CBF (in various species) reported in the literature. Differences in study methodology undoubtedly contribute to this variation and should be taken into consideration when reviewing studies and interpreting their results.

Like anesthetics, the effect of vasoactive agents may be species-dependent. Use of phenylephrine does not seem to change CBF or ICP in dogs but can increase CBF in rats, rabbits, and lambs [64,67–73]. Use of norepinephrine and epinephrine resulted in no significant change in CBF, ICP, and cerebral oxygen utilization, but dopamine caused an increase in all these parameters in sheep [74]. However, CBF was not changed after dopamine administration in young rabbits and monkeys [71]. Additionally, the effect of epinephrine and norepinephrine on CBF and cerebral metabolic rate of oxygen ($CMRO_2$) was dependent on the status of the BBB in dogs, where no change was noted with an intact BBB but increases in CBF and $CMRO_2$ were observed with increased BBB permeability [75].

The effects of β-adrenergic agonists seem to be dose- and species-dependent. At clinically relevant doses, dobutamine and dopamine do not seem to change CBF and $CMRO_2$ in monkeys but cause a dose-dependent decrease in CBF in dogs [76,77].

Sedatives and anesthetics

Anesthetic and sedative drugs can negatively interfere with CBF, CMR, and the electrophysiology of the brain; therefore, knowledge of these effects and how to modify them to improve clinical outcomes is crucial for better patient care. Typically, CBF and CBV vary in parallel; however, there are some clinical situations (i.e., cerebral ischemia) where they can change independently [78]. Furthermore, there are some cases where the magnitude of change in CBF may be less than that of CBV [79]. Most acute anesthetic-induced changes in ICP occur due to changes in CBV [80]. Thus, it is important to note that anesthetic-mediated CBF changes do not necessarily predict their impact on ICP because they may not be accompanied by similar changes in CBV [80,81]. Ideally, understanding drug-related impacts on CPP is more important than potential isolated changes in CBF and ICP. Generally, most anesthetic drugs cause decreases in CBF and CMR, and autoregulation and CO_2 responsiveness are maintained with injectable anesthetics.

Opioids

Usually, the direct effects of opioids on CBF, $CMRO_2$, CBV, and ICP are minimal and CO_2 responsiveness is typically preserved [82–84]. Most opioids cause a decrease in CBF and CBV and a decrease or no change in ICP [79,82,85–87]. However, there are conflicting results in the literature regarding the effects of some opioids, such as sufentanil and remifentanil. Some studies involving sufentanil demonstrate a transient increase in CBF and $CMRO_2$, but minimal effects or a decrease in ICP [88]; others describe a decrease or no change in CBF and $CMRO_2$ with no change in ICP in veterinary species [82,86]. In humans, a dose-dependent increase in regional CBF has been shown with remifentanil [89]. The type of anesthetic protocol or the lack of general anesthesia (e.g., use of opioid alone or opioid with nitrous oxide only) may have contributed to some of this variation and, in general, sufentanil and remifentanil are not considered contraindicated in neuroanesthesia.

Nonetheless, indirect increases in ICP due to hypoventilation and hypercapnia associated with opioid administration need to be prevented in certain clinical neurological patients (i.e., traumatic brain injury and space-occupying brain lesions). Sudden decreases in MAP that may accompany bolus doses of potent opioids in certain species should also be prevented or corrected as they may be associated with transient reductions in CPP and increases in ICP [90].

In addition, the systemic effects that may accompany administration of some opioids can have adverse impacts on the CNS. For instance, histamine release associated with administration of morphine or meperidine can result in cerebral vasodilation and an increase in CBV and ICP, while vomiting associated with initial administration of morphine or hydromorphone may lead to an increase in ICP.

α_2-Adrenergic receptor agonists

Xylazine produces a dose-dependent and transient decrease in ICP in dogs with increased ICP due to subarachnoid hemorrhage [69]. Xylazine did not change ICP in horses anesthetized with pentobarbital [91], and decreased ICP in conscious horses [92]. A more recent study with normocapnic, healthy horses anesthetized with isoflurane and lidocaine constant rate infusion demonstrated a decrease in ICP and an increase in CPP following xylazine bolus administration but no change in ICP following administration of xylazine in conscious horses [93]. Lowering the head is a common characteristic of sedation with α_2-adrenergic receptor agonists; however, head height does not seem to correlate with ICP in the conscious horse, likely due to active compensatory changes in cerebral vascular resistance to maintain CBV and CBF [94]. In general, one should prevent lowering of the head in anesthetized animals because anesthetic drugs may impair normal physiologic regulation. Lowering of the head below the level of the heart in the anesthetized horse was associated with a significant increase in ICP and a decrease in CBF, which could potentially predispose the animal to ischemia; spinal cord blood flow values were very low, but unaffected by head-down positioning in anesthetized horses [17].

Dexmedetomidine has been shown to decrease CBF with little to no effect on $CMRO_2$ in isoflurane-anesthetized dogs [95,96]. This decrease in CBF is likely related to α_2-adrenergic receptor-mediated vasoconstriction of cerebral vessels [95] and decreased cerebral metabolism associated with reduced brain activity [97]. In healthy piglets anesthetized with propofol–remifentanil total intravenous anesthesia (TIVA), the addition of dexmedetomidine resulted in a significant decrease in cerebral oxygenation when blood pressure was low, but cerebral perfusion and oxygenation were not affected when blood pressure was normal [98], again demonstrating the importance of blood pressure on cerebral dynamics. In dogs anesthetized with isoflurane, no change in ICP and an increase in CPP was reported following medetomidine administration [99].

The effects of α_2-adrenergic receptor agonists on CBF, CBV, ICP, or CPP in animals with different underlying neurologic diseases have not been well studied, but based on data from healthy animals, their use seems reasonable. However, reversal with the α_2-adrenergic receptor antagonist tolazoline has been shown to increase CBF and ICP [69]; therefore, in situations where increased ICP is a concern, α_2-adrenergic receptor agonists should be used with caution as reversal of sedation may impact ICP.

Phenothiazines

The use of acepromazine in dogs with a history of seizures or those prone to seizures (e.g., myelography) is controversial. Despite older literature suggesting acepromazine is contraindicated in these patients, recent studies using clinical doses of acepromazine in dogs indicate no increased seizure risk [100–102]. However, the drug can increase CBV (35–56% above control) in dogs [103], so its use should be avoided in patients with high ICP. As with all anesthetic agents, hemodynamic effects (i.e., vasodilation and hypotension) are possible so blood pressure should be monitored, and hypotension treated to maintain MAP within a range consistent with physiologic cerebral autoregulation.

Benzodiazepines

In general, benzodiazepines are considered to be safe agents with few hemodynamic effects. At clinically relevant doses, midazolam and diazepam decrease CBF (approximately 50–60% below control) and EEG activity, and $CMRO_2$ either decreases or remains unchanged depending on the species [87,104,105]. In a hypoxic model in dogs, midazolam provided greater neuroprotection than diazepam but less than pentobarbital [104].

The effects of the benzodiazepine antagonist flumazenil on CBF and $CMRO_2$ are transient (lasting only between 15–30 min) and dose-dependent when administered following midazolam in dogs [105]. At low doses (0.0025 mg/kg), administration resulted in an increase in CSF pressure and reversal of the reduction in EEG activity and $CMRO_2$ produced by midazolam; while administration of higher doses (0.01–0.16 mg/kg) resulted in decreased cerebral vascular resistance, an increase in CBF and CSF pressure, but no change in CPP [105]. Much higher doses of flumazenil (1 mg/kg) can result in a more profound increase in CBF and ICP and a decrease in MAP in dogs [106]. Use of flumazenil alone (i.e., independent of midazolam) or in dogs that received midazolam but also had high CSF pressure did not result in the changes noted above [105]. In humans sedated with midazolam with traumatic brain injury and poorly controlled ICP, flumazenil resulted in a marked increase in ICP and a decrease in CPP [107]. Therefore, flumazenil should be used with caution in patients for whom increased ICP would be detrimental.

Lidocaine

Lidocaine administration results in dose-dependent decreases in EEG activity and $CMRO_2$ [108]. At a clinically relevant dose (3 mg/kg), it has minimal effect on CBF and cerebral vascular resistance and induces only a transient decrease in $CMRO_2$ [108]. A lidocaine bolus can be used as an adjunct treatment to prevent an acute increase in ICP during craniotomy and endotracheal tube suctioning [109,110]. A cough reflex during endotracheal intubation may result in increased ICP [111]. In dogs, topical lidocaine (0.4 mg/kg) applied to the larynx was insufficient to prevent the cough reflex, but IV lidocaine (1.5–2 mg/kg) was effective [112–114]; however, IV fentanyl was superior to IV lidocaine for cough reflex suppression [113]. In cats, an IV fentanyl bolus associated with topical laryngeal lidocaine application was more effective at decreasing the cough reflex than topical lidocaine alone [115]. Despite the cough-suppressing effect of lidocaine, a study in humans showed that IV lidocaine was unable to completely prevent the increase in ICP associated with endotracheal intubation in neurosurgical patients [116].

Pretreatment with lidocaine has been shown to attenuate acute hypertension and an increase in ICP, as well as increase the recovery of neural function after acute cerebral ischemia induced by air embolism in cats [117]. Intravenous lidocaine has also been shown to have beneficial effects on cortical ischemia and electrophysiologic activity in injured feline brains [118,119]. Careful attention to the dose of lidocaine, with cautious consideration of species differences, is necessary to avoid systemic toxicity and associated detrimental CNS effects (i.e., seizures) [108].

Barbiturates

Barbiturates cause a decrease in CBF, $CMRO_2$, and ICP, and maintain cerebrovascular reactivity to CO_2, but ventilation should be controlled in patients where increases in ICP are contraindicated due to the potential for hypoventilation/apnea leading to hypercapnia and increased ICP [26,120–122]. Additionally, the anticonvulsant properties of thiobarbiturates are potentially beneficial in epileptics or in patients undergoing procedures such as myelography where seizures are a possible complication [120]. However, barbiturate anesthesia is commonly associated with longer recoveries from anesthesia compared to other agents such as propofol, which may be problematic in neurosurgical patients as it may significantly delay postoperative neurologic evaluations.

Propofol

Propofol administration results in decreased EEG activity, CBF, $CMRO_2$, and ICP, while maintaining cerebrovascular reactivity to CO_2 similar to barbiturates [70,123–125]. However, at very high infusion rates (0.8 mg/kg/min), propofol can result in decreased CPP in dogs [70]. The decreased CBF and cerebrovascular reactivity to CO_2 during a hypocapnic challenge from propofol was not statistically significant when compared to isoflurane anesthesia in dogs, though the authors suggested this could be due to small sample size [126]. In humans, a propofol bolus before endotracheal tube suctioning in patients with severe brain disease reduced the cough response, reduced the intracranial hypertensive response, and improved long-term prognosis [127].

Propofol can cause myoclonus in dogs which may be related to its antagonist actions at glycine receptors in the spinal cord and brainstem [128]. Propofol has been shown to be effective at managing seizures following surgical treatment of portosystemic shunts and may be effective at controlling status epilepticus resistant to conventional therapy (i.e., benzodiazepines and barbiturates) in dogs and cats [129,130].

The effect of different intravenous anesthetics including propofol (as well as methohexital and ketamine) in two feline models of brain edema revealed that all drugs studied were effective at decreasing ICP in a space-occupying lesion model (mimicking vasogenic brain edema), likely because a large volume of brain tissue was still viable and the drug-induced decrease in $CMRO_2$ resulted in vasoconstriction and a decrease in ICP [131]. However, administration using a different model, cytotoxic brain edema with diffuse intracellular damage, resulted in no drug-induced change in ICP, likely because autoregulation of the cerebral vasculature was impaired in this model.

Alfaxalone

Alfaxalone was previously manufactured in a formulation containing alfadolone in Cremophor EL®, and its use was discontinued due to severe side effects. Most of the studies in the literature associated with cerebral metabolism and dynamics involve this previous formulation and show decreases in CBF, $CMRO_2$, and ICP while maintaining cerebrovascular reactivity to CO_2 [111,132,133]. More recent studies using the current formulation of alfaxalone (in cyclodextrin) also show a decrease in CBF [126,134]. The CBF was significantly lower following alfaxalone total intravenous anesthesia (TIVA) when compared to anesthesia with isoflurane [126]. Additionally, alfaxalone TIVA was associated with greater cerebrovascular reactivity to CO_2 during hypocapnic challenge compared to isoflurane and propofol, which could represent an advantage when adjustments in ventilation to decrease CO_2 are performed under anesthesia in patients with increased ICP [126].

Etomidate

Etomidate administration results in significant decreases in CBF, $CMRO_2$, and ICP, and maintenance of cerebrovascular reactivity to CO_2 [132,135,136]. The cerebral metabolic effects (e.g., decreased $CMRO_2$) of etomidate are secondary to its effects on neuronal function, like many other anesthetics including thiopental and isoflurane [135,137,138]. In addition, etomidate seems to be a potent direct cerebral vasoconstrictor, independent of its effect on $CMRO_2$ [135].

Etomidate has the advantage of providing good hemodynamic stability, seems to preserve the cerebral metabolic state even in the face of hypotension [139], and is effective in decreasing ICP with minimal change in CPP in patients with intracranial space-occupying lesions and traumatic brain injury [132,140].

Myoclonus that may be observed during etomidate induction is not associated with epileptiform activity on EEG in humans [141]. However, etomidate should be avoided in epileptic patients because it can precipitate EEG epileptic activity in humans [142]. Furthermore, myoclonus in some species may resemble retching, theoretically leading to an increase in ICP. Co-administration with agents such as benzodiazepines may prevent or attenuate these effects.

Ketamine

Compared to other intravenous anesthetics, ketamine produces unique effects in various body systems (e.g., stimulation of the cardiovascular system and minimal respiratory depression), and its effects on cerebral metabolism and hemodynamics are no exception. Ketamine can cause increases in CBF, $CMRO_2$, and ICP but autoregulation seems to be maintained and CO_2 responsiveness preserved [143–145]; however, its effects are not necessarily straightforward. Increased CBF and ICP have only been demonstrated in spontaneously ventilating animals; in animals where ventilation was controlled, decreased CBF and variable effects on $CMRO_2$ (either decreased or increased) have been observed [146–148]. In addition, when compared to other intravenous anesthetics such as alfaxalone, ketamine resulted in significantly higher CBF in monkeys [134]. In healthy dogs, ketamine was reported to increase CBF in some areas of the brain (parietal, occipital, and thalamic regions) but not in others (frontal cortex) [149]; however, increases and decreases in different brain regions have been reported in various studies with different doses of ketamine in both dogs and cats [150,151]. Regardless, potential increases in $CMRO_2$ and decreases in CBF (i.e., dissociation of cerebral oxygen demand and supply) could increase the risk of cerebral ischemia [152].

Despite the controversy in the literature regarding the impact of ketamine on brain physiology and dynamics; some authors discourage its use in patients with a history of seizures and patients with space-occupying lesions, closed-head traumatic injuries, and other conditions associated with high ICP [153]. However, a retrospective study in humans with increased ICP showed that use of ketamine in these patients was associated with lower mortality rates compared to etomidate and midazolam, and the authors suggested that its use should be considered in these patients without concern for worsening outcomes [154]. The combination of drugs that depress cerebral metabolism, such as midazolam or thiopental, with ketamine, prevented the increase in CBF, $CMRO_2$, and ICP but did not change ketamine's effect on MAP or the EEG [143,152]. Additionally, subanesthetic doses of ketamine (2 mg/kg) did not have any significant effects on CBF, $CMRO_2$, or the EEG in mechanically ventilated pigs [147] and were associated with decreased ICP and increased CPP in a feline space-occupying lesion model of brain edema [131]. Ketamine has neuroprotective properties and its use in combination with other sedatives has recently been proposed as a safe and effective protocol for sedation/anesthesia and analgesia in neurocritical human patients (e.g., traumatic brain injury) [155,156].

EEG activity increases following ketamine administration [157]. Seizure-like activity has been reported when ketamine was used in sedation/anesthetic protocols in dogs; however, it was not possible to rule out other causes for this abnormal activity [158,159]. Conversely, in cats, ketamine did not induce convulsant activity but had mild antiepileptic effects instead [157]. In fact, ketamine has been reported as a treatment for status epilepticus and cluster seizures in veterinary patients [160–162].

Inhalation anesthetics

Inhalation anesthetics generally result in dose-dependent decreases in CMR, however, the net effect on CBF is a balance between decreases caused by reduced CMR and increases due to direct cerebral vasodilation. This varies depending on the inhalant anesthetic used and the concentration delivered. Typically, with isoflurane, there is minimal effect on CBF if the inhalant concentration remains at or below the minimum alveolar concentration (MAC); at concentrations above 1 MAC, vasodilatory effects predominate and CBF may increase or remain unchanged despite CMR decreases [163–166]. Additionally, inhalation anesthetics cause a dose-dependent decrease in MAP and CPP in dogs, cats, and horses [166–169]. The CO_2 responsiveness of the cerebral circulation is preserved or enhanced with inhalant anesthetics [38,170]. The addition of nitrous oxide to other inhalant anesthetics produces an increase in CBF and ICP and either no change or an increase in $CMRO_2$ in animals [171–173].

The effect on ICP is variable depending on the inhalant anesthetic used. Enflurane above 1 MAC produced EEG and motor evidence of seizure activity [163]. In dogs, halothane and enflurane at approximately 1 MAC increased CBV and ICP for over 3 h [174]. On the other hand, isoflurane at approximately 1 MAC also increased CBV for over 3 h, but the increase in ICP was short-lived (approximately 20 min) [79]. Additionally, in an intracranial mass model in dogs, the CSF pressure-lowering effect of 4 h of hypocapnia was sustained with isoflurane but not with halothane or enflurane [175]. Desflurane resulted in greater increases in CSF pressure and CBF when compared to isoflurane during normocapnia [176,177]. In a study comparing isoflurane and sevoflurane at different MAC multiples (1, 1.5, and 2 MAC) in normocapnic healthy dogs, ICP did not change significantly at different MAC multiples and was similar between the inhalants; however, at higher concentrations (2 MAC), CPP was better maintained with sevoflurane compared to isoflurane [178]. Conversely, in rats with diffuse brain injury, sevoflurane anesthesia resulted in higher ICP and lower CPP values when compared to isoflurane [179]. Therefore, isoflurane or sevoflurane may be better inhalant choices for patients at risk of intracranial hypertension, but when ICP is persistently increased, inhalation anesthetics should be replaced by intravenous anesthetics [180]. Injectable anesthetics, such as propofol, preserve autoregulation better when compared to inhalants (including isoflurane, sevoflurane, and desflurane) [181,182]. Additionally, when isoflurane anesthesia was compared to propofol TIVA in dogs with intracranial disease, propofol anesthesia resulted in higher MAP (and potentially higher CPP), decreased requirements for dopamine, and better recovery quality [183].

Neuromuscular blocking agents

Nondepolarizing neuromuscular blocking agents generally have minimal direct effects on the CNS, although indirect effects may occur. Laudanosine, a metabolite of atracurium, may be epileptogenic and is likely linked to the EEG evidence of cerebral arousal noted in dogs following high dose of atracurium (1–2.5 mg/kg IV); however, this cerebral stimulation was not accompanied by increases in CBF, $CMRO_2$, and ICP [184]. Atracurium has the potential to stimulate histamine release and could, theoretically, decrease CPP due to decreased MAP or increased ICP; however, this has not been demonstrated in the literature [184,185]. Pancuronium, vecuronium, and atracurium administration to anesthetized animals resulted in no change in CBF, $CMRO_2$, ICP, and CPP [184,186,187]. Similarly, rocuronium and vecuronium were not associated with changes in ICP or CPP in human neurosurgical patients [188].

Depolarizing neuromuscular blocking agents, such as succinylcholine and suxamethonium, can increase ICP due to muscle fasciculations leading to increased CBF and CBV [187,189,190]; therefore, their use is contraindicated in patients at risk of intracranial hypertension.

Pathophysiology and anesthetic management of specific neurological conditions

Central nervous system conditions

Intracranial hypertension

Several neurological conditions including intracranial tumors, traumatic brain injury (TBI), meningoencephalitis, and hemorrhage can present with intracranial hypertension or high ICP [191–195], and restoration and maintenance of normal ICP and CPP are crucial to improving outcomes [194,196]. A comprehensive discussion of the prognostics, signs, and management of these patients is beyond the scope of this chapter; however, the reader can find recent publications on these subjects elsewhere [193,194,197–199]. Anesthesia for imaging and/or surgery is required for many of these patients. It is important to note any changes in a patient's neurological status before anesthesia that may be indicative of increased ICP including mentation (i.e., obtunded, stuporous, or comatose), brainstem reflexes (i.e., abnormal pupillary light reflex with or without other cranial nerve deficits), and gait abnormalities including opisthotonos postures [3]. In addition, it is important to note cardiopulmonary status in general (i.e., potential neurogenic pulmonary edema and cardiovascular instability/arrhythmias) and measure preanesthetic arterial blood pressure [197,200]. Often, but not always, patients with intracranial hypertension will present with systemic hypertension (i.e., Cushing reflex, discussed earlier), which is a compensatory mechanism to maintain CPP. Cerebral herniation may be detected on magnetic resonance imaging and may occur at one of several locations (foramen magnum, subfalcine, and rostral and caudal transtentorial) or via a skull defect (Fig. 39.2B) [201].

Guidelines for managing blood pressure in anesthetized patients with intracranial hypertension are scarce in the literature, especially in veterinary medicine. In human patients following acute CNS injury (i.e., TBI) or those with intracranial masses, it is recommended to maintain CPP and MAP at normal or high-normal levels because CBF may be low in certain regions of the brain and the autoregulatory response to hypotension may not be preserved in all areas [180]. Therefore, even MAP values in the range of 60–70 mmHg may predispose these patients to cerebral ischemia, and higher blood pressures may be required to ensure appropriate cerebral perfusion [202–204]. On the other hand, arterial hypertension could predispose the patient to increased ICP, potential cerebral edema, and in cases of intracranial procedures, hemorrhage in the perioperative period [205–207].

Hypercapnia causes an increase in CBF, CBV, and ICP [37,38, 91,168]. Therefore, controlled ventilation of patients with high ICP (to achieve low-normal $PaCO_2$ between 35 and 40 mmHg) is important and should be instituted immediately after induction of anesthesia and continued until extubation to prevent hypercapnia and further increases in ICP with potential decreased CPP during anesthesia. Controlled ventilation can be a useful tool to manage ICP in patients with intracranial hypertension. Hyperventilation (i.e., hypocapnia) can decrease CBF and ICP and help reduce acute brain swelling, as well as prevent herniation or reduce brain bulk to facilitate surgical access [153,180]. However, the use of hyperventilation remains controversial, especially in hypotensive patients and those with pathological brain conditions associated with inadequate perfusion and hypoxia (i.e., ischemic stroke, tumor, and TBI). Hyperventilation and hypocapnia can lead to increased cerebral vascular resistance which may result in shunting of blood from normal areas of the brain to affected areas (i.e., areas of vasomotor paralysis); this is known as "inverse intracerebral steal" (discussed earlier) and could potentially lead to ischemia of normal areas of the brain [51,54,57,208]. Additionally, hyperventilation cannot result in a sustained decrease in CBF as brain interstitial pH drops during prolonged hyperventilation (5–6 h) due to increasing lactate and decreasing bicarbonate levels, leading to a return of CBF to baseline [39–41]. Furthermore, periods of sustained hyperventilation may put the patient at risk of a significant increase in ICP upon restoration of normocapnia, and the increase in $PaCO_2$ should be allowed to happen very gradually [180].

Along with preventing hypercapnia and maintaining adequate blood pressure (i.e., avoiding both hypotension and hypertension), other important strategies in patients with elevated ICP include avoiding increases in CBF associated with inadequate oxygenation/hypoxia which may exacerbate intracranial hypertension (Fig. 39.6). Patients should be preoxygenated before induction of anesthesia and administered oxygen supplementation post-extubation as needed. In addition, mechanical increases in ICP should be avoided through careful handling, positioning, and perianesthetic management. This includes positioning the head above the heart, avoiding flexion or rotation of the neck, avoiding pressure on the neck (e.g., neck leads or jugular venous occlusion), avoiding excessive positive end-expiratory pressure during controlled ventilation, preventing vomiting (after premedication and during recovery from anesthesia), preventing coughing (during intubation, suctioning of airway, and extubation), and providing a smooth anesthetic recovery overall [14,17,42,111,197].

As discussed previously, most sedatives and injectable anesthetics will contribute to decreases in CBF and ICP. In general, premedication with a non-emetogenic opioid and benzodiazepine is considered the safest option. There is some controversy regarding the use of α_2-adrenergic receptor agonists in this patient population due to their cardiovascular effects (i.e., bradycardia, hypertension, and decreased cardiac output) [95,204,209]. However, dexmedetomidine seems to have neuroprotective effects [210,211] and appears to be safe in human neurocritical patients, including those with TBI [212–214]. In dogs, dexmedetomidine has also been administered during intracranial surgeries and resulted in similar outcomes compared to opioid-based protocols [215]; however, further investigation in veterinary patients with high ICP is warranted.

For induction of anesthesia, the use of propofol is considered safe in patients with high ICP; however, doses should be carefully titrated to avoid hypotension, minimize respiratory depression, and prevent prolonged recoveries, especially if propofol is used for TIVA in cats [216]. While etomidate provides excellent cardiovascular stability, it may cause cortisol suppression and potentially induce myoclonus, nausea, and vomiting [217], which are undesirable in this population of patients. Etomidate administration has also been shown to increase the risk of cerebral hypoxia in the setting of cerebral ischemia [218], so other options for induction of anesthesia are recommended in such patients. Information on cerebral dynamics following alfaxalone (with cyclodextrin) administration is scarce. In a study involving healthy dogs, alfaxalone TIVA resulted in similar CBF values to propofol TIVA and better-maintained CO_2 responsiveness to hypocapnia [126]. However, further investigation is required before alfaxalone can be recommended in veterinary patients with high ICP. The use of ketamine remains controversial, as described in the previous section. While not historically recommended for use in this patient population, recent studies in humans with neurological conditions causing high ICP (i.e., TBI) suggest ketamine may be appropriate when combined with other sedatives/anesthetics because of its positive cardiopulmonary effects, minimal effect on ICP, and positive effect on CPP [155,156,209]. While more studies in veterinary medicine involving neurocritical patients are warranted, subanesthetic doses of ketamine appear to be safe [131,147,209].

Avoiding or minimizing agents that increase ICP and decrease CPP (i.e., inhalation anesthetics) is advisable in patients with persistently increased ICP (i.e., patients with large intracranial tumors or signs of brain herniation and TBI patients with an expanding mass lesion), and the use of TIVA for maintenance of anesthesia is preferable. Administration of an IV lidocaine bolus (topical lidocaine in cats) or IV fentanyl bolus prior to endotracheal intubation to prevent coughing should be considered [112–115]. In addition, the use of IV lidocaine as an adjunct intraoperatively has been shown to prevent acute increases in ICP during craniotomy and has other beneficial effects in models of cerebral ischemia [109,117–119]. Even though some analgesics, such as opioids, can cause respiratory depression (hypercapnia) and an increase in ICP, it is important to recognize that pain itself can contribute to increases in CBF and potentially ICP, and analgesics such as opioids can attenuate this effect [219]. Therefore, analgesics should not be withheld in painful patients (i.e., TBI) and should be administered to those undergoing painful procedures such as craniotomies.

Patient monitoring is critical as hypoventilation and/or hypotension resulting from the use of sedatives, analgesics, or injectable and inhalation anesthetics could lead to further increases in ICP and decreases in CPP [82,90,98]. Overall, use of short-acting drugs and/or low, titrated doses in a balanced anesthetic technique is recommended because some of these patients, especially those undergoing long procedures such as craniotomies, may experience prolonged recoveries and the antagonism of sedative agents (i.e., α_2-adrenergic receptor agonists and benzodiazepines) may precipitate an increase in ICP and a decrease in CPP [69,105–107]. Even if seizures were not previously reported, it is important to monitor for signs of seizure activity; patients with TBI, intracranial neoplasia, or any intracranial disease process affecting the prosencephalon may develop seizure activity in the perianesthetic period.

Diligent monitoring of patients with suspected or confirmed intracranial hypertension during general anesthesia is essential, and should include body temperature, electrocardiography, capnography, pulse oximetry, and ideally invasive blood pressure and arterial blood gases ($PaCO_2$ and PaO_2). Intravenous fluid administration to maintain euvolemia is advisable but excessive fluid administration (leading to increased central venous pressure, decreased venous outflow, and potentially increased ICP and decreased CPP) and use of fluids that reduce serum osmolarity should be avoided due to the potential risk of cerebral edema [14,220]. In the case of intraoperative hemorrhage requiring administration of large fluid volumes (e.g., during a craniotomy), the combination of crystalloids with colloids or blood products may be appropriate [180].

Hyperosmolar therapy with mannitol or hypertonic saline is the primary tool for pharmacologic management of acute elevations in ICP (e.g., TBI, edema secondary to tumor, or intracerebral hemorrhage). These osmotic agents decrease brain tissue volume by removing free water from normal brain tissue [194,195]. Mannitol can have several undesirable side effects including diuresis and volume depletion, hypotension, electrolyte disturbances (transient decreases in sodium and chloride, and increases in potassium), and rebound cerebral edema. With repeated mannitol use, serum osmolality should be monitored and maintained at or below 320 mOsm/L, and its use should be avoided in patients with renal disease (due to potential risk of acute renal failure), congestive heart failure, and hypovolemia [194,195,221,222]. The ICP lowering dose of mannitol is 0.5 to 1 g/kg over 10–20 min and no more than three boluses should be administered in a 24-h period to minimize side effects [195,222]. As mannitol may crystallize at room temperature, crystalized preparations should be warmed to approximately 37 °C (99 °F) and administered using an in-line filter or by using filter needles [222].

Hypertonic saline is another hyperosmolar treatment option with several advantages over mannitol including increased MAP and CPP, enhanced microcirculation, and anti-inflammatory effects [194,197]. However, it can also be associated with undesirable side effects including electrolyte disturbances (sustained hypernatremia and hyperchloremia), rebound cerebral edema, and hyperchloremic metabolic acidosis [194,195,221]. It should be avoided in patients with congestive heart failure and renal failure [194,195]. The recommended dose of hypertonic saline is 4 mL/kg (7.2%) or 5.4 mL/kg (3%) over 15–20 min [195,204]. Comparison of these two hyperosmolar agents for treatment of intracranial hypertension in humans yielded mixed results regarding efficacy with no significant difference in clinical neurological outcome between treatments [223–226]. In summary, there is no consensus in the literature regarding which hyperosmolar agent is the best choice in this patient population, but hypertonic saline is usually recommended over mannitol in hypovolemic patients [195,197,222,227]. In any case, careful monitoring of volume status, electrolytes, and acid–base parameters should be performed when using hyperosmolar agents [197,221].

The use of steroids in patients with TBI has been associated with increased mortality and is not recommended in this population [197,228]. Steroids, however, can limit the formation of cerebral edema and attenuate ICP increases in patients with intracranial tumors and are indicated for this purpose, including in the perioperative period (i.e., during craniotomies) [229–231].

Seizures

Generalized seizure activity is associated with a marked increase in CBF and CMR, with systemic and cerebral acidosis and potential decreases in PaO_2 and increases in $PaCO_2$ and ICP [232–234]. While idiopathic epilepsy is the most common cause of seizures in dogs, other etiologies including structural epilepsy and reactive seizures are possible [235]. Structural epilepsy includes neoplasia, infectious and immune-mediated disease, TBI, congenital malformations, vascular lesions (strokes), and degenerative diseases. Reactive seizures include toxin ingestion, nutritional deficits, and metabolic derangements. A comprehensive review of etiopathogenesis, treatment, and prognosis of patients with seizures is beyond the scope of this chapter, but recent publications on these subjects are available elsewhere [199,235–238].

Anesthesia for diagnostic imaging and/or surgery may be required for patients with a history of seizures. While seizures can happen at any point in the perianesthetic period, they are uncommon during the maintenance phase of anesthesia [239,240]. It is important to know which antiepileptic drugs the patient is receiving before anesthesia and continue these medications in the perianesthetic period. Some older-generation antiepileptic drugs, such as phenytoin, phenobarbital, and primidone, have important drug interactions relevant to the anesthetist including the induction of cytochrome P450 enzymes, but that is not the case for the newer antiepileptic drugs, gabapentin and levetiracetam [240]. In addition to understanding potential drug interactions, it is also important to know the anticonvulsant properties of sedatives and anesthetics and take this into account when designing anesthetic protocols for these patients. Benzodiazepines, barbiturates, and propofol are safe drugs to use in patients with a history of seizures, and they can be used to treat status epilepticus [129,130,241]. As discussed earlier, acepromazine use remains controversial in patients with a seizure history, though it is generally considered to be safe. Many opioids are associated with reports of myoclonus and/or seizures, especially alfentanil [242–245]. Alfaxalone can produce myoclonus, but it has been shown to have anticonvulsant effects [246,247]. Etomidate should probably be avoided in patients with a history of seizures, especially in epileptic patients [142,241]. The use of ketamine is controversial, but in general, its use in patients with seizures appears to be safe, and it can be used to treat status epilepticus and cluster seizures [157,160–162]. Regarding inhalation anesthetics precipitating seizure activity, enflurane has been most commonly implicated [163]; however, seizure activity in humans has also been reported following anesthesia with sevoflurane [248,249]. Thus, isoflurane is probably the best choice of inhalation anesthetic in patients with a history of seizures and has been utilized in cases of refractory status epilepticus in humans [250].

A recent review did not find evidence to support a reduction in the risk of late seizures or mortality rate with the prophylactic use of anticonvulsants in humans following TBI [251]. There is no consensus on this matter in veterinary medicine, but if seizures happen, prompt treatment is required and can be accomplished with barbiturates, benzodiazepines, or other potent anticonvulsants such as levetiracetam [238,240]. It is also important to ensure adequate ventilation, oxygenation, and appropriate blood pressure to maintain CBF and CPP [180].

In cases where horses experience seizures in the anesthesia recovery period, as may occur following myelography, administration of benzodiazepines (0.1–0.2 mg/kg IV) and xylazine (0.1–0.2 mg/kg IV) has been suggested as treatment. If seizures are not controlled by these interventions, re-anesthetizing the animal has been recommended [153,252].

Spinal cord injury and spine surgery

Specific considerations pertaining to the different advanced imaging modalities are reviewed elsewhere and are largely centered around individual patient comorbidities. Myelography can be performed to confirm and localize the site of disk herniation [253]. In these cases, the administration of contrast into the subarachnoid space has been associated with potential seizures [102,254]. In general, the anesthetic/sedative drug choices do not seem to influence the likelihood of seizures post-myelography although a limited number of drugs were used in a clinical assessment of myelography complications [255]. Nonetheless, drugs that are associated with seizure activity should be avoided or used with caution. Large-breed dogs, cervical lesions, large total volumes of iohexol, and injection into the cerebellomedullary cistern were associated with higher risk of seizures following myelography [102,255]. The incidence of seizures was also increased with shorter anesthesia times and in dogs that did not have surgery after the myelogram, most likely because the length of time between injection of contrast and recovery from anesthesia was shorter [102]. Other complications during anesthesia include apnea (likely due to contrast reaching the brainstem), bradycardia, bradyarrhythmias, and asystole. Complications in the postanesthetic period include intensification of pre-existing neurologic signs, prolonged recovery, hyperthermia, and vomiting [255,256]; therefore, vigilant monitoring of these patients is warranted. Appropriate anesthetic depth to avoid patient movement during manipulation of the needle is essential to prevent further trauma to the spinal cord. In addition, hyperflexion of the neck for cerebellomedullary cistern puncture can result in kinking of the endotracheal tube and airway obstruction, so careful monitoring of ventilation is also important in these cases. After cervical myelography, the head should be kept elevated to minimize cranial flow of the contrast agent [257].

A discussion of the mechanisms of spinal injury, emergency care procedures, diagnosis, and management of acute spinal cord injury is beyond the scope of this chapter, but reviews of these topics in dogs and cats are available elsewhere [258,259]. Some important considerations for the anesthetist will be covered here.

In veterinary medicine, advanced imaging and/or surgery may be required for several disease processes including intervertebral disk herniation, fibrocartilaginous embolism, myelitis, spinal tumors, and spinal trauma (fractures and luxation). While the location of the lesion plays a role, general perianesthetic complications related to spinal surgery include moderate to severe hemorrhage from the vertebral sinus or vertebral artery and severe and/or persistent pain (i.e., neuropathic pain) [254,260–264]. Pneumothorax/hemothorax has been reported with surgeries in the thoracic region specifically and careful intraoperative monitoring is necessary to identify this complication and facilitate early intervention [260,261]. Complications specific to procedures involving a ventral cervical approach include profound bradycardia and hypotension which may be unresponsive to treatment (potentially due to the surgical approach causing traction of carotid arteries and vagal trunks), recurrent laryngeal nerve injury, aspiration pneumonia, airway obstruction due to endotracheal tube compression by surgical instruments, and hypoventilation leading to respiratory failure or apnea [254,263,265–270]. Some of these complications may even occur in anesthetized patients with cervical spinal lesions that are not undergoing surgery. It is important to closely monitor these patients throughout the anesthetic period and beyond recovery as many complications may develop or worsen in the postoperative period.

Respiratory depression ranging from hypoventilation to complete respiratory failure can occur in patients with cervical spinal injuries (either on presentation or after surgery) or ascending myelomalacia, necessitating mechanical ventilation [254,269–271]. Temporary tracheostomy may be considered for such patients as this will allow mechanical ventilation for prolonged periods with minimal sedation requirements [269]. The mechanisms of hypoventilation are not well understood and are likely multifactorial. It is possible that pathways (reticulospinal tracts) from the respiratory centers in the brainstem to neurons innervating the muscles of respiration (diaphragm, intercostal, and extrathoracic airway muscles) are disrupted by the spinal lesion, by surgery, or by progressive postoperative edema from surgical manipulation [263,269,270,272]. Furthermore, the phrenic nerve may be compromised by the pathology itself or by surgical trauma to its nerve roots leading to impaired diaphragmatic function [263,269]. The phrenic nerve in dogs arises from cervical spinal cord segments 5 through 7 (corresponding to cervical vertebral bodies 4 through 6) [3,273]; because projections from the reticulospinal tracts are bilateral, even unilateral lesions may result in bilateral clinical manifestations of autonomic motor dysfunction [273]. Patients with spinal cord lesions cranial to the origin of motor neurons responsible for innervating the muscles of respiration may be more likely to present with clinical respiratory difficulties. In fact, dogs with lesions between C2–C4 were more likely to need mechanical ventilation in a retrospective study [269]. In these cases, patients are unable to maintain alveolar ventilation due to respiratory muscle paralysis or paresis and hypoxemia develops secondary to hypoventilation [269,274]. Monitoring end-tidal carbon dioxide in the immediate postoperative period while the patient remains intubated is indicated to ensure normocapnia in patients with cervical lesions. Following extubation, arterial blood gas assessment should be performed to evaluate both $PaCO_2$ and PaO_2. Additionally, patients with cervical lesions may develop aspiration pneumonia. In such cases, the ability to ventilate may not be compromised but patients will present with abnormal gas exchange and hypoxemia due to lung pathology [269,274].

Patients with severe spinal cord injuries can also experience spinal shock, which occurs when both ascending and descending nerve fibers caudal to the site of injury are affected, resulting in flaccid paralysis of the limbs and loss of reflexes [275,276]. In addition, patients with cervical spinal cord injuries can experience impaired sympathetic outflow (at the level of the cranial thoracic spine) which disrupts the balance between sympathetic and parasympathetic activity and results in increased parasympathetic tone. This affects not only the respiratory system (resulting in cholinergic bronchoconstriction and related respiratory complications), but also the cardiovascular system leading to significant cardiovascular instability (bradycardia, bradyarrhythmias, hypotension, ventricular arrhythmias, and asystole) [263,270,277,278]. Therefore, in addition to complications associated with the surgical approach (traction of carotid arteries and vagal trunks), impaired sympathetic outflow constitutes another important cause of cardiovascular instability in patients with cervical spinal cord injuries and may contribute to morbidity and mortality [254,263,265,270].

Intraoperative management should be focused on addressing individual complications as described while providing optimal, multimodal analgesia. Careful attention should be paid to positioning the patient prior to placement of surgical drapes to avoid positional interference with monitoring equipment or the anesthetic breathing system or predisposing the patient to neuropathy or myopathy. Fluid therapy should be tailored to the patient with the goal of euvolemia; hemorrhage may be managed with fluid replacement as indicated. Hypotension in this patient population can predispose to impaired perfusion and ischemia of the spinal cord so blood pressure should be closely monitored, and hypotension aggressively treated if it occurs [180,254,259,279,280].

Patients with suspected vertebral fractures and/or luxation may need to be immobilized in lateral recumbency on a backboard before induction and intubation to minimize movement and further injury to the spinal cord [259,281]. Discussion with the neurosurgeon prior to immobilization and/or positioning and manipulation of the patient for these procedures is warranted. Additional considerations and complications are the same as those outlined above and are specific to the region of the spinal cord affected. Analgesia is an important component in management of any trauma patient and in those with painful spinal cord injuries.

Horses and cervical spondylomyelopathy

Cervical spondylomyelopathy, also known as "wobbler syndrome," is a spinal cord condition in horses involving compression of the spinal cord due to cervical vertebral malformation resulting in ataxia, dysmetria, paresis, and an abnormal gait [282,283]. Horses with this condition may undergo anesthesia for myelography (with radiography, computed tomography, or magnetic resonance imaging) and/or surgery [282,284–286]. Complications associated with cervical myelography in horses include arrhythmias and dramatic changes in blood pressure (decrease or increase) during the procedure, as well as worsening of ataxia, pneumonia, neck pain, muscle fasciculations, seizures, hyperesthesia, head shaking, obtundation or dull mentation, myopathies, prolonged recoveries, and catastrophic recoveries with fracture [252,284,287–289]. Injection of higher volumes of contrast agent and prolonged anesthesia time has been associated with increased risk of adverse neurological events in a multicenter retrospective study [287]. Reported postoperative complications of relevance to the anesthetist include vertebral fracture, implant failure or breakage, pain, spinal cord edema, postanesthetic upper respiratory tract obstruction (and pulmonary edema), and laryngeal hemiplegia; both latter complications required tracheostomy [282,290]. Patient positioning with overextension of the neck seems to be correlated to postanesthetic upper respiratory tract obstruction [282]. Supplies for an emergent tracheostomy procedure should be available near the recovery stall in addition to supplies to re-induce anesthesia in the event of a fracture.

Careful cardiorespiratory monitoring (electrocardiography, invasive arterial blood pressure, capnography, and arterial blood gases) and controlled ventilation during cervical myelography is recommended. Changes in the positioning of the patient during radiographs, such as elevation of the head and extension and flexion of the neck after contrast administration, may be required during the procedure [252,291]. These positional changes can result in inadvertent extubation or anesthesia circuit disconnection, potential airway obstruction (especially with flexion of the neck), tracheal injury due to endotracheal tube movement during manipulation of the neck, and exacerbation of spinal cord injury and neurological signs due to anesthetic-induced muscle relaxation combined with positional changes [252,289,292]. Careful positioning, avoiding overinflation of the endotracheal tube cuff (and potentially deflating the cuff before moving the head and neck), keeping the head elevated as long as possible, and diligent post-myelography patient monitoring are important considerations [252,284,287,292].

A variety of protocols have been reported in the literature for anesthesia of horses undergoing cervical myelography, but no systematic comparison has been performed evaluating the quality of induction and recovery as well as the incidence of complications. Preanesthetic evaluation should include assessment of the patient's degree of ataxia. Light premedication (i.e., low, titrated doses) with xylazine (0.2–0.5 mg/kg) with or without butorphanol (0.02 mg/kg) is typically recommended to avoid excessive ataxia or recumbency before anesthesia induction. However, higher doses of xylazine, other α_2-adrenergic receptor agonists, and acepromazine have also been reported as premedication before cervical myelography in horses [284,285]. Some horses may have to be anesthetized in their stalls and returned to the same location for recovery due to severe ataxia and/or recumbency, but if the horse can be safely moved to the induction area, this should be done before administration of any sedatives. The use of guaifenesin in combination with barbiturates (thiopental or thiamylal) or guaifenesin and/or ketamine and a benzodiazepine (midazolam or diazepam) has been reported or recommended by different authors for induction of anesthesia [153,252,282,285,292]. Anesthesia induction protocols involving propofol and ketamine have been shown to produce better recovery qualities when compared to ketamine and midazolam induction in healthy horses anesthetized for short periods (60 min) [293]; however, it is difficult to predict if this would be the case for horses with wobbler syndrome. Maintenance of anesthesia with inhalant agents (preferably isoflurane or sevoflurane) is most common; however, use of TIVA (i.e., a combination of guaifenesin, ketamine, and an α_2-adrenergic receptor agonist) for maintenance of anesthesia has also been reported [284,285].

During recovery, the use of ropes or other methods of assistance, padded recovery stalls, thick foam pads, and padded helmets have been recommended to limit potential injuries in these patients [252,284,285]. A sling recovery system could be considered in cases of severe ataxia or for horses that are recumbent prior to anesthesia [153,252]. Administration of non-steroidal anti-inflammatories or steroids has been recommended by different authors to minimize complications [153,252,288].

Peripheral nervous system conditions

Myasthenia gravis

Myasthenia gravis (MG) is an acquired autoimmune neuromuscular disease characterized by autoantibody-mediated destruction of postsynaptic nicotinic ACh receptors at the neuromuscular junction [294–296]. A congenital form of MG, characterized by structural or functional defects at the neuromuscular junction (without autoimmunity), is part of a larger clinically heterogeneous group of disorders known as "congenital myasthenic syndromes" and is now considered a separate entity [295,297]. Both diseases (autoimmune and congenital) result in focal or generalized clinical muscle weakness and fatigability [294,296]. The focus of this section will be anesthetic management of patients with the more common autoimmune version of the disease.

Hyperthyroid cats receiving methimazole can develop drug-induced autoimmune MG [298]. Some patients with MG (cats more frequently than dogs) have concurrent thymoma and may need anesthesia for surgical procedures and/or radiation therapy [296,297,299,300]. Treatment of MG patients can involve anticholinesterase agents (also known as acetylcholinesterase inhibitors) such as pyridostigmine to prolong the action of ACh at the neuromuscular junction, as well as steroids [294,296,299]. Some authors recommend continuation of the anticholinesterase agents until the day of surgery to avoid respiratory distress postoperatively; however, this is controversial [301,302]. A potential side effect of anticholinesterase therapy in MG patients is excessive accumulation of ACh at the neuromuscular junction resulting in weakness due to desensitization of the postsynaptic membrane, known as "cholinergic crisis" [294,296]. The ACh will also affect muscarinic receptors, potentially leading to bradycardia, bronchospasm, miosis, intestinal hyperperistalsis, and hypersalivation [302].

Aspiration pneumonia and respiratory failure are frequent causes of death in cats and dogs with MG [294]. Patients with acute fulminant MG, those with worsening skeletal muscle weakness due to surgical stress and anesthesia, or those with severe aspiration pneumonia may require intubation and mechanical ventilation in the perioperative period [296]. Anesthesia for the MG patient carries a high risk due to the presence of megaesophagus and potential regurgitation, the risk of upper airway obstruction and aspiration pneumonia (due to decreased laryngeal and pharyngeal muscle function and protective airway reflexes), respiratory failure (due to intercostal muscle and diaphragmatic weakness and/or aspiration pneumonia), and potential drug interactions. Some drugs can negatively affect neuromuscular transmission and should be avoided in patients with MG including aminoglycoside, quinolone, and macrolide antibiotics, β-adrenergic blockers, calcium channel blockers, phenothiazines, iodinated contrast agents, quinidine and procainamide, phenytoin, and magnesium salts [296,302,303].

Due to their compromised respiratory muscle strength and decreased respiratory reserve, anesthetic considerations for MG patients include selection of drugs associated with minimal respiratory depression, preoxygenation prior to induction of anesthesia, prevention of hypothermia which can enhance neuromuscular blockade, and provision of ventilatory monitoring and support during and potentially after anesthesia [301,302]. Elevating the patient's head during induction of anesthesia, rapid endotracheal intubation and inflation of the cuff to protect the airway, and suctioning the esophagus as soon as possible are recommended to reduce the risk of complications associated with regurgitation and aspiration. The use of metoclopramide or histamine type-2 receptor antagonists may be considered in these patients [301,302]. There is no consensus in the human or veterinary medical literature on the ideal anesthetic protocol for MG patients to decrease the incidence of complications or the need for ventilation in the postoperative period [301,302,304].

Benzodiazepines can contribute to muscle weakness and their use in MG patients is questionable [305]. Opioids provide excellent analgesia with potential sedation but should be used cautiously. Small doses of short-acting opioids with careful monitoring are recommended to reduce risks associated with respiratory depression [301,302]. The use of intravenous anesthetics to rapidly induce anesthesia and gain control of the airway (i.e., propofol, etomidate, alfaxalone, or ketamine) is recommended [301,302]. While inhalation anesthetics have potent neuromuscular blocking effects and cause significant respiratory depressants, they facilitate rapid adjustments in anesthetic depth and undergo rapid elimination, making them good options for maintenance of anesthesia [306,307]. Locoregional and systemic adjunctive techniques (i.e., ketamine constant rate infusion) can be considered to decrease inhalant and opioid requirements. In general, local anesthetics decrease the sensitivity of the postjunctional membrane to ACh, but ester local anesthetics should be avoided in patients receiving anticholinesterase agents because they are metabolized by plasma cholinesterases. Therefore, the use of low doses of amide local anesthetics are recommended in MG patients [301,302,305,308]. The use of anticholinergics is controversial. If an anticholinergic is required intraoperatively to treat bradycardia in an MG patient, atropine is recommended over glycopyrrolate because the latter produces greater nicotinic receptor blockade and is, therefore, more likely to affect neuromuscular transmission [309].

Neuromuscular blocking agents should generally be avoided in MG patients as they are resistant to the effects of depolarizing agents and potentially very sensitive to the effects of nondepolarizing agents, resulting in profound and prolonged blockade [301,308,310]. If neuromuscular blockade is required, it is important to use lower doses of a nondepolarizing agent and quantitative monitoring of neuromuscular function (i.e., train of four with acceleromyography) at the end of anesthesia to ensure that no residual blockade persists [311,312]. The use of reversal agents such as neostigmine to reverse nondepolarizing neuromuscular blockade in MG patients is controversial [301,302].

Patients with MG are at risk of serious complications in the perioperative period. Cholinergic crisis, as described above, is related to excessive accumulation of ACh (due to anticholinesterase agent therapy) causing desensitization of the postsynaptic membrane. Myasthenic crisis, caused by further reductions in ACh receptor function with acute aggravation of muscular weakness, can happen in the postoperative period due to surgery, anesthesia, pain, and stress [301,302]. Both cholinergic and myasthenic crises result in similar clinical signs (generalized muscle weakness and potential respiratory failure) and emergency intubation and ventilatory support may be required. The use of an anticholinesterase agent test (historically referred to as the "Tensilon test") may help differentiate between myasthenic and cholinergic crises because muscle strength will improve in the case of myasthenic crisis. In the case of a cholinergic crisis, the anticholinesterase agent test may lead to muscle fasciculations, miosis, and exacerbation of respiratory signs [301,302,308].

The patient's ability to maintain appropriate spontaneous ventilation with normal end-tidal carbon dioxide levels (and ideally $PaCO_2$) should be assessed before extubation. Suction should always be available in case of regurgitation. In the immediate postanesthetic period, once the patient is extubated, the anesthetist should continue monitoring oxygenation and ventilation while watching for signs of airway obstruction and assessing respiratory rate, breathing pattern, appropriate chest excursions, pulse oximetry, and ideally, arterial blood gases (PaO_2 and $PaCO_2$). Anticholinesterase agent therapy should be resumed as soon as possible [301,308]. Postoperative analgesia is critical, but caution is warranted to avoid respiratory depression and exacerbation of muscle weakness; therefore, use of balanced analgesic techniques with drugs such as non-steroidal anti-inflammatory agents (if the patient is not receiving steroids), and regional anesthesia/analgesia to minimize opioid use is important [305]. Other drugs with analgesic properties that should be used with caution in MG patients include tricyclic antidepressants, pregabalin, and gabapentin [305].

References

1 Jenkins TW. *Functional Mammalian Neuroanatomy*, 2nd edn. Philadelphia, PA: Lea and Febiger, 1978: 480.

2 Becker S, Selby LA. Canine hydrocephalus. *Compend Contin Educ Pract Vet* 1980; **11**(8): 647–652.

3 de Lahunta A, Glass E, Kent M. Cerebrospinal fluid and hydrocephalus. In: de Lahunta A, Glass E, Kent M, eds. *Veterinary Neuroanatomy and Clinical Neurology*, 4th edn. St. Louis, MO: Elsevier, 2014: 78–101.
4 Hall JE, Hall ME. Cerebral blood flow, cerebrospinal fluid, and brain metabolism. In: Hall JE, Hall ME, eds. *Guyton and Hall Textbook of Medical Physiology*, 14th edn. Philadelphia, PA: Elsevier, 2020: 777–786.
5 Jurk IR, Thibodeau MS, Whitney K, *et al.* Acute vision loss after general anesthesia in a cat. *Vet Ophthalmol* 2001; **4**(2): 155–158.
6 Stiles J, Weil AB, Packer RA, *et al.* Post-anesthetic cortical blindness in cats: twenty cases. *Vet J* 2012; **193**(2): 367–373.
7 Martin-Flores M, Scrivani PV, Loew E, *et al.* Maximal and submaximal mouth opening with mouth gags in cats: implications for maxillary artery blood flow. *Vet J* 2014; **200**(1): 60–64.
8 Barton-Lamb AL, Martin-Flores M, Scrivani PV, *et al.* Evaluation of maxillary arterial blood flow in anesthetized cats with the mouth closed and open. *Vet J* 2013; **196**(3): 325–331.
9 Marcus ML, Heistad DD, Ehrhardt JC, *et al.* Regulation of total and regional spinal cord blood flow. *Circ Res* 1977; **41**(1): 128–134.
10 Scott CM, Marlin DJ, Schroter RC. Quantification of the response of equine apocrine sweat glands to beta2-adrenergic stimulation. *Equine Vet J* 2001; **33**(6): 605–612.
11 Pohorecky L, Wurtman R. Adrenocortical control of epinephrine synthesis. *Pharmacol Rev* 1971; **23**(1): 1–35.
12 Glick D. The autonomic nervous system. In: Miller RD, Eriksson LI, Fleisher LA, *et al.*, eds. *Miller's Anesthesia*, 8th edn. Philadelphia, PA: Elsevier Saunders, 2015: 346–386.
13 Mokri B. The Monro–Kellie hypothesis: applications in CSF volume depletion. *Neurology* 2001; **56**(12): 1746–1748.
14 Wilson MH. 2.0: the dynamic vascular and venous pathophysiological components of intracranial pressure. *J Cereb Blood Flow Metab* 2016; **36**(8): 1338–1350.
15 Shapiro HM. Intracranial hypertension: therapeutic and anesthetic considerations. *Anesthesiology* 1975; **43**(4): 445–471.
16 Tameem A, Krovvidi H. Cerebral physiology. *Contin Educ Anaesth Crit Care Pain* 2013; **13**(4): 113–118.
17 Brosnan RJ, Esteller-Vico A, Steffey EP, *et al.* Effects of head-down positioning on regional central nervous system perfusion in isoflurane-anesthetized horses. *Am J Vet Res* 2008; **69**(6): 737–743.
18 Fodstad H, Kelly PJ, Buchfelder M. History of the Cushing reflex. *Neurosurgery* 2006; **59**(5): 1132–1137.
19 Cushing H. Some experimental and clinical observations concerning states of increased intracranial tension. The Miitter Lecture for 1901. *Am J Med Sci* 1902; **124**: 375–400.
20 Cushing H. Concerning a definite regulatory mechanism of the vaso-motor centre which controls blood pressure during cerebral compression. *Johns Hopkins Hosp Bull* 1901; **12**: 290–292.
21 Cushing H. The blood pressure reaction of acute cerebral compression illustrated by cases of intracranial hemorrhage: a sequel to the Miitter Lecture for 1901. *Am J Med Sci* 1903; **125**: 1017–1044.
22 Heymans C. The control of heart rate consequent to changes in the cephalic blood pressure and in the intracranial pressure. *Am J Physiol (Legacy Content)* 1928; **85**(3): 498–506.
23 Schmidt EA, Despas F, Pavy-Le Traon A, *et al.* Intracranial pressure is a determinant of sympathetic activity. *Front Physiol* 2018; **9**: 11.
24 Tsai YH, Lin JY, Huang YY, *et al.* Cushing response-based warning system for intensive care of brain-injured patients. *Clin Neurophysiol* 2018; **129**(12): 2602–2612.
25 Kalmar AF, Van Aken J, Caemaert J, *et al.* Value of Cushing reflex as warning sign for brain ischaemia during neuroendoscopy. *Br J Anaesth* 2005; **94**(6): 791–799.
26 Patel PM, Drummond JC, Lemkuil BP. Cerebral physiology and the effects of anesthetic drugs. In: Miller RD, Eriksson LI, Fleisher LA, *et al.*, eds. *Miller's Anesthesia*, 8th edn. Philadelphia, PA: Elsevier Saunders, 2015: 387–422.
27 Claassen JAHR, Thijssen DHJ, Panerai RB, *et al.* Regulation of cerebral blood flow in humans: physiology and clinical implications of autoregulation. *Physiol Rev* 2021; **101**(4): 1487–1559.
28 Papasilekas T, Themistoklis KM, Melanis K, *et al.* A brief review of brain's blood flow-metabolism coupling and pressure autoregulation. *J Neurol Surg A Cent Eur Neurosurg* 2021; **82**(3): 257–261.
29 Iadecola C. The neurovascular unit coming of age: a journey through neurovascular coupling in health and disease. *Neuron* 2017; **96**(1): 17–42.
30 Attwell D, Buchan AM, Charpak S, *et al.* Glial and neuronal control of brain blood flow. *Nature* 2010; **468**(7321): 232–243.
31 Willie CK, Tzeng YC, Fisher JA, *et al.* Integrative regulation of human brain blood flow. *J Physiol* 2014; **592**(5): 841–859.
32 Michenfelder JD, Milde JH. The relationship among canine brain temperature, metabolism, and function during hypothermia. *Anesthesiology* 1991; **75**(1): 130–136.
33 Michenfelder JD, Theye RA. Hypothermia: effect on canine brain and whole-body metabolism. *Anesthesiology* 1968; **29**(6): 1107–1112.
34 Busija DW, Leffler CW. Hypothermia reduces cerebral metabolic rate and cerebral blood flow in newborn pigs. *Am J Physiol Heart Circ Physiol* 1987; **253**(4): H869–H873.
35 Michenfelder JD, Milde JH, Katušić ZS. Postischemic canine cerebral blood flow is coupled to cerebral metabolic rate. *J Cereb Blood Flow Metab* 1991; **11**(4): 611–616.
36 Arrich J, Herkner H, Müllner D, *et al.* Targeted temperature management after cardiac arrest. A systematic review and meta-analysis of animal studies. *Resuscitation* 2021; **162**: 47–55.
37 Grubb RL, Raichle ME, Eichling JO, *et al.* The effects of changes in PaCO2 on cerebral blood volume, blood flow, and vascular mean transit time. *Stroke* 1974; **5**(5): 630–639.
38 McPherson RW, Brian JE Jr., Traystman RJ. Cerebrovascular responsiveness to carbon dioxide in dogs with 1.4% and 2.8% isoflurane. *Anesthesiology* 1989; **70**(5): 843–850.
39 Raichle ME, Posner JB, Plum F. Cerebral blood flow during and after hyperventilation. *Arch Neurol* 1970; **23**(5): 394–403.
40 Kontos HA, Raper AJ, Patterson JL. Analysis of vasoactivity of local pH, PCO_2 and bicarbonate on pial vessels. *Stroke* 1977; **8**(3): 358–360.
41 Albrecht RF, Miletich DJ, Ruttle M. Cerebral effects of extended hyperventilation in unanesthetized goats. *Stroke* 1987; **18**(3): 649–655.
42 Mardimae A, Balaban DY, Machina MA, *et al.* The interaction of carbon dioxide and hypoxia in the control of cerebral blood flow. *Pflüg Arch* 2012; **464**(4): 345–351.
43 Brown MM, Wade JP, Marshall J. Fundamental importance of arterial oxygen content in the regulation of cerebral blood flow in man. *Brain J Neurol* 1985; **108**: 81–93.
44 Jones MD, Traystman RJ, Simmons MA, *et al.* Effects of changes in arterial O_2 content on cerebral blood flow in the lamb. *Am J Physiol* 1981; **240**(2): H209–H215.
45 Crystal GJ, Czinn EA, Salem MR. The mechanism of increased blood flow in the brain and spinal cord during hemodilution. *Anesth Analg* 2014; **118**(3): 637–643.
46 Tomiyama Y, Brian JE, Todd MM. Plasma viscosity and cerebral blood flow. *Am J Physiol Heart Circ Physiol* 2000; **279**(4): H1949–H1954.
47 Lassen NA. Cerebral blood flow and oxygen consumption in man. *Physiol Rev* 1959; **39**(2): 183–238.
48 Drummond JC. Blood pressure and the brain: how low can you go? *Anesth Analg* 2019; **128**(4): 759–771.
49 Drummond JC. The lower limit of autoregulation: time to revise our thinking. *Anesthesiology* 1997; **86**(6): 1431–1433.
50 Harper AM, Glass HI. Effect of alterations in the arterial carbon dioxide tension on the blood flow through the cerebral cortex at normal and low arterial blood pressures. *J Neurol Neurosurg Psychiatry* 1965; **28**(5): 449–452.
51 Lassen NA, Christensen MS. Physiology of cerebral blood flow. *Br J Anaesth* 1976; **48**(8): 719–734.
52 Messick JM, Newberg LA, Nugent M, *et al.* Principles of neuroanesthesia for the nonneurosurgical patient with CNS pathophysiology. *Anesth Analg* 1985; **64**(2): 143–174.
53 Langfitt TW, Weinstein JD, Kassell NF. Cerebral vasomotor paralysis produced by intracranial hypertension. *Neurology* 1965; **15**: 622–641.
54 Sharma VK, Teoh HL, Paliwal PR, *et al.* Reversed Robin Hood syndrome in a patient with luxury perfusion after acute ischemic stroke. *Circulation* 2011; **123**(7): e243–e244.
55 Lassen NA. The luxury-perfusion syndrome and its possible relation to acute metabolic acidosis localised within the brain. *Lancet Lond Engl* 1966; **2**(7473): 1113–1115.
56 Lassen NA. The luxury perfusion syndrome. *Scand J Clin Lab Investig Suppl* 1968; **102**: X: A.
57 Smith AL, Wollman H. Cerebral blood flow and metabolism: effects of anesthetic drugs and techniques. *Anesthesiology* 1972; **36**(4): 378–400.
58 Griffiths IR. Spinal cord blood flow in dogs: the effect of blood pressure. *J Neurol Neurosurg Psychiatry* 1973; **36**(6): 914–920.
59 Trim CM. Postanesthetic hemorrhagic myelopathy or myelomalacia. *Vet Clin North Am Equine Pract* 1997; **13**(1): 73–77.
60 Brosnan RJ, Steffey EP, LeCouteur RA, *et al.* Effects of isoflurane anesthesia on cerebrovascular autoregulation in horses. *Am J Vet Res* 2011; **72**(1): 18–24.
61 Dohi S, Takeshima R, Naito H. Spinal cord blood flow during spinal anesthesia in dogs: the effects of tetracaine, epinephrine, acute blood loss, and hypercapnia. *Anesth Analg* 1987; **66**(7): 599–606.
62 Griffiths IR. Spinal cord blood flow in dogs: 2. The effect of the blood gases. *J Neurol Neurosurg Psychiatry* 1973; **36**(1): 42–49.
63 Kazama S, Masaki Y, Maruyama S, *et al.* Effect of altering cerebrospinal fluid pressure on spinal cord blood flow. *Ann Thorac Surg* 1994; **58**(1): 112–115.
64 Ong BY, MacIntyre C, Bose D, *et al.* Comparison of two methods of altering blood pressures for assessing neonatal cerebral blood flow autoregulation. *Can J Physiol Pharmacol* 1986; **64**(7): 1023–1026.

65 Pearce WJ, Bevan JA. Diltiazem and autoregulation of canine cerebral blood flow. *J Pharmacol Exp Ther* 1987; **242**(3): 812–817.

66 Tanaka M, Yoshida Y, Mitomi A, *et al.* Effects of calcium antagonists, felodipine and nicardipine, on cerebral circulation in dogs. *Jpn J Pharmacol* 1990; **52**(2): 273–279.

67 Johnston WE, DeWitt DS, Vinten-Johansen J, *et al.* Phenylephrine does not reduce cerebral perfusion during canine cardiopulmonary bypass. *Anesth Analg* 1994; **79**(1): 14–18.

68 Chikovani O, Corkill G, McLeish I, *et al.* Effect on canine cerebral blood flow of two common pressor agents during prolonged halothane anesthesia. *Surg Neurol* 1978; **9**(3): 211–213.

69 McCormick JM, McCormick PW, Zabramski JM, *et al.* Intracranial pressure reduction by a central α2-adrenoreceptor agonist after subarachnoid hemorrhage. *Neurosurgery* 1993; **32**(6): 974–979.

70 Artru AA, Shapira Y, Bowdle TA. Electroencephalogram, cerebral metabolic, and vascular responses to propofol anesthesia in dogs. *J Neurosurg Anesthesiol* 1992; **4**(2): 99–109.

71 Koyama K, Mito T, Takashima S, *et al.* Effects of phenylephrine and dopamine on cerebral blood flow, blood volume, and oxygenation in young rabbits. *Pediatr Neurol* 1990; **6**(2): 87–90.

72 Mutch WAC, Mato LA, Ringaert KRA. Phenylephrine increases regional cerebral blood flow following hemorrhage during isoflurane-oxygen anesthesia. *Anesthesiology* 1989; **70**(2): 276–279.

73 Patel PM, Mutch WA. The cerebral pressure-flow relationship during 1.0 MAC isoflurane anesthesia in the rabbit: the effect of different vasopressors. *Anesthesiology* 1990; **72**(1): 118–124.

74 Myburgh JA, Upton RN, Grant C, *et al.* A comparison of the effects of norepinephrine, epinephrine, and dopamine on cerebral blood flow and oxygen utilisation. *Acta Neurochir* 1998; **71**(Suppl): 19–21.

75 Artru AA, Nugent M, Michenfelder JD. Anesthetics affect the cerebral metabolic response to circulatory catecholamines. *J Neurochem* 1981; **36**(6): 1941–1946.

76 Bandres J, Yao L, Nemoto EM, *et al.* Effects of dobutamine and dopamine on whole brain blood flow and metabolism in unanesthetized monkeys. *J Neurosurg Anesthesiol* 1992; **4**(4): 250–256.

77 Tobata D, Takao K, Mochizuki M, *et al.* Effects of dopamine, dobutamine, amrinone and milrinone on regional blood flow in isoflurane anesthetized dogs. *J Vet Med Sci* 2004; **66**(9): 1097–1105.

78 Gibbs JM, Leenders KL, Wise RJ, *et al.* Evaluation of cerebral perfusion reserve in patients with carotid-artery occlusion. *Lancet* 1984; **1**(8370): 182–186.

79 Artru AA. Relationship between cerebral blood volume and CSF pressure during anesthesia with isoflurane or fentanyl in dogs. *Anesthesiology* 1984; **60**(6): 575–579.

80 Todd MM, Weeks J. Comparative effects of propofol, pentobarbital, and isoflurane on cerebral blood flow and blood volume. *J Neurosurg Anesthesiol* 1996; **8**(4): 296–303.

81 Todd MM, Weeks JB, Warner DS. The influence of intravascular volume expansion on cerebral blood flow and blood volume in normal rats. *Anesthesiology* 1993; **78**(5): 945–953.

82 Sheehan PB, Zornow MH, Scheller MS, *et al.* The effects of fentanyl and sufentanil on intracranial pressure and cerebral blood flow in rabbits with an acute cryogenic brain injury. *J Neurosurg Anesthesiol* 1992; **4**(4): 261–267.

83 Yaster M, Koehler RC, Traystman RJ. Interaction of fentanyl and nitrous oxide on peripheral and cerebral hemodynamics in newborn lambs. *Anesthesiology* 1994; **80**(2): 364–371.

84 Milde LN, Milde JH, Gallagher WJ. Cerebral effects of fentanyl in dogs. *Br J Anaesth* 1989; **63**(6): 710–715.

85 Hoffman WE, Cunningham F, James MK, *et al.* Effects of remifentanil, a new short-acting opioid, on cerebral blood flow, brain electrical activity, and intracranial pressure in dogs anesthetized with isoflurane and nitrous oxide. *Anesthesiology* 1993; **79**(1): 107–113.

86 Werner C, Hoffman WE, Baughman VL, *et al.* Effects of sufentanil on cerebral blood flow, cerebral blood flow velocity, and metabolism in dogs. *Anesth Analg* 1991; **72**(2): 177–181.

87 Baughman VL, Hoffman WE, Albrecht RF, *et al.* Cerebral vascular and metabolic effects of fentanyl and midazolam in young and aged rats. *Anesthesiology* 1987; **67**(3): 314–319.

88 Milde LN, Milde JH, Gallagher WJ. Effects of sufentanil on cerebral circulation and metabolism in dogs. *Anesth Analg* 1990; **70**(2): 138–146.

89 Wagner KJ, Willoch F, Kochs EF, *et al.* Dose-dependent regional cerebral blood flow changes during remifentanil infusion in humans: a positron emission tomography study. *Anesthesiology* 2001; **94**(5): 732–739.

90 Werner C, Kochs E, Bause H, *et al.* Effects of sufentanil on cerebral hemodynamics and intracranial pressure in patients with brain injury. *Anesthesiology* 1995; **83**(4): 721–726.

91 Moore RM, Trim CM. Effect of hypercapnia or xylazine on lateral ventricle and lumbosacral cerebrospinal fluid pressures in pentobarbital-anesthetized horses. *Vet Surg* 1993; **22**(2): 151–158.

92 Moore RM, Trim CM. Effect of xylazine on cerebrospinal fluid pressure in conscious horses. *Am J Vet Res* 1992; **53**(9): 1558–1561.

93 Reed RA, Epstein KL, Bramski JH, *et al.* The effect of xylazine on intracranial pressure in anesthetized and standing horses. *J Vet Emerg Crit Care* 2021; **31**(4): 476–482.

94 Brosnan RJ, LeCouteur RA, Steffey EP, *et al.* Direct measurement of intracranial pressure in adult horses. *Am J Vet Res* 2002; **63**(9): 1252–1256.

95 Zornow MH, Fleischer JE, Scheller MS, *et al.* Dexmedetomidine, an alpha 2-adrenergic agonist, decreases cerebral blood flow in the isoflurane-anesthetized dog. *Anesth Analg* 1990; **70**(6): 624–630.

96 Karlsson BR, Forsman M, Roald OK, *et al.* Effect of dexmedetomidine, a selective and potent alpha2-agonist, on cerebral blood flow and oxygen consumption during halothane anesthesia in dogs. *Anesth Analg* 1990; **71**(2): 125–129.

97 Prielipp RC, Wall MH, Tobin JR, *et al.* Dexmedetomidine-induced sedation in volunteers decreases regional and global cerebral blood flow. *Anesth Analg* 2002; **95**(4): 1052–1059.

98 Mikkelsen MLG, Ambrus R, Rasmussen R, *et al.* The effect of dexmedetomidine on cerebral perfusion and oxygenation in healthy piglets with normal and lowered blood pressure anaesthetized with propofol-remifentanil total intravenous anaesthesia. *Acta Vet Scand* 2017; **59**(1): 27.

99 Keegan RD, Greene SA, Bagley RS, *et al.* Effects of medetomidine administration on intracranial pressure and cardiovascular variables of isoflurane-anesthetized dogs. *Am J Vet Res* 1995; **56**(2): 193–198.

100 Tobias KM, Marioni-Henry K, Wagner R. A retrospective study on the use of acepromazine maleate in dogs with seizures. *J Am Anim Hosp Assoc* 2006; **42**(4): 283–289.

101 Drynan EA, Gray P, Raisis AL. Incidence of seizures associated with the use of acepromazine in dogs undergoing myelography. *J Vet Emerg Crit Care (San Antonio)* 2012; **22**(2): 262–266.

102 da Costa RC, Parent JM, Dobson H. Incidence of and risk factors for seizures after myelography performed with iohexol in dogs: 503 cases (2002–2004). *J Am Vet Med Assoc* 2011; **238**(10): 1296–1300.

103 Tudorica A, Fang Li H, Hospod F, *et al.* Cerebral blood volume measurements by rapid contrast infusion and T-weighted echo planar MRI. *Magn Reson Med* 2002; **47**(6): 1145–1457.

104 Nugent M, Artru AA, Michenfelder JD. Cerebral metabolic, vascular and protective effects of midazolam maleate: comparison to diazepam. *Anesthesiology* 1982; **56**(3): 172–176.

105 Artru AA. Flumazenil reversal of midazolam in dogs: dose-related changes in cerebral blood flow, metabolism, EEG, and CSF pressure. *J Neurosurg Anesthesiol* 1989; **1**(1): 46–55.

106 Fleischer JE, Milde JH, Moyer TP, *et al.* Cerebral effects of high-dose midazolam and subsequent reversal with RO 15-1788 in dogs. *Anesthesiology* 1988; **68**(2): 234–242.

107 Chiolero RL, Ravussin P, Anderes JP, *et al.* The effects of midazolam reversal by RO 15-1788 on cerebral perfusion pressure in patients with severe head injury. *Intensive Care Med* 1988; **14**(3): 196–200.

108 Sakabe T, Maekawa T, Ishikawa T, *et al.* The effects of lidocaine on canine cerebral metabolism and circulation related to the electroencephalogram. *Anesthesiology* 1974; **40**(5): 433–441.

109 Bedford RF, Persing JA, Pobereskin L, *et al.* Lidocaine or thiopental for rapid control of intracranial hypertension? *Anesth Analg* 1980; **59**(6): 435–437.

110 Donegan MF, Bedford RF. Intravenously administered lidocaine prevents intracranial hypertension during endotracheal suctioning. *Anesthesiology* 1980; **52**(6): 516–518.

111 Moss E, Powell D, Gibson RM, *et al.* Effects of tracheal intubation on intracranial pressure following induction of anaesthesia with thiopentone or althesin in patients undergoing neurosurgery. *Br J Anaesth* 1978; **50**(4): 353–360.

112 Panti A, Cafrita IC, Clark L. Effect of intravenous lidocaine on cough response to endotracheal intubation in propofol-anaesthetized dogs. *Vet Anaesth Analg* 2016; **43**(4): 405–411.

113 Bravo VR, Palomba N, Corletto F, *et al.* Comparison between intravenous lidocaine and fentanyl on cough reflex and sympathetic response during endotracheal intubation in dogs. *Vet Anaesth Analg* 2020; **47**(4): 481–489.

114 Thompson KR, Rioja E. Effects of intravenous and topical laryngeal lidocaine on heart rate, mean arterial pressure and cough response to endotracheal intubation in dogs. *Vet Anaesth Analg* 2016; **43**(4): 371–378.

115 Martín Bellido V, Martínez I Ferré B, McDonald H, *et al.* Effect of intravenous fentanyl on cough reflex and quality of endotracheal intubation in cats. *Vet Anaesth Analg* 2023; **50**(3): 230–237.

116 Samaha T, Ravussin P, Claquin C, *et al.* Prevention of increase of blood pressure and intracranial pressure during endotracheal intubation in neurosurgery: esmolol versus lidocaine. *Ann Fr Anesth Réanimation* 1996; **15**(1): 36–40.

117 Evans DE, Kobrine AI, LeGrys DC, *et al.* Protective effect of lidocaine in acute cerebral ischemia induced by air embolism. *J Neurosurg* 1984; **60**(2): 257–263.

118 Nagao S, Murota T, Momma F, *et al.* The effect of intravenous lidocaine on experimental brain edema and neural activities. *J Trauma* 1988; **28**(12): 1650–1655.

119 Shokunbi MT, Gelb AW, Wu XM, *et al.* Continuous lidocaine infusion and focal feline cerebral ischemia. *Stroke* 1990; **21**(1): 107–111.

120 Ilkiw JE. Advantages and guidelines for using ultrashort barbiturates for induction of anesthesia. *Vet Clin North Am Small Anim Pract* 1992; **22**(2): 261–264.

121 Shores A. Neuroanesthesia: a review of the effects of anesthetic agents on cerebral blood flow and intracranial pressure in the dog. *Vet Surg* 1985; **14**(3): 257–263.

122 Quandt JE, Robinson EP, Rivers WJ, *et al.* Cardiorespiratory and anesthetic effects of propofol and thiopental in dogs. *Am J Vet Res* 1998; **59**(9): 1137–1143.

123 Wooten TL, Lowrie CT. Comparison of cerebrospinal fluid pressure in propofol- and thiopental-anesthetized eucapnic dogs. *Vet Surg* 1993; **22**(2): 148–150.

124 Haberer JP, Audibert G, Saunier CG, *et al.* Effect of propofol and thiopentone on regional blood flow in brain and peripheral tissues during normoxia and hypoxia in the dog. *Clin Physiol* 1993; **13**(2): 197–207.

125 Werner C, Hoffman WE, Kochs E, *et al.* The effects of propofol on cerebral blood flow in correlation to cerebral blood flow velocity in dogs. *J Neurosurg Anesthesiol* 1992; **4**(1): 41–46.

126 Bini G, Bailey KM, Voyvodic JT, *et al.* Effects of alfaxalone, propofol and isoflurane on cerebral blood flow and cerebrovascular reactivity to carbon dioxide in dogs: a pilot study. *Vet J* 2023; **291**: 105939.

127 Wu M, Yin X, Chen M, *et al.* Effects of propofol on intracranial pressure and prognosis in patients with severe brain diseases undergoing endotracheal suctioning. *BMC Neurol* 2020; **20**(1): 394.

128 Cattai A, Rabozzi R, Natale V, *et al.* The incidence of spontaneous movements (myoclonus) in dogs undergoing total intravenous anaesthesia with propofol. *Vet Anaesth Analg* 2015; **42**(1): 93–98.

129 Steffen F, Grasmueck S. Propofol for treatment of refractory seizures in dogs and a cat with intracranial disorders. *J Small Anim Pract* 2000; **41**(11): 496–499.

130 Heldmann E, Holt DE, Brockman DJ, *et al.* Use of propofol to manage seizure activity after surgical treatment of portosystemic shunts. *J Small Anim Pract* 1999; **40**(12): 590–594.

131 Nimkoff L, Quinn C, Silver P, *et al.* The effects of intravenous anesthetics on intracranial pressure and cerebral perfusion pressure in two feline models of brain edema. *J Crit Care* 1997; **12**(3): 132–136.

132 Dearden NM, McDowall DG. Comparison of etomidate and althesin in the reduction of increased intracranial pressure after head injury. *Br J Anaesth* 1985; **57**(4): 361–368.

133 Sari A, Maekawa T, Tohjo M, *et al.* Effects of althesin on cerebral blood flow and oxygen consumption in man. *Br J Anaesth* 1976; **48**(6): 545–550.

134 Li CX, Kempf D, Howell L, *et al.* Effects of alfaxalone on cerebral blood flow and intrinsic neural activity of rhesus monkeys: a comparison study with ketamine. *Magn Reson Imaging* 2021; **75**: 134–140.

135 Milde LN, Milde JH, Michenfelder JD. Cerebral functional, metabolic, and hemodynamic effects of etomidate in dogs. *Anesthesiology* 1985; **63**(4): 371–377.

136 Renou AM, Vernhiet J, Macrez P, *et al.* Cerebral blood flow and metabolism during etomidate anaesthesia in man. *Br J Anaesth* 1978; **50**(10): 1047–1051.

137 Newberg LA, Milde JH, Michenfelder JD. The cerebral metabolic effects of isoflurane at and above concentrations that suppress cortical electrical activity. *Anesthesiology* 1983; **59**(1): 23–28.

138 Michenfelder JD. The interdependency of cerebral functional and metabolic effects following massive doses of thiopental in the dog. *Anesthesiology* 1974; **41**(3): 231–236.

139 Frizzell RT, Meyer YJ, Borchers DJ, *et al.* The effects of etomidate on cerebral metabolism and blood flow in a canine model for hypoperfusion. *J Neurosurg* 1991; **74**(2): 263–269.

140 Modica PA, Tempelhoff R. Intracranial pressure during induction of anaesthesia and tracheal intubation with etomidate-induced EEG burst suppression. *Can J Anaesth* 1992; **39**(3): 236–241.

141 Ghoneim MM, Yamada T. Etomidate: a clinical and electroencephalographic comparison with thiopental. *Anesth Analg* 1977; **56**(4): 479–485.

142 Ebrahim ZY, DeBoer GE, Luders H, *et al.* Effect of etomidate on the electroencephalogram of patients with epilepsy. *Anesth Analg* 1986; **65**(10): 1004–1006.

143 Dawson B, Michenfelder JD, Theye RA. Effects of ketamine on canine cerebral blood flow and metabolism: modification by prior administration of thiopental. *Anesth Analg* 1971; **50**(3): 443–447.

144 Långsjö JW, Maksimow A, Salmi E, *et al.* S-ketamine anesthesia increases cerebral blood flow in excess of the metabolic needs in humans. *Anesthesiology* 2005; **103**(2): 258–268.

145 Långsjö JW, Kaisti KK, Aalto S, *et al.* Effects of subanesthetic doses of ketamine on regional cerebral blood flow, oxygen consumption, and blood volume in humans. *Anesthesiology* 2003; **99**(3): 614–623.

146 Schwedler M, Miletich DJ, Albrecht RF. Cerebral blood flow and metabolism following ketamine administration. *Can Anaesth Soc J* 1982; **29**(3): 222–226.

147 Akeson J, Björkman S, Messeter K, *et al.* Cerebral pharmacodynamics of anaesthetic and subanaesthetic doses of ketamine in the normoventilated pig. *Acta Anaesthesiol Scand* 1993; **37**(2): 211–218.

148 Tranquilli WJ, Thurmon JC, Benson GJ. Organ blood flow and distribution of cardiac output in hypocapnic ketamine-anesthetized swine. *Am J Vet Res* 1983; **44**(8): 1578–1582.

149 Vlerick L, Peremans K, Dockx R, *et al.* The long-term effects of single and repeated subanaesthetic ketamine administration on regional cerebral blood flow in healthy dogs measured with 99mTc-HMPAO SPECT. *Psychiatry Res Neuroimaging* 2019; **285**: 18–24.

150 Waelbers T, Polis I, Vermeire S, *et al.* 5-HT$_{2A}$ Receptors in the feline brain: ^{123}I-5-I-R91150 kinetics and the influence of ketamine measured with micro-SPECT. *J Nucl Med* 2013; **54**(8): 1428–1433.

151 Waelbers T, Polis I, Vermeire S, *et al.* Effect of ketamine on the regional cerebral blood flow and binding index of the 5-HT2A receptor radioligand 123I-R91150 in the canine brain. *J Vet Behav* 2015; **10**(4): 332–337.

152 Akeson J, Björkman S, Messeter K, *et al.* Low-dose midazolam antagonizes cerebral metabolic stimulation by ketamine in the pig. *Acta Anaesthesiol Scand* 1993; **37**(6): 525–531.

153 Harvey RC, Greene SA, Thomas WB. Neurological disease. In: Tranquilli WJ, Thurmon JC, Grimm KA, eds. *Lumb & Jones' Veterinary Anesthesia and Analgesia*, 4th edn. Ames, IA: Blackwell Publishing, 2007: 903–914.

154 Cornelius BG, Webb E, Cornelius A, *et al.* Effect of sedative agent selection on morbidity, mortality and length of stay in patients with increase in intracranial pressure. *World J Emerg Med* 2018; **9**(4): 256–261.

155 Godoy DA, Badenes R, Pelosi P, *et al.* Ketamine in acute phase of severe traumatic brain injury "an old drug for new uses?" *Crit Care* 2021; **25**(1): 19.

156 Rueda Carrillo L, Garcia KA, Yalcin N, *et al.* Ketamine and its emergence in the field of neurology. *Cureus* 2022; **14**(7): e27389.

157 Celesia GG, Chen RC. Effects of ketamine on EEG activity in cats and monkeys. *Electroencephalogr Clin Neurophysiol* 1974; **37**(4): 354–353.

158 Adami C, Spadavecchia C, Casoni D. Seizure activity occurring in two dogs after S-ketamine-induction. *Schweiz Arch Tierheilkd* 2013; **155**(10): 569–572.

159 Lervik A, Haga HA, Becker M. Abnormal motor activity during anaesthesia in a dog: a case report. *Acta Vet Scand* 2010; **52**(1): 64.

160 Roynard P, Bilderback A, Dewey CW. Intravenous ketamine bolus(es) for the treatment of status epilepticus, refractory status epilepticus, and cluster seizures: a retrospective study of 15 dogs. *Front Vet Sci* 2021; **8**: 547279.

161 Sánchez Fernández I, Goodkin HP, Scott RC. Pathophysiology of convulsive status epilepticus. *Seizure* 2019; **68**: 16–21.

162 Coles L, Rosenthal ES, Bleck TP, *et al. Why ketamine. Epilepsy Behav EB* 2023; **141**: 109066.

163 Scheller MS, Nakakimura K, Fleischer JE, *et al.* Cerebral effects of sevoflurane in the dog: comparison with isoflurane and enflurane. *Br J Anaesth* 1990; **65**(3): 388–392.

164 Roald OK, Forsman M, Steen PA. The effects of prolonged isoflurane anaesthesia on cerebral blood flow and metabolism in the dog. *Acta Anaesthesiol Scand* 1989; **33**(3): 210–213.

165 Maekawa T, Tommasino C, Shapiro HM, *et al.* Local cerebral blood flow and glucose utilization during isoflurane anesthesia in the rat. *Anesthesiology* 1986; **65**(2): 144–151.

166 Todd MM, Drummond JC. A comparison of the cerebrovascular and metabolic effects of halothane and isoflurane in the cat. *Anesthesiology* 1984; **60**(4): 276–282.

167 Takahashi H, Murata K, Ikeda K. Sevoflurane does not increase intracranial pressure in hyperventilated dogs. *Br J Anaesth* 1993; **71**(4): 551–555.

168 Brosnan RJ, Steffey EP, LeCouteur RA, *et al.* Effects of ventilation and isoflurane end-tidal concentration on intracranial and cerebral perfusion pressures in horses. *Am J Vet Res* 2003; **64**(1): 21–25.

169 Hans P, Dethier JC, Godin D, *et al.* Compared effects of enflurane and of halothane on the intracranial pressure and the cerebral perfusion pressure in the dog. *Acta Anaesthesiol Belg* 1980; **31**(Suppl): 49–59.

170 Drummond JC, Todd MM. The response of the feline cerebral circulation to $PaCO_2$ during anesthesia with isoflurane and halothane and during sedation with nitrous oxide. *Anesthesiology* 1985; **62**(3): 268–273.

171 Kaieda R, Todd MM, Warner DS. The effects of anesthetics and $PaCO_2$ on the cerebrovascular, metabolic, and electroencephalographic responses to nitrous oxide in the rabbit. *Anesth Analg* 1989; **68**(2): 135–143.

172 Sakabe T, Kuramoto T, Inoue S, *et al.* Cerebral effects of nitrous oxide in the dog. *Anesthesiology* 1978; **48**(3): 195–200.

173 Tsai YC, Lin SS, Lee KC, *et al.* Cerebral effects of nitrous oxide during isoflurane-induced hypotension in the pig. *Br J Anaesth* 1994; **73**(5): 667–672.

174 Artru AA. Relationship between cerebral blood volume and CSF pressure during anesthesia with halothane or enflurane in dogs. *Anesthesiology* 1983; **58**(6): 533–539.

175 Artru AA. Reduction of cerebrospinal fluid pressure by hypocapnia: changes in cerebral blood volume, cerebrospinal fluid volume and brain tissue water and electrolytes. II. Effects of anesthetics. *J Cereb Blood Flow Metab* 1988; **8**(5): 750–756.

176 Artru AA, Powers K, Doepfner P. CSF, sagittal sinus, and jugular venous pressures during desflurane or isoflurane anesthesia in dogs. *J Neurosurg Anesthesiol* 1994; **6**(4): 239–248.

177 Holmström A, Akeson J. Cerebral blood flow at 0.5 and 1.0 minimal alveolar concentrations of desflurane or sevoflurane compared with isoflurane in normoventilated pigs. *J Neurosurg Anesthesiol* 2003; **15**(2): 90–97.

178 Chohan AS, Greene SA, Keegan RD, *et al.* Intracranial pressure and cardiopulmonary variables during isoflurane or sevoflurane anesthesia at various minimum alveolar concentration multiples in normocapnic dogs. *Am J Vet Res* 2013; **74**(3): 369–374.

179 Goren S, Kahveci N, Alkan T, *et al.* The effects of sevoflurane and isoflurane on intracranial pressure and cerebral perfusion pressure after diffuse brain injury in rats. *J Neurosurg Anesthesiol* 2001; **13**(2): 113–119.

180 Lemkuil BP, Drummond JC, Patel PM, *et al.* Anesthesia for neurologic surgery and neurointerventions. In: Gropper MA, Cohen NH, Eriksson LI, *et al.*, eds. *Miller's Anesthesia*, 9th edn. Philadelphia, PA: Elsevier Saunders, 2019: 1868–1910.

181 Strebel S, Lam AM, Matta B, *et al.* Dynamic and static cerebral autoregulation during isoflurane, desflurane, and propofol anesthesia. *Anesthesiology* 1995; **83**(1): 66–76.

182 McCulloch TJ, Visco E, Lam AM. Graded hypercapnia and cerebral autoregulation during sevoflurane or propofol anesthesia. *Anesthesiology* 2000; **93**(5): 1205–1209.

183 Caines D, Sinclair M, Valverde A, *et al.* Comparison of isoflurane and propofol for maintenance of anesthesia in dogs with intracranial disease undergoing magnetic resonance imaging. *Vet Anaesth Analg* 2014; **41**(5): 468–479.

184 Lanier WL, Milde JH, Michenfelder JD. The cerebral effects of pancuronium and atracurium in halothane-anesthetized dogs. *Anesthesiology* 1985; **63**(6): 589–597.

185 Tarkkanen L, Laitinen L, Johansson G. Effects of d-tubocurarine on intracranial pressure and thalamic electrical impedance. *Anesthesiology* 1974; **40**(3): 247–251.

186 Giffin JP, Hartung J, Cottrell JE, *et al.* Effect of vecuronium on intracranial pressure, mean arterial pressure and heart rate in cats. *Br J Anaesth* 1986; **58**(4): 441–443.

187 Ducey JP, Deppe SA, Foley KT. A Comparison of the effects of suxamethonium, atracurium and vecuronium on intracranial haemodynamics in swine. *Anaesth Intensive Care* 1989; **17**(4): 448–455.

188 Schramm WM, Strasser K, Bartunek A, *et al.* Effects of rocuronium and vecuronium on intracranial pressure, mean arterial pressure and heart rate in neurosurgical patients. *Br J Anaesth* 1996; **77**(5): 607–611.

189 Lanier WL, Milde JH, Michenfelder JD. Cerebral stimulation following succinylcholine in dogs. *Anesthesiology* 1986; **64**(5): 551–559.

190 Thiagarajah S, Sophie S, Lear E, *et al.* Effect of suxamethonium on the ICP of cats with and without thiopentone pretreatment. *Br J Anaesth* 1988; **60**(2): 157–160.

191 Cherubini GB, Mantis P, Martinez TA, *et al.* Utility of magnetic resonance imaging for distinguishing neoplastic from non-neoplastic brain lesions in dogs and cats. *Vet Radiol Ultrasound* 2005; **46**(5): 384–387.

192 Palmer AC, Malinowski W, Barnett KC. Clinical signs including papilloedema associated with brain tumours in twenty-one dogs. *J Small Anim Pract* 1974; **15**(6): 359–386.

193 Cameron S, Weltman JG, Fletcher DJ. The prognostic value of admission point-of-care testing and modified Glasgow Coma Scale score in dogs and cats with traumatic brain injuries (2007–2010): 212 cases. *J Vet Emerg Crit Care (San Antonio)* 2022; **32**(1): 75–82.

194 Schizodimos T, Soulountsi V, Iasonidou C, *et al.* An overview of management of intracranial hypertension in the intensive care unit. *J Anesth* 2020; **34**(5): 741–757.

195 DiFazio J, Fletcher DJ. Updates in the management of the small animal patient with neurologic trauma. *Vet Clin North Am Small Anim Pract* 2013; **43**(4): 915–940.

196 Seki S, Teshima K, Ito D, *et al.* Impact of intracranial hypertension on the short-term prognosis in dogs undergoing brain tumor surgery. *J Vet Med Sci* 2019; **81**(8): 1205–1210.

197 Kuo KW, Bacek LM, Taylor AR. Head trauma. *Vet Clin North Am Small Anim Pract* 2018; **48**(1): 111–128.

198 Evans EK, Fernandez AL. Current trends in the management of canine traumatic brain injury: an internet-based survey. *Can Vet J* 2019; **60**(1): 73–79.

199 Nout-Lomas YS. Traumatic nervous system injury. *Vet Clin North Am Equine Pract* 2022; **38**(2): 363–377.

200 Chen HI. Hemodynamic mechanisms of neurogenic pulmonary edema. *Biol Signals* 1995; **4**(3): 186–192.

201 Bagley RS. Pathophysiologic sequelae of intracranial disease. *Vet Clin North Am Small Anim Pract* 1996; **26**(4): 711–733.

202 El-Beheiry H. Protecting the brain during neurosurgical procedures: strategies that can work. *Curr Opin Anaesthesiol* 2012; **25**(5): 548–555.

203 Jellish WS. Anesthetic issues and perioperative blood pressure management in patients who have cerebrovascular diseases undergoing surgical procedures. *Neurol Clin* 2006; **24**(4): 647–659.

204 Armitage-Chan EA, Wetmore LA, Chan DL. Anesthetic management of the head trauma patient. *J Vet Emerg Crit Care* 2007; **17**(1): 5–14.

205 Kalfas IH, Little JR. Postoperative hemorrhage: a survey of 4992 intracranial procedures. *Neurosurgery* 1988; **23**(3): 343–347.

206 Hatashita S, Hoff JT, Ishii S. Focal brain edema associated with acute arterial hypertension. *J Neurosurg* 1986; **64**(4): 643–649.

207 Mayhan WG. Disruption of blood–brain barrier during acute hypertension in adult and aged rats. *Am J Physiol* 1990; **258**: H1735–H1738.

208 Harp JR, Wollman H. Cerebral metabolic effects of hyperventilation and deliberate hypotension. *Br J Anaesth* 1973; **45**(3): 256–262.

209 Flower O, Hellings S. Sedation in traumatic brain injury. *Emerg Med Int* 2012; **2012**: 637171.

210 Maier C, Steinberg GK, Sun GH, *et al.* Neuroprotection by the alpha 2-adrenoreceptor agonist dexmedetomidine in a focal model of cerebral ischemia. *Anesthesiology* 1993; **79**(2): 306–312.

211 Cosar M, Eser O, Fidan H, *et al.* The neuroprotective effect of dexmedetomidine in the hippocampus of rabbits after subarachnoid hemorrhage. *Surg Neurol* 2009; **71**(1): 54–59.

212 Tsaousi GG, Lamperti M, Bilotta F. Role of dexmedetomidine for sedation in neurocritical care patients: a qualitative systematic review and meta-analysis of current evidence. *Clin Neuropharmacol* 2016; **39**(3): 144–151.

213 Hatfield J, Soto AL, Kelly-Hedrick M, *et al.* Safety, efficacy, and clinical outcomes of dexmedetomidine for sedation in traumatic brain injury: a scoping review. *J Neurosurg Anesthesiol* 2023; 10.1097/ANA.0000000000000907.

214 Aryan HE, Box KW, Ibrahim D, *et al.* Safety and efficacy of dexmedetomidine in neurosurgical patients. *Brain Inj* 2006; **20**(8): 791–798.

215 Marquez-Grados F, Vettorato E, Corletto F. Sevoflurane with opioid or dexmedetomidine infusions in dogs undergoing intracranial surgery: a retrospective observational study. *J Vet Sci* 2020; **21**(1): e8.

216 Pascoe PJ, Ilkiw JE, Frischmeyer KJ. The effect of the duration of propofol administration on recovery from anesthesia in cats. *Vet Anaesth Analg* 2006; **33**(1): 2–7.

217 Forman SA. Clinical and molecular pharmacology of etomidate. *Anesthesiology* 2011; **114**(3): 695–707.

218 Edelman GJ, Hoffman WE, Charbel FT. Cerebral hypoxia after etomidate administration and temporary cerebral artery occlusion. *Anesth Analg* 1997; **85**(4): 821–825.

219 Lorenz IH, Kolbitsch C, Hinteregger M, *et al.* Remifentanil and nitrous oxide reduce changes in cerebral blood flow velocity in the middle cerebral artery caused by pain. *Br J Anaesth* 2003; **90**(3): 296–299.

220 Tommasino C, Moore S, Todd MM. Cerebral effects of isovolemic hemodilution with crystalloid or colloid solutions. *Crit Care Med* 1988; **16**(9): 862–868.

221 Hoehne SN, Yozova ID, Vidondo B, *et al.* Comparison of the effects of 7.2% hypertonic saline and 20% mannitol on electrolyte and acid–base variables in dogs with suspected intracranial hypertension. *J Vet Intern Med* 2021; **35**(1): 341–351.

222 Dewey CW. Emergency management of the head trauma patient. Principles and practice. *Vet Clin North Am Small Anim Pract* 2000; **30**(1): 207–225.

223 Kamel H, Navi BB, Nakagawa K, *et al.* Hypertonic saline versus mannitol for the treatment of elevated intracranial pressure: a meta-analysis of randomized clinical trials. *Crit Care Med* 2011; **39**(3): 554–559.

224 Wakai A, McCabe A, Roberts I, *et al.* Mannitol for acute traumatic brain injury. *Cochrane Database Syst Rev* 2013; **2013**(8): CD001049.

225 Mortazavi MM, Romeo AK, Deep A, *et al.* Hypertonic saline for treating raised intracranial pressure: literature review with meta-analysis. *J Neurosurg* 2012; **116**(1): 210–221.

226 Chen H, Song Z, Dennis JA. Hypertonic saline versus other intracranial pressure-lowering agents for people with acute traumatic brain injury. *Cochrane Database Syst Rev* 2020; **1**(1): CD010904.

227 Carney N, Totten AM, O'Reilly C, *et al.* *Guidelines for the management of severe traumatic brain injury*, fourth edition. *Neurosurgery* 2017; **80**(1): 6–15.

228 Edwards P, Arango M, Balica L, *et al.* Final results of MRC CRASH, a randomised placebo-controlled trial of intravenous corticosteroid in adults with head injury-outcomes at 6 months. *Lancet* 2005; **365**(9475): 1957–1959.

229 Hu H, Barker A, Harcourt-Brown T, *et al.* Systematic review of brain tumor treatment in dogs. *J Vet Intern Med* 2015; **29**(6): 1456–1463.

230 Bebawy JF. Perioperative steroids for peritumoral intracranial edema: a review of mechanisms, efficacy, and side effects. *J Neurosurg Anesthesiol* 2012; **24**(3): 173–177.

231 Ryken TC, Kuo JS, Prabhu RS, *et al.* Congress of Neurological Surgeons systematic review and evidence-based guidelines on the role of steroids in the treatment of adults with metastatic brain tumors. *Neurosurgery* 2019; **84**(3): E189–E191.

232 Plum F, Posner JB, Troy B. Cerebral metabolic and circulatory responses to induced convulsions in animals. *Arch Neurol* 1968; **18**(1): 1–13.

233 Bolwig TG, Quistorff B. In vivo concentration of lactate in the brain of conscious rats before and during seizures: a new ultra-rapid technique for the freeze-sampling of brain tissue. *J Neurochem* 1973; **21**(5): 1345–1348.

234 Perlman JM, Volpe JJ. Seizures in the preterm infant: effects on cerebral blood flow velocity, intracranial pressure, and arterial blood pressure. *J Pediatr* 1983; **102**(2): 288–293.

235 Berendt M, Farquhar RG, Mandigers PJ, *et al.* International veterinary epilepsy task force consensus report on epilepsy definition, classification and terminology in companion animals. *BMC Vet Res* 2015; **11**: 182.

236 Blades Golubovic S, Rossmeisl JH. Status epilepticus in dogs and cats, part 1: etiopathogenesis, epidemiology, and diagnosis. *J Vet Emerg Crit Care (San Antonio)* 2017; **27**(3): 278–287.

237 Blades Golubovic S, Rossmeisl JH. Status epilepticus in dogs and cats, part 2: treatment, monitoring, and prognosis. *J Vet Emerg Crit Care (San Antonio)* 2017; **27**(3): 288–300.

238 Podell M, Volk HA, Berendt M, *et al.* 2015 ACVIM Small animal consensus statement on seizure management in dogs. *J Vet Intern Med* 2016; **30**(2): 477–490.

239 Hymes JA. Seizure activity during isoflurane anesthesia. *Anesth Analg* 1985; **64**(3): 367–368.

240 Perks A, Cheema S, Mohanraj R. Anaesthesia and epilepsy. *Br J Anaesth* 2012; **108**(4): 562–571.

241 Reddy RV, Moorthy SS, Dierdorf SF, *et al.* Excitatory effects and electroencephalographic correlation of etomidate, thiopental, methohexital, and propofol. *Anesth Analg* 1993; **77**(5): 1008–1011.

242 Tortella FC. Endogenous opioid peptides and epilepsy: quieting the seizing brain? *Trends Pharmacol Sci* 1988; **9**(10): 366–372.

243 Saboory E, Derchansky M, Ismaili M, *et al.* Mechanisms of morphine enhancement of spontaneous seizure activity. *Anesth Analg* 2007; **105**(6): 1729–1735.

244 McGuire G, El-Beheiry H, Manninen P, *et al.* Activation of electrocorticographic activity with remifentanil and alfentanil during neurosurgical excision of epileptogenic focus. *Br J Anaesth* 2003; **91**(5): 651–655.

245 Shih CJ, Doufas AG, Chang HC, *et al.* Recurrent seizure activity after epidural morphine in a post-partum woman. *Can J Anaesth* 2005; **52**(7): 727–729.

246 Miziak B, Chrościńska-Krawczyk M, Czuczwar SJ. *Neurosteroids and seizure activity. Front Endocrinol (Lausanne)* 2020; **11**: 541802.

247 Hansen SL, Sperling BB, Sánchez C. Anticonvulsant and antiepileptogenic effects of GABAA receptor ligands in pentylenetetrazole-kindled mice. *Prog Neuropsychopharmacol Biol Psychiatry* 2004; **28**(1): 105–113.

248 Constant I, Seeman R, Murat I. Sevoflurane and epileptiform EEG changes. *Paediatr Anaesth* 2005; **15**(4): 266–274.

249 Mohanram A, Kumar V, Iqbal Z, *et al.* Repetitive generalized seizure-like activity during emergence from sevoflurane anesthesia. *Can J Anaesth* 2007; **54**(8): 657–661.

250 Zeiler FA, Zeiler KJ, Teitelbaum J, *et al.* Modern inhalational anesthetics for refractory status epilepticus. *Can J Neurol Sci* 2015; **42**(2): 106–115.

251 Thompson K, Pohlmann-Eden B, Campbell LA, *et al.* Pharmacological treatments for preventing epilepsy following traumatic head injury. *Cochrane Database Syst Rev* 2015; **2015**(8): CD009900.

252 Hodgson DS, Dunlop CI. General anesthesia for horses with specific problems. *Vet Clin North Am Equine Pract* 1990; **6**(3): 625–650.

253 Israel SK, Levine JM, Kerwin SC, *et al.* The relative sensitivity of computed tomography and myelography for identification of thoracolumbar intervertebral disk herniations in dogs. *Vet Radiol Ultrasound* 2009; **50**(3): 247–252.

254 Rossmeisl JH, White C, Pancotto TE, *et al.* Acute adverse events associated with ventral slot decompression in 546 dogs with cervical intervertebral disc disease. *Vet Surg* 2013; **42**(7): 795–806.

255 Lewis DD, Hosgood G. Complications associated with the use of iohexol for myelography of the cervical vertebral column in dogs: 66 cases (1988–1990). *J Am Vet Med Assoc* 1992; **200**(9): 1381–1384.

256 Carroll GL, Keene BW, Forrest LJ. Asystole associated with iohexol myelography in a dog. *Vet Radiol Ultrasound* 1997; **38**(4): 284–287.

257 Widmer WR, Blevins W. Veterinary myelography: a review of contrast media, adverse effects, and technique. *J Am Anim Hosp Assoc* 1991; **27**(2): 163–177.

258 Olby NJ, Moore SA, Brisson B, *et al.* ACVIM consensus statement on diagnosis and management of acute canine thoracolumbar intervertebral disc extrusion. *J Vet Intern Med* 2022; **36**(5): 1570–1596.

259 Park EH, White GA, Tieber LM. Mechanisms of injury and emergency care of acute spinal cord injury in dogs and cats. *J Vet Emerg Crit Care (San Antonio)* 2012; **22**(2): 160–178.

260 Brisson BA, Moffatt SL, Swayne SL, *et al.* Recurrence of thoracolumbar intervertebral disk extrusion in chondrodystrophic dogs after surgical decompression with or without prophylactic fenestration: 265 cases (1995–1999). *J Am Vet Med Assoc* 2004; **224**(11): 1808–1814.

261 Bartels KE, Creed JE, Yturraspe DJ. Complications associated with the dorsolateral muscle-separating approach for thoracolumbar disk fenestration in the dog. *J Am Vet Med Assoc* 1983; **183**(10): 1081–1083.

262 Brisson BA, Holmberg DL, Parent J, *et al.* Comparison of the effect of single-site and multiple-site disk fenestration on the rate of recurrence of thoracolumbar intervertebral disk herniation in dogs. *J Am Vet Med Assoc* 2011; **238**(12): 1593–1600.

263 Clark D. An analysis of intraoperative and early postoperative mortality associated with cervical spinal decompressive surgery in the dog. *J Am Anim Hosp Assoc* 1986; **22**(6): 739–744.

264 Zidan N, Medland J, Olby N. Long-term postoperative pain evaluation in dogs with thoracolumbar intervertebral disk herniation after hemilaminectomy. *J Vet Intern Med* 2020; **34**(4): 1547–1555.

265 Stauffer JL, Gleed RD, Short CE, *et al.* Cardiac dysrhythmias during anesthesia for cervical decompression in the dog. *Am J Vet Res* 1988; **49**(7): 1143–1146.

266 Lemarié RJ, Kerwin SC, Partington BP, *et al.* Vertebral subluxation following ventral cervical decompression in the dog. *J Am Anim Hosp Assoc* 2000; **36**(4): 348–358.

267 Pasternak JJ, Lanier WL. Neuroanesthesiology update 2010. *J Neurosurg Anesthesiol* 2011; **23**(2): 67–99.

268 Java MA, Drobatz KJ, Gilley RS, *et al.* Incidence of and risk factors for postoperative pneumonia in dogs anesthetized for diagnosis or treatment of intervertebral disk disease. *J Am Vet Med Assoc* 2009; **235**(3): 281–287.

269 Beal MW, Paglia DT, Griffin GM, *et al.* Ventilatory failure, ventilator management, and outcome in dogs with cervical spinal disorders: 14 cases (1991–1999). *J Am Vet Med Assoc* 2001; **218**(10): 1598–1602.

270 Kube S, Owen T, Hanson S. Severe respiratory compromise secondary to cervical disk herniation in two dogs. *J Am Anim Hosp Assoc* 2003; **39**(6): 513–517.

271 Okada M, Kitagawa M, Ito D, *et al.* Magnetic resonance imaging features and clinical signs associated with presumptive and confirmed progressive myelomalacia in dogs: 12 cases (1997–2008). *J Am Vet Med Assoc* 2010; **237**(10): 1160–1165.

272 Krieger AJ. Respiratory failure after ventral spinal surgery: a clinical and experimental study. *J Surg Res* 1973; **14**(6): 512–517.

273 King A. Autonomic components of the central nervous system. In: King A, ed. *Physiological and Clinical Anatomy of the Domestic Mammals*. Oxford, UK: Oxford University Press, 1987: 189–192.

274 Ramsey J, DeBlieux P. Respiratory failure. In: Ali J, Summer W, Levitzky M, eds. *Pulmonary Pathophysiology – a Clinical Approach*, 3rd edn. New York, NY: McGraw-Hill Medical, 2010: 227–247.

275 Atkinson PP, Atkinson JL. Spinal shock. *Mayo Clin Proc* 1996; **71**(4): 384–389.

276 Ditunno JF, Little JW, Tessler A, *et al.* Spinal shock revisited: a four-phase model. *Spinal Cord* 2004; **42**(7): 383–395.

277 Spungen AM, Dicpinigaitis PV, Almenoff PL, *et al.* Pulmonary obstruction in individuals with cervical spinal cord lesions unmasked by bronchodilator administration. *Paraplegia* 1993; **31**(6): 404–407.

278 Dicpinigaitis PV, Spungen AM, Bauman WA, *et al.* Bronchial hyperresponsiveness after cervical spinal cord injury. *Chest* 1994; **105**(4): 1073–1076.

279 Griffiths IR, Trench JG, Crawford RA. Spinal cord blood flow and conduction during experimental cord compression in normotensive and hypotensive dogs. *J Neurosurg* 1979; **50**(3): 353–360.

280 Olby N. The pathogenesis and treatment of acute spinal cord injuries in dogs. *Vet Clin North Am Small Anim Pract* 2010; **40**(5): 791–807.

281 Hawthorne JC, Blevins WE, Wallace LJ, *et al.* Cervical vertebral fractures in 56 dogs: a retrospective study. *J Am Anim Hosp Assoc* 1999; **35**(2): 135–146.

282 Pezzanite LM, Easley JT, Bayless R, *et al.* Outcomes after cervical vertebral interbody fusion using an interbody fusion device and polyaxial pedicle screw and rod construct in 10 horses (2015–2019). *Equine Vet J* 2022; **54**(2): 347–358.

283 Mannaa M, Shamaa AA, Shawky A, *et al.* A novel surgical technique for treatment of cervical vertebral stenotic myelopathy (wobbler syndrome) in a filly. *J Equine Vet Sci* 2023; **126**: 104493.

284 Gough SL, Anderson JDC, Dixon JJ. Computed tomographic cervical myelography in horses: technique and findings in 51 clinical cases. *J Vet Intern Med* 2020; **34**(5): 2142–2151.

285 Kondo T, Sato F, Tsuzuki N, *et al.* Characteristic computed tomographic myelography findings in 23 Thoroughbred horses. *J Vet Med Sci* 2022; **84**(4): 525–532.

286 Garrett KS. Special diagnostic techniques in equine neurology (radiography, ultrasonography, computed tomography, and magnetic resonance imaging). *Vet Clin North Am Equine Pract* 2022; **38**(2): 171–188.

287 Mullen KR, Furness MC, Johnson AL, *et al.* Adverse reactions in horses that underwent general anesthesia and cervical myelography. *J Vet Intern Med* 2015; **29**(3): 954–960.

288 Nelson BB, Goodrich LR, Barrett MF, *et al.* Use of contrast media in computed tomography and magnetic resonance imaging in horses: techniques, adverse events and opportunities. *Equine Vet J* 2017; **49**(4): 410–424.

289 Hubbell JA, Reed SM, Myer CW, *et al.* Sequelae of myelography in the horse. *Equine Vet J* 1988; **20**(6): 438–440.
290 Moore BR, Reed SM, Robertson JT. Surgical treatment of cervical stenotic myelopathy in horses: 73 cases (1983–1992). *J Am Vet Med Assoc* 1993; **203**(1): 108–112.
291 Rantanen N, Gavin P, Barbee D, *et al.* Ataxia and paresis in horses. Part II. Radiographic and myelographic examination of the cervical column. *Compend Contin Educ Pract Vet* 1981; **3**: S161–S171.
292 Rainger JE, Hughes KJ, Kessell A, Dart CM. Pleuropneumonia as a sequela of myelography and general anaesthesia in a Thoroughbred colt. *Aust Vet J* 2006; **84**(4): 138–140.
293 Jarrett MA, Bailey KM, Messenger KM, *et al.* Recovery of horses from general anesthesia after induction with propofol and ketamine versus midazolam and ketamine. *J Am Vet Med Assoc* 2018; **253**(1): 101–107.
294 Mignan T, Targett M, Lowrie M. Classification of myasthenia gravis and congenital myasthenic syndromes in dogs and cats. *J Vet Intern Med* 2020; **34**(5): 1707–1717.
295 Shelton GD. Muscular disorders. In: Ettinger S, Feldman E, Côté E, eds. *Textbook of Veterinary Internal Medicine: Diseases of the Dog and the Cat*, 8th edn. St. Louis, MO: Elsevier Saunders, 2017: 2149.
296 Shelton GD. Myasthenia gravis and disorders of neuromuscular transmission. *Vet Clin North Am Small Anim Pract* 2002; **32**(1): 189–206.
297 Shelton GD. Myasthenia gravis and congenital myasthenic syndromes in dogs and cats: a history and mini-review. *Neuromuscul Disord* 2016; **26**(6): 331–334.
298 Shelton GD, Ho M, Kass PH. Risk factors for acquired myasthenia gravis in cats: 105 cases (1986–1998). *J Am Vet Med Assoc* 2000; **216**(1): 55–57.
299 Hague DW, Humphries HD, Mitchell MA, *et al.* Risk factors and outcomes in cats with acquired myasthenia gravis (2001–2012). *J Vet Intern Med* 2015; **29**(5): 1307–1312.
300 Smith AN, Wright JC, Brawner WR, *et al.* Radiation therapy in the treatment of canine and feline thymomas: a retrospective study (1985–1999). *J Am Anim Hosp Assoc* 2001; **37**(5): 489–496.
301 Muckler VC, O'Brien JM, Matson SE, *et al.* Perianesthetic implications and considerations for myasthenia gravis. *J Perianesthesia Nurs* 2019; **34**(1): 4–15.
302 Shilo Y, Pypendop BH, Barter LS, *et al.* Thymoma removal in a cat with acquired myasthenia gravis: a case report and literature review of anesthetic techniques. *Vet Anaesth Analg* 2011; **38**(6): 603–613.
303 Howard JF Jr. Myasthenia Gravis – a Manual for the Health Care Provider. *Myasthenia Gravis Foundation of America.* www.myasthenia.org (accessed August 2023).
304 Naguib M, el Dawlatly AA, Ashour M, *et al.* Multivariate determinants of the need for postoperative ventilation in myasthenia gravis. *Can J Anaesth* 1996; **43**(10): 1006–1013.
305 Haroutiunian S, Lecht S, Zur AA, *et al.* The challenge of pain management in patients with myasthenia gravis. *J Pain Palliat Care Pharmacother* 2009; **23**(3): 242–260.
306 Nilsson E, Muller K. Neuromuscular effects of isoflurane in patients with myasthenia gravis. *Acta Anaesthesiol Scand* 1990; **34**(2): 126–131.
307 Vanlinthout LE, Booij LH, van Egmond J, *et al.* Effect of isoflurane and sevoflurane on the magnitude and time course of neuromuscular block produced by vecuronium, pancuronium and atracurium. *Br J Anaesth* 1996; **76**(3): 389–395.
308 Abel M, Eisenkraft JB. Anesthetic implications of myasthenia gravis. *Mt Sinai J Med N Y* 2002; **69**(1–2): 31–37.
309 Brown J, Laiken N. Muscarinic receptor agonists and antagonists. In: Brunton L, Chabner B, Knollmann B, eds. *Goodman & Gilman's the Pharmacological Basis of Ttherapeutics*, 12th edn. New York, NY: McGraw-Hill, 2011: 219–238.
310 Paterson IG, Hood JR, Russell SH, *et al.* Mivacurium in the myasthenic patient. *Br J Anaesth* 1994; **73**(4): 494–498.
311 Jones RS, Sharp NJ. Use of the muscle relaxant atracurium in a myasthenic dog. *Vet Rec* 1985; **117**(19): 500–501.
312 Jones RS, Brown A, Watkins PE. Use of the muscle relaxant vecuronium in a myasthenic dog. *Vet Rec* 1988; **122**(25): 611.

40 Physiology, Pathophysiology, and Anesthetic Management of Patients with Hepatic Disease

Vaidehi V. Paranjape[1] **and Fernando Garcia-Pereira**[2]

[1] Department of Small Animal Clinical Sciences, Virginia-Maryland College of Veterinary Medicine, Virginia Tech University, Blacksburg, Virginia, USA

[2] Pet Urgent Response and Emergency, Jacksonville, Florida, USA

Chapter contents

Introduction, 847
Functional anatomy and physiology, 847
  Structural organization of the liver, 847
  Hepatic blood flow, 848
  Hepatic functions, 850
Assessment of hepatic function, 851
  Biochemical derangements in liver pathology, 851
  Interpretation of liver enzymes, 852
  Assessment of coagulation, 852
Anesthetics and hepatic disease, 853
  Sedatives, 853
  Injectable anesthetic agents, 854
  Inhalant anesthetic agents, 854
  Neuromuscular blocking agents, 855
Hepatic pathophysiology and anesthetic management, 855
  Hepatitis, 855
  Portosystemic shunt, 856
  Hepatic neoplasia, 856
  Hepatic lobe torsion, 857
  Gallbladder and extrahepatic biliary tract pathology, 857
Anesthetic considerations for diagnostic or minimally invasive procedures, 857
  Ultrasound-guided biopsy, 857
  Laparoscopic procedures, 857
  Laparotomy, 858
  Interventional radiology, 858
Pain management in hepatobiliary diseases, 858
References, 858

Introduction

The liver is centrally located between the diaphragm and abdominal viscera and receives 20–30% of total cardiac output (CO) via the portal vein and hepatic artery. The liver plays a vital role in homeostasis and is responsible for the biotransformation and excretion of endogenous and exogenous substances. Significant exogenous physiologic support may be necessary for patients with clinically relevant hepatic dysfunction. In addition, consideration must be given to anesthetic and adjunct drug selection to avoid delayed recovery. Anesthetic and surgical procedures involving the liver may cause ischemia and reperfusion injury, inducing acute and chronic hepatic dysfunction. Hence, it is crucial to maintain adequate hepatic blood flow and oxygen delivery during general anesthesia. Clinical application of anatomic and physiologic knowledge is necessary to optimize anesthetic management during hepatic and extrahepatic biliary disease interventions.

Functional anatomy and physiology

The liver is the largest gland in the body, comprising 1.5–4% of total body weight, and is anatomically and physiologically similar among species. The liver can be divided into four main lobes (left, right, quadrate, and caudate lobes). The right and left lobes may be further subdivided into separate lateral and medial lobes. A gallbladder is present in most domestic species with the exception of the horse and the rat, in which large bile ducts compensate for the absence of the gallbladder. In some species, the bile duct terminates directly on the duodenum (e.g., canine and bovine), but in others, it shares a common duct with the pancreas (e.g., cat, horse, and small ruminants). This can be of importance, as some hepatobiliary diseases can also affect the pancreas of those species [1].

Structural organization of the liver

The hexagonal hepatic lobule is the basic anatomic unit of the liver. Cylindrical plates of hepatocytes are separated by venous sinusoids (fenestrated capillaries) and radiate around a central vein like spokes in wheel. The portal triad (hepatic arterioles, portal venules, bile canaliculi, lymphatics, and nerves) is present at each corner of the hexagon. The perisinusoidal space (or space of Disse) lies between the sinusoids and hepatocytes, containing plasma and allowing hepatocytes to absorb nutrients and waste products. Macrophage-derived Kupffer cells line the perisinusoidal space (Fig. 40.1). These cells have phagocytic function and are active in hepatic inflammatory responses. The hepatic arterial (HA) blood

Veterinary Anesthesia and Analgesia: The Sixth Edition of Lumb and Jones. Edited by Leigh Lamont, Kurt Grimm, Sheilah Robertson, Lydia Love and Carrie Schroeder.
© 2024 John Wiley & Sons, Inc. Published 2024 by John Wiley & Sons, Inc.
Companion website: www.wiley.com/go/lamont/anesthesia

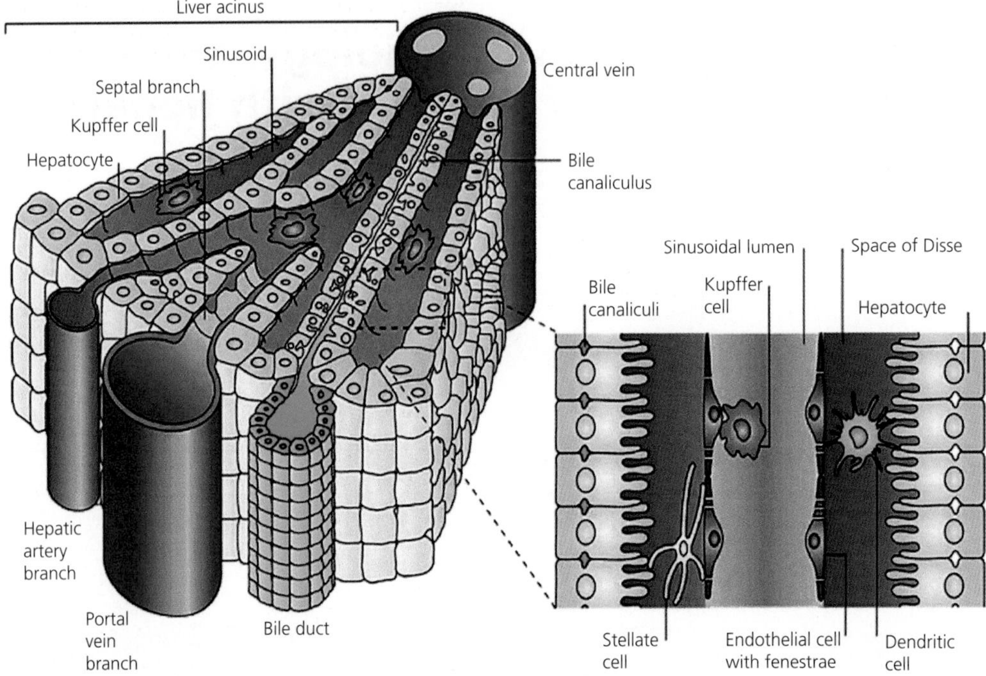

Figure 40.1 Structures of the liver lobule and liver acinus. Source: Du *et al.* [2], with permission.

enters the sinusoid either directly or through the peribiliary capillary plexus and mixes with portal venous blood in the low-pressure sinusoid microvasculature.

Although the hepatic lobule is the traditional organizational unit of the liver, a more logical functional unit is the acinus, which comprises three different zones (Fig. 40.2). Zone 1, known as the periportal area is centered around the portal triad, making it oxygen rich due to its close proximity with the hepatic artery. Zone 1 is most adaptable to hemodynamic stressors, least susceptible to necrosis, and first to undergo regeneration. The hepatocytes in this zone contain many mitochondria, and most oxidative metabolic processes occur here. Zone 2 is a transitional zone between zones 1 and 3. Zone 3 is the pericentral zone, located in close proximity to the central vein (centrilobular), where blood leaves the organ to join the central circulation. This zone has the lowest oxygen tension, is most susceptible to hemodynamic and toxic stress, and is the last to regenerate. The hepatocytes in this zone contain a large amount of smooth endoplasmic reticulum and microsomal enzyme activity, and therefore play a major role in drug detoxification, or Phase I and II metabolism.

Hepatic blood flow

Afferent blood supply to the liver is composed of both arterial and portal venous blood and all the blood exits the liver via the hepatic veins. The arrangement of hepatic structures is centered on the caudal vena cava and portal vein. The portal vein supplies 75% of the hepatic blood flow (HBF) and is formed by blood returning from the splanchnic circulation, including most of the gastrointestinal tract and spleen (Fig. 40.3). The splenic vein contribution to the portal blood is rich in pancreatic hormones and cytokines, while the superior mesenteric vein brings nutrients, toxins, and bacteria that are absorbed from the gastrointestinal tract. The HA provides the remaining 25% of HBF; however, it supplies 45–50% of the liver's oxygen requirements. Although the portal vein carries blood with a lower oxygen content than the HA, its contribution to the organ's oxygenation is significant due to the large volume of blood that it delivers [4].

HBF is regulated via intrinsic and extrinsic mechanisms. The HA supplies arterial blood via a high-pressure system and mean pressure in the HA is similar to that in the aorta. The HA possesses α_1-, α_2-, and β_2-adrenergic receptors. Sympathetic activation constricts HA smooth muscle, increases arterial resistance, and reduces blood flow. β-Adrenergic stimulation vasodilates hepatic arterioles, decreases vascular resistance, and increases flow through the HA. However, this effect may be blocked by non-selective β-adrenergic receptor antagonists administered to decrease portal pressure in human patients with liver cirrhosis [5]. In contrast, the portal vein contains α-adrenergic but not β_2-adrenergic receptors [6]. Minor changes in hepatic venous tone and hepatic venous pressure can result in large changes in hepatic blood volume, favoring the liver's ability to act as a blood reservoir. For example, during hemorrhage, hepatic venous pressure decreases, shifting blood into the central venous circulation and augmenting circulating blood volume. Blood loss can be reduced during liver surgery by lowering the central venous pressure, thereby reducing hepatic venous pressure and hepatic blood volume.

The liver's high blood flow is due to low vascular resistance in the portal vein. Normally, the portal vein pressure is about 7–10 mmHg. However, with hepatocellular injury, fibrous tissue can form in the affected areas, impeding blood flow and causing portal hypertension [6]. An increase in portal pressure can promote neovascularization of splanchnic vasculature and development of acquired portosystemic shunts. An increase in portal flow must be compensated such that portal venous pressure is minimally affected. In order to preserve adequate sinusoidal perfusion pressure while maintaining low portal venous pressure, HBF is regulated by mechanisms targeting HA inflow, portal venous inflow, and the interrelationship between HA and portal venous inflow circuits [7]. Several

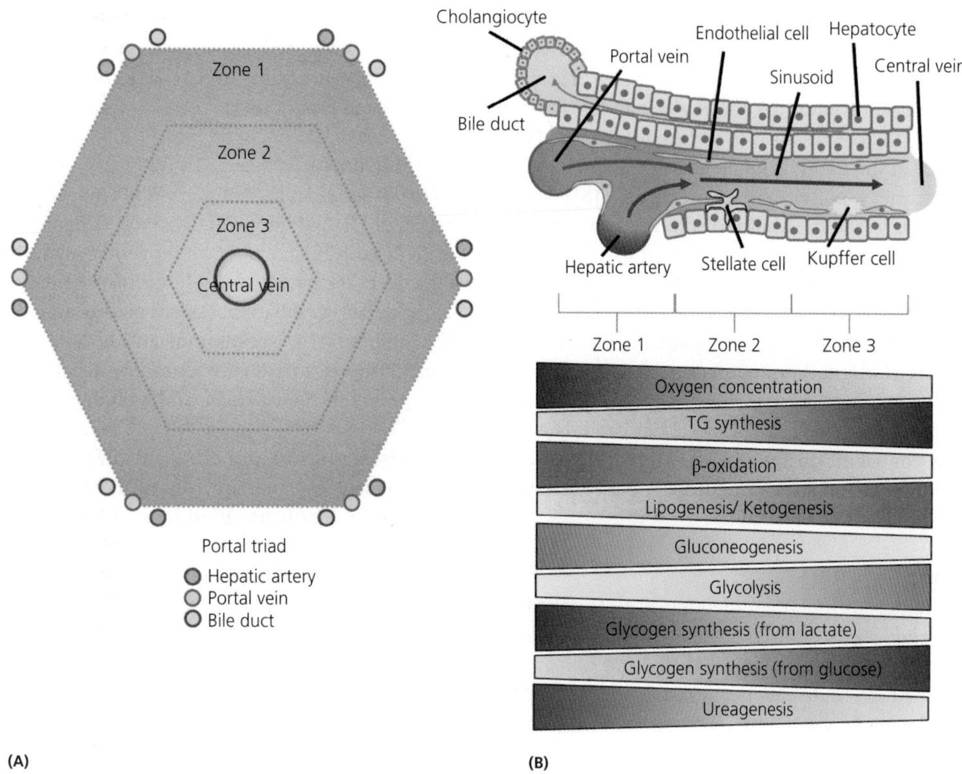

Figure 40.2 **A.** Microanatomy of the hepatic parenchyma within a hepatic lobule: Zone 1, periportal; zone 3, pericentral; zone 2, between zones 1 and 3. **B.** A schematic representation of a liver acinus and the corresponding zonation of several metabolic processes across the acinus. The gradients depicted below the scheme pertain to both essential hemostasis and metabolic processes along the acinus. Source: Trefts *et al.* [3], with permission.

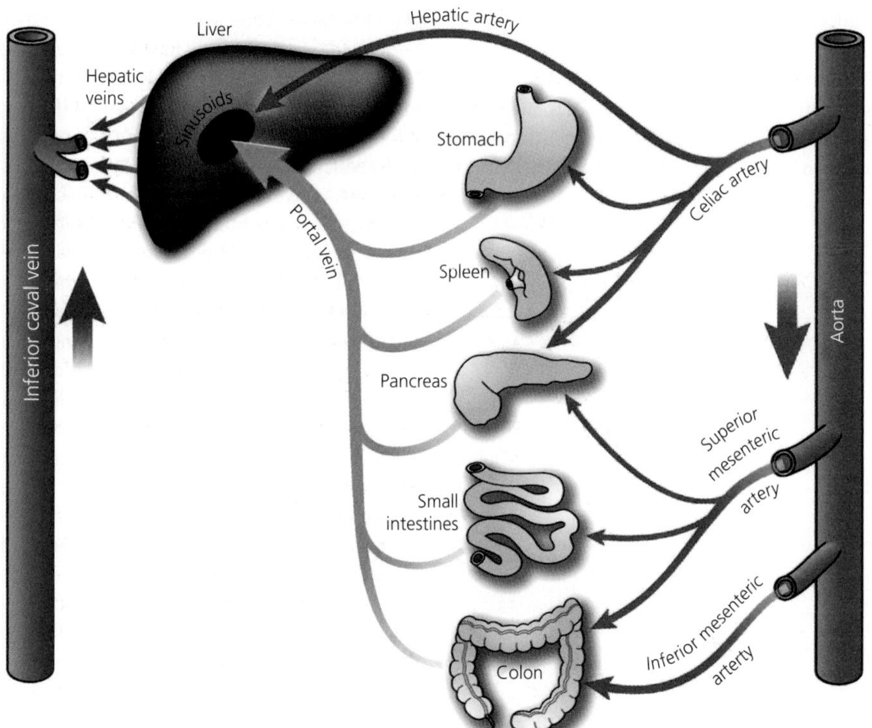

Figure 40.3 The splanchnic circulation. Source: Gelman and Mushlin [4], with permission.

intrinsic mechanisms are responsible for maintaining adequate sinusoidal perfusion pressure while maintaining low portal venous pressure, including (1) low basal resistance, (2) distensible pre- and post-sinusoid resistance sites, (3) the myogenic constrictive response of the HA, (4) the HA response to oxygen tension or pH of portal venous blood, (5) the highly compliant hepatic vasculature, and (6) the hepatic artery buffer response (HABR) [8]. These unique mechanisms represent the ability of the hepatic artery to produce compensatory flow changes in response to changes in portal venous flow. The HABR is mechanistically associated with adenosine because as portal blood flow decreases, adenosine accumulates, causing vasodilation of nearby hepatic arterioles. This dilation increases arterial blood flow and maintains hepatic perfusion [8]. Other vasoactive mediators such as nitric oxide, carbon monoxide, and hydrogen sulfide may be potential candidates to affect HA flow and contribute to the HABR. Moreover, sensory innervation (neurokinin-1) and sensory neuropeptides (calcitonin gene-related peptide) may also be related to HABR [7].

Hepatic functions

The liver performs numerous functions affecting all systems of the body (Table 40.1). It plays a major role in protein synthesis and degradation, including albumin, coagulation proteins, and numerous peptides. Glycogen storage, nutrient metabolism, detoxification, and excretion of endogenous waste products and xenobiotics are other important functions.

Protein homeostasis

Normally, plasma protein availability is abundant relative to daily consumption. Albumin is the most abundant protein produced by the liver and is involved in several homeostatic processes. Notably, albumin is a major contributor to plasma oncotic pressure. Albumin production is regulated (via feedback) in part through plasma oncotic pressure in addition to its plasma concentration [10]. Albumin is a low-affinity/high-capacity major plasma transport protein, and it plays a significant role in drug binding of acidic anesthetic drugs (e.g., barbiturates). In contrast, alpha-1 acid glycoprotein (AAG) represents a relatively smaller percentage of total plasma proteins. It is considered a high-affinity/low-capacity plasma protein, and mainly binds to basic drugs (e.g., local anesthetics). In most disease states such as inflammation, infection, and neoplasia, AAG levels have been shown to increase in humans and animals. This promotes the utility of AAG as a clinical biomarker for disease diagnosis and prognosis [11].

Table 40.1 Pertinent functions of the liver.

Metabolic	Synthetic	Homeostatic
Xenobiotic metabolism	Coagulation and anticoagulation proteins	Intravascular volume regulation (RAAS)
Protein metabolism (ammonia, urea)	Plasma proteins (albumin, alpha-1 acid glycoprotein)	Glucose homeostasis
Lipid metabolism (triglyceride)	Steroid hormones (cholesterol)	Regulation of portal blood flow (HABR)
Glucose metabolism (gluconeogenesis, glycogenolysis, and glycogenesis)	Thrombopoietin	Liver regeneration and growth
Carbohydrate metabolism	Angiotensinogen	Plasma oncotic pressure
Nutrient metabolism (amino acids, lipids, and vitamins)	Insulin-like growth factor	Innate and adaptive immunity
Bile production and secretion	Fetal and extramedullary hematopoiesis	
Biotransformation and biliary excretion	Acute phase proteins	
	Plasma cholinesterases	

RAAS, renin–angiotensin–aldosterone system; HABR, hepatic artery buffer response.
Source: Adapted from Mulaikal and Emond [9].

Coagulation

Several coagulation factors, such as fibrinogen (factor I), prothrombin (factor II), factors V, VII, IX, X, XI, XII, and XIII, prekallikrein, and high molecular weight kininogen are synthesized or activated by the liver. The liver is also responsible for the synthesis of proteins that modulate coagulation, such as plasminogen, plasminogen activator inhibitor-1, α_2-antiplasmin, antithrombin, and proteins C and S. Furthermore, it performs vitamin K-dependent carboxylation of prothrombin, factors VII, IX, and X, and proteins C and S [9].

Biotransformation and elimination of xenobiotics

The enzymatic systems involved in the biotransformation of substances are generally localized to the liver. However, other tissues, such as the lungs, kidneys, and gastrointestinal tract, have significant metabolic capabilities for some drugs. The route of administration and subsequent drug distribution to these sites must be considered when administering sedatives, analgesics, and anesthetics [12]. First-pass hepatic metabolism significantly reduces the bioavailability of several drugs, especially after enteral, and in some species rectal, administration.

Xenobiotic biotransformation can be divided into Phase I (oxidation, reduction, or hydrolysis) and Phase II (conjugation) reactions. Phase I transformation introduces a polar group (e.g., OH^- and NH_2^-) to the parent drug typically via the cytochrome P450 system (CYPs). While such reactions often inactivate the drug, the addition of these functional radicals may result in formation of active metabolites for some drugs, or cause activation of a prodrug. One example of a prodrug is codeine, which is catalyzed by CYP2D6 and *O*-demethylated to form morphine. Local codeine *O*-demethylation in the central nervous system could explain the analgesic effect of codeine despite relatively low plasma levels of morphine [13].

The CYP450 system is the most important group of metabolizing enzymes in the body. They are found in several tissues, such as the liver, kidney, and intestines, and are responsible for the oxidation and reduction of xenobiotics and endogenous substances. These reactions convert relatively lipophilic compounds into hydrophilic metabolites to facilitate their elimination through the urine or bile. They are mostly carried out intracellularly in the microsomes of the smooth endoplasmic reticulum (i.e., microsomal enzymes). Zone 3 hepatocytes have the highest content of CYP450 enzymes. Their localization is important in predicting the region where hepatic damage will be most evident when a drug is metabolized to toxic substances. An example is severe centrilobular necrosis and cholangiohepatitis observed in some cats following administration of oral diazepam [14]. Although the same families and subfamilies of P450 enzymes are present in most domestic species, different individual enzymes might be encountered in each species. Additionally, the same enzyme may be present but act on a different substrate range compared with humans [15]. Therefore, it becomes problematic to extrapolate drug doses, intervals, effects, and metabolic fate from human-derived data to veterinary species. Differences in CYP activity exist not only among species but also among different breeds and genders. For example, Beagles have greater propofol hydroxylase activity (CYP2B) than Greyhounds [16]. Gender variability in dogs and cats for different CYP families has also been described [17].

Phase II reactions are responsible for conferring further hydrophilicity to a drug, facilitating its excretion. These reactions occur mostly in the cytosol. The domestic cat has been recognized to have a reduced ability to form glucuronide conjugates of many xenobiotics (e.g., propofol) [18]. Therefore, when low molecular weight phenolic derivatives are given to cats, they are biotransformed slowly, or are biotransformed and eliminated by other mechanisms [19]. Defects of the UDP-glucuronosyltransferase (UGT)1A6 gene seem to be responsible for the poor glucuronidation of some drugs in cats, such as acetaminophen [20]. However, cats have other UGT enzymes that can biotransform some xenobiotics [21].

Acting as the most diverse catalysts, CYPs contribute to interindividual variations in drug responses, resulting from genetic and epigenetic variants, as well as factors such as gender, age, nutritional status, disease states, and pathophysiological states. The CYPs can be inhibited or induced by concomitant drugs and circulating metabolites, which can influence treatment outcomes through drug–drug interaction, drug–gene interaction, and drug–drug–gene interaction [22]. Some xenobiotics can induce CYP and glucuronosyltransferase activity. Ketamine can induce both enzyme types, contributing to the development of its own tolerance in rats [23].

Reduced protein activity results in decreased removal of certain drugs from brain to blood, and from blood to bile on the hepatocellular surface in humans [24]. This may be related to some adverse effects of ivermectins and morphine-like derivatives from brain to systemic circulation in MDR1 (ABCB1) mutant dogs [25]. In the last two decades, a large amount of information on the metabolism and interaction of specific drugs in veterinary species has been published [26]. However, further research is warranted to characterize individual CYPs for each species and their substrates.

Immune and inflammatory response

The liver has a large role in host defenses. Of the nonparenchymal cells in the liver, four types of antigen-presenting cells serve as immunologic gatekeepers. These are Kupffer cells, dendritic cells, stellate cells, and sinusoidal endothelial cells, all responsible for innate immunity. Bacteria and toxins that gain access to the portal circulation are routinely phagocytized and processed by Kupffer cells in the sinusoids [27]. Kupffer cells are also scavengers of inflammatory mediators, appearing to limit the extent of the inflammatory response [28]. However, when an overwhelming amount of endotoxin is present, activated Kupffer cells can produce reductive oxygen radicals and cytokines. These processes allow Kupffer cells to signal hepatocytes and endothelial cells, changing their transcription products, in addition to recruiting circulating neutrophils. This hepatic immunologic response can be responsible for hepatocellular injury seen in some disease conditions. The close interaction between the inflammatory response and coagulation also plays a role in the pathogenesis of hepatic and multiorgan failure. For example, during endotoxemia and hypoperfusion, the activated hepatic cells (Kupffer cells, hepatocytes, and endothelial cells) promote an inflammatory, hypercoagulable state [29].

Assessment of hepatic function

Whenever a patient's hepatic function is questioned, a biochemical profile, coagulation panel, and substrate metabolism tests should be requested. However, a reduction of approximately 70–80% of hepatic function must be present before observing abnormalities in biochemical parameters; hence, these disturbances are not sensitive indicators of hepatic dysfunction. Limitations of conventional coagulation tests have led to increased interest in viscoelastic testing systems and their use in global hemostasis assays.

Biochemical derangements in liver pathology

Substrate metabolism tests such as serum bilirubin, ammonia, and pre- and postprandial bile acids are better indicators of hepatic function than serum liver enzyme concentrations [30]. Hyperbilirubinemia can be caused by prehepatic disease (e.g., hemolysis), primary hepatic disease (e.g., decreased hepatocyte function), and post-hepatic disease (e.g., extrahepatic biliary obstruction). Hyperbilirubinemia is reported in approximately 50% of dogs with chronic hepatitis (CH) and is a negative prognostic indicator [31]. Measurement of serum conjugated (direct) and unconjugated (indirect) bilirubin to distinguish between prehepatic, hepatic, or post-hepatic hyperbilirubinemia is not clinically reliable [32]. A study evaluating the sensitivity and specificity of fasting ammonia and serum bile acids for diagnosis of portosystemic shunt (PSS) in dogs and cats found the tests to have high sensitivity and specificity in both species [33]. Indocyanine green and sulfobromophthalein clearance tests are quantitative measures of hepatic function, reflecting blood flow-dependent clearance, hepatocyte uptake, and biliary excretion. Hepatic clearance of indocyanine green can change in direct proportion to variations in liver blood flow, as seen in isoflurane-anesthetized dogs where a 63% reduction in CO resulted in a 26% decline in clearance [34]. In human patients, the hepatic metabolism of lidocaine is considered as a dynamic liver function test. It is non-invasive, easy, and quick to perform. Lidocaine is converted to monoethylglycinexylidide (MEGX) and subsequently to glycinexylidide (GX) by the hepatic cytochrome P450 enzyme system. As MEGX accurately reflects the severity of hepatic dysfunction, it is valuable for quantitative evaluation of liver dysfunction along with being a prognostic predictor of liver disease in adults [35]. In dogs, MEGX testing has been shown to successfully differentiate closed extrahepatic PSS from persistent shunting after gradual attenuation surgery [36].

Hepatobiliary disease also results in decreased protein synthesis as well as altered glucose, urea nitrogen, and lipid metabolism. Because the liver normally produces albumin at one-third of its capacity, hypoalbuminemia is seen only in severe cases of hepatic dysfunction or severe protein loss [32]. Glomerular disease, protein-losing enteropathies, and hemorrhage are non-hepatic causes and should be ruled out when hypoalbuminemia is present. Alpha and beta globulins may also be diminished with hepatic dysfunction. Reduction in plasma protein concentrations will decrease the bound fraction of some drugs, which can result in changes in volume of distribution, plasma concentration, and drug effect. Patients with PSS or acute hepatic failure are often hypoglycemic, or at risk for clinical hypoglycemia during the perianesthetic period. Mechanisms of hypoglycemia in hepatic dysfunction include one or a combination of the following: (1) decreased gluconeogenesis, (2) decreased glycogen storage, and (3) diminished response to glucagon. Monitoring and maintenance of normoglycemia should be a priority during anesthesia.

Serum cholesterol concentrations can be increased, normal, or decreased in patients with hepatobiliary disease. A recent canine study identified a significant positive association between hyperlipidemia (specifically hypercholesterolemia), liver enzymes, and total serum bile acid (TSBA) concentrations in dogs suffering from CH [37]. Decreased concentrations of blood urea nitrogen and cholesterol were seen to develop in approximately 40% of dogs with CH, occurring most commonly in those with cirrhosis.

Hypoglycemia is rare in CH and is more often associated with acute liver failure. The TSBA concentrations are uniformly increased when portosystemic shunting is present, and their sensitivity for detecting cirrhosis and the presence of an acquired PSS is high. Dogs with cholestasis (i.e., hyperbilirubinemia) associated with hepatic disease will always have increased TSBA concentrations. Hyperammonemia has similar sensitivity for detection of CH or cirrhosis and acquired PSS as TSBA and is somewhat more specific because it is not affected by cholestasis [31].

Interpretation of liver enzymes

Enzyme concentration abnormalities are common, but their relation to patient risk is often difficult to interpret. The serum concentration of alanine aminotransferase (ALT), aspartate aminotransferase (AST), alkaline phosphatase (ALP), lactate dehydrogenase (LDH), and γ-glutamyl transpeptidase (GGT) are the most commonly measured hepatocellular enzymes in biochemical profiles. Hepatobiliary tissue damage can cause cellular leakage, resulting in increased plasma concentration of hepatocellular enzymes. However, this rise does not necessarily indicate the degree of hepatic dysfunction. This is especially true for chronic liver diseases, where reduced hepatocellular numbers secondary to fibrosis may result in near-normal liver enzyme values in the face of severely compromised function. Additionally, elevation of enzymes may represent cellular insult, but may not correlate with any inability to biotransform drugs used for anesthesia and pain management.

In several retrospective canine studies, serum ALT activity has shown reliability during CH screening. However, histopathologic evidence of CH can exist in the absence of increased serum liver enzyme activity. As CH progresses and hepatic parenchyma decreases, ALP and GGT activities increase compared to ALT [31]. Even though ALP can be associated with biliary obstruction or injury, its elevation may originate in other locations such as placenta (during pregnancy) and bone. Diagnostic efficacy of serum ALP and GGT was higher (91%) when used together in dogs with histologically confirmed hepatobiliary disease (e.g., cholestasis) [38]. The position of the liver between the splanchnic and systemic circulation creates the potential for diseases of other organ systems to involve the liver, and consequently cause an increase in circulating liver enzymes. Additionally, several enzymes are found in tissue outside the liver (e.g., AST in skeletal muscle, heart, kidney, pancreas, adipose tissue, and brain) and injury to these tissues may be falsely interpreted as hepatic injury. Elevation of liver enzymes, although highly sensitive for hepatocellular injury, is not specific to liver dysfunction.

Assessment of coagulation

Coagulation status should be considered in patients with liver disease undergoing a surgical procedure, including laparoscopic liver biopsy. CH patients may show no clinical signs of a coagulopathy but may be hypocoagulable and be at a greater risk of coagulopathy after an insult such as surgery [39]. Hepatobiliary disease can give rise to complex alterations in coagulation. These alterations involve changes in pro- and anticoagulants, as well as factors participating in fibrinolysis. The net effect of this is that patients with liver dysfunction can have laboratory and clinical features of both hypo- and hypercoagulability. This is well demonstrated in dogs with congenital PSS that can be in a hypercoagulable or hypocoagulable state [40,41]. The concomitant changes in both pro- and antihemostatic pathways result in a "rebalanced" hemostatic state in these patients. This new hemostatic balance appears to be much more fragile than the hemostatic balance in healthy individuals, and hence, patients with liver disease can readily experience both hemostasis-related bleeding and thrombotic events. These insights into the hemostatic balance during liver disease warrant revised recommendations for clinical management of hemostasis [42]. Emerging evidence states that such a "rebalanced" state of coagulation also occurs in dogs with liver disease. Whether canine patients have clinical bleeding or thrombosis depends on factors that shift the coagulation state one way or the other. Hemorrhage can be induced by uremia, infection, hypervolemia, or acidosis, whereas thrombosis is precipitated with aggravated portal hypertension, use of corticosteroids, proinflammatory states, or with simultaneously occurring pro-thrombotic conditions [43].

Prolongations in prothrombin time (PT) and activated partial thromboplastin time (aPTT) and bleeding from provocative procedures suggest hypocoagulable tendencies. Increases in clot strength, D-dimers, von Willebrand's factor, and factor VIII activity; decreases in antithrombin and protein C activity; and an increased incidence of thrombosis in the splanchnic circulation suggest hypercoagulable tendencies [44,45]. Fibrinogen also plays several key roles in maintaining both primary and secondary hemostasis and is converted by thrombin into an insoluble fibrin network that, together with platelet aggregates, induces hemostasis in response to rupture of the endothelium. In humans and dogs, plasma fibrinogen concentration during liver cirrhosis progressively decreased with worsening disease, indicating a close relationship between the severity of cirrhosis and hemostatic changes [46,47]. Thrombocytopenia can develop with hepatic disease and is due to mechanisms including decreased platelet production due to thrombopoietin deficiency and direct megakaryocyte toxicity, decreased platelet half-life due to splenomegaly and hypersplenism, and possibly autoantibodies. Consumption of platelets by intrahepatic or systemic platelet activation may also contribute to decreased platelet counts [42]. In addition, vitamin K malabsorption may develop secondary to certain hepatic diseases (e.g., hepatic lipidosis) or cholestasis (e.g., complete biliary obstruction). Vitamin K acts as a cofactor for the enzyme γ-glutamyl carboxylase, which activates coagulation factors II (prothrombin), VII, IX, and X. Hence, hepatobiliary diseases can result in secondary hemostasis defects through decreased vitamin K-mediated carboxylation of coagulation factors [48]. Vitamin K supplementation may be recommended for some liver diseases and could be administered prior to invasive procedures such as liver biopsy or feeding tube placement, due to increased risk of bleeding.

Blood typing and crossmatching may be warranted if the coagulation profile is abnormal or if a blood transfusion is anticipated. Fresh frozen plasma (FFP) or cryoprecipitate may be transfused in liver diseases both therapeutically and prophylactically to correct deranged coagulation. However, as the etiology of coagulation defects in liver disease is highly complex, the clinical benefit of prophylactic administration of FFP on the basis of abnormal coagulation tests alone, is questionable [49]. The constituents of FFP include all coagulation factors that are essential to clot formation (i.e., factors II, V, VII, VIII, IX, X, and XI). Repletion of coagulation factors with FFP bypasses the need for vitamin K carboxylation in the liver for coagulation factor formation. In spite of these benefits, FFP transfusion comes with the risk of increasing portal hypertension, hypervolemia, and assorted other risks, including immune-mediated reactions. Risk of exacerbating portal hypertension and transfusion-related lung injury argues against routine use of FFP in this population [50].

Other than the conventional coagulation tests, viscoelastic testing systems (VETs) for clot detection are increasingly being used in veterinary medicine for diagnosis of the hemostatic states: normocoagulable, hypercoagulable, hypocoagulable, excessive fibrinolysis, or decreased fibrinolysis. These methods can also evaluate platelet inhibition, functional fibrinogen measurement, and fibrinolysis [51]. Because VETs assess cellular and protein components of hemostasis (platelets and coagulation factors), as well as fibrinolysis, they are referred to as the "global assays of hemostasis." The VETs provide (1) graphical and numerical results that reflect the dynamic nature of fibrin formation and breakdown, and (2) information on the time of onset of fibrin formation, rate of fibrin formation, strength of fibrin clot, and fibrinolysis at defined intervals. Currently, commercially available VETs include the Sonoclot® Coagulation and Platelet Function Analyzer, thromboelastography (TEG), and rotational thromboelastometry. A novel portable handheld analyzer, the Viscoelastic Coagulation Monitor (VCM Vet™) has been recently introduced for use in dogs and cats to fulfill the clinical need for bedside testing in emergency suites, intensive care units, operating rooms, and field examinations [52,53]. In patients suffering from hepatic disease, VETs may be a superior tool to pinpoint coagulation abnormalities, monitor hemostasis during resuscitation of clinical bleeding disorders, evaluate anticoagulant use, and optimize treatment plans. The diagnostic utility of TEG has been recognized in dogs suffering from acute liver disease, gallbladder mucocele, congenital PSS, and chronic hepatopathies, as well as in cats with cholestatic liver disease [41,43,45,54,55].

Anesthetics and hepatic disease

Sedatives

Frequently, opioid administration is sufficient to provide adequate sedation and analgesia for diagnostic and surgical procedures in obtunded patients suffering from liver disease. Hydromorphone, oxymorphone, fentanyl, and methadone are full μ-opioid receptor agonists that provide good sedation and analgesia. Compared with morphine and meperidine, they present some potential advantages, as they are not associated with elevations in plasma histamine concentrations and decreased blood pressure after intravenous administration [56,57]. Metabolic pathways for most opioids such as oxidation via the CYP system (CYP2D6 and 3A4) or glucuronidation can be impaired in the setting of severe liver disease. The CYP system is not only affected by liver dysfunction but is also influenced by malnutrition and suboptimal protein consumption, which are common issues in cirrhotic patients [58].

Morphine is metabolized by the liver to morphine-6-glucuronide (active metabolite with analgesic effects) and morphine-3-glucuronide (inactive metabolite with potential neurotoxic effects), which are then cleared renally. With reduced first-pass metabolism in cirrhotic patients, morphine is likely more bioavailable and lower oral doses are recommended. Human studies show that morphine has a decreased plasma clearance and a prolonged elimination half-life in patients with severe cirrhosis. Similarly, in cirrhotic patients, the analgesic effects of codeine may be more variable due to reduced conversion to morphine via CYP2D6 [58,59]. Drug elimination capacity of other opioids can also decrease in liver disease, but drug bioavailability may increase. These changes may be secondary to reductions in HBF or reductions in CYP450 enzyme activity. In clinical scenarios of hypoalbuminemia, alterations in opioid distribution volumes will also impact drug accumulation [60]. Opioids with short elimination half-lives such as fentanyl can be used as intravenous infusions in the face of liver dysfunction, but careful dose titration is required because the context-sensitive half-life of opioid infusions will be longer than in normal patients. Remifentanil is a synthetic opioid that allows for high clearance, rapid elimination, and recovery independent of dose or duration of infusion. It is metabolized by plasma esterase and shows no accumulation after continuous infusion in humans presenting with severe liver disease [61]. Other synthetic lipophilic opioids such as sufentanil and alfentanil, although short-acting, may also pose risks for accumulation due to extended half-lives during liver dysfunction [60]. The reversibility of opioids is an advantage in the face of hepatic dysfunction.

Most sedatives used in veterinary medicine can be categorized into one of three groups: phenothiazines, benzodiazepines, and α_2-adrenergic receptor agonists. Acepromazine may be used in patients with liver disease, but careful assessment of the patient and conservative dosing is necessary. Acepromazine causes vasodilation due to antagonism of α_1-adrenergic receptors. Acepromazine vasodilation may be beneficial to increase renal blood flow in anesthetized dogs [62], but experimental verification that it has the same effect on the hepatic circulation is lacking. When a patient has diminished intravascular oncotic pressure (e.g., hypoalbuminemia), hypovolemia and hypotension can be present even before sedation. In these cases where preoperative volume resuscitation is vital, acepromazine should be avoided due to its potent vasodilatory effects. Acepromazine is also known to affect platelet aggregation in dogs and should be avoided if significant coagulation abnormalities are present [63]. Moreover, its long-lasting effects, which could be further prolonged in the face of liver disease, as well as its irreversibility make acepromazine a less popular choice as a sedative in the face of hepatic dysfunction.

Benzodiazepine sedative drugs are often advocated in cases where there is significant disease because they tend to have fewer adverse cardiovascular effects. However, their use in patients with liver disease may be less advantageous. Advanced liver disease may result in hepatic encephalopathy (HE) due to accumulation of ammonium, *N*-methyl-D-aspartate (NMDA) receptor hyperactivity, and decreased adenosine triphosphate, among other causes [64,65]. In humans, the benzodiazepine antagonist flumazenil has been shown to minimize clinical signs associated with HE in the short-term [66]. The use of benzodiazepines in veterinary patients presenting with HE is controversial as they may exhibit increased response to these drugs, resulting in profound sedation and aggravation of the HE [64,67]. In the absence of HE, benzodiazepines can be used safely in patients with liver disease, although hepatic elimination is likely reduced and prolonged effects may occur [68,69]. Unwanted effects such as prolonged sedation can be antagonized by flumazenil if needed.

Dexmedetomidine provides excellent sedative, analgesic, and muscle relaxant effects yet may be associated with significant cardiovascular depression characterized by decreases in CO of as much as 50% [70]. Despite this, HBF is unchanged in normal dogs after intravenous administration of up to 10 μg/kg, based on radioactive microsphere methodology [71]. On the contrary, an increase in HA blood flow was reported with increasing medetomidine concentrations in sheep, which was attributed to the significant reduction in CO causing a subsequent fall in portal vein blood flow [72]. Medetomidine and dexmedetomidine have been shown to decrease hepatic enzymatic activity *in vitro*. It could be speculated that they would have clinically relevant pharmacokinetic drug interactions that would be more apparent in animals with liver disease. However, it is likely that their sparing effects on doses of other anesthetic agents (pharmacodynamic drug interaction) may be more clinically relevant than any direct effects on liver metabolic capacity [73]. Antagonism of α_2-adrenergic receptor agonists can speed recovery in animals with liver disease and would minimize the impact of impaired metabolism on the duration of α_2-adrenergic receptor agonist action. Keeping these factors in mind, authors of this chapter cautiously use dexmedetomidine at doses of 0.5–2 μg/kg IV titrable to effect, or 2–5 μg/kg IM, dependent on the level of sedation required and severity of hepatic disease.

Injectable anesthetic agents

Numerous studies have evaluated the effects of inhalant anesthetics on hepatic function and blood flow. However, relatively few studies have examined the impact of injectable anesthetics. Ketamine appears to cause a modest decrease in HBF compared to thiopental and etomidate [74,75]. Propofol has been shown to maintain HBF via arterial vasodilation in dogs and thiopental appears to have similar effects [76,77]. In rabbits, propofol attenuated hepatic reperfusion injury, caused oxidative radical formation, increased total HBF, and preserved oxygen balance [78–80]. As a general rule, most agents have minimal direct effects on HBF if systemic arterial blood pressure is maintained within normal limits. Propofol clearance exceeds HBF, suggesting an extra-hepatic site of metabolism and making it a reasonable choice for patients with liver disease [81,82]. A retrospective study found no increase in morbidity or mortality in cats with hepatic lipidosis that were anesthetized with propofol for feeding tube placement [83]. However, like most anesthetic drugs, it has dose-dependent cardiac depressant and systemic vasodilatory effects that may alter HBF in some cases [84]. A recent human study found no comparable differences in HBF with propofol-based and sevoflurane-based anesthetic regimens [85]. On the other hand, there is a lack of literature on alfaxalone and its effects on hepatic physiology. However, use of Althesin® (i.e., alfadolone and alfaxalone mixture) in Greyhounds was shown to decrease HBF and hepatic oxygen supply despite relatively unchanged hepatic oxygen consumption [75], while in humans it was shown to negatively affect liver function tests [86].

Thiopental decreases HBF either from increased HA vascular resistance or from reduced CO and blood pressure [75]. Thiopental undergoes metabolism by the liver, has several active metabolites, and its administration may result in the induction of microsomal enzyme activity [87,88]. Termination of its anesthetic effects results mostly from redistribution to non-target tissues, suggesting that it may be acceptable to use it as a single bolus for induction.

Etomidate causes minimal cardiovascular effects compared with propofol during anesthetic induction [84]. However, etomidate is in a propylene glycol-based vehicle. Propylene glycol is a hyperosmolar molecule and may cause erythrocyte rupture [89]. Because some patients presenting with hepatobiliary disease may have bilirubinemia and icterus due to biliary obstruction or decreased hepatic conjugation, the potential hemolysis caused by etomidate could further overload the liver. Although hemolysis does not appear to be significant in normal dogs after a single bolus, the clinical consequences in animals with liver disease have not been studied [90]. Etomidate clearance did not seem to change in human patients with hepatic cirrhosis compared with healthy patients, but the volume of distribution and elimination half-life doubled [91]. This increase in volume of distribution can mostly be explained by the inverse correlation between the plasma albumin concentration and protein binding but may also be due to a slight decrease in albumin-binding properties in the presence of hepatic cirrhosis or renal failure [92]. Etomidate has been demonstrated to inhibit cortisol synthesis by inhibiting adrenal mitochondrial 11β-hydroxylase and is generally not recommended in critical illness-related corticosteroid insufficiency of sepsis [93]. Human patients with non-septic acute and chronic liver diseases have shown lower baseline and stimulated cortisol levels (hepatoadrenal syndrome) [94]. Furthermore, when ACTH stimulation tests were performed in these patients, the presence of etomidate in the anesthetic protocol increased the presence of adrenal insufficiency from 38 to 57% [93]. Hepatoadrenal syndrome has not yet been reported in the veterinary literature; however, care should be taken regarding the presence of concomitant adrenal insufficiency when using etomidate in liver patients. Etomidate is primarily metabolized by esterase hydrolysis in the rat. However, this route does not seem to play a significant role in the drug's breakdown in several other species studied, pointing to hepatic metabolism [95]. Its hepatic extraction ratio is 0.5, or 50% of the HBF, which indicates that small changes in HBF or function will have only moderate effects on etomidate clearance [96]. Overall, etomidate seems to be a reasonable induction agent for patient with hepatic dysfunction owing to its minimal cardiovascular effects, which preserve systemic and hepatic blood flow.

Dissociative anesthetics such as ketamine and tiletamine are acceptable choices for the induction of anesthesia in patients with hepatic disease, though dosing should be carefully titrated to effect. The co-administration of a benzodiazepine (e.g., zolazepam with tiletamine in Telazol®) may result in prolonged effects in animals with impaired hepatic function. In dogs, dissociative anesthetics are metabolized mostly by the liver; however, termination of effect would be expected to be minimally affected after administration of a single dose used for induction due to drug redistribution to muscular and adipose tissues [97]. A study in rats and a report in humans have shown ketamine infusions to cause hepatic injury after prolonged use, especially when repeated within a short interval between treatments [98,99]. The authors of the human report recommended that liver enzymes be routinely measured during chronic treatment using ketamine [98]. In dogs, ketamine did not result in improved hepatic circulation, hepatic oxygen metabolism, or hepatic mitochondrial redox state during serious hypoxemia [100]. Also, ketamine increased HA blood flow in pigs [101] and decreased hepatic oxygen delivery in Greyhounds [74].

Inhalant anesthetic agents

Inhalant anesthetics alter HBF in a dose-dependent fashion. In general, inhalants impair autoregulatory mechanisms (i.e., HABR) that would otherwise maintain total HBF. Studies in dogs have shown that isoflurane, sevoflurane, and desflurane better maintain total HBF, oxygen supply, and delivery–consumption ratios than halothane or enflurane (Fig. 40.4) [102,103]. Although sevoflurane and desflurane appear to have the least effect on HBF, it is important to note that, among the commonly used agents (isoflurane, sevoflurane, and desflurane), these effects are dose-dependent. Consequently, efforts to reduce the dose administered will have a significantly greater impact than choice of inhalant anesthetic.

Halothane hepatotoxicity can be subdivided into type 1 (mild) and type 2 (fulminant). The causes of type 1 and type 2 hepatotoxicities are not fully understood but they are thought to be completely separate disease processes. Type 1 hepatotoxicity is much more common and has a self-limiting course. The hypothesized mechanism is that when halothane is broken down via the CYP450 system, it biotransforms into reactive intermediates. Metabolism

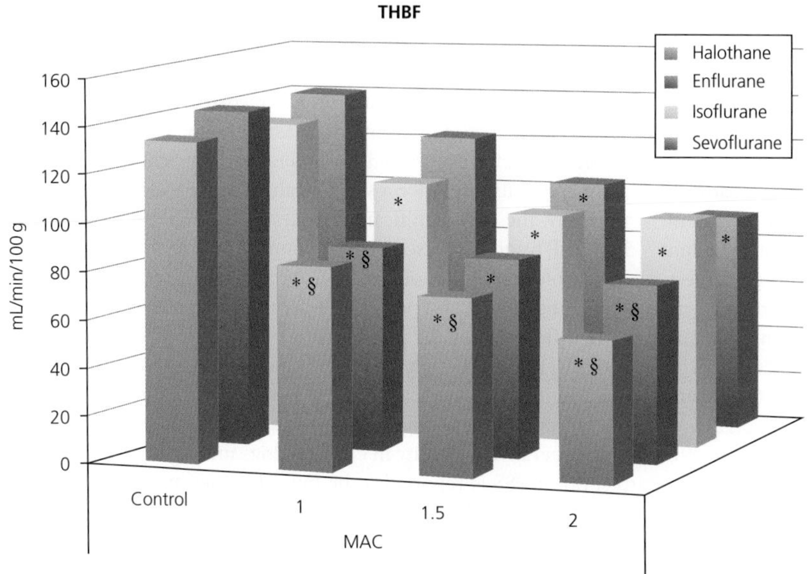

Figure 40.4 Effect of inhalant anesthetics on total hepatic blood flow (THBF) in Greyhound dogs. Bars marked with * are significantly different ($p<0.05$) from their respective control group (awake dogs). Bars marked with § are significantly different ($p<0.05$) from THBF values for isoflurane and sevoflurane at comparable minimum alveolar concentration (MAC) levels. Source: Adapted from Hartman *et al.* [102]; Frink *et al.* [103].

via oxidation and reduction are simultaneous via CYP2E1/CYP2A6 and CYP3A4/CYP2A6 pathways, respectively, dependent on oxygen tension. Metabolism via the reductive pathway causes increased hepatocyte hypoxemia and subsequent injury. Free radical intermediates, chlorotrifluoroethane or chlorodifluoroethene, are created in this pathway. These free radicals can lead to inactivation and destruction of CYP450, resulting in elevation of aminotransferases. Apart from type 1 hepatotoxicity, which occurs in approximately 20–30% of patients, halothane may also induce fulminant hepatitis (i.e., type 2 hepatotoxicity). The immune system plays a key role in the development of halothane hepatitis. Liver trifluoroacetyl protein adducts are created via the oxidative biotransformation of halothane, resulting in an antibody-mediated reaction triggering hepatitis [104].

Isoflurane in a lipid emulsion was demonstrated to have a protective effect on hepatic ischemia/reperfusion injury (IRI) when injected intravenously into rats. The mechanism for such protection seemed to be related to Kupffer cell inhibition [105]. Conversely, another study found protective effects of inhaling sevoflurane when given before, during, and after injury, but failed to find any beneficial effect of isoflurane administered by the same route on a rat model of IRI [106]. Perhaps inhalant preconditioning may have beneficial effects during hepatic surgery if IRI is predicted. For infants with obstructive jaundice that had reduced portal blood flow and compensatory increases in HA blood flow, sevoflurane displayed a protective effect on HBF [107]. Moreover, it exhibited anti-inflammatory and tissue-protective properties during liver IRI [108].

Neuromuscular blocking agents

The disposition of neuromuscular blocking agents (NMBAs) may be affected by liver disease. Vecuronium, rocuronium, and mivacurium all have increased volumes of distribution, prolonged elimination half-lives, and prolonged durations of effect in human patients with hepatic cirrhosis [109–111]. Atracurium and cisatracurium undergo liver-independent elimination (by non-specific ester hydrolysis or Hofmann elimination) and have similar pharmacokinetics and pharmacodynamics in both healthy and liver-diseased patients [112,113]. A study evaluating cisatracurium found no difference in onset and duration of action between healthy and PSS-affected dogs [114]. Exclusion of liver from the circulation resulted in significantly reduced requirement of rocuronium during orthotopic liver transplantation in humans; however, sugammadex could rapidly reverse the blockade in patients with liver dysfunction undergoing hepatic surgery [115,116].

Hepatic pathophysiology and anesthetic management

The management of patients with hepatic dysfunction centers around three main concerns: hepatic synthetic function (e.g., albumin, blood glucose, and coagulation proteins), hepatic metabolic function (Phase I and II reactions), and maintenance of hepatic oxygen delivery to avoid further hepatic insult. Preanesthetic evaluation and diagnostic testing can help define the degree of impairment and provide information about how the anesthetic plan should be altered and how much anesthetic risk is increased.

Hepatitis

Patients with acute or chronic hepatitis (CH) can present clinical signs and laboratory abnormalities that may be correlated with prognosis. Generally, the clinical signs and laboratory results for patients with liver dysfunction are non-specific (e.g., anorexia, diarrhea, weight loss, polyuria/polydipsia, fever, and fatigue). Jaundice, coagulation abnormalities, HE, and ascites can also be present, representing significant hepatic insufficiency. Ascites is a negative prognostic factor in dogs and humans with hepatitis [117]. Interestingly, one study found no relationship between the biochemical parameter results and severity of liver disease [118]. In another study investigating CH in Labrador Retrievers, it was demonstrated that 45% of these dogs presented with hyperbilirubinemia and 21% with hypoalbuminemia. Also, it was shown that prolongation of PT and aPTT, thrombocytopenia, anorexia, and hypoglobulinemia were associated with shorter survival times [39]. Another single-center study found that 57% of patients with hepatic diseases had at least one abnormal coagulation parameter at presentation. Furthermore, the presence of cirrhosis in addition to CH was associated with the worst coagulation abnormalities among all liver diseases. Most of the coagulation abnormalities found in this study were related to a decrease in coagulation factor synthesis, and not due to increased consumption of factors [119]. Therefore, the simple presence of hepatic disease demonstrated by biochemical abnormalities with or without clinical signs should be taken into consideration by the anesthetist, independent of the degree of abnormality, as the blood work changes do not necessarily correlate with disease severity. Also, in CH, coagulopathies are often absent, probably due to the balanced decrease in pro- and anticoagulant factors. However, in the presence of an insult, such as surgery, decompensation can occur, and postoperative coagulopathy can result. This is particularly problematic in hypotensive patients where large volumes of fluid therapy are used to maintain perfusion. Volume expansion dilutes circulating coagulation factors and can cause decompensation and clinical abnormalities [120,121].

Portosystemic shunt

Portosystemic shunts (PSSs) are anomalous vessels flowing from the portal circulation (e.g., splenic, phrenic, cranial mesenteric, caudal mesenteric, gastric, or gastroduodenal veins) to the central circulation (e.g., vena cava or azygous vein) without first passing through the liver [122]. The blood bypassing the liver allows substances normally metabolized there (e.g., ammonia, bile acids, and short-chain fatty acids) to accumulate in the systemic circulation [123]. When shunts are present at birth, blood flow to the liver is decreased and hepatotropic substances are not effectively delivered. This results in a liver that fails to develop normally and that is often undersized with abnormal intrahepatic vascular structure.

PSS patients may present with non-specific signs such as hypoglycemia, hypoalbuminemia, coagulopathies, and altered response to substances metabolized and excreted by the liver [122,123]. Hypoglycemia and prolonged recoveries from anesthesia were reported in dogs with a congenital PSS [124], although postoperative administration of acepromazine may have contributed to the prolonged recoveries seen in those patients. Many patients are undiagnosed until they are anesthetized for surgical sterilization and fail to recover normally from anesthesia.

It has been hypothesized that refractory hypoglycemia in dogs with PSS could be due to relative adrenal insufficiency, similar to that commonly seen with sepsis. In one study, no difference was found in preoperative baseline or post-ACTH stimulation testing among healthy dogs presenting for ovariohysterectomy and dogs with PSS. However, 30% of the PSS dogs presented with preoperative hypoglycemia and over 40% developed hypoglycemia within 4 h after surgery. Although inadequate adrenal response was not found in this population of PSS dogs, animals that presented with postoperative refractory hypoglycemia or prolonged anesthetic recoveries usually responded to the administration of dexamethasone (0.1 mg/kg, IV) [124].

Seizures and HE may occur in PSS cases and are considered poor prognostic indicators [64]. Flumazenil has been used to improve mental status in humans with HE and it is hypothesized that intrinsic benzodiazepine-like compounds are important in this syndrome [125]. However, in dogs with chronic HE 8 to 12 weeks after placement of a portocaval shunt and 40% hepatectomy, sarmazenil caused significant improvement of encephalopathy signs, while flumazenil had no effect [126]. Recently, C-reactive protein plasma levels were shown to be elevated in PSS dogs presenting with HE [127]. These findings reinforce the similarities in the pathogenesis of HE in humans and PSS dogs and the involvement of an inflammatory process in its pathogenesis.

In a prospective study, platelet count, packed cell volume, and factor II, V, VII, and X concentrations were lower prior to surgery and aPTT was prolonged in PSS dogs compared with healthy dogs. The postoperative hemostatic profile revealed further alterations such as an increase in PT and decrease in factor I, IX, and XI concentrations. However, when postoperative hemostatic values were compared with those for a set of healthy patients undergoing ovariectomy, the only significant changes in the PSS group were prolonged PT and decreased platelet count. Additionally, even though the absolute activities of factors II, V, VII, and X were lower in the PSS group, the relative percentage changes from preoperative values were different only for platelet count and factor II (prothrombin) activity [128]. Although the *in vitro* coagulation tests of PSS patients are commonly abnormal, clinical signs of bleeding disorders are uncommon in these dogs during and after shunt attenuation.

Preoperative mortality in cats and dogs undergoing surgical correction of PSS is reported to be low. However, postoperative outcomes have variable results in both species, including deterioration of patients' neurologic signs and death [129,130]. It is difficult to determine what role the anesthetic technique plays in postoperative outcomes. Many patients recover normally from anesthesia and begin to experience problems in the same time frame as the expected shunt closure, implying a greater role of altered blood flow in producing neurologic signs and death.

Hepatic neoplasia

Severe and uncontrollable hemorrhage is a potentially catastrophic complication during and following hepatic lobe resection. Immediate availability of blood products, including plasma, packed red blood cells, and whole blood, should be considered. Blood typing and cross-matching may be helpful in determining which donors are suitable for emergency transfusion. Preoperative autologous blood transfusion is also a feasible alternative to allogenic transfusions for dogs undergoing surgical procedures with a high risk of intraoperative hemorrhage (e.g., liver lobectomy) [131]. Other blood-saving strategies incorporated to minimize intraoperative blood loss during major surgery in human patients include use of antifibrinolytics (e.g., tranexamic acid, ε-aminocaproic acid), acute normovolemic hemodilution, cell salvage, surgical-site drains, laparoscopic and robotic surgery, diathermy, and topical agents (e.g., fibrin sealants, gelatin-thrombin matrices, and oxidized cellulose) [114].

Neoplasia may be associated with preoperative hemoabdomen, and a preanesthetic transfusion may be necessary to improve perfusion and oxygen delivery during anesthesia. Quantification of the volume of blood lost before hemostasis is achieved can be helpful in determining the need for blood replacement, but the chronicity of blood loss will usually result in varying hemodynamic consequences. Therefore, decisions to transfuse are often based on several factors, including hematocrit, rate of blood loss, volume of blood loss, and hemodynamic stability. Blood flow and oxygen uptake by the liver may be impaired by hemodynamic instability, manipulation of the liver, endogenous and exogenous vasoconstrictors, and anesthetic agents. Central venous catheterization can be helpful when substantial fluid shifts or large-volume transfusions are anticipated.

The major goal of fluid therapy is to optimize tissue perfusion, which is usually achieved by an increase in CO. Whether the latter will occur after a fluid challenge depends mostly on where the individual patient lies on the cardiac function (Frank–Starling) curve. If the patient lies on the steep side of this curve, CO should increase after preload augmentation (i.e., the patient is fluid-responsive). However, after the plateau is reached, further increases in preload do not lead to significant increases in CO (i.e., the patient is fluid non-responsive). Thus, fluid loading in this setting may be hazardous. Over the past two decades, many studies have been performed in human and veterinary medicine to search for the best index to predict fluid responsiveness in a variety of clinical situations and to optimize volume resuscitation of critically ill patients undergoing major surgeries. Dynamic indexes (e.g., pulse pressure variation, stroke volume variation, systolic pressure variation, and superior and inferior vena cava diameter variations) have been shown to be clearly superior to the traditional static preload variables (e.g., pulmonary artery occlusion pressure and central venous pressure) [132–134]. During hepatic retraction, compression of the major abdominal vessels by the surgeon is possible. Effective communication between the anesthetist and surgeon is extremely important to facilitate diagnosis of major hemodynamic complications versus temporary insults necessary for surgical access. Both hypo- and hypercarbia decrease portal blood flow, and vigilant monitoring is necessary to prevent and promptly treat these complications. Coagulopathies and poor liver function are often confounding factors in these surgical cases and prognosis worsens as the percentage of hepatic mass excised increases.

Studies of the effects of general anesthesia and types of anesthetics on surgical outcomes are lacking. General anesthesia is known to cause dose-dependent cardiovascular and immune suppression. In an attempt to minimize such complications, Yamamoto *et al.* reported a case series in which all patients had partial hepatectomies under only sedation and epidural anesthesia. After following 10 human patients, it was concluded that epidural techniques can be used for partial hepatectomies and also for other abdominal surgeries [135]. Recently, thoracolumbar epidural anesthesia with lidocaine resulted in either steady or increased HBF compared to saline control in propofol-anesthetized dogs, probably due to vasodilation of the HA induced by selective blockade of sympathetic ganglia [136].

Hepatic lobe torsion

Hepatic lobe torsion has been described in dogs, horses, cats, and rabbits. The outcome is reported to be mostly favorable if recognition and surgical correction are made early. Canine patients may show relatively mild non-specific clinical signs such as increased liver enzymes. Similar to dogs, horses present with non-specific clinical signs and laboratory results, including peritoneal fluid accumulation, colic, inappetence, lethargy, and increased liver enzymes, which makes diagnosis difficult, potentially resulting in poor prognosis [137]. Surgical removal of the liver lobe is indicated, and anesthetic management is similar to hepatic lobe resection for neoplasia. In the rabbit, medical management may be viable, but these patients may still need to be anesthetized for diagnostic imaging [138].

Gallbladder and extrahepatic biliary tract pathology

Extrahepatic biliary obstruction (EHBO) and cholecystectomy are associated with relatively high perioperative morbidity and mortality. In one study, preoperative elevation of plasma creatinine and hypotension in the immediate postoperative period were associated with increased mortality, especially in the presence of pancreatitis and septic bile peritonitis [139]. The earlier assumption of hypocoagulability in canine patients with EHBO should be re-evaluated. Hypercoagulability in dogs with gallbladder mucoceles has also been demonstrated by thromboelastography (TEG) [45]. As in humans with EHBO, it is possible that either hyper- or hypocoagulation can be present and should be investigated to provide the appropriate support or treatment [140]. In a study investigating the association of gallbladder mucoceles and endocrinopathies, dogs with hyperadrenocorticism were 29 times more likely to have a biliary mucocele [141]. These findings are important to the anesthesiologist as hyperadrenocorticism may also be associated with hypercoagulable states.

Anesthetic considerations for diagnostic or minimally invasive procedures

Liver biopsy may be necessary to determine the etiology and prognosis of hepatic disease. Samples can be obtained by ultrasound guidance, laparoscopy, and laparotomy. Laparoscopy and laparotomy can also be used for the staging and resection of neoplasia or hepatobiliary repair. Knowledge of the specific implications of each technique is vital for the anesthetist.

Ultrasound-guided biopsy

Biopsies can often be accomplished with sedation alone. For this technique, the patient needs to lie still and not react to the sound or sensation of device activation. There is a chance that bleeding will occur after the biopsy, so the technique is not advisable in animals with significant coagulation abnormalities. The patient's clinical signs and laboratory results, in addition to their demeanor and mentation, will determine drug combination and dose selection. Administration of an opioid alone or in combination with midazolam or dexmedetomidine is often sufficient to facilitate ultrasound-guided biopsies in a range of mildly to severely obtunded patients. Flumazenil can be administered to reverse the sedative effects of benzodiazepines if necessary. When dexmedetomidine is used, atipamezole administration usually results in rapid and complete reversal of sedation and cardiovascular effects. In the absence of pain, naloxone may be administered to improve mentation and ventilation when opioid analgesia is no longer required or desirable. Vasovagal hypotension shortly after percutaneous liver biopsy has been reported [142]. Post-procedure monitoring for signs of hemorrhage (e.g., mucous membrane color, blood pressure, hematocrit, or repeat ultrasound) is warranted when the risk of bleeding is significant.

Laparoscopic procedures

In addition to the possibility of bleeding and potential difficulties in achieving hemostasis, laparoscopy introduces concerns related to insufflation of gases into the abdomen. The infusion of carbon dioxide to distend the abdomen and improve visualization can decrease cardiac venous return and impair ventilation. Cranial displacement of the diaphragm can make it more difficult for the spontaneously breathing animal to maintain adequate minute ventilation due to decreased pulmonary functional residual capacity and tidal volume. Reduction in functional residual capacity may also increase the risk of perianesthetic hypoxemia. Intermittent positive-pressure ventilation (IPPV) may be required to maintain adequate oxygenation and ventilation. The anesthetist should also communicate with the surgeon to monitor the intra-abdominal pressure, which should range from 10–16 mmHg with allowance for species differences [143]. In dogs, pneumoperitoneum can cause transient increases in hepatic transaminases that last up to 48 h after desufflation. The increases in ALT and AST were directly proportional to the intra-abdominal pressure and duration of insufflation [144]. The use of IPPV can decrease HBF, probably by decreasing venous return and CO, so ventilator settings must be vigilantly monitored. A reversed Trendelenburg position can help to minimize the effect of carboperitoneum on ventilation; however, body position is usually dictated by the need of the surgeon to ensure adequate visualization. Capnography, although helpful, can be misleading because the difference between end-tidal ($P_{ET}CO_2$) and arterial ($PaCO_2$) carbon dioxide tensions can be significant due to ventilation–perfusion mismatching in some patients. Arterial blood gas analysis may be more indicative of ventilatory status.

Laparotomy

In addition to the concerns already mentioned for hepatic patients (e.g., hypoglycemia, hypoproteinemia, coagulopathies, and decreased drug metabolism), universal complications associated with any general anesthetic episode and open abdominal surgery must be taken into consideration. Hypothermia (which can exacerbate coagulopathies) is common in these cases and body temperature should be monitored and supportive measures instituted.

Interventional radiology

This technique uses fluoroscopy to guide an intravenous catheter to the site where an anomalous vessel (PSS) joins the systemic circulation. An expandable stent is placed in the caudal vena cava next to the anomalous insertion. This stent will prevent the thrombotic coils deployed into the shunt vessel from becoming lost in the systemic circulation if they dislodge [145]. The challenge for the anesthetist is to ensure complete immobilization of the patient at the critical stage of stent placement. During general anesthesia, an NMBA (e.g., rocuronium or atracurium) bolus or infusion can facilitate immobilization if mechanical ventilation is available. In some situations, the interventionalist may require an inspiratory hold to decrease the patient's abdominal movement during critical periods (e.g., measuring the anomalous vessel and placement of the stent). Hypothermia is a common problem, and the use of a radiolucent heating pad is essential. Monitoring of cardiovascular (i.e., arterial blood pressure, heart rate and rhythm, and central venous pressure) and respiratory parameters (i.e., $P_{ET}CO_2$ and SpO_2) is required. Invasive arterial blood pressure monitoring is ideal, but not mandatory, and central venous pressure can be measured by connecting a sterile electronic transducer to the jugular catheter used by the surgeon to place the stent. Central venous pressure measurements will help assess patient blood volume and guide fluid therapy based on trends, and also inform the surgeon of the abdominal caval pressure as the catheter is advanced. As in other patients with hepatic disease, volume, pressor, and inotropic support may be needed.

Pain management in hepatobiliary diseases

The goals of analgesia during hepatic surgery are similar to other types of surgery, but unique considerations such as altered pharmacokinetics and pharmacodynamics and altered mental status are included in planning of the analgesic regimen. Opioids remain the mainstay of analgesia in the perioperative period. Frequent assessments of analgesia are required to determine appropriate administration intervals. In humans, morphine can cause spasms of the common bile duct by constriction of the sphincter of Oddi, which increases the size and pressure in the gallbladder. This effect has not been demonstrated or observed in veterinary patients [146]. Sufentanil, alfentanil, fentanyl, and remifentanil are shorter-acting opioids with pharmacokinetics that are minimally affected by liver disease. If a continuous infusion is not practical or desired, intermittent administration of hydromorphone, morphine, buprenorphine, methadone, and oxymorphone can be used, but a reduced dose or prolonged dosing interval may be needed. Opioid-induced gastrointestinal disturbances (e.g., nausea, vomiting, gastrointestinal reflux, and ileus) should be managed with antiemetics and prokinetics.

Infiltration of the surgical incision or performing regional blockade using thoracic epidural analgesia, transversus abdominis plane block, rectus sheath block, or quadratus lumborum block with long-acting local anesthetics such as bupivacaine 0.25–0.5% or liposomal bupivacaine suspension can be strategies for multimodal analgesia for hepatic surgery. Benefits of regional techniques include adequate postoperative pain management, enhanced recovery and surgical outcomes, intraoperative inhalant-sparing effects, and reduced need for opioids during the perioperative period [147]. Non-steroidal anti-inflammatory drugs (NSAIDs) are also a viable option, however, they have the potential to cause hepatic injury, either intrinsically (e.g., aspirin and acetaminophen) or idiosyncratically (e.g., COX-2-selective agents). Idiosyncratic toxic reactions are rare, unpredictable, and not related to dose or pre-existing liver disease. Clinical signs include inappetence, vomiting, and icterus associated with elevations in serum hepatic enzymes and bilirubin. Any unexplained increase in these biochemical parameters after initiation of NSAID therapy should be investigated. Additionally, NSAIDs may impair coagulation and hemostasis by affecting clot formation and platelet aggregation. Owing to the potential for adverse effects, the administration of NSAIDs to patients with hepatic dysfunction, especially those with coagulopathies, should be avoided or very closely monitored.

References

1 Weiss DJ, Gagne JM, Armstrong PJ. Relationship between inflammatory hepatic disease and inflammatory bowel disease, pancreatitis, and nephritis in cats. *J Am Vet Med Assoc* 1996; **209**(6): 1114–1116.

2 Du Y, Li N, Long M. Liver sinusoid on a chip. In: Doh J, Fletcher D, Piel M, eds. *Methods in Cell Biology*. Cambridge, MA: Elsevier, 2018; **146**: 105–134.

3 Trefts E, Gannon M, Wasserman DH. The liver. *Curr Biol* 2017; **27**(21): R1147–R1151.

4 Charbon GA, Anderson MF. Hepatic haemodynamics as related to blood flow through gut, spleen, and pancreas. *Gut* 1989; **30**(2): 265–278.

5 Ljubicic N, Bilic A. The effects of selective and non-selective adrenoceptor blockade on the portal blood flow in patients with liver cirrhosis. *Scand J Gastroenterol* 1991; **26**(7): 751–757.

6 Gelman S, Mushlin PS. Catecholamine-induced changes in the splanchnic circulation affecting systemic hemodynamics. *Anesthesiology* 2004; **100**(2): 434–439.

7 Eipel C, Abshagen K, Vollmar B. Regulation of hepatic blood flow: the hepatic arterial buffer response revisited. *World J Gastroenterol* 2010; **16**(48): 6046–6057.

8 Lautt WW, Legare DJ, d'Almeida MS. Adenosine as putative regulator of hepatic arterial flow (the buffer response). *Am J Physiol* 1985; **248**(3 Pt 2): H331–H338.

9 Mulaikal T, Emond JC. Physiology and anatomy of the liver. In: Wagener G, ed. *Liver Anesthesiology and Critical Care Medicine*, 2nd edn. Switzerland: Springer International Publishing AG, part of Springer Nature, 2018: 3–18.

10 Schreiber G, Urban J. The synthesis and secretion of albumin. *Rev Physiol Biochem Pharmacol* 1978; **82**: 27–95.

11 Smith SA, Waters NJ. Pharmacokinetic and Pharmacodynamic considerations for drugs binding to alpha-1-acid glycoprotein. *Pharm Res* 2018; **36**(2): 30.

12 Hunter RP, Mahmood I, Martinez MN. Prediction of xenobiotic clearance in avian species using mammalian or avian data: how accurate is the prediction? *J Vet Pharmacol Ther* 2008; **31**(3): 281–284.

13 Sindrup SH, Brosen K. The pharmacogenetics of codeine hypoalgesia. *Pharmacogenetics* 1995; **5**(6): 335–346.

14 Center SA, Elston TH, Rowland PH, *et al.* Fulminant hepatic failure associated with oral administration of diazepam in 11 cats. *J Am Vet Med Assoc* 1996; **209**(3): 618–625.

15 Shimada T, Mimura M, Inoue K, *et al.* Cytochrome P450-dependent drug oxidation activities in liver microsomes of various animal species including rats, guinea pigs, dogs, monkeys, and humans. *Arch Toxicol* 1997; **71**(6): 401–408.
16 Court MH, Hay-Kraus BL, Hill DW, *et al.* Propofol hydroxylation by dog liver microsomes: assay development and dog breed differences. *Drug Metab Dispos* 1999; **27**(11): 1293–1299.
17 van Beusekom CD, Schipper L, Fink-Gremmels J. Cytochrome P450-mediated hepatic metabolism of new fluorescent substrates in cats and dogs. *J Vet Pharmacol Ther* 2010; **33**(6): 519–527.
18 Capel ID, Millburn P, Williams RT. The conjugation of 1- and 2-naphthols and other phenols in the cat and pig. *Xenobiotica* 1974; **4**(10): 601–615.
19 Capel ID, French MR, Millburn P, *et al.* Species variations in the metabolism of phenol. *Biochem J* 1972; **127**(2): 25P–26P.
20 Court MH, Greenblatt DJ. Molecular basis for deficient acetaminophen glucuronidation in cats. An interspecies comparison of enzyme kinetics in liver microsomes. *Biochem Pharmacol* 1997; **53**(7): 1041–1047.
21 Ebner T, Schanzle G, Weber W, *et al.* In vitro glucuronidation of the angiotensin II receptor antagonist telmisartan in the cat: a comparison with other species. *J Vet Pharmacol Ther* 2013; **36**(2): 154–160.
22 Zhao M, Ma J, Li M, *et al.* Cytochrome P450 enzymes and drug metabolism in humans. *Int J Mol Sci* 2021; **22**(23): 12808.
23 Livingston A, Waterman AE. The development of tolerance to ketamine in rats and the significance of hepatic metabolism. *Br J Pharmacol* 1978; **64**(1): 63–69.
24 Lee J, Boyer JL. Molecular alterations in hepatocyte transport mechanisms in acquired cholestatic liver disorders. *Semin Liver Dis* 2000; **20**(3): 373–384.
25 Mealey KL, Northrup NC, Bentjen SA. Increased toxicity of P-glycoprotein-substrate chemotherapeutic agents in a dog with the MDR1 deletion mutation associated with ivermectin sensitivity. *J Am Vet Med Assoc* 2003; **223**(10): 1434, 1453–1455.
26 Fink-Gremmels J. Implications of hepatic cytochrome P450-related biotransformation processes in veterinary sciences. *Eur J Pharmacol* 2008; **585**(2–3): 502–509.
27 Laskin DL. Nonparenchymal cells and hepatotoxicity. *Semin Liver Dis* 1990; **10**(4): 293–304.
28 Katz S, Jimenez MA, Lehmkuhler WE, *et al.* Liver bacterial clearance following hepatic artery ligation and portacaval shunt. *J Surg Res* 1991; **51**(3): 267–270.
29 Dhainaut JF, Marin N, Mignon A, *et al.* Hepatic response to sepsis: interaction between coagulation and inflammatory processes. *Crit Care Med* 2001; **29**(7 Suppl): S42–S47.
30 Center SA, Erb HN, Joseph SA. Measurement of serum bile acids concentrations for diagnosis of hepatobiliary disease in cats. *J Am Vet Med Assoc* 1995; **207**(8): 1048–1054.
31 Webster CRL, Center SA, Cullen JM, *et al.* ACVIM consensus statement on the diagnosis and treatment of chronic hepatitis in dogs. *J Vet Intern Med* 2019; **33**(3): 1173–1200.
32 Lawrence YA, Steiner JM. Laboratory evaluation of the liver. *Vet Clin North Am Small Anim Pract* 2017; **47**(3): 539–553.
33 Ruland K, Fischer A, Hartmann K. Sensitivity and specificity of fasting ammonia and serum bile acids in the diagnosis of portosystemic shunts in dogs and cats. *Vet Clin Pathol* 2010; **39**(1): 57–64.
34 Weiss M, Krejcie TC, Avram MJ. A physiologically based model of hepatic ICG clearance: interplay between sinusoidal uptake and biliary excretion. *Eur J Pharm Sci* 2011; **44**(3): 359–365.
35 Ercolani G, Grazi GL, Calliva R, *et al.* The lidocaine (MEGX) test as an index of hepatic function: its clinical usefulness in liver surgery. *Surgery* 2000; **127**(4): 464–471.
36 Devriendt N, Serrano G, Croubels S, *et al.* Evaluation of serum lidocaine/monoethylglycylxylidide concentration to assess shunt closure in dogs with extrahepatic portosystemic shunts. *J Vet Intern Med* 2021; **35**(1): 261–268.
37 Assawarachan SN, Chuchalermporn P, Maneesaay P, *et al.* Changes in serum lipid profiles among canine patients suffering from chronic hepatitis. *Vet Sci* 2021; **8**(10): 221.
38 Center SA, Slater MR, Manwarren T, *et al.* Diagnostic efficacy of serum alkaline phosphatase and gamma-glutamyltransferase in dogs with histologically confirmed hepatobiliary disease: 270 cases (1980–1990). *J Am Vet Med Assoc* 1992; **201**(8): 1258–1264.
39 Shih JL, Keating JH, Freeman LM, *et al.* Chronic hepatitis in Labrador Retrievers: clinical presentation and prognostic factors. *J Vet Intern Med* 2007; **21**(1): 33–39.
40 Niles JD, Williams JM, Cripps PJ. Hemostatic profiles in 39 dogs with congenital portosystemic shunts. *Vet Surg* 2001; **30**(1): 97–104.
41 Kelley D, Lester C, DeLaforcade A, *et al.* Thromboelastographic evaluation of dogs with congenital portosystemic shunts. *J Vet Intern Med* 2013; **27**(5): 1262–1267.
42 Lisman T, Hernandez-Gea V, Magnusson M, *et al.* The concept of rebalanced hemostasis in patients with liver disease: communication from the ISTH SSC working group on hemostatic management of patients with liver disease. *J Thromb Haemost* 2021; **19**(4): 1116–1122.
43 Fry W, Lester C, Etedali NM, *et al.* Thromboelastography in dogs with chronic hepatopathies. *J Vet Intern Med* 2017; **31**(2): 419–426.
44 Webster CR. Hemostatic disorders associated with hepatobiliary disease. *Vet Clin North Am Small Anim Pract* 2017; **47**(3): 601–615.
45 Pavlick M, DeLaforcade A, Penninck DG, *et al.* Evaluation of coagulation parameters in dogs with gallbladder mucoceles. *J Vet Intern Med* 2021; **35**(4): 1763–1772.
46 Shao Z, Zhao Y, Feng L, *et al.* Association between plasma fibrinogen levels and mortality in acute-on-chronic hepatitis B liver failure. *Dis Markers* 2015; **2015**: 468596.
47 Elhiblu MA, Dua K, Mohindroo J, *et al.* Clinico-hemato-biochemical profile of dogs with liver cirrhosis. *Vet World* 2015; **8**(4): 487–491.
48 Girolami A, Ferrari S, Cosi E, *et al.* Vitamin K-dependent coagulation factors that may be responsible for both bleeding and thrombosis (FII, FVII, and FIX). *Clin Appl Thromb Hemost* 2018; **24**(Suppl 9): 42S–47S.
49 Stanworth SJ. The evidence-based use of FFP and cryoprecipitate for abnormalities of coagulation tests and clinical coagulopathy. *Hematology Am Soc Hematol Educ Program* 2007: 179–186.
50 Shah NL, Intagliata NM, Northup PG, *et al.* Procoagulant therapeutics in liver disease: a critique and clinical rationale. *Nat Rev Gastroenterol Hepatol* 2014; **11**(11): 675–682.
51 Wei H, Child LJ. Clinical utility of viscoelastic testing in chronic liver disease: a systematic review. *World J Hepatol* 2020; **12**(11): 1115–1127.
52 Buriko Y, Drobatz K, Silverstein DC. Establishment of normal reference intervals in dogs using a viscoelastic point-of-care coagulation monitor and its comparison with thromboelastography. *Vet Clin Pathol* 2020; **49**(4): 567–573.
53 Rosati T, Jandrey KE, Burges JW, *et al.* Establishment of a reference interval for a novel viscoelastic coagulometer and comparison with thromboelastography in healthy cats. *Vet Clin Pathol* 2020; **49**(4): 660–664.
54 Kelley D, Lester C, Shaw S, *et al.* Thromboelastographic evaluation of dogs with acute liver disease. *J Vet Intern Med* 2015; **29**(4): 1053–1062.
55 Kakar N, Daniel G, Fellman C, *et al.* Thromboelastography in cats with cholestatic liver disease. *J Feline Med Surg* 2021; **23**(2): 160–167.
56 Guedes AG, Papich MG, Rude EP, *et al.* Comparison of plasma histamine levels after intravenous administration of hydromorphone and morphine in dogs. *J Vet Pharmacol Ther* 2007; **30**(6): 516–522.
57 Robinson EP, Faggella AM, Henry DP, *et al.* Comparison of histamine release induced by morphine and oxymorphone administration in dogs. *Am J Vet Res* 1988; **49**(10): 1699–1701.
58 Imani F, Motavaf M, Safari S, *et al.* The therapeutic use of analgesics in patients with liver cirrhosis: a literature review and evidence-based recommendations. *Hepat Mon* 2014; **14**(10): e23539.
59 Rakoski M, Goyal P, Spencer-Safier M, *et al.* Pain management in patients with cirrhosis. *Clin Liver Dis (Hoboken)* 2018; **11**(6): 135–140.
60 Soleimanpour H, Safari S, Shahsavari Nia K, *et al.* Opioid drugs in patients with liver disease: a systematic review. *Hepat Mon* 2016; **16**(4): e32636.
61 Dershwitz M, Hoke JF, Rosow CE, *et al.* Pharmacokinetics and Pharmacodynamics of remifentanil in volunteer subjects with severe liver disease. *Anesthesiology* 1996; **84**(4): 812–820.
62 Bostrom I, Nyman G, Kampa N, *et al.* Effects of acepromazine on renal function in anesthetized dogs. *Am J Vet Res* 2003; **64**(5): 590–598.
63 Barr SC, Ludders JW, Looney AL, *et al.* Platelet aggregation in dogs after sedation with acepromazine and atropine and during subsequent general anesthesia and surgery. *Am J Vet Res* 1992; **53**(11): 2067–2070.
64 Lidbury JA, Cook AK, Steiner JM. Hepatic encephalopathy in dogs and cats. *J Vet Emerg Crit Care (San Antonio)* 2016; **26**(4): 471–487.
65 Palomero-Gallagher N, Zilles K. Neurotransmitter receptor alterations in hepatic encephalopathy: a review. *Arch Biochem Biophys* 2013; **536**(2): 109–121.
66 Als-Nielsen B, Gluud LL, Gluud C. Benzodiazepine receptor antagonists for hepatic encephalopathy. *Cochrane Database Syst Rev* 2004; **(2)**: CD002798.
67 Jones EA, Yurdaydin C, Basile AS. The role of endogenous benzodiazepines in hepatic encephalopathy: animal studies. *Alcohol Alcohol Suppl* 1993; **2**: 175–180.
68 Nishiyama T, Hirasaki A, Toda N, *et al.* Pharmacokinetics of midazolam in patients with liver damage for hepatectomy. *Masui* 1993; **42**(6): 871–875.
69 Bozkurt P, Kaya G, Suzer O, *et al.* Diazepam serum concentration-sedative effect relationship in patients with liver disease. *Middle East J Anaesthesiol* 1996; **13**(4): 405–413.
70 Flacke WE, Flacke JW, Bloor BC, *et al.* Effects of dexmedetomidine on systemic and coronary hemodynamics in the anesthetized dog. *J Cardiothorac Vasc Anesth* 1993; **7**(1): 41–49.
71 Lawrence CJ, Prinzen FW, de Lange S. The effect of dexmedetomidine on nutrient organ blood flow. *Anesth Analg* 1996; **83**(6): 1160–1165.
72 Talke PO, Traber DL, Richardson CA, *et al.* The effect of alpha(2) agonist-induced sedation and its reversal with an alpha(2) antagonist on organ blood flow in sheep. *Anesth Analg* 2000; **90**(5): 1060–1066.

73 Baratta MT, Zaya MJ, White JA, *et al.* Canine CYP2B11 metabolizes and is inhibited by anesthetic agents often co-administered in dogs. *J Vet Pharmacol Ther* 2010; **33**(1): 50–55.
74 Thomson IA, Fitch W, Campbell D, *et al.* Effects of ketamine on liver blood flow and hepatic oxygen consumption. Studies in the anaesthetised greyhound. *Acta Anaesthesiol Scand* 1988; **32**(1): 10–14.
75 Thomson IA, Fitch W, Hughes RL, *et al.* Effects of certain i.v. anaesthetics on liver blood flow and hepatic oxygen consumption in the greyhound. *Br J Anaesth* 1986; **58**(1): 69–80.
76 Wouters PF, Van de Velde MA, Marcus MA, *et al.* Hemodynamic changes during induction of anesthesia with eltanolone and propofol in dogs. *Anesth Analg* 1995; **81**(1): 125–131.
77 Haberer JP, Audibert G, Saunier CG, *et al.* Effect of propofol and thiopentone on regional blood flow in brain and peripheral tissues during normoxia and hypoxia in the dog. *Clin Physiol* 1993; **13**(2): 197–207.
78 Zhu T, Pang Q, McCluskey SA, *et al.* Effect of propofol on hepatic blood flow and oxygen balance in rabbits. *Can J Anaesth* 2008; **55**(6): 364–370.
79 Ye L, Luo CZ, McCluskey SA, *et al.* Propofol attenuates hepatic ischemia/reperfusion injury in an in vivo rabbit model. *J Surg Res* 2012; **178**(2): e65–e70.
80 Chan KC, Lin CJ, Lee PH, *et al.* Propofol attenuates the decrease of dynamic compliance and water content in the lung by decreasing oxidative radicals released from the reperfused liver. *Anesth Analg* 2008; **107**(4): 1284–1289.
81 Zoran DL, Riedesel DH, Dyer DC. Pharmacokinetics of propofol in mixed-breed dogs and Greyhounds. *Am J Vet Res* 1993; **54**(5): 755–760.
82 Servin F, Farinotti R, Haberer JP, *et al.* Propofol infusion for maintenance of anesthesia in morbidly obese patients receiving nitrous oxide. A clinical and pharmacokinetic study. *Anesthesiology* 1993; **78**(4): 657–665.
83 Posner LP, Asakawa M, Erb HN. Use of propofol for anesthesia in cats with primary hepatic lipidosis: 44 cases (1995–2004). *J Am Vet Med Assoc* 2008; **232**(12): 1841–1843.
84 Sams L, Braun C, Allman D, *et al.* A comparison of the effects of propofol and etomidate on the induction of anesthesia and on cardiopulmonary parameters in dogs. *Vet Anaesth Analg* 2008; **35**(6): 488–494.
85 van Limmen J, Wyffels P, Berrevoet F, *et al.* Effects of propofol and sevoflurane on hepatic blood flow: a randomized controlled trial. *BMC Anesthesiol* 2020; **20**(1): 241.
86 Blunnie WP, Zacharias M, Dundee JW, *et al.* Liver enzyme studies with continuous intravenous anaesthesia. *Anaesthesia* 1981; **36**(2): 152–156.
87 Sams RA, Muir WW. Effects of phenobarbital on thiopental pharmacokinetics in Greyhounds. *Am J Vet Res* 1988; **49**(2): 245–249.
88 Taylor JD, Richards RK, Tabern DL. Metabolism of S35 thiopental (Pentothal); chemical and paper chromatographic studies of S35 excretion by the rat and monkey. *J Pharmacol Exp Ther* 1952; **104**(1): 93–102.
89 Nebauer AE, Doenicke A, Hoernecke R, *et al.* Does etomidate cause haemolysis? *Br J Anaesth* 1992; **69**(1): 58–60.
90 Moon PF. Acute toxicosis in two dogs associated with etomidate-propylene glycol infusion. *Lab Anim Sci* 1994; **44**(6): 590–594.
91 Bonnardot JP, Levron JC, Deslauriers M, *et al.* Pharmacokinetics of continuous infusion of etomidate in cirrhotic patients. *Ann Fr Anesth Reanim* 1991; **10**(5): 443–449.
92 Carlos R, Calvo R, Erill S. Plasma protein binding of etomidate in patients with renal failure or hepatic cirrhosis. *Clin Pharmacokinet* 1979; **4**(2): 144–148.
93 Molenaar N, Bijkerk RM, Beishuizen A, *et al.* Steroidogenesis in the adrenal dysfunction of critical illness: impact of etomidate. *Crit Care* 2012; **16**(4): R121.
94 Hauser GJ, Brotzman HM, Kaufman SS. Hepatoadrenal syndrome in pediatric patients with end-stage liver disease. *Pediatr Crit Care Med* 2012; **13**(3): e145–e149.
95 Calvo R, Carlos R, Erill S. Etomidate and plasma esterase activity in man and experimental animals. *Pharmacology* 1979; **18**(6): 294–298.
96 Van Hamme MJ, Ghoneim MM, Ambre JJ. Pharmacokinetics of etomidate, a new intravenous anesthetic. *Anesthesiology* 1978; **49**(4): 274–277.
97 Kaka JS, Hayton WL. Pharmacokinetics of ketamine and two metabolites in the dog. *J Pharmacokinet Biopharm* 1980; **8**(2): 193–202.
98 Noppers IM, Niesters M, Aarts L, *et al.* Drug-induced liver injury following a repeated course of ketamine treatment for chronic pain in CRPS type 1 patients: a report of 3 cases. *Pain* 2011; **152**(9): 2173–2178.
99 Wai MS, Chan WM, Zhang AQ, *et al.* Long-term ketamine and ketamine plus alcohol treatments produced damages in liver and kidney. *Hum Exp Toxicol* 2012; **31**(9): 877–886.
100 Oohara K. Effect of ketamine on hepatic circulation and oxygen metabolism during hypoxia in dog. *Masui* 1993; **42**(10): 1440–1447.
101 Tranquilli WJ, Thurmon JC, Benson GJ. Organ blood flow and distribution of cardiac output in hypocapnic ketamine-anesthetized swine. *Am J Vet Res* 1983; **44**(8): 1578–1582.
102 Hartman JC, Pagel PS, Proctor LT, *et al.* Influence of desflurane, isoflurane and halothane on regional tissue perfusion in dogs. *Can J Anaesth* 1992; **39**(8): 877–887.
103 Frink EJ Jr., Morgan SE, Coetzee A, *et al.* The effects of sevoflurane, halothane, enflurane, and isoflurane on hepatic blood flow and oxygenation in chronically instrumented greyhound dogs. *Anesthesiology* 1992; **76**(1): 85–90.
104 Safari S, Motavaf M, Seyed Siamdoust SA, *et al.* Hepatotoxicity of halogenated inhalational anesthetics. *Iran Red Crescent Med J* 2014; **16**(9): e20153.
105 Lu H, Yang LQ, Yu WF, *et al.* Protection of liver against ischemia/reperfusion injury by Kupffer cell mediated emulsified isoflurane preconditioning: experiment with rats. *Zhonghua Yi Xue Za Zhi* 2007; **87**(35): 2468–2471.
106 Bedirli N, Ofluoglu E, Kerem M, *et al.* Hepatic energy metabolism and the differential protective effects of sevoflurane and isoflurane anesthesia in a rat hepatic ischemia-reperfusion injury model. *Anesth Analg* 2008; **106**(3): 830–837, table of contents.
107 Zhou ZJ, Wang X, Song Z, *et al.* Effect of sevoflurane anaesthesia on hepatic blood flow in infants with obstructive hepatobiliary disease. *Acta Anaesthesiol Scand* 2016; **60**(8): 1067–1074.
108 Granja TF, Kohler D, Schad J, *et al.* Adenosine receptor Adora2b plays a mechanistic role in the protective effect of the volatile anesthetic sevoflurane during liver ischemia/reperfusion. *Anesthesiology* 2016; **125**(3): 547–560.
109 Lebrault C, Berger JL, D'Hollander AA, *et al.* Pharmacokinetics and pharmacodynamics of vecuronium (ORG NC 45) in patients with cirrhosis. *Anesthesiology* 1985; **62**(5): 601–605.
110 Devlin JC, Head-Rapson AG, Parker CJ, *et al.* Pharmacodynamics of mivacurium chloride in patients with hepatic cirrhosis. *Br J Anaesth* 1993; **71**(2): 227–231.
111 van Miert MM, Eastwood NB, Boyd AH, *et al.* The pharmacokinetics and pharmacodynamics of rocuronium in patients with hepatic cirrhosis. *Br J Clin Pharmacol* 1997; **44**(2): 139–144.
112 De Wolf AM, Freeman JA, Scott VL, *et al.* Pharmacokinetics and pharmacodynamics of cisatracurium in patients with end-stage liver disease undergoing liver transplantation. *Br J Anaesth* 1996; **76**(5): 624–628.
113 Ward S, Neill EA. Pharmacokinetics of atracurium in acute hepatic failure (with acute renal failure). *Br J Anaesth* 1983; **55**(12): 1169–1172.
114 Adams WA, Mark Senior J, Jones RS, *et al.* cis-Atracurium in dogs with and without porto-systemic shunts. *Vet Anaesth Analg* 2006; **33**(1): 17–23.
115 Weng XC, Zhou L, Fu YY, *et al.* Dose requirements of continuous infusion of rocuronium and atracurium throughout orthotopic liver transplantation in humans. *J Zhejiang Univ Sci B* 2005; **6**(9): 869–872.
116 Fujita A, Ishibe N, Yoshihara T, *et al.* Rapid reversal of neuromuscular blockade by sugammadex after continuous infusion of rocuronium in patients with liver dysfunction undergoing hepatic surgery. *Acta Anaesthesiol Taiwan* 2014; **52**(2): 54–58.
117 Raffan E, McCallum A, Scase TJ, *et al.* Ascites is a negative prognostic indicator in chronic hepatitis in dogs. *J Vet Intern Med* 2009; **23**(1): 63–66.
118 Fuentealba C, Guest S, Haywood S, *et al.* Chronic hepatitis: a retrospective study in 34 dogs. *Can Vet J* 1997; **38**(6): 365–373.
119 Prins M, Schellens CJ, van Leeuwen MW, *et al.* Coagulation disorders in dogs with hepatic disease. *Vet J* 2010; **185**(2): 163–168.
120 118. Stellingwerff M, Brandsma A, Lisman T, *et al.* Prohemostatic interventions in liver surgery. *Semin Thromb Hemost* 2012; **38**(3): 244–249.
121 Rogers CL, O'Toole TE, Keating JH, *et al.* Portal vein thrombosis in cats: 6 cases (2001–2006). *J Vet Intern Med* 2008; **22**(2): 282–287.
122 Center SA, Magne ML. Historical, physical examination, and clinicopathologic features of portosystemic vascular anomalies in the dog and cat. *Semin Vet Med Surg Small Anim* 1990; **5**(2): 83–93.
123 Vallarino N, Pil S, Devriendt N, *et al.* Diagnostic value of blood variables following attenuation of congenital extrahepatic portosystemic shunt in dogs. *Vet Rec* 2020; **187**(7): e48.
124 Holford AL, Tobias KM, Bartges JW, *et al.* Adrenal response to adrenocorticotropic hormone in dogs before and after surgical attenuation of a single congenital portosystemic shunt. *J Vet Intern Med* 2008; **22**(4): 832–838.
125 Aronson LR, Gacad RC, Kaminsky-Russ K, *et al.* Endogenous benzodiazepine activity in the peripheral and portal blood of dogs with congenital portosystemic shunts. *Vet Surg* 1997; **26**(3): 189–194.
126 Meyer HP, Legemate DA, van den Brom W, *et al.* Improvement of chronic hepatic encephalopathy in dogs by the benzodiazepine-receptor partial inverse agonist sarmazenil, but not by the antagonist flumazenil. *Metab Brain Dis* 1998; **13**(3): 241–251.
127 Gow AG, Marques AI, Yool DA, *et al.* Dogs with congenital porto-systemic shunting (cPSS) and hepatic encephalopathy have higher serum concentrations of C-reactive protein than asymptomatic dogs with cPSS. *Metab Brain Dis* 2012; **27**(2): 227–229.
128 Kummeling A, Teske E, Rothuizen J, *et al.* Coagulation profiles in dogs with congenital portosystemic shunts before and after surgical attenuation. *J Vet Intern Med* 2006; **20**(6): 1319–1326.

129 Tisdall PL, Hunt GB, Youmans KR, *et al.* Neurological dysfunction in dogs following attenuation of congenital extrahepatic portosystemic shunts. *J Small Anim Pract* 2000; **41**(12): 539–546.
130 Lipscomb VJ, Jones HJ, Brockman DJ. Complications and long-term outcomes of the ligation of congenital portosystemic shunts in 49 cats. *Vet Rec* 2007; **160**(14): 465–470.
131 Sharma S, Boston SE, Kotlowski J, *et al.* Preoperative autologous blood donation and transfusion in dogs undergoing elective surgical oncology procedures with high risk of hemorrhage. *Vet Surg* 2021; **50**(3): 607–614.
132 Monnet X, Marik PE, Teboul JL. Prediction of fluid responsiveness: an update. *Ann Intensive Care* 2016; **6**(1): 111.
133 Araos J, Kenny JS, Rousseau-Blass F, *et al.* Dynamic prediction of fluid responsiveness during positive pressure ventilation: a review of the physiology underlying heart-lung interactions and a critical interpretation. *Vet Anaesth Analg* 2020; **47**(1): 3–14.
134 Boysen SR, Gommeren K. Assessment of volume status and fluid responsiveness in small animals. *Front Vet Sci* 2021; **8**: 630643.
135 Yamamoto K, Fukumori D, Yamamoto F, *et al.* First report of hepatectomy without endotracheal general anesthesia. *J Am Coll Surg* 2013; **216**(5): 908–914.
136 Iseri T, Nakamori M, Fujimoto Y. Effects of thoracolumbar epidural anesthesia with lidocaine on the systemic hemodynamics and hepatic blood flow in propofol anesthetized dogs. *J Vet Med Sci* 2021; **83**(12): 1877–1884.
137 Tennent-Brown BS, Mudge MC, Hardy J, *et al.* Liver lobe torsion in six horses. *J Am Vet Med Assoc* 2012; **241**(5): 615–620.
138 Sheen JC, Vella D, Hung L. Retrospective analysis of liver lobe torsion in pet rabbits: 40 cases (2016–2021). *Vet Rec* 2022: e1971.
139 Mehler SJ, Mayhew PD, Drobatz KJ, *et al.* Variables associated with outcome in dogs undergoing extrahepatic biliary surgery: 60 cases (1988–2002). *Vet Surg* 2004; **33**(6): 644–649.
140 Cakir T, Cingi A, Yegen C. Coagulation dynamics and platelet functions in obstructive jaundiced patients. *J Gastroenterol Hepatol* 2009; **24**(5): 748–751.
141 Mesich ML, Mayhew PD, Paek M, *et al.* Gall bladder mucoceles and their association with endocrinopathies in dogs: a retrospective case-control study. *J Small Anim Pract* 2009; **50**(12): 630–635.
142 Proot SJ, Rothuizen J. High complication rate of an automatic Tru-Cut biopsy gun device for liver biopsy in cats. *J Vet Intern Med* 2006; **20**(6): 1327–1333.
143 Mayhew PD. Advanced laparoscopic procedures (hepatobiliary, endocrine) in dogs and cats. *Vet Clin North Am Small Anim Pract* 2009; **39**(5): 925–939.
144 Nesek-Adam V, Rasic Z, Kos J, *et al.* Aminotransferases after experimental pneumoperitoneum in dogs. *Acta Anaesthesiol Scand* 2004; **48**(7): 862–866.
145 Bussadori R, Bussadori C, Millan L, *et al.* Transvenous coil embolisation for the treatment of single congenital portosystemic shunts in six dogs. *Vet J* 2008; **176**(2): 221–226.
146 Helm JF, Venu RP, Geenen JE, *et al.* Effects of morphine on the human sphincter of Oddi. *Gut* 1988; **29**(10): 1402–1407.
147 Dieu A, Huynen P, Lavand'homme P, *et al.* Pain management after open liver resection: Procedure-Specific Postoperative Pain Management (PROSPECT) recommendations. *Reg Anesth Pain Med* 2021; **46**(5): 433–445.

41 Physiology, Pathophysiology, and Anesthetic Management of Patients with Gastrointestinal Disease

Jennifer G. Adams
Hull, Georgia, USA

Chapter contents

Anatomy of the gastrointestinal tract, 862
Effects of anesthetic agents on gastrointestinal function, 863
- Nausea and vomiting, 864
- Gastroesophageal reflux, 865
- Esophagitis and esophageal stricture, 868
- Aspiration, 868
- Gastrointestinal motility/postoperative ileus, 869

Gastrointestinal conditions requiring anesthesia, 871
- Laparotomy, 871
- Megaesophagus, 873
- Gastric dilation–volvulus, 874
- Hemoabdomen, 876
- Intestinal neoplasia, 877
- Septic peritonitis, 879
- Foreign body removal and other abdominal procedures, 882

References, 882

Anatomy of the gastrointestinal tract

The gastrointestinal tract (GIT) of small animals is a continuous multilayered tube with variations in size, shape, and function for each organ. It includes the oropharynx, esophagus, stomach, small intestine, colon, and rectum. The liver, biliary tract, and exocrine pancreas are also part of the GIT; however, hepatic and pancreatic function and disease are addressed in Chapters 40 and 42, respectively.

The intestinal wall has four main layers (from inside to outside): the mucosa, the submucosa, the muscularis with two layers of smooth muscle (an inner circular layer and outer longitudinal layer), and the serosa. The muscular layers of the esophagus are an exception to this basic structure. The entire esophagus of the dog is composed of striated muscle, whereas cats, horses, pigs, and primates have striated muscle in the proximal two-thirds and smooth muscle in the distal portion, including the esophago–gastric junction. The composition of the specialized epithelium of the mucosal layer varies with each organ, but all organs perform transport, digestive, secretory, and absorptive functions in addition to providing immune protection and surveillance. Controlled rhythmic contractions of the muscular layers mix and transport ingesta throughout the GIT. The external serosal layer is a thin membrane made up of secretory cells that produce and secrete serous fluid. This fluid lubricates the surface, facilitating motility by decreasing friction due to contact with itself and other abdominal organs [1–3].

The design of the control system of the GIT is remarkably large and complex, with a total number of enteric neurons similar to that of the spinal cord [2]. Intestinal function relies on input from both the enteric nervous system (ENS) and the central nervous system (CNS), as well as endocrine and immune support. The ENS has extrinsic and intrinsic components that are supplied with parasympathetic and sympathetic input via the autonomic nervous system (ANS). The intrinsic component includes the myenteric and submucosal plexuses. The myenteric plexus controls intestinal motility and is located between the circular and longitudinal muscle layers. The submucosal plexus coordinates motion of the luminal epithelium and is found between the submucosa and the inner circular muscle layer. Other minor plexuses are also found within the muscle and submucosal layers [1–4].

The extrinsic ENS consists of parasympathetic innervation to the upper and lower GIT via the vagus and pelvic nerves, respectively, and sympathetic innervation via spinal segments T1-L3. Both afferent and efferent nerve fibers are contained within the same nerves. Preganglionic parasympathetic neurons have long axons that synapse with ganglia of the myenteric or submucosal plexuses *within* the GIT. Whereas preganglionic sympathetic fibers synapse with ganglia just *outside* the GIT, the postganglionic sympathetic neurons travel into the GIT itself, synapsing with the intrinsic plexuses and/or directly onto targets in the intestine. Acetylcholine (ACh) is the neurotransmitter released by all preganglionic fibers. Postganglionic parasympathetic neurons may utilize ACh, nitric oxide, adenosine triphosphate, serotonin, or various peptides such as substance P, vasoactive intestinal peptide (VIP), neuropeptide Y (NPY), or gastrin-releasing peptide (GRP). Postganglionic sympathetic neurons release norepinephrine. In addition to the cholinergic, adrenergic, and peptidergic receptors, many other receptor types are found in the GIT

Veterinary Anesthesia and Analgesia: The Sixth Edition of Lumb and Jones. Edited by Leigh Lamont, Kurt Grimm, Sheilah Robertson, Lydia Love and Carrie Schroeder.
© 2024 John Wiley & Sons, Inc. Published 2024 by John Wiley & Sons, Inc.
Companion website: www.wiley.com/go/lamont/anesthesia

that modify secretory, endocrine, and muscular activity. Receptors for μ- and δ-opioids, several serotonin types, and histamine are just a few. Gastrin, secretin, cholecystokinin, gastric inhibitory peptide, motilin, and ghrelin are hormones with significant secretory and/or motility effects within the GIT [1–7].

Intestinal motility relies on two major patterns of muscular activity, the migrating motor complexes (MMC) seen during fasting, and a digestive pattern that begins when foodstuffs enter the stomach. MMCs are seen in dogs and humans, but motility in cats is controlled by a migrating spike complex pattern that is somewhat weaker than the MMC. The interstitial cells of Cajal, located within the myenteric plexuses, are specialized pacemaker cells that create and maintain MMCs. These are so-called "slow waves" of depolarization that spread via gap junctions between smooth muscle cells over large sections of intestine but remain below the depolarization threshold for propulsive contractions. This activity provides an effective housekeeping function for the intestine, moving residual fluid, mucus, bacteria, and cellular debris aborally during the interdigestive period. As a food bolus arrives, electrical activity increases, and the digestive pattern begins. Sphincters and sections of intestine in the path of the bolus relax to allow entry as other sections contract in a segmental or propulsive fashion. Ingesta is mixed and moved along the GIT using the circular and longitudinal muscles, respectively. Feedback inhibition also occurs along the tract to "brake" the intestine, providing longer and more thorough contact for digestion. Both the digestive and interdigestive patterns are controlled by the parasympathetic nervous system, with ACh and substance P responsible for contraction and VIP and nitric oxide producing relaxation. Sympathetic input is primarily inhibitory, seen during times of stress, excitement, anxiety, fear, or pain. Numerous neurotransmitters and hormones are involved in the initiation and processing of the digestive phase, affecting motility, secretion, digestion, absorption, and blood flow [1,2,4–7].

Effects of anesthetic agents on gastrointestinal function

In healthy patients, the effects on the GIT of most anesthetic agents are usually short-lived as normal function returns with the decline of drug levels. Some adjunctive agents may have a longer duration, so decisions about their use should be made with an understanding of the primary GI problem, pre-existing or concurrent illness or organ dysfunction, and effects of surgery since these may obscure and/or compound the effects of the anesthetic drugs. Prolonged effects into the postoperative period have the potential to affect outcomes. Gastrointestinal disorders during or following anesthesia are not infrequent in veterinary patients. Bloat and regurgitation in ruminants, colic in horses, as well as anorexia, diarrhea, and ileus in rabbits, are common [8–14]. Vomiting, regurgitation, and diarrhea in dogs and cats are not common but do occur perioperatively. Davies *et al.* [14] identified postoperative regurgitation and/or vomiting (PORV) in 30/244 dogs (12.3%) presenting for non-elective procedures. GI and neurologic surgery, the American Society of Anesthesiologists (ASA) score of 4, emergency presentation, history of vomiting or regurgitation, use of sevoflurane, and intact gender were significantly associated with PORV.

Physiologic abnormalities encountered perioperatively may produce signs of GI dysfunction and can be confused with direct effects of anesthetic drugs. These include dehydration, hypovolemia, hypotension, anemia, protein and electrolyte abnormalities, acid–base derangements, hypoxia, myocardial dysfunction, hypothermia, and changes in ANS tone. Vomiting patients may be alkalotic due to loss of H^+ and Cl^- but eventually become acidotic with significant volume loss and/or tissue ischemia. As with all patients, preanesthetic evaluation of and treatment for any abnormalities of patient status are necessary to minimize the effects of anesthesia and maximize the potential for a positive outcome.

Effects of surgery that may significantly affect perioperative GI function (and often anesthetic management) include tissue manipulation/handling, hemorrhage, and correction of the underlying GI problem (e.g., reperfusion of the stomach following derotation of a gastric dilation and volvulus). The surgeon and anesthetist should work together to minimize the effects of both surgery and anesthesia on perioperative GI function.

The effects of anesthetic agents on the GIT include changes in saliva and its production, nausea, vomiting, ileus, regurgitation, gastroesophageal reflux (GER), constipation, reduced secretion or alteration of digestive fluids, and aerophagia (associated with panting). Salivation and panting can lead to fluid loss and contribute to hemoconcentration/dehydration. Although there is considerable overlap of the effects of many drugs (e.g., opioids, α_2-adrenergic receptor agonists, anticholinergics, and inhalants all reduce motility), some effects tend to be more specific (e.g., anticholinergics reduce the volume of saliva but increase viscosity). Ileus can result in tympany, especially if microbial gas production continues at a high rate as seen in ruminants and equine patients. In small animals, some suggest that this could be a contributing factor to the rare occurrence of gastric dilation (GD) or gastric dilation–volvulus, (GDV) seen in dogs postoperatively. Anesthesia is often implicated as a risk factor for the development of GDV, and anecdotal reports are common. GD following sedation [15] or injectable anesthesia [16] are reported, however, published reports of GDV following anesthesia could not be found.

Concurrent or chronic illness may complicate the clinical picture. For example, diabetic patients may suffer from gastroparesis and delayed gastric emptying secondary to autonomic neuropathy [17] and may be more likely to develop reflux, esophagitis, and/or vomiting postoperatively. Anemic or hypoproteinemic patients present treatment challenges with fluid therapy, especially if hypotension occurs. Stress of disease, pain, and hospitalization also predispose patients to GI dysfunction, especially anorexia, gastric ulceration, digestive disturbance, and diarrhea [5,7,12]. If anesthetic drugs are the primary cause of GI dysfunction in patients, many of these signs (e.g., ileus, nausea, vomiting) should resolve relatively quickly following cessation of drug administration. If they persist or are severe, further evaluation of the patient is warranted to ensure that another cause is not present (e.g., acid–base or electrolyte abnormalities, hypotension, GI foreign body, GDV, GI ulceration, and internal hemorrhage).

The most significant perianesthetic complications associated with GI dysfunction include pulmonary aspiration and/or esophagitis following vomiting, regurgitation or GER, and postoperative ileus (POI). Aspiration may cause pneumonitis, pneumonia, and severe hypoxemia, which can result in cardiac arrest. An episode of general anesthesia is reported to be a very common risk factor for esophagitis and aspiration pneumonia or pneumonitis in small animals. Positioning and duration of anesthesia are reported risk factors for the latter. When severe or unrecognized/untreated, stricture of the esophageal mucosa can develop, which can lead to persistent vomiting, regurgitation, dysphagia, weight loss, and debilitation [17–20].

POI greatly affects patient comfort following surgery and can affect outcomes. A greater incidence of nausea and vomiting, poor wound healing, and delayed oral intake and mobility are seen with persistent ileus. The risk of respiratory and other system complications is increased; longer hospital stays are seen and subsequently, greater financial burden [9,10,20–23].

Nausea and vomiting

Nausea and vomiting are common adverse effects of anesthetic agents, especially in human patients. The underlying mechanisms of emesis are complex, as several mechanisms result in vomiting, and two target areas exist in the CNS. A humoral pathway is stimulated by blood-borne substances that affect the chemoreceptor trigger zone (CTZ), whereas the vomiting center (VC) is activated by a neural pathway. Vomiting occurs when the VC is directly stimulated by one or more neurotransmitters. Histamine, ACh, dopamine, serotonin (5HT and $5HT_3$), and neurokinin-1 (NK_1 or substance P) are important neurotransmitters in the VC. Dopamine, serotonin, and α_2-adrenergic receptors are found in the CTZ. Located outside the blood–brain barrier, the CTZ is sensitive to low levels of emetic agents in the circulation. Input from the cerebral cortex (anxiety and anticipation), the vestibular apparatus (motion sickness), and local damage to the GIT stimulate the VC. Mucosal irritation and damage or distention of GI tissues produce emesis via the release of serotonin and/or stimulation of vagal afferent receptors [6,24–28]. Vasopressin has also been shown to cause nausea and vomiting, possibly via effects on central opioid receptors [29–31].

While many opioids are associated with a high incidence of vomiting (e.g., morphine and hydromorphone), antiemesis has also been reported. This effect is thought to occur when increased numbers of opioid receptors in the VC are stimulated, as with very lipophilic opioids (fentanyl and congeners) or when given intravenously, especially at higher doses (butorphanol). This may also explain why vomiting is seen primarily after the first dose of opioids and is uncommon following subsequent doses [32,33].

The incidence of vomiting seen with anesthetic drugs is variable and depends on species, drugs used, dosage, route and timing of administration, presence/absence of pain, and concurrent medical problems. Aerophagia and repeated swallowing of blood and saliva (especially following dentistry procedures) can also significantly increase the risk of vomiting during recovery. Most instances of vomiting occur with premedication in dogs and cats. Since vomiting is an active process, it usually does not occur during maintenance of surgical anesthesia but can be seen during light planes or at intubation as the vomiting reflex in dogs and cats is not abolished until Stage 3/Plane II [34]. Inhalant anesthetics are a significant cause of postoperative nausea and vomiting (PONV) in humans [28,35,36], but this incidence is much lower in veterinary species. Vomiting occurs occasionally at induction with propofol [37] and often with etomidate [38] when used alone in dogs, and in recovery following continuous infusion of propofol [39]. A clinical study that compared the incidence of adverse effects in dogs maintained with propofol versus isoflurane after propofol induction reported a very low incidence of vomiting or retching, with 4/91 in the isoflurane group and 1/58 in the propofol group. However, a high incidence of hypersalivation was seen in recovery, affecting just over 20% of both groups. No other signs of nausea were seen, and the dogs did not appear painful. A cause for the salivation was not identified [40]. Another study reported salivation in 7/40 (17.5%) and vomiting during recovery in 6/40 (15%) when propofol was used for induction following four different premedication protocols. Most (12/13) of these were dogs not given acepromazine. The one dog given acepromazine presented for vomiting and had been anesthetized for gastroscopy [41]. Anticholinergics were not used in either study. Although emesis occurred in one dog and one cat during field studies of Alfaxan® [42], it is rarely seen clinically and was not reported in multi-dose research studies in small animals [43,44].

α_2-Adrenergic receptor agonists and μ-opioid receptor agonists cause vomiting in dogs and cats [32,45–50]. The incidence of vomiting clinically appears to be more common at higher doses and is generally greater in cats than dogs. Vomiting was not reported with continuous infusions of very low doses of dexmedetomidine or medetomidine in healthy dogs and cats [51–53]. There is minimal difference in the incidence of vomiting between the different α_2-adrenergic receptor agonists; however, a significant difference is seen with different opioids. Vomiting is less frequent with lower dosages and when patients are fasted prior to administration. Morphine, meperidine, and hydromorphone (especially in cats), and to a lesser extent oxymorphone, are associated with the highest risk of vomiting. Vomiting is much less frequent with fentanyl and its derivatives, and is uncommon with methadone, butorphanol, and buprenorphine [32,54,55]. However, two reports investigating the use of methadone in dogs with local analgesia for stifle surgery showed an unexpected incidence of vomiting. Although other mechanisms could not be eliminated, both authors suggested that the analgesia produced by the nerve blocks may have allowed this adverse effect of methadone to predominate, whereas when pain is present, side effects of opioids are less common [56,57].

Acepromazine has a mild antiemetic effect via dopamine antagonism in the CTZ. It decreases vomiting significantly, especially when given prior to opioids in dogs. Its antihistamine effects may also contribute when morphine or meperidine is given concurrently [54,55,58]. The incidence of vomiting/nausea also varies when different opioids are combined with α_2-adrenergic receptor agonists. Eleven of 18 cats vomited after dexmedetomidine with buprenorphine while only one of 19 given dexmedetomidine and butorphanol vomited [59].

Adjunct drugs given during anesthesia may also cause vomiting. Up to 75% of dogs administered a high dose of lidocaine (200 μg/kg/min) as a continuous infusion during sevoflurane anesthesia vomited in recovery. When the dose was reduced (50 μg/kg/min), vomiting did not occur postoperatively [60]. In contrast, decreased nausea and vomiting were seen in humans treated with a lidocaine continuous rate infusion (CRI) for abdominal surgery [61,62].

Antiemetic therapy

Metoclopramide is a central dopamine (D_2) receptor antagonist that has been used for many years as an antiemetic in dogs. It also has prokinetic effects on the stomach, duodenum, and jejunum, and has some muscarinic and serotonin receptor (5-HT_3 receptor antagonist/5-HT_4 receptor agonist) actions at higher doses [7]. When given subcutaneously 30 min prior to premedication with morphine and dexmedetomidine in dogs, metoclopramide prevented nausea and vomiting and greatly reduced these signs when given concurrently [63]. The serotonin antagonist group (e.g., ondansetron, dolasetron, and palonosetron) and the NK_1 receptor antagonist, maropitant, have proven useful to prevent or decrease emesis caused by chemotherapeutic agents [30,64,65], α_2-adrenergic receptor agonists [66,67], and opioids [67–70]. Maropitant affects receptors in both the VC and the CTZ, as well as in the GIT and other organs. It has been shown to reduce perioperative vomiting and nausea very effectively in dogs and cats and is now widely used in clinical practice. There is some evidence it produces inhalant anesthetic-sparing effects and investigations into potential analgesic and anti-inflammatory effects are ongoing. The anti-nausea effect of maropitant is reportedly not as strong as that produced with ondansetron in dogs [30,67,71,72]. Swallow *et al.* did not find improvement in signs of PONV when given to 24 dogs for ovariectomy although the isoflurane requirement was reduced [73]. However, when given to 40 dogs for ovariohysterectomy, the incidence of pre- and postoperative emesis was almost eliminated, fewer patients required rescue analgesia, and improvement in appetite and the quality of recovery was seen; the addition of omeprazole did not provide any further benefit [74]. Hay-Kraus *et al.* and Sharun *et al.* have published reviews of the many actions and uses of maropitant in veterinary medicine [75,76].

Dexamethasone is an effective antiemetic in humans for the prophylactic treatment of PONV [28,36,77]. It decreases the frequency of vomiting in cats induced by xylazine, but only at high doses [78]. The anti-inflammatory, anti-immune, and adverse endocrine and GI effects probably preclude its routine use as a prophylactic antiemetic in veterinary patients.

Benzodiazepines, phenothiazines, and butyrophenones have been shown to have antiemetic effects in humans. Formerly, droperidol was used frequently in small animals as a sedative, especially in combination with fentanyl (Innovar Vet®). Droperidol is considered a highly effective antiemetic in humans; however, the risk of cardiac arrhythmias precluded its use for a time [28,36]. It has since been determined that the cardiovascular effects are minimized when lower doses are used [28]; however, other adverse effects such as sedation, excitement, extrapyramidal effects, and the availability of better alternatives preclude the routine use of butyrophenones as antiemetics in veterinary patients.

Non-pharmacologic interventions for PONV in humans include acupuncture or acupressure [28,36]. Needling at acupuncture point Pericardium-6 (PC6) decreased the incidence of nausea and vomiting with hydromorphone in dogs [79], while electroacupuncture at PC6 was shown to prevent emesis induced by vasopressin in dogs. Pretreatment with naloxone prevented antiemesis, suggesting that opioid pathways may be involved [31].

Gastroesophageal reflux

Gastroesophageal reflux disease (GERD) is a common syndrome in humans. It is reported to occur in 5–20% of adults but may be as high as 40% in some areas [80]. The proposed mechanisms of reflux include abnormally low lower esophageal sphincter (LES) pressure (LESP), increased frequency and duration of transient lower esophageal sphincter relaxations (TLSRs), and alteration of the anti-reflux barrier. TLSRs are normal events that occur with swallowing and vent gas formed in the stomach. They are most often seen following ingestion of food. TLSRs do not occur during general anesthesia in dogs and humans or during deep sleep in people. Relaxation of the diaphragmatic crus and the LES must be present for normal TLSRs to occur [80–85].

Although the specific mechanism of anesthetic-induced GER is unclear, reflux occurs when intragastric pressure exceeds or equals the LESP, and the barrier pressure normally present between the two areas is lost [80–85]. Intra-abdominal and intrathoracic pressure also contribute to LESP and the incidence of GER. The anti-reflux barrier is created by the anatomical arrangement of the LES, the right crus of the diaphragm, and the oblique angle at the junction of the esophagus and the cardia. The LES is actually located above and below the hiatus of the diaphragm and is several centimeters in length. Functionally, it is a high-pressure zone just above the cardia created by a variable arrangement of muscle layers in the distal esophagus in combination with the angle of the crura of the diaphragm. To prevent retrograde flow of gastric contents, the LES remains in a tonically contracted state until stimulated to relax via relaxation of the upper esophageal sphincter and/or waves of peristaltic contractions higher in the esophagus [80–85].

Table 41.1 Neurotransmitters and hormones that affect lower esophageal sphincter (LES) tone.

Decrease LES tone	Increase LES tone
Nitric oxide and nitrates	Prostaglandin E
Vasoactive intestinal peptide	Muscarinic M_2, M_3 receptor agonists
Nicotine	Gastrin
β-Adrenergic receptor agonists	Substance P
Dopamine	α-Adrenergic receptor agonists
Cholecystokinin	Prostaglandin Fα
Secretin	Motilin
Calcitonin gene-related peptide	
Adenosine	

Source: Compiled from Washabau [1]; Hershcovici *et al.* [83].

Although primarily controlled by the parasympathetic nervous system, numerous neurotransmitters and hormones are involved in regulation of LES tone (Table 41.1) [1,83].

Clinical GERD is less common in dogs and cats than in humans but has been identified in both species [86–89]. Brachycephalic dog breeds are predisposed to GER [90–96]. Functional and anatomical abnormalities of the esophagus and LES, and inflammatory lesions of the upper GIT have been identified in brachycephalic breeds [19,91,92]. Eivers *et al.* evaluated 26 dogs for esophageal dysfunction using videofluoroscopy and identified esophageal dysmotility, GER, and hiatal hernia; 77% were brachycephalic [92]. GERD is likely underdiagnosed since mild cases may not result in clinical signs [86,88,89]. "Silent reflux" events are known to occur in people without consequence [80]. These have recently been identified in healthy dogs using nuclear scintigraphy [97].

Numerous anesthetic drugs and adjunct medications, including sedatives, analgesics, induction agents, inhalants, and anticholinergics, have been shown to decrease LESP in humans, dogs, and cats, predisposing anesthetized patients to GER (Table 41.2) [82,85,98–106].

Perioperative GER is common; incidence varies from 0 to 71% of cases. Numerous studies have investigated the occurrence of GER under many conditions and with many anesthetic and/or adjunct agents (Table 41.3) [107–127].

GER is more frequent with intra-abdominal and orthopedic procedures in dogs and may be more common in dogs than cats [12,101,104,116–118]. GER occurred in 9/27 cats anesthetized for dental procedures [120], but was not more common during intra-abdominal procedures in 44 cats compared to 30 controls [121]. Vomiting associated with premedication prior to anesthesia was not associated with increased GER in dogs [123–125]; however, the occurrence of GER under anesthesia is variable and unpredictable.

In spite of numerous investigations, the mechanism of GER seen with general anesthesia has not been proven. Loss of the barrier pressure (gastric pressure – LESP) between the distal esophagus and the stomach must occur [80–85], but it is not clear what specifically triggers this phenomenon. Most cases of anesthesia-related

Table 41.2 Effects of various anesthetics, analgesics, sedatives, adjunct medications, and miscellaneous factors on lower esophageal sphincter pressure (LESP) reported in dogs, cats, and/or humans.

Decrease LESP	Increase LESP	No Change
β-Adrenergic agonists	α-Adrenergic agonists	Atracurium
Acepromazine	Acetylcholine	Dexmedetomidine
Alfaxalone–alfadolone[b]	Antacids	Histamine (H_2) antagonists (cimetidine, ranitidine)
Aminophylline	Anticholinesterases	Metoprolol
Atropine, glycopyrrolate	Domperidone	Nitrous oxide[a]
Benzodiazepines	Edrophonium	NMBA reversal with neostigmine and glycopyrrolate
Calcium channel antagonists	Gastric acidification	Propofol
Change from lateral to dorsal recumbency	Histamine	Propranolol
Cisapride	Increased gastric or abdominal pressure	Proton pump inhibitors
Cricoid pressure	Metoclopramide	Remifentanil
Dexmedetomidine (high doses)	Neostigmine	
Dorsal versus lateral recumbency	Pancuronium	
Fentanyl–droperidol	Succinylcholine	
Hiatal hernia	Vecuronium (small increase)	
Inhalant anesthetics		
Ketamine[c]		
Laryngeal mask airway		
Meperidine		
Morphine		
Nitroprusside		
Nitrous oxide[a]		
Obesity		
Oxymorphone		
Pregnancy		
Propofol (high doses)		
Residual neuromuscular blockade		
Thiopental		
Tricyclic antidepressants		
Xylazine		
Xylazine–ketamine[c]		

NMBA, neuromuscular blocking agent.
[a] Conflicting results concerning nitrous oxide.
[b] Reported with Saffan®, not Alfaxan®.
[c] Ketamine decreased LESP compared with awake values, but it remained much higher compared to other drugs.
Source: Compiled from Cotton and Smith [85]; Ogunnaike and Whitten [98]; Open Anesthesia [99]; Strombeck and Harrold [100]; Hall *et al.* [101]; Waterman and Hashim [102]; van der Hoeven *et al.* [103]; Hashim and Waterman [104]; Hashim and Waterman [105]; Hashim *et al.* [106].

Table 41.3 Anesthetic protocols, procedures, and other factors reported to impact the incidence of regurgitation or gastroesophageal reflex (GER).

Increased incidence of GER	No difference	Decreased incidence of GER
Abdominal procedures	Decreased fasting times/small meal	Dexmedetomidine–hydromorphone compared to acepromazine–hydromorphone
Brachycephalic breed	Halothane versus isoflurane versus sevoflurane	Diazepam compared to atropine–propionylpromazine
Dorsal recumbency	Recumbency or head tilt	High-dose metoclopramide infusion
Esophageal disorders, dysmotility	Standard fast compared to short fast (17.3 h versus 4.7 h)	Meperidine compared to morphine
Gastric acidity	Vomiting following premedication	Short fast (3 h versus 10 h)
Hiatal hernia		
Imaging studies		
Large deep-chested dogs (spinal surgery)		
LMA compared to ET tube (kittens)		
Longer anesthetic duration		
Medetomidine compared to acepromazine–opioid		
Morphine (increased incidence with higher doses)		
Neurologic surgery		
Older dogs, sicker dogs (ASA ≥ 3)		
Orthopedic surgery		
Prolonged fast		
Propofol compared to thiopental		
Shorter fasting		
Factors associated with increased incidence of GER in humans		
Altered consciousness		
Full stomach		
Late pregnancy		
LMA (some types)		
NSAID use		
Other factors		
Dogs that reflux early more often regurgitate		
Increased gastric pH, no difference with gastric volume		
Prolonged fasting increases gastric acidity		
Type, volume of food		

LMA, laryngeal mask airway; ET, endotracheal; NSAID, non-steroidal anti-inflammatory drug.
Source: Compiled from Savvas *et al.* [107]; Savvas *et al.* [108]; Savvas *et al.* [109]; Galatos and Raptopoulos [110]; Savvas and Raptopoulos [111]; Wilson and Evans [112]; Tsompanidou *et al.* [113]; Viskjer and Sjöström [114]; Anagnostou *et al.* [115]; Wilson [116]; Galatos and Raptopoulos [117]; Wilson *et al.* [118]; Raptopoulos and Galatos [119]; Garcia *et al.* [120]; Sideri *et al.* [121]; Galatos *et al.* [122]; Wilson *et al.* [123]; Wilson *et al.* [124]; Wilson *et al.* [125]; Costa *et al.* [126]; Flouraki *et al.* [127].

GER in dogs and cats develop fairly soon following induction, usually before 30 min [116,117]. Choice of premedication plays a role in some cases [126] but not in others [127]. GER is frequent with opioids [112,127] especially μ-opioid receptor agonists such as morphine and hydromorphone [116,123,126]. Dosage may also be a factor, as higher doses of morphine cause more GER than lower doses [123]. Induction with propofol has resulted in greater incidence of GER in dogs [107,119] but not in cats [121]. Pharyngeal stimulation may be a factor as it decreases pressure at the LES. Minor pharyngeal stimulation elicited relaxation of the LES more than 50% of the time in opossums anesthetized with pentobarbital [128], while subthreshold stimulus of the pharynx produced longitudinal esophageal muscle contraction and LES relaxation in humans [129]. Interestingly, GER was seen in 50% of kittens managed with an LMA versus 14% with an endotracheal tube [130]. Perhaps the combination of pharyngeal stimulation at induction combined with the effects of multiple anesthetic drugs during the transition into deeper levels of anesthesia is significant; however, this does not explain episodes of reflux that occur later during anesthesia or in those without endotracheal intubation [121]. GER is seen with virtually all inhalants; no difference was seen in dogs anesthetized with halothane, isoflurane, or sevoflurane [125]. Numerous factors are certainly involved in the mechanism of GER; specific triggers may be multiple and vary with patients, drugs used, procedures, ASA status, and other circumstances.

In spite of the high frequency of GER detected using pH or impedance monitoring in dogs and cats, the incidence of visible regurgitation (i.e., oral drainage of fluid) is much lower. In a large study of 4257 dogs at a referral practice over a 2-year period, regurgitation was visually confirmed in only 27 or 0.63% of cases, with large dogs and orthopedic procedures at highest risk [131].

Regurgitation was observed in 75 or 1.3% of 5736 dogs in another large study [132], where greater risk was seen with an ASA status ≥ 3, abdominal or imaging procedures, long anesthetic duration, and larger size. Dogs anesthetized for all types of procedures regurgitated less than 1% of the time, even though GER was identified in 16.3 and 17.4% of cases in two other reports [110,117]. During orthopedic procedures in dogs following administration of various anesthetics agents, regurgitation occurred in 0–17% of the cases, while GER was identified in 25–71% of the cases [114,118,123–125]. In several studies involving cats, regurgitation was reported in 0, 2%, 0, and 0 cases with an incidence of GER of 18, 16, 33.3, and 50% [120–122,130].

Prevention of GER in anesthetized dogs has been investigated with H_2 receptor antagonists, proton pump inhibitors (PPIs), and prokinetic drugs. Although H_2 receptor antagonists increase gastric pH in dogs, they are not as effective at maintaining increased pH as PPIs; and even with PPIs, multiple doses are required [133–137]. Omeprazole given preoperatively to 47 dogs decreased the frequency of acidic reflux (4 with omeprazole versus 13 without); however, as lower esophageal pH was the only parameter measured, some reflux events may have been missed [136]. When two doses of omeprazole were given preoperatively to dogs, the incidence of GER was not different, but a much higher pH of the reflux, 6.3 ± 1.5 versus 4.1 ± 1.5 versus 3.8 ± 1.1, was seen [137]. When dogs were given maropitant, omeprazole, or both, no difference was seen in the occurrence of GER or the pH of the reflux [138]. The incidence of GER was significantly lower in cats given two doses of omeprazole, but some treated cats still had multiple episodes of reflux [120]. A study in 61 dogs using both impedance and pH monitors found that esomeprazole alone increased pH, and the addition of cisapride decreased the incidence of reflux significantly from 8/21 with placebo to 2/18 in the combination group [139]. When an infusion of cisapride was given preoperatively to dogs anesthetized for surgical treatment of laryngeal paralysis fewer cases of aspiration pneumonia were seen, which is thought to be caused by GER [140].

Metoclopramide alone decreased the incidence of GER, but did not completely prevent it in dogs. This effect was seen only when given via continuous infusion at a high dose [141]. Intravenous metoclopramide, and/or ranitidine prior to anesthesia followed by a metoclopramide infusion, did not decrease the incidence of GER in dogs anesthetized for ovariohysterectomy [142]. Maropitant given prior to induction in combination with an infusion of metoclopramide for 24 h did not prevent clinical signs of GER in the postoperative period [143].

The effect of several palliative treatments for GER has been examined. Esophageal lavage in 32/48 dogs with reflux pH < 4 using water, or two bicarbonate solutions increased the pH to > 4 in 78.6% with water and 100% with bicarbonate. Interestingly, the pH improved in 16/48 dogs without treatment [144]. Removal of reflux fluid from the esophagus via suctioning in 10 dogs did not significantly change the esophageal pH, lavage with tap water increased the pH to > 4.0, and the infusion of a small volume of sodium bicarbonate increased the pH to > 6.0, an effect that lasted from 1.5 to 3 h [145]. Repeated suctioning and tap water lavage followed by bicarbonate therapy were also evaluated in dogs [146]. Lavage was determined to be unnecessary as the final esophageal pH did not differ once bicarbonate was applied. Bicarbonate therapy may not prevent further reflux/regurgitation and may not help with non-acidic reflux. However, it could be beneficial with acidic reflux to reduce the risk or severity of esophagitis. Suctioning and lavage can be useful in cases with a large volume of regurgitation.

Several authors have examined the effects of fasting duration and types of food on the incidence of GER, gastric volume, and pH in dogs, with somewhat variable results. Some have shown that a short fast utilizing small volumes of canned food results in decreased incidence of GER [108–111], higher gastric pH, and lower gastric volume [106]. Others have not seen a difference with shorter fasting times [112,113] and another found a greater incidence of GER and regurgitation with a shorter fast and a higher pH with a longer fasting time [114].

Actual fasting times are often much longer than recommended in humans and animals. In people, fasting is associated with hunger, thirst, decreased satisfaction, and sometimes nausea, vomiting, or dehydration postoperatively. Because research has not shown a decreased incidence of aspiration pneumonia with long fasting times, the guidelines used by the ASA were revised in 2017 for healthy patients [147]. The minimum fasting guidelines for adults and children with a low risk of aspiration include: (1) clear liquids, 2 h; (2) breast milk, 2 h; (3) milk-type liquids, 6 h; and (4) a light meal 6 h prior to anesthesia. Eight hours or more is recommended if meat or a fatty meal is ingested [147]. In 2023, further revision included the recommendation that healthy adults should drink a carbohydrate-type clear liquid up to 2 h prior to the procedure, and clear liquids in children be allowed/encouraged up to 2 h prior to anesthesia as well [148]. In 2020, the American Animal Hospital Association (AAHA) published revised guidelines on fasting in a similar fashion. Water is not withheld, and food is allowed up to 4–6 h prior to the procedure in healthy adults. Very young (< 8 weeks) or small (< 2 kg) patients should have food withheld for no more than 1–2 h [149].

Prevention of GER is difficult; however, vigilant monitoring to identify when it has occurred and appropriate intervention will minimize complications. General management recommendations to treat GER in the perianesthetic period are summarized in Box 41.1.

Box 41.1 Recommendations for management of gastroesophageal reflex (GER) in the perianesthetic period.

1. Observe patients following premedication, especially with heavy sedation and drugs that cause emesis (e.g., morphine and α_2-adrenergic receptor agonists).
2. Maintain sedated patients in sternal recumbency whenever possible and attain a secure airway quickly following induction.
3. Select and place an appropriate endotracheal tube:
   i. Correctly sized.
   ii. Properly lubricated.
   iii. Appropriate cuff inflation.
4. Recheck tube placement and cuff inflation, especially with transport and re-positioning.
5. Keep head tipped downward to encourage drainage of GER away from the airway.
6. Have supplies close by for suctioning and cleaning of the pharynx and esophagus.
7. If vomiting or regurgitation occurs – direct the patient's head downward.
8. Manage recovery:
   i. Examine pharynx before extubation.
   ii. Lavage esophagus when large-volume GER has occurred.
   iii. Extubate with the endotracheal tube cuff partially inflated.
   iv. Position patient with head/nose down, lower than shoulder at all times.

Esophagitis and esophageal stricture

Esophagitis can occur when the esophageal mucosa is exposed to caustic substances for prolonged periods and/or when esophageal defense mechanisms are impaired or overwhelmed. Esophageal defense mechanisms include a superficial mucus/bicarbonate barrier on the mucosal surface, tight junctions between epithelial cells, and an intracellular and interstitial buffering capacity that is dependent on blood flow. Lack of clearance of esophageal contents via intermittent swallowing is also a factor in anesthetized patients. Saliva is often decreased under anesthesia and, of course, anesthetized patients cannot swallow. Saliva provides dilution, bicarbonate to neutralize acid, and volume to flush the lumen of the esophagus. Resistance to 30 min of exposure to acid has been demonstrated; however, pepsin, trypsin, bile salts, and possibly other irritating or caustic substances may be as important as acids in causing esophageal damage. Exposure to acidic reflux also induces release of inflammatory mediators that contact and damage nerve endings resulting in decreased LESP, which predisposes to further GER and perpetuates the cycle [18,19,81,150].

Esophagitis and subsequent esophageal stricture are secondary illnesses, caused by damage from exposure to gastric/intestinal fluids. GER, vomiting and/or regurgitation, ingestion of foreign bodies or caustic substances (including some medications such as doxycycline and clindamycin), motility disorders, congenital or anatomic abnormalities (e.g., hiatal hernia and megaesophagus), trauma, neoplasia, infection, neuromuscular disease, and any cause of altered mentation are contributing factors. Hypergastrinemia with resultant hyperacidity, delayed gastric emptying due to pyloric outflow obstruction, pancreatitis, or diabetes are also reported causes [18,19, 87,88,151–156]. An inflammatory cause of eosinophilic esophagitis known to occur in people has been reported in a dog and a kitten [157,158]. Cats with chronic gingivostomatitis have also been found to have concurrent esophagitis [159].

A history of recent general anesthesia is very common in dogs and cats diagnosed with esophagitis, with perianesthetic GER as the most likely underlying cause. Retrospective studies have examined the incidence, risk factors, and outcome of esophagitis/stricture [87,89,151–158]. Leib *et al.* [89] identified 18 of 28 (64%), Adamama-Moraitou *et al.* [160] found 13 of 20 (65%), and Kushner and Shofer [161] reported 25 of 30 (83%) patients with esophageal stricture diagnosed soon following general anesthesia. Overall mortality in these reports was 21, 30, and 30%, respectively. Greater risk of esophagitis was seen in patients anesthetized for intra-abdominal procedures, especially ovariohysterectomy [160]. Manipulation of abdominal structures is presumed to increase gastric pressure, while LESP is decreased by anesthetic agents. Progesterone levels in intact females were thought to contribute to decreased LESP; however, a study of barrier pressure and GER in female dogs anesthetized during four different phases of their reproductive cycle showed no effect of hormone levels on barrier pressure, the incidence of GER, or esophagitis [162]. In contrast to dogs, a study of esophageal disease in cats over a 7.5-year period found anesthesia to be involved in only one of 33 cases [154]. This may not reflect the true incidence in cats since signs may be readily overlooked.

When all cases presented for anesthesia over a 10-year period were examined retrospectively, a very low incidence of postanesthetic esophageal dysfunction was reported. Twenty-five patients with esophageal stricture following anesthesia were identified at one institution (0.1% of 23,295 cases) [161], 3 cases of esophagitis and 10 cases of esophageal stricture (13 total cases, 0.07% of caseload) occurred over 8 years at another [163]. Mortality associated with the esophageal complications was 30 and 23%, respectively. Vomiting and regurgitation occurred postoperatively in most or all of these patients. Four of the 13 dogs also had aspiration pneumonia. Weight loss, debilitation, and chronic cough were seen in some dogs (Fig. 41.1). A case report of two young cats that had exhibited vomiting and/or regurgitation, and dysphagia soon after elective general anesthesia developed rupture of the esophagus and were euthanized, one at 6 days, the other at 14 days postoperatively [164].

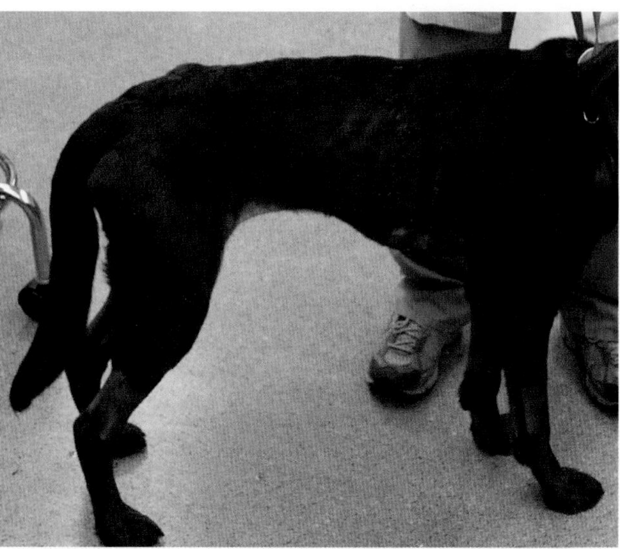

Figure 41.1 Patients with esophageal stricture may be debilitated due to dysphagia and aspiration pneumonia. Source: Dr. Jennifer Adams, with permission.

Although esophageal dysfunction following anesthesia is uncommon overall, the history of many cases includes an episode of general anesthesia. This is a devastating complication with a high mortality. Any patient that exhibits vomiting, regurgitation, nausea, salivation, dysphagia, and/or anorexia postoperatively should be monitored closely. When signs persist, these patients should be thoroughly evaluated for esophageal disease.

Aspiration

Aspiration of GI contents can occur perioperatively following GER, vomiting, and/or regurgitation. It can also occur during heavy sedation that impairs protective airway reflexes. Respiratory complications following aspiration include hypoventilation and/or hypoxemia, pneumonitis, bacterial pneumonia, and sometimes cardiac arrest. The extent of airway pathology depends on the volume and type of fluid aspirated. Three phases of damage have been identified. Stage 1 is immediate and is caused by direct damage to the epithelium. This injury to the lung is actually like a chemical burn due to the effect of gastric fluid on tissue, with greater damage seen with low pH, even if the volume is small. Varying degrees of atelectasis, decreased compliance, ventilation–perfusion mismatch, and decreased oxygenation develop at this point. Stage 2 is an inflammatory reaction that follows within 4–6 h, causing pneumonitis. If not severe, this lesion may resolve. However, with more significant injury, alveolar macrophages and Type II pneumocytes release cytokines that stimulate the influx of neutrophils, which release other inflammatory mediators, causing acute lung injury even without bacterial involvement. Surfactant is also altered by inflammation, contributing to impairment of gas exchange. Stage 3 is seen when bacteria invade damaged tissue, producing aspiration pneumonia (AP) [19,165–167].

Incidents of aspiration are not commonly witnessed, but early recognition and intervention are paramount to limiting the severity of pneumonitis/pneumonia. Signs of aspiration range from "silent" with no apparent abnormalities to obvious airway obstruction following visible regurgitation of gastric contents. Increased risk is seen with anesthesia, especially in patients with laryngeal and esophageal disorders, vomiting, neurologic disease, and GER [19,20,164–174]. People with AP more often have altered mental status, dysphagia, and esophageal disorders as common pre-existing conditions [167]. Brachycephalic breeds are predisposed to aspiration due to an increased incidence of GER, vomiting, and regurgitation that is common in these breeds. The underlying cause is likely an increased negative pressure that is caused by the upper airway obstruction secondary to their brachycephalic anatomy [19,93,96,167,175].

Clinical signs in anesthetized patients include unexplained oxygen desaturation, hypercarbia, tachypnea, dyspnea or irregular respiratory patterns, auscultable abnormalities, and blanching of mucous membranes. Oxygen (100%) should be administered and the patient immediately positioned with the head down for drainage of aspirated material; removal should be instituted as soon as possible. Suction of the airways can be used for liquid aspiration, but bronchoscopy is often required when particulate matter is present. Bronchodilator therapy and mechanical ventilation with positive end-expiratory pressure (PEEP) may be needed to improve oxygenation. Prophylactic antibiotics are not usually recommended for pneumonitis cases owing to the potential for emergence of resistant bacteria [19,165,166,170]. Since bacterial colonization occurs later in the process, in humans antibiotics are recommended only in those with confirmed infection, especially in otherwise healthy patients. However, patients with GI obstruction or on chronic antacid therapy may be an exception owing to the potential for enteric organisms to be found in reflux fluid [165,166,170]. It can be difficult to document the presence of infection quickly in veterinary patients, so antibiotic therapy is often instituted early in the course of treatment [167,168].

A very large multicenter study evaluated the anesthesia caseload at six veterinary institutions over an 11-year period to determine the incidence and risk factors for AP following anesthesia or sedation in dogs [20]. The criteria included radiographic or necropsy evidence of AP within 72 h of sedation or general anesthesia. Multivariate analysis of numerous patients, procedures, and anesthetic factors was performed for 240 cases along with 488 controls. The incidence varied significantly between institutions, from 0.04–0.26%, with an overall incidence of 0.17%. Of 12 dogs who were given sedation only, three developed AP. Multivariate analysis revealed the following to be associated with anesthetic-related AP: (1) patient factors including megaesophagus (ME) and pre-existing respiratory or neurologic disease; (2) procedural factors including upper airway surgery, endoscopy, thoracotomy, laparotomy, and neurosurgery; and (3) anesthetic events, including regurgitation during or after anesthesia and hydromorphone given intravenously at induction. Some factors were significantly associated with AP but did not remain following the multivariate analysis (odds ratio, OR < 2). These included the male gender and increasing ASA patient score, age, and body weight. Use of continuous infusion of analgesics or anesthetic agents was associated with a greater incidence of AP (OR 1.8) when utilized during anesthesia but not when given postoperatively. ME, in spite of a low occurrence, had the highest OR of 22.3, and upper airway surgery was next with OR 9.2. No specific breed was identified. Time of day, extubation during anesthesia, and the use of anticholinergics, positive-pressure ventilation, or epidural analgesia were not associated with AP. Regurgitation was witnessed in only two cases with AP. Forty-six of the 240 dogs (19.2%) were euthanized or died prior to discharge. However, an association of death with AP could not be identified from the available data, so mortality was not determined [20].

A smaller retrospective study found a 16% incidence of anesthesia-associated AP in 125 dogs diagnosed over a 3.5-year period. They also found AP following sedation in 16% of these cases as well [176]. A retrospective case-control study examined AP within 48 h of anesthesia in dogs with intervertebral disk disease. Significant risk factors for postoperative AP included preanesthetic tetraparesis, a cervical lesion, MRI study, multiple anesthetic episodes, longer duration of anesthesia, and postanesthetic vomiting or regurgitation [171]. Although AP appears to be less common in cats, it does occur. Levy *et al.* evaluated the cases of 28 cats diagnosed with AP that presented over a 12-year period. Vomiting was the most common predisposing factor identified. Anesthesia was important in 18%; enteral nutrition (18%), neurologic disease (7%), and laryngeal disease (3.6%) were also identified [177]. In 33 cats with AP, Dear *et al.* found that GI disease was the most common risk factor (25/33); 27% (9) of these cats had been anesthetized within 3 days of the diagnosis [178]. Dogs with laryngeal paralysis often develop AP, especially following surgical intervention [174].

Even though the overall incidence of aspiration occurring perioperatively is low, predisposing factors are common and AP carries a high risk of mortality. Vigilant monitoring for signs of aspiration is necessary, especially since most cases are subclinical, similar to GER and esophagitis. Perioperative management to prevent these complications with appropriate intervention as soon as possible is always indicated. These strategies are described in the GER section. Cisapride may be useful as a preventive treatment for AP. The incidence of AP was significantly less in dogs given a 90-min infusion of cispride prior to laryngeal surgery [140]. Anesthetic management with attention to preventive measures has shown good success. Baetge *et al.* altered several aspects of the anesthetic protocol for 149 patients that were repeatedly anesthetized for radiation therapy. The incidence of pneumonia in 146 cases performed prior to the modifications was 10 times greater than in the study group. They kept patients in sternal as much as possible and always in recovery, avoided anticholinergics, did not use μ-opioid receptor agonists, kept the head elevated above the shoulders, maintained endotracheal tube cuff inflation until just before extubation, and aseptically handled all anesthesia supplies [179]. Of 105 geriatric dogs given famotidine, maropitant, and fentanyl for anesthesia, none vomited, four showed nausea, two regurgitated, and one developed AP postoperatively [180].

Gastrointestinal motility/postoperative ileus

Rabbits, horses, ruminants, and humans appear to be especially sensitive to the effects of anesthetic agents on GI motility [21,22,181–185]. Postoperative nausea and vomiting (PONV) and ileus are very common in humans, and postoperative ileus (POI) is one of the most common reasons for prolonged hospitalization in humans [21–24,185]. Although most frequent following GI surgery, POI is seen with other procedures in humans [21] and with many types of surgery in horses. It is also seen in critical care patients that have not had anesthesia or surgery [5,7,186]. POI is associated with increased mortality following colic surgery in horses [23,183], while colic in general and cecal impaction, in particular, are potentially serious complications seen following routine anesthesia and surgery in horses and may be associated with the development of ileus [9,184]. Rabbits are prone to GI stasis following stressful situations, including anesthesia [13,181,182]. Dogs and cats certainly suffer from disruption of normal motility during and after anesthesia; however, related clinical problems are not frequently reported. Numerous researchers have used the dog as a model for the investigation of POI, but there are few specific reports of the incidence seen in clinical patients [186]. In fact, POI is rarely mentioned in veterinary surgery textbooks or reviews of abdominal surgery in small animals. With the advent of intensive multimodal pain management protocols and more diverse and challenging surgical procedures, the potential of these interventions to negatively affect motility has only increased.

Prolonged gastric emptying time has been identified in dogs during hospitalization using a wireless capsule to measure intestinal motility. Median emptying time was 17.6 h at home versus 71.8 h in hospital. Other parts of the intestine were not affected in this study [187]. Decreased motility in dogs that were fasted for 12–24 h was identified using ultrasound [188]. Intestinal function is temporarily disrupted by most anesthetic/analgesic agents, including anticholinergics, μ-opioid receptor agonists, α_2-adrenergic receptor agonists, inhalants, nitrous oxide, and induction agents other than ketamine [24,26,32,189–195]. Xylazine and medetomidine can inhibit motility of the stomach, small intestine [191,192], and colon [193] for hours in the dog. Anticholinergic drugs profoundly reduce GI motility in most species [196–203]. The effects of opioids on motility are many and varied. μ-Opioid receptor agonists given systemically delay gastric emptying, increase sphincter tone, and variably affect intestinal smooth muscle contraction. Propulsive motility is inhibited and segmental contractions are enhanced, especially in the colon; absorption is increased while secretion is decreased. Constipation is a frequent complication with systemic opioids, from the combined effects on fluid transport and prolonged transit time [32,195,203]. In contrast, when morphine is administered epidurally, GI motility returns much faster in both dogs and humans [204,205]. Following general anesthesia in humans, motility generally returns to the small intestine first, then the stomach, and eventually the colon, which may require 5 days or more [206]. In experimental dogs with ileus, motility of the distal intestine and colon recovered first, followed by the proximal intestine and the stomach [207].

Torrente *et al.* evaluated 237 dogs that were anesthetized for diagnostics or surgery and found that 33.4% of these developed GI issues post-anesthesia [12]. 17.3% had GER, 5.5% vomited, and 10.5% developed diarrhea. Duration of anesthesia, intra-abdominal surgery, and positioning changes were significantly associated with GER; treatment with colloids for hypotension, anesthetic duration, and altering the mode of ventilation increased the risk of vomiting postoperatively. Dogs that were given acepromazine for premedication vomited less frequently. Diarrhea was seen more often with longer anesthetic duration, body position or mode of ventilation changes, and hypoxemia. A recent report of 82 dogs anesthetized for emergency abdominal surgery found that 50% were anorexic, 21% developed diarrhea, and 26% had decreased motility postoperatively [208].

A 2014 investigation examined the effect of laparoscopy and prolonged sevoflurane anesthesia on propulsive motility and transit time in dogs anesthetized for ovariohysterectomy [209]. Following oral administration, a wireless sensor continuously measured intraluminal pressure, pH, and temperature as it traversed the GIT. The pressures created by gastric and small intestinal contractions and their frequency were recorded, and a motility index and emptying or transit time were calculated. The frequency of contraction was not different from awake controls; however, changes in motility were seen within 20 minutes of induction. The motility index and the amplitudes of contraction of both the stomach and small bowel decreased significantly. Emptying and transit times were prolonged, with means of 49 and 11.5 hours and maxima of 59 and 14 h, respectively. Laparoscopy and ovariohysterectomy were performed in all the dogs, so it is unclear what specific effects these procedures may have had on GI function. All dogs were given hydromorphone and cephalexin for recovery, which could have affected the postoperative results, especially the opioid. The results of this study found a decrease in the force of intestinal contraction, inhibition of propulsive motility, and prolonged gastric emptying and small intestinal transit time.

The mechanism of POI is multifactorial, with neural, hormonal, inflammatory, and pharmacologic components, but the inflammatory response seen in the muscularis externa is considered the most important and likely the primary cause of prolonged POI. Activation of the sympathetic nervous system via a reflex arc between splanchnic afferents and adrenergic neurons in the spinal cord inhibits motility very soon following the surgical incision, but this effect is short-lived without other insult to the GIT. Handling of the intestine stimulates neural pathways that involve the brainstem and the hypothalamus to inhibit motility with activation of the hypothalamic–pituitary–adrenal axis. Corticotropin-releasing factor (CRF), calcitonin gene-related peptide, and substance P are released, resulting in production of multiple inflammatory mediators. CRF release in the hypothalamus affects function of the ANS in the brain, resulting in decreased activity of vagal efferents, which inhibits GI motility. Tissue handling also incites a local inflammatory response within the intestine that is proportional to the intensity of intestinal damage. Mast cells, primarily located in the mucosa and submucosa are activated as well as the resident macrophages that are located near the myenteric plexus of the muscularis layer. Activation of macrophages is an important step in the inflammatory phase as influx of other leukocytes follows and release of inflammatory mediators is stimulated. Enteric glial cells are very sensitive to mechanical stimuli with direct handling of intestine, pressure from distension, and tissue damage caused by edema and inflammation. These cells are normally involved in modulation of motility and glial dysfunction has been identified in many GI diseases, including POI. Alteration of the intestinal microbiome also occurs and contributes to the inflammation and loss of barrier function seen with POI. Surgically induced peritoneal inflammation also occurs that contributes to the local and systemic effects seen. POI is further exacerbated by the effects of anesthetic agents on motility, the use of opioids, and also the presence of peritonitis and sepsis [195,206,210–214].

Numerous interventions have been attempted in people to reduce or ameliorate the incidence of POI. The Enhanced Recovery Society has published guidelines for most every body system based on current best practice protocols to prevent or minimize the occurrence of POI following elective and emergent procedures. Good success has been seen, with improved outcomes, shorter hospitalization, decreased costs, and improved patient well-being and satisfaction (Table 41.4). Enhanced recovery after surgery (ERAS) protocols involve all members of the surgery/anesthesia/recovery team and address all aspects of the perioperative period. Use of less-invasive surgical techniques whenever possible, short fasting times, preanesthetic carbohydrate loading, avoidance of opioids, epidural anesthesia–analgesia, careful fluid therapy to avoid overhydration, early ambulation, and enteral intake are just some of the components of an ERAS protocol. Detailed descriptions can be found at

Table 41.4 Recommendations for prevention and treatment of postoperative ileus (POI).

Goal	Interventions
Maintain intestinal blood flow and oxygenation	Fluid therapy – goal-oriented, restricted (avoid excessive volume) Avoid saline, use balanced solutions ± colloids Prevention, prompt treatment of hypotension Prevention, treatment of low protein, albumin Maintain oxygen therapy, use higher F_IO_2 throughout
Perioperative analgesia	Systemic opioid-sparing protocols Thoracic epidural with local anesthetic – block sympathetic input Epidural morphine – less inhibition of motility Peripheral nerve blocks – transverse abdominis plane block NSAIDs – COX-2 inhibitors[a] – reduce inflammation Lidocaine infusion – anti-inflammatory, less/shorter POI Dexmedetomidine infusion postoperatively Electroacupuncture at ST_{36}
Surgical techniques	Minimize handling of intestine Laparoscopy whenever possible – less inflammation, shorter POI • Helium is better – CO_2 promotes infection via tissue acidosis • Air actually stimulates inflammation • Use lower insufflation pressure
Postoperative care	Maintain oxygenation and blood volume/arterial blood pressure Enteral nutrition and ambulation as soon as possible Avoid nasogastric tubes Laxative therapy to treat, prevent constipation
Prokinetic medication/therapeutics	
Alvimopan, Methylnaltrexone	Peripheral opioid receptor antagonists
Erythromycin, Azithromycin	Motilin/ghrelin receptor agonists
Metoclopramide	Dopamine (D_2) receptor antagonist, serotonin receptor agonist ($5HT_4$)
Domperidone	Dopamine (D_2) receptor antagonist
Ranitidine, Nizatidine	H_2 receptor antagonists
Mosapride, Prucalopride,	Act on serotonin receptors
Cisapride	No longer used in people but is used in animals, compounded
Anti-inflammatory and prokinetic	Daikenchuto – Japanese herbal preparation; ginger, ginseng, zanthoxylum fruit

F_IO_2, inspired concentration of oxygen; NSAID, non-steroidal anti-inflammatory drug; COX-2, prostaglandin synthase-2.

[a] COX-2 inhibitors are avoided in patients where risk of anastomotic leakage or sepsis is present.

Source: Compiled from Whitehead *et al.* [5]; Grocott *et al.* [21]; Mythen [185]; Boysen [186]; DeHaven-Hudkins *et al.* [203]; Nakayoshi *et al.* [204]; Pöpping *et al.* [205]; Lubawski and Saclarides [206]; Sido *et al.* [210]; van Bree *et al.* [211]; Vather and Bissett [212]; Hussain and Park [213]; Mazzotta *et al.* [214]; Campoy [215]; Yang *et al.* [216]; Kaye *et al.* [217]; Chen *et al.* [218]; Cooke *et al.* [219]; Leslie *et al.* [220]; Rimbäck *et al.* [221]; Malone *et al.* [222].

https://erassociety.org. Campoy has reviewed the application of ERAS protocols in veterinary medicine with an emphasis on local anesthesia–analgesia [215].

Gastrointestinal conditions requiring anesthesia

Many patients that require anesthesia for GI disease are emergent and/or may be critically ill. Thorough preanesthetic evaluation and preparation prior to anesthesia help to minimize complications; however, this is not always possible in extremely emergent patients. Recommendations for a basic workup include measurement of hematocrit, total protein, blood urea nitrogen (BUN), creatinine, serum alkaline phosphatase (ALP), alanine aminotransferase (ALT), aspartate aminotransferase (AST), bilirubin, albumin, electrolytes, and total carbon dioxide. Blood gas analysis and lactate are important in sick patients. Additional diagnostics appropriate to the problem at hand should be evaluated, such as radiographs or abdominal ultrasound. Computed tomography or MRI is sometimes used in stable patients for determination of diagnosis and prognosis prior to surgery.

General guidelines for the management of anesthesia for abdominal procedures are similar to those for other disease conditions. Preservation of tissue oxygen delivery through the maintenance of blood flow and avoidance of hypoxemia are paramount. Additional consideration should be given to predictable complications (e.g., endotoxemia with damaged intestine, reperfusion injury following derotation of twisted segments of intestine, cardiac dysrhythmias during splenectomy, or GDV), and appropriate treatments planned/prepared. Finally, administration of adjunctive drugs to provide pain management, speed return of GI function, and limit adverse effects such as nausea and vomiting will improve patient care and outcomes.

Laparotomy

The plan for an exploratory laparotomy varies more with the patient's condition than with the primary GI problem. All levels of patient status using the ASA I–V +/- E classification may be seen. Some patients are healthy (e.g., gastropexy) and their management is similar to that of other elective abdominal procedures (e.g., ovariohysterectomy). Other patients may be severely ill and require laparotomy as a life-saving intervention. Fluid deficits, electrolyte abnormalities, and acid–base imbalance should be corrected as much as is reasonable prior to induction. All equipment for anesthesia and monitoring should be assembled and tested for proper function prior to induction.

Some patients may have pre-existing organ dysfunction that may or may not be related to the reason for exploratory laparotomy. Ketamine, especially as a prolonged continuous infusion, should probably not be used in patients with renal dysfunction, especially cats since they excrete ketamine and its metabolites to a significant extent in the urine. Where available, thiopental should be avoided in debilitated patients and those with severe liver dysfunction. It should also not be used in sighthounds. Both thiopental and propofol can sensitize the myocardium to catecholamine-associated arrhythmias and should be used cautiously in patients with pre-existing dysrhythmias or cardiac disease, or when arrhythmias are highly likely such as with GDV or splenic masses. In both research and clinical studies, alfaxalone has not been reported to cause arrhythmias [43,44,223]. Etomidate is often preferred for patients with pre-existing myocardial dysfunction (e.g., poor contractility) who are otherwise healthy as it has minimal effects on cardiovascular function. A dose of midazolam or diazepam, 0.2 mg/kg IV, just prior to etomidate will improve muscle relaxation and facilitate intubation. Historically, etomidate was not recommended in sick patients as it causes adrenal suppression and has been associated with greater mortality in humans [224–227]. Some reports have not found greater mortality when used only for induction [228,229], however, a tendency toward adrenal insufficiency or hospital-acquired pneumonia and sepsis has been identified [227–229]. Qin *et al.* found significantly decreasing levels of cortisol and aldosterone during a 3-h infusion of etomidate in dogs [230]. Also, a recent clinical study of etomidate for induction in healthy dogs was stopped due to the development of pigmenturia [231]. Inhalant induction is not recommended for exploratory laparotomy, especially in patients with frequent emesis. Following effective premedication, healthy patients and those in good overall condition (ASA I, II) can be induced with titration of usual doses of ketamine, propofol, and alfaxalone separately or in combination [232]. In healthy dogs, ketamine increases heart rate, blood pressure, and cardiac output, while these parameters are decreased by propofol and thiopental in a dose-dependent manner. Propofol interferes with baroreceptor responses and is more often associated with bradycardia and hypoxemia [226,233]. Alfaxalone increased heart rate and decreased cardiac output, arterial blood pressure, and systemic vascular resistance in healthy cats and dogs without premedication [43,44]; however, in clinical settings, hypotension following induction is not common. No differences were found when induction with alfaxalone was compared to diazepam–fentanyl with or without propofol in ASA III–V dogs [223]. Ketamine is often suggested for induction due to its cardiovascular-stimulating effects. However, since this is due to centrally mediated increases in sympathetic tone, the opposite effect can be seen in very ill patients with poor sympathetic reserve [233–235]. Intramuscular premedication can be used in healthy patients anesthetized for elective procedures; however, intravenous premedication is preferred for higher-risk patients. Combination of a benzodiazepine and an opioid is most often utilized. Midazolam or diazepam with hydromorphone, methadone, oxymorphone, or fentanyl (or its congeners) are titrated intravenously to effect. Since the incidence of vomiting is greater with hydromorphone, other opioids should be used in patients with frequent emesis. The pharmacokinetic profile of remifentanil makes it a good choice for compromised patients. It is used in dogs and cats [236,237]; however, it is quite expensive and not available in some areas. To avoid traditional induction drugs entirely in compromised patients, additional doses of premedicants (opioid and benzodiazepine) can be titrated IV until intubation is possible. Bradycardia and respiratory depression may be significant following high doses of opioids used for induction, so supplies and equipment for intubation, ventilation, and monitoring should be immediately available.

Isoflurane or sevoflurane are preferred for maintenance of anesthesia for exploratory laparotomy over halothane as the latter sensitizes the myocardium to arrhythmias and decreases tissue blood flow to a greater extent. Desflurane can be useful for its rapid induction and recovery characteristics, however, it is not commonly used and is unavailable in some countries. It requires a special heated vaporizer to produce consistent concentration of vapor and is more expensive. Nitrous oxide (N_2O) is not recommended since it diffuses readily into intestinal organs, causing or exacerbating distention and potentially compromising ventilation. N_2O also has significant side effects in humans, including interference with vitamin B_{12} metabolism, damage to the CNS, and abortion [238]. All the halogenated anesthetics used currently have deleterious effects on the environment; however, those associated with N_2O and especially desflurane are much greater. The "carbon footprint" of N_2O is reportedly 310 times that of CO_2, while desflurane is 2500 times. N_2O also contributes to depletion of the ozone layer in the atmosphere [238,239]. Use of desflurane was recently banned by the National Health Service in Scotland [240]. N_2O is not commonly used in veterinary medicine and its use in people has greatly decreased.

The respiratory and cardiovascular effects of all the inhalants are more pronounced in debilitated patients; hypoventilation and hypotension are common. Pre-existing cardiovascular depression decreases the minimum alveolar concentration (MAC) required to maintain anesthetic depth. Vaporizer settings should be kept as low as possible to minimize hypotension. Occasionally, discontinuation of inhalant anesthesia and transition to injectable maintenance is necessary to maintain blood pressure in patients with severe sepsis that do not respond to fluid and/or inotropic and/or vasopressor therapy. Patients with a distended GIT, especially those that are obese, are more likely to become hypoxemic, especially in recovery when oxygen is discontinued, due to hypoventilation and atelectasis. Non-invasive monitoring of blood pressure should be initiated prior to induction, arterial catheterization should be considered soon following induction. Monitoring of blood pressure and oxygen saturation should be continued into recovery; oxygen supplementation is often required postoperatively [172], and cardiovascular support may sometimes be needed as well.

To minimize the amount of inhalant needed or if anesthetic depth is inadequate, additional sedatives and/or analgesics are given intermittently or as a CRI. Continuous infusion provides a more constant level of drug delivery, and greatly reduces MAC. Infusions are initially set at a specific rate and the inhalant setting is varied to maintain the desired anesthetic depth, although infusion rates may be varied as well. An opioid, lidocaine, and/or ketamine can be administered in combination or separately as CRIs [241–247], though lidocaine is not recommended for use in cats [248]. α_2-Adrenergic agonists can also be given as infusions. Dexmedetomidine has been evaluated both during and after anesthesia in healthy small animals and found to be useful and without serious side effects, although close monitoring of cardiovascular parameters is warranted [247–249]. Recent reviews of anesthesia of septic human patients do not mention use of dexmedetomidine intraoperatively [229], however, it is used routinely for sedation in critically ill patients, and has been associated with improved outcomes in some cases [250].

In patients without hypovolemia, sepsis, coagulopathy, or dermatitis in the lumbosacral area, epidural administration of a local anesthetic with or without morphine can also provide intra- and postoperative analgesia. Local anesthesia using transversus abdominis plane blocks and/or intercostal blocks can be very helpful to provide analgesia and minimize opioid use, especially in the postoperative period [251–253].

Fluid therapy is continued during anesthesia; the type of fluids and the rate necessary will vary depending on the patient's status. Regular assessment of fluid status is necessary as fluid overload has deleterious effects on the efficacy of fluid exchange in the interstitium, resulting in edema, dysfunction of the glycocalyx, and further damage to tissues [254–257]. Hypotension is common in exploratory laparotomy cases and has been consistently associated with greater mortality in patients with sepsis, peritonitis, and emergency abdominal surgery [226,258–260]. The GIT lacks an autoregulatory response to blood pressure as seen in the brain and kidney and prolonged hypotension can be more damaging to intestinal tissues and should therefore be vigorously treated [226]. If hypotension persists despite correction of volume deficits, infusions of inotropes such as dobutamine and/or dopamine may increase cardiac output and improve blood pressure. Vasopressors are considered when decreased systemic vascular resistance is a significant component of hypotension. Ephedrine is a sympathomimetic which can be given as a bolus; it is effective primarily for mild transient decreases in blood pressure. Phenylephrine, norepinephrine, vasopressin, and epinephrine are given as infusions and titrated to effect. These drugs are potent vasoconstrictors and should be used at the lowest effective dose to minimize tissue ischemia despite improved blood pressure [245,255,260–263] (see Chapter 21 for dosages).

Monitoring patients for exploratory laparotomy should include the usual parameters of anesthetic depth, mucous membrane color and refill time, heart rate and rhythm, respiratory rate/effort/pulse strength, and arterial blood pressure. Invasive blood pressure measurement is preferred by anesthesiologists for most laparotomies since changes in cardiac output and pressure can be rapid and/or severe. Pulse oximetry and capnography provide valuable information on patient status with continuous real-time evaluation of ventilation and gas exchange and are commonly used. Arterial blood gas analysis is used to document respiratory and metabolic status and to periodically evaluate the results of therapy. Lactate measurement is an indirect estimate of tissue perfusion and oxygenation status [264]. Changes in lactate lag behind alterations of tissue metabolism, but measurement at presentation and over time is of value in the evaluation of therapy and prognosis of patients with severe disease [208,265–269]. Because of the variability of blood pressure measurement in hypovolemic, unstable patients, measurement of cardiac output would be very helpful in the assessment of cardiovascular status; however, this is not commonly available for clinical patients. Monitoring of the variation of the pulse pressure or the systolic arterial pressure waveform during mechanical ventilation has been found to be a reliable parameter that infers the presence of hypovolemia [254,270,271], suggesting a need for fluid/volume therapy (Fig. 41.2). Close attention to volume loss and the actions of the surgeon during laparotomy helps to avoid hemodynamic compromise by enabling the anesthetist to anticipate and treat problems in a timely fashion. For example, cardiovascular function is greatly affected by blood loss or removal of large volumes of effusion, and with handling of large masses. Manipulation and derotation of ischemic bowel leads to the release of numerous inflammatory mediators that cause vasodilation and possibly cardiac dysfunction (Fig. 41.3).

Monitoring should continue throughout anesthesia and into recovery. Signs of anesthetic depth, heart and respiratory rate, mucous membrane color and capillary refill time, temperature, blood pressure, and electrocardiography should be periodically evaluated. Postoperative pain management is important for the

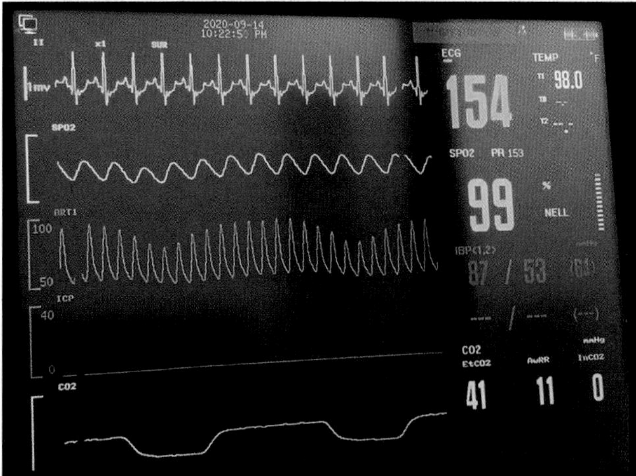

Figure 41.2 Patient monitor showing systolic pressure (or pulse pressure) variation of the arterial waveform in an anesthetized mechanically ventilated dog. The presence of systolic pressure or pulse pressure variation is associated with hypovolemia and fluid responsiveness. Source: Dr. Juliana Figueiredo, VCA West Coast Specialty and Emergency Animal Hospital, Fountain Valley, CA.

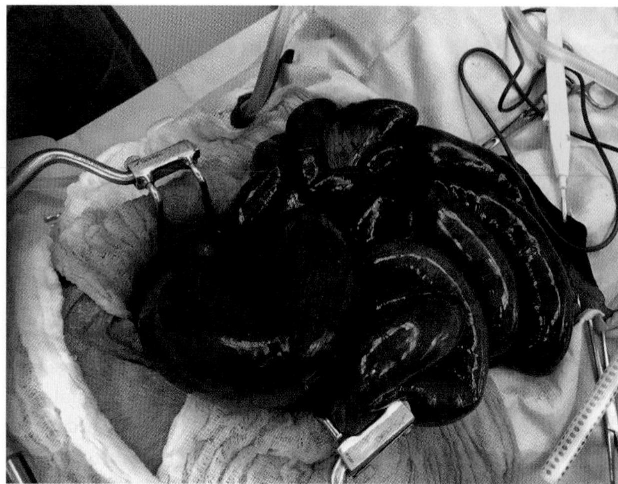

Figure 41.3 Mesenteric torsion in a dog presenting for acute onset of abdominal discomfort/pain and profound depression. Manipulation and derotation of ischemic bowel leads to release of inflammatory mediators resulting in vasodilation and potential cardiac dysfunction. Source:. Dr. Jane Quandt, Department of Small Animal Medicine and Surgery, College of Veterinary Medicine, University of Georgia, Athens, GA.

comfort and the outcome of patients with GI disease. Opioids are continued as intermittent boluses intravenously or intramuscularly, or via continuous infusion. Infusions of lidocaine and/or ketamine are also effective. Lidocaine causes nausea and vomiting in dogs at high infusion rates [60,272] but was associated with improved outcomes in humans following abdominal surgery [61,62,218,219], and in dogs with GDV [273] and peritonitis [274]. Lidocaine given intraoperatively has also been shown to decrease postoperative pain in humans [61,62,218,219]. Higher dosing and use of multiple modes of analgesia are often required in the first 24 h postoperatively. These should be decreased as soon as possible so that enteral feeding and ambulation can be instituted and to minimize the incidence of ileus. Infusions of low doses of α_2-adrenergic receptor agonists can be useful, especially in patients with high analgesic requirements or opioid dysphoria. Valtolina *et al.* found that dexmedetomidine infusion provided effective postoperative analgesia similar to morphine without significant adverse effects in ill dogs [275]. However, infusions of α_2-adrenergic receptor agonists can have significant cardiovascular side effects, so their use should be carefully considered in the individual patient [249].

Non-steroidal anti-inflammatory drugs (NSAIDs) are used in human, ruminant, and equine patients following GI surgery with minimal complications [220,276–283], although a greater risk of dehiscence of anastomosis was associated with NSAID use in humans [284]. Dogs and cats are relatively sensitive to the GI side-effects of NSAIDs such as ulceration and hemorrhage [280–282]. Although useful in healthy patients anesthetized for elective procedures such as gastropexy, the risks and benefits should be considered and it may be best to avoid NSAIDs in patients with GI disease, renal compromise, hypotension, liver disease, coagulopathy, and other conditions that could be exacerbated by NSAID administration [283].

Megaesophagus

Regurgitation, food retention, and defective peristalsis of the esophagus are seen in patients with primary esophageal dysmotility *without* dilation or persistent megaesophagus (ME) [285]. ME is a persistent dilation caused by damage to the esophageal musculature or defective peristalsis. Classified as congenital or acquired, regurgitation is the most frequent clinical sign, with weight loss and poor body condition in adults, intolerance of solid food, and failure to thrive in young patients. Aspiration pneumonia (AP) is common, and cough and abnormal lung sounds may be present. ME is rare in cats but not uncommon in dogs. However, cats with dysautonomia, an acquired abnormality of autonomic ganglia that leads to GI dysfunction, usually have ME. Congenital idiopathic ME has been reported in several breeds of dogs and a few cats. A lack of vagal sensory input is presumed to be the underlying mechanism. Peristalsis of the esophagus does not occur because the presence of a food bolus is not detected. Acquired ME is idiopathic, caused by esophageal obstruction, and secondary to other diseases. Vascular ring anomaly, esophageal stricture, hiatal hernia, tumor, granuloma, and foreign bodies cause obstruction. With time, muscular damage caused by dilation proximal to the lesion becomes irreversible. Idiopathic ME is the most common cause of the acquired form in adult dogs. The mechanism is thought to be similar to the congenital form; with loss of normal motility, ingesta remains in the esophagus and eventually results in dilation. Acquired ME is secondary to or associated with peripheral neuropathy, neuromuscular disease, laryngeal paralysis, severe esophagitis, lead poisoning, lupus myositis, and hypoadrenocorticism. Hypothyroidism is reported but has been discounted by some authors [285–287]. Chronic or recurrent gastric dilation with or without volvulus was also identified as a risk factor in a retrospective evaluation of 136 dogs diagnosed with ME. Evidence for concurrent hypothyroidism in these cases was evaluated but was not found [287]. Myasthenia gravis (MG) is a very common cause of ME, reported to occur in 25–30% of cases. ME is often the first clinical sign of MG in dogs [285,288]. MG is reported in cats, but is more common in dogs likely due to the higher proportion of striated muscle in the canine esophagus. ME is only rarely seen in cats with MG [289]. A recent retrospective study of 99 dogs with ME not associated with a structural lesion found a high proportion of idiopathic cases; 10 were congenital, 89 were acquired, with 42.7% of the latter idiopathic, and 38.2% due to MG [290]. Transient ME was seen in three dogs with coral snake envenomation. All three dogs had respiratory difficulty, two developed AP, and two required ventilation [291]. An unusual outbreak of ME occurred in 398 dogs in Latvia and Australia from 2014 to 2018. The feeding of two different brands of dry dog food was incriminated in each country, although a specific ingredient could not be identified and the underlying physiologic defect was not determined [292].

Patients with ME may be anesthetized for diagnostics or treatment, such as endoscopy, computed tomography, electromyography, nerve conduction studies, muscle/nerve biopsy, bougienage, foreign body removal, and vascular ring anomaly correction. ME may also be a concurrent disease in patients anesthetized/sedated for unrelated procedures such as dentistry or radiographs. Since ME is often associated with neurologic disease, these patients should be closely monitored for esophageal dysfunction and possibly respiratory insufficiency [290]. GER, regurgitation, and aspiration are the primary concerns when anesthetizing patients with ME. Prolonged fasting is not advised as the dilation prevents complete emptying of esophageal contents and an increased incidence of GER has been seen with long fasting times in normal dogs [110,111]. Some patients with chronic disease may be thin or debilitated due to malnutrition and some may be dehydrated if unable to retain adequate fluid intake. Many have repeated episodes of AP and are at greater risk of hypoxemia perioperatively. Patients should be stabilized prior to elective anesthesia with IV fluid therapy and appropriate treatment for pneumonia. A dedicated anesthetist is important for patients with ME, as airway management and constant monitoring for leakage of esophageal contents are necessary. Suction of esophageal contents should be performed immediately after intubation and just before discontinuation of anesthesia to reduce the risk of aspiration. Sternal recumbency and elevation of the neck with the nose tipped down may also help decrease the incidence. If regurgitation occurs, the nose and head should be lowered immediately to allow drainage. Preoxygenation is recommended for those with active pneumonia; these patients should be restrained cautiously to avoid struggling and excessive stress. Anesthetic drugs should be chosen based on the patient's status, with rapid IV induction and intubation necessary to secure and protect the airway as quickly as possible. Avoidance of drugs that cause vomiting such as some opioids (e.g., morphine or hydromorphone) and α_2-adrenergic receptor agonists is also recommended. Reversible and shorter-acting agents are preferred. In recovery, extubation should be delayed as long as possible, and oxygen should be supplemented in recovery until oxygen saturation is consistently normal. Gastroprotectants, antacids, and antiemetics given preoperatively are recommended.

Patients with ME due to MG may be treated with pyridostigmine bromide, which increases levels of ACh by inhibiting anticholinesterase that would normally break down ACh. Cholinergic crisis is therefore possible, but this is rare. The effect of neuromuscular blocking agents (NMBAs) is unpredictable in myasthenic patients and possibly others with idiopathic ME. They do not respond to depolarizing agents but are quite sensitive to nondepolarizing agents. Very low doses of NMBAs should be utilized if paralysis is necessary. Specific monitoring of the extent of blockade must be available. Sugammadex is effective as a reversal agent for NMBAs [293].

Gastric dilation–volvulus

The incidence of gastric dilation–volvulus (GDV) at 50 emergency clinics in the United Kingdom over a 17-month period was 0.64% (492/77,088 cases) [294]. Approximately, 10 cases per clinic per month is an underestimation, however, as it does not include cases presenting during regular hours at day clinic practices. Acute GDV is life-threatening, seen most often in adult large or giant breed dogs, especially those with a deep-chested conformation. However, it can occur in small breed dogs and puppies, and has been reported in five cats, three with concurrent diaphragmatic hernias [295–297]. Although an underlying motility disorder is presumed to be important in the pathogenesis and altered motility patterns have been identified *after* GDV in patients and research subjects with created GDV, the actual pathogenesis of the condition has not been elucidated [298–303]. The etiology is multifactorial with numerous risk factors identified, including large/giant breed; deep-chested conformation; "slim" body condition; middle to older age; close relative that has experienced GDV; multiple diets, feeding, and exercise routines; aerophagia; stress; hospitalization; nervous, anxious, or aggressive demeanor; and gastric foreign body [294,295,304–307]. Recent studies have identified specific genetic immune system variants in Great Danes with GDV [308]. Inflammatory bowel disease and dysbiosis of the GI microbiome may also be associated with increased risk of GDV [305,309]. Mortality has decreased since the 1980s but is still high. Studies have reported mortality rates of 10–26.8% [294,304,306,310–316], but these refer to dogs treated surgically and do not reflect the actual case numbers seen. Unfortunately, many cases are euthanized at presentation because of prognosis, cost, or other factors [314,315]; clinical practices aimed at prevention and early recognition would likely have the most significant effect overall [306,315]. Gastropexy has proven to be preventive in dogs at high risk and those following GDV. Reported recurrence rates are 0–5% with most developing dilation but not volvulus [306,316,317]. Improved survival is likely associated with improvements in medical therapy, especially fluid resuscitation, early decompression of the stomach whenever possible, and timely surgical intervention. Mortality is correlated with damage to the stomach and surrounding organs, gastric perforation, sepsis, peritonitis, the presence of cardiac dysrhythmias pre- or postoperatively, both hypo- and hyperthermia at presentation, postoperative acute renal failure, hypotension at any time during hospitalization, the duration from onset to presentation or surgery, the time from presentation to surgery, and the severity of systemic compromise at presentation [306,310–314]. Reperfusion injury has also been implicated as a significant factor associated with mortality with GDV [318–320].

GDV is always an emergency. Blood flow to the stomach and surrounding organs is compromised as abdominal veins become obstructed, greatly decreasing venous return to the heart, and producing severe relative hypovolemia and distributive shock. Distention of the stomach also restricts ventilation via interference with diaphragmatic excursion. Early clinical signs include restlessness and anxiety, followed by hypersalivation, vomiting and/or retching, and distention of the abdomen (Fig. 41.4) Eventually, depression, weakness, and dyspnea develop if distention is not relieved. Vomiting, salivation, and sequestration of hydrogen and chloride ions that occur with gastric outflow obstruction initially cause metabolic alkalosis. Metabolic acidosis develops later, secondary to the effects of ischemia and decreased hydration, with increased lactate production and the release of inflammatory mediators. Endotoxemia can also develop with damage to the portal system. Reperfusion injury occurs when ischemia is reversed with gastric decompression/derotation and redistribution of fluid volume [306,318–320].

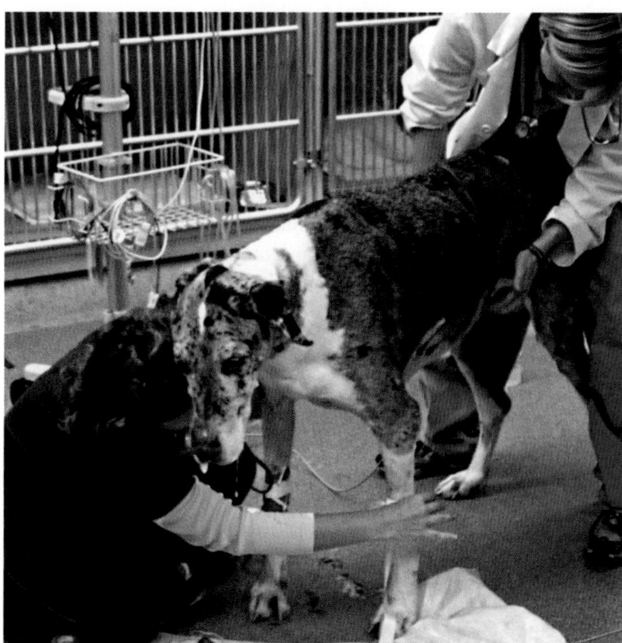

Figure 41.4 Preparation of a Great Dane with gastric dilation–volvulus, (GDV) for anesthesia and surgery. Intravenous access has been secured and fluid resuscitation initiated, ECG leads have been attached to evaluate cardiac rhythm, and the degree of abdominal distension is assessed. Note the salivation and depressed mentation of the dog. Source: Dr. Jennifer Adams, with permission.

Intravenous fluid therapy and gastric decompression should be initiated as quickly as possible. Baseline laboratory evaluation should include packed cell volume (PCV), total solids (TS), electrolytes, creatinine, and acid–base status. A clotting profile and venous lactate are useful to evaluate prognosis and guide therapy but generally should not delay surgical intervention if the owners would proceed regardless of the results. Gastric necrosis is likely present when more than one hemostatic test is abnormal and when lactate is greatly elevated at presentation [321–323] and/or fails to decrease significantly with fluid resuscitation. Increased lactate at presentation [265,321–324] and decreased clearance were associated with higher mortality [265,325]. Radiography to distinguish between dilation and dilation–volvulus, should be delayed until cardiovascular resuscitation is well under way. Anesthetic personnel, equipment, and supplies should be made ready prior to arrival of the patient so that surgical intervention may commence as soon as possible. Previous emergent therapy was to administer "shock" doses (80–90 mL/kg) of crystalloid solution via large-bore catheters, using multiple venous access points. However, use of goal-directed resuscitation guidelines to achieve appropriate clinical endpoints rather than a specific volume avoids hypervolemia and tissue edema and may improve outcomes [254,255,326–330]. Portions of the estimated deficit are given over 15–30 min and the patient's response is determined. Clinical parameters to monitor include heart rate, arterial blood pressure, mucous membrane color and perfusion, tissue oxygenation, and mentation. PCV, TS or total protein, blood gases, and venous oxygen saturation should be measured as needed. Use of balanced crystalloid solutions is useful; however, faster and longer-lasting resuscitation is achieved with the addition of small volumes of hypertonic saline 7.5% at 2–4 mL/kg over 15 min, or colloids at 5–10 mL/kg over 30 min. Alternatively, a combination of colloid and hypertonic saline is given at 4–6 mL/ kg [328]. This simultaneous use of hypertonic saline and colloid has been shown to improve cardiovascular status in both experimental and clinical cases of GDV [331,332]. As previously mentioned, acute kidney injury has been seen in people following treatment with colloids, so their use is not recommended in human medicine.

Thoracic auscultation and electrocardiography should be performed soon following presentation, as cardiac arrhythmias are common with GDV. Most are ventricular in origin, although sinus tachycardia, atrial fibrillation, and atrioventricular block can also occur, and the "R on T" phenomenon is sometimes seen (Fig. 41.5) [304,306,311,333]. Specific antiarrhythmic therapy may not be necessary if the dysrhythmia is of minimal cardiovascular consequence or correction of hypovolemia, hypoxemia, hypercarbia, acid–base status, and/or electrolyte abnormalities provide resolution. Treatment of ventricular tachycardia is often needed when extrasystoles are numerous or multifocal, the sustained rate is very high (> 160 beats/min), extrasystoles are very early such that an "R on T" phenomenon is possible, and always when hemodynamic status is affected by the arrhythmia. Lidocaine bolus is given slowly IV at 1–2 mg/kg followed by CRI at 25–100 μg/kg/min [334]. Postoperative therapy for cardiac arrhythmias is often necessary. A lidocaine CRI is particularly useful as it decreases anesthetic requirements in dogs by as much as 37–43% [60,335] and may have positive effects on outcome. When lidocaine was given preemptively in dogs with GDV, significantly fewer cases with cardiac dysrhythmias, less renal impairment, and shorter hospitalization time were found as

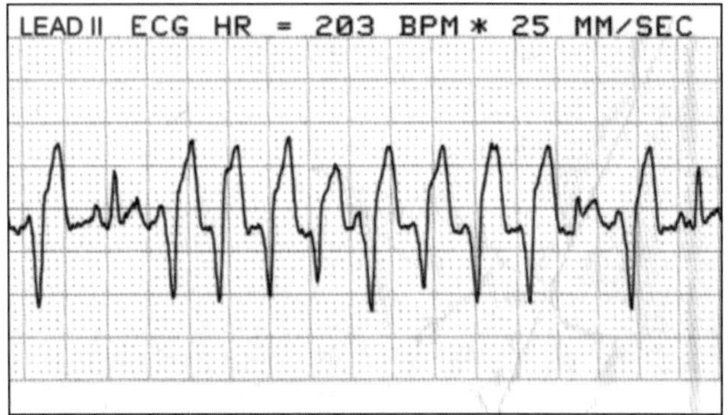

Figure 41.5 Ventricular tachycardia seen postoperatively in a dog anesthetized for correction of gastric dilation–volvulus (GDV). Source: Dr. Jennifer Adams, with permission.

compared to a historical control group [273]. Lidocaine has also been shown to have numerous anti-inflammatory effects [336–338] and may have prokinetic effects [61,218,221,222,339]. Improved survival has also been seen in dogs with septic peritonitis [274] and horses treated surgically for small intestinal colic [340].

Despite much research devoted to the effects of ischemia/reperfusion injury and its prevention or treatment, few therapies have been adopted in clinical practice. Avoidance of hyperoxia may be useful since greater damage was seen following reperfusion in cardiac arrest patients maintained at higher-than-normal PaO_2 levels [341]. Inhibition of oxygen-free radical formation with antioxidants and iron-chelating drugs such as deferoxamine has been shown to reduce reperfusion injury in dogs with GDV [318,342]. Ethyl pyruvate has been shown to preserve, protect, and even improve cellular function in many tissues and species with ischemia/reperfusion injury and may prove useful as a treatment for dogs with GDV or other ischemic lesions [343].

Gastric lavage is sometimes necessary during correction of a GDV. Considerations for lavage are similar to those for GER, upper GI endoscopy, and ME. Leakage of gastric contents is common and the endotracheal tube can be displaced. The head should be tipped downwards to direct gastric contents away from the pharynx. The pharynx should be examined and cleaned of any fluid or debris that may have leaked around the nasogastric tube prior to recovery. Postoperative dysmotility is reported in GDV patients; they should be monitored closely in recovery for regurgitation, vomiting, ileus, and aspiration [299,303,305,320].

Hemoabdomen

Causes of hemorrhage into the peritoneal cavity are traumatic or atraumatic. Trauma is most often due to injury from impact with motor vehicles or penetrating objects. It can also be caused by a fall and during fights with other animals. Abdominal organs, especially liver and spleen, vasculature, and/or the abdominal wall are affected. Atraumatic lesions include hematoma or neoplasia of abdominal organs, organ displacement or torsion, and coagulation abnormalities (e.g., rodenticide toxicity and autoimmune thrombocytopenia) [344–348]. Anaphylaxis was also recently reported as a cause of hemoperitoneum in 11 dogs [349].

Coagulopathy can also result from acute trauma and has been suggested to contribute to 25% of deaths due to uncontrolled hemorrhage in people [350]. Initially, a hypocoagulable state caused by the inflammation produced by tissue injury and shock develops, followed later by hypercoagulation with thromboembolism and organ failure. Hypothermia and acidemia are often present and contribute to coagulopathy. Acute traumatic coagulopathy is diagnosed using routine clotting profiles and viscoelastic measures such as thromboelastography [344–346,350]. It was identified in 11/33 dogs with severe trauma [351] and in 1/18 dogs and 1/19 cats with lesser injury [352].

Hemorrhage due to neoplasia is common, especially in dogs. Potential sites include the liver, spleen, mesentery, and adrenal glands, with the spleen being most often affected. Hemangiosarcoma is the most common abdominal neoplasm in both dogs and cats and usually affects the spleen and/or liver. Long-term prognosis is guarded to poor [347,348,353], but a high percentage of canine cases with abdominal hemorrhage survive anesthesia and surgery to discharge [353]. A retrospective investigation of spontaneous atraumatic hemoperitoneum in 65 cats found that 46% had abdominal neoplasia and 54% had non-neoplastic disease; hepatic necrosis and coagulopathy accounted for most of the latter cases. Only eight of the cats (12.3%) survived to discharge [354].

Hemorrhage into the abdomen can be gradual or sudden, and can quickly become life-threatening. Clinical signs are similar to blood loss from any cause with progressive signs of hypovolemic shock such as increasing tachycardia, pale mucous membranes, weak pulses, weakness and/or lethargy, decreased mentation, and cold extremities. Compensatory mechanisms such as splanchnic vasoconstriction and reflex tachycardia may initially mask clinical signs of hypovolemia; however, as blood loss approaches 30% of the blood volume, these mechanisms are exhausted [345]. Hypothermia is seen in dogs and is common in cats at presentation. Abdominal distention, a palpable fluid wave, abdominal pain, and subcutaneous discoloration at the umbilicus and scrotum are also sometimes seen. Radiography may show loss of abdominal detail with a "ground-glass" appearance. Ultrasound will reveal the presence of free fluid and may reveal a mass or metastatic disease. Abdominocentesis produces a bloody sample that does not clot and that has a PCV similar to the systemic PCV is diagnostic for hemorrhage [344]. Peritoneal lavage may be necessary with smaller volumes of blood loss or when ultrasound is not available [347,348]; a PCV of 2–5% in lavage samples is indicative of hemorrhage [347]. Depending on the severity of volume lost, the systemic PCV, TS/TP, and platelet count may be normal or decreased, and, as lactate increases, base excess becomes more negative, and central venous oxygen tension decreases [345].

Anesthetic considerations for hemoabdomen include hypovolemia, anemia, respiratory compromise associated with large masses or fluid volumes compressing the diaphragm, and any organ dysfunction that may be present. Ideally, the patient is stabilized prior to surgery with intravenous fluids and sometimes transfusion. The rate of blood loss is important, and some prefer to replace erythrocyte losses after the source of bleeding is stopped if the patient is stable enough to delay transfusion. It is not necessary to correct the entire RBC deficit preoperatively; however, the patient should be treated to achieve normovolemia and a PCV $\geq$ 30% in dogs or 20% in cats, as oxygen delivery is usually adequate above these levels. "Hypotensive" resuscitation to an endpoint less than ideal, such as systolic arterial pressure of 90 mmHg or mean arterial pressure of 60 mmHg, is sometimes pursued when control of the source of hemorrhage can be achieved quickly [346]. Lower PCVs are often tolerated during anesthesia when they are a result of chronic blood loss rather than acute hemorrhage. Patients with anaphylaxis require treatment with an antihistamine and/or epinephrine and may not require surgical intervention [349].

The volume of prior and ongoing blood loss must be estimated and replaced to limit effects on cardiac output. Estimating loss is often difficult; techniques include weighing bloody sponges and towels, tracking the volume of lavage fluid used, and estimating the volume of blood and fluid collected in suction bottles.

Isotonic crystalloids are used for initial volume replacement. The specific volume required is unknown and depends on the speed of loss, but multiples of the volume lost are recommended (e.g., 1.5–3 times the loss for acute hemorrhage and up to eight times for gradual loss affecting the intracellular volume). When intracellular volume is affected, replacement can proceed more slowly than when acute hemorrhage is present. Boluses of 10–20 mL/kg for dogs and 5–10 mL/kg for cats are given, the patient is reassessed, and boluses are repeated as needed up to appropriate endpoints. Colloids were considered a rational replacement for plasma loss, given at a ratio close to 1:1, if PCV and protein levels were adequate. However, concerns about renal damage with colloid therapy have decreased their use [355–357]. Losses greater than 20–30% of the patient's total blood volume should be replaced with whole blood, plasma and packed RBCs, or an RBC substitute such as Oxyglobin®, if available, to ensure adequate oxygen delivery. Autotransfusion is useful in some cases but not recommended with septic peritonitis, urinary rupture, and neoplastic lesions. Catecholamine and inotrope infusions are used for other procedures when needed, but vasopressin may produce better results in patients with hemorrhagic shock [358].

TS or total protein levels should be maintained at greater than 4–4.5 g/dL. PCV and TS are measured intermittently to monitor the efficacy of therapy and the speed of blood loss, realizing that hemodilution will be present and that colloids will interfere with refractometer readings. Response to volume restoration and increased oxygen-carrying capacity (e.g., normalization of heart rate and blood pressure) are useful guides to fluid therapy during anesthesia. Improvement of variation of the systolic arterial pressure waveform or pulse pressure may also be seen. Lactate is a useful indicator of tissue oxygen delivery as it increases with severe hypovolemia and decreases as volume, cardiovascular function, and perfusion improve [264]. Although rapid volume replacement is sometimes necessary for extremely hypovolemic patients, large volumes cause hypocoagulability and result in "dilutional coagulopathy" [345,346,353].

Evacuation of blood and manipulation of organs or abdominal masses can cause significant hemodynamic instability. Sequestration of a portion of the blood volume in the exteriorized tissues and/or redistribution of blood volume affects cardiac output and peripheral perfusion. In humans, anesthetized for abdominal surgery, a syndrome of tachycardia, hypotension, and cutaneous hyperemia has been reported, called "mesenteric traction syndrome" [98,358,359]. This has not been described or perhaps not investigated in animals, but prostacyclin, histamine, and other vasoactive substances are released, causing fluctuations in hemodynamic status when tension is placed on mesenteric vasculature. The review of 38 studies with 1102 patients by Olsen *et al.* found mesenteric traction syndrome developed in 76% of patients anesthetized for major abdominal surgery that included procedures on the GIT, aorta, and large organs.

Cardiac arrhythmias are common with splenic masses and other functional neoplasms (e.g., pheochromocytoma). Ventricular premature contractions and tachycardias are seen most often in dogs. The cause is uncertain, and they may persist during recovery. Predisposing factors such as hypovolemia, hypotension, hypoxemia, hypercarbia, and electrolyte abnormalities are other causes of dysrhythmias under anesthesia.

Anesthetic and analgesic drug choices are based on patient status. Those with shorter duration and reversibility are preferred. The MAC of inhalants is decreased with volume loss; vaporizer settings should be as low as possible and decreased in anticipation of this when sudden hemorrhage occurs. Although the use of dexmedetomidine in hemorrhaged dogs did not compromise global perfusion significantly [360], it did prevent the pulse pressure variation normally associated with hypovolemia [361]. This effect could interfere with monitoring and volume resuscitation of hemorrhaging patients. Dogs in this study were also given atropine to block the cardiac effects of dexmedetomidine and allow vascular effects to be identified. Atropine is not recommended when dexmedetomidine is used in clinical patients, so the effects of dexmedetomidine alone are not known when hemorrhage is present. Consequently, this drug should be avoided or used very judiciously in those with less significant blood loss.

Intestinal neoplasia

Overall, cancer of the GIT is not common (< 10%) when compared to all types of neoplasms in dogs and cats. Most patients are middle-aged dogs or older cats, and many are male. Lymphoma, carcinoma, leiomyoma, and gastrointestinal stromal tumors are found in the GIT of dogs and cats and malignancy is very common. Adenocarcinoma is most common in the lesser curvature and pyloric area of the stomach and large intestine (especially the rectum) of dogs. Lymphoma is most frequent in the small intestine but adenocarcinoma and sarcomas, including GI stromal tumors and leiomyosarcoma, also occur. Gastrointestinal stromal tumors are also seen in the cecum and large intestine. In cats, lymphoma is the most common intestinal neoplasm, primarily found in the jejunum and ileum, but adenocarcinoma and mast cell tumors also occur. Feline adenocarcinoma is an aggressive neoplasm that frequently metastasizes to lymph nodes and lungs and sometimes results in carcinomatosis [362–367].

Specific etiologies of GI neoplasia in animals have not been determined. Risk factors for GI lymphoma in cats include exposure to cigarette smoke, the presence of *Helicobacter* spp on biopsy, and infection with feline leukemia (FeLV) and feline immunodeficiency (FIV) viruses. Unlike other types of lymphoma, cats with GI lymphoma usually test negative for FeLV and FIV, but underlying retroviral infection is still suspect. Chronic inflammation as seen with GERD and inflammatory bowel disease, disruption of hormonal pathways as with gastrinomas, and chronic inflammation caused by infection (*Spirocerca lupi, Helicobacter* spp) are proposed underlying mechanisms. Hereditary predisposition to intestinal carcinoma is reported in Chow, Staffordshire Terrier, and German and Belgian Shepherd dogs, as well as in Siamese cats [363,364,366,368].

Esophageal neoplasia is rare in small animals; squamous cell carcinoma, fibrosarcoma, osteosarcoma, and leiomyoma are seen. Squamous cell carcinoma is most common in cats. Infection with *S. lupi* is reported to cause fibrosarcoma, osteosarcoma, and other undifferentiated sarcomas. Melanoma is seen in the esophagus; it is more common in canine breeds with black mucous membranes [362,363,369].

Rare neuroendocrine tumors (or carcinoids) arise from enterochromaffin cells found in the mucosa of the GIT. Previously called "amine precursor uptake and decarboxylation tumors" (APUDomas), carcinoids are rare in animals. Carcinoid syndrome occurs occasionally in humans; one report of ventricular tachycardia and melena in a Boxer dog was associated with an intestinal carcinoid [370]. Serotonin, histamine, substance P, various kinins, catecholamines, and prostaglandins are just some of the chemicals secreted by carcinoid tumors. Usually, these substances are transported to the liver and metabolized; however, if they gain access to the circulation or the lumen of the bowel, clinical signs of hemodynamic instability and pulmonary and GI dysfunction follow. Arrhythmias, hypo- or hypertension, vasodilation, bronchospasm, diarrhea, and hypersecretion of intestinal fluid may occur. Anesthesia for such tumors should avoid the use of drugs that encourage histamine release such as morphine, meperidine, atracurium, and succinylcholine. Dopamine, ephedrine, epinephrine, norepinephrine, histamine, and isoproterenol have been associated with carcinoid episodes in humans. Pretreatment with antihistamines and serotonin antagonists may be beneficial. Somatostatin receptors are found in some carcinoid tumors; the somatostatin analog octreotide is used to decrease secretion of serotonin and other substances. This has minimized clinical signs in humans and allowed the use of sympathomimetics under anesthesia [98,362].

Clinical signs of GI neoplasia usually reflect the area affected; malaise, weight loss, and anorexia may be the only signs. Vomiting, diarrhea, and melena are also common with gastric and small intestinal lesions. Regurgitation is frequent with esophageal disease. Tenesmus, hematochezia, and constipation occur with lesions of the rectum. Abdominal pain, distention, hemorrhage, obstruction, perforation, and intussusception also occur with GI neoplasia [362, 363,365–367,369,370]. Mechanical effects of neoplasia may be seen with large tumors potentially compromising diaphragmatic excursion and causing or contributing to hypoventilation. Esophageal masses may affect respiration via pressure on the trachea.

Anemia, hypoproteinemia, increased alkaline phosphatase, and increased BUN are the most common laboratory abnormalities seen with neoplasia of the GIT. Anemia can be due to multiple mechanisms including blood loss, lack of red blood cell production, or increased destruction of red cells. Protein-losing enteropathy is common, causing hypoproteinemia due to hypoalbuminemia. BUN increases with chronic intraluminal blood loss due to recycling of protein [371]. Other enzyme changes are variable. White blood cell counts vary from normal to extremely elevated in patients with lymphoma and leukemia.

Abdominal palpation may suggest the presence of neoplasia. Lesions are identified most often with radiography and ultrasonography. Aspirates and/or biopsies needed for definitive diagnosis may be obtained in conscious patients with ultrasound guidance; however, endoscopy and/or laparotomy under general anesthesia are sometimes necessary.

Paraneoplastic syndromes (PNS) sometimes occur with GI neoplasia and can affect anesthetic management. PNS are caused by production of substances that affect tissues distant to the primary tumor. Numerous PNS exist, but not all patients exhibit signs of PNS. Some PNS are associated with a few particular types of neoplasia, others may be seen in many. A PNS may be the initial sign of cancer in some patients and lead to the diagnosis. Improvement of the PNS suggests a positive response to treatment, while recurrence is seen with loss of remission [372,373].

In addition to general clinical signs of GI dysfunction, weight loss is often seen with GI neoplasia. Although anorexia is an important cause of weight loss, cachexia is also significant. Cachexia is a loss of body condition in spite of a reasonable intake of calories. Decreased appetite is due to direct effects of neoplastic tissue but is also from inflammation that causes release of several cytokines, including interleukin-1 (IL-1) and interleukin-6 (IL-6), that affect the balance between appetite stimulation and inhibition. Cachexia is actually a destructive syndrome that alters fat and carbohydrate metabolism and interferes with growth and anabolic pathways to produce muscle wasting commonly seen in cancer patients. Effects are again produced by mediators of inflammation including tumor necrosis factor-α, IL-1, IL-6, nuclear factor κB, and others. Even though some patients may actually be overweight at diagnosis, muscle wasting is often present and loss of body condition and weight continues with time. Both body weight and low body condition score have been associated with non-survival in cancer patients [372,373].

Hypercalcemia of malignancy in dogs is common with T-cell lymphoma (35–55%) and anal sac apocrine gland adenocarcinoma (25%) but is less frequent with GI adenocarcinoma. It is most common in cats with lymphoma, squamous cell carcinoma, and multiple myeloma. Secretion of parathyroid hormone (PTH) or a PTH-related-peptide affects pathways in bone and kidney, resulting in increased serum calcium and eventually mineralization of tissues, especially the kidney. Numerous other factors have also been identified that contribute to hypercalcemia of malignancy, including inflammatory cytokines and calcitriol. Osteolysis that occurs with lesions of bone also increases serum calcium [372,373].

Hypoglycemia is seen with leiomyoma/leiomyosarcoma, lymphoma, and GI stromal tumors. It can be due to secretion of insulin, but it is often from excessive use of glucose by neoplastic tissue, and interference with gluconeogenesis and glycogenolysis. Thrombocytopenia and/or coagulopathy are seen with hemangiosarcoma, lymphoma, and mast cell tumors. Histamine release from mast cell tumors and gastrinomas can lead to gastric ulceration and hemorrhage. Histamine release can also occur under anesthesia, causing vasodilation and hypotension. Although most common with renal tumors, erythrocytosis is reported with lymphoma and hepatic tumors. Mucous membranes are erythematous and polydipsia and neurologic signs can be seen. The elevated PCV complicates fluid therapy management, as patients are not necessarily hypovolemic or dehydrated and the PCV does not decrease as expected with fluids. Hyperglobulinemia is seen with all types of myelomas. Both erythrocytosis and hyperglobulinemia can cause hyperviscosity syndrome, which alters blood flow in tissues, resulting in inadequate delivery of oxygen and nutrients. Coagulopathy and damage to heart, brain, and ocular tissues may occur. Hypertrophic osteopathy is sometimes seen with esophageal tumors, thought to be caused by increased periosteal blood flow; the effects on bone can be extremely painful [363,369,372,373].

Anesthetic management for patients with GI neoplasia is similar to that described for laparotomy and hemoabdomen with attention to therapy for hypoproteinemia and PNS. Plasma and/or colloid administration may be needed when total protein is < 4.5 mg/dL or albumin is < 2.0 mg/dL. Infusion of human albumin has been used but severe side effects, including death, have been seen in some dogs [374–378]. Although not without side effects, canine-specific albumin is available and is a better choice than human albumin [379]. Hypercalcemia may cause muscle tremors or weakness and arrhythmias, and can affect blood pressure. Correction of hypercalcemia in animals displaying clinical signs is beneficial prior to anesthesia; however, treatment is not pursued in asymptomatic animals with minimal hypercalcemia. Therapy to decrease calcium levels relatively quickly prior to surgery includes dilution via fluid therapy using 0.9% sodium chloride, which also encourages renal excretion, diuresis with furosemide, and calcitonin to inhibit osteoclastic activity in bone. Glucocorticoids can also be given; bisphosphonates are used for long-term management [372,380]. Glucose should be monitored in patients with hypoglycemia and dextrose administered as needed to maintain serum glucose above 80 mg/dL. Intermittent monitoring of glucose is facilitated by use of an embedded monitor. This modality has been used under anesthesia to evaluate the completeness of surgical excision of functional tumors such as insulinoma [381]. See Chapter 42 for further information on glucose and calcium therapy. Treatment of anemia is described above in the hemoabdomen section.

Patients with mast cell tumors should be premedicated with antihistamines and avoidance of drugs that stimulate histamine release, such as morphine and meperidine, is recommended. Mechanical effects on ventilation can be seen with obstructive intestinal lesions or large abdominal masses due to compromise of diaphragmatic excursions. Esophageal tumors can affect intubation and ventilation via pressure on the trachea. Paraneoplastic fever is not uncommon, especially with cancer of hematopoietic cells. The immune response to antigens presented by neoplastic cells as well as inflammation from necrotic tumors produces fever. Fever due to secondary infection may also occur in damaged tissue and must be distinguished from paraneoplastic fever. Effects of chemotherapy may also produce fever. Sepsis can occur with immunosuppression and peritonitis caused by GIT cancers [372,373]. Hemorrhage is common in patients with neoplasia and management is described above in the hemoabdomen section.

Septic peritonitis

Several authors have reviewed septic peritonitis in dogs [382–384], cats [267,385–389], or both [258,390–393]. It is categorized as localized or diffuse, and primary, secondary, or tertiary depending on the extent of disease and source of infection, respectively. *Tertiary* peritonitis is the recurrence or persistence of infection following treatment via surgery and antibiotics for an initial episode. *Secondary* peritonitis is most common in animals, due to perforation/leakage from the GIT. Foreign bodies, ulcers, obstruction, ischemic lesions, abscess/infection of organs or masses, trauma from motor vehicle impact, bite wounds, other penetrating injuries, and sometimes blunt trauma are causes. Some injuries may not break the skin but still damage intestine enough to cause leakage and induce septic peritonitis. Iatrogenic causes include dehiscence of intestinal anastamoses or incisions, inadvertent puncture of intestine, leakage around feeding tubes, and contamination of the abdomen at surgery. Spontaneous perforation of the GIT occurs occasionally with steroid or NSAID therapy. Aseptic secondary peritonitis is seen with leakage of urine, bile, gastric fluid, or pancreatic secretions. In *primary* septic peritonitis, an intra-abdominal source of infection cannot be identified [386,387,390,391,393]. Variable mortality has been reported in small animals (31–69%) [267,383,387–389]. Patients with secondary peritonitis treated surgically have higher survival rates than those treated medically or those with primary peritonitis [267,392]. Pre-existing peritonitis, low albumin and protein levels, and intraoperative hypotension were risk factors for postoperative septic peritonitis and death in dogs [383]. A study of mortality and dehiscence in dogs following GI surgery found that the rate of dehiscence was low at 5.3% (9/170); however, ASA status ≥ 3 and high lactate concentration were factors associated with dehiscence, septic peritonitis, and nonsurvival [384]. A *higher* blood glucose level was associated with increased mortality in one study [389]. Early use of antibiotics was found to be associated with greater survival in a report of 83 cats with septic peritonitis [388].

Anorexia, lethargy, and vomiting are the most common clinical signs in dogs and cats. Diarrhea and abdominal pain are also seen in dogs; discomfort is reported but often vague or inapparent in cats. Signs of sepsis relate to the severity of abdominal contamination in most cases. Unlike dogs, bradycardia and hypothermia are frequently seen in cats with sepsis [385–387]. Diagnosis is suggested by history and physical examination, while abdominal radiographs and ultrasonography may reveal a specific lesion with or without effusion [394]. Pneumoperitoneum is diagnostic for intestinal leakage or infection with gas-forming bacteria [391,392]. A septic infiltrate seen on cytology of peritoneal effusion or lavage fluid confirms the diagnosis of septic peritonitis. Increased lactate can be seen in serum and/or in the abdominal fluid. Peritoneal lactate and its comparison to serum lactate was diagnostic in ≥ 90% of dogs, but not in cats [395]. Although factors identified with prognosis vary, hypotension, hypoalbuminemia, and hyperlactatemia are consistently associated with mortality [382–384,386,387,392,393,395,396].

Patients with peritonitis are some of the most challenging cases presented for anesthesia. Clinical signs may suggest the presence of a septic focus, and confirmation may be obtained prior to laparotomy via diagnostics such as abdominocentesis, radiographs, and/or ultrasound. However, exploratory laparotomy can be a diagnostic as well as a therapeutic procedure. Septic patients are more sensitive to the depressant effects of anesthetic agents, so a thorough evaluation of the severity of cardiovascular compromise should be performed. Many cases are urgent or emergent, which may not permit a complete diagnostic evaluation; however, clinical signs and laboratory parameters have been evaluated in combination to allow early identification of sepsis. In 1991, human critical care physicians sought terminology to better define and describe *inflammation* and *sepsis* in critically ill patients. They agreed that systemic inflammation may occur with any severe insult, including trauma, hemorrhage, ischemia, and immune disease, as well as infection, and called it the "systemic inflammatory response syndrome" (SIRS). *Sepsis* was defined as SIRS in response to infection, most often bacterial, but fungal, protozoal, and viral infections also occur [397–400]. Criteria developed to identify SIRS included heart rate, respiratory rate or $PaCO_2$, and temperature, combined with total white blood cell count (Table 41.5); evaluation of the mucous membranes was added later as an estimate of tissue perfusion. Sepsis was identified when two or more SIRS criteria were present in response to infection. Severe sepsis was present with poor perfusion, hypotension, and organ dysfunction. Septic shock was described as persistent hypotension and elevated lactate in spite of appropriate fluid resuscitation, requiring vasopressor therapy [398–405]. Some patients may be normotensive but exhibit signs of decreased perfusion such as cool extremities, poor capillary refill time and abnormal mucous membrane color, lactic acidosis, decreased urine output, and depressed mental status. While

Table 41.5 Criteria for systemic inflammatory response syndrome (SIRS)/sepsis in dogs, cats, and humans.

Parameter	Dog	Cat	Human
Heart rate (beats/min)	> 120	< 140 or > 225	> 90
Respiratory rate (breaths/min)	> 40	> 40	> 20
or $PaCO_2$ (mmHg)	< 30		< 32
Temperature (°F)	< 100.4 or > 104.0	< 100 or > 104	< 96.8 or > 100.4
Leukogram white blood cells/μL	> 18,000 or < 5000	> 19,000 or < 5000	> 12,000 or < 4000
or % immature band cells	> 5%	> 5%	> 10%
Prolonged CRT, abnormal mucous membrane color			

Source: Compiled from Bone *et al.* [397]; Nunnally [399]; Singer *et al.* [401]; Rank and Hansen [403]; Purvis and Kirby [404]; Hardie [405].

definitions have changed somewhat over the years, terminology has returned to more simplified versions in some respects. According to the "Sepsis 3" consensus conference in 2016 [401], "severe sepsis" has been abandoned, while *sepsis* is now defined as "life-threatening organ dysfunction caused by a dysregulated host response to infection." Septic shock remains as "persisting hypotension requiring vasopressors to maintain MAP ≥ 65 mmHg with a serum lactate level > 2 mmol/L despite adequate volume resuscitation" [398–402].

The pathophysiology of sepsis and septic shock is quite complex, and the knowledge base has vastly expanded since SIRS criteria were first developed. The body's response to an insult is designed to ensure/restore oxygen delivery to vital tissues. Multiple systems participate in the inflammatory response, and although some cases may progress from SIRS to sepsis to multiple organ dysfunction syndrome (MODS), most do not proceed along a continuum. Early accounts describe an immune response triggered by organisms, their byproducts, and/or the resultant tissue damage, that then injures the patient as well. The primary components that trigger an inflammatory response are now called "pathogen-associated molecular patterns" (PAMPs) and/or damage-associated molecular patterns (DAMPs). PAMPs include the classic endotoxins and exotoxins from gram-negative or gram-positive bacteria and many other substances that alert innate immune cells to a foreign presence. DAMPs are endogenous structures/substances derived from damaged host cells and can arise from non-infectious sources such as injury and toxins. Pattern recognition receptors interact with PAMPs/DAMPs to initiate the immune response, and are located inside or outside cells, in the bloodstream or body fluids. Pattern recognition receptors are located on neutrophils, macrophages, dendritic cells, platelets, complement, natural killer cells, fibroblasts, some epithelial cells including those of the GIT, and many others. Signaling pathways are triggered that result in activation of multiple genes to produce pro- and anti-inflammatory effects. If the source is eliminated, the immune response subsides and saves appropriate information for future insults. However, with sepsis, "dysregulation" develops. Normal intrinsic responses are uncontrolled and proinflammatory effects overwhelm anti-inflammatory activities; actual suppression of the immune system also occurs [406]. A myriad of inflammatory mediators is involved, including tumor necrosis factor-α, interleukins, leukotrienes, prostaglandins, cytokines, various peptides, the potent vasodilator nitric oxide (NO), oxygen radicals, and platelet-activating factor. Any/all organ systems may suffer, but in addition to the source location, the cardiovascular, respiratory, neurologic, and hemostatic systems are most profoundly affected. The net result is hypotension caused by vasodilation and a relative or absolute hypovolemia with shifting of volume to the venous side of the circulation. Damage to the glycocalyx occurs, causing loss of endothelial barrier function. Fluid leaks into cells and the interstitium, resulting in edema, cellular damage, and protein loss. Normal or increased cardiac output is present initially, but myocardial contractility is eventually impaired. Coagulopathy also develops that contributes to tissue ischemia. Adrenal insufficiency and decreased endogenous vasopressin levels also exacerbate hypotension. The net result is septic shock, also called "vasoplegic" or "distributive shock," with hypotension in spite of appropriate fluid resuscitation. Vasopressor therapy is required as well as inotropic support for cardiac dysfunction [255,398–400,402,407].

The GIT is the most common source of sepsis in animals and is also the "shock organ" in dogs. However, it plays a role in the generation of SIRS/sepsis even when the intestinal serosa is intact or the primary source is elsewhere. Inflammatory damage to the barrier functions of the GI mucosa allows absorption of non-microbial factors into the lymphatic system, which then drain into the venous system via the thoracic duct. Ongoing SIRS is magnified, and respiratory dysfunction/distress and multiple organ failure may ensue via this pathway. Translocation of bacteria and bacterial products also occurs in some patients and is also thought to occur via lymphatics rather than the portal system. However, bacterial translocation is not necessary for the development of SIRS and MODS [408,409]. There is also evidence that alteration of the GI microbiome contributes to sepsis pathophysiology as well [410].

Although early identification of SIRS/sepsis is vital to survival, SIRS is a clinical diagnosis. Signs are not always obvious in animals, especially cats, and may overlap with non-septic illness. Anaphylaxis causes similar signs with abnormal mucous membrane color, hypotension, altered mentation, and so on and must be differentiated from sepsis [349,411]. In humans, the SIRS criteria were ultimately considered inadequate for many patients, and other scoring systems were developed. The Sequential Organ Failure Assessment (SOFA) score is used to screen patients for organ dysfunction. It includes measures of neurologic, cardiovascular, renal, hepatic, and hematologic function. A shorter variation, the quick-SOFA (qSOFA), eliminates laboratory data and focuses on mental status, low systolic blood pressure, and increased respiratory rate. The Acute Patient Physiologic and Laboratory Evaluation (APPLE) and its modification, fastAPPLE, were developed to be used in hospitalized patients, and include more laboratory parameters [402,412]. Other scoring systems exist that apply to specific patient categories, but all are designed to help identify sepsis, assess the severity of illness, and infer risks of morbidity as well as mortality. SIRS criteria, SOFA, APPLE, and modifications have been adapted and used in critically ill dogs and cats [385,398,402,413–419]. They have all been shown to perform well in some groups but no scoring system is 100% reliable. It is not recommended to rely on one scoring system alone to infer the presence of sepsis [402,403,417,418,420]. However, their use prompts clinicians to look more closely when a septic source is not obvious and enables discussions of prognosis and survival with owners and other veterinarians.

In 2002, the Surviving Sepsis Campaign (SSC) [421] was launched globally to educate medical professionals and governments about the increasing incidence of sepsis and offer guidelines for identification and treatment. It also recommended methods for early diagnosis and provided guidance for management of these difficult cases. Updates have been published periodically [421,422]; veterinary recommendations are similar [326,404], but further study is needed to determine specific protocols for animals. The SSC promotes guidelines as care "bundles." According to 2021 SSC guidelines [420,421], the initial bundle should be instituted within *1 h* of the recognition of sepsis (Box 41.2). Collection of samples for blood cultures is performed prior to administration of broad-spectrum antibiotics,

Box 41.2 Hour-1 care bundle for septic patients.

When sepsis is likely, begin the following within 1 h of recognition:

1 Measure lactate level and recheck if initial measurement is > 2 mmol/L.
2 Obtain blood cultures and then administer antibiotics.
3 Begin IV crystalloid therapy at 30 mL/kg if hypotensive or lactate ≥ 4 mmol/L.
4 Initiate vasopressor therapy if hypotension persists and maintain MAP ≥ 65 mmHg.

MAP, mean arterial pressure.
Source: Adapted from the Surviving Sepsis Website [421].

Table 41.6 Goals of therapy for sepsis to achieve within 3 h of initiating treatment.

Parameter	Goal
Mean arterial pressure (MAP)	> 65 mmHg
Central venous oxygen saturation ($ScvO_2$)	> 70%
Central venous pressure (CVP)	8–12 mmHg
Urine output	> 0.5 mL/kg/h

Source: Compiled from Butler [326]; Rivers *et al.* [327]; Nunnally [399]; Evans *et al.* [420].

which should also be given within the first hour. Fluid resuscitation should begin immediately with intravenous isotonic crystalloids. Diagnostics to identify an infective source should begin as soon as possible, and lactate should be measured at admission and repeated intermittently to evaluate response to therapy. Goals of initial therapy should be achieved within 3 h (Table 41.6), with central venous oxygen saturation ($ScvO_2$) > 70%, urine output > 0.5 mL/kg/h, central venous pressure of 8–12 mmHg, and mean arterial pressure (MAP) of > 65 mmHg. This MAP is lower than previous recommendations, as no difference in outcome was seen when a higher pressure was used. Measurement of mixed venous oxygen saturation ($S\bar{v}O_2$) requires catheterization of the pulmonary artery, but the use of the central venous oxygen saturation ($ScvO_2$) from the cranial vena cava is an acceptable alternative [423]. Lactate can also be used to estimate oxygen delivery when central catheterization is not available [420,423].

Elimination or treatment of an infective focus, or "source control," should be pursued as soon as possible as well. This is often where the anesthetist is needed. Prior to anesthesia, patients with SIRS/sepsis have hopefully been stabilized via vigorous fluid resuscitation and with vasopressors and/or inotropes when necessary to correct hypovolemia/hypotension. Unfortunately, controversy still exists as to appropriate fluid therapy protocols for septic patients. Since the introduction of the SSC, there has been a switch to goal-oriented therapy with clinical endpoints of fluid resuscitation protocols, as better outcomes were identified using lower rates of crystalloids with earlier use of vasopressors [326,327,420]. Kuttab *et al.* found greater mortality in septic patients that did not receive the 30 mL/kg dose of fluids by 3 h as recommended by the 2016 SSC guidelines [424]. However, recent clinical trials and meta-analyses of restrictive versus liberal fluid therapy protocols in hypotensive septic patients [425] and in patients anesthetized for major abdominal surgery [426] have not found differences in mortality. The latter study also found fewer renal complications with higher fluid volumes. Perhaps close attention to the entire bundle of recommendations has resulted in better outcomes rather than specific fluid rates, however, this remains to be determined.

Isotonic crystalloids are preferred over saline or colloids [330,420,427]. The use of synthetic colloids in critically ill patients is controversial. Meta-analyses of the use of hetastarch (hydroxyethyl starch) in septic human patients have shown evidence of acute kidney injury and greater mortality [355,356]; colloid or gelatin use is not recommended by the SSC [420]. Studies in dogs and cats have shown no difference or some negative effects [330,357,428], but further study is required to make firm recommendations. Many still utilize synthetic colloids as alternatives, such as albumin or plasma, are not always available or are expensive. However, it is likely wise to avoid colloids whenever possible. The volume-expanding effects of colloids are not as great as expected in septic patients, they are associated with coagulopathy, and they may actually result in greater tissue edema in ill patients [429]. The long-standing concept that vascular permeability is dependent on the balance between colloid osmotic and hydrostatic pressures on either side of the endothelium has been challenged. Revision of the Starling principle of fluid dynamics explains that permeability is more dependent on the endothelial glycocalyx, which is a layer of complex carbohydrates arranged in a thick gel-like mesh lining the surface of the vascular endothelium. It is negatively charged and traps albumin and proteins, and serves as a barrier to movement of fluid and substances into the interstitium. It has been shown that the differences between capillary blood and the glycocalyx, rather than the interstitium, are most important. Damage to the glycocalyx that occurs with inflammation, ischemia, and even high fluid rates results in further tissue edema as the protection it normally provides is compromised [429–434]. Macdonald *et al.* [434] found no correlation between markers of endothelial glycocalyx shedding and total volume of fluids administered over the first 24 h in septic patients, while others have identified greater mortality with higher fluid volumes and damage to the endothelial glycocalyx [435]. Infusion of albumin or plasma is recommended when severe hypoalbuminemia/hypoproteinemia is present and when large volumes of crystalloids have been utilized [330,420], as these minimize damage to the glycocalyx. Human albumin has been used in animals but adverse effects, including anaphylaxis and death, are reported [330,374–378,433]; canine-specific albumin is now available [380]. Albumin can also be administered as a hypertonic solution to expand volume but must be given slowly via a central line [328,379].

Vasopressors are administered when patients remain hypotensive following fluid resuscitation. Norepinephrine is the first choice in humans and small animals, followed by vasopressin, then epinephrine [261–263,420]. As very potent vasoconstrictors, these drugs should be given at the lowest effective dose to avoid ischemia and masking of persistent hypovolemia. Inotropes are used when myocardial dysfunction is identified or suspected, and dobutamine is preferred over dopamine [420]. Inotropes are often necessary during anesthesia to offset the depressant effects of inhalants.

Relative adrenal insufficiency also occurs in SIRS/sepsis [436–438]. Corticosteroids are necessary for patients to respond to vasopressor therapy; therefore, physiologic doses are recommended for patients who are still hypotensive following volume replacement and vasopressor therapy [420]. A recent Cochrane review found treatment with corticosteroids reduced duration of intensive care, overall length of hospitalization, and mortality in humans [439]. Reversal of hypotension was seen following corticosteroid treatment in a dog with septic shock due to pneumonia [437]. A prospective study of low-dose corticosteroid treatment in 21 dogs with SIRS did not find an effect on survival [438]. Similarly, a retrospective study compared treatment with or without corticosteroids in 47 dogs with sepsis and did not find an effect on survival [440]. However, more of the treated patients were sicker, and likely had a higher baseline risk of mortality. Further study is required to determine the effect of corticosteroid treatment in septic veterinary patients. Septic patients may exhibit hyper- or hypoglycemia. A blood glucose concentration > 180 mg/dL [420] is the trigger for insulin therapy in humans which is higher than previous recommendations. Hypoglycemia is treated with dextrose as needed [271] and is discussed further in Chapter 42.

Anesthetic choices and management for patients with septic peritonitis are similar to those described for exploratory laparotomy and GDV. Dosage requirements are greatly decreased in these patients, and combinations of low levels of inhalant with infusions of intravenous agents and adjunctive medications are utilized, titrating to effect at the lowest effective dose rates [234,235,271]. Ketamine is suggested for induction since its sympathomimetic effects support blood pressure; however, catecholamine depletion in severely ill patients would negate this effect [234,235,271]. Combinations of two drugs such as ketamine with propofol or alfaxalone may be useful [232]. Etomidate has been combined with propofol for total intravenous anesthesia in older humans with good results [441]; however, concerns about negative outcomes exist with use of etomidate [228,229]. Lidocaine has been shown to improve short-term survival in dogs with peritonitis [274] and horses with small intestinal lesions [340]; it has also been associated with better outcomes in humans [61,62,219]. Close attention to clinical signs, oxygenation, and perfusion is always necessary in anesthetized patients, but anesthetic management can directly affect outcomes in septic patients as intraoperative hypotension has been repeatedly associated with mortality [208,226,258]. Monitoring has been described previously and, for septic patients in particular, measurement of cardiac output is very useful. Lung injury is not uncommon in septic patients and ventilator settings should be altered as needed, according to arterial blood gas evaluation. Lower tidal volumes are recommended (6–8 mL/kg) with a maximum end-inspiratory plateau pressure of $\leq$ 30 cmH_2O [234,271,420,442]. PEEP may also be needed. Postoperatively, cardiovascular support and monitoring are continued, and oxygen insufflation or ventilatory support may be needed in cases with inadequate gas exchange.

Foreign body removal and other abdominal procedures

Anesthetic considerations for intestinal obstruction, removal or biopsy of abdominal masses and/or the intestine, and colectomy are similar to those for exploratory laparotomy discussed above. Hemorrhage is often associated with removal of abdominal masses as discussed previously; however, it may occur with dissection of adhesions or fibrous tissue, which can be insidious and should be monitored closely to identify significant blood loss. A non-linear foreign body of the GIT was the most common reason for emergency abdominal surgery in a retrospective analysis of 82 dogs over a three-year period (31 dogs, 39%). Other reasons included pyometra (15 dogs, 18.3%), GDV (15 dogs, 18.3%), and hemoperitoneum (8 dogs, 6.5%); only three dogs presented with a linear foreign body [208]. Surveys of foreign body obstruction in dogs and cats consistently show overall good outcomes with over 90% survival in both dogs and cats [443,444]; however, mortality was higher with linear foreign bodies and the need for multiple intestinal procedures in one report [445].

Ischemic lesions of intestine also occur in dogs and cats. A report of 153 dogs with small intestinal intussusception found that most dogs were young, with a median age of 10 months. No cause was identified in most cases, the most common location was ileocolic, resection and anastomosis were required in 84%, and mortality was 6% after 14 days. Postoperative complications were seen in 35%, most often diarrhea, regurgitation, and septic peritonitis [446]. Of 20 cats identified with intussusception, 10 were less than one year of age and 9 were over six years of age. The most common location was jejuno-jejunal; diagnosis was idiopathic in seven of the young cats, while lymphoma or inflammatory bowel disease was identified in seven of the older cats [447]. Some patients with intussusception present with a prolonged history of vomiting, weight loss, and significant debilitation as lesions may produce partial as opposed to complete obstruction.

Anorexia, depression, nausea and persistent vomiting, and abdominal pain are common clinical signs in patients with obstruction, with subsequent fluid deficits and electrolyte abnormalities. Although exploratory laparotomy for foreign body removal and other lesions of the intestine is often straight forward, duration of these procedures may be long, as meticulous dissection, multiple resections, and anastamoses may be required. Perforation, dehiscence, or leakage are common complications that can lead to or exacerbate peritonitis and sepsis. Repeat laparotomy is sometimes required for treatment of peritonitis and other complications. Some patients, especially dogs, present repeatedly for foreign body removal. Hemorrhage can be seen in these patients due to the presence of scar tissue. Periodic reassessment of blood gases, PCV, TS, electrolytes, lactate, and glucose is performed as needed. Overall fluid requirements must be considered when duration is prolonged to avoid hypervolemia. Anesthetic management and postoperative concerns are similar to other laparotomy patients, with attention to analgesia, and treatment and prevention of vomiting, reflux, and aspiration.

References

1 Washabau RJ. Integration of gastrointestinal function. In: Washabau RJ, Day MJ, eds. *Canine and Feline Gastroenterology*. St. Louis, MO: Saunders Elsevier, 2013: 1–29.

2 Herdt TH. Regulation of gastrointestinal function. In: Klein BG, ed. *Cunningham's Textbook of Veterinary Physiology*, 6th edn. St. Louis, MO: Elsevier, 2020: 284–292.

3 Bowen R. Fundamental physiology and anatomy of the digestive system. In: *Pathophysiology of the Digestive System*. http://www.vivo.colostate.edu/hbooks/pathphys/digestion/basics/gi_microanatomy.html (accessed June 2022).

4 Herdt TH. Motility patterns of the gastrointestinal tract. In: Klein BG, ed. *Cunningham's Textbook of Veterinary Physiology*, 6th edn. St. Louis, MO: Saunders Elsevier, 2020: 293–306.

5 Whitehead K, Cortes Y, Eirmann L. Gastrointestinal dysmotility disorders in critically ill dogs and cats. *J Vet Emerg Crit Care* 2016; **26**(2): 234–253.

6 Bowen R. Control of digestive system function. In: *Pathophysiology of the Digestive System. Colorado State University*.http://www.vivo.colostate.edu/hbooks/pathphys/digestion/basics/control.html (accessed June 2022).

7 Husnik R, Gaschen F. Gastric motility disorders in dogs and cats. *Vet Clin North Am Small Anim Pract* 2021; **51**: 43–59.

8 Lin HC. Preanesthetic considerations. In: Lin HC, Passler T, Clark-Price S, eds. *Farm Animal Anesthesia: Cattle, Small Ruminants, Camelids, and Pigs*, 2nd edn. Hoboken, NJ: John Wiley and Sons, 2022: 1–4.

9 Jago RC, Corletto F, Wright IM. Peri-anaesthetic complications in an equine referral hospital: risk factors for post anaesthetic colic. *Equine Vet* 2015; **47**: 635–640.

10 Mehra JM, Tolbert MK, Moore GE, *et al.* Clinical features and risk factors for gastrointestinal complications in dogs treated surgically for thoracolumbar intervertebral disc extrusion. *Front Vet Sci* 2021; **8**: 785228.

11 Andersen MS, Clark L, Dyson SJ, *et al.* Risk factors for colic in horses after general anaesthesia for MRI or nonabdominal surgery: absence of evidence of effect from perianaesthetic morphine. *Equine Vet J* 2006; **38**: 368–374.

12 Torrente C, Vigueras I, Manzanilla EG, *et al.* Prevalence of and risk factors for intraoperative gastroesophageal reflux and postanesthetic vomiting and diarrhea in dogs undergoing general anesthesia. *J Vet Emerg Crit Care (San Antonio)* 2017; **27**: 397–408.

13 Lee HW, Machin H, Adami C. Peri-anaesthetic mortality and nonfatal gastrointestinal complications in pet rabbits: a retrospective study on 210 cases. *Vet Anaesth Analg* 2018; **45**: 520–528.

14 Davies JA, Fransson BA, Davis AM. Incidence of and risk factors for postoperative regurgitation and vomiting in dogs – 244 cases (2000–2012). *J Am Vet Med Assoc* 2015; **246**: 327–335.

15 Totta E, Pavlidou K, Savvas I. Gastric dilatation during sedation in a Doberman with intranasal malignancy. *Hellen J Companion Anim Med* 2020; **9**: 111–117.

16 Savas I, Plevraki, Raptopoulos D. Aerophagia and gastric dilation following tiletamine/zolazepam anaesthesia in a dog. *Vet Rec* 2001; **149**: 20–21.

17 Washabau RJ, Hall JA. Stomach: dysmotility. In: Washabau RJ, Day MJ, eds. *Canine and Feline Gastroenterology*. St. Louis, MO: Saunders Elsevier, 2013: 630–634.

18 Kook PH. Esophagitis in cats and dogs. *Vet Clin North Am Small Anim Pract* 2021; **51**: 1–15.

19 Grobman M. Aerodigestive disease in dogs. *Vet Clin North Am Small Anim Pract* 2021; **51**: 17–32.

20 Ovbey DH, Wilson DV, Bednarski RM, *et al.* Prevalence and risk factors for canine post-anesthetic aspiration pneumonia (1999–2009): a multicenter study. *Vet Anaesth Analg* 2014; **41**: 127–136.

21 Grocott MP, Browne JP, Van der Meulen J, *et al.* The Postoperative Morbidity Survey was validated and used to describe morbidity after major surgery. *J Clin Epidemiol* 2007; **60**: 919–928.

22 Buscail E, Deraison C. Postoperative ileus: a pharmacological perspective. *Br J Pharmacol* 2022; **179**: 3283–3305.

23 Hellstrom EA, Ziegler AL, Blikslager AT. Postoperative ileus: comparative pathophysiology and future therapies. *Front Vet Sci* 2021; **8**: 714800.

24 Washabau RJ. Vomiting: pathophysiology and mechanisms. In: Washabau RJ, Day MJ, eds. *Canine and Feline Gastroenterology*. St. Louis, MO: Saunders Elsevier, 2013: 167–169.

25 Bowen R. Physiology of vomiting. In: *Pathophysiology of the Digestive System. Colorado State University*. http://www.vivo.colostate.edu/hbooks/pathphys/digestion/stomach/vomiting.html (accessed February 2023).

26 Papich MG. Drugs affecting GI function. In: Riviere JE, Papich MG, eds. *Veterinary Pharmacology and Therapeutics*, 9th edn. Ames, IA: Wiley-Blackwell, 2009: 1247–1251.

27 Elwood C, Devauchelle P, Elliott J, *et al.* Emesis in dogs: a review. *J Small Anim Pract* 2010; **51**: 4–22.

28 Shaikh SI, Nagarekha D, Hegade G, *et al.* Postoperative nausea and vomiting: a simple yet complex problem. *Anesth Essays Res* 2016; **10**: 388–396.

29 Henze L, Foth S, Meller S, *et al.* Ondansetron in dogs with nausea associated with vestibular disease: a double-blinded, randomized placebo-controlled crossover study. *J Vet Int Med* 2022; **36**: 1726–1732.

30 Kenward H, Elliott J, Lee T, *et al.* Anti-nausea effects and pharmacokinetics of ondansetron, maropitant and metoclopramide in a low-dose cisplatin model of nausea and vomiting in the dog: a blinded crossover study. *BMC Vet Res* 2017; **13**: 244.

31 Tatewaki M, Strickland C, Fukuda H, *et al.* Effects of acupuncture on vasopressin-induced emesis in conscious dogs. *Am J Physiol Regul Integr Comp Physiol* 2005; **288**: R401–R408.

32 KuKanich B, Papich MG. Opioid analgesic drugs. In: Riviere JE, Papich MG, eds. *Veterinary Pharmacology and Therapeutics*, 9th edn. Ames, IA: Wiley-Blackwell, 2009: 308–319.

33 Johnston KD. The potential for mu-opioid receptor agonists to be anti-emetic in humans: a review of clinical data. *Acta Anaesthesiol Scand* 2010; **54**: 132–140.

34 Muir WW III. General considerations for anesthesia. In: Tranquilli WJ, Thurmon JC, Grimm KA, eds. *Lumb and Jones' Veterinary Anesthesia and Analgesia*, 4th edn. Ames, IA: Blackwell Publishing, 2007: 13–14.

35 Apfel CC, Kranke P, Katz MH, *et al.* Volatile anaesthetics may be the main cause of early but not delayed postoperative vomiting: a randomized controlled trial of factorial design. *Br J Anaesth* 2002; **88**: 659–668.

36 Gan TJ, Belani KG, Bergese S, *et al.* Fourth consensus guidelines for the management of postoperative nausea and vomiting. *Anesth Analg* 2020; **131**: 411–448.

37 Redondo García JI. Clinical evaluation of a new formulation of propofol in a medium-chain and long-chain triglycerides emulsion in dogs. *J Vet Pharmacol Ther* 2007; **30**: 288–294.

38 Muir WW III, Mason DE. Side effects of etomidate in dogs. *J Am Vet Med Assoc* 1989; **194**: 1430–1434.

39 Hall LW, Chambers JP. A clinical trial of propofol infusion anaesthesia in dogs. *J Small Anim Pract* 1987; **28**: 623–637.

40 Tsai YC, Wang LY, Yeh LS. Clinical comparison of recovery from total intravenous anesthesia with propofol and inhalation anesthesia with isoflurane in dogs. *J Vet Med Sci* 2007; **69**: 1179–1182.

41 Smith JA, Gaynor JS, Bednarski RM, *et al.* Adverse effects of administration of propofol with various preanesthetic regimens in dogs. *J Am Vet Assoc* 1993; **202**: 1111–1118.

42 Alfaxan® Multidose Package Insert (Pdf Version). https://dailymed.nlm.nih.gov/dailymed/getFile.cfm?setid=2a8e4d17-3ff3-4aa3-a990-7cb012a3123a&type=pdf (accessed February 2023).

43 Lerche P, Wiese A, Nelson L, *et al.* The cardiorespiratory and anesthetic effects of clinical and supraclinical doses of alfaxalone in cats. *Vet Anaesth Analg* 2009; **36**: 42–54.

44 Muir W, Lerche P, Wiese A, *et al.* Cardiorespiratory and anesthetic effects of clinical and supraclinical doses of alfaxalone in dogs. *Vet Anaesth Analg* 2008; **5**: 451–462.

45 Vaha-Vahe T. Clinical evaluation of medetomidine, a novel sedative and analgesic drug for dogs and cats. *Acta Vet Scand* 1989; **30**: 267–273.

46 Cullen LK. Medetomidine sedation in dogs and cats: a review of its pharmacology, antagonism and dose. *Br Vet J* 1996; **152**: 519–535.

47 Sinclair MD. A review of the physiological effects of α_2-agonists related to the clinical use of medetomidine in small animal practice. *Can Vet J* 2003; **44**: 885–897.

48 Posner LP, Burns P. Sedative agents: tranquilizers, alpha-2 agonists and related agents. In: Riviere JE, Papich MG, eds. *Veterinary Pharmacology and Therapeutics*, 9th edn. Ames, IA: Wiley-Blackwell, 2009: 344.

49 Granholm M, McKusick BC, Westerholm FC, *et al.* Evaluation of the clinical efficacy and safety of dexmedetomidine or medetomidine in cats and their reversal with atipamezole. *Vet Anaesth Analg* 2006; **33**: 214–223.

50 Zoetis Dexdomitor® (Dexmedetomidine) Package Insert. https://www.zoetisus.com/content/_assets/docs/Petcare/dexdomitor05-pi.pdf (accessed February 2023).

51 Lamont L, Burton S, Caines D, *et al.* Effects of 2 different medetomidine infusion rates on selected neurohormonal and metabolic parameters in dogs. *Can J Vet Res* 2012; **76**: 143–144.

52 van Oostrom H, Doornenbal A, Schot A, *et al.* Neurophysiological assessment of the sedative and analgesic effects of a constant rate infusion of dexmedetomidine in the dog. *Vet J* 2010; **190**: 338–344.

53 Ansah OB, Raekallio M, Vainio O. Correlation between serum concentrations following continuous intravenous infusion of dexmedetomidine or medetomidine in cats and their sedative and analgesic effects. *J Vet Pharmacol Ther* 2000; **23**: 1–8.

54 Valverde A, Cantwell S, Hernández J, *et al.* Effects of acepromazine on the incidence of vomiting associated with opioid administration in dogs. *Vet Anaesth Analg* 2004; **31**: 40–45.

55 Monteiro ER, Junior AR, Assis HMQ, *et al.* Comparative study on the sedative effects of morphine, methadone, butorphanol or tramadol, in combination with acepromazine, in dogs. *Vet Anaesth Analg* 2009; **36**: 25–33.

56 Ryan AC, Murrell JC, Gurney MA. Post-Operative Nausea and Vomiting (PONV) observed in a clinical study designed to assess the analgesic effects of intravenous and subcutaneous methadone in dogs. *Vet J* 2022; **287**: 105876

57 Bini G, Vettorato E, De Gennaro C, *et al.* A retrospective comparison of two analgesic strategies after uncomplicated tibial plateau levelling osteotomy in dogs. *Vet Anaesth Analg* 2018; **45**: 557–565.

58 Karaccas Y, Teixeira-Neto FJ, Giordano T, *et al.* Incidence of emesis after different doses of morphine and the effects of three phenothiazine premedications on morphine induced vomiting in dogs. *Presented at the World Congress of Veterinary Anaesthesiology*, Santos, Brazil, September 12–16, 2006.

59 Bhalla RJ, Trimble TA, Leece EA, *et al.* Comparison of intramuscular butorphanol and buprenorphine combined with dexmedetomidine for sedation in cats. *J Feline Med Surg* 2018; **20**: 325–331.

60 Matsubara LM, Oliva VN, Gabas DT, *et al.* Effect of lidocaine on the minimum alveolar concentration of sevoflurane in dogs. *Vet Anaesth Analg* 2009; **36**: 407–413.

61 McCarthy GC, Megalla SA, Habib AS. Impact of intravenous lidocaine infusion on postoperative analgesia and recovery from surgery: a systematic review of randomized controlled trials. *Drugs* 2010; **70**: 1149–1163.

62 Marret E, Rolin M, Beaussier M, *et al.* Meta-analysis of intravenous lidocaine and postoperative recovery after abdominal surgery. *Br J Surg* 2008; **95**: 1331–1338.

63 Brioschi FA, Gioeni D, Jacchetti A, *et al.* Effect of metoclopramide on nausea and emesis in dogs premedicated with morphine and dexmedetomidine. *Vet Anaesth Analg* 2018; **45**: 190–194.

64 Rau SE, Barber LG, Burgess KE. Efficacy of maropitant in the prevention of delayed vomiting associated with administration of doxorubicin to dogs. *J Vet Intern Med* 2010; **24**: 12–17.

65 de la Puente-Redondo VA, Tilt N, Rowan TG, *et al.* Efficacy of maropitant for treatment and prevention of emesis caused by intravenous infusion of cisplatin in dogs. *Am J Vet Res* 2007; **68**: 48–56.

66 Santos LCP, Ludders JW, Erb HN, *et al.* A randomized, blinded, controlled trial of the antiemetic effect of ondansetron on dexmedetomidine-induced emesis in cats. *Vet Anaesth Analg* 2011; **38**: 320–327.

67 Martin-Flores M, Mastrocco A, Lorenzutti AM, *et al.* Maropitant administered orally 2–2.5 h prior to morphine and dexmedetomidine reduces the incidence of emesis in cats. *J Feline Med Surg* 2017; **19**: 876–879.

68 Hay-Kraus BL. Efficacy of maropitant in preventing vomiting in dogs premedicated with hydromorphone. *Vet Anaesth Analg* 2013; **40**: 28–34.

69 Burke JE, Hess RS, Silverstein DC. Effectiveness of orally administered maropitant and ondansetron in preventing preoperative emesis and nausea in healthy dogs premedicated with a combination of hydromorphone, acepromazine, and glycopyrrolate. *J Am Vet Med Assoc* 2021; **260**: S40–S45.

70 Mathis A, Lee K, Alibhai HI. The use of maropitant to prevent vomiting induced by epidural administration of preservative free morphine through an epidural catheter in a dog. *Vet Anaesth Analg* 2011; **38**: 516–517.

71 Claude AK, Dedeaux A, Chiavaccini L, *et al.* Effects of maropitant citrate or acepromazine on the incidence of adverse events associated with hydromorphone premedication in dogs. *J Vet Intern Med* 2014; **28**: 1414–1417.

72 Foth S, Meller S, Kenward H, *et al.* The use of ondansetron for the treatment of nausea in dogs with vestibular syndrome. *BMC Vet Res* 2021; **17**: 222.

73 Swallow A, Rioja E, Elmer T, *et al.* The effect of maropitant on intraoperative isoflurane requirements and postoperative nausea and vomiting in dogs: a randomized clinical trial. *Vet Anaesth Analg* 2017; **44**: 785–793.

74 Lotti F, Boscan P, Twedt D, *et al.* Effect of oral maropitant and omeprazole on emesis, appetite and anesthesia recovery quality in dogs. *Vet Anaesth Analg* 2018; **45**: 855.e9.

75 Hay-Kraus BL. Spotlight on the perioperative use of maropitant citrate. *Vet Med (Auckl)* 2017; **8**: 41–51.

76 Sharun K, Jambagi K, Arya M, *et al.* Clinical applications of substance p (neurokinin-1 receptor) antagonist in canine medicine. *Arch Razi Inst* 2021; **76**: 1175–1182.

77 Karanicolas PJ, Smith SE, Kanbur B, *et al.* The impact of prophylactic dexamethasone on nausea and vomiting after laparoscopic cholecystectomy: a systematic review and meta-analysis. *Ann Surg* 2008; **248**: 751–762.

78 Topal A, Gül NY. Effects of dexamethasone, metoclopramide or acepromazine on emesis in cats sedated with xylazine hydrochloride. *Acta Vet Brno* 2006; **75**: 299–303.

79 Scallan EM, Simon BT. The effects of acupuncture point Pericardium 6 on hydromorphone-induced nausea and vomiting in healthy dogs. *Vet Anaesth Analg* 2016; **43**: 495–501.

80 Fass R, Boeckxstaens GE, El-Serag H, *et al.* Gastro-oesophageal reflux disease. *Nat Rev Dis Primers* 2021; **7**: 55.

81 Holloway RH. The anti-reflux barrier and mechanisms of gastro-oesophageal reflux. *Clin Gastroenterol* 2000; **14**: 681–699.

82 Cox MR, Martin CJ, Dent J, *et al.* Effect of general anaesthesia on transient lower oesophageal sphincter relaxations in the dog. *Aust N Z J Surg* 1988; **58**: 825–830.

83 Hershcovici T, Mashimo H, Fass R. The lower esophageal sphincter. *Neurogastroenterol Motil* 2011; **23**: 819–830.

84 Martin CJ, Dodds WJ, Liem HH, *et al.* Diaphragmatic contribution to gastroesophageal competence and reflux in dogs. *Am J Physiol* 1992; **263**: G551–G557.

85 Cotton BR, Smith G. The lower oesophageal sphincter and anaesthesia. *Br J Anaesth* 1984; **56**: 37–46.

86 Muenster M, Hoerauf A, Vieth M. Gastro-oesophageal reflux disease in 20 dogs (2012 to 2014). *J Small Anim Pract* 2017; **58**: 276–283.

87 Han E, Broussard J, Baer KE. Feline esophagitis secondary to gastroesophageal reflux disease: clinical signs and radiographic, endoscopic, and histopathological findings. *J Am Anim Hosp Assoc* 2003; **39**: 161–167.

88 Washabau RJ. Esophagus. In: Washabau RJ, Day MJ, eds. *Canine and Feline Gastroenterology*. St. Louis, MO: Saunders Elsevier, 2013: 580–594.

89 Leib MS, Dinnel H, Ward DL, *et al.* Endoscopic balloon dilation of benign esophageal strictures in dogs and cats. *J Vet Intern Med* 2001; **15**: 547–552.

90 Shaver SL, Barbur LA, Jimenez DA, *et al.* Evaluation of gastroesophageal reflux in anesthetized dogs with brachycephalic syndrome. *J Am Anim Hosp Assoc* 2017; **53**: 24–31.

91 Freiche V, German AJ. Digestive diseases in brachycephalic dogs. *Vet Clin North Am Small Anim Pract* 2021; **51**: 61–78.

92 Eivers C, Rueda RC, Liuti T, *et al.* Retrospective analysis of esophageal imaging features in brachycephalic versus non-brachycephalic dogs based on videofluoroscopic swallowing studies. *J Vet Intern Med* 2019; **33**: 1740–1746.

93 Downing F, Gibson S. Anaesthesia of brachycephalic dogs. *J Small Anim Pract* 2018; **59**: 725–733.

94 Gruenheid M, Aarnes TK, McLoughlin MA, *et al.* Risk of anesthesia-related complications in brachycephalic dogs. *J Am Vet Med Assoc* 2018; **253**: 301–306.

95 Oda A, Wang WH, Hampton AK, *et al.* Perianesthetic mortality in English Bulldogs: a retrospective analysis in 2010–2017. *BMC Vet Res* 2022; **18**: 198.

96 Poncet CM, Dupré GP, Freiche VG, *et al.* Prevalence of gastrointestinal tract lesions in 73 brachycephalic dogs with upper respiratory syndrome. *J Small Anim Pract* 2005; **46**: 273–279.

97 Grobman ME, Maitz CA, Reinero CR. Detection of silent reflux events by nuclear scintigraphy in healthy dogs. *J Vet Intern Med* 2020; **34**: 1432–1439.

98 Ogunnaike BO, Whitten CW. Gastrointestinal disorders. In: Barash PG, Cullen BF, Stoelting RK, *et al.*, eds. *Clinical Anesthesia*, 6th edn. Philadelphia, PA: Lippincott, Williams & Wilkins, 2009: 1221–1228.

99 Open Anesthesia. Anesthetic Drugs Affecting Lower Esophageal Sphincter Tone. https://www.openanesthesia.org/keywords/anesthetic-drugs-affecting-lower-esophageal-sphincter-tone (accessed March 2023).

100 Strombeck DR, Harrold D. Effects of atropine, acepromazine, meperidine and xylazine on gastroesophageal sphincter pressure in the dog. *Am J Vet Res* 1985; **46**: 963–965.

101 Hall JA, Magne ML, Twedt DC. Effect of acepromazine, diazepam, fentanyl-droperidol, and oxymorphone on gastroesophageal sphincter pressure in healthy dogs. *Am J Vet Res* 1987; **48**: 556–557.

102 Waterman AE, Hashim MA. Effects of thiopentone and propofol on lower oesophageal sphincter and barrier pressure in the dog. *J Small Anim Pract* 1992; **33**: 530–533.

103 van der Hoeven CW, Attia A, Deen L, *et al.* The influence of anaesthetic drugs on the LOS in propofol/nitrous oxide anaesthetized dogs. Pressure profilometry in an animal model. *Acta Anaesthesiol Scand* 1995; **39**: 822–826.

104 Hashim MA, Waterman AE. Effect of acepromazine, pethidine and atropine premedication on lower oesophageal sphincter pressure and barrier pressure in anaesthetized cats. *Vet Rec* 1993; **133**:158–160.

105 Hashim MA, Waterman AE. Effects of thiopentone, propofol, alphaxalone-alphadolone, ketamine and xylazine-ketamine on lower oesophageal sphincter pressure and barrier pressure in cats. *Vet Rec* 1991; **129**: 137–139.

106 Hashim MA, Waterman AE, Pearson H. Effect of body position on oesophageal and gastric pressures in the anaesthetized dog. *J Small Anim Pract* 1995; **36**: 196–200.

107 Savvas I, Pavlidou K, Anagnostou T, *et al.* factors affecting intraoperative gastro-oesophageal reflux in dogs and cats. *Animals (Basel)* 2022; **12**: 247.

108 Savvas I, Raptopoulos D, Rallis T. A "light meal" three hours preoperatively decreases the incidence of gastro-esophageal reflux in dogs. *J Am Anim Hosp Assoc* 2016; **52**: 357–363.

109 Savvas I, Rallia T, Raptopoulos D. The effect of pre-anaesthetic fasting time and type of food on gastric content volume and acidity in dogs. *Vet Anaesth Analg* 2009; **36**: 539–546.

110 Galatos A, Raptopoulos D. Gastro-oesophageal reflux during anaesthesia in the dog: the effect of preoperative fasting and premedication. *Vet Rec* 1995; **137**: 479–483.

111 Savvas I, Raptopoulos D. Incidence of gastro-oesophageal reflux during anaesthesia, following two different fasting times in dogs. *Vet Anaesth Analg* 2000; **27**: 54–62.

112 Wilson DV, Evans AT. Effect of a short preanesthetic fast on risk of gastroesophageal reflux during anesthesia in dogs. *Presented at the Annual Meeting of the American College of Veterinary Anesthesiologists*, Chicago, IL, September 12–13, 2006.

113 Tsompanidou P, Robben JH, Savvas I. The effect of the preoperative fasting regimen on the incidence of gastro-oesophageal reflux in 90 dogs. *Animals (Basel)* 2021; **12**: 64.

114 Viskjer S, Sjöström L. Effect of the duration of food withholding prior to anesthesia on gastroesophageal reflux and regurgitation in healthy dogs undergoing elective orthopedic surgery. *Am J Vet Res* 2017; **78**: 144–150.

115 Anagnostou TL, Kazakos GM, I Savvas I, *et al.* Gastro-oesophageal reflux in large-sized, deep-chested versus small-sized, barrel-chested dogs undergoing spinal surgery in sternal recumbency. *Vet Anaesth Analg* 2017; **44**: 35–41.

116 Wilson DV. Peri-anesthetic gastroesophageal reflux. *Presented at the International Veterinary Emergency and Critical Care Symposium*, Nashville, TN, September 14–18, 2011.

117 Galatos A, Raptopoulos D. Gastro-oesophageal reflux during anaesthesia in the dog: the effect of age, positioning and type of surgical procedure. *Vet Rec* 1995; **137**: 513–516.

118 Wilson DV, Boruta DT, Dhanjal JK, *et al.* The prevalence of anesthetic-related gastroesophageal reflux during fracture repair in dogs. *Presented at the American College of Veterinary Anesthesia Autumn Conference, International Veterinary Emergency and Critical Care Symposium, Phoenix*, AZ, September 18–21, 2008.

119 Raptopoulos D, Galatos AD. Gastro-oesophageal reflux during anaesthesia induced with either thiopentone or propofol in the dog. *J Vet Anaesth* 1997; **24**: 20–21.

120 Garcia RS, Belafsky PC, Maggiore AD, *et al.* Prevalence of gastroesophageal reflux in cats during anesthesia and effect of omeprazole on gastric pH. *J Vet Intern Med* 2017; **31**: 734–742.

121 Sideri AI, Galatos AD, Gouletsou PG, *et al.* Gastro-oesophageal reflux during anaesthesia in the cat: the effect of intra-abdominal surgery. *Presented at the Association of Veterinary Anaesthetists Autumn meeting*, September 3rd–4th, 2010. *Vet Anaesth Analg* 2011; **38**: 1–28.

122 Galatos AD, Savas I, Prassinos NN, *et al.* Gastro-oesophageal reflux during thiopentone or propofol anaesthesia in the cat. *J Vet Med A Physiol Pathol Clin Med* 2001; **48**: 287–294.

123 Wilson DV, Evans AT, Miller R. Effects of preanesthetic administration of morphine on gastroesophageal reflux and regurgitation during anesthesia in dogs. *Am J Vet Res* 2005; **66**: 386–390.

124 Wilson DV, Evans AT, Mauer WA. Pre-anesthetic meperidine: associated vomiting and gastroesophageal reflux during the subsequent anesthetic in dogs. *Vet Anaesth Analg* 2007; **34**: 15–22.

125 Wilson DV, Boruta DT, Evans AT. Influence of halothane, isoflurane, and sevoflurane on gastroesophageal reflux during anesthesia in dogs. *Am J Vet Res* 2006; **67**: 1821–1825.

126 Costa RS, Wetmore LA, Stein A. Randomized, blinded, controlled clinical trial to assess gastroesophageal reflux and regurgitation in dogs undergoing general anesthesia after hydromorphone premedication with or without acepromazine or dexmedetomidine. *Am J Vet Res* 2021; **82**: 695–700.

127 Flouraki ES, Savvas I, Kazakos G, *et al.* The effect of premedication on the incidence of gastroesophageal reflux in 270 dogs undergoing general anesthesia. *Animals* 2022; **12**: 2667.

128 Paterson WG, Rattan S, Goyal RK. Experimental induction of isolated lower esophageal sphincter relaxation in anesthetized opossums. *J Clin Invest* 1986; **77**: 1187–1193.

129 Leslie E, Bhargava V, Mittal RK. A novel pattern of longitudinal muscle contraction with subthreshold pharyngeal stimulus: a possible mechanism of lower esophageal sphincter relaxation. *Am J Physiol Gastrointest Liver Physiol* 2012; **302**: G542–G547.

130 Sideri AI, Apostolos D, Galatos AD, *et al.* Gastro-oesophageal reflux during anaesthesia in the kitten: comparison between use of a laryngeal mask airway or an endotracheal tube. *Vet Anaesth Analg* 2009; **36**: 547–554.

131 Lamata C, Loughton V, Jones M, *et al.* The risk of passive regurgitation during general anaesthesia in a population of referred dogs in the UK. *Vet Anaesth Analg* 2012; **39**: 266–274.

132 De Miguel García C, Pinchbeck GL, Dugdale A, *et al.* Retrospective study of the risk factors and prevalence of regurgitation in dogs undergoing general anaesthesia. *Open Vet Sci J* 2013; **7**: 6–11.

133 Mansfield CS, Hyndman T. Gastric cytoprotective agents. In: Washabau RJ, Day MJ, eds. *Canine and Feline Gastroenterology*. St. Louis, MO: Saunders Elsevier, 2013: 500–504.

134 Bersenas AME, Mathews KA, Allen DG, *et al.* Effects of ranitidine, famotidine, pantoprazole, and omeprazole on intragastric pH in dogs. *Am J Vet Res* 2005; **66**: 425–431.

135 Tolbert K, Bissett S, King A, *et al.* Efficacy of oral famotidine and 2 omeprazole formulations for the control of intragastric pH in dogs. *J Vet Intern Med* 2011; **25**: 47–54.

136 Panti A, Bennett RC, Corletto F, *et al.* The effect of omeprazole on oesophageal pH in dogs during anaesthesia. *J Small Anim Pract* 2009; **50**: 540–544.

137 Lotti F, Twedt D, Warrit K, *et al.* Effect of two different pre-anaesthetic omeprazole protocols on gastroesophageal reflux incidence and pH in dogs. *J Small Anim Pract* 2021; **62**: 677–682.

138 Lotti F, Boscan P, Twedt D, *et al.* Effect of maropitant, maropitant with omeprazole and esophageal lavage on gastroesophageal reflux in anesthetized dogs. *Vet Anaesth Analg* 2018; **45**: 885e8–885e9.

139 Zacuto AC, Marks SL, Osborn J, *et al.* The influence of esomeprazole and cisapride on gastroesophageal reflux during anesthesia in dogs. *J Vet Intern Med* 2012; **26**: 518–525.

140 Ogden J, Ovbey D, Saile K. Effects of preoperative cisapride on postoperative aspiration pneumonia in dogs with laryngeal paralysis. *J Small Anim Pract* 2019; **60**: 83–190.

141 Wilson DV, Evans AT, Mauer WA. Influence of metoclopramide on gastroesophageal reflux in anesthetized dogs. *Am J Vet Res* 2006; **67**: 26–31.

142 Favarato ES, Souza MV, Costa PR, *et al.* Evaluation of metoclopramide and ranitidine on the prevention of gastroesophageal reflux episodes in anesthetized dogs. *Res Vet Sci* 2012; **93**: 466–467.

143 Jones CT, Fransson BA. Evaluation of the effectiveness of preoperative administration of maropitant citrate and metoclopramide hydrochloride in preventing postoperative clinical gastroesophageal reflux in dogs. *J Am Vet Med Assoc* 2019; **255**: 437–445.

144 Lotti F, Boscan P, Warrit K, *et al.* Strongly acidic gastroesophageal reflux and esophageal lumen pH before and after esophageal lavage with water or two bicarbonate concentrations in anesthetized dogs. *Am J Vet Res* 2022; **83**: 1–5.

145 Wilson DV, Evans AT. The effect of topical treatment on esophageal pH during acid reflux in dogs. *Vet Anaesth Analg* 2007; **34**: 339–343.

146 Allison A, Italiano M, Robinson R. Comparison of two topical treatments of gastro-oesophageal regurgitation in dogs during general anaesthesia. *Vet Anaesth Analg* 2020; **47**: 672–675.

147 Practice guidelines for preoperative fasting and the use of pharmacologic agents to reduce the risk of pulmonary aspiration: application to healthy patients undergoing elective procedures. An updated report by the American Society of Anesthesiologists Task Force on Preoperative fasting and the use of pharmacologic agents to reduce the risk of pulmonary aspiration. *Anesthesiology* 2017; **126**: 376–393.

148 Joshi GP, Abdelmalak BB, Weigel WA, *et al.* 2023 American Society of Anesthesiologists practice guidelines for preoperative fasting: carbohydrate-containing clear liquids with or without protein, chewing gum, and pediatric fasting duration – a modular update of the 2017 American Society of Anesthesiologists practice guidelines for preoperative fasting. *Anesthesiology* 2023; **138**: 132–151.

149 Grubb T, Sager J, Gaynor JS, *et al.* 2020 American Animal Hospital Association (AAHA) Anesthesia and monitoring guidelines for dogs and cats. *J Am Anim Hosp Assoc* 2020; **56**: 59–82.

150 Evander A, Little AG, Riddell RH, *et al.* Composition of the refluxed material determines the degree of reflux esophagitis in the dog. *Gastroenterology* 1987; **93**: 280–286.

151 Glazer A, Walters P. Esophagitis and esophageal strictures. *Compend Contin Educ Vet* 2008; **30**: 281–292.

152 Han E. Diagnosis and management of reflux esophagitis. *Clin Tech Small Anim Pract* 2003; **18**: 231–238.

153 Sellon RK, Willard MD. Esophagitis and esophageal strictures. *Vet Clin North Am Small Anim Pract* 2003; **33**: 945–967.

154 Frowde PE, Battersby IA, Whitley NT, *et al.* Oesophageal disease in 33 cats. *J Feline Med Surg* 2011; **13**: 564–569.

155 Gal A, Ridgway MD, Fredrickson RL. An unusual clinical presentation of a dog with gastrinoma. *Can Vet J* 2011; **52**: 641–644.

156 Bissett SA, Davis J, Subler K, *et al.* Risk factors and outcome of bougienage for treatment of benign esophageal strictures in dogs and cats: 28 cases (1995–2004). *J Am Vet Med Assoc* 2009; **235**: 844–850.

157 Mazzei MJ, Bissett SA, Murphy KM, *et al.* Eosinophilic esophagitis in a dog. *J Am Vet Med Assoc* 2009; **235**: 61–65.

158 Pera J, Palma D, Donovan TA. Eosinophilic esophagitis in a kitten. *J Am Anim Hosp Assoc* 2017; **53**: 214–220.

159 Kouki MI, Papadimitriou SA, Psalla D, *et al.* Chronic gingivostomatitis with esophagitis in cats. *J Vet Intern Med* 2017; **31**: 1673–1679.

160 Adamama-Moraitou KK, Rallis TS, Prassinos NN, *et al.* Benign esophageal stricture in the dog and cat: a retrospective study of 20 cases. *Can J Vet Res* 2002; **66**: 55–59.

161 Kushner LI, Shofer FS. Incidence of esophageal strictures and esophagitis after general anesthesia. *Presented at the World Congress of Veterinary Anaesthesiology*, Knoxville, TN, September 17–20, 2003.

162 Anagnostou TL, Savvas I, Kazakos GM, *et al.* Effect of endogenous progesterone and oestradiol-17β on the incidence of gastro-oesophageal reflux and on the barrier pressure during general anaesthesia in the female dog. *Vet Anaesth Analg* 2009; **36**: 308–318.

163 Wilson DV, Walshaw R. Postanesthetic esophageal dysfunction in 13 dogs. *J Am Anim Hosp Assoc* 2004; **40**: 455–460.

164 Adami C, Di Palma S, Gendron K, *et al.* Severe esophageal injuries occurring after general anesthesia in two cats: case report and literature review. *J Am Anim Hosp Assoc* 2011; **47**: 436–442.

165 Janda M, Scheeren TWL, Nöldge-Schomburg GF. Management of pulmonary aspiration. *Best Pract Res Clin Anaesthesiol* 2006; **20**: 409–427.

166 Marik PE. Pulmonary aspiration syndromes. *Curr Opin Pulm Med* 2011; **17**: 149–154.

167 Sherman R, Karagiannis M. Aspiration pneumonia in the dog: a review. *Top Companion Anim Med* 2017; **3**: 21–27.

168 Dear JD. Bacterial pneumonia in dogs and cats: an update. *Vet Clin North Am Small Anim Pract* 2020; **50**: 447–465.

169 Schulze HM, Rahilly LJ. Aspiration pneumonia in dogs: pathophysiology, prevention, and diagnosis. *Compend Contin Educ Vet* 2012; **34**: E5.

170 Schulze HM, Rahilly LJ. Aspiration pneumonia in dogs: treatment, monitoring, and prognosis. *Compend Contin Educ Vet* 2012; **34**: E1.

171 Java MA, Drobatz KJ, Gilley RS, *et al.* Incidence of and risk factors for postoperative pneumonia in dogs anesthetized for diagnosis or treatment of intervertebral disk disease. *J Am Vet Med Assoc* 2009; **235**: 281–287.

172 Alwood AJ, Brainard BM, LaFond E, *et al.* Postoperative pulmonary complications in dogs undergoing laparotomy: frequency, characterization and disease-related risk factors. *J Vet Emerg Crit Care* 2006; **16**: 176–183.

173 Kogan DA, Johnson LR, Sturges BK, *et al.* Etiology and clinical outcome in dogs with aspiration pneumonia: 88 cases (2004–2006). *J Am Vet Med Assoc* 2008; **233**: 1748–1755.

174 Wilson D, Monnet E. Risk factors for the development of aspiration pneumonia after unilateral arytenoid lateralization in dogs with laryngeal paralysis: 232 cases (1987–2012). *J Am Vet Med Assoc* 2016; **248**: 188–194.

175 Krainer D, Gilles Dupré G. Brachycephalic obstructive airway syndrome. *Vet Clin North Am Small Anim Pract* 2022; **52**: 749–780.

176 Tart KM, Babski DM, Lee JA. Potential risks, prognostic indicators, and diagnostic and treatment modalities affecting survival in dogs with presumptive aspiration pneumonia: 125 cases (2005–2008). *J Vet Emerg Crit Care* 2010; **20**: 319–329.

177 Levy N, Ballegeer E, Koenigshof A. Clinical and radiographic findings in cats with aspiration pneumonia: retrospective evaluation of 28 cases. *J Small Anim Pract* 2019; **60**: 356–360.

178 Dear JD, Vernau W, Johnson EG, *et al.* Clinicopathologic and radiographic features in 33 cats with aspiration and 26 cats with bronchopneumonia (2007–2017). *J Vet Intern Med* 2021; **35**: 480–489.

179 Baetge C, Cummings KJ, Deveau M. Reduced risk of pneumonia after changes in anesthetic procedures for dogs receiving repeated anesthesia for radiation treatment. *Vet Radiol Ultrasound* 2019; **60**: 241–245.

180 Moyer AL, McKee TS, Bergman PJ, *et al.* Low incidence of postoperative nausea, vomiting, regurgitation, and aspiration pneumonia in geriatric dogs receiving maropitant, famotidine, and fentanyl as part of an anesthesia protocol. *J Am Vet Med Assoc* 2021; **260**: S46–S51.

181 Flecknell P. Analgesia and post-operative care. In: *Laboratory Animal Anesthesia*, 3rd edn. San Diego, CA: Elsevier Academic Press, 2009: 171–172.

182 Hawkins MG, Pascoe PJ. Anesthesia, analgesia and sedation of small mammals. In: Quesenberry KE, Carpenter JW, eds. *Ferrets, Rabbits, and Rodents Clinical Medicine and Surgery*, 3rd edn. St. Louis, MO: Saunders Elsevier, 2012: 430–445.

183 Morton AJ, Blikslager AT. Surgical and postoperative factors influencing short-term survival of horses following small intestinal resection: 92 cases (1994–2001). *Equine Vet J* 2002; **34**: 450–454.

184 Senior JM, Pinchbeck GL, Allister R, *et al.* Post anaesthetic colic in horses: a preventable complication? *Equine Vet J* 2006; **38**: 479–484.

185 Mythen MG. Postoperative gastrointestinal tract dysfunction: an overview of causes and management strategies. *Cleve Clin J Med* 2009; **76**(Suppl 4): S66–S71.

186 Boysen S. GI motility and ileus in the ICU: should we be worried about it? *Presented at the European Veterinary Emergency and Critical Care Congress*, Ghent, Belgium, June 6–8, 2019.

187 Warrit K, Boscan P, Ferguson LE, *et al.* Effect of hospitalization on gastrointestinal motility and pH in dogs. *J Am Vet Med Assoc* 2017; **251**: 65–70.

188 Sanderson JJ, Boysen SR, McMurray JM, *et al.* The effect of fasting on gastrointestinal motility in healthy dogs as assessed by sonography. *J Vet Emerg Crit Care (San Antonio)* 2017; **27**: 645–650.

189 Healy TE, Foster GE, Evans EF, *et al.* Effect of some i.v. anaesthetic agents on canine gastrointestinal motility. *Br J Anaesth* 1981; **53**: 229–233.

190 Steinbrook RA. Epidural anesthesia and gastrointestinal motility. *Anesth Analg* 1998; **86**: 837–844.

191 Nakamura K, Hara S, Tomizawa N. The effects of medetomidine and xylazine on gastrointestinal motility and gastrin release in the dog. *J Vet Pharmacol Ther* 1997; **20**: 290–295.

192 Hsu WH, McNeel SV. Effect of yohimbine on xylazine-induced prolongation of gastrointestinal transit in dogs. *J Am Vet Med Assoc* 1983; **183**: 297–300.

193 Maugeri S, Ferrè JP, Intorre L, *et al.* Effects of medetomidine on intestinal and colonic motility in the dog. *J Vet Pharmacol Ther* 1994; **17**: 148–154.

194 Boscan P, Van Hoogmoed LM, Farver TB, *et al.* Evaluation of the effects of the opioid agonist morphine on gastrointestinal tract function in horses. *Am J Vet Res* 2006; **67**: 992–997.

195 Washabau RJ. Small intestine: dysmotility. In: Washabau RJ, Day MJ, eds. *Canine and Feline Gastroenterology*. St. Louis, MO: Saunders Elsevier, 2013: 707–709.

196 Washabau RJ. Gastrointestinal motility disorders and gastrointestinal prokinetic therapy. *Vet Clin North Am Small Anim Pract* 2003; **33**: 1007–1028.

197 Ali-Melkkilä T, Kanto J, Iisalo E. Pharmacokinetics and related pharmacodynamics of anticholinergic drugs. *Acta Anaesthesiol Scand* 1993; **37**: 633–642.

198 Eger EI II. Atropine, scopolamine, and related compounds. *Anesthesiology* 1962; **23**: 365–383.

199 Burger DM, Wiestner T, Hubler M, *et al.* Effect of anticholinergics (atropine, glycopyrrolate) and prokinetics (metoclopramide, cisapride) on gastric motility in Beagles and Labrador Retrievers. *J Vet Med A Physiol Pathol Clin Med* 2006; **53**: 97–107.

200 Braun U, Gansohr B, Haessig M. Ultrasonographic evaluation of reticular motility in cows after administration of atropine, scopolamine and xylazine. *J Vet Med A Physiol Pathol Clin Med* 2002; **49**: 299–302.

201 Teixeira-Neto FJ, McDonell WN, Black WD, *et al.* Effects of glycopyrrolate on cardiorespiratory function in horses anesthetized with halothane and xylazine. *Am J Vet Res* 2004; **65**: 456–463.

202 Short, CE, Paddleford, RR, Cloyd GD. Glycopyrrolate for prevention of pulmonary complications during anesthesia. *Mod Vet Pract* 1974; **55**: 194–196.

203 DeHaven-Hudkins DL, DeHaven RN, Little PJ, *et al.* The involvement of the mu-opioid receptor in gastrointestinal pathophysiology: therapeutic opportunities for antagonism at this receptor. *Pharmacol Ther* 2008; **117**: 162–187.

204 Nakayoshi T, Kawasaki N, Suzuki Y, *et al.* Epidural administration of morphine facilitates time of appearance of first gastric interdigestive migrating complex in dogs with paralytic ileus after open abdominal surgery. *J Gastrointest Surg* 2007; **11**: 648–654.

205 Pöpping DM, Elia N, Van Aken HK, *et al.* Impact of epidural analgesia on mortality and morbidity after surgery: systematic review and meta-analysis of randomized controlled trials. *Ann Surg* 2014; **259**: 1056–1067.

206 Lubawski J, Saclarides T. Postoperative ileus: strategies for reduction. *Ther Clin Risk Manag* 2008; **4**: 913–917.

207 Yokoyama T, Kitazawa T, Takasaki K, *et al.* Recovery of gastrointestinal motility from post-operative ileus in dogs: effects of Leu13-motilin (KW-5139) and PGF2 alpha. *Neurogastroenterol Motil* 1995; **7**: 199–210.

208 Fages A, Soler C, Fernández-Salesa N, *et al.* Perioperative outcome in dogs undergoing emergency abdominal surgery: a retrospective study on 82 cases (2018–2020). *Vet Sci* 2021; **8**: 209.

209 Boscan P, Cochran S, Monnet E, *et al.* Effect of prolonged general anesthesia with sevoflurane and laparoscopic surgery on gastric and small bowel propulsive motility and pH in dogs. *Vet Anaesth Analg* 2014; **41**: 73–81.

210 Sido B, Teklote JR, Hartel M, *et al.* Inflammatory response after abdominal surgery. *Best Pract Res Clin Anaesthesiol* 2004; **18**: 439–454.

211 van Bree SH, Nemethova A, Cailotto C, *et al.* New therapeutic strategies for post-operative ileus. *Nat Rev Gastroenterol Hepatol* 2012; **9**: 675–683.

212 Vather R, Bissett I. Management of prolonged post-operative ileus: evidence-based recommendations. *Aust N Z J Surg* 2013; **83**: 319–324.

213 Hussain Z, Park H. Inflammation and impaired gut physiology in post-operative ileus: mechanisms and the treatment options. *J Neurogastroenterol Motil* 2022; **28**: 517–530.

214 Mazzotta E, Villalobos-Hernandez EC, Fiorda-Diaz J, *et al.* Postoperative ileus and postoperative gastrointestinal tract dysfunction: pathogenic mechanisms and novel treatment strategies beyond colorectal enhanced recovery after surgery protocols. *Front Pharmacol* 2020; **11**: 583422.

215 Campoy C. Development of Enhanced Recovery After Surgery (ERAS) protocols in veterinary medicine through a one-health approach: the role of anesthesia and locoregional techniques. *J Am Vet Med Assoc* 2022; **260**: 1751–1759.

216 Yang J-W, Shao J-K, Wang Y. Effect of acupuncture on postoperative ileus after laparoscopic elective colorectal surgery: a prospective, randomised, controlled trial. *E Clinical Medicine* 2022; **49**: 101472.

217 Kaye AD, Chernobylsky DJ, Thakur P. Dexmedetomidine in Enhanced Recovery after Surgery (ERAS) protocols for postoperative pain. *Curr Pain Headache Rep* 2020; **24**: 21.

218 Chen P-C, Lai C-H, Fang C-J, *et al.* Intravenous infusion of lidocaine for bowel function recovery after major colorectal surgery: a critical appraisal through updated meta-analysis, trial sequential analysis, certainty of evidence, and meta-regression. *Front Med (Lausanne)* 2022; **8**: 759215.

219 Cooke C, Kennedy ED, Foo I. Meta-analysis of the effect of perioperative intravenous lidocaine on return of gastrointestinal function after colorectal surgery. *Tech Coloproctol* 2019; **23**: 15–24.

220 Leslie JB, Viscusi ER, Pergolizzi JV Jr., *et al.* Anesthetic routines: the anesthesiologist's role in GI recovery and postoperative ileus. *Adv Prev Med* 2011; **2011**: 976904.

221 Rimbäck G, Cassuto J, Tollesson PO. Treatment of postoperative paralytic ileus by intravenous lidocaine infusion. *Anesth Analg* 1990; **70**: 414–419.

222 Malone E, Ensink J, Turner T, *et al.* Intravenous continuous infusion of lidocaine for treatment of equine ileus. *Vet Surg* 2006; **35**: 60–66.

223 Psatha E, Alibhai H IK, Jimenez-Lozano A, *et al.* Clinical efficacy and cardiorespiratory effects of alfaxalone, or diazepam/fentanyl for induction of anaesthesia in dogs that are a poor anaesthetic risk. *Vet Anaesth Analg* 2011; **38**: 24–36.

224 Chan CM, Mitchell AL, Shorr AF. Etomidate is associated with mortality and adrenal insufficiency in sepsis: a meta-analysis. *Crit Care Med* 2012; **40**: 2945–2953.

225 Gu W-J, Wang F, Tang L, *et al.* Single-dose etomidate does not increase mortality in patients with sepsis: a systematic review and meta-analysis of randomized controlled trials and observational studies. *Chest* 2015; **147**: 335–346.

226 Duke-Novakovski T, Carr A. Perioperative blood pressure control and management. *Vet Clin North Am Small Anim Pract* 2015; **45**: 965–981.

227 Pansiritanachot W, Ruangsomboon O, Limsuwat C. Independent risk factors of mortality in patients with sepsis receiving single-dose etomidate as an induction agent during rapid sequence intubation in a large tertiary emergency department in Thailand. *BMC Emerg Med* 2022; **22**: 94.

228 Cagliani JA, Ruhemann A, Molmenti E, *et al.* Association between etomidate use for rapid sequence intubation and adrenal insufficiency in sepsis. *Cureus* 2021; **13**: e13445.

229 Weiss B, Schiefenhövel F, Grunow JJ, *et al.* Infectious complications after etomidate vs. propofol for induction of general anesthesia in cardiac surgery – results of a retrospective, before-after study. *J Clin Med* 2021; **10**: 2908.

230 Qin B, Hu H, Cao B, *et al.* Effects of continuous infusion of etomidate at various dose rates on adrenal function in dogs. *BMC Anesthesiol* 2016; **8**: 2.

231 Jones TL, Calbay R, da Cunha AF, *et al.* Descriptive assessment of adverse events associated with midazolam-etomidate versus saline-etomidate in healthy hydromorphone premedicated dogs. *J Small Anim Pract* 2021; **62**: 437–441.

232 Martinez-Taboada F, Leece EA. Comparison of propofol with ketofol, a propofol-ketamine admixture, for induction of anaesthesia in healthy dogs. *Vet Anaesth Analg* 2014; **41**: 575–582.

233 Ilkiw JE. Injectable anesthesia in dogs – Part 2: comparative pharmacology. In: Gleed R, Ludders J, eds. *Recent Advances in Veterinary Anesthesia and Analgesia: Companion Animals*, updated July 18, 2002.

234 Bughrara N, Cha S, Safa R, *et al.* Perioperative management of patients with sepsis and septic shock, part 1 – systematic approach. *Anesthesiol Clinics* 2020; **38**: 107–122.

235 Quandt J. Anesthesia in the critically ill patient. In: Silverstein DC, Hopper K, eds. *Small Animal Critical Care Medicine*, 3rd edn. St. Louis, MO: Saunders Elsevier, 2023: 778–786.

236 Murahata Y, Hikasa Y, Hayashi S, *et al.* The effect of remifentanil on the minimum alveolar concentration (MAC) and MAC derivatives of sevoflurane in dogs. *J Vet Med Sci* 2018; **80**: 1086–1093.

237 Steagall PVM, Aucoin M, Monteiro BP, *et al.* Clinical effects of a constant rate infusion of remifentanil, alone or in combination with ketamine, in cats anesthetized with isoflurane. *J Am Vet Med Assoc* 2015; **246**: 976–981.

238 Brown SM, Sneyd JR. Nitrous oxide in modern anaesthetic practice. *BJA Educ* 2016; **16**: 87–91.

239 Jones RS, West E. Environmental sustainability in veterinary anaesthesia. *Vet Anaesth Analg* 2019; **46**: 409–420.

240 National Health Service Scotland, Centre for Sustainable Delivery. News Release, NHS Scotland First In World To 'Clean Up' Anaesthetic Gases. https://www.nhscfsd.co.uk/news/nhs-scotland-first-in-world-to-clean-up-anaesthetic-gases (accessed March 2023).

241 Duke T. Partial intravenous anesthesia in cats and dogs. *Can Vet J* 2013; **54**: 276–282.

242 Aguado D, Benito J, Gómez de Segura IA. Reduction of the minimum alveolar concentration of isoflurane in dogs using a constant rate of infusion of lidocaine-ketamine in combination with either morphine or fentanyl. *Vet J* 2011; **189**: 63–66.

243 Muir WW III, Wiese AJ, March PA. Effects of morphine, lidocaine, ketamine, and morphine-lidocaine-ketamine drug combination on minimum alveolar concentration in dogs anesthetized with isoflurane. *Am J Vet Res* 2003; **64**: 1155–1160.

244 Wilson J, Doherty TJ, Egger CM, *et al.* Effects of intravenous lidocaine, ketamine, and the combination on the minimum alveolar concentration of sevoflurane in dogs. *Vet Anaesth Analg* 2008; **35**: 289–296.

245 Quandt J. Analgesia and constant rate infusions. In: Silverstein DC, Hopper K, eds. *Small Animal Critical Care Medicine*, 3rd edn. St. Louis, MO: Saunders Elsevier, 2023: 787–794.

246 Pypendop BH, Ilkiw JE. Assessment of the hemodynamic effects of lidocaine administered IV in isoflurane-anesthetized cats. *Am J Vet Res* 2005; **66**: 661–668.

247 Pascoe PJ. The cardiopulmonary effects of dexmedetomidine infusions in dogs during isoflurane anesthesia. *Vet Anaesth Analg* 2015; **42**: 360–368.

248 Pypendop BH, Barter LS, Stanley SD. Hemodynamic effects of dexmedetomidine in isoflurane-anesthetized cats. *Vet Anaesth Analg* 2011; **38**: 555–567.

249 Pypendop BH. α-Agonists and antagonists. In: Silverstein DC, Hopper K, eds. *Small Animal Critical Care Medicine*, 3rd edn. St. Louis, MO: Elsevier, 2023: 905–910.

250 Ramos D, Benavente R, Torres DH, *et al.* Dexmedetomidine improves cardiovascular and ventilatory outcomes in critically ill patients: basic and clinical approaches. *Front Pharmacol* 2020; **10**: 1641.

251 Portelaa DA, Verdierb N, Oterob PE. Regional anesthetic techniques for the pelvic limb and abdominal wall in small animals: a review of the literature and technique description. *Vet J* 2018; **238**: 27–40.

252 Viderman D, Aubakirova M, Abdildin YG. Transversus abdominis plane block in colorectal surgery: a meta-analysis. *Front Med (Lausanne)* 2022; **8**: 802039.

253 Cavaco JS, Otero PO, Ambrósio AM, *et al.* Analgesic efficacy of ultrasound-guided transversus abdominis plane block in dogs undergoing ovariectomy. *Front Vet Sci* 2022; **9**: 1031345.

254 Boysen SR, Kris Gommeren K. Assessment of volume status and fluid responsiveness in small animals. *Front Vet Sci* 2021; **8**: 630643.

255 Montcalgre F, Lyons BM. Fluid therapy in dogs and cats with sepsis. *Front Vet Sci* 2021; **8**: 622127.

256 Cooper ES, Silverstein DC. Fluid therapy and the microcirculation in health and critical illness. *Front Vet Sci* 2021; **8**: 625708.

257 Smart L, Silverstein DC. The endothelial surface layer. In: Silverstein DC, Hopper K, eds. *Small Animal Critical Care Medicine*, 3rd edn. St. Louis, MO: Saunders Elsevier, 2023: 55–60.

258 King LG. Postoperative complications and prognostic indicators in dogs and cats with septic peritonitis: 23 cases (1989–1992). *J Am Vet Med Assoc* 1994; **204**: 407–414.

259 Anderson T, Beever L, Hall J, *et al.* Outcome following surgery to treat septic peritonitis in 95 cats in the United Kingdom. *J Small Anim Pract* 2021; **62**: 744–749.

260 Valverde A. Fluid resuscitation for refractory hypotension. *Front Vet Sci* 2021; **8**: 621696.

261 Murphy KM, Rishniw M, Silverstein DC. Use of vasopressors for treatment of vasodilatory hypotension in dogs and cats by Diplomates of the American College of Veterinary Emergency and Critical Care. *J Vet Emerg Crit Care (San Antonio)* 2022; **32**: 714–722.

262 Hart S, Silverstein DC. Catecholamines. In: Silverstein DC, Hopper K, eds. *Small Animal Critical Care Medicine*, 3rd edn. St. Louis, MO: Saunders Elsevier, 2023: 855–860.

263 Silverstein DC, Hart S. Vasopressin. In: Silverstein DC, Hopper K, eds. *Small Animal Critical Care Medicine*, 3rd edn. St. Louis, MO: Saunders Elsevier, 2023: 861–866.

264 Pang DS, Boysen S. Lactate in veterinary critical care: pathophysiology and management. *J Am Anim Hosp Assoc* 2007; **43**: 270–279.

265 Mooney E, Raw C, Hughes D. Plasma lactate concentration as a prognostic biomarker in dogs with gastric dilation and volvulus. *Top Companion Anim Med* 2014; **29**: 71–76.

266 Cortellini S, Seth M, Kellett-Gregory LM. Plasma lactate concentrations in septic peritonitis: a retrospective study of 83 dogs (2007–2012). *J Vet Emerg Crit Care (San Antonio)* 2015; **25**: 388–395.

267 Parsons KJ, Owen LJ, Lee K, *et al.* A retrospective study of surgically treated cases of septic peritonitis in the cat (2000–2007). *J Small Anim Pract* 2009; **50**: 518–524.

268 Blutinger AL, Zollo AM, Weltman J, *et al.* Prospective evaluation of plasma lactate parameters for prognosticating dogs with shock. *J Vet Emerg Crit Care (San Antonio)* 2021; **31**(3): 351–359.

269 Kohen CJ, Hopper K, Kass PH, *et al.* Retrospective evaluation of the prognostic utility of plasma lactate concentration, base deficit, pH, and anion gap in canine and feline emergency patients. *J Vet Emerg Crit Care (San Antonio)* 2018; **28**: 54–61.

270 Dalmagro TL, Teixeira-Neto FJ, Celeita-Rodrıguez N, *et al.* Comparison between pulse pressure variation and systolic pressure variation measured from a peripheral artery for accurately predicting fluid responsiveness in mechanically ventilated dogs. *Vet Anaesth Analg* 2021; **48**: 501–508.

271 Patel A, Nunnally ME. The septic patient. *Anesthesiol Clin* 2020; **38**: 889–899.

272 MacDougall LM, Hethey JA, Livingston A, *et al.* Antinociceptive, cardiopulmonary, and sedative effects of five intravenous infusion rates of lidocaine in conscious dogs. *Vet Anaesth Analg* 2009; **36**: 512–522.

273 Bruchim Y, Itay S, Shira BH, *et al.* Evaluation of lidocaine treatment on frequency of cardiac arrhythmias, acute kidney injury, and hospitalization time in dogs with gastric dilatation volvulus. *J Vet Emerg Crit Care* 2012; **22**: 419–427.

274 Bellini L, Seymour CJ. Effect of intraoperative constant rate infusion of lidocaine on short-term survival of dogs with septic peritonitis: 75 cases (2007–2011). *J Am Vet Med Assoc* 2016; **248**: 422–429.

275 Valtolina C, Robben JH, Uilenreef J, *et al.* Clinical evaluation of the efficacy and safety of a constant rate infusion of dexmedetomidine for postoperative pain management in dogs. *Vet Anaesth Analg* 2009; **36**: 369–383.

276 PROSPECT. Procedure Specific Postoperative Pain Management. https://esraeurope.org/prospect/ (accessed April 2023).

277 Chapman SJ, Garner JJ, Drake, TM. Systematic review and meta-analysis of nonsteroidal anti-inflammatory drugs to improve GI recovery after colorectal surgery. *Dis Colon Rectum* 2019; **62**: 248–256.

278 Lin HC. Pain management for farm animals. In: Lin HC, Passler T, Clark-Price S, eds. *Farm Animal Anesthesia: Cattle, Small Ruminants, Camelids, and Pigs*, 2nd edn. Hoboken, NJ: John Wiley and Sons, 2022: 215–219.

279 Robertson SA, Sanchez LC. Treatment of visceral pain in horses. *Vet Clin North Am Equine Pract* 2010; **26**: 603–617.

280 KuKanich B, Bidgood T, Knesl O. Clinical pharmacology of nonsteroidal anti-inflammatory drugs in dogs. *Vet Anaesth Analg* 2012; **39**: 69–90.

281 Lascelles BD, Court MH, Hardie EM, *et al.* Nonsteroidal anti-inflammatory drugs in cats: a review. *Vet Anaesth Analg* 2007; **34**: 228–250.

282 Papich MG. An update on nonsteroidal anti-inflammatory drugs (NSAIDs) in small animals. *Vet Clin North Am Small Anim Pract* 2008; **38**: 1243–1266.

283 Monteiro B, Steagall PV. Non-steroidal anti-inflammatory drugs. In: Silverstein DC, Hopper K, eds. *Small Animal Critical Care Medicine*, 3rd edn. St. Louis, MO: Elsevier, 2023: 911–918.

284 Smith SA, Roberts DJ, Lipson ME, *et al.* Postoperative nonsteroidal anti-inflammatory drug use and intestinal anastomotic dehiscence: a systematic review and meta-analysis. *Dis Colon Rectum* 2016; **59**: 1087–1097.

285 Washabau RJ. Esophagus, dysmotility. In: Washabau RJ, Day MJ, eds. *Canine and Feline Gastroenterology*. St. Louis, MO: Saunders Elsevier, 2013: 591–595.

286 Mace S, Shelton GD, Eddlestone S. Megaesophagus. *Compend Contin Educ Vet* 2012; **34**: E1–E8.

287 Gaynor AR, Shofer FS, Washabau RJ. Risk factors for acquired megaesophagus in dogs. *J Am Vet Med Assoc* 1997; **211**: 1406–1412.

288 Forgash JT, Chang YM, Mittelman NS. Clinical features and outcome of acquired myasthenia gravis in 94 dogs. *J Vet Intern Med* 2021; **35**: 2315–2326.

289 Hague DW, Humphries HD, Mitchell MA, *et al.* Risk factors and outcomes in cats with acquired myasthenia gravis (2001–2012). *J Vet Intern Med* 2015; **29**: 1307–1312.

290 Gomes SA, Van Ham L, Van Ham A. Canine nonstructural megaesophagus as a clinical sign of potential neurological disease: 99 cases. *J Am Anim Hosp Assoc* 2020; **56**: 7–16.

291 Heinz JA, Mankin J, Pashmakova M. Transient megaesophagus following coral snake envenomation in three dogs (2013–2018). *J Am Anim Hosp Assoc* 2020; **56**: 320.

292 Hurley KJ, Mansfield C, VanHoutan IM, *et al.* A comparative analysis of two unrelated outbreaks in Latvia and Australia of acquired idiopathic megaesophagus in dogs fed two brands of commercial dry dog foods: 398 cases (2014–2018). *J Am Vet Med Assoc* 2021; **259**: 172–183.

293 Daum P, Smelt J, Ibrahim IR. Perioperative management of myasthenia gravis. *BJA Educ* 2021; **21**: 414–419.

294 O'Neill DG, Case J, Boag AK, *et al.* Gastric dilation-volvulus in dogs attending UK emergency-care veterinary practices: prevalence, risk factors and survival. *J Small Anim Pract* 2017; **58**: 629–638.

295 Glickman L, Glickman NW, Perez CM. Analysis of risk factors for gastric dilatation and dilatation-volvulus in dogs. *J Am Vet Med Assoc* 1994; **204**: 23–31.

296 Leary ML, Sinnott-Stutzman V. Spontaneous gastric dilatation-volvulus in two cats. *J Vet Emerg Crit Care (San Antonio)* 2018; **28**: 346–355.

297 Formaggini L, Schmidt K, Lorenzi D. Gastric dilatation-volvulus associated with diaphragmatic hernia in three cats: clinical presentation, surgical treatment and presumptive aetiology. *J Feline Med Surg* 2008; **10**: 198–201.

298 Brockman DJ, Holt DE, Washabau RJ. Pathogenesis of acute canine gastric dilatation-volvulus syndrome: is there a unifying hypothesis? *Compend Contin Educ Vet* 2000; **22**: 1108–1114.

299 Hall JA, Solie TN, Seim HB III, *et al.* Gastric myoelectric and motor activity in dogs with gastric dilatation-volvulus. *Am J Physiol* 1993; **265**(4 Pt 1): G646–G653.

300 Hall JA, Willer RL, Solie TN, Twedt DC. Effect of circumcostal gastropexy on gastric myoelectric and motor activity in dogs. *J Small Anim Pract* 1997; **38**: 200–207.

301 Coleman KA, Boscan P, Ferguson L, *et al.* Evaluation of gastric motility in nine dogs before and after prophylactic laparoscopic gastropexy: a pilot study. *Aust Vet J* 2019; **97**: 225–230.

302 Gazzola KM, Nelson LL. The relationship between gastrointestinal motility and gastric dilatation-volvulus in dogs. *Top Companion Anim Med* 2014; **29**: 64–66.

303 Washabau RJ, Hall JA. Stomach: obstruction. In: Washabau RJ, Day MJ, eds. *Canine and Feline Gastroenterology*. St. Louis, MO: Saunders Elsevier, 2013: 624–628.

304 Brockman DJ, Washabau RJ, Drobatz KJ. Canine gastric dilatation/volvulus syndrome in a veterinary critical care unit: 295 cases (1986–1992). *J Am Vet Med Assoc* 1995; **207**: 460–464.

305 Bell JS. Inherited and predisposing factors in the development of gastric dilatation volvulus in dogs. *Top Companion Anim Med* 2014; **29**: 60–63.

306 Rosselli D. Updated information on gastric dilatation and volvulus and gastropexy in dogs. *Vet Clin North Am Small Anim Pract* 2022; **52**: 317–337.

307 de Battisti A, Toscano MJ, Formaggini L. Gastric foreign body as a risk factor for gastric dilatation and volvulus in dogs. *J Am Vet Med Assoc* 2012; **241**: 1190–1193.

308 Harkey MA, Villagran AM, Venkataraman GM, *et al.* Associations between gastric dilatation-volvulus in Great Danes and specific alleles of the canine immune-system genes DLA88, DRB1, and TLR5. *Am J Vet Res* 2017; **78**: 934–945.

309 Hullar MAJ, Lampe JW, Torok-Storb BJ, *et al.* The canine gut microbiome is associated with higher risk of gastric dilatation-volvulus and high risk genetic variants of the immune system. *PLOS ONE* 2018; **13**: e0197686.

310 Brourman JD, Schertel ER, Allen DA, *et al.* Factors associated with perioperative mortality in dogs with surgically managed gastric dilatation-volvulus: 137 cases (1988–1993). *J Am Vet Med Assoc* 1996; **208**: 1855–1858.

311 Beck J, Staatz A, Pelsue D, *et al.* Risk factors associated with short-term outcome and development of perioperative complications in dogs undergoing surgery because of gastric dilatation-volvulus: 166 cases (1992–2003). *J Am Vet Med Assoc* 2006; **229**: 1934–1939.

312 Buber T, Saragusty J, Ranen E, *et al.* Evaluation of lidocaine treatment and risk factors for death associated with gastric dilatation and volvulus in dogs: 112 cases (1997–2005). *J Am Vet Med Assoc* 2007; **230**: 1334–1339.

313 Mackenzie G, Barnhart M, Kennedy S, *et al.* A retrospective study of factors influencing survival following surgery for gastric dilatation-volvulus syndrome in 306 dogs. *J Am Anim Hosp Assoc* 2010; **46**: 97–102.

314 Song KK, Goldsmid SE, Lee J, *et al.* Retrospective analysis of 736 cases of canine gastric dilatation volvulus. *Aust Vet J* 2020; **98**: 232–238.

315 Sharp CR, Rozanski EA, Finn E, *et al.* The pattern of mortality in dogs with gastric dilatation and volvulus. *J Vet Emerg Crit Care (San Antonio)* 2020; **30**: 232–238.

316 Przywara JF, Abel SB, Peacock JT, *et al.* Occurrence and recurrence of gastric dilatation with or without volvulus after incisional gastropexy. *Can Vet J* 2014; **55**: 981–984.

317 Allen P, Paul A. Gastropexy for prevention of gastric dilatation-volvulus in dogs: history and techniques. *Top Companion Anim Med* 2014; **29**: 77–80.

318 Lantz GC, Badylak SF, Hiles MC, *et al.* Treatment of reperfusion injury in dogs with experimentally induced gastric dilatation-volvulus. *Am J Vet Res* 1992; **53**: 1594–1598.

319 Sharp CR, Rozanski EA. Cardiovascular and systemic effects of gastric dilatation and volvulus in dogs. *Top Companion Anim Med* 2014; **29**: 67–70.

320 Bruchim Y, Kelmer E. Postoperative management of dogs with gastric dilatation and volvulus. *Top Companion Anim Med* 2014; **29**: 81–85.

321 de Papp E, Drobatz KJ, Hughes D. Plasma lactate concentration as a predictor of gastric necrosis and survival among dogs with gastric dilatation-volvulus: 102 cases (1995–1998). *J Am Vet Med Assoc* 1999; **215**: 49–52.

322 Santoro Beer KA, Syring RS, Drobatz KJ. Evaluation of plasma lactate concentration and base excess at the time of hospital admission as predictors of gastric necrosis and outcome and correlation between those variables in dogs with gastric dilatation-volvulus: 78 cases (2004–2009). *J Am Vet Med Assoc* 2013; **242**: 54–58.

323 Rauserova-Lexmaulova L, Vanova-Uhrikova I, Rehakova K. Acid–Base, electrolyte and lactate abnormalities as well as gastric necrosis and survival in dogs with gastric dilation-volvulus syndrome. A retrospective study in 75 dogs. *Top Companion Anim Med* 2020; **39**: 100403.

324 Millis DL, Hauptman JG, Fulton RB Jr. Abnormal hemostatic profiles and gastric necrosis in canine gastric dilatation-volvulus. *Vet Surg* 1993; **22**: 93–97.

325 Zacher LA, Berg J, Shaw SP, *et al.* Association between outcome and changes in plasma lactate concentration during presurgical treatment in dogs with gastric dilatation-volvulus: 64 cases (2002–2008). *J Am Vet Med Assoc* 2010; **236**: 892–897.

326 Butler AL. Goal-directed therapy in small animal critical illness. *Vet Clin North Am Small Anim Pract* 2011; **41**: 817–838.

327 Rivers EP, Katranji M, Jaehne KA, *et al.* Early interventions in severe sepsis and septic shock: a review of the evidence one decade later. *Minerva Anestesiol* 2012; **78**: 712–724.

328 Mazzaferro E, Powell LL. Fluid therapy for the emergent small animal patient: crystalloids, colloids, and albumin products. *Vet Clin North Am Small Anim Pract* 2022; **52**: 781–796.

329 Levinson AT, Casserly BP, Levy MM. Reducing mortality in severe sepsis and septic shock. *Semin Resp Crit Care Med* 2011; **32**: 195–205.

330 Balakrishnan A, Silverstein DC. Shock fluids and fluid challenge. In: Silverstein DC, Hopper K, eds. *Small Animal Critical Care Medicine*, 3rd edn. St. Louis, MO: Elsevier, 2023: 402–408.

331 Allen DA, Schertel ER, Muir WW III, *et al.* Hypertonic saline/dextran resuscitation of dogs with experimentally induced gastric dilatation-volvulus shock. *Am J Vet Res* 1991; **52**: 92–96.

332 Schertel ER, Allen DA, Muir WW, *et al.* Evaluation of a hypertonic saline-dextran solution for treatment of dogs with shock induced by gastric dilatation-volvulus. *J Am Vet Med Assoc* 1997; **210**: 226–230.

333 Muir WW, Lipowitz AJ. Cardiac dysrhythmias associated with gastric dilatation-volvulus in the dog. *J Am Anim Hosp Assoc* 1978; **172**: 683–689.

334 Cole S, Drobatz K. Emergency management and critical care. In: Tilley LP, Smith FWK Jr., Oyama MA, Sleeper MM, eds. *Manual of Canine and Feline Cardiology*, 4th edn. St. Louis, MO: Saunders Elsevier, 2008: 352.

335 Valverde A, Doherty TJ, Hernández J, *et al.* Effect of lidocaine on the minimum alveolar concentration of isoflurane in dogs. *Vet Anaesth Analg* 2004; **31**: 264–271.

336 Cook VL, Jones Shults J, McDowell MR, *et al.* Anti-inflammatory effects of intravenously administered lidocaine hydrochloride on ischemia-injured jejunum in horses. *Am J Vet Res* 2009; **70**: 1259–1268.

337 Lahav M, Levite M, Bassani L, *et al.* Lidocaine inhibits secretion of IL-8 and IL-1β and stimulates secretion of IL-1 receptor antagonist by epithelial cells. *Clin Exp Immunol* 2002; **127**: 226–233.

338 Yardeni IZ, Beilin B, Mayburd E, *et al.* The effect of perioperative intravenous lidocaine on postoperative pain and immune function. *Anesth Analg* 2009; **109**: 24–29.

339 Torfs S, Delesalle C, Dewulf J, *et al.* Risk factors for equine postoperative ileus and effectiveness of prophylactic lidocaine. *J Vet Intern Med* 2009; **23**: 606–611.

340 Durket E, Gillen A, Kittwitz J. Meta-analysis of the effects of lidocaine on postoperative reflux in the horse. *Vet Surg* 2020; **49**: 44–52.

341 Kilgannon JH, Jones AE, Shapiro NI, *et al.* Association between arterial hyperoxia following resuscitation from cardiac arrest and in-hospital mortality. *J Am Med Assoc* 2010; **303**: 2165–2171.

342 Badylak SF, Lantz GC, Jeffries M. Prevention of reperfusion injury in surgically induced gastric dilatation-volvulus in dogs. *Am J Vet Res* 1990; **51**: 294–299.

343 Lu C, Wang C, Xiao H, *et al.* Ethyl pyruvate: a newly discovered compound against ischemia-reperfusion injury in multiple organs. *Pharm Res* 2021; **171**: 105757.

344 Pratschke K. Approach to haemoabdomen in small animal patients. *In Pract* 2020; **42**: 5–19.

345 Hall K, Drobatz K. Volume resuscitation in the acutely hemorrhaging patient: historic use to current applications. *Front Vet Sci* 2021; **8**: 638104.

346 Boyd C, Smart L. Hemorrhagic shock In: Silverstein DC, Hopper K, eds. *Small Animal Critical Care Medicine*, 3rd edn. St. Louis, MO: Elsevier, 2023: 422–427.

347 Vinayak A, Krahwinkel DJ. Managing blunt trauma-induced hemoperitoneum in dogs and cats. *Compend Contin Educ Vet* 2004; **26**: 276–291.

348 Herold LV, Devey JJ, Kirby R, *et al.* Clinical evaluation and management of hemoperitoneum dogs. *J Vet Emerg Crit Care* 2008; **18**: 40–53.
349 Hnatusko AL, Gicking JC, Lisciandro GR. Anaphylaxis-related hemoperitoneum in 11 dogs. *J Vet Emerg Crit Care (San Antonio)* 2021; **31**: 80–85.
350 Moore EE, Moore HB, Kornblith LZ, *et al. Trauma-induced coagulopathy. Nat Rev Dis Primers* 2021; **7**: 30.
351 Herrero Y, Schefer RJ, Muri BM, *et al.* Prevalence of acute traumatic coagulopathy in acutely traumatized dogs and association with clinical and laboratory parameters at presentation. *Vet Comp Orthop Traumatol* 2021; **34**: 214–222.
352 Gottlieb DL, Prittie J, Buriko Y, *et al.* Evaluation of acute traumatic coagulopathy in dogs and cats following blunt force trauma. *J Vet Emerg Crit Care (San Antonio)* 2017; **27**: 35–43.
353 Lux CN, Culp WTN, Mayhew PD, *et al.* Perioperative outcome in dogs with hemoperitoneum: 83 cases (2005–2010). *J Am Vet Med Assoc* 2013; **242**: 1385–1391.
354 Culp WT, Weisse C, Kellogg ME, *et al.* Spontaneous hemoperitoneum in cats: 65 cases (1994–2006). *J Am Vet Med Assoc* 2010; **236**: 978–982.
355 Mutter TC, Ruth CA, Dart AB. Hydroxyethyl starch (HES) versus other fluid therapies: effects on kidney function. *Cochrane Database Syst Rev* 2013; **7**: CD007594.
356 Haase N, Perner A, Hennings LI, *et al.* Hydroxyethyl starch 130/0.38–0.45 versus crystalloid or albumin in patients with sepsis: systematic review with meta-analysis and trial sequential analysis. *BMJ* 2013; **346**: f839.
357 Boyd CJ, Sharp CR, Claus MA. Prospective randomized controlled blinded clinical trial evaluating biomarkers of acute kidney injury following 6% hydroxyethyl starch 130/0.4 or Hartmann's solution in dogs. *J Vet Emerg Crit Care (San Antonio)* 2021; **31**: 306–314.
358 Avgerinos DV, Theoharides TC. Mesenteric traction syndrome or gut in distress. *Int J Immunopathol Pharmacol* 2005; **18**: 195–199.
359 Olsen AO, Bazancir LA, Dahl S, *et al.* Mesenteric traction syndrome-incidence, impact, and treatment: a systematic scoping review of the literature. *Anaesth Crit Care Pain Med* 2023; **42**: 101162.
360 Cândido TD, Teixeira-Neto FJ, Diniz MS, *et al.* Effects of a dexmedetomidine constant rate infusion and atropine on changes in global perfusion variables induced by hemorrhage followed by volume replacement in isoflurane-anesthetized dogs. *Am J Vet Res* 2014; **75**: 964–973.
361 Diniz MS, Teixeira-Neto FJ, Cândido TD, *et al.* Effects of dexmedetomidine on pulse pressure variation changes induced by hemorrhage followed by volume replacement in isoflurane-anesthetized dogs. *J Vet Emerg Crit Care (San Antonio)* 2014; **24**: 681–692.
362 Selmic LE, Selting KA, Reagan JK. Cancer of the gastrointestinal tract. In: Vail DM, Thamm DH, Liptak JM, eds. *Withrow and McEwen's Small Animal Clinical Oncology*, 6th edn. St. Louis, MO: Saunders Elsevier, 2020: 452–468.
363 Willard MD. Alimentary neoplasia in geriatric dogs and cats. *Vet Clin North Am Small Anim Pract* 2012; **42**: 693–706.
364 Matsuyama A. Gastrointestinal Neoplasia in Dogs and Cats, Merck Veterinary Manual. https://www.merckvetmanual.com/digestive-system/diseases-of-the-stomach-and-intestines-in-small-animals/gastrointestinal-neoplasia-in-dogs-and-cats (accessed February 2023).
365 Minami T. Stomach neoplasia. In: Washabau RJ, Day MJ, eds. *Canine and Feline Gastroenterology*. St. Louis, MO: Saunders Elsevier, 2013: 634–637.
366 Bergman PJ. Small intestine neoplasia. In: Washabau RJ, Day MJ, eds. *Canine and Feline Gastroenterology*. St. Louis, MO: Saunders Elsevier, 2013: 710–714.
367 Washabau RJ, Hall JA. Large intestine. In: Washabau RJ, Day MJ, eds. *Canine and Feline Gastroenterology*. St. Louis, MO: Saunders Elsevier, 2013: 764–767.
368 Sahora A, Khanna C. Cellular growth/neoplasia. In: Washabau RJ, Day MJ, eds. *Canine and Feline Gastroenterology*. St. Louis, MO: Saunders Elsevier, 2013: 61–69.
369 Willard MD. Esophagus: neoplasia. In: Washabau RJ, Day MJ, eds. *Canine and Feline Gastroenterology*. St. Louis, MO: Saunders Elsevier, 2013: 595–598.
370 Tappin S, Brown P, Ferasin L. An intestinal neuroendocrine tumour associated with paroxysmal ventricular tachycardia and melena in a 10-year-old Boxer. *J Small Anim Pract* 2008; **49**: 33–37.
371 Tripathi NK, Gregory CR, Latimer KS. Urinary system. In: Latimer KS, ed. *Duncan and Prasse's Veterinary Laboratory Medicine: Clinical Pathology*, 5th edn. Ames, IA: Wiley-Blackwell, 2011: 275.
372 Bailey DB. Paraneoplastic syndromes. In: Vail DM, Thamm DH, Liptak JM, eds. *Withrow and McEwen's Small Animal Clinical Oncology*, 6th edn. St. Louis, MO: Saunders Elsevier, 2020: 98–112.
373 Elliott J. Paraneoplastic syndromes in dogs and cats. *In Pract* 2014; **36**: 443–452.
374 Trow AV, Rozanski EA, Delaforcade AM, *et al.* Evaluation of use of human albumin in critically ill dogs: 73 cases (2003–2006). *J Am Vet Assoc* 2008; **233**: 607–612.
375 Mathews KA, Barry M. The use of 25% human serum albumin: outcome and efficacy in raising serum albumin and systemic blood pressure in critically ill dogs and cats. *J Vet Emerg Crit Care* 2005; **15**: 110–118.
376 Mathews KA. The therapeutic use of 25% human serum albumin in critically ill dogs and cats. *Vet Clin North Am Small Anim Pract* 2008; **38**: 595–605.
377 Francis AH, Martin LG, Haldorson GJ, *et al.* Adverse reactions suggestive of type III hypersensitivity in six healthy dogs given human albumin. *J Am Vet Med Assoc* 2007; **230**: 873–879.
378 Powell C, Thompson L, Murtaugh RJ. Type III hypersensitivity reaction with immune complex deposition in 2 critically ill dogs administered human serum albumin. *J Vet Emerg Crit Care* 2013; **23**: 598–604.
379 Sahagian MJ, Mastrocco A, Weltman JG, *et al.* Retrospective analysis of the use of canine-specific albumin in 125 critically ill dogs. *J Vet Emerg Crit Care (San Antonio)* 2023; **33**: 192–200.
380 Trepanier LA. Pharmacologic management of feline hyperthyroidism. *Vet Clin North Am Small Anim Pract* 2007; **37**: 775–788.
381 Collgros NC, Bray JP. Blood glucose monitoring during surgery in dogs to assess completeness of surgical resection of insulinoma: 11 cases. *J Am Vet Med Assoc* 2022; **261**: 229–236.
382 Bentley AM, Otto CM, Shofer FS. Comparison of dogs with septic peritonitis: 1988–1993 versus 1999–2003. *J Vet Emerg Crit Care* 2007; **17**: 391–398.
383 Grimes JA, Schmiedt CW, Cornell KK, *et al.* Identification of risk factors for septic peritonitis and failure to survive following gastrointestinal surgery in dogs. *J Am Vet Med Assoc* 2011; **238**: 486–494.
384 Gill S, Buote NJ, Peterson NW, *et al.* Factors associated with dehiscence and mortality rates following gastrointestinal surgery in dogs. *J Am Vet Med Assoc* 2019; **255**: 569–573.
385 Brady CA, Otto CM, Van Winkle TJ, *et al.* Severe sepsis in cats: 29 cases (1986–1998). *J Am Vet Med Assoc* 2000; **217**: 531–535.
386 Costello MF, Drobatz KJ, Aronson LR, *et al.* Underlying cause, pathophysiologic abnormalities, and response to treatment in cats with septic peritonitis: 51 cases (1990–2001). *J Am Vet Med Assoc* 2004; **225**: 897–902.
387 Ruthrauff CM, Smith J, Glerum L. Primary bacterial septic peritonitis in cats: 13 cases. *J Am Anim Hosp Assoc* 2009; **45**: 268–276.
388 Scotti KM, Koenigshof A, Sri-Jayantha LSH, *et al.* Prognostic indicators in cats with septic peritonitis (2002–2015): 83 cases. *J Vet Emerg Crit Care (San Antonio)* 2019; **29**: 647–652.
389 Anderson T, Beever L, Hall J, *et al.* Outcome following surgery to treat septic peritonitis in 95 cats in the United Kingdom. *J Small Anim Pract* 2021; **62**: 744–749.
390 Culp WT, Holt DE. Septic peritonitis. *Compend Contin Educ Vet* 2010; **32**: E1–E14.
391 Ragetly GR, Bennett RA, Ragetly CA. Septic peritonitis: etiology, pathophysiology, and diagnosis. *Compend Contin Educ Vet* 2011; **33**: E1–E6.
392 Culp WT, Zeldis TE, Reese MS, *et al.* Primary bacterial peritonitis in dogs and cats: 24 cases (1990–2006). *J Am Vet Med Assoc* 2009; **234**: 906–913.
393 Tart K. Peritonitis. In: Silverstein DC, Hopper K, eds. *Small Animal Critical Care Medicine*, 3rd edn. St. Louis, MO: Elsevier, 2023: 701–704.
394 Anderson, KL, Feeney DA. Diagnostic imaging of the gastrointestinal tract. In: Washabau RJ, Day MJ, eds. *Canine and Feline Gastroenterology*. St. Louis, MO: Saunders Elsevier, 2013: 205–244.
395 Levin GM, Bonczynski JJ, Ludwig LL, *et al.* Lactate as a diagnostic test for septic peritoneal effusions in dogs and cats. *J Am Anim Hosp Assoc* 2004; **40**: 364–371.
396 Kenney EM, Rozanski EA, Rush JE, *et al.* Association between outcome and organ system dysfunction in dogs with sepsis: 114 cases (2003–2007). *J Am Vet Med Assoc* 2010; **236**: 83–87.
397 Bone RC, Sibbald WJ, Sprung CL. The ACCP-SCCM Consensus Conference on sepsis and organ failure. *Chest* 1992; **101**: 1480–1483.
398 Gyawali B, Ramakrishna K, Dhamoon AS. Sepsis: the evolution in definition, pathophysiology, and management. *SAGE Open Med* 2019; **7**: 1–13.
399 Nunnally ME. Sepsis for the anesthetist. *Br J of Anaesth* 2016; **117**: iii44–iii51.
400 Lambden S, Creagh-Brown BC, Hunt J, *et al.* Definitions and pathophysiology of vasoplegic shock. *Critical Care* 2018; **2**: 174.
401 Singer M, Deutschman CS, Seymour CW. The third international consensus definitions for sepsis and septic shock (Sepsis-3). *JAMA* 2016; **315**: 801–810.
402 Boller EM, Silverstein DC. Sepsis and septic shock. In: Silverstein DC, Hopper K, eds. *Small Animal Critical Care Medicine*, 3rd edn. St. Louis, MO: Elsevier, 2023: 519–526.
403 Rank K, Hansen B. SIRS, MODS, and sepsis. In: Silverstein DC, Hopper K, eds. *Small Animal Critical Care Medicine*, 3rd edn. St. Louis, MO: Elsevier, 2023: 42–48.
404 Purvis D, Kirby R. Systemic inflammatory response syndrome: septic shock. *Vet Clin North Am Small Anim Pract* 1994; **24**: 1225–1247.
405 Hardie EM. Life threatening bacterial infection. *Compen Cont Educ Pract Vet* 1995; **17**: 763–778.
406 Hotchkiss RS, Monneret G, Payen D. Sepsis-induced immunosuppression: from cellular dysfunctions to immunotherapy. *Nat Rev Immunol* 2013; **13**: 862–874.
407 Montealegre-Golcher F. Surviving Sepsis in Veterinary Medicine. https://www.isvma.org/wp-content/uploads/2018/10/SurvivingsepsisinVeterinary-Medicine.pdf (accessed March 2023).

408 Deitch EA. Gut-origin sepsis: evolution of a concept. *Surgeon* 2012; **10**: 350–356.

409 Assimakopoulos SF, Triantos C, Thomopoulos K, *et al.* Gut-origin sepsis in the critically ill patient: pathophysiology and treatment. *Infection* 2018; **46**: 751–760.

410 Adelman MW, Woodworth MH, Langelier C, *et al.* The gut microbiome's role in the development, maintenance, and outcomes of sepsis. *Critical Care* 2020; **24**: 278.

411 Walters AM, O'Brien MA, Selmic LE. Comparison of clinical findings between dogs with suspected anaphylaxis and dogs with confirmed sepsis. *J Am Vet Med Assoc* 2017; **251**: 681–688.

412 Lambden S, Laterre PF, Levy MM, *et al.* The SOFA score-development, utility and challenges of accurate assessment in clinical trials. *Critical Care* 2019; **23**: 374.

413 Troia R, Mascalzoni G, Calipa S, *et al.* Multiorgan dysfunction syndrome in feline sepsis: prevalence and prognostic implication. *J Feline Med Surg* 2019; **21**: 559–565.

414 Hayes G, Mathews K, Doig G, *et al.* The Acute Patient Physiologic and Laboratory Evaluation (APPLE) score: a severity of illness stratification system for hospitalized dogs. *J Vet Intern Med* 2010; **24**: 1034–1047.

415 Hayes G, Mathews K, Doig G, *et al.* The Feline Acute Patient Physiologic and Laboratory Evaluation (Feline APPLE) Score: a severity of illness stratification system for hospitalized cats. *J Vet Intern Med* 2011; **25**: 26–38.

416 Summers AM, Vezzi N, Gravelyn T, *et al.* Clinical features and outcome of septic shock in dogs: 37 Cases (2008–2015). *J Vet Emerg Crit Care (San Antonio)* 2021; **31**: 360–370.

417 Osgood AM, Hollenbeck D, Yankin I. Evaluation of quick sequential organ failure scores in dogs with severe sepsis and septic shock. *J Small Anim Pract* 2022; **63**: 739–746.

418 Ortolani JM, Bellis TJ. Evaluation of the quick Sequential Organ Failure Assessment score plus lactate in critically ill dogs. *J Small Anim Pract* 2021; **62**: 874–880.

419 Babyak JM, Sharp CR. Epidemiology of systemic inflammatory response syndrome and sepsis in cats hospitalized in a veterinary teaching hospital. *J Am Vet Med Assoc* 2016; **249**: 65–71.

420 Evans L, Rhodes A, Alhazzani W, *et al.* Surviving sepsis campaign: international guidelines for management of sepsis and septic shock. *Intensive Care Med* 2021; **47**: 1181–1247.

421 Surviving Sepsis Campaign Website. www.sccm.org/SurvivingSepsisCampaign/Home (accessed April 2023).

422 Dellinger RP, Rhodes A, Evans L, *et al.* Surviving Sepsis Campaign. *Crit Care Med* 2023; **51**: 431–444.

423 Conti-Patara A, de Araújo Caldeira J, de Mattos-Junior E, *et al.* Changes in tissue perfusion parameters in dogs with severe sepsis/septic shock in response to goal-directed hemodynamic optimization at admission to ICU and the relation to outcome. *J Vet Emerg Crit Care* 2012; **22**: 409–418.

424 Kuttab HI, Lykins JD, Hughes MD, *et al.* Evaluation and predictors of fluid resuscitation in patients with severe sepsis and septic shock. *Crit Care Med* 2019; **47**: 1582–1590.

425 Shapiro NI, Douglas IS, Brower RG, *et al.* Early restrictive or liberal fluid management for sepsis-induced hypotension. *N Engl J Med* 2023; **388**: 499–510.

426 Messina A, Robba C, Calabrò L, *et al.* Perioperative liberal versus restrictive fluid strategies and postoperative outcomes: a systematic review and metanalysis on randomised-controlled trials in major abdominal elective surgery. *Crit Care* 2021; **25**: 205.

427 Stephens R, Mythen M. Resuscitation fluids and hyperchloraemic metabolic acidosis. *Trauma* 2003; **5**: 141–143.

428 Sigrist NE, Kälin N, Dreyfus A. Effects of hydroxyethyl starch 130/0.4 on serum creatinine concentration and development of acute kidney injury in nonazotemic cats. *J Vet Intern Med* 2017; **31**: 1749–1756.

429 Smart L, Hughes D. The effects of resuscitative fluid therapy on the endothelial surface layer. *Front Vet Sci* 2021; **8**: 661660.

430 Milford EM, Reade MC. Resuscitation fluid choices to preserve the endothelial glycocalyx. *Crit Care* 2019; **23**: 77.

431 Woodcock TE, Michel CC. Advances in the starling principle and microvascular fluid exchange; consequences and implications for fluid therapy. *Front Vet Sci* 2021; **8**: 623671.

432 Adamik K-N, Yozova ID. Colloids Yes or No? - a "Gretchen Question" Answered. *Front Vet Sci* 2021; **8**: 624049.

433 Centola SJ. Colloid solutions. In: Silverstein DC, Hopper K, eds. *Small Animal Critical Care Medicine*, 3rd edn. St. Louis, MO: Elsevier, 2023: 391–395.

434 Macdonald S, Bosio E, Shapiro NI, *et al.* No association between intravenous fluid volume and endothelial glycocalyx shedding in patients undergoing resuscitation for sepsis in the emergency department. *Sci Rep* 2022; **12**: 8733.

435 Hippensteel JA, Uchimido R, Tyler PD, *et al.* Intravenous fluid resuscitation is associated with septic endothelial glycocalyx degradation. *Crit Care* 2019; **23**: 259.

436 Martin LG. Critical illness-related corticosteroid insufficiency in small animals. *Vet Clin North Am Small Anim Pract* 2011; **41**: 767–782.

437 Peyton JL, Burkitt JM. Critical illness-related corticosteroid insufficiency in a dog with septic shock. *J Vet Emerg Crit Care* 2009; **19**: 262–268.

438 Marchetti M, Pierini A, Favilla G, *et al.* Critical illness-related corticosteroid insufficiency in dogs with systemic inflammatory response syndrome: a pilot study in 21 dogs. *Vet J* 2021; **273**: 105677.

439 Annane D, Bellissant E, Bollaert PE, *et al.* Corticosteroids for treating sepsis in children and adults. *Cochrane Database Syst Rev* 2019; **12**: CD002243.

440 Summers AM, Culler C, Yaxley PE, *et al.* Retrospective evaluation of the use of hydrocortisone for treatment of suspected critical illness-related corticosteroid insufficiency (CIRCI) in dogs with septic shock (2010–2017): 47 cases. *J Vet Emerg Crit Care (San Antonio)* 2021; **31**: 371–379.

441 Chen L, Liang X, Tan X, *et al.* Safety and efficacy of combined use of propofol and etomidate for sedation during gastroscopy: systematic review and meta-analysis. *Med (Baltimore)* 2019; **98**: e15712.

442 Hopper K. Mechanical ventilation-core concepts. In: Silverstein DC, Hopper K, eds. *Small Animal Critical Care Medicine*, 3rd edn. St. Louis, MO: Elsevier, 2023: 185–192.

443 Kan T, Hess RS, Clarke DL. Clinical findings and patient outcomes following surgical treatment of chronic gastrointestinal FB obstructions in dogs and cats: 72 cases (2010–2020). *Can J Vet Res* 2022; **86**: 311–315.

444 Hobday MM, Pachtinger GE, Drobatz KJ, *et al.* Linear versus non-linear gastrointestinal foreign bodies in 499 dogs: clinical presentation, management and short-term outcome. *J Small Anim Pract* 2014; **55**: 560–565.

445 Hayes G. Gastrointestinal foreign bodies in dogs and cats: a retrospective study of 208 cases. *J Small Anim Pract* 2009; **50**: 576–583.

446 Larose PC, Singh A, Giuffrida MA, *et al.* Clinical findings and outcomes of 153 dogs surgically treated for intestinal intussusceptions. *Vet Surg* 2020; **49**: 870–878.

447 Burkitt JM, Drobatz KJ, Saunders HM, *et al.* Signalment, history, and outcome of cats with gastrointestinal tract intussusception: 20 cases (1986–2000). *J Am Vet Med Assoc* 2009; **234**: 771–776.

42 Physiology, Pathophysiology, and Anesthetic Management of Patients with Endocrine Disease

Renata S. Costa[1], Teela Jones[2] and Thomas K. Graves[3]

[1] Section of Anaesthesia and Analgesia, School of Veterinary Medicine, Murdoch University, Murdoch, Western Australia, Australia
[2] Summit Veterinary Referral Center, Tacoma, Washington, USA
[3] Professor and Dean Emeritus, College of Veterinary Medicine, Midwestern University, Glendale, Arizona, USA

Chapter contents

Introduction, 891
Anatomy and physiology, 891
Adrenal gland, 893
Hypoadrenocorticism, 893
Hyperadrenocorticism, 895
Pheochromocytoma, 898
Pancreas and kidney, 900
Diabetes mellitus, 901
Diabetes insipidus, 904
Insulinoma, 906
Pancreatitis, 908
Thyroid gland, 908
Hypothyroidism, 908
Hyperthyroidism, 909
Thyroid neoplasia, 912
Parathyroid gland, 913
Hyperparathyroidism, 914
References, 915

Introduction

The endocrine system plays an important role in homeostasis through secretion of hormones that function in metabolism, growth, reproduction, and digestion. In patients with endocrine disorders, an understanding of the physiology and pathophysiology of the disease process is imperative to provide adequate perianesthetic management.

The endocrine system regulates the secretion of hormones from several peripheral organs under the direction of the hypothalamus together with the hypophysis (pituitary gland) (Fig. 42.1). Hormones are substances secreted into the circulation in small amounts to produce a biologic effect at distant target organs or cells. Hormones may be proteins (corticotropin, growth hormone, and insulin), peptides (oxytocin and vasopressin), steroids (glucocorticoids, mineralocorticoids, and sex hormones), or amines (dopamine, melatonin, and epinephrine). Other hypothalamic hormones include oxytocin, and prolactin-releasing hormone, while other pituitary hormones include gonadotropin (GH), somatostatin, prolactin, luteinizing hormone, and follicle-stimulating hormone.

Anatomy and physiology

The hypothalamus is a small area located in the ventral aspect of the diencephalon flanking each side of the third ventricle, almost directly above the caudal pharynx. In addition to endocrine control of metabolism, growth, and reproduction, the hypothalamus helps to coordinate other vital aspects of mammalian physiology including the autonomic nervous system, behavior, emotion, and digestion [1]. A physiologic stress response may be activated during sedation, anesthesia, or following noxious stimuli ultimately activating the hypothalamic–pituitary–adrenal axis [2]. Activation of this axis leads to release of cortisol and catecholamines from the adrenal gland resulting in increases in heart rate, blood pressure, and systemic vascular resistance. Increases in metabolic rate, oxygen consumption, and hyperglycemia, as well as release of cytokines, vasopressin, and insulin also occur [2].

The pituitary gland is located just below the hypothalamus. It has two main lobes, distinct in both anatomic composition and function: the adenohypophysis or anterior pituitary (AP) and the neurohypophysis or posterior pituitary (PP).

The AP functions like a true endocrine gland, producing and secreting peptide and glycoprotein hormones that target the pancreas, thyroid gland, adrenal glands, reproductive organs, and the intestine. These hormones regulate various cellular processes including growth, metabolism, reproduction, and response to stress. The AP has three distinct areas – the pars tuberalis, the pars intermedia, and the pars distalis. Hypothalamic-releasing hormones, such as thyrotropin-releasing hormone and corticotropin-releasing hormone, regulate AP hormonal secretion. Once the hypothalamic hormones reach their target cells in the AP, they may stimulate or inhibit the synthesis and secretion of AP hormones (e.g., thyroid-stimulating hormone [TSH]).

The PP is primarily a conduit between the hypothalamus and the peripheral circulation. It is composed of the pars nervosa and

Veterinary Anesthesia and Analgesia: The Sixth Edition of Lumb and Jones. Edited by Leigh Lamont, Kurt Grimm, Sheilah Robertson, Lydia Love and Carrie Schroeder.
© 2024 John Wiley & Sons, Inc. Published 2024 by John Wiley & Sons, Inc.
Companion website: www.wiley.com/go/lamont/anesthesia

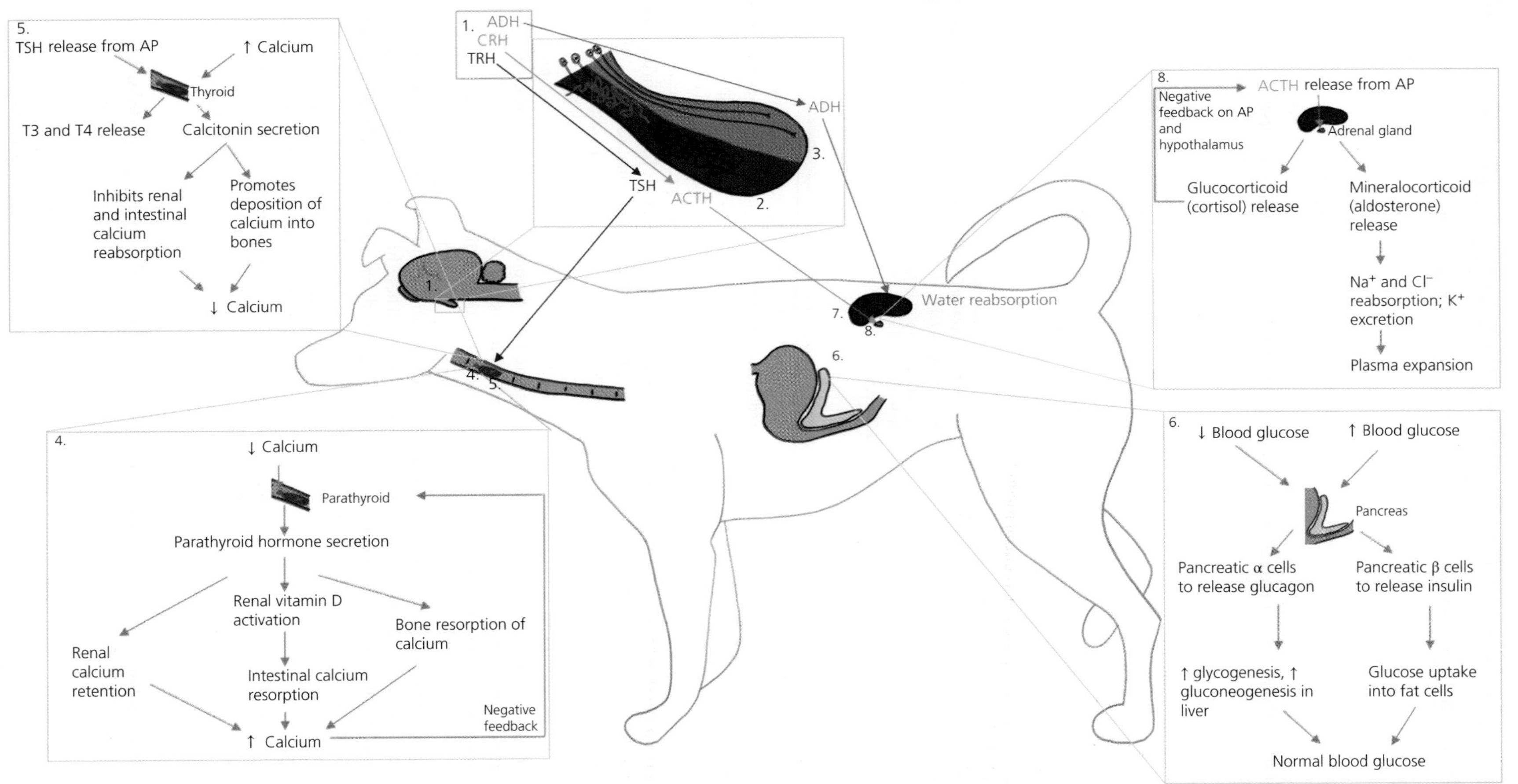

Figure 42.1 Summary of important hormones in the hypothalamic–pituitary axis, target tissues, and physiologic responses [1–3]. 1. Hypothalamus; 2. Anterior pituitary gland (AP); 3. Posterior pituitary gland; 4. Parathyroid gland; 5. Thyroid gland; 6. Pancreas; 7. Kidney; 8. Adrenal gland. TRH, thyrotropin-releasing hormone; CRH, corticotropin-releasing hormone; ADH, antidiuretic hormone; TSH, thyroid-stimulating hormone (thyrotropin); ACTH, adrenocorticotropic hormone (corticotropin); PTH, parathyroid hormone. Source: Dr. Teela Jones; with permission.

infundibular stalk. Axons in the supraoptic and paraventricular nuclei of the hypothalamus extend into the pars nervosa. Hormones that are produced by the hypothalamus, such as oxytocin and vasopressin, are secreted into the peripheral circulation by these specialized neurosecretory cells [1]. In contrast to the AP that produces hormones that stimulate the production of other hormones, the PP secretes hormones that directly affect target tissues [1]. For example, vasopressin or antidiuretic hormone (ADH) acts on the kidneys to control water reabsorption.

Relevant anatomy, physiology, and pathophysiology of common endocrine disorders affecting the adrenal gland, pancreas, kidney, thyroid gland, and parathyroid glands are described below. Specific anesthetic considerations and appropriate perianesthetic management of small animals presenting with endocrinopathies are also discussed.

Adrenal gland

The two adrenal glands are located retroperitoneally; each gland is craniomedial to the kidney. They are composed of a central medulla and outer cortex. The medulla is densely innervated with preganglionic sympathetic fibers and is considered part of the autonomic nervous system. Its main cell type, the chromaffin cell, produces epinephrine and norepinephrine, which are important in emergent and stressful circumstances [3]. The adrenal cortex is an important endocrine organ with three distinct zones (zona glomerulosa, zona fasciculata, and zona reticularis). The zona glomerulosa is the most superficial, and it secretes mineralocorticoids, mainly aldosterone. Deep to this area is the zona fasciculata, which secretes glucocorticoid hormones, primarily cortisol in the dog and cat. The deepest zone of the adrenal cortex is the zona reticularis, which secretes sex hormones (Fig. 42.2) [3].

Aldosterone, secreted by the zona glomerulosa, stimulates sodium and chloride reabsorption and potassium excretion in the cortical collecting ducts of the renal tubules. Because water follows sodium, it is also reabsorbed, which promotes plasma volume expansion [4]. Cortisol, secreted by the zona fasciculata, affects endothelial integrity, vascular permeability, and sensitivity to catecholamines, ultimately regulating vascular tone and blood pressure. Cortisol is also involved in the modulation of inflammation by stabilizing lysosomal membranes, decreasing leukocyte migration, reducing capillary permeability, and altering circulating leukocyte levels and antibody production.

Hypoadrenocorticism

Diminished function of the adrenal cortex resulting in glucocorticoid and/or mineralocorticoid deficiency produces hypoadrenocorticism or Addison's disease. Dogs with Addison's disease are usually presented for complications associated with deficiency of both aldosterone and cortisol. However, a form of the disease characterized by signs of cortisol deficiency only ("atypical" hypoadrenocorticism) has been recognized [5].

Primary hypoadrenocorticism due to failure of the adrenal gland is the most common form of the disease and most likely occurs due to immune-mediated destruction of the adrenal cortex [6,7]. Causes of secondary hypoadrenocorticism include lack of production of adrenocorticotropic hormone (ACTH) by the pituitary gland, iatrogenic disease following treatment for hyperadrenocorticism, or when high-dose steroid therapy is abruptly withdrawn. Tertiary hypoadrenocorticism caused by hypothalamic malfunction also exists.

Hypoadrenocorticism occurs most often in young- to middle-aged female dogs (median age 4 years). Most commonly affected purebred dogs include Standard Poodles, West Highland White Terriers, Great Danes, Rottweilers, and Portuguese Water Dogs. There are no known breed predilections in cats, but most are also middle-aged at the time of diagnosis [8].

Clinical presentation

Clinical signs of hypoadrenocorticism are usually non-specific and may include anorexia, lethargy, vomiting, diarrhea, weight loss, and polyuria/polydipsia (PU/PD). Whenever a patient, especially a middle-aged female dog, is presented with vague gastrointestinal clinical signs and/or lethargy, Addison's disease should be suspected. Signs of the disease range from mild to severe, and those patients presenting in an acute Addisonian crisis are at risk of death.

Glucocorticoid deficiency is responsible for many of the vague, chronic, waxing and waning clinical signs. Mineralocorticoid (e.g., aldosterone) deficiency leads to potassium retention and urinary sodium and water loss. Hyperkalemia due to potassium retention can lead to myocardial excitability, muscle weakness, inability to

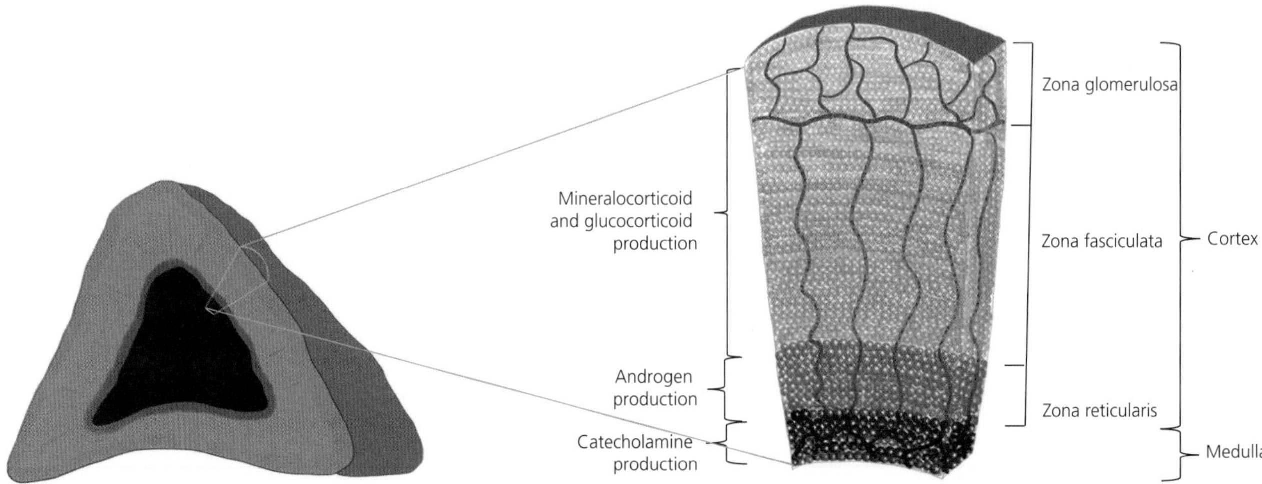

Figure 42.2 Diagrammatic cross-section of the adrenal gland [3]. Source: Dr. Teela Jones; with permission.

retain bicarbonate and chloride, and loss of renal concentrating ability. Impaired sodium retention can result in decreased extracellular fluid and plasma volume, low cardiac output, and impaired renal blood flow. When severe, these changes result in dehydration, azotemia, hypotension, bradycardia, collapse, and hypovolemic shock.

Clinical pathology

Anemia, lymphocytosis, or eosinophilia may be present on a complete blood count (CBC). The lack of a stress leukogram in an ill patient should also lead the clinician to suspect glucocorticoid deficiency and possibly hypoadrenocorticism [9].

Serum biochemistry findings can include hyperkalemia and hyponatremia (Na^+:K^+ < 27:1), hypoalbuminemia, mild hypercalcemia, and, in dehydrated patients, prerenal azotemia due to decreased blood flow to the kidneys [9]. Even though the azotemia is prerenal in origin, a low urine specific gravity (i.e., < 1.030 in the dog and < 1.040 in the cat) may be evident owing to the inability to retain sodium [10,11]. Mild to moderate hypoglycemia may also be apparent in some animals. This is mainly due to decreased levels of glucocorticoid resulting in a reduction of gluconeogenesis and an increased sensitivity to insulin.

Diagnosis and treatment

Definitive diagnosis of hypoadrenocorticism requires measurement of serum concentrations of cortisol before and after stimulation with ACTH [12]; however, the CBC and serum biochemistry findings listed above are helpful when a diagnosis of hypoadrenocorticism is suspected. Once the diagnosis is made, treatment carries a good prognosis [6,7,13].

Dogs and cats in non-critical condition are treated with mineralocorticoid and glucocorticoid supplementation. Mineralocorticoid treatment can be with injectable desoxycorticosterone pivalate (DOCP) or oral fludrocortisone. Fludrocortisone has mild glucocorticoid activity; thus, glucocorticoid supplementation is not always needed. Patients treated with DOCP should also receive low maintenance doses of a glucocorticoid.

Addisonian patients in adrenal crisis require intravenous (IV) fluid therapy and monitoring of electrolytes. Normal saline ([Na^+] 154 mEq/L) is commonly administered for the initial treatment to replace circulatory volume and sodium deficits [10,11]. However, sodium concentrations should be raised gradually, not exceeding 0.5 mEq/kg/h, to avoid neurological signs caused by osmotic demyelination syndrome [14,15]. Note that the most appropriate fluid or fluid combination to administer should be based on each animal's baseline sodium concentration. In cases of severe hyponatremia, a balanced electrolyte solution such as Lactated Ringer's solution (LRS) ([Na^+] 130 mEq/L) may be a more appropriate treatment. Although balanced electrolyte solutions such as LRS contain potassium (4 mEq/L), it appears that fluid resuscitation and the increase in glomerular filtration rate alone will still initiate kaliuresis [11].

Another important aspect of stabilization of an animal in Addisonian crisis is evaluation of the electrocardiogram (ECG) and management of hyperkalemia if necessary. Common treatments for life-threatening hyperkalemia include administration of IV calcium gluconate (as a cardioprotective agent) and dextrose, insulin, and sodium bicarbonate (to lower serum potassium) [16]. Suggested management of hyperkalemia is presented in Table 42.1. Dexamethasone, 0.25 mg/kg IV, can be administered before the completion of the ACTH stimulation test [16]. Hydrocortisone and prednisolone cross-react with some cortisol assays and should be withheld until after ACTH stimulation testing is complete.

Anesthetic considerations and management

Unstable or poorly controlled animals with hypoadrenocorticism may require anesthesia for emergency procedures. These animals must be evaluated for hyperkalemia and hyponatremia, prerenal azotemia, hypovolemia and hypotension, metabolic acidosis, and hypoglycemia [17–19]. These abnormalities should be managed prior to anesthesia. A baseline blood pressure and ECG should also be obtained. Goal-directed volume replacement can be accomplished with IV isotonic crystalloids, and this may be adequate to correct electrolyte abnormalities and stabilize vascular volume and blood pressure. Electrocardiography may show evidence of hyperkalemia including tall, narrow T waves, prolonged QRS complexes, and atrial standstill, usually when serum concentrations exceed 5.5 mEq/L, although this is variable [20]. If hyperkalemia persists, especially if bradycardia and/or arrhythmias are present, specific therapy as described in the previous section is warranted. After initial stabilization, sedation and anesthesia are performed utilizing balanced anesthetic protocols and multimodal analgesia. Premedication with intravenous opioids is commonly

Table 42.1 Suggested management of hyperkalemia.

Treatment	Dose	Mechanism	Comments
Replacement crystalloid fluids	Shock dose (dogs 90 mL/kg; cats 60 mL/kg) in aliquots of ⅓ of total dose based on patient reassessment	Correction of hypovolemia, dilution of K^+, and diuresis	K^+ in balanced crystalloids has not been reported to exacerbate hyperkalemia
Calcium gluconate 10% solution	0.5–1.5 mL/kg IV over 10–20 min	Increases cardiac myocyte threshold potential, restores normal gradient between threshold potential and resting membrane potential, reduces myocardial irritability	Monitor ECG and slow/discontinue if bradycardia or arrhythmias occur Does not lower K^+; antagonizes effect of hyperkalemia on myocardium Rapid onset of action
Regular insulin followed by dextrose	0.2–0.5 U/kg insulin IV followed by 4 mL dextrose (12.5–25%) IV per unit of insulin	Insulin stimulates transport of glucose and K^+ into cells	Rapid onset of action Monitor blood glucose levels
Dextrose	0.5–1 mL/kg IV bolus followed by dextrose (2.5%–5%) IV CRI	May stimulate endogenous insulin secretion	Monitor blood glucose levels
Sodium bicarbonate	1–3 mEq/kg IV over 30 min	Corrects metabolic acidosis; promotes K^+ uptake into cell in exchange for H^+ via Na^+-K^+ ATPase	Reserved for severe metabolic acidosis; controversial as first-line therapy

CRI, constant rate infusion.
Source: Koenig [4]; Lathan and Thompson [16]; Kintzer and Peterson [17]; Stafford and Bartges [18]; Koenig [19].

recommended. Butorphanol is often administered for non-painful procedures, whereas full μ-opioid receptor agonists are preferred for invasive or painful procedures. In these cases, short-acting full μ-opioid receptor agonists may also be administered as a constant rate infusion (CRI) to provide analgesia, dose-dependent sedation, and minimum alveolar concentration (MAC)-sparing effects. Anesthesia may be induced with drugs such as propofol, alfaxalone, ketamine–benzodiazepine, and other combinations such as propofol and midazolam. It is important to note that induction of anesthesia with etomidate is usually avoided in animals with hypoadrenocorticism, especially when critically ill, as cortisol synthesis may be depressed from inhibition of 11β-hydroxylase in dogs and cats [21–26].

Many animals with hypoadrenocorticism will undergo anesthesia for surgical procedures unrelated to the disease and have been previously managed with medical therapy at the time of surgery [2,17]. The choice of anesthetic protocol in these patients is not as critical as the perioperative medical management. However, anesthetic protocol selection should reflect the patient's health status and stability, and procedure being performed. Provision of locoregional anesthesia whenever possible is recommended due to desirable effects such as reliable analgesia, decreased systemic drug requirements, and MAC-sparing effects, which may help maintain normal blood pressure intraoperatively. Even for animals with well-controlled hypoadrenocorticism, it is recommended to assess hydration status, blood pressure, and ECG prior to anesthesia.

The normal mineralocorticoid supplementation regimen of animals with Addison's disease undergoing anesthesia should be continued. Glucocorticoid doses, however, may require adjustment because these animals have inappropriate responses to stressful situations including hospitalization, surgery, and anesthesia. In addition to baseline steroid therapy, several preoperative glucocorticoid supplementation protocols have been recommended for people with hypoadrenocorticism to prevent adrenal crisis and refractory hypotension in the perioperative period [27]. There have been no studies proving the benefits of additional preoperative steroid supplementation in dogs undergoing surgery; however, it has been suggested that prednisone is doubled the day before and 1–2 days following the stressful event [16]. Recommended doses of glucocorticoids include 0.1–0.5 mg/kg of dexamethasone sodium phosphate IV or up to 1–2 mg/kg of prednisolone sodium succinate IV, with lower doses repeated as necessary [4,28]. Postoperatively, additional glucocorticoids are administered as needed.

Due to the negative fluid balance and electrolyte abnormalities, hypotension is a common intraoperative complication of animals with hypoadrenocorticism. Addisonian patients may not respond adequately to basic interventions or may present in hypovolemic shock; therefore, advanced monitoring techniques including invasive (direct) blood pressure may be beneficial. If invasive blood pressure is measured, variation in the amplitude of the systolic pressure waveform during positive-pressure ventilation may be seen when hypovolemia is present [29]. A balanced electrolyte solution should be administered intraoperatively at a rate of 5–10 mL/kg/h. This rate should be adjusted or supplemental boluses administered depending on the patient's hydration status [27,30]. Positive inotropes may also be necessary to maintain adequate blood pressure intraoperatively [27,30]. As previously discussed, insufficient glucocorticoid secretion may result in cardiovascular consequences including hypotension. Although there is little evidence in veterinary medicine, hypotension refractory to vasopressor administration has been successfully treated with hydrocortisone in a dog [31].

Hyperadrenocorticism

Excess circulating concentrations of cortisol produces hyperadrenocorticism (HAC) or Cushing's syndrome [32]. In 80–85% of spontaneous or naturally occurring cases, the disease is due to increased secretion of ACTH from a pituitary tumor, usually an adenoma of the corticotropes in the pars distalis of the pituitary, resulting in bilateral adrenocortical hyperplasia and excessive cortisol secretion. This is known as "pituitary-dependent hyperadrenocorticism." Albeit less common, a cortisol-secreting tumor of the adrenal gland can also lead to hyperadrenocorticism. Chronic administration of glucocorticoids may result in iatrogenic Cushing's syndrome [33,34].

Spontaneous HAC generally occurs in middle-aged and older dogs. Although the literature is conflicting, female and neutered dogs appear to be at a higher risk [35]. Any purebred or mixed-breed dog can be affected, but Standard Schnauzers and Fox Terriers appear to be predisposed. Although this chapter focuses on small animal patients, it is important to note that HAC is also a common endocrine disease of older horses and ponies and is referred to as "pituitary pars intermedia dysfunction" (PPID) [36]. There is no sex predilection, and the incidence has been reported as 15–30% in older horses [37].

Clinical presentation

Clinical signs of dogs with hyperadrenocorticism include bilaterally symmetrical alopecia, comedones, recurrent skin infections, thin skin, dermal hyperpigmentation, dermal and muscle atrophy, PU/PD, polyphagia, pendulous abdomen, hepatomegaly, panting, hypertension, and lethargy (Fig. 42.3) [32]. Albeit not common, large pituitary tumors can result in neurological signs.

The clinical signs observed are due to the increased circulating concentrations of cortisol. Cortisol stimulates gluconeogenesis, protein and fat catabolism, leading to redistribution of adipose tissue both dorsally and within the abdomen and the resultant pendulous abdomen. Polyuria occurs because cortisol inhibits ADH release. Systemic hypertension may occur due to increased vascular responsiveness to catecholamines, increased activation of the renin–angiotensin system and increased angiotensin II, and decreased release of vasodilatory prostaglandins and hyperaldosteronism [38,39].

Clinical pathology

Findings on CBC are non-specific, however, dogs with HAC often exhibit changes consistent with a stress leukogram (neutrophilia, monocytosis, lymphopenia, and eosinopenia) [32].

Serum biochemistry findings include increased alkaline phosphatase (ALP) activity in 90% or more of cases, increased alanine aminotransferase (ALT) activity, hypercholesterolemia, and hyperglycemia [32,40]. ALP activity increases as a result of a steroid-induced isoform of the enzyme. This steroid-induced ALP isoform has not been demonstrated in cats. Hyperglycemia may be due to increased gluconeogenesis and decreased peripheral tissue utilization through insulin antagonists [38]. Excess glucocorticoid secretion may result in concurrent diabetes mellitus characterized by insulin resistance [41]. Serum phosphorus may be decreased due to polyuria. Urinalysis typically reveals low urine specific gravity with or without mild proteinuria. Concurrent urinary tract infection is common in dogs with HAC [42].

Diagnosis and treatment

The diagnosis of HAC should be based on history and clinical findings and can be confirmed by one or a combination of the following screening tests: ACTH stimulation test, low-dose dexamethasone

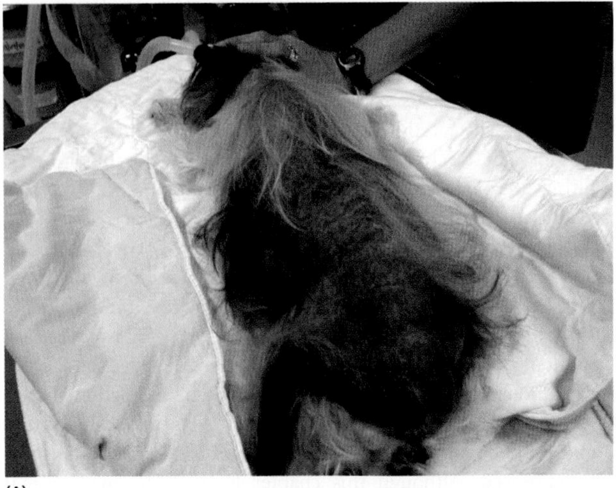
(A)

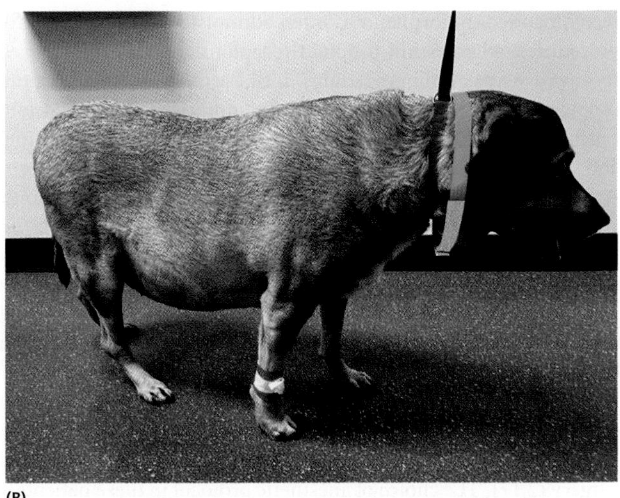
(B)

Figure 42.3 **A.** Mixed-breed dog diagnosed with hyperadrenocorticism and diabetes mellitus with alopecia and abdominal distension. Patient is placed on a conductive heating device and is being preoxygenated in preparation for induction of anesthesia. Source: Dr. Tanya Duke-Novakovski; with permission. **B.** Mixed-breed dog with diabetes mellitus and hyperadrenocorticism exhibiting classic signs of pendulous abdomen, organomegaly, and panting. Source: Dr. Renata S. Costa, with permission.

suppression test (LDDS), urine cortisol:creatinine ratio (UCCR), and dexamethasone-suppressed UCCR [43,44]. According to some reports, the diagnostic accuracies of the dexamethasone-suppressed UCCR and LDDS are greater than that of the ACTH stimulation test and may, therefore, be preferred [45]. In addition to screening tests for HAC, tests to differentiate the cause of the condition are also recommended. High-dose dexamethasone suppression test can confirm pituitary-dependent HAC, and adrenal tumors can be investigated by abdominal ultrasound. Diagnostic imaging modalities such as computed tomography (CT) or magnetic resonance imaging (MRI) can confirm the presence of a pituitary tumor.

Most canine patients with pituitary-dependent disease are treated with the adrenocorticostatic drug, trilostane. Trilostane causes reversible, competitive inhibition of the 3β-hydroxysteroid dehydrogenase enzyme necessary for the production of cortisol, aldosterone, and androgens in the adrenal cortex. The adrencorticolytic drug, mitotane, is still prescribed in some cases [46,47]. Mitotane causes necrosis of the deeper zones of the adrenal cortex, sparing the superficial mineralocorticoid-producing zone. Both treatments can precipitate an acute Addisonian crisis (see hypoadrenocorticism).

In addition to medical management, surgical resection of tumors by transsphenoidal hypophysectomy [48] or adrenalectomy [49] has been successful. For elective procedures, animals should be treated with trilostane for 3–4 weeks prior to surgery in an effort to reverse the metabolic derangements of HAC and minimize the risk of complications associated with adrenalectomy [50]. Treating HAC in cats is challenging and less predictable. Optimal treatments for HAC in cats have not been established [51].

Animals with HAC are predisposed to hypertension [52], which should be managed with antihypertensive drugs such as angiotensin-converting enzyme (ACE) inhibitors, in conjunction with trilostane or mitotane prior to surgery [2,53]. Hypertension may lead to cardiac changes including pressure and volume overload, left ventricular hypertrophy, and congestive heart failure. Persistent high blood pressure can cause kidney injury, and volume overload may occur due to renal sodium retention and increased circulating volume. Hypercoagulability and subsequent pulmonary thromboembolism resulting from excess production of vitamin K-dependent clotting factors is a potentially life-threatening complication of HAC [38]. However, it appears that only a small subset of dogs with HAC develop thrombosis and current guidelines only support antithrombotic therapy (i.e., heparin and clopidogrel) if HAC is accompanied by other risk factors for thrombosis [54].

Anesthetic considerations

Dogs with pituitary-dependent HAC often require anesthesia for other concurrent diseases [2], elective procedures, and diagnostic imaging. These animals should be carefully evaluated and stabilized prior to sedation or any anesthetic event. A CBC and serum biochemistry are recommended to assess hydration status, electrolytes, and hepatic and renal function, especially when dealing with geriatric patients. A thorough physical examination should be performed and baseline blood pressure measured to determine if concurrent hypertension is present.

When adrenal neoplasia is suspected, the extent of local vascular invasion is usually determined with abdominal ultrasound and/or CT prior to the surgical procedure. Animals with cortisol-secreting adrenocortical tumors may undergo adrenalectomy [17]. Blood type should be determined and a crossmatch performed if the animal is to undergo an invasive procedure such as an adrenalectomy, especially if the tumor is in close proximity to or is invading the aorta or vena cava. Blood or packed red blood cells (RBCs) should be available as excessive intraoperative hemorrhage may occur [55,56].

Animals with HAC may be prothrombotic and hypercoagulable and if hypercoagulability is suspected, thromboelastography (TEG) can help guide the most appropriate treatment perioperatively. When an antithrombotic agent is being administered, clotting times should also be evaluated. Measurement of activated partial thromboplastin time (aPTT) may be indicated to ensure that the patient is receiving an appropriate dose and is not at increased risk for excessive bleeding during surgery. The goal is an (aPTT) that is increased by no more than 1.5–2-fold [2,55,57–59].

If the patient is hypertensive and the planned procedure is elective, it should be postponed until this comorbidity is further assessed and managed. Hypertensive dogs may be treated with ACE inhibitors and, although there have been no studies investigating the effects of withholding these agents prior to anesthesia, a study with 12 healthy female Beagle dogs receiving oral enalapril 90 min prior to isoflurane anesthesia showed an increase in the severity of intraoperative hypotension [60]. Therefore, some anesthesiologists discontinue ACE inhibitors 24 h prior to the scheduled procedure.

Animals with Cushing's syndrome, even those undergoing medical management, may develop PU/PD. Reduced total water intake attributed to both the stress of an unusual environment and fasting could result in rapid dehydration in those animals. Hydration status should be carefully assessed using both physical examination and laboratory parameters (e.g., capillary refill time, mucous membrane color, skin turgor, heart rate, blood pressure, and PCV/TS). Goal-directed perianesthetic fluid therapy should be instituted to prevent or treat dehydration and hypotension [2].

Animals treated with mitotane or trilostane may lack functional adrenocortical reserve, and their lower cortisol levels may impair their ability to handle stressful anesthetic or surgical events appropriately. These cases should be managed as iatrogenic Addisonians and may require preoperative glucocorticoid supplementation with 0.1–0.2 mg/kg of dexamethasone sodium phosphate IV [4,28]. In addition, serum sodium and potassium concentrations should be monitored in these patients [2,16].

Anesthetic management

No specific anesthetic protocol is contraindicated for patients with Cushing's syndrome; however, drug choices should be based on the patient's health status and concurrent comorbidities. Patients may be geriatric and/or in poor condition and lethargy is common [2]; therefore, intense sedation may not be required. The anesthesiologist should aim to select drugs and dosages that allow for a smooth and quick recovery to promote movement within 4 h of surgery to improve blood flow. This is particularly important when thrombosis is a concern [52].

Opioids are generally administered to provide analgesia and because they induce minimal dose-dependent cardiorespiratory effects. Sedatives and tranquilizers may not be needed, but a benzodiazepine or a low dose of acepromazine may be administered in conjunction with the opioid. Note that acepromazine may result in worsening of intraoperative hypotension due to its vasodilatory effects, especially in dogs managed with antihypertensive drugs; thus, the authors usually reserve its administration to otherwise healthy but nervous animals. α_2-Adrenergic receptor agonists inhibit pancreatic β-cells resulting in a transient increase in blood glucose [61–63]. Although their use is unlikely to cause clinically relevant adverse effects, there are no published, evidence-based guidelines for use of α_2-adrenergic receptor agonists in animals with HAC or diabetes mellitus. As pain and stress will also result in a physiological and transient increase in blood glucose, a balanced anesthetic protocol is recommended. If α_2-adrenergic receptor agonists are used in patients with concurrent diabetes mellitus, judicious use of additional insulin is warranted to avoid hypoglycemia once the effects of the α_2-adrenergic receptor agonists have waned.

For patients undergoing adrenalectomies, administration of hydrocortisone 2 mg/kg IV or dexamethasone 0.07–0.2 mg/kg IV has been recommended immediately after induction of anesthesia [64,65]. Administration of non-steroidal anti-inflammatory drugs (NSAIDs) is often avoided in HAC patients owing to the potential risk of gastrointestinal ulceration, nephropathy, and hepatopathy in dogs with high endogenous cortisol concentrations [2,66,67]. Use of NSAIDs must be carefully considered based on how well-controlled the disease is, the patient's clinical signs and cortisol levels, and potential concurrent renal or hepatic disease.

If a dog with uncontrolled HAC and hypertension presents for an emergency procedure, a balanced anesthetic and multimodal analgesic protocol may reduce fluctuations in blood pressure intraoperatively. Additionally, as in cases of pheochromocytomas, sodium nitroprusside, β-adrenergic blockers, magnesium sulfate, or increasing inhalant concentrations may be used to control fluctuations in heart rate and blood pressure (see pheochromocytoma) [68].

Animals with HAC often have thin skin and fragile veins, which may present challenges for intravenous catheterization. They may also have delayed primary wound healing and should be handled gently. Minimal hair clipping is advised to reduce the risk of skin trauma, which could become a source of infection, and to minimize heat loss. However, there is limited evidence demonstrating the correlation of area shaved and rectal temperature during anesthesia [69].

Preoxygenation is indicated prior to induction, especially in patients with large pendulous abdomens (Fig. 42.3A). Studies in healthy patients have demonstrated prolongation of the time to desaturation when oxygen is supplemented via face mask [70,71]. Dogs with HAC commonly hypoventilate during anesthesia due to increased abdominal fat, hepatomegaly, respiratory muscle weakness, and bladder distension [2]. Hypoventilation and poor respiratory function may lead to ventilation–perfusion mismatch, atelectasis, hypercapnia, and respiratory acidosis. Hypoxemia may result if oxygen is not supplemented, especially during recovery. These animals may also develop pulmonary mineralization and pulmonary thromboembolism [38,72–74]. Animals with HAC may also be more prone to developing hypothermia under anesthesia due to muscle and dermal atrophy and alopecia. During anesthesia, ventilatory support is often required using intermittent positive-pressure ventilation, especially in animals positioned in dorsal recumbency. Close monitoring of ventilation and oxygenation via end-tidal carbon dioxide, pulse oximetry, and/or arterial blood gas analysis is warranted. In the postoperative period, ventilation and hemoglobin saturation should continue to be monitored, especially if the animal is hypothermic. Severe hypothermia decreases cellular metabolism and lowers carbon dioxide production, resulting in diminished stimulation of ventilation and reduced respiratory rate and tidal volume [75]. Rewarming results in increased metabolic rate and oxygen consumption [76,77]; thus, oxygen supplementation is recommended. Temperature should be monitored and supplemental warming devices employed, but care must be taken to avoid thermal burns.

Blood pressure should be monitored, and direct measurement via an arterial line is recommended for animals anesthetized for invasive procedures such as an adrenalectomy due to the high risk of hemorrhage [2,27]. Furthermore, when an enlarged abdomen and/or hepatomegaly is present, venous return to the heart may be compromised, which could result in intraoperative hypotension. Hypotension may be exacerbated by the presence of hypovolemia, the use of positive-pressure ventilation, and positioning in dorsal recumbency [29].

Following adrenalectomy, especially with invasion of the vena cava, animals are at even greater risk of thromboembolic complications in recovery. Based on the rational use of antithrombotics in veterinary critical care (CURATIVE) guidelines [54], antithrombotic drugs should not be discontinued prior to invasive procedures in animals at high risk for thrombosis; however, these drugs may be withheld in animals at low-to-moderate risk for thrombosis. In animals where antithrombotic therapy was discontinued prior to surgery, therapy can be restarted immediately after the procedure as long as there is no evidence of ongoing bleeding. If signs of thrombosis develop at any point, antithrombotic therapy should be initiated immediately. Clinical signs of thromboembolic events are often non-specific and highly variable [78]; however, acute onset of dyspnea, tachypnea, cyanosis, and collapse should prompt suspicion of pulmonary thromboembolism. Arterial blood gas analysis usually reveals hypoxemia, hypocapnia, and an increased alveolar to arterial oxygen gradient. Treatment is symptomatic and should be instituted immediately, with increased inspired oxygen concentrations and cardiovascular support as needed [2]. Postoperative dexamethasone 0.05–0.15 mg/kg IV has been administered to prevent the development of hypoadrenocorticism [64,79]. Sodium and potassium should also be monitored and mineralocorticoid therapy instituted if the sodium:potassium ratio decreases dramatically [56].

Pheochromocytoma

Pheochromocytoma (PHEO) is a catecholamine-secreting tumor that arises from chromaffin cells of the adrenal medulla. Chromaffin cells synthesize, store, and release catecholamines in response to sympathetic stimulation. In PHEO, catecholamine release may be episodic or continuous and may or may not be related to physiologic stressors such as fear, stress, tumor manipulation, and drugs [80]. This malignant or locally invasive tumor has been reported in several species including dogs, cats, and people [81–83]. Approximately 15–38% of dogs with PHEO have neoplastic invasion of the caudal vena cava; however, clinical signs are not associated with the extent or presence of vena caval invasion (Fig. 42.4) [79,84,85]. Invasive PHEOs have been reported to affect not only the vena cava, but also the aorta, renal veins, and hepatic veins [4,86].

In veterinary species, there are limited data regarding the specific catecholamines released from these tumors. Higher concentrations of plasma metabolites of norepinephrine in comparison to epinephrine have been reported in dogs [86]. In cats, norepinephrine is typically the catecholamine released by PHEO [80].

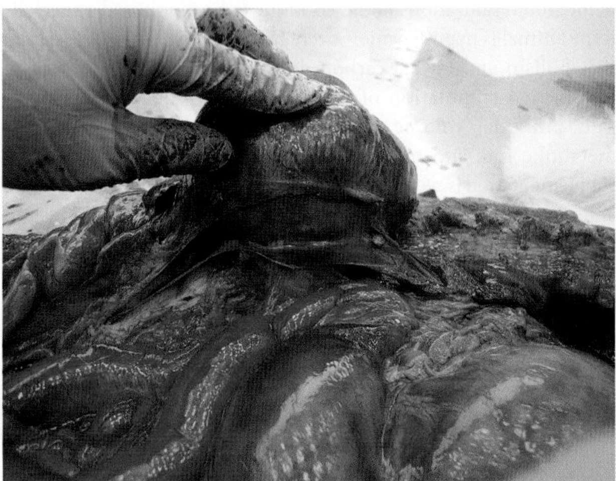

Figure 42.4 A 12-year-old Siberian husky with a pheochromocytoma (10 cm × 7 cm × 6 cm) of the right adrenal gland severely compressing and invading the caudal vena cava. Source: Dr. Jung Keun Lee, Diagnostic Pathology Center, Midwestern University, Glendale, AZ; with permission.

PHEO tends to occur in older dogs (10–12 years), and there is no known breed or sex predilection [82,86–89]. Note that many small animals with PHEO may be asymptomatic, which explains the high number of cases (48–80%) diagnosed postmortem or as an incidental finding on abdominal ultrasound [81,82].

Clinical presentation

Clinical signs of PHEO may be dramatic but are often intermittent and paroxysmal due to the episodic release of catecholamines [17]. The most common signs are weakness, syncope, tachypnea, tachyarrhythmia, hypertension, and seizures [4]. Underlying disorders secondary to chronic hypertension may be observed including retinal detachment, pulmonary venous congestion or pulmonary edema, and congestive heart failure (82,83).

Animals with PHEO may also have other concurrent endocrinopathies such as hyperadrenocorticism (HAC). Therefore, this disorder should be ruled out and/or managed, especially in dogs where HAC is more commonly seen (see hyperadrenocorticism) [88,90].

Clinical pathology

Findings on CBC and serum biochemistry are usually non-specific. Urinalysis in 10 out of 20 dogs with PHEO showed proteinuria, likely caused by a hypertensive glomerulopathy [91]. If HAC is also present, liver enzymes may be elevated, and a stress leukogram may be present (see hyperadrenocorticism).

Diagnosis and treatment

Clinical signs of episodic weakness, collapse, hypertension, and arrhythmias are suggestive of PHEO. Abdominal ultrasound is commonly used to diagnose the presence of an adrenal mass, local metastasis, and thrombi, as it is readily available and does not require general anesthesia [91–94]. Contrast-enhanced ultrasonography may aid in the differentiation of adrenal tumors [95]. Advanced imaging including CT and MRI can also be used and are useful in evaluation of tumor architecture, metastasis, degree of invasion, and thrombi [80,92,93].

Diagnosis of PHEO can be determined via biopsy, but this is rarely performed owing to the difficulty in obtaining good samples and the risk of hemorrhage or a hypertensive crisis. Additionally, there is not clear evidence of histopathological features predictive of metastasis [93]. Other diagnostic tools used to confirm PHEO in dogs and cats include urinary catecholamines and the metanephrine-to-creatinine ratio, and plasma metanephrine and normetanephrine analysis [96,97]. However, these biomarkers may also be elevated in dogs with HAC, due to non-adrenal illness, and other factors such as excitement [97].

Definitive treatment for PHEO is surgical resection of the tumor. To determine the feasibility and complexity of the surgery, it is advised to assess the origin, architecture, vascularity, and invasiveness of the mass via CT or MRI [55,56,86,91–93].

Anesthetic considerations

Preoperative evaluation and stabilization is of the utmost importance in animals with suspected PHEO. Thoracic radiographs prior to surgery should be considered as metastasis to the lung may occur [88]. Further advanced diagnostic imaging will help determine the feasibility of surgical removal in addition to the probable need for crossmatching and blood transfusion [55,56,86,91]. Preanesthetic blood pressure and ECG evaluation is indicated, and medical management to stabilize these animals should be performed prior to anesthesia.

Catecholamine-induced hypertension can be managed with phenoxybenzamine, a long-acting non-competitive α_1-adrenergic receptor antagonist with some α_2-adrenergic receptor antagonism. It is recommended to start phenoxybenzamine treatment 1–2 weeks before surgery. An oral dose of 0.25 mg/kg twice daily is often prescribed, but higher doses may be required, up to 2.5 mg/kg twice daily. Serial blood pressure measurements should be performed to evaluate response to therapy [4,55,56,86,89,98,99]. It has been reported that although preoperative administration of phenoxybenzamine did not decrease the frequency or severity of perioperative hypertension in dogs with PHEO, the mortality rate decreased from 43% to 13%. This improved outcome may be due to the reduction in vasoconstriction and improvement of intravascular volume [89].

Prazosin, a competitive, reversible α_1-adrenergic receptor antagonist, is an alternative agent to manage catecholamine-induced hypertension when phenoxybenzamine is not available [100]. Oral doses range from 0.25 to 1 mg/kg twice daily. In contrast to phenoxybenzamine, prazosin's effects can be overcome by high concentrations of catecholamines. Therefore, phenoxybenzamine is considered the drug of choice for animals undergoing surgery for PHEO excision. Doxazosin is another alternative to phenoxybenzamine, but reports of its clinical use in veterinary medicine are limited. [101,102]. Doxazosin has been used at a dosage of 0.5 mg/kg orally every 24 h to manage hypertension in an HAC dog with a PHEO [103].

Atrial and ventricular tachycardia and, less often, atrioventricular block may occur with these tumors [2,86,104]. Severe tachycardia can be treated with oral β-adrenergic receptor antagonists, such as propranolol (0.2–1 mg/kg every 8 h) or atenolol (0.2–1 mg/kg every 12 h). However, better results are seen when α-adrenergic receptor blockade, usually with phenoxybenzamine, is instituted first because administration of a β-adrenergic receptor blocker alone may lead to unopposed α-adrenergic receptor-mediated vasoconstriction, which may exacerbate hypertension [2,17,27,86,105]. The risk of bradyarrhythmias may also be reduced by preoperative management of hypertension.

Cardiac evaluation is an important determinant of whether surgical treatment for PHEO should be pursued. Third-degree atrioventricular block in dogs with PHEO has been related to myocardial damage and atrioventricular nodal fibrosis from chronic catecholamine exposure [104].

Anesthetic management

Animals undergoing adrenalectomy are often classified as ASA III, IV, or V, and risk factors associated with the surgical procedure include significant hemorrhage, precipitation of a hypertensive crisis, cardiac arrhythmias, and intraoperative/postoperative hypotension following tumor excision. A minimum database consisting of a CBC, serum biochemistry profile, urinalysis, baseline ECG, and blood pressure should be evaluated prior to anesthesia. Hydration status should be assessed and appropriate preoperative fluid therapy instituted to correct any signs of dehydration or hypovolemia. Chronic sympathetic stimulation and vasoconstriction seen with PHEO may cause intravascular volume depletion [17,86]. Factors that could stimulate further catecholamine release such as fear, stress, pain, hypothermia, shivering, hypoxia, and hypercapnia should be minimized as much as possible.

Blood type should be determined and crossmatch considered prior to surgery. There is significant potential for intraoperative blood loss, particularly for tumors involving the right adrenal gland due to its proximity to the caudal vena cava. Therefore, packed RBCs, fresh frozen plasma, or whole blood should be available for immediate volume resuscitation if needed [2,55,56,86,91,106]. LRS and hypertonic saline can be used in the initial resuscitation of hemorrhagic shock and may stabilize cardiovascular parameters until a blood transfusion can be initiated [107,108]. Effects of hypertonic saline outlast those of LRS [108]. Continuous ECG and invasive arterial blood pressure measurement should be performed to identify and manage cardiac arrhythmias and abrupt changes in blood pressure [17,86]. Multiple intravenous access sites should be available to promptly manage intraoperative complications. Central venous access may be beneficial for intraoperative and postoperative management.

Although most anesthetic drugs have been used in animals with PHEO with some success, drugs with sympathomimetic or vagolytic effects, such as ketamine and anticholinergics, are often avoided to prevent possible adverse hemodynamic responses. Histamine release associated with morphine and atracurium administration may result in sympathetic stimulation in response to vasodilation. Thiobarbiturates and halothane, though no longer available in many countries, have historically been avoided owing to their tendency to cause ventricular arrhythmias, especially in the presence of high catecholamine levels. Acepromazine may complicate the treatment of hypotension due to its α-adrenergic receptor blocking effects, particularly if the animal has been pretreated with phenoxybenzamine [2,27,56,86].

Case reports in humans and dogs suggest that dexmedetomidine could aid in controlling hypertensive surges during anesthesia of patients undergoing PHEO excision. Catecholamine release and sympathetic response may be reduced by dexmedetomidine binding to presynaptic α_2-adrenergic receptors resulting in inhibition of norepinephrine release [109]. Based on the authors' experience, administration of dexmedetomidine (0.5–1 μg/kg/h) IV as a CRI is helpful to stabilize blood pressure changes intraoperatively. There is, however, a lack of controlled studies investigating the effects of dexmedetomidine on physiological variables and perioperative outcomes of animals undergoing adrenalectomies [110–113].

A suggested balanced anesthetic protocol for animals with PHEO includes IV premedication with an opioid that does not promote histamine release (e.g., hydromorphone, methadone, or fentanyl) combined with a benzodiazepine. Induction of anesthesia may be accomplished with IV propofol, alfaxalone, or etomidate [55,89,98]. Isoflurane or sevoflurane is preferred for anesthetic maintenance as opposed to desflurane, which can cause sympathetic stimulation [114]. Inhalant agents should be supplemented with a potent, rapid-acting opioid CRI (e.g., fentanyl, sulfentanil, or remifentanil) and potentially other MAC-sparing agents combined in a balanced anesthetic protocol [2,86,89].

Drugs for the treatment of perioperative complications must be readily available for administration when an emergency arises, especially during induction of anesthesia or tumor manipulation. The authors recommend calculation of all emergency drugs prior to anesthesia, and it may be beneficial to prepare syringes of those most likely to be needed in advance. Table 42.2 provides drug dosages for antiarrhythmic therapy and blood pressure support. Profound fluctuations in blood pressure are often observed during PHEO surgery. Sodium nitroprusside, a direct-acting vasodilator, is the agent of choice to treat severe hypertension due to its potency,

Table 42.2 Treatments for intraoperative complications in animals with pheochromocytoma.

Complication	Drug	Dose	Comments
Hypertension	Nitroprusside	0.1–10 μg/kg/min IV	Dilates arterioles and veins independent of catecholamines; direct BP monitoring preferred
	Phentolamine	0.1 mg/kg IV followed by at 1–2 μg/kg/min CRI	Induces short-acting α-adrenergic blockade
	Magnesium sulfate ($MgSO_4$)	50 mg/kg (diluted) over 15 min, followed by 15 mg/kg/h CRI	Inhibits catecholamine release, induces α-adrenergic blockade, directly dilates arterioles
Tachyarrhythmia	Lidocaine	2 mg/kg IV, followed by 50–80 μg/kg/min CRI	For management of ventricular arrhythmias
	Esmolol	0.25–0.5 mg/kg IV over 1–2 min followed by 10–200 μg/kg/min CRI	Only after α-adrenergic blockade or may precipitate hypertensive crisis; induces short-acting β_1-adrenergic blockade; for sinus or supraventricular tachycardia
Refractory hypotension	Phenylephrine	0.4–4 μg/kg/min CRI	Induces potent α_1-adrenergic agonism; may cause vagally mediated bradycardia; use lowest effective dose
	Norepinephrine	0.05–1 μg/kg/min CRI	Use lowest effective dose
	Vasopressin	0.2–0.8 IU/kg IV and/or 0.002–0.006 IU/kg/min CRI	Indicated if patient has reduced sensitivity to catecholamines; works in acidic environment; use lowest effective dose

BP, blood pressure; CRI, constant rate infusion.
Source: Veres-Nyéki [2]; Koenig [4]; Kyles *et al.* [55]; Santoro-Beer and Mandell [86]; Viilman and Vettorato [113]; Robinson [115]; Pedro *et al.* [116]; Nazari *et al.* [117].

rapid onset, and short duration of action. Phentolamine, a short-acting competitive α-adrenergic receptor antagonist and direct vasodilator, is an alternative for the treatment of intraoperative hypertension [17,27,55,86,89]. Another commonly administered agent is magnesium sulfate ($MgSO_4$). In human patients, $MgSO_4$ has been used for the treatment of hypertension and arrhythmias during anesthesia. $MgSO_4$ inhibits the release of catecholamines from the adrenal medulla and peripheral nerve terminals, reduces the sensitivity of α-adrenergic receptors to catecholamines, is a direct vasodilator, and has antiarrhythmic effects [4,27].

Arrhythmias are another common perioperative complication of animals with PHEO. Tachyarrhythmias are usually managed with lidocaine or β-adrenergic receptor antagonists. Esmolol, a β-adrenergic blocker, has a rapid onset, a short duration of action, and readily controls heart rate [2,4,17,27,86]. Supraventricular and ventricular rhythm disturbances are sometimes managed with the class III antiarrhythmic agent, amiodarone, that blocks potassium channels but also inhibits β-adrenergic receptors, calcium channels, and sodium channels [115–117]. Reflex bradycardia may also occur secondary to hypertension. Appropriate management of blood pressure usually corrects the changes in heart rate. However, if bradycardia is accompanied by hypotension, anticholinergics may be required.

Intraoperative and postoperative hypotension following PHEO excision is common. It is multifactorial due to an immediate decrease in catecholamine concentrations, vasodilation from residual α-adrenergic receptor blockade caused by phenoxybenzamine, impaired sympathetic reflexes, and hypovolemia. Treatment includes reduction of inhalant concentration, reduction or discontinuation of nitroprusside/phentolamine/magnesium sulfate, and volume expansion with isotonic crystalloid or colloid fluids. Vasopressor (e.g., phenylephrine and norepinephrine) and inotropic drugs are used to treat refractory hypotension, although patients treated with phenoxybenzamine may be less responsive to vasopressor therapy [2,17,27,86,118]. Treatment with a non-catecholamine pressor, such as vasopressin, may be necessary to maintain adequate blood pressure [118].

To protect vital organs from reduced oxygen delivery, surface-induced hypothermia to a temperature of 32 °C (89.6 °F) has been advocated for animals requiring temporary vascular occlusion during PHEO resection [55,89,119]. Additionally, during anesthesia, blood pressure values should be maintained close to the animal's baseline blood pressure to prevent renal hypoperfusion and ischemia. If bilateral adrenalectomy has been performed, glucocorticoid and mineralocorticoid replacement therapy will be necessary. In addition, blood glucose should be monitored postoperatively because hypoglycemia may occur when plasma catecholamine concentrations decrease suddenly. Continuous ECG and blood pressure monitoring should be maintained for at least 24 h postoperatively [27,86].

During the recovery period, thromboembolic events may occur. Antithrombotic drugs should not be discontinued in animals at high risk for thrombosis; however, they may be withheld in cases of low to moderate risk. In these cases, antithrombotic drugs can be restarted immediately after the procedure if there is no evidence of ongoing bleeding or if development of a thrombosis occurs [54].

Pancreas and kidney

The pancreas is a nodular, bilobed gland located within the mesentery at the angle where the duodenum meets the stomach. The pancreas is composed of acini and pancreatic islets, previously known as "islets of Langerhans." The acinar cells produce and secrete digestive enzymes via the pancreatic duct into the duodenum. Two pancreatic ducts are usually found in the dog but only one in the cat. The pancreatic or dorsal duct drains the left lobe and joins the main bile duct before entering the duodenum at the major duodenal papilla; the ventral or accessory duct drains the right lobe into the duodenum at the minor duodenal papilla. The cat has only the dorsal duct to drain both areas [120]. The pancreatic islets secrete hormones such as insulin (β-cells), glucagon (α-cells), somatostatin (δ-cells), and pancreatic polypeptide (pancreatic polypeptide cells) into the bloodstream, thereby exerting critical endocrine effects. Pancreatic endocrine disorders involving insulin include diabetes mellitus and insulinoma.

The kidneys are essential for maintenance of extracellular fluid homeostasis. When they are unable to adequately concentrate urine and maintain fluid balance either due to impaired production of ADH or impaired renal response to ADH, the resulting endocrine disorder is known as "diabetes insipidus."

Diabetes mellitus

Diabetes mellitus (DM) occurs due to inadequate insulin secretion or resistance to the effects of insulin, which culminates in the development of hyperglycemia. Hyperglycemia occurs following impairment of glucose uptake into tissues and increased hepatic gluconeogenesis. It results in fluid shifting from the intracellular space into the intravascular space thus causing cellular dehydration.

In dogs, the predominant form of DM is caused by β-cell destruction resulting in insulin deficiency and hyperglycemia. This is homologous to type 1 DM in people [121,122]. In cats, insulin resistance is most common. Insulin is available, but target tissues have an impaired ability to respond to its metabolic effects, and eventual exhaustion of β-cells ensues [123]. This is homologous to type 2 DM in humans [121,123–125]. In approximately ¼ of cats, DM is secondary to hypersomatotropism.

DM occurs most often in middle-aged or older animals. In dogs, there is a female sex predilection, whereas in cats, it is more frequently diagnosed in neutered males [121,123,126]. There are several canine breeds at increased risk for DM, including the Australian Terrier, Miniature and Standard Schnauzers, Samoyed, Miniature and Toy Poodles, Cairn Terrier, Keeshond, Bichon Frise, and Finnish Spitz [127]. Reports indicate that Burmese cats may be at a higher risk in some geographical areas [123]. Because cats primarily have the type 2 form, obesity increases the risk of diabetes dramatically in this species [123,128].

Clinical presentation

The clinical presentation of animals with DM may be non-specific, but a common reported sign is polyuria/polydipsia (PU/PD). When the concentration of glucose in the plasma exceeds the renal threshold for proximal tubular reabsorption of glucose from the filtrate, glucosuria ensues, causing osmotic diuresis and PU/PD. Animals may also be dehydrated or hypovolemic. Because DM is a catabolic condition, dogs with insulin deficiency may have severe depletion of both energy stores and protein mass. Clinical signs such as lethargy, polyphagia, and weight loss may be seen. Older cats (> 7 years) with weight loss and polyphagia should be tested for hyperthyroidism as clinical signs of both diseases are similar and can occur concurrently [129].

Other signs of DM depend on the severity and chronicity of hyperglycemia. Cataracts are common in dogs with DM due to disruption of normal lens metabolism (Fig. 42.5), and some cats with chronic DM develop a peripheral neuropathy that results in a plantigrade posture (Fig. 42.6).

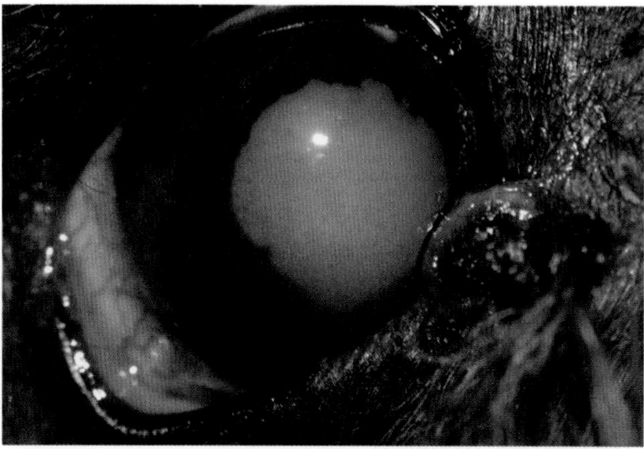

Figure 42.5 A 9-year-old diabetic Schnauzer with cataract-associated uveitis. The dog required general anesthesia for phacoemulsification. Source: Dr. Stephanie Pumphrey, Veterinary Ophthalmology, Cummings School of Veterinary Medicine at Tufts University, North Grafton, MA; with permission.

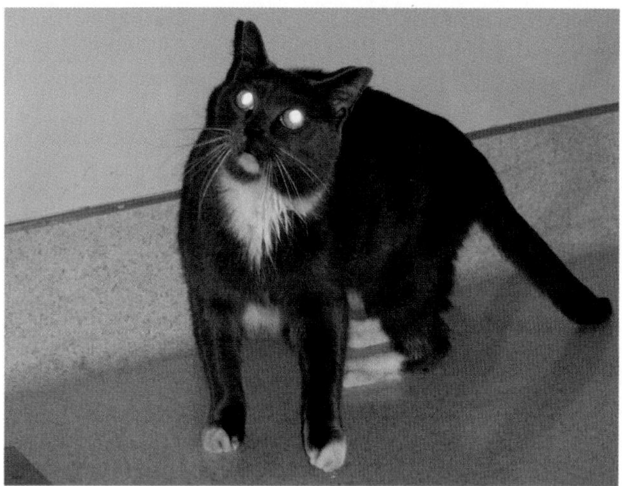

Figure 42.6 Plantigrade posture in a cat with DM is caused by peripheral neuropathy. The posture itself may not represent a complicating factor for anesthesia; however, it does suggest chronic and/or uncontrolled diabetes. Serial measurements of blood glucose during anesthesia, ± insulin/dextrose administration, are warranted perioperatively. Source: Dr. Todd Green, Department of Small Animal Medicine and Surgery, St. George's University, St. George's, Grenada; with permission.

In severe manifestations of DM such as diabetic ketoacidosis (DKA) or hyperglycemic hyperosmolar syndrome (HHS), patients can present in critical condition with clinical signs of vomiting, anorexia, severe dehydration, depression, coma, or death. Ketones are synthesized from fatty acids as a substitute form of energy because glucose is not transported into the cells. Excess ketoacids results in acidosis and severe electrolyte abnormalities, which can be life-threatening. HHS is an uncommon form of diabetic crisis marked by severe hyperglycemia, minimal or no urine ketones, hypovolemia, decreased glomerular filtration rate (GFR), weakness, and possible coma. Animals with DKA often have other concurrent diseases such as acute pancreatitis, urinary tract infection, and hyperadrenocorticism [130]. Animals with DKA and HHS should be stabilized prior to undergoing sedation or anesthesia.

Clinical pathology

Findings on CBC are often normal, but dogs and cats with DKA may present with a non-regenerative anemia. Leukocytosis may occur in animals with concurrent infection, which is common in DM and DKA.

The most important serum biochemistry finding in animals with DM is hyperglycemia, but elevated liver enzyme activity and hypercholesterolemia may also occur [131]. In dehydrated patients, azotemia and electrolyte disorders including hypokalemia, hypernatremia, hyponatremia, hypophosphatemia, and hypochloremia can be observed. Pseudohyponatremia may be caused by hyperglycemia resulting in increased water retention in the intravascular space.

Urinalysis should also be performed and glucosuria can be identified when the blood glucose (BG) exceeds the renal threshold, approximately 200 mg/dL in dogs and 250 mg/dL in cats [129,132]. Proteinuria and ketonuria may also be seen. Nitroprusside reagent urine test strips do not detect the dominant ketone produced in DKA, 3-hydroxybutyrate (3-HB); therefore, ketonuria may not be detected [133]. A 3-HB ketone meter or serum 3-HB could be used to identify the presence of this ketone. In dogs and cats with DKA, blood gas analysis reveals a low concentration of bicarbonate and, with the increased production of ketoacid anions, a high anion gap [134].

Diagnosis and treatment

The hallmarks of diagnosis of DM are persistent hyperglycemia (BG > 200 mg/dL in dogs and > 270 mg/dL in cats with classic clinical signs of hyperglycemia) and glucosuria. In cats, stress hyperglycemia should be ruled out by reassessing BG in a calmer environment and/or measuring serum fructosamine concentrations [129].

Although treatment protocols are constantly evolving, dogs are commonly treated with either porcine lente (Vetsulin®) or neutral protamine Hagedorn (NPH) insulin, and cats with either glargine (Lantus®) or NPH insulin [129]. In cats, dietary management with diets low in carbohydrates and high in protein has been advocated [135]. Oral hypoglycemic drugs have been advocated to control hyperglycemia in diabetic cats, but the use of these drugs is not commonplace [136].

Treatment of DKA often requires hospitalization and critical care, including IV fluid therapy, insulin CRI, and intensive monitoring of acid–base status, fluid balance, glucose, and electrolytes [123,137,138]. Fluid therapy usually involves administration of an isotonic crystalloid. In animals with hypernatremia, 0.9% sodium chloride could be administered to minimize the risk of rapid sodium changes (> 0.5 mEq/h) and transcellular fluid shifts; however, it may result in increased chloride concentration and may not correct acidemia as well as other balanced electrolyte solutions [133,139]. Fluids such as Hartmann's solution or polyionic hypotonic maintenance solution may be advantageous due to a resultant increase in bicarbonate and base excess [139]. LRS is avoided by some clinicians due to the hepatic conversion of lactate to ketones, whereas the buffers in Plasma-Lyte® and Normosol-R® are acetate and gluconate, which are metabolized by skeletal muscle [133,139]. Rapid-acting insulins, such as regular insulin, are usually administered as CRIs, and close and regular monitoring of BG is required.

Monitoring treatment success is somewhat controversial, but measurement of serum fructosamine concentrations may be used to evaluate long-term control of hyperglycemia. Although serial BG curves have traditionally been recommended to assess the effects of insulin therapy, their use is called into question by studies in both dogs and cats showing their poor reliability for predicting glycemic control [140,141]. In cases of DKA and during anesthesia of animals with DM, serial BG measurements should be performed. Continuous glucose monitors that measure rapid changes in interstitial glucose levels have been used with success in dogs with DKA.

Anesthetic considerations

In well-regulated diabetic dogs, the BG concentration measured within 1–4 h of insulin administration should be between 150 and 250 mg/dL. An early morning BG concentration greater than 300 mg/dL could suggest poor glycemic control. However, a single measurement does not confirm this because BG concentrations even in well-controlled diabetic dogs may vary throughout the day and excursions of 400–600 mg/dL could be observed. In cases of high BG levels, inadequate glycemic control is more likely present if the fructosamine concentration is greater than 500 mg/dL [142].

Hyperglycemia has been associated with higher morbidity, depression of leukocyte function, increased wound infections, and decreased tissue perfusion in dogs and people [143,144]. Additionally, animals with unregulated diabetes can have marked fluctuation of BG concentrations during anesthesia. Anesthesia for elective procedures should be postponed in patients with poorly regulated DM. One exception to this recommendation is intact females with insulin resistance that require ovariohysterectomy before the disease can be controlled [142].

Fluid therapy to correct water losses and electrolyte imbalances should be instituted before anesthesia. In any hyperglycemic and DKA animal, hydration status, acid–base status, and electrolyte imbalances should be assessed and corrected as preoperative hyperglycemia can contribute to hyperosmolar diuresis with subsequent dehydration, hypovolemia, and increased risk for intraoperative hypotension [2,30,145].

When dogs and cats with diabetes require anesthesia for medical and surgical procedures, these may not be directly related to DM or may be due to comorbidities secondary to DM. For example, many diabetic dogs develop cataracts, which require removal via phacoemulsification under anesthesia [2]. Timely monitoring of serum BG during the perioperative period and appropriate intervention (e.g., with regular insulin or dextrose administration) can help prevent severe hyper- and hypoglycemia during the perioperative period. Patients with DKA should not be anesthetized until clinical signs have subsided and the animal has been stabilized.

Anesthetic management

Whenever possible, anesthetic procedures for patients with DM should be performed early in the day to reduce the need for prolonged fasting times, to allow for a rapid return to normal activity and insulin regimen, and to allow for close monitoring postoperatively. Although preoperative fasting times can vary, food is often withheld after 10 pm for morning procedures. On the day of anesthesia, numerous fasting and insulin administration protocols have been recommended (Table 42.3). Although glycemic control was achieved with most protocols, withholding insulin completely was associated with greater increases in intraoperative BG levels [146,147]. In animals receiving basal insulin, dose reduction prior to anesthesia may not be necessary. However, intermediate-acting insulin dose may need to be decreased pending fasting duration. Note that there is no consensus statement in veterinary medicine on fasting times and insulin regimens preoperatively. Additionally, there are no data on the association between level of glycemic control and postprocedural or long-term outcome.

Serial BG measurements before and after induction of anesthesia, every 30–60 min throughout anesthesia, and postoperatively are often required. However, the time and frequency of rechecks may vary depending on the BG results obtained. If BG values are consistently stable, measurements may be performed less often. If BG fluctuations are moderate to severe, this should prompt the clinician to monitor the values closely and undertake more frequent sampling. Dextrose solutions may be provided to maintain BG levels within the patient's normal or clinically acceptable range. It is important to remember that stress-induced increases in BG may

Table 42.3 Summary of suggested guidelines for preoperative insulin management of diabetic patients based on retrospective studies, clinical studies, and textbooks.

Fasting time	Preoperative insulin regimen	Dextrose administration	Outcome and/or comments	Reference
6 and 12 h	½ usual insulin dose SC morning of surgery	No dextrose administered	Lower intraoperative increases in BG in groups receiving insulin compared to group where insulin was withheld; No dogs became hypoglycemic	Adami C, *et al.*, 2020 [146]; retrospective study
12 h	Full insulin dose SC morning of surgery			
12 h	No insulin morning of surgery			
7–7.5 h	¼ usual insulin dose SC morning of surgery	ND or not administered	No dogs became hypoglycemic; Normoglycemia in 4% of samples; Severe hyperglycemia in 58% of samples	Kronen P, *et al.*, 2001 [147]; prospective clinical study
	Full insulin dose SC morning of surgery		Hypoglycemia in 25% of dogs; Normoglycemia in 15% of samples; Severe hyperglycemia in 57% of samples	
6 h	Full usual intermediate-acting insulin dose SC in the afternoon prior to surgery	No dextrose administered	No dogs became hypoglycemic intraoperatively; hyperglycemia (> 300 mg/dL) in 65% of dogs	Norgate DJ, *et al.*, 2021 [157], prospective clinical study
12 h	½ usual intermediate-acting insulin dose SC morning of surgery		No dogs became hypoglycemic intraoperatively; hyperglycemia (> 300 mg/dL) in 67% of dogs	
Recommendations from textbooks				
ND	BG < 100 mg/dL: administer no insulin	2.5–5% dextrose infusion at 1–2 mL/kg/h	Monitor BG q 30 min	Behrend E, *et al.*, 2018 [129]
	BG 100–200 mg/dL: administer ¼ usual dose	2.5–5% dextrose infusion at 1–2 mL/kg/h	Monitor BG q 30–60 min	
	BG > 200 mg/dL: administer ½ usual dose	If BG < 150 mg/dL: dextrose infusion	Monitor BG q 30–60 min; may evaluate for ketonuria	
	BG > 300 mg/dL: administer full dose or regular insulin	Do not administer dextrose infusion	Monitor BG q 30–60 min; may evaluate for ketonuria	
ND	BG < 145 mg/dL: administer no insulin	If BG < 145 mg/dL: 0.9% saline with 5% dextrose;	Monitor BG q 30–60 min	Veres-Nyéki KO, 2016 [2]
	BG 145–270 mg/dL: administer ½ usual dose	If BG 145–250 mg/dL: 0.9% saline with 2.5% dextrose;		
	BG > 270 mg/dL: administer full usual dose	If BG > 250 mg/dL: 0.9% saline with no dextrose		
Food withheld after 10 pm	BG < 100 mg/dL: administer no insulin	2.5–5% dextrose infusion	Monitor BG q 30–60 min; Maintain BG between 150–250 mg/dL (dextrose and insulin as needed)	Nelson RW, 2015 [142]
	BG 100–200 mg/dL: administer ¼ usual dose	2.5–5% dextrose infusion		
	BG > 200 mg/dL: administer ½ usual dose	If BG < 150 mg/dL: dextrose infusion		

ND, no data; BG, blood glucose.

occur due to anesthesia and surgery and should also be taken into consideration when evaluating BG levels.

Although continued insulin administration during preoperative fasting potentially increases the risk of hypoglycemia, insulin activity is important even during fasting to allow tissue uptake of nutrients. In addition, stress associated with anesthesia and surgery causes the release of hormones such as corticosteroids and catecholamines. These hormones promote glycogenolysis, gluconeogenesis, and ketogenesis, all of which increase the insulin requirement. Therefore, perioperative insulin administration is indicated to prevent severe hyperglycemia and minimize ketone formation perioperatively [142]. It is imperative to resume the patient's usual insulin regimen and monitor clinical signs in the days following the procedure to ensure appropriate management of DM and prevent DKA.

Balanced anesthesia with reversible, short-acting drugs such as full μ-opioid receptor agonists and benzodiazepines will allow for a fast recovery after anesthesia [2]. Locoregional anesthesia should be considered whenever possible due to its MAC-sparing effects, reliability in managing intra- and postoperative pain, and minimal systemic side effects. Local anesthetics are the only class of drugs that block transduction and transmission of nociceptive input and provide complete analgesia; thus, these techniques are an integral part of a multimodal analgesic protocol. Ophthalmic nerve blocks could be considered for animals undergoing anesthesia for ocular procedures including enucleation, entropion, corneal laceration repair, and phacoemulsification [148]. These local anesthetic techniques need to be carefully performed by trained personnel to minimize the risk of complications such as hemorrhage, globe perforation, and nerve damage. The anesthetist should also be aware of the risk of initiating the oculocardiac reflex; therefore, heart rate and/or ECG should be monitored when performing ophthalmic blocks. As previously mentioned, some animals with DM may have peripheral neuropathies, and regional techniques should not be performed on the affected limb(s). However, other local blocks and techniques, including infiltration with liposome-encapsulated bupivacaine (Nocita®), should still be considered. As locoregional techniques are associated with few systemic effects, they may help promote faster anesthetic recoveries. Other agents that also provide analgesia and MAC-sparing effects should be utilized if there are no contraindications. The authors routinely administer ketamine as a CRI (loading dose 1–2 mg/kg IV followed by 0.6–1.2 mg/kg/h) to dogs and cats undergoing invasive and painful procedures [149]. In dogs, a lidocaine CRI can also be administered (loading dose 1–2 mg/kg IV followed by 50 μg/kg/min) to provide balanced anesthesia [150].

Although there are no absolute drug contraindications in diabetic patients, anesthetic protocols should be chosen based on each individual patient, their concurrent comorbidities, and the specific procedure. For example, animals with DM undergoing ocular procedures may have suspected or confirmed increased intraocular pressures (IOP). Drugs known to cause a high incidence of vomiting, such as hydromorphone and morphine, should be avoided as they can further increase IOP. The anesthetist may also consider administering an antiemetic drug such as maropitant prior to premedication.

Extreme β-cell deficiency is often seen in diabetic dogs by the time clinical disease is apparent; therefore, while the endocrine effects of the α_2-adrenergic receptor agonists are unlikely to be clinically relevant, they should be noted. α_2-Adrenergic receptor agonists, such as dexmedetomidine, inhibit the release of insulin likely via stimulation of islet β-cell α_2-adrenergic receptors, resulting in a transient increase in plasma glucose [63,151]. Knowledge of this possible endocrine effect of α_2-adrenergic receptor agonists may be important when assessing BG levels in the intra- and postoperative periods. Caution is advised when administering additional insulin in this situation as hypoglycemia could develop once the effects of the α_2-adrenergic receptor agonist wane.

Neuromuscular blocking agents (NMBAs) are commonly administered to animals with DM undergoing ophthalmic procedures to provide centralization and immobilization of the globe. Differences between NMBAs have been reported. Vecuronium appears to have a shorter duration of action in patients with DM [152], whereas atracurium's duration is similar in diabetics and non-diabetic dogs [153]. Higher infusion rates of rocuronium seem to be required for neuromuscular blockade of diabetic versus non-diabetic dogs undergoing phacoemulsification [154].

During anesthetic maintenance of any patient with DM, frequent perioperative monitoring of BG is recommended every 30–60 min [2,147]. Fluctuations in BG concentration may be affected by several factors including the efficacy of current medical management and the complexity of surgery, preoperative glucocorticoid administration, and the presence of infection [27]. As with preoperative fasting and insulin administration, multiple protocols to control hypo- and hyperglycemia have been recommended. It has been reported that if a BG concentration greater than 300 mg/dL persists, regular insulin could be administered IV or IM at 20% of the patient's usual dosage of long-acting insulin [142]. Subsequent doses of regular insulin should be timed to avoid hypoglycemia, and the dosage should be adjusted based on the effect of the first injection [142]. When BG is less than 100 mg/dL, IV dextrose may be required during anesthesia and BG monitored every 30 min [129]. In the authors' clinical experience, persistent and severe hyperglycemia may be treated in accordance with recommendations for stabilization of DKA patients with the administration of 0.1 U/kg IM regular insulin [133]. Although the optimal target for BG in the perioperative period has not been defined, maintaining levels between 150 and 250 mg/dL until the patient recovers and starts to eat is advised [142]. Dextrose infusions are formulated by adding the appropriate amount of 50% dextrose to an isotonic fluid such as LRS to obtain a final concentration of 2.5–5% dextrose. At these concentrations, dextrose can be administered via a peripheral vessel, but dextrose concentrations higher than 5% should be administered via a central line. Dextrose should be stopped when/if the BG reaches 250 mg/dL in dogs or 300 mg/dL in cats, as this level is likely to promote glycosuria and diuresis [142].

The BP and ECG should be closely and continuously monitored during anesthesia due to possible marked derangements intraoperatively [155]. It is also recommended to obtain a baseline BP prior to anesthesia as diabetes is a risk factor for hypertension in dogs. Another aspect to consider is that hypertensive animals may be receiving BP medication, and the vasodilatory effects of these drugs can predispose animals to developing severe and often refractory hypotension during anesthesia [27,155]. In people with DM, the cardiovascular effects of autonomic diabetic neuropathy can predispose these patients to developing perioperative dysrhythmias and intraoperative hypotension [27]. In veterinary medicine, one study concluded that there were differences in vagal tone between diabetic and non-diabetic dogs [156]; however, it is unknown if this condition is associated with intraoperative hypotension or other cardiovascular complications. Diabetic dogs appear to be more likely to become hypotensive than non-diabetic dogs undergoing phacoemulsification. The increased incidence and severity of intraoperative hypotension was attributed to hypovolemia secondary to hyperglycemia and the resultant osmotic diuresis and not to any systemic medication [145]. As mentioned previously, appropriate goal-directed fluid therapy to correct dehydration and/or hypovolemia should be instituted. Intraoperative fluid rates of LRS at 5–10 mL/kg/h for dogs and 3–5 mL/kg/h for cats may be adequate in most cases. The authors recommend that dextrose supplementation be performed using a separate syringe pump or separate fluid bag to avoid iatrogenic hyperglycemia. The total amount of fluids being administered should be calculated to remain within the rate previously described. Also note that intraoperative hyperkalemia, a potentially life-threatening complication, has been reported in dogs with DM undergoing bilateral phacoemulsification [157]. If ECG changes are noted, assessment of plasma potassium concentration is recommended.

Hypoglycemia can result in prolonged anesthetic recovery and central nervous system dysfunction. Lack of insulin or insulin resistance may initiate energy production from fatty acids due to insufficient glucose transport into the cell. Subsequent ketone production may result in DKA. Several of the clinical signs associated with these complications may go unnoticed until the end of anesthesia [2]. In non-diabetic dogs, hyperglycemic patients had longer hospital stays and higher incidence of septic complications [144]. Other reports demonstrate a negative association between hyperglycemia and disease states including congestive heart failure and severity of head trauma. Therefore, monitoring and management of BG levels are required. It is recommended to feed the patient a small amount of food once recovered from anesthesia and return to the routine schedule for insulin administration the following day [2]. Continued monitoring with dextrose and insulin administration as needed should be continued for patients that are not eating [142].

Diabetes insipidus

Antidiuretic hormone (ADH) or vasopressin is produced in the hypothalamus and stored and released from the posterior pituitary gland. This hormone is important for water, osmolar, and blood pressure homeostasis. Increased plasma osmolality or decreased blood volume stimulates the release of ADH into the bloodstream. It then acts on the kidneys, specifically in the distal convoluted tubule and collecting ducts controlling urinary water excretion. To normalize plasma osmolality and increase blood volume, ADH binds to vasopressin V_2 receptors in the kidneys, increasing expression of aquaporin-2 water channels. This allows water to move down its concentration gradient, out of the nephron, and back into the bloodstream. In high concentrations, ADH causes vasoconstriction via binding of V_1 receptors in vascular smooth muscle and activation of G-protein-coupled receptors. The increased peripheral vascular resistance helps normalize blood pressure [158].

Diabetes insipidus (DI) is an endocrine disorder characterized by an inadequate renal response to ADH (nephrogenic DI) or impaired hypothalamic production of ADH (central DI). Nephrogenic DI may be primary/congenital possibly due to mutations in either vasopressin V_2 receptors or aquaporin-2 water channels [159]. It may also be secondary to disorders such as hypoadrenocorticism, sepsis, pyelonephritis, and liver insufficiency. This decreased renal response to ADH may also be iatrogenic following glucocorticoid and α_2-adrenergic receptor agonist administration, or secondary to hypokalemia or hypercalcemia likely due to downregulation of aquaporin-2 water channels in the kidney. Central DI may be a congenital disorder or manifest after damage to the hypothalamus or pituitary gland (e.g., brain tumor and traumatic brain injury).

Central and nephrogenic DI are uncommon in dogs and rare in cats. Familial or congenital DI has been reported in a family of Siberian huskies, a Miniature Poodle, and a German Shepherd Dog [160,161]. Secondary nephrogenic DI is often seen in critically ill animals.

There is no known age or sex predilection. In a retrospective study of 20 dogs, central DI was observed in middle-aged to older animals [162]. In a case report of five cats with central DI, all animals were under 3 years of age with a history of prior trauma present or possible in all of them [163].

Clinical presentation

The most common clinical signs of DI are marked polyuria (urine production of > 50 mL/kg/day) and polydipsia (water consumption of > 100 mL/kg/day). Dehydration, urinary bladder distension, lethargy, anorexia, and neurological signs such as seizures may also occur. Neurological signs may occur due to acute and profound hypernatremia [161].

Clinical pathology

Findings on CBC are often normal, but increases in hematocrit and hyperproteinemia may be observed in dehydrated or hypovolemic animals with DI. Serum biochemistry findings may include prerenal azotemia, hypernatremia, and increased serum osmolarity (> 375 mOsm/L). Decreased blood urea nitrogen (BUN) concentration may be due to polyuria and ADH deficiency [164]. Urine specific gravity (USG) often reveals consistently low USG (hyposthenuria). In cats, hyposthenuria with a USG between 1.003 and 1.006 has been reported [163]. In dogs with central DI, consistently low USG, either hyposthenuria or isosthenuria, may be seen due to the inability to concentrate urine [162].

Diagnosis and treatment

Persistent inability to concentrate urine during a water deprivation test and a history of severe PU/PD are diagnostic findings of DI. Animals with central DI will be hyposthenuric despite being dehydrated due to the lack of ADH. A definitive diagnosis may be obtained following a modified water deprivation test. Desmopressin acetate (exogenous vasopressin, DDAVP®) is administered intramuscularly, and USG response is evaluated. An increase in USG after desmopressin indicates central DI. Lack of response to desmopressin is suggestive of nephrogenic DI [162,163]. Care should be taken with these diagnostic tests to avoid side effects such as severe dehydration and development of acute hypernatremia. A maximum of 5% dehydration is advised. Diagnostic imaging (CT or MRI) is recommended when central DI is suspected and may reveal a mass or tumor near the pituitary gland [158,162]. Diagnosis of DI may also be reached by ruling out common causes of PU/PD such as DM and HAC. In addition to standard hematology and biochemistry, other tests commonly performed include measurement of serum osmolality, urine electrolytes and culture, and thyroid, adrenal, and liver function tests.

Animals with DI may present with severe dehydration, evidence of free fluid loss, and/or hypernatremia. Emergency treatment includes aggressive fluid therapy, treatment of hypernatremia, and possible administrations of desmopressin. Sodium concentrations should be corrected slowly to prevent cellular swelling and neuronal edema; mild to moderate and/or acute hypernatremia (Na^+ < 180 mEq/L) should be corrected at a rate of $\leq$ 1 mEq/L/h, and severe and/or chronic hypernatremia (Na^+ > 180 mEq/L) should be corrected at a rate of $\leq$ 0.5 mEq/L/h [165]. Free water deficits may be corrected with 5% dextrose in water at a rate of 3–6 mL/kg/h or 0.45% dextrose in water administered at a rate relative to the calculated free water loss [165,166]. If volume resuscitation is required to treat hypovolemia, which may be the case with DI, a crystalloid solution with a sodium concentration similar to the patient's sodium concentration is recommended. This may require making a patient-specific solution by combining crystalloid fluids and hypertonic saline [166]. Exogenous ADH can be provided in the form of desmopressin, 1 drop (1.5–4 μL) of the 100 μg/mL nasal spray, instilled into the conjunctival sac OU every 8–12 h; however, this will be ineffective in patients with nephrogenic DI [167]. Plasma sodium concentrations should be monitored at least every 4 h and central nervous system (CNS) status monitored continuously [165].

Treatment of animals with central DI is accomplished with administration of desmopressin orally or by conjunctival drops [166]. Treatment for nephrogenic DI involves treatment of the underlying cause. Antidiuretic agents such as thiazides and low-sodium and low-protein diets may be used in an attempt to decrease serum sodium concentrations [159,166]. Avoid water restriction in animals with DI to minimize the risk of dehydration and hypovolemia.

Anesthetic considerations and management

Animals with DI may require anesthesia or sedation for elective or urgent procedures not related to the primary disease process. When anesthetizing or sedating animals with DI, animals should be allowed free access to water until premedication to avoid dehydration, hypovolemia, and intraoperative hypotension. For animals treated with desmopressin, the normal desmopressin regimen can be administered prior to anesthesia [2]. Fluid therapy to correct water losses and electrolyte imbalances is required based on the patient's hydration and electrolyte status (see above). Isotonic fluid therapy to avoid development of water depletion and hypernatremia (> 160 mEq/L) may be preferred in some cases.

Balanced anesthesia with reversible, short-acting drugs (e.g., full μ-opioid receptor agonists and benzodiazepines) to allow for a fast recovery after anesthesia is ideal [2]. Although there are no absolute drug contraindications in patients with DI, anesthetic protocols should be based on each individual patient, their comorbidities, and the specific procedure. For example, animals with brain tumors or a history of trauma may have or may develop increased intracranial pressure (ICP). Techniques and agents considered neuroprotective should be instituted, and care should be taken to minimize further increases in ICP, for example, by avoiding drugs known to cause vomiting such as hydromorphone. The clinical relevance of the endocrine effects of α_2-adrenergic receptor agonists is unclear but should be noted. α_2-Adrenergic receptor agonists, such as medetomidine, induce often profound diuresis in dogs and cats likely due to inhibition of ADH release from the CNS [167,168]. These agents should be avoided in hypovolemic or dehydrated patients.

Blood pressure and ECG should be closely monitored as electrolyte derangements are possible [155]. Note that desmopressin does not act on vascular smooth muscle V_1 receptors and, therefore, should not cause excessive vasoconstriction and hypertension. Ventilation should also be carefully monitored and end-tidal carbon dioxide maintained in the low normal range (35–38 mmHg) when there is any suspicion of trauma, a space-occupying brain lesion, and/or when neurological signs such as seizures are present prior to anesthesia. Additionally, recovery should occur in a quiet environment, and drugs such as midazolam should be readily available to treat neurological signs. Placement of a urinary catheter before anesthesia or prior to recovery can facilitate accurate urinary output quantification and assessment of hydration status. Hydration status, plasma sodium concentrations, and neurologic status should be closely monitored throughout recovery.

Insulinoma

Insulinoma is a functional tumor of pancreatic β-cells that secretes insulin and is unresponsive to changes in BG [169]. The hypersecretion of insulin leads to episodes of severe hypoglycemia and/or chronic hypoglycemia. Hypoglycemia and accompanying clinical signs can occur when BG is $\leq$ 60 mg/dL. However, animals with chronic hypoglycemia may have even lower BG concentrations and remain asymptomatic. These tumors, which are often malignant, tend to occur in either limb of the pancreas rather than in the body, and most have metastasized at the time of diagnosis [169,170]. In dogs, metastasis is often found within abdominal lymph nodes, liver, and lungs [171–173].

Insulin-secreting tumors are rare in cats [174] and uncommon in dogs [168,173]. In dogs, insulinomas often occur in middle-aged and older dogs (8.5–10 years old) and with a mean bodyweight of > 25 kg [169,175–177]. Insulinoma is the most common pancreatic tumor found in middle-aged and older ferrets (median 4 and 5 years old) [178–180].

Clinical presentation

Clinical signs of insulinoma are often non-specific, may occur intermittently, and are due to severe and/or prolonged hypoglycemia. Signs may be precipitated by fasting, excitement, or exercise. Neurological signs are common and are due to cerebral hypoglycemia (neuroglycopenia). Lack of clinical signs in animals with insulinoma may be due to chronic hypoglycemia resulting in upregulation of cerebral glucose uptake.

The most commonly reported clinical signs associated with insulinoma include seizures, weakness, and changes in consciousness and behavior. Other signs such as collapse, obtundation, tremors, and ataxia may also be observed [181,182]. In ferrets, clinical signs include behavioral changes, irritability, ptyalism, and weakness [181,183]. Seizures occur less commonly in this species compared to dogs and usually only with severe hypoglycemia [184].

Clinical pathology

Hypoglycemia is the most consistent and often the only abnormality noted in animals with insulinoma. Serial blood samples may be required due to BG fluctuation throughout the day. BG concentrations are affected by counter-regulatory mechanisms and feeding. Another possible finding is non-specific increases in liver enzyme activity. Additionally, hypokalemia due to insulin driving potassium into cells may be observed [175,176,185].

Diagnosis and treatment

Fasting hypoglycemia is the hallmark for diagnosis of insulinoma. It occurs due to hyperinsulinism resulting in increased glucose uptake and decreased hepatic glucose output [186]. A normal or increased serum insulin concentration during a hypoglycemic episode (BG < 60 mg/dL) is suggestive of an insulinoma. The insulin:glucose ratio is no longer recommended for diagnosis of insulinoma because of poor accuracy and the potential for abnormal ratios in animals with other causes of hypoglycemia [175,176]. Once insulinoma is suspected or confirmed, abdominal ultrasound and/or CT are indicated for the identification of a pancreatic tumor [187]. Thoracic radiographs should be taken to screen for pulmonary metastases.

Surgical removal of the pancreatic tumor is usually recommended and may improve survival [188]. However, surgery is rarely curative due to tumor malignancy. Metastases to lymph nodes and liver are commonly observed. Overall survival rate reported in dogs undergoing surgery is approximately 20 months (7–42 months), while medically treated dogs have survival rates of approximately 8 months [170,188]. Survival rates for cats are thought to be considerably lower. In ferrets, the mean survival rate reported in one study was 668 days following pancreatic nodulectomy with partial pancreatectomy and 186 days with medical management [188].

Medical management of animals with insulinoma focuses on treating hypoglycemia and reducing the risk of hypoglycemic crisis. Treatment includes feeding small, frequent meals, and/or administering glucocorticoids. Prednisone is the most used corticosteroid, and it is administered to antagonize the effects of insulin and increase gluconeogenesis [173]. Other possible treatments include administration of diazoxide, a benzothiadiazide, that reduces insulin secretion by preventing closure of K^+ ATP channels on the β-cell plasma membrane, preventing depolarization of the cell. Gastrointestinal side effects are common in dogs receiving diazoxide. Streptozotocin, a nitrosourea compound that is toxic to β-cells, has been used occasionally for medical treatment of insulinoma in dogs [189]. Treatment of hypoglycemic crisis involves administration of glucose at 0.5–1 mL/kg of 50% dextrose diluted for IV administration. The typical dextrose dilution used is 2.5–5%, and this can be achieved by adding 50–100 mL of 50% dextrose to a 1-L bag of crystalloids. However, care must be taken to monitor response to therapy closely in animals with insulinoma. Intravenous dextrose can stimulate further insulin secretion and exacerbate hypoglycemia. Blood glucose concentration should be monitored hourly to identify unpredictable changes in BG. Intravenous infusion of glucagon has been reported to help stabilize BG concentrations in a dog with an insulinoma-associated hypoglycemic crisis [190].

Anesthetic considerations

Hypoglycemia should be managed prior to anesthesia. The target BG concentration is 50–60 mg/dL [2,191,192], although animals with insulinomas frequently tolerate resting BG concentrations of

30–40 mg/dL without clinical signs [30]. Preoperative hypoglycemia can be managed with oral glucose supplementation (e.g., corn syrup and dextrose) and/or IV supplementation with 2.5–5% dextrose solution if clinical signs are observed [2]. Additionally, infusion of glucagon at 5–40 ng/kg/min IV CRI following a bolus of 50 ng/kg IV [4,190] or in conjunction with infusion of a low concentration of dextrose [56] could be considered.

Clinical signs of hypoglycemia may be masked by anesthesia and only observed in the postoperative period [27]. Therefore, frequent BG measurements are required when anesthetizing an animal with insulinoma, starting with a baseline preoperative BG concentration [30,169]. Serial intraoperative BG monitoring every 30–60 min is recommended [2,147]. The goal is to maintain intraoperative BG concentrations at or near the baseline concentration that prevented clinical signs associated with neuroglycopenia prior to anesthesia [4,27]. It is important to note that tumor manipulation during surgery may lead to insulin spikes, which may exacerbate hypoglycemia [27]. However, these effects are often transient, and treatment may not be required.

Anesthetic management

Prolonged preoperative fasting in animals with insulinoma must be avoided, and a maximum 8 h fast should be adequate. Patients should be closely monitored, and BG concentrations assessed [56]. Dextrose ($\leq$ 5%) supplementation may be required perioperatively, and BG concentrations should be increased gradually [2,4,191,193]. A separate fluid bag with added dextrose is recommended to minimize the risk of delivering an inadvertent IV bolus. The volume of other fluids administered should be decreased to maintain the overall rate desired (usually 5–10 mL/kg/h of crystalloid) and avoid fluid overload. Serial BG measurements and dextrose titration are critical to avoid hypo- and hyperglycemia. Hyperglycemia should be avoided so that the tumor is not stimulated to release more insulin, which can result in refractory hypoglycemia [2,4,30,169,190,194].

No specific anesthetic protocol is contraindicated for patients with insulinoma, and drug choices should be based on patients' health status and concurrent comorbidities. Adequate analgesia is critical in animals with insulinoma because sympathetic stimulation may result in hyperglycemia, tumor stimulation, and rebound hypoglycemia [169]. Animals undergoing abdominal surgery, including pancreatic tumor excision, require balanced anesthetic and multimodal analgesic protocols. Full μ-opioid receptor agonists are usually part of the premedication and are also administered intraoperatively to provide analgesia and MAC-sparing effects. Administration of low doses of α_2-adrenergic receptor agonists as part of the premedication protocol may be considered. In one study of dogs with insulinoma, a perioperative dose of 5 μg/kg of medetomidine resulted in decreases in plasma insulin concentrations and increases in BG concentrations. The study also reported more stable BG and blood pressures intraoperatively and a decrease in glucose supplementation required during anesthesia. The stable blood pressure observed may be due to the analgesic properties and anesthetic-sparing effects of the α_2-adrenergic receptor agonist [194]. α_2-Adrenergic receptor agonists inhibit pancreatic β-cells resulting in a transient increase in BG [63,151]. Care should be taken when evaluating BG levels after administration of α_2-adrenergic receptor agonists. Locoregional anesthetic techniques, such as epidurals and transversus abdominis plane (TAP) blocks, should be considered to provide multimodal analgesia and further anesthetic-sparing effects. NSAIDs may be beneficial in patients that are not receiving glucocorticoids for medical management. Concurrent administration of NSAIDs and steroids is not recommended due to possible adverse renal and gastrointestinal effects [195]. There are no specific contraindications for induction agents or maintenance of anesthesia. Induction of anesthesia can be performed with agents such as propofol, alfaxalone, ketamine, and midazolam or diazepam, and maintenance with inhalants such as isoflurane or sevoflurane is acceptable.

During anesthetic maintenance, blood pressure, heart rate, ECG, hemoglobin saturation (SpO_2), respiratory rate, end-tidal carbon dioxide, and temperature should be continuously monitored. Maintenance of mean arterial blood pressure above 60 mmHg and prevention of hypoxemia are anesthetic goals [191]. Neuroglycopenic animals are prone to intraoperative hypotension [196–198]. Adequate organ perfusion may help reduce the risk of postoperative complications such as pancreatitis, which is one of the most common complications following partial pancreatectomy. In addition to hypoglycemia, hypothermia is another common complication [194], and active patient warming techniques are advised (Fig. 42.7).

Serial BG measurement should be continued postoperatively. Animals with advanced stages of the disease, with gross metastasis at the time of surgery or with partially resected primary tumors, are likely to have persistent signs of hypoglycemia postoperatively [179,181,183,199]. Persistent postoperative hypoglycemia is associated with decreased survival times in dogs and ferrets [181,199]. Transient hyperglycemia may also occur in some animals due to atrophy of the remaining pancreatic β-cells, and it appears to be a positive prognostic factor [172,181]. Temporary insulin administration may be needed until BG concentrations stabilize [169,191]. Development of DM following insulinoma resection has also been reported and, in these cases, permanent

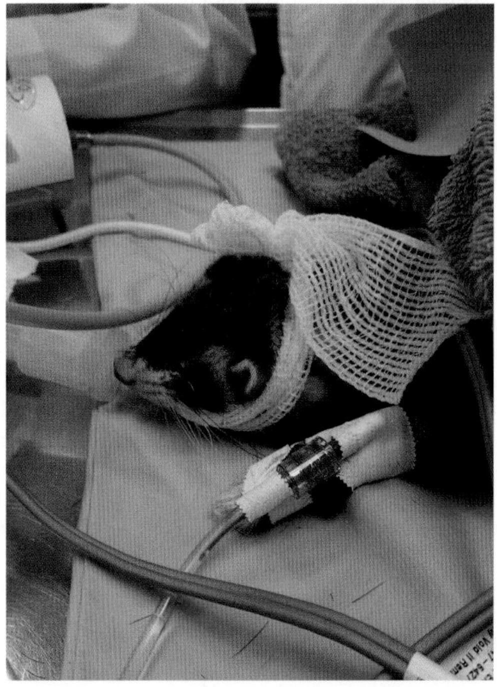

Figure 42.7 Ferret under inhalant anesthesia being monitored with Doppler, oscillometric blood pressure, ECG, pulse oximetry, and capnography. A circulating warm water blanket is used for thermoregulatory support. Source: Dr. Teela Jones, with permission.

insulin treatment may be required [181]. Other potential postoperative complications include duodenal necrosis due to vascular compromise, ventricular arrhythmias, and CNS dysfunction secondary to prolonged hypoglycemia [56,105,191].

Pancreatitis

Although pancreatitis is not considered a endocrinopathy *per se*, the disease may affect both exocrine and endocrine pancreatic functions. While patients are not frequently anesthetized for surgical or medical intervention of pancreatitis, it may be necessary to anesthetize or sedate an animal with concurrent pancreatitis. Pancreatitis is a painful condition and multimodal analgesic protocols are paramount. Sedation with an IV opioid and an analgesic CRI including an opioid, lidocaine, and/or ketamine are recommended. Advanced analgesic techniques may be required due to uncontrolled or refractory pain. A continuous TAP block using bupivacaine administered through a catheter was reported to reduce pain scores in dogs with acute pancreatitis and abdominal pain [200]. The authors routinely perform a combination of caudal intercostal nerve blocks in conjunction with bilateral, cranial TAP blocks and/or epidural regional anesthesia for animals with refractory pain. In people, regional anesthesia with bupivacaine and liposomal-encapsulated bupivacaine has shown promising results for management of pancreatitis and postoperative pain [201–203]. Anecdotally, off-label use of liposomal bupivacaine (Nocita®) for TAP and intercostal nerve blocks can provide efficient and longer lasting analgesia in dogs and cats, but no published data are currently available in veterinary medicine.

Thyroid gland

The thyroid gland has two lobes, one on each side of the trachea. Each lobe is located distal to the larynx, ventrolateral to the trachea, and extending from the fifth to eighth tracheal rings. The thyroid gland is composed of numerous follicles lined by epithelial cells that produce and secrete hormones. These follicles serve as a storage area for precursors of thyroid hormones. Interspersed between the follicles, clusters of parafollicular or C cells are found that produce calcitonin. The parathyroid glands are located in very close proximity to the thyroid gland [3].

The thyroid gland is regulated by the hypothalamic–pituitary–thyroid axis, which is an endocrine negative feedback loop. When thyroid hormone (TH) is needed, the hypothalamus releases thyrotropin-releasing hormone (TRH) that triggers the anterior pituitary gland to secrete thyroid-stimulating hormone (TSH) (also known as "thyrotropin"). TSH stimulates the thyroid gland to release hormones, most importantly thyroxine (T4) and triiodothyronine (T3) (Fig. 42.1). In the liver, kidney, brain, and skeletal muscle, T4 is converted to T3. T3 and, to a lesser extent, T4 control the secretion of TRH and TSH through negative feedback [204,205]. Physiologic concentrations of TH are anabolic and vital to nervous system development, growth, basal metabolism, and thermogenesis.

Hypothyroidism

Reduction of circulating concentrations of the active thyroid hormones T3 and T4 results in hypothyroidism. This clinical syndrome may be congenital or acquired and occurs due to a defect in any part of the hypothalamic–pituitary–thyroid axis. Primary hypothyroidism occurs commonly in dogs, where it is most often an immune-mediated disease caused by lymphocytic infiltration of the thyroid gland with eventual destruction of thyroid tissue [206]. Idiopathic atrophy of the thyroid gland, with no associated inflammatory component, is also described in the dog as a cause of clinical hypothyroidism [206].

Hypothyroidism occurs most often in middle-aged to older dogs (median age 7 years) [206–208]. There is no known sex predilection [209]. Large purebred dogs such as Doberman Pinschers, Great Danes, Irish Setters, English Setters, and Golden Retrievers appear to be predisposed.

Clinical presentation

Clinical signs of hypothyroidism are caused by a decrease in metabolic rate. Signs are vague and non-specific and include weight gain, hair loss, dry skin and hair coat, and decreased activity [207,210]. Other abnormalities such as pyoderma, otitis, seizures, facial paralysis, laryngeal paralysis, megaesophagus, and myopathies have been anecdotally observed in animals with hypothyroidism [210,211].

In severe forms of the disease, myxedema can develop. Myxedema occurs when abnormally high amounts of mucin accumulate in the skin and other tissues resulting in edematous skin. Myxedema coma is a rare syndrome characterized by myxedema, severe lethargy, hypotension, hypoventilation, and hypothermia [212].

Clinical pathology

Mild normocytic normochromic anemia is the most common hematological abnormality present. It is likely due to decreased production of erythropoietin and lack of TH effects on bone marrow [207,210,213].

Serum biochemistry findings include hypercholesterolemia and hypertriglyceridemia [207,210,213]. These abnormalities are common in hypothyroid dogs because inadequate TH levels impact lipid metabolism, including impaired degradation (lipolysis).

Diagnosis and treatment

Routine screening tests to assess total T4 may not be reliable. Factors such as systemic illness (i.e., euthyroid sick syndrome) or the administration of drugs such as corticosteroids, carprofen, and sulfonamides, may decrease total T4 concentrations resulting in an erroneous diagnosis of hypothyroidism [214–216]. A more accurate test is the evaluation of serum free T4 in combination with canine thyroid-stimulating hormone (cTSH) concentrations. However, considerable overlap of test results may still occur in dogs with hypothyroidism compared to dogs with non-thyroid disease [217]. Circulating antibodies against thyroglobulin may be a marker for lymphocytic thyroiditis and could help support the diagnosis [213]. Additionally, TSH stimulation testing could also be performed, but the expense and unavailability of TSH limits the use of this test.

Treatment of hypothyroidism involves daily supplementation with L-thyroxine (levothyroxine, synthetic T4). Follow-up measurement of total T4 approximately 6 h postadministration can be used to monitor treatment success [210]. Therapy may also be monitored based on clinical response and normalization of hematological and biochemical abnormalities.

Anesthetic considerations

Prior to sedation or anesthesia for elective procedures, hypothyroid animals should be appropriately treated with synthetic hormones [2]. Blood work should be performed to assess the possible presence of mild to moderate anemia. In most cases, however, the anemia observed in animals with hypothyroidism is not clinically significant [218]. Severe hypothyroidism resulting in profound cardiovascular and/or neurological effects is rare, but stabilization of these patients prior to anesthesia is critical [4,218]. Stabilization of cases of myxedema coma involves administration of IV thyroid supplementation and cardiovascular support [219].

Muscle weakness and obesity are often present, which may compromise the animal's ability to ventilate spontaneously and oxygenate appropriately during the perioperative period. Markedly obese dogs have reduced function residual capacity and compression and absorption atelectasis due to increased thoracic fat deposition can exacerbate ventilation–perfusion (V/Q) mismatch during anesthesia [220,221]. Positioning the patient in sternal recumbency is recommended when feasible as dorsal recumbency may result in further V/Q mismatch [222]. Ideally, mechanical ventilation should be available to support ventilation intraoperatively when needed. Hair thinning or alopecia is common in hypothyroid animals, which may result in marked intraoperative hypothermia if thermoregulatory support is not provided. Temperature should be closely monitored, and active warming devices utilized.

Dogs with hypothyroidism may also have comorbidities such as laryngeal paralysis and megaesophagus, making them more prone to regurgitation and aspiration pneumonia [27]. Adequate fasting prior to any procedure and rapid airway capture following induction of anesthesia is recommended. Appropriate equipment such as suction canisters with tubing should be readily available to manage regurgitation if it occurs.

Untreated and inadequately treated hypothyroid patients have reduced metabolic rates and decreased hepatic metabolism of drugs, which could potentially prolong recovery after sedation or anesthesia [2,27]. Recoveries may be further delayed in hypothermic patients.

Anesthetic management

No specific drug protocol is contraindicated in well-managed, otherwise healthy animals that are euthyroid at the time of anesthesia. However, patients with poorly controlled or uncontrolled hypothyroidism may present with comorbidities that necessitate anesthesia. Short-acting drugs that are rapidly metabolized or reversible are usually preferred. Especially in a lethargic geriatric animal, an opioid such as methadone or hydromorphone combined with a benzodiazepine such as midazolam generally produces adequate preanesthetic sedation. Acepromazine is an irreversible drug that can exacerbate hypotension and hypothermia; thus, it should not be administered to hypovolemic and/or anemic animals. α_2-Adrenergic receptor agonists may cause or exacerbate hypothermia, bradyarrhythmias, and decreased cardiac output. Since cardiac output may already be impaired in dogs with poorly controlled hypothyroidism due to reduced myocardial contractility, α_2-adrenergic receptor agonists are not usually a first-line choice in these patients [209]. For stable, previously hypothyroid animals, acepromazine and dexmedetomidine are often administered in conjunction with an opioid.

In obese animals, body composition changes may affect the pharmacokinetics and pharmacodynamics of administered drugs [223]. Reduction of anesthetic drug dose or dose calculation based on lean/ideal body weight should be considered in obese hypothyroid dogs [224,225]. Heavy sedation in obese dogs results in poor oxygenation variables and, thus, should be avoided [221], or supplemental oxygen should be provided. Prior to induction of anesthesia, preoxygenation of the hypothyroid dog is recommended. Preoxygenation with a tight-fitting face mask has been shown to prolong the time to desaturation [70,71].

Although it is likely that most anesthetic agents have been used in hypothyroid animals without any perceived increase in anesthetic risk, propofol or alfaxalone and inhalant agents are often recommended for anesthetic induction and maintenance, respectively [2]. Isoflurane produces similar dose-dependent decreases in cardiac output and blood pressure in both euthyroid and hypothyroid dogs and, thus, is a suitable anesthetic in these patients. As with any patient, isoflurane-induced cardiovascular depression can be minimized by using balanced anesthetic techniques [226]. Halothane, though no longer available in many countries, has direct myocardial depressant effects and should be avoided to preserve cardiac output [2,227]. Studies have shown that the MAC of halothane and isoflurane in both euthyroid and hypothyroid dogs are clinically similar [226,228]. Anecdotally, hypothyroid dogs appear to have reduced requirements for anesthetic drugs. This clinical impression may be related to hypothyroid dogs being more prone to hypothermia, which has MAC-sparing effects, as well as inadvertent administration of higher doses of injectable drugs in obese patients. Euthyroid obese dogs have been shown to require smaller effective propofol doses for induction of anesthesia compared to ideal weight dogs when the dosage was calculated based on total body weight [226].

Continuous monitoring of heart rate and rhythm, blood pressure, ventilation, oxygenation, and temperature is important for the anesthetic management of these patients. Fluid therapy rate may be adjusted based on ideal body weight in obese patients [229,230]. Sinus bradycardia, low QRS amplitude, inverted T waves, and decreased left ventricular function have been observed in hypothyroid dogs [210]. Bradycardia and hypotension are common intraoperative complications and should be treated with anticholinergics, crystalloid or synthetic colloid fluid therapy, and positive inotropes [2,4]. Rewarming hypothermic patients may also improve or correct bradycardia and hypotension. Hypoventilation is common, especially when obesity is present, and mechanical ventilation may be required to maintain normocapnia and adequate oxygenation. Thermoregulatory support should be provided to prevent and treat hypothermia.

Slow recoveries may occur as mentioned previously. Diligent monitoring with pulse oximetry, provision of ventilatory support, oxygen supplementation, and active warming, when indicated, are vital during the recovery period. Patients with myxedema coma may require IV hormone replacement therapy with L-thyroxine postoperatively [27,231].

Hyperthyroidism

Excessive circulating concentrations of active T3 and T4 result in hyperthyroidism. This clinical syndrome is usually caused by poorly controlled hypersecretion of TH from autonomously hyperfunctional nodules of the thyroid gland [232]. The etiology of this disease is unknown but, similar to human patients with toxic nodular goiter, activating mutations of TSH receptors may be involved [233].

In cats, the most common thyroid gland disease resulting in hyperthyroidism is benign adenomatous hyperplasia [234,235]. In rare cases (only 1–2% of cats with thyrotoxicosis), thyroid carcinoma is the cause. Hyperthyroidism occurs much less commonly in dogs compared to cats, and thyroid carcinoma is the most common cause in this species. Hyperthyroidism is documented in less than 20% of dogs diagnosed with thyroid carcinoma [236]. In contrast to thyroid adenomas in cats, thyroid carcinomas in dogs are usually large and invasive [237].

Hyperthyroidism is one of the most common disorders of middle-aged and older cats (mean age 12 years) [238,239]. There is no sex or breed predilection [234,238,239].

Clinical presentation

Clinical signs of hyperthyroidism are multisystemic and caused by pathologically high metabolism due to sustained excessive circulating TH concentrations. High levels of TH are catabolic and cause increased gluconeogenesis, protein breakdown, and nitrogen wasting. Common clinical signs include weight loss with normal or increased appetite, polyphagia, vomiting, diarrhea, PU/PD, hyperactivity, and behavioral changes that can range from depression to aggression.

Hypertension, myocardial hypertrophy, chronic cellular malnutrition, hepatocellular stress, and decreased gastrointestinal transit time are also observed in animals with hyperthyroidism [234,238,239]. Physical examination findings include poor body condition, tachycardia, heart murmur, gallop rhythm, palpable unilateral or bilateral thyroid nodules, and an unkempt hair coat (Fig. 42.8) [238,239].

Thyrotoxic storm, described as a syndrome of severe hyperthyroidism, occurs rarely in cats and dogs [240–242]. This life-threatening manifestation of the disease results in severe tachycardia, fever, gastrointestinal signs, and CNS signs. Thyrotoxic storm is not well described in veterinary medicine, and specific triggers are unknown.

Clinical pathology

Mild erythrocytosis is the most common hematological finding in cats with hyperthyroidism [239]. This is likely mediated through TH effects (β-adrenergic stimulation) on the bone marrow and an increase in oxygen consumption resulting in increased erythropoietin levels.

Serum biochemistry findings include mild to marked elevation of liver-derived enzyme activity, a mild increase in BUN without a concurrent increase in creatinine concentrations, and hypokalemia. Elevations in alanine aminotransferase (ALT) and/or serum ALP activity are found in approximately 75% of hyperthyroid cats. A study of hyperthyroid cats with severe elevations in liver enzymes showed normal liver function [243]. Increased BUN occurs due to increased protein catabolism. Elevations in both BUN and creatinine levels may indicate the presence of concurrent renal disease [234,235,239,243,244]. Hypokalemia may be observed in hyperthyroid cats due to movement of potassium from the extracellular space into the intracellular space stimulated by high TH levels and stress-induced release of catecholamines [245,246].

Animals with thyrotoxic storm have similar clinical pathology findings to those described above. However, these animals also present with extremely high concentrations of TH [242].

Diagnosis and treatment

Enlargement of one or both thyroid glands can be detected during physical examination in many cats with hyperthyroidism; however, this is not a pathognomonic finding. Diagnosis is based on clinical presentation, as described above, and measurement of total T4 levels. High serum total T4 concentration confirms the diagnosis in most cases [247]. Some hyperthyroid cats may have occult hyperthyroidism with normal total T4 concentrations. This may be due to fluctuations in hormone concentrations or concurrent non-thyroidal disease. In these cases, other diagnostic tests such as measurement of free T4, repeated measurements of total T4, thyroid scintigraphy, or T3 suppression testing may be required [247,248].

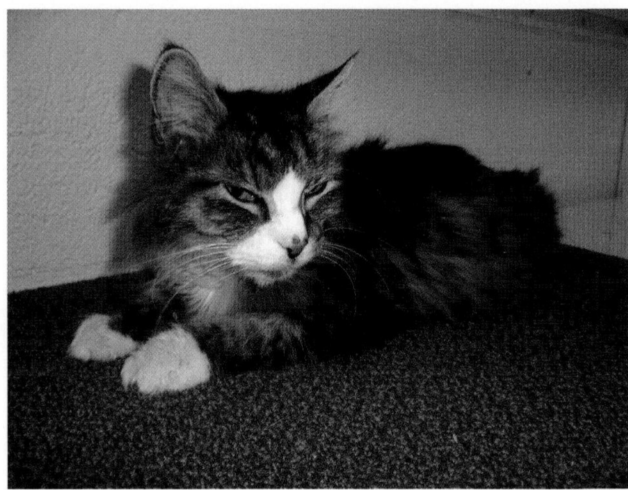

(A)

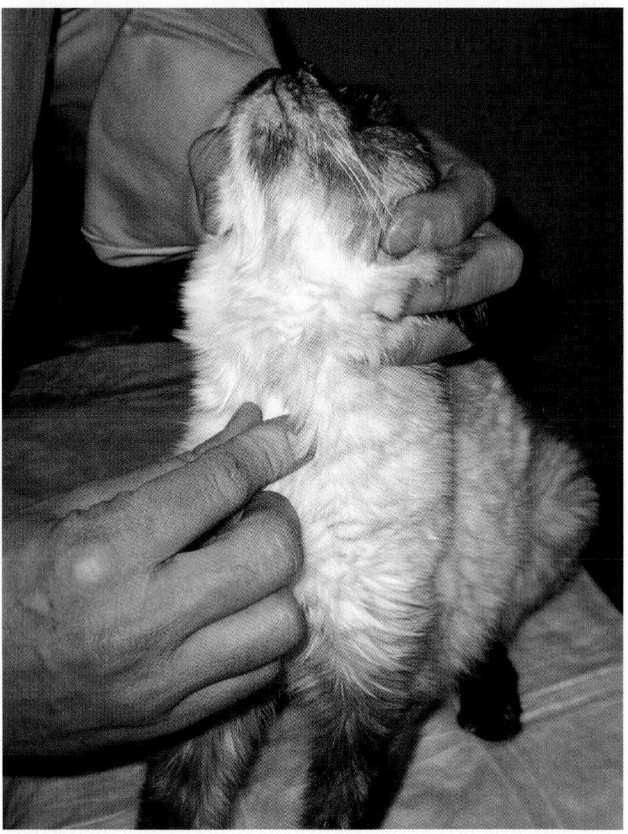

(B)

Figure 42.8 **A.** A cat with hyperthyroidism presented with weight loss and depression. These signs suggest that poorly controlled hyperthyroidism and elective anesthesia should be delayed. Source: Dr. Todd Green, Department of Small Animal Medicine and Surgery, St. George's University, St. George's, Grenada; with permission. **B.** Thyroid nodule palpation in a cat with hyperthyroidism. Source: Dr. Thomas Graves, with permission.

Heart murmurs and gallop sounds are often detected during physical examination of cats with hyperthyroidism and concurrent comorbidities such as hypertrophic cardiomyopathy (HCM) may be present. Therefore, thoracic imaging and echocardiography may be useful in assessing the cardiovascular system of these patients.

The cardiac biomarkers N-terminal pro-brain natriuretic peptide (NTproBNP) and cardiac troponin I were elevated in cats with hyperthyroidism before treatment but were not able to distinguish between thyrotoxic myopathy and primary feline HCM [238]. In hyperthyroid dogs, thoracic radiographs are recommended to investigate the presence of pulmonary metastases. Abdominal ultrasound may be performed in hyperthyroid cats to assess renal architecture and size, although further renal testing may better define renal function.

The treatment of choice for feline hyperthyroidism is radioiodine therapy. It is non-invasive, has few side effects, and is effective in most cases [249]. Another effective treatment option is medical management with methimazole or carbimazole [250]. However, these antithyroid drugs often cause side effects such as vomiting, self-induced facial excoriation, and anorexia. Surgical thyroidectomy is less common in cats but is still performed in some cases [246]. Surgical complications include iatrogenic hypoparathyroidism, laryngeal paralysis, and hypothyroidism. Approximately 30% of cats with hyperthyroidism develop mild but stable renal failure following medical treatment [251]. β-Adrenergic receptor antagonists, amlodipine, or ACE inhibitors may be used to manage tachycardia and hypertension in cats with hyperthyroidism [27,156,252].

Management of thyroid carcinoma in dogs is dependent on the size and stage of the tumor [236]. Surgery may be a viable option for small non-invasive tumors. Large or non-resectable tumors may require radiation and chemotherapy; however, treatment is rarely curative.

Although uncommon, thyroid storm is usually treated with antithyroid drugs to decrease hormone synthesis. TH secretion may be inhibited by administration of iodine (oral potassium iodide, oral ipodate, or IV sodium iodide). Additionally, corticosteroids may be administered to inhibit the peripheral conversion of T4 to the active hormone T3. Hyperthermia should be treated and fluid therapy used to correct dehydration. If the patient presents in heart failure, appropriate management (e.g., diuretic agents) should be initiated. Tachyarrhythmias may be treated with β-adrenergic blockers.

Anesthetic considerations

Whenever possible, hyperthyroidism should be treated prior to sedation or general anesthesia. Medications including methimazole can be administered on the morning of surgery. A preoperative thyroid panel can confirm a euthyroid state. If total T4 or free T4 are above the reference range, elective procedures should be postponed, and treatment with carbimazole or methimazole for 6–12 weeks may be indicated to minimize anesthetic and surgical complications [253].

A thorough examination should be performed to assess the cardiorespiratory system and hydration status. Blood work will help assess hydration (PCV and TS) and renal function (BUN and creatinine) and reveal any electrolyte abnormalities (e.g., potassium and calcium) [156]. Baseline ECG and blood pressure measurements should be obtained, especially if a heart murmur, gallop rhythm, HCM, or azotemia is present or suspected. Hypertension may be seen in animals with untreated or unregulated hyperthyroidism and/or with chronic kidney disease (CKD). In hypertensive animals with CKD, renal autoregulatory mechanisms that normally stabilize GFR over a wide range of blood pressures (80–180 mmHg) may be impaired and shifted to a higher range. Therefore, even mild decreases in blood pressure during anesthesia may decrease renal blood flow and GFR. The authors recommend maintaining the arterial blood pressure within 20% of resting blood pressure measurements as a goal. Additionally, preanesthetic fluids to restore normovolemia and hydration may be considered [254], but caution is advised in animals with cardiac abnormalities. Correcting dehydration preoperatively and preserving cardiac output through use of anesthetic-sparing techniques may help reduce episodes of intraoperative hypotension.

Intraoperative hypotension may be exacerbated in hypertensive animals treated with drugs such as atenolol, amlodipine, or ACE inhibitors. A study in healthy dogs treated with enalapril showed increased severity of intraoperative hypotension. Extrapolating from these data, withholding ACE inhibitors for 24 h prior to the scheduled procedure could be considered [60].

Hemorrhage during surgical excision of thyroid tumors may occur. Many of these tumors are highly vascularized and, especially in dogs, they are often large and invasive. Patients with larger tumors should be blood typed and crossmatched prior to anesthesia, and blood products should be readily available to manage intraoperative blood loss.

A possible postoperative complication, especially following bilateral thyroidectomy, is the development of transient hypocalcemia. Hypocalcemia may occur due to removal, damage, or local edema of the parathyroid glands. Postoperative measurement of calcium levels is advised, and supplementation may be required [246,255,256].

Anesthetic management

If emergency surgery is required in an untreated hyperthyroid cat, cardiovascular stabilization is paramount. Fluid resuscitation and electrolyte supplementation may be required, especially in cats experiencing PU/PD and vomiting. Cats with concurrent hypertrophic cardiomyopathy, tachyarrhythmias, or hypertension should be managed as described previously.

No specific drug protocol is contraindicated in treated, otherwise healthy cats that are euthyroid on the time of anesthesia. However, many cats with hyperthyroidism are presented with comorbidities requiring specific anesthetic management. When sedating or anesthetizing these animals, the goal should be to minimize increases in oxygen consumption, hypertension, tachycardia, and arrhythmias. Pain- and stress-induced catecholamine release should be avoided or minimized; therefore, multimodal analgesia and low-stress handling techniques are paramount.

Premedication of hyperthyroid cats generally includes administration of an opioid. Opioids cause dose-dependent decreases in heart rate and, thus, myocardial oxygen consumption. If dogs and cats are undergoing non-painful procedures, butorphanol is often the agent of choice. For surgical or painful procedures, a full μ-opioid receptor agonist is generally used. Benzodiazepines or acepromazine may be included in the preanesthetic protocol [257]. Benzodiazepines are good choices for sick, unstable animals due to minimal cardiorespiratory effects, but in healthy animals, paradoxical excitement or disinhibition may ensue. Acepromazine, an α-adrenergic receptor antagonist, causes vasodilation and could help counteract pre-existing hypertension. It may also reduce the sensitivity of the myocardium to catecholamines thus decreasing the occurrence of catecholamine-induced arrhythmias. Acepromazine, however, has long-lasting, irreversible effects and may worsen intraoperative hypotension. Its use should be avoided when the patient is hypovolemic, on antihypertensive medication, or when tumors are large or invasive with increased risk of blood loss. In cats with HCM, acepromazine is usually avoided because it may reduce preload and increase the pressure gradient across the left ventricular outflow tract in these patients. Low doses of α_2-adrenergic receptor agonists such as dexmedetomidine may increase preload, reduce heart rate, and enhance diastolic filling in some patients with HCM [258], but this must be weighed against the potential for reduced cardiac output. In fractious cats, alfaxalone could be added to the preanesthetic protocol to improve sedation. It causes dose-dependent immobilization with minimal cardiorespiratory depression [258–260].

Intravenous propofol or alfaxalone are common agents used to induce anesthesia but can cause dose-dependent hypotension and hypoventilation [261]. Etomidate can also be used, especially for cats with advanced heart disease. This agent has minimal cardiovascular effects and is usually co-administered with a benzodiazepine. However, etomidate may not be the drug of choice for systemically ill patients undergoing invasive procedures due to its transient suppression of cortisol secretion. Propofol and alfaxalone can also be co-administered with a benzodiazepine, which reduces the required dose of the primary anesthetic agent, potentially reducing side effects [262].

Induction doses of dissociative, sympathomimetic anesthetic agents such as ketamine stimulate sympathetic output resulting in an increase in heart rate and a decrease in ventricular filling [2,257]. Telazol® also increases sympathetic tone resulting in an increase in heart rate and mean arterial pressure [263]. Drugs known to increase heart rate and myocardial oxygen demand or consumption should be avoided or used with caution in hyperthyroid cats, especially if HCM is also present. Chamber induction of anesthesia with an inhalant agent is also not recommended due to the high stress levels associated with this technique, environmental contamination, and limited monitoring ability.

Anesthesia is generally maintained with inhalant anesthetics such as isoflurane or sevoflurane. Halothane, though no longer available in many countries, was historically avoided in these patients as it could sensitize the myocardium to catecholamines and produce arrhythmias [264]. A balanced anesthesia protocol with short-acting opioid infusions and locoregional anesthetic techniques will help maintain adequate anesthetic depth, supplement analgesia, and avoid exaggerated sympathetic nervous system responses [27].

Blood pressure, heart rate, and ECG should be closely monitored. Invasive (direct) blood pressure monitoring is considered the gold standard and should be performed in patients that are critically ill, have renal or cardiac disease, or are undergoing surgery for large or invasive tumor resection. Fluid rates should be tailored to the patients' health status; they should be decreased in patients with cardiac disease or congestive heart failure, or marginally increased in patients with renal disease [265]. The increased metabolic rate associated with feline hyperthyroidism increases demand for oxygen and glucose, and production of carbon dioxide. This, combined with poor body condition and possible muscle weakness, makes these animals more prone to hypoxemia, hypercapnia, and hypothermia. Preoxygenation, provision of thermoregulatory support, continuous monitoring with pulse oximetry and capnography, and ventilatory support are recommended.

Hyperthyroid animals, especially if receiving antihypertensive drugs, may have refractory hypotension intraoperatively, requiring positive inotropes. In cats with nonobstructive HCM, dopamine was reported to increase cardiac output. However, in HCM cats with outflow tract obstruction, positive inotropes may increase obstruction to blood flow further decreasing cardiac output. Management of hypotension in cats with HCM is often challenging [266]. Phenylephrine was reported to increase blood pressure in cats with HCM but did not increase cardiac output [266]. If profound bradycardia and hypotension persist despite adequate anesthetic depth, normothermia, and provision of MAC-sparing drugs, a low-dose dobutamine infusion or anticholinergic may be required. Anticholinergics may reduce diastolic filling due to tachycardia [267] and are usually avoided by the authors, except in emergency situations. These agents cause parasympathetic blockade leading to an increase in myocardial oxygen consumption and increased arrhythmogenicity. Dobutamine in hypovolemic patients or at high infusion rates may result in tachyarrhythmias and should be used with caution. However, dobutamine may be a more favorable option in this situation due to its short duration of action.

Anesthetic recovery should occur in a quiet place and sedation may be administered. To smooth recovery and decrease stress-related catecholamine release, a low dose of a sedative such as acepromazine (0.005–0.01 mg/kg IV) may be administered if there are no contraindications. Thyrotoxic storm may be seen in the postanesthetic period. This is rare but may occur in untreated or poorly managed hyperthyroid patients. Monitoring of heart rate and rhythm, respiratory rate, blood pressure, body temperature, and, ideally, pulse oximetry should be continued throughout recovery.

Thyroid neoplasia

In dogs, most thyroid tumors are non-functional carcinomas, and they do not secrete excessive TH. Pulmonary metastases are common, and local invasion of tissues such as the trachea, esophagus, musculature, and vasculature may occur [268]. Dogs with thyroid tumors usually present with a large space-occupying lesion in the ventral cervical region (Fig. 42.9).

Clinical signs are associated with the size of the thyroid tumor and secondary damage to the cervical tissues. These may include stridor, dyspnea, coughing, gagging, dysphagia, anorexia, weight loss, and concurrent laryngeal paralysis [268,269].

Diagnostic evaluation of thyroid tumors includes biopsy of the mass and serum TH measurement. Thoracic radiographs are indicated to identify pulmonary metastases [268]. Other imaging modalities, such as CT or MRI, may identify the extent of local invasion. Thyroidectomy is preferred for mobile, well-differentiated tumors, whereas unresectable tumors can sometimes be treated with radiation or radioactive iodine-131 [268].

Anesthetic considerations and management

Maintenance of a patent airway, provision of analgesia, and readiness to manage possible sudden blood loss are the main goals of anesthesia. Hemorrhage has been reported as the most common intraoperative complication in thyroidectomies [268]. Blood products should be available and, ideally, preanesthetic evaluation should include a coagulation panel, blood type, and cross-match [270]. Aspiration pneumonia has been the most reported postoperative complication following tumor resection [269]. Laryngeal paralysis may be identified postoperatively; therefore, airway examination at the time of intubation and extubation is warranted [269].

Combinations of dexmedetomidine or acepromazine with hydromorphone or butorphanol have been studied for provision of sedation while maintaining laryngeal function for airway evaluation [271,272]. Heavy sedation should be performed cautiously in patients with respiratory compromise, and equipment for intubation along with an injectable induction agent, such as

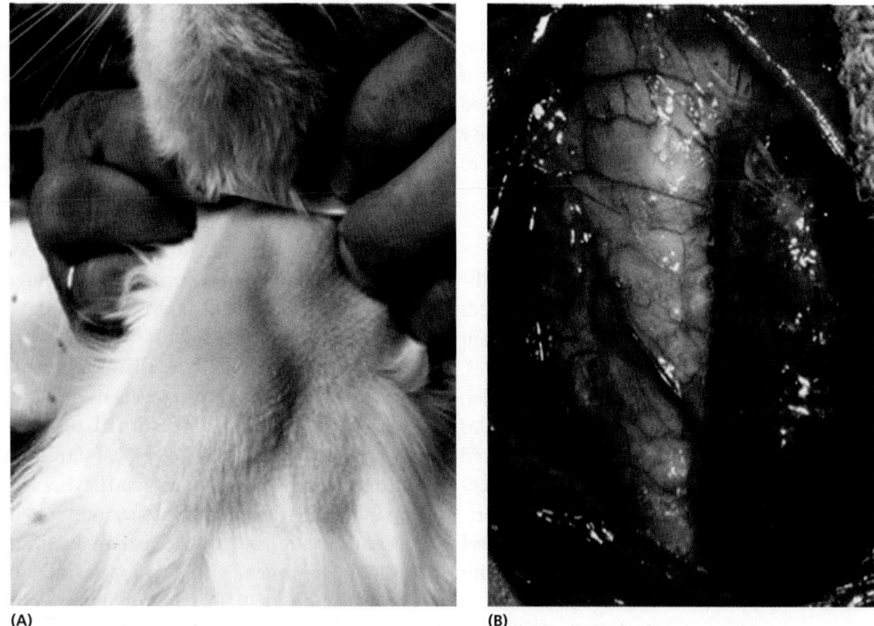

Figure 42.9 **A.** Although large thyroid masses are most common in dogs, cats are occasionally diagnosed with this disease. Large space-occupying masses can be associated with respiratory distress prior to anesthesia and may represent a challenge for endotracheal intubation. Source: Dr. Robert Sherding, Department of Veterinary Clinical Sciences, The Ohio State University, Columbus, OH; with permission. **B.** Large mass in the ventral neck compressing the trachea. Airway obstruction may occur in recovery due to edema and hemorrhage. Source: Dr. Stephen Birchard, Circle City Veterinary Specialty and Emergency Hospital, Carmel, IN; with permission.

propofol, should be readily available. Although full μ-opioid receptor agonists can cause dose-related respiratory depression, they are routinely administered for invasive and/or painful procedures and are still considered the gold standard for analgesia. However, opioids associated with high incidences of gastroesophageal reflux and/or regurgitation, such as morphine and hydromorphone [273,274], may be best avoided.

Prior to induction of anesthesia, preoxygenation is recommended to prolong the time to desaturation [71]. If tracheal invasion is present, multiple endotracheal tubes, guarded endotracheal tubes, and tracheostomy supplies should be available. Propofol or alfaxalone is often administered for induction of anesthesia, especially if airway evaluation is being performed prior to endotracheal intubation [272]. Alternatively, a ketamine–benzodiazepine combination may be administered to induce anesthesia and will provide additional analgesia. All induction agents should be administered to effect as they cause dose-dependent respiratory depression. Inhalant anesthetics such as isoflurane or sevoflurane are typically used for maintenance of anesthesia.

Direct arterial blood pressure, pulse oximetry, ECG, and capnography should be monitored intraoperatively. Volume resuscitation during acute hemorrhage may include isotonic crystalloids, artificial colloids, and/or blood products, preferably whole blood transfusion, depending on the magnitude of blood lost [106]. Hypertonic saline 7.5% (4 mL/kg IV over 10–20 min) has been shown to improve hemodynamic performance without inducing signs of volume overload in a canine model of hemorrhagic shock [108]. Multimodal analgesia and anesthetic-sparing techniques will allow reduction of delivered inhalant concentrations and thereby minimize adverse cardiovascular side effects. Alterations in renal blood flow and renal injury may occur in patients receiving NSAIDs that experience hypotension/hypovolemia during anesthesia [275]. Therefore, it is recommended to delay NSAID administration until the postoperative period when the patient's hemodynamic status has been re-evaluated and determined to be stable.

Complications during recovery may be related to laryngeal paralysis, aspiration pneumonia, tracheal compression, and hemorrhage. To reduce the incidence of aspiration pneumonia during extubation and promote adequate ventilation, the patient should recover in sternal recumbency with the head slightly elevated. A strong swallow should be evident before removing the endotracheal tube. If regurgitation is observed or suspected, leaving the endotracheal tube cuff partially inflated during extubation may further protect the airway from gastric contents. Supplies for induction of anesthesia and rapid re-intubation should be readily available in the event of airway obstruction.

Hypocalcemia may develop in cases where the parathyroid gland was not preserved, requiring supplementation with calcium and vitamin D [276]. Serial measurements of ionized calcium should be considered in cases where preservation of the parathyroid gland was not possible or is uncertain.

Parathyroid gland

The parathyroid glands are located near the thyroid gland [3]. Dogs and cats have four parathyroid glands, two embedded near the caudomedial pole of each lobe of the thyroid and two external glands typically on the cranial dorsolateral surface of the thyroid lobe. Ectopic parathyroid tissue is common in cats, less so in dogs [277]. The parathyroid glands have densely packed cells surrounding capillary vessels [3].

Parathyroid glands produce and secrete parathyroid hormone (PTH) in response to decreased serum calcium concentrations. There are no PTH releasing or stimulating hormones. PTH increases serum calcium via three main mechanisms: (1) it stimulates activity of osteoclasts to reabsorb bone; (2) it results in absorption of calcium from the gastrointestinal tract (GIT) via the activated form of vitamin D, which is produced in the kidney; and (3) it reduces excretion of calcium in the urine [3]. In healthy animals, normal or increased serum ionized calcium (*i*Ca) concentrations have a strong negative feedback effect on PTH secretion and also stimulate the thyroid to release calcitonin which has opposite effects of PTH (Fig. 42.1).

Hyperparathyroidism

Increased concentrations of circulating PTH result in hyperparathyroidism. When excessive amounts of PTH are produced, persistent hypercalcemia occurs and calcification of soft tissues, with resultant dysfunction of affected structures or organs, ensues. Hyperparathyroidism can be a primary or secondary disorder. Primary hyperparathyroidism is generally caused by a singular benign adenoma of an extracapsular parathyroid gland. Parathyroid adenomas autonomously secrete PTH, causing hypercalcemia [278,279]. Parathyroid adenocarcinomas are very rare. Secondary hyperparathyroidism is an adaptive increase in PTH induced by hypocalcemia and hyperphosphatemia associated with CKD or an unbalanced diet [280]. The following discussion is focused on primary hyperparathyroidism in the dog.

Primary hyperparathyroidism is an uncommon disorder of middle-aged and older dogs (mean age 10.2 years) and is a rare condition in cats. There is no known breed or sex predilection [278,281–283]. However, a genetic predisposition for parathyroid tumors has been found in Keeshonds [284].

Clinical presentation

Clinical signs of primary hyperparathyroidism are often lacking. In many cases, an incidental finding of increased total calcium (*t*Ca) concentration on routine blood work warrants further investigation and measurement of ionized calcium (*i*Ca) concentration. Ionized calcium is the physiologic active form and is a superior measurement compared with *t*Ca in patients with hyperparathyroidism [285]. Furthermore, prediction of *i*Ca based on *t*Ca concentration was less accurate in patients with concurrent diseases such as CKD [285]. On physical examination, parathyroid adenomas are small and rarely palpable in dogs, but they may be palpable in cats [286,287]. Some animals may display mild clinical signs because of severity or chronicity of hypercalcemia.

Polyuria and polydipsia are the most commonly reported clinical signs. Hypercalcemia interferes with the ability of the kidneys to concentrate urine resulting in polyuria. There is an impaired response to ADH due to calcium interference with vasopressin V_2 receptors in the renal tubules. Activation of calcium-sensing receptors decreases reabsorption of sodium, potassium, and chloride and causes downregulation of aquaporin-2 water channels. Polydipsia follows to compensate for fluid loss from frequent urination [278,288]. In severe cases, or with chronic hypercalcemia, animals may present dehydrated or hypovolemic.

Lower urinary tract inflammation and urolithiases (calcium-containing urinary stones) in the bladder, ureters, or kidneys may also be identified in animals with hyperparathyroidism. In addition, hypercalcemia affects intestinal function, and animals may present for vomiting, weight loss, constipation, or anorexia.

Clinical pathology

Hypercalcemia is the most consistent finding in animals with hyperparathyroidism. High calcium causes increased excretion of other electrolytes such as phosphorus, sodium, and potassium. Serum biochemistry may reveal hypophosphatemia and azotemia. Urinalysis may reveal low USG. These findings may be due to the diuretic effects of hypercalcemia; however, chronic hypercalcemia may cause renal damage resulting in CKD in some dogs [27,279]. Acid–base status and urea and creatinine concentrations should be assessed in patients with suspected CKD.

Diagnosis and treatment

Diagnosis of hyperparathyroidism is based on elevated *i*Ca, a history of PU/PD, a low or low-normal serum phosphorus concentration, and an inappropriately high serum concentration of PTH. A "normal" concentration of PTH in the presence of hypercalcemia is also indicative of hyperparathyroidism because PTH secretion should be suppressed by increased levels of calcium [289]. PTH has been reported to be within the normal reference range in cats with hyperparathyroidism [285]. Cervical ultrasonography correlates well with direct tumor measurements and has been recommended [287,290]. Urinalysis and abdominal ultrasound often reveal urinary tract infections, cystic calculi, and renal mineralization [278,287].

Initial treatment of hypercalcemia includes intravenous administration of 0.9% sodium chloride (100–125 mL/kg/day) aimed at improving GFR, increasing renal calcium and sodium excretion, and thus decreasing calcium reabsorption [291,292]. Additionally, some animals may also be hypovolemic due to urinary and gastrointestinal water losses, and fluid resuscitation is paramount. Water *ad libitum* should be available to animals with hypercalcemia. Once normovolemic, furosemide, a loop diuretic, can be administered (2–4 mg/kg twice or three times daily) to help increase renal calcium excretion. To further decrease calcium concentrations in animals with persistent hypercalcemia, prednisolone or dexamethasone may be used to reduce bone and intestinal absorption of calcium and increase renal calcium excretion (Table 42.4) [27,291,293]. In cases with life-threatening hypercalcemia [*t*Ca > 17–20 mg/dL (4.3–5.0 mmol/dL)], sodium bicarbonate, administered IV as a slow bolus, can decrease *i*Ca by promoting binding of calcium to albumin [279].

Surgical parathyroidectomy is curative and is the most commonly performed treatment option. It allows for direct excision of the tumor while sparing the thyroid gland and the remaining healthy parathyroid gland. Ultrasound-guided ethanol ablation is a minimally invasive alternative to surgical parathyroidectomy, but

Table 42.4 Treatments for hypercalcemia in dogs with hyperparathyroidism.

Treatment	Dose	Comments
0.9% saline	90–120 mL/kg q 24 h IV	Volume expansion dilutes serum Ca^{2+}, extra Na^+ in renal tubules ↓ Ca^{2+} reabsorption
Furosemide[a]	2–4 mg/kg q 8–12 h IV	↑ Ca^{2+} loss in urine ↓ reabsorption in bone
Prednisone	1–2 mg/kg q 12 h PO	↓ intestinal absorption
Dexamethasone	0.1–0.2 mg/kg q 12 h IV	↑ excretion in urine
Calcitonin	4–6 IU/kg q 8–12 h SC	↓ activity of osteoclasts
Pamidronate	1.3–2 mg/kg in 150 mL of 0.9% NaCl IV over 2–4 h	Inhibits osteoclast-mediated bone resorption ↑ Ca^{2+} uptake by bone
Sodium bicarbonate	1 mEq/kg IV slowly up to 4 mEq/kg	↑ binding of Ca^{2+} to albumin Emergency situations only

↑, increase; ↓, decrease; q, every.
[a] Not all diuretics are useful; for example, thiazides should be avoided as they cause acidosis which increases ionized Ca^{2+}.
Source: Schenk and Chew [291]; Green and Chew [293].

ethanol may not destroy the entire tumor and repeat administration may be needed. Percutaneous ultrasound-guided radiofrequency heat ablation has also been reported and resulted in few short- or long-term complications [288,294]. Coughing, change in bark, and Horner's syndrome have been reported as postoperative complications after ethanol and heat ablation [294].

Anesthetic considerations and management

Although administration of calcitriol (active vitamin D metabolite) 3–5 days prior to anesthesia has been reported, a more recent retrospective study found no protective value in its prophylactic administration to prevent hypocalcemia in the postoperative period (48 h) after parathyroidectomy [279,295]. If calcitriol is administered, careful monitoring of serum calcium and clinical signs should be performed, and therapy discontinued if hypercalcemia worsens [291].

A thorough preanesthetic evaluation is required, and hydration status and electrolyte imbalances corrected. Serum calcium concentration should be measured, and symptomatic animals treated appropriately, as described above. Anesthesia should be postponed when *t*Ca is greater than 15–16 mg/dL (3.75–4 mmol/L) due to the increased risk of side effects such as arrhythmias. Although there are conflicting data regarding predictors of postoperative hypocalcemia, high *i*Ca concentrations may increase the risk of postoperative hypocalcemia after surgical removal or heat ablation in dogs with primary hyperparathyroidism [283,291,296,297].

Absolute hypovolemia due to volume depletion in addition to the relative hypovolemia caused by drug-induced vasodilation can greatly affect maintenance of normal blood pressures intraoperatively. The presence or suspicion of CKD is another reason to maintain adequate hydration status and ensure normovolemia before anesthesia [56]. Perioperatively, a calcium-free isotonic crystalloid solution is preferred (e.g., Normosol-R®) in animals with high *i*Ca. If renal dysfunction is present, fluid rates up to 20–30 mL/kg/h during anesthesia may be required [298,299]. The authors usually maintain fluid rates at approximately 10 mL/kg/h. Especially in dogs with higher preoperative calcium concentrations, renal failure may be unmasked postoperatively, and renal values should be closely monitored [279]. Consider placing a urinary catheter to measure urine output intra- and postoperatively.

Anesthetic drug choices should be based on the animal health status and concurrent comorbidities. There are no anesthetic drugs or techniques specifically contraindicated for euvolemic dogs with primary hyperparathyroidism undergoing elective procedures. Animals with a history of vomiting may benefit from administration of an antiemetic agent such as maropitant 30–60 min prior to opioid premedication. Alternatively, opioids associated with lower incidences of vomiting, such as methadone, meperidine, and fentanyl, could be used as part of the premedication protocol. Full μ-opioid receptor agonists are generally administered to provide appropriate analgesia. α_2-Adrenergic receptor agonists, such as dexmedetomidine and medetomidine, benzodiazepines, and/or phenothiazines (acepromazine), are often included in the intramuscular protocol to provide sedation. Induction of anesthesia can be accomplished with propofol, alfaxalone, ketamine–benzodiazepine, or etomidate, and anesthesia is generally maintained with an inhalant anesthetic. Constant rate infusions of lidocaine, dexmedetomidine, ketamine, and/or short-acting full μ-opioid receptor agonists may be delivered intraoperatively for MAC-sparing effects. For further multimodal analgesia, NSAIDs may be beneficial in animals without renal dysfunction and that are not receiving glucocorticoids. Although there are no reports in the veterinary literature, humans with hyperparathyroidism and hypercalcemia required higher doses of vecuronium than patients without hyperparathyroidism [297]. However, non-depolarizing muscle relaxants are rarely required for parathyroidectomies in veterinary patients.

Heart rate, ECG, and blood pressure should be closely monitored. Hypercalcemia is associated with increased myocardial contractility and, in severe cases, can progress to incomplete or complete atrioventricular block and cardiac arrest. ECG changes are characterized by slowed conduction and include bradycardia, a prolonged PR interval, a widened QRS complex, and a shortened QT interval [291,293]. Blood gas analysis is warranted to monitor electrolytes and acid–base status and may be indicated intraoperatively if ECG and/or blood pressure changes are noted.

Invasive (direct) blood pressure monitoring is preferred for hemodynamically unstable patients, those with concurrent renal disease, and those with large tumors. Respiratory rate and effort, end-tidal carbon dioxide, and pulse oximetry should also be monitored continuously. Although parathyroid tumors are usually not large, hemorrhage and airway compromise are still possible complications of parathyroidectomy. Hypertonic saline and blood products should be available to manage hemorrhage. Multiple large bore IV catheters or a central line are recommended if a large or invasive tumor is present. Ventilation should be closely monitored whenever surgery is performed in the vicinity of the larynx or trachea. Damage to the recurrent laryngeal nerve is possible due to its proximity to the thyroid and parathyroid glands [300]. Pulse oximetry monitoring should be continued until the animal is fully recovered.

Intraoperative PTH measurements can help confirm successful tumor excision. A > 50% decrease in PTH concentrations 20–45 min post-excision indicates removal of the affected tissue [301,302].

The most common complication following parathyroidectomy is hypocalcemia due to hypercalcemia-induced atrophy of the remaining parathyroid gland. Therefore, inadequate serum PTH concentration results in hypocalcemia that is usually transient [283,296,297]. The median time to the lowest calcium concentration reported was at 48 h and clinical hypocalcemia developed on average 4 days postoperatively [303]. Mild postoperative hypocalcemia without clinical signs is usually not treated. However, acute decreases in calcium levels, *t*Ca < 6 mg/dL (< 1.5 mmol/L), and development of clinical signs such as muscle cramping or tremors, seizures, tetany, anorexia, pain, and coma must be treated. Parenteral or oral calcium supplementation and administration of calcitriol are common treatments for animals with hypocalcemia [279,297]. Intravenous calcium should be administered slowly to effect via a dedicated IV catheter. Calcium gluconate (10%) solution can be administered at 0.5–1.5 mL/kg/h, while heart rate and ECG are closely monitored. Infusion rates should be decreased or discontinued if bradycardia, shortening of the QT interval, or development of arrhythmias is observed. Frequent monitoring of *i*Ca is required in these patients postoperatively [291].

References

1 Petroff BK, Greco DS. The endocrine system. In: Klein BG, ed. *Cunningham's Textbook of Veterinary Physiology*, 6th edn. St. Louis, MO: Saunders Elsevier, 2020: 378–393.

2 Veres-Nyéki KO. Endocrine disease. In: Duke-Novakovski T, de Vries M, Seymour C, eds. *BSAVA Manual of Canine and Feline Anaesthesia and Analgesia*, 3rd edn. Quedgeley, UK: British Small Animal Veterinary Association, 2016: 375–390.

3 Petroff BK, Greco DS. The endocrine glands and their function. In: Klein BG, ed. *Cunningham's Textbook of Veterinary Physiology*, 6th edn. St. Louis, MO: Saunders Elsevier, 2020: 394–427.

4 Koenig A. Endocrine emergencies in dogs and cats. *Vet Clin North Am Small Anim Pract* 2013; **43**: 869–897.
5 Thompson AL, Scott-Moncrieff JC, Anderson JD. Comparison of classic hypoadrenocorticism with glucocorticoid-deficient hypoadrenocorticism in dogs: 46 cases (1985–2005). *J Am Vet Med Assoc* 2007; **230**: 1190–1194.
6 Klein SC, Peterson ME. Canine hypoadrenocorticism. *Part I. Can Vet J* 2010; **51**: 63–69.
7 Klein SC, Peterson ME. Canine hypoadrenocorticism. *Part II. Can Vet J* 2010; **51**: 179–184.
8 Peterson ME, Greco DS, Orth DN. Primary hypoadrenocorticism in ten cats. *J Vet Intern Med* 1989; **3**: 55–58.
9 Peterson ME, Kintzer PP, Kass PH. Pretreatment clinical and laboratory findings in dogs with hypoadrenocorticism: 225 cases (1979–1993). *J Am Vet Med Assoc* 1996; **208**: 85–91.
10 Tyler RD, Qualls CW Jr, Heald RD, *et al.* Renal concentrating ability in dehydrated hyponatremic dogs. *J Am Vet Med Assoc* 1987; **191**: 1095–1100.
11 Burkitt Creedon JM. Hypoadrenocorticism. In: Silverstein D, Hopper K, eds. *Small Animal Critical Care Medicine*, 2nd edn. St. Louis, MO: Saunders Elsevier, 2015: 380–384.
12 Lathan P, Moore GE, Zambon S, *et al.* Use of a low-dose ACTH stimulation test for diagnosis of hypoadrenocorticism in dogs. *J Vet Small Intern Med* 2008; **22**: 1070–1073.
13 Kintzer PP, Peterson ME. Treatment and long-term follow-up of 205 dogs with hypoadrenocorticism. *J Vet Intern Med* 1997; **11**: 43–49.
14 Brady CA, Vite CH, Drobatz KJ. Severe neurologic sequelae in a dog after treatment of hypoadrenal crisis. *J Am Vet Med Assoc* 1999; **215**: 210, 222–225.
15 MacMillan KL. Neurologic complications following treatment of canine hypoadrenocorticism. *Can Vet J* 2003; **44**: 490–492.
16 Lathan P, Thompson AL. Management of hypoadrenocorticism (Addison's disease) in dogs. *Vet Med: Res Rep* 2018; **9**: 1–10.
17 Kintzer PP, Peterson ME. Diseases of the adrenal gland. In: Birchard SJ, Sherding RG, eds. *Saunders Manual of Small Animal Practice*, 3rd edn. St. Louis, MO: Saunders Elsevier, 2006: 357–375.
18 Stafford JR, Bartges JW. A clinical review of pathophysiology, diagnosis and treatment of uroabdomen in the dog and cat. *J Vet Emergency Crit Care* 2013; **23**: 216–229.
19 Koenig A. Hypoglycemia. In: Silverstein and Hopper, eds. *Small Animal Critical Care Medicine*, 2nd edn. St. Louis, MO: Saunders Elsevier, 2015: 352–34.
20 Riordan LL, Shaer M. Potassium disorders. In: Silverstein and Hopper, eds. *Small Animal Critical Care Medicine*, 2nd edn. St. Louis, MO: Saunders Elsevier, 2015: 269–273.
21 Dodam JR, Kruse-Elliott KT, Aucoin DP, *et al.* Duration of etomidate-induced adrenocortical suppression during surgery in dogs. *Am J Vet Res* 1990; **51**: 786–788.
22 Moon PF. Cortisol suppression in cats after induction of anesthesia with etomidate, compared with ketamine–diazepam combination. *Am J Vet Res* 1997; **58**: 868–871.
23 Sams L, Braun C, Allman D, *et al.* A comparison of the effects of propofol and etomidate on the induction of anesthesia and on cardiopulmonary parameters in dogs. *Vet Anaesth Analg* 2008; **35**: 488–494.
24 Qin B, Hu H, Cao B, *et al.* Effects of continuous infusion of etomidate at various dose rates on adrenal function in dogs. *BMC Anesthesiology* 2016; **16**: 1–6.
25 Van der Linden P, Schmartz D, Gilbart E, *et al.* Effects of propofol, etomidate, and pentobarbital on critical oxygen delivery. *Crit Care Med* 2000; **28**: 2492–2499.
26 Xu X, Wei Y, Dong Y, *et al.* A novel etomidate analog EL-0052 retains potent hypnotic effect and stable hemodynamics without suppressing adrenocortical function. *J Pharmacol Exp Ther* 2021; **379**: 324–330.
27 Zuo L, Dillman D. Endocrine disease. In: Hines RL, Jones SB, eds. *Stoelting's Anesthesia and Co-Existing Disease*, 8th edn. Philadelphia, PA: Saunders Elsevier, 2022: 439–464.
28 Scott-Moncrieff JC. Hypoadrenocorticism. In: Feldman EC, Nelson RW, Reusch C, *et al.* eds. *Canine and Feline Endocrinology and Reproduction*, 4th edn. St. Louis, MO: Saunders Elsevier, 2015: 485–520.
29 Berkenstadt H, Friedman Z, Preisman S, *et al.* Pulse pressure and stroke volume variations during severe hemorrhage in ventilated dogs. *Br J Anaesth* 2005; **94**: 721–726.
30 Pascoe PJ. Perioperative management of fluid therapy. In: DiBartola SP, ed. *Fluid, Electrolyte, and Acid-Base Disorders in Small Animal Practice*, 4th edn. St. Louis, MO: Saunders Elsevier, 2012: 405–435.
31 Peyton JL, Burkitt JM. Critical illness-related corticosteroid insufficiency in a dog with septic shock. *J Vet Emerg Crit Care* 2009; **19**: 262–268.
32 Melián C, Perez-Alenza MD, Peterson ME. Hyperadrenocorticism in dogs. In: Ettinger SJ, Feldman EC, eds. *Textbook of Veterinary Internal Medicine*, 7th edn. St. Louis, MO: Saunders Elsevier, 2010: 1816–1840.
33 Behrend EN, Kennis R. Atypical Cushing's syndrome in dogs: arguments for and against. *Vet Clin North Am Small Anim Pract* 2010; **40**: 285–296.
34 Frank LA, Henry GA, Whittemore JC, *et al.* Serum cortisol concentrations in dogs with pituitary-dependent hyperadrenocorticism and atypical hyperadrenocorticism. *J Vet Intern Med* 2015; **29**: 193–199.
35 Carotenuto G, Malerba A, Dolfini C, *et al.* Cushing's syndrome – an epidemiological study based on a canine population of 21, 821 dogs. *Open Vet J* 2019; **9**: 27–32.
36 Perkins GA, Lamb S, Erb HN, *et al.* Plasma adrenocorticotropin (ACTH) concentrations and clinical response in horses treated for quine Cushing's disease with cyproheptadine or pergolide. *Equine Vet J* 2002; **34**: 679–685.
37 Hatazoe T, Kawaguchi H, Hobo S, *et al.* Pituitary pars intermedia dysfunction (Equine Cushing's disease) in a Thoroughbred stallion: a single report. *J Equine Sci* 2015; **26**: 125–128.
38 Nichols R. Complications and concurrent disease associated with canine hyperadrenocorticism. *Vet Clin North Am Small Anim Pract* 1997; **27**: 309–320.
39 Van der Pas R, van Esch JHM, de Bruin C, *et al.* Cushing's disease and hypertension: in vivo and in vitro study of the role of the renin-angiotensin-aldosterone system and effects of medical therapy. *Eur J Endocrinol* 2014; **170**: 181–191.
40 Peterson ME. Diagnosis of hyperadrenocorticism in dogs. *Vet Clin North Am Small Anim Pract* 1984; **14**: 731–749.
41 Ishino H, Hara Y, Teshima T, *et al.* Hypophysectomy for a dog with coexisting Cushing's disease and diabetes mellitus. *J Vet Med Sci* 2010; **72**: 343–348.
42 Forrester SD, Troy GC, Dalton MN, *et al.* Retrospective evaluation of urinary tract infection in 42 dogs with hyperadrenocorticism or diabetes mellitus or both. *J Vet Intern Med* 1999; **13**: 557–560.
43 Kooistra HS, Galac S. Recent advances in the diagnosis of Cushing's syndrome in dogs. *Vet Clin North Am Small Anim Pract* 2010; **40**: 259–267.
44 Gilor C, Graves TK. Interpretation of laboratory tests for canine Cushing's syndrome. *Top Compan Anim Med* 2011; **26**: 98–108.
45 Kooistra HS, Galac S. Recent advances in the diagnosis of Cushing's syndrome in dogs. *Top Compan Anim Med* 2012; **27**: 21–24.
46 Barker EN, Campbell S, Tebb AJ, *et al.* A comparison of the survival times of dogs treated with mitotane or trilostane for pituitary-dependent hyperadrenocorticism. *J Vet Intern Med* 2005; **19**: 810–815.
47 Brown CG, Graves TK. Hyperadrenocorticism: treating dogs. *Compend Contin Educ Pract Vet* 2007; **29**: 132–134.
48 Meij B, Voorhout G, Rijnberk A. Progress in transsphenoidal hypophysectomy for treatment of pituitary-dependent hyperadrenocorticism in dogs and cats. *Mol Cell Endocrinol* 2002; **197**: 89–96.
49 Jiménez Peláez M, Bouvy BM, Dupré GP. Laparoscopic adrenalectomy for treatment of unilateral adrenocortical carcinomas: technique, complications, and results in seven dogs. *Vet Surg* 2008; **37**: 444–453.
50 Vaughan MA, Feldman EC, Hoar BR, *et al.* Evaluation of twice-daily, low-dose trilostane treatment administered orally in dogs with naturally occurring hyperadrenocorticism. *J Am Vet Med Assoc* 2008; **232**: 1321–1328.
51 Graves TK. Hypercortisolism in cats (feline Cushing's syndrome). In: Ettinger SJ, Feldman EC eds. *Textbook of Veterinary Internal Medicine*, 7th edn. St. Louis, MO: Saunders Elsevier, 2010: 1840–1847.
52 Adin CA, Nelson RW. Adrenal glands. In: Tobias KM, Johnston SA, eds. *Veterinary Surgery: Small Animal*. St. Louis, MO: Saunders Elsevier, 2012: 2033–2042.
53 Behrend EN. Canine hyperadrenocorticism. In: Feldman EC, Nelson RW, Reusch C, *et al.* eds. *Canine and Feline Endocrinology and Reproduction*, 4th edn. St. Louis, MO: Saunders Elsevier, 2015: 377–451.
54 Goggs R, Blais M-C, Brainard BM, *et al.* American College of Veterinary Emergency and Critical Care (ACVECC) consensus on the rational use of antithrombotics in veterinary critical care (CURATIVE) guidelines: small animal. *J Vet Emerg Crit Care* 2019; **29**: 12–36.
55 Kyles AE, Feldman EC, De Cock HE, *et al.* Surgical management of adrenal gland tumors with and without associated tumor thrombi in dogs: 40 cases (1994–2001). *J Am Vet Med Assoc* 2003; **223**: 654–662.
56 de Brito Galvão JF, Chew DJ. Metabolic complications of endocrine surgery in companion animals. *Vet Clin North Am Small Anim Pract* 2011; **41**: 847–868.
57 Scavelli TD, Peterson ME, Matthiesen DT. Results of surgical treatment for hyperadrenocorticism caused by adrenocortical neoplasia in the dog: 25 cases (1980–1984). *J Am Vet Med Assoc* 1986; **189**: 1360–1364.
58 Anderson CR, Birchard SJ, Powers BE, *et al.* Surgical treatment of adrenocortical tumors: 21 cases (1990–1996). *J Am Anim Hosp Assoc* 2001; **37**: 93–97.
59 Schwartz P, Kovak JR, Koprowski A, *et al.* Evaluation of prognostic factors in the surgical treatment of adrenal gland tumors in dogs: 41 cases (1999–2005). *J Am Vet Med Assoc* 2008; **232**: 77–84.
60 Coleman AE, Shepard MK, Schmiedt CW, *et al.* Effects of orally administered enalapril on blood pressure and hemodynamic response to vasopressors during isoflurane anesthesia in healthy dogs. *Vet Anaesth Analg* 2016; **43**: 482–494.

61 Burton SA, Lemke KA, Ihle SL, *et al.* Effects of medetomidine on serum insulin and plasma glucose concentrations in clinically normal dogs. *Am J Vet Res* 1997; **58**: 1440–1442.

62 Sinclair MD. A review of the physiological effects of alpha2-agonists related to the clinical use of medetomidine in small animal practice. *Can Vet J* 2003; **44**: 885–897.

63 Bouillon J, Duke T, Focken AP, *et al.* Effects of dexmedetomidine on glucose homeostasis in healthy cats. *J Feline Med Surg* 2020; **22**: 344–349.

64 Peláez MJ, Bouvy BM, Dupré GP. Laparoscopic adrenalectomy for treatment of unilateral adrenocortical carcinomas: technique, complications, and results in seven dogs. *Vet Surg* 2008; **37**: 444–453.

65 Naan EC, Kirpensteijn J, Dupré GP, *et al.* Innovative approach to laparoscopic adrenalectomy for treatment of unilateral adrenal gland tumors in dogs. *Vet Surg* 2013; **42**: 710–715.

66 Trepanier LA. Drug interactions and differential toxicity of NSAIDs. In: *Proceedings of the 22nd Annual Veterinary Medical Forum – American College of Veterinary Internal Medicine*, 2004: 535–537.

67 KuKanich B. Outpatient oral analgesics in dogs and cats beyond nonsteroidal antiinflammatory drugs: an evidence-based approach. *Vet Clin North Am Small Anim Pract* 2013; **43**: 1109–1125.

68 Gupta A, Garg R, Gupta N. Update in perioperative anesthetic management of pheochromocytoma. *World J Anes* 2015; **4**: 83–90.

69 Isaza D, DiGangi BA, Isaza N, *et al.* Impact of surgical preparatory rinses with isopropyl alcohol or water on perioperative body temperature in pediatric female dogs and cats. *Vet Anaesth Analg* 2021; **48**: 198–204.

70 McNally EM, Robertson SA, Pablo LS. Comparison of time to desaturation between preoxygenated and nonpreoxygenated dogs following sedation with acepromazine maleate and morphine and induction of anesthesia with propofol. *Am J Vet Res* 2009; **70**: 1333–1338.

71 Ambros B, Carrozzo MV, Jones T. Desaturation times between dogs preoxygenated via face mask or flow-by technique before induction of anesthesia. *Vet Anaesth Analg* 2018; **45**: 452–458.

72 Burns MG, Kelly AB, Hornof WJ, *et al.* Pulmonary artery thrombosis in three dogs with hyperadrenocorticism. *JAMA* 1981; **178**: 388–393.

73 Berry CR, Hawkins EC, Huerley KJ, *et al.* Frequency of pulmonary mineralization and hypoxemia in 21 dogs with pituitary-dependent hyperadrenocorticism. *J Vet Intern Med* 2000; **14**: 151–156.

74 Dorrestein E, Peda A, Thrall MA, *et al.* Fatal pulmonary thromboembolism in a two-year-old dog receiving long-term corticosteroid therapy. *Vet Rec Case Rep* 2019; **7**: 1–4.

75 Beilin B, Shavit Y, Razumovsky J, *et al.* Effects of mild perioperative hypothermia on cellular immune response. *Anesthesiology* 1998; **89**: 1133–1140.

76 Oncken A, Kirby R, Rudloff E. Hypothermia in critically ill dogs and cats. *Compend Contin Educ Pract Vet* 2001; **23**: 506–520.

77 Armstrong SR, Roberts BK, Aronsohn M. Perioperative hypothermia. *J Vet Emerg Crit Care* 2005; **15**: 32–37.

78 Goggs R, Benigni L, Fuentes VL, *et al.* Pulmonary thromboembolism. *J Vet Emerg Crit Care (San Antonio)* 2009; **19**: 30–52.

79 Lang JM, Schertel E, Kennedy S, *et al.* Elective and emergency surgical management of adrenal gland tumors: 60 cases (1999–2006). *JAHA* 2011; **47**: 428–435.

80 Gunn-Moore D, Simpson K. Pheochromocytoma in cats. In: Rand J, ed. *Clinical Endocrinology of Companion Animals*. Ames, IA: Wiley-Blackwell, 2013: 137–142.

81 Barthez PY, Nyland TG, Feldman EC. Ultrasonographic evaluation of the adrenal gland in dogs. *J Am Vet Med Assoc* 1995; **207**: 1180–1183.

82 Platt SR, Sheppard BJ, Graham J, *et al.* Pheochromocytoma in the vertebral canal of two dogs. *J Am Anim Hosp Assoc* 1998; **34**: 365–371.

83 Reusch CE. Pheochromocytoma and multiple endocrine neoplasia. In: Feldman EC, Nelson RW, Reusch C, *et al.*, eds. *Canine and Feline Endocrinology and Reproduction*, 4th edn. St. Louis, MO: Saunders Elsevier, 2015: 521–554.

84 Bouayad H, Feeney DA, Caywood DD, *et al.* Pheochromocytoma in dogs: 13 cases (1980–1985). *J Am Vet Med Assoc* 1987; **191**: 1610–1615.

85 Santamarina G, Espino L, Vila M, *et al.* Aortic thromboembolism and retroperitoneal hemorrhage associated with a pheochromocytoma in a dog. *J Vet Intern Med* 2003; **17**: 917–922.

86 Santoro-Beer K, Mandell DC. Pheochromocytoma. In: Silverstein and Hopper, eds. *Small Animal Critical Care Medicine*, 2nd edn. St. Louis, MO: Elsevier Saunders, 2015: 371–375.

87 Gilson SD, Withrow SJ, Wheeler SL, *et al.* Pheochromocytoma in 50 dogs. *J Vet Intern Med* 1994; **8**: 228–232.

88 Barthez PY, Marks SL, Woo J, *et al.* Pheochromocytoma in dogs: 61 cases (1984–1995). *J Vet Intern Med* 1997; **11**: 272–278.

89 Herrera MA, Mehl ML, Kass PH, *et al.* Predictive factors and the effect of phenoxybenzamine on outcome in dogs undergoing adrenalectomy for pheochromocytoma. *J Vet Intern Med* 2008; **22**: 1333–1339.

90 Von Dehn J, Nelson RW, Feldman EC, *et al.* Pheochromocytoma and hyperadrenocorticism in dogs: six cases (1982–1992). *J Am Vet Med Assoc* 1995; **207**: 322–324.

91 Maher ER, McNiel EA. Pheochromocytoma in dogs and cats. *Vet Clin North Am Small Anim Pract* 1997; **27**: 359–380.

92 Rosenstein DA. Diagnostic imaging in canine pheochromocytoma. *Vet Radiol Ultrasound* 2000; **41**: 499–506.

93 Galac S, Korpershoek E. Pheochromocytomas and paragangliomas in humans and dogs. *Vet Comp Oncol* 2017; **15**: 1158–1170.

94 Besso JG, Penninck DG, Gliatto JM. Retrospective ultrasonographic evaluation of adrenal lesions in 26 dogs. *Vet Radiol Ultrasound* 1997; **38**: 448–455.

95 Bargellini P, Orlani R, Dentini A, *et al.* Use of contrast-enhanced ultrasound in the differential diagnosis of adrenal tumors in dogs. *J Am Anim Hosp Assoc* 2016; **52**: 132–143.

96 Gostelow R, Bridger N, Syme HM. Plasma-free metanephrine and free normetanephrine measurement for the diagnosis of pheochromocytoma in dogs. *J Vet Intern Med* 2013; **27**: 83–90.

97 Quante S, Boretti FS, Kook PH, *et al.* Urinary catecholamine and metanephrine to creatinine ratios in dogs with hyperadrenocorticism or pheochromocytoma, and in healthy dogs. *J Vet Intern Med* 2010; **24**: 1093–1097.

98 Massari F, Nicoli S, Romanelli G, *et al.* Adrenalectomy in dogs with adrenal tumors: 52 cases (2002–2008). *J Am Vet Med Assoc* 2011; **239**: 216–221.

99 Barrera J, Bernard F, Ehrhart EJ, *et al.* Evaluation of risk factors for outcome associated with adrenal gland tumors with or without invasion of the caudal vena cava and treated via adrenalectomy in dogs: 86 cases (1993–2009). *J Am Vet Med Assoc* 2013; **242**: 1715–1721.

100 Fischer J, Lane IF, Cribb AE. Urethral pressure profile and hemodynamic effects of phenoxybenzamine and prazosin in non-sedated male beagle dogs. *Can J Vet Res* 2003; **67**: 30–38.

101 Ramakrishna H. Pheochromocytoma resection: current concepts in anesthetic management. *J Anaes Clin Pharm* 2015; **31**: 317–323.

102 Berends AMA, Kerstens MN, Lenders JWM, *et al.* Approach to the patient: perioperative management of the patient with pheochromocytoma or sympathetic paraganglioma. *J Clin Endocrinol Metab* 2020; **105**: 3088–3102.

103 Soler Arias EA, Castillo VA, Louiset E, *et al.* Cushing's syndrome cause by intraadrenocortical adrenocorticotropic hormone in a dog. *J Vet Intern Med* 2021; **36**: 264–271.

104 Mak G, Allen J. Simultaneous pheochromocytoma and third-degree atrioventricular block in 2 dogs. *J Vet Emerg Crit Care* 2013; **23**: 610–614.

105 Shimada A, Morita T, Ikeda N, *et al.* Hypoglycaemic brain lesions in a dog with insulinoma. *J Comp Pathol* 2000; **122**: 67–71.

106 Hall K, Drobatz K. Volume Resuscitation in the acutely hemorrhaging patient: historic use to current applications. *Front Vet Sci* 2021; **8**: 1–12.

107 Us MH, Özkan S, Oral L, *et al.* Comparison of the effects of hypertonic saline and crystalloid infusions on haemodynamic parameters during haemorrhagic shock in dogs. *J Int Med Res* 2001; **29**: 508–515.

108 Seliskar A, Svete AN, Kozelj M. Haemodynamic and renal effects of resuscitation of dogs from haemorrhagic shock with hypertonic saline or Lactated Ringer's solution combined with whole blood. *Veterinarni Medicina* 2011; **4**: 187–201.

109 Ebert TJ, Hall JE, Barney JA. The effects of increasing plasma concentrations of dexmedetomidine in humans. *Anesthesiology* 2000; **93**: 382–394.

110 Wong AYC, Cheung CW. Dexmedetomidine for resection of a large phaeochromocytoma with invasion into the inferior vena cava. *Br J Anaesth* 2004; **93**: 873.

111 Polavarapu HV, Kurian AA, Josloff R. Is dexmedetomidine the agent of choice in the resection of pheochromocytoma? *Am Surg* 2012; **78**: 127–128.

112 Singh S, Singh A. Dexmedetomidine induced catecholamine suppression in pheochromocytoma. *J Nat Sci Biol Med* 2014; **5**: 182–183.

113 Viilman I, Vettorato E. Perioperative use of thoracic epidural anesthesia, dexmedetomidine and magnesium sulphate infusion in a dog undergoing neuroendocrine tumor resection. *Vet Rec Case Rep* 2021; **9**: 1–6.

114 Clarke KW. Desflurane and sevoflurane: new volatile anesthetic agents. *Vet Clin North Am Small Anim Pract* 1999; **29**: 793–810.

115 Robinson JL. Effect of vasopressin and phenylephrine on arterial blood pressure and heart rate in conscious dogs. *Am J Physiol* 1986; **251**: H253–H260.

116 Pedro B, López-Alvarez J, Fonfara S, *et al.* Retrospective evaluation of the use of amiodarone in dogs with arrhythmias (from 2003 to 2010). *J Small Anim Pract* 2012; **53**: 19–26.

117 Nazari MA, Rosenblum JS, Haigney MC, *et al.* Pathophysiology and acute management of tachyarrhythmias in pheochromocytoma. JACC review topic of the week. *J Amer Coll Cardiol* 2020; **76**: 451–464.

118 Augoustides JG, Abrams M, Berkowitz D, *et al.* Vasopressin for hemodynamic rescue in catecholamine-resistant vasoplegic shock after resection of massive pheochromocytoma. *Anesthesiology* 2004; **101**: 1022–1024.

119 Moon PF, Ilkiw JE. Surface-induced hypothermia in dogs: 19 cases (1987–1989). *J Am Vet Med Assoc* 1993; **202**: 437–444.

120 Washabau RJ. Pancreas. In: Washabau RJ, Day MJ, eds. *Canine and Feline Gastroenterology*. St. Louis, MO: Saunders Elsevier, 2013: 799–802.

121 Hoenig M. Comparative aspects of diabetes mellitus in dogs and cats. *Mol Cell Endocrinol* 2002; **197**: 221–229.

122 Nelson RW. Canine diabetes mellitus. In: Ettinger SJ, Feldman EC, eds. *Textbook of Veterinary Internal Medicine*, 7th edn. St. Louis, MO: Saunders Elsevier, 2010: 1782–1796.

123 Sparkes AH, Cannon M, Church D, *et al.* ISFM Consensus guidelines on the practical management of diabetes mellitus in cats. *J Feline Med Surg* 2015; **17**: 235–250.

124 Reusch C. Feline diabetes mellitus. In: Ettinger SJ, Feldman EC, eds. *Textbook of Veterinary Internal Medicine*, 7th edn. St. Louis, MO: Saunders Elsevier, 2010: 1796–1816.

125 O'Brien TD. Pathogenesis of feline diabetes mellitus. *Mol Cell Endocrinol* 2002; **197**: 213–219.

126 Mattin M, O'Neill D, Church D, *et al.* An epidemiological study of diabetes mellitus in dogs attending first opinion practice in the UK. *Vet Rec* 2014; **174**: 349.

127 Guptill L, Glickman L, Glickman N. Time trends and risk factors for diabetes mellitus in dogs: analysis of veterinary medical data base records (1970–1999). *Vet J* 2003; **165**: 240–247.

128 Rand JS, Fleeman LM, Farrow HA, *et al.* Canine and feline diabetes mellitus: nature or nurture? *J Nutr* 2004; **134**: 2072S–2080S.

129 Behrend E, Holford A, Lathan P, *et al.* 2018 AAHA diabetes managements guidelines for dogs and cats. *J Amer Anim Hosp Assoc* 2018; **54**: 1–21.

130 Hume DZ, Drobatz KJ, Hess RS. Outcome of dogs with diabetic ketoacidosis: 127 dogs (1993–2003). *J Vet Intern Med* 2006; **20**: 547–555.

131 Greco DS. Diagnosis of diabetes mellitus in cats and dogs. *Vet Clin North Am Small Anim Pract* 2001; **31**: 845–853.

132 Kerl ME. Renal tubular disease. In: Ettinger SJ, Feldman EC, eds. *Canine and Feline Endocrinology*, 4th edn. St. Louis, MO: Saunders, 2015: 2062–2068.

133 Rudloff E. Diabetic ketoacidosis in the cat. Recognition and essential treatment. *J Feline Med Surg* 2017; **19**: 1167–1174.

134 Chong SK, Reineke EL. Point of care glucose and ketone monitoring. *Top Companion Anim Med* 2016; **31**: 18–26.

135 Frank G, Anderson W, Pazak H, *et al.* Use of high-protein diet in the management of feline diabetes mellitus. *Vet Ther* 2001; **2**: 238–246.

136 Palm CA, Feldman EC. Oral hypoglycemics in cats with diabetes mellitus. *Vet Clin North Am Small Anim Pract* 2013; **43**: 407–415.

137 O'Brien MA. Diabetic emergencies in small animals. *Vet Clin North Am Small Anim Pract* 2010; **40**: 317–333.

138 Malerba E, Cattani C, Del Baldo F, *et al.* Accuracy of a flash glucose monitoring system in dogs with diabetic ketoacidosis. *J Vet Intern Med* 2020; **34**: 83–91.

139 West E, Pettitt R, Jones RS, *et al.* Acid–base electrolyte balance following administration of three crystalloid solutions in dogs undergoing elective orthopaedic surgery. *Vet Anaesth Analg* 2013; **40**: 482–493.

140 Fleeman LM, Rand JS. Evaluation of day-to-day variability of serial blood glucose concentration curves in diabetic dogs. *J Am Vet Med Assoc* 2003; **222**: 317–321.

141 Alt N, Kley S, Haessig M, *et al.* Day-to-day variability of blood glucose concentration curves generated at home in cats with diabetes mellitus. *J Am Vet Med Assoc* 2007; **230**: 1011–1017.

142 Nelson RW. Canine diabetes mellitus. In: Feldman EC, Nelson RW, eds. *Canine and Feline Endocrinology and Reproduction*, 4th edn. St. Louis, MO: Saunders Elsevier, 2015: 213–257.

143 Nishikawa T, Ederlstein D, Brownlee M. The missing link: a single unifying mechanism for diabetic complications. *Kidney Int Suppl* 2000; **77**: S26–S30.

144 Torre DM, deLaforcade AM, Chan DL. Incidence and clinical relevance of hyperglycemia in critically ill dogs. *J Vet Intern Med* 2007; **21**: 971–975.

145 Oliver JA, Clark L, Corletto F, *et al.* A comparison of anesthetic complications between diabetic and nondiabetic dogs undergoing phacoemulsification cataract surgery: a retrospective study. *Vet Ophthalmol* 2010; **13**: 244–250.

146 Adami C, Haynes RS, Sanchez RF, *et al.* Effect of insulin and fasting regimen on blood glucose concentrations of diabetic dogs during phacoemulsification. *J Am Anim Hosp Assoc* 2020; **56**: 1–6.

147 Kronen PWM, Moon-Massat RF, Ludders JW, *et al.* Comparison of two insulin protocols for diabetic dogs undergoing cataract surgery. *Vet Anaesth Analg* 2001; **28**: 146–155.

148 Shilo-Benjamini Y. A review of ophthalmic local and regional anesthesia in dogs and cats. *Vet Anaesth Analg* 2019; **46**: 14–27.

149 Pascoe PJ, Ilkiw JE, Craig C, *et al.* The effects of ketamine on the minimum alveolar concentration of isoflurane in cats. *Vet Anaesth Analg* 2007; **34**: 31–39.

150 Ortega M, Cruz I. Evaluation of a constant rate infusion of lidocaine for balanced anesthesia in dogs undergoing surgery. *Can Vet J* 2011; **52**: 856–860.

151 Restitutti F, Raekallio M, Vainiopää M, *et al.* Plasma glucose, insulin, free fatty acids, lactate and cortisol concentration in dexmedetomidine-sedated dogs with or without MK-467: a peripheral α-2 adrenoreceptor antagonist. *Vet J* 2012; **193**: 481–485.

152 Clark L, Leece EA, Brearly JC. Diabetes mellitus affects the duration of action vecuronium in dog. *Vet Anaesth Analg* 2012; **39**: 472–479.

153 Leece EA, Clark L. Diabetes mellitus does not affect the neuromuscular blocking action of atracurium in dogs. *Vet Anaesth Analg* 2017; **44**: 697–702.

154 Haga HA, Bettembourg V, Lervik A. Rocuronium infusion: a higher rate is needed in diabetic than nondiabetic dogs. *Vet Anaesth Analg* 2019; **46**: 28–35.

155 Hopper K, Brown S. Hypertensive crisis. In: Silverstein D, Hopper K, eds. *Small Animal Critical Care Medicine*, 2nd edn. St. Louis, MO: Saunders Elsevier, 2015: 51–54.

156 Kenefick S, Parker N, Slater L, *et al.* Evidence of cardiac autonomic neuropathy in dogs with diabetes mellitus. *Vet Rec* 2007; **161**: 83–88.

157 Norgate DJ, Nicholss D, Gueddes RF, *et al.* Comparison of two protocols for insulin administration and fasting time in diabetic dogs anaesthetized for phacoemulsification: a prospective clinical trial. *Vet Rec* 2021; **188**: e81.

158 Cohen M, Post GS. Water transport in the kidney and nephrogenic diabetes insipidus. *J Vet Intern Med* 2002; **16**: 510–517.

159 Wesche D, Deen PMT, Knoers NVAM. Congenital nephrogenic diabetes insipidus: the current state of affairs. *Pediatr Nephrol* 2012; **27**: 2183–2204.

160 Luzius H, Jans DA, Grünbaum EG, *et al.* A low affinity vasopressin V2-receptor in inherited nephrogenic diabetes insipidus. *J Recept Res* 1992; **12**: 351–368.

161 Goldstein RE. Diabetes insipidus. In: Silverstein DC, Hopper K, eds. *Small Animal Critical Care Medicine*, 2nd edn. St. Louis, MO: Saunders Elsevier, 2015: 357–362.

162 Harb MF, Nelson RW, Feldman EC, *et al.* Central diabetes insipidus in dogs: 20 cases (1986–1995). *J Am Vet Med Assoc* 1996; **209**: 1884–1888.

163 Aroch I, Mazaki-Tovi M, Shemesh O, *et al.* Central diabetes insipidus in five cats: clinical presentation, diagnosis and oral desmopressin therapy. *J Feline Med Surg* 2005; **7**: 333–339.

164 Comtois R, Bertrand S, Beauregard H, *et al.* Low serum urea level in dehydrated patients with central diabetes insipidus. *Canadian Med Assoc J* 1988; **139**: 965–969.

165 Burkitt Creedon JM. Sodium disorders. In: Silverstein, DC, Hopper K, eds. *Small Animal Critical Care Medicine*, 2nd edn. St. Louis, MO: Elsevier Saunders, 2015: 263–268.

166 Ueda Y, Hopper K. Sodium and water balance. In: Drobatz KJ, Hopper K, Rozanki E, *et al.*, eds. *Textbook of Small Animal Emergency Medicine, I&II*. Hoboken, NJ: Wiley-Blackwell, 2019: 690–699.

167 Saleh N, Aoki M, Shimada T, *et al.* Renal effects of medetomidine in isoflurane-anesthetized dogs with special reference to its diuretic action. *J Vet Med Sci* 2005; **67**: 461–465.

168 Murahata Y, Hikasa Y. Comparison of the diuretic effects of medetomidine hydrochloride and xylazine hydrochloride in healthy cats. *Am J Vet Res* 2012; **73**: 1871–1880.

169 Goutal CM, Brugmann BL, Ryan KA. Insulinoma in dogs: a review. *J Am Anim Hosp Assoc* 2012; **48**: 151–163.

170 Hess RS. Insulin-secreting islet cell neoplasia. In: Ettinger SJ, Feldman EC, eds. *Textbook of Veterinary Internal Medicine*, 7th edn. St. Louis, MO: Saunders Elsevier, 2010: 1779–1782.

171 Shahar R, Rousseaux C, Steiss J. Peripheral polyneuropathy in a dog with functional islet B-cell tumor and widespread metastasis. *J Am Vet Med Assoc* 1985; **187**: 175–177.

172 Trifondou MA, Kirpensteijn J, Robben JH. A retrospective evaluation of 51 dogs with insulinoma. *Vet Q* 1998; **20**: 114–115.

173 Goutal CM, Brugmann BL, Ryan KA, *et al.* Insulinoma in dogs: a review. *J Am Anim Hosp Assoc* 2012; **48**: 151–163.

174 Greene SN, Bright RM. Insulinoma in a cat. *J Small Anim Pract* 2008; **49**: 38–40.

175 Leifer CE, Peterson ME, Matus RE. Insulin-secreting tumor: diagnosis and medical and surgical management in 55 dogs. *J Am Vet Med Assoc* 1986; **188**: 60–64.

176 Caywood DD, Klausner JS, O'Leary TP, *et al.* Pancreatic insulin secreting neoplasms: clinical, diagnostic and prognostic features in 73 dogs. *J Am Anim Hosp Assoc* 1988; **24**: 577–584.

177 Polton GA, White RN, Brearley MJ. Improved survival in a retrospective cohort of 28 dogs with insulinoma. *J Small Anim Pract* 2007; **48**: 151–156.

178 Li X, Fox JG, Padrid PA. Neoplastic diseases in ferrets: 574 cases (1968–1997). *J Am Vet Med Assoc* 1998; **212**: 1402–1406.

179 Weiss CA, Williams BH, Scott MV. Insulinoma in the ferret: clinical findings and treatment comparison of 66 cases. *J Am Anim Hosp Assoc* 1998; **34**: 471–475.

180 Avallone G, Forlani A, Tecilla M, *et al.* Neoplastic diseases in the domestic ferret (Mustela putorius furo) in Italy: classification and tissue distribution of 856 cases (2000–2010). *BMC Vet Res* 2016; **12**: 1–8.

181 Del Dusto I, German AJ, Treggiari E, *et al.* Incidence of postoperative complications and outcome of 48 dogs undergoing surgical management of insulinoma. *J Vet Intern Med* 2020; **34**: 1135–1143.

182 Ryan D, Pérez-Accino J, Gonçalves R, *et al.* Clinical findings, neurological manifestations and survival of dogs with insulinoma: 116 cases (2009–2020). *J Small Anim Pract* 2021; **62**: 531–539.

183 Ehrhart N, Withrow SJ, Ehrhart EJ, *et al.* Pancreatic beta cell tumor in ferrets: 20 cases (1986–1994). *J Am Vet Med Assoc* 1996; **209**: 1737–1740.

184 Elie MS, Zerbe CA. Insulinoma in dogs, cats and ferrets. *Compend Contin Educ Pract Vet* 1995; **17**: 51–59.

185 Dunn JK, Bostock DE, Herrtage ME, *et al.* Insulin-secreting tumors of the canine pancreas: clinical and pathological features of 11 cases. *J Small Anim Pract* 1993; **34**: 325–331.

186 Idowu O, Heading K. Hypoglycemia in dogs: causes, management, and diagnosis. *Can Vet J* 2018; **59**: 642–649.

187 Robben JH, Pollak YW, Kirpensteijn J, *et al.* Comparison of ultrasonography, computed tomography, and single-photon emission computed tomography for the detection and localization of canine insulinoma. *J Vet Intern Med* 2005; **19**: 15–22.

188 Cleland NT, Morton J, Delisser PJ. Outcomes after surgical management of canine insulinoma in 49 cases. *Vet Comp Oncol* 2021; **19**: 428–441.

189 Moore AS, Nelson RW, Henry CJ, *et al.* Streptozocin for treatment of pancreatic islet cell tumors in dogs: 17 cases (1989–1999). *J Am Vet Med Assoc* 2002; **221**: 811–818.

190 Fischer JR, Smith SA, Harkin KR. Glucagon constant-rate infusion: a novel strategy for the management of hyperinsulinemic–hypoglycemic crisis in the dog. *J Am Anim Hosp Assoc* 2000; **36**: 27–32.

191 Reine NJ, Bonczynski J. Pancreatic beta cell neoplasia. In: Birchard SJ, Sherding RG, eds. *Saunders Manual of Small Animal Practice*, 3rd edn. St. Louis, MO: Saunders Elsevier, 2006: 390–397.

192 Koenig A. Chapter 66: hypoglycemia. In: Silverstein D, Hopper K, eds. *Small Animal Critical Care Medicine*, 2nd edn. St. Louis, MO: Saunders Elsevier, 2015: 352–357.

193 Meleo KA, Peterson ME. Treatment of insulinoma in dogs, cats, and ferrets. In: Bonagura JD, Twedt DC, eds. *Kirk's Current Veterinary Therapy XV*. St. Louis, MO: Saunders Elsevier, 2014: E130–E134.

194 Guedes AG, Rude EP. Effects of pre-operative administration of medetomidine on plasma insulin and glucose concentrations in healthy dogs and dogs with insulinoma. *Vet Anaesth Analg* 2013; **40**: 472–481.

195 Narita T, Sato R, Motoishi K, *et al.* The interaction between orally administered non-steroidal anti-inflammatory drugs and prednisolone in healthy dogs. *J Vet Med Sci* 2007; **69**: 353–363.

196 Meleo K. Management of insulinoma patients with refractory hypoglycemia. *Probl Vet Med* 1990; **2**: 602–609.

197 Dougherty TB, Cronau LH Jr. Anesthetic implications for surgical patients with endocrine tumors. *Int Anesthesiol Clin* 1998; **36**: 31–44.

198 Lurye JC, Behrend EN. Endocrine tumors. *Vet Clin North Am Small Anim Pract* 2001; **31**: 1083–1110.

199 Caplan ER, Peterson ME, Mullen HS, *et al.* Diagnosis and treatment of insulin-secreting pancreatic islet cell tumors in ferrets: 57 cases (1986–1994). *J Am Vet Med Assoc* 1996; **209**: 1741–1745.

200 Freitag FA, Bozak VL, do Carmo MP, *et al.* Continuous transverse abdominis plane block for analgesia in three dogs with abdominal pain. *Vet Anaesth Analg* 2018; **45**: 581–583.

201 Gress F, Schmitt C, Sherman S, *et al.* A prospective randomized comparison of endoscopic, ultrasound- and computed tomography-guided celiac plexus block for management chronic pancreatitis pain. *Am J Gastroenterol* 1999; **94**: 900–905.

202 Morales R Jr, Mentz H III, Newall G, *et al.* Use of abdominal field block injection with liposomal bupivacaine to control postoperative pain after abdominoplasty. *Aesthetic Surg J* 2013; **33**: 1148–1153.

203 Mojtaba F, Arnab M, Neupane R, *et al.* Efficacy of transversus abdominis plane block with liposomal wall reconstruction. *Am J Surg* 2015; **212**: 399–405.

204 Ortiga-Carvalho TM, Chiamolera MI, Pazos-Moura CC, *et al.* Hypothalamus-pituitary-thyroid axis. *Compr Physiol* 2016; **6**: 1387–1428.

205 Feldt-Rasmussen U, Effraimidis G, Klose M. The hypothalamus-pituitary-thyroid (HPT)-axis and its roles in the physiology and pathophysiology of other hypothalamus-pituitary function. *Mol Cell Endocrinol* 2021; **525**: 1–5.

206 Mooney CT. Canine hypothyroidism: a review of aetiology and diagnosis. *N Z Vet J* 2011; **59**: 105–114.

207 Panciera DL. Hypothyroidism in dogs: 66 cases (1987–1992). *J Am Vet Med Assoc* 1994; **204**: 761–767.

208 Dixon RM, Reid SWJ, Mooney CT. Epidemiological, clinical, haematological and biochemical characteristics of canine hypothyroidism. *Vet Rec 999*; **145**: 481–487.

209 Panciera D. Hypothyroidism in dogs. In: Rand J, Behrend E, Gunn-Moore D, Campbell-Ward M, eds. *Clinical Endocrinology of Companion Animals*. Ames, IA: Wiley-Blackwell, 2012: 263–272.

210 Scott-Moncrieff JC. Hypothyroidism. In: Feldman EC, Nelson RW, Reusch CE, *et al.* eds. *Canine and Feline Endocrinology*, 4th edn St. Louis, MO: Saunders Elsevier, 2015: 77–135.

211 Roopali B, Roy S, Ali SL. Haematological alteration in hypothyroidism dogs. *Pharm Innov J* 2020; **9**: 49–52.

212 Finora K, Greco D. Hypothyroidism and myxedema coma. *Compend Contin Educ Pract Vet* 2007; **29**: 19–31.

213 Ferguson DC. Testing for hypothyroidism in dogs. *Vet Clin North Am Small Anim Pract* 2007; **37**: 647–669.

214 Daminet S, Ferguson DC. Influence of drugs on thyroid function in dogs. *J Vet Intern Med* 2003; **17**: 463–472.

215 Peterson ME, Melián C, Nichols R. Measurement of serum total thyroxine, triiodothyronine, free thyroxine, and thyrotropin concentrations for diagnosis of hypothyroidism in dogs. *J Am Vet Med Assoc* 1997; **211**: 1396–1402.

216 Scott-Moncrieff JC, Nelson RW, Bruner JM, *et al.* Comparison of serum concentrations of thyroid-stimulating hormone in healthy dogs, hypothyroid dogs, and euthyroid dogs with concurrent disease. *J Am Vet Med Assoc* 1998; **212**: 387–391.

217 Kantrowitz LB, Peterson ME, Melián C, *et al.* Serum total thyroxine, total triiodothyronine, free thyroxine, and thyrotropin concentrations in dogs with nonthyroidal disease. *J Am Vet Med Assoc* 2001; **219**: 765–769.

218 Panciera DL, Peterson ME, Birchard SJ. Diseases of the thyroid gland. In: Birchard SJ, Sherding RG, eds. *Saunders Manual of Small Animal Practice*, 3rd edn. St. Louis, MO: Saunders Elsevier, 2006: 327–342.

219 Pullen WH, Hess RS. Hypothyroid dogs treated with intravenous levothyroxine. *J Vet Intern Med* 2006; **20**: 32–37.

220 Bach JF, Rozanski EA, Bedenice D, *et al.* Association of expiratory airways dysfunction with marked obesity in healthy adult dogs. *Am J Vet Res* 2007; **68**: 670–675.

221 Mosing M, German AJ, Holden SL, *et al.* Oxygenation and ventilation characteristics in obese sedated dogs before and after weight loss: a clinical trial. *Vet J* 2013; **198**: 367–371.

222 Sarlis NJ, Gourgiotis L. Thyroid emergencies. *Rev Endocr Metab Disord* 2003; **4**: 129–136.

223 Love L, Cline MG. Perioperative physiology and pharmacology in the obese small animal patient. *Vet Anaesth Analg* 2015; **42**: 119–132.

224 Lemmens HJM. Perioperative pharmacology in morbid obesity. *Curr Opin Anaesthesiol* 2010; **23**: 485–491.

225 Correa Devito FC, Cristina G, Patricio F, *et al.* Comparative study of anaesthesia induction in obese dogs using propofol dosages based on lean body weight of total body weight. *Vet Anim Sci* 2020; **10**: 1–5.

226 Berry SH, Panciera DL. The effect of experimentally induced hypothyroidism on the isoflurane minimum alveolar concentration in dogs. *Vet Anaesth Analg* 2015; **42**: 50–54.

227 McMurphy RM, Hodgson DS, Bruyette DS, *et al.* Cardiovascular effects of 1.0, 1.5, and 2.0 minimum alveolar concentrations of isoflurane in experimentally induced hypothyroidism in dogs. *Vet Surg* 1996; **25**: 171–178.

228 Babad AA, Eger EI II. The effects of hyperthyroidism and hypothyroidism on halothane and oxygen requirement in dogs. *Anesthesiology* 1968; **29**: 1087–1093.

229 Jain AK, Dutta A. Stroke volume variation as a guide to fluid administration in morbidly obese patients undergoing laparoscopic bariatric surgery. *Obes Surg* 2010; **20**: 709–715.

230 Davis H, Jensen T, Johnson A, *et al.* American Animal Hospital Association (AAHA); American Association of Feline Practitioners (AAFP; 2013). 2013 AAHA/AAFP fluid therapy guidelines for dogs and cats. *J Am Anim Hosp Assoc* 2013; **49**: 149–159.

231 Papi G, Corsello SM, Pontecorvi A. Clinical concepts on thyroid emergencies. *Front Endocrinol (Lausanne)* 2014; **5**: 102.

232 Mooney CT. Hyperthyroidism. In: Ettinger SJ, Feldman EC, eds. *Textbook of Veterinary Internal Medicine*, 7th edn. St. Louis, MO: Saunders Elsevier, 2010: 1761–1778.

233 Peterson ME, Ward CR. Etiopathologic findings of hyperthyroidism in cats. *Vet Clin North Am Small Anim Pract* 2007; **37**: 633–645.

234 Peterson ME, Kintzer PP, Cavanagh PG, *et al.* Feline hyperthyroidism: pretreatment clinical and laboratory evaluation of 131 cases. *J Am Vet Med Assoc* 1983; **183**: 103–110.

235 Thoday KL, Mooney CT. Historical, clinical and laboratory features of 126 hyperthyroid cats. *Vet Rec* 1992; **131**: 257–264.

236 Barber LG. Thyroid tumors in dogs and cats. *Vet Clin North Am Small Anim Pract* 2007; **37**: 755–773.

237 Harari J, Patterson JS, Roenthal RC. Clinical and pathological features of thyroid tumors in 26 dogs. *J Am Vet Med Assoc* 1986; **188**: 1160–1164.

238 Sangster JK, Panciera DL, Abbott JA, *et al.* Cardiac biomarkers in hyperthyroid cats. *J Vet Intern Med* 2014; **28**: 465–472.
239 Broussard JD, Peterson ME, Fox PR. Changes in clinical and laboratory findings in cats with hyperthyroidism from 1983 to 1993. *J Am Vet Med Assoc* 1995; **206**: 302–305.
240 Tolbert MK, Ward CR. Feline focus – feline thyroid storm: rapid recognition to improve patient survival. *Compend Contin Educ Pract Vet* 2010; **32**: E1–E6.
241 Klubo-Gwiezdzinska J, Wartofsky L. Thyroid emergencies. *Med Clin North Am* 2012; **96**: 385–403.
242 Merkle JE, Boudreaux B, Langohr I, *et al.* Thyroid storm in a dog secondary to thyroid carcinoma. *J Vet Emerg Crit Care* 2021; **31**: 428–431.
243 Berent AC, Drobatz KJ, Ziemer, *et al.* Liver function in cats with hyperthyroidism before and after 131I therapy. *J Vet Intern Med* 2007; **21**: 1217–1223.
244 Graves TK. Hyperthyroidism and the kidneys. In: August JR, ed. *Consultations in Feline Internal Medicine*, 6th edn. St. Louis, MO: Saunders Elsevier, 2010: 268–273.
245 Nemzek JA, Kruger JM, Walshaw R, *et al.* Acute onset of hypokalemia and muscular weakness in four hyperthyroid cats. *J Am Vet Assoc* 1994; **205**: 65–67.
246 Naan EC, Kirpensteijn J, Kooistra HS, *et al.* Results of thyroidectomy in 101 cats with hyperthyroidism. *Vet Surg* 2006; **35**: 287–293.
247 Peterson ME. Diagnostic tests for hyperthyroidism in cats. *Clin Tech Small Anim Pract* 2006; **21**: 2–9.
248 Graves TK, Peterson ME. Diagnosis of occult hyperthyroidism in cats. *Probl Vet Med* 1990; **2**: 683–692.
249 Peterson ME. Radioiodine treatment of hyperthyroidism. *Clin Tech Small Anim Pract* 2006; **21**: 34–39.
250 Trepanier LA. Pharmacologic management of feline hyperthyroidism. *Vet Clin North Am Small Anim Pract* 2007; **37**: 775–788.
251 Langston CE, Reine N. Hyperthyroidism and the kidney. *Clin Tech Small Anim Pract* 2006; **21**: 17–21.
252 Henik RA, Stepien RL, Wenholz LJ, *et al.* Efficacy of atenolol as a single antihypertensive agent in hyperthyroid cats. *J Feline Med Surg* 2008; **10**: 577–582.
253 Birchard SJ. Thyroidectomy in the cat. *Clin Tech Small Anim Pract* 2006; **21**: 29–33.
254 Robertson SA, Gogolski SM, Pascoe P, *et al.* AAFP feline anesthesia guidelines. *J Feline Med Surg* 2018; **20**: 602–634.
255 Welches CD, Scavelli TD, Matthiesen DT, *et al.* Occurrence of problems after three techniques of bilateral thyroidectomy in cats. *Vet Surg* 1989; **18**: 392–396.
256 Touhy JL, Worley DR, Withrow SJ. Outcome following simultaneous bilateral thyroid lobectomy for treatment of thyroid gland carcinoma in dogs: 15 cases (1994–2010). *J Am Vet Med Assoc* 2012; **241**: 95–103.
257 Robinson R, Borgeat K. Cardiovascular disease. In: Duke-Novakovski T, de Vries M, Seymour C, eds. *BSAVA Manual of Canine and Feline Anaesthesia and Analgesia*, 3rd edn. Quedgeley, UK: British Small Animal Veterinary Association, 2016: 282–312.
258 Steinbacher R, Dörfelt R. Anesthesia in dogs and cats with cardiac disease – an impossible endeavour or a challenge with manageable risk? *Eur J Companion Anim Pract* 2013; **23**: 4–22.
259 Ramoo S, Bradbury LA, Anderson GA, *et al.* Sedation of hyperthyroid cats with subcutaneous administration of a combination of alfaxalone and butorphanol. *Aust Vet J* 2013; **91**: 131–136.
260 Tamura J, Ishizuka T, Fukui S, *et al.* Sedative effects of intramuscular alfaxalone administered to cats. *J Vet Med Sci* 2015; **77**: 897–904.
261 Warne LN, Beths T, Whittem T, *et al.* A review of the pharmacology and clinical application of alfaxalone in cats. *Vet J* 2015; **203**: 141–148.
262 Robinson R, Borer-Weir K. The effects of diazepam or midazolam on the dose of propofol required to induce anaesthesia in cats. *Vet Anaesth Analg* 2015; **42**: 493–501.
263 Saha DC, Saha AC, Malik G, *et al.* Comparison of cardiovascular effects of tiletamine-zolazepam, pentobarbital, and ketamine-xylazine in male rats. *J Amer Assoc Lab Anim Sci* 2007; **46**: 74–80.
264 Purchase IFH. Cardiac arrhythmias occurring during halothane anaesthesia in cats. *Br J Anaesth* 1966; **38**: 13–22.
265 De Vries M, Putter G. Perioperative anaesthetic care of the cat undergoing dental and oral procedures: key considerations. *J Feline Med Surg* 2015; **17**: 23–36.
266 Wiese AJ, Barter LS, Kittleson MD, *et al.* Cardiovascular and respiratory effects of incremental doses of dopamine and phenylephrine in the management of isoflurane-induced hypotension in cats with hypertrophic cardiomyopathy. *Am J Vet Res* 2012; **73**: 908–916.
267 Pang D, Rondenay Y, Héile P, *et al.* Sudden cardiac death associated with occult hypertrophic cardiomyopathy in a dog under anesthesia. *Can Vet J* 2005; **46**: 1122–1125.
268 Campos M, Ductalle R, Rutteman G, *et al.* Clinical, pathologic, and immunohistochemical prognostic factors in dogs with thyroid carcinoma. *J Vet Intern Med* 2014; **28**: 1805–1813.
269 Reagan JK, Selmic LE, Fallon C, *et al.* Complications and outcomes associated with unilateral thyroidectomy in dogs with naturally occurring thyroid tumors: 156 cases (2003–2015). *J Am Vet Med Assoc* 2019; **255**: 926–932.
270 Liptak JM. Canine thyroid carcinoma. *Clin Tech Small Anim Pract* 2007; **22**: 75–81.
271 DeGroot WD, Tobias KM, Browning DC. Examination of laryngeal function of healthy dogs by using sedation protocol with dexmedetomidine. *Vet Surg* 2020; **49**: 124–130.
272 Radkey DI, Hardie RJ, Smith LJ. Comparison of the effects of alfaxalone and propofol with acepromazine, butorphanol and/or doxapram on laryngeal motion and quality of examination in dogs. *Vet Anaesth Analg* 2018; **45**: 241–249.
273 Wilson DV, Evans AT, Miller R. Effects of preanesthetic administration of morphine on gastroesophageal reflux and regurgitation during anesthesia in dogs. *Am J Vet Res* 2005; **66**: 386–390.
274 Costa RS, Wetmore LA, Stein A. Randomized, blinded, controlled clinical trial to assess gastroesophageal reflux and regurgitation in dogs undergoing general anesthesia after hydromorphone premedication with or without acepromazine or dexmedetomidine. *Am J Vet Res* 2021; **82**: 695–700.
275 KuKanich B, Bidgood T, Knesl O. Clinical pharmacology of nonsteroidal anti-inflammatory drugs in dogs. *Vet Anaesth Analg* 2012; **39**: 69–90.
276 Fukui S, Endo Y, Hirayama K, *et al.* Identification and preservation of the parathyroid gland during total thyroidectomy in dogs with bilateral thyroid carcinoma: a report of six cases. *J Vet Med Sci* 2015; **77**: 747.
277 Seguin B, Bronlee L. Thyroid and parathyroid glands. In: Tobias KN, Johnston SA, eds. *Veterinary Surgery Small Animal*, 1st edn. St. Louis, MO: Saunder Elsevier, 2012: 2050–2053.
278 Feldman EC, Hoar B, Pollard R, *et al.* Pretreatment clinical and laboratory findings in dogs with primary hyperparathyroidism: 210 cases (1987–2004). *J Am Vet Med Assoc* 2005; **227**: 756–761.
279 Gear RN, Neiger R, Skelly BJ, *et al.* Primary hyperparathyroidism in 29 dogs: diagnosis, treatment, outcome and associated renal failure. *J Small Anim Pract* 2005; **46**: 10–16.
280 Parker VJ, Gilor C, Chew DJ. Feline hyperparathyroidism: pathophysiology, diagnosis and treatment of primary and secondary disease. *J Feline Med Surg* 2015; **17**: 427–439.
281 Bonczynski J. Primary hyperparathyroidism in dogs and cats. *Clin Tech Small Anim Pract* 2007; **22**: 70–74.
282 Schaefer C, Goldstein RE. Canine primary hyperparathyroidism. *Compend Contin Educ Pract Vet* 2009; **31**: 382–390.
283 Milovancev M, Schmiedt CW. Preoperative factors associated with postoperative hypocalcemia in dogs with primary hyperparathyroidism that underwent parathyroidectomy: 62 cases (2004–2009). *J Am Vet Med Assoc* 2013; **242**: 507–515.
284 Goldstein RE, Atwater CZ, Cazolli DM, *et al.* Inheritance, mode of inheritance, and candidate genes for primary hyperparathyroidism in Keeshonden. *J Vet Intern Med* 2007; **21**: 199–203.
285 Schenck PA, Chew DJ. Calcium: total or ionized? *Vet Clin North Am Small Anim Pract* 2008; **38**: 497–502.
286 Savary KCM, Price GS, Vaden SL. Hypercalcemia in cats: a retrospective study of 71 cases: (1991–1997). *J Vet Intern Med* 2000; **14**: 184–189.
287 Sawyer ES, Northrup NC, Schmiedt CW, *et al.* Outcome of 19 dogs with parathyroid carcinoma after surgical excision. *Vet Comp Oncol* 2011; **10**: 57–64.
288 Leal RO, Pascual LF, Hernandez J. The use of percutaneous ultrasound-guided radiofrequency heat ablation for treatment of primary hyperparathyroidism in eight dogs: outcome and complications. *Vet Sci* 2018; **5**: 91.
289 Graves TK. When normal is abnormal: keys to laboratory diagnosis of hidden endocrine disease. *Top Comp Anim Med* 2011; **26**: 45–51.
290 Wisner ER, Penninck D, Biller DS, *et al.* High resolution parathyroid sonography. *Vet Radiol Ultrasound* 1997; **38**: 462–466.
291 Schenk PA, Chew DJ. Diseases of the parathyroid gland and calcium disorders. In: Birchard SJ, Sherding RG, eds. *Saunders Manual of Small Animal Practice*, 3rd edn. St. Louis, MO: Saunders Elsevier, 2006: 343–356.
292 Schenk PA, Chew DJ, Nagode LA, *et al.* Disorders of calcium: hypercalcemia and hypocalcemia. In: DiBartola SP, ed. *Fluid, Electrolyte, and Acid–Base Disorders in Small Animal Practice*, 4th edn. St. Louis, MO: Saunders Elsevier, 2012: 137–163.
293 Green T, Chew DJ. Calcium disorders. In: Silverstein D, Hopper K, eds. *Small Animal Critical Care Medicine*. St. Louis, MO: Saunders Elsevier, 2009: 233–239.
294 Rasor L, Pollard R, Feldman EC. Retrospective evaluation of three treatment methods for primary hyperparathyroidism in dogs. *J Am Anim Hosp Assoc* 2007; **43**: 70–77.
295 Armstrong AJ, Hauptman JG, Stanley BJ, *et al.* Effect of prophylactic calcitriol administration of serum ionized calcium concentrations after parathyroidectomy: 78 cases (2005–2015). *J Vet Intern Med* 2018; **32**: 99–106.

296 Arbaugh M, Smeak D, Monnet E. Evaluation of preoperative serum concentrations of ionized calcium and parathyroid hormone as predictors of hypocalcemia following parathyroidectomy in dogs with primary hyperparathyroidism: 17 cases (2001–2009). *J Am Vet Med Assoc* 2012; **24**: 233–236.
297 Roland EJL, Wierda JMKH, Eurin BG, *et al.* Pharmacodynamic behaviour of vecuronium in primary hyperparathyroidism. *Can J Anaesth* 1994; **41**: 694–698.
298 Dear JD, Kass PH, Della Maggiore AM, *et al.* Association of hypercalcemia before treatment with hypocalcemia after treatment in dogs with primary hyperparathyroidism. *J Vet Intern Med* 2017; **31**: 349–354.
299 Brezis M, Rosen S. Hypoxia of the renal medulla – its implications for disease. *N Engl J Med* 1995; **332**: 647–655.
300 Radlinsky MG. Thyroid surgery in dogs and cats. *Vet Clin North Am Small Anim Pract* 2007; **37**: 789–798.
301 Ham K, Greenfield CL, Barger A, *et al.* Validation of a rapid parathyroid hormone assay and intraoperative measurement of parathyroid hormone in dogs with benign naturally occurring parathyroidism. *Vet Surg* 2009; **38**: 122–132.
302 Graham KJ, Wilkinson M, Culvenor J, *et al.* Intraoperative parathyroid hormone concentration to confirm removal of hypersecretory parathyroid tissue and time to postoperative normocalcaemia in nine dogs with primary hyperparathyroidism. *Aust Vet J* 2012; **90**: 203–209.
303 Burkhardt SJ, Sumner JP, Mann S. Ambidirectional cohort study on the agreement of ultrasonography and surgery in the identification of parathyroid pathology, and predictors of postoperative hypocalcemia in 47 dogs undergoing parathyroidectomy due to primary parathyroidism. *Vet Surg* 2021; **50**: 1379–1388.

43 Physiology, Pathophysiology, and Anesthetic Management of Patients with Renal Disease

Stuart C. Clark-Price[1] **and Julie R. Fischer**[2]

[1] Department of Clinical Sciences, College of Veterinary Medicine, Auburn University, Auburn, Alabama, USA

[2] Veterinary Specialty Hospital of North County (Ethos Veterinary Health), San Marcos, California, USA

Chapter contents

Introduction, 922
Normal anatomy and physiology, 922
  Anatomy of the urinary tract, 923
  Physiologic function, 924
Testing and monitoring renal function, 926
  Canine and feline, 926
  Equine, 928
  Ruminant, 929
Acute kidney injury/acute renal failure, 929
  Etiology and pathogenesis, 929
  Clinical features and diagnosis, 931
Chronic kidney disease, 931
  Etiology and pathogenesis, 931
  Clinical features and diagnosis, 932
  Staging chronic kidney disease, 932
  Further diagnostics and treatment, 932
Anesthetic drugs and renal disease, 933
Anesthetic management of patients with renal disease, 936
  Adjunctive treatments for patients with renal disease, 936
Anesthetic management of patients with urethral or bilateral ureteral obstruction, 937
Anesthetic management of patients with urinary bladder rupture and uroabdomen, 938
Postanesthesia oliguria and acute kidney injury, 939
Acknowledgment, 939
References, 939

Introduction

The kidneys receive and require 20–25% of cardiac output to appropriately perform their intricate and multifaceted role in the maintenance of physiologic homeostasis. By its nature, general anesthesia alters hemodynamics and organ perfusion, thus inherently posing specific potential risk to healthy kidneys and even more so to diseased or compromised kidneys. Renal disease and functional impairment occur frequently in veterinary patients, particularly in geriatric ones, with a 1–3% overall prevalence in cats, up to 20% of cats having chronic kidney disease (CKD) during their lifetime, and 35–80% of cats older than 15 years affected [1–3]. The prevalence of CKD in dogs is lower and has been reported at 0.05–3.74% depending on inclusion criteria, with the largest and most recent study reporting a 0.21–0.37% overall prevalence [4]. Histopathologic examination of the kidneys of nonazotemic cats shows chronic degenerative changes including glomerulosclerosis, tubular atrophy, interstitial inflammation, and fibrosis that increases in severity with age [5]. Similar chronic changes have been shown in aged canine kidneys as well, suggesting that geriatric patients may be at heightened risk of renal damage from nephrotoxic drugs and hemodynamic shifts, even when these patients are nonazotemic [6].

Equine and ruminant patients have a much lower overall prevalence of renal disease than cats and will be discussed less in this chapter. The overall prevalence of CKD in horses is 0.12% with a prevalence of 0.23% in horses older than 15 years of age, increasing to 0.51% in stallions older than 15 years of age [7]. Acute kidney injury occurs more commonly than CKD in horses, with 23% of horses presenting for colic having evidence of injury and as many as 25% of neonatal foals presenting for intensive care [8].

Because animals with renal disease will routinely require anesthesia, clinicians must have a working knowledge of renal physiology and pathophysiology, as well as a thorough understanding of both the potential renal effects of the sedative, analgesic, and anesthetic drugs they select and how best to protect kidney health and function during their use.

Normal anatomy and physiology

A complete in-depth overview of the anatomy and physiology of the renal system is beyond the scope of this chapter; the reader is referred to medical anatomy and physiology textbooks for further detailed descriptions [9–11].

Veterinary Anesthesia and Analgesia: The Sixth Edition of Lumb and Jones. Edited by Leigh Lamont, Kurt Grimm, Sheilah Robertson, Lydia Love and Carrie Schroeder.
© 2024 John Wiley & Sons, Inc. Published 2024 by John Wiley & Sons, Inc.
Companion website: www.wiley.com/go/lamont/anesthesia

Anatomy of the urinary tract

Grossly, the urinary system can be divided into the kidneys, the ureters, the urinary bladder, and the urethra. The kidney can be further divided into the cortex, medulla, and renal pelvis. The renal pelvis is essentially the expanded proximal portion of the ureters, which carry urine from the kidney to the urinary bladder. Between species, there are several anatomic differences that exist within the kidney. Dogs, cats, horses, and small ruminants have unilobar kidneys that contain a renal crest or basin within the renal pelvis that collects urine and empties into the proximal urethra. Additionally, gland-like structures in the wall of the horse's renal pelvis secrete a mucous-like substance that is responsible for the cloudy and foamy nature of normal horse urine. Swine and bovine kidneys are multilobar kidneys that contain renal papillae (medullary extensions or pyramids) that empty into cup-like calyces that then empty into the renal pelvis. The gross shape of the kidney is fairly similar in that most species have the classic kidney shape with a smooth surface and two poles. The exceptions are the right kidney of the horse, which tends to have a heart-like shape, and the lobulated kidneys of the bovine species, due to incomplete fusion of the kidney lobes. The ureters are smooth muscle-lined tubes that carry urine from the kidney to the bladder. The urinary bladder can be anatomically divided into the body and the neck or trigone region. The body consists of a compliant three-layered muscular wall that can accommodate incoming urine for storage and later voiding. This allows the bladder to vary greatly in shape, size, and position within the pelvis and abdomen. The urethra is a muscular tube that connects the bladder to the genitals, allowing transit of urine from the bladder to the external environment. Anatomic variations of the urethra exist based on gender and species.

The functional units of the kidneys are nephrons (Fig. 43.1), which consist of a renal corpuscle and associated tubule, span the cortex and medulla of the kidney, and exist within a vital milieu called the renal interstitium. The renal interstitium is composed of cellular components ("interstitial cells") residing in a loose glycosaminoglycan matrix. The majority of interstitial cells are specialized fibroblasts that structurally stabilize the kidney by weaving around and between nephrons, and by connecting to each other via intermediate-like junctions. These fibroblasts have very well developed rough endoplasmic reticulum, ribosomes, and Golgi apparatus to support their many synthetic functions. A smaller population of marrow-derived cells migrates through the interstitium; in healthy kidneys, most of these are major histocompatibility complex (MHC) class II-expressing dendritic cells, but in disease states, particularly inflammatory states, invasion by other mononuclear cells (e.g., lymphocytes, monocytes/macrophages, and other dendritic cells) is common. The interstitial matrix is a living interconnection among the three chief functional components of the kidney, that is, the vasculature, the tubules, and the glomeruli, and serves as a thoroughfare between the renal tubules and the peritubular capillaries. Solute and water transport occurs from the tubular lumina through the interstitium and into the peritubular capillaries, while oxygen and nutrients travel from

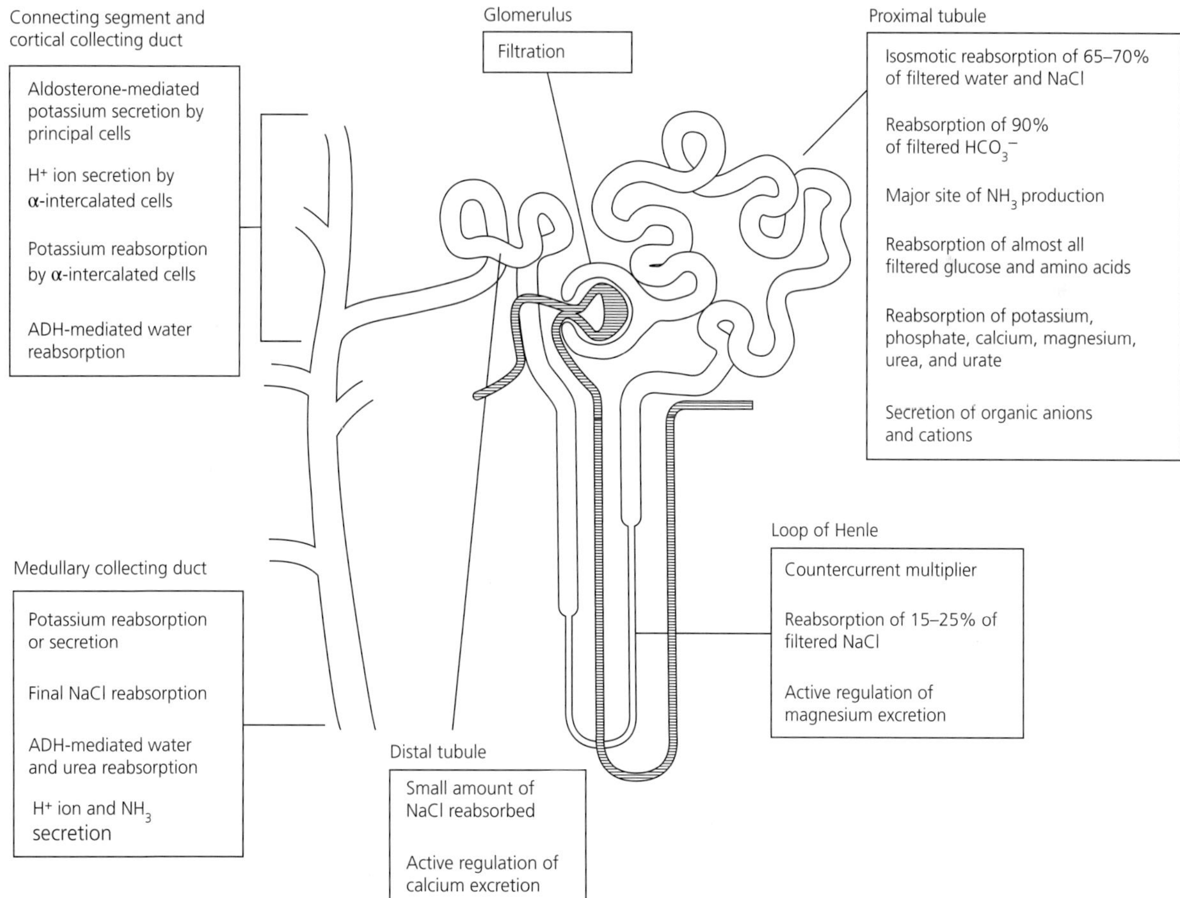

Figure 43.1 Anatomy and physiologic function of each portion of the nephron. Source: DiBartola [11], reproduced with permission of Elsevier.

the capillaries through the interstitium to nourish the tubular cells [12].

Renal tubules are responsible for modification of plasma filtrate into urine and are described in functional segments termed the proximal tubule, loop of Henle, distal tubule, and collecting duct. Tubules comprise the substantial majority of renal mass, with blood vessels, interstitium, and renal corpuscles present in much smaller quantities. The cortex contains the corpuscles, which are tight, spherical convolutions of glomerular capillaries surrounded by a specialized proximal tubular outpouching called Bowman's capsule. Initial filtration of plasma occurs at the glomerulus across the glomerular filtration barrier (described later in the chapter); the filtrate then flows into Bowman's capsule and from there into the proximal renal tubule. The cortical parenchyma consists of renal tubules and capillaries packed around glomeruli in seemingly random fashion, surrounded by small amounts of intercalated interstitium. The medulla consists entirely of tubules, arterioles, capillaries, and interstitium, packed tightly together with the tubules and vessel networks arranged radially in near-parallel formation within the parenchyma and in much more organized fashion than in the cortex. The final tubular product, urine, flows into the renal pelvis in transit to the ureter, which then propels the urine by peristaltic waves into the bladder [13].

Physiologic function

The kidneys govern or play a significant role in a myriad of homeostatic processes, chiefly maintaining water and electrolyte balance, acid–base regulation, systemic blood pressure management, extracellular fluid volume composition, excretion of dissolved foreign substances and metabolic wastes, vitamin D production and calcium–phosphorus balance, hormone secretion, metabolism and excretion, erythrocyte production, and even gluconeogenesis. They accomplish many of these functions through generation of urine by the processes of filtration, reabsorption, and secretion and receive about 25% of the cardiac output in order to do so. In fact, the renal arteries branch directly from the caudal aorta, providing the high percentage of cardiac output necessary to facilitate filtration and maintain the kidneys' high metabolic activity (i.e., very high oxygen and substrate consumption). Kidneys, especially the proximal tubules, are particularly susceptible to hypoxic damage and even short-term renal ischemia can lead to acute kidney injury (AKI).

Renal blood flow (RBF) is regulated by extrinsic nervous and hormonal control and by intrinsic autoregulation. The renal vasculature is highly innervated by sympathetic constrictor fibers originating in the spinal cord segments between T4 and L1, yet the kidneys lack sympathetic vasodilating fibers and parasympathetic innervation. Dopamine receptors in the renal vasculature and tubules help regulate vasodilation and blood flow. There are two known subtypes of dopamine receptors, D_1 and D_2. Both of these receptors have been identified in dogs, rats, rabbits, and other animals. It was thought that cats did not possess renal dopamine receptors; however, in 2003, a D_1-like receptor was identified that is considered to be different from receptors found in rats, dogs, or humans [14]. Intrinsic autoregulation of RBF is demonstrated by a constant flow when the mean arterial blood pressure ranges from 80 to 180 mmHg. When the mean arterial blood pressure is in this range, the kidney can control blood flow via alteration of resistance in the glomerular afferent arterioles. Although the exact mechanism of renal autoregulation is not known, the phenomenon protects glomerular capillaries during hypertension and preserves renal function during hypotension. In addition to renal autoregulation, extrinsic forces (e.g., neural, hormonal, and pharmacologic) and intrinsic forces (e.g., kidney disease) may cause alterations in RBF. Catecholamines are major hormonal regulators of RBF. Epinephrine and norepinephrine cause dose-dependent changes in RBF. Low doses increase arterial blood pressure and increase RBF through increased cardiac output, whereas higher doses cause a decreased RBF through increased vascular resistance. The renin–angiotensin–aldosterone system, discussed later in this chapter, is also an important regulator of RBF. In addition, prostaglandins play an important role in the regulation of RBF. Prostaglandin-E_2 (PGE_2) and prostaglandin-I_2 (PGI_2 or prostacyclin) cause vasodilation within the kidney. Generation of PGE_2 and PGI_2 occurs through the upregulation of cyclo-oxygenase enzymes; in particular, the cyclo-oxygenase-2 (COX-2) enzyme plays a largely constitutive and protective role. The COX-2 enzyme is found mainly in the macula densa but can also be found in other areas of the cortex and the medulla. During low blood flow or hypotensive states, COX-2-derived prostaglandins promote natriuresis, renin release, and vasodilation of afferent arterioles to preserve RBF.

Although the kidney receives a high percentage of the cardiac output, blood flow is not evenly distributed throughout the kidney. The renal cortex receives the majority of the blood (90–95%), thus leaving the medulla relatively hypoperfused and hypoxic. This dichotomous blood flow strategy maximizes flow-dependent activities in areas of the kidney that specialize in high-efficiency filtration.

Hydrostatic pressure drives plasma filtration across the glomerular filtration barrier and into the proximal convoluted tubules. The filtration barrier consists of the glomerular capillaries, the glomerular basement membrane, and specialized epithelial cells called "podocytes." The glomerular capillaries consist of a single layer of endothelial cells with small fenestrations that provide the filtration surface and allow only fluid, very small proteins, and electrolytes to be filtered. Under these cells is the glomerular basement membrane, an acellular, trilaminar structure composed of various proteins and proteoglycans, that provides a scaffold for the epithelial cells and a negatively charged barrier that excludes larger negatively charged molecules (chiefly proteins). The last layer of the glomerular filtration barrier is formed by the network of extensively branching podocytes that cover the entire glomerular surface. The tiny spaces between the interdigitating processes of these cells are specialized junctions called "slit pores" or "slit diaphragms," which provide the most size-restrictive portion of the filtration barrier. With the exception of albumin and larger proteins, the glomerular filtrate received by Bowman's capsule is very similar in composition to plasma (Table 43.1).

The rate of formation of the filtrate, or glomerular filtration rate (GFR), is a measurable parameter that can be evaluated clinically to determine renal excretory function. GFR is expressed as milliliters of glomerular filtrate per kilogram of body weight formed per minute (mL/kg/min). Blood flow into the glomeruli for filtration is under pressure and is regulated by afferent (preglomerular) and efferent (postglomerular) arterioles. The amount of filtrate formed is directly related to the pressure across the capillaries, and this pressure can be described mathematically using Starling's equation:

$$Q = K_f\left[(P_c - P_i) - \sigma(\pi_c - \pi_i)\right]$$

where Q is the net fluid movement across the capillaries, K_f is the filtration coefficient (which depends on the permeability and length of the filtration surface), P_c is the capillary hydrostatic pressure, P_i is the interstitial hydrostatic pressure, σ is the reflection or filtration coefficient, π_c is the capillary oncotic pressure, and π_i is the interstitial oncotic pressure. When measured at the afferent arteriole

Table 43.1 Major activity and filtrate composition in the nephron.

Nephron structure	Major activity	Filtrate composition	Comments
Glomerulus	Filtration of plasma	Isotonic	Cell-free filtrate containing only fluid, electrolytes, and small proteins
Proximal convoluted tubule	45–55% of filtrate is reabsorbed	Isotonic	90% of HCO_3^- is reabsorbed and filtrate becomes acidic
Descending loop of Henle	25–40% of filtrate H_2O is reabsorbed	Hypertonic	H_2O reabsorption via osmosis
Ascending loop of Henle	Major area of solute reabsorption	Hypotonic	Active transport via Na^+-K^+ ATPase, cells are impermeable to H_2O
Distal convoluted tubule	5% of filtrate is reabsorbed	Hypotonic	Less than 10% of originally filtered H_2O is present
Collecting duct	0.5–10% of H_2O reabsorption	Hyper-, iso-, or hypotonic (urine)	Under the influence of arginine vasopressin

end of the glomerulus, the net filtration pressure is about 10 mmHg, resulting in a net outflow. When measured at the efferent arteriole end of the glomerulus, the net filtration pressure is about 0 mmHg, resulting in zero net outflow.

RBF and, thus, usually GFR are maintained within a consistent range in spite of changes in systemic blood pressure by an autoregulation system controlled in large part by the renin–angiotensin–aldosterone hormone system (RAAS). When blood pressure and subsequent renal perfusion decrease, the enzyme renin is released from specialized juxtaglomerular cells located in the walls of the afferent arterioles, just proximal to the glomeruli. Renin acts on angiotensinogen (produced by the liver) to release angiotensin I, which is swiftly converted to angiotensin II (AT-II, a potent vasoconstrictor) by angiotensin-converting enzyme (ACE). This conversion occurs chiefly while blood flows through the small vessels in the lungs, since most ACE is produced by the pulmonary small vascular endothelium. The kidneys and other blood vessels also produce some ACE and generate a smaller amount of AT-II locally. AT-II directly increases blood pressure through constriction of smooth muscle in arterioles but also has multiple endocrine and paracrine effects. Locally within the kidney, AT-II activates sodium uptake in the tubules of the nephron, promoting fluid retention and increased blood volume. At the adrenal gland, AT-II increases release of the steroid hormone aldosterone, which promotes sodium conservation, potassium elimination, and increased fluid retention and blood pressure. At the pituitary gland, AT-II enhances vasopressin (also known as antidiuretic hormone) release, which increases water reabsorption in the kidneys through the insertion of water channels (aquaporin-2) into the membrane of the distal tubules of the nephron. Vasopressin also has direct vasoconstrictive properties through G-protein-coupled V receptors in vascular endothelium. Additionally, AT-II induces intrarenal release of the vasodilating prostaglandins PGE_2 and prostacyclin (PGI_2) that counteract the vasoconstricting effects of AT-II, thereby preventing excessive intrarenal vascular resistance and local ischemia. A second intrinsic system, called "tubuloglomerular feedback," also contributes to the autoregulatory system that helps maintain GFR. A distinct group of epithelial cells within the distal convoluted tubule (DCT), the macula densa, contact the glomerulus between the afferent and efferent arterioles as part of the juxtaglomerular apparatus (JGA). Osmoreceptors within the macula densa cells sense decreased sodium concentrations within the tubular lumen and initiate a cascade of events resulting in renin release from the juxtaglomerular cells. Alternatively, increased sodium chloride concentrations result in an undefined cascade of events that suppresses renin release and leads to production of vasoactive factors (nitric oxide, adenosine triphosphate, prostaglandins) that reduce GFR and promote free water conservation.

Filtered fluid that leaves the glomerulus next enters the proximal convoluted tubules (PCTs). The major function of the PCT is to reabsorb the majority of the filtrate; in fact, more than 60% of the filtered substances are reabsorbed in the PCT. Transport across the PCT membrane into the interstitial tissues and then into the vascular space occurs via both active and passive transport with Starling's forces dictating the passive phases. The majority of ions filtered at the glomerulus (Na^+, K^+, Ca^{2+}, Cl^-, and HCO_3^-) are reabsorbed in the PCT so that filtrate leaving the PCT and entering the loop of Henle has lower levels of electrolytes than plasma. Water passively follows the active reabsorption of electrolytes so that the osmolality of the tubular fluid is similar to that of plasma at both ends of the PCT. Organic low-molecular-weight proteins (insulin, glucagon, parathyroid hormone, etc.) that were filtered are also actively reabsorbed in the PCT. Secretion of substances also occurs in the PCT. Organic ionic wastes are eliminated via secretion into the filtrate; these include protein-bound exogenous substances that are not filtered at the glomerulus, for example, endotoxins, antibiotics, and anesthetic and analgesic drugs such as morphine and ketamine, and endogenous wastes such as bile salts, urates, and prostaglandins. PCT secretion is exceptionally important for endogenous waste removal in birds and reptiles. In mammals, one of the main waste products from muscle metabolism is urea, which is freely filtered at the glomerulus; however, uric acid is the waste product from muscle metabolism in birds and reptiles. Uric acid is not filtered at the glomeruli, and its removal is dependent upon active mechanisms in the PCT in these species.

Next, the remaining filtrate enters the descending loop of Henle (DloH). Metabolic activity within the DloH is minimal, and little to no active transport process occurs. Pure water reabsorption and minimal solute drag occur as the filtrate travels through the DloH to the highly active ascending (AloH) or thick portion of the loop of Henle.

The AloH is one of the most metabolically active parts of the tubule and the entire kidney. It is composed of simple cuboidal epithelium with many mitochondria, which provide the energy for high-capacity active transport. Here, the filtrate is further modified as the majority of electrolyte reabsorption within the loop of Henle takes place in the AloH. An abundant concentration of Na^+-K^+ ATPase pumps can be found on the luminal surface of the tubules, which are responsible for the active transport of Na^+, K^+, and Cl^- into the cell and out of the filtrate. Other ions such as Mg^{2+} and Ca^{2+} move down a cation-selective paracellular pathway into the interstitium. In the case of K^+ in particular, hyperkalemia can result in electrical conduction pathology, and therefore, both apical and basolateral K^+ channels exist to increase secretion into the filtrate for eventual removal in the urine. As the AloH is highly metabolically active, it has a high demand for substrates such as oxygen and, therefore, has increased sensitivity to damage during hypoxemia or hypotension. Additionally, several medications can exert their effects both therapeutically and pathologically at the AloH. For example, furosemide works as a diuretic by inhibiting Na^+-K^+ ATPase pumps and preventing electrolyte and fluid reabsorption while aminoglycoside antibiotics such as gentamicin can inhibit protein synthesis and result in acute tubular necrosis in the PCT and the AloH. The AloH is impermeable to water so that filtrate entering the DCT is hypotonic; this is, in fact, how the kidney forms dilute urine in the absence of antidiuretic hormone (ADH).

After the AloH, the highly modified hypotonic filtrate enters the DCTs. Electrolyte and water reabsorption occurs to modify the filtrate further; however, K^+ and H^+ secretion is of major importance in the DCT. Because the majority of HCO_3^- was reabsorbed in the PCT, only a very small amount of HCO_3^- remains, and therefore, both K^+ and H^+ must be actively pumped into the lumen to counter an imbalance between negatively and positively charged ions. This can result in K^+ and H^+ competing with each other for secretion and is often the reason why hyperkalemia is associated with acidemia.

Finally, the filtrate enters the collecting duct where it can be modified one more time before being classified as urine. Collecting duct tubular cells must be impermeable to water when patients are overhydrated and permeable to H_2O during dehydration. This is accomplished via the actions of the hormone vasopressin (ADH). When states of dehydration exist, vasopressin is released from the neurohypophysis, stimulated by increased plasma osmolality, and its presence at the level of the kidneys induces the translocation and insertion of water channels (aquaporin-2) into the cells of the DCT and collecting duct. Water is then allowed to be reabsorbed, resulting in a more concentrated urine. Interestingly, α_2-adrenergic receptor agonist drugs, such as xylazine, block the vasopressin receptors located within the collecting ducts, preventing water reabsorption. This can be observed clinically as animals voiding large amounts of dilute urine after sedation with an α_2-adrenergic receptor agonist and can result in worsening dehydration in animals with a negative fluid balance.

On leaving the collecting duct, the filtrate is considered to be urine, where it is gathered in the renal pelvis and transported to the urinary bladder via the ureters for storage and voiding.

Testing and monitoring renal function

Canine and feline

Biochemical testing

Any determination of intrinsic renal dysfunction must start by identifying/excluding and/or correcting any prerenal (i.e., anything that decreases RBF) and postrenal (i.e., anything that blocks normal transit of urine from the kidney to the urethral orifice) causes of azotemia. Evaluation of blood urea nitrogen (BUN) and serum creatinine concentrations in combination with urine specific gravity has long served as the chief method of routine clinical diagnosis and serial monitoring of renal function in dogs and cats. As GFR declines, serum creatinine increases (though in nonlinear fashion) and, since it is affected by fewer extrarenal factors than BUN, serum creatinine measurement is the most commonly employed indirect estimate of GFR. Unfortunately, neither BUN nor serum creatinine is particularly sensitive or specific for intrinsic renal disease and, at best, provides a rough index of GFR [15–19].

Decreased diagnostic accuracy for these analytes results in part because BUN and serum creatinine generally do not rise out of the reference range before roughly 75% of functional renal mass has been lost; however, many other factors influence this as well. In dogs and cats with CKD, compensatory hypertrophy and hyperfiltration in the remaining functional nephrons can also mask the degree of degeneration present. The relationship between GFR and the inverse of serum creatinine concentration is logarithmic rather than linear and can, therefore, lead to overestimation of renal function in early CKD and underestimation in later-stage disease. Because creatinine is a breakdown product of creatine phosphate generated during normal myocyte metabolism, serum creatinine concentration can vary greatly relative to an individual animal's muscle mass. Heavily muscled dogs, such as Greyhounds, may have serum creatinine measurements that fall above the reference range in spite of normal kidney function, while sarcopenic animals often have serum creatinine measurements that significantly under-represent the severity of kidney disease present. Total ingested protein load, among other extrarenal factors, can markedly increase BUN concentration (and to a lesser extent, serum creatinine), while hepatic insufficiency or a very low protein diet may decrease it, irrespective of kidney function.

The limitations of BUN and serum creatinine in assessing renal function have led to investigation of other biomarkers for this purpose, one of which is symmetric dimethylarginine (SDMA) [20,21]. This molecule is an endogenous product of intracellular protein methylation and degradation that is chiefly renally excreted and freely filtered at the glomerulus. Serum concentration of SDMA has been shown by clearance studies in azotemic and nonazotemic cats [17] and in dogs with hereditary nephropathy [18] to be strongly inversely correlated with GFR (in linear fashion). Serum SDMA concentration increases when approximately 40% of functional renal mass is lost, making it a more sensitive marker of early CKD in dogs and cats than serum creatinine, which increases after approximately 75% functional decrement, as mentioned above. Unlike serum creatinine, SDMA is not affected by increased or decreased muscle mass in a given animal, and studies specifically examining non-renal modifiers of SDMA in dogs have shown that asymptomatic mitral regurgitation, age, breed, sex, and vigorous exercise have no influence on serum SDMA concentrations [22,23]. On average, monitoring of SDMA permits detection of CKD 17 months earlier in cats and 9 months earlier in dogs than does assessment of serum creatinine [19,21,24,25]. As with BUN and creatinine, any process that results in decreased GFR can increase SDMA concentration; thus, although it will also be elevated in animals with decreased GFR due to AKI, SDMA concentration cannot be used to distinguish between AKI and CKD [26]. Currently, the International Renal Interest Society (IRIS) recommends using both serum creatinine and SDMA as complementary parameters in the staging of CKD. Regardless of which biochemical parameters are used, their longitudinal/serial monitoring in the same patient will improve detection of declining renal function, even if values remain within normal limits. For example, a serum creatinine concentration that increases from 0.6 to 1.2 mg/dL over time may indicate a ≥ 50% reduction in renal function (assuming that muscle mass has not changed, and hydration status is normal).

Since normal kidneys regulate total body water by adjusting the amount excreted in urine, measurement of urine specific gravity (USG, comparison of the weight of a solution to the weight of water) can help assess renal tubular function; however, like BUN and serum creatinine, USG is neither a sensitive nor specific measure of function. The normal dog kidney can produce a USG > 1.030, while a normal feline kidney can produce a USG of > 1.035, depending on water balance at any given time, though a physiologically appropriate USG can vary from 1.001 to up to 1.075 in the dog and 1.085 in the cat. When renal function declines beyond a certain point, the kidneys lose the capacity to concentrate and dilute filtrate; thus, the urine produced remains in a fixed range called the isosthenuric range (1.008–1.012), which is the USG range of unmodified glomerular filtrate entering the proximal tubule. In dogs, decrements in urine-concentrating ability are not detectable until approximately two-thirds of the nephrons are non-functional. In cats, this proportion is thought to be higher, since it is not uncommon for cats with renal azotemia (and thus more than 75% loss of renal function) to retain the ability to produce significantly hypersthenuric urine. In addition to this lack of sensitivity, extrarenal influences can compromise urine-concentrating ability, as seen with decreased ADH secretion or responsiveness (e.g., hypercalcemia, hyperadrenocorticism, glucocorticoid exposure, etc.), use of diuretic medications, renal medullary washout, significant glucosuria, and other causes. Hypovolemia and consequent decreased GFR in these patients can thus result in azotemia with inappropriate isosthenuria, in spite of underlying normal renal functional capacity [27].

As an alternative or complement to standard clinicopathologic tests, the detection and quantification of multiple urine biomarkers, including clusterin, cystatin C, γ-glutamyl transpeptidase (GGT), *N*-acetylglucosaminidase (NAG), and neutrophil gelatinase-associated lipocalin (NGAL), have been proven able to indicate pre-azotemic nephron damage in the dog [28–31]. These biomarkers may be useful both in the acute (NAG, GGT, NGAL, cystatin C, and clusterin), and chronic (cystatin C, NGAL, and SDMA) setting [29,32,33]. Since some enzymes originate from specific cellular organelles, those enzymurias mark damage to a specific anatomic site. For example, γ-glutamyl transpeptidase (GGT) originates from the proximal tubular brush border and *N*-acetylglucosaminidase (NAG) is a lysosomal enzyme. Enzymuria usually precedes azotemia and decreased urine-concentrating ability associated with nephrotoxic proximal tubular injury by several days. Urine GGT:creatinine and NAG:creatinine ratios have been shown to reflect accurately 24-h urine GGT and NAG excretion in dogs, if determined before the onset of azotemia [28]. Determination of baseline urine GGT:creatinine and NAG:creatinine ratios, therefore, could be considered in dogs with possible pre-existing acute renal insult that are to receive potentially nephrotoxic drugs. Two- to threefold increases in the GGT:creatinine or NAG:creatinine ratio over the baseline are suggestive of clinically relevant tubular damage. Drug therapy should be discontinued if this occurs.

The repeatable presence of renal proteinuria is both a marker of renal disease and also a negative prognostic factor when identified in animals with CKD [34–37]. Detection of greater than normal amounts of protein in the urine, usually initially by dipstick analysis, should prompt classification by identification of origin: physiologic (e.g., from fever, extreme heat/cold, and seizure), prerenal (e.g., due to hyperglobulinemia), postrenal (e.g., from genital or lower urinary tract inflammation), or renal, due to intrinsic tubular or glomerular disease. Significant proteinuria of renal origin is persistent (multiple assessments above reference range, separated by 7–14 days) and associated with a normal/inactive urine sediment. Urine protein concentration is quantitated in a ratio with the concentration of creatinine (urine protein:creatinine, UPC); a UPC > 0.4 is considered abnormal in the cat and a UPC > 0.5 is considered abnormal in the dog. Renal proteinuria can be associated with increased filtration through damaged glomerular capillary walls (i.e., glomerular proteinuria, UPC usually > 2.0) and/or decreased reabsorption by tubular epithelial cells (i.e., tubular proteinuria, UPC usually < 2.0). Tubular lesions in patients with AKI may result in proteinuria; however, most often this is a transient finding directly related to tubular epithelial damage and resolves with regeneration of the tubular epithelium if the patient recovers. When renal proteinuria is seen in patients with CKD, it is generally a chronic finding. The sensitivity of renal proteinuria as a marker of CKD is high, especially if the UPC or species-specific albuminuria is serially monitored [35,36,38–40]. Documenting persistent renal proteinuria with a UPC > 2.0 often signals the presence of glomerular disease, full discussion of which is beyond the scope of this chapter, but renal proteinuria of any magnitude above reference range can induce ongoing tubulointerstitial inflammation and fibrosis, nephron loss, and accelerated progression of CKD [36,40,41]. The variety of mechanisms by which this happens are not fully understood, but proximal renal tubular overload/damage from high-protein filtrate and the resulting ongoing interstitial inflammation, renal oxidative stress, and hypoxic renal environment are among them [42]. Patients with significant renal proteinuria, even nonazotemic ones, should thus be considered likely more vulnerable to renal damage from nephrotoxic substances and abnormal hemodynamic states than similar nonproteinuric patients would be.

Renal clearance and glomerular filtration rate

Renal clearance is the rate at which a substance is completely cleared from a specified volume of plasma. Substances used to measure renal clearance must be freely filtered by the glomerulus (not protein bound) and not be affected by tubular reabsorption or secretion, or by metabolism elsewhere in the body. In addition, the substance used must not alter renal function. Measurement of GFR by clearance studies, generally accepted as the most sensitive and specific method to assess renal function, may be performed to achieve greater diagnostic accuracy than routine laboratory testing provides. This process can be particularly useful when renal disease is suspected prior to the onset of renal azotemia. Though GFR measurement using plasma clearance of creatinine or iohexol, and also via technetium-based renal scintigraphy, has been validated in dogs and cats and is described below, these procedures are significantly more cumbersome, time consuming, and expensive than standard blood and urine testing, plus availability of nuclear medicine is particularly limited. For those reasons, clearance studies are not commonly performed for routine assessment of renal function, even at specialty centers. Specific, detailed instructions for clinical GFR assessment via iohexol or creatinine clearance can be found on the IRIS website.

Renal clearance of inulin is the gold standard method for the determination of GFR; however, it is difficult to measure inulin in plasma and urine. On the other hand, it is relatively easy and therefore more practical to determine the renal clearance of creatinine (*CrCl*) as an approximation of GFR. *CrCl* is the volume of plasma cleared of creatinine per minute and is calculated by multiplying the concentration of creatinine in urine by the rate of urine production and then dividing the product by the serum creatinine concentration:

$$CrCl\left(\text{mL/min}\right)=\frac{\left[\text{urine creatinine}\left(\text{mg/dL}\right)\times\text{urine volume}\left(\text{mL/min}\right)\right]}{\text{serum creatinine}\left(\text{mg/dL}\right)}$$

For example, if the urine creatinine concentration is 60 mg/dL, urine production is 3 mL/min, and the serum creatinine concentration is 1.8 mg/ dL, then 100 mL of plasma is cleared of creatinine per minute. This value is divided by the animal's body weight in kilograms and expressed in milliliters per minute per kilogram. Note that prerenal and postrenal factors, and also renal parenchymal lesions, will influence GFR. The major disadvantage of renal clearance studies is the requirement for timed urine collections.

From a clinical standpoint, plasma clearance studies are less invasive and less time consuming. For example, plasma clearance of iohexol, an iodinated radiographic contrast agent, has been shown to estimate GFR reliably in dogs and cats. Iohexol plasma clearance is ideally performed in patients that are well hydrated and fasted for 12 h prior to the study. Iohexol is administered IV at a dosage of 300 mg iodine/kg body weight and then blood samples are collected at 2, 3, and 4 h after the IV injection from a separate vein. Serum from each blood sample is harvested (~1.5 mL of serum is needed per sample) and then transported either chilled or frozen to the specialized reference laboratory (e.g., Diagnostic Center for Population and Animal Health, Toxicology Section, Michigan State University) for measurement and calculation of GFR.

Renal scintigraphy using ^{99m}Tc-labeled diethylenetriamine-pentaacetic acid also allows the GFR to be measured and is available at several universities in the United States and at major referral centers. This is a quick, non-invasive method that does not require urine collection and has the advantage of being able to quantitatively evaluate individual kidney function. Disadvantages of this procedure include its limited availability, exposure of the animal to radioisotopes, the need for radioisotope disposal, and poorer correlation with inulin clearance compared with plasma iohexol clearance.

Urine output measurement

Measuring the volume of urine produced is most frequently used as an aid in determining the maintenance fluid requirements of dogs and cats with AKI. Since these patients can range from markedly polyuric to completely anuric, actual quantification rather than estimation of output increases precision of assessment and fluid therapy. One major goal of fluid therapy in patients with AKI is to restore and/or maintain euvolemia to assure appropriate tissue (particularly renal) perfusion, while avoiding volume overload and its clinical consequences. Fluid therapy should be tailored to match urine volume plus other losses, including insensible losses (e.g., water loss due to respiration) and continuing losses (e.g., fluid loss due to vomiting or diarrhea). Insensible losses are estimated at 20 mL/kg/day. Urine output is quantitated at 6–8-h intervals (best accomplished with indwelling or intermittent urinary catheterization) and that volume plus insensible loss is replaced over an equivalent subsequent time period. The volume of fluid loss due to vomiting and/or diarrhea may be estimated, and that amount is added to the 24-h fluid needs of the patient. Fluid losses or gains can also be indirectly estimated by weighing the patient two to three times per day on the same scale.

Renal biopsy

Biopsy and histopathologic evaluation of renal tissue are valuable diagnostic and prognostic tools, most often performed in cases of significant renal proteinuria or AKI. Though most management strategies for renal disease are broadly applicable to animals with nephropathies based on laboratory and physiologic parameters combined with measurable responses to therapy, applicability of certain targeted treatments depends on direct tissue examination. In addition, the prognosis for animals with renal disease will be most accurate and clinically useful when severity of dysfunction, renal histopathologic findings, and response to treatment can be examined together. Renal biopsy should be considered only after less invasive tests, often including response to therapies, have been carried out and coagulation/hemostasis has been assessed. Acquisition and examination of renal tissue is appropriate if the diagnosis is in question (e.g., glomerulonephritis versus amyloidosis), if treatment may be altered based on results (e.g., confirmation of and culture in bacterial pyelonephritis, immune-mediated versus non-immune-mediated glomerulonephritis), or if the prognosis or client inclination to pursue further treatment may vary depending on findings (e.g., evidence of reversible tubular lesions in a dog or cat with AKI or presence of extensive fibrosis). Contraindications to renal biopsy include a solitary kidney, coagulopathy, severe systemic hypertension, late stage 3 and stage 4 CKD, and renal lesions associated with fluid accumulation (e.g., hydronephrosis, renal cysts, and abscesses). Very small patients (< 5 kg) may present additional challenge and risk for percutaneous biopsy procedures due to the smaller biopsy target, proximity of large vessels, and greater clinical impact of a given volume of hemorrhage [43]. Renal biopsy should not be attempted by inexperienced clinicians or in animals that are not adequately restrained.

Specimens can be obtained percutaneously using the keyhole technique, or under laparoscopic or ultrasonographic guidance. Frequently, the best way to obtain renal tissue is at laparotomy when both kidneys can be visualized, postbiopsy hemorrhage can be accurately assessed and treated, and an adequate biopsy specimen assured. The cortical region of the kidney should be biopsied to obtain an adequate number of glomeruli in the specimen and to avoid renal nerves and major vessels at the corticomedullary junction and in the medullary region. Most animals will have microscopic hematuria for 1–3 days after the biopsy procedure, and transient gross hematuria is not uncommon. Severe hemorrhage is rare and is almost always the result of faulty technique.

The International Veterinary Renal Pathology Service (IVRPS) housed at Texas A&M University is currently considered the nephropathologic standard for veterinary renal biopsy analysis. The IVRPS provides comprehensive sample analysis (light microscopy, transmission electron microscopy, and immunofluorescence evaluation), as well as histopathologic and clinical interpretation of results and their implications by nephropathologists and nephrologists. Information on ordering biopsy specimen collection kits, determining adequacy of samples acquired, and proper sample preparation and submission, as well as detailed information on when and how to appropriately biopsy a kidney is available online. Though they chiefly handle canine and feline samples, renal biopsies from other species are accepted. Even if a different pathology service is used, use of immunofluorescence and transmission electron microscopic assessment in addition to light microscopy is strongly recommended when evaluating renal tissue. Communication with the laboratory pathologist prior to biopsy will help determine which analytic modalities are available and which fixatives should be used to maximize utility of the biopsy sample.

Equine

Prior to laboratory testing, physical exam findings can indicate renal dysfunction in horses. Common findings in horses with CKD include weight loss, polyuria/polydipsia, and ventral edema [8]. As in small animal patients, serum creatinine is a commonly used index to assess renal function (GFR). Similar to small animals, it is expected that serum creatinine elevations associated with renal lesions will not be observed until approximately 60–75% of the nephrons become non-functional, and measurement of serum creatinine in early renal disease is of little value [44]. Breed may play a role in normal serum creatinine concentrations as heavily muscled breeds such as quarter horses have a greater upper limit in their normal reference range [44]. However, individual horses have minimal variation in serum creatinine concentrations making historical values particularly valuable for assessing change over time [45]. BUN measurement as a single test of renal function in horses has minimal diagnostic value. In horses, BUN is reabsorbed after filtration at the collecting ducts in a rate-dependent manner based on the rate of fluid movement. As fluid rates and volumes increase in the collecting duct, less urea is reabsorbed; as fluid rates decrease, more urea is reabsorbed independent of the filtration rate of urea. Therefore, fluid therapy in horses with renal disease may reduce BUN but not in a manner that reflects improvement in GFR. Because serum creatinine is not reabsorbed, it is the most commonly used single test of renal function in horses. Azotemia, elevated serum creatinine and BUN, can be further divided into prerenal, renal, and postrenal in origin. The use of a BUN to serum creatinine (BUN:creatinine) ratio has been described for use in characterizing azotemia in horses and to separate acute and chronic forms of renal failure. The ratio is theoretically higher for prerenal azotemia because of increased urea reabsorption due to dehydration and low tubular flow rates compared with azotemia secondary to intrinsic renal disease. In horses with acute renal failure, BUN:creatinine ratios are less than 10:1, whereas in chronic disease, ratios can be expected to be greater than 10:1 [46].

GFR can also be measured in equine patients, providing a quantitative assessment of renal function; however, measurement of urine output is challenging in horses as an indwelling urinary catheter for urine collection is impractical.

Serum electrolyte concentration measurements should also be considered in the diagnostic plan for horses with renal disease. Na^+ and Cl^- levels are often decreased in horses with renal disease, whereas K^+ can be elevated, decreased, or normal. Hyperkalemia is most often observed with disease states associated with urine outflow obstructions or urinary bladder ruptures and subsequent uroperitoneum. Serum Ca^{2+} should also be monitored as horses with AKI are often hypocalcemic whereas those with CKD are often hypercalcemic.

Urine samples should be obtained from horses with suspected renal disease for a complete urinalysis, including sediment examination. As in small animal patients, specific gravity should be measured along with microscopic examination for cells, casts, and crystals. The brush borders of the proximal tubular cells are rich in enzymes that play a role in the metabolic activity of the endothelium. Measured urinary GGT has been used, as a ratio with urine creatinine to determine and monitor the extent of acute tubular damage. GGT to urine creatinine ratios greater than 100 IU/g are considered to be clinically important, but lower ratios should be interpreted with caution as GGT release from the proximal tubules can occur with minor insults that may be clinically irrelevant.

Fractional clearance of electrolytes may hold better diagnostic utility than urinary GGT for acute tubular damage [46]. The nephrons, as a collective group, work to conserve more than 99% of filtered Na^+ and Cl^- ions in the normal horse (supplemented salts or intravenous fluid administration will artificially increase the amount of excreted electrolytes in urine and, thus, complicate the utility of fractional clearance calculations). Increases in fractional clearance may be an indicator of early tubular damage. Serum and urine samples are collected simultaneously, and Na^+, Cl^-, and creatinine levels are determined. Using the following equation, a clearance value can be determined for sodium and chloride:

$$Cl_A/Cl_{Cr} = \frac{\text{serum}[\text{Cr}]}{\text{urine}[\text{Cr}]} \times \frac{\text{urine}[\text{A}]}{\text{serum}[\text{A}]} \times 100$$

where Cl_A/Cl_{Cr} is the fractional clearance ratio, [A] is the measured electrolyte A (either Na^+ or Cl^-), and [Cr] is creatinine concentration.

Symmetric dimethylarginine assays have been validated for use in horses, and reference ranges have been reported for adult horses and neonatal foals [47–49]. However, clinical utility in horses continues to be investigated and, to date, SDMA has not gained widespread use in equine patients.

Renal biopsy via ultrasound guidance is easily performed in horses, and use of a needle biopsy instrument minimizes the risks (e.g., hemorrhage, bowel penetration, and peritonitis). Biopsy and histopathology can identify the type of lesion, location, and severity and provide guidance for prognosis.

Ruminant

Many of the same diagnostic procedures performed in small animals and horses can be performed in ruminant species. However, for economic concerns, renal function testing is often limited to findings on routine chemistry analysis and urinalysis strips.

Acute kidney injury/acute renal failure

Etiology and pathogenesis

The two major causes of AKI are toxic and ischemic injury, and the kidneys are highly susceptible to both due to their unique anatomic and physiologic features. For example, the large RBF (approximately 20% of the cardiac output) results in the increased delivery of bloodborne toxicants to the kidney compared to other organs. Within the renal cortex, the epithelial cells of the proximal tubule and thick ascending loop of Henle are most frequently affected by ischemic and toxicant-induced injury. These particular susceptibilities occur, respectively, due to the many transport functions and consequent high metabolic rates of these cells, and to increased exposure from the combination of disproportionately high blood flow (the cortex receives 90% of the blood supplied by the renal artery) and the large endothelial surface area created by the glomerular capillaries. Toxicants disrupt the metabolic pathways that generate ATP, and ischemia can rapidly deplete cellular ATP stores. With the resulting loss of energy, the Na^+-K^+ pump fails, leading to cell swelling and death. By resorbing water and electrolytes from the glomerular filtrate, tubular epithelial cells may be exposed to increasingly higher concentrations of toxicants within the tubular lumen. Toxicants that are either secreted or resorbed by tubular epithelial cells (e.g., gentamicin) may accumulate in high concentrations within these cells; similarly, the countercurrent multiplier system may concentrate toxicants in the medulla. Finally, the kidneys also play a role in the biotransformation of many drugs and toxicants. This usually results in the formation of metabolites that are less toxic than the parent compound; however, in some cases (e.g., the oxidation of ethylene glycol to glycolate and oxalate), the metabolites are more toxic than the parent compound.

Toxic insults to the kidney are often caused by therapeutic agents, in addition to nephrotoxicants such as ethylene glycol and grapes/raisins. Similarly, ischemic insults to the kidney can occur in the hospital setting in conjunction with anesthesia and surgery or with the use of vasoactive agents or non-steroidal anti-inflammatory drugs (NSAIDs) [50]. Prolonged anesthesia with inadequate fluid therapy in older animals with pre-existing, subclinical CKD is a frequent cause of renal ischemia and AKI in the hospital setting. Normal kidneys can maintain adequate renal perfusion pressure by autoregulation provided that the mean arterial blood pressure exceeds approximately 60–70 mmHg. This autoregulation may be compromised, however, in patients with pre-existing CKD, especially during anesthesia. The resulting decline in RBF and perfusion pressure can adversely affect GFR and delivery of oxygen and nutrients to the metabolically active tubular epithelial cells. Tubular cell swelling secondary to decreased Na^+-K^+ pump activity occurs due to osmotic extraction of water from the extracellular space, which, in turn, can cause the amount of water in the plasma to decrease. The consequences of decreased plasma water in the renal vasculature are red blood cell aggregation and vascular congestion and stasis, which tend to potentiate and perpetuate decreased glomerular blood flow and decreased oxygen and nutrient delivery.

In AKI, tubular dysfunction and reduced glomerular filtration occur at the individual nephron level as a result of a combination of tubular obstruction, tubular backleak, renal arteriolar vasoconstriction, and decreased glomerular capillary permeability. Specifically, cellular debris within the tubule may inspissate and obstruct the flow of filtrate through the nephron. Alternatively, interstitial edema (e.g., secondary to overhydration) may compress and obstruct renal tubules. Tubular backleak is enhanced by tubular obstruction and consequent increased intratubular pressures proximal to the obstruction. The decreased reabsorption of solute and water by damaged proximal tubule segments results in the increased delivery of solutes and fluid to the distal nephron and macula densa in many nephrons, which causes afferent glomerular arteriole constriction. The exact mediators of this vasoconstriction are not known, but natriuretic factor, the renin–angiotensin–aldosterone system, and thromboxane may be involved. A decrease in the permeability of the glomerular capillary wall also leads to a reduction in glomerular filtration. The impaired glomerular capillary permeability that occurs in AKI often persists after vasoconstriction and RBF have been corrected.

Several classification systems have been developed for humans to describe and stratify the continuum of renal injury represented by AKI (e.g., RIFLE, AKIN, and KDIGO). Recently, IRIS has created a similar staging system for use in dogs and cats based on serum creatinine, urine production, and need for renal replacement therapy (Table 43.2). Because AKI by its nature is a fluid, evolving condition, this grading system is intended to characterize a point in the course of disease, and a given patient's grade of AKI is expected to change as the disease state evolves over time. The IRIS CKD staging system (described below) is intended to better characterize and group veterinary patients with AKI to aid therapeutic recommendations and prognostication. Patients who stabilize into a chronically azotemic state can then be reclassified into a CKD stage. A detailed description of the IRIS AKI grading system is available online [51].

Acute tubular damage leading to AKI has four distinct phases: (1) initiation; (2) extension; (3) maintenance; and (4) recovery. The initiation phase includes the time of and immediately following initial renal insult, when sublethal cellular insult has occurred but the basement membrane remains unaffected and renal function remains relatively normal. During initiation, therapeutic interventions that remove or interrupt the inciting process and reduce ongoing additional damage can prevent development of established AKI. During the extension phase, original mechanisms of cellular injury may be combined with or replaced by the inflammation, ischemia, and direct tissue damage from release of proteolytic enzymes and proinflammatory cytokines, decreased endothelial nitric oxide, and many other mechanisms. The sublethal injuries may then induce necrotic or apoptotic cellular death. During extension, routine laboratory testing will begin to show loss of concentrating ability and usually azotemia. The maintenance phase is characterized by the development of a critical amount of renal parenchymal damage; this phase is variable in length but generally lasts 1–3 weeks. Endothelial cytoskeletal damage leads to release of tight junctions and adhesion to the basement membrane, resulting in cellular desquamation and backleak of filtrate through the basement membrane into the interstitium where it causes additional inflammatory response. Tubular epithelial cells and cellular or granular casts are often seen at this point of the process. The sloughed epithelial cells may obstruct tubules, leading to oliguria or anuria. Although therapeutic interventions during maintenance (whether supportive care, diuretics, or extracorporeal renal replacement therapies) may be lifesaving, they cannot change the severity of existing lesions, improve function, or hasten recovery. The aim of patient management during maintenance is to create stability for long enough that renal recovery has an opportunity to occur. In the recovery phase, renal lesions are repaired and function improves; in oligoanuric animals, this is usually heralded by increasing urine output and in non-oliguric animals by decreasing azotemia. Tubular damage may be reversible if the basement membrane remains intact and viable epithelial cells are present to repopulate the tubule. Although new nephrons cannot be produced and irreversibly damaged nephrons cannot be repaired, functional hypertrophy of surviving nephrons may sufficiently compensate for

Table 43.2 International Renal Interest Society (IRIS) acute kidney injury (AKI) grading criteria.

AKI grade	Serum creatinine (mg/dL)	Serum creatinine (μmol/L)	Clinical description
Grade I	< 1.6	< 140	Nonazotemic AKI: a. Documented AKI (historical, clinical, laboratory, or imaging evidence of AKI, clinical oliguria/anuria, volume responsiveness[a]) and/or b. Progressive nonazotemic increase in blood creatinine; ≥ 0.3 mg/dL (≥ 26.4 mmol/L) within 48 h c. Measured oliguria (< 1 mL/kg/h) or anuria over 6 h
Grade II	1.7–2.5	141–220	Mild AKI: a. Documented AKI and static or progressive azotemia b. Progressive azotemic increase in blood creatinine; ≥ 0.3 mg/dL (≥ 26.4 mmol/L) within 48 h, or volume responsiveness[a] c. Measured oliguria (< 1 mL/kg/h) or anuria over 6 h
Grade III	2.6–5.0	221–439	Moderate to severe AKI:
Grade IV	5.1–10.0	440–880	a. Documented AKI and increasing severities
Grade V	> 10.0	> 880	of azotemia and functional renal failure

[a] Volume responsiveness is considered an increase in urine production to greater than 1 mL/kg/h over 6 h and/or a decrease in serum creatinine to baseline over 48 h.

the decrease in nephron numbers, so that even if renal functional recovery remains incomplete, adequate function may be re-established. Length of the recovery phase is also highly variable and may last for weeks or many months [52–55].

Clinical features and diagnosis

Clinical signs of AKI are often non-specific and include lethargy, depressed mentation, hypo/anorexia, vomiting, diarrhea, and dehydration; occasionally, uremic breath, oral ulcers, or tongue-tip necrosis may be present. A diagnosis of AKI is suspected if azotemia develops acutely and is associated with persistent isosthenuria or minimally concentrated urine, or if progressive but nonazotemic elevation of creatinine ≥ 0.3 mg/dL (≥ 26.4 mmol/L) within 48 h is observed. Animals with AKI may initially have normal urine output but usually become polyuric, oliguric, or anuric. Dehydration and prerenal azotemia superimposed on an inability to concentrate urine (e.g., Addison's disease, hypercalcemia, or overzealous use of furosemide) initially mimics renal failure; however, in these prerenal cases, volume replacement results in resolution of the azotemia.

Acute renal failure occurs within hours or days of exposure to an insult. Clinical signs and clinicopathologic findings more frequently associated with AKI include enlarged or swollen kidneys, hemoconcentration, good body condition, active urine sediment (e.g., granular casts, renal epithelial cells, and pyuria), and relatively severe hyperkalemia and metabolic acidosis (usually in the face of oliguria/anuria). Clinical signs in an animal with AKI tend to be severe relative to those seen in an animal with CKD and a similar magnitude of azotemia. Renal ultrasound in dogs and cats with AKI usually shows normal sized to enlarged kidneys, often with diffusely normal to slightly hypoechoic renal cortices. In animals with grape/raisin or lily toxicity, however, the renal cortices are often bright; with calcium oxalate nephrosis associated with ethylene glycol ingestion, this change is usually marked (with cortices hyperechoic to normal splenic tissue). Kidneys of animals with pyelonephritis usually have bilateral mild to moderate pyelectasia, often with increased renal pelvic echogenicity and sometimes with mild proximal ureteral dilation. In cases of ureteral obstruction, dilation of both the renal pelvis and the ureter to the point of the obstruction are often present. Perirenal fluid is often seen with leptospirosis (dogs) or renal lymphoma (usually cats) and occasionally with other causes of AKI as well [52,54,56].

A recent study found the ratio of renal cortical thickness to abdominal aortic diameter (at the left renal arterial branch) to be significantly increased in dogs with AKI compared with normal dogs and dogs with CKD; thus, calculation of this ratio could serve as a method of identifying AKI on ultrasound [57]. The resistive index (ratio between the peak systolic velocity and the end diastolic velocity) in renal interlobar arteries (renal resistive index; RRI) can also be calculated via ultrasound and Doppler interrogation and is significantly increased in both humans and dogs with AKI. A positive correlation between creatinine and RRI has been demonstrated in dogs with AKI, as well as a correlation between reduction in RRI and a favorable prognosis [58].

Renal biopsy specimens from dogs and cats with AKI show proximal tubular cell degeneration, ranging from cloudy swelling to necrosis, with edema and mononuclear and polymorphonuclear leukocyte infiltration in the interstitium. Ethylene glycol and melamine-associated nephrotoxicity are frequently associated with intratubular crystals. Although toxicant-induced AKI cannot be differentiated histopathologically from AKI caused by ischemia in all cases, renal histologic findings are often helpful in establishing a prognosis. Evidence of tubular regeneration (e.g., flattened, basophilic epithelial cells with irregular nuclear size, mitotic figures, and high nuclear-to-cytoplasmic ratios) and the finding of generally intact tubular basement membranes are good prognostic findings and may be observed as early as 3 days post-insult. Conversely, large numbers of granular casts, extensive tubular necrosis, interstitial mineralization and fibrosis, and disrupted tubular basement membranes are poor prognostic indicators. In addition to the renal histopathologic changes, the degree of functional impairment and, even more importantly, the response to therapy should be considered when formulating a prognosis.

Chronic kidney disease

Etiology and pathogenesis

Most of the time, the term "chronic kidney disease" (CKD) is intended to mean self-perpetuating chronic tubulointerstitial nephritis, though proteinuric and other types of kidney disease may be involved as well. Interstitial diseases usually stem mechanistically from injury to one of the other major functional components of the kidney (tubules, vasculature, and glomeruli); injury to any one component has the ready potential to affect the other two through their common contact with the interstitium. Because of the interdependence and physical intercalation of the vascular, glomerular, tubular, and interstitial components of the kidney, the endpoint of severe or ongoing damage to any of these components will be marked interstitial fibrosis with varying degrees of inflammation and will appear histopathologically as indistinguishable end-stage tubulointerstitial nephritis and fibrosis. For instance, as discussed above in AKI, direct tubular insult (usually toxic or ischemic) results in renal tubular epithelial injury, disruption of the barrier between the tubular lumen and the interstitial space, and production of proinflammatory cytokines. Cytokine production and backleak of ultrafiltrate from the tubule into the interstitium lead to chemotaxis of proinflammatory cells and, thus, to interstitial inflammation and eventual fibrosis. Alternatively, initial direct injury to the vasculature results in diminished interstitial perfusion and thus hypoxia, leading to cellular swelling and death. The resulting edema and inflammation lead eventually to interstitial fibrosis. Finally, primary glomerular lesions classically cause decreased permselectivity and thus protein-rich ultrafiltrate enters the tubule. Increased protein transit through the interstitium occurs as the proximal renal tubular epithelial cells reclaim as much of the filtered proteins as possible and return them to the bloodstream. Increased protein trafficking through the interstitium leads to production of proinflammatory cytokines, interstitial inflammation, and eventually to interstitial fibrosis. Interstitial diseases cause injury to the renal vasculature and tubules chiefly by compromising perfusion and diffusion; they cause injury to glomeruli by producing local inflammation. The final common pathway of severe and/or enduring insult to any single renal functional component is interstitial inflammation and fibrosis, with consequent damage to the other functional components. The nephrons of chronically diseased kidneys are morphologically heterogeneous, with changes ranging from severe atrophy and fibrous connective tissue replacement to marked hypertrophy. The histopathologic changes, however, are not process-specific, and thus, the underlying cause of chronic tubulointerstitial nephritis is usually not elucidated by direct tissue examination [59–61].

The pathophysiology of CKD can be considered at both the organ and systemic levels. At the level of the kidney, the fundamental pathologic change that occurs is a loss of nephrons and decreased GFR. The resulting derangements in water and electrolyte balance, accumulation of normally renally excreted organic solutes, and impaired renal hormone synthesis cumulatively result in the variable clinical constellation known as "uremic syndrome." The most common signs associated with the uremic syndrome are gastrointestinal (e.g., dysrexia, nausea, vomiting, halitosis, oral ulceration, stomatitis, diarrhea, and melena); weight loss, lethargy, hypothermia, hypertension, sarcopenia, anemia, and weakness frequently also occur. Altered behavior or seizures may be present secondary to uremic or hypertensive encephalopathy; less commonly, pneumonitis, pericarditis, bleeding diatheses, or osteodystrophy occur [1,59,62,63].

In addition to excreting metabolic wastes and maintaining fluid and electrolyte balance, the kidneys function as endocrine organs and also catabolize several peptide hormones; both hormonal synthesis and catabolism are deranged in animals with CKD, usually in proportion to severity of disease. For example, decreased renal production of erythropoietin and calcitriol contributes to the development of non-regenerative anemia and hyperparathyroidism, respectively. Conversely, decreased metabolism and excretion of parathyroid hormone and gastrin leads to increased serum concentrations of these hormones, contributing to development of hyperparathyroidism and gastritis, respectively. Some pathophysiologic changes that occur in CKD are brought about by initially physiologic compensatory mechanisms. The osteodystrophy of CKD occurs secondary to hyperparathyroidism, which develops in an attempt to maintain normal plasma calcium and phosphorus concentrations. Similarly, the GFR of intact hypertrophied nephrons increases in animals with CKD in an attempt to maintain adequate renal function, but proteinuria and glomerulosclerosis consequent to hyperfiltration in these individual nephrons cause additional tubulointerstitial damage.

Clinical features and diagnosis

In contrast to AKI, CKD develops over a period of months or years, and its clinical signs are often relatively mild for the magnitude of the azotemia. Unique signs of CKD include a long-standing history of weight loss, polyuria/polydipsia, poor body condition, non-regenerative anemia, and small and irregularly shaped kidneys. A diagnosis of CKD is usually based on a combination of compatible historical, physical examination, and clinicopathologic findings. Plain radiographs can confirm the presence of small kidneys in small animal patients but is usually not feasible in larger horses and ruminants. Renal ultrasonography will usually show diffusely hyperechoic and often thinned renal cortices with loss of the normal corticomedullary distinction and overall decrease in size; mild pyelectasia is also a common finding [64,65]. The increased cortical echogenicity results from replacement of the irreversibly damaged nephrons with fibrous connective tissue. Chronic cortical infarcts are common, appearing as radially oriented, hyperechoic wedges or bands, extending from the corticomedullary junction to the capsular surface. Frequently, the cortical collapse and fibrosis associated with infarcts results in irregularity of renal shape. Radiographic studies and ultrasonography can identify other changes associated with CKD, such as cysts or mineralization and can also help identify or rule out potentially treatable causes of CKD, such as pyelonephritis and nephrolithiasis [65,66]. As mentioned for AKI, the ratio of renal cortical thickness to abdominal aortic diameter measured ultrasonographically may be useful in identifying CKD, since this ratio was shown to be significantly decreased in dogs with CKD compared with normal dogs and dogs with AKI [57]. Renal biopsy is not routinely performed in animals with CKD unless the diagnosis is in question and the disease is not advanced. Renal histopathologic preparations will show some combination of a loss of tubules with replacement fibrosis and mineralization, glomerulosclerosis and glomerular atrophy, and foci of mononuclear cells (small lymphocytes, plasma cells, and macrophages) within the interstitium in association with fibrous connective tissue replacement.

Staging chronic kidney disease

Once prerenal and/or postrenal azotemia are resolved and a diagnosis of CKD has been established (i.e., the disease is stable), staging is appropriate to help clinicians refine and focus diagnostic and therapeutic efforts in a consistent fashion. Table 43.3 details the staging system for canine and feline CKD developed by IRIS, with initial staging determined by serum creatinine and ideally also SDMA, and substaging delineated by the presence or absence of proteinuria and systemic hypertension (Tables 43.4 and 43.5). The classic diagnosis of CKD based on renal azotemia (persistent renal azotemia superimposed on the inability to concentrate urine) pertains to CKD stages 2–4. Stage 1 CKD (non-azotemic CKD) may be diagnosed in cats and dogs with persistent proteinuria of renal origin, urine-concentrating deficits due to renal parenchymal disease, increases in serum creatinine or SDMA concentration over time (even if values remain in the normal range), abnormal renal palpation, or renal imaging abnormalities. A detailed description of IRIS guidelines for staging dogs and cats with CKD as well as condensed pocket guides may be found online [51].

Further diagnostics and treatment

In general, the diagnostic approach to a patient once CKD has been identified and staged is focused on three areas: (1) characterization of the renal disease; (2) characterization of the stability of the renal disease and renal function; and (3) characterization of the patient's problems associated with the decreased renal function. Evaluation of canine and feline CKD patients ideally includes identification/quantification of proteinuria, measurement of systemic blood pressure, urine culture, and kidney imaging. The stability of renal

Table 43.3 International Renal Interest Society (IRIS) chronic kidney disease (CKD) staging system for cats and dogs.

	Stage 1			Stage 2			Stage 3			Stage 4		
	Serum creatinine		SDMA	Serum creatinine		SDMA	Serum creatinine		SDMA	Serum creatinine		SDMA
	mg/dL	μmol/L	μg/dL	mg/dL	μmol/L	μg/dL	mg/dL	μmol/L	μg/dL	mg/dL	μmol/L	μg/dL
Cats	< 1.6	< 140	< 18	1.6–2.8	140–250	18–25	2.9–5.0	251–440	26–38	> 5.0	> 440	> 38
Dogs	< 1.4	< 125	< 18	1.4–2.8	125–250	18–35	2.9–5.0	251–440	36–54	> 5.0	> 440	> 54

Table 43.4 International Renal Interest Society (IRIS) chronic kidney disease (CKD) substaging for proteinuria in cats and dogs.

Urine protein:creatinine	Substage
< 0.2 (cats and dogs)	Nonproteinuric
0.2–0.4 (cats), 0.2–0.5 (dogs)	Borderline proteinuric
> 0.4 (cats), > 0.5 (dogs)	Proteinuric

Table 43.5 International Renal Interest Society (IRIS) chronic kidney disease (CKD) substaging for hypertension for cats and dogs.

Systolic blood pressure (mmHg)	Blood pressure substage	Risk of target organ damage
< 140	Normotensive	Minimal
140–159	Prehypertensive	Low
160–179	Hypertensive	Moderate
> 179	Severely hypertensive	High

function may be assessed by serial monitoring of abnormalities identified during the initial evaluation of renal disease. This monitoring should always include serial serum biochemistry profiles, urinalyses, surveillance for and quantification of proteinuria (e.g., urine protein:creatinine [UPC]), fundic exam, and measurement of blood pressure, but may also include follow-up urine cultures and ultrasonographic examinations. Characterization of the renal disease and its stability are most important in the earlier stages of CKD when appropriate treatment has the greatest potential to improve or stabilize renal function. Identification of mitigatable sequela of CKD becomes the more important focus in later stages, when clinical signs tend to be more severe. In the later stages of CKD, diagnostic (and subsequent therapeutic) efforts should be directed at the anorexia, vomiting, acidosis, hypokalemia, hypertension, anemia, and other disease consequences that adversely affect the patient's quality of life.

Treatment recommendations for early-stage CKD focus on proactive surveillance to identify and treat modifiable disease factors (e.g., proteinuria, hypertension, urinary infection, and urolithiasis) in an effort to preserve remaining renal function. Discontinuation of potentially nephrotoxic medications, maintenance of euhydration, and (generally at stage 2 disease) institution of diets designed for renal disease are the cornerstones of management. Renoprotective diets have been conclusively shown to markedly decrease uremic crises and decrease mortality in both dogs and cats with naturally occurring CKD [67]. These diets are formulated to limit phosphorus and minimize the waste products of protein catabolism, which are thought to play a primary role in uremia. Fortification of these diets with omega-3 polyunsaturated fatty acids and antioxidants decreases proteinuria, cholesterol, number of renal lesions, and overall mortality in dogs. Other modifications include increased B vitamins to replace increased renal loss, buffers (e.g., potassium citrate and sodium bicarbonate) to mitigate metabolic acidosis, potassium supplementation in feline diets to counter renal losses, and avoidance of excess sodium to potentially decrease risk of hypertension [59,62,67,68].

For animals with late stage 2–4 CKD, treatment focuses on amelioration of the clinical consequences of further declining renal function in addition to continuing the interventions already recommended in earlier stages of disease. Usually, this entails the use of antiemetics (e.g., ondansetron and maropitant) and appetite stimulants (e.g., mirtazapine and capromorelin). Administration of additional buffers (usually sodium bicarbonate) to mitigate metabolic acidosis or ACE inhibitors, angiotensin receptor blockers, and/or calcium channel blockers to manage hypertension may be needed. Esophageal feeding tubes enable provision of low-stress ideal nutrition, hydration, and medications to patients and can be excellent life-improving and life-extending tools when patients cannot maintain appropriate oral intake. Anemia of CKD develops chiefly due to decreased numbers of erythropoietin-producing renal fibroblasts, but gastric ulceration, uremia-induced platelet dysfunction, and shortened erythrocyte lifespan are also contributory factors, and timely administration of erythropoiesis-stimulating agents (e.g., darbepoetin alfa) when anemia begins to develop can improve appetite, energy, and quality of life, as well as prevent need for transfusion [59,62,68,69]. Detailed stage-specific CKD treatment recommendations for dogs and cats may be found on the IRIS website [51].

Anesthetic drugs and renal disease

Renal disease and injury can result in alterations in the pharmacokinetics and pharmacodynamics of drugs administered during the perianesthetic period. Many of the drugs (or their metabolites) commonly used have some degree of renal metabolism and/or excretion (e.g., ketamine, benzodiazepines, and some opioids), and potential alterations in pharmacokinetic parameters should be considered in the anesthetic plan for these patients. Additionally, comorbidities associated with renal diseases, including azotemia, acid–base disturbances, electrolyte imbalances, dehydration, anemia, coagulopathy, hypertension, and encephalopathy, should be considered and appropriate alterations made in drug and therapy choices.

Azotemia is often associated with a decrease in plasma pH and can decrease plasma protein binding of administered drugs, resulting in higher concentrations of active free drug and increased risk of relative overdose. However, the clinical significance of this effect may be of minor importance. Regarding the effects of anesthetics on RBF, all anesthetics are likely to decrease the rate of glomerular filtration. Anesthetic drugs may directly affect RBF, or they may indirectly alter renal function via changes in cardiovascular and/or neuroendocrine activity [70]. Sedative and analgesic drugs have varying effects on RBF and GFR and generally relate to individual drug effects on cardiac output and vasomotor tone. Most anesthetics that decrease GFR do so as a consequence of decreased RBF (Table 43.6). Anesthetics that alter catecholamine release and systemic concentrations may have variable effects on RBF and, thus, GFR and renal function. For example, intramuscular administration of a combination of medetomidine and butorphanol increased GFR in healthy dogs, whereas that of a combination of medetomidine, butorphanol, and atropine did not [71]. However, in another study,

Table 43.6 Generalized effects of anesthetics on renal blood flow (RBF) and glomerular filtration rate (GFR).

Drug	RBF	GFR
Acepromazine	No change	No change
α_2-Adrenergic agonists	Decrease	No change
Benzodiazepines	No change	No change
Isoflurane	Slight decrease	Decrease
Sevoflurane	Slight decrease	Decrease
Ketamine	Increase	Decrease or no change
Propofol	No change	No change
Alfaxalone	–	–
Etomidate	No change	No change

medetomidine significantly decreased GFR in healthy dogs, whereas a combination of xylazine, ketamine, and halothane or propofol did not affect GFR [72].

Knowledge of the adverse effects of drugs used in the perianesthetic period is essential; it is often the results of magnification of these side effects in the face of renal disease that poses the greatest risk for these patients. Phenothiazine tranquilizers (e.g., acepromazine) produce dose-dependent hypotension by antagonism of vascular α-adrenergic receptors. Phenothiazines may also antagonize dopamine receptors and therefore may prevent dopamine-induced increases in RBF during surgery. However, RBF and GFR do not change significantly in the face of mild hypotension and may actually impart protection of renal function after low-dose acepromazine administration [73]. Additionally, the use of phenothiazines as a renal preconditioning agent reduced the histopathologic damage in kidneys subject to ischemia and reperfusion [74]. A relatively low dose of acepromazine (0.01–0.02 mg/kg) in patients with stable kidney disease has been recommended [75]. Acepromazine use should probably be restricted to patients with stable and compensated renal disease and avoided in patients in acute crises or in which maintenance of adequate perfusion pressure during anesthesia is a concern.

α_2-Adrenergic receptor agonist drugs, such as dexmedetomidine and xylazine, can have significant dose-dependent depressant effects on heart rate and cardiac output and increase systemic vascular resistance. These effects could be expected to reduce RBF and subsequently GFR; in fact, in a study using a short-term controlled-rate infusion, dexmedetomidine was shown to decrease RBF by up to 30% [76]. However, there is evidence that medetomidine in combination with anticholinergic and opioid agents has minimal effects on GFR in dogs [71]. Additionally, dexmedetomidine may be renal protective in the face of ischemia and reperfusion injury. Dexmedetomidine reduced metabolic activity and demonstrated antioxidant effects in rabbits undergoing experimental renal ischemia and reperfusion injury [77]. For patients at risk for acute renal injury due to hypoperfusion, dexmedetomidine use may have some benefit, but α_2-adrenergic receptor agonist administration is accompanied by profound diuresis. The mechanism is likely multifactorial, including inhibition of vasopressin release, inhibition of cyclic adenosine monophosphate (cAMP) formation in the kidney, redistribution of aquaporin-2 receptors, inhibition of renin release, increased atrial natriuretic peptide, inhibition of renal sympathetic activity, osmotic diuresis due to increased plasma glucose, and inhibition of tubular sodium reabsorption [78]. Interestingly, these mechanisms differ in importance between individual agents and species [78–81]. For instance, xylazine had a greater diuretic effect than medetomidine in dogs, and medetomidine decreased plasma vasopressin whereas xylazine did not [79]. The increased production of dilute urine may be detrimental in patients with postrenal urinary tract obstruction or dehydration and hypovolemia [80,81]. The addition of vatinoxan, a peripheral α_2-adrenergic receptor antagonist, to a sedative protocol utilizing dexmedetomidine may attenuate the hemodynamic effects and maintain abdominal organ blood flow, including to the kidneys [82].

Benzodiazepines are a commonly used class of drugs within veterinary medicine, primarily for their muscle relaxant and mild sedative properties. Diazepam and midazolam have minimal effects on cardiac output, systemic vascular resistance, and blood pressure. Consequently, their use has little impact on RBF and GFR. However, benzodiazepines, like most injectable anesthetic and analgesic drugs, are protein bound in the plasma, and their use in azotemic patients may consequently result in more active free drug. Reduction in initial dosage is probably warranted in patients with acute kidney disease or those which are severely acidotic, azotemic, or hypoproteinemic. Patients with stable disease may not need any adjustment in dosage. Additionally, in patients with AKI, midazolam may have reduced hepatic metabolism. Through an unknown mechanism, as the severity and duration of AKI increases, the activity of CYP3A, an enzyme associated with the P450 system in the liver, is decreased, delaying metabolism and prolonging the effect of drugs such as midazolam [83]. Diazepam and lorazepam are not water soluble and, therefore, are delivered in propylene glycol for injection. Propylene glycol can induce proximal renal tubular cell injury and necrosis, particularly with drugs administered as infusions [84–86]. Midazolam is water soluble and delivered in an aqueous solution and may be a more appropriate benzodiazepine for use in patients with significant kidney disease.

Anesthetic and analgesic protocols for patients with kidney disease are often built around the use of opioids [75]. Opioids will provide sedation and analgesia to patients with minimal impact on cardiac output and thus RBF [87]. It should be noted, however, that the pharmacokinetics of opioids can be altered in patients with renal disease or failure [88]. Longer acting opioids with active metabolites, such as morphine and meperidine (pethidine), should be used with caution as the metabolites have a delayed clearance. In humans, it has been recommended to avoid the use of agents such as morphine and meperidine altogether in patients with renal dysfunction to avoid prolonged narcosis [88]. However, species differences in the metabolism of morphine may reduce the risk of these drugs in veterinary patients. The pharmacokinetics of buprenorphine, alfentanil, sufentanil, and remifentanil, at least in human patients with renal dysfunction, are minimally changed. Fentanyl, administered as a single dose, shows little change in its pharmacokinetic profile; however, significant tissue accumulation and prolonged effect can occur with continuous infusion [89]. Remifentanil is a short-acting opioid that undergoes complete metabolism within the plasma and, although a metabolite GR90291 can accumulate in patients with renal failure, it does not produce significant opioid effects. It is, therefore, one of the most recommended opioids for use in human patients with renal dysfunction [90]. Clinicians should also be cognizant of the fact that opioids can cause urine retention when administered systemically or as an epidural injection.

Injectable anesthetic agents can also have an effect on renal parameters. Although rarely used in modern anesthesia, thiobarbiturates increase systemic vascular resistance but decrease renal vascular resistance with no net change in RBF. Of interest, a serious concern with barbiturates is the change in pharmacodynamics associated with this class of drugs in patients with renal disease. Barbiturates (like many other drugs) are highly protein bound, and this protein binding can be altered in states of severe azotemia. It is well documented that animals with azotemia have decreased protein binding of thiopental and are at a higher risk of relative overdose when using thiopental [91,92]. Additionally, the central nervous system of azotemic animals is more susceptible to the effects of thiopental when measured by electroencephalogram [93,94]. This is thought to occur from allosteric endogenous compounds that enhance thiopental effects that are normally inhibited in nonazotemic animals. It is probably best practice to avoid the use of thiopental in patients with azotemia or renal disease; however, if necessary, total dosages should be reduced.

Ketamine (and likely tiletamine) increases RBF and renal vascular resistance [95]. Even though there can be an increase in RBF, ketamine administration may result in an abnormal distribution of blood flow within the kidney. Additionally, as the dose of ketamine increases, renal sympathetic nerve activity increases, RBF decreases, and renal vascular resistance increases [96]. Ketamine also directly inhibits dopamine transporter proteins in the kidney, but the clinical relevance of this is unclear [97]. Ketamine and its metabolites are highly dependent on renal excretion. In cats, it has been said that the majority of the drug is excreted unchanged and, therefore, should be avoided in cats with renal insufficiency [98]. In fact, ketamine is metabolized to norketamine, a first-step metabolite, in the liver of cats; however, unlike in other species, norketamine is not further metabolized [99]. Ketamine is 53% protein bound, and higher levels of free drug can be expected in azotemic animals, although the increase in free drug may be clinically unimportant [100]. Interestingly, in humans after long-term abuse, the development of two syndromes involving the urinary system, ketamine-induced ulcerative cystitis and ketamine-induced vesicopathy, has been reported [101,102].

Propofol is one of the most commonly used induction agents in human and veterinary anesthesia. Propofol demonstrates a dose- and rate-dependent reduction in arterial blood pressure. However, it has minimal effects on RBF and GFR at low-to-moderate doses and is frequently used for the induction of anesthesia in patients with kidney disease [103,104]. In sheep, propofol caused minor hemodynamic changes in RBF that were not considered to be clinically important [105], and GFR was not significantly affected in dogs administered propofol at clinically used dosages [72,106]. In human patients with CKD and uremia, the pharmacokinetics of propofol were similar to those of healthy control patients, and recovery from propofol anesthesia was no different to that of controls [108,109]. Propofol is considered to be a suitable agent for induction and total intravenous anesthesia in human patients with uremia, although reduced doses may be required [110].

While current studies that evaluate the direct effects of the current formulation of alfaxalone on RBF and GFR are lacking, the hemodynamic effects of this agent have been assessed. Administration of alfaxalone to healthy patients results in hemodynamic effects that are relatively insignificant [111–115]. Furthermore, like many anesthetics, biotransformation occurs primarily via the liver, and renal insufficiency is not expected to result in substantial differences in anesthetic recovery when used for induction. As such, titration of alfaxalone for anesthetic induction or intramuscular administration for sedation of patients would be an appropriate choice for patients presenting with renal insufficiency.

Etomidate is an anesthetic agent known for its minimal effects on heart rate, blood pressure, and cardiac output. Etomidate has also been shown to have no significant effect on renal function and urine output in anesthetized rats [116]. Like propofol, etomidate does not significantly affect GFR in dogs [106]. However, as with diazepam, propylene glycol is used as a solvent in most etomidate preparations.

Inhalant anesthetics can cause systemic hypotension, especially during excessive depth, which can result in renal ischemia secondary to reduced RBF and GFR. This is a result of one of the major side effects of potent volatile anesthetics, peripheral vasodilation, in addition to a dose-dependent depression of myocardial contractility and cardiac output. Concurrently, inhalation anesthetics also tend to decrease RBF and GFR in a dose-dependent manner. Light planes of inhalation anesthesia preserve renal autoregulation of blood flow, whereas deep planes are associated with depression of autoregulation and decreases in RBF. Although isoflurane has minor direct effects on RBF, it decreases GFR and urine output in dogs under experimental conditions [117]. Sevoflurane, although not well studied, seems to have similar effects to isoflurane on RBF [118]. However, when sevoflurane comes into contact with certain carbon dioxide absorbents, it degrades to a nephrotoxic substance called "compound A." Compound A has been shown to cause permanent damage to the kidneys of rats but has not been shown to cause problems in humans with renal insufficiency or in dogs with normal renal function [119,120]. Desflurane has no effect on RBF at concentrations up to twice the minimum alveolar concentration (MAC), but it decreases renal vascular resistance at concentrations greater than 1.75 MAC [121]. For most human patients, and most likely for veterinary patients, the effects of inhaled anesthetics on renal function are reversed at the termination of anesthesia. However, some patients may not regain the ability to regulate urine production for several days [122]. Any patient that demonstrates postanesthetic oliguria should be evaluated immediately for AKI.

As stated previously, COX-1 and COX-2 are necessary for the normal functioning of the healthy kidney. In fact, of the two enzymes, COX-2 may be more important for renal development and preservation of RBF and GFR, particularly during hypovolemia [123]. NSAIDs exert their effects through suppression of these enzymes, reducing the production of proinflammatory prostaglandins. Unfortunately, NSAIDs also suppress the production of prostaglandins necessary for constitutive functions. NSAIDs that preferentially suppress COX-2 may be more detrimental to renal function than more mixed-profile NSAIDs in patients with kidney disease [123]. In healthy dogs, the use of perioperative carprofen or meloxicam did not result in adverse effects or alterations of renal function [124]. Additionally, in dogs undergoing repair of traumatic fractures, the administration of perioperative carprofen did not cause any clinically relevant adverse effects. However, even in healthy patients, the use of NSAIDs may result in fatal renal injury in dogs and cats [125,126]. Historically, the use of NSAIDs in cats with CKD was avoided. However, newer research indicates that use in these cats may not be as harmful as once believed. Long-term use of low-dose meloxicam (0.02 mg/kg/day) in cats with CKD does not appear to result in decreased renal function; however, proteinuria may increase [127]. In cats with CKD (IRIS stage < 4), 4–12 weeks of oral robenacoxib was no different than placebo in the number of adverse events that occurred with no overall increase in risk [128]. When considering the use of NSAIDs in animals with CKD, obtaining informed owner consent and thorough patient monitoring are essential. A review of this topic as well as recommendations for long-term therapy with NSAIDs in cats with CKD has been published [129].

Anesthesia and the stress associated with surgery can cause the release of aldosterone, vasopressin, renin, and catecholamines. Accordingly, RBF and GFR (and, therefore, urine production) are generally decreased with surgery in any patient. In fact, in a study involving the administration of intravenous fluid (10 mL/kg/h) to dogs with normal kidney function undergoing routine orthopedic surgical procedures, evidence of both reduced urine output (below the usual range of 1–2 mL/kg/h) and significant fluid retention was documented [130]. This decrease in urine output may be a normal compensatory mechanism that occurs during reduced metabolic activity of the kidney or during a period when the kidneys are working to conserve solutes and fluid during insults to the body. It is, therefore, recommended to use additional parameters rather than only urine output as an indicator of fluid balance and renal function in anesthetized animals [130].

Anesthetic management of patients with renal disease

Patients with suspected or known renal disease or dysfunction should have a complete physical examination, biochemical testing, baseline arterial blood pressure measurement, and renal function evaluation prior to any anesthetic event. Additionally, renal diseases are often accompanied by dysfunction of other organ systems and should be considered in any anesthetic plan. Concomitant drug therapy should also be accounted for and incorporated into the anesthetic plan. For example, cats with hyperthyroidism may have CKD, hypertension, and hypertrophic cardiomyopathy. Antihypertensive and antiarrhythmic drugs can result in patients having an increased response to drugs that affect the central nervous system, leading to relative overdose.

Preanesthetic stabilization of patients with renal disease may be more critical to a successful outcome than the anesthetic drugs that are administered. Overall, the most important parameters for a patient with renal disease are hydration status and circulating blood volume. Maintaining RBF and GFR through adequate hydration will reduce the likelihood of further renal injury and preserve renal function [131]. Hydration has been shown to be effective in the treatment of renal injury and is a good strategy to prevent the progression of early-stage kidney disease to more advanced-stage kidney disease [132]. Azotemic patients can be administered intravenous fluids before surgery to achieve euhydration and diuresis. If azotemia is severe and is accompanied by electrolyte abnormalities or acid–base imbalances, hospitalization and diuresis can be performed over several hours prior to anesthesia. Anemic patients undergoing anesthesia and procedures with the potential for blood loss should have a red blood cell transfusion if the hematocrit is less than 18–20%.

Once a patient is deemed stable, anesthesia can be performed. In order to minimize significant shifts in cardiac output, blood pressure, and perfusion, a balanced anesthetic plan with agents that have minimal effects on the cardiovascular system is recommended. Premedication in small animal patients can be achieved with an opioid–benzodiazepine combination, either intramuscularly or titrated to effect intravenously; induction of anesthesia can be accomplished with alfaxalone, propofol, etomidate, benzodiazepine-dissociative, or benzodiazepine–opioid combinations. It is important to remember that all of these anesthetic drugs can cause some degree of reduced RBF and/or GFR and that using these drugs "to effect" is recommended. Anesthesia can be maintained with either isoflurane or sevoflurane. In addition, constant rate infusions using opioid agonists such as remifentanil or fentanyl for inhalant anesthetic reduction will reduce the dose-dependent side effects of inhalant anesthetics and may improve RBF and GFR. In adult horses, anesthetic premedication without an α_2-adrenergic receptor agonist is impractical; hence, using reduced doses and combining with butorphanol may allow for adequate sedation. Induction with a benzodiazepine–ketamine or propofol–ketamine combination can be performed. Using a reduced dose of ketamine may limit the induction agent's adverse effects on RBF and GFR. In smaller horses or ponies, propofol can be used as an induction agent.

Continuing intravenous fluid therapy throughout the anesthetic period is recommended to maintain fluid volume and hydration. While optimal perianesthetic fluid administration rates in veterinary patients have not been assessed in large-scale clinical studies, a good starting point would be to administer an initial rate of 10 mL/kg for the first hour followed by a rate of 5 mL/kg/h thereafter. These rates may be altered based on the patient's physiologic state and comorbidities, including dehydration, hypovolemia, heart disease, hypoproteinemia, or severe anemia. The choice of intravenous fluid is based on the animal's electrolyte and acid–base status. In general, animals with mild-to-moderate renal insufficiency/failure that are well prepared for surgery or anesthesia can be administered a replacement crystalloid intravenous fluid. If there is potential for urinary tract obstruction or the patient is anuric, intravenous fluids should be used cautiously to prevent fluid overload until the obstruction is relieved or the anuria resolves.

Vigilant monitoring of a patient will help the anesthetist to identify hypotension, arrhythmias, hypoxemia, or hypoventilation that could negatively impact renal function. Continuous electrocardiography (ECG) can detect changes in cardiac electrical activity that can be associated with electrolyte abnormalities such as hyperkalemia. Arterial blood pressure (ABP) should be measured to detect systemic hypotension and decreased renal perfusion pressure. Indirect ABP measurement can be easily performed with an oscillometric or Doppler technique; however, direct arterial catheterization is preferred as it is a more accurate and immediate measurement. Additionally, arterial blood gas samples can be obtained from the arterial catheter for analysis. Mean ABP should be maintained above 70–80 mmHg. In patients exhibiting hypertension when evaluated prior to anesthesia, maintenance of mean ABP closer to preanesthetic levels (i.e., within ~20%) may be necessary to preserve renal perfusion. Pulse oximetry (SpO_2) can be used to detect hemoglobin desaturation rapidly and alert the anesthetist to the potential for a decrease in tissue oxygen delivery. Continuous end-tidal carbon dioxide ($P_{ET}CO_2$) measurement can be used to detect hypoventilation and the need for assisted ventilation. Excessive arterial carbon dioxide can lead to acidemia, which may exacerbate acute renal disease [133]. Periodic arterial blood gas analysis can be useful for following trends in pH, oxygen content, and electrolytes. Advanced monitoring can be performed, particularly in critically ill animals. For example, central venous pressure (CVP) can be measured via a jugular catheter as one indirect measurement of blood volume to evaluate the rate of intravenous fluid administration. Normal CVP should be between 3 and 5 cmH_2O in dogs and cats. If the CVP rises more than 10 cmH_2O, fluid administration should be slowed or stopped. If the CVP falls in response to the fluids being stopped, they may be resumed at a slower rate. An elevated CVP of more than 10 cmH_2O indicates inadequate myocardial function or volume overload. Cardiac output measurement can give indications of preload, stroke volume, system vascular resistance, and patient response to inotropic and pressor agents that can have an effect on RBF and GFR. Less invasive assessments of volume status, discussed elsewhere, may include pulse pressure waveform analysis.

Adjunctive treatments for patients with renal disease

During the perianesthetic period, pharmacologic manipulation of cardiovascular and renal physiology may be beneficial in renal disease patients. Dopamine infusions (3–20 μg/kg/min) have long been considered useful in improving myocardial function and cardiac output. In human patients with renal disease, lower (e.g., renal) doses of dopamine (2 μg/kg/min) have historically been shown to increase urinary output but do not improve overall outcome compared with IV fluid therapy [132]. In dogs, low doses (1–3 μg/kg/min) were once used to promote RBF and GFR, but studies showing benefit are lacking and this strategy has fallen out of favor. Controversy exists regarding the use of dopamine to improve renal function in cats. Questions remain as to whether or not cats have appropriate dopamine receptors in their kidneys and low-dose dopamine has not been shown to have a diuretic effect in cats [134]. In fact, dopamine infusions of 10–100 μg/kg/min may increase urine output without changing GFR, suggesting that this diuresis is due to decreased tubular reabsorption and that dopamine receptors appear to have a minimal role in RBF or GFR in cats [135]. Doses of dopamine above approximately 10 μg/kg/min may cause α-adrenergic renal vasoconstriction and decreased RBF. An alternative inotrope for use during anesthesia is dobutamine (2–20 μg/kg/min). Dobutamine can increase cardiac output and potentially blood pressure without significant vasoconstrictive and dopaminergic actions.

Furosemide has also been investigated during anesthesia in patients with renal dysfunction. As a loop diuretic, furosemide decreases the metabolic activity of the renal tubules; however, furosemide infusion has been shown to result in elevated creatinine levels in anesthetized human patients, and its use is not recommended [132,136,137].

The osmotic diuretic mannitol has several potentially beneficial effects on the kidney. Mannitol is freely filtered and not reabsorbed by the kidney and, therefore, acts as an osmotic agent in the renal tubules and also in the systemic circulation. Administration of mannitol can induce renal arteriole dilation, decrease vascular resistance and blood viscosity, and scavenge oxygen free radicals. Mannitol has been used as a renal protective solution during kidney transplant in humans leading to a lower incidence of acute renal failure and delayed graft function [138]. Mannitol has also been used to reduce the incidence of contrast-induced nephropathy by preventing tubular necrosis [139,140]. RBF in cats may be improved by administering an intravenous loading dose of mannitol (500 mg/kg) and continuing a constant rate infusion (1 mg/kg/min) during the anesthetic period [141]. In a canine study where dogs underwent a 50% reduction in renal blood flow, mannitol (loading dose 500 mg/kg, infusion 20 mg/kg/min) improved RBF, GFR, and effective renal plasma flow [142]. However, in healthy dogs, a 500 mg/kg bolus dose increased fractional excretion of both sodium and urea but did not appear to increase GFR, even when followed by a 1 mg/kg/min infusion [143]. Repeated boluses rather than an infusion may be more clinically useful in dogs. In AKI, mannitol induced the redistribution of systemic blood flow to the kidneys and increased urine flow [144]. In an experimental model of hypoxia in rabbit kidneys, mannitol reduced tubular cell swelling and prevented proximal intratubular hypertension, resulting in improved blood flow [145]. Mannitol should be used cautiously in patients that are receiving other diuretics such as acetazolamide, as excessive use can result in hyponatremic acute renal failure [146]. Additionally, osmotic nephrosis has been reported with excessively high doses, with administration to hypovolemic patients, when combined with furosemide, or when administered to diabetic patients [147,148].

Fenoldopam is a dopamine receptor agonist at the D_1 receptor that has renal vasodilating properties. Fenoldopam has no effect on D_2 or α-adrenergic receptors that can cause vasoconstriction and result in decreased RBF and GFR. In fact, fenoldopam increases RBF and may assist in preserving renal function. Fenoldopam has been shown to decrease creatinine and improve renal function in humans at a dose of 0.1 μg/kg/min compared with dopamine infusion and may be effective in decreasing renal hypoperfusion [149]. In dogs, fenoldopam at a dose of 0.8 μg/kg/min resulted in a steady-state plasma concentration of 20 ± 17 ng/mL. Heart rate and systolic blood pressure were unaffected by the infusion in any of the dogs [150]. However, in a canine model of rhabdomyolysis, fenoldopam administration decreased creatinine clearance and increased the severity of renal injury and, in dogs with AKI secondary to heatstroke, it failed to increase urine output, GFR, fractional excretion of sodium, or odds of survival [151,152]. In awake, healthy cats, fenoldopam at 0.5 μg/kg/min increased urine output only after 6 h of infusion and increased sodium excretion. Additionally, fenoldopam administration had a biphasic effect on GFR, decreasing in the first 6 h and then increasing subsequently [153].

Anesthetic management of patients with urethral or bilateral ureteral obstruction

Species commonly presenting for obstruction and correction of urethral obstruction are cats, dogs, sheep, and goats; however, horses and cattle can also be affected. Cats are the species most commonly affected by acute bilateral or sequential bilateral ureteral obstruction. Both clinical conditions can cause mild to life-threatening postrenal uremic crisis. These patients often present with metabolic and acid–base abnormalities, including hyperkalemia, azotemia, acidemia, hyperphosphatemia, hyperglycemia, hypocalcemia, hyponatremia, and hypochloremia. Hyponatremia and hypochloremia are often associated with urine leakage into the abdominal cavity, and any patient presenting with these abnormalities should be examined for urinary tract rupture. Hyperkalemia is perhaps of greatest concern and should be addressed immediately. In general, patients having a serum potassium concentration greater than 5.5–6.0 mEq/L should not be anesthetized until the potassium levels can be normalized. Electrocardiographic abnormalities are commonly observed with potassium concentrations exceeding 7 mEq/L. The presence of ECG abnormalities at a given plasma concentration can also be related to the chronicity of the change, suggesting that preanesthetic ECG may be of value any time potassium abnormalities are present. The resting membrane potential of cardiac muscle depends on the permeability and extracellular concentration of potassium (Fig. 43.2). During hyperkalemia, the membrane's resting potential is raised (partially depolarized), and fewer sodium channels are available to participate in the action potential. As the serum potassium concentration increases, repolarization occurs more rapidly and automaticity, conductivity, contractility, and excitability are decreased. These changes produce the classic ECG appearance of a peaked T wave with a prolonged PR interval progressing to wide QRS complexes and loss of P waves.

Mild chronic hyperkalemia may not require treatment prior to anesthesia. If treatment is instituted for chronic hyperkalemia, serum potassium should be lowered gradually to allow intracellular potassium time to reestablish physiological transmembrane concentration gradients. If hyperkalemia is acute or ECG abnormalities are noted,

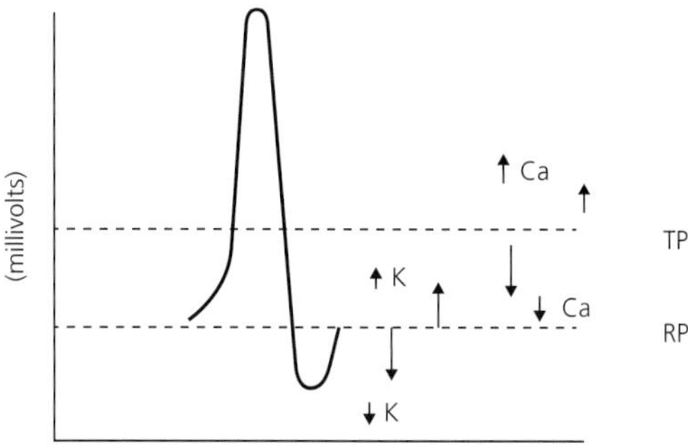

Figure 43.2 Relationships between extracellular concentrations of potassium and calcium and the resting potential (RP) and threshold potential (TP). An action potential is generated when there is sufficient depolarization to reach the TP. Increased extracellular potassium will result in raised (less negative) RP, whereas increased extracellular calcium will result in raised TP.

treatment should be initiated prior to induction of anesthesia. The most rapid treatment for the cardiac effects associated with hyperkalemia is 10% calcium chloride (0.1 mg/kg IV). Calcium will increase the membrane's threshold potential, resulting in increased myocardial conduction and contractility. Because increased serum potassium concentration causes the resting potential to be less negative (partially depolarized), the calcium ion-induced increase in threshold potential temporarily restores the normal gradient between resting and threshold potentials. It should be recognized that administration of calcium will not affect the serum potassium concentration, and its effects will, therefore, be short-lived. Regimens to decrease the serum potassium concentration by shifting potassium intracellularly include combined infusion of dextrose and insulin and bicarbonate administration (Table 43.7). Because acidemia favors extracellular movement of potassium and worsens hyperkalemia, intermittent positive-pressure ventilation may be required to prevent anesthetic drug-induced hypercapnia and respiratory acidosis.

In most appropriately restrained or sedated small animal patients, decompressive percutaneous cystocentesis can be safely performed by palpation or with ultrasound guidance to drain urine and reduce patient discomfort. When complications occur, they are usually associated with improper technique or inadequate patient restraint. Although rare bladder injury and rupture and aortic laceration have been reported, studies specifically examining the safety of this procedure in cats with urethral obstruction did not demonstrate clinically significant complications [154–158]. Intravenous fluid therapy should be instituted to correct dehydration and acid–base and electrolyte abnormalities. Once the patient is stabilized, anesthesia can be provided with a protocol similar to that discussed previously for small animal patients and small ruminants, and standard protocols for larger patients. Horses with urethral obstruction have been reported to rupture their bladder during induction of anesthesia, presumably due to increased abdominal compartment pressure from recumbency [159]. Perineal urethrostomy can be performed in male horses using sedation and epidural anesthesia to relieve the obstruction. Intravenous fluid therapy using potassium-free fluids has been considered the treatment of choice for animals with urethral obstruction. However, particularly in cats, compared with physiologic saline (0.9% NaCl), Lactated Ringer's solution is a better choice as animals have a decreased duration of metabolic and electrolyte imbalances after the obstruction is cleared [160].

Cats with oligoanuric acute ureteral obstruction (usually from stone disease, stricture, intraluminal concretions, or luminal inflammation, edema, hypertrophy, or fibrosis) usually are presented with the same metabolic derangements as animals with urethral obstruction and similar care is appropriate. Management is complicated, however, by several factors including: (1) correction of the obstruction usually requires surgical intervention (e.g., placement of a ureteral stent or subcutaneous ureteral bypass system, ureterotomy, or ureteral reimplantation); (2) oligoanuria may limit the utility of intravenous fluid therapy; and (3) presurgical (and sometimes also postsurgical) stabilization may require hemodialysis. These cats also usually experience AKI secondary to the hemodynamic, inflammatory, and apoptotic effects of the obstruction and, consequently, frequently sustain some degree of permanent loss of renal function after the obstruction is relieved [161–164].

In cats with mild or partial urethral obstruction, only sedation may be needed to facilitate passing a urethral catheter and clearing the obstruction. In these cases, after fluid therapy and stabilization, an opioid can be administered for analgesia followed by subanesthetic doses of propofol (0.25–1.0 mg/kg, IV) for sedation. Supplemental oxygen should be provided during propofol sedation. In male cats, intraurethral administration of 4 mL of diluted atracurium (0.5 mg/mL) significantly increased the chance and reduced the time necessary to relieve an obstruction [165]. Another approach is the use of a coccygeal epidural, described in Chapter 60, with a local anesthetic such as lidocaine for reducing pain and discomfort during and after unblocking of the urethra [166]. However, intravesicular administration of lidocaine and sodium bicarbonate has no beneficial effects and does not reduce the recurrence rate or severity of clinical signs in cats with urethral obstruction [167].

Careful postanesthetic care of these patients is essential as marked and/or prolonged diuresis after the obstruction has been relieved is common. Urine output of greater than 2 mL/kg/h can be expected in about 46% of cats within the first 6 h of treatment, which will require higher fluid therapy rates that should be tapered off over the following few days [168].

In sheep or goats with urethral obstruction, sedation or anesthesia may be needed to extrude the penis and examine the urethral process, one of the most common sites for urethral obstruction in these species. Preanesthetic stabilization to correct acid–base, fluid, and electrolyte imbalances should occur in a manner similar to that mentioned previously for small animal patients. α_2-Adrenergic receptor agonists, such as xylazine, should be avoided owing to their diuretic effects [169]. A benzodiazepine in combination with an opioid may provide adequate sedation for initial examination, particularly in painful animals. Anesthesia can be induced with injectable propofol or a benzodiazepine–dissociative combination, or with an inhalant anesthetic delivered by face mask. Additionally, adjunctive anesthesia can be provided with epidural administration of a local anesthetic.

Anesthetic management of patients with urinary bladder rupture and uroabdomen

Uroabdomen is defined as urine in the peritoneal cavity and can occur in any species of animal. In small animals, uroabdomen is most commonly caused by vehicular trauma but can also result from rupture of ureters, bladder, or urethra secondary to obstruction

Table 43.7 Treatment options for patients with hyperkalemia.

Treatment	Dosage	Use	Comments
Calcium chloride	0.1 mg/kg, IV	Raises threshold potential	Administer slowly; temporary effect only
50% Dextrose	1–2 mL/kg, IV	Increases endogenous insulin release to drive K^+ into cells	Dilute to 5–10% solution to reduce osmotic damage
Regular insulin	0.25–1 U/kg, IV	Drives K^+ into cells	Administer with dextrose and monitor blood glucose to prevent hypoglycemia
Sodium bicarbonate	1–2 mEq/kg, IV	Increases pH to cause exchange of intracellular H^+ for K^+	Monitor ventilation; CO_2 retention can result in worsening of acidemia

or neoplasia, or from iatrogenic injury. In large animal species, uroabdomen is most commonly associated with urethral obstruction; however, in neonatal foals, it is most commonly found in males and is thought to occur when the foal passes through the birth canal with a full bladder or secondary to umbilical infection and necrosis of the urachus [170].

In any species, it is important to recognize that uroabdomen is not a surgical emergency. Correction of postrenal azotemia, acid–base, and electrolyte abnormalities is paramount, and surgical correction can usually be delayed for several hours until the patient is stabilized [171]. Hyponatremia, hypochloremia, and hyperkalemia are common abnormalities. Hyponatremia and hypochloremia develop as a result of dilution from excess free water that is unable to be excreted, and hyperkalemia develops because excess potassium is unable to be excreted in the face of liberation from intracellular stores, particularly during acidosis [172]. Fluid and electrolyte replacement therapy is recommended, and hyperkalemia can be treated as previously indicated. Abdominocentesis can be performed to remove accumulating urine and reduce the azotemic and potassium loads. Peritoneal fluid creatinine can be compared with serum creatinine and ratios greater than 2:1 confirm uroperitoneum. Once a patient's serum abnormalities are normalized, and potassium in particular is reduced, animals can be anesthetized with previously mentioned protocols for surgical correction.

Postanesthesia oliguria and acute kidney injury

Decreased urine output and AKI are important complications that can develop after anesthesia and include the development of incidental kidney disease in addition to acute progression of CKD. Postanesthesia oliguria (< 0.5 mL/kg/h) can occur in patients after prolonged anesthesia or after a major surgical procedure and should prompt consideration and evaluation of causes of oliguria or AKI [173]. Some degree of oliguria can be expected in patients that have fluid or blood loss and secondary to the stress response of the adrenal cortex. In human patients, increased aldosterone and vasopressin release has been documented in the first 24 h after surgery. These increases result in increased salt and water reabsorption, thereby reducing urine production. However, this oliguria should be temporary and generally does not last for more than 24 h.

Pathologic causes of postanesthesia oliguria and AKI can be divided into prerenal, renal, and postrenal categories [173]. Prerenal causes include hypotension and hypovolemia. Renal causes include acute tubular necrosis (ischemia and reperfusion) and acute interstitial nephritis (drug toxicity associated with NSAIDs, antibiotics, or diuretics). Postrenal abnormalities can result from physical obstruction of urine flow.

Techniques designed for the prevention of postanesthesia oliguria and AKI are recommended, particularly in high-risk patients. Physiologic monitoring of vital signs for identification of hypotension and decreased perfusion includes mucous membrane color, capillary refill time, measurement of blood pressure, pulse oximetry, $P_{ET}CO_2$, and electrocardiography. Advanced monitoring techniques such as CVP and cardiac output measurements may be warranted in critical patients. Administration of intravenous fluids to maintain or expand intravascular volume is the mainstay of therapy for the prevention of AKI [173]. Historically, synthetic colloidal therapy with hydroxyethyl starch was considered potentially beneficial in maintaining vascular expansion; however, there is some evidence that it may be nephrotoxic [174]. As mentioned previously, the use of mannitol may be appropriate for maintenance of RBF and GFR during anesthesia in cases with high risk of postanesthetic oliguria or AKI. Techniques to maintain mean arterial pressures greater than 60–65 mmHg in small animal patients and smaller horses and ruminants and greater than 70–75 mmHg in adult horses and ruminants are of paramount importance for adequate perfusion of the kidneys. The level of acceptable hypotension is dependent on baseline blood pressure, and mean arterial pressures may need to be maintained at higher levels in patients with chronic hypertension [175]. In human patients, it is recommended that mean arterial pressure be maintained within 20% of awake baseline values, since this is within the range of blood pressure drop during sleep [173,176]. The use of inotropic agents or anesthetic-sparing techniques (MAC reduction) to achieve these desired pressures should be standard practice for patients with conditions that predispose to AKI.

Management of the postanesthetic patient in which oliguria or AKI is diagnosed should start with determining the cause. Reversible causes such as obstruction, hypotension, and hypovolemia should be ruled out or corrected. Measurement of blood pressure and intravenous fluid challenges can be useful. If the oliguria is determined to be of renal origin (not pre- or postrenal), function and diagnostic testing as described previously should be performed.

Treatment of postanesthesia oliguria and AKI is centered on judicious and closely monitored intravenous fluid and electrolyte therapy. The use of diuretic and vasoactive drugs is controversial. Dopamine has traditionally been used in patients with oliguria and AKI. Historically, lower doses ranging from 1 to 3 μg/kg/min had been used to increase RBF, GFR, urine output, and sodium excretion and decrease renal vascular resistance in several species [177]. In humans, low-dose dopamine therapy in patients with renal dysfunction resulted in transient improvements in urine output and creatinine levels; however, mortality and long-term outcomes did not improve [178]. The use of diuretics such as furosemide has also failed to show any improvement in clinical outcomes and may even worsen renal injury [168]. In hypovolemic patients, furosemide may increase the nephrotoxicity of other drugs by increasing their contact time in the renal tubules [179]. Diuretics may, however, be useful in patients that develop pulmonary edema and fluid overload secondary to AKI [180]. Mannitol, as stated previously, may have beneficial effects in patients with AKI and can also be used in patients with volume overload and pulmonary edema.

Once postanesthetic oliguria and AKI have been identified and reversible conditions have been treated, the goal of therapy is to minimize ongoing or long-term renal damage. Long-term monitoring of renal function may be necessary.

Acknowledgment

The authors wish to acknowledge Dr. Gregory F. Grauer for his contributions to the previous edition that have been carried forward into this chapter.

References

1 Bartges JW. Chronic kidney disease in dogs and cats. *Vet Clin North Am Small Anim Pract* 2012; **42**(4): 669–692.

2 Conroy M, Brodbelt DC, O'Neill D, *et al.* Chronic kidney disease in cats attending primary care practice in the UK: a VetCompass™ study. *Vet Rec* 2019; **184**(17): 526.

3 Roura X. Risk Factors in Dogs and Cats for Development of Chronic Kidney Disease. International Renal Interest Society (IRIS), 2019. www.iris-kidney.com/education/education/index.html (accessed July 2023).

4 O'Neill DG, Elliott J, Church DB, *et al.* Chronic kidney disease in dogs in UK veterinary practices: prevalence, risk factors, and survival. *J Vet Int Med* 2013; **27**(4): 814–821.

5 Quimby JM, McLeland SM, Cianciolo RE, *et al.* Frequency of histologic lesions in the kidneys of cats without kidney disease. *J Feline Med Surg* 2022; **24**(12): e472–e480.

6 Cianciolo R, Hokamp J, Naabity M. Advances in the evaluation of canine renal disease. *Vet J* 2016; **215**: 21–29.

7 Schott HC, Waldridge B, Bayly WM. Examination of the urinary system. In: Reed SM, Bayly WM, Sellon DC, eds. *Equine Internal Medicine*, 4th edn. St. Louis, MO: Saunders Elsevier, 2010: 888–990.

8 Olsen E, van Galen G. Chronic renal failure – causes, clinical findings, treatments and prognosis. *Vet Clin North Am Equine Pract* 2022; **38**(1): 25–46.

9 Rose DB, Post T, Stokes J. *Clinical Physiology of Acid–Base and Electrolyte Disorders*, 6th edn. New York, NY: McGraw-Hill, 2013.

10 Hall JE, Hall ME. The urinary system: functional anatomy and urine formation by the kidneys. In: *Guyton and Hall Textbook of Medical Physiology*, 14th edn. Philadelphia, PA: Saunders Elsevier, 2021: 321–330.

11 DiBartola SP. Applied renal physiology. In: DiBartola SP, ed. *Fluid, Electrolyte, and Acid–Base Disorders in Small Animal Practice*, 4th edn. St. Louis, MO: Saunders Elsevier, 2012: 26–43.

12 Zeisberg M, Kalluri R. Physiology of the renal interstitium. *Clin J Am Soc Nephrol* 2015; **10**(10): 1831–1840.

13 Hall JE, Hall ME. Glomerular filtration, renal blood flow, and their control. In: Hall JE, Hall ME, eds. *Guyton and Hall Textbook of Medical Physiology*, 14th edn. Philadelphia, PA: Elsevier, 2021: 321–330.

14 Flournoy WS, Wohl JS, Albrecht-Schmitt TJ, *et al.* Pharmacologic identification of putative D1 dopamine receptors in feline kidneys. *J Vet Pharmacol Ther* 2003; **26**(4): 283–290.

15 Boozer L, Cartier L, Sheldon S, *et al.* Lack of utility of laboratory "normal" ranges for serum creatinine concentration for the diagnosis of feline chronic renal insufficiency. *J Vet Intern Med* 2002; **16**: 354.

16 Nabity MB, Lees GE, Boggess M, *et al.* Week-to week variability of iohexol clearance, serum creatinine, and symmetric dimethylarginine in dogs with stable chronic renal disease. *J Vet Intern Med* 2013; **27**(3): 734.

17 Braff J, Obare E, Yerramilli M, *et al.* Relationship between serum symmetric dimethylarginine concentration and glomerular filtration rate in cats. *J Vet Intern Med* 2014; **28**(6): 1699–1701.

18 Nabity MB, Lees GE, Boggess M, *et al.* Symmetric dimethylarginine assay validation, stability, and evaluation as a marker for early detection of chronic kidney disease in dogs. *J Vet Intern Med* 2015; **29**(4): 1036–1044.

19 Grauer G. Early diagnosis of chronic kidney disease in dogs & cats: use of serum creatinine & symmetric dimethylarginine. *Today's Vet Pract* 2016; **6**(2): 68–72.

20 Relford R, Robertson J, Clements C. Symmetric dimethylarginine: improving the diagnosis and staging of chronic kidney disease in small animals. *Vet Clin North Am Small Anim Pract* 2016; **46**(6): 941–960.

21 Hall JA, Yerramilli M, Obare E, *et al.* Serum concentrations of symmetric dimethylarginine and creatinine in dogs with naturally occurring chronic kidney disease. *J Vet Intern Med* 2016; **30**(3): 794–802.

22 Pedersen LG, Tarnow I, Olsen LH, *et al.* Body size, but neither age nor asymptomatic mitral regurgitation, influences plasma concentrations of dimethylarginines in dogs. *Res Vet Sci* 2006; **80**(3): 336–342.

23 Moesgaard SG, Holte AV, Mogensen T, *et al.* Effects of breed, gender, exercise, and white-coat effect on markers of endothelial function in dogs. *Res Vet Sci* 2007; **82**(3): 409–415.

24 Hall JA, Yerramilli M, Obare E, *et al.* Comparison of serum concentrations of symmetric dimethylarginine and creatinine as kidney function biomarkers in cats with chronic kidney disease. *J Vet Intern Med* 2014; **28**(6): 1676–1683.

25 Yerramilli M, Yerramilli M, Obare E, *et al.* Symmetric dimethylarginine (SDMA) increases earlier than serum creatinine in dogs with chronic kidney disease (CKD). *J Vet Intern Med* 2014; **28**(3): 1084–1085.

26 Dahlem DP, Neiger R, Schweighauser A. Plasma symmetric dimethylarginine concentration in dogs with acute kidney injury and chronic kidney disease. *J Vet Intern Med* 2017; **31**(3): 799–804.

27 Peich TL, Wycislo KL. Importance of urinalysis. *Vet Clin North Am Small Anim Pract* 2019; **49**(2): 233–245.

28 Grauer GF, Greco DS, Behrend EN, *et al.* Estimation of quantitative enzymuria in dogs with gentamicin-induced nephrotoxicosis using urine enzyme/creatinine ratios from spot urine samples. *J Vet Intern Med* 1995; **9**(5): 324–327.

29 Adedeji AO, Sonee M, Chen Y, *et al.* Evaluation of novel urinary biomarkers in beagle dogs with amphotericin B-induced kidney injury. *Int J Toxicol* 2023; **42**(2): 146–155.

30 Ruiz P, Durán Á, Duque FJ, *et al.* Urinary cystatin C and N-acetyl-beta-D-glucosaminidase (NAG) as early biomarkers for renal disease in dogs with leishmaniosis. *Vet Parasitol* 2023; **318**: 109930.

31 Ko HY, Kim J, Geum M, *et al.* Cystatin C and neutrophil gelatinase-associated lipocalin as early biomarkers for chronic kidney disease in dogs. *Top Companion Anim Med* 2021; **45**: 100580.

32 Harjen HJ, Nicolaysen TV, Negard T, *et al.* Serial serum creatinine, SDMA and urinary acute kidney injury biomarker measurements in dogs envenomated by the European adder (*Vipera berus*). *BMC Vet Res* 2021; **17**(1): 154.

33 Davis J, Rossi G, Cianciolo RE, *et al.* Early diagnosis of acute kidney injury subsequent to severe hypotension and fluid resuscitation in anaesthetized dogs. *Vet Anaesth Analg* 2022; **49**(4): 344–353.

34 Jacob F, Polzin DJ, Osborne CA, *et al.* Evaluation of the association between initial proteinuria and morbidity rate or death in dogs with naturally occurring chronic renal failure. *J Am Vet Med Assoc* 2005; **226**(3): 393–400.

35 Syme HM, Markwell PJ, Pfeiffer D, *et al.* Survival of cats with naturally occurring chronic renal failure is related to severity of proteinuria. *J Vet Intern Med* 2006; **29**(3): 528–535.

36 Grauer G. Measurement, interpretation, and implications of proteinuria and albuminuria. *Vet Clin North Am Small Anim Pract* 2007; **37**(2): 283–295.

37 Wehner A, Hartmann K, Hirschberger J. Associations between proteinuria, systemic hypertension and glomerular filtration rate in dogs with renal and nonrenal diseases. *Vet Rec* 2008; **162**(5): 141–147.

38 Lees GE, Brown SA, Elliott J, *et al.* Assessment and management of proteinuria in dogs and cats; 2004 ACVIM Forum Consensus Statement (small animal). *J Vet Intern Med* 2005; **19**(3): 377–385.

39 Chakrabarti S, Syme HM, Elliott J. Clinicopathological variables predicting progression of azotemia in cats with chronic kidney disease. *J Vet Intern Med* 2012; **26**(2): 275–281.

40 Jepson RE, Brodbelt D, Vallance C, *et al.* Evaluation of predictors of the development of azotemia in cats. *J Vet Intern Med* 2009; **23**(4): 806–813.

41 Vaden SL. Glomerular diseases. In: Ettinger SJ, Feldman EC, Cote E, eds. *Textbook of Veterinary Internal Medicine*, 8th edn. Philadelphia, PA: WB Saunders, 2017: 1959–1972.

42 Toblli JE, Bevione P, DiGennaro F, *et al.* Understanding the mechanisms of proteinuria: therapeutic implications. *Int J Nephrol* 2012: 546039.

43 Lees GE, Cianciolo RE, Clubb FJ Jr. Renal biopsy and pathologic evaluation of glomerular disease. *Top Companion Anim Med* 2011; **26**(3): 143–153.

44 Schott HC, Esser MM. The sick adult horse: renal clinical pathologic testing and urinalysis. *Vet Clin North Am Equine Pract* 2020; **36**(1): 121–134.

45 Hokamp JA, Nabity MB. Renal biomarkers in domestic species. *Vet Clin Pathol* 2016; **45**(1): 28–56.

46 Schott HC. Chronic renal failure. In: Reed SM, Bayly WM, Sellon DC, eds. *Equine Internal Medicine*, 3rd edn. St. Louis, MO: Saunders Elsevier, 2010: 1183–1198.

47 Gough RL, McGovern KF. Serum symmetric dimthylarginine concentration in healthy neonatal Thoroughbred foals. *Equine Vet J* 2022; **54**(5): 958–964.

48 Bozorgmanesh R, Thornton J, Snyder J, *et al.* Symmetric dimethylarginine concentrations in healthy neonatal foals and mares. *J Vet Intern Med* 2021; **35**(6): 2891–2896.

49 Schott HC, Gallant LR, Coyne M, *et al.* Symmetric dimethylarginine and creatinine concentrations in serum of healthy draft horses. *J Vet Intern Med* 2021; **35**(2): 1147–1154.

50 Surdyk KK, Sloan DL, Brown SA. Renal effects of carprofen and etodolac in euvolemic and volume-depleted dogs. *Am J Vet Res* 2012; **73**(9): 1485–1490.

51 International Renal Interest Society (IRIS) Guidelines. www.iris-kidney.com/guidelines/index.html (accessed July 2023).

52 Ross L. Acute kidney injury in dogs and cats. *Vet Clin North Am Small Anim Pract* 2022; **52**(3): 659–672.

53 Cowgill LD, Langston C. Acute kidney insufficiency. In: Bartges J, Polzin DJ, eds. *Small Animal Nephrology and Urology*. West Sussex, UK: Wiley Blackwell, 2011: 472–523.

54 Langston C. Acute kidney injury. In: Ettinger SJ, Feldman EC, Cote E, eds. *Textbook of Veterinary Internal Medicine*, 8th edn. Philadelphia, PA: WB Saunders, 2017: 1919–1934.

55 Hall JE, Hall ME. Acute kidney injury. In: Hall JE, Hall ME, eds. *Guyton and Hall Textbook of Medical Physiology*, 14th edn. Philadelphia, PA: Elsevier, 2021: 429–432.

56 Huynh E, Berry CR. Ultrasonography of the urinary tract: kidneys and ureters. *Today's Vet Pract* 2017; **7**(6): 31–45.

57 Choo D, Kim SS, Kwon D, *et al.* Ultrasonographic quantitative evaluation of acute and chronic renal disease using the renal cortical thickness to aorta ratio in dogs. *Vet Radiol Ultrasound* 2023; **64**(1): 140–148.

58 Rohini BG, George A, Usha NP, *et al.* A retrospective study of acute kidney injury in dogs with renal resistive index as a prognostic indicator. *J Vet Anim Sci* 2022; **53**(4): 583–591.

59 Polzin DJ. Chronic kidney disease. In: Ettinger SJ, Feldman EC, Cote E, eds. *Textbook of Veterinary Internal Medicine*, 8th edn. Philadelphia, PA: WB Saunders, 2017: 1938–1959.

60 Brown CA, Elliott J, Schmiedt CW, *et al.* Chronic kidney disease in aged cats: clinical features, morphology, and proposed pathogeneses. *Vet Pathol* 2016; **53**(2): 309–326.

61 Jepsen RE. Current understanding of the pathogenesis of progressive chronic kidney disease in cats. *Vet Clin North Am Small Anim Pract* 2016; **46**(6): 1015–1048.

62 Quimby JM. Update on medical management of clinical manifestations of chronic kidney disease. *Vet Clin North Am Small Anim Pract* 2016; **46**(6): 1163–1181.

63 Kabatchnick E, Langston C, Olson B, *et al.* Hypothermia in uremic dogs and cats. *J Vet Intern Med* 2016; **30**(5): 1648–1654.

64 Yan GY, Chen KY, Wang HC, *et al.* Relationship between ultrasonographically determined renal dimensions and International Renal Interest Society stages in cats with chronic kidney disease. *J Vet Intern Med* 2020; **34**(4): 1464–1475.

65 Perondi F, Lippi I, Marchetti V, *et al.* How ultrasound can be useful for staging chronic kidney disease in dogs: ultrasound findings in 855 cases. *Vet Sci* 2020; 7(4): 147.

66 Huguet EE, Berry CR, Cole CC. Ultrasonography for diagnosing chronic kidney disease in dogs and cats. *Today's Vet Pract* 2023; **2**: 56–65.

67 Polzin DJ. A step-wise approach to managing chronic kidney disease: application of evidence based medicine. *J Vet Emerg Crit Care* 2013; **23**(2): 205–215.

68 Parker VJ. Nutritional management for dogs and cats with chronic kidney disease. *Vet Clin North Am Small Anim Pract* 2021; **51**(3): 685–710.

69 Chalhoub S, Langston CE, Farrelly J. The use of darbepoetin to stimulate erythropoiesis in anemia of chronic kidney disease in cats: 25 cases. *J Vet Intern Med* 2012; **26**(2): 363–369.

70 Hall JA. Renal effects of the inhalation agents. In: Faust RJ, ed. *Anesthesiology Review*, 3rd edn. Philadelphia, PA: Churchill Livingstone, 2002: 103–104.

71 Grimm JB, Grimm KA, Kneller SK, *et al.* The effect of a combination of medetomidine– butorphanol and medetomidine, butorphanol, atropine on glomerular filtration rate in dogs. *Vet Radiol Ultrasound* 2001; **42**(5): 458–462.

72 Fusellier M, Desfontis JC, Madec S, *et al.* Influence of three anesthetic protocols on glomerular filtration rate in dogs. *Am J Vet Res* 2007; **68**(8): 807–811.

73 Bostrom I, Nyman G, Kampa N, *et al.* Effects of acepromazine on renal function in anesthetized dogs. *Am J Vet Res* 2003; **64**(5): 590–598.

74 Pazoki-Toroudi HR, Ajami M, Habibey R. Premedication and renal preconditioning: a role for alprazolam, atropine, morphine and promethazine. *Fundam Clin Pharmacol* 2010; **24**(2): 189–198.

75 Weil AB. Anesthesia for patients with renal/hepatic disease. *Top Companion Anim Med* 2010; **25**(2): 87–91.

76 Lawrence CJ, Prinzen FW, de Lange S. The effect of dexmedetomidine on nutrient organ blood flow. *Anesth Analg* 1996; **83**(6): 1160–1165.

77 Kilic K, Hanci V, Selek S, *et al.* The effects of dexmedetomidine on mesenteric arterial occlusion-associated gut ischemia and reperfusion-induced gut and kidney injury in rabbits. *J Surg Res* 2012; **178**(1): 223–232.

78 Murahata Y, Hikasa Y. Comparison of the diuretic effects of medetomidine hydrochloride and xylazine hydrochloride in healthy cats. *Am J Vet Res* 2012; **73**(12): 1871–1880.

79 Talukder MH, Hikasa Y. Diuretic effects of medetomidine compared with xylazine in healthy dogs. *Can J Vet Res* 2009; **73**(3): 224–236.

80 Nunez E, Steffey EP, Ocampo L, *et al.* Effects of α_2-adrenergic receptor agonists on urine production in horses deprived of food and water. *Am J Vet Res* 2004; **65**(10): 1342–1346.

81 Saleh N, Aoki M, Shimada T, *et al.* Renal effects of medetomidine in isoflurane anesthetized dogs with special reference to its diuretic action. *J Vet Med Sci* 2005; **67**(5): 461–465.

82 Restitutti F, Laitinen MR, Raekallio MR, *et al.* Effect of MK-467 on organ blood flow parameters detected by contrast-enhanced ultrasound in dogs treated with dexmedetomidine. *Vet Anaesth Analg* 2013; **40**(6): e48–e56.

83 Kirwan CJ, MacPhee IA, Lee T, *et al.* Acute kidney injury reduces the hepatic metabolism of midazolam in critically ill patients. *Intensive Care Med* 2012; **38**(1): 76–84.

84 Yorgin PD, Theodorou AA, Al-Uzri A, *et al.* Propylene glycol-induced proximal renal tubular cell injury. *Am J Kidney Dis* 1997; **30**(1): 134–139.

85 Hayman M, Seidl EC, Ali M, *et al.* Acute tubular necrosis associated with propylene glycol from concomitant administration of intravenous lorazepam and trimethoprim– sulfamethoxazole. *Pharmacotherapy* 2003; **23**(9): 1190–1194.

86 Zar T, Yusufzai I, Sullivan A, *et al.* Acute kidney injury, hyperosmolality and metabolic acidosis associated with lorazepam. *Nat Clin Pract Nephrol* 2007; **3**(9): 515–520.

87 Cummings K, Naguib MA. Opioid agonists and antagonists. In: Flood P, Rathmell JP, Shafer S, eds. *Pharmacology and Physiology in Anesthetic Practice*, 5th edn. Philadelphia, PA: Wolters Kluwer, 2015: 217–256.

88 Hohne C, Donaubauer B, Kaisers U. Opioids during anesthesia in liver and renal failure. *Anaesthesist* 2004; **53**(3): 291–303.

89 Davies G, Kingswood C, Street M. Pharmacokinetics of opioids in renal dysfunction. *Clin Pharmacokinet* 1996; **31**(6): 410–422.

90 Hoke JF, Shulgman D, Dershwitz M, *et al.* Pharmacokinetics and pharmacodynamics of remifentanil in persons with renal failure compared with healthy volunteers. *Anesthesiology* 1997; **87**(3): 533–541.

91 Danhof M, Levy G. Kinetics of drug action in disease states. V. Acute effect of urea infusion on phenobarbital concentrations in rats at onset of loss of righting reflex. *J Pharmacol Exp Ther* 1985; **232**(2): 430–434.

92 Ghoneim MM, Pandya H. Plasma protein binding of thiopental in patients with impaired renal or hepatic function. *Anesthesiology* 1975; **42**(5): 545–549.

93 Srıvastava K, Hatanaka T, Katayama K, *et al.* Influence of plasma dialysate from normal and renal dysfunction rats on the electroencephalogram and gamma-aminobutyric acid A receptor complex modulation of thiopental. *Biol Pharm Bull* 1999; **22**(3): 288–294.

94 Srirastava K, Hatanaka T, Katayama K, *et al.* Pharmacokinetic and pharmacodynamic consequences of thiopental in renal dysfunction rats: evaluation with electroencephalography. *Biol Pharm Bull* 1998; **21**(12): 1327–1333.

95 Priano LL. Alteration of renal hemodynamics by thiopental, diazepam, and ketamine in conscious dogs. *Anesth Analg* 1928; **61**(10): 853–862.

96 Chien CT, Cheng YJ, Chen CF, *et al.* Differentiation of ketamine effects on renal nerve activity and renal blood flow in rats. *Acta Anaesthesiol Taiwan* 2004; **42**(4): 185–189.

97 Nishimura M, Sato K. Ketamine stereoselectively inhibits rat dopamine transporter. *Neurosci Lett* 1999; **274**(2): 131–134.

98 Flecknell PA. Injectable anaesthetics. In: Hall LW, Taylor PM, eds. *Anaesthesia of the Cat*. London, UK: Baillière Tindall, 1994: 129–156.

99 Waterman AE. Influence of premedication with xylazine on the distribution and metabolism of intramuscularly administered ketamine in cats. *Res Vet Sci* 1983; **35**(3): 285–290.

100 Baggott JD, Blake JW. Disposition kinetics of ketamine in the domestic cat. *Arch Int Pharmacodyn Ther* 1976; **220**(1): 115–124.

101 Morgan CJ, Curran HV. Ketamine use: a review. *Addiction* 2012; **107**(1): 27–38.

102 Middela S, Pearce I. Ketamine-induced vesicopathy: a literature review. *Int J Clin Pract* 2010; **65**(1): 27–30.

103 Wouters PF, Van de Velde MA, Marcus MA, *et al.* Hemodynamic changes during induction of anesthesia with eltanolone and propofol in dogs. *Anesth Analg* 1995; **81**(1): 125–131.

104 Shiga Y, Minami K, Uezono Y, *et al.* Effects of the intravenously administered anaesthetics ketamine, propofol, and thiamylal on the cortical renal blood flow in rats. *Pharmacology* 2003; **68**(1): 17–23.

105 Booke M, Armstrong C, Hinder F, *et al.* The effects of propofol on hemodynamics and renal blood flow in healthy and in septic sheep, and combined with fentanyl in septic sheep. *Anesth Analg* 1996; **82**(4): 738–743.

106 Chang J, Kim S, Jung J, *et al.* Evaluation of the effects of thiopental, propofol, and etomidate on glomerular filtration rate measured by the use of dynamic computed tomography in dogs. *Am J Vet Res* 2011; **72**(1): 146–151.

108 Kirvela M, Olkkola KT, Rosenberg PH, *et al.* Pharmacokinetics of propofol and haemodynamic changes during induction of anaesthesia in uraemic patients. *Br J Anaesth* 1992; **68**(2): 178–182.

109 Nathan N, Debord J, Narcisse F, *et al.* Pharmacokinetics of propofol and its conjugates after continuous infusion in normal and in renal failure patients: a preliminary study. *Acta Anaesthesiol Belg* 1993; **44**(3): 77–85.

110 de Gasperi A, Mazza E, Noe L, *et al.* Pharmacokinetic profile of the induction dose of propofol in chronic renal failure patients undergoing renal transplantation. *Minerva Anesthesiol* 1996; **62**(1): 25–31.

111 Whittem T, Pasloske KS, Heit MC, *et al.* The pharmacokinetics and pharmacodynamics of alfaxalone in cats after single and multiple intravenous administration of Alfaxan at clinical and supraclinical doses. *J Vet Pharmacol Ther* 2008; **31**(6): 571–579.

112 Taboada FM, Murison PJ. Induction of anaesthesia with alfaxalone or propofol before isoflurane maintenance in cats. *Vet Rec* 2010; **167**(3): 85–89.

113 Psatha E, Alibhai HI, Jimenez-Lozano A, *et al.* Clinical efficacy and cardiorespiratory effects of alfaxalone, or diazepam/fentanyl for induction of anaesthesia in dogs that are a poor anaesthetic risk. *Vet Anaesth Analg* 2011; **38**(1): 24–36.

114 Warne LN, Beths T, Whittem T, *et al.* A review of the pharmacology and clinical application of alfaxalone in cats. *Vet J* 2015; **203**(2): 141–148.

115 Tamura J, Oyama N, Fukui S, *et al.* Comparison of the anesthetic effects between 5 mg/kg of alfaxalone and 10 mg/kg of propofol administered intravenously in cats. *J Vet Med Sci* 2021; **83**(1): 73–77.

116 Petersen JS, Shalmi M, Christensen S, *et al.* Comparison of the renal effects of six sedating agents in rats. *Physiol Behav* 1996; **60**(3): 759–765.

117 Gelman S, Fowler KC, Smith LR. Regional blood flow during isoflurane and halothane anesthesia. *Anesth Analg* 1984; **63**(6): 557–565.

118 Bernard JM, Doursout MF, Wouters P, *et al.* Effects of sevoflurane and isoflurane on hepatic circulation in the chronically instrumented dog. *Anesthesiology* 1992; **77**(3): 541–545.

119 Conzen PF, Kharasch ED, Czerner SFA, *et al.* Low-flow sevoflurane compared with low-flow isoflurane anesthesia in patients with stable renal insufficiency. *Anesthesiology* 2002; **97**(3): 578–584.

120 Sun L, Suzuki Y, Takata M, *et al.* Repeated low-flow sevoflurane anesthesia: effects on hepatic and renal function in beagles. *Masui* 1997; **46**(3): 351–357.

121 Merin RG, Bernard JM, Doursout MF, *et al.* Comparison of the effects of isoflurane and desflurane on cardiovascular dynamics and regional blood flow in the chronically instrumented dog. *Anesthesiology* 1991; **74**(3): 568–574.

122 Hayes MA, Goldenberg IS. Renal effects of anesthesia and operation mediated by endocrines. *Anesthesiology* 1963; **24**: 487–499.

123 Kramer BK, Kammerl MC, Komhoff M. Renal cyclooxygenase-2 (COX-2). Physiological, pathophysiological, and clinical implications. *Kidney Blood Press Res* 2004; **27**(1): 43–62.

124 Crandell DE, Mathews KA, Dyson DH. Effect of meloxicam and carprofen on renal function when administered to healthy dogs prior to anesthesia and painful stimulation. *Am J Vet Res* 2004; **65**(10): 1384–1390.

125 Pages JP. Néphropathies dues aux anti-inflammatoires non stéroïdiens (AINS) chez le chat: 21 observations (1993–2001). *Prat Méd Chir Anim Compagnie* 2005; **40**: 177–181.

126 Dyer F, Diesel G, Cooles S, *et al.* Suspected adverse reactions, 2009. *Vet Rec* 2010; **167**(4): 118–121.

127 KuKanich K, George C, Roush JK, *et al.* Effects of low-dose meloxicam in cats with chronic kidney disease. *J Feline Med Surg* 2021; **23**(2): 138–148.

128 King JN, Seewald W, Forster S, *et al.* Clinical safety of robenacoxib in cats with chronic musculoskeletal disease. *J Vet Intern Med* 2021; **35**(5): 2384–2394.

129 Monteiro B, Steagall PVM, Lascelles BDX, *et al.* Long-term use of non-steroidal anti-inflammatory drugs in cats with chronic kidney disease: from controversy to optimism. *J Small Anim Pract* 2019; **60**(8): 459–462.

130 Boscan P, Pypendop BH, Siao DT, *et al.* Fluid balance, glomerular filtration rate, and urine output in dogs anesthetized for an orthopedic surgical procedure. *Am J Vet Res* 2010; **71**(5): 501–507.

131 Wagener G, Brentjens TE. Anesthetic concerns in patients presenting with renal failure. *Anesthesiol Clin* 2010; **28**(1): 39–54.

132 Lassnigg A, Donner E, Grubhofer G, *et al.* Lack of renoprotective effects of dopamine and furosemide during cardiac surgery. *J Am Soc Nephrol* 2000; **11**(1): 97–104.

133 Kazory A, Ducloux D. Successful management of respiratory failure can improve renal function. *Am J Crit Care* 2009; **18**(1): 10–11.

134 Wohl JS, Schwartz DD, Flournoy S, *et al.* Renal hemodynamic and diuretic effects of low-dosage dopamine in anesthetized cats. *J Vet Emerg Crit Care* 2007; **17**(1): 45–52.

135 Clark KL, Roberson MJ, Drew GM. Do renal tubular dopamine receptors mediate dopamine-induced diuresis in the anesthetized cat? *J Cardiovasc Pharmacol* 1991; **17**(2): 267–276.

136 Langston CE. Acute kidney injury. In: Ettinger SJ, Feldman EC, Cote E, eds. *Textbook of Veterinary Internal Medicine*, 8th edn. St. Louis, MO: Elsevier, 2017: 1615–1633.

137 Ho KM, Power BM. Benefits and risks of furosemide in acute kidney injury. *Anaesthesia* 2010; **65**(3): 283–293.

138 Van de Laar SC, Schouten GN, Ijzermans JN, *et al.* Effect of mannitol on kidney function after kidney transplantation: a systemic review and meta-analysis. *Transplant Proc* 2021; **53**(7): 2122–2132.

139 Yang B, Xu J, Fengying X, *et al.* Intravascular administration of mannitol for acute kidney injury prevention: a systematic review and meta-analysis. *PLoS ONE* 2014; **9**(1): e85029.

140 Kalogirou TE, Meditoshou S, Davidopoulou S, *et al.* Investigating the possible protective role of direct intra-arterial administration of mannitol and N-acetylcysteine and *Per Os* administration of simvastatin against contrast-induced nephropathy: an experimental study in a rabbit model. *Cardiovasc Intervent Radiol* 2019; **42**(12): 1777–1785.

141 McClellan JM, Goldstein RE, Erb HN, *et al.* Effects of administration of fluids and diuretics on glomerular filtration rate, renal blood flow, and urine output in healthy awake cats. *Am J Vet Res* 2006; **67**(4): 715–722.

142 Behnia R, Koushanpour E, Brunner EA. Effects of hyperosmotic mannitol infusion on hemodynamics of dog kidney. *Anesth Analg* 1996; **82**(5): 902–908.

143 Segev G, Stafford C, Kirby J, *et al.* Sequential changes in urine production, glomerular filtration rate, and electrolyte excretion after mannitol administration. *J Vet Intern Med* 2019; **33**(3): 1362–1367.

144 Braqadottir G, Redfors B, Ricksten SE. Mannitol increases renal blood flow and maintains filtration fraction and oxygenation in postoperative acute kidney injury: a prospective interventional study. *Crit Care* 2012; **16**(4): R159.

145 Bipat R, Steels P, Cuypers Y, *et al.* Mannitol reduces the hydrostatic pressure in the proximal tubule of the isolated blood-perfused rabbit kidney during hypoxic stress and improves its function. *Nephron Extra* 2011; **1**(1): 201–211.

146 Tsai SF, Shu KH. Mannitol-induced acute renal failure. *Clin Nephrol* 2010; **74**(1): 70–73.

147 Nair SM, Power NE, Coleman JA. Examining mannitol use in kidney cancer surgery: a cautionary tale of extrapolated surgical data. *Eur Urol Focus* 2019; **5**(6): 930–934.

148 Agarwal RC, Jain RK, Anurag Y. Prevention of perioperative renal failure. *JAPI* 2008; **56**: 956–964.

149 Brienza N, Malcangi V, Dalfino L, *et al.* A comparison between fenoldopam and low-dose dopamine in early renal dysfunction of critically ill patients. *Crit Care Med* 2006; **34**(3): 707–714.

150 Bloom CA, Labato MA, Hazarika S, *et al.* Preliminary pharmacokinetics and cardiovascular effects of fenoldopam continuous rate infusion in six healthy dogs. *J Vet Pharmacol Ther* 2012; **35**(3): 224–230.

151 Murray C, Markos F, Snow HM, *et al.* Effects of fenoldopam on renal blood flow and its function in a canine model of rhabdomyolysis. *Eur J Anaesthesiol* 2003; **20**(9): 711–718.

152 Segev G, Bruchim Y, Berl N, *et al.* Effects of fenoldopam on kidney function parameters and its therapeutic efficacy in the management of acute kidney injury in dogs with heatstroke. *J Vet Intern Med* 2018; **32**(3): 1109–1115.

153 Simmons JP, Wohl JS, Schwartz DD, *et al.* Diuretic effects of fenoldopam in healthy cats. *J Vet Emerg Crit Care* 2006; **16**(2): 96–103.

154 Buckely GJ, Aktay SA, Rozanski EA. Massive transfusion and surgical management of iatrogenic aortic laceration associated with cystocentesis in a dog. *J Am Vet Med Assoc* 2009; **235**(3): 288–291.

155 Hall J, Hall K, Powell LL, *et al.* Outcome of male cats managed for urethral obstruction with decompressive cystocentesis and urinary catheterization: 47 cats (2009–2012). *J Vet Emerg Crit Care* 2015; **25**(2): 256–262.

156 Reineke E, Cooper ES, Takacs JD, *et al.* Multicenter evaluation of decompressive cystocentesis in the treatment of cats with urethral obstruction. *J Am Vet Med Assoc* 2021; **258**(5): 483–492.

157 Cooper ES, Owens TJ, Chew DJ, *et al.* A protocol for managing urethral obstruction in male cats without urethral catheterization. *J Am Vet Med Assoc* 2010; **237**(11): 1261–1266.

158 Gerken KK, Cooper ES, Butler AL, *et al.* Association of abdominal effusion with a single decompressive cystocentesis prior to catheterization in male cats with urethral obstruction. *J Vet Emerg Crit Care* 2020; **30**(1): 11–17.

159 Pankowski RL, Fubini SL. Urinary bladder rupture in a two-year-old horse: sequel to a surgically repaired neonatal injury. *J Am Vet Med Assoc* 1987; **191**(5): 560–562.

160 Cunha MG, Freitas GC, Carregaro AB, *et al.* Renal and cardiorespiratory effects of treatment with lactated Ringer's solution or physiologic saline (0.9% NaCl) solution in cats with experimentally induced urethral obstruction. *Am J Vet Res* 2010; **71**(7): 840–846.

161 Adams LG. Ureteral disorders. In: Ettinger SJ, Feldman EC, Cote E, eds. *Textbook of Veterinary Internal Medicine*, 8th edn. Philadelphia, PA: WB Saunders, 2017: 1985–1991.

162 Langston C, Eatroff A. Acute kidney injury. In: Little SE, ed. *August's Consultations in Feline Internal Medicine*, Vol. 7. St. Louis, MO: Elsevier, 2016: 483–498.

163 Fischer JR. Acute ureteral obstruction. In: August JR, ed. *Consultations in Feline Internal Medicine*, 5th edn. St. Louis, MO: Elsevier Health Sciences, 2005: 379–386.

164 Fischer J, Lane I, Stokes J. Acute postrenal azotemia: etiology, clinicopathology, and pathophysiology. *Compend Contin Educ Vet* 2009; **31**(11): 520–533.

165 Galluzzi F, De Rensis F, Menozzi A, *et al.* Effect of intraurethral administration of atracurium besylate in male cats with urethral plugs. *J Small Anim Pract* 2012; **53**(7): 411–415.

166 O'Hearn AK, Wright BD. Coccygeal epidural with local anesthetic for catheterization and pain management in the treatment of feline urethral obstruction. *J Vet Emerg Crit Care* 2011; **21**(1): 50–52.

167 Zezza L, Reusch CE, Gerber B. Intravesical application of lidocaine and sodium bicarbonate in the treatment of obstructive idiopathic lower urinary tract disease in cats. *J Vet Intern Med* 2012; **26**(3): 526–531.

168 Francis BJ, Wells RJ, Rao S, *et al.* Retrospective study to characterize postobstructive diuresis in cats with urethral obstruction. *J Feline Med Surg* 2010; **12**(8): 606–608.

169 Saulez MN. Urolithiasis and obstructive disease. In: Smith BP, Van Metre DC, Pusterla N, eds. *Large Animal Internal Medicine*, 6th edn. St. Louis, MO: Elsevier, 2020: 973.

170 Hardy J. Uroabdomen in foals. *Equine Vet Educ* 1998; **10**(1): 21–25.

171 Divers TJ, Dawson-Soto DR, Fulz LE. Urinary system disorders in the foal. In: Smith BP, Van Metre DC, Pusterla N, eds. *Large Animal Internal Medicine*, 6th edn. St. Louis, MO: Elsevier, 2020: 981.

172 Behr MJ, Hackett RP, Bentinck-Smith J, *et al.* Metabolic abnormalities associated with rupture of the urinary bladder in neonatal foals. *J Am Vet Med Assoc* 1981; **178**(3): 255.

173 Chenitz KB, Lane-Fall MG. Decreased urine output and acute kidney injury in the postanesthesia care unit. *Anesthesiol Clin* 2012; **30**(3): 513–526.
174 Groeneveld AB, Navickis RJ, Wilkes MM. Update on the comparative safety of colloids: a systemic review of clinical studies. *Ann Surg* 2011; **253**(3): 470–483.
175 Venkataraman R, Kellum JA. Prevention of acute renal failure. *Chest* 2007; **131**(1): 300–308.
176 Loredo JS, Nelesen R, Ancoli-Israel S, *et al.* Sleep quality and blood pressure dipping in normal adults. *Sleep* 2004; **27**(6): 1097–1103.
177 Schwartz LB, Bissell MG, Murphy M, *et al.* Renal effects of dopamine in vascular surgical patients. *J Vasc Surg* 1988; **8**(4): 367–374.
178 Friedrich JO, Adhikari N, Herridge MS, *et al.* Meta-analysis: low-dose dopamine increases urine output but does not prevent renal dysfunction or death. *Ann Intern Med* 2005; **142**(7): 510–524.
179 Hastie MJ, Shanewise JS. Diuretics. In: Flood P, Rathmell JP, Shafer S, eds. *Pharmacology and Physiology in Anesthetic Practice*, 5th edn. Philadelphia, PA: Wolters Kluwer, 2015: 533–541.
180 Karajala V, Mansour W, Kellum JA. Diuretics in acute kidney injury. *Minerva Anestesiol* 2009; **75**(5): 251–257.

44 Anesthetic Considerations for Renal Replacement Therapy

Rebecca A. Johnson
Department of Surgical Sciences, School of Veterinary Medicine, University of Wisconsin, Madison, Wisconsin, USA

Chapter contents

Introduction, 944
Intracorporeal techniques, 944
Renal transplantation, 944
Peritoneal dialysis, 948
Extracorporeal techniques, 950
Intermittent hemodialysis and continuous renal replacement therapy, 950
References, 952

Introduction

The kidneys are responsible for numerous essential biological functions, such as maintaining acid–base, electrolyte, and endocrine balance, regulating blood pressure, and forming urine by filtering hematologic nitrogenous end-products while retaining solutes, proteins, and blood cells [1]. Acute kidney injury (AKI) and chronic kidney disease (CKD) are common clinical entities that are associated with impaired kidney function (see Chapter 43). Depending on etiology and chronicity, patients may exhibit clinical signs such as vomiting, diarrhea, oral ulceration, anorexia, weight loss, polydipsia, and urine output changes such as polyuria, oliguria, or anuria. Patients also commonly present with electrolyte and acid–base disturbances (e.g., hyperkalemia and metabolic acidosis) and/or volume overload. To relieve these severe clinical signs, stabilize patient condition, improve quality of life, and extend lifespan, renal replacement therapies are utilized, especially if medical therapy has been unsuccessful.

Renal replacement therapies include both intracorporeal (renal transplantation and peritoneal dialysis [PD]) and extracorporeal (intermittent hemodialysis [IHD] and continuous renal replacement therapy [CRRT]) techniques. Although these therapies are associated with significant financial, ethical, and emotional considerations, they have progressed from non-traditional, infrequent clinical entities to more common, progressive therapeutic options for companion animals with renal impairment. In this chapter, first, the unique principles used in the critical anesthetic management of dogs and cats undergoing renal transplantation are discussed, followed by a brief discussion of anesthetic considerations for specific dialysis techniques.

Intracorporeal techniques

Renal transplantation

In the mid-1950s, Guild *et al.* performed the first successful renal transplantation on identical twin humans [2]. Although the first renal transplant in clinical veterinary medicine occurred in 1984, only in the last few decades has renal transplantation gained popularity in clinical veterinary medicine as a therapy for companion animals with CKD [3]. Morbidity and mortality rates associated with renal transplantation differ significantly between dogs and cats. For example, mean survival time for clinical canine patients is variable, reported to be from 18 days [4] up to 8 months [5]. In contrast, 70–93% of cats are discharged after surgery [3], and mean survival times in clinical feline patients are between 360 and 653 days, with 59–79% still alive after 6 months and 32–45% after 3 years [3,6–8]. The exact reasons for lower success rates in dogs compared with cats are not entirely clear. However, strong canine host immune responses require that potent immunosuppressive therapy is administered to prevent rejection, thereby increasing the possibility of adverse events [4,9–11]; thromboembolism, allograft rejection, and respiratory, neurologic, skin, and urinary tract infections are commonly reported [3]. Although thromboembolism is associated with immunosuppression (among other factors) and is reported as a complication in human transplantation, it is infrequently seen in cats [11,12]. Increasing age of both canine and feline patients is associated with decreased survival rates following transplantation [4,8,13], whereas severe preoperative azotemia, hypertension, and increased left ventricular wall thickness are also associated with increased mortality in cats [8]. Thus, although renal transplantation appears to be a promising treatment for CKD in

Veterinary Anesthesia and Analgesia: The Sixth Edition of Lumb and Jones. Edited by Leigh Lamont, Kurt Grimm, Sheilah Robertson, Lydia Love and Carrie Schroeder.
© 2024 John Wiley & Sons, Inc. Published 2024 by John Wiley & Sons, Inc.
Companion website: www.wiley.com/go/lamont/anesthesia

animals, discriminant patient selection and preoperative risk assessment may enhance the survival of kidney transplant recipients. Since the majority of current clinical patients undergoing transplantation are cats, this chapter focuses on feline techniques.

Ethical considerations

Currently, debate exists concerning the ethics surrounding renal transplantation in veterinary medicine (for review, see [14] and [15]). For example, in 2003, the Royal College of Veterinary Surgeons (RCVS) in the United Kingdom approved guidelines for feline renal transplantation based on procedures being done in other countries such as the United States, New Zealand, and Australia [14]. The guidelines were set up using strict standards and included using source animals that were siblings or cohorts screened for compatibility to the recipient. However, in 2013, the procedure was suspended in the UK pending review and in 2016 deliberations were ongoing, as the RCVS began considering feline renal transplantation as a possible "mutilation" procedure in the living source cat making it less "cat-like." In addition, the Royal Society for the Prevention of Cruelty to Animals suggests that renal transplantation is potentially illegal as it causes unnecessary feline suffering, among various other debatable issues [14]. The term "donor cat" is also under debate by the RCVS as the source cat cannot freely make the choice to give up the organ themself [15]. Thus, although renal transplantation in cats appears to be medically feasible and advantageous in some instances as cats may live longer following renal transplantation when compared with cats medically managed for CKD [8], many perspectives and much debate still exist regarding its place in veterinary medicine.

Preoperative considerations

Many patients with CKD that present for renal transplantation will have acid–base and electrolyte abnormalities. A complete blood count and serum biochemistry should be performed as the magnitude of the elevations in blood urea nitrogen (BUN) and creatinine levels is associated with increased mortality in cats [8], but not in dogs [4]. In addition, urinalysis and urine culture, blood typing, thoracic and abdominal radiographs, cardiac and abdominal ultrasound, and systemic blood pressure measurements should be performed to screen for any pre-existing comorbidities and to ensure compatible blood types. Comorbidities such as hypertension and cardiovascular disease are common and are associated with a higher postoperative mortality in feline patients as previously mentioned [8]. Thus, perioperative treatment of these disorders may reduce complication rates and patients should be medically managed before transplantation.

Preoperative patient preparation includes placement of a double- or triple-lumen central venous catheter for chronic administration of balanced electrolyte solutions to correct electrolyte and acid–base abnormalities, to measure central venous pressure (CVP), and to facilitate blood sampling (Fig. 44.1).

The right jugular is preferred in the event that an esophagostomy tube is required to facilitate nutritional support following surgery. Immunosuppressive and antihypertensive therapy may also be instituted, and hemo- or peritoneal dialysis may be performed prior to transplantation, particulary in anuric, profoundly azotemic, and edematous cats (see below) [3]. Depending on patient needs, red blood cell transfusion, whole blood transfusion, or erythropoietin, replacement therapy may also be administered to enhance oxygen-carrying capacity if the patient is severely anemic (PCV < 20%). However, the transfusion trigger point for

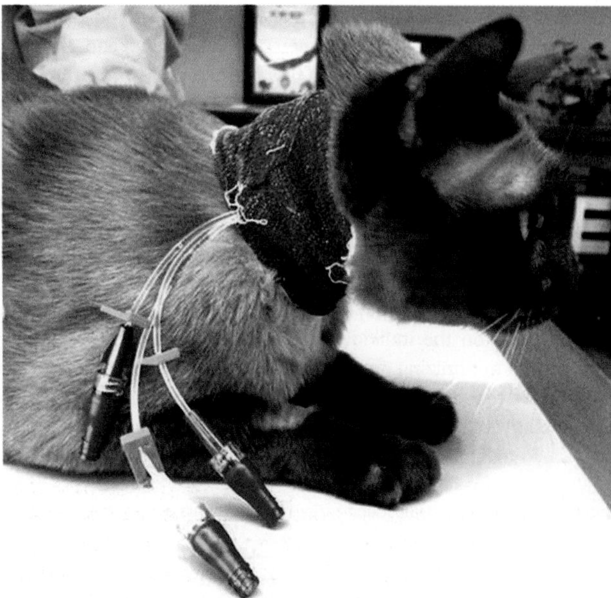

Figure 44.1 An example of a triple-lumen intravenous catheter inserted in the right jugular vein of a cat. These catheters may be placed preoperatively under sedation using the Seldinger technique and are subsequently used for hemodialysis techniques, fluid therapy, blood administration, and blood sampling perioperatively. Source: Dr. Rebecca Johnson, with permission.

patients with CKD is often lower than for healthier patients owing to compensatory mechanisms associated with chronic disease; therefore, patients should be assessed on an individual basis. The use of autogenous mesenchymal stem cells to improve long-term outcomes by reducing the possibility of acute rejection and/or systemic infection is currently under investigation [3]. Although stem cell work is promising in humans [16] and *in vitro* feline studies are favorable [17], additional *in vivo* feline investigations are needed, especially since complications associated with the addition of a surgical harvesting procedure in an already compromised cat may preclude its use [3].

Donor animals are routinely screened with a serum chemistry, complete blood count, blood typing, urinalysis and culture, and infectious disease testing (toxoplasmosis, feline leukemia virus, and feline immunodeficiency virus in cats; heartworm in dogs). Computed tomography to characterize renal tissue and vasculature is frequently performed. Approximately 84% of feline donors had no associated long-term effects associated with nephrectomy, whereas 7% developed renal insufficiency or died of urinary tract disease [18].

Anesthetic management

The ultimate goal of the anesthetic period is to provide acceptable anesthesia, analgesia, and muscle relaxation to patients without compromising existing renal function or function of the new kidney. Hence, the anesthetic plan includes agents that have minimal cardiovascular depression, are not directly nephrotoxic, and minimally rely on the kidneys for their excretion. In addition, prudent anesthetic techniques required for any patient anesthetized for prolonged periods such as adequate padding, generous and repeated application of ocular lubricant, consistent core body temperature monitoring, and active warming with a forced-air warmer to reduce hypothermia should be employed for both the donor and the recipient. All attempts to reduce anesthetic time should be made, and good communication between the anesthetic and surgical teams is imperative throughout the perioperative procedures as prolonged anesthetic times (median = 300 min) are associated with reduced overall survival rates in cats [13].

Kidney donor management

Currently, live kidney donors are already owned or are adopted by the recipient's owner prior to any surgical procedure. They are young, healthy animals with normal cardiovascular and renal function; anesthetic procedures for kidney removal are generally routine and are chosen based on the individual donor's disposition and anesthetic needs while minimizing any cardiovascular depression (Table 44.1). Specific to the donor, acepromazine is frequently used pre- or intraoperatively to promote renal vasculature dilation through α_1-adrenergic receptor blockade [19,20]; any associated hypotension must be quickly addressed to ensure that kidney perfusion pressure is supported. Vasoconstrictive agents such as α_2-adrenergic receptor agonists are avoided if possible to reduce potential increases in vascular resistance [21–26]. Appropriate analgesic techniques are used as required; epidurals with preservative-free morphine, with or without a local anesthetic such as bupivacaine or ropivacaine, and other systemic μ-opioid receptor agonists are commonly used as adjunctive analgesic agents. Other agents to improve renal perfusion such as mannitol can also be administered. Anesthetic monitoring is routine but focuses on the cardiovascular system; pulse oximetry, electrocardiography, direct (dorsal pedal, coccygeal, or femoral arterial catheter) or indirect (oscillometric or Doppler ultrasonic) arterial blood pressure, end-tidal carbon dioxide/anesthetic gases, and core body temperature are monitored continuously. Blood gas analyses, including electrolytes, and packed cell volumes are performed perioperatively.

Table 44.1 Suggested anesthetic and analgesic agents for renal replacement therapy patients.

Agent			Dose/Route
Preanesthetic sedatives/analgesics			
	Benzodiazepines	Midazolam	0.05–0.2 mg/kg IV, IM
		Diazepam	0.05–0.2 mg/kg IV
	Opioids	Fentanyl	1.0–5.0 μg/kg IV
		Hydromorphone	0.05–0.1 mg/kg IV, IM
		Methadone	0.2–0.5 mg/kg IV, IM
Induction agents			
		Propofol	1.0–6.0 mg/kg IV to effect
		Alfaxalone	0.5–2.0 mg/kg IV to effect
Maintenance agents			
	Inhalants	Desflurane	Minimal concentrations to effect
		Isoflurane	
		Sevoflurane	
	Opioids	Fentanyl	2–20 μg/kg/h IV
Postoperative analgesics			
	Opioids	Fentanyl	1–2 μg/kg/h IV with careful monitoring
		Buprenorphine	20–30 μg/kg IV, TM
		Methadone	0.2–0.5 mg/kg IV, IM

IV, intravenous; IM, intramuscular; TM, transmucosal.

Kidney recipient management

Kidney recipient anesthesia is handled similarly to that for other patients with CKD (see Chapter 43). However, recipients present unique challenges as they accept a new kidney (graft) that has been removed from a donor and stored in hypoxic conditions for minutes to hours (Fig. 44.2A) (for microsurgical and storage techniques, see [3,4,27–30]). Although few currently used anesthetic agents are directly nephrotoxic, and no specific anesthetic agents are associated with changes to short-term or overall survival rates [13], many anesthetics alter renal function through decreases in cardiac output, systemic vascular resistance and blood pressure, neuroendocrine status, and renal blood flow (RBF), which will subsequently affect the glomerular filtration rate (GFR). The stress response to surgery can release aldosterone, vasopressin, renin, and endogenous catecholamines, which can increase renal vascular resistance and subsequently reduce GFR [31–33]. Hence, the objectives of the anesthetic period include reducing patient stress and maintaining systemic blood pressure (and, therefore, GFR) to the greatest extent possible via the use of anesthetic agents with minimal cardiovascular depression.

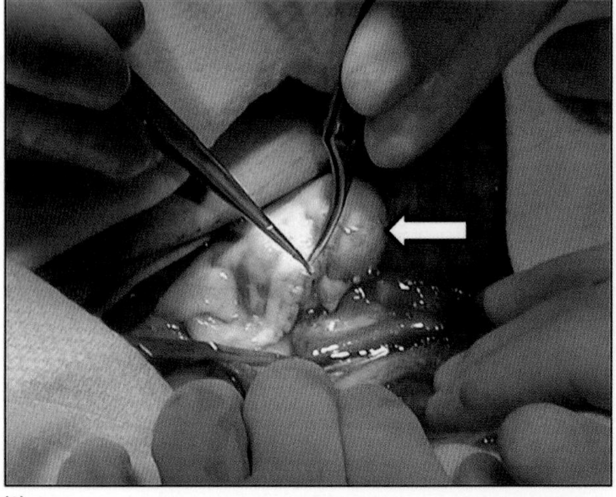
(A)

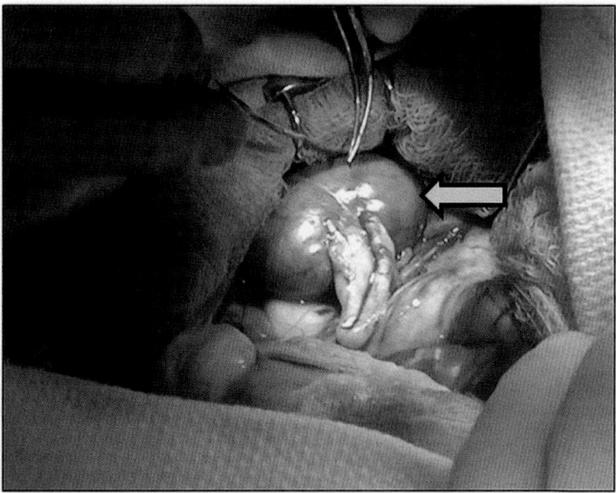
(B)

Figure 44.2 Intraoperative renal transplantation. **A.** Donor kidney (white arrow) placed in the abdomen of the recipient following extracorporeal storage. Note the pale color of the stored kidney as the anastomoses are not yet completed in this photograph. **B.** Donor kidney (gray arrow) following renal artery and vein anastomoses and application of chlorpromazine to the renal artery. Note the pink (perfused) color of the kidney compared with the kidney in **A.** Source: Dr. Jon McAnulty, Department of Surgical Sciences, School of Veterinary Medicine, University of Wisconsin, Madison, WI, USA, with permission.

Similar to the kidney donor, anesthetic and analgesic agents must be chosen according to the individual patient's physiologic status and signalment as each transplant patient is unique; there is no universal protocol that can be used for every patient. Preoperative medication using a combination of the μ-opioid receptor agonist, fentanyl, and a benzodiazepine is common since neither fentanyl nor the benzodiazepine class of drugs substantially affects cardiovascular function at clinically acceptable doses (Table 44.1) [34–37]. For example, fentanyl or a fentanyl analog (including sufentanil, alfentanil, and remifentanil) and midazolam are commonly used intravenously to facilitate anesthetic induction, provide analgesia, and reduce the stress response to surgery. Fentanyl is also advantageous since it has a relatively short duration of action, which facilitates rapid adjustments, does not release histamine, and is minimally excreted (< 10%) unchanged by the kidneys [38–40]. Although other opioids, such as hydromorphone, may be acceptable for use as analgesics, systemic morphine is not recommended. Systemic morphine administration increases plasma histamine levels, which can be associated with systemic hypotension [38]. In addition, morphine-6-glucuronide is an active metabolic product of morphine in dogs and humans, and delayed elimination of this metabolite in patients with renal insufficiency may prolong drug effects [41–45]. Although cats have low levels of glucuronyl transferase and morphine undergoes a different type of conjugation reaction in this species, the pharmacokinetics of morphine are somewhat similar to those of dogs and humans, but clearance rates may be slightly slower [46–48]. Hence, systemic morphine administration in feline kidney recipients is not routinely recommended when other opioids are available. Similarly, α_2-adrenergic receptor agonists, such as dexmedetomidine, should be avoided as they reduce cardiac output with increases in systemic vascular resistance [21–26]. Phenothiazines are also not recommended as a routine premedication in recipients since administration can reduce systemic vascular resistance and potentially decrease arterial blood pressure in dogs and cats via peripheral α-adrenergic receptor blockade [20,49,50].

Anesthetic induction can be accomplished with slow administration of small doses of propofol as it is rapidly metabolized by both hepatic and extra-hepatic means and RBF and GFR are minimally affected (Table 44.1) [51,52]. Although the effects of alfaxalone on RBF and GFR are not specifically reported in cats, small boluses of alfaxalone may also be used since postinduction cardiovascular effects appear similar to those of propofol (for review, see [53]). Although significantly metabolized in the liver, ketamine is usually avoided since its active metabolite, norketamine, is excreted unchanged by the kidney [54] and may contribute to prolonged drug effects in animals with decreased renal function. If ketamine is required as a premedication or induction agent (for example, due to animal behavior or lack of an alternative), doses should be reduced as much as possible by combination with appropriate coinduction agents. Etomidate may be used but is not commonly recommended since, although it has minimal cardiovascular effects, it induces transient adrenal suppression, which has been associated with increased postoperative mortality in critically ill humans [55,56]. Etomidate's effect on postoperative mortality in compromised cats is unknown.

During anesthetic maintenance (Table 44.1), most inhalant anesthetics reduce GFR (isoflurane, sevoflurane, and desflurane), and attempts to reduce levels and maintain systemic blood pressure should be made [52,57]. Therefore, it is common to use a constant rate infusion of fentanyl or another fentanyl analog throughout the surgical procedure to reduce inhalant levels and enhance antinociception [58–60]. In addition, an epidural containing preservative-free morphine may be used; addition of local anesthetics to the epidural is usually avoided to reduce any further hypotension from profound decreases in vascular resistance due to sympathetic nervous system blockade. Following such epidural techniques, cats should be closely monitored for associated hypotension. Although there have been concerns that sevoflurane may not be safe for use in AKI or CKD due to the production of potentially nephrotoxic compound A (in rodents) and inorganic fluoride, no adverse effects have been shown in clinical patients and sevoflurane can be used in these patients, as can isoflurane and desflurane [57,61–63].

Intraoperative anesthetic monitoring is essential for the risk management of renal transplant patients. For example, intraoperative hypoxemia is associated with reduced overall survival rates [13]. Thus, monitoring includes pulse oximetry, capnometry, inhalant agent levels, electrocardiography, and core body temperature. In addition, intraoperative hemodynamic monitoring and management are imperative to ensure reasonable organ perfusion pressure, yet not subject the patient to fluid overload. Although CVP does not always correlate well with the patient's overall fluid status, acute CVP changes may indicate impending fluid overload. However, this relationship is still debated [64]. Pulse pressure variation or pleth variability index may be better indices of fluid status in the mechanically ventilated patient, although their usefulness in cats have not been fully investigated [65]. Invasive blood pressure should be closely monitored since patients may experience normo-, hypo-, or hypertension throughout the procedure and into the postoperative period. An arterial catheter should be placed in the dorsal pedal or femoral artery; however, the descending aorta or its major branches may be occluded during renal artery anastomosis, and the signal will be lost during this period. The coccygeal artery may be used but can be difficult to keep clean postoperatively, which may negate its use in an immunosuppressed patient. Care in handling these catheters is essential as patients may be purposely heparinized and excessive bleeding at the puncture site may occur. Indirect blood pressure measurement using an ultrasonic Doppler flow detector or oscillometric technique applied to the front limb should be performed concurrently with invasive monitoring as these indirect techniques can be used during aortic occlusion and/or if an artery cannot be catheterized; however, they can be less accurate depending on circumstances [66–70].

Intravenous fluid therapy in human transplant surgeries has recently been addressed [71]. Large crystalloid volumes are not recommended, but accelerated fluid administration during the initial period of graft ischemia may improve subsequent kidney function. Thus, feline fluid rates of 3–5 mL/kg/h based on the individual patient's needs and comorbidities (e.g., heart disease) with small, accelerated (3–5 mL/kg) fluid boluses over approximately 15 min as needed during ischemia are recommended. These guidelines also suggest that a balanced electrolyte solution should be used; 0.9% sodium chloride is not recommended due to extracellular shifts in serum potassium, increases in serum chloride, and a decrease in pH (hyperchloremic acidosis) [71–74]. In fact, hyperkalemia does not worsen with balanced solutions, and 0.9% sodium chloride can actually result in significant metabolic disorders [71–74]. Synthetic colloids such as hydroxyethyl starches should not be used due to potential adverse effects such as coagulopathies, reticuloendothelial system dysfunction, and delayed or impaired renal function [71,75].

If patients are normovolemic during surgery, yet remain hypotensive under general anesthesia, β-adrenergic receptor agonists, such as dobutamine, can be used to increase cardiac output. The use of dopamine remains controversial because of species differences in receptor pharmacology and potential increases in systemic vascular resistance with higher doses [45]. If the patient cannot tolerate further fluid loading, titrated vasopressors, such as norepinephrine, may be considered to treat hypotension, despite the risk of renal vasoconstriction. In humans, norepinephrine use does not have a negative effect on recipient graft function since the harmful effects of systemic hypotension likely outweigh the potential renal vasoconstriction caused by norepinephrine [76,77]. However, this has yet to be tested in clinical veterinary transplant patients.

During surgery, other pharmaceutical agents may be administered to aid in graft survival. For example, mannitol (0.25–1.0 g/kg) may be administered intravenously as the vascular anastomosis is nearly completed to increase renal perfusion pressure, reduce ischemia–reperfusion injury, and diminish the delay in graft function [4,45,78]. Heparin may be administered once adequate hemostasis is maintained since patients are often prothrombotic due to hypercoagulability and hypofibrinolysis [12,79]. If the newly anastomosed renal artery exhibits profound vasoconstriction, chlorpromazine may be used topically as a peripheral α-adrenergic receptor antagonist and direct vascular smooth muscle relaxant to initiate vasodilation of the artery and likely enhance RBF (Fig. 44.2B) [80]. Prior to the end of the surgical procedure in cats, the fentanyl infusion may be discontinued and buprenorphine administered intravenously for postoperative analgesia (Table 44.1) as reversal of pure μ-opioid receptor agonists increases 30-day survival rates [13]. Although buprenorphine is classified as a partial opioid receptor agonist, partial receptor activation (versus antagonism) may reduce any cardiorespiratory depression associated with full μ-opioid receptor agonists, yet still provide analgesia. Alternatively, fentanyl (or fentanyl analog) infusions may be carefully titrated in cats, and also in dogs, at lower dosages for postoperative analgesia. However, intensive postoperative cardiovascular monitoring is recommended if these agents are used. Non-steroidal anti-inflammatory agents (NSAIDs) are not recommended owing to their potential nephrotoxic, hepatotoxic, and gastrointestinal effects [81]. Appropriately placed local or regional anesthetic techniques in the body wall using liposomal bupivacaine (≤ 5.3 mg/kg) or bupivacaine solution (up to 1–2 mg/kg) may also be advantageous as part of multimodal analgesia therapy, although they have not been specifically studied in renal transplant patients.

Surgical recovery and complications

The recovery period requires intensive monitoring for associated complications [3]. Patient stress should be minimized and the patient kept warm as hypothermia is common in the postoperative period. Electrolytes and packed call volume should be monitored and imbalances corrected with fluid therapy and/or blood products as needed. Patients should undergo frequent pain scoring with validated systems [82], and multimodal analgesic techniques used to minimize side effects associated with any one analgesic agent. Nutritional support is imperative; esophagostomy tubes can be placed if required.

Hypertension can be present throughout the procedure or can occur following vascular clamp removal from the new kidney. It may persist or even worsen postoperatively [3,4,7,8,28,83,84]. The pathogenesis of postoperative hypertension is likely multifactorial, possibly due to a combination of primary renal disease and calcineurin inhibitors (such as the immunosuppressive agent cyclosporine), but it does not appear to be related to increased renin or angiotensin II levels after kidney reperfusion [4,7,8,83–86]. Although intraoperative hypertension can be quickly managed with increasing inhalant concentrations and/or nitroprusside infusions, postoperative management is usually accomplished with the continued administration of antihypertensive agents such as hydralazine, acepromazine, or amlodipine. Therefore, frequent or continuous arterial blood pressure monitoring is essential in the postoperative period, ideally with an arterial line. Indirect blood pressures using an ultrasonic Doppler flow detector may also be used if arterial catheterization is not possible or cannot be maintained [66–70]. Cats that have close monitoring and management of postoperative blood pressure have reduced rates of postoperative neurologic disease, including seizures, stupor, ataxia, and central blindness [87], although no link was found in one study between postoperative seizures and hypertension [8]. However, it is possible that postoperative ischemic events may be likely in postoperative hypertensive cats that lead to overt neurologic signs.

Other postoperative complications can include rejection, infection, retroperitoneal fibrosis, thromboembolic disease (dogs), congestive heart failure, delayed graft function, neurologic disease, uroabdomen, gingival hyperplasia associated with cyclosporine, and intestinal intussusception [3,4,8]. In some cases, postoperative hemodialysis can be used to manage delayed graft function, acute rejection, pyelonephritis, and other complications until the problem is resolved [88]. Although these significant complications remain, surgical and anesthetic techniques are consistently improving as additional information regarding preoperative patient stabilization and the mechanisms underlying such complications becomes available.

Peritoneal dialysis

Peritoneal dialysis (PD) is an alternative renal replacement therapy used to temporarily remove solutes and excess fluid and to control electrolyte and acid–base balance until renal function recovers sufficiently, especially in AKI. Comprehensive reviews of the techniques and equipment have been published [89–91]. In PD, the exchange of solutes and fluid occurs between two compartments: the peritoneal capillary blood and the dialysate placed in the peritoneal cavity. Fluid and solutes are transported via diffusion and osmosis/ultrafiltration, with a minor role played by convection (Fig. 44.3) [92]. More specifically, solutes are removed as they diffuse across the semipermeable peritoneal membranes, the rate being determined by the membrane permeability of the molecules (size and charge), available surface area, and concentration gradient. Fluids are removed by osmosis/ultrafiltration as water moves from areas with low osmolar concentrations into the dialysate, which has high osmolality (e.g., dextrose) or by using pressure gradients. Convection of solutes also occurs as they are trapped in the flow of water, although this process is more important in hemodialysis (see the section titled "Extracorporeal techniques" later in text) than in PD [92]. Overall transport across the peritoneal membrane is commonly explained by the three-pore theory, where large pores (100–200 Å in diameter) allow the transport of macromolecules such as albumin, small pores (20–25 Å) allow low-molecular-weight substances such as urea, creatinine, and glucose to pass, and ultrasmall pores (4–6 Å) transport only water [93].

Case selection

Typically, PD is used for veterinary patients with AKI associated with oliguria or anuria refractory to fluid therapy and in patients with severe acute uremia with BUN > 100 mg/dL or creatinine

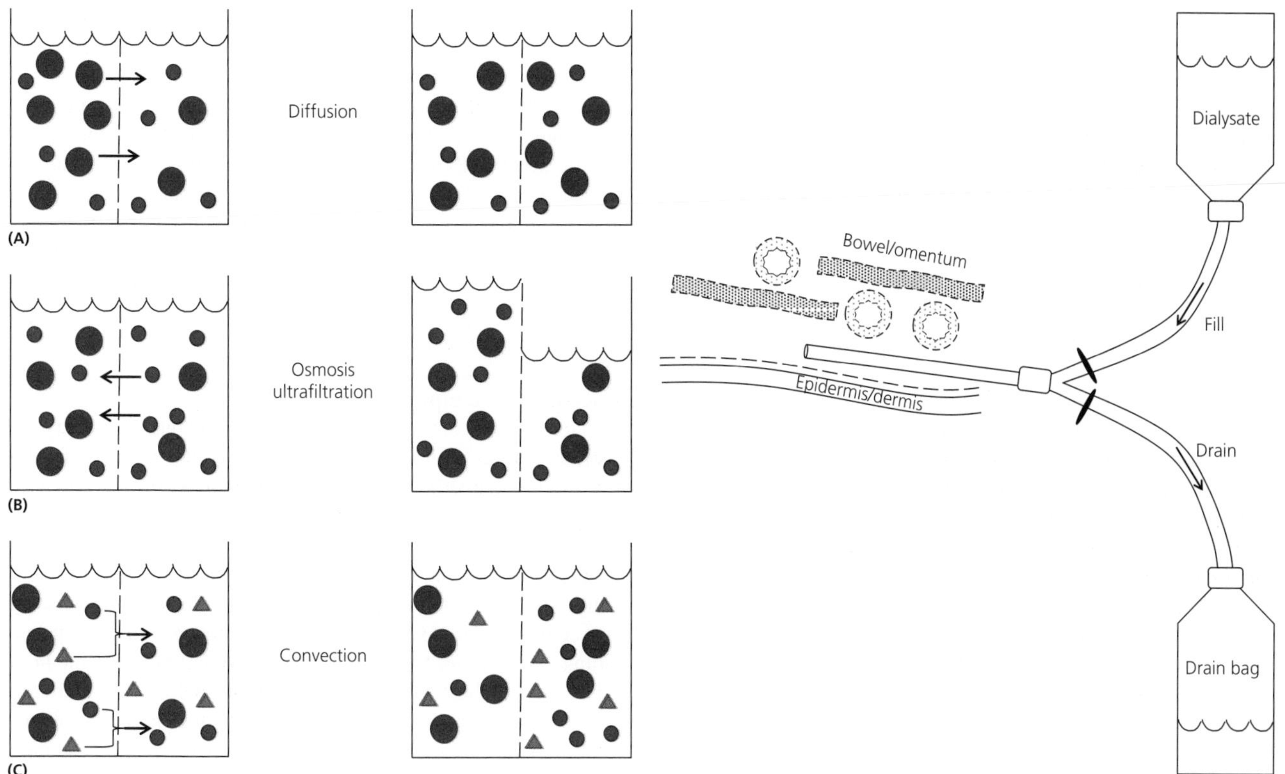

Figure 44.3 Schematic representation of processes involved in dialysis techniques. **A.** *Diffusion.* Diffusion occurs when solutes travel across a semipermeable membrane based on their concentration gradient; solutes move from a higher concentration to areas with lower concentrations. **B.** *Osmosis/ultrafiltration.* Osmosis is the net movement of water (solvent) across a semipermeable membrane into a region of higher solute concentration in an attempt to equalize the relative solute concentration. With ultrafiltration, hydrostatic pressure is used to force solvent across the membrane. **C.** *Convection.* Convection occurs as the solute travels within the mass movement of the solvent.

Figure 44.4 Drain-and-fill technique for peritoneal dialysis. The peritoneal cavity is initially infused by gravity or pump with fresh dialysate through a preplaced peritoneal catheter. During the dwell time, neither the fresh dialysate bag nor the drain bag is opened, and fluids and solutes are exchanged from the blood within the peritoneal capillaries into the dialysate across the semipermeable peritoneal membrane (dashed lines). The dialysate is then drained from within the peritoneal cavity and discarded.

> 10 mg/dL [91,94]. PD is also used for the treatment of exposure to diffusible toxins such as ethylene glycol and barbiturates, severe metabolic abnormalities (e.g., hypercalcemia and hyperkalemia), and extreme core body temperature derangements [91,93]. Although PD is less efficient than hemodialysis in reducing uremia [93], several case reports have shown the efficacy of PD in veterinary patients [95–98]. The advantages include minimal technical skill required, no requirement for vascular access, good cardiovascular tolerance, lack of expensive extracorporeal equipment, and decreased risk of bleeding [91,99]. However, it is not recommended for patients with severe coagulopathy, peritoneal adhesions, peritonitis, diaphragmatic or abdominal hernias, or severe hypoalbuminemia [89,91].

Procedures and equipment

PD is accomplished through a fill-and-drain system using an indwelling peritoneal catheter (Fig. 44.4). The catheter and its placement are absolutely critical for successful PD. The catheter should allow sufficient inflow and outflow volumes, be biocompatible, resist infection, and reduce leakage [91,93]. Catheters come in various brands and types and can be aseptically placed percutaneously using the Seldinger technique, through a mini-surgical approach, or by direct visualization through a laparotomy or laparoscopy [89–93]. When using the percutaneous or mini-surgical approach, the patient should be clipped and aseptically prepared; sedation and a local anesthetic block of the skin ± peritoneum is required (Table 44.1). Commonly, a μ-opioid receptor agonist such as fentanyl, with or without a benzodiazepine such as midazolam, administered intravenously is adequate to complete the procedure. Intravenous buprenorphine, butorphanol, or hydromorphone may alternatively be used. Lidocaine infiltration around the tube insertion site is recommended. If surgical catheter implantation is required, animals can be managed similarly to other AKI cases, taking care to maintain blood pressure without further fluid overloading of the patient.

Following catheter placement, a variety of dialysates containing glucose as an osmotic agent can be used for the exchange procedures, each with their own advantages and disadvantages (for reviews, see [89–93]). The goal is not to normalize the azotemia immediately but gradually to correct the patient's hemodynamic status and acid–base and electrolyte derangements while reducing BUN to 60–100 mg/dL and creatinine to 4.0–6.0 mg/dL over 24–48 h [94]. First, a small amount of fresh dialysate is initially directed into the drainage bag, and the peritoneal cavity is drained so that any contaminants introduced during the catheterization procedure are flushed into the drainage bag and not the peritoneal cavity.

Warmed (38–39 °C) dialysate solution is placed in the peritoneal cavity by gravity or infusion pump over 5–10 min, where it remains for approximately 30–45 min (the "dwell time"). Following the exchange of fluid and solutes across the membrane, the dialysis fluid is removed over 15 min and discarded. This is repeated hourly until the patient stabilizes [89]. Initial infusion volumes are small (10–20 mL/kg) but may be increased after 24 h to 30–40 mL/kg. Once the goals have been met, patients are frequently changed to chronic dialysis protocols where the dialysate remains in the peritoneal cavity for longer periods and three to four exchanges per day are performed [91,93]. Patients should be continuously monitored for acute blood volume and electrolyte changes. Catheter outflow obstructions are common and body weight, systemic arterial blood pressure, urine output, and pulmonary status are monitored extremely closely. Other complications also occur but are usually manageable, and include dialysate retention, subcutaneous sequestration of dialysate, hypoalbuminemia, peritonitis, and pleural effusion (for reviews, see [89–91]).

In summary, PD is an effective tool in managing AKI or dialysable toxin exposure and may even be used in cases where hemodialysis and/or transplantation are not feasible. The PD procedures frequently require sedation, and/or general anesthesia and patients should be treated similarly to others with renal impairment.

Extracorporeal techniques

Intermittent hemodialysis and continuous renal replacement therapy

The first attempt at hemodialysis was performed in 1914 by Abel *et al.*, who removed blood from animals, passed it through a device with semipermeable membranes, and then placed it back into the animal [100]. They termed this process "vividiffusion," which has become the fundamental process upon which current hemodialysis techniques are based. Both intermittent hemodialysis (IHD) and continuous renal replacement therapy (CRRT) use hollow-fiber semipermeable membranes. Historically, IHD was used to quickly reduce small solutes (such as uremic toxins), whereas CRRT was mainly used over a longer period of time and was particularly applied to patients with hemodynamic instability (for review, see [101]). Currently, a variety of dialyzer options are available, and overlap exists between them; slower treatments can now be attained on IHD machines and CRRT equipment can be used for intermittent techniques as well.

Although four mechanisms are used to remove solutes (diffusion, convection, adsorption, and separation), IHD mainly uses the principle of diffusion to normalize acid–base and electrolyte abnormalities and to remove uremic toxins from the blood through a semipermeable membrane, thus improving clinical status. The solute concentration gradient, molecular weight, and membrane permeability all affect the rate of transfer across the dialysis membrane [102]. Since the molecular size of the solute is the main determinant of its ability to be removed by dialysis, conventional dialyzers are most effective at removing low-molecular-weight substances (< 500 Da) such as urea, creatinine, and electrolytes. However, they can remove solutes up to 1000 Da, while high-flux dialyzers can remove solutes up to 11,000 Da [103]. CRRT uses convection or combinations of diffusion/convection, and to a lesser extent, adsorption, to remove solutes. Convection (also called "solvent drag"), using a pressure gradient, physically moves water and solutes across a membrane, which allows removal of larger solvents (up to 40,000 Da) compared to diffusion alone.

In veterinary medicine, extracorporeal therapy is primary used in AKI where renal function is expected to return quickly or as indefinite renal replacement therapy during CKD [88,104,105]. Patients for extracorporeal therapy commonly present with hypervolemia, refractory hyperkalemia with acidemia, and symptomatic uremia (BUN > 80–120 mg/dL, creatinine > 6–8 mg/dL) refractory to medical treatment [101]. IHD can also be performed prior to renal transplantation to stabilize a high-risk patient further [102,106–108]. Modified current human dialysis techniques have been used in many diverse animal species, including tortoises, rabbits, sheep, and horses [109], but it is only routinely used clinically in cats and dogs.

Procedures and equipment

A reliable, double- or triple-lumen intravenous jugular catheter (preferably a dialysis catheter) is imperative for the success of IHD (Fig. 44.1). These catheters can be temporary or permanent and have been described in detail elsewhere [101,110]. The right jugular is preferred due to its straight path to the cranial vena cava, right atrium, and caudal vena cava; the catheter tip should be located in the right atrium [101]. Temporary (noncuffed, non-tunneled) catheters are most commonly used for IHD and are routinely placed employing a Seldinger or modified Seldinger technique using sedation (Table 44.1) and a local anesthetic block of the catheter site. Ultrasound guidance or a surgical approach may be required in patients with edema, thrombosis, or changes in volume status. Permanent catheters are often cuffed, with a portion located subcutaneously. Insertion often requires a short period of general anesthesia and patients are treated similarly to others with AKI or CKD (Table 44.1).

The dialyzer (i.e., artificial kidney) is a small, disposable, sealed compartment containing thousands of hollow straws (called the "hollow-fiber design") (Fig. 44.5A) [102]. The blood flows within the straws and the dialysate flows in a concurrent or countercurrent direction around the straws. The membranes are semipermeable, allowing transfer of fluid and solutes by diffusion and convection [102]. There are many types of dialyzer units, differing in chamber, tubing, and pore size. The selection of the hemodialyzer is based on the amount of extracorporeal blood volume and also on its diffusive, connective, and biocompatibility features (Fig. 44.5B) [88]. In some IHD machines, the extracorporeal circuit holds less blood volume than in some CRRT machines [101] and may be advantageous in smaller patients. CRRT machines usually use prepackaged dialysate and replacement fluid, allowing them to be more portable but more expensive as well [101].

Anticoagulation is an essential part of extracorporeal therapy. It is accomplished either by delivery of unfractionated heparin into the extracorporeal circuit with an integrated syringe pump or by adding sodium citrate to the circuit, thereby decreasing the ionized calcium to < 0.4 mmol/L [101]. In the latter, patient hypocalcemia is avoided by administering calcium citrate or gluconate at the return/venous catheter site [101].

Hemodialysis machines (Fig. 44.6) come in several brands, are fairly expensive, and have been reviewed elsewhere [111]. The machine allows manipulations of blood flow rate, dialysate flow rate, direction of blood flow and dialysate flow, dialysate composition, treatment length, sodium profiling to regulate plasma osmolality, anticoagulant administration rate, returning blood temperature, and fluid removal from the blood [102]. Although these machines can remove wastes extremely efficiently and fairly quickly, as previously mentioned, the goal is not to decrease BUN and creatinine rapidly but to return the patient's homeostasis

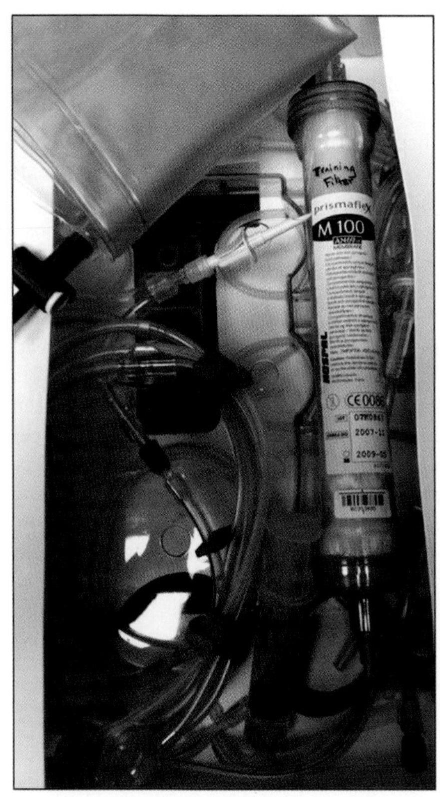

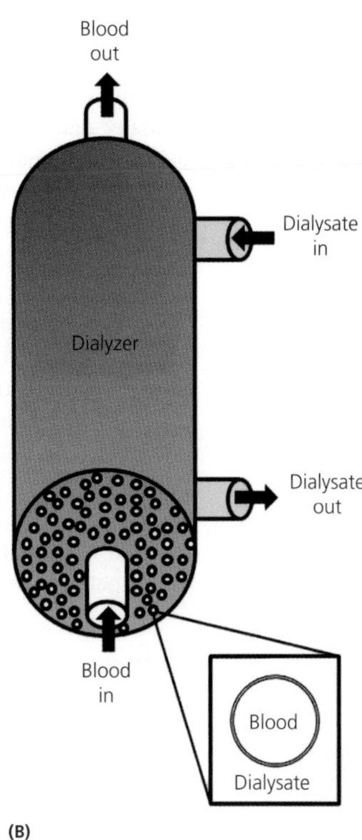

(A) (B)

Figure 44.5 The hemodialyzer. **A.** An example of a currently used hemodialyzer set (Prismaflex® System Hemofilter Set, Gambro, Lakewood, CO, USA). Sets are sterile and prepackaged with all the necessary filtration and tubing required by the hemodialysis machine. Multiple types are commercially available that can provide diffusion, convection and adsorption, depending on the dialysis prescription. Source: Dr. Rebecca Johnson, with permission. **B.** Schematic representation of the "hollow-fiber" design within the hemodialyzer. It consists of numerous straws for blood transport separated from the dialysate by a semipermeable membrane through which exchange of solutes and water occurs. Dialyzed blood is then returned to the patient through a centrally placed intravenous catheter.

gradually over multiple sessions. Sessions are usually planned at two to three times per week and are 1–6 h in length, but can be longer depending on patient need.

Patient monitoring

The ultimate goal for extracorporeal therapy is to either significantly improve uremic states in AKI or to prolong patient survival and improve patient stability in CKD, since, in most cases, renal function does not recover without renal transplantation. Individualized, intensive patient monitoring is imperative since complications frequently occur. Coagulation testing, complete blood counts, and serum chemistries, including hematocrit and ionized calcium levels, should be performed. Critical parameters, including blood pressure measurements, should be obtained prior to, throughout, and following therapy. Pre-existing hypotension should be corrected prior to dialysis, especially in patients where the extracorporeal circuit volume is greater than 20% of the patient's blood volume. During treatment, patients may decompensate quickly, potentially resulting in cardiac arrhythmias, hypotension, and hypoxemia, among others, especially within the first 15 min of dialysis. Following therapy, dialysis disequilibrium syndrome (and corresponding neurologic dysfunction from cerebral edema) and hemorrhage associated with anticoagulation are common issues potentially leading to mortality. Although prolonged complications are infrequently fatal, they do occur and consist of hypotension, hypovolemia, venous thrombosis, pulmonary thromboembolism, pulmonary edema, pleural effusion, anemia, thrombocytopenia, leukopenia, nausea, vomiting, and inappetence [88,106,112–114]. Despite complications with the technique, extracorporeal therapies appear to be a viable treatment modality to improve outcomes in dogs and cats that do not respond adequately to medical management of their renal impairment.

Pharmacologic agent clearance in dialysis

One goal of renal replacement therapy is to enhance the clearance of potential endogenous or exogenous toxins within the blood. However, plasma levels of drugs being administered to the patient can also be affected by these therapies and can make dosing protocols challenging. Although the type of dialysis technique chosen affects the extent of drug removal from the blood, other factors, such as membrane, solute, and patient characteristics, also affect drug clearance [115].

Membrane properties

The filter age, material, surface area, and pore size influence drug filtration, with higher permeability filters and filters with larger surface areas allowing for more drug clearance in dialysis. The effects are more pronounced for intermediate molecular weight drugs [116]. In addition, the choice of dialysis technique will affect the amount of drug removal. The ultrafiltration rate, dialysis rate, blood flow rate, and, for convective processes, the selection of pre- versus postdialyzer replacement fluids can also change drug clearance rates based on the protocol chosen for a specific patient [117].

Drug characteristics

The solubility, volume of distribution, molecular weight, protein binding, pK_a, and degree of renal and extrarenal elimination of the specific drug will affect its clearance rate [117]. For example, drugs with a large volume of distribution usually have a high affinity for tissues with a smaller proportion found in the intravascular space. The lower blood concentration results in a smaller concentration gradient to drive clearance by dialysis. In contrast, drugs with smaller volumes of distribution are more likely to remain intravascular and be quickly cleared by dialysis techniques [118,119].

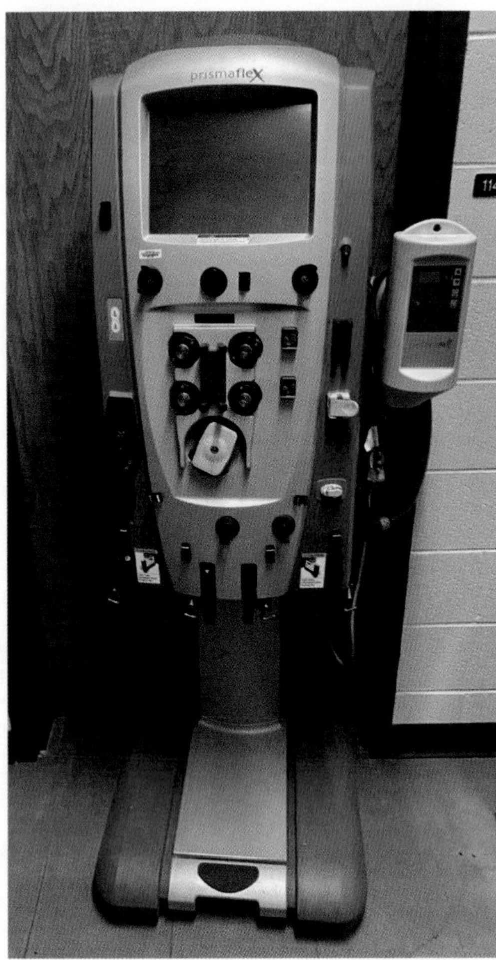

Figure 44.6 The hemodialysis machine. This is an example of a hemodialysis machine (Prismaflex® System, Gambro, Lakewood, CO, USA) that can accommodate the hemodialysis equipment described in Fig. 44.5. The machine should be able to deliver a wide range of extracorporeal blood purification therapies that can be individualized to each patient's needs and should be compatible with a range of hemofiltration sets supplied by the specific company. Source: Dr. Rebecca Johnson, with permission.

Highly protein-bound drugs are less likely to be removed by dialysis than unbound drugs since bound drugs cannot cross dialysis membranes as easily as free drugs [119]. An important caveat is that disease states such as uremia, hypoalbuminemia, and nephrotic syndrome are associated with reduced protein binding of drugs, potentially allowing for more to be cleared by dialysis [120]. In addition, according to the Gibbs–Donnan effect, anionic proteins within the blood decrease the availability of cationic drugs available for clearance [118]. Therefore, if an anesthetic or analgesic drug has a relatively small volume of distribution (e.g., alfentanil versus fentanyl) and/or has relatively low protein binding (e.g., ketamine versus thiopental), its clearance may be hastened during dialysis.

Patient factors

Several patient factors affect drug clearance during dialysis. Patient age, gender, residual renal function, and cardiovascular and liver reserve function may directly or indirectly alter the amount of free drug available for filtration by dialysis [121]. In addition, changes in acid–base status of the animal that are associated with concurrent (renal) disease also affect the ionization of some pharmacologic agents, which can change the volume of drug distribution, protein binding, and renal or hepatic drug clearance [117].

Many data have been collected on drug protocols in patients undergoing renal replacement therapies, especially with regard to antibiotics (for review, see [115]). However, studies on the disposition of anesthetic or analgesic agents, especially in veterinary patients, are lacking. Since most dialysis techniques in veterinary medicine are intermittent in nature (PD or IHD), it may be prudent to administer analgesic agents immediately after the dialysis treatment is completed to ensure that adequate levels are achieved before the next dialysis treatment and to try to extend the time between doses. Until detailed investigations on the pharmacokinetics of specific anesthetic and analgesic agents in veterinary patients undergoing dialysis have been performed, we must extrapolate our drug dosing schedules based on available human drug information, monitor the patient's status closely, and dose according to the individual patient's needs.

References

1 Syme HM, Jepson R. Clinical approach and laboratory evaluation of renal disease. In: Ettinger SJ, Feldman EC, Cote E, eds. *Textbook of Veterinary Internal Medicine*, 8th edn. Philadelphia, PA: Elsevier, 2017: 4603–4649.

2 Merrill JP, Murray JE, Harrison JH, *et al.* Successful homotransplantation of the human kidney between identical twins. *J Am Med Assoc* 1956; **160**(4): 1364–1380.

3 Aronson LR. Update on the current status of kidney transplantation for chronic kidney disease in animals. *Vet Clin North Am Small Anim Pract* 2016; **46**(6): 1193–1218.

4 Hopper K, Mehl ML, Kass PH, *et al.* Outcome after renal transplantation in 26 dogs. *Vet Surg* 2012; **41**(3): 316–327.

5 Mathews KA, Holmberg DL. Kidney transplantation in dogs with naturally occurring end-stage renal disease. *J Am Anim Hosp Assoc* 2000; **36**(6): 475.

6 Mathews KA, Gregory CR. Renal transplants in cats: 66 cases (1987–1996). *J Am Vet Med Assoc* 1997; **211**(11): 1432–1436.

7 Adin CA, Gregory CR, Kyles AE, *et al.* Diagnostic predictors of complications and survival after renal transplantation in cats. *Vet Surg* 2001; **30**(6): 515–521.

8 Schmiedt CW, Holzman G, Schwartz T, *et al.* Survival, complications, and analysis of risk factors after renal transplantation in cats. *Vet Surg* 2008; **37**(7): 683–695.

9 Kyles AE, Gregory CR, Griffey SM, *et al.* Immunosuppression with a combination of the leflunomide analog, FK778, and microemulsified cyclosporine for renal transplantation in mongrel dogs. *Transplantation* 2003; **75**(8): 1128–1133.

10 Bernsteen L, Gregory CR, Kyles A, *et al.* Microemulsified cyclosporine-based immunosuppression for the prevention of acute renal allograft rejection in unrelated dogs: preliminary experimental study. *Vet Surg* 2003; **32**(3): 213–219.

11 Gregory CR, Kyles A, Bernsteen L, *et al.* Results of clinical renal transplantation in 15 dogs using triple drug immunosuppressive therapy. *Vet Surg* 2006; **35**(2): 105–112.

12 Friedman GS, Meier-Kriesche HU, Kaplan B, *et al.* Hypercoagulable states in renal transplant candidates: impact of anticoagulation upon incidence of renal allograft thrombosis. *Transplantation* 2001; **72**(6): 1073–1078.

13 Snell W, Aronson L, Phillips H, *et al.* Influence of anesthetic variables on short-term and overall survival rates in cats undergoing renal transplantation surgery. *Am Vet Med Assoc* 2015; **247**(3): 267–277.

14 Yeates JW. Ethical considerations in feline renal transplantations. *Vet J* 2014; **202**(3): 405–407.

15 RCVS Council. Kidney transplants in cats: RCVS considers its guidance. *Vet Record* 2016 April **2**: 332–333.

16 Tan J, Wu W, Xu X. Induction therapy with autologous mesenchymal stem cells in living-related kidney transplants: a randomized controlled trial. *J Am Med Assoc* 2012; **307**(11): 1169–1177.

17 Mumaw JL, Schmiedt CW, Breidling S, *et al.* Feline mesenchymal stem cells and supernatant inhibit reactive oxygen species production in cultured feline neutrophils. *Res Vet Sci* 2015; **103**: 60–69.

18 Wormser C, Aronson LR. Perioperative morbidity and long-term outcome of unilateral nephrectomy in feline kidney donors: 141 cases (1998–2013). *J Am Vet Med Assoc* 2016; **248**(3): 275–281.

19 Popovic NA, Mullane JF, Yhap EO. Effects of acetylpromazine maleate on certain cardiorespiratory responses in dogs. *Am J Vet Res* 1972; **33**(9): 1819–1824.

20 Ludders JW, Reitan JA, Martucci R, *et al.* Blood pressure response to phenylephrine infusion in halothane-anesthetized dogs given acetylpromazine maleate. *Am J Vet Res* 1983; **44**(6): 996–999.
21 Lawrence CJ, Prinzen FW, de Lange S. The effects of dexmedetomidine on nutrient organ blood flow. *Anesth Analg* 1996; **83**(6): 1160–1165.
22 Ansah OB, Raekallio M, Vainio O. Comparison of three doses of dexmedetomidine with medetomidine in cats following intramuscular administration. *J Vet Pharmacol Ther* 1998; **21**(5): 380–387.
23 Pypendop BH, Verstegen JP. Hemodynamic effects of medetomidine in the dog: a dose titration study. *Vet Surg* 1998; **27**(6): 612–622.
24 Lamont LA, Bulmer BJ, Grimm KA, *et al.* Cardiopulmonary evaluation of the use of medetomidine hydrochloride in cats. *Am J Vet Res* 2001; **62**(11): 1745–1749.
25 Mendes GM, Selmi AL, Barbudo-Selmi GR, *et al.* Clinical use of dexmedetomidine as premedicant in cats undergoing propofol–sevoflurane. *J Feline Med Surg* 2003; **5**(5): 265–270.
26 Murrell JC, Hellebrekers LJ. Medetomidine and dexmedetomidine: a review of the cardiovascular effects and antinociceptive properties in the dog. *Vet Anaesth Analg* 2005; **32**(3): 117–127.
27 McAnulty JF. Hypothermic storage of feline kidneys for transplantation: successful ex vivo storage up to 7 hours. *Vet Surg* 1998; **27**(4): 312–320.
28 Bernsteen L, Gregory CR, Pollard RE, *et al.* Comparison of two surgical techniques for renal transplantation in cats. *Vet Surg* 1999; **28**(6): 417–420.
29 Bernsteen L., Gregory CR, Kyles A, *et al.* Renal transplantation in cats. *Clin Tech Small Anim Pract* 2000; **15**(1): 40–45.
30 Philips H, Aronson LR. Use of end-to-side arterial and venous anastomosis techniques for renal transplantation in two dogs. *J Am Vet Med Assoc* 2012; **240**(3): 298–303.
31 Hayes MA, Goldenberg IS. Renal effects of anesthesia and operation mediated by endocrines. *Anesthesiology* 1963; **24**: 487–499.
32 Walker LA, Buscemi-Bergin M, Gellai M. Renal hemodynamics in conscious rats: effects of anesthesia, surgery, and recovery. *Am J Physiol* 1983; **245**(1): F67–F74.
33 Koepke JP. Renal responses to stressful environmental stimuli. *Fed Proc* 1985; **44**(13): 2823–2827.
34 Chai CY, Wang CS. Cardiovascular actions of diazepam in the cat. *J Pharmacol Exp Ther* 1966; **154**(2): 271–280.
35 Freye E. Effect of high doses of fentanyl on myocardial infarction and cardiogenic shock in the dog. *Resuscitation* 1974; **3**(2): 105–113.
36 Liu W, Bidway AV, Stanley TH, *et al.* Cardiovascular dynamics after large doses of fentanyl and fentanyl plus N_2O in the dog. *Anesth Analg* 1976; **55**(2): 168–172.
37 Jones DJ, Stehling LC, Zauder HL. Cardiovascular responses to diazepam and midazolam maleate in the dog. *Anesthesiology* 1979; **51**(5): 430–434.
38 Rosow CE, Moss J, Philbin DM, *et al.* Histamine release during morphine and fentanyl anesthesia. *Anesthesiology* 1982; **56**(2): 93–96.
39 Peng P, Sandler AN. A review of the use of fentanyl analgesia in the management of acute pain in adults. *Anesthesiology* 1999; **90**(2): 576–599.
40 Cummings III K, Naguib MA. Opioid agonists and antagonists. In: Flood P, Rathmell JP, Shafer S, *et al.*, eds. *Stoelting's Pharmacology and Physiology in Anesthetic Practice*, 5th edn. Philadelphia, PA: Wolters Kluwer Health, 2015: 217–256.
41 Chauvin M, Sandouk P, Scherrmann JM, *et al.* Morphine pharmacokinetics in renal failure. *Anesthesiology* 1987; **66**(3): 327–331.
42 Sear JW, Hand CW, Moore RA, *et al.* Studies on morphine disposition: influence of general anesthesia on plasma concentrations of morphine and its metabolites. *Br J Anaesth* 1989; **62**(1): 22–27.
43 Sear JW, Hand CW, Moore RA, *et al.* Studies on morphine disposition: influence of renal failure on the kinetics of morphine and its metabolites. *Br J Anaesth* 1989; **62**(1): 22–27.
44 Osborne R, Joel S, Grebenik K, *et al.* The pharmacokinetics of morphine and morphine glucuronides in kidney failure. *Clin Pharmacol Ther* 1993; **54**(2): 158–167.
45 Schmidt S, Jungwirth B. Anesthesia for renal transplant surgery: an update. *Eur J Anesthesiol* 2012; **29**(12): 552–558.
46 Davis LE, Donnelly EJ. Analgesic drugs in the cat. *J Am Vet Med Assoc* 1968; **153**(9): 1161–1167.
47 Faura CC, Collins SL, Moore RA, *et al.* Systematic review of factors affecting the ratios of morphine and its major metabolites. *Pain* 1998; **74**(1): 43–53.
48 Taylor PM, Robertson SA, Dixon MJ, *et al.* Morphine, pethidine and buprenorphine disposition in the cat. *J Vet Pharmacol Ther* 2001; **24**(6): 391–398.
49 Colby ED, Sanford TD. Blood pressure and heart and respiratory rates of cats under ketamine/xylazine, ketamine/acepromazine anesthesia. *Feline Pract* 1981; **11**(5): 19–21.
50 Stepien RL, Bonagura JD, Bednarski RM, *et al.* Cardiorespiratory effects of acepromazine maleate and buprenorphine hydrochloride in clinically normal dogs. *Am J Vet Res* 1995; **56**(1): 78–84.
51 Shiga Y, Minami K, Uezono Y, *et al.* Effects of the intravenously administered anaesthetics ketamine, propofol and thiamylal on the cortical renal blood flow in rats. *Pharmacology* 2003; **68**(1): 17–23.
52 Schroeder CA. Renal disease. In: Johnson RA, Snyder LB, Schroeder CA, eds. *Canine and Feline Anesthesia and Coexisting Disease*, 2nd edn. Hoboken, NJ: John Wiley & Sons, Inc, 2022: 202–224.
53 Chiu KW, Robson S, Devi JL, *et al.* The cardiopulmonary effects and quality of anesthesia after induction with alfaxalone in 2-hydroxypropyl-β-cyclodextrin in dogs and cats: a systematic review. *J Vet Phamacol Ther* 2016; **39**(6): 525–538.
54 Hanna RM, Borchard RE, Schmidt SL. Pharmacokinetics of ketamine HCl and metabolite I in the cat: a comparison of i.v., i.m., and rectal administration. *J Vet Pharmacol Ther* 1988; **11**(1): 84–93.
55 Kruse-Elliott KT, Swanson CR, Aucoin DP. Effects of etomidate on adrenocortical function in canine surgical patients. *Am J Vet Res* 1987; **48**(7): 1098–1100.
56 Albert SG, Ariyan S, Rather A. The effect of etomidate on adrenal function in critical illness: a systematic review. *Intensive Care Med* 2011; **37**(6): 901–910.
57 Flood P, Shafer S. Inhaled anesthetics. In: Flood P, Rathmell JP, Shafer S, *et al.*, eds. *Stoelting's Pharmacology and Physiology in Anesthetic Practice*, 5th edn. Philadelphia, PA: Wolters Kluwer Health, 2015: 98–159.
58 Murphy MR, Hug CC Jr. The anesthetic potency of fentanyl in terms of its reduction of enflurane MAC. *Anesthesiology* 1982; **57**(6): 485–488.
59 Ilkiw JE, Pascoe PJ, Fisher LD. Effect of alfentanil on the minimum alveolar concentration of isoflurane in cats. *Am J Vet Res* 1997; **58**(11): 1267–1273.
60 Murphy EJ. Acute pain management pharmacology for the patient with concurrent renal or hepatic disease. *Anaesth Intensive Care* 2005; **33**(3): 311–322.
61 Cronnelly R, Salvatierra O, Feduska NJ. Renal allograft function following halothane, enflurane, or isoflurane anesthesia. *Anesth Analg* 1984; **63**: 202.
62 Litz RJ, Hübler M, Lorenz W, *et al.* Renal responses to desflurane and isoflurane in patients with renal insufficiency. *Anesthesiology* 2002; **97**(5): 1133–1136.
63 Teixeira S, Costa G, Costa F, *et al.* Sevoflurane versus isoflurane: does it matter in renal transplantation? *Transplant Proc* 2007; **39**(8): 2486–2488.
64 Marik PE, Baram M, Vahid B. Does central venous pressure predict fluid responsiveness? A systematic review of the literature and the tale of seven mares. *Chest* 2008; **134**(1): 172–178.
65 Sano H, Seo J, Wightman P, *et al.* Evaluation of pulse pressure variation and pleth variability index to predict fluid responsiveness in mechanically ventilated isoflurane-anesthetized dogs. *J Vet Emerg Crit Care* 2018; **28**(4): 301–309.
66 Grandy JL, Dunlop CI, Hodgeson DS, *et al.* Evaluation of the Doppler ultrasonic method of measuring systolic arterial blood pressure in cats. *Am J Vet Res* 1992; **53**(7): 1166–1169.
67 Binns SH, Sisson DD, Buoscio DA, *et al.* Doppler ultrasonographic, oscillometric sphygmomanometric, and photoplethysmographic techniques for noninvasive blood pressure measurement in anesthetized cats. *J Vet Intern Med* 1995; **9**(6): 405–414.
68 Caulkett NA, Cantwell SL, Houston DM. A comparison of indirect blood pressure monitoring techniques in the anesthetized cat. *Vet Surg* 1998; **27**(4): 370–377.
69 Bosiack AP, Mann FA, Dodam JR, *et al.* Comparison of ultrasonic Doppler flow monitor, oscillometric, and direct arterial blood pressure measurements in ill dogs. *J Vet Emerg Crit Care* 2010; **20**(2): 207–215.
70 Shih A, Robertson S, Vigani A, *et al.* Evaluation of an indirect oscillometric blood pressure monitor in normotensive and hypotensive anesthetized dogs. *J Vet Emerg Crit Care* 2010; **20**(3): 313–318.
71 Wagener G, Bezinover D, Wang C, *et al.* Fluid management during kidney transplantation: a consensus statement of the Committee on Transplant Anesthesia of the American Society of Anesthesiologists. *Transplantation* 2021; **105**(8): 1677–1683.
72 O'Malley CM, Frumento RJ, Hardy MA, *et al.* A randomized, double-blind comparison of lactated Ringer's solution and 0.9% NaCl during renal transplantation. *Anesth Analg* 2005; **100**(5): 1518–1524.
73 Hadimioglu N, Saadawy I, Saglam T, *et al.* The effect of different crystalloid solutions on acid–base balance and early kidney function after kidney transplantation. *Anesth Analg* 2008; **107**(1): 264–269.
74 Khajavi MR, Etezadi F, Moharari RS, *et al.* Effects of normal saline vs. lactated Ringer's during renal transplantation. *Ren Fail* 2008; **30**(5): 535–539.
75 Davidson IJ. Renal impact of fluid management with colloids: a comparative review. *Eur J Anaesthesiol* 2006; **23**(9): 721–738.
76 Bellomo R, Wan L, May C. Vasoactive drugs and acute kidney injury. *Crit Care Med* 2008; **36**(Suppl 4): S179–S186.
77 Kim JM, Kim SJ, Joh JW, *et al.* Is it safe to use a kidney from an expanded criteria donor? *Transplant Proc* 2011; **43**(6): 2359–2362.
78 Schnuelle J, Johannes van der Woude F. Perioperative fluid management in renal transplantation: a narrative review of the literature. *Transpl Int* 2006; **19**(12): 947–959.
79 Irish A. Hypercoagulability in renal transplant recipients. Identifying patients at risk of renal allograft thrombosis and evaluating strategies for prevention. *Am J Cardiovasc Drugs* 2004; **4**(3): 139–149.
80 Kwok J, Flood P. Drugs used for psychopharmacologic therapy. In: Flood P, Rathmell JP, Shafer S, *et al.*, eds. *Staoelting's Pharmacology and Physiology in Anesthetic Practice*, 5th edn. Philadelphia, PA: Wolters Kluwer Health, 2015: 822–844.

81 KuKanich B, Bidgood T, Knesl O. Clinical pharmacology of nonsteroidal antiinflammatory drugs in dogs. *Vet Anaesth Analg* 2012; **39**(1): 69–90.

82 Gruen ME, Lascelles BDX, Colleran E, *et al.* 2022 pain management guidelines for dogs and cats. *J Am Anim Hosp Assoc* 2022; **58**(2): 55–76.

83 Kyles AE, Gregory CR, Wooldridge JD, *et al.* Management of hypertension controls postoperative neurologic disorders after renal transplantation in cats. *Vet Surg* 1999; **28**(6): 436–441.

84 Tutone VK, Mark PB, Stewart GA, *et al.* Hypertension, antihypertensive agents and outcomes following renal transplantation. *Clin Transplant* 2005; **19**(2): 181–192.

85 Schmiedt CW, Mercurio A, Glassman M, *et al.* Effects of renal autograft ischemic and reperfusion associated with renal transplantation on arterial blood pressure variables in clinically normal cats. *Am J Vet Res* 2009; **70**: 1426–1432.

86 Schmiedt CW, Mercurio A, Vandenplas M, *et al.* Effects of renal autograftischemic storage and reperfusion on intraoperative hemodynamic patterns andplasma renin concentrations in clinically normal cats undergoing renal autotransplantation and contralateral nephrectomy. *Am J Vet Res* 2010; **71**: 1220–1227.

87 Kyles AE, Gregory CR, Wooldridge JD, *et al.* Management of hypertension controls postoperative neurologic disorders after renal transplantation in cats. *Vet Surg* 1999; **28**(6): 436–441.

88 Cowgill LD, Francey T. Hemodialysis and extracorporeal blood purification. In: DiBartola SP, ed. *Fluid, Electrolyte, and Acid-Base Disorders in Small Animal Practice*, 4th edn. St Louis, MO: Saunders Elsevier, 2012: 680–709.

89 Bersenas AME. A clinical review of peritoneal dialysis. *J Vet Emerg Crit Care* 2011; **21**(6): 605–617.

90 Cooper RL, Labato MA. Peritoneal dialysis in veterinary medicine. *Vet Clin North Am Small Anim Pract* 2011; **41**(1): 91–113.

91 Vitalaru A. Peritoneal dialysis in dogs and cats. *J Hell Vet Medical Soc* 2021; **71**(4): 2419–2424.

92 Blowey DL, Alon US. Dialysis principles for primary health-care providers. *Clin Pediatr* 2005; **44**(1): 19–29.

93 Ross LA, Labato MA. Peritoneal dialysis. In: DiBartola SP, ed. *Fluid, Electrolyte, and Acid-Base Disorders in Small Animal Practice*, 4th edn. St Louis, MO: Saunders Elsevier, 2012: 665–679.

94 Cowgill LD. Application of peritoneal dialysis and hemodialysis in the management of renal failure. In: Osborne CA, ed. *Canine and Feline Nephrology and Urology*. Baltimore, MD: Lee & Febiger, 1995: 573–584.

95 Fox LE, Grauer FG, Dubielzig RR, *et al.* Reversal of ethylene glycol-induced nephrotoxicosis in a dog. *J Am Vet Med Assoc* 1987; **191**(11): 1433–1435.

96 Crisp MS, Chew DJ, DiBartola SP, *et al.* Peritoneal dialysis in dogs and cats: 27 cases (1976–1987). *J Am Vet Med Assoc* 1989; **195**(9): 1262–1266.

97 Beckel NF, O'Toole TE, Rozanski EA, *et al.* Peritoneal dialysis in the management of acute renal failure in 5 dogs with leptospirosis. *J Vet Emerg Crit Care* 2005; **15**(3): 201–205.

98 Dorval P, Boysen SR. Management of acute renal failure in cats using peritoneal dialysis: a retrospective study of six cases (2003–2007). *Feline Med Surg* 2009; **11**(2): 107–115.

99 Gabriel DP, Nascimento GVR, Caramori JT, *et al.* Peritoneal dialysis in acute renal failure. *Renal Failure* 2006; **28**(6): 451–456.

100 Abel J, Rowntree L, Turner B. On the removal of diffusible substances from the circulating blood of living animals by dialysis. *J Pharmacol Exp Ther* 1914; **5**(3): 275–316.

101 Foster JD. Extracorporeal therapies in the emergency room and intensive care unit. *Vet Clin North Am Small Anim Pract* 2020; **50**(6): 1215–1236.

102 Bloom CA, Labato MA. Intermittent hemodialysis for small animals. *Vet Clin North Am Small Anim Pract* 2011; **41**(1): 115133.

103 Ghannoum M, Roberts DM, Hoffman RS, *et al.* A stepwise approach for the management of poisoning with extracorporeal treatments. *Semin Dial* 2014; **27**(4): 362–370.

104 Eatroff AE, Langston CE, Chalhoub S, *et al.* Long-term outcome of cats and dogs with acute kidney injury treated with intermittent hemodialysis: 135 cases (1997–2010). *J Am Vet Med Assoc* 2012; **241**(11): 1471–1478.

105 Acierno MJ. Continuous renal replacement therapy in dogs and cats. *Vet Clin North Am Small Anim Pract* 2011; **41**(1): 135–146.

106 Elliott DA. Hemodialysis. *Clin Tech Small Anim Pract* 2000; **15**(3): 136–148.

107 Langston C. Hemodialysis in dogs and cats. *Compend Contin Educ Pract Vet* 2002; **24**(7): 540–549.

108 Groman R. Apheresis in veterinary medicine: therapy in search of a disease. In: *Proceedings of the Advanced Renal Therapies Symposium*. New York, NY: Animal Medical Center, 2010: 26–32.

109 Cowgill LD, Langston CE. History of hemodialysis in dogs and companion animals. In: Ing TS, Rahman MA, Kjellstrand CM, eds. *Dialysis: History, Development and Promise*. Singapore: World Scientific, 2012: 901–914.

110 Chalhoub S, Langston CE. Vascular access for extracorporeal renal replacement therapy in veterinary patients. *Vet Clin North Am Small Anim Pract* 2011; **41**(1): 147–161.

111 Poeppel K, Langston CE, Chalhoub S. Equipment commonly used in veterinary renal replacement therapy. *Vet Clin North Am Small Anim Pract* 2011; **41**(1): 177–191.

112 Langston CE, Cowgill LD, Spano JA. Applications and outcomes of hemodialysis in cats: a review of 29 cases. *J Vet Intern Med* 1997; **11**(6): 348–355.

113 Fischer JR, Pantaleo V, Francey T, *et al.* Veterinary hemodialysis: advances in management and technology. *Vet Clin North Am Small Anim Pract* 2004; **34**(4): 935–967.

114 Langston CE, Poeppel K, Mitelberg E. *AMC DIALYSIS HANDBOOK*. New York: Animal Medical Center, 2010: 3.

115 Monaghan KN, Acierno MJ. Extracorporeal removal of drugs and toxins. *Vet Clin Noth Am Small Anim Pract* 2011; **41**(1): 227–238.

116 Joy MS, Matzke GR, Frye RF, *et al.* Determinants of vancomycin clearance by continuous venovenous hemofiltration and continuous venovenous hemodialysis. *Am J Kidney Dis* 1998; **31**(6): 1019–1027.

117 Bouman CS. Antimicrobial dosing strategies in critically ill patients with acute kidney injury and high-dose continuous veno-venous hemofiltration. *Curr Opin Crit Care* 2008; **14**(6): 654–659.

118 Bugge JF. Pharmacokinetics and drug dosing adjustments during continuous venovenous hemofiltration or hemodiafiltration in critically ill patients. *Acta Anaesthesiol Scand* 2001; **45**(8): 929–934.

119 Churchwell MD, Mueller BA. Drug dosing during continuous renal replacement therapy. *Semin Dial* 2009; **22**(2): 185–188.

120 Choi G, Gomersall CD, Tian Q, *et al.* Principles of antibacterial dosing in continuous renal replacement therapy. *Crit Care Med* 2009; **37**(7): 2268–2282.

121 Bayliss G. Dialysis in the poisoned patient. *Hemodial Int* 2010; **14**(2): 158–167.

45 Anesthetic Considerations During Pregnancy and for the Newborn

Marc R. Raffe[1] **and Elizabeth Goudie-DeAngelis**[2]

[1] Veterinary Anesthesia and Critical Care Associates, LLC, St. Paul, Minnesota, USA

[2] Tristate Veterinary Anesthesia, PLLC, White Plains, New York, USA

Chapter contents

Introduction, 955
Pregnancy-associated changes in maternal physiology, 955
  Cardiovascular, 955
  Coagulation, 956
  Pulmonary, 956
  Gastrointestinal, 957
  Liver and kidney, 957
  Uterine blood flow, 957
  Neuroendocrine, 957
Pharmacologic alterations induced by pregnancy, 957
Anesthesia during pregnancy, 958
Anesthetic drugs and cesarean section, 959
  Anticholinergics, 959
  Tranquilizers and sedatives, 959
  Opioids, 959
  Injectable anesthetics, 960
  Dissociatives, 960
  Neuroleptanalgesia, 960
  Inhalation anesthetics, 960
  Neuromuscular blocking agents, 961
  Guaifenesin, 961
  Local anesthetics, 961
  Supplemental agents, 961
Anesthetic techniques for cesarean section, 961
  General anesthesia, 961
  Regional anesthesia, 964
  Local anesthesia, 965
Care of the newborn, 965
Postoperative pain management, 965
References, 966

Introduction

The ideal anesthetic protocol for pregnant or periparturient (usually defined as labor and the time within a few weeks of labor) patients provides analgesia, muscle relaxation, and sedation/narcosis without endangering either mother or fetus. By their very nature, anesthetics, analgesics, tranquilizers, and sedatives cross the blood–brain barrier. The physicochemical properties that allow drugs to cross the blood–brain barrier also facilitate placental transfer.

Factors in decision-making regarding anesthesia protocols in these patients include the unique physiology of the mother during pregnancy and labor, the impact of selected drugs on the mother and fetus, carryover effects of administered drugs on the neonate following separation from the mother, and the effect of commonly observed anesthesia-related complications on the fetus and mother. General anesthesia is needed for commonly performed periparturient procedures, but it is not possible to selectively anesthetize the mother because all agents that affect the maternal central nervous system will also affect the fetus. All drugs that change the maternal physiology will affect fetal homeostasis. This is especially pertinent during anesthesia for cesarean section when separation of the fetus from the uteroplacental attachment occurs. A complete understanding of the physiologic changes present in the gravid patient and the potential impact of anesthetic drugs is essential to navigate both mother and fetus safely through the perioperative period.

Pregnancy-associated changes in maternal physiology

Metabolic demands during gestation and parturition are met by physiologic adaptation, which is unique to this period (Table 45.1). Most of the data describing physiologic adaptation to pregnancy has been obtained from humans and ewes. Although little work has been done in other species, the changes should be comparable, if not greater, in magnitude because birth weight expressed as a percentage of maternal weight for people, sheep, dogs, and cats is 5.7%, 11.4%, 16.1%, and 13.2%, respectively [1]. This suggests that the physiologic burden and, therefore, physiologic adaptation may actually be greater in animals than humans.

Cardiovascular

During pregnancy, maternal blood volume increases by approximately 40%; plasma volume increases by 40–50%, which is more than the 20% increase in red cell mass, resulting in decreased

Veterinary Anesthesia and Analgesia: The Sixth Edition of Lumb and Jones. Edited by Leigh Lamont, Kurt Grimm, Sheilah Robertson, Lydia Love and Carrie Schroeder.
© 2024 John Wiley & Sons, Inc. Published 2024 by John Wiley & Sons, Inc.
Companion website: www.wiley.com/go/lamont/anesthesia

Table 45.1 Physiological alterations induced by pregnancy.

Variable	Change
Heart rate	↑
Cardiac output	↑
Blood volume	↑
Plasma volume	↑
Packed cell volume, hemoglobin, and plasma protein	↓
Arterial blood pressure	unchanged
Central venous pressure	unchanged; ↑ during labor
Minute volume of ventilation	↑
Oxygen consumption	↑
pHa and PaO_2	unchanged
$PaCO_2$	↓
Total lung and vital capacity	unchanged
Functional residual capacity	↓
Gastric emptying time and intragastric pressure	↑
Gastric motility and pH of gastric secretions	↓
Gastric chloride ion and enzyme concentration	↑
AST, LDH, and BSP retention time	↑
Plasma cholinesterase	↓
Renal plasma flow and glomerular filtration rate	↑
Blood urea nitrogen and creatinine	↓
Sodium ion and water balance	unchanged

hemoglobin concentration and packed cell volume [2]. This results in a dilutional physiologic anemia. Increased heart rate and stroke volume cause cardiac output to increase 30–50% above normal [3,4]. Plasma estrogens decrease peripheral vascular resistance producing an increase in cardiac output, while systolic and diastolic blood pressures remain unchanged. Cardiac output is also influenced during labor by body position, pain, and apprehension [2]. During labor, systolic pressure increases by 10–30 mmHg. Cardiac output increases an additional 10–25% during labor and the immediate postpartum period, as a result of blood extrusion from the contracting uterus [5]. Although central venous pressure does not change during pregnancy, it increases slightly (4–6 cmH_2O) during labor and has been reported to increase by up to 50 cmH_2O during painful fetal extraction [6]. The posterior vena cava and aorta can be compressed by the enlarged uterus and its contents during dorsal recumbency. This can cause decreased venous return and cardiac output with concurrent reduction in uterine and renal blood flow [7,8]. Although this does not appear to be as serious a problem in dogs and cats, time spent restrained or positioned in dorsal recumbency should be kept to a minimum [7,8,9].

Because cardiac work is increased during pregnancy and parturition, cardiac reserve is decreased. Patients with previously well-compensated heart disease may suffer pulmonary congestion and heart failure caused by a gestation induced increase in cardiac workload and hemodynamic demand secondary to parturition-associated pain [10]. In such patients, pain and anxiety control is a key component of successful patient management during the periparturient period. However, care must be taken to avoid additional cardiac depression and decompensation induced by excessive doses of sedatives or anesthetics. The use of ecbolic agents during or after parturition can adversely affect cardiovascular function. Oxytocin in large or repeated doses induces peripheral vasodilation and hypotension, which can adversely affect both mother and fetus through decreased tissue perfusion. Ergot derivatives used to control uterine bleeding can induce vasoconstriction and hypertension [11].

Coagulation

In humans, major changes to the coagulation system occur throughout pregnancy with the greatest changes noted at term [12]. There is often a mild, non-clinically significant thrombocytopenia due to dilution, destruction, and consumption of platelets. The concentrations of clotting factors VII, VIII, IX, X, XI, Von Willebrand factor (VWF), and fibrinogen increase throughout pregnancy, while factors XI and XIII decrease, leading to a nearly doubling of coagulation activity at the end of pregnancy. Plasma fibrinolytic activity decreases until after placental delivery then returns to normal. There is a general increase in clotting ability at the time of parturition, which may increase the risk of perianesthetic clot formation in the dam.

Pulmonary

In humans, increased serum progesterone concentration during pregnancy increases respiratory center sensitivity to carbon dioxide. Increased minute volume during gestation produces a progressive reduction in $PaCO_2$ during gestation; this value approaches 30 mmHg at parturition. Metabolic compensation for respiratory alkalosis maintains arterial pH within normal values. Hyperventilation may further be stimulated during labor by pain, apprehension, and anxiety. During pregnancy, oxygen consumption increases by 20% as a result of the demands imposed by the developing fetus, placenta, uterine muscle, and mammary tissue. Arterial oxygen tension remains unchanged [2].

Pregnancy also affects the mechanics of ventilation. Airway conductance is increased and total pulmonary resistance is decreased by progesterone-induced relaxation of bronchial smooth muscle. Lung compliance is unaffected. Functional residual capacity (FRC) is decreased by displacement of the diaphragm and abdominal organs by the gravid uterus. In addition, FRC further decreases during labor because of increased pulmonary blood volume secondary to uterine contraction. Because FRC is reduced, small airway closure develops at end-exhalation in approximately one-third of human parturients [2]. Tidal volume increases by 45%, but total lung capacity and vital capacity are unaltered [13]. In addition, hypoventilation produces hypoxemia and hypercapnia more frequently in pregnant than non-pregnant patients. Hypoxemia is exacerbated by increased oxygen consumption during labor. Oxygen administration prior to anesthetic induction increases oxygen reserve by facilitating pulmonary denitrogenation [14]. Preoxygenation is advisable if the patient is tolerant of this procedure.

Induction of anesthesia with inhalation agents is more rapid in pregnant than non-pregnant patients. The equilibration rate between inspired and alveolar anesthetic partial pressure is accelerated by increased alveolar ventilation via increased minute ventilation and decreased FRC.

In the fetus, gas exchange occurs via the placenta. Carbon dioxide and oxygen move across the placental barrier by passive diffusion. Movement of carbon dioxide is facilitated by the Haldane effect; as the maternal blood releases oxygen to the fetus, its carbon dioxide carrying capacity is increased. As the fetal hemoglobin releases the carbon dioxide, its hemoglobin then becomes more able to bind to oxygen, referred to as the "double Haldane effect" [15]. Oxygen movement is facilitated by the Bohr effect. As maternal hemoglobin binds to carbon dioxide, the pH is decreased, which causes a right shift of the oxyhemoglobin dissociation curve. On the fetal side, the release of carbon dioxide from fetal hemoglobin results in a left shift of the oxyhemoglobin saturation curve, thus enhancing its binding affinity for oxygen; this is called the "double Bohr effect" [16]. In addition, fetal hemoglobin has a lower P_{50} than adult hemoglobin, enhancing its oxygen binding [17].

Gastrointestinal

A number of functional changes in gastrointestinal physiology occur during gestation and parturition. Physical displacement of the stomach by the gravid uterus, decreased gastric motility, and changes in serum progesterone level contribute to delayed gastric emptying and are most pronounced during the last trimester. Acid, chloride, and enzyme concentrations in gastric secretions are increased due to changes in hormone physiology present during gestation. Lower esophageal sphincter tone is decreased, and intragastric pressure is increased. Pain and anxiety during labor have been shown to further decrease gastric motility [2].

These changes increase the risk of regurgitation (both active and passive), and aspiration is increased in parturients [18]. Frequently, patients presented for cesarean section have recently eaten or the time of the last feeding is unknown. Parturients should be regarded as having a full stomach, and anesthesia techniques should be selected that produce rapid airway management and control to prevent aspiration of foreign material. Because the risk of regurgitation and aspiration is considered high in periparturient patients, prophylactic measures are recommended. Metoclopramide and an H_2-receptor antagonist drug (e.g., cimetidine, ranitidine, or famotidine) may be administered as part of the preanesthetic protocol [19]. Prophylactic administration of antiemetics, such as maropitant and ondansetron, is a common practice in companion animals.

Risk of vomiting increases with hypotension, hypoxia, and toxic reactions to local anesthetics. Smooth induction of general anesthesia and preventing hypotension during epidural anesthesia will decrease the incidence of vomiting. Because silent regurgitation can occur when the intragastric pressure is high, a cuffed endotracheal tube with adequate airway seal is preferred for airway management during general anesthesia. Passive regurgitation can be induced by positive-pressure ventilation with a face mask or by manipulation of abdominal viscera. Although atropine reduces the lower esophageal sphincter (LES) pressure, it may decrease reflux by reducing the frequency of LES relaxation, but it may also inhibit the actions of metoclopramide that increase gastric motility and emptying by sensitizing gastric smooth muscle to acetylcholine [6,19]. The clinician should always be cognizant that gastroesophageal reflux can occur in the anesthetized patient (see Chapters 2 and 41 for further details).

Liver and kidney

Pregnancy induces minor changes in hepatic function. Plasma protein concentration decreases slightly, but total plasma volume is increased because of the increase in blood volume. Bilirubin concentration is unaltered. Serum enzyme concentrations (serum alanine aminotransferase and alkaline phosphatase) can be slightly increased. Plasma cholinesterase (also known as pseudocholinesterase) concentration decreases, which may lead to prolonged action of succinylcholine in pregnant patients, particularly if they have been recently exposed to organophosphate parasiticides (e.g., anthelmintics, flea collars, or dips). Despite these alterations, overall liver function is generally well maintained [2].

Renal plasma flow and glomerular filtration rate are increased by approximately 60% in pregnant patients; blood urea nitrogen (BUN) and creatinine concentrations are lower than in non-pregnant patients [6]. Sodium and water balance are unaffected. Elevated BUN or creatinine levels may indicate renal pathology or compromise in parturient patients. In these patients, drugs with known nephrotoxic potential, such as aminoglycoside antibiotics, and non-steroidal anti-inflammatory drugs (NSAIDs), should be avoided.

Uterine blood flow

Stable uteroplacental circulation is important to fetal and maternal homeostasis and neonatal survival. Uterine blood flow is directly proportional to systemic perfusion pressure and inversely proportional to vascular resistance in myometrial blood vessels. Placental perfusion is dependent on uteroplacental perfusion pressure, and there is no significant autoregulation in the uteroplacental circulation; however, placental vessels do have rudimentary mechanisms for changing vascular resistance and contain α-adrenergic and β_2-adrenergic receptors [20]. Placental perfusion is directly linked to mean uterine perfusion pressure and uterine vascular resistance. Anesthesia may decrease uterine blood flow; in addition, uterine vascular resistance is increased by uterine contractions and hypertonia (oxytocic response). Placental hypotension is associated with hypovolemia, anesthetic-induced cardiovascular depression, or sympathetic blockade resulting in reduced uterine perfusion pressure. Uterine vasoconstriction is induced by endogenous sympathetic discharge or by exogenous sympathomimetic drugs having α_1-adrenergic effects (e.g., epinephrine, norepinephrine, methoxamine, phenylephrine, and metaraminol) [2,20,21,22]. Hypotension induced by adjunctive drugs combined with increased uterine tone induced by ecbolics should be avoided.

Neuroendocrine

In humans, it has been reported that increased progesterone levels at term contribute to reduced anesthesia requirements. This observation may not be consistent in veterinary species; it is well-documented in the dog and cat that progesterone levels decrease during gestation to basal, or slightly above basal, levels at term [23–27]. Horses have low blood progesterone levels at term; progesterone is undetectable in the blood during the second half of gestation as its source shifts from the corpus lutea in the ovary [28,29]. It is unlikely that progesterone has a significant impact on anesthesia requirements if cesarean section is warranted.

The fetus' capacity for gluconeogenesis is very limited. Therefore, as the fetal blood glucose source is from the mother, it is important to maintain normal maternal blood glucose concentrations. In the bitch, induction of labor results in a drop in core body temperature of at least 1.2 °C [23].

Summary

Pregnant (gravid) patients are at greater anesthetic risk because of pregnancy-associated physiologic alterations. Cardiac reserve diminishes during pregnancy; high-risk patients can suffer acute cardiac decompensation or failure. Gravid patients are prone to hypoventilation, hypoxia, and hypercapnia because of altered pulmonary function. The risk of embolism in the perianesthetic period is greater for these patients. Anesthetic requirements may be decreased, and the likelihood of a relative overdose and cardiorespiratory depression is greater than in non-gravid patients. Emesis or regurgitation and aspiration can occur if induction of anesthesia is not immediately followed by rapid airway control.

Pharmacologic alterations induced by pregnancy

Pregnancy affects the uptake, distribution, and disposition of anesthetic agents and adjuncts. The concentration of free (non-ionized, unbound) drug in maternal plasma is affected by changes in protein binding, placental transfer, distribution in fetal tissues, and biotransformation by the maternal and fetal liver. The effect of pregnancy on anesthetic agents has been studied [30]. The rate of barbiturate biotransformation appears to be decreased in pregnancy [30]. Succinylcholine and procaine metabolism are decreased because of decreased plasma cholinesterase concentration [30]. Increased renal blood flow and glomerular filtration associated with pregnancy favor renal drug excretion. In certain species, the minimum alveolar concentration (MAC) is reduced for all volatile agents [31]. MAC values are reduced in pregnant versus non-pregnant ewes but not in canines [32]. Reduced MAC requirement coupled with a decreased FRC results in rapid anesthetic induction requiring as little as one-fourth to one-fifth of induction time compared to non-pregnant patients [33]. Due to the increased rate of uptake, care must be taken to prevent volatile agent overdose in pregnant patients.

The placenta is highly permeable to anesthetic drugs, and most anesthetics and anesthetic adjuncts diffuse quickly across the placental barrier. Placental transfer of drugs can occur by four mechanisms; the most important mechanism is simple diffusion (Fick's law of diffusion). Other mechanisms include facilitated diffusion (glucocorticoids), active transport (norepinephrine and dopamine), and pinocytosis [33]. Diffusion across the placenta is determined by the drug's molecular weight, the percentage of drug bound to maternal plasma protein, lipid solubility, and degree of ionization. Drugs with low molecular weight (MW < 500 Daltons [Da]), low degree of protein binding, high lipid solubility, and those that are non-ionized at maternal blood pH diffuse rapidly across the placenta. Conversely, drugs that are larger (MW > 1000 Da), are highly protein bound, have low lipid solubility, and are mostly ionized generally cross the placenta slowly [30,33,34]. Neuromuscular blocking drugs, unlike other anesthetic and anesthetic adjunctive drugs, are highly ionized and have low lipid solubility. Although they can be recovered from fetal blood, they are generally regarded as having minimal placental transfer and negligible fetal effect [31,33]. The placenta does not appear to metabolize anesthetic drugs or adjuncts.

Physiochemical properties within the fetus and mother also affect placental drug transfer [33]. The degree to which a drug is ionized is determined by its pK_a and the pH of the maternal body fluids. Normal fetal pH is 0.1 unit less than that of the mother [30]. Drugs that are weak acids will be less ionized as pH decreases. For example, thiopental is a weak acid with a pK_a of 7.6. In acidemic patients (pH < 7.4), a greater proportion of the administered dose is in the non-ionized form. As the proportion of the non-ionized form of the drug increases, the drug fraction that is protein bound is reduced, thus effectively increasing the clinical response on a milligram per kg basis. As a result, it is well recognized that acidemia decreases the required anesthetic dose of thiopental and other barbiturates. For weak basic drugs, lower fetal pH increases ionized drug concentration, thereby reducing the maternal–fetal concentration gradient and non-ionized drug transfer across the placenta to the fetus. Weak basic drugs with pK_a values near 7.4 such as opioids and local anesthetics are more highly ionized at pH values less than their pK_a. Local anesthetics move across the placenta but do not easily diffuse back due to the lower pH of the fetus. Therefore, they are found in higher concentrations in fetal tissues and plasma compared to those of the mother because of "ion trapping." Hence, their effect on the mother and fetus is less on a milligram per kg basis [30,33].

Fetal drug concentration is also affected by redistribution, metabolism, and protein binding. Drug concentration in the umbilical vein is greater than in fetal organs (brain, heart, and other vital organs). Approximately 85% of umbilical venous blood initially passes through the fetal liver where drugs may be sequestered or metabolized. In addition, umbilical venous blood containing drug enters the inferior vena cava via the ductus venosus and mixes with drug-free blood returning from the lower extremities and pelvic viscera [30,33] (Fig. 45.1). Due to these mechanisms, it appears that fetal circulation buffers vital fetal tissues from sudden changes in drug concentration. Drug binding to fetal proteins may also reduce free-drug availability [30,33]. Drugs dynamically redistribute out of the fetus into the mother as maternal plasma levels decrease, making clinical estimation of fetal plasma concentrations difficult. Additional variables in fetal drug concentration include slower drug metabolism contributing to a prolonged *in vivo* drug presence. Toxicity can be enhanced by fetal or maternal metabolism to more toxic metabolites and by drug–metabolite and drug–drug interactions [34].

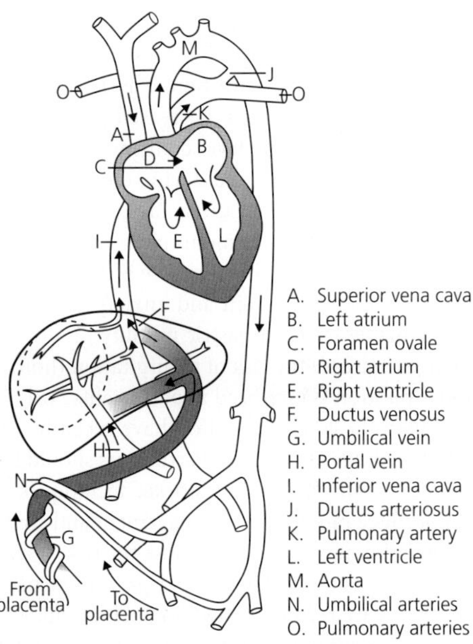

Figure 45.1 The direction of blood flow in the fetal vascular system is indicated by arrows. The darkened vascular segments represent the umbilical blood and its path of flow into the liver and inferior vena cava via the ductus venosus. Blood flow through the foramen ovale and ductus arteriosus provides a direct path to the arterial system, bypassing the lungs. In neonates, the ductus arteriosus and foramen ovale close shortly after birth. This functional closure redirects blood flow through the neonate's lungs where it is arterialized, as in the adult. The time required for complete anatomic closure of the foramen ovale varies by species and typically takes several months (but may require as many as 12 months in foals).

Administration of a fixed dose of drugs with rapidly decreasing plasma concentration (e.g., thiopental, propofol, or succinylcholine) briefly exposes the fetus and placenta to a high maternal blood drug concentration. This is in contrast to the sustained maternal blood levels of drugs administered by continuous infusion or inhalation, which result in continuous placental transfer of drug to the fetus [30,34].

Anesthesia during pregnancy

Maternal exposure to general anesthesia has potential consequences for the unborn fetus. Fetal risks change during development and are categorized by gestational trimester. General anesthesia during the first trimester of pregnancy is associated with fetal teratogenesis, spontaneous abortion, and fetal death. Anesthesia exposure during the middle trimester is generally considered the safest period of gestation; however, spontaneous abortion and fetal death have been reported during this period [35]. Anesthesia exposure during the last trimester carries a risk of premature labor and fetal death. There appears to be species variability with respect to anesthesia-associated risk. This may be due to placental anatomy, uteroplacental perfusion, and maternal homeostasis. There does not appear to be a specific drug-linked risk associated with increased fetal morbidity/mortality [35].

Care must be taken to ensure that maternal physiology is maintained during the anesthesia episode. Critical attention to support of maternal cardiorespiratory physiology, oxygen delivery, and acid–base balance ensures undisturbed uteroplacental perfusion and oxygen delivery; these are of paramount importance for postanesthetic fetal viability. In the human literature, it is recommended that NSAIDs be avoided after the first trimester to prevent premature closure of the ductus arteriosus [36,37].

Anesthetic drugs and cesarean section

Anesthetic drugs should be carefully chosen and properly administered to avoid excessive maternal depression and to maximize neonatal vigor and viability. As noted above, the specific characteristics that make a drug an excellent anesthetic agent are also those that facilitate rapid transplacental transfer and neonatal depression. Therefore, it is prudent to consider that no agent should be used unless distinctly indicated. A brief overview of anesthetic drug classes in periparturient anesthesia follows.

Anticholinergics

Anticholinergic drugs, such as atropine and glycopyrrolate, have been historically used to decrease salivation and inhibit excessive vagal efferent activity that may occur when traction is applied to the uterus [38]. Their risk-reducing value varies with species; they are more effective in dogs and cats, with less impact in other species. Glycopyrrolate may actually increase the viscosity of secretions via its drying properties, resulting in viscous saliva [39]. Many expectant mothers have eaten immediately before delivery. The presence of gastric contents increases the likelihood of regurgitation, which is enhanced by hypoxia or hypotension. The influence of anticholinergics upon emesis is variable [6,38]. In women, atropine has not been shown to decrease the incidence of emesis at parturition [34]. Glycopyrrolate has been shown to be equivalent to ondansetron in prevention of postoperative nausea and vomiting [39]. Additionally, because glycopyrrolate does not readily cross the placenta, it does not affect the fetus to the same extent as atropine.

Tranquilizers and sedatives

Because of their long duration of action, there is no indication for the routine use of these agents in parturients [6,33]. They should be restricted to markedly apprehensive or excited patients and only in doses sufficient to induce a calming effect. Acepromazine can induce significant maternal and fetal depression even at relatively low doses. Diazepam and midazolam can induce neonatal depression characterized by the absence of vocalization, lethargy, hypotonus, apnea, and hypothermia immediately following birth [40–42]. It has been suggested that these effects are dose related and can be minimized by administering low doses of diazepam (< 0.14 mg/kg IV), although no safe dose has been established in domestic animals [42]. Residual benzodiazepine-induced lethargy and muscle relaxation in either the mother or neonate can be antagonized with flumazenil, a specific benzodiazepine antagonist administered to effect [43].

α_2-Adrenergic receptor agonists have significant effects on both maternal and fetal homeostasis. Xylazine rapidly crosses the placenta and induces both maternal and fetal respiratory and circulatory depression. When used with ketamine, xylazine produces significant cardiopulmonary changes, resulting in decreased tissue perfusion in healthy dogs [44]. The use of xylazine or xylazine–ketamine combinations should be avoided in small animal patients presented for cesarean section [45]. However, combinations of xylazine and ketamine have often been used in mares presenting with dystocia.

Detomidine appears to be well tolerated when administered to pregnant mares at 20–60 µg/kg IV. Two studies demonstrated no increase in drug-related change in uterine activity or increased incidence of spontaneous abortion following repeated dosing [46,47]. Similar results have been reported in cattle [48]. Limited information is available regarding the effect of medetomidine on pregnancy. In dogs, there appears to be a dose-related effect on uterine muscle activity that was documented during the parturient and immediate post-parturient period [49]. A study in which medetomidine was used as a premedicant in canine cesarean section reported a high percentage of viable puppies following surgery [50]. All puppies and bitches were prophylactically administered atipamezole following delivery. Similar results were reported when dexmedetomidine was used as a premedicant in canine cesarean section [51]. There are case reports of dexmedetomidine use in human cesarean section patients with good success [52]. Romifidine induces a transient increase in intrauterine pressure following administration [53].

There is very little information on trazodone use in pregnancy; one small multicenter study evaluating trazodone use in humans during both the first trimester and throughout gestation did not find a higher incidence of major malformations, but there may have been an increase in spontaneous abortion [54]. There were no data on neonatal vigor within this study. More data are available on gabapentin; exposure both early and late in gestation resulted in cardiac defects, increased risk of preterm birth, and increased need for neonatal intensive care [55]. Gabapentin is minimally secreted into milk with no side effects noted in suckling infants. Similarly, studies of infants whose mothers were taking trazodone during breastfeeding found very low levels within milk and few side effects in the infants [56]. Both trazodone and gabapentin should be used with caution during gestation and only as needed in the periparturient period.

Opioids

Opioids rapidly cross the placenta and can cause neonatal respiratory and neurobehavioral depression [34,57,58]. In addition, fetal elimination may require 2–6 days. It appears that equianalgesic doses of opioids induce an equal degree of central nervous system depression. Therefore, choice is based on the desired duration of opioid action. Commonly used µ-opioid receptor agonists include morphine, fentanyl, meperidine, oxymorphone, hydromorphone, and methadone [34]. Agents having opioid agonist–antagonist or partial agonist activity include butorphanol and buprenorphine, respectively. Butorphanol provides mild to moderate sedation but less intense analgesia than a full agonist. Buprenorphine produces mild sedation plus good to excellent analgesia.

One of the advantages of opioid agonists is that direct antagonists are available to reverse their action. Of the antagonist agents, naloxone (0.04 mg/kg IV) appears to be the most effective. Naloxone is a pure antagonist without agonist action. Nalorphine and levallorphan, two other antagonist agents, have opioid activity of their own and can increase respiratory depression induced by other non-opioid agents (e.g., barbiturates, phenothiazines, and inhalation agents). Because all opioid antagonists rapidly cross the placenta, maternal administration before delivery has been advocated to reverse opioid induced neonatal depression. However, this technique deprives the mother of analgesia at the time when it is needed most; therefore, antagonist agents should be administered directly to neonates. Finally, because the action of naloxone is shorter than that of most opioid agonists, renarcotization may occur as naloxone is metabolized and excreted. Therefore, both mother and neonates should be carefully monitored for recurring signs of narcosis after opioid reversal with naloxone [34]. Should this occur, additional naloxone can be given Additional information on opioids is available in Chapter 23.

Injectable anesthetics

Intravenous propofol administration produces rapid induction of anesthesia, suitable for intubation followed by inhalation anesthesia. Propofol rapidly crosses the placenta but is rapidly cleared from the neonatal circulation. In dogs, propofol followed by isoflurane anesthesia resulted in newborn survival rates comparable to those with epidural anesthesia and superior to those with general anesthesia induced with thiopental [59]. Cohort retrospective studies by Moon *et al.* indicated that administration of propofol intravenously followed by isoflurane resulted in good puppy vigor, vocalization, and survival following delivery [42]. Their findings were similar to those in a previously reported study [59]. Constant rate infusion of propofol as a sole anesthetic agent in pregnant ewes demonstrated maternal hemodynamics superior to those of isoflurane anesthesia [60]. The uterine blood flow profile was similar in both techniques. Propofol–sevoflurane anesthesia in pregnant ewes and goats demonstrated that fetal physiology was maintained following propofol administration, but hemodynamic indices decreased after exposure to sevoflurane [60,61]. These studies support the use of propofol in a balanced general anesthesia protocol for cesarean section.

Etomidate is a short-acting non-barbiturate hypnotic. In dosages suitable for anesthetic induction, etomidate induces rapid anesthesia with minimal cardiovascular effects in dogs [62,63]. Etomidate is rapidly redistributed and metabolized by hepatic microsomal enzymes and by plasma esterase. Based on its rapid elimination profile in cats, etomidate may be suitable for repeated intravenous administration in low doses in this species [63]. However, repeated administration of etomidate may also cause acute hemolysis, as has been reported in dogs [64]. Etomidate frequently causes pain on intravenous injection in non-premedicated patients [65]. In addition, myoclonus or involuntary movements can occur upon injection; these side effects can be prevented by premedication with benzodiazepines and/or opioids; however, these drugs may exacerbate neonatal depression.

Alfaxalone is a widely used short-acting hypnotic used for anesthetic induction in companion animals. There have been a series of reports comparing its use to propofol in cesarean section anesthesia [66–70]. Several studies compare the use of either propofol or alfaxalone in combination with inhalant (isoflurane, sevoflurane) anesthesia. Puppy vigor immediately following delivery and two-day survival are equal to, or better, with an alfaxalone-based protocol compared to a propofol-based protocol [66,69]. Greater puppy depression and lower Apgar scores at time of delivery were noted when alfaxalone was used as the sole anesthetic agent compared to when it was used for induction and followed by isoflurane [68].

Dissociatives

Ketamine has been used in general anesthesia for cesarean section. In women, doses of less than 1 mg/kg induced minimal neonatal depression [38]. Alternatively, thiopental (2–3 mg/kg) and ketamine (0.5 mg/kg) have been co-administered to induce anesthesia in parturient women [38]. Low doses of ketamine (3–5 mg/kg IV in dogs, 2–4 mg/kg IV in cats, and 2 mg/kg IV in horses) may be used for anesthetic induction [71,72]. Because effective induction doses for these agents are higher in companion animals than humans, neonatal depression is more likely to be associated with their use. A retrospective cohort study in dogs indicated that ketamine use leads to increased incidence of respiratory depression, apnea, decreased vocalization, and increased mortality in newborn puppies [41,42]. For these reasons, ketamine should be used cautiously in this species. A case report describes the use of ketamine for anesthesia in a late-term gravid cow that required a metacarpal repair; anesthesia was induced with 2 mg/kg ketamine IV and 0.6 mg/kg/h continuous ketamine infusion (in combination with xylazine infusion and isoflurane) and the dam delivered a healthy calf 1 month after the procedure [73]. No data for comparative fetal viability are available in other species.

Little information is available regarding the use of tiletamine–zolazepam for cesarean section. Based on its pharmacologic profile, the characteristics of this proprietary drug mixture are qualitatively similar to those of other dissociative–benzodiazepine mixtures. *In vivo* characteristics of these agents suggest that caution should be exercised in companion animal cesarean section anesthesia because of their rapid and extensive transplacental transfer and absence of a specific dissociative antagonist.

Neuroleptanalgesia

The combination of opioid and tranquilizer class drugs can induce anesthesia effectively in depressed and exhausted patients. As noted above, both opioids and tranquilizers extensively cross the utero-placental interface and may cause significant fetal depression. These agents are usually used as an anesthetic supplement following fetal removal, although they have been successfully used for induction and maintenance prior to fetal extraction. If fetal depression is noted after administration of these agents, sublingual or intranasal administration of 0.4 mg/mL naloxone (10–20 μg, 1–2 drops) rapidly reverses opioid effects in neonates; alternatively, 0.1 mg/kg IV or intraosseous can be administered. Continuous monitoring for neonatal renarcotization is warranted [63].

Inhalation anesthetics

Inhalation anesthetics may be used to maintain general anesthesia. These agents readily cross the placenta with rapid fetal and maternal equilibration. The degree of neonatal depression is proportional to the depth of anesthesia induced in the mother. Deep levels of maternal anesthesia cause maternal hypotension, decreased uterine blood flow, and fetal acidosis. Isoflurane, sevoflurane, and desflurane are preferred because induction and recovery of mother and neonate are more rapid. Nitrous oxide can be used to potentiate their effects, thus decreasing the total amount of volatile agent administered; however, this effect is less in animals compared to humans because of the difference in the MAC of nitrous oxide. In humans, nitrous oxide administered at 60% or less has minimal effect on fetal depression. Neonatal diffusion hypoxia does not occur upon delivery [33,34].

Neuromuscular blocking agents

Neuromuscular blocking agents are infrequently used in veterinary medicine during pregnancy or at parturition. These drugs cross the placenta to a very limited extent and have little effect on neonates when used in clinical doses. Because of this property, these drugs can be useful in balanced anesthesia techniques for cesarean section to facilitate rapid airway management and provide surgical site relaxation [30,33,34]. If a neuromuscular blocking agent is selected, atracurium and vecuronium are preferred due to their intermediate duration of action. Long-acting agents, such as pancuronium and doxacurium, are avoided because of their length of action compared with procedure time [34]. Whenever neuromuscular blocking agents are administered, controlled positive-pressure ventilation must be utilized and nondepolarizing agents should be reversed.

Guaifenesin

Guaifenesin is a centrally acting muscle relaxant used to relax skeletal muscle in horses, cattle, and small ruminants. Although reports are limited, clinical impressions indicate that transplacental transfer is minimal based on vigor of the newborn after delivery.

Local anesthetics

Local anesthetics are frequently used in combination with other agents or as the sole anesthetic agent for regional techniques. Esters of *para*-aminobenzoic acid (procaine or tetracaine) are metabolized by maternal and fetal plasma cholinesterase (also known variably as butyrylcholinesterase or pseudocholinesterase). Hence, there is little accumulation of these agents in the fetus. Amide derivatives (e.g., lidocaine, mepivacaine, bupivacaine, etidocaine, and ropivacaine) are metabolized by hepatic microsomal enzymes. After absorption from the injection site, blood levels decrease slowly but can reach significant concentrations in the fetus. Neonatal blood concentrations in excess of 3 μg/mL of lidocaine or mepivacaine can cause neonatal depression at delivery. These concentrations rarely occur after epidural administration but can occur with excessive drug volumes when used for local infiltration [30].

Sympathetic blockade resulting in maternal hypotension and decreased uteroplacental perfusion may occur after epidural injection. This can be controlled by judicious administration of IV fluids to offset the increased capacity of the vascular system [74,75]. In addition to IV fluids, vasopressors can be used to treat maternal hypotension caused by sympathetic blockade. Because ephedrine acts centrally and has minimal arterial vasoconstrictor properties while increasing venous tone and preload, it can be used to treat maternal hypotension, thus restoring uterine blood flow [75]. Mephentermine acts in a similar manner. Other agents with α_1-adrenergic receptor activity increase maternal blood pressure by increasing systemic vascular resistance. However, they may cause uterine blood flow to decrease, and fetal deterioration often occurs. In addition, these agents can stimulate hypertonic uterine contractions, further decreasing uteroplacental perfusion.

Supplemental agents

Antiemetics

Concerns regarding emesis or passive regurgitation immediately following anesthesia induction have been reported in human obstetric literature. This concern arises from recent food ingestion coupled with delayed gastrointestinal transit time noted with pregnancy. To reduce patient risk of regurgitation and aspiration, several drug classes have been recommended. The recommended drugs are targeted to modify one or more of the following: gastroesophageal sphincter tone, gastric pH, downstream movement of gastrointestinal contents, or the vomiting reflex. Currently, recommendations for parturient human patients include administration of an H_2-receptor antagonist, non-particulate antacid, and a prokinetic prior to anesthesia induction. Reports suggest that maropitant, a central-acting antiemetic, is highly effective in reducing emesis in dogs during the perioperative period [76]. Its application in veterinary obstetric anesthesia is still not defined.

Inotropes and vasopressors

Inotropic and vasopressor agents may be required during general anesthesia, especially in a physiologically compromised dam. A meta-analysis from 2020 in humans evaluated several vasopressors for the treatment of hypotension during cesarean section in humans and found that norepinephrine better preserved umbilical acid–base status compared with phenylephrine and ephedrine [74]. A previous meta-analysis demonstrated the superiority of phenylephrine to ephedrine in maintenance of umbilical pH and fetal acidosis [75]. These studies both support the use of norepinephrine or phenylephrine for maternal hypotension; however, norepinephrine may be associated with better fetal outcomes.

Anesthetic techniques for cesarean section

Selection of an anesthetic protocol for cesarean section should prioritize the safety of the mother and fetus, patient comfort, and the veterinarian's familiarity with the selected anesthetic drugs. A major goal of drug selection should be to maintain maternal homeostasis and minimize fetal depression. Fetal depression may result from changes in placental perfusion associated with uterine contractions, thereby increasing the risk of fetal hypoxemia, acidosis, and stress. The veterinarian is faced with the dilemma of having to anesthetize a physiologically compromised mother without adversely affecting the fetus.

General anesthesia

Cesarean section anesthesia can be accomplished by either regional or general anesthesia. General anesthesia is often selected for performing cesarean sections in dogs, cats, and horses. Advantages of general anesthesia include speed and ease of induction, reliability, reproducibility, and control. General anesthesia provides optimum operating conditions with relaxed immobile patients. Tracheal intubation ensures control of the maternal airway, thereby preventing aspiration of vomitus or regurgitated gastrointestinal tract contents. In addition, it provides a route for maternal oxygen administration and ventilation if needed. When general anesthesia is administered and monitored properly, maternal cardiopulmonary function is well maintained [38,72].

General anesthesia may be more appropriate than regional anesthesia in selected clinical situations. These include severe maternal hypovolemia, prolonged dystocia in which the mother is exhausted and the fetus is severely stressed, maternal cardiac disease or failure, morbid obesity, brachycephalic dogs with upper airway obstruction, and cases in which the mother is so aggressive or fractious as to preclude regional anesthesia. Additionally, if the safety or value of the mother is more important than that of the offspring to the client, general anesthesia will likely allow more intensive anesthetic management of maternal problems. Finally, most veterinarians are more confident in their ability to induce general anesthesia safely than to use regional anesthesia techniques alone. Ideally, a combination of general anesthesia with a local anesthetic technique is used.

General anesthesia does, however, have certain disadvantages. It will likely produce greater neonatal depression than regional anesthesia. Inadequate anesthetic depth may induce maternal catecholamine release, which may result in hypertension and decreased uteroplacental perfusion, leading to both maternal and fetal stress and deterioration of cardiopulmonary function [30,41]. Loss of airway protective reflexes following anesthetic induction may result in aspiration and airway management challenges if the trachea is not properly intubated. Aspiration and inability to intubate the trachea successfully are the leading causes of maternal mortality associated with cesarean section in women. Fortunately, most dogs, cats, and horses are relatively easy to intubate because of their anatomic features. Brachycephalic breeds often pose a challenge due to anatomical abnormalities of the upper airway. Swine are relatively difficult to intubate, and this may present a challenge to the anesthetist.

Horses

Dystocia in mares has a profound effect on the survival of foals [77–79]. Foals are normally delivered within 20–30 min after chorioallantoic membrane rupture. Few foals survive when the duration is increased to 40 min, and none are likely to survive when the duration is 90 min or longer [78,79]. The time from chorioallantoic rupture to delivery is significantly different in surviving versus non-surviving foals [77,80]. This makes dystocia in mares more of an emergency than it is for most species [78–80].

Physical examination, anesthetic induction, and delivery should be accomplished in the shortest period possible when there is the chance of delivering a live foal [78]. Time-consuming techniques for anesthetic induction should be abandoned in favor of methods that provide reliable sedation and smooth, controlled induction with favorable recoveries. Goals for anesthesia are no different than for performing cesarean section in other species, but with a greater emphasis placed on rapid procedure completion. Laboring mares are typically agitated and distressed prior to anesthetic induction; good sedation is, therefore, important to ensure a smooth and safe induction. Xylazine and detomidine will provide sufficient sedation and can be reversed in the foal after delivery. Detomidine may cause less increase in uterine tone than xylazine and has been suggested by some as the sedative of choice in mares [47]. When butorphanol is combined with xylazine or detomidine, reliable restraint and analgesia occur. The dose of xylazine or detomidine can be lowered when combined with butorphanol, minimizing potential side effects of the α_2-adrenergic receptor agonists.

Anesthesia induction can be rapidly achieved with ketamine and diazepam (Table 45.2). Anesthesia is then maintained with isoflurane or sevoflurane in 100% oxygen [78]. While vaginal delivery is attempted, the ventral abdomen is clipped and prepared so that, if needed, cesarean section may be accomplished rapidly. In one report, this approach to dystocia resulted in 94% of vaginal delivery mares and 89% of cesarean section mares surviving to discharge with a 42% delivery of live foals and nearly 30% of foals surviving to discharge [81]. In this scenario, specific choice of anesthetic agent is probably less important than the time to induction and delivery of the foal. Studies have been carried out comparing the effects of isoflurane and halothane in pregnant mares, and no marked differences in outcome were noted [82]. Less soluble agents (such as isoflurane and sevoflurane) have the advantage of being more rapidly cleared from foals after delivery than halothane [83]. In pony mares premedicated with acepromazine, butorphanol, and detomidine, induced with detomidine–ketamine, and maintained with propofol, cardiovascular function was preserved in both the mare and the fetus [84]. In the field, where equipment is not readily available for delivering inhalation anesthesia, a guaifenesin–ketamine–xylazine mixture has been infused to effect for up to 1 h to maintain an adequate level of central nervous system depression [85].

Monitoring and support of an anesthetized pregnant mare are no different than for any anesthetized horse. Care should be taken to avoid maternal hypoxemia in order to preserve fetal oxygenation until delivery; arterial blood gases should be assessed. Mechanical ventilation should be considered to help offset the ventilation–perfusion mismatching that occurs under general anesthesia. Positive-pressure ventilation in a mare with severe abdominal distension has the potential to drastically decrease cardiac output and to compromise perfusion of all tissues including the uterus and placenta. Arterial blood pressure should be monitored directly and ideally kept above a mean value of 70 mmHg by adjusting anesthetic depth, rate of fluid delivery, and judicious use of inotropes and/or vasopressors when indicated.

Mares recovering from dystocia or cesarean section may have a difficult time regaining the strength needed to stand. Special attention should be given to the condition of the recovery area. The recovery floor should be cleaned of all obstetric lubricant and dried. Mares should be placed on a well-padded surface and may be rope-assisted during recovery when necessary.

Dogs and cats

Many general anesthesia techniques for cesarean section in dogs and cats have been reported to be satisfactory (Table 45.2) [86,87]. All reported techniques have common strategies for successful patient management, which include the following: (1) induction of anesthesia must be smooth and rapid; (2) intubation should be accomplished quickly, and ventilation supported to ensure adequate oxygenation; and (3) the drugs and technique selected should maintain fetal viability as much as possible.

As previously noted, studies have compared the outcome on maternal safety and fetal vitality of several commonly used anesthesia protocols used in cesarean section. The results of these studies indicated that, in dogs, propofol or alfaxalone followed by isoflurane anesthesia resulted in newborn survival rates comparable to those using epidural anesthesia and superior to those with general anesthesia induced with thiopental [41,42,67,69,70]. Sevoflurane has also been reported to result in viable newborns when used in cesarean section anesthesia protocols [88]. Comparable studies have not been performed in cats; however, their maternal–fetal anatomy and physiology support similar success with this strategy [89].

Supplemental oxygen administration to the newborn can significantly increase viability following surgical extraction. Supplemental oxygen administration to the mother is not associated with a decrease in uterine blood flow or fetal acidosis [34]. Fetal red blood cells have a lower 2,3-diphosphoglycerate concentration than do adult red blood cells; hence, fetal hemoglobin can carry more oxygen at low oxygen tensions than can adult hemoglobin. Physiologically, this is important because it ensures a higher level of hemoglobin saturation at the normally low oxygen partial pressures (PO_2 of umbilical vein blood is 30 mmHg) to which the fetus is exposed. Inspired oxygen concentrations of 50% or more during general anesthesia result in more vigorous neonates because of

Table 45.2 Selected anesthesia techniques for elective and emergency cesarean section anesthesia in common domestic species. Each case will require individual assessment so that the most suitable protocol is chosen.

	Drug or technique		
	Elective cesarean section	**Emergency cesarean section**	**General comments**
Dog	1. Propofol 4–8 mg/kg *or* Alfaxalone 1.5–2.5 mg/kg Isoflurane or sevoflurane +/– Lumbosacral epidural[a] Post-delivery analgesics 2. Fentanyl 3–5 μg/kg Propofol 2–3 mg/kg *or* Alfaxalone 1–2 mg/kg *or* Etomidate 1–2 mg/kg Isoflurane or sevoflurane +/– Lumbosacral epidural[a] Post-delivery analgesics 3. Dexmedetomidine 2 μg/kg Propofol 2–3 mg/kg *or* Alfaxalone 1–2 mg/kg *or* Etomidate 1–2 mg/kg Isoflurane or sevoflurane +/– Lumbosacral epidural[a] Post-delivery analgesics	1. +/– Sedation Lumbosacral epidural[a] 2. Propofol 4–8 mg/kg *or* Alfaxalone 1.5–2.5 mg/kg Isoflurane or sevoflurane +/– Lumbosacral epidural[a] Post-delivery analgesics 3. Fentanyl 3–5 μg/kg Propofol 2–3 mg/kg *or* Alfaxalone 1–2 mg/kg *or* Etomidate 1–2 mg/kg Isoflurane or sevoflurane +/– Lumbosacral epidural[a] Post-delivery analgesics 4. Dexmedetomidine 2 μg/kg Propofol 2–3 mg/kg *or* Alfaxalone 1–2 mg/kg *or* Etomidate 1–2 mg/kg Isoflurane or sevoflurane +/– Lumbosacral epidural[a] Post-delivery analgesics	Epidural patients not under general anesthesia may need to be restrained by an assistant; induction of general anesthesia may be required if the patient resists restraint Preoxygenate mother if possible and administer oxygen to neonates post-delivery Minimal inhalant agent use until all fetuses are delivered Reverse dexmedetomidine with sublingual atipamezole if fetal depression is evident Reverse fentanyl with sublingual naloxone if fetal depression is evident
Cat	1. Propofol 4–8 mg/kg *or* Alfaxalone 1.5–2.5 mg/kg Isoflurane or sevoflurane +/– Lumbosacral epidural[a] Post-delivery analgesics 2. Fentanyl 3–5 μg/kg Propofol 2–4 mg/kg *or* Alfaxalone 1–2 mg/kg Isoflurane or sevoflurane +/– Lumbosacral epidural[a] Post-delivery analgesics 3. Ketamine 3 mg/kg Propofol 2–4 mg/kg *or* Alfaxalone 1–2 mg/kg Isoflurane or sevoflurane +/– Lumbosacral epidural[a] Post-delivery analgesics	1. Propofol 2–4 mg/kg *or* Alfaxalone 1–2 mg/kg Lumbosacral epidural[a] +/– Isoflurane or sevoflurane via face mask 2. Propofol 4–8 mg/kg *or* Alfaxalone 1.5–2.5 mg/kg Isoflurane or sevoflurane +/– Lumbosacral epidural[a] Post-delivery analgesics 3. Fentanyl 3–5 μg/kg Propofol 2–4 mg/kg *or* Alfaxalone 1–2 mg/kg Isoflurane or sevoflurane +/– Lumbosacral epidural[a] Post-delivery analgesics 4. Ketamine 3 mg/kg Propofol 2–4 mg/kg *or* Alfaxalone 1–2 mg/kg Isoflurane or sevoflurane +/– Lumbosacral epidural[a] Post-delivery analgesics	Epidural patients not under general anesthesia may need to be restrained by an assistant; induction of general anesthesia may be required if the patient resists restraint Preoxygenate mother if possible and administer oxygen to neonates post-delivery Minimal inhalant agent dose until all fetuses are delivered Reverse fentanyl with sublingual naloxone if fetal depression is evident

	Drug or technique	General comments
Horse	1. +/– Xylazine 0.5 mg/kg Guaifenesin to effect Ketamine 2 mg/kg Isoflurane or sevoflurane Caudal epidural for pain management 2. Xylazine 0.8 mg/kg Ketamine 2.2 mg/kg Diazepam 0.08 mg/kg Isoflurane or sevoflurane Caudal epidural for pain management	Standing restraint and regional anesthesia is not performed in cesarean section in horses Postoperative pain management plan similar to that used for colic patients

(*Continued*)

Table 45.2 (Continued)

	Drug or technique	General comments
Cattle	1. Xylazine 10 mg Distal paravertebral block 2. Xylazine 10 mg Inverted L-block 3. Xylazine 10 mg Incisional line block 4. Xylazine 10 mg Guaifenesin to recumbency Isoflurane or sevoflurane following intubation	Avoid recumbency with regional block Reverse xylazine in newborns if depression is noted Supplemental analgesia in postoperative period as warranted Caudal epidural to decrease post-parturient "straining"
Sheep/ Goat	1. Xylazine 0.05–0.1 mg/kg *or* Dexmedetomidine 5–20 μg/kg Lumbosacral epidural 2. Xylazine 0.05–0.1 mg/kg *or* Dexmedetomidine 5–20 μg/kg Incisional line block 3. Propofol 3–5 mg/kg Isoflurane or sevoflurane following intubation	Variable and inconsistent response to opioids for pain management α_2-Adrenergic receptor agonists are frequently used for supplemental analgesia
Pig	1. Dexmedetomidine 5–20 μg/kg *or* Romifidine 60–100 μg/kg Lumbosacral epidural 2. Dexmedetomidine 5–20 μg/kg *or* Romifidine 60–100 μg/kg Incisional line block 3. Propofol 4–6 mg/kg Isoflurane or sevoflurane	Will require sedation in addition to regional analgesia for elective cesarean section in pigs Good response to opioid analgesic agents following fetal removal
Llama	1. Guaifenesin to effect Propofol 2–4 mg/kg Isoflurane or sevoflurane following intubation	Limited reports in literature Pain management following fetal removal

[a] Dog/cat lumbosacral epidural = 1 mg/kg lidocaine or 0.5 mg/kg bupivacaine + 0.1 mg/kg morphine

improved oxygenation [34]. Therefore, oxygen administration is indicated regardless of the anesthetic protocol.

Tidal and minute ventilation must be critically evaluated during the anesthetic period to avoid either hypoventilation or hyperventilation. The overall effect of carbon dioxide on the fetus is not clear, but passive hyperventilation of the mother causes hypocapnia with decreased uterine artery blood flow [90]. Decreased placental perfusion may result in fetal hypoxia, hypercapnia, and acidosis. When a physiologically normal arterial oxygen level is present, a modest increase in $PaCO_2$ is well tolerated by the fetus [34]. Adequacy of ventilation and oxygenation may be assessed by observing rate of respiration, excursion of the chest wall and/or reservoir bag, and color of mucous membranes, as well as monitoring hemoglobin saturation using pulse oximetry, end-tidal CO_2 using capnography, and arterial PaO_2 and $PaCO_2$ measurement using blood gas analysis.

Maintaining hemodynamic perfusion indices is essential for the safety and vitality of both the mother and fetus. Blood pressure should be monitored and kept above a mean arterial pressure of 70 mmHg by adjusting anesthetic depth and rate of fluid delivery, and by administering inotropes and vasopressors, as needed.

Regional anesthesia

Regional anesthesia techniques are well established for cesarean section. There is increased sensitivity to, and distribution of, local anesthetic agents during gestation and parturition. This is due, in part, to changes in regional blood flow whereby vertebral venous sinuses assume an increased role in venous drainage compared to other veins closer to the gravid uterus. Increased venous flow and distention results in reduced epidural space volume, thereby increasing distribution of an equivolume epidural injection to a greater area than in non-gravid patients. Because of this change, the dose and/or volume of local anesthetic for epidural or spinal anesthesia can be reduced by approximately one-third in pregnant patients as compared with non-parturients to achieve an equivalent distribution and regional nerve block.

Neuraxial anesthesia (epidural or subarachnoid) has the advantages of technique simplicity, minimal exposure of the fetus to maternally administered drugs, and less intraoperative bleeding. In addition, muscle relaxation and analgesia are optimal. Caudal spinal anatomy in the lumbosacral region varies by species. The spinal cord terminates at the level of the sixth lumbar vertebra in dogs, reducing the risk of subarachnoid (true spinal) injection of the anesthetic agent. The spinal cord terminates variably between L7 and mid-sacrum in cats, making subarachnoid injection a greater possibility [89]. In swine and ruminants, the spinal cord terminates at the mid-sacrum, making subarachnoid injection a possibility at the lumbosacral junction.

Disadvantages of epidural or subarachnoid anesthesia include hypotension secondary to sympathetic blockade. Hypotension induced by epidural anesthesia can be managed with IV fluid and vasopressor administration. Lactated Ringer's solution or 0.9 or 0.45% sodium chloride mixed with equal volumes of 5% dextrose solution can be administered at approximately 20 mL/kg over 15–20 min to maintain arterial blood pressure. When hypotension is severe (MAP < 60 mm Hg), vasopressors should be administered [74,75]. Hypotension and visceral manipulation during the procedure can cause nausea and vomiting. Because the mother remains conscious, the forelimbs and head often move and may interfere with surgery. Epidural or subarachnoid techniques cannot be used in highly excited or fractious patients or in mares because they panic when they are unable to stand.

The combination of an epidural with a general anesthetic technique allows for reduction in inhalant and analgesic or sedative agent requirements resulting in a reduced incidence of hypotension, bradycardia, and hypoventilation. In addition, the dam is provided analgesia without the need for sedating agents in the postoperative period allowing for more rapid nursing and discharge.

Dogs and cats

Epidural anesthesia has been successfully used in dogs and cats for cesarean section anesthesia [77,78]. Traditionally, a short-acting local anesthetic drug is administered at a dose of 1 mL per 3.25–4.5 kg of body weight in the epidural space to provide surgical site anesthesia. The local anesthetic may be supplemented with epidural opioids and α_2-adrenergic receptor agonists to extend the postoperative analgesic period. Epidural morphine may also be administered as a sole adjunct to general anesthesia to provide extended analgesia in the postoperative period.

Pigs

Epidural and spinal techniques work well in sows. The technique is well established and not difficult to perform (Chapter 66). When using this technique, it is sometimes necessary to restrain the head and forelimbs. If sows are sedated and restrained in lateral recumbency with the head extended, the soft palate may occlude the airway and the patient may suffocate. Because cesarean section in swine is often viewed as a last-ditch effort by producers, it is often delayed until the sow's overall condition has severely deteriorated. Therefore, a high percentage of sows presented for cesarean section demonstrate hypovolemia and hypotension. Fluids can be readily administered to sows via indwelling venous catheters placed prior to anesthetic administration. This will restore circulating volume and offset hypotension induced by neuraxial techniques.

Cattle, sheep, and goats

Epidural anesthesia may be safely used in ewes, does, and cows. Epidural and spinal anesthesia often induces recumbency, which is undesirable in large ruminants. An alternative is to perform a standing cesarean section in cattle using either a proximal or distal paravertebral block or inverted L-block of the left flank (Chapter 66) [91]. In cows that are in poor condition, exhausted, or in shock, the distal technique is preferred because it does not induce a scoliosis-like position and the cow is more likely to remain standing throughout the procedure. Acepromazine does not cause uterine contractions and can be used with or without xylazine for minor sedation during standing procedures in cows [91]. In llamas and alpacas, the majority of fetuses reside in the left uterine horn, so the dam should be restrained in right lateral recumbency [92]. A combination of butorphanol with xylazine has been used successfully [93]. An epidural, spinal, or local infusion technique should be incorporated for analgesia.

Local anesthesia

An infiltrative "field block" technique may be used but has several disadvantages compared with regional techniques. Infiltration requires larger amounts of local anesthetic agent, which is systemically absorbed and can create fetal depression. In addition, muscle relaxation and analgesia are not as profound or as uniform compared with regional anesthesia. In many cases, field block anesthesia is supplemented with heavy sedation or tranquilization and these agents further contribute to maternal and fetal depression. For these reasons, field block techniques are often abandoned for either general or epidural anesthesia.

Care of the newborn

Following delivery, the newborn's head and face are manually cleared of fetal membranes, and the oropharynx is suctioned to remove fluid. The umbilical vessels should be milked toward the fetus to empty them of blood, clamped or ligated approximately 2–5 cm from the body wall, and severed from the placenta. Neonates can then be gently rubbed with a towel to dry them and stimulate breathing. Vigorous motion should be avoided to prevent amniotic fluid displacement from the lungs as this is critical for normal distribution of pulmonary surfactant in the alveoli. The head and neck should be supported and not shaken to avoid whiplash and prevent cerebral injury [94]. Flow-by oxygen administration in the vicinity of the muzzle is helpful to increase heart rate and oxygen delivery to tissues in distressed, exhausted neonates. Reversal of opioids by sublingual or intranasal administration of 1–2 drops (10–20 μg) of naloxone is warranted in cases where opioids were administered as part of the general anesthesia technique. An oral dose of 2.5% dextrose (0.1–0.5 mL) is helpful to improve energy substrates required for initial breathing effort in stressed neonates. Finally, maintaining warmth is vital because hypothermia can occur rapidly after birth [95].

A small IV catheter may be used to intubate and deliver oxygen in small neonates that do not begin to spontaneously breathe. Ventilatory support can be provided by using a syringe as a ventilator and three-way valve attached to an oxygen source. Oxygen is aspirated into the syringe and the valve repositioned so that small breaths can be given to the neonate. As a final option, doxapram can be used to stimulate breathing in neonates. In puppies, a dosage of 1–5 mg (approximately 1–5 drops from a 20–22 gauge needle) is topically administered onto the oral mucosa or injected intramuscularly or subcutaneously. In kittens, the dosage is 1–2 mg (approximately 1–2 drops from a 20–22 gauge needle). Airways must be cleared before doxapram administration.

External thoracic compressions may be warranted if the heart rate is slow and does not respond to support measures [95]. The use of atropine in the neonate is controversial as neonatal bradycardia is likely due to hypoxemia. The 2020 American Heart Association cardiopulmonary resuscitation (CPR) guidelines for neonates do not include the use of atropine but instead recommend epinephrine if there is no response to basic life support measures. A rapid physical examination to identify potential genetic defects (i.e., cleft palate, chest deformity, or abdominal wall fusion) is also important to determine viability of the neonate. Newborn puppy viability has been correlated with umbilical vein blood lactate concentrations [96]. Umbilical vein lactate levels > 5 mmol/L were correlated with increased neonatal mortality within 48 h of delivery. Five-minute Apgar scores have also been evaluated in puppies as a prognostic indicator of early survival [97]. Puppies with scores in the 7–10 range had greater 48-h survival rates compared to those with lower scores.

When general anesthesia is used in ruminants or horses, the oropharynx can be cleared of fluid, and the trachea intubated after the fetal head is delivered through the uterine incision. The fetus can then be delivered and the umbilical cord severed. Because the uteroplacental and umbilical circulation is preserved until the airway is secured, hypoxia is prevented. Once the fetus is delivered, ventilation can be supported, if necessary, via a bag valve mask (Ambu®) resuscitator.

After completion of surgery and recovery from anesthesia, the newborn can be introduced to the mother. If introduction is delayed, the neonates should be exposed briefly to the mother to allow intake of colostrum and then kept in a warm environment until anesthesia recovery is complete to avoid accidental crushing. If regional anesthesia was used, newborns can be placed with their mother as soon as the surgery is complete.

Postoperative pain management

This represents a challenge in cesarean section patients because of concerns regarding transfer of anesthetic and analgesic drugs into milk and its impact on neonates. This area has been extensively studied in people and in food-producing species. Most of the current information is from humans and cattle; however, because of the similarity of the lactation process in all mammals, the information may be extrapolated to other species.

Codeine, propoxyphene, and morphine are well tolerated by newborns when used in maternal pain management, even when repeat doses are administered over several days [98]. Meperidine (pethidine) has been reported to cause decreased suckling behavior and sedation when used in serial doses [98,99]. Fentanyl and sufentanil are not detectable in breast milk after epidural administration in humans [100].

NSAIDs appear to reach only limited levels in milk after maternal administration. In humans, acetaminophen and aspirin are considered compatible with breastfeeding [98]. Studies evaluating carprofen in cattle indicated that milk levels were below detectable limits (< 0.022 μg/mL) after a single-dose administration. After experimental induction of mastitis, carprofen was detected at low levels (0.16 μg/mL) for 12 h following single-bolus administration and decreased to undetectable levels (< 0.022 μg/mL) by 24 h [101]. Similar results have recently been reported in the dog [102]. Following a single dose of ketoprofen (3.3 mg/kg) in cattle, detectable but non-quantifiable concentrations were present in milk for only 2 h [103]. Similar results have been reported in lactating goats [104]. Meloxicam is approved in the European Union and Canada for use in dairy cows [105]. Based on the evidence available, there is no contraindication for NSAID use in postpartum dams except where NSAIDs are contraindicated for other reasons (e.g., hypovolemia, renal disease). NSAID transfer from the dam to neonates is minimal and clinically insignificant [102,105].

Interest in locoregional pain control for post-cesarean section patients has gained momentum with the introduction of bupivacaine liposome injectable suspension (BLIS). In humans, BLIS is labeled for postoperative anesthesia in any surgical site [106]. It is used for postoperative cesarean section analgesia with the goals of extended duration pain control and reduced opioid requirement [106–109]. A randomized controlled clinical study found that BLIS wound infusion decreased incisional pain, motion pain, and opioid consumption for the first 48 h following surgery [110]. Another study evaluated BLIS use in transversus abdominis plane (TAP) block with and without intrathecal morphine for elective cesarean section in women. The combination of a BLIS TAP block and intrathecal morphine was superior for pain control at 24, 48, and 72 h compared to TAP block or intrathecal morphine alone [111]. Currently, BLIS is labeled for orthopedic procedures and onychectomy in companion animals [112]. Off-label use for abdominal and thoracic surgery in small animal patients is common in clinical practice.

Local anesthetic drugs (e.g., lidocaine and bupivacaine) and first-generation bupivacaine metabolites are excreted in milk after epidural administration in humans. Although these agents are detectable in milk, their influence on neonates is negligible based on maximum Apgar (activity, pulse, grimace, appearance, and respiration) scores after delivery [113]. A prospective cohort study evaluating the level of bupivacaine in breast milk after the use of BLIS for postoperative TAP blocks following elective cesarean sections found that bupivacaine was present in all plasma and milk samples. However, it was calculated that neonates would have consumed less than 1% of the maternal dose at any time point during the 96 hour study and this was not considered to be of clinical concern [114].

Based on current evidence, it appears that most commonly used analgesic drug classes may be safely administered during the lactation period without adverse effects on newborns.

References

1 Dawes GS. *Foetal and Neonatal Physiology: Comparative Study of the Changes at Birth*. Chicago, IL: Year Book Medical, 1968: 15.
2 Shnider SM. The physiology of pregnancy. *In: Annual Refresher Course Lectures American Society of Anesthesiologists.* 1978: 1251–1258.
3 Kerr MG. Cardiovascular dynamics in pregnancy and labor. *Br Med Bull* 1968; **24**(1): 19–24.
4 Ueland K, Parer JT. Effects of estrogens on the cardiovascular system of the ewe. *Am J Obstet Gynecol* 1966; **96**(3): 400–406.
5 Ueland K, Hansen JM. Maternal cardiovascular dynamics. II. Posture and uterine contractions. *Am J Obstet Gynecol* 1969; **103**(1): 1–7.
6 James EM. Physiologic changes during pregnancy. In: *Annual Refresher Course American Society of Anesthesiologists.* 1980: 1251–1255.
7 Humphries A, Mirjalili SA, Tarr GP, *et al.* Hemodynamic changes in women with symptoms of supine hypotensive syndrome. *Acta Obstet Gynecol Scand* 2019; **99**: 631–636.
8 Pei-Shan Zhao. Supine hypotensive syndrome: a comprehensive review of literature. *Transl Perioper & Pain Med* 2014; **1**(2): 22–26.
9 Scott DB. Inferior vena caval occlusion in late pregnancy. *Clin Anesth* 1974; **10**(2): 37–50.
10 Stoneham AE, Graham J, Rozanski EA, *et al.* Pregnancy-associated congestive heart failure in a cat. *J Am Anim Hosp Assoc* 2006; **42**(6): 457–461.
11 Lipton B, Hershey SC, Baez S. Compatibility of oxytocics with anesthetic agents. *JAMA* 1962; **179**(6): 410–416.
12 Katz D, Beilin Y. Disorders of coagulation in pregnancy. *Br J Anaesth* 2015; **115**(Suppl 2): ii75–ii88.
13 LoMauro A, Aliverti A. Respiratory physiology of pregnancy: physiology masterclass. *Breathe (Sheff)* 2015; **11**(4): 297–301.
14 Ambros B, Carrozzo MV, Jones T. Desaturation times between dogs preoxygenated via face mask or flow-by technique before induction of anesthesia. *Vet Anaesth Analg* 2018; **45**(4): 452–458.
15 Thomas C, Lumb AB. Physiology of haemoglobin. *Contin Educ Anaesth Crit Care & Pain* 2012; **12**: 251–256.
16 Benner A, Patel AK, Singh K, *et al.* Physiology, Bohr Effect. StatPearls 2022 PMID: 30252284.
17 Griffiths SK, Campbell JP. Placental structure, function and drug transfer. *Contin Educ Anaesth Crit Care & Pain* 2015; **15**: 84–89.
18 Anagnostou, TL, Savvas I, Kazakos GM, *et al.* The effect of the stage of the ovarian cycle (anoestrus or dioestrus) and of pregnancy on the incidence of gastro-

oesophageal reflux in dogs undergoing ovariohysterectomy. *Vet Anaesth Analg* 2015; **42**(5): 502–511.

19 Paddleford RR. Anesthesia for cesarean section in the dog. *Vet Clin North Am Small Anim Pract* 1992; **22**(2): 481–484.

20 Resch BE, Ducza E, Gáspár R, *et al.* Role of adrenergic receptor subtypes in the control of human placental blood vessels. *Mol Reprod Dev* 2003; **66**(2): 166–171.

21 Chooi C, Cox JJ, Lumb RS, *et al.* Techniques for preventing hypotension during spinal anaesthesia for caesarean section. *Cochrane Database Syst Rev* 2017; **8**(8): CD002251.

22 Resch BE, Ducza E, Gáspár R, *et al.* Role of adrenergic receptor subtypes in the control of human placental blood vessels. *Mol Reprod Dev* 2003; **66**(2): 166–171.

23 Hoffmann B. Hormonal control of pregnancy and parturition in the dog. *In: Proceedings of the WSAVA.* 2004: 1–4.

24 Concannon PW. Understanding and monitoring canine pregnancy. *In: Proceedings of the WSAVA.* 2005: 1–7.

25 Verhage HG, Beamer NB, Brenner RM. Plasma levels of estradiol and progesterone in the cat during polyestrus, pregnancy and pseudopregnancy. *Biol Reprod* 1976; **14**(5): 579–585.

26 Root-Kustriz MV. Clinical management of pregnancy in cats. *Theriogenology* 2006; **66**(1): 145–150.

27 Taverne M, Noakes DE. Parturition and the care of parturient animals and the newborn. In: Noakes DE, Parkinson TJ, England GCW, eds. *Veterinary Reproduction and Obstetrics*, 10th edn. St. Louis, MO: WB Saunders, 2018: 115–147.

28 Kelleman AA. Equine pregnancy and clinical applied physiology. *In: Proceedings of the American Association of Equine Practitioners.* 2013; **59**: 350–358.

29 Conley AJ. Review of the reproductive endocrinology of the pregnant and parturient mare. *Theriogenology.* 2016; **86**(1): 355–365.

30 Alper MH. Perinatal pharmacology. *In: Annual Refresher Course American Society of Anesthesiologists.* 1979: 1261–1267.

31 Palahniuk RJ, Shnider SM, Eger EI. Pregnancy decreases the requirement for inhaled anesthetic agents. *Anesthesiology* 1974; **41**(1): 82–83.

32 Kostakis C, Anagnostou T, Savvas I, *et al.* The effect of progesterone on the anesthetic and analgesic requirements for ovariohysterectomy in the dog. *J Hel Vet Med Soc* 2019; **70**(3): 1717–1726.

33 Einster M. Perinatal pharmacology. In: *Annual Refresher Course Lectures American Society of Anesthesiologists.* 1980: 1261–1264.

34 Gutsche B. Perinatal pharmacology. *In: Annual Refresher Course American Society of Anesthesiologists.* 1978: 1291–1299.

35 Rosen MA, Weiskopf RB. Management of anesthesia for the pregnant surgical patient. *Anesthesiology* 1999; **91**: 1159–1164.

36 Theis JCW. Acetylsalicylic acid (ASA) and non-steroidal drugs (NSAIDS) during pregnancy: are they safe? *Can Fam Physician* 1996; **42**: 2347–2349.

37 Malm H, Borisch C. Analgesics, non-steroidal anti-inflammatory drugs (NSAIDs), muscle relaxants, and antigout medications. In: Schaefer C, Peters P, Miller R, eds. *Drugs During Pregnancy and Lactation Treatment Options and Risk Assessment*, 3rd edn. London, UK: Elsevier, 2015: 27–58.

38 Datta S, Alper MH. Anesthesia for cesarean section. *Anesthesiology* 1980; **53**(2): 142–160.

39 Jain R, Sharma R. A comparative study of effects of glycopyrrolate and ondansetron on nausea and vomiting in cesarean section under spinal anesthesia. *Anesth Essays Res* 2015; **9**(3): 348–352.

40 Moon PF, Erb HN, Ludders JW. Perioperative management and mortality rates of dogs undergoing cesarean section in the United States and Canada. *J Am Vet Med Assoc* 1998; **213**(3): 365–369.

41 Moon P, Erb H, Ludders J, *et al.* Perioperative risk factors for puppies delivered by cesarean section in the United States and Canada. *J Am Anim Hosp Assoc* 2000; **36**(4): 359–368.

42 Moon-Massat PF, Erb HN. Perioperative factors associated with puppy vigor after delivery by cesarean section. *J Am Anim Hosp Assoc* 2002; **38**(1): 90–96.

43 Tranquilli WJ, Lemke KA, Williams LL, *et al.* Flumazenil efficacy in reversing diazepam or midazolam overdose in dogs. *J Vet Pharmacol Ther* 1992; **19**: 65–68.

44 McDonnell W, Van Corder I. Cardiopulmonary effects of xylazine/ketamine in dogs [Abstract]. In: *Annual Scientific Meeting of the American College of Veterinary Anesthesiologists*, Las Vegas, NV, 1982.

45 Ryan SD, Wagner AE. Cesarean section in dogs: anesthetic management. *Compend Contin Educ Pract Vet* 2006; **28**(1): 44–45.

46 Terttu K, Oijala M. The effect of detomidine (Domosedan) on the maintenance of equine pregnancy and foetal development: ten cases. *Equine Vet J* 1988; **20**(5): 323–326.

47 Jedruch J, Gajewski Z, Kuussaari J. The effect of detomidine hydrochloride on the electrical activity of the uterus in pregnant mares. *Acta Vet Scand* 1989; **30**(3): 307–311.

48 Pyorala E, Koppinen J, Vainio O, *et al.* Detomidine in pregnant cows. *Nord Vet Med* 1986; **38**(4): 237–240.

49 Jedruch J, Gajewski Z, Ratajska-Michalczak K. Uterine motor responses to an alpha 2-adrenergic agonist medetomidine hydrochloride in the bitches during the end of gestation and the post-partum period. *Acta Vet Scand Suppl* 1989; **85**: 129–134.

50 De Cramer KGM, Joubert KE, Nöthling JO. Puppy survival and vigor associated with the use of low dose medetomidine premedication, propofol induction and maintenance of anesthesia using sevoflurane gas-inhalation for cesarean section in the bitch. *Theriogenology* 2017; **96**: 10–15.

51 Groppetti D, Di Cesare F, Pecile A, *et al.* Maternal and neonatal wellbeing during elective C-section induced with a combination of propofol and dexmedetomidine: how effective is the placental barrier in dogs? *Theriogenology* 2019; **129**: 90–98.

52 El-Tahan MR, Mowafi HA, Al Sheikh IH, *et al.* Efficacy of dexmedetomidine in suppressing cardiovascular and hormonal responses to general anaesthesia for cesarean delivery: a dose-response study. *Int J Obstet Anesth* 2012; **21**(3): 222–229.

53 Schatzmann U, Josseck H, Stauffer J-L, *et al.* Effects of α2-agonists on intrauterine pressure and sedation in horses: comparison between detomidine, romifidine and xylazine. *Zentralbl Veterinarmed A* 1994; **41**(7): 523–529.

54 Einarson A, Bonari L, Voyer-Lavigne S, *et al.* A multicentre prospective controlled study to determine the safety of trazodone and nefazodone use during pregnancy. *Can J Psychiatry* 2003; **48**(2): 106–110.

55 Patomo E, Hernandez-Diaz S, Huybrechts KF, *et al.* Gabapentin in pregnancy and the risk of adverse neonatal and maternal outcomes: a population-based cohort study nested in the US Medicaid Analytic eXtract dataset. *PLoS Med* 2020; **17**(9): e1003322.

56 Davanzo R, Dal Bo S, Bua J, *et al.* Antiepileptic drugs and breastfeeding. *Ital J Pediatr* 2013; **39**: 50.

57 Palahniuk RJ. Obstetric anesthesia in the healthy parturient. *In: Annual Refresher Course American Society of Anesthesiologists.* 1979: 1271–1274.

58 Hodgkinson R, Bhatt M, Wang CN. Double-blind comparison of the neurobehaviour of neonates following the administration of different doses of meperidine to the mother. *Can Anaesth Soc J* 1978; **25**(5): 405–411.

59 Funkquist PM, Nyman GC, Lofgren AJ, *et al.* Use of propofol-isoflurane as an anesthetic regimen for cesarean section in dogs. *J Am Vet Med Assoc* 1997; **211**(3): 313–317.

60 Gaynor JS, Wertz EM, Alvis M, *et al.* A comparison of the haemodynamic effects of propofol and isoflurane in pregnant ewes. *J Vet Pharmacol Ther* 1998; **21**(1): 69–73.

61 Setoyama K, Shinzato T, Misumi K, *et al.* Effects of propofol–sevoflurane anesthesia on the maternal and fetal hemodynamics blood gases, and uterine activity in pregnant goats. *J Vet Med Sci* 2003; **65**(10): 1075–1081.

62 Sams L, Braun C, Allman D, *et al.* A comparison of the effects of propofol and etomidate on the induction of anesthesia and on cardiopulmonary parameters in dogs. *Vet Anaesth Analg* 2008; **35**(6): 488–494.

63 Muir WW, Swanson CR. Principles, techniques, and complications of feline anesthesia and chemical restraint. In: Sherding R, ed. *The Cat: Diseases and Clinical Management.* New York, NY: Churchill Livingstone, 1989: 81–116.

64 Ko JCH, Thurmon JC, Benson GJ, *et al.* Acute haemolysis associated with etomidate-propylene glycol infusion in dogs. *Vet Anaesth Analg* 1993; **20**(2): 92–94.

65 Niedermirtl F, Eberhardt M, Namer B, *et al.* Etomidate and propylene glycol activate nociceptive TRP ion channels. *Mol Pain* 2018; **14**: 1744806918811699.

66 Doebeli A, Michel E, Bettschart R, *et al.* Apgar score after induction of anesthesia for canine cesarean section with alfaxalone versus propofol. *Theriogenology* 2013; **80**(8): 850–854.

67 Metcalfe S, Hulands-Nave A, Bell M, *et al.* Multicentre, randomised clinical trial evaluating the efficacy and safety of alfaxalone administered to bitches for induction of anaesthesia prior to cesarean section. *Aust Vet J* 2014; **92**(9): 333–338.

68 Conde Ruiz C, Del Carro AP, Rosset E, *et al.* Alfaxalone for total intravenous anaesthesia in bitches undergoing elective caesarean section and its effects on puppies: a randomized clinical trial. *Vet Anaesth Analg* 2016; **43**(3): 281–290.

69 Melandri M, Alonge S, Peric T, *et al.* Effects of alfaxalone or propofol on giant-breed dog neonates' viability during elective caesarean sections. *Animals* 2019; **9**(11): 962.

70 Haythornthwaite B. Comparison of the safety of alfaxalone and propofol as anaesthetic induction agents in bitches undergoing C-section. *Vet Evid* 2020; **5**(3).

71 Bidwell LA. Anesthesia for dystocia and anesthesia of the equine neonate. *Vet Clin North Am Equine Pract* 2013; **29**(1): 215–222.

72 Rankin D. Neonatal anesthesia. In: Greene SA, ed. *Veterinary Anesthesia and Pain Management Secrets.* Philadelphia, PA: Hanley & Belfus, 2002: 229–233.

73 Martin Jurado O, Jud R, Muggli E, *et al.* Balanced anaesthetic approach in a late-term gravid cow undergoing metacarpal fracture repair. *Case Rep Vet* 2011; **743827**: 1–5.

74 Singh PM, Singh NP, Reschke M, *et al.* Vasopressor drugs for the prevention and treatment of hypotension during neuraxial anaesthesia for Cesarean delivery: a

Bayesian network meta-analysis of fetal and maternal outcomes. *Br J Anaesth* 2020; **124**(3): e95–e107.

75 Xu C, Liu S, Huang Y, *et al.* Phenylephrine vs. ephedrine in cesarean delivery under spinal anesthesia: a systematic literature review and meta-analysis. *Int J Surg* 2018; **60**: 48–59.

76 Hay Kraus BL. Efficacy of maropitant in preventing vomiting in dogs premedicated with hydromorphone. *Vet Anaesth Analg* 2013; **40**(1): 28–34.

77 Youngquist RS. Equine obstetrics. In: Morrow DA, ed. *Current Therapy in Theriogenology*, 2nd edn. Philadelphia, PA: Saunders, 1986: 693–699.

78 Byron CR, Embertson RM, Bernard WV, *et al.* Dystocia in a referral hospital setting: approach and results. *Equine Vet J* 2010; **35**(1): 82–85.

79 Embertson RM. Dystocia and caesarean sections: the importance of duration and good judgment. *Equine Vet J* 1999; **31**(3): 179–180.

80 Freeman DE, Hungerford LL, Schaeffer D, *et al.* Cesarean section and other methods for assisted delivery: comparison of effects on mare mortality and complications. *Equine Vet J* 1999; **31**(3): 203–207.

81 Abernathy-Young KK, LeBlanc MM, Embertson RM, *et al.* Survival rates of mares and foals and postoperative complications and fertility of mares after cesarean section: 95 cases (1986–2000). *J Am Vet Med Assoc* 2012; **241**(7): 927–934.

82 Daunt DA, Steffey EP, Pascoe JR. Actions of isoflurane and halothane in pregnant mares. *J Am Vet Med Assoc* 1992; **201**(9): 1367–1374.

83 Wilson DV. Anesthesia and sedation for late-term mares. *Vet Clin North Am Equine Pract* 1994; **10**: 219–236.

84 Taylor PM, White KL, Fowden AL, *et al.* Propofol anaesthesia for surgery in late gestation pony mares. *Vet Anaesth Analg* 2001; **28**(4): 177–187.

85 Lin HC, Wallace RL, Harrison IW, *et al.* A case report on the use of guaifenesin-ketamine-xylazine anesthesia for equine dystocia. *Cornell Vet* 1994; **84**(1): 61–66.

86 Gilson SD. Cesarean section. In: Slatter D, ed. *Slatter's Textbook of Small Animal Surgery*, 3rd edn. Philadelphia, PA: Elsevier Science, 2003; **2**: 1517–1520.

87 Ryan SD, Wagner AE. Cesarean section in dogs: anesthetic management. *Compend Contin Educ Pract Vet* 2006; **28**(1): 44–45.

88 Vilar JM, Batista M, Perez R, *et al.* Comparison of three anesthetic protocols for the elective cesarean section in the dog: effects on the bitch and the newborn puppies. *Anim Reprod Sci* 2018; **190**: 53–62.

89 Hall LW, Taylor PM. *Anaesthesia of the Cat*. London, UK: Baillière Tindall, 1994.

90 Behrman RE, Parer JT, Novy MJ. Acute maternal respiratory alkalosis (hyperventilation) in the pregnant rhesus monkey. *Pediatr Res* 1967; **1**: 354–1363.

91 Seddighi R, Dougherty T. Field sedation and anesthesia of ruminants. *Vet Clin North Am Food Animal Pract* 2016; **32**(3): 553–570.

92 Ratto M, Urra F, Silva M. Laterality of ovulation and presence of the embryo do not affect uterine horn blood flow during the first month of gestation in llamas. *Front Vet Sci* 2020; **7**: 598117.

93 Vermunt JJ, Parkinson TJ, Noakes DE. Defects of presentation, position and posture in livestock: delivery by cesarean hysterotomy. In: Noakes DE, Parkinson TJ, England GCW, eds. *Veterinary Reproduction and Obstetrics*, 10th edn. St. Louis, MO: WB Saunders, 2018: 291–314.

94 Goericke-Pesch S, Wehrend A. New method for removing mucus from the upper respiratory tract of newborn puppies following cesarean section. *Vet Rec* 2012; **170**(11): 289.

95 Traas AM. Resuscitation of canine and feline neonates. *Theriogenology* 2008; **70**(3): 343–348.

96 Groppetti D, Pecile A, Del Carro AP, *et al.* Evaluation of newborn canine viability by means of umbilical vein lactate measurement, *Apgar score and uterine tocodynamometry. Theriogenology* 2010; **74**(7): 1187–1196.

97 Veronesi MC, Panzani S, Faustini M, *et al.* An Apgar scoring system for routine assessment of newborn puppy viability and short-term survival prognosis. *Theriogenology* 2009; **72**(3): 401–407.

98 Bar-Oz B, Bulkowstein M, Benyamini L, *et al.* Use of antibiotic and analgesic drugs during lactation. *Drug Saf* 2003; **26**(13): 925–935.

99 Wittels B, Glosten B, Faure EAM, *et al.* Postcesarean analgesia with both epidural morphine and intravenous patient-controlled analgesia. *Anesth Analg* 1997; **85**(3): 600–606.

100 Madej TH, Strunin L. Comparison of epidural fentanyl with sufentanil. *Anaesthesia* 1987; **42**(11): 1156–1161.

101 Lohuis JACM, Werven T, Brand A, *et al.* Pharmacodynamics and pharmacokinetics of carprofen, a non-steroidal anti-inflammatory drug, in healthy cows and cows with Escherichia coli endotoxin-induced mastitis. *J Vet Pharmacol Ther* 1991; **14**(3): 219–229.

102 Ferrari D, Lundgren S, Holmberg J, *et al.* Concentration of carprofen in the milk of lactating bitches after cesarean section and during inflammatory conditions. *Theriogenology* 2022; **181**: 59–68.

103 De Graves FJ, Riddell MG, Schumacher J. Ketoprofen concentrations in plasma and milk after intravenous administration in dairy cattle. *Am J Vet Res* 1996; **57**(7): 1031–1034.

104 Musser JMB, Anderson KL, Tyczkowska KL. Pharmacokinetic parameters and milk concentrations of ketoprofen after administration as a single intravenous bolus dose to lactating goats. *J Vet Pharmacol Ther* 1998; **21**(5): 358–363.

105 Warner R, Ydstie JA, Wulf LW, *et al.* Comparative pharmacokinetics of meloxicam between healthy postpartum vs. mid-lactation dairy cattle. *Front Vet Sci* 2020; **7**: 548.

106 University of Illinois Chicago Monthly FAQs. What Efficacy Supports the Use of Liposomal Bupivacaine for post-cesarean pain control? August 2020. https://dig.pharmacy.uic.edu/faqs/2020-2/august-2020-faqs/what-efficacy-supports-the-use-of-liposomal-bupivacaine-for-post-cesarean-pain-control/ (accessed May 2023).

107 Prabhu M, Clapp MA, McQuaid-Hanson E, *et al.* Liposomal bupivacaine block at the time of cesarean delivery to decrease postoperative pain. *Obstet Gynecol* 2018; **132**(1): 70–78.

108 United States National Library of Medicine, ClinicalTrials.gov. Efficacy and Safety of EXPAREL versus Standard of Care (SoC) in Subjects Undergoing Elective Cesarean Section (CHOICE). January 2020. www.clinicaltrials.gov/ct2/show/NCT03853694 (accessed May 2023).

109 Pacira Bioscience News Release. EXPAREL Achieves Primary and Key Secondary Endpoints in Phase 4 CHOICE Study in Cesarean Section Patients, January 2020. www.globenewswire.com/en/news-release/2020/01/07/1967140/0/en/EXPAREL-Achieves-Primary-and-Key-Secondary-Endpoints-in-Phase-4-CHOICE-Study-in-Cesarean-Section-Patients.html (accessed May 2023).

110 United States National Library of Medicine, ClinicalTrials.gov. Evaluate the Safety and Efficacy of EXPAREL When Administered via Infiltration into the TAP vs. Bupivacaine Alone in Subjects Undergoing Elective C-Sections (C-Section). April 2019. www.clinicaltrials.gov/ct2/show/NCT03176459 (accessed May 2023).

111 Habib AS, Nedeljkovic SS, Horn J-L, *et al.* Randomized trial of transversus abdominis plane block with liposomal bupivacaine after cesarean delivery with or without intrathecal morphine. *J Clin Anesth* 2021; **75**: 110527.

112 Nocita® Product Website. www.elanco.us/products-services/dogs/nocita (accessed May 2023).

113 Ortega D, Viviand X, Lorec AM, *et al.* Excretion of lidocaine and bupivacaine in breast milk following epidural anesthesia for cesarean delivery. *Acta Anaesthesiol Scand* 1999; **43**(4): 394–397.

114 Mustafa HJ, Wong HL, Al-Kofahi M, *et al.* Bupivacaine pharmacokinetics and breast milk excretion of liposomal bupivacaine administered after cesarean birth. *Obstet Gynecol* 2020; **136**(1): 70–76.

SECTION 6

Nociception and Pain

46 Physiology and Pathophysiology of Pain

Kate L. White
School of Veterinary Medicine and Science, University of Nottingham, Nottingham, UK

Chapter contents

Introduction, 971
Receipt, encoding, and transmission of nociceptive information, 972
  Biology of sensory transduction, 972
Sensitization, 972
Initiation of a generator potential, 973
  Transmission of the action potential, 973
Anatomy of the dorsal horn, 973
Pharmacology of descending controls, 976
  Norepinephrine, 976
  Serotonin (5-HT), 976
  Dopamine, 976
  The role of the opioids, 976
  Endocannabinoids, 977
  GABA and glycine, 977
Tonic control, 977
The spino-bulbo-spinal loop, 977
Models of nociception and analgesic testing, 977
  Limitations of current animal models, 978
  Experimental animal (subject), 978
  Nociceptive assay, 978
  Biomarkers, 978
  Translational pain models, 978
  Nociceptive and pain assays, 978
  Phasic pain tests, 978
  Stimulus modalities, 979
  Site of stimulus application, 979
Outcome measures, 979
  Behavior, 979
  Neurophysiologic endpoints, 979
Ethical considerations, 983
  Maximum stimulus intensity, 984
Measurement of nociceptive withdrawal thresholds in companion animals, 984
  Pain models – tonic tests, 984
  Induced pain models, 985
Behavior, 985
  Abdominal muscle contraction, 990
  Physiologic responses, 990
  Neuronal activity, 990
Naturally occurring disease models, 990
Recent trends in pain evaluation in rodents, 990
  Place preference paradigm, 990
  Operant response paradigms, 990
  Assessment of spontaneous behaviors, 991
  Facial expression, 991
References, 991

Introduction

Pain is a complex, multidimensional experience involving sensory and affective components. In layperson terms, "pain is not just about how it feels, but how it makes you feel," and it is the unpleasant feelings that cause the suffering we associate with pain. Pain is a uniquely individual experience in humans, the pain that one individual feels associated with an injury may differ greatly from that experienced by another, both in its intensity and in how it is perceived and felt. This is evidenced from almost every clinical trial report of a new analgesic regimen, even when confounding factors are well controlled.

Pain is officially defined by the International Association for the Study of Pain (IASP) as *an unpleasant sensory and emotional experience associated with, or resembling that associated with, actual or potential tissue damage.* The definition is expanded upon with the addition of six key notes and etymology of the word pain for further context [1]. Furthermore, the nature of pain is variable across many situations. The stories of pain experienced in traumatic situations clearly illustrate that the time course of pain and its impact on our feelings and how we behave are not directly linked in time. This is well explored by Patrick Wall in *Pain: The Science of Suffering* [2]. Among many illustrations of the complexities of pain, he describes the experience of Harry Beecher, a young medical officer treating wounded troops admitted to a hospital on the beachhead at Anzio in 1944 during the Second World War. Seriously wounded soldiers admitted to the hospital over a period of 4 months were asked "are you in pain; do you want something for it." The answer was "no" to both questions in 70% of cases. Later, after the War, he asked the same two questions of a group of age-matched men who had undergone surgery at the Massachusetts General Hospital in Boston and 70% answered "yes" to both questions. He concluded that something about the context in which tissue damage occurred

Veterinary Anesthesia and Analgesia: The Sixth Edition of Lumb and Jones. Edited by Leigh Lamont, Kurt Grimm, Sheilah Robertson, Lydia Love and Carrie Schroeder.
© 2024 John Wiley & Sons, Inc. Published 2024 by John Wiley & Sons, Inc.
Companion website: www.wiley.com/go/lamont/anesthesia

influenced the degree of pain suffered. The lack of pain in the early time course of some traumatic injuries is often followed by pain reports within 24 hours; pain is rarely absent over time. The well-known phenomenon of phantom limb pain reveals the contrary position – in a large percentage of people who have amputations, pain is present chronically in the area of the amputated limb, although healing is complete. Clearly, the onset of disease and pain as a consequence of this is less dramatic and immediate than in the traumatic situations described above and reflects the more common triggers and causes of pain in humans.

The nature of pain is equally complex in animals, although all aspects of its experience and expression are not likely to be identical. The physiology and pathophysiology of pain are remarkably similar and well conserved across mammalian species, and the capacity of animals to suffer as sentient creatures is well established and enshrined in law in many countries.

Receipt, encoding, and transmission of nociceptive information

Biology of sensory transduction

The majority of pain experiences stem from activity in nociceptive primary afferent (sensory) neurons caused by thermal, mechanical, or/and chemical stimuli. The membrane of the peripheral terminal is populated with transduction proteins capable of responding to the stimuli. *Transduction* is defined as the process where a harmful stimulus is converted into an electrical signal [3–6]. The transducers or ionotropic receptors can crudely be described by the type and origin of stimulus (mechanical, thermal, and chemical), their tissue type association, and whether they are extrinsic or intrinsic to the primary afferent. However, thereafter the classification breaks down because these transducers lack a single criterion to reliably identify them [7,8]. Additionally, as a population they share anatomical, biochemical, physical, and functional heterogeneity, which may have hindered efficacy of therapy and contributed to a failure of translation of preclinical data to clinical use.

So, for example, a selection of the mechanosensory and thermosensory transduction channels in mammalian skin is outlined in Table 46.1. The activators and modality of the channels is characterized in the table but *in vivo* the activator may also initiate other types of cells to release chemicals and the functional implications of these concurrent events are still to be properly understood. This area of research is rapidly expanding, and the polymodality of receptors makes classification challenging. Chemical or chemo tranducers are well characterized, numerous, and can respond to exogenous and endogenous compounds. The direct form of chemotransducer is an ion channel that has a binding site for a ligand; also known as ionotropic receptors. An indirect form known as a metabotropic receptor also exists, which is slower, with the chemotransduction driven by an intracellular signaling cascade [9]; see below.

The cloning of the transient receptor potential cation vanilloid subfamily member 1 (TRPV1) was pivotal not only in furthering the understanding of chemotransduction in nociceptive afferents, but also in thermotransduction [10,11]. Other mammalian transient receptor potential (TRP) family receptors, TRP subfamily ankyrin (TRPA), and TRP subfamily melastatin (TRPM), share a thermotransduction role with a number of the two-pore potassium channels (K2P) [12,13], as well as the $Na_v1.8$ channel [14]. Despite the overwhelming evidence that mechanosensation is the most common component of somatosensation, it is the least well understood. The transducers known to play a role in mammalian mechanotransduction include the Piezo channels, TRPA1 and TRPV4, transient Ca^{2+} channels, and at least three K2P channels [15–20]. There will be overlap of the contribution of the mechanosensitive properties with the chemosensitive properties as chemicals are released from cells in response to mechanical stimuli. This overlap and lack of transducer specificity makes interpretation from intact preparations difficult.

Sensitization

The definition of *sensitization* is a decreased threshold for response, and/or can also be characterized by an increased response to a suprathreshold stimulus. Additionally, an increase in spontaneous activity can occur in the nociceptors, and an increase in receptor field size in the dorsal horn can be detected [21,22]. Peripheral sensitization refers to an increased responsiveness in the nociceptive neurons in the periphery, whereas central sensitization refers to an increased responsiveness of nociceptive neurons in the central nervous system (CNS) to their normal or subthreshold afferent input. It is within these spinal neurons that "wind-up" (the progressive repeated stimulation of C fibers) occurs [23,24]. All primary afferents release glutamate, and the three inotropic receptors for glutamate (*N*-methyl-D-aspartate [NMDA], α-amino-3-hydroxy-5-methyl-4-isoxazoleproprionic acid [AMPA], and kainate) are present in the dorsal horn. Wind-up can be considered a product of the temporal summation of NMDA and neurokinin-1 (NK_1) receptor-mediated cumulative depolarizations caused by primary afferent release of glutamate and the excitatory neuropeptide substance P, respectively [25–27]. Temporal summation describes an increased perception of pain in response to repetitive painful stimuli. Sensitization is a neurophysiological construct that can only definitively be determined if both the neural input and output are known. Clinically, the term sensitization is inferred in cases of reported *allodynia* (pain due to a stimulus that would not normally provoke pain) and *hyperalgesia* (increased pain from a stimulus that normally provokes pain). Both these terms do not infer a mechanism *per se* [28,29].

In inflammatory states, a large number of endogenous factors released in the vicinity of the free endings of the nociceptors can cause sensitization [25]. The nociceptors express characteristic patterns of the different inflammatory mediator receptors; guanine nucleotide binding protein- (G-protein) coupled receptors (GPCRs), ligand-gated ion channels, tyrosine kinase, or cytokine receptors in response to the inflammation. These indirect forms of chemotransducers known as metabotropic receptors operate more slowly (compared to the inotropic receptors), with the chemotransduction driven by an intracellular signaling cascade [9]. The commonest example of this metabotropic receptor is the GPCR, which includes the μ-, κ-, and δ-opioid receptors, which can be targeted for pain relief [30]. There is plentiful evidence of chemicals being released from thermally and mechanically stimulated tissue too, making this an overlapping and complicated area of study that is being fervently researched. There is an ever-increasing list of metabotropic receptors in the sensory neurons. These include receptors for cytokines, chemokines, and neurotrophins, albeit the number normally active is small, including those for bradykinin (B_1 and B_2) [31], histamine (H_1) [32], ATP [33,34], endothelin-1 [35], proteases (PAR-2) [36], and prostacyclin (PGI_2) [37]. This area of study is further complicated by the fact that a neuron can express ionotropic and metabotropic receptors for the same ligand [38].

Table 46.1 A selection of mammalian mechanosensory and thermosensory transduction channels associated with the skin.

Family	Identity	Modality	Activators	Temperature range	Location	References
TRPA	TRPA1	Thermal, Mechanical	Isothiocyanates, Ca^{2+}, icilin	< 18 °C	C fibers	[39,40]
TRPC	TRPC1	Mechanical	Receptor/store-operated	N/A	C and Aδ fibers	[41,42]
	TRPC5	Thermal	Thioredoxin	25–37 °C		[43]
TRPM	TRPM3	Thermal	Pregnenolone sulfate	> 30 °C	C and Aδ fibers	[44]
	TRPM8		Menthol, icilin	< 28 °C	C fibers	[45–48]
TRPV	TRPV1	Thermal, Osmotic	Capsaicin, H^+	> 42 °C	C and Aδ fibers, keratinocytes	[49–51]
	TRPV2	Thermal, Osmotic, Mechanical	Endocannabinoids, diphenyl compounds 2-aminoethoxydiphenyl borate	> 52 °C	Aδ and Aβ fibers, immune cells	[52,53]
	TRPV3	Thermal	Camphor, carvacrol, diphenyl compounds	> 34–39 °C	C fibers, keratinocytes	[54]
	TRPV4	Thermal, Osmotic, Mechanical (in injury)	PUFAs, 4αPDD, epoxyeicosatrienoic acids	> 27–34 °C	C and Aδ fibers, keratinocytes, Merkel cells	[15,55]
DEG/ ENaC	ASIC1	Mechanical (touch)	H^+	N/A	Aδ, Aβ, and C fibers	[56,57]
	ASIC2					[58,59]
	ASIC3					[60]
K2P channel	TREK-1	Thermal, Mechanical	PUFAs, H^+	Noxious cold and noxious heat 40–46 °C 20–25 °C	Aδ and C fibers, Aβ?	[61–63]
	TREK-2			Noxious cold and noxious heat	C fibers Dorsal root ganglia	[47,64]
	TRAAK				C fibers Dorsal root ganglia	[13,65]
VGNC	Na_v 1.8	Thermal	No subfamily activator	Noxious cold	C fibers Dorsal root ganglia	[66–68]
Piezo	Piezo 1	Mechanical	Pyrazine?	N/A	Dorsal root ganglia (less than Piezo 2) Merkel cells	[69–71]
	Piezo 2				Dorsal root ganglia Aδ fibers	

TRP, transient receptor potential; TRPA, transient receptor potential subfamily ankyrin; TRPC, transient receptor potential subfamily canonical; TRPM, transient receptor potential subfamily melastatin; TRPV, transient receptor potential subfamily vanilloid; DEG/ENaC, degenerin/epithelial sodium channel; ASIC, acid-sensing ion channel; VGNC, voltage-gated sodium channel; PUFA, polyunsaturated fatty acid; 4αPDD, 4α-phorbol 12,13-didecanoate; K2P channel, two-pore domain potassium channel; TREK, TWIK subfamily K (where TWIK, tandem of P-domains in a weak inward rectifying channel); TRAAK, TWIK subfamily K member 4; H^+, protons. Source: Adapted from Lumpkin and Caterina [7].

Initiation of a generator potential

The resting potential of the nociceptive afferent is −40 mV, decreasing to between −50 and −75 mV at the cell body. The action potential (AP) threshold range is between −35mV and −55mV [72]. For the sensory information to be propagated to the CNS, an AP must be generated by membrane depolarization caused by the transduction process. This event is termed a "generator potential" (GP) and can be initiated in three main different ways. First, via the opening of an ion channel which pushes the membrane potential above threshold and causes an AP that can be propagated toward the CNS. One such example of this is the TRPV1 channel, which can be activated by both thermal and chemical stimuli [7,73]. Second, the GP can be indirectly elicited by the closing of K^+ channels (potassium family subfamily K member 2 (TREK-1), potassium family subfamily K member 3 (TASK-1), and others) normally responsible for hyperpolarizing currents. TREK-1 channels can be activated by mechanical stimulation, hydrogen ions, and warm temperature demonstrating their polymodal behavior [63]. Third, also indirectly, via activation of low-threshold voltage-gated ion channels that are in close association with ion channels capable of driving membrane depolarization [74].

Transduction at the nociceptor terminal results in a GP that travels passively to the spike initiation zone. At this point, an AP can be generated that is transmitted via nociceptive afferents.

Transmission of the action potential

Propagation of the AP along the axon of the nociceptor is caused by the initial depolarization that spreads in one direction as adjacent voltage-gated sodium channels (VGSCs) open. Primary sensory neurons exhibit a rich heterogenous morphology and the most common way to classify these neurons is based upon their speed of conduction [75]. The Aα/β group are myelinated axons with the fastest speed of conduction (33–75 m/s). The Aδ group are thinner myelinated fibers with an intermediate speed (5–30 m/s), and the C fibers are the smallest unmyelinated fibers with the slowest conducting speed (0.5–2 m/s). Most of the neurons conducting within the Aα/β group do not encode noxious stimuli but respond to innocuous mechanical stimuli and are classified as low-threshold mechanoreceptors. Most of the Aδ and C fibers encode noxious stimuli and are classified as nociceptors.

Anatomy of the dorsal horn

The dorsal horn is divided into parallel laminae based on the packing density of the neurons [76]. The termination of the primary afferents in the dorsal horn laminae is determined by fiber diameter and receptive field modality [77,78]. Smaller diameter nociceptive afferents synapse with nociceptive-specific (NS) cells in laminae I–II of the superficial dorsal horn, with a small number terminating deeper in the spinal cord. Lamina I neurons contribute to the spinothalamic and spinoreticular tracts both responsible for processing pain and temperature information [79,80]. Lamina II (substantia gelatinosa) is the major site for nociceptive inputs (C and Aδ fibers) arriving at the spinal cord [81] and consists mainly of densely packed unmyelinated interneurons [82]. Lamina II has been shown to have explicit organization of modules of neurons that differentially modify and transmit the afferent input from the Aδ and C fibers [83]. Lamina II central neurons, with C fiber input, were shown to excite lamina II vertical neurons with Aδ input. Lamina II outer vertical neurons with Aδ input excited lamina I neurons [84]. The function of this arrangement is postulated to be an ability of the afferent input to be amplified or modulated. C fibers can be divided into two groups, based on phenotype and sensitivity to neurotrophins, although functionally the differentiation is less clear. One group is sensitive to nerve growth factor (NGF) and usually contains substance P, calcitonin gene-related peptide (CGRP), and galanin (peptidergic fibers); the second group is distinguished by binding sites for lectin isolectin B4 and usually possesses the purinergic receptors $P2X_3$ and $P2Y_1$ (non-peptidergic fibers) [85–87]. The central projections of these two populations of C fibers differ in their arborization, the peptidergic C fibers branching in lamina I and the outer portion of lamina II with a small number extending to deeper terminals. The non-peptidergic fibers project to the central portion of lamina II [88]. The non-peptidergic C fibers are chiefly associated with the superficial layers of the skin [89], whereas peptidergic fibers tend to innervate other tissues in addition to the deeper layers of the skin [90]. In summary, the simplistic classification of C and A fiber nociceptors on morphology and conduction speed fails to capture the extensive diversity of primary afferents.

Laminae III–VI are known as the deep dorsal horn and receive less nociceptive input. Transmission of innocuous stimuli is predominantly through large diameter, myelinated Aβ fibers, which terminate in laminae III–VI, hence within these laminae are proprioceptive neurons responding exclusively to touch [78]. In addition to the NS and the proprioceptive neurons, a third class of spinal neurons is described, known as wide dynamic range (WDR). The WDR neurons can receive noxious or non-noxious input from Aδ, Aβ, or C fibers and respond in a graded manner (i.e., frequency of APs) from low through to high threshold noxious input. The WDR neurons (also known as trigger, lamina V type, Class 2, multireceptive, or convergent neurons) are found in superficial layers but more so in lamina V and include interneurons involved in the polysynaptic reflexes and projection neurons [91]. For Aδ fibers terminating in lamina V, the interneurons they synapse with decussate and ascend in the spinothalamic tract, while those terminating more superficially synapse with interneurons forming the spinoparabrachial tract (Fig. 46.1). The ventral and intermediate laminae are less important in terms of inputs from primary afferents. Laminae VII and X receive a proportion of nociceptive input that is mainly visceral in origin [92,93]. Muscle afferents feed into laminae V, VI, and VII.

The primary afferents form excitatory synapses with either WDR projection cells (convey information to various parts of the brain) or interneurons (responsible for local circuitry within the spinal cord; an example is represented in Fig. 46.1 connecting the WDR neurons of lamina V with the superficial dorsal horn). All primary afferents use glutamate as their primary excitatory synaptic transmitter, although arrangements do differ. Interneurons can be classified as either excitatory (predominantly glutaminergic) or inhibitory (mainly γ-aminobutyric acid- (GABA-) or glycinergic). The morphology of the interneurons has been most closely studied in lamina II, with a classification scheme that includes islet, central, radial, and vertical interneurons [83,94–96].

An alternative approach to classification is to use immunocytochemistry and stratify the interneurons based on neuropeptide and protein localization [97,98]. Many neuropeptides have been identified, and consequently, several neuropeptide receptors expressed by the interneurons are being studied, including the tachykinin receptors, neurokinin-1 (NK_1) and neurokinin-3 (NK_3); the μ-opioid receptor-1 (MOR-1); the somatostatin-2A receptor (sst_{2A}); and the neuropeptide Y-1 receptor (Y_1). It is not possible to use the neuropeptides to definitively define populations of interneurons, although some markers show a restricted distribution. The dorsal horn also receives input from axons descending from various parts of the brain (Fig. 46.1). All three glutamate receptors (AMPA, NMDA, and kainate) are found in the dorsal horn. The $GABA_A$ and glycine receptors are distributed throughout the spinal cord and are most likely expressed on all dorsal horn neurons. Many studies do not distinguish between the interneurons and the projection neurons when describing receptors for glutamate, GABA, and glycine. GABA is present in ~25%, 30%, and 40% of neurons in laminae I, II, and III, respectively [99]. Spinal cord wiring is complex and little understood, the main spinal signaling pathways in the rodent are comprehensively reviewed elsewhere [100].

It is within the spinal cord that substantial transformation and modulation of the nociceptive signal can occur before it ascends to higher centers [101], due to the discrete populations of intrinsic interneurons that can alter responses of NS and WDR neurons, with astrocytes and microglia also modulating, particularly in disease states [102–104]. Superficially in lamina I of the dorsal horn, there is a large population of projection neurons, which preferentially express the NK_1 receptor for substance P [105,106] and are thereby nociceptive neurons. These neurons project to the periaqueductal gray (PAG), thalamus, and particularly the parabrachial area (PA). These cells also project to the rostral ventral medulla (RVM) and can influence descending controls [107,108].

The ascending tracts are typically named according to where they terminate in the brain [109]. The *spinothalamic tract* (terminating in the thalamus) integrates the thalamic traffic (and other signals) and is responsible for the discriminative/localization component of pain via projections to the sensorimotor cortex, insular cortex, and the anterior cingulate originating mainly from laminae I, IV, V, and X [110,111]. The *spinobulbar tract* (terminating in both the hindbrain and midbrain regions associated with pain processing) conveys the affective/intensity component, and projects to the amygdala and hypothalamus via the parabrachial nucleus [112]. This spinobulbar pathway can influence and recruit descending pathways via the PAG, pontine locus coeruleus (LC), and RVM, thereby dictating the output passing through the spinal cord [113,114] (Fig. 46.1).

The PAG is one of the most important structures associated with the descending pain control system [115,116] and receives information from the somatosensory and cingulate cortices, the thalamus, amygdala, and hypothalamus, and from the ascending pathways. The PAG–RVM exerts a degree of selective inhibition of C fiber-mediated nociceptive impulses but preserves A fiber messages coding sensory and discriminatory information [117–119] and the RVM can be considered the final relay point through which facilitation or inhibition of the nociceptive message passes [120,121]. The degree of inhibition or facilitation is controlled in the RVM by at

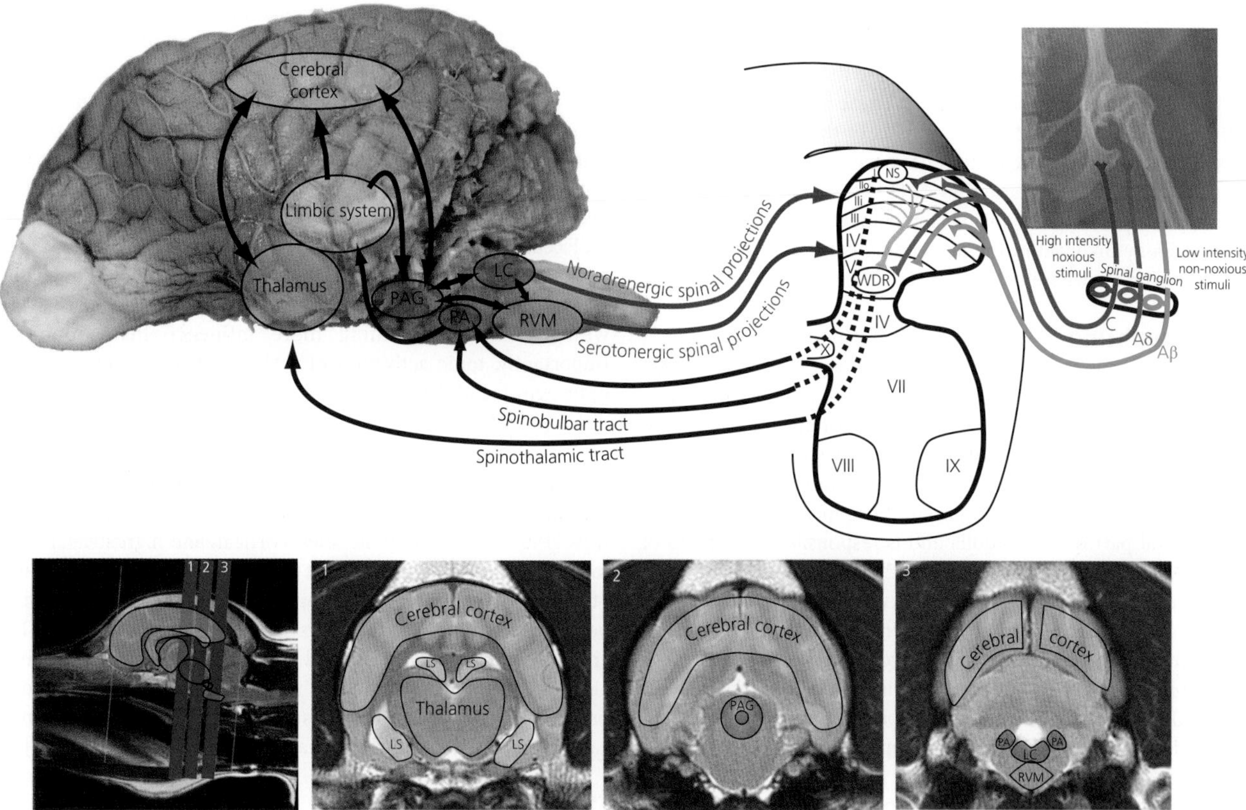

Figure 46.1 Schematic diagram of pain pathway from periphery to brain including sagittal midline T2 weighted MRI images from a dog brain with selected transverse images at the level of the (1) thalamus, (2) midbrain, and (3) rostral medulla annotated to indicate the anatomical localization of regions involved in descending modulation. Primary afferent fibers (Aβ, Aδ, and C fibers) transmit impulses from the periphery (osteoarthritic hip joint) to the dorsal horn of the spinal cord. Secondary NS cells are predominantly located in the superficial dorsal horn (laminae I–II), with most WDR neurons located in the deeper dorsal horn (e.g., lamina V). Lamina V neurons in particular project to the thalamus (via the spinothalamic tract) where there are subsequent neuronal projections to various cortical regions that form part of a "pain matrix" (primary and secondary somatosensory, insular, anterior cingulate, and prefrontal cortices). The descending pathways originate from brainstem nuclei such as the rostral ventromedial medulla (RVM) and the locus coeruleus (LC), which are directly influenced by the ascending spinobulbar projections and higher centers to modulate spinal processing. PAG, periaqueductal gray; DRG, dorsal route ganglion; RVM, rostroventromedial medulla; LC, locus coeruleus; LS, limbic system; NS, nociceptive-specific; PA, parabrachial nucleus; WDR, wide dynamic range. Source: White *et al.* [122], with permission from Elsevier.

least two different types of neurons known as "ON cells" and "OFF cells." Briefly, the ON, OFF, and neutral cells are defined by their response to nociceptive input [123]. The ON cells show a burst of activity prior to nociceptive input and are considered a component of excitatory drive. The OFF cells show a short-lived decrease in firing rate before nociceptive input and are considered inhibitory. Neutral cells do not respond to nociceptive input. The role of these cells may be more complicated than previously thought [124–126]. The RVM can be considered a relay station but requires a forebrain loop [127]. Furthermore, the anterior cingulate cortex (ACC) projections regulating spinal neurons [128,129] can also modulate the pain experience. The ACC potentially offers a further target for manipulating the pain signature but understanding its role requires more sophisticated paradigms. The role of the ACC and pain processing has been comprehensively described [130].

In the mature adult rat, descending inhibition is targeted to spinal neurons with a strong afferent C fiber input. However, in the first few weeks postnatally, the system is controlled differently with greater descending facilitation particularly targeted to the A fiber input [131]. The evolutionary reason proposed for this A fiber input is to provide the dorsal horn with low-level, non-noxious, tactile input, thereby promoting the development of the animal's sensory networks. The switch from facilitation to inhibition as the animal matures is primarily dependent on endogenous opioid levels in the RVM [132] with GABA and endocannabinoid levels also playing a role [133,134]. It is possible that immature nervous systems could be at risk of excessive sensory overload and peripheral injury in the first few weeks of life where facilitation is favored [135].

In summary, this balance of inhibition and facilitation of descending pathways is a dynamic product of the afferent evoked activity, the age of the animal, but also the excitability of the dorsal horn cell [131]. The descending pathways appear to lack specificity, influencing all portions of the spinal cord and it is this widespread and intrinsic influence that is responsible for the ability to facilitate or inhibit transmission but other senses too, potentially explaining why some chronic pain states have clinical signs distinct from pain alone but can manifest with debilitating effects on sleep and other emotions [136,137]. Moreover, the perception of pain is sensitive to many mental processes therefore not exclusively driven by or maintained by the noxious input [138]; heightened anxiety and fear, for example, can then often exacerbate the suffering of pain [139].

Pharmacology of descending controls

The monoamines norepinephrine (noradrenaline) and 5-hydroxytryptamine (serotonin, 5HT) are the major transmitters in the descending controls [127,140]. These bidirectional monoaminergic systems modulate the outputs of the dorsal horn neurons. The inhibition or facilitation has been shown to be mediated by distinctly different receptors [141–143], but the output is determined by the type of noxious input and the response to it. The pharmacology involved in the descending controls is comprehensively covered elsewhere [127].

Norepinephrine

Norepinephrine is the major neurotransmitter released by sympathetic postganglionic nerve fibers and is involved in autonomic regulation of numerous organs. These noradrenergic cell groups were mapped in 1964 and are prefixed by the letter A (for aminergic) [144]. Areas A1 to A7 inclusive contain norepinephrine; areas A8 to A14 contain dopamine. Group A1 is located in the caudal ventrolateral part of the medulla and is responsible for aspects of body fluid metabolism [145], group A2 plays a role in stress and food intake and is located in the solitary nucleus [146]. Group A5 (close to the superior olivary complex) and A7 (in the pontine reticular formation) project to the spinal cord [147].

Norepinephrine plays a major role in modulating nociception [148–150]; the majority of descending projections originating from the pontine nucleus LC contain norepinephrine (areas A6 and adjoining A4) and microstimulation of this nucleus was shown to produce antinociceptive effects via spinal α_2-adrenergic receptors [151]. In healthy subjects, the noradrenergic system serves to regulate pain thresholds, with its role becoming more prominent in cases of injury or inflammation [150]. Norepinephrine released from the LC is also involved in the regulation of vigilance, attention, and cognitive functions but it is still not possible to surmise the net effect of the noradrenergic system on supraspinal structures; evidence exists for both antinociceptive and pronociceptive actions [152]. However, in the LC-spinal descending pathway, the central noradrenergic system inhibits pain, and drugs acting on the α_2-adrenergic receptor (alone or as an adjuvant) have proven effective to varying degrees as analgesics. In humans, topically applied α_2-adrenergic receptor agonists may have a role in treating neuropathies [153], and intra-articular administration has reduced postoperative knee pain [154]. Patients with intractable cancer pain have benefited from intrathecal administration [155]. The α_2-adrenergic receptor agonists are widely utilized in wild, domestic, and laboratory animals for sedation, analgesia, and muscle relaxation. In general, spinally administered α_2-adrenergic receptor agonists have an enhanced antinociceptive potency in animal models with a persistent injury [156–158], and the intensity, duration, and type of noxious injury will ultimately determine the response [159–162]. Likewise, altered noradrenergic activity (for example, a reduction in the inhibitory influences) can lead to the hypersensitivity seen in models of both acute inflammation and nerve injury [158,163–165], hence the interest in targeting this system. This central role is further evidenced by studies that have demonstrated restoration of diminished noradrenergic control after use of intrathecal reboxetine, a selective norepinephrine reuptake inhibitor, following the development of a neuropathic pain phenotype [166].

Serotonin (5-HT)

Serotonin is commonly considered one of the most important neurotransmitters. Studies have shown that ~20% of the neurons in the RVM are serotonergic, and there was early evidence for 5-HT involvement in descending modulation [167]. These descending pain modulatory pathways influence nociception through activation of different serotonergic receptors in the spinal cord [168]. Both acute and chronic noxious stimuli can activate these RVM 5-HT neurons and increase the expression of 5-HT receptors in the spinal cord [169,170]. The 5-HT neurons can also influence non-serotonergic neurons. The collaterals of the 5-HT neurons have been shown to regulate the bidirectional control from the ON and OFF cells in the RVM [171]. The serotonergic/5-HT system is more complex than the adrenergic system with pain inhibition or facilitation attributable to different subtypes of 5-HT receptors [172–174] with facilitation assuming more influence than inhibition. Importantly, tonic activation of 5-HT (and non-5-HT)-mediated brainstem facilitatory influences is one of the contributors to the development and maintenance of central sensitization [175,176].

Dopamine

The monoamine dopamine is also involved in descending controls [140] with mesolimbic, mesocortical, and nigrostriatal dopaminergic pathways able to inhibit primarily the affective component of nociception [177,178]. The dopamine system is embedded in the pain matrix circuitry [179] but is also needed for movement [180] and is associated with reward [181], learning, and cognition [182,183]. Studies have shown that dopamine therapies may offer promise as analgesics but efforts to develop therapies are complicated by its intrinsic role in so many other modalities [184,185].

The role of the opioids

The descending pathways can also be considered components of an opioid-sensitive matrix. Experiments have shown that numerous drugs interacting with components of the descending pathways can influence or mimic the production of endogenously produced opioids, indeed there is evidence of a bulbospinal opioidergic pathway [186].

The PAG is one of the major sources of opioid-mediated inhibition of ascending nociceptive impulses [187]. Cortical inputs synapse at the PAG mediating a "top-down" endogenous pain inhibition system. The projections from the PAG extend to the RVM and noradrenergic pontine nuclei which in turn modulate nociceptive input at the spinal cord through the release of norepinephrine and serotonin. The dorsal-dorsolateral portions of the PAG play a role in stress-induced analgesia, which is independent of opioids but depends on endocannabinoids, whereas the lateral-ventrolateral portions of the PAG are implicated in analgesia induced by opioids and non-steroidal anti-inflammatory drugs (NSAIDs) [188].

The placebo effect is one example of this "top-down" modulating pathway. This refers to an analgesic construct that can be elicited in certain people that has its mechanisms associated with activation of the μ-opioid receptor and changes in blood flow to the rostral anterior and pregenual cingulate cortices, the dorsolateral prefrontal cortex, and anterior insular cortex [189,190]. In the case of placebo, it is now apparent that a complex web of interwoven processes is responsible rather than the once simplistic view that the μ-opioid receptor was solely responsible [191]. The opioidergic descending tracts are also implicated in distraction and hypnosis and offer potential for developing further analgesic interventions. Functional magnetic resonance imaging (fMRI) studies have shown (particularly in placebo and nocebo studies) that the descending pathways are the conduits through which the cognitive influences affect a pain experience. This experience is also subsequently modulated by the individual's control and ongoing response to the pain experience exerted by prefrontal limbic brain regions [138,192]. The exact mechanisms involved in the descending controls are not yet fully understood, but a consensus on their importance is without doubt, and research into recruitment of their endogenous modulating attributes is ongoing.

Endocannabinoids

The endocannabinoids are involved in the processing of nociceptive inputs [193]. The expression of endocannabinoid receptors and the presence of ligands and metabolites are dynamic and dependent on the type of pain being expressed. The system offers attractive targets for analgesic opportunities, although the isolation of the analgesic properties of molecules without psychoactive side effects is a challenging conundrum. The analgesia produced by NSAIDs in the descending pain control system also requires activation of the cannabinoid-1 (CB_1) receptor [188]. Furthermore, numerous experiments suggest that opioids, NSAIDs, and the cannabinoids in the PAG and RVM interact to potentially decrease GABAergic inhibition and thus enhance the descending flow of impulses that inhibit pain as a mechanism of analgesia [194–196]. The endocannabinoid system can adapt in the face of persistent pain states such as osteoarthritis offering a potential target of spinal hyperexcitability [197]. However, the drugs trialed so far modulate the affective component but not the sensory component of the pain [198].

GABA and glycine

GABA and glycine are inhibitory transmitters and influence nociception via their presence within interneurons [199–201]. These GABAergic or glycinergic projections can inhibit noxious inputs into the dorsal horn of the spinal cord and the neurons can express either or both neurotransmitters [202]. Studies have also demonstrated that the ON, OFF, and neutral cells have varying expression of GABA and glycine, but the expression is determined by the context of the pain experience; for example, in one study using a model of peripheral inflammation, the gene expression and the phenotype of the ON and OFF cells was altered [203].

Tonic control

In the absence of nociceptive input, spinal nociceptive neurons are under both tonic and stimulus-evoked (phasic) descending controls [204,205]. Characterization of the receptors involved in the tonic control mechanisms has been undertaken [206–208]. One important caveat to these experiments involving discrete lesions and anesthesia is they may inadvertently overlook the contribution of the plasticity of the spinal cord in response to inflammation, or indeed the differences in the free-ranging conscious animal compared to the anesthetized animal, and these should be considered when drawing conclusions.

The spino-bulbo-spinal loop

Pain consists of a somatosensory component and a psychological, affective component. The term "nociception" refers to the neural activity in the peripheral and central nervous systems caused by a painful stimulus and the term "pain" itself is used to describe both this and the emotional and autonomic responses to the insult. These different components of pain are processed in separate, discrete areas of the brain. The nociceptive insult is the cause of pain, but in some cases this insult is absent, and its magnitude is not linearly related to the pain that is reported or behaviors that are displayed [209]. This is, in part, a consequence of a feedback loop between the brain and spinal cord. This spino-bulbo-spinal loop can alter the extent to which pain signals are amplified or inhibited within the spinal cord.

Models of nociception and analgesic testing

Although significant advances have been made in the basic understanding of pain processing and modulation in recent years, large gaps in our knowledge remain, particularly in the fields of anatomic, biochemical, and physiologic mechanisms of pain. The current situation in animals with respect to adequacy of pain management is less well documented. Drugs with proven efficacy for the treatment of acute surgical pain are available for companion animals (e.g., licensed opioids and NSAIDs). However, with the exception of NSAIDs, the repertoire of licensed drugs for the management of chronic pain (e.g., pain caused by degenerative joint disease) in companion animals is very limited. Acute and chronic pain remain poorly treated in farm animals and exotic species.

It is widely accepted that research in animals is pivotal to an increased understanding of nociceptive and pain mechanisms and the development of new analgesic drugs, for both humans and animals. Pain studies in humans generally focus on characterizing pain states, with few studies investigating underlying pain mechanisms, and studies in humans are inevitably hampered by ethical constraints. Although in humans the advent of advanced neuroimaging techniques allows the *in vivo* study of patterns of CNS activity concurrent with self-report of pain perception, ethical considerations surrounding induced pain models in humans, combined with current technological limitations, means that neuroimaging cannot replace the need for animal pain models. In addition, neuroimaging lacks cellular resolution and poor temporal resolution; fMRI may not distinguish between very high levels of neuronal activity in the brain (and therefore may not be sensitive to different pain intensities) because the blood oxygen level-dependent (BOLD) signal can reach a ceiling. Neuroimaging does not allow the interrogation of small areas of the CNS such as the dorsal horn of the spinal cord or the peripheral nervous system with any precision, as the technique relies on integrating electrical signals across large sampling regions such as the brain.

Two main approaches have been adopted when studying pain in animals. The first approach is to study responses to brief noxious stimuli (defined as stimuli that are damaging to, or threaten to damage, normal tissues) in naive animals. In other words, brief phasic noxious thermal, electrical, or mechanical stimuli are delivered to healthy animals and the magnitude of the stimulus threshold required to elicit a response is measured (e.g., nociceptive threshold testing), or changes in neuronal activity, animal behavior, or body systems are studied during delivery of the stimulus. Response to brief phasic stimuli is commonly utilized as the outcome measure in analgesic drug testing (i.e., as an integral component of pain models), although it should be viewed as having limited applicability owing to the previously naive (normal) state of the nervous system and singular nociceptive modality (e.g., thermal nociceptors), which differs from most clinical pain syndromes.

The second approach is to induce pain in the animal by delivery of a tonic, sustained noxious stimulus that induces peripheral or central sensitization and subsequently to study pain mechanisms (e.g., by recording changes in behavioral or neuronal activity) or test analgesic drugs. In this chapter, the broad term "pain model" is used to refer to the second approach. There is interest in using companion animals with naturally occurring disease conditions that cause pain (e.g., spontaneous osteoarthritis [OA] in dogs) [210] to study pain mechanisms and evaluate analgesic drug efficacy for both humans and animals. However, there are disadvantages when using nonhuman subjects in analgesic studies, such as the lack of verbal feedback about the "feelings" of the patient's pain and the vulnerability to observer bias.

Within any pain model, there are three distinct components that must be differentiated [211]. First, there is the study subject (variables include species, strain, sex, and age); second, there is the stimulus or type of tissue damage that is used to initiate pain (e.g., an injection of an irritant substance into a joint versus measuring cutaneous thermal threshold); and third, there is the outcome measure (e.g., behavior or physiological parameter) used as the surrogate biomarker for pain. Significant interest has arisen recently in trying to improve pain biomarkers in animal models with the recognition that endpoints such as a tail flick in response to a noxious stimulus may be largely reflexive and not an indicator of higher brain perception. This is of particular relevance in the development of pain models for analgesic drug development.

Limitations of current animal models

Despite significant efforts in analgesic drug discovery, there has been limited success in developing and marketing new analgesic drugs with efficacy and acceptable adverse effect profiles for clinical patients with pain. Putative new analgesic drugs undergo screening and preclinical testing in animal models; therefore, it is important that the performance of a new analgesic in animal models is successfully translated to the human pain model and clinical patients. Although the reasons for failure of new drugs at the preclinical–clinical interface are multifactorial, there is a general agreement that limitations of available animal models play a major role in the current bottleneck in analgesic drug development. Recognized general limitations of animal pain models occur at the level of the experimental animal (subject) and the pain assay or biomarker used to assess pain.

Experimental animal (subject)

The majority of preclinical pain research is carried out in young adult, healthy, intact male laboratory mice and rats of a specific strain. Although useful as a cost-effective and rapid screening method for *in vivo* testing of candidate molecules, this does not always translate well to the clinical population of pain patients. Therefore, it has been recommended that pain studies include more diverse and heterogeneous groups of animals comprising both genders and a variety of strains [212].

Nociceptive assay

Many nociceptive (pain) assays are currently available that aim to model nociceptive, inflammatory, and neuropathic pain. However, it is immediately apparent that there is a mismatch between the underlying pathophysiologic changes induced in experimental assays and the etiology of clinical pain conditions. For example, nerve ligation is commonly used as a model of neuropathic pain, yet diseases associated with neuropathic pain in humans rarely result from complete nerve ligation or nerve compression. There are often co-existing abnormalities that also contribute to the perceived pain, such as neuropathy and inflammation. Most pain assays do not mimic the complexity of clinical pain states. Induced models of OA in rats and mice usually focus on the stifle joint and are induced by sterile inflammation or surgical disruption of the joint, leading to a rapid progression of OA that does not consider the effect(s) of aging itself on perceived pain [213].

Biomarkers

Until recently, most behavioral biomarkers used to measure analgesic drug effect in animal pain models relied on either evoked spinal reflexes (e.g., limb withdrawal from a von Frey filament) or innate behaviors such as vocalization or guarding that can also be performed by decerebrate animals [214]. Evoked withdrawal responses detect hyperalgesia and allodynia (although the two are difficult to distinguish from each other in animals) and therefore only provide information on the sensory and discriminative components of pain. They do not provide information about the emotional (affective) component, which is critical to the experience of pain in humans and animals, although more difficult to define in the latter. Although many patients with chronic neuropathic pain experience hyperalgesia and allodynia, they commonly report spontaneous pain (i.e., non-evoked pain) as the most debilitating and distressing aspect of their condition [215]. Therefore, unless biomarkers that evaluate spontaneous pain are employed in an assay, the effect on spontaneous pain may go undetected. New biomarkers sensitive to spontaneous pain that can detect changes in behavior associated with emotion are being developed.

Translational pain models

In recent years, the importance of translational approaches to animal research, which aim to bridge gaps between basic animal research and medical practice, has been recognized. As such, efforts are under way to develop assays and biomarkers that directly translate to experimental human pain models. This increases the likelihood that analgesics found to be effective in preclinical studies will remain efficacious in human clinical trials. Currently, there are very few assays that are translatable, although intradermal or cutaneous application of capsaicin and the ultraviolet B (UVB) pain model are notable exceptions. The use of spontaneous disease models in companion animals is another approach to improving translatability of pain assays between humans and animals. Experimental pain studies in humans rely largely on psychophysics to quantify pain and therefore analgesic drug efficacy, but self-reporting of pain is inherently subjective. Commonly used behavioral biomarkers such as reflex withdrawal are also vulnerable to observer subjectivity. Considerable variability of reported results among researchers and laboratories is therefore common. Clearly, objective biomarkers directly translatable to humans that reflect the underlying neurobiology of perceived pain are needed to improve pain models.

Nociceptive and pain assays

In the following sections, the term "pain" is used to describe all assays carried out in awake animals; if the animal is anesthetized during the assay, the term "nociception" is used.

Phasic pain tests

Brief noxious (phasic) stimuli are widely used to elicit responses in order to study nociceptive pathways and increase the understanding of the neurobiology of pain in experimental animals and also for the purposes of analgesiometry (i.e., measuring changes in biomarkers to study the action of analgesic drugs). Broadly, "nociceptive threshold testing" in animals and "quantitative sensory testing" (QST) in humans are the terms used to describe the application of tests utilizing brief phasic stimuli. The stimuli might be applied to naive animals or animals with induced pain, thus allowing the study of nociceptive pathways and drug efficacy in normal animals and animals with altered pain sensitivity caused by central and/or peripheral sensitization. For a complete review of phasic pain tests, see Le Bars *et al.* [216].

Beecher [217] was one of the first authors to set out ideal criteria for producing acute pain experimentally, and some of the optimal characteristics are as follows:

- The stimulus is applied to a body part where neurohistologic variations are at a minimum between different individuals and the stimulus can be measured and closely associated with the changes that produce pain.
- Quantitative data can be collected in response to a given stimulus under given conditions.
- There is little tissue damage at the pain threshold level and the hazard to the subject is small at high intensities.
- There is a relationship between the magnitude of the stimulus and the intensity of the pain experienced.
- It is possible to carry out repeat measurements without interfering with subsequent measurements.
- The stimulus is easy to apply and there is a clearly identifiable endpoint.
- The test should be applicable to both humans and animals.

Stimulus modalities

Four modalities of noxious stimulation are commonly used in phasic acute nociceptive tests: electrical, thermal, mechanical, and chemical. The advantages and disadvantages of these different modalities when used to generate acute pain are shown in Table 46.2. Chemical stimulation is considered separately because it causes a slower, progressive, and non-escapable noxious stimulus. Commonly used phasic tests in awake animals are described in Table 46.3 (thermal stimuli), Table 46.4 (mechanical stimuli), and Table 46.5 (electrical stimuli).

Site of stimulus application

For practical reasons, phasic nociceptive stimuli are usually applied to the skin to activate cutaneous nociceptors, although stimuli are also applied to viscera in some models. The predominance of tests involving cutaneous nociceptors reflects the ease of access to the skin and the ability to stimulate the skin with minimal restraint of the animal. In awake laboratory animals, the plantar surface of the hind paw is often used as the site of stimulation because it is readily accessible for application of heat and mechanical stimuli. Awareness of the differences in cutaneous sensitivity between haired (found on most of the body) and glabrous skin (the plantar paw) in laboratory animals is important as it alters the translatability of pain tests between rats and humans [218]. The tail is commonly used as the site of stimulus application in acute pain tests in rats (e.g., thermal nociceptive stimuli). However, the tail is also essential for thermoregulation and balance, which can influence threshold responses measured following stimulation [216]. Concurrent noxious stimulation of more than one body part at the same time recruits endogenous inhibitory mechanisms and confounds measured threshold responses, so is best avoided [219]. Another consideration is the potential for repeated stimulation of the same body site to cause peripheral and central sensitization, thereby causing a reduction in threshold over time.

Outcome measures

Behavior

Laboratory animals generate a range of behavioral responses to delivery of phasic noxious stimuli classified by the underlying nociceptive pathways that are activated. The endpoints classically used for each assay are detailed below; however, a few general comments are outlined here. Many phasic tests rely on the detection of motor withdrawal responses; therefore, impaired motor function (e.g., during administration of analgesic drugs that have concurrent effects on locomotion) will confound threshold responses. It is important to differentiate between withdrawal responses that are reflex (governed predominantly by spinal mechanisms) and more complex behaviors such as escape, avoidance, or licking of the body part where the stimulus was applied. The complexity of the endpoint behavior will to some extent reflect recruitment of underlying nociceptive or pain mechanisms and therefore are commonly differentially sensitive to analgesic drugs [220]. Endpoint behaviors used in nociceptive tests should ideally be nociceptive specific, reliable, reproducible, and sensitive to administration of analgesic drugs.

Neurophysiologic endpoints

Neurophysiologic techniques are increasingly important in studies to elucidate ascending pain pathways and cortical representation of pain [221–223]. Techniques that afford a direct window on the function of the CNS, such as electroencephalography, provide a unique insight into pain processing and how activation of nociceptive pathways results in pain perception in a conscious animal. The electroencephalogram (EEG) is the electrical activity recorded from electrodes placed at various locations on the scalp (human) or head (other species) [224–226]. It consists of the summated electrical activity of populations of neurons together with a contribution from the glial cells. Neurons are excitable cells with intrinsic electrical properties that result in the production of electrical and magnetic fields. These fields may be recorded at a distance from their sources and are termed "far-field potentials." Fields recorded a short distance from their source are termed "near-field" or "local field potentials." Activity recorded from the surface of the cortex is described as the electrocorticogram (ECoG), whereas electrical activity recorded from the scalp is the EEG. The EEG and ECoG are both far-field potentials. An evoked potential (EP) is generated by recording the EEG time-locked to a sensory stimulus, such as presentation of an auditory tone. Averaging the EEG over a sequence of responses allows the electrical activity specific to the stimulus to be extracted and presented by a plot of voltage (amplitude) against time. Somatosensory-evoked potentials (SEPs) recorded from the dura at various loci in animals in response to repetitive noxious stimuli are used extensively to study pain and analgesia. Table 46.6 outlines the advantages and limitations of EEG and EPs in phasic pain tests.

Nociceptive withdrawal reflexes (NWRs) are an established neurophysiologic measure used in rodent models as a direct measure of spinal cord hyperexcitability and thus a biomarker of central sensitization [227,228]. They have also been translated to humans to quantify spinal cord excitability in patients with chronic pain, including pain caused by OA [229]. The *NWR threshold* is defined as the magnitude of the stimulus (e.g., electrical current) that is required to elicit an electromyographic (EMG) response remembering that central sensitization causes a decrease in this threshold. Temporal summation (amplification of the magnitude of the EMG signal in response to repetitive noxious stimulation) of the NWR is also measured to probe changes in the spinal nociceptive processing. Use of these techniques in rodents requires anesthesia. NWR thresholds and temporal summation have been measured in awake dogs and horses using electrical stimuli and used to characterize the antinociceptive effects of analgesic drugs [230–232].

The third major neurophysiologic endpoint used in phasic pain tests in laboratory animals is direct recording of neuronal activity during stimulus application, for example, recording from peripheral afferent sensory fibers or dorsal horn neurons using *in vivo* electrophysiology. These studies are usually carried out under terminal anesthesia.

Table 46.2 Advantages and disadvantages of different stimulus modalities used to study acute pain.

Stimulus modality	Characteristics of the stimulus	Advantages	Disadvantages
Electrical	Direct activation of all nerve fibers, thereby bypassing transduction mechanisms at the peripheral nociceptor.	1. Quantifiable. 2. Brief; controlled onset and offset. 3. Reproducible. 4. Non-invasive. 5. Bypasses peripheral nociceptor transduction mechanisms that may be advantageous in the study of central pain mechanisms. 6. Elicits a synchronized pattern of neuronal activity that is sufficient to generate reflex responses. 7. Graded behavioral responses to increasing stimulus intensities. 8. Translatable between humans and animals.	1. Not a natural stimulus. 2. Indiscriminate activation of all fiber types (therefore not selective for Aδ or C fibers). 3. Bypasses peripheral nociceptor transduction mechanisms, therefore of limited use for the study of peripheral pain mechanisms. 4. Elicits a synchronized pattern of neuronal activity that does not replicate patterns of activity that occur in clinical pain states. 5. Impedance of the tissue will determine the magnitude of the delivered stimulus – care must be taken to standardize the stimulus magnitude as much as possible.
Thermal: general comments	Selective activation of cutaneous thermosensitive and nociceptive fibers. Rate of heating can be altered to selectively activate Aδ or C fibers.	1. Natural stimulus. 2. Most thermal stimuli deliver slow rates of heating of nociceptors and therefore selectively activate C fibers; efficient for revealing the activity of opioid analgesics.	1. Surface skin temperature can be measured easily, but more difficult to measure the temperature at the level of the nociceptor. Thermocouples placed in the deeper tissues to measure temperature often disturb heat transfer. 2. Thermal hyperalgesia is clinically less problematic than mechanical hyperalgesia in clinical pain patients.
Thermal: radiant heat source	Conventional radiant heat sources emit light in the visible or adjacent infrared spectra.	1. Easy to build. 2. Selective; no concurrent stimulation of non-nociceptive neurons (e.g., low-threshold mechanosensitive neurons).	1. Conventional radiant heat sources often lack power to cause synchronized neuronal activity and therefore generate reflex responses. 2. Infrared light sources in the wavelengths generated by radiant heat sources are poorly absorbed by skin. 3. Variability in stimulus magnitude determined by: a. reflectance, transmittance, and absorption; properties of the skin and the electromagnetic spectrum emitted by the source of radiation, b. conduction properties of the skin, c. initial temperature of the skin, d. the amount of caloric energy delivered to the surface of the skin.
Thermal: contact thermode	Heat thermosensitive receptors by means of the conduction properties of the skin.	1. Can deliver a slope of heating that grows linearly with time and can be precisely controlled. 2. Difficult to secure laboratory animals, widely used in companion and farm animals.	1. Concurrent activation of low-threshold non-nociceptive nerves that exert an inhibitory influence on pain mechanisms. 2. Thermode surface is usually flat and rigid and therefore does not conform very well to the skin surface. 3. Rate of thermal transfer is dependent on the quality of the thermode–skin contact.
Thermal: immersion in a temperature-controlled water bath		1. Rapid, although not instantaneous increase in skin temperature.	
Thermal: CO_2 laser	Long-wavelength infrared source of radiation.	1. Near-total absorption of the light by the skin, irrespective of skin pigmentation or radiation from the skin surface. 2. Thermal energy is maintained in the superficial surface of the skin where thermosensitive nerve terminals are located, limiting damage and therefore pain in deeper tissues. 3. A highly focused beam can be generated, good spatial discrimination. 4. Very rapid rates of heating can be achieved, allowing rapid onset and offset of the stimulus while meeting target temperature. 5. No contact between the laser and the skin is necessary, therefore there is no concurrent activation of mechanosensitive non-nociceptive nerves.	1. Expensive to buy. 2. Safety precautions must be adopted during use (e.g., humans should wear protective eye goggles to prevent retinal damage from stray laser light).
Mechanical	Activation of Aδ and C fiber mechanoreceptors (e.g., von Frey filaments). Visceral pain can also be triggered by mechanical distension (e.g., colonic distension with a balloon).	1. Mechanical hyperalgesia is a cardinal feature of chronic pain, therefore testing mechanical sensitivity is clinically relevant.	1. Low-threshold mechanoreceptors are always co-stimulated; therefore, the stimulus is not specific. 2. Conventional mechanical stimuli, e.g., von Frey filaments, do not allow delivery of brief mechanical stimuli with a rapid onset and offset. 3. Difficult to apply in a controlled manner to laboratory animals.

Table 46.3 Phasic tests utilizing thermal stimuli.

Test	Brief description of methods including activation of nociceptive/ pain pathways	Species in which tests are commonly applied	Behavioral endpoint	"Cut-Off"	Advantages	Disadvantages
Tail-flick test (radiant heat)	Radiant heat applied to a small area on the tail; reaction time before a tail flick occurs is measured ("tail-flick latency"). Radiant heat emission can be controlled to adjust tail-flick latency to alter sensitivity of the assay. A photoelectric cell timer switches off the lamp (heat source) when the tail is withdrawn. Selective activation of cutaneous thermosensitive and nociceptive fibers.	Rodents	Tail-flick. Generally considered to be a spinal reflex when high-intensity power is used to generate the radiant heat and the tail-flick latency is short. Will be subject to control by supraspinal structures. When the rate of heating is slower, then tail flick probably involves higher neural structures.	Maximum latency (usually estimated to be 4–5 times the latency in naive animals)	Simple to carry out. Clearly identifiable endpoint response, limits variability between animals under controlled experimental conditions.	Tail is the predominant organ of thermoregulation in the rat. Factors that can affect tail-flick latency and must be controlled for within an experiment include: 1. The rate of heating (determined by the power of the radiant heat source), 2. The area of tail stimulated (including site, proximal or distal, and total area). Prone to habituation (i.e., increase in latency) with shortened inter-stimulus interval and increased stimulus intensity.
Tail-flick test (immersion method)	Immersion of the tail in a hot liquid to produce a very rapid and linear increase in tail temperature. Greater area of the tail stimulated than for the radiant heat method. Latency to tail movement is measured. A noxious cold stimulus can be used instead of a heat stimulus. Selective activation of cutaneous thermosensitive and nociceptive fibers.	Rodents Monkeys	Sudden movement of the tail that may be associated with whole-body movements.	Maximum latency (see above)	Simple to carry out. Reflexes and higher neural structures generate the endpoint behavior. Capability to change the temperature of the water bath and therefore alter the sensitivity of the test (e.g., to study analgesics of different efficacies).	Tail is the predominant organ of thermoregulation in the rat. Latency will be modulated by the surface area of the tail stimulated.
Paw withdrawal test	Radiant heat is applied to the plantar surface of the hind paw. Latency to paw withdrawal is measured, a photoelectric cell timer switches off the lamp (heat source) when the paw is withdrawn. Termed the "Hargreaves test" when combined with inflammation to study hyperalgesia. Selective activation of cutaneous thermosensitive and nociceptive fibers.	Rodents Dogs	Paw withdrawal. Complex behavioral response.	Maximum latency (see above)	Simple. Animal is freely moving, readily able to perform withdrawal responses.	Baseline temperature of the skin will affect the latency to withdrawal. Freely moving animal, background level of activity in the flexor muscles of the leg varies with the position of the animal and this can alter speed of withdrawal response.
Radiant heat	Heat source applied to a distinct body part on the animal, e.g., coronary band in horses, flank in pigs. Radiant heat may be generated by a light source or CO_2 laser. Selective activation of cutaneous thermosensitive and nociceptive fibers.	Horses Pigs Cats	Withdrawal response to move the body part away from the stimulus, e.g., foot lift.	Maximum latency (see above)	Simple.	Some restraint is necessary to allow the heat to be focused on the selected body part. Baseline temperature of the skin will affect the latency to withdrawal.
Hot-plate test	Animal is introduced to an open-ended cylindrical space with a floor consisting of a metallic plate that is heated to a constant temperature (most commonly by a thermode). Reaction time (latency) to a behavioral response is measured. Activation of cutaneous thermosensitive and nociceptive fibers, coactivation of low-threshold mechanoreceptors.	Rodents Birds (adapted, e.g., heated perch)	Paw licking. Jumping. Other complex behaviors such as sniffing or washing may be observed. Complex behavioral responses that are supraspinally integrated.	Maximum latency (see above)	Various behavioral endpoints may be differentially sensitive to analgesic drugs (increases sensitivity of the assay).	Stimulates all four limbs and the tail simultaneously; may therefore recruit descending endogenous analgesia mechanisms. Complexity of behavioral responses that vary between animals can make it difficult to define the endpoint. Reaction times decrease with increased testing of the same animal, therefore difficult to obtain a stable baseline.

(Continued)

Table 46.3 (Continued)

Test	Brief description of methods including activation of nociceptive/ pain pathways	Species in which tests are commonly applied	Behavioral endpoint	"Cut-Off"	Advantages	Disadvantages
Contact thermode secured to the skin of the animal over a body part that is relatively flat to ensure sustained contact at the same pressure	Conventional thermodes have slow (< 1 °C/s) rates of heating and selectively activate C fibers rather than Aδ fibers. Temperature at which a behavioral response occurs is the "threshold" temperature. Activation of cutaneous thermosensitive and nociceptive fibers, coactivation of low-threshold mechanoreceptors.	Horses Cats Dogs Birds Reptiles	*Nature* of the response varies between species, time of the response (early or late), and the site of application of the stimulus. Repertoire of behavioral endpoints may be documented, e.g., skin twitch, head turn, movement to try to avoid the stimulus, leg lift (if stimulus is applied to the distal limb). Reflex and organized complex responses occur.	Maximum temperature varies depending on species and type of thermode	Equipment is relatively simple to build. Can apply to freely moving animal and well tolerated.	*Nature* of the endpoint may vary between animals, can be difficult to compare data between animals and between different experimenters. Limited sites of application of the thermode dependent on species. Threshold temperature affected by factors such as starting skin temperature and environmental temperature.
Cold (rarely used in phasic tests of acute pain in naive animals, commonly used to assess neuropathic pain)	Application of a droplet of acetone or ethyl chloride spray to the hind paw to provide localized cooling of the skin. Use of ice-water baths (tail or foot immersion) or cold plates (e.g., Peltier cooled plate) on which the animal stands.	Rodents Dogs	Behavioral response (e.g., withdrawal) from the cold stimulus is typically observed, such as foot lifting, latency to lift the paw from a cold plate.	Maximum latency (usually estimated to be 4–5 times the latency in naive animals)	Abnormal sensory responses to cold are a common feature of clinical neuropathic pain states in humans.	Magnitude of the cold stimulus is difficult to control and is affected by the ambient temperature and the temperature of the animal's skin.

Table 46.4 Phasic tests utilizing mechanical stimuli.

Test	Brief description of methods including activation of nociceptive/pain pathways	Species in which tests are commonly applied	Behavioral endpoint	"Cut-Off"	Advantages	Disadvantages
von Frey	von Frey filaments are blunt-ended plastic hairs of various diameters on fixed applicators. They are applied locally (most commonly to the plantar surface of the hind paw in rats) until they bend, at which point they exert a calibrated pressure. Filaments may also be used to assess responses to dynamic mechanical stimuli (e.g., brush allodynia). Automated and electronic von Frey devices are also available that provide a continuous scale of application (e.g., electronic esthesiometer). Site of application is variable in animals other than rodents. Activates Aδ and C fibers (depending on filament diameter), coactivation of low-threshold mechanoreceptors.	Rodents Dogs Horses Cattle Sheep	Withdrawal response to move away from the stimulus. May be accompanied by behaviors such as licking (e.g., of the paw) in animals with inflammatory or neuropathic pain arising from the stimulated area. The von Frey filament weight or the pressure applied by an electronic device required to elicit withdrawal is recorded.	Manual von Frey filament systems do not employ a "cut-off," although this may be imposed by the experimenter. Automated devices allow a maximum preset pressure to be attained and the stimulus application is stopped. Maximum force (usually estimated to be 4–5 times the force in naive animals)	Easy to apply. May evaluate mechanical hyperalgesia and allodynia (although difficult to distinguish between them). Widely used, large body of published reference data.	No "gold standard" protocol for application, data generated between different experimenters and labs are very variable. Not nociceptive specific due to coactivation of low-threshold mechanoreceptors. Debate about whether stimulus application elicits pain or nociception/ mechanical sensations (e.g., touch) only. Rate of application of force not standardized in manual von Frey testing.
Randall–Selitto test	Hind paw is placed between a fixed element (e.g., surface or blunt point) and a mobile blunt point exerting controlled pressure. The pressure is usually provided by a sliding counterweight system. Activates predominantly Aδ fibers, coactivation of low-threshold mechanoreceptors.	Rats	Threshold (in grams) for appearance of a given behavior. The behavior may be a reflex withdrawal, struggling, or vocalization depending on the protocol.	Imposed by the experimenter, should be below the level at which stimulus application causes tissue damage (usually estimated to be 4–5 times the force in naive animals)	When carried out correctly, can give reproducible and reliable readings.	Requires the animal to be restrained in an unnatural position, which requires training and prehabituation.
Strain gauges	Strain gauges are fixed on blunt forceps. The animal is loosely restrained, the forceps are placed around the hind paw and an incremental force is applied until the paw is withdrawn. Predominantly activates Aδ fibers (dependent on probe type), coactivation of low-threshold mechanoreceptors.	Rats	Withdrawal response.	Imposed by the experimenter, should be below the level at which stimulus application causes tissue damage (usually estimated to be 4–5 times the force in naive animals)	When carried out correctly, can give reproducible and reliable readings.	Rate of application of force is variable depending on the experimenter; careful standardization is required.

Table 46.4 (Continued)

Test	Brief description of methods including activation of nociceptive/pain pathways	Species in which tests are commonly applied	Behavioral endpoint	"Cut-Off"	Advantages	Disadvantages
Mechanical devices used in species other than rodents	A variety of devices have been described, in general, force is applied to a body part via a blunt-ended pin/probe that is advanced against the skin and tissues using pneumatic devices that may be manually or electronically controlled. Nociceptive fiber activation will be determined by the type of pin/probe; sharp tips are more likely to activate Aδ fibers, larger diameter blunt-ended pins will more likely activate C fibers, coactivation of low-threshold mechanoreceptors.	Dogs Cats Horses Chickens	Withdrawal response. Stimuli commonly applied to the limb hence limb withdrawal is a common endpoint.	Imposed by the experimenter, should be below the level at which stimulus application causes tissue damage (usually estimated to be 4–5 times the force in naive animals)	Devices are secured to the animal allowing it to move freely. Well tolerated by animals. Rate of application of force can be controlled.	Prehabituation may be required to give repeatable responses within the same individual. Repertoire of behavioral responses may be shown that signal the "endpoint" of the test, can lead to variability between different experimenters.

Table 46.5 Phasic tests utilizing electrical stimuli.

Test	Brief description of methods including activation of nociceptive/pain pathways	Species in which tests are commonly applied	Behavioral endpoint	"Cut-Off"	Advantages	Disadvantages
Application of long-lasting trains of electrical stimuli applied to the tail and/or paw	Electrical stimuli of gradually increasing intensities are delivered in trains lasting hundreds of milliseconds using subcutaneous electrodes or via the floor of a cage in which the animal is placed.	Rodents	Sequence of responses depending on intensity from reflex movement/withdrawal, vocalization during stimulation, and vocalization that persists after the end of the stimulus. Responses are organized on a hierarchical basis dependent on the level of integration of the nociceptive and pain pathways.	Maximum current intensity (estimated to be 4–5 times the intensity in naive animals)	Complex behavioral responses can be elicited.	Concurrent stimulation of the paws and tail (electrical stimulation delivered through the floor) will likely recruit endogenous analgesia mechanisms.
Use of single shocks or short chains of electrical stimulation of the tail	Threshold current intensity at which a defined behavioral response is displayed (± latency to the response). Stimuli delivered via subcutaneous electrodes.	Rodents Monkeys	Sequence of behaviors; twitching, escape behaviors, vocalizations, and biting of the electrodes that are hierarchically organized (see above). Vocalizations may be recorded electronically and analyzed (e.g., spectrum, reaction time, threshold to vocalization).	Maximum current intensity (estimated to be 4–5 times the intensity in naive animals)	Complex behavioral responses can be elicited.	
Electrical stimulation of the dental pulp	Some evidence to indicate that most of the afferent nerve fibers in dental pulp are nociceptive, thus allowing selective activation of nociceptive fibers using electrical stimuli. The experimental paradigm varies depending on the physiology of the tooth being stimulated (i.e., whether the tooth is continuously erupting, e.g., rat incisors, or has limited growth, e.g., cat and dog).	Rodents Dogs Cats Monkeys	Disynaptic jaw-opening reflex that can be recorded electromyographically from the digastric muscle in awake animals. Coordinate behavioral responses such as licking, chewing, or changes in facial expression.	Maximum current intensity (estimated to be 4–5 times the intensity in naive animals)	Reflex response is easily quantifiable. Can reveal the activity of non-opioid analgesics that cannot be detected by the hot-plate test.	Debate over the selectivity of the electrical stimulus to activate nociceptive fibers. Not sensitive to the effects of NSAIDs.

Ethical considerations

It is widely acknowledged that studies in animals have played, and will continue to play, a pivotal role in advancing knowledge and developing new analgesic molecules in pain research. However, the majority [233] of pain studies require the delivery of painful stimuli to the animal, and therefore are associated with ethical concerns and constraints that must be respected by the research community. The IASP published guidelines on the ethical use of animals in pain research and the updated ARRIVE 2.0 guidelines for reporting research are good reference sources for those working in this field [233]. The key points of the guidelines with respect to ethics in pain research are summarized as follows:

- Understand moral and ethical issues and arguments associated with the use of animals in experimentation.
- Understand how to design experiments that minimize the numbers of animals used, that maximize statistical inferences, and

Table 46.6 Advantages and limitations of neurophysiologic techniques used to measure pain in awake animals.

Technique	Advantages	Limitations
Raw electroencephalogram (EEG)	Flexible; the user can manipulate the recording equipment in order to optimize signal quality. All EEG data are retained, allowing comprehensive and detailed analysis. Data are recorded in real time rather than provision of discontinuous data points.	Large quantities of data are generated that can hinder interpretation. Data require complex mathematical processing after collection; therefore, they cannot be immediately interpreted. Definition of an *endpoint* to a ramped stimulus is therefore problematic. A basic understanding of EEG recording is required. Subcutaneous needle electrodes or surface electrodes usually give a poor signal-to-noise ratio in awake animals; implantation of dural electrodes for awake recordings is invasive.
Evoked potentials, e.g., somatosensory-evoked potentials (SEPs)	Evoked potentials generated from high-intensity noxious stimuli provide specific information on the neural processing of noxious stimuli. Targeted placement of electrodes at specific intracerebral loci allows the brain structures involved in the neural processing of pain to be identified. The SEP waveform is relatively easy to interpret.	Signal averaging is required to generate a SEP; therefore, noxious stimuli must be repeatedly applied. The amplitude of the SEP signal is small compared with the EEG or electrical noise. Some skill is required to generate a SEP with an acceptable signal-to-noise ratio. The stimuli used to generate a SEP should only stimulate nociceptive fibers or the SEP will include non-nociceptive components. This is challenging and has only been achieved using radiant heat generated by lasers. Laser-evoked potentials reflect predominately Aδ fiber-mediated activity rather than C fiber activity. Owing to the difficulties in generating a noxious stimulus that is time-locked to allow EEG recording, SEPs are most commonly generated by heat (laser-evoked potentials) or electrical stimuli only.

that maximize the recording of variables relevant to the assessment of pain experienced by animals.

- Know how to employ a nociceptive stimulus or condition that is minimal in intensity and duration (tested on the investigator when possible) so as to shorten the duration of an experiment consistent with the attainment of justifiable, ethical research objectives.
- Know reasons why unanesthetized animals should be minimally exposed to nociceptive stimuli from which they cannot escape or which they cannot avoid or terminate.
- Know reasons why pharmacologically paralyzed animals are anesthetized or rendered neurosurgically insensate.

Maximum stimulus intensity

All phasic pain tests should incorporate a maximum stimulus intensity that is not exceeded in any test and is below the threshold intensity for that stimulus modality that is sufficient to cause lasting tissue damage. This is fundamental to carrying out pain experiments ethically in animals. It is important to maintain the physiologic well-being of the animal to ensure that collected data are valid, since tissue damage at the site of stimulation will induce peripheral and central sensitization that will result in a change in responsiveness in the pain test over time. The time interval between the application of each repeat test should be selected in order to prevent upregulation of nociceptive pathways. These factors are particularly important in tests involving the administration of analgesic drugs, where behavioral responses to the assay may be obtunded until high stimulus intensities would be otherwise attained.

Measurement of nociceptive withdrawal thresholds in companion animals

In recent years, numerous studies have been published in which nociceptive withdrawal thresholds were utilized to investigate the analgesic efficacy of drugs in companion animals [234–238] and to probe upregulation of nociceptive processes in clinical conditions causing pain (e.g., after surgery or as a result of chronic inflammatory diseases such as foot rot in sheep) [239–242]. Undoubtedly, measurement of nociceptive withdrawal thresholds to assess analgesic drug efficacy has a number of advantages. However, the effect of confounding factors must be understood in order to maximize the quality of the collected data. For example, environmental temperature, skin temperature, and level of distraction of the animal can all affect measured thresholds. Some advantages of the measurement of nociceptive withdrawal thresholds to quantify analgesic drug efficacy include the following:

- It is applied to naive animals to study the test drug in the target species.
- It is an objective measure of drug effect against a standardized noxious stimulus, thereby eliminating the variability associated with measuring drug effect in a clinical pain model.
- The methodology is ethically acceptable; imposing a maximum stimulus intensity below the level required to cause tissue damage prevents lasting harm.

However, there are several important limitations associated with the measurement of nociceptive withdrawal thresholds that must be considered during data interpretation:

- The technique relies on the detection of an endpoint behavior that may be reflexive (e.g., skin twitch) or more complex (whole-body movement away from the stimulus). When measuring responses to analgesic drug administration, it is important that the endpoint response is standardized to reduce variability in the collected data.
- It is problematic to relate a change in threshold to the clinical efficacy of the drug with any certainty.
- Owing to the requirement to impose a maximum stimulus intensity, data are very commonly censored following administration of an analgesic drug, so that the relative efficacies of different drugs (where censorship occurs for more than one drug) cannot be determined.
- There is a minimal time interval required between subsequent tests in order to prevent sensitization, which is problematic for pharmacokinetic–pharmacodynamic studies where frequent measurement of nociceptive thresholds is advantageous.
- Measurement of nociceptive withdrawal thresholds in naive animals allows the measurement of the analgesic effect of the drug (e.g., analgesic efficacy of opioids) but does not allow the assessment of the antihyperalgesic effects of drugs such as NSAIDs unless an inflammatory focus is introduced.

Pain models – tonic tests

Some pain models induce pain created by tissue or nerve injury and are therefore associated with medium- to long-lasting pain. Naturally occurring disease models of pain in animals are attractive because of their greater translatability to clinical pain conditions in humans; however, the number of conditions for which a well-characterized, spontaneous pain model exists is currently limited.

Animal models of pain should fulfill a multidimensional set of criteria of validity to be considered relevant for human pathophysiology, of which face, mechanistic, and predictive validity are considered pivotal [243]. Face validity is the similarity of what is observed in the animal model to the human and is considered in terms of both ethologic validity (i.e., similarity in behaviors) and biomarker validity (i.e., the function of the biomarker in representing underlying neurobiological mechanisms). Mechanistic validity assesses the similarity of the mechanism working in the animal model to the mechanism that is presumed to be working in the human disease, referring at the same time to the mechanism that is considered to produce changes in a biological biomarker and the mechanism that is sensitive to the action of effective therapeutic agents. Predictive validity is the performance of a therapeutic agent in the animal model compared with the therapeutic efficacy in clinical patients. It is widely acknowledged that current animal pain models fail to meet these criteria fully.

Induced pain models

Many different pain models have been developed with the primary aim of increasing understanding and treatment of clinical pain states. The majority of these have been developed in rodents, but some have been translated to companion and farm animals. Models are broadly divided into inflammatory or neuropathic pain models, although some newer models trigger both inflammatory and neuropathic pain mechanisms because it is recognized that many clinical pain conditions in humans have both a neuropathic and an inflammatory component [244]. Induced disease models have also been developed to replicate some disease conditions in humans, such as painful diabetic neuropathy and postherpetic neuralgia [245–247]. A large repertoire of biomarkers is used to assay pain in animal models. Broadly, these biomarkers can be classified based on whether the biomarker involves (1) measurement of phasic responses to acute noxious stimuli in awake animals (see above); (2) measurement of changes in spontaneous behavior; (3) assessment of affective state in more complex behavioral tests; or (4) measurements conducted in anesthetized animals (e.g., nociceptive withdrawal reflexes [NWRs]).

Models of inflammatory pain

Most models of inflammatory pain involve the injection of inflammatory mediators themselves or of chemical substances that provoke an immune response. The substances may be injected intradermally or subcutaneously, intraperitoneally, or into the joint capsule. Common cutaneous models of inflammatory pain and their advantages and disadvantages are shown in Table 46.7. Recognition that pain elicited from muscle has different characteristics from cutaneous pain has led to the development of models of muscle pain and hyperalgesia to better understand the mechanisms underlying the development of chronic muscle pain. Stimuli used to elicit muscle pain include injection of low-pH saline (pH 5.2–6.9), carrageenan, cytokines (e.g., tumor necrosis factor-α and interleukin-6), mustard oil, zymogen, and hypertonic saline.

Arthritis is one of the most prevalent chronic health conditions and is a leading cause of disability in humans. Therefore, arthritis pain has long been a major area of research in biomedical science and different animal models of arthritis are available for the assessment of joint pain and analgesic drug effects. Commonly the knee (stifle) joint is studied in OA models. Animal models of OA include spontaneous OA in specific strains of mice and guinea pigs, intra-articular injections of compounds to induce joint inflammation, or surgical disruption of the joint. Common models of arthritis (OA and rheumatoid arthritis) and their advantages and disadvantages are summarized in Table 46.8. Common methods of assessing arthritic knee joint pain are given in Table 46.9, including their advantages and disadvantages.

Models of neuropathic pain

Neuropathic pain is characterized by sensory abnormalities such as unpleasant abnormal sensation (dysesthesia), hyperalgesia, and allodynia. A battery of neuropathic pain models have been developed in animals in an attempt to simulate the diverse etiology of clinical neuropathic pain conditions in humans. These models cause substantial suffering to the animal, in terms of both pain severity and duration. As such, predefined endpoints are usually imposed that can be used to indicate when euthanasia of the animal is required. These endpoints are often relatively crude and relate to the general health status of the animal, for example, weight loss. There are no translational neuropathic pain models because the nerve damage required to produce neuropathic pain is irreversible. Table 46.10 gives an overview of the characteristics of commonly used models of neuropathic pain, with their advantages and disadvantages. Until recently, neuropathic pain in these models was most commonly assessed by application of phasic pain tests and assessment of behavior.

Models of visceral pain

Visceral pain, particularly arising from the bowel, is one of the most common reasons for medical presentation in humans and an area of unmet clinical need. Models of visceral pain in animals have been developed to better understand both the underlying neurophysiology of visceral pain pathways as well as the dysregulations of visceral hypersensitivity that occur with functional bowel disorders, such as irritable bowel syndrome (IBS). However, modeling IBS is particularly challenging because it is a functional disorder and therefore lacks significant pathology around which an animal model is based. An overview of methods used to induce visceral pain or visceral sensitivity in animals is given in Table 46.11. These methods are broadly divided into phasic stimuli that cause transient visceral stimulation (e.g., colorectal distension) and methods that produce tonic pain by inducing sensitization of the viscera (e.g., injection of irritant substances into the peritoneum or sensitization of the gut via instillation of irritant substances into the gut lumen). A range of different outcome measures is used to evaluate visceral pain in animals, ranging from behavior in awake animals to evoked reflexes and physiologic responses.

Behavior

Behavioral endpoints that are species-specific have been developed to quantify visceral nociception. The behavior of the rat has been scored during colorectal distension [248], where a graded score is given dependent on whether behavioral responses are confined to a brief head movement followed by immobility (score 1) through to body arching and lifting of pelvic structures (score 4). Referred somatic hyperalgesia associated with a noxious visceral stimulus is also used as a criterion for visceral pain, evaluated by, for example, application of von Frey hairs to the abdomen and scoring of subsequent behavioral responses. Owing to the prevalence of colic as a clinical manifestation of visceral pain in the horse, a number of methods are used to evaluate visceral pain in this species following visceral distension. Endpoint behaviors include expulsion of the balloon from the rectum (colorectal distension) associated with flank watching [249,250] and signs of abdominal pain such as pawing at the ground, kicking of the abdomen, and weight shifting of the hind limbs following duodenal distension [251]. Writhing

Table 46.7 Common models of cutaneous inflammatory pain.

Name	Model description	Species	Biomarker	Advantages	Disadvantages
Formalin test	0.5–0.1 5% formalin (37% formaldehyde) is injected intradermally (in rodents it is injected into the dorsal surface of the rat forepaw). Injection initially activates nociceptors (phase 1, 3 minutes after injection); the late phase (phase 2, 20–30 min after injection) involves a period of sensitization during which inflammatory phenomena (including paw edema) occur. Both phase 1 and 2 are considered to be triggered by peripheral mechanisms; phase 2 involves central sensitization.	Rodents	Change in complex behaviors (licking, paw lifting). Behavioral reaction is biphasic, accompanying the biphasic nature of the underlying neurophysiologic mechanisms that evoke pain. Application of phasic pain tests. Paw volume.	Neurophysiology is well understood. Widely used as a pain assay, a large database to describe effects of different analgesics in the formalin model is available. Pain is of short duration (1–2 h), although inflammation may persist for a longer period.	Difficult to quantify the pain-related behaviors, therefore outcome assessment can be variable between experimenters. Short-duration inflammatory pain model only.
Carrageenan	Carrageenan is made from sulfated polysaccharides extracted from red seaweed. It is injected to elicit localized inflammation through induction of an immune response and activation of nociceptors.	Rodents (commonly injected intradermally in the paw). Cats, horses (tissue cage models)	Behavioral changes associated with inflammatory pain, generally less well defined than following injection of formalin. Application of phasic pain tests. Paw volume.	Well-established pain model. Does not elicit a systemic immune response.	Site of injection may remain thickened for a long duration, precluding repeat testing at the same site. Difficult to solubilize; thick, viscous substance that can make injection difficult.
Complete Freund's adjuvant (CFA)	Suspension of heat-killed *Mycobacterium butyricum* or *Mycobacterium tuberculosum* in an adjuvant. Doses used in rodent pain models produce cutaneous inflammation that appears in minutes to hours and peaks within 5–8 h; duration of inflammation is ~ 24 h, hyperalgesia can persist for 1–2 weeks.	Rodents (commonly injected intradermally in the paw)	See carrageenan	See carrageenan	See carrageenan
Mustard oil	Elicits inflammatory pain by activating transient receptor potential cation channel, subfamily A (TRPA1), an excitatory ion channel of primary afferent nociceptors. Usually applied topically to the skin; effects are of short duration.	Rodents	See carrageenan		
Zymogen	A glucan from the cell walls of yeast; activates primary afferent nociceptors.	Rodents	See carrageenan		
Kaolin	A suspension of kaolin is injected subcutaneously; may be mixed with carrageenan. Duration of inflammatory pain is ~ 1–2 days.	Cats Rodents	Application of phasic pain tests.	Well-established pain model.	See carrageenan
Capsaicin	Pungent component of chilies that activates the transient receptor potential vanilloid type 1 (TRPV1), a heat-sensitive cation on nociceptor terminals. Used to study neurogenic inflammation and hyperalgesia. Intradermal injection of capsaicin results in a flare reaction (neurogenic inflammation), allodynia, and hyperalgesia, the areas of which extend beyond the injection site. Duration of thermal and mechanical hyperalgesia is dose-dependent but can be up to 24 h.	Rodents Humans	Application of phasic pain tests. Area of flare.	Translational. Well-established pain model, underlying neurophysiologic mechanisms are well described.	Poor relationship between underlying pain mechanisms following capsaicin and clinical pain states. Repeated application of capsaicin results in desensitization of nociceptors to capsaicin and other noxious stimuli (which is reversible). At high concentrations, capsaicin will cause sensory neuron toxicity and cell death.
Skin incision	A surgical skin incision is used to generate inflammation.	Rodents	Application of phasic pain tests. Behavioral changes associated with inflammatory pain.	Triggers inflammatory pain mechanisms that are identical to those triggered by surgical trauma.	Invasive. Cannot repeat in individual animals. Care must be taken to ensure asepsis.
Surgery (e.g., castration and OHE)	Animals undergoing routine neutering are recruited for analgesia studies.	Cats Dogs Horses Deer (e.g., velvet antler removal)	Behavior. Application of phasic pain tests. EEG and EPs.	Animals would be undergoing surgery regardless, therefore adheres to the experimental principle of reduction. Clinically relevant pain model to allow study of pain mechanisms and efficacy of analgesic drugs.	Magnitude of the surgical stimulus may vary depending on patient factors and the skill of the surgeon. Requires case recruitment (i.e., owner consent).
UVB irradiation	Exposure to a UVB light source to produce a localized burn injury characterized by sterile inflammation.	Rats Pigs	Application of phasic pain tests.	Translational. Induces central and peripheral sensitization.	Characteristics of the skin will affect the magnitude of the injury induced by a standardized exposure to UVB radiation.

UVB, ultraviolet B.

Table 46.8 Models of osteoarthritis (OA) and rheumatoid arthritis.

Name	Model description	Species	Advantages	Disadvantages
Spontaneous OA in specific (e.g., Hartley albino) guinea pig strains	Bilateral disease of the knee joint that involves cartilage degeneration, subchondral sclerosis, and bone cysts. The pathogenesis is not fully understood.	Guinea pigs	Predictable onset and progression of the disease. Many similarities in disease progression to human OA.	The strains of guinea pigs are expensive to buy and must be housed for a long period before severe OA changes develop (up to 2 years).
Spontaneous OA in other laboratory animals	See above	Hamsters Mice	See above	See above, although progression of the disease will be more rapid in animals with a shorter life span, such as mice.
Surgically induced OA	Surgically induced trauma to the joint caused by creation of a meniscal tear or meniscectomy. Progressive changes in the knee joint occur relatively rapidly post-surgery	Rats Mice Guinea pigs Dogs Rabbits	Reproducible. Mimics pathologic changes and pain of OA in humans.	Depending on the size of the animal (species), the surgery can be technically challenging. Rapid progression of lesions after surgery, therefore insensitive in the detection of new compounds with protective effects against the development of OA.
Intra-articular monosodium iodoacetate (MIA) injection into the knee	Induces degeneration of cartilage by inhibition of aerobic glycolysis, which kills chondrocytes. Joint pathology is characterized by chondrocyte necrosis resulting in decreased thickness of articular cartilage and fibrillation of the cartilage surface, separation of necrotic cartilage from the underlying bone, and exposure of subchondral bone.	Can be induced in many species, commonly used in rats	Induced pathology is similar to human OA.	Arthritic changes take several weeks to develop.
Inflammatory monoarthritis (knee joint)	Injection of kaolin and carrageenan into the joint to produce an aseptic use-dependent monoarthritis with damage to the cartilage, inflammation of the synovia, and synovial fluid exudate. Other irritants that may be injected include zymosan and complete Freund's adjuvant (CFA).	Predominantly rats and mice; cats, primates.	Joint inflammation develops rapidly and persists for weeks. Large database relating to use of the model in laboratory animals.	Only mimics the acute inflammatory phase of human OA.
Rheumatoid arthritis	Polyarthritis induced by injection of immunogenic adjuvants (e.g., CFA). The adjuvant is usually injected intradermally or subcutaneously into the footpad or base of the tail to generate a polyarthritis.	Predominantly rats and mice	Well established and reproducible.	Systemic nature of the arthritis can affect the overall condition and well-being of the animals and confound pain assessment.
	Immunogenic adjuvant arthritis induced by intradermal injection of cartilage-derived proteins.	Rats Mice	See above	See above
	Non-immunogenic adjuvant arthritis induced by injection of compounds that do not contain major histocompatibility complex-binding peptides but involve T-cell activation, e.g., mineral oil injected intradermally or subcutaneously.	Rats Mice	See above	See above
Gouty arthritis	Injection of monosodium urate crystals dissolved in saline or uric acid or suspended in mineral oil into the knee joint to produce acute inflammation.	Rats Mice Dogs Chickens Cats	Acute synovitis generated within a few hours that resolves rapidly (within 3–7 days). No signs of systemic disease.	

Table 46.9 Common methods of assessing knee joint pain in arthritis.

Name	Brief description of the biomarker	Species in which the outcome measure is commonly utilized	Advantages	Disadvantages
Weight bearing on the hind paws	Weight distribution between the two hind paws is measured as the force exerted by each hind limb on a transducer plate in the floor over a given period. Weight borne by each hind limb is expressed as a percentage of bodyweight. A weight-bearing deficit on the affected limb is taken as an indicator of pain.	Rodents	Simple. Translational.	Requires restraint of the animal and does not assess weight distribution to the forelimbs as occurs with hind limb arthritis. Indirect measure of knee pain.
Weight bearing across all four paws	Weight load is detected while the animal is walking across four pairs of force sensor plates on the floor of an enclosed walkway.	Rodents Dogs Assessment of arthritis in other joints in chickens, cats, horses	Simple. Does not require restraint of the animal although a constant walking speed is usually necessary to facilitate data interpretation. Translational.	Animals are required to move, which can be affected by motivation (and is integrally linked to pain).
Posture and gait analysis	Static and dynamic behaviors have been quantified using subjective rating scales. Gait analysis using kinematic techniques.	Rodents Large animal species, including dogs, cats, horses, chickens	Subjective scales are simple to use and cost-effective. Gait analysis techniques are objective. Translational.	Subjective scales are inherently variable and unvalidated. Gait analysis data can be difficult to interpret and requires the animal to walk at a constant speed. Willingness to walk is affected by motivation (and is integrally linked to pain).

(*Continued*)

Table 46.9 (Continued)

Name	Brief description of the biomarker	Species in which the outcome measure is commonly utilized	Advantages	Disadvantages
Spontaneous mobility	Automated systems are available (e.g., biotelemetry, activity boxes for rodents, or continuous video of behavior and pattern recognition). Collar-mounted accelerometers to track movement over time along three axes. Assessment of willingness to perform spontaneous behavioral tasks, e.g., willingness of dogs to walk upstairs or cats to jump up or down from a raised surface.	Rodents Large animal species including dogs, cats, horses, chickens	Objective. Use of automated systems speeds and simplifies data analysis.	Willingness to move is affected by motivation (and is integrally linked to pain).
Mechanical or heat sensitivity of the paw	See phasic pain tests (Tables 46.3 and 46.4).			
Mechanical sensitivity of the knee	Knee joint is compressed using calibrated forceps equipped with force transducers. Force required to evoke a reflex withdrawal is measured.	Rats Mice	Measures sensitivity of the knee joint that is not confounded by the hind paw. Translational.	Requires restraint of the animal.
Struggling threshold angle of knee extension	Tibia is extended until the animal displays struggling behavior while the femur is held in position; the extension angle is then calculated.	Rats	Measures sensitivity of the knee joint that is not confounded by the hind paw.	Requires restraint of the animal.
Vocalizations evoked by compression of the knee	Audible and ultrasonic vocalizations are measured, representing nociceptive and emotional-affective responses, respectively.	Rats Mice	Ultrasonic vocalizations may give a better indication of joint pain than other reflexive measures such as withdrawal thresholds.	Use of vocalizations has not been fully validated in rodent OA models.
Neurophysiologic measures	Measurement of nociceptive withdrawal reflexes to electrical and mechanical stimuli in anesthetized animals to measure upregulation of central pain pathways. Direct recording from dorsal horn neurons to map peripheral receptive field size and neuronal activity (threshold and firing frequency) in response to non-noxious and noxious stimuli applied in the receptive field of the cell. Recording of spontaneous firing in peripheral sensory nerve fibers.	Rats Mice	Allows detailed investigation of the neurophysiologic changes accompanying pain caused by OA.	Requires anesthesia; experiments are non-recovery. Technically challenging.

Table 46.10 Examples of common models of neuropathic pain, all of which are commonly induced in rats and mice.

Name	Model description	Induced behavioral changes	Advantages	Disadvantages
Peripheral nerve injury models				
Axotomy model	Complete transection of the sciatic nerve at the mid-thigh level combined with lesioning of the saphenous nerve to induce complete denervation of the hind limb. A neuroma develops at the proximal nerve stump.	Pain is produced in the absence of any sensory input to the area. Autotomy is often observed, although whether this is an indication of spontaneous pain or a result of excessive grooming in the absence of sensory feedback is debated.		Complete nerve transection is uncommon in humans. Severe ethical issues associated with autotomy.
Chronic constriction injury	3–4 loose silk ligatures are placed around the sciatic nerve. Constriction of the sciatic nerve is associated with intraneural edema, focal ischemia, and Wallerian degeneration.	Mild-to-moderate autotomy, guarding, excessive licking, and altered weight bearing. These features persist for at least 7 weeks after surgery.	Clinical features correspond to complex regional pain syndrome in humans and the model has been used extensively for research on spontaneous pain and abnormal sensations.	Variable outcomes between different animals likely associated with the tightness of the ligatures placed around the nerve and type of suture material.
Partial sciatic nerve ligation	Tight ligation of half to one-third of the sciatic nerve using a single ligature.	Paw guarding and licking, not associated with autotomy.	Immediate onset and long-lasting duration of allodynia and hyperalgesia parallel pain in humans with causalgia.	
Spared nerve injury	The tibial and common peroneal nerves are tightly ligated followed by axotomy of the distal nerve, the sural nerve remains undamaged (hence spared nerve injury model). Allows the comparison of difference in mechanical and thermal sensitivities of non-injured skin territories adjoining denervated areas.	See above	Surgical model is relatively easy to create compared with other models and has lesser variability in the degree of damage. Allows simultaneous investigational changes in both injured primary sensory neurons and unharmed sensory neurons so that their relative contribution to the pathophysiology of pain can be determined.	

Table 46.10 (Continued)

Name	Model description	Induced behavioral changes	Advantages	Disadvantages
Sciatic inflammatory neuritis	A catheter is implanted around the sciatic nerve (under anesthesia), which is used to inject zymosan in awake, freely moving rats.	See above	Human neuropathies are commonly caused by inflammation or infection rather than trauma, and inflammatory events occur after trauma. This model may better mimic many human conditions causing neuropathic pain.	
Cuffing of the sciatic nerve	Placement of a polyethylene cuff around the sciatic nerve.	See above	High reproducibility associated with a more consistent magnitude of nerve injury compared with nerve ligation or axotomy.	
Central pain models				
Weight drop or contusion model	Spinal cord is exposed at the thoracolumbar level and a constant weight is dropped on the spinal cord to induce injury.	Severe paraplegia and complete segmental necrosis. Dysthesia, spontaneous, and evoked pain.		Ethical considerations associated with paraplegia.
Excitotoxic spinal cord injury	Intraspinal injections of excitatory amino acids to simulate injury-induced elevations of excitatory amino acids.	See above	Progressive pathologic changes associated with the injection closely resemble those induced by ischemic and traumatic spinal cord injury.	
Spinal hemisection	Spinal cord is hemisected just cranial to L1 with a blade.	See above	Number and type of injured fibers are controlled in each animal. The injured and intact sides of the animal are completely separated.	
Drug-induced neuropathy models				
Drug-induced neuropathy	Systemic injection of drugs that induce neuropathy such as vincristine and cisplatin.	Induce neuropathy; the clinical features are determined by the nerve type targeted by the drug.	Non-surgical.	Drugs often produce concurrent effects on the general health of the animal that can confound pain assessment.
Disease-induced neuropathy models				
Diabetes-induced neuropathy	Diabetes is induced in the animal, e.g., by administration of pancreatic β-cell toxins such as streptozotocin (STZ) or use of transgenic animals (mice) with type I and II diabetes.	Induce a peripheral neuropathy with associated signs of neuropathic pain.	Depending on the model can replicate clinical signs associated with painful diabetic neuropathy in humans.	Animals develop other metabolic derangements associated with diabetes that can confound pain assessment.
Cancer pain models, e.g., bone cancer pain	Bone cancer is induced in the animal, e.g., by inoculation of osteolytic fibrosarcoma cells into the femur of specific strains of mice.	Produce behavioral changes attributed to neuropathic and inflammatory pain.	Demonstrate the distinct pharmacologic and neurochemical aspects of cancer pain, suggesting the involvement of inflammatory, neuropathic, and tumorigenic components in the pathogenesis of pain.	May induce systemic changes in the animal associated with tumor growth that can compromise well-being and confound pain assessment.

Table 46.11 Common models of visceral pain.

Name	Model description	Advantages	Disadvantages
Visceral distension	Overfilling the bladder with fluid, pressure distension of the colon, duodenum, esophagus, or ureter. Distension pressure is usually controlled by a barostat (computer-controlled pump).	"Natural"' type of stimulus. Mechanical distension is relatively easy to control.	Challenging to develop devices that provide a rapid distension (square-wave stimulus); increasing ramp distension profile is more common. Type and predictability of the distension predict outcome, independent of the distension pressure. Repeated distension does not result in visceral hypersensitivity; therefore, cannot replicate pain and the heightened visceral sensitivity that occurs in people with inflammatory bowel disease (IBD).
Chemical irritation to induce hypersensitivity of the colon prior to mechanical distension	Application of chemical irritants to the colon (e.g., instillation of acetic acid, mustard oil, turpentine, zymosan).	Induce peripheral and central sensitization and increase responses to mechanical distension.	Debate over whether chemical irritation prior to distension induces changes similar to the functional changes that occur in people with IBD.
Chronic irrigation of the bladder to induce cystitis using compounds such as mustard oil and cyclophosphamide	Acute or chronic instillation of compounds that are known irritants.	Chronic administration of compounds causes histologic and neurophysiologic bladder changes that are similar to pathologic changes induced by clinical conditions resulting in chronic cystitis.	
Intraperitoneal injections of irritant agents, e.g., acetic or hydrochloric acid, bradykinin, mustard oil		Well-established pain model.	Parietal peritoneum receives somatic innervation; therefore, model causes visceral and somatic pain. Latency to writhing and duration are dependent on the chemical properties of the injected irritant.
Models of acute pancreatitis pain	Induction of pancreatic damage using systemic injection (IV) of dibutyltin dichloride; pancreatic injection of capsaicin or bradykinin.	Histologic changes resembling acute pancreatitis in humans develop.	There are almost no models of chronic pancreatitis.

(i.e., stereotyped abdominal contractions, movements of the whole body, twisting of the dorsoabdominal muscles, reduction in motor activity, and motor incoordination) are evoked in response to intraperitoneal administration of irritants and are collectively used as the outcome measure in the abdominal writhing test (rodents). The movements are considered reflex responses and are quantified in terms of their frequency. However, the frequency of cramps decreases spontaneously over time and therefore the writhing test is not used to assess the duration of action of putative analgesics. The number of cramps is also extremely variable between individual animals.

Abdominal muscle contraction

A common endpoint in rodent studies of visceral nociception is contraction of the abdominal muscles in response to colorectal distension, usually recorded using electromyography in both awake (by prior implantation of EMG wires) and anesthetized animals [252,253]. There is a correlation between the distending pressure and the integrated EMG signal or the number of spike bursts during the period of distension. EMG responses in neck muscles can also be recorded as a measure of nociceptive response to gastric distension. To avoid implanting EMG wires in muscles, abdominal contraction following balloon distension can be detected by amplifying rapid changes in pressure that are induced in the balloon.

Physiologic responses

In awake rats, visceral distension causes an increase in blood pressure and tachycardia, whereas, during deep anesthesia, a depressor response and bradycardia are generally noted (although the magnitude of the depressor/bradycardia response is modulated by the anesthetic agent used) [254].

Neuronal activity

The most direct approach to evaluate the effects of visceral distension is the recording of the neuronal activity of afferent or second-order neurons in anesthetized animals in acute electrophysiologic studies. Longer-term neuronal responses are also evaluated by measuring c-*fos* expression in different areas of the spinal cord in response to mechanical distension. Visceral evoked potentials (EPs) following colorectal distension are used to evaluate visceral nociception in awake rats [254,255].

Naturally occurring disease models

The study of naturally occurring or spontaneous diseases in animals has great potential because the underlying etiopathogenesis of the pain more likely replicates the mechanisms that result in clinical pain states in humans. With the exception of spontaneous OA in some species of guinea pigs and rodents, spontaneous disease models are most relevant to large animals. Spontaneous OA in the dog is a commonly used and appropriate (although perhaps not ideal) model for translational and comparative studies based on animal size, anatomy, disease mechanisms, clinical similarities, and response to therapy. OA in dogs occurs as a result of trauma, degenerative changes, and overuse, as it does in humans [256]. There is also interest in exploiting naturally occurring OA in cats as a translational model for human OA. However, with the exception of OA in dogs, there are few other naturally occurring animal disease models that are validated as translatable pain models for human clinical pain conditions. Bone cancer pain (dogs) [257] and pain caused by idiopathic cystitis in cats [258] are notable exceptions. Using naturally occurring diseases in companion animals requires that validated outcome measures to assess pain are available (e.g., Canine Brief Pain Inventory) [259,260]. This approach overcomes the ethical considerations associated with creating experimental pain in animals. However, limitations include: (1) ethical constraints imposed by studying pet dogs, and (2) lack of homogeneity of the disease processes. Companion animal disease models are likely to be most useful as an intermediate step to study pain mechanisms or analgesic drug efficacy that sit between preclinical rodent models and experimental pain studies in humans.

Recent trends in pain evaluation in rodents

There is a growing trend in preclinical research to develop better methods for assessing pain rather than nociception in rodents, thus attempting to record and "take into account" the affective or emotional component of pain in pain measurement. Although this area of research is still in its infancy, significant efforts have been made to develop novel measures of animal affect, many of them developed from the fields of ethology and animal welfare science. Some examples of new approaches to measuring pain in rodents are described below.

Place preference paradigm

The (conditioned) place preference paradigm is commonly used to evaluate the affective/motivational properties of drugs. The paradigm involves the pairing of a drug state with environments that have distinctive stimuli (i.e., a place). During a period of learning, the animal learns to associate one environment with treatment and the test drug and a second environment with a control treatment (e.g., saline). Subsequently, the animal's place preference is determined by allowing the animal to choose between these two environments, with the choice being made when the animal has not received the drug treatment. This paradigm is used to evaluate the effect of analgesic drugs on animals in chronic pain, with the underpinning rationale that animals in chronic pain should show a place preference for the environment that is paired with an analgesic drug. Place preference tests require animal training and must be carried out carefully to avoid confounding factors, for example, ensuring there are no factors inherent in the test environment that might induce a place preference other than the drug treatment. This type of test has been used to show the analgesic effects of different classes of drugs in the complete Freund's adjuvant (CFA) inflammatory pain model in rats, bladder cancer model in mice [261,262], and analgesic effects of butorphanol in chickens with naturally occurring keel bone fractures [263] and in calves undergoing disbudding [264,265].

Operant response paradigms

Operant response paradigms are commonly used in behavioral pharmacology and have been adapted to study the analgesic efficacy of different drugs in rodents. Operant conditioning relies on training animals to associate making a particular response with receiving either a reward (e.g., a sugar pellet) or a punishment (e.g., a foot shock). Operant paradigms allow the animal to exert control over the outcome, which is one of the key differences between operant and Pavlovian conditioning, where an outcome is associated with a stimulus over which the animal has no control. An example of an operant paradigm is one that gives a rat a choice between receiving a reward (e.g., sweet condensed milk) or preventing receipt of an aversive painful stimulus [266–268]. To receive the reward, the animal must poke its nose through an opening equipped with a thermode, so that the aversive stimulus (e.g., heat or cold) is obtained at the same time as the reward. Reward-seeking behavior is reduced following peripheral inflammation, an observation that is reversed with analgesic drugs. The operant behavior paradigms allow the observation of more spontaneous types of behaviors when compared with stimulus-evoked studies but require considerable training and also have a motivational component that can complicate the interpretation of pain-related behavior.

Assessment of spontaneous behaviors

Quantification of spontaneous behavior has long been recognized as a useful tool for studying pain severity and analgesic drug efficacy in rodents [269]. However, traditional behavioral analysis is limited because it is extremely time-consuming, so only a limited range of behaviors tend to be studied for a short period. The recent development of automated systems to quantify behaviors in rodents has significantly enhanced the capability of behavioral analysis in the study of pain. These systems have the capacity to collect data continuously and in a standardized way so that variation and error are minimized, to provide information about the movement of individual animals, and to track complex changes in behavior. Therefore, they offer the opportunity to detect very subtle changes in the behavior of individual animals in terms of both mobility and interactive behaviors such as play, nesting, and lying with cage mates. This significantly increases the sensitivity of behavioral assessment to detect pain and the effects of analgesic drug administration.

Willingness to burrow (rats and mice) and to build nests in the home cage (mice) are used as pain bioassays in experimental models of pain in these species. These tests use the principle that rodents are highly motivated to perform these behaviors in their home cage if given the means to do so (i.e., burrowing and nesting substrate); therefore, quantifying an altered willingness to carry out these behaviors offers a means to probe changes in affective state following pain induction and subsequent administration of analgesic drugs. Spontaneous burrowing behavior in rats is reduced by peripheral nerve injury or inflammatory pain and the effect is reversed by the administration of some analgesic drugs, showing the utility of this assay in assessing pain-associated behavior [270]. Similar studies have been carried out in mice using burrowing behavior [271] and nest-making [272], although not all pain models result in burrowing deficits [273] and the administration of analgesics minimally affects the complexity of nest building [274].

Facial expression

Emotions are associated with specific facial expression signatures in humans and this premise has been translated to animals to quantify changes in facial expression as a biomarker for pain. Langford *et al.* [275] were the first group to formally develop a facial coding scale for pain in mice (Mouse Grimace Scale [MGS]). The scale was developed by capturing still images of mouse faces before and after induction of abdominal pain caused by peritoneal injection of acetic acid. Facial action units that were altered by pain included orbital tightening, nose bulge, cheek bulge, ear position, and whisker change. Importantly, following a formal training session, blinded observers were able to discriminate between "in pain" and "no pain" mice using the MGS. Langford *et al.* applied the MGS to mice that had undergone different nociceptive tests and found that the MGS was sensitive for some nociceptive assays but not others. Noxious stimuli of moderate duration (10 min to 4 h) were most likely to be associated with a "pain face," whereas very brief noxious stimuli (e.g., phasic pain tests) and neuropathic pain states were not detected by the MGS. This may reflect the nociceptive nature of phasic pain tests, and the fact that pain of a longer duration is not accompanied by a persistent change in facial expression. Importantly, chemical lesioning of the rostral anterior insula, a structure that is activated in humans by pain with an important emotional component, produced attenuation of the pain face. Pain scales using facial expressions have been extended to other experimental animals, including rats, rabbits, horses, cows, and pigs [276–280], and have been incorporated into clinical pain assessment by many clinicians.

References

1 Raja SN, Carr DB, Cohen M, *et al.* The revised International Association for the Study of Pain definition of pain: concepts, challenges, and compromises. *Pain* 2020; **161**(9): 1976–1982.
2 Wall PD. *Pain: The Science of Suffering.* New York, NY: Columbia University Press, 2000.
3 Cesare P, McNaughton P. A novel heat-activated current in nociceptive neurons and its sensitization by bradykinin. *Proc Natl Acad Sci USA* 1996; **93**(26): 15435–15439.
4 Reichling DB, Levine JD. Heat transduction in rat sensory neurons by calcium-dependent activation of a cation channel. *Proc Natl Acad Sci USA* 1997; **94**(13): 7006–7011.
5 Thut PD, Wrigley D, Gold MS. Cold transduction in rat trigeminal ganglia neurons in vitro. *Neuroscience* 2003; **119**(4): 1071–1083.
6 Gold MS, Gebhart GF. Nociceptor sensitization in pain pathogenesis. *Nat Med* 2010; **16**(11): 1248–1257.
7 Lumpkin EA, Caterina MJ. Mechanisms of sensory transduction in the skin. *Nature* 2007; **445**(7130): 858–865.
8 Jordt SE, McKemy DD, Julius D. Lessons from peppers and peppermint: the molecular logic of thermosensation. *Curr Opin Neurobiol* 2003; **13**(4): 487–492.
9 Goudet C, Magnaghi V, Landry M, *et al.* Metabotropic receptors for glutamate and GABA in pain. *Brain Res Rev* 2009; **60**(1): 43–56.
10 Messeguer A, Planells-Cases R, Ferrer-Montiel A. Physiology and pharmacology of the vanilloid receptor. *Curr Neuropharmacol* 2005; **4**: 1–15.
11 Holzer P, Izzo AA. The pharmacology of TRP channels. *Br J Pharmacol* 2014; **171**: 2469–2473.
12 Nikolaev YA, Cox CD, Ridone P, *et al.* Mammalian TRP ion channels are insensitive to membrane stretch. *J Cell Sci* 2019; **132**: jcs238360.
13 Noël J, Zimmermann K, Busserolles J, *et al.* The mechano-activated K^+ channels TRAAK and TREK-1 control both warm and cold perception. *EMBO J* 2009; **28**: 1308–1318.
14 Zimmermann K, Leffler A, Babes A, *et al.* Sensory neuron sodium channel Nav1.8 is essential for pain at low temperatures. *Nature* 2007; **447**: 855–858.
15 Liedtke W. TRPV4 as osmosensor: a transgenic approach. *Pflugers Arch* 2005; **451**(1): 176–180.
16 Gottlieb PA, Sachs F. Piezo1: properties of a cation selective mechanical channel. *Channels (Austin)* 2012; **6**(4): 214–219.
17 Woo SH, Lukacs V, De Nooij JC, *et al.* Piezo2 is the principal mechanotransduction channel for proprioception. *Nat Neurosci* 2015; **18**(12): 1756–1762.
18 Amato V, Viña E, Calavia MG, *et al.* TRPV4 in the sensory organs of adult zebrafish. *Microsc Res Tech* 2012; **75**(1): 89–96.
19 François A, Schüetter N, Laffray S, *et al.* The low-threshold calcium channel Cav3.2 determines low-threshold mechanoreceptor function. *Cell Rep* 2015; **10**(3): 370–382.
20 Maingret F, Fosset M, Lesage F, *et al.* TRAAK is a mammalian neuronal mechano-gated K+ channel. *J Bio Chem* 1999; **274**(3): 1381–1387.
21 Cook AJ, Woolf CJ, Wall PD, *et al.* Dynamic receptive field plasticity in rat spinal cord dorsal horn following C-primary afferent input. *Nature* 1987; **325**(7000): 151–153.
22 Woolf CJ, King AE. Dynamic alterations in the cutaneous mechanoreceptive fields of dorsal horn neurons in the rat spinal cord. *J Neurosci* 1990; **10**(8): 2717–2726.
23 Cuellar JM, Dutton RC, Antognini JF, *et al.* Differential effects of halothane and isoflurane on lumbar dorsal horn neuronal windup and excitability. *Br J Anaesth* 2005; **94**(5): 617–625.
24 Staud R, Cannon RC, Mauderli AP, *et al.* Temporal summation of pain from mechanical stimulation of muscle tissue in normal controls and subjects with fibromyalgia syndrome. *Pain* 2003; **102**(1–2): 87–95.
25 Herrero JF, Laird JMA, Lopez-Garcia JA. Wind-up of spinal cord neurones and pain sensation: much ado about something? *Prog Neurobiol* 2000; **61**(2): 169–203.
26 Dickenson AH, Sullivan AF. Evidence for a role of the NMDA receptor in the frequency dependent potentiation of deep rat dorsal horn nociceptive neurones following C-fibre stimulation. *Neuropharmacology* 1987; **26**(8): 1235–1238.
27 Davies SN, Lodge D. Evidence for involvement of N-methylaspartate receptors in "wind-up" of class 2 neurones in the dorsal horn of the rat. *Brain Res* 1987; **424**(2): 402–406.
28 International Association for the Study of Pain (IASP) Revised Definition of *Pain*, 2020. www.iasp-pain.org/resources/terminology/#pain (accessed June 2023).
29 Treede RD, Rief W, Barke A, *et al.* A classification of chronic pain for ICD-11. *Pain* 2015; **156**(6): 1003–1007.
30 Malfait AM, Miller RJ. Emerging targets for the management of osteoarthritis pain. *Curr Osteoporos Rep* 2016; **14**(6): 260–268.
31 Maurer M, Bader M, Bas M, *et al.* New topics in bradykinin research. *Allergy* 2011; **66**(11): 1397–1406.
32 Mobarakeh JI, Sakurada S, Katsuyama S, *et al.* Role of histamine H1 receptor in pain perception: a study of the receptor gene knockout mice. *Eur J Pharmacol* 2000; **391**(1–2): 81–89.
33 Burnstock G. Purinergic mechanisms and pain – an update. *Eur J Pharmacol* 2013; **716**(1–3): 24–40.
34 Bodin P, Burnstock G. Purinergic signalling: ATP release. *Neurochem Res* 2001; **26**(8–9): 959–969.
35 Gokin AP, Fareed MU, Pan HL, *et al.* Local injection of endothelin-1 produces pain-like behavior and excitation of nociceptors in rats. *J Neurosci* 2001; **21**(14): 5358–5366.

36 Rattenholl A, Steinhoff M. Role of proteinase-activated receptors in cutaneous biology and disease. *Drug Dev Res* 2003; **59**(4): 408–416.

37 Smith JAM, Amagasu SM, Eglen RM, *et al.* Characterization of prostanoid receptor-evoked responses in rat sensory neurones. *Br J Pharmacol* 1998; **124**(3): 513–523.

38 Nandigama R, Bonitz M, Papadakis T, *et al.* Muscarinic acetylcholine receptor subtypes expressed by mouse bladder afferent neurons. *Neuroscience* 2010; **168**(3): 842–850.

39 Bandell M, Story GM, Hwang SW, *et al.* Noxious cold ion channel TRPA1 is activated by pungent compounds and bradykinin. *Neuron* 2004; **41**: 849–857.

40 Karashima Y, Damann N, Prenen J, *et al.* Bimodal action of menthol on the transient receptor potential channel TRPA1. *J Neurosci* 2007; **27**: 9874–9884.

41 Garrison SR, Dietrich A, Stucky CL. TRPC1 contributes to light-touch sensation and mechanical responses in low-threshold cutaneous sensory neurons. *J Neurophysiol* 2012; **107**: 913–922.

42 Maroto R, Raso A, Wood TG, et al. TRPC1 forms the stretch-activated cation channel in vertebrate cells. *Nat Cell Biol* 2005; **7**: 179–185.

43 Zimmermann K, Lennerz JK, Hein A, *et al.* Transient receptor potential cation channel, subfamily C, member 5 (TRPC5) is a cold-transducer in the peripheral nervous system. *Proc Natl Acad Sci USA* 2011; **108**: 18114–1819.

44 Paricio-Montesinos R, Schwaller F, Udhayachandran A, *et al.* The sensory coding of warm perception. *Neuron* 2020; **106**: 830–841.

45 Tajino K, Hosokawa H, Maegawa S, *et al.* Cooling-sensitive TRPM8 is thermostat of skin temperature against cooling. *PLoS One* 2011; **6**: e17504.

46 McKemy DD, Neuhausser WM, Julius D. Identification of a cold receptor reveals a general role for TRP channels in thermosensation. *Nature* 2002; **416**: 52–58.

47 Acosta C, Djouhri L, Watkins R, *et al.* TREK2 expressed selectively in IB4-binding C-fiber nociceptors hyperpolarizes their membrane potentials and limits spontaneous pain. *J Neurosci* 2014; **34**: 1494–1509

48 Bautista DM, Siemens J, Glazer JM, et al. The menthol receptor TRPM8 is the principal detector of environmental cold. *Nature* 2007; **448**: 204–209.

49 Caterina MJ, Julius D. The vanilloid receptor: a molecular gateway to the pain pathway. *Annu Rev Neurosci* 2001; **24**: 487–517.

50 Woodbury CJ, Zwick M, Wang S, *et al.* Nociceptors lacking TRPV1 and TRPV2 have normal heat responses. *J Neurosci* 2004; **24**: 6410–6415.

51 Szallasi A, Cruz F, Geppetti P. TRPV1: a therapeutic target for novel analgesic drugs? *Trends Mol Med* 2006; **12**: 545–554.

52 Lee H, Caterina MJ. TRPV channels as thermosensory receptors in epithelial cells. *Pflugers Arch* 2005; **151**: 160–167.

53 Peier AM, Moqrich A, Hergarden AC, *et al.* A TRP channel that senses cold stimuli and menthol. *Cell* 2002; **108**: 705–715.

54 Moqrich A, Hwang SW, Earley TJ, *et al.* Impaired thermosensation in mice lacking TRPV3, a heat and camphor sensor in the skin. *Science* 2005; **307**: 1468–1472.

55 Güler AD, Lee H, Iida T, *et al.* Heat-evoked activation of the ion channel, TRPV4. *J Neurosci* 2002; **22**: 6408–6414.

56 Page AJ, Brierley SM, Martin CM, *et al.* The ion channel ASIC1 contributes to visceral but not cutaneous mechanoreceptor function. *Gastroenterology* 2004; **127**: 1739–1747.

57 Calavia MG, Montaño JA, García-Suárez O, *et al.* Differential localization of acid-sensing ion channels 1 and 2 in human cutaneus pacinian corpuscles. *Cell Mol Neurobiol* 2010; **30**: 841–848.

58 Drew LJ, Rohrer DK, Price MP, *et al.* Acid-sensing ion channels ASIC2 and ASIC3 do not contribute to mechanically activated currents in mammalian sensory neurones. *J Physiol* 2004; **556**: 691–710.

59 Bianchi L, Driscoll M. Protons at the gate: DEG/ENaC ion channels help us feel and remember. *Neuron* 2002; **34**: 337–340.

60 Mogil JS, Breese NM, Witty MF, *et al.* Transgenic expression of a dominant-negative ASIC3 subunit leads to increased sensitivity to mechanical and inflammatory stimuli. *J Neurosci* 2005; **25**: 9893–9901.

61 Maingret F. TREK-1 is a heat-activated background K+ channel. *EMBO J* 2000; **19**: 2483-2491.

62 Franks NP, Honoré E. The TREK K2P channels and their role in general anaesthesia and neuroprotection. *Trends Pharmacol Sci* 2004; **25**: 601-608.

63 Honoré E. The neuronal background K2P channels: focus on TREK1. *Nat Rev Neurosci* 2007; **8**(4): 251–261.

64 Pereira V, Busserolles J, Christin M, *et al.* Role of the TREK2 potassium channel in cold and warm thermosensation and in pain perception. *Pain* 2014; **155**: 2534–2544.

65 Schneider ER, Anderson EO, Gracheva EO, *et al.* Temperature sensitivity of two-pore (K2P) potassium channels. *Curr Top Membr* 2014; **74**: 113–115.

66 Luiz AP, MacDonald DI, Santana-Varela S, *et al.* Cold sensing by Na V 1.8-positive and Na V 1.8-negative sensory neurons. *Proc Natl Acad Sci USA* 2019; **116**: 3811–3816.

67 Wood JN, Boorman JP, Okuse K, *et al.* Voltage-gated sodium channels and pain pathways. *J Neurobiol* 2004; **61**: 55–71.

68 Akopian AN, Souslova V, England S, *et al.* The tetrodotoxin-resistant sodium channel SNS has a specialized function in pain pathways. *Nat Neurosci* 1999; **2**: 541–548.

69 Parpaite T, Coste B. Piezo channels. *Curr Biol* 2017; **27**: R250–R252.

70 Coste B, Mathur J, Schmidt M, *et al.* Piezo1 and Piezo2 are essential components of distinct mechanically activated cation channels. *Science* 2010; **330**: 55–60.

71 Volkers L, Mechioukhi Y, Coste B. Piezo channels: from structure to function. *Pflugers Arch* 2014; **467**: 95–99.

72 Baccaglini PI, Hogan PG. Some rat sensory neurons in culture express characteristics of differentiated pain sensory cells. *Proc Natl Acad Sci USA* 1983; **80**(2): 594–598.

73 Caterina MJ, Schumacher MA, Tominaga M, *et al.* The capsaicin receptor: a heat-activated ion channel in the pain pathway. *Nature* 1997; **389**(6653): 816–824.

74 Liu B, Linley JE, Du X, *et al.* The acute nociceptive signals induced by bradykinin in rat sensory neurons are mediated by inhibition of M-type K+ channels and activation of Ca2+-activated Cl– channels. *J Clin Invest* 2010; **120**(4): 1240–1252.

75 Koerber HR, Druzinsky RE, Mendell LM. Properties of somata of spinal dorsal root ganglion cells differ according to peripheral receptor innervated. *J Neurophysiol* 1988; **60**(5): 1584–1596.

76 Rexed B. The cytoarchitectonic organization of the spinal cord of the cat. *J Comp Neurol* 1952; **96**(3): 415–495.

77 Wall PD. The laminar organization of dorsal horn and effects of descending impulses. *J Physiol* 1967; **188**(3): 403–423.

78 Light AR, Perl ER. Spinal termination of functionally identified primary afferent neurons with slowly conducting myelinated fibers. *J Comp Neurol* 1979; **186**(2): 133–150.

79 Ikeda H, Heinke B, Ruscheweyh R, *et al.* Synaptic plasticity in spinal lamina I projection neurons that mediate hyperalgesia. *Science* 2003; **299**(5610): 1237–1240.

80 Craig AD, Kniffki KD. Spinothalamic lumbosacral Lamina I cells responsive to skin and muscle stimulation in the cat. *J Physiol* 1985; **365**: 197–221.

81 Swett JE, Woolf CJ. The somatotopic organization of primary afferent terminals in the superficial laminae of the dorsal horn of the rat spinal cord. *J Comp Neurol* 1985; **231**(1): 66–77.

82 Woodbury JC, Ritter AM, Koerber HR. Central anatomy of individual rapidly adapting low-threshold mechanoreceptors innervating the "Hairy" skin of newborn mice: early maturation of hair follicle afferents. *J Comp Neurol* 2001; **436**(3): 304–323.

83 Lu Y, Perl ER. Modular organization of excitatory circuits between neurons of the spinal superficial dorsal horn (laminae I and II). *J Neurosci* 2005; **25**(15): 3900–3907.

84 Lu Y, Perl ER. A specific inhibitory pathway between substantia gelatinosa neurons receiving direct C-fiber input. *J Neurosci* 2003; **23**(25): 8752–8758.

85 Zhang X, Ju G, Elde R, *et al.* Effect of peripheral nerve cut on neuropeptides in dorsal root ganglia and the spinal cord of monkey with special reference to galanin. *J Neurocytol* 1993; **22**(5): 342–381.

86 Zhang X, Ji RR, Nilsson S, *et al.* Neuropeptide Y and galanin binding sites in rat and monkey lumbar dorsal root ganglia and spinal cord and effect of peripheral axotomy. *Eur J Neurosci* 1995; **7**(3): 367–380.

87 Molliver DC, Radeke MJ, Feinstein SC, *et al.* Presence or absence of TrKA protein distinguishes subsets of small sensory neurons with unique cytochemical characteristics and dorsal horn projections. *J Comp Neurol* 1995; **361**(3): 404–416.

88 Saeed AW, Ribeiro-da-Silva A. Non-peptidergic primary afferents are presynaptic to neurokinin-1 receptor immunoreactive lamina I projection neurons in rat spinal cord. *Mol Pain* 2012; **8**: 64.

89 Taylor AMW, Peleshok JC, Ribeiro-Da-Silva A. Distribution of P2X3-immunoreactive fibers in hairy and glabrous skin of the rat. *J Comp Neurol* 2009; **514**(6): 555–566.

90 Perry MJ, Lawson SN. Differences in expression of oligosaccharides neuropeptides, carbonic anhydrase and neurofilament in rat primary afferent neurons retrogradely labelled via skin, muscle or visceral nerves. *Neuroscience* 1998; **85**(1): 293–310.

91 Le Bars D, Cadden SW. What is a Wide-Dynamic-Range cell? *Pain* 2010; **5**: 331–338.

92 Sugiura Y, Terui N, Hosoya Y. Difference in distribution of central terminals between visceral and somatic unmyelinated (C) primary afferent fibers. *J Neurophysiol* 1989; **62**(4): 834–840.

93 Olivar T, Cervero F, Laird JMA. Responses of rat spinal neurones to natural and electrical stimulation of colonic afferents: effect of inflammation. *Brain Res* 2000; **866**(1–2): 168–177.

94 Grudt TJ, Perl ER. Correlations between neuronal morphology and electrophysiological features in the rodent superficial dorsal horn. *J Physiol* 2002; **540**(Pt 1): 189–207.

95 Maxwell DJ, Belle MD, Cheunsuang O, *et al.* Morphology of inhibitory and excitatory interneurons in superficial laminae of the rat dorsal horn. *J Physiol* 2007; **584**(Pt 2): 521–533.

96 Yasaka T, Tiong SYX, Hughes DI, *et al.* Populations of inhibitory and excitatory interneurons in lamina II of the adult rat spinal dorsal horn revealed by a combined electrophysiological and anatomical approach. *Pain* 2010; **151**(2): 475–588.

97 Todd AJ, Spike RC. The localization of classical transmitters and neuropeptides within neurons in laminae I-III of the mammalian spinal dorsal horn. *Prog Neurobiol* 1993; **41**(5): 609–645.

98 Todd AJ. Neuronal circuitry for pain processing in the dorsal horn. *Nat Rev Neurosci* 2010; **11**(12): 823–836.

99 Polgár E, Hughes DI, Riddell JS, *et al.* Selective loss of spinal GABAergic or glycinergic neurons is not necessary for development of thermal hyperalgesia in the chronic constriction injury model of neuropathic pain. *Pain* 2003; **104**(1–2): 229–239.

100 Chédotal A. Roles of axon guidance molecules in neuronal wiring in the developing spinal cord. *Nat Rev Neurosci* 2019; **20**(7): 380–396.

101 Kayalioglu G. Projections from the spinal cord to the brain. In: Watson C, Paxinos G, Kayalioglu G, eds. *The Spinal Cord: A Christopher and Dana Reeve Foundation Text and Atlas*, 3rd edn. New York, NY: Elsevier/Academic Press, 2009: 148–167.

102 Hains BC, Waxman SG. Activated microglia contribute to the maintenance of chronic pain after spinal cord injury. *J Neurosci* 2006; **26**(16): 4308–4317.

103 Scholz J, Woolf CJ. The neuropathic pain triad: neurons, immune cells and glia. *Nat Neurosci* 2007; **10**(11): 1361–1368.

104 Ji RR, Berta T, Nedergaard M. Glia and pain: is chronic pain a gliopathy? *Pain* 2013; **154**(Suppl 1): S10–S28.

105 Todd AJ. Anatomy of primary afferents and projection neurones in the rat spinal dorsal horn with particular emphasis on substance P and the neurokinin 1 receptor. *Exp Physiol* 2002; **87**(2): 245–249.

106 Doyle CA, Hunt SP. Substance P receptor (neurokinin-1)-expressing neurons in lamina I of the spinal cord encode for the intensity of noxious stimulation: a c-Fos study in rat. *Neuroscience* 1999; **89**(1): 17–28.

107 Suzuki R, Morcuende S, Webber M, *et al.* Superficial NK1-expressing neurons control spinal excitability through activation of descending pathways. *Nat Neurosci* 2002; **5**(12): 1319–1326.

108 Gauriau C, Bernard JF. Pain pathways and parabrachial circuits in the rat. *Exp Physiol* 2010; **87**(2): 251–258.

109 Dostrovsky J, Craig A. Ascending projection systems. In: McMahon S, Koltzenburg M, Tracey I, Turk D, eds. *Textbook of Pain*, 6th edn. Philadelphia, PA: Elsevier Saunders, 2013: 182–197.

110 Dum RP, Levinthal DJ, Strick PL. The spinothalamic system targets motor and sensory areas in the cerebral cortex of monkeys. *J Neurosci* 2009; **29**(45): 14223–14235.

111 Sengul G, Watson C. Ascending and descending pathways in the spinal cord. In: Paxinos G, ed. *The Rat Nervous System*, 4th edn. New York, NY: Academic Press, 2014: 115–130.

112 Craig AD. Pain Mechanisms: labeled lines versus convergence in central processing. *Annu Rev Neurosci* 2003; **26**: 1–30.

113 Waters AJ, Lumb BM. Descending control of spinal nociception from the periaqueductal grey distinguishes between neurons with and without C-fibre inputs. *Pain* 2008; **134**(1–2): 32–40.

114 Benarroch EE. Descending monoaminergic pain modulation: bidirectional control and clinical relevance. *Neurology* 2008; **71**(3): 217–221.

115 Keay KA, Bandler R. Periaqueductal gray. In: Paxinos G, ed. *The Rat Nervous System*. New York, NY: Elsevier, 2015: 207–221.

116 Behbehani MM. Functional characteristics of the midbrain periaqueductal gray. *Prog Neurobiol* 1995; **46**(6): 575–605.

117 Lu Y, Sweitzer SM, Laurito CE, *et al.* Differential opioid inhibition of C- and A delta- fiber mediated thermonociception after stimulation of the nucleus raphe magnus. *Anesth Analg* 2004; **98**: 414-419.

118 McMullan S, Lumb BM. Midbrain control of spinal nociception discriminates between responses evoked by myelinated and unmyelinated heat nociceptors in the rat. *Pain* 2006; **124**: 59-68.

119 Heinricher MM, Tavares I, Leith JL, *et al.* Descending control of nociception: Specificity, recruitment and plasticity. *Brain Res Rev* 2009; **60**: 214-225.

120 Villanueva L, Le Bars D. The activation of bulbo-spinal controls by peripheral nociceptive inputs: Diffuse noxious inhibitory controls. *Biol Res* 1995; **28**: 113-125.

121 Calejesan AA, Kim SJ, Zhuo M. Descending facilitatory modulation of a behavioral nociceptive response by stimulation in the adult rat anterior cingulate cortex. *Eur J Pain* 2000; **4**: 83-96.

122 White K, Targett M, Harris J. Gainfully employing descending controls in acute and chronic pain management. *Vet J* 2018; **237**: 16–25.

123 Fields HL, Vanegas H, Hentall ID, *et al.* Evidence that disinhibition of brain stem neurones contributes to morphine analgesia. *Nature* 1983; **306**(5944): 684–686.

124 Cleary DR, Neubert MJ, Heinricher MM. Are opioid-sensitive neurons in the rostral ventromedial medulla inhibitory interneurons? *Neuroscience* 2008; **151**(2): 564–571.

125 Lau BK, Vaughan CW. Descending modulation of pain: the GABA disinhibition hypothesis of analgesia. *Curr Opin Neurobiol* 2014; **29**: 159–164.

126 Salas R, Ramirez K, Vanegas H, *et al.* Activity correlations between on-like and off-like cells of the rostral ventromedial medulla and simultaneously recorded wide-dynamic-range neurons of the spinal dorsal horn in rats. *Brain Res* 2016; **1652**: 103–110.

127 Millan MJ. Descending control of pain. *Prog Neurobiol* 2002; **66**(6): 355–474.

128 Gu L, Uhelski ML, Anand S, *et al.* Pain inhibition by optogenetic activation of specific anterior cingulate cortical neurons. *PLoS ONE* 2015; **10**(2): e0117746.

129 Kang SJ, Kwak C, Lee J, *et al.* Bidirectional modulation of hyperalgesia via the specific control of excitatory and inhibitory neuronal activity in the ACC. *Mol Brain* 2015; **8**(1): 81.

130 Fuchs PN, Peng YB, Boyette-Davis JA, *et al.* The anterior cingulate cortex and pain processing. *Front Integr Neurosci* 2014; **8**: 35.

131 Koch SC, Fitzgerald M. The selectivity of rostroventral medulla descending control of spinal sensory inputs shifts postnatally from A fibre to C fibre evoked activity. *J Physiol* 2014; **592**(7): 1535–1544.

132 Hathway GJ, Koch S, Low L, *et al.* The changing balance of brainstem-spinal cord modulation of pain processing over the first weeks of rat postnatal life. *J Physiol* 2009; **587**(Pt 12): 2927–2935.

133 Li MH, Suchland KL, Ingram SL. GABAergic transmission and enhanced modulation by opioids and endocannabinoids in adult rat rostral ventromedial medulla. *J Physiol* 2015; **593**(1): 217–230.

134 Hathway GJ, Vega-Avelaira D, Fitzgerald M. A critical period in the supraspinal control of pain: opioid-dependent changes in brainstem rostroventral medulla function in preadolescence. *Pain* 2012; **153**(4): 775–783.

135 Schwaller F, Kwok C, Fitzgerald M. Postnatal maturation of the spinal-bulbo-spinal loop: brainstem control of spinal nociception is independent of sensory input in neonatal rats. *Pain* 2016; **157**(3): 677–686.

136 Tracey I. Getting the pain you expect: mechanisms of placebo, nocebo and reappraisal effects in humans. *Nat Med* 2010; **16**(11): 1277–1283.

137 Zhuo M. Neural mechanisms underlying anxiety-chronic pain interactions. *Trends Neurosci* 2016; **39**(3): 136–145.

138 Wiech K, Ploner M, Tracey I. Neurocognitive aspects of pain perception. *Trends Cogn Sci* 2008; **12**(8): 306–313.

139 Wiech K, Tracey I. The influence of negative emotions on pain: behavioral effects and neural mechanisms. *Neuroimage* 2009; **47**(3): 987–994.

140 Bannister K, Dickenson AH. What do monoamines do in pain modulation? *Curr Opin Support Palliat Care* 2016; **10**(20): 143–148.

141 Zhuo M, Gebhart G. Characterization of descending inhibition and facilitation from the nuclei reticularis-gigantocellularis and gigantocellularis pars alpha in the rat. *Pain* 1990; **42**(3): 337–350.

142 Zhuo M, Gebhart GE. Spinal cholinergic and monoaminergic receptors mediate descending inhibition from the nuclei reticularis gigantocellularis and gigantocellularis pars alpha in the rat. *Brain Res* 1990; **535**(1): 67–78.

143 Zhuo M, Gebhart GF. Spinal serotonin receptors mediate descending facilitation of a nociceptive reflex from the nuclei reticularis gigantocellularis and gigantocellularis pars alpha in the rat. *Brain Res* 1991; **550**(1): 35–48.

144 Dahlstroem A, Fuxe K. Evidence for the existence of monoamine-containing neurons in the central nervous system. I. Demonstration of monoamines in the cell bodies of brain stem neurons. *Acta Physiol Scand Suppl* 1964; **232**(Suppl): 1–55.

145 Antunes-Rodrigues J, De Castro M, Elias LLK, *et al.* Neuroendocrine control of body fluid metabolism. *Physiol Rev* 2004; **84**(1): 169–208.

146 Rinaman L. Hindbrain noradrenergic A2 neurons: diverse roles in autonomic, endocrine, cognitive, and behavioral functions. *Am J Physiol Regul Integr Comp Physiol* 2011; **300**(2): R222–R235.

147 Felten DL, Sladek JR. Monoamine distribution in primate brain V. Monoaminergic nuclei: anatomy, pathways and local organization. *Brain Res Bull* 1983; **10**(2): 171–284.

148 Pertovaara A. Noradrenergic pain modulation. *Prog Neurobiol* 2006; **80**(2): 53–83.

149 Gyires K, Zádori ZS, Török T, *et al.* Alpha(2) Adrenoceptor subtypes-mediated physiological, pharmacological actions. *Neurochem Int* 2009; **55**(7): 447–453.

150 Pertovaara A. The noradrenergic pain regulation system: a potential target for pain therapy. *Eur J Pharmacol* 2013; **716**(1–3): 2–7.

151 Jones SL, Gebhart GF. Characterization of coeruleospinal inhibition of the nociceptive tail-flick reflex in the rat: mediation by spinal alpha 2-adrenoceptors. *Brain Res* 1986; **364**(2): 315–330.

152 Llorca-Torralba M, Borges G, Neto F, *et al.* Noradrenergic locus coeruleus pathways in pain modulation. *Neuroscience* 2016; **338**: 93–113.

153 Wrzosek A, Woron J, Dobrogowski J, *et al.* Topical clonidine for neuropathic pain. *Cochrane Database Syst Rev* 2015; **8**(8): CD010967.

154 Al-Metwalli RR, Mowafi HA, Ismail SA, *et al.* Effect of intra-articular dexmedetomidine on postoperative analgesia after arthroscopic knee surgery. *Br J Anaesth* 2008; **101**(3): 395–399.

155 Eisenach JC, DuPen S, Dubois M, *et al.* Epidural clonidine analgesia for intractable cancer pain. *Pain* 1995; **61**(3): 391–399.

156 Yaksh TL, Pogrel JW, Lee YW, *et al.* Reversal of nerve ligation-induced allodynia by spinal alpha-2 adrenoceptor agonists. *J Pharmacol Exp Ther* 1995; **272**(1): 207–214.

157 Mansikka H, Idänpään-Heikkilä JJ, Pertovaara A. Different roles of α2-adrenoceptors of the medulla versus the spinal cord in modulation of mustard oil-induced central hyperalgesia in rats. *Eur J Pharmacol* 1996; **297**(1): 19–26.

158 Xu M, Kontinen VK, Kalso E. Endogenous noradrenergic tone controls symptoms of allodynia in the spinal nerve ligation model of neuropathic pain. *Eur J Pharmacol* 1999; **366**(1): 41–45.

159 Poree LR, Guo TZ, Kingery WS, *et al.* The analgesic potency of dexmedetomidine is enhanced after nerve injury: a possible role for peripheral alpha-2-adrenoceptors. *Anesth Analg* 1998; **87**(4): 941–948.

160 Kingery WS, Guo TZ, Davies MF, *et al.* The α(2A) adrenoceptor and the sympathetic postganglionic neuron contribute to the development of neuropathic heat hyperalgesia in mice. *Pain* 2000; **85**(3): 345–358.

161 Malmberg AB, Hedley LR, Jasper JR, *et al.* Contribution of α_2 receptor subtypes to nerve injury-induced pain and its regulation by dexmedetomidine. *Br J Pharmacol* 2001; **132**(8): 1827–1836.

162 Lähdesmäki J, Scheinin M, Pertovaara A, *et al.* The α2A-adrenoceptor subtype is not involved in inflammatory hyperalgesia or morphine-induced antinociception. *Eur J Pharmacol* 2003; **468**(3): 183–189.
163 Green GM, Lyons L, Dickenson AH. Alpha-2-Adrenoceptor antagonists enhance responses of dorsal horn neurones to formalin induced inflammation. *Eur J Pharmacol* 1998; **347**(2–3): 201–204.
164 Rahman W, D'Mello R, Dickenson AH. Peripheral nerve injury-induced changes in spinal alpha(2)-adrenoceptor-mediated modulation of mechanically evoked dorsal horn neuronal responses. *J Pain* 2008; **9**(4): 350–359.
165 De Felice M, Sanoja R, Wang R, *et al.* Engagement of descending inhibition from the rostral ventromedial medulla protects against chronic neuropathic pain. *Pain* 2011; **152**(12): 2701–2709.
166 Hughes S, Hickey L, Donaldson LF, *et al.* Intrathecal reboxetine suppresses evoked and ongoing neuropathic pain behaviours by restoring spinal noradrenergic inhibitory tone. *Pain* 2015; **156**(2): 328–334.
167 Le Bars D. Serotonin and pain. In: Osborne NN, Hamon M, eds. *Neuronal Serotonin*. New York, NY: Wiley, 1988: 171–229.
168 Dogrul A, Ossipov MH, Porreca F. Differential mediation of descending pain facilitation and inhibition by spinal 5HT-3 and 5HT-7 receptors. *Brain Res* 2009; **1280**: 52–59.
169 Zhang YQ, Gao X, Huang YL, *et al.* Expression of 5-HT1A receptor mRNA in rat dorsal raphe nucleus and ventrolateral periaqueductal gray neurons after peripheral inflammation. *Neuroreport* 2000; **11**(15): 3361–3365.
170 Cai YQ, Wang W, Hou YY, *et al.* Optogenetic activation of brainstem serotonergic neurons induces persistent pain sensitization. *Mol Pain* 2014; **10**: 70.
171 Braz JM, Basbaum AI. Genetically expressed transneuronal tracer reveals direct and indirect serotonergic descending control circuits. *J Comp Neurol* 2008; **507**(6): 1990–2003.
172 Suzuki R, Rahman W, Hunt SP, *et al.* Descending facilitatory control of mechanically evoked responses is enhanced in deep dorsal horn neurones following peripheral nerve injury. *Brain Res* 2004; **1019**(1–2): 68–76.
173 Dogrul A, Ossipov MH, Porreca F. Differential mediation of descending pain facilitation and inhibition by spinal 5HT-3 and 5HT-7 receptors. *Brain Res* 2009; **1280**: 52–59.
174 Viguier F, Michot B, Hamon M, *et al.* Multiple roles of serotonin in pain control mechanisms-implications of 5-HT$_7$ and other 5-HT receptor types. *Eur J Pharmacol* 2013; **716**(1–3): 8–16.
175 Urban MO, Gebhart GF. Supraspinal contributions to hyperalgesia. *Proc Natl Acad Sci USA* 1999; **96**(14): 7687–7692.
176 Porreca F, Ossipov MH, Gebhart GF. Chronic pain and medullary descending facilitation. *Trends Neurosci* 2002; **25**(6): 319–325.
177 Magnusson JE, Fisher K. The involvement of dopamine in nociception: the role of D1 and D2 receptors in the dorsolateral striatum. *Brain Res* 2000; **855**(2): 260–266.
178 Gao X, Zhang Y, Wu G. Effects of dopaminergic agents on carrageenan hyperalgesia after intrathecal administration to rats. *Eur J Pharmacol* 2001; **418**(1–3): 73–77.
179 Wood PB. Role of central dopamine in pain and analgesia. *Expert Rev Neurother* 2008; **8**(5): 781–797.
180 Cenci MA. Dopamine dysregulation of movement control in l-DOPA-induced dyskinesia. *Trends Neurosci* 2007; **30**(5): 236–243.
181 Baik JH. Dopamine signaling in reward-related behaviors. *Front Neural Circuits* 2013; **7**: 152.
182 Robbins TW, Arnsten AFT. The neuropsychopharmacology of fronto-executive function: monoaminergic modulation. *Annu Rev Neurosci* 2009; **32**: 267–287.
183 Werlen E, Jones MW. Modulating the map: dopaminergic tuning of hippocampal spatial coding and interactions. *Prog Brain Res* 2015; **219**: 187–216.
184 Evans MS, Lysakowski C, Tramèr MR. Nefopam for the prevention of postoperative pain: quantitative systematic review. *Br J Anaesth* 2008; **101**(5): 610–617.
185 Park HJ, Park JU, Yoo W, *et al.* Analgesic effects of nefopam in patients undergoing bimaxillary osteotomy: a double-blind, randomized, placebo-controlled study. *J Craniomaxillofac Surg* 2016; **44**(2): 210–214.
186 Gjerstad J, Tjølsen A, Svendsen F, *et al.* Inhibition of spinal nociceptive responses after intramuscular injection of capsaicin involves activation of noradrenergic and opioid systems. *Brain Res* 2000; **859**(1): 132–136.
187 Waters AJ, Lumb BM. Inhibitory effects evoked from both the lateral and ventrolateral periaqueductal grey are selective for the nociceptive responses of rat dorsal horn neurones. *Brain Res* 1997; **752**(1–2): 239–249.
188 Vanegas H, Vazquez E, Tortorici V. NSAIDS, opioids, cannabinoids and the control of pain by the central nervous system. *Pharmaceuticals* 2010; **3**(5): 1335–1347.
189 Zubieta J-K, Bueller JA, Jackson LR, *et al.* Placebo effects mediated by endogenous opioid activity on μ-opioid receptors. *J Neurosci* 2005; **25**(34): 7754–7762.
190 Petrovic P, Kalso E, Petersson KM, *et al.* A prefrontal non-opioid mechanism in placebo analgesia. *Pain* 2010; **150**(1): 59–65.
191 Eippert F, Bingel U, Schoell ED, *et al.* Activation of the opioidergic descending pain control system underlies placebo analgesia. *Neuron* 2009; **63**(4): 533–543.
192 Krummenacher P, Candia V, Folkers G, *et al.* Prefrontal cortex modulates placebo analgesia. *Pain* 2010; **148**(3): 368–374.
193 Jenkins S, Worthington M, Harris J, *et al.* Differential modulation of withdrawal reflexes by a cannabinoid in the rabbit. *Brain Res* 2004; **1012**(1–2): 146–153.
194 Tham SM, Angus JA, Tudor EM, *et al.* Synergistic and additive interactions of the cannabinoid agonist CP55,940 with μ opioid receptor and alpha2-adrenoceptor agonists in acute pain models in mice. *Br J Pharmacol* 2005; **144**(6): 875–884.
195 Guindon J, Beaulieu P. Antihyperalgesic effects of local injections of anandamide, ibuprofen, rofecoxib and their combinations in a model of neuropathic pain. *Neuropharmacology* 2006; **50**(7): 814–823.
196 Guindon J, Hohmann AG. The endocannabinoid system and pain. *CNS Neurol Disord Drug Target* 2009; **8**(6): 403–421.
197 Sagar DR, Staniaszek LE, Okine BN, *et al.* Tonic modulation of spinal hyperexcitability by the endocannabinoid receptor system in a rat model of osteoarthritis pain. *Arthritis Rheum* 2010; **62**(12): 3666–3676.
198 Lötsch J, Weyer-Menkhoff I, Tegeder I. Current evidence of cannabinoid-based analgesia obtained in preclinical and human experimental settings. *Eur J Pain* 2018; **22**(3): 471–484.
199 McLaughlin BJ, Barber R, Saito K, *et al.* Immunocytochemical localization of glutamate decarboxylase in rat spinal cord. *J Comp Neurol* 1975; **164**(3): 305–321.
200 Harvey RJ, Rigo J-M. Glycinergic transmission: physiological, developmental and pathological implications. *Front Mol Neurosci* 2010; **3**: 115.
201 Harvey R, Depner U, Wässle H, *et al.* GlyR alpha3: an essential target for spinal PGE2-mediated inflammatory pain sensitization. *Science* 2004; **304**(5672): 884–887.
202 Hossaini M, Goos JAC, Kohli SK, *et al.* Distribution of glycine/GABA neurons in the ventromedial medulla with descending spinal projections and evidence for an ascending glycine/GABA projection. *PLoS ONE* 2012; 7(4): e35293.
203 Miki K, Zhou QQ, Guo W, *et al.* Changes in gene expression and neuronal phenotype in brain stem pain modulatory circuitry after inflammation. *J Neurophysiol* 2002; **87**(2): 750–760.
204 Sandkuhler J, Fu QG, Zimmermann M. Spinal pathways mediating tonic or stimulation-produced descending inhibition from the periaqueductal gray or nucleus raphe magnus are separate in the cat. *J Neurophysiol* 1987; **58**(2): 327–341.
205 Gilbert AK, Franklin KBJ. GABAergic modulation of descending inhibitory systems from the rostral ventromedial medulla (RVM). Dose-response analysis of nociception and neurological deficits. *Pain* 2001; **90**(1–2): 25–36.
206 Soja PJ, Sinclair JG. Evidence that noradrenaline reduces tonic descending inhibition of cat spinal cord nociceptor-driven neurones. *Pain* 1983; **15**(1–4): 71–81.
207 Rivot JP, Calvino B, Besson JM. Is there a serotonergic tonic descending inhibition on the responses of dorsal horn convergent neurons to C-fibre inputs? *Brain Res* 1987; **403**(1): 142–146.
208 Clarke RW, Harris J. The organization of motor responses to noxious stimuli. *Brain Res Rev* 2004; **46**(2): 163–172.
209 Loeser JD, Treede RD. The Kyoto protocol of IASP basic pain terminology. *Pain* 2008; **137**(30): 473–477.
210 Garner B, Stoker A, Kuroki K, *et al.* Using animal models in osteoarthritis biomarker research. *J Knee Surg* 2011; **24**(40): 251–264.
211 Mogil JS. Animal models of pain: progress and challenges. *Nat Rev Neurosci* 2009; **10**(4): 283–294.
212 Rice ASC, Cimino-Brown D, Eisenach JC, *et al.* Animal models and the prediction of efficacy in clinical trials of analgesic drugs: a critical appraisal and call for uniform reporting standards. *Pain* 2008; **139**(2): 243–247.
213 Vincent TL, Williams RO, Maciewicz R, *et al.* Arthritis Research UK animal models working group. Mapping pathogenesis of arthritis through small animal models. *Rheumatology* 2012; **51**(11): 1931–1941.
214 Matthies BK, Franklin KBJ. Effects of partial decortication on opioid analgesia in the formalin test. *Behav Brain Res* 1995; **67**(1): 59–66.
215 Backonja MM, Stacey B. Neuropathic pain symptoms relative to overall pain rating. *J Pain* 2004; **5**(9): 491–497.
216 Le Bars D, Gozariu M, Cadden SW. Animal models of nociception. *Pharmacol Rev* 2001; **53**(4): 597–652.
217 Beecher HK. The measurement of pain; prototype for the quantitative study of subjective responses. *Pharmacol Rev* 1957; **9**(1): 59–209.
218 Treede RD. Neurophysiological studies of pain pathways in peripheral and central nervous system disorders. *J Neurol* 2003; **250**(10): 1152–1161.
219 Villanueva L, Peschanski M, Calvino B, *et al.* Ascending pathways in the spinal cord involved in triggering of diffuse noxious inhibitory controls in the rat. *J Neurophysiol* 1986; **55**(1): 34–55.
220 Barrot M. Tests and models of nociception and pain in rodents. *Neuroscience* 2012; **211**: 39–50.
221 Valeriani M, Pazzaglia C, Cruccu G, *et al.* Clinical usefulness of laser evoked potentials. *Neurophysiol Clin* 2012; **42**(5): 345–353.
222 Baumgärtner U, Greffrath W, Treede RD. Contact heat and cold, mechanical, electrical and chemical stimuli to elicit small fiber-evoked potentials: merits and limitations for basic science and clinical use. *Neurophysiol Clin* 2012; **42**(5): 267–280.
223 Garcia-Larrea L. Objective pain diagnostics. *Neurophysiol Clin* 2012; **42**(4): 187–197.

224 Murrell JC, Johnson CB. Neurophysiological techniques to assess pain in animals. *J Vet Pharmacol Ther* 2006; **29**(5): 325–335.
225 van Oostrom H, Stienen PJ, van den Bos R, *et al.* Somatosensory-evoked potentials indicate increased unpleasantness of noxious stimuli in response to increasing stimulus intensities in the rat. *Brain Res Bull* 2007; **71**(4): 404–409.
226 van Oostrom H, Stienen PJ, van den Bos R, *et al.* Development of a rat model to assess the efficacy of the somatosensory-evoked potential as indicator of analgesia. *Brain Res Protoc* 2005; **15**(1): 14–20.
227 Kimura S, Tanabe M, Honda M, *et al.* Enhanced wind-up of the C-fiber-mediated nociceptive flexor reflex movement following painful diabetic neuropathy in mice. *J Pharmacol Sci* 2005; **97**(2): 195–202.
228 Kelly S, Dobson KL, Harris J. Spinal nociceptive reflexes are sensitized in the monosodium iodoacetate model of osteoarthritis pain in the rat. *Osteoarthritis Cartilage* 2013; **21**(9): 1327–1335.
229 Courtney CA, Witte PO, Chmell SJ, *et al.* Heightened flexor withdrawal response in individuals with knee osteoarthritis is modulated by joint compression and joint mobilization. *J Pain* 2010; **11**(2): 179–185.
230 Peterbauer C, Larenza PM, Knobloch M, *et al.* Effects of a low dose infusion of racemic and S-ketamine on the nociceptive withdrawal reflex in standing ponies. *Vet Anaesth Analg* 2008; **35**(5): 414–423.
231 Rohrbach H, Korpivaara T, Schatzmann U, *et al.* Comparison of the effects of the alpha-2 agonists detomidine, romifidine and xylazine on nociceptive withdrawal reflex and temporal summation in horses. *Vet Anaesth Analg* 2009; **36**(4): 384–395.
232 Spadavecchia C, Arendt-Nielsen L, Spadavecchia L, *et al.* Effects of butorphanol on the withdrawal reflex using threshold, suprathreshold and repeated subthreshold electrical stimuli in conscious horses. *Vet Anaesth Analg* 2007; **34**(1): 48–58.
233 Percie du Sert N, Hurst V, Ahluwalia A, *et al.* The ARRIVE guidelines 2.0: updated guidelines for reporting animal research. *PLoS Biol* 2020; **18**(7): e3000410.
234 Hoffmann MV, Kästner SBR, Kietzmann M, *et al.* Contact heat thermal threshold testing in beagle dogs: baseline reproducibility and the effect of acepromazine, levomethadone and fenpipramide. *BMC Vet Res* 2012; **8**: 206.
235 Slingsby LS, Taylor PM, Monroe T. Thermal antinociception after dexmedetomidine administration in cats: a comparison between intramuscular and oral transmucosal administration. *J Feline Med Surg* 2009; **11**(10): 829–834.
236 Pypendop B, Siao K, Ilkiw JE. Thermal antinociceptive effect of orally administered gabapentin in healthy cats. *Am J Vet Res* 2010; **71**(9): 1027–1032.
237 Love EJ, Murrell J, Whay HR. Thermal and mechanical nociceptive threshold testing in horses: a review. *Vet Anaesth Analg* 2011; **38**(1): 3–14.
238 Ambros B, Duke T. Effect of low dose rate ketamine infusions on thermal and mechanical thresholds in conscious cats. *Vet Anaesth Analg* 2013; **40**(6): e76–e82.
239 Ley SJ, Livingston A, Waterman AE. The effect of chronic clinical pain on thermal and mechanical thresholds in sheep. *Pain* 1989; **39**(3): 353–357.
240 Ley SJ, Waterman AE, Livingston A. A field study of the effect of lameness on mechanical nociceptive thresholds in sheep. *Vet Rec* 1995; **137**(4): 85–87.
241 Slingsby LS, Jones A, Waterman-Pearson AE. Use of a new finger-mounted device to compare mechanical nociceptive thresholds in cats given pethidine or no medication after castration. *Res Vet Sci* 2001; **70**(3): 243–246.
242 Lascelles BD, Cripps PJ, Jones A, *et al.* Efficacy and kinetics of carprofen, administered preoperatively or postoperatively, for the prevention of pain in dogs undergoing ovariohysterectomy. *Vet Surg* 1998; **27**(6): 568–582.
243 Willner P. The validity of animal models of depression. *Psychopharmacology* 1984; **83**(1): 1–16.
244 Sacerdote P, Franchi S, Moretti S, *et al.* Cytokine modulation is necessary for efficacious treatment of experimental neuropathic pain. *J Neuroimmune Pharmacol* 2013; **8**(1): 202–211.
245 Fleetwood-Walker S, Quinn J, Wallace C, *et al.* Behavioural changes in the rat following infection with varicella-zoster virus. *J Gen Virol* 1999; **80**(Pt 9): 2433–2436.
246 Lynch JL, Gallus NJ, Ericson ME, *et al.* Analysis of nociception, sex and peripheral nerve innervation in the TMEV animal model of multiple sclerosis. *Pain* 2008; **136**(3): 293–304.
247 Lee BH, Seong J, Kim UJ. Behavioral characteristics of a mouse model of cancer pain. *Yonsei Med J* 2005; **46**(2): 252–259.
248 Al-Chaer ED, Kawasaki M, Pasricha PJ. A new model of chronic visceral hypersensitivity in adult rats induced by colon irritation during postnatal development. *Gastroenterology* 2000; **119**(5): 1276–1285.
249 Sanchez LC, Merritt AM. Colorectal distention in the horse: visceral sensitivity, rectal compliance and effect of i.v. xylazine or intrarectal lidocaine. *Equine Vet J* 2005; **37**(1): 70–74.
250 Robertson SA, Sanchez LC, Merritt AM, *et al.* Effect of systemic lidocaine on visceral and somatic nociception in conscious horses. *Equine Vet J* 2005; **37**(2): 122–127.
251 Sanchez L, Elfenbein JR, Robertson SA. Effect of acepromazine, butorphanol, or N-butylscopolammonium bromide on visceral and somatic nociception and duodenal motility in conscious horses. *Am J Vet Res* 2008; **69**(5): 579–585.
252 Willis WD, Al-Chaer ED, Quast MJ, *et al.* A visceral pain pathway in the dorsal column of the spinal cord. *Proc Natl Acad Sci USA* 1999; **96**(14): 7675–7679.
253 Laird JMA, Martinez-Caro L, Garcia-Nicas E, *et al.* A new model of visceral pain and referred hyperalgesia in the mouse. *Pain* 2001; **92**(3): 335–342.
254 Ness TJ, Gebhart GF. Colorectal distension as a noxious visceral stimulus: physiologic and pharmacologic characterization of pseudaffective reflexes in the rat. *Brain Res* 1988; **450**(1–2): 153–169.
255 Hultin L, Nissen TD, Kakol-Palm D, *et al.* Colorectal distension-evoked potentials in awake rats: a novel method for studies of visceral sensitivity. *Neurogastroenterol Motil* 2012; **24**(10): 964–e466.
256 Cook JL, Kuroki K, Visco D, *et al.* The OARSI histopathology initiative – recommendations for histological assessments of osteoarthritis in the dog. *Osteoarthritis Cartilage* 2010; **18**(3): 66–79.
257 Brown DC, Boston R, Coyne JC, *et al.* A novel approach to the use of animals in studies of pain: validation of the canine brief pain inventory in canine bone cancer. *Pain Med* 2009; **10**(1): 133–142.
258 Hague DW, Stella JL, Buffington CAT. Effects of interstitial cystitis on the acoustic startle reflex in cats. *Am J Vet Res* 2013; **74**(1): 144–147.
259 Brown DC, Boston RC, Coyne JC, *et al.* Ability of the Canine Brief Pain Inventory to detect response to treatment in dogs with osteoarthritis. *J Am Vet Med Assoc* 2008; **233**(8): 1278–1283.
260 Brown DC, Boston RC, Farrar JT. Comparison of force plate gait analysis and owner assessment of pain using the Canine Brief Pain Inventory in dogs with osteoarthritis. *J Vet Intern Med* 2013; **27**(1): 22–30.
261 Roughan JV, Coulter CA, Flecknell PA, *et al.* The conditioned place preference test for assessing welfare consequences and potential refinements in a mouse bladder cancer model. *PLoS ONE* 2014; **9**: 103362.
262 Sufka KJ. Conditioned place preference paradigm: a novel approach for analgesic drug assessment against chronic pain. *Pain* 1994; **58**(3): 355–366.
263 Nasr MAF, Murrell J, Nicol CJ. The effect of keel fractures on egg production, feed and water consumption in individual laying hens. *Br Poult Sci* 2013; **54**(2): 165–170.
264 Adcock SJJ, Tucker CB. Conditioned place preference reveals ongoing pain in calves 3 weeks after disbudding. *Sci Rep* 2020; **10**(1): 3849.
265 Ede T, von Keyserlingk MAG, Weary DM. Conditioned place aversion of caustic paste and hot-iron disbudding in dairy calves. *J Dairy Sci* 2020; **103**(12): 11653–11658.
266 Rossi HL, Vierck CJ, Caudle RM, *et al.* Characterization of cold sensitivity and thermal preference using an operant orofacial assay. *Mol Pain* 2006; **2**: 37.
267 Nolan TA, Hester J, Bokrand-Donatelli Y, *et al.* Adaptation of a novel operant orofacial testing system to characterize both mechanical and thermal pain. *Behav Brain Res* 2011; **217**(2): 477–480.
268 Neubert JK, Widmer CG, Malphurs W, *et al.* Use of a novel thermal operant behavioral assay for characterization of orofacial pain sensitivity. *Pain* 2005; **116**(3): 386–395.
269 Flecknell PA. Refinement of animal use-assessment and alleviation of pain and distress. *Lab Anim* 1994; **28**(3): 222–231.
270 Zhang XY, Barakat A, Diaz-Delcastillo M, *et al.* Systematic review and meta-analysis of studies in which burrowing behavior was assessed in rodent models of disease-associated persistent pain. *Pain* 2022; **163**(11): 2076–2102.
271 Deacon RMJ. Burrowing in rodents: a sensitive method for detecting behavioral dysfunction. *Nat Protoc* 2006; **1**(1): 118–121.
272 Deacon R. Assessing burrowing, nest construction, and hoarding in mice. *J Vis Exp* 2012; **59**: e2607.
273 Shepherd AJ, Cloud ME, Cao YQ, *et al.* Deficits in burrowing behaviors are associated with mouse models of neuropathic but not inflammatory pain or migraine. *Front Behav Neurosci* 2018; **12**: 124.
274 Jirkof P, Fleischmann T, Cesarovic N, *et al.* Assessment of postsurgical distress and pain in laboratory mice by nest complexity scoring. *Lab Anim* 2013; **47**(3): 153–161.
275 Langford DJ, Bailey AL, Chanda ML, *et al.* Coding of facial expressions of pain in the laboratory mouse. *Nat Methods* 2010; **7**(6): 447–449.
276 Gleerup KB, Andersen PH, Munksgaard L, *et al.* Pain evaluation in dairy cattle. *Appl Anim Behav Sci* 2015; **171**: 25–32.
277 Sotocinal SG, Sorge RE, Zaloum A, *et al.* The Rat Grimace Scale: a partially automated method for quantifying pain in the laboratory rat via facial expressions. *Mol Pain* 2011; **7**: 55.
278 Keating SCJ, Thomas AA, Flecknell PA. Evaluation of EMLA cream for preventing pain during tattooing of rabbits: changes in physiological, behavioral and facial expression responses. *PLoS ONE* 2012; **7**(9): e44437.
279 Dalla Costa E, Minero M, Lebelt D, *et al.* Development of the Horse Grimace Scale (HGS) as a pain assessment tool in horses undergoing routine castration. *PLoS ONE* 2014; **9**(3): e92281.
280 Vullo C, Barbieri S, Catone G, *et al.* Is the Piglet Grimace Scale (PGS) a useful welfare indicator to assess pain after cryptorchidectomy in growing pigs? *Animals* 2020; **10**(3): 412.

47 Recognition and Quantification of Acute and Chronic Pain

Jo C. Murrell
Bristol Veterinary Specialists, Severn Beach, Bristol, UK

Chapter contents

Introduction, 996
Recognition of acute pain, 996
Changes in behavior, 996
Physiological parameters, 998
Electroencephalogram, 999
Functional magnetic resonance imaging, 999
Infrared thermography, 1000
Accelerometry and step-counts, 1000
Recognition of chronic pain, 1000
Changes in behavior, 1000
Physiological parameters, 1000
Visual observation of gait, 1001
Force plate gait analysis, 1001
Kinematic gait analysis, 1001
Accelerometry, 1001
Quantification of acute pain, 1001
Unidimensional pain assessment scales, 1002
Simple descriptive scales, 1002
Numerical rating scale, 1002
Visual analog scale, 1002
Multidimensional pain assessment scales, 1003
Grimace scales, 1003
How often should you conduct acute pain assessment in animals?, 1003
Who should conduct pain assessment?, 1005
Factors confounding use of pain assessment tools, 1005
Quantification of chronic pain, 1005
References, 1007

Introduction

There is an ever-increasing understanding of the signs associated with acute and chronic pain as well as ways in which these phenomena can be measured. There is also now a plethora of validated tools to measure acute and chronic pain although the evidence suggests that they have not been widely adopted in general practice. This is unfortunate because unless pain is quantified it is very difficult to treat it effectively without falling into the trap of over or undertreating pain, with both scenarios having a negative impact on the animal.

Recognition of acute pain

The various methods available to recognize acute pain are discussed below. Table 47.1 provides a summary of the principal advantages and disadvantages of each.

Changes in behavior

Changes in spontaneous behavior form the cornerstone of methods to recognize acute pain across species. Behavioral changes can be used to detect both the sensory (e.g., how much does it hurt? and where does it hurt?) and the emotional component (e.g., depression, anxiety) of pain. The detection of behavioral changes is facilitated if the normal (pain-free) behavior of the animal is known, therefore pet owners or carers can play a key role in the detection of acute pain. Similarly, animal care staff such as veterinary nurses or technicians who spend a lot of time with the animal can be pivotal to detecting changes in behavior throughout the day and in response to the administration of analgesic drugs. Formal assessment of behavior can be achieved by using an ethogram (a catalog of behaviors) specifically related to pain in the species being observed, however, careful observation of behavior is also sufficient to detect signs of pain.

Characteristic changes in behavior associated with different types of pain have been described. Behavioral changes that have been described in dogs with abdominal pain include a hunched appearance and adoption of a praying position where the animal appears to stretch out with the front legs positioned near the ground and the back legs in a more upright position (Fig. 47.1, Video 47.1).

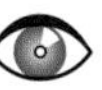

Dogs with abdominal pain do not look comfortable and relaxed and often cannot sleep, showing an inability to settle and a tense abdomen when palpated. Cats with abdominal pain also show a tense abdomen on palpation and a hunched appearance (Fig. 47.2). Behavioral changes have also been noted in cats by owners in the three days following surgery for ovariohysterectomy and include decreased playfulness, increased time spent sleeping, and an altered

Veterinary Anesthesia and Analgesia: The Sixth Edition of Lumb and Jones. Edited by Leigh Lamont, Kurt Grimm, Sheilah Robertson, Lydia Love and Carrie Schroeder.
© 2024 John Wiley & Sons, Inc. Published 2024 by John Wiley & Sons, Inc.
Companion website: www.wiley.com/go/lamont/anesthesia

Table 47.1 Summary of the advantages and disadvantages of different methods used to recognize acute pain.

Method to recognize acute pain	Advantages	Disadvantages
Behavior	Can provide a good insight into how the animal "feels" about their pain "Gold standard" measure of acute pain	Can be time consuming to collect data Presence of an observer may influence the behavior of an animal Risk of confounding factors changing the behavior of an animal
Physiology	Objective means to measure pain	Many biomarkers are related to stress and are not pain-specific Some biomarkers are invasive to measure e.g., blood samples for serum cortisol
Electroencephalogram	Direct assessment of brain activity may provide insights into pain perception Objective means to measure pain	Generates a large amount of data that can be difficult to interpret Requires knowledge of data acquisition and signal-processing techniques Anesthesia can facilitate a high signal-to-noise ratio for the data but may also influence the recorded data
Functional magnetic resonance imaging	Direct assessment of brain activity may provide insights into pain perception	Changes in brain activity may not be specific to pain Currently requires anesthesia for pain studies in animals Requires access to an appropriate scanner
Infrared thermography	Quick to carry out Non-invasive	Skin surface temperature can be affected by stress and is not specific to pain
Accelerometry	Accelerometers are inexpensive to purchase Easy to use Placing them on the animal is unlikely to change the behavior of the animal	Generates a large amount of data Activity may be increased for reasons that are not specific to pain e.g., during administration of potent opioids to horses

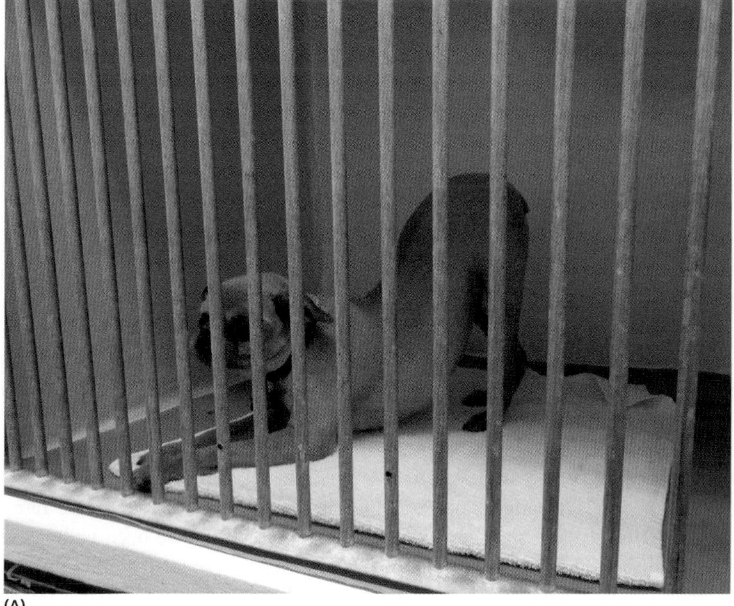
(A)

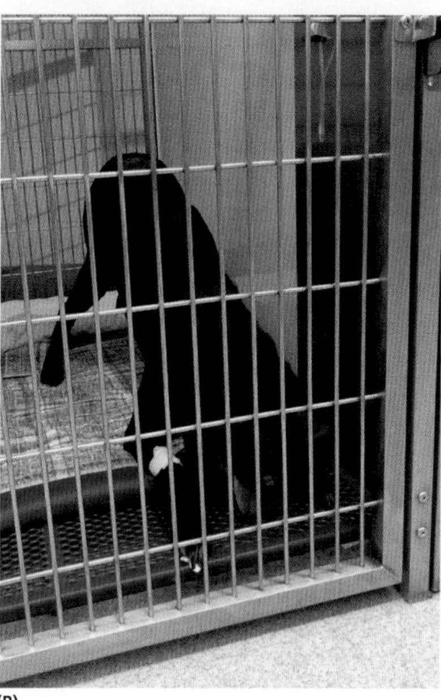
(B)

Figure 47.1 In dogs, adoption of a "praying posture" is suggestive of abdominal pain. **A.** Praying position in a dog diagnosed with acute pancreatitis. **B.** Praying position in a dog that had undergone surgery for a splenectomy. Source: Dr. Sheilah Robertson, with permission.

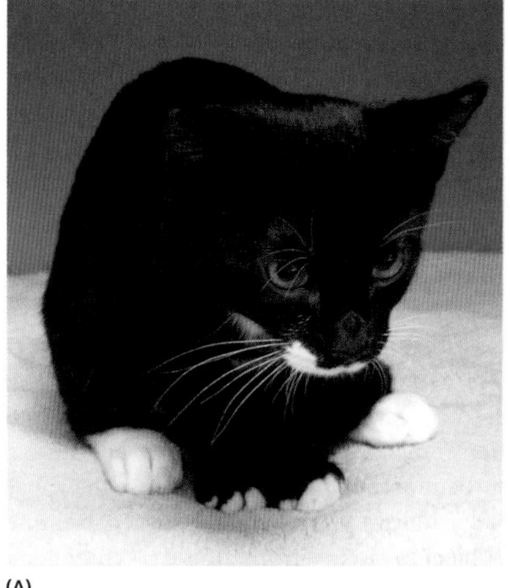
(A)

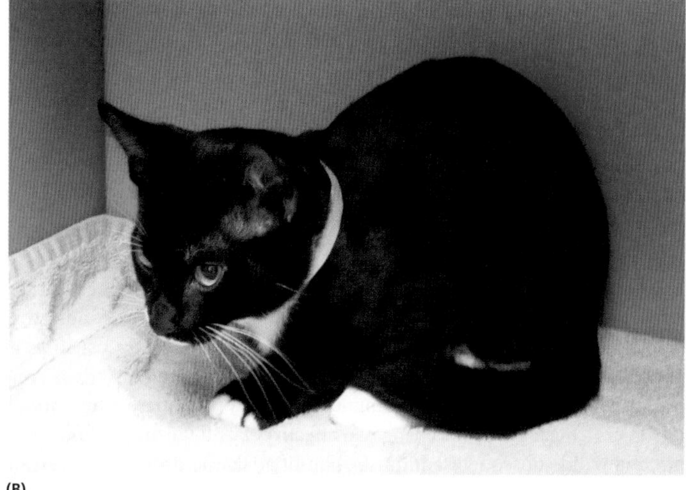
(B)

Figure 47.2 In cats, a hunched or "tucked up" posture is suggestive of abdominal pain. This cat had undergone an elective ovariohysterectomy 6 h earlier. Source: Dr. Sheilah Robertson, with permission.

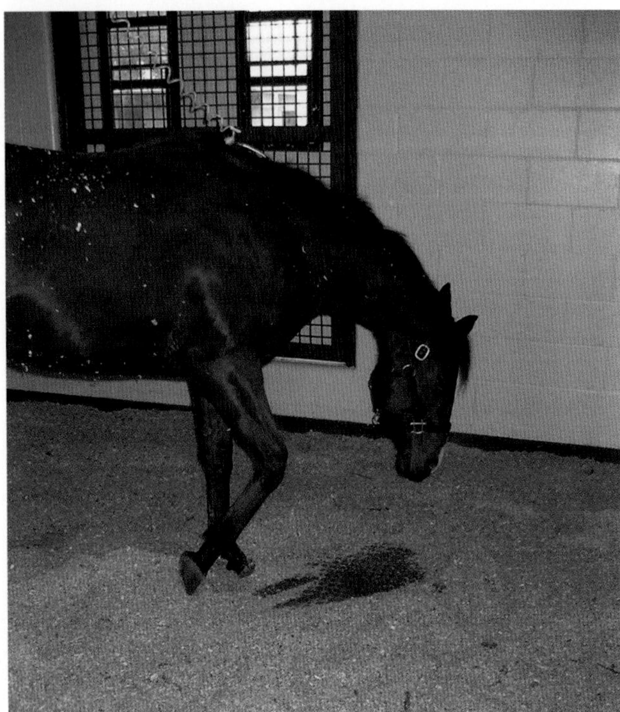

Figure 47.3 This horse is pawing at the ground, a behavior that is related to abdominal pain. Source: Dr. Sheilah Robertson, with permission.

way of moving, suggestive of abdominal pain [1]. Horses with colic may be restless, depressed, show flank watching, weight shifting, kicking of the abdomen, pawing at the ground (Fig. 47.3), and stretching [2].

An important part of behavioral assessment of pain is interaction with the animal, particularly the application of gentle pressure around any wound or painful area in order to detect secondary hyperalgesia and allodynia. This should be done gently so as not to cause the animal more pain, but it is an essential part of behavioral pain assessment and is included as part of many tools used to quantify pain.

Changes in facial expression have received a significant amount of attention as a biomarker for acute pain across species. This has largely stemmed from work in neonates which showed that reliable changes in facial expression could be detected during painful interventions such as heel lancing for blood sample collection [3]. The first work in animals was carried out in mice and led to the development of the Mouse Grimace Scale [4]. The detection of pain using facial expression across species largely relies on recognizing changes in facial action units, which are a set of facial muscle movements which correspond to a displayed emotion. Typically, changes in ear position and eye-opening are included in the scoring system, with other changes being largely species-dependent. Details of specific grimace scales used to quantify pain are given later in this chapter.

Changes in complex patterns of behavior such as burrowing and nest-making have been used in rats and mice, respectively, as indicators of pain that may be a more sensitive biomarker of affective state or how the animal is feeling about their pain than traditional nociceptive tests. These tests use the principle that rodents are highly motivated to perform these behaviors in their home cage if given the means to do so (i.e., burrowing and nesting substrate); therefore, quantifying an altered willingness to carry out these behaviors offers a means to probe changes in affective state following pain induction and subsequent administration of analgesic drugs. Spontaneous burrowing behavior in rats is reduced by peripheral nerve injury or inflammatory pain [5], an effect that is reversed by the administration of analgesic drugs, showing the utility of this assay in analgesic drug development. Similar studies have been carried out in mice using burrowing behavior [6]. The complexity of nest-making has been shown to relate to postoperative pain in mice, although the complexity of nest-making was not restored by treatment with carprofen [7], suggesting that it may not be a good biomarker for efficacy of analgesic treatment.

Advantages of using behavior to assess pain are that it may provide direct insight into how the animal is feeling and therefore how painful the animal is. Disadvantages include that it is time consuming to carry out and requires careful observation of the animal. The presence of an observer may also change the behavior of the animals being observed. Questions have also been raised about the objectivity of behavior as a tool to recognize pain. However, behavior can be an objective means depending on how it is measured.

Factors confounding behavioral assessment of acute pain

Although behavior can be a reliable tool to assess acute pain, a number of confounding factors can interfere with behavioral pain assessment, especially in the immediate postoperative period during recovery from anesthesia. A full bladder can make animals restless and unwilling to settle and this can confound pain assessment. Similarly, it is difficult to behaviorally assess a fear-aggressive animal, especially because interaction with such animals is often limited. Sedation is a big confounder of behavioral pain assessment; animals that are sedated can appear very comfortable and settled, but it is important to be aware that sedation does not necessarily equate to adequate analgesia. It is advisable to wait until 30–40 min after the end of anesthesia to assess pain when the patient is more rousable and less sedated. Emergence delirium and dysphoria from the overzealous use of opioids during anesthesia can also cause behavioral changes such as agitation and vocalization that can be confused with pain.

Physiological parameters

Changes in physiological parameters such as heart rate, blood pressure, respiratory rate, and cortisol have been widely used as a biomarker for acute pain, particularly in farm animal studies where changes in these parameters have been used to assess pain caused by husbandry procedures such as castration [8,9]. Generally, pain can cause an increase in heart rate, blood pressure, and respiratory rate through stimulation of the sympathetic nervous system due to an interaction between pathways that transmit sensory information and the central autonomic nervous system in the brain. Pain also causes activation of the hypothalamo–pituitary–adrenal axis, which is the neuroendocrine stress pathway. Cortisol is one of the end products of this pathway and therefore has been widely used as a biomarker for stress caused by acute pain in farm animals, particularly pain caused by castration in lambs and calves and tail docking in lambs [10]. Another neuroendocrine biomarker of pain that has been studied is β-endorphin [11]. Blood biomarkers of pain and distress are considered objective biomarkers of pain. However, a big caveat to their use is that neuroendocrine biomarkers are primarily indicators of stress, and although pain is a stressor, other stressors such as handling to collect a blood sample can cause elevations in their concentrations. In horses, anesthesia alone will cause marked elevations in neuroendocrine biomarkers, so that the capacity for further increases due to pain associated with surgery is limited [12]. Cortisol is also subject to circadian rhythms in secretion and there may be a ceiling effect on cortisol secretion. Heart rate, respiratory rate, and blood pressure, although relatively easy to measure, are also considered to be non-specific for pain. Blood pressure and heart rate may change intraoperatively due to blood loss or the effects of surgical manipulation of nerves such as the vagus nerve, rather than being specific biomarkers of nociception. Similarly, postoperative changes in these parameters may indicate stress caused by factors other than pain.

Heart rate variability assesses beat-to-beat variability in the timing between one heartbeat and the next [13]. Heart rate variability is used to investigate the balance between sympathetic and parasympathetic nervous system activity, with a decrease in heart rate variability shown with nociception or pain due to a shift in balance toward sympathetic nervous system activity. Heart rate variability data are generally analyzed using frequency domain measures calculated using fast Fourier transformation, such as high- and low-frequency power and the low-frequency/high-frequency ratio [13]. Monitors designed to detect intraoperative nociception have been developed for animals based on heart rate variability data, for example, the Parasympathetic Tone Activity (PTA) monitor (MDoloris Medical Systems, Loos, France) [14].

Production parameters such as average daily weight gain have been used to assess pain following castration in calves [10]; however, they are often too imprecise to detect acute changes in pain after castration. Furthermore, weight gain after castration may be negatively influenced by a decrease in testosterone after removal of the testes [15].

Electroencephalogram

The electroencephalogram (EEG) can be recorded from the surface of the head of animals and has been widely used as a measure of acute pain following surgical interventions such as castration. Fig. 47.4 shows EEG recording in an anesthetized deer. Measurement of the EEG relies on recording the summated electrical activity of populations of neurons together with glial cells (for a review see Murrell and Johnson [16]). These electrical potentials can be recorded from the surface of the head using electrodes connected to amplifiers and an EEG recording system, including an analog-to-digital converter. The raw EEG signal is recorded in real time, but this can be difficult to interpret and generates a large amount of data in a short space of time. Commonly, fast Fourier transformation is applied to raw EEG data, off-line at the end of an experiment, changing the signal from the time domain to the frequency domain to produce a power spectrum. Simple descriptors can be derived from the power spectrum, including the median frequency, spectral edge frequency 95%, and total power. EEG changes during nociception are frequently reported as percentage changes in these descriptors compared with an unstimulated baseline period [17,18]. Commonly a change in the level of synchronization of the EEG is described. Desynchronization is characterized as increased high-frequency activity and decreased power in the low-frequency bands of the EEG and is associated with an increased level of arousal due to noxious stimuli. Conversely, synchronization refers to an EEG pattern of high-amplitude, low-frequency activity. In human studies, the frequency of EEG activity has been denoted by δ (0–4 Hz), θ (4–8 Hz), α (8–12 Hz), and β (> 12 Hz), and the relative amount of activity in each frequency band is reported. These frequency bands also have functionality associated with them in man, and this method has been adopted by some authors investigating EEG in animals [19]. However, it is important to be aware that the division of the EEG into these frequency bands in animals is completely arbitrary and may be inappropriate in animals as compared to humans. Advantages of using the EEG as a marker of nociception in animals include its objectivity and the fact that signals are being recorded directly from the brain, which can be considered the seat of pain perception. Disadvantages include the need to understand the complex nature of the EEG acquisition equipment and the underlying signal-processing techniques. It can also be difficult to record high-quality EEG signals in awake animals while anesthesia may interfere with EEG data acquisition depending on the anesthetic agent used [20]. Many of the studies investigating EEG changes with nociception in anesthetized animals have been carried out using halothane as an inhalant anesthetic agent because it is less depressant to the EEG compared with isoflurane or sevoflurane [20–22].

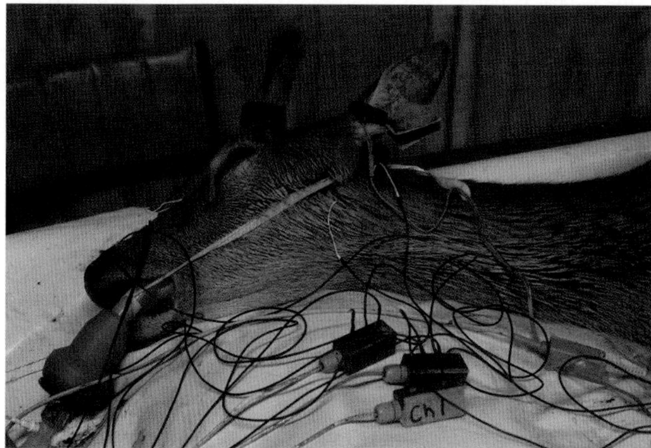

Figure 47.4 This image shows EEG recording in an anesthetized deer. The needle electrodes are placed subcutaneously and attached to pre-amplifiers (the metal boxes in the foreground of the picture). Source: Dr. Jo Murrell, with permission.

Functional magnetic resonance imaging

Functional magnetic resonance imaging (fMRI) uses blood oxygen level-dependent imaging (BOLD) to detect changes in blood flow to different regions of the brain. Hemoglobin is diamagnetic when oxygenated but paramagnetic when deoxygenated. This difference in magnetic properties leads to small differences in the magnetic resonance signal of blood depending on the degree of oxygenation. When areas of the brain are activated, such as during application of a noxious stimulus, blood flow to these areas will usually increase, which can be seen on the fMRI image. There are many studies in humans that have investigated which areas of the brain are activated during application of noxious thermal and mechanical stimuli [23]. These studies have led to identification of the so-called "pain matrix," the complex pattern of areas of the brain that are activated when a noxious stimulus is processed [24]. However, it is important to be aware that the pain matrix may not be specific to pain and similar areas of the brain may be activated by loud auditory, startling visual, and salient non-painful mechanical stimuli [25]. This has led to the suggestion that the pain matrix is in fact a saliency detection system [25]. Although there have been numerous studies elucidating path pathways in rats and mice using fMRI, studies using fMRI to detect pain or noxious stimuli in companion and farm animals are currently nonexistent. This is largely because of difficulties associated with training an animal to lie still in the scanner while a noxious or painful stimulus is delivered.

Infrared thermography

Infrared thermography can be used to measure changes in skin surface temperature before and after a noxious intervention such as castration. It is hypothesized that release of hormones such as epinephrine and norepinephrine associated with noxious stimulation causes peripheral vasoconstriction and therefore a decrease in skin temperature that can be quantified using a thermal imaging camera. Eye temperature has also been used as a biomarker for pain, with a decrease in eye temperature noted after castration without local anesthetic in calves, attributed to sympathetically driven changes in tone in the eye capillary beds [26]. Changes in comb temperature have been measured in poultry and the temperature changes in the head, snout, and vulva have been measured in pigs [27]. Although monitoring of skin surface temperature at different sites is non-invasive and quick to conduct it also has limitations. Thermal imaging cameras are expensive to purchase and the area which has to be measured must be defined and analyzed in a standardized way. Skin surface temperature is affected by stress and disease; therefore, it is a measure that is non-specific for pain.

Accelerometry and step-counts

Accelerometry has been widely used as a measure of acute pain in calves following castration or dehorning [28,29]. They have also been used as a marker of acute postoperative pain after ovariohysterectomy in dogs [30]. Triaxial accelerometers estimate acceleration along the *x*, *y*, and *z* axes, allowing measurement of position relative to the ground, and the direction and speed of movement. Some accelerometers will allow measurement of time spent standing, lying, and walking as well as giving an accurate step count. Advantages of accelerometry are that it is non-invasive, accelerometers are relatively inexpensive to purchase, and they can record high-resolution data over a relatively long period of time. Attaching pedometers is also unlikely to influence the behavior of the animal because they are small and lightweight to wear. Step-counts can also be used as a surrogate marker for pain, measured using pedometers. Like accelerometers, these are inexpensive to purchase, and can be easily attached and used. Fig. 47.5 shows a pedometer attached to a horse's forelimb.

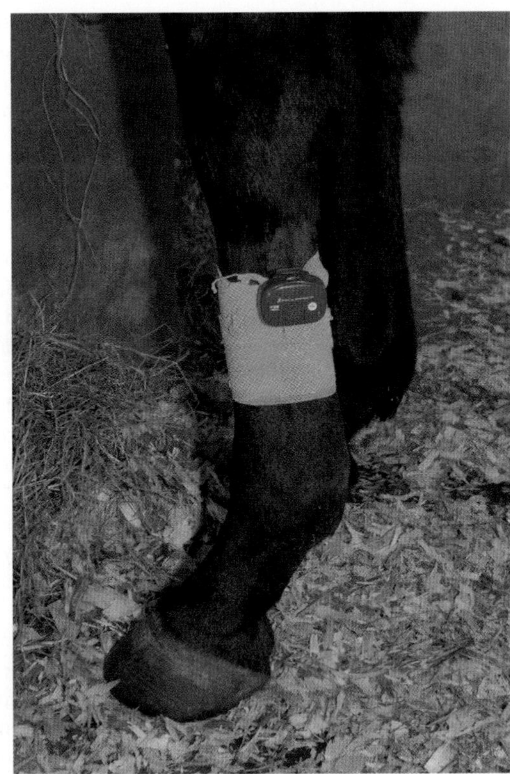

Figure 47.5 A pedometer attached to the forelimb of a horse to measure step count. Source: Dr. Jo Murrell, with permission.

Recognition of chronic pain

Detection of chronic pain is challenging across all species and is probably more difficult than the detection of acute pain. Behavioral changes can be very subtle and vary according to the species, pain condition, and individual. Many of the techniques used to assess acute pain are not appropriate for the detection of chronic pain in animals or have not been trialed for this purpose. The reason for this may be that, unlike acute pain where established clinical pain models exist (e.g., castration or tail docking), common clinical chronic pain models are lacking. Exceptions to this may be osteoarthritis, Chiari-like malformation and syringomyelia in dogs, or laminitis in horses, which are relatively well-characterized clinical models of chronic pain. A summary of the advantages and disadvantages of the various methods to recognize chronic pain that are discussed below is provided in Table 47.2.

Changes in behavior

Changes in behavior associated with osteoarthritis have been characterized in dogs and cats and there is evidence that these behavioral changes can be detected by owners [31,32], although the detected changes in behavior may not always be attributed to osteoarthritis by the owner. Enomoto *et al.* [31] have developed a checklist for owners of cats which asks questions about whether their cat can jump up normally, jump down normally, the ability of the cat to climb up and down stairs, run, and chase objects. The role of owners in detecting chronic pain caused by osteoarthritis in cats and dogs is emphasized by the importance of clinical metrology instruments in measuring pain caused by this condition as discussed later in this chapter. Chiari-like malformation and syringomyelia are common conditions in small and toy breed dogs such as the Cavalier King Charles Spaniel. They commonly co-exist and are believed to cause clinical signs indicative of neuropathic pain such as allodynia or dysesthesia. Dogs appear to dislike being touched over areas of skin around the neck and may not tolerate a neck collar. Phantom scratching, where dogs appear to scratch the air without making skin contact, sometimes while walking may be suggestive of dysesthesia [33]. Chronic laminitis is a painful and debilitating condition in horses that results in severe pain with a neuropathic component [34]. Characteristic behavioral changes associated with laminitis in horses include lameness, which most commonly affects at least two limbs, leaning back onto the heels to take the weight off the painful toe area, and shifting weight between feet when resting.

Physiological parameters

Generally, physiological biomarkers are less helpful in the recognition of chronic pain than they are for the recognition of acute pain. Changes in heart rate, respiratory rate, and blood pressure do not

Table 47.2 Summary of the advantages and disadvantages of different methods used to recognize chronic pain.

Method to recognize chronic pain	Advantages	Disadvantages
Behavior	Can provide a good insight into how the animal "feels" about their pain "Gold standard" measure of chronic pain	Can be time consuming to collect data Presence of an observer may influence the behavior of an animal Risk of confounding factors changing the behavior of an animal
Physiology	Objective means to measure pain	Less helpful in the assessment of chronic compared to acute pain May be invasive
Force plate gait analysis	Objective means to measure pain associated with lameness	Cannot measure step or stride length More useful when the animal has a single-limb lameness Requires an understanding of the complex software required for data analysis
Kinematic gait analysis	Objective means to measure pain associated with lameness	Requires an understanding of the complex software required for data analysis Markers on the body can shift in position rendering data collection inaccurate
Accelerometry	Accelerometers are inexpensive to purchase Easy to use Placing them on the animal is unlikely to change the behavior of the animal	Generates a large amount of data Activity may be increased for reasons that are not specific to pain e.g., during administration of potent opioids to horses

persist in chronic pain states and changes in neuroendocrine biomarkers have largely not been assessed in chronic states. An exception may be heart rate variability which has been shown to return to more normal resting conditions when horses with laminitis were treated with analgesics [35].

Visual observation of gait

Visual observation of gait, or lameness scoring is commonly used to assess lameness in companion animals. Techniques to facilitate visual observation of lameness include choosing a surface for observation that is even and flat, observing the animal at a walk and trot, watching the animal both going away from and coming toward you, and when it moves in a circle. Generally, an animal that is lame on the forelimb will shift weight caudally and lift the head on the lame limb, or "nod" the head down on the sound limb. With hindlimb lameness, weight tends to be shifted cranially with the head and neck lowered and extended to offset weight from the hind end. Numerical rating scales and visual analog scales are used to quantify lameness, although visual observation is recognized to be less sensitive at detecting lameness than force plate or kinematic gait analysis techniques [36].

Force plate gait analysis

With force plate gait analysis metal plates are mounted on the floor or walkway to measure ground reaction forces. Force plate gait analysis is viewed as the gold standard for evaluation of lameness with peak vertical force (PVF) (maximal force applied during the stance phase) in the vertical axis the most commonly used variable to assess lameness [37]. The vertical impulse (VI) can be derived by calculating the area under the vertical force curve over time. In general, a lame animal has a lower PVF and VI in the lame limb. Although force plate gait analysis is more sensitive than observation to detect lameness there are limitations to this technique. These include an inability to measure stride or step length, the need for the animal to transverse the force plate at a constant velocity, the need for a long walkway, multiple trials, and the complexity of software and data analysis.

Kinematic gait analysis

Kinematic gait analysis quantifies the positions, velocities, acceleration, and deceleration, and angles of anatomical structures in space. Generally, kinematic gait analysis systems use colored or reflective markers that identify specific anatomical landmarks, and these markers are tracked as the animal moves by a series of cameras. Outputs from kinematic gait analysis include displacement, which is the distance recorded when a marker changes position; angular velocity, which is the speed at which this change occurs; and range of motion, which is calculated from the displacement of a specific joint. Kinematic gait analysis has been applied to dogs, horses, and chickens; in the latter, it was used to quantify gait abnormalities associated with lameness in broiler chickens and identify evolutionary gait differences between broiler chickens and jungle fowl [38]. Limitations of kinematic gait analysis include the potential for skin movement altering marker placement, accuracy, and repeatability of marker placement, as well as the complexity of software and data analysis.

Accelerometry

In addition to its role in acute pain assessment, accelerometry has been widely used to assess pain associated with osteoarthritis in cats [39] and dogs [40], and to document a treatment effect when animals are administered an analgesic [41]. Advantages of accelerometry for chronic pain are similar to those for acute pain.

Quantification of acute pain

A number of different tools have been developed to try and measure acute pain across different species. However, where data are available, it shows that adoption of these tools in general practice is low. In a 2021 study in Australia, only 14% of respondents in small animal practices used validated pain scales to quantify pain [42]. This finding is also supported by an older study in the UK where only 14% of small animal general practitioners were using pain assessment tools [43]. Interestingly the percentage of respondents using pain assessment tools was significantly higher (60–80%) among respondents who were members of the Association of Veterinary Anaesthetists [43].

There are a number of excellent reasons to use tools to try and quantify pain across different species. Unless you use a pain assessment tool it is difficult to know what level of pain the animal is experiencing and therefore treat it appropriately with analgesics. It is also difficult to objectively assess the response to analgesic drug administration to determine whether it has been adequate or whether more analgesic drugs are required. Tools also help with the actual assessment of pain, because using a structured instrument to assess pain aids in coming to some sort of conclusion about whether the animal is experiencing pain or not. They also help standardize the process of pain assessment between individuals in a clinical setting so that when more than one person is assessing pain in an individual animal interobserver variability should be reduced.

It is essential that tools used for the quantification of acute and chronic pain are validated. Validity provides evidence that the tool is measuring what it is intended to measure; there are a number of different types of validity that are outlined below.

- ***Criterion validity*** is assessed by statistically testing a new measurement technique against a "gold standard." However, with pain scales in animals, this can often be problematic because no gold standard exists, that is, it is impossible to know how much pain an animal is experiencing because self-report is not possible.
- ***Content validity*** relates to the appropriateness and completeness of the items comprising the instrument. Generally, content validity is assessed using expert judgment, whereby experts are requested to rate the relevance and clarity of items using a rating scale. These ratings are then used to calculate a content validity index for the scale, which objectively allows the developers of the scale to remove items that are not relevant.
- ***Construct validity*** is the extent to which the new instrument or pain scale behaves in a way that is consistent with theoretical hypotheses. For example, you would expect pain scores on a new scale to decrease after the administration of analgesics. This is termed a "known groups approach" to construct validation.
- ***Reliability*** of a measurement instrument is the extent to which it yields consistent reproducible estimates of what is assumed to be an underlying true score. Inter-rater reliability is when two individuals measure the same subject at the same time and intra-rater reliability is when an unchanging subject is measured at two time points by the same individual; both forms of reliability are important for a pain assessment tool. Cronbach's alpha is also a measure of reliability. It measures internal consistency or how closely a set of items are related as a group.
- ***Responsiveness*** is the property of a clinical instrument that ensures that it can detect differences in pain that are important to the clinician or the patient. If the instrument is not very responsive, it may not be able to detect clinically relevant changes in pain level.
- ***Clinical utility*** is the final property of an instrument that should be considered. This can be described as the "user-friendliness" of the tool. For example, to be useful in practice a pain assessment tool must be easy to use and quick to complete, otherwise it is not likely to be widely adopted.

Unidimensional pain assessment scales

Unidimensional pain scales take into account the "How much does it hurt?" aspect of pain but are very poor at measuring the emotional component of pain. They are useful because they are easy to understand and quick to use but they have typically not undergone any of the different methods of validation described above. In clinical practice, they have been largely superseded by the application of multidimensional pain scales which measure both the sensory and emotional components of pain.

Simple descriptive scales

Simple descriptive scales (SDSs) are basic and highly subjective pain scales that typically have four or five descriptors. These scale types do not demonstrate sensitivity in detecting small changes in pain intensity, but they are simple and quick to use.

Numerical rating scale

The numerical rating scale (NRS) uses numbers rather than descriptors to score pain. This scale type is discontinuous with unequal weighting between the categories (sometimes leading to incorrect statistical analysis of research data). It is often used when scoring individual behavioral characteristics within multidimensional scales. Although numerical scales are quick to use and complete, they tend to show greater intra- and interobserver variability than composite pain scales [2].

Visual analog scale

The visual analog scale (VAS) is a simple continuous scale that is widely used and consists of a 100 mm line anchored at either end with (0) no pain and (100) worst imaginable pain (for this procedure or condition). The observer places a mark on the line at a point that correlates with their assessment of the pain. Training is necessary to reduce variation between assessors. One of the much-debated questions about the VAS is the linearity of the scale (e.g., Does a score of 60 mm represent twice as much pain as 30 mm?). This is obviously important when determining an appropriate statistical test for evaluating the data generated. One survey demonstrated that approximately 50% of studies involving VAS measurements applied parametric statistics [44]. However, other researchers advocate the use of nonparametric statistics for nonlinear data. Use of confidence intervals may assist in the interpretation of the data from a VAS but do not solve the problem of violation of the underlying assumptions of the statistical test [44,45].

Studies have shown significant observer variability with all three of the aforementioned scales [46]. Hewetson *et al.* investigated the use of an NRS and verbal rating scale to describe lameness in horses and found 55–60% interobserver variability with the two scales [47]. Intraobserver variability was of a similar magnitude of 58–60%. This highlights the subjective nature of the lameness examination and the variability that occurs when using these subjective scales. When one trained observer performs all observations, the NRS becomes a more reliable scale.

Lascelles *et al.* reported the refinement of the VAS, which involves a dynamic and interactive assessment of the patient (DIVAS). Numerous studies adopted this approach [48,49]. This additional component of the VAS involves observing the animal from a distance, then approaching and interacting with the patient, and finally palpating the wound and surrounding area. VAS scales for questionnaires have also been investigated for assessing pain and lameness in dogs [50].

Multidimensional pain assessment scales

A large number of multidimensional or composite pain scales have been developed for use in different species. Many of these scales have undergone a significant degree of validation making them preferred tools over unidimensional pain scales. The first composite pain scale to be developed was the Glasgow Composite Pain Scale-Canine and its Short Form [51] which was developed using a psychometric approach. The instrument requires that the observer looks at the dog from outside of the kennel, then goes inside the kennel and interacts with the dog, palpates around any wound or painful area, and finally asks questions about comfort level and demeanor. The maximum possible score is dependent on whether the dog can be walked outside or not; if the dog is nonambulatory the maximum possible score is 20, while if it can be walked then the maximum possible score is 24. An intervention level has been established as 5 or greater out of 20 or 6 or greater out of 24 [52]. This scale has also been translated and validated in the Italian language [53]. The Short Form of the Glasgow Composite Pain Scale-Canine is quick and simple to use, giving it good clinical utility. However, it is important to note that sedation is a big confounder to the scale, with dogs that are heavily sedated scoring highly. It is advisable to wait until dogs are fully recovered from anesthesia before the scale is applied. A recent review suggested that although the English version of the scale had been widely used in research studies it was sometimes modified, or the intervention level was adjusted, invalidating the scale [54].

The same research group that developed the canine Glasgow scale has also developed a multidimensional scale to assess acute pain in cats; the Glasgow Composite Pain Scale-Feline [55] (Web resource 47.1). This scale has been validated in cats and has a similar look and feel to the composite scoring system in dogs, with the same pattern of looking at the cat from outside of the cage, interacting with the cat, and palpating gently around any wound or painful area. One difference from the dog instrument is the inclusion of facial expressions in the cat scale. The maximum possible score for the scale is 20, with an intervention level defined as a score of 5 or greater out of 20 [56]. One recent study suggested that training in using the scale did not significantly change analgesia decision-making, suggesting that scale is still relatively robust to use, even by naive individuals [57]. 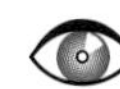 Videos 47.2, 47.3, and 47.4, along with their accompanying score sheets, illustrate how the Glasgow Composite Pain Scale-Feline is used.

The UNESP-Botucatu multidimensional pain scale for cats is an alternative to the Glasgow Composite Pain Scale-Feline. It was first developed in 2011 [58], and although only validated in cats undergoing ovariohysterectomy, it was found to be reliable, but the clinical utility of the instrument was poor, being time consuming to complete. It also required measurement of blood pressure which may not be practicable in a clinical setting. More recently, a short form of the UNESP-Botucatu scale has been developed [59]. This was evaluated in cats undergoing various orthopedic and soft tissue procedures and showed good construct validity, responsiveness reliability, and sensitivity and specificity for feline acute pain assessment. The short form also showed good clinical utility, being easier to use than the original longer version.

A number of different composite pain scales have been validated in horses for different types of pain. The first scale to be developed and validated was an instrument to measure orthopedic pain [60]. Later, this pain scale was also validated for acute pain after gastrointestinal surgery [61]. van Loon and van Dierendonck [62] developed the EQUUS-COMPASS pain scale for measurement of pain caused by acute colic in horses. This scale showed good sensitivity and specificity for discrimination between healthy controls and horses with acute colic, as well as good reproducibility. It also showed good clinical utility. Other composite pain scales in horses include the UNESP-Botucatu multidimensional pain scale for assessing pain in horses after castration [63].

For an overview of multidimensional pain scales that have been developed for measurement of acute pain in different species and their validation see Table 47.3.

Grimace scales

The use of grimace scales to quantify pain has risen in popularity recently, largely because the scales are quick and simple to use and many of them have undergone validation. They also do not require interaction with the animal and assessments can be made from a distance, which can be helpful for wild or feral animals. Facial Action Coding Systems (FACS) were originally developed in humans as a methodology to formally interrogate facial expressions. FACS provides a systematic methodology to identify and code facial expressions on the basis of underlying muscle movement. These may be used to determine whether a combination of facial action units is involved in a certain type of emotion such as the expression of pain. The Equine Facial Action Coding System has been described [64]. However, in the context of pain, what has been more commonly described rather than FACS, is facial expressions or grimace scales associated with pain. Grimace scales exist for mice [65], rats [66], rabbits [67], horses [68], lambs [69], sheep [70,71], piglets [72], ferrets [73], cats [74], and donkeys [75]. A recent systematic review evaluated the measurement properties (reliability, validity, and responsiveness) of these grimace scales [76]. The instruments that demonstrated a high level of evidence for measurement properties were the grimace scales developed for the mouse, rat, horse, and cat. A moderate level of evidence was shown for the rabbit, lamb, sheep [71], ferret, and piglet grimace scales, while a low level of evidence was shown for the other sheep [70] and donkey grimace scales. The most reported measurement property for the grimace scales in general was construct validity followed by responsiveness to analgesic interventions. However, reliability, internal consistency, and criterion validity have been less widely reported for the grimace scales. For a summary of grimace scales that have been developed for different species see Table 47.4. Fig. 47.6 shows a "feline pain face." This can be scored using the Feline Grimace Scale [74]. Guidance on using the Feline Grimace Scale can be found at: www.felinegrimacescale.com.

How often should you conduct acute pain assessment in animals?

The frequency of acute pain assessment in the perioperative period depends on a number of factors. It is important not to assess pain too frequently or the animal may not be able to rest, although this is less of a problem when using grimace scales because direct interaction with the animal is not necessary. However, pain assessment needs to be frequent enough to detect an animal that is in pain. Assessing pain every 4 h is reasonable, and this correlates with the duration of action of methadone, a commonly used analgesic in cats and dogs. In these species, assessing pain 30 min after administration of methadone is sensible to detect animals that are experiencing

Table 47.3 List of multidimensional pain scales developed for quantification of acute pain.

Species	Scale abbreviation	Scale name	Reference(s)	Outcome measures	Type of pain assessed	Validation studies conducted
Cats	CSU-FAPS	Colorado State University Feline Acute Pain Scale	Shipley *et al.* 2021 [77]	Behavior	Acute	No
	UNESP-Botucatu-MCPS	UNESP-Botucatu-multidimensional composite pain scale	Brondani *et al.* 2011 [58]	Behavior, Physiology	Acute	Yes
	UNESP-Botucatu-MCPS-SF	UNESP-Botucatu-multidimensional composite pain scale-Short Form	Belli *et al.* 2021 [59]	Behavior	Acute	Yes
	GCPS-F	Glasgow Composite Pain Scale-Feline	Calvo *et al.* 2014 [55]	Behavior	Acute	Yes
Dogs	Melbourne	University of Melbourne Pain Scale	Firth and Haldane 1999 [78]	Behavior, Physiology	Acute	No
	GCPS-C	Glasgow Composite Pain Scale-Canine	Holton *et al.* 2001 [51]	Behavior	Acute	Yes
	GCPS-C-SF	Glasgow Composite Pain Scale-Canine – Short Form	Reid *et al.* 2007 [52]	Behavior	Acute	Yes
	4A Vet Pain Scale	4A Vet Pain Scale	Holopherne-Doran *et al.* 2010 [79]	Behavior	Acute	Yes
	CSU	Colorado State University Canine Acute Pain Scale		Behavior	Acute	No
Horses	ECPS	Equine Composite Measure Pain Scale	Bussieres *et al.* 2008 [60]	Behavior, Physiology	Acute – orthopedic and colic	Yes
	CMPS	Composite Measure Pain Scale	Gleerup and Lindegaard 2016 [80]	Behavior	Acute – LPS-induced transient synovitis	No
	PASPAS	Post Abdominal Surgery Pain Assessment Scale	Graubner *et al.* 2011 [81]	Behavior, Physiology	Acute – post-abdominal surgery	Yes
	EAAPS	Equine Acute Abdominal Pain Scale	Sutton *et al.* 2013 [2]	Behavior	Acute colic	Yes
	EQUUS-COMPASS	EQUUS-Composite Pain Assessment	van Loon and van Dierendonck 2015 [62]	Behavior, Physiology	Acute colic	Yes
	UNESP-Botucatu	UNESP-Botucatu	Taffarel *et al.* 2015 [63]	Behavior	Acute – post-castration	Yes
Donkeys	EQUUS-DONKEY-COMPASS	EQUUS-Donkeys-Composite Pain Assessment	Van Dierendonck 2020 [75]	Behavior	Acute – colic and orthopedic	Yes
Cattle	UNESP-Botucatu	UNESP-Botucatu	De Oliveira *et al.* 2014 [82]	Behavior	Acute	Yes
Sheep	UNESP-Botucatu	UNESP-Botucatu	Silva *et al.* 2020 [83]	Behavior	Acute	Yes
Pigs	UPAPS	UNESP-Botucatu Pig Composite Acute Pain Scale	Luna *et al.* 2020 [84]	Behavior	Acute	Yes
Rabbits	CANCRS	Composite Pain Scale for assessment and quantification of pain in rabbits	Banchi *et al.* 2020 [85]	Behavior, Physiology	Acute	Yes
	BRPS	Bristol Rabbit Pain Scale	Benato *et al.* 2021 [86]	Behavior	Acute	Yes

Table 47.4 List of facial grimace scales developed for quantification of acute pain.

Species	Scale abbreviation	Scale name	Reference(s)	Outcome measures	Type of pain assessed	Validation studies conducted
Cats	FGS	Facial Grimace Scale	Evangelista *et al.* 2019 [74]	Facial expressions	Acute	Yes
Horses	HGS	Horse Grimace Scale	Dalla Costa *et al.* 2014, 2016 [87,88]	Facial expressions	Acute – post-castration and laminitis	Yes
	EPF	Equine Pain Face	Gleerup *et al.* 2015 [89]	Facial expressions	Acute – clinical and experimental pain	No
	EquiFACS	Facial Action Coding System	Wathan *et al.* 2015 [64]	Facial expressions	Not evaluated in acute pain states	Not applicable
	RHpE	Facial Expressions of Ridden Horses	Dyson *et al.* 2018 [90]	Facial expressions and head carriage	Acute – orthopedic pain	No
	EQUUS-FAP	EQUUS Facial Expression of Pain	van Loon and van Dierendonck 2017 [91]	Facial expressions	Acute – colic and head-related	Yes
	EQUUS-FAP-FOALS	EQUUS Facial Expression of Pain in Foals	van Loon *et al.* 2020 [92]	Facial expressions	Acute	No
Donkeys	EQUUS-DONKEY-FAP	EQUUS-Donkeys-Facial Assessment of Pain	van Dierendonck 2020 [75]	Facial expressions	Acute – head-related	No
Sheep	SGS	Sheep Grimace Scale	Hager *et al.* 2017 [70]	Facial expressions	Acute	Yes
		Facial expression for pain in lambs	Guesgen *et al.* 2016 [69]	Facial expressions	Acute	No
		Sheep facial expression scale	McLennan *et al.* 2016 [71]	Facial expressions	Acute	No
Pigs		Piglet Grimace Scale	Viscardi *et al.* 2017, [72]	Facial expressions	Acute	No
Ferrets		Ferret Grimace Scale	Reijgwart *et al.* 2016 [73]	Facial expressions	Acute	Yes
Rabbits and rodents	RbtGS	Rabbit facial grimace scale	Keating *et al.* 2011 [67]	Facial expressions	Acute	Yes
	RGS	Rat grimace scale	Sotocinal *et al.* 2011 [66]	Facial expressions	Acute	Yes
	MGS	Mouse grimace scale	Langford *et al.* 2010 [65]	Facial expressions	Acute	Yes

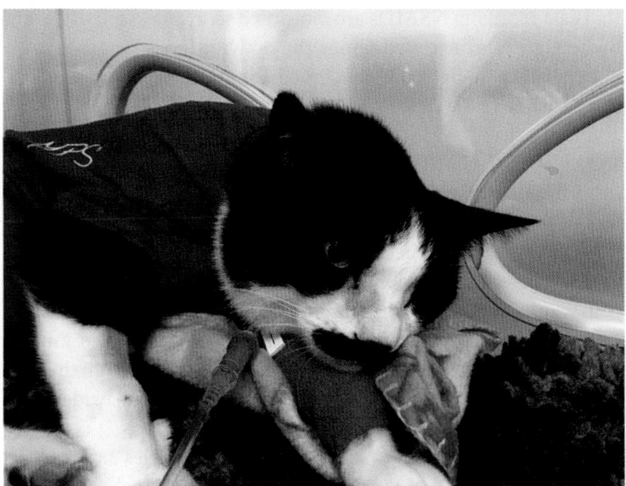

Figure 47.6 This cat is displaying changes in its facial expression indicative of pain. Using the Feline Grimace Scale this cat scores 6 or 7 out of 10, indicating that rescue analgesia is required. Source: Dr. Jo Murrell.

breakthrough pain. If analgesia is only to be administered on the basis of quantification of pain, then an interval of every 2 h is recommended. Although this is time consuming and labor-intensive, this frequency is important to ensure that animals that become painful do not get missed and become painful between assessments. If a rescue dose of analgesic is required, then it is important to check that a single dose of analgesic is sufficient by reassessing pain 30 min later and giving further doses of analgesic if required.

Who should conduct pain assessment?

Individuals conducting pain assessments should be trained in applying the tool that they are using to score pain. However, it is important to note that for many pain quantification tools, formal training does not exist. Exceptions are the Feline Grimace Scale (FGS) for which a website is available with training in using the tool (www.felinegrimacescale.com, accessed June 2023), and the Botucatu Multidimensional pain scale for which training in using the tool is also available on a website (www.animalpain.org/en/home-en/, accessed June 2023). Veterinary surgeons are not necessarily the best placed to conduct pain scoring and often this task is better delegated to animal care staff or veterinary nurses or technicians. The animal care staff generally spend more time with the animals than veterinary surgeons and are therefore better placed to detect changes in behavior over time and with administration of analgesic drugs. Use of the FGS by owners has been formally evaluated and it was found to be a reliable tool for owners to score acute pain in cats, with good agreement with pain scores assigned by veterinary surgeons. This makes the FGS a useful tool for owners to use to assess pain in cats after discharge from the hospital [93].

Factors confounding use of pain assessment tools

The factors confounding use of pain assessment tools are similar to those confounding behavioral assessments of pain and were discussed previously.

Quantification of chronic pain

Similar to acute pain, quantification of chronic pain is also imperative to measure the impact of pain on the animal and monitor the effect of analgesic treatment. Unless pain is measured it cannot be treated and managed effectively. It is also important to monitor Quality of Life (QoL) in animals with chronic pain because living with a painful condition long-term can have an enormous negative impact on QoL.

Tools devised for assessment of chronic pain are heavily dependent on owner assessment with interpretation and decision-making done in conjunction with the veterinarian. The same caveats about using a pain scale that is validated and reliable apply to chronic pain assessment as acute pain assessment. In fact, recent studies demonstrate little correlation between the owner assessment and force plate gait analysis when evaluating response to treatment in osteoarthritic dogs [37]. This is not to suggest that sophisticated evaluation methods are not useful but emphasizes that treatment efficacy in the eyes of the owners likely includes overall QoL [94].

A number of tools or clinical metrology instruments have been developed for the measurement of chronic pain and QoL in dogs [95,96]. These have been designed to some extent from existing QoL instruments for humans and mainly focus on the measurement of pain caused by osteoarthritis. QoL assessments aid in decision-making with respect to painful treatment interventions and the need for euthanasia [97,98]. QoL is an abstract construct used in human medicine that seems wholly appropriate when applied to the welfare of animals [99,100], although there is no general consensus on the definition of QoL in veterinary medicine [101]. One proposed definition is that it represents the aspects of an animal's life that make life better or worse for that specific animal [101]. Health-Related Quality of Life (HRQoL) is a narrower term that defines the specific effect of a medical condition on an individual's health [102].

Recently, a framework for assessment of HRQoL in dogs has been constructed [103]. The aim of this work was to inform the development of reliable instruments to measure HRQoL in dogs with osteoarthritis that are applicable to general veterinary practice and can be used to assess treatment outcomes in clinical veterinary studies. The four domains of HRQoL which were suggested were capability (e.g., lameness, stiffness, difficulty jumping), physical appearance (e.g., abnormal posture), mood (e.g., quiet and withdrawn), and behavior (e.g., attention seeking). All four categories were considered to be influenced by pain caused by osteoarthritis.

A web-based tool has also been developed to measure HRQoL in dogs [104]. The instrument comprises 22 items with four domains identified in this tool: energetic/enthusiastic, happy/content, active/comfortable, and calm/relaxed. The tool showed good discriminative ability to differentiate between healthy and sick dogs. One limitation to this tool is that it requires a fee to access it which may prevent widespread adoption in clinical practice.

Since there is no "gold standard" of chronic pain assessment with which to compare QoL or other clinical metrology instrument scales, psychometric testing of various scales has been undertaken. The Liverpool Osteoarthritis in Dogs (LOAD) scale, the Helsinki Chronic Pain Index (HCPI), and the Canine Brief Pain Inventory (CBPI) were comparatively evaluated in 222 dogs with OA [105]. There were moderate correlations between all instruments, implying construct validity for all of them. Significant but weak correlations were found between LOAD scores and "symmetry index" (calculated from force-platform analysis for peak vertical force) and between CBPI scores and symmetry index. The CBPI is a multifactorial tool composed of a Pain Severity Score, Pain Interference Score, and an Overall Quality of Life Score. Studies by Walton *et al.* [105] and others addressed criterion validity for the CPBI, as did a study by Brown *et al.* comparing the CPBI with force plate analysis [37]. For the CBPI, meaningful treatment differences have been defined as a decrease of ≥ 1 in Pain Severity Score and a decrease of ≥ 2 in Pain Interference Score [37], with Pain Interference Score being more sensitive at detecting treatment success than Pain Severity Score. The authors hypothesized that this is because the questions in the pain interference score section are more specific, relating to the dog's activity and playfulness, rather than the questions in the Pain Severity Score section that are more difficult to define.

The HCPI is an 11-item single-construct index of chronic pain [106]. Changes in the HCPI correlated well with changes in QoL and mobility VAS. It appears to provide a valid, reliable, and responsive method of assessing treatment response in osteoarthritic dogs. The HCPI has criterion validity on the basis of a correlation between HCPI and a QoL score on a VAS [107]. Interestingly, when the VAS and HCPI were compared using owner evaluation of pain in arthritic dogs, the conclusion was that a VAS was a poor tool for untrained owners because of poor face validity (i.e., owners could not identify their dogs' behavior as signs of pain). Only after the owners had seen pain diminish and then return (after completing a course of NSAIDs) did the VAS have face validity. The HCPI did not correlate with symmetry index from force plate analysis in the study undertaken by Walton *et al.* [105]. The reasons for this are unclear, but likely a function of wording and the weighting of descriptors.

An alternative to using a structured questionnaire to measure pain caused by osteoarthritis in dogs and cats is to use a tool called the Client-Specific Outcome Measures (CSOM) scale [108]. The CSOM uses three items tailored to each animal that the owners are asked to follow and assess. At the first appointment, the pet owner decides on the activity and rates the difficulty in performing the activity and these activities are then tracked over time. This approach can overcome the limitations of some questions in structured questionnaires, which may not apply to all animals (e.g., whether the animal can walk upstairs when the owner lives in a one-story home).

The feline musculoskeletal pain index (FMPI) is a client questionnaire with good readability, internal consistency–reliability, and repeatability [109,110]. The FMPI did not, however, demonstrate responsiveness or criterion validity in subsequent testing [111]. Responsiveness describes whether changes in a parameter can be detected following treatment, ideally in a blinded placebo-controlled design. The lack of responsiveness may have been a result of many factors, such as a large placebo effect. In a novel study, Gruen *et al.* [112] used the FMPI and CSOM and were able to circumvent the placebo effect by demonstrating recurrence of clinical signs after withdrawal of treatment compared with placebo. Criterion validity describes whether the results generated correlate with another validated measure. The FMPI did not show criterion validity either; however, this was correlated with activity measured by accelerometry [110]. This lack of correlation challenges the assumption that degenerative joint disease decreases activity, and that cats receiving NSAIDs are motivated to increase activity. Some owners are unconcerned about the activity levels *per se* in their elderly cats and are more concerned about other potential indicators of pain. These findings highlight a need to include both active and non-active terms to assess cat pain and QoL better.

As well as the FMPI, another instrument has recently been developed to quantify pain in cats with osteoarthritis; the MI-CAT (C) was developed for owners or caregivers to assess pain [113] while the MI-CAT (V) has been developed for veterinarians [114]. The tool for veterinarians contains 25 items involving body posture, gait, willingness, and ease of horizontal movements, jumping, and a general lameness score. A commercial company has also initially validated a tool to measure HRQoL in cats [115], although this tool requires payment of a fee to use it which may limit widespread uptake of the scoring system.

Multidimensional scales do not exist for all species and may not be appropriate in some cases. Some unidimensional scales have been used for chronic pain with some success. For example, Welsh *et al.* used the VAS and SDS to assess pain from "footrot" lameness in sheep [116].

One problem with clinical metrology instruments, in general, is a large placebo effect when completed by owners. In clinical research studies assessing new analgesics, this hinders the ability of an instrument to demonstrate a treatment effect which is disadvantageous, with placebo effects of up to nearly 50% for treatment success in some studies of dogs with osteoarthritis [117]. This also highlights the importance of including a placebo in analgesia studies of chronic pain using currently available tools to quantify pain. There are a number of recommendations that have been made to encourage accurate results when an owner is completing a clinical metrology instrument. First, it is important that the person who spends most time with the animal completes the instrument because they are likely to know the animal best. Second, the instrument should be completed before the consultation with the veterinarian because this avoids biasing the results. For example, if the veterinarian says they think the animal looks good today, then this may bias the results of the owner. Third, in order to avoid regression to the mean, it is recommended to omit the first pain assessment score on recruitment to clinical trials. This is because animals are often recruited to clinical trials by their owners when pain levels are high. This gives an initial high score for the instrument, then over time, due to the waxing and waning nature of chronic pain, scores will naturally decrease. Unless the first score is discarded, this will falsely show an effect of treatment. A similar effect can be seen with the CSOM [108]. Another reason that could contribute to the regression to the mean with the CSOM is that when the owners go home and track the three chosen activities over time, the owner realizes that the pet is not as impaired at performing the activities as they initially thought [108]. There is some discussion over whether to use a dependent or non-dependent interviewing technique with clinical metrology instruments [108]. Independent interviewing is when a questionnaire is answered without access to previous questionnaire data, whereas dependent interviewing is when access to previous answers is allowed. There is some evidence that dependent interviewing may increase treatment effect and effect size which would be advantageous in a clinical trial [108].

For an overview of different scales that have been developed to measure chronic pain and their validation see Table 47.5.

Table 47.5 List of clinical metrology instruments and pain scales, including quality of life assessments, developed for quantification of chronic pain.

Species	Scale abbreviation	Scale name	Reference(s)	Outcome measures	Type of pain assessed	Validation studies conducted
Dogs	HCPI	Helsinki Chronic Pain Index	Hielm-Björkman *et al.* 2009 [106]	Behavior, Locomotion	Orthopedic	Yes
	CBPI	Canine Brief Pain Inventory	Brown *et al.* 2007 [96]	Behavior, Locomotion	Orthopedic and bone cancer	Yes
	LOAD	Liverpool Osteoarthritis in Dogs	Walton *et al.* 2013 [105]	Behavior, Locomotion	Orthopedic	Yes
	HRQL instruments	Health-Related Quality of Life Instruments	Reid *et al.* 2013 [118]	Behavior	–	No
	Short form-HRQL instruments	Short form-Health-Related Quality of Life Instruments	Reid *et al.* 2018 [104]	Behavior	–	Yes
	COAST	Canine Osteoarthritis Staging Tool	Cachon *et al.* 2018 [119]	Clinical metrology instrument, clinical examination, radiography	Orthopedic	Yes
Cats	FMPI	Feline Musculoskeletal Pain Index	Benito *et al.* 2013 [110]	Behavior, Locomotion	Orthopedic	Yes
	MI-Cat (V)	Montreal Instrument for Cat Arthritis Testing-Veterinarian	Klinck *et al.* 2018 [114]	Behavior	Orthopedic	Yes
	MI-Cat (C)	Montreal Instrument for Cat Arthritis Testing-Caretaker/Owner	Klinck *et al.* 2017 [113]	Behavior	Orthopedic	Yes
	HRQL instruments	Health-Related Quality of Life Instruments	Noble *et al.* 2019 [115]	Behavior	–	Yes

References

1 Vaisanen MA-M, Tuomikoski SK, Vainio OM. Behavioral alterations and severity of pain in cats recovering at home following elective ovariohysterectomy or castration. *J Am Vet Med Assoc* 2007; **231**(2): 236–242.

2 Sutton GA, Paltiel O, Soffer M, *et al.* Validation of two behavior-based pain scales for horses with acute colic. *Vet J* 2013; **197**(3): 646–650.

3 Grunau RVE, Craig KD. Pain expression in neonates: facial action and cry. *Pain* 1987; **28**(3): 395–410.

4 Langford DJ, Bailey AL, Chanda AL, *et al.* Coding of facial expressions of pain in the laboratory mouse. *Nat Methods* 2010; **7**(6): 447–449.

5 Andrews N, Legg E, Lisak D, *et al.* Spontaneous burrowing behavior in the rat is reduced by peripheral nerve injury or inflammation associated pain. *Eur J Pain* 2012; **16**(6): 485–495.

6 Jirkof P. Burrowing and nest building behavior as indicators of well-being in mice. *J Neurosci Methods* 2014; **234**: 139–146.

7 Jirkof P, Fleischmann T, Cesarovic N, *et al.* Assessment of postsurgical distress and pain in laboratory mice by nest complexity scoring. *Lab Anim* 2013; **47**(3): 153–161.

8 Lester SJ, Mellor DJ, Holmes RJ, *et al.* Behavioral and cortisol responses of lambs to castration and tailing using different methods. *NZ Vet J* 1996; **44**(2): 45–54.

9 Olson ME, Ralston B, Burwash L, *et al.* Efficacy of oral meloxicam suspension for prevention of pain and inflammation following band and surgical castration in calves. *BMC Vet Res* 2016; **12**(1): 102.

10 Stafford KJ, Mellor DJ. The welfare significance of the castration of cattle: a review. *NZ Vet J* 2005; **53**(5): 271–278.

11 Shutt DA, Fell LR, Connell R, *et al.* Stress responses in lambs docked and castrated surgically or by the application of rubber rings. *Aust Vet J* 1988; **65**(1): 5–7.

12 Taylor PM. Equine stress responses to anesthesia. *Br J Anaesth* 1989; **63**(6): 702–709.

13 Von Borell E, Langbein J, Despres G, *et al.* Heart rate variability as a measure of autonomic regulation of cardiac activity for assessing stress and welfare in farm animals – a review. *Physiol Behav* 2007; **92**(3): 293–316.

14 Mansour C, Mocci R, Santangelo B, *et al.* Performance of the Parasympathetic Tone Activity (PTA) index to predict changes in mean arterial pressure in anaesthetized horses with different health conditions. *Res Vet Sci* 2021; **139**: 43–50.

15 King BD, Cohen RD, Guenther CL, *et al.* The effect of age and method of castration on plasma cortisol in beef calves. *Can J Anim Sci* 1991; **71**: 257–263.

16 Murrell JC, Johnson CB. Neurophysiological techniques to assess pain in animals. *J Vet Pharmacol Ther* 2006; **29**(5): 325–335.

17 Murrell JC, Johnson CB, White KL, *et al.* Changes in the EEG during castration in horses and ponies anaesthetized with halothane. *Vet Anaesth Analg* 2003; **30**(3): 138–146.

18 Murrell JC, White KL, Johnson CB. Investigation of the EEG effects of intravenous lidocaine during halothane anesthesia in ponies. *Vet Anaesth Analg* 2005; **32**(4): 212–221.

19 Otto KA, Voigt S, Piepenbrock S, *et al.* Differences in quantitated electroencephalographic variables during surgical stimulation of horses anaesthetized with isoflurane. *Vet Surg* 1996; **25**(3): 249–255.

20 Murrell JC, Waters D, Johnson CB. Comparative effects of halothane, isoflurane, sevoflurane and desflurane on the electroencephalogram of the rat. *Lab Anim* 2008; **42**(2): 161–170.

21 Lehmann HS, Musk GC, Laurence M, *et al.* Mitigation of electroencephalographic and cardiovascular responses to castration in Bos indicus bulls following the administration of either lidocaine or meloxicam. *Vet Anaesth Analg* 2017; **44**(6): 1341–1352.

22 McIlhone AE, Beausoleil NJ, Kells NJ, *et al.* Effects of halothane on the electroencephalogram of the chicken. *Vet Med Sci* 2018; **4**(2): 98–105.

23 Iannetti GD, Mouraux A. From the neuromatrix to the pain matrix (and back). *Exp Brain Res* 2010; **205**(1): 1–12.

24 Fomberstein K, Qadri S, Ramani R. Functional MRI and pain. *Curr Opin Anaesthesiol* 2013; **26**(5): 588–593.

25 Legrain V, Iannetti GD, Plaghki L, *et al.* The pain matrix reloaded: a salience detection system for the body. *Prog Neurobiol* 2011; **93**(1): 111–124.

26 Stewart M, Stafford KJ, Dowling SK, *et al.* Eye temperature and heart rate variability of calves disbudded with our without local anaesthetic. *Physiol Behav* 2008; **93**(4–5); 789–797.

27 Baysinger A, Webb SR, Brown J, *et al.* Proposed multidimensional pain outcome methodology to demonstrate analgesic drug efficacy and facilitate future drug approval for piglet castration. *Anim Health Res Rev* 2021; **22**(2): 163–176.

28 Heinrich A, Duffield TF, Lissemore KD, *et al.* The effect of meloxicam on behavior and pain sensitivity of dairy calves following cautery dehorning with local anaesthetic. *J Dairy Sci* 2010; **93**(6): 2450–2457.

29 Coetzee JF, Mosher RA, KuKanich B, *et al.* Pharmacokinetics and effects of intravenous meloxicam in weaned Holstein claves following scoop dehorning without local anesthesia. *BMC Vet Res* 2012; **8**: 153.

30 Culp WTN, Mayhew PD, Brown DC. The effect of laparoscopic versus open ovariectomy on postsurgical activity in small dogs. *Vet Surg* 2009; **38**(7): 811–817.

31 Enomoto M, Lascelles BDX, Gruen ME. Development of a checklist for the detection of degenerative joint disease-associated pain in cats. *J Feline Med Surg* 2020; **22**(12): 1137–1147.

32 Belshaw Z, Dean R, Asher L. Could it be osteoarthritis? How dog owners and veterinary surgeons describe identifying canine osteoarthritis in a general practice setting. *Prev Vet Med* 2020; **185**: 105198.

33 Rusbridge C, Jeffery ND. Pathophysiology and treatment of neuropathic pain associated with syringomyelia. *Vet J* 2008; **175**(2): 164–172.

34 Driessen B, Bauquier SH, Zarucco L. Neuropathic pain management in chronic laminitis. *Vet Clin North Am Equine Pract* 2010; **26**(2): 315–337.

35 Rietmann TR, Stauffacher M, Bernasconi P, *et al.* The association between heart rate, heart rate variability, endocrine and behavioral pain measures in horses suffering from laminitis. *J Vet Med A Physiol Pathol Clin Med* 2004; **51**(5): 218–225.

36 Evans R, Horstman C, Conzemius M. Accuracy and optimization of force platform gait analysis in Labradors with cranial cruciate disease evaluated at a walking gait. *Vet Surg* 2005; **34**(5): 445–449.

37 Brown DC, Boston RC, Farrar JT. Comparison of force plate gait analysis with owner assessment of pain using the Canine Brief Pain Inventory in dogs with osteoarthritis. *J Vet Intern Med* 2013; **27**(1): 22–30.

38 Caplen G, Hothersall B, Murrell JC, *et al.* Kinematic analysis quantified gait abnormalities associated with lameness in broiler chickens and identifies evolutionary gait differences. *PLoS ONE* 2012; **7**(7): e40800.

39 Gruen ME, Alfaro-Cordoba M, Thomson AE, *et al.* The use of functional data analysis to evaluate activity in a spontaneous model of degenerative joint disease associated pain in cats. *PLoS ONE* 2017; **12**(1): e0169576.

40 Smith M, Mendl M, Murrell JC. Associations between osteoarthritis and duration and quality of night-time rest in dogs. *Appl Anim Behav Sci* 2022; **253**: 105661.

41 Muller C, Gines JA, Conzemius M, *et al.* Evaluation of the effect of signalment and owner-reported impairment level on accelerometer-measured changes in activity in osteoarthritic dogs receiving a non-steroidal anti-inflammatory. *Vet J* 2018; **242**: 48–52.

42 Rae L, MacNab N, Bidner S, *et al.* Attitudes and practices of veterinarians in Australia to acute pain management in cats. *J Feline Med Surg* 2022; **24**(8): 715–725.

43 Hunt JR, Knowles TG, Lascelles BD, *et al.* Prescription of perioperative analgesics by UK small animal veterinary surgeons in 2013. *Vet Rec* 2015; **176**(19): 493.

44 Mantha S, Thisted R, Foss J, *et al.* A proposal to use confidence intervals for visual analog scale data for pain measurement to determine clinical significance. *Anesth Analg* 1993; **77**(5): 1041–1047.

45 Coulter CA, Flecknell PA, Leach MC, *et al.* Reported analgesic administration to rabbits undergoing experimental surgical procedures. *BMC Vet Res* 2011; **7**: 12.

46 Holton LL, Scott EM, Nolan AM, *et al.* Comparison of three methods used for assessment of pain in dogs. *J Am Vet Med Assoc* 1998; **212**(1): 61–66.

47 Hewetson M, Christley RM, Hunt ID, *et al.* Investigations of the reliability of observational gait analysis for the assessment of lameness in horses. *Vet Rec* 2006; **158**(25): 852–858.

48 Lascelles B, Cripps P, Mirchandani S, *et al.* Carprofen as an analgesic for postoperative pain in cats: dose titration and assessment of efficacy in comparison to pethidine hydrochloride. *J Small Anim Pract* 1995; **36**(12): 535–541.

49 Slingsby L, Waterman-Pearson A. Comparison of pethidine, buprenorphine and ketoprofen for postoperative analgesia after ovariohysterectomy in the cat. *Vet Rec* 1998; **143**(7): 185–189.

50 Hudson JT, Slater MR, Taylor L, *et al.* Assessing repeatability and validity of a visual analogue scale questionnaire for use in assessing pain and lameness in dogs. *Am J Vet Res* 2004; **65**(12): 1634–1643.

51 Holton L, Reid J, Scott EM, *et al.* Development of a behavior-based scale to measure acute pain in dogs. *Vet Rec* 2001; **148**(17): 525–531.

52 Reid J, Nolan AM, Hughes JML, *et al.* Development of the short-form Glasgow Composite Measure Pain Scale (CMPS-SF) and derivation of an analgesic intervention score. *Anim Welf* 2007; **16**(S): 97–104.

53 Della Rocca G, Colpo R, Reid J, *et al.* Creation and validation of the Italian version of the Glasgow Composite Measure Pain Scale-Short Form (ICMPS-SF). *Vet Ital* 2018; **54**(3): 251–260.

54 Testa B, Reid J, Scott ME, *et al.* The Short Form of the Glasgow Composite Measure Pain Scale in post-operative analgesia studies in dogs: a scoping review. *Front Vet Sci* 2021; **8**: 751949.

55 Calvo G, Holden E, Reid J, *et al.* Development of a behavior-based measurement tool with defined intervention level for assessing acute pain in cats. *J Small Anim Pract* 2014; **55**(12): 622–629.

56 Reid J, Scott EM, Calvo G, *et al.* Definitive Glasgow acute pain scale for cats: validation and intervention level. *Vet Rec* 2017; **180**(18): 449.

57 Moody CM, Niel L, Pang DJ. Is training necessary for efficacious use of the Glasgow Feline Composite Measure Pain Scale. *Can Vet J* 2022; **63**(6): 609–616.

58 Brondani JT, Luna SPL, Padovani CR. Refinement and initial validation of a multidimensional composite scale for use in assessing acute postoperative pain in cats. *Am J Vet Res* 2011; **72**(2): 174–183.

59 Belli M, de Oliveira AR, de Lima MT, *et al.* Clinical validation of the short and long UNESP-Botucatu scales for feline pain assessment. *Peer J* 2021; **9**: e11225.

60 Bussieres G, Jacques C, Lainay O. Development of a composite orthopaedic pain scale in horses. *Res Vet Sci* 2008; **85**(2): 294–306.

61 van Loon JP, Jonckheer-Sheehy VS, Back W, *et al.* Monitoring equine visceral pain with a composite pain scale score and correlation with survival after emergency gastrointestinal surgery. *Vet J* 2014; **200**(1); 109–115.

62 van Loon JP, Van Dierendonck MC. Monitoring acute equine visceral pain with the Equine Utrecht University Scale for Composite Pain Assessment (EQUUS-COMPASS) and the Equine Utrecht University Scale for Facial Assessment of Pain (EQUUS-FAP): a scale construction study. *Vet J* 2015; **206**(3): 356–364.

63 Taffarel MO, Luna SP, de Oliveira FA, *et al.* Refinement and partial validation of the UNESP-Botucatu multidimensional composite pain scale for assessing postoperative pain in horses. *BMC Vet Res* 2015; **11**: 83.

64 Wathan J, Burrows AM, Waller BM, *et al.* EquiFACS: the Equine Facial Action Coding System. *PLoS ONE* 2015; **10**: e0131738.

65 Langford DJ, Bailey AL, Chanda ML, *et al.* Coding of facial expressions of pain in the laboratory mouse. *Nat Methods* 2010; **7**(6): 447–449.

66 Sotocinal SG, Sorge RE, Zaloum A, *et al.* The Rat Grimace Scale: a partially automated method for quantifying pain in the laboratory rat via facial expressions. *Mol Pain* 2011; **7**: 55.

67 Keating SCJ, Thomas AA, Flecknell PA, *et al.* Evaluation of EMLA cream for preventing pain during tattooing of rabbits: changes in physiological, behavioral and facial expression responses. *PLoS ONE* 2012; **7**(9): e44437.

68 Dalla Costa E, Dai F, Lecchi C, *et al.* Towards and improved pain assessment in castrated horses using facial expressions (HGS) and circulating miRNAs. *Vet Rec* 2021; **188**(9): e82.

69 Guesgen MJ, Beausoleil NJ, Leach M, *et al.* Coding and quantification of a facial expression for pain in lambs. *Behav Processes* 2016; **132**: 49–56.

70 Hager C, Biernot S, Buettner M, *et al.* The Sheep Grimace Scale as an indicator of post-operative distress and pain in laboratory sheep. *PLoS ONE* 2017; **12**(4): e0175839.

71 McLennan K, Mahmoud M. Development of an Automated Pain Facial Expression Detection System for sheep (*Ovies Aries*). *Animals (Basel)* 2019; **9**(4): 196.

72 Viscardi AV, Hunniford M, Lawlis P, *et al.* Development of a Piglet Grimace Scale to evaluate piglet pain using facial expressions following castration and tail docking: a pilot study. *Front Vet Sci* 2017; **4**: 51.

73 Riejgwart ML, Schoemaker NJ, Pascuzzo R, *et al.* The composition and initial validation of a grimace scale in ferrets after surgical implantation of a telemetry probe. *PLoS ONE* 2017; **12**(11): e0187986.

74 Evangelista MC, Watanabe R, Leung V, *et al.* Facial expressions of pain in cats: the development and validation of a Feline Grimace Scale. *Sci Rep* 2019: **9**(1): 19128.

75 van Dierendonck MC, Burden FA, Rickards K, *et al.* Monitoring acute pain in donkeys with the Equine Utrecht University Scale for Donkeys Composite Pain Assessment (EQUUS-DONKEY-COMPASS) and the Equine Utrecht University Scale for Donkey Facial Assessment of Pain (EQUUS-DONKEY-FAP). *Animals (Basel)* 2020; **10**(2): 354.

76 Evangelista MC, Monteiro BP, Steagall PV. Measurement properties of grimace scales for pain assessment in nonhuman mammals: a systematic review. *Pain* 2022; **163**(6): e697–e714.

77 Shipley H, Guedes A, Graham L, *et al.* Preliminary appraisal of the reliability and validity of the Colorado State University Feline Acute Pain Scale. *J Feline Med Surg* 2021; **21**(4): 335–339.

78 Firth AM, Haldane SL. Development of a scale to evaluate postoperative pain in dogs. *J Am Vet Med Assoc* 1999; **214**(5): 651–659.

79 Holopherne-Doran D, Laboissiere B, Gogny M. Validation of the 4A-VET postoperative pain scale in dogs and cats. *Vet Anaesth Analg* 2010; **37**(4): 383 (abstract).

80 Gleerup KB, Lindegaard C. Recognition and quantification of pain in horses: a tutorial review. *Equine Vet Educ* 2016; **28**: 47–57.

81 Graubner C, Gerber V, Doherr M, *et al.* Clinical application and reliability of a post abdominal surgery pain assessment scale (PASPAS) in horses. *Vet J* 2011; **188**(2): 178–183.

82 de Oliveira FA, Luna SP, do Amaral JB, *et al.* Validation of the UNESP-Botucatu unidimensional composite pain scale for assessing postoperative pain in cattle. *BMC Vet Res* 2014; **10**: 200.

83 Silva NEOF, Trindade PHE, Oliveira AR, *et al.* Validation of the UNESP-Botucatu composite scale to assess acute postoperative abdominal pain in sheep (USAPS). *PLoS ONE* 2020; **15**(10): e0239622.

84 Luna SPL, Lucelia de Araujo A, da Nobrega Neto PI, *et al.* Validation of the UNESP-Botucatu pig composite acute pain scale (UPAPS). *PLoS ONE* 2020; **15**(6): e0233552.

85 Banchi P, Quaranta G, Ricci A, *et al.* Reliability and construct validity of a composite pain scale for rabbits (CANCRS) in a clinical environment. *PLoS ONE* 2020; **15**(4): e0221377.

86 Benato L, Murrell J, Knowles TG, *et al.* Development of the Bristol Rabbit Pain Scale (BRPS): a multidimensional composite pain scale specific to rabbits (*Oryctolagus caniculus*). *PLoS ONE* 2021; **16**(6): e0252417.

87 Dalla Costa E, Minero M, Lebelt D, *et al.* Development of the Horse Grimace Scale (HGS) as a pain assessment tool in horses undergoing routine castration. *PLoS ONE* 2014; **9**(3): e92281.

88 Dalla Costa E, Stucke E, Dai F, *et al.* Using the Horse Grimace Scale (HGS) to assess pain associated with acute laminitis in horses (*Equus caballus*). *Animals (Basel)* 2016; **6**(8): 47.

89 Gleerup KB, Forkman B, Lindegaard C, *et al.* An equine pain face. *Vet Anaesth Analg* 2015; **42**(1): 103–114.

90 Dyson S, Berger J, Ellis A, *et al.* Development of an ethogram for a pain scoring system in ridden horses and its application to determine the presence of musculoskeletal pain. *J Vet Behav Clin Appl Res* 2018; **23**: 47–57.

91 van Loon JP, Van Dierendonck MC. Monitoring equine head related pain with the Equine Utrecht University Scale for Facial Assessment of Pain (EQUUS-FAP). *Vet J* 2017; **220**: 88–90.

92 van Loon JP, Verhaar N, van den Berg, *et al.* Objective assessment of acute pain in foals using a facial expression-based pain scale. *Animals (Basel)* 2020; **10**(9): 1610.

93 Evangelista MC, Steagall PV. Agreement and reliability of the Feline Grimace Scale among cat owners, veterinarians, veterinary students and nurses. *Sci Rep* 2021; **11**(1): 5262.

94 Hercock CA, Pinchbeck G, Giejda A, *et al.* Validation of a client-based clinical metrology instrument for the evaluation of canine elbow arthritis. *J Small Anim Pract* 2009; **50**(6): 266–271.

95 Wiseman-Orr ML, Nolan AM, Reid J, *et al.* Development of a questionnaire to measure the effects of chronic pain on health-related quality of life in dogs. *Am J Vet Res* 2004; **65**(8): 1077–1084.

96 Brown DC, Royston RC, Coyne JC, *et al.* Development and psychometric testing of an instrument designed to measure chronic pain in dogs with osteoarthritis. *Am J Vet Res* 2007; **68**(6): 631–637.

97 Lynch S, Savary-Bataille L, Leeuw B, *et al.* Development of a questionnaire assessing health-related quality-of-life in dogs and cats with cancer. *Vet Comp Oncol* 2011; **9**(3): 172–182.

98 Noli C, Minafo G, Galzerano M. Quality of life of dogs with skin diseases and their owners. Part 1: development and validation of a questionnaire. *Vet Dermatol* 2011; **22**(4): 335–343.

99 Birnbacher D. Quality of life – evaluation or description? *Ethical Theory Moral Pract* 1999; **2**(1): 25–36.

100 Wiseman-Orr ML, Scott EM, Reid J, *et al.* Validation of a structured questionnaire as an instrument to measure chronic pain in dogs on the basis of effects on health-related quality of life. *Am J Vet Res* 2006; **67**(11): 1826–1836.

101 Belshaw Z, Yeates J. Assessment of quality of life and chronic pain in dogs. *Vet J* 2018; **239**: 59–64.

102 Cella DF. Quality of life: the concept. *J Palliat Care* 1992; **8**(3): 8–13.

103 Roberts C, Armson B, Bartram D, *et al.* Construction of a conceptual framework for assessment of quality of life in dogs with osteoarthritis. *Front Vet Sci* 2021; **8**: 741864.

104 Reid J, Wiseman-Orr L, Scott M. Shortening of an existing generic online health-related quality of life instrument for dogs. *J Small Anim Pract* 2018; **59**(6): 334–342.

105 Walton MB, Cowderoy E, Lascelles D, *et al.* Evaluation of construct and criterion validity for the "Liverpool Osteoarthritis in dogs" (LOAD) clinical metrology instrument and comparison to two other instruments. *PLoS ONE* 2013; **8**(3): e58125.

106 Hielm-Björkman AK, Rita H, Tulamo RM. Psychometric testing of the Helsinki Chronic Pain Index by completion of a questionnaire in Finnish by owners of dogs with chronic signs of pain caused by osteoarthritis. *Am J Vet Res* 2009; **70**(6): 727–734.

107 Hielm-Björkman AK, Kapatkin AS, Rita HJ. Reliability and validity of a visual analogue scale used by owners to measure chronic pain attributable to osteoarthritis in their dogs. *Am J Vet Res* 2011; **72**(5): 601–607.

108 Muller C, Gaines B, Gruen M, *et al.* Evaluation of clinical metrology instrument in dogs with osteoarthritis. *J Vet Intern Med* 2016; **30**(3): 836–846.

109 Zamprogno H, Hansen BD, Bondell HD. Item generation and design testing of a questionnaire to assess degenerative joint disease-associated pain in cats. *Am J Vet Res* 2010; **71**(12): 1417–1424.

110 Benito J, Depuy V, Hardie E, *et al.* Reliability and discriminatory testing of a client-based clinical metrology instrument, feline musculoskeletal pain index (FMPI) for the evaluation of degenerative joint disease associated pain in cats. *Vet J* 2013; **196**(3): 368–373.

111 Benito J, Hansen B, Depuy V, *et al.* Feline musculoskeletal pain index: responsiveness and testing of criterion validity. *J Vet Intern Med* 2013; **27**(3): 474–482.

112 Gruen ME, Griffith E, Thomson A, *et al.* Detection of clinically relevant pain relief in cats with degenerative joint disease associated pain. *J Vet Intern Med* 2014; **28**(2): 346–350.

113 Klinck MP, Gruen ME, Del Castillo JRE, *et al.* Development and preliminary validity and reliability of the Montreal Instrument for Cat Arthritis Testing, for use by Caretaker/Owner, MI-CAT(C), via a randomized clinical trial. *Appl Anim Behav Sci* 2017; **200**: 96–105.

114 Klinck MP, Monteiro BP, Lussier B, *et al.* Refinement of the Montreal Instrument for Cat Arthritis Testing, for use by veterinarians: detection of naturally occurring osteoarthritis in laboratory cats. *J Feline Med Surg* 2018; **20**(8): 728–740.

115 Noble CE, Wiseman-Orr LM, Scott ME, *et al.* Development, initial validation, and reliability testing of a web-based generic feline health-related quality-of-life instrument. *J Feline Med Surg* 2019; **21**(2): 84–94.

116 Welsh EM, Gettinby G, Nolan AM. Comparison of a visual analogue scale and a numerical rating scale for assessment of lameness, using sheep as a model. *Am J Vet Res* 1993; **54**(6): 976–983.

117 Rausch-Derra L, Huebner M, Wofford J, *et al.* A prospective, randomized, masked, placebo-controlled multisite clinical study of grapiprant, an EP4 Prostaglandin Receptor Antagonist (PRA) in dogs with osteoarthritis. *J Vet Intern Med* 2016; **30**(3): 756–763.

118 Reid J, Wiseman-Orr ML, Scott EM, *et al.* Development, validation and reliability of a web-based questionnaire to measure health-related quality of life in dogs. *J Small Anim Pract* 2013; **54**(5): 227–233.

119 Cachon T, Frykman O, Innes JF, *et al.* Face validity of a proposed tool for staging canine osteoarthritis: Canine Osteoarthritis Staging Tool (COAST). *Vet J* 2018; **235**: 1–8.

48 Clinical Management and Pharmacologic Treatment of Pain

Carolyn M. McKune
Mythos Veterinary, LLC, Gainesville, Florida, USA

Chapter contents

Introduction, 1010
Anticipation of pain, 1010
Assessment of pain, 1011
Alleviation of pain, 1011
Decision-making tools, 1011
Tiers of the decision-making tree, 1011
First-tier, acute pain, 1011
First-tier, chronic pain, 1013
Second tier, 1014
Third tier, 1016
Evidence for agents that modify osteoarthritis in companion animals, 1016
Evidence for biologic agents in companion animals, 1017
Novel concept drugs, 1017
References, 1017

Introduction

According to the International Association for the Study of Pain (IASP), pain is "an unpleasant sensory and emotional experience associated with, or resembling that associated with, actual or potential tissue damage" [1]. This definition has been subtly but critically altered from its previous 1979 definition, which implied through words such as "described" instead of "associated," that the ability to speak was a prerequisite for pain. The current definition includes the accompanying note: "verbal description is only one of several behaviors to express pain; inability to communicate does not negate the possibility that a human or a nonhuman animal experiences pain."

It is beyond the scope of a single chapter to address the clinical management and pharmacologic treatment of pain in its entirety. As such, this chapter focuses on initiatives to "anticipate, assess, and alleviate pain" [2]. The goals of the chapter are to:

1 Define a *proactive/preventive* [3] and *multimodal approach* to pain, and highlight the most effective approach utilizing the entire veterinary team and the owner.
2 Introduce a recently proposed "tiered decision tree" to help prioritize the use of evidence-based therapies [3].
3 Critically evaluate the differences in approach to treatment plans among common companion animal species.

Anticipation of pain

The concept of proactive pain management begins with acknowledging that pain is a sequela to many invasive and even some minimally invasive procedures. It is now accepted that proactivity is essential to effectively advocate for the patient. Harnessing the power of proactivity allows the clinician to engage in a plan to address pain before it occurs, rather than simply reacting to its presence. Education of the entire veterinary team is a key component in this strategy and different approaches are required depending on the type of pain being addressed. Foundational understanding of acute (adaptive) versus chronic (maladaptive) pain management allows us to employ an approach that is suitable for each patient. For example, acute pain is best managed as early as possible in the process. For elective procedures, such as castration or ovariohysterectomy, pain management is instituted prior to the start of surgery. However, in other situations, proactivity includes identifying diseases, such as osteoarthritis (OA) or laminitis, which are likely to cause long-term pain and implementing a pain mitigation strategy as early as possible, with a focus on improving quality of life.

Each member of the pain management team has a different role to play in the educational continuum with contributions from researchers, clinicians, and educators leading to enhanced standards of care for veterinary patients. While experts publish evidence-based information to validate pain assessment and alleviation strategies, everyone must be well-informed regarding current developments and continually update themselves so information can be disseminated to those directly responsible for patient care. This requires good communication skills, a structured approach, and a foundation of evidence-based information.

Suggestions for providing a coordinated pain management framework include having a case coordinator, for example, a trained technician or nurse, who is responsible for reaching out to follow-up

Veterinary Anesthesia and Analgesia: The Sixth Edition of Lumb and Jones. Edited by Leigh Lamont, Kurt Grimm, Sheilah Robertson, Lydia Love and Carrie Schroeder.
© 2024 John Wiley & Sons, Inc. Published 2024 by John Wiley & Sons, Inc.
Companion website: www.wiley.com/go/lamont/anesthesia

on a patient's progress and facilitate additional re-checks as necessary [3]. Successful pain management also includes education of the owner about the characteristics of their animal that may predispose them to chronic pain (e.g., breed, diet, body weight, body condition score, and age), the behavioral indicators of pain they should look for, and the importance of administering prescribed pain medications.

Assessment of pain

Assessment of pain is critically important and this is covered in detail in Chapter 47. Pain assessment using validated tools is an essential outcome measure of any pain management protocol. Unfortunately, validated pain assessment tools are not available for all species, including most captive species in zoos, wildlife, fish, and amphibians. In the absence of a validated pain assessment tool, the practitioner must use their familiarity with these animals, including their natural behaviors, to make an educated assessment.

Alleviation of pain

The practitioner should prepare analgesic plans with a realistic goal in mind. In many cases, reduction of pain so that quality of life is improved is achievable, whereas complete absence of pain is not. The plan is deemed effective if reassessment of pain, using a chosen outcome measure, confirms this goal.

Analgesic plans for acute pain are often successful because the animal usually has a diagnosis, a planned procedure, or known trauma, which allows targeted interventions. Inflammation is a core component of acute pain, and this is amenable to preventive or preemptive therapy. *Preventive* and *preemptive* analgesia, while often used interchangeably, are not the same. Preemptive analgesia alludes to the timing of analgesic administration – usually prior to noxious stimuli occurring [4]. Katz *et al.* [5] describe preventive analgesia as "minimizing the deleterious immediate and long-term effects of noxious perioperative afferent input." The key to this concept is preventing peripheral and central sensitization, which will reduce pain and analgesic requirements.

Analgesic plans should match the degree (intensity) of anticipated or existing pain and its duration. Patients are assessed and reassessed for pain while in the clinic and after discharge by hospital staff (preferably the case coordinator) and owners, respectively. Treatment plans should also address patient anxiety. Children may experience significant anxiety related to painful medical procedures resulting in a greater perception of pain with subsequent procedures [6]. To reduce procedural pain and anxiety both pharmacologic (analgesics, anxiolytics, and sedatives) and non-pharmacologic (distraction and play) interventions are used, many of which could be adapted for veterinary patients.

Chronic pain is challenging in that it must start with an acknowledgment that it may be present, and it should be assessed or screened for during physical examinations. For example, older dogs and cats should be screened for OA and owners educated that changes in behavior can be due to pain and not the pet slowing down with age. Managing chronic pain can be challenging due to its complex etiology, lack of efficacious therapies, and potential limitations related to the owner's ability to care for the animal due to financial, time, and physical constraints. As with acute pain, anxiety should be addressed. Fig. 48.1 demonstrates the challenges owners may face when caring for pets with chronic pain and other comorbidities.

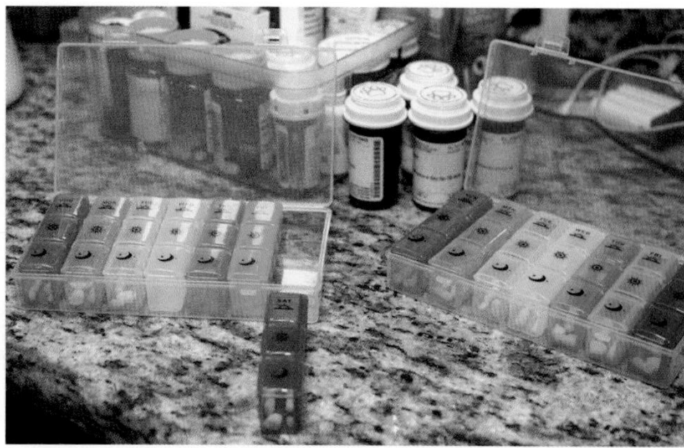

Figure 48.1 This image shows the medication box for a single canine patient with chronic otitis externa. Not pictured are the refrigerated medications, such as the allergy injections. In the background, there are also pills for the other household pets with osteoarthritis. The owner of this patient hired a separate care giver just to assist with the mid-day routine and basic care of the patient. Not all owners have this financial freedom. Source: Dr. Carolyn McKune, with permission.

Decision-making tools

Gruen *et al.* [3] have proposed an evidence-based "decision-making tree" for the treatment of acute and chronic pain in dogs and cats (Fig. 48.2).

While Fig. 48.2 focuses on canine and feline patients, a similar approach can be used in other species based on species-specific evidence (treatments in the first tier have robust evidence supporting use in that species, treatments in the second tier have moderate evidence, and those in the third tier have limited evidence). Additional information on pain management in particular species is available in species-specific chapters elsewhere in this book.

Tiers of the decision-making tree

First-tier, acute pain

When acute pain is present, but a definitive diagnosis is not confirmed, the clinician most often relies on first-tier drugs, which will provide reliable analgesia with minimal side effects. For small companion animal species (e.g., dogs, cats, and some pocket pets), opioids are a logical choice (see Chapter 23). For large animal species, non-steroidal anti-inflammatory drugs (NSAIDs) (see Chapter 24) and α_2-adrenergic receptor agonists (Chapter 22) are commonly used; opioids are administered by both systemic and epidural routes [7–9].

For acute pain of a known cause, the first tier of therapy often includes analgesia that targets the source of pain. For example, acute pain that is inflammatory in nature (e.g., a skin incision) will respond well to an NSAID. There are very few patients that do not benefit from a local anesthetic block and many techniques are applicable to surgical procedures. Please refer to other chapters dedicated to local anesthetic techniques in specific species for more information on these techniques. Supportive and nursing care, including nutrition, keeping patients warm and dry, and ensuring dressings are comfortable and clean are also important components of patient care. The International Society of Feline Medicine and the American Association of Feline Practitioners have created nursing care guidelines specific to the needs of cats [10]. Certain modalities, such as cold therapy, are also appropriate in many species [11–13]. Further information on non-pharmacologic management of pain is available in Chapter 49.

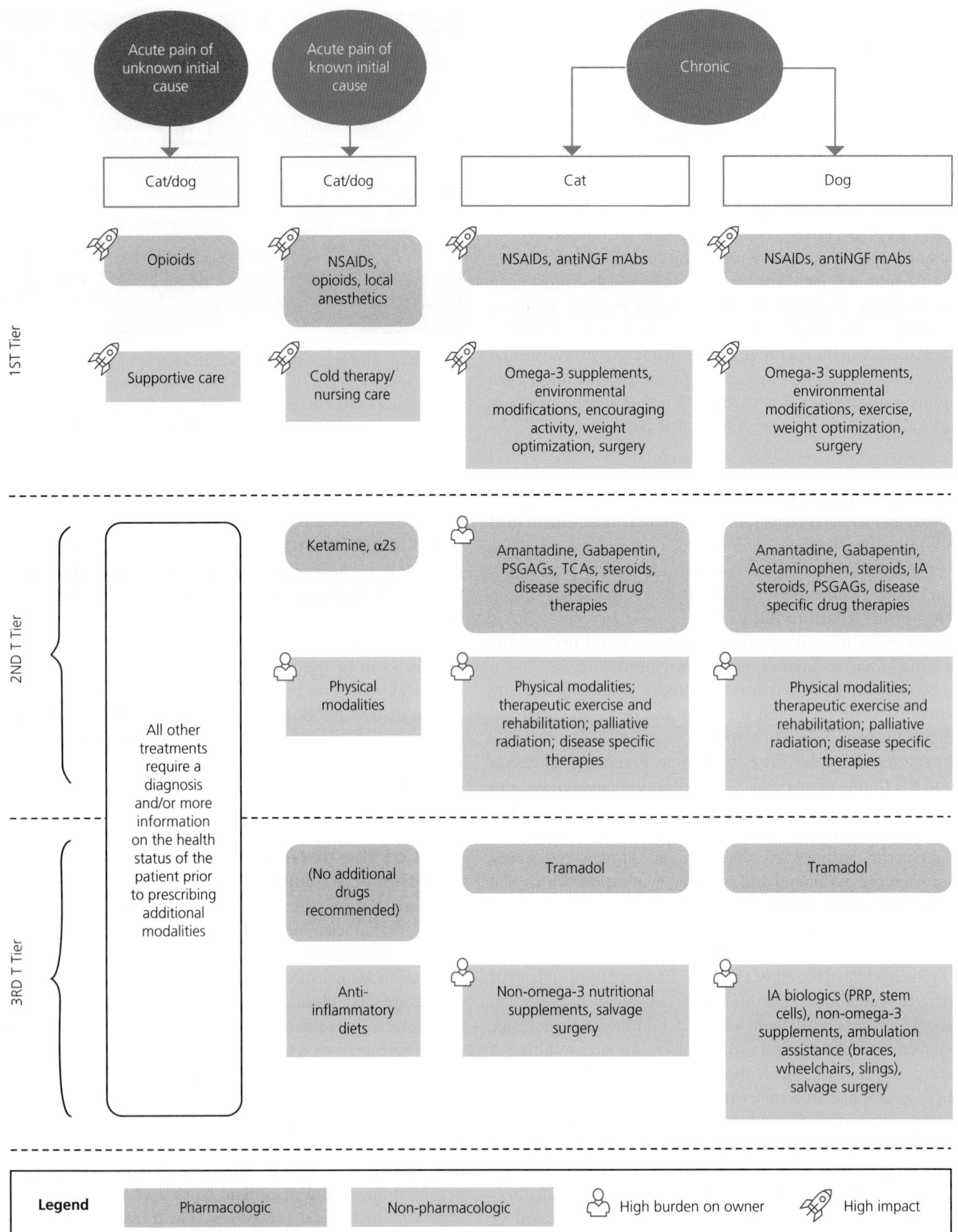

Figure 48.2 Decision tree for prioritizing pain management therapies. This figure outlines a tiered approach to pain management in cats and dogs for acute and chronic pain. Tiers are presented from highest recommendation (most evidence for effectiveness) to lowest, although all therapies presented have some evidence to support their use. Physical modalities include laser therapy, pulsed electromagnetic field therapy, acupuncture, and transcutaneous electrical nerve stimulation. Surgical procedures for chronic pain include top-tier treatments such as dental procedures, removal of painful lesions, joint stabilization and replacement, and amputation; lower-tier (salvage) procedures include arthrodesis, denervation, and excision arthroplasty. NSAIDs, non-steroidal anti-inflammatories; antiNGF mAbs, anti-nerve growth factor monoclonal antibodies; α2s, α_2-adrenergic receptor agonists; PSGAGs, polysulfated glycosaminoglycans; TCAs, tricyclic antidepressants; IA; intra-articular; PRP, platelet-rich plasma. Source: Gruen *et al.* [3], with permission of the American Animal Hospital Association.

First-tier, chronic pain

NSAIDs have traditionally been used as first-line drugs for chronic pain such as OA in many species. Chapter 24 provides information on the pharmacology of NSAIDs, and Chapter 71 is dedicated specifically to management of canine and feline OA patients.

There is evidence to support the use of omega-3-fatty acids, which contain alpha-linolenic acid (ALA), eicosapentaenoic acid (EPA), and docosahexaenoic acid (DHA), for some types of chronic pain, with their mode of action presumed to be via reducing oxidative stress [14]. Cats with degenerative joint disease that were fed a diet high in EPA and DHA (which also included glucosamine–chondroitin sulfate and green-lipped mussel extract) demonstrated significant improvement in activity compared to a control group [15,16], as did dogs in a similar study [17]. Omega-3 fatty acid-supplemented diets have been shown to improve weight bearing in dogs with OA [18]. A range of omega-3-fatty acid dosages are reported in the literature, and it is important to follow recommended doses [19]. Evidence for the benefits of omega-3 fatty acids is strong and, in some studies, they have allowed a reduction in NSAID dosage [20]. A comprehensive meta-analysis reviewing the quality and efficacy of omega-3 fatty acid supplementation supported its use for both canine and feline OA [16]. Omega-3 fatty acids may also be beneficial in horses. *In vitro* studies suggest equine synoviocytes readily incorporate omega-3 fatty acids to modulate inflammatory responses [21].

Locally administered corticosteroids have been used in horses with chronic joint pain for many years for their anti-inflammatory effects [22,23]. In horses, evidence suggests that steroids may help them to return to normal function [24–26]. However, the specific steroid used was a significant factor, with horses administered methylprednisolone in the sacroiliac joint more likely to return to work than those administered triamcinolone [24]. Conversely, methylprednisolone leads to more cartilage damage in articular joints than triamcinolone [27]. There is less evidence supporting this intervention in other species and this class of drug is considered "second tier" in dogs and cats.

Anti-nerve growth factor monoclonal antibodies (anti-NGF mAbs) are a breakthrough therapy for the control of OA pain in dogs and cats. Nerve growth factor (NGF), which is essential during development of the nervous system, appears to alter neuronal plasticity in conditions of chronic pain after the nervous system has matured [28]. In response to noxious stimuli, peripheral NGF protein is produced and released to facilitate binding to tropomyosin-receptor kinase A (TrkA) receptors, which are present in nerve endings in subchondral bone [29]. Once this binding occurs, the complex becomes internalized and is transported to the dorsal root ganglion where, through binding to a multitude of different receptors, it ultimately leads to central sensitization. Peripherally, the binding of NGF to the TrkA receptor results in inflammatory mediator release, including histamine from mast cells and serotonin, as well as other pro-inflammatory effects [30]. Synovial fluid from dogs with OA demonstrates increased NGF concentrations [31]. Pharmacotherapies, in the form of biological agents, target this growth factor peripherally. Anti-NGF monoclonal antibodies are not chemically synthesized, but rather derived from natural sources. Specifically, monoclonal antibodies are produced through recombinant engineering or single B-lymphocyte clones in laboratory animals [30] and, as they are species-specific, they are recognized as native. A proposed benefit and important feature of anti-NGF mAbs is that they do not block endogenous signaling as is seen with traditional analgesics [32]. NGF controls various endogenous ion channels, receptors, and signaling molecules and if anti-NGF mAbs were to block these pathways, undesirable side effects could result [33]. In clinical trials, some human patients receiving anti-NGF mAbs developed rapidly progressing OA, characterized by increased pain and radiographic changes. This adverse effect was linked to high doses of anti-NGF mAbs or their combination with NSAIDs [34]; as a result, anti-NGF mAbs are not currently approved for use in humans. These adverse effects have not been reported in animals.

Bedinvetmab is a commercially available anti-NGF mAb formulation for use in dogs. It is administered subcutaneously at a dose of 1 mg/kg and has a terminal elimination half-life of 9.5 ± 1.8 days, primarily due to antibody recycling at the FcRn receptor [35]. It is intended as a once-a-month therapeutic and this duration of action is corroborated by a study evaluating another anti-NGF mAb (ranevetmab) where owners used a clinical metrology instrument (the Canine Brief Pain Inventory) to score pain in their dogs for a period of four weeks following an injection of the anti-NGF mAb versus saline [36]. Another study involving 26 dogs included an objective measurement of function (accelerometry) in addition to clinical metrology instruments. Compared to the placebo group, dogs administered ranevetmab showed significant improvement versus pretreatment based on pain scores as well as activity measured by an accelerometer [37]. Previous anti-NGF mAbs were associated with a reduction in inflammatory pain in a canine kaolin model [38]. In studies looking at the safety of bedinvetmab, the drug was well tolerated in Beagle dogs over a period of 6 months. Clinical evaluations, including neurologic, ophthalmic, and joint evaluations found no adverse effects, nor were there any concerns with a two-week concurrent administration of NSAIDs [35]. Treatment-related immunogenicity has not been reported [35].

Frunevetmab is a felinized anti-NGF mAb labeled for the control of OA-related pain in cats. Minimum dosage is 1 mg/kg, administered subcutaneously, although significantly higher doses (up to 28 mg/kg) are well tolerated [39]. In a multicenter, randomized, placebo-controlled, double-blinded study of 275 cats, significant improvement was noted in client-specific outcome measures as well as owner-assessed global treatment response with frunevetmab versus placebo. Three doses were given 28 days apart and cats were assessed on days 28 and 56. Veterinarians assessed joint pain as improved, although this was not significant until later in the evaluation process at days 56 and 84 [40]. These improvements were consistent with reports from pilot studies looking at frunevetmab [41,42]. In the same study, evaluating 275 cats, adverse events did not differ between placebo and treatment groups, except for a variety of dermatologic issues, including dermatitis, alopecia, pruritis, and scabbing, which occurred significantly more frequently in cats that received frunevetmab [40]. This was also noted in the pilot study [42]. At the time of writing, areas in need of further research include the degree and duration of analgesic effect a patient may have from frunevetmab, as well as the necessary time to determine possible adverse events and/or immunogenicity, which may occur [30]. Future studies may expand the list of painful conditions that respond to anti-NGF mAbs.

Non-pharmacologic tier-one strategies for the management of chronic pain include encouraging activity, environmental modification, and weight management (Fig. 48.2). The approach to chronic pain management is integrative; therefore, the reader is encouraged to combine treatment strategies from this chapter with those described in Chapter 49.

Second tier

Second-tier pain management treatments are best used in addition to tier-one modalities or when first-tier modalities do not meet the needs of the patient. It is appropriate that a more definitive diagnosis of the origin of pain is confirmed before these methods are employed. Suggestions for second-tier modalities have less robust data to support their use and this section will review the information that is available. Evidence for second-tier drugs used for *chronic* pain is particularly difficult to evaluate because chronic pain is complex and has many unique clinical presentations. For example, chronic pain can originate from multiple different organs, have a variety of stages, involve multiple pathways, and create varying degrees of emotional distress and reduction in quality of life. More than one chronic condition can exist at one time, so it is unlikely we will ever find a single "silver bullet" to use in these patients. We have an ethical obligation to use agents, which we currently have access to, and which have potential benefits with limited adverse effects when administered appropriately [43].

Ketamine, a *N*-methyl-D-aspartate (NMDA) receptor antagonist, is a versatile drug with a place in anesthesia and pain management. In people, ketamine has been used to manage acute and chronic pain, in burn and cancer patients, and for alleviation of neuropathic pain [44–48]. Ketamine is often regarded as a more effective analgesic for somatic rather than visceral pain [49], especially when pain is inflammatory in origin. In people, the dose of ketamine required for analgesia is much lower than that required for anesthesia, especially when it is combined with an opioid [50]. These low doses do not appear effective in the cat or dog when assessed by mechanical and thermal threshold testing in non-painful animals [51,52]. This may reflect the pain model used as, in the absence of clinical pain, it is unlikely that NMDA receptors were activated. Ketamine has been disappointing as a sole analgesic agent when administered as a constant rate infusion (CRI) [51,53], with only a single study in the dog [54] and cat [55] showing benefit, and several studies showing none. However, with the difficulty in recent years of accessing opioids reliably in some countries, ketamine infusions combined with lidocaine and/or opioids and/or α_2-adrenergic receptor agonists, have become commonplace in veterinary anesthesia, providing perioperative analgesia for a variety of procedures [56–61]. Clinical studies suggest that ketamine in combination with lidocaine is superior to tramadol alone [62]. However, when compared to a local anesthetic nerve block for patients undergoing cranial cruciate repair, the combination of an opioid, ketamine, and lidocaine was not as effective as the block for postoperative analgesia [63], thus reinforcing the importance of first-tier analgesic choices (e.g., local blocks). This theory is also supported in one study in cats, where the addition of targeted local blocks to an anesthesia protocol that included ketamine showed benefits [64]. In addition to analgesic benefits, low-dose infusions of ketamine appear to have few adverse cardiopulmonary effects in dogs [65,66]. No data exists on the cardiac effects of ketamine when used as a CRI in cats, leaving some clinicians unsure of its role in this species given the prevalence of subclinical cardiac disease [67,68]. However, when ketamine was administered at 23 μg/kg/min after a 2 mg/kg loading dose, to reduce propofol CRI requirements in a small number of cats, cardiovascular variables were not changed [69]. In the cat, ketamine is a component of various popular injectable drug combinations used to produce general anesthesia (e.g., "kitty magic") [70], and likely contributes a degree of analgesia to these protocols [71].

Non-traditional routes of administration of ketamine have been studied including its use as a regional and topical analgesic [72,73], or given in the epidural space [74–77]; however, these techniques are not common in clinical practice.

In the horse, subanesthetic doses of ketamine combined with tramadol provided analgesia in cases of chronic laminitis [78], although caution is warranted when gastrointestinal transit time is a concern [79].

A large meta-analysis of human studies concluded that magnesium, likely through its antagonism at NDMA receptors and calcium channels, reduced postoperative opioid use and resulted in lower pain scores [80]; however, the evidence supporting this is modest at best [81]. It is therefore not surprising that there is little work to support the use of magnesium as an analgesic strategy in animals.

Two oral NMDA receptor antagonists, amantadine and memantine (an amantadine derivative), have been studied for their potential analgesic properties. Further information about these drugs is available in Chapter 25.

In addition to targeted administration, systemic administration of local anesthetics for provision of analgesia has been studied with varying results. In conscious dogs, there was no change in nociceptive threshold using electrical cutaneous stimulation over a range of doses of systemically administered lidocaine [82]; however, this may reflect the model used in the study. Investigators using a thermal threshold model reported that systemically administered lidocaine had variable and species-specific effects [83]. Clinical procedures, which may serve as better models, yield different results with systemic lidocaine administration [84]. Similarly, work done by Tsai *et al.* suggests that systemic administration of lidocaine provided comparable analgesia to meloxicam in dogs undergoing ovariohysterectomy [85]. In a meta-analysis of human patients who received systemic lidocaine, the evidence was weak to moderate for pain reduction, and the studies that reported an effect found this only during early time points; however, the same meta-analysis suggested that gastrointestinal recovery from anesthesia was positively impacted by use of systemic lidocaine [86]. Some veterinary patients (particularly those at risk for decreased gastrointestinal transit time or ileus, such as horses) may benefit from the prokinetic effects of systemic lidocaine [87]. By minimizing development of ileus, which is painful, lidocaine may have indirect analgesic effects. Unfortunately, the use of lidocaine did not translate into improved survival for horses with small intestinal lesions [88], and may indeed negatively impact their recovery from anesthesia [89–91]. Therefore, careful patient selection and judicious use of lidocaine in horses is advised.

At the dose necessary for reduction of inhalant requirements in cats, significant cardiovascular depression occurs [92], and although there may be analgesic benefits [55], the risks of lidocaine infusions in cats may outweigh the benefits.

Topical administration of eutectic mixtures of local anesthetics produces analgesia and reduces inflammation, with minimal systemic uptake [93–96]. Novel formulations of bupivacaine, including liposome-encapsulated bupivacaine, which is released over 72 h, may be useful in multiple species [97–99]. The utility of this formulation is limited to infiltrative techniques using a moving-needle injection technique in order to infiltrate deep and superficial layers of the surgical site. The product license in the United States is limited to regional analgesia for feline onychectomy and infiltration for canine stifle surgery [98], but continued research may expand its clinical application.

Targeted nerve blocks, such as the transversus abdominis plane (TAP) block, showed no additional benefit of using liposome-encapsulated bupivacaine compared to a dexmedetomidine–bupivacaine infiltration, although both techniques resulted in lower pain scores compared to the control group which did not receive a TAP block [100]. Caution is advised with incorporation of liposome-encapsulated bupivacaine into targeted blocks that may impact critical neurologic pathways, as prolonged effects may occur [101]. For example, a brachial plexus block performed bilaterally with liposome-encapsulated bupivacaine could last up to 72 h. If the drug diffused rostrally and desensitized cervical spinal nerves C3–C5, blockade of the phrenic nerve could necessitate the use of mechanical ventilation. In addition to patient side effects, client communication is equally important. For example, owners may perceive a reduction in motor function as detrimental, when in fact the extended effect of the block may contribute to better pain relief.

There are case reports of side effects when blocks were performed with unencapsulated bupivacaine, such as Horner's syndrome secondary to a brachial plexus block [102].

α_2-Adrenergic receptor agonists are discussed in greater detail in Chapter 22. Xylazine, detomidine, romifidine, medetomidine, and dexmedetomidine are commercially available veterinary α_2-adrenergic receptor agonists that provide analgesia in a variety of species [103–107]. A relatively new agent is a combination of the α_2-adrenergic receptor agonist, medetomidine, and a peripheral antagonist, vatinoxan, with the aim of eliminating the unwanted effects of medetomidine, such as vasoconstriction and bradycardia. Further work is necessary to assess this combination as an analgesic since α_2-adrenergic receptor agonists mediate analgesia both peripherally and centrally [108–112].

Benefit versus risk must be assessed before including any drugs in a pain management plan. In certain patients, the benefits of α_2-adrenergic receptor agonists are significant. In horses, xylazine provides significant relief of visceral and somatic pain, perhaps even more so than opioids or NSAIDs [113,114]. This species difference may be the result of α_2-adrenergic receptor distribution in the central nervous system [115]. Calves undergoing castration had a reduction in serum cortisol (one physiologic marker of pain) and improved behavior when a combination of low-dose xylazine and ketamine was administered prior to the procedure [116]. Antinociception was improved in llamas receiving tiletamine–zolazepam when xylazine was concurrently administered [117]. Alternative routes of administration may provide varied benefits, such as the caudal epidural administration of detomidine in horses [118].

Regurgitant cardiac disease, which is prevalent in older dogs, is an example of a situation where there may be more risk than benefit to using α_2-adrenergic receptor agonists. Likewise, in a critically ill patient who is already obtunded, the use of systemic α_2-adrenergic receptor agonists may not be appropriate. When used as a component of an analgesic plan, this class of drug is more suited to healthy patients. The medetomidine–vatinoxan combination may help to ameliorate these concerns; however, as stated previously, the analgesic properties of this combination have not been studied.

Gel oromucosal formulations of α_2-adrenergic receptor agonists (e.g., dexmedetomidine and detomidine) are available and labeled for use in several species for noise aversion in dogs and sedation in horses, respectively. At the time of writing, the use of these agents as analgesic adjuvants has not been reported. In human patients, topical clonidine has undergone a Cochrane review and was found to have limited efficacy [119]; therefore, it warrants little attention as an analgesic in veterinary medicine.

Acetaminophen (paracetamol) is used in dogs and horses as a primary or adjunct analgesic. Unlike traditional NSAIDs, acetaminophen may target a COX-1 splice variant (COX-3). In equine patients [120], acetaminophen has a high oral bioavailability [121,122], with clinical reports suggesting it provides analgesia.

Inhibitors of soluble epoxide hydrolase are a new class of non-NSAID anti-inflammatory and analgesic drugs, which increase endogenous concentrations of epoxy fatty acids by blocking their hydrolysis [123]. Epoxy fatty acids are analgesic and anti-inflammatory signaling molecules, thus applicable to inflammatory diseases such as OA. The inhibitor with the most stability and potency across species seems to be *trans*-4-{4-[3-(4-trifluromethoxy-phenyl)-ureido]-cyclohexyloxy}-benzoic acid (*t*-TUCB) [123]. In horses, reduced lameness after intravenous injection of *t*-TUCB has been demonstrated [124,125]. Pharmacokinetic work in the horse suggests that a dose of 1 mg/kg is most suitable to achieve an anti-inflammatory effect [126], although in a small study, a dose of 0.1 mg/kg resulted in statistically significant improvement in pain scores for horses with chronic and severe laminitis [127]. The drug is relatively well tolerated, but gas colic was reported in a single horse [127]. There can be large species variations in drug bioavailability and metabolism, and inhibitors of soluble epoxide hydrolase are no exception [128]. Studies suggest a high oral bioavailability in dogs [129] and, when administered orally, they appear to reduce pain in dogs with naturally occurring arthritis [130]. While this work is preliminary, further investigation is warranted. Little to no clinical data is available regarding these agents in cats.

Bisphosphonates decrease osteoclast activity by reducing development of osteoclast progenitors as well as by increasing osteoclast apoptosis [131]. This limits bone resorption and may have positive effects in horses with arthritis, lumbar spinal pain from cauda equina syndrome, and navicular disease [132–135]. Bisphosphonates also resulted in improved lameness scores in horses with bone fragility disease [136]. However, because of the effects on osteoclast activity, bisphosphonates can also perpetuate or exacerbate microfractures, and have detrimental effects in juvenile horses [131].

Dogs appear to tolerate the bisphosphonate zoledronic acid used for bone pain [137], although a small number developed azotemia [138,139]. Other bisphosphonates, such as tiludronate, also appear to improve bone pain in dogs [140,141]. This is an improvement over the historic use of pamidronate, which provided modest to no improvement for pain in dogs associated with diseases such as osteosarcoma [142–144]. Zoledronate was well tolerated in cats [145]; however, at the time of writing, there is no clinical data evaluating the drug's efficacy in cancer-associated pain. A comprehensive review and species comparison is available [146].

Canine patients may benefit from intra-articular injections of steroids or other agents [147,148]. Small-scale studies evaluating slow-release triamcinolone acetonide show encouraging results in dogs [149]. Comprehensive reviews on this topic are available [150], and additional reading is imperative because novel therapies with promise receive approval intermittently and may offer effective pain relief for challenging conditions. One such intervention is ^{117m}Sn radiocolloid, which appears effective for debilitating conditions such as low to intermediate-grade elbow OA in dogs [151,152].

Additional drugs in the second tier include amitriptyline, nortriptyline, pregabalin, and gabapentin. These drugs and evidence for their role in pain management are reviewed in Chapter 25.

Third tier

Third-tier agents have either minimal evidence for their use, or evidence suggests they are unlikely to be useful. Tramadol use in dogs falls into this category, with a recent systematic review and meta-analysis finding low to very low analgesic benefits [153]. Maropitant, a neurokinin-1 (NK_1) receptor antagonist is an excellent anti-emetic, but there is limited evidence to support any anti-inflammatory or analgesic effect [154].

Other third-tier agents include polysulfated glycosaminoglycans (PSGAGs), chondroitin, hyaluronic acid (HA) and high molecular weight derivatives, pentosan polysulfate, polyacrylamide hydrogel, avocado–soybean unsaponifiables (ASUs), eggshell membrane (ESM), and *Boswellia serrata*, among others. As with chondroitin sulfate, the theoretical benefits of glucosamine stem from its role in the regulation of collagen synthesis and its contribution to glycosaminoglycan and proteoglycan synthesis [155]. Chondroitin sulfate also contributes to the cartilage matrix and enhances its resistance and elasticity [156]. However, because both of these agents fall outside the jurisdiction of regulatory agencies (e.g., government drug regulatory bodies), which require accountability for claims, formulations are highly variable in their concentrations and compositions; this may be the reason the information on their use in veterinary patients is inconsistent. These agents, despite their mixed efficacy, are unlikely to have adverse gastrointestinal, renal, or hepatic effects. However, if one is choosing a supplement on this basis, it may be more beneficial to choose marine-based fatty acid compounds, which demonstrate subjective and objective improvement in OA measures [16]. Side effects of PSGAGs are considered mild [43]. Both HA and polyacrylamide hydrogel reduce the force of impact on joints as well as provide lubrication, preventing further deterioration of the joint. ASUs appear to provide their beneficial effect through inhibition of inflammatory mediators, thus promoting cartilage repair [157]. Eggshell membrane, which is found between the albumin and outer calcified layer of chicken eggs, may be beneficial to joints. The proposed benefits stem from the membranes being a Type I collagen, as well as containing some of the glycosaminoglycans discussed here. Additionally, they may also reduce pro-inflammatory cytokines [158]. *Boswellia serrata* has been used for its anti-inflammatory properties for many years [159].

Evidence for agents that modify osteoarthritis in companion animals

PSGAGs have been studied extensively in the horse with various *in vivo*, *ex vivo*, *in vitro*, and *in situ* models with either clinical or histological outcomes as metrics for improvement or lack thereof. Most studies involved relatively few subjects. Reported results vary from minimal effects [160], to mixed effects [161], to improvement [162–165]. Combination administration (rather than administration of a single agent) is considered most effective for prophylaxis or treatment for OA in horses, although the cost of this approach limits its practical application [166]. Newer formulations of HA, including functionalized nanogels [167,168], have shown promise in bench-top experiments. Prolonged residence time has been demonstrated, which has built on the foundation of success in arthritis treatment that HA is known for [169,170]. Pentosan polysulfate has limited evidence to support its use. A small study of 18 horses [171] suggested efficacy, while other small studies showed limited improvement but minimal harm [172], as long as dosage was appropriate [173]. Although it has limited evidence for use in the horse, it continues to be popular [166]. Likewise, there is *in vitro* work suggesting polyacrylamide hydrogel is efficacious in improving joint disease [174]. There was also significant long-term improvement in clinical patients [175,176] and this conclusion was supported by meta-analysis of the literature [169]. ASUs have shown promise in some studies looking at inflammatory mediator reduction [177–179], although clinical pain was not significantly reduced in an experimental model of OA in the horse [180]. While *B. serrata* appears safe as a feed additive for horses [181], no clinical studies of its efficacy were available at the time of writing.

Like the horse, a significant amount of canine work evaluating PSGAGs is *in vitro* work and results are mixed. Some cell preparation studies demonstrated characteristics that may be beneficial in OA [182,183], while others reported less conclusive results [184,185]. Older clinical studies demonstrate improvement in lameness scores [186]. Route of administration makes a difference, with parenteral administration having more positive outcomes than enteral administration [187,188]. Although the evidence is weak, when using a mixture of these agents as dietary supplements, improvement in clinical signs was reported [189]. In a double-blind, randomized prospective clinical trial, dogs with OA receiving intra-articular high molecular weight hyaluronic acid showed greater improvement than those receiving allogenic mesenchymal stromal cells [190]. At least one other study supports improvement in function and reduced impairment after HA injection [191]. Alternative methods for HA administration include the oral route, and there was an increase in HA concentration in synovial fluid in patients administered oral HA [192]. These studies add to the data that supports the use of HA in dogs with joint disease [193,194]. Bench work supports the use of pentosan polysulfate in dogs [182,195,196]. In a canine cruciate model, pentosan polysulfate had favorable effects [187], with minimal side effects. Work done in dogs with ASUs suggests dosage is an important factor for improvement, with dogs dosed at 10 to 12 mg/kg/day [197,198] demonstrating more positive outcomes than those given 5 mg/kg/day [199]. Studies have evaluated osteochondral defects [200], as well as the potentiating effects of anti-inflammatory drugs with these agents [201]. Clinical studies involving eggshell membranes that assessed anti-inflammatory effects and clinical improvement came close, but failed, to show statistically relevant benefits [202,203]. This could be related to dosage, as dogs with hip dysplasia experienced clinical improvement with these agents [204]. The majority of work with *B. serrata* has been done with dogs. Unfortunately, optimum dosing is unknown. Clinical studies show efficacy at a dosage of 40 mg/kg/day [205], although no pharmacokinetic data is available to confirm if more or less is appropriate. This is further complicated by a lack of regulation ensuring supplements of *B. serrata* contain what they claim to, and studies demonstrate a huge range of concentrations within various formulations [206]. There is also work demonstrating efficacy when it is used as part of a combination of interventions [189,207–209].

Work done with PSGAGs in cats is unimpressive, with a strong placebo effect demonstrating improvement in both control and treatment groups [210]. Pentosan polysulfate was also evaluated in the cat for obstructive feline idiopathic cystitis and was found to have no impact on recurrence of the obstruction or clinical signs [211]. Pentosan polysulfate use in the cat is not benign, as evidenced by a single report of a 14-year-old cat developing acute and spontaneous subcutaneous and intramuscular hemorrhage after administration [212].

Evidence for biologic agents in companion animals

Intra-articular biologic agents, such as stem cell therapies or platelet-rich plasma, reside in the third tier due to limited evidence for their efficacy and (unlike orally administered disease-modifying agents) the inherent risks associated with intra-articular administration [213,214]. This inferior risk-to-benefit ratio places these agents lower on a list of recommendations. Issues such as variability in their preparation make quantifying improvements challenging [215–217]. In horses, there is evidence for improvement with stem cells both in case reports and large studies [218,219]. The source of the biologics made a difference as some patients worsened after repeated exposure to products from an allogenic source versus an autologous source [220–222]. These agents appear to have minimal adverse events in multiple species; in fact, many of the studies suggest they are well tolerated but fall short of reporting evidence of improvement [223–225]. At low doses, biologics such as adult mesenchymal stem cells may be enhanced by concomitant use of steroids [226].

Owners reported an improvement in dogs receiving stem cells after intra-articular injections, although objective analysis such as orthopedic examination, radiographs, synovial fluid analysis, and pressure plate analysis could not demonstrate a benefit [227]. One study examining owner outcome measures as well as scoring by a veterinarian demonstrated improvement in dogs receiving stem cells [228]. For specific disorders, such as trochlear groove reconstruction for patellar ligament deviation or in combination with surgery for lumbosacral spinal cord disease, stem cells could prove beneficial [229,230]. However, dogs with OA showed a greater improvement with intra-articular HA as opposed to allogenic stem cells [231]. Autologous stem cell therapy may yield better results [232]. Little to no information is available on feline subjects using intra-articular biologic therapies. A comprehensive review is available for those with interest in implementing stem therapy in their canine patients [233].

Autologous conditioned serum has been used as a therapy in horses with OA to improve lameness scores through generation of interleukin-1 receptor antagonist (IRAP), which inhibits the cytokine interleukin-1 [234–237]. Like many biologic products, preparation had a significant impact on the consistency of the product [238–240]. There was no clear evidence that IRAP was more beneficial than treatment with corticosteroids and HA [147], as all patients improved in one study comparing the two agents. Retrospective studies that looked at long-term improvement (six months after therapy) did not demonstrate an effect of IRAP [241]. Modest, gradual reductions in lameness and joint pathology in horses were found in one study [242] in the short term, with another small clinical study of 16 horses also suggesting improvement [243] over the course of 35 days. While *in vitro* studies in dogs suggest autologous serum may be useful [244], more clinical work is necessary to draw any conclusions. No work is available on use of this modality in cats.

Novel concept drugs

There are several drugs that have gained recent attention for their potential role in pain management, including those that act in the endocannabinoid system. Until more information is widely available, it is difficult to assign these agents to a tier.

Other non-pharmacologic options, such as acupuncture, corrective shoeing, fractionated radiation, and salvage procedures are discussed in other chapters. Further information on non-pharmacologic management of pain is available in Chapter 49.

References

1 Raja SNC, Cohen M, Finnerup NB, *et al.* The revised International Association for the Study of Pain definition of pain: concepts, challenges, and compromises. *Pain* 2020; **161**(9): 1976–1982.

2 Schug SA. 2011 – the global year against acute pain. *Anaesth Intensive Care* 2011; **39**(1): 11–14.

3 Gruen ME, Lascelles BDX, Colleran E, *et al.* 2022 AAHA pain management guidelines for dogs and cats. *J Am Anim Hosp Assoc* 2022; **58**(2): 55–76.

4 Rosero EB, Joshi GP. Preemptive, preventive, multimodal analgesia: what do they really mean? *Plast Reconstr Surg* 2014; **134**(4 Suppl 2): 85S–93S.

5 Katz J, Clarke H, Seltzer Z. Review article: preventive analgesia: quo vadimus? *Anesth Analg* 2011; **113**(5): 1242–1253.

6 Sajeev MF, Kelada L, Yahya Nur AB, *et al.* Interactive video games to reduce paediatric procedural pain and anxiety: a systematic review and meta-analysis. *Br J Anaesth* 2021; **127**(4): 608–619.

7 Van Hoogmoed LM, Galuppo LD. Laparoscopic ovariectomy using the endo-GIA stapling device and endo-catch pouches and evaluation of analgesic efficacy of epidural morphine sulfate in 10 mares. *Vet Surg* 2005; **34**(6): 646–650.

8 Bennett R, Steffey E. Use of opioids for pain and anesthetic management in horses. *Vet Clin North Am Equine Pract* 2002; **18**(1): 47–60.

9 Martin-Flores M, Campoy L, Kinsley MA, *et al.* Analgesic and gastrointestinal effects of epidural morphine in horses after laparoscopic cryptorchidectomy under general anesthesia. *Vet Anaesth Analg* 2014; **41**(4): 430–437.

10 Carney HC, Little S, Brownlee-Tomasso D, *et al.* AAFP and ISFM feline-friendly nursing care guidelines. *J Feline Med Surg* 2012; **14**(5): 337–349.

11 von Freeden N, Duerr F, Fehr M, *et al.* Comparison of two cold compression therapy protocols after tibial plateau leveling osteotomy in dogs. *Tierarztl Prax Ausg K Kleintiere Heimtiere* 2017; **45**(4): 226–233.

12 Luethy D. Cryotherapy techniques: best protocols to support the foot in health and disease. *Vet Clin North Am Equine Pract* 2021; **37**(3): 685–693.

13 Wang ZR, Ni GX. Is it time to put traditional cold therapy in rehabilitation of soft-tissue injuries out to pasture? *World J Clin Cases* 2021; **9**(17): 4116–4122.

14 Barrouin-Melo SM, Anturaniemi J, Sankari S, *et al.* Evaluating oxidative stress, serological- and haematological status of dogs suffering from osteoarthritis, after supplementing their diet with fish or corn oil. *Lipids Health Dis* 2016; **15**(1): 139.

15 Lascelles BD, DePuy V, Thomson A, *et al.* Evaluation of a therapeutic diet for feline degenerative joint disease. *J Vet Intern Med* 2010; **24**(3): 487–495.

16 Barbeau-Gregoire M, Otis C, Cournoyer A, *et al.* A 2022 Systematic review and meta-analysis of enriched therapeutic diets and nutraceuticals in canine and feline osteoarthritis. *Int J Mol Sci* 2022; **23**(18): 10384.

17 Roush JK, Dodd CE, Fritsch DA, *et al.* Multicenter veterinary practice assessment of the effects of omega-3 fatty acids on osteoarthritis in dogs. *J Am Vet Med Assoc* 2010; **236**(1): 59–66.

18 Roush JK, Cross AR, Renberg WC, *et al.* Evaluation of the effects of dietary supplementation with fish oil omega-3 fatty acids on weight bearing in dogs with osteoarthritis. *J Am Vet Med Assoc* 2010; **236**(1): 67–73.

19 Fritsch DA, Allen TA, Dodd CE, *et al.* Dose-titration effects of fish oil in osteoarthritic dogs. *J Vet Intern Med* 2010; **24**(5): 1020–1026.

20 Fritsch DA, Allen TA, Dodd CE, *et al.* A multicenter study of the effect of dietary supplementation with fish oil omega-3 fatty acids on carprofen dosage in dogs with osteoarthritis. *J Am Vet Med Assoc* 2010; **236**(5): 535–539.

21 Caron JP, Gandy JC, Brown JL, *et al.* Omega-3 fatty acids and docosahexaenoic acid oxymetabolites modulate the inflammatory response of equine recombinant interleukin1beta-stimulated equine synoviocytes. *Prostaglandins Other Lipid Mediat* 2019; **142**: 1–8.

22 Brommer H, Schipper P, Barneveld A, *et al.* Systemic or intrasynovial medication as singular or as combination treatment in horses with (peri-)synovial pain. *Vet Rec* 2012; **171**(21): 527.

23 Mangal D, Uboh CE, Soma LR, *et al.* Inhibitory effect of triamcinolone acetonide on synthesis of inflammatory mediators in the equine. *Eur J Pharmacol* 2014; **736**: 1–9.

24 Ellis KL, Seabaugh K, King MR. Retrospective analysis of horses with ultrasound evaluation of the sacroiliac region and response to local corticosteroid injection: 42 cases. *J Equine Vet Sci* 2021; **102**: 103634.

25 Marsh CA, Schneider RK, Sampson SN, *et al.* Response to injection of the navicular bursa with corticosteroid and hyaluronan following high-field magnetic resonance imaging in horses with signs of navicular syndrome: 101 cases (2000–2008). *J Am Vet Med Assoc* 2012; **241**(10): 1353–1364.

26 de Grauw JC, Visser-Meijer MC, Lashley F, *et al.* Intra-articular treatment with triamcinolone compared with triamcinolone with hyaluronate: a randomised open-label multicentre clinical trial in 80 lame horses. *Equine Vet J* 2016; **48**(2): 152–158.

27 McIlwraith CW, Lattermann C. Intra-articular corticosteroids for knee pain – what have we learned from the equine athlete and current best practice. *J Knee Surg* 2019; **32**(1): 9–25.

28 Lewin GR, Rueff A, Mendell LM. Peripheral and central mechanisms of NGF-induced hyperalgesia. *Eur J Neurosci* 1994; **6**(12): 1903–1912.

29 Michael GJ, Kaya E, Averill S, *et al.* TrkA immunoreactive neurones in the rat spinal cord. *J Comp Neurol* 1997; **385**(3): 441–455.

30 Enomoto M, Mantyh PW, Murrell J, *et al.* Anti-nerve growth factor monoclonal antibodies for the control of pain in dogs and cats. *Vet Rec* 2019; **184**(1): 23.

31 Isola M, Ferrari V, Miolo A, *et al.* Nerve growth factor concentrations in the synovial fluid from healthy dogs and dogs with secondary osteoarthritis. *Vet Comp Orthop Traumatol* 2011; **24**(4): 279–284.

32 Cheppudira BP, Trevino AV, Petz LN, *et al.* Anti-nerve growth factor antibody attenuates chronic morphine treatment-induced tolerance in the rat. *BMC Anesthesiol* 2016; **16**(1): 73.

33 Mantyh PW, Koltzenburg M, Mendell LM, *et al.* Antagonism of nerve growth factor-TrkA signaling and the relief of pain. *Anesthesiology* 2011; **115**(1): 189–204.

34 Miller RE, Block JA, Malfait AM. Nerve growth factor blockade for the management of osteoarthritis pain: what can we learn from clinical trials and preclinical models? *Curr Opin Rheumatol* 2017; **29**(1): 110–118.

35 Krautmann M, Walters R, Cole P, *et al.* Laboratory safety evaluation of bedinvetmab, a canine anti-nerve growth factor monoclonal antibody, in dogs. *Vet J* 2021; **276**: 105733.

36 Webster RP, Anderson GI, Gearing DP. Canine Brief Pain Inventory scores for dogs with osteoarthritis before and after administration of a monoclonal antibody against nerve growth factor. *Am J Vet Res* 2014; **75**(6): 532–535.

37 Lascelles BD, Knazovicky D, Case B, *et al.* A canine-specific anti-nerve growth factor antibody alleviates pain and improves mobility and function in dogs with degenerative joint disease-associated pain. *BMC Vet Res* 2015; **11**: 101.

38 Gearing DP, Virtue ER, Gearing RP, *et al.* A fully caninised anti-NGF monoclonal antibody for pain relief in dogs. *BMC Vet Res* 2013; **9**: 226.

39 Gearing DP, Huebner M, Virtue ER, *et al.* In vitro and in vivo characterization of a fully felinized therapeutic anti-nerve growth factor monoclonal antibody for the treatment of pain in cats. *J Vet Intern Med* 2016; **30**(4): 1129–1137.

40 Gruen ME, Myers JAE, Tena JS, *et al.* Frunevetmab, a felinized anti-nerve growth factor monoclonal antibody, for the treatment of pain from osteoarthritis in cats. *J Vet Intern Med* 2021; **35**(6): 2752–2762.

41 Gruen ME, Thomson AE, Griffith EH, *et al.* A feline-specific anti-nerve growth factor antibody improves mobility in cats with degenerative joint disease-associated pain: a pilot proof of concept study. *J Vet Intern Med* 2016; **30**(4): 1138–1148.

42 Gruen ME, Myers JAE, Lascelles BDX. Efficacy and safety of an anti-nerve growth factor antibody (frunevetmab) for the treatment of degenerative joint disease-associated chronic pain in cats: a multisite pilot field study. *Front Vet Sci* 2021; **8**: 610028.

43 Varcoe G, Tomlinson J, Manfredi J. Owner perceptions of long-term systemic use of subcutaneous administration of polysulfated glycosaminoglycan. *J Am Anim Hosp Assoc* 2021; **57**(5): 205–211.

44 Kosharskyy B, Almonte W, Shaparin N, *et al.* Intravenous infusions in chronic pain management. *Pain Physician* 2013; **16**(3): 231–249.

45 Elia N, Tramèr MR. Ketamine and postoperative pain – a quantitative systematic review of randomised trials. *Pain* 2005; **113**(1–2): 61–70.

46 White PF, Way WL, Trevor AJ. Ketamine – its pharmacology and therapeutic uses. *Anesthesiology* 1982; **56**(2): 119–136.

47 Bell RF. Ketamine for chronic non-cancer pain. *Pain* 2009; **141**(3): 210–214.

48 Leppert W. Ketamine in the management of cancer pain. *J Clin Oncol* 2013; **31**(10): 1374.

49 Alam S, Saito Y, Kosaka Y. Antinociceptive effects of epidural and intravenous ketamine to somatic and visceral stimuli in rats. *Can J Anaesth* 1996; **43**(4): 408–413.

50 Ahern TL, Herring AA, Stone MB, *et al.* Effective analgesia with low-dose ketamine and reduced dose hydromorphone in ED patients with severe pain. *Am J Emerg Med* 2013; **31**(5): 847–851.

51 Bergadano A, Andersen OK, Arendt-Nielsen L, *et al.* Plasma levels of a low-dose constant-rate-infusion of ketamine and its effect on single and repeated nociceptive stimuli in conscious dogs. *Vet J* 2009; **182**(2): 252–260.

52 Ambros B, Duke T. Effect of low dose rate ketamine infusions on thermal and mechanical thresholds in conscious cats. *Vet Anaesth Analg* 2013; **40**(6): e76–e82.

53 Sarrau S, Jourdan J, Dupuis-Soyris F, *et al.* Effects of postoperative ketamine infusion on pain control and feeding behaviour in bitches undergoing mastectomy. *J Small Anim Pract* 2007; **48**(12): 670–676.

54 Wagner AE, Walton JA, Hellyer PW, *et al.* Use of low doses of ketamine administered by constant rate infusion as an adjunct for postoperative analgesia in dogs. *J Am Vet Med Assoc* 2002; **221**(1): 72–75.

55 Correa JMX, Niella RV, Oliveira JNS, *et al.* Antinociceptive and analgesic effect of continuous intravenous infusion of maropitant, lidocaine and ketamine alone or in combination in cats undergoing ovariohysterectomy. *Acta Vet Scand* 2021; **63**(1): 49.

56 Skelding AM, Valverde A, Kilburn G. Evaluation of the analgesic effect of fentanyl-ketamine and fentanyl-lidocaine constant rate infusions in isoflurane-anesthetized dogs undergoing thoracolumbar hemilaminectomy. *Vet Anaesth Analg* 2021; **48**(3): 407–414.

57 Van Wijnsberghe AS, Marolf V, Claeys S, *et al.* Effects of fentanyl-lidocaine-ketamine versus sufentanil-lidocaine-ketamine on the isoflurane requirements in dogs undergoing total ear canal ablation and lateral bulla osteotomy. *Vet Anaesth Analg* 2020; **47**(5): 595–603.

58 Lewis KA, Bednarski RM, Aarnes TK, *et al.* Postoperative comparison of four perioperative analgesia protocols in dogs undergoing stifle joint surgery. *J Am Vet Med Assoc* 2014; **244**(9): 1041–1046.

59 Steagall PV, Aucoin M, Monteiro BP, *et al.* Clinical effects of a constant rate infusion of remifentanil, alone or in combination with ketamine, in cats anesthetized with isoflurane. *J Am Vet Med Assoc* 2015; **246**(9): 976–981.

60 Gutierrez-Blanco E, Victoria-Mora JM, Ibancovichi-Camarillo JA, *et al.* Evaluation of the isoflurane-sparing effects of fentanyl, lidocaine, ketamine, dexmedetomidine, or the combination lidocaine-ketamine-dexmedetomidine during ovariohysterectomy in dogs. *Vet Anaesth Analg* 2013; **40**(6): 599–609.

61 Gutierrez-Blanco E, Victoria-Mora JM, Ibancovichi-Camarillo JA, *et al.* Postoperative analgesic effects of either a constant rate infusion of fentanyl, lidocaine, ketamine, dexmedetomidine, or the combination lidocaine-ketamine-dexmedetomidine after ovariohysterectomy in dogs. *Vet Anaesth Analg* 2015; **42**(3): 309–318.

62 Kaka U, Rahman NA, Abubakar AA, *et al.* Pre-emptive multimodal analgesia with tramadol and ketamine-lidocaine infusion for suppression of central sensitization in a dog model of ovariohysterectomy. *J Pain Res* 2018; **11**: 743–752.

63 Kalamaras AB, Aarnes TK, Moore SA, *et al.* Effects of perioperative saphenous and sciatic nerve blocks, lumbosacral epidural or morphine-lidocaine-ketamine infusion on postoperative pain and sedation in dogs undergoing tibial plateau leveling osteotomy. *Vet Anaesth Analg* 2021; **48**(3): 415–421.

64 Fudge JM, Page B, Mackrell A, *et al.* Evaluation of targeted bupivacaine for reducing acute postoperative pain in cats undergoing routine ovariohysterectomy. *J Feline Med Surg* 2020; **22**(2): 91–99.

65 de Moura RS, Bittar IP, Gomes JH, *et al.* Plasma concentration, cardiorespiratory and analgesic effects of ketamine-fentanyl infusion in dogs submitted to mastectomy. *BMC Vet Res* 2022; **18**(1): 225.

66 Franco LG, Wilges CHM, Junior DP, *et al.* Effects of ketamine constant rate infusions on cardiac biomarkers and cardiac function in dogs. *Vet Anaesth Analg* 2018; **45**(3): 250–259.

67 Payne JR, Brodbelt DC, Luis Fuentes V. Cardiomyopathy prevalence in 780 apparently healthy cats in rehoming centres (the CatScan study). *J Vet Cardiol* 2015; **17**(Suppl 1): S244–S257.

68 Paige CF, Abbott JA, Elvinger F, *et al.* Prevalence of cardiomyopathy in apparently healthy cats. *J Am Vet Med Assoc* 2009; **234**(11): 1398–1403.

69 Ilkiw JE, Pascoe PJ. Cardiovascular effects of propofol alone and in combination with ketamine for total intravenous anesthesia in cats. *Am J Vet Res* 2003; **64**(7): 913–917.

70 Gates MC, Littlewood KE, Kongara K, *et al.* Cross-sectional survey of anaesthesia and analgesia protocols used to perform routine canine and feline ovariohysterectomies. *Vet Anaesth Analg* 2020; **47**(1): 38–46.

71 Kalchofner Guerrero KS, Reichler IM, Schwarz A, *et al.* Alfaxalone or ketamine-medetomidine in cats undergoing ovariohysterectomy: a comparison of intra-operative parameters and post-operative pain. *Vet Anaesth Analg* 2014; **41**(6): 644–653.

72 Kumar A, Sharma D, Datta B. Addition of ketamine or dexmedetomidine to lignocaine in intravenous regional anesthesia: a randomized controlled study. *J Anaesthesiol Clin Pharmacol* 2012; **28**(4): 501–504.

73 Uzaraga I, Gerbis B, Holwerda E, *et al.* Topical amitriptyline, ketamine, and lidocaine in neuropathic pain caused by radiation skin reaction: a pilot study. *Support Care Cancer* 2012; **20**(7): 1515–1524.

74 Gómez de Segura IA, De Rossi R, Santos M, *et al.* Epidural injection of ketamine for perineal analgesia in the horse. *Vet Surg* 1998; **27**(4): 384–391.

75 DeRossi R, Benites A, Ferreira J, *et al.* Effects of lumbosacral epidural ketamine and lidocaine in xylazine-sedated cats. *J S Afr Vet Assoc* 2009; **80**(2): 79–83.

76 Rojas AC, Alves JG, Moreira E Lima R, *et al.* The effects of subarachnoid administration of preservative-free S(+)-ketamine on spinal cord and meninges in dogs. *Anesth Analg* 2012; **114**(2): 450–455.

77 Song XJ, Zhao ZQ. NMDA and non-NMDA receptors mediating nociceptive and non-nociceptive transmission in spinal cord of cat. *Zhongguo Yao Li Xue Bao* 1993; **14**(6): 481–485.

78 Guedes AG, Matthews NS, Hood DM. Effect of ketamine hydrochloride on the analgesic effects of tramadol hydrochloride in horses with signs of chronic laminitis-associated pain. *Am J Vet Res* 2012; **73**(5): 610–619.

79 Hocking G, Cousins MJ. Ketamine in chronic pain management: an evidence-based review. *Anesth Analg* 2003; **97**(6): 1730–1739.

80 Albrecht E, Kirkham KR, Liu SS, *et al.* Peri-operative intravenous administration of magnesium sulphate and postoperative pain: a meta-analysis. *Anaesthesia* 2013; **68**(1): 79–90.

81 Morel V, Pickering ME, Goubayon J, *et al.* Magnesium for pain treatment in 2021? State of the art. *Nutrients* 2021; **13**(5).

82 MacDougall LM, Hethey JA, Livingston A, *et al.* Antinociceptive, cardiopulmonary, and sedative effects of five intravenous infusion rates of lidocaine in conscious dogs. *Vet Anaesth Analg* 2009; **36**(5): 512–522.

83 Pypendop BH, Ilkiw JE, Robertson SA. Effects of intravenous administration of lidocaine on the thermal threshold in cats. *Am J Vet Res* 2006; **67**(1): 16–20.

84 Smith LJ, Bentley E, Shih A, *et al.* Systemic lidocaine infusion as an analgesic for intraocular surgery in dogs: a pilot study. *Vet Anaesth Analg* 2004; **31**(1): 53–63.

85 Tsai TY, Chang SK, Chou PY, *et al.* Comparison of postoperative effects between lidocaine infusion, meloxicam, and their combination in dogs undergoing ovariohysterectomy. *Vet Anaesth Analg* 2013; **40**(6): 615–622.

86 Kranke P, Jokinen J, Pace NL, *et al.* Continuous intravenous perioperative lidocaine infusion for postoperative pain and recovery. *Cochrane Database Syst Rev* 2015; **(7)**: CD009642.

87 Cook VL, Blikslager AT. Use of systemically administered lidocaine in horses with gastrointestinal tract disease. *J Am Vet Med Assoc* 2008; **232**(8): 1144–1148.

88 Salem SE, Proudman CJ, Archer DC. Has intravenous lidocaine improved the outcome in horses following surgical management of small intestinal lesions in a UK hospital population? *BMC Vet Res* 2016; **12**(1): 157.

89 Valverde A, Gunkelt C, Doherty TJ, *et al.* Effect of a constant rate infusion of lidocaine on the quality of recovery from sevoflurane or isoflurane general anaesthesia in horses. *Equine Vet J* 2005; **37**(6): 559–564.

90 Wagner AE, Mama KR, Steffey EP, *et al.* Comparison of the cardiovascular effects of equipotent anesthetic doses of sevoflurane alone and sevoflurane plus an intravenous infusion of lidocaine in horses. *Am J Vet Res* 2011; **72**(4): 452–460.

91 Valverde A, Rickey E, Sinclair M, *et al.* Comparison of cardiovascular function and quality of recovery in isoflurane-anaesthetised horses administered a constant rate infusion of lidocaine or lidocaine and medetomidine during elective surgery. *Equine Vet J* 2010; **42**(3): 192–199.

92 Pypendop B, Ilkiw J. Assessment of the hemodynamic effects of lidocaine administered IV in isoflurane-anesthetized cats. *Am J Vet Res* 2005; **66**(4): 661–668.

93 Crisi PE, De Santis F, Giordano MV, *et al.* Evaluation of eutectic lidocaine/prilocaine cream for jugular blood sampling in cats. *J Feline Med Surg* 2021; **23**(2): 185–189.

94 Gibbon K, Cyborski J, Guzinski M, *et al.* Evaluation of adverse effects of EMLA (lidocaine/prilocaine) cream for the placement of jugular catheters in healthy cats. *J Vet Pharmacol Ther* 2003; **26**(6): 439–441.

95 Keating SC, Thomas AA, Flecknell PA, *et al.* Evaluation of EMLA cream for preventing pain during tattooing of rabbits: changes in physiological, behavioural and facial expression responses. *PLoS ONE* 2012; **7**(9): e44437.

96 Wagner K, Gibbon K, Strom T, *et al.* Adverse effects of EMLA (lidocaine/prilocaine) cream and efficacy for the placement of jugular catheters in hospitalized cats. *J Feline Med Surg* 2006; **8**(2): 141–144.

97 Gordon-Evans WJ, Suh HY, Guedes AG. Controlled, non-inferiority trial of bupivacaine liposome injectable suspension. *J Feline Med Surg* 2020; **22**(10): 916–921.

98 Reader RC, McCarthy RJ, Schultz KL, *et al.* Comparison of liposomal bupivacaine and 0.5% bupivacaine hydrochloride for control of postoperative pain in dogs undergoing tibial plateau leveling osteotomy. *J Am Vet Med Assoc* 2020; **256**(9): 1011–1019.

99 Richard BM, Newton P, Ott LR, *et al.* The safety of EXPAREL (R) (bupivacaine liposome injectable suspension) administered by peripheral nerve block in rabbits and dogs. *J Drug Deliv* 2012; **2012**: 962101.

100 Campoy L, Martin-Flores M, Boesch JM, *et al.* Transverse abdominis plane injection of bupivacaine with dexmedetomidine or a bupivacaine liposomal suspension yielded lower pain scores and requirement for rescue analgesia in a controlled, randomized trial in dogs undergoing elective ovariohysterectomy. *Am J Vet Res* 2022; **83**(9).

101 Campoy L, Martin-Flores M, Gleed RD, *et al.* Block duration is substantially longer with a liposomal suspension of bupivacaine than with 0.5% bupivacaine HCl potentiated with dexmedetomidine following an ultrasound-guided sciatic nerve block in Beagles. *Am J Vet Res* 2022; **83**(8).

102 Santoro F, Kaartinen J. Ultrasound-guided brachial plexus block and suspected Horner's syndrome in an alpaca (*Vicugna pacos*) undergoing traumatic scapulohumeral luxation reduction and articular capsule reconstruction. *Open Vet J* 2022; **12**(6): 1035–1038.

103 Valverde A. Alpha-2 agonists as pain therapy in horses. *Vet Clin North Am Equine Pract* 2010; **26**(3): 515–532.

104 Kästner SB. A2-agonists in sheep: a review. *Vet Anaesth Analg* 2006; **33**(2): 79–96.

105 Murrell JC, Hellebrekers LJ. Medetomidine and dexmedetomidine: a review of cardiovascular effects and antinociceptive properties in the dog. *Vet Anaesth Analg* 2005; **32**(3): 117–127.

106 Meyer H, Starke A, Kehler W, *et al.* High caudal epidural anaesthesia with local anaesthetics or alpha(2)-agonists in calves. *J Vet Med A Physiol Pathol Clin Med* 2007; **54**(7): 384–389.

107 Slingsby L, Taylor P, Monroe T. Thermal antinociception after dexmedetomidine administration in cats: a comparison between intramuscular and oral transmucosal administration. *J Feline Med Surg* 2009; **11**(10): 829–834.

108 Paalzow L. Analgesia produced by clonidine in mice and rats. *J Pharm Pharmacol* 1974; **26**(5): 361–363.

109 Fehrenbacher JC, Loverme J, Clarke W, *et al.* Rapid pain modulation with nuclear receptor ligands. *Brain Res Rev* 2009; **60**(1): 114–124.

110 Ishii H, Kohno T, Yamakura T, *et al.* Action of dexmedetomidine on the substantia gelatinosa neurons of the rat spinal cord. *Eur J Neurosci* 2008; **27**(12): 3182–3190.

111 Guo TZ, Jiang JY, Buttermann AE, *et al.* Dexmedetomidine injection into the locus ceruleus produces antinociception. *Anesthesiology* 1996; **84**(4): 873–881.

112 Dogrul A, Coskun I, Uzbay T. The contribution of alpha-1 and alpha-2 adrenoceptors in peripheral imidazoline and adrenoceptor agonist-induced nociception. *Anesth Analg* 2006; **103**(2): 471–477.

113 Pippi NL, Lumb WV. Objective tests of analgesic drugs in ponies. *Am J Vet Res* 1979; **40**(8): 1082–1086.

114 Muir WW, Robertson JT. Visceral analgesia: effects of xylazine, butorphanol, meperidine, and pentazocine in horses. *Am J Vet Res* 1985; **46**(10): 2081–2084.

115 Hellyer PW, Bai L, Supon J, *et al.* Comparison of opioid and alpha-2 adrenergic receptor binding in horse and dog brain using radioligand autoradiography. *Vet Anaesth Analg* 2003; **30**(3): 172–182.

116 Coetzee JF, Gehring R, Tarus-Sang J, *et al.* Effect of sub-anesthetic xylazine and ketamine ('ketamine stun') administered to calves immediately prior to castration. *Vet Anaesth Analg* 2010; **37**(6): 566–578.

117 Seddighi R, Elliot SB, Whitlock BK, *et al.* Physiologic and antinociceptive effects following intramuscular administration of xylazine hydrochloride in combination with tiletamine–zolazepam in llamas. *Am J Vet Res* 2013; **74**(4): 530–534.

118 Goodrich LR, Nixon AJ, Fubini SL, *et al.* Epidural morphine and detomidine decreases postoperative hindlimb lameness in horses after bilateral stifle arthroscopy. *Vet Surg* 2002; **31**(3): 232–239.

119 Serednicki WT, Wrzosek A, Woron J, *et al.* Topical clonidine for neuropathic pain in adults. *Cochrane Database Syst Rev* 2022; **5**: CD010967.

120 Kohn CW, Muir WW. Selected aspects of the clinical pharmacology of visceral analgesics and gut motility modifying drugs in the horse. *J Vet Intern Med* 1988; **2**(2): 85–91.

121 West E, Bardell D, Morgan R, *et al.* Use of acetaminophen (paracetamol) as a short-term adjunctive analgesic in a laminitic pony. *Vet Anaesth Analg* 2011; **38**(5): 521–522.

122 Tavanaeimanesh H, Azarnoosh A, Ashar FS, *et al.* Comparison of analgesic effects of a constant rate infusion of both tramadol and acetaminophen versus those of infusions of each individual drug in horses. *J Equine Vet Sci* 2018; **64**: 101–106.

123 Shihadih DS, Harris TR, Kodani SD, *et al.* Selection of potent inhibitors of soluble epoxide hydrolase for usage in veterinary medicine. *Front Vet Sci* 2020; **7**: 580.

124 Carlson A, Johnson PJ, Lei Z, *et al.* Anti-nociceptive efficacy of the soluble epoxide hydrolase inhibitor t-TUCB in horses with mechanically induced lameness. *Res Vet Sci* 2022; **152**: 504–509.

125 Guedes AG, Morisseau C, Sole A, *et al.* Use of a soluble epoxide hydrolase inhibitor as an adjunctive analgesic in a horse with laminitis. *Vet Anaesth Analg* 2013; **40**(4): 440–448.

126 Guedes AGP, Aristizabal F, Sole A, *et al.* Pharmacokinetics and antinociceptive effects of the soluble epoxide hydrolase inhibitor t-TUCB in horses with experimentally induced radiocarpal synovitis. *J Vet Pharmacol Ther* 2018; **41**(2): 230–238.

127 Guedes A, Galuppo L, Hood D, *et al.* Soluble epoxide hydrolase activity and pharmacologic inhibition in horses with chronic severe laminitis. *Equine Vet J* 2017; **49**(3): 345–351.

128 McReynolds CB, Yang J, Guedes A, *et al.* Species differences in metabolism of soluble epoxide hydrolase inhibitor, EC1728, highlight the importance of clinically relevant screening mechanisms in drug development. *Molecules* 2021; **26**(16): 5034.

129 Tsai HJ, Hwang SH, Morisseau C, *et al.* Pharmacokinetic screening of soluble epoxide hydrolase inhibitors in dogs. *Eur J Pharm Sci* 2010; **40**(3): 222–238.

130 McReynolds CB, Hwang SH, Yang J, *et al.* Pharmaceutical effects of inhibiting the soluble epoxide hydrolase in canine osteoarthritis. *Front Pharmacol* 2019; **10**: 533.

131 Vergara-Hernandez FB, Nielsen BD, Colbath AC. Is the use of bisphosphonates putting horses at risk? An osteoclast perspective. *Animals (Basel)* 2022; **12**(13): 1722.

132 Kamm L, McIlwraith W, Kawcak C. A review of the efficacy of tiludronate in the horse. *J Equine Vet Sci* 2008; **28**(4): 209–214.

133 Gough MR, Thibaud D, Smith RKW. Tiludronate infusion in the treatment of bone spavin: a double blind placebo-controlled trial. *Equine Vet J* 2010; **42**(5): 381–387.

134 Hadgaonkar S, Patwardhan S, Bhilare P, *et al.* A polyostotic Paget's Disease involving lumbar spine presenting with cauda equina syndrome: an unusual entity. *J Orthop Case Rep* 2021; **11**(10): 1–5.

135 Coudry V, Thibaud D, Riccio B, *et al.* Efficacy of tiludronate in the treatment of horses with signs of pain associated with osteoarthritic lesions of the thoracolumbar vertebral column. *Am J Vet Res* 2007; **68**(3): 329–337.

136 Katzman SA, Nieto JE, Arens AM, *et al.* Use of zoledronate for treatment of a bone fragility disorder in horses. *J Am Vet Med Assoc* 2012; **240**(11): 1323–1328.

137 Fan TM, de Lorimier LP, Garrett LD, *et al.* The bone biologic effects of zoledronate in healthy dogs and dogs with malignant osteolysis. *J Vet Intern Med* 2008; **22**(2): 380–387.

138 Brewer DJ, Macfarlane M, O'Connell E, *et al.* Toxicity of zoledronic acid after intravenous administration: a retrospective study of 95 dogs. *J Vet Intern Med* 2022; **36**(1): 253–258.

139 Vidal SA, Skorupski KA, Willcox JL, *et al.* Retrospective evaluation of acute kidney injury after zoledronic acid administration to dogs with malignant osteolysis. *Front Vet Sci* 2021; **8**: 647846.

140 Rialland P, Otis C, Moreau M, *et al.* Association between sensitisation and pain-related behaviours in an experimental canine model of osteoarthritis. *Pain* 2014; **155**(10): 2071–2079.

141 Moreau M, Rialland P, Pelletier JP, *et al.* Tiludronate treatment improves structural changes and symptoms of osteoarthritis in the canine anterior cruciate ligament model. *Arthritis Res Ther* 2011; **13**(3): R98.

142 Fan TM, de Lorimier LP, Charney SC, *et al.* Evaluation of intravenous pamidronate administration in 33 cancer-bearing dogs with primary or secondary bone involvement. *J Vet Intern Med* 2005; **19**(1): 74–80.

143 Fan TM, de Lorimier LP, O'Dell-Anderson K, *et al.* Single-agent pamidronate for palliative therapy of canine appendicular osteosarcoma bone pain. *J Vet Intern Med* 2007; **21**(3): 431–439.

144 Fan TM, Charney SC, de Lorimier LP, *et al.* Double-blind placebo-controlled trial of adjuvant pamidronate with palliative radiotherapy and intravenous doxorubicin for canine appendicular osteosarcoma bone pain. *J Vet Intern Med* 2009; **23**(1): 152–160.

145 Lundberg AP, Tran Hoang C, Billhymer A, *et al.* Combining radiation therapy with zoledronate for the treatment of osteo-invasive feline oral squamous cell carcinoma. *Vet Comp Oncol* 2022; **20**(4): 788–796.

146 Suva LJ, Cooper A, Watts AE, *et al.* Bisphosphonates in veterinary medicine: the new horizon for use. *Bone* 2021; **142**: 115711.

147 Franklin SP, Franklin AL. Randomized controlled trial comparing autologous protein solution to hyaluronic acid plus triamcinolone for treating hip osteoarthritis in dogs. *Front Vet Sci* 2021; **8**: 713768.

148 Kinzel S, Hein S, Buecker A, *et al.* Diagnosis and treatment of arthrosis of cervical articular facet joints in Scottish Deerhounds: 9 cases (1998–2002). *J Am Vet Med Assoc* 2003; **223**(9): 1311–1315.

149 Tellegen A, Beukers M, Rudnik-Jansen I, *et al.* Intra-articular slow-release triamcinolone acetonide from polyesteramide microspheres as a treatment for osteoarthritis. *Pharmaceutics* 2021; **13**(3): 372.

150 Lotsikas PJ. Intra-articular injectates: what to use and why. *Vet Clin North Am Small Anim Pract* 2022; **52**(4): 967–975.

151 Donecker J, Fabiani M, Gaschen L, *et al.* Treatment response in dogs with naturally occurring grade 3 elbow osteoarthritis following intra-articular injection of 117mSn (tin) colloid. *PLoS ONE* 2021; **16**(7): e0254613.

152 Lattimer J, Fabiani M, Gaschen L, *et al.* Clinical effectiveness and safety of intraarticular administration of a (117m) Tin radiocolloid (Synovetin OA(TM)) for treatment of early and intermediate grade osteoarthritis of the elbow in a dose finding study conducted in 44 dogs. *Vet Radiol Ultrasound* 2023; **64**(2): 351–359.

153 Donati PA, Tarragona L, Franco JVA, *et al.* Efficacy of tramadol for postoperative pain management in dogs: systematic review and meta-analysis. *Vet Anaesth Analg* 2021; **48**(3): 283–296.

154 Kinobe RT, Miyake Y. Evaluating the anti-inflammatory and analgesic properties of maropitant: a systematic review and meta-analysis. *Vet J* 2020; **259–260**: 105471.

155 Anderson CC, Cook JL, Kreeger JM, *et al.* In vitro effects of glucosamine and acetylsalicylate on canine chondrocytes in three-dimensional culture. *Am J Vet Res* 1999; **60**(12): 1546–1551.

156 Henrotin Y, Sanchez C, Balligand M. Pharmaceutical and nutraceutical management of canine osteoarthritis: present and future perspectives. *Vet J* 2005; **170**(1): 113–123.

157 Christensen R, Bartels EM, Astrup A, *et al.* Symptomatic efficacy of avocado–soybean unsaponifiables (ASU) in osteoarthritis (OA) patients: a meta-analysis of randomized controlled trials. *Osteoarthritis Cartilage* 2008; **16**(4): 399–408.

158 Ruff KJ, DeVore DP, Leu MD, *et al.* Eggshell membrane: a possible new natural therapeutic for joint and connective tissue disorders. Results from two open-label human clinical studies. *Clin Interv Aging* 2009; **4**: 235–240.

159 Hosain NA, Ghosh R, Bryant DL, *et al.* Isolation, structure elucidation, and immunostimulatory activity of polysaccharide fractions from Boswellia carterii frankincense resin. *Int J Biol Macromol* 2019; **133**: 76–85.

160 Kawcak CE, Frisbie DD, McIlwraith CW. Effects of extracorporeal shock wave therapy and polysulfated glycosaminoglycan treatment on subchondral bone, serum biomarkers, and synovial fluid biomarkers in horses with induced osteoarthritis. *Am J Vet Res* 2011; **72**(6): 772–779.

161 Frean SP, Cambridge H, Lees P. Effects of anti-arthritic drugs on proteoglycan synthesis by equine cartilage. *J Vet Pharmacol Ther* 2002; **25**(4): 289–298.

162 Verde C, Ferrante M, Simpson MI, *et al.* Efficacy of intramuscular polysulfated glycosaminoglycan in a controlled study of equine carpitis. *J Vet Pharmacol Ther* 2010; **33**(4): 357–362.

163 Moraes JR, Facco GG, Moraes FR, *et al.* Effects of glycosaminoglycan polysulphate on the organisation of collagen fibres in experimentally induced tendonitis in horses. *Vet Rec* 2009; **165**(7): 203–205.

164 Frisbie DD, Kawcak CE, McIlwraith CW, *et al.* Evaluation of polysulfated glycosaminoglycan or sodium hyaluronan administered intra-articularly for treatment of horses with experimentally induced osteoarthritis. *Am J Vet Res* 2009; **70**(2): 203–209.

165 Kristiansen KK, Kold SE. Multivariable analysis of factors influencing outcome of 2 treatment protocols in 128 cases of horses responding positively to intra-articular analgesia of the distal interphalangeal joint. *Equine Vet J* 2007; **39**(2): 150–156.

166 Kramer CM, Tsang AS, Koenig T, *et al.* Survey of the therapeutic approach and efficacy of pentosan polysulfate for the prevention and treatment of equine osteoarthritis in veterinary practice in Australia. *Aust Vet J* 2014; **92**(12): 482–487.

167 Cullier A, Casse F, Manivong S, *et al.* Functionalized nanogels with endothelin-1 and bradykinin receptor antagonist peptides decrease inflammatory and cartilage degradation markers of osteoarthritis in a horse organoid model of cartilage. *Int J Mol Sci* 2022; **23**(16): 8949.

168 Porcello A, Gonzalez-Fernandez P, Jordan O, *et al.* Nanoforming hyaluronan-based thermoresponsive hydrogels: optimized and tunable functionality in osteoarthritis management. *Pharmaceutics* 2022; **14**(3): 659.

169 da Silva Xavier AA, da Rosa PP, de Brum Mackmill L, *et al.* An assessment of the effectiveness of hyaluronic acid and polyacrylamide hydrogel in horses with osteoarthritis: systematic review and network meta-analysis. *Res Vet Sci* 2021; **134**: 42–50.

170 de Souza AF, Paretsis NF, De Zoppa A. What is the evidence of hyaluronic acid and polyacrylamide hydrogel in intra-articular therapy in equines? Systematic literature review. *J Equine Vet Sci* 2020; **86**: 102909.

171 McIlwraith CW, Frisbie DD, Kawcak CE. Evaluation of intramuscularly administered sodium pentosan polysulfate for treatment of experimentally induced osteoarthritis in horses. *Am J Vet Res* 2012; **73**(5): 628–633.

172 Kwan C, Bell R, Koenig T, *et al.* Effects of intra-articular sodium pentosan polysulfate and glucosamine on the cytology, total protein concentration and viscosity of synovial fluid in horses. *Aust Vet J* 2012; **90**(8): 315–320.

173 Dart A, Perkins N, Dowling P, *et al.* The effect of three different doses of sodium pentosan polysulphate on haematological and haemostatic variables in adult horses. *Aust Vet J* 2001; **79**(9): 624–627.

174 Vishwanath K, McClure SR, Bonassar LJ. Polyacrylamide hydrogel lubricates cartilage after biochemical degradation and mechanical injury. *J Orthop Res* 2023; **41**(1): 63–71.

175 de Clifford LT, Lowe JN, McKellar CD, *et al.* A double-blinded positive control study comparing the relative efficacy of 2.5% polyacrylamide hydrogel (paag) against triamcinolone acetonide (ta) and sodium hyaluronate (ha) in the management of middle carpal joint lameness in racing Thoroughbreds. *J Equine Vet Sci* 2021; **107**: 103780.

176 Tnibar A, Schougaard H, Camitz L, *et al.* An international multi-centre prospective study on the efficacy of an intraarticular polyacrylamide hydrogel in horses with osteoarthritis: a 24 months follow-up. *Acta Vet Scand* 2015; **57**: 20.

177 Grzanna MW, Au RY, Au AY, *et al.* Avocado/soybean unsaponifiables, glucosamine and chondroitin sulfate combination inhibits proinflammatory COX-2 expression and prostaglandin e2 production in tendon-derived cells. *J Med Food* 2020; **23**(2): 139–146.

178 Ownby SL, Fortuno LV, Au AY, *et al.* Expression of pro-inflammatory mediators is inhibited by an avocado/soybean unsaponifiables and epigallocatechin gallate combination. *J Inflamm (Lond)* 2014; **11**(1): 8.

179 Heinecke LF, Grzanna MW, Au AY, *et al.* Inhibition of cyclooxygenase-2 expression and prostaglandin E2 production in chondrocytes by avocado soybean unsaponifiables and epigallocatechin gallate. *Osteoarthritis Cartilage* 2010; **18**(2): 220–227.

180 Kawcak CE, Frisbie DD, McIlwraith CW, *et al.* Evaluation of avocado and soybean unsaponifiable extracts for treatment of horses with experimentally induced osteoarthritis. *Am J Vet Res* 2007; **68**(6): 598–604.

181 Bampidis V, Azimonti G, de Lourdes Bastos M, *et al.* Safety and efficacy of a feed additive consisting of an extract of olibanum from *Boswellia serrata* Roxb. ex Colebr. for use in dogs and horses (FEFANA asbl). *EFSA J* 2022; **20**(3): e07158.

182 Akaraphutiporn E, Bwalya EC, Kim S, *et al.* Effects of pentosan polysulfate on cell proliferation, cell cycle progression and cyclin-dependent kinases expression in canine articular chondrocytes. *J Vet Med Sci* 2020; **82**(8): 1209–1218.

183 Sevalla K, Todhunter RJ, Vernier-Singer M, *et al.* Effect of polysulfated glycosaminoglycan on DNA content and proteoglycan metabolism in normal and osteoarthritic canine articular cartilage explants. *Vet Surg* 2000; **29**(5): 407–414.

184 Bwalya EC, Kim S, Fang J, *et al.* Effects of pentosan polysulfate and polysulfated glycosaminoglycan on chondrogenesis of canine bone marrow-derived mesenchymal stem cells in alginate and micromass culture. *J Vet Med Sci* 2017; **79**(7): 1182–1190.

185 de Haan JJ, Goring RL, Beale BS. Evaluation of polysulfated glycosaminoglycan for the treatment of hip dysplasia in dogs. *Vet Surg* 1994; **23**(3): 177–181.

186 Fujiki M, Shineha J, Yamanokuchi K, *et al.* Effects of treatment with polysulfated glycosaminoglycan on serum cartilage oligomeric matrix protein and C-reactive protein concentrations, serum matrix metalloproteinase-2 and -9 activities, and lameness in dogs with osteoarthritis. *Am J Vet Res* 2007; **68**(8): 827–833.

187 Budsberg SC, Bergh MS, Reynolds LR, *et al.* Evaluation of pentosan polysulfate sodium in the postoperative recovery from cranial cruciate injury in dogs: a randomized, placebo-controlled clinical trial. *Vet Surg* 2007; **36**(3): 234–244.

188 Innes JF, Barr AR, Sharif M. Efficacy of oral calcium pentosan polysulphate for the treatment of osteoarthritis of the canine stifle joint secondary to cranial cruciate ligament deficiency. *Vet Rec* 2000; **146**(15): 433–437.

189 Martello E, Bigliati M, Adami R, *et al.* Efficacy of a dietary supplement in dogs with osteoarthritis: a randomized placebo-controlled, double-blind clinical trial. *PLoS ONE* 2022; **17**(2): e0263971.

190 Kim S, Elam L, Johnson V, *et al.* Intra-articular injections of allogeneic mesenchymal stromal cells vs. high molecular weight hyaluronic acid in dogs with osteoarthritis: exploratory data from a double-blind, randomized, prospective clinical trial. *Front Vet Sci* 2022; **9**: 890704.

191 Alves JC, Santos A, Jorge P, *et al.* Intraarticular triamcinolone hexacetonide, stanozolol, Hylan G-F 20 and platelet concentrate in a naturally occurring canine osteoarthritis model. *Sci Rep* 2021; **11**(1): 3118.

192 Serra Aguado CI, Ramos-Pla JJ, Soler C, *et al.* Effects of oral hyaluronic acid administration in dogs following tibial tuberosity advancement surgery for cranial cruciate ligament injury. *Animals (Basel)* 2021; **11**(5): 1264.

193 Chen LH, Xue JF, Zheng ZY, *et al.* Hyaluronic acid, an efficient biomacromolecule for treatment of inflammatory skin and joint diseases: a review of recent developments and critical appraisal of preclinical and clinical investigations. *Int J Biol Macromol* 2018; **116**: 572–584.

194 Aragon CL, Hofmeister EH, Budsberg SC. Systematic review of clinical trials of treatments for osteoarthritis in dogs. *J Am Vet Med Assoc* 2007; **230**(4): 514–521.

195 Wijekoon HMS, Bwalya EC, Fang J, *et al.* Inhibitory effects of sodium pentosan polysulfate on formation and function of osteoclasts derived from canine bone marrow. *BMC Vet Res* 2018; **14**(1): 152.

196 Bwalya EC, Kim S, Fang J, *et al.* Pentosan polysulfate inhibits IL-1β-induced iNOS, c-Jun and HIF-1α upregulation in canine articular chondrocytes. *PLoS ONE* 2017; **12**(5): e0177144.

197 Altinel L, Saritas ZK, Kose KC, *et al.* Treatment with unsaponifiable extracts of avocado and soybean increases TGF-beta1 and TGF-beta2 levels in canine joint fluid. *Tohoku J Exp Med* 2007; **211**(2): 181–186.

198 Boileau C, Martel-Pelletier J, Caron J, *et al.* Protective effects of total fraction of avocado/soybean unsaponifiables on the structural changes in experimental dog osteoarthritis: inhibition of nitric oxide synthase and matrix metalloproteinase-13. *Arthritis Res Ther* 2009; **11**(2): R41.

199 Scott RM, Evans R, Conzemius MG. Efficacy of an oral nutraceutical for the treatment of canine osteoarthritis. A double-blind, randomized, placebo-controlled prospective clinical trial. *Vet Comp Orthop Traumatol* 2017; **30**(5): 318–323.

200 Altinel L, Sahin O, Kose KC, *et al.* Healing of osteochondral defects in canine knee with avocado/soybean unsaponifiables: a morphometric comparative analysis. *Eklem Hastalik Cerrahisi* 2011; **22**(1): 48–53.

201 Grzanna MW, Secor EJ, Fortuno LV, *et al.* Anti-inflammatory effect of carprofen is enhanced by avocado/soybean unsaponifiables, glucosamine and chondroitin sulfate combination in chondrocyte microcarrier spinner culture. *Cartilage* 2020; **11**(1): 108–116.

202 Muller C, Enomoto M, Buono A, *et al.* Placebo-controlled pilot study of the effects of an eggshell membrane-based supplement on mobility and serum biomarkers in dogs with osteoarthritis. *Vet J* 2019; **253**: 105379.

203 Ruff KJ, Kopp KJ, Von Behrens P, *et al.* Effectiveness of NEM((R)) brand eggshell membrane in the treatment of suboptimal joint function in dogs: a multicenter, randomized, double-blind, placebo-controlled study. *Vet Med (Auckl)* 2016; **7**: 113–121.

204 Aguirre A G-QE, Fenaux M, Sanchez N, *et al.* The efficacy of Ovopet® in the treatment of hip dysplasia in dogs. *J Vet Med Anim Health* 2018; **10**: 198–207.

205 Reichling J, Schmokel H, Fitzi J, *et al.* Dietary support with Boswellia resin in canine inflammatory joint and spinal disease. *Schweiz Arch Tierheilkd* 2004; **146**(2): 71–79.

206 Miscioscia E, Shmalberg J, Scott KC. Measurement of 3-acetyl-11-keto-beta-boswellic acid and 11-keto-beta-boswellic acid in *Boswellia serrata* Supplements Administered to Dogs. *BMC Vet Res* 2019; **15**(1): 270.

207 Gabriele V, Bisanzio D, Riva A, *et al.* Long-term effects of a diet supplement containing Cannabis sativa oil and *Boswellia serrata* in dogs with osteoarthritis following physiotherapy treatments: a randomised, placebo-controlled and double-blind clinical trial. *Nat Prod Res* 2022: 1–5.

208 Caterino C, Aragosa F, Della Valle G, *et al.* Clinical efficacy of Curcuvet and Boswellic acid combined with conventional nutraceutical product: an aid to canine osteoarthritis. *PLoS ONE* 2021; **16**(5): e0252279.

209 Omura Y, Horiuchi N, Jones MK, *et al.* Temporary anti-cancer & anti-pain effects of mechanical stimulation of any one of 3 front teeth (1st incisor, 2nd incisor, & canine) of right & left side of upper & lower jaws and their possible mechanism, & relatively long term disappearance of pain & cancer parameters by one optimal dose of DHEA, Astragalus, *Boswellia serrata*, often with press needle stimulation of True ST. 36. *Acupunct Electrother Res* 2009; **34**(3–4): 175–203.

210 Cunningham R, Gruen ME, Thomson A, *et al.* Evaluation of a nutritional supplement for the alleviation of pain associated with feline degenerative joint disease: a prospective, randomized, stratified, double-blind, placebo-controlled clinical trial. *J Feline Med Surg* 2022; **24**(10): 962–974.

211 Delille M, Frohlich L, Muller RS, *et al.* Efficacy of intravesical pentosan polysulfate sodium in cats with obstructive feline idiopathic cystitis. *J Feline Med Surg* 2016; **18**(6): 492–500.

212 Tong MX, Romine JF, Hardcastle MR. Acute and severe haemorrhage following pentosan polysulfate injection in a Cornish Rex. *JFMS Open Rep* 2021; **7**(2): 20551169211058650.

213 Bertoni L, Branly T, Jacquet S, *et al.* Intra-articular injection of 2 different dosages of autologous and allogeneic bone marrow- and umbilical cord-derived mesenchymal stem cells triggers a variable inflammatory response of the fetlock joint on 12 sound experimental horses. *Stem Cells Int* 2019; **2019**: 9431894.

214 Ursini TL, Amelse LL, Elkhenany HA, *et al.* Retrospective analysis of local injection site adverse reactions associated with 230 allogenic administrations of bone marrow-derived mesenchymal stem cells in 164 horses. *Equine Vet J* 2019; **51**(2): 198–205.

215 Rowland AL, Burns ME, Levine GJ, *et al.* Preparation technique affects recipient immune targeting of autologous mesenchymal stem cells. *Front Vet Sci* 2021; **8**: 724041.

216 Bertoni L, Jacquet-Guibon S, Branly T, *et al.* Evaluation of allogeneic bone-marrow-derived and umbilical cord blood-derived mesenchymal stem cells to prevent the development of osteoarthritis in an equine model. *Int J Mol Sci* 2021; **22**(5): 2499.

217 De Francesco F, Riccio V, Biswas R, *et al.* In vitro characterization of canine microfragmented adipose tissue non-enzymatically extracted from the thigh and lumbar regions. *Animals (Basel)* 2021; **11**(11): 3231.

218 Melotti L, Carolo A, Elshazly N, *et al.* Case report: repeated intralesional injections of autologous mesenchymal stem cells combined with platelet-rich plasma for superficial digital flexor tendon healing in a show jumping horse. *Front Vet Sci* 2022; **9**: 843131.

219 Marinas-Pardo L, Garcia-Castro J, Rodriguez-Hurtado I, *et al.* Allogeneic adipose-derived mesenchymal stem cells (Horse Allo 20) for the treatment of osteoarthritis-associated lameness in horses: characterization, safety, and efficacy of intra-articular treatment. *Stem Cells Dev* 2018; **27**(17): 1147–1160.

220 Joswig AJ, Mitchell A, Cummings KJ, *et al.* Repeated intra-articular injection of allogeneic mesenchymal stem cells causes an adverse response compared to autologous cells in the equine model. *Stem Cell Res Ther* 2017; **8**(1): 42.

221 Frisbie DD, McCarthy HE, Archer CW, *et al.* Evaluation of articular cartilage progenitor cells for the repair of articular defects in an equine model. *J Bone Joint Surg Am* 2015; **97**(6): 484–493.

222 Pigott JH, Ishihara A, Wellman ML, *et al.* Inflammatory effects of autologous, genetically modified autologous, allogeneic, and xenogeneic mesenchymal stem cells after intra-articular injection in horses. *Vet Comp Orthop Traumatol* 2013; **26**(6): 453–460.

223 Van Hecke L, Magri C, Duchateau L, *et al.* Repeated intra-articular administration of equine allogeneic peripheral blood-derived mesenchymal stem cells does not induce a cellular and humoral immune response in horses. *Vet Immunol Immunopathol* 2021; **239**: 110306.

224 Depuydt E, Broeckx SY, Van Hecke L, *et al.* The evaluation of equine allogeneic tenogenic primed mesenchymal stem cells in a surgically induced superficial digital flexor tendon lesion model. *Front Vet Sci* 2021; **8**: 641441.

225 Mocchi M, Bari E, Dotti S, *et al.* Canine mesenchymal cell lyosecretome production and safety evaluation after allogenic intraarticular injection in osteoarthritic dogs. *Animals (Basel)* 2021; **11**(11): 3271.

226 Marycz K, Smieszek A, Grzesiak J, *et al.* Effects of steroids on the morphology and proliferation of canine and equine mesenchymal stem cells of adipose origin – in vitro research. *Acta Vet Hung* 2014; **62**(3): 317–333.

227 Daems R, Van Hecke L, Schwarzkopf I, *et al.* A feasibility study on the use of equine chondrogenic induced mesenchymal stem cells as a treatment for natural occurring osteoarthritis in dogs. *Stem Cells Int* 2019; **2019**: 4587594.

228 Harman R, Carlson K, Gaynor J, *et al.* A Prospective, randomized, masked, and placebo-controlled efficacy study of intraarticular allogeneic adipose stem cells for the treatment of osteoarthritis in dogs. *Front Vet Sci* 2016; **3**: 81.

229 He S, Zhang J, Chen W, *et al.* Umbilical cord mesenchymal stem cells promote the repair of trochlear groove reconstruction in dogs. *Front Vet Sci* 2022; **9**: 922390.

230 Chen CC, Yang SF, Wang IK, *et al.* The long-term efficacy study of multiple allogeneic canine adipose tissue-derived mesenchymal stem cells transplantations combined with surgery in four dogs with lumbosacral spinal cord injury. *Cell Transplant* 2022; **31**: 9636897221081487.

231 Kim S, Elam L, Johnson V, *et al.* Intra-articular injections of allogeneic mesenchymal stromal cells vs. high molecular weight hyaluronic acid in dogs with osteoarthritis: exploratory data from a double-blind, randomized, prospective clinical trial. *Front Vet Sci* 2022; **9**: 890704.

232 Sanghani-Kerai A, Black C, Cheng SO, *et al.* Clinical outcomes following intra-articular injection of autologous adipose-derived mesenchymal stem cells for the treatment of osteoarthritis in dogs characterized by weight-bearing asymmetry. *Bone Joint Res* 2021; **10**(10): 650–658.

233 Brondeel C, Pauwelyn G, de Bakker E, *et al.* Review: mesenchymal stem cell therapy in canine osteoarthritis research: "Experientia Docet" (Experience Will Teach Us). *Front Vet Sci* 2021; **8**: 668881.

234 Evans CH, Chevalier X, Wehling P. Autologous conditioned serum. *Phys Med Rehabil Clin N Am* 2016; **27**(4): 893–908.

235 Frisbie DD, McIlwraith CW. Evaluation of gene therapy as a treatment for equine traumatic arthritis and osteoarthritis. *Clin Orthop Relat Res* 2000; (379 Suppl): S273–S287.

236 Nixon AJ, Grol MW, Lang HM, *et al.* Disease-modifying osteoarthritis treatment with interleukin-1 receptor antagonist gene therapy in small and large animal models. *Arthritis Rheumatol* 2018; **70**(11): 1757–1768.

237 Pelletier JP, Caron JP, Evans C, *et al.* In vivo suppression of early experimental osteoarthritis by interleukin-1 receptor antagonist using gene therapy. *Arthritis Rheum* 1997; **40**(6): 1012–1019.

238 Muir SM, Reisbig N, Baria M, *et al.* The concentration of plasma provides additional bioactive proteins in platelet and autologous protein solutions. *Am J Sports Med* 2019; **47**(8): 1955–1963.

239 Lasarzik de Ascurra J, Ehrle A, Einspanier R, *et al.* Influence of incubation time and incubation tube on the cytokine and growth factor concentrations of autologous conditioned serum in horses. *J Equine Vet Sci* 2019; **75**: 30–34.

240 Watson Levings RS, Broome TA, Smith AD, *et al.* Gene therapy for osteoarthritis: pharmacokinetics of intra-articular self-complementary adeno-associated virus interleukin-1 receptor antagonist delivery in an equine model. *Hum Gene Ther Clin Dev* 2018; **29**(2): 90–100.

241 Bertuglia A, Basano I, Pagliara E, *et al.* Effect of intravenous tiludronate disodium administration on the radiographic progression of osteoarthritis of the fetlock joint in Standardbred racehorses. *J Am Vet Med Assoc* 2021; **259**(6): 651–661.

242 Watson Levings RS, Smith AD, Broome TA, *et al.* Self-complementary adeno-associated virus-mediated interleukin-1 receptor antagonist gene delivery for the treatment of osteoarthritis: test of efficacy in an equine model. *Hum Gene Ther Clin Dev* 2018; **29**(2): 101–112.

243 Frisbie DD, Kawcak CE, Werpy NM, *et al.* Clinical, biochemical, and histologic effects of intra-articular administration of autologous conditioned serum in horses with experimentally induced osteoarthritis. *Am J Vet Res* 2007; **68**(3): 290–296.

244 Huggins SS, Suchodolski JS, Bearden RN, *et al.* Serum concentrations of canine interleukin-1 receptor antagonist protein in healthy dogs after incubation using an autologous serum processing system. *Res Vet Sci* 2015; **101**: 28–33.

49 Non-Pharmacologic Management of Pain

Bonnie D. Wright
MistralVet, Johnstown, Colorado, USA

Chapter contents

Introduction, 1023
Physiology of non-pharmacologic pain medicine, 1023
Peripheral cutaneous sensory receptors, 1024
Temperature-related modalities, 1024
Acupuncture – peripheral neuromodulation, 1024
Massage, touch, stretching, exercise, 1024
Photobiomodulation therapy, 1025
Electromagnetic therapies, 1025
Extracorporeal shockwave therapies, 1025
Central neuromodulation – spinal and supraspinal locations, 1025
Mechanotransduction, 1025
Metabolism, blood flow, and immune modulation, 1026
Body weight and obesity, 1026
References, 1026

Introduction

Treatment of pain, both the acute self-limiting and especially the longer-duration or ongoing varieties, greatly benefits from therapies that alter the body's potent homeostatic and neuroimmune modulatory capacity. Non-pharmacologic therapies target the extensive and effective endogenous analgesic systems housed within the nervous system as well as the myofascial system.

Understanding the physiology of neuroimmune and fascial modulation facilitates applying discrete therapies to augment the pharmacologic treatment of pain conditions. These therapies may be machine-based, practitioner-applied, or self-applied through directed forms of motion. Although most of these therapies lack the research base of pharmacologic therapies, they are firmly rooted in the science of physiology, and are potent tools for comprehensive treatment of pain in veterinary medicine.

Physiology of non-pharmacologic pain medicine

Physiology provides a complex, multifaceted tapestry for both pain sensing and modification of transmitted signals. Non-pharmacologic interventions for the treatment of pain interface with these pre-existing structures and receptors in many of the same ways as pharmaceuticals, including but not limited to endogenous opioids, 5-hydroxytryptamine, glutamate, norepinephrine (noradrenaline), dopamine, γ-aminobutyric acid, endocannabinoids, acetylcholine, and purines [1]. Understanding the physiology of nervous system wiring, which is reviewed in Chapter 46, is the first step toward understanding methods to intervene in these endogenous systems and help modify them toward homeostasis. In addition to modification of pain, there is overlap between the nervous system and other endogenous, homeostatic systems such as the immune state, gastrointestinal motility and enteric control, vasomotor tone and fluid balance, and hormonal and reproductive balance [2–4]. Due to their global (entire organism) effects, non-pharmaceutical therapies often have overlapping actions on several homeostatic systems.

The database for non-pharmacologic treatments is rapidly expanding in the wake of scientific discovery and the response to the human opioid epidemic [5,6]. At the time of writing, the most researched and accepted techniques of non-pharmacologic pain control can be grouped into those that influence peripheral cutaneous sensory tissues through delivery of energy (light or acoustic) or sensory stimuli [7], those that modify central (spinal and supraspinal) neurotransmitters, including modulation of vagal activity and other components of the autonomic nervous system [1,8,9], and those that utilize the physiology of mechanosensitive tissues to elicit physiologic changes [9,10]. Most modalities work through a combination of these mechanisms.

In addition to provision of non-pharmacologic therapies to patients, compelling data suggests their overall metabolic state is also important. Obesity is a proinflammatory state, and there is strong evidence that appropriate body condition is integral to pain control [11]. Similarly, dietary management may reduce proinflammatory products, and administration of omega-3 fatty acids may reduce inflammatory states in dogs [12].

Veterinary Anesthesia and Analgesia: The Sixth Edition of Lumb and Jones. Edited by Leigh Lamont, Kurt Grimm, Sheilah Robertson, Lydia Love and Carrie Schroeder.
© 2024 John Wiley & Sons, Inc. Published 2024 by John Wiley & Sons, Inc.
Companion website: www.wiley.com/go/lamont/anesthesia

Peripheral cutaneous sensory receptors

Temperature-related modalities, such as application of ice and heat, work primarily through peripheral cutaneous sensory tissues and transient receptor potential (TRP) channels [7]. Other sources of peripheral cutaneous tissue modulation include acupuncture, massage, stretching, photobiomodulation, electromagnetic therapies, and extracorporeal shockwave therapy (ESWT).

While much focus is placed on the nociceptive role of cutaneous innervation, it is important to note that many peripheral analgesic modalities also work through sensory receptors other than nociceptors, which underlies the importance of touch in the treatment of pain [13].

Temperature-related modalities

Applying cold to skin decreases temperature up to a depth of 2–4 cm. This results in decreased activation of tissue nociceptors and slows conduction velocity along peripheral axons (cold-induced neuropraxia) [14]. Specific cold-sensitive ion channels, TRPM8 channels, contribute to analgesia by decreasing signaling through other pain-sensitizing channels as well as reducing incoming painful stimuli via central inhibitory interneurons [15]. Cold therapy also decreases edema formation via sympathetically mediated vasoconstriction and decreased delivery of inflammatory mediators to injured tissues. Another contribution to pain relief comes from reduced muscle spasms. Cold applied directly to muscles inhibits the motor reflex loops that maintain contraction and spasticity, thereby reducing the latter and relieving muscle spasms [16]. Muscle spasm may be present in patients with both acute and chronic pain and is a major cause of discomfort [14]. Ice is generally considered for acute injuries (up to three days postoperatively or postinjury) but, due to its analgesic effects, may also be used long term [7].

Unlike coolness, heat (or chemical mediators such as capsaicin or ginger) is not considered directly analgesic at the level of nerve endings but, because it increases blood flow and collagen distensibility (which reduces stiffness), it may provide some analgesia [17]. TRPV1 channels on afferent nerve endings sense heat. This can result in a proinflammatory or anti-inflammatory state via interleukin (IL)-6 in muscle tissue [18]. In general, heat is used more frequently for chronic conditions associated with fibrous or musculotendinous restrictions, or to help drain edema after it has formed which usually occurs on approximately the third day after an injury [17].

Acupuncture – peripheral neuromodulation

Acupuncture and related therapies utilize discrete neuroanatomic points on the body. These have effects in each of the three physiologic pathways described in this chapter: neuromodulation at peripheral, spinal, dorsal root ganglion, and supraspinal levels; myofascial mechanotransduction; and temperature-related changes. The cutaneous sensory system is critical to efficacy, as many studies have shown that these effects are abolished by local anesthetic drugs [19]. Most recognized acupuncture points are anatomically rich and characterized by myelinated and unmyelinated nerves, low-threshold mechanoreceptors (LTMRs), fibroblasts and the collagen matrix, mast cells, and microcirculatory complexes [20]. Needle placement causes direct nerve stimulation as well as secondary stimulation through mechanical forces applied to the fascia and cellular milieu in the region surrounding the point.

It has long been recognized that acupuncture points are found in cutaneous regions that show high levels of diverse innervation [20]. This occurs where groups of nerves emerge through bone, muscle, and fascia from their origins, where they branch or join, and where they attenuate distally. These nerve fibers are made up of Aβ and Aγ (myelinated) and C (non-myelinated) fibers, as well as autonomic fibers; acupoints generally have greater neural density compared to non-acupoint regions [21].

In general, myelinated somatic sensory fibers are most prevalent near acupuncture points, with most being Aβ and Aγ fibers, except in strong motor or Golgi tendon points. While there is often a focus in acupuncture research on the modification of high-threshold (HT) pain-sensing nerve types, it is likely that LTMRs play an important role in this modality [13]. Acupuncture needle sensation is seldom painful, and many of the sensations typically associated with acupuncture (such as warmth, coolness, pressure, and movement) are probably associated with LTMR activation and the engagement of TRP channels, rather than nociceptor activation.

These peripheral components, which are located in the skin and along peripheral nerve bundles, help explain why neuromodulation is the primary mechanism mediating acupuncture analgesia. Acupuncture stimulates afferent nerve fibers, and this has been demonstrated with manual acupuncture as well as with electroacupuncture. Both manual and electrical forms of stimulation activate all four types of nerves, Aα, Aβ, Aδ, and C fibers, although at unique discharge frequencies [22].

Acupuncture effects may also be enhanced by the reflex activity of axons, providing a cutaneous autocrine response at afferent sensory nerves simultaneous with the signal traveling along the previously recognized prodromal nerve pathway. This provides a potential anatomic explanation for the sensation of energy moving along "meridians," which are the sensory pathways long recognized in traditional acupuncture [9,21].

When evaluating the similarities and divergent characteristics between the recognized acupuncture points on the body, an important consideration is the global position of the point on the patient. For example, stimulation of distal points tends to be associated with greater homeostatic effects, such as regulation of immune function, organ function, and sympathetic/parasympathetic balance. This observation is partially explained by the fact that autonomic fiber density increases in the distal limbs and in association with nerves and blood vessels, and these areas are replete with acupuncture points. Many of these peripheral autonomic fibers are sympathetic noradrenergic fibers which play key roles in neuroimmune homeostasis [9,21]. At the point of an acupuncture needle, the release of neurochemicals such as purines and histamines contribute to this small, local response, which is amplified and ultimately results in systemic, homeostasis-modifying, gene transcription-modifying effects.

Massage, touch, stretching, exercise

Non-painful touch, body movement, and exercise can invoke analgesia through peripheral mechanisms [13,23–25]. Peripheral neuromodulation through various touch-related sensory receptors, Aβ and low-threshold C fibers, and TRP channels all play a role in reducing painful input from the peripheral nervous system. The autonomic nervous system is also deeply involved in pain and immune processing [26,27]. Exercise is one of several physical medicine methods utilized for pain reduction and its ability to modify autonomic nervous system activity appears to be one of the potential explanations for its hypoalgesic effects [28]. A discussion of the various types, methods, and limitations of therapeutic exercise is beyond the scope of this chapter.

Photobiomodulation therapy

When photobiomodulation (PBMT) is applied to peripheral nerves, depolymerization of the microtubules in Aδ and C fibers occurs, and the electrophysiological gradient within nociceptive nerves is degraded [29].

Nociceptor activity is decreased within 10 to 20 minutes of treatment. Reductions in proinflammatory mediators such as prostaglandin-E_2 (PGE_2), IL-6, and tumor necrosis factor-α (TNFα) occur, and reductions in acetylcholine decrease muscle spasm activity. Increased blood flow and stimulation of mitochondria contribute to the tissue healing effects of PBMT at clinically appropriate doses.

Electromagnetic therapies

Various therapies use electrical or magnetic frequencies to reduce pain and manage increased pain states [30]. The precise mechanisms are not fully elucidated, but interference with the electrical transmission of pain signals is postulated [31]. This field of treatment is based on both the ability of living cells to produce electrical fields (as measured by electrocardiography, electroencephalography, and bioimpedance), as well as respond to exogenously applied electrical fields. Direct healing effects have been documented and are attributed to mitochondrial activation, chemical changes (mediated by receptors including calcitonin gene-related peptide, nerve growth factor, and substance P), mechanotransduction, and thermal effects [32]. These changes, as with tissue deformation, have been found at the cellular, tissue, spinal segmental, and supraspinal levels. Electromagnetic fields may reduce acute and chronic pain and can be provided in a targeted manner with transcutaneous or percutaneous electrical nerve stimulation (TENS or PENS), pulsed electromagnetic field (PEMF) loops or beds, as well as other larger devices that provide a field of energy to the entire patient [33]. Implanted electromagnetic stimulators are being used to treat various chronic pain conditions in humans [34].

Extracorporeal shockwave therapies

Similar to other forms of movement for reduced pain transmission, extracorporeal shockwave therapies (ESWT) may be effective for both acute and chronic pain conditions. Local tissue effects on peripheral nerve endings mediate a portion of this effect, and ESWT therapies also work through tissue mechanotransduction to increase neurochemical mediators of pain and immunity [10,35].

Central neuromodulation – spinal and supraspinal locations

Neuromodulation is such a large category that it encompasses nearly all non-pharmaceutical therapies but includes modalities that modify pain homeostasis through recognized nervous system receptors and autonomic activities. Most of the modalities discussed under the peripheral nervous system will also induce upstream changes in the central nervous system at spinal and supraspinal locations. The modalities that have been studied that act on specific central pain receptors include acupuncture, PBMT, electromagnetic therapies, touch, stretching, and exercise [1,9,28]. Management of stress and modalities that reduce negative experiences also work through neuromodulation at the level of central pain regulation [36].

Drugs and management techniques that reduce anxiety can reduce pain sensitivity and awareness through their central effects. A variety of soothing olfactory and auditory tools have been studied to reduce pain and anxiety in hospitalized veterinary patients [37–39].

Mechanotransduction

Mechanotransduction is emerging as an important regulator of pain, metabolic, and cellular activity [35]. The effects can be seen directly in pain sensitivity in osteoarthritis where motion, stretching, and movement-based therapies are hypoalgesic [28]. This modulatory system also contributes to the supportive role of exercise and weight-bearing on cartilage health, bone and tendon formation, and the effects of acupuncture on the nervous system [17,40,41]. While there is considerable overlap between mechanotransduction in peripheral tissues and cutaneous sensory processing, this section will be limited to the effects of cellular mechanotransduction separate from those influencing the peripheral nervous system, which was covered previously.

Tissue traction or mobilization is a powerful modulator of intrinsic healing in soft tissues such as skin, muscle, ligaments, tendons, fascia, cartilage, and periosteum. When tissue is deformed, growth factors and a variety of proteins and neurotransmitters are released, leading to changes in pain processing, metabolic processes, inflammation, blood flow, and healing capacity [42]. Various methods such as provider-applied techniques (acupuncture, massage, and myofascial trigger point release), self-applied motion (stretching, exercise, and physical therapy), and mechanical devices (ESWT) depend heavily on these physiologic networks. Changes in the "loose" connective tissue of the body have a dramatic influence on fluid movement through tissues as reticular connective tissue forms the structural framework of the lymphatic system. The lymphatic system is central to immune homeostasis as demonstrated by the coalescing of lymphocytes and other immune cells into lymph nodes along these lymphatic chains. Thus, connective tissue fibroblasts are integral to both immune and neural homeostasis and these cells may be stimulated by acupuncture.

As an example of fascial mechanotransduction, when an acupuncture needle is placed, a dynamic and self-sustaining change occurs in the fascia that can be identified microscopically, but also by measuring chemical mediators and gene transcription [42]. This change radiates along the fascial network of an organism, creating far-reaching effects. Of note, these impacts are self-sustaining as fibroblasts exert force on their neighbors, which changes the local neurochemistry and creates a new population of activated fibroblasts, which exert similar effects on cells in a widening radius, thereby spreading the signal over both space and time.

Meanwhile, fascia is integral to the movement of fluid through the tissues. Fascia surrounding organs and appendicular structures form fluid highways and even exert regulatory functions over the movement of this fluid [43]. Fascia has also been found to have significant independent innervation, allowing it to provide a proprioceptive, body-wide sense of awareness [44]. Furthermore, fascia is involved in coordination of movement, both protecting joints from uncoordinated stresses as well as integrating communication between similar muscle groups that are not in direct muscular contact (such as coordinating extension between the quadriceps and gastrocnemius muscles) [27].

Thus, fascia plays a critical role in the efficacy of many non-pharmacologic movement-based treatments. In the periphery, this is primarily tied to the microcirculation and microscopic nerve and vasodilatory influences. Elsewhere in the body, this is related to macroscopic structures through integration of nerve and motor communication, body awareness, and facilitation of delivery and removal of life-sustaining fluids to extravascular body compartments.

Metabolism, blood flow, and immune modulation

A discussion of metabolism, blood flow, and immunity previously seemed unrelated to the discussion of pain. Through recent advances in the study of the neuroimmune–inflammatory axis, however, these homeostatic systems are now considered part of a larger central regulatory syncytium [26]. Pain influences the autonomic nervous system, and the autonomic nervous system influences pain. Likewise, treatment of the peripheral loci of the autonomic nervous system through the fascia (home of the lymphatics and extracellular fluid space) and the peripheral sensory system will influence the autonomic nervous system, and thus the intrinsic pain regulatory systems of the body [44]. It is not possible to separate out non-pharmacologic treatment of pain from modulation of the autonomic nervous system, and the endogenous ability to inhibit and stimulate these inseparable homeostatic systems.

Body weight and obesity

Osteoarthritis studies in dogs and cats have consistently shown a high correlation between obesity and clinical lameness. Adipose cells are proinflammatory and may change the kinematics of motion leading to worsening of pain conditions. Likewise, adipose-related systemic inflammation has been shown to contribute to signs associated with intervertebral disk disease. Thus, weight loss and exercise are critical components of non-pharmacologic pain management, both for their direct effects on the neuroimmune–endocrine system, and for their role in reducing inflammation [45].

References

1 Chen T, Zhang WW, Chu YX, *et al.* Acupuncture for pain management: molecular mechanisms of action. *Am J Chin Med* 2020; **48**(4): 793–811.

2 Yeater TD, Cruz CJ, Cruz-Almeida Y, *et al.* Autonomic nervous system dysregulation and osteoarthritis pain: mechanisms, measurement, and future outlook. *Curr Rheumatol Rep* 2022; **24**(6): 175–183.

3 Jacobson A, Yang D, Vella M, *et al.* The intestinal neuroimmune axis: crosstalk between neurons, immune cells, and microbes. *Mucosal Immunol* 2021; **14**(3): 555–565.

4 Pavlov VA, Chavan SS, Tracey KJ. Molecular and functional neuroscience in immunity. *Annu Rev Immunol* 2018; **36**: 783–812.

5 Ghai B, Jafra A, Bhatia N, *et al.* Opioid sparing strategies for perioperative pain management other than regional anaesthesia: a narrative review. *J Anaesthesiol Clin Pharmacol* 2022; **38**(1): 3–10.

6 Tick H, Nielsen A, Pelletier KR, *et al.* Evidence-based nonpharmacologic strategies for comprehensive pain care: The Consortium Pain Task Force White Paper. *Explore (NY)* 2018; **14**(3): 177–211.

7 Wright B, Kronen PW, Lascelles D, *et al.* Ice therapy: cool, current and complicated. *J Small Anim Pract* 2020; **61**(5): 267–271.

8 Huntingford JL, Petty MC. Evidence-based application of acupuncture for pain management in companion animal medicine. *Vet Sci* 2022; **9**(6): 252.

9 Wright BD. Acupuncture for the treatment of animal pain. *Vet Clin North Am Small Anim Pract* 2019; **49**(6): 1029–1039.

10 Simplicio CL, Purita J, Murrell W, *et al.* Extracorporeal shock wave therapy mechanisms in musculoskeletal regenerative medicine. *J Clin Orthop Trauma* 2020; **11**(Suppl 3): S309–S318.

11 Marshall W, Bockstahler B, Hulse D, *et al.* A review of osteoarthritis and obesity: current understanding of the relationship and benefit of obesity treatment and prevention in the dog. *Vet Comp Orthop Traumatol* 2009; **22**(5): 339–345.

12 Tsuruta K, Backus RC, DeClue AE, *et al.* Effects of parenteral fish oil on plasma nonesterified fatty acids and systemic inflammatory mediators in dogs following ovariohysterectomy. *J Vet Emerg Crit Care (San Antonio)* 2017; **27**(5): 512–523.

13 Zimmerman A, Bai L, Ginty DD. The gentle touch receptors of mammalian skin. *Science* 2014; **346**(6212): 950–954.

14 Malanga GA, Yan N, Stark J. Mechanisms and efficacy of heat and cold therapies for musculoskeletal injury. *Postgrad Med* 2015; **127**(1): 57–65.

15 Liu B, Fan L, Balakrishna S, *et al.* TRPM8 is the principal mediator of menthol-induced analgesia of acute and inflammatory pain. *Pain* 2013; **154**(10): 2169–2177.

16 Lee SU, Bang MS, Han TR. Effect of cold air therapy in relieving spasticity: applied to spinalized rabbits. *Spinal Cord* 2002; **40**(4): 167–173.

17 Millis DL, Ciuperca IA. Evidence for canine rehabilitation and physical therapy. *Vet Clin North Am Small Anim Pract* 2015; **45**(1): 1–27.

18 Obi S, Nakajima T, Hasegawa T, *et al.* Heat induces interleukin-6 in skeletal muscle cells via TRPV1/PKC/CREB pathways. *J Appl Physiol (1985)* 2017; **122**(3): 683–694.

19 Dundee JW, Ghaly G. Local anesthesia blocks the antiemetic action of P6 acupuncture. *Clin Pharmacol Ther* 1991; **50**(1): 78–80.

20 Zhang ZJ, Wang XM, McAlonan GM. Neural acupuncture unit: a new concept for interpreting effects and mechanisms of acupuncture. *Evid Based Complement Alternat Med* 2012; **2012**: 429412.

21 Zhao ZQ. Neural mechanism underlying acupuncture analgesia. *Prog Neurobiol* 2008; **85**(4): 355–375.

22 Kagitani F, Uchida S, Hotta H. Afferent nerve fibers and acupuncture. *Auton Neurosci* 2010; **157**(1–2): 2–8.

23 Fidanza F, Polimeni E, Pierangeli V, *et al.* A better touch: C-tactile fibers related activity is associated to pain reduction during temporal summation of second pain. *J Pain* 2021; **22**(5): 567–576.

24 Tomschi F, Lieverkus D, Hilberg T. Exercise-induced hypoalgesia (EIH) in response to different exercise intensities. *Eur J Appl Physiol* 2022; **122**(10): 2213–2222.

25 Stove MP, Hirata RP, Palsson TS. The tolerance to stretch is linked with endogenous modulation of pain. *Scand J Pain* 2021; **21**(2): 355–363.

26 Yeater TD, Cruz CJ, Cruz-Almeida Y, *et al.* Autonomic nervous system dysregulation and osteoarthritis pain: mechanisms, measurement, and future outlook. *Curr Rheumatol Rep* 2022; **24**(6): 175–183.

27 Zügel M, Maganaris CN, Wilke J, *et al.* Fascial tissue research in sports medicine: from molecules to tissue adaptation, injury and diagnostics: consensus statement. *Br J Sports Med* 2018; **52**(23): 1497.

28 Naugle KM, Fillingim RB, Riley JL III. A meta-analytic review of the hypoalgesic effects of exercise. *J Pain* 2012; **13**(12): 1139–1150.

29 DE Oliveira MF, Johnson DS, Demchak T, *et al.* Low-intensity LASER and LED (photobiomodulation therapy) for pain control of the most common musculoskeletal conditions. *Eur J Phys Rehabil Med* 2022; **58**(2): 282–289.

30 Paolucci T, Pezzi L, Centra AM, *et al.* Electromagnetic field therapy: a rehabilitative perspective in the management of musculoskeletal pain – a systematic review. *J Pain Res* 2020; **13**: 1385–1400.

31 Vuka I, Marcius T, Dosenovic S, *et al.* Neuromodulation with electrical field stimulation of dorsal root ganglion in various pain syndromes: a systematic review with focus on participant selection. *J Pain Res* 2019; **12**: 803–830.

32 Gaynor JS, Hagberg S, Gurfein BT. Veterinary applications of pulsed electromagnetic field therapy. *Res Vet Sci* 2018; **119**: 1–8.

33 Hellyer PW, Crump K, Shafford HL, *et al.* The use of pulsed electromagnetic field (PEMF) therapy to provide post-operative analgesia in the dog. *Vet Anaesth Analg* 2000; **27**(2): 104.

34 Knotkova H, Hamani C, Sivanesan E, *et al.* Neuromodulation for chronic pain. *Lancet* 2021; **397**(10289): 2111–2124.

35 Murthy SE, Loud MC, Daou I, *et al.* The mechanosensitive ion channel Piezo2 mediates sensitivity to mechanical pain in mice. *Sci Transl Med* 2018; **10**(462): eaat9897.

36 Hernández-Avalos I, Flores-Gasca E, Mota-Rojas D, *et al.* Neurobiology of anesthetic-surgical stress and induced behavioral changes in dogs and cats: a review. *Vet World* 2021; **14**(2): 393–404.

37 Frank D, Beauchamp G, Palestrini C. Systematic review of the use of pheromones for treatment of undesirable behavior in cats and dogs. *J Am Vet Med Assoc* 2010; **236**(12): 1308–1316.

38 Lindig AM, McGreevy PD, Crean AJ. Musical dogs: a review of the influence of auditory enrichment on canine health and behavior. *Animals (Basel)* 2020; **10**(1): 127.

39 Lefman SH, Prittie JE. Psychogenic stress in hospitalized veterinary patients: causation, implications, and therapies. *J Vet Emerg Crit Care (San Antonio)* 2019; **29**(2): 107–120.

40 Murthy SE, Loud MC, Daou I, *et al.* The mechanosensitive ion channel Piezo2 mediates sensitivity to mechanical pain in mice. *Sci Transl Med* 2018; **10**(462): eaat9897.

41 Bramson MTK, Van Houten SK, Corr DT. Mechanobiology in tendon, ligament, and skeletal muscle tissue engineering. *J Biomech Eng* 2021; **143**(7): 070801.

42 Langevin HM, Nedergaard M, Howe AK. Cellular control of connective tissue matrix tension. *J Cell Biochem* 2013; **114**(8): 1714–1719.

43 Findley TW. Fascia research from a clinician/scientist's perspective. *Int J Ther Massage Bodywork* 2011; **4**(4): 1–6.

44 Langevin HM. Fascia mobility, proprioception, and myofascial pain. *Life (Basel)* 2021; **11**(7): 668.

45 Frye CW, Shmalberg JW, Wakshlag JJ. obesity, exercise and orthopedic disease. *Vet Clin North Am Small Anim Pract* 2016; **46**(5): 831–841.

SECTION 7

Comparative Anesthesia and Analgesia

50 Comparative Anesthesia and Analgesia – Dogs and Cats

Peter J. Pascoe[1] and Bruno H. Pypendop[2]

[1] Emeritus Professor, Department of Surgical and Radiological Sciences, School of Veterinary Medicine, University of California–Davis, Davis, California, USA

[2] Department of Surgical and Radiological Sciences, School of Veterinary Medicine, University of California–Davis, Davis, California, USA

Chapter contents

Dogs, 1029
- Range of sizes, 1029
- Sighthounds, 1030
- Other breed sensitivities to anesthesia, 1031
- Histamine release, 1031
- Brachycephalic breeds, 1032
- Tracheal collapse, 1032
- Red blood cell potassium, 1033

Cats, 1033
- Handling and behavior, 1033
- Drug metabolism in cats, 1034
- Inhalant anesthetics, 1034
- Opioids, 1034
- Non-steroidal anti-inflammatory drugs, 1035
- Endotracheal intubation, 1035
- Cortical blindness, 1035
- Fluid therapy and blood volume, 1036
- Blood groups, 1036
- Dopamine and dopamine receptors, 1036

References, 1036

Dogs

Range of sizes

The domestic dog has been manipulated by selective breeding into a bewildering variety of shapes and sizes, originally with some functional purpose, but more recently with appearance as a major driving force of breed standards. This has led to an array of adult dog weights ranging from < 1 kg (e.g., teacup Yorkshire terrier) to > 100 kg (e.g., St. Bernard). Clinical experience suggests that smaller dogs generally require larger doses, on a mg/kg basis, of many drugs used in the perioperative period compared with large dogs. However, there is no scientific basis for calculating these relative dose rates. One common approach to this issue is to use an exponent based on metabolic activity. Within a species, this is usually thought to be two-thirds, and a common formula used for calculation of body surface area (BSA) based on body mass (BM) is as follows: BSA (m^2) = 0.101 × (BM in kg)$^{2/3}$. This formula has been criticized and a number of other multipliers and exponents have been proposed [1]. The use of BSA is historical; BSA happens to also vary as a function of $BM^{2/3}$, so BSA started being used to index various functions. While its exact calculation has been, and still is, debated, it is actually irrelevant to allometric scaling, including scaling of drug dose. The relevant information is the slope of the relationship between size (i.e., BM) and the variable to be corrected (e.g., dose); this slope is determined by the exponent, and therefore scaling to $BM^{0.67}$ instead of BSA would be as effective (provided that dose actually varies with that function of body size) and would avoid the criticism that exact BSA may not be known. Nevertheless, use of BSA to adjust dose has been used extensively with chemotherapeutic agents but this does not reduce the toxic side effects of these drugs, as smaller dogs seem to be more likely to suffer from adverse effects [2]. The inclusion of a body length factor may help to reduce the variability associated with different breeds and a recent study using computerized tomography (CT) scanning included this in their final model to calculate BSA [3]. The manufacturers of medetomidine and dexmedetomidine decided to use BSA and the product monograph for the dog provides doses in mg/m^2. Using their recommendation, a 1 kg dog would receive 37 μg/kg and an 80 kg dog would get 9 μg/kg of dexmedetomidine administered intravenously (IV). In clinical practice, many people have found that the dose for the bigger dogs is inadequate, suggesting that $BM^{0.67}$ may not be the correct function of BM for these drugs. Most drugs used for anesthesia and sedation are targeting the central nervous system and are metabolized in the liver. When we use drugs IV, they are distributed to the body by the cardiac output and when we use inhalants, they are taken up through the lungs. Accordingly, should drug dose be scaled to brain mass, hepatic metabolism, cardiac output, lung capacity, or some complex interaction of these body attributes that also accounts for the lipid solubility or hydrophobicity of the drug, assuming the latter would affect uptake by many of the tissues mentioned [1]? Table 50.1 shows how the dose might be affected by scaling it to some of these different tissues and attributes. Perhaps a more rational approach would be to base it on pharmacokinetics using virtual parameters to define the passage and distribution of a drug throughout the body. While the "central compartment," as defined in a pharmacokinetic analysis, is likely to include the blood

Veterinary Anesthesia and Analgesia: The Sixth Edition of Lumb and Jones. Edited by Leigh Lamont, Kurt Grimm, Sheilah Robertson, Lydia Love and Carrie Schroeder.
© 2024 John Wiley & Sons, Inc. Published 2024 by John Wiley & Sons, Inc.
Companion website: www.wiley.com/go/lamont/anesthesia

Table 50.1 Doses of a drug scaled to various metabolic activities or organ weights based on a 20 μg/kg dose for a 20 kg dog.

kg	BSA dose (dose/kg)	BMR dose (dose/kg)	Renal clearance dose (dose/kg)	Kidney weight dose (dose/kg)	Hepatic blood flow dose (dose/kg)	Liver weight dose (dose/kg)	Hepatic function dose (dose/kg)	Heart weight dose (dose/kg)	Brain weight dose (dose/kg)
Formula	$0.0484 \times BM^{0.67}$	$3.8 \times BM^{0.734}$	$4.2 \times (BMx1000)^{0.69}$	$0.0212 \times (BM \times 1000)^{0.85}$	$0.0554 \times BM^{0.894}$	$0.037 \times BM^{0.849}$	$0.00816 \times BM^{0.885}$	$0.0066 \times (BM \times 1000)^{0.98}$	$39 \times BM^{0.27}$
1	54 (54)	44 (44)	51 (51)	31 (31)	27 (27)	31 (31)	28 (28)	21 (21)	178 (178)
5	158 (32)	145 (29)	154 (31)	123 (25)	116 (23)	123 (25)	117 (23)	103 (21)	275 (55)
10	251 (25)	240 (24)	248 (25)	222 (22)	215 (22)	222 (22)	217 (22)	203 (21)	332 (33)
20	400 (20)	400 (20)	400 (20)	400 (20)	400 (20)	400 (20)	400 (20)	400 (20)	400 (20)
30	525 (18)	539 (18)	529 (18)	565 (19)	575 (19)	564 (19)	573 (19)	595 (20)	446 (15)
50	739 (15)	784 (16)	753 (15)	872 (17)	907 (18)	871 (17)	900 (18)	982 (20)	512 (10)
80	1013 (13)	1107 (14)	1041 (13)	1300 (16)	1381 (17)	1298 (16)	1364 (17)	1556 (19)	582 (7)
100	1176 (12)	1303 (13)	1214 (12)	1571 (16)	1686 (17)	1569 (16)	1662 (17)	1937 (19)	618 (6)

BM, body mass in kg; BSA, body surface area; BMR, basal metabolic rate.
The scaling factors are drawn from [14–17]. Note that the exponent (slope) contains the relevant information, as identical doses would be calculated by the relationships with similar exponents, regardless of the difference in the multiplier (e.g., kidney weight and liver weight doses). Values in parentheses are the equivalent dose/kg for that body weight to illustrate the decreasing dose/kg with increase in body mass.

volume and some of the vessel-rich tissues (e.g., brain, kidney, and heart), empirical pharmacokinetic models do not try to relate compartment volumes to actual, physical volumes in the body, and use changes in plasma concentration to describe the movement of the drug in the body. Initial distribution of a drug is into this central compartment and that appears to generally scale to body weight [4]. Because at least some drugs used in anesthesia, in particular the induction agents, but possibly also some of the analgesics, produce an effect with a rapid onset and short duration, concentrations immediately after administration (i.e., after dilution in the central compartment) are likely highly relevant to the effect [5]. Based on these considerations, it would appear that, at least for these drugs, calculation of the dose based on body weight is most appropriate. The relationship between dose and body size, and between dosing interval and body size is more complicated, as other pharmacokinetic parameters, such as clearance, appear to scale to a range of functions (exponents) of body weight, depending on the drug [4].

A further complication for both canine and feline patients is the current increase in pet obesity with estimates that over 50% of cats and dogs are overweight or obese [6–8]. This presents a challenge for the anesthetist because the brain of the animal is still the same size as that of the lean animal but there are no simple techniques available to estimate what that lean weight would be. Although adipose tissue has a low blood supply, it will obviously begin to affect the volume of distribution of a drug if there is a large amount in the body and it is likely that the blood volume of the animal may have increased as well [9]. Experience in humans indicates that the dose of induction drugs is greater than the dose expected for the predicted lean body weight but not as high as the dose required for the actual body weight of the patient. For example, in a study of propofol dose in obese and non-obese children, the total dose for the obese children was only 7% greater, even though the average weight of the obese children was 170% of the non-obese children [10]. In dogs, propofol was infused at 2.5 mg/kg/min and the dose at loss of consciousness was compared between a control group (Body Condition Score [BCS] 4–5 on a nine-point scale) and an obese group (BCS 8–9). The total dose was 19% higher in the obese group when these animals weighed 170% of the non-obese dogs [11]. The dose of propofol adjusted to an estimate of lean BM was not statistically different from the control group. This study was performed in dogs less than 10 kg so the data may not apply to larger obese dogs. Such relative changes in dose can be accounted for, in clinical practice, by titrating the drug to the desired effect. Obesity has many other medical implications for our patients that need to be addressed before and during anesthesia [12,13].

Sighthounds

These are dogs that hunt based on being able to see their prey rather than using scent. Phenotypically these dogs are deep-chested and have long legs and relatively narrow bodies. The muscles on the pelvic limbs are well developed and powerful to provide the thrust required to attain the high speeds necessary to outrun their prey. As hunters, they are also very lean animals. In an article on anesthesia in sighthounds, the Afghan, Borzoi, Saluki, Greyhound, Italian Greyhound, Whippet, Irish Wolfhound, Scottish Deerhound, Ibizan hound, Basenji, and Rhodesian Ridgeback, as well as a number of other rarer breeds were included [18]. However, it is now clear, on the basis of genetic analysis, that these breeds do not all share the same lineage [19]. In the most recent analysis, the sighthounds can be split into two groups. The first group includes the Greyhound, Italian Greyhound, Whippet, Borzoi, Deerhound, and Irish Wolfhound, while the Saluki, Afghan Hound, Ibizan Hound, and Pharoah Hound comprise a distinctly different genetic group. Published studies related to the topic of anesthesia and sighthounds relate specifically to the Greyhound and show that these dogs have a longer recovery from thiobarbiturates than other breeds [20,21]. There are also data showing slightly longer recoveries following both propofol and alfaxalone in Greyhounds [22,23]. This was initially ascribed to the phenotype of these dogs with regard to their large muscle mass and minimal adipose tissue and hence the generalization to all sighthounds. However, more recent data have suggested that the Greyhound may have some relative deficiencies in hepatic metabolism. One study examined the pharmacokinetics of thiopental in Greyhounds and showed that the plasma concentrations plateaued after an initial distribution phase. The Greyhounds were then administered phenobarbital in order to increase hepatic microsomal enzymes and then given thiopental again. The plasma concentrations of thiopental decreased at rates similar to those of mixed-breed dogs after this treatment [24]. These data do not prove that there is a hepatic deficiency in this breed, they merely show that if the rate of hepatic metabolism is increased, it will lead to a more rapid recovery. However, it has now been shown that Greyhounds have polymorphisms in their CYP2B11 cytochrome gene (H2, H3) that lead to slower metabolism of substrates for this enzyme. This polymorphism has been shown to be highest in the American Kennel Club-registered Greyhounds but is present in sighthounds in the first group above, but not the second group. This implies that this delayed recovery is less likely to affect the second group despite their lean body type. There are no published reports of significantly delayed anesthetic recoveries in sighthounds other than Greyhounds, although there are many anecdotes regarding such events. With this in mind, and until we have better information, it is probably best to avoid the use of thiobarbiturates in group one sighthounds and expect slightly longer recoveries from other anesthetic induction agents. Some drugs have been used to inhibit CYP2B11 in order to prolong the activity of known substrates for this enzyme. An example of this is the inclusion of fluconazole with methadone, which can increase the peak plasma concentration of methadone 17- to 30-fold and prolong its duration of action from minutes to hours [25].

Other breed sensitivities to anesthesia

Information obtained from the World Wide Web suggests that many purebred dogs have increased "sensitivity" to anesthetics. This is a subject that is constantly referred to by clients in veterinary practice who have been advised by a breeder or have looked up information themselves [26]. The origin of these "sensitivities" is unclear and very few of them have been consistently reported in any particular breed. An abnormal response to an anesthetic could be related to an individual strain within a breed whereby a particular breeder or group of breeders have produced animals that have a characteristic that they want to promote at the expense of alterations in response to anesthetics. Such a trait may not be present in all members of the breed, but the breed may earn that reputation. An abnormal response could also be related to a genetic trait that has been promoted over time and has become more generalized. The multidrug resistance (MDR)-1 or ABCB1 gene polymorphism has been found in a number of herding breeds and some others (http://prime.vetmed.wsu.edu/2021/10/19/breeds-commonly-affected-by-mdr1-mutation/). This gene controls the production of P-glycoprotein, which is an intracellular transporter protein that removes substances from the inside of the cell. This is a member of the adenosine-5′-triphosphate (ATP) binding cassette (ABC) family of proteins and so is one of several proteins that perform this function [27]. These proteins are found in many areas of the body but their presence in the intestine and the blood–brain barrier are most important for the anesthetist. Some drugs inhibit the action of P-glycoprotein and so may be associated with increased uptake of other drugs, others are removed from the cell by P-glycoprotein and so an animal with minimal production of this protein may show increased sensitivity to that drug. Acepromazine is a P-glycoprotein inhibitor, so even under normal circumstances, it may enhance the uptake of other drugs into the brain or through the intestine following oral administration. It is also suggested that it will cause more profound sedation in dogs with the ABCB1 (MDR1) mutation. Many of the opioids interact with P-glycoprotein and so their uptake into the brain is increased in ABCB1-deficient dogs. From experiments in ABCB1-deficient mice, there is about a 25% increase in the uptake of morphine and fentanyl and more than a twofold increase in the uptake of methadone [28,29]. Meperidine does not appear to interact with P-glycoprotein [30]. *In vitro* data would suggest that sufentanil, alfentanil, oxymorphone, and butorphanol [29,31] do not have significant interactions with P-glycoprotein, although it has been suggested that butorphanol may have some increased effect in ABCB1-deficient dogs. Buprenorphine appears to have minimal interaction with P-glycoprotein but its metabolite, norbuprenorphine, is ejected from the brain by this transporter. Norbuprenorphine is a potent respiratory depressant and so repeated administration of buprenorphine to ABCB1-deficient dogs may increase the risk of this adverse event [32]. The drugs used for the induction and maintenance of anesthesia do not appear to interact with P-glycoprotein.

Other breed "sensitivities" may have more to do with prevalent pathology in that breed rather than something inherent in the breed as a whole. Boxers appear to be sensitive to the effects of acepromazine, something that has been "well known" without any documented information (it is often quoted as being restricted to British Boxers but these authors have seen problems in North American Boxers too). This sensitivity tends to take the form of collapse following acepromazine and has been associated with profound bradycardia (authors' observations) but it is not known if this is related to the prevalence of arrhythmogenic right ventricular cardiomyopathy in this breed or an enhancement of a vagal response to the drug, as reported in a number of brachycephalic breeds [33]. The authors have also observed greater than expected sedation in Boxers administered acepromazine. Given the plethora of other drugs available for premedication, it seems unnecessary to use acepromazine in this breed or, if used, it seems prudent to administer very low doses (0.01–0.03 mg/kg) in combination with an anticholinergic (to prevent bradycardia) and monitor the animal carefully after administration.

The sense from the internet is that most breeds are "sensitive" to anesthetics yet very few anesthesiologists recognize such differences in purebred animals. However, a number of breeds have emerged from morbidity/mortality studies as having higher risks based on univariate analysis. These effects did not appear to survive a multivariate analysis indicating that other factors may have more strongly influenced the observed complication rate (e.g., a greater incidence of complications in small breed dogs) [34,35]. In one study, the "pastoral" or herding dogs were found to have a high mortality rate and it is possible that this is related to the ABCB1 (MDR1) gene polymorphism mentioned above [34]. Obviously, breeds that have a predisposition to cardiac disease may have greater risks for anesthesia. Despite the unreliability of internet reports of breed sensitivities, it is incumbent on the anesthetist to investigate specific concerns that are presented by an owner. If the last two of the owner's same-breed dogs died under anesthesia, it would be foolhardy to dismiss this without obtaining more details of the circumstances.

Histamine release

This appears to be greater in dogs than in other species, but the specific mechanism is unclear. The most notorious example of this was the spectacular release of histamine following the administration of alfaxalone–alfadolone in its original Cremophor base. This resulted in the deaths of a number of dogs [36] before pretreatment with antihistamines was advocated [37]. The drug in this formulation was never licensed for use in dogs, although many practitioners continued to use it in conjunction with antihistamines [38]. Morphine and meperidine are two opioids known to release histamine and, although it is difficult to make direct comparisons between species, the plasma concentrations of histamine in dogs appear to be considerably higher than those found in humans [39–41]. Of note in one experiment in humans is that the hemodynamic effects of the histamine release were not entirely blocked by administration of H_1 or H_2 blockers but were abolished when both were co-administered [41]. Cetirizine appears to be more effective than diphenhydramine at preventing the effect of histamine in a skin wheal but this was after a 6-day course of the drug so it is not known if this would be true with a single dose [42]. Recently, a study tested the histamine release in dogs with mast cell tumors (MCT) administered 0.5 mg/kg morphine intramuscular (IM) and in two MCT cell lines [43]. Unsurprisingly, there was no statistical difference in histamine release, but the authors concluded that morphine administration would be "safe" in dogs with MCT. However, their study only included 10 animals and they did not include the route of administration in this statement. This is an unfortunate overstatement of their results.

Brachycephalic breeds

Of the breeds in this class, there are various degrees of the manifestation of the typical brachycephalic obstructive airway syndrome (BOAS) – stenotic nares, elongated soft palate, everted lateral ventricles, hypoplastic trachea, and bronchial collapse [44]. The addition of conchal shortening to these anatomical abnormalities, with effects on both rostral and caudal obstruction of the nasal passages, has been described [45]. This constellation of anatomic changes leads to a higher-than-normal potential for airway obstruction, especially if the animal is not fully conscious and it is likely that these dogs suffer from something similar to sleep apnea in humans. Brachycephalic dogs have been shown to have higher $PaCO_2$ and lower PaO_2 values than meso- or dolicocephalic dogs [46]. Important considerations for the anesthetist are summarized in Box 50.1.

These authors' preference is that any brachycephalic dog that is to be anesthetized should have its upper airway examined immediately after induction and surgical correction performed if deemed necessary. Ideally, this should be done before any other procedure so that any bleeding has stopped by the time the animal is recovering. This reduces the risk of postoperative airway obstruction by removing some of the contributing factors.

Box 50.1 Important considerations for anesthetic management of brachycephalic breeds.

1. Avoid oversedation in the preanesthetic period since this may increase the likelihood of airway obstruction.
2. Have a range of endotracheal tubes (ETTs) available down to some very small diameters in relation to the size of the animal. For example, it is not unusual, in a 25 kg English Bulldog, to find that a 6.5 mm ETT, is the largest one that can be used (compared to a 10–12 mm ETT in a similar-sized non-brachycephalic dog).
3. Preoxygenate the patient if possible.
4. Use an induction technique that provides the shortest time between the start of injection and the ability to intubate. A mask induction with an inhalant is not recommended.
5. Use induction and maintenance drugs that allow for a rapid return of consciousness.
6. Maintain the airway for as long as possible during recovery. As the dentition of these animals is also abnormal, it is rare for a brachycephalic dog to be able to really damage an ETT with its teeth, so it is relatively safe to leave an ETT in place when the animal starts to chew, compared with most other dogs. In the authors' experience, these animals also take longer to recover than normal dogs, possibly because of their sleep apnea, making them stay asleep when they have a clear airway.
7. Observe the patient for paradoxical ventilation immediately after extubation to diagnose obstruction as quickly as possible. When the airway is obstructed, the thorax will collapse during inspiration while the abdomen expands.
8. Attempt to clear the airway by placing the animal in sternal recumbency and extending the head, opening the mouth, and pulling the tongue forward. Sometimes just propping the head up so that the neck is extended will be enough to maintain an open airway during the early period after extubation. The authors have also used an oral airway (consisting of a large bore ETT that has been cut off to a length that will reach the larynx but not enter it) in dogs that tolerate it.
9. Reintubate the patient and wait longer if the animal obstructs when the ETT is first removed. Sometimes it can take an hour or more beyond the point where the dog has tongue tone and can swallow.

Tracheal collapse

Some breeds such as Yorkshire Terriers are well known for this, and it can be very difficult to manage. Clinical signs include coughing, honking, hacking, wheezing, and dyspnea, although some dogs can have a degree of collapse with no clinical signs other than exercise intolerance. Tracheal collapse is also commonly associated with collapse in the lower airways making it even more difficult to manage perioperatively [47]. In theory, an extrathoracic tracheal collapse should be associated with increased inspiratory effort while an intrathoracic collapse is associated with an increased expiratory effort, but clinically, this is often not that distinct. Although, traditionally, radiographs have been used as part of the diagnostic workup for these cases, it has been shown that this is a relatively insensitive test compared with bronchoscopy [47]. Tidal breathing flow–volume loops are also a useful diagnostic tool and can be used to separate those dogs with and without tracheal collapse and those with severe collapse compared with mild/moderate disease. The variables used in this diagnosis are (1) the expiratory time divided by the inspiratory time, (2) the inspiratory time divided by the total respiratory time, and (3) the expiratory flow at end-tidal volume plus 75% end-tidal volume divided by the same inspiratory variable [48].

Medical management of these patients is often possible with the use of antibiotics to treat respiratory infections, weight loss, antisecretory agents, antitussives, and diuretics [49]. Anabolic steroids such as stanozolol may also improve the airway of these animals and could be used as a preoperative treatment to decrease the risk to these patients [50]. However, mean survival times have been much greater with the addition of a stent than with medical management alone [51].

The anesthetic management of these patients is, in many ways, similar to that used for brachycephalic breeds. In setting up for these animals, it is important to have endotracheal tubes (ETTs) available that are long enough to reach the carina if there is expected to be intrathoracic tracheal collapse. Once an airway has been secured and the tracheal collapse bypassed the patient may breathe spontaneously or be put on positive-pressure ventilation with or without continuous positive airway pressure (CPAP)/positive end-expiratory pressure (PEEP) if there is bronchomalacia involved. Recovery is the most dangerous period if the airway has not been stented, as collapse may reoccur and cause airway obstruction. It is therefore important to try to provide a calm recovery with a slow return to consciousness so that there are no sudden increases in activity that require increased respiratory effort or that will stimulate coughing. Antitussives, acepromazine, and α_2-adrenergic receptor agonists can be extremely helpful if administered close to the time of extubation. In order to reduce the risk of coughing, it may be prudent to remove the ETT earlier than normal. A technique for applying CPAP via facemask has been described, which may prove useful for these patients [52].

Many extra- or intra-luminal stents have been inserted in dogs with tracheal collapse [53]. With the placement of extraluminal stents, the anesthetic management is as above. For intraluminal stents, the dog must be intubated initially for tracheal size measurement. This is achieved by placing an ETT just past the larynx and inflating the lungs to 20 cm H_2O. The relevant tracheal diameter is then measured using known measurement markers in the image (e.g., fluoroscopy with image capture). In small patients, it is not possible to deploy the stent through the ETT so anesthesia must be maintained using injectable anesthetics such as propofol or alfaxalone and oxygen supplemented by insufflation or jet ventilation during placement.

Red blood cell potassium

Dogs are unusual in having low potassium concentrations in their erythrocytes. Concentrations around 5–6 mmol/L are usually found in most canine erythrocytes but there are a number of breeds, including the Akita, Shiba Inu, and some other Japanese breeds, that may have high potassium concentrations. This only becomes a concern when blood is stored. In citrate-phosphate-dextrose-adenine (CPDA-1) stored canine blood, plasma potassium increased to over 8 mmol/L after 30 days of storage but in human stored red cells (where the erythrocytes contain higher concentrations of potassium), the plasma potassium increased to 30 mmol/L at 3 weeks and to 44 mmol/L by 6 weeks [54,55]. Even with these higher concentrations of potassium, it is unlikely to significantly raise plasma potassium during a single unit transfusion in humans but when multiple units are used, it can result in hyperkalemia [56].

Cats

Handling and behavior

Recommendations for feline-friendly handling have been developed by the American Association of Feline Practitioners and the International Society of Feline Medicine and endorsed by the American Animal Hospital Association [57,58]. In particular, handling a fearful or aggressive cat may be challenging. Recommendations for managing these cats include training prior to the visit to get them used to the cat carrier and being in the vehicle. A number of drugs have been used to calm animals prior to transportation and these include gabapentin, trazodone, α_2-adrenergic receptor agonists, acepromazine, alprazolam, and melatonin [59,60] (Table 50.2). Gabapentin has been examined in a number of studies and has been shown to reduce the stress of transport, sedate the cat, and facilitate handling at the clinic [61–63]. The pharmacokinetics of the drug are significantly altered in cats with chronic kidney disease, suggesting that lower doses should be used in these animals [64]. Presedating a cat with gabapentin does not appear to alter acute antinociception [65]. Gabapentin administered IV to cats did not appear to affect inhalant anesthetic minimum alveolar concentration (MAC), but oral administration resulted in a 32% reduction in MAC [66,67]. These different results may be simply due to dose, although this is deemed unlikely. The highest plasma concentration in the IV study maintained the peak plasma concentration expected after approximately 25 mg/kg orally for the duration of MAC determination. Although the oral study used 30 mg/kg, the plasma concentration would be expected to gradually decrease below its peak over time, likely resulting in limited differences between the IV and oral studies at the time of MAC measurement [66]. A dose of 10–20 mg/kg can be used as a starting point and it has been suggested that it be given the night before and on the day of the visit, ideally 2–3 h before travel. Trazodone can also decrease anxiety associated with transportation and entering the clinic and it may ensure that the cat is easier to manage in the clinic [68]. A number of behavioral side effects are reported with trazodone, including vomiting, diarrhea, hypersalivation, excitation, and ataxia. Dexmedetomidine, in the form of Sileo® gel for mucosal application, which is licensed in dogs to treat fear of loud noises, has been used off-label in cats. Use of the injectable solution of dexmedetomidine for buccal administration has also been examined [69]. As with any α_2-adrenergic receptor agonist, it can produce profound sedation and may induce vomiting. Alprazolam is a benzodiazepine but there are no studies in cats showing its value in this setting. Although it is classified as an anxiolytic, excitation has been reported with the use of two other benzodiazepines in cats (midazolam and diazepam), so it may not be the most reliable drug to use for this purpose [70]. Acepromazine is usually criticized by behaviorists as not being an anxiolytic, but it is an ataractic that tends to decrease the animal's awareness of its surroundings. It is best to use the injectable solution for buccal administration, which facilitates administration by the owner. Although the sedation with

Table 50.2 Drugs used for decreasing anxiety and/or causing sedation in cats in preparation for visits to a veterinary hospital.

Medication	Form and concentration	Feline dose and route	Onset	Duration	Adverse effects
Dexmedetomidine	Injectable solution 0.5 mg/mL	20–40 μg/kg Buccal	30–40 min	1.5–2 h	Vomiting Hypersalivation
Dexmedetomidine	Gel (Sileo® 0.1 mg/mL)	20–40 μg/kg Buccal	30–40 min	1.5–2 h	Vomiting Hypersalivation
Trazodone	Tablets 50 or 100 mg	50–100 mg per cat Oral	90–150 min	3–4 h	Ataxia Vomiting, gagging, diarrhea Salivation Paradoxical excitation Behavioral disinhibition
Gabapentin	Capsules 100 or 300 mg	100 mg/cat (may increase to 30 or 40 mg/kg if needed) Oral	90–180 min	8 h	Ataxia Vomiting Salivation
Alprazolam	Tablets 0.25 mg	0.0125–0.025 mg/kg 0.125 mg/cat Oral	30–60 min	Not reported	Ataxia Paradoxical excitation Behavioral disinhibition
Melatonin	Tablets 1, 3, or 5 mg	3–5 mg/cat Oral		Not reported	
Acepromazine	Injectable solution 10 mg/mL	0.01–0.05 mg/kg Buccal	20–30 min	Variable	

acepromazine in cats is rarely profound, it may decrease the animal's reactiveness to transportation and examination, but there are no studies supporting this application. Acepromazine may decrease the dose of drug needed for induction and maintenance of anesthesia [71]. Melatonin has been shown to have a calming effect in some cats [72]. One group has been using a combination of gabapentin and melatonin for preoperative sedation and has anecdotally reported positive effects with this combination [59].

Fractious cats may require sedation prior to handling. Several agents and combinations have been reported to be effective. In particular, α_2-adrenergic receptor agonists alone or combined with opioids or dissociative anesthetics, and dissociative anesthetics usually combined with acepromazine or a benzodiazepine, appear to produce consistent, dose-dependent sedation in cats [73–79]. α_2-Adrenergic receptor agonist–ketamine combinations have been shown to be effective following oral administration [80–82] and tiletamine–zolazepam produced profound sedation following buccal administration [83]. Alfaxalone alone or in combination with α_2-adrenergic receptor agonists, ketamine, midazolam, and/or opioids produces sedation following intramuscular administration, although the quality of sedation may be variable [84–89].

Behaviors associated with acute and chronic pain may be difficult to detect in cats. Particular attention should be given to loss of normal behavior, such as decreased appetite, decreased grooming, or decreased activity; expression of abnormal behaviors, such as inappropriate elimination, vocalization, aggression, altered facial expression, or hiding; and reaction to touch or palpation of the painful area [90]. A few tools for the assessment of acute pain have recently been validated in cats. These include the short and long UNESP-Botucatu scales for feline pain assessment, the Feline Grimace Scale, and the Glasgow composite measure pain scale – feline [91–93]. All have limitations that are important to recognize when making decisions on whether analgesic treatment is warranted [94].

Drug metabolism in cats

It is documented that important metabolic differences exist between cats and dogs or humans; dose extrapolation from these latter species to cats should therefore be done with caution. In particular, the activity of UDP-glucuronosyltransferase (UGT), an enzyme involved in the conjugation of many substrates, is much lower in cats than in dogs and humans [95–97]. This results, for example, in a reduced ability to eliminate acetaminophen (paracetamol), with a high potential for toxicity. The genetic cause for this low enzymatic activity has been identified; cats have a nonfunctional pseudogene for UGT1A6 [95]. In addition, cats may also have reduced Phase I metabolism (oxidation, reduction, and hydrolysis) compared to other species, due to lower activity of some hepatic cytochrome P450 (CYP) enzymes. It has been reported that the activities of CYP1A, CYP2C, CYP2D, CYP2E, and CYP3A were lower in feline than in canine and human hepatic microsomes, but the activity of CYP2B was comparable [98]. This may contribute to the differences in drug metabolism observed in cats, compared to dogs or humans. For example, a study on the pharmacokinetics of tramadol, reported that the rate at which *O*-desmethyltramadol (the metabolite likely responsible for the opioid effect of tramadol) was produced appeared to be similar to that of humans deficient in CYP2D6, who get less pain relief from this drug compared to "good metabolizers" [99]. Another example of interest in anesthesia is propofol. The clearance of propofol was reported to be at least twice as fast in dogs than in cats [100–102]. Propofol is metabolized through glucuronidation by UGT and hydrolysis by CYP2B6 and CYP2C in humans [103]; in dogs, the rate-limiting step was reported to be mediated by CYP2B11 [104]. It is therefore unclear, based on the study cited above reporting similar activities of CYP2B in dogs and cats, why cats clear propofol much more slowly than dogs. The differences in metabolism of propofol may have clinical consequences, as increasing the duration of propofol infusion has been reported to significantly prolong recovery in cats [105].

Inhalant anesthetics

The potency of inhalant anesthetics, as characterized by their MAC, tends to be higher in cats than in many other species, including dogs and horses [67,106–117]. Nitrous oxide was found to decrease the MAC of halothane, but when combined with isoflurane, the effect was inconsistent [107,117]. While, to these authors' knowledge, there is no study directly comparing the effects of inhalant anesthetics in dogs and cats, clinical experience suggests that at similar anesthetic depth, blood pressure tends to be lower in cats than in dogs. Some evidence for this can be found by comparing studies in which inhalant anesthetics were administered at similar multiples of their MAC in both species. Such studies show that, at moderate inhalant anesthetic concentrations, blood pressure and cardiac index are more depressed in cats than in dogs [115,118–121].

Opioids

In cats, opioids cause pupillary dilation and sometimes excitation [122]. Opioid-induced manic behavior in cats is only seen following administration of very high doses, that are not clinically relevant. In one study, the intraperitoneal administration of morphine at 1 mg/kg did not induce manic response, whereas 5, 10, and 20 mg/kg induced excitement in 1, 2, and 5 out of 5 cats, respectively [123]. At clinical doses, opioids cause analgesia and euphoria, and sometimes dysphoria [124–126]. It has been suggested that the effects of high-dose morphine may be characterized by a non-opioid receptor-mediated effect [127]. There is evidence that the manic response in cats is not due to the action of opioids *per se* but related to the release of monoamines [123].

Opioids may have biphasic effects on the cardiovascular system in cats. At low doses, they may lower heart rate and blood pressure, while large doses increase heart rate, cardiac output, and blood pressure [122,128]. These latter effects seem to be related to increased concentrations of circulating catecholamines, and do not occur in adrenalectomized cats [122,129]. Catecholamine-induced hemodynamic effects appear to be mediated centrally through opioid receptors, as they are prevented by naloxone [130].

Hyperthermia following opioid administration has been reported in cats [131–134]. *Severe hyperthermia* has been defined as a body temperature greater than 41.7 °C [133]. The effect may be dose-dependent and appears more consistent when higher doses are administered. In a retrospective clinical study, the administration of hydromorphone at doses between 0.05 and 0.1 mg/kg was strongly associated with rectal temperatures > 40 °C; this association was confirmed in a prospective clinical study [131,132]. In the research setting, a prospective study showed that clinically relevant doses of several opioids result in increased body temperature; however, in that study, the increase was mild-to-moderate, and body temperature remained < 40 °C in most cases [133].

Opioids decrease the dose of inhalant anesthetic required to produce immobility in cats [135]. However, the magnitude of the effect of full μ-opioid receptor agonists appears to be smaller in cats than in some other species and may be inconsistent; to the authors' knowledge, the largest reduction in MAC of an inhalant anesthetic induced by a full μ-opioid receptor agonist in cats was approximately 35%, following administration of alfentanil to produce very high plasma concentrations (500 ng/mL) [136]. For comparison, plasma alfentanil concentrations close to half the value targeted in the cat study (223 ng/mL) reduced MAC by 68.5% in dogs [137]. While different inhalant anesthetics were used in the dog and cat studies (enflurane and isoflurane, respectively), the difference in effect suggests a large difference in potency of alfentanil in the two species. Moreover, 35% was the maximum MAC reduction observed in cats (higher plasma concentrations did not result in a further decrease in MAC), whereas in dogs, the maximum mean MAC reduction induced by alfentanil was 72.5%. The variability in MAC reduction may also be larger in cats than in dogs, as illustrated by the fact that studies on the effect of the same opioid do not consistently detect a decrease in MAC [126,138]. A study comparing the effects of high plasma concentrations of fentanyl, alfentanil, and sufentanil on the MAC of isoflurane in cats found significant MAC reduction only during administration of alfentanil; the effect was antagonized by administration of naltrexone, suggesting that it is mediated by opioid receptors [139]. It has been suggested that this small effect of full μ-opioid receptor agonists on MAC may be related to the central sympathetic stimulation mentioned above, as combining fentanyl with acepromazine (a dopamine and α_1-adrenergic receptor antagonist) results in a large MAC reduction that is at least partially reversible with naltrexone [140]. In addition, butorphanol, a κ-opioid receptor agonist and μ-opioid receptor antagonist was reported to produce a plasma concentration-dependent reduction in MAC by up to 68% [141]. Butorphanol does not appear to result in sympathetic stimulation, providing additional support to the hypothesis that such stimulation is responsible for the limited effect of μ-opioid receptor agonists on MAC in cats.

Buprenorphine is commonly used in cats, based on studies reporting good efficacy and initial data suggesting excellent bioavailability and efficacy following buccal administration and oral transmucosal absorption [142–144]. However, more recent studies have reported lower bioavailability and limited efficacy of buccal buprenorphine in nociceptive threshold models [145]. Subcutaneous administration of low to moderate doses of buprenorphine is reported to result in erratic absorption [146]. However, subcutaneous administration of a high dose of a concentrated (1.8 mg/mL) formulation of buprenorphine (Simbadol®) to cats resulted in consistent and prolonged absorption, providing antinociception for a minimum of 24 h [147]. The label dose of this formulation appears to result in a high incidence of hyperthermia [148]. We have also observed a high incidence of dysphoria. A transdermal buprenorphine formulation (Zorbium®) was approved in the United States in 2022 for the control of postoperative pain in cats. A single administration results in analgesia with an onset of 2 h and a duration of up to 4 days. This formulation appears to result in a high incidence of hyperthermia, although the clinical significance of this finding has been questioned [149–151].

Non-steroidal anti-inflammatory drugs

The use of non-steroidal anti-inflammatory drugs (NSAIDs) in cats has been reviewed [152–155]. These drugs are commonly used in cats for their anti-inflammatory and analgesic properties; however, caution is recommended, since glucuronide conjugation is a major metabolic pathway for many of these drugs [153]. The incidence of adverse effects (renal injury, hepatotoxicity, gastrointestinal ulceration, and abnormal hemostasis) in cats may therefore be higher than in some other species, due to larger exposure following a given dose. The use of prostaglandin synthase-2 (COX-2) selective or specific agents may decrease the risk for some, but not all of these adverse effects. Nevertheless, there is favorable evidence for the short-term, typically perioperative use of several NSAIDs in cats, including carprofen [156–163], ketoprofen [156,159,164–166], tolfenamic acid [156,167,168], and robenacoxib [164,165,169–171]. With the exception of carprofen, these drugs are licensed for repeated administration in cats in some countries; in the United States, meloxicam is licensed for single administration, and robenacoxib for up to 3 days in that species.

Recommendations have been issued by a panel of experts on the long-term use of NSAIDs in cats [152]. A retrospective study suggested that meloxicam could be administered long term to cats at 0.02 mg/kg once daily, even if they have stable chronic kidney disease [172]. In that study, there was less progression of kidney disease in treated cats than in untreated cats. A few studies have evaluated the use of grapiprant, an EP4 prostaglandin receptor antagonist in cats [173,174]. Analgesic efficacy appeared inferior to that of carprofen following ovariohysterectomy [174].

Endotracheal intubation

The Confidential Enquiry into Perioperative Small Animal Fatalities found that endotracheal intubation increased the odds of anesthetic-related death in cats by a factor of approximately two [175]. Previous studies have also suggested that endotracheal intubation was associated with major complications in cats [176,177]. The reasons for these findings are not entirely clear; however, they may be related to the small size of the cat's upper airway, and to the laryngeal responsiveness to mechanical stimulation in that species. Laryngeal spasms can be produced in anesthetized and decerebrate cats by mechanical stimulation of the soft palate, pharynx, larynx, and trachea [178,179]. It has been recommended to desensitize the larynx with a local anesthetic or to use a short-acting neuromuscular blocking agent prior to intubation in cats in order to decrease the incidence of laryngeal spasm [180–182]; nevertheless, it is possible that improper intubation technique would be more likely to cause complications in cats than in dogs.

Tracheal avulsion or rupture and bronchial rupture have been reported in cats [183–188]. In the majority of cases, tracheal rupture was associated with intubation. It was hypothesized that cuff overinflation, possibly in combination with multiple position changes, was likely the mechanism. Associated clinical signs were subcutaneous emphysema, coughing, gagging, dyspnea, anorexia, and fever. Surgical and conservative management were successful unless the injury extended to the carina.

Cortical blindness

Postanesthetic cortical blindness has been reported in cats [189,190]. According to one case series, the blindness is temporary in the majority of cases, and the use of mouth gags may be a risk factor for postanesthetic blindness, due to cerebral ischemia [189]. A study evaluating blood flow in the maxillary artery (the main source of blood supply to the retinae and brain) in anesthetized cats using imaging techniques showed that the use of spring-loaded mouth gags to open the mouth maximally resulted in alterations in blood flow and the electroretinogram in some cats [191]. The authors concluded that mechanical occlusion of blood flow through the maxillary artery during maximal opening of the mouth may contribute to the pathogenesis of postanesthetic blindness due to reduced blood flow to the retina.

Fluid therapy and blood volume

The Confidential Enquiry into Perioperative Small Animal Fatalities suggested that the administration of intravenous fluids during anesthesia resulted in an approximately fourfold increase in the risk of death [175]. While the reasons for this finding are not entirely clear, excessive fluid administration resulting in fluid overload was suspected to be at least partly responsible. Cats may be at higher risk of fluid overload and/or excessive dilution of blood components than dogs, particularly when large amounts of fluids are rapidly administered, because their blood volume is somewhat smaller. Blood volume in cats has been reported to be 56–67 mL/kg [192–194]. Rapid fluid administration during inhalant anesthesia may also be more frequent in cats than in dogs, since blood pressure tends to be lower at similar anesthetic concentrations (see inhalant anesthetics above). Moreover, due to their small size, cats may be more likely to inadvertently receive excessive fluid volumes than larger species. Rate of fluid administration is typically based on body weight; based on the considerations above, it may be preferable to adjust these rates based on some fraction of blood volume. Expert consensus recommendations of 3 mL/kg/h of isotonic crystalloid for fluid therapy during anesthesia have been published [195].

Blood groups

Three blood groups – A, B, and AB – have been identified in cats [196,197]. Cats with type B blood have naturally occurring, strong hemagglutinating antibodies against type A cells, whereas cats with type A blood have naturally occurring, weak hemolyzing and hemagglutinating antibodies against type B cells [198]. Severe transfusion reactions of the anaphylactic type, with almost immediate destruction of the transfused red blood cells, are therefore commonly observed if type A blood is transfused to a cat with type B blood; cats with type A blood receiving type B blood typically only develop mild transfusion reactions [198,199]. In addition, naturally occurring antibodies against a common antigen, Mik, has been found to be involved in acute hemolytic transfusion reactions following an AB-matched transfusion [200]. Typing and cross-matching are therefore essential prior to blood transfusion in cats [201,202]. Consensus statements on prevention and monitoring of transfusion reactions have been developed [203,204].

Prevalence of the different blood types has been reported for various geographical locations [197,198,205–218]. Type A blood has the highest prevalence, ranging from 62 to 99.6%; in the United States, close to 100% of domestic cats are type A. The prevalence of type B blood ranges from 0.4 to 36%, the latter being reported for the Sydney area of Australia. Cats with type AB blood are rare, representing 5% or less of the feline population (less than 0.2% in North America).

Prevalence of B blood is moderate-to-high (15–60%) in some cat breeds, including British shorthair, Abyssinian, Birman, Devon Rex, Himalayan, Persian, Scottish Fold, Somali, Angora, and Turkish Van, whereas it is very low (close to 0%) in other breeds, including American shorthair, Siamese, and Norwegian Forest [198,211,219].

Dopamine and dopamine receptors

Dopamine is commonly used in anesthetized cats to treat hypotension. Within the range of clinical doses, its effect is believed to be due to an increase in cardiac contractility, mediated by activation of β_1-adrenergic receptors. A study demonstrated increases in cardiac index without significant increase in vascular resistance at doses, ranging from 2.5 to 20 μg/kg/min [220]. Another, more controversial indication for low doses of dopamine is to increase renal blood flow, particularly in acute renal failure. The effect is postulated to be due to activation of dopamine D_1 receptors, causing renal vasodilation and increased renal blood flow. It is unclear whether cats would respond to dopamine in that manner. D_1 receptors have been identified in feline kidneys; however, they appear different from the human and canine D_1 receptors [221]. Regardless, studies in humans have failed to demonstrate benefits of low-dose dopamine in acute renal failure and suggest that some effects may actually be detrimental [222,223]. In cats with renal failure, the use of dopamine may be indicated at doses that increase cardiac output, particularly during hypotension, rather than at doses targeting D_1 receptors.

References

1 Price GS, Frazier DL. Use of body surface area (BSA)-based dosages to calculate chemotherapeutic drug dose in dogs: I. Potential problems with current BSA formulae. *J Vet Intern Med* 1998; **12**(4): 267–271.
2 Coffee C, Roush JK, Higginbotham ML. Carboplatin-induced myelosuppression as related to body weight in dogs. *Vet Comp Oncol* 2020; **18**(4): 804–810.
3 Girens R, Bukoski A, Maitz CA, *et al.* Use of computed tomography and radiation therapy planning software to develop a novel formula for body surface area calculation in dogs. *J Vet Intern Med* 2019; **33**(2): 792–799.
4 Mahmood I. Application of allometric principles for the prediction of pharmacokinetics in human and veterinary drug development. *Adv Drug Deliv Rev* 2007; **59**(11): 1177–1192.
5 Krejcie TC, Avram MJ. What determines anesthetic induction dose? It's the front-end kinetics, doctor! *Anesth Analg* 1999; **89**(3): 541–544.
6 McGreevy PD, Thomson PC, Pride C, *et al.* Prevalence of obesity in dogs examined by Australian veterinary practices and the risk factors involved. *Vet Rec* 2005; **156**(22): 695–702.
7 Scarlett JM, Donoghue S, Saidla J, *et al.* Overweight cats: prevalence and risk factors. *Int J Obes Relat Metab Disord* 1994; **18**(Suppl 1): S22–S28.
8 Association for Prevention of Pet Obesity. https://petobesityprevention.org/2018
9 Kaltman AJ, Goldring RM. Role of circulatory congestion in the cardiorespiratory failure of obesity. *Am J Med* 1976; **60**(5): 645–653.
10 Olutoye OA, Yu X, Govindan K, *et al.* The effect of obesity on the ED(95) of propofol for loss of consciousness in children and adolescents. *Anesth Analg* 2012; **115**(1): 147–153.
11 Devito FC, Patricio GCF, Flor PB, *et al.* Comparative study of anaesthesia induction in obese dogs using propofol dosages based on lean body weight or total body weight. *Vet Anim Sci* 2020; **10**: 100131.
12 Clutton RE. The medical implications of canine obesity and their relevance to anaesthesia. *Brit Vet J* 1988; **144**(1): 21–28.
13 Love L, Cline MG. Perioperative physiology and pharmacology in the obese small animal patient. *Vet Anaesth Analg* 2015; **42**(2): 119–132.
14 Davidson IW, Parker JC, Beliles RP. Biological basis for extrapolation across mammalian species. *Regul Toxicol Pharmacol* 1986; **6**(3): 211–237.
15 Adolph EF. Quantitative relations in the physiological constitutions of mammals. *Science* 1949; **109**(2841): 579–585.
16 Boxenbaum H. Interspecies variation in liver weight, hepatic blood flow, and antipyrine intrinsic clearance: extrapolation of data to benzodiazepines and phenytoin. *J Pharmacokinet Biopharm* 1980; **8**(2): 165–176.
17 Bronson RT. Brain weight-body weight scaling in breeds of dogs and cats. *Brain Behav Evol* 1979; **16**(3): 227–236.
18 Court MH. Anesthesia of the sighthound. *Clin Tech Small Anim Pract* 1999; **14**(1): 38–43.
19 Parker HG, Kim LV, Sutter NB, *et al.* Genetic structure of the purebred domestic dog. *Science* 2004; **304**(5674): 1160–1164.
20 Bogan J. Factors affecting duration of thiopentone anaesthesia in dogs, with particular reference to greyhounds. *Proc Assoc Vet Anaesth Gr Br Ir* 1970; **1**: 18–24.
21 Sams RA, Muir WW, Detra RL, *et al.* Comparative pharmacokinetics and anesthetic effects of methohexital, pentobarbital, thiamylal, and thiopental in Greyhound dogs and non- Greyhound, mixed-breed dogs. *Am J Vet Res* 1985; **46**(8): 1677–1683.
22 Pasloske K, Sauer B, Perkins N, *et al.* Plasma pharmacokinetics of alfaxalone in both premedicated and unpremedicated Greyhound dogs after single, intravenous administration of Alfaxan at a clinical dose. *J Vet Pharmacol Ther* 2009; **32**(5): 510–513.
23 Zoran DL, Riedesel DH, Dyer DC. Pharmacokinetics of propofol in mixed-breed dogs and greyhounds. *Am J Vet Res* 1993; **54**(5): 755–760.

24 Sams RA, Muir WW. Effects of phenobarbital on thiopental pharmacokinetics in greyhounds. *Am J Vet Res* 1988; **49**(2): 245–249.

25 KuKanich B, KuKanich K, Rankin D, *et al.* The effect of fluconazole on oral methadone in dogs. *Vet Anaesth Analg* 2019; **46**(4): 501–509.

26 Hofmeister EH, Watson V, Snyder LB, *et al.* Validity and client use of information from the World Wide Web regarding veterinary anesthesia in dogs. *J Am Vet Med Assoc* 2008; **233**(12): 1860–1864.

27 Tournier N, Decleves X, Saubamea B, *et al.* Opioid transport by ATP-binding cassette transporters at the blood–brain barrier: implications for neuropsychopharmacology. *Curr Pharm Des* 2011; **17**(26): 2829–2842.

28 Hassan HE, Myers AL, Coop A, *et al.* Differential involvement of P-glycoprotein (ABCB1) in permeability, tissue distribution, and antinociceptive activity of methadone, buprenorphine, and diprenorphine: in vitro and in vivo evaluation. *J Pharm Sci* 2009; **98**(12): 4928–2940.

29 Dagenais C, Graff CL, Pollack GM. Variable modulation of opioid brain uptake by P-glycoprotein in mice. *Biochem Pharmacol* 2004; **67**(2): 269–276.

30 Hassan HE, Mercer SL, Cunningham CW, *et al.* Evaluation of the P-glycoprotein (ABCB1) affinity status of a series of morphine analogs: comparative study with meperidine analogs to identify opioids with minimal P-glycoprotein interactions. *Int J Pharm* 2009; **375**(1–2): 48–54.

31 Groenendaal D, Freijer J, Rosier A, *et al.* Pharmacokinetic/pharmacodynamic modelling of the EEG effects of opioids: the role of complex biophase distribution kinetics. *Eur J Pharm Sci* 2008; **34**(2–3): 149–163.

32 Brown SM, Campbell SD, Crafford A, *et al.* P-glycoprotein is a major determinant of norbuprenorphine brain exposure and antinociception. *J Pharmacol Exp Ther* 2012; **343**(1): 53–61.

33 Popovic NA, Mullane JF, Yhap EO. Effects of acetylpromazine maleate on certain cardiorespiratory responses in dogs. *Am J Vet Res* 1972; **33**(9): 1819–1824.

34 Brodbelt DC, Pfeiffer DU, Young LE, *et al.* Results of the Confidential Enquiry into Perioperative Small Animal Fatalities regarding risk factors for anesthetic-related death in dogs. *J Am Vet Med Assoc* 2008; **233**(7): 1096–1104.

35 Dyson DH, Maxie MG, Schnurr D. Morbidity and mortality associated with anesthetic management in small animal veterinary practice in Ontario. *J Am Anim Hosp Assoc* 1998; **34**(4): 325–335.

36 Denton TG, Du Toit DF, Reece-Smith H. Reactions to Althesin in dogs. *Anaesthesia* 1980; **35**(6): 615–616.

37 Bomzon L. A limited trial of Saffan in the dog. *J Small Anim Pract* 1981; **22**(12): 769–773.

38 Corbett HR. The use of Saffan in the dog. *Aust Vet Pract* 1977; **7**(3): 184–188.

39 Robinson EP, Faggella AM, Henry DP, *et al.* Comparison of histamine release induced by morphine and oxymorphone administration in dogs. *Am J Vet Res* 1988; **49**(10): 1699–1701.

40 Flacke JW, Flacke WE, Bloor BC, *et al.* Histamine release by four narcotics: a double-blind study in humans. *Anesth Analg* 1987; **66**(8): 723–730.

41 Philbin DM, Moss J, Rosow CE, *et al.* Histamine release with intravenous narcotics: protective effects of H1 and H2-receptor antagonists. *Klin Wochenschr* 1982; **60**(17): 1056–1059.

42 Banovic F, Denley T, Blubaugh A, *et al.* Effect of diphenhydramine and cetirizine on immediate and late-phase cutaneous allergic reactions in healthy dogs: a randomized, double-blinded crossover study. *Vet Dermatol* 2020; **31**(4): 256–258.

43 Curley TL, Thamm DH, Johnson SW, *et al.* Effects of morphine on histamine release from two cell lines of canine mast cell tumor and on plasma histamine concentrations in dogs with cutaneous mast cell tumor. *Am J Vet Res* 2021; **82**(12): 1013–1018.

44 De Lorenzi D, Bertoncello D, Drigo M. Bronchial abnormalities found in a consecutive series of 40 brachycephalic dogs. *J Am Vet Med Assoc* 2009; **235**(7): 835–840.

45 Oechtering TH, Oechtering GU, Noller C. Structural characteristics of the nose in brachycephalic dog breeds analysed by computed tomography. *Tierarztl Prax Ausg K Kleintiere Heimtiere* 2007; **35**(3): 177–187.

46 Hoareau GL, Jourdan G, Mellema M, *et al.* Evaluation of arterial blood gases and arterial blood pressures in brachycephalic dogs. *J Vet Intern Med* 2012; **26**(4): 897–904.

47 Johnson LR, Pollard RE. Tracheal collapse and bronchomalacia in dogs: 58 cases (7 /2001–1 /2008). *J Vet Intern Med* 2010; **24**(2): 298–305.

48 Pardali D, Adamama-Moraitou KK, Rallis TS, *et al.* Tidal breathing flow-volume loop analysis for the diagnosis and staging of tracheal collapse in dogs. *J Vet Intern Med* 2010; **24**(4): 832–842.

49 White RAS, Williams JM. Tracheal collapse in the dog – is there really a role for surgery? A survey of 100 cases. *J Small Anim Pract* 1994; **35**(4): 191–196.

50 Adamama-Moraitou KK, Pardali D, Athanasiou LV, *et al.* Conservative management of canine tracheal collapse with stanozolol: a double blinded, placebo control clinical trial. *Int J Immunopathol Pharmacol* 2011; **24**(1): 111–118.

51 Congiusta M, Weisse C, Berent AC, *et al.* Comparison of short-, intermediate-, and long-term results between dogs with tracheal collapse that underwent multimodal medical management alone and those that underwent tracheal endoluminal stent placement. *J Am Vet Med Assoc* 2021; **258**(3): 279–289.

52 Briganti A, Melanie P, Portela D, *et al.* Continuous positive airway pressure administered via face mask in tranquilized dogs. *J Vet Emerg Crit Care* 2010; **20**(5): 503–508.

53 Sun F, Uson J, Ezquerra J, *et al.* Endotracheal stenting therapy in dogs with tracheal collapse. *Vet J* 2008; **175**(2): 186–193.

54 Karon BS, van Buskirk CM, Jaben EA, *et al.* Temporal sequence of major biochemical events during blood bank storage of packed red blood cells. *Blood Transfus* 2012; **10**(4): 453–461.

55 Maede Y, Amano Y, Nishida A, *et al.* Hereditary high-potassium erythrocytes with high Na, K-ATPase activity in Japanese shiba dogs. *Res Vet Sci* 1991; **50**(1): 123–125.

56 Vraets A, Lin Y, Callum JL. Transfusion-associated hyperkalemia. *Transfus Med Rev* 2011; **25**(3): 184–196.

57 Rodan I, Sundahl E, Carney H, *et al.* AAFP and ISFM feline-friendly handling guidelines. *J Feline Med Surg* 2011; **13**(5): 364–375.

58 Rodan I, Dowgray N, Carney HC, *et al.* 2022 AAFP/ISFM cat friendly veterinary interaction guidelines: approach and handling techniques. *J Feline Med Surg* 2022; **24**(11): 1093–1132.

59 Karas A. Reducing patient anxiety: orally administered agents for reducing the impact of hospital visits. *IVECCS* 2021 (Abtract); 39–43.

60 Erickson A, Harbin K, MacPherson J, *et al.* A review of pre-appointment medications to reduce fear and anxiety in dogs and cats at veterinary visits. *Can Vet J* 2021; **62**(9): 952–960.

61 Allen ME, LeBlanc NL, Scollan KF. Hemodynamic, echocardiographic, and sedative effects of oral gabapentin in healthy cats. *J Am Anim Hosp Assoc* 2021; **57**(6): 278–284.

62 van Haaften KA, Forsythe LRE, Stelow EA, *et al.* Effects of a single preappointment dose of gabapentin on signs of stress in cats during transportation and veterinary examination. *J Am Vet Med Assoc* 2017; **251**(10): 1175–1181.

63 Hudec CP, Griffin CE. Changes in the stress markers cortisol and glucose before and during intradermal testing in cats after single administration of pre-appointment gabapentin. *J Feline Med Surg* 2020; **22**(2): 138–145.

64 Quimby JM, Lorbach SK, Saffire A, *et al.* Serum concentrations of gabapentin in cats with chronic kidney disease. *J Feline Med Surg* 2022; **24**(12): 1260–1266.

65 Pypendop BH, Siao KT, Ilkiw JE. Thermal antinociceptive effect of orally administered gabapentin in healthy cats. *Am J Vet Res* 2010; **71**(9): 1027–1032.

66 Chen H, Yang H, Li M, *et al.* Effect of oral administration of gabapentin on the minimum alveolar concentration of isoflurane in cats. *Front Vet Sci* 2023; **10**: 1117313.

67 Reid P, Pypendop BH, Ilkiw JE. The effects of intravenous gabapentin administration on the minimum alveolar concentration of isoflurane in cats. *Anesth Analg* 2010; **111**(3): 633–637.

68 Stevens BJ, Frantz EM, Orlando JM, *et al.* Efficacy of a single dose of trazodone hydrochloride given to cats prior to veterinary visits to reduce signs of transport- and examination-related anxiety. *J Am Vet Med Assoc* 2016; **249**(2): 202–207.

69 Slingsby LS, Taylor PM, Monroe T. Thermal antinociception after dexmedetomidine administration in cats: a comparison between intramuscular and oral transmucosal administration. *J Feline Med Surg* 2009; **11**(10): 829–834.

70 Ilkiw JE, Suter CM, Farver TB, *et al.* The behaviour of healthy awake cats following intravenous and intramuscular administration of midazolam. *J Vet Pharmacol Ther* 1996; **19**(3): 205–216.

71 Heard DJ, Webb AI, Daniels RT. Effect of acepromazine on the anesthetic requirement of halothane in the dog. *Am J Vet Res* 1986; **47**(10): 2113–2115.

72 Ruviaro Tuleski GL, Silveira MF, Bastos RF, *et al.* Behavioral and cardiovascular effects of a single dose of gabapentin or melatonin in cats: a randomized, double-blind, placebo-controlled trial. *J Feline Med Surg* 2022; **24**(12): e524–e534.

73 Biermann K, Hungerbuhler S, Mischke R, *et al.* Sedative, cardiovascular, haematologic and biochemical effects of four different drug combinations administered intramuscularly in cats. *Vet Anaesth Analg* 2012; **39**(2): 137–150.

74 Selmi AL, Mendes GM, Lins BT, *et al.* Evaluation of the sedative and cardiorespiratory effects of dexmedetomidine, dexmedetomidine-butorphanol, and dexmedetomidine-ketamine in cats. *J Am Vet Med Assoc* 2003; **222**(1): 37–41.

75 Nagore L, Soler C, Gil L, *et al.* Sedative effects of dexmedetomidine, dexmedetomidine-pethidine and dexmedetomidine-butorphanol in cats. *J Vet Pharmacol Ther* 2013; **36**(3): 222–228.

76 Navarrete R, Dominguez JM, Granados Mdel M, *et al.* Sedative effects of three doses of romifidine in comparison with medetomidine in cats. *Vet Anaesth Analg* 2011; **38**(3): 178–185.

77 Selmi AL, Barbudo-Selmi GR, Mendes GM, *et al.* Sedative, analgesic and cardiorespiratory effects of romifidine in cats. *Vet Anaesth Analg* 2004; **31**(3): 195–206.

78 Ansah OB, Raekallio M, Vainio O. Comparison of three doses of dexmedetomidine with medetomidine in cats following intramuscular administration. *J Vet Pharmacol Ther* 1998; **21**(5): 380–387.

79 Dyson DH, Atilola M. A clinical comparison of oxymorphone-acepromazine and butorphanol-acepromazine sedation in dogs. *Vet Surg* 1992; **21**(5): 418–421.

80 Santos LC, Ludders JW, Erb HN, *et al.* Sedative and cardiorespiratory effects of dexmedetomidine and buprenorphine administered to cats via oral transmucosal or intramuscular routes. *Vet Anaesth Analg* 2010; **37**(5): 417–424.

81 Grove DM, Ramsay EC. Sedative and physiologic effects of orally administered alpha 2-adrenoceptor agonists and ketamine in cats. *J Am Vet Med Assoc* 2000; **216**(12): 1929–1932.

82 Wetzel RW, Ramsay EC. Comparison of four regimens for intraoral administration of medication to induce sedation in cats prior to euthanasia. *J Am Vet Med Assoc* 1998; **213**(2): 243–245.

83 Nejamkin P, Cavilla V, Clausse M, *et al.* Sedative and physiologic effects of tiletamine–zolazepam following buccal administration in cats. *J Feline Med Surg* 2020; **22**(2): 108–113.

84 Deutsch J, Jolliffe C, Archer E, *et al.* Intramuscular injection of alfaxalone in combination with butorphanol for sedation in cats. *Vet Anaesth Analg* 2017; **44**(4): 794–802.

85 Lazzarini E, Martinelli E, Brioschi FA, *et al.* Intramuscular alfaxalone and methadone with or without ketamine in healthy cats: effects on sedation and echocardiographic measurements. *Vet Anaesth Analg* 2020; **47**(5): 621–630.

86 Tamura J, Ishizuka T, Fukui S, *et al.* Sedative effects of intramuscular alfaxalone administered to cats. *J Vet Med Sci* 2015; **77**(8): 897–904.

87 Rodrigo-Mocholi D, Belda E, Bosmans T, *et al.* Clinical efficacy and cardiorespiratory effects of intramuscular administration of alfaxalone alone or in combination with dexmedetomidine in cats. *Vet Anaesth Analg* 2016; **43**(3): 291–300.

88 Cremer J, Ricco CH. Cardiovascular, respiratory and sedative effects of intramuscular alfaxalone, butorphanol and dexmedetomidine compared with ketamine, butorphanol and dexmedetomidine in healthy cats. *J Feline Med Surg* 2018; **20**(10): 973–979.

89 Wheeler EP, Abelson AL, Lindsey JC, *et al.* Sedative effects of alfaxalone and hydromorphone with or without midazolam in cats: a pilot study. *J Feline Med Surg* 2021; **23**(12): 1109–1116.

90 Hellyer P, Rodan I, Brunt J, *et al.* AAHA/AAFP pain management guidelines for dogs and cats. *J Feline Med Surg* 2007; **9**(6): 466–480.

91 Belli M, de Oliveira AR, de Lima MT, *et al.* Clinical validation of the short and long UNESP-Botucatu scales for feline pain assessment. *Peer J* 2021; **9**: e11225.

92 Evangelista MC, Watanabe R, Leung VSY, *et al.* Facial expressions of pain in cats: the development and validation of a Feline Grimace Scale. *Sci Rep* 2019; **9**(1): 19128.

93 Reid J, Scott EM, Calvo G, *et al.* Definitive Glasgow acute pain scale for cats: validation and intervention level. *Vet Rec* 2017; **180**(18): 449.

94 Steagall PV, Monteiro BP. Acute pain in cats: recent advances in clinical assessment. *J Feline Med Surg* 2019; **21**(1): 25–34.

95 Court MH, Greenblatt DJ. Molecular genetic basis for deficient acetaminophen glucuronidation by cats: UGT1A6 is a pseudogene, and evidence for reduced diversity of expressed hepatic UGT1A isoforms. *Pharmacogenetics* 2000; **10**(4): 355–369.

96 Court MH, Greenblatt DJ. Molecular basis for deficient acetaminophen glucuronidation in cats. An interspecies comparison of enzyme kinetics in liver microsomes. *Biochem Pharmacol* 1997; **53**(7): 1041–1047.

97 Court MH, Greenblatt DJ. Biochemical basis for deficient paracetamol glucuronidation in cats: an interspecies comparison of enzyme constraint in liver microsomes. *J Pharm Pharmacol* 1997; **49**(4): 446–449.

98 van Beusekom CD, Schipper L, Fink-Gremmels J. Cytochrome P450-mediated hepatic metabolism of new fluorescent substrates in cats and dogs. *J Vet Pharmacol Ther* 2010; **33**(6): 519–527.

99 Pypendop BH, Ilkiw JE. Pharmacokinetics of tramadol, and its metabolite O-desmethyl-tramadol, in cats. *J Vet Pharmacol Ther* 2008; **31**(1): 52–59.

100 Cleale RM, Muir WW, Waselau AC, *et al.* Pharmacokinetic and pharmacodynamic evaluation of propofol administered to cats in a novel, aqueous, nano-droplet formulation or as an oil-in-water macroemulsion. *J Vet Pharmacol Ther* 2009; **32**(5): 436–445.

101 Hughes JM, Nolan AM. Total intravenous anesthesia in greyhounds: pharmacokinetics of propofol and fentanyl--a preliminary study. *Vet Surg* 1999; **28**(6): 513–524.

102 Cockshott ID, Douglas EJ, Plummer GF, *et al.* The pharmacokinetics of propofol in laboratory animals. *Xenobiotica* 1992; **22**(3): 369–375.

103 Restrepo JG, Garcia-Martin E, Martinez C, *et al.* Polymorphic drug metabolism in anaesthesia. *Curr Drug Metab* 2009; **10**(3): 236–246.

104 Hay Kraus BL, Greenblatt DJ, Venkatakrishnan K, *et al.* Evidence for propofol hydroxylation by cytochrome P4502B11 in canine liver microsomes: breed and gender differences. *Xenobiotica* 2000; **30**(6): 575–588.

105 Pascoe PJ, Ilkiw JE, Frischmeyer KJ. The effect of the duration of propofol administration on recovery from anesthesia in cats. *Vet Anaesth Analg* 2006; **33**(1): 2–7.

106 Brown BR Jr., Crout JR. A comparative study of the effects of five general anesthetics on myocardial contractility. *I. Isometric conditions. Anesthesiology* 1971; **34**(3): 236–245.

107 Steffey EP, Gillespie JR, Berry JD, *et al.* Anesthetic potency (MAC) of nitrous oxide in the dog, cat, and stump-tail monkey. *J Appl Physiol* 1974; **36**(5): 530–532.

108 Drummond JC, Todd MM, Shapiro HM. Minimal alveolar concentrations for halothane, enflurane, and isoflurane in the cat. *J Am Vet Med Assoc* 1983; **182**(10): 1099–1101.

109 Webb AI, McMurphy RM. Effect of anticholinergic preanesthetic medicaments on the requirements of halothane for anesthesia in the cat. *Am J Vet Res* 1987; **48**(12): 1733–1735.

110 Steffey EP, Howland D Jr., Giri S, *et al.* Enflurane, halothane, and isoflurane potency in horses. *Am J Vet Res* 1977; **38**(7): 1037–1039.

111 Doi M, Yunoki H, Ikeda K. The minimum alveolar concentration of sevoflurane in cats. *J Anesth* 1988; **2**(1): 113–114.

112 McMurphy R, Hodgson D. The minimum alveolar concentration of desflurane in cats. *Vet Surg* 1995; **24**(5): 453–455.

113 Barter LS, Ilkiw JE, Steffey EP, *et al.* Animal dependence of inhaled anaesthetic requirements in cats. *Br J Anaesth* 2004; **92**(2): 275–277.

114 Pypendop BH, Ilkiw JE. The effects of intravenous lidocaine administration on the minimum alveolar concentration of isoflurane in cats. *Anesth Analg* 2005; **100**(1): 97–101.

115 Pypendop BH, Ilkiw JE. Hemodynamic effects of sevoflurane in cats. *Am J Vet Res* 2004; **65**(1): 20–25.

116 Escobar A, Pypendop BH, Siao KT, *et al.* Effect of dexmedetomidine on the minimum alveolar concentration of isoflurane in cats. *J Vet Pharmacol Ther* 2012; **35**(2): 163–168.

117 Imai A, Ilkiw JE, Pypendop BH, *et al.* Nitorus oxide does not consistently reduce isoflurane requirement in cats. *Vet Anaesth Analg* 2002; **19**(2): 98.

118 Mutoh T, Nishimura R, Kim HY, *et al.* Cardiopulmonary effects of sevoflurane, compared with halothane, enflurane, and isoflurane, in dogs. *Am J Vet Res* 1997; **58**(8): 885–890.

119 Grandy JL, Hodgson DS, Dunlop CI, *et al.* Cardiopulmonary effects of halothane anesthesia in cats. *Am J Vet Res* 1989; **50**(10): 1729–1732.

120 Hodgson DS, Dunlop CI, Chapman PL, *et al.* Cardiopulmonary effects of anesthesia induced and maintained with isoflurane in cats. *Am J Vet Res* 1998; **59**(2): 182–185.

121 McMurphy R, Hodgson D. Cardiopulmonary effects of desflurane in cats. *Am J Vet Res* 1996; **57**(3): 367–370.

122 Wallenstein MC. Biphasic effects of morphine on cardiovascular system of the cat. *Eur J Pharmacol* 1979; **59**(3–4): 253–260.

123 Dhasmana KM, Dixit KS, Jaju BP, *et al.* Role of central dopaminergic receptors in manic response of cats to morphine. *Psychopharmacologia* 1972; **24**(3): 380–383.

124 Robertson SA, Wegner K, Lascelles BDX. Antinociceptive and side-effects of hydromorphone after subcutaneous administration in cats. *J Feline Med Surg* 2009; **11**(2): 76–81.

125 Lascelles BD, Robertson SA. Antinociceptive effects of hydromorphone, butorphanol, or the combination in cats. *J Vet Intern Med* 2004; **18**(2): 190–195.

126 Brosnan RJ, Pypendop BH, Siao KT, *et al.* Effects of remifentanil on measures of anesthetic immobility and analgesia in cats. *Am J Vet Res* 2009; **70**(9): 1065–1071.

127 Yaksh TL, Harty GJ, Onofrio BM. High dose of spinal morphine produce a nonopiate receptor-mediated hyperesthesia: clinical and theoretic implications. *Anesthesiology* 1986; **64**(5): 590–597.

128 Pascoe PJ, Ilkiw JE, Fisher LD. The cardiovascular effects of equipotent isoflurane and alfentanil/isoflurane MAC multiple in cats. *Am J Vet Res* 1997; **58**(11): 1274–1279.

129 Pascoe PJ, Ilkiw JE, Fisher LD. Cardiovascular effects of equipotent isoflurane and alfentanil/isoflurane minimum alveolar concentration multiple in cats. *Am J Vet Res* 1997; **58**(11): 1267–1273.

130 Gaumann DM, Yaksh TL, Tyce GM, *et al.* Sympathetic stimulating effects of sufentanil in the cat are mediated centrally. *Neurosci Lett* 1988; **91**(1): 30–35.

131 Niedfeldt RL, Robertson SA. Postanesthetic hyperthermia in cats: a retrospective comparison between hydromorphone and buprenorphine. *Vet Anaesth Analg* 2006; **33**(6): 381–389.

132 Posner LP, Gleed RD, Erb HN, *et al.* Post-anesthetic hyperthermia in cats. *Vet Anaesth Analg* 2007; **34**(1): 40–47.

133 Posner LP, Pavuk AA, Rokshar JL, *et al.* Effects of opioids and anesthetic drugs on body temperature in cats. *Vet Anaesth Analg* 2010; **37**(1): 35–43.

134 Clark WG, Cumby HR. Hyperthermic responses to central and peripheral injections of morphine sulphate in the cat. *Br J Pharmacol* 1978; **63**(1): 65–71.

135 Ilkiw JE, Pascoe PJ, Tripp LD. Effects of morphine, butorphanol, buprenorphine, and U50488H on the minimum alveolar concentration of isoflurane in cats. *Am J Vet Res* 2002; **63**(8): 1198–1202.

136 Ilkiw JE, Pascoe PJ, Fisher LD. Effect of alfentanil on the minimum alveolar concentration of isoflurane in cats. *Am J Vet Res* 1997; **58**(11): 1274–1279.
137 Hall RI, Szlam F, Hug CC Jr. The enflurane-sparing effect of alfentanil in dogs. *Anesth Analg* 1987; **66**(12): 1287–1291.
138 Ferreira TH, Aguiar AJ, Valverde A, *et al.* Effect of remifentanil hydrochloride administered via constant rate infusion on the minimum alveolar concentration of isoflurane in cats. *Am J Vet Res* 2009; **70**(5): 581–588.
139 Brosnan RJ, Pypendop BH, Stanley SD. Phenylpiperidine opioid effects on isoflurane minimum alveolar concentration in cats. *J Vet Pharmacol Ther* 2020; **43**(6): 533–537.
140 Brosnan RJ, Pypendop BH. Evaluation of whether acepromazine maleate causes fentanyl to decrease the minimum alveolar concentration of isoflurane in cats. *Am J Vet Res* 2021; **82**(5): 352–357.
141 Pypendop BH, Goich M, Shilo-Benjamini Y. Effect of intravenous butorphanol infusion on the minimum alveolar concentration of isoflurane in cats. *Vet Anaesth Analg* 2022; **49**(2): 165–172.
142 Robertson SA, Lascelles BD, Taylor PM, *et al.* PK-PD modeling of buprenorphine in cats: intravenous and oral transmucosal administration. *J Vet Pharmacol Ther* 2005; **28**(5): 453–460.
143 Robertson SA, Taylor PM, Sear JW. Systemic uptake of buprenorphine by cats after oral mucosal administration. *Vet Rec* 2003; **152**(22): 675–678.
144 Robertson SA, Taylor PM, Lascelles BD, *et al.* Changes in thermal threshold response in eight cats after administration of buprenorphine, butorphanol and morphine. *Vet Rec* 2003; **153**(15): 462–465.
145 Steagall PV, Monteiro BP, Lavoie AM, *et al.* Preliminary investigation of the thermal antinociceptive effects of codeine in cats. *J Feline Med Surg* 2015; **17**(12): 1061–1064.
146 Steagall PV, Pelligand L, Giordano T, *et al.* Pharmacokinetic and pharmacodynamic modelling of intravenous, intramuscular and subcutaneous buprenorphine in conscious cats. *Vet Anaesth Analg* 2013; **40**(1): 83–95.
147 Doodnaught GM, Monteiro BP, Benito J, *et al.* Pharmacokinetic and pharmacodynamic modelling after subcutaneous, intravenous and buccal administration of a high-concentration formulation of buprenorphine in conscious cats. *PLoS ONE* 2017; **12**(4): e0176443.
148 Martin-Flores M, Lorenzutti AM, Nugen SA, *et al.* High-dose buprenorphine results in a greater occurrence of postoperative hyperthermia than morphine in a randomized clinical trial in cats undergoing ovariohysterectomy. *Am J Vet Res* 2022; **83**(6).
149 Freise KJ, Reinemeyer C, Warren K, *et al.* Single-dose pharmacokinetics and bioavailability of a novel extended duration transdermal buprenorphine solution in cats. *J Vet Pharmacol Ther* 2022; **45**(Suppl 1): S31–S39.
150 Clark TP, Linton DD, Freise KJ, *et al.* Multicentered masked placebo-controlled phase 3 clinical study of an extended duration transdermal buprenorphine solution for post-operative pain in cats. *J Vet Pharmacol Ther* 2022; **45**(Suppl 1): S52–S66.
151 Clark TP, Linton DD, Freise KJ, *et al.* Margin of safety of extended-duration transdermal buprenorphine solution following multiple-dose administrations to cats. *J Vet Pharmacol Ther* 2022; **45**(Suppl 1): S67–S84.
152 Sparkes AH, Heiene R, Lascelles BD, *et al.* ISFM and AAFP consensus guidelines: long-term use of NSAIDs in cats. *J Feline Med Surg* 2010; **12**(7): 521–538.
153 Lascelles BD, Court MH, Hardie EM, *et al.* Nonsteroidal anti-inflammatory drugs in cats: a review. *Vet Anaesth Analg* 2007; **34**(4): 228–250.
154 Robertson SA. Managing pain in feline patients. *Vet Clin North Am Small Anim Pract* 2008; **38**(6): 1267–1290, vi.
155 Gruen ME, Lascelles BDX, Colleran E, *et al.* 2022 AAHA Pain management guidelines for dogs and cats. *J Am Anim Hosp Assoc* 2022; **58**(2): 55–76.
156 Slingsby LS, Waterman-Pearson AE. Postoperative analgesia in the cat after ovariohysterectomy by use of carprofen, ketoprofen, meloxicam or tolfenamic acid. *J Small Anim Pract* 2000; **41**(10): 447–450.
157 Polson S, Taylor PM, Yates D. Analgesia after feline ovariohysterectomy under midazolam-medetomidine-ketamine anaesthesia with buprenorphine or butorphanol, and carprofen or meloxicam: a prospective, randomised clinical trial. *J Feline Med Surg* 2012; **14**(8): 553–559.
158 Taylor PM, Steagall PV, Dixon MJ, *et al.* Carprofen and buprenorphine prevent hyperalgesia in a model of inflammatory pain in cats. *Res Vet Sci* 2007; **83**(3): 369–375.
159 Tobias KM, Harvey RC, Byarlay JM. A comparison of four methods of analgesia in cats following ovariohysterectomy. *Vet Anaesth Analg* 2006; **33**(6): 390–398.
160 Mollenhoff A, Nolte I, Kramer S. Anti-nociceptive efficacy of carprofen, levomethadone and buprenorphine for pain relief in cats following major orthopaedic surgery. *J Vet Med A Physiol Pathol Clin Med* 2005; **52**(4): 186–198.
161 Al-Gizawiy MM, Rudé EP. Comparison of preoperative carprofen and postoperative butorphanol as postsurgical analgesics in cats undergoing ovariohysterectomy. *Vet Anaesth Analg* 2004; **31**(3): 164–174.
162 Balmer TV, Irvine D, Jones RS, *et al.* Comparison of carprofen and pethidine as postoperative analgesics in the cat. *J Small Anim Pract* 1998; **39**(4): 158–164.
163 Lascelles BD, Cripps P, Mirchandani S, *et al.* Carprofen as an analgesic for postoperative pain in cats: dose titration and assessment of efficacy in comparison to pethidine hydrochloride. *J Small Anim Pract* 1995; **36**(12): 535–541.
164 Sano T, King JN, Seewald W, *et al.* Comparison of oral robenacoxib and ketoprofen for the treatment of acute pain and inflammation associated with musculoskeletal disorders in cats: a randomised clinical trial. *Vet J* 2012; **193**(2): 397–403.
165 Giraudel JM, Gruet P, Alexander DG, *et al.* Evaluation of orally administered robenacoxib versus ketoprofen for treatment of acute pain and inflammation associated with musculoskeletal disorders in cats. *Am J Vet Res* 2010; **71**(7): 710–719.
166 Morton CM, Grant D, Johnston L, *et al.* Clinical evaluation of meloxicam versus ketoprofen in cats suffering from painful acute locomotor disorders. *J Feline Med Surg* 2011; **13**(4): 237–243.
167 Murison PJ, Tacke S, Wondratschek C, *et al.* Postoperative analgesic efficacy of meloxicam compared to tolfenamic acid in cats undergoing orthopaedic surgery. *J Small Anim Pract* 2010; **51**(10): 526–532.
168 Benito-de-la-Vibora J, Lascelles BD, Garcia-Fernandez P, *et al.* Efficacy of tolfenamic acid and meloxicam in the control of postoperative pain following ovariohysterectomy in the cat. *Vet Anaesth Analg* 2008; **35**(6): 501–510.
169 Kamata M, King JN, Seewald W, *et al.* Comparison of injectable robenacoxib versus meloxicam for peri-operative use in cats: results of a randomised clinical trial. *Vet J* 2012; **193**(1): 114–118.
170 Pelligand L, House AK, Summers BA, *et al.* Development and validation of a tissue cage model of acute inflammation in the cat. *J Vet Pharmacol Ther* 2012; **35**(3): 239–248.
171 Giraudel JM, King JN, Jeunesse EC, *et al.* Use of a pharmacokinetic/pharmacodynamic approach in the cat to determine a dosage regimen for the COX-2 selective drug robenacoxib. *J Vet Pharmacol Ther* 2009; **32**(1): 18–30.
172 Gowan RA, Lingard AE, Johnston L, *et al.* Retrospective case-control study of the effects of long-term dosing with meloxicam on renal function in aged cats with degenerative joint disease. *J Feline Med Surg* 2011; **13**(10): 752–761.
173 Rausch-Derra LC, Rhodes L. Safety and toxicokinetic profiles associated with daily oral administration of grapiprant, a selective antagonist of the prostaglandin E2 EP4 receptor, to cats. *Am J Vet Res* 2016; **77**(7): 688–692.
174 Teixeira LG, Vaccarin CV, Schimites PI, *et al.* Grapiprant or carprofen following ovariohysterectomy in the cat: analgesic efficacy, hematological, biochemical and urinalysis evaluation. *J Feline Med Surg* 2022; **24**(8): e153–e162.
175 Brodbelt DC, Pfeiffer DU, Young LE, *et al.* Risk factors for anaesthetic-related death in cats: results from the Confidential Enquiry into Perioperative Small Animal Fatalities (CEPSAF). *Brit J Anaesth* 2007; **99**(5): 617–623.
176 Dyson DH, Maxie MG, Schnurr D. Morbidity and mortality associated with anesthetic management in small animal veterinary practice in Ontario. *J Am Anim Hosp Assoc* 1998; **34**(4): 325–335.
177 Clarke KW, Hall LW. A survey of anaesthesia in small animal practice: AVA/BSAVA report. *J Assoc Vet Anaesth* 1990; **17**(1): 4–10.
178 Rex MA. Laryngospasm and respiratory changes in the cat produced by mechanical stimulation of the pharynx and respiratory tract: problems of intubation in the cat. *Br J Anaesth* 1971; **43**(1): 54–57.
179 Rex MA. A review of the structural and functional basis of laryngospasm and a discussion of the nerve pathways involved in the reflex and its clinical significance in man and animals. *Br J Anaesth* 1970; **42**(10): 891–899.
180 Jones TL, Boyer K, Chapman K, *et al.* Evaluation of the time to desensitization of the larynx of cats following topical lidocaine application. *J Feline Med Surg* 2021; **23**(6): 563–567.
181 Moreno-Sala A, Ortiz-Martinez R, Valdivia AG, *et al.* Use of neuromuscular blockade with rocuronium bromide for intubation in cats. *Vet Anaesth Analg* 2013; **40**(4): 351–358.
182 Sakai DM, Zornow KA, Campoy L, *et al.* Intravenous rocuronium 0.3 mg/kg improves the conditions for tracheal intubation in cats: a randomized, placebo-controlled trial. *J Feline Med Surg* 2018; **20**(12): 1124–1129.
183 White RN, Oakley MR. Left principal bronchus rupture in a cat. *J Small Anim Pract* 2001; **42**(10): 495–498.
184 White RN, Burton CA. Surgical management of intrathoracic tracheal avulsion in cats: long-term results in 9 consecutive cases. *Vet Surg* 2000; **29**(5): 430–435.
185 Mitchell SL, McCarthy R, Rudloff E, *et al.* Tracheal rupture associated with intubation in cats: 20 cases (1996–1998). *J Am Vet Med Assoc* 2000; **216**(10): 1592–1595.
186 Hardie EM, Spodnick GJ, Gilson SD, *et al.* Tracheal rupture in cats: 16 cases (1983–1998). *J Am Vet Med Assoc* 1999; **214**(4): 508–512.
187 White RN, Milner HR. Intrathoracic tracheal avulsion in three cats. *J Small Anim Pract* 1995; **36**(8): 343–347.
188 Lawrence DT, Lang J, Culvenor J, *et al.* Intrathoracic tracheal rupture. *J Feline Med Surg* 1999; **1**(1): 43–51.

189 Stiles J, Weil AB, Packer RA, *et al.* Post-anesthetic cortical blindness in cats: twenty cases. *Vet J* 2012; **193**(2): 367–373.

190 Jurk IR, Thibodeau MS, Whitney K, *et al.* Acute vision loss after general anesthesia in a cat. *Vet Ophthalmol* 2001; **4**(2): 155–158.

191 Barton-Lamb AL, Martin-Flores M, Scrivani PV, *et al.* Evaluation of maxillary arterial blood flow in anesthetized cats with the mouth closed and open. *Vet J* 2013; **196**(3): 325–331.

192 Breznock EM, Strack D. Effects of the spleen, epinephrine, and splenectomy on determination of blood volume in cats. *Am J Vet Res* 1982; **43**(11): 2062–2066.

193 Breznock EM, Strack D. Blood volume of nonsplenectomized and splenectomized cats before and after acute hemorrhage. *Am J Vet Res* 1982; **43**(10): 1811–1814.

194 Spink RR, Malvin RL, Cohen BJ. Determination of erythrocyte half life and blood volume in cats. *Am J Vet Res* 1966; **27**(119): 1041–1043.

195 Davis H, Jensen T, Johnson A, *et al.* 2013 AAHA/AAFP fluid therapy guidelines for dogs and cats. *J Am Anim Hosp Assoc* 2013; **49**(3): 149–159.

196 Eyquem A, Podliachouk L, Millot P. Blood groups in chimpanzees, horses, sheep, pigs, and other mammals. *Ann N Y Acad Sci* 1962; **97**: 320–328.

197 Griot-Wenk ME, Callan MB, Casal ML, *et al.* Blood type AB in the feline AB blood group system. *Am J Vet Res* 1996; **57**(10): 1438–1442.

198 Giger U, Bucheler J. Transfusion of type-A and type-B blood to cats. *J Am Vet Med Assoc* 1991; **198**(3): 411–418.

199 Lanevschi A, Wardrop KJ. Principles of transfusion medicine in small animals. *Can Vet J* 2001; **42**(6): 447–454.

200 Weinstein NM, Blais MC, Harris K, *et al.* A newly recognized blood group in domestic shorthair cats: the Mik red cell antigen. *J Vet Intern Med* 2007; **21**(2): 287–292.

201 Taylor S, Spada E, Callan MB, *et al.* 2021 ISFM consensus guidelines on the collection and administration of blood and blood products in cats. *J Feline Med Surg* 2021; **23**(5): 410–432.

202 McClosky ME, Cimino Brown D, Weinstein NM, *et al.* Prevalence of naturally occurring non-AB blood type incompatibilities in cats and influence of crossmatch on transfusion outcomes. *J Vet Intern Med* 2018; **32**(6): 1934–1942.

203 Davidow EB, Blois SL, Goy-Thollot I, *et al.* Association of Veterinary Hematology and Transfusion Medicine (AVHTM) Transfusion Reaction Small Animal Consensus Statement (TRACS). Part 1: definitions and clinical signs. *J Vet Emerg Crit Care (San Antonio)* 2021; **31**(2): 141–166.

204 Davidow EB, Spada E, Proverbio D. Editorial: blood groups in companion animals. *Front Vet Sci* 2021; **8**: 792720.

205 Bagdi N, Magdus M, Leidinger E, *et al.* Frequencies of feline blood types in Hungary. *Acta Vet Hung* 2001; **49**(4): 369–375.

206 Medeiros MA, Soares AM, Alviano DS, *et al.* Frequencies of feline blood types in the Rio de Janeiro area of Brazil. *Vet Clin Pathol* 2008; **37**(3): 272–276.

207 Giger U, Kilrain CG, Filippich LJ, *et al.* Frequencies of feline blood groups in the United States. *J Am Vet Med Assoc* 1989; **195**(9): 1230–1232.

208 Zheng L, Zhong Y, Shi Z, *et al.* Frequencies of blood types A, B, and AB in non-pedigree domestic cats in Beijing. *Vet Clin Pathol* 2011; **40**(4): 513–517.

209 Hubler M, Arnold S, Casal M, *et al.* The blood group distribution in domestic cats in Switzerland. *Schweiz Arch Tierheilkd* 1993; **135**(8): 231–235.

210 Jensen AL, Olesen AB, Arnbjerg J. Distribution of feline blood types detected in the Copenhagen area of Denmark. *Acta Vet Scand* 1994; **35**(2): 121–124.

211 Knottenbelt CM, Addie DD, Day MJ, *et al.* Determination of the prevalence of feline blood types in the UK. *J Small Anim Pract* 1999; **40**(3): 115–118.

212 Mylonakis ME, Koutinas AF, Saridomichelakis M, *et al.* Determination of the prevalence of blood types in the non-pedigree feline population in Greece. *Vet Rec* 2001; **149**(7): 213–214.

213 Ruiz de Gopegui R, Velasquez M, Espada Y. Survey of feline blood types in the Barcelona area of Spain. *Vet Rec* 2004; **154**(25): 794–795.

214 Silvestre-Ferreira AC, Pastor J, Almeida O, *et al.* Frequencies of feline blood types in northern Portugal. *Vet Clin Pathol* 2004; **33**(4): 240–243.

215 Malik R, Griffin DL, White JD, *et al.* The prevalence of feline A/B blood types in the Sydney region. *Aust Vet J* 2005; **83**(1–2): 38–44.

216 Arikan S, Gurkan M, Ozaytekin E, *et al.* Frequencies of blood type A, B and AB in non-pedigree domestic cats in Turkey. *J Small Anim Pract* 2006; **47**(1): 10–13.

217 Forcada Y, Guitian J, Gibson G. Frequencies of feline blood types at a referral hospital in the south east of England. *J Small Anim Pract* 2007; **48**(10): 570–573.

218 Marques C, Ferreira M, Gomes JF, *et al.* Frequency of blood type A, B, and AB in 515 domestic shorthair cats from the Lisbon area. *Vet Clin Pathol* 2011; **40**(2): 185–187.

219 Arikan S, Duru SY, Gurkan M, *et al.* Blood type A and B frequencies in Turkish Van and Angora cats in Turkey. *J Vet Med A Physiol Pathol Clin Med* 2003; **50**(6): 303–306.

220 Pascoe PJ, Ilkiw JE, Pypendop BH. Effects of increasing infusion rates of dopamine, dobutamine, epinephrine, and phenylephrine in healthy anesthetized cats. *Am J Vet Res* 2006; **67**(9): 1491–1499.

221 Flournoy WS, Wohl JS, Albrecht-Schmitt TJ, *et al.* Pharmacologic identification of putative D1 dopamine receptor in feline kidneys. *J Vet Pharmacol Ther* 2003; **26**(4): 283–290.

222 Jones D, Bellomo R. Renal-dose dopamine: from hypothesis to paradigm to dogma to myth and, finally, superstition? *J Intensive Care Med* 2005; **20**(4): 199–211.

223 Schenarts PJ, Sagraves SG, Bard MR, *et al.* Low-dose dopamine: a physiologically based review. *Curr Surg* 2006; **63**(3): 219–225.

51 Comparative Anesthesia and Analgesia – Community Medicine Settings

Emily McCobb
Department of Clinical Sciences, Cummings School of Veterinary Medicine, Tufts University, North Grafton, Massachusetts, USA

Chapter contents

Introduction, 1041
High-quality high-volume spay-neuter, 1041
Clinical situations requiring anesthesia, 1041
HQHVSN – healthy dogs, cats, and rabbits, 1041
Spay-neuter for higher risk patients, 1045
Anesthesia for non-spay-neuter procedures in shelters, 1045
References, 1046

Introduction

Over the past 10 years, the scope of medicine practiced within animal shelters and other settings within the animal welfare industry has greatly evolved, as evidenced by the establishment of shelter medicine as an American Board of Veterinary Practitioners specialty in 2014 [1]. Veterinarians working in animal shelters and associated clinics provide care to a variety of patients, including animals in the shelter, newly adopted animals, and animals belonging to members of the public, as well as animals involved in cruelty investigations. Within shelter populations, many animals present with unknown health status and a range of behavior challenges such as fear, anxiety, and aggression. Patients may include victims of animal cruelty or neglect. Spay and neuter of shelter animals prior to adoption is standard policy, and these patients include pediatric and juvenile as well as geriatric patients [2–8]. The care provided must balance the needs of the individual animal with those of the entire population, often while working with budget or equipment limitations.

High-quality high-volume spay-neuter

In addition to caring for shelter animals, many organizations also provide low-cost spay and neuter services for members of the public [9]. Most organizations employ high-quality high-volume spay-neuter (HQHVSN) practice which the Association of Shelter Veterinarians (ASV) defines as "efficient surgical initiatives that meet or exceed veterinary medical standards of care in providing accessible, targeted sterilization of large numbers of cats and dogs to reduce their overpopulation and subsequent euthanasia [10]." While many spay or neuter patients are young and healthy (ASA I), members of the public may also present higher risk patients such as geriatric or brachycephalic dogs and cats for surgery. Morbidity and mortality rates in sterilization programs are remarkably low [11], due to thorough staff training, short procedure times, and the large numbers of young and healthy patients, although the impact of a balanced anesthesia protocol cannot be discounted. Thoughtful, practical, and reliable protocols for all aspects of the patient's peri-anesthetic care are essential to allow safe and efficient processing of large numbers of patients [10,12].

HQHVSN programs can be successful in a variety of settings including standing clinics, "MASH style" or mobile units, and field clinics, and operate both domestically and internationally (Fig. 51.1). In such settings, the available equipment may be limited, and flexibility and creativity are often required to maximize the patient experience while minimizing resource utilization. Available drugs may also be limited. Many HQHVSN programs rely on total injectable anesthesia [13–18].

Clinical situations requiring anesthesia

Whether in the shelter or at a community clinic, a variety of patients present for anesthesia in shelter medicine.

HQHVSN – healthy dogs, cats, and rabbits

A large proportion of the patients in shelter medicine anesthesia are healthy dogs, cats, and rabbits presenting for elective spaying or neutering. It is the standard of care for shelter animals to be sterilized prior to adoption and this policy may even be legally required in some states. In addition, spay-neuter outreach to local communities as well as Trap Neuter Return (TNR) programs for free roaming cats are essential to reduce shelter intake and thus shelter euthanasia [9]. The ASV has published guidelines for spay-neuter programs [11,12], and a textbook devoted to HQHVSN practice is also available [19].

Veterinary Anesthesia and Analgesia: The Sixth Edition of Lumb and Jones. Edited by Leigh Lamont, Kurt Grimm, Sheilah Robertson, Lydia Love and Carrie Schroeder.
© 2024 John Wiley & Sons, Inc. Published 2024 by John Wiley & Sons, Inc.
Companion website: www.wiley.com/go/lamont/anesthesia

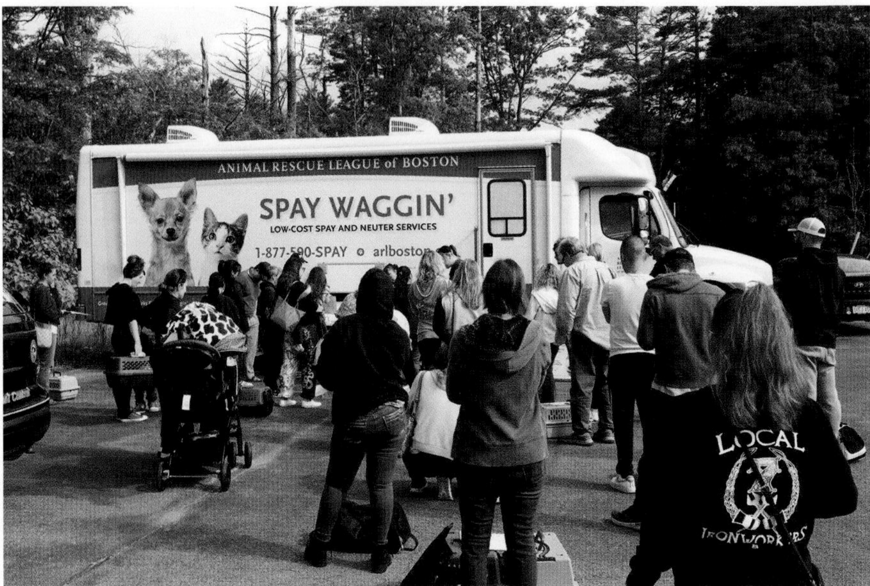

Figure 51.1 Mobile spay-neuter clinic.

Preoperative considerations

Each program determines which patients are suitable candidates for the spay-neuter clinic, depending on staff training and clinic capabilities. According to the ASV guidelines, a veterinarian should make the final decision regarding acceptance of any patient for surgery based on historical and physical examination findings [10]. Veterinarians must weigh the risks and benefits of anesthetizing patients with mild infectious or noninfectious medical conditions, such as upper respiratory tract disease, parasite infestation, or subclinical heartworm infection against the risk of the animal not returning for surgery. Patient history should include current health status, current clinical signs of disease, current medications and supplements, previous vaccinations, pre-existing medical conditions, and previous adverse reactions. In addition, clients should be instructed to appropriately withhold food from their animals prior to surgery. Fasting times and other preanesthetic recommendations are the same as for patients of similar species and age presenting for anesthesia in other clinical settings. Clients must be informed of surgical and anesthetic risks and must consent to the anticipated procedures.

Prior to anesthesia, a brief screening physical exam should be performed on every patient with a focus on the cardiorespiratory systems. Animals that are anxious or unsocialized should be sedated as soon as the physical examination is completed. Feral animals are examined after anesthesia induction. Routine preanesthetic laboratory screening is not generally performed in HQHVSN clinics for apparently healthy patients and indeed is likely unnecessary for healthy patients presenting for anesthesia in most circumstances [20]. Routine laboratory screening testing for patients with normal physical exam findings is unlikely to change the patient's ASA status, recommended anesthetic protocol, or affect patient outcome after anesthesia [20,21]. Using a spectrum of care approach [22], the costs of any diagnostic tests must be carefully weighed against potential benefits.

Drug protocols for HQHVSN

Selecting an appropriate protocol for an HQHVSN program depends on several factors such as the number and type of patients presenting each day, technician skill level, drug availability, and the timing of and competence in performing various surgical and anesthetic techniques. A variety of protocols are safe, humane, efficient, and cost effective but all must provide the following: (1) analgesia, (2) stress reduction or anxiolysis, (3) immobility and muscle relaxation, and (4) controlled, reversible depression of the central nervous system resulting in unconsciousness. Numerous cost-effective protocols, combining multiple anesthetic and analgesic drugs, including injectable and inhalant agents, exist for achieving balanced anesthesia in pediatric and adult patients [13–17,23–35]. A few examples of common protocols are given in Table 51.1. Anesthetic drugs should be calculated for each individual patient using an actual or estimated (for intractable patients) body weight. The use of a chart that expresses drug doses as a function of body weight may help prevent calculation errors [10]. However, when using a dose chart, caution is advised for patient weights at both extremes of the range provided (i.e., very small and very large patients). In these cases, dosing based on body surface area or metabolic scaling is recommended to improve accuracy (i.e., larger patients usually require lower drug doses on a per weight basis). For situations in which an accurate body weight cannot be obtained prior to drug administration, such as programs serving community cats, safety is increased by using reversible agents, avoiding drugs that result in marked cardiorespiratory depression, and estimating body weight as accurately as possible. Close physical monitoring of the patients following drug administration can also allow timely recognition of adverse physiologic side effects.

Equipment

The anesthesia equipment used in HQHVSN clinics is generally the same as that used in any veterinary practice setting. However, in a high-volume setting, special consideration should be given to equipment use and maintenance to enhance patient safety. All anesthesia equipment including endotracheal tubes, laryngoscopes, anesthesia machines, and monitors should be prepared and checked daily prior to use [40,41]. A machine safety checklist is available in Chapter 6. Any time the anesthesia circuit is changed (such as switching back and forth from a rebreathing to a non-rebreathing system), the machine checklist should be repeated to ensure that the circuit has been connected correctly. Anesthesia equipment in

Table 51.1 Common injectable anesthesia protocols used in HQHVSN clinics.

Protocol	Dose/Recipe	Comments	Reference
Hydromorphone–acepromazine	Hydromorphone 0.1 mg/kg, Acepromazine 0.05 mg/kg IM	Common premedication for dogs; can also be used for cats Induction can be via Telazol®, propofol, or ketamine–midazolam combinations	[36]
TTDex	Combine 2.5 mL Butorphanol (10 mg/mL) and 2.5 mL Dexmedetomidine (0.5 mg/mL) into one bottle of Telazol® Administer at 0.035 mL/kg IM to provide surgical anesthesia	Used for cats and dogs Dose recommendations range from 0.01 mL/kg to 0.035 mL/kg IM, depending on level of sedation/anesthesia required	[37,38]
DKB	Dexmedetomidine 10–20 μg/kg, Ketamine 3–10 mg/kg, Buprenorphine 0.01–0.02 mg/kg IM	Many variations for cats, rabbits, and dogs Butorphanol can also be substituted for buprenorphine which provides superior sedation but less analgesia	[17,38]
TKX	Combine 4 mL of Ketamine (100 mg/mL) and 1 mL of Xylazine (100 mg/mL) into one bottle of Telazol® Administer 0.25 mL IM per "average" (~ 4 kg) cat	May be used in some feral cat programs Does not provide lasting analgesia	[39]
Quad combination	Ketamine 60 mg/m^2, Midazolam 3 mg/m^2, Buprenorphine μg/m^2, Dexmedetomidine 300 μg/m^2 IM	Common protocol for cats in the UK Body surface area = (10.4 × BW$^{0.67}$)/100 (a smart phone app is available)	[14]

high-volume programs undergoes intense use, often by multiple personnel, which can put additional strain on equipment. Heavily used equipment in high-volume programs should be serviced frequently. Anesthesia machines and monitors should be maintained in accordance with manufacturers' recommendations through regularly performed in-house procedures or outsourcing to equipment service companies [41].

Carbon dioxide absorbents should be checked and changed regularly; high patient volumes dictate increased frequency for changing and cleaning of canisters. Soda lime should be changed after an appropriate period of use according to canister size. Anesthesia circuits, masks, and endotracheal tubes should be cleaned by soaking in a dilute chlorhexidine solution, taking care to rinse thoroughly. A waste gas scavenging system should be used; both active and passive systems are acceptable. Use of charcoal canisters in high-volume clinics is discouraged as they are acceptable for only short periods of time, typically < 6–8 h or as determined by the weight gain of the canister, and are variably effective [10,42].

Monitoring and patient support

Each individual patient should be carefully monitored from the time of drug administration until recovery. Identification of changes in vital parameters is essential for accurate assessment [43]. The most reliable means to ensure ongoing patient assessment and safety during anesthesia is vigilant "hands-on" observation by trained staff [10]. Monitoring should involve assessment of various combinations of vital parameters using an objective means of monitoring in accordance with current veterinary anesthesia monitoring guidelines [44,45]. Options include but are not limited to pulse detection via palpation or Doppler ultrasound, auscultation of the heartbeat, pulse oximetry, capnography, and blood pressure monitoring. The use of pulse oximetry is highly encouraged because this modality provides an objective auditory and visual means of determining the presence of a pulse, pulse rate, and adequacy of oxygenation [46]. Use of pulse oximetry monitors has been associated with a decreased risk of anesthetic death in cats [47].

While some patients will oxygenate adequately while breathing room air, oxygen supplementation, including pre- and postoperatively, is recommended for high-risk patients such as brachycephalic animals as well as those that are frail, ill, or in advanced stages of pregnancy. In addition, oxygen supplementation should be immediately available as needed for all heavily sedated or anesthetized patients. Ventilation can be accomplished in anesthetized patients by connecting the anesthesia machine to a rebreathing circuit with a functional carbon dioxide absorbent or to a non-rebreathing circuit with appropriate oxygen flow rates. Alternatively, a manual resuscitator (e.g., Ambu® bag) connected to an oxygen source with a regulator can be used as a means of oxygen supplementation and ventilation. Ventilation is compromised when carbon dioxide absorbents are depleted or exhausted; therefore, vigilance in monitoring carbon dioxide absorbent adequacy is necessary. Capnography is a useful tool for judging adequacy of ventilation, detecting carbon dioxide absorbent exhaustion or other causes of rebreathing, and assessing patient circulatory status [48].

General anesthesia may be maintained using a mask, endotracheal tube, or laryngeal mask airway device. When balanced anesthesia is achieved using injectable drug protocols, routine intubation of all patients undergoing spay-neuter surgery should be considered [10]. However, the benefits of intubation (i.e., protection of the airway, ability to ventilate, and reduced waste gas exposure for staff) should be weighed against the risks, particularly airway trauma, with some species being more likely to sustain tracheal injuries (rabbits, cats). If intubation is performed as a standard part of an anesthetic protocol, having an anesthesia team that possesses the required skills for this maneuver is critical to success [49]. The ability to perform intubation when medically indicated, including rapid intubation in emergency situations, is a requirement for all spay-neuter programs [10,49–52]. The anesthetist must verify the placement of the endotracheal tube by direct visualization or via capnography. Specific patients that may benefit from intubation include all brachycephalic breeds, overweight or obese patients, animals in advanced stages of gestation, patients with pre-existing severe upper respiratory disease, and patients for which procedures are anticipated to require a long duration of anesthesia (e.g., greater than 30 min).

Intravenous (IV) access is typically obtained in patients undergoing general anesthesia by placement of an IV catheter, which allows for the immediate administration of resuscitation drugs, IV fluids, reversal agents, and supplemental doses of analgesics or anesthetics if necessary. However, in HQHVSN settings where surgery times are very short and especially when general anesthesia is induced via intramuscular injection, an IV catheter is often not placed. In all

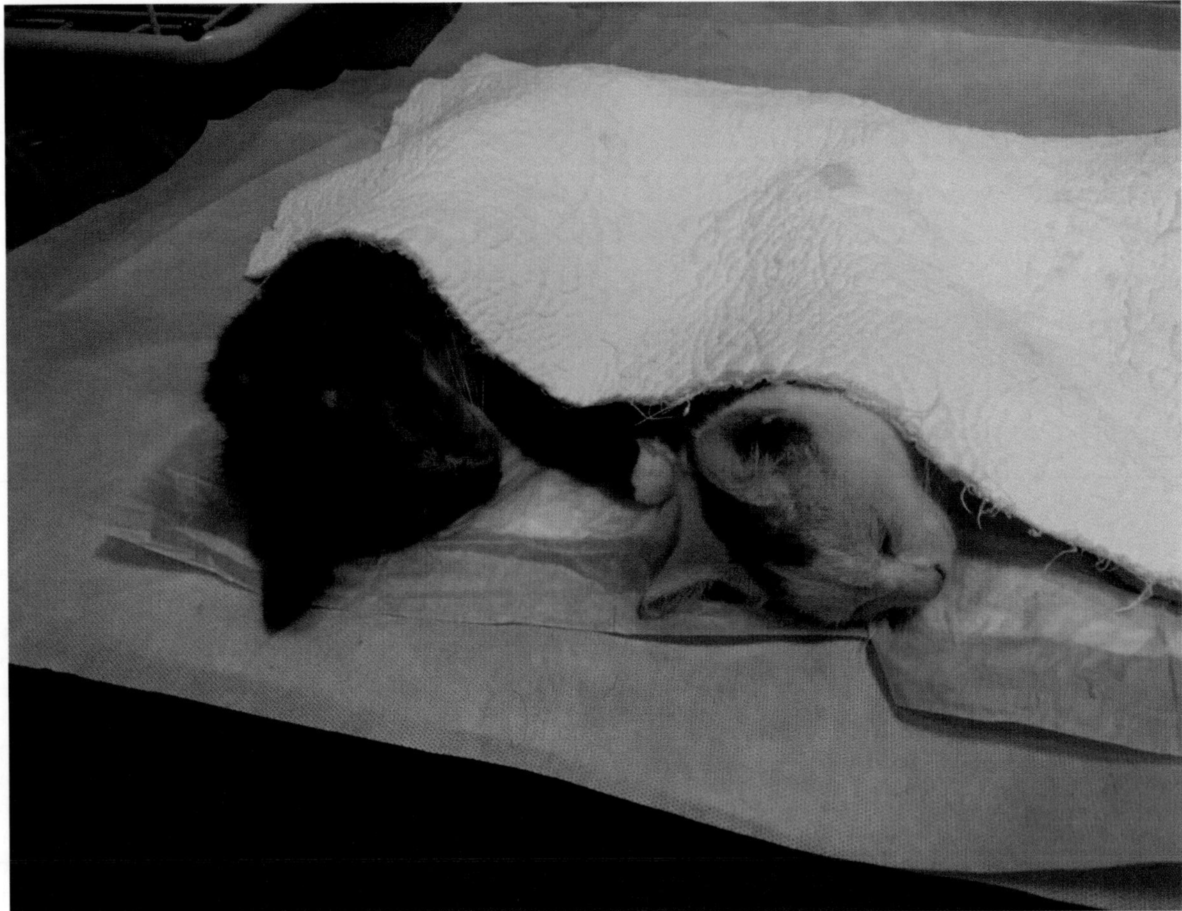

Figure 51.2 "Beach style" setup consisting of a warm padded area for managing recovery of multiple patients simultaneously in an HQHVSN program.

cases, the team should be prepared to obtain IV access in an emergency. IV fluid administration is not required for all elective surgical procedures especially when surgical times are brief [10,53]. For routine fluid support for many patients, subcutaneous administration may be adequate. IV fluid supplementation is recommended for high-risk patients, such as those that may be presented for ovariohysterectomy in advanced stages of pregnancy or with evidence of pyometra, and when significant blood loss or prolonged surgery times are anticipated or encountered.

Patient temperature should be monitored to prevent hypo- or hyperthermia. Prewarming patients prior to administration of premedication and anesthetic agents may reduce perioperative hypothermia [54]. Contact with cold surfaces should be minimized to the extent possible. The use of low oxygen flow rates with rebreathing anesthetic circuits can also help conserve body heat. Intraoperative heat loss can be further minimized by limiting body cavity exposure, increasing environmental temperature, and providing additional insulation for the patient (e.g., by wrapping extremities in materials such as bubble wrap, newspaper, and polystyrene) [55]. Active patient warming can be achieved using heated surgical tables, semiconductive polymer fabric heating blankets, circulating warm water blankets, and warm air blankets [56,57]. Warmth in the patient's microenvironment can be provided by use of carefully protected warmed containers. In contrast, unprotected contact with or careless use of blow dryers, heat lamps, drying cages, electric heating pads, and hot water or heated materials must be avoided to prevent thermal injury [10,55].

Recovery

Patients should be continuously attended while intubated. Many programs use a "beach style" (Fig. 51.2) setup for recovery, which consists of a warm padded area where groups of patients can be placed. Precautions for biosecurity and patient safety are important when using a recovery beach. Once patients are extubated and/or capable of maintaining their airway, they can be returned to their home cage, a clinic cage, or a carrier. Patients should be alert, oriented, warm, ambulatory, and pain-free prior to discharge from the clinic. Many clinics use reversal agents for α_2-adrenergic receptor agonists that are part of the anesthetic protocol. At least one study demonstrated that α_2-adrenergic receptor antagonists can hasten recovery without decreasing the quality of analgesia when full μ-opioid receptor agonists and non-steroidal anti-inflammatory drugs (NSAIDs) are also administered [58].

Analgesia for spay-neuter programs

Published guidelines for spay-neuter programs state explicitly that appropriate analgesia must be provided [10]. Acceptable choices include opioids, α_2-adrenergic receptor agonists, NSAIDs, and local anesthetics [59–83]. Multimodal analgesia involves the use of multiple analgesic agents with different pharmacologic mechanisms to control pain and should include the use of local blocks [84]. Additional information about local blocks is provided in Table 51.2. The use and timing of NSAID administration should be based on the specific drug and individual patient. In particular, consideration should be given to patient hydration status and the presence of pre-existing hepatic, renal, or gastrointestinal disease, or clotting

Table 51.2 Suggested local blocks for surgeries common in shelter medicine.

Procedure	Regional block	Dose	Reference
Enucleation	Peribulbar block	Bupivacaine 2 mg/kg total dose Cats: dilute with saline to 3.5–4 mL total volume for "average" (~ 4 kg) cat Dogs: dilute with saline to 0.2–0.8 mL/kg total volume for dogs	[86]
Dental extractions	Infraorbital, mandibular, and maxillary blocks	Bupivacaine 1–2 mg/kg total dose	[87]
Femoral head and neck osteotomy or hindlimb amputation	Lumbosacral epidural	Morphine (preservative-free) 0.1 mg/kg or Buprenorphine 0.005 mg/kg combined with Bupivacaine 0.5 mg/kg	[86]
Perineal urethrostomy	Caudal epidural	Bupivacaine 0.25 mg/kg, dilute 1:1 with saline	[88]
Castration	Intratesticular block	Lidocaine 1–4 mg/kg or Bupivacaine 2 mg/kg	[89]
Ovariohysterectomy	Intraperitoneal block	Bupivacaine 2 mg/kg, dilute to 1 mL/kg with saline	[89]
Total ear canal ablation	Auricular block	Bupivacaine 2 mg/kg	[90]
General soft tissue or orthopedic surgery	Infiltrative block Infiltrative block	Bupivacaine 2 mg/kg infused in all layers of closure Liposome-encapsulated bupivacaine (Nocita®) 5.3 mg/kg, can be diluted 1:1 with saline or 0.5% bupivacaine	[86,91]
	Wound soaker catheter	Bupivacaine 1–2 mg/kg q 6–8 hours or Lidocaine 1.5–3 mg/kg/hour	

abnormalities [85]. If objective monitoring is limited or lacking (e.g., blood pressure), it may be safest to wait and administer NSAIDs in the recovery period while preemptively managing pain with opioids, local anesthetics, and adjuncts such as ketamine. Administration of NSAIDs to patients that are clinically or subclinically dehydrated should be avoided due to the increased risk of adverse effects including nephrotoxicity.

Additional analgesics to be given after discharge are not always required for spay-neuter surgeries when incisions are small and a multimodal preventive protocol with an NSAID is used perioperatively. However, all patients are individuals and clinicians should consider that some patients may require continued analgesia after discharge. For example, patients such as very large dogs or those having additional surgeries in combination with spay-neuter (mass removals, etc.) are likely to be more painful postoperatively than a routine puppy or kitten patient might be. Options for discharge medications are presented in Table 51.3.

Table 51.3 Analgesic and anxiolytic medication options for discharge.

Class	Medication	Notes
NSAIDs	Carprofen	Dogs only (in the United States) Oral and injectable formulations available
	Meloxicam	Cats and dogs Oral and injectable formulations available Recommend dosing at lower than label recommendations (0.1 mg/kg once perioperatively for cats)
	Robenacoxib	Cats and dogs Oral and injectable formulations available
Local anesthetics	Liposome-encapsulated bupivacaine	Nocita® can be diluted 1:1 with saline or 0.5% bupivacaine
Anxiolytics	Gabapentin	10–20 mg/kg q8 hours, orally
	Trazodone	5–10 mg/kg q6 hours, orally
Opioids	Oral transmucosal (OTM) buprenorphine	0.02–0.04 mg/kg Either "standard" (0.3 mg/mL) or concentrated (1.8 mg/mL; Simbadol®) formulations can be administered via this route OTM administration can be used in both cats and dogs but absorption of buprenorphine via this route is lower in dogs versus cats
	Subcutaneous concentrated buprenorphine	Simbadol® 0.12–0.24 mg/kg SC, for use in cats only at this high dose
	Topical buprenorphine	Zorbium® for use in cats only
	Fentanyl transdermal patch	1–4 μg/kg/hour Can prescribe a box of five patches from a pharmacy
	Tramadol	2–10 mg/kg q8 hours, orally May not provide effective analgesia in dogs
Over the counter	Acetaminophen	15–30 mg/kg q8 hours, orally For use in *dogs only*

Spay-neuter for higher risk patients

Higher risk patients may present for spay-neuter surgery at a high-volume or shelter clinic. Within shelter populations, neutering before adoption policies generally apply regardless of patient age. Pediatric spay-neuter is routine in HQHVSN clinics and surgery in patients as young as 6 weeks is supported by published guidelines [10]. Information on anesthesia for pediatric patients is available in Chapter 68 as well as in numerous other articles [2,23,24,31–35]. Special attention is also warranted for geriatric patients who present for spaying or neutering due to the increased risk of underlying disease. Shelter or welfare clinics may also have other higher risk patients present for neutering such as patients with pyometra or brachycephalic airway disease. Other patients may have been victims of cruelty or neglect and have pre-existing pain and/or be in poor condition. Community clinic programs are encouraged to develop individualized anesthesia protocols for higher risk patients. For example, protocols with large doses of α_2-adrenergic receptor agonists may not be appropriate for geriatric patients or those with advanced underlying cardiac disease [92]. Veterinarians should communicate with the pet owner or legal agents for these animals about the increased risk of anesthesia. However, despite this increased risk, most patients can be neutered successfully with attention to detail and close monitoring.

Anesthesia for non-spay-neuter procedures in shelters

Shelter animals and patients at community clinics may present for surgeries other than spay or neuter. For example, traumatized animals often require surgeries such as fracture repair, enucleation, limb amputation, or femoral head ostectomy. As shelter populations age (due to decreasing need for euthanasia) and more underserved pets are able to access veterinary care, a need for low-cost dentistry procedures under anesthesia has also emerged. While most of these cases are not inherently different from those presenting to regular general practice, they require additional time and attention in a resource scarce environment where staff are more used to protocol-based medicine.

Patients presenting for non-spay-neuter surgery should be worked up as much as clinic equipment and resources allow. The preanesthetic work up for such cases generally includes laboratory work and imaging as indicated where available. Each patient should receive an individually designed anesthetic protocol with balanced anesthesia and appropriate analgesia. For most surgical procedures, a pure μ-opioid receptor agonist such as hydromorphone or methadone is indicated, in accordance with current pain management guidelines [85]. IV catheters should be placed, and anesthesia can be induced with any number of medications commonly available in shelters such as Telazol®, ketamine, or propofol [37,38]. For analgesia, a balanced protocol should include appropriate local blocks. Non-steroidal anti-inflammatory medications should be given unless contraindicated [85]. Patients undergoing invasive or longer (greater than 30 min) procedures should be individually monitored according to American College of Veterinary Anesthesia and Analgesia monitoring guidelines [45].

References

1 Nolen RS. A specialty whose time has come – shelter medicine recognized as veterinary specialty. *J Am Vet Med Assoc* 2014; **244**(11): 1219–1221.

2 Bushby P, Griffin B. An Overview of Pediatric Spay and Neuter Benefits and Techniques. DVM 360, February 1, 2011. www.dvm360.com/view/overview-pediatric-spay-and-neuter-benefits-and-techniques (accessed June 2023).

3 Howe LM. Short term results and complications of prepubertal gonadectomy in cats and dogs. *J Am Vet Med Assoc* 1997; **211**(1): 57–62.

4 Howe LM, Slater MR, Boothe HW, *et al.* Long term outcome of gonadectomy performed at an early age or traditional age in cats. *J Am Vet Med Assoc* 2000; **217**(11): 1661–1665.

5 Joyce A, Yates D. Help stop teenage pregnancy! Early-age neutering in cats. *J Feline Med Surg* 2011; **13**(1): 3–10.

6 Root Kustritz MV. Early spay-neuter: clinical considerations. *Clin Tech Small Anim Pract* 2002; **17**(3): 124–128.

7 Spain CV, Scarlett JM, Houpt KA. Long term risks and benefits of early age neutering in cats. *J Am Vet Med Assoc* 2004; **224**(3): 372–380.

8 Kustritz MVR. Determining the optimal age for gonadectomy of dogs and cats. *J Am Vet Med Assoc* 2007; **231**: 1665–1675.

9 Griffin B. High-quality, high-volume sterilization programs. *Clin Theriogenol* 2013; **5**: 183–189.

10 Griffin B, Bushby PA, McCobb E, *et al.* The Association of Shelter Veterinarians' 2016 veterinary medical care guidelines for spay-neuter programs. *J Am Vet Med Assoc* 2016; **249**(2): 165–188.

11 Levy JK, Bard KM, Tucker SJ, *et al.* Perioperative mortality in cats and dogs undergoing spay- or castration at a high-volume clinic. *Vet J* 2017; **224**: 11–15.

12 Looney A, Bohling MW, Bushby PA, *et al.* The Association of Shelter Veterinarians veterinary medical care guidelines for spay-neuter programs. *J Am Vet Med Assoc* 2008; **223**(1): 74–86.

13 Ko JCH, Abbo LA, Weil AB, *et al.* A comparison of anesthetic and cardiorespiratory effects of tiletamine-zolazepam-butorphanol and tiletamine-zolazepam-butorphanol-medetomidine in cats. *Vet Ther* 2007; **8**: 164–176.

14 Polson S, Taylor PM, Yates D. Analgesia after feline ovariohysterectomy under midazolam-medetomidine-ketamine anaesthesia with buprenorphine or butorphanol, and carprofen or meloxicam: a prospective, randomized clinical trial. *J Feline Med Surg* 2012; **14**: 553–559.

15 Barletta M, Austin BR, Ko JC, *et al.* Evaluation of dexmedetomidine and ketamine in combination with opioids as injectable anesthesia for castration in dogs. *J Am Vet Med Assoc* 2011; **238**: 1159–1167.

16 Krimins RA, Ko JC, Weil AB, *et al.* Evaluation of anesthetic, analgesic, and cardiorespiratory effects in dogs after intramuscular administration of dexmedetomidine-butorphanol-tiletamine-zolazepam or dexmedetomidine-tramadol-ketamine drug combinations. *Am J Vet Res* 2012; **73**: 1707–1714.

17 Harrison KA, Robertson SA, Levy JK, *et al.* Evaluation of medetomidine, ketamine and buprenorphine for neutering feral cats. *J Feline Med Surg* 2011; **13**: 896–902.

18 Posner LP, Applegate J, Cannedy A, *et al.* Total injectable anesthesia of dogs and cats for remote location veterinary sterilization clinic. *BMC Vet Res* 2020; **16**: 304.

19 White S. *High-Quality, High-Volume Spay and Neuter and Other Shelter Surgeries*. Hoboken, NJ: Wiley-Blackwell, 2020.

20 Alef M, Von Praun F, Oechtering G. Is routine pre-anaesthetic haematological and biochemical screening justified in dogs? *Vet Anaesth and Analg* 2008; **35**(2): 132–140.

21 Del Mar Díaz M, Kaartinen J, Allison A. Preanaesthetic blood tests in cats and dogs older than 8 years: anaesthetists' prediction and peri-anaesthetic changes. *Vet Anaesth Analg* 2021; **48**(6): 854–860.

22 Brown CR, Garrett LD, Gilles WK, *et al.* Spectrum of care: more than treatment options. *J Am Vet Med Assoc* 2021; **259**(7): 712–717.

23 Faggella AM, Aronsohn MG. Anesthetic techniques for neutering 6- to 14-week-old-kittens. *J Am Vet Med Assoc* 1993; **202**: 56–62.

24 Faggella AM, Aronsohn MG. Evaluation of anesthetic protocols for neutering 6- to 14-week-old pups. *J Am Vet Med Assoc* 1994; **205**: 308–314.

25 Selmi AL, Mendes GM, Lins BT, *et al.* Comparison of xylazine and medetomidine as premedicants for cats being anaesthetized with propofol-sevoflurane. *Vet Rec* 2005; **157**: 139–143.

26 Joubert RM. Routine veterinary anaesthetic management practices in South Africa. *J S Afr Vet Assoc* 2000; **71**: 166–172.

27 Joubert RM. Anaesthesia and analgesia for dogs and cats in South Africa undergoing sterilisation and with osteoarthrities – an update from 2000. *J S Afr Vet Assoc* 2006; **77**: 224–228.

28 Mendes GM, Selmi AL, Barbudo-Selmi GR, *et al.* Clinical use of dexmedetomidine as premedicant in cats undergoing propofol-sevoflurane anaesthesia. *J Feline Med Surg* 2003; **5**: 265–270.

29 O'Hagan B, Pasloske K, McKinnon C, *et al.* Clinical evaluation of alfaxalone as an anaesthetic induction agent in dogs less than 12 weeks of age. *Aust Vet J* 2012; **90**: 346–350.

30 O'Hagan BJ, Pasloske K, McKinnon C, *et al.* Clinical evaluation of alfaxalone as an anaesthetic induction agent in cats less than 12 weeks of age. *Aust Vet J* 2012; **90**: 395–401.

31 Patel CM, Yates D. Evaluation of an anesthetic protocol for the neutering of eight to twelve week-old puppies. *Vet Rec* 2003; **152**(14): 439–440.

32 Polson S, Taylor PM, Yates D. Effects of age and reproductive status on postoperative pain after routine ovariohysterectomy in cats. *J Feline Med Surg* 2014; **16**: 170–176.

33 Porters N, deRooster H, Moons CPH, *et al.* Prepubertal gonadectomy in cats: different injectable anesthetic combinations and comparison with gonadectomy at traditional age. *J Feline Med Surg* 2015; **17**(6): 458–467.

34 Robertson SA, Levy J, Gunkel C, *et al.* Comparison of isoflurane and butorphanol with medetomidine, ketamine and buprenorphine for anesthesia of 7–12 week old kittens for surgical sterilization (abstract). In: *Proceedings of the Association Veterinary Anaesthetists Spring Meeting*. Doorwerth, Netherlands; May 27–30, 2003.

35 Robertson SA. Anaesthesia and analgesia for kittens and puppies. In: *Proceedings of the European Veterinary Conference*. Voorjaarsdagen, Amsterdam, Netherlands; April 27–29, 2007.

36 ASPCApro. Pharmacology for Spay/Neuter Clinics. www.aspcapro.org/resource/pharmacology-spayneuter-clinics (accessed June 2023).

37 Ko JC, Berman, AG. Anesthesia in shelter medicine. *Top Companion Anim Med* 2010; **25**(2): 92–97.

38 Ko JC, Krimins RA. Anesthesia in shelter medicine and high-volume/high-quality spay and neuter programs. In: Ko JC, ed. *Small Animal Anesthesia and Pain Management*, 2nd edn. Boca Raton, FL: CRC Press/Taylor and Francis Group, 2019: 419–427.

39 Williams LS, Levy JK, Robertson SA, *et al.* Use of the anesthetic combination of tiletamine, zolazepam, ketamine, and xylazine for neutering feral cats. *J Am Vet Med Assoc* 2002; **220**(10): 1491–1495.

40 American Society of Anesthesiologists (ASA). Recommendations for Pre-Anesthesia Checkout, 2008. www.asahq.org/standards-and-practice-parameters/2008-asa-recommendations-for-pre-anesthesia-checkout (accessed February 2023).

41 Dorsch JA, Dorsch SE. Equipment checkout and maintenance. In: Dorsch JA, Dorsch SE, eds. *Understanding Anesthesia Equipment*, 5th edn. Philadelphia, PA: Lippincott Williams and Wilkins, 2008: 931–954.

42 Smith JC, Bolon B. Comparison of three commercially available activated charcoal canisters for passive scavenging of waste isoflurane during conventional rodent anesthesia. *Contemp Top Lab Anim Sci* 2003; **42**: 10–15.

43 Haskins SC. Monitoring the anesthetized patient. In: Grimm K, Lamont L, Tranquilli W, *et al.*, eds. *Veterinary Anesthesia and Analgesia*, 5th edn. Ames, IA: Wiley Blackwell, 2015: 86–113.

44 Grubb T, Sager J, Gaynor JS, *et al.* 2020 AAHA Anesthesia and monitoring guidelines for dogs and cats. *J Am Anim Hosp Assoc* 2020; **56**: 59–82.

45 American College of Veterinary Anesthesia and Analgesia (ACVAA). *Small Animal Monitoring Guidelines*. www.acvaa.org/veterinarians/guidelines (accessed June 2023).

46 Robertson SA. Oxygenation and ventilation. In: Green SA, ed. *Veterinary Anesthesia and Pain Management Secrets*. Philadelphia, PA: Hanley and Belfus, 2002: 15–20.

47 Brodbelt DC, Pfeiffer DU, Young LE, *et al.* Risk factors for anaesthetic-related death in cats: results from the Confidential Enquiry into Perioperative Small Animal Fatalities (CEPSAF). *Br J Anaesth* 2007; **99**: 617–623.

48 Dorsch JA, Dorsch SE. Gas monitoring. In: Dorsch JA, Dorsch SE, eds. *Understanding Anesthesia Equipment*, 5th edn. Philadelphia, PA: Wolters Kluwer Health-Lippincott Williams & Wilkins, 2007: 685.

49 McKelvey D. Anesthetic problems and emergencies. In: McKelvey D, Hollingshead KS, eds. *Small Animal Anesthesia and Analgesia*, 2nd edn. St. Louis, MO: Mosby, 2000: 225–251.

50 The Reassessment Campaign on Veterinary Resuscitation (RECOVER) initiative. *RECOVER Guidelines*. www.recoverinitiative.org/cpr-guidelines/current-recover-guideline (accessed March 2023).

51 Cole SG, Otto CM, Hughes D. Cardiopulmonary cerebral resuscitation in small animals – a clinical practice review Part II. *J Vet Emerg Crit Care* 2003; **13**: 13–23.

52 Muir WW. Cardiovascular emergencies. In: Muir WW, Hubbell JAE, Skarda RT, eds. *Handbook of Veterinary Anesthesia*, 4th edn. St. Louis, MO: Mosby, 2007: 557–575.

53 Davis H, Jensen T, Johnson A, *et al.* 2013 AAHA/AAFP fluid therapy guidelines for dogs and cats. *J Am Anim Hosp Assoc* 2013; **49**: 149–159.

54 Andrzejowski J, Hoyle J, Eapen G, *et al.* Effect of prewarming on post-induction core temperature and the incidence of inadvertent perioperative hypothermia in patients undergoing general anaesthesia. *Br J Anaesth* 2008; **101**: 627–631.

55 Harvey RC. Hypothermia. In: Greene SA, ed. *Veterinary Anesthesia and Pain Management Secrets*. Philadelphia, PA: Hanley and Belfus, 2002: 149–152.

56 Clark-Price SC, Dossin O, Jones KR, *et al.* Comparison of three different methods to prevent heat loss in healthy dogs undergoing 90 minutes of general anesthesia. *Vet Anaesth Analg* 2013; **40**: 280–284.

57 Machon RG, Raffe MR, Robinson EP. Warming with a forced air warming blanket minimizes anesthetic-induced hypothermia in cats. *Vet Surg* 1999; **28**: 301–310.

58 Hasiuk MM, Brown D, Cooney C, *et al.* Application of fast-track surgery principles to evaluate effects of atipamezole on recovery and analgesia following ovariohysterectomy in cats anesthetized with dexmedetomidine-ketamine-hydromorphone. *J Am Vet Med Assoc* 2015; **246**(6): 645–653.

59 Dobbins S, Brown NO, Shofer FS. Comparison of the effects of buprenorphine, oxymorphone hydrochloride, and ketoprofen for postoperative analgesia after onychectomy or onychectomy and sterilizatioin in cats. *J Am Anim Hosp Assoc* 2002; **38**: 507–514.

60 Campbell VL, Drobatz KJ, Perkowski SZ. Postoperative hypoxemia and hypercarbia in healthy dogs undergoing routine ovariohysterectomy or castration and receiving butorphanol or hydromorphone for analgesia. *J Am Vet Med Assoc* 2003; **222**: 330–336.

61 Ko JC, Mandsager RE, Lange DN, *et al.* Cardiorespiratory responses and plasma cortisol concentrations in dogs treated with medetomidine before undergoing ovariohysterectomy. *J Am Vet Med Assoc* 2000; **217**: 509–514.

62 Al-Gizawiy MM, P Rudé E. Comparison of preoperative carprofen and postoperative butorphanol as postsurgical analgesics in cats undergoing ovariohysterectomy. *Vet Anaesth Analg* 2004; **31**: 164–174.

63 Caulkett N, Read M, Fowler D, *et al.* A comparison of the analgesic effects of butorphanol with those of meloxicam after elective ovariohysterectomy in dogs. *Can Vet J* 2003; **44**: 565–570.

64 Dzikiti TB, Joubert KE, Venter LJ, *et al.* Comparison of morphine and carprofen administered alone or in combination for analgesia in dogs undergoing overiohysterectomy. *J S Afr Vet Assoc* 2006; **77**: 120–126.

65 Fresno L, Moll J, Peñalba B, *et al.* Effects of preoperative administration of meloxicam on whole blood platelet aggregation, buccal musocal bleeding time, and haematological indices in dogs undergoing elective ovariohysterectomy. *Vet J* 2006; **170**: 138–140.

66 Lobetti RG, Joubert KE. Effect of administration of nonsteroidal anti-inflammatory drugs before surgery on renal function in clinically normal dogs. *Am J Vet Res* 2000; **61**: 1501–1507.

67 Leece EA, Brearley JC, Harding EF. Comparison of carprofen and meloxicam for 72 hours following ovariohysterectomy in dogs. *Vet Anaesth Analg* 2005; **32**: 184–192.

68 Lemke KA, Runyon CL, Horney BS. Effects of preoperative administration of ketoprofen on anesthetic requirements and signs of postoperative pain in dogs undergoing elective ovariohysterectoomy. *J Am Vet Med Assoc* 2002; **221**: 1268–1275.

69 Slingsby LS, Waterman-Pearson AE. The post-operative analgesic effects of ketamine after canine ovariohysterectomy – a comparison between pre- or post-operative administration. *Res Vet Sci* 2000; **69**: 147–152.

70 Slingsby LS, Waterman-Pearson AE. Postoperative analgesia in the cat after ovariohysterectomy by use of carprofen, ketoprofen, meloxicam or tolfenamic acid. *J Small Anim Pract* 2000; **41**: 447–450.

71 Slingsby LS, Waterman-Pearson AE. Comparison between meloxicam and carprofen for postoperative analgesia after feline ovariohysterectomy. *J Small Anim Pract* 2002; **43**: 286–289.

72 Carpenter RE, Wilson DV, Evans AT. Evaluation of intraperitoneal and incisional lidocaine or bupivacaine for analgesia following ovariohysterectomy in the dog. *Vet Anaesth Analg* 2004; **31**: 46–52.

73 Wilson DV, Barnes KS, Hauptman JG. Pharmacokinetics of combined intraperitoneal and incisional lidocaine in the dog following ovariohysterectomy. *J Vet Pharmacol Ther* 2004; **27**: 105–109.

74 Tobias KM, Harvey RC, Byarlay JM. A comparison of four methods of analgesia in cats following ovariohysterectomy. *Vet Anaesth Analg* 2006; **33**: 390–398.

75 Huuskonen V, Hughes JM, Estaca Banon E, *et al.* Intratesticular lidocaine reduces the response to surgical castration in dogs. *Vet Anaesth Analg* 2013; **40**: 74–82.

76 Moldal ER, Eriksen T, Kirpensteijn J, *et al.* Intratesticular and subcutaneous lidocaine alters the intraoperative haemodynamic responses and heart rate variability in male cats undergoing castration. *Vet Anaesth Analg* 2013; **40**: 63–73.

77 Morgaz J, Navarrete R, Munoz-Rascon P, *et al.* Postoperative analgesic effects of dexketoprofen, buprenorphine and tramadol in dogs undergoing ovariohysterectomy. *Res Vet Sci* 2013; **95**: 278–282.

78 Staffieri F, Centonze P, Gigante G, *et al.* Comparison of the analgesic effects of robenacoxib, buprenorphine and their combination in cats after ovariohysterectomy. *Vet J* 2013; **197**: 363–367.

79 Steagall PV, Taylor PM, Rodrigues LC, *et al.* Analgesia for cats after ovariohysterectomy with either buprenorphine or carprofen alone or in combination. *Vet Rec* 2009; **164**: 359–363.

80 Giordano T, Steagall PV, Ferreira TH, *et al.* Postoperative analgesic effects of intravenous, intramuscular, subcutaneous or oral transmucosal buprenorphine administered to cats undergoing ovariohysterectomy. *Vet Anaesth Analg* 2010; **37**: 357–366.

81 Shih AC, Robertson S, Isaza N, *et al.* Comparison between analgesic effects of buprenorphine, carprofen, and buprenorphine with carprofen for canine ovariohysterectomy. *Vet Anaesth Analg* 2008; **35**: 69–79.

82 Ko JC, Freeman LJ, Barletta M, *et al.* Efficacy of oral transmucosal and intravenous administration of buprenorphine before surgery for postoperative analgesia in dogs undergoing ovariohysterectomy. *J Am Vet Med Assoc* 2011; **238**: 318–328.

83 Stevens BJ, Posner, LP, Jones CA, *et al.* Comparison of the effect of intratesticular lidocaine/bupivacaine vs. saline placebo on pain scores and incision site reactions in dogs undergoing routine castration. *Vet J* 2013; **196**(3): 499–503.

84 Corletto F. Multimodal and balanced analgesia. *Vet Res Commun* 2007; **31**: 59–63.

85 Epstein ME, Rodan I, Griffenhagen G, *et al.* AAHA/AAFP pain management guidelines for dogs and cats. *J Feline Med Surg* 2015; **17**: 251–272.

86 Campoy L, Read M. *Small Animal Regional Anesthesia and Analgesia*. Ames, IA: Wiley-Blackwell, 2013.

87 Beckman B, Legendre L. Regional nerve blocks for oral surgery in companion animals. *Compend Contin Educ Pract Vet* 2002; **24**(6): 429–444.

88 Pratt CL, Blakrishna A, McGowan E, *et al.* A prospective randomized, double-blinded clinical study evaluating the efficacy and safety of bupivacaine versus morphine-bupivacaine in caudal epidurals in cats with urethral obstruction. *J Vet Emerg Crit Care* 2020; **30**(2): 170–178.

89 Steagall PVM, Benito J, Monteiro B, *et al.* Intraperitoneal and incisional analgesia in small animals: simple, cost-effective techniques. *J Small Anim Pract* 2020; **61**: 19–23.

90 Gaynor J, Muir WW. *Handbook of Veterinary Pain Management*, 3rd edn. St. Louis, MO: Elsevier Health Sciences, 2015.

91 Abelson AA, McCobb E, Shaw S, *et al.* Use of wound soaker catheters for the administration of local anesthetic for post-operative analgesia: 56 cases. *Vet Anaesth Analg* 2009; **36**(6): 597–602.

92 Lemke KA. Perioperative use of selective alpha-2 agonists and antagonists in small animals. *Can Vet J* 2004; **45**(6): 475–480.

52 Comparative Anesthesia and Analgesia – Horses

Lori A. Bidwell
East West Equine Sports Medicine, Lexington, Kentucky, USA

Chapter contents

Introduction, 1048
Anesthetic risk, 1048
Variation in size, 1048
Cardiopulmonary resuscitation, 1049
Considerations for equine induction, 1049
Effect of recumbency in equine patients, 1049
Heart rate considerations, 1049
Equine neonate versus foal, 1049
The pregnant mare, 1050
Fluid therapy considerations, 1050
Recovery, 1050
References, 1050

Introduction

Equine anesthesia has always been associated with greater patient risk compared to other common domestic species. Delivery of anesthesia is complicated by many factors including the large patient size range, the need to induce controlled recumbency during anesthetic induction, specialized equipment requirements, perfusion issues related to large body mass, and instinctive behaviors. In addition, drug dosages are often extrapolated from those of other species and many of the drugs are used in an extra-label manner. Understanding the unique factors associated with equine anesthesia compared to other species is the first step in improving patient safety.

Anesthetic risk

The risk of anesthetic mortality is greater in equine species compared to other domestic animals. Studies have reported overall mortality rates between 0.24% and 2.24% for horses [1–7] compared to the widely reported rates for dogs (0.05%) and cats (0.11%) [8]. However, other smaller studies from other countries have reported higher small animal mortality rates that are similar to those reported for equine patients [9–11]. A mortality rate of 1% is commonly referenced in most surgical facilities when discussing the risk of anesthesia with horse owners; however, the percentage can increase considerably with metabolically unstable patients such as those with colic, where mortality has been reported to be as high as 38.3% [12]. The primary complications associated with death are cardiac arrest, orthopedic injuries in recovery, and myopathy or neuropathy in the postanesthesia period. Complication rates as high as 17.5% have been reported [13]. Postanesthetic colic is an additional concern. The use of opioid analgesics, time of surgery, choice of anesthetics, breed, and concurrent use of certain antibiotics have been implicated as risk factors for developing postoperative colic, although specific mechanisms have not been definitively determined [13–19].

Variation in size

Horses come in a broad range of sizes. A miniature horse foal can weigh less than 10 kg, while a draft horse used for competition pulling can weigh up to 1300 kg. Because of this size variation, specific equipment must be purchased to move these animals, deliver anesthetic, and assist or control ventilation. A small animal anesthetic machine can be used for most miniature horses, neonates, and foals up to 150 kg, but large animal anesthetic systems must be purchased for older foals and horses. The limiting factors with most small animal systems include the volume of the carbon dioxide absorbent canister, the volume of the reservoir bag, and the diameter of the breathing system tubing and adaptor that connects to the endotracheal tube. Endotracheal tubes, reservoir bags, and anesthetic tubing are specifically designed for equine patients and are, therefore, more expensive than equipment used in small animal patients (much of which is repurposed from the human market). Much of the monitoring equipment designed for human patients can be adapted for use on larger species. One common problem is that human monitors often consider normal heart rates in adult horses to be bradycardic with default alarms set for rates below 40 beats/min.

Surgical tables and hoisting mechanisms must be designed specifically for equine or large animal patients. If a practice regularly sees large draft breed horses, it is wise to purchase a 2-ton hoist rather than the typical 1-ton hoist as larger horses can overstress

Veterinary Anesthesia and Analgesia: The Sixth Edition of Lumb and Jones. Edited by Leigh Lamont, Kurt Grimm, Sheilah Robertson, Lydia Love and Carrie Schroeder.
© 2024 John Wiley & Sons, Inc. Published 2024 by John Wiley & Sons, Inc.
Companion website: www.wiley.com/go/lamont/anesthesia

inappropriate equipment. In addition, the typical surgical table designed for an adult equine is not big enough to support the mass of a 1000 kg patient for a procedure requiring lateral recumbency. Therefore, two surgical tables may need to be used together to provide adequate support. If two tables are not available, the use of stacked pads or mats can substitute under limbs, head, and neck. Many of the draft breeds do not have long enough tails to attach a rope for assisted recovery. Fortunately, most draft horses are relatively cooperative regarding recovery.

Size is also a factor in determining peripheral (skeletal muscle) perfusion. Mean arterial blood pressure requirements increase as muscle mass (and muscle compartment/compression pressure) increases [5]. The risk of postanesthetic neuropathy and myopathy is higher in equine patients, particularly draft and large warmblood breeds. While recommendations on minimum mean arterial pressures during anesthesia vary, this author recommends a minimum mean arterial blood pressure in horses greater than 500 kg of at least 80 mmHg based on personal experience. Maintaining a mean arterial blood pressure of greater than 70 mmHg in normal adult horses has been shown to minimize postoperative complications associated with hypotension [20,21]. Neonates and foals have lower normal resting mean arterial blood pressure (47–50 mmHg in neonates and 55–70 mmHg in foals), but there has been a report of a neonate developing postanesthetic myositis after an anesthetic event with average mean arterial blood pressure between 45 and 65 mmHg [22]. Therefore, the goal with all ages and sizes of horses should be to maintain blood pressure above 60 mmHg in foals and 70–80 mmHg in adults depending on body size. Adjuncts to increase mean arterial blood pressure include inotropes, vasopressors, and catecholamines. Dobutamine is used most often in equine patients, but dopamine, ephedrine, phenylephrine, vasopressin, norepinephrine, epinephrine, and calcium salts are alternative options if used appropriately. Of the inotropes, dobutamine has been found to be the most useful for increasing mean arterial blood pressure in neonates, foals, and adult horses under general anesthesia [23–28].

Cardiopulmonary resuscitation

Anatomic variation complicates cardiopulmonary resuscitation. An equine neonate or older foal can be managed similar to a canine but adult equine ribs are narrow and impossible to separate by hand if open chest cardiac compressions are required. A rib resection is required for open chest compressions, and this is not practical in most situations. Therefore, chest compressions on an adult equine patient require use of the anesthetist's full body weight concentrated on either both knees or feet. External chest compressions must be performed at a minimum of 80 compressions/min in an adult to produce a cardiac output near 50% of that of a deeply anesthetized horse [29]. However, external compressions of 20/min in ponies have been shown to produce a cardiac output of approximately 50% normal baseline values [30]. As an alternative to external compressions, when a horse suffers cardiopulmonary arrest during general anesthesia for abdominal exploration, the surgeon can make an incision through the diaphragm and perform direct cardiac compression.

Although cardiac arrhythmias are common in horses during exercise and after anesthesia, ventricular fibrillation is uncommon in horses prior to arrest [31–33]. Even if ventricular fibrillation is present, most electrical cardiac defibrillators are not designed to deliver a large enough electrical output required to defibrillate an adult equine heart.

Considerations for equine induction

Inducing recumbency in horses from the standing position can be dangerous. In order to minimize the risk, appropriate sedation and muscle relaxation should be administered prior to induction. Ketamine is one of the primary induction drugs used in horses, but it has minimal muscle relaxant properties. Muscle relaxation and induction quality can be improved by increasing the dose of premedication, adding an opioid or phenothiazine to an α_2-adrenergic receptor agonist, and/or administering ketamine with a coinduction agent (commonly either a benzodiazepine or propofol) [34–37].

There are differences in induction doses between horses, donkeys, and mules. Donkeys are typically less affected by premedication and induction drugs when compared to horses. Mules appear to be intermediate between donkeys and horses. A starting point for dosing drugs for donkeys can be based on 1.5 times the dose of a horse. The exception to this rule is guaifenesin, as donkeys are more sensitive to the central effects of the drug, resulting in hypotension and apnea with bolus administration. The difference in response to drugs in donkeys appears to be due to variation in body water distribution and drug metabolism [38,39].

Effect of recumbency in equine patients

Prolonged recumbency in equine patients is not benign. Ventilation–perfusion mismatch and shunting are inevitable when an equine patient is recumbent. Lateral recumbency results in atelectasis of the dependent lung and dorsal recumbency results in progressive atelectasis of the dorsal lung fields [40]. Controlled ventilation can improve arterial oxygenation, but in a patient with abdominal distension associated with colic, ruptured bladder, or pregnancy, cardiac output can be compromised during periods of high intrathoracic pressure. In contrast to small animal patients, a recent study performed with horses found that decreasing the inspired oxygen concentration to 50% from > 95% resulted in significant reductions in arterial oxygen saturation; therefore, the use of lower inspired oxygen concentrations to reduce atelectasis is not recommended [41–45].

Heart rate considerations

Sedation with an α_2-adrenergic receptor agonist in horses results in bradycardia. This can be further compounded by the concurrent administration of many anesthetic drugs. However, the dissociative agents ketamine and tiletamine have sympathomimetic properties and administration often produces transient increases in heart rate. Typically, once heart rate returns to baseline levels under anesthesia, there are no peaks or large changes in heart rate that are indicative of arousal as is seen in small animal patients. Increased heart rate in response to surgical stimulation is unusual in the healthy adult equine under general anesthesia.

Equine neonate versus foal

A neonate is less equipped to alter stroke volume in response to hypovolemia and bradycardia. In neonates, heart rate has a primary function in controlling cardiac output. The most commonly used agents for premedication in horses are α_2-adrenergic receptor agonists, and one effect associated with these drugs is bradycardia. Therefore, it seems prudent to minimize the use of α_2-adrenergic receptor agonists in neonates or compromised older foals. Older foals can have variable responses to drugs and should be dosed individually based on behavior [46,47].

The pregnant mare

A pregnant mare presenting for an emergency procedure requiring general anesthesia has several physiologic differences that challenge the anesthetist. Vasodilation induced by inhalant anesthetic is enhanced by circulating hormones induced by pregnancy and parturition [48]. In human females, endothelial-derived hyperpolarizing factor and nitric oxide are responsible for decreased vascular tone [49]. Oxygenation in the mare is complicated by the gravid uterus and abdominal contents placing pressure on the diaphragm, resulting in reduced functional residual capacity. Controlled or assisted ventilation is often necessary to allow the mare to receive an appropriate tidal volume. Tipping the mare slightly off dorsal recumbency also facilitates venous return by reducing direct compression of the caudal vena cava. In order to appropriately ventilate the pregnant mare, airway pressures often exceed 30 cmH_2O, particularly when the mare is in the Trendelenburg position for manipulation of the fetus. In this situation, airway pressures reaching 60 cmH_2O are often required to deliver a tidal volume of 10 mL/kg. In addition to ventilation concerns, endotracheal intubation is recommended to prevent aspiration of gastrointestinal contents. Due to the emergency nature of dystocia or cesarean section, fasting prior to the procedure rarely occurs. In human medicine, elevated intragastric pressure, delayed gastric emptying, and circulating progesterone relaxing the gastroesophageal sphincter are blamed for the increased risk of aspiration pneumonia [50–51].

Fluid therapy considerations

A discussion involving fluid therapy in horses under general anesthesia can be controversial. The traditional thought process regarding fluid therapy involves administration of isotonic fluids at a rate of 5–15 mL/kg/h with fluid boluses delivered as needed during periods of hypotension. This rate of administration has been found to be ineffective in preventing hypotension induced by inhaled anesthetics [52]. The plasma volume expansion from crystalloids is less than 20–25% of the volume administered. In addition, the traditional practice of administering crystalloids for blood loss in a 3:1 ratio is not as effective as once thought. Rather than using a prescribed fluid rate for every patient, crystalloids and colloids should be administered on a patient-specific basis by using goal-directed fluid therapy endpoints (e.g., blood gases, capillary refill time, mucous membrane color, and pulse variation) for evaluation [53–55].

Recovery

The true challenge of equine anesthesia compared to other domestic species is safely returning the patient to the standing position without injury. The role of the anesthetist continues through the recovery period by appropriate selection of sedatives and often assisting the horse in attempts to stand. Horses have a flight instinct that prevents most of them from remaining recumbent in the recovery stall. In addition, some patients will prematurely attempt to stand because of the need to urinate following administration of large volumes of intravenous fluids and increased urine production following α_2-adrenergic receptor agonist administration.

The transition of a horse receiving anesthetic in 100% oxygen with vascular and ventilatory support to a recovery stall without monitoring or oxygen supplementation is not one in which heavy sedation is recommended. However, sedation may smooth the recovery from inhalant anesthesia. It is important to use a balance of technique and sedation for a safe recovery. Ideally, the adult horse should be maintained in recumbency until there is loss of nystagmus, response to sound, and return of menace and tongue tone in response to gentle traction. Menace response is a learned behavior, so foals typically will not respond to stimulation over the eye unless there is direct contact with the lids or cornea (the latter is not recommended unless in an emergency situation). Sedation can be administered just prior to moving the horse into recovery. Depending on the depth of anesthesia, 50–150 mg of xylazine or 5–20 mg of romifidine or detomidine, with or without 2–5 mg of acepromazine, can be administered intramuscularly prior to moving the horse into recovery. An additional small dose of a sedative can be administered intravenously if needed [56–59]. A towel over the eyes and cotton in the ears aids in minimizing stimulation from outside the stall, particularly in horses that are sound sensitive.

There are several recovery techniques that can be utilized depending on the specific case: unassisted recovery or "self-recovery," rope recovery utilizing ropes on the halter and tail as a pulley system through rings on the walls, pool recovery, sling recovery, and recovery on a tilt table [60]. Personnel safety should be considered when developing a recovery plan for any particular situation [61]. Self-recovery is practical for young healthy horses after elective procedures. Rope, pool, sling, and tilt table recovery are utilized for patients in whom instability or weakness is a concern. Rope recovery requires a stall with rings in the walls, strong cotton or web rope and two people to pull the ropes to assist the horse at the appropriate time, but may reduce the number of attempts at standing [62,63]. Some finesse is needed in that the head rope should be used for support and the tail rope is used for the majority of assistance (where the most effort is required by the handler). Horses need to have freedom in their front end to get momentum to stand; therefore, the head rope should not be pulled tightly until the horse is standing. Pool, sling, and tilt table recovery are typically reserved for fractures and horses with neurologic concerns. Recovering a foal from anesthesia is a very different process from that of adults. Foals should be assisted in recovery until approximately 5–6 months of age.

References

1 Johnston GM, Taylor PM, Holmes MA, *et al.* Confidential Enquiry into Perioperative Equine Fatalities (CEPEF-1): preliminary results. *Equine Vet J* 1995; **27**: 193–200.
2 Bidwell LA, Bramlage LR, Rood WA. Equine perioperative fatalities associated with general anesthesia at a private practice: a retrospective case series. *Vet Anaesth Analg* 2007; **34**: 23–30.
3 Johnston GM, Eastman JK, Wood JL, *et al.* The Confidential Enquiry into Perioperative Equine Fatalities (CEPEF): mortality results of Phases 1 and 2. *Vet Anaesth Analg* 2002; **29**: 159–170.
4 Young SS, Taylor PM. Factors influencing the outcome of equine anaesthesia: a review of 1,314 cases. *Equine Vet J* 1993; **25**: 147–151.
5 O'Donovan KA, Aarnes TK, Hubbell JA, *et al.* Risk of anesthesia-related complications in draft horses: a retrospective, single-center analysis. *Vet Anaesth Analg* 2023; **50**: 157–162.
6 Gozalo-Marcilla M, Bettschart-Wolfensberger R, Johnston M, *et al.* Data collection for the fourth multicentre confidential enquiry into perioperative equine fatalities (CEPEF4) study: new technology and preliminary results. *Animals (Basel)* 2021; **11**: 2549.
7 Laurenza C, Ansart L, Portier K. Risk factors of anesthesia-related mortality and morbidity in one equine hospital: a retrospective study on 1,161 cases undergoing elective or emergency surgeries. *Front Vet Sci* 2020; **6**: 514.

8 Brodbelt DC, Bissitt KJ, Hammond RA, *et al.* The risk of death: the confidential enquiry into perioperative small animal fatalities. *Vet Anaesth Analg* 2008; **35**: 365–373.
9 Bille C, Auvigne V, Libermann S, *et al.* Risk of anaesthetic mortality in dogs and cats: an observational cohort study of 3546 cases. *Vet Anaesth Analg* 2012; **39**: 59–68.
10 Gil L, Redondo JI. Canine anaesthetic death in Spain: a multicentre prospective cohort study of 2012 cases. *Vet Anaesth Analg* 2013; **40**: e57–e67.
11 Itami T, Aida H, Asakawa M, *et al.* Association between preoperative characteristics and risk of anaesthesia-related death in dogs in small-animal referral hospitals in Japan. *Vet Anaesth Analg* 2017; **44**: 461–472.
12 Adami C, Westwood-Hearn H, Bolt DM, *et al.* Prevalence of electrolyte disturbances and perianesthetic death risk factors in 120 horses undergoing colic surgery. *J Equine Vet Sci* 2020; **84**: 102843.
13 Jago RC, Corletto F, Wright IM. Peri-anaesthetic complications in an equine referral hospital: risk factors for post anaesthetic colic. *Equine Vet J* 2015; **47**: 635–640.
14 Nelson BB, Lordan EE, Hassel DM. Risk factors associated with gastrointestinal dysfunction in horses undergoing elective procedures under general anaesthesia. *Equine Vet J Suppl* 2013; **45**: 8–14.
15 Senior JM, Pinchbeck GL, Allister R, *et al.* Post anaesthetic colic in horses: a preventable complication? *Equine Vet J* 2006; **33**: 479–484.
16 Little D, Redding WR, Blikslager AT. Risk factors for reduced perioperative fecal output in horses: 37 cases (1997–1998). *J Am Vet Med Assoc* 2001; **218**: 414–420.
17 Mircica E, Clutton RE, Kyles KW, *et al.* Problems associated with perioperative morphine in horses: a retrospective cases analysis. *Vet Anaesth Analg* 2003; **30**: 147–155.
18 Senior JM, Pinchbeck G, Dugdale AHA, *et al.* A retrospective study of the risk factors and prevalence of colic in horses after orthopaedic surgery. *Vet Rec* 2004; **155**: 321–325.
19 Anderson MS, Clark L, Dyson S, *et al.* Risk factors for colic in horses after general anaesthesia for MRI or nonabdominal surgery: absence of evidence of effect from perianaesthetic morphine. *Equine Vet J* 2006; **38**: 368–374.
20 Duke T, Filzek U, Read MR, *et al.* Clinical observations surrounding an increased incidence of postanesthetic myopathy in halothane-anesthetized horses. *Vet Anaesth Analg* 2006; **33**: 122–127.
21 Grandy JL, Steffey EP, Hodgson DS, *et al.* Arterial hypotension and the development of postanesthetic myopathy in halothane-anesthetized horses. *Am J Vet Res* 1987; **48**: 192–197.
22 Manning M, Dubielzig R, McGuirk S. Postoperative myositis in a neonatal foal: a case report. *Vet Surg* 1996; **24**: 69–72.
23 Craig CA, Haskens SC, Hildebrand SV. The cardiopulmonary effects of dobutamine and norepinephrine in isoflurane-anesthetized foals. *Vet Anaesth Analg* 2007; **34**: 377–387.
24 Valverde A, Giguere S, Sanchez LC, *et al.* Effects of dobutamine, norepinephrine and vasopressin on cardiovascular function in anesthetized neonatal foals with induced hypotension. *Am J Vet Res* 2006; **67**: 1730–1737.
25 deVries A, Brearly JC, Taylor PM. Effects of dobutamine on cardiac index and arterial blood pressure in isoflurane-anesthetized horses under clinical conditions. *J Vet Pharmacol Ther* 2009; **32**: 353–358.
26 Dancker C, Hopster K, Rohn K, *et al.* Effects of dobutamine, dopamine, phenylephrine and noradrenaline on systemic haemodynamics and intestinal perfusion in isoflurane anaesthetised horses. *Equine Vet J* 2018; **50**: 104–110.
27 Schier MF, Raisis AL, Secombe CJ, *et al.* Effects of dobutamine hydrochloride on cardiovascular function in horses anesthetized with isoflurane with or without acepromazine maleate premedication. *Am J Vet Res* 2016; **77**: 1318–1324.
28 Ohta M, Kurimoto S, Ishikawa Y, *et al.* Cardiovascular effects of dobutamine and phenylephrine infusion in sevoflurane-anesthetized Thoroughbred horses. *J Vet Med Sci* 2013; **75**: 1443–1448.
29 Hubbell JA, Muir WW, Gaynor JS. Cardiovascular effects of thoracic compression in horses subjected to euthanasia. *Equine Vet J* 1993; **25**: 282–284.
30 Frauenfelder HC, Fessler JF, Latshaw HS, *et al.* External cardiovascular resuscitation of the anesthetized pony. *J Am Vet Med Assoc* 1981; **179**: 673–676.
31 Morgan RA, Raftery AG, Cripps P, *et al.* The prevalence and nature of cardiac arrhythmias in horses following general anaesthesia and surgery. *Acta Vet Scand* 2011; **23**: 53–62.
32 Buhl R, Meldgaard C, Barbesgaard L. Cardiac arrhythmias in clinically healthy showjumping horses. *Equine Vet J* 2010; **38**(Suppl): 196–201.
33 Barbesgaard L, Buhl R, Meldgaard C. Prevalence of exercise-associated arrhythmias in normal performing dressage horses. *Equine Vet J* 2010; **38**(Suppl): 202–207.
34 Mantrell S, Nyman G. Effects of additional premedication on romifidine and ketamine anesthesia in horses. *Acta Vet Scand* 1996; **37**: 315–325.
35 Hubbell JA, Hinchcliff KW, Schmall LM, *et al.* Anesthetic, cardiorespiratory and metabolic effects of four intravenous anesthetic regimens induced in horses immediately after maximal exercise. *Am J Vet Res* 2000; **61**: 1545–1552.
36 Posner LP, Kasten JI, Kata C. Propofol with ketamine following sedation with xylazine for routine induction of general anaesthesia in horses. *Vet Rec* 2013 Dec 7; **173**(22): 550.
37 Jarrett MA, Bailey KM, Messenger KM, *et al.* Recovery of horses from general anesthesia after induction with propofol and ketamine versus midazolam and ketamine. *J Am Vet Med Assoc* 2018 Jul 1; **253**(1): 101–107.
38 Maloiy GMO. Water economy of the Somali donkey. *Am J Physiol* 1970; **219**: 1522–1527.
39 Matthews NS, Taylor TS, Hartsfield SM, *et al.* Pharmacokinetics of ketamine in mules and mammoth asses premedicated with xylazine. *Equine Vet J* 1994; **26**: 241–243.
40 Nyman G, Funkquist B, Kyart C, *et al.* Atelectasis causes gas exchange impairment in the anaesthetized horse. *Equine Vet J* 1990; **22**: 317–324.
41 Gonçalves Dias LG, Nunes N, Lopes PC, *et al.* The effects of 2 levels of inspired oxygen fraction in blood gas variables in propofol-anesthetized dogs with high intracranial pressure. *Can J Vet Res* 2009; **73**: 111–116.
42 Crumley MN, McMurphy RM, Hodgson DS, Kreider SE. Effects of inspired oxygen concentration in ventilation, ventilatory rhythm, and gas exchange in isoflurane-anesthetized horses. *Am J Vet Res* 2013; **74**: 183–190.
43 Calero Rodriguez A, de Grauw JC, van Loon JPAM. Effect of different inspired fractions of oxygen on F-shunt and arterial partial pressure of oxygen in isoflurane-anaesthetized and mechanically ventilated Shetland ponies. *Vet Anaesth Analg* 2021; **48**: 930–934.
44 Savvas I, Pavlidou K, Braun C, *et al.* Evaluation of the effect of the inspired oxygen fraction on blood oxygenation during inhalant anaesthesia in horses: a systematic review with meta-analysis. *Animals (Basel)* 2021; **11**: 2245.
45 Schauvliege S, Savvas I, Gasthuys F. The effect of the inspired oxygen fraction on arterial blood oxygenation in spontaneously breathing, isoflurane anaesthetized horses: a retrospective study. *Vet Anaesth Analg* 2015; **42**: 280–285.
46 O'Connor SJ, Gardner DS, Ousey JC, *et al.* Development of baroreflex and endocrine responses to hypotensive stress in newborn foals and lambs. *Pflurgers Arch* 2005; **450**: 298–306.
47 Lombard CW, Evans M, Martin L, *et al.* Blood pressure, electrocardiogram and echocardiogram measurements in the growing pony foal. *Equine Vet J* 1984; **16**: 342–347.
48 Fowden AL, Forhead AJ, Ousey JC. The endocrinology of equine parturition. *Exp Clin Endocrinol Diabetes* 2008; **116**: 393–403.
49 Morton JS, Davidge ST. Arterial endothelium-derived hyperpolarization – potential role in pregnancy adaptations and complications. *J Cardiovasc Pharmacol* 2013; **61**: 197–203.
50 American College of Obstetricians and Gynecologists. ACOG Technical Bulletin: pulmonary disease in pregnancy. *J Gynecol Obstet* 1996; **54**: 187–196.
51 Baggish MS, Hooper S. Aspiration as a cause of maternal death. *Obstet Gynecol* 1974; **43**: 327–336.
52 Valverde A, Gianotti G, Rioja-Garcia E, *et al.* Effects of high-volume, rapid fluid therapy on cardiovascular function and hematological values during isoflurane-induced hypotension in healthy dogs. *Can J Vet Res* 2012; **76**: 99–108.
53 Muir WW III, Wiese AJ. Comparison of lactated Ringer's solution and a physiologically balanced 6% hetastarch plasma expander for the treatment of hypotension induced via blood withdrawal in isoflurane-anesthetized dogs. *Am J Vet Res* 2004; **65**: 1189–1194.
54 Jacob M, Chappell D, Homann-Kiefer K, *et al.* The intravascular volume effect of Ringer's lactate is below 20%: a prospective study in humans. *Crit Care* 2012; **16**: R86.
55 Araos J, Kenny JS, Rousseau-Blass F, *et al.* Dynamic prediction of fluid responsiveness during positive pressure ventilation: a review of the physiology underlying heart-lung interactions and a critical interpretation. *Vet Anaesth Analg* 2020; **47**: 3–14.
56 Oijala M, Katila T. Detomidine (Domosedan) in foals: sedative and analgesic effects. *Equine Vet J* 1988; **20**: 327–330.
57 Valverde A, Black B, Cribb NC, *et al.* Assessment of unassisted recovery from repeated general isoflurane anesthesia in horses following post-anesthetic administration of xylazine or acepromazine or a combination of xylazine and ketamine. *Vet Anaesth Analg* 2013; **40**: 3–12.
58 Woodhouse KJ, Brosnan RJ, Nguyen KQ, *et al.* Effects of postanesthetic sedation with romifidine or xylazine on quality of recovery from isoflurane anesthesia in horses. *J Am Vet Med Assoc* 2013; **15**: 242–244.
59 Loomes K, Louro LF. Recovery of horses from general anaesthesia: a systematic review (2000–2020) of risk factors and influence of interventions during the recovery period. *Equine Vet J* 2022; **54**: 201–218.
60 Banquler SH, Kona-Brown JJ. Comparison of the effects of xylazine and romifidine administered perioperatively on the recovery of anesthetized horses. *Can Vet J* 2011; **52**: 987–993.
61 de Miguel Garcia C, Campoy L, Parry S, *et al.* Questionnaire on the process of recovering horses from general anesthesia and associated personnel injury in equine practice. *Vet Anaesth Analg* 2021; **48**: 223–229.
62 Arndt S, Hopster K, Sill V, *et al.* Comparison between head-tail-rope assisted and unassisted recoveries in healthy horses undergoing general anesthesia for elective surgeries. *Vet Surg* 2020; **49**: 329–338.
63 Louro LF, Robson K, Hughes J, *et al.* Head and tail rope-assisted recovery improves quality of recovery from general anaesthesia in horses undergoing emergency exploratory laparotomy. *Equine Vet J* 2022; **54**: 875–884.

53 Comparative Anesthesia and Analgesia – Ruminants and Swine

HuiChu Lin
Department of Clinical Sciences, College of Veterinary Medicine, Auburn University, Auburn, Alabama, USA

Chapter contents

Introduction, 1052
Drug administration, 1054
Positioning during anesthesia, 1056
Cardiovascular system, 1056
Respiratory system, 1057
Gastrointestinal tract, 1057
Ruminal tympany, 1057
Regurgitation, 1057
Salivation, 1058
Endotracheal intubation, 1058
Thermoregulation, 1060
Hypothermia, 1060
Malignant hyperthermia, 1060
Species differences in anesthetic dose requirements, 1061
Airway management during recovery, 1061
Acknowledgment, 1062
References, 1062

Introduction

Special considerations exist for general anesthesia in farm animals, such as cattle, small ruminants, camelids, and pigs, due to their unique anatomy and physiology as well as their normal behaviors. Cattle, sheep, and goats have a stomach that is divided into four compartments, whereas llamas and alpacas have three compartments. Though anatomically different, the digestive system of these animals functions similarly. Significant size and body weight differences exist, varying from 2–3 kg immediately after birth to 500–1000 kg when fully grown. Accurate dosing of injectable drugs and appropriately sized anesthetic equipment and accessories should be available. Ruminants are generally docile and tolerate physical restraint well, allowing many minor surgical procedures to be performed in the conscious patient with regional anesthesia. Because camelids and swine are less tolerant of physical restraint, general anesthesia is more frequently performed for even minor surgical procedures.

Farm animals share nociceptive pathway anatomy and physiology with other mammals and, therefore, have the ability to process information similarly. Analgesia is an essential part of surgical and anesthetic management. When surgical procedures require general anesthesia, balanced anesthetic techniques should be employed to provide unconsciousness, amnesia, and muscle relaxation. Minimizing the stress response induced by handling, surgery, and anesthesia is also important.

Anesthesia and surgery can be costly relative to the value of the animal whose ultimate purpose is slaughter for human consumption. In addition, anesthetics, sedatives, and analgesics commonly used in farm animal practice may not have regulatory approval for use in ruminants, camelids, and swine [1,2]. In the United States, the Animal Medicinal Drug Use Clarification Act (AMDUCA) of 1994 codifies the requirements for extra-label drug use (ELDU). In general, ELDU is permitted when animal health is threatened or death may result if a condition is untreated; however, the prescribing veterinarian is responsible for advising owners to ensure that no residual drug reaches processors or consumers [3].

Many anesthetics have short plasma elimination half-lives ($t_{½}$) and achieve general anesthesia at low tissue concentrations due to their potency. Nevertheless, veterinarians should consult the Food Animal Residual Avoidance Databank (FARAD) for guidance on estimated meat and milk withdrawal intervals for ELDU of analgesics, tranquilizers, and injectable anesthetics as well as for updates on drugs where extra-label use is prohibited [1,2,4,5] (Table 53.1). Practitioners working outside the United States should consult the appropriate regulations for their practice area to determine the specific requirements for drug use in animals intended for food production. Camelids are considered fiber animals, so concerns for withdrawal times and violative drug residues are minimal.

In addition to use as food, farm animal species of all types are often kept as companion animal pets. In particular, pot-bellied pigs have become popular house pets in the last two decades. There are many anatomic and physiologic characteristics of pigs that make anesthetic management challenging. Although the commercial value of these pets may not be extraordinary, their owners are often willing to spend more for veterinary care. Although it is unlikely for a companion animal to end up in the food chain, the possibility of a pot-bellied pig being slaughtered for food consumption does

Veterinary Anesthesia and Analgesia: The Sixth Edition of Lumb and Jones. Edited by Leigh Lamont, Kurt Grimm, Sheilah Robertson, Lydia Love and Carrie Schroeder.
© 2024 John Wiley & Sons, Inc. Published 2024 by John Wiley & Sons, Inc.
Companion website: www.wiley.com/go/lamont/anesthesia

Table 53.1 The recommended withdrawal interval for ruminants for single and multiple treatments of anesthetic and analgesic drugs.

Drug	Species	Dose (mg/kg)	Milk withdrawal interval (hours)	Meat withdrawal interval (days)	Country
Acepromazine	Cattle, sheep, goats	≤ 0.13 IV ≤ 0.44 IM	48	7	United States
Acepromazine	Swine	≤ 0.055 IV ≤ 0.44 IM	–	7	United States
Acepromazine	Cattle	0.13 IV 0.27 IM	48	2	Australia
Acepromazine	Cattle	0.055 IV 0.13–0.44 IM 0.13–0.26 PO	48	7	Canada
Acepromazine	Swine	≤ 0.13 IM	–	7	Canada
Aspirin	Cattle, sheep, goats	≤ 100 q 12 h	24	1	United States
Atropine	Cattle, sheep, goats	Anesthetic adjunct	24	7	United States
Atropine	Cattle Sheep	0.03–0.06 IV, IM, SC, q 24 h 0.08–0.16 IV, IM, SC, q 24 h Multiple doses, ≤ 0.2 mg/kg	72 144	14 28	United Kingdom Antidote
Atropine	Swine	0.02–0.04 IV, IM, SC, q 24 h Multiple doses, ≤ 0.2 mg/kg	72 144	14 28	United Kingdom Antidote
Bupivacaine	Cattle Sheep, goats	0.05 1.5–1.8	Cleared rapidly	Cleared rapidly	United States
Butorphanol	Cattle	0.02–0.25 IV	72	4 or 5	United States
Butorphanol	Sheep	0.022–0.05 IV, IM	48	2	United States
Detomidine	Cattle, sheep, goats	≤ 0.08 IV or IM	72	3	United States
Detomidine	Cattle	0.02–0.08 IV or IM	72	1	Switzerland
Diazepam	Cattle, sheep, goats	≤ 0.1 IV		10	United States
DMSO	Cattle, sheep, goats	Not specified	96	4	United States
Fentanyl	Goats	50 μg/h, transdermal patch	48–96	2–4	United States
Flunixin meglumine	Cattle	≤ 2.2 IV q 24 h for ≤ 3 days ≤ 2.2 IV once ≤ 2.2 IM, SC, PO, once ≤ 2.2 IM, SC, PO, multiple doses	36 84 96 ≤ 60	4 7 10 –	United States
Flunixin meglumine	Swine	2.2 IM 2.2 IV or PO, ≥ 1 dose 2.2 IM, if product not labeled for swine	12 21 13–15	–	United States
Guaifenesin	Cattle, sheep, goats	≤ 100 IV	48	3	United States
Guaifenesin	Cattle	60–100 IV	Not specified	Not specified	Switzerland
Ketamine	Cattle, sheep, goats	≤ 2 IV 10 IM	48	3	United States
Ketamine	Swine	≤ 10 IV or IM 20	–	2 4	United States
Ketamine	Cattle	5 IV 10–20 IM	0	0	France
Ketamine	Cattle	Adult: 2 IV Calves: ≤ 10 IV	72	1	Switzerland
Ketoprofen	Cattle, sheep, goats	≤ 3.3 q 24 h for ≤ 3 days	24	7	United States
Lidocaine (with epinephrine)	Cattle, sheep, goats	Infiltration epidural	24	1	United States
Lidocaine (2%)	Cattle	≤ 15 mL epidural ≤ 100 mL SC	24 72	1 4	United States
Meloxicam	Cattle	0.5 IM, SC	120	15	European countries
Meloxicam	Swine	–	–	5	European countries
Meloxicam	Cattle, sheep, goats	0.5–1 PO, single dose ≤ 1 PO, multiple doses 1 PO, single dose	21 30 15	–	United States
Meloxicam	Cattle Sheep	Injectable formulation	96 11 *days*	20 11	Australia, New Zealand
Meloxicam	Swine	Injectable formulation	–	5	Australia, New Zealand
Meloxicam	Cattle Sheep	Injectable formulation	96 11 *days*	20 11	Canada
Meloxicam	Cattle (not in lactating animals)	Oral formulation	–	35	Canada
Meloxicam	Swine	Injectable formulation	–	5	Canada
Meperidine	Cattle, sheep, goats	2–4	48–96	2–4	United States
Morphine	Cattle, sheep, goats	0.1 once, IV, IM, epidural	48	14	United States
Phenylbutazone	Cattle, sheep, goats	Not recommended, prolonged excretion. In the United States, it is illegal to use phenylbutazone in female dairy cattle ≥ 20 months of age.	–	–	United States

(*Continued*)

Table 53.1 (Continued)

Drug	Species	Dose (mg/kg)	Milk withdrawal interval (hours)	Meat withdrawal interval (days)	Country
Propofol	Calves	3 IV	Cannot be determined	3	United States
Telazol®	Swine	≤ 2 IM	30	–	United States
Tolazoline	Cattle	2–4 IV	48	8	New Zealand, United States
Ultrashort-acting barbiturates	Cattle, sheep, goats	Thiamylal: ≤ 5.5 Thiopental: ≤ 9.4	24	1	United States
Xylazine	Cattle Sheep Goats	0.016–0.1 IV 0.05–0.3 IM 0.2 IM	72 24 120	5 4 10	United States
Xylazine	Cattle	0.11–0.33 IM	48	3	Canada
Xylazine	Cattle	0.025–0.15 IV 0.025–0.3 IM	0	2	France
Xylazine	Cattle	0.016–0.1 IV 0.01–0.3 IM 1.2–2 IM	72 120	3 7	Germany
Xylazine	Cattle	0.05–0.4 IM	24	4	New Zealand
Xylazine	Cattle	0.016–0.1 IV 0.05–0.3 IM	72	3	Switzerland
Xylazine	Cattle	0.05–0.3 IM	48	14	United Kingdom
Yohimbine	Cattle, sheep, goats	≤ 0.3 IV	72	7	United States

IM, intramuscular; IV, intravenous; PO, per os; SC, subcutaneous.
Source: Craigmill *et al.* [1]; Fajt [5]; Coetzee [9]; Haskel *et al.* [10]; Valverde and Doherty [11]; Passler [12].

exist [6]. Therefore, it is important that owners be educated about the potential drug residues in the meat. Special considerations for laboratory swine are discussed extensively elsewhere [7,8].

Drug administration

Oral administration of a tranquilizer or sedative is sometimes needed to facilitate capture and/or reduce stress associated with restraint. In ruminants and camelids, oral medication is absorbed primarily via the rumen. Absorption is affected by motility and the pH of the ruminal fluid. Reticuloruminal motility is primarily controlled by the medullary gastric center in the brain. Physical conditions like central nervous system depression, pain, fear, excitement, pyrexia, endotoxemia, hypocalcemia, and extreme wall distension (e.g., rumen tympany) tend to reduce rumen motility. Analgesics and anesthetics like opioids, α_2-adrenergic receptor agonists, and general anesthetics also decrease gastric motility, resulting in prolonged gastric emptying time and enhanced drug absorption [13]. The pH difference of saliva (8.2), plasma (7.4), and ruminal contents (5.5–6.5) affects drug absorption by altering drug ionization. Ionization and the amount of drug in saliva, plasma, and the rumen are constantly changing, making it difficult to predict bioavailability and distribution of orally administered drugs (e.g., tranquilizers, sedatives, or injectable anesthetics) [13]. In monogastric animals like pigs, the pH in the stomach is acidic (1.5–2.5) [14]. As a result, absorption from the gastrointestinal tract is more predictable in these species leading to greater bioavailability of orally administered sedative drugs. Oral administration of trazodone (8–10 mg/kg) and gabapentin (20 mg/kg) can be given to pet miniature pigs the night before and again 2 h prior to the veterinary visit to reduce stress and ease restraint for minor procedures such as hoof trim [15]. Intranasal administration of a sedative such as midazolam (0.4 mg/kg) has been reported to produce calming effects in pigs with a bioavailability of 64% and a terminal $t_{½}$ of 145 min, compared to 158 min following intravenous (IV) administration. Rapid anxiolytic effects and sedation occurred within 3–4 min following administration of either 0.2 or 0.4 mg/kg [16].

The external jugular veins of ruminants are easily palpable and visualized when occluded. A 14 gauge, 2–3 inch needle can be placed in the jugular vein of adult cattle for administration of injectable anesthetics and fluids during surgery. A 14 gauge, 5¼-inch over-the-needle indwelling catheter may be placed and secured for longer duration IV medication or fluid therapy. A surgical cutdown can be performed to facilitate insertion of the catheter through the thick skin of adult cattle. A 16 or 18 gauge IV catheter is appropriate for calves and small ruminants. The technique for IV catheterization in smaller ruminant species is similar to that used in calves. However, skin incision is generally not needed in smaller ruminants and the jugular vein is easily visualized when occluded.

Venipuncture and catheterization can be difficult in camelids because these animals have thick fiber coats and neck skin. More importantly, they do not have a jugular furrow, and the external jugular veins lie deep to the sternomandibularis and brachiocephalicus muscles, ventral to the cervical vertebral transverse processes, and superficial to the carotid artery and vagosympathetic trunk within the carotid sheath for most of their length [17–21]. External jugular veins of camelids are not always visible even with occlusion of the vessels, particularly in adult males. Camelids, like other long-necked animals, have four or five jugular vein valves located at irregular intervals to prevent blood pooling in the head when the animal grazes. The presence of these valves can hinder the advancement of an IV catheter, even when correct catheter placement is confirmed by blood flowing into the stylet of the catheter. The right external jugular vein is preferred for venipuncture and catheterization to avoid damage to the esophagus, which runs on the left side of the neck. The landmarks for venipuncture in camelids are the cranial portion of the neck at the level of the mandible, on the caudoventral aspect of the neck, medial to the fifth cervical vertebral transverse process [19] (Fig. 53.1). Care should be taken to verify that a catheter is not accidentally placed in the carotid artery before injection of medications.

Venous blood of camelids appears to be bright red and, thus, may be mistaken for arterial blood. It has been suggested that the adaptations essential to high altitude existence are responsible for the bright red color of camelid venous blood, including the elliptical

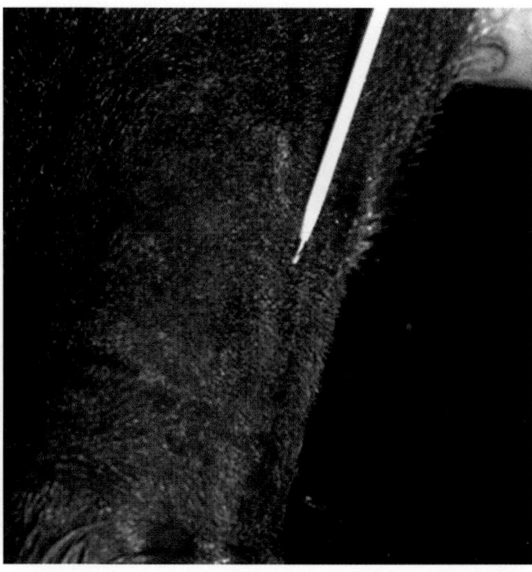

Figure 53.1 Intravenous catheterization in a llama. Source: Dr. HuiChu Lin, with permission.

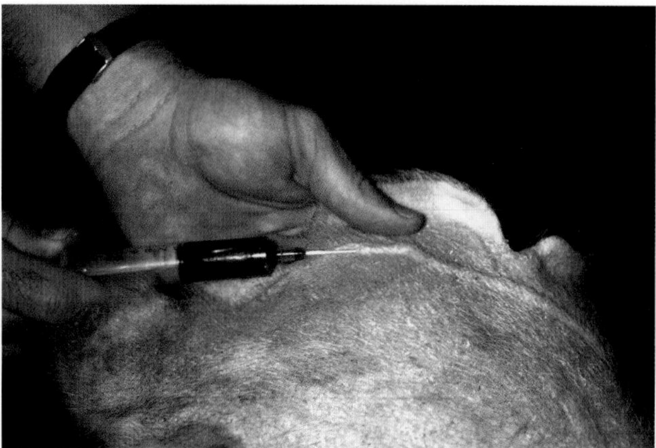

Figure 53.2 Intravenous injection in the auricular vein in a pig. Source: Dr. HuiChu Lin, with permission.

shape of their red blood cells, the relatively high concentration of hemoglobin in red cells, and a left-shifted oxygen–hemoglobin dissociation curve [22]. Attention to an absence of characteristic pulsatile arterial flow will help prevent inadvertent carotid arterial injection [19]. A 14 gauge indwelling catheter is appropriate for adult camelids, and a 16 or 18 gauge catheter is suitable for crias. The catheter should be secured with suture or a bandage. Skin cutdown is helpful in passing the catheter into the jugular vein [23,24]. Distension of the jugular vein with sterile saline facilitates advancement. If distension of the vessel is unsuccessful, relocate the placement site 1–2 cm cranially or caudally from the previous site [24]. The auricular (ear) vein is an alternative site for IV injection using a 25 gauge needle or butterfly catheter to deliver a small volume of sedative drug to cooperative camelids.

Pigs usually resist physical restraint. They are easily stressed when restrained and generally respond by constant struggling and vocalization [25–27]. Preanesthetic physical examination and evaluation should be as stress-free as possible, especially since some pigs are susceptible to the genetic disorder, malignant hyperthermia (MH), or porcine stress syndrome (see below). Hog boards or crowd/sorting boards (36.5 × 30.5 inches) can be used to confine a pig to a small area in order to facilitate physical examination or drug administration by limiting the pig's movement. A "forking" technique has been used in pigs to reduce anxiety, produce calming effects, and minimize stress prior to intramuscular (IM) injection of drugs [28]. IM administration of midazolam (0.1–0.5 mg/kg) [15,29]; midazolam (0.1–0.3 mg/kg) and butorphanol (0.1–0.3 mg/kg) [30]; midazolam (0.2 mg/kg), butorphanol (0.2–0.4 mg/kg), and xylazine (1 mg/kg) [29]; or dexmedetomidine (0.01–0.04 mg/kg) [30] have been administered for preanesthetic chemical restraint and sedation.

In general, rapid IM administration tends to be less stressful than IV administration for pigs. Most pigs have a thick layer of subcutaneous fat, especially pot-bellied pigs. The adipose tissue layers in the neck and rump are particularly thick. Accurate deposition of preanesthetics or anesthetics into the muscle layer requires a needle of adequate length. Too short a needle will result in depositing the drug into the adipose tissue and slowed onset of action. It is recommended that the IM injection be made in the divot behind the base of the ear near the lateral aspect of the second cervical vertebra where the fat layer overlying the muscle is thin [31]. This author prefers a 23 gauge, 1½ inch needle for IM injection in these muscles as it appears to induce less pain and pigs often do not respond. At the cervical or thoracic areas of the trapezius muscle, at least a 2 inch long needle will be required to ensure drug injection into muscle tissue. Inconsistent effects are observed more frequently if shorter needles are used in these areas [25]. Alternatively, IM injection can be made at the semimembranosus and semitendinosus muscles located just above the hock or in the caudal portion of the biceps femoris muscle [25]. In pigs intended as food, IM injection into the "ham" muscles including gluteal, semimembranosus, and semitendinosus muscles is not recommended because of the potential for muscle inflammation and fibrosis [32].

IV injection of preanesthetics or anesthetics in pigs can be very difficult, particularly in pot-bellied pigs, because of the lack of visible superficial veins. On occasion, an auricular vein can be used for IV injection if the pig cooperates or is easily restrained (Fig. 53.2). Ideally, deep sedation and immobilization is achieved first with IM injection. The jugular vein or anterior vena cava can be used for IV injection, but this technique is difficult due to the thick neck and abundant jowls.

Auricular veins, especially lateral auricular veins, are common sites for IV injection because they are superficial and easily accessible. However, in dark-colored ears, IV injection remains challenging (e.g., pot-bellied pigs). In larger adults, the central dorsal auricular vein is often utilized. An 18 or 20 gauge, 1–1½ inch hypodermic needle, indwelling catheter, or butterfly catheter can be used, while a 21 or 23 gauge needle is suitable for smaller ears. A butterfly catheter has a shorter needle and tends to stay in the vessel better than hypodermic needles, especially when the animal struggles during the injection. An indwelling catheter can be placed in an auricular, cephalic, or superficial abdominal/mammary vein if postoperative IV medication and/or fluid therapy are needed. In debilitated pigs, when repeated administration of medications or continuous fluid therapy is required, a central venous catheter can be placed in the jugular vein via the Seldinger technique using a large animal long-term venous catheterization kit (e.g., Mila International Inc.) with the pig under general anesthesia (Fig. 53.3) [33].

Intramedullary cannulation has been used for fluid and drug administration when other vascular access cannot be established. An 18 gauge cannula can be placed into either the greater tubercle of the humerus or the trochanteric fossa of the femur. Although this technique is performed easily in immature pigs, rate of fluid administration may be limited in older pigs due to the presence of fat and fibrosis of the medullary canal [34].

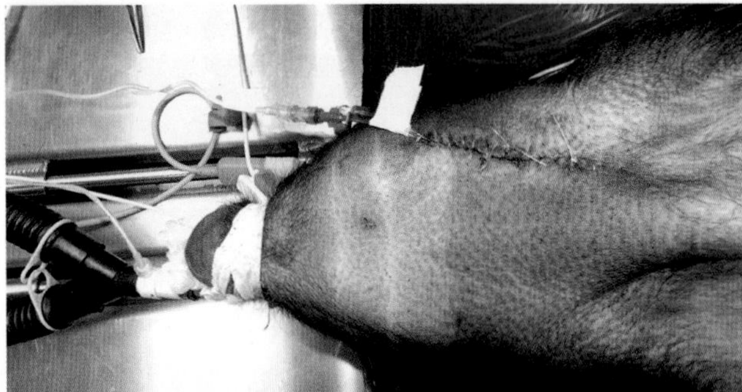

Figure 53.3 Jugular catheterization in a pig. Source: Dr. HuiChu Lin, with permission.

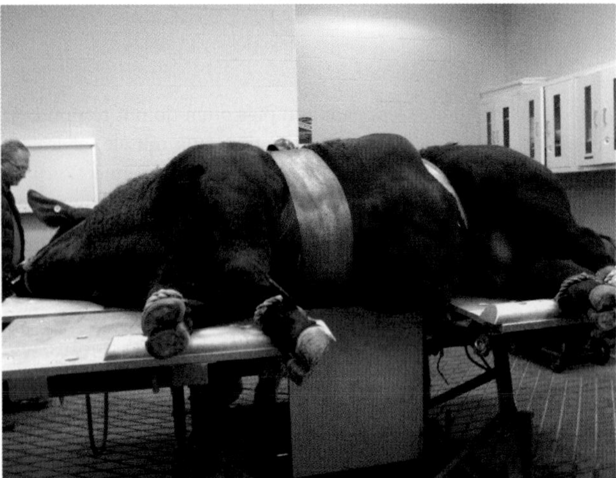

Figure 53.4 Positioning of the head and neck during lateral recumbency in a bull. Source: Dr. HuiChu Lin, with permission.

Positioning during anesthesia

Neuromyopathy has been associated with improper positioning and inadequate padding of the surgery table. Myopathy does not occur readily in large ruminants, but nerve paralysis has been observed. Adult cattle should be placed on a 10-cm-thick high-density foam pad, whereas a 5-cm-thick foam pad is sufficient for calves, small ruminants, and camelids. When placing adult cattle in dorsal recumbency, the animal should be balanced squarely on its back with the gluteal areas bearing equal weight. All limbs should be flexed and relaxed. In lateral recumbency, an automotive inner tube (valve stem pointed down) can be placed under the elbow of the dependent (lower) forelimb to prevent radial nerve paralysis. The dependent forelimb is placed through the inner tube and the tube positioned directly under the shoulder, which prevents pressure on the radial nerve as it traverses the musculospiral groove of the humerus. The bony point of the shoulder should be positioned within the hollow center of the inner tube. Non-elastic or duct tape can be wrapped over the part of the inner tube not under the weight of the shoulder (opposite the valve stem) to prevent the tube from collapsing under the shoulder thereby ensuring support.

Once the inner tube is in place, pull the dependent forelimb anteriorly so the weight of the thorax rests on the triceps but not the humerus. Both uppermost limbs (front and hindlimbs) should be elevated and parallel to the table surface to minimize the pressure on the radial, femoral, or peroneal nerve of the dependent limb and

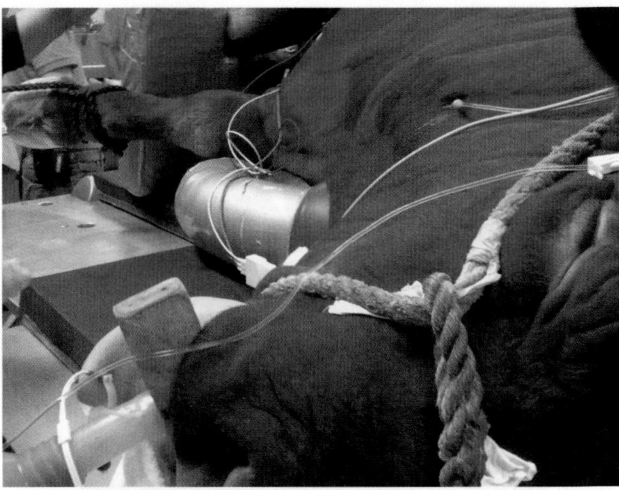

Figure 53.5 Supportive H block and inner tube to prevent neuromyopathy during lateral recumbency in a bull. Source: Dr. HuiChu Lin, with permission.

prevent nerve paralysis. The head and neck should be at a slightly extended position (Figs. 53.4 and 53.5). The dependent eye needs to be protected by administration of ophthalmic ointment and ensuring closure of the eye to minimize the risk of corneal ulcer [35,36]. For camelids, similar precautions should be instituted to prevent radial nerve paralysis. A padded, supporting "H block" made of styrofoam with duct tape around the exterior can be used to support the upper, non-dependent limbs and keep pressure off the lower, dependent limbs. In dorsal recumbency, overflexion or overstretching of the limbs to clear the limbs from the operative site with ropes should be avoided. Camelids have prominent eyes and administration of ophthalmic ointment and additional padding with gauze or soft towels under the dependent eye will minimize the potential for corneal laceration or ulceration [37].

Cardiovascular system

Cardiopulmonary depression associated with commonly used anesthetics tends to result in hypoventilation and hypoxemia [38]. Furthermore, compression of the great vessels such as the vena cava by the weight of abdominal viscera while in lateral or dorsal recumbency can result in decreased venous return, cardiac output, arterial blood pressures, and tissue perfusion [39]. Studies have shown that ventilation, cardiac output, and arterial blood pressure are better maintained when animals are positioned in sternal recumbency [40,41]. Unfortunately, many surgical procedures performed under general anesthesia require the animal to be placed in lateral or dorsal recumbency for easy surgical access. Nevertheless, arterial blood pressure in cattle in most instances is maintained within acceptable limits during anesthesia [35].

In calves during isoflurane anesthesia, heart rate was reported to be 92 beats/min, and systolic, mean, and diastolic arterial blood pressures were 87, 63, and 49 mmHg, respectively [42]. These values were similar to those reported in calves anesthetized with xylazine–ketamine and isoflurane [43]. In 8–12-week-old Holstein calves anesthetized with sevoflurane, heart rate was 72 beats/min with a mean arterial blood pressure of 91 mmHg [44], whereas in calves anesthetized with desflurane, heart rate was 87 beats/min and mean arterial blood pressure was 75 mmHg [45]. Arnes *et al.* reported that invasive (direct) measurements of systolic, mean, and diastolic arterial blood pressures in isoflurane-anesthetized sheep and goats, cattle < 150 kg, and cattle > 150 kg were 101, 78, and 64 mmHg; 116, 91, and 74 mmHg; and 131, 107, and 91 mmHg, respectively [46]. This report demonstrated that non-invasive oscillometric blood pressure measurements did not accurately represent the true blood pressure and, thus, cannot be used to predict directly measured arterial blood pressures. Therefore, it is important to monitor direct arterial blood pressure using invasive blood pressure techniques whenever possible in clinical practice. The auricular artery in ruminants and camelids can be used for arterial catheter placement for direct arterial blood pressure measurements. In pot-bellied pigs, arterial catheterization may be more difficult due to the small size of the auricular artery. However, a small gauge catheter (e.g., 22 gauge) may be placed successfully.

Hypertension is sometimes observed in bulls and adult cows positioned in lateral recumbency during inhalational anesthesia with systolic blood pressures > 200 mmHg and diastolic pressures > 120 mmHg [47,48]. This hypertension was observed frequently when thiopental was used for induction of anesthesia in healthy adult cattle. The animals appeared to be under an appropriate plane of anesthesia and no intervention was undertaken (personal observation). Administration of xylazine or acepromazine preanesthetically or as part of the induction anesthetic regimen tends to decrease arterial blood pressures [49].

Respiratory system

Positional changes required for anesthesia and surgery can result in significant mismatching of ventilation and perfusion and cattle tend to have greater differences between alveolar and arterial O_2 partial pressures (P_AO_2 – PaO_2) than horses, particularly if placed in dorsal recumbency (even in the conscious state) [50–52]. This is a result of gravity and the weight of the chest wall on pulmonary blood flow and alveolar ventilation [50,51]. Normal, conscious cattle breathe with a smaller tidal volume and faster respiratory rate than do horses. Factors thought to be responsible for this include smaller and completely separated bovine lung lobes [53]; lower work of breathing due to a greater maximum change in pleural pressure and the non-elastic work of breathing as well as lower dynamic lung compliance [54,55]; decreased breathing efficiency due to a diaphragm that is flatter and more vertical in conformation [56]; a large, easily expandable stomach which sits immediately caudal to the diaphragm and, when filled to its maximum, occupies three-quarters of the abdominal cavity [57–59]; and, finally, a tendency to greater alveolar ventilation and higher O_2 consumption [60].

Lateral or dorsal recumbency causes the weight of the abdominal viscera to shift downward and forward, pushing the diaphragm further into the thoracic cavity, resulting in decreased functional residual capacity. The rumen of adult cattle is a large fermentation chamber with a capacity of 115–150 L or 250–300 g/kg of body weight. Preanesthetic fasting may reduce the degree of fermentation, but fermentation continues during anesthesia and gas accumulates in the rumen due to prohibition of eructation, resulting in increased intragastric pressure. As a result, lung compliance, tidal volume, and minute ventilation decrease significantly. This, in turn, increases the degree of ventilation–perfusion mismatch and the subsequent development of hypoventilation and hypoxemia [40,41].

Lateral recumbency has been reported to cause a significant decrease in PaO_2 in conscious sheep [61]. Severe hypoxemia and pulmonary edema have been implicated as the cause of death in sheep that die under anesthesia when xylazine has been administered [62–64]. Hypoxemia has also been observed in standing sheep during xylazine sedation [65,66]. All α_2-adrenergic receptor agonists cause significant decreases in PaO_2 in sheep without affecting $PaCO_2$ [67]. Increased airway pressure [68], severe pulmonary parenchymal damage [69], as well as bronchospasm and venospasm [70] occur as a result of peripheral α_2-adrenergic stimulation and activation of pulmonary intravascular macrophages.

Gastrointestinal tract

Ruminal tympany

Ruminal tympany may occur during general anesthesia of ruminants because fermentation continues in anesthetized animals. Postprandial gas production of an average of 30 L/h has been reported in cattle [71]. Normal, conscious animals are able to relieve the gas produced by fermentation through the esophagus. However, sedatives, anesthetics, and some body positions inhibit gastrointestinal motility and inhibit eructation. Placement of an orogastric tube helps to minimize accumulation of gas and bloating as a result of fermentation and ruminal tympany during anesthesia.

Regurgitation

Regurgitation and aspiration of stomach contents can occur in ruminants and camelids during anesthesia, particularly in non-fasted animals. The chance of regurgitation decreases significantly when water is restricted for 6–12 h and feed withheld for 12–24 h prior to anesthesia. Adult cattle have a large rumen that is usually full of liquid material and does not empty completely even after 24–48 h of fasting. Regurgitation tends to occur more frequently when animals are in left lateral compared to right lateral recumbency. It can occur during either light (active regurgitation) or deep (passive regurgitation) anesthesia in spite of preanesthetic fasting and water withholding. Active regurgitation occurs during light anesthesia and is characterized by explosive discharge of large quantities of ruminal material. Passive regurgitation occurs during deep planes of anesthesia when the esophageal muscles and transluminal pressure gradients relax. If the airway is not protected, a large amount of ruminal material can be inhaled into the trachea and reach the small airways. Consequences of aspiration of acidic ruminal content may include aspiration pneumonia. Aspiration pneumonia is often characterized by reflex airway closure, bronchospasm, destruction of type II alveolar cells and pulmonary capillary lining cells, pulmonary edema and hemorrhage, dyspnea, hypoxemia, and cyanosis.

The prognosis following aspiration depends on the amount and the pH of the ruminal material [71]. Pigs tend to have very acidic stomach contents with pH values as low as 1.5–2.5 [10], but pH values remain between 5.5 and 6.5 for the rumen [13] and between 6.4 and 7.0 for the C-1 compartment of camelids [37]. Thus, in ruminants and camelids, the impact of aspiration depends more on the amount of bacterial microflora and solid food materials aspirated, whereas in pigs the acidity of the aspirate is directly damaging to pulmonary tissues. Nevertheless, reflex airway constriction, mechanical airway obstruction, and aspiration of bacteria occur and can be life threatening in ruminants [71]. In extreme cases, the animal dies before an endotracheal tube can be placed to protect the airway. Preoperative withholding of feed and water and keeping the animal in sternal recumbency with the head elevated until an endotracheal tube is securely in place and the cuff inflated following induction are recommended in all anesthetized ruminants and camelids. Active suction can be used to remove regurgitant from the oral cavity if necessary.

Pigs are monogastric, and regurgitation does not occur as commonly as in ruminants. However, vomiting can result if pigs are not fasted before anesthesia and following the administration of xylazine. Maropitant, a neurokinin-1 receptor antagonist, is licensed for use as an antiemetic drug in dogs and cats. Maropitant has oral bioavailability of 20% and 50% in dogs and cats, respectively [72]. In addition, maropitant infusions reduce the minimum alveolar concentration of sevoflurane [73,74]. Maropitant is reported to prevent vomiting effectively in dogs and cats [72,75,76]. However, its effectiveness for postoperative nausea and vomiting in dogs is controversial [77,78]. In cats receiving 0.44 mg/kg of xylazine, maropitant was reported to be effective in reducing emesis and motion sickness by 76%, 90%, and 100%, following SC, PO, and IV administration, respectively [72]. There are no reports of the use of maropitant in pigs, but its administration may be useful in preventing vomiting during the perianesthetic period. In pigs, withholding food for 12 h is sufficient for most elective surgeries, while 24 h may be required for stomach or small intestinal surgeries [27,79]. Water can be allowed until the time of preanesthetic administration although some authors recommend withholding water for 2 h for most elective surgeries [80] and 4–6 h for stomach or small intestinal surgeries [79,81]. It has been recommended to remove hay, alfalfa, or straw from the diet and environment for a minimum of 2–3 days prior to anesthesia to avoid prolonged gastric emptying time and minimize the potential for postoperative vomiting.

Salivation

Ruminants normally salivate profusely during anesthesia. Total amounts of salivary secretion in conscious adult cattle and sheep have been reported to be 50 and 6–16 L per 24 h, respectively [82,83]. If the trachea is left unprotected during anesthesia, aspiration of large amounts of saliva can cause complications. Thus, tracheal intubation with appropriate inflation of the cuff should be instituted immediately following induction. For large ruminants, positioning the animal on the surgery table in a way that the throat latch is elevated relative to the mouth and thoracic inlet helps to drain and prevent pooling of saliva and regurgitant in the oral cavity (see Fig. 53.4). Placing a sandbag or rolled towel under the neck of smaller ruminants or camelids to elevate the throat latch allows saliva and regurgitant to flow away from the airway opening [84] (Fig. 53.6). In addition, active suction can be used to remove excessive saliva from the oral cavity and avoid accumulation and potential aspiration of the saliva and/or regurgitant.

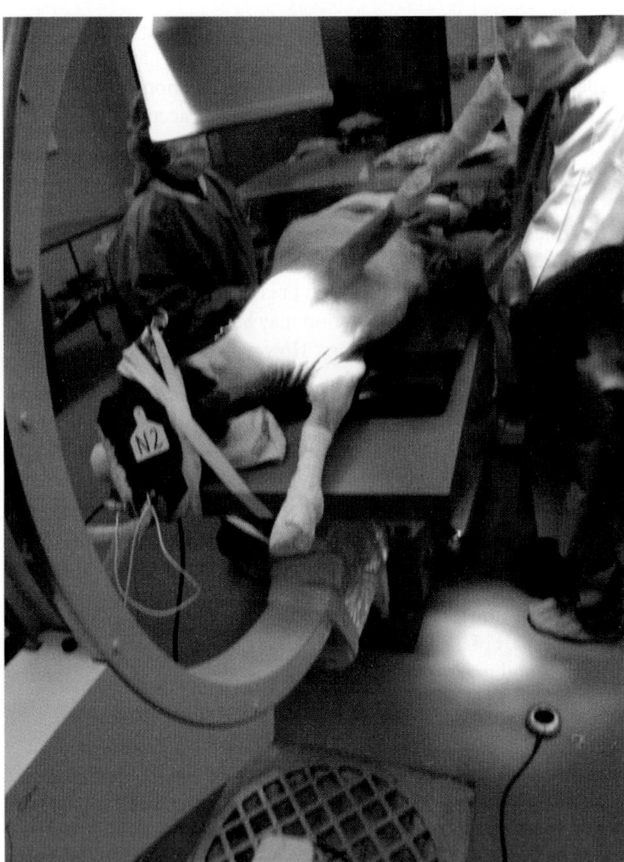

Figure 53.6 Elevation of the throat latch during lateral recumbency in a goat. Source: Dr. HuiChu Lin, with permission.

Endotracheal intubation

Tracheal intubation is relatively difficult to accomplish in farm animals. Blind intubation, as performed in horses, is less likely to succeed. For large ruminants, this author's preference is to use the digital palpation technique to guide the endotracheal tube into the trachea with the animal in either sternal or lateral recumbency immediately following induction of anesthesia. Another technique is to use a stomach tube as stylet and, with the aid of digital palpation, to place the stomach tube in the trachea. The anesthetist then threads the endotracheal tube into the trachea and removes the stomach tube once the endotracheal tube is in place.

In calves, intubation is easier when the animal is placed in sternal recumbency and an assistant pulls the mouth open by placing a loop of gauze around the upper jaw and a second loop around the lower jaw. An assistant should lift the head up and keep the head and the neck in a straight line to allow visualization of the epiglottis and the larynx. If the larynx cannot be visualized, the neck should be extended further. A laryngoscope with a long blade (250–350 mm) can be used to depress the tongue base and the epiglottis to enable visualization of the larynx. A "guide tube" or "stylet" (e.g., two 10 French, 22 inch long polyethylene canine urethral catheters taped together to make up three times the length of the endotracheal tube) can be used (Figs. 53.7 and 53.8). A cuffed endotracheal tube will prevent regurgitation and aspiration of ruminal contents, and the calf should be maintained in sternal recumbency until the cuff is inflated.

Intubation in small ruminants and camelids is more difficult when compared to carnivores, because their jaws cannot be opened as widely, their intermandibular space is narrow, and the laryngeal opening is invisible behind the thick base of the tongue. In addition, the elongated soft palate may be situated either ventral or dorsal to the epiglottis in llamas and alpacas [37]. In general, the technique used for tracheal intubation of small ruminants and camelids is similar to that used in calves. With the animal in sternal recumbency, intubation is accomplished with the help of a guide tube or stylet and a long-bladed laryngoscope (250–350 mm) as described for calves previously. Hyperextending the animal's neck is sometimes helpful in visualizing the larynx (see Figs 53.7 and 53.8). If difficulty is encountered in advancing the endotracheal tube through the larynx into the trachea, repositioning of the head, fixing the larynx from the exterior, and gently rotating the tube 360° while advancing the tube are recommended. Most importantly, the animal must be adequately anesthetized, and lidocaine may be

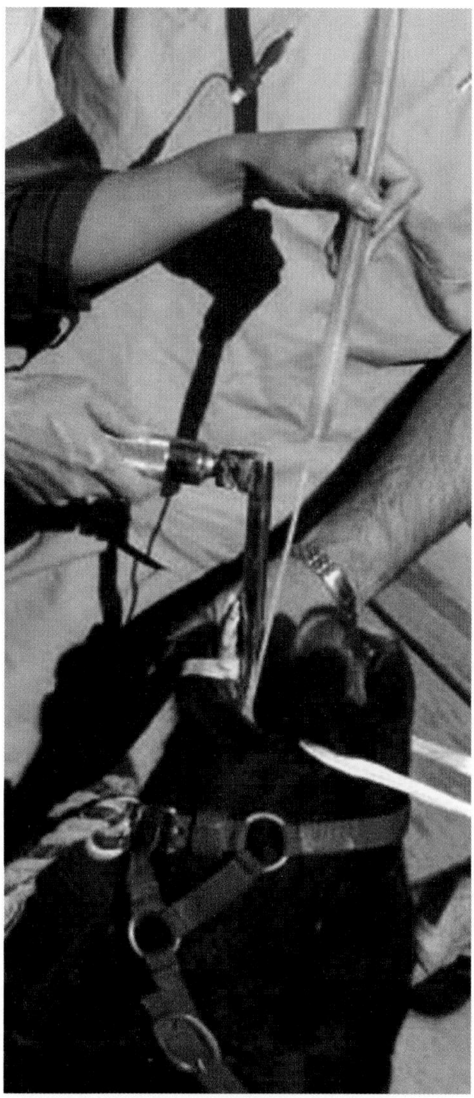

Figure 53.7 Endotracheal intubation of a llama. Source: Dr. HuiChu Lin, with permission.

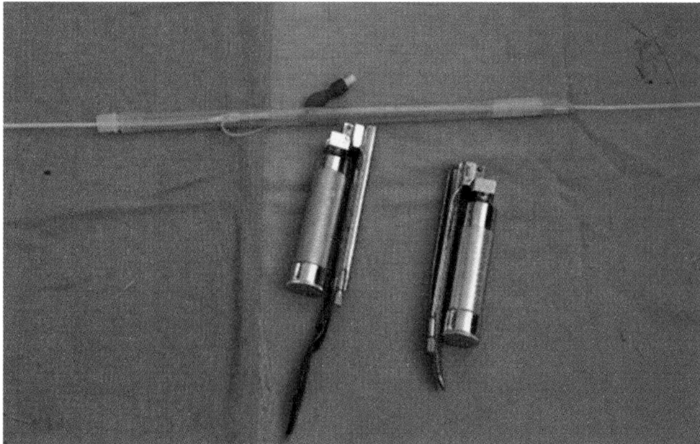

Figure 53.8 Endotracheal tracheal tube, "guide tube" (stylet), and laryngoscope used for calves, small ruminants, camelids, and pigs. Source: Dr. HuiChu Lin, with permission.

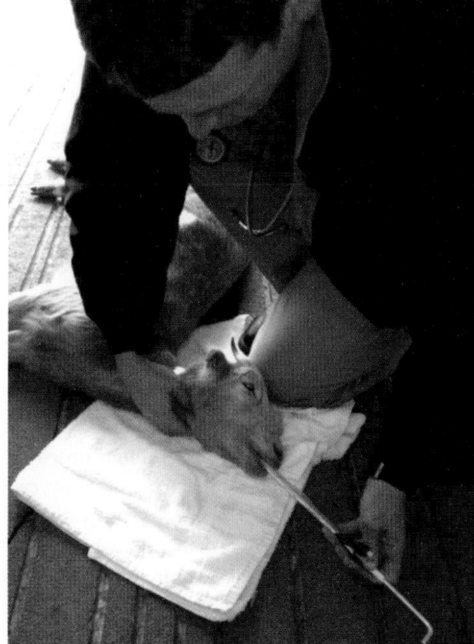

Figure 53.9 "Stick intubation" technique in a goat. Source: Dr. HuiChu Lin, with permission.

applied to the arytenoids to prevent laryngospasms. Similar to calves, a cuffed endotracheal tube should be used, and the animal should be maintained in sternal recumbency until the cuff is inflated appropriately. Blind intubation, similar to that used in horses, has been used for intubation in sheep and goats. However, this technique may require multiple attempts in order to successfully place the endotracheal tube in the trachea.

Another technique described as "stick intubation" has been used effectively in small ruminants in the field. With the animal in lateral recumbency, a small-diameter rod made of wood or stainless steel can be used as a stylet to stiffen the endotracheal tube, with one hand occluding the esophagus, while the other hand manipulates the endotracheal tube into the trachea (Fig. 53.9). Care and gentle maneuvering should always be used to prevent laryngeal spasm and minimize trauma to the oral mucous membranes.

Of all domestic species, endotracheal intubation has proven to be most difficult in pigs because the mouth cannot be widely opened, the epiglottis is often entrapped behind the soft palate, the prominent dorsal protrusion of the base of the tongue obstructs the view for direct visualization of the larynx, the small larynx slopes downward creating an acute angle to the tracheal opening (ventral floor fornix), and they are prone to laryngeal spasm. Vomiting can also occur if intubation is attempted when the pig is under a light plane of anesthesia, especially when the animal is not appropriately fasted prior to anesthesia. Application of a small amount of a local anesthetic (e.g., 2% lidocaine solution) to desensitize the larynx may reduce the potential for laryngeal spasm. In larger or adult pigs, tracheal intubation is easier to accomplish with the pig in sternal recumbency. Using the same technique as in small ruminants and camelids with the aid of a laryngoscope and stylet, the epiglottis and laryngeal aperture can be visualized. Keeping in mind the acute angle between the larynx and tracheal opening, it is helpful to put some dorsal pressure at the end of the endotracheal tube as it enters the larynx. This technique keeps the tip of the tube slightly elevated as it advances into the trachea. Other helpful tips for successful endotracheal intubation in pigs are to spin the tube 180° or use a screw-like approach and advance it in a dorsal direction as the tube passes through the arytenoid cartilages and enters the trachea [8,25,85,86]. Correct placement of the tube in the trachea should be confirmed by capnography.

Thermoregulation

Hypothermia

Decreased heat production and increased heat loss are the primary causes of hypothermia observed during anesthesia and surgery [87]. Hypothermia is a common anesthetic complication in small companion animals but is rarely an issue for adult cattle and camelids because of their large body mass to surface area ratio. The body temperature of adult cattle and camelids seldom drops more than 0.5 °C during anesthesia if none of the major body cavities are opened. However, hypothermia can be a significant problem in small ruminants, particularly in pediatric patients. Hypothermia results in reduction of anesthetic requirements and prolonged recoveries [88]. Although often obese, pigs lack an insulating hair coat and, thus, are prone to hypothermia and must be protected from temperature extremes and insensible heat loss during anesthesia [27]. In pediatric pigs, a long duration of anesthesia without supplemental heat has resulted in hypothermia with body temperatures of 92 °F/33 °C and subsequent prolonged recovery (personal observation). Therefore, supplemental heat with a forced warm air unit, circulating warm water blanket, or resistive foam electric heating pad (e.g., HotDog Patient Warming System) can be used to minimize reduction of body temperature. Supplemental heat sources specifically designed for use in anesthetized patients should be used to reduce the risk of thermal burns.

Malignant hyperthermia

Malignant hyperthermia (MH), also referred to as "porcine stress syndrome," is a genetic disorder with mutation of the ryanodine receptor gene (RyR1), which encodes calcium channels in the sarcoplasmic reticulum of skeletal muscles [89–91]. The presence of mutated ryanodine receptors allows a massive amount of calcium to be released from the sarcoplasmic reticulum into the cytoplasm, resulting in excessive generalized skeletal muscle contraction [92]. MH has been reported in other animal species, but pigs and humans seem overrepresented [89,91,92]. Certain breeds of pigs, such as Pietrain, Poland China, and Landrace, have a higher prevalence of this syndrome compared to other breeds, such as Large White, Yorkshire, and Hampshire, where the incidence is much less [79,93].

In pigs, the clinical signs of MH syndrome are manifested as a sudden and dramatic rise in body temperature and end-tidal carbon dioxide ($P_{ET}CO_2$) followed by excessive muscle fasciculations, muscle rigidity, tachypnea, tachycardia, arrhythmias, myoglobinuria, metabolic acidosis, renal failure, and often death. Prognosis is usually poor once the episode is initiated in spite of immediate aggressive treatments. The triggering agents of MH include stress (induced by excitement, transportation, or preanesthetic handling and restraint), halogenated inhalational anesthetics (e.g., halothane, isoflurane, sevoflurane, and desflurane), and succinylcholine. Lidocaine and ketamine have been suggested as triggering agents, but there is no evidence to support this theory [94]. Treatments for MH are primarily symptomatic. Early recognition of symptoms (e.g., muscle rigidity, sudden rise in body temperature and $P_{ET}CO_2$) and aggressive treatments (e.g., immediate discontinuation of inhalation anesthetics and institution of ice packs and alcohol baths) are the foundations of therapy. Dantrolene sodium has been effective as a treatment (1–3 mg/kg IV) and prophylaxis (5 mg/kg PO) for MH [34]. In 1981, McGrath *et al.* [95] reported that acepromazine at 1.1 mg/kg IM and 1.65 mg/kg IM reduced the incidence of MH by 40% and 73%, respectively. A lower dose of 0.55 mg/kg IM was only able to delay but not prevent the onset of the episode.

Halogenated inhalational anesthetics are a known trigger for MH, and halothane is most frequently reported as an initiator in pigs [96]. Only one incidence of isoflurane-induced MH has been reported in a pot-bellied pig [97]. The pig received isoflurane for induction and maintenance of anesthesia. A significant increase in heart rate and intense shivering occurred 90 min after induction. The pig recovered from anesthesia and was standing within 10 min. However, intense shivering persisted, and rectal temperature rose from 99 °F/37.2 °C to 104 °F/40.1 °C. Oral dantrolene (5 mg/kg) was administered. The rectal temperature continued to rise to 106.7 °F/41.5 °C over the next 30 min but decreased to 100.4 °F/53 °C and 103.4 °F/39.7 °C over the next 18 h. Administration of oral dantrolene continued for 24 h (5 mg/kg, q8h). Body temperature returned to normal 24 h after recovery from anesthesia and remained normal for the remainder of hospitalization. The pig was discharged and sent home with close observation. Physical examination of the pig performed two weeks after the episode appeared to be normal and MH was not confirmed with genetic testing [97]. In an isoflurane-anesthetized Angus bull, an MH episode with fatal outcome was reported [98]. Progressive increases in heart rate, $P_{ET}CO_2$, as well as $PaCO_2$ were observed 76 min after induction of anesthesia. Isoflurane was discontinued and another anesthesia machine was used to provide 100% O_2 and continuation of resuscitation. Heart rate and $P_{ET}CO_2$ continued to rise, and the body temperature also increased from 103.1 °F/39.5 °C to 110.3 °F/43.5 °C at 140 min following induction. The resuscitation effort was unsuccessful, and the bull developed ventricular fibrillation followed by asystole. The clinical signs of the MH episode in the pot-bellied pig and the bull described here are unlike the clinical signs typically observed in pigs in which muscle rigidity, and sudden increases in body temperature and $P_{ET}CO_2$ normally develop within minutes after exposure to a triggering agent. Clinical signs of MH were not observed until 90 min in the pot-bellied pig and 75 min in the Angus bull after initiation of isoflurane. This delayed onset of clinical signs has been reported in horses [99], dogs [100], and cats [101].

There are no reports of sevoflurane-induced MH episodes in cattle. Analysis of muscular contracture in frogs showed that the augmentation of caffeine-induced contractures of sartorius muscle by isoflurane is three times, enflurane is four times, and halothane is 11 times baseline [102]. A human study showed that in a total of 75 MH cases, 42 were isoflurane-related, 12 were sevoflurane-related, 11 were halothane-related, and 8 were enflurane-related [103]. The lower incidence associated with halothane in humans likely represents its limited use in people. Definitive diagnosis of MH susceptibility in pigs requires *in vitro* contracture testing, which is based on the contracture of muscle fibers in the presence of halothane or caffeine. This technique is expensive and requires a surgical muscle biopsy and sophisticated equipment [104]. The halothane–succinylcholine challenge was employed by direct administration of 3–5% halothane via face mask for 3–5 min to young pigs. Positive results were indicated by appearance of muscle rigidity of the hindlimbs, hyperthermia, or death [105]. Formerly, the halothane challenge test was used in the field (barnyard halothane challenge) to guide appropriate culling from swine breeding herds [106]. Seeler *et al.* [107] further recommended that animals that did not react to 5 min of halothane be given a dose of succinylcholine (0.75 mg/kg IV), another trigger of MH, along with halothane and positive-pressure ventilation for 8 min. A negative response to this challenge confirmed that the pig was not an MH carrier [107]. At the time, the halothane–succinylcholine challenge test was considered to be the best way to accurately identify potential carriers of MH, and producers were able to eliminate susceptible pigs from their breeding herds. Recently, the development of a DNA-based polymerase chain reaction (PCR) test allows for definitive diagnosis of the gene mutation in skeletal muscle ryanodine receptors in MH-susceptible pigs. This DNA test requires the producer to collect a blood sample in a sterile-heparinized test tube or on a specialized absorbent card. As a result, swine producers are able to separate carriers of the mutated gene from non-carriers and successfully eliminate MH from their breeding stock. Therefore, fewer cases of MH have been reported recently [108–110]. The DNA test is commercially available and is inexpensive, costing US$20–35 per sample. At the time of publication, Marsfield Clinic in Wisconsin, PE AgGen in California, Prairie State Semen in Illinois [111], and NEOGEN in Michigan [112] all perform this DNA test.

Species differences in anesthetic dose requirements

Xylazine is a potent sedative, analgesic, and muscle relaxant that is frequently used as a preanesthetic agent or anesthetic adjunct in ruminants and camelids. Cattle require only one-tenth of the dose needed in horses to produce equipotent sedation [113]. It appears that Brahmans have the lowest dose requirement, Herefords are intermediate, and Holsteins are the least sensitive [114,115].

Administration of xylazine to pregnant ruminants in the final trimester may cause altered uterine motility and may be associated with premature parturition and retention of fetal membranes [116,117]. In pregnant dairy cows during late gestation, administration of xylazine (0.04 mg/kg IV) resulted in a significant increase in uterine vascular resistance (118–156%) and a decrease in uterine blood flow (25–59%) which resulted in a significant decrease in O_2 delivery (59%) [118]. Therefore, the use of xylazine during late gestation in pregnant ruminants is not routinely recommended to avoid detrimental effects to the fetus.

Pronounced and prolonged responses have been observed when xylazine was administered to cattle under high ambient temperature [119]. Interestingly, camelids require more xylazine than ruminants, so higher doses are required to produce similar sedation and the dose requirement is even higher for alpacas than llamas. Compared to other farm animal species, pigs have the highest dose requirement for α_2-adrenergic agonist-induced sedation. α_2-Adrenergic receptor agonists alone may not produce adequate sedation in some pigs. Pigs also appear less responsive to the pharmacologic effects of opioids [120,121]. Though benzodiazepines may not consistently produce sedation in other species, they are reliably effective in pigs [26].

Ruminants and camelids require less tolazoline (an α_2-adrenergic receptor antagonist) than other species [122,123]. Lower doses of tolazoline at 0.5–1.5 mg/kg IV are recommended for use in ruminants. Others have suggested that IV administration of tolazoline should be avoided, except in emergency situations, to prevent adverse effects such as hypotension and cardiac asystole [124].

Statements by owners and breeders regarding anesthetic management such as "injectable anesthetics should not be used in young pigs" and "ketamine in particular should not be used in pot-bellied pigs of any age" are common [125]. These statements are not supported by controlled, scientific studies. Furthermore, the clinical experiences of this author and most practicing veterinarians indicate otherwise.

Ruminants recover gradually but smoothly from Telazol® anesthesia as a result of the slower metabolism and longer lasting effect of zolazepam [126,127]. Pigs, on the other hand, often experience prolonged and rough recoveries characterized by swimming motions with repeated attempts to right themselves when recovering from Telazol® anesthesia, similar to that observed when ketamine is used alone [26,128]. Tiletamine and zolazepam are eliminated more slowly in pigs than in other species [128] and tiletamine apparently has a longer effect than zolazepam in pigs [127].

Ruminants reportedly have extremely low levels of pseudocholinesterase, the enzyme responsible for metabolism and inactivation of depolarizing neuromuscular blocking drugs such as succinylcholine. Therefore, administration of succinylcholine to ruminants often results in prolonged duration of muscle paralysis and is contraindicated [129].

Airway management during recovery

Prior to removal of the endotracheal tube, manual removal of regurgitant material and saliva from the buccal cavity or by lavaging with water may be performed. During recovery, displacement of the soft palate can occur in camelids, causing the soft palate to situate dorsally to the epiglottis and hinder air flow into the larynx. This is a serious condition and may result in upper airway obstruction and eventually cardiac arrest since camelids are obligate nasal breathers. If the animal has regained consciousness and the swallowing reflex, the problem can be corrected by encouraging the animal to swallow. Otherwise, the animal needs to be reintubated until the swallowing reflex returns [130].

Prolonged duration of dorsal recumbency in camelids often results in severe nasal edema, which can cause airway obstruction following extubation during recovery [131]. Keeping the animal in sternal recumbency with the head elevated, administration of a nasal spray containing phenylephrine, and providing O_2 insufflation with a demand valve should be instituted until the nasal edema diminishes and adequate air flow through the nasal cavity resumes.

Pigs are more difficult to intubate until one becomes accustomed to their anatomic differences. Laryngeal edema and laryngospasm caused by failed intubation attempts can potentially result in airway obstruction in lightly anesthetized pigs. Topical lidocaine applied to the larynx and an adequate plane of anesthesia during the intubation process will allow smooth and successful intubation and minimize laryngeal trauma [132]. In sows receiving spinal anesthesia and placed in lateral recumbency for cesarean section, restraint of the head with rope may be necessary to prevent head movement. Care should be taken to avoid placing the head in extension. Unlike most other species, extension of the head can complicate rather than resolve upper airway obstruction in swine. Similar to camelids, dorsal displacement of soft palate resulting in airway obstruction and suffocation has been reported in swine due to their long soft palate engaging the larynx [132]. This complication occurs in non-intubated pigs during anesthesia or following extubation as a result of dorsal displacement of the long soft palate [130]. Noisy respiration after extubation indicates possible laryngeal spasm or upper airway obstruction and should be investigated immediately [25].

Acknowledgment

Portions of this chapter also appear in the text *Farm Animal Anesthesia: Cattle, Small Ruminants, Camelids, and Pigs.*

References

1 Craigmill AL, Rangel-Lugo M, Damian P, *et al.* Extralabel use of tranquilizers and general anesthetics. *J Am Vet Med Assoc* 1997; **211**: 302–304.

2 Davis JL, Smith GW, Baynes RE, *et al.* Update on drug prohibited for extralabel use in food animals. *J Am Vet Med Assoc* 2009; **235**: 528–534.

3 US Food and Drug Administration. Animal Medicinal Drug Use Clarification Act of 1994 (AMDUCA). www.fda.gov/animal-veterinary/guidance-regulations/animal-medicinal-drug-use-clarification-act-1994-amduca (accessed January 2023).

4 Papich MG. Drug residue considerations for anesthetics and adjunctive drugs in food-producing animals. *Vet Clin North Am Food Animal Pract* 1996; **12**: 693–706.

5 Fajt VR. Label and extralabel drug use in small ruminants. *Vet Clin North Am Food Anim Pract* 2001; **17**: 403–420.

6 Lord LK, Wittum T. Survey of humana organizations and slaughter plants regarding experiences with Vietnamese potbellied pigs. *J Am Vet Med Assoc* 1997; **211**: 562–565.

7 Smith AC, Ehler W, Swindle MM. Anesthesia and analgesia in swine. In: Kohn DH, Wixson SK, White WJ, Benson GJ, eds. *Anesthesia and Analgesia in Laboratory Animals.* New York, NY: Academic Press, 1997: 313–336.

8 Swindle MM. Anesthesia and analgesia. In: *Surgery, Anesthesia, and Experimental Techniques in Swine.* Ames, IA: Iowa State University Press, 1998: 33–63.

9 Coetzee JF. A review of pain assessment techniques and pharmacological approach to pain relief after bovine castration: practical implications for cattle production within the United States. *Appl Anim Behav Sci* 2011; **135**: 192–213.

10 Haskel SRR, Gehing R, Payne MA, *et al.* Update on FARAD food animal drug withholding recommendation. *J Am Vet Med Assoc* 2003; **223**: 1277–2003.

11 Valverde A, Doherty TJ. Pain management in cattle and small ruminants. In: Anderson DE, Rings DM, eds. *Current Veterinary Therapy: Food Animal Medicine,* 5th edn. St Louis, MO: Saunders/Elsevier, 2009: 534–574.

12 Passler T. Regulatory and legal considerations of anesthetics and analgesics used in food-producing animals. In: Lin HC, Walz P, eds. *Farm Animal Anesthesia: Cattle, Small Ruminants, Camelids, and Pigs.* Ames, IA: Wiley-Blackwell, 2014: 228–247.

13 Hinchcliff KW, Jernigan AD, Upson DW, *et al.* Ruminant pharmacology. *Vet Clin North Am Food Anim Pract* 1991; **7**: 633–649.

14 DeRouchey J, Goodband B, Tokach M, *et al.* Digestive system of the pig – anatomy and function. *Proceedings of the North American Veterinary Conference*, 2009: 375–376.

15 Mozzachio C. Handling and Restraint and Routine Veterinary Care of the Miniature Pigs. LafeberVet AAVSB RACE Provider #776-36251, https://lafeber.com/vet/wp-content/uploads/2019/04/Routine-Vet-Care-Mini-Pig-LV-reduced-size.pdf (updated April 8, 2019).

16 Lacoste L, Bouquet S, Ingrand P, *et al.* Intranasal midazolam in piglets: pharmacodynamics (0.2 vs 0.4 mg/kg) and pharmacokinetics (0.4 mg/kg) with bioavailiability determination. *Lab Anim* 2000; **34**: 29–35.

17 Fowler ME. The jugular vein (*Lama peruna*): a clinical note. *J Zoo Anim Med* 1983; **14**: 77–78.

18 Fowler ME. *Anatomy information. Camelid Medicine Workshop Syllabus* 1984: 5–16.

19 Amsel SI, Kainer RA, Johnson LW. Choosing the best site to perform venipuncture in a llama. *Vet Med* 1987; **82**: 535–536.

20 Riebold TW, Kaneps AJ, Schmotzer WB. Anesthesia in the llama. *Vet Surg* 1989; **18**: 400–404.

21 Pugh DG, Navarre CB, Ruffin DC, *et al.* A review of diagnostic procedures in llamas and alpacas. *Vet Med* 1999; **94**: 654–659.

22 Grint N, Dugdale A. Brightness of venous blood in South American camelids: implications for jugular catheterization. *Vet Anaesth Analg* 2009; **36**: 63–66.

23 Heath RB. Llama anesthetic programs. *Vet Clin North Am Food Anim Pract* 1989; **5**: 71–80.

24 Davis IA, McGaffin JR, Kuchinka GD. Intravenous catheterization of the external jugular vein in llamas. *Compend Contin Educ Pract Vet* 1996; **18**: 330–335.

25 Ko JCH, Thurmon JC, Tranquilli WJ, *et al.* Problems encountered when anesthetizing potbellied pigs. *Vet Med* 1993; **88**: 435–440.

26 Moon PF, Smith LJ. General anesthetic techniques in swine. *Vet Clin North Am Food Anim Pract* 1996; **12**: 663–691.

27 Wolff P. Pet pig problems. *Proceedings of the North American Veterinary Conference* 2009: 416–419.

28 'Forking Technique' to Minimize Stress and Facilitate Injection in Pigs. http://www.youtube.com/watch?v=p6LiZVgk6nc

29 Lin HC. Standing sedation and chemical restraint. In: Lin HC, Walz P, eds. *Farm Animal Anesthesia: Cattle, Small Ruminants, Camelids, and Pigs.* Ames, IA: Wiley-Blackwell, 2014: 39–59.

30 Lin HC. Injectable anesthetics and field anesthesia. In: Lin HC, Walz P, eds. *Farm Animal Anesthesia: Cattle, Small Ruminants, Camelids, and Pigs.* Ames, IA: Wiley-Blackwell, 2014: 60–94.

31 SOP: Intramuscular Injection in Swine. University Veterinarian and Animal Resources, Virginia Tech Institutional Animal Care and Use Committee, December 12, 2017. https://ouv.vt.edu/content/dam/ouv_vt_edu/sops/large-animal/sop-swine-intramuscular-injection.pdf

32 Ivany JM, Muir WW. Farm animal anesthesia. In: Fubini SL, Ducharme NG, eds. *Farm Animal Surgery.* St. Louis, MO: Saunders, 2004: 97–112.

33 Maxwell H, Kennedy S. Technique for jugular catheterization of swine using the Seldinger technique. *Proceedings of the Auburn University CVM Annual Conference, Auburn, AL.* Virtual, 2020.

34 Anderson DE, St. Jean G. Anesthesia and surgical procedures in swine. In: Zimmerman JJ, Karriker LA, Ramirez A, *et al.*, eds. *Diseases of Swine*, 10th edn. Ames, IA: Wiley-Blackwell, 2012: 119–140.

35 Thurmon JC, Benson GJ. Anesthesia in ruminants and swine. In: Howard JC, ed. *Current Veterinary Therapy: Food Animal Practice*, 3rd edn. Philadelphia, PA: WB Saunders, 1993: 58–76.

36 Riebold TW. Ruminants. In: Tranquilli WJ, Thurmon JC, Grimm KA, eds. *Lumb and Jones' Veterinary Anesthesia and Analgesia*, 4th edn. Ames, IA: Blackwell Publishing, 2007: 731–746.

37 Fowler ME. Anesthesia. In: *Medicine and Surgery of Camelids*, 3rd edn. Ames, IA: Wiley-Blackwell, 2010: 111–127.

38 Lin HC, Tyler JW, Welles EG, *et al.* Effects of anesthesia induced and maintained by continuous intravenous administration of guaifenesin, ketamine, and xylazine in spontaneously breathing sheep. *Am J Vet Res* 1993; **54**: 1913–1916.

39 Klein L, Fisher N. Cardiopulmonary effects of restraint in dorsal recumbency on awake cattle. *Am J Vet Res* 1988; **49**: 1605–1608.

40 Musewe VO, Gillespie JR, Berry JD. Influence of ruminal insufflation on pulmonary function and diaphragmatic electromyography in cattle. *Am J Vet Res* 1979; **40**: 26–31.

41 Desmecht D, Linden A, Lekeux P. Pathophysiological response of bovine diaphragm function to gastric distension. *J Appl Physiol* 1995; **78**: 1537–1546.

42 Kerr CL, Windeyer C, Bouré LP, *et al.* Cardiopulmonary effects of administration of a combination solution of xylazine, guaifenesin and ketamine or inhaled isoflurane in mechanically ventilated calves. *Am J Vet Res* 2007; **68**: 1287–1293.

43 Offinger J, Meyer H, Fischer J, *et al.* Comparison of isoflurane inhalation anaesthesia, injection anaesthesia and high volume caudal epidural anaesthesia for umbilical surgery in calves; metabolic, endocrine and cardiopulmonary effects. *Vet Anaesth Analg* 2012; **39**: 123–136.

44 Greene SA, Keegan RD, Valdez RA, *et al.* Cardiovascular effects of sevoflurane in Holstein calves. *Vet Anaesth Analg* 2002; **29**: 59–63.

45 Keegan RD, Greene SA, Valdez RA, *et al.* Cardiovascular effects of desflurane in mechanically ventilated calves. *Am J Vet Res* 2006; **67**: 537–391.

46 Aarnes TK, Hubbell JAE, Lerche P, *et al.* Comparison of invasive and oscillometric blood pressure measurement techniques in anesthetized sheep, goats, and cattle. *Vet Anaesth Analg* 2015; **41**: 174–185.

47 Semrad SD, Trim CM, Hardee GE. Hypertension in bulls and steers anesthetized with guaifenesin-thiobarbiturate-halothane combinations. *Am J Vet Res* 1985; **47**: 1477–1582.

48 Clarke KW, Trim CM, Hall LW. Anaesthesia of cattle. In: Clarke KW, Trim CM, Hall LW, eds. *Veterinary Anaesthesia*, 11th edn. Edinburgh: Saunders/Elsevier. 2014: 313–343.

49 Warren RG, McDonell W, Adetuni A, *et al.* Cardiopulmonary effects of xylazine/halothane anesthesia in mature cows. *Proceedings of the Annual Meeting of the American College of Veterinary Anesthesiologists* 1983: 35–36.

50 McDonell W. Respiratory system. In: Thurmon JC, Tranquilli WJ, Benson GJ, eds. *Lumb and Jones' Veterinary Anesthesia*, 3rd edn. Baltimore, MD: Williams & Wilkins, 1996: 115–147.

51 Tagawa M, Okano S, Sako T, *et al.* Effect of change in body position on cardiopulmonary function and plasma cortisol in cattle. *J Vet Med Sci* 1994; **56**: 131–134.

52 Wagner AE, Muir WW, Brospitch BJ. Cardiopulmonary effects of position in conscious cattle. *Am J Vet Res* 1990; **51**: 7–10.

53 McLaughlin RF, Tyler WS, Canada RO. A study of the subgross pulmonary anatomy in various mammals. *Am J Vet Res* 1961; **108**: 149–165.

54 Musewe VO. Respiration mechanics, breathing patterns, ventilation, and diaphragmatic electromyogram (EMG) in normal, unsedated adult, domestic cattle (*Bos Taurus*) breathing spontaneously in the standing and the sternal-recumbent body positions, and during inflation of the rumen with air. PhD thesis. Davis, CA: University of California Davis, 1978.

55 Gallivan GJ, McDonell WN, Forrest JB. Comparative pulmonary mechanics in the horse and the cow. *Res Vet Sci* 1989; **46**: 322–330.

56 Lumb AB. Pulmonary ventilation: mechanisms and the work of breathing. In: Lumb AB, ed. *Nunn's Applied Respiratory Physiology*. Oxford: Butterworth Heinemann, 2000: 112–137.

57 Dyce KM, Sack WO, Wensing CJG. The abdomen of the ruminants. In: *Textbook of Veterinary Anatomy*. Philadelphia, PA: WB Saunders, 1987: 633–656.

58 Habel RE. Ruminant digestive system. In: Getty R, ed. *Sisson and Grossman's The Anatomy of the Domestic Animals*, 5th edn. Philadelphia, PA: WB Saunders, 1975: 861–915.

59 Kesler EM, Ronning M, Knodt CB. Functional and structural development of the ruminant forestomach. *J Anim Sci* 1951; **10**: 969–975.

60 Gallivan GJ, McDonell WN, Forrest JB. Comparative ventilation and gas exchange in the horse and the cow. *Res Vet Sci* 1989; **46**: 331–336.

61 Mitchell B, Williams JT. Respiratory function changes in sheep associated with lying in lateral recumbency and with sedation by xylazine. *Proceedings of the Association of Veterinary Anaesthetists of Great Britain and Ireland*, 1976–77; **6**: 30–36.

62 Hsu WH, Schaffer DD, Hanson CE. Effects of tolazoline and yohimbine on xylazine induced central nervous system depression, bradycardia, and tachypnea in sheep. *J Am Vet Med Assoc* 1987; **190**: 423–426.

63 Hsu WH, Hanson CE, Hembrough FB, *et al.* Effects of idazoxan, tolazoline, and yohimbine on xylazine-induced respiratory changes and central nervous system depression in ewes. *Am J Vet Res* 1989; **50**: 1570–1573.

64 Lin HC, Tyler JW, Wallace SS, *et al.* Telazol and xylazine anesthesia in sheep. *Cornell Vet* 1993; **83**: 117–124.

65 Doherty TJ, Ballinger JA, McDonnell WN, *et al.* Antagonism of xylazine-induced sedation by a new alpha-2 adrenergic receptor antagonist idazoxan. *Can J Vet Res* 1987; **55**: 244–248.

66 Waterman AE, Nolan A, Livingston A. Influence of idazoxan on respiratory blood gas changes induced by alpha-2 adrenergic receptor adrenoceptor agonist drugs in conscious sheep. *Vet Rec* 1987; **121**: 105–107.

67 Celly CS, McDonell WN, Black WD. The comparative hypoxaemic effect of four alpha-2 adrenergic receptor adrenoceptor agonists (xylazine, romifidine, detomidine, and medetomidine) in sheep. *J Vet Pharmacol Ther* 1997; **20**: 464–471.

68 Nolan A, Livingston A, Waterman A. The effects of alpha-2 adrenoceptor agonists on airway pressure in anaesthetized sheep. *J Vet Pharmacol Ther* 1986; **9**: 157–163.

69 Celly CS, Atwal OS, McDonell WN, *et al.* The histopathologic alterations induced in the lungs of sheep by use of alpha-2 adrenergic receptor-adrenergic receptor agonists. *Am J Vet Res* 1999; **60**: 154–161.

70 Kästner SBR. Alpha-2 adrenergic receptor-agonists in sheep: a review. *Vet Anaesth Analg* 2006; **33**: 79–96.

71 Steffey EP. Some characteristics of ruminants and swine that complicate management of general anesthesia. *Vet Clin North Am Food Animal Pract* 1986; **2**: 507–516.

72 Hickman MA, Cox SR, Mahabir S, *et al.* Safety, pharmacokinetics and use of the novel NK-1 receptor antagonist maropitant (Cerenia) for the prevention of emesis and motion sickness in cats. *J Vet Pharmacol Ther* 2008; **31**: 220–229.

73 Boscan P, Monnet E, Mama K, *et al.* Effect of maropitant, a neurokinin-I receptor antagonist, on anesthetic requirement during noxious visceral stimulation of the ovary in dogs. *Am J Vet Res* 2011; **72**: 1576–1579.

74 Niyom S, Boscan P, Twedt DC, *et al.* Effect of maropitant, a neurokinin-I receptor antagonist, on the minimum alveolar concentration of sevoflurane during stimulation of the ovarian ligament in cats. *Vet Anaesth Analg* 2013; **40**: 435–431.

75 de la Puente-Redondon VA, Siedek EM, Benchaoui HA, *et al.* The antiemetic efficacy of maropitant (Cerenia) in the treatment of ongoing emesis caused by a wide range of underlying clinical aetiologies in canine patients in Europe. *J Small Anim Pract* 2007; **48**: 93–98.

76 Ramsey DS, Kincaid K, Watkins JA, *et al.* Safety and efficacy of injectable and oral maropitant, a selective neurokinin I receptor antagonist, in a randomized clinical trial for treatment of vomiting in dogs. *J Vet Pharmacol Ther* 2008; **31**: 553–543.

77 Swallow A, Rioja E, Elmer T, *et al.* The effect of maropitant on intraoperative isoflurane requirements and postoperative nausea and vomiting in dogs : a randomized clinical trial. *Vet Anaesth Analg* 2017; **44**: 785–793.

78 McCormack R, Olley L, Glanemann B, *et al.* Prospective observational study of the use of omeprazole and maropitant citrate in veterinary specialist care. *Sci Rep* 2020; **10**: 15727.

79 Thurmon JC, Benson GJ. Special anesthesia considerations of swine. In: Short CE, ed. *Principles & Practice: Veterinary Anesthesia*. Baltimore, MD: Williams & Wilkins, 1987: 308–322.

80 Clarke KW, Trim CM, Hall LW. Anesthesia of the pig. In: Clarke KW, Trim CM, Hall LW, eds. *Veterinary Anaesthesia*, 11th edn. Edinburgh, UK: Saunders/Elsevier, 2014: 535–403.

81 Malavasi LM. Swine. In: Grimm KA, Lamont LA, Tranquilli WJ, *et al.*, eds. *Lumb & Jones' Veterinary Anesthesia and Analgesia*, 5th edn. Ames, IA: Wiley-Blackwell, 2015: 928–940.

82 Somers M. Saliva secretion and its functions in ruminants. *Aust Vet J* 1957; **33**: 297–301.

83 Kay RNR. The rate of flow and composition of various salivary secretion in sheep and calves. *J Physiol* 1960; **150**: 515–537.

84 Thurmon JC, Benson GJ. Anesthesia in ruminants. In: Howard JL, ed. *Current Veterinary Therapy: Food Animal Practice*. Philadelphia, PA: WB Saunders, 1983: 58–81.

85 Swindle MM. *Anesthetic and Perioperative Techniques in Swine*. Andover, MA: Charles River Laboratories, 1991.

86 Wilbers AM. Routine veterinary care of pot-bellied pigs. *Proceedings of the North American Veterinary Conference*, 2009: 410–412.

87 Haskins SC. Monitoring the anesthetized patients. In: Short CE, ed. *Principles & Practice: Veterinary Anesthesia*. Baltimore, MD: Williams & Wilkins, 1987: 455–477.

88 Hall LW, Clarke KW. Accident and emergencies associated with anesthesia. In: *Veterinary Anaesthesia*, 8th edn. London: Baillière Tindall: London, 1983: 367–538.

89 Fuji J, Otsu K, Zorzato F, *et al.* Identification of a mutation in porcine ryanodine receptor associated with malignant hyperthermia. *Science* 1991; **253**: 448–451.

90 Geer R, Decanniere C, Ville H, *et al.* Identification of halothane gene carriers by use of an in vivo 3IP nuclear magnetic resonance spectroscopy in pigs. *Am J Vet Res* 1992; **53**: 1711–1714.

91 Houde A, Pomnier SA, Roy R. Detection of the ryanodine receptor mutation associated with malignant hyperthermia in purebred swine populations. *J Anim Sci* 1993; **71**: 1414–1418.

92 Stoelting RK, Dierdorf SF, McCammon RL. Pediatric patients. In: *Anesthesia and Coexisting Disease*, 2nd edn. New York, NY: Churchill Livingstone, 1988: 807–883.

93 Jorgensen JS, Cannedy AL. Physiologic and pathologic considerations for ruminants and swine anesthesia. *Vet Clin North Am Food Anim Pract* 1996; **12**: 481–500.

94 Hildebrand SV. Hyperthermia, malignant hyperthermia, and myopathy. In: Short CE, ed. *Principles & Practice: Veterinary Anesthesia*. Baltimore, MD: Williams & Wilkins, 1987: 517–532.

95 McGrath CJ, Rempel WE, Addis PB, *et al.* Acepromazine and droperidol inhibition of halothane-induced malignant hyperthermia (porcine stress syndrome) in swine. *Am J Vet Res* 1981; **42**: 195–198.

96 Stoelting RK, Hillier SC. Inhaled anesthetics. In: *Pharmacology & Physiology in Anesthetic Practice*, 4th edn. Philadelphia, PA: Lippincott Williams & Wilkins, 2005: 42–86.

97 Claxton-Gill MS, Cornick-Seahorn JL, Gamboa JC, *et al.* Suspected malignant hyperthermia syndrome in a miniature pot-bellied pig anesthetized with isoflurane. *J Am Vet Med Assoc* 1993; **203**: 1434–1436.

98 Skelding A, Valverde A. Intra-operative hyperthermia in a young Angus bull with a fatal outcome. *Can Vet J* 2017; **58**: 614–616.

99 Aleman M, Nieto J, Magdesian K. Malignant hyperthermia associated with ryanodine receptor 1 (C7360G) mutation in quarter horses. *J Vet Int Med* 2009; **23**: 329–334.

100 Chohan A, Greene S. Anesthesia case of the month: malignant hyperthermia. *J Am Vet Med Assoc* 2011; **239**: 936–940.

101 Thomas S, Burton C, Armitage-Chan E. Intra-operative hyperthermia in a cat with a fatal outcome. *Vet Anaesth Analg* 2014; **41**: 290–296.

102 Reed SB, Strobel GE. An in vitro model of malignant hyperthermia: differential effects of inhalation anesthetics on caffeine-induced muscle contractures. *Anesthesiology* 1978; **48**: 254–259.

103 Hopkins PM. Malignant hyperthermia: pharmacology of triggering. *Br J Anaesth* 2011; **107**: 48–56.

104 Hildebrand SV. Hyperthermia, malignant hyperthermia, and myopathy. In: Short CE ed. *Principle & Practice of Veterinary Anesthesia*. Baltimore, MD: Williams & Wilkins, 1987: 517–532.

105 McGrath CJ, Lee JC, Rempel WE. Halothane testing for malignant hyperthermia in swine: dose-response effects. *Am J Vet Res* 1984; **45**: 1734–1736.

106 Webb AI, Gordon CHC. Halothane sensitivity as a field test for stress susceptibility in the pig. *Anim Prod* 1978; **26**: 157–168.

107 Seeler DC, McDonnell WN, Basrur PK. Halothane and halothane succinylcholine induced malignant hyperthermia (porcine stress syndrome) in a population of Ontario boars. *Can J Comp Med* 1983; **47**: 284–290.

108 Monin G, Larzul C, le Roy P, *et al.* Effects of the halothanegenotype and slaughter weight on texture of pork. *J Anim Sci* 1999; **77**: 408–415.

109 Wendt M, Bickhardt K, Herzog A, *et al.* Porcine stress syndrome and PsE meat: clinical symptoms, pathogenesis, etiology and animal right aspects. *Berlinber und Münchener Tierärztliche Wochenschrift* 2000; **113**: 173–190.

110 Lahucky R, Baulain U, Henning M, *et al.* In vivo PNMR studies on biopsy skeletal muscle samples compared with meat quality of normal and heterozygous malignant hyperthermia in pigs. *Meat Sci* 2002; **61**: 233–241.

111 Stalder K. Porcine Stress Syndrome and its Effects on Maternal, Feedlot and Carcass Quantitatives and Qualitative Traits. Agriculture Extension Service, University of Tennessee. www.extension.tennessee.edu/publications/Documents/PB1606.pdf

112 Neogen Corporation Website. Porcine Stress Syndrome (PSS) Testing. www.neogen.com/categories/livestock-genetic-traits-conditions/porcine-stress-syndrome/

113 Greene SA, Thurmon JC. Xylazine – a review of its pharmacology and use in veterinary medicine. *J Vet Pharmacol Ther* 1988; **11**: 295–313.

114 Raptopoulos D, Weaver BMQ. Observations following intravenous xylazine administration in steers. *Vet Rec* 1984; **114**: 567–569.

115 Trim CM. Special anesthesia considerations in the ruminant. In: Short CE, ed. *Principles & Practice: Veterinary Anesthesia*. Baltimore, MD: Williams & Wilkins, 1987: 285–300.

116 LeBlanc MM, Hubbell JAE, Smith HC. The effect of xylazine hydrochloride on intrauterine pressure in the cow and the mare. *Proceedings of the Annual Meeting of the Society of Theriogenology* 1984: 211–220.

117 Jansen CAM, Lowe KC, Nathanielsz PW. The effects of xylazine on uterine activity, fetal and maternal oxygenation, cardiovascular function, and fetal breathing. *Am J Obstet Gynecol* 1984; **148**: 386–390.

118 Hodgson DS, Dunlop CI, Chapman PL, *et al.* Cardiopulmonary effects of xylazine and acepromazine in pregnant cows in late gestation. *Am J Vet Res* 2002; **63**: 1695–1699.

119 Fayed AH, Abdalla EB, Anderson RR, *et al.* Effect of xylazine in heifers under thermoneutral or heat stress conditions. *Am J Vet Res* 1989; **50**: 151–153.

120 Steffey EP, Baggot JD, Eisele JH, *et al.* Morphine-isoflurane interaction in dogs, swine and Rhesus monkeys. *J Vet Pharmacol Ther* 1994; **17**: 202–210.

121 Moon PF, Scarlett JM, Ludders JW, *et al.* The effect of fentanyl on the minimum alveolar concentration of isoflurane in swine. *Anesthesiology* 1995; **83**: 535–542.

122 Read MR, Duke T, Towes AR. Suspected tolazoline toxicosis in a llama. *J Am Vet Med Assoc* 2000; **216**: 227–229.

123 Lin HC, Riddell MG. Tolazoline: dose responses and side effects in non-sedated Holstein calves. *Bov Practitioner* 2008; **42**: 86–92.

124 Anderson DE. New methods for chemical restraint and field anesthesia in cattle. *Proceedings of the North American Veterinary Conference* 2011: 6–11.

125 Pigs 4 Ever Website. www.pigs4ever.com/pot_belly_pig_information (accessed September 2014).

126 Lin HC, Thurmon JC, Benson GJ, *et al.* The hemodynamic response of calves to tiletamine-zolazepam anesthesia. *Vet Surg* 1989; **18**: 328–334.

127 Lin HC, Thurmon JC, Benson GJ, *et al.* Telazol – a review of its pharmacology and use in veterinary medicine. *J Vet Pharmacol Ther* 1992; **16**: 383–418.

128 Kumar AH, Mann J, Remmel RP. Pharmacokinetics of tiletamine and zolazepam (Telazol) in anesthetized pigs. *J Vet Pharmacol Ther* 2006; **129**: 587–589.

129 Adams HR. Cholinergic pharmacology: neuromuscular blocking agents. In: Booth NH, McDonald LE, eds. *Veterinary Pharmacology and Therapeutics*, 6th edn. Ames, IA: Iowa State University Press, 1998: 137–151.

130 Riebold TW. Management of intraoperative and postoperative anesthetic complications in ruminants and swine. *Vet Clin North Am Food Animal Pract* 1986; **2**: 665–676.

131 Abrahamsen EJ. Chemical restraint, anesthesia, and analgesia for camelids. *Vet Clin North Am Food Animal Pract* 2009; **25**: 455–494.

132 Benson GJ. Anesthetic management of ruminants and swine with selected pathophysiologic alteration. *Vet Clin North Am Food Anim Pract* 1986; **2**: 677–691.

54 Comparative Anesthesia and Analgesia – Laboratory Animals

Henri G.M.J. Bertrand[1] and Aurélie A. Thomas[2]
[1]Agenda Veterinary Services, Kingston Upon Hull, East Riding of Yorkshire, UK
[2]Clinical Pharmacology and Safety Sciences, AstraZeneca, Cambridge, UK

Chapter contents

Introduction, 1065
Anesthetics and analgesics, 1065
  Inhalant anesthetics, 1065
  Injectable anesthetics, 1067
  Opioids, 1068
  Anti-inflammatory drugs, 1069
  Local and regional analgesia and anesthesia, 1069
  Gabapentin and pregabalin, 1070
Laboratory rodents and lagomorphs, 1070
  Anatomic and physiologic considerations, 1070
  Handling, restraint, and drug administration, 1070
  Airway management, 1070
  Breathing systems, 1071
  Fluid therapy, 1072
  Maintenance of body temperature, 1072
  Postoperative care, 1072
Non-human primates, 1073
  Anesthetic considerations, 1073
  Preanesthetic considerations, 1073
  Endotracheal intubation, 1073
  Equipment and monitoring, 1073
  Recovery, 1073
  Non-human primates in neuroscience, 1074
  Pain assessment and management, 1074
References, 1074

Introduction

With up to 100 million animals used in research annually worldwide, including 1 million animals anesthetized annually in the United Kingdom alone [1], laboratory animal medicine and anesthesia are an important area requiring veterinary involvement. With the implementation of the principles of the 3Rs – *Reduction, Replacement, Refinement* [2] – and increased awareness of the importance of the public's perception of the use of animal models for research, the involvement of veterinary anesthetists in this field has been steadily increasing. There is now a general acceptance of the need to refine experiments, that is, to reduce to a minimum the pain and distress that might be experienced when animals are used in research. However, a 2009 survey indicated that less than 25% of laboratory rodents received postoperative analgesics, while less than 40% were anesthetized with agents likely to have some analgesic properties [3]. Encouraging greater use of postoperative analgesics and implementing improvements in anesthesia and intraoperative care require veterinary anesthetists to become aware of the unique challenges posed by working in a research environment. In addition to working with less familiar species, under constraints that are specific to the research project and the local legislative framework, the anesthetist may also be asked to work with agents that are not usually encountered in clinical practice (e.g., chloralose and urethane), to advise researchers on the most appropriate anesthetic and analgesic protocols in light of study goals, to accommodate animals with appropriate anesthesia lasting as short as a few seconds or as long as a few days, and to provide expertise on the ethical aspects of research projects. Although dealing with these issues may seem daunting, the involvement of veterinary anesthetists is essential to help promote improvements in anesthesia and perioperative care as well as enhancing the standards of animal welfare.

Anesthetics and analgesics

Commonly used drug doses for laboratory animals are listed in Tables 54.1–54.3. Unless specified below, the reader should assume that the drugs' pharmacokinetics in laboratory animals are broadly similar to those described in companion animals. Some particularly relevant properties of commonly used sedative, anesthetic, and analgesic agents are described in this section.

Inhalant anesthetics

Inhalants (mainly isoflurane and sevoflurane) continue to be popular in laboratory animal anesthesia for a number of reasons. Their adverse effects are well documented, they can be administered to all commonly used laboratory rodents, and one agent (isoflurane) undergoes virtually no biotransformation [10]. Consequently, isoflurane represents a good option for most commonly used research protocols when avoidance of metabolic confounding factors is required. Second, using inhalants allows rapid induction and

Veterinary Anesthesia and Analgesia: The Sixth Edition of Lumb and Jones. Edited by Leigh Lamont, Kurt Grimm, Sheilah Robertson, Lydia Love and Carrie Schroeder.
© 2024 John Wiley & Sons, Inc. Published 2024 by John Wiley & Sons, Inc.
Companion website: www.wiley.com/go/lamont/anesthesia

Table 54.1 Commonly used drugs and dosages in commonly encountered small mammals.

	Mice	Rats	Guinea pigs	Rabbits	Comments	References
Atropine	0.04 mg/kg SC	0.05 mg/kg IP, SC	0.05 mg/kg IM, IP	50–250 µg/kg IM, SC		[4]
Glycopyrrolate	??	0.5 mg/kg IM	??	0.1 mg/kg IM, IV		[4]
Acepromazine	2–5 mg/kg IP, SC	2.5 mg/kg IM, IP	0.5–1 mg/kg IM	1 mg/kg IM		[4]
Xylazine	5–10 mg/kg IP	1–5 mg/kg IP	5 mg/kg IP	2–5 mg/kg IM, SC		[4]
Medetomidine	30–100 µg/kg SC	30–100 µg/kg SC	0.5 mg/kg IM, IP	0.1–0.5 mg/kg IM, SC		[4]
Dexmedetomidine	15–50 µg/kg SC	15–50 µg/kg SC	0.25 mg/kg IM, IP	50–250 µg/kg, IM, SC		[4]
Diazepam	5 mg/kg IP	2.5–5 mg/kg IP	2.5 mg/kg IP, IM	1–2 mg/kg IM		[4]
Midazolam	5 mg/kg IP	5 mg/kg IP	5 mg/kg IP	0.5–2 mg/kg IV, IM, IP		[4]
Alfaxalone	80 mg/kg IP	2–5 mg/kg IV, 20 mg/kg IP	40 mg/kg IM, IP	9–12 mg/kg IM		[4–6]
Ketamine	100–200 mg/kg IM	50–100 mg/kg IM, IP	40–100 mg/kg IM, IP	25–50 mg/kg IM		[4]
Ketamine plus acepromazine	100 mg/kg, 5 mg/kg IP	75 mg/kg, 2.5 mg/kg IP	100 mg/kg, 5 mg/kg IP	50 mg/kg, 1 mg/kg IM	Light anesthesia	[4]
Ketamine plus dexmedetomidine	100 mg/kg, 0.25 mg/kg IP	60–75 mg/kg, 0.125–0.25 mg/kg IP	40 mg/kg, 0.25 mg/kg IP	15 mg/kg, 0.125 mg/kg SC	Surgical plane of anesthesia, but more variable effects in mice	[4]
Medetomidine plus midazolam plus fentanyl	0.5 mg/kg, 5 mg/kg, 50 µg/kg SC	0.15 mg/kg, 2 mg/kg, 5 µg/kg SC	0.2 mg/kg, 1 mg/kg, 25 µg/kg SC	0.2 mg/kg, 1 mg/kg, 20 µg/kg IM		[4]
Alfaxalone plus dexmedetomidine	30 mg/kg, 0.3 mg/kg IP	30 mg/kg, 0.05 mg/kg IP	??	6 mg/kg, 0.2 mg/kg IM		[4,7]
Urethane	??	1000 mg/kg IP	1500 mg/kg IV, IP	1000–2000 mg/kg IV	Non-recovery procedures only	[4]

IM, intramuscular; IP, intraperitoneal; IV, intravenous; SC, subcutaneous; ??, unknown.

Table 54.2 Commonly used drugs and dosages for selected primate species.

	Macaque *spp*	Marmosets	Comments	References
Atropine	0.04 mg/kg SC	0.05 mg/kg IP, SC		[4]
Glycopyrrolate	??	0.5 mg/kg IM		[4]
Diazepam	5 mg/kg IP	2.5–5 mg/kg IP		[4]
Xylazine	5–10 mg/kg IP	1–5 mg/kg IP		[4]
Medetomidine	30–100 µg/kg SC	30–100 µg/kg SC		[4]
Dexmedetomidine	15–50 µg/kg SC	15–50 µg/kg SC		[4]
Ketamine	5–25 mg/kg IM	15–50 mg/kg IM	Immobilization	[4,8]
Ketamine plus dexmedetomidine	5–10 mg/kg, 0.01–0.03 mg/kg IM	5 mg/kg, 0.05 mg/kg IM	Light to moderate anesthesia	[4]
Ketamine plus xylazine	10 mg/kg, 0.15–0.5 mg/kg IM	10 mg/kg, 0.15–0.5 mg/kg IM	Light to moderate anesthesia	[4]
Alfaxalone	1–3 mg/kg IV (after initial ketamine sedation)	10 mg/kg IM, 2–5 mg/kg IV	Immobilization (IM), light–medium anesthesia	[4]
Medetomidine plus midazolam plus alfaxalone	0.02 mg/kg, 0.3 mg/kg, 2 mg/kg SC	??		[9]
Medetomidine plus midazolam plus fentanyl	0.02 mg/kg, 0.5 mg/kg, 10 µg/kg SC	??		[4]

IM, intramuscular; IP, intraperitoneal; IV, intravenous; SC, subcutaneous; ??, unknown.

Table 54.3 Neuromuscular junction blocking agents and dosages for selected laboratory animal species.

	Mice	Rats	Guinea pigs	Rabbits	Non-human primates	References
Alcuronium	??	??	??	0.1–0.2 mg/kg IV	??	[4]
Atracurium	??	??	??	??	0.3–0.6 mg/kg IV	[4]
Pancuronium	??	2 mg/kg IV	0.06 mg/kg IV	0.1 mg/kg, IV	0.08–0.1 mg/kg IV	[4]
Vecuronium	??	1 mg/kg IV	??	??	0.04–0.06 mg/kg IV	[4]

IV, intravenous; ??, unknown.

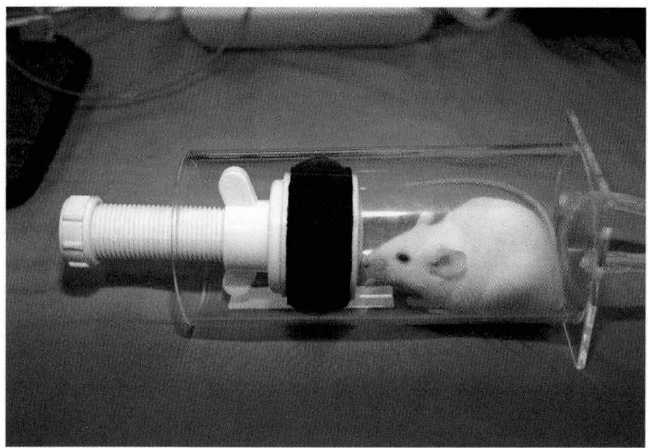

Figure 54.1 Induction chamber for use with small (< 100 g) mammals. The chamber size is appropriate to the size of animal, allowing the concentration of anesthetic agent to be increased rapidly without the use of high fresh gas flows.

easy adjustment of the anesthetic depth to a standard, predetermined level, therefore reducing the variation between subjects and subsequently minimizing the number of animals to be used in a particular study. Third, inhalants are commonly used for induction of small mammals in an anesthetic chamber (Fig. 54.1), a simple and easy method of anesthesia induction. Finally, recovery from isoflurane and sevoflurane anesthesia is usually rapid compared to injectable anesthetic combinations given by subcutaneous (SC) or intramuscular (IM) injection.

Minimum alveolar concentration (MAC) values in smaller mammals are broadly similar to those in other species, with relatively little variation across rodent inbred strains or genotypes [11]. Although modern inhalant agents are widely considered to be both effective and non-irritant [12,13], they vary in their pungency, and this may affect an animal's willingness to breathe normally [14,15]. Apneic episodes can occur in rabbits with all of the commonly used agents, and this, coupled with possible catecholamine release, could increase the anesthetic risk and also introduce some intersubject variability. When inducing anesthesia in rabbits with a face mask, briefly removing the mask if an episode of apnea occurs and replacing the mask when respiration resumes will avoid the risks associated with prolonged breath holding. Some degree of aversion to volatile agents has been demonstrated in rats and mice, with isoflurane being more aversive than sevoflurane or halothane [16], and sevoflurane less aversive than isoflurane [17]. This aversion increases with repeated exposure to volatile anesthetics [18,19].

Isoflurane appears particularly irritant to guinea pigs, triggering pronounced ocular and nasal discharge. In the authors' experience, sevoflurane appears less irritating but still causes lacrimation. Halothane is much less irritating in guinea pigs, but this needs to be balanced against the risk of other adverse effects [20,21]. The manufacture of halothane was discontinued in most Western countries such as the Unites States; however, it remains available from specialist sources for use in defined research projects. In all species, stress associated with induction of anesthesia can be minimized by use of preanesthetic medication.

Inhalants anesthetic agents are fluorocarbons and act like greenhouse gases, contributing to global warming. Isoflurane has a 100-year Global Warming Potential (GWP_{100}) of 510, and vaporization of one 250 mL bottle of isoflurane has a similar global warming effect as 190 kg of CO_2 [22]. The environmental impact of inhalants can be mitigated by using low-flow anesthesia techniques (with a precise rodent flowmeter) and combining the use of inhalants with injectable agents for their "MAC-sparing" effects.

Injectable anesthetics

Ketamine remains the agent most widely used for anesthetizing laboratory rodents. It is most frequently used in combination with sedatives or sedative–analgesics, because when administered as the sole agent to rodents, it does not produce even light anesthesia. In combination with xylazine and acepromazine, ketamine produces a safe, long-lasting (e.g., 54 ± 6 min (mean ± SEM)), and stable surgical plane of anesthesia in mice [23]. When ketamine is combined with either medetomidine or dexmedetomidine, the depth of anesthesia is less consistent than in other non-rodent species, but this is still a useful combination in many mouse strains [23,24]. The most reliable combination for producing a surgical plane of anesthesia in rats and most other rodents is ketamine in combination with an α_2-adrenergic receptor agonist [4].

Unlike in other species, ketamine used alone in non-human primates (NHPs) produces heavy sedation (10 mg/kg) to light surgical anesthesia (25 mg/kg) [4], with good relaxation of skeletal and laryngeal muscles. Repeated use of ketamine in NHPs, however, raises a few concerns. First, ketamine has been shown to be associated with long-term cognitive impairment in NHPs if administered during a sensitive period for brain development (*in utero* or during the first week of life) [25,26]. This is a significant concern given that most NHPs are used as animal models for neuroscience studies. Repeated ketamine administrations are associated with anesthetic tolerance. Anesthetic doses administered for three consecutive days are sufficient to increase the time to recumbency by approximately 35% [27], and this is comparable with human data. Ketamine has also been reported to cause local myotoxic effects in New World primates [28], such that other injectable agents such as alfaxalone may be preferred for IM injection in these species.

Alternatives to ketamine use in primates (using α_2-adrenergic receptor agonists, benzodiazepines, and/or opioids) have been described [29–31]. Although the magnitude of sedation may be unsuitable for surgical procedures, a combination of fentanyl–midazolam–medetomidine (10 μg/kg, 0.5 mg/kg, and 20 μg/kg, respectively) administered IM provides reliable sedation and can be easily reversed with atipamezole–naloxone (0.2 mg/kg and 10 μg/kg, respectively), providing rapid and good quality recovery [31]. It is of interest that NHPs are notably resistant to sedation with benzodiazepines. Doses as high as 3 mg/kg, administered orally, merely produce light sedation and anxiolysis, without inducing recumbency [30].

Most injectable anesthetic agents have similar properties in small rodents and companion animals and, therefore, are not discussed in depth here. One noteworthy difference relating to the use of injectable anesthetics in small rodents is the difficulty of obtaining intravenous access. This results in anesthetic combinations being administered as a single injection by the intraperitoneal (IP), SC, or IM route, rather than intravenously, to effect. Although this is a simple and rapid means of producing anesthesia, it has inevitable consequences in relation to the safety of certain anesthetic agents, especially those with a narrow safety margin. Since there is considerable variation between different strains of rodents in their response to injectable anesthetic agents, anesthetic combinations that have a broad safety margin or are wholly or partially reversible are preferred. If a neuroleptanalgesic combination is used (typically, fentanyl combined with either medetomidine/dexmedetomidine or acepromazine), fentanyl can be partially antagonized with small doses of buprenorphine, butorphanol, or even nalbuphine instead of complete reversal with naloxone [32]. By doing so, the respiratory depressant effects and some of the sedative effects induced by the potent μ-opioid receptor agonist are reversed, but some analgesia is preserved for the immediate recovery period. Note that the formulation Hypnorm® (fentanyl–fluanisone) is not readily commercially available anymore.

As in other species, the potent, short-acting opioids (e.g., phenylpiperidines including alfentanil, sufentanil, and remifentanil) are effective agents for multimodal anesthesia in laboratory animals and can significantly reduce required inhalant anesthetic concentrations. However, their respiratory depressant effects may necessitate respiratory support (i.e., intubation and ventilation), which can be more challenging in rodents. When suitable apparatus and expertise are available, their use combined with medetomidine can constitute a refinement to more classic injectable protocols in rats [33].

Alfaxalone, a neurosteroid, has attracted attention in laboratory animal anesthesia. Laboratory mice and rats administered alfaxalone alone IP or SC never reached a surgical plane of anesthesia and the addition of opioids and/or α_2-adrenergic receptor agonists is necessary to facilitate invasive procedures. It is important to note that doses and effects of alfaxalone vary greatly between sex and rodent strain and pilot studies are highly recommended to refine the anesthesia protocol before initiating the experiment [5,34–36]. In NHPs, similar effects of a single dose of alfaxalone have been observed, and co-administration with other anesthetics is necessary to induce deep sedation or general anesthesia [9,37,38]. Alfaxalone does not produce muscle damage, as does ketamine, and this can be very beneficial in small primates [39].

Some injectable anesthetic agents remain in research settings due to scientific reasons or ease of use but are no longer used in veterinary clinical practice. Urethane is an ethyl carbamate producing long-lasting and stable (6–10 h) surgical anesthesia with few adverse cardiovascular or respiratory effects [40,41]. Urethane is still used for non-recovery procedures involving recording of certain central nervous system (CNS) responses and for neuropharmacology studies. Spinal reflexes are depressed, but it has virtually no depressant action on the brain itself (EEG comparable to sleep patterns), and most autonomic reflexes are well preserved [42]. It is a water-soluble compound metabolized by the liver into ethanol and carbamic acid before renal excretion. Despite initial studies suggesting that urethane mainly acts on $GABA_A$ receptors, it is now established that only 23% of urethane's action is $GABA_A$ mediated. Urethane interacts at a multitude of receptors including the α_1-glycine receptor (agonist, 33%), the NMDA and AMPA receptors (antagonist, 10% and 18%, respectively), and possibly acetylcholine receptors, but with only weak effects at each target [43]. When administered IP, it has profound endocrine and metabolic effects, producing peritonitis, necrosis of the abdominal contents, and massive leakage of plasma into the peritoneal cavity [41], so must only be used for non-recovery procedures. Urethane is a carcinogen and protective equipment should be worn when it is handled [44].

α-Chloralose is an anesthetic that has numerous dose-dependent CNS effects, both excitatory and inhibitory. It provides long-lasting light anesthesia (8–10 h), with minimal cardiovascular side effects. However, induction and recovery are very prolonged and accompanied by excitement, so the agent is usually restricted to terminal procedures after induction of anesthesia with another agent (typically an inhalant). A further disadvantage of chloralose is that anesthetic depth is not usually sufficient for surgical manipulations to be performed, and it has poor analgesic properties.

Chloral hydrate is used occasionally in rodent anesthesia for neuropharmacology studies. Surgical depth of anesthesia can be achieved [40], but in some strains of rats, chloral hydrate causes postanesthetic ileus that can be fatal [45]. Using a dilute solution of chloral hydrate may help reduce the incidence of ileus.

Tribromoethanol is used primarily in mice although its popularity has declined markedly because of undesirable side effects. If incorrectly prepared or stored, administration is associated with high mortality. This can also occur when freshly prepared solutions are used [46]. The incidence of adverse effects varies greatly in different research facilities, perhaps due to the agent itself not being supplied as a commercial pharmaceutical product. For this reason, decisions as to whether to use the agent should be made on a case-by-case basis. When used successfully, tribromoethanol produces 15–20 min of surgical anesthesia, with reasonably rapid recovery.

Opioids

Despite growing emphasis on animal welfare and refinement of animal models, less than 25% of laboratory rodents undergoing surgical procedures are given analgesic drugs (35% of those that are, receive buprenorphine [3]). This might be partially explained by a number of largely unfounded concerns related to potential interactions of opioids and other analgesics and specific types of research projects. For example, despite a lack of convincing clinical data in humans, opioids are commonly associated with immunodepression in critical care patients. This has led to concerns that use of these agents in a research setting could cause immunomodulation, and this could introduce confounding factors in some research models. In laboratory animals, this phenomenon is subject to major inter-strain variability [47], and immunodepression is only evident when animals receive doses that are significantly greater than those used for postoperative pain relief (e.g., 300 mg/kg morphine) for prolonged periods of time [48–50]. Opioids have also been shown to influence tumor growth and metastasis, and this has been considered a contraindication for their use when implanting or transplanting tumors for cancer research studies. Published data are conflicting in this area, suggesting that morphine can either promote or slow down tumor growth and metastatic spread. The mechanisms involved remain poorly understood and, in addition to their potential immunomodulating effects, opioids may impact tumor cell aggressiveness and angiogenesis [51].

In each of these examples, a proper appraisal of the available literature in consultation with the researchers involved should lead to an evidence-based decision as to whether to use opioids or whether an alternative analgesic strategy should be adopted. When making these decisions, it is also important to include a consideration of the various effects of unalleviated pain. In the authors' experience, there are almost no circumstances in which an analgesic regimen of some type cannot be implemented and untreated pain can be a greater confounder of scientific results [52,53].

Among the opioids, buprenorphine remains the analgesic agent most frequently administered to laboratory animals, both to rodents [3] and to larger species [54]. Buprenorphine is 35 times more potent than morphine when administered IM in rats [55] and has a long duration of action (3–5 h in mice, 6–8 h in rats). Its poor oral bioavailability (5–10%), coupled with a significant hepatic first-pass metabolism, renders oral administration of buprenorphine of limited value in rodents as its duration of action decreases to 1–2 h (0.5 mg/kg, rats) [56], although this may still provide sufficient analgesia following some surgical procedures [57]. Although use of buprenorphine in palatable oral formulations remains popular, we recommend it is only given by this route when effective methods of pain assessment are being used.

Buprenorphine's ceiling effect has been well-described in the literature and occurs only when doses exceeding about 3 mg/kg are administered in rats [58]; therefore, it is of little concern when using this agent for postoperative pain relief. Clinically relevant adverse effects of opioids are similar to those in other animal species. Interestingly, studies in rats showed that even at large IV doses, buprenorphine failed to produce clinically significant respiratory depression [59,60]. An unusual effect of opioids in rodents is the production of pica behavior. This is thought to be analogous to vomiting in other species and has been reported following use of buprenorphine in rats [61]. The incidence of pica appears to be low, but, if noted, analgesia should be provided using a non-opioid analgesic.

Other opioids can be used in laboratory animals. Methadone, for instance, has proven antinociceptive properties in mice and rats [62] and was shown to attenuate signs of neuropathic pain for 2 h in mice (3 mg/kg SC) [63]. This effect may be due to μ-opioid receptor agonist actions on peripheral opioid receptors [62], in combination with antagonism of NMDA receptors. Although species-specific studies documenting the efficacy of this agent in alleviating postsurgical pain are lacking, methadone has been used by the authors in NHPs (0.3–0.5 mg/kg IM) when the surgical procedure renders the animal at risk of experiencing chronic or neuropathic pain. Compared to other full μ-opioid receptor agonists, methadone seems to produce less sedation and inappetence.

Managing pain in laboratory rodents can be difficult because of the large numbers of animals that may need to be treated (e.g., 20–30 animals all undergoing surgery in one day). In addition, the relatively short action of some analgesics requires repeated handling and injections, which in itself can be stressful. Possible approaches to these problems are the use of slow-release preparations and transdermal delivery (e.g., cutaneous patch) technology. Fentanyl patches or transdermal solutions can be used in larger laboratory animals, with the same concerns and indications for use as in other species. It is important to securely attach the patch to the animal to reduce the risk of ingestion. Ingestion of a patch can be fatal since fentanyl is readily absorbed by the oropharyngeal mucosa [64]. Alternatively, if the patch is rapidly ingested with minimal oropharyngeal contact, there may be few clinical signs since there appears to be a high first-pass metabolism following gastrointestinal absorption. Transdermal fentanyl diffuses well into the milk of pregnant rats. It can be an alternative route to administer analgesic to pups, but high doses (200 μg/kg/h) can result in slower growth and corneal opacity [65]. A few studies documented that the application of transdermal fentanyl solution relieved pain in a paw incisional model and complete Freund's adjuvant-induced arthritis, but the duration of efficacy was variable [66,67]. In smaller rodents, the use of transdermal fentanyl may be limited for practical reasons.

Slow-release formulations of a number of analgesics have been compounded (e.g., Buprenorphine SR®, Veterinary Technologies, LLC, Windsor, CO, United States). This formulation appears to provide sustained release for up to 72 h in rats and mice. Preliminary studies suggested up to 12 h of pain reduction can be provided in mice [68] and a longer duration in rats [69]. The latter study did not report any problems with pica, but up to 40% of the rats developed some skin irritation following SC injection. A modified formulation appears to have resolved problems of irritancy following injection. Pharmacokinetic studies performed in NHPs suggest that Buprenorphine SR® plasma concentrations remain above a possible analgesic threshold for approximately 5 days, but no pharmacodynamics tests were performed [70]. As with rats, injection site reactions have been reported in NHPs, but they can be limited by the administration of a highly concentrated solution (10 mg/mL) [71].

Anti-inflammatory drugs

Non-steroidal anti-inflammatory drugs (NSAIDs) are the second most commonly administered agents for pain relief in rodents and other laboratory animal species [3,54]. All of the NSAIDs licensed for use in animals or people can be administered in laboratory rodent and NHP species. Of the agents available, the oral preparation of meloxicam is of particular value as it is highly palatable to many small rodents and to NHPs, particularly if added to their favorite foodstuff. The efficacy of NSAIDs in relieving postoperative pain in rodents has been widely reported [57,72,73], but their duration of action remains uncertain. Carprofen and meloxicam appear to have a duration of at least 8 and possibly 24 h. The general considerations related to their use in other veterinary species apply equally to laboratory animal species; however, since most laboratory animals undergoing surgery are young, healthy adults, concerns related to pre-existing diseases are usually reduced.

Specific concerns related to the use of NSAIDs in animal models are sparse and poorly understood. Given the link between inflammation and carcinogenesis, recent studies have attempted to characterize the relationship between NSAIDs and cancer models. The results suggest that, in addition to the mechanism of action (degree of COX-1 versus COX-2 inhibition), the type of cancer and the dose and frequency of NSAID administration (U-shaped response curve) correlate to efficacy [74–76].

A meta-analysis of clinical studies suggested that steroids might be useful adjuncts to a multimodal analgesic approach to managing surgical pain. A single preoperative dose of dexamethasone, administered to people, contributed to a reduction in postoperative pain as well as opioid consumption, without any steroid-associated adverse effects [77]. The analgesic mechanism of dexamethasone remains obscure and may be related to its general anti-inflammatory properties as well as interactions with opioid receptors [78]. Since steroids may be administered routinely to laboratory animals following neurosurgery procedures, it may be necessary to factor their potential analgesic effects into a postoperative care protocol. When not indicated for other purposes, steroids may not be a first-line choice of analgesia provision because of their negative effect on wound healing and immunomodulation [79].

Local and regional analgesia and anesthesia

Local anesthetic techniques are underutilized in laboratory species, and regional analgesia (spinal or epidural techniques) have been used primarily as research techniques [80]. The same general principles and approaches used in larger species can be applied in laboratory rodents, but their small size makes overdose more likely. Local anesthesia is most often used in conjunction with general anesthesia, since small rodents are likely to be stressed by the physical restraint needed if local anesthesia is used alone. Use of local anesthetics enables the dosage of general anesthetic agents to be reduced, usually minimizing adverse effects and potential interactions with research variables. Infiltration of the surgical site can be a means of prolonging the duration of surgical anesthesia, rather than administering additional doses of injectable anesthetic agents. Aside from local infiltration, topical local anesthesia (e.g., using local anesthetic creams) can be used to prevent pain or discomfort associated with venipuncture [81] or to provide anesthesia for minor procedures (e.g., ethyl chloride for tail biopsy in mice) [82]. Maximum safe doses of local anesthetics have not been well documented but, as a guide, total dose should not exceed 10 mg/kg of lidocaine or 2 mg/kg of bupivacaine.

Gabapentin and pregabalin

Despite their abundant use in animal models of chronic pain, very few studies have looked at the benefit of gabapentin and pregabalin in laboratory animals as part of postsurgical pain management. A study anecdotally reports prolonged analgesia in a mouse model of fibromyalgia 4 days after gabapentin administration [83]. More recently, the MAC-sparing effect of gabapentin was demonstrated in rats with both sevoflurane and isoflurane [84,85]. There appear to be no reports of the use of these drugs for clinical pain relief in NHPs.

Laboratory rodents and lagomorphs

Anatomic and physiologic considerations

In order to anesthetize these species safely and effectively, and to manage their perioperative care, it is important to become familiar with their normal behavior, anatomy, and physiology. Rats, mice, and hamsters are active primarily during the dark phase of their photoperiod, while rabbits are most active at dawn and dusk (i.e., crepuscular). This should be remembered when assessing normal behavior during what would usually be an inactive phase of their diurnal rhythm. Almost all feeding and drinking by rats and mice occurs during the dark phase and postsurgical pain or stress following procedures undertaken during the light phase can suppress these activities. Consequently, voluntary oral intake may not resume for 24 h or more. This can have significant detrimental effects in these small animals, since relatively short periods of fasting can result in hypoglycemia and moderate dehydration. For similar reasons, preanesthetic fasting should be avoided, and since these species do not vomit, fasting does not reduce the incidence of aspiration.

Withholding food from rabbits and guinea pigs should also be avoided, since it can result in gastrointestinal disturbances, which can have serious consequences (e.g., alterations to gut flora, ileus, and enterotoxemia). Since these species do not vomit, there is no advantage to withholding food. All of these species exhibit a degree of neophobia, so their normal diet should always be offered postsurgically along with palatable high-energy and high-water content supplements. All of these species are coprophagic, a normal activity that is important for adequate nutrition. Inadvertent prevention of this activity by use of Elizabethan collars, to prevent interference with wounds, for example, should be avoided.

The small size of rodents makes clinical examination difficult, and since these species often regard people as a threat, they often show elevated heart and respiratory rates. These rates may exceed 200–250 breaths or heart beats per minute, so they are too fast to accurately record on clinical examination (Table 54.4). The small size also restricts venous access, except in the rabbit where access via the marginal auricular, saphenous, or cephalic veins is relatively easy. The most important consequence of the small size of these animals is their high surface-area-to-body-weight ratio, which greatly increases heat loss during anesthesia. Even short periods of anesthesia are associated with significant cooling unless efforts are made to minimize hypothermia.

The metabolic rate of most species varies with body mass raised to the three-quarters power. Small mammals have a high metabolic rate resulting in a relatively high dose requirement of many of the agents commonly used in anesthesia and pain management. For example, the commonly recommended dose of buprenorphine in a dog is 0.01–0.03 mg/kg, whereas in a mouse, the dose rate is 0.05–0.1 mg/kg [55]. Calculations of a dose for mice, based on the dose in dogs, using allometric scaling provides a similar dose (0.05 mg/kg). If a validated dose rate is not available, a calculation using allometric scaling is more likely to provide an appropriate dose than simple extrapolation based on the animal's weight.

Handling, restraint, and drug administration

General principles of good handling should be applied to rodents and lagomorphs. It is currently well recognized in rodents that tunnel handling for husbandry and observation purposes decreases overall animal anxiety [86]. This handling method uses tunnels, usually made of plastic or cardboard, that form part of the animals' cage enrichment and can be used to gently pick up mice. However, as the administration of anesthetics may require transient restraint of the animals, it is important that the anesthetist or an assistant is familiar with restraint methods to prevent unnecessary suffering and distress. Illustrations of methods of restraint are widely available (e.g., www.researchanimaltraining.com). Drug administration is safer and easier if an assistant restrains the animal, while a second person administers the drug. IM injections are best avoided if a large volume of agent is required since it can cause muscle damage [87]. IP administration of injectable anesthetics is widely practiced in research facilities. It is simple and convenient but is associated with a relatively high failure rate because of inadvertent drug delivery into the fat, SC, or gut tissue [88]. When possible, it is preferable to use the SC route, which is simple to undertake in all of these species. Common sites for SC injection are either in the scruff or the flank. As in other species, the volume administered should be the lowest possible, and suggested doses are listed in Table 54.1.

Airway management

In most research facilities, oxygen and volatile anesthetics are delivered to small rodents and rabbits using a face mask. This makes support of ventilation difficult to achieve, and where there is a need for this, endotracheal intubation should be considered. With practice, intubation is straightforward in rabbits [4], but more difficult

Table 54.4 Normal physiologic parameter values for common laboratory animal species.

	Mice	Rats	Guinea pigs	Rabbits	Non-human primates (rhesus)	References
Heart rate (beats/min)	570	350	155	220	150	[4]
Respiratory rate (breaths/min)	180	80	120	55	35	[4]
Body temperature	37 °C	38 °C	38 °C	38 °C	39 °C	[4]
Adult body weight	30–40 g	250–450 g	500–1500 g	0.5–8 kg	6–12 kg	[4]
Food consumption (complete pelleted diet)	10–20 g/100 g	10 g/100 g	6 g/100 g	5 g/100 g	–	[4]
Water consumption	10–20 mL/100 g	10–12 mL/100 g	100 mL/kg	120 mL/kg	50–100 mL/kg	[4]

in guinea pigs and small rodents. It is made easier if a purpose-designed apparatus is used (Figs. 54.2 and 54.3), which allows direct visualization of the larynx during intubation. Since rats are obligate nasal breathers, the use of a nose cone tightly applied on the nose can be an alternative to intubation when mechanical ventilation is required [89] and intubation unsuccessful.

Breathing systems

Once intubated, the animal should be connected to a breathing system. Unmodified Bain circuits and T-pieces can be used when animals are breathing spontaneously, but care must be taken to minimize equipment deadspace. It is reasonable to assume that tidal volume is approximately 5–10 mL/kg (e.g., a mouse will have a tidal volume of only 0.2–0.3 mL). Significant rebreathing of expired gases can only be avoided by using low-deadspace connectors for the breathing system.

Fresh gas flow rates needed to minimize rebreathing can be calculated for these breathing systems using standard formulas; however, in many research facilities, flow rates when using face masks are often greatly in excess of requirements (e.g., 1–2 L/min for a mouse, rather than 30–50 mL/min). This may be because the vaporizer is not accurate at very low flows, but additional reasons include the use of active scavenging systems (Fig. 54.4) that over-extract from the mask, drawing in room air. Delivered anesthetic gas (concentration) dilution results in animals becoming inadequately anesthetized at lower fresh gas flows. These problems can be avoided by using specifically designed low-flow, passive scavenged masks (Fig. 54.5) or purpose-designed equipment such as that shown in Fig. 54.6.

The low tidal volumes of rodents often require use of purpose-designed ventilators although "T-piece occluder" designs can

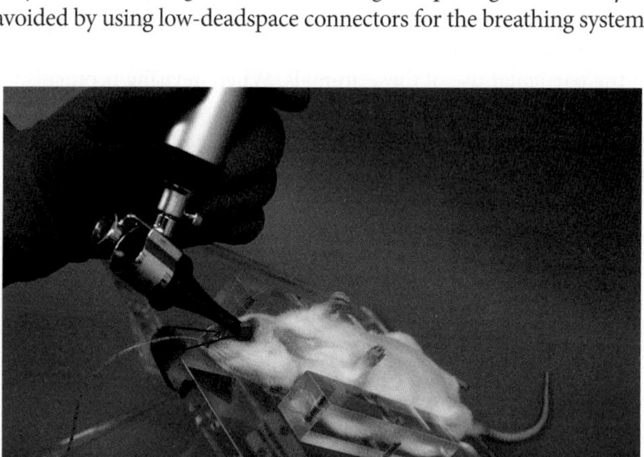

Figure 54.2 Visualization of the larynx in a rat using a modified otoscope speculum (Hallowell EMC) to enable intubation. A nasal catheter is used to deliver oxygen or volatile anesthetic during the procedure.

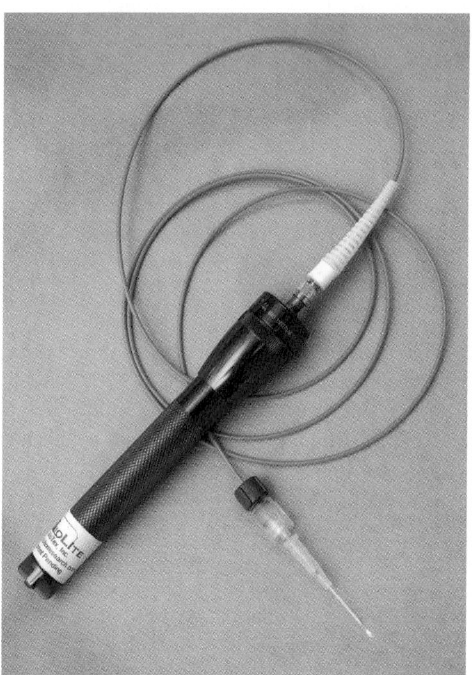

Figure 54.3 Fiberoptic guide for intubation of rats and mice (Kent Scientific). An intravenous catheter is used as the endotracheal tube.

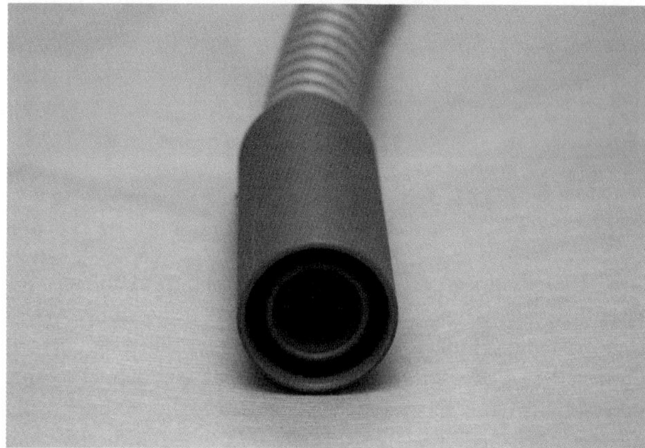

Figure 54.4 Rodent face mask with active scavenge system. The outer mask is attached to an extraction system.

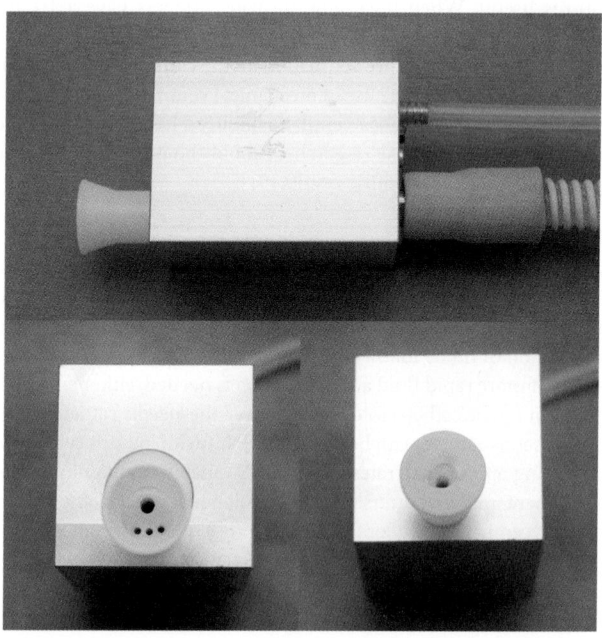

Figure 54.5 Low-deadspace passively scavenged rodent mask (Advanced Anesthesia Specialists). Side view showing metal block that stabilizes the mask and provides warming of the anesthetic gases (top). View of mask to show gas delivery and scavenging ports (lower left). Mask with rubber membrane in place, to provide a seal around the mouse's nose (lower right).

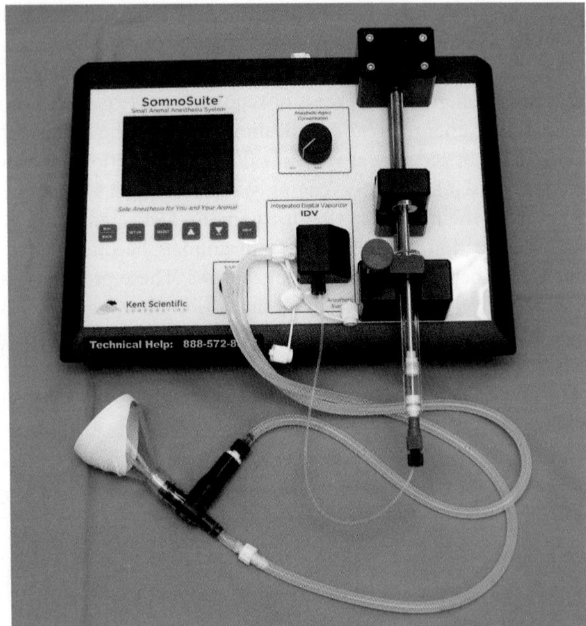

Figure 54.6 Rodent electronic vaporizer, mask, and ventilator system (Kent Scientific).

function well. In larger species such as rabbits, ventilators and breathing systems used in cats can be used successfully. A wide range of rodent ventilators are available from specialist suppliers. As in other species, key factors to consider are the range of tidal volumes and respiratory frequencies that can be delivered, whether positive end-expiratory pressure (PEEP) is required, whether the ventilator requires a compressed gas source to operate, whether it is mechanically driven, and what safety features and alarms are provided. As in other species, the ability to alter the inspiratory:expiratory (I:E) ratio is useful. When breathing normally, rodents have a 1:1 I:E ratio [90]; however, extending this to 1:2 or 1:3 to minimize the effects of positive-pressure ventilation on the cardiovascular system can be an advantage. The use of mechanical ventilation by inexperienced operators may cause ventilator-induced lung injury, and the anesthetist should advise researchers about the potential influence of this outcome on scientific results [91].

Fluid therapy

General principles of fluid therapy apply to rodents and lagomorphs. However, small patient size limits the use of intravenous fluid administration. If animals are not clinically dehydrated, then absorption of fluids following IP or SC administration occurs over 4–6 h. If more rapid fluid administration is needed, either a peripheral vein can be catheterized using an over-the-needle catheter or an intraosseous catheter can be placed [92]. Infusion pumps capable of delivering appropriate rates are readily available from a number of equipment manufacturers. During prolonged general anesthesia, hypoglycemia is a frequent complication [93], and the administration of dextrose 5% solution as fluid therapy is advisable [94].

Maintenance of body temperature

Hypothermia is a frequent complication of anesthesia, especially in small mammals due to their high surface-area-to-mass ratio. Preventing hypothermia early and aggressively is required; otherwise, mice can lose several degrees of core temperature within the first 15 min after induction of anesthesia [95]. Electrical heating pads suitable for use in small rodents are available, as well as circulating warm water blankets and thermogenic pads. Devices that adjust the temperature of the blanket depending upon the body temperature of the animal are preferred, but it is important to check that the temperature sensor probe tip is sufficiently small for use in rodents. It is also advisable to monitor the temperature of the blanket directly, using an additional thermometer. Forced air warming systems can be used in rabbits but are usually impractical for use in mice and rats. Following anesthesia, animals should be placed in a suitable incubator to maintain body temperature during recovery.

Postoperative care

Postsurgical pain management, together with other supportive care, is essential if recovery from surgery and anesthesia is to be rapid and uneventful. When dealing with laboratory animals, anesthetists must be aware of the additional considerations that arise as a result of the particular use of these animals. When devising protocols for postoperative pain relief, the potential interactions of the agents chosen on research protocols can be minimized by use of appropriate dose rates for an appropriate period of time. This requires accurate assessment of the degree of pain that is present and its duration in order to determine the efficacy of analgesic therapy.

A number of pain assessment tools have been developed, including those which track simple and objective clinical measures such as body weight and food and water consumption [96], complex behavioral measures such as nest building [97], or specific pain-related behaviors [72,73]. Rodents express a series of pain behaviors specific to the surgery they have undergone. Those behaviors constitute an ethogram validated for pain assessment in rats and mice and used to assess the efficacy of analgesic therapy [98]. The changes in facial expression can be scored (Grimace scales) to assess laboratory animal pain, and this has been a rapidly growing field of study [99–101]. Grimace scales have been used successfully to assess pain and the efficacy of analgesics in pain studies across species [102,103]; however, their use for clinical cage-side assessments in rodents has limitations. It is recognized that observers tend to underestimate pain, and adjustments must also be made to account for the significant variations in baseline (pain-free) scores across different strains and between sexes [104]. In light of these factors, it is preferable to use facial expression instruments alongside other measures such as clinical or behavioral scoring [105].

Once the need for analgesic therapy has been established, all of the options used in veterinary clinical practice can be applied in rodents and lagomorphs. Many of the analgesic agents used in humans, dogs, and cats were originally assessed for efficacy and safety in laboratory rodents, so a great deal of basic information is available to guide clinical decision-making. In addition, there are a growing number of clinical trials that provide more reliable clinical data (Table 54.5). In addition to the use of NSAIDs and opioids by injection, oral preparations have been recommended, but when dosing via food or drinking water, care must be taken to ensure animals consume sufficient amounts at appropriate time intervals. As discussed above, since animals often do not eat during the light phase of their photoperiod, this may interfere with effective medication. Recording body weight preoperatively, and monitoring it in the postoperative period, is a simple means of assessing the adequacy of fluid and food intake and, thus, drug administration. Analgesia can also be provided by infiltration of the surgical site with local anesthetic, and by epidural and intrathecal administration of analgesics, although practical constraints may limit this approach in small rodents [106,107].

Table 54.5 Analgesic drugs and dosages for common laboratory animal species.

	Mice	Rats	Guinea pigs	Rabbits	Non-human primates	References
Buprenorphine	0.05–0.1 mg/kg IP, SC q6–8 h	0.01–0.05 mg/kg IP, SC q6–8 h	0.05 mg/kg IP, SC q6–8 h	0.01–0.05 mg/kg SC, IM q6–8 h	0.005–0.05 mg/kg SC, IM q6–12 h	[4,108]
Butorphanol	1–2 mg/kg IP, SC q2 h	1–2 mg/kg IP, SC q2 h	1–2 mg/kg IP, SC q3 h	0.1–0.5 mg/kg SC q3 h	0.1 mg/kg SC, IM q3 h	[4]
Carprofen	5 mg/kg SC, PO q12 h	5 mg/kg SC, PO q12 h	4 mg/kg SC q24 h	4 mg/kg SC q24 h	3–4 mg/kg SC q24 h	[4]
Meloxicam	5 mg/kg SC q24 h	1 mg/kg IP, SC, PO q24 h	0.5–1.0 mg/kg SC q24 h	0.6 mg/kg SC, IM q24 h	0.1–0.2 mg/kg IP, SC, PO q24 h	[4]
Morphine	2.5 mg/kg IP, SC q2–4 h	2.5 mg/kg IP, SC q2–4 h	2.5 mg/kg IP, SC q2–4 h	2–5 mg/kg SC, IM q2–4 h	1–2 mg/kg SC, IM q2–4 h	[4]
Tramadol	5 mg/kg IP, SC q6–12 h	5 mg/kg IP, SC q6–12 h	??	??	1–2 mg/kg SC, IM q2–4 h; 2 mg/kg PO q12 h	[4]

IM, intramuscular; IP, intraperitoneal; SC, subcutaneous; PO, oral; ??, unknown.

Non-human primates

A variety of non-human primates (NHPs) are used worldwide for biomedical research. The species used range from New World primates (capuchins, marmosets, squirrel monkeys) to Old World primates (macaques, baboons). NHPs are used in a wide range of biomedical studies, primarily for neuroscience, immunology, and infectious diseases research [109]. Given the highly sensitive nature of NHPs for biomedical research, any proposed project should take particular care to apply the 3Rs principle to minimize potential pain and distress caused by the experiments.

Anesthetic considerations

Handling any conscious NHP should be avoided not only because of the stress caused to the animal, but also because of the risk of physical injuries to the operator (mainly bites and scratches). In addition to the risk of traumatic injury, NHPs can carry several hazardous and, in some cases, potentially fatal zoonotic diseases (i.e., herpes B virus) [110]. Appropriate personal protective equipment, usually comprising gloves, eye protection, and a laboratory coat or gown, should be worn when working with NHPs.

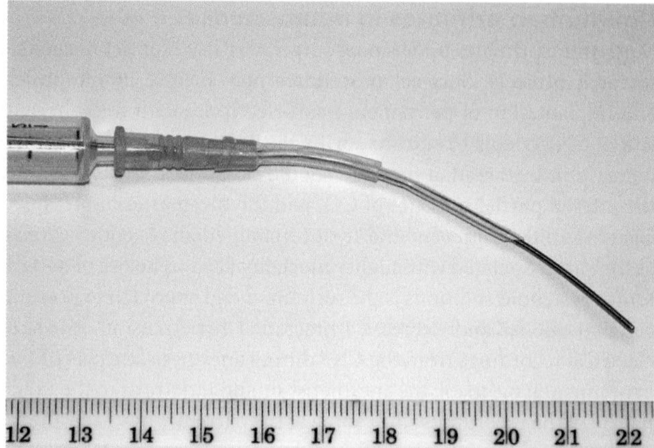

Figure 54.7 Modified catheter for intubation of marmosets or other small primates. The silastic tubing provides a seal at the larynx, and also reduces the risk of kinking of the catheter at the hub. A Seldinger catheter guidewire, anchored in a syringe, is used to aid intubation (Hallowell EMC).

Preanesthetic considerations

Primates are social animals and should be group housed whenever possible in a cage containing retreat areas. Assessing the health condition of a freely moving primate in its home cage is challenging, reducing any preanesthetic examination to a simple visual check. Consequently, the preanesthetic physical examination is commonly performed under sedation (usually ketamine based) [108]. Intravenous access is achieved via superficial veins (e.g., cephalic or saphenous veins) using a 20–22 gauge catheter. The caudal (tail) vein is a more suitable option for New World monkeys using a 22–24 gauge catheter.

Endotracheal intubation

Primates should be fasted 6–12 h prior to anesthesia because of their ability to regurgitate or vomit. Following induction, intubation is recommended to prevent aspiration. In NHPs, the descent of the larynx causes a large part of the tongue to be in the hypopharynx, potentially restricting visualization of the entrance to the larynx. The larynx is richly vascularized and seems to be particularly prone to tissue trauma compared to non-primate species, so care should be taken while introducing the endotracheal tube. The diameter of the larynx and trachea is smaller in primates than in other species of equivalent weight. For instance, a 3–3.5 mm outer diameter (OD) endotracheal tube is appropriate for a 6 kg macaque, and a 5.5 mm OD tube would be suitable for an adult male macaque (15 kg). In New World monkeys, the animal is best placed in dorsal recumbency on a tilting table to maximize the alignment of the oral cavity with the larynx. Marmosets or capuchins are best intubated with a modified over-the-needle catheter mounted on a stylet (Fig. 54.7) [111]. Marmosets, like pigs, have a pronounced laryngotracheal angle, and the tube should be gently rotated 180° once it has passed between the vocal folds [111]. Lastly, special attention should be paid to the length of the tube, as NHPs have shorter tracheas than other species. The distal end of the tube should not be advanced past the points of the scapula on a macaque to avoid endobronchial intubation or trauma to the carina [112]. In marmosets, the length of the trachea can be predicted by multiplying the craniosacral length of the marmoset by a factor of 0.42 [111].

Equipment and monitoring

New World monkeys often appear heavier than they actually are (by a few hundred grams). In these smaller species, a rodent ventilator, breathing system, and monitoring devices are appropriate. Larger primate species can easily be anesthetized and monitored with similar apparatus to that used in cats and small dogs. Physiological support during anesthesia is similar to other domestic species. A mixture of medical air and oxygen for prolonged anesthesia will prevent complications arising from oxygen toxicity.

Recovery

Recovery from anesthesia should be as rapid and smooth as possible. Gentle extubation is usually performed as soon as protective reflexes begin to return and hemoglobin saturation remains within normal limits without supplemental oxygen. Primates are usually recovered in purpose-built cages at high ambient temperature to prevent hypothermia. The recovery cage design should minimize the risk of the anesthetist or nursing staff being bitten while monitoring the animal's recovery. Important benchmarks of anesthetic recovery in NHP's include the ability to maintain a sitting position and recovery of motor coordination. Food and water should be gradually reintroduced over the first several hours following extubation. Keeping the NHP separate from its social group for 6–12 h is preferable to ensure that all anesthetic effects have dissipated to prevent social conflict. However, the decision to prolong separation should be carefully assessed in light of potential negative impacts on the group structure, animal welfare, and scientific results [113,114].

Non-human primates in neuroscience

Most of the primates undergoing surgery are used for neuroscience research projects. Surgical procedures may involve craniotomies and implantation of permanent neuroelectrodes with the inherent risk of CNS edema or seizure during the postoperative period. Any increase in intracranial pressure should be avoided by controlling the arterial partial pressure of CO_2 and the mean arterial pressure. Using steroids to prevent and treat cerebral edema is controversial as they are associated with higher mortality [115]. The use of hypertonic crystalloid solutions is the recommended approach to prevent cerebral edema and decrease intracranial hypertension [116]. If electrical recordings from the CNS during anesthesia are part of the experimental protocol, the anesthetist should inquire as to the exact nature of the recordings since some of the currently used anesthetic agents (i.e., propofol and isoflurane) are known to modulate specific types of CNS activity [117,118]. Finally, the anesthetist may be asked to maintain a primate in a stable plane of anesthesia for prolonged non-recovery procedures (> 24 h). During these prolonged periods of anesthesia, special care should be taken to avoid negative energy balance and electrolyte disturbances, and support urinary voiding by catheterization, as for non-experimental species.

Pain assessment and management

Humane and ethical concerns, as well as animal welfare regulations, stipulate the use of appropriate analgesics for procedures that may cause pain or distress to laboratory animals. However, no scale definitively assesses pain in NHPs in a clinical setting. Both clinical impression and numerical pain scores (usually visual analogue or numerical rating scales) are used despite the paucity of validation studies. As in any other species, behavioral indicators of pain are expected (e.g., decreased food intake and activity) and are attenuated by the administration of analgesics [119,120]. Primates tend to hide behavioral signs of mild or moderate pain from unfamiliar observers, so animals are best assessed by a familiar handler or remotely via cameras. The development of the Facial Action Coding System for the macaque [121] and common marmoset [122] has introduced the possibility of using facial expressions to assess pain in these species [108,123,124]. It is important to note that the available scales were validated by retrospectively analyzing images or recorded videos, and their value for cage-side pain assessment requires further study.

All of the commonly available analgesics can be used in primates, but long-lasting drugs/formulations are preferred to avoid the stress induced by repeated physical restraint and drug injection (see Table 54.5). Because of the lack of validated methods for assessing pain, a wide range of doses and frequencies have been reported in the literature [108]. The use of a fentanyl transdermal formulation has proven to adequately diffuse and distribute systemically [125,126]. In the authors' experience, fentanyl patches can be applied to NHPs to provide relief from moderate to severe pain. Applied fentanyl patches should be protected (e.g., protective jacket), and the primate group should be closely monitored to avoid the risk of fentanyl overdose following oral ingestion of the patch [64]. As in other species, multimodal analgesic approaches combining opioids and NSAIDs appear to be particularly useful in controlling postsurgical pain [108].

References

1 Great Britain Home Office. Statistics of Scientific Procedures on Living Animals, 2021. http://www.gov.uk/government/statistics/statistics-of-scientific-procedures-on-living-animals-great-britain-2021

2 Russel W, Burch L. *The Principles of Humane Experimental Technique*. London, UK: Universities Federation for Animal Welfare, 1992.

3 Stokes EL, Flecknell PA, Richardson CA. Reported analgesic and anaesthetic administration to rodents undergoing experimental surgical procedures. *Lab Anim* 2009; **43**(2): 149–154.

4 Flecknell P. *Laboratory Animal Anaesthesia and Analgesia*, 5th edn. London, UK: Academic Press, 2023.

5 West SE, Lee JC, Johns TN, *et al.* Intraperitoneal alfaxalone and alfaxalone-dexmedetomidine anesthesia in Sprague-Dawley rats (*Rattus norvegicus*). *J Am Assoc Lab Anim Sci* 2020; **59**(5): 531–538.

6 Siriarchavatana P, Ayers JD, Kendall LV. Anesthetic activity of alfaxalone compared with ketamine in mice. *J Am Assoc Lab Anim Sci* 2016; **55**(4): 426–430.

7 Bradley MP, Doerning CM, Nowland MH, *et al.* Intramuscular administration of alfaxalone alone and in combination for sedation and anesthesia of rabbits (*Oryctolagus cuniculus*). *J Am Assoc Lab Anim Sci* 2019; **58**(2): 216–222.

8 Goodroe A, Fitz C, Bakker J. Current topics in marmoset anesthesia and analgesia. *ILAR J* 2020; **61**(2): 218–229.

9 Bertrand HGMJ, Sandersen C, Murray J, *et al.* A combination of alfaxalone, medetomidine and midazolam for the chemical immobilization of rhesus macaque (*Macaca mulatta*): Preliminary results. *J Med Primatol* 2017; **46**(6): 332–336.

10 Eger EI. Isoflurane: a review. *Anesthesiology* 1981; **55**(5): 559–576.

11 Sonner JM, Gong D, Eger EI. Naturally occurring variability in anesthetic potency among inbred mouse strains. *Anesth Analg* 2000; **91**(3): 720–726.

12 Atkinson RS, Rushman GB. *Lee's Synopsis of Anesthesia*. Oxford, UK: Butterworth Heinemann, 1993.

13 Jones RM. Desflurane and sevoflurane: inhalation anaesthetics for this decade? *Br J Anaesth* 1990; **65**(4): 527–536.

14 Flecknell PA, Liles JH. Halothane anaesthesia in the rabbit: a comparison of the effects of medetomidine, acepromazine and midazolam on breath-holding during induction. *J Vet Anaesth* 1996; **23**(1): 11–14.

15 Hedenqvist P, Roughan JV, Antunes L, *et al.* Induction of anaesthesia with desflurane and isoflurane in the rabbit. *Lab Anim* 2001; **35**(2): 172–179.

16 Leach MC, Bowell VA, Allan TF, *et al.* Measurement of aversion to determine humane methods of anaesthesia and euthanasia. *Anim Welf* 2004; **13**(S1): S77–S86.

17 Guedes SR, Valentim AM, Antunes LM. Mice aversion to sevoflurane, isoflurane and carbon dioxide using an approach-avoidance task. *Appl Anim Behav Sci* 2017; **189**: 91–97.

18 Frost K, Shah M, Leung VSY, *et al.* Aversion to desflurane and isoflurane in Sprague-Dawley rats (*Rattus norvegicus*). *Animals (Basel)* 2020; **10**(6): 950.

19 Kulkarni S, Hickman D. Isoflurane and carbon dioxide elicit similar behavioral responses in rats. *Animals (Basel)* 2020; **10**(8): 1–18.

20 Furst SM, Luedke D, Gaw HH, *et al.* Demonstration of a Cellular immune response in halothane-exposed guinea pigs. *Toxicol Appl Pharmacol* 1997; **143**(2): 245–255.

21 Shenton JM, Chen J, Uetrecht JP. Animal models of idiosyncratic drug reactions. *Chem Biol Interact* 2004; **150**(1): 53–70.

22 Campbell M, Pierce JMT. Atmospheric science, anaesthesia, and the environment. *BJA Educ* 2015; **15**(4): 173–179.

23 Arras M, Autenried P, Rettich A, *et al.* Optimization of intraperitoneal injection anesthesia in mice: drugs, dosages, adverse effects, and anesthesia depth. *Comp Med* 2001; **51**(5): 443–456.

24 Burnside WM, Flecknell PA, Cameron AI, *et al.* A comparison of medetomidine and its active enantiomer dexmedetomidine when administered with ketamine in mice. *BMC Vet Res* 2013; **9**(1): 48.

25 Paule MG, Li M, Allen RR, *et al.* Ketamine anesthesia during the first week of life can cause long-lasting cognitive deficits in rhesus monkeys. *Neurotoxicol Teratol* 2011; **33**(2): 220–230.

26 Slikker W Jr, Zou X, Hotchkiss CE, *et al.* Ketamine-induced neuronal cell death in the perinatal rhesus monkey. *Toxicol Sci* 2007; **98**(1): 145–158.

27 Settle TL, Rico PJ, Lugo-Roman LA. The effect of daily repeated sedation using ketamine or ketamine combined with medetomidine on physiology and anesthetic characteristics in rhesus macaques. *J Med Primatol* 2010; **39**(1): 50–57.

28 Davy CW, Trennery PN, Edmunds JG, *et al.* Local myotoxicity of ketamine hydrochloride in the marmoset. *Lab Anim* 1987; **21**(1):60–67.

29 Miyabe T, Nishimura R, Mochizuki M, *et al.* Chemical restraint by medetomidine and medetomidine-midazolam and its reversal by atipamezole in Japanese macaques (*Macaca fuscata*). *Vet Anaesth Analg* 2001; **28**(3): 168–174.

30 Pulley ACS, Roberts JA, Lerche NW. Four preanesthetic oral sedation protocol for rhesus macaques (*Macaca mulatta*). *J Zoo Wildl Med* 2004; **35**(4): 497–502.

31 Bertrand HGMJ, Ellen YC, O'Keefe S, *et al.* Comparison of the effects of ketamine and fentanyl-midazolam-medetomidine for sedation of rhesus macaques (*Macaca mulatta*). *BMC Vet Res* 2016; **12**(1): 93.

32 Hu C, Flecknell PA, Liles JH. Fentanyl and medetomidine anaesthesia in the rat and its reversal using atipamazole and either nalbuphine or butorphanol. *Lab Anim* 1992; **26**(1): 15–22.

33 Ter Horst EN, Krijnen PAJ, Flecknell P, *et al.* Sufentanil-medetomidine anaesthesia compared with fentanyl/fluanisone-midazolam is associated with fewer ventricular arrhythmias and death during experimental myocardial infarction in rats and limits infarct size following reperfusion. *Lab Anim* 2018; **52**(3): 271–279.

34 Arenillas M, Gomez de Segura IA. Anaesthetic effects of alfaxalone administered intraperitoneally alone or combined with dexmedetomidine and fentanyl in the rat. *Lab Anim* 2018; **52**(6): 588–598.

35 Erickson RL, Blevins CE, De Souza Dyer C, *et al.* Alfaxalone-xylazine anesthesia in laboratory mice (*Mus musculus*). *J Am Assoc Lab Anim Sci* 2019; **58**(1): 30–39.

36 Ferrini E, Mecozzi L, Corsi L, *et al.* Alfaxalone and dexmedetomidine as an alternative to gas anesthesia for micro-CT lung imaging in a bleomycin-induced pulmonary fibrosis murine model. *Front Vet Sci* 2020; **7**: 588592.

37 Wada S, Koyama H, Yamashita K. Sedative and physiological effects of alfaxalone intramuscular administration in cynomolgus monkeys (*Macaca fascicularis*). *J Vet Med Sci* 2020; **82**(7): 1021–1029.

38 Marion BM, Ghering JM, Dixon BC, *et al.* Comparison of alfaxalone-midazolam, tiletamine-zolazepam, and ketamine-acepromazine anesthesia during plethysmography in cynomolgus macaques (*Macaca fascicularis*) and rhesus macaques (*Macaca mulatta*). *Comp Med* 2022; **72**(4): 248–256.

39 Bakker J, Uilenreef JJ, Pelt ERJ, *et al.* Comparison of three different sedative-anaesthetic protocols (ketamine, ketamine-medetomidine and alphaxalone) in common marmosets (*Callithrix jacchus*). *BMC Vet Res* 2013; **9**: 113.

40 Field KJ, White WJ, Lang M, *et al.* Anaesthetic effects of chloral hydrate, pentobarbitone and urethane in adult male rats. *Lab Anim* 1993; **27**(3): 258–269.

41 Maggi CA, Meli A. Suitability of urethane anesthesia for physiopharmacological investigations in various systems. Part 1: general considerations. *Experientia* 1986; **42**(2): 109–114.

42 Pagliardini S, Gosgnach S, Dickson CT. Spontaneous sleep-like brain state alternations and breathing characteristics in urethane anesthetized mice. *PLoS ONE* 2013; **8**(7): e70411.

43 Hara K, Harris RA. The anesthetic mechanism of urethane: the effects on neurotransmitter-gated ion channels. *Anesth Analg* 2002; **94**(2): 313–318.

44 Field KJ, Lang CM. Hazards of urethane (ethyl carbamate): a review of the literature. *Lab Anim* 1988; **22**(3): 255–262.

45 Fleischman RW, McCracken D, Forbes W. Adynamic ileus in the rat induced by chloral hydrate. *Lab Anim Sci* 1977; **27**(2): 238–243.

46 Lieggi CC, Artwohl JE, Leszczynski JK, *et al.* Efficacy and safety of stored and newly prepared tribromoethanol in ICR mice. *Contemp Top Lab Anim Sci* 2005; **44**(1): 17–22.

47 Eisenstein TK, Meissler JJ, Rogers TJ, *et al.* Mouse strain differences in immunosuppression by opioids in vitro. *J Pharmacol Exp Ther* 1995; **275**(3): 1484–1489.

48 Chao CC, Hu S, Molitor TW, *et al.* Morphine potentiates transforming growth factor-beta release from human peripheral blood mononuclear cell cultures. *J Pharmacol Exp Ther* 1992; **262**(1): 19–24.

49 MacFarlane AS, Peng X, Meissler JJ, *et al.* Morphine increases susceptibility to oral Salmonella typhimurium infection. *J Infect Dis* 2000; **181**(4): 1350–1358.

50 Wang J, Barke RA, Charboneau R, *et al.* Morphine induces defects in early response of alveolar macrophages to Streptococcus pneumoniae by modulating TLR9-NF-kappa B signaling. *J Immunol* 2008; **180**(5): 3594–3600.

51 Afsharimani B, Cabot P, Parat MO. Morphine and tumor growth and metastasis. *Cancer Metastasis Rev* 2011; **30**(2): 225–238.

52 Jirkof P. Side effects of pain and analgesia in animal experimentation. *Lab Anim (NY)* 2017; **46**(4): 123–128.

53 Lofgren J, Miller AL, Lee CCS, *et al.* Analgesics promote welfare and sustain tumour growth in orthotopic 4T1 and B16 mouse cancer models. *Lab Anim* 2018; **52**(4): 351–364.

54 Coulter CA, Flecknell PA, Richardson CA. Reported analgesic administration to rabbits, pigs, sheep, dogs and non-human primates undergoing experimental surgical procedures. *Lab Anim* 2009; **43**(3): 232–238.

55 Roughan JV, Flecknell PA. Buprenorphine: a reappraisal of its antinociceptive effects and therapeutic use in alleviating post-operative pain in animals. *Lab Anim* 2002; **36**(3): 322–343.

56 Leach MC, Forrester AR, Flecknell PA. Influence of preferred foodstuffs on the antinociceptive effects of orally administered buprenorphine in laboratory rats. *Lab Anim* 2010; **44**(1): 54–58.

57 Roughan JV, Flecknell PA. Evaluation of a short duration behaviour-based post-operative pain scoring system in rats. *Eur J Pain* 2003; **7**(5): 397–406.

58 Raffa RB, Ding Z. Examination of the preclinical antinociceptive efficacy of buprenorphine and its designation as full- or partial-agonist. *Acute Pain* 2007; **9**(3): 145–152.

59 Ohtani M, Kotaki H, Nishitateno K, *et al.* Kinetics of respiratory depression in rats induced by buprenorphine and its metabolite, norbuprenorphine. *J Pharmacol Exp Ther* 1997; **281**(1): 428–433.

60 Gueye PN, Borron SW, Risède P, *et al.* Buprenorphine and midazolam act in combination to depress respiration in rats. *Toxicol Sci* 2002; **65**(1): 107–114.

61 Clark JA, Myers PH, Goelz MF, *et al.* Pica behavior associated with buprenorphine administration in the rat. *Lab Anim Sci* 1997; **47**(3): 300–303.

62 He L, Kim J, Ou C, *et al.* Methadone antinociception is dependent on peripheral opioid receptors. *J Pain* 2009; **10**(4): 369–379.

63 Erichsen HK, Hao JX, Xu XJ, *et al.* Comparative actions of the opioid analgesics morphine, methadone and codeine in rat models of peripheral and central neuropathic pain. *Pain* 2005; **116**(3): 347–358.

64 Deschamps JY, Gaulier JM, Podevin G, *et al.* Fatal overdose after ingestion of a transdermal fentanyl patch in two non-human primates. *Vet Anaesth Analg* 2012; **39**(6): 653–656.

65 Dutriez-Casteloot I, Emmanuelli V, Wiart JF, *et al.* Long-lasting analgesia with transdermal fentanyl: a new approach in rat neonatal research. *Front Pharmacol* 2022; **13**: 798011.

66 Clemensen J, Rasmussen LV, Abelson KSP. Transdermal fentanyl solution provides long-term analgesia in the hind-paw incisional model of postoperative pain in male rats. *In Vivo* 2018; **32**(4): 713–719.

67 Berke MS, Colding-Jørgensen P, Pedersen LG, *et al.* Effects of transdermal fentanyl treatment on acute pain and inflammation in rats with adjuvant-induced monoarthritis. *Comp Med* 2022; **72**(5): 320–329.

68 Carbone ET, Lindstrom KE, Diep S, *et al.* Duration of action of sustained-release buprenorphine in 2 strains of mice. *J Am Assoc Lab Anim Sci* 2012; **51**(6): 815–819.

69 Foley PL, Liang H, Crichlow AR. Evaluation of a sustained-release formulation of buprenorphine for analgesia in rats. *J Am Assoc Lab Anim Sci* 2011; **50**(2): 198–204.

70 Nunamaker EA, Halliday LC, Moody DE, *et al.* Pharmacokinetics of 2 formulations of buprenorphine in macaques (*Macaca mulatta* and *Macaca fascicularis*). *J Am Assoc Lab Anim Sci* 2013; **52**(1): 48–56.

71 Haertel AJ, Schultz MA, Colgin LM, *et al.* Predictors of subcutaneous injection site reactions to sustained-release buprenorphine in rhesus macaques (*Macaca mulatta*). *J Am Assoc Lab Anim Sci* 2021; **60**(3): 329–336.

72 Wright-Williams SL, Courade JP, Richardson CA, *et al.* Effects of vasectomy surgery and meloxicam treatment on faecal corticosterone levels and behaviour in two strains of laboratory mouse. *Pain* 2007; **130**(1–2): 108–118.

73 Roughan JV, Flecknell PA. Behavioural effects of laparotomy and analgesic effects of ketoprofen and carprofen in rats. *Pain* 2001; **90**(1–2): 65–74.

74 Nadda N, Setia S, Vaish V, *et al.* Role of cytokines in experimentally induced lung cancer and chemoprevention by COX-2 selective inhibitor, etoricoxib. *Mol Cell Biochem* 2013; **372**(1–2): 101–112.

75 Williams JL, Ji P, Ouyang N, *et al.* NO-donating aspirin inhibits the activation of NF-kappaB in human cancer cell lines and Min mice. *Carcinogenesis* 2008; **29**(2): 390–397.

76 Shukoor MI, Tiwari S, Sankpal UT, *et al.* Tolfenamic acid suppresses cytochrome P450 2E1 expression in mouse liver. *Integr Biol (Camb)* 2012; **4**(9): 1122–1129.

77 De Oliveira GS, Almeida MD, Benzon HT, *et al.* Perioperative single dose systemic dexamethasone for postoperative pain: a meta-analysis of randomized controlled trials. *Anesthesiology* 2011; **115**(3): 575–588.

78 Pieretti S, Di Giannuario A, Domenici MR, *et al.* Dexamethasone-induced selective inhibition of the central mu opioid receptor: functional in vivo and in vitro evidence in rodents. *Br J Pharmacol* 1994; **113**(4): 1416–1422.

79 Durmus M, Karaaslan E, Ozturk E, *et al.* The effects of single-dose dexamethasone on wound healing in rats. *Anesth Analg* 2003; **97**(5): 1377–1380.

80 Fairbanks CA. Spinal delivery of analgesics in experimental models of pain and analgesia. *Adv Drug Deliv Rev* 2003; **55**(8): 1007–1041.

81 Flecknell PA, Liles JH, Williamson HA. The use of lignocaine-prilocaine local anaesthetic cream for pain-free venepuncture in laboratory animals. *Lab Anim* 1990; **24**(2): 142–146.

82 Jones CP, Carver S, Kendall LV. Evaluation of common anesthetic and analgesic techniques for tail biopsy in mice. *J Am Assoc Lab Anim Sci* 2012; **51**(6): 808–814.
83 Nishiyori M, Ueda H. Prolonged gabapentin analgesia in an experimental mouse model of fibromyalgia. *Mol Pain* 2008; **4**: 52.
84 Boruta DT, Sotgiu G, Golder FJ. Effects of intraperitoneal administration of gabapentin on the minimum alveolar concentration of isoflurane in adult male rats. *Lab Anim* 2012; **46**(2): 108–113.
85 Aguado D, Abreu M, Benito J, *et al.* The effects of gabapentin on acute opioid tolerance to remifentanil under sevoflurane anesthesia in rats. *Anesth Analg* 2012; **115**(1): 40–45.
86 Henderson LJ, Dani B, Serrano EMN, *et al.* Benefits of tunnel handling persist after repeated restraint, injection and anaesthesia. *Sci Rep* 2020; **10**(1): 14562.
87 Smiler KL, Stein S, Hrapkiewicz KL, *et al.* Tissue response to intramuscular and intraperitoneal injections of ketamine and xylazine in rats. *Lab Anim Sci* 1990; **40**(1): 60–64.
88 Gaines Das R, North D. Implications of experimental technique for analysis and interpretation of data from animal experiments: outliers and increased variability resulting from failure of intraperitoneal injection procedures. *Lab Anim* 2007; **41**(3): 312–320.
89 Krutrök N, Pehrsson S, Van Zuydam N, *et al.* Ventilation via nose cone results in similar hemodynamic parameters and blood gas levels as endotracheal intubation during open chest surgery in rats. *Lab Anim* 2022; **56**(2): 157–164.
90 Schwarte LA, Zuurbier CJ, Ince C. Mechanical ventilation of mice. *Basic Res Cardiol* 2000; **95**(6): 510–520.
91 Wolthuis EK, Vlaar APJ, Choi G, *et al.* Mechanical ventilation using non-injurious ventilation settings causes lung injury in the absence of pre-existing lung injury in healthy mice. *Crit Care* 2009; **13**(1): R1.
92 Briscoe JA, Syring R. Techniques for emergency airway and vascular access in special species. *Semin Avian Exot Pet Med* 2004; **13**(3): 118–131.
93 Albrecht M, Henke J, Tacke S, *et al.* Effects of isoflurane, ketamine-xylazine and a combination of medetomidine, midazolam and fentanyl on physiological variables continuously measured by telemetry in Wistar rats. *BMC Vet Res* 2014; **10**: 198.
94 Navarro KL, Huss M, Smith JC, *et al.* Mouse anesthesia: the art and science. *ILAR J* 2021; **62**(1–2): 238–273.
95 Caro AC, Hankenson FC, Marx JO. Comparison of thermoregulatory devices used during anesthesia of C57BL/6 mice and correlations between body temperature and physiologic parameters. *J Am Assoc Lab Anim Sci* 2013; **52**(5): 577–583.
96 Liles JH, Flecknell PA. The influence of buprenorphine or bupivacaine on the post-operative effects of laparotomy and bile-duct ligation in rats. *Lab Anim* 1993; **27**(4): 374–380.
97 Pham TM, Hagman B, Codita A, *et al.* Housing environment influences the need for pain relief during post-operative recovery in mice. *Physiol Behav* 2010; **99**(5): 663–668.
98 Roughan JV, Flecknell PA. Behaviour-based assessment of the duration of laparotomy-induced abdominal pain and the analgesic effects of carprofen and buprenorphine in rats. *Behav Pharmacol* 2004; **15**(7): 461–472.
99 Langford DJ, Bailey AL, Chanda ML, *et al.* Coding of facial expressions of pain in the laboratory mouse. *Nat Methods* 2010; 7(6): 447–449.
100 Keating SCJ, Thomas AA, Flecknell PA, *et al.* Evaluation of EMLA cream for preventing pain during tattooing of rabbits: changes in physiological, behavioural and facial expression responses. *PLoS ONE* 2012; **7**(9): e44437.
101 Leach MC, Klaus K, Miller AL, *et al.* The assessment of post-vasectomy pain in mice using behaviour and the Mouse Grimace Scale. *PLoS ONE* 2012; **7**(4): e35656.
102 Faller KME, McAndrew DJ, Schneider JE, *et al.* Refinement of analgesia following thoracotomy and experimental myocardial infarction using the Mouse Grimace Scale. *Exp Physiol* 2015; **100**(2): 164–172.
103 Roughan JV, Bertrand HGMJ, Isles HM. Meloxicam prevents COX-2-mediated post-surgical inflammation but not pain following laparotomy in mice. *Eur J Pain* 2016; **20**(2): 231–240.
104 Miller AL, Leach MC. The Mouse Grimace Scale: a clinically useful tool? *PLoS ONE* 2015; **10**(9): e0136000.
105 Mota-Rojas D, Olmos-Hernández A, Verduzco-Mendoza A, *et al.* The utility of grimace scales for practical pain assessment in laboratory animals. *Animals (Basel)* 2020; **10**(10): 1838.
106 Thomas AA, Detilleux J, Sandersen CF, *et al.* Minimally invasive technique for intrathecal administration of morphine in rats: practicality and antinociceptive properties. *Lab Anim* 2017; **51**(5): 479–489.
107 Thomas A, Miller A, Roughan J, *et al.* Efficacy of intrathecal morphine in a model of surgical pain in rats. *PLoS ONE* 2016; **11**(10): e0163909.
108 Bertrand HGMJ, Sandersen C, Flecknell PA. Reported analgesic and anaesthetic administration to non-human primates undergoing experimental surgical procedure: 2010–2015. *J Med Primatol* 2018; **47**(4): 217–225.
109 Carlsson HE, Schapiro SJ, Farah I, *et al.* Use of primates in research: a global overview. *Am J Primatol* 2004; **63**(4): 225–237.
110 Jiang X, Fan Z, Li S, *et al.* A review on zoonotic pathogens associated with non-human primates: understanding the potential threats to humans. *Microorganisms* 2023; **11**(2): 246.
111 Thomas AA, Leach MC, Flecknell PA. An alternative method of endotracheal intubation of common marmosets (*Callithrix jacchus*). *Lab Anim* 2012; **46**(1): 71–76.
112 Murphy KL, Baxter MG, Flecknell PA. Anesthesia and analgesia in nonhuman primates. In: Abee CR, Mansfield K, Tardif SD, Morris T, eds. *Nonhuman Primates in Biomedical Research*, 2nd edn. Philadelphia, PA: Academic Press, 2012: 403–435.
113 Truelove MA, Martin AL, Perlman JE, *et al.* Pair housing of macaques: a review of partner selection, introduction techniques, monitoring for compatibility, and methods for long-term maintenance of pairs. *Am J Primatol* 2017; **79**(1): 1–15.
114 Hannibal DL, Bliss-Moreau E, Vandeleest J, *et al.* Laboratory rhesus macaque social housing and social changes: implications for research. *Am J Primatol* 2017; **79**(1): 1–14.
115 Edwards P, Arango M, Balica L, *et al.* Final results of MRC CRASH, a randomised placebo-controlled trial of intravenous corticosteroid in adults with head injury-outcomes at 6 months. *Lancet* 2005; **365**(9475): 1957–1959.
116 Rangel-Castillo L, Gopinath S, Robertson CS. Management of intracranial hypertension. *Neurol Clin* 2008; **26**(2): 521–541.
117 Bovill JG, Antognini JF, Atherley R, *et al.* Isoflurane action in spinal cord indirectly depresses cortical activity associated with electrical stimulation of the reticular formation. *Anesth Analg* 2003; **96**(4): 999–1003.
118 Mahon S, Deniau JM, Charpier S. Relationship between EEG potentials and intracellular activity of striatal and cortico-striatal neurons: an in vivo study under different anesthetics. *Cereb Cortex* 2001; **11**(4): 360–373.
119 Allison SO, Halliday LC, French JA, *et al.* Assessment of buprenorphine, carprofen, and their combination for postoperative analgesia in olive baboons (*Papio anubis*). *J Am Assoc Lab Anim Sci* 2007; **46**(3): 24–31.
120 Descovich KA, Richmond SE, Leach MC, *et al.* Opportunities for refinement in neuroscience: indicators of wellness and post-operative pain in laboratory macaques. *ALTEX* 2019; **36**(4): 535–554.
121 Parr LA, Waller BM, Burrows AM, *et al.* Brief communication: MaqFACS: a muscle-based facial movement coding system for the rhesus macaque. *Am J Phys Anthropol* 2010; **143**(4): 625–630.
122 Correia-Caeiro C, Burrows A, Wilson DA, *et al.* CalliFACS: the common marmoset Facial Action Coding System. *PLoS ONE* 2022; **17**(5): e0266442.
123 Gris VN, Broche N, Kaneko A, *et al.* Investigating subtle changes in facial expression to assess acute pain in Japanese macaques. *Sci Rep* 2022; **12**(1): 19675.
124 Paterson EA, O'Malley CI, Moody C, *et al.* Development and validation of a cynomolgus macaque grimace scale for acute pain assessment. *Sci Rep* 2023; **13**(1): 3209.
125 Smith AA, Halliday LC, Lindeblad MO, *et al.* Evaluation of analgesic patches in cynomolgus macaques (*Macaca fascicularis*). *J Am Assoc Lab Anim Sci* 2019; **58**(3): 356–361.
126 Carlson AM, Kelly R, Fetterer DP, *et al.* Pharmacokinetics of 2 formulations of transdermal fentanyl in cynomolgus macaques (*Macaca fascicularis*). *J Am Assoc Lab Anim Sci* 2016; **55**(4): 436–442.

55 Comparative Immobilization and Anesthesia – Free-Ranging Terrestrial Mammals

Nigel Caulkett[1] and Jon M. Arnemo[2]

[1] Faculty of Veterinary Medicine, University of Calgary, Calgary, Alberta, Canada

[2] Inland Norway University of Applied Sciences, Campus Evenstad, Norway and Swedish University of Agricultural Sciences, Umeå, Sweden

Chapter contents

Introduction, 1077
Field anesthesia, 1077
General considerations, 1077
Weather, 1078
Equipment, 1078
Capture technique, 1078
Hazards, 1079
Remote drug delivery equipment, 1079
Darts, 1080
Pharmacology, 1080
Ideal drug combination for wildlife capture, 1080
Opioids, 1081
Opioid antagonists, 1082
Cyclohexamines, 1082
α_2-Adrenergic receptor agonists,1083
α_2-Adrenergic receptor antagonists, 1083
Neuroleptic drugs, 1084
Neurosteroids (alfaxalone), 1084
Drug combinations, 1084
The capture event, 1084
Precapture planning, 1084
Induction, 1085
Monitoring and supportive care, 1085
Recovery, 1087
Complications related to wildlife capture, 1087
Physical trauma, 1087
Hyperthermia, 1087
Hypothermia, 1088
Exertional myopathy, 1088
Respiratory depression and hypoxemia, 1088
Capture-associated mortality, 1088
Protocols and doses, 1088
References, 1088

Introduction

Chemical immobilization of free-ranging wildlife can be challenging. The nature of the procedure dictates that veterinarians must alter or even ignore many of the principles that underlie good anesthetic practice in other settings. It is generally not possible to access the patients for a preanesthetic physical examination or laboratory work. Physical status of the patients cannot be accurately assessed, and animals are usually assumed to be healthy. Even if physical status and anesthetic risk could be determined, generally only a few effective protocols are available [1–3].

Induction of anesthesia in wildlife can be extremely stressful, and stress-related conditions or injuries can result. Free-ranging wildlife are subject to environmental hazards and are often at risk for hypothermia or hyperthermia. Appropriate supportive care, such as controlled ventilation, intravenous (IV) fluid therapy, or inotropic support, is often not possible in field situations. Veterinarians may be required to work on species for which there is very little information about their physiology or pharmacologic response to drugs. Extrapolation between similar species may be required but can result in unexpected complications. Issues of human safety must also be considered. Given the challenges that are encountered during wildlife capture, it is not surprising that morbidity and mortality of animals can be high and injury to people engaged in the capturing procedure more common.

This chapter focuses on the major principles of wildlife capture and handling. It is beyond the scope of a single chapter to provide complete dose recommendations for terrestrial mammals. *The Handbook of Wildlife Chemical Immobilization* [1] and *Zoo Animal and Wildlife Immobilization and Anesthesia* [3] can be used to find detailed drug and dose information for individual species.

Field anesthesia

General considerations

Wildlife capture is often required for both research and management purposes. Capture events should be carefully planned because complications can often be anticipated and responses better prepared. Capture sites may be chosen based on their suitability and the timing chosen in an appropriate season of the year when environmental hazards are minimized. For example, ungulates may be captured in late winter or spring to decrease the risk of hyperthermia and enable tracking in snow or visualization of animals in

Veterinary Anesthesia and Analgesia: The Sixth Edition of Lumb and Jones. Edited by Leigh Lamont, Kurt Grimm, Sheilah Robertson, Lydia Love and Carrie Schroeder.
© 2024 John Wiley & Sons, Inc. Published 2024 by John Wiley & Sons, Inc.
Companion website: www.wiley.com/go/lamont/anesthesia

deciduous forest. Often individual animals do not have to be targeted in management projects, and the capture team can choose any animal in a relatively safe capture environment. It is generally possible to adhere to strict pursuit time limits. If it is not absolutely necessary to capture the target animal, pursuit can be terminated to decrease the risk of stress-related disease, such as exertional myopathy. Current literature and experts in the field can be consulted prior to the capture event to ensure that the most suitable technique is used. It may also be possible to close areas to the public where wildlife are captured. Finally, appropriate equipment for monitoring and supportive care should be obtained and taken into the field when possible.

Weather

Weather conditions may dictate whether wildlife capture is possible. Safe helicopter flight is generally not possible in high winds or foggy conditions. Snow and rain can lead to hypothermia, particularly if wind is also present to enhance convective heat loss. Smaller mammals may be particularly prone to hypothermia. Hyperthermia is a serious complication that can be difficult to treat in field situations. Several of the drug regimens used for wildlife capture can impede thermoregulation and lead to hypothermia or hyperthermia [3,4]. When possible, captures should be planned for the cooler hours of the day during summer months. In remote locations, sudden changes in weather may also be a hazard to personnel. It is important to keep track of current and forecasted conditions during planned events. Capture for management purposes may occur at any time. Provisions should be made to prevent heat loss and actively cool animals, if required.

Equipment

Logistics generally dictate what type of equipment can be carried in a field situation. It is often difficult to carry all but the most necessary pieces. Fortunately, there are compact ambulatory monitors suitable for field use.

Equipment should withstand field use and be as lightweight and compact as possible. Hypoxemia is a common complication of wildlife anesthesia, particularly with ruminants [3–7]. Oxygen is fundamental supportive care during field anesthesia. Aluminum E and D cylinders, combined with a sturdy regulator and flowmeter, are ideal for field use (Fig. 55.1). Oxygen concentrators may provide an attractive alternative to compressed oxygen cylinders as they do not require refilling and eliminate many of the risks of working with compressed gas [8] (Fig. 55.2). Often, nasal insufflation of oxygen is adequate to treat hypoxemia. However, equipment for airway management and ventilatory support is recommended for many scenarios. It is difficult to carry a wide range of emergency drugs or an adequate volume of crystalloid fluids to treat shock, but a basic emergency kit containing epinephrine, atropine, lidocaine, and reversal agents should always be carried. Ruminants are predisposed to ruminal tympany, so a suitably sized tube to desufflate the rumen should be available. Equipment should also be carried to treat lacerations and other incidental injuries during capture.

Capture technique

An animal may be captured initially by physical or chemical means. The choice of capture technique depends on the species, the terrain, the facilities, and the experience of the capture crew. Many species of ungulates can be effectively captured and handled by experienced teams with physical techniques such as net guns [4,9]. Physical restraint can be very stressful for wild animals, but

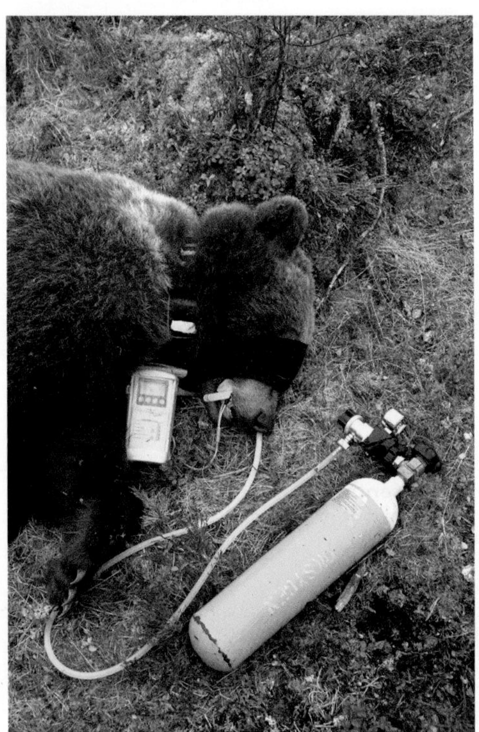

Figure 55.1 Oxygen delivery via intranasal supplementation in a brown bear

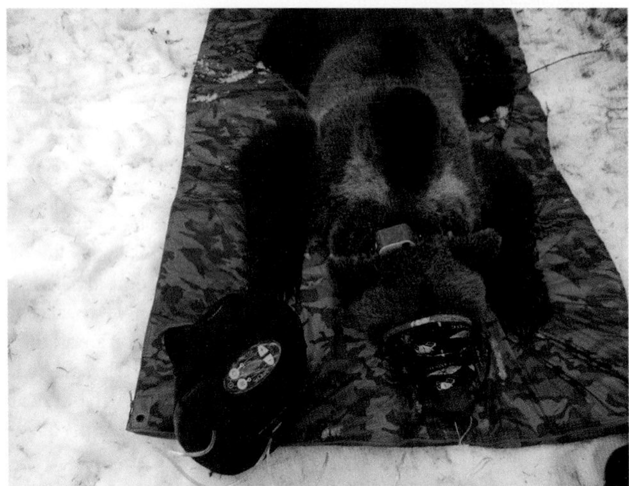

Figure 55.2 Portable oxygen concentrators can be used instead of compressed gas cylinders in field situations. They have some advantages for use in remote locations.

sedatives or anesthetics can be used to decrease the stress of handling once animals have been netted [4,9].

Net gunning can cause high rates of mortality if it is performed by inexperienced personnel. The risk to capture personnel can also be high. During a 10-year period in New Zealand, there were 127 helicopter crashes and 25 human fatalities during net gun capture of red deer [10]. These figures stress the need for experienced pilots and capture personnel.

The use of physical restraint will confine an animal's movements during the induction of anesthesia, which may be a positive when terrain dictates a limited escape route. Physical restraint can induce greater stress than chemical restraint [11]. Generally, physical restraint should be of brief duration to avoid stress-related complications.

Hazards

A number of hazards can be encountered during anesthesia of free-ranging wildlife. It is important to perform a risk assessment prior to embarking on a project to identify and minimize the risks. The target species can pose a risk to personnel. In addition to the obvious risks of serious personnel injury from carnivores, ungulates can also act aggressively. Many deer species undergo a period of rut during the breeding season, during which stags are often more aggressive. Injury may also occur from flailing limbs or heads in lightly anesthetized animals. It is important to know how a species will act in a stressful situation, and to leave an exit for the animal (and for the capture personnel) if things do not go according to plan. The best way to avoid injury is to work with people who are familiar with animal behavior. Many species carry zoonotic disease, so capture personnel should be aware of this potential and handle the animal appropriately.

During capture, the focus tends to be on the captured animal. It is always important to be aware of the surrounding environment because other animals may approach. This is particularly important with social carnivores, such as lions. It is also important with bears, particularly if members of a family group are captured. In these situations, an armed lookout should be posted to protect the capture team.

A firearm backup is important with more dangerous species. The primary person performing the backup should be trained and experienced in the use of firearms, and an appropriate firearm should be used. If firearms are commonly used, all members of the capture team should receive firearm safety training. Similar training is advisable for people using dart rifles or pistols. Pepper spray may be considered as a non-lethal alternative to firearms. Recent studies have demonstrated that pepper spray is as effective as a firearm in many situations [12] (Fig. 55.3).

The environment itself can be hazardous since capture may occur in remote and rugged locations. In these situations, personnel must be prepared to look after themselves if they cannot return to a base area. A method of communication with rescue services should be established. In some environments, weather can change rapidly and often dictates whether capture should take place. There are hazards specific to the terrain and region; for instance, capture personnel should receive avalanche training before working in mountainous regions during winter when there is an avalanche risk. It is important to anticipate risks in any environment.

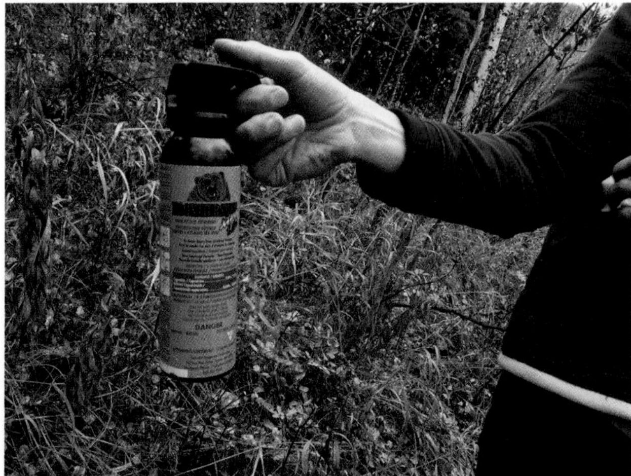

Figure 55.3 Pepper spray has been proven to effectively deter bear attacks. It is a potential less-lethal option for personal defense against dangerous wildlife.

Pharmaceuticals used for wildlife immobilization and anesthesia can present a serious human health hazard because of their high potency and concentrated formulations. Handling of potent opioids, such as etorphine and thiafentanil, carries the risk of lethal toxicity in people [1,13]. These drugs must be handled with extreme caution. Protective clothing, such as disposable gloves and face shields, should be used to prevent skin or mucous membrane contact. A pharmacologic antagonist should be available to treat human exposure. Potent opioids receive a great deal of attention, but any concentrated sedative or anesthetic must also be handled carefully. Medetomidine can be formulated at a concentration of 40 mg/mL for use in wildlife. Dexmedetomidine, which is used at a dose of 0.5–1 μg/kg IV in people [14], is twice as potent as medetomidine [15]. This dose is equivalent to 1–2 μg of medetomidine per 1 kg of body weight or a total of 75–150 μg in a 75 kg person. The high end of this dose range is equivalent to a 0.0038 mL volume of concentrated medetomidine. Obviously, there is serious risk of toxicity from exposure to a very low volume of a 40 mg/mL medetomidine formulation. Tiletamine–zolazepam is another immobilizing mixture that can be delivered in a concentrated form and therefore must be handled with caution. Everyone working on a capture team should be trained in first aid, and equipment should be available to provide respiratory and airway support.

Wildlife anesthesia should never be performed by a single person. At least two trained people should be present whenever potent drugs are handled. Loading and charging of darts is a time of high risk for exposure to drugs. Darts should be charged under a protective cover to decrease the risk of accidental drug exposure. Antagonists, such as naloxone or naltrexone, should always be immediately available in case of inadvertent human exposure.

Dart delivery equipment should be handled with care and only by trained individuals. Darts have the potential to induce significant tissue injury and death. Firearm safety rules apply to darting equipment, and individuals handling this equipment should be appropriately trained.

Helicopters present a significant hazard. Wildlife capture requires a very skilled pilot to decrease the risk of injury to the target animal and the capture personnel. Anyone working around a helicopter must receive training in helicopter safety [16].

Prior to any capture, it is advisable to meet with local medical personnel and discuss an evacuation and treatment plan in case of inadvertent human exposure. A meeting of this nature will familiarize physicians and emergency medical services personnel with the drugs that are being used and the potential treatments. In the event of an emergency, this can save valuable time and someone's life.

Remote drug delivery equipment

Wildlife capture often requires drug delivery over relatively long distances. Generally, it is difficult to deliver drugs accurately at distances greater than 40 m, but there have been major advances in the equipment available for remote drug delivery. It is important to realize that these systems have the potential to produce serious injury or death if they are used inappropriately. The major sources of injury arise from dart impact trauma, high-velocity injection of dart contents, and inaccurate dart placement.

Dart impact trauma results from dispersion of energy on dart impact. Impact kinetic energy (KE) is represented by the following equation:

$$KE = \frac{1}{2} M \times V^2$$

where M is mass (kg), and V is velocity (m/s) [1]. High velocity is the major factor that will cause trauma. A good general rule is to use the lowest velocity that will provide an accurate trajectory at a given distance. Practice with a darting system at a variety of distances is vital to minimize velocity. The other major factor is the mass of the dart. Darts with a lower mass will have less impact energy at a given velocity. This should be a consideration in the choice of a darting system, particularly when dealing with smaller animals that are more prone to trauma.

Inaccurate dart placement can cause injury. This most frequently occurs if the dart penetrates the abdomen, thorax, or other vital structures of the head and neck. The major factors that can lead to inaccurate dart placement include lack of practice with the darting system, an attempt to place a dart over an excessive range, inherent inaccuracy of the darting system, and wind, including down-wash from the helicopter rotor during aerial darting.

The final source of injury is related to high-velocity injection of dart contents. Systems that expel drug via an explosive charge can disrupt tissue and produce trauma. These systems should only be used on large, well-muscled animals (Fig. 55.4). Injection volume should be minimized to decrease the degree of tissue trauma. When possible, the use of darts that deliver their contents via compressed air should be considered. The choice of system depends on the range required, the dart size, and individual characteristics of the target animal. A more complete review and manufacturer information can be found elsewhere [1,3,16].

Darts

Darts must deliver their contents into a muscle group on impact for induction to be rapid and smooth. Choice of a system will depend on the situation and the size of the animal.

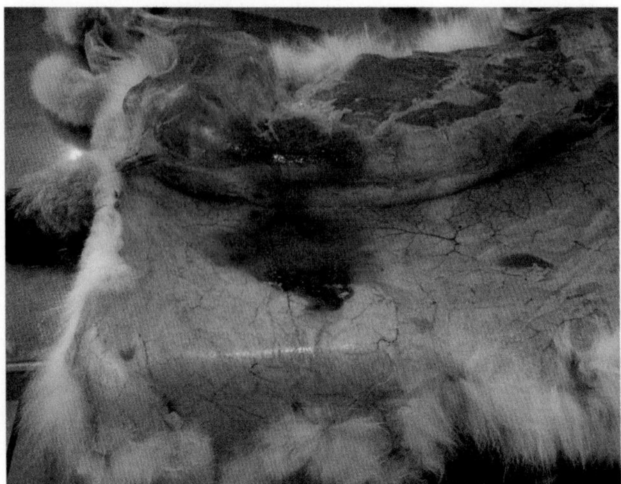

Figure 55.4 Dart-induced trauma in a lynx; note the extensive subcutaneous hemorrhage at the dart site.

Explosive discharge mechanisms

Darts that use an explosive discharge mechanism can produce considerable muscle trauma and should be reserved for large, well-muscled animals. These darts have an aluminum or plastic body into which a small explosive cap is placed between the plunger and the tail. Upon impact, a firing pin inside the cap is forced forward, against the resistance of a spring, detonating the charge. The expanding gas pushes the plunger forward and the drug is expelled through the needle. The short duration of injection (e.g., 0.001 s) can result in high injectate velocity, which may cause tissue damage [16]. The explosive caps are very sensitive to moisture and must be kept dry. When placed in the dart, the cap must have its open end against the tail. If it is turned around, detonation and expulsion of the drug will occur at the moment the projector is fired.

If reusable darts are used, the fit of the dart should be tested by inserting the dart in the muzzle. If it slides in and out with ease, the dart is not significantly deformed, and it can be reloaded. If the dart jams in the muzzle, the dart should not be reused. With repeated use, the dart body may expand to the point where the aluminum is weakened by the threads cut into it. This is caused by the high pressure created in the dart when gases from the explosive charge push the plunger forward.

All of the darts with explosive discharge mechanisms inject through the tip of the needle. The needle should be barbed so that it stays in the animal during injection. If there is no barb or if the barb is removed, the force of the frontal expulsion of the drug is often sufficiently powerful to drive the dart out of the animal, resulting in only partial injection.

Air-activated mechanisms

These darts consist of an aluminum or plastic body into which compressed air is introduced through a one-way valve in the tail piece. At impact, a silicone seal is displaced, exposing a port in the side of the needle. The plunger is pushed forward by air pressure, and the drug is expelled through the open port. Depending on the type and usage, plastic darts can be used repeatedly, but will eventually begin to leak or lose air pressure. In extreme cold, the drug may freeze inside the dart; therefore, darts should be kept warm in a secure container placed in an inside pocket or in a heated vehicle or helicopter.

Pharmacology

Ideal drug combination for wildlife capture

Wildlife immobilization has progressed a great deal in recent years. A variety of drugs are available to facilitate capture and handling, and new techniques continue to develop. An ideal drug or combination thereof would possess the following properties.

Rapid onset of activity

A rapid effect is one of the most important attributes required in a capture drug. The induction period is a hazardous time. Handlers and bystanders may be at risk of injury if induction is prolonged. Rapid onset will limit the risks of trauma, hyperthermia, and possibly capture myopathy. Ideally, the animal should be immobilized within 1–5 min after injection. Practically, most current combinations can take longer than 5 min to induce anesthesia.

High margin of safety

Drugs used for wildlife capture must have a high margin of safety. It is difficult to transport supportive equipment into the field so capture drugs should produce minimal cardiopulmonary depression.

Wild animals are not weighed prior to capture, and it is common to overestimate weight. Capture drugs must have high safety margins or therapeutic indices to decrease the risk of mortality from overdose.

Handler safety

Precautions must always be taken to avoid human exposure to drugs. Ideally, drugs should be relatively safe to handle, with minimum risks of intoxication if the handler contacts the drug. The ability to antagonize the effects of any drug is also desirable in field situations.

Small volume of delivery

Capture drugs should be potent and concentrated enough to facilitate delivery at low volumes, ideally less than 3 mL. This decreases the risk of injection trauma from high-velocity injection and facilitates accurate dart flight.

Level of central nervous system effect

The animal should rapidly lose motor function and ideally become unconscious and unaware of its surroundings.

Ability to antagonize immobilization

Free-ranging wildlife often live in an environment full of potential hazards, so they must be cared for until they are fully awake. A pharmacologic antagonist will speed recovery and is also of value in emergency situations. Because it can be difficult to provide supportive care, complications such as hyperthermia can quickly become life-threatening and drug antagonism may be the only viable option in managing unexpected complications.

Species versatility

Wildlife managers often deal with a variety of species. Thus, an ideal drug or combinations thereof should have predictable effects in a wide range of species. The use of a single protocol in a variety of species limits the variety of drugs required to be kept on hand and increases familiarity with the pharmacodynamics of the drug or drug combination.

Drug stability

Wildlife capture may need to be performed in a wide range of ambient temperatures. Ideally, drugs should remain stable, in solution, over a wide range of temperatures.

Analgesia

It has become more common to perform potentially painful procedures during wildlife handling. These procedures can include ear tagging, tooth removal, biopsies, and even surgery for abdominal or subcutaneous implant placement. These procedures dictate that appropriate intraoperative and postoperative analgesia be provided.

Opioids

A variety of opioids have been used for wildlife capture. Opioids can be used in a wide range of species but are particularly effective in ungulates. The opioids produce analgesia and sedation but lack muscle-relaxant properties. They have been used alone or, more often, with a neuroleptic agent, the inclusion of which potentiates the opioid's sedative effects, resulting in a smoother induction and decreased muscle rigidity. Opioids are predictable, act relatively fast, and can be reversed with the administration of a suitable antagonist. If not reversed, the duration of immobilization is lengthy, often several hours, during which the animal is at risk from opioid-induced respiratory depression, thermoregulatory problems, and environmental hazards. Underdosing of opioids can result in a prolonged induction time characterized by central nervous system (CNS) excitation, which can cause hyperthermia, exhaustion, lost animals, and/or death of the animal. The adverse effects of opioid-induced immobilization include:

1. Excitation after administration, resulting in aimless running, pacing, or walking, which may lead to hyperthermia or capture myopathy [17]
2. Regurgitation of ruminal content or vomiting; the risk of regurgitation appears increased when an opioid is combined with xylazine [18]
3. Severe respiratory depression and hypoxemia [7,8]
4. Muscle rigidity [17]
5. Resedation [17]

Potent opioids, such as etorphine and thiafentanil, are several thousand times more potent than morphine in humans and must be handled carefully to avoid accidental exposure [1–3,13].

Carfentanil

Carfentanil was used for capture of free-ranging ungulates and some large carnivores beginning in the early 1980s but is no longer available due to human drug abuse.

Etorphine

Etorphine has been used successfully in many species, but has been particularly effective in ungulates, rhinoceroses, and elephants. Etorphine can be used alone or in combination with a suitable neuroleptic or sedative agent. Induction course and immobilization duration are dose dependent. Underdosing can cause excitation with its associated problems. At optimum doses, the first effects may be observed 3–8 min after intramuscular (IM) injection. The full effect may be reached in 20–30 min. Recovery is slow (up to 7 or 8 h) if no antagonist is given. When an antagonist is administered, animals will recover in 1–3 min after IV injection and in 5–10 min following IM injection. The most serious adverse effect is respiratory depression. For that reason, an animal should not be kept immobilized longer than necessary, and drug effect should be reversed as soon as possible. Other side effects are often dose or species dependent and may include excitement, muscle tremors, convulsions, regurgitation, bloat, bradycardia, tachycardia, hypertension, hyperthermia, and resedation.

Thiafentanil

Thiafentanil has some potential advantages over etorphine, such as rapid induction, greater therapeutic index, shorter half-life, lower incidence of resedation, and less respiratory and cardiac depression [19]. Thiafentanil is commercially available only in South Africa and the United States, but its use has been described in a variety of species [1,3,19]. It has been used alone or in combination with an α_2-adrenergic receptor agonist. Reports have detailed the use of thiafentanil combined with medetomidine and ketamine [20]. This is a promising drug combination that appears to be efficacious and have fewer side effects than high-dose single opioid immobilization [3,20].

Butorphanol

Butorphanol has agonist activity at the κ-opioid receptor and is generally antagonistic at μ-opioid receptors. It is commercially available in concentrations of 30 and 50 mg/mL. These high-concentration formulations greatly increase the utility of this drug for remote delivery. In North America, butorphanol is commonly used in combination with medetomidine and azaperone for capture of wild ungulates [21–25]. The combination of butorphanol–azaperone–medetomidine is known as "BAM" and has the advantage of a small volume for remote drug delivery, and the ability to antagonize sedation with naltrexone and atipamezole [21–26]. The major adverse side effect is hypoxemia [24]. Supplemental inspired oxygen can offset hypoxemia [24]. This combination has proven to be reliable in most ungulate species, however, some challenges have been encountered with helicopter-based capture of bison [25]. BAM has been used successfully for immobilization of black bears [26]. Its use has not been described in larger more dangerous bear species, and it may be advisable to incorporate a dissociative anesthetic, such as tiletamine, into the protocol to decrease the risk of sudden arousal from sedation. Butorphanol administered in combination with etorphine improved ventilatory function and oxygenation during immobilization of rhinos [7,27].

Opioid antagonists

A major advantage of opioid-based immobilization is the ability to antagonize the opioid. To be effective, the antagonist's effect should outlast the agonist drug's sedation, and ideally be highly selective for the desired receptor type(s). The three drugs commonly used for this purpose are naltrexone, naloxone, and diprenorphine. Naltrexone is probably the most versatile drug, with the lowest risk of resedation. Naloxone and naltrexone are the preferred antagonists for opioid overdose in humans.

Naltrexone

Naltrexone is commercially available in a 50 mg/mL concentration. It is a pure opioid antagonist (i.e., it has no known agonistic properties) that will produce rapid antagonism of opioid receptor agonists. The major advantage of naltrexone is that it will produce reliable antagonism due to its long duration of action [1,3]. Naltrexone has been recommended at a dose of 10–30 mg per 1 mg of etorphine or thiafentanil administered. The drug is effective following IM and IV administration. A more rapid antagonism will occur if it is administered intravenously.

Naloxone

Naloxone is also a pure opioid antagonist. It may be used to reverse the effects of all the aforementioned opioids, and reversal occurs within 1–3 min of IV injection. Naloxone has a short half-life so animals may revert to a state of motor impairment within a few hours due to resedation and require repeated treatment.

Diprenorphine

Diprenorphine used to be the antagonist for reversal of the effects of etorphine. While it does have agonistic properties of its own, when given following etorphine, diprenorphine acts as an antagonist. Reversal is rapid following IV injection, with animals becoming ambulatory in 1–3 min. If the antagonist is injected intramuscularly, reversal takes longer (up to 15–20 min). Adverse effects are rare, although overdosing may cause continued immobilization because of its partial agonist activity. The preferred opioid antagonist is now naltrexone.

Cyclohexamines

This class of drugs produce a state of dissociative anesthesia. When used alone, the cyclohexamines produce muscle rigidity or twitching. Other adverse effects are hyperthermia, excessive salivation, catecholamine release, and convulsions. The cyclohexamines act fast, have a relatively wide margin of safety, and depress respiration and circulation only moderately at optimum doses. Laryngeal reflexes are somewhat preserved with these agents.

Cyclohexamines are used in combination with a benzodiazepine or α_2-adrenergic receptor agonist, which will be additive or synergistic, produce a smoother induction and recovery, and alleviate the muscle rigidity common with dissociative anesthetics [3]. Potent selective α_2-adrenergic receptor agonists, such as medetomidine or dexmedetomidine, used at high doses will significantly reduce the dose requirements of cyclohexamines. The reduced cyclohexamine dose will result in more rapid and better-quality recoveries following antagonism of the α_2-adrenergic receptor agonist drug [1,3]. The cyclohexamines have been used in a wide variety of species, but are particularly known for their effectiveness in carnivores, primates, and birds. There are no known antagonists for this class of drugs. The drugs in this category include ketamine and the tiletamine–zolazepam combination.

Ketamine

Ketamine is commercially available aqueous solutions up to 200 mg/mL. Ketamine should never be used as the sole immobilizing agent. A tranquilizer/sedative should be co-administered in almost all cases to reduce or prevent its hypertonic effects. Ketamine has been used successfully in many species, and doses vary widely from one species to another. Induction time and immobilization duration are dose and species dependent. At optimum doses, the first effects are observed in 2–5 min following IM injection, with the full effects usually attained in 5–10 min. Immobilization usually lasts from 45 min to 2 h.

Adverse effects of ketamine may include convulsions, catatonia, apnea, excessive salivation, and hyperthermia. Many of these effects can be negated by adding a benzodiazepine or α_2-adrenergic receptor agonist. Medetomidine–ketamine combinations have some advantages over xylazine use because a lower dose of ketamine is usually required [1,3,28]. This will result in smaller injection volumes and the ability to antagonize medetomidine with fewer adverse side effects from the remaining ketamine. It is noteworthy that ketamine-based combinations are unreliable in bears. Sudden recoveries have been encountered with xylazine–ketamine and medetomidine–ketamine in brown and polar bears [29].

Tiletamine–zolazepam

A commercial preparation of tiletamine, a dissociative anesthetic, and zolazepam, a benzodiazepine agonist, is available as a freeze-dried powder product. It is effective in a variety of species and at optimum doses its first effects may be noticeable within 1 or 2 min following IM injection. Full effects can be reached within 15–30 min. The onset is usually smooth, with good muscle relaxation and somatic analgesia. The duration of effect, quality of emergence, and duration of recovery vary with species because tiletamine and zolazepam are metabolized at different rates in various species. Recovery occurs in 3–8 h in most cases but may be prolonged in some species.

The tiletamine–zolazepam combination may cause hypertension and increase heart rate and cardiac output. Other effects are salivation, occasional muscle rigidity and ataxia, and hyperthermia (particularly if the mixture is combined with an α_2-adrenergic receptor agonist) [29–32]. Tiletamine–zolazepam has been used alone in a variety of species [33]. It is effective in carnivores, and recovery tends to be smooth, but can be prolonged. The use of this combination alone in ungulates can result in rough recoveries. Reconstitution of tiletamine–zolazepam with an α_2-adrenergic receptor agonist will decrease the volume injected, enhance analgesia, and decrease recovery times following antagonism of the α_2-adrenergic receptor agonist [29–32,34–37].

α_2-Adrenergic receptor agonists

α_2-Adrenergic receptor agonists are CNS depressants with sedative, muscle-relaxant, and analgesic properties. Used alone, α_2-adrenergic receptor agonists produce unreliable immobilization in most wild species. They are best used in combination with opioids or dissociative anesthetics. When used in high doses, α_2-adrenergic receptor agonists may critically depress respiration and circulation. Commonly encountered adverse effects include hypoxemia in ungulates and hypertension with or without bradycardia [5,6,22–25,28–32,35–37]. These agents can also contribute to ruminal tympany and regurgitation in ungulates [18,35]. In very excited animals (capture situations), they do not produce a predictable level of immobilization. They also disrupt thermoregulatory mechanisms, leading to hyperthermia or hypothermia [28,29,38]. Recovery without reversal from high doses is usually prolonged and difficult. In field situations, it is generally recommended that the effects of α_2-adrenergic receptor agonists be antagonized at the completion of the procedure to help minimize adverse physiologic actions and capture outcomes.

There are five α_2-adrenergic receptor agonists on the market: xylazine, romifidine, detomidine, medetomidine, and dexmedetomidine. The difference in potency between these drugs is species dependent [1]. Xylazine and medetomidine have been widely used in wildlife.

Xylazine

Xylazine is commonly available in 20 and 100 mg/mL aqueous solutions. It is also available in powder form and as a 300 mg/mL solution specifically for use in wildlife capture. The 20 mg/mL solution is too dilute to be useful for remote injection.

When administered alone, xylazine does not produce reliably immobilized free-ranging wildlife. It may appear to induce a recumbent, sleep-like state but stimulation may cause rapid arousal with defense responses intact. In calm animals, the initial sedative effect may be seen within 4–5 min of IM injection, with full effect reached within 15–20 min. Adverse effects can include hypoxemia, bradycardia, hypotension, ruminal tympany, and decreased thermoregulatory ability.

Xylazine has been used effectively in combination with opioids and cyclohexamines. The response to high doses of xylazine may conceal a recovery from the primary immobilizing drug and place workers at risk if the animal is suddenly aroused by noises, touch, or other stimulation.

The effects of xylazine may be reversed with the administration of several α_2-adrenergic receptor antagonists. Approximately 1 mg of atipamezole administered intramuscularly is required to antagonize 10 mg of xylazine. If xylazine is used in combination with a cyclohexamine, its effects should not be reversed before the animal has metabolized a significant fraction of the latter in an attempt to minimize the adverse effects of the cyclohexamine.

Xylazine is typically used intramuscularly for wildlife immobilization. Intranasal administration can be beneficial to decrease stress and struggling following net gun capture [9]. This route has a relatively rapid onset of activity and is simple to administer in physically restrained animals [9].

Detomidine

Detomidine is commercially available in a 10 mg/mL solution. The effects of detomidine have been well studied in horses, but information on its use for immobilization of captive and free-ranging equids and wild animals is limited. It has been combined with etorphine in rhinoceros and has proven to be effective in zebras when combined with carfentanil and ketamine [39,40]. The action of detomidine is much like that of xylazine. Its effects may be reversed by an appropriate α_2-adrenergic receptor antagonist. In general, 5 mg of atipamezole, administered by IM injection, should be used to antagonize 1 mg of detomidine.

Medetomidine

Medetomidine is a potent α_2-adrenergic receptor agonist that has proven useful for wildlife capture. The 1 mg/mL formulation suitable for use in small mammals is too dilute for use in larger species. Medetomidine is also commercially available in 10, 20, and 40 mg/mL concentrations, which are more adequate for capture of most large land mammals. Medetomidine will produce sedation, analgesia, and muscle relaxation. Medetomidine should not be used alone because, as with xylazine, immobilization is unreliable. Medetomidine can be combined with a low dose of ketamine or tiletamine–zolazepam. A relatively low dose of the dissociative drug is required in combination with medetomidine, and antagonism of medetomidine with atipamezole (at three to five times the medetomidine dose) will hasten recovery [1,28]. Similar to all α_2-adrenergic receptor agonists, adverse effects of medetomidine include hypertension, bradycardia, and hypoxemia [6,24,28–30,35,37]. Hypoxemia may be particularly pronounced in ruminants [6,41]. Medetomidine can also impair thermoregulatory ability, resulting in hyperthermia [28,29,38].

Dexmedetomidine

Dexmedetomidine is approximately twice as potent as medetomidine; currently, it is commercially available only in 0.5 mg/mL for small animal use, but compounded formulations of up to 20 mg/mL can be sourced. It can be used interchangeably with medetomidine at approximately half the dose (on a microgram basis) [42].

α_2-Adrenergic receptor antagonists

The utility of α_2-adrenergic receptor agonist-induced sedation is greatly increased by the availability of specific antagonists. Atipamezole is the most selective of the three currently available antagonists and can be used in all species. There are apparent species-dependent differences in response to yohimbine and tolazoline but less so with atipamezole. Yohimbine, for example, is not particularly effective in wild bovids, and either tolazoline or atipamezole reversal is preferred in these species. Antagonists should generally be administered intramuscularly unless the situation is an emergency. CNS excitement, tachycardia, and hypotension followed by hypertension may be seen with IV antagonist administration [28,41]. Animals may arouse rapidly and without warning from immobilization following IV administration of atipamezole [29,35,37]. With potentially dangerous species, this may not allow adequate time to retreat to a safe distance.

Vatinoxan (MK-467) is an α_2-adrenergic receptor antagonist that does not cross the blood–brain barrier, i.e., the agent might be used to antagonize peripheral effects of new α_2-adrenergic receptor agonists. Studies in wildlife indicate that vatinoxan has potential for preventing cardiovascular and other side effects of α_2-adrenergic receptor agonists, without significantly compromising their analgesic or sedative effects [43].

Neuroleptic drugs

Neuroleptic agents, such as acepromazine and droperidol, have been used as adjunctive agents in wildlife capture for many years. Typically, they have been used in combination with potent opioids such as etorphine. A more recent application of these agents is the use of long-acting tranquilizers to facilitate translocation of wild animals. Long-acting neuroleptics have been developed to treat human psychosis. Depending on the formulation, these drugs may have effects for days to weeks. They will produce an overall reduction in stress of handling, which should decrease the incidence of trauma and myopathy and facilitate adaptation to a novel environment. Typically, these agents are of the phenothiazine, butyrophenone, or benzodiazepine drug classes [44,45]. A short-acting agent, such as haloperidol, may be combined with a long-acting agent, such as perphenazine enanthate, to produce a rapid onset of action and prolonged activity [45].

Perphenazine enanthate

Perphenazine is a slow-onset, long-acting phenothiazine derivative formulated in a sesame oil vehicle. The onset of perphenazine is 12–16 h, and its effects can last up to 10 days. The use of this drug has been reported in a variety of species, including red deer and Przewalski's horses [45,46]. Flight distance is decreased in red deer, and animals maintain better body condition than controls during changes in environment [46]. In Przewalski's horses, the drug has been used to effectively decrease dominance aggression during the establishment of a bachelor herd [46].

Zuclopenthixol acetate

This drug is a thioxanthine derivative that has been used in a variety of species with effects lasting up to 3–4 days [47–50]. Treated animals have a decreased flight distance and are easier to manipulate. Animals spend more time eating and drinking compared with controls and spend less time pacing. A dose of 1 mg/kg IM has been used in most studies. Occasionally, extrapyramidal signs have been noted [49] but typically resolved without treatment [49]. A study in caribou demonstrated that zuclopenthixol acetate could be used to decrease stress and mortality during translocation [50]. In this study, three animals demonstrated side effects within 24 h of dosing (backing up when walking, rapid jaw movement, excessive pawing, panting, muscle twitches, and low head carriage). These symptoms rapidly resolved following IM administration of midazolam at a dose of 0.2 mg/kg [50].

Azaperone

This butyrophenone drug has classically been used for tranquilization of swine. It has been used in combination with α_2-adrenergic receptor agonists and opioids for anesthesia and immobilization of wild and farmed ungulates [47]. In pigs, it has a duration of approximately 6 h. Its duration of action has not been reported in wildlife species. Azaperone has been used in wild ungulates to provide tranquilization for short translocations.

Neurosteroids (alfaxalone)

Alfaxalone is a neuroactive steroid formulated in 2-hydroxypropyl-β-cyclodextrin. Alfaxalone is typically used as an induction agent or as an anesthetic agent in total IV anesthesia protocols. When administered via the IM route, it will induce dose-dependent effects ranging from sedation to anesthesia. Alfaxalone has the advantage of being useful in a wide variety of wildlife species and is often combined with other drugs to facilitate chemical restraint or light anesthesia. It has been successfully used in combination with medetomidine and azaperone to successfully immobilize wild mule deer and bighorn sheep [51,52]. The major side effects of this combination are hypoxemia and respiratory depression [51–53]. A major limitation of alfaxalone is that the current commercially available formulation has a concentration of 10 mg/mL, necessitating the use of large drug volumes that may not be suitable for remote drug delivery in some species. A novel formulation at a concentration of 40 mg/mL has been developed and effectively used in wild bighorn sheep [53]. Once it is commercially available, it should prove to be useful for immobilization of a variety of wildlife species.

Drug combinations

As stated previously, it is uncommon to use single agents for wildlife capture. Typically, agents are combined either for their synergistic immobilizing effects or to counter adverse physiologic effects of singular agents. The combination of an opioid with an α_2-adrenergic receptor agonist has already been discussed. Xylazine–ketamine has been used for many years and has the advantage of versatility (i.e., it is effective in many ungulate and carnivore species). Medetomidine–ketamine shares the versatility of xylazine–ketamine, with the advantages of decreased volume and lower ketamine requirement. Antagonism of medetomidine will likely cause fewer side effects from residual ketamine, because its dose requirement is lower [1,3,28].

Medetomidine–ketamine is useful in a wide range of species. Nevertheless, it should always be used cautiously. Its use is even avoided in bears, because sudden recoveries have been reported in brown and polar bears [29]. Xylazine–tiletamine–zolazepam and medetomidine–tiletamine–zolazepam can be delivered in small volumes and are useful in a wide range of wildlife species, as well. Antagonism of the α_2-adrenergic receptor agonist will hasten recovery. Time to sternal recumbency and standing is generally more rapid after antagonism of medetomidine compared with xylazine because of the lower dose requirement of tiletamine–zolazepam when combined with medetomidine [29–32].

The combination of butorphanol, azaperone, and medetomidine (BAM) has been used to successfully capture a variety of wild and captive species [21–26]. Sedation is reversible with atipamezole and naltrexone in combination.

Alfaxalone is typically used in combination with other drugs [51–53]. The utility of alfaxalone for wildlife capture will be increased once a more concentrated formulation becomes readily available [53].

The capture event

Precapture planning

Before undertaking any wildlife capture, an appropriate plan of action must be devised. The target species should be researched to determine the most effective and current techniques. A decision needs to be made as to the use of physical or chemical restraint. Logistical considerations are important and include establishing communication and evacuation plans. Equipment must be carefully selected for use in the field. Drug needs must be anticipated, and it is generally wise to budget for at least 50% more drug than is actually needed. This will help to offset any drug wasted from lost darts or poor dart placement.

In the immediate precapture period, the target animal is located, and weight is estimated. The terrain, weather, and other factors must be evaluated to determine whether capture should be attempted. Occasionally, the drug dart is loaded after the target animal has been located and observed; however, in most situations, it is more practical to load the darts beforehand. Drug doses may be calculated for specific sizes or age groups, and the darts are preloaded and marked accordingly. However, metal darts should not be kept loaded for longer than a 12 h period because of the possibility that corrosive action of the drugs may impair the injection mechanism. Preloaded darts with air-activated discharge mechanisms should not be pressurized because they have a tendency to lose pressure if armed for an extended period.

Generally, the animal will need to be approached to within a distance of 30–40 m for accurate dart delivery. There are many methods to facilitate approaching to within this distance. Animals may be stalked, baited, approached in a vehicle or helicopter, or trapped or snared prior to approach. Trapping has the advantage of limiting movement during the capture event, but it may prove to be more stressful than helicopter capture [11]. Pursuit of animals should generally be limited to no more than 2–5 min. The incidence of capture myopathy, hyperthermia, and trauma will increase with prolonged chase times. In management situations, pursuit may often be required until the animal is captured. It is beyond the scope of this chapter to thoroughly discuss species-specific considerations. It is advisable to include experienced personnel on the capture team and to consult with experienced wildlife managers, biologists, and veterinarians to determine anticipated complications, animal behavior when stressed, and the current approaches to dealing with the target species.

Induction

Many factors may influence induction time. These include the drug dose received, the animal's physical condition, its age and gender, and its sensitivity to the immobilizing drug. Dart placement is probably the most important determinant of induction time. To facilitate quick absorption of the drug, the muscle masses of the neck, shoulder, or hindquarter must be injected (Fig. 55.5). Animals that are excited or stressed can have induction times that are considerably longer than in calm animals.

Some animals will put on considerable fat deposits prior to denning and fasting and must be dealt with in a different manner during these periods of the year. Brown bears, for example, can generally be darted in the hindquarter when they emerge from spring dens. In the fall, these animals have considerable fat deposits overlying the rump and must be darted in the shoulder or neck. As soon as the dart is placed, the time should be recorded, and the animal must be carefully observed to ensure that it is not lost during the induction period.

The initial approach to a darted animal can be dangerous. The animal should be observed from a safe distance to determine that there is no purposeful movement. When α_2-adrenergic receptor agonist-based protocols are used (e.g., medetomidine–ketamine or xylazine–tiletamine–zolazepam), the animal's head or limbs should not move prior to approach. If tiletamine–zolazepam alone or opioids are used, there may be some involuntary movement in adequately immobilized animals.

Once it has been determined that the animal is immobilized, it should be cautiously approached accompanied by a firearm backup if necessary. It is important to leave safe exits for the capture team and the animal. To gauge the animal's response, auditory stimulation such as clapping or shouting should be employed. If there is no response to auditory stimulation, the response to tactile stimulation should be gauged. It is advisable to use a stick or pole syringe to extend reach when stimulating the animal (Fig. 55.6). When it is safe, the palpebral reflex and airway can be checked. A set of vital signs, including rectal temperature, respiratory rate, and heart rate, should be monitored. The animal's eyes can be lubricated with an ophthalmic solution or gel, and a blindfold can be placed to decrease visual stimulation. At this point, hobbles may be considered to limit movement in the event of sudden recovery in ungulates.

Monitoring and supportive care

Following capture, the animal should be positioned to avoid pressure points and ensure optimum ventilation in a recumbent animal. Carnivores may be positioned in lateral or sternal recumbency, but ruminants should be positioned in sternal recumbency whenever possible. The head and neck should be extended to maintain a patent airway. A stretcher system may be employed to facilitate movement of the animal and to keep it elevated above the ground. Vital signs should be monitored every 5–10 min. Painful procedures such as tooth extraction or biopsies should be performed soon after induction when the animal is in the deepest plane of anesthesia.

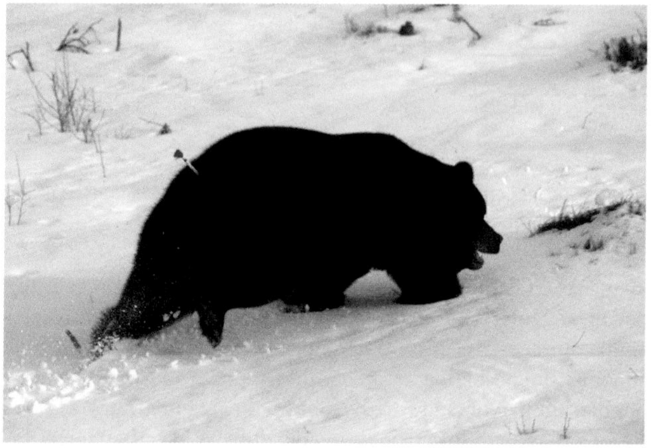

Figure 55.5 Correct dart placement in a brown bear. The dart has been placed into the well-muscled hindquarter of the bear.

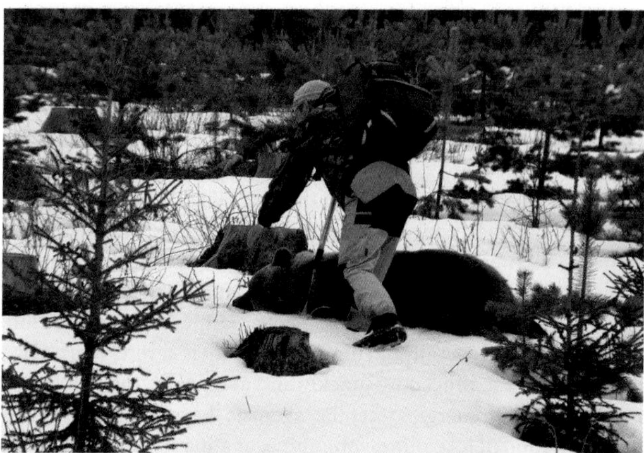

Figure 55.6 Cautious approach to a bear. It is important to extend your reach and have an escape route planned during the initial approach to dangerous wildlife.

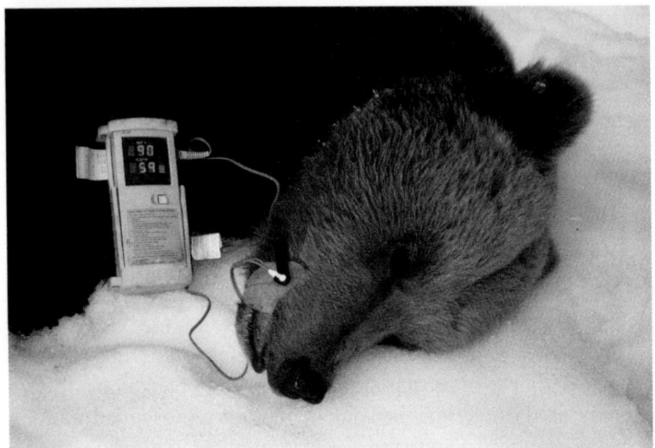

Figure 55.7 Pulse oximeter used to measure percent hemoglobin saturation in a brown bear.

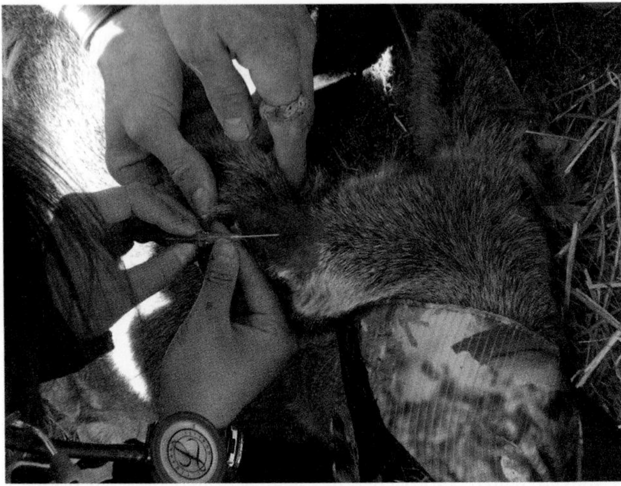

Figure 55.8 Placement of an arterial catheter into the auricular artery of a white-tailed deer.

If animals are manipulated to determine body mass, it is best to do this during a deeper plane of immobilization–anesthesia because stimulus can hasten arousal [54].

Hypoxemia is common during wildlife immobilization and anesthesia [1–6]. Hypoxemia in the face of hyperthermia is particularly serious. Hyperthermia and increased metabolic rate increase tissue oxygen demand. This can increase the risk of inducing exertional myopathy or even cause acute mortality. Hypoxemia can often be prevented or treated in the field with the administration of supplemental oxygen. The animal should ideally be monitored with a pulse oximeter. Normal hemoglobin saturation should be 95–98%. If a pulse oximeter is not available, the mucous membranes should be monitored closely for cyanosis. Severely hypoxemic animals are often tachycardic. Tachycardia followed by severe bradycardia (heart rate < 30 beats/min) is often a warning sign that hypoxemia is very severe. The occurrence of hypoxemia has been linked to prolongation of recovery times in ungulates [55,56].

Portable equipment is available to facilitate oxygen delivery. An ambulatory regulator and an aluminum D cylinder are lightweight, portable, and sturdy. They can provide a 10 L/min flow for up to 30 min. An E cylinder will provide this flow for 1 h or more. Portable oxygen concentrators have been used effectively as well. A nasal catheter can be used for insufflation in most animals. The catheter should be threaded as far as the medial canthus of the eye. The flow rate should be adjusted to maintain a saturation of greater than 95% (Fig. 55.7).

Heart rate and pulse quality should be monitored every 5–10 min. The auricular artery is easily palpated in many ungulate species but if it cannot be palpated, a femoral pulse can usually be used. Equipment is available to measure direct or indirect blood pressure and electrocardiographic status in the field (Figs. 55.8 and 55.9).

In ruminants, sternal recumbency will help to prevent ruminal tympany. If ruminal tympany is a problem, the animal may be rocked gently to stimulate eructation. A tube passed nasally or orally to the rumen can be used but may predispose to regurgitation and aspiration. Generally, if ruminal tympany is severe, it is advisable to finish the procedure quickly and antagonize the anesthetic agents. If α_2-adrenergic receptor agonists have been used, the administration of tolazoline, yohimbine, or atipamezole will help to reinitiate ruminal activity and facilitate the correction of tympany.

Rectal temperature should be monitored every 5–10 min. Ungulates are particularly prone to hyperthermia, especially after a long chase. Planning immobilization during cooler periods of the day or at cooler times of the year should be considered. A rectal temperature ≥ 2 °C greater than normal is cause for concern, and attempts should be made to cool the animal. Cold water sprayed on the animal or snow packed into the inguinal and axillary regions may help lower body temperature. A rectal temperature ≥ 3 °C greater than normal is an emergency and should be treated aggressively.

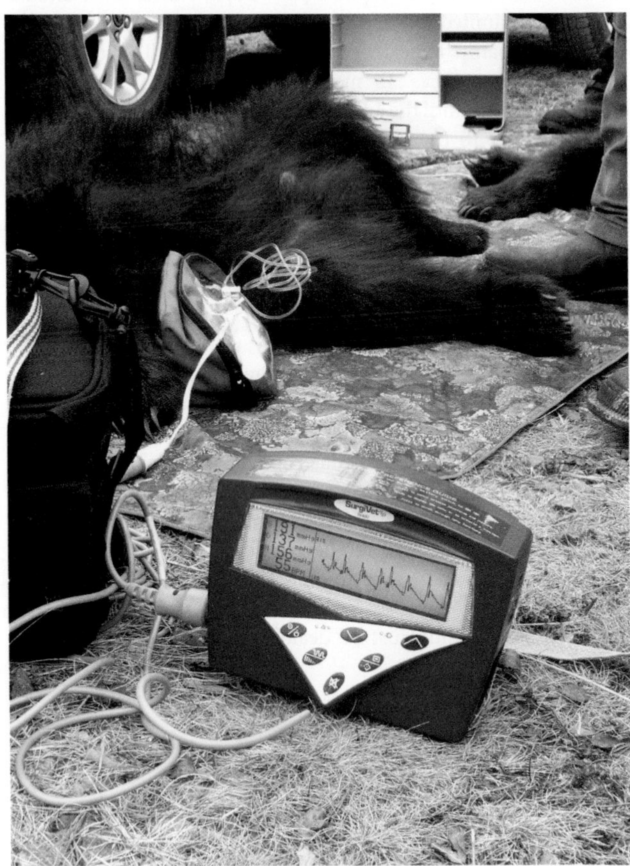

Figure 55.9 Direct pressure measurement in a brown bear. The arterial catheter has been placed in the femoral artery of the bear.

Loud noises increase the risk of sudden arousal, especially the vocalizations of distressed offspring. Other factors to consider are movement (i.e., changing the body position of a bear or location of the anesthetized animal) or degree of painful stimuli. Signs for assessing CNS depression will depend on the agent used. As drug effects lessen, spontaneous blinking will occur. Carnivores often develop chewing and paw movements. They will start to lift their head and may attempt to raise themselves with their forelimbs. Animals with significant head movement generally require a "top-up" dose of tiletamine–zolazepam or ketamine unless they are to be left to recover. Small additional doses of tiletamine–zolazepam can significantly prolong recovery and should be used only if longer than 30 min of additional immobilization is required. Ketamine is a better "top-up" choice if only 5–20 min of additional time is needed.

With xylazine–ketamine, or medetomidine–ketamine, immobilization, head lifting or limb movement signals that the animal is minimally obtunded and should not be approached or manipulated. Increased intensity of the palpebral reflex or nystagmus are generally good indicators that CNS depression is lessening. When procedures are completed, the area should be cleared of equipment, and personnel should retreat to a safe area and observe the recovery.

Recovery

Considerations for recovery vary depending on the drugs used and the circumstances at hand. If a reversible drug combination was not used, the animal should be observed until it can ambulate. The animal should be placed in a comfortable position and its airway cleared. A final set of vital signs are obtained. Typically, two people remain with the animal to administer the reversal drug(s). Antagonists are typically administered IM unless there is an immediate physiologic need for rapid IV drug reversal.

Complications related to wildlife capture

Physical trauma

During immobilization and capture, physical injuries such as contusions, lacerations, abrasions, punctures, and fractures may occur. Minor injuries can be treated successfully in the field, but fractures and other serious conditions are difficult to treat effectively and often require that the animal be euthanized.

Minor lacerations may be cleaned, treated with a topical antibiotic ointment, and protected with an insect repellant. An appropriate antibiotic may be given intramuscularly to help prevent infection. Closure may be considered for large lacerations, which should be cleaned and debrided as much as possible. These lacerations are often contaminated and, if they are closed, appropriate drainage and administration of long-acting antibiotics must be considered.

The potential for physical trauma may be reduced by taking careful notice of any hazard in the environment that may increase the likelihood of injury during capture. Traps, snares, nets, or other forms of manual restraint should be appropriate for the species and set by trained individuals.

Hyperthermia

The most immediate sign is a critical rise in rectal temperature to above 40–41 °C (depending on the species). It is important to note that rectal temperature measurement has been shown to underestimate core temperature by up to 1 °C [57]. This should be taken into consideration when deciding if hyperthermia should be treated. Symptoms of severe hyperthermia include rapid shallow breathing, panting, and weak, rapid, or irregular heart rate. Treatment includes moving the animal into shade or spraying it with cold water. Room temperature IV fluid administration and/or cold water enemas may also be indicated [38] (Fig. 55.10). Packing ice or snow around the animal in the winter may also be helpful. Antagonism of α_2-adrenergic receptor agonists should also be considered to normalize body temperature [38].

The risk of hyperthermia may be reduced by avoiding warm days, limiting activities to the coolest part of the day, avoiding prolonged pursuits, and minimizing physical restraint (Fig. 55.11).

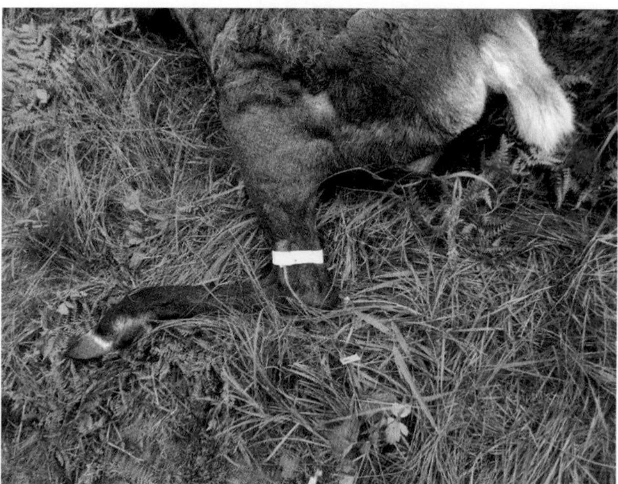

Figure 55.10 Catheter placed into the lateral saphenous vein of a mountain caribou. Venous access is recommended to facilitate intravenous fluid administration to treat hypovolemia or hyperthermia.

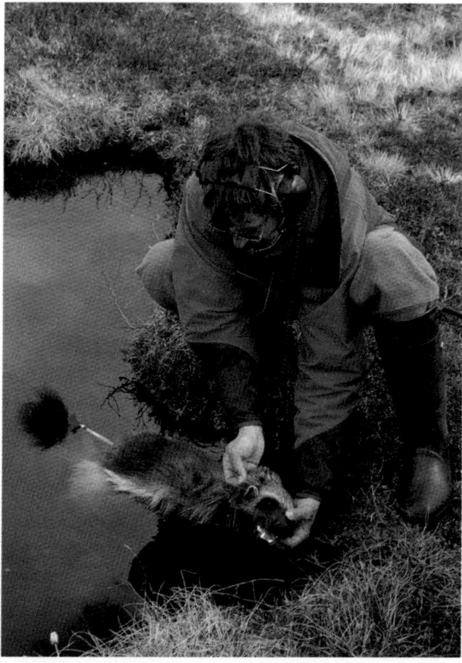

Figure 55.11 Active cooling of a hyperthermic wolverine. In a field situation, immersion in cold water can be a good option to treat severe hyperthermia in smaller wildlife species.

Hypothermia

Hypothermia is of most concern when ambient temperatures are low. It occurs most commonly in young animals, animals with small body mass, and those in poor body condition. Hypothermia is generally characterized by a rectal temperature ≥ 2 °C below normal. It may result in prolonged recovery, acidosis, coagulopathies, and arrhythmias. Supportive procedures consist of drying and covering the animal and providing external heat sources such as hot water bottles.

Exertional myopathy

Most free-ranging animals exert themselves infrequently. They are not conditioned for running at full effort over long distances. Chasing wild animals with a helicopter or motor vehicle imposes a tremendous amount of stress. The effects of sympathetic exhaustion from sustained stress combined with intense muscular exertion can cause a life-threatening syndrome known as "exertional myopathy" [3,58].

Intense sustained muscular exertion leads to the production and buildup of lactate in muscle cells and metabolic acidosis. Severe lactate accumulation may cause metabolic dysfunction or death of skeletal muscle cells, resulting in the release of intracellular potassium ions (K^+), calcium ions (Ca^{2+}), and myoglobin. High plasma concentrations of myoglobin and ultrafiltrate within the renal tubules can cause acute renal failure. Hyperkalemia and acidosis cause acute arrhythmias and circulatory failure.

Exertional myopathy is difficult to treat, so prevention is of the utmost importance. Chase time should be limited to 2 min and, if the capture effort fails, it should not be resumed for at least 1 day. In situations where several individuals from the same herd require capture (often the situation with net gunning), it is advisable to have enough handlers to capture multiple individuals at the same time rather than repeatedly stressing the herd. Visual and auditory stimulation, handling, and restraint of the captured animal should be kept to a minimum. Four common clinical syndromes of exertional myopathy have been identified: acute death syndrome, delayed peracute death syndrome, ataxic-myoglobinuric syndrome, and muscle rupture syndrome.

Respiratory depression and hypoxemia

Major causative factors include immobilizing agents (particularly potent opioids), ventilation–perfusion mismatching, and airway obstruction.

The best technique for preventing hypoventilation is endotracheal intubation and controlled ventilation with supplemental inspired oxygen. This can be difficult in field situations, however, particularly with larger animals. The partial reversal of opioids has been used to treat respiratory depression when intubation was impractical [7,27].

Hypoxemia due to hypoventilation and/or ventilation–perfusion mismatch generally responds to supplemental inspired oxygen delivery [3,8,24,55,56], although arterial CO_2 partial pressure can increase and respiratory acidemia often becomes more severe during the administration of supplemental inspired oxygen [56,59]. Other causes of acute respiratory compromise include aspiration and pneumothorax (secondary to dart penetration of the thoracic cavity). Pneumothorax requires thoracocentesis, so equipment to perform this procedure should be available if at all possible.

Capture-associated mortality

There is no doubt that the chemical immobilization of free-ranging mammals is a minimal form of veterinary anesthesia conducted under the most extreme circumstances. Anesthetic risk is influenced by the capture protocols chosen to meet the challenges unique to each species and its environment. Typically, most deaths are observed in the early phase of a large capture project before immobilization methods have been refined, drug doses have been adjusted, and team members are experienced. Moreover, an increased risk of mortality accompanies health evaluation of animals under environmental or pathogenic stress. Overall, capture mortality of free-ranging mammals can be grouped into three categories:

1. Direct effects of the immobilizing drug itself (e.g., respiratory depression, shock, hyperthermia, and asphyxia caused by tympany or vomiting)
2. Indirect effects (e.g., drowning, pneumothorax due to misplacement of darts, and trauma from dart impact) or indirect consequences of the drug used (e.g., etorphine often induces hyperthermia, which may cause the animal to seek water for cooling, with drowning as a possible sequela)
3. Secondary effects caused by the capture process itself (e.g., trauma from traps, long-term effects from chasing or stress, separation of family groups, and various problems with radio collars or implantable transmitters). Secondary effects have nothing to do with the anesthetic risk *per se* and should be treated as a separate entity.

By using immobilizing drugs and doses with proven safety, proper remote drug delivery systems, and established capture methods and techniques, an experienced capture team decreases the risk of mortality [2].

Protocols and doses

Readers are referred to the *Handbook of Wildlife Chemical Immobilization* and *Zoo Animal and Wildlife Immobilization and Anesthesia* for complete dosing information and a reference list by species [1,3]. It should be appreciated that doses required for immobilization of free-ranging animals are generally higher than those required in captive individuals [1,60]. This factor must be kept in mind when doses are planned for wildlife capture, or a relative underdose may occur. Obviously, injection site and method of drug delivery also affect dose requirements. Comparison of hand injection versus dart delivery demonstrated that 50% more drug was required when animals were darted [61]. Dart needle length also has a major impact on induction times and time to retrieval of the darted animal, with longer 40 mm needles resulting in more rapid induction when compared to 30 mm needles in ground darted fallow deer [62]. It is important to consider these factors when attempting to extrapolate doses used in captive wildlife to dose requirements in free-ranging animals.

References

1 Kreeger TJ, Arnemo JM. *Handbook of Wildlife Chemical Immobilization*, 5th edn. South Freeport, ME: Center for Wildlife Studies Press, 2018.

2 Chinnadurai SK, Strahl-Heldreth D, Fiorello CV, *et al.* Best-practice guidelines for field-based surgery and anesthesia of free-ranging wildlife. I. Anesthesia and analgesia. *J Wildl Dis* 2016; **52**: 14–27.

3 West G, Heard D, Caulkett NA, eds. *Zoo Animal and Wildlife Immobilization and Anesthesia*, 2nd edn. Ames, IA: Wiley-Blackwell, 2014.

4 Lian M, Evans AE, Beckmen KB, *et al.* Restraint and immobilization. In: Tryland M, Kutz S, eds. *Reindeer and Caribou. Health and Disease.* Boca Raton, FL: Taylor & Francis Group, 2019: 465–491.

5 Read MR. A review of alpha-2 adrenoceptor agonists and the development of hypoxemia in domestic and wild ruminants. *J Zoo Wildl Med* 2003; **34**: 134–138.

6 Lakhdhir S, Caulkett N, Duke-Novakovski T, *et al.* Evaluation of intramuscular sodium nitroprusside injection to improve oxygenation in medetomidine-alfaxalone-azaperone anesthetized white-tailed deer (*Odocoileus virginianus*). *J Vet Anaesth Analg* 2021; **48**: 65–73.

7 Buss P, Miller M, Fuller A, *et al.* Postinduction butorphanol administration alters oxygen consumption to improve blood gases in etorphine-immobilized white rhinoceros. *J Vet Anaesth Analg* 2018; **45**: 57–67.

8 Fahlman Å, Caulkett N, Arnemo JM, *et al.* Efficacy of a portable oxygen concentrator with pulsed delivery for treatment of hypoxemia during anesthesia of wildlife. *J Zoo Wildl Med* 2012; **43**: 67–76.

9 Cattet MRL, Caulkett NA, Wilson C, *et al.* Intranasal administration of xylazine to reduce stress in elk captured by net gun. *J Wildl Dis* 2004; **40**: 562–565.

10 Jessup DA, Clark RK, Weaver RA, *et al.* The safety and cost-effectiveness of net-gun capture of desert bighorn sheep (*Ovis canadensis nelsoni*). *J Zoo Anim Med* 1988; **19**: 208–213.

11 Cattet MRL, Christison K, Caulkett NA, *et al.* Physiologic responses of grizzly bears to different methods of capture. *J Wildl Dis* 2003; **39**: 649–654.

12 Smith T, Herrero S, Debruyn T, *et al.* Efficacy of bear deterrent spray in Alaska. *J Wildl Manage* 2008; **72**: 640–645.

13 Haymerle A, Fahlman Å, Walzer C. Human exposures to immobilizing agents: results of an online survey. *Vet Rec* 2010; **167**: 327–332.

14 Hoy SM, Keating GM. Dexmedetomidine: a review of its use for sedation in mechanically ventilated patients in an intensive care setting and for procedural sedation. *Drugs* 2011; **71**: 1481–1501.

15 Kallio A, Ponkilainen R, Scheinin H. Effects of dexmedetomidine, a selective alpha-2 adrenoceptor agonist on hemodynamic control mechanisms. *Clin Pharmacol Ther* 1989; **46**: 33–42.

16 Kock MD, Burroughs R, *eds. Chemical and Physical Restraint of Wild Animals. A Training and Field Manual for African Species, 2nd edn.* Greyton, South Africa: International Wildlife Veterinary Services, 2012.

17 Haigh JC. Opioids in zoological medicine. *J Zoo Wildl Med* 1990; **21**: 391–413.

18 Kreeger TJ. Xylazine-induced aspiration pneumonia in Shira's moose. *Wildl Soc Bull* 2000; **28**: 751–753.

19 Lance BR, Kenny DE. Thiafentanil oxalate (A3080) in domestic ungulate species. In: Miller RE, Fowler ME, eds. *Fowler's Zoo and Wild Animal Medicine*, vol. **7**. St. Louis, MO: Elsevier, 2012: 589–595.

20 Grobler D, Bush M, Jessup D, *et al.* Anaesthesia of gemsbok (Oryx gazelle) with a combination of A3080, medetomidine and ketamine. *J S Afr Vet Assoc* 2001; **72**: 81–83.

21 Miller BF, Osborn DA, Lance WR, *et al.* Butorphanol-azaperone-medetomidine for immobilization of captive white-tailed deer. *J Wildl Dis* 2009; **45**: 457–467.

22 Siegal-Willet JSB, Citino SB, Wade S, *et al.* Butorphanol, azaperone and medetomidine anesthesia in free-ranging white-tailed deer (*Odocoileus virginianus*) using radio transmitter darts. *J Wildl Dis* 2009; **45**: 468–480.

23 Wolfe LL, Fisher MC, Davis TR, *et al.* Efficacy of a low-dosage combination of butorphanol, azaperone, and medetomidine (BAM) to immobilize Rocky Mountain elk. *J Wildl Dis* 2014; **50**: 676–680.

24 Mich PH, Wolfe LL, Sirochman TM, *et al.* Evaluation of intramuscular butorphanol, azaperone, and medetomidine and nasal oxygen insufflation for the chemical immobilization of white-tailed deer (*Odocoilius virginianus*). *J Zoo Wildl Med* 2008; **39**: 480–487.

25 Harms JN, Jung TS, Hallock M, *et al.* Efficacy of a butorphanol, azaperone, and medetomidine combination for helicopter-based immobilization of bison (*Bison bison*). *J Wildl Dis* 2018; **54**: 819–824.

26 Williamson RH, Muller LI, Blair CD. The use of xylazine-ketamine or butorphanol-azaperone-medetomidine to immobilize American black bears (*Ursus americanus*). *J Wildl Dis* 2018; **54**: 503–510.

27 Miller M, Buss P, Joubert J, *et al.* Use of butorphanol during immobilization of free-ranging white rhinoceros (*Ceratotherium simum*). *J Zoo Wildl Med* 2013; **44**: 55–61.

28 Jalanka HH, Roeken BO. The use of medetomidine, medetomidine-ketamine combinations, and atipamezole in nondomestic mammals: a review. *J Zoo Wildl Med* 1990; **21**: 259–282.

29 Cattet MRL, Caulkett NA, Polischuk SC, *et al.* Anesthesia of polar bears with zolazepam-tiletamine, medetomidine-ketamine, and medetomidine-zolazepam-tiletamine. *J Zoo Wildl Med* 1999; **30**: 354–360.

30 Caulkett NA, Cattet MRL, Caulkett JM, *et al.* Comparative physiological effects of Telazol, medetomidine-ketamine, and medetomidine-Telazol in polar bears (*Ursus maritimus*). *J Zoo Wildl Med* 1999; **30**: 504–509.

31 Cattet MRL, Caulkett NA, Lunn NJ. Anesthesia of polar bears using xylazine-zolazepam- tiletamine or zolazepam-tiletamine. *J Wildl Dis* 2003; **39**: 655–664.

32 Cattet MRL, Caulkett NA, Stenhouse GB. Anesthesia of grizzly bears using xylazine- zolazepam-tiletamine or zolazepam-tiletamine. *Ursus* 2003; **14**: 88–93.

33 Schobert E. Telazol use in wild and exotic animals. *Vet Med* 1987; **82**: 1080–1088.

34 Murray SSL, Monfort SL, Ware L, *et al.* Anesthesia in female white-tailed deer using Telazol and xylazine. *J Wildl Dis* 2000; **36**: 670–675.

35 Caulkett NA, Cattet MRL, Cantwell S, *et al.* Anesthesia of wood bison with medetomidine-Telazol and xylazine-Telazol combinations. *Can Vet J* 2000; **41**: 49–53.

36 Millspaugh JJ, Brundige GC, Jenks JA, *et al.* Immobilization of Rocky Mountain elk with Telazol and xylazine hydrochloride, and antagonism by yohimbine hydrochloride. *J Wildl Dis* 1995; **31**: 259–262.

37 Caulkett NA, Cattet MRL. Physiological effects of medetomidine-zolazepam-tiletamine immobilization in black bears (*Ursus americanus*). *J Wildl Dis* 1997; **33**: 618–622.

38 Ozeki LM, Caulkett N, Stenhouse G, *et al.* Effect of active cooling and alpha-2 adrenoceptor antagonism on core temperature in anesthetized brown bears (*Ursus arctos*). *J Zoo Wildl Med* 2015; **46**: 279–285.

39 Kock MD, Morkel P, Atkinson M, *et al.* Chemical immobilization of free-ranging white rhinoceros (*Ceratotherium simum simum*) in Hwange and Matobo National Parks, Zimbabwe, using combinations of etorphine (M99), fentanyl, xylazine and detomidine. *J Zoo Wildl Med* 1995; **26**: 207–219.

40 Klein L, Citino SB. Comparison of detomidine/carfentanil/ketamine and medetomidine/ ketamine anesthesia in Grevy's zebra. In: *Proceedings of the Joint Conference of the American Association of Zoo Veterinarians, Wildlife Disease Association, and American Association of Wildlife Veterinarians*, East Lansing, MI: 1995: 290–293.

41 Caulkett NA, Duke T, Cribb PH. Cardiopulmonary effects of medetomidine-ketamine in domestic sheep (*Ovis ovis*) maintained in sternal recumbency. *J Zoo Wildl Med* 1996; **27**: 217–226.

42 Fandos Esteruelas N, Cattet M, Zedrosser A, *et al.* A double-blinded, randomized comparison of medetomidine-tiletamine-zolazepam and dexmedetomidine-tiletamine-zolazepam in free-ranging brown bears (*Ursus arctos*). *PLoS ONE* 2017; **12**: e0170764.

43 Einwaller J, Painer J, Raekallio M, *et al.* Cardiovascular effects of intravenous vatinoxan (MK-467) in medetomidine–tiletamine–zolazepam anaesthetised red deer (*Cervus elaphus*). *J Vet Anaesth Analg* 2020; **47**: 518–527.

44 Ebedes H. The use of long-acting tranquilizers in captive wild animals. In: McKenzie A, ed. *The Capture and Care Manual: Capture, Care, Accommodation and Transportation of Wild African Animals.* Pretoria, South Africa: Wildlife Decision Services and the South African Veterinary Foundation, 1993: 71–99.

45 Diverio S, Goddard PJ, Gordon IJ, *et al.* The effect of management practices on stress in farmed red deer (*Cervus elaphus*) and its modulation by long-acting neuroleptics: behavioural responses. *Appl Anim Behav Sci* 1993; **36**: 363–376.

46 Atkinson MW, Blumer ES. The use of a long-acting neuroleptic in the Mongolian wild horse (*Equus przewalskii przewalskii*) to facilitate the establishment of a bachelor herd. In: *Proceedings of the Annual Meeting of the American Association of Zoo Veterinarians*, Houston, TX, 1997: 199–200.

47 Shury TK. Use of azaperone with zuclopenthixol acetate for tranquilization of free ranging wood bison and immobilization with carfentanil and xylazine. In: *Proceedings of the Annual Meeting of the American Association of Zoo Veterinarians*, Omaha, NE: 1998: 408–409.

48 Clippinger TL, Citino SB, Wade S. Behavioral and physiologic response to an intermediate- acting tranquilizer, zuclopenthixol, in captive Nile lechwe (*Kobus megaceros*). In: *Proceedings of the Annual Meeting of the American Association of Zoo Veterinarians*, Omaha, NE: 1998: 38–40.

49 Read M, Caulkett N, McCallister M. Evaluation of zuclopenthixol acetate to decrease handling stress in wapiti. *J Wildl Dis* 2000; **36**: 450–459.

50 Slater O, Backwell A, Cook R, *et al.* The use of a long-acting tranquilizer (*zuclopenthixol acetate*) and live video monitoring for successful long-distance transport of caribou (*Rangifer tarandus*). *Rangifer* 2021; **41**: 13–26.

51 Mathieu A, Caulkett N, Stent PM, *et al.* Capture of free-ranging mule deer (*Odocoileus hemonius*) with a combination of medetomidine-azaperone and alfaxalone. *J Wildl Dis* 2017; **53**: 296–303.

52 Williams M, Caulkett N, Neuhaus P, *et al.* Comparison of the efficacy and safety of medetomidine-ketamine versus medetomidine-alfaxalone-azaparone combination in free-ranging Rocky Mountain Bighorn Sheep (*Ovis Canadensis*). *J Zoo Wildl Med* 2018; **49**: 662–670.

53 Patterson M, Caulkett N, Neuhaus P, *et al.* The utility of a novel formulation of alfaxalone in a remote delivery system. *J Vet Anaesth Analg* 2021; **48**: 537–540.

54 Cattet MRL, Caulkett NA, Streib KA, *et al.* Cardiopulmonary response of anesthetized polar bears to suspension by net and sling. *J Wildl Dis* 1999; **35**: 548–556.

55 Risling TE, Fahlman Å, Caulkett NA, *et al.* Physiological and behavioral effects of hypoxemia in reindeer immobilized with xylazine-etorphine. *Anim Prod Science* 2011; **51**: 1–4.

56 Paterson JM, Caulkett NA, Woodbury MR. Physiologic effects of nasal oxygen or medical air administered prior to and during carfentanil-xylazine anesthesia in North American elk (*Cervus canadensis manitobensis*). *J Zoo Wildl Med* 2009; **40**: 39–50.

57 Ozeki L, Fahlman A, Stenhouse G, *et al.* Evaluation of the accuracy of different methods of monitoring body temperature in anesthetized brown bears (*Ursus arctos*). *J Zoo Wildl Med* 2014; **45**: 819–824.

58 Breed D, Meyer L, Steyl J, *et al.* Conserving wildlife in a changing world: understanding capture myopathy – a malignant outcome of stress during capture and translocation. *Conserv Physiol* 2019; **7**: coz027.
59 Lian M, Björck S, Arnemo J, *et al.* Severe hypoxemia in muskoxen (*Ovibos moschatus*) immobilized with etorphine and xylazine corrected with supplemental nasal oxygen. *J Wildl Dis* 2017; **53**: 356–360.
60 Heard DJ. Chemical immobilization of felids, ursids, and small ungulates. *Vet Clin North Am Exot Anim Pract* 2001; **4**: 267–298.
61 Ryeng KA, Arnemo JM, Larsen S. Determination of optimal immobilizing doses of a medetomidine hydrochloride and ketamine hydrochloride combination in captive reindeer. *Am J Vet Res* 2001; **62**: 119–126.
62 Bergvall UA, Kjellander P, Ahlqvist P, *et al.* Chemical immobilization of free-ranging fallow deer (*Dama dama*): effect of needle length on induction time. *J Wildl Dis* 2015; **51**: 484–487.

56 Comparative Anesthesia and Analgesia – Marine Mammals

Julie A. Balko[1] and James E. Bailey[2]

[1]Department of Molecular Biomedical Sciences, College of Veterinary Medicine, North Carolina State University, Raleigh, North Carolina, USA
[2]Innovative Veterinary Medicine, Inc., Ponte Vedra, Florida, USA

Chapter contents

Introduction, 1091
Breathing, sleep, and ventilation, 1092
  Breathing, 1092
  Sleep, 1093
  Ventilation, 1093
Preanesthetic assessment and planning, 1095
Protocol selection, 1097
  Sedation and anesthesia, 1097
  Cetacean anesthesia, 1098
  Pinniped anesthesia, 1098
  Sirenian anesthesia, 1099
Vascular access, 1099
  Cetacean vascular access, 1099
  Pinniped vascular access, 1101
  Manatee vascular access, 1102
Airway management, 1102
  Cetacean intubation, 1103
  Pinniped intubation, 1104
  Manatee intubation, 1104
Monitoring and support, 1105
Dive reflex, 1106
Anesthetic recovery, 1106
Acknowledgment, 1107
References, 1107

Introduction

Marine mammals are a diverse group of mammals that have evolved physically and physiologically to survive and thrive in varied marine environments, often at extremes of temperature, water depth, and pressure, and in limited daylight. Marine mammals are classified into four different taxonomic groups: cetaceans (whales, dolphins, and porpoises), pinnipeds (seals, sea lions, and walruses), sirenians (manatees and dugongs), and marine fissipeds (polar bears and sea otters). Anesthetic considerations for fissipeds (carnivorous mammals with separated toes) are discussed elsewhere.

The ancestors of Cetacea developed on land, returning to the water 55 million years ago to evolve anatomically, physiologically, and behaviorally for a completely aquatic existence today [1]. Most clinical experience has been with the bottlenose dolphin (*Tursiops truncatus, Tursiops truncatus gilli*, and *Tursiops truncatus aduncus*), the most common cetacean managed in research, exhibit, and rehabilitation facilities. Other odontocete species have also been successfully managed in zoos and aquaria for many years, including killer whales (*Orcinus orca*), beluga or white whales (*Delphinapterus leucas*), Pacific white-sided dolphins (*Lagenorhynchus obliquidens*), false killer whales (*Pseudorca crassidens*), rough-toothed dolphins (*Steno bredanensis*), as well as several hybrid delphinoid species [2,3]. With increasing longevity in managed care, dolphins 50 years of age or older are not uncommon, with a median age of 32.0 years versus 19.9 years in free-ranging counterparts, demonstrating the overall health of managed care populations [4,5].

Pinnipeds are aquatic, carnivorous marine mammals with streamlined torpedo-shaped bodies, and limbs modified into flippers (pinniped meaning "feather" or "wing"-footed). The living representatives of the order Pinnipedia include three families: Phocidae, the earless or "true" seals, Otariidae, the eared seals (fur seals and sea lions), and Odobenidae, the tusked seals (walruses). Pinnipeds are quite variable in body conformation with head-to-tail lengths ranging from 1.5 m to 6.5 m and body weights ranging from 35 to 3500 kg. Most clinical experience has been with the harbor seal (*Phoca vitulina*), the California sea lion (*Zalophus californianus*), and Pacific walrus (*Odobenus rosmarus divergens*), as these are the most common species in managed populations [6]. Fortunately, these species are not at conservation risk, and most pinnipeds in captivity are not captured from the wild, but rather the result of managed care breeding programs [7]. Many other pinnipeds species have been successfully managed in zoos and aquaria as part of conservation efforts, including gray seals, harp seals, Hawaiian monk seals, Stellar sea lions, and Atlantic walruses, to name a few. Unfortunately, anesthetic expertise is lacking for the many other species that will likely require conservation measures in the future.

Sirenians, commonly called "sea cows," are fully aquatic marine mammals comprised of three species of manatees (Trichechidae) and one species of dugong (Dugongidae), distributed throughout fresh, brackish, and marine tropical waters of North and South America, Africa, and Australia [8,9]. These hindgut fermenters,

Veterinary Anesthesia and Analgesia: The Sixth Edition of Lumb and Jones. Edited by Leigh Lamont, Kurt Grimm, Sheilah Robertson, Lydia Love and Carrie Schroeder.
© 2024 John Wiley & Sons, Inc. Published 2024 by John Wiley & Sons, Inc.
Companion website: www.wiley.com/go/lamont/anesthesia

genetically related to elephants, are the sole obligate herbivores of the marine mammal world, although they have been observed to ingest invertebrates [10]. Sirenians are currently listed internationally as vulnerable or threatened, with some species considered endangered [9–13]. Habitat loss, natural disease, and human interaction mishaps (e.g., boat strikes) have resulted in this state of duress for the species and have, at times, necessitated advanced surgical and anesthetic intervention.

Advancements in medical and surgical interventions for managed marine mammals have necessitated increasingly frequent application of sedation and general anesthesia in this cohort. While this has improved the longevity and well-being of this mature and relatively closed population, it has also resulted in a growing amount of clinical anesthesia experience. As these techniques develop and translate to application in a field setting, free-living marine mammals too will benefit.

Breathing, sleep, and ventilation

As the 1956 Nobel laureate in Medicine, Dr. Dickenson Richards, once said, "Breathing is truly a strange phenomenon of life, caught midway between the conscious and the unconscious, and peculiarly sensitive to both" [14]. Too often, anesthesia textbooks are dedicated to drug combinations and protocols rather than understanding the consequences of those choices and the management of expected (and unexpected) physiologic fallout. Of particular importance to marine mammal species is an understanding of the influence of drug choices on breathing and ventilation.

Breathing

Pinnipeds, cetaceans, and sirenians have an apneustic breathing pattern; the normal conscious breathing pattern of many marine mammals involves exhalation followed immediately by inhalation and a breath-hold or apneustic interval. The rhythm for breathing is generated by a complex neural network in the brainstem involving both excitatory and inhibitory circuits. The medulla oblongata is the lower half of the brainstem and contains the dorsal and ventral respiratory groups. *In vivo* and *in vitro* experiments suggest a site in the rostral ventrolateral medulla, the preBötzinger Complex (preBötC), as the site of excitatory neurons both driving inspiration and generating the respiratory pattern [15,16]. Expiratory activity is regulated primarily by the Bötzinger complex (BötC), also located in the rostral ventrolateral medulla; in contrast, it contains mostly inhibitory neurons. The BötC has direct projections to and from the preBötC. The retrotrapezoid nucleus (RTN) of the central respiratory network, which has direct connection to the BötC, contains pH-sensitive neurons. These neurons express the transcription factor paired-like homeobox 2B (Phox2B); subjects with naturally occurring or induced mutations of Phox2B do not respond to CO_2 or the pH change induced by CO_2 [17]. As such, these Phox2B-expressing neurons are fundamental to the generation and coordination of inspiration and expiration related to chemosensory control of breathing. Although the overall central respiratory network is far more complex than described here, it should be clear that perturbations of the function of this network severely disrupt breathing.

Inhalation anesthetic agents alter the folding, localization, and aggregation of the Phox2B protein structure, thus affecting its ability to trigger breathing in response to rising blood CO_2 concentrations [18,19]. Phox2B has been identified in the medulla of a wide variety of species [20,21], but it is theorized that the degree of expression, intrinsic functionality, degree of protein structural change, and localization when exposed to anesthetic agents may vary by species. As a result, this may alter each species' CO_2 responsiveness during equipotent anesthetic exposure.

Inhalation anesthetic agents produce dose-dependent depression of respiration, with a decrease in responsiveness to blood CO_2 concentrations as the anesthetic concentration rises; this appears to relate to RTN responsiveness to changes in CO_2 (or associated pH changes) [22]. This depression varies with species and clinically appears to follow the trend: human ~ canid < equid < otariid < phocid ~ cetacean [23]. The shift in the response to CO_2 is such that, anecdotally, anesthetized otariids will not spontaneously ventilate until the arterial partial pressure of CO_2 ($PaCO_2$) is 60–80 mmHg. This appears even more pronounced in phocids, cetaceans, and sirenians, which are unlikely to spontaneously ventilate at equipotent levels of anesthetic exposure, even when the $PaCO_2$ rises to the point of becoming anesthetic itself ($PaCO_2 \geq$ 90–95 mmHg). Additionally, these species are likely to be apneic at light planes of anesthesia, where even gross purposeful movement may be evident.

It has long been recognized that exogenously administered opioids are potent depressants of ventilation [24]. This is the result of a number of mechanisms, mainly activation of μ-opioid receptors at multiple neuronal sites including BötC, preBötC, and other locations within the central respiratory network. The end result is decreased respiratory rate, tidal volume, and response to hypercapnia and hypoxemia, as well as loss of upper airway control (i.e., swallowing and prevention of aspiration); these effects are reversible with μ-opioid receptor antagonists [25,26]. Interestingly, the respiratory depression of inhalation anesthetic agents is, at least in part, due to the influence of endogenous opioids [26]. As marine mammal species are anecdotally sensitive to opioids and prone to respiratory depression, further investigation of the endogenous opioid systems (β-endorphins, enkephalins, and dynorphins) and their receptors (μ or MOR, δ or DOR, and κ or KOR) is warranted.

γ-Aminobutyric acid (GABA) is the most abundant inhibitory neurotransmitter in the mammalian central nervous system (CNS) with $GABA_A$ receptors distributed throughout cortical and subcortical areas. Considering its bounty, the receptor's importance to memory, awareness, and consciousness becomes evident. Generally speaking, most modern anesthetic agents enhance the function of GABA and $GABA_A$ receptors which is important to anesthesia and emergence [27,28]. $GABA_A$ receptors are also present in the preBötC and stimulation can depress breathing, in part explaining the respiratory depressive effects of GABA agonist anesthetic drugs seen in some species [29]. Similar to terrestrial mammals, this effect appears to be both rate- and dose-dependent in many marine mammal species, and overly rapid delivery of most modern anesthetic agents may cause apnea prior to sufficient relaxation of the jaw and upper airway, complicating intubation.

Not all anesthetic agents exert their effect through action on GABA and $GABA_A$ receptors. While ketamine possesses some GABA effects, it primarily acts through the *N*-methyl-D-aspartate (NMDA) glutamate receptors. Clinically, ketamine commonly alters the respiratory pattern, but infrequently interrupts spontaneous breathing at clinically relevant dosages. Ketamine has been successfully used to induce anesthesia of pinnipeds, mainly in free-ranging settings. However, it has rarely been used in cetaceans and sirenians [30,31]; this is likely due to historical investigators' needs to emulate sleep, as ketamine enhances cortical cholinergic tone and alters electroencephalographic (EEG) activity, interfering with sleep studies.

As ketamine likely produces less respiratory depression than opioids in marine mammals and modulates pain through NMDA glutamate receptor inhibition, it remains a candidate for further investigation in marine mammals.

To summarize, anesthetic agents depress the adequacy of spontaneous, involuntary ventilation in marine mammals, and even subanesthetic dosages may cause significant respiratory depression or apnea, especially in phocids, cetaceans, and sirenians.

Sleep

Biologists and veterinarians have long been fascinated by the interplay of sleep and breathing in fully aquatic mammals. *Sleep* might be simply defined as a state of immobility that is rapidly reversible and is best conducted in a place perceived as comfortable and safe. The superficial appearance of sleep and anesthesia led many investigators to equate drug-induced unconsciousness with sleep; however, significant differences between the two states exist. Sleep involves the brainstem and frontal lobe function, while anesthetic drugs, such as propofol, have widespread or global influence on the brain [32]. In the 1960s, John Lilly observed that bottlenose dolphins slept with one eye open [33]. While he never produced any EEGs to support this hypothesis, he proposed from these observations what we now know as unihemispheric sleep. Unfortunately, he also misinterpreted barbiturate-induced respiratory depression as the absence of involuntary breathing in cetaceans, leading to death [34]. Misinformed and misguided, many still reference Lilly believing that dolphins only breathe voluntarily, only undergo unihemispheric sleep, and must "wake" for every breath. Instead, the existing literature supports the conclusion that ventilation in marine mammals is automatic or involuntary, albeit sensitive to anesthetic drugs, and marine mammals are capable of bihemispheric sleep in the aquatic environment.

Bihemispheric (both cerebral hemispheres) slow-wave sleep is the traditional sleep pattern of most mammals in which both eyes are shut and both halves of the brain are simultaneously unconscious. In contrast, unihemispheric slow-wave sleep is a sleep pattern in which one-half of the brain is at rest while the other half remains vigilant. The concept of sleep, breathing, thermoregulation, and vigilance while in action was first described in birds "on the wing" [35] and has since been documented in marine mammals. In the 1970s, Serafetinides reported the first EEG evidence of unihemispheric sleep in cetaceans using subcutaneous needle electrodes in a pilot whale (*Globicephala scammoni*) [36]. Mukhametov used screw electrodes that allowed a degree of free movement around a small, shallow pool to record EEG readings of multiple, isolated dolphins over 24-h periods [37,38]. These dolphins demonstrated that the vast majority of their slow waves were unihemispheric (with the contralateral eye held open), appearing first in one hemisphere and then the other. Remarkably, each hemisphere appeared to accumulate a separate sleep debt and when deprived of slow-wave sleep for several days, only that hemisphere showed the typical sleep rebound; the non-deprived hemisphere continued to alternate its slow-wave sleep in the usual amount [39]. Using a small implantable telemetry unit, Ridgway replicated these earlier unihemispheric EEG findings and also recorded symmetrical EEG readings in both hemispheres during anesthesia and the recovery period after thiopental and halothane [40]. Short periods of EEG slow waves were identified days later in both hemispheres in the unanesthetized state.

Pinnipeds can sleep on land and in water, with species differences in time spent sleeping in the water. Pinnipeds demonstrate a slower respiratory frequency when in water and when compared with terrestrial mammals of similar size [41]. Respiration during sleep, both in the water and on land, has been examined in a number of pinniped species including the gray seal, walrus, northern fur seal, southern sea lion, northern elephant seals, and Caspian seals [38,42–49]. The first variant of sleep in pinnipeds, and the predominant pattern for pinniped sleep studied on land, is bilaterally symmetrical slow-wave sleep (BSWS) and rapid eye movement (REM) sleep, similar to that observed in terrestrial mammals [45,47]. The second pattern is characterized by a striking interhemispheric EEG asymmetry during slow-wave sleep (SWS) and a very small amount of REM sleep. This pattern is recorded when fur seals sleep in water and is somewhat similar to cetacean unihemispheric slow-wave sleep [36–40,50]. Sleep varies significantly between otariids and phocids; for example, respiratory pauses increase significantly during sleep of some phocids (e.g., ringed seal) [51]. Generally speaking, it has been theorized these differences relate to their respective ecological niches or range of living conditions.

Although previous reports in the Antillean manatee (*Trichechus manatus manatus*) demonstrated bilateral δ waves with no unihemispheric sleep, a later study in a separate species, the Amazonian manatee (*Trichechus inunguis*) using EEG readings collected over a longer period of time (5 days) demonstrated a different pattern [52]. That is, unihemispheric slow waves occupied approximately one-quarter of all waves, and bihemispheric slow waves characterized the majority of sleep. Sleep was characterized by short arousals for the act of respiration, followed by a rapid return to sleep during respiratory pauses. Overall, results demonstrated a circadian rhythm for sleep and wakefulness, and similar slow-wave sleep to that evident in other aquatic species.

In humans, home methods have been developed to study sleep as laboratory settings are uncomfortable and produce a barrier to accurate study [53]. Unfortunately, historic marine mammal laboratory sleep studies were often performed in wild-caught subjects which were minimally acclimated, held in isolation in a very restricted space, had surgically implanted wires, and were frequently under the influence of barbiturates, benzodiazepines, or propofol to induce a "sleeplike" state. Even in these suboptimal conditions, marine mammal subjects clearly demonstrated bihemispheric and slow-wave sleep for a portion of the time and none experienced respiratory arrest.

In short, marine mammals are capable of both unihemispheric and bihemispheric sleep and appear to be involuntary breathers that can bring breathing under voluntary control as needed, similar to terrestrial mammals. Unihemispheric sleep affords them the benefits of sleep, breathing, thermoregulation, and vigilance while remaining in their aquatic environment.

Ventilation

Unfortunately, there is limited evidence-based data on the respiratory mechanics of anesthetized marine mammals. The elastic properties of excised lungs of marine mammals have been examined and the static inflation and deflation, pressure–volume curves have been measured. Inflation curves of excised dolphin and sea lion lungs were similar to dog lungs [54–56]. However, the deflation curves for the dolphin demonstrated greater recoil with smaller residual volumes compared with terrestrial mammals [54,57]. This may be due to the greater abundance of elastic fibers and muscle in the supportive tissue of the lung and conducting airways in the dolphin; however, possible biochemical differences must still be examined. Pulmonary morphology and mechanics of actively breathing dolphins have been reviewed [58], but data on the mechanics of ventilation for the unconscious and anesthetized dolphin remains unstudied.

In general, there is a tendency for the lungs and chest wall of mammals to return to their original shape after being inflated mechanically, secondary to elastance. For air to flow into the lungs, the elastic resistance of the lungs and the chest wall must be overcome. This elastic impedance of the lungs and chest wall is additive. The inverse of elastance is compliance, or the ease with which the chest wall and lungs are distended. When the chest wall and lungs are very stiff and resist expansion (low compliance), there is a greater tendency for the lungs and thorax to collapse, and extra work is necessary to deliver a normal volume of air to the apneic patient when using a mechanical ventilator. In marine mammals, the extensive cartilaginous reinforcement of the airways from the trachea to the level of the alveolar sac (respiratory bronchioles are absent) should allow higher flow rates and faster gas exchange during the brief surface intervals of these animals [56]; however, this also contributes to elastic recoil and alters total compliance in the anesthetized, mechanically ventilated animal. This overall elastic recoil is so profound that it is the sole driving force for expiration in the surfacing pilot whale [59]. Others have recently noted that the chest wall of larger marine mammals appears to be much less compliant than terrestrial large animals [54,60]. Although studies are needed to confirm these observations of low total compliance, low compliance is particularly evident in anesthetized dolphins when out of water (beached). Specific respiratory mechanical data of unconscious marine mammals, in both beached and neutral buoyant states, is needed. It is theorized that total compliance will be significantly increased where large marine mammals, particularly cetaceans, can be maintained near-neutral buoyant under anesthesia, such as applied in the past [61]. Investigations into methods of neutral buoyant (simulated microgravity) anesthesia are underway.

Controlled mechanical ventilation (CMV) is the mechanical ventilation method available on nearly all veterinary anesthesia ventilators. It has often been treated as merely a convenience, taking the place of squeezing the anesthetic reservoir bag by hand to deliver a breath. However, new modes of ventilation, previously used only in intensive care units, are becoming available not only to mechanically ventilate the anesthetized patient, but to be used as therapeutic tools. The conventional CMV mode begins the ventilator cycle at a baseline (ambient) airway pressure and elevates it to deliver a resultant tidal volume (Fig. 56.1). Disadvantages of CMV include the need for application of relatively high peak inspiratory pressures (PIP) compared with other ventilation methods. This may lead to reduced venous return and cardiac output, and poor distribution of inspired gas flow with subsequent development of atelectasis and ventilation–perfusion mismatch. The addition of extrinsic positive end-expiratory pressure (PEEP) to CMV in an attempt to reopen small airways and collapsed alveoli has been applied to large animal patients, but has proven minimally effective except at very high pressures that consequently significantly reduce cardiac output [62]. Early research in dolphins attempted to overcome the inadequacy of CMV for dolphin anesthesia by mimicking the normal respiratory pattern of dolphins with apneustic plateau ventilation (APV) [61,63–69]. With this mode, a prolonged inspiratory pause (apneustic plateau) is used and airway pressures then return to ambient pressure (0 cmH_2O) at the end of expiration. Though a significant improvement in ventilation methodology, APV still failed to mitigate the development of significant atelectasis by allowing excessive time for lung deflation at ambient pressure [66].

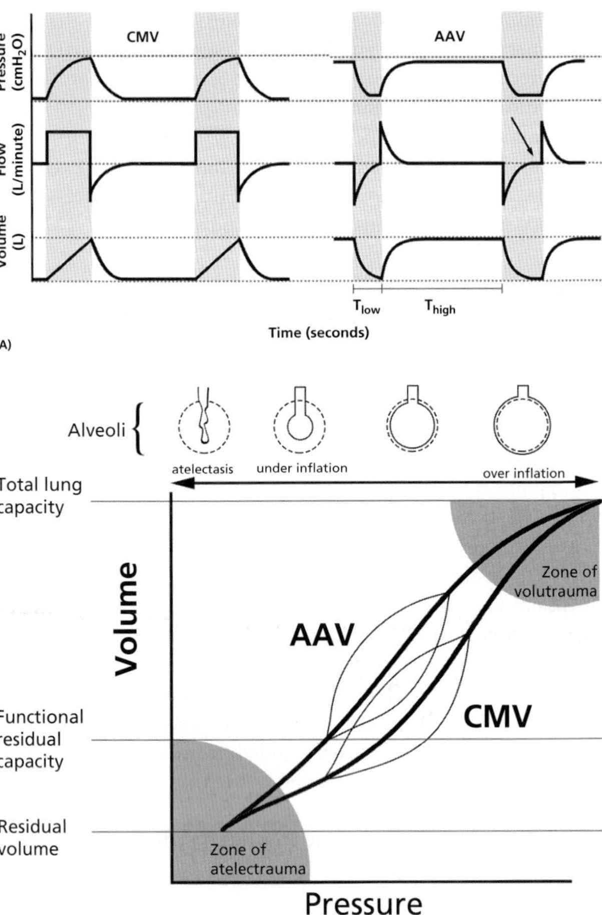

Figure 56.1 **A.** Schematic idealized illustrations of observed pressure, flow, and volume versus time waveforms for controlled mechanical ventilation (CMV) and apneustic anesthesia ventilation (AAV). The gray background indicates periods of tidal ventilation corresponding to inspiratory time during CMV and the time (T_{low}) at the low-pressure setting (P_{low}) during AAV. The white background indicates expiratory time during CMV and the time (T_{high}) of applied high pressure (P_{high}) during AAV. CMV intermittently raises pressure from ambient to peak inspiratory pressure with most of the cycle time spent at ambient pressure. AAV intermittently releases pressure from P_{high} to P_{low} to preserve lung volume. Importantly, the duration of each AAV release (T_{low}) is limited to prevent expiratory flow stagnation (i.e., an expiratory flow of zero). Above, the first AAV release illustrates proper limitation of release time whereas the second illustrates excessively long release time with flow stagnation (arrow). **B.** Theoretical schematic illustration of dynamic pressure–volume curves (thin lines) for controlled mechanical ventilation (CMV) and apneustic anesthesia ventilation (AAV) superimposed on individual pressure–volume curves (bold lines) for the respiratory system. AAV was designed to preserve lung architecture and compliance in the anesthetized human by periodically releasing airway pressure from a high to low level while maintaining lung volume at or above functional residual capacity (FRC). By contrast, CMV ventilates the lung from below FRC leading to the development of atelectasis, shifting of the pressure–volume curve to the right, and lower compliance. In this scenario, higher pressures are required during CMV to achieve the same tidal volume. Source: Dr. James Bailey, Innovative Veterinary Medicine Inc., 2023; with permission.

Unlike CMV, airway pressure release ventilation (APRV) employs an elevated baseline pressure followed by a drop in airway pressure to accomplish tidal ventilation. As first described in 1987, APRV involves continuous positive airway pressure (CPAP) with an intermittent pressure release phase [70,71]. More specifically, APRV is better described as applying continuous airway pressure (P_{high}) identical to CPAP to maintain adequate lung volume and promote alveolar recruitment, with a time-cycled release phase to a lower pressure (P_{low}) very transiently. Mechanically, this is not too dissimilar from the early APV mode used on dolphins, however, APV uses a P_{low} of 0 cmH_2O and time sufficient for alveoli to collapse. APRV was developed to maintain functional residual capacity (FRC, the volume of gas remaining in the lung after a normal expiration) at a level that would optimize gas exchange and lung compliance in the spontaneously ventilating patient in respiratory failure. Unfortunately, when APRV is applied to the unconscious, non-spontaneously ventilating patient (e.g., marine mammals), it allows lung volume to drop below FRC and may promote the development of atelectasis.

Apneustic anesthesia ventilation (AAV) was developed to maintain lung volume at a level slightly greater than FRC. In this mode of ventilation, tidal ventilation occurs when airway pressure is transiently reduced from P_{high} (CPAP) to P_{low} (the release pressure), allowing lung volume to decrease to no lower than FRC and supporting partial inflation of alveoli (Fig. 56.1). Immediate reapplication of P_{high} leads to the alveoli remaining partially inflated (at a volume above FRC) prior to the lung volume increase. This intermittent pressure release and reapplication permits tidal breathing to occur without allowing development of atelectasis. Target P_{high} and P_{low} are determined by optimizing compliance and the desired tidal volume. Note that mechanically, AAV and APV modes of ventilation are similar. However, the key distinction is that exhalation to lower airway pressures for a longer duration during APV can result in atelectasis, decreased compliance, derangement of ventilation and perfusion (V/Q mismatch), and hypoxemia. During AAV application, V/Q matching is maintained at baseline levels in anesthetized patients, and lung mechanics are normalized [72–74]. Of note, published studies in horses indicate AAV should not be applied in a static mode and is best used clinically as a dynamic mode of ventilation involving regular adjustments [74]. That said, it might better be described as a continuum of recruitment maneuvers. When applied in this dynamic mode, the advantages of AAV over other modes of ventilation include lower mean intrathoracic (pleural) pressure, augmented venous return, improved cardiovascular performance, and better distribution of inspired gas flow resulting in improved ventilation–perfusion matching [75]. The AAV mode is specifically indicated in patients with low lung and thoracic compliance, as may be the case in large marine mammal species, particularly the "beached," anesthetized dolphin.

APV, APRV, and AAV will each mimic the breathing patterns of conscious, actively breathing marine mammals, and live subject testing is needed to elucidate their role in the target marine mammal population. Of these modes, AAV would be anticipated to provide superior ventilatory support to the anesthetized, non-spontaneously ventilating marine mammal and is actively under evaluation in California sea lions and bottlenose dolphins [76]. Additional testing of these modes of ventilation, including the evaluation of lower inspired oxygen concentrations, is currently underway and is producing promising results in both terrestrial and marine mammal species [68,74,76,77].

Permissive or intentional hypercapnia

In theory, "lung protective" ventilation strategies that utilize lower tidal volumes may limit alveolar overdistension and minimize lung injury; however, they will concurrently lead to hypercapnia, commonly referred to as "permissive hypercapnia" in medical literature [78]. Fundamentally, when properly performed, AAV will produce a degree of intentional hypercapnia. Both intentional hypercapnia (whereby hypercapnia is intentionally implemented as part of the ventilation mode such as in AAV) and permissive hypercapnia (whereby hypercapnia is accepted in avoidance of potentially negative ventilatory effects) are generally well tolerated and are described in greater detail elsewhere in this textbook.

Allowing a degree of intentional or permissive hypercapnia will allow implementation of lung protective ventilatory strategies and can both increase cardiac output and promote offloading of oxygen to tissues if held to a reasonable level. Although one may rationalize a degree of benefit of hypercapnia, recent work has suggested that high levels of CO_2 are not beneficial to pinnipeds and indicate a need for enhanced monitoring and support [79]. If intentional or permissive hypercapnia is used, the following parameters are suggested limits: $PaCO_2 < 80$ mmHg; pH > 7.20; and $PaO_2 > 80$ mmHg. The authors apply both intentional hypercapnia and eucapnia, situationally dependent. Since hypercapnia increases cardiac output and blood pressure, individuals accustomed to use of permissive hypercapnia who achieve eucapnia, as a choice or out of necessity, may need to be prepared to manage hypotension they may not routinely observe. Additionally, hypercapnia may increase pulmonary vascular resistance of the ventilated lung, which can result in increased shunt fraction. Interestingly, sea lions appear to undergo hypoxic pulmonary vasodilation rather than vasoconstriction, perhaps increasing shunt fraction in improperly ventilated marine mammal species under anesthesia [80].

Preanesthetic assessment and planning

The first step in any sedation or anesthetic event is determination of whether chemical restraint is even necessary. Many minimally invasive procedures (e.g., blood sampling and diagnostic imaging) can be completed under behavioral control alone and addition of simple local anesthetic blocks may even facilitate more invasive procedures (e.g., tissue biopsy). If needed, this can be combined with mild sedation for short, minimally invasive procedures. Immobilization or general anesthesia will be warranted for longer or more invasive procedures (e.g., surgery), in free-ranging species or those without behavioral control, or with large, potentially hazardous marine mammal subjects. While true anesthetic risk is still largely unknown for the vast majority of marine mammal species, it is likely higher than traditional domestic species due to a number of factors, including unknown health status, extrapolated pharmacology, and challenges with monitoring; a single retrospective study reported a perianesthetic mortality rate of 4.3% for free-ranging pinnipeds undergoing sedation or anesthesia at a renowned rescue and rehabilitation facility [81].

In managed populations where a voluntary preanesthetic health assessment is feasible, examination and laboratory tests can provide an overview of the animal's current health status and identify concurrent disease states. This is especially relevant when considering that many anesthetic procedures in managed populations are performed on geriatric patients. Where possible, this should include, at minimum, a physical examination, complete blood count and serum chemistry panel with a urinalysis, and imaging (e.g., radiographs, abdominal ultrasound, and echocardiography) performed where appropriate. Trainers must be vigilant to maintain necessary medical behaviors, but the anesthetist must recognize how disease (e.g., decreased vision), pain, and medications (e.g., preoperative opioids) can alter or lead to loss of medical behaviors. In situations in which a preanesthetic health assessment is limited (e.g., behaviorally non-compliant patients, and free-ranging subjects), visual inspection from a distance and interview of the managing trainers and veterinarians where possible should be performed. A limited preanesthetic assessment could put subjects at greater risk for negative outcomes and the anesthetist should prepare accordingly.

When tailoring an anesthetic protocol, the anesthetist must consider the species, size, age, demeanor, training, as well as the working environment. Anesthesia of marine mammals requires a balance of behavioral, mechanical (physical), and chemical restraint. Though often useful, excessive reliance on mechanical restraint may lead to physical injury to the patient (e.g., improper desensitization, "off behaviors" due to illness), hyperthermia, or exertional myopathic conditions [82]. Similarly, even though darting an animal with ultrapotent anesthetic agents to cause immobilization can be efficacious, it may result in severe negative physiologic effects. As such, emphasis should be placed on preprocedural behavioral training for voluntary medical procedures whenever time and resources exist, as these may reduce the need for mechanical or aggressive chemical restraint. When mechanical restraint is needed, desensitization training to mechanical restraint devices, such as netting, slings, and squeeze cages is recommended. With proper desensitization training and chemical sedation, mechanical devices may be used to improve the safety of anesthetic procedures for both the patient and personnel, without undue added risk.

The choices of anesthetic and perianesthetic drugs applied to marine mammal species have actually been rather limited, yet have been reviewed many times over the years, with focus primarily on immobilization cocktails and field applications of anesthetic drugs [83–90]. Induction of anesthesia of marine mammals requires a balance of behavioral, mechanical, and chemical restraint (Fig. 56.2). For instance, the process of anesthesia for pinnipeds has ranged from heavy mechanical restraint by lasso of juvenile Stellar sea lions followed by dowel and board squeeze/entrapment and mask induction with inhalation anesthetic alone [91,92], to solely chemical

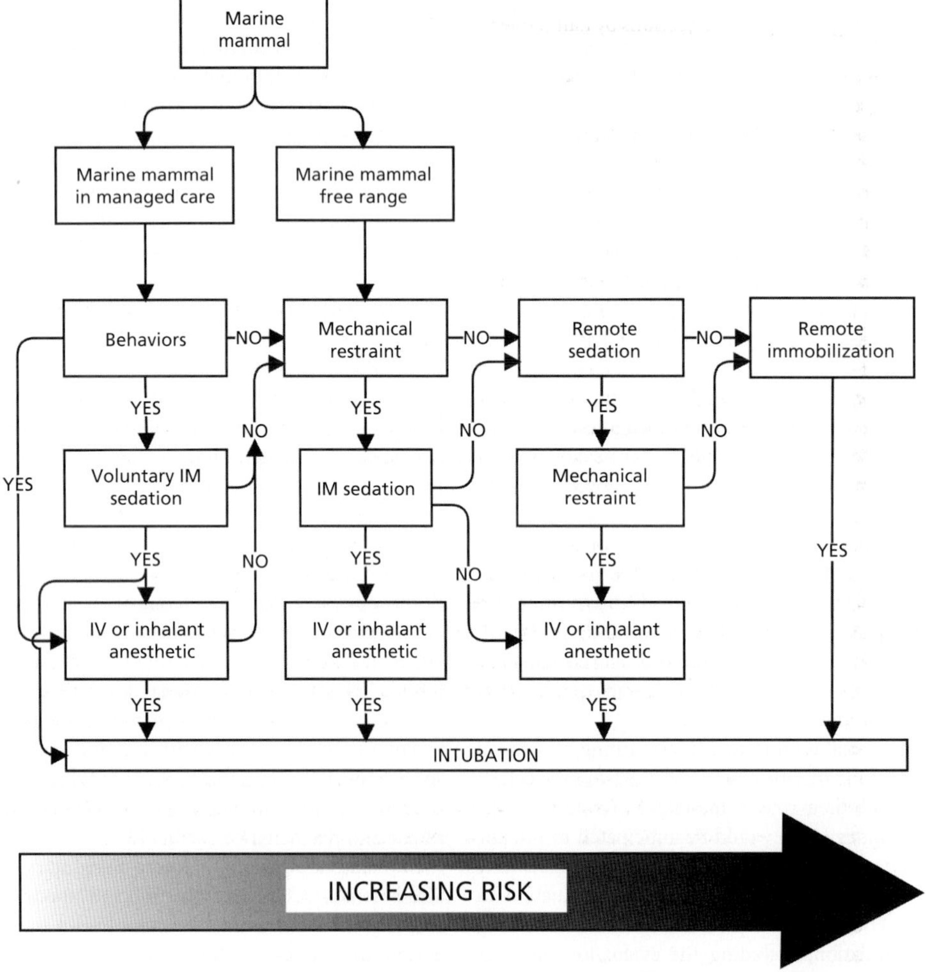

Figure 56.2 Anesthesia of marine mammal species requires a balance of behaviors, mechanical restraint, and chemical restraint. Behaviors are useful responses taught to marine mammals by qualified trainers. Although free-living subjects may have natural behaviors that can be leveraged for capture, behavioral control will be poor. Mechanical restraint is the physical control of the subject by devices such as nets, slings, husbandry boxes, or squeeze cages. Chemical restraint is the application of pharmacologic agents (drugs) to bring the subject to a manageable state by producing tranquilization, sedation, neuroleptanalgesia, immobilization, or anesthesia. Sedation is not immobilization; however, immobilization is anesthesia. Immobilization cocktails should be considered higher risk. Risk increases as we move from behavioral control to chemical immobilization, particularly delivered by remote means leading to lack of proximity to the subject and delayed support. Source: Dr. James Bailey, Innovative Veterinary Medicine Inc., 2023; with permission.

restraint by various potent and efficacious combinations of anesthetic agents delivered by dart, to remarkable behavior control by training for mask induction with an inhalation anesthetic agent alone under trainer command. In any situation, the concept of balanced anesthesia (use of a combination of drugs and techniques at lower individual doses to minimize dose-dependent side effects) should be employed. Additionally, for marine mammals, a balanced approach to anesthesia usually includes considerations beyond anesthetic drug selection. For example, with sufficient personnel, it is feasible to manually restrain small cetaceans and sirenians, but pinnipeds of size will require additional tools for restraint.

The rationale for the anesthetic protocol begins with assessment of behaviors. Behaviors are useful responses taught to marine mammals by qualified trainers. Desensitization training and voluntary medical behaviors contribute in no small part to more positive outcomes in managed populations, eliminating the need for aggressive restraint methods or potent cocktails with severe physiologic consequences. Skilled trainers and animal handlers are necessary to support safe anesthesia, and they must be given both the opportunity and time required for training where possible. Examples of useful medical behaviors are holding on target for injections by hand, tolerance of mechanical restraint in a squeeze cage, self-beaching of dolphins, or acceptance of an anesthetic mask for inhalation anesthetic delivery. Even in subjects that could be very difficult to restrain, such behaviors can be sufficiently robust to allow free-standing application of anesthetic agents without physical restraint. Without medical behaviors, there is greater reliance on both mechanical restraint, which can become dangerous and lead to injury, and chemical restraint, which often needs to be more profound.

With chemical restraint, *ut est rerum omnium magister usus* or, experience is the best teacher [93]. Anesthesia methods applied to free-living subjects are highly variable and often depend on the experience of the personnel, as well as the historical success of the method applied. For example, though less commonly used in managed species, the combination of tiletamine and zolazepam (Telazol® or Zoletil®) is still the preferred immobilization method for free-living elephant seals. As most free-living subjects are anesthetized to facilitate study of the species as a whole, these subjects are usually healthy individuals that may better tolerate the physiological challenges of a broader range of necessary mechanical and chemical restraint methods. On the contrary, rescued free-living subjects are often debilitated or otherwise unhealthy and are at greater risk of negative outcomes in the face of immobilization methods necessary for the safety of human caretakers. The authors recognize the broad range of sedation and anesthesia methods applied to the wide variety of marine mammal species over the past many decades, and offer only to provide some general, repeatable methods in hopes of improved outcomes for all the species under our care, particularly the growing geriatric populations.

Protocol selection

Historically, drugs used in the anesthetic and perianesthetic period in marine mammals have been quite limited. These have been extensively reviewed in other texts and primarily focus on immobilization cocktails and field applications of anesthetic drugs [83–86]. To tabulate that historical information again here would not serve the anesthetist well and, instead, a brief summary of common drug choices for each species is provided below. As noted previously, anesthesia of marine mammals requires a balance of behavioral, physical/mechanical, and chemical restraint, although various combinations of the above have been used. Managed populations do not generally require aggressive restraint methods or potent cocktails for induction, especially if preprocedural behavioral training is implemented. When selecting an anesthetic protocol, the risk-benefit ratio for each drug and technique should be carefully considered and the anesthetist should be reminded that, "There are no safe anesthetic agents; there are no safe anesthetic procedures; there are only safe anesthetists" (Robert Smith) [94,95]. The importance of vigilant perianesthetic monitoring and support in conjunction with any anesthetic protocol cannot be overstated and will be discussed further.

While specific drugs will not be discussed in detail, α_2-adrenergic receptor agonist use in pinnipeds warrants discussion. One of the most commonly administered drug combinations in this cohort involves various combinations of midazolam, butorphanol, and medetomidine, and has proven effective in field immobilization of young, healthy otariids for short procedures [96]. While useful in certain situations, the authors have anecdotally appreciated a higher incidence of negative outcomes in some managed populations with use of an α_2-adrenergic receptor agonist. Medetomidine was used in > 50% of induction protocols reported in a retrospective assessment of anesthetic mortality in a cohort of rescued, untrained, free-living otariids of variable disease condition and severity; perianesthetic mortality in that study was 4.3% [81]. Additionally, a high negative outcome rate (e.g., ciliary body hemorrhage, hyphema, and death) was anecdotally reported in pinnipeds following medetomidine or dexmedetomidine administration for ophthalmologic procedures. In a series of 13 prolonged ophthalmologic procedures on geriatric California sea lions (median age 22.5 years) immobilized with a combination of midazolam, butorphanol, and dexmedetomidine, one subject vomited, two had arrhythmias, two had prolonged recoveries, and three died during anesthesia or within 72 h of recovery [86,97]. For these reasons, α_2-adrenergic receptor agonists, despite their reversibility, may not be a reasonable choice in geriatric marine mammals or those undergoing lengthy procedures, and would be ill-advised in phocids and odobenids [98]. This is not to say the α_2-adrenergic receptor agonists are not effective or on occasion necessary; however, the anesthetist must recall Maslow's Axiom that "it is tempting, if the only tool you have is a hammer, to treat everything as if it were a nail" [99]. While it is easy, and sometimes necessary, to dart an animal with potent efficacious anesthetic agents (including α_2-adrenergic receptor agonists), all options should be explored and the physiologic consequences for this convenience should be considered. That being said, more judicious use of α_2-adrenergic receptor agonists may yet prove beneficial.

Sedation and anesthesia

Relatively few pharmacologic agents have gained acceptance for use in managed populations of marine mammals. In brief, benzodiazepines (diazepam 0.05–0.3 mg/kg PO, IM, IV; midazolam 0.05–0.3 mg/kg IM, IV) are commonly used, often in combination with opioids (butorphanol 0.1–0.4 mg/kg IM; meperidine 0.1–2 mg/kg IM) to produce sedation or neuroleptanalgesia. Immobilization can be achieved with the addition of medetomidine (0.01–0.03 mg/kg IM) or dexmedetomidine (0.002–0.01 mg/kg IM) in some otariid pinnipeds, but not cetaceans or sirenians. Concentrated versions of midazolam, butorphanol, and medetomidine assist with remote delivery by dart or pole syringe by minimizing volume. Alternatively, alfaxalone (0.5–2 mg/kg IM, IV) has been introduced for immobilization where larger volumes or multiple intramuscular injections are feasible in pinnipeds. An experimental, concentrated (40 mg/mL) alfaxalone formulation, RD0387, which allows for reduced volumes has recently been used successfully for immobilization of large otariids in lieu of medetomidine [100]. Other parenteral anesthetic agents have been used for immobilization or induction of general anesthesia. The cyclohexamines, ketamine (1–10 mg/kg IM, IV), or tiletamine (in Telazol® or Zoletil®; 1–2 mg/kg IM, IV), have been used but are not reversible and are less favored. The phenolic compound propofol (1–6 mg/kg IV) is used routinely in the extradural vein for induction of anesthesia of phocids and odobenids for rapid airway control and ease of intubation in preference over slower mask induction with inhalation anesthetics. Behaviorally non-compliant patients can be injected remotely by pole syringe or dart, but it is imperative the drug is delivered into muscle and not fat, or uptake will be poor. Repeat dosing from presumed "failed delivery" can lead to eventual cumulative drug uptake and overdose with sudden onset of CNS depression and respiratory depression.

Inhalation anesthetics (e.g., isoflurane and sevoflurane) have been used successfully in marine mammals. They are low-solubility agents and are minimally metabolized. For mask induction, sevoflurane has a faster onset and lesser pungency, thus, it has become preferred. The minimum alveolar concentration (MAC) of inhalant anesthetics has not yet been determined for any marine mammal species, making comparison of equipotent concentrations to other species imprecise. However, the effect of inhalation anesthetic agents is well preserved over the wide variety of mammalian species tested, so the dose of inhalation anesthetic for marine mammals will likely differ little from other mammalian species. Anecdotally, the authors use MAC estimations of 1.3% for isoflurane and 2.3% for sevoflurane. In the authors' experience performing marine mammal anesthesia over the past decade, with similar preanesthetic drugs (i.e., benzodiazepine and opioid), the end-expired sevoflurane concentration usually needs to be maintained at approximately 1.8 to 2.0% to prevent gross, purposeful movement in response to a surgical stimulus.

An in-depth discussion of anesthetic agents and their effects to be used for all orders of marine mammals is beyond the scope of this chapter. Instead, a brief summary of commonly used agents and their administration in each order is presented below.

Cetacean anesthesia

The first attempt to anesthetize a dolphin was made in the 1930s in which a dolphin was administered "ether by cone" over the blowhole, became apneic, and died [101]. After concurrent dolphin deaths associated with intraperitoneal barbiturate anesthesia [102], Nagel successfully developed an endotracheal intubation method and induced a state where the dolphins were "largely insensitive to noxious stimuli" with nitrous oxide (N_2O) and O_2 (70%:30%) delivered by a ventilator and using neuromuscular blockade with succinylcholine [63,69]. Although this method appeared "safe," it was inadequate for major surgery. Ridgway and McCormick used combinations of inhaled halothane and intravascular thiopental for induction and maintenance of anesthesia sufficient for major surgery [65,66]. However, uncertain about the effects of injectable agents, the early successful anesthetic inductions involved manual restraint and conscious intubation followed by halothane administered via endotracheal tube. This produced excitement and dysphoria characterized by significant swimming motions, a physical response less commonly observed with current methods of balanced anesthesia.

In managed care settings, cetacean sedation and anesthesia are heavily supported by behavioral training. These intelligent species are amenable to desensitization or other behavioral training and, ideally, this is incorporated into routine medical or husbandry training. Fasting of food for at least 12 h duration is typically practiced as regurgitation can occur. The target animal is often separated from conspecifics and preanesthetic sedation is often used to reduce stress and facilitate patient compliance. Currently, benzodiazepines alone (either diazepam 0.25 mg/kg PO or midazolam 0.08 mg/kg IM) or in combination with opioids (butorphanol 0.1 mg/kg IM or meperidine 0.1 mg/kg IM) are used for preanesthetic sedation. Midazolam 0.1 mg/kg IM (0.05–0.2 mg/kg IM) with butorphanol 0.1 mg/kg IM (0.1–0.3 mg/kg IM) has provided sedation for minor procedures in bottlenose dolphins, killer whales, and even 20,000 kg North Atlantic right whales (*Eubalaena glacialis*) [103,104]. Propofol (2–3 mg/kg IV) is used, often with supplemental midazolam (0.02 mg/kg IV) for induction of anesthesia in the lateral caudal subcutaneous vein (LCSV). Anesthesia of dolphins has been maintained with the inhalation anesthetics halothane, isoflurane, and more recently, sevoflurane in oxygen [31,64,65,105–108]. Controlled mechanical ventilation (CMV) has been applied with variable success, as well as the alternative mode, apneustic anesthesia ventilation (AAV), which is currently undergoing clinical trials.

Pinniped anesthesia

Phocid anesthesia

Similar to other marine mammals, desensitization and behavioral training when possible are keys to phocid health in managed care; this includes desensitization to use of a "blood collection box" for extradural anesthetic drug administration and, for larger pinnipeds, use of a squeeze cage. In brief, benzodiazepines are very effective in tranquilizing phocids. In wild captures, intravenous diazepam 0.25 mg/kg in combination with mechanical restraint using a simple hoop-net prior to mask induction with inhalation anesthetic is not uncommon. In managed populations, subjects can be trained to accept an intramuscular injection of midazolam and inhalation anesthetic via mask under behavioral restraint alone. Free-living phocids remain somewhat excitable with a concurrent elevated respiratory rate, resulting in successful mask induction using inhalant anesthetics. In contrast, animals in managed populations tend to breath-hold, which can delay induction. These subjects can also become apneic from anesthetic exposure before sufficiently relaxed for smooth intubation, thus, induction with IV anesthetic agents is often pursued. This usually includes behavioral or mechanical restraint (e.g., blood collection box) for extradural venous puncture and IV administration of propofol (1–2 mg/kg titrated to effect); this is often in combination with IM premedication (e.g., midazolam 0.2 mg/kg IM and butorphanol 0.2 mg/kg IM) to reduce induction drug requirements. Butorphanol is often sufficient for the purpose of control without significant respiratory depression; however, full μ-opioid receptor agonists (e.g., meperidine) have been used for greater sedation of larger phocid species where there is inadequate behavioral control. Due to the likelihood of apnea following any induction protocol, the anesthetist should be prepared for prompt intubation, usually performed under direct laryngoscopy. In field settings where inhalation anesthesia may not be readily available, heavy sedation can be maintained for longer procedures with repeated dosing of midazolam, butorphanol, and ketamine IV, alone or in combination.

Otariid anesthesia

Training robust medical behaviors is crucial to reducing anesthetic risk in otariids. Behaviors, such as free-standing anesthetic induction by mask, have been trained even in extremely large otariid species. Benzodiazepines are anxiolytic, but further sedation with opioids is generally needed for most otariid subjects, even when properly trained for mechanical restraint. A scissor-style squeeze cage is commonly used for mechanical restraint in managed populations, and has been used for some free-living capture and longer-term holding situations [109,110]. Subjects are trained to accept temporary restraint by squeeze allowing for injection of sedative agents. Accurate intramuscular delivery of drugs is necessary, or uptake will be poor. The intramuscular sedative combination (midazolam 0.2 mg/kg and butorphanol 0.2 mg/kg or meperidine 2 mg/kg) is administered, and time allowed for uptake and full effect (20–25 min). Sedation is followed with mechanical restraint by squeeze to facilitate mask induction. Mechanical restraint significantly enhances control and human safety but is not without risk. Inadequately trained or sedated subjects may attempt to resist mask induction or bite at the bars, the latter of which can break teeth and fracture jaws. Even subjects known to tolerate a squeeze cage can become intolerant when ill. Only properly designed squeeze cages with padded bars should be used for this method of restraint. Boat bumpers and rolled towels can be used to center the head for mask induction and act as safe bite "toy." It is preferred that the anesthetic mask be malleable to move between cage bars, if necessary, mold to the face of the subject, and tolerate biting without injury to the subject. A modified traffic cone has proven ideal for this purpose [111]. The combination of intramuscular midazolam (0.2–0.3 mg/kg) and meperidine (1–2 mg/kg) may produce neuroleptanalgesia in some species, such as southern sea lions, and result in marked sedation. A squeeze cage is not always available or may be of inadequate size for larger subjects making mechanical restraint impractical and improvised squeezes have been created, but efficacy and response are often variable. Large custom walrus restraint nets can be effective for large sea lions and fur seals. Where mechanical restraint is not possible, a greater reliance is placed on pharmacologic agents. A combination of concentrated intramuscular midazolam 0.2 mg/kg, butorphanol 0.2 mg/kg, and medetomidine 0.01 mg/kg is commonly used, but results in bradycardia, vasoconstriction, and a reduction in cardiac output, complicating vascular access and challenging debilitated and geriatric patients physiologically. A combination of medetomidine and the peripheral α_2-adrenergic receptor antagonist vatinoxan (Zenalpha®) has recently been used in otariids, but clear benefit is not yet evident. Alternatively, the combination of concentrated intramuscular midazolam 0.2 mg/kg, butorphanol 0.2 mg/kg, and alfaxalone 1 mg/kg is currently under review with promising results [100].

Odobenid anesthesia

Walrus subjects in managed population can be very well trained such that delivery of intramuscular midazolam (0.2 mg/kg) or even direct extradural or saphenous venous needle placement for delivery of propofol (2–4 mg/kg) can be performed under behavioral control. However, most walruses will need additional intramuscular sedation and analgesia using an opioid, particularly when not participating in medical behaviors due to illness and/or discomfort; meperidine (2 mg/kg) is often chosen, but butorphanol (0.2 mg/kg) has also been used. In young patients, the combination of midazolam and meperidine can produce a state of neuroleptanalgesia sufficient to permit intubation. If this combination is not sufficient for intubation, the authors have used a low dose of alfaxalone (< 0.5 mg/kg) to bridge control, but further evaluation is needed before recommending this drug. As noted previously, induction is performed using propofol (0.5–4 mg/kg) delivered in the extradural or saphenous vein. Intubation is performed blindly via manual palpation and, as these species often experience apnea following propofol administration, the anesthetist must be well prepared for intubation.

Sirenian anesthesia

To our knowledge, no dugong has ever undergone anesthesia and most anesthesia experience has been with the Florida manatee (*Trichechus manatus latirostris*). Many manatees needing anesthesia for surgical procedures come from rescue and rehabilitation facilities that perform lifesaving work on untrained subjects. It is recommended that only trained personnel participate in the handling and restraint of sirenians, and we emphasize here that quality trainers and animal handlers are necessary for safe anesthesia of these marine mammals. The strong thrust of sirenian tails and large body size make injury to both handlers and animals possible. For this reason, it is preferred that manatees are removed from the water for procedures and personnel wear helmets for safety. In captive environments, physical restraint is accomplished by corralling the animal using nets, dry-docking within a pool by draining the water, or raising a medical pool floor above the water level; the animal is then placed within a stretcher for transport.

As the sole obligate herbivores of the marine mammal world, preanesthetic fasting is often extended to 24 h. Historically, manatees were sedated with midazolam (0.08 mg/kg IM) and mask induced with isoflurane via a modified 5-gallon plastic water bottle [112,113], but this was tedious and time consuming. Currently, midazolam (0.05–0.2 mg/kg IM) has been used in combination with butorphanol (0.05–0.15 mg/kg IM) to achieve neuroleptanalgesia sufficient to facilitate conscious nasotracheal intubation. When necessary, this can be supplemented with sevoflurane via a nasal mask, as manatees are obligate nasal breathers. Meperidine (0.05–0.2 mg/kg) had been used in place of butorphanol for greater analgesia but has fallen from favor as, anecdotally, there has been prolongation in the time to achieve a level of recovery sufficient for the manatee to raise its head to breathe when submerged.

Vascular access

Cetacean vascular access

There are several peripheral sites from which blood may be collected in the cetacean. The arteriovenous nature of the peripheral vasculature in these species, however, means very few of these sites allow rapid drug or fluid administration or clear differentiation of arterial and venous blood. Consequently, true venous and arterial access are desirable, and have become increasingly attainable as imaging and vascular access methodology have improved. In this section, we describe common clinically accessible sites for blood sampling and both arterial and venous catheter placement.

Braun's 1905 angiograms of the arteries of the fluke and pectoral flipper of the harbor porpoise helped begin documentation of the extensively branching network of the peripheral vasculature of cetaceans [114]. In 1941, the complex arterial and venous blood supply of the dolphin and manatee were described [115] and, in 1951, Tomilin first described the closely adhering venous reticulum associated with the arteries involved in temperature regulation which he called "complex vessels" [116]. We now know these as the periarterial vascular rete (PAVR). Shortly thereafter, the countercurrent heat exchange function of this "artery-within-vein arrangement" of the PAVR was first hypothesized [117]. The radiographic, gross,

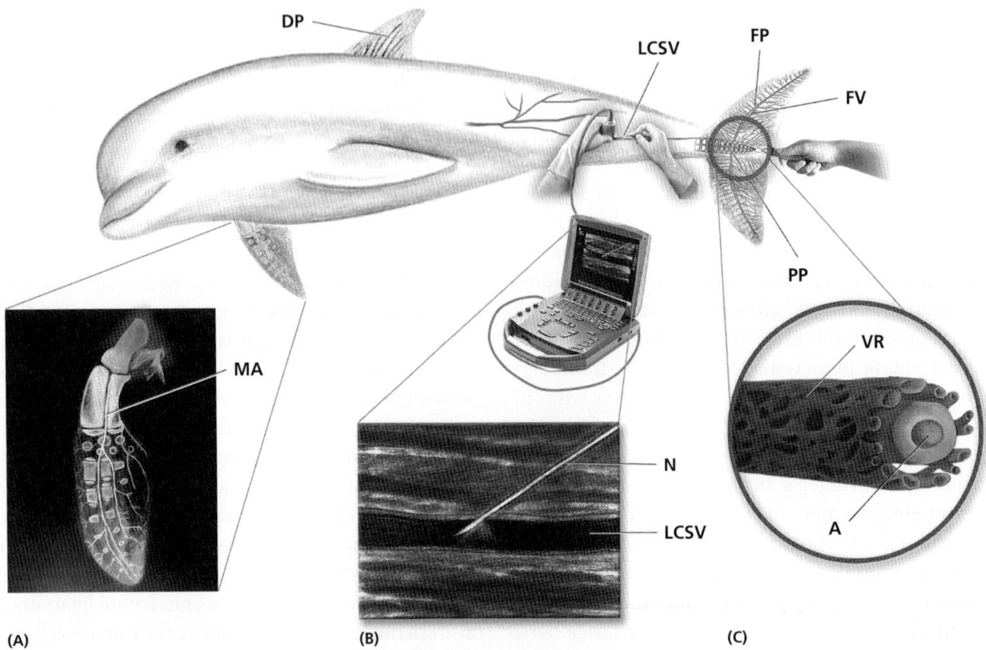

Figure 56.3 Bottlenose dolphin vascular access locations. **A.** Illustrates angiography of the median artery (MA) in the pectoral flipper. **B.** Illustrates a longitudinal plane ultrasound image of the lateral caudal subcutaneous vein (LCSV) with an echogenic needle (N) placed. **C.** Illustrates the periarterial venous rete (VR) surrounding an artery (A) together comprising the periarterial vascular rete (PAVR). DP, dorsal fin PAVR; LCSV, lateral caudal subcutaneous vein; FP, fluke PAVR; FV, fluke veins; PP, peduncle PAVR. Source: **A.** Adapted and modified from Fawcett [115]; Dr. James Bailey, Innovative Veterinary Medicine Inc., 2023. **C.** Adapted and modified from Elsner *et al.* [118]; Dr. James Bailey, Innovative Veterinary Medicine Inc., 2023.

and histologic anatomy of the PAVR was further detailed via corrosion casting of its architecture (Fig. 56.3C) [118].

Armed with this knowledge, it must be noted that when performing "venipuncture" at a PAVR location, it is the artery (surrounded by the venous reticulum, the periarterial venous rete) that is most probably penetrated by the needle. This may be evidenced by rapid passive outflow of blood. Depending on the location and angle of incidence, the needle lumen may communicate with the artery, venous reticulum, or the perivascular space or channels through the firm collagenous matrix surrounding the PAVR. This imprecise positioning, and the likelihood of needle migration, can result in blood source mixing and possible perivascular leakage. With proper aseptic technique, this is an acceptable location for blood collection and delivery of isotonic crystalloid fluids, but caution is advised in delivering other medication. Arteries are muscular and will respond to changes in pH or osmolarity, direct cytotoxicity, or known vasopressor activity through vasospasm, thrombosis, or direct vascular injury. Accordingly, there are a number of anecdotal reports of fluke injury and circumferential sloughing after delivery of medications, such as insufficiently diluted antibiotics, into the peduncle or fluke PAVR [119]. As noted above, it is documented that drugs of extreme pH (e.g., the barbiturate anesthetic thiopental) will cause vascular injury and severe complications when injected into arteries [120]. That said, thiopental delivery has been reported (10 mg/kg IV, 50 mg/mL) in the peduncle PAVR without complication on multiple occasions [61,64–66]. However, it should be noted that these injections were usually delivered in crystalloid perianesthetic fluids, thus, diluting the drug prior to entry into the PAVR [personal communication: Dr. Sam H. Ridgway, 2020]. Common anesthetic drugs administered intravascularly in cetaceans include midazolam and propofol. There are some reports of vasculitis and vascular impairment after intraarterial delivery of the midazolam in human subjects, but symptoms resolved without sequelae with no specific intervention. Propofol is well known to cause pain on injection, but it has not been associated with any vascular injury when inadvertently delivered intraarterial. If true venous access is not acquired for anesthetic drug delivery, we advise careful drug selection and use of crystalloid fluids during induction for the purpose of dilution. True venous access in the lateral caudal subcutaneous vein as described below is now routine and will enhance safety.

Lateral caudal subcutaneous vein

First proposed in 1997 and attempted in 1998 [107,121], catheterization of the lateral caudal subcutaneous vein (LCSV), also known as "lateral subcutaneous caudal vein" and historically referred to as the "caudal ventral peduncle," "caudal superficial peduncle," "superficial caudal peduncle vein," or "superficial lateral peduncle vein," was not perfected until 2011 [122]. The LCSV is now the first choice for true venous access in the dolphin and catheterization of this vessel is a routine procedure. It is commonly performed with the animal in modified sternal recumbency, with the peduncle tilted approximately 10–15 degrees from midline to expose the area of interest (Fig. 56.3B). The authors have had the greatest success catheterizing the LCSV with ultrasound guidance using a linear transducer (10-5 MHz) and a single lumen, 4 to 5 French micro-introducer catheter kit utilizing a modified Seldinger method [123]. When necessary, longer peripherally inserted central catheters (PICCs) with one or more lumens can be placed. In a transverse ultrasound view, the ventral branch of the LCSV lies just dorsolateral to the levator ani (pubocaudalis) muscle and ventromedial to the hypaxialis lumborum (supracoccygeus) muscle. In the longitudinal view, the vein travels caudal to cranial under the blubber, becoming larger and diving deeper as it travels craniad. Further caudad, as the vessel diameter becomes smaller, the subdermal sheath connective tissue thickens, making catheter placement more difficult. The optimal catheter placement site should be a balance between vessel depth (more superficial), vessel diameter (larger), and minimized perivascular connective tissue. Even in more cranial locations, perivascular connective tissue is quite dense, making a stiffened micro-introducer dilator cannula preferred for placement. For patient comfort and compliance, a local anesthetic block (subcutaneous lidocaine) with or without sedation is used prior to catheter placement. Pressure cranial to the site of venipuncture may help increase the diameter of the vessel and facilitate cannulation as can warm wet towels placed over the vessel. Attempts have been made to maintain an LCSV catheter in the postanesthetic aquatic environment, with some limited success [124].

Median artery

It is feasible to catheterize many arteries of the cetacean PAVR. Used for collection of blood in early studies, the median artery of the pectoral flipper of dolphins is now a commonly acceptable location for cannulation [125,126]. The median artery sits snuggly between the radius and ulna, slightly palmar, under the dense connective tissue of the flipper (Fig. 56.3A). Doppler flow probes and ultrasound can facilitate identification and cannulation of the median artery, but the location is also digitally palpable. The authors have had the greatest success catheterizing the median artery with ultrasound guidance using a linear transducer (10-5 MHz) and a 4 to 5 French micro-introducer catheter kit utilizing a modified Seldinger method similar to those used for venous access. For placement, the dolphin is positioned in lateral recumbency, and the dependent pectoral flipper is pulled laterally and slightly cranial for placement. In a transverse view across the palmar surface of the flipper, the artery sits slightly superficial to the notch formed by the convergence of the radius and ulna. To maintain patency of the cannula, 2–5 unit/mL of heparinized 0.9% NaCl is used to regularly flush the catheter. Modern disposable blood pressure transducers with integrated, pressurized flush mechanisms can be used to simplify maintenance of the catheter. The transducer is zeroed to the level of the right atrium (physiologic zero) and invasive blood pressures are continuously monitored. Blood can also be collected from this site for analysis of arterial blood gases or other hematologic or biochemical indices.

Pinniped vascular access

Vascular access is feasible in pinnipeds, with ultrasound facilitating visualization in the majority of locations. Venipuncture of the extradural vein of phocids and odobenids can be performed using a spinal or Tuohy needle inserted perpendicularly between the dorsal spinous processes of lumbar vertebrae 3 and 4. The needle can be maintained throughout a procedure or converted to a small-diameter cannula using commercially available epidural catheter kits. Though small in diameter, thus limiting fluid volume delivery, such extradural venous catheters have been aseptically maintained for up to a week postoperatively for drug delivery. Venous access of the external jugular vein, though visible on smaller subjects, is facilitated by ultrasound and is more commonly performed in otariids than phocids and odobenids (Fig. 56.4A). Commercially available longer PICCs may be more easily maintained in the jugular vein of larger subjects. Cannulation of pectoral and pelvic flipper veins is also possible and most often performed with the animal positioned in lateral or modified dorsal recumbency. Visualization of the pectoral flipper antebrachial vein (also referred to as the "brachial vein" or "superficial palmar vein") and occasionally the cephalic vein do not require ultrasound, but this tool can be useful, especially in hypotensive, hypovolemic, or smaller patients (Fig. 56.4B). Branches of the pelvic flipper medial saphenous veins (Fig 56.4C), particularly in phocids and odobenids, are best visualized with

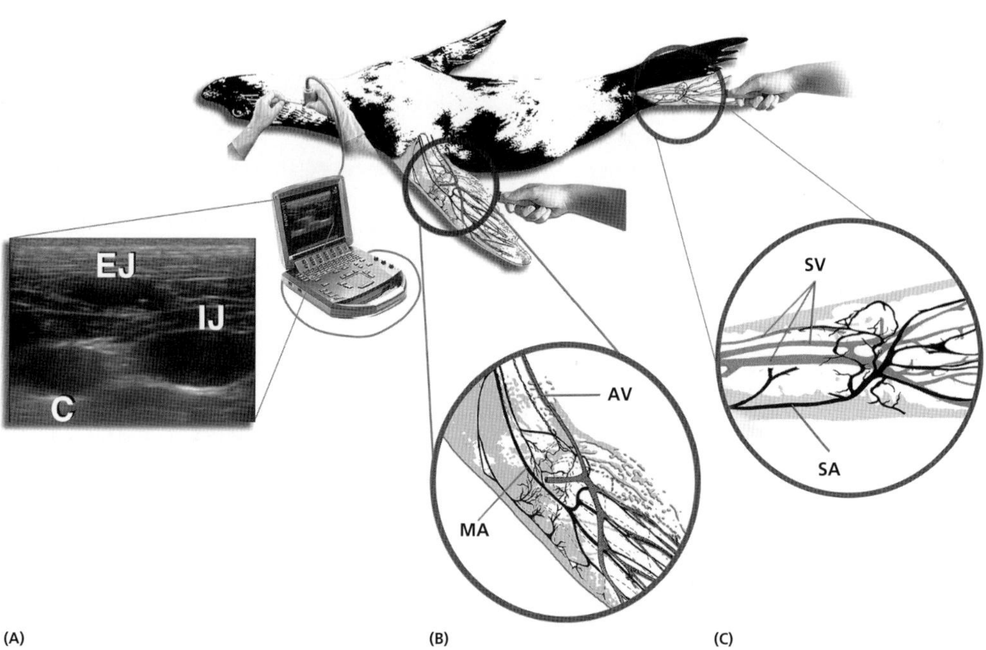

Figure 56.4 Pinniped jugular, pectoral flipper, and pelvic flipper vasculature. **A.** Transverse ultrasound image of the external jugular vein (EJ), internal jugular vein (IJ), and carotid artery (C). **B.** Diagram of the median artery (MA) and antebrachial vein (AV). **C.** Diagram of the saphenous artery (SA) and plantar branches of the saphenous vein (SV). Source: Adapted with permission from St. Pierre [127]; Dr. James Bailey, Innovative Veterinary Medicine Inc., 2023.

ultrasound guidance on the plantar aspect of the limb. The median artery is positioned at the convergence of the radius and ulna (as described for dolphins) and, anecdotally, is best accessed at the junction between the haired and non-haired portion of the pectoral flipper. Doppler flow probes and ultrasound can facilitate identification and cannulation of the median artery, but the location is also digitally palpable. Standard over-the-needle catheters can be used to cannulate both arteries and veins to reduce cost, but modern micro-introducer kits using a modified Seldinger technique simplify and expedite cannulation. Venous cannulation of pinnipeds, ultrasound-guided or otherwise, may be complicated by α_2-adrenergic receptor agonist administration, hypovolemia, disease, or drug-induced hypotension.

Manatee vascular access

As Fawcett wrote, "The most characteristic feature of the circulatory system of the manatee is the complete subdivision of the larger arteries, usually near their sources, into great numbers of small arteries which run parallel for considerable distances without any significant diminution in caliber." This is "most highly developed in the vascularization of the pectoral limb" and "resembles rather the arrangement of a broom" [115]. As such, the typical site for blood sampling in manatees of all ages is the interosseous space between the radius and ulna, which contains a vascular bundle of veins and arteries (Fig 56.5B). It can be accessed from the medial or lateral sides of the pectoral flippers, usually based on personal preference, using an 18 gauge, 5 cm (2 inch) needle in adults or a 20 gauge, 3.75 cm (1.5 inch) needle in juveniles [128]. Cannulation of the brachial vascular bundle is complicated by the perpendicular placement of the needle relative to the arteriovenous plexus. A vascular bundle is also available for venipuncture under the fluke (paddle) in the ventral vertebral arch. This technique is particularly useful in younger animals where pectoral vessels are small, but has also been used in anesthetized adult manatees using spinal or Tuohy needles. While these techniques have been used in conscious individuals, subjects can move and displace the needle or produce explosive forward thrust of the fluke and injure the phlebotomist as well as the vascular bundle. Perivascular leakage of drugs can also occur in these vascular bundle venipuncture sites, potentially resulting in local tissue inflammation or necrosis.

"Cephalic" and "caudal" veins have also been described and diagramed for the pectoral flipper of manatee (Fig. 56.5A) [129]. The cephalic vein was cannulated using a "cut-down" technique and a standard over-the-needle catheter during anesthesia of one Florida manatee [113]. However, in recent years, transcutaneous cannulation has become feasible in the palmar digital veins, as well as the median artery of the manatee pectoral flipper (Fig. 56.5D). Similar to other discussed species, the median artery sits snuggly in the interosseous space between the radius and ulna, slightly palmar on the flipper, under the thick dermis and connective tissue. Doppler flow probes or ultrasound are mandatory to facilitate identification and cannulation of the artery, as it is not externally palpable. The authors have had success catheterizing the median artery of six adult Florida manatees with ultrasound guidance using a linear transducer (10-5 MHz) and a 4 to 5 French micro-introducer catheter kit utilizing a modified Seldinger technique, similar to methods used for vascular access in other marine mammals.

Airway management

Orotracheal or nasotracheal intubation should be considered in every immobilized or anesthetized marine mammal for reasons similar to other species, including maintenance of airway patency, delivery of assisted ventilation, and protection from regurgitation. Unique risk factors in marine mammal species, including redundant pharyngeal tissue and risk of apnea with induction agents, further emphasize the importance of rapid intubation. This is especially true if using remotely delivered drugs or mechanical restraint

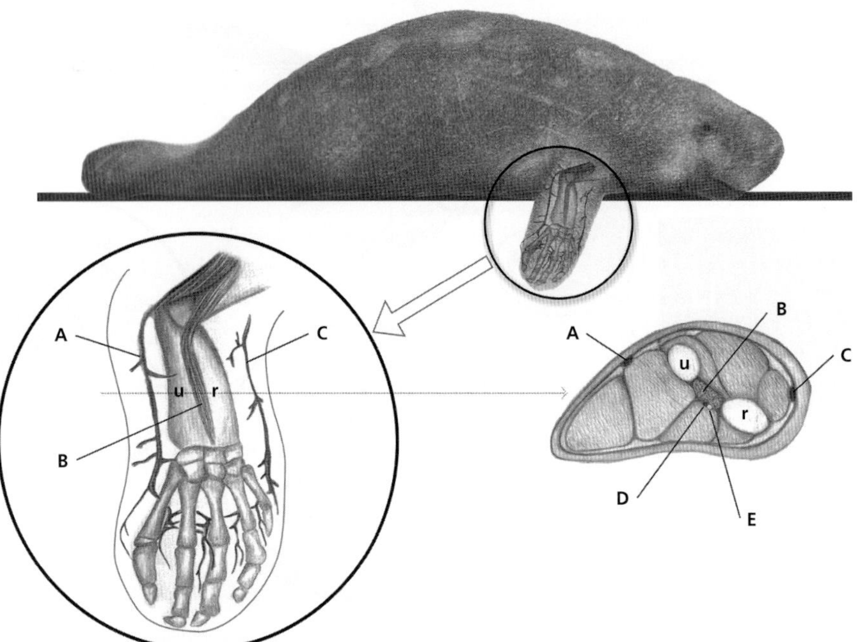

Figure 56.5 Florida manatee (*Trichechus manatus latirostris*) pectoral flipper vasculature position including caudal vein (A), brachial vascular bundle (B), cephalic vein (C), median artery (D), median nerve (E), radius (r), and ulna (u). On the right is a cross-sectional view with the palmar surface facing down. Source: Adapted with permission from White [129]; Rommel and Caplan [130]; Dr. James Bailey, Innovative Veterinary Medicine Inc., 2023.

devices that may logistically delay "hands-on" access to the patient or in situations in which airway patency is compromised. Regardless of induction technique, careful observation for both continued spontaneous ventilation and airway patency is necessary and will guide the urgency of intubation. Proper airway management requires consideration of the logistics of anesthetic induction, knowledge of airway anatomy and the physical condition of the target species, as well as preparation of necessary equipment. Many species are obligate nasal breathers (e.g., Cetaceans and manatees), which may influence the approach to both intubation and extubation. Tools used in intubation such as elongated laryngoscopes, malleable stylets, and flexible fiberoptic bronchoscopes must be available as required; in some species, alternate methods of airway management, such as nasotracheal intubation, must also be considered. Similarly, as many marine mammals may become apneic prior to sufficient relaxation for simple intubation, advanced planning for and experience in alternative options for airway management is necessary.

Cetacean intubation

Endotracheal intubation of adult bottlenose dolphins and larger odontocete species is usually performed using an oral approach to the larynx (Fig. 56.6). While less ideal, this can be accomplished in a conscious animal in an emergency situation, but is preferably performed following heavy sedation or anesthetic induction. Size 16 to 30 mm ID endotracheal tubes with inflatable, high-volume, low-pressure cuffs are appropriate for most adult bottlenose dolphins. Soft, rolled towels are used to hold open the mandible and maxilla and the larynx is accessed blindly by palpation. The elongated epiglottal and cricoarytenoid cartilages of the larynx ("goose-beak") are manually displaced from their connection to the nasopharyngeal sphincter and oriented in a rostral direction. Two fingers of one hand are placed into the glottis and, using the other hand, the endotracheal tube is guided through the glottis. Care should be taken to shield the cuff with the palm and forearm when advancing the endotracheal tube to prevent cuff damage by the sharp teeth. Tracheal intubation should be confirmed using a capnograph. The trachea is very short in most odontocetes and a right-sided accessory bronchus precedes the carina [131]; awareness of the depth of insertion is necessary to prevent blockade of this bronchus. Use of a flexible endoscope can both facilitate intubation and assure proper depth of insertion. Once positioned in place, similar to terrestrial mammals, the tube should be secured to the maxilla using a tie, and the cuff inflated to a minimum occlusive volume. Intubation through the blowhole is possible, but usually reserved for smaller odontocetes in which the oral approach is prohibitive due to their small mouth and oropharynx. Similar to orotracheal intubation, this technique can be performed in conscious, sedated,

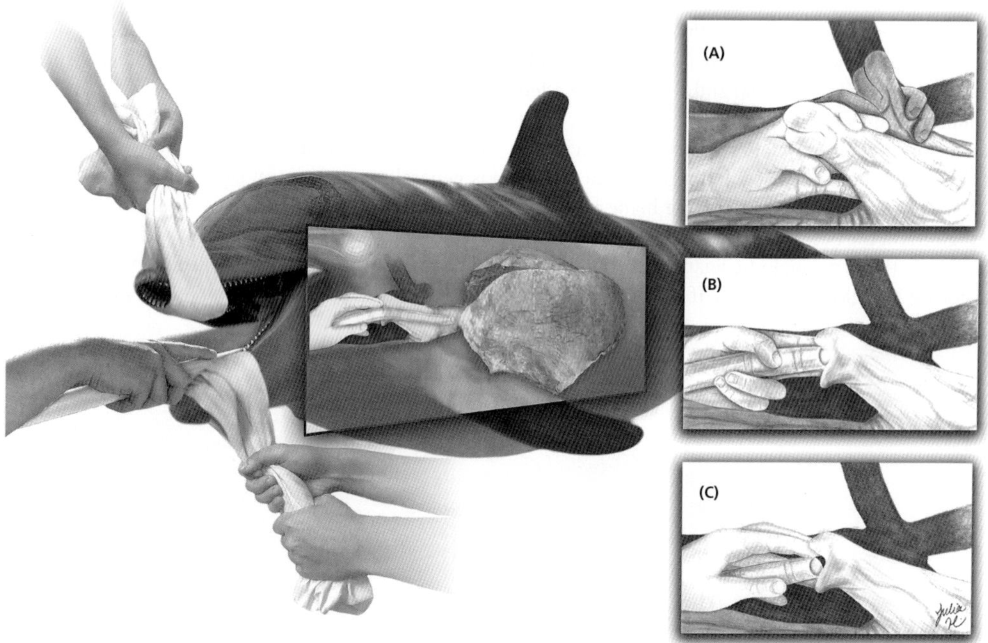

Figure 56.6 Endotracheal intubation of a dolphin in sternal recumbency. Blowhole response to touch, palpebral reflex, and jaw tone are vigilantly monitored during anesthetic induction. Classically, two soft, towels are placed between the mandible and maxilla to hold the mouth open. A hand of the anesthetist is inserted into the oropharynx. **A.** The larynx resembling the beak of a goose ("goosebeak') is gently grasped and pulled cranioventrally from its location in the nasopharynx. **B.** Classically, one or two fingers are inserted into the glottis to guide endotracheal tube placement, as the endotracheal tube is passed over the palm of the hand. The endotracheal tube is pushed forward and advanced by the second hand still outside the mouth. Using two fingers, the anesthetist can spread the fingers apart to open the larynx further. This method may be mandatory for conscious or inadequately anesthetized patients having excessive muscular control of the larynx. Unfortunately, this approach involves fingers that in part obstruct the larynx and, thus, may limit endotracheal tube size options. **C.** Alternatively, in the adequately relaxed patient, a single digit can depress the epiglottis without entering the larynx. This author depresses the epiglottis with the fourth digit (ring finger) as the first, second, and third digits (thumb, index, and middle fingers, respectively) control the tip of the endotracheal tube to redirect and position the beveled edge of the tube and facilitate advancement through the larynx. Keeping fingers out of the larynx may allow for larger endotracheal tube placement. The endotracheal tube can be rotated to position the Murphy eye of the tube to the right of the patient to minimize the likelihood of obstructing the accessory bronchus. The "x-ray' view above demonstrates this positioning relative to the trachea and lungs. Source: Dr. James Bailey, Innovative Veterinary Medicine Inc. 2023; with permission.

and anesthetized animals. In all situations, a relatively smaller endotracheal tube is inserted into the blowhole and advanced through the left or right nasal cavity into the trachea. This approach is greatly facilitated by the use of a flexible endoscope for both visualization of the laryngeal opening and as a stylet to guide advancement of the tube. While this method seems straightforward, it is subjectively more complicated than oral intubation due to redundant tissue and muscular folds between the blowhole and larynx that are used for vocalization and echolocation. Not surprisingly, this limits the size of the tube that can be used. While it has not been attempted to the authors' knowledge, theoretically, intubation of the blowhole could be maintained in a conscious animal beyond anesthetic recovery if necessitated by the animal's medical needs. That said, prolonged blowhole intubation could create inflammation or result in abnormal blowhole function, which would be problematic once the animal is returned to the water. Blowhole intubation has been used in small dolphins (*Stenella styx* and *Delphinus delphis*) under experimental conditions at sea [132]. To facilitate laryngeal anesthesia for conscious intubation, lidocaine (2%) was applied to the blowhole, nasal passages, and larynx using a small metal cannula prior to passing the uncuffed endotracheal tube.

Pinniped intubation

Subjectively, compared to other marine mammal species, the adequately anesthetized pinniped is less difficult to intubate since the larynx can be visualized and the vocal cords are relatively immobile. Cuffed endotracheal tubes of sizes 8 to 22 mm ID are suitable. An oral approach is used. After induction of anesthesia, the patient is positioned in sternal recumbency with the mandible and maxilla pulled apart with rope or webbing material and the neck extended in a straight orientation. Care should be taken not to twist the head or neck as this can distort the normal anatomy, particularly in larger pinnipeds. A laryngoscope should be used, but a good light source (e.g., headlamp) can be useful. The laryngoscope blade is placed underneath the epiglottis at the base of the tongue and gently forced downward; this stretches the hypoepiglottic ligament, dropping the epiglottis and exposing the glottic opening. If needed, a second laryngoscope blade rotated 180 degrees or similar device (e.g., silicone spatula) can be used to push upwards on the soft palate and improve visualization; this can also be achieved with the tip of the endotracheal tube. Advancement of the tube timed with inspiration (e.g., abduction of the arytenoid cartilages) may ease the process.

Larger pinnipeds often have excessive soft palate and pharyngeal tissues and physically heavy heads, both of which can impede positioning and visualization. In these situations, blind intubation via palpation is usually selected and is similar to intubation of domestic large animal species such as cattle. An appropriate level of anesthesia is crucial for safety, but a bite block can also be used to protect the individual's arm. With the animal positioned as described above, the anesthetist's hand is cupped around the distal aspect of the endotracheal tube and inserted into the oropharynx. The epiglottis is digitally retracted, the arytenoids are identified, and the endotracheal tube is manually guided into the trachea. In larger species or with smaller arms, this can be accomplished using a two-hand technique and the digits can be used to gently hold the arytenoids open. In lieu of this palpation method, fiberoptic intubation scopes can be used to improve human safety, but may be logistically complicated. Using either technique, tracheal insertion should be confirmed with a capnograph. If unavailable, bilateral thoracic auscultation should be performed to confirm placement and concurrently rule out one-lung intubation. The tube should also be secured to the maxilla using a tie and the cuff inflated to a minimum occlusive volume.

Manatee intubation

The manatee has several anatomic characteristics that make visualization of the caudal pharynx and larynx using an oral approach extremely difficult, including a curved angle of the tongue, a narrow buccal cavity, and a long soft palate. As a result, oral intubation is generally unsuccessful and, instead, the glottis and trachea are best accessed from the nasal cavities. While nasotracheal tubes have occasionally been passed blindly with success, dependable tracheal intubation is best accomplished with endoscopic assistance (Fig. 56.7). This visualization helps in wild sirenians which are

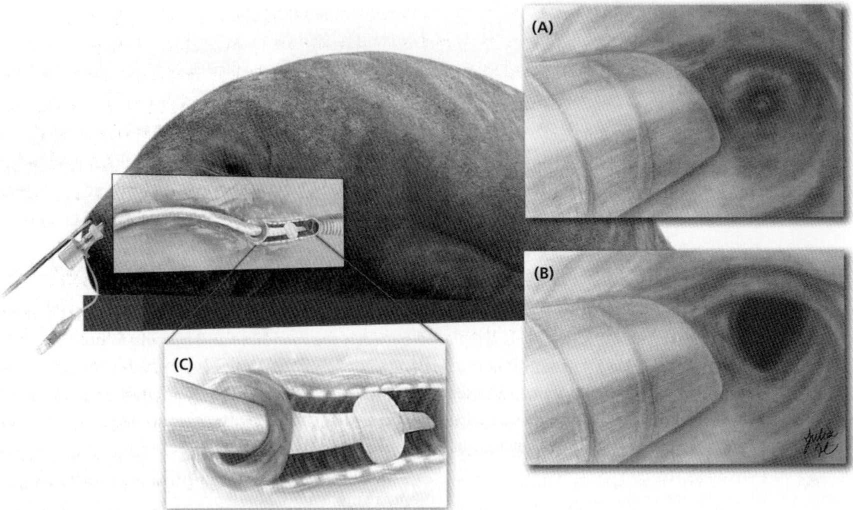

Figure 56.7 Endoscopic-assisted nasal intubation of the Florida manatee (*Trichechus manatus latirostris*). **A.** and **B.** Endoscope placement through the nasal passage allows visualization of the glottis to time intubation with glottal opening. **C.** Note the final positioning of the endotracheal tube tip cranial to the carina after advancement of the endotracheal tube into the trachea. Source: Dr. James Bailey, Innovative Veterinary Medicine Inc., 2023; with permission.

commonly infested with nasopharyngeal trematodes and occasionally have severe rhinitis or tracheitis [133,134]. Use of a scope can also aid in maneuvering around caudal pharyngeal tissue which can impede glottal visualization, especially during breath-holding in heavily sedated manatees. Stylets may be used to assist passage of the endotracheal tube through the glottis if using the scope separately, though preplacing the endotracheal tube over the end of a scope usually results in quicker intubation and confirmation of accurate placement [128,135]. Application of lidocaine gel or spray to the nares and glottis prior to intubation attempts can also be helpful. In Florida manatees, it is recommended to use relatively long cuffed endotracheal tubes (8 to 14 mm ID) designed for foals. Due to the short length of the manatee trachea, intubation of a single bronchus can occur; bronchoscopy can confirm proper positioning of the endotracheal tube cranial to the carina. Once placed, the nasotracheal tube should be secured in place and the cuff inflated to a minimum occlusive volume.

Monitoring and support

The importance of vigilant monitoring during marine mammal anesthesia cannot be overstated and this extends throughout all four phases of the anesthetic episode (premedication, induction, maintenance, and recovery), during any sedation episode, and during any period of mechanical/physical restraint. Monitoring is a challenging, complex process which requires superb critical thinking skills and should involve at least one dedicated anesthetist. Arguably, the most important monitor is the anesthetist themself as a wealth of information can be collected using the human eyes and ears and a basic stethoscope (e.g., anesthetic depth, mucous membrane color, respiratory rate and effort, and auscultation). Even during situations of limited patient access, observation of the thoracic wall can confirm both ventilation and myocardial contraction (e.g., apex beat). Productive ventilation and a patent airway are important to confirm, particularly when using aggressive immobilization cocktails, with physically large species, or with fully aquatic species (cetaceans, sirenians) that are "beached," as partial or complete airway obstruction can occur. In some situations, subjects will flare their nostrils and attempt to move their diaphragm and thoracic wall, but ventilation will be suboptimal and consistent with partial or complete airway obstruction. Thus, ventilation with evidence of air flow must be monitored from the time of first handling to after full recovery. Monitoring should be continuously performed, and physiologic values ideally recorded every 5 min. The anesthetist should understand acceptable or "normal" physiologic parameters for the target species prior to the anesthetic event. Historically, most anesthetic monitoring in marine mammal anesthesia was non-invasive in nature. While this is appropriate in some situations (e.g., sedation), advances in technology and vascular access techniques have laid the groundwork for routine use of more invasive monitoring techniques (e.g., invasive blood pressure and arterial blood gas analysis).

In addition to visual assessment of the patient as discussed above, additional non-invasive monitoring tools (i.e., electrocardiogram, pulse oximetry, temperature, end-tidal gas analysis, and non-invasive blood pressure) should be considered for every sedation or anesthetic event. The decision to exclude a monitoring tool should be based on patient compliance and the consideration for personnel safety, among other factors. A 3-lead electrocardiogram allows assessment of heart rate and rhythm and should be placed as soon as access to the patient is safe. The marine mammals discussed here have a type 2/category B cardiac conduction system, similar to the horse, with a diffuse Purkinje network and an overall axis of depolarization that is different than domestic dogs and cats [78]. As such, a modified base apex lead is frequently used in larger subjects to simplify electrode placement and optimize the ECG tracing. Pulse oximetry probes provide an assessment of the oxygen saturation of hemoglobin; as this technology relies on pulsatile arterial flow, a concurrent pulse rate is also obtained and should always be compared to the heart rate generated on an ECG. Reusable clip-type transmittance probes (originally designed for the human ear) are frequently placed on the tongue or mucous membranes of the oral or urogenital regions with reflectance probes allowing placement in additional areas (e.g., dorsal aspect of the rectal cavity). Hypoxemia is a potential anesthetic complication, especially in spontaneously ventilating or larger marine mammals, thus, continuous assessment of oxygenation is a necessity. Monitoring of temperature is paramount in both managed care and free-ranging settings as hypo- or hyperthermia can frequently occur. Temperature probes should be inserted at least 30 cm into the esophagus or rectum and, thus, hand-held style thermometers common in domestic animal anesthesia are usually not sufficient. While often forgotten until well into the anesthetic episode, prioritization of temperature assessment and thermoregulatory support should occur. End-tidal gas analysis (i.e., CO_2, O_2, and inhalant concentration) can provide a wealth of information (e.g., confirm intubation, assess ventilation and perfusion, and guide vaporizer management during induction, maintenance, and recovery) and is discussed in detail in Chapters 14, 15, and 16. Both intubated and non-intubated patients should have a gas analyzer attached between the breathing circuit and the patient, as even a tight-fitting facemask will usually allow assessment of ventilatory trends through gas analysis. Blood pressure measurement is performed to obtain an objective measurement of systemic perfusion and is standard of care in veterinary anesthesia. Non-invasive blood pressure assessment is limited by patient size and limb anatomy, among other factors. While non-invasive blood pressure monitors have yet to be validated in marine mammal species, the use of oscillometric cuffs on the pectoral and occasionally pelvic flippers of small to medium-sized pinnipeds have been used to identify trends and contribute to assessment of the overall clinical picture. With that in mind, if an appropriate cuff size is available (i.e., width of the cuff approximately 40% of the circumference of the limb) for the target species, the authors encourage its use in pinnipeds. Even in situations in which invasive blood pressure monitoring is planned, cannulation of an artery takes time and may not always be successful, thus, non-invasive blood pressure measurement should still be used. Unfortunately, no non-invasive blood pressure measurement has yet proven successful in cetaceans or sirenians. "Normal" arterial blood pressure values in marine mammal species are largely unknown, but the authors anecdotally define hypotension as a mean arterial pressure (MAP) < 70 mmHg in pinnipeds and sirenians and < 90–100 mmHg in cetaceans (conscious MAP range 115–142 mmHg) [136,137].

Invasive blood pressure monitoring has become a standard of care for marine mammals in managed care, but can be technically challenging in manatees and small phocids [137]. Placement of arterial catheters is discussed in the vascular access section of this chapter. This monitoring tool should be used whenever possible in immobilized or anesthetized marine mammals, especially for longer procedures, compromised or geriatric patients, or when significant anesthetic or procedural complications are expected (e.g., hypoxemia and hemorrhage). Principles of hypotension management are similar to domestic species and include a reduction in inhalant delivery, techniques for MAC reduction, volume loading where appropriate, and intravenous use of inotropes (e.g., dobutamine 0.2–2 μg/kg/min, ephedrine 0.05–0.1 mg/kg) or vasopressors (e.g., phenylephrine 0.1–1 μg/kg/min, norepinephrine 0.01–0.1 μg/kg/min).

Similar to invasive blood pressure monitoring, blood gas, electrolyte, and lactate analyses should be used whenever possible in immobilized or anesthetized marine mammals, especially for lengthy anesthetic procedures, in compromised or geriatric subjects, or when significant anesthetic or procedural complications are expected (e.g., hypoxemia and hypotension). Interpretation of blood gas data is reviewed elsewhere in this textbook. However, early testing of even venous blood can warn of excessive exertion during the process of anesthetic induction and the potential for developing rhabdomyolysis [82].

Cushioning with thick (4 to 8 inch) medium-density, open-cell foam padding similar to that used for large terrestrial mammals is necessary to minimize development of myopathy and neuropathy, especially during longer procedures [138]. Waterproof closed-cell foam padding provides minimal cushioning and should be reserved for short procedures. The insulating effect of foam padding also minimizes conductive heat loss. As discussed previously, thermoregulatory support is necessary as hypo- or hyperthermia may occur. Control of environmental temperature (if possible), minimization of stress or excitement in the preanesthetic period, use of external patient warming devices (i.e., circulating warm water or forced air blankets), and dry-docking or towel-drying patients prior to anesthesia can be useful adjuncts. For cetaceans, near-neutral buoyant liquid suspension systems have been used [61] and are currently being reevaluated for positioning support and thermoregulation.

Dive reflex

When discussing the dive reflex or dive response in marine mammals handled for sedation and anesthesia, it is generally directed at concerns for breath-holding and circulatory adjustments, specifically apnea, bradycardia, and regional vasoconstriction. Studies have convincingly proven that pinnipeds demonstrate a profound "dive reflex" when forced to dive [139]. Furthermore, these same animals when allowed to dive voluntarily do not demonstrate the same degree of bradycardia as when forced into a dive [140–142]. As such, the normal dive response of pinnipeds appears to be more graded and under conscious control while the response is more exaggerated if the animal does not know when the dive will end. Importantly, none of the studied animals died as a result of the dive reflex during forced or voluntary dives, and there is no evidence to suggest this is a potential outcome (as long as they are allowed the opportunity to surface and breathe). There is also no evidence that the dive reflex remains intact in pinnipeds during chemically induced unconsciousness. On the contrary, there is evidence that anesthesia depresses or eliminates the dive reflex [143,144]. A wealth of anecdotal evidence supports the notion that the heart rate of a marine mammal stabilizes during general anesthesia when proper physiologic support is provided. Although activation of the dive reflex has quite often been blamed for negative outcomes in marine mammal anesthesia over many decades, it is more likely that the *lack* of a dive response is the issue. That is, during drug- and disease-induced physiologic derangements (e.g., apnea, hypoxemia, vasodilation, and hypoperfusion), the lack of this elegant reflex control and lack of ability to direct blood flow to vital organs may precipitate negative consequences. Indeed, an intact dive response might well enhance the probability of positive outcomes in anesthetized pinnipeds. This significantly underscores the need for mindful anesthetic monitoring and support of sedated or anesthetized marine mammals.

There are some physiologic reflexes, including the laryngeal, oculocardiac, and other trigeminocardiac and vagally induced reflexes that may occur in the anesthetized marine mammal, especially at light planes of anesthesia (e.g., induction and recovery). Occurrence of these reflexes and resultant bradycardia may well be confused with a "dive reflex." Bradycardia during sedation, immobilization, or anesthesia can also result from inadequate respiratory support in that severe hypoxemia and myocardial hypoxia can cause terminal bradycardia. While the true occurrence of a "dive reflex" during general anesthesia of marine mammals is questionable, monitoring for bradycardia of any etiology or other physiologic disturbances is important.

Anesthetic recovery

Anesthetic vigilance, monitoring, and support do not end just because the anesthetic vaporizer has been turned off as anesthetic complications can occur into and beyond the recovery period. This is especially important to highlight in situations involving free-ranging or dangerous animals where monitoring capabilities and human safety are sometimes at odds. Ventilatory support (e.g., mechanical ventilator, manual resuscitator bag, and demand valve) may be necessary well into recovery. As alluded to earlier, monitoring the end-expired anesthetic concentration in recovery can guide administration of reversal agents. More specifically, the authors administer reversal agents when the inhalant anesthetic is at a concentration that is expected to produce minimal effect on awareness (approximate MAC_{awake} of isoflurane < 0.4%, sevoflurane < 0.8%); this strategy theoretically promotes arousal at a timepoint when unwanted dysphoria from the inhalant is minimal.

Limited pharmacokinetic data on opioids and non-steroidal anti-inflammatory drugs in marine mammals suggest the half-life of many useful anesthetic and perianesthetic drugs will have a surprisingly long duration of action when compared to terrestrial species [145–148]. For this reason, it is preferable to use anesthetic drugs that can be eliminated easily without metabolism (i.e., inhalation anesthetics) or are reversible. As such, it is common to reverse benzodiazepines, opioids, and α_2-adrenergic receptor agonists to speed recovery and promote the return of effective spontaneous ventilation in marine mammals.

Full reversal of clinically used benzodiazepines, on a milligram-for-milligram basis, requires 1 part flumazenil for every 13 parts of midazolam or every 26 parts diazepam [149]. The functional half-life of flumazenil can be estimated from terrestrial animal models as at least one hour. As intravenous administration may result in an abrupt and excitable recovery and large volumes are often needed, the authors recommend half the calculated dose of flumazenil be delivered intramuscularly and, 5 min later, half the calculated dose is administered intravenously. The response is then evaluated before any redosing.

Full reversal of opioids can be achieved with naloxone 0.01 mg/kg or naltrexone 0.05–0.1 mg/kg (0.5–1 mg/kg for ultrapotent opioids). The half-life of naloxone is variable in terrestrial species but can be approximated at 20–30 min, where naltrexone can be anticipated to have a much longer species-dependent half-life of 7–8 h and a slow terminal elimination-phase half-life of around 24 h. Naloxone can be used at a full or partial dosage to attenuate the level of opioid-induced postoperative depression, theoretically allowing return of residual opioid analgesia. Where analgesia is not necessary, or the subject is perceived to have excessive opioid-induced respiratory depression, naltrexone can be used to provide sustained reversal of opioid effects. The authors use a partial IM and IV strategy as described above for flumazenil. As, anecdotally, opioid reversal tends to greatly increase arousal, it is usually administered as the final drug in any IV reversal strategy.

Reversal of concentrated medetomidine is dependent on the ratio of milligrams of antagonist drug to milligrams of α_2-adrenergic receptor agonist, not the volume. Atipamezole is delivered at 5 and 10 times the milligram dose of medetomidine and dexmedetomidine, respectively, for full reversal via the intramuscular route to avoid rapid arousal and/or potential hypotension. When α_2-adrenergic receptor agonists are absolutely necessary for induction of anesthesia, but the cardiovascular effects of the α_2-adrenergic receptor agonists are deemed undesirable for the target patient, the authors will administer atipamezole after achieving an appropriate end-expired anesthetic level and, preferably, after gaining vascular access for provision of necessary support.

The endotracheal tube should be maintained in the airway as long as possible within the safety guidelines for the species involved. Protective contact restrictions for large pinnipeds can influence this decision-making process in favor of human safety. Subjects will routinely attempt to extubate prematurely or cough and inadvertently extubate as they regain reflex control of their airway. Given the respiratory depressant effect of anesthetic agents in marine mammals, it is possible for these species to extubate prematurely and either develop airway obstruction or become apneic; this is particularly true of phocids, cetaceans, and sirenians. For this reason, the authors try to maintain IV access as long as safely possible into the recovery period as reintubation may not be possible without reinduction of anesthesia. It is also advisable to have an additional endotracheal tube (usually one size smaller) on hand as well as both drugs and tools for reintubation. Phenylephrine (0.5–1%) nasal spray can be used to reduce nasal cavity edema that can develop from recumbency and endotracheal tube ties around the muzzle. Respiratory stimulants, such as the nonspecific central nervous stimulant doxapram (1 mg/kg IM, IV), are generally unnecessary, but worthy of mention as a tool for managing respiratory depression when there is lack of airway control in a semi-conscious animal. Unfortunately, this only increases cerebral oxygen consumption in the face of inadequate ventilation and may do more harm than good in most instances.

Acknowledgment

The authors would like to extend sincere thanks to Ms. Julia Hudson for her work creating the illustrations that appear in this chapter.

References

1 Gingerich PD, Wells NA, Russell DE, *et al.* Origin of whales in epicontinental remnant seas: new evidence from the early eocene of Pakistan. *Science* 1983; **220**: 403–405.

2 Nishiwaki M, Tobayama T. Morphological study of the hybrid between *Tursiops* and *Pseudorca*. *Sci Rep Whales Res Inst* 1982; **34**: 109–121.

3 Zornetzer HR, Duffield DA. Captive-born bottlenose dolphin × common dolphin (*Tursiops truncatus* × *Delphinus capensis*) intergeneric hybrids. *Can J Zool* 2003; **81**(10): 1755–1762.

4 Venn-Watson S, Jensen ED, Ridgway SH. Effects of age and sex on clinicopathologic reference ranges in a healthy managed Atlantic bottlenose dolphin population. *J Am Vet Med Assoc* 2007; **231**(4): 596–601.

5 Venn-Watson SK, Jensen ED, Ridgway SH. Evaluation of population health among bottlenose dolphins (*Turiops truncatus*) at the United States Navy Marine Mammal Program. *J Am Vet Med Assoc* 2011; **238**(3): 356–360.

6 Lawson P, Buck EH. *Marine Mammals in Captivity: Background and Management Issues in the United States*. Washington, DC: Congressional Research Service, 1997: 1–19.

7 Corkeron P. Captivity. In: Corkeron P, ed. *Encyclopedia of Marine Mammals*, 2nd edn. New York, NY: Elsevier, 2009: 183–188.

8 Domning DP, Hayek LC. Interspecific and intraspecific morphological variation in manatees (Sirenia: Trichechus). *Mar Mammal Sci* 1986; **2**(2): 87–144.

9 Reynolds JE, Odell DK. *Manatees and Dugongs*. New York, NY: Facts on File, 1991: 1–192.

10 Courbis SS, Worthy GAJ. Opportunistic carnivory by Florida manatees (*Trichechus manatus latirostris*). *Aquat Mamm* 2003; **29**(1): 104–107.

11 Convention on International Trade in Endangered Species (CITES). Appendices I, II and III. www.cites.org/sites/default/files/eng/app/2023/E-Appendices-2023-02-23.pdf (accessed July 2023).

12 International Union for Conservation of Nature (IUCN). Redlist of Threatened Species 2022. www.iucnredlist.org (accessed April 2023).

13 Environmental Conservation Online System (ECOS). United States Fish & Wildlife Service, 2023. https://ecos.fws.gov/ecp/species/4469 (accessed July 2023).

14 Richards DW Jr. The Lewis A. Conner memorial lecture, the nature of cardiac and of pulmonary dyspnea. *Circulation* 1953; **7**(1): 15–29.

15 Smith JC, Ellenberger HH, Ballanyi K, *et al.* Pre-Bötzinger complex: a brainstem region that may generate respiratory rhythm in mammals. *Science* 1991; **254**(5032): 726–729.

16 Kam K, Worrell JW, Janczewski WA, *et al.* Distinct inspiratory rhythm and pattern generating mechanisms in the preBötzinger complex. *J Neurosci* 2013; **33**(22): 9235–9245.

17 Marina N, Abdala AP, Trapp S, *et al.* Essential role of Phox2b-expressing ventrolateral brainstem neurons in the chemosensory control of inspiration and expiration. *J Neurosci* 2010; **30**(37): 12466–12473.

18 Dubreuil V, Barhanin J, Goridis C, *et al.* Breathing with Phox2b. *Philos Trans R Soc Lond B Biol Sci* 2009; **364**: 2477–2483.

19 Coghlan M, Richards E, Shaik S, *et al.* Inhalational anesthetics induce neuronal protein aggregation and affect ER trafficking. *Sci Rep* 2018; **8**: 5275.

20 Albersheim-Carter J, Blubaum A, Ballagh IH, *et al.* Testing the evolutionary conservation of vocal motoneurons in vertebrates. *Respir Physiol Neurobiol* 2016; **224**: 2–10.

21 Nomaksteinsky M, Kassabov S, Chettouh Z, *et al.* Ancient origin of somatic and visceral neurons. *BMC Biol* 2013; **11**: 53.

22 Munson Edwin S, Larson Philip C, Babad Arthur A, *et al.* The effects of halothane, fluroxene and cyclopropane on ventilation: a comparative study in man. *Anesthesiology* 1966; **27**(6): 716–728.

23 Colitz CMH, Bailey JE. Lens diseases and anesthetic considerations for ophthalmologic procedures in pinnipeds. In: Miller RE, Lamberski N, Calle PP, eds. *Fowler's Zoo and Wild Animal Medicine Current Therapy*, Vol. **9**. St. Louis, MO: Elsevier, 2019: 610–617.

24 Weil JV, McCullough RE, Kline JS, *et al.* Diminished ventilatory response to hypoxia and hypercapnia after morphine in normal man. *N Engl J Med* 1975; **292**(21): 1103–1106.

25 Pattinson KT. Opioids and the control of respiration. *Br J Anaesth* 2008; **100**(6): 747–758.

26 Dahan A, Sarton E, Teppema L, *et al.* Anesthetic potency and influence of morphine and sevoflurane on respiration in μ-opioid receptor knockout mice. *Anesthesiology* 2001; **94**(5): 824–832.

27 Garcia PS, Kolesky SE, Jenkins A. General anesthetic actions on GABA(A) receptors. *Curr Neuropharmacol* 2010; **8**(1): 2–9.

28 Kelz MB, García PS, Mashour GA, *et al.* Escape from oblivion: neural mechanisms of emergence from general anesthesia. *Anesth Analg* 2019; **128**(4): 726–736.

29 Montandon G, Wu H, Liu H, *et al.* Delta-subunit containing GABA(A) receptors modulate respiratory networks. *Sci Rep* 2017; **7**(1): 18105.

30 Walsh M RT, McBain J, Dalton L, *et al.* Sedation and anesthesia techniques in cetaceans. In: *Proceedings of the American Association of Zoo Veterinarians Annual Conference*. Tampa, FL, 2006.

31 Reidarson T. Cetacean medicine. In: Fowler M, Miller ER, eds. *Zoo and Wild Animal Medicine*, 5th edn. Orlando, FL: WB Saunders, 2003: 442–459.

32 Li Y, Wang S, Pan C, *et al.* Comparison of NREM sleep and intravenous sedation through local information processing and whole brain network to explore the mechanism of general anesthesia. *PLoS ONE* 2018; **13**(2): e0192358.

33 Lilly JC. Animals in aquatic environments: adaptation of mammals to the ocean. In: Baker PT, ed. *Handbook of Physiology: Adaptation to the Environment*. Washington, DC: American Physiology Society, 1964: 741–747.

34 Bailey J, Ridgway S, Dold C. Cetaceans. In: West G, Heard D, Caulkett N, eds. *Zoo Animal and Wildlife Immobilization and Anesthesia*, 2nd edn. Ames, IA: Wiley, 2014: 679–692.

35 Edwards A. *Swifts. Nature* 1887; **36**(939): 605.

36 Serafetinides EA, Shurley JT, Brooks RE. Electroencephalogram of the pilot whale, *Globicephala scammoni*, in wakefulness and sleep: lateralization aspects. *Int J Psychobiol* 1972; **2**(2): 129–135.

37 Mukhametov LM, Supin AY, Polyakova IG. Interhemispheric asymmetry of the electroencephalographic sleep patterns in dolphins. *Brain Res* 1977; **134**: 581–584.

38 Mukhametov LM. Sleep in marine mammals. *Exp Brain Res* 1984; **8**: 227–238.

39 Oleksenko A, Mukhametov L, Polyakova I, *et al.* Unihemispheric sleep deprivation in bottlenose dolphins. *J Sleep Res* 1992; **1**(1): 40–44.

40 Ridgway SH. Asymmetry and symmetry in brain waves from dolphin left and right hemispheres: some observations after anesthesia, during quiescent hanging behavior, and during visual obstruction. *Brain Behav Evol* 2002; **60**(5): 265–274.

41 Mortola JP, Limoges M-J. Resting breathing frequency in aquatic mammals: a comparative analysis with terrestrial species. *Respir Physiol Neurobiol* 2006; **154**: 500–514.

42 Ridgway SH, Harrison RJ, Joyce PL. Sleep and cardiac rhythm in the grey seal. *Science* 1975; **187**: 553–554.

43 Lyamin OI, Kosenko PO, Vyssotski AL, *et al.* Study of sleep in a walrus. *Dokl Biol Sci* 2012; **444**: 188–191.

44 Pryaslova JP, Lyamin OI, Siegel JM, *et al.* Behavioral sleep in the walrus. *Behav Brain Rese* 2009; **201**: 80–87.

45 Mukhametov LM, Lyamin OI, Polyakova IG. Interhemispheric asynchrony of the sleep EEG in northern fur seals. *Experientia* 1985; **41**(8): 1034–1035.

46 Lapierre JL, Kosenko PO, Lyamin OI, *et al.* Cortical acetylcholine release is lateralized during asymmetrical slow-wave sleep in northern fur seals. *J Neurosci* 2007; **27**(44): 11999–12006.

47 Lyamin OI, Lapierre JL, Kosenko PO, *et al.* Electroencephalogram asymmetry and spectral power during sleep in the northern fur seal. *J Sleep Res* 2008; **17**: 154–165.

48 Lyamin OI, Mukhametov LM, Chetyrbok IS, *et al.* Sleep and wakefulness in the southern sea lion. *Behav Brain Res* 2002; **128**: 129–138.

49 Kendall-Bar JM, Williams TM, Mukherji R, *et al.* Brain activity of diving seals reveals short sleep cycles at depth. *Science* 2023; **380**(6642): 260–265.

50 Lyamin OI, Kosenko PO, Lapierre JL, *et al.* Fur seals display a strong drive for bilateral slow-wave sleep while on land. *J Neurosci* 2008; **28**(48): 12614–12621.

51 Matishov GG, Voynov VB, Verbitsky EV, *et al.* The cardiorespiratory function and electrical activity of the brain of the ringed seal during the transition from wakefulness to sleep. *Dokl Biol Sci* 2012; **442**: 1–6.

52 Mukhametov LM, Lyamin OI, Chetyrbok IS, *et al.* Sleep in an Amazonian manatee, *Trichechus inunguis*. *Experientia* 1992; **48**(4): 417–419.

53 Zancanella E, do Prado LF, de Carvalho LB, *et al.* Home sleep apnea testing: an accuracy study. *Sleep Breath* 2022; **26**(1): 117–123.

54 Fahlman A, Loring SH, Ferrigno M, *et al.* Static inflation and deflation pressure–volume curves from excised lungs of marine mammals. *J Exp Biol* 2011; **214**(22): 3822–3828.

55 Denison D, Warrell DA, West JB. Airway structure and alveolar emptying in the lungs of sea lions and dogs. *Respir Physiol* 1972; **13**: 253–261.

56 Ponganis PJ. Diving mammals. *Compr Phys* 2011; **1**(1): 447–465.

57 Kooyman GL, Sinnett EE. Mechanical properties of the harbor porpoise lung, *Phocoena phocoena*. *Respir Physiol* 1979; **36**: 287–300.

58 Piscitelli M, Raverty SA, Lillie MA, *et al.* A review of cetacean lung morphology and mechanics. *J Morphol* 2013; **274**: 1425–1440.

59 Olsen CR, Hale FC, Elsner R. Mechanics of ventilation in the pilot whale. *Respir Physiol* 1969; **7**: 137–149.

60 Moore MJ, Hammar T, Arruda J, *et al.* Hyperbaric computed tomographic measurement of lung compression in seals and dolphins. *J Exper Biol* 2011; **214**: 2390–2397.

61 Ridgway SH, McCormick JG, Wever EG. Surgical approach to the dolphin's ear. *J Exp Zool* 1974; **188**: 265–276.

62 Kerr CL, McDonell WN. Oxygen supplementation and ventilatory assist devices. In: Muir WH, Hubbell JAE, eds. *Equine Anesthesia: Monitoring and Emergency Therapy*, 2nd edn. St. Louis, MO: Saunders Elsevier, 2009: 332–352.

63 Nagel EL, Morgane PJ, McFarland WL. Anesthesia for the bottlenose dolphin. *Science* 1964; **146**: 1591–1593.

64 Ridgway SH. Medical care of marine mammals. *J Am Vet Med Assoc* 1965; **147**(10): 1077–1085.

65 Ridgway SH, McCormick JG. Anesthetization of porpoises for major surgery. *Science* 1967; **158**(3800): 510–512.

66 Ridgway SH, McCormick JG. Anesthesia of the porpoise. In: Soma LR, ed. *Textbook of Veterinary Anesthesia*. Baltimore, MD: Williams and Wilkins Co, 1971: 394–403.

67 Nagel EL, Morgane PJ, McFarland WL. Anesthesia for the bottlenose dolphin. *Vet Med Small Anim Clin* 1966; **61**(3): 6.

68 McCormick JG, Ridgway SH. History of the development of anesthesia for the dolphin: a quest to study a brain as large as man's. *Anesthesiology* 2018; **129**(1): 11–21.

69 Nagel EL, Morgane PJ, McFarland WL. Anesthesia for the bottlenose dolphin, *Tursiops truncatus*. *Surv Anesthesiol* 1966; **10**(2): 149.

70 Downs JB, Stock MC. Airway pressure release ventilation: a new concept in ventilatory support. *Crit Care Med* 1987; **15**(5): 459–461.

71 Stock MC, Downs JB, Frolicher DA. Airway pressure release ventilation. *Crit Care Med* 1987; **15**(5): 462–466.

72 Bratzke E, Downs JB, Smith RA. Intermittent CPAP: a new mode of ventilation during general anesthesia. *Anesthesiology* 1998; **89**(2): 334–340.

73 Downs JB, Robinson LA, Steighner ML, *et al.* Open lung ventilation optimizes pulmonary function during lung surgery. *J Surg Res* 2014; **192**(2): 242–249.

74 Bukoski A, Hodgson D, Downs J, *et al.* An implementation of apneustic anesthesia ventilation in the horse: comparison with conventional mechanical ventilation. *Vet Anaesth Analg* 2022; **49**(4): 372–381.

75 Downs John B, inventor. Method and apparatus for breathing during anesthesia. Patent WO1998010818A1. 1996.

76 Bailey J, Ridgway S. Anesthesia ventilator for Atlantic bottlenose dolphins and California sea lions. Navy STTR FY2014A-Topic N14A-T015. Office of Naval Research, 2020.

77 Le-Bert C, Bukoski A, Downs J, *et al.* Comparison of cardiopulmonary effects of controlled mechanical ventilation and apneustic anesthesia ventilation in bottlenose dolphins, *Tursiops truncatus* and California sea lions, *Zalophus californianus*. In: *Proceedings of the 52nd Annual American Association of Zoo Veterinarians Conference*. Nashville, TN, 2020.

78 Bailey J, Pablo LS. Anesthetic and physiologic considerations for veterinary endosurgery. In: Freeman LJ, ed. *Veterinary Endosurgery*. St. Louis, MO: Mosby, 1999.

79 Ponganis PJ, McDonald BI, Tift MS, *et al.* Effects of inhalational anesthesia on blood gases and pH in California sea lions. *Mar Mammal Sci* 2017; **33**(3): 1–12.

80 Olson KR, Whitfield NL, Bearden SE, *et al.* Hypoxic pulmonary vasodilation: a paradigm shift with a hydrogen sulfide mechanism. *Am J Physiol Regul Integr Comp Physiol* 2010; **298**(1): R51–R60.

81 Stringer EM, Van Bonn W, Chinnadurai SK, *et al.* Risk factors associated with perianesthetic mortality of stranded free-ranging California sea lions (*Zalophus californianus*) undergoing rehabilitation. *Zoo and Wildl Med* 2012; **43**(2): 233–239.

82 Bailey JE, Flanagan C, Meegan J, *et al.* Cogent evidence of rhabdomyolysis in a California sea lion (*Zalophus californianus*) and a South African fur seal (*Arctocephalus pusillus pusillus*) during anesthesia. In: *Proceedings of the 43rd Annual International Association for Aquatic Animal Medicine Conference*. Atlanta, GA, 2012.

83 Haulena M, Heath RB. Marine mammal anesthesia. In: Dierauf LA, Gulland FMD, eds. *Marine Mammal Medicine*, 2nd edn. Boca Raton, FL: CRC Press, 2001: 655–688.

84 Brunson DB. Comparative anesthesia and analgesia of aquatic mammals. In: Grimm KA, Lamont LA, Tranquilli WJ, *et al.*, eds. *Veterinary Anesthesia and Analgesia*, 5th edn. Ames, IA: Wiley Blackwell, 2015: 777–783.

85 Haulena M. Otariid seals. In: West G, Heard D, Caulkett N, eds. *Zoo Animal and Wildlife Immobilization and Anesthesia*. Ames, IA: Wiley Blackwell, 2007: 469–478.

86 Gulland FMD, Dierauf LA, Whitman KL, eds. *CRC Handbook of Marine Mammal Medicine*. Boca Raton, FL: CRC Press, 2018.

87 Brunson DB. Walrus. In: West G, Heard D, Caulkett N, eds. *Zoo Animal and Wildlife Immobilization and Anesthesia*. Ames, IA: Wiley Blackwell, 2007: 479–483.

88 Chittick EJ, Walsh MT. Sirenians (Manatees and Dugongs). In: West G, Heard D, Caulkett N, eds. *Zoo Animal and Wildlife Immobilization and Anesthesia*. Ames, IA: Wiley Blackwell, 2007: 497–505.

89 Dold C, Ridgway SH. Cetaceans. In: West G, Heard D, Caulkett N, eds. *Zoo Animal and Wildlife Immobilization and Anesthesia*. Ames, IA: Wiley Blackwell, 2007: 485–496.

90 Lynch M, Bodley K. Phocid seals. In: West G, Heard D, Caulkett N, eds. *Zoo Animal and Wildlife Immobilization and Anesthesia*. Ames, IA: Wiley Blackwell, 2007: 459–468.

91 McAllister D, ed. Underwater capture of juvenile Steller sea lions with scuba: a narrated video presentation. *21st Annual Scientific Diving Symposium of the American Academy of Underwater Sciences*. Seward, Alaska, 2001.

92 Mellish J, Calkins DG, Christen DR, *et al.* Temporary captivity as a research tool: comprehensive study of wild pinnipeds under controlled conditions. *Aquat Mamm* 2006; **32**(1): 58.

93 Dinter, B. Gaius Julius Caesar. *Commentarii de bello civili*. Leipzig, Germany: B.G. Teubner, 1876.

94 Muir WW, Hubbell JAE, Bednarski RM. *Handbook of Veterinary Anesthesia*, 4th edn. Maryland Heights, MO: Mosby Elsevier, 2000.

95 Smith RM. *Anesthesia for Infants and Children*. St. Louis, MO: Mosby, 1959.

96 Spelman LH. Reversible anesthesia of captive California sea lions (*Zalophus californianus*) with medetomidine, midozolam, butorphanol, and isoflurane. *J Zoo Wildl Med* 2004; **35**(1): 65–69.

97 Colitz CMH, Bailey JE. Lens diseases and anesthetic considerations for ophthalmologic procedures in pinnipeds. In: Miller RE, Lamberski N, Calle PP, eds. *Fowler's Zoo and Wild Animal Medicine Current Therapy*, Vol. **9**. St. Louis, MO: Elsevier, 2019: 610–617.
98 Li J. Comparison of anaesthetic protocols and outcomes in largha seals (*Phoca largha*), harbor seals (*Phoca vitulina*) and California sea lions (*Zalophus cailfornianus*) at Ocean Park Hong Kong. In: *Proceedings of the 54th Annual International Association for Aquatic Animal Medicine Conference*. Salt Lake City, UT, 2023.
99 Maslow AH. *The Psychology of Science, a Reconnaissance*. New York, NY: Harper & Row, 1966.
100 Madden CBJ, Johnson SP, Pasloske K. Case series evaluating the efficacy of alfaxalone 4% injection in pinnipeds. In: *Proceedings of the 14th World Congress of Veterinary Anaesthesia and Analgesia*. Sydney, Australia, 2023.
101 Langworthy OR. A description of the central nervous system of the porpoise (Tursiops truncatus). *J Comp Neurol* 1932; **52**(2): 437–498.
102 Lilly JC. My first experiments with dolphins. In: *Man and Dolphin*. New York, NY: Doubleday & Company, 1961: 48–61.
103 Moore M, Walsh M, Bailey J, *et al*. Sedation at sea of entangled North Atlantic right whales (*Eubalaena glacialis*) to enhance disentanglement. *PLoS ONE* 2010; **5**(3): e9597.
104 Moore M, Andrews R, Austin T, *et al*. Rope trauma, sedation, disentanglement, and monitoring-tag associated lesions in a terminally entangled North Atlantic right whale (*Eubalaena glacialis*). *Mar Mammal Sci* 2012; **29**(2): E98–E113.
105 Medway W, McCormick JG, Ridgway SH, *et al*. Effects of prolonged halothane anesthesia on some cetaceans. *J Am Vet Med Assoc* 1970; **157**(5): 576–582.
106 Linnehan R, MacMillan A. Propofol/isoflurane anesthesia and debridement of a corneal ulcer in an Atlantic bottlenose dolphin (*Tursiops truncatus*). In: *Proceedings of the American Association of Zoo Veterinarians*. Calgary, AB, 1991.
107 Dover SR, Beusse D, Walsh T, *et al*. Laparoscopic techniques for the bottlenose dolphin (*Tursiops truncatus*). In: *Proceedings of the 30th Annual International Association for Aquatic Animal Medicine Conference*. 1999; **30**: 128–129.
108 Bailey J. Cetacean anesthesia: a review of 10 clinical anesthesia events, lessons learned and future plans. In: *Proceedings of the 47th Annual International Association for Aquatic Animal Medicine Conference*. Virginia Beach, VA, 2016.
109 Ridgway SH, Simpson JG. Anesthesia and restraint for the California sea lion, *Zalophus californianus*. *J Am Vet Med Assoc* 1969; **155**: 1059–1063.
110 Skinner JP, Tuomi PA, Mellish JA. The influence of time in captivity, food intake and acute trauma on blood analytes of juvenile Steller sea lions, *Eumetopias jubatus*. *Conserv Physiol* 2015; **3**(1): cov008.
111 Heath RB, DeLong R, Jameson V, *et al*. Isoflurane anesthesia in free ranging sea lion pups. *J Wildl Dis* 1997; **33**(2): 206–210.
112 Walsh M, Webb A, Bailey J, *et al*. Sedation and anesthesia of the Florida manatee. *Int Assoc Aquat Anim Med* 1997.
113 Bailey J, Walsh MT, Webb AI, *et al*. Anesthesia of the Florida manatee (*Trichechus manatus*). In: *Proceedings of the 23rd Annual Meeting of the American College of Veterinary Anesthesiology*. Orlando, FL, 1998.
114 Braun M. Einiges über phocaena communis less. [harbour porpoise]. *Zoologischer Anzeiger* 1905; **29**(5): 145–149.
115 Fawcett D. A comparative study of blood vascular bundles in the Florida manatee (*Trichechus latirostris*) and in certain cetaceans and edentates. *J Morphol* 1942; **71**: 105–124.
116 Tomilin AG. Temperature regulation in cetaceans. *Priroda* 1951; **6**: 55–58.
117 Scholander PF, Schevill WE. Counter-current vascular heat exchange in the fins of whales. *J App Physiol* 1955; **8**(3): 279–282.
118 Elsner R, Pirie J, Kenney DD, *et al*. Functional circulatory anatomy of cetacean appendages. In: Harrison RJ, ed. *Functional Anatomy of Marine Mammals*, 2nd edn. London, UK: Academic Press, 1974: 143–159.
119 Lowenstine LJ, Groff J, Rideout B, *et al*. Necropsy findings in two juvenile beaked whales (*Mesoplodon* spp.) maintained in captivity for rehabilitation after stranding. In: *Proceedings of the 21st Annual International Association for Aquatic Animal Medicine Conference*. Vancouver, British Columbia, 1990.
120 Sen S, Chini EN, Brown MJ. Complications after unintentional intra-arterial injection of drugs: risks, outcomes, and management strategies. *Mayo Clin Proc* 2005; **80**(6): 783–795.
121 Stetter MD, McClave C, Cook RA. Marine mammal intravenous catheterization techniques. In: *Proceedings of the 29th Annual American Association of Zoo Veterinarians Conference*. Houston, TX, 1997.
122 Ivančić M, Johnson S, Costidis AM, *et al*. A technique for ultrasound-guided catheterization of a peripheral vein in the bottlenose dolphin (*Tursiops truncatus*). In: *Proceedings of the 46th Annual American Association of Zoo Veterinarians Conference*. Chicago, IL, 2015.
123 Seldinger SI. Catheter replacement of the needle in percutaneous arteriography: a new technique. *Acta Radiologica* 1953; **39**(5): 368–376.
124 Daly A, Mooney L, Peters B, *et al*. Catheter fixation and isolation in bottlenose dolphins (*Tursiops truncatus*). In: *Proceedings of the 44th Annual International Association for Aquatic Animal Medicine Conference*. Sausalito, CA, 2013.
125 Medway W, Geraci JR. Hematology of the bottlenose dolphin (*Tursiops truncatus*). *Am J Physiol* 1964; **207**: 1367–1370.
126 Ivančić M, Bailey JE, Costidis AM. Technique for ultrasound-guided arterial catheter placement in the pectoral flipper of the bottlenose dolphin (*Tursiops truncatus*). In: *Proceedings of the 46th Annual International Association for Aquatic Animal Medicine Conference*. Chicago, IL, 2014.
127 St. Pierre H. The topographical splanchnology and the superficial vascular system of the harp seal (*Pagophilus groenlandicus*) (Erxleben JCP, 1777). In: Harrison RJ, ed. *Functional Anatomy of Marine Mammals*, Vol. **2**. London, UK: Academic Press, 1974: 161–195.
128 Murphy D. Sirenia. In: Fowler ME, ed. *Zoo and Wild Animal Medicine*, 5th edn. St. Louis, MO: Elsevier Science, 2003: 476–482.
129 White JR. Manatee biology and medicine. In: Dierauf LA, ed. *CRC Handbook of Marine Mammal Medicine: Health, Disease, and Rehabilitation*. Boca Raton, FL: CRC Press, 1990: 601–623.
130 Rommel SA, Caplan H. Vascular adaptations for heat conservation in the tail of Florida manatees (*Trichechus manatus latirostris*). *J Anat* 2003; **202**(4): 343–353.
131 Green R. Observations on the anatomy of some cetaceans and pinnipeds. In: Ridgeway SH, ed. *Mammals of the Sea: Biology and Medicine*. Springfield, IL: Charles C. Thomas Publishers, 1972: 247–297.
132 Rieu M, Gautheron B. Preliminary observations concerning a method for introduction of a tube for anaesthesia in small delphinids. *Life Sci* 1968; **7**: 1141–1146.
133 Beck C, Forrester D. Helminths of the Florida manatee, *Trichechus manatus latirostris*, with a discussion and summary of the parasites of sirenians. *J Parasit* 1988; **74**: 628–637.
134 Bossart GD. Manatees. In: Dierauf LA, Gulland FMD, eds. *Marine Mammal Medicine*, 2nd edn. Boca Raton, FL: CRC Press, 2001: 939–960.
135 Walsh MT. Manatee medicine. In: Fowler ME, Miller ER, eds. *Zoo & Wild Animal Medicine, Current Therapy*, 4th edn. Philadelphia, PA: Saunders Company, 1999: 507–516.
136 Sommer L, McFarland W, Galliano R, *et al*. Hemodynamic and coronary angiographic studies in the bottlenose dolphin (*Tursiops truncatus*). *Amer J Physiol-Legacy Content* 1968; **215**(6): 1498–1505.
137 Bailey J. Arterial blood pressure monitoring of select pinnipeds: multi-case presentation. In: *Proceedings of the 44th Annual International Association for Aquatic Animal Medicine Conference*. Sausalito, CA, 2013.
138 Bednarski R. Anesthesia equipment. In: Muir WH, Hubbell JAE, eds. *Equine Anesthesia: Monitoring and Emergency Therapy*. St. Louis, MO: Mosby Year Book, 1991: 325–351.
139 Irving L, Scholander PF, Grinnell SW. Significance of the heart rate to the diving ability of seals. *J Cell Comp Physiol* 1941; **18**(3): 283–297.
140 Thompson D, Fedak MA. Cardiac responses of grey seals during diving at sea. *J Exp Biol* 1993; **174**: 139–154.
141 Kooyman GL, Ponganis PJ. The physiological basis of diving to depth: birds and mammals. *Annu Rev of Physiol* 1998; **60**: 19–32.
142 Davis RW, Castellini MA, Kooyman GL, *et al*. Renal glomerular filtration rate and hepatic blood flow during voluntary diving in Weddell seals. *Am J Physiol* 1983; **245**(5): R743–R748.
143 Whayne T, Smith N, Eger E, *et al*. The effects of halothane anesthesia on reflex cardiovascular responses to simulated diving and the Valsalva maneuver. *Anesthesiology* 1971; **34**(3): 262–270.
144 Elsner R, Franklin DL, Van Citters RL, *et al*. Cardiovascular defense against asphyxia. *Science* 1966; **153**: 941–949.
145 Nutter FB, Haulena, M, Bai SA. Preliminary pharmacokinetics of single-dose intramuscular butorphanol in elephant seals (*Mirounga angustirostris*). In: *Proceedings of the 30th Annual American Association of Zoo Veterinarians Conference*. Omaha, NE, 1998.
146 Molter CM, Barbosa L, Johnson S, *et al*. Pharmacokinetics of a single subcutaneous dose of sustained release buprenorphine in northern elephant seals (*Mirounga angustirostris*). *J Zoo Wildl Med* 2015; **46**(1): 52–61.
147 Trumbull E. Comparative pharmacokinetics of a single dose of meloxicam in the California sea lion (*Zalophus californianus*) and Pacific harbor seal (*Phoca vitulina richardii*). In: *Proceedings of the 54th Annual International Association for Aquatic Animal Medicine Conference*. Salt Lake City, UT, 2023.
148 Simeone CA, Nollens HH, Meegan JM, *et al*. Pharmacokinetics of single dose oral meloxicam in bottlenose dolphins (*Tursiops truncatus*). *J Zoo Wildl Med* 2014; **45**(3): 594–599.
149 Pawson P. Sedatives. In: Maddison JE, Page SW, Church DB, eds. *Small Animal Clinical Pharmacology*, 2nd edn. Edinburgh, UK: WB Saunders, 2008: 113–125.

57 Comparative Anesthesia and Analgesia – Reptiles, Amphibians, and Fishes

Sathya K. Chinnadurai[1] **and Cornelia I. Mosley**[2]
[1] Chicago Zoological Society/Brookfield Zoo, Brookfield, Illinois, USA
[2] Elanco Animal Health, Mississauga, Ontario, Canada

Chapter contents

Introduction, 1110
Reptile anesthesia, 1110
Anatomy and physiology, 1110
Metabolism and thermoregulation, 1111
Cardiovascular system, 1111
Pulmonary system, 1112
Renal system, 1113
Hepatic system, 1113
Clinical anesthesia, 1114
Pain, nociception, and analgesia, 1114
Amphibian anesthesia, 1116
Anatomy and physiology, 1117
Clinical anesthesia, 1118
Anesthetic agents, 1118
Monitoring, 1119
Recovery, 1119
Fish anesthesia, 1120
Anatomy and physiology, 1120
Overview of clinical anesthesia of fish, 1122
References, 1123

Introduction

Reptiles, amphibians, and fishes are unique animal classes encountered in veterinary medicine and are very different in terms of anatomy, physiology, and behavioral adaptations from the more familiar mammals. Regardless of the differences among these animal classes, by using sound anesthetic principles reasonably safe and effective anesthesia can be performed, even in the absence of species-specific information. In the following sections, emphasis has been placed on providing comparative anatomic and physiologic information relevant to the anesthetic management of each class of animals. A comprehensive review of the anesthetic and analgesic literature is beyond the scope of this text but is available elsewhere and should be consulted for additional detail [1–6].

Reptile anesthesia

Anesthetic management of reptiles is associated with many challenges. Reptilia represents a diverse class of animals in terms of size, environmental requirements, behavior, physiology, and anatomy. There are over 7800 species represented by four main orders (Crocodylia, Testudines, Squamata, and Rhynchocephalia). Compounding the difficulties created by these inherent species differences, historically there was relatively little peer-reviewed research investigating anesthesia and analgesia in reptiles and much of the earlier literature is anecdotal in nature and persists as accepted fact despite contradictory evidence. Fortunately, there has been considerable interest in this area recently and scientific studies investigating anesthesia and analgesia in reptiles are becoming more available.

Applying generalized anesthetic recommendations to such a large and varying group of animals is difficult. Clinical application of various techniques is often ascribed to one of the three principal orders: the crocodilians (crocodiles and alligators), the chelonians (tortoises and turtles), and the squamates (snakes and lizards). An understanding of normal physiology, pathophysiology, the action and disposition of anesthetic and related drugs, and a familiarity with the design and use of related anesthetic equipment are important considerations. A thorough preanesthetic assessment and carefully designed anesthetic plan with attention to premedication, induction, maintenance, monitoring, supportive care, recovery, and ongoing postoperative support and analgesia all contribute to the reduction of risk associated with anesthesia.

Anatomy and physiology

Reptiles have long been considered to be the class of vertebrates that reflect the evolutionary transition between the aquatic and amphibious ectothermic vertebrates, and endothermic birds and mammals. Reptiles arguably represent one of the most ancient, successful, and well-adapted classes of animals, with some species surviving essentially unchanged for hundreds of millions of years. Recent investigations recognize reptilian physiologic evolutionary

Veterinary Anesthesia and Analgesia: The Sixth Edition of Lumb and Jones. Edited by Leigh Lamont, Kurt Grimm, Sheilah Robertson, Lydia Love and Carrie Schroeder.
© 2024 John Wiley & Sons, Inc. Published 2024 by John Wiley & Sons, Inc.
Companion website: www.wiley.com/go/lamont/anesthesia

adaptations as "optimal or advantageous," enabling exothermic animals to inhabit almost all of the available non-polar ecological niches.

Although many aspects of reptilian physiology are similar to those of endothermic vertebrates, significant differences are present. Such differences may alter both the action and disposition of anesthetics and analgesics.

Metabolism and thermoregulation

The ectothermic nature of reptiles and their generally lower metabolic rates are probably the two most striking differences between mammals and reptiles that impede extrapolation of anesthetic principles and practices between the two groups. Reptiles derive much of their body heat from the surrounding environment and use behaviors such as basking or burrowing to regulate their body temperatures. Reptiles can also alter their body temperature through changes in their cardiovascular physiology. During periods of warming, some reptiles increase their heart rate and the degree of right-to-left cardiac shunting to increase the fraction of blood flow that is directed to the periphery for heating and ultimate return to the body core [7]. This adaptation facilitates more rapid and efficient warming of the animal.

Reptiles will tend to choose a preferred optimal temperature zone (POTZ) maintaining a body temperature that is presumably ideal for the animal. In most instances, reptiles undergoing anesthesia should be maintained at the average or the high end of their POTZ to ensure optimal metabolic function. Species-specific ranges can often be found in general husbandry references or extrapolated from known species, which are found in similar natural habitats. In general, 20–25 °C is recommended for most aquatic and temperate reptile species, and 25–35 °C for most tropical species [8].

Although ambient temperature is one of the main determinants of metabolic rate in resting reptiles, and consequently the metabolism and excretion of drugs [9], there are significant interspecies and intraindividual variations. Minimum and maximum oxygen consumption rates of individual reptilian species range from almost zero to values similar to a resting mammal [10]. The oxygen consumption of any individual is a function of the species, the temperature, and the individual. In general, the varanid and lacertid lizards tend to have relatively high metabolic rates, and boid snakes and chelonians have lower rates. Surface-dwelling squamates have higher metabolic rates than burrowing species, and species of lizards that eat insects or other vertebrates have higher metabolic rates than herbivorous species [11]. Those species with higher inherent metabolic rates may be expected to more rapidly metabolize and excrete drugs compared to those with lower metabolic rates, but this has not been demonstrated conclusively.

Cardiovascular system

The non-crocodilian reptile heart has three chambers: two completely separate atria and a single anatomically continuous ventricle. The crocodilian heart is more typical of that seen in mammals and birds with two completely divided atria and two ventricles. In the crocodilian heart, the foramen of Panizza allows for some intravascular shunting under circumstances of breath holding, such as diving. In non-crocodilian reptiles, the ventricle is divided into two main chambers by a septum-like structure called the "Muskelleiste" or "muscular ridge" (Fig. 57.1). This ridge originates from the ventral ventricular wall and runs from the ventricular apex to the base, dividing the ventricle into two anatomically defined but connected chambers: the cavum pulmonale and the cavum dorsale [12,13], comparable in function to the right and left ventricles of mammals, respectively. The cavum dorsale is sometimes further subdivided into the cavum venosum and cavum arteriosum. The dorsolateral border of the muscular ridge is free, permitting the flow of blood between the cavum pulmonale and cavum dorsale. However, during ventricular systole, the muscular ridge presses against the dorsal wall of the ventricle and separates the cavum pulmonale from the cavum dorsale; thus, in a functional sense, the heart is capable of acting as a two-circuit pump. The pulmonary artery arises from the cavum pulmonale, and two aortic arches arise from the cavum venosum of the cavum dorsale. The left aortic arch becomes the dorsal aorta while the right aortic arch forms the subclavian and carotid arteries and a third branch joins the dorsal aorta. However, there is considerable anatomic variation among species.

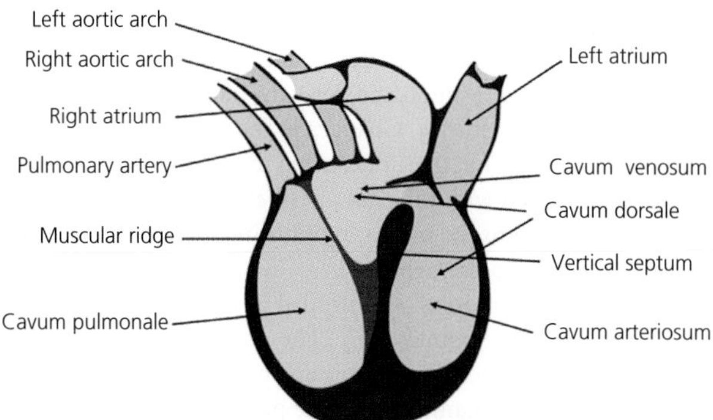

Figure 57.1 A generalized schematic demonstrating the anatomy and separation of blood flow in the non-crocodilian reptile heart. The cavum venosum is the region of the heart where mixing of oxygenated and deoxygenated blood may occur. Deoxygenated blood returning to the heart via the right atrium passes through the cavum venosum to the cavum pulmonale. The volume of blood remaining in the cavum venosum after the muscular ridge contacts the dorsal wall of the heart (during systole), relative to the volume of oxygenated blood in the cavum arteriosum, will determine the magnitude of the shunted fraction of blood. The shunt fraction is ultimately controlled by pressure differences between the systemic and pulmonary circulations resulting in larger or smaller volumes of deoxygenated blood remaining in the cavum venosum during systole.

Cardiac shunting occurs commonly in reptiles [14–16]. Cardiac shunts can occur in both directions, and under some circumstances may occur simultaneously in both directions [14,17,18]. The direction of the net shunt determines whether the systemic or pulmonary circulation receives the majority of the cardiac output. Intracardiac shunting has three important functions. First, shunting serves to stabilize the oxygen content of the blood during respiratory pauses. Second, the right-to-left shunt is partly responsible for facilitating heating by increasing systemic blood flow. Third, a right-to-left shunt directs blood away from the lungs during breath holding.

During anesthesia, cardiac shunting can affect systemic arterial oxygen content and the uptake and elimination of inhaled anesthetics. The size and direction of the shunts are ultimately controlled by pressure differences between the pulmonary and systemic circulations and the washout of blood remaining in the cavum venosum (an anatomic subchamber of the cavum dorsale described in many reptiles) [14,16,18,19]. The pressure differences are principally controlled by cholinergic and adrenergic factors that regulate the vascular resistance of the pulmonary and systemic circulation [14,20–25].

Large right-to-left shunts limit the amount of anesthetic uptake early in the anesthetic period and slow anesthetic elimination at the end of anesthesia. Such shunts can delay the induction to and recovery from inhaled anesthesia. Changes in the level and direction of shunts may account for the unexpected awakening seen in some reptiles anesthetized with inhalant anesthetics. Intracardiac shunts also have implications for patient monitoring, in particular airway gas monitoring and pulse oximetry.

Blood pressure in reptiles is controlled by mechanisms similar to those described in mammals [26]. The cardiovascular system of reptiles responds to both cholinergic and adrenergic stimulation in a manner similar to mammals and the presence of a baroreceptor reflex has been described [27]. The resting blood pressures of reptiles tend to be stable in the absence of external stimuli but may vary with temperature, activity, or state of arousal [28,29]. In contrast to mammals, systemic arterial blood pressures vary greatly among various reptilian species, making it difficult to identify a "normal" arterial blood pressure [26]. "Normal" blood pressure in reptiles may be more profoundly affected by environmental stresses such as habitat and temperature, species activity level, and size compared to the role of these factors in influencing blood pressure in mammals. This greater variability may originate from a reptile's poor ability to regulate normal homeostasis independent of temperature and environment.

Chelonians tend to have the lowest mean arterial pressures (15–30 mmHg) while some varanids have resting arterial pressures similar to mammals (60–80 mmHg) [30]. In the green iguana, normal resting mean arterial blood pressures are reported to be in the range of 40–50 mmHg while mean pulmonary arterial pressures are in the range of 15–30 mmHg [30]. The systemic blood pressures in snakes correspond to the gravitational stress they are likely to experience [31–33]. Snakes from arboreal habitats tend to have higher arterial pressures than those that are primarily aquatic. An allometric relationship between arterial blood pressure and body mass has also been described in snakes. As body mass increases, so does blood pressure. Several anesthetics, such as sevoflurane, isoflurane, halothane, propofol, tiletamine–zolazepam, and ketamine, have been shown to induce cardiopulmonary changes in reptiles similar to those seen in mammals [34–42].

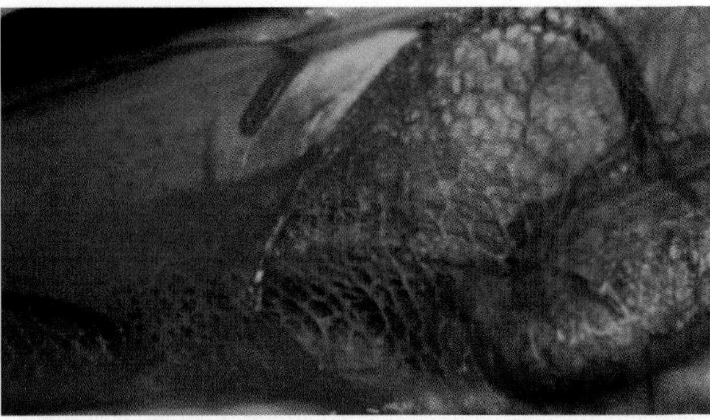

Figure 57.2 The lungs of many reptiles tend to be "sac-like" with a comparatively low respiratory surface area relative to total lung volume. However, lung structure varies markedly among species with highly aerobic species having more partitions and invaginations to increase respiratory surface area. The image shows the dissection of the lung in a boid snake demonstrating the sac-like structure.

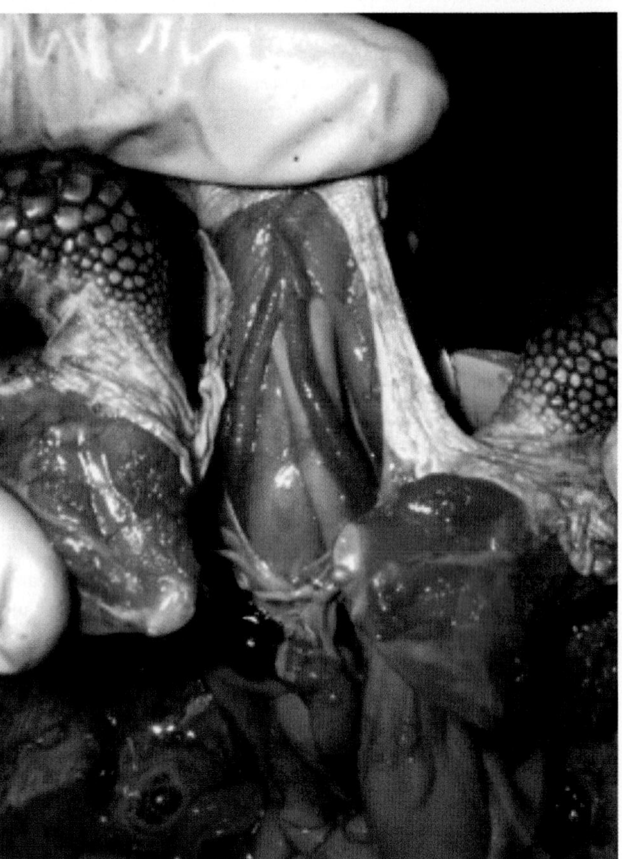

Figure 57.3 The trachea of many chelonians bifurcates quite proximally, increasing the risk of unilateral bronchial intubation.

Pulmonary system

The most significant difference between the respiratory physiology of reptiles, mammals, and birds is the lower oxygen consumption rate of reptiles. This difference reflects the lower reptilian metabolic rate. Both reptile respiratory anatomy and physiology vary markedly across species. The lungs of non-crocodilian reptiles are suspended freely in the common pleuroperitoneal cavity and are not located in a closed pleural space. In reptiles, the lungs tend to be sac-like with varying degrees of partitioning (Fig. 57.2). Highly aerobic species such as the varanids tend to have highly partitioned lungs with numerous septae and invaginations that increase the surface area for gas exchange. Chelonians and lizards tend to have paired lungs while most snakes have a single functional right lung. The functional units of the lung are referred to as "ediculi" and "faveoli," which are structures analogous to mammalian alveoli. Most reptile lungs exhibit areas of both types of parenchyma. There is little detail regarding the trachea and extrapulmonary bronchial tree system in reptiles. The tracheal rings of chelonians tend to be complete, necessitating care when placing an endotracheal tube. In addition, the trachea may bifurcate quite proximally, so inadvertent endobronchial intubation may occur (Fig. 57.3). Many snakes also possess a tracheal lung, the significance of which is unclear. The lungs of reptiles tend to have a smaller respiratory surface area relative to lung volume.

Because reptiles lack a diaphragm, they rely on the thoracic musculature for ventilation. Both inspiration and expiration are active processes so the respiratory depression associated with anesthesia may be more profound than that observed in mammalian species where expiration is a passive process. Because the muscles of ventilation include many of the same muscles used for locomotion, these two functions are relatively incompatible. Chelonians are faced with additional respiratory challenges since expansion of the thoracic cavity by movement of the ribs is not possible. The dorsal surface of the lungs is attached to the carapace and the ventral surface is attached to the abdominal viscera. Inspiration is accomplished by enlarging the visceral cavity, and expiration occurs by forcing the viscera up against the lungs, driving air out. This is accomplished by contraction of various posterior abdominal muscles and several pectoral girdle muscles.

Control of respiration

The control of respiration in reptiles is poorly understood. Both peripheral receptor and centrally mediated control have been proposed. It seems most likely that there is an interaction between a central system, which generates the pattern of respiration and afferent chemoreceptor input [43,44]. Both carbon dioxide partial pressure and pH appear important for stimulating normal ventilation but there is evidence that oxygen tension may play a role in normal ventilation, even under normoxic conditions [45]. Although there are some species variations, reptiles are generally viewed as episodic breathers [46–48]. Breathing occurs in respiratory "bursts" of activity followed by a pause of varying duration. Pulmonary vascular perfusion is also intermittent and changes in perfusion are in concert with respiratory rate and rhythm [22,49,50]. Ambient temperature has variable effects on the frequency, tidal volume, and minute ventilation [51] and due consideration should be given to maintaining the optimal temperature for a particular species.

Effects of inspired carbon dioxide and oxygen

The response of reptiles to inspired carbon dioxide (CO_2) is quite variable. Inspiration of greater than 4% CO_2 in snakes and lizards produces an increase in tidal volume, a decrease in respiratory frequency, and an overall decrease in minute ventilation [52,53]. In turtles, specifically *Pseudemys scripta* and *Chrysemys picta*, the response to an increase in CO_2 is an increase in minute ventilation as a result of increases in both respiratory frequency and tidal volume [26,54–56]. In turtles, breathing less than 21% but more than 10% oxygen produces little change in the respiratory pattern. At fractional inspired oxygen concentrations below 10%, some species increase ventilation while others retain their resting minute ventilation. Others may decrease ventilation [48,52,57–59]. In those species in which minute ventilation decreases or remains unchanged, metabolic oxygen consumption decreases.

During anesthesia, most reptiles are maintained using an inhalant anesthetic delivered in nearly 100% oxygen. The delivery of a high oxygen concentration may further compound respiratory depression by blunting the contribution of oxygen for the stimulation of normal ventilation. In several reptile species, exposure to 100% oxygen significantly decreases minute ventilation [52,54,60–62], suggesting that high inspired oxygen may be responsible for at least some of the respiratory depression seen during anesthesia. The magnitude of this effect is likely small compared to the effects of anesthetics on central control of respiration and the muscles of respiration. However, there is some evidence that in the green iguana, recoveries from isoflurane anesthesia may be faster when the animal is breathing room air rather than 100% oxygen, possibly by improving ventilation and the subsequent removal of the inhalant from the body [63]. Interestingly, in studies using Dumeril's monitors (*Varanus dumerili*) and bearded dragons (*Pogona vitticeps*), no significant differences in recovery times from either isoflurane or sevoflurane anesthesia were found between animals ventilated with room air or those ventilated with 100% oxygen [64].

A newer method described to shorten the time of anesthetic recovery from inhalant anesthesia is administration of intramuscular epinephrine. Epinephrine administered at 0.1 mg/kg IM was shown to significantly reduce the time from cessation of inhalant anesthesia to spontaneous ventilation and recovery in snapping turtles [65]. The authors of these studies proposed that the sympathomimetic effects of epinephrine may speed inhalant expulsion from the lungs, by reducing cardiopulmonary shunting. These findings may be relevant to other reptilian taxa.

Renal system

Reptiles cannot produce urine more concentrated than plasma, making the excretion of nitrogenous wastes more challenging for terrestrial reptiles. Most reptiles excrete nitrogenous waste as uric acid (uricotelic). Some turtles and crocodilians can also excrete urea. Uric acid is produced in the liver, and, unlike ammonia and urea, it is very insoluble in water and is excreted as a semi-solid in dilute urine. In the reptilian kidney tubule, urine is very dilute so uric acid remains in solution. The cloaca forms a common conduit for products of the urogenital and gastrointestinal systems. It is often described as three distinct compartments but the actual degree of anatomic separation of these compartments varies by species. The most craniad portion is the coprodeum, which is a continuation of the terminal colon followed by the urodeum that receives connections from the urogenital system and urinary bladder (if present; not all reptiles have a urinary bladder, e.g., snakes) and the proctodeum, which is the most caudal section also commonly described as the vent. Dilute urine empties into the urodeum and then into the bladder or large intestine (via the coprodeum) where water is reabsorbed causing the uric acid to precipitate. This results in the excretion of nitrogenous waste with relatively little water. The bladder of some reptiles can be used for the storage of water. Reptilian urine is not a good indicator of renal function.

Many reptiles also have specialized salt-excreting glands that allow for the excretion of very high concentrations of sodium, potassium, and chloride. Many reptiles living in extremely arid locations can tolerate the marked fluctuations in total body water and plasma osmolarity that can occur in these environments. When faced with limited water supplies, plasma osmolarity can rise to levels higher than those known in any other vertebrate species. Many reptiles also have a renal portal system where blood from the hind legs and tail will pass through the kidneys before returning to the heart [66]. The effect of this system on the pharmacokinetics of drugs seems to be of little clinical significance in healthy animals. However, it is probably still best to avoid injection of nephrotoxic drugs or those that are likely to be significantly metabolized by the kidney into the hindlimbs and tail of reptiles [67].

Hepatic system

The reptilian liver appears to be similar in structure and function to the liver of other vertebrates. Although there is little detail known about the reptilian liver, it is assumed that it probably plays important roles in tolerance to anaerobic metabolism, hypothermia, and adaptation to the physical environment. The liver of reptiles has a lower metabolic capacity compared to mammalian livers [68] and the metabolic rate is very sensitive to changes in temperature [69]. The lower metabolic rates for the reptilian liver probably account for at least some of the prolonged effects commonly seen with drugs such as antibiotics. The lower metabolic capacity of the liver may partly contribute to the prolonged anesthetic recoveries seen when using drugs that require extensive hepatic metabolism for termination of their clinical effect.

Clinical anesthesia

Detailed information regarding clinical anesthesia in reptiles has been reviewed elsewhere and the reader should consult these references for specific information on anesthetic and analgesic techniques, drugs, dosage, and patient monitoring recommendations [1–6]. A few general concepts regarding reptile anesthesia will be presented below.

Patient presentation/assessment

Regardless of species or procedure, a preanesthetic assessment should be performed on all patients. Patient assessment should include a complete history, species identification, and physical examination. Any additional diagnostic tests such as blood work and imaging should be performed as indicated. Because most anesthetics produce some degree of cardiopulmonary depression, animals should be physiologically stable prior to the induction of anesthesia if possible. In some reptiles, the size, disposition, or anatomy may prevent the performance of a physical examination. In these animals, an assessment of body weight and general appearance may assist in determining the general health status of the animal. Species identification and information on their natural habitat may be useful. All animals should be kept at their preferred body temperature (PBT) throughout the anesthetic period and recovery. Performing anesthetic procedures early in the day allows animals predisposed to prolonged recoveries to recover during regular working hours rather than late into the night when support staff and patient supervision may be reduced.

Routes of drug administration

Intramuscular drug administration is most common in reptiles. Historically, hindlimb and tail sites have been avoided because of concerns related to the first-pass effect associated with passage of administered drugs through the kidneys via the renal portal system during absorption. However, studies in some reptiles (turtles and green iguanas) suggest that this may be more of a theoretical than practical concern because only a small fraction of blood from the hindlimbs and tail passes through the kidney [66,67]. However, it is probably best to avoid hindlimb and tail administration of nephrotoxic drugs. The epaxial muscles provide a suitable injection site in most snakes. In lizards, the muscle mass of the forelimb (triceps and biceps), hindlimb (quadriceps, semimembranosus, and semitendinosus), and tail can be used. Caution should be used in species known to autotomize (drop) their tails (many geckos), because it is possible for an animal to "shed" their tail during handling. In chelonians, injections are most often administered in the triceps muscle. The cranial surface of the foreleg should be avoided since the proximity of the radial nerve to injection sites in this area increases the risk of damage to this nerve. The pectoral muscles can also be used, though in many chelonian species, there is a lack of significant muscle mass in this area.

While intravenous drug administration is not always feasible in reptiles, the combination of good technique, practice, appropriate patient selection, and skilled physical restraint can facilitate predictable access to the ventral coccygeal vein in even very small snakes and lizards and the dorsal coccygeal vein in tortoises and freshwater turtles. In sea turtles, the dorsal cervical sinus has also been used for intravenous administration of drugs [70]. Intravascular injection decreases the latency of onset of action of an administered drug. It also decreases the variability in uptake and tissue irritation that is associated with intramuscular injections in reptiles. Techniques for catheterization of the coccygeal vein in both lizards and crocodilians have been described [71].

Intravenous catheterization of the coccygeal or abdominal veins is most often performed without direct visualization. In some species of turtles and tortoises, the jugular vein can be visualized but this technique often requires a skin incision and blunt dissection. Venous sinus sites are not ideal for intravenous catheter placement, but over-the-needle catheters can be used. A small gauge wire stylet through a needle (Seldinger technique) can be used to facilitate difficult catheterization. When required, cut-down procedures should be performed in conjunction with a local or general anesthetic. Lidocaine diluted down to a 1% solution with sterile saline can be used for local infiltration. Although toxic doses have not been determined in reptiles, it is probably best to use less than 8–10 mg/kg. The most common sites for vascular access and associated technical tips are presented in Box 57.1.

Intraosseous catheterization has been described in the green iguana (*Iguana iguana*), sea turtles, and desert tortoises [72–75]. Studies in green iguanas found similar renal uptake of the radioactive substance whether administered intraosseously or intravenously [72]. In desert tortoises, intraosseous administration via the humerus resulted in delivery to the systemic circulation (84%) that was similar to jugular administration, followed by the femur, plastocarpacial junction, and the gular region of the plastron [75]. This suggests that intraosseous drug administration is a suitable alternative to intravenous administration. To the authors' knowledge, propofol is the only anesthetic drug that has been studied with intraosseous administration, but many other anesthetic and non-anesthetic drugs have been administered successfully via this route.

Endotracheal intubation

Intubation is easily accomplished in most reptiles because the glottis is in a relatively rostral position in the mouth at the base of the tongue. A small drop of lidocaine (diluted to 1%) can be used to desensitize the glottis and may facilitate tracheal intubation. In some aquatic reptiles, anatomic modifications of glottal folds may obscure direct visualization. The animal should be intubated with the largest diameter tube that can be placed easily. The mucus of reptiles tends to be very viscous and mucoid plugs can form in endotracheal tubes during longer procedures. It is important that this be recognized quickly as an inability of the lungs to fully deflate during expiration will occur. The trachea of some chelonians bifurcates quite rostrally, and endobronchial intubation is possible. The tracheal rings in chelonians and crocodiles are complete, and in most reptiles cuffed endotracheal tubes are avoided to prevent accidental overinflation and damage to the tracheal structures.

Pain, nociception, and analgesia

Analgesic management of reptiles is challenging as a result of their unique physiologic, anatomic, and behavioral adaptations. Reptile pain and nociception have not been extensively studied, although there is compelling evidence that reptiles are capable of nociception. However, the sensory significance of nociception to the individual is poorly understood. *Pain* is normally defined as "an unpleasant sensory and emotional experience associated with, or resembling that associated with, actual or potential tissue damage" [76]. By this definition, pain is essentially an emotional experience. Arguably, it is impossible to describe this experience in

Box 57.1 Sites for intravascular access in reptiles.

Squamates (snakes)

- The coccygeal vein is located on the ventral midline of the tail. The needle should be inserted sufficiently caudal to the vent in order to avoid the hemipenes and anal sacs. The vessel is entered via a ventral midline approach and the needle is advanced with gentle suction until either the vein or the vertebral body is contacted.
- The jugular vein can be used but requires a skin incision to visualize. An incision is made 4–7 scutes cranial to the heart at the junction of the ventral scutes and lateral body scales. The vein is then identified using blunt dissection just medial to the tips of the ribs.
- The palatine vein is easily visualized in larger snakes and is located medial to the palatine teeth in the roof of the mouth. The technique is greatly facilitated by short-term anesthesia, but it is possible to collect blood from these vessels in awake animals using a mouth speculum.
- Use of the heart for drug administration is not recommended except for emergency situations.
- There are to our knowledge no intraosseous sites described for drug administration in snakes.

Squamates (lizards)

- The coccygeal vein is located on the ventral midline of the tail. The needle should be inserted sufficiently caudal to the vent in order to avoid the hemipenes. The vessel can be entered from either a ventral midline approach or laterally. The ventral approach is simple to perform: the needle is advanced with gentle suction until the vein, or a vertebral body is contacted. The lateral technique involves inserting the needle just ventral to the transverse process of the vertebral body and walking the needle ventral until the vein is contacted.
- The ventral abdominal vein is located on the ventral midline of the abdomen and can be entered percutaneously or via a small skin incision for direct visualization of the vessel.
- The cephalic vein is located on the dorsal surface of the distal foreleg. A skin incision is generally required for visualization.
- The jugular vein is located on the lateral surface of the neck at about the level of the tympanum. It may be palpated in some species but is generally difficult to visualize. A small skin incision is often required for direct visualization. The jugular veins tend to be located more dorsal than those in mammals. There is a large lymphatic sinus close to the vein and contamination with this lymph fluid occurs frequently.
- Intraosseous techniques have been described for the distal femur, proximal tibia, and proximal humerus. The techniques are similar to those described for other small animal patients.

Chelonians (turtles and tortoises)

- The dorsal coccygeal vein is located midline dorsal to the coccygeal vertebrae. It is a technique requiring minimal restraint. The needle is introduced in a craniad direction at a 45–90° angle from the skin.
- The dorsal cervical sinus (supravertebral) is located on the dorsolateral aspect of the neck in sea turtles. It is located one-third the distance from the carapace to the head, cranial to the cranial edge of the carapace. The head is directed forward and down, and the needle is introduced lateral to the midline on either side.
- The occipital venous sinus has been described in freshwater turtles and is located on midline ventral to the supraoccipital crest. It requires that the head be restrained firmly and in an extended ventroflexed (45–90° angle from the carapace) position. The needle is then introduced midline just caudal to the occiput and nearly perpendicular to the spine. Lymph contamination is a possibility.
- The subcarpacal sinus or supravertebral sinus is located under the carapace, just caudal to the last cervical vertebra and craniad to the first thoracic vertebra. This sinus can be approached by pressing the head into the shell and palpating for the first thoracic vertebra (incorporated into the carapace). The needle should be directed through the skin just caudal to the juncture of the last cervical vertebra up toward the carapace and first thoracic vertebra.
- The jugular veins are located on the lateral sides of the neck at about the level of the tympanum. In some species, venipuncture of the jugular vein is relatively straightforward and can be visualized or a small skin incision can be made to facilitate direct visualization. Unfortunately, this technique requires the neck to be fully extended, and in uncooperative animals, a short-acting anesthetic or tranquilizer may be required.
- Intraosseous techniques have been described using the plastron/plastron bridge, but needles/catheters may end up in an intracoelomic rather than intraosseous position. The technique is described as passing a needle at an angle through the bony bridge between the plastron and carapace.

reptiles given our current level of understanding and available technology. However, undoubtedly reptiles experience noxious insults as some sort of negative event and modify their behavior to escape such insults. A more robust and inclusive definition of *pain* may be more appropriate when describing pain in non-human animals. For example, the following definition of *pain* would avoid the emotional aspects associated with the human definition and yet is suitably robust to encompass a range of experiences reasonably expected to result in what we might refer to as pain in a human: "a sensory experience representing awareness of damage or the potential for tissue damage that results in a behavioral and physiologic response to minimize/prevent the recurrence and promote healing of damage" (modified from Molony [77]). The experience of pain in non-human animals may be similar to the experience in humans but it is important to consider that among classes and species of animals, pain may differ quantitatively and qualitatively.

There are many gaps present in our understanding of reptile nociception, pain, consciousness, and suffering and although tempting, extrapolation from other vertebrate lineages should be undertaken cautiously. Reptiles have undergone millions of years of independent biologic evolution, separate from other vertebrate classes. While it is appealing to assume that all lineages of vertebrates have evolved similar survival strategies, it may also be somewhat presumptuous. It is true that the ability to sense noxious stimulus or potentially damaging stimuli is arguably necessary for the survival of all animals (invertebrates and vertebrates), but it is the significance of this sensation to the individual that remains less clear. Does the ability to perceive and suffer from pain, as defined in human terms, offer an evolutionary or biologic advantage to all animals or only some animals (i.e., humans)? Unfortunately, this is a complex and elusive question but one that nonetheless merits investigation. Regardless of an animal's ability to experience pain and suffering as a negative emotional response, the aim should be to limit the biologic perturbations associated with the physiologic (nociceptive) processing accompanying a noxious stimulus.

Evidence for pain in reptiles

Various criteria have been used to evaluate the balance of evidence for the presence or absence of pain in animals. These criteria as they pertain to reptiles are briefly described below.

Presence of nociceptors

The origination of the sensation associated with a noxious stimulus, transduction, occurs in specialized sensory nerve endings called "nociceptors." Primarily nociceptive neurons (slowly adapting polymodal C fibers) have not been identified in reptiles. However, there is no evidence in the literature that they have been sought and not found but rather no one has looked specifically for these types of fibers. However, high-threshold Aδ mechanical nociceptors [78] and C fiber mechanical nociceptors [79] have been identified in one species of snake. These fibers are nociceptors capable of transmitting nociceptive information.

Ascending transmission pathways

Spinothalamic projections analogous to the neospinothalamic (fast pain) and paleospinothalamic (slow pain) tracts have been identified [80] in reptiles and are presumed to be capable of transmitting nociceptive information from the body to the brain. Trigeminal tracts have also been identified [78,81] that may be capable of transmitting pain from the head to the brain. Unfortunately, there are no functional studies examining the role of these pathways in nociceptive processing.

Brain structures

Reptiles appear to possess brain structures necessary for experiencing pain (neocortex) and morphologically there are direct spinal connections to the brainstem and dorsal thalamus in the midbrain. However, once again functional studies are lacking, and it is possible and even likely that brain processing of information may occur differently in different animals. For example, in some animals, smell and vision are highly developed and vast regions of the brain are dedicated to these activities, possibly producing sensations far beyond those a human could experience or even imagine.

It has been suggested that differences in reptiles' brain systems compared to birds and mammals may be ones of degrees of elaboration rather than presence or absence [82]. It is possible that the response to a noxious stimulus in reptiles is associated with less fidelity and scope compared to mammals. Perhaps a reptile's "emotions" and the experience of pain are an "all or none" phenomena (rage or no rage, pain or no pain) rather than the graded experiences of human emotions (rage, anger, irritation, discontent, neutral, happiness, etc.). Certainly, humans describe a range of painful experiences from those that are simply a mild irritant to those that are intolerable.

Nociceptive receptors and substances

The opioid system has been well studied in reptiles and the presence of opioid receptors and endogenous opioids has been described [83–85]. Their exact role, receptor subtypes present, and their anatomic locations are somewhat less clear. Although opioids are important for modulating the neural processing of noxious stimuli, they also play roles in many other body systems, such as the reproductive, thermoregulatory, gastrointestinal, and circadian systems. In addition, several nociceptive-related neuropeptides (i.e., glutamate, substance P, and calcitonin gene-related peptide) have been identified in reptiles but their functions are not well elucidated.

Known analgesic actions on nociceptive or nocifensive behaviors

It is important to note that behavioral evidence does not always suggest awareness or conscious recognition of the nociceptive stimulus (i.e., pain perception). Many of the tests used to examine an animal's response to a known or presumptive analgesic are actually measuring the effect the substance has on the animal's nociceptive or nocifensive response. "Nocifensive" is a poorly defined term that is sometimes used to describe the unconscious withdrawal or movement away from a noxious stimulus. It is a response that can occur below the level of consciousness and hence differs from the response associated specifically with pain perception.

Several experimental studies have examined the response of reptiles to substances known to be analgesic in mammals, primarily opioids. These studies have involved evaluating responses to various types of noxious stimuli, including thermal, mechanical, and chemical irritation. In general, these studies suggest that opioids reduce the response to some of these stimuli, although there is inconsistency among the different experimental nociceptive models used, the response of different reptile species to similar testing situations, and the drugs themselves.

It must be noted that the inability to demonstrate a reduction in the nociceptive responses of an animal when administered a substance known to be analgesic in humans, or other animals, does not necessarily mean the substance has no effect on nociception, only that it did not have an effect given the specific experimental design used. There are numerous factors (i.e., dose, specific nociceptive model used, species, personnel involved, and experimental conditions) that can affect the results, and broad generalizations based on a single experiment should be made cautiously. For example, when reptiles are in the presence of something or someone that might be perceived as a threat (e.g., human), the reptile may appear to "ignore" or minimize the significance of the noxious stimulus (e.g., heat) and hence their measurable responses to this insult. Tonic immobility is often used to describe the antipredator behavior demonstrated by many prey species. This response is associated with modulation of ascending nociceptive pathways that appear to have an antinociceptive effect [86–88]. The lack of normal response to a noxious stimulus could certainly influence the results of an experiment and should be considered when designing and evaluating experiments. However, with accumulating work and evidence, some trends useful for clinical decision-making are being discovered.

Avoidance learning

There are no known studies of avoidance learning in response to a noxious stimulus in reptiles.

Suspension of normal behavior

Although there are no specific studies that have examined the suspension of normal behaviors in reptiles, experiencing what one might call pain, there is reasonable anecdotal information from clinicians and reptile owners. These experiences suggest that a reptile's normal behaviors (eating, basking, and social interaction) are altered by animal pain and the provision of an appropriate analgesic will hasten the resumption of these normal behaviors compared to allowing the animal's discomfort to diminish naturally. Of course, this is anecdotal, and the observations are undoubtedly influenced by preconceived biases and beliefs, including a belief that analgesics can hasten recovery from pain.

Amphibian anesthesia

Providing anesthesia and analgesia for amphibians is a challenge for most clinicians but due to the growing popularity of amphibians as pets, it is an increasingly needed service. Amphibians are also used extensively in laboratory research and display exhibitions and from an animal welfare aspect, it is necessary to provide this service with knowledge and skill. A solid understanding of anatomy and physiology of the wide variety of species in this group of animals is essential for providing good perioperative anesthesia care.

The class Amphibia has three orders with over 4500 species and newly discovered species are added every year [89,90]. The order

Anura represents frogs and toads (over 3500 living species), the order Caudata (around 375 species) includes salamanders, newts, and sirens, and the order Gymnophiona includes the caecilians (88 species) [89]. Each species has its own anatomic and physiologically unique features and extrapolations from one species to the other are not always possible. In addition, there are a limited number of studies to help guide anesthesia and pain management in amphibians.

Anatomy and physiology

Metamorphosis

Amphibians change significantly throughout their life with a metamorphosis from strictly aquatic egg and larval stages to an adult stage that can be terrestrial, semi-aquatic, or aquatic [91]. This metamorphosis includes the loss of the tail and gills, development of lungs, transformation from a two-chambered to a three-chambered heart, and development of four legs [91–93]. The unique features that stand out in amphibians are the multiple forms of breathing (gills, lungs, skin, and buccopharyngeal), the three-chambered heart, semipermeable skin, a renal portal system, and ectothermic temperature regulation.

Metabolism and thermoregulation

Amphibians are ectotherms. Each species has a preferred optimum temperature and has limited tolerance to temperature changes. Changes will affect metabolism, fluid regulation, and activity levels [94]. In general, amphibians require cooler temperatures than reptiles, and ambient temperatures of 23.8–26.7 °C (75–80 °F) are reported to be an acceptable range for most species during the peri-anesthetic period [92,94]. Species-specific needs (tropical versus subtropical species) should be identified, and temperatures adjusted. To optimize ambient humidity, levels should be maintained above 70% [92].

Cardiovascular system

The cardiovascular system of adult amphibians is composed of a three-chambered heart, an arterial/venous vascular system, and an extensive lymphatic system, in comparison to tadpoles that only have a two-chambered heart and a single loop circulation system, similar to fish [93]. The adult amphibian heart has two atria and one ventricle and is considered to have an incomplete double circulation [95,96]. The heart lies internally underneath the pectoral girdle and sternum and a heartbeat can be visualized on the ventral surface (midline just caudal to the level of the animal's shoulder) [91,93]. The right atrium is larger than the left atrium in all amphibians and the ventricle is thick-walled with numerous trabeculae found in many species [93]. In caudatans, the interatrial septum can be incomplete (fenestrated) but in anurans it is complete [92,93].

All of the venous blood arrives at the sinus venosus and enters the right atrium [95,96]. The arterialized blood flows into the left atrium and both atria empty into the one ventricle. During ventricular systole, the blood is pumped into the bulbus cordis from where three main arteries leave (carotid artery, aorta, and pulmocutaneous artery) [95–97]. The carotid artery sends oxygenated blood to the head, the aorta sends oxygenated mixed blood to the body, and the pulmocutaneous artery sends mostly venous blood to skin and lungs to pick up oxygen [96–98]. The ventricle in frogs, toads, and salamanders is anatomically one ventricle but is functionally divided due to the slit-like trabecular meshwork, that keeps arterial (oxygenated) blood on the left side of the ventricle and venous (desaturated) blood on the right side by creating a laminar flow pattern and preventing mixing during contraction [96–100]. Additionally, a spiral valve in the bulbus cordis will create spiral streaming of blood flow and direction of more oxygenated blood to the carotid artery and aorta from the left side of the ventricle, while the pulmocutaneous arteries receive more venous blood [96]. The septa between the three different arteries also help guide the blood flow, depending on cardiac output [96,100].

The amphibian lymphatic system is characterized by a high rate of lymph production and flow and functions to drain fluid from tissues and return it to the circulation [101]. The lymphatic system includes lymph hearts that lie in junctions of veins, and which beat irregularly or synchronously at 50–60 beats per min depending on the fluid status of the animal [101]. Various numbers of lymph hearts are present depending on species. Frogs and salamanders have fewer (i.e., 4–20) than caecilians (i.e., 100–200) [93]. These lymph hearts function to preserve unidirectional flow of lymph back to the heart and to return proteins to the circulation [93,101]. Lymph is mainly formed from plasma filtration as well as transcutaneous water uptake. Lymph collects in large subcutaneous lymph sacs (especially in anurans) and flows through afferent pores into the lymph hearts [101]. The lymph sacs can give indications of disease and fluid load when enlarged [92,94,101].

Both salamanders and anurans have a renal portal system and a hepatic portal system [93,94,97,102]. For the renal portal system, the veins from the hindlegs of the animal unite into the Jacobson's veins, which are paired and flow through the kidneys before entering the postcaval vein. Blood that flows through the hepatic portal vein system will flow from the ventral abdominal vein through the liver before entering the postcaval vein and returning to the heart. The factors that regulate the renal portal system are not fully understood, but the renal portal and hepatic portal systems may impact the pharmacokinetics of drugs that are administered in the hindlegs or tail (first-pass effect), so anesthetics are in some instances preferentially injected into the front end of the animal.

Specific vessels for venipuncture in amphibians are the ventral abdominal vein, the femoral and lingual veins (lingual venous plexus on underside of tongue in anurans), and the tail vein in caudatans [90,103]. Depending on the size of the animal, these can be used for blood collection or administration of anesthetic agents.

Respiratory system

Adult amphibians have up to four different modes of respiration. Most prominent are pulmonic and cutaneous gas exchange and buccopharyngeal (gular or guttural) breathing [93]. Aquatic salamanders also breathe via external gills (branchial mode) [93]. The buccal cavity and pharynx are used for gas exchange and can either be viewed as an extension of cutaneous respiration or its own entity due to its specific muscular pumping activity and unique vascular supply [93]. Cutaneous respiration is possible due to a large surface area (often increased via skinfolds), a very thin and semi-permeable epidermis, and a dermis that is highly vascularized [93]. This form of breathing is important as it is an efficient form of respiration during anesthesia.

The anatomic lungs in amphibians come in various shapes and sizes from small simple sac-like structures (aquatic species) to sacculated forms with alveoli in the anterior lung area (terrestrial species) [93]. The lungs are located cranially in amphibians following a short trachea with cartilaginous rings. The lungs have pulmonic epithelium that can easily be damaged with overventilation, or an endotracheal tube placed too far distally [91,104]. Endotracheal tubes should be advanced just past the larynx [90,91,93,104]. The mode of respiration may change in various species depending on environmental oxygen and carbon dioxide tensions [103,105]. When administered 100% oxygen, the animal commonly stops breathing through their lungs or via the buccopharyngeal movements and primarily relies on cutaneous respiration [103]. This complicates assessment of anesthetic depth, ventilation, and oxygenation. For cutaneous respiration to be efficient, the skin must be kept moist [94]. The permeability of the skin for gas exchange varies in different species (toads have thicker and less permeable skin).

Cutaneous system and fluid regulation

Amphibian skin is an important organ for immune functions and water regulation [92]. Evaporation through the skin is a major contributing factor to water loss (particularly on the dorsal surface) [92,94]. Uptake of water from the environment is managed from the ventral surface, including a functional structure in the pelvic area called the "drinking patch," which contributes 80% of water uptake in anurans [94]. Only a very small percentage of water intake is from gastrointestinal uptake; therefore, oral fluid supplementation will be less effective than keeping an animal moist by soaking in an appropriate fluid (e.g., isotonic or hypotonic water) [92,94]. Osmolality of the environmental fluid is particularly important in aquatic amphibians as the difference between external fluid and plasma osmolality will determine water regulation and movement. Amphibians can change the composition of their plasma to tolerate fluctuations in water osmolality, but an imbalance can lead to volume overload when the kidneys are compromised [94]. The high permeability of amphibian skin allows for absorption of exogenous compounds such as drugs and toxic substances.

Clinical anesthesia

Preanesthetic considerations

Species-specific knowledge about the particular amphibian patient is helpful for anesthesia planning and delivery. Using hypothermia is outdated and providing adequate anesthesia and analgesia is the standard of care. There is still a need for species-specific studies for amphibians as well as clinical anesthesia publications.

Physical examination and restraint

The amphibian patient should be evaluated before anesthesia, similar to any other species, to detect abnormalities that may increase the risk of anesthetic complications. Observation in its enclosure will provide information on general activity level and demeanor, breathing pattern, and hydration. Due to the sensitivity of the amphibian skin, premoistened and talc-free latex or nitrile gloves should be worn when handling to reduce the risk of skin damage and transfer of pathogens and toxins to or from both handler and animal [90,92,103]. Secretion of toxins from the skin is common in many amphibian species and can lead to irritation, various degrees of illness, and potentially death (some poisonous frogs can produce lethal toxins) [92,103]. Other skin secretions of some species can be gluey or foul-smelling, which are difficult to remove from the handler and cause discomfort [103]. Some species are able to expel their secretion over quite a distance and protective eyewear should be considered [103].

The water/fluids used to moisten the gloves and the water used to keep the animal wet should be distilled and dechlorinated to prevent chlorine uptake via the skin [90–92,103]. Some handlers also suggest coating the gloves with a non-toxic water-soluble gel to provide better skin protection in species with delicate skin [103].

Amphibians often show an instinctive flight response and should be gently restrained to prevent falling or escape. Restraint should be as brief, efficient, stress-free, comfortable, and safe for the animal as possible. Some species struggle, others cease in resignation, although a potential sudden burst of activity to escape should always be anticipated [103]. In animals that seem very stressed and difficult to restrain, a clear plastic or glass jar or plastic bag can be used to facilitate the handling. Many anurans tend to fill themselves with air when they are stressed, which can make a physical examination more difficult [92]. Often amphibians urinate when stressed or handled and the lack of this behavior may be an indication of dehydration [92]. Dehydrated amphibians show skin tenting and sunken eyes, feel tacky, and show decreased activity and mentation, so rehydration is important before attempting anesthesia [92].

Restraint is successfully performed in caudatans by encircling the animal behind their forelimbs with the index finger and thumb with the remaining fingers enclosing the body [90,103]. Salamanders have a tail autotomy reflex so the tail should be handled with care [90,103]. Some anurans can bite, and bigger species can be held by grasping them on a skinfold on their back behind the front legs or by holding them immediately anterior to the hindlegs with one hand and around the front legs with the second hand [90,103]. Sometimes chemical immobilization is necessary for a thorough physical examination.

Hypocalcemia is a common problem in amphibians and the hypocalcemic animal may present with tetany, muscle fasciculations, paresis, gastrointestinal stasis, and bloating [94]. Hypocalcemia can be treated with calcium gluconate in a bath as calcium is readily taken up via the skin [92,94]. Blood chemistry analysis is not generally done before anesthesia to minimize stress of restraint but can be done after induction if a more thorough clinical evaluation is desired.

Fasting

In general, fasting is not necessary as amphibians can maintain a closed larynx and risk of aspiration is minimal. Fasting is reserved for species that eat large rodent prey, and recommendations are to fast these species for 24–48 h prior to anesthesia to decrease risk of ileus and facilitate visualization during coelomic procedures [91].

Anesthetic agents

There are various anesthetic drugs that can be used in amphibians. Selection depends on the procedure to be performed, level of immobilization needed, and duration of anesthesia. Options for topical/cutaneous administration include immersion in tricaine methanesulfonate (MS-222), clove oil and its derivatives, volatile anesthetics, and less commonly, benzocaine. Injectable agents, including alfaxalone, have gained popularity and allowed for a controlled administration of individual bolus doses.

MS-222 is the most commonly used immersion agent and seems to have a wide margin of safety in most species. Due to the acidic pH of MS-222, it does require buffering with sodium bicarbonate in amphibians to avoid pain or tissue damage [91,106,107]. Despite the wide use of MS-222 in anurans, objective evaluation of the drug's physiologic effects is limited. In African clawed frogs (*Xenopus laevis*), MS-222 at 1 g/L provided surgical anesthesia for 30 min and 2 g/L for 60 min. Both concentrations caused pronounced respiratory depression, but no decrease in heart rate or oxygen saturation and no histological organ damage [108].

Clove oil and its derivative compounds eugenol and isoeugenol exhibit different species-specific responses in amphibians [109]. A common side-effect is gastric prolapse, which might be due to the pungent taste of clove oil [110]. Clove oil is administered via immersion and might cause cutaneous necrosis in some species when administered directly on the skin of the animal [111].

When comparing the effects of MS-222, clove oil, and ketamine–diazepam on the stress response in cane toads (*Rhinella marina*) [112], it was noted that clove oil resulted in a much greater elevation in serum corticosterone compared to the other two protocols. When comparing clove oil (450 ppm) to injectable propofol (25 or 35 mg/kg intracoelomic) in tiger salamanders (*Ambystoma tigrinum*), both drugs provided surgical anesthesia, while clove oil had a faster onset of action and longer duration [110]. When propofol (35 mg/kg intracoelomic) was compared to MS-222 (1 g/L as a bath) in Sonoran desert toads (*Bufo alvarius*), MS-222 produced surgical anesthesia in 100% of toads, whereas propofol produced surgical anesthesia in 11% [113].

Topical (cutaneous) administration of various agents such as sevoflurane or isoflurane liquid mixed in KY jelly has been reported and seems to have species-specific variability in effect [114]. Isoflurane can also be bubbled through the water via an anesthetic delivery system (routine anesthesia machine) [114]. This method has the disadvantage of high exposure levels of waste gases for humans in the surrounding environment. To decrease the risk, sealed containers should be used, which conversely makes handling the patient difficult. Induction times are slow and recovery times are rapid as soon as the patient is removed from the bath [91].

Parenteral injections of propofol, alfaxalone, ketamine, or α_2-adrenergic receptor agonists have been reported, but show wide species-specific variability, unpredictable inductions and recoveries, and undesirable mortality rates [91,115]. Propofol can be used in the form of an immersion bath for chemical restraint and sedation (but not surgical anesthesia) [116]. In recent years, alfaxalone anesthesia has had considerable appeal to amphibian anesthetists due to the ease of intramuscular administration and short duration of action. In American bullfrogs, intramuscular alfaxalone produced immobilization in frogs but did not provide sufficient anesthesia to prevent response to noxious stimuli. In the same study, bath immersion in alfaxalone (2 g/L) for up to 30 min did not result in anesthesia [115]. Neither propofol nor alfaxalone are appropriate sole agents for painful procedures and additional analgesic drugs should be used. Premedication can be done in some species but is not routinely performed. However, the administration of an analgesic with or without a sedative before induction may be beneficial, particularly in larger species.

Monitoring

Heart rate (HR), respiration rate, and anesthetic depth are most commonly monitored during amphibian anesthesia. As normal HRs differ between species, a baseline HR should ideally be obtained in the individual before anesthesia. If this is not practical due to stress on the animal, a baseline HR should be taken immediately after induction so trends can be identified. HR can be obtained by visualization or with the help of a small Doppler probe placed over the heart (at the xiphoid process of the sternum). An electrocardiogram can show good tracings of electrical events, but care should be taken to avoid skin damage with alligator clips or electrode patches. Hypodermic needles (27 gauge) can be inserted through the skin and alligator clips then fastened to the needles. The esophageal ECG (single probe) is an excellent alternative to the external ECG set up [107]. Knowledge of normal HRs in specific amphibian species is limited, although it is generally accepted that, overall, amphibians have relatively low HR values (approximately 50 beats per min) [94].

Under anesthesia, HR trends will provide information about the animal's status. A sudden drop or a slow decrease in HR over time suggests an increase in depth and adjustments to anesthetic administration should be made. Adjustments are made by changing the anesthetic concentration of the bath (diluting or, in case of a desired increase in depth, concentrating the anesthetic agent in the solution). Alternatively, syringes filled with desired anesthetic concentrations can be premade and used as needed to lighten or deepen the anesthetic depth via flushing the solution over the skin of the amphibian [91].

The stages of anesthesia have been reported by various clinicians [91,103,104]. Cessation of movement and loss of the righting reflex is often the first indication that anesthetic induction is complete. A light stage is assumed when the righting reflex is lost, and abdominal breathing movement stopped. Surgical anesthetic depth is reached when the withdrawal reflex is lost (e.g., no response to toe pinch in hindleg) and no gular respiration is present. Gular respiration can be visualized as the movement under the mandible and along the ventral neck. Although apnea is common (i.e., no visible gular and/or abdominal breathing), cutaneous respiration is still present as long as the dermis is kept moist to enable gas exchange [91]. Intubation is commonly not necessary unless it is a larger species with poor permeability of the dermis or other concerns about oxygenation are present [91]. A narrow glottis can make intubation challenging [107]. Due to the short trachea, the endotracheal tube should not be advanced too far beyond the larynx. Pulse oximetry has not yet been validated in amphibians, so it is primarily used to monitor trends (Fig. 57.4). Intraoperative support is provided by assuring that adequate thermal support, adequate fluid uptake, and adequate analgesia for painful procedures are addressed.

Recovery

The recovery phase in amphibians can be prolonged and close monitoring may reduce complications. Any residual topical anesthetic should be rinsed off and the animal should be recovered on room air. The surface and skin should be kept moist with fluid. Withdrawal reflexes will return first with an increase in gular respiration. The righting reflex should strengthen, and the animal should start moving around with improving coordination. Most recoveries are smooth and rather slow, but some amphibians may go through a phase of excitement and erratic movements and require monitoring to prevent injuries. The animal should only be returned to its normal environment when fully recovered to prevent accidental drowning [90,107].

Analgesia is an important aspect of adequate anesthesia management in any species, including amphibians. Research has demonstrated that amphibians have a well-established endogenous opioid system and that opioids are effective in providing pain relief [117–120]. Behavior studies demonstrate an alteration of behavior and avoidance of painful stimuli, suggesting that amphibians have a sense of discomfort [121,122]. The nociceptive structures and pathways present in some amphibian species are comparable to those in mammals [123,124]. The afferent sensory fibers of frogs show the same characteristics as mammalian sensory afferent fibers: large and medium myelinated A fibers, small myelinated B fibers, and small unmyelinated C fibers, [122,123,125]. The sensory afferent fibers then connect in the dorsal area of the frog's spinal cord [123,126]. Neurotransmitters associated with nociceptive transmission (e.g., substance P and glutamate) and endorphinergic neurons to inhibit the release of substance P are also present in the amphibian spinal cord. It has also been recognized that peripheral sensitization to noxious stimuli can occur [122,127,128]. Opioid

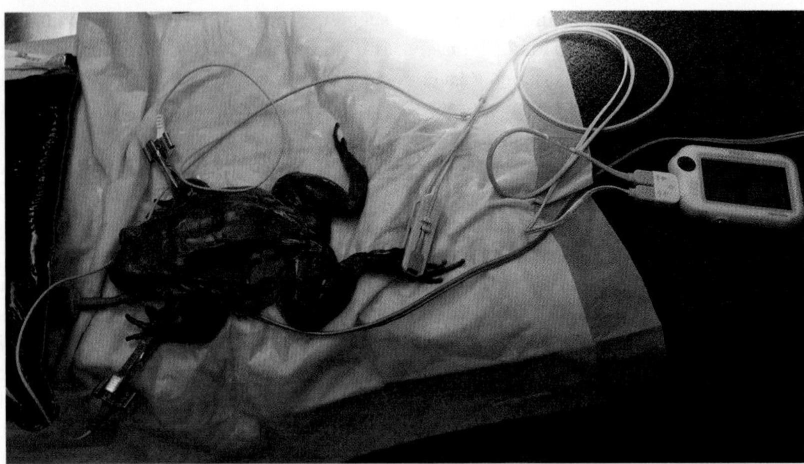

Figure 57.4 Surgical monitoring of a Smokey jungle frog (*Leptodactylus pentodactylus*). A two-lead ECG is used to monitor heart rate and rhythm, and a pulse oximeter has been placed on the left hind foot for approximation of hemoglobin oxygen saturation. The animal is tracheally intubated and monitored with capnography. Capnography and pulse oximetry have not yet been validated for many reptile and amphibian species, but have been used to monitor trends. Source: Dr. Sathya Chinnadurai, with permission.

receptors and endogenous opioid peptides are highly evolved in the amphibian brain and spinal cord [120,122,123,129].

Dermorphin is a potent amphibian-specific opioid compound that is present in the skin of certain South American frog species [122,130–132]. It is considered to be 40 times more potent than morphine with its main activity as a full μ-opioid receptor agonist [131]. Deltorphine, another endogenous opioid peptide produced in the skin of another frog genus, acts as a potent δ-opioid receptor agonist [131]. The functional role of dermorphin in amphibians is not clear, but it has been speculated to play a role in protection from predators or be involved in hibernation.

The ascending nociceptive pathways from the spinal cord to the brain are not fully understood in amphibians [123] and the projection to the telencephalon seems less organized but is recognized [107]. The perception of pain and subsequent suffering in amphibians is an ongoing debate due to the lack of a cerebral and/or limbic cortex [122,123,125]. Independent of that debate, nociception appears to be well developed and analgesics should be used when painful procedures are performed to prevent any physiologic and pathophysiologic consequences of the upregulation of the nociceptive pathway, including a significant stress response.

Various studies have been performed to assess efficacy of different analgesic agents [92,121,124,133–137]. Most recommendations come from studies conducted with acetic acid applied to the skin as the noxious stimulus [124]. Very little research has focused on clinical analgesia, but some recommendations have been made by clinicians who perform amphibian anesthesia in clinical settings. It should be kept in mind that species-specific differences are likely present and that extrapolation from one species to the next may be associated with varying effects in onset, duration, and efficacy.

All opioids (including butorphanol, morphine, buprenorphine, and fentanyl) seem to have a dose-dependent effect with relatively long durations and lower margins of safety at high doses compared to other domesticated species [92,121,124,133,134]. The α_2-adrenergic receptor agonists (e.g., xylazine and dexmedetomidine) also provide long-lasting analgesia and can be used without producing immobilization [124,135–137].

Fish anesthesia

There have been significant advances in fish anesthesia over the past 15 to 20 years with enhanced understanding of species-specific physiology in response to anesthesia [138,139]. To date, there are over 30,000 different species of fish with dissimilar anatomy and physiology that are adapted to various diverse aquatic ecosystems. Their classification is constantly changing but currently, 4500 genera, 515 families, and 62 orders are recognized.

The teleosts (jawed fish) are the biggest group among fish. Other less common groups are the ray-finned fishes (Acinopteryii), lobe-finned fishes (Sarcopterygii), and jawless fishes (Agnatha) [139,140]. A daunting number of differences in relation to water temperature, water quality and salinity, behavior, and response to drugs make anesthesia in fish a challenge [139].

Anatomy and physiology

Respiratory system

Most fish use gills for respiration, but various adaptations have been made in many fish species depending on oxygen (O_2) availability and demand. The gills are located behind the head in the buccal cavity and are covered by a sturdy flap (e.g., the operculum in bony fish) for protection. A gill consists of a gill arch, a filament, and a comprehensive vascular system. These highly folded, highly vascular, and very thin membranes make for efficient gas exchange. The vascular anatomy consists of a branchial basket, that arises from the aorta, and afferent branchial arteries that branch off to supply the arch and bifurcate further into afferent filamental arteries, which end at the tip of the filament [141]. The afferent filamental arteries then branch into afferent lamellar arterioles to supply the lamella. Blood flows through the lamella via various channels and blood gases (O_2 and CO_2) are variably exchanged depending on maximal surface area contact, changes in blood flow velocity, and optimal O_2 gradient tensions. The short efferent lamellar arterioles arise and provide blood flow back into efferent filamental arteries and at the base of the filament the blood flows into the efferent branchial arteries that later form the lateral aorta [141]. These vessels are the arterio-arterial circulation. A countercurrent system to optimize oxygen uptake is present in many fish. The venous blood moves in the opposite direction to the water, to create a more favorable gradient between the oxygen in the blood and water to maximize uptake [141]. The fish will draw in water through its mouth (flap over the gills is closed) and the water is pushed out over the gills by closing the mouth and opening the gill cover. Some species force water over the gills to achieve more efficient ventilation for increased metabolic demand and varying degrees of this ram ventilation are used in specific species (rhythmic movements of lower jaw and opercula or consistent movement through water) [139,142]. The number of gills varies in different species (e.g., 3–7 arches). Additional functions of the gills include osmoregulation, nitrogen excretion, hormone metabolism, and acid–base regulation [141].

The skin also functions as a respiratory organ. Highly vascular skin, particularly in the young, can facilitate diffusion of gases. This ability is species-dependent but can constitute up to 30% of respiration in some [143]. Therefore, skin should be handled carefully and with wet gloves to prevent damage. Various other modifications and adaptations have evolved in different fish species and a thorough knowledge of these species-specific respiratory functions is crucial to understand their potential impact on anesthesia [139].

Cardiovascular system

The cardiovascular system in fish is considered a single-cycle closed-loop circulation system. This means that the four-chambered heart pumps blood in a single circuit through the body, picking up oxygen on the way through the gills. The heart itself consists of a sinus venosus, a single atrium, a ventricle, and a bulbus arteriosus. It is commonly referred to as a "two-chambered heart" or a "four-chambered heart arranged in series" [144]. Blood is pumped out of the single-chambered ventricle into the bulbus arteriosus through a pair of ventricular-bulbar valves at the ventricular-bulbar junction. The bulbus arteriosus in most fish is non-contractile but elastic and resembles a bulge at the base of the aorta [144]. In sharks, this bulbus arteriosus is called the "conus arteriosus" with contractile cardiac muscle fibers and several rows of valves [144]. Blood flows from the aorta to the gills for oxygenation and then to the body. The hepatic and the common cardinal veins drain blood returning from the body into the sinus venosus (a sac-like contractile structure) [144] before blood flows into the atrium. At the sinoatrial junction, the atrium and the sinus venosus are separated by a sinoatrial valve that regulates the flow into the atrium. From the thin-walled but muscular atrium, the blood is pumped back into the ventricle through a pair of atrioventricular valves at the atrioventricular junction. The valves ensure unidirectional blood flow [144].

On an ECG (pre- and postcordial leads), the P wave represents the onset of atrial (auricular) contraction. The QRS represents depolarization of the ventricle, with the P-R interval corresponding to the time for the impulse to cross the atrium and the atrioventricular junction. The T wave represents repolarization of the ventricle [145]. Fish do seem to have a baroreceptor reflex that slows HR when arterial blood pressure increases [145]. A branchiocardiac reflex exists (increasing HR with increasing respiratory rate) to ensure optimal oxygen uptake. This reflex can be utilized with the described "buccal flow/HR reflex," which increases HR by increasing water flow rate through the buccal cavity (either by moving fish through the water or flowing anesthetic-free water through the buccal cavity/gills to hasten elimination of anesthetics) [139,146,147].

Nervous system

Fish, like vertebrates, have a peripheral and a central nervous system. The peripheral nervous system can be functionally divided into a somatic division (responsible for motor and sensory activity) and an autonomic division, which includes sympathetic, parasympathetic, and enteric nervous systems [148]. The central nervous system includes a spinal cord, medulla oblongata, and a brain that has a telencephalon, diencephalon (epithalamus, thalamus, and hypothalamus), mesencephalon, and cerebellum. Fish possess an archipallium but, like amphibians, lack a neopallium in the cerebrum [148].

Fish are easily stressed, resulting in high morbidity and mortality [148–150]. Main stressors are water quality changes (e.g., temperature, pH, and nitrogenous waste concentration), handling, transportation, disease, noise and light abnormalities, inadequate nutrition, stocking, and many more [148]. Fish react to stress via a neuroendocrine response that includes the adrenergic system and the hypothalamic–pituitary–interrenal axis [148]. Various factors and neurotransmitters play a role, including corticotropin-releasing factor, adrenocorticotropic hormone, catecholamines, etc. [148]. Fish show three stages of the stress response depending on duration and intensity of the stressing factor (e.g., primary, secondary, and tertiary stress response) [148,151,152]. The primary response is similar to mammals via a neuroendocrine pathway resulting in a fight or flight response through catecholamine release [148,153]. With persistent stress, consistent circulation of cortisol and catecholamines will lead to the secondary response resulting in increases in cardiac output, metabolic rate, respiration, lactic acid, and fatty acids [148,154]. Continuing chronic stress leads to the tertiary stress response, which manifests as physiologic exhaustion, including decreased immune function, reproduction, growth rate, changes in behavior, and increased mortality [148,151,152,155].

Nociception in fish is considered a stress factor that elicits a strong response. After reception of nociceptive signals from nociceptors, signals travel via the peripheral nerves (C or Aδ fibers, depending on species and pain stimulus) [148]. Similar to mammals, the signal is sent via the spinothalamic and trigeminal tracts to the brain. Fish have a functional endogenous opioid system and all four opioid receptor types have been identified [117,119,148,154,156–158]. Ongoing debate continues to drive research into whether fish are able to experience pain or a pain-like state [148,159–164]. Even though this question remains largely unanswered, it is accepted that fish have a functional nociceptive system and are capable of nociception and respond with stress to a noxious stimulus [147,148,160]. Since this response to noxious stimulation is evident, scientists and clinicians should aim to provide analgesia to alleviate the stress response [148,165–167]. Recommendations have been published for analgesics used in fish that undergo surgical procedures. Focus has been on NSAIDs, local anesthetics, and opioids [104, 139,148,149,168,169].

Thermoregulation

Almost all fish are ectothermic, meaning that anesthesia is impacted when water temperatures are outside their optimal temperature ranges. Induction time and recovery are usually prolonged in lower temperatures due to decreased respiratory rates and cardiac output, and slower metabolism [168,170]. Acidosis and hypercapnia occur at higher temperatures, leading to hyperventilation and subsequently decreased induction and recovery times [170]. Tuna and some shark species have developed the ability of endothermy by conserving heat and increasing body temperature above ambient water temperatures.

Overview of clinical anesthesia of fish

Mylniczenko *et al.* have provided an excellent description of fish anesthesia in *Zoo Animal and Wildlife Immobilization and Anesthesia, 2nd edn.* [139], with detailed species-specific drug information. The following will provide a general overview of fish anesthesia and the reader is directed to the above chapter for specific details on bony fish anesthesia.

Considerations for fish anesthesia

All fish are anesthetized or sedated in water. Anesthesia is commonly performed via immersion in a water bath and subsequently maintained in flow-by systems. In larger species, injectable anesthesia can be used to facilitate smooth induction. It is important that all water quality parameters are similar to the water of the fish's normal environment. This includes the water temperature, salinity, pH, and mineral composition (hardness) [167]. Water from the fish's tank (environment) is commonly used for induction and anesthesia.

The equipment, drug concentrations, and dosing depend on the species, size, and condition. Similar to mammals, bigger fish need less drug per unit weight.

Anesthetic drugs used for fish anesthesia include tricaine methanesulfonate (MS-222), benzocaine, metomidate, isoeugenol, 2-pheoxyethanol, and quinaldine. Simplistically, MS-222 is a local anesthetic that blocks voltage-gated sodium channels leading to the inhibition of action potentials and nerve conduction [171]. Its anesthetic mechanism of action is not fully understood but has been attributed to peripheral and central effects of Na^+ channel and, to a lesser extent, K^+ and Ca^{2+} channel blockade, as well as activation of second messengers via membrane-bound protein activation [171]. Muscle relaxation, sedation, and cardiovascular and respiratory depression occur in a dose-dependent manner. MS-222 is administered by immersion and uptake is via the gills and skin. MS-222 is rapidly biotransformed via acetylation into polar and non-polar metabolites [172] and is excreted via the gills and kidneys. Continual administration of MS-222 via flow-through to the gills can be used to maintain anesthesia. The concentration can be changed to adjust depth of anesthesia. MS-222 is water soluble and the dissolution of the drug into water may decrease pH. Depending on the optimal water pH for a specific fish species, water may need to be buffered to ensure ideal water quality. Buffer requirements depend on the anesthetic concentration used and the alkalinity of the water source [173]. Salt water is usually more alkaline and has a natural buffering capacity [169]. MS-222 is the only United States Food and Drug Administration (FDA) approved anesthetic for fish with a withdrawal time of 21 days [174].

Benzocaine is also a local anesthetic but has the disadvantage that it needs to be dissolved in an organic solvent (ethanol or acetone) before adding it to water to use as an immersion anesthetic. Metomidate is a non-barbiturate hypnotic that inhibits $GABA_A$ receptors. Metomidate decreases cortisol release by blocking activation of the hypothalamus–pituitary–interrenal axis [175]. Administration of metomidate is by immersion or oral administration. Isoeugenol is a compound of clove oil and has become a commonly used fish anesthetic (Aqui-S™). Its use is associated with cardiorespiratory depression and induction of a stress response and the agent has been controversial due to its potential carcinogenic properties.

Combinations of drugs have been explored to decrease the adverse effects associated with the use of a single anesthetic in higher doses. Adjunctive drugs that have been combined with the anesthetic agents include benzodiazepines, opioids, and NSAIDs. Morphine has been used as an analgesic in fish and shows promising effectiveness in some species. It appears to have a long duration of action [176–178]. Butorphanol and buprenorphine appear to have limited analgesic effects in the species studied [165,179].

Parenteral administration of anesthetic agents (intravenous, intramuscular, and intracoelomic), in addition to enteral (oral) administration, can be used as an alternative to immersion in some larger species. The most practical method with the least potential for damage is intramuscular administration. The ideal injection site in most species is the dorsal saddle area, which is located around the dorsal fin [138]. Problems associated with intramuscular anesthetic use include unreliable response, prolonged recovery, and the need for ventilatory support [147,169,180]. These problems may be influenced by health conditions, age, stress, body condition, and others, that can lead to varying degrees of response. This form of anesthetic administration can help in circumstances where tank induction is not practical (big species, big holding facilities, and personal safety requirements such as for sharks, rays, etc.) [180,181]. Injections can be performed with a pole syringe or an underwater dart gun, or by hand injection [182]. Injectable anesthetic agents used are species-dependent and include azaperone, medetomidine, or dexmedetomidine with ketamine, alfaxalone, or propofol.

Preanesthetic considerations

Fasting fish for 12–24 h is recommended when possible to reduce the amount of nitrogenous waste production (ammonia and nitrite). High levels of nitrogenous waste compounds may decrease oxygenation, lead to acidemia and methemoglobinemia, and may affect uptake and metabolism of anesthetic agents [147]. The risk of regurgitation can be reduced when the fish is fasted. Regurgitation can lead to obstruction of gills [147,183].

Anesthetic depth can be monitored by assessing muscle relaxation via jaw tone and body muscle tone in addition to monitoring HR and respiratory rate. Evaluating loss of righting reflex and responsiveness to stimuli is also important. Fish show similar signs and stages of anesthetic depth as mammals and various descriptions have been published throughout the literature [147,167,184].

In general, fish anesthesia is subdivided into three levels or stages (light, surgical, and deep). Depending on the fish species, the characteristics of a specific level might have different attributes. Surgical anesthesia will be associated with a loss of equilibrium, loss of reaction to pressure on the peduncle, and loss of reaction to emersion with no activity and relaxed muscles. Respiratory rate and HR consistently decrease with increasing depth. Heart beats can be directly visualized in thin body-walled species, but most species require a Doppler probe or an ECG to evaluate HR. The Doppler probe can be placed directly over the heart or into the opercular slit. ECG clips can be placed on the fins or attached to hypodermic needles placed through the skin. ECG electrode patches are not recommended due to concern for damaging the skin. Respiratory rate is monitored by observing gill movements. With increasing depth of anesthesia movements will become reduced. If cardiac output is adequate, flow-by of water through the gills will provide adequate gas exchange, but it is recommended to decrease the anesthetic concentration. Flowing water through the gills is easily achieved by moving the fish through the water, but in most situations where surgery is performed, a recirculating water system is required to allow procedures on the fish while it remains out of the water.

The technique for performing flow-by anesthesia of fish can vary with the available equipment, but in general, fish are induced in a tank with anesthetic added to the water. After achieving adequate depth of anesthesia, the fish is taken out of the water tank and placed on an elevated foam holder or padded fenestrated shelf inside a container, which can collect circulated water. The buccal cavity is intubated with a bifurcated plastic tube (size depending on species) and connected to a non-recirculating or recirculating system (dependent on fish size) to supply aerated water containing anesthetics. Recirculating systems will reuse the collected water via a submersible variable-flow aquarium pump or manually via a syringe.

An example of a non-recirculating system is an intravenous fluid bag filled with water, which contains anesthetic and an air stone for aeration. The bag (reservoir) is connected with a drip-set to tubing inserted into the buccal cavity [104,139,140,147]. Recommended flow rates are influenced by drug concentration, but 1–3 L/kg/min is common to ensure the gills remain wet for optimal gas exchange but prevent gastric dilation which can occur at higher flows [147]. The fish's skin and cornea remain moistened by gently spraying water over the fish with a syringe.

At the end of the procedure, the depth of anesthesia is lightened. Providing the fish has strong pulses and is ventilating well by itself, it is placed into a dedicated aerated recovery tank void of any anesthetics. The fish is held in an upright position and moved through the water to provide flow of oxygenated water across the gills for washout. The fish will gradually be able to hold itself up and start swimming with decreasing degrees of incoordination. The fish should be monitored during recovery to prevent injury.

References

1 Sladky KK, Mans C. Clinical anesthesia in reptiles. *J Exot Pet Med* 2012; **21**: 17–31.

2 Fleming GJ. Crocodilians (crocodiles, alligators, caimans, gharial). In: West G, Heard DJ, Caulkett N, eds. *Zoo Animal and Wildlife Immobilization and Anesthesia*, 2nd edn. Ames, IA: Wiley Blackwell, 2014: 325–336.

3 Bertelsen MF. Squamates (snakes and lizards). In: West G, Heard DJ, Caulkett N, eds. *Zoo Animal and Wildlife Immobilization and Anesthesia*, 2nd edn. Ames, IA: Wiley Blackwell, 2014: 351–364.

4 Vigani A. Chelonians (turtles, tortoises, and terrapins). In: West G, Heard DJ, Caulkett N, eds. *Zoo Animal and Wildlife Immobilization and Anesthesia*, 2nd edn. Ames, IA: Wiley Blackwell, 2014: 365–387.

5 Schumacher J, Yelen T. Anesthesia and analgesia. In: Mader DR, ed. *Reptile Medicine and Surgery*, 2nd edn. St. Louis, MO: Saunders Elsevier, 2006: 442–452.

6 Schumacher J, Mans C. Anesthesia. In: Mader DR, Divers SJ, eds. *Current Therapy in Reptile Medicine and Surgery*. St. Louis, MO: Elsevier Saunders, 2014: 134–153.

7 Baker LA, White FN. Redistribution of cardiac output in response to heating in *Iguana iguana*. *Comp Biochem Physiol* 1970; **35**: 253–262.

8 Varga M. Captive maintenance and welfare. In: Girling SJ, Raiti P, eds. *BSAVA Manual of Reptiles*, 2nd edn. Gloucester, UK: BSAVA Press, 2004: 6–17.

9 Preston DL, Mosley CA, Mason RT. Sources of variability in recovery time from methohexital sodium anesthesia in snakes. *Copeia* 2010; **3**: 496–501.

10 Ultsch GR, Jackson DC. Long-term submergence at 3 degrees C of the turtle Chrysemys picta bellii in normoxic and severely hypoxic water. III. Effects of changes in ambient PO2 and subsequent air breathing. *J Exp Biol* 1982; **97**: 87–99.

11 Andrews RM, Pough FH. Metabolism of squamate reptiles: allometric and ecological relationships. *Physiol Zool* 1985; **58**: 214–231.

12 Van Mierop LHS, Kutsche M. Some aspects of comparative anatomy of the heart. In: Johansen K, Burggren WW, eds. *Cardiovascular Shunts: Phylogenetic, Ontogenic and Clinical Aspects*. Copenhagen, Denmark: Munksgaard, 1985: 38–56.

13 Van Mierop LHS, Kutsche M. Comparative anatomy of the ventricular septum. In: Wenick ACG, ed. *The Ventricular Septum in the Heart*. Boston, MA: Martinus Nijhoff, 1981: 35–46.

14 Comeau SG, Hicks JW. Regulation of central vascular blood flow in the turtle. *Am J Physiol* 1994; **267**: R569–R578.

15 Herman J, Wang T, Smits AW, *et al.* The effects of artificial lung inflation on pulmonary blood flow and heart rate in the turtle *Trachemys scripta*. *J Exp Biol* 1997; **200**: 2539–2545.

16 Hicks JW, Ishimatsu A, Molloi S, *et al.* The mechanism of cardiac shunting in reptiles: a new synthesis. *J Exp Biol* 1996; **199**: 1435–1446.

17 Ishimatsu A, Hicks JW, Heisler N. Analysis of intracardiac shunting in the lizard, *Varanus niloticus*: a new model based on blood oxygen levels and microsphere distribution. *Respir Physiol* 1988; **71**: 83–100.

18 Heisler N, Neumann P, Maloiy GM. The mechanism of intracardiac shunting in the lizard *Varanus exanthematicus*. *J Exp Biol* 1983; **105**: 15–31.

19 Hicks JW, Malvin GM. Mechanism of intracardiac shunting in the turtle *Pseudemys scripta*. *Am J Physiol* 1992; **262**: R986–R992.

20 Luckhardt AB, Carlson AJ. Studies on the visceral sensory nervous system. *Am J Physiol* 1921; **56**: 72–112.

21 White FN. Circulation. In: Gans C, Dawson WR, eds. *Biology of the Reptilia, Physiology A*. New York, NY: Academic Press, 1976: 275–334.

22 Burggren WW, Glass ML, Johansen K. Pulmonary ventilation: perfusion relationships in terrestrial and aquatic chelonian reptiles. *Can J Zool* 1977; **55**: 2024–2034.

23 Milsom WK, Langille BL, Jones DR. Vagal control of pulmonary vascular resistance in the turtle *Chrysemys scripta*. *Can J Zool* 1977; **55**: 359–367.

24 Berger PJ, Burnstock G. Autonomic nervous system. In: Gans C, ed. *Biology of the Reptilia*. New York, NY: Academic Press, 1979: 1–57.

25 Lillywhite HB, Donald JA. Pulmonary blood flow regulation in an aquatic snake. *Science* 1989; **245**: 293–295.

26 Burggren W, Farrell A, Lillywhite HB. Vertebrate cardiovascular systems. In: Dantzler WH, ed. *Handbook of Physiology*. New York, NY: Oxford University Press, 1997: 254–267.

27 Berger PJ. The reptilian baroreceptor and its role in cardiovascular control. *Am Zool* 1987; **27**: 111–120.

28 Stinner JN. Cardiovascular and metabolic responses to temperature in *Coluber constrictor*. *Am J Physiol* 1987; **253**: R222–R227.

29 Stinner JN, Ely DL. Blood pressure during routine activity, stress, and feeding in black racer snakes (*Coluber constrictor*). *Am J Physiol* 1993; **264**: R79–R84.

30 Farrell AP. Introduction to cardica scope in lower vertebrates. *Can J Zool* 1991; **69**: 1981–1984.

31 Seymour RS, Lillywhite HB. Blood pressure in snakes from different habitats. *Nature* 1976; **264**: 664–666.

32 Lillywhite HB, Pough FH. Control of arterial pressure in aquatic sea snakes. *Am J Physiol* 1983; **244**: R66–R73.

33 Lillywhite HB, Gallagher KP. Hemodynamic adjustments to head-up posture in the partly arboreal snake, *Elaphe obsoleta*. *J Exp Zool* 1985; **235**: 325–334.

34 Bennett RA, Schumacher J, Hedjazi-Haring K, *et al.* Cardiopulmonary and anesthetic effects of propofol administered intraosseously to green iguanas. *J Am Vet Med Assoc* 1998; **212**: 93–98.

35 Schumacher J, Lillywhite HB, Norman WM, *et al.* Effects of ketamine HCl on cardiopulmonary function in snakes. *Copeia* 1997: 395–400.

36 Custer RS, Bush M. Physiologic and acid–base measures of gopher snakes during ketamine or halothane-nitrous oxide anesthesia. *J Am Vet Med Assoc* 1980; **177**: 870–874.

37 Bonath K. Halothane inhalation anaesthesia in reptiles and its clinical control. *Int Zoo Yearb* 1979; **19**: 112–125.

38 Rooney MB, Levine G, Gaynor J, *et al.* Sevoflurane anesthesia in desert tortoises (*Gopherus agassizii*). *J Zoo Wildl Med* 1999; **30**: 64–69.

39 Stirl R, Bonath KH. Cardiovascular, pulmonary and acid–base measurements in boa constrictors during tiletamine-zolazepam sedation. In: *Proceedings of the 5th International Congress of Veterinary Anesthesia*, 1994.

40 Arena PC, Richardson KC, Cullen LK. Anaesthesia in two species of large Australian skink. *Vet Rec* 1988; **123**: 155–158.

41 Anderson NL, Wack RF, Calloway L, *et al.* Cardiopulmonary effects and efficacy of propofol as an anesthetic in brown tree snakes (*Boiga irregularis*). *Bull Assoc Reptil Amphib Vet* 1999; **9**: 9–15.

42 Mosley CA, Dyson D, Smith DA. The cardiovascular dose-response effects of isoflurane alone and combined with butorphanol in the green iguana (*Iguana iguana*). *Vet Anaesth Analg* 2004; **31**: 64–72.

43 Milsom WK. Mechanoreceptor modulation of endogenous respiratory rhythms in vertebrates. *Am J Physiol* 1990; **259**: R898–R910.

44 Smatresk NJ. Chemoreceptor modulation of endogenous respiratory rhythms in vertebrates. *Am J Physiol* 1990; **259**: R887–R897.

45 Wang T, Smits AW, Burggren W. Pulmonary function in reptiles. In: Gans C, Gaunt AS, eds. *Biology of the Reptilia*. Ithaca, NY: Society for the Study of Amphibians and Reptiles, 1998: 319.

46 Wood SC, Lenfant CJM. Respiration: mechanics, control and gas exchange. In: Gans C, Dawson WR, eds. *Biology of the Reptilia, Physiology A*. New York, NY: Academic Press, 1976: 225–274.

47 Shelton G, Jones DR, Milsom WK. Control of breathing in ectothermic vertebrates. In: Geiger SR, Widdicombe JG, eds. *Handbook of Physiology. Section 3: The Respiratory System*. Bethesda, MD: American Physiological Society, 1986.

48 Glass ML, Wood SC. Gas exchange and control of breathing in reptiles. *Physiol Rev* 1983; **63**: 232–260.

49 Johansen K, Hanson D, Lenfant C. Respiration in a primitive air breather, *Amia calva. Respir Physiol* 1970; **9**: 162–174.
50 Shelton G, Burggren W. Cardiovascular dynamics of the chelonia during apnoea and lung ventilation. *J Exp Biol* 1976; **64**: 323–343.
51 Perry SF. Structure and function of the reptilian respiratory system. In: Lenfant C, Wood CM, eds. *Comparative Pulmonary Physiology. Current Concepts.* New York, NY: Marcel Dekker, 1989: 193–236.
52 Glass ML, Johansen K. Control of breathing in *Acrochordus javanicus*, an aquatic snake. *Physiol Zool* 1976; **49**: 328–340.
53 Templeton JR, Dawson WR. Respiration in the lizard *Crotaphytus collaris. Physiol Zool* 1963; **36**: 104–121.
54 Glass ML, Burggren W, Johansen K. Ventilation in an aquatic and a terrestrial helonian reptile. *J Exp Biol* 1978; **72**: 165–179.
55 Jackson DC, Palmer SE, Meadow WL. The effects of temperature and carbon dioxide breathing on ventilation and acid–base status of turtles. *Respir Physiol* 1974; **20**: 131–146.
56 Jackson DC, Kraus DR, Prange HD. Ventilatory response to inspired CO2 in the sea turtle: effects of body size and temperature. *Respir Physiol* 1979; **38**: 71–81.
57 Boyer DR. Comparative effects of hypoxia on respiratory and cardiac function in reptiles. *Physiol Zool* 1966; **39**: 307–316.
58 Jackson DC. Ventilatory response to hypoxia in turtles at various temperatures. *Respir Physiol* 1973; **18**: 178–187.
59 Hitzig BM, Allen JC, Jackson DC. Central chemical control of ventilation and response of turtles to inspired CO2. *Am J Physiol* 1985; **249**: R323–R328.
60 Benchetrit G, Armand J, Dejours P. Ventilatory chemoreflex drive in the tortoise, *Testudo horsfieldi. Respir Physiol* 1977; **31**: 183–191.
61 Benchetrit G, Dejours P. Ventilatory CO2 drive in the tortoise *Testudo horsfieldi. J Exp Biol* 1980; **87**: 229–236.
62 Frankel HM, Spitzer A, Blaine J, *et al.* Respiratory response of turtles (*Pseudemys scripta*) to changes in arterial blood gas composition. *Comp Biochem Physiol* 1969; **31**: 535–546.
63 Diethelm G. *The effect of oxygen content of inspiratory air (FIO_2) on recovery times in the green iguana (Iguana iguana).* Doctor of Veterinary Medicine thesis, *University of Zurich*, 2001.
64 Bertelsen MF, Mosley CA, Crawshaw GJ, *et al.* Inhalation anesthesia in Dumeril's monitor (*Varanus dumerili*) with isoflurane, sevoflurane, and nitrous oxide: effects of inspired gases on inducion and recovery. *J Zoo Wildl Med* 2005; **36**: 62–68.
65 Goe A, Shmalberg J, Gatson B, *et al.* Epinephrine or GV-26 electrical stimulation reduces inhalant anesthetic recovery time in common snapping turtles (*Chelydra serpentina*). *J Zoo Wildl Med* 2016; **47**:501–507.
66 Holz P, Barker IK, Crawshaw GJ, *et al.* The anatomy and perfusion of the renal portal system in the red-eared slider (*Trachemys scripta elegans*). *J Zoo Wildl Med* 1997; **28**: 378–385.
67 Holz P, Barker IK, Burger JP, *et al.* The effect of the renal portal system on pharmacokinetic parameters in the red-eared slider (*Trachemys scripta elegans*). *J Zoo Wildl Med* 1997; **28**: 386–393.
68 Berner NJ. Oxygen consumption by mitochondria from an endotherm and an ectotherm. *Comp Biochem Physiol B Biochem Mol Biol* 1999; **124**: 25–31.
69 Penick DN, Paladino FV, Steyermark AC, *et al.* Thermal dependence of tissue metabolism in the green turtle (*Chelonia mydas*). *Comp Biochem Physiol* 1996; **113A**: 293–296.
70 Chittick EJ, Stamper MA, Beasley JF, *et al.* Medetomidine, ketamine, and sevoflurane for anesthesia of injured loggerhead sea turtles: 13 cases (1996–2000). *J Am Vet Med Assoc* 2002; **221**: 1019–1025.
71 Wellehan JFX, Lafortune M, Gunkel C, *et al.* Coccygeal vascular catheterization in lizards and crocodilians. *J Herpetol Med Surg* 2004; **14**: 26–28.
72 Maxwell LK, Jacobson ER. Allometric scaling of kidney function in green iguanas. *Comp Biochem Physiol A Mol Integr Physiol* 2004; **138**: 383–390.
73 Bennett RA. Reptile anesthesia. *Semin Avian Exot Pet Med* 1998; **7**: 30–40.
74 Whitaker BR, Krum H. Medical management of sea turtles. In: Fowler ME, Miller RE, eds. *Zoo and Wild Animal Medicine*, 4th edn. Philadelphia, PA: WB Saunders, 1999: 217.
75 Young BD, Stegeman N, Norby B, *et al.* Comparison of intraosseous and peripheral venous fluid dynamics in the desert tortoise (*Gopherus agassizii*). *J Zoo Wildl Med* 2012; **43**: 59–66.
76 International Association for the Study of Pain (IASP) Terminology. www.iasp-pain.org/resources/terminology/ (accessed September 2022).
77 Molony V. Comments on Anand and Craig, PAIN, 67 (1996) 3–6. *Pain* 1997; **70**: 293.
78 Liang YF, Terashima S, Zhu AQ. Distinct morphological characteristics of touch, temperature, and mechanical nociceptive neurons in the crotaline trigeminal ganglia. *J Comp Neurol* 1995; **360**: 621–633.
79 Terashima S, Liang YF. C mechanical nociceptive neurons in the crotaline trigeminal ganglia. *Neurosci Lett* 1994; **179**: 33–36.
80 Kevetter GA, Willis WD. Collateralization in the spinothalamic tract: new methodology to support or deny phylogenetic theories. *Brain Res* 1984; **319**: 1–14.
81 Desfilis E, Font E, Garcia-Verdugo JM. Trigeminal projections to the dorsal thalamus in a lacertid lizard, *Podarcis hispanica. Brain Behav Evol* 1998; **52**: 99–110.
82 Butler AB, Cotterill RM. Mammalian and avian neuroanatomy and the question of consciousness in birds. *Biol Bull* 2006; **211**: 106–127.
83 De la Iglesia JA, Martinez-Guijarro FI, Lopez-Garcia C. Neurons of the medial cortex outer plexiform layer of the lizard *Podarcis hispanica*: Golgi and immunocytochemical studies. *J Comp Neurol* 1994; **341**: 184–203.
84 Lindberg I, White L. Reptilian enkephalins: implications for the evolution of proenkephalin. *Arch Biochem Biophys* 1986; **245**: 1–7.
85 Ng TB, Hon WK, Cheng CH, *et al.* Evidence for the presence of adrenocorticotropic and opiate-like hormones in the brains of two sea snakes, *Hydrophis cyanocinctus* and *Lapemis hardwickii. Gen Comp Endocrinol* 1986; **63**: 31–37.
86 Mauk MD, Olson RD, LaHoste GJ, *et al.* Tonic immobility produces hyperalgesia and antagonizes morphine analgesia. *Science* 1981; **213**: 353–354.
87 Porro CA, Carli G. Immobilization and restraint effects on pain reactions in animals. *Pain* 1988; **32**: 289–307.
88 Tambeli CH, Fischer L, Monaliza SL, *et al.* The functional role of ascending nociceptive control in defensive behavior. *Brain Res* 2012; **1464**: 24–29.
89 Wright KM. Taxonomy of amphibians kept in captivity. In: Wright KM, Whitaker BR, eds. *Amphibian Medicine and Captive Husbandry*. Malabar, FL: Krieger, 2001: 3–14.
90 Mitchell MA. Anesthetic considerations for amphibians. *J Exot Pet Med* 2009; **18**: 40–49.
91 Baitchman E, Stetter MD. Amphibians. In: West G, Heard DJ, Caulkett N, eds. *Zoo Animal and Wildlife Immobilization and Anesthesia*, 2nd edn. Ames, IA: Wiley Blackwell, 2014: 303–311.
92 Clayton LA, Gore SR. Amphibian emergency medicine. *Vet Clin North Am Exot Anim Pract* 2007; **10**: 587–620.
93 Wright KM. Anatomy for the clinician. In: Wright KM, Whitaker BR, eds. *Amphibian Medicine and Captive Husbandry*. Malabar, FL: Krieger, 2001: 15–30.
94 Wright KM. Applied physiology. In: Wright KM, Whitaker BR, eds. *Amphibian Medicine and Captive Husbandry*. Malabar, FL: Krieger, 2001: 31–34.
95 Haberich FJ. Demonstration of the functional separation of venous and arterial blood in the frog circulation by x-ray angiography. *Pflugers Arch Gesamte Physiol Menschen Tiere* 1967; **293**: 193–198.
96 Haberich FJ. The functional separation of venous and arterial blood in the univentricular frog heart. *Ann NY Acad Sci* 1965; **127**: 459–475.
97 Heinz-Taheny KM. Cardiovascular physiology and disease of amphibians. *Vet Clin North Am Exot Anim Pract* 2009; **12**: 39–50.
98 Langille BL, Jones DR. Dynamics of blood flow through the hearts and arterial systems of anuran amphibia. *J Exp Biol* 1977; **68**: 1–17.
99 Johansen K, Hanson D. Functional anatomy of the hearts of lungfishes and amphibians. *Am Zool* 1968; **8**: 191–210.
100 Johansen K. Cardiovascular dynamics in the amphibian *Amphiuma tridactylum* Cuvier. *Acta Physiol Scand* 1964; **217**: 1–82.
101 Jones JM, Wentzell LA, Toews DP. Posterior lymph heart pressure and rate and lymph flow in the toad *Bufo marinus* in response to hydrated and dehydrated conditions. *J Exp Biol* 1992; **169**: 207–220.
102 Duellman WE, Trueb L. *Biology of Amphibians*. Baltimore, MD: Johns Hopkins University Press, 1994.
103 Wright KM. Restraint techniques and euthanasia. In: Wright KM, Whitaker BR, eds. *Amphibian Medicine and Captive Husbandry*. Malabar, FL: Krieger, 2001: 111–122.
104 Stetter MD. Fish and amphibian anesthesia. *Vet Clin North Am Exot Anim Pract* 2001; **4**: 69–82.
105 West NH, van Vliet BH. Sensory mechanism regulaing the cardiovascular and respiratory systems. In: Feder ME, Burggren WW, eds. *Environmental Physiology of the Amphibians*. Chicago, IL: University of Chicago Press, 1992: 151–182.
106 Downes U. Tricaine (MS222) is a safe anesthetic compound compared to benzocaine and pentobarbital to induce anesthesia in leopard frogs (*Rana pipiens*). *Pharmacol Rep* 2005; **57**: 467–474.
107 Guenette SA, Giroux MC, Vachon P. Pain perception and anaesthesia in research frogs. *Exp Anim* 2013; **62**: 87–92.
108 Lalonde-Robert V, Beaudry F, Vachon P. Pharmacologic parameters of MS-222 and physiologic changes in frogs (*Xenopus laevis*) after immersion at anesthetic doses. *J Am Assoc Lab Anim Sci* 2012; **51**: 464–468.
109 Goulet F, Vachon P, Helie P. Evaluation of the toxicity of eugenol at anesthetic doses in African clawed frogs (*Xenopus laevis*). *Toxicol Pathol* 2011; **39**: 471–477.
110 Mitchell MA, Riggs S, Singleton B. Evaluating the clinical and cardiopulmonary effects of clove oil and propofol in tiger salamanders (*Ambystoma tigrinum*). *J Exot Pet Med* 2009; **18**: 50–56.
111 Ross A, Guenette SA, Helie P, *et al.* Case of cutaneous necrosis in African clawed frogs *Xenopus laevis* after the topical application of eugenol. *Can Vet J* 2006; **47**: 1115–1117.

112 Hernández SE, Sernia C, Bradley AJ. The effect of three anaesthetic protocols on the stress response in cane toads (*Rhinella marina*). *Vet Anaesth Analg* 2012; **39**(6): 584–590.

113 Wojick KB, Langan JN, Mitchell MA. Evaluation of MS-222 (Tricaine Methanesulfonate) and propofol as anesthetic agents in Sonoran desert toads (*Bufo alvarius*). *J Herpetol Med Surg* 2010; **20**(2): 79–83.

114 Stetter MD, Raphael B, Indiviglio F, *et al.* Isoflurane anesthesia in amphibians: comparison of five application methods. In: *Proceedings of the American Association of Zoo Veterinarians*, 1996; 255–257.

115 Posner LP, Bailey KM, Richardson EY, *et al.* Alfaxalone anesthesia in bullfrogs (*Lithobates catesbeiana*) by injection or immersion. *J Zoo Wildl Med* 2013; **44**: 965–971.

116 Guenette SA, Beaudry F, Vachon P. Anesthetic properties of propofol in African clawed frogs (*Xenopus laevis*). *J Am Assoc Lab Anim Sci* 2008; **47**: 35–38.

117 Rosenblum PM, Peter RE. Evidence for the involvement of endogenous opioids in the regulation of gonadotropin secretion in male goldfish, *Carassius auratus*. *Gen Comp Endocrinol* 1989; **73**: 21–27.

118 Stevens CW, Klopp AJ, Facello JA. Analgesic potency of mu and kappa opioids after systemic administration in amphibians. *J Pharmacol Exp Ther* 1994; **269**: 1086–1093.

119 Rosenblum PM, Callard IP. Endogenous opioid peptide system in male brown bullhead catfish, *Ictalurus nebulosus* Lesueur: characterization of naloxone binding and the response to naloxone during the annual reproductive cycle. *J Exp Zool* 1988; **245**: 244–255.

120 Stevens CW. Opioid research in amphibians: an alternative pain model yielding insights on the evolution of opioid receptors. *Brain Res Brain Res Rev* 2004; **46**: 204–215.

121 Koeller CA. Comparison of buprenorphine and butorphanol analgesia in the eastern red-spotted newt (*Notophthalmus viridescens*). *J Am Assoc Lab Anim Sci* 2009; **48**: 171–175.

122 Machin KL. Amphibian pain and analgesia. *J Zoo Wildl Med* 1999; **30**: 2–10.

123 Stevens CW. Analgesia in amphibians: preclinical studies and clinical applications. *Vet Clin North Am Exot Anim Pract* 2011; **14**: 33–44.

124 Duncan A. Reptile and amphibian analgesia. In: Fowler ME, Miller RE, eds. *Zoo and Wild Animal Medicine*, 7th edn. Philadelphia, PA: Elsevier, 2012: 247–253.

125 Machin KL. Fish, amphibian, and reptile analgesia. *Vet Clin North Am Exot Anim Pract* 2001; **4**: 19–33.

126 Nikundiwe AM, de Boer-van Huizen R, ten Donkelaar HJ. Dorsal root projections in the clawed toad (*Xenopus laevis*) as demonstrated by anterograde labeling with horseradish peroxidase. *Neuroscience* 1982; **7**: 2089–2103.

127 Echlin F, Propper N. 'Sensitization' by injury of the cutaneous nerve endings in the frog. *J Physiol* 1937; **88**: 388–400.

128 Habgood JS. Sensitization of sensory receptors in the frog's skin. *J Physiol* 1950; **111**: 195–213.

129 Stevens CW. Opioid antinociception in amphibians. *Brain Res Bull* 1988; **21**: 959–962.

130 Braga PC, Tiengo M, Biella G, *et al.* Dermorphin, a new peptide from amphibian skin, inhibits the nociceptive thalamic neurons firing rate evoked by noxious stimuli. *Neurosci Lett* 1984; **52**: 165–169.

131 Erspamer V. The opioid peptides of the amphibian skin. *Int J Devl Neuroscience* 1992; **10**: 3–30.

132 Stevens CW, Yaksh TL. Spinal action of dermorphin, an extremely potent opioid peptide from frog skin. *Brain Res* 1986; **385**: 300–304.

133 Mettam JJ, Oulton LJ, McCrohan CR, *et al.* The efficacy of three types of analgesic drugs in reducing pain in the rainbow trout, *Oncorhynchus mykiss*. *Appl Anim Behav Sci* 2011; **133**: 265–274.

134 Mohan S, Stevens CW. Systemic and spinal administration of the mu opioid, remifentanil, produces antinociception in amphibians. *Eur J Pharmacol* 2006; **534**: 89–94.

135 Brenner GM, Klopp AJ, Deason LL, *et al.* Analgesic potency of alpha adrenergic agents after systemic administration in amphibians. *J Pharmacol Exp Ther* 1994; **270**: 540–545.

136 Stevens CW, MacIver DN, Newman LC. Testing and comparison of non-opioid analgesics in amphibians. *Contemp Top Lab Anim Sci* 2001; **40**: 23–27.

137 Willenbring S, Stevens CW. Thermal, mechanical and chemical peripheral sensation in amphibians: opioid and adrenergic effects. *Life Sci* 1996; **58**: 125–133.

138 Neiffer DL, Stamper MA. Fish sedation, analgesia, anesthesia, and euthanasia: considerations, methods, and types of drugs. *ILAR J* 2009; **50**: 343–360.

139 Mylniczenko ND, Neiffer DL, Clauss TM. Boney fish (lungfish, sturgeon, teleosts). In: West G, Heard DJ, Caulkett N, eds. *Zoo Animal and Wildlife Immobilization and Anesthesia*, 2nd edn. Ames, IA: Wiley Blackwell, 2014: 209–260.

140 Harms CA. Anesthesia in fish. In: Fowler ME, Miller RE, eds. *Zoo and Wild Animal Medicine*, 5th edn. St. Louis, MO: WB Saunders, 2003: 2–20.

141 Olson KR. Vascular anatomy of the fish gill. *J Exper Zool* 2002; **293**: 214–231.

142 Bushnell PG, Jones DR. Cardiovascular and respiratory physiology of tuna: adaptations for support of exceptionaly high metabolic rates. *Environ Biol Fishes* 1994; **40**: 303–318.

143 Bruecker P, Graham M. The effects of the anesthetic ketamine hydrochloride on oxygen consumption rates and behaviour in the fish Heros *(Cichlasoma) citrinellum*. *Comp Biochem Physiol* 1993; **104C**: 57–59.

144 Sherrill J, Weber ES, Marty GD, *et al.* Fish cardiovascular physiology and disease. *Vet Clin North Am Exot Anim Pract* 2009; **12**: 11–38.

145 Satchell GH. The reflex co-ordination of the heart beat with respiration in the dogfish. *J Exp Biol* 1960; **37**: 719–731.

146 Ross L, Ross B. *Anaesthetic and Sedative Techniques for Aquatic Animals*, 3rd edn. Oxford, UK: Wiley Blackwell, 2008.

147 Neiffer DL, Stamper MA. Fish sedation, analgesia, anesthesia, and euthanasia: considerations, methods, and types of drugs. *ILAR J* 2009; **50**: 343–360.

148 Weber ES. Fish analgesia: pain, stress, fear aversion, or nociception? *Vet Clin North Am Exot Anim Pract* 2011; **14**: 21–32.

149 Weber EP III, Weisse C, Schwarz T, *et al.* Anesthesia, diagnostic imaging, and surgery of fish. *Compend Contin Educ Vet* 2009; **31**: E11.

150 Laitinen M, Valtonen T. Cardiovascular, ventilatory and total activity responses of brown trout to handling stress. *J Fish Biol* 1994; **45**: 933–942.

151 Barton BA, Iwama G. Physiological changes in fish from stress in aquaculture with emphasis on the response and effects of corticsterioids. *Annu Rev Fish Dis* 1991; **1**: 3–26.

152 Barton BA, Morgan JD, Vijayan MN. Physiological and condition-related indicators of environmental stress in fish. In: Adams SM, ed. *Biological Indicators of Aquatic Ecosystem Stress*. Bethesda, MD: American Fisheries Society, 2002: 111–148.

153 Donaldson EM. The pituitary–interrenal axis as an indicator of stress in fish. In: Pickering AD, ed. *Stress and Fish*. London, UK: Academic Press, 1981: 11–47.

154 Ackerman PA, Forsyth RB, Mazur CF, *et al.* Stress hormones and the cellular stress response in salmonids. *Fish Physiol Biochem* 2000; **23**: 327–336.

155 Gregory TR, Wood CM. The effects of chronic plasma cortisol elevation on the feeding behavior, growth, competitive ability, and swimming performance of juvenile rainbow trout. *Physiol Biochem Zool* 1999; **72**: 286–295.

156 Dreborg S, Sundstrom G, Larsson TA, *et al.* Evolution of vertebrate opioid receptors. *Proc Natl Acad Sci USA* 2008; **105**: 15487–15492.

157 McDonald LK, Joss JM, Dores RM. The phylogeny of Met-enkephalin and Leuenkephalin: studies on the holostean fish *Lepisosteus platyrhincus* and the Australian lungfish, *Neoceratodus forsteri*. *Gen Comp Endocrinol* 1991; **84**: 228–236.

158 Vallarino M. Occurrence of β-endorphin-like immunoreactivity in the brain of the teleost, *Boops boops*. *Gen Comp Endocrinol* 1995; **60**: 63–69.

159 Posner LP. Introduction: pain and distress in fish: a review of the evidence. *ILAR J* 2009; **50**: 327–328.

160 Sneddon LU. Pain perception in fish: indicators and endpoints. *ILAR J* 2009; **50**: 338–342.

161 Sneddon LU, Braithwaite VA, Gentle MJ. Do fishes have nociceptors? Evidence for the evolution of a vertebrate sensory system. *Proc Biol Sci* 2003; **270**: 1115–1121.

162 Sneddon LU. Evolution of nociception in vertebrates: comparative analysis of lower vertebrates. *Brain Res* 2004; **46**: 123–130.

163 Rose JD. The neurobehavioral nature of fishes and the question of awareness of pain. *Rev Fish Sci* 2002; **10**: 1–38.

164 Rose D, Woodbury CJ. Animal models of nociception and pain. In: Conn PM, ed. *Sourcebook of Models for Biomedical Research*. Totoway, NJ: Humana Press, 2008: 333–339.

165 Harms CA, Lewbart GA, Swanson CR, *et al.* Behavioral and clinical pathology changes in koi carp (*Cyprinus carpio*) subjected to anesthesia and surgery with and without intra-operative analgesics. *Comp Med* 2005; **55**: 221–226.

166 Smith SA. Pain and distress in fish. *ILAR J* 2009; **50**: 327–415.

167 Sneddon LU. Clinical anesthesia and analgesia in fish. *J Exot Pet Med* 2012; **21**: 32–43.

168 Neiffer DL, Stamper MA. Fish sedation, analgesia, anesthesia, and euthanasia: considerations, methods, and types of drugs. *ILAR J* 2009; **50**: 343–360.

169 Harms CA. Anesthesia in fish. In: Fowler ME, Miller RE, eds. *Zoo and Wild Animal Medicine, Current Therapy*, 4th edn. Philadelphia, PA: WB Saunders, 1999: 158–163.

170 Aguiar LH, Kalinin AL, Rantin FT. The effects of temperature on the cardio-respiratory function of the neotropical fish *Piaractus mesopotamicus*. *J Therm Biol* 2002; **27**: 299–308.

171 Butterworth JF IV, Strichartz GR. Molecular mechanisms of local anesthesia: a review. *Anesthesiology* 1990; **72**: 711–734.

172 Wayson KA, Downes H, Lynn RK, *et al.* Studies on the comparative pharmacology and selective toxicity of tricaine methanesulfonate: metabolism as a basis of the selective toxicity in poikilotherms. *J Pharmacol Exp Ther* 1976; **198**: 695–708.

173 Carter KM, Woodley CM, Brown RS. A review of tricaine methanesulfonate for anesthesia of fish. *Rev Fish Biol Fisheries* 2011; **21**: 51–59.

174 Rub AM, Jepsen N, Liedtke TL, *et al.* Surgical insertion of transmitters and telemetry methods in fisheries research. *Am J Vet Res* 2014; **75**: 402–416.
175 Davis KB, Griffin BR. Physiological responses of hybrid striped bass under sedation of several anesthetics. *Aquaculture* 2004; **233**: 531–548.
176 Baker TR, Baker BB, Johnson SM, *et al.* Comparative analgesic efficacy of morphine sulfate and butorphanol tartrate in koi (*Cyprinus carpio*) undergoing unilateral gonadectomy. *J Am Vet Med Assoc* 2013; **243**: 882–890.
177 Newby NC, Gamper AK, Stevens ED. Cardiorespiratory effects and efficacy of morphine sulfate in winter flounder (*Pseudopleuronectes americanus*). *Am J Vet Res* 2007; **68**: 592–597.
178 Newby NC, Wilkie MP, Stevens ED. Morphine uptake, disposition, and analgesic efficacy in the common goldfish (*Carassius auratus*). *Can J Zool* 2009; **87**: 388–399.
179 Davis MR, Mylniczenko N, Storm T, *et al.* Evaluation of intramuscular ketoprofen and butorphanol as analgesics in chain dogfish (*Scyliorhinus rotifer*). *Zoo Biol* 2006; **25**: 491–500.
180 Mylniczenko ND, Clauss TM, Stamper MA. Elasmobranchs and holocephalans. In: West G, Heard DJ, Caulkett N, eds. *Zoo Animal and Wildlife Immobilization and Anesthesia*, 2nd edn. Ames, IA: Wiley Blackwell, 2014: 261–301.
181 Flemming GJ, Heard DJ, Floyd RF, *et al.* Evaluation of propfol and medetomidine-ketamine for short-term immobilization of Gulf of Mexico sturgeon (*Acipenser oxyrinchus de soti*). *J Zoo Wildl Med* 2003; **34**: 153–158.
182 Harvey B, Denny C, Kaiser S, *et al.* Remote intramuscular injection of immobilizing drugs into fish using a laser-aimed underwater dart gun. *Vet Rec* 1988; **122**: 174–177.
183 Harms CA, Bakal RS. Techniques in fish anesthesia. *J Sm Exot Anim Med* 1995; **3**: 19–25.
184 Oikawa S, Takeda T, Itazawa Y. Scale effects of MS-222 on a marine teleost, porgy *Pagrus* major. *Aquaculture* 1994; **121**: 369–379.

58 Comparative Anesthesia and Analgesia – Birds

John W. Ludders[1] and David Sanchez-Migallon Guzman[2]

[1]Emeritus Professor, Department of Clinical Sciences, College of Veterinary Medicine, Cornell University, Ithaca, New York, USA
[2]Department of Medicine and Epidemiology, School of Veterinary Medicine, University of California–Davis, Davis, California, USA

Chapter contents

Introduction, 1127
Respiratory system, 1127
  Ventilation components, 1128
  Gas exchange component, 1129
  Control of ventilation, 1134
Cardiovascular system, 1134
  Renal portal system, 1134
Preanesthetic patient evaluation and preparation, 1135
  Physical restraint, 1135
  Physical examination, 1135
  Fasting, 1135
General pharmacologic considerations, 1135
  Routes of drug administration, 1135
  Allometric scaling and pharmacokinetics, 1136
Drugs used for analgesia and anesthesia, 1137
  Opioids, 1137
  Non-steroidal anti-inflammatory drugs, 1139
  Local anesthetics, 1141
  Injectable induction drugs, 1141
  Inhalant anesthetics, 1142
  Adjuncts to general anesthesia, 1143
  Drugs of historical interest, 1143
Anesthetic management, 1144
  Airway management, 1144
  Breathing circuits and fresh gas flows, 1144
  Induction methods, 1144
  Monitoring and support, 1145
  Recovery, 1148
References, 1148

Introduction

The class Aves consists of 27 Orders, 168 Families, and approximately 10,000 species worldwide. Birds, regarded as the only clade of dinosaurs that survived the Cretaceous–Paleogene extinction event 66 million years ago [1], inhabit every continent on this planet and live in a wide range of environmental niches. For example, emperor penguins (*Aptenodytes forsteri*) live in the Antarctic, and one study recorded an individual ocean dive record of 540 m (1772 ft) lasting 18 min [2]. A Ruppell's griffon (*Gyps rueppelli*), the highest-flying bird, encountered a jet at 11,485 m (37,900 feet) over the west African country of Côte d'Ivoire. Bar-headed geese (*Anser indicus*) routinely fly over the Himalayas, some as high as 7290 m (23,917 ft), when migrating between central and south Asia [1]. The burrowing owl (*Athene cunicularia*) nests underground while wandering albatrosses spend most of their life in soaring flight over the Southern Ocean. The weight and size of birds vary greatly. Bee hummingbirds (*Mellisuga helenae*) measure 5–6 cm (2–2.4 in) in length and weigh 1.6–2 g while the ostrich (*Struthio camelus*) has a height of 2.75 m (9 ft) and weighs up to 145 kg.

Throughout time, humans have had a practical interest in birds as a source of food. In domesticating and selecting for desirable production characteristics, such as rapid weight gain or high egg production, a number of structural and functional changes have occurred in domesticated species, changes not seen in their wild relatives. For example, domesticated turkeys and chickens have smaller lung volumes and less gas exchange surface area compared to their wild counterparts.

The tremendous diversity in form, function, and mode of life existing across avian orders and between wild and domesticated species, as well as variation that exists within any given species, pose challenges to the anesthetic management of birds. Indeed, the risk of anesthesia-related death of birds is as high as 3.9% [3–5]. Challenges associated with anesthetizing birds can be lessened by considering and applying basic principles of avian anatomy, physiology, and pharmacology.

Respiratory system

The avian respiratory system consists of two separate and distinct functional components: one for ventilation (larynx, trachea, syrinx, bronchi, air sacs, thoracic skeleton, muscles of respiration), and one for gas exchange (parabronchial lung). These two components can be used to advantage when anesthetizing birds, especially when using inhalant anesthetics.

Veterinary Anesthesia and Analgesia: The Sixth Edition of Lumb and Jones. Edited by Leigh Lamont, Kurt Grimm, Sheilah Robertson, Lydia Love and Carrie Schroeder.
© 2024 John Wiley & Sons, Inc. Published 2024 by John Wiley & Sons, Inc.
Companion website: www.wiley.com/go/lamont/anesthesia

Ventilation components

Larynx, trachea, syrinx

The avian larynx is located at the base of the tongue and protrudes into the pharynx as a somewhat heart-shaped mound [6]. Birds do not have an epiglottis, so when the tongue is pulled gently forward the larynx is easily visualized in most birds (Fig. 58.1). A notable exception is the flamingo with its ventroflexed beak and large fleshy tongue that make it difficult to visualize the larynx.

The avian trachea, which consists of complete cartilaginous rings, conducts air from the nares and mouth to the bronchi while warming, moisturizing, and screening particulate matter from inspired gas [6]. From one avian class to another, there are tracheal anatomical differences that have significant implications for ventilation. For example, emu and ruddy ducks have an inflatable sac-like diverticulum that opens from the trachea. In emu of both sexes, the sac arises from the ventral surface of the trachea approximately three-quarters of the way down the neck where the tracheal rings are incomplete and form a slit-like opening (Fig 58.2) [6]. This sac is responsible for the characteristic booming call of the emu. In male ruddy ducks, the sac opens in a depression on the dorsal wall of the trachea immediately caudal to the larynx, thus lying between the trachea and esophagus [6]. The sac may act as a sounding board for the bill-drumming display of the males [6].

Some penguins and petrels possess a double trachea consisting of a median septum dividing part of the trachea into right and left channels [6]. In both groups of birds, the septum extends cranially from the bronchial bifurcation, but its length is variable; in the jackass penguin (*Spheniscus demersus*), it extends to within a centimeter of the larynx [7], whereas in the rockhopper penguin (Eudyptes *spp.*), the septum is only 5 mm in length [6].

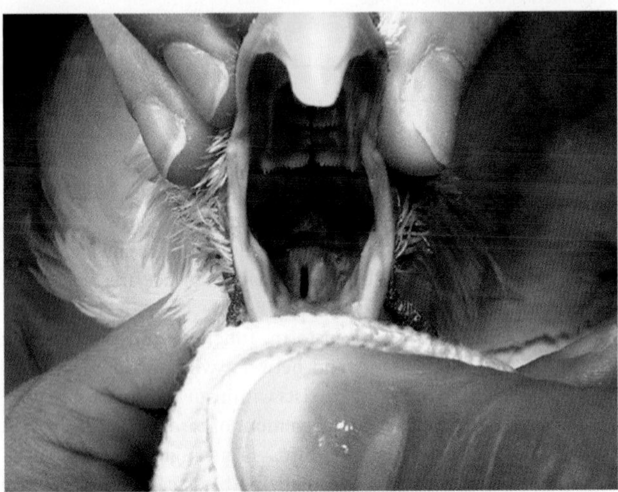

Figure 58.1 Larynx of a chicken.

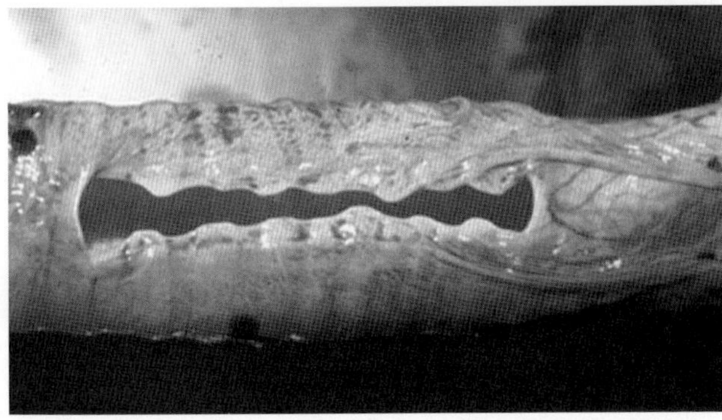

Figure 58.2 Tracheal slit of an emu (*Dromaius novaehollandiae*). Source: Dr. Julie A. Smith, with permission.

Other classes of birds have complex tracheal loops or coils in the caudal neck, within the keel, or within the thorax and keel (Fig. 58.3). Studies in cranes (Grus *spp.*) have demonstrated that tracheal coiling enables these birds to produce extremely loud calls using very low driving pressures [8].

Birds generally have relatively long necks, not to mention tracheal loops and coils, which affect tracheal deadspace, an important consideration during general anesthesia. The typical avian trachea is 2.7 times longer than that of comparably sized mammals, but it is 1.29 times wider, so tracheal resistance to gas flow is comparable in birds and mammals [6]. Tracheal deadspace volume in birds is about 4.5 times larger than that of comparably sized mammals, but the relatively low respiratory frequency (about one-third that of mammals) and larger tidal volume of birds (about four times larger than in a comparably sized mammal) ensure that the effect of the larger tracheal deadspace volume is decreased [6]. The net effect is that avian tracheal minute ventilation is only about 1.5 to 1.9 times that of mammals [6].

The syrinx, the sound-producing organ in birds, is located at the junction of the trachea and mainstem bronchi and the details of its structure vary among avian species. Its location and structure (a number of variably ossified cartilages, muscles, and vibrating soft structures) explain why gas flowing through the trachea, especially during positive-pressure ventilation, can produce sound in an anesthetized, intubated bird.

Primary and secondary bronchi

Mammals have 23 orders of bronchial branching leading to the gas exchange area of the lung (the alveoli), but birds have only three orders of branching before reaching gas exchange tissue [9]. The avian bronchial system consists of a primary bronchus (extrapulmonary and intrapulmonary), secondary bronchi, and tertiary

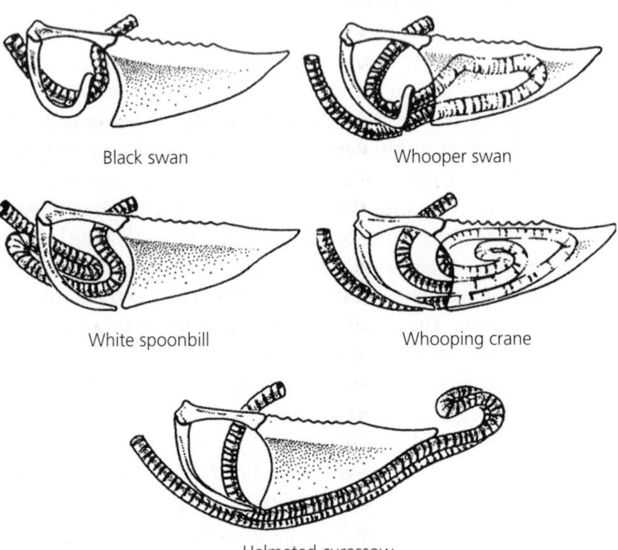

Figure 58.3 Different forms of tracheal loops: black swan (*Cygnus atratus*); whooper swan (*Cygnus cygnus*); white spoonbill (*Platalea leucorodia*); whooping crane (*Grus americana*); helmeted curassow (*Crax Pauxi*). Source: Adapted from McLelland [6].

bronchi (referred to as "parabronchi"). The parabronchi and their surrounding mantle of tissue (the peri-parabronchial mantle) is where gas exchange occurs [6,9].

The primary bronchus enters the lung ventrally and obliquely at the junction of the cranial and middle thirds of the lung, then passes dorsolaterally to the lung surface where it turns caudally in a dorsally curved direction until, at the caudal lung margin, it opens into the abdominal air sac [10]. The primary bronchi have low columnar, pseudostratified epithelium overlying a well-developed internal circular smooth muscle layer, and longitudinally oriented smooth muscles [11] that can change the internal diameter of the primary bronchus. Acetylcholine, pilocarpine, and histamine contract bronchial smooth muscles; atropine blocks the effects of these drugs but has no effect when given alone [12].

A secondary bronchus is any bronchus arising from a primary bronchus; for a short distance, they have the same histologic structure as the primary bronchus, but subsequently develop simple squamous epithelium [13,14]. In most birds, the secondary bronchi are arranged into four groups: medioventral, mediodorsal, lateroventral, and laterodorsal secondary bronchi [15]. The medioventral secondary bronchi arise from the primary intrapulmonary bronchus close to where it enters the lung and occupy the ventral surface of the lung [16]. The mediodorsal, lateroventral, and laterodorsal secondary bronchi arise from the caudal curved portion of the primary intrapulmonary bronchus. Many medioventral and lateroventral secondary bronchi open through ostia into the cervical, clavicular, cranial thoracic, caudal thoracic, and abdominal air sacs.

Air sacs

With a few notable exceptions, most birds have nine pulmonary air sacs that connect to the lungs: two cervical, an unpaired clavicular, two cranial and two caudal thoracic, and two abdominal air sacs. Some exceptions include storks, where each caudal thoracic air sac is divided in two, making 11 air sacs; domestic fowl, where the cervical air sacs are fused, making eight air sacs; songbirds, where the cranial thoracic air sacs are fused to the single median clavicular sac, making seven air sacs in all; and turkeys, where the caudal thoracic air sacs are absent and they have a fused cervicoclavicular air sac, making seven definitive air sacs [15]. In contrast to the pulmonary air sacs, the cervicocephalic air sacs are not connected to the lung and are divided into cephalic and cervical portions; they connect to caudal aspects of the infraorbital sinus. Extensive cervicocephalic air sac development has been noted in budgerigars, cockatiels, conures, Amazon parrots, macaws, and cockatoos.

Air sacs are thin-walled, vessel-poor structures composed of simple squamous epithelium; they do not significantly contribute to gas exchange [17,18]. In chickens (*Gallus gallus domesticus*), adrenergic and cholinergic nerve plexuses have been described in the walls of air sacs, along with vasoactive intestinal peptide and fibers containing substance P, somatostatin, and enkephalin-immunoreactive fibers [18]. To a varying extent, depending upon the species, diverticula from the pulmonary air sacs aerate the cervical vertebrae, some of the thoracic vertebrae, vertebral ribs, sternum, humerus, pelvis, and head and body of the femur [15].

The pulmonary air sacs functionally provide a flow of air to the relatively rigid avian lung which changes in volume by only 1.4% [19]. Based on their bronchial connections, air sacs are grouped into a cranial group consisting of the cervical, clavicular, and cranial thoracic air sacs, and a caudal group consisting of the caudal thoracic and abdominal air sacs [20]. The volume is distributed approximately equally between the cranial and caudal groups [21]. During ventilation, all air sacs are effectively ventilated, with the possible exception of the cervical air sacs; the ratio of ventilation to volume is similar for each air sac [21,22].

Muscles of respiration and the thoracic skeleton

In birds, unlike in mammals, inspiration and expiration are active processes requiring muscular activity. Birds lack a muscular diaphragm, so pressures do not differ between the thoracic and abdominal cavities [11,15,16,23]. Inspiration and expiration occur through movement of the sternum by contraction of the cervical, thoracic, and abdominal muscles [16,23]. As the inspiratory muscles contract, the internal volume of the thoracoabdominal cavity increases (Fig. 58.4). Since air sacs are the only volume-compliant structures in the body cavity [19], pressure within the air sacs becomes negative relative to ambient atmospheric pressure, and air flows from the atmosphere into the pulmonary system, specifically into the pulmonary air sacs and across the gas exchange surfaces of the lungs. During expiration, pressure within the air sacs becomes positive relative to ambient atmospheric pressure, and air flows from the air sacs and pulmonary system to the environment.

Gas exchange component

Tertiary bronchi (parabronchi) and air capillaries

A parabronchus (tertiary bronchus) and its mantle of surrounding tissue, consisting of air capillaries and blood capillaries, is the basic unit of gas exchange. Paleopulmonic parabronchi are long, narrow tubes that anastomose and connect the medioventral to the

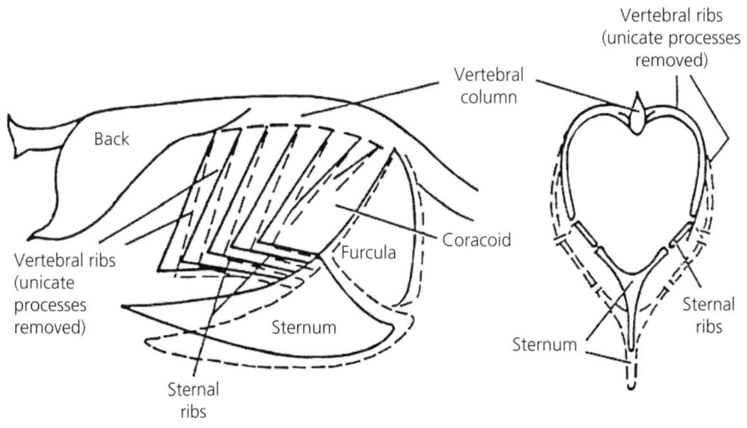

Figure 58.4 Changes in the position of the thoracic skeleton during breathing in a bird. The solid lines represent the thoracic position at the end of expiration while the dotted lines show the thoracic position at the end of inspiration. Source: Fedde MR. Respiration. In: Sturkie PD, ed. *Avian Physiology*, 4th edn. New York, NY: Springer-Verlag, 1986; 191–220.

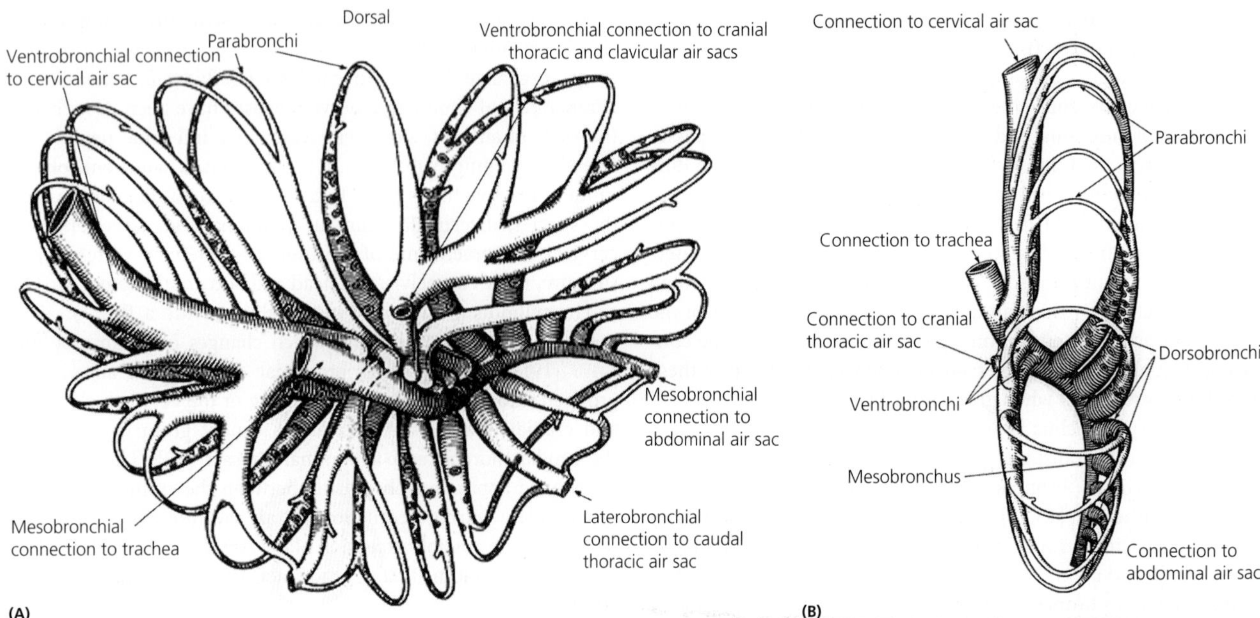

Figure 58.5 Two views of secondary bronchi and parabronchi in the right lung of a goose. **A.** Medial view. **B.** Dorsal view. Source: Brackenbury, JH. Ventilation of the lung-air sac system. In: Seller TJ, ed. *Bird Respiration*, Vol I. Boca Raton, FL: CRC Press, 1987; with permission.

mediodorsal secondary bronchi; the neopulmonic parabronchi profusely interconnect mainly the laterodorsal and lateroventral secondary bronchi [19] (Fig. 58.5A and B). There is a network of smooth muscle surrounding the entrances to the parabronchi; electrical stimulation of the vagus nerve causes the smooth muscle to contract, thus narrowing the parabronchial openings [24]. The inner surfaces of the tubular parabronchi are pierced by numerous openings into chambers called "atria" that are separated from each other by inter-atrial septa (Fig. 58.6A and B) covered by a thin epithelial layer with a core of densely packed bundles of smooth muscle framing the atrial openings [15]. Since the avian lung is richly innervated with vagal and sympathetic nerves, it is possible that afferent and efferent neural pathways exist for controlling pulmonary smooth muscle, thus varying airflow through the parabronchial lung in response to a variety of stimuli [20].

Arising from the abluminal floor of each atrium are funnel-shaped ducts (infundibulae) that lead to air capillaries measuring 3 to 20 μm in diameter, and which are globular in shape, not tubular as previously alleged, and that interconnect via short, narrow passageways; the blood capillaries with which the air capillaries entwine consist of segments that are about as long as they are wide and form an anastomosing three-dimensional network spatially arranged in the exchange tissue [19]. It is in this highly compact tissue of air and blood capillaries that gas exchange occurs [19] (Fig. 58.7A–C).

The law of Laplace ($P = \gamma/r$; where P is opening pressure, γ is surface tension, and r is radius of tubule) applied to small-diameter tubules, such as air capillaries, indicates that high surface tensions result and generate significant negative pressure across the blood–gas barrier that could lead to influx of fluid or collapse the tubules [25]. However, air and blood capillaries possess innate structural elements that preserve their anatomic and gas exchange integrity [26]. These elements form an interdependent, tightly coupled network of tension and compression – a tensegrity state – in the avian lung that gives the lungs their shape while strengthening the air and blood capillaries, thus preserving their function [19].

Paleopulmonic and neopulmonic parabronchi: lung volumes and direction of gas flow

There are two types of parabronchial tissue: (1) paleopulmonic parabronchial tissue (paleopulmonic lung), found in all birds, consisting of parallel stacks of profusely anastomosing parabronchi; and (2) neopulmonic parabronchial tissue (neopulmonic lung), a meshwork of anastomosing parabronchi located in the caudolateral portion of the lung, the degree of development of which is species-dependent (Fig. 58.8A–C). Penguins and emu have only paleopulmonic parabronchi. Pigeons, ducks, and cranes have both paleopulmonic and neopulmonic parabronchi with the neopulmonic parabronchi accounting for 10–12% of the total lung volume. In fowl-like and song birds, the neopulmonic parabronchi are more developed and may account for 20–25% of total lung volume. Paleopulmonic and neopulmonic parabronchi are histologically indistinguishable from each other [19].

Compared to mammals, specific total lung volume in birds is about 27% smaller, but specific surface area of the blood–gas (tissue) barrier is ~15% greater; the ratio of the tissue surface area to the volume of the exchange tissue is 170–305% greater [27]. The harmonic mean thickness of the tissue barrier in birds is 56–67% less (less resistance to gas diffusion) and the pulmonary capillary blood volume is 22% greater. With the exception of specific total lung volume, these morphometric parameters favor the gas exchange capacity of birds [27].

The specific volume (respiratory gas volume per unit body mass) of the avian pulmonary system is between 100 and 200 mL/kg, but the volume of gas in the parabronchi and air capillaries where gas exchange occurs accounts for only 10% of the total specific volume [21]. By comparison, a dog's specific volume is 45 mL/kg, and the pulmonary gas volume in the mammalian lung is 96% of the total specific volume. Because the ratio of residual gas volume (i.e., gas in the lungs) to tidal volume is so much smaller in birds than in mammals, it has been suggested that cyclic changes in the direction of parabronchial gas flow (i.e., tidal flow) could produce significant and intolerable cyclic changes in gas exchange analogous to breath

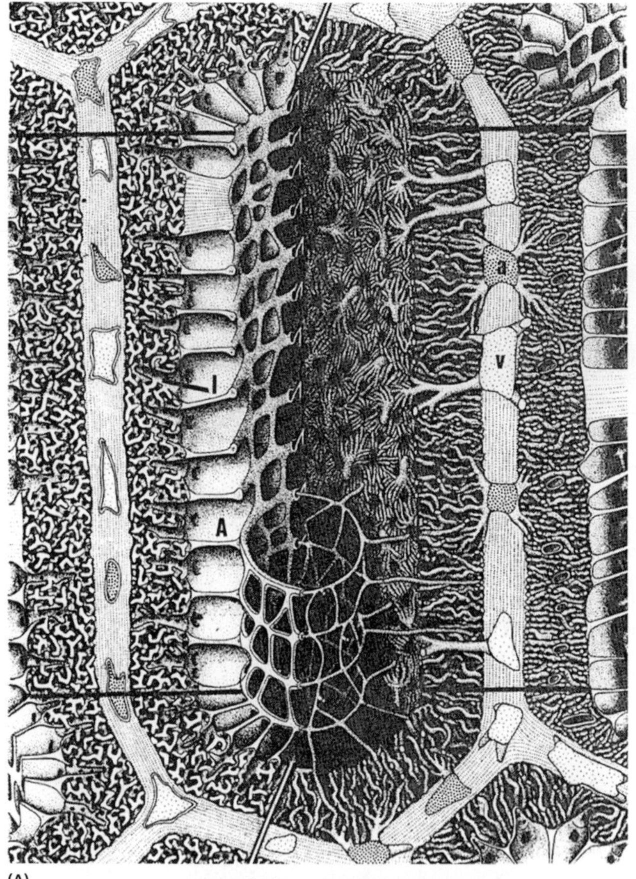

(A)

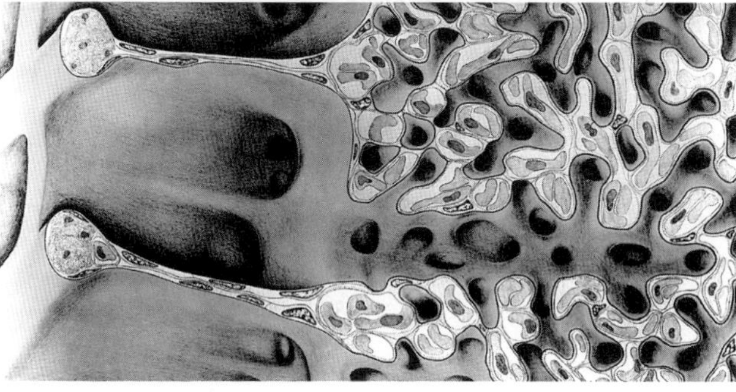

(B)

Figure 58.6 Three-dimensional drawings of a parabronchus and an atrium. **A.** Sagittal section of a parabronchus. On the left side are atria with infundibula departing from them and the three-dimensional air capillary meshwork arising from the infundibula. On the right side within the interparabronchial septa are the arterioles *(dense stippling)* from which the capillaries originate and run radially to the lumen. The infundibula lie between the capillaries which are surrounded by a well-developed three-dimensional air capillary network. **B.** Atrium and infundibulum. At the left, two of the circular smooth muscle bundles surrounding the lumen of the parabronchus are shown in cross-section. The atria are separated by septa running horizontally and vertically. Originating from each atrium a few infundibula pass perpendicularly into the parabronchial mantle. At the right, an infundibulum is shown in longitudinal section with air capillaries arising from it at all levels. The air capillaries cross-link and interlace, making up a three-dimensional meshwork around the blood capillaries. The very thin epithelium of the air capillaries and its surfactant film are shown as a single dark line. Source: Duncker [11], reproduced with permission from Elsevier.

holding [28]. The unidirectional flow of gas within the paleopulmonic lung solves this problem.

Direction of gas flow and gas exchange

During a respiratory cycle, the direction of gas flow in the paleopulmonic parabronchi is caudocranial, continuous, and unidirectional, but in the neopulmonic parabronchi it is tidal (i.e., the direction of flow changes during the respiratory cycle [19] (Fig. 58.9A and B). The exact course of inspired air through the avian respiratory system has been debated for years, but now a general consensus exists on its route during respiratory cycles [19]. It takes two inspiratory and two expiratory cycles for inspired air to pass through the lung–air sac system [19]. During the first inspiratory cycle, the air flows through the trachea and the extrapulmonary and intrapulmonary primary bronchi (mesobronchus) and then the caudal air sacs; in the next breathing cycle (the first expiratory cycle), the air is expelled from the caudal air sacs and directed into the parabronchial system of the lung via the mediodorsal secondary bronchi; during the next breathing cycle, (the second inspiratory cycle), the air in the parabronchial system moves to the cranial air sacs; and in the subsequent breathing cycle (the second expiratory cycle), the air in the cranial air sacs is expelled to the outside through the extrapulmonary primary bronchus and the trachea. The unidirectional flow of gas through the paleopulmonic parabronchi is probably due to aerodynamic valves, not mechanical valves [19]. Although poorly understood, the mechanisms involved probably include the orientation of secondary bronchial and air sac orifices to the direction of gas flow, elastic pressure differences between the cranial and caudal group of air sacs, and gas convective inertial forces [18].

Cross-current model of gas exchange

The movement of gas within the parabronchi and outwards into the atria and infundibulae is by convective flow and then by diffusion into the air capillaries [29,30]. Blood flows from the periphery via the interparabronchial artery and arterioles, ultimately flowing into the blood capillaries where it meets the outward-moving air capillaries. The cross-current model and its multicapillary serial arterialization system best describe gas exchange in the avian lung. The multicapillary serial arterialization system increases the duration over which the respiratory media (air and blood) are exposed to each other [18]. Thus, the quantity of oxygen and carbon dioxide in the oxygenated blood that ultimately returns to the heart via the pulmonary vein is derived from an aggregate effect of very small quantities exchanged at the infinitely many points where the air and blood capillaries contact [19]. Reversing the direction of air or blood flow in a multicapillary serial arterialization system only changes the sequence in which the blood is arterialized in the blood capillaries; the overall amount of oxygen that is exchanged does not change [19]. Within the avian lung is a counter-current system created by the centripetal (inward) flow of deoxygenated blood and the centrifugal (radial, outward) flow of air from the parabronchial lumen [18,19]. However, since the air and blood capillaries entwine very closely, at any one point they contact over very short distances that may fall far short of the critical lengths needed for efficient gas exchange in a "conventional counter-current system." (Fig. 58.10). The significance of this counter-current system for gas exchange under normal physiologic conditions is uncertain; under extreme conditions (flight at altitude), such an arrangement may contribute to gas exchange.

The efficiency of the avian lung can be put into perspective by considering what happens to the partial pressures of carbon dioxide

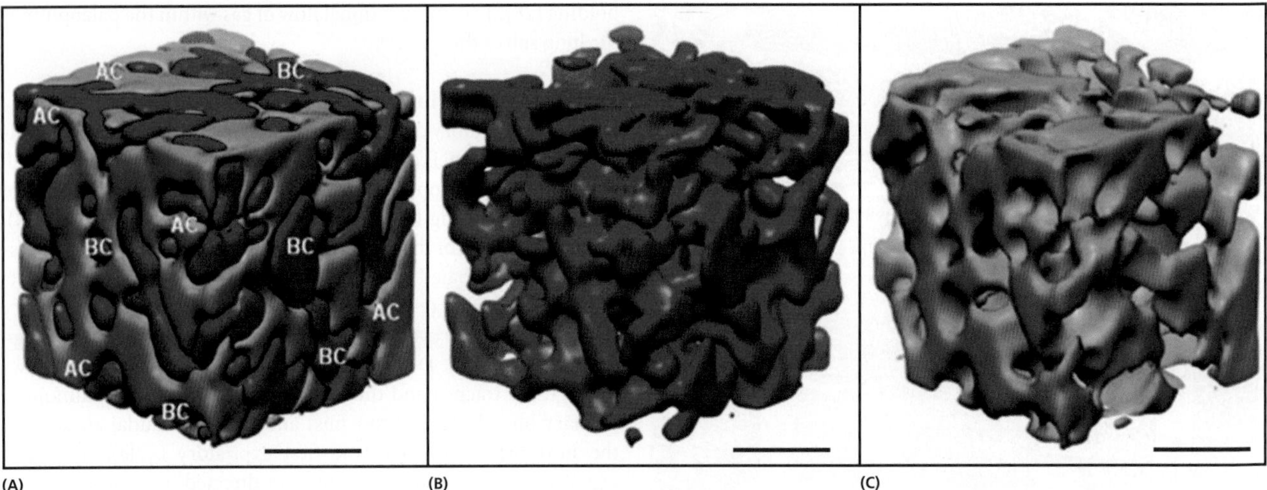

Figure 58.7 Three-dimensional reconstruction showing the intimate intertwining of blood and air capillaries in the paleopulmonic lung of the ostrich (*Struthio camelus*). **A.** Combined three-dimensional reconstructions of the blood capillary (BC, red) and air capillary (AC, cyan) systems. **B.** Three-dimensional reconstruction of the blood capillaries. **C.** Three-dimensional reconstruction of the air capillaries. Scale bars = 20 μm. Source: Maina JN, Woodward JD. Three-dimensional serial section computer reconstruction of the arrangement of the structural components of the parabronchus of the ostrich, *Struthio camelus* lung. *Anat Rec (Hoboken)* 2009; **292**(11): 1685–1698, with permission.

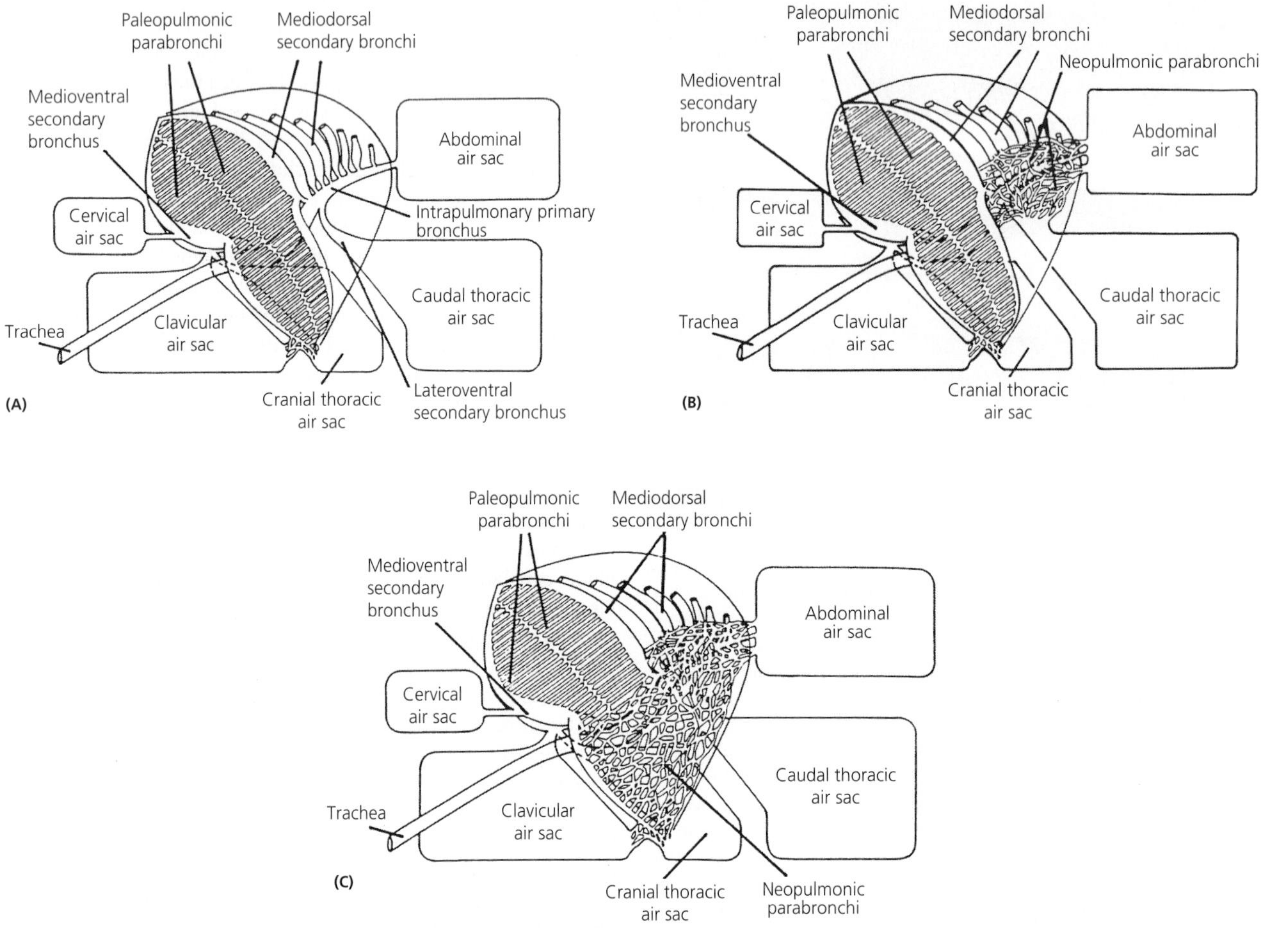

Figure 58.8 Diagram of paleopulmonic and neopulmonic lungs. **A.** The paleopulmonic lung found in penguins and emus. **B.** The paleopulmonic and neopulmonic lung found in storks, ducks, and geese. **C.** The paleopulmonic and the more highly developed neopulmonic lung found in chickens, sparrows, and other songbirds. Source: Fedde [20], with permission of Elsevier.

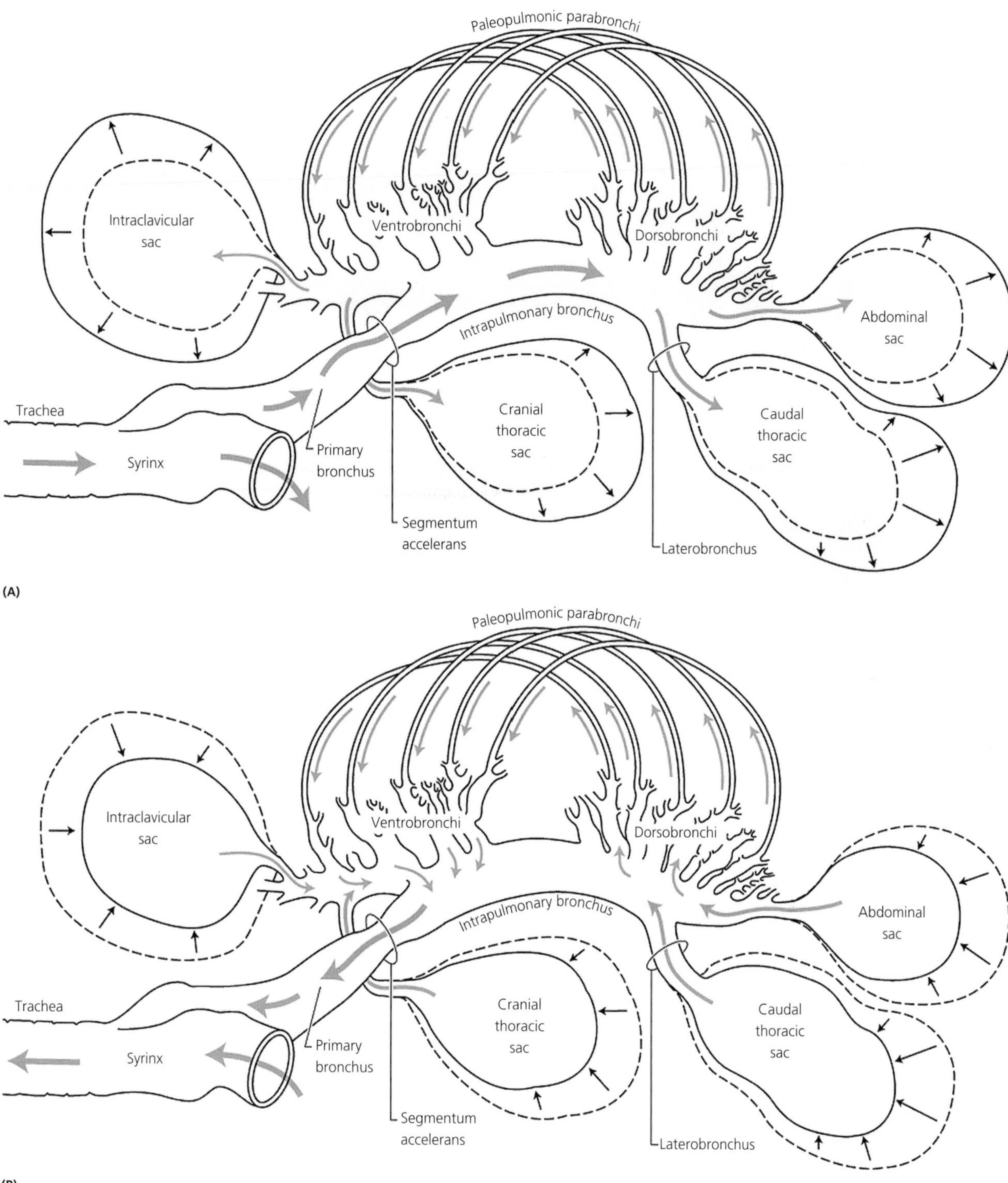

Figure 58.9 Schematic representation of gas flow through the avian pulmonary system during inspiration and expiration. The neopulmonic lung has been removed for clarity. **A.** Inspiration. **B.** Expiration. Source: Adapted from Brown *et al.* [9]; Fedde [20].

(CO_2) and oxygen (O_2) both in respired gas flowing through the lung and in blood perfusing the lung. As gas flows along a parabronchus, it receives CO_2 and gives off O_2 such that gas at the inflow end of the parabronchus has the lowest partial pressure of CO_2, while gas at the outflow end has the highest partial pressure of CO_2; the reverse is true of O_2. The overall result, under hypoxic conditions and during exercise, is that the partial pressure of CO_2 in end-parabronchial gas (P_ECO_2) can exceed the partial pressure of CO_2 in arterial blood ($PaCO_2$), and the partial pressure of O_2 in end-parabronchial gas (P_EO_2) can be lower than the partial pressure of O_2 in arterial blood (PaO_2) [31–33]. This potential overlap of blood and gas partial pressure ranges for both CO_2 and O_2 demonstrates the high gas exchange efficiency of the avian lung [31,32]. Thus, there is no equivalent of alveolar gas because parabronchial

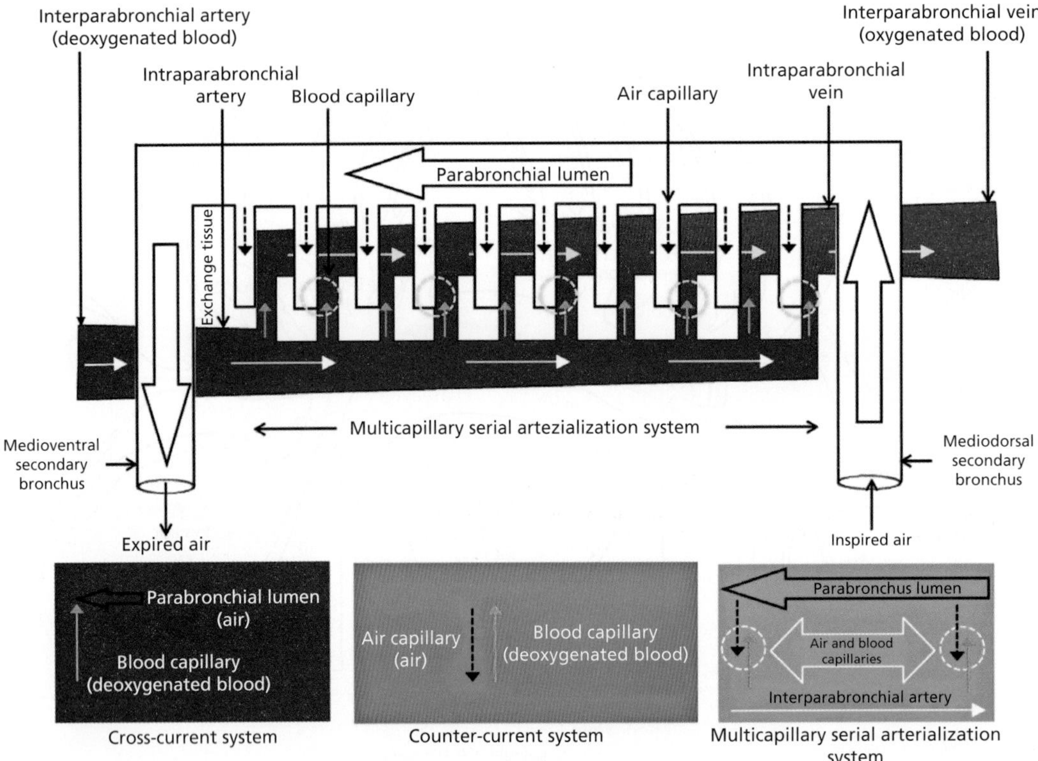

Figure 58.10 Diagram depicting the three intertwined systems involved in gas exchange in the avian parabronchus: cross-current, counter-current, and multicapillary serial arterialization. The cross-current system consists of air flowing in the parabronchial lumen at right angles to that of deoxygenated blood flowing from the periphery of the parabronchus *(small pink arrows)*. The counter-current system is formed by the centripetal flow of deoxygenated blood in the blood capillaries relative to the centrifugal diffusion of air in the air capillaries *(black dashed arrows)*. The multicapillary serial arterialization system is formed by multiple successive contacts between the air and blood capillaries in the gas exchange tissue *(dashed yellow circles)*. For clarity, the atria and infundibula are not shown. The shading of blood from blue to red in the intraparabronchial vein reflects the increasing oxygenation of blood as it passes through the parabronchial gas exchange tissue. Source: Maina [19], with permission.

gas continuously changes in composition as it flows along the length of the parabronchus [34]. Practically speaking, this means the avian lung can extract 40 cm^3 of oxygen from each liter of inspired air, whereas the mammalian lung can extract 30 cm^3 of oxygen [19].

Control of ventilation

Birds have many of the same physiologic components for respiratory control as mammals, such as a central respiratory pattern generator, central chemoreceptors sensitive to PCO_2, and many similar peripheral chemoreceptors [35]. Birds have a unique group of peripheral receptors located in the lung called "intrapulmonary chemoreceptors" (IPCs) that are vagal respiratory afferents inhibited by high lung PCO_2 and excited by low lung PCO_2, thus providing phasic feedback for the control of breathing, specifically rate and depth of breathing [35–38]. They are not mechanoreceptors and they are insensitive to hypoxia [39,40]. However, IPCs are not the sole receptors stimulated by inhaled gas containing low partial pressures of CO_2; arterial and central chemoreceptors are also stimulated [41].

There may be species differences in CO_2 responsiveness depending upon the ecologic niche a given species occupies. The CO_2 responsiveness of IPCs in chickens, ducks, emus, and pigeons is greater than that of burrowing owls that live underground where the CO_2 concentration is higher than that of above-ground-dwelling birds [42,43].

Cardiovascular system

The avian heart is a four-chambered muscular pump that separates venous blood from arterial blood. Birds have larger hearts, larger stroke volumes, lower heart rates, and higher cardiac output than mammals of comparable body mass [44]. Birds also have higher blood pressure than mammals [44,45]. The atria and ventricles are innervated by sympathetic and parasympathetic nerves [46], and norepinephrine and epinephrine are the principal sympathetic neurotransmitters while acetylcholine is the principal parasympathetic neurotransmitter.

The conduction system of the avian heart consists of the sinoatrial node, the atrioventricular node and its branches, and Purkinje fibers [46]. Two groups of animals can be identified by the depth and degree to which Purkinje fibers ramify within the ventricular myocardium, and the pattern of ramification is classified as type 1 or 2 (or category A or B) [47]. The pattern of Purkinje fiber distribution within the ventricular myocardium is responsible for QRS morphology. In birds, Purkinje fibers completely penetrate the ventricular myocardium from endocardium to epicardium and the pattern of ventricular activation is described as type 2b, a pattern that may facilitate synchronous beating at high heart rates [48].

Renal portal system

The avian kidney receives venous blood from the legs via the renal portal circulation, and arterial blood via the arterial circulation [49,50]. The flow of afferent venous blood, unlike in other non-mammalian vertebrates, is not obligatory; venous blood can either perfuse the renal parenchyma or bypass it and enter the central circulation. A unique valve-like structure, the shape of which varies from species to species, is located within the external iliac vein where the efferent renal vein joins it [49]. The valve contains smooth muscle innervated by adrenergic and cholinergic nerves. Epinephrine causes the valve to relax (open) and venous blood from the legs enters the central circulation, whereas acetylcholine causes it to contract (close) and venous blood perfuses the kidney [49,51]. The control of renal valve activity is complex and its effects on drug uptake are not fully understood.

Preanesthetic patient evaluation and preparation

Physical restraint

Proper physical restraint of a bird is a crucial aspect of anesthetic management. In general, a bird is restrained so that its wings and legs are controlled and not allowed to flap or kick about. For long-necked birds such as herons and cranes, the neck must be gently controlled so that the bird does not suffer head, eye, or neck trauma; restraining the bird's head and neck also protects the handler. Improper restraint can cause a variety of problems for a bird, including physical trauma (wing or leg fractures), or physiological stress with increased levels of catecholamines, especially epinephrine, which may predispose to cardiovascular instability [46,52]. Physical restraint can cause significant changes in heart and respiratory rates, and body temperature.

Because birds cannot dissipate heat through the skin, they can become stressed and easily overheated with prolonged restraint. For example, during 15 min of restraint of Amazon parrots (Amazona *spp.*), the average cloacal temperature increased significantly by 4.3 °F while mean respiratory rates increased significantly from 129 to 252 breaths/min [53]. This emphasizes the importance of limiting restraint time and watching for tachypnea, even in healthy birds, so as to avoid potentially life-threatening increases in body temperature [53]. However, in restrained birds, the behavioral indicators of stress – increased respiratory and heart rates – may vary by species.

In barred owls (*Strix varia*), heart and respiratory rates decreased significantly during 15 min of restraint while body temperature significantly increased [54]. In a study of red-tailed hawks (*Buteo jamaicensis*) manually restrained for 15 min while hooded or not hooded, heart and respiratory rates decreased significantly while cloacal temperature increased significantly regardless of hooding; when hooded, the hawks had significantly lower heart and respiratory rates than when not hooded [55]. Thus, hooding amplified the decrease in heart rate and respiratory rate compared to nonhooding but had no effect on stress-induced hyperthermia [55]. It would seem that barred owls and red-tailed hawks cope differently with restraint-associated stress when compared to psittacine species [54].

In a study of geese conditioned over several weeks to 5 min of physical restraint, the humoral indices of stress – catecholamines, corticosterone, and lactate – significantly increased within 2 min after the start of physical restraint despite weeks of conditioning to restraint and the fact that the birds appeared outwardly calm [56]. Thus, the absence of stress cannot be deduced from behavioral observations only [56].

Anesthesia and sedation may ameliorate the humoral stress response. Awake and manually restrained Hispaniolan Amazon parrots had significantly higher serum corticosterone levels (33.7 ± 2.83 ng/mL) than when anesthetized with isoflurane (19.8 ± 1.97 ng/mL) [57]. In manually restrained Hispaniolan Amazon parrots (*Amazona ventralis*) administered midazolam (2 mg/kg) intranasally, the mean rate of cloacal temperature increase was significantly slower and remained significantly lower in birds that received midazolam compared with controls [58].

Understanding the physical characteristics and defense mechanisms birds possess is crucial for effective restraint that protects both the bird and handler. Each avian species has its own unique and effective means of defense and attack. Birds of prey will use their talons and inflict severe physical trauma on a handler or assistant, and the risk of infection from such wounds is quite real. Although most birds of prey do not bite, they can and will use their talons and beak to great effect. Psittacines have very strong beaks that can cause severe soft tissue injury. Cranes and herons use their long, pointed beaks in a spearing manner, and they tend to strike at eyes, a reason for wearing eye protection when working with these birds. Cranes and ratites, such as emus and ostriches, also will jump and strike forward with their legs and clawed feet; an adult ratite can produce a very powerful and dangerous strike-kick.

Physical examination

Every bird should be given a thorough physical examination prior to anesthesia. A number of excellent texts describe in detail the techniques for physical examination and what to look for in specific avian species [59–61]. In general, quiet observation of a bird in its cage will provide a great deal of information. A bird's awareness of and attention to its surrounding environment, body form, and posture, feather condition, and respiratory rate provide clues to its physical condition. Birds should be removed from their cage and examined, with particular attention given to the respiratory and cardiovascular systems. For small species, a stethoscope with a pediatric head should be used for cardiopulmonary examinations. For those species with a crop, it should be palpated in the thoracic inlet to make sure it is empty. The pectoral muscles over the keel should be assessed as they are a good indicator of body condition.

Fasting

A reasonable approach for healthy birds is to withhold food long enough for the upper gastrointestinal tract to empty, usually overnight in large birds and 4 to 6 h in smaller birds [62]. For raptorial species, a 24 h fast is recommended. In an emergency, a bird with a full crop should be held upright during induction with a finger positioned just below the mandible so as to block the esophagus [62]. Once the bird is anesthetized, the crop can be emptied by placing a finger covered with gauze over the choanal slits to prevent food from entering the nasal cavity and then milking the food contents out of the crop and esophagus [62]. At the end of anesthesia, the oral cavity should be checked for and cleaned of food material to prevent aspiration.

General pharmacologic considerations

Routes of drug administration

Sedation offers numerous benefits in avian medicine, including attenuation of stress responses caused by manual restraint and ease of diagnostic sample collection and imaging, and it may decrease the risk of morbidity and mortality in critically ill patients [63,64]. There are a number of routes by which sedative and anesthetic drugs can be administered to birds. Subcutaneous injection sites include the area over the back between the wings, the wing web, and the skin fold in the inguinal region.

Intramuscular injections can be made in the pectoral and thigh muscles. In birds, drugs injected intramuscularly in the hind limb or caudal body might be carried in the blood through the renal portal system and perfuse the kidneys such that some portion of the injected drug may be excreted by the kidney without reaching the general systemic circulation, or it may bypass the kidneys and undergo first-pass hepatic metabolism [65]. In great horned owls administered butorphanol either via the jugular vein or the medial metatarsal vein, the $AUC_{0\rightarrow\infty}$ after medial metatarsal vein administration was significantly less than the $AUC_{0\rightarrow\infty}$ after jugular vein administration of the drug, results indicating a possible renal portal first-pass effect, but no other kinetic parameters were significantly different [66]. In a pharmacokinetic study of florfenicol, an antibiotic, there was no evidence of an influence of the renal portal system on its kinetic parameters when injected into the leg muscles [65].

For intravenous injections as well as for catheterization, the ulnar vein, dorsal metatarsal vein, and jugular vein can be used; the right jugular vein is larger and easier to visualize than the left jugular vein. The ulnar vein can be catheterized in birds as small as cockatiels. An alternative non-invasive route that is safe and rapidly induces sedation in birds (first effect within 3–5 min) is the intranasal route [64]. When using this route, tissue trauma associated with IM injections and subsequent elevations of muscle enzymes in clinical chemistry tests are avoided, and it is not painful. Its limitations are that there may be incomplete drug delivery to a bird due to sneezing, physiologically narrowed nostrils, such as in cockatoos, and upper airway disease, such as blocked or stenotic nostrils [64]. Intranasal delivery of drugs is made with either an insulin syringe (0.5 mL) or tuberculin syringe (1.0 mL) [64].

The intranasal route (IN) has been used to administer a variety of sedative and analgesic drugs to facilitate minor therapeutic procedures in a variety of birds. Xylazine, diazepam, and midazolam have been administered IN to budgerigars (*Melopsittacus undulatus*) and finches [67,68], and juvenile ostriches (*Struthio camelus*) weighing 50–61 kg and aged 4–5 months [69]. Midazolam, detomidine, or combinations of midazolam, xylazine, and ketamine have been administered IN to ring-necked parakeets and successfully reversed with flumazenil, yohimbine, or atipamezole [70]. Intranasal midazolam and diazepam produced rapid and effective sedation in canaries, and xylazine and detomidine produced sedation but not sustained recumbency; specific antagonists (flumazenil and yohimbine) effectively reversed sedation [71]. In pigeons, a combination of midazolam and dexmedetomidine administered IN produced an effective degree of immobilization lasting 20 to 30 min, which was partially antagonized with atipamezole 10 min after its application [72]. In wild blue-and-yellow macaws (*Ara ararauna*), midazolam (2 mg/kg) divided into two equal volumes, was administered IN over 3–5 s via a 24 gauge catheter inserted approximately 2–5 mm into each nostril; sedation occurred in 77% of the macaws and lasted on average 20 min without adverse side effects [73]. In a project involving implantation of intracoelomic satellite transmitters in female surf scoters (*Melanitta perspicillata*), 26 were administered midazolam (4.6–5.9 mg/kg) intranasally, and the same volume of saline (1 mL) was given to another 26 adult female surf scoters [74]. The odds of presumed death in the saline group were 5.3 times higher than in the midazolam-treated group; the presumed mortality at 30 days for the midazolam group (23%) was lower than for the saline group (61%) [74].

Allometric scaling and pharmacokinetics

There is a large number of avian species, each one of which has species-specific pharmacokinetic and pharmacodynamic profiles for each injectable drug [52]. Recognizing this reality, the following discussion of anesthetic and analgesic drugs will highlight a few key pharmacological realties pertaining to birds and focus primarily on drugs for which there are pharmacokinetic and pharmacodynamic data. The rational use of drugs is based primarily on our understanding of pharmacokinetic behavior coupled with information on pharmacodynamic activity, an approach that advances avian anesthesia and analgesia [75]. The reader is referred elsewhere for a more comprehensive review of anesthetic and analgesic drugs used in birds [76].

There are many reasons for using injectable drugs for anesthesia and analgesia in birds, including low cost, ease of use, rapidity of anesthetic inductions, no need for expensive equipment to deliver or maintain anesthesia, minimal if any anesthetic pollution of the work environment, and possible reduction of inhalant anesthetic requirements when used in combination. However, injectables also have inherent disadvantages including: (1) difficulty in delivering a safe volume to small birds, (2) ease in overdosing by any route, (3) difficulty in maintaining surgical anesthesia without severe cardiopulmonary depression, (4) the potential for prolonged, violent recoveries, and (5) significant variation in dose and response among and within species [52,77].

Allometric scaling has been used to determine doses of drugs used in birds [78–81]. Indeed, in the absence of pharmacokinetic data for a drug, general principles of allometric scaling may serve as a rational basis for understanding how body mass or metabolic rate affects drug doses, but there are limitations in its application. Allometric equations, with some exceptions, are based on the assumption that all birds are pharmacologically similar, and only distinguish between two large groups of birds – passerines and non-passerines – a distinction that ignores the many structural and functional differences in the kidneys of birds within these two groups [51]. Drugs used in birds are formulated primarily for mammals. Differences in anatomy and physiology of the two classes of animals make it difficult to achieve pharmacokinetic equivalency between birds and mammals using allometric equations that do not take these differences into consideration [51,82]. Using allometric scaling, it may be possible to derive some pharmacokinetic parameters for a drug, but not all necessary parameters that would allow for safe administration of a drug [83,84]. Allometric scaling is not useful for extrapolating doses of non-steroidal anti-inflammatory drugs (NSAIDs) between avian species [85]. The pharmacologic reality is that for safe use of drugs in birds, we need pharmacokinetic and pharmacodynamic data.

Early pharmacodynamic studies identified significant differences in response among avian species administered the same drug [52,86,87]. For example, the commercially available form of ketamine, which consists of a racemic mixture of *S*(+)- and *R*(−)-enantiomers, produces poor-quality chemical restraint and anesthesia in great horned and snowy owls [87]. When great horned owls receive only the *S*(+)-enantiomer of ketamine, anesthesia induction is smoother and there are fewer cardiac arrhythmias, whereas the *R*(−)-enantiomer is associated with inadequate muscle relaxation, cardiac arrhythmias, and excitement during recovery [87]. It is unknown whether these differences are due to differing metabolic pathways among birds, production of pharmacologically active metabolites, or differences in types of receptors or receptor sensitivity.

Drugs used for analgesia and anesthesia

Opioids

Recognizing and assessing pain in birds can be difficult because it relies on an understanding of species and individual normal behaviors that could be masked in the presence of an observer. Birds tend to respond to noxious stimuli with a fight-or-flight response (i.e., escape reactions, vocalization, and excessive movement), and/or conservation–withdrawal responses (i.e., no escape attempts or minimal vocalization and immobility). Pain can change a bird's social interactions, such as perching away from the flock, reduction in social grooming, or interactions with the owner. Grooming activity may decrease when a bird is painful, but conversely overgrooming and feather-destructive behaviors have been associated with chronic pain, which may include neuropathic pain [88]. These behavioral signs coupled with studies involving psittacines, raptors, domestic fowl, and pigeons, and using a variety of analgesiometric techniques and pharmacokinetic studies, have been used to determine the plasma concentrations of drugs that produce analgesia in birds (for examples, see [89–94]).

Few studies have been conducted regarding the distribution, quantity, structure, and function of each opioid receptor type in birds. In an earlier study in pigeons, the regional distribution of μ (mu), κ (kappa), and δ (delta) opioid receptors in the forebrain and midbrain were similar to mammals, but the κ- and δ-opioid receptors were more prominent in the pigeon forebrain and midbrain than μ-opioid receptors and 76% of opioid receptors in the forebrain were determined to be κ-type [95]. These findings, together with earlier studies in opioids in birds, led to a paradigm in which κ-opioid receptor agonists such as butorphanol were considered the drugs of choice for pain management in birds. More recent studies of opioid receptors in chicks [96], pigeons, and cockatiels [97] challenge this paradigm and suggest that μ-opioid receptor agonist drugs might actually be better choices for some avian species when treating pain. The results of recent studies are described in the following paragraphs. Interestingly, when looking at the structure of opioid receptors (μ, κ, and δ) in the peregrine falcon (*Falco peregrinus*), snowy owl (*Bubo scandiacus*), and blue-fronted Amazon parrot (*Amazona aestiva*), nucleotide homologies with humans ranging from 77–82% were found, which might account for some of the differences seen in the efficacy of these drugs [98]. Most importantly, the large variability in pharmacokinetics and pharmacodynamics between species, and in some cases significant age- and sex-dependent variability, has clearly shown that making pharmacologic generalizations across the class Aves, and extrapolating drug doses from one avian species to another must be exercised cautiously [75].

Butorphanol

Butorphanol has been studied in gray parrots and Timneh parrots (*Psittacus erithacus* and *Psittacus timneh*) [89], domestic pigeons [99], red-tailed hawks (*Buteo jamaicensis*) and great horned owls (*Bubo virginianus*) [66], Hispaniolan Amazon parrots (*Amazona ventralis*) [90,100–104], broiler chickens (*Gallus gallus domesticus*) [105,106], Indian peafowl (*Pavo cristatus*) [107], sulphur-crested cockatoos and yellow-crested cockatoos (*Cacatua galerita, Cacatua sulphurea cintrinocristata* and *Cacatua sulphurea sulphurea*) [108], green-cheeked conures (*Pyrrhura molinae*) [101], American kestrels (*Falco sparverius*) [109], and orange-winged Amazon parrots (*Amazona amazonica*) [104]. Most of these studies have evaluated the pharmacokinetics of the standard butorphanol tartrate formulation and some sustained-release formulations, but only a few have evaluated the potential analgesic effects. The pharmacokinetic studies have shown that butorphanol has excellent parenteral and poor oral bioavailability (less than 10%), is quickly absorbed following SC and IM injection, and has a very short half-life (e.g., Hispaniolan Amazon parrots 0.51 h, red-tailed hawks 0.93 h, great horned owls 1.78 h, American kestrels 1.48 h, and chickens 1.19 h), which makes frequent intermittent administration (every 2–3 h) or administration by constant rate infusion (CRI) necessary. Pharmacodynamic studies have shown that relatively high doses are required in psittacines (e.g., 1 mg/kg in gray parrots when assessed using electrical antinociception and 5 mg/kg in Amazon parrots when using thermal antinociception) and are associated with a very short duration of action (between 20 min and 1.5 h) and a relatively small effect; however, studies are lacking to evaluate the effect of different doses.

A study involving gray parrots, white cockatoos (*Cacatua alba*), and blue-fronted Amazon parrots (*Amazona aestiva aestiva*) and using the minimum anesthetic concentration (MAC)-sparing technique to determine the analgesic properties of butorphanol (1 mg/kg IM) resulted in a reduction of isoflurane MAC in cockatoos and gray parrots, but not in the blue-fronted Amazon parrots indicating species variability to either the dose or the drug itself [110]. In white cockatoos, butorphanol significantly reduced isoflurane MAC from 1.44 ± 0.07% to 1.08 ± 0.05% [108,110]. Based upon these studies, doses of 1–5 mg/kg have been recommended in psittacines [111].

In raptors, results of the only pharmacodynamic study of butorphanol have been very different from those in psittacines. In American kestrels, doses of 1, 3, and 6 mg/kg IM had no thermal antinociceptive effects and males showed hyperalgesia at the higher dose [109]. These results discourage the use of butorphanol for analgesia in American kestrels and other birds of the Falco genus; it is unknown if these findings can be extrapolated to other raptors.

Lame broiler chickens receiving butorphanol 2 mg/kg IV finished an obstacle course faster than the control group, and together with the latency-to-lie results reported in the same study, this suggests that butorphanol may be analgesic for up to 2 h [106]. The butorphanol sustained-release formulations used with osmotic pumps, while promising, unfortunately, are not readily available to clinicians and are not frequently used.

Nalbuphine

Nalbuphine has been studied in Hispaniolan Amazon parrots with standard and sustained-release formulations. The pharmacokinetic studies have shown that the standard formulation of nalbuphine hydrochloride has a similar profile as butorphanol, with a slightly shorter half-life. The pharmacodynamic studies using thermal antinociception resulted in significant results at 12.5 mg/kg for up to 3 h, while higher doses of 25 and 50 mg/kg were not different from control [92,112]. A sustained-release formulation of nalbuphine had a longer half-life and duration of effect (up to 12 h) [113], but it is not readily available at this time.

Hydromorphone

Hydromorphone has been studied in American kestrels, cockatiels, and orange-winged Amazon parrots. The pharmacokinetic studies demonstrated that hydromorphone has good parenteral (IM) bioavailability, is quickly absorbed, and has a longer half-life (e.g., 1.26 h in American kestrels [114], 0.99 h in cockatiels [115], and 1.74 h in orange-winged Amazon parrots [116]) than butorphanol in these species, indicating that frequent administration (approximately every 3–6 h) would be required. The analgesiometry studies have shown that relatively high doses are required in psittacines when compared to raptors. In raptors, the studies in American kestrels have shown that hydromorphone at 0.1, 0.3, and 0.6 mg/kg IM had a dose-dependent effect using the thermal antinociception model [117]. In psittacines, in contrast, studies in cockatiels using the same antinociceptive dose as in kestrels showed no significant effect [115]. In orange-winged Amazon parrots, higher doses of hydromorphone at 1 and 2 mg/kg showed thermal antinociception for 3–6 h, respectively [118]. Agitation, nausea-like behavior (including vomiting in one bird), ataxia, and pupillary constriction were observed following administration of the 1 and 2 mg/kg hydromorphone doses which suggest that lower doses be used in this species.

Morphine

Morphine has been evaluated in multiple studies involving chickens (*Gallus gallus domesticus*). The only pharmacokinetic study has followed IV administration of 2 mg/kg IV and resulted in a half-life of 68 min, with a large volume of distribution and rapid clearance [119]. Pharmacodynamic results from earlier studies have been conflicting and difficult to interpret likely due to the high doses evaluated, but more recent studies suggest that morphine might have analgesic and MAC-sparing effects in avian species. In an early study, 200 mg/kg of morphine was injected to suppress nociception in chicks using the toe pinch test [120], but in a later study using noxious electrical stimulation, morphine produced analgesia in chicks at 30 mg/kg [121]. Further investigations using noxious thermal stimulation reported strain-dependent analgesic effects of morphine, requiring doses of 15, 30, and 100 mg/kg for two different White Leghorn lines and a cross of Rhode Island Red × Light Sussex, respectively [122]; analgesic and hyperalgesic effects were reported with a 30 mg/kg dose in the Rhode Island Red cross, and White Leghorn and Cal White strains, respectively [123]. In a MAC reduction study in chickens, three doses of morphine injected IV caused a dose-dependent decrease in isoflurane MAC in all birds. The baseline isoflurane MAC of 1.24 ± 0.05% was reduced 15.1 ± 2.7%, 39.7 ± 3.1%, and 52.4 ± 4.0% at doses of 0.1, 1.0, and 3.0 mg/kg, respectively [124]. In a recent study evaluating the analgesic efficacy of morphine, lame broiler chickens underwent an obstacle course and latency-to-lie test before and at 30 min and 2 h after injection of 2 mg/kg IV of morphine to assess their walking and standing abilities [106]. Morphine treatment caused sedation even in the sound chickens and resulted in an increased time to finish the obstacle course as the chicks tended to sit down rather than walk thereby confounding assessment of its analgesic effects [106].

Fentanyl

Fentanyl has been evaluated in white cockatoos [125], red-tailed hawks [75,126], helmeted guineafowl (*Numida meleagris*) [127], chickens [128,129], and Hispaniolan Amazon parrots [75,130]. The pharmacokinetic studies have shown significant differences in the half-life, ranging from 30–90 min, a fact that discourages extrapolating drug doses between avian species. In chickens, 25 μg/h transdermal fentanyl patches have a large variability in plasma concentrations, but all chickens reached the human target plasma concentrations of 0.2–1.2 ng/mL within 2–4 h and maintained concentrations above that target for 72 h with a rapid decrease in plasma concentrations following removal of the patch [129]. The transdermal veterinary formulation evaluated in helmeted guineafowl was discontinued [127]. Pharmacodynamic studies have shown that significantly higher fentanyl doses or rates of infusion are needed to achieve desired analgesic or MAC-sparing effects in psittacines as compared to other species. However, adverse effects occur at these higher doses or rates, such as agitation in awake white cockatoos receiving 0.2 mg/kg IM [125], or dose-dependent decreases in heart rate and blood pressure in anesthetized Hispaniolan Amazon parrots [130].

In raptors, the findings have been very different, and the rates required to achieve the same MAC-sparing effects have been 17 times lower than in psittacines, and without any significant negative effects on heart rate or blood pressure. Rates of 10–30 μg/kg/h IV decreased isoflurane MAC in a dose-dependent manner by 31–55% [126].

Methadone

Methadone has been studied in orange-winged Amazon parrots [118] and chickens [131,132]. The pharmacokinetic studies have shown a longer half-life than other opioid drugs but with differences between species (e.g., orange-winged Amazon parrots 2.3 h, chickens under anesthesia 3 h). The pharmacodynamic study assessing thermal antinociception suggests that relatively high doses are required in orange-winged Amazon parrots with an IM dose of 6 mg/kg, but not 1 or 3 mg/kg, resulting in thermal antinociception. Agitation, ataxia, and nausea-like behavior were observed following administration, and consideration of lower doses for clinical use in this species is warranted. In chickens, isoflurane MAC-sparing effects were documented after IM administration of 6 mg/kg, but not 3 mg/kg, with reductions of 29%, 27%, and 10% noted at 15, 30, and 45 min after methadone administration, respectively [132].

Buprenorphine

Buprenorphine has been studied in gray parrots [89,133], domestic pigeons [99], American kestrels [134–137], red-tailed hawks [138], cockatiels [94], and orange-winged Amazon parrots [Guzman, unpublished data]. The pharmacokinetic studies have been performed with standard, sustained-released, and concentrated formulations. Those studies have shown major differences in the half-life between species (e.g., 1.5 h in American kestrels [135] and 6.23 h in red-tailed hawks [138]). In red-tailed hawks, 0.3 mg/kg and 1.8 mg/kg doses using concentrated buprenorphine resulted in plasma concentrations being maintained above 1 ng/mL for at least 24 and 48 h, respectively [138]. Results of pharmacodynamic studies in psittacines have been discouraging because of the lack of significant effect with electrical and thermal antinociception in the species and doses evaluated (e.g., 0.1 mg/kg IM in gray parrots [89] and 0.6, 1.2, and 1.8 mg/kg IM in cockatiels [94]). Recent unpublished studies have shown a small but significant effect in orange-winged Amazon parrots following 2 mg/kg IM, but not at 1 and 0.1 mg/kg doses [Guzman, unpublished data]. In contrast, pharmacodynamic studies in raptors have shown a longer duration of action than other opioids (e.g., up to 6 to 9 h in American kestrels following 0.6 mg/kg IM [134]) with mild sedation. High doses have been shown to be well tolerated and provide longer analgesic effects with moderate sedation. Sustained-release formulations are commercially available (e.g., Buprenorphine SR-LAB™) and have also been shown to be well tolerated and associated with prolonged effects (e.g., 24 h following 1.8 mg/kg SC in American kestrels), thus minimizing handling and the need for repeated injections [137].

Tramadol

Tramadol has been evaluated in bald eagles (*Haliaeetus leucocephalus*) [139], peafowl (*Pavo cristatus*) [140], red-tailed hawks [141], Hispaniolan Amazon parrots [142–145], American kestrels [146], African penguins (*Spheniscus demersus*) [147], and Muscovy ducks (*Cairina moschata domestica*) [148]. Tramadol half-life varies significantly between avian species (e.g., red-tailed hawks 1.3 h versus African penguins 7.3 h). In those species for which pharmacokinetics studies have been published, the primary active metabolite *O*-desmethyltramadol (M_1) has also been measured and at concentrations that would be analgesic in other species; in most cases, it also has a longer half-life than the parent drug. As there are large differences in oral bioavailability between species, such as 24% in Hispaniolan Amazon parrots [144] and almost 98% in bald eagles [139], pharmacokinetic realities must be taken into consideration when extrapolating doses between studies and routes of administration. Following oral administration, pharmacodynamic studies of psittacine and raptor species have shown large differences in the doses required for thermal antinociception, which could be explained by differences in pharmacokinetics alone. For example, Hispaniolan Amazon parrots showed thermal antinociception at 30 mg/kg PO and 5 mg/kg IV [144], but not at 10 or 20 mg/kg PO [145]. On the other hand, American kestrels treated with 5 mg/kg PO had significant antinociception while higher doses of 15 and 30 mg/kg PO resulted in a shorter duration of action and gastrointestinal adverse effects in a few birds [146]. No sedation or agitation was seen in these psittacine and raptor studies. In Muscovy ducks, 30 mg/kg PO effectively improved a number of pain-associated variables in a temporary intertarsal joint arthritis model as assessed by ground-reactive forces measured by a pressure-sensitive walkway system [148].

Non-steroidal anti-inflammatory drugs

Over the past two decades the advances in avian pharmacology, especially pharmacokinetics and pharmacodynamics, have been impressive. Studies of analgesics have provided insights as to which drugs in which species are efficacious, and which drugs are ineffective or potentially toxic. This reality is especially true of non-steroidal anti-inflammatory drugs (NSAIDs). To present a laundry list of NSAIDs and their doses would detract from the central message of this section which is that NSAIDs can be effective analgesics in birds, but they have potential for toxicity. This spectrum of activity varies with the drug, the dose, and the avian species in question. The following provides a historical perspective of NSAIDs and discusses a few select drugs that highlight the challenges inherent to their use in birds.

A 2004 report in *Nature* documented that > 95% of old-world vultures (Gyps *spp.*) died in India, Nepal, and Pakistan as a result of consuming carcasses of animals dosed with the veterinary drug diclofenac, an NSAID [149–151]. Cows are sacred in India and Hindu religion, and they often die naturally rather than being slaughtered for meat; open disposal of livestock carcasses is the norm. Scavengers, including vultures which are considered nature's most successful scavengers and provide an array of ecological, economic, and cultural services [150], have year-round widespread access to carrion. Studies of the vulture deaths subsequently documented that the carcasses contained high levels of diclofenac and other NSAID residues [151] that cause renal failure in birds. NSAID toxicity has been reported for raptors, storks, cranes, and owls, suggesting that the potential conservation impact of NSAIDs may extend beyond Gyps vultures and could be significant for New World vultures [152]. However, there are no reported mortalities for the NSAID meloxicam, which has been administered to over 700 birds from 60 species, a finding that supports other studies indicating the suitability of this NSAID to replace diclofenac in Asia [152].

Meloxicam

Meloxicam, the most frequently used NSAID in birds, has a highly variable elimination half-life among avian species when administered orally or intravenously (Tables 58.1 and 58.2) [82,85,153,154].

Table 58.1 Pharmacokinetic parameters of a single dose of meloxicam administered orally to a variety of avian species.

Group and species	C_{max} (μg/mL)	T_{max} (h)	$t_{1/2el}$ (h)	$AUC_{0\text{–last}}$ (μg·h/mL)	$AUC_{0\text{–}\infty}$ (μg·h/mL)	Oral bioavailability (%)	Reference
Psittacines							
Hispaniolan Amazon parrots (*n* = 8; 1 mg/kg)	3.7 ± 1.1	5.0 ± 3.2	15.8 ± 8.6	102	113 ± 71	49 to 75 (range)	[155]
Gray parrots (*n* = 6; 1 mg/kg)	4.69 ± 0.75	13.2 ± 3.5	33.3 ± 3.1	81.0 (SE 5.73)	97.3	38.1 ± 3.6	[156]
Cockatiels (*n* = 24; 1 mg/kg)	0.102 (0.019)[a]	1.27 (17.32)[a]	0.90 (32.34)[a]	–	0.295 (0.019)[a]	11	[82]
Raptors							
Great horned owls (*n* = 5; 0.5 mg/kg)	0.36 ± 0.08	7.8 ± 4.2	5.07 ± 4.5	–	–	62 ± 0.15	[157]
Red-tailed hawks (*n* = 5; 0.5 mg/kg)	0.18 ± 0.16	0.73 ± 0.23	3.97 ± 3.32	–	–	74 ± 0.48	[157]
Poultry							
White Leghorn (*n* = 8; 1 mg/kg)	7.21 ± 3.29	2.0 ± 0.92	2.79 ± 1.01	–	37.92 ± 6.91	–	[158]
Wyandotte (*n* = 8; 1 mg/kg)	6.25 ± 1.53	3.25 ± 2.12	5.53 ± 1.37	–	61.84 ± 14.92	–	[158]
Bilgorajska geese (*n* = 8; 0.5 mg/kg)	5.19 ± 1.25	2 (1-4)	3.65 ± 1.74	–	38.1 ± 20.0	64.2 ± 24.0	[159]
Other							
African penguins (*n* = 8; 1 mg/kg)	10.8[b] (7.06–21.98)	12.0[b] (8.0–24.0)	28.6[b] (25.4–60.6)	432.3[b] (345.5–763.7)	520.7[b] (354.1–856.7)	–	[160]
American flamingos (*n* = 14; 1.0 mg/kg)	1.00 ± 0.88	1.33 ± 1.32	3.83 ± 2.64	–	2.54 ± 1.48	–	[161]
Caribbean flamingos (*n* = 5; 3 mg/kg)	1.52[b] (0.84–2.38)	3.0[b] (1.0–4.0)	1.85[b] (0.90–3.24)	–		–	[162]
Brown pelicans (*n* = 6; 0.2 mg/kg)	1.22 (SE 0.25)	24	36.3[c]	81.0 (SE 5.73)		44.7	[163]

All data are mean ± SD unless otherwise indicated.

[a] Population pharmacokinetic study using a sparse sampling protocol; fixed effect parameter; no measurement of individual variability.

[b] Data are median (min–max).

[c] Longest elimination half-life reported to date in any avian species.

C_{max}, maximum concentration; T_{max}, time to maximum concentration; $t_{1/2\ el}$, elimination half-life; AUC, area under the curve.

Table 58.2 Pharmacokinetic parameters of meloxicam in plasma after intravenous administration of 0.5 mg/kg in ostriches, ducks, turkeys, pigeons, and chickens (n = 6), and 1 mg/kg in Hispaniolan Amazon parrots (n = 11) and gray parrots (n = 6).

Parameter	Ostriches	Ducks	Turkeys	Pigeons	Chickens	Hispaniolan Amazon parrots	Gray parrots
AUC (mg·h/L)	0.73 ± 0.18	8.38 ± 1.32	9.40 ± 1.60	18.35 ± 9.84	40.79 ± 5.87	0.104 ± 0.054	0.024 ± 0.002
Cl (L/h·kg)	0.72 ± 0.2	0.06 ± 0.010	0.05 ± 0.011	0.03 ± 0.030	0.01 ± 0.002	0.012 ± 0.014	0.002
$V_{d(area)}$ (L/kg)	0.58 ± 0.19	0.06 ± 0.017	0.07 ± 0.015	0.14 ± 0.10	0.05 ± 0.005	0.232 ± 0.22	0.091 ± 0.004
$t_{1/2\ el}$ (h)	0.5	0.72	0.99	2.40	3.21	15.9	31.4
k_{el}	6.09 ± 4.58	1.62 ± 0.61	1.45 ± 0.79	0.29 ± 0.10	0.22 ± 0.04	–	–
MRT (h)	0.41 ± 0.25	0.77 ± 0.20	1.47 ± 0.27	3.89 ± 1.49	4.41 ± 0.84	–	49.9 ± 5.7

Data are mean ± SD.
AUC, area under the curve; *Cl*, clearance; V_d, volume of distribution; $t_{1/2\ el}$, elimination half-life (harmonic mean); k_{el}, elimination constant; MRT, mean resident time.
Source: Adapted from Baert and De Backer [85] (ostriches, ducks, turkeys, pigeons, chickens), Molter *et al.* [155] (Hispaniolan Amazon parrots), and Montesinos *et al.* [156] (gray parrots).

For example, the elimination half-life ($t_{1/2el}$) after oral administration of meloxicam (1 mg/kg) ranges from a low of 3.83 h in American flamingos to a high of 36.3 h in brown pelicans [155–157,160,163]. The clearance (in L/kg/h) of meloxicam can also vary significantly within the same species. For example, IV administration to three different age groups of emus yielded significantly faster clearance in emu chicks (1.32 L/kg/h) compared to adults (0.387 L/kg/h) [164]. Thus, from species to species and within species, there are clinically significant variations in meloxicam metabolism and elimination. As previously stated, this large variability in pharmacokinetics and pharmacodynamics from one avian species to another, and even significant age- and sex-dependent variability, show that making pharmacologic generalizations across the class Aves must be exercised cautiously [75].

The renal and analgesic effects of meloxicam have been evaluated in gray and Hispaniolan Amazon parrots [165,166]. In gray parrots, no significant differences were found between hematologic and plasma biochemical values before and after 14 days of treatment with meloxicam (0.5 mg/kg IM every 12 h); renal lesions were absent in 9 of 10 representative post-treatment biopsy samples [165]. In another study involving gray parrots, the pharmacokinetic and long-term renal effects of meloxicam were assessed via several treatment regimens: 1 mg/kg IM every 24 h for 7 days; 1 mg/kg PO every 24 h for 12 days; and 1.6 mg/kg IM every 24 h for 7 days. Meloxicam plasma concentrations were maintained at values greater than effective analgesic concentrations described for other avian species and no adverse clinical renal effects were detected in this population [166]. However, the authors expressed concern about the clinical relevance of plasma drug accumulation and stated that this issue needs further investigation to assess the safety of prolonged treatment with meloxicam in gray parrots and other avian species [166].

In gray parrots, the pharmacokinetics of meloxicam (1 mg/kg) were determined following single IV, IM, and PO administrations [156]. Oral administration resulted in slower absorption (T_{max} of 13.2 ± 3.5 h, and C_{max} of 4.69 ± 0.75 µg/mL), and lower bioavailability (38.1 ± 3.6%) compared to the IM route (78.4 ± 5.5%) [156]. At 24 h, plasma concentrations following IV, IM, and PO administrations were higher than those reported for Hispaniolan Amazon parrots at 12 h with predicted analgesic effects [156].

Hispaniolan parrots with experimentally induced arthritis had significantly better return to baseline weight bearing on the arthritic pelvic limb when treated with meloxicam (1 mg/kg IM) than control parrots or parrots treated with lower doses of meloxicam. All fecal samples collected from the parrots following induction of arthritis and treatment with meloxicam were negative for occult blood [91].

A pharmacokinetic study in Hispaniolan Amazon parrots administered meloxicam (1 mg/kg IV, IM, and PO) resulted in mean plasma concentrations of 3.7 ± 2.5 µg/mL following IV administration and 3.5 ± 2.2 µg/mL following IM administration [155]. Six hours after oral administration, the peak mean plasma concentration was 3.5 ± 1.2 µg/mL. The authors speculated that a mean plasma concentration of 3.5 µg/mL would provide analgesia in Hispaniolan Amazon parrots, but the individual variation that was observed may result in some birds having low plasma meloxicam concentrations after IV, IM, or oral administration [155].

Carprofen

Much of the literature concerning carprofen describes its positive analgesic effects in poultry with husbandry-associated painful conditions [167–171] or experimentally induced arthritis [172,173].

A few articles have described its effects in non-poultry species. In Hispaniolan parrots with microcrystalline sodium urate-induced arthritis, carprofen by itself did not provide effective analgesia [174]. Pigeons administered carprofen at 2, 5, or 10 mg/kg IM once daily for 7 days had increased aspartate aminotransferase and alanine aminotransferase enzyme concentrations, gross lesions in muscle injection sites and liver, and histologic lesions in liver and muscle [175]. The results of a survey of veterinarians and zoos documented the outcomes of NSAID treatments of over 870 scavenging birds from 79 species; carprofen was associated with 13% mortality of treated birds [152].

Grapiprant

Grapiprant is classified as a prostaglandin-E_2 receptor antagonist that does not inhibit COX enzymes and is approved for use in dogs [154,176]. The pharmacokinetics of grapiprant have been determined in fasted and fed red-tailed hawks [154,177]. In fasted birds treated with grapiprant (30 mg/kg PO, and advanced to the crop), plasma grapiprant concentrations were > 164 ng/mL, which is a level considered to be therapeutic in dogs with osteoarthritis [154]. Adverse effects included some regurgitation during the initial phase of the study to determine an effective dose for grapiprant, but no regurgitation during the single-dose phase of the study. Food consumption was reduced in five of the six red-tailed hawks over the course of the study and was managed by force-feeding the hawks. In a follow-up study of the hawks when the drug was administered orally with food, plasma grapiprant mean C_{max}

was 88% lower and median T_{max} was 16 h, about eight times longer than when the hawks were fasted [177]. The analgesic effects of grapiprant have not yet been determined in birds.

Local anesthetics

In the past, local anesthetics used in avian species, especially in small birds, had unfortunate consequences including seizures and cardiac arrest due to the use of high doses [77,178]. For example, 0.1 mL of 2% lidocaine administered intramuscularly or subcutaneously to a 30 g parakeet is equivalent to 67 mg/kg, a toxic dose in any animal. More recent studies of lidocaine and bupivacaine indicate that these drugs can be used safely and effectively in birds, even at doses higher than previously thought to be safe [179]. For example, in a study in which bupivacaine was administered IV to isoflurane-anesthetized chickens, the median effective dose (ED_{50}) of 1.96 mg/kg was associated with a 50% probability of causing clinically relevant cardiovascular effects, defined as ≥ 30% change in heart rate or mean arterial pressure [180].

Lidocaine and bupivacaine have been assessed for their efficacy in producing brachial plexus blockade. In chickens, lidocaine (20 mg/kg), or bupivacaine (5 mg/kg), both with epinephrine, were injected after nerve stimulator localization of the brachial plexus; only 66% of 18 blocks produced sensory blockade [181]. In isoflurane-anesthetized female mallard ducks (*Anas platyrhynchos*), axillary and dorsal approaches to the brachial plexus were evaluated after either bupivacaine (2 or 8 mg/kg), or a combination of lidocaine (15 mg/kg) and epinephrine (3.8 μg/kg) were injected around the brachial plexus following nerve stimulator localization [182]. Blockade was assessed using electrodiagnostic methods and by monitoring birds for the presence of wing droop and change in motor function on recovery from anesthesia. Results were highly variable for all techniques. No technique significantly affected electrodiagnostic results or produced consistent wing droop [182]. Brachial plexus blockade using either a palpation-guided technique or an ultrasound-guided technique and administering lidocaine (2 mg/kg) in a total volume of 0.3 mL, was attempted in isoflurane-anesthetized Hispaniolan Amazon parrots, but neither technique produced an effective block at the lidocaine doses used [183]. Although the brachial plexus blockades of these three reports were unsuccessful, none of the birds had adverse effects attributable to the local anesthetic drug doses.

Lidocaine (8 mg total dose) was used to provide additional analgesia to an isoflurane-anesthetized mallard duck (*Anas platyrhynchos*) undergoing surgical repair of a pelvic limb fracture. Using both ultrasound and nerve stimulator localization techniques, lidocaine was injected around the femoral nerve (0.4 mL, 2% solution) when extension of the stifle was observed, and around the sciatic nerve (0.3 mL, 2% solution) when flexion of the stifle was elicited [184]. No adverse drug effects were reported.

Bupivacaine doses as high as 10 mg/kg were used in a field study involving implantation of satellite transmitters in male and female free-ranging spectacled eiders (*Somateria fischeri*), king eiders (*Somateria spectabilis*), and common eiders (*Somateria mollissima*), where all received propofol, bupivacaine, and postoperative ketoprofen for analgesia [185]. None of the female spectacled or common eiders, and only 1 of the 5 female king eiders died during the postoperative period, but 4 of 10 male spectacled eiders and 5 of 6 male king eiders died within 1–4 days after surgery [185]. Based on histopathologic findings, the authors reported that the perioperative use of ketoprofen caused lethal renal damage in the male eiders, and that bupivacaine did not cause the deaths [185].

Spinal anesthesia with lidocaine or bupivacaine has been reported in chickens [186,187]. An anatomic study identified the space between the synsacrum and first free coccygeal vertebra (synsacrococcygeal space) as the most suitable site for spinal injection. At this location, the dura mater adheres to the internal wall of the spinal canal and the subarachnoid space is large, so injections at this site are into the subarachnoid space, not the epidural space [186]. Subarachnoid injections of lidocaine (0.5, 1, or 2 mg/kg) resulted in analgesia that was similar for all doses; the authors deemed this a feasible, practical, inexpensive, and simple technique for pericloacal regional anesthesia [186]. A subsequent study reported the spinal effects of lidocaine (2 mg/kg) and bupivacaine (0.1, 0.25, and 0.5 mg/kg) with both drugs administered using the loss of resistance technique. The highest dose of bupivacaine (0.5 mg/kg) had a slower onset of action (3.33 ± 1.23 min) compared to lidocaine (1.37 ± 0.52 min) and resulted in a longer duration of spinal anesthesia (54 ± 6.08 min) compared to that provided by lidocaine (17.87 ± 3.18 min) [187].

Although local anesthetics may provide sufficient local analgesia in birds, they do not relieve the stress associated with physical restraint of an awake bird. In all of the studies cited above, all birds were sedated prior to general and local anesthesia.

Injectable induction drugs

Propofol

Propofol has been used clinically in a variety of avian species including a barn owl [188], domestic pigeons [189], red-tailed hawks and great horned owls [190], Hispaniolan parrots [191], mallard and canvasback ducks [192,193], eiders [185], mute swans [194], chickens [195,196], wild turkeys [197], rheas [198], a king penguin undergoing magnetic resonance imaging [199], and in field research involving bar-tailed godwits and bristle-thigh curlews [200]. These studies demonstrate that propofol can be a useful injectable anesthetic, but with two important caveats: it is devoid of antinociceptive properties so it cannot be used as the sole anesthetic for painful procedures and must be used with appropriate analgesic drugs and techniques, either pre-, intra-, or postoperatively. It can produce apnea of sufficient duration as to cause death so being prepared to intubate and assist ventilation is a requirement and, when possible, providing oxygen-enriched inspired gas is strongly encouraged. In a pharmacokinetic study of propofol in great horned owls, the induction dose was lower than typically used for dogs, pigs, rats, and rabbits, a finding explained by the lower volume of the central compartment [190]. In an orthopedic research project, the propofol-sparing effects of methadone, fentanyl, or nalbuphine were investigated in domestic chickens undergoing ulnar osteotomy [196]. Methadone and nalbuphine, but not fentanyl, significantly decreased the propofol infusion rate required to maintain anesthesia [196].

Alfaxalone

Alfaxalone (Alfaxan®), a neuroactive steroid anesthetic with activity at γ-aminobutyric acid (GABA) receptors, is a re-formulation of alfaxalone and alfadolone, a drug combination released as Saffan in 1970 for veterinary use. The solubilizing agent in that drug combination was polyethylated castor oil which accounted for its adverse effects in mammals and birds, including cardiac arrhythmias and allergic reactions, that subsequently led to its withdrawal from the market. Alfaxalone, the new formulation, is water soluble and available as an injectable solution that can be administered IV, IM, or SC in birds, and produces dose-dependent immobilization without analgesia [63]. It has been used in parakeets [201–203], Quaker parrots (*Myiopsitta monachus*) [204], black-cheeked lovebirds (*Agapornis nigrigenis*) [205], chickens [206,207], peafowl [208], ducks [209], mute swans (*Cygnus olor*) [210], and common buzzards (*Buteo buteo*) [211]. When used alone it can have a rapid onset of action, a short duration of effect, and produce variable degrees of hyperactivity during induction and recovery.

Alfaxalone has been administered IM to parakeets at doses ranging from 5 to 20 mg/kg. Sedation without and with recumbency was achieved with 5 mg/kg and 10 mg/kg doses, respectively [202]. In one study, the sedative effects of alfaxalone (15 mg/kg IM) were compared to those of butorphanol–midazolam [201] and alfaxalone produced a shorter but more consistent duration of sedation (28 ± 6 min) than butorphanol–midazolam (72 ± 57 min) [201]. In another study, 15 mg/kg produced mild to moderate sedation while 20 mg/kg produced moderate to profound sedation; both doses caused statistically significant but clinically mild cardiorespiratory effects and a significant decrease in body temperature [203].

A majority of black-cheeked lovebirds administered only alfaxalone (12.6 ± 0.9 mg/kg SC) had rough inductions and recoveries, effects the authors believed could have been minimized if the birds had been placed in a more confined space [205]. The authors further stated that alfaxalone provided nearly 1 h of stable, non-analgesic sedation appropriate for non-invasive procedures in this species [205]. Hyperexcitement and muscle tremors also occurred in Quaker parrots when alfaxalone (10 or 25 mg/kg IM) was administered as the sole sedative agent, and these effects were attenuated by combining alfaxalone (10 mg/kg IM) with midazolam (1 mg/kg IM) [204].

In chickens, alfaxalone administered IV for anesthesia was associated with hyperactivity during induction and recovery [206,212], effects that may be lessened by premedicating with butorphanol–midazolam [212] or ketamine or xylazine [207]. In an LD_{50} intraperitoneal injection model involving chicks, the ED_{50} of alfaxalone was 32.9 mg/kg and the LD_{50} was 102.4 mg/kg; the ED_{50} was decreased by combining alfaxalone with ketamine or xylazine [207].

Alfaxalone in mute swans [210] and buzzards [211] has been described as producing acceptable sedation or anesthesia with a few notable caveats. In the swan study, the anesthetic effects of alfaxalone were compared to those of ketamine–xylazine, and a greater incidence of postinduction apnea and a higher incidence of agitation on recovery were reported with alfaxalone compared to ketamine–xylazine [210]. In the buzzard study, alfaxalone produced good to excellent anesthesia characterized by rapid induction of anesthesia, excellent muscle relaxation, unresponsiveness to noxious stimuli, and smooth, uneventful recovery. Hypoventilation and apnea were uncommon at clinically relevant doses but became important adverse effects when larger doses were administered rapidly IV [211].

In peafowl [208] and mallard ducks [209], alfaxalone when used alone did not produce acceptable anesthesia. Whether this is a dose issue or species issue remains to be determined.

Inhalant anesthetics

Inhalant anesthetics possess several advantages for patient management, including rapid induction and recovery of anesthesia, more precise control of anesthetic depth, concurrent provision of oxygen for respiratory support, and recovery that is not dependent on metabolic or excretory pathways. A disadvantage is the need for special equipment such as a source of oxygen, a vaporizer, a breathing circuit, and a mechanism for scavenging waste anesthetic gases. Currently, isoflurane and sevoflurane are considered the inhalant anesthetics of choice for use in birds, with the latter providing faster induction and recovery times [213–215]. In bald eagles, isoflurane administration resulted in tachycardia, hypertension, and more arrhythmias compared with sevoflurane [213]. In red-tailed hawks, isoflurane significantly depressed spontaneous ventilation compared to hawks anesthetized with sevoflurane [214]. Cardiopulmonary differences between isoflurane and sevoflurane have not been fully evaluated in psittacine birds. Desflurane has been used in birds, but less so than isoflurane or sevoflurane. Sevoflurane has a less pungent odor than isoflurane and is generally better tolerated during mask induction, but it is more expensive than isoflurane.

Minimum anesthetic concentration

The concepts guiding our use of inhalant anesthetics are as applicable to birds as they are to mammals. One such concept is the minimum alveolar concentration (MAC) of an inhalant anesthetic that prevents gross purposeful movement in 50% of anesthetized mammals exposed to a maximal noxious stimulus. MAC provides a description of concentration and effect across a wide range of animal species, allows us to quantify factors which influence anesthetic requirements, and is equally applicable to all inhalation anesthetics [216]. The term, as defined, is not appropriate in discussions concerning birds because they do not have an alveolar lung. For birds, "MAC" has been defined as the "minimum anesthetic concentration" required to prevent gross purposeful movement in response to a painful stimulus [217], and it is usually determined via a bracketing technique.

MAC values of halothane, isoflurane, and sevoflurane in birds are shown in Table 58.3 and are similar to MAC values reported for

Table 58.3 Minimum anesthetic concentration (MAC) for halothane, isoflurane, and sevoflurane in birds.

Species	Halothane	Isoflurane	Sevoflurane
Amazon parrot (*Amazona aestiva*)	–	–	2.4% [220]
Blue-fronted Amazon parrot (*Amazona aestiva aestiva*)	–	1.46% [110]	–
Cockatoos (Cacatua *spp.*)	–	1.44% [108]	–
Hispaniolan Amazon parrot (*Amazona ventralis*)	–	2.09% [130]	–
Thick-billed parrot (*Rhynchopsitta pachyrhyncha*)	–	1.07% [221]	2.39–3.94%[a] [222]
White-eyed parakeet (*Psittacara leucophthalmus*)	–	2.47%[a] [223]	–
Quaker parrot (*Myiopsitta monachus*)	–	2.52%[a]224]	–
Chicken (*Gallus gallus*)	0.85% [225]	1.25% [226] 1.1% [132]	2.21% [227]
Cinereous vulture (*Aegypius monachus*)	–	1.06% [228]	–
Crested serpent eagle (*Spilornis cheela hoya*)	–	1.46% [215]	2.03% [215]
Red-tailed hawk (*Buteo jamaicensis*)	–	2.05% [126]	–
Duck (*Anas platyrhynchos*)	1.05% [229]	1.32% [230]	–
Guineafowl (*Numida meleagris*)	–	–	2.90% [231]
Rock pigeon (*Columba livia*)	–	–	3.0% [232]
Sandhill crane (*Grus canadensis*)	–	1.35% [217]	–

[a] MAC determined using a cross-over design.

mammals [218,219]. This lends support to the observation that different classes or species of animals do not show large variations in effective concentrations of inhalant anesthetics [216].

Hypoventilation makes it difficult to control the plane of anesthesia, and it can have a variety of adverse effects on cardiac function. For example, unifocal and multifocal cardiac arrhythmias occurred in 50% of ducks anesthetized and maintained at a constant end-tidal halothane concentration of 1.5%, and in which $PaCO_2$ was varied from 40 to 80 mm Hg through addition of CO_2 to the inspired oxygen [233]. The mean $PaCO_2$ at which arrhythmias developed was 67 ± 12 mm Hg; in five of six ducks, the arrhythmias disappeared after CO_2 inhalation was terminated [233]. To avoid the adverse effects of hypercarbia on cardiac function in anesthetized birds, ventilation should be supported by maintaining a light plane of anesthesia and, when possible, by assisting or controlling ventilation.

Adjuncts to general anesthesia

Nitrous oxide

Nitrous oxide can be used as an adjunct to general anesthesia but is not suitable as the sole anesthetic [234]. Nitrous oxide (50%) may decrease the concentration of isoflurane necessary to maintain a suitable plane of anesthesia by only 11% [235]. As with other anesthetic gases and vapors, nitrous oxide is not uniquely sequestered or concentrated in the air sacs. The considerations for using nitrous oxide are the same as for its use in mammals, such as adequate pulmonary function and delivery of sufficient oxygen to meet the patient's metabolic demands. Thirty percent oxygen is generally accepted as the minimum fraction of inspired oxygen that should be provided. Nitrous oxide may pose problems in some birds with normal subcutaneous air pockets [236]. For example, pelicans have subcutaneous pockets of air that do not communicate with the respiratory system and the use of N_2O in these birds can result in subcutaneous emphysema [237].

Neuromuscular blocking drugs

Neuromuscular paralytic drugs have two purposes in birds: whole-body skeletal muscle paralysis to facilitate surgical procedures, and to produce mydriasis. The neuromuscular and cardiovascular effects of atracurium used as a muscle paralytic, have been reported in chickens [238]. The effective dose associated with 95% twitch depression in 50% of the birds ($ED_{95/50}$) was 0.25 mg/kg IV, and the $ED_{95/95}$ was calculated by probit analysis to be 0.46 mg/kg IV. The duration of action for the 0.25 mg/kg and 0.45 mg/kg doses was 34.5 ± 5.8 and 47.8 ± 10.3 min, respectively, and these durations are similar to those reported in dogs [239,240]. Edrophonium (0.5 mg/kg IV) reversed muscle paralysis. There were small but statistically significant changes in cardiovascular variables (i.e., heart rate decreased, and blood pressure increased) after administering atracurium, but these changes were considered clinically unimportant [238].

Avian pupillary diameter is controlled primarily by skeletal muscles and neuromuscular blocking drugs may be applied topically to produce mydriasis with two notable exceptions, alcuronium and pancuronium, which do not produce safe or consistently effective mydriasis in some species [241]. In adult cockatoos (*Cacatua sulphurea*), gray parrots (*Psittacus erithacus*), and blue-fronted Amazon parrots (*Amazona aestivate*), vecuronium (injectable formulation; 0.8 mg/mL) alone and diluted in sterile sodium chloride solution (0.9% NaCl), consistently produced the greatest pupillary dilation, and did so with few systemic side effects with one notable exception – a cockatoo collapsed and died soon after a combination of vecuronium and saponin (a surface-acting penetrating agent) was topically applied to its eye [242]. This suggests that vecuronium administered topically as a mydriatic should not be combined with an agent that promotes corneal penetration, as enhanced systemic uptake may have potentially fatal effects. It also reinforces the reality that avian species differ significantly in their responses to any given drug. For neuromuscular blocking drugs, a contributing factor may be the tremendous variation in acetylcholinesterase levels from one avian species to another: from 0.87 μmol of substrate hydrolyzed/min/mL in cormorants to 7.89 μmol of substrate hydrolyzed/min/mL in mallard ducks [243].

In juvenile double-crested cormorants (*Phalacrocorax auritus*), vecuronium alone or in combination with atropine and phenylephrine was evaluated as a mydriatic [244]. The drug combination produced the most consistent and greatest dilation and longest average duration; no side effects from vecuronium were observed [244]. However, in a study involving adult double-crested cormorants, vecuronium by itself produced much better dilation than was observed in the juvenile double-crested cormorants [244]. The difference between the juvenile birds and the adults was the very blue irides of the adults compared to the brown irides of the young cormorants; the authors speculated that the ability of melanin to bind drugs may explain the difference in response [244]. Indeed, a study investigating the mydriatic effect of rocuronium in pigeons reported that the iris of birds with grayish brown-colored irides ("bull eye") did not dilate after a single application of rocuronium and only two out of eight did so after a second application [245].

In European kestrels (*Falco tinnunculus*), rocuronium (0.12 mg in each eye) [246], or vecuronium (4 mg/mL; two drops in each eye, three times, at 15-min intervals) [241], effectively produced mydriasis. Rocuronium has been shown to be effective in a number of raptorial species, including common buzzards (*Buteo buteo*; 0.40 mg in each eye), little owls (*Athene noctua*; 0.20 mg in each eye) [247], tawny owls (*Strix aluco*; single topical administration of 0.35 mg in each eye) [248], and scops owls (*Otus scops*; 0.15 mg in each eye) [249]. Rocuronium also significantly decreases intraocular pressure in kestrels and little owls [250].

Rocuronium produces mydriasis in Hispaniolan Amazon parrots (*Amazona ventralis*) [251,252]. In the study by Baine *et al.*, topically applied rocuronium (0.15 mg per eye) rapidly produced mydriasis and had a prolonged duration of action; 24 h after treatment 2 of the 10 birds had superficial corneal ulceration as determined by fluorescein staining [251]. The authors speculated that the low pH of the rocuronium solution could account for the ulceration. In the Petritz *et al.* study, rocuronium (20 μL/eye, 10 mg/mL solution) applied topically produced mydriasis lasting up to 360 min after drug administration with minimal adverse effects noted other than three birds having transient inferior eyelid paresis that resolved within 24 h [252]. Baine speculated that in addition to acidic pH, eyelid paresis could be a contributing causative factor of the corneal ulceration [251].

Drugs of historical interest

In the past, barbiturates, the combination drug Equithesin, and α-chloralose have been used for sedating or anesthetizing birds, sometimes in clinical settings, but more often in research or field situations. Surgical anesthesia can be maintained for relatively long periods of time (1 to 12 h) by using intermediate- to long-acting barbiturates or combinations of drugs with intermediate durations of effect. Pentobarbital, when injected intravenously, requires 10 to 15 min for full onset of action and produces anesthesia lasting several hours [178]. Because of its slow onset of action, the drug should be administered initially as a bolus consisting of half the total dose and the remainder titrated over several minutes until the desired plane of anesthesia is achieved. Phenobarbital is a long-acting barbiturate that produces anesthesia lasting up to 24 h when administered intravenously [178]. Its onset of action is very slow, requiring as much as 30 min before surgical anesthesia is achieved.

Equithesin is a combination of pentobarbital, chloral hydrate, and magnesium sulfate. It does not produce a surgical plane of anesthesia when used alone but produces surgical anesthesia lasting as long as 90 min when combined with diazepam [253].

α-Chloralose, a general depressant and tranquilizer, is used to capture birds in the wild, such as cranes, crows, storks, wild turkeys, and Canada geese. The drug is usually mixed with a bait that is attractive to the birds to be captured. When using corn to capture cranes, each kernel is drilled out and the α-chloralose is packed into the kernel, not sprinkled on top of the corn as the cranes will not eat it. The amount of drug mixed with the bait depends on the avian species to be captured and the number of birds at the bait site that are likely to eat the baited food. For some species, date, time of day, temperature, and humidity must be taken into consideration when planning bait-and-capture sessions [254–256]. Capture myopathy has occurred after α-chloralose baiting and physical capture of sandhill cranes during a banding study [257].

Anesthetic management

Airway management

Intubation may be difficult in species with unique oropharyngeal anatomy, or very small birds. For example, psittacine species, such as budgerigar parakeets (*Melopsittacus undulatus*), can be difficult to intubate because of the difficult-to-visualize location of the glottis at the base of the humped, fleshy tongue [258]. Appropriately sized Cole endotracheal tubes can be used in small birds, and commercially manufactured (Jorgensen Labs®) endotracheal tubes as small as 1.0 mm ID for budgerigars and 1.5 mm ID for lovebirds do exist. Red-rubber catheters can also be cut-to-size and used for intubation. However, compliant tubes < 2 mm ID are often highly flexible and kink easily, so they must be secured properly to prevent occlusion. Intravenous catheters can be used as endotracheal tubes [259] but are a less desirable alternative for intubating and delivering inhalant anesthetics to very small birds because of their lack of flexibility that can cause tracheal trauma. If an IV catheter is used for intubation it must be appropriately sized and secured to the head with the neck extended to prevent injury to the trachea [259].

Another hazard of small-diameter endotracheal tubes is the resistance they impose on gas flow, a hazard that increases when tubes become partially or completely obstructed as a result of mucus accumulation or plugs. Resistance to flow through a tube is inversely proportional to the tube's radius raised to the fourth power. For example, decreasing the radius from 3 to 2 mm or 2 to 1 mm would increase resistance approximately 5 and 15 times, respectively. Mucus production during anesthesia can be copious and the cold, non-humidified fresh gas used to deliver inhalant anesthesia has a drying effect that makes the mucus thick and tenacious. Endotracheal tube obstruction can be detected by observing the bird's pattern of ventilation. As the airway becomes progressively occluded, the expiratory phase becomes prolonged. An artificial sigh of the bird usually confirms the presence of an obstruction because the keel will move and the abdominal wall will expand in a seemingly normal manner, but they will return slowly or not at all to their end-expiratory positions. Airway noises, especially gurgling, may be heard as the tube becomes more obstructed with mucus. Airway obstructions must be corrected quickly either by extubating the bird, cleaning the tube, and re-inserting it, by replacing it with a fresh tube, or by gently suctioning it with a small red-rubber tube. An anticholinergic, such as atropine (0.04 mg/kg) or glycopyrrolate (0.01 mg/kg), administered intramuscularly, may reduce mucus production and lessen the risk of developing mucus plugs, but it may also increase mucus viscosity thus making it harder to clear secretions from the tube.

If a cuffed endotracheal tube is used, the cuff should either not be inflated or must be inflated with extreme caution; in small birds, it is better not to inflate the cuff. Because of the complete cartilaginous tracheal rings, an overly inflated cuff will injure the tracheal mucosa, or rupture the tracheal rings at the site of the cuff; when a cuff is over inflated, the tracheal rings tend to rupture longitudinally rather than circumferentially. On average, intubation-induced tracheal trauma and obstruction becomes evident 16 days post-intubation when the processes of healing and fibrotic narrowing of the trachea cause signs of dyspnea [260].

As mentioned previously, flamingos with their ventroflexed beaks and large fleshy tongues, can be difficult to intubate. One strategy is to reduce the amount of equipment in the mouth during intubation. This can be accomplished by shining a transilluminator light from the outside of the mouth into the oral cavity; a cotton-tipped applicator can be used to bring the tongue forward so as to visualize the laryngeal opening into which the endotracheal tube is inserted [personal communication: Dr. Noha Abou-Madi, Cornell University; November 1, 2012].

The double trachea in jackass penguins (*Spheniscus demersus*) poses a challenge for intubation. One technique for intubating these birds is to use two Cole tubes attached to a double-pronged circuit adapter, the type used for double-lumen endotracheal tubes [personal communication: Dr. Frank Golder; July 2, 2013]. Ostriches can be intubated using endotracheal tubes with internal diameters of 10 to 18 mm, while emus generally require endotracheal tubes measuring 9 to 14 mm [261]. Careful inflation of the cuff is usually necessary to enable effective ventilation of adult ratites. The tracheal cleft in emus does not complicate intubation, but makes effective positive-pressure ventilation difficult, a problem overcome by wrapping a towel snuggly around the middle and distal thirds of the neck [261].

Breathing circuits and fresh gas flows

Nonrebreathing circuits, such as the Bain circuit or Norman elbow, rather than circle breathing circuits, are ideal for use in small birds with small tidal volumes because they do not have to overcome the resistance to ventilation imposed by unidirectional valves. An additional advantage of all-plastic nonrebreathing circuits is their light weight, a desirable feature when used in very small birds. Oxygen flow for a nonrebreathing circuit should be two to three times minute ventilation, or 150 to 200 mL/kg/min. For larger birds, such as ratites, the breathing circuit should be commensurate with the size of the bird. Emus and ostriches weighing less than 130 kg can be maintained on a small animal breathing circuit while larger ostriches can be maintained on a large animal breathing circuit [261].

Induction methods

The number and variety of techniques for inducing gas anesthesia in birds are only limited by the anesthetist's imagination. Birds can be induced with commercially available small animal masks, or with homemade masks fabricated from plastic bottles, syringe cases, syringes, or breathing hose connectors. Mask induction techniques can be used in a wide variety and sizes of birds, from the very small up to and including the emu. Mask inductions are unsatisfactory in adult ostriches [261].

Other techniques include the use of plastic bags or chambers. Birds can be induced by inserting their heads into plastic bags (preferably clear plastic) into which oxygen and anesthetic vapor are introduced via a nonrebreathing circuit. Plastic bags have been used to completely enclose a bird cage in order to induce anesthesia in a difficult-to-manage bird [262].

An anesthetic chamber can be used to induce anesthesia. A disadvantage of this technique is that the anesthetist is not in physical contact with the bird and is unable to get a feel for how the bird is responding to the anesthetic. In addition, birds can injure themselves as they pass through stage 2 (involuntary excitement) anesthesia.

Whatever technique is used, the anesthetist must take precautions to control and eliminate anesthetic gas pollution in the work environment. If a mask is used it should fit snugly over the bird's beak and face, or over its entire head. If a plastic bag or chamber is used, it should be free of leaks. Once induction is completed, the bag or chamber must be removed from the area without the contents being released into the workplace environment.

Monitoring and support

The 2008 Confidential Enquiry into Perioperative Small Animal Fatalities provided some data regarding perianesthetic mortality in birds [3]. In that study, the perianesthetic mortality rate was 3.94 % for parrots which is approximately 20 times higher than rates for dogs and cats. The mortality rate was 16.3% for budgerigars, and 1.76% for "other birds." That study did not provide further information as to what species were included as "other birds," the health status of the patients, anesthetic protocols, or degree of monitoring and support during the procedures. A subsequent study found that 3.4% of birds died during anesthesia [4]. Unfortunately, none of the variables investigated in that study were associated with an increased risk of anesthesia-related death; absent such information makes it difficult to predict which birds might have an anesthesia-related death [4]. A 2021 study defined *anesthesia-related mortality* in birds as those deaths occurring during anesthesia and up to 7 days post anesthesia; by this definition, anesthesia-related mortality was 3.88% [5]. Birds with an abnormal health status had a 15.53-fold increased risk of death compared with those with a normal health status. The duration of anesthesia was a statistically significant risk factor in the univariable analysis, but not when combined with health status [5]. A more recent study looked at avian mortality rate based on ASA physical status [263] and found that patients assigned an ASA status of I and II had a rate of 0% (95% CI 0.0–0.2) and 0.6% (CI 0.2–1.3), respectively, while patients assigned a status of III, IV, and V had rates of 5.9% (CI 4.3–8.0), 18.8% (CI 13.4–25.7), and 50.0% (CI 29.9–70.1), respectively. Investigation into timing of death showed that the majority of patients died following cessation of general anesthesia (81.48%), with a majority of postanesthetic deaths occurring within 3 h of anesthetic recovery.

Avian anesthesia is fraught with challenges, not the least of which is size; it is difficult to obtain preoperative blood work, secure the airway, obtain IV access, and monitor blood pressure in very small patients. Nonetheless, the above-cited studies make a strong case for monitoring birds during and following anesthesia. Physiologic variables to monitor include respiratory rate and tidal volume, oxygenation, expired CO_2, heart rate and rhythm, body temperature, and muscle relaxation.

Central nervous system

Anesthetic depth can be assessed by checking muscle tone and various reflexes. The loss of muscle tone in the legs or wings can denote transition from a light to a medium plane of anesthesia. The withdraw reflex in response to a toe pinch is lost when the bird is in a medium (surgical) plane of anesthesia. Palpebral reflexes are usually lost at a medium plane of anesthesia, but corneal reflexes persist until a deep plane of anesthesia. Heart and respiratory rates increase when birds experience pain, or when the depth of anesthesia is too light; conversely, they may decrease at a deep plane of anesthesia, signaling the need to lighten the plane of anesthesia.

Respiratory system

The gas exchange efficiency of the avian lung is not limited to O_2 and CO_2, but also applies to the exchange of inhalant anesthetics.

The avian lung lacks a significant functional residual volume, a feature that limits how long a bird can remain apneic during anesthesia. This is a concern during induction of anesthesia of birds, especially waterfowl, because apnea and bradycardia can occur and may last for up to five minutes. Although referred to as a "dive response," in diving ducks under experimental conditions it is a stress response mediated by stimulation of trigeminal receptors in the beak and nares [264–267]. Anesthetic gases are not required to elicit this response as it can be triggered by placing a mask snugly over a bird's beak and face. During this stress response, blood flow is preferentially distributed to the kidneys, heart, and brain [268,269]. This stress response makes safe induction of anesthesia challenging and raises the question, would premedicants such as butorphanol or midazolam ameliorate or eliminate the dive response and shorten the time to intubation in birds likely to experience a dive response, such as waterfowl? In non-divers, specifically adult Hispaniolan Amazon parrots (*Amazona ventralis*), butorphanol did not shorten the time between induction with sevoflurane and intubation compared to birds not sedated with butorphanol [100]. Other indicators of stress in birds due to manual restraint include increases in body temperature and respiratory rate. Using those measures of stress, Hispaniolan Amazon parrots sedated with midazolam (2 mg/kg) administered intranasally had a slower rate of rise in cloacal temperature compared to the same birds when administered saline, and mean respiratory rates were significantly lower for up to 12 min [58].

In mammalian species, it is well recognized that anesthetics, through their effects on the central nervous system and peripheral chemoreceptors, significantly depress ventilatory responses to hypoxia and hypercapnia [270–272]. Since birds have many of the same mechanisms for controlling ventilation, one must assume that anesthetics will similarly depress avian ventilatory control mechanisms. Several studies have shown that inhalants depress the responsiveness of a number of peripheral control mechanisms in birds, including intrapulmonary chemoreceptors, that directly or indirectly affect ventilation [273–275].

General anesthesia disrupts ventilatory control mechanisms in birds, thus whenever possible a bird's ventilation should be assisted or controlled so as to minimize or prevent anesthesia-induced hypoventilation. During positive-pressure ventilation, the direction of gas flow within the avian lung may be reversed, but the efficiency of the cross-current and multicapillary serial arterialization system is independent of the direction of air flow relative to blood flow [19]. Studies of mechanically, bi-directionally ventilated birds from which arterial blood samples were collected and analyzed, did not show adverse effects of mechanical ventilation on gas exchange [217,276,277].

Because of the flow-through nature of the avian pulmonary system, it is possible to ventilate birds by flowing a continuous stream of gas through the trachea and lungs, and out through a ruptured or cannulated air sac [217,276–279]. It is also possible to cannulate an abdominal or caudal thoracic air sac and flow inhalant anesthetic through the air sac, across the lung, and out via the trachea. This same technique can be used to induce and maintain anesthesia in birds [269,278,280,281] and offers a unique, effective means by which to maintain anesthesia for procedures that require full, unimpeded access to the head. This technique has been used in birds as small as zebra finches [282]. In one study of ducks in which arterial blood gases were compared before and after cannulation of the clavicular air sac, both PaO_2 and $PaCO_2$ remained unchanged, but tidal volume increased, and minute ventilation doubled [283]. However, a study involving sulphur-crested cockatoos (*Cacatua galerita*) reported that anesthesia could not be maintained in this species when isoflurane was insufflated through the clavicular air sac [280]. This suggests that there may be species differences as to which air sac is best cannulated for delivery of inhalant anesthetics.

Monitoring respiratory rate and tidal volume by visually observing the frequency and degree of motion of the sternum or movements of the breathing circuit reservoir bag, give a general sense of the adequacy of ventilation and the depth of anesthesia. However, assessing the adequacy of ventilation solely on respiratory frequency can be misleading. High respiratory frequencies in an anesthetized bird do not necessarily indicate the bird is light and hyperventilating but are often associated with small tidal volumes and a greater proportion of deadspace ventilation than effective ventilation [217].

In general, halothane, isoflurane, and sevoflurane, in a dose-dependent manner, depress ventilation in birds [217,225,229,230, 284–287]. The anesthetic or apneic index (AI) is a measure of the tendency of an inhalant anesthetic to cause respiratory depression and apnea. It is derived by dividing the end-tidal concentration of an anesthetic at apnea by the MAC for the anesthetic [288]. The lower the AI for an anesthetic, the greater its depressant effect on ventilation. In ducks anesthetized with halothane the AI was 1.51 [229] and for isoflurane it was 1.65 [230], values considerably lower than those reported for dogs (2.5) and cats (2.4) [289], and horses (2.3) [290]. This suggests that isoflurane depresses ventilation more in birds than in mammals. However, in a study of isoflurane in chickens (*Gallus gallus domesticus*), AI was similar to that reported for mammals [291]. Species differences (ducks versus chickens) or differences in how apnea was assessed may account for the differences in results.

Capnography should be used to monitor ventilation in anesthetized birds, while understanding its limitations. In birds, capnography measures the partial pressure of end-expired carbon dioxide (P_ECO_2), not end-tidal carbon dioxide ($P_{ET}CO_2$), and it provides information regarding ventilatory status. Accurate sampling of airway gas may require adjustments in sampling flow rate or technique [292]. In intubated birds during positive-pressure ventilation, there is acceptable correlation between P_ECO_2 and $PaCO_2$, with P_ECO_2 slightly exceeding $PaCO_2$ [292,293]. A P_ECO_2 of 30 to 45 mm Hg indicates adequate ventilation during inhalation anesthesia in most birds and approximates a normal physiologic range of 25 to 40 mmHg for $PaCO_2$ in awake birds. In contrast, during air sac insufflation anesthesia of chickens, P_ECO_2 was not strongly associated with $PaCO_2$ [294]. This latter study also demonstrated that

Table 58.4 Arterial blood gases in birds spontaneously breathing air (F_IO_2 = 21%) unless otherwise indicated.

Species	pHa	$PaCO_2$ (mmHg)	PaO_2 (mmHg)
Chicken – Domestic (Gallus *spp.*)[a]	7.48–7.53	29–33	82
Duck – Mallard (*Anas platyrhynchos*)[a]	7.56	31	81
Duck – Muscovy (*Cairina moschata*)[a]	7.46–7.49	37–38	82–96
Duck – Pekin (*Anas platyrhynchos*)[a]	7.46–7.48	28–34	94–100
Duck – Pekin (*Anas platyrhynchos*)[b]	7.40	40	84
Emu (*Dromaius novaehollandiae*)[a]	7.45	34	100
Falcon – Gyrfalcon (*Falco rusticolus*)[b]	7.42	37	204
Goose – Bar-headed (*Anser indicus*)[a]	7.47	32	93
Goose – Domestic (*Anser anser*)[a]	7.52	32	97
Hawk – Red-tailed (*Buteo jamaicensis*)[a]	7.49	27	108
Owl – Burrowing (*Athene cunicularia*)[a]	7.46	33	98
Parrot – Amazon (*Amazona aestiva*)[c]	7.43–7.46	22	96–100
Penguin – Adelie (*Pygoscelis adeliae*)[a]	7.51	37	84
Penguin – Chinstrap (*Pygoscelis antarctica*)[a]	7.52	37	89
Penguin – Gentoo (*Pygoscelis papua*)[a]	7.49	41	77
Pigeon (*Columba livia*)[a]	7.50	30	95
Swan – Mute (*Cygnus olor*)[a]	7.5	27	91

[a] Not anesthetized; data derived from Powell [22] (various species).
[b] Anesthetized; data derived from Rode *et al.* [283] (duck) and Raghav *et al.* [295] (gyrfalcon; F_IO_2 > 95%).
[c] Not anesthetized; data derived from de Paula *et al.* [220] (parrot).

P_ECO_2 cannot be used to determine optimum insufflation gas flow rates solely based on weight and previously derived values for minute ventilation [294]. When feasible, arterial blood gases, specifically $PaCO_2$, should be the preferred method for monitoring CO_2 during air sac insufflation anesthesia to verify patient ventilation (Table 58.4).

Respiratory pauses longer than 10 to 15 s should be treated by lightening the plane of anesthesia and, when possible, ventilating the bird by either periodically squeezing the reservoir bag or using a positive-pressure mechanical ventilator. Intermittent positive-pressure ventilation (IPPV) is recommended at 2 breaths/min in spontaneously ventilating birds, and 10–20 breaths/min in apneic birds. A maximum pressure of 10–20 cm H_2O is recommended to prevent air sac volutrauma. If used in combination with capnography, IPPV rate should be adjusted to maintain P_ECO_2 between 30 and 45 mmHg.

Pulse oximetry can be used to monitor oxygenation, but typical pulse oximeters are designed to measure oxygenated and deoxygenated mammalian hemoglobin, not avian hemoglobin. Critical incidents in birds, such as cardiac dysrhythmias, severe blood loss, or movement artifacts, cause fluctuations and discontinuity of displayed values and failure to record actual values [296]. Oximeters also tend to underestimate oxygenation levels at high oxygen saturation levels and overestimate oxygenation levels at lower saturation levels [296]. Recent development of pulse oximeters for use in small animals, such as mice, has addressed some of the shortcomings of early pulse oximeters [297]. The adequacy of cardiopulmonary function and oxygenation can also be assessed visually by noting the color and capillary refill time of mucous membranes, the color of the cere, beak, or bill, as well as coloration on the head where there is a lack of feathers.

An early study reported that dorsal recumbency of anesthetized chickens, especially of "heavy breeds," may adversely affect ventilation [298]. At least two factors may explain this phenomenon: (1) the weight of the abdominal viscera may compress the abdominal air sacs thereby effectively reducing a bird's tidal volume; and (2) during anesthesia there is some degree of muscle relaxation such that a bird with large, heavy pectoral muscles may not be able to generate sufficient muscular effort to lift the keel against gravity, again reducing tidal volume. In a computed tomographic study of isoflurane-anesthetized red-tailed hawks (*Buteo jamaicensis*), one that did not measure physiologic variables, such as $PaCO_2$ and PaO_2, mean partial air sac volume was smallest in dorsal recumbency compared to lateral and sternal recumbency [299]. Sternal recumbency resulted in the greatest lung and air sac volumes and lowest lung density compared to right lateral or dorsal recumbency [299]. In another study that measured respiratory rate and volume as well as physiologic variables in isoflurane-anesthetized red-tailed hawks, dorsal recumbency did not compromise minute ventilation or oxygen transport more than when the birds were in lateral recumbency [300]. However, the birds hypoventilated in both positions, and $PaCO_2$ differed with time, and the position by time interaction. Despite similar minute ventilation in both positions, birds in dorsal recumbency hypoventilated more yet maintained higher PaO_2, suggesting parabronchial ventilatory or pulmonary blood flow distribution changes with position [300]. The effect of body position has also been investigated in isoflurane-anesthetized Humboldt penguins (*Spheniscus humboldti*) where air sac volume was lowest in dorsal recumbency, and lung density was highest compared to lateral recumbency [301]. All of these studies suggest that body position during anesthesia may affect the avian pulmonary system. Thus, as with any anesthetized patient, to overcome ventilation problems in birds associated with anesthesia-induced muscle relaxation, it is reasonable to provide IPPV.

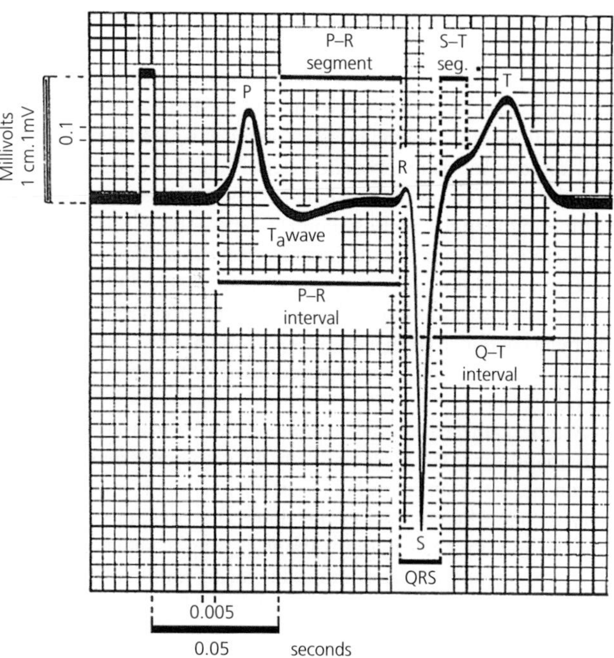

Figure 58.11 An ECG from a pigeon. The ECG trace from a normal bird may have the appearance of ventricular tachycardia primarily because of the large negative S wave. Source: Nap *et al.* [302], Taylor & Francis.

Cardiovascular system

The heart is an electromechanical pump. Its function can be assessed by monitoring heart rate and rhythm, mucous membrane color and refill time, palpation of peripheral pulses, ECG monitoring, and indirect or direct arterial blood pressure monitoring. A stethoscope can be used to monitor heart rate and rhythm, and an esophageal stethoscope can facilitate this mode of cardiac monitoring. The esophageal probe should be inserted into the thoracic esophagus using digital manipulation to bypass the crop. The ultrasonic Doppler flow detector can be used to monitor heart rate and rhythm by placing the sensor over one of several arteries: the cranial tibial artery, palpable on the cranial aspect of the hock joint; the superficial ulnar artery, palpable on the ventral surface of the elbow joint; the deep radial artery, palpable on the ventral surface of the distal radius near the carpal joint; or the palatal artery in the dorsal oropharynx.

Standard bipolar and augmented limb leads can be used to monitor and record the avian ECG. To assure adequate skin contact for an interference-free signal, ECG clips can be attached to hypodermic needles inserted through the skin at the base of each wing and through the skin at the level of each stifle. An alternative technique is to attach the ECG clips to stainless steel wires that have been inserted through the prepatagium of each wing and the skin at the lateral side of each stifle. The wire size selected depends on the size of the bird. 20 or 22 gauge wire can be used in birds larger than 500 g. Appropriately sized hypodermic needles are used to insert the wires through the skin.

The morphometry of the normal avian ECG has been mistaken for ventricular tachycardia (Fig. 58.11) [48] so it is incumbent on an anesthetist to be familiar with avian electrocardiograms in order to distinguish between normal and abnormal cardiac rhythms encountered during anesthesia. Electrocardiograms have been described for a number of avian species, including gray (*Psittacus erithacus*) and Amazon (Amazona *spp.*) parrots [302], Pekin duck [303], peregrine falcon (*Falco peregrinus brookei*) [304], Eurasian kestrel, griffon vulture, little owl, and Eurasian eagle owl [305], and golden (*Chrysolophus pictus*) and silver (*Lophura nycthemera*) pheasants [306].

The effect of halothane on blood pressure can be variable. In chickens and ducks, increasing concentrations of halothane can cause a decrease in mean arterial blood pressure [225,307], or no change [229]. In contrast, isoflurane appears to consistently cause a dose-dependent decrease in mean arterial blood pressure [217,230,307,308], possibly because of isoflurane-associated peripheral vasodilation. Sevoflurane has been reported to decrease blood pressure in chickens in a dose-dependent manner during controlled ventilation [227,286], but not during spontaneous ventilation probably because of hypercapnia due to hypoventilation [286]. In crested caracara (*Caracara plancus*), sevoflurane moderately depressed blood pressure and did so without producing cardiac arrhythmias [284]. In red-tailed hawks anesthetized with sevoflurane, blood pressure was significantly lower compared to when they were awake and physically restrained [309].

In mammals, positive-pressure ventilation depresses mean arterial blood pressure by creating positive intrathoracic pressures that compress the great vessels, thus impeding the venous return of blood to the heart. In sandhill cranes anesthetized with isoflurane, mean arterial blood pressure was actually higher during positive-pressure ventilation than during spontaneous ventilation [217].

Blood pressure can be monitored and measured either indirectly or directly, but avian anatomy and physiology make either technique challenging. Indirect methods include using a Doppler flow probe (Parks Electronics, Aloha, Oregon, USA) to monitor pulsatile blood flow in small birds, or blood pressure when used with a sphygmomanometer in either moderate or large-size birds. However, in awake birds representing 17 commonly kept psittacine species weighing between 230 and 1263 g, Doppler-derived blood pressure measurements were imprecise [310]. Attempts to measure blood pressure with an oscillometric device in Hispaniolan Amazon parrots (*Amazona ventralis*) proved unsuccessful [311]. In those same birds, there was substantial disagreement between indirectly measured blood pressure obtained with a Doppler device and directly measured systolic arterial blood pressure [311]. In anesthetized and awake red-tailed hawks, the results of a study comparing Doppler and oscillometric methods of indirect blood pressure measurement with direct arterial measurement indicated that the oscillometric technique was unreliable [309]. Using a Doppler device and a cuff of 40–50% of limb circumference, measurements obtained from either the pectoral or pelvic limbs yielded values closer to mean arterial blood pressure than systolic arterial blood pressure [309].

Arterial catheterization is required for direct arterial blood pressure monitoring. For birds less than 200 g, the preferred catheterization site is the superficial ulnar artery, one that is prominent but very mobile where it crosses the elbow, thus making catheterization technically challenging without causing a hematoma [312]. Furthermore, the anatomy of the wing makes it difficult to secure a catheter at this location. For medium to large birds, the deep radial artery is the preferred site [312,313] due to its minimal mobility as it lies between the tendons of the *extensor digitorum longus* and the *flexor digitorum profundus* in the distal wing of most birds [312]. Catheterization should occur where the artery is most superficial at the ulnar carpal bone or the distal head of the ulna [312]. For aquatic or long-legged birds, the cranial tibial or dorsal metatarsal arteries can be catheterized [313]. The external carotid artery can be catheterized, but surgical dissection is required for visualization and catheterization [294].

Monitoring a physiological variable such as arterial blood pressure implies that action will be taken if blood pressure differs from the expected. This touches on the concept of action limits: in an anesthetized patient, what blood pressure requires intervention? What constitutes hypotension, and what constitutes hypertension? For birds, there are no clear answers since cited blood pressures vary across avian species. For example, direct blood pressure measurements are higher in psittacines, cranes, raptors, and owls than in pigeons, chickens, and ducks [314]. In chickens, normal mean arterial blood pressure (MAP) is approximately 84 ± 13 mm Hg, and in conscious red-tailed hawks, it is 187 ± 42 mm Hg [314]. In humans, a 30% decrease from baseline MAP is one indicator of hypotension [315], and this metric has been used to define hypotension in birds [314]. As such, hypotension in chickens would be a MAP ≤ 59 mmHg, and ≤ 131 mmHg in red-tailed hawks, both of which would require intervention, such as lightening the plane of anesthesia, administering fluids, and cardiac inotropes, including dopamine or dobutamine.

In general, birds tend to have a higher plasma osmolality compared to mammals [316]. For this reason, fluids with an osmolarity close to 300–320 mOsm/L, such as Normosol®-R, Plasma-Lyte®-R, Plasma-Lyte®-A, and 0.9% NaCl, have been recommended for fluid therapy in birds, specifically parrots [178], and are reasonable choices for fluid support of any bird during anesthesia [316].

In a dose-dependent manner, dobutamine at 5, 10, and 15 μg/kg/min and dopamine at 5, 7, and 10 μg/kg/min increased arterial blood pressure in Hispaniolan Amazon parrots [314]. However, 4 out of 12 parrots receiving dobutamine at 15 μg/kg/min developed marked second-degree atrioventricular block accompanied by a dramatic decrease in blood pressure, a situation that quickly resolved after the dobutamine infusion was discontinued [314].

Body temperature

Body temperature must be monitored as hypothermia is the most commonly encountered problem during anesthesia [317]. The stress associated with anesthesia and surgery is minimized when birds are maintained at or near their normal body temperature which is 40 to 41 °C (104 to 106 °F) [318]. During anesthesia, it is not unusual to see major fluctuations in body temperature, but hypothermia decreases the amount of anesthetic needed to maintain anesthesia, causes cardiac instability, and prolongs recovery. In well-insulated birds (feathers, drapes, and warming devices), hyperthermia can also occur and cause cardiac instability and increased oxygen demand. Body temperature can be monitored with an electronic thermometer and a long flexible thermistor probe inserted into the esophagus to the level of the heart. Temperature monitored via the cloaca can vary significantly over time owing to cloacal movements that affect the position of the thermometer or thermistor probe.

Methods for warming birds during anesthesia include convective (forced warm air), conductive, and radiant heat sources. In anesthetized Hispaniolan Amazon parrots (*Amazona ventralis*) covered with a clear plastic drape, a forced air warming device was used to maintain body temperature. The device did not prevent an initial drop in core body temperature, but it maintained body temperature within a clinically acceptable range [319]. A disadvantage to using a forced air warming device is that it can blow air into the surgical site. The type of anesthetic delivery system, with or without heated air, does not appear to affect core body temperature in isoflurane-anesthetized pigeons [320]. Electric heating pads and gloves filled with hot water are not appropriate warming methods for birds as they can cause thermal injury.

Recovery

Precautions should be taken to protect birds while they recover from anesthesia. During recovery, birds should be in a warm (25 °C/77 °F) incubator until fully recovered. Birds must be kept from flopping around, as this can lead to serious neck, wing, or leg injuries. Struggling and flopping behavior can be prevented by lightly wrapping a bird with a towel but wrapping poses its own hazards. If a bird is wrapped too tightly, sternal movements will be impeded, and breathing will be difficult if not impossible. Wrapping can lead to excessive retention of body heat and cause hyperthermia. If a bird has not been fasted prior to anesthesia, regurgitation can occur during recovery. Keeping a bird intubated during the recovery phase helps to maintain a patent airway.

References

1 Scott GR, Hawkes LA, Frappell PB, *et al.* How bar-headed geese fly over the Himalayas. *Physiology* 2015; **30**(2): 107–115.
2 Handrich Y, Bevan RM, Charrassin JB, *et al.* Hypothermia in foraging king penguins. *Nature* 1997; **388**(6637): 64–67.
3 Brodbelt DC, Blissitt KJ, Hammond RA, *et al.* The risk of death: the Confidential Enquiry into Perioperative Small Animal Fatalities. *Vet Anaesth Analg* 2008; **35**(5): 365–373.
4 Seamon AB, Hofmeister EH, Divers SJ. Outcome following inhalation anesthesia in birds at a veterinary referral hospital: 352 cases (2004–2014). *J Am Vet Med Assoc* 2017; **251**(7): 814–817.
5 Dobbs P, Moittié S, Liptovszky M. Avian anaesthesia related mortality and the associated risk factors in a UK zoological collection. *Vet Anaesth Analg* 2021; **48**(6): 922–929.
6 McLelland J. Larynx and trachea. In: King AS, McLelland J, eds. *Form and Function in Birds*, 4th edn. London, UK: Academic Press, 1989: 69–103.
7 Zeek PM. Double trachea in penguins and sea lions. *Anat Rec* 1951; **111**(3): 327–343.

8 Gaunt AS, Gaunt SLL, Prange HD, *et al.* The effects of tracheal coiling on the vocalizations of cranes (Aves; Gruidae). *J Comp Physiol* 1987; **161**(1): 43–58.
9 Brown RE, Brain JD, Wang N. The avian respiratory system: a unique model for studies of respiratory toxicosis and for monitoring air quality. *Environ Health Perspect* 1997; **105**(2): 188–200.
10 Duncker HR. Structure of avian lungs. *Respir Physiol* 1972; **14**(1): 44–63.
11 Duncker HR. Structure of the avian respiratory tract. *Respir Physiol* 1974; **22**(1–2): 1–19.
12 King AS, Cowie AF. The functional anatomy of the bronchial muscle of the bird. *J Anat* 1969; **105**: 323–336.
13 Hodges RD. *The Histology of the Fowl.* London, UK: Academic Press, 1974: 648.
14 King AS, McLelland J. *Birds – Their Structure and Function*, 2nd edn. London, UK: Bailliere Tindall, 1984: 334.
15 McLelland J. Anatomy of the lungs and air sacs. In: King AS, McLelland J, eds. *Form and Function in Birds*, 4th edn. London, UK: Academic Press, 1989: 221–279.
16 Scheid P, Piiper J. Gas exchange and transport. In: Seller TJ, ed. *Bird Respiration*, 1st edn. Boca Raton, FL: CRC Press, 1987: 97–129.
17 Magnussen H, Willmer H, Scheid P. Gas exchange in air sacs: contribution to respiratory gas exchange in ducks. *Respir Physiol* 1976; **26**(1): 129–146.
18 Maina JN. Development, structure, and function of a novel respiratory organ, the lung-air sac system of birds: to go where no other vertebrate has gone. *Biol Rev Camb Philos Soc* 2006; **81**(4): 545–579.
19 Maina JN. Pivotal debates and controversies on the structure and function of the avian respiratory system: setting the record straight. *Biol Rev Camb Philos Soc* 2017; **92**(3): 1475–1504.
20 Fedde MR. Structure and gas-flow pattern in the avian respiratory system. *Poult Sci* 1980; **59**(12): 2642–2653.
21 Scheid P, Piiper J. Respiratory mechanics and air flow in birds. *Form and Function in Birds*, 4th edn. London, UK: Academic Press, 1989: 369–391.
22 Powell FL. Respiration. In: Scanes CG, Sturkie PD, eds. *Sturkie's Avian Physiology*, 6th edn. London, UK: Academic Press/Elsevier, 2014: 301–336.
23 Duncker HR. The lung air sac system of birds. A contribution to the functional anatomy of the respiratory apparatus. *Ergeb Anat Entwicklungsgesch* 1971; **45**(6): 7–171.
24 Barnas GM, Mather FB, Fedde MR. Response of avian intrapulmonary smooth muscle to changes in carbon dioxide concentration. *Poult Sci* 1978; **57**(5): 1400–1407.
25 Bernhard W, Gebert A, Vieten G, *et al.* Pulmonary surfactant in birds: coping with surface tension in a tubular lung. *Am J Physiol Regul Integr Comp Physiol* 2001; **281**(1): R327–R337.
26 Maina JN, Jimoh SA, Hosie M. Implicit mechanistic role of the collagen, smooth muscle, and elastic tissue components in strengthening the air and blood capillaries of the avian lung. *J Anat* 2010; **217**(5): 597–608.
27 Maina JN, King AS, Settle G. An allometric study of pulmonary morphometric parameters in birds, with mammalian comparisons. *Philos Trans R Soc Lond B Biol Sci* 1989; **326**(1231): 1–57.
28 Scheid P. Mechanisms of gas exchange in bird lungs. *Rev Physiol Biochem Pharmacol* 1979; **86**: 138–186.
29 Crank WD, Gallagher RR. Theory of gas exchange in the avian parabronchus. *Respir Physiol* 1978; **35**(1): 9–25.
30 Woodward JD, Maina JN. Study of the structure of the air and blood capillaries of the gas exchange tissue of the avian lung by serial section three-dimensional reconstruction. *J Microsc* 2008; **230**(Pt 1): 84–93.
31 Piiper J, Scheid P. Gas exchange in avian lungs: models and experimental evidence. In: Bolis L, Schmidt-Nielsen K, Maddrell SHP, eds. *Comparative Physiology*. Amsterdam, NL: North-Holland Publishing Company, 1973.
32 Powell FL, Scheid P. Physiology of gas exchange in the avian respiratory system. In: King AS, McLelland J, eds. *Form and Function in Birds*, 4th edn. London, UK: Academic Press, 1989: 393–437.
33 Powell FL, Shams H, Hempleman SC, *et al.* Breathing in thin air: acclimatization to altitude in ducks. *Respir Physiol Neurobiol* 2004; **144**(2–3): 225–235.
34 Scheid P, Piiper J. Analysis of gas exchange in the avian lung: theory and experiments in the domestic fowl. *Respir Physiol* 1970; **9**(2): 246–262.
35 Gleeson M, Molony V. Control of breathing. In: King AS, McLelland J, eds. *Form and Function in Birds*, 4th edn. London, UK: Academic Press, 1989; 439–484.
36 Hempleman SC, Adamson TP, Begay RS, *et al.* CO2 transduction in avian intrapulmonary chemoreceptors is critically dependent on transmembrane Na+/H+ exchange. *Am J Physiol Regul Integr Comp Physiol* 2003; **284**(6): R1551–R1559.
37 Hempleman SC, Rodriguez TA, Bhagat YA, *et al.* Benzolamide, acetazolamide, and signal transduction in avian intrapulmonary chemoreceptors. *Am J Physiol Regul Integr Comp Physiol* 2000; **279**(6): R1988–R1995.
38 Shoemaker JM, Hempleman SC. Avian intrapulmonary chemoreceptor discharge rate is increased by anion exchange blocker 'DIDS'. *Respir Physiol* 2001; **128**(2): 195–204.
39 Barnas GM, Mather FB, Fedde MR. Are avian intrapulmonary CO2 receptors chemically modulated mechanoreceptors or chemoreceptors? *Respir Physiol* 1978; **35**(2): 237–243.
40 Hempleman SC, Burger RE. Receptive fields of intrapulmonary chemoreceptors in the Pekin duck. *Respir Physiol* 1984; **57**(3): 317–330.
41 Fedde MR, Nelson PI, Kuhlmann WD. Ventilatory sensitivity to changes in inspired and arterial carbon dioxide partial pressures in the chicken. *Poult Sci* 2002; **81**(6): 869–876.
42 Hempleman SC, Burger RE. Comparison of intrapulmonary chemoreceptor response to PCO2 in the duck and chicken. *Respir Physiol* 1985; **61**(2): 179–184.
43 Kilgore DL, Faraci FM, Fedde MR. Static response characteristics of intrapulmonary chemoreceptors in the pigeon and burrowing owl, a species with a blunted ventilatory sensitivity to carbon dioxide. *Fed Proc* 1984; **43**: 638.
44 Grubb BR. Allometric relations of cardiovascular function in birds. *Am J Physiol* 1983; **245**: H567–H572.
45 Sturkie PD. Heart and circulation: anatomy, hemodynamics, blood pressure, blood flow. In: Sturkie PD, ed. *Avian Physiology*, 4th edn. New York, NY: Springer-Verlag, 1986: 130–166.
46 Sturkie PD. Heart: contraction, conduction, and electrocardiography. In: Sturkie PD, ed. *Avian Physiology*, 4th edn. New York, NY: Springer-Verlag, 1986: 167–190.
47 O'Callaghan MW. Regulation of heart beat. In: Phillipson AT, Hall LW, Pritchard WR, eds. *Scientific Foundations of Veterinary Medicine*. London, UK: William Heinemann Medical Books Limited, 1980: 303–312.
48 Keene BW, Flammer K. ECG of the month. *J Am Vet Med Assoc* 1991; **198**(3): 408–409.
49 Burrows ME, Braun EJ, Duckles SP. Avian renal portal valve: a reexamination of its innervation. *Am J Physiol* 1983; **245**(4): H628–H634.
50 Palmore WP, Ackerman N. Blood flow in the renal portal circulation of the turkey: effect of epinephrine. *Am J Vet Res* 1985; **46**(7): 1589–1592.
51 Frazier DL, Jones MP, Orosz SE. Pharmacokinetic considerations of the renal system in birds: Part I. anatomic and physiologic principles of allometric scaling. *J Avian Med Surg* 1995; **9**(2): 92–103.
52 Hawkins MG, Paul-Murphy JR. Avian analgesia. *Vet Clin North Am Exot Anim Pract* 2011; **14**(1): 61–80.
53 Greenacre CB, Lusby AL. Physiologic responses of Amazon Parrots (Amazona species) to manual restraint. *J Avian Med Surg* 2004; **18**(1): 19–22.
54 Doss GA, Mans C. The effect of manual restraint on physiological parameters in barred owls (*Strix varia*). *J Avian Med Surg* 2016; **31**(1): 1–5.
55 Doss GA, Mans C. Changes in physiologic parameters and effects of hooding in red-tailed hawks (*Buteo jamaicensis*) during manual restraint. *J Avian Med Surg* 2016; **30**(2): 127–132.
56 Le Maho Y, Karmann H, Briot D, *et al.* Stress in birds due to routine handling and a technique to avoid it. *Am J Physiol* 1992; **263**(4 Pt 2): R775–R781.
57 Heatley JJ, Oliver JW, Hosgood G, *et al.* Serum corticosterone concentrations in response to restraint, anesthesia, and skin testing in Hispaniolan Amazon parrots (*Amazona ventralis*). *J Avian Med Surg* 2000; **14**(3): 172–176.
58 Mans C, Guzman DS, Lahner LL, *et al.* Sedation and physiologic response to manual restraint after intranasal administration of midazolam in Hispaniolan Amazon parrots (*Amazona ventralis*). *J Avian Med Surg* 2012; **26**(3): 130–139.
59 Cooper JE. *Birds of Prey: Health and Disease*, 3rd edn. Oxford, UK: Blackwell Science, 2002: 345.
60 Miller RE, Fowler ME. *Fowler's Zoo and Wild Animal Medicine Current Therapy*, 7th edn. St. Louis, MO: Elsevier/Saunders, 2012.
61 Ritchie BW, Harrison GJ, Harrison LR. *Avian Medicine: Principles and Application.* Lake Worth, FL: Wingers Publishing, 1994: 1384.
62 Sinn LC. Anesthesiology. In: Zantop DW, ed. *Avian Medicine: Principles and Application*. Lake Worth, FL: Wingers Publishing, 1997: 589–599.
63 Doss G, Mans C. Avian sedation. *J Avian Med Surg* 2021; **35**(3): 253–268.
64 Mans C. Sedation of pet birds. *J Exot Pet Med* 2014; **23**(2): 152–157.
65 Bello A, Poźniak B, Smutkiewicz A, *et al.* The influence of the site of drug administration on florfenicol pharmacokinetics in turkeys. *Poult Sci* 2022; **101**(1): 101536.
66 Riggs SM, Hawkins MG, Craigmill AL, *et al.* Pharmacokinetics of butorphanol tartrate in red-tailed hawks (*Buteo jamaicensis*) and great horned owls (*Bubo virginianus*). *Am J Vet Res* 2008; **69**(5): 596–603.
67 Bigham AS, Zamani Moghaddam AK. Finch (*Taeneopygia guttata*) sedation with intranasal administration of diazepam, midazolam or xylazine. *J Vet Pharmacol Ther* 2013; **36**(1): 102–104.
68 Sadegh AB. Comparison of intranasal administration of xylazine, diazepam, and midazolam in budgerigars (*melopsittacus undulatus*) clinical evaluation. *J Zoo Wildl Med* 2013; **44**(2): 241–244.
69 Araghi M, Azizi S, Vesal N, *et al.* Evaluation of the sedative effects of diazepam, midazolam, and xylazine after intranasal administration in juvenile ostriches (*Struthio camelus*). *J Avian Med Surg* 2016; **30**(3): 221–226.
70 Vesal N, Eskandari MH. Sedative effects of midazolam and xylazine with or without ketamine and detomidine alone following intranasal administration in ring-necked parakeets. *J Am Vet Med Assoc* 2006; **228**(3): 383–388.

71 Vesal N, Zare P. Clinical evaluation of intranasal benzodiazepines, alpha-agonists and their antagonists in canaries. *Vet Anaesth Analg* 2006; **33**(3): 143–148.

72 Hornak S, Liptak T, Ledecky V, *et al*. A preliminary trial of the sedation induced by intranasal administration of midazolam alone or in combination with dexmedetomidine and reversal by atipamezole for a short-term immobilization in pigeons. *Vet Anaesth Analg* 2015; **42**(2): 192–196.

73 Schaffer DP, Raposo AC, Liborio FA, *et al*. Intranasal administration of midazolam in blue-and-yellow macaws (*Ara ararauna*): evaluation of sedative effects. *Vet Anaesth Analg* 2016; **43**(4): 459–460.

74 Net RL, Mulcahy DM, Santamaria-Bouvier A, *et al*. Intranasal administration of midazolam hydrochloride improves survival in female surf scoters (*melanitta perspicillata*) surgically implanted with intracoelomic transmitters. *J Zoo Wildl Med* 2019; **50**(1): 167–175.

75 Pascoe PJ, Pypendop BH, Pavez Phillips JC, *et al*. Pharmacokinetics of fentanyl after intravenous administration in isoflurane-anesthetized red-tailed hawks (*Buteo jamaicensis*) and Hispaniolan Amazon parrots (*Amazona ventralis*). *Am J Vet Res* 2018; **79**(6): 606–613.

76 Sanchez-Migallon Guzman D, Beaufrère H, Welle KR, *et al*. Birds. In: Carpenter JW, Harms CA, eds. *Carpenter's Exotic Animal Formulary*, 6th edn. Philadelphia, PA: Saunders/Elsevier, 2022.

77 Franchetti DR, Klide AM. Restraint and anesthesia. In: Fowler ME, ed. *Zoo and Wild Animal Medicine*. Philadelphia, PA: WB Saunders, 1978: 359–364.

78 Boxenbaum H. Interspecies scaling, allometry, physiological time, and the ground plan of pharmacokinetics. *J Pharmacokinet Biopharm* 1982; **10**(2): 201–227.

79 Dorrestein GM. The pharmacokinetics of avian therapeutics. *Vet Clin North Am Small Anim Pract* 1991; **21**(6): 1241–1264.

80 Schmidt-Nielsen K. *Scaling, Why is Animal Size so Important? Cambridge*, UK: Cambridge University Press, 1984.

81 Sedgwick CJ, Pokras MA. Extrapolating rational drug doses and treatment periods by allometric scaling. In: *Proceedings of the 55th Annual Meeting of the American Animal Hospital Association*, 1988: 156–161.

82 Dhondt L, Devreese M, Croubels S, *et al*. Comparative population pharmacokinetics and absolute oral bioavailability of COX-2 selective inhibitors celecoxib, mavacoxib and meloxicam in cockatiels (*Nymphicus hollandicus*). *Sci Rep* 2017; **7**(1): 12043.

83 Pinheiro BC, A Silva Dantas Lima D, Lima WC, *et al*. Allometric scaling for chemical restraint in greater rheas (*Rhea americana*) with tiletamine and zolazepam. *BMC Vet Res* 2014; **10**: 66–72.

84 Waxman S, Prados AP, De Lucas JJ, *et al*. Evaluation of allometric scaling as a tool for extrapolation of the enrofloxacin dose in American black vultures (*Coragyps atratus*). *Am J Vet Res* 2019; **80**(8): 727–735.

85 Baert K, De Backer P. Comparative pharmacokinetics of three non steroidal anti inflammatory drugs in five bird species. *Comp Biochem Physiol C Toxicol Pharmacol* 2003; **134**(1): 25–33.

86 Dorrestein GM, van Miert AS. Pharmacotherapeutic aspects of medication of birds. *J Vet Pharmacol Ther* 1988; **11**(1): 33–44.

87 Redig PT, Larson AA, Duke GE. Response of great horned owls given the optical isomers of ketamine. *Am J Vet Res* 1984; **45**(1): 125–127.

88 Hawkins MG, Paul-Murphy J, Sanchez-Migallon Guzman D. Recognition, assessment and management of pain in birds. In: Speer BL, ed. *Current Therapy in Avian Medicine and Surgery*, 1st edn. St. Louis, MO: Elsevier, 2016: 616–630.

89 Paul-Murphy JR, Brunson DB, Miletic V. Analgesic effects of butorphanol and buprenorphine in conscious African grey parrots (*Psittacus erithacus erithacus* and *Psittacus erithacus timneh*). *Am J Vet Res* 1999; **60**(10): 1218–1221.

90 Sladky KK, Krugner-Higby L, Meek-Walker E, *et al*. Serum concentrations and analgesic effects of liposome-encapsulated and standard butorphanol tartrate in parrots. *Am J Vet Res* 2006; **67**(5): 775–781.

91 Cole GA, Paul-Murphy JR, Krugner-Higby L, *et al*. Analgesic effects of intramuscular administration of meloxicam in Hispaniolan parrots (*Amazona ventralis*) with experimentally induced arthritis. *Am J Vet Res* 2009; **70**(12): 1471–1476.

92 Sanchez-Migallon Guzman D, KuKanich B, Keuler NS, *et al*. Antinociceptive effects of nalbuphine hydrochloride in Hispaniolan Amazon parrots (*Amazona ventralis*). *Am J Vet Res* 2011; **72**(6): 736–740.

93 Desmarchelier M, Troncy E, Fitzgerald G, *et al*. Analgesic effects of meloxicam administration on postoperative orthopedic pain in domestic pigeons (*Columba livia*). *Am J Vet Res* 2012; **73**(3): 361–367.

94 Guzman DSM, Houck EL, Knych HKD, *et al*. Evaluation of the thermal antinociceptive effects and pharmacokinetics after intramuscular administration of buprenorphine hydrochloride to cockatiels (*Nymphicus hollandicus*). *Am J Vet Res* 2018; **79**(12): 1239–1245.

95 Mansour A, Khachaturian H, Lewis ME, *et al*. Anatomy of CNS opioid receptors. *Trends Neurosci* 1988; **11**(7): 308–314.

96 Csillag A, Bourne RC, Stewart MG. Distribution of mu, delta, and kappa opioid receptor binding sites in the brain of the one-day-old domestic chick (*Gallus domesticus*): an in vitro quantitative autoradiographic study. *J Comp Neurol* 1990; **302**(3): 543–551.

97 Fousse SL, Golsen BM, Sanchez-Migallon Guzman D, *et al*. Varying expression of Mu and kappa opioid receptors in cockatiels (*Nymphicus hollandicus*) and domestic pigeons (*Columba livia domestica*). *Front Genet* 2020; **11**: 549558.

98 Duhamelle A, Raiwet DL, Langlois I, *et al*. Preliminary findings of structure and expression of opioid receptor genes in a peregrine falcon (*Falco peregrinus*), a snowy owl (*Bubo scandiacus*), and a blue-fronted Amazon parrot (*Amazona aestiva*). *J Avian Med Surg* 2018; **32**(3): 173–184.

99 Gaggermeier B, Henke J, Schatzmann U, eds. Investigations on analgesia in domestic pigeons (*C. livia*) using buprenorphine and butorphanol. *Proceedings of European Association of Avian Veterinarians*. Munich, Germany: German Veterinary Medical Society, March 7–10, 2001.

100 Klaphake E, Schumacher J, Greenacre C, *et al*. Comparative anesthetic and cardiopulmonary effects of pre- versus postoperative butorphanol administration in Hispaniolan Amazon Parrots (*Amazona ventralis*) anesthetized with sevoflurane. *J Avian Med Surg* 2006; **20**(1): 2–7.

101 Paul-Murphy JR, Krugner-Higby LA, Tourdot RL, *et al*. Evaluation of liposome-encapsulated butorphanol tartrate for alleviation of experimentally induced arthritic pain in green-cheeked conures (*Pyrrhura molinae*). *Am J Vet Res* 2009; **70**(10): 1211–1219.

102 Guzman DS, Flammer K, Paul-Murphy JR, *et al*. Pharmacokinetics of butorphanol after intravenous, intramuscular, and oral administration in Hispaniolan Amazon parrots (*Amazona ventralis*). *J Avian Med Surg* 2011; **25**(3): 185–191.

103 Laniesse D, Guzman DSM, Knych HK, *et al*. Pharmacokinetics of butorphanol tartrate in a long-acting poloxamer 407 gel formulation administered to Hispaniolan Amazon parrots (*Amazona ventralis*). *Am J Vet Res* 2017; **78**(6): 688–694.

104 Laniesse D, Sanchez-Migallon Guzman D, Smith DA, *et al*. Evaluation of the thermal antinociceptive effects of subcutaneous administration of butorphanol tartrate or butorphanol tartrate in a sustained-release poloxamer 407 gel formulation to orange-winged Amazon parrots (*Amazona amazonica*). *Am J Vet Res* 2020; **81**(7): 543–550.

105 Singh PM, Johnson C, Gartrell B, *et al*. Pharmacokinetics of butorphanol in broiler chickens. *Vet Rec* 2011; **168**(22): 588.

106 Singh PM, Johnson CB, Gartrell B, *et al*. Analgesic effects of morphine and butorphanol in broiler chickens. *Vet Anaesth Analg* 2017; **44**(3): 538–545.

107 Clancy MM, KuKanich B, Sykes JM. Pharmacokinetics of butorphanol delivered with an osmotic pump during a seven-day period in common peafowl (*Pavo cristatus*). *Am J Vet Res* 2015; **76**(12): 1070–1076.

108 Curro TG, Brunson DB, Paul-Murphy JR. Determination of the ED50 of isoflurane and evaluation of the isoflurane-sparing effect of butorphanol in cockatoos (*Cacatua spp.*). *Vet Surg* 1994; **23**(5): 429–433.

109 Guzman DS, Drazenovich TL, Kukanich B, *et al*. Evaluation of thermal antinociceptive effects and pharmacokinetics after intramuscular administration of butorphanol tartrate to American kestrels (*Falco sparverius*). *Am J Vet Res* 2014; **75**(1): 11–18.

110 Curro TG, ed. Evaluation of the isoflurane-sparing effects of butorphanol and flunixin in Psittaciformes. *Proceedings of Association of Avian Veterinarians*. Reno, NV: Association of Avian Veterinarians, 1994.

111 Lichtenberger M, Lennox A, Chavez W, *et al*. The use of butorphanol constant rate infusion in psittacines. *Proceedings of Association of Avian Veterinarians*. Milwaukee, WI: Association of Avian Veterinarians, 2009.

112 Keller DL, Sanchez-Migallon Guzman D, Klauer JM, *et al*. Pharmacokinetics of nalbuphine hydrochloride after intravenous and intramuscular administration to Hispaniolan Amazon parrots (*Amazona ventralis*). *Am J Vet Res* 2011; **72**(6): 741–745.

113 Sanchez-Migallon Guzman D, Braun JM, Steagall PV, *et al*. Antinociceptive effects of long-acting nalbuphine decanoate after intramuscular administration to Hispaniolan Amazon parrots (*Amazona ventralis*). *Am J Vet Res* 2013; **74**(2): 196–200.

114 Guzman DS, KuKanich B, Drazenovich TL, *et al*. Pharmacokinetics of hydromorphone hydrochloride after intravenous and intramuscular administration of a single dose to American kestrels (*Falco sparverius*). *Am J Vet Res* 2014; **75**(6): 527–531.

115 Houck EL, Guzman DS, Beaufrère H, *et al*. Evaluation of the thermal antinociceptive effects and pharmacokinetics of hydromorphone hydrochloride after intramuscular administration to cockatiels (*Nymphicus hollandicus*). *Am J Vet Res* 2018; **79**(8): 820–827.

116 Sanchez-Migallon Guzman D, Knych H, Douglas J, *et al*. Pharmacokinetics of hydromorphone hydrochloride after intramuscular and intravenous administration of a single dose to orange-winged Amazon parrots (*Amazona amazonica*). *Am J Vet Res* 2020; **81**(11): 894–898.

117 Guzman DS, Drazenovich TL, Olsen GH, *et al*. Evaluation of thermal antinociceptive effects after intramuscular administration of hydromorphone hydrochloride to American kestrels (*Falco sparverius*). *Am J Vet Res* 2013; **74**(6): 817–822.

118 Guzman DSM, Douglas JM, Beaufrère H, *et al*. Evaluation of the thermal antinociceptive effects of hydromorphone hydrochloride after intramuscular administration to orange-winged Amazon parrots (*Amazona amazonica*). *Am J Vet Res* 2020; **81**(10): 775–782.

119 Singh PM, Johnson C, Gartrell B, *et al.* Pharmacokinetics of morphine after intravenous administration in broiler chickens. *J Vet Pharmacol Ther* 2010; **33**(5): 515–518.

120 Schneider C. Effects of morphine-like drugs in chicks. *Nature* 1961; **191**: 607–608.

121 Bardo MT, Hughes RA. Brief communication. Shock-elicited flight response in chickens as an index of morphine analgesia. *Pharmacol Biochem Behav* 1978; **9**(1): 147–149.

122 Fan SG, Shutt AJ, Vogt M. The importance of 5-hydroxytryptamine turnover for the analgesic effect of morphine in the chicken. *Neuroscience* 1981; **6**(11): 2223–2227.

123 Hughes RA. Codeine analgesic and morphine hyperalgesic effects on thermal nociception in domestic fowl. *Pharmacol Biochem Behav* 1990; **35**(3): 567–570.

124 Concannon KT, Dodam JR, Hellyer PW. Influence of a Mu- and kappa-opioid agonist on isoflurane minimal anesthetic concentration in chickens. *Am J Vet Res* 1995; **56**(6): 806–811.

125 Hoppes S, Flammer K, Hoersch L, *et al.* Disposition and analgesic effects of fentanyl in white cockatoos (*Cacatua alba*). *J Avian Med Surg* 2003; **17**(3): 124–130.

126 Pavez JC, Hawkins MG, Pascoe PJ, *et al.* Effect of fentanyl target-controlled infusions on isoflurane minimum anaesthetic concentration and cardiovascular function in red-tailed hawks (*Buteo jamaicensis*). *Vet Anaesth Analg* 2011; **38**(4): 344–351.

127 Waugh L, Knych H, Cole G, *et al.* Pharmacokinetic evaluation of a long-acting fentanyl solution after transdermal administration in helmeted guineafowl (*Numida meleagris*). *J Zoo Wildl Med* 2016; **47**(2): 468–473.

128 da Rocha RW, Escobar A, Pypendop BH, *et al.* Effects of a single intravenous bolus of fentanyl on the minimum anesthetic concentration of isoflurane in chickens (*Gallus gallus domesticus*). *Vet Anaesth Analg* 2017; **44**(3): 546–554.

129 Delaski KM, Gehring R, Heffron BT, *et al.* Plasma concentrations of fentanyl achieved with transdermal application in chickens. *J Avian Med Surg* 2017; **31**(1): 6–15.

130 Hawkins MG, Pascoe PJ, DiMaio Knych HK, *et al.* Effects of three fentanyl plasma concentrations on the minimum alveolar concentration of isoflurane in Hispaniolan Amazon parrots (*Amazona ventralis*). *Am J Vet Res* 2018; **79**(6): 600–605.

131 Escobar A, Barletta M, Pypendop BH, *et al.* Pharmacokinetics and pharmacodynamics of methadone administered intravenously and intramuscularly to isoflurane-anesthetized chickens. *Am J Vet Res* 2021; **82**(3): 181–188.

132 Escobar A, da Rocha RW, Pypendop BH, *et al.* Effects of methadone on the minimum anesthetic concentration of isoflurane, and its effects on heart rate, blood pressure and ventilation during isoflurane anesthesia in hens (*Gallus gallus domesticus*). *PLoS ONE* 2016; **11**(3): e0152546.

133 Paul-Murphy J, Hess JC, Fialkowski JP. Pharmacokinetic properties of a single intramuscular dose of buprenorphine in African grey parrots (*Psittacus erithacus erithacus*). *J Avian Med Surg* 2004; **18**(4): 224–228.

134 Ceulemans SM, Guzman DS, Olsen GH, *et al.* Evaluation of thermal antinociceptive effects after intramuscular administration of buprenorphine hydrochloride to American kestrels (*Falco sparverius*). *Am J Vet Res* 2014; **75**(8): 705–710.

135 Gustavsen KA, Guzman DS, Knych HK, *et al.* Pharmacokinetics of buprenorphine hydrochloride following intramuscular and intravenous administration to American kestrels (*Falco sparverius*). *Am J Vet Res* 2014; **75**(8): 711–715.

136 Guzman DS, Knych HK, Olsen GH, *et al.* Pharmacokinetics of a sustained release formulation of buprenorphine after intramuscular and subcutaneous administration to American kestrels (*Falco sparverius*). *J Avian Med Surg* 2017; **31**(2): 102–107.

137 Guzman DSM, Ceulemans SM, Beaufrère H, *et al.* Evaluation of the thermal antinociceptive effects of a sustained-release buprenorphine formulation after intramuscular administration to American kestrels (*Falco sparverius*). *J Avian Med Surg* 2018; **32**(1): 1–7.

138 Gleeson MD, Guzman DSM, Knych HK, *et al.* Pharmacokinetics of a concentrated buprenorphine formulation in red-tailed hawks (*Buteo jamaicensis*). *Am J Vet Res* 2018; **79**(1): 13–20.

139 Souza MJ, Martin-Jimenez T, Jones MP, *et al.* Pharmacokinetics of intravenous and oral tramadol in the bald eagle (*Haliaeetus leucocephalus*). *J Avian Med Surg* 2009; **23**(4): 247–252.

140 Black PA, Cox SK, Macek M, *et al.* Pharmacokinetics of tramadol hydrochloride and its metabolite O-desmethyltramadol in peafowl (*Pavo cristatus*). *J Zoo Wildl Med* 2010; **41**(4): 671–676.

141 Souza MJ, Martin-Jimenez T, Jones MP, *et al.* Pharmacokinetics of oral tramadol in red-tailed hawks (*Buteo jamaicensis*). *J Vet Pharmacol Ther* 2011; **34**(1): 86–88.

142 Souza MJ, Gerhardt L, Cox S. Pharmacokinetics of repeated oral administration of tramadol hydrochloride in Hispaniolan Amazon parrots (*Amazona ventralis*). *Am J Vet Res* 2013; **74**(7): 957–962.

143 Geelen S, Sanchez-Migallon Guzman D, Souza MJ, *et al.* Antinociceptive effects of tramadol hydrochloride after intravenous administration to Hispaniolan Amazon parrots (*Amazona ventralis*). *Am J Vet Res* 2013; **74**(2): 201–206.

144 Souza MJ, Sanchez-Migallon Guzman D, Paul-Murphy JR, *et al.* Pharmacokinetics after oral and intravenous administration of a single dose of tramadol hydrochloride to Hispaniolan Amazon parrots (*Amazona ventralis*). *Am J Vet Res* 2012; **73**(8): 1142–1147.

145 Sanchez-Migallon Guzman D, Braun JM, Cox SK, *et al.* Antinociceptive effects after oral administration of tramadol hydrochloride in Hispaniolan Amazon parrots (*Amazona ventralis*). *Am J Vet Res* 2012; **73**(8): 1148–1152.

146 Guzman DS, Drazenovich TL, Olsen GH, *et al.* Evaluation of thermal antinociceptive effects after oral administration of tramadol hydrochloride to American kestrels (*Falco sparverius*). *Am J Vet Res* 2014; **75**(2): 117–123.

147 Kilburn JJ, Cox SK, Kottyan J, *et al.* Pharmacokinetics of tramadol and its primary metabolite O-desmethyltramadol in African penguins (*Spheniscus demersus*). *J Zoo Wildl Med* 2014; **45**(1): 93–99.

148 Bailey RS, Sheldon JD, Allender MC, *et al.* Analgesic efficacy of tramadol compared with meloxicam in ducks (*Cairina moschata domestica*) evaluated by ground-reactive forces. *J Avian Med Surg* 2019; **33**(2): 133–140.

149 Oaks JL, Gilbert M, Virani MZ, *et al.* Diclofenac residues as the cause of vulture population decline in Pakistan. *Nature* 2004; **427**(6975): 630–633.

150 Ogada DL, Keesing F, Virani MZ. Dropping dead: causes and consequences of vulture population declines worldwide. *Ann N Y Acad Sci* 2012; **1249**: 57–71.

151 Naidoo V, Mompati KF, Duncan N, *et al.* The Pied Crow (*Corvus albus*) is insensitive to diclofenac at concentrations present in carrion. *J Wildl Dis* 2011; **47**(4): 936–944.

152 Cuthbert R, Parry-Jones J, Green RE, *et al.* NSAIDs and scavenging birds: potential impacts beyond Asia's critically endangered vultures. *Biol Lett* 2007; **3**(1): 90–93.

153 Miller KA, Hill NJ, Carrasco SE, *et al.* Pharmacokinetics and safety of intramuscular meloxicam in zebra finches (*Taeniopygia guttata*). *J Am Assoc Lab Anim Sci* 2019; **58**(5): 589–593.

154 Rodriguez P, Paul-Murphy JR, Knych HK, *et al.* Pharmacokinetics of grapiprant administered to red-tailed hawks (*Buteo jamaicensis*) after food was withheld for 24 hours. *Am J Vet Res* 2021; **82**(11): 912–919.

155 Molter CM, Court MH, Cole GA, *et al.* Pharmacokinetics of meloxicam after intravenous, intramuscular, and oral administration of a single dose to Hispaniolan Amazon parrots (*Amazona ventralis*). *Am J Vet Res* 2013; **74**(3): 375–380.

156 Montesinos A, Ardiaca M, Gilabert JA, *et al.* Pharmacokinetics of meloxicam after intravenous, intramuscular and oral administration of a single dose to African grey parrots (*Psittacus erithacus*). *J Vet Pharmacol Ther* 2017; **40**(3): 279–284.

157 Lacasse C, Gamble KC, Boothe DM. Pharmacokinetics of a single dose of intravenous and oral meloxicam in red-tailed hawks (*Buteo jamaicensis*) and great horned owls (*Bubo virginianus*). *J Avian Med Surg* 2013; **27**(3): 204–210.

158 Souza MJ, Gerhardt LE, Shannon L, *et al.* Breed differences in the pharmacokinetics of orally administered meloxicam in domestic chickens (*Gallus domesticus*). *J Am Vet Med Assoc* 2021; **259**(1): 84–87.

159 Sartini I, Łebkowska-Wieruszewska B, Lisowski A, *et al.* Pharmacokinetic profiles of meloxicam after single IV and PO administration in Bilgorajska geese. *J Vet Pharmacol Ther* 2020; **43**(1): 26–32.

160 Morrison J, Greenacre CB, George R, *et al.* Pharmacokinetics of a Single dose of oral and intramuscular meloxicam in African penguins (*Spheniscus demersus*). *J Avian Med Surg* 2018; **32**(2): 102–108.

161 Boonstra JL, Cox SK, Martin-Jimenez T. Pharmacokinetics of meloxicam after intramuscular and oral administration of a single dose to American flamingos (*Phoenicopertus ruber*). *Am J Vet Res* 2017; **78**(3): 267–273.

162 Lindemann DM, Carpenter JW, KuKanich B. Pharmacokinetics of a single dose of oral and subcutaneous meloxicam in Caribbean flamingos (*Phoenicopterus ruber ruber*). *J Avian Med Surg* 2016; **30**(1): 14–22.

163 Horgan MD, Knych HK, Siksay SE, *et al.* Pharmacokinetics of a single dose of oral meloxicam in rehabilitated wild brown pelicans (*Pelecanus occidentalis*). *J Avian Med Surg* 2020; **34**(4): 329–337.

164 Castineiras D, Armitage L, Lamas LP, *et al.* Perioperative pharmacokinetics and pharmacodynamics of meloxicam in emus (*Dromaius novaehollandiae*) of different age groups using nonlinear mixed effect modelling. *J Vet Pharmacol Ther* 2021; **44**(4): 603–618.

165 Montesinos A, Ardiaca M, Juan-Sallés C, *et al.* Effects of meloxicam on hematologic and plasma biochemical analyte values and results of histologic examination of kidney biopsy specimens of African grey parrots (*Psittacus erithacus*). *J Avian Med Surg* 2015; **29**(1): 1–8.

166 Montesinos A, Encinas T, Ardiaca M, *et al.* Pharmacokinetics of meloxicam during multiple oral or intramuscular dose administration to African grey parrots (*Psittacus erithacus*). *Am J Vet Res* 2019; **80**(2): 201–207.

167 McGeown D, Danbury TC, Waterman-Pearson AE, *et al.* Effect of carprofen on lameness in broiler chickens. *Vet Rec* 1999; **144**(24): 668–671.

168 Danbury TC, Weeks CA, Chambers JP, *et al.* Self-selection of the analgesic drug carprofen by lame broiler chickens. *Vet Rec* 2000; **146**(11): 307–311.

169 Caplen G, Colborne GR, Hothersall B, *et al.* Lame broiler chickens respond to non-steroidal anti-inflammatory drugs with objective changes in gait function: a controlled clinical trial. *Vet J* 2013; **196**(3): 477–482.

170 Nasr MA, Nicol CJ, Wilkins L, *et al.* The effects of two non-steroidal anti-inflammatory drugs on the mobility of laying hens with keel bone fractures. *Vet Anaesth Analg* 2015; **42**(2): 197–204.

171 Riber AB, Herskin MS, Foldager L, *et al.* Are changes in behavior of fast-growing broilers with slight gait impairment (GS0-2) related to pain? *Poult Sci* 2021; **100**(3): 100948.

172 Hocking PM, Robertson GW, Gentle MJ. Effects of non-steroidal anti-inflammatory drugs on pain-related behaviour in a model of articular pain in the domestic fowl. *Res Vet Sci* 2005; **78**(1): 69–75.

173 Caplen G, Baker L, Hothersall B, *et al.* Thermal nociception as a measure of non-steroidal anti-inflammatory drug effectiveness in broiler chickens with articular pain. *Vet J* 2013; **198**(3): 616–619.

174 Paul-Murphy JR, Sladky KK, Krugner-Higby LA, *et al.* Analgesic effects of carprofen and liposome-encapsulated butorphanol tartrate in Hispaniolan parrots (*Amazona ventralis*) with experimentally induced arthritis. *Am J Vet Res* 2009; **70**(10): 1201–1210.

175 Zollinger TJ, Hoover JP, Payton ME, *et al.* Clinicopathologic, gross necropsy, and histologic findings after intramuscular injection of carprofen in a pigeon (*Columba livia*) model. *J Avian Med Surg* 2011; **25**(3): 173–184.

176 Sartini I, Giorgi M. Grapiprant: a snapshot of the current knowledge. *J Vet Pharmacol Ther* 2021; **44**(5): 679–688.

177 Rodriguez P, Paul-Murphy JR, Knych HK, *et al.* Absorption of grapiprant in red-tailed hawks (*Buteo jamaicensis*) is decreased when administered with food. *Am J Vet Res* 2022; **83**(6).

178 Fedde MR. Drugs used for avian anesthesia: a review. *Poult Sci* 1978; **57**(5): 1376–1399.

179 DiGeronimo PM, da Cunha AF. Local and regional anesthesia in zoological companion animal practice. *Vet Clin North Am Exot Anim Pract* 2022; **25**(1): 321–336.

180 DiGeronimo PM, da Cunha AF, Pypendop B, *et al.* Cardiovascular tolerance of intravenous bupivacaine in broiler chickens (*Gallus gallus domesticus*) anesthetized with isoflurane. *Vet Anaesth Analg* 2017; **44**(2): 287–294.

181 Figueiredo JP, Cruz ML, Mendes GM, *et al.* Assessment of brachial plexus blockade in chickens by an axillary approach. *Vet Anaesth Analg* 2008; **35**(6): 511–518.

182 Brenner DJ, Larsen RS, Dickinson PJ, *et al.* Development of an avian brachial plexus nerve block technique for perioperative analgesia in mallard ducks (*Anas platyrhynchos*). *J Avian Med Surg* 2010; **24**(1): 24–34.

183 da Cunha AF, Strain GM, Rademacher N, *et al.* Palpation- and ultrasound-guided brachial plexus blockade in Hispaniolan Amazon parrots (*Amazona ventralis*). *Vet Anaesth Analg* 2013; **40**(1): 96–102.

184 Trujanovic R, Otero PE, Larenza-Menzies MP. Ultrasound- and nerve stimulation-guided femoral and sciatic nerve block in a duck (*Anas platyrhynchos*) undergoing surgical fixation of a tibiotarsal fracture. *Vet Anaesth Analg* 2021; **48**(2): 277–278.

185 Mulcahy DM, Tuomi P, Larsen SR. Differential mortality for male spectacled eiders (*Somateria fischeri*) and king eiders (*Somateria spectabilis*) subsequent to anesthesia with propofol, bupivacaine, and ketoprofen. *J Avian Med Surg* 2003; **17**(3): 117–123.

186 Kazemi-Darabadi S, Akbari G, Shokrollahi S. Development and evaluation of a technique for spinal anaesthesia in broiler chickens. *N Z Vet J* 2019; **67**(5): 241–248.

187 Khamisabadi A, Kazemi-Darabadi S, Akbari G. Comparison of anesthetic efficacy of lidocaine and bupivacaine in spinal anesthesia in chickens. *J Avian Med Surg* 2021; **35**(1): 60–67.

188 Mama KR, Phillips LG Jr., Pascoe PJ. Use of propofol for induction and maintenance of anesthesia in a barn owl (*Tyto alba*) undergoing tracheal resection. *J Zoo Wildl Med* 1996; **27**(3): 397–401.

189 Fitzgerald G, Cooper JE. Preliminary studies on the use of propofol in the domestic pigeon (*Columba livia*). *Res Vet Sci* 1990; **49**(3): 334–338.

190 Hawkins MG, Wright BD, Pascoe PJ, *et al.* Pharmacokinetics and anesthetic and cardiopulmonary effects of propofol in red-tailed hawks (*Buteo jamaicensis*) and great horned owls (*Bubo virginianus*). *Am J Vet Res* 2003; **64**(6): 677–683.

191 Langlois I, Harvey RC, Jones MP, *et al.* Cardiopulmonary and anesthetic effects of isoflurane and propofol in Hispaniolan Parrots (*Amazona ventralis*). *J Avian Med Surg* 2003; **17**(1): 4–10.

192 Machin KL, Caulkett NA. Cardiopulmonary effects of propofol and a medetomidine-midazolam-ketamine combination in mallard ducks. *Am J Vet Res* 1998; **59**(5): 598–602.

193 Machin KL, Caulkett NA. Evaluation of isoflurane and propofol anesthesia for intraabdominal transmitter placement in nesting female canvasback ducks. *J Wildl Dis* 2000; **36**(2): 324–334.

194 Muller K, Holzapfel J, Brunnberg L. Total intravenous anaesthesia by boluses or by continuous rate infusion of propofol in mute swans (*Cygnus olor*). *Vet Anaesth Analg* 2011; **38**(4): 286–291.

195 Lukasik VM, Gentz EJ, Erb HN, *et al.* Cardiopulmonary effecs of propofol anesthesia in chickens (*Gallus gallus*). *J Avian Med Surg* 1997; **11**: 93–97.

196 Santos EA, Monteiro ER, Herrera JR, *et al.* Total intravenous anesthesia in domestic chicken (*Gallus gallus domesticus*) with propofol alone or in combination with methadone, nalbuphine or fentanyl for ulna osteotomy. *Vet Anaesth Analg* 2020; **47**(3): 347–355.

197 Schumacher J, Citino SB, Hernandez K, *et al.* Cardiopulmonary and anesthetic effects of propofol in wild turkeys. *Am J Vet Res* 1997; **58**(9): 1014–1017.

198 Clippinger TL, Platt SR, Bennett RA, *et al.* Electrodiagnostic evaluation of peripheral nerve function in rheas and barred owls. *Am J Vet Res* 2000; **61**(4): 469–472.

199 Bigby SE, Carter JE, Bauquier S, *et al.* Use of propofol for induction and maintenance of anesthesia in a king penguin (*Aptenodytes patagonicus*) undergoing magnetic resonance imaging. *J Avian Med Surg* 2016; **30**(3): 237–242.

200 Mulcahy DM, Gartrell B, Gill RE, *et al.* Coelomic implantation of satellite transmitters in the bar-tailed godwit (*Limosa lapponica*) and the bristle-thighed curlew (*numenius tahitiensis*) using propofol, bupivacaine, and lidocaine. *J Zoo Wildl Med* 2011; **42**(1): 54–64.

201 Escalante GC, Balko JA, Chinnadurai SK. Comparison of the sedative effects of alfaxalone and butorphanol–midazolam administered intramuscularly in budgerigars (*Melopsittacus undulatus*). *J Avian Med Surg* 2018; **32**(4): 279–285.

202 Balko JA, Lindemann DM, Allender MC, *et al.* Evaluation of the anesthetic and cardiorespiratory effects of intramuscular alfaxalone administration and isoflurane in budgerigars (*Melopsittacus undulatus*) and comparison with manual restraint. *J Am Vet Med Assoc* 2019; **254**(12): 1427–1435.

203 Romano J, Hasse K, Johnston M. Sedative, cardiorespiratory, and thermoregulatory effects of alfaxalone on budgerigars (*Melopsittacus undulatus*). *J Zoo Wildl Med* 2020; **51**(1): 96–101.

204 Whitehead MC, Hoppes SM, Musser JMB, *et al.* The use of alfaxalone in Quaker parrots (*Myiopsitta monachus*). *J Avian Med Surg* 2019; **33**(4): 340–348.

205 Greunz EM, Limon D, Bertelsen MF. Alfaxalone sedation in black-cheeked lovebirds (*Agapornis nigrigenis*) for non-invasive procedures. *J Avian Med Surg* 2021; **35**(2): 161–166.

206 White DM, Martinez-Taboada F. Induction of anesthesia with intravenous alfaxalone in two Isa brown chickens (*Gallus gallus domesticus*). *J Exot Pet Med* 2019; **29**: 119–122.

207 Alatrushi AN, Naser AS. The safety profile of the anesthetic effect of alfaxalone and its interaction with xylazine and ketamine in chick's model (*Gallus gallus domesticus*). *Mac Vet Rev* 2021; **44**(2): 203–209.

208 Hasse K, Crawford A, Gustafson D, *et al.* Plasma concentration and pharmacodynamics of intramuscular administration of alfaxalone in Indian peafowl (*Pavo cristatus*). *J Zoo Wildl Med* 2022; **53**(1): 108–115.

209 Kruse TN, Messenger KM, Bowman AS, *et al.* Pharmacokinetics and pharmacodynamics of alfaxalone after a single intramuscular or intravascular injection in mallard ducks (*Anas platyrhynchos*). *J Vet Pharmacol Ther* 2019; **42**(6): 713–721.

210 Baldrey V, Stanford M, Bacon H. A comparison of the pharmacodynamic effects of intravenous ketamine–xylazine with alfaxalone in mute swans (*Cygnus olor*) presenting at a wildlife veterinary hospital. *Vet Anaesth Analg* 2021; **48**(5): 716–724.

211 Kilic N. Clinical evaluation of alfaxalone in cyclodextrin as an intravenous anesthetic in the common buzzards (*Buteo buteo*). *Iran J Vet Surg* 2021; **16**(1): 24–28.

212 Mastakov A, Henning J, de Gier R, *et al.* Induction of general anesthesia with alfaxalone in the domestic chicken. *J Avian Med Surg* 2021; **35**(3): 269–279.

213 Joyner PH, Jones MP, Ward D, *et al.* Induction and recovery characteristics and cardiopulmonary effects of sevoflurane and isoflurane in bald eagles. *Am J Vet Res* 2008; **69**(1): 13–22.

214 Granone TD, de Francisco ON, Killos MB, *et al.* Comparison of three different inhalant anesthetic agents (isoflurane, sevoflurane, desflurane) in red-tailed hawks (*Buteo jamaicensis*). *Vet Anaesth Analg* 2012; **39**(1): 29–37.

215 Chan FT, Chang GR, Wang HC, *et al.* Anesthesia with isoflurane and sevoflurane in the crested serpent eagle (*Spilornis cheela hoya*): minimum anesthetic concentration, physiological effects, hematocrit, plasma chemistry and behavioral effects. *J Vet Med Sci* 2013; **75**(12): 1591–1600.

216 Quasha AL, Eger EI II, Tinker JH. Determination and applications of MAC. *Anesthesiology* 1980; **53**(4): 315–334.

217 Ludders JW, Rode J, Mitchell GS. Isoflurane anesthesia in sandhill cranes (*Grus canadensis*): minimal anesthetic concentration and cardiopulmonary dose-response during spontaneous and controlled breathing. *Anesth Analg* 1989; **68**(4): 511–516.

218 Eger EI. *Isoflurane: A Compendium and Reference*. Madison, WI: Anaquest, a Division of BOC, 1985: 143.

219 Steffey EP. Inhalation anesthetics. In: Thurmon JC, Tranquilli WJ, Benson GJ, eds. *Lumb & Jones' Veterinary Anesthesia*, 3rd edn. Baltimore, MD: Williams & Wilkins, 1996: 297–329.

220 de Paula VV, Otsuki DA, Auler Jo J, *et al.* The effect of premedication with ketamine, alone or with diazepam, on anaesthesia with sevoflurane in parrots (*Amazona aestiva*). *BMC Vet Res* 2013; **9**(1): 142.

221 Mercado JA, Larsen RS, Wack RF, *et al.* Minimum anesthetic concentration of isoflurane in captive thick-billed parrots (*Rhynchopsitta pachyrhyncha*). *Am J Vet Res* 2008; **69**(2): 189–194.

222 Phair KA, Larsen RS, Wack RF, *et al.* Determination of the minimum anesthetic concentration of sevoflurane in thick-billed parrots (*Rhynchopsitta pachyrhyncha*). *Am J Vet Res* 2012; **73**(9): 1350–1355.

223 Escobar A, da Rocha RW, Midon M, *et al.* Effects of tramadol on the minimum anesthetic concentration of isoflurane in white-eyed parakeets (*psittacara leucophthalmus*). *J Zoo Wildl Med* 2017; **48**(2): 380–387.

224 Zaheer OA, Sanchez A, Beaufrère H. Minimum anesthetic concentration of isoflurane and sparing effect of midazolam in Quaker parrots (*Myiopsitta monachus*). *Vet Anaesth Analg* 2020; **47**(3): 341–346.

225 Ludders JW, Mitchell GS, Schaefer SL. Minimum anesthetic dose and cardiopulmonary dose response for halothane in chickens. *Am J Vet Res* 1988; **49**(6): 929–932.

226 Naganobu K, Hagio M. Dose-related cardiovascular effects of isoflurane in chickens during controlled ventilation. *J Vet Med Sci* 2000; **62**(4): 435–437.

227 Naganobu K, Fujisawa Y, Ohde H, *et al.* Determination of the minimum anesthetic concentration and cardiovascular dose response for sevoflurane in chickens during controlled ventilation. *Vet Surg* 2000; **29**(1): 102–105.

228 Kim YK, Lee SS, Suh EH, *et al.* Minimum anesthetic concentration and cardiovascular dose-response relationship of isoflurane in cinereous vultures (*Aegypius monachus*). *J Zoo Wildl Med* 2011; **42**(3): 499–503.

229 Ludders JW. Minimal anesthetic concentration and cardiopulmonary dose-response of halothane in ducks. *Vet Surg* 1992; **21**(4): 319–324.

230 Ludders JW, Mitchell GS, Rode J. Minimal anesthetic concentration and cardiopulmonary dose response of isoflurane in ducks. *Vet Surg* 1990; **19**(4): 304–307.

231 Escobar A, Valadao CA, Brosnan RJ, *et al.* Effects of butorphanol on the minimum anesthetic concentration for sevoflurane in guineafowl (*Numida meleagris*). *Am J Vet Res* 2012; **73**(2): 183–188.

232 Botman J, Gabriel F, Dugdale AH, *et al.* Anaesthesia with sevoflurane in pigeons: minimal anaesthetic concentration (MAC) determination and investigation of cardiorespiratory variables at 1 MAC. *Vet Rec* 2016; **178**(22): 560–565.

233 Naganobu K, Hagio M, Sonoda T, *et al.* Arrhythmogenic effect of hypercapnia in ducks anesthetized with halothane. *Am J Vet Res* 2001; **62**(1): 127–129.

234 Arnall L. Anaesthesia and surgery in cage and aviary birds (I). *Vet Rec* 1961; **73**: 139.

235 Korbel R, Burike S, Erhardt W, *et al.* Effects of nitrous oxide application in racing pigeons (*Columbia livia* gmel., 1789, var. dom.) A study using the air sac perfusion technique. *Israel J Vet Med* 1996; **51**(3/4): 133–139.

236 Hawkins MG, Guzman DS-M, Beaufrère H, *et al.* Birds. In: Carpenter JW, Marion CJ, eds. *Exotic Animal Formulary*, 5th edn: WB Saunders, 2018: 167–375.

237 Reynold WT. Unusual anesthetic complication in a pelican. *Vet Rec* 1983; **113**: 204.

238 Nicholson A, Ilkiw JE. Neuromuscular and cardiovascular effects of atracurium in isoflurane-anesthetized chickens. *Am J Vet Res* 1992; **53**(12): 2337–2342.

239 Martin-Flores M, Lau EJ, Campoy L, *et al.* Twitch potentiation: a potential source of error during neuromuscular monitoring with acceleromyography in anesthetized dogs. *Vet Anaesth Analg* 2011; **38**(4): 328–335.

240 McMurphy RM, Davidson HJ, Hodgson DS. Effects of atracurium on intraocular pressure, eye position, and blood pressure in eucapnic and hypocapnic isoflurane-anesthetized dogs. *Am J Vet Res* 2004; **65**(2): 179–182.

241 Mikaelian I, Paillet I, Williams D. Comparative use of various mydriatic drugs in kestrels (*Falco tinnunculus*). *Am J Vet Res* 1994; **55**(2): 270–272.

242 Ramer JC, Paul-Murphy JR, Brunson D, *et al.* Effects of mydriatic agents in cockatoos, African gray parrots, and Blue-fronted Amazon parrots. *J Am Vet Med Assoc* 1996; **208**(2): 227–230.

243 Thompson HM. Avian serum esterases: species and temporal variations and their possible consequences. *Chem Biol Interact* 1993; **87**(1–3): 329–338.

244 Loerzel SM, Smith PJ, Howe A, *et al.* Vecuronium bromide, phenylephrine and atropine combinations as mydriatics in juvenile double-crested cormorants (*Phalacrocorax auritus*). *Vet Ophthalmol* 2002; **5**(3): 149–154.

245 Susanti L, Kang S, Lee E, *et al.* Efficacy of topical rocuronium bromide as a mydriatic agent in domestic pigeons (*Columba livia*). *J Vet Med Sci* 2021; **83**(3): 501–506.

246 Barsotti G, Briganti A, Spratte JR, *et al.* Safety and *Efficacy of Bilateral Topical Application of Rocuronium Bromide for Mydriasis in* European kestrels (*Falco tinnunculus*). *J Avian Med Surg* 2012; **26**(1): 1–5.

247 Barsotti G, Briganti A, Spratte JR, *et al.* Bilateral mydriasis in common buzzards (*Buteo buteo*) and little owls (*Athene noctua*) induced by concurrent topical administration of rocuronium bromide. *Vet Ophthalmol* 2010; **13**(Suppl): 35–40.

248 Barsotti G, Briganti A, Spratte JR, *et al.* Mydriatic effect of topically applied rocuronium bromide in tawny owls (*Strix aluco*): comparison between two protocols. *Vet Ophthalmol* 2010; **13**(Suppl): 9–13.

249 Cantero F, Ortillés Á, Peña MT, *et al.* Safety and efficacy of unilateral topical application of rocuronium bromide in healthy scops owls (*Otus scops*). *Vet Ophthalmol* 2021; **24**(2): 169–176.

250 Barsotti G, Asti M, Giani E, *et al.* Effect of topical ophthalmic instillation of rocuronium bromide on the intraocular pressure of kestrels (*Falco tinnunculus*) and little owls (*Athene noctuae*). *J Am Vet Med Assoc* 2019; **255**(12): 1359–1364.

251 Baine K, Hendrix DV, Kuhn SE, *et al.* The efficacy and safety of topical rocuronium bromide to induce bilateral mydriasis in Hispaniolan Amazon parrots (*Amazona ventralis*). *J Avian Med Surg* 2016; **30**(1): 8–13.

252 Petritz OA, Guzman DS, Gustavsen K, *et al.* Evaluation of the mydriatic effects of topical administration of rocuronium bromide in Hispaniolan Amazon parrots (*Amazona ventralis*). *J Am Vet Med Assoc* 2016; **248**(1): 67–71.

253 Christensen J, Fosse RT, Halvorsen OJ, *et al.* Comparison of various anesthetic regimens in the domestic fowl. *Am J Vet Res* 1987; **48**(11): 1649–1657.

254 Belant JL, Seamans TW. Comparison of three formulations of alpha-chloralose for immobilization of Canada geese. *J Wildl Dis* 1997; **33**(3): 606–610.

255 Belant JL, Seamans TW. Alpha-chloralose immobilization of rock doves in Ohio. *J Wildl Dis* 1999; **35**(2): 239–242.

256 Hartup BK, Schneider L, Engels JM, *et al.* Capture of sandhill cranes using alpha-chloralose: a 10-year follow-up. *J Wildl Dis* 2014; **50**(1): 143–145.

257 Businga NK, Langenberg J, Carlson L. Successful treatment of capture myopathy in three wild greater sandhill cranes (*Grus canadensis tabida*). *J Avian Med Surg* 2007; **21**(4): 294–298.

258 Sedgwick CJ. Anesthesia of caged birds. In: Kirk R, ed. *Current Veterinary Therapy VII*, 7th edn. Philadelphia, PA: WB Saunders, 1980: 653–656.

259 Roberson DW, Alosi JA, Messana EP, *et al.* Endotracheal isoflurane anesthesia for chick auditory surgery. *Hear Res* 2000; **141**: 165–168.

260 Sykes JM, Neiffer D, Terrell S, *et al.* Review of 23 cases of postintubation tracheal obstructions in birds. *J Zoo Wildl Med* 2013; **44**(3): 700–713.

261 Ludders JW, Matthews N. Avian anesthesia. In: Thurmon J, Benson J, Tranquilli W, eds. *Lumb and Jones' Veterinary Anesthesia*, 3rd edn. Baltimore, MD: Williams & Wilkins, 1996: 645–669.

262 Bednarski RM, Ludders JW, LeBlanc PH, *et al.* Isoflurane-nitrous oxide-oxygen anesthesia in an Andean condor. *J Am Vet Med Assoc* 1985; **187**(11): 1209–1210.

263 Hollwarth AJ, Pestell ST, Byron-Chance DH, *et al.* Mortality outcomes based on ASA grade in avian patients undergoing general anesthesia. *J Exot Pet Med* 2022; **41**: 14–19.

264 Butler PJ. The exercise response and the "classical" diving response during natural submersion in birds and mammals. *Can J Zool* 1988; **66**: 29–39.

265 Furilla RA, Jones DR. The contribution of nasal receptors to the cardiac response to diving in restrained and unrestrained redhead ducks (*Aythya americana*). *J Exp Biol* 1986; **121**(1): 227–238.

266 Jones DR, Furilla RA, Heieis MRA, *et al.* Forced and voluntary diving in ducks: cardiovascular adjustments and their control. *Can J Zool* 1988; **66**(1): 75–83.

267 Woakes AJ. Metabolism in diving birds: studies in the laboratory and the field. *Can J Zool* 1988; **66**: 138.

268 Jones DR, Bryan RM, West NH, *et al.* Regional distribution of blood flow during diving in the duck (*Anas platyrhynchos*). *Can J Zool* 1979; **57**(5): 995–1002.

269 Wijnberg ID, Lagerweij E, Zwart P. Inhalation anaesthesia in birds through the abdominal air sac, using a unidirectional, continuous flow. *4th International Congress of Veterinary Anaesthesia*. Utrecht, NL, 1991.

270 Hirshman CA, McCullough RE, Cohen PJ, *et al.* Hypoxic ventilatory drive in dogs during thiopental, ketamine, or pentobarbital anesthesia. *Anesthesiology* 1975; **43**(6): 628–634.

271 Hirshman CA, McCullough RE, Cohen PJ, *et al.* Depression of hypoxic ventilatory response by halothane, enflurane and isoflurane in dogs. *Br J Anaesth* 1977; **49**(10): 957–963.

272 Pavlin EG, Hornbein TF. Anesthesia and the control of ventilation. In: Cherniak NS, Widdicombe JG, eds. *Handbook of Physiology: The Respiratory System*. Bethesda, MA: American Physiological Society, 1986: 972.

273 Bagshaw RJ, Cox RH. Baroreceptor control of heart rate in chickens (*Gallus domesticus*). *Am J Vet Res* 1986; **47**: 293.

274 Molony V. Classification of vagal afferents firing in phase with breathing in Gallus domesticus. *Respir Physiol* 1974; **22**(1–2): 57–76.

275 Pizarro J, Ludders JW, Douse MA, *et al.* Halothane effects on ventilatory responses to changes in intrapulmonary CO2 in geese. *Respir Physiol* 1990; **82**(3): 337–347.

276 Pettifer GR, Cornick-Seahorn J, Smith JA, *et al.* The comparative cardiopulmonary effects of spontaneous and controlled ventilation by using the Hallowell EMC Anesthesia Work Station in Hispaniolan Amazon parrots (*Amazona ventralis*). *J Avian Med Surg* 2002; **16**(4): 268–276.

277 Piiper J, Drees F, Scheid P. Gas exchange in the domestic fowl during spontaneous breathing and artificial ventilation. *Respir Physiol* 1970; **9**: 234.

278 Burger RE, Lorenz FW. Artificial respiration in birds by unidirectional air flow. *Poult Sci* 1960; **39**: 236–237.

279 Burger RE, Meyer M, Graf W, *et al.* Gas exchange in the parabronchial lung of birds: experiments in unidirectionally ventilated ducks. *Respir Physiol* 1979; **36**(1): 19–37.

280 Jaensch SM, Cullen L, Raidal SR. Air sac functional anatomy of the sulphur-crested cockatoo (Cacatua galerita) during isoflurane anesthesia. *J Avian Med Surg* 2002; **16**(1): 2–9.

281 Whittow GC, Ossorio N. A new technic for anesthetizing birds. *Lab Anim Care* 1970; **20**(4 Pt 1): 651–656.

282 Nilson PC, Teramitsu I, White SA. Caudal thoracic air sac cannulation in zebra finches for isoflurane anesthesia. *J Neurosci Methods* 2005; **143**(2): 107–115.

283 Rode J, Bartholow S, Ludders JW. Ventilation through an air sac cannula during tracheal obstruction in ducks. *J Assoc Avian Vet* 1990; **4**(2): 98–102.

284 Escobar A, Thiesen R, Vitaliano SN, *et al.* Some cardiopulmonary effects of sevoflurane in crested caracara (*Caracara plancus*). *Vet Anaesth Analg* 2009; **36**(5): 436–441.

285 Jaensch SM, Cullen L, Raidal SR. Comparative cardiopulmonary effects of halothane and isoflurane in galahs (*Eolophus roseicapillus*). *J Avian Med Surg* 1999; **13**(1): 15–22.

286 Naganobu K, Ise K, Miyamoto T, *et al.* Sevoflurane anaesthesia in chickens during spontaneous and controlled ventilation. *Vet Rec* 2003; **152**(2): 45–48.

287 Seok SH, Jeong DH, Hong IH, *et al.* Cardiorespiratory dose-response relationship of isoflurane in Cinereous vulture (*Aegypius monachus*) during spontaneous ventilation. *J Vet Med Sci* 2017; **79**(1): 160–165.

288 Regan MJ, Eger EI. Effect of hypothermia in dogs on anesthetizing and apneic doses of inhalation agents. Determination of the anesthetic index (Apnea/MAC). *Anesthesiology* 1967; **28**(4): 689–700.

289 Steffey EP, Howland D Jr. Isoflurane potency in the dog and cat. *Am J Vet Res* 1977; **38**(11): 1833–1836.

290 Steffey EP, Howland D Jr., Giri S, *et al.* Enflurane, halothane, and isoflurane potency in horses. *Am J Vet Res* 1977; **38**(7): 1037–1039.

291 Midon M, Escobar A, Yamada DI, *et al.* Isoflurane respiratory anesthetic index in chickens (*gallus gallus domesticus*). *J Zoo Wildl Med* 2021; **52**(1): 327–331.

292 Edling TM, Degernes LA, Flammer K, *et al.* Capnographic monitoring of anesthetized African grey parrots receiving intermittent positive pressure ventilation. *J Am Vet Med Assoc* 2001; **219**(12): 1714–1718.

293 Desmarchelier M, Rondenay Y, Fitzgerald G, *et al.* Monitoring of the ventilatory status of anesthetized birds of prey by using end-tidal carbon dioxide measured with a microstream capnometer. *J Zoo Wildl Med* 2007; **38**(1): 1–6.

294 Pare M, Ludders JW, Erb HN. Association of partial pressure of carbon dioxide in expired gas and arterial blood at three different ventilation states in apneic chickens (*Gallus domesticus*) during air sac insufflation anesthesia. *Vet Anaesth Analg* 2013; **40**(3): 245–256.

295 Raghav R, Middleton R, Ahamed R, *et al.* Analysis of arterial and venous blood gases in healthy Gyr Falcons (*Falco rusticolus*) under anesthesia. *J Avian Med Surg* 2015; **29**(4): 290–297.

296 Schmitt PM, Gobel T, Trautvetter E. Evaluation of pulse oximetry as a monitoring method in avian anesthesia. *J Avian Med Surg* 1998; **12**(2): 91–99.

297 Ivy CM, York JM, Lague SL, *et al.* Validation of a pulse oximetry system for high-altitude waterfowl by examining the hypoxia responses of the Andean goose (*Chloephaga melanoptera*). *Physiol Biochem Zool* 2018; **91**(3): 859–867.

298 King AS, Payne DC. Normal breathing and the effects of posture in *Gallus domesticus*. *J Physiol* 1964; **174**: 340–347.

299 Malka S, Hawkins MG, Jones JH, *et al.* Effect of body position on respiratory system volumes in anesthetized red-tailed hawks (*Buteo jamaicensis*) as measured via computed tomography. *Am J Vet Res* 2009; **70**(9): 1155–1160.

300 Hawkins MG, Malka S, Pascoe PJ, *et al.* Evaluation of the effects of dorsal versus lateral recumbency on the cardiopulmonary system during anesthesia with isoflurane in red-tailed hawks (*Buteo jamaicensis*). *Am J Vet Res* 2013; **74**(1): 136–143.

301 Nevitt BN, Langan JN, Adkesson MJ, *et al.* Comparison of air sac volume, lung volume, and lung densities determined by use of computed tomography in conscious and anesthetized Humboldt penguins (*Spheniscus humboldti*) positioned in ventral, dorsal, and right lateral recumbency. *Am J Vet Res* 2014; **75**(8): 739–745.

302 Nap AMP, Lumeij JT, Stokhof AA. Electrocardiogram of the African grey (*Psittacus erithacus*) and Amazon (*Amazona spp.*) parrot. *Avian Pathol* 1992; **21**(1): 45–53.

303 Cinar A, Bagci C, Belge F, *et al.* The electrocardiogram of the Pekin duck. *Avian Dis* 1996; **40**(4): 919–923.

304 Rodriguez R, Prieto-Montana F, Montes AM, *et al.* The normal electrocardiogram of the unanesthetized peregrine falcon (Falco peregrinus brookei). *Avian Dis* 2004; **48**(2): 405–409.

305 Talavera J, Guzman MJ, del Palacio MJ, *et al.* The normal electrocardiogram of four species of conscious raptors. *Res Vet Sci* 2008; **84**(1): 119–125.

306 Hassanpour H, Zarei H, Nasiri L, *et al.* Electrocardiogram analysis of the golden (*Chrysolophus pictus*) and silver (*Lophura nycthemera*) pheasants. *J Zoo Wildl Med* 2018; **49**(4): 881–886.

307 Goelz MF, Hahn AW, Kelley ST. Effects of halothane and isoflurane on mean arterial blood pressure, heart rate, and respiratory rate in adult Pekin ducks. *Am J Vet Res* 1990; **51**(3): 458–460.

308 Greenlees KJ, Clutton RE, Larsen CT, *et al.* Effect of halothane, isoflurane, and pentobarbital anesthesia on myocardial irritability in chickens. *Am J Vet Res* 1990; **51**(5): 757–758.

309 Zehnder AM, Hawkins MG, Pascoe PJ, *et al.* Evaluation of indirect blood pressure monitoring in awake and anesthetized red-tailed hawks (*Buteo jamaicensis*): effects of cuff size, cuff placement, and monitoring equipment. *Vet Anaesth Analg* 2009; **36**(5): 464–479.

310 Johnston MS, Davidowski LA, Rao S, *et al.* Precision of repeated, Doppler-derived indirect blood pressure measurements in conscious psittacine birds. *J Avian Med Surg* 2011; **25**(2): 83–90.

311 Acierno MJ, da Cunha A, Smith J, *et al.* Agreement between direct and indirect blood pressure measurements obtained from anesthetized Hispaniolan Amazon parrots. *J Am Vet Med Assoc* 2008; **233**(10): 1587–1590.

312 Schnellbacher R, da Cunha A, Olson EE, *et al.* Arterial catheterization, interpretation, and treatment of arterial blood pressures and blood gases in birds. *J Exot Pet Med* 2014; **23**(2): 129–141.

313 Comolli J, d'Ovidio D, Adami C, *et al.* Technological advances in exotic pet anesthesia and analgesia. *Vet Clin North Am Exot Anim Pract* 2019; **22**(3): 419–439.

314 Schnellbacher RW, da Cunha AF, Beaufrère H, *et al.* Effects of dopamine and dobutamine on isoflurane-induced hypotension in Hispaniolan Amazon parrots (*Amazona ventralis*). *Am J Vet Res* 2012; **73**(7): 952–958.

315 Brady K, Hudson A, Hood R, *et al.* Personalizing the definition of hypotension to protect the brain. *Anesthesiology* 2020; **132**(1): 170–179.

316 Beaufrère H, Acierno MJ, Mitchell M, *et al.* Plasma osmolality reference values in African grey parrots (*Psittacus erithacus erithacus*), Hispaniolan Amazon parrots (*Amazona ventralis*), and red-fronted macaws (*Ara rubrogenys*). *J Avian Med Surg* 2011; **25**(2): 91–96.

317 Hawkins MG, Griffenhagen GM. Raptor sedation and anesthesia. *Vet Clin North Am Exotic Anim Pract* 2022; **25**(1): 135–161.

318 Phalen DN, Mitchell ME, Cavazos-Martinez ML. Evaluation of three heat sources for their ability to maintain core body temperature in the anesthetized avian patient. *J Avian Med Surg* 1996; **10**(3): 174–178.

319 Rembert MS, Smith JA, Hosgood G, *et al.* Comparison of traditional thermal support devices with the forced-air warmer system in anesthetized Hispaniolan Amazon parrots (*Amazona ventralis*). *J Avian Med Surg* 2001; **15**(3): 187–193.

320 Boedeker NC, Carpenter JW, Mason DE. Comparison of body temperatures of pigeons (*Columba livia*) anesthetized by three different anesthetic delivery systems. *J Avian Med Surg* 2005; **19**(1): 1–6.

SECTION 8

Anesthesia and Analgesia for Domestic Species

59 Dogs and Cats

Carolina H. Riccó Pereira and Phillip Lerche
Department of Veterinary Clinical Sciences, College of Veterinary Medicine, The Ohio State University, Columbus, Ohio, USA

Chapter contents

Introduction, 1157
Preanesthetic considerations, 1158
  Signalment, 1158
  History, 1158
  Physical examination, 1158
  Laboratory evaluation, 1158
  Physical status, 1159
Patient preparation, 1159
  Fasting, 1159
  Patient stabilization, 1159
Anesthetic and analgesic plan, 1159
  Short-term anesthesia (less than 15 min), 1159
  Intermediate-term anesthesia (15 min to 1 h), 1162
  Long-term anesthesia (longer than 1 h), 1162
Premedication, 1162
Induction, 1162
  Chamber or mask inhalant induction, 1163
  Intravenous high-dose opioid induction, 1163
Anesthetic maintenance, 1163
The anesthetic record, 1163
Perioperative analgesia, 1163
Recovery, 1164
Delayed anesthetic recovery, 1164
Acknowledgment, 1165
References, 1165

Introduction

The selection of a particular anesthetic plan is predicated upon the patient's physical status and temperament, the type of procedure for which anesthesia is being considered, anticipated degree of perioperative pain, the familiarity of the anesthetist with the anesthetic drugs, the type of facility and equipment available, the personnel available for assistance, and the cost of anesthetic drugs [1,2]. There is no single best method for anesthetizing dogs or cats, and familiarity with just one anesthetic technique at best limits a veterinarian's ability to perform the myriad of surgical and diagnostic procedures commonly performed in a modern veterinary practice and at worst results in unnecessary risk to the patient. A debilitated dog or cat undergoing extensive repair of a fractured limb will require a different anesthetic regimen than one undergoing routine neutering, one requiring short-term restraint for radiography, or a geriatric patient requiring extensive dental surgery.

General anesthesia is characterized by muscle relaxation, unconsciousness, amnesia, and analgesia. It is difficult for a single drug to provide all of these elements without causing significant disturbances to patient homeostasis. Inhalant anesthetics come closest to satisfying all of these conditions, but even they are more useful when co-administered with anesthetic adjunctive drugs such as sedatives, opioids, local anesthetics, or hypnotics. As a general rule, when formulating an anesthetic plan, it is best to consider using relatively low doses of several different drugs rather than a large dose of a single drug. For example, apnea resulting from a large bolus of propofol can be eliminated, or its duration shortened, by prior administration of opioids, acepromazine, benzodiazepines, or α_2-adrenergic receptor agonists, which allows administration of a lower propofol dose [3]. The opioid drugs, while important components of modern anesthetic regimens, by themselves do not produce general anesthesia [4]. Muscle rigidity, salivation, and long recoveries associated with large dosages of ketamine can be lessened when the latter is combined in reduced doses with opioids, α_2-adrenergic receptor agonists, and hypnotic drugs such as benzodiazepines [5].

Any plan for procedural sedation or general anesthesia must include a provision to control pain if it is present or anticipated. A good analgesic regimen should include drugs sufficient to ensure analgesia during and after the procedure. The one aspect that should not vary among anesthetic procedures is the degree of vigilance associated with monitoring an anesthetized dog or cat. Early warning of impending anesthetic difficulty is the single most important factor responsible for decreasing anesthetic-related morbidity and mortality.

Consideration should also be given to the use of anesthetic checklists to improve patient outcomes [1].

Veterinary Anesthesia and Analgesia: The Sixth Edition of Lumb and Jones. Edited by Leigh Lamont, Kurt Grimm, Sheilah Robertson, Lydia Love and Carrie Schroeder.
© 2024 John Wiley & Sons, Inc. Published 2024 by John Wiley & Sons, Inc.
Companion website: www.wiley.com/go/lamont/anesthesia

Preanesthetic considerations

Recording a thorough history and conducting the physical and laboratory evaluation are the most important components of a preanesthetic evaluation. Even young, seemingly healthy, animals presenting for routine procedures, such as neutering, require both. These animals may have never been examined previously by a veterinarian, and congenital disorders, severe parasitism, or heartworm disease may be discovered.

Signalment

Review of patient signalment is a key preanesthetic consideration (Box 59.1). Anesthesiologists are often questioned about "sensitivity to anesthesia" in a variety of dog and cat breeds. Although several breed-associated anesthesia concerns (e.g., predisposition to hereditary diseases that increase anesthetic risk) have been documented, all breeds have been successfully anesthetized by using standard anesthetic regimens, and most reports of "sensitivities" are anecdotal. An assessment of the validity of information relating to anesthesia in dogs on the World Wide Web reported that information was often incomplete, and that breed sensitivities mentioned were not supported by scientific evidence [6]. One well-documented breed-associated anesthetic concern is the altered pharmacokinetics of barbiturates and propofol in certain sighthounds, which is associated with a mutation in cytochrome P450 CYB2B11 enzyme expression [7–9]. Another is brachycephalic breeds and their associated airway anatomic malformations. This presents a concern for ensuring a patent airway throughout the perianesthetic period. There is also evidence that these breeds possess greater resting vagal tone, heightening the concern for anesthetic-induced bradycardia [10]. Anesthetic risk has been shown to increase in these breeds as body weight decreases and as duration of anesthetic increases, with the incidence of intra- and postoperative complications being 1.6 and 4.3 times greater than in non-brachycephalic dogs, respectively [11]. Since toy breeds have a greater surface area to body mass ratio and have a relatively greater metabolic rate, they require careful attention to maintenance of body heat and blood glucose concentrations. Additionally, they require a relatively greater dose of drugs on a per-kilogram basis than larger dogs. Reduced doses of some drugs (acepromazine, butorphanol, maropitant, and ondansetron) should be used in breeds that are known to have the ABCB1 gene (formerly known as "MDR1") [12]. Further information about canine breed-specific anesthetic considerations is available in Chapter 50. Generally, there are no sex-related differences in the response to anesthesia. However, a history of the estrus cycle will often identify recent estrus and thus alert the clinician to the concerns associated with an enlarged and vascularized uterus. This would potentially cause concern regarding blood loss during an ovariohysterectomy. Additionally, the owner of an intact female animal should be queried about the possibility of their animal being pregnant because the stress of surgery and anesthesia may adversely affect the fetus(es), and pregnancy can affect multiple body systems (see Chapter 45).

Age is an important anesthetic consideration. Generally, the very young (less than 8 weeks old) and the aged (more than 80% of their expected lifespan) do not metabolize anesthetic drugs as rapidly as healthy adult animals [13]. Healthy geriatric patients may only require 25–50% of the dose of sedatives, hypnotics, tranquilizers, and opioids given to comparable young, healthy animals.

Box 59.1 Signalment and history, including questions of organ system function.

1 **Signalment**
 i Age
 ii Breed
 iii Sex
2 **Body weight**
3 **Duration of ongoing complaint**
4 **Concurrent medications**
 i Angiotensin-converting enzyme inhibitors
 ii H_2 blockers
 iii Antibiotics: aminoglycosides
 iv Cardiac glycosides
 v Phenobarbital
 vi Non-steroidal anti-inflammatory drugs
 vii Calcium channel blockers
 viii β-blockers
 ix Tricyclic antidepressants
5 **Signs of organ system disease**
 i Diarrhea
 ii Vomiting
 iii Polyuria–polydipsia
 iv Seizures and personality change
 v Exercise intolerance
 vi Coughing and stridor
 vii Weight loss and loss of body condition
6 **Previous anesthesia and allergies**
7 **Duration since last meal**

History

In addition to questions concerning organ system function (Box 59.1), the owner should also be asked about any previous anesthetic episodes, past and present illnesses, and past and current medication history, including history of heartworm prophylaxis [14]. The time elapsed since the last feeding should be noted.

Physical examination

The preanesthetic physical examination should be thorough, with all body systems considered (Box 59.2). Any abnormality discovered by physical examination or suggested by the medical history should be followed with appropriate laboratory or other suitable diagnostic testing. The assessment of an animal's temperament is critical. Vicious or aggressive animals will require a different approach to anesthesia than quiet, cooperative individuals.

Laboratory evaluation

There is no objective evidence supporting age-based or American Society of Anesthesiologists (ASA) physical-status-based (see below) minimum laboratory evaluation requirements [1]. Regardless, the minimum preanesthetic laboratory data suggested for young, healthy dogs are hematocrit and plasma protein. These tests are easy, quick, and inexpensive to perform. Hematocrit is an indicator of hemoglobin concentration, which directly relates to the ability of the blood to transport oxygen to tissues. As a general rule, a hematocrit of less than 20% indicates the need for perioperative administration of blood. Hemoglobin concentration (g/dL) can be approximated by dividing the hematocrit by three.

For elective procedures in middle-aged to older animals, or animals treated chronically with medications that could alter liver or renal function (e.g., non-steroidal anti-inflammatory drugs, phenobarbital, or antineoplastic chemotherapeutics), a complete blood count, urinalysis, and biochemistry profile is recommended. Other laboratory tests should be performed (e.g., thoracic radiographs and/or echocardiography, abdominal radiographs, and/or ultrasound) if the history or physical examination suggests specific organ system disease. A minimum laboratory database prior to emergency anesthesia for a debilitated dog or cat should include packed cell volume, total protein, and electrolytes (sodium, potassium, and chloride).

Box 59.2 Preanesthetic physical examination.

1 **Body weight and body condition**
  i Obesity
  ii Cachexia
  iii Dehydration
2 **Cardiopulmonary**
  i Heart rate and rhythm
  ii Respiratory rate and effort
  iii Auscultation
    a Heart sounds and murmurs
    b Breath sounds
  iv Capillary refill time
  v Mucous membrane color
    a Pallor
    b Cyanosis
  vi Pulse character
3 **Central nervous system and special senses**
  i Temperament
  ii Seizure, coma, and stupor
  iii Vision and hearing
4 **Gastrointestinal**
  i Parasites
  ii Abdominal palpation
5 **Hepatic**
  i Icterus
  ii Abnormal bleeding
6 **Renal**
  i Palpation of kidneys and bladder
7 **Integument**
  i Tumors
  ii Flea infestation
8 **Musculoskeletal**
  i Lameness
  ii Fractures
9 **Pain assessment**
10 **Patient temperament**

Box 59.3 List of conditions that should be corrected prior to anesthesia.

1 **Severe dehydration**
2 **Anemia or hypoproteinemia**
  i Packed cell volume < 20% with acute blood loss
  ii Serum albumin concentration < 2.0 g/dL
3 **Acid–base and electrolyte disturbances**
  i pH < 7.2
  ii Serum potassium concentration < 2.5–3.0 or > 6.0 mEq/L
4 **Pneumothorax**
5 **Cyanosis**
6 **Oliguria or anuria**
7 **Congestive heart failure**
8 **Severe, life-threatening cardiac arrhythmias**

Table 59.1 Physical status classification of veterinary patients.

ASA physical status[a]	Patient description
I	Normal healthy patient
II	Non-incapacitating systemic disease (e.g., obesity, mild dehydration, and simple fractures)
III	Severe systemic disease not incapacitating (e.g., compensated renal insufficiency, stable congestive heart failure, controlled diabetes mellitus, or cesarean section)
IV	Severe systemic disease that is a constant threat to life (e.g., gastric dilation and volvulus)
V	Moribund, not expected to live 24 h irrespective of intervention (e.g., severe uncompensated systemic disturbance)

ASA, American Society of Anesthesiologists.
[a] Procedures performed under emergency conditions are denoted by placing an *E* after the physical status number.

Physical status

Many factors (e.g., age, breed, concurrent disease, surgical procedure, surgeon skill, and available equipment) contribute to the overall anesthetic risk for a given patient. One risk factor is the physical status of the patient. A convenient system of status classification for veterinary patients has been adapted from the ASA [1]. In general, physical status I and II patients appear to be at less risk for anesthetic complications. Physical statuses III–V are usually at greater anesthetic risk. However, this is not to imply that category I and II patients are at no risk from unanticipated anesthetic mishaps (Table 59.1).

Patient preparation

Fasting

Healthy dogs and cats should be fasted for 4–6 h prior to being anesthetized, if possible [1]. Water can be allowed until just prior to anesthesia for most procedures. Dogs and cats less than 8 weeks old should not be fasted longer than 1–2 h because they are at a greater risk for perianesthetic hypoglycemia. They should receive dextrose-containing intravenous (IV) fluids during any prolonged anesthesia (longer than 15 min) and/or serial blood glucose measurements until fully recovered.

Patient stabilization

When possible, life-threatening physiological disturbances should be medically addressed prior to anesthesia (Box 59.3). This may, however, not always be possible, and anesthesia should never be delayed if immediate surgical or medical intervention is needed to save the patient's life.

Anesthetic and analgesic plan

Several aspects should be considered when formulating an anesthetic plan (Box 59.4). In general, techniques for procedural sedation or general anesthesia rely primarily on local anesthesia, injectable anesthesia, or inhalation anesthesia. Regardless, these primary techniques are typically supplemented with some degree of drug-induced sedation and systemically administered analgesics. Techniques frequently overlap. For example, inhalant anesthesia is usually initiated with injectable anesthetics. Local anesthetic nerve blocks are typically performed under general anesthesia or sedation.

The remainder of the discussion regarding the choice of anesthetic and analgesic drugs assumes that the reader has reviewed and is familiar with the clinical pharmacology of the various anesthetic drugs as presented elsewhere in this text. Although the drug combinations described are suitable for a variety of patients, the reader should refer to the appropriate sections of this text or consult a veterinary anesthesiologist if questions remain about how to anesthetize and monitor specific patients. Drug availability can be an issue, so it is best to become familiar with a variety of techniques.

Short-term anesthesia (less than 15 min)

By themselves, sedative–opioid combinations are suitable for short-term restraint for minimally invasive procedures or those procedures not requiring general anesthesia, such as radiography or physical examination in an intractable animal (Tables 59.2 and 59.3). An advantage is that one or both of these components are reversible, allowing a rapid return to preanesthetic mentation and

Box 59.4 Considerations for selecting an anesthetic plan.

1 Procedure to be performed
- **i** Duration
  - **a** < 15 min
  - **b** 15 min – 1 h
  - **c** > 1 h
- **ii** Type of procedure
  - **a** Minor medical or surgical
  - **b** Major invasive surgery
- **iii** Anticipated perioperative pain

2 Available assistance and equipment
- **i** Assistance
  - **a** Ventilatory assist or control
  - **b** Restraint
- **ii** Equipment
  - **a** Anesthetic machine
  - **b** Ventilator
- **iii** Type of inhalant anesthetic
- **iv** Appropriate monitoring and supportive care devices

3 Patient's temperament
- **i** Quiet, relaxed, or calm
- **ii** Nervous and/or excitable
- **iii** Vicious
- **iv** Moribund or comatose

4 Physical status
- **i** ASA category I through V

5 Breed
- **i** Sighthound
- **ii** Brachycephalic
- **iii** Toy/giant breed

Table 59.2 Sedatives and tranquilizers for procedural sedation or premedication.

Drug	Dosage (mg/kg)[a]	Comments
Dexmedetomidine	Dogs, 0.002–0.02 IV, IM Cats, 0.003–0.04 IV, IM	Moderate to deep sedation Duration 60–180 min
Medetomidine–vatinoxan (Zenalpha®)	Dogs, 0.01–0.03 IM	Moderate to deep sedation Duration 30–90 min
Acepromazine	Dogs, 0.02–0.1 IV, IM, SC (3 mg maximum) Cats, 0.02–0.1 IV, IM (1 mg maximum)	Mild to moderate sedation Duration 30–90 min
Midazolam	Dogs, 0.1–0.3 IV, IM (7 mg maximum) Cats, 0.1–0.2 IV, IM	Minimal sedation Most useful when combined with other sedatives, opioids, or ketamine Can cause excitation when given as the sole agent

IM, intramuscular; IV, intravenous; SC, subcutaneous.
[a] Generally the low end of the dosage range is used IV and in sick or debilitated patients.

function (Table 59.4). Any of the short-term injectable drugs discussed below can be added to the sedative–opioid regimen when complete immobilization or general anesthesia is necessary. If potentially painful surgical procedures are attempted under heavy sedation (e.g., laceration repair following dexmedetomidine–butorphanol), a local anesthetic should be incorporated in the plan to reduce the risk of animal arousal due to surgical stimulation.

Several drugs are available for procedural sedation or short-term anesthesia (Tables 59.2, 59.3, 59.5, 59.6, and 59.7). Immobilization for a short duration where strong analgesia is not required (e.g., radiography, suture removal, and otoscopic examination) can be performed most simply with IV injectable drugs such as propofol, alfaxalone, ketamine–propofol, ketamine–midazolam, tiletamine–zolazepam, or etomidate. These drugs induce rapid and predictable short-term loss of consciousness. The duration of action following a single-bolus dose of these drugs is generally less than 15 min, except tiletamine–zolazepam which provides approximately 30 min of chemical restraint, with animals becoming ambulatory 30–60 min post administration. Prior administration of sedative or tranquilizer drugs generally improves the quality of immobilization [15,16].

Table 59.3 Opioids and sedative–opioid combinations.

Drug(s)	Dosage (mg/kg)	Comments
Morphine	Dogs and cats[a], 0.1–0.5 IV (slow), IM, SC	Duration 3–5 h Vomiting Mild sedation Dysphoria can occur when used alone in young, healthy dogs or cats Can precipitate histamine release
Hydromorphone	Dogs and cats[a], 0.1–0.2 IV, IM, SC	Duration 3–5 h Vomiting Mild sedation Dysphoria can occur when used alone in young, healthy dogs or cats
Oxymorphone	Dogs and cats[a], 0.05–0.1 IV, IM, SC	Same as for hydromorphone; less incidence of vomiting
Methadone	Dogs and cats[a], 0.3–0.5 IV, IM, SC	Same as for oxymorphone; minimal incidence of vomiting
Butorphanol	Dogs and cats, 0.2–0.4 IV, IM, SC	Duration 1 hour in dogs; up to 2–3 h in cats Opioid agonist–antagonist Minimal sedation when used alone
Buprenorphine (various formulations)		Partial opioid agonist
0.3 mg/mL injectable	Dogs and cats, 0.01–0.02 IV, IM, SC; oral transmucosal (cats)	Duration 6–8 h
Simbadol® 1.8 mg/mL injectable *(cats only)*	Cats, 0.24 mg/kg SC	Duration 24 h
Zorbium® 20 mg/mL topical/transdermal *(cats only)*	Cats, 1.2–3 kg: 0.4 mL (8 mg); 3–7.5 kg: 1 mL (20 mg), topically	Duration 4 days See manufacturer's guidelines for administration and safe handling practices of this product
Dexmedetomidine–opioid[b]	Dogs, 0.002–0.007 IV, IM Cats, 0.003–0.01 IV, IM	Duration of sedation 30–90 min Both drugs are reversible Can be combined in the same syringe Observe for bradycardia Useful for immobilization of fractious or vicious animals
Acepromazine–opioid[b]	Dogs, 0.02–0.1 IV, IM Cats, 0.02–0.1 IV, IM	Duration of sedation 30–120 min Can be combined in the same syringe Useful for immobilization of fractious or vicious animals
Midazolam–opioid[b]	Dogs, 0.1–0.3 IV, IM Cats, 0.1–0.2 IV, IM	Duration of sedation 40 min Can be combined in the same syringe Generally produces poor results in young, healthy animals Not recommended for immobilization of fractious or vicious animals Better quality restraint in older or debilitated animals

IM, intramuscular; IV, intravenous; SC, subcutaneous.
[a] Use lower end of dosage for this opioid in cats.
[b] Use dosage ranges for opioids listed above.

Table 59.4 Antagonists of various classes of anesthetic drugs.

Drug class being antagonized	Antagonist drug	Dosage (mg/kg)
α_2-Adrenergic receptor agonists	Yohimbine	0.1 IM
	Atipamezole	Dogs, equal volume of administered dose[a] of medetomidine or dexmedetomidine, IM Cats, half the volume of administered dose of medetomidine or dexmedetomidine, IM
Benzodiazepines	Flumazenil	0.01–0.2[b] IV
Opioids	Naloxone	0.002–0.02[c] IV, IM

IM, intramuscular; IV, intravenous.
[a] Dosage in milligrams equals 5 times the previously administered dosage of medetomidine or 10 times the previously administered dosage of dexmedetomidine and Zenalpha®.
[b] Begin with lowest dosage and repeat, if necessary, to effect.
[c] Use lowest dosage for "partial" reversal and highest dosage for complete reversal (see text for explanation).

Table 59.5 Injectable anesthetic drugs.

Drug	Dosage (mg/kg)	Comments
Propofol	4.0–6.0 IV to effect	Duration 5–10 min after single-bolus dose Apnea for several minutes with rapid injection
	0.2–0.8 mg/kg/min CRI	Can be used for maintenance of anesthesia as part of a TIVA protocol
Alfaxalone	1.0–5.0 IV, IM	Duration 5–10 min after single-bolus dose Use lower end of dosage IV after premedication and for anesthetic induction Use larger dosages IM for longer-term immobilization
	0.1–0.2 mg/kg/min CRI	Can be used for maintenance of anesthesia as part of a TIVA protocol
Etomidate	0.5–2.0 IV	Duration 5–10 min Myoclonus, gagging/retching
Ketamine[a]	5.0–10 IV, IM	Duration 10–20 min Typically combined with a benzodiazepine for muscle relaxation (diazepam or midazolam 0.25–0.5 mg/kg)
Telazol® (tiletamine–zolazepam)[a]	1.0–4.0 IV, IM	Duration 30–60 min Muscle relaxation, emergence delirium, hypersalivation, tachycardia
Propofol, Ketamine	2.0 IV, 2.0 IV	Duration 5–10 min after single-bolus dose Less hypotension than with propofol alone
Thiopental[b]	8.0–20.0 IV	Use lower dosage after premedication
Methohexital[c]	3.0–8.0 IV	Duration 3–5 min Muscle rigidity Best if preceded by a sedative or tranquilizer

IM, intramuscular; IV, intravenous; CRI, constant rate infusion; TIVA, total intravenous anesthesia.
[a] Intramuscular ketamine and Telazol®-based combinations for use in cats are provided in Table 59.7.
[b] Thiopental is no longer available in a number of countries, including the United States; it is listed here for completeness.
[c] Methohexital is not commonly used in veterinary anesthesia in the United States; it is listed here for completeness.

Currently, propofol is widely used for short-term immobilization in cats and dogs. Because of its rapid plasma clearance, multiple boluses of propofol, or a propofol constant rate infusion (CRI), can be used to prolong the duration of restraint without significantly prolonging the duration of recovery [15]. Respiratory depression may be significant and ventilatory assistance should be available.

Alfaxalone is a neurosteroid anesthetic drug that produces hypnosis and muscle relaxation by enhancing conduction of the $GABA_A$ receptor. Immobilization is characterized by excellent muscle relaxation and hypnosis in dogs and cats. Although labeled in the United States

Table 59.6 Options for premedication in healthy dogs and cats[a].

Patient type	Premedication
Young, normal, healthy	Acepromazine Dexmedetomidine Either of the above sedatives with an opioid agonist if moderate to severe perioperative pain is anticipated, or for moderate restraint Either of the above with buprenorphine if less intense pain is anticipated, or for moderate restraint Either of the above with butorphanol if minimal pain is anticipated, or for moderate restraint
Aggressive/unpredictable behavior[b]	Acepromazine–opioid agonist combination Dexmedetomidine–opioid agonist combination
Geriatric	Acepromazine (low end of dosage range)–opioid combination Midazolam–opioid combination
Painful procedures	Acepromazine–opioid agonist combination Dexmedetomidine–opioid agonist combination Midazolam–opioid agonist combination

[a] These drugs or drug combinations should be administered intramuscularly 15 to 30 min prior to anesthetic induction.
[b] Can add ketamine 2–5 mg/kg IM to these combinations for additional restraint.

Table 59.7 Examples of intramuscular injectable anesthesia in cats.

Drug	Dosage (mg/kg)	Comments
Telazol®, Dexmedetomidine, Buprenorphine, ± Ketamine (for very aggressive cats)	1–3, 0.005–0.02, 0.01–0.02, 3–5	Duration 30–60 min Adequate protocol for short invasive procedures (ovariohysterectomy, laceration repair, enucleation, wound cleaning, etc.) May result in residual drowsiness for over 24 h
Ketamine, Dexmedetomidine, Opioid, (e.g., Buprenorphine)	5–10, 0.01–0.02, 0.01–0.02	Duration 15–30 min Adequate protocol for minor surgical procedures (castration, small laceration repair, suture removal, etc.), diagnostic procedures (radiographs, ultrasound, blood draw, computed tomography, skin biopsy, etc.), or physical exams in aggressive patients May result in excitement/hyperactivity during recovery phase

for IV induction of anesthesia, it can also be administered intramuscularly (IM) for sedation of dogs and cats. Alfaxalone administered either as a single agent (IM or IV) or combined with other sedatives at higher dosages (5 mg/kg IM) is not recommended given its poor recovery quality [17–19]. However, when lower dosages (1–3 mg/kg IM) combined with additional sedatives are used, these effects are much improved [20–22]. Its duration of action is dose-dependent, and it provides good cardiovascular stability in healthy patients [23,24]. Like propofol, it is compatible for use following commonly used preanesthetic sedatives and tranquilizers to maintain general anesthesia as a CRI [25,26]. Respiratory depression may, however, be significant, and ventilatory assistance should be available [25,26].

A combination of ketamine and midazolam produces less muscle relaxation than propofol, alfaxalone, or propofol–ketamine. In dosages typically used, ketamine–midazolam is also associated with increased salivation and dysphoria upon recovery [5]. However, dissociative anesthetic combinations generally produce less respiratory and cardiovascular depression than other available short-acting injectable anesthetics. Muscle relaxation and recovery quality are improved, and salivation is lessened when dissociatives are given with, or preceded by, a sedative or tranquilizer [5].

While thiopental is no longer available in a number of countries, including the United States, it is relatively inexpensive and suitable for short-term restraint of most healthy dogs and cats. A disadvantage to its use as a sole anesthetic is that relatively large doses are required, full recovery can take up to 1 h, and recovery can be associated with ataxia and disorientation. These undesirable characteristics are reduced when its administration is preceded by a tranquilizer such as acepromazine or a sedative such as dexmedetomidine. Another disadvantage is that it must be administered IV, a problem with fractious or uncooperative animals. Perivascular thiopental administration is associated with local tissue inflammation, pain, and potential tissue necrosis. Perivascular administration should be attended to by infiltrating the area with a crystalloid fluid (e.g., 0.9% sodium chloride) at a volume equal to 3–5 times the volume of perivascularly administered thiopental. Additionally, a local anesthetic such as lidocaine and an anti-inflammatory (e.g., methylprednisolone) may be infiltrated near the site of perivascular injection. Another important side effect of thiopental is the significant respiratory depression that can accompany its use.

The relatively cumbersome nature of inhalation anesthetic delivery makes it inconvenient for use in very short procedures, and its use solely for routine induction of unconsciousness and anesthesia is not recommended. On occasion, it can prove useful for chamber induction of feral or fractious cats. It can also be useful for short-term anesthesia in neonates or those animals with severe organ system compromise and a reduced ability to clear drugs through the kidney or liver. Mask induction with inhalant anesthetics should be preceded by preanesthetic administration whenever possible to reduce the stress and anxiety (and catecholamine release) associated with initial inspiration of high concentrations of inhalant anesthetics. Care should also be taken to minimize environmental contamination and subsequent exposure of veterinary staff to inhalant anesthetic.

Intermediate-term anesthesia (15 min to 1 h)

For procedures of intermediate duration that do not require significant analgesia, the previously discussed drugs suitable for short-term restraint can be used and re-dosed to effect. Typically, one-third to half of the induction dose is administered slowly to prolong the anesthetic effect. Thiopental and ketamine–midazolam should not be re-dosed multiple times. Their initial duration of action following bolus administration depends primarily on redistribution away from the brain to other tissues, such as muscle. However, when these tissues are saturated with drug, redistribution greatly slows, and metabolism becomes the rate-limiting factor for awakening. Propofol and alfaxalone, because of their relatively rapid clearances and large volumes of distribution, can be administered repeatedly to dogs by using small boluses or by CRI (Table 59.5).

Invasive surgical procedures such as canine and feline gonadectomy typically require 15 min to 1 h of anesthesia, accompanied by good perioperative analgesia. Several options are available. Total injectable anesthesia, where a drug combination is injected IV or IM and will last for the duration of the procedure, is suitable for short-term anesthesia in healthy animals, and is frequently used in cats for procedures such as castration and wound care (Table 59.7). A combination of Telazol®, ketamine, and xylazine is suitable for cats, although its use has been associated with relatively prolonged recoveries and it provides minimal postoperative analgesia [27]. An alternative is the combination of dexmedetomidine, ketamine, and an opioid agonist. Inclusion of dexmedetomidine in the combination facilitates antagonism of the α_2-adrenergic agonist's hypnotic and analgesic effects with atipamezole, if required. Inhalation anesthesia following sedation and induction of anesthesia with a rapidly acting injectable drug such as propofol is also appropriate for procedures of intermediate duration and may be the most convenient and most controllable option. Inhalant anesthetic delivery of this duration usually requires endotracheal intubation and careful monitoring but offers the benefit of enabling a rapid adjustment of anesthetic depth should anesthetic conditions change unexpectedly (e.g., loss of blood or respiratory arrest).

Long-term anesthesia (longer than 1 h)

Long procedures are best managed by maintenance with inhalation anesthesia. Awakening from sevoflurane and isoflurane anesthesia is predictably rapid. Even sick and debilitated patients recover from prolonged periods of inhalation anesthesia relatively quickly, and liver or renal impairment does not preclude drug clearance. As an alternative, injectable anesthesia using drugs administered IM or IV has been described (see above) [25–31].

Total intravenous anesthesia (TIVA) can also be used for longer-term anesthetic maintenance. Techniques that involve infusion of propofol or alfaxalone, often in combination with opioids and/or reversible sedatives, are most suited for prolonged anesthesia because propofol and alfaxalone undergo rapid and predictable clearance. Techniques involving infusion or repeated administration of longer-acting, non-reversible drugs, such as Telazol®, are less suited for long procedures as they result in protracted recoveries. Most anesthetic techniques are associated with some degree of respiratory depression and a loss of the protective swallowing reflex, so tracheal intubation and a means to assist ventilation are essential for reducing anesthetic risk.

Premedication

While inhalation anesthesia can be initiated without premedication, administration of a sedative or tranquilizer often in combination with an opioid is recommended prior to induction of anesthesia (Tables 59.2 and 59.3). Preanesthetic drugs aid in restraint, reduce apprehension, decrease the quantity of potentially more depressant drugs used to produce general anesthesia, facilitate induction, enhance perioperative analgesia, and reduce arrhythmogenic autonomic reflex activity. Premedications are usually administered IM or SC 15–30 min before induction. The choice of premedication depends on signalment, temperament, physical status, concurrent disease, the procedure to be performed, drug availability, and personal preference (Table 59.6). For procedures associated with postoperative pain, premedication should include an analgesic such as an opioid and possibly a non-steroidal anti-inflammatory drug. Fewer analgesics are typically needed postoperatively when analgesics are administered preemptively [32]. Repeated and frequent patient assessment following surgery is needed to assess the adequacy of analgesia. Additional analgesics should be administered when needed (see Chapter 47).

Induction

Induction of anesthesia is most easily accomplished in most cats and dogs with propofol, alfaxalone, ketamine–midazolam, propofol–ketamine, or etomidate (Table 59.5). Advantages of an IV method of induction include rapid loss of consciousness and ability to intubate the trachea quickly. Alternatives to these rapid IV induction protocols include administration of a higher dose IM dissociative (cyclohexamine) anesthetic–benzodiazepine combination (e.g.,

Telazol®), chamber or mask inhalant induction, or high-dose IV opioid induction. These techniques can be useful in special circumstances, but for routine use in healthy dogs and cats, their disadvantages generally outweigh their advantages.

Chamber or mask inhalant induction

One disadvantage to chamber and mask induction is the associated waste-gas pollution. Another is the struggling and associated stress that some animals experience during the induction phase [33]. Mask induction is most easily accomplished in moribund animals and small tractable dogs. Prior tranquilization or sedation enhances the quality and speed of induction, as does the use of a non-rebreathing system to deliver the anesthetic agent initially [34]. Chamber induction is most useful in intractable cats and very small dogs. Isoflurane and sevoflurane are the most suitable inhalants for this technique because they produce a relatively rapid induction [35]. Relatively high oxygen flow rates (4 L/min for chamber and 3 L/min for mask) and vaporizer settings (3–5% isoflurane and 5–7% sevoflurane in healthy animals) are used. The use of nitrous oxide is not necessary during chamber or mask induction with currently used agents [36]. With chamber induction, once the animal has lost its righting reflex and is unresponsive to the chamber being tilted from side to side, it is removed from the chamber and induction is continued using an appropriately sized mask. Mask induction is begun by exposing the animal to the mask and oxygen. The inhalation concentration is slowly increased to 3–5% for isoflurane and 5–7% for sevoflurane. This is accomplished with a non-rebreathing or rebreathing circuit by gradually increasing the vaporizer setting over 2–4 min. Use of a non-rebreathing anesthetic system to deliver gas to the chamber or mask will facilitate rapid induction because exchange of the room air, which is present in the reservoir bag, breathing circuit, and carbon dioxide absorber prior to starting induction, with anesthetic-laden gas from the vaporizer is not necessary.

Intravenous high-dose opioid induction

A disadvantage to opioid induction is the accompanying relatively slow loss of consciousness. Advantages include good cardiovascular stability (although severe bradycardia may be seen when anticholinergics are not co-administered) and the attenuation of the stress response associated with anesthesia and surgery. Opioid induction works best in debilitated dogs and is not recommended in cats or young, healthy dogs that are not well sedated. Incremental doses of an opioid agonist (Table 59.3) are alternated with small incremental doses of midazolam (Table 59.2) until the dog can be intubated. This technique does not always result in a patient that can be intubated; therefore, an IV induction agent should be available, and given to effect if needed.

Anesthetic maintenance

The maintenance phase of anesthesia begins when unconsciousness is induced and ends with discontinuation of anesthetic delivery. After the loss of consciousness, a properly sized, cuffed endotracheal tube or alternative airway (e.g., supraglottic airway device) is usually inserted to allow assisted ventilation, if necessary, and protect against aspiration of oropharyngeal contents. Adequate cardiovascular function is rapidly verified, and the anesthetic vaporizer is turned on. The initial and subsequent anesthetic vaporizer settings (percentage concentration of inhalant) vary with the condition of the patient, the type of breathing circuit used, and the fresh-gas flow rate (Table 59.8). The relatively high fresh-gas flow rate and vaporizer setting that are initially used after induction are decreased to maintenance settings when the patient nears the desired anesthetic plane (usually when palpebral reflexes disappear, and the heart rate begins to decrease). The vaporizer setting is adjusted according to signs of anesthetic depth. The most useful signs of anesthetic depth in dogs and cats include a combination of ocular signs (palpebral reflex and position of the globe), muscle tone (assessed by opening the mouth to its full extent), heart and respiratory rates, and systemic arterial blood pressure. Other monitors that may be used include a pulse oximeter and a capnometer. Pulse oximetry non-invasively provides an estimate of hemoglobin's oxygen saturation (normal is greater than 95%). This information along with packed cell volume or hemoglobin concentration indicates the oxygen content of arterial blood. A capnometer non-invasively assesses ventilation by monitoring respiratory rate and end-tidal expired carbon dioxide (CO_2) partial pressure, which is related to arterial CO_2. End-tidal CO_2 monitors can also identify problems with the gas delivery system such as rebreathing due to malfunctioning one-way valves and exhausted CO_2 absorbent, especially when graphic display of the CO_2 time profile is provided (i.e., a capnogram). Additional information on patient monitoring is available in Chapters 10, 11, 12, 13, 14, 15, and 16.

Table 59.8 Vaporizer settings[a].

Drug	Induction phase (%)	Maintenance phase (%)
Isoflurane	3	1–3
Sevoflurane	4–5	2–4

[a] Listed vaporizer settings are for a rebreathing (circle) system assuming a fresh gas flow rate of 1–2 L/min during the inhalant induction phase (i.e., the first several minutes following anesthetic induction with an injectable drug), and a fresh-gas flow rate of at least 10 mL/kg/min during the maintenance phase. Vaporizer settings for closed rebreathing systems are typically 1–2% higher. See the text for discussion of mask or chamber induction.

The anesthetic record

This is part of the patient's permanent record and should include notation of patient status, the anesthetic drugs used (including time of administration, dose, and effect), duration of the surgery, and notation of significant perioperative events. Ideally, heart rate, respiratory rate, blood pressure, and any other variables monitored should be recorded at regular intervals (every 5 min). Recording these data at regular intervals creates a visual aid that assists in determining the change in patient status during the anesthetic period. For example, a steadily increasing heart rate accompanied by a steadily decreasing blood pressure during a 15-min interval could signal hypotension caused by fluid loss or excessive anesthetic depth. This is easily observed on the anesthetic record but may not be noticed without the visual prompt of the data recorded over time.

Perioperative analgesia

Concurrent administration of various analgesic drugs during inhalation anesthesia is useful to enhance intraoperative and postoperative analgesia. These drugs can be continued into the postanesthetic period to maintain analgesia. Infusions of low doses of ketamine, lidocaine, opioids, and their combinations have been described as adjuncts to inhalation anesthesia [37–39] (Table 59.9). When using these drugs, the concentration of inhalant anesthetic can often be significantly reduced. Increased respiratory depression is a concern,

Table 59.9 Drugs and drug combinations administered by constant rate infusion (CRI) to enhance intraoperative analgesia.

Drug(s)	Infusion rate (IV)	Comments
Ketamine	0.6–1.2 mg/kg/h	Useful as an adjunct to other perioperative analgesics
Fentanyl	5–15 μg/kg/h	Useful alone or with other perioperative analgesics
Remifentanil	4–60 μg/kg/h	Has a very short half-life, therefore once CRI is terminated additional opioids are likely to be needed to control pain
Hydromorphone	0.02–0.04 mg/kg/h	Useful alone or with other perioperative analgesics
Lidocaine[a]	1.5–4.5 mg/kg/h	Useful alone or with other perioperative analgesics; first administer a loading dose of 2 mg/kg
Morphine, Lidocaine[a], Ketamine	0.24 mg/kg/h, 3.0 mg/kg/h, 0.6 mg/kg/h	Useful alone or with other perioperative analgesics; first administer loading doses of 2 mg/kg lidocaine, 0.5 mg/kg ketamine, and 0.1 mg/kg morphine[b] IV
		Delivery of each drug separately via syringe pumps facilitates individual adjustment of drug infusion rates without impacting IV fluid delivery
		Alternatively, all three drugs can be added to a bag of isotonic crystalloids (LRS, Plasma-Lyte®, 0.9% NaCl, etc.) and administered at 5 mL/kg/h as follows: • To a 500 mL bag of IV fluids, add 24 mg of morphine, 300 mg of lidocaine, and 60 mg of ketamine. • To a 1 L bag of IV fluids, add 48 mg of morphine, 600 mg of lidocaine, and 120 mg of ketamine.
		Drug concentrations in the bag need to be adjusted to facilitate changes to the delivered fluid and/or drug infusion rate

[a] Avoid lidocaine in cats.
[b] A morphine loading dose is not necessary if a full agonist opioid was administered during premedication.

and the adequacy of ventilation should be closely monitored, with ventilation being assisted as needed.

Local and regional anesthetic techniques can and should be used when indicated to enhance analgesia and decrease general anesthetic requirements intraoperatively. Many different techniques are available for dogs and cats with reasonable safety and efficacy and are presented in Chapter 60.

Recovery

Recovery begins when the procedure for which a patient has been anesthetized is finished and the anesthetic drugs have been discontinued. Patient status should be monitored regularly during recovery until the patient is conscious and extubated, and heart rate, respiratory rate, and body temperature have returned to normal. Young, healthy animals undergoing routine procedures usually do not need supplemental oxygen during recovery, although it should always be immediately available. Continuous use of pulse oximetry is helpful to identify unexpected postanesthetic hypoxemia. Hypoxemia caused by respiratory depression, atelectasis-related ventilation–perfusion mismatch, and/or rapidly decreased fraction of inspired oxygen (e.g., near 100% oxygen when attached to an anesthetic breathing system to 21% when breathing room air) is easily addressed if detected early. If nitrous oxide was used during anesthetic maintenance, the breathing system should be repeatedly filled with oxygen, and the patient allowed to breathe an oxygen-enriched gas mixture for 5–10 min after discontinuation of nitrous oxide. This helps prevent the diffusion hypoxia that can develop if the inspired oxygen concentration suddenly decreases while nitrous oxide is rapidly moving from the blood into the alveolar gas. Sick or debilitated dogs and cats benefit from supplemental oxygen during recovery, particularly if hypothermic, because shivering can significantly increase oxygen consumption. The endotracheal tube cuff should be partially deflated and endotracheal tube untied when a patient is disconnected from the anesthetic machine. This permits extubation in the event that the patient rapidly awakens and begins chewing, but care should be exercised when moving the animal to the recovery area so premature accidental extubation does not occur. At this time the animal's nose should be positioned downwards slightly to allow drainage of any accumulated oral or pharyngeal fluid that accumulated during the procedure. If an esophageal stethoscope or temperature probe was used, it should be removed prior to terminating anesthetic delivery. Dogs and cats should be extubated as soon as swallowing occurs, unless there is a specific contraindication to removing the endotracheal tube at this time (e.g., brachycephalic airway syndrome). Dogs and cats should never be left to recover unobserved. Patients should recover in a well-ventilated area to minimize pollution of the workspace by exhaled anesthetic gas.

Occasionally, a dog or cat will suddenly awaken from anesthesia disoriented and will vocalize, paddle, and appear incoherent. This sudden arousal can be caused by emergence delirium, opioid dysphoria, or pain, and it is important to distinguish between them. Emergence delirium occurs most frequently in poorly or non-premedicated animals and in particular those awakening rapidly from inhalant anesthesia. With emergence delirium, the dog or cat will become quiet and more comfortable, usually within 10 min. A quiet, reassuring voice and gentle restraint can guide the animal through this period of excitement. Alternatively, a low dosage of IV propofol (0.25–1 mg/kg) can dramatically lessen the dysphoric behavior, allowing a smooth recovery. Occasionally, a low dose of dexmedetomidine (0.5–1 μg/kg IV) or acepromazine (0.005–0.02 mg/kg IV) is necessary to quiet an excited, dysphoric animal. If pain is believed to be the cause of the rough recovery, rapidly acting opioid analgesics (e.g., fentanyl) should be administered IV. Postoperative pain control is managed best with preanesthetic analgesic administration of relatively long-lasting analgesics, perioperative analgesic infusion, local anesthetics, and attention to signs of pain. Dogs and cats can become dysphoric during recovery, related to perioperative opioid administration [40]. Opioid dysphoria can be diminished with partial opioid reversal using the opioid antagonist naloxone (1–2 μg/kg IV).

Dogs or cats receiving perioperative fluids can develop a fully distended or overdistended urinary bladder that can cause signs of discomfort. If a full bladder is palpated, it can be gently expressed prior to recovery.

Delayed anesthetic recovery

Occasionally, a dog or cat that received several drugs (especially opioids) during the anesthetic episode will remain mildly hypothermic and unresponsive. In these instances, consideration should be given to antagonism of reversible drugs (α_2-adrenergic receptor agonists or opioids) that were given as part of the anesthetic regimen. Relatively small IV boluses of naloxone (1–2 μg/kg) can be used to reverse the central nervous system (CNS) and thermoregulatory depression associated with the opioids while leaving opioid analgesia mostly intact. Atipamezole can be used to reverse α_2-adrenergic receptor agonist-related CNS depression.

Severe hypoglycemia is an easily corrected problem that can result in delayed anesthetic recovery. Blood glucose concentration should be measured if hypoglycemia is suspected, and IV dextrose-containing fluids given until blood glucose concentrations normalize. Arterial hypotension associated with blood loss or poor cardiac function can cause altered mentation and slow recovery. Periodic measurement of arterial blood pressure during recovery, especially in debilitated patients, is warranted. Hypercapnia ($PaCO_2$ approaching 100 mmHg) associated with respiratory-depressant anesthetic and adjunctive drugs may cause severe mental impairment and possibly respiratory arrest. Use of capnometry or arterial blood gas analysis during the anesthetic maintenance and recovery period helps facilitate early detection and correction of respiratory depression. Occasionally, animals with undiagnosed, compensated CNS disease (e.g., hydrocephalus) may decompensate under anesthesia, resulting in impaired brain function. Prevention of hypercapnia, hypoxemia, and hypotension, and rapid implementation of resuscitative measures (e.g., mannitol and controlled positive-pressure ventilation) may limit brain injury and speed recovery. Many problems that lead to delayed recovery from anesthesia can be prevented or otherwise managed with appropriate patient monitoring during and after anesthetic drug delivery.

Acknowledgment

The authors would like to acknowledge the invaluable contribution of our colleague, Richard M. Bednarski, whose original work serves as the foundation for this chapter.

References

1 Grubb T, Sager J, Gaynor JS, *et al.* AAHA anesthesia and monitoring guidelines for dogs and cats. *J Am Anim Hosp Assoc* 2020; **56**(2): 59–82.
2 Robertson SA, Gogolski SM, Pascoe P, *et al.* AAFP feline anesthesia guidelines. *J Feline Med Surg* 2018; **20**: 602–634.
3 Kojima K, Nishimura R, Mutoh T, *et al.* Effects of medetomidine-midazolam, acepromazine-butorphanol, and midazolam-butorphanol on induction dose of thiopental and propofol and on cardiopulmonary changes in dogs. *Am J Vet Res* 2002; **63**: 1671–1679.
4 Hall R, Szlam F, Hug C. The enflurane sparing effect of alfentanil in dogs. *Anesth Analg* 1987; **66**: 1287–1291.
5 Haskins S, Farver T, Patz J. Cardiovascular changes in dogs given diazepam and diazepam-ketamine. *Am J Vet Res* 1986; **47**: 795–798.
6 Hofmeister EH, Watson V, Snyder LBC, *et al.* Validity and client use of information from the World Wide Web regarding veterinary anesthesia in dogs. *J Am Vet Med Assoc* 2008; **233**: 1860–1864.
7 Robinson EP, Sams RA, Muir WW. Barbiturate anesthesia in greyhound and mixed breed dogs: comparative cardiopulmonary effects, anesthetic effects, and recovery rates. *Am J Vet Res* 1986; **47**: 2105–2112.
8 Hay Kraus BL, Greenblatt DJ, Venkatakrishnan K, *et al.* Evidence for propofol hydroxylation by cytochrome P4502B11 in canine liver microsomes: breed and gender differences. *Xenobiotica* 2000; **30**: 575–588.
9 Martinez SE, Andresen MC, Zhu Z, *et al.* Pharmacogenomics of poor drug metabolism in Greyhounds: cytochrome P450 (CYP) 2B11 genetic variation, breed distribution, and functional characterization. *Sci Rep* 2020; **10**: 69.
10 Doxey S, Boswood A. Differences between breeds of dog in a measure of heart rate variability. *Vet Rec* 2004; **154**: 713–717.
11 Grunheid M, Aarnes TK, McLoughlin MA, *et al.* Risk of anesthesia-related complications in brachycephalic dogs. *J Am Vet Med Assoc* 2018; **253**: 301–306.
12 Washington State University Clinical Pharmacology Laboratory. Drugs that Have Been Documented to Cause Problems in Dogs with the MDR1 Mutation. Available at: www.vcpl.vetmed.wsu.edu/problem-drugs (accessed June 2022).
13 Tavoloni N. Postnatal changes in hepatic microsomal enzyme activities in the puppy. *Biol Neonate* 1985; **47**: 305–316.
14 Seahorn J, Robertson S. Concurrent medications and their impact on anesthetic management. *Vet Forum* 2002; **119**: 50–67.
15 Nolan AM, Reid J. Pharmacokinetics of propofol administered by infusion in dogs undergoing surgery. *Br J Anaesth* 1993; **70**: 546–551.
16 Smith JA, Gaynor JS, Bednarski RM, *et al.* Adverse effects of administration of propofol with various preanesthetic regimens in dogs. *J Am Vet Med Assoc* 1993; **202**: 1111–1115.
17 Grubb TL, Greene SA, Perez TE. Cardiovascular and respiratory effects, and quality of anesthesia produced by alfaxalone administered intramuscularly to cats sedated with dexmedetomidine and hydromorphone. *J Feline Med Surg* 2013; **15**: 858–865.
18 Tamura J, Ishizuka T, Fukui S, *et al.* The pharmacological effects of the anesthetic alfaxalone after intramuscular administration in dogs. *J Vet Med Sci* 2015; **77**: 289–296.
19 Rodrigo-Mocholi D, Belda E, Bosmans T, *et al.* Clinical efficacy and cardiorespiratory effects of intramuscular administration of alfaxalone alone or in combination with dexmedetomidine in cats. *Vet Anaesth Analg* 2016; **43**: 291–300.
20 Khenissi L, Nikolayenkova-Topie O, Broussaud S, *et al.* Comparison of intramuscular alfaxalone and ketamine combined with dexmedetomidine and butorphanol for castration in cats. *J Feline Med Surg* 2017; **19**: 791–797.
21 Cremer J, Riccó CH. Cardiovascular, respiratory and sedative effects of intramuscular alfaxalone, butorphanol and dexmedetomidine compared with ketamine, butorphanol and dexmedetomidine in healthy cats. *J Feline Med Surg* 2018; **20**: 973–979.
22 Murdock MA, Riccó Pereira CH, Aarnes TK, *et al.* Sedative and cardiorespiratory effects of intramuscular administration of alfaxalone and butorphanol combined with acepromazine, midazolam, or dexmedetomidine in dogs. *Am J Vet Res* 2020; **81**: 65–76.
23 Ribas T, Bublot I, Junot S, *et al.* Effects of intramuscular sedation with alfaxalone and butorphanol on echocardiographic measurements in healthy cats. *J Feline Med Surg* 2015; **17**: 530–536.
24 Lazzarini E, Martinelli E, Brioschi FA, *et al.* Intramuscular alfaxalone and methadone with or without ketamine in healthy cats: effects on sedation and echocardiographic measurements. *Vet Anaesth Analg* 2020; **47**: 621–630.
25 Suarez MA, Dzikit BT, Stegmann FG, *et al.* Comparison of alfaxalone and propofol administered as total intravenous anesthesia for ovariohysterectomy in dogs. *Vet Anaesth Analg* 2012; **39**: 236–244.
26 Herbert GL, Bowlt KL, Ford-Fennah V, *et al.* Alfaxalone for total intravenous anesthesia in dogs undergoing ovariohysterectomy: a comparison of premedication with acepromazine and dexmedetomidine. *Vet Anaesth Analg* 2013; **40**: 124–133.
27 Williams LS, Levy JK, Robertson SA, *et al.* Use of the anesthetic combination of tiletamine, zolazepam, ketamine, and xylazine for neutering feral cats. *J Am Vet Med Assoc* 2002; **220**: 1491–1495.
28 Hughes JM, Nolan AM. Total intravenous anesthesia in greyhounds: pharmacokinetics of propofol and fentanyl – a preliminary study. *Vet Surg* 1999; **28**: 513–524.
29 Ilkiw JE, Pascoe PJ. Effect of variable-dose propofol alone and in combination with two fixed doses of ketamine for total intravenous anesthesia in cats. *Am J Vet Res* 2003; **64**: 907–912.
30 Ilkiw JE, Pascoe PJ. Cardiovascular effects of propofol alone and in combination with ketamine for total intravenous anesthesia in cats. *Am J Vet Res* 2003; **64**: 913–915.
31 Mendes G, Selmi A. Use of a combination of propofol and fentanyl, alfentanil, or sufentanil for total intravenous anesthesia in cats. *J Am Vet Med Assoc* 2003; **223**: 1608–1613.
32 Woolf CF, Chong M. Preemptive analgesia: treating postoperative pain by preventing the establishment of central sensitization. *Anesth Analg* 1993; **77**: 362–379.
33 Mutoh T, Nishimura R, Kim H. Rapid inhalation induction of anesthesia by halothane, enflurane, isoflurane, and sevoflurane and their cardiopulmonary effects in dogs. *J Vet Med Sci* 1995; **57**: 1007–1013.
34 Mutoh T, Nishimura R, Sasaki N. Effects of medetomidine-midazolam, midazolam-butorphanol, or acepromazine-butorphanol as premedicants for mask induction of anesthesia with sevoflurane in dogs. *Am J Vet Res* 2002; **63**: 1022–1028.
35 Lerche P, Muir WW, Grubb T. Mask induction of anaesthesia with isoflurane or sevoflurane in premedicated cats. *J Small Anim Pract* 2002; **43**: 12–15.
36 Mutoh T, Nishimura R, Sasaki N. Effects of nitrous oxide on mask induction of anesthesia with sevoflurane or isoflurane in dogs. *Am J Vet Res* 2001; **62**: 1727–1733.
37 Wagner A, Walaton J, Hellyer P, *et al.* Use of low doses of ketamine administered by constant rate infusion as an adjunct for postoperative analgesia in dogs. *J Am Vet Med Assoc* 2002; **221**: 72–75.
38 Muir W, Wiese A, March P. Effects of morphine, lidocaine, ketamine, and morphine-lidocaine-ketamine drug combination on minimum alveolar concentration in dogs anesthetized with isoflurane. *Am J Vet Res* 2003; **64**: 1155–1160.
39 Nunes de Moraes A, Dyson D, O'Grady M, *et al.* Plasma concentrations and cardiovascular influence of lidocaine infusions during isoflurane anesthesia in healthy dogs and dogs with subaortic stenosis. *Vet Surg* 1998; **27**: 486–497.
40 Becker WM, Mama KR, Rao S, *et al.* Prevalence of dysphoria after fentanyl in dogs undergoing stifle surgery. *Vet Surg* 2013; **42**: 302–307.

60 Canine and Feline Local Anesthetic and Analgesic Techniques

Raphaël Vézina Audette[1], Alexander C.S. Thomson[2], Ciara A. Barr[3], Luis Campoy[4], Matt Read[5] and Santiago Peralta[4]

[1] Portland Veterinary Emergency and Specialty Care, Portland, Maine, USA
[2] City University of Hong Kong Veterinary Medical Centre, Hong Kong SAR, China
[3] Department of Clinical Sciences and Advanced Medicine, School of Veterinary Medicine, University of Pennsylvania, Philadelphia, Pennsylvania, USA
[4] Department of Clinical Sciences, College of Veterinary Medicine, Cornell University, Ithaca, New York, USA
[5] MedVet Columbus, Worthington, Ohio, USA

Chapter contents

Introduction, 1166
Classification of locoregional anesthesia, 1167
  Topical anesthesia, 1167
  Local infiltration, 1167
  Intravenous regional anesthesia, 1167
  Neuraxial anesthesia, 1168
  Peripheral nerve blocks, 1168
Physiology of nerve blockade, 1168
  Anatomy of the peripheral nerve, 1168
  Local anesthetic pharmacology, 1169
  Differential blockade, 1169
  Local anesthetic additives, 1169
Patient preparation, 1169
Equipment, 1170
  Needles, 1170
  Catheters, 1171
  Injection pressure monitors, 1172
  Peripheral nerve stimulators, 1172
  Ultrasound, 1173
Blocks of the head, 1174
  Maxillary techniques, 1174
  Mandibular techniques, 1175
  Local tissue dental blocks, 1177
  Anesthesia for ophthalmic procedures, 1177
  Auricular techniques, 1178
  Trigeminal nerve block, 1178
Blocks of the thorax and abdomen, 1178
  Thoracic paravertebral block, 1179
  Intercostal nerve block, 1179
  Interpleural regional analgesia, 1181
  Fascial plane block techniques, 1182
Blocks of the thoracic limb, 1185
  Anatomy of sensory innervation, 1185
  Cervical paravertebral block, 1186
  Subscalenic brachial plexus block, 1186
  Axillary brachial plexus block, 1186
  Proximal radial, ulnar, median, and musculocutaneous nerve block, 1187
  Distal radial, ulnar, median, and musculocutaneous nerve block, 1188
  Radial, ulnar, and median nerve block (ring block), 1188
Blocks of the pelvic limb, 1188
  Anatomy, 1188
  Lumbar plexus block, 1188
  Femoral/saphenous nerve block, 1189
  Sciatic nerve block, 1190
  Intra-articular blocks, 1191
Neuraxial techniques, 1192
  Contraindications, 1192
  Anatomy, 1192
  Epidural technique, 1194
  Catheter placement, 1197
  Intrathecal (spinal) anesthesia, 1197
Complications of locoregional anesthesia, 1197
  Local anesthetic systemic toxicity, 1198
  Neuronal damage, 1198
References, 1198

Introduction

Local and regional (locoregional) anesthetic and analgesic techniques are a cornerstone of modern veterinary anesthetic and analgesic protocols. However, the relevance of locoregional anesthesia extends beyond the perioperative setting to include applications in interventional pain management, both acute and chronic. Due to their unique mechanism of action targeting voltage-gated sodium channels along nerve fibers, local anesthetics interrupt transmission of neural impulses along axons and contribute significantly to decreasing nociceptive traffic along the pain pathways in both the peripheral and central nervous systems. The benefits of incorporating local or regional blocks into analgesic protocols are many, ranging from profound surgical anesthesia and analgesia, inhibition of central sensitization, a decreased reliance on systemically administered opioids and their associated adverse effects, lowering of inhaled anesthetic requirements for maintenance of a desired surgical plane of anesthesia and, ultimately, a potential for better surgical outcomes with a significant decrease in patient morbidity and mortality.

Locoregional anesthetic techniques range in complexity, from simple local infiltration techniques needing minimal equipment and training (e.g., ventral midline infiltration or "line blocks," ring

Veterinary Anesthesia and Analgesia: The Sixth Edition of Lumb and Jones. Edited by Leigh Lamont, Kurt Grimm, Sheilah Robertson, Lydia Love and Carrie Schroeder.
© 2024 John Wiley & Sons, Inc. Published 2024 by John Wiley & Sons, Inc.
Companion website: www.wiley.com/go/lamont/anesthesia

blocks, and testicular blocks), to more complex ultrasound-guided regional anesthesia techniques requiring advanced training and mastery of applied functional musculoskeletal and neuroanatomy. Ultrasound guidance has recently been described for a wide variety of peripheral nerve and fascial plane block techniques, allowing for a more precise and targeted delivery of local anesthetic solutions and decreased risks of nerve injury or vascular puncture. In some techniques, ultrasound guidance may be used in conjunction with peripheral neurostimulation to provide further confirmation that targeted structures are properly identified. In veterinary medicine, species-specific anatomic studies are needed to determine the relevance and safety of various locoregional anesthetic techniques. Extrapolating from descriptions of blocks described in human medical textbooks, or even from one animal species to another, may lead to treatment failures since the comparative neuroanatomy often contains important differences. Preliminary cadaveric studies assessing distribution of injectate and staining of target nerve fibers must be followed by well-designed, blinded, randomized, controlled clinical trials to evaluate analgesic efficacy. The past decade has seen exponential growth in the number of publications on locoregional anesthesia in veterinary medicine. The low cost of local anesthetics and the positive impact of these techniques on patient welfare make locoregional anesthesia a vital component of many balanced anesthetic protocols.

Classification of locoregional anesthesia

Topical anesthesia

Topical anesthesia is the oldest form of locoregional anesthesia and refers to the direct application of a local anesthetic agent to skin or mucosa to produce superficial desensitization. Topical anesthesia is still commonly used in companion animals; proparacaine and tetracaine are used for short-term corneal desensitization, and atomized lidocaine is routinely used to desensitize the arytenoids prior to tracheal intubation, particularly in cats [1,2]. However, application of local anesthetics to intact skin is complicated by the presence of the stratum corneum, which limits absorption. Skin preparations of local anesthetics may contain higher concentrations and permeation enhancers such as eucalyptol or propylene glycol [3]. Application of heat, ultrasonic waves, and electrical energy has also been reported to increase absorption of local anesthetics across the skin [3].

In companion animals, a eutectic mixture of lidocaine and prilocaine (EMLA™ cream) is commonly used for venipuncture and superficial skin procedures. The combination of local anesthetics reduces the melting point of each, permitting a higher local anesthetic concentration in the liquid phase. The efficacy and depth of desensitization are dependent on contact time; placing an occlusive dressing over the application site is often recommended to enhance absorption. The use of EMLA™ cream has been reported to significantly reduce stress in cats when applied 30 min prior to jugular venipuncture [4]. In dogs, application of EMLA™ cream 60 min before IV catheter placement reduced behavioral reactions without affecting catheter placement success rate [5].

Transdermal lidocaine patches have been evaluated in dogs, cats, and horses [6–11]. Human studies have demonstrated an analgesic effect and reduced postoperative opioid consumption in patients with lidocaine patches applied [12,13]. However, extrapolation of human data to animals is tenuous due to differences in skin composition that may affect drug absorption and controlled clinical trials have not yet demonstrated a significant analgesic benefit in veterinary patients [8]. Lidocaine patches appear to be well tolerated in dogs and cats with few side effects, low systemic absorption, and a low risk of systemic toxicity [6,9]. It is important to note, however, that the systemic absorption of lidocaine from patches increases in the presence of surgical wounds compared to intact skin [14].

Local infiltration

Local infiltration is the deposition of local anesthetic into and around a surgical site, rather than targeting specific neural structures. It may be particularly useful when a regional nerve block is difficult or contraindicated, or when the required equipment for more advanced techniques is not available. However, local infiltration may result in incomplete blockade of sensory fibers supplying the target site due to imprecision and the inhibitory effect of tissue inflammation on local anesthetic efficacy. As a result, clinical studies evaluating the analgesic efficacy of incisional and peri-incisional blocks in companion animals have demonstrated mixed results [15–19].

Local infiltration is most commonly delivered by injection, but multi-fenestrated catheters (i.e., "soaker catheters") may be implanted for repeated or continuous infiltration of a surgical site. In humans, local anesthetic wound infiltration has been associated with a reduction in postoperative opioid requirements, reduced postoperative nausea and vomiting, and a reduced length of hospital stay [20]. A retrospective study in dogs identified catheter disconnection, seroma formation, and local anesthetic systemic toxicity (LAST) as potential complications associated with infiltration catheters but did not find an increased incidence of surgical site infection compared to historical controls [21]. However, controversy remains about the effect of high concentrations of local anesthetics on wound healing. This effect may vary by the specific local anesthetic used, as well as the stage of wound healing. For example, some studies have indicated no effect of lidocaine on wound healing, while levobupivacaine may have a beneficial effect in the early phase and a detrimental effect thereafter [22]. The clinical implications of these studies are unclear in companion animals but, in general, local infiltration appears to be well tolerated with a low incidence of adverse effects.

Tumescent anesthesia is a type of local infiltration first developed for liposuction in humans. A large volume of dilute local anesthetic, combined with epinephrine and sodium bicarbonate, is infused into the subcutaneous tissues by a blunt-ended, multi-fenestrated Klein cannula [23]. Though high total doses of local anesthetic may be used (up to 55 mg/kg lidocaine in obese humans), the addition of a vasoconstrictor to the tumescent solution limits systemic absorption and reduces the risk of LAST [24]. Tumescent anesthesia has been reported in dogs and cats undergoing mastectomy [25–27]. Dogs receiving 15 mL/kg of a tumescent solution containing 0.16% lidocaine with epinephrine showed no difference in physiologic parameters from dogs receiving an epidural and intercostal nerve block; neither group required rescue analgesia for at least 6 h after surgery [27]. Similarly, tumescent anesthesia consisting of 15 mL/kg of 0.32% lidocaine with epinephrine was effective and well tolerated in a study of 12 cats [26]. The total lidocaine doses reported for tumescent anesthesia were 24 mg/kg in dogs and 48 mg/kg in cats.

Intravenous regional anesthesia

Intravenous regional anesthesia (IVRA), also known as a Bier block, involves administration of local anesthetic into a peripheral vein, where it is distributed to the tissues served by the local venous drainage. Once the target vein has been catheterized, the limb is elevated, and a tight bandage is placed to exsanguinate the area. A tourniquet is applied proximal to the bandage and the area to be anesthetized and the bandage is removed. Lidocaine 0.5% (0.6 mL/kg) is then injected into the catheter, resulting in desensitization of tissues distal to the tourniquet.

IVRA can be used for short (< 90 min) procedures of the distal extremities, particularly when minimal hemorrhage is desirable. In one canine study, IVRA with lidocaine was found to provide equivalent intraoperative analgesia to a brachial plexus block for carpal arthrodesis [28]; however, IVRA is better suited to surgeries of shorter duration, such as digit amputation.

Application of the tourniquet itself may be a source of pain, particularly ischemic pain transmitted by sympathetic fibers in the adventitia of major arteries [29]. In addition, once the tourniquet is released, transient increases in local anesthetic plasma concentrations can result in signs of systemic toxicity. Strategies to minimize or prevent these complications include limiting the time the tourniquet is in place, releasing the tourniquet slowly at the end of the procedure, and avoiding the use of cardiotoxic local anesthetics such as bupivacaine for this technique.

Neuraxial anesthesia

Neuraxial anesthesia dates back to 1885, when neurologist James Corning injected 26 mg of cocaine into the space between two vertebrae of a young dog, resulting in anesthesia of the pelvic limbs lasting 4 h [30]. Further refinement of this experiment led to the development of techniques for administering anesthetic agents into the epidural or subarachnoid spaces. These techniques remain in wide use today in both human and veterinary anesthesia.

Epidural anesthesia and analgesia refer to administration of anesthetic agents into the space immediately superficial to the dura mater of the spinal cord. This space is normally occupied by loose connective tissue, adipose tissue, blood vessels, and lymphatics. Subarachnoid anesthesia, also known as spinal or intrathecal anesthesia, refers to administration of drug into the subarachnoid space, between the arachnoid membrane and the pia mater. Unlike the epidural space, the subarachnoid space contains cerebrospinal fluid.

Both epidural and subarachnoid anesthesia work by bathing the spinal nerve roots in anesthetic as they leave the spinal cord, inhibiting neural transmission. The magnitude and duration of analgesia are dependent on the physical and chemical characteristics of the anesthetics used, as well as their concentration. However, the mechanism of drug distribution differs between epidural and spinal anesthesia. Whereas the distribution of anesthesia from an epidural injection predominantly depends on the injection site and the volume injected, the distribution of a spinal injection is also dependent on patient positioning and the baricity of the injectate. Baricity refers to the density of the solution compared to the density of cerebrospinal fluid.

While commonly performed in veterinary medicine, neuraxial anesthesia requires operator skill and is reliant on somewhat subjective criteria for determining correct placement of the needle, which may vary based on conformation and body condition. As a result, epidural failure rates of 12–30% have been estimated in companion animals [31]. A variety of techniques have been investigated for improving epidural success rate, including use of a nerve stimulator and ultrasound guidance [32–34].

Peripheral nerve blocks

Nerve blocks involve the administration of a local anesthetic adjacent to a peripheral nerve to block conduction. This results in sensory and/or motor deficits, depending on the nerve fiber composition, in the targeted anatomic region due to loss of both afferent and efferent nerve function. A variety of techniques may be used to identify the location of the target nerve(s), including palpation, anatomical landmarks, nerve stimulators, or ultrasound guidance. Although regional anesthesia may be provided utilizing any of these techniques, ultrasound guidance has been shown to improve the anatomical accuracy and success rate of a variety of nerve blocks in both human and veterinary medicine [35–38].

Fascial plane blocks are a relatively new subset of regional anesthetic techniques that involve deposition of a local anesthetic solution in between two layers of fascia, relying on spread of injectate volume within a fascial plane that contains nerves, rather than identification of and injection around discrete nerves [39]. The mechanism by which fascial plane blocks provide analgesia is still not well understood as studies in human medicine have found significant variability in the distribution of analgesia, sometimes even at sites distant from the expected distribution [40]. While most evidence clearly supports an analgesic benefit of fascial plane blocks, these results may indicate additional mechanisms of action are at play, such as systemic absorption of large doses of local anesthetic [41].

When successful, nerve blocks provide complete analgesia by preventing transmission of nociceptive signals to the central nervous system. Due to their superior analgesic effect, regional anesthetic techniques are associated with a greater reduction in the surgical stress response and improved postoperative analgesia when compared to opioid-based protocols [42–45]. A variety of excellent texts and other tools are available for teaching and learning regional anesthetic techniques in veterinary patients.

Physiology of nerve blockade

Anatomy of the peripheral nerve

Nerve impulses are carried by axons (often referred to as fibers) which are long, thin projections of neurons whose cell bodies reside in the sensory/dorsal root ganglia (afferent neurons) or brainstem/spinal cord (efferent neurons). Axons vary in diameter and myelination based on their function and required conduction speed. For example, the Aδ fibers responsible for fast, sharp pain are myelinated and much larger in diameter than the unmyelinated C fibers responsible for slow, aching pain. Each axon is surrounded by a loose, elastic connective tissue structure called the endoneurium, which consists mostly of collagen. Axons are bundled together in fascicles, which are surrounded by a more robust connective tissue sheath called the perineurium. Fascicles divide and converge with each other every few millimeters along the length of the nerve [46]. The outer sheath of the nerve, a continuation of the dura mater containing the nerve's blood supply, is the epineurium.

The relevance of this microanatomy to locoregional anesthesia has been the subject of much research and debate. Intraneural, extrafascicular injection of local anesthetic is associated with extensive longitudinal spread along the nerve without significant nerve damage [47–49]. However, intrafascicular injection of volumes as low as 0.05 mL have been associated with fascicular rupture, demyelination, and nerve damage in rodent models [50], and larger volumes injected proximally may cause inadvertent spinal anesthesia [47]. Though intraneural, extrafascicular injection may result in profound, long-lasting nerve block, it is not recommended due to the risk of inadvertent intrafascicular injection, as well as the risk of disrupting epineurial blood vessels and compromising nerve perfusion.

Nerves are loosely mobile and contain elastic elements, so they can be stretched without damaging the individual axons. They are loosely connected to surrounding structures by a connective tissue meshwork called the paraneurium. Blunt instruments, such as nerve block needles, will often push nerves to the side rather than perforating them. When performing a peripheral nerve block, it is preferable to avoid unnatural positioning that stretches the nerve, as this may increase the risk of inadvertent nerve puncture.

Local anesthetic pharmacology

A more in-depth discussion of local anesthetics is presented in Chapter 29. In short, local anesthetics are amphipathic molecules that exert their effects through use-dependent blockade of voltage-gated sodium channels. The sodium channels $Na_V1.7$, $Na_V1.8$, and $Na_V1.9$ are implicated in propagating action potentials along nociceptive nerve axons [51], although local anesthetics do not bind exclusively to these subtypes. The relative affinity of local anesthetics for off-target receptors, such as cardiac ion channels, accounts for the differences in their pharmacologic and toxic effects [52].

Local anesthetics are weak bases with pK_a values greater than 7.4, meaning they are partially ionized at physiologic pH. Because uncharged local anesthetic molecules must cross the lipid membrane to access their intracellular binding sites on sodium ion channels, their onset of action is influenced by pK_a. For example, local anesthetics with a high pK_a, such as bupivacaine ($pK_a = 8.1$), have a longer onset time than those with a low pK_a, such as lidocaine ($pK_a = 7.8$). Molecular weight, concentration, and lipid solubility also contribute to local anesthetic onset time and potency. High concentration, lipid solubility, and low molecular weight facilitate diffusion across cell membranes, decreasing onset time [52].

Duration of local anesthetic effect is determined by several factors, including protein binding, site of injection, vasoactivity, and regional vascularity. Drugs with a long duration of action often have a long onset time. Mixing different local anesthetics together to produce both short onset time and long duration has occasionally been advocated, particularly with dental nerve blocks. However, this practice results in unpredictable blockade, as the concentration and pH of each local anesthetic in the mixture are altered. Most literature evaluating local anesthetic mixtures has demonstrated a reduction in block duration without an appreciable improvement in onset time, and this practice is therefore of little value and is not recommended [53,54].

Differential blockade

Differential blockade describes the phenomenon that different types of nerve fibers demonstrate variable susceptibility to local anesthetics. This was first demonstrated by Gasser and Erlanger in 1929, who found that sensory fibers were more easily depressed by cocaine than motor fibers [55]. While this effect was initially attributed to the smaller size of sensory fibers, subsequent research demonstrated that A fibers are more susceptible to local anesthetic block than C fibers, seemingly at odds with clinical observations [56,57]. In practice, sympathetic fibers are most susceptible to blockade, followed by pain, touch/proprioception, and finally motor fibers. This indicates that several factors besides fiber diameter contribute to local anesthetic susceptibility, including the position of the fibers within the nerve (mantle effect), myelination, and density of ion channels in the axonal membrane. Small, unmyelinated nerve fibers may have a shorter critical length of local anesthetic exposure required to produce conduction block [58]. In addition, some local anesthetics, such as bupivacaine and ropivacaine, exhibit intrinsic differential blocking properties at low concentrations, preferentially producing sensory blockade [59,60].

Local anesthetic additives

Adjunctive medications may be added to local anesthetic to potentiate or prolong sensory blockade or reduce the total dose or concentration of local anesthetic required for locoregional anesthetic techniques. High total doses and concentrations of local anesthetics are associated with increased incidence of nerve block-associated complications and neurotoxicity, so multimodal perineural analgesia is desirable [61]. A wide variety of different drugs, such as opioids, adrenergic agonists, corticosteroids, buffers, ketamine, and hyaluronidase have been studied as local anesthetic adjuvants.

Opioids

Opioid receptors are synthesized in the dorsal root ganglia and transported peripherally along the axons of afferent nerves, especially after inflammation or tissue injury [62]. These peripheral opioid receptors may serve as analgesic targets for locoregional anesthetic techniques since their activation decreases the excitability of nociceptor terminals. However, not all opioids are equally effective in prolonging the duration of peripheral nerve blocks. Lipid solubility and ionization state likely influence the ability of a particular opioid to penetrate the nerve sheaths and access opioid receptors at the axonal membrane [63]. Buprenorphine, a highly lipid-soluble opioid, has been demonstrated to significantly prolong the effect of peripheral nerve blocks in humans [64–66]; however, opioids with lower lipid solubility, such as morphine, or a higher degree of ionization, such as fentanyl, are less likely to be effective. The synergistic effect of buprenorphine may also be attributable to its local anesthetic effects, as it produces use-dependent blockade of voltage-gated sodium ion channels [67].

Adrenergic agonists

Epinephrine has a long history as an additive to local anesthetics. Its vasoconstrictive effect counteracts the vasodilation produced by many local anesthetics, therefore decreasing systemic absorption and prolonging the duration of blockade. It may also contribute directly to analgesia through activation of α_2-adrenergic receptors in the axons of peripheral nerves. Epinephrine is commonly added in a concentration of 2.5–5 μg/mL. In combination with local anesthetics, epinephrine may reduce blood flow to peripheral nerves, although this effect varies with the dose and specific local anesthetic used [68]. It should be used with caution in extremities as, in rare cases, local vasoconstriction may impair perfusion in areas with limited collateral circulation [69].

α_2-Adrenergic receptor agonists are commonly added to local anesthetics. While α_2-adrenergic receptor agonists may also produce local vasoconstriction, plasma concentrations of local anesthetic are similar with and without the addition of an α_2-adrenergic receptor agonist, suggesting similar systemic absorption [70]. Additional mechanisms, such as direct suppression of A and C fiber activity, likely account for their synergistic analgesic effect [71]. Clonidine is widely used in human regional anesthetic techniques and is associated with improved quality and duration of blockade [70–72]. Dexmedetomidine is more commonly used in veterinary medicine and has demonstrated similar beneficial effects in human patients [73].

Patient preparation

The majority of nerve blocks in dogs and cats are performed under either sedation or general anesthesia. Patients should be relaxed, easy to manipulate and position, and either minimally or completely unresponsive to needle advancement, electrolocation, and injection. Patient positioning is an important aspect of any regional anesthetic procedure since nerves are flexible structures whose locations can vary depending on the patient's position. Recommended approaches for different nerve blocks may or may not be possible depending on the patient's position and, in some instances, patient positioning may also influence the distribution of drugs following injection. Using described and standardized positioning may minimize complications.

Thorough medical history-taking and physical examination should be performed prior to sedation or anesthesia on candidates for regional anesthetic techniques to document any pre-existing condition that may complicate or contraindicate locoregional blocks, such as known or presumed hypersensitivities, peripheral neuropathies or, in the case of neuraxial blocks, hypovolemia, coagulation disorders, or infection or neoplasia involving the puncture site. Clinicians should evaluate sensory and motor function prior to performing any nerve block. An overview of the regional anesthesia technique should be provided to the patient's owners when obtaining informed consent. The anesthetist should also discuss the risk of potential complications with the members of the healthcare team, including the patient's owners. Injection sites should be aseptically prepared to decrease the risk of infection. Equipment and agents for the locoregional technique should be selected and readied ahead of time to limit unnecessary delays and improve patient safety.

Equipment

Historically, equipment for companion animal regional anesthesia has often been sourced from human medical supply companies. However, as interest in advanced pain management techniques for animals expands, specialized equipment designed for veterinary use is becoming more commonly available. A wide variety of equipment may be encountered in veterinary practice, with variable price and quality. Continued development of veterinary-specific products is likely to improve utility and patient safety.

Needles

Needles are used to deliver local anesthetic and other drugs, but they may serve additional purposes, such as aiding in nerve location or catheter implantation. The utility of a particular needle for these purposes is dependent on its design and physical characteristics. Needles are available in many different lengths and gauges with varying tip designs and, in the case of ultrasound-guided techniques, echogenicity. They may be insulated or non-insulated, depending on whether they have a plastic, non-conducting sheath coating the shaft of the needle. In general, longer needles are used when targeting deeper structures, but they may be more challenging to manipulate and prone to bending. Selecting a larger gauge needle reduces the flexibility of the needle, but larger gauges are associated with more tissue trauma and injury of nerves that are inadvertently punctured [74,75]. Smaller needles may be prone to breaking or bending, especially if manufacturing defects are present, the patient moves during the procedure, or an incorrect technique is used [76,77].

The design of the needle tip may aid the anesthetist in estimating the position of the needle (Fig. 60.1). Hypodermic needles have long, acutely angled (12–15°) bevels designed to easily cut through tissue. This is not a desirable feature of a needle used for peripheral nerve blocks since this tip design provides little tactile feedback and is more likely to injure delicate nerves [78]. Needles designed for peripheral nerve blocks have short, blunt (30–45°) bevels that encounter variable resistance as the needle is advanced through tissue layers. This design is less likely to cut or puncture through the perineurium if a nerve is accidentally contacted [79]. The tip of Tuohy needles is blunt and rounded which, when used to perform an epidural injection, may convey a popping sensation when the needle passes through the ligamentum flavum and enters the epidural space.

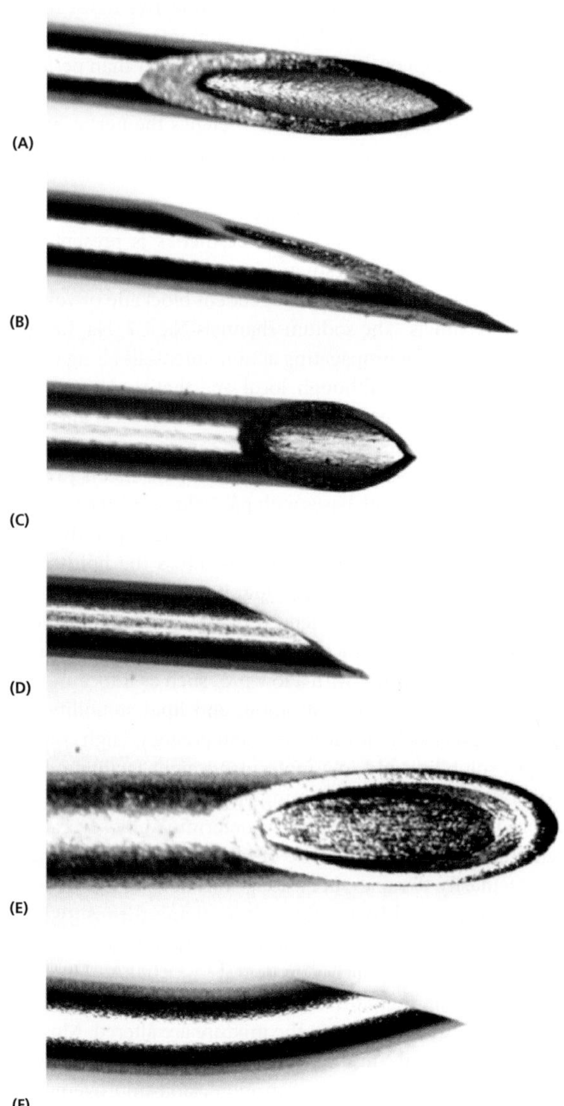

Figure 60.1 Needle tips at 25× magnification. **A.** and **B.** 22 gauge hypodermic needle; **C.** and **D.** 20 gauge insulated nerve block needle; **E.** and **F.** 20 gauge Tuohy needle. Note the short bevel of the insulated needle and the round, blunt tip of the Tuohy needle when compared with the hypodermic needle.

Insulated stimulating needles are coated with a non-conducting material along the entire length of the shaft, which allows precise application of electrical current at the tip of the needle for nerve location. Whereas a non-insulated needle may cause muscle or nerve stimulation along the entire length of its shaft, an insulated needle only stimulates structures in close proximity to the tip. Non-insulated needles are therefore less precise in terms of confirming that the tip is close to the target nerve and require a higher threshold stimulation current to elicit a motor response. Stimulating needles are manufactured with a cable that connects to a nerve stimulator and often have an extension line that may be connected to a syringe.

During ultrasound-guided procedures, visualization of the needle is important both for the success of the nerve block and patient safety. Poor visibility of the needle tip may result in inadvertent damage to the nerve or other nearby structures. Various methods of mechanical and optical needle guidance have been developed to improve accuracy, such as needle guides that attach directly to the ultrasound transducer. Echogenic needles have etched textures along their shafts, providing multiple reflective angles that increase ultrasonic visibility [80]. This is particularly helpful when a steep insertion angle is required to reach the target nerve, since visibility decreases as ultrasound waves are reflected away from the transducer [81]. Advances in both ultrasound and needle technology promise further improvement in needle visualization. Ultrasound-actuated needles that vibrate and produce a color Doppler signal are currently under investigation [82]. A photoacoustic needle that produces its own ultrasound waves via pulsed laser and an intraluminal optical fiber has also been reported [83].

Spinal needles are designed to puncture the dura mater and access the subarachnoid space for delivery of drugs or to sample cerebrospinal fluid. While more blunt than hypodermic needles, spinal needles are sharper than needles that are specifically designed for epidural use; therefore, using spinal needles for epidural injection may increase the risk of inadvertent dural puncture depending on the site of injection. Most spinal needles contain a close-fitting stylet that prevents occlusion of the lumen with a tissue plug as the needle is advanced. The hub of a spinal needle is usually transparent, allowing the operator to watch for the appearance of spinal fluid or blood as the needle is advanced. Many different tip designs have been developed, but the most common currently in use are Quincke, Sprotte, and Atraucan® spinal needles. The Quincke needle, first developed by German surgeon Heinrich Quincke in 1891, has a short V-shaped cutting bevel [84]. It remains the most common spinal needle in use today but may be associated with a higher incidence of post-dural puncture headache due to transdural fluid leakage [85]. The Sprotte needle is a modification of the earlier Whitacre (or pencil-point) spinal needle, and has a long, blunt conical shape tapering to a sharp point. The distal orifice is on the side of the tip, rather than at the point, and is larger than the original Whitacre design. This design is intended to separate dural fibers laterally, rather than cutting through them, allowing them to seal over the puncture site when the needle is withdrawn [86]. However, because the distal orifice is proximal to the tip of the needle, it is possible for the tip and the orifice to be located in separate compartments, especially in very small patients. The Atraucan® spinal needle is a proprietary Huber-type design introduced in 1993. The Atraucan® needle produces a small, linear cut in the dura, rather than the V-shaped cut produced by Quincke needles, resulting in less transdural fluid leakage. Unlike the Sprotte needle, the distal orifice of the Atraucan® needle is located at the tip. However, it has a sharp, delicate tip that is prone to being damaged [86].

Tuohy needles are designed specifically for epidural use, but they can also be used for peripheral nerve blocks or catheter insertion. As with spinal needles, Tuohy needles have a close-fitting removable stylet and a transparent hub. Tuohy needles have a curved, blunt bevel and are typically marked every 10 mm along the shaft. This design provides high-fidelity tactile feedback, minimizes the risk of inadvertent dural puncture, and directs catheter insertion. Both uninsulated and insulated Tuohy needles are available. The Weiss epidural needle is a modification of the Tuohy needle that adds wings to the needle hub. These wings are grasped between the thumb and index finger during placement to stabilize and direct the needle. Some needle designs have removable wings that slot into place on the hub.

Catheters

Many different types and brands of catheters are available for continuous or intermittent locoregional anesthetic techniques. They may be characterized by their material, length, gauge, method of insertion, number of fenestrations, and additional functions such as electrical stimulation.

Most catheters used in locoregional anesthesia are through-the-needle, but over-the-needle catheters are also commercially available, as well as systems that use an over-the-needle cannula as an introducer for the catheter. A variety of needle types and designs are used as described above. Once inserted using aseptic technique, the needle is removed, and the catheter is connected to an injection port and 0.2 μm bacterial filter, secured with suture, and covered with a protective dressing. The catheter may be tunneled subcutaneously near the insertion site for additional security.

Complications related to the use of catheters in locoregional anesthesia may be equipment- or drug-related. Catheter dislodgement, disconnection, and occlusion are relatively minor incidents that may require removal or replacement of the catheter. Breakage of catheters is a rare but potentially problematic complication, although surgical removal of the broken fragment is not usually indicated if the fragment is sterile and inert [87]. Withdrawing a catheter through the needle during placement may increase the risk of catheter breakage, since the catheter may shear on the needle bevel. Drug-related complications may be more serious, especially if cumulative local anesthetic doses exceed toxic doses. Careful calculation and confirmation of local anesthetic doses is essential to minimize these risks and, although it is a rare event, care providers should be well versed in the signs and treatments for local anesthetic systemic toxicity (LAST).

Modern epidural catheters are often composed of materials with high melting points, high tensile strength, and low friction, such as nylon blends or polytetrafluoroethylene (Teflon). Most are radiopaque, and some brands contain coiled wire for added strength and kink resistance [88]. MRI compatibility varies by manufacturer. Epidural catheters are often supplied in kits containing the catheter itself, a Tuohy needle, an adapter, an injection port, and a bacterial filter. Epidural catheters are usually long and thin, so resistance to injection is much higher than would be expected with a normal epidural injection. Microcatheters are available for spinal use; however, continuous spinal anesthesia is less commonly performed due to the higher risk of neurotoxicity and detrimental hemodynamic effects [89].

Continuous nerve block catheters evolved from epidural catheters, and share similar qualities of heat resistance, strength, and low friction. Like epidural catheters, these catheters are commonly supplied in kits containing all necessary equipment for implantation. Some kits contain an insulated needle with an attached port through which the catheter can be passed. This allows simultaneous nerve stimulation, injection, and feeding of the catheter without disconnecting the extension line and potentially moving the position of the needle. Nerve block catheters may have additional features, such as incorporated stimulating wires to verify correct positioning and echogenic reflectors to improve ultrasound visibility. Self-coiling "pigtail" catheters have been described for some types of continuous nerve blocks to prevent displacement of the catheter from the target injection site [90].

Multi-fenestrated catheters have many small openings at the distal end of the catheter, providing better dispersion of local anesthetic in the target area. Dispersion is primarily dependent on the number, size, and position of fenestrations [91]. Rate of drug administration may also affect dispersion, as bolus doses tend to disperse more homogeneously than slow infusions [92].

Wound soaker catheters are typically long, flexible, closed-end polyurethane catheters with multiple side fenestrations to allow for wide distribution of injected local anesthetic. They allow for continuous or intermittent delivery of local anesthetic as part of a multimodal postoperative analgesic strategy [21]. In dogs, the use of bupivacaine through wound soaker catheters has been associated with lower pain scores and analgesic requirements and improved appetite compared to a saline control [93]. Typically, wound soaker catheters are implanted with the tip positioned in the deepest layer of the surgical site during closure, with the proximal end exiting dorsally through a separate skin incision. However, they may be placed in a variety of locations, including subcutaneous, subfascial, intra-articular, periosteal, and peripleural. While purpose-made wound soaker catheters are commercially available, they can also be improvised from red rubber and other similar catheters by heat sealing the distal opening and creating fenestrations with a small (25–27 gauge) needle. However, cutting additional fenestrations into a red rubber catheter may compromise its structural integrity, increasing the risk of breakage within the patient.

Injection pressure monitors

While injection pressure is partially dependent on equipment variables such as needle gauge and length, changes in injection pressure may be associated with injection into different tissues [94]. Nerve injury due to intrafascicular injection has been associated with high injection pressure (25–45 psi), while perineural and epidural injections are associated with relatively low injection pressure [95–97]. Therefore, monitoring injection pressure may be useful for both safety and accuracy of locoregional techniques. Three major types of injection pressure monitors are currently available [98]. The first is the loss of resistance syringe, which relies on Boyle's law where the compression of a known volume of air in the syringe is used to estimate injection pressure; greater bubble compression is associated with higher injection pressure [98]. This method is commonly used for epidural techniques, as a significant drop in injection pressure occurs as the tip of the needle crosses the ligamentum flavum and enters the epidural space. Saline is commonly added to the syringe as well to prevent injection of air into the epidural space, which may be associated with complications such as venous air embolism or nerve root compression [99]. The second type of injection pressure monitor is the electronic manometer in syringe pumps; these devices are primarily used to detect occlusions during constant rate infusions and may have adjustable alarm thresholds. A syringe pump designed for regional anesthesia procedures, the Medovate SAFIRA®, is operated by a foot pedal and injects local anesthetic automatically while monitoring injection pressure. The third category of injection pressure monitors is inline devices. Two inline pressure monitors that are commercially available are the B. Braun B-Smart™ and the PAJUNK® NerveGuard. Both devices are attached between the syringe and the extension line of the needle. The B-Smart™ consists of a rising piston which displays the approximate pressure in psi, while the NerveGuard has a spring device that automatically blocks injection once a threshold pressure is exceeded. An injection pressure monitor integrated into the needle tip has been described but is not yet commercially available [100].

Peripheral nerve stimulators

Peripheral nerve stimulators deliver intermittent square-wave electrical currents via stimulating needles, eliciting specific muscular twitch responses to aid nerve location. They can be used in conjunction with ultrasound guidance. The minimum current required to elicit a response depends on the distance between the tip of the needle and the nerve. This relationship is described by Coulomb's law, where the required stimulating charge is related to the electrode-to-nerve distance [101]. Therefore, as the tip of the stimulating needle approaches the nerve, a lower current is required to stimulate it, and current can be used to approximate needle-to-nerve distance. It was previously thought that intraneural injections could be avoided by closely monitoring the minimum stimulating current. However, studies evaluating simultaneous nerve stimulation and ultrasound guidance have found that the minimum stimulating current actually increases when the needle is in direct contact with the nerve; therefore, relatively high minimum stimulating currents do not rule out the possibility of intraneural injection [102–104]. Current channeling has been proposed as an explanation for this phenomenon [105].

The susceptibility of a particular nerve fiber to stimulation can be described by two basic properties, rheobase and chronaxie. Rheobase is the minimum electrical current required to produce a sustained action potential and reflects membrane excitability. Chronaxie is the minimum impulse duration required to stimulate the nerve at a current twice the rheobase. Because chronaxie is influenced by axon diameter and myelination, chronaxie is typically shorter for motor fibers compared to sensory fibers. This difference allows peripheral nerve stimulators to selectively stimulate motor fibers using short-duration impulses. Impulse duration delivered by most peripheral nerve stimulators used for locoregional anesthesia is approximately 0.1 ms.

Peripheral nerve stimulators should have an easily readable display and the ability to adjust the current (0.1–1.0 mA) and frequency of stimulation. Some peripheral nerve stimulators incorporate a remote control or foot pedal to allow the operator to make adjustments without breaking sterility. Because currents as low as 0.2–0.3 mA may be used when locating peripheral nerves, nerve stimulators used for monitoring neuromuscular blockade may not be suitable for use in regional anesthesia.

Terminology describing the polarity of peripheral nerve stimulator components may be confusing and counterintuitive at first. Peripheral nerve stimulators use cathodal stimulation, meaning the negative electrode (cathode) is the searching electrode (i.e., the stimulating needle or catheter), and the positive electrode (anode) is the returning electrode. Current in the form of electrons flows from the cathode to the anode; as the cathode approaches the nerve, the density of negative charges on the outer surface axonal membrane increases, inducing nerve depolarization. If the electrodes were reversed, hyperpolarization of the nerve would occur due to accumulation of positive extracellular charge [106]. In the case of modern peripheral nerve stimulators, the cathode and anode have non-interchangeable connectors to prevent them from being inadvertently switched.

The electrical resistance encountered by the stimulating needle changes as it passes through body tissue. Therefore, peripheral nerve stimulators must continuously adjust their voltage to maintain a constant current in accordance with Ohm's law. However, the electrical characteristics and performance of commercially available peripheral nerve stimulators are highly variable, and anesthetists should be aware of the limitations of the equipment they are using [107–109]. Error often increases with high resistance and low current [109]. Modern peripheral nerve stimulators often incorporate a flashing light or audible tone change if the circuit is disconnected or for some other reason the indicated current cannot be delivered [106].

Peripheral nerve stimulators should be used with insulated needles so that the application of electrical current is precise. The negative electrode (i.e., black, cathode) connects to the stimulating needle, while the positive electrode (i.e., red, anode) attaches to the patient's skin, usually by an alligator clip or electrode patch. With modern nerve stimulators, the positive electrode can be attached anywhere on the patient provided good contact is achieved. The frequency of the nerve stimulator should be set to 2 Hz if the stimulator is being used alone, or 1 Hz if used in conjunction with an ultrasound to minimize disruption of the image.

The insulated needle is inserted through the skin using anatomic landmarks or ultrasound guidance, depending on the specific technique being used. The initial current should be set to 1.0–1.5 mA, depending on the depth of the targeted structure. The needle is then slowly advanced, while observing for the desired muscular response(s); twitches elicited by direct muscle stimulation should not be interpreted as success. If no twitches are observed, the needle is withdrawn to the level of the skin and redirected. Once a twitch is obtained, the current is slowly decreased to zero, making small adjustments to maintain the muscular response. The current is then slowly increased until a minimum stimulating current of < 0.5 mA is achieved, at which point the local anesthetic can be delivered. The syringe is gently aspirated to check for blood and local anesthetic solution is injected, monitoring closely for high injection pressure. If blood is aspirated or resistance to injection is encountered, the needle should be repositioned before injecting.

As local anesthetic solution is injected, the conductive area around the tip of the needle expands, and the low current used for stimulation is dispersed. This usually leads to a loss of the muscular response and does not indicate that the block has taken immediate effect.

Ultrasound

Nerve blockade performed using visual ultrasound guidance was first reported in 1994 when Kapral *et al.* used the technique for supraclavicular brachial plexus block in humans [110]. Since then, ultrasound guidance has revolutionized the field of locoregional anesthesia, improving the safety and accuracy of many different nerve blocks in both human and veterinary medicine. Ultrasound is now commonly used to identify peripheral nerves, as well as other anatomic landmarks such as blood vessels, bones, muscles, and fascial planes. It may be used in conjunction with nerve stimulation to further enhance safety and accuracy. Besides regional anesthesia, ultrasound has many useful roles in anesthesia, such as aiding vascular access, assessment of cardiac and diaphragmatic function, diagnosis of pneumothorax or effusions, and others. However, its utility is dependent on selection of an appropriate ultrasound machine, transducer, and settings, as well as the skill and ability of the operator to correctly identify anatomy.

Ultrasound transducers convert electrical energy into sound waves using piezoelectric materials, such as quartz crystals, that vibrate when current is applied. These sound waves are transmitted into the body at a particular frequency and are then reflected back toward the transducer. The reflected information is simultaneously processed to create an image [111]. Transducers may be linear or curved, and are available in a wide variety of frequencies, shapes, and widths. Frequency is directly related to axial resolution and inversely related to penetration depth [111]. High-frequency linear transducers are most commonly used to perform ultrasound-guided nerve blocks, as they produce high-resolution images; however, lower-frequency curved transducers are occasionally used when targeting deeper structures.

Conventional B-mode ultrasound generates an image based on a single beam angle at a frequency designated by the transducer. However, this mode of imaging is particularly susceptible to speckle, reflection, and shadowing artifacts [112]. These artifacts may make small structures difficult or impossible to distinguish when ultrasound machines that employ conventional B-mode imaging are used. Advances in ultrasound technology have led to the creation of spatial compound and tissue harmonic imaging to reduce artifacts and improve image quality. Spatial compound imaging acquires overlapping frames from multiple frequencies or beam angles, collating them into a single image. In practice, this leads to an averaging of artifacts across the multiple images acquired, reducing noise and clutter in the compound image. Tissue harmonic imaging collects information from harmonic frequencies, which are multiples of the fundamental transducer frequency [113]. Combining tissue harmonic and compound imaging produces better axial resolution and image quality than either modality alone [114–116].

Doppler ultrasonography uses shifts in ultrasound wave frequency to detect movement, as with blood flow in vascular structures or spread of local anesthetic during injection. It is displayed as a color signal overlying the grayscale ultrasound image, with the color indicating the direction of movement with respect to the transducer. Doppler ultrasound is often used in regional anesthesia to identify vascular structures and distinguish them from nerves; however, it may reduce temporal resolution due to its low frame rate. Reducing the size of the color window may minimize this effect [111]. To reduce color artifact, Doppler velocity should be set between 15 and 35 cm/s [112].

Ultrasound transducers should be held with a low grip to facilitate fine movements. Hydrophilic gel or alcohol is used for acoustic coupling, and enough pressure should be applied to maintain adequate contact without collapsing veins or distorting anatomic landmarks. Movements to scan the anatomy may include sliding, rotating, or tilting the transducer [117]. The ultrasound machine should be positioned ergonomically within the operator's direct line of vision. Depending on the specific technique used, the needle may be introduced in-plane, in which the long axis of the needle is aligned with the transducer, or out-of-plane, in which the long axis of the needle is perpendicular to the transducer. Shallow insertion angles provide better needle visualization than steep angles due to reflection of more ultrasound waves back toward the transducer [118].

The region of interest should be positioned in the center of the ultrasound image, where surrounding structures and their spatial relationships can be seen clearly, and within the transducer's focal zone. The gain, or brightness of the image, should be adjusted to provide the best contrast between the nerve and surrounding structures. Peripheral nerves are variable in appearance on ultrasound, but generally consist of a hyperechoic epineurium surrounding a hypoechoic center. The short axis may be round, oval, or spindle-shaped, depending on the location and the nerve. Individual

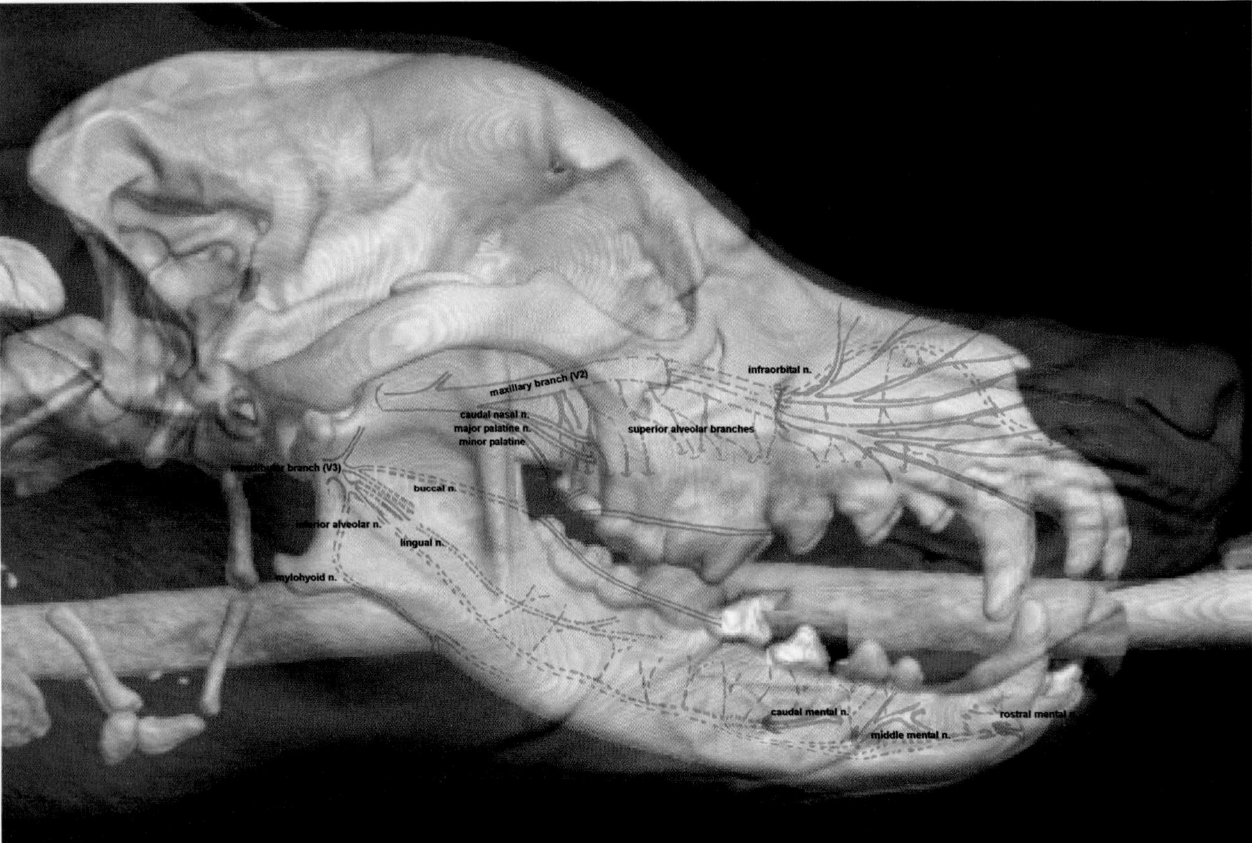

Figure 60.2 Distribution of the maxillary (V_2) and mandibular (V_3) branches of the trigeminal nerve (cranial nerve V).

hypoechoic nerve fascicles surrounded by hyperechoic perineurium are sometimes seen with high-resolution ultrasound. Nerves often lie in close proximity to blood vessels, which are readily identifiable with color Doppler. Anatomic variation and imaging artifacts may be disorienting to novice operators; therefore, a thorough understanding of regional anatomy and familiarity with ultrasound imaging is essential for the safety and success of ultrasound-guided techniques [119,120].

Blocks of the head

Oral, maxillofacial, ophthalmic, and auricular diseases requiring surgical intervention are common in small animals. Nerve blocks are widely used and indicated for the prevention and relief of pain associated with maxillofacial and dental surgery [121,122]. Correctly administered regional anesthesia reduces systemic anesthetic and analgesic requirements and is associated with improved postoperative analgesia and attenuation of the surgical stress response [44,123,124]. Common indications for local and regional anesthesia of the head in small animals include dental and oral surgery, maxillomandibular fracture repair, and ophthalmic surgery.

The implementation of local and regional anesthesia requires a thorough understanding of the relevant anatomy. The majority of sensory innervation to the head is supplied by the trigeminal nerve (cranial nerve V), with small caudal contributions from branches of the facial nerve (cranial nerve VII), and cervical spinal nerves [125]. The trigeminal nerve divides into the ophthalmic (V_1), maxillary (V_2), and mandibular (V_3) branches. The sensory innervation to the oral cavity, including all the intraoral structures, is provided by the mandibular and maxillary divisions and their corresponding branches (Fig. 60.2). Selection of a regional anesthetic technique should be predicated on the procedure and anatomy of the individual patient. Advanced imaging, such as computed tomography, may aid in both surgical planning and the selection of a regional anesthetic technique. As with any technique, care should be taken to avoid passing the needle through diseased or neoplastic tissue. All patients receiving regional anesthesia should be monitored for signs of systemic local anesthetic toxicity, though it is rare with appropriate dosing and aspiration to avoid intravascular injection [126].

Needle sizes ranging from 1 to 1.5 inch, 25 to 27 gauge, have been recommended [121]; needles should be flexible and ideally have a short, atraumatic bevel [127]. Because the tips of these needles become easily blunt or bent, the needle that is used to draw the anesthetic from the vial should not be used to administer the block [128]. Additionally, a new needle should be used for each site when performing more than one block.

Maxillary techniques

Anatomy

The maxillary nerve provides sensory innervation to the maxillary teeth and associated hard and soft tissues, hard and soft palates, nose, and lower eyelids. It exits the cranium via the round foramen and courses rostrally along the dorsal surface of the medial pterygoid muscle toward the pterygopalatine fossa (Fig. 60.3). At that point, the zygomatic and pterygopalatine nerves arise, and the maxillary nerve continues its course as the infraorbital nerve, entering the infraorbital canal via the maxillary foramen. The pterygopalatine nerve gives rise to the minor and major palatine nerves. These

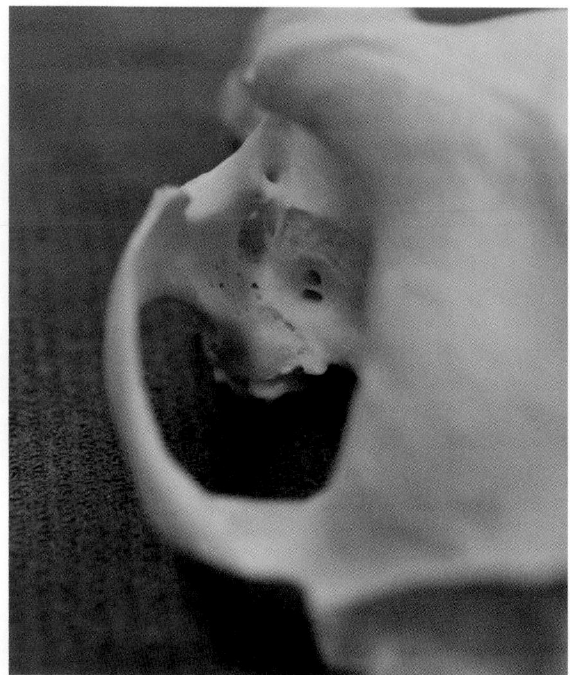

Figure 60.3 Caudal view of the pterygopalatine fossa. The maxillary foramen is the larger oval-shaped foramen in the center of the fossa and represents the caudal opening of the infraorbital canal.

emerge at the palatal area via the corresponding foramina, and provide innervation to the soft and hard palate, respectively [125]. The caudal, middle, and rostral superior alveolar nerves arise from the infraorbital nerve. The caudal superior alveolar nerves arise in the pterygopalatine fossa before the infraorbital nerve enters the canal, and they supply the first and second molar teeth. Within the infraorbital canal, the middle and rostral superior alveolar nerves emerge; these nerves supply the rostral premolars via numerous foramina located on the floor of the canal, and the canine and incisor teeth via the maxillary incisive canal. The infraorbital nerve exits the infraorbital canal via the infraorbital foramen, and gives rise to the external nasal, internal nasal, and superior labial branches [125].

Indications

When the maxillary nerve is blocked, the entire ipsilateral maxillary quadrant is anesthetized, including all teeth, associated gingiva, alveolar bone, dental pulp, and the hard and soft palates. Other maxillofacial structures anesthetized include part of the nasal mucosa (excluding the septal mucosa served by the ethmoidal nerve) and the upper lip [129–131]. The indications for a maxillary block or rostral blockade of the infraorbital nerve depend on the area of desired local anesthetic coverage and include ipsilateral maxillary dental extractions, oral surgery, and endodontic therapy, maxillectomy, incisivectomy, rhinotomy, rhinoscopy, and palatal surgery [121,132].

Technique

Several techniques have been described to block the maxillary nerve and its more distal branches and detailed descriptions are provided elsewhere [121,130,132]. Some of the techniques approach the nerve extraorally while others utilize an intraoral approach. Dependent on the technique utilized, the patient may be positioned in dorsal, sternal, or lateral recumbency.

A subzygomatic approach to the maxillary nerve has been described; however, the authors recommend caution with this advanced technique due to the risk of salivary gland and maxillary artery puncture, as well as nerve trauma, associated with the perpendicular approach to the nerve [121,131,133]. Similarly, the approach to the maxillary nerve via the maxillary tuberosity (or caudal intraoral) approach is associated with risks of accidental penetration of the orbit, possible perpendicular contact with the maxillary nerve, and injury to the maxillary artery and zygomatic salivary gland [132]. There are no clinical studies documenting the efficacy and safety of the maxillary tuberosity technique.

The rostral branches of the maxillary nerve can also be blocked using an infraorbital approach. The infraorbital foramen may be palpated extra- or intraorally. In dogs, the foramen is consistently located dorsal to the maxillary third premolar tooth and is easily palpated as an oval-shaped structure. In cats, the foramen is located immediately medial to the prominent rostral end of the zygomatic arch [121,134]. After the infraorbital foramen has been identified, the dominant hand is used to advance the needle caudally on a horizontal plane, maintaining it parallel to the hard palate (Fig. 60.4A) [132]. Following careful aspiration to ensure an absence of vascular puncture, a volume ranging from 0.1–1 mL, dependent upon size and conformation, of 0.5% bupivacaine may be injected. In cats and brachycephalic dogs, a short needle is recommended. Larger dogs may have a canal longer than 2 cm, so a longer needle or catheter is necessary to reach the targeted area [121]. It is important to note that insertion of the needle into the full length of the infraorbital canal should be avoided due to the risk of damage to the vascular structures within the canal or, in the case of brachycephalic or feline patients, orbital structures. One safe alternative is to advance an intravenous catheter off the stylet following entrance into the canal to deliver local anesthetic (Fig. 60.4B).

The infraorbital approach offers several advantages over other techniques used to block the maxillary nerve. First, it ensures that the needle is advanced accurately to the desired location. Also, the tip of the needle advances parallel to nerves, decreasing the risk of nerve damage by avoiding perpendicular contact. Moreover, because the canal guides the needle, damage to the zygomatic salivary gland is unlikely. Evidence suggests that this technique is safer and more effective than the lateral approach in both cats and dogs; however, the infraorbital approach may not consistently anesthetize the maxillary molar area if the anesthetic agent is deposited in the infraorbital canal and not in the pterygopalatine fossa [121,135]. It is also possible that this is due to collateral innervation to the associated alveolar mucosa and gingiva via the buccal nerve (branch of the mandibular nerve) [129]. A technique to block the buccal nerve in small animals has not been documented. Hematoma formation at the infraorbital foramen area is a frequent but usually minor complication that results from accidental laceration of the infraorbital artery or one of its branches, or the accompanying vein [121,134]. Immediate treatment is usually limited to applying manual pressure over the area to promote hemostasis.

Mandibular techniques

Anatomy

The mandibular nerve exits the cranium via the oval foramen and courses rostrally on the medial aspect of the temporomandibular joint, giving rise to the buccal and masticatory nerves. The masticatory nerve provides motor innervation to the rostral belly of the digastricus muscle; the buccal nerve crosses the pterygoid muscles toward the lateral aspect of the ramus and provides sensory

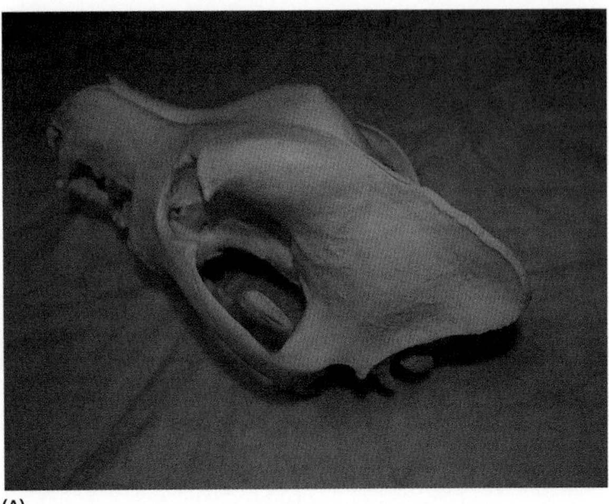

(A)

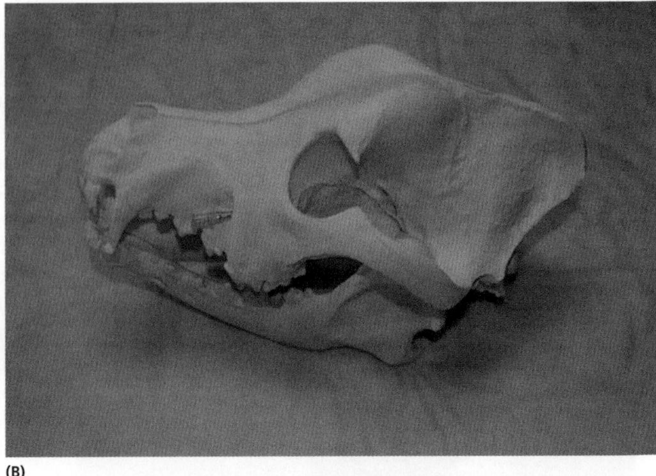

(B)

Figure 60.4 **A.** Caudal view of the infraorbital canal with a hypodermic needle inserted into the canal. **B.** Lateral view of the infraorbital canal with an intravenous catheter threaded into the canal for single delivery of local anesthetics. Source: Dr. Raphaël Vézina Audette.

innervation to the vestibular mucosa and skin ventral to the zygomatic bone. As the mandibular nerve continues its course rostrally, it gives rise to the lingual, mylohyoid, and inferior alveolar nerves. The mylohyoid nerve supplies the rostral belly of the digastricus muscle and the mylohyoid muscle. The lingual nerve supplies the rostral two-thirds of the tongue while the sublingual nerve, a branch of the lingual nerve, supplies the sublingual mucosa. On the lateral aspect of the medial pterygoid muscle, the mandibular nerve becomes the inferior alveolar nerve, coursing rostrally toward the mandibular foramen. At that point, the inferior alveolar nerve penetrates the mandibular canal via the mandibular foramen, where it provides sensory fibers to the teeth before further ramifying into the caudal, middle, and rostral mental nerves, which exit the mandibular canal via the corresponding mental foramen [125].

Indications

Blocking the inferior alveolar nerve provides regional anesthesia to the ipsilateral mandibular quadrant, including teeth, alveolar bone, and gingiva. The indications for an inferior alveolar nerve block include ipsilateral mandibular dental extractions and oral surgery, endodontic therapy, biopsies, and mandibulectomy [121,132]. The mental nerves supply the lower lip and rostral intermandibular area [125].

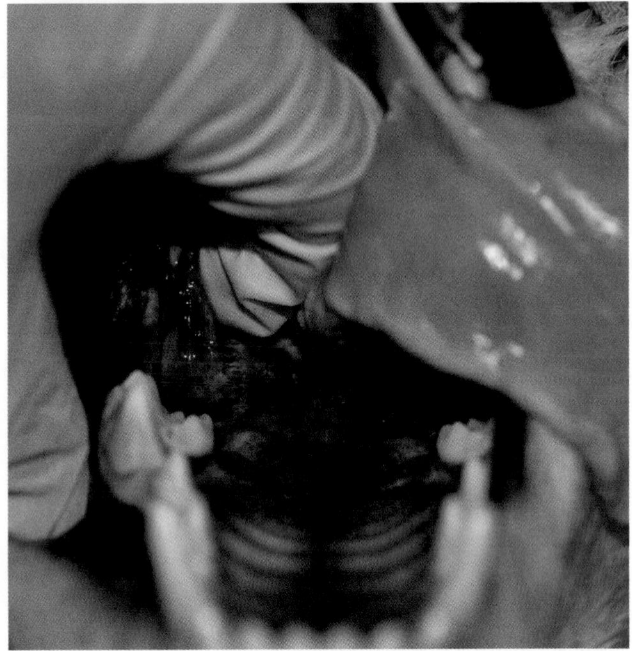

Figure 60.5 Palpation of the mandibular foramen of a dog cadaver. The index finger of the nondominant hand is used to locate the foramen intraorally at a point between the mandibular third molar tooth and the angular process, on the medial aspect of the ramus.

Technique

Ideally, the patient should be placed in dorsal or lateral recumbency to allow for successful palpation of landmarks as well as needle advancement. The mandibular foramen can be palpated intraorally using the index finger of the non-dominant hand (Fig. 60.5). The foramen is located on the medial and ventral portion of the ramus, between the third mandibular molar tooth and the angular process (Fig. 60.6). Alternatively, gentle palpation can be used to identify the inferior alveolar nerve and artery before it enters the canal [121,132]. While maintaining the index finger on the mandibular foramen, the other hand is used to advance the needle. The needle can be introduced intraorally under the mucosa, or extraorally through the skin of the ventral aspect of the mandible (Fig. 60.7). For both techniques, the needle must be slowly advanced along the medial aspect of the mandible until the tip is located over the mandibular foramen and 0.1–0.5 mL of 0.5% bupivacaine is injected [121]. Hematoma formation at the mandibular foramen may be a frequent but usually minor complication that results from laceration of the local blood vessels [134]. Immediate treatment is applying manual pressure over the area to promote hemostasis. Another reported, but apparently infrequent, complication is self-mutilation of the tongue during recovery from general anesthesia [133]. It has been suggested that this is due to diffusion of the local anesthetic solution onto the lingual nerve when attempting an inferior alveolar block using the caudal approach [121]. Deep tongue lacerations can occur very quickly and may bleed profusely; if severe, the patient may require immediate surgical repair under general anesthesia.

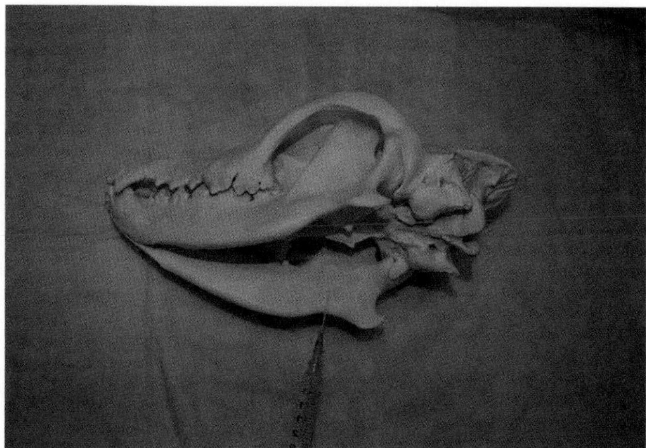

Figure 60.6 Location of the mandibular foramen, located on the medial and ventral portion of the ramus, between the third mandibular molar tooth and the angular process. Source: Dr. Raphaël Vézina Audette.

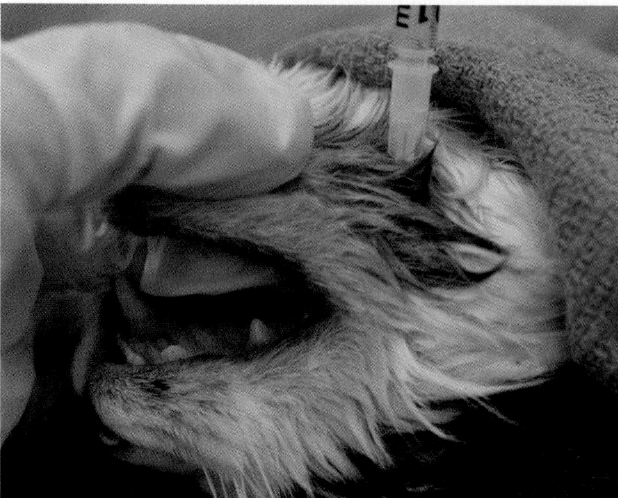

Figure 60.7 Extraoral caudal approach to the inferior alveolar nerve of a cat cadaver. The needle is introduced through the skin of the ventral mandibular area and is slowly advanced along the medial aspect of the ramus toward the mandibular foramen, where the anesthetic agent will be deposited.

The rostral approach consists of blocking the inferior alveolar nerve directly in the mandibular canal via the middle mental foramen (Fig. 60.8). The area anesthetized is variable and likely depends on how caudal within the canal the local anesthetic agent diffuses [136–138]. In general, the applicability of this technique may be limited to the rostral premolar, canine, and incisor teeth, and the rostral area of the lower lip. The middle mental foramen is palpated either intra- or extraorally using the non-dominant hand. The foramen is typically located between the roots of the canine and the first premolar teeth. Intraorally, the area is covered by the labial frenulum; it may be necessary to displace it rostrally or caudally. Owing to its small size, the middle mental foramen is generally not palpable in small dogs and cats. Once the foramen has been identified, a needle is introduced at a 45° angle and advanced until it is engaged in the mental foramen and 0.1–0.3 mL of 0.5% bupivacaine is injected; this can be done intra- or extraorally. Significant needle manipulation may be necessary, and damage to the middle mental and inferior alveolar nerve and artery is possible.

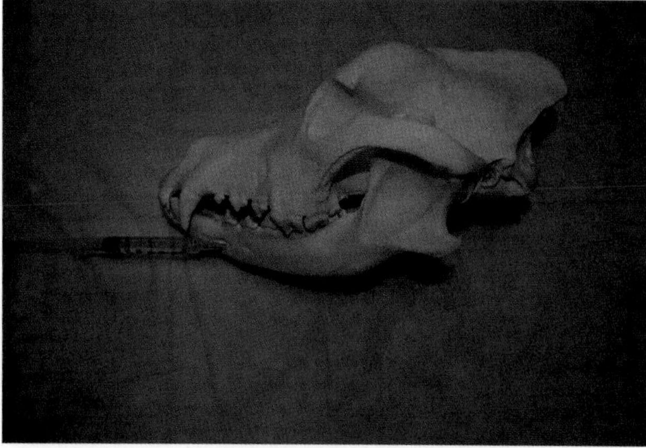

Figure 60.8 Insertion of a hypodermic needle into the mental foramen for blockade of the inferior alveolar nerve. Source: Dr. Raphaël Vézina Audette.

Local tissue dental blocks

Local dental infiltrative blocks are routinely used in human dentistry either as the sole means to achieve anesthesia for dental and oral procedures or to supplement regional anesthesia techniques [139]. Common local block techniques include intraosseous, intraligamentary (periodontal ligament), supraperiosteal, and intrapulpal injection [121,132]. Local anesthesia for dental procedures in dogs and cats has been reviewed in several publications [129,140]; however, no published clinical data are available on the use of these techniques in dogs and cats. Some local block techniques (e.g., intraligamentary) have been tested in dogs under experimental conditions [141], while others (e.g., supraperiosteal) are hypothetically considered ineffective owing to the thickness of the associated cortical bone [132]. Some local blocks require specialized equipment, representing an additional cost [141]. In addition, the duration of action of local dental blocks is shorter than that of regional blocks [132]. As a result, local dental blocks are infrequently used in dogs and cats.

Anesthesia for ophthalmic procedures

Anatomy

The orbit and surrounding tissues receive sensory innervation from the ophthalmic division of the trigeminal nerve (V_1), which emerges through the orbital fissure and divides into the frontal, lacrimal, and nasociliary nerves. The lower eyelid receives sensory innervation from the zygomatic nerve, which branches from the maxillary division of the trigeminal nerve (V_2) [125]. Motor innervation to the globe is provided by the oculomotor, trochlear, and abducens nerves. These nerves and their branches are located within the retrobulbar musculofascial cone, a tapering structure behind the globe consisting of the four rectus muscles and their associated connective tissues. The musculofascial cone tapers posteriorly to the annular tendon, which surrounds the optic nerve as it emerges from the skull through the optic foramen. Ophthalmic nerve blocks in this region are indicated for the prevention and relief of ophthalmic pain and to prevent the oculocardiac reflex during procedures involving the eye [142–144]. Preoperative administration of a retrobulbar nerve block is associated with a reduced incidence of the oculocardiac reflex during enucleation and superior analgesia when compared to an intraoperative splash block [144,145].

Techniques

Several different techniques have been described to provide regional anesthesia of the eye and orbital tissues, which vary in their ability to produce akinesia of the globe. These techniques may be classified as extraconal or intraconal (outside or within the musculofascial cone), or retrobulbar or peribulbar (behind or around the eye). Retrobulbar blocks are more invasive and carry a risk of damaging the optic nerve; therefore, they are almost exclusively performed for enucleation, while less invasive peribulbar techniques or topical anesthesia are preferred for other types of ophthalmic procedures.

Classically, a retrobulbar block is performed by inserting a curved needle at the junction of the middle and temporal third of the lower eyelid, directing the tip behind the globe until a popping sensation is appreciated and the eye rolls dorsally, indicating puncture into the musculofascial cone. Volume of injectate is dependent on the size of the patient, ranging from approximately 2–3 mL of 0.5% bupivacaine [143]. Alternatively, a supratemporal approach modeled on the technique used in horses has also been developed in dogs [146]. In this technique, the needle is inserted between the posterior aspect of the orbital ligament and the zygomatic process of the temporal bone and advanced ventromedially until the musculofascial cone is punctured. Deposition of local anesthetic within the musculofascial cone results in complete analgesia and akinesia of the globe. It is important to note that the optic nerve sheath contains cerebrospinal fluid (CSF) that is contiguous with intracranial CSF; accidental injection of local anesthetic within the optic nerve sheath can result in severe complications, such as total brainstem anesthesia [147–149]. As with all regional anesthetic techniques, cautious needle advancement and aspiration prior to injection of local anesthetic should be used.

Peribulbar and extraconal techniques are less invasive than intraconal techniques and carry a lower risk of damage to the optic nerve. They rely on diffusion of local anesthetic from the extraconal space into the intraconal space and may produce akinesia less reliably than intraconal techniques. Using a blind technique, the needle is inserted percutaneously at the anterior dorsomedial and ventrolateral margins of the eye and advanced until the tip of the needle is level with the equator of the globe, being careful not to puncture the globe itself [150]. Ultrasound guidance may aid the operator in positioning the needle within the extraconal space. An ultrasound-guided in-plane peribulbar technique has been described in canine cadavers, in which the ultrasound transducer is positioned caudal to the orbital ligament, and the needle is introduced caudally, guiding the tip into the extraconal space. Peribulbar spread of injectate was successful in all attempts [151]. A similar posterior ultrasound-guided approach with the transducer oriented transversely was less consistent in delivering injectate to the targeted structures [152].

Sub-Tenon's anesthesia refers to infiltration of local anesthetic within Tenon's capsule, the fibrous sheath surrounding the eyeball. It requires a specialized sub-Tenon's cannula, several different types of which have been described with similar characteristics [153]. Sub-Tenon's anesthesia, described in depth elsewhere, has been reported to produce analgesia and akinesia for cataract surgery in dogs [154].

Auricular techniques

Anatomy

Nerve blocks of the auricular region may be indicated for pain management or surgeries involving the ear canal, tympanic bulla, or pinna. Sensory innervation of the external ear canal is provided by the auriculotemporal nerve and the auricular branches of the facial nerve, while the pinna is innervated by the caudal auricular and the greater occipital nerves [150]. The auriculotemporal nerve arises from the mandibular division of the trigeminal nerve (V_3), running cranially to the external ear canal along the caudodorsal border of the masseter muscle and in close proximity to the facial nerve. The caudal auricular nerve is a branch of the facial nerve, and the greater occipital nerve is the largest branch of the second cervical spinal nerve.

Techniques

A blind approach to the great auricular nerve has been described in which the needle is inserted ventral to the transverse process of the atlas and advanced 0.3 cm ventromedially toward the jugular groove [155]. The auriculotemporal nerve can be blocked by inserting a needle perpendicular to the skin at the caudolateral border of the zygomatic arch and advancing toward the temporomandibular junction [155]. Alternatively, ultrasound guidance may be used to block the auriculotemporal and caudal auricular nerves; an ultrasound transducer is positioned in the coronal plane over the parotid salivary gland, perpendicular to the ramus of the mandible [150]. The auriculotemporal and caudal auricular nerves can be visualized between the external acoustic meatus and parotid salivary gland caudally and the condyloid process of the mandible cranially. The needle is introduced out-of-plane ventral to the transducer and advanced dorsomedially at an approximately 45° angle until the tip is positioned caudal to the condyloid process. The great auricular nerve is located superficially, cranial to the bifurcation of the jugular vein into the maxillary and linguofacial veins. It is easily visualized on ultrasound with the transducer oriented in the transverse plane at the level of the atlas. The great auricular nerve is a small, oval structure dorsal to the maxillary vein and mandibular salivary gland. Blocking the great auricular nerve provides analgesia to the skin overlying the caudal ramus of the mandible and on the dorsal surface of the pinna. Akinesia of the eyelid is possible due to the relationship between the auriculotemporal nerve and the facial nerve and should be treated with ophthalmic lubricants until palpebral function has returned.

Trigeminal nerve block

Ultrasound-guided trigeminal nerve block has been reported in a dog undergoing extensive head surgery involving exenteration, caudal maxillectomy, and zygomatic arch resection [156]. Proximal blockade of the trigeminal nerve provides a broad area of desensitization in a single injection site, including areas innervated by the ophthalmic branch (V_1) such as the orbit and nasal septum. However, the block is technically challenging compared to more peripheral techniques. The needle is introduced in-plane to the ultrasound transducer immediately caudal to the orbital ligament and advanced ventrally toward the caudal pterygopalatine fossa, where the three branches of the trigeminal nerve and the maxillary artery can be visualized lateral to the frontal bone and overlying the sphenoid bone [150,156]. Doppler ultrasonography can aid in identification of the maxillary artery. The volume delivered is 0.1 mL/cm of the cranium length from the inion to the nasion.

Blocks of the thorax and abdomen

Dependent upon the region that requires blockade, there are a number of techniques that may be used to provide regional anesthesia to the thoracic walls, with or without visceral analgesia. In general, the innervation of the thorax and abdomen is provided by branches of spinal nerves. Dorsal branches of thoracic spinal nerves extend dorsally and divide into medial and lateral branches to innervate the epaxial muscles and the skin near the dorsal midline. The sensory innervation of the lateral and ventral thoracic wall is provided by the ventral branches of the thoracic spinal nerves via the intercostal nerves [125]. The skin of the thorax is innervated by dorsal, lateral, and ventral cutaneous branches of the spinal nerves [157].

Thoracic paravertebral block

The thoracic paravertebral space in dogs has been described as a wedge-shaped area bordered ventrally by the parietal pleura, medially by the vertebral bodies, intervertebral discs, and foramina, laterally by the intercostal muscles, and dorsally incompletely by the costotransverse ligament [158]. Ventral branches of the spinal nerves travel distally via the dorsal compartment of the thoracic paravertebral space. Before the advent of technologies such as neurostimulation or ultrasonography to guide injections of local anesthetics, the standard approach to the thoracic paravertebral space consisted of a blind technique guided by anatomical landmarks [159]. Loss of resistance to injection performed with a loss of resistance syringe and the characteristic pop-like feeling perceived by the operator once the endothoracic fascia is pierced by the tip of a Tuohy needle were long considered confirmatory for locating the thoracic paravertebral space. Portela *et al.* described a nerve stimulator-guided method for injections into the thoracic paravertebral space; however, this technique was associated with a complication rate of 20%, which included instances of epidural spread and intrapleural migration of injectate from accidental puncture of the parietal pleura [158]. This technique, though imperfect, brought about a level of objectivity beyond that of blind injections where the subjective pop-like feeling of the needle through the internal intercostal membrane guided the injection. The sonoanatomy of the canine thoracic paravertebral space in dog cadavers was subsequently described, along with a method to perform a thoracic paravertebral block with ultrasound guidance, further decreasing risks associated with the thoracic paravertebral block [160,161]. In addition to enabling the use of a lower volume of injectate, ultrasound guidance afforded a superior level of safety as direct visualization of the needle during injection prevented the puncture of the parietal pleura. Single injection points of diluted dye injectate in cadaveric studies resulted in staining beyond the thoracic paravertebral space despite correctly located injections, suggesting that local anesthetic spread outside of the immediate paravertebral space may play a role in the regional anesthesia observed with this technique. Based on inconsistent staining of multiple levels of spinal nerves under cadaveric conditions, complete thoracic anesthesia may require injection at multiple spaces.

Another canine cadaveric study suggests the utility of this technique may extend beyond the thorax. Spinal nerves originating from T10 to L1 contribute sensory innervation to the cranial abdomen; caudal thoracic paravertebral spaces can also be injected to provide somatic and visceral analgesia at the level of the cranial abdomen [162]. Though this technique was associated with mediastinal contamination in 80% of injections, no other complications were noted.

Clinically, a single injection at the level of the caudal thoracic paravertebral space has been shown to provide adequate analgesia in radical mastectomy [163], lateral thoracotomy [164], and adrenalectomy via midline laparotomy [165]. The thoracic paravertebral block was also described in other animal species (*Vulpes vulpes*) [166]. Together, the evidence suggests thoracic paravertebral blocks are useful for the provision of perioperative analgesia in thoracic and cranial abdominal surgeries. It is important to note that ultrasound-guided thoracic paravertebral block is a technically challenging technique and is recommended for more advanced practitioners of ultrasound-guided regional anesthesia.

Intercostal nerve block

Caudal to each rib, the intercostal nerve runs as part of a neurovascular bundle that also includes the intercostal artery and vein (Figs. 60.9 and 60.10). The neurovascular bundles are bordered by the endothoracic fascia medially and the internal intercostal muscles laterally [125]. The intercostal nerves provide sensory and motor innervation to the parietal pleura and lateral thoracic body wall and give rise to the lateral and ventral cutaneous branches that supply the skin of the mid- to ventral thorax [157]. Intercostal nerve blocks have been described as a technique to provide superior analgesia for dogs undergoing thoracic surgery [167–169].

The safety and utility of intercostal blocks is well supported in the literature. Berg and Orton compared the effects of different analgesic modalities on the respiratory function of dogs following thoracotomies [170]. Intravenous administration of opioids caused significant respiratory depression in dogs due to a concomitant decrease in minute volume and respiratory frequency and led to clinically significant hypoventilation and hypoxemia; however, a treatment group that received intercostal nerve blocks with bupivacaine exhibited no such respiratory depression in the immediate postoperative period. Similarly, Thompson and Johnson compared selective intercostal nerve blocks to interpleural instillation of bupivacaine and systemic morphine administration in dogs undergoing lateral thoracotomies and assessed respiratory function and analgesia postoperatively [168]. Dogs treated with systemic opioids experienced more complications than dogs in the other treatment groups such as perioperative hypothermia, with slower return to normal temperature and blood gas alterations suggestive of poor respiratory function. Though all groups showed a downward trend in PaO_2, only the morphine and interpleural bupivacaine groups had significantly lower PaO_2 compared to baseline. Another study of the effect of intercostal nerve blocks on arterial blood gas tensions in dogs that underwent thoracotomies noted that PaO_2 and $PaCO_2$ were not different before and after treatment at 4 and 8 h postoperatively, suggesting that intercostal nerve blocks with bupivacaine afforded postoperative analgesia sufficient to normalize respiratory function in dogs [169].

As innervation of the cranial abdomen involves thoracic dermatomes, the addition of selective (e.g., T8–T10) intercostal nerve blocks may provide adjunctive coverage to other abdominal regional anesthetic techniques. A study comparing the analgesic efficacy of a combination of intercostal nerve blocks and spinal anesthesia to a sufentanil constant rate infusion in cats undergoing unilateral radical mastectomies showed that both intraoperative and postoperative analgesia was superior in patients that received locoregional anesthesia as part of their anesthetic protocol [171].

The sternum and associated tissues may be blocked via various ultrasound-guided parasternal blocks, described elsewhere [172,173] These techniques aim to desensitize the terminal branches of the intercostal nerves, distal to where the lateral cutaneous branches bifurcate off the intercostal nerves, thus providing analgesia solely at the level of the thoracic ventral midline (i.e., for median sternotomies). In theory, this technique would be expected to spare intercostal muscle function and preserve ventilatory function, though

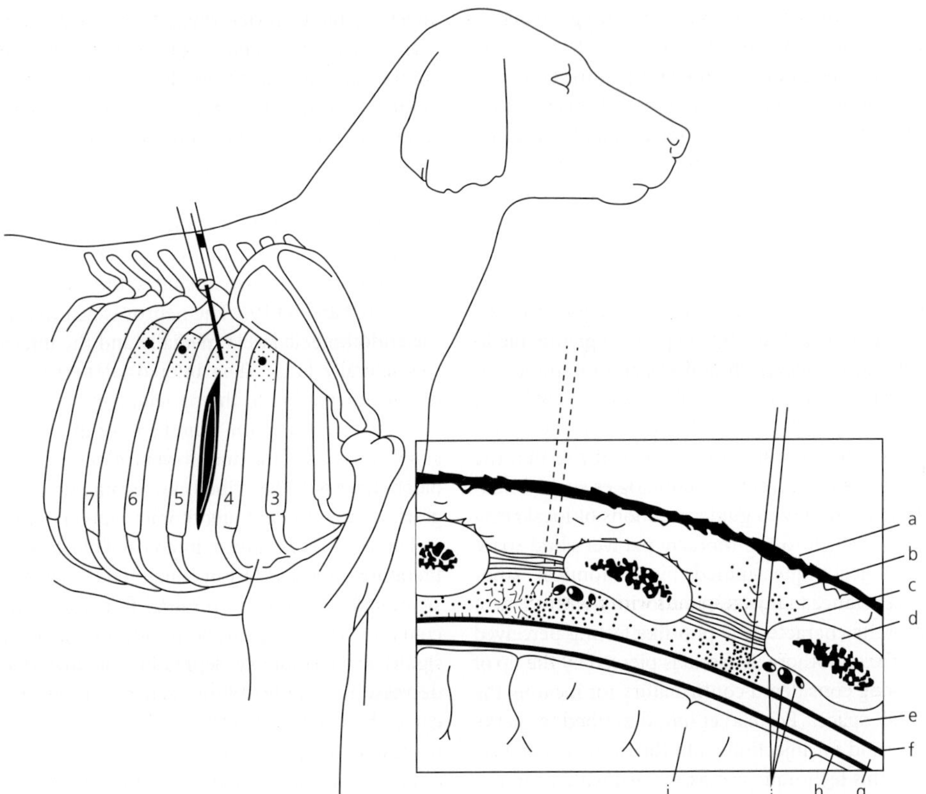

Figure 60.9 Needle placement for inducing intercostal nerve blocks in a dog, showing the lateral aspect and the sagittal section. Inset: (a) skin, (b) subcutaneous tissue, (c) intercostal muscles, (d) rib, (e) subcostal space, (f) parietal pleura and fascia, (g) interpleural space, (h) visceral pleura, (i) intercostal artery, vein, and nerve, and (j) lung.

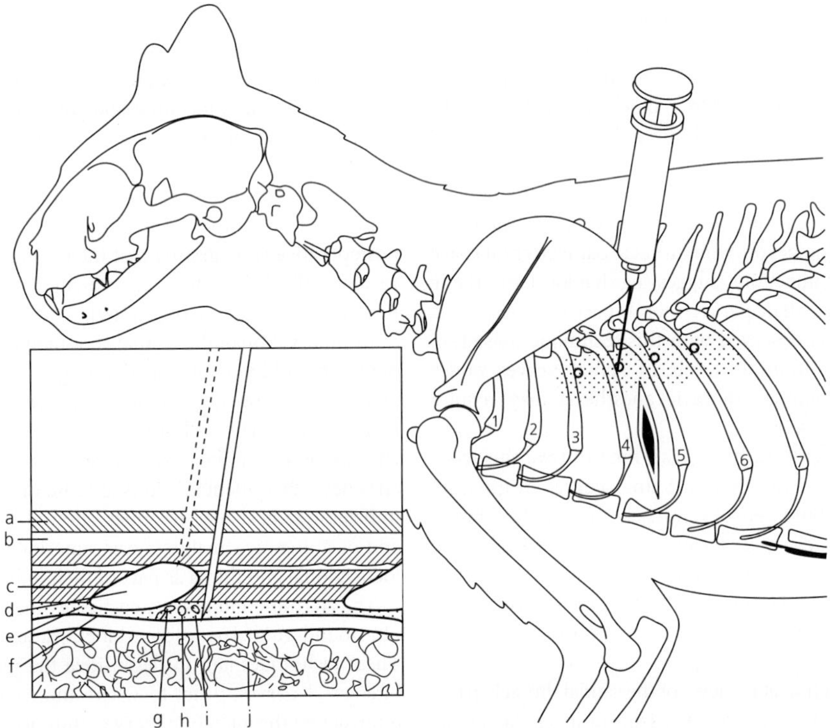

Figure 60.10 Needle placement for inducing intercostal nerve blocks in a cat, showing the lateral aspect and the sagittal section. Inset: (a) skin, (b) subcutaneous tissue, (c) intercostal muscles, (d) rib, (e) subcostal space, (f) parietal pleura and fascia, (g) intercostal vein, (h) intercostal artery, (i) intercostal nerve, and (j) lung.

clinical trials have yet to be conducted to assess the clinical efficacy of this technique in veterinary patients.

In order to decrease the risks of block failure secondary to inaccuracy of blind injections and reduce the risks of complications associated with potential pleural puncture, Thomson *et al.* studied the sonoanatomy of the intercostal space and described a novel ultrasound-guided technique for intercostal nerve blocks [35]. Though slightly more time consuming than blind injections, the authors reported a significant improvement in the accuracy of intercostal nerve staining with ultrasound guidance compared with the blind technique with 68/70 (97%) successful injections versus 45/70 (64%).

Interpleural regional analgesia

Interpleural regional analgesia involves infiltration of a local anesthetic solution into the potential space between the parietal and visceral pleura. Multiple studies in dogs have shown that interpleurally administered local anesthetics work by diffusion across the parietal pleura to block the underlying intercostal nerves, resulting in multidermatomal blockade [174]. The distribution of blockade is gravity-dependent and corresponds with the lowermost part of pleural space where pooling of the local anesthetic solution occurs [175]. Interpleural administration of local anesthetics has proven useful for providing pain relief not only for thoracic surgeries, but also for painful disorders of the cranial abdomen (e.g., pancreatitis) [176].

While effective, it is important to note the possible complications of this technique. The large surface area of the pleura can potentially result in rapid absorption of the administered local anesthetic solution and high plasma levels of the local anesthetic can result, potentially leading to local anesthetic systemic toxicity (LAST) [177]. No adverse cardiovascular effects were reported when local anesthetic was administered interpleurally to patients with or without an open pericardium [178]. While direct lung trauma is unlikely with careful technique, a small volume of air can be aspirated into the pleural space due to the negative intrathoracic pressure. This can result in an insignificant pneumothorax and is not considered to be of clinical significance. Potentially more significant is a potential loss of diaphragmatic function on the injection side after administration of interpleural bupivacaine [179]. Dogs that received bilateral blockade demonstrated paradoxical respirations and generated negative intra-abdominal pressures upon inspiration. Patients at increased risk of cardiovascular and respiratory complications may be better treated with alternative methods of pain relief (e.g., intercostal nerve blocks and thoracic epidural anesthesia).

With the patient positioned in lateral recumbency, an over-the-needle catheter connected to a syringe filled with 2–3 mL of saline via a three-way stopcock is advanced onto the lateral aspect of the seventh or eighth rib at its midpoint between the dorsal and ventral midline. The needle is then walked off the cranial border of the rib until it can be advanced through the intercostal space. Entering the thorax at the cranial border of the rib helps minimize the risk of traumatizing the intercostal nerve and vascular bundle that lies caudal to each rib. Once the parietal pleura has been penetrated (often with a palpable "pop" or "click"), the column of saline in the syringe will slowly decrease in volume as the negative interpleural pressure aspirates the saline into the interpleural space. Once the needle tip has been confirmed to be in the interpleural space, the catheter is gently advanced off the needle stylet into the interpleural space (Fig. 60.11). The preloaded syringe with local anesthetic solution is then attached to the catheter and the calculated volume of local anesthetic is slowly injected over 1–2 min into the interpleural space. Following injection of the local anesthetic, the catheter is withdrawn and the patient is positioned with the operative side down for at least 10 min, allowing the local anesthetic to pool and block the underlying intercostal nerves.

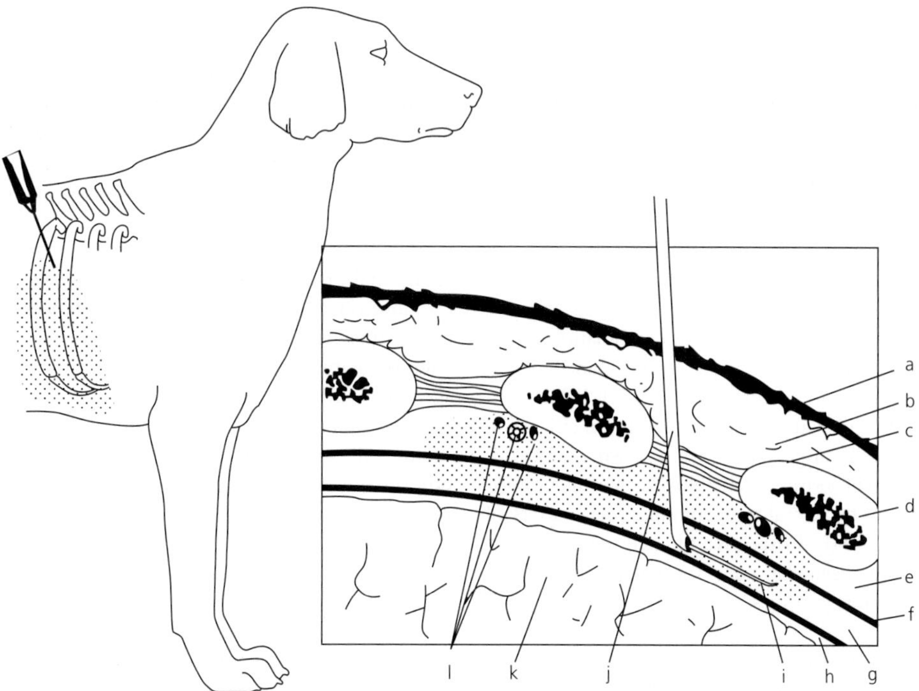

Figure 60.11 Interpleural catheter placement in a dog. Inset: (a) skin, (b) subcutaneous tissue, (c) intercostal muscles, (d) rib, (e) subcostal space, (f) parietal pleura and fascia, (g) interpleural space, (h) visceral pleura, (i) catheter, (j) Tuohy needle, (k) lung, and (l) intercostal artery, vein, and nerve.

Alternatively, an indwelling catheter or chest tube can be placed into the interpleural space to facilitate repeated injections. Catheter dislodgement can occur whenever an indwelling catheter is placed at any site in the body; after correctly positioning the catheter in the interpleural space, it should be secured to the patient by means of adhesive patches, tissue glue, suture, and/or bandages. Subcutaneous tunneling of larger gauge interpleural catheters can be used as a further means to reduce the likelihood of dislodgment and to prevent air from inadvertently entering the interpleural space around the catheter. A C-clamp or other similar device may be used to reduce the possibility of air being aspirated through the chest tube or catheter following inadvertent dislodgment or other issues.

Fascial plane block techniques

Fascial plane blocks represent a relatively novel class of ultrasound-guided regional anesthetic techniques in veterinary medicine. They rely on the deposition of higher volumes of dilute local anesthetic into a fascial plane that contains nerves, rather than targeting discrete nerves. In both human and veterinary medicine, there has been an explosion of descriptions of novel techniques with accompanying cadaveric studies. In most cases, prospective, controlled trials are lacking yet many practitioners of regional anesthesia utilize these techniques frequently as part of a balanced analgesic plan. Each technique described below has been detailed in initial cadaveric studies; the reader is directed to the referenced literature for more complete descriptions of individual techniques.

Serratus plane block

The serratus plane block, also known as the serratus ventralis or serratus anterior plane block, is a fascial plane block that was originally proposed in human patients as an alternative method to providing locoregional anesthesia to the thoracic body wall via desensitization of the lateral cutaneous branches of T2 to T9 [180]. A veterinary adaptation of this ultrasound-guided technique has been described in canine cadavers [181]. The technique consists of injecting a volume of local anesthetic solution in the fascial plane between the serratus ventralis thoracis and the latissimus dorsi muscles or, in the alternative deep technique, between the serratus ventralis thoracis and the external intercostal muscles. As it is usually recommended to desensitize up to two dermatomes cranial and caudal to the site of surgery due to the significant overlap in receptive fields on the thorax, the serratus plane block is expected to only produce partial thoracic anesthesia involving the cranial thoracic dermatomes based on spread of injectate in cadaver subjects.

Despite questionable efficacy for complete thoracic anesthesia in cadaveric studies, there is clinical evidence that suggests effective perioperative analgesia may be afforded by a combination of the transversus abdominis plane block with the serratus plane block in dogs undergoing unilateral radical mastectomy [182]. While prospective randomized clinical trials evaluating the clinical efficacy of this technique in thoracic surgery are lacking, two case series describe the effective use of serratus plane block as part of a multimodal analgesic protocol for lateral thoracotomies for a variety of surgical conditions [183,184]. Prospective blinded and appropriately controlled studies are needed to assess the utility of this locoregional technique in veterinary species.

Quadratus lumborum block

Upon exiting through their respective intervertebral foramina, the ventral rami of the twelfth and thirteenth thoracic spinal nerves (T12, T13) run within the bundles of the quadratus lumborum (QL) muscle while the first three lumbar spinal nerves (L1–L3) course between the QL muscle and the psoas muscle. Lumbar spinal nerves course through the transverse fascia that separates the retroperitoneum from the sublumbar musculature. They penetrate the transversus abdominis muscle to continue their course within the fascial plane that exists between the transversus abdominis muscle and the internal abdominal oblique muscle. Together with the caudal thoracic spinal nerves (T9–T13), these lumbar spinal nerves provide motor and sensory innervation to the abdomen. In addition, sympathetic ganglia are present alongside the vertebral bodies from T13–L5 and are responsible for autonomic innervation of the abdominal viscera [185]. There are several different approaches that may be utilized to deposit local anesthetic into the fascial planes that surround the QL muscle to provide regional anesthesia suitable for abdominal procedures. These have been described extensively in the human literature and have more recently been described and evaluated in veterinary patients.

An initial canine cadaveric study provided a thorough assessment of the anatomy and sonoanatomy of the canine QL plane and evaluated the feasibility of an in-plane ultrasound-guided injection technique [185]. Injections of 0.3 mL/kg of dye–lidocaine injectate performed at the level of L1 were associated with successful cranial lumbar nerve and splanchnic nerve staining. However, inconsistent staining was found for more cranial (i.e., T13) spinal nerve segments, indicating that surgery of the cranial abdomen may require either a higher volume of injectate or that the QL block would need to be combined with another technique. Furthermore, injections into the intermuscular plane between the psoas major and the QL muscles using the described technique were less likely to be feasible in larger breed dogs due to the excessive depth. Two alternative approaches to delivering injections lateral to the QL were then assessed, the transverse or longitudinal needle approaches [186]. The authors determined that a transverse approach to the lateral QL plane with 0.3 mL/kg of injectate per hemiabdomen was feasible and resulted in more consistent spread of injectate. No complications such as intra-abdominal or epidural contamination were noted in either technique. In both studies, the approach to the QL was performed from a ventrolateral to dorsomedial direction.

Due to concern about the risk of making an intra-abdominal injection or causing inadvertent injury to adjacent abdominal organs, another approach to the QL block was described whereby the needle was advanced in a dorsolateral to ventromedial trajectory targeting the medial aspect of the QL [187]. This technique yielded results similar to those described previously and no ectopic abdominal or epidural injectate was observed. When assessed by CT, however, there were important differences noted in the craniocaudal injectate spread. Another study evaluated use of a higher volume of injectate consisting of dye and a radiopaque contrast agent (0.6 mL/kg) and also found distinct patterns of reach as assessed by anatomic dissection and CT evaluation [188]. These findings illustrate how different evaluation methods (e.g., dissection versus advanced imaging) or injectate solution types (e.g., dye versus local anesthetic combined with contrast agent) can be an important source of variation in studies of ultrasound-guided blocks, and that the relationship between cadaveric studies involving contrast media or tissue dyes may not equate to clinical block efficacy when techniques are performed in live patients using different local anesthetic solutions.

Cadaveric studies in cats have also been performed and, similar to previous studies in dogs, the results varied between assessment techniques and found staining that could potentially be associated with incomplete regional anesthesia of the abdomen [189,190]. A QL block as part of multimodal analgesia protocol was described in a case report involving a cat undergoing exploratory laparotomy and cystotomy [191]. Those authors reported the need for intraoperative administration of rescue analgesia at the beginning of surgery, but none thereafter, and the patient was reportedly comfortable with pain scores consistently below the suggested intervention threshold using a validated pain scoring instrument. Like many fascial plane techniques, no clinical studies have been published to date evaluating the efficacy of QL blocks in companion animals for perioperative analgesia, and more research is needed to bridge the gap between the findings of laboratory cadaveric studies and pain management in clinical cases.

Transversus abdominis plane block

The abdominal wall is innervated by thoracolumbar spinal nerves including T9 to T12, the costoabdominalis nerve (T13), and the three most cranial lumbar nerves (iliohypogastricus cranialis nerve [L1], iliohypogastricus caudalis nerve [L2], and ilioinguinalis nerve [L3]). Nerves course along the fascial plane in between the internal abdominal oblique muscle and the transversus abdominis muscle, underneath a thin sheet of connective tissue that is tightly adhered to the transversus abdominis muscle [192]. Thus, sensory blockade to the abdominal wall can be achieved by injecting local anesthetic solution in the intermuscular plane known as the transversus abdominis plane (TAP). Occasionally, additional thoracic nerves located more cranially may be found in the TAP.

Several cadaveric studies aimed at characterizing the spread of injectates within the TAP have been published [193–196]. Variable staining of sensory nerve fibers with even the highest volumes of injectate tested (0.25–1 mL/kg of 0.25% bupivacaine and dye solutions) suggest that a combination of a subcostal and mid or caudal abdominal approach may be necessary to effectively desensitize the ventral abdominal midline. Interestingly, most studies appear to indicate that a ceiling effect exists. While craniocaudal spread increases up to a volume of 0.5 mL/kg; doubling the volume to 1 mL/kg does not result in a greater reach. Interestingly, one study reported no significant difference in number of ventral spinal nerves stained between dogs receiving a single-point TAP block per side as compared to two injections per side, though the area of injectate spread did differ significantly between groups [197]. Beyond the volume of the injectate, variables that may affect spread include cadaver condition, position, and duration between injection and dissection. Additionally, the composition of the dye may account for interstudy variability since the physical and chemical properties of the solutions may change their ability to penetrate tissues [198]. Different injection techniques have also revealed different patterns of staining, with a combination of subcostal and lateral injections yielding a better craniocaudal staining pattern than a combination of cranial and caudal lateral injections [199].

To perform an ultrasound-guided TAP block in canine and feline patients undergoing exploratory laparotomy with incisions extending from the xiphoid to the caudal abdomen, the authors recommend a four-point technique combining the lateral and subcostal approaches. The authors' preference is to draw up 0.35 mL/kg of bupivacaine 0.5%, diluted in a 1:1 ratio with sterile saline 0.9%. Dexmedetomidine can be added to the final solution in a ratio of 1 μg/mL of solution. The resulting solution is split evenly to perform a total of four injections.

For the lateral approach, a linear high-frequency transducer is placed in either a transverse or longitudinal orientation, midway between the last rib and the iliac crest, and midway between the ventral and dorsal midline (Fig. 60.12). The body wall is identified as the first hyperechoic line superficial to the peritoneum. The muscle immediately superficial to the peritoneum is the transversus abdominis which lies deep to the internal abdominal oblique muscle. The TAP is the potential space between these two muscles, appearing as a hyperechoic line that can be hydrodissected by injecting a local anesthetic. The procedure is repeated on both sides.

For the subcostal approach, the transducer is placed in a transverse orientation, perpendicular to the linea alba just caudal to the xiphoid process. The probe is then rotated 10–15° with the marker located cranially. The resulting position of the transducer is parallel to the costal arch and oblique to the midline. The rectus abdominis and transversus abdominis muscles are visualized, and the peritoneum is again identified as a thick hyperechoic structure separating the peritoneal cavity and the body wall. The overlying transversus abdominis muscle is separated from the more superficial rectus abdominis muscle by the fascia of the transversus abdominis muscle (superficial), which can be identified as a characteristic triangle. When these structures have been identified, the needle is inserted from the cranial aspect of the transducer, using an in-plane technique, with a 20° angle, so that the tip is located in the fascial plane between the rectus abdominis and transversus abdominis muscles.

The first report of clinical use of a TAP block in a veterinary species described an uneventful anesthetic event to facilitate the surgical excision of a gastrointestinal foreign body in a Canadian lynx [200]. In that report, the bilateral TAP block was performed with one injection of 0.4 mL/kg of 0.125% bupivacaine on each side (a total of 1 mg/kg) as part of a multimodal analgesic plan. The patient exhibited no signs of discomfort up to 10 h postoperatively. A retrospective study evaluated the use of a cranial and caudal TAP block (0.3 to 0.35 mL/kg per injection) combined with intercostal nerve blocks in dogs undergoing mastectomy [201]. The combination of TAP and intercostal blocks as part of a balanced multimodal analgesic protocol in combination with low doses of systemic opioids produced adequate intraoperative and immediate postoperative analgesia. In an assessment of duration of analgesic effect, TAP blocks were performed with either a liposome-encapsulated formulation of bupivacaine or 0.25% bupivacaine potentiated with dexmedetomidine [202]. The authors did not find a significant advantage to liposome-encapsulated bupivacaine in that the duration of analgesia afforded by the technique was equivalent in each group and was limited to approximately 24 h. It is important to consider that, given the low fraction of free bupivacaine in the commercially available liposome-encapsulated bupivacaine suspension, its use in preoperative locoregional blocks may not provide sufficient intraoperative analgesia. Consequently, consideration may be given to mixing the suspension with standard bupivacaine (though no other agents should be combined with liposomal formulations of bupivacaine).

Though locoregional blocks are best performed in the context of preemptive analgesia, TAP blocks may be performed postoperatively in certain situations where time is of the essence and performance of a preoperative block is not feasible (e.g., such as emergent celiotomies for rapidly bleeding abdominal masses or cesarean sections where fetal stress is documented) or when ultrasound equipment is not readily available. However, in such cases, the presence of a pneumoperitoneum may cause a mirroring artifact that would make the identification of the TAP more difficult and may lead to

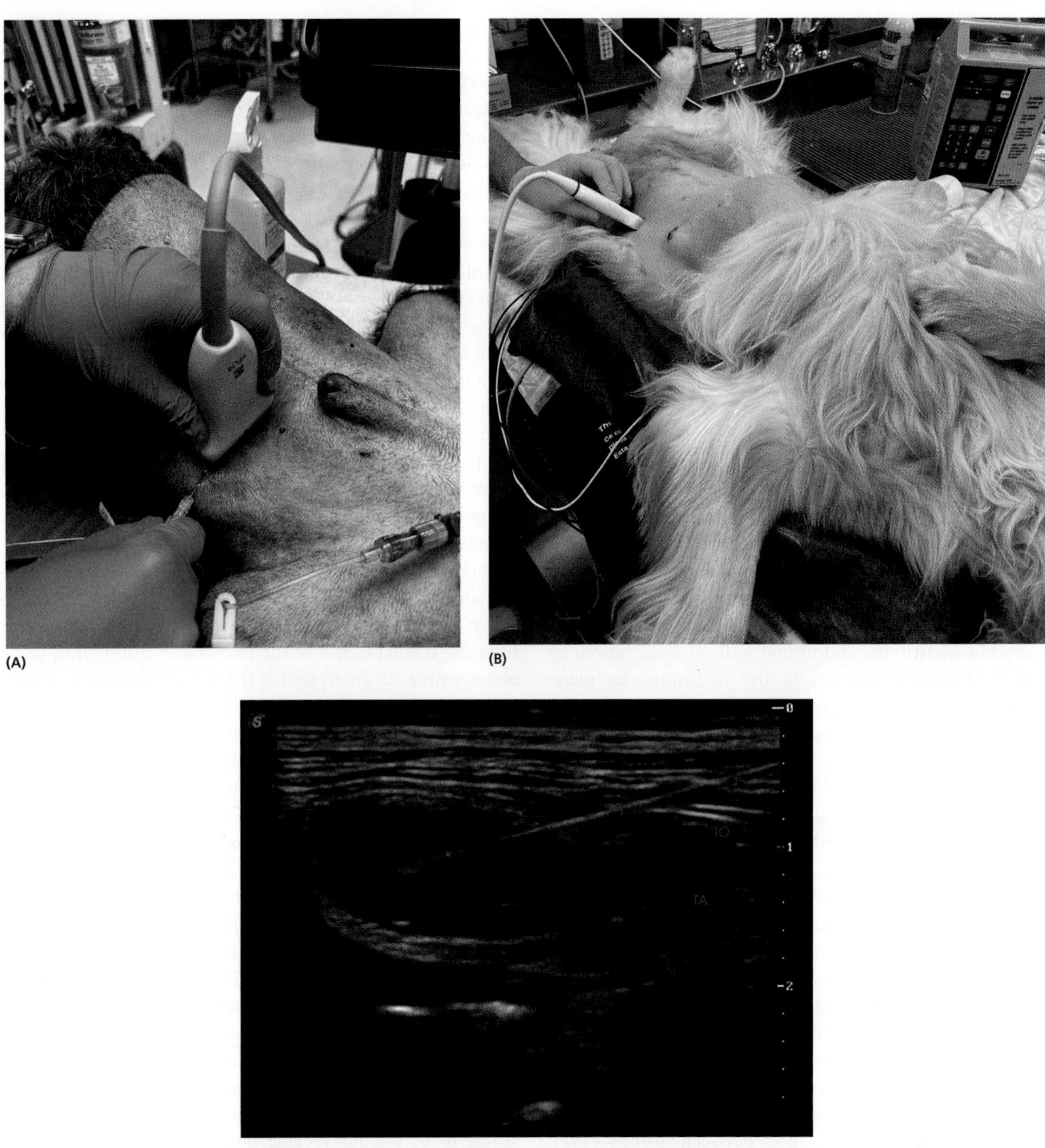

Figure 60.12 Ultrasound probe positioning for the lateral approach to the transversus abdominis plane (TAP) block in either **A.** transverse, or **B.** longitudinal positioning. **C.** Ultrasound image of local anesthetic solution within the transversus abdominis plane, between the transversus abdominis (TA) and internal abdominal oblique (IO) muscles. Source: Dr. Carrie Schroeder (A); Dr. Raphaël Vézina Audette (B and C.).

abdominal puncture and/or organ damage if the artifact is not correctly recognized [120]. An alternative to ultrasound-guided blocks consists of an open surgeon-assisted approach where local anesthetic solution is injected at the level of the aponeurosis of the transversus abdominis muscle [203].

Erector spinae plane block

Motor and sensory innervation to the epaxial muscles and dorsum is provided by the dorsal rami of the thoracic and lumbar spinal nerves while the lateral branches of the dorsal rami provide motor innervation to the longissimus thoracis, levatores costarum, and iliocostalis thoracis muscles. These lateral extensions are known as dorsal cutaneous branches, and they supply sensory innervation from the dorsal midline to the lateral axillary limit of the thoracic body wall [157]. Motor innervation to the transversospinalis muscle group and sensory innervation to the vertebral laminae, ligaments, and facet joints are derived from the medial branches of the dorsal rami of the spinal nerves [204].

The erector spinae plane (ESP) block is a fascial plane block in which a local anesthetic is deposited deep to the erector spinae muscles, resulting in spread of local anesthetic solution in the epaxial compartment that involves the lateral and medial branches of the dorsal rami [205]. The original landmark for ESP injections is the dorsolateral edge of the transverse process, which corresponds to the ventromedial aspect of the longissimus thoracis muscle. Single injections along the thoracolumbar spine result in variable and unpredictable craniocaudal spread according to the results of various cadaver studies [206–208]. Medial and lateral branches of the dorsal rami are consistently targeted by ESP injections and the injectate appears to remain confined to the epaxial compartment. More recently, a cadaveric study comparing injections aimed at the lateral process or mamillary processes of the thoracolumbar spine caudal to T11 indicated that medial branches of the dorsal branches of the spinal nerves were more reliably stained when the needle is directed at the mamillary processes [209]. This technique is thus preferred since innervation of the vertebral laminae, facet joints, and epaxial muscles of dogs comes from the medial branches. Cadaveric canine studies of the ESP block have only rarely identified hypaxial spread of injectate, and epidural and/or thoracic paravertebral space contamination have not been reported in cadaveric studies involving thoracic ESP blocks [206–208]. Epidural migration was observed in 11.7% of cadavers injected with a transverse approach to the L4 vertebra [208] and may be responsible for rare complications such as sympathetic blockade and subsequent sinus arrest when performed at the T13 or L1 segment in dogs [210]. It is thus anticipated that ESP blocks would provide regional anesthesia to the dorsolateral aspect of the body wall and would be a suitable technique to use in the context of neurosurgery such as hemilaminectomies. This is supported by the findings of a retrospective study in dogs in which there was a significant reduction of perioperative opioid administration and more stable cardiovascular status in patients undergoing hemilaminectomies that received an ESP block [211].

Further support for application of this block comes from a case report of a dog undergoing opioid-free anesthesia for hemilaminectomy surgery [212]. The ESP block may also prove useful in the context of interventional pain management practice for treatment of chronic pain associated with vertebral articular facet degeneration [207]. The potential versatility of this block was highlighted in a case report involving a dog with acute pancreatitis and intractable pain despite systemic infusions of fentanyl, lidocaine, ketamine, and dexmedetomidine that responded favorably to ESP block [213]. A small retrospective study evaluating the addition of ultrasound-guided ESP block at T5–T9 to multimodal analgesic protocols in dogs undergoing median sternotomies suggested the technique may also be of some benefit in this context [214]. Since anatomic studies have not identified a clear path for distribution of injectate toward the ventral branches of the spinal nerves, the exact mechanism whereby the ESP block may provide analgesia for cranial abdominal pain remains unknown.

Blocks of the thoracic limb

Anatomy of sensory innervation

Spinal nerves emerge from the intervertebral canals of the cervical, thoracic, and lumbar vertebral column as postganglionic fibers that contain both sensory and motor nerves that originate from the dorsal and ventral horns of the spinal cord, respectively. Except in the thoracic region, the ventral branches of the spinal nerves form plexi, networks of nerve fibers that ultimately combine to form the specific motor and sensory peripheral nerves that serve the thoracic and pelvic limbs.

While species and individual variations may exist, the brachial plexus is generally formed by the ventral branches of the C6 to T1 spinal nerves [215]. Although early anatomic studies of the canine brachial plexus identified occasional contributions from the C5 and/or T2 nerves, more recent studies have failed to corroborate these observations [216]. The brachial plexus includes the following nerves (with respective contributing cervical ventral rami): pectoral (C6),

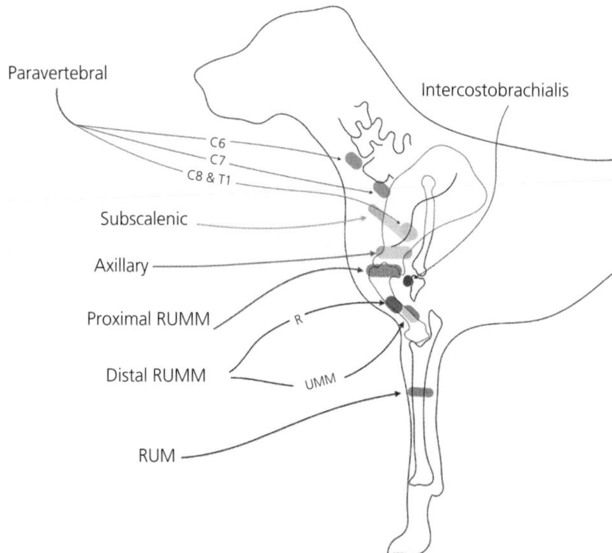

Figure 60.13 Various approaches to the brachial plexus and distal branches. RUMM, radial, ulnar, median, and musculocutaneous nerves; RUM, radial, ulnar, and median nerves. Source: Otero *et al.* [253], with permission.

suprascapular (C6 and C7), subscapular (C6 and C7), musculocutaneous (C7 and C8), axillary (C7 and C8), radial (C7, C8, and T1), median (C7, C8, and T1), ulnar (C7, C8, and T1), long thoracic (C7), thoracodorsal (C8 and T1), and lateral thoracic (T1) nerves [215,216]. Various approaches may be utilized to provide regional anesthesia to the brachial plexus and its distal branches (Fig. 60.13).

The brachial plexus provides motor, sensory, and autonomic innervation to the thoracic limb, including four extrinsic muscles. The ventral rami of the cervical spinal nerves emerge from their respective intervertebral foramina and pass through the intertransversarius muscles to course distally between the scalenus and subscapularis muscles. The phrenic nerve, which supplies motor innervation to the diaphragm, primarily originates from the ventral branches of C5, C6, and C7 and thus is anatomically related to the brachial plexus [125]. The spinal nerve T1 emerges from the first thoracic intervertebral space and contributes a primary branch to the brachial plexus that innervates the elbow and antebrachium, and a minor branch that innervates the first intercostal space. The T2 spinal nerve rarely contributes fibers to the brachial plexus. Instead, its ventral ramus forms the intercostobrachial nerve that innervates the pectoral ventral dermatomes and its dorsal ramus innervates the caudal cervical region. Lateral cutaneous branches of T2 provide sensory innervation to the lateral aspect of the shoulder.

The radial, ulnar, musculocutaneous, and median nerves course distally through the axilla in a sheath of connective tissue bordered cranially by the biceps brachii and coracobrachialis muscles, medially by the pectoralis muscle, and laterally by the triceps muscle. Within the axillary sheath, multiple layers of connective tissues separate individual components of the neurovascular bundle. Beyond the proximal third of the humerus, the radial nerve separates from the median, ulnar, and musculocutaneous nerves to assume its final position between the brachialis muscle and the triceps. The median, ulnar, and musculocutaneous nerves remain with the brachial artery and vein, deep to the pectoralis muscles and the thin fibrous sheet that serves as an insertion tendon to the humerus for the deep pectoralis, latissimus dorsi, cutaneous trunci, and tensor fascia antebrachii muscles, medial to the triceps.

Mid-humerus, the musculocutaneous nerve innervates the coracobrachialis, biceps brachii, and brachialis muscles and, at the level of the forearm, gives off the medial cutaneous antebrachial nerve. At the level of the forearm, the radial nerve courses superficially and branches into a medial and a lateral superficial radial nerve on either side of the cephalic vein. The median nerve travels alongside the median artery and vein, caudal to the pronator teres, and cranial to the flexor carpi radialis. The ulnar nerve courses laterocaudally deep to the flexor carpi ulnaris and gives off lateral and palmar branches at the carpus to innervate the dorsolateral and palmar aspects of the manus.

Cervical paravertebral block

The cervical paravertebral block in dogs is an advanced-level technique originally described by Lemke and Dawson that provides surgical anesthesia to the thoracic limb's most proximal structures including the scapula, the shoulder, and the humerus which cannot be blocked with the traditional axillary approach to the brachial plexus [130]. Since then, revised techniques have been proposed using alternative landmarks, neurostimulation, and ultrasound guidance, but most have failed to yield significant improvements in accuracy and safety [217–226]. Overall, the technique appears to be associated with an unacceptably high rate of complications relative to the potential benefits of the block. Anatomic landmark (i.e., "blind" approaches) and nerve stimulator-guided techniques are associated with inherent risks, including technical failure, nerve damage from direct needle trauma, or inadvertent puncture of blood vessels in the area. Although ultrasound guidance allows for direct visualization of the target nerves and surrounding structures and thus may be considered safer, ultrasound-guided paravertebral brachial plexus blocks can be associated with Horner's syndrome (caused by epidural spread of local anesthetic or blockade of the cervicothoracic ganglia); in addition, extraneous injectate spread involving the mediastinum or the phrenic nerve is also possible leading to hemidiaphragmatic paralysis [224,225]. Potentially deleterious complications include epidural spread of injectate, intravascular injection with associated local anesthetic toxicity, and pneumothorax secondary to needle penetration into the thoracic inlet. Based on these risks and the ability to use other, safer techniques to achieve comparable levels of anesthesia and/or analgesia for procedures of the thoracic limb, use of cervical paravertebral blocks is not recommended.

Subscalenic brachial plexus block

Before reaching the axillary space, the ventral branches of the C6, C7, C8, and T1 spinal nerves course caudoventrally within a fascial plane that is bordered by the scalenus muscle and the longus colli muscle. Using ultrasound guidance, the more proximal aspect of the brachial plexus can be blocked by injecting local anesthetic solution within the fascial plane at this location with minimal risk of epidural, mediastinal, or intrapleural spread [227]. The extent of blockade would be expected to include all parts of the thoracic limb distal to the scapulohumeral joint; indications for this technique may include forelimb amputation and surgical approaches to the humerus and elbow. Potential risks of this technique include incidental blockade of the phrenic nerve and Horner's syndrome [228].

Axillary brachial plexus block

The traditional "blind" approach to performing a brachial plexus block consists of manually palpating the axillary artery and the greater tubercle of the humerus and injecting a solution of local anesthetic in the general vicinity of the nerves that make up the brachial plexus. This technique was originally described by Tufvesson in 1951 [229]. Many years later, Futema *et al.* described the use of nerve stimulator guidance to perform axillary brachial plexus blocks in dogs undergoing surgical procedures of the mid-humerus [230]. A prospective, randomized, controlled study demonstrated that successful surgical anesthesia of the thoracic limb could be achieved in dogs undergoing carpal arthrodesis or surgery of the radius/ulna following nerve stimulator-guided axillary brachial plexus blocks with mixtures of local anesthetics [231]. Dogs that received brachial plexus blocks with a local anesthetic required lower postoperative rescue analgesia and lower intraoperative opioid administration guided by autonomic nociceptive responses or absence thereof. Following these landmark studies, assessments of nerve stimulation to guide brachial plexus blockade continued to develop. The neurostimulation of individual nerves of the brachial plexus and associated muscular responses were meticulously mapped in dogs [232]. A subsequent evaluation of nerve staining with different volumes of a lidocaine and methylene blue solution injected via neurostimulation guidance in the axillary space revealed satisfactory staining of the target nerves with the use of at least 0.3 mL/kg in medium-sized dogs (16–40 kg, median 22 kg) [233]. Indeed, in a comparison of the clinical features of nerve stimulator-guided brachial plexus block with a traditional approach guided by anatomical landmarks, it was concluded that neurostimulation improved the success rate of this block in dogs [234].

Subsequently, Campoy *et al.* performed a terminal prospective study to describe a new combined nerve stimulator- and ultrasound-guided technique to block the brachial plexus at the level of the axilla [235]. Their technique differed from previous descriptions in that the dogs were positioned in dorsal recumbency and the needle inserted in a craniocaudal direction, in-plane with the ultrasound probe (Fig. 60.14). With this technique, though the nerve roots of C7 to T1 were consistently stained with a low volume of lidocaine and methylene blue solution (0.15 mL/kg), the root of C6 was missed or insufficiently stained in most cases. A subsequent anatomic (i.e., "blind technique") evaluation of the axillary brachial plexus performed via anatomic landmarks with twice the volume of dye–local anesthetic solution only achieved complete staining of main nerves (musculocutaneous, ulnar, median, and radial) or of the ventral nerve rami from which these nerves originate (C7, C8, and T1) in 58% of cases [216]. These findings support the use of ultrasound guidance to increase success rates as well as reduce the volumes of local anesthetic that are required to achieve successful axillary brachial plexus blocks.

The sonoanatomy of the brachial plexus is dependent on patient positioning because neurovascular bundles that course through sheaths of connective tissue between musculofascial planes are somewhat mobile [236]. In a study assessing the location of the nerves of the brachial plexus with canine subjects positioned in dorsal recumbency, the radial nerve was located caudolateral to the axillary artery, the median and ulnar nerves caudomedial to the axillary artery (in more than 90% of cases), and the musculocutaneous nerve was consistently located cranial to the axillary artery. These findings highlight the importance of patient positioning when it comes to successful ultrasound identification of nerves and the advantage of placing patients in dorsal recumbency rather than lateral recumbency for this block as the musculocutaneous nerve was more easily identified. Similarly in cats, despite direct visualization of the nerve roots by ultrasound, patient positioning was found to significantly impact the success of the block. Axillary brachial

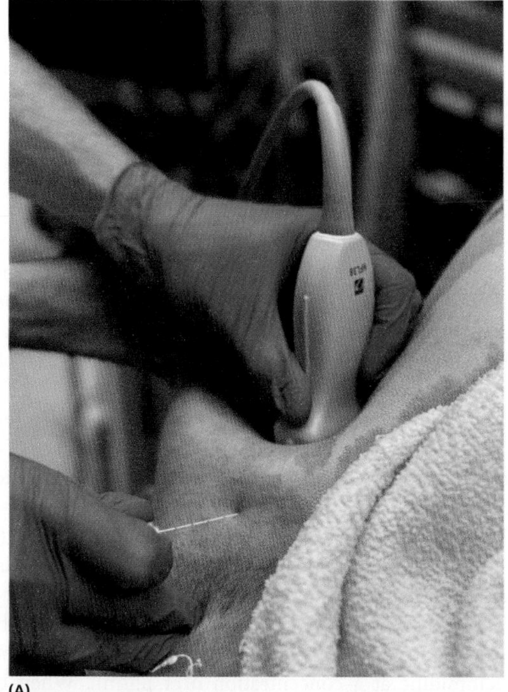

(A)

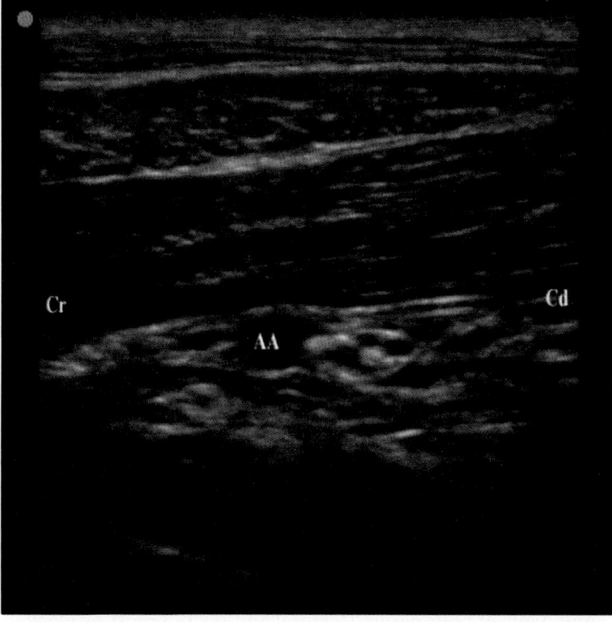

(B)

Figure 60.14 Ultrasound-guided regional anesthesia of the brachial plexus using the axillary approach. **A.** The patient is positioned in dorsal recumbency with the needle inserted using an in-plane approach. **B.** Prior to needle insertion, nerve roots of C6–T1 can be visualized surrounding the axillary artery (AA) on the ultrasound image. Cr, cranial; Cd, caudal. Source: Dr. Carrie Schroeder.

plexus blockade in cats positioned in dorsal recumbency with the limb held in abduction at a 90° angle had more success as compared to positioning in dorsal recumbency with the thoracic limbs extended caudally [237].

Clinically, the axillary approach to the brachial plexus can also be performed with the use of anatomic landmarks, without advanced equipment such as ultrasound or nerve stimulators, yielding clinically acceptable success rates when higher volumes of local anesthetics are used [238]. The increase in sophistication of the technique may come at the cost of efficiency when inexperienced operators perform the techniques, but evidence toward increased safety such as decreased risks for vascular puncture or direct nerve trauma supports the use of combined techniques. Akasaka *et al.* compared ultrasound-guided and nerve stimulator-guided axillary brachial plexus blocks in dogs and found that though the success rates did not differ between each group, ultrasound guidance resulted in faster blocks compared to nerve stimulator guidance [239]. Complications may still occur despite ultrasound guidance or nerve stimulation. There are isolated reports of serious complications including life-threatening cardiac arrhythmias following nerve stimulator-guided axillary brachial plexus block [240], in addition to pneumothorax [241], and phrenic nerve blockade with resulting hemidiaphragmatic paralysis [237]. More likely potential complications include direct nerve damage or vascular puncture with subsequent hematoma formation. As with all techniques, diligent patient monitoring during and after the block is performed is recommended.

As duration of motor blockade may last longer than sensory blockade, inference of the analgesic effects of nerve blocks should not be made on the basis of continued motor deficits. Rather, pain scoring using a validated pain assessment instrument is recommended. To provide an extended duration of analgesia, catheterization of the axillary brachial plexus has been described in awake dogs; though feasible, concerns about dislocation of the catheter and evidence of local anesthetic channeling resulting in uneven distribution among target nerves have curbed the enthusiasm of clinicians for this technique [242].

Proximal radial, ulnar, median, and musculocutaneous nerve block

The radial, ulnar, median, and musculocutaneous (RUMM) nerves can be blocked at the level of the proximal medial humerus within the axilla (proximal RUMM block or distal brachial plexus block). This provides motor and sensory block of the elbow and distal thoracic limb. At this location, these four nerves are contained within a connective tissue sheath, the axillary sheath, that is derived from the deep cervical fasciae. In a preliminary cadaver study, due to the presence of the axillary sheath, the four target nerves contained within the sheath were adequately stained without extravasation of the dye solution into the surrounding tissues or complications such as phrenic nerve or intrathoracic contamination [243]. In a cohort of 15 client-owned dogs, an in-plane approach to an ultrasound-guided injection of local anesthetic solution (0.15 mL/kg of 0.5% ropivacaine) provided intraoperative analgesia associated with significant opioid-sparing effects and postoperative analgesia for up to 8 h [243]. The approach described in this study is performed distal to the axillary brachial plexus block and specifically targets the RUMM nerves as opposed to the spinal nerve roots located more proximally.

In cats, an ultrasound-guided lateral approach to block the radial, ulnar, median, and musculocutaneous nerves was recently described. A single injection technique was unsuccessful at consistently blocking the musculocutaneous nerve when the tip of the needle was directed at the radial nerve, and a second injection directed at the musculocutaneous nerve proved necessary due to the presence of interrupted layers of connective tissue that separate the different components of the neurovascular bundle [244].

Distal radial, ulnar, median, and musculocutaneous nerve block

An alternative to the traditional axillary brachial plexus block consists of targeting individual RUMM nerves at the level of the mid- to distal humerus (distal RUMM block). This technique was initially evaluated in dogs in a study that involved anatomic evaluation of injectate distribution in canine cadavers followed by a placebo-controlled, prospective, crossover clinical evaluation of the technique [245]. The radial nerve courses laterally and separates from the ulnar, median, and musculocutaneous nerves at the level of the proximal third of the humerus and thus, this technique was described as two separate injections in order to successfully reach all of the target nerves. Though their pilot study demonstrated adequate staining of all but one of targeted nerves when sufficient volumes of injectate were used (0.1 mL/kg and 0.15 mL/kg for the lateral and medial approach, respectively), complete sensory blockade was not obtained in all limbs tested. They found that the degree and duration of sensory deficits varied across the different dermatomes that were tested and the extent and duration of motor deficits differed from the sensory blockade.

The distal RUMM block technique can be performed with nerve stimulation guidance; the successful application of this technique was described in a clinical case report as part of a multimodal analgesic plan consisting of systemic opioids and regional anesthesia (0.5% bupivacaine) for a muscle biopsy in the distal thoracic limb of a dog in which general anesthesia was considered to have an increased risk of complications [246]. Descriptions of ultrasound-guided mid-humeral RUMM block techniques in dogs undergoing distal limb surgical procedures have also been published [247,248]. An ultrasound-guided lateral approach to the RUMM block in cats has been described and found that target nerves were more successfully stained with 0.4 mL of methylene blue using an in-plane approach [249]. The clinical efficacy of the technique remains to be confirmed in cats.

Radial, ulnar, and median nerve block (ring block)

To selectively block structures distal to the elbow, perineural injections of local anesthetics around the radial, ulnar, and median (RUM) nerves can be performed anywhere along the course of the nerves. However, surgical procedures involving the manus and/or digits do not require the entire thoracic limb to be blocked. While regional anesthetic techniques applied more proximally will result in acceptable analgesia, they typically also result in motor blockade, which is often unnecessary for procedures involving the distal limb and can result in trauma due to decreased mobility and proprioceptive deficits.

The somatic organization of individual nerve fibers within plexi is such that afferent nerve fibers from the distalmost aspects of a limb are found in the center of nerves, while the more peripheral fibers innervate more proximal dermatomes. Furthermore, the size of nerves can adversely influence the success and duration of sensory blocks. This theoretically raises the issue that attempting to block the manus with a brachial plexus or proximal RUMM block may carry a greater risk of failure, though no study exists comparing the intensity or duration of analgesia at the distal limb with ring blocks versus more proximal blocks [250]. For this reason, the radial, ulnar, and median nerves are commonly blocked at a location immediately proximal to the carpus by means of a four-point block that will selectively desensitize the superficial branches of the radial nerve (dorsomedially), the dorsal branch of the ulnar nerve (laterally), the palmar branch of the ulnar nerve (palmaromedially), and the median nerve (palmarolaterally) (RUM block). The technique can be simplified to a ring block where the target nerves are all successfully blocked following a circumferential subcutaneous infiltration of local anesthetic proximal to the carpus, as previously described [251,252].

Blocks of the pelvic limb

Until relatively recently, local anesthetic techniques for the pelvic limb of small companion animals were limited mainly to epidural or spinal anesthesia or intra-articular injections. However, peripheral nerve blockade can provide highly effective analgesia with potentially less morbidity than neuraxial anesthesia [254]. When compared with epidural anesthesia, peripheral nerve blockade of the pelvic limb for orthopedic surgery provided similar requirements for postoperative analgesia with a lower incidence of intraoperative hypotension and postoperative urinary retention in dogs [254,255].

Bupivacaine (0.5%) with or without dexmedetomidine (0.5–2 μg/mL of injectate solution) is commonly used to provide surgical anesthesia, although 0.5% ropivacaine may also be used. The addition of 50 μg of dexmedetomidine to a 50 mL vial of 0.5% bupivacaine will create a solution that contains 0.5% bupivacaine and dexmedetomidine at a concentration of 1 μg/mL. When bupivacaine alone (0.15 mL/kg) was used for femoral and sciatic nerve blocks, the duration of action for sensory blockade was found to be 15 and 10 h, respectively [256]. The addition of dexmedetomidine may further prolong sensory blockade; however, this has not been demonstrated in all studies [257,258].

Anatomy

The pelvic limb is served by two nerve plexi (lumbar and sacral) and both must be partly or entirely blocked to provide surgical anesthesia and analgesia to the entire pelvic limb (including the hemipelvis). The lumbar plexus supplies the lateral femoral cutaneous nerve (L3, L4), the genitofemoral nerve (L3, L4), the femoral nerve (L4, L5, L6), and the obturator nerve (L4, L5, L6) [259]. The sacral plexus supplies the sciatic nerve (L6, L7, S1), the cranial and caudal gluteal nerves (L6, L7, S1), and the caudal cutaneous femoral nerve (S1, S2) [256].

Blocking the femoral nerve (or its distal sensory continuation, the saphenous nerve) will provide anesthesia of the femur (mid-diaphysis to distal), the femorotibial joint (medial aspect of the femorotibial joint capsule and intra-articular structures), the skin of the dorsomedial tarsus, and the first digit. Blocking the sciatic nerve alone is sufficient to perform surgery involving the foot or hock. Components of both nerves (femoral and sciatic) must be blocked for almost any stifle or proximal tibial surgical procedure (e.g., tibial plateau leveling osteotomy).

Lumbar plexus block

The lumbar plexus is formed via the ventral branches of L4, L5, and L6 within the psoas compartment, a sheath formed by the iliopsoas and psoas minor muscles [260]. Regional blockade of the nerves of the lumbar plexus can be achieved using either nerve stimulator or ultrasound guidance [42,45]. When a psoas compartment block is combined with a parasacral lumbosacral trunk block, regional anesthesia to the entire limb can result, sufficient for pelvic limb amputation, hip surgery, or femur surgery [259].

Three different approaches to nerve stimulation-guided lumbar plexus blocks have been described: a single-injection paravertebral approach [233], a three-point paravertebral approach [261], and a lateral pre-iliac approach [260]. Using the single-injection paravertebral approach, a stimulating needle is introduced through the epaxial muscles at the L5–L6 intervertebral level toward the iliopsoas muscle until a quadriceps femoris muscle twitch is elicited [233]. Epidural and abdominal spread of contrast injected at this location occurred in a small proportion of subjects [233]; indeed, in a retrospective study examining this technique, one of 95 cases showed bilateral motor deficit, consistent with epidural spread [262].

While the single-injection approach utilizes a large volume of local anesthetic (0.4 mL/kg) to desensitize the lumbar plexus, the three-point approach aims to utilize a smaller volume (0.05 mL/kg) at each of three sites to block the individual ventral branches of the L4, L5, and L6 nerve roots prior to them forming the lumbar plexus [261]. Using this approach, when combined with a parasacral lumbosacral trunk block, less rescue analgesia was needed for pelvic limb amputations in dogs [42].

The lateral pre-iliac approach aims to block the femoral nerve caudally within the psoas compartment where it is further from the vasculature [260]. This approach utilizes a stimulating needle inserted through the lateral aspect of the lumbar muscles, cranial to the wing of the ilium. Comparison of the effect of blocking the lumbar plexus via the sagittal paravertebral or lateral pre-iliac approach in dogs undergoing pelvic limb orthopedic surgery failed to show a statistically significant difference in success rate (74.7% versus 82.3%) or rescue analgesia (33.7% versus 27.1%), although the volume used for the paravertebral approach was lower than that previously described (0.15 mL/kg versus 0.4 mL/kg) [262]. The lumbosacral plexus block, when combined with sciatic nerve block, has also been shown to be effective in cats undergoing hindlimb orthopedic procedures [263].

The lumbar plexus block can also be achieved via combined ultrasound–nerve stimulator guidance or under ultrasound guidance alone. In either situation, a linear, high-frequency transducer is positioned on the ventral aspect of the abdomen and lumbar muscles, cranial to the iliac crest. At this location, the femoral nerve can be identified as a hypoechoic, round structure within the body of the iliopsoas muscle [259]. The needle can be advanced toward the femoral nerve using several different approaches in dogs; however, when introduced from the lateral aspect of the lumbar muscles there is less risk of inadvertent vascular puncture (e.g., the external iliac artery) [264]. When combined with a sciatic nerve block, ultrasound-guided lumbar plexus block improves analgesia and recovery quality for dogs undergoing tibial plateau leveling osteotomy [265].

Using nerve stimulation and/or ultrasound guidance, the sciatic nerve may also be blocked more proximally utilizing a parasacral approach at the lumbosacral trunk. At this location, anesthesia/analgesia can be provided to the proximal femur and pelvis that is sufficient for hind limb amputation and hip and femur surgery when combined with a lumbar plexus block [42,259].

Femoral/saphenous nerve block

At the caudal aspect of the iliopsoas muscle, the femoral nerve exits the muscle and courses across the femoral triangle (Fig. 60.15). The femoral triangle is demarcated by the iliopsoas muscle cranially, the pectineus muscle caudally, and the sartorius muscle cranially. Within the triangle, the femoral nerve is located cranial to the femoral artery and vein, running deep to the caudal belly of the sartorius muscle. At this level, the femoral nerve gives rise to the saphenous nerve and

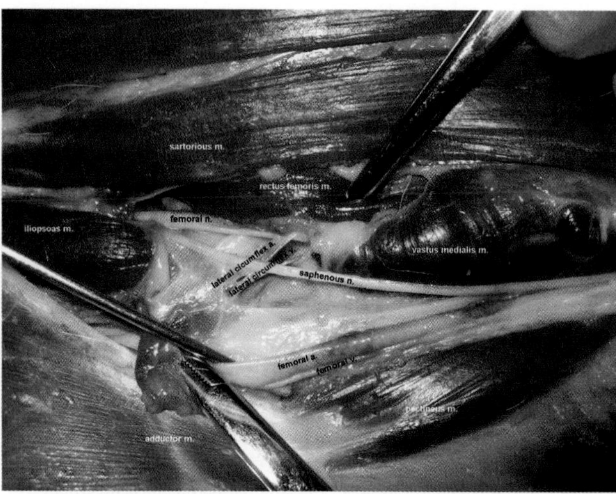

Figure 60.15 Dissection of the femoral triangle of the left pelvic limb of a dog cadaver. The caudal belly of the sartorius muscle has been displaced cranially to allow for visualization of the femoral nerve. Note the anatomic relationship of the femoral vessels to the femoral nerve.

the lateral circumflex vessels originate from the femoral artery and vein. These vessels cross the femoral triangle in a craniocaudal direction, disappearing between the vastus medialis and rectus femoris muscles. The femoral nerve then continues distally, entering the quadriceps muscle between the vastus medialis and rectus femoris. The saphenous nerve is the sensory branch of the femoral nerve and, when it is blocked in combination with a sciatic nerve block, anesthesia for stifle surgery will be achieved while still preserving quadriceps muscle function [259]. While other branches of the femoral and obturator nerve may contribute some sensory innervation to the stifle in dogs [266], a recent retrospective analysis found no difference in intraoperative or postoperative analgesic requirements between a saphenous–sciatic and a lumbar plexus–sciatic nerve block in dogs undergoing stifle surgery [254].

For nerve stimulator-guided blockade of the femoral nerve, the patient should be positioned in lateral recumbency with the limb to be blocked positioned uppermost. The limb should be abducted 90° and extended caudally, making it easier to palpate and identify the pectineus and iliopsoas muscles and to palpate the pulse of the femoral artery. Since the femoral nerve will be located cranial to the femoral artery, the puncture site is located cranial to the femoral artery within the femoral triangle (Fig. 60.16). An insulated needle (e.g., 22 gauge, 50 mm) is advanced toward the iliopsoas muscle, maintaining a 20–30° angle with respect to the skin. As the needle is advanced, the fascia iliaca will be penetrated (a "pop" can usually be appreciated). Once the tip of the needle is near the femoral nerve, contractions of the quadriceps muscle will result in stifle extension. Bupivacaine (0.5%, 0.1 mL/kg) combined with dexmedetomidine (0.5 μg/mL) provides approximately 14 (range 6–24) h of effect until rescue analgesia may be needed following stifle surgery [255,267,268].

Alternatively, nerve stimulation can be combined with ultrasound with the transducer placed over the femoral triangle in a craniocaudal direction. Doing this will provide a short-axis view of the femoral artery and the nerve. Since it is usually compressed by the pressure that is being exerted by the ultrasound transducer, the femoral vein is rarely seen adjacent to the artery (Fig. 60.17). The femoral nerve is located cranial and deep to the femoral artery and is identifiable as a small, hyperechoic structure directly beneath the thin caudal belly of the sartorius muscle and the fascia iliaca

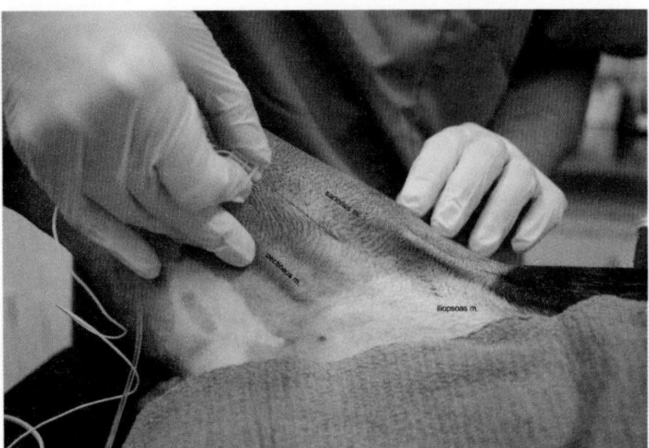

Figure 60.16 Performance of a right-sided femoral nerve block in a dog using a femoral triangle approach. The stimulating needle is inserted cranial to the femoral artery and advanced toward the iliopsoas muscle, maintaining a 20–30° angle to the skin.

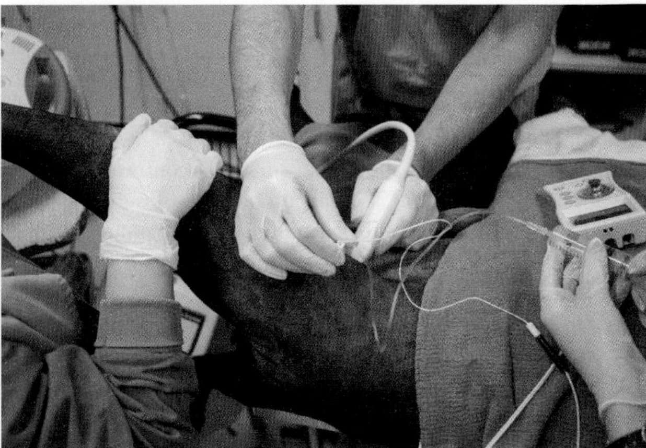

Figure 60.18 Performance of a left-sided femoral nerve block in a dog. The ultrasound transducer is positioned to visualize the femoral triangle in short-axis in the inguinal area, and the stimulating needle is advanced in-plane in a cranial-to-caudal direction through the sartorius and rectus femoris muscles toward the femoral nerve.

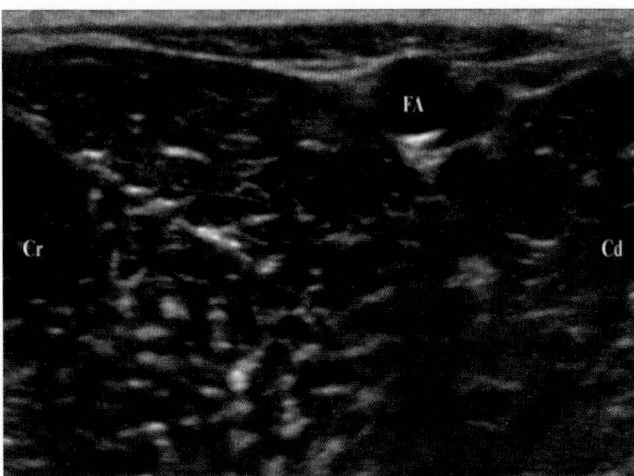

Figure 60.17 Ultrasonographic cross-sectional (short-axis) view of the femoral triangle of a dog. FA, femoral artery; Cr, cranial; Cd, caudal. Source: Dr. Carrie Schroeder.

(which appears as a thin hyperechoic line superficial to the femoral nerve). The rectus femoris muscle can be seen cranial to the femoral nerve. The puncture site is located in the proximal and cranial aspect of the thigh (cranial belly of the sartorius muscle) in-plane with the transducer (Fig. 60.18). The recommended volume to be injected is 0.1 mL/kg [235]. However, the final injection volume can be assessed by monitoring the ultrasound image.

The saphenous nerve may be blocked distally along the medial femur to minimize motor blockade of the quadriceps. As this nerve is sensory, nerve stimulator-guidance is not feasible. Instead, the saphenous nerve may be identified under ultrasound guidance at the level of the middle-third of the femur, in a triangular fascial plane located immediately cranial to the femoral artery (Fig. 60.19) [36,123].

Sciatic nerve block

The sciatic nerve courses from its points of origin distally down the pelvic limb between the greater trochanter of the femur and the ischiatic tuberosity (Fig. 60.20). In this region, the sciatic nerve gives rise to muscular branches that supply the semitendinosus and semimembranosus muscles. The caudal gluteal vessels lie just caudal to these muscular branches and must be avoided when the needle is placed close to the sciatic nerve at this location. Immediately distal to the greater trochanter and ischiatic tuberosity, the sciatic nerve lies between the biceps femoris muscle laterally, and the semimembranosus/semitendinosus muscles caudally, and the adductor muscle medially. The sciatic nerve then divides into its two main branches, the tibial nerve medially and the common peroneal nerve laterally. The location of this division is variable and can occur anywhere from the level of the hip joint to just proximal to the stifle joint.

Sciatic nerve blocks may be performed utilizing nerve stimulation and/or ultrasound guidance. For either technique, the patient should be positioned in lateral recumbency with the limb to be blocked positioned uppermost in a natural position. For a nerve stimulator-guided approach, the greater trochanter and ischiatic tuberosity should first be identified. The puncture site is located at a point between the cranial and the middle thirds of a line that could be drawn between these two bony landmarks. An insulated needle (22 gauge, 50 mm) is inserted through the skin and is advanced ventromedially at a 45° angle to the skin (Fig. 60.21). Once the tip of the needle is near the sciatic nerve, dorsiflexion or plantar extension of the foot will be elicited. The recommended volume to be injected is 0.1 mL/kg. Contractions of the semimembranosus or semitendinosus muscles should not be considered an acceptable endpoint. If stimulation of the hamstring muscles is observed without movement of the foot, the needle is likely stimulating the muscular branches of the sciatic nerve and not the sciatic nerve itself. Injection of a local anesthetic at this location will miss the sensory components of the sciatic nerve and may result in block failure.

If performing the sciatic nerve block using ultrasound guidance, the transducer should be placed in a craniocaudal orientation over the biceps femoris muscle on the lateral aspect of the thigh, distal to the ischiatic tuberosity (Fig. 60.22). Using this approach, a short-axis view of the sciatic nerve should be obtained (Fig. 60.23). An insulated needle (22 gauge, 50–100 mm) will enter the skin from the caudal aspect of the thigh, in-plane with the ultrasound transducer. The needle should be advanced toward the sciatic nerve in a

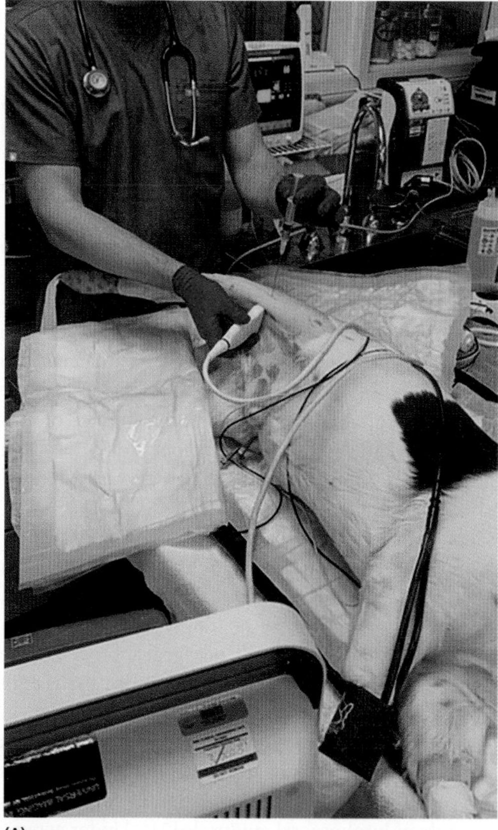

(A)

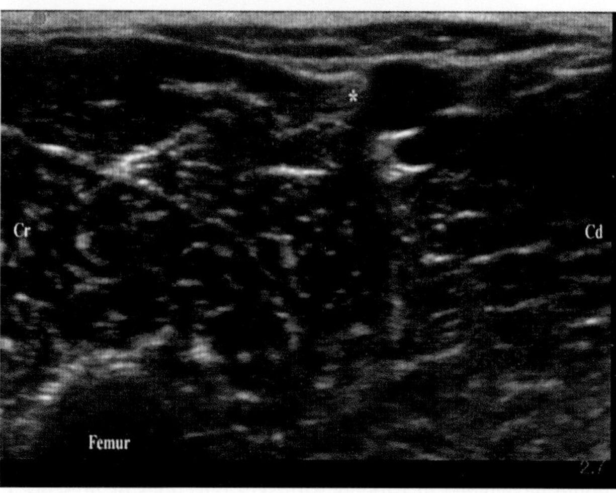

(B)

Figure 60.19 Ultrasound-guided saphenous nerve block. **A.** The saphenous nerve may be identified under ultrasound guidance at the level of the middle-third of the femur. **B.** It is visualized in a triangular fascial plane (*) located immediately cranial to the femoral artery. Cr, cranial; Cd, caudal. Source: Dr. Raphaël Vézina Audette (A); Dr. Carrie Schroeder (B).

caudo-cranial direction through the semimembranosus muscle, medial to the fascia of the biceps femoris muscle. As is the case with all ultrasound-guided blocks, the needle tip should be kept in the field of view at all times. If nerve stimulation is used along with ultrasound guidance, plantar extension (from tibial nerve stimulation), or dorsiflexion (from peroneal nerve stimulation) of the foot will be elicited when the needle approaches the sciatic nerve.

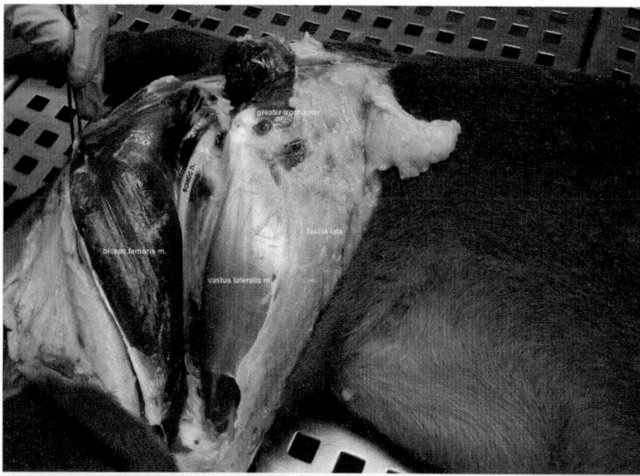

Figure 60.20 Dissection of lateral thigh of a canine cadaver showing the right sciatic nerve. The biceps femoris muscle has been reflected caudally and the gluteal muscle has been transected to allow for easier visualization of the sciatic nerve and its surrounding structures. Methylene blue dye has been used to stain the proximal aspect of the sciatic nerve.

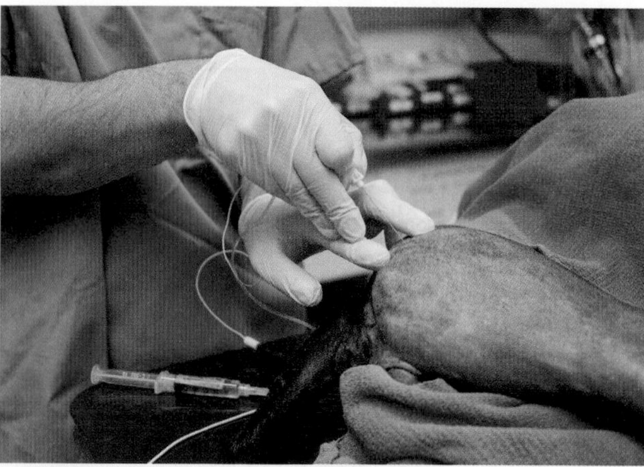

Figure 60.21 Performance of a right-sided sciatic nerve block in a dog using the lateral approach. The index and middle fingers of the nondominant hand are used to palpate the greater trochanter and ischiatic tuberosity. The puncture site is located one-third of the distance from the greater trochanter to the ischiatic tuberosity.

The recommended volume of local anesthetic to be injected is 0.1 mL/kg, although the final injection volume can be assessed by monitoring the ultrasound image [235].

Intra-articular blocks

An additional strategy for pain management following joint surgery is the intra-articular administration of analgesics such as local anesthetics or opioids. The intra-articular injection of local anesthetics desensitizes intra-articular structures only and may reduce the dose and interval for administering supplemental analgesic therapy [269].

Stifle technique

The patient is positioned in dorsal or lateral recumbency. The stifle joint is held in a flexed position. The needle is inserted lateral to the patellar ligament, midway between the cranial pole of the patella and the tibial tuberosity, and the hub of the needle is observed for the presence of synovial fluid (confirming correct needle position). However, absence of synovial fluid does not necessarily rule out

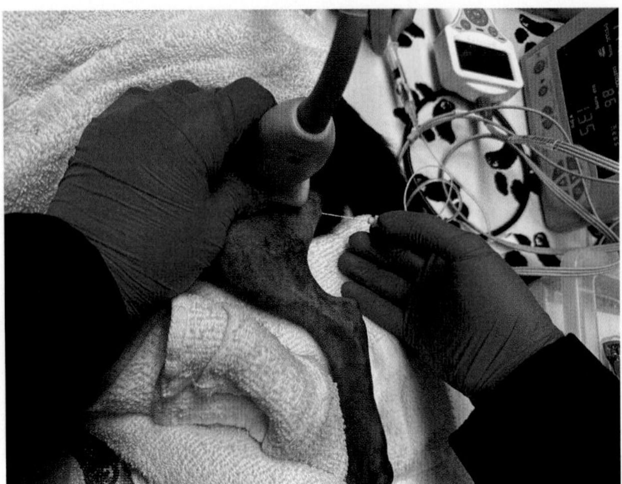

Figure 60.22 Performance of a left-sided sciatic nerve block in a dog. The ultrasound transducer is placed over the area immediately distal to the greater trochanter and ischiatic tuberosity. The stimulating needle follows a caudo-cranial direction toward the sciatic nerve through the semimembranosus muscle, medial to the fascia of the biceps femoris muscle. Source: Dr. Carrie Schroeder.

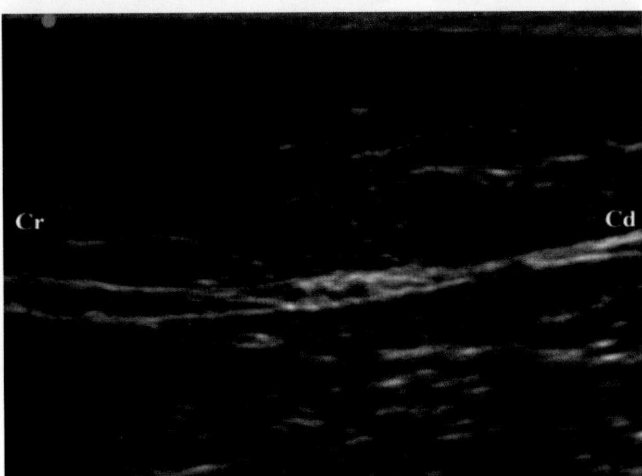

Figure 60.23 Ultrasonographic cross-sectional (short-axis) view of the sciatic nerve deep to the biceps femoris muscle. Cr, cranial; Cd, caudal. Source: Dr. Carrie Schroeder.

correct needle location. Depending on the size of the patient, 1–6 mL of local anesthetic solution may be injected into the joint. Lack of resistance during injection confirms correct intra-articular position of the needle tip and excludes injection into periarticular soft tissue or a fat pad.

The stifle may also be blocked utilizing ultrasound-guided local anesthetic injection of the popliteal fossa utilizing the "infiltrating around genicular structures" or "FLAGS" technique, described in dogs [270]. This technique may provide sufficient analgesia for stifle surgery while maintaining motor function; however, further studies are needed to assess its clinical safety and utility.

Coxofemoral joint technique

The patient should be positioned in lateral recumbency with the coxofemoral joint to be injected uppermost; the limb should be slightly flexed, with the stifle in a neutral position. The puncture site is located cranial and proximal to the greater trochanter. Once the needle has entered the joint, the hub of the needle should be observed for evidence of synovial fluid to confirm correct needle positioning. However, absence of synovial fluid does not rule out correct needle positioning. Depending on the size of the patient, 1–6 mL of local anesthetic solution can be injected into the joint [271]. Lack of resistance during injection confirms correct intra-articular position of the needle tip and excludes injection into periarticular soft tissue or a fat pad.

Neuraxial techniques

The administration of agents with analgesic properties via the epidural or spinal routes provides effective anesthesia and analgesia for procedures involving the pelvis and pelvic limbs, as well as the tail, perineum, and caudal abdomen. In addition, the use of epidural anesthesia for blockade of thoracic segments in dogs has been extensively studied [272]. Epidural analgesia can also be extended by using an indwelling catheter.

The lumbosacral approach (L7–S1) to performing epidural anesthesia in dogs and cats is technically straightfoward to perform owing to the relatively wide intervertebral space at this location, although more cranial approaches in dogs have also been described [273,274]. Alternatively, a sacrococcygeal approach to the epidural space has been described in cats to minimize the risk of dural puncture and help facilitate urethral catheterization in blocked cats [275,276] and a sacrococcygeal approach in dogs has been described to minimize the risk of accidental dural puncture, as a high frequency of "subarachnoid contamination of contrast" was reported in one study of lumbosacral epidurals [31]. Under experimental conditions in canine cadavers, the cranial extent of contrast spread in the epidural space appears similar between the lumbosacral and sacrococcygeal locations [277].

Contraindications

There are several contraindications to the use of epidural anesthesia in small animal patients. Alternatives to epidural anesthesia should be considered in patients with bleeding disorders (e.g., thrombocytopenia). Since placing a needle in the vertebral canal can result in inadvertent puncture of an epidural venous sinus, hemorrhage may result in the formation of an epidural hematoma compressing neural structures such as the cauda equina, different spinal nerve roots, dural sac, or even the spinal cord. Epidural anesthesia using a local anesthetic should be avoided in patients with uncorrected hypovolemia and hypotension since they will be at further risk due to vasodilation following sympathetic nerve blockade. Opioids may continue to be used in these patients. Finally, epidural anesthesia should be avoided in patients with skin infections or presence of neoplasia or other lesions at the site of injection. In these patients, alternative routes for performing the epidural injection (e.g., sacrococcygeal route) or selection of a different regional anesthetic technique should be considered. Potential complications associated with neuraxial administration (single dose or continuous infusion) and strategies to avoid them are summarized in Table 60.1.

Anatomy

The vertebral canal contains the epidural space and the intrathecal structures. The roof of the canal is formed by the vertebral laminae and the interarcuate ligament (also known as the ligamentum flavum or yellow ligament). This ligament widens at the level of the intervertebral openings. The epidural space in the dog is largest at the lumbosacral level where the dural sac tapers (Fig. 60.24).

Table 60.1 Potential complications associated with neuraxial techniques.

Complication	Possible explanation	Comments and strategies for avoidance
Related to the technique		
Accidental drug administration		Correct syringe labeling and implementation of "time-outs/ checklists" are recommended to prevent this type of operator error from occurring
Neural damage/neurotoxicity		Appropriate techniques and equipment should be used to minimize tissue trauma The use of preservative-free, "for epidural use" solutions is recommended
Infections		Strict adherence to best practice and standard of care in terms of skin preparation and technique is recommended
Inadvertent subarachnoid/spinal or subdural injection	Subarachnoid (intrathecal, spinal) needle location	Check for absence of CSF and deliver a test dose before delivering the full dose to rule out intrathecal or subdural needle insertion
Inadvertent intravascular injection	Intravascular needle location such as the ventral venous plexus	Check for absence of blood and deliver a test dose before delivering the full dose to rule out intravascular needle insertion
Related to local anesthetic solutions		
Hypotension/bradycardia	Sympathetic blockade	Intravenous fluids, vasopressors, and anticholinergic drugs should be used as needed
Horner's syndrome	Blockade of sympathetic trunk at cervical dermatomes	Can be observed if local anesthetic reaches cervical dermatomes
Respiratory depression	Extensive migration of the injectate, resulting in intercostal nerve blockade, and rarely, anesthetic effects on the brainstem or phrenic nerve	Avoid excessive cranial migration of local anesthetic Opioids can cause delayed respiratory depression
Total spinal anesthesia	Local anesthetic-induced depression of the cervical spinal cord and the brainstem Excessive spread of an intrathecal injection of local anesthetic Inadvertent spinal injection	Avoid excessive cranial migration of local anesthetic
Local anesthetic systemic toxicity		Careful calculation of drug dosing Aspiration prior to local anesthetic administration to avoid intravascular administration
Related to opioids		
Urinary retention	Detrusor muscle relaxation, interruption of sacral parasympathetic outflow, bladder atony	Patients should be monitored over the first 24–48 h following epidural morphine, and treated symptomatically as needed Urinary catheterization or bladder expression, as needed

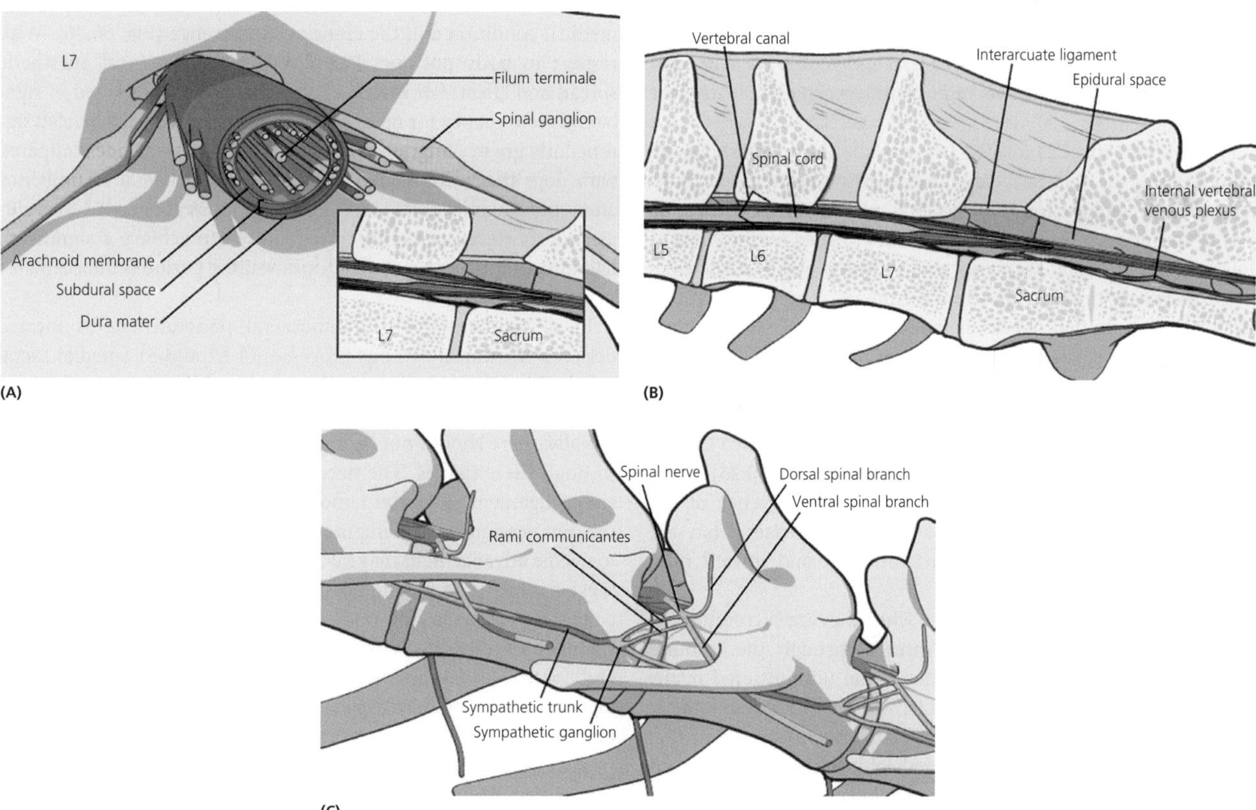

Figure 60.24 **A.** and **B.** Spinal anatomy at the lumbosacral level. Note that the interarcuate ligament is also known as the ligamentum flavum. **C.** Sympathetic trunk and its relationship to the vertebrae.

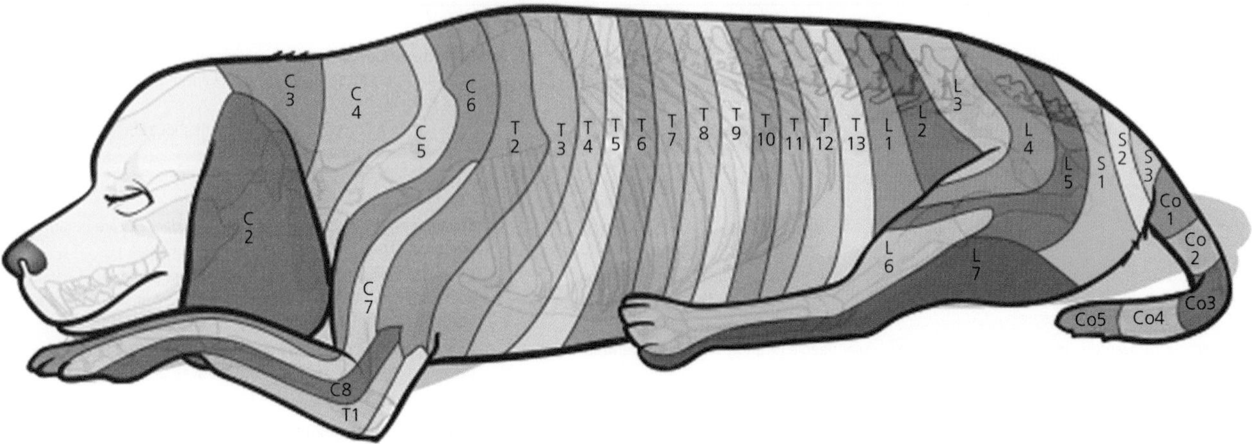

Figure 60.25 Dermatome map of sensory innervation to the skin in the dog.

At this level (L7–S1), the supraspinous and interspinous ligaments are relegated to the fibrous and connective tissue in between where the two epaxial muscles meet. Caudally, the spinal cord tapers into a conical structure called the conus medullaris. In most dogs, the dural sac typically ends at the level of L6–L7 while the conus medullaris is located at the lumbosacral space in smaller breeds and younger patients. In cats, however, the dural sac extends caudally as far as the first sacral segment. The dorsal and ventral rootlets emerge bilaterally from each segment of the spinal cord and bind together to form the dorsal and ventral roots. Each root progresses separately toward the intervertebral foramen, at which point the dorsal and ventral roots merge to form the corresponding spinal nerve. The dura mater (dura mater spinalis) forms a cylindrical tube with lateral extensions accompanying the roots and spinal nerves as they exit the vertebral canal through intervertebral foramina. Each spinal nerve divides into dorsal and ventral branches and (in the region of T1–L4) two rami communicantes that join the sympathetic trunk.

The epidural space is located between the dura mater and the boundaries of the vertebral canal. It contains adipose tissue, connective tissue, and the internal vertebral venous plexus. The cauda equina comprises a bundle of nerve fibers formed by the roots of the sacrum and caudal segments and is located within and caudal to the dural sac around the filum terminale. The pelvic limb is supplied by the spinal nerves at the level of L3–S1 (lumbosacral plexus). Therefore, segmental blockade at this level is necessary to block the entire pelvic limb. Innervation to the canine abdominal wall and peritoneum is provided by the branches of T11, T12, and T13 cranially and branches of L1, L2, and L3 caudally via sympathetic and ilioepigastric–ilioinguinal nerves (Fig. 60.25) [125]. Innervation of the thorax is provided by the branches of the T2–T13 spinal nerves. The sympathetic chain arises from the T1–L4 segments of the spinal cord (outward and inward rami communicantes) (Fig. 60.24C).

Spinal nerve roots become blocked when they are surrounded by a local anesthetic solution as it spreads through the epidural space [278]. Cranial migration of a solution administered in the epidural space is related to the injected volume of local anesthetic solution [279–281]. However, several studies have reported that the same total drug mass administered epidurally in different concentrations and volumes produces a similar spread of sensory blockade; this has been observed in humans [282,283] and in dogs [284,285]. It appears that once a sufficient volume of drug has reached a particular location (dermatome), the intensity and duration of the resulting block will depend on the concentration of the local anesthetic administered. Put simply, once the nerves are blocked, a greater concentration serves to increase the intensity and duration of effect. These effects include sensory and motor blockade; additionally, preganglionic sympathetic blockade will result in vasodilation in the blocked dermatomes and, in some cases, may contribute to arterial hypotension. The degree of sympathetic nerve blockade caused by epidural anesthesia is related to the extent of local anesthetic spread.

Epidural technique

To perform an epidural injection, the patient may be placed in either sternal or lateral recumbency, depending on the patient's medical condition and the clinician's preference (Fig. 60.26). With respect to body position, laterality may impact local anesthetic spread and effect. For instance, dogs that were maintained in right lateral recumbency for up to 40 min after injection experienced significantly greater migration of injectate on the right side compared with dogs that were turned from left to right lateral recumbency after epidural injections [280]. Further studies are needed to evaluate the shortest amount of time required to achieve a significant laterality of the block since a 40-min waiting period is unacceptable in clinical situations.

In dogs, the standard lumbosacral puncture site is located between the dorsal spinous processes of L7 and S1 (medial sacral crest) (Fig. 60.26). The needle (spinal or Tuohy) is advanced through the skin and into the subcutaneous tissue (Fig. 60.27). Usually, there should not be any resistance to needle advancement through these tissues. The needle is then engaged into the suprasinous ligament, the stylet removed, and further advanced through the supraspinous and interspinous ligaments (Fig. 60.28). Resistance to needle advancement may be appreciated as the needle penetrates these ligaments. If during any of these manipulations, the needle comes into contact with bony structures, it should be withdrawn slightly and redirected cranial or caudal as appropriate in a gentle and controlled manner. Several methods have been developed for identifying the epidural space, including the use of a "hanging drop," "loss of resistance," electrostimulation, and ultrasonography. In cats, since the dural sac extends caudally beyond the lumbosacral space, the authors recommend performing sacrococcygeal epidurals to avoid complications. If lumbosacral injection is desired, cautious and slow advancement of the needle should be utilized to

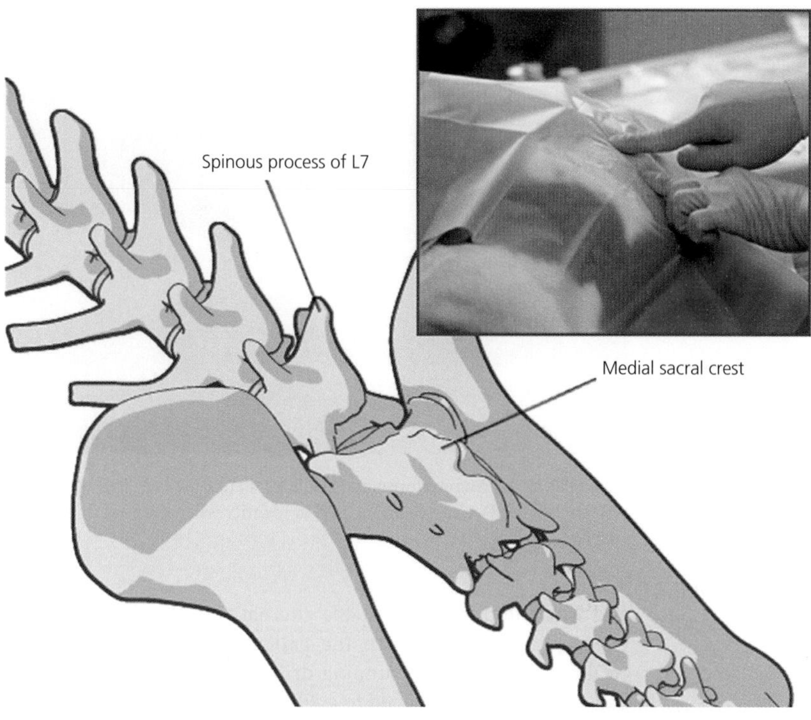

Figure 60.26 The typical puncture site for performing epidural anesthesia in the dog is located between the spinous process of L7 and the medial sacral crest of S1.

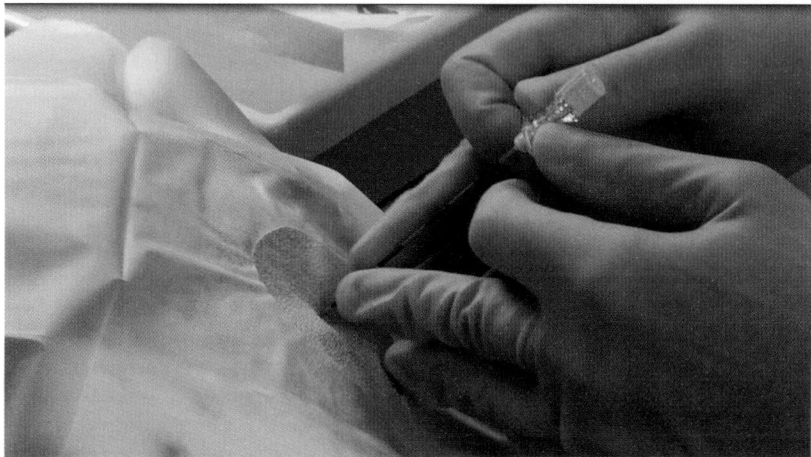

Figure 60.27 A Tuohy needle is advanced toward the epidural space at the lumbosacral space of a dog. Note that the index fingers and thumbs of each hand are used to hold the wings while the middle fingers are used to stabilize the needle shaft.

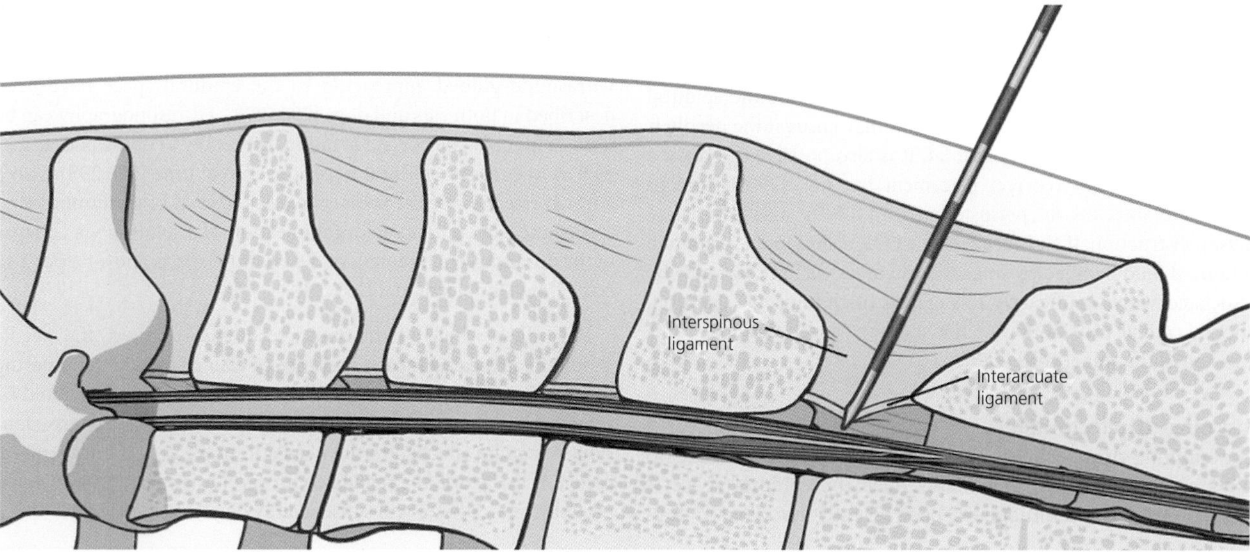

Figure 60.28 Illustration showing a Tuohy needle entering the epidural space at the lumbosacral junction. Note the recoil of the interarcuate ligament (ligamentum flavum).

Table 60.2 Volumes of local anesthetics used for epidural anesthesia in dogs.

Drug	Puncture site	Dermatome	Volume (mL/kg)	Reference
Bupivacaine 0.25%	Lumbosacral	L3	0.2	[281]
Bupivacaine 0.5%	Lumbosacral	Adequate for ovariohysterectomy[a]	0.36	[286]
Bupivacaine 0.25%	Lumbosacral	T9	0.4	[281]

[a] The ovaries are supplied by the sympathetic chain via the hypogastric nerves (T10–L1).

Table 60.3 Volumes of local anesthetics (based on dye-staining studies) used for epidural anesthesia in cats.

Drug	Puncture site	Dermatome	Volume (mL/kg)
Methylene blue solution	Lumbosacral	L1–L2	0.2
Methylene blue solution	Lumbosacral	Up to T7	0.3
Methylene blue solution	Lumbosacral	T6–T10	0.4

Source: Adapted from Lee *et al.* [279].

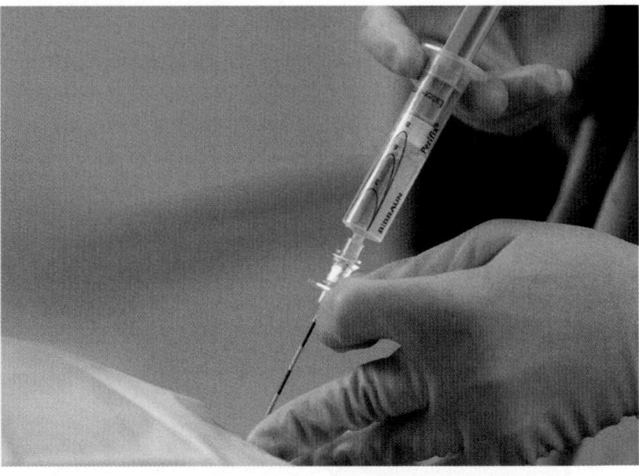

Figure 60.29 During performance of epidural anesthesia, a "loss of resistance" (LOR) syringe can be used to identify when the epidural space is entered.

avoid dural puncture. The typical doses that are recommended for epidural anesthesia in dogs and cats are presented in Tables 60.2 and 60.3.

Hanging drop

To perform an epidural with the hanging drop technique, a drop of saline or local anesthetic solution is placed in the hub of a spinal or Tuohy needle; as the needle penetrates the epidural space, it will usually be aspirated into the needle. In dogs, pressure within the epidural space has been reported to be anywhere from −6 to +15 mmHg [287]. It seems that gravity and the possible subatmospheric pressure within the epidural space and mainly the recoil of the ligamentum flavum when pierced by a blunt needle such as a Tuohy needle may play a role in the efficacy of this technique. One study reported 100% false negatives (i.e., the needle tip is located within the epidural space, but saline remains in the hub) with the hanging drop technique when the spinal needle was placed during lateral recumbency, compared with a positive aspiration in seven out of eight dogs positioned in sternal recumbency [288].

Loss of resistance

Resistance to injection of air or fluid may be felt while the needle is advanced through the intervertebral ligaments. If slight pressure is being applied to the plunger of a "loss of resistance" (LOR) syringe, a sudden loss of resistance to injection will be appreciated when the needle punctures the ligamentum flavum and enters the epidural space (Fig. 60.29). A false-positive result may ensue if the needle is located within the intervertebral fat. It is also possible to obtain a false-negative result (correct placement but no LOR) if foreign material (blood clots, fat, periosteum, skin) fills the needle bore and causes obstruction. If air is used for the LOR technique, a very small volume should be injected since the use of air (0.3 mL/kg) may be associated with significantly less spread of the injected solution, uneven cranial distribution of the solution, and occasional compression of the spinal cord [289].

Running-drip technique

The running-drip technique relies on hydrostatic pressure to allow a saline drip to run reliably once the epidural space is entered [290]. The technique has been recently described in dogs and was found to be a suitable alternative to the hanging drop technique, especially when the patient is positioned in lateral recumbency [291]. The running-drip technique utilizes a 100 mL bag of 0.9% saline attached to a 20 drop/mL drip set attached via a three-way stopcock to a Tuohy needle. The drip set chamber is then elevated 60 cm above the dog and opened. Once an unequivocal increase in the dripping rate is observed, the three-way stopcock is opened to the atmosphere and examined for the presence of CSF or blood. This technique has also been shown to identify entry of the needle into epidural space at the sacrococcygeal space in dogs [32].

Electrolocation

Several studies have demonstrated that each layer of the spinal cord requires a different threshold current to elicit a motor response [292,293]. Nerve stimulation may, therefore, be useful for identifying the lumbosacral epidural space in dogs. When the needle tip is located in the epidural space, twitches in the pelvic limbs and tail will be observed [294,295]. Nerve stimulation can also be helpful in identifying the epidural space when performing sacrococcygeal epidural injections in both dogs and cats, with a distinctive tail twitch appreciated when the needle is located in the epidural space [34].

Ultrasound-guided

Ultrasound-guided approaches to the epidural space have been described in both cats and dogs [296–298]. Ultrasonography can be used to identify the correct location, especially in obese patients, as well as to confirm epidural injections in real time [296,299]. Using a transverse view of the spinal canal at the level of the lumbosacral space, one can confirm epidural injection of a solution via collapse of the dural sac, enlargement of the epidural space, and/or a positive color flow Doppler signal [297,298].

Regardless which of the above techniques is used, the needle should be inspected for the presence of CSF or blood after entering the epidural space. If either fluid is observed, the needle should be removed and the procedure should be repeated. If desired, an extension set can be attached to the needle to make drug administration easier. At this point, the calculated drug volume can be administered partially (if a catheter will subsequently be placed) or totally.

Catheter placement

An indwelling catheter may be placed into the epidural space to facilitate drug administration. Epidural catheters are typically found in a commercially available kit that may contain a Touhy needle, epidural catheter, threading assist guide, catheter connector, and bacterial filter. When using a Tuohy needle, the bevel of the needle should be directed cranially to assist with placement of the catheter. Once in the epidural space, if the needle hub is tipped caudally, it will further facilitate the catheter exiting the needle and being advanced into the epidural space. A threading assist guide can be attached to the needle hub to aid with catheter insertion. The epidural catheter should be threaded with the dominant hand through the needle, paying attention to the depth markings on the catheter (four solid marks indicate the point at which the catheter should be exiting the needle tip) (Fig. 60.30). Slight resistance to advancement may be appreciated as the catheter is passing beyond the tip of the needle. The catheter should be advanced (1 cm at a time) past the final desired location to account for needle withdrawal. In most cases, the catheter should not be advanced into the epidural space more than 5 cm owing to the risk of the catheter curling back on itself. The catheter should never be withdrawn with the needle left in place owing to the risk of shearing the catheter with the bevel of the needle. If the catheter is accidentally sheared off or broken, it is usually left in place and surgical retrieval is not usually recommended. To withdraw the needle, the catheter is held at its point of entry between the thumb and index fingers while the needle is removed. The catheter should be sterilely secured via a preferred technique; subcutaneous tunneling of the catheter several centimeters away from its point of entry provides good fixation while at the same time minimizing potential catheter site contamination. After having checked for the absence of spontaneous flow of CSF or blood from the catheter when the end of the catheter is held in a dependent position, a catheter connector and a bacterial filter can be attached. Following negative aspiration, the remainder of the initial bolus of solution can be administered.

Drugs for continuous epidural anesthesia and analgesia

The analgesics that are most frequently used by the authors for continuous epidural anesthesia are bupivacaine (0.06%–0.25%) with or without the addition of morphine (0.1 mg/kg per 12–24 h), buprenorphine (4 µg/kg in a total volume of 0.2 mL/kg), or fentanyl (2–4 µg/mL solution with 20–40 µg of fentanyl per 10 mL of bupivacaine mixed in the same syringe). The recommended infusion rate through the catheter is 0.02–0.05 mL/kg/h. If analgesia is inadequate, a bolus of a more concentrated solution can be given (e.g., 0.5% bupivacaine) and the rate of the infusion can be increased while maintaining the original concentrations. If the extension of blockade is found to be excessive, the rate should be subsequently reduced. If signs of muscle weakness appear, the concentration is reduced while maintaining the same infusion rate. If signs of deep sedation appear, the opioid dose can be reduced. Alternatively, bolus dosing of the catheter may be utilized using similar agents and volumes to single-injection techniques. Note that the tip of the epidural catheter may be located several segments more cranially than with typical lumbosacral injection, depending on the length of the catheter threaded into the epidural space.

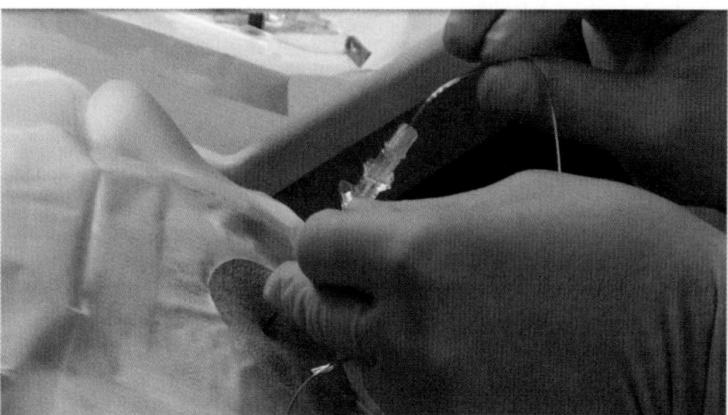

Figure 60.30 An epidural catheter is advanced into the hub of a Tuohy needle. Four solid marks are used to indicate the point at which the catheter should be exiting the needle tip.

Intrathecal (spinal) anesthesia

While epidural anesthesia is commonly used for hind limb procedures in small animals, recent literature has documented the use of intrathecal anesthesia as an alternative, where a more profound blockade with a shorter duration of effect may be preferable [300]. A direct comparison of epidural to spinal anesthesia for pelvic limb orthopedic surgery in dogs found a lower procedural failure rate and decreased intraoperative rescue analgesia requirement in dogs receiving intrathecal anesthesia [300]. Typically, the dose of local anesthetic is reduced by 30% as compared to epidural administration [300]. Utilization of a hyperbaric local anesthetic solution can be useful to produce unilateral blockade with reduced hemodynamic impact by placing the patient with the affected side down following intrathecal injection [301]. While a large study in humans has documented increased serious complication rates, such as cardiac arrest and neurologic damage, associated with spinal anesthesia as compared to epidural anesthesia [302], no such studies exist in veterinary medicine. A retrospective study examining the effects of intrathecal bupivacaine or levobupivacaine in 82 dogs found minimal side effects, with the most common being hypotension (29%) [303]. Less common side effects reported were bradycardia (8.5%), hypersalivation (7%), and urinary retention (5%). In a similar retrospective study of 58 cats, hypotension (50%) and bradycardia (39%) were the only reported complications [304].

In dogs, intrathecal anesthesia can be performed at the level of L5–L6 using a spinal needle. The needle is advanced slowly into the subarachnoid space, at which point CSF outflow becomes visible in the hub of the needle. In cats, intrathecal anesthesia can be performed either with a median approach at L7–S1 or a paramedian approach with cephalad angulation at L5–6 or L6–L7 [304]. The paramedian approach at L5–L6 or L6–L7 may have a higher success rate in cats as compared to the median approach at L7–S1 due to lower CSF pressure needed for CSF outflow into the hub of the spinal needle.

Complications of locoregional anesthesia

While the use of locoregional anesthesia has many benefits and is gaining traction in small animal practice, one must be aware of the potential complications associated with these procedures. Unfortunately, there are no large-scale multicenter studies in small animals demonstrating the incidence of complications related to the use of locoregional anesthesia. Smaller scale studies documenting side effects associated with epidural, intrathecal, and regional anesthesia reported a low incidence of complications [254,303–306]. Serious complications associated with locoregional anesthesia include local anesthetic systemic toxicity, neuronal damage, inadvertent trauma to surrounding structures, and infection. Additional side effects associated with neuraxial blockade are presented in Table 60.1.

Local anesthetic systemic toxicity

High plasma concentrations can result in local anesthetic systemic toxicity (LAST) which can be manifested as central nervous system (CNS) and cardiovascular complications, including nystagmus, twitching, seizures, CNS depression, hypotension, arrhythmias, and cardiac arrest. Typically, the onset of CNS complications occurs first; however, these can be masked by anesthesia, leading to progression to cardiovascular compromise. Elevated plasma concentrations can occur due to local anesthetic overdose or inadvertent intravascular injection. The total amount of local anesthetic to be used should be calculated to remain below the toxic dose and aspiration prior to injections should be performed to reduce the likelihood of intravascular injection.

While LAST symptoms are likely to occur shortly after injection of local anesthetic, with a median time of 53 s (interquartile range 30–180 s) in one human study, some cases may present over 15 min later, thus it is important to continue to closely monitor patients following locoregional anesthesia [307]. Should unexplained signs of cardiovascular compromise such as progressive hypotension, bradycardia, or ventricular arrhythmia develop following local anesthetic administration, LAST should be considered as a likely diagnosis. LAST should be treated with lipid emulsion therapy (1.5 mL/kg of 20% lipid emulsion) while providing supportive care to maintain cardiovascular function, oxygenation, and prevent seizures. If not already intubated, the patient should be intubated and ventilated with 100% oxygen to prevent hypoxia and acidosis which can potentiate LAST [307]. If seizures occur, they should be treated with benzodiazepines. Should cardiac arrest occur, the RECOVER CPR protocol should be followed in addition to the administration of lipid emulsion, however, amiodarone and not lidocaine should be administered to treat ventricular tachycardia [307]. The American Society of Regional Anesthesia (ASRA) provides multiple resources for providers of regional anesthesia, including LAST treatment guidelines.

Neuronal damage

Neurologic injury can range from short-term complications such as temporary dysesthesias to long-term neuropraxia. Neuronal damage is thought to result from mechanical trauma, neuronal ischemia, neurotoxicity, and/or infection. Neuronal trauma can result from excessive pressures exerted from subdural hematoma formation during neuraxial anesthesia or due to intraneural injection peripherally. While subepineural injections can result in prolonged blockade, these are not associated with long-term neuronal damage [95,308,309]. However, intraneural (within the perineurium) injection, typically associated with high injection pressures, results in nerve damage [95]. While a retrospective study in dogs receiving sciatic nerve blocks showed no neurologic complications at 6 weeks [305], larger scale studies in humans reported a rate of long-term injury of 2–4 per 10,000 blocks [310]. Although these appear to be rare complications, the consequences are severe, so one should attempt to minimize risk by avoiding high-pressure injections, utilizing specialized needles, and ultrasound guidance when possible [311]. While the use of nerve stimulation may also help guide proximity to the nerve, thereby reducing the chances of intraneural injection, studies have demonstrated that low current intensities (< 0.3 mA) may not always elicit a motor response and thus nerve stimulation alone does not appear sufficient to detect nerve contact and intraneural injection [312].

References

1 Kim J, Kim NS, Lee KC, *et al.* Effect of topical anesthesia on evaluation of corneal sensitivity and intraocular pressure in rats and dogs. *Vet Ophthalmol* 2013; **16**(1): 43–46.
2 Jones TL, Boyer K, Chapman K, *et al.* Evaluation of the time to desensitization of the larynx of cats following topical lidocaine application. *J Feline Med Surg* 2021; **23**(6): 563–567.
3 Kumar M, Chawla R, Goyal M. Topical anesthesia. *J Anaesthesiol Clin Pharmacol* 2015; **31**(4): 450–456.
4 Crisi PE, De Santis F, Giordano MV, *et al.* Evaluation of eutectic lidocaine/prilocaine cream for jugular blood sampling in cats. *J Feline Med Surg* 2021; **23**(2): 185–189.
5 van Oostrom H, Knowles TG. The clinical efficacy of EMLA cream for intravenous catheter placement in client-owned dogs. *Vet Anaesth Analg* 2018; **45**(5): 604–608.
6 Ko J, Weil A, Maxwell L, *et al.* Plasma concentrations of lidocaine in dogs following lidocaine patch application. *J Am Anim Hosp Assoc* 2007; **43**(5): 280–283.
7 Bidwell LA, Wilson DV, Caron JP. Lack of systemic absorption of lidocaine from 5% patches placed on horses. *Vet Anaesth Analg* 2007; **34**(6): 443–446.
8 Re Bravo V, Aprea F, Bhalla RJ, *et al.* Effect of 5% transdermal lidocaine patches on postoperative analgesia in dogs undergoing hemilaminectomy. *J Small Anim Pract* 2019; **60**(3): 161–166.
9 Ko JC, Maxwell LK, Abbo LA, *et al.* Pharmacokinetics of lidocaine following the application of 5% lidocaine patches to cats. *J Vet Pharmacol Ther* 2008; **31**(4): 359–367.
10 Weiland L, Croubels S, Baert K, *et al.* Pharmacokinetics of a lidocaine patch 5% in dogs. *J Vet Med A Physiol Pathol Clin Med* 2006; **53**(1): 34–39.
11 Merema DK, Schoenrock EK, Le Boedec K, *et al.* Effects of a transdermal lidocaine patch on indicators of postoperative pain in dogs undergoing midline ovariohysterectomy. *J Am Vet Med Assoc* 2017; **250**(10): 1140–1147.
12 Saber AA, Elgamal MH, Rao AJ, *et al.* Early experience with lidocaine patch for postoperative pain control after laparoscopic ventral hernia repair. *Int J Surg* 2009; **7**(1): 36–38.
13 Habib AS, Polascik TJ, Weizer AZ, *et al.* Lidocaine patch for postoperative analgesia after radical retropubic prostatectomy. *Anesth Analg* 2009; **108**(6): 1950–1953.
14 Joudrey SD, Robinson DA, Kearney MT, *et al.* Plasma concentrations of lidocaine in dogs following lidocaine patch application over an incision compared to intact skin. *J Vet Pharmacol Ther* 2015; **38**(6): 575–580.
15 McFadzean WJM, Macfarlane P, Granger N, *et al.* Influence of peri-incisional epaxial muscle infiltration with bupivacaine pre- or post-surgery on opioid administration in dogs undergoing thoraco-lumbar hemilaminectomy. *Vet J* 2021; **270**: 105622.
16 Kiriaki PP. The effect of pre-emptive incisional bupivacaine block on postoperative pain after coeliotomy in dogs. *Veterinary Evidence* 2021; **6**(1).
17 Campagnol D, Teixeira-Neto FJ, Monteiro ER, *et al.* Effect of intraperitoneal or incisional bupivacaine on pain and the analgesic requirement after ovariohysterectomy in dogs. *Vet Anaesth Analg* 2012; **39**(4): 426–430.
18 Savvas I, Papazoglou LG, Kazakos G, *et al.* Incisional block with bupivacaine for analgesia after celiotomy in dogs. *J Am Anim Hosp Assoc* 2008; **44**(2): 60–66.
19 Fitzpatrick CL, Weir HL, Monnet E. Effects of infiltration of the incision site with bupivacaine on postoperative pain and incisional healing in dogs undergoing ovariohysterectomy. *J Am Vet Med Assoc* 2010; **237**(4): 395–401.
20 Whiteman A, Bajaj S, Hasan M. Novel techniques of local anaesthetic infiltration. *Contin Educ Anaesth Crit Care Pain* 2011; **11**(5): 167–171.
21 Abelson AL, McCobb EC, Shaw S, *et al.* Use of wound soaker catheters for the administration of local anesthetic for post-operative analgesia: 56 cases. *Vet Anaesth Analg* 2009; **36**(6): 597–602.
22 Zeren S, Kesici S, Kesici U, *et al.* Effects of levobupivacaine on wound healing. *Anesth Analg* 2013; **116**(2): 495–499.
23 Klein JA. Tumescent technique for local anesthesia improves safety in large-volume liposuction. *Plast Reconstr Surg* 1993; **92**(6): 1085–1098, discussion 99–100.
24 Klein JA. Anesthetic formulation of tumescent solutions. *Dermatol Clin* 1999; **17**(4): 751–759, v–vi.
25 Credie Lde F, Luna SP, Futema F, *et al.* Perioperative evaluation of tumescent anaesthesia technique in bitches submitted to unilateral mastectomy. *BMC Vet Res* 2013; **9**: 178.
26 Moreira CM, Oliveira RL, Costa GA, *et al.* Evaluation of tumescent local anesthesia in cats undergoing unilateral mastectomy. *Vet Anaesth Analg* 2021; **48**(1): 134–141.
27 Sanches MC, Maroneze BP, Salame JP, *et al.* Tumescent anesthesia or epidural anesthesia combined with intercostal block in bitches submitted to mastectomy. *Ciência Animal Brasileira* 2020; **21**(4): e53552.
28 De Marzo C, Crovace A, De Monte V, *et al.* Comparison of intra-operative analgesia provided by intravenous regional anesthesia or brachial plexus block for pancarpal arthrodesis in dogs. *Res Vet Sci* 2012; **93**(3): 1493–1497.

29 Boezaart A, Smith C, Zasimovich Y, *et al.* Femoral artery block: the relationship between visceral and ischemic pain. *Reg Anesth Pain Med* 2022; **47**(1): 70–71.

30 Looseley A. Corning and cocaine: the advent of spinal anaesthesia. *Grand Rounds* 2009; **9**: L1–L4.

31 Liotta A, Busoni V, Carrozzo MV, *et al.* Feasibility of ultrasound-guided epidural access at the lumbo-sacral space in dogs. *Vet Radiol Ultrasound* 2015; **56**(2): 220–228.

32 Martinez-Taboada F, Otero PE, Laredo F, *et al.* Identification of the sacrococcygeal epidural space using the nerve stimulation test or the running-drip method in dogs. *Vet Anaesth Analg* 2020; **47**(3): 385–390.

33 Credie L, Luna SPL. Real-time ultrasound-guided lumbosacral epidural anaesthesia in obese or appropriate body condition score dogs: a randomized clinical trial. *Vet J* 2022; **280**: 105791.

34 Verdier N, Martinez-Taboada F, Otero PE, *et al.* Evaluation of electrical nerve stimulation to confirm sacrococcygeal epidural needle placement in dogs. *Vet Anaesth Analg* 2021; **48**(4): 612–616.

35 Thomson ACS, Portela DA, Romano M, *et al.* Evaluation of the effect of ultrasound guidance on the accuracy of intercostal nerve injection: a canine cadaveric study. *Vet Anaesth Analg* 2021; **48**(2): 256–263.

36 Costa-Farre C, Blanch XS, Cruz JI, *et al.* Ultrasound guidance for the performance of sciatic and saphenous nerve blocks in dogs. *Vet J* 2011; **187**(2): 221–224.

37 Sala-Blanch X, De Andres J. Image-guided techniques for peripheral nerve blocks. *Curr Opin Anaesthesiol* 2004; **17**(5): 409–415.

38 Marhofer P, Greher M, Kapral S. Ultrasound guidance in regional anaesthesia. *Br J Anaesth* 2005; **94**(1): 7–17.

39 Chin KJ, Versyck B, Elsharkawy H, *et al.* Anatomical basis of fascial plane blocks. *Reg Anesth Pain Med* 2021; **46**(7): 581–599.

40 Chin KJ, Lirk P, Hollmann MW, *et al.* Mechanisms of action of fascial plane blocks: a narrative review. *Reg Anesth Pain Med* 2021; **46**(7): 618–628.

41 Byrne K, Smith C. Erector spinae plane block: systemic local anesthetic by proxy? *Reg Anesth Pain Med* 2021; **46**(7): 639–640.

42 Congdon JM, Boscan P, Goh CSS, *et al.* Psoas compartment and sacral plexus block via electrostimulation for pelvic limb amputation in dogs. *Vet Anaesth Analg* 2017; **44**(4): 915–924.

43 Mosing M, Reich H, Moens Y. Clinical evaluation of the anaesthetic sparing effect of brachial plexus block in cats. *Vet Anaesth Analg* 2010; **37**(2): 154–161.

44 Romano M, Portela DA, Breghi G, *et al.* Stress-related biomarkers in dogs administered regional anaesthesia or fentanyl for analgesia during stifle surgery. *Vet Anaesth Analg* 2016; **43**(1): 44–54.

45 Portela D, Melanie P, Briganti A, Breghi G. Nerve stimulator-guided paravertebral lumbar plexus anaesthesia in dogs. *Vet Res Commun* 2008; **32**(Suppl 1): S307–S310.

46 Stewart JD. Peripheral nerve fascicles: anatomy and clinical relevance. *Muscle Nerve* 2003; **28**(5): 525–541.

47 Selander D, Sjostrand J. Longitudinal spread of intraneurally injected local anesthetics. An experimental study of the initial neural distribution following intraneural injections. *Acta Anaesthesiol Scand* 1978; **22**(6): 622–634.

48 Jeng CL, Rosenblatt MA. Intraneural injections and regional anesthesia: the known and the unknown. *Minerva Anestesiol* 2011; **77**(1): 54–58.

49 Bigeleisen PE. Nerve puncture and apparent intraneural injection during ultrasound-guided axillary block does not invariably result in neurologic injury. *Anesthesiology* 2006; **105**(4): 779–783.

50 Whitlock EL, Brenner MJ, Fox IK, *et al.* Ropivacaine-induced peripheral nerve injection injury in the rodent model. *Anesth Analg* 2010; **111**(1): 214–220.

51 Cummins TR, Sheets PL, Waxman SG. The roles of sodium channels in nociception: implications for mechanisms of pain. *Pain* 2007; **131**(3): 243–257.

52 Becker DE, Reed KL. Local anesthetics: review of pharmacological considerations. *Anesth Prog* 2012; **59**(2): 90–101; quiz 2–3.

53 Ribotsky BM, Berkowitz KD, Montague JR. Local anesthetics. Is there an advantage to mixing solutions? *J Am Podiatr Med Assoc* 1996; **86**(10): 487–491.

54 Sepehripour S, Dheansa BS. Is there an advantage in onset of action with mixing lignocaine and bupivacaine? *J Plast Reconstr Aesthet Surg* 2017; **70**(12): 1782.

55 Gasser HS, Erlanger J. The role of fiber size in the establishment of a nerve block by pressure or cocaine. *Am J Physiol Legacy Content* 1929; **88**(4): 581–591.

56 Gokin AP, Philip B, Strichartz GR. Preferential block of small myelinated sensory and motor fibers by lidocaine: in vivo electrophysiology in the rat sciatic nerve. *Anesthesiology* 2001; **95**(6): 1441–1454.

57 Gissen AJ, Covino BG, Gregus J. Differential sensitivities of mammalian nerve fibers to local anesthetic agents. *Anesthesiology* 1980; **53**(6): 467–474.

58 Raymond SA, Steffensen SC, Gugino LD, *et al.* The role of length of nerve exposed to local anesthetics in impulse blocking action. *Anesth Analg* 1989; **68**(5): 563–570.

59 Liu SS, Ware PD. Differential sensory block after spinal bupivacaine in volunteers. *Anesth Analg* 1997; **84**(1): 115–119.

60 Oda A, Ohashi H, Komori S, *et al.* Characteristics of ropivacaine block of Na+ channels in rat dorsal root ganglion neurons. *Anesth Analg* 2000; **91**(5): 1213–1220.

61 Krishna Prasad GV, Khanna S, Jaishree SV. Review of adjuvants to local anesthetics in peripheral nerve blocks: current and future trends. *Saudi J Anaesth* 2020; **14**(1): 77–84.

62 Stein C. Targeting pain and inflammation by peripherally acting opioids. *Front Pharmacol* 2013; **4**: 123.

63 Bazin JE, Massoni C, Bruelle P, *et al.* The addition of opioids to local anaesthetics in brachial plexus block: the comparative effects of morphine, buprenorphine and sufentanil. *Anaesthesia* 1997; **52**(9): 858–862.

64 Schnabel A, Reichl SU, Zahn PK, *et al.* Efficacy and safety of buprenorphine in peripheral nerve blocks: a meta-analysis of randomised controlled trials. *Eur J Anaesthesiol* 2017; **34**(9): 576–586.

65 Candido KD, Winnie AP, Ghaleb AH, *et al.* Buprenorphine added to the local anesthetic for axillary brachial plexus block prolongs postoperative analgesia. *Reg Anesth Pain Med* 2002; **27**(2): 162–167.

66 Candido KD, Hennes J, Gonzalez S, *et al.* Buprenorphine enhances and prolongs the postoperative analgesic effect of bupivacaine in patients receiving infragluteal sciatic nerve block. *Anesthesiology* 2010; **113**(6): 1419–1426.

67 Leffler A, Frank G, Kistner K, *et al.* Local anesthetic-like inhibition of voltage-gated Na(+) channels by the partial mu-opioid receptor agonist buprenorphine. *Anesthesiology* 2012; **116**(6): 1335–1346.

68 Neal JM. Effects of epinephrine in local anesthetics on the central and peripheral nervous systems: neurotoxicity and neural blood flow. *Reg Anesth Pain Med* 2003; **28**(2): 124–134.

69 Zhu AF, Hood BR, Morris MS, *et al.* Delayed-onset digital ischemia after local anesthetic with epinephrine injection requiring phentolamine reversal. *J Hand Surg Am* 2017; **42**(6): 479 e1–e4.

70 Nishikawa T, Dohi S. Clinical evaluation of clonidine added to lidocaine solution for epidural anesthesia. *Anesthesiology* 1990; **73**(5): 853–859.

71 Eisenach JC, De Kock M, Klimscha W. Alpha(2)-adrenergic agonists for regional anesthesia. A clinical review of clonidine (1984–1995). *Anesthesiology* 1996; **85**(3): 655–674.

72 Popping DM, Elia N, Marret E, *et al.* Clonidine as an adjuvant to local anesthetics for peripheral nerve and plexus blocks: a meta-analysis of randomized trials. *Anesthesiology* 2009; **111**(2): 406–415.

73 El-Boghdadly K, Brull R, Sehmbi H, *et al.* Perineural dexmedetomidine is more effective than clonidine when added to local anesthetic for supraclavicular brachial plexus lock: a systematic review and meta-analysis. *Anesth Analg* 2017; **124**(6): 2008–2020.

74 Steinfeldt T, Graf J, Schneider J, *et al.* Histological consequences of needle-nerve contact following nerve stimulation in a pig model. *Anesthesiol Res Pract* 2011; **2011**: 591851.

75 Steinfeldt T, Nimphius W, Werner T, *et al.* Nerve injury by needle nerve perforation in regional anaesthesia: does size matter? *Br J Anaesth* 2010; **104**(2): 245–253.

76 Ethunandan M, Tran AL, Anand R, *et al.* Needle breakage following inferior alveolar nerve block: implications and management. *Br Dent J* 2007; **202**(7): 395–397.

77 Shapiro DM, Ye Y, Burnett G, *et al.* Broken peripheral nerve block needles with considerations and recommendations. *J Clin Anesth* 2020; **60**: 17–18.

78 Prakash S, Kumar A. Needle tip and peripheral nerve blocks. *J Anaesthesiol Clin Pharmacol* 2018; **34**(1): 129–130.

79 Steinfeldt T, Nimphius W, Wurps M, *et al.* Nerve perforation with pencil point or short bevelled needles: histological outcome. *Acta Anaesthesiol Scand* 2010; **54**(8): 993–999.

80 Munirama S, Joy J, Columb M, *et al.* A randomised, single-blind technical study comparing the ultrasonic visibility of smooth-surfaced and textured needles in a soft embalmed cadaver model. *Anaesthesia* 2015; **70**(5): 537–542.

81 Hebard S, Hocking G. Echogenic technology can improve needle visibility during ultrasound-guided regional anesthesia. *Reg Anesth Pain Med* 2011; **36**(2): 185–189.

82 Jiang T, Zhu X, Jiao Y, *et al.* Localization accuracy of ultrasound-actuated needle with color Doppler imaging. *Diagnostics (Basel)* 2020; **10**(12): 1020.

83 Watanabe K, Tokumine J, Lefor AK, *et al.* Photoacoustic needle improves needle tip visibility during deep peripheral nerve block. *Sci Rep* 2021; **11**(1): 8432.

84 Quincke H. Die lumbalpunction des hydrocephalus. *Berliner Klinische Wochenschrift* 1891; **28**: 929–933.

85 Morrison LM, McCrae AF, Foo I, *et al.* An in vitro comparison of fluid leakage after dural puncture with Atraucan, Sprotte, Whitacre, and Quincke needles. *Reg Anesth* 1996; **21**(2): 139–143.

86 Calthorpe N. The history of spinal needles: getting to the point. *Anaesthesia* 2004; **59**(12): 1231–1241.

87 Usar P, Kar AA, Citak G, *et al.* Breakage of an epidural catheter inserted for labor analgesia. *Turk J Anaesthesiol Reanim* 2015; **43**(4): 282–284.

88 Toledano RD, Tsen LC. Epidural catheter design: history, innovations, and clinical implications. *Anesthesiology* 2014; **121**(1): 9–17.

89 Moore JM. Continuous spinal anesthesia. *Am J Ther* 2009; **16**(4): 289–294.

90 Luyet C, Seiler R, Herrmann G, *et al.* Newly designed, self-coiling catheters for regional anesthesia--an imaging study. *Reg Anesth Pain Med* 2011; **36**(2): 171–176.

91 Campolo M, Molin D, Rawal N, *et al.* Protocols to compare infusion distribution of wound catheters. *Med Eng Phys* 2012; **34**(3): 326–332.

92 Mowat I, Tang R, Vaghadia H, *et al.* Epidural distribution of dye administered via an epidural catheter in a porcine model. *Br J Anaesth* 2016; **116**(2): 277–281.

93 Hardie EM, Lascelles BDX, Meuten T, *et al.* Evaluation of intermittent infusion of bupivacaine into surgical wounds of dogs postoperatively. *Vet J* 2011; **190**(2): 287–289.

94 Claudio R, Hadzic A, Shih H, *et al.* Injection pressures by anesthesiologists during simulated peripheral nerve block. *Reg Anesth Pain Med* 2004; **29**(3): 201–205.

95 Hadzic A, Dilberovic F, Shah S, *et al.* Combination of intraneural injection and high injection pressure leads to fascicular injury and neurologic deficits in dogs. *Reg Anesth Pain Med* 2004; **29**(5): 417–423.

96 Son WG, Jang M, Yoon J, *et al.* The effect of epidural injection speed on epidural pressure and distribution of solution in anesthetized dogs. *Vet Anaesth Analg* 2014; **41**(5): 526–533.

97 Kapur E, Vuckovic I, Dilberovic F, *et al.* Neurologic and histologic outcome after intraneural injections of lidocaine in canine sciatic nerves. *Acta Anaesthesiol Scand* 2007; **51**(1): 101–107.

98 Gadsden J. Current devices used for the monitoring of injection pressure during peripheral nerve blocks. *Expert Rev Med Devices* 2018; **15**(8): 571–578.

99 Saberski LR, Kondamuri S, Osinubi OY. Identification of the epidural space: is loss of resistance to air a safe technique? A review of the complications related to the use of air. *Reg Anesth* 1997; **22**(1): 3–15.

100 Quadri C, Saporito A, Capdevila X. Real-time continuous monitoring of injection pressure at the needle tip for peripheral nerve blocks: description of a new method. *Anaesthesia* 2018; **73**(2): 187–194.

101 Urmey WF. Using the nerve stimulator for peripheral or plexus nerve blocks. *Minerva Anestesiol* 2006; **72**(6): 467–471.

102 Sauter AR, Dodgson MS, Stubhaug A, *et al.* Ultrasound controlled nerve stimulation in the elbow region: high currents and short distances needed to obtain motor responses. *Acta Anaesthesiol Scand* 2007; **51**(7): 942–948.

103 Perlas A, Niazi A, McCartney C, *et al.* The sensitivity of motor response to nerve stimulation and paresthesia for nerve localization as evaluated by ultrasound. *Reg Anesth Pain Med* 2006; **31**(5): 445–450.

104 Chan VW, Brull R, McCartney CJ, *et al.* An ultrasonographic and histological study of intraneural injection and electrical stimulation in pigs. *Anesth Analg* 2007; **104**(5): 1281–1284.

105 Ben-David B, Chelly JE. Current channeling: a theory of nerve stimulator failure. *Anesth Analg* 2003; **96**(5): 1531–1532.

106 Klein SM, Melton MS, Grill WM, *et al.* Peripheral nerve stimulation in regional anesthesia. *Reg Anesth Pain Med* 2012; **37**(4): 383–392.

107 Barthram CN. Nerve stimulators for nerve location – are they all the same? *A study of stimulator performance. Anaesthesia* 1997; **52**(8): 761–764.

108 Jochum D, Iohom G, Diarra DP, *et al.* An objective assessment of nerve stimulators used for peripheral nerve blockade*. *Anaesthesia* 2006; **61**(6): 557–564.

109 Hadzic A, Vloka J, Hadzic N, *et al.* Nerve stimulators used for peripheral nerve blocks vary in their electrical characteristics. *Anesthesiology* 2003; **98**(4): 969–974.

110 Kapral S, Krafft P, Eibenberger K, *et al.* Ultrasound-guided supraclavicular approach for regional anesthesia of the brachial plexus. *Anesth Analg* 1994; **78**(3): 507–513.

111 Ng A, Swanevelder J. Resolution in ultrasound imaging. *Cont Educ Anaesth Crit Care Pain* 2011; **11**(5): 186–192.

112 Xu D, De Meirsman S, Schreurs R. Optimizing an ultrasound image. In: Hadzic A, ed. *Hadzic's Textbook of Regional Anesthesia and Acute Pain Management*, 2nd edn. New York, NY: McGraw-Hill Education, 2017.

113 Chan V, Perlas A. Basics of ultrasound imaging. In: Narouze S, ed. *Atlas of Ultrasound-Guided Procedures in Interventional Pain Management*. New York, NY: Springer, 2010: 13–19.

114 Oktar SO, Yucel C, Ozdemir H, *et al.* Comparison of conventional sonography, real-time compound sonography, tissue harmonic sonography, and tissue harmonic compound sonography of abdominal and pelvic lesions. *Am J Roentgenol* 2003; **181**(5): 1341–1347.

115 Bozzato A, Loika A, Hornung J, *et al.* Comparison of conventional B-scan, tissue harmonic imaging, compound imaging and tissue harmonic compound imaging in neck lesion characterisation. *Eur Arch Otorhinolaryngol* 2010; **267**(10): 1593–1598.

116 Yen CL, Jeng CM, Yang SS. The benefits of comparing conventional sonography, real-time spatial compound sonography, tissue harmonic sonography, and tissue harmonic compound sonography of hepatic lesions. *Clin Imaging* 2008; **32**(1): 11–15.

117 Marhofer P, Chan VW. Ultrasound-guided regional anesthesia: current concepts and future trends. *Anesth Analg* 2007; **104**(5): 1265–1269.

118 Chin KJ, Perlas A, Chan VW, *et al.* Needle visualization in ultrasound-guided regional anesthesia: challenges and solutions. *Reg Anesth Pain Med* 2008; **33**(6): 532–544.

119 Sites BD, Brull R, Chan VW, *et al.* Artifacts and pitfall errors associated with ultrasound-guided regional anesthesia. Part I: understanding the basic principles of ultrasound physics and machine operations. *Reg Anesth Pain Med* 2007; **32**(5): 412–418.

120 Romano M, Portela DA, Otero PE, *et al.* Mirroring artefact [sic] during postoperative transversus abdominis plane (TAP) block in two dogs. *Vet Anaesth Analg* 2020; **47**(5): 727–728.

121 Pascoe PJ. Anesthesia and pain management. In: Verstraete FJM, Lommer MJ, eds. *Oral and Maxillofacial Surgery in Dogs and Cats*. Oxford, UK: W.B. Saunders, 2012: 23–42.

122 Bellows J, Berg ML, Dennis S, *et al.* 2019 AAHA Dental Care Guidelines for dogs and cats. *J Am Anim Hosp Assoc* 2019; **55**(2): 49–69.

123 Kalamaras AB, Aarnes TK, Moore SA, *et al.* Effects of perioperative saphenous and sciatic nerve blocks, lumbosacral epidural or morphine-lidocaine-ketamine infusion on postoperative pain and sedation in dogs undergoing tibial plateau leveling osteotomy. *Vet Anaesth Analg* 2021; **48**(3): 415–421.

124 Tavakoli A, Tazik ME, Abbasi A. Comparison of production of pain and oxidative stress after induction of local nerve block or use of NSAIDs following painful dental procedures in dogs. *Iran J Vet Surg* 2021; **16**(1): 29–33.

125 Hermanson JW, de Lahunta A. *Miller and Evans' Anatomy of the Dog*, 5th ed. New York, NY: Elsevier Health Sciences, 2018.

126 Aprea F, Vettorato E, Corletto F. Severe cardiovascular depression in a cat following a mandibular nerve block with bupivacaine. *Vet Anaesth Analg* 2011; **38**(6): 614–618.

127 Selander D, Dhuner KG, Lundborg G. Peripheral nerve injury due to injection needles used for regional anesthesia. An experimental study of the acute effects of needle point trauma. *Acta Anaesthesiol Scand* 1977; **21**(3): 182–188.

128 Rout PG, Saksena A, Fisher SE. An investigation of the effect on 27-gauge needle tips following a single local anaesthetic injection. *Dent Update* 2003; **30**(7): 370–374.

129 O'Morrow C. Advanced dental local nerve block anesthesia. *Can Vet J* 2010; **51**(12): 1411–1415.

130 Lemke KA, Dawson SD. Local and regional anesthesia. *Vet Clin North Am Small Anim Pract* 2000; **30**(4): 839–857.

131 Viscasillas J, Seymour CJ, Brodbelt DC. A cadaver study comparing two approaches for performing maxillary nerve block in dogs. *Vet Anaesth Analg* 2013; **40**(2): 212–219.

132 Rochette J. Regional anesthesia and analgesia for oral and dental procedures. *Vet Clin North Am Small Anim Pract* 2005; **35**(4): 1041–1058, viii–ix.

133 Chau A. Tongue lacerations in a geriatric dog after bilateral inferior alveolar nerve blocks with bupivacaine. *Vet Rec Case Rep* 2017; **5**: e000433.

134 Woodward TM. Pain management and regional anesthesia for the dental patient. *Top Companion Anim Med* 2008; **23**(2): 106–114.

135 Shilo-Benjamini Y, Letz S, Peery D, *et al.* Comparison of three regional anaesthetic techniques for infraorbital or maxillary nerve block in cats: a cadaveric study. *J Feline Med Surg* 2022; **24**(4): 322–327.

136 Gross ME, Pope ER, O'Brien D, *et al.* Regional anesthesia of the infraorbital and inferior alveolar nerves during noninvasive tooth pulp stimulation in halothane-anesthetized dogs. *J Am Vet Med Assoc* 1997; **211**(11): 1403–1405.

137 Gross ME, Pope ER, Jarboe JM, *et al.* Regional anesthesia of the infraorbital and inferior alveolar nerves during noninvasive tooth pulp stimulation in halothane-anesthetized cats. *Am J Vet Res* 2000; **61**(10): 1245–1247.

138 Krug W, Losey J. Area of desensitization following mental nerve block in dogs. *J Vet Dent* 2011; **28**(3): 146–150.

139 Reader ANJ, Hargreave K, Cohen S. Local anesthesia in endodontics. In: Hargreaves KM, Cohen S, Berman LH, eds. *Cohen's Pathways of the Pulp*, 10th edn. St. Louis, MO: Mosby Elsevier, 2011: 671–719.

140 Gracis M. The oral cavity. In: Campoy LR, Read MR, eds. *Small Animal Regional Anesthesia and Analgesia*. Ames, IA: Wiley-Blackwell, 2013: 119–140.

141 Moore PA, Cuddy MA, Cooke MR, *et al.* Periodontal ligament and intraosseous anesthetic injection techniques: alternatives to mandibular nerve blocks. *J Am Dent Assoc* 2011; **142**(Suppl 3): 13S–18S.

142 Accola PJ, Bentley E, Smith LJ, *et al.* Development of a retrobulbar injection technique for ocular surgery and analgesia in dogs. *J Am Vet Med Assoc* 2006; **229**(2): 220–225.

143 Myrna KE, Bentley E, Smith LJ. Effectiveness of injection of local anesthetic into the retrobulbar space for postoperative analgesia following eye enucleation in dogs. *J Am Vet Med Assoc* 2010; **237**(2): 174–177.

144 Vézina-Audette R, Steagall PVM, Gianotti G. Prevalence of and covariates associated with the oculocardiac reflex occurring in dogs during enucleation. *J Am Vet Med Assoc* 2019; **255**(4): 454–458.

145 Zibura AE, Posner LP, Ru H, *et al.* A preoperative bupivacaine retrobulbar block offers superior antinociception compared with an intraoperative splash block in dogs undergoing enucleation. *Vet Ophthalmol* 2020; **23**(2): 225–233.

146 Chiavaccini L, Micieli F, Meomartino L, *et al.* A novel supra-temporal approach to retrobulbar anaesthesia in dogs: preliminary study in cadavers. *Vet J* 2017; **223**: 68–70.

147 Kostadinov I, Hostnik A, Cvenkel B, *et al.* Brainstem anaesthesia after retrobulbar block. *Open Med (Wars)* 2019; **14**: 287–291.

148 Tolesa K, Gebreal GW. Brainstem anesthesia after retrobulbar block: a case report and review of literature. *Ethiop J Health Sci* 2016; **26**(6): 589–594.

149 Javitt JC, Addiego R, Friedberg HL, *et al.* Brainstem anesthesia after retrobulbar block. *Ophthalmology* 1987; **94**(6): 718–724.

150 Klaumann PR, Menzies RA, Briganti A, *et al.* Perineural anesthesia of the head, eye and ear. In: Otero PE, Portela DA, eds. *Manual of Small Animal Regional Anesthesia*, 2nd edn. Buenos Aires, Argentina: Editorial Inter-Médica, 2019: 313–374.

151 Foster A, Medina-Serra R, Sanchis-Mora S, *et al.* In-plane ultrasound-guided peribulbar block in the dog: an anatomical cadaver study. *Vet Anaesth Analg* 2021; **48**(2): 272–276.

152 Viscasillas J, Everson R, Mapletoft EK, *et al.* Ultrasound-guided posterior extraconal block in the dog: anatomical study in cadavers. *Vet Anaesth Analg* 2019; **46**(2): 246–250.

153 Kumar CM, Dodds C, McLure H, *et al.* A comparison of three sub-Tenon's cannulae. *Eye (Lond)* 2004; **18**(9): 873–876.

154 Bayley KD, Read RA. Sub-Tenon's anesthesia for canine cataract surgery. *Vet Ophthalmol* 2018; **21**(6): 601–611.

155 Stathopoulou TR, Pinelas R, Haar GT, *et al.* Description of a new approach for great auricular and auriculotemporal nerve blocks: a cadaveric study in foxes and dogs. *Vet Med Sci* 2018; **4**(2): 91–97.

156 Viscasillas J, Ter Haar G. Ultrasound-guided trigeminal nerve block as local anaesthetic technique for exenteration and excision of the zygomatic arch with partial caudal maxillectomy in a dog. *Vet Anaesth Analg* 2017; **44**(3): 688–690.

157 Bailey CS, Kitchell RL, Haghighi SS, *et al.* Cutaneous innervation of the thorax and abdomen of the dog. *Am J Vet Res* 1984; **45**(9): 1689–1698.

158 Portela DA, Otero PE, Sclocco M, *et al.* Anatomical and radiological study of the thoracic paravertebral space in dogs: iohexol distribution pattern and use of the nerve stimulator. *Vet Anaesth Analg* 2012; **39**(4): 398–408.

159 Santoro F, Franci P, Grandis A, *et al.* Distribution of injectates in the thoracic paravertebral space of the dog and cat: a cadaveric study. *Open Vet J* 2021; **11**(1): 27–35.

160 Portela DA, Campoy L, Otero PE, *et al.* Ultrasound-guided thoracic paravertebral injection in dogs: a cadaveric study. *Vet Anaesth Analg* 2017; **44**(3): 636–645.

161 Ferreira TH, Teixeira LBC, Schroeder CA, *et al.* Description of an ultrasound-guided thoracic paravertebral block technique and the spread of dye in dog cadavers. *Vet Anaesth Analg* 2018; **45**(6): 811–819.

162 Serra RM, Jimenez CP, Monticelli P, *et al.* Assessment of an ultrasound-guided technique for catheterization of the caudal thoracic paravertebral space in dog cadavers. *Open Vet J* 2019; **9**(3): 230–237.

163 Santoro F, Debidda P, Franci P. Single-injection caudal thoracic paravertebral block improves pain control and recovery quality in female dogs undergoing unilateral radical mastectomy: a randomized controlled trial. *J Am Vet Med Assoc* 2021; **260**(S1): S53–S58.

164 Garbin M, Bertolizio G, Portela DA. Thoracic paravertebral block for an opioid-free thoracotomy in a dog. *Vet Anaesth Analg* 2021; **48**(4): 622–623.

165 Lopez-Ramis V, Canfran S, Gomez de Segura IA. Caudal thoracic paravertebral block in a dog undergoing surgical adrenalectomy. *Vet Anaesth Analg* 2022; **49**(2): 219–220.

166 Monticelli P, Jones I, Viscasillas J. Ultrasound-guided thoracic paravertebral block: cadaveric study in foxes (Vulpes vulpes). *Vet Anaesth Analg* 2017; **44**(4): 968–972.

167 Pascoe PJ, Dyson DH. Analgesia after lateral thoracotomy in dogs. Epidural morphine vs. intercostal bupivacaine. *Vet Surg* 1993; **22**(2): 141–147.

168 Thompson SE, Johnson JM. Analgesia in dogs after intercostal thoracotomy. A comparison of morphine, selective intercostal nerve block, and interpleural regional analgesia with bupivacaine. *Vet Surg* 1991; **20**(1): 73–77.

169 Flecknell PA, Kirk AJ, Liles JH, *et al.* Post-operative analgesia following thoracotomy in the dog: an evaluation of the effects of bupivacaine intercostal nerve block and nalbuphine on respiratory function. *Lab Anim* 1991; **25**(4): 319–324.

170 Berg RJ, Orton EC. Pulmonary function in dogs after intercostal thoracotomy: comparison of morphine, oxymorphone, and selective intercostal nerve block. *Am J Vet Res* 1986; **47**(2): 471–474.

171 Cicirelli V, Debidda P, Maggio N, *et al.* Use of spinal anaesthesia with anaesthetic block of intercostal nerves compared to a continuous infusion of sufentanyl [sic] to improve analgesia in cats undergoing unilateral mastectomy. *Animals (Basel)* 2021; **11**(3): 887.

172 Zublena F, Briganti A, De Gennaro C, *et al.* Ultrasound-guided parasternal injection in dogs: a cadaver study. *Vet Anaesth Analg* 2021; **48**(4): 563–569.

173 Escalante GE, Ferreira TH, Hershberger-Braker KL, *et al.* Evaluation of ultrasound-guided pecto-intercostal block in canine cadavers. *Vet Anaesth Analg* 2022; **49**(2): 182–188.

174 Stobie D, Caywood DD, Rozanski EA, *et al.* Evaluation of pulmonary function and analgesia in dogs after intercostal thoracotomy and use of morphine administered intramuscularly or intrapleurally and bupivacaine administered intrapleurally. *Am J Vet Res* 1995; **56**(8): 1098–1109.

175 Riegler FX, VadeBoncouer TR, Pelligrino DA. Interpleural anesthetics in the dog: differential somatic neural blockade. *Anesthesiology* 1989; **71**(5): 744–750.

176 Dravid RM, Paul RE. Interpleural block – part 1. *Anaesthesia* 2007; **62**(10): 1039–1049.

177 Kushner LI, Trim CM, Madhusudhan S, *et al.* Evaluation of the hemodynamic effects of interpleural bupivacaine in dogs. *Vet Surg* 1995; **24**(2): 180–187.

178 Bernard F, Kudnig ST, Monnet E. Hemodynamic effects of interpleural lidocaine and bupivacaine combination in anesthetized dogs with and without an open pericardium. *Vet Surg* 2006; **35**(3): 252–258.

179 Kowalski SE, Bradley BD, Greengrass RA, *et al.* Effects of interpleural bupivacaine (0.5%) on canine diaphragmatic function. *Anesth Analg* 1992; **75**(3): 400–404.

180 Blanco R, Parras T, McDonnell JG, *et al.* Serratus plane block: a novel ultrasound-guided thoracic wall nerve block. *Anaesthesia* 2013; **68**(11): 1107–1113.

181 Freitag FA, Gaio TS, Dos Santos AA, *et al.* Ultrasound-guided superficial serratus plane block in dog cadavers: an anatomical evaluation and volume dispersion study. *Vet Anaesth Analg* 2020; **47**(1): 88–94.

182 Teixeira LG, Pujol DM, Pazzim AF, *et al.* Combination of Transversus abdominis plane block and Serratus plane block anesthesia in dogs submitted to masctetomy. *Pesquisa Veterinária Brasileira* 2018; **38**(2): 315–319.

183 Asorey I, Sambugaro B, Bhalla RJ, *et al.* Ultrasound-guided serratus plane block as an effective adjunct to systemic analgesia in four dogs undergoing thoracotomy. *Open Vet J* 2021; **10**(4): 407–411.

184 Bosak VL, Piontkovsky RJ, Mazur Dos Santos A, *et al.* Ultrasound-guided superficial serratus plane block in multimodal analgesia for three dogs undergoing surgical correction of persistent ductus arteriosus. *Vet Anaesth Analg* 2022; **49**(3): 330–332.

185 Garbin M, Portela DA, Bertolizio G, *et al.* Description of ultrasound-guided quadratus lumborum block technique and evaluation of injectate spread in canine cadavers. *Vet Anaesth Analg* 2020; **47**(2): 249–258.

186 Garbin M, Portela DA, Bertolizio G, *et al.* A novel ultrasound-guided lateral quadratus lumborum block in dogs: a comparative cadaveric study of two approaches. *Vet Anaesth Analg* 2020; **47**(6): 810–818.

187 Viscasillas J, Terrado J, Marti-Schaffhausen R, *et al.* A modified approach for the ultrasound-guided quadratus lumborum block in dogs: a cadaveric study. *Animals (Basel)* 2021; **11**(10): 2945.

188 Marchina-Goncalves A, Gil F, Laredo FG, *et al.* Evaluation of high-volume injections using a modified dorsal quadratus lumborum block approach in canine cadavers. *Animals (Basel)* 2021; **12**(1): 18.

189 Dos-Santos JD, Ginja M, Alves-Pimenta S, *et al.* A description of an ultrasound-guided technique for a quadratus lumborum block in the cat: a cadaver study. *Vet Anaesth Analg* 2021; **48**(5): 804–808.

190 Dos-Santos JD, Ginja M, Alves-Pimenta S, *et al.* Comparison of dorsoventral and ventrodorsal approaches for ultrasound-guided quadratus lumborum block in cats: a cadaver study. *Vet Anaesth Analg* 2022; **49**(5): 481–489.

191 Argus APV, Freitag FAV, Bassetto JE, *et al.* Quadratus lumbar block for intraoperative and postoperative analgesia in a cat. *Vet Anaesth Analg* 2020; **47**(3): 415–417.

192 Castaneda-Herrera FE, Buritica-Gaviria EF, Echeverry-Bonilla DF. Anatomical evaluation of the thoracolumbar nerves related to the transversus abdominis plane block technique in the dog. *Anat Histol Embryol* 2017; **46**(4): 373–377.

193 Schroeder CA, Snyder LB, Tearney CC, *et al.* Ultrasound-guided transversus abdominis plane block in the dog: an anatomical evaluation. *Vet Anaesth Analg* 2011; **38**(3): 267–271.

194 Bruggink SM, Schroeder KM, Baker-Herman TL, *et al.* Weight-based volume of injection influences cranial to caudal spread of local anesthetic solution in ultrasound-guided transversus abdominis plane blocks in canine cadavers. *Vet Surg* 2012; **41**(4): 455–457.

195 Zoff A, Laborda-Vidal P, Mortier J, *et al.* Comparison of the spread of two different volumes of contrast medium when performing ultrasound-guided transversus abdominis plane injection in dog cadavers. *J Small Anim Pract* 2017; **58**(5): 269–275.

196 Drozdzynska M, Monticelli P, Neilson D, *et al.* Ultrasound-guided subcostal oblique transversus abdominis plane block in canine cadavers. *Vet Anaesth Analg* 2017; **44**(1): 183–186.

197 Freitag FAV, Muehlbauer E, Gaio TD, *et al.* Evaluation of injection volumes for the transversus abdominis plane block in dog cadavers: a preliminary trial. *Vet Anaesth Analg* 2021; **48**(1): 142–146.

198 de Miguel Garcia C, Whyte M, St James M, *et al.* Effect of contrast and local anesthetic on dye spread following transversus abdominis plane injection in dog cadavers. *Vet Anaesth Analg* 2020; **47**(3): 391–395.

199 Romano M, Portela DA, Thomson A, *et al.* Comparison between two approaches for the transversus abdominis plane block in canine cadavers. *Vet Anaesth Analg* 2021; **48**(1): 101–106.

200 Schroeder CA, Schroeder KM, Johnson RA. Transversus abdominis plane block for exploratory laparotomy in a Canadian lynx (*Lynx canadensis*). *J Zoo Wildl Med* 2010; **41**(2): 338–341.

201 Portela DA, Romano M, Briganti A. Retrospective clinical evaluation of ultrasound-guided transverse abdominis plane block in dogs undergoing mastectomy. *Vet Anaesth Analg* 2014; **41**(3): 319–324.

202 Campoy L, Martin-Flores M, Boesch JM, *et al.* Transverse abdominis plane injection of bupivacaine with dexmedetomidine or a bupivacaine liposomal suspension yielded lower pain scores and requirement for rescue analgesia in a controlled, randomized trial in dogs undergoing elective ovariohysterectomy. *Am J Vet Res* 2022; **83**(9): ajvr.22.03.0037.

203 Harfoush M, Wilson D, Kim SY, Claude A. Open approach to the ventral transversus abdominis plane in the dog: evaluation and injectate dispersion in cadavers. *Vet Anaesth Analg* 2021; **48**(5): 767–774.

204 Forsythe WB, Ghoshal NG. Innervation of the canine thoracolumbar vertebral column. *Anat Rec* 1984; **208**(1): 57–63.

205 Otero PE, Fuensalida SE, Russo PC, *et al.* Mechanism of action of the erector spinae plane block: distribution of dye in a porcine model. *Reg Anesth Pain Med* 2020; **45**(3): 198–203.

206 Ferreira TH, St James M, Schroeder CA, *et al.* Description of an ultrasound-guided erector spinae plane block and the spread of dye in dog cadavers. *Vet Anaesth Analg* 2019; **46**(4): 516–22.

207 Portela DA, Castro D, Romano M, *et al.* Ultrasound-guided erector spinae plane block in canine cadavers: relevant anatomy and injectate distribution. *Vet Anaesth Analg* 2020; **47**(2): 229–237.

208 Medina-Serra R, Foster A, Plested M, *et al.* Lumbar erector spinae plane block: an anatomical and dye distribution evaluation of two ultrasound-guided approaches in canine cadavers. *Vet Anaesth Analg* 2021; **48**(1): 125–133.

209 Cavalcanti M, Teixeira JG, Medina-Serra R, *et al.* Erector spinae plane block at the thoracolumbar spine: a canine cadaveric study. *Vet Anaesth Analg* 2022; **49**(6): 656–663.

210 Sambugaro B, Campbell N, Drozdzynska MJ. Two cases of sinus arrest following erector spinae plane block in dogs. *Vet Anaesth Analg* 2022; **49**(5): 510–511.

211 Portela DA, Romano M, Zamora GA, *et al.* The effect of erector spinae plane block on perioperative analgesic consumption and complications in dogs undergoing hemilaminectomy surgery: a retrospective cohort study. *Vet Anaesth Analg* 2021; **48**(1): 116–124.

212 Zannin D, Isaka LJ, Pereira RH, *et al.* Opioid-free total intravenous anesthesia with bilateral ultrasound-guided erector spinae plane block for perioperative pain control in a dog undergoing dorsal hemilaminectomy. *Vet Anaesth Analg* 2020; **47**(5): 728–731.

213 Bartholomew KJ, Ferreira TH. Ultrasound-guided erector spinae plane block as part of a multimodal analgesic approach in a dog with acute pancreatitis. *Vet Anaesth Analg* 2021; **48**(4): 629–632.

214 Ferre BMI, Drozdzynska M, Vettorato E. Ultrasound-guided bilateral erector spinae plane block in dogs undergoing sternotomies anaesthetised with propofol-dexmedetomidine continuous infusion. *Vet Res Commun* 2022; **46**(4): 1331–1337.

215 Allam MW, Lee DG, Nulsen FE, *et al.* The anatomy of the brachial plexus of the dog. *Anat Rec* 1952; **114**(2): 173–179.

216 Skelding A, Valverde A, Sinclair M, *et al.* Anatomical characterization of the brachial plexus in dog cadavers and comparison of three blind techniques for blockade. *Vet Anaesth Analg* 2018; **45**(2): 203–211.

217 Hofmeister EH, Kent M, Read MR. Paravertebral block for forelimb anesthesia in the dog-an anatomic study. *Vet Anaesth Analg* 2007; **34**(2): 139–142.

218 Podsiedlik M, Hofmeister EH, Duke-Novakovski T. Comparison of 2 blind approaches to the paravertebral brachial plexus regional block in canine cadavers. *Can J Vet Res* 2022; **86**(1): 20–26.

219 Lemke KA, Creighton CM. Paravertebral blockade of the brachial plexus in dogs. *Vet Clin North Am Small Anim Pract* 2008; **38**(6): 1231–1241.

220 Guilherme S, Benigni L. Ultrasonographic anatomy of the brachial plexus and major nerves of the canine thoracic limb. *Vet Radiol Ultrasound* 2008; **49**(6): 577–583.

221 Bagshaw HS, Larenza MP, Seiler GS. A technique for ultrasound-guided paravertebral brachial plexus injections in dogs. *Vet Radiol Ultrasound* 2009; **50**(6): 649–654.

222 Rioja E, Sinclair M, Chalmers H, *et al.* Comparison of three techniques for paravertebral brachial plexus blockade in dogs. *Vet Anaesth Analg* 2012; **39**(2): 190–200.

223 Choquette A, Del Castillo JRE, Moreau M, *et al.* Comparison of lidocaine and lidocaine-epinephrine for the paravertebral brachial plexus block in dogs. *Vet Anaesth Analg* 2017; **44**(2): 317–328.

224 Monticelli P, Fitzgerald E, Viscasillas J. A sonographic investigation for the development of ultrasound-guided paravertebral brachial plexus block in dogs: cadaveric study. *Vet Anaesth Analg* 2018; **45**(2): 195–202.

225 Benigni L, Lafuente P, Viscasillas J. Clinical comparison of two techniques of brachial plexus block for forelimb surgery in dogs. *Vet J* 2019; **244**: 23–27.

226 Evangelista MC, Monteiro BP, Doodnaught GM, *et al.* Paravertebral brachial plexus blockade in cats: a cadaver study. *J Feline Med Surg* 2018; **20**(6): 591–595.

227 Portela DA, Romano M, Otero PE. Locoregional anesthesia of the thoracic limbs and thorax in small animals. *Vet Clin North Am Small Anim Pract* 2019; **49**(6): 1063–1083.

228 Chohan A. Anesthesia case of the month. *J Am Vet Med Assoc* 2019; **255**(9): 1016–1018.

229 Tufvesson G. Anestesi av plexus brachialis. *Nord Vet Med* 1951; **3**: 183–193.

229 Nutt P. Brachial plexus analgesia in dog. *Vet Rec* 1962; **74**: 874–876.

230 Futema F, Fantoni DT, Auler JO Jr., *et al.* A new brachial plexus block technique in dogs. *Vet Anaesth Analg* 2002; **29**(3): 133–139.

231 Wenger S, Moens Y, Jaggin N, *et al.* Evaluation of the analgesic effect of lidocaine and bupivacaine used to provide a brachial plexus block for forelimb surgery in 10 dogs. *Vet Rec* 2005; **156**(20): 639–642.

232 Mahler SP, Adogwa AO. Anatomical and experimental studies of brachial plexus, sciatic, and femoral nerve-location using peripheral nerve stimulation in the dog. *Vet Anaesth Analg* 2008; **35**(1): 80–89.

233 Campoy L, Martin-Flores M, Looney AL, *et al.* Distribution of a lidocaine-methylene blue solution staining in brachial plexus, lumbar plexus and sciatic nerve blocks in the dog. *Vet Anaesth Analg* 2008; **35**(4): 348–354.

234 Sakonju I, Maeda K, Maekawa R, *et al.* Relative nerve blocking properties of bupivacaine and ropivacaine in dogs undergoing brachial plexus block using a nerve stimulator. *J Vet Med Sci* 2009; **71**(10): 1279–1284.

235 Campoy L, Bezuidenhout AJ, Gleed RD, *et al.* Ultrasound-guided approach for axillary brachial plexus, femoral nerve, and sciatic nerve blocks in dogs. *Vet Anaesth Analg* 2010; **37**(2): 144–153.

236 da Silva LC, Futema F, Cortopassi SR. Ultrasonographic study of a modified axillary approach to block the major branches of the brachial plexus in dogs. *Vet Anaesth Analg* 2020; **47**(1): 82–87.

237 Anson A, Laredo FG, Gil F, *et al.* Comparison of two techniques for ultrasound-guided axillary brachial plexus blockade in cats. *J Feline Med Surg* 2015; **17**(6): 476–485.

238 Skelding A, Valverde A, Aguilera R, *et al.* Comparison of 3 blind brachial plexus block techniques during maintenance of anesthesia and postoperative pain scores in dogs undergoing surgical procedures of the thoracic limb. *Can J Vet Res* 2019; **83**(3): 197–205.

239 Akasaka M, Shimizu M. Comparison of ultrasound- and electrostimulation-guided nerve blocks of brachial plexus in dogs. *Vet Anaesth Analg* 2017; **44**(3): 625–635.

240 Adami C, Studer N. A case of severe ventricular arrhythmias occurring as a complication of nerve-stimulator guided brachial plexus location. *Vet Anaesth Analg* 2015; **42**(2): 230–231.

241 Bhalla RJ, Leece EA. Pneumothorax following nerve stimulator-guided axillary brachial plexus block in a dog. *Vet Anaesth Analg* 2015; **42**(6): 658–659.

242 Moens NM, Caulkett NA. The use of a catheter to provide brachial plexus block in dogs. *Can Vet J* 2000; **41**(9): 685–689.

243 Tayari H, Otero P, Rossetti A, *et al.* Proximal RUMM block in dogs: preliminary results of cadaveric and clinical studies. *Vet Anaesth Analg* 2019; **46**(3): 384–394.

244 Otero PE, Fuensalida SE, Sanchez F, *et al.* Development of a lateral ultrasound-guided approach for the proximal radial, ulnar, median and musculocutaneous (RUMM) nerve block in cats. *Vet Anaesth Analg* 2020; **47**(5): 686–693.

245 Trumpatori BJ, Carter JE, Hash J, *et al.* Evaluation of a midhumeral block of the radial, ulnar, musculocutaneous and median (RUMM block) nerves for analgesia of the distal aspect of the thoracic limb in dogs. *Vet Surg* 2010; **39**(7): 785–796.

246 Bortolami E, Love EJ, Harcourt-Brown TR, *et al.* Use of mid-humeral block of the radial, ulnar, musculocutaneous and median (RUMM block) nerves for extensor carpi radialis muscle biopsy in a conscious dog with generalized neuro-muscular disease. *Vet Anaesth Analg* 2012; **39**(4): 446–447.

247 Portela DA, Raschi A, Otero PE. Ultrasound-guided mid-humeral block of the radial, ulnar, median and musculocutaneous (RUMM block) nerves in a dog with traumatic exposed metacarpal luxation. *Vet Anaesth Analg* 2013; **40**(5): 552–554.

248 Castineiras D, Viscasillas J, Seymour C. A modified approach for performing ultrasound-guided radial, ulnar, median and musculocutaneous nerve block in a dog. *Vet Anaesth Analg* 2015; **42**(6): 659–661.

249 Leung JBY, Rodrigo-Mocholi D, Martinez-Taboada F. In-plane and out-of-plane needle insertion comparison for a novel lateral block of the radial, ulnar, median and musculocutaneous nerves in cats. *Vet Anaesth Analg* 2019; **46**(4): 523–528.

250 Enomoto M, Lascelles BD, Gerard MP. Defining the local nerve blocks for feline distal thoracic limb surgery: a cadaveric study. *J Feline Med Surg* 2016; **18**(10): 838–845.

251 Douglas H, Welsh S, Barr C. Clinical techniques in veterinary dermatology: regional anaesthesia of the canine and feline distal limb. *Vet Dermatol* 2021; **32**(1): 90–e17.

252 Grubb T, Lobprise H. Local and regional anaesthesia in dogs and cats: descriptions of specific local and regional techniques (Part 2). *Vet Med Sci* 2020; **6**(2): 218–234.

253 Otero PE, Fuensalida SE, Verdier N, *et al.* Peripheral nerve blocks of the thoracic limb. In: Otero P, Portela DA, eds. *Manual of Small Animal Regional Anesthesia, Illustrated Anatomy for Nerve Stimulation and Ultrasound-Guided Nerve Blocks*, 2nd edn. Cuidad Autonoma de Buenos Aires, Argentina: Editorial Inter-Médica, 2019

254 Ferrero C, Borland K, Rioja E. Retrospective comparison of three locoregional techniques for pelvic limb surgery in dogs. *Vet Anaesth Analg* 2021; **48**(4): 554-562.

255 Campoy L, Martin-Flores M, Ludders JW, *et al.* Comparison of bupivacaine femoral and sciatic nerve block versus bupivacaine and morphine epidural for stifle surgery in dogs. *Vet Anaesth Analg* 2012; **39**(1): 91–98.

256 Portela DA, Verdier N, Otero PE. Regional anesthetic techniques for the pelvic limb and abdominal wall in small animals: a review of the literature and technique description. *Vet J* 2018; **238**: 27–40.

257 Cathasaigh MO, Read MR, Atilla A, *et al.* Blood concentration of bupivacaine and duration of sensory and motor block following ultrasound-guided femoral and sciatic nerve blocks in dogs. *PLoS ONE* 2018; **13**(3): e0193400.

258 Trein TA, Floriano BP, Wagatsuma JT, *et al.* Effects of dexmedetomidine combined with ropivacaine on sciatic and femoral nerve blockade in dogs. *Vet Anaesth Analg* 2017; **44**(1): 144–153.

259 Evangelista MC, Doodnaught GM, Fantoni DT, *et al.* Sciatic and femoral nerve blockade using bupivacaine alone, or in combination with dexmedetomidine or buprenorphine in cats. *Vet Rec* 2017; **180**(24): 592.

260 Portela DA, Otero PE, Briganti A, *et al.* Femoral nerve block: a novel psoas compartment lateral pre-iliac approach in dogs. *Vet Anaesth Analg* 2013; **40**(2): 194–204.

261 Portela DA, Otero PE, Tarragona L, *et al.* Combined paravertebral plexus block and parasacral sciatic block in healthy dogs. *Vet Anaesth Analg* 2010; **37**(6): 531–541.

262 Vettorato E, De Gennaro C, Okushima S, *et al.* Retrospective comparison of two peripheral lumbosacral plexus blocks in dogs undergoing pelvic limb orthopaedic surgery. *J Small Anim Pract* 2013; **54**(12): 630–637.

263 Vettorato E, Corletto F. Retrospective assessment of peripheral nerve block techniques used in cats undergoing hindlimb orthopaedic surgery. *J Feline Med Surg* 2016; **18**(10): 826–833.

264 Mahler SP. Ultrasound guidance to approach the femoral nerve in the iliopsoas muscle: a preliminary study in the dog. *Vet Anaesth Analg* 2012; **39**(5): 550–554.

265 Warrit K, Griffenhagen G, Goh C, *et al.* Comparison of ultrasound-guided lumbar plexus and sciatic nerve blocks with ropivacaine and sham blocks with saline on perianesthetic analgesia and recovery in dogs undergoing tibial plateau leveling osteotomy surgery. *Vet Anaesth Analg* 2019; **46**(5): 673–681.

266 O'Connor BL, Woodbury P. The primary articular nerves to the dog knee. *J Anat* 1982; **134**(Pt 3): 563–572.

267 Bartel AK, Campoy L, Martin-Flores M, *et al.* Comparison of bupivacaine and dexmedetomidine femoral and sciatic nerve blocks with bupivacaine and buprenorphine epidural injection for stifle arthroplasty in dogs. *Vet Anaesth Analg* 2016; **43**(4): 435–443.

268 Campoy L, Martin-Flores M, Gleed RD, *et al.* Block duration is substantially longer with a liposomal suspension of bupivacaine than with 0.5% bupivacaine HCl potentiated with dexmedetomidine following an ultrasound-guided sciatic nerve block in Beagles. *Am J Vet Res* 2022; **83**(8): ajvr.22.01.0007.

269 Day TK, Pepper WT, Tobias TA, *et al.* Comparison of intra-articular and epidural morphine for analgesia following stifle arthrotomy in dogs. *Vet Surg* 1995; **24**(6): 522–530.

270 Gingold BM, Milloway MC, Morgan MJ. A novel motor-sparing locoregional nerve block technique for stifle surgery in dogs. *Vet Anaesth Analg* 2020; **47**(5): 731–732.

271 Saunders WB, Hulse DA, Schulz KS. Evaluation of portal locations and periarticular structures in canine coxofemoral arthroscopy: a cadaver study. *Vet Comp Orthop Traumatol* 2004; **17**(04): 184–188.

272 Hotvedt R, Platou ES, Refsum H. Effects of thoracic epidural analgesia on cardiovascular function and plasma concentration of free fatty acids and catecholamines in the dog. *Acta Anaesthesiol Scand* 1984; **28**(2): 132–137.

273 Valverde A. Epidural analgesia and anesthesia in dogs and cats. *Vet Clin North Am Small Anim Pract* 2008; **38**(6): 1205–1230.

274 Zhang D, Nishimura R, Nagahama S, *et al.* Comparison of feasibility and safety of epidural catheterization between cranial and caudal lumbar vertebral segments in dogs. *J Vet Med Sci* 2011; **73**(12): 1573–1577.

275 Maierl J, Reindl S, Knospe C. Observations on epidural anesthesia in cats from the anatomical viewpoint. *Tierarztl Prax* 1997; **25**(3): 267–270.

276 O'Hearn AK, Wright BD. Coccygeal epidural with local anesthetic for catheterization and pain management in the treatment of feline urethral obstruction. *J Vet Emerg Crit Care (San Antonio)* 2011; **21**(1): 50–52.

277 Vesovski S, Makara M, Martinez-Taboada F. Computer tomographic comparison of cranial spread of contrast in lumbosacral and sacrococcygeal epidural injections in dog cadavers. *Vet Anaesth Analg* 2019; **46**(4): 510–515.

278 Liu SS, Bernards CM. Exploring the epidural trail. *Reg Anesth Pain Med* 2002; **27**(2): 122–124.

279 Lee I, Yamagishi N, Oboshi K, *et al.* Distribution of new methylene blue injected into the lumbosacral epidural space in cats. *Vet Anaesth Analg* 2004; **31**(3): 190–194.

280 Gorgi AA, Hofmeister EH, Higginbotham MJ, *et al.* Effect of body position on cranial migration of epidurally injected methylene blue in recumbent dogs. *Am J Vet Res* 2006; **67**(2): 219–221.

281 Freire CD, Torres ML, Fantoni DT, *et al.* Bupivacaine 0.25% and methylene blue spread with epidural anesthesia in dog. *Vet Anaesth Analg* 2010; **37**(1): 63–69.

282 Nakayama M, Yamamoto J, Ichinose H, *et al.* Effects of volume and concentration of lidocaine on epidural anaesthesia in pregnant females. *Eur J Anaesthesiol* 2002; **19**(11): 808–811.

283 Duggan J, Bowler GM, McClure JH, *et al.* Extradural block with bupivacaine: influence of dose, volume, concentration and patient characteristics. *Br J Anaesth* 1988; **61**(3): 324–331.

284 Otero PE, Tarragona L, Ceballos M, *et al.* Epidural cephalic spread of a local anaesthetic in dogs: a mathematical model using the column length [Abstract]. *Vet Anaesth Analg* 2010; **37**(3): P1–P88.

285 Otero PE, Tarragona L, Waxman Dova S. Effects of epidurally administered ropivacaine at three different concentrations in dogs [Abstract]. *Vet Anaesth Analg* 2006; **34**(4): 69.

286 Almeida TF, Fantoni DT, Mastrocinque S, *et al.* Epidural anesthesia with bupivacaine, bupivacaine and fentanyl, or bupivacaine and sufentanil during intravenous administration of propofol for ovariohysterectomy in dogs. *J Am Vet Med Assoc* 2007; **230**(1): 45–51.

287 Iff I, Moens Y, Schatzmann U. Use of pressure waves to confirm the correct placement of epidural needles in dogs. *Vet Rec* 2007; **161**(1): 22–25.

288 Naganobu K, Hagio M. The effect of body position on the 'hanging drop' method for identifying the extradural space in anaesthetized dogs. *Vet Anaesth Analg* 2007; **34**(1): 59–62.

289 Iseri T, Nishimura R, Nagahama S, *et al.* Epidural spread of iohexol following the use of air or saline in the 'loss of resistance' test. *Vet Anaesth Analg* 2010; **37**(6): 526–530.

290 Baraka A. Identification of the peridural space by a running infusion drip. *Br J Anaesth* 1972; **44**(1): 122.

291 Martinez-Taboada F, Redondo JI. Comparison of the hanging drop technique and running-drip method for identifying the epidural space in dogs. *Vet Anaesth Analg* 2017; **44**(2): 329–336.

292 Tsui BC, Gupta S, Finucane B. Detection of subarachnoid and intravascular epidural catheter placement. *Can J Anaesth* 1999; **46**(7): 675–678.

293 Tsui BCH, Wagner A, Cave D, *et al.* Threshold current for an insulated epidural needle in pediatric patients. *Anesth Analg* 2004; **99**(3): 694–696.

294 Garcia-Pereira FL, Hauptman J, Shih AC, *et al.* Evaluation of electric neurostimulation to confirm correct placement of lumbosacral epidural injections in dogs. *Am J Vet Res* 2010; **71**(2): 157–160.

295 Read MR. Confirmation of epidural needle placement using nerve stimulation in dogs. *Vet Anaesth Analg* 2005; **32**(4): 13.

296 Gregori T, Viscasillas J, Benigni L. Ultrasonographic anatomy of the sacrococcygeal region and ultrasound-guided epidural injection at the sacrococcygeal space in dogs. *Vet Rec* 2014; **175**(3): 68.

297 Credie L, Luna S. The use of ultrasound to evaluate sacrococcygeal epidural injections in cats. *Can Vet J* 2018; **59**(2): 143–146.

298 Otero PE, Verdier N, Zaccagnini AS, *et al.* Sonographic evaluation of epidural and intrathecal injections in cats. *Vet Anaesth Analg* 2016; **43**(6): 652–661.

299 Castro D, Portela DA, Otero PE. Positive color flow Doppler test used to confirm sacrococcygeal epidural injection in a dog. *Vet Anaesth Analg* 2020; **47**(2): 280–281.

300 Sarotti D, Rabozzi R, Franci P. Comparison of epidural versus intrathecal anaesthesia in dogs undergoing pelvic limb orthopaedic surgery. *Vet Anaesth Analg* 2015; **42**(4): 405–413.

301 Di Cianni S, Rossi M, Casati A, *et al.* Spinal anesthesia: an evergreen technique. *Acta Biomed* 2008; **79**(1): 9–17.

302 Auroy Y, Narchi P, Messiah A, *et al.* Serious complications related to regional anesthesia: results of a prospective survey in France. *Anesthesiology* 1997; **87**(3): 479–486.

303 Sarotti D, Rabozzi R, Corletto F. Efficacy and side effects of intraoperative analgesia with intrathecal bupivacaine and levobupivacaine: a retrospective study in 82 dogs. *Vet Anaesth Analg* 2011; **38**(3): 240–251.

304 Sarotti D, Cattai A, Franci P. Combined spinal and general anaesthesia in 58 cats undergoing various surgical procedures: description of technique and retrospective perioperative evaluation. *J Feline Med Surg* 2019; **21**(12): 1127–1133.

305 Vettorato E, Bradbrook C, Gurney M, *et al.* Peripheral nerve blocks of the pelvic limb in dogs: a retrospective clinical study. *Vet Comp Orthop Traumatol* 2012; **25**(4): 314–320.

306 Kalchofner Guerrero KS, Guerrero TG, Schweizer-Kolliker M, *et al.* Incidence of delayed hair re-growth, pruritus, and urinary retention after epidural anaesthesia in dogs. *Tierarztl Prax Ausg K Kleintiere Heimtiere* 2014; **42**(2): 94–100.

307 Neal JM, Bernards CM, Butterworth JFT, *et al.* ASRA practice advisory on local anesthetic systemic toxicity. *Reg Anesth Pain Med* 2010; **35**(2): 152–161.

308 Sala-Blanch X, Ribalta T, Rivas E, *et al.* Structural injury to the human sciatic nerve after intraneural needle insertion. *Reg Anesth Pain Med* 2009; **34**(3): 201–205.

309 Sala-Blanch X, Lopez AM, Pomes J, *et al.* No clinical or electrophysiologic evidence of nerve injury after intraneural injection during sciatic popliteal block. *Anesthesiology* 2011; **115**(3): 589–595.

310 Neal JM, Kopp SL, Pasternak JJ, *et al.* Anatomy and pathophysiology of spinal cord injury associated with regional anesthesia and pain medicine: 2015 update. *Reg Anesth Pain Med* 2015; **40**(5): 506–525.

311 Boselli E, Hopkins P, Lamperti M, *et al.* European Society of Anaesthesiology and Intensive Care guidelines on peri-operative use of ultrasound for regional anaesthesia (PERSEUS regional anesthesia): peripheral nerves blocks and neuraxial anaesthesia. *Eur J Anaesthesiol* 2021; **38**(3): 219–250.

312 Portela DA, Otero PE, Biondi M, *et al.* Peripheral nerve stimulation under ultrasonographic control to determine the needle-to-nerve relationship. *Vet Anaesth Analg* 2013; **40**(6): e91–e99.

61 Horses

Regula Bettschart-Wolfensberger
Department of Diagnostics and Clinical Sciences, Vetsuisse Faculty, University of Zürich, Zürich, Switzerland

Chapter contents

Introduction, 1205
Preanesthetic considerations, 1205
Standing sedation, 1206
Preanesthetic sedation, 1206
Induction of anesthesia, 1206
Maintenance of general anesthesia, 1208
  α_2-Adrenergic receptor agonists, 1208
  Lidocaine, 1209
  Ketamine, 1209
  Opioids, 1209
  Muscle relaxants – benzodiazepines and guaifenesin, 1209
Field anesthesia, 1210
Monitoring, 1210
Adequate cardiovascular function and tissue oxygenation, 1210
Anesthesia recovery, 1211
  Environmental considerations, 1211
  Timing of recovery, 1212
  Additional sedation and analgesia, 1212
  Recovery assist systems, 1213
References, 1214

Introduction

General anesthesia in horses is challenging. Nevertheless, a recent multicenter [1] and some single-center surveys [2–4] indicate that general-anesthesia-related mortality has decreased compared to studies performed 20 years ago [5]. To avoid the risks of general anesthesia, there is a growing tendency to perform as many surgical interventions as possible in standing sedated horses [6]. Sedative techniques, along with better local anesthetic techniques, have been developed for this purpose. The risks of standing surgeries, however, remain to be determined and compared to those of general anesthesia [1,7]. There are still many unstudied and unanswered questions about how to best perform equine anesthesia for an optimal outcome. This chapter aims to provide an overview of peculiarities associated with horses and a focus on the management of anesthesia and solutions for common problems.

Preanesthetic considerations

Guidelines on how adult horses should be prepared prior to anesthesia, including transport, fasting, and behavioral considerations, have varied, and little evidence-based guidance addressing these concerns is available. Horses that were transported the morning before surgery showed higher cortisol levels than horses that were kept in the clinic the night before [8], so stress might be reduced if preoperative transport of the animal is avoided.

In adult horses, the patient's nutritional status before elective general anesthesia may influence intraoperative oxygenation and potentially impact the risk of postoperative colic. Postoperative colic is a significant problem [9,10], but the literature is mostly retrospective, and reported effects are confounded by the many factors involved. In horses where mainly dissociative-based anesthesia induction protocols (e.g., ketamine) are used, unlike in other species, regurgitation and aspiration of gastric contents is uncommon as long as the horse is not suffering from colic. Since horses typically browse for their food, prolonged fasting can cause stress in individual horses, which will negatively influence motility of the gastrointestinal tract [11] or potentiate ulceration [12]. A negative energy balance might impair normal metabolism and derange oxygen–glucose physiology during the perioperative period, although that is usually not a concern for healthy adult horses. In foals up to about 4 weeks of age, however, fasting is best avoided.

Preanesthetic fasting also has potential benefits. Less material in the gastrointestinal (GI) tract places less pressure on the major abdominal vessels and causes less cranial displacement of the diaphragm. This may lessen impairment of venous return to the heart and improve ventilation via an increase in functional residual capacity, likely providing better oxygenation and oxygen delivery to the tissues. Further, ongoing microbial gas production within the GI tract is probably decreased in fasted horses. Since postoperative colic can be a major complication following anesthesia and surgery in horses, reduced gas production can limit ileus. This effect on

Veterinary Anesthesia and Analgesia: The Sixth Edition of Lumb and Jones. Edited by Leigh Lamont, Kurt Grimm, Sheilah Robertson, Lydia Love and Carrie Schroeder.
© 2024 John Wiley & Sons, Inc. Published 2024 by John Wiley & Sons, Inc.
Companion website: www.wiley.com/go/lamont/anesthesia

colic rates has been shown in fasted in comparison with unfasted horses [10]. However, the use of a muzzle to limit oral intake of solid feed has been associated with more postoperative colic than the simple avoidance of preoperative feeding while allowing the horse to consume some of its bedding [13]. Many anesthesiologists are convinced that preoperative overnight fasting for 8–12 h is beneficial for most horses. Easy access to water is important and may be impaired by a muzzle; however, for certain horses, this will necessitate limiting the amount of edible bedding available.

Horses instinctively tend to flee when they are threatened or frightened. Therefore, the periods immediately before losing and after regaining consciousness can be difficult to manage in horses unaccustomed to close human contact, those experiencing injuries, or simply due to the unusual environment. Once a horse is excited or frightened, it can be very difficult to calm it down again. Often, higher sedative doses (with potentially more untoward side effects) will be needed. Therefore, it is important to avoid excitement and reduce pain and stress through proper use of sedative and analgesic drugs before anesthesia induction and during the recovery period.

In addition to the judicious use of sedatives, common principles of physical restraint should be applied to the handling of horses. Some degree of physical restraint is combined with appropriate sedatives to yield a tractable horse. The method of physical restraint will be based on a number of factors, including the size and temperament of the horse, the availability of personnel, and the duration or type of procedure.

Standing sedation

Sedation of horses for physical examination or standing procedures is commonly performed using readily available sedatives and analgesics (Table 61.1). Intravenous (IV) administration of α_2-adrenergic receptor agonists (e.g., xylazine, detomidine, romifidine, medetomidine, or dexmedetomidine) forms the basis of most drug combinations used to achieve moderate or heavy sedation in horses. Their combination with opioid analgesic drugs will lead to more reliable sedation and, therefore, is strongly recommended. Sublingual administration of detomidine (Dormosedan Gel®, Zoetis) may be useful for horses that cannot be given injections. For standing surgeries, use of sedation is combined with administration of both systemic and local analgesics. Epidural injection of local anesthetics in combination with xylazine or detomidine at the first intercoccygeal space is recommended for perineal surgeries. Various combinations of epidural α_2-adrenergic receptor agonists, local anesthetics, and opioids have been proposed for perioperative pain control for surgeries distal to the thoracic region [14].

Preanesthetic sedation

For most cases, it is possible to catheterize a jugular vein using local anesthetic infiltration with or without prior administration of a sedative. Intramuscular (IM) acepromazine (e.g., 0.03–0.05 mg/kg) at least 30 min before placement of an IV catheter may help calm some horses [17]. In uncooperative animals where catheter placement is difficult, acepromazine alone at the above-mentioned dose rates does not usually result in adequate sedation. In those horses, it can be beneficial to sedate them with IM injection of a longer acting α_2-adrenergic receptor agonist (e.g., 0.04 mg/kg romifidine, or 0.01 mg/kg detomidine) and subsequently add an opioid such as butorphanol (0.02 mg/kg). Yearlings, thoroughbreds, and Arabians tend to need higher dosages and, in very difficult horses, doubling the initial dose of the sedative will avoid the repetitive stress of injection and resulting stimulation. Most important is to leave horses given IM sedation (detomidine at least 20 min, and romifidine 30 min) in an undisturbed environment to allow peak effects to develop before handling. If further doses of sedatives are needed to achieve satisfactory calming effects, long-lasting cardiopulmonary effects dominated by reduced cardiac output, peripheral vasoconstriction and reduced tissue perfusion may result [18,19]. This might be detrimental in the case of general anesthesia. Myopathies and neuropathies are a consequence of inadequate tissue blood flow and contribute to the incidence of equine perioperative fatalities [20]. As acepromazine is relatively long acting, cannot be antagonized, and has numerous potential adverse effects, the anesthetist should avoid its use in cases involving pre-existing hypotension, anemia, hypothermia, or moderate to severe liver impairment.

Following catheter placement, unsedated horses are ideally left undisturbed for at least 5–10 min. Stress-free transfer of the horse to the surgical area is facilitated by administering approximately one-third of the total intended IV dose of chosen α_2-adrenergic receptor agonist. (Table 61.1). As soon as some sedation becomes apparent, horses can usually be walked into the anesthesia induction area with minimal resistance.

Once in the induction area, the remainder of the sedative is administered slowly to reach the desired depth of sedation (i.e., the horse becomes unresponsive to surrounding stimuli). In horses that do not become heavily sedated within 5–10 min, depending on the choice of α_2-adrenergic receptor agonist, an additional injection of approximately 25% of the initial dose may be administered, or an opioid may be added, to enhance sedation and analgesia. Generally, reduction of the dose of α_2-adrenergic receptor agonists is reserved only for severely compromised horses that cannot be stabilized before anesthesia induction. In such patients, a higher dose of benzodiazepine during anesthesia induction (up to 0.1 mg/kg instead of 0.02 mg/kg) or the use of guaifenesin may improve muscle relaxation.

Some veterinarians consider sedation before general anesthesia with shorter acting α_2-adrenergic receptor agonists such as xylazine (0.5–1.0 mg/kg), medetomidine (7 μg/kg), or dexmedetomidine (3–5 μg/kg) safer. Their untoward cardiopulmonary effects are shorter lasting than those associated with detomidine or romifidine, and peak intensity of adverse effects is less pronounced [21,22].

Some anesthetists prefer to combine sedatives with opioids. The combination of α_2-adrenergic receptor agonists with an opioid receptor agonist improves quality of sedation [23–25], and better analgesia is provided. In horses, the minimum alveolar concentration (MAC) of inhaled anesthetics is not consistently decreased following opioids [26], but if α_2-adrenergic receptor agonists are used together with opioids, the effect of the α_2-adrenergic receptor agonist on MAC is consistent and more pronounced [27]. Opioids might contribute to respiratory depression caused by general anesthetics [28] and also carry the potential to reduce fecal output and predispose to colic after anesthesia [29]. However, evidence supporting this contention is poor [30], and a more recent study showed that hydromorphone did not increase incidence of postoperative colic [31]. Still, some anesthetists do not routinely administer opioids before anesthesia induction, and intraoperative analgesia is provided by other means.

Induction of anesthesia

For most veterinarians, the preferred anesthetic induction agent in horses is ketamine. Other induction drugs are available and may be used in horses (Table 61.2). When used appropriately, the

Table 61.1 Drugs used for standing chemical restraint, for analgesia, or as preanesthetics in horses.

Drug	Dose and route	Onset of optimal effect	Comments
Sedatives			
Acepromazine	0.02–0.05 mg/kg, IM, IV	30–40 min	Only sedative that causes no ataxia Very long-acting (dose-dependent duration of 2–4 h) Causes sequestration of erythrocytes in spleen, vasodilation, and decreased arterial blood pressure Avoid use in neonates, hypotensive, hypothermic, or stressed horses Ideally combine with α_2-adrenergic receptor agonists
α_2-Adrenergic receptor agonists Cause dose-dependent ataxia, analgesia, peripheral vasoconstriction, and bradycardia (less during CRI) Negative impact on digestion Increased urine output, hyperglycemia			
Detomidine	0.01–0.02 mg/kg, IV	3–5 min	Relatively long-acting sedative, head-down posture
	0.02–0.04 mg/kg, IM	20 min	Start with a low dose, repeat as needed (but not before 20 min) Allow adequate time for onset; can also be given orally
	0.0125–0.0198 mg/kg/h, IV CRI	Use after bolus	Some authors suggest reducing the dose over time
Dexmedetomidine	0.003–0.005 mg/kg, IV	3–5 min	Shortest acting sedative, premedication dose
	0.00175–0.002 mg/kg/h, IV CRI	Use after bolus	Produces excellent analgesia during general anesthesia
Medetomidine	0.005–0.007 mg/kg, IV	3–5 min	Relatively short-acting sedative, premedication dose; marginally longer duration than dexmedetomidine
	0.0035–0.005 mg/kg/h, IV CRI	Use after bolus	Produces excellent analgesia during general anesthesia
Romifidine	0.04–0.1 mg/kg, IV	5–10 min	Relatively long-acting sedative; produces head-down posture
	0.08–0.12 mg/kg, IM	15–25 min	Start with a low dose, repeat as needed (but not before 30 min)
	0.018–0.040 mg/kg/h, IV CRI	Use after bolus	
Xylazine	0.5–1.0 mg/kg, IV	3–5 min	Relatively short-acting sedative, head-down posture
Analgesics			
Opioids Produce potent to very potent analgesia Potential for behavioral side effects if used without sedatives or at excessive dose rates More potent opioids will impair ventilation dose-dependently Negative influence on propulsive gastrointestinal motility			
Butorphanol	0.01–0.03 mg/kg, IV	3–5 min	Analgesic; usually given in combination with a sedative
Buprenorphine	0.005–0.01 mg/kg, IV		Analgesic; sedate with α_2-adrenergic receptor agonist prior to administration
	0.06 mg/kg, SL		Longer acting than other opioids, can be administered SL
Morphine	0.1–0.2 mg/kg, IM, IV	3–5 min	Analgesic; sedate with α_2-adrenergic receptor agonist prior to administration Has potential for excitation, especially in non-painful horses or at higher dose rates
Methadone	0.2–0.5 mg/kg, IM, IV		Similar to morphine
Non-steroidal anti-inflammatories[a] Reduce inflammation and produce analgesia Can cause gastrointestinal ulceration and impair maintenance of renal perfusion (avoid use in dehydrated horses) May impair bone healing			
Phenylbutazone	1.1–4.4 mg/kg, IV, PO	8–12–24 h	Analgesic; extreme perivascular irritant
Flunixin meglumine	1.1 mg/kg, IV, IM, PO 0.25 mg/kg, IV	12–24 h 8 h	Analgesic; local tissue reactions when administered IM; negative effect on mucosal repair
Meloxicam	0.6 mg/kg, IV, PO	24 h	Does not impede mucosal repair; well tolerated by foals
Ketoprofen	2.2 mg/kg, IV	24 h	Less effective for orthopedic pain than phenylbutazone
Firocoxib	0.09 mg/kg, IV	24 h	Well tolerated by foals
	0.1 mg/kg, PO	24 h	Start with a loading dose of 0.3 mg/kg to reach steady state within 1 day

IV, intravenous; IM, intramuscular; PO, oral; CRI, constant rate infusion; SL, sublingual.
[a] [15,16].

Table 61.2 Drugs used for induction and maintenance of anesthesia in sedated horses.

Drug	Dose and route	Comments
Diazepam	0.02–0.06 mg/kg, IV	Used for muscle relaxation; combined with ketamine
Guaifenesin	50 mg/kg, IV to effect	Muscle relaxant, must be used in combination with anesthetics such as ketamine or propofol
Ketamine	2.0–3.0 mg/kg, IV	Requires maximal sedation prior to administration to induce anesthesia
Midazolam	0.02–0.06 mg/kg, IV	Used for muscle relaxation; combined with ketamine
Tiletamine–zolazepam	0.7–1.0 mg/kg, IV	Requires maximal sedation prior to administration to induce anesthesia; may be reconstituted with ketamine and either xylazine or detomidine in various combinations of "TKX" or "TKD" Recovery quality often not ideal
"Triple drip"	1–2 mL/kg/h	Mixture of guaifenesin 5%, ketamine 0.1–0.2%, and xylazine 0.05% Xylazine can be replaced with detomidine (10 mg in 500 mL) Do not use to induce anesthesia in adult horses Used for extending injectable anesthesia induced by xylazine–ketamine

horse will slowly assume sternal and then lateral recumbency. A significant disadvantage of ketamine in comparison with other alternatives (propofol, alfaxalone, and barbiturates) is poor muscle relaxation and hypnosis when used alone. To minimize these undesirable effects, horses should be deeply sedated before anesthetic induction with ketamine. Additionally, the use of centrally acting muscle relaxants significantly enhances the quality of equine anesthesia induction. Guaifenesin (35–50 mg/kg) can be given intravenously to effect (until the horse becomes ataxic and buckles its knees) just prior to the bolus of ketamine (with or without additional muscle relaxants such as the benzodiazepines, diazepam or midazolam). These drugs reduce muscle hypertonus and reflex activity, which facilitates endotracheal intubation. Guaifenesin administration can be cumbersome in adult horses as effective dosages result in the need for relatively large volumes to be administered. Furthermore, it can cause phlebitis even if used at a relatively low concentration of 5% [32]. For this reason, many prefer to use a benzodiazepine for muscle relaxation. An additional advantage of benzodiazepine use is the availability of an antagonist, flumazenil. It has not been extensively studied or routinely used in equine anesthesia because of expense, but in cases of emergency a dose of 0.02 mg/kg IV can reverse the respiratory side effects of benzodiazepines and eventually shorten recovery [33]. A more recent study compared the use of ketamine in combination with propofol (0.5 mg/kg) or midazolam (0.1 mg/kg) for anesthesia induction [34] and found slightly better recoveries with propofol following 1 h of isoflurane anesthesia.

Some anesthetists prefer to keep the dose of the benzodiazepines for co-induction low (0.02 mg/kg), which minimizes the impact on respiration and reduces ataxia during recovery. An IV bolus of ketamine of 2–3 mg/kg in combination with diazepam or midazolam results in recumbency within 1.5–2 min and is associated with relatively deep anesthesia for about 8–15 min. Nevertheless, for surgical manipulations, the use of additional local or systemic analgesia is advised. If the surgical procedure is not successfully performed within this time frame, or if the trachea is intubated and maintenance of anesthesia with an inhalation agent is begun, additional ketamine (1–1.5 mg/kg IV) may be administered. If a short-acting α_2-adrenergic receptor agonist was used for sedation (xylazine, medetomidine, or dexmedetomidine), it should also be readministered at 50% of the initial dose.

Following anesthesia induction with ketamine, some animals will have rapid nystagmus, limb movements, or muscle tremors. Under such circumstances, additional anesthetic drug(s) should be given without delay to prevent emergence from anesthesia during critical periods such as hoisting onto the surgical table. As short-acting barbiturates have the fastest onset of action, many anesthetists prefer thiopental for this purpose when it is available. A dose of 0.5 mg/kg in most horses will relax muscles without causing apnea, and intubation can be easily performed. Other alternatives to barbiturates with good hypnotic properties that have been described for anesthesia in horses are alfaxalone and propofol. Propofol induction of an adult horse requires a large volume of drug that may prove cost prohibitive [35]. Alfaxalone (1 mg/kg IV) has been compared with ketamine or thiopental for induction of anesthesia [36] and showed similar induction and recovery qualities; however, in another study, horses receiving alfaxalone had a higher incidence (5/6 horses) of muscle tremors during induction [37]. Similar to the use of propofol, alfaxalone induction requires administration of a large volume, and, to date, this remains expensive.

Maintenance of general anesthesia

The use of several drugs in combination is called "balanced anesthesia" if their net effects produce unconsciousness, muscle relaxation, amnesia, and antinociception. In modern equine practice, there are multiple combinations that can achieve this balance. The use of inhalant-only anesthesia for maintenance has largely been replaced by the use of inhalation anesthesia in combination with sedatives, analgesics, and muscle relaxants, given either by infusion or by repetitive bolus administration. This type of anesthesia is called "partial intravenous anesthesia" (PIVA). If no inhalation agent is used and only IV drugs are administered, it is called "total intravenous anesthesia" (TIVA).

The aim of PIVA is to provide analgesia and reduce inhalation anesthetic requirements. By modulating antinociception intraoperatively, a balanced anesthesia protocol is expected to reduce postoperative pain while better maintaining cardiopulmonary function compared to inhalation anesthesia alone. While PIVA with lidocaine [38] compared to pure inhalant anesthesia did not result in improved cardiopulmonary function, there is general agreement among practitioners that PIVA is, under most circumstances, superior to the use of inhalation anesthesia alone. Preliminary results of a large multicenter study (CEPEF 4) reported that the use of PIVA has increased from 38% to 62% over the last two decades [1]. For surgeries where the surgical field can be locally or regionally anesthetized, the use of PIVA is not mandatory. However, the use of such techniques is limited in horses compared to other species because regional desensitization of extremities persisting into the recovery phase can result in injuries during the horse's attempts to stand.

For PIVA, lidocaine, ketamine, different α_2-adrenergic receptor agonists, and various opioids (alone or in combination with each other) have been used as adjuncts to inhalation anesthesia [39,40]. Some anesthetists have also advocated additional midazolam or guaifenesin to enhance muscle relaxation, although the impact of muscle relaxants on recovery needs to be considered carefully. The problem with all these polypharmacy combinations is that the pharmacokinetic and pharmacodynamic interactions can be difficult to predict in individual animals [41]. During clinical anesthesia, plasma levels cannot be rapidly measured, so some drugs with a narrow therapeutic window (e.g., lidocaine) might result in toxic levels when standard dose rates are used under certain circumstances [41,42], for example in colics with compromised hepatic blood flow.

The half-life of most drugs will be prolonged with increased infusion time (so-called "context-sensitive half-life"). Also, the pathophysiologic status of the individual horse can influence half-lives of drugs, in particular differences in cardiac output and hepatic blood flow. Metabolites with pharmacological activity, such as norketamine, that are metabolized more slowly than the parent drug [43], can potentially accumulate and influence recovery after longer infusions. If PIVA is used, the anesthetist has to be aware of the pharmacokinetic and pharmacodynamics effects of all the drugs used.

A discussion of some of the drugs that are used for PIVA and important aspects of their use follows. Additional reviews, including dose rates for common drugs, are available [39,40,44].

α_2-Adrenergic receptor agonists

All available α_2-adrenergic receptor agonists have been used successfully for PIVA in horses and cause reliable sedation, good analgesia, and inhalant anesthetic dose reduction. Accumulation will not lead to excitement in recovery but to prolonged sedation, eventually leading to a longer but smoother recovery phase. α_2-Adrenergic receptor agonists are used for sedation prior to induction of anesthesia in almost all horses, and this acts as an effective loading dose, thereby reducing the time required to achieve a target plasma concentration without the need to administer an intraoperative loading dose.

Dexmedetomidine, medetomidine, and xylazine [45,46] are shorter acting than detomidine or romifidine [47], making them better suited for titration of effect during PIVA. Numerous PIVA studies involving α_2-adrenergic receptor agonists have been published. Because dose and study designs varied widely, with only two different protocols compared or only successful use of a single protocol reported [48,49], it remains difficult to determine which α_2-adrenergic receptor agonist is superior. Interestingly, most reports involve dexmedetomidine or medetomidine, both of which are not licensed for horses in Europe or North America.

Anesthesia-associated fatalities in horses are mostly related to recovery from general anesthesia. Studies investigating the effects of anesthesia protocols on recovery are important to consider. PIVA, including medetomidine infusion, has been shown to result in better recovery quality compared with a lidocaine [50] or *S*(+)-ketamine infusion [51] and similar quality, but longer duration recovery, than with xylazine constant rate infusion (CRI) [45,52]. In one study, recovery quality was better with dexmedetomidine CRI compared to medetomidine CRI [46]. No accumulation of medetomidine (3.5 µg/kg/h) or its metabolites has been noted [53], even with CRIs up to 9 h, resulting in recoveries (time to standing) no longer than 1.5 h [54]. Clinical use of a dexmedetomidine CRI (1–2 µg/kg/h) administered at half of the dose of a medetomidine CRI appears to have similar adjunctive anesthetic properties in horses undergoing inhalant anesthesia.

An IV bolus of an α_2-adrenergic receptor agonist causes vasoconstriction, bradycardia, and a decrease in cardiac output – adverse effects that can be undesirable during equine anesthesia. However, during CRI of lower doses of xylazine or medetomidine, these adverse cardiopulmonary effects are minimized [21,55]. In one study involving experimental horses administered dexmedetomidine CRIs, reduced cardiopulmonary function and oxygen delivery were noted compared to isoflurane alone [56]. However, a clinical study was not able to identify any negative effects associated with dexmedetomidine PIVA [57]. In the future, the use of peripherally acting α_2-adrenergic receptor antagonists may reduce vasoconstriction and optimize perfusion of the anesthetized horse [58].

Urine production is increased with administration of α_2-adrenergic receptor agonists; therefore, placement of a urinary catheter during surgeries lasting longer than 30 min is recommended to avoid overdistension of the bladder intraoperatively and to prevent urination during the recovery period. Replacement of fluids lost via increased urine production should be included in the fluid therapy plan.

Different opioids have been used for balanced anesthesia in combination with medetomidine and dexmedetomidine CRIs [41]. Whereas butorphanol (25 µg/kg IV loading dose followed by 25 µg/kg/h CRI) during isoflurane-medetomidine anesthesia failed to show any effect other than prolonged time to swallowing following anesthesia [59], morphine (0.15 mg/kg bolus followed by 0.1 mg/kg/h) in combination with a dexmedetomidine CRI resulted in a 67% decrease in inhalant anesthetic requirements [60].

Lidocaine

Lidocaine is frequently used as part of balanced anesthesia in horses due to its numerous useful effects [39]. Cardiovascular safety seems to be good, as the horse is not particularly prone to adverse cardiovascular effects of low-dose lidocaine [61]. The inhalant anesthetic requirement (MAC) decreases in a dose-dependent fashion [62], and at clinically used dose rates (1.2 mg/kg bolus given over 10 min, followed by 35–60 µg/kg/min) the MAC reduction is about 25–27% [63], with resultant plasma lidocaine levels of around 2000 ng/mL. Since plasma levels of 1850–4530 ng/mL have been associated with visual dysfunction, tremors, or ataxia [61], lidocaine administration should be stopped 30 min before the end of inhalation anesthesia to minimize problems in recovery [64]. Lidocaine clearance is reduced by general anesthesia and some disease processes [41,42], so careful or reduced dosing is advocated in compromised horses.

Ketamine

Ketamine is a dissociative anesthetic and analgesic that is a noncompetitive antagonist at *N*-methyl-D-aspartate (NMDA) receptors and is, therefore, potentially useful as an analgesic in cases of chronic or neuropathic pain [65]. Ketamine can cause sympathetic nervous system stimulation rather than the depression that is seen with most other anesthetic drugs, and its use in patients with cardiovascular compromise is reasonable in many cases. Ketamine in PIVA (0.6–1.0 mg/kg/h) can reduce inhalant requirements by up to 25%. A potential problem during prolonged infusions of ketamine (e.g., longer than 2 h) is the accumulation of active metabolites, including norketamine [43], with considerably longer half-lives than ketamine. Even if ketamine administration is stopped before the inhalation agent is turned off, some residual effects causing excitement during recovery may persist. A reduction in inhalant anesthetic requirement of up to 49% has been achieved when ketamine was combined with lidocaine [66,67], although the influence on recovery following prolonged use (> 2 h) remains to be tested.

Opioids

There is no doubt that µ-opioid receptor agonists are analgesics in horses as in other species, but they do not provide a reliable intraoperative effect [26]. Morphine has been shown to improve recovery [28,68] if the dose used is not too high (0.1 mg/kg IM). Therefore, some clinicians choose to administer morphine before recovery. The sole use of morphine for PIVA does not seem advantageous [69], but if it is combined with dexmedetomidine, a dramatic and probably beneficial reduction in MAC was reported [60]. Also, when shorter acting opioids such as fentanyl were tested for PIVA in clinical cases [70], no MAC-sparing effect was reported. Only an experimental study involving relatively high dose rates of fentanyl reported a consistent MAC-reducing effect [71]; however, another report showed no reliable MAC reduction but a very high incidence of poor recoveries [72]. On the other hand, when remifentanil [73] and fentanyl [74] were combined with medetomidine or dexmedetomidine for PIVA, the outcome was good. More studies are needed before this can be recommended. Intra-articular morphine is safe and causes good and long-lasting pain relief [75] and may also be administered to provide postoperative analgesia following arthroscopic procedures.

Muscle relaxants – benzodiazepines and guaifenesin

Various reports have included benzodiazepines or guaifenesin as adjuncts during equine anesthesia. Benzodiazepines can provide MAC reduction [76], and intraoperative anesthesia is improved by muscle relaxation without a negative impact on cardiovascular function. Midazolam CRI (0.5 mg/kg/h) in combination with ketamine, medetomidine, and sevoflurane has been advocated because of its minimal effects on cardiopulmonary function compared with other protocols [77]. Guaifenesin, ketamine, and medetomidine in combination with sevoflurane have resulted in similar outcomes [78]. However, midazolam or guaifenesin CRIs during inhalation anesthesia may result in severe ataxia and difficult recoveries after prolonged surgeries (e.g., longer than 2 h).

Field anesthesia

Common protocols for providing anesthesia to horses and ponies under field conditions include combinations of ketamine and an α_2-adrenergic receptor agonist [79]. Topping off xylazine–ketamine anesthesia by administering one-quarter to half the induction dose of each is a common practice. Addition of butorphanol (0.02 mg/kg IV) or an IV infusion of guaifenesin may aid in attaining appropriate levels of analgesia or skeletal muscle relaxation, respectively. Guaifenesin should not be given as the sole agent to horses because it provides no analgesic effect and has minimal hypnotic effect. Alternatively, diazepam (0.1 mg/kg IV) and midazolam (0.1 mg/kg IV) have been used to replace guaifenesin when enhanced skeletal muscle relaxation is desired.

The combination of guaifenesin, ketamine, and xylazine (often referred to as "triple drip") has been described when IV maintenance of anesthesia is needed for a longer procedure [80]. Briefly, solutions of 0.1% or 0.2% ketamine, 0.05% xylazine, and 5% guaifenesin are prepared. Alternatively, other α_2-adrenergic receptor agonists may be substituted for xylazine. The mixture is administered to horses already anesthetized with xylazine and ketamine (or a similar protocol using another α_2-adrenergic receptor agonist and ketamine) in order to extend anesthesia following attainment of recumbency. Typical doses of triple drip for field anesthesia are 1–2 mL/kg/h IV. Some anesthetists prefer to administer 50–100 mL of triple drip after every 7–10 min of anesthesia. If the respiration rate increases, it indicates that the anesthetic plane is lightening and a shorter interval between boluses is needed. Deeper or slower respirations indicate that the interval between boluses should be increased. For most horses weighing around 450 kg, approximately 1 h of general anesthesia is provided by 1 L of triple drip. For simple "topping off" of xylazine–ketamine anesthesia, triple drip solution offers a satisfactory alternative. Intubation and availability of supplemental oxygen are prudent during triple drip anesthesia. Respiratory depression and bradycardia may occur during administration; hence, respiration and heart rate should be monitored closely during anesthesia.

Monitoring

Monitoring of anesthesia in horses, distilled to its essence, consists of the collection of data that allows the anesthetist to judge whether the depth of anesthesia (requiring both hypnosis and analgesia) is sufficient and cardiopulmonary function is adequate to meet the oxygen demands of all tissues. To ascertain the level of anesthesia that is ideal for an individual horse can be difficult since the two (anesthetic depth versus cardiopulmonary function) are often competing. Inhalation anesthetics dose-dependently depress cardiopulmonary function, which is why anesthetists attempt to maintain anesthesia at as light a level as possible. However, unstable anesthesia dominated by repetitive movement of the horse followed by hasty drug administration should be avoided. During inhalation-based anesthesia, a sluggish palpebral reflex should usually be present without nystagmus. However, some horses will not retain palpebral reflexes despite being at a light anesthetic level. In spontaneously breathing horses, respiration should be regular and not influenced by surgical stimulation. During TIVA with alfaxalone- or propofol-based protocols, judgment of depth of anesthesia is similar to that for inhalation anesthesia. Ketamine-based anesthesia is influenced by concurrently administered drugs but may be more difficult to assess as ocular reflexes often are stronger (spontaneous blinking), and the presence of nystagmus is not necessarily indicative of insufficient anesthetic depth. Ketamine-anesthetized horses should show no reaction to surgical stimulation and should have a regular breathing pattern, although apneustic breathing may be seen.

Various parameters can be measured for assessment of cardiopulmonary function during anesthesia [81]. Commonly monitored parameters include heart rate, arterial blood pressures, respiratory rate, hemoglobin saturation (measured by pulse oximetry), and end-tidal CO_2. Modern monitoring during equine anesthesia should also include the composition of inspired and expired gases, capnometry, body temperature, and urine production. Capillary refill time, mucous membrane color, heart rate, respiration rate and pattern, as well as pulse quality are useful measures that can be easily assessed under field conditions. In addition, the use of a pulse oximeter, at a minimum, is strongly encouraged in the field. Arterial blood gases, pH, packed cell volume, plasma proteins, lactate, or relevant electrolytes can be measured repeatedly, especially during long or complicated anesthesia. Although these parameters have ranges that are considered clinically acceptable, a single normal value does not necessarily assure that oxygenation of vital tissues is adequate. The measurement of cardiac output, muscle lactate concentration [82], or tissue perfusion [83,84] is not currently routine, but improved technology may improve their clinical utility in the future and may give more insight as to what is happening at the tissue level.

Adequate cardiovascular function and tissue oxygenation

It is well recognized that one of the most important aspects of equine anesthesia is maintenance of adequate cardiovascular function and tissue oxygenation. Optimal positioning of horses on soft padding will evenly distribute the horse's weight and prevent focal areas of hypoperfusion. Care should be taken to avoid positioning that might stretch or compress nerves (such as flexing limbs under tension or extending the neck in dorsal recumbency). Most studies investigating factors affecting the development of postanesthetic myopathy were performed using halothane anesthesia [85,86]. From these studies, it was learned that minimal mean arterial blood pressures of $\geq$ 70 mmHg appear important to maintain perfusion of large muscles during recumbency. Since halothane is not a vasodilator like modern inhalation anesthetics (e.g., isoflurane and sevoflurane), tissue perfusion is likely maintained at slightly lower mean arterial blood pressures with the more modern agents, provided that local compression of tissues does not prevent flow. This is logical since perfusion is also a function of cardiac output and vascular resistance, not arterial blood pressure alone.

Under clinical circumstances, arterial blood pressure is usually the primary cardiovascular parameter measured, even though it does not allow direct assessment of tissue perfusion. This is due to the ease with which relatively accurate data can be gathered and the relationship between arterial blood pressure and tissue blood flow (although many confounders exist). When mean arterial blood pressure is low (< 60 mmHg), interventions are required in any case. However, if the mean arterial pressure is 70 mmHg or greater, it does not necessarily ensure that all tissues are well perfused. Other parameters should be assessed concurrently (e.g., mucous membrane color, heart rate, serum lactate, and fluid status) to determine whether vasoconstriction may be impairing tissue perfusion despite "normal" arterial pressures at or above 70 mmHg.

Impaired cardiopulmonary function will result in decreased peripheral tissue oxygenation. Cardiopulmonary function is usually reduced more as the dose of inhalation agent increases [87]. Therefore, careful titration of inhalation anesthetics is warranted. Despite adequate fluid therapy and a light depth of anesthesia, perfusion may not be adequate, requiring administration of sympathomimetics, especially in critically ill horses [88]. Dobutamine (up to 1.5 μg/kg/min) can increase arterial blood pressures and cardiac output with minimal undesired effects such as tachyarrhythmias. In the case of low systemic vascular resistance (e.g., endotoxemia), ephedrine (0.06 mg/kg), norepinephrine (0.1–0.5 μg/kg/min), and phenylephrine (0.25–2 μg/kg/min) are reasonable options [88]. However, the use of vasoconstrictors without concurrent increases in cardiac output may raise blood pressure but decrease tissue perfusion [84], so careful titration and monitoring are important with their use. Once more advanced cardiovascular monitoring equipment becomes available and practical for clinical use in horses, goal-directed vasopressor and fluid therapy will hopefully help further optimize anesthetic management and outcome [89].

Another important factor for the anesthetist to monitor and manage is ventilation. Two thorough reviews have recently been published [90,91]. Adequate ventilation is crucial to maintain arterial oxygenation and elimination of carbon dioxide. However, indiscriminate use of mechanical ventilation may have detrimental cardiovascular ramifications. During spontaneous ventilation, mean intrapleural pressures are subatmospheric, which facilitates venous return, cardiac output, and oxygen delivery. In contrast, controlled mechanical ventilation using intermittent positive-pressure ventilation, especially using high airway pressures and short expiratory times, can induce the opposite.

Anesthesia of spontaneously ventilating horses often results in relatively high arterial CO_2 partial pressures ($PaCO_2$ > 65 mmHg) [92]. The level of acceptable hypercapnia in horses is debatable and may depend on several factors, including cardiovascular function and acid–base status. One study in mechanically ventilated horses reported beneficial cardiopulmonary stimulation with moderate ($PaCO_2$ ~60 mmHg) and severe ($PaCO_2$ > 80 mmHg) hypercapnia (i.e., permissive hypercapnia) [93]. However, other anesthetists have stated that a $PaCO_2$ above 70 mmHg is unacceptably high in most patients [94]. In a prospective study of elective clinical cases, no difference in cardiopulmonary function (including cardiac output measurements) between spontaneous and controlled ventilation groups could be demonstrated ($PaCO_2$ 50–60 mmHg in both groups) [92]. Yet, others have reported cardiovascular function and muscle perfusion to be clearly worse with controlled ventilation in comparison with spontaneous breathing [95]. In clinical practice where cardiac output is usually not measured, it is sometimes difficult to decide whether controlled or spontaneous ventilation is best. In horses with poor cardiovascular function that cannot be stabilized before anesthesia, or in colic cases with severe abdominal distension resulting in reduced venous return that is further exacerbated by dorsal recumbency, it may be better to allow spontaneous ventilation in an effort to maintain cardiac output. In athletic horses and thoroughbreds, however, mechanical ventilation is often necessary. If mechanical ventilation is planned, it should be initiated soon after induction of anesthesia with the goal of reducing the alveolar–arterial oxygen gradient ($P(A\text{-}a)O_2$) [96]. To optimize ventilation further, various positive end-expiratory pressure (PEEP) levels (5–30 cmH_2O) have been used in horses [91]. PEEP should be initiated at the outset of anesthesia to reduce the intrapulmonary shunt fraction and increase functional residual capacity; however, pharmacologic support of the cardiovascular system is needed to counteract reductions in cardiac output and impaired tissue oxygen delivery [91]. When PEEP (10 cmH_2O) was combined with repetitive recruitment maneuvers in horses with colic, arterial oxygenation improved, but PEEP's influence on oxygen delivery was not evaluated as cardiac output was not measured [97]. Continuous positive airway pressure (CPAP) of 8 cmH_2O in spontaneously breathing horses increased arterial oxygenation, but its influence on oxygen delivery remains to be thoroughly evaluated [91].

Anesthesia recovery

Recovery is a multifactorial event [98]. It is the result of both factors that are fixed and others that can be influenced. Important factors include the construction and size of the recovery box, the personnel and equipment available, the type and duration of surgery performed, as well as the age, sex, breed, behavior, and the health status of the horse. Also, intraoperative factors such as hypotension, hypoxemia, body temperature, and drugs used for anesthesia induction, maintenance, and recovery all play key roles. The following paragraphs aim at giving some guidelines to optimize recovery.

Environmental considerations

For optimal recovery, it is important to provide the horse with a warm and quiet environment. For foals, the best recovery option may be in the stall with its mother (Fig. 61.1). It is usually not beneficial for horses to recover in a dimly lit recovery stall [99], but the eyes can be covered with a towel to reduce light stimuli if desired (Fig. 61.2). This allows the horse to see once it achieves sternal recumbency. Ear plugs (either commercially available or made of cotton) may reduce auditory stimuli or, more commonly, ambient noise is kept to a minimum. With the aid of a soft, deflatable pillow

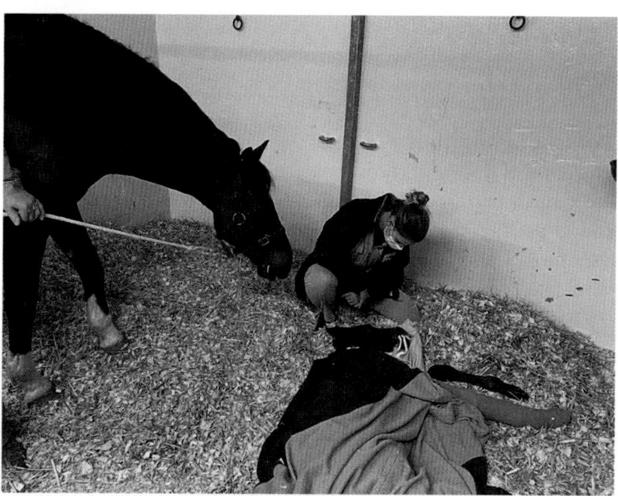

Figure 61.1 Foal recovering in the stall with its mother.

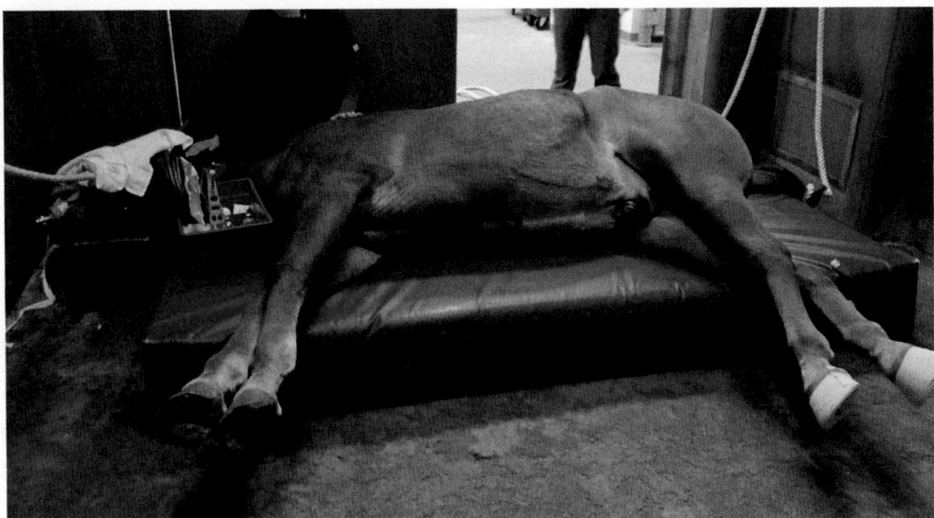

Figure 61.2 Horse positioned for recovery from general anesthesia. Source: Dr. Tania Perez, Veterinary Teaching Hospital, Washington State University, Pullman, WA, with permission.

or mattress, horses can to some extent be discouraged from attempting to stand too early [100].

By allowing additional time for anesthetic drug elimination, better and more coordinated recoveries are usually achieved. Most horses do not readily accept the endotracheal tube remaining in place once they have begun to regain consciousness, although various techniques have been used to maintain airway patency and allow oxygen administration during the recovery phase. Delayed extubation may be associated with increased risk of laryngeal spasm and this should be weighed against the benefit of maintaining an airway during recovery. In fasted horses, some clinicians prefer to extubate slightly before swallowing is expected (especially in young, difficult horses). The administration of 0.25% phenylephrine [101] into the nasal passages results in rapid local vasoconstriction, decongestion, and improved air flow. Upper airway obstruction may lead to pulmonary edema [102], possibly with fatal consequences. If there is any potential for upper airway obstruction (due to, for example, laryngeal surgery or long recumbency in combination with low plasma albumin concentration), the cuffed endotracheal tube can be fixed to the mandible and extubation delayed until the horse is standing. Care should be taken that nothing can be aspirated through the tube. If horses have a nasogastric tube in place (as is often the case in patients undergoing colic surgery), this should be removed before recovery to prevent complications [103].

Timing of recovery

The optimal timing of recovery is dependent on the anesthetic and the surgery performed. Recumbency is often irksome to the horse and is usually kept to a minimum. However, following general anesthesia lasting 1 h or longer, a horse may take 30–45 min to eliminate the anesthetic adequately. Ideally, the horse assumes a sternal position and then waits a further 10–15 min to stand up. If it chooses to remain in sternal recumbency longer, this is not harmful. However, if the horse is still in lateral recumbency after 60 min, it should be carefully evaluated, and necessary measures taken to minimize the risk of neuropathy or myopathy. If there is no obvious explanation for the prolonged period of recumbency or inability to maintain sternal recumbency, hand clapping or other stimuli may persuade it to rise.

Additional sedation and analgesia

Optimal sedation and analgesia facilitate a good recovery. All aspects named in the following paragraph have been described recently in more detail [98]. Horses will recover better with postanesthetic sedation, and this effect seems to be dose dependent. All sedatives impair cardiopulmonary function to some extent. During recovery when the cardiopulmonary effects of other anesthetic agents are rapidly dissipating, the effects of α_2-adrenergic receptor agonists are well tolerated, provided that low doses are used and administration is slow (over 3–5 min). In one study utilizing research horses, no differences among recovery parameters were demonstrated between xylazine (0.1 mg/kg IV), detomidine (2 μg/kg IV), and romifidine (8 μg/kg IV) [104]. However, a clinical study in healthy horses comparing xylazine (0.1 or 0.2 mg/kg IV) with romifidine (10 or 20 μg/kg IV) following isoflurane anesthesia demonstrated that 20 μg/kg romifidine resulted in the best quality recoveries, and it was speculated that higher dose rates could be beneficial in difficult horses [105]. Other experimental studies have also investigated if a 15–30-min prolongation of anesthesia with ketamine or propofol in combination with xylazine after discontinuation of inhalant anesthetic administration would result in improved recovery [106,107]. In those studies, the use of injectable anesthesia at the end of anesthesia improved recovery quality; however, propofol combinations resulted in apnea and low arterial oxygenation, which was deemed a significant complication. A single bolus of xylazine in comparison with xylazine combined with ketamine following isoflurane anesthesia resulted in better recoveries in another group of experimental horses [108]. This study also tested acepromazine (0.02 mg/kg IV), which resulted in a similar recovery quality to xylazine–ketamine.

The ideal time to administer the sedative is dependent on the status and character of the horse, the duration of anesthesia, and the drug selected as the time to achieve a maximal effect differs between various α_2-adrenergic receptor agonists (e.g., romifidine takes longer than xylazine) [109]. If the sedative is given too early in recovery or at too high a dose, and significant levels of inhalant anesthetic remain, spontaneous ventilation might be impaired. On the other hand, if a difficult horse has already started to move, it will be more difficult to prevent attempts to stand with only a small bolus of an α_2-adrenergic receptor agonist. Of course, the optimum time point of administration of the sedative is also dependent on the inhalant anesthetic used and the use of other concurrent drugs. Following isoflurane or sevoflurane anesthesia, the horse can be allowed to breathe oxygen for about 3–5 min. When the first signs of a reduced depth of anesthesia become apparent (spontaneous blinking, slow nystagmus, and increased respiratory rate), xylazine, dexmedetomidine, or medetomidine can be given. If romifidine is chosen, it is administered as soon as spontaneous breathing is present owing to the longer onset of action. Horses that show nystagmus or limb movements can be given the sedative without delay.

Although opioids provide good analgesia, their effect on recovery seems dependent on the type of opioid, the dose used, and the study design [98]. The use of morphine (0.1 or 0.2 mg/kg IM given 20 min after induction of anesthesia) in a clinical setting involving short duration upper airway surgery was shown to improve recovery quality. However, it also reduced arterial oxygenation in spontaneously breathing horses [28]. Therefore, some anesthetists prefer to administer morphine (0.1 mg/kg IM) 10 min before the end of surgery.

Recovery assist systems

Catastrophic injuries during recovery lead to the majority of equine anesthetic fatalities. Horses with long bone fractures, geriatric horses, and exhausted horses (such as pregnant mares or horses with colic following extensive surgeries) often do not have the strength to safely resume standing and may require assistance. Several systems aimed at helping horses during this crucial phase have been tested. Evidence has shown that average recovery quality is better if horses are helped with head and tail ropes, but in no report was the fatality rate reduced with assisted recovery [98]. On the contrary, one report involving horses recovering from colic surgery detected an increased risk of fatal trauma [110] when head and tail ropes were used compared to no help during recovery. The decision whether to assist recovery or not should be made based on recovery box design, availability of trained personnel, availability of adequate assist systems, and the severity of surgery along with the horse's weight, age, temperament, and fitness status.

Numerous systems have been described. Tail ropes with or without head ropes can be used to assist most horses. Experienced personnel will aid in success since timing is important to avoid pulling the horse off balance. The ropes can be used to stabilize the horse but should not be used to attempt to lift it. For recovery of horses with specific concerns (e.g., long bone fractures), slings or nets have been used [111]. Ideally, the horse would be made accustomed to such a device before anesthesia to increase acceptance during recovery. Hydropools [112] (Figs. 61.3 and 61.4) or pools with a supporting raft system [113] are other options for safe recovery of horses that are not capable of regaining a standing position without risk of severe injury.

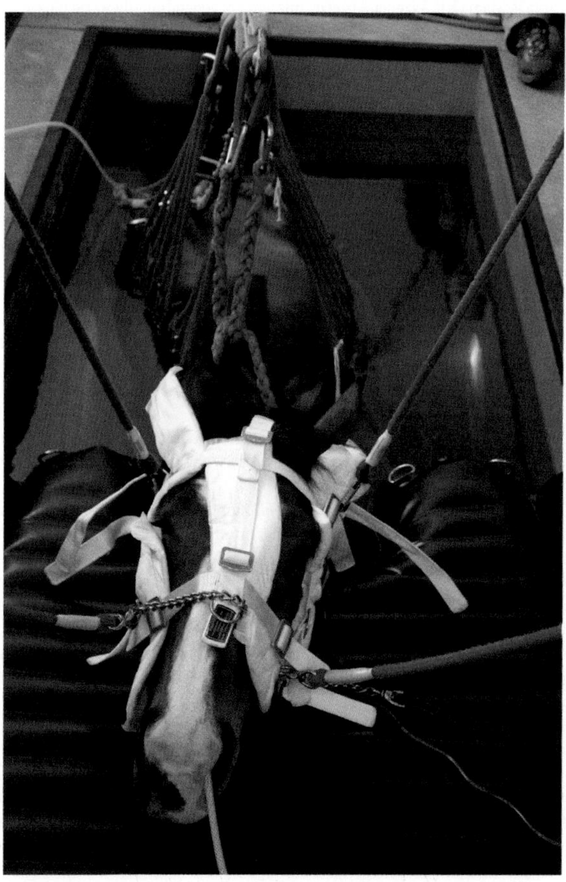

Figure 61.3 Horse recovering from general anesthesia in a hydropool.

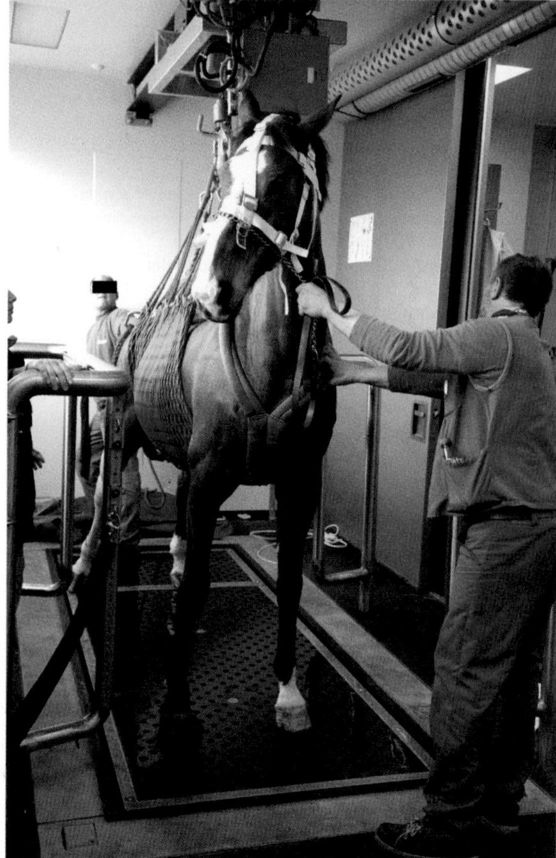

Figure 61.4 Standing horse after hydropool floor has been raised to ground level.

References

1 Gozalo-Marcilla M, Bettschart-Wolfensberger R, Johnston M, *et al.* Data collection for the fourth multicentre Confidential Enquiry into Perioperative Equine Fatalities (CEPEF4) study: new technology and preliminary results. *Animals* 2021; **11**(9): 2549.

2 Bidwell LA, Bramlage LR, Rood WA. Equine perioperative fatalities associated with general anaesthesia at a private practice – a retrospective case series. *Vet Anaesth Analg* 2007; **34**(1): 23–30.

3 Dugdale AHA, Obhrai J, Cripps PJ. Twenty years later: a single-centre repeat retrospective analysis of equine perioperative mortality and investigation of recovery quality. *Vet Anaesth Analg* 2016; **43**(2): 171–178.

4 Laurenza C, Ansart L, Portier K. Risk factors of anesthesia-related mortality and morbidity in one equine hospital: a retrospective study on 1161 cases undergoing elective or emergency surgeries. *Front Vet Sci* 2020; **6**: 514.

5 Johnston GM, Eastment JK, Wood JL, *et al.* The Confidential Enquiry into Perioperative Equine Fatalities (CEPEF): mortality results of Phases 1 and 2. *Vet Anaesth Analg* 2002; **29**(4): 159–170.

6 Lesté-Lasserre C. Standing fast: standing surgeries for horses. The Horse [Internet], May 26, 2020. www.thehorse.com/171463/standing-fast-standing-surgeries-for-horses/

7 Vigani A, Garda-Pereira FL. Anesthesia and analgesia for standing equine surgery. *Vet Clin North Am Equine Pract* 2014; **30**(1): 1–7.

8 Fujiyama M, Jones T, Duke-Novakovski T. Evaluation of the perioperative stress response from dexmedetomidine infusion alone with butorphanol bolus or remifentanil infusion compared with ketamine and morphine infusions in isoflurane-anesthetized horses. *Vet Anaesth Analg* 2021; **48**(3): 344–355.

9 Bailey PA, Hague BA, Davis M, *et al.* Incidence of post-anesthetic colic in non-fasted adult equine patients. *Can Vet J* 2016; **57**(12): 1263–1266.

10 Senior JM, Pinchbeck GL, Allister R, *et al.* Post anaesthetic colic in horses: a preventable complication? *Equine Vet J* 2006; **38**(5): 479–484.

11 Hospes R, Bleul U. The effect of extended preoperative fasting in mares undergoing surgery of the perineal region. *J Equine Vet Sci* 2007; **27**(12): 542–545.

12 Murray MJ, Eichorn ES. Effects of intermittent feed deprivation, intermittent feed deprivation with ranitidine administration, and stall confinement with ad libitum access to hay on gastric ulceration in horses. *Am J Vet Res* 1996; **57**(11): 1599–1603.

13 Jones RS, Edwards GB, Brearley JC. Commentary on prolonged starvation as a factor associated with post operative colic. *Equine Vet Educ* 1991; **3**(1): 16–18.

14 Natalini C, Driessen B. Epidural and spinal anesthesia and analgesia in the equine. *Clin Tech Equine Pract* 2007; **6**: 145–153.

15 Cook VL, Blikslager AT. The use of nonsteroidal anti-inflammatory drugs in critically ill horses. *J Vet Emerg Crit Care (San Antonio)* 2015; **25**(1): 76–88.

16 Knych HK. Nonsteroidal anti-inflammatory drug use in horses. *Vet Clin North Am Equine Pract* 2017; **33**(1): 1–15.

17 Driessen B, Zarucco L, Kalir B, *et al.* Contemporary use of acepromazine in the anaesthetic management of male horses and ponies: a retrospective study and opinion poll. *Equine Vet J* 2011; **43**(1): 88–98.

18 Daunt DA, Dunlop CI, Chapman PL, *et al.* Cardiopulmonary and behavioral-responses to computer-driven infusion of detomidine in standing horses. *Am J Vet Res* 1993; **54**(12): 2075–2082.

19 Edner A, Nyman G, Essen-Gustavsson B. The relationship of muscle perfusion and metabolism with cardiovascular variables before and after detomidine injection during propofol-ketamine anaesthesia in horses. *Vet Anaesth Analg* 2002; **29**(4): 182–199.

20 Raisis AL. Skeletal muscle blood flow in anaesthetized horses Part II: effects of anaesthetics and vasoactive agents. *Vet Anaesth Analg* 2005; **32**(6): 331–337.

21 Ringer SK, Schwarzwald CC, Portier KG, *et al.* Effects on cardiopulmonary function and oxygen delivery of doses of romifidine and xylazine followed by constant rate infusions in standing horses. *Vet J* 2013; **195**(2): 228–234.

22 Yamashita K, Tsubakishita S, Futaok S, *et al.* Cardiovascular effects of medetomidine detomidine and xylazine in horses. *J Vet Med Sci* 2000; **62**(10): 1025–1032.

23 Ringer SK, Portier KG, Fourel I, *et al.* Development of a xylazine constant rate infusion with or without butorphanol for standing sedation of horses. *Vet Anaesth Analg* 2012; **39**(1): 1–11.

24 Ringer SK, Portier KG, Fourel I, *et al.* Development of a romifidine constant rate infusion with or without butorphanol for standing sedation of horses. *Vet Anaesth Analg* 2012; **39**(1): 12–20.

25 Gozalo-Marcilla M, Luna SP, Crosignani N, *et al.* Sedative and antinociceptive effects of different combinations of detomidine and methadone in standing horses. *Vet Anaesth Analg* 2017; **44**(5): 1116–1127.

26 Bennett RC, Steffey E. Use of opioids for pain and anesthetic management in horses. *Vet Clin North Am Equine Pract* 2002; **18**(1): 47–60.

27 Gozalo-Marcilla M, Hopster K, Gasthuys F, *et al.* Minimum end-tidal sevoflurane concentration necessary to prevent movement during a constant rate infusion of morphine or morphine plus dexmedetomidine in ponies. *Vet Anaesth Analg* 2014; **41**(2): 212–219.

28 Love EJ, Lane JG, Murison PJ. Morphine administration in horses anaesthetized for upper respiratory tract surgery. *Vet Anaesth Analg* 2006; **33**(3): 179–188.

29 Senior JM, Pinchbeck GL, Dugdale AHA, *et al.* Retrospective study of the risk factors and prevalence of colic horses after orthopaedic surgery. *Vet Rec* 2004; **155**: 321–325.

30 Mackenzie C. Do opioids cause colic? *Equine Vet Educ* 2017; **29**(7): 401–402.

31 Skrzypczak H, Reed, R, Barletta M, *et al.* A retrospective evaluation of the effect of perianesthetic hydromorphone administration on the incidence of postanesthetic signs of colic in horses. *Vet Anaesth Analg* 2020; **47**(6): 757–762.

32 Herschl MA, Trim CM, Mahaffey EA. Effects of 5 % and 10 % guaifenesin infusion on equine vascular endothelium. *Vet Surg* 1992; **21**: 494–497.

33 Douglas H, Hopster K, Cerullo M, *et al.* The effects of flumazenil on ventilatory and recovery characteristics in horses following midazolam-ketamine induction and isoflurane anaesthesia. *Equine Vet J* 2021; **53**(6): 1257–1267.

34 Jarrett MA, Bailey KM, Messenger KM, *et al.* Recovery of horses from general anesthesia after induction with propofol and ketamine versus midazolam and ketamine. *J Am Vet Med Assoc* 2018; **253**(1): 101–107.

35 Brosnan RJ, Steffey EP, Escobar A, *et al.* Anesthetic induction with guaifenesin and propofol in adult horses. *Am J Vet Res* 2011; **72**(12): 1569–1575.

36 Wakuno A, Aoki M, Kushiro A, *et al.* Comparison of alfaxalone, ketamine and thiopental for anaesthetic induction and recovery in Thoroughbred horses premedicated with medetomidine and midazolam. *Equine Vet J* 2017; **49**(1): 94–98.

37 Keates HL, van Eps AW, Pearson MRB. Alfaxalone compared with ketamine for induction of anaesthesia in horses following xylazine and guaifenesin. *Vet Anaesth Analg* 2012; **39**(6): 591–598.

38 Wagner AE, Mama KR, Steffey EP, *et al.* Comparison of the cardiovascular effects of equipotent anesthetic doses of sevoflurane alone and sevoflurane plus an intravenous infusion of lidocaine in horses. *Am J Vet Res* 2011; **72**(4): 452–460.

39 Gozalo-Marcilla M, Gasthuys F, Schauvliege S. Partial intravenous anaesthesia in the horse: a review of intravenous agents used to supplement equine inhalation anaesthesia Part 1: lidocaine and ketamine. *Vet Anaesth Analg* 2014; **41**(4): 335–345.

40 Gozalo-Marcilla M, Gasthuys F, Schauvliege S. Partial intravenous anaesthesia in the horse: a review of intravenous agents used to supplement equine inhalation anaesthesia Part 2: opioids and alpha-2 adrenoceptor agonists. *Vet Anaesth Analg* 2015; **42**(1): 1–16.

41 Feary DJ, Mama KR, Wagner AE, *et al.* Influence of general anesthesia on pharmacokinetics of intravenous lidocaine infusion in horses. *Am J Vet Res* 2005; **66**: 574–580.

42 Feary DJ, Mama KR, Thomasy SM, *et al.* Influence of gastrointestinal tract disease on pharmacokinetics of lidocaine after intravenous infusion in anesthetized horses. *Am J Vet Res* 2006; **67**: 317–322.

43 Lankveld DPK, Driessen B, Soma LR, *et al.* Pharmacodynamic effects and pharmacokinetic profile of a long-term continuous rate infusion of racemic ketamine in healthy conscious horses. *J Vet Pharmacol Therap* 2006; **29**: 477–488.

44 Valverde A. Balanced anesthesia and constant-rate infusions in horses. *Vet Clin North Am Equine Pract* 2013; **29**(1): 89–122.

45 Wiederkehr A, Barbarossa A, Ringer SK, *et al.* Clinical randomized comparison of medetomidine and xylazine for isoflurane balanced anesthesia in horses. *Front Vet Sci* 2021; **8**: 603695.

46 Sacks M, Ringer SK, Bishofberger AS, *et al.* Clinical comparison of dexmedetomidine and medetomidine for isoflurane balanced anaesthesia in horses. *Vet Anaesth Analg* 2017; **44**(5): 1128–1138.

47 England GC, Clarke KW. Alpha 2 adrenoceptor agonists in the horse – a review. *Br Vet J* 1996; **152**(6): 641–657.

48 Wagner AE, Dunlop CI, Heath RB, *et al.* Hemodynamic function during neurectomy in halothane-anesthetized horses with or without constant dose detomidine infusion. *Vet Surg* 1992; **21**(3): 248–255.

49 Devisscher L, Schauvliege S, Dewulf J, *et al.* Romifidine as a constant rate infusion in isoflurane anaesthetized horses: a clinical study. *Vet Anaesth Analg* 2010; **37**(5): 425–433.

50 Ringer SK, Kalchofner K, Boller J, *et al.* A clinical comparison of two anaesthetic protocols using lidocaine or medetomidine in horses. *Vet Anaesth Analg* 2007; **34**(4): 257–268.

51 Menzies MPL, Ringer SK, Conrot A, *et al.* Cardiopulmonary effects and anaesthesia recovery quality in horses anaesthetized with isoflurane and low-dose S-ketamine or medetomidine infusions. *Vet Anaesth Analg* 2016; **43**(6): 623–634.

52 Kalin I, Henze IS, Ringer SK, *et al.* Comparison of recovery quality following medetomidine versus xylazine balanced isoflurane anaesthesia in horses: a retrospective analysis. *Animals* 2021; **11**(8): 2440.

53 Bettschart-Wolfensberger R, Clarke KW, Vainio O, *et al.* Pharmacokinetics of medetomidine in ponies and elaboration of a medetomidine infusion regime which provides a constant level of sedation. *Res Vet Sci* 1999; **67**(1): 41–46.

54 Kalchofner KS, Ringer SK, Boller J, *et al.* Clinical assessment of anesthesia with isoflurane and medetomidine in 300 equidae. *Pferdeheilkunde* 2006; **22**(3): 301–308.

55 Bettschart-Wolfensberger R, Bettschart R, Vainio O, *et al.* Cardiopulmonary effects of a two hour infusion of medetomidine and its reversal by atipamezole in horses and ponies. *Vet Anaesth Analg* 1999; **26**: 8–12.

56 Risberg AI, Ranheim B, Krontveit RI, *et al.* The cardiovascular status of isoflurane-anaesthetized horses with and without dexmedetomidine constant rate infusion evaluated at equivalent depths of anaesthesia. *Vet Anaesth Analg* 2016; **43**(4): 412–423.

57 Marcilla MG, Schauvliege S, Segaert S, *et al.* Influence of a constant rate infusion of dexmedetomidine on cardiopulmonary function and recovery quality in isoflurane anaesthetized horses. *Vet Anaesth Analg* 2012; **39**(1): 49–58.

58 Neudeck S, Twele L, Kopp V, *et al.* Pharmacodynamics and plasma concentrations of dexmedetomidine with or without vatinoxan as a constant-rate infusion in horses anaesthetized with isoflurane – a pilot study. *J Vet Pharmacol Ther* 2021; **44**(5): 754–765.

59 Bettschart-Wolfensberger R, Dicht S, Vullo C, *et al.* A clinical study on the effect in horses during medetomidine-isoflurane anaesthesia, of butorphanol constant rate infusion on isoflurane requirements, on cardiopulmonary function and on recovery characteristics. *Vet Anaesth Analg* 2011; **38**(3): 186–194.

60 Gozalo-Marcilla M, Hopster K, Gasthuys F, *et al.* Minimum end-tidal sevoflurane concentration necessary to prevent movement during a constant rate infusion of morphine or morphine plus dexmedetomidine in ponies. *Vet Anaesth Analg* 2014; **41**(2): 212–219.

61 Meyer GA, Lin HC, Hanson RR, *et al.* Effects of intravenous lidocaine overdose on cardiac electrical activity and blood pressure in the horse. *Equine Vet J* 2001; **33**: 434–437.

62 Doherty TJ, Frazier DL. Effect of intravenous lidocaine on halothane minimum alveolar concentration in ponies. *Equine Vet J* 1998; **30**: 300–303.

63 Rezende ML, Wagner AE, Mama KR, *et al.* Effects of intravenous administration of lidocaine on the minimum alveolar concentration of sevoflurane in horses. *Am J Vet Res* 2011; **72**(4): 446–451.

64 Valverde A, Gunkel C, Doherty TJ, *et al.* Effect of a constant rate infusion of lidocaine on the quality of recovery from sevoflurane or isoflurane general anaesthesia in horses. *Equine Vet J* 2005; **37**: 559–564.

65 Muir WW. NMDA receptor antagonists and pain: ketamine. *Vet Clin North Am Equine Pract* 2010; **26**(3): 565–578.

66 Enderle AK, Levionnois OL, Kuhn M, *et al.* Clinical evaluation of ketamine and lidocaine intravenous infusions to reduce isoflurane requirements in horses under general anaesthesia. *J Vet Anaesth Analg* 2008; **35**: 297–305.

67 Villalba M, Santiago I, Gomez de Segura IA. Effects of constant rate infusion of lidocaine and ketamine with or without morphine on isoflurane MAC in horses. *Equine Vet J* 2011; **43**(6): 721–726.

68 Clark L, Clutton RE, Blissitt KJ, *et al.* The effects of morphine on recovery of horses from halothane anaesthesia. *Vet Anaesth Analg* 2008; **35**: 22–29.

69 Gozalo-Marcilla M, Steblaj B, Schauvliege S, *et al.* Comparison of the influence of two different constant-rate infusions (dexmedetomidine versus morphine) on anaesthetic requirements, cardiopulmonary function and recovery quality in isoflurane anaesthetized horses. *Res Vet Sci* 2013; **95**(3): 1186–1194.

70 Dmitrovic P, Vanaga J, Dupont J, *et al.* Effect of fentanyl infusion on heart rate variability and anaesthetic requirements in isoflurane-anaesthetized horses. *Animals* 2021; **11**(10): 2922.

71 Thomasy SM, Steffey EP, Mama KR, *et al.* The effects of i.v. fentanyl administration on the minimum alveolar concentration of isoflurane in horses. *Br J Anaesth* 2006; **97**(2): 232–237.

72 Knych HK, Steffey EP, Mama KR, *et al.* Effects of high plasma fentanyl concentrations on minimum alveolar concentration of isoflurane in horses. *Am J Vet Res* 2009; **70**(10): 1193–1200.

73 Benmansour P, Duke-Novakovski T. Prolonged anesthesia using sevoflurane remifentanil and dexmedetomidine in a horse. *Vet Anaesth Analg* 2013; **40**(5): 521–526.

74 Mizobe F, Wakuno A, Okada J, *et al.* Clinical usefulness of intravenous constant rate infusion of fentanyl and medetomidine under sevoflurane anesthesia in Thoroughbred racehorses undergoing internal fixation surgery. *J Equine Sci* 2017; **28**(4): 143–147.

75 Di Salvo A, Chiaradia E, Nannarone S, *et al.* Intra-articular use of analgesic/antinflammatory drugs in dogs and horses. *Res Vet Sci* 2021; **134**: 159–170.

76 Matthews NS, Dollar NS, Shawley RV. Halothane-sparing effect of benzodiazepines in ponies. *Cornell Vet* 1990; **80**(3): 259–265.

77 Kushiro T, Yamashita K, Umar MA, *et al.* Anesthetic and cardiovascular effects of balanced anesthesia using constant rate infusion of midazolam-ketamine-medetomidine with inhalation of oxygen-sevoflurane (MKM-OS anesthesia) in horses. *J Vet Med Sci* 2005; **67**(4): 379–384.

78 Yamashita K, Satoh M, Umikawa A, *et al.* Combination of continuous intravenous infusion using a mixture of guaifenesin-ketamine-medetomidine and sevoflurane anesthesia in horses. *J Vet Med Sci* 2000; **62**(3): 229–235.

79 Lerche P. Total intravenous anesthesia in horses. *Vet Clin North Am Equine Pract* 2013; **29**(1): 123–129.

80 Davidson GS. Equine anesthesia: triple drip. *Int J Pharm Compd* 2008; **12**(5): 402–404.

81 Dagnall C, Khenissi L, Love E. Monitoring techniques for equine anaesthesia. *Equine Vet Edu* 2021: 13581.

82 Edner AH, Essen-Gustavsson B, Nyman GC. Metabolism during anaesthesia and recovery in colic and healthy horses: a microdialysis study. *Acta Veterinaria Scandinavica* 2009; **51**(1): 10.

83 Raisis AL. Skeletal muscle blood flow in anaesthetized horses Part I: measurement techniques. *Vet Anaesth Analg* 2005; **32**(6): 324–330.

84 Dancker C, Hopster K, Rohn K, *et al.* Effects of dobutamine, dopamine, phenylephrine, and noradrenaline on systemic haemodynamics and intestinal perfusion in isoflurane anaesthetised horses. *Equine Vet J* 2018; **50**(1): 104–110.

85 Duke T, Filzek U, Read MR, *et al.* Clinical observations surrounding an increased incidence of postanaesthetic myopathy in halothane-anaesthetized horses. *Pferdeheilkunde* 2006; **22**(4): 467–467.

86 Grandy JL, Steffey EP, Hodgson DS, *et al.* Arterial hypotension and the development of postanesthetic myopathy in halothane-anesthetized horses. *Am J Vet Res* 1987; **48**(2): 192–197.

87 Brosnan RJ. Inhaled anesthetics in horses. *Vet Clin North Am Equine Pract* 2013; **29**(1): 69–87.

88 Schauvliege S, Gasthuys F. Drugs for cardiovascular support in anesthetized horses. *Vet Clin North Am Equine Pract* 2013; **29**(1): 19–49.

89 Teixeira-Neto FJ, Valverde A. Clinical application of the fluid challenge approach in goal-directed fluid therapy: what can we learn from human studies? *Front in Vet Sci* 2021; **8**: 701377.

90 Stefanik E, Drewnowska O, Lisowka B, *et al.* Causes, effects and methods of monitoring gas exchange disturbances during equine general anaesthesia. *Animals (Basel)* 2021; **11**(7): 2049.

91 Mosing M, Senior JM. Maintenance of equine anaesthesia over the last 50 years: controlled inhalation of volatile anaesthetics and pulmonary ventilation. *Equine Vet J* 2018; **50**(3): 282–291.

92 Kalchofner KS, Picek S, Ringer SK, *et al.* A study of cardiovascular function under controlled and spontaneous ventilation in isoflurane-medetomidine anaesthetized horses. *Vet Anaesth Analg* 2009; **36**(5): 426–435.

93 Khanna AK, McDonell WN, Dyson DH, *et al.* Cardiopulmonary effects of hypercapnia during controlled intermittent positive pressure ventilation in the horse. *Can J Vet Res* 1995; **59**(3): 213–221.

94 Moens Y. Mechanical ventilation and respiratory mechanics during equine anesthesia. *Vet Clin North Am Equine Pract* 2013; **29**(1): 51–67.

95 Edner A, Nyman G, Essen-Gustavsson B. The effects of spontaneous and mechanical ventilation on central cardiovascular function and peripheral perfusion during isoflurane anaesthesia in horses. *Vet Anaesth Analg* 2005; **32**(3): 136–146.

96 Nyman G, Funkquist B, Kvart C, *et al.* Atelectasis causes gas exchange impairment in the anaesthetised horse. *Equine Vet J* 1990; **22**(5): 317–324.

97 Hopster K, Lastner SBR, Rohn K, *et al.* Intermittent positive pressure ventilation with constant positive end-expiratory pressure and alveolar recruitment manoeuvre during inhalation anaesthesia in horses undergoing surgery for colic and its influence on the early recovery period. *Vet Anaesth Analg* 2011; **38**(3): 169–177.

98 Gozalo-Marcilla M, Ringer SK. Recovery after general anaesthesia in adult horses: a structured summary of the literature. *Animals* 2021; **11**(6): 1777.

99 Clark-Price SC, Posner L, Gleed RD. Recovery of horses from general anesthesia in a darkened or illuminated recovery stall. *Vet Anaesth Analg* 2008; **35**(6): 473–479.

100 Ray-Miller WM, Hodgson DS, McMurphy RM, *et al.* Comparison of recoveries from anesthesia of horses placed on a rapidly inflating-deflating air pillow or the floor of a padded stall. *J Am Vet Med Assoc* 2006; **229**(5): 711–716.

101 Lukasik VM, Gleed RD, Scarlett JM, *et al.* Intranasal phenylephrine reduces post anesthetic upper airway obstruction in horses. *Equine Vet J* 1997; **29**(3): 236–238.

102 Senior M. Post-anaesthetic pulmonary oedema in horses: a review. *Vet Anaesth Analg* 2005; **32**(4): 193–200.

103 Veres-Nyeki KO, Graubner C, Aloisio F, *et al.* Pulmonary edema at recovery after colic operation with in-situ nasogastric tube in a horse. *Schweiz Arch Tierheilkd* 2011; **153**(9): 401–404.

104 Santos M, Fuente M, Garcia-Iturralde R, *et al.* Effects of alpha-2 adrenoceptor agonists during recovery from isoflurane anaesthesia in horses. *Equine Vet J* 2003; **35**(2): 170–175.

105 Woodhouse KJ, Brosnan RJ, Nguyen KO, *et al.* Effects of postanesthetic sedation with romifidine or xylazine on quality of recovery from isoflurane anesthesia in horses. *J Am Vet Med Assoc* 2013; **242**(4): 533–539.

106 Wagner AE, Mama KR, Steffey EP, *et al.* Evaluation of infusions of xylazine with ketamine or propofol to modulate recovery following sevoflurane anesthesia in horses. *Am J Vet Res* 2012; **73**(3): 346–352.

107 Steffey EP, Mama KR, Brosnan RJ, *et al.* Effect of administration of propofol and xylazine hydrochloride on recovery of horses after four hours of anesthesia with desflurane. *Am J Vet Res* 2009; **70**(8): 956–963.

108 Valverde A, Black B, Cribb NC, *et al.* Assessment of unassisted recovery from repeated general isoflurane anesthesia in horses following post-anesthetic administration of xylazine or acepromazine or a combination of xylazine and ketamine. *Vet Anaesth Analg* 2013; **40**(1): 3–12.
109 Ringer SK, Portier K, Torgerson PR, *et al.* The effects of a loading dose followed by constant rate infusion of xylazine compared with romifidine on sedation, ataxia and response to stimuli in horses. *Vet Anaesth Analg* 2013; **40**(2): 157–165.
110 Rüegg M, Bettschart-Wolfensberger, Hartnack, *et al.* Comparison of non-assisted and tail rope-assisted recovery after abdominal surgery in horses. *Pferdeheilkunde* 2016; **32**: 469–478.
111 Steffey EP, Brosnan RJ, Galuppo LD, *et al.* Use of propofol-xylazine and the Anderson Sling Suspension System for recovery of horses from desflurane anesthesia. *Vet Surg* 2009; **38**(8): 927–933.
112 Picek S, Kalchofner KS, Ringer SK, *et al.* Anaesthetic management for hydropool recovery in 50 horses. *Pferdeheilkunde* 2010; **26**: 515–522.
113 Sullivan EK, Klein LV, Richardson DW, *et al.* Use of a pool-raft system for recovery of horses from general anesthesia: 393 horses (1984–2000). *J Am Vet Med Assoc* 2002; **221**(7): 1014–1018.

62 Horses with Colic

Ludovica Chiavaccini[1] **and Lauren R. Duffee**[2]

[1] Department of Comparative, Diagnostic and Population Medicine, College of Veterinary Medicine, University of Florida, Gainesville, Florida, USA
[2] Massachusetts Veterinary Referral Hospital, Woburn, Massachusetts, USA

Chapter contents

Introduction, 1217
Endotoxemia and systemic inflammatory response syndrome, 1217
Preanesthetic considerations, 1218
  Clinical history, 1218
  Physical examination, 1219
  Diagnostics, 1219
Anesthetic risks and anticipated complications, 1219
  Hypotension, 1219
  Impaired ventilation–perfusion matching, 1220
  Arrhythmias, 1221
  Postanesthetic myopathy and neuropathy, 1221
Preparation of the surgical area, 1221
Stabilization and fluid resuscitation, 1222
Anesthetic protocol, 1224
  Premedication, 1224
  Induction and intubation, 1224
Maintenance of anesthesia, 1225
  Adjunct agents, 1225
  Locoregional anesthesia, 1227
  Monitoring, 1227
  Ventilation strategies, 1228
Recovery, 1228
References, 1229

Introduction

"Colic" is a term used to describe abdominal pain in the horse. The underlying pathology typically occurs in the gastrointestinal tract but can also be caused by disease in the kidneys, bladder, or other viscera. Colic is a significant cause of morbidity and mortality in equine practice. Most horses with colic are treated with medical management, and only a minority of cases require surgical intervention. In a 1997 epidemiological study, approximately 11 colic cases occurred for every 100 horse-years. While 75% of these were mild and resolved with no treatment or a single farm visit, 4% of all cases needed surgical intervention [1]. The percentage increases when considering horses hospitalized for colic. Of 1588 horses with colic presenting to a veterinary hospital in Denmark for inpatient care, 31% needed exploratory laparotomy [2]. Similarly, in another study on 649 horses hospitalized for colic, 28% received abdominal surgery [3]. Recent epidemiological studies have found an average survival to discharge rate of 42–54% for colic surgery [2,4]. Patients that present with colic that require surgical intervention represent a high-risk population that necessitates careful preparation and intensive perioperative management. This chapter will focus on the anesthetic management of surgical colic cases, including the practical and theoretical aspects of preparing for an emergent exploratory laparotomy. After discussing the management concerns and anticipated anesthetic complications, the authors will describe the stabilization of the patient and selection of an appropriate anesthetic protocol.

Endotoxemia and systemic inflammatory response syndrome

Endotoxemia in the colic horse presents a significant challenge to the anesthetist. Recent studies estimate that 30% of all horses with colic [5,6] and 55% of horses needing colic surgery [6] meet systemic inflammatory response syndrome (SIRS) criteria. The clinical effects of sepsis, often exacerbated during general anesthesia due to sympathetic suppression and the pharmacologic effects of anesthetic drugs, underlie many anticipated anesthetic complications encountered in horses undergoing colic surgery. Therefore, the anesthetist should understand the etiopathogenesis and the therapeutic strategies to manage the endotoxemic horse.

Endotoxemia occurs when gram-negative bacteria or their cell wall components, such as lipopolysaccharide (LPS), enter the bloodstream. With strangulating colic lesions, the impaired blood supply to the entrapped bowel leads to segments of ischemic gastrointestinal mucosa and consequent impairment of epithelial integrity that allow for translocation of these bacterial components [7,8]. LPS is bound by circulating LPS-binding protein; this complex then binds to the CD14 protein on the surface of

Veterinary Anesthesia and Analgesia: The Sixth Edition of Lumb and Jones. Edited by Leigh Lamont, Kurt Grimm, Sheilah Robertson, Lydia Love and Carrie Schroeder.
© 2024 John Wiley & Sons, Inc. Published 2024 by John Wiley & Sons, Inc.
Companion website: www.wiley.com/go/lamont/anesthesia

circulating macrophages. Activated macrophages then secrete numerous proinflammatory cytokines that initiate a signaling cascade, leading to the onset of SIRS [9,10]. Interleukin-1 (IL-1) induces fever, increases circulating neutrophils, reduces albumin synthesis, and increases acute phase protein production. Tumor necrosis factor-α (TNFα) stimulates further IL-1 production, neutrophil adhesion, and extravasation and plays a role in the coagulopathy seen during endotoxemia. Interleukin-6 (IL-6) leads to the differentiation of B-lymphocytes into antibody-producing cells and increases the production of acute phase proteins [7]. The release of epinephrine and norepinephrine into the systemic circulation is triggered by LPS, which increases cardiac output and causes tachycardia, pulmonary hypertension, arterial hypoxemia, and tachypnea. Splenic contraction contributes to hemoconcentration in dogs and, likely, in horses [11]. Myocardial dysfunction, characterized by biventricular dilation and reduced ejection fraction, is attributed to increased circulating TNFα [12]. The release of reactive oxygen species by neutrophils increases circulating inflammatory cytokines, like TNFα, and matrix metalloproteinases (MMPs), leading to endothelial glycocalyx degradation. Degradation of the glycocalyx increases vascular permeability to fluid and plasma proteins [12,13]. Circulating inflammatory mediators also result in vascular dysregulation and decreased systemic vascular resistance, leading to systemic hypotension [12]. Increased lactate concentrations, metabolic acidosis, and perfusion-dependent oxygen consumption suggest disruptions in oxygen delivery and cellular metabolism, although the mechanism is not entirely understood [12]. Thus, septic shock has hypovolemic, cardiogenic, and distributive components, contributing to a state of hypoperfusion. Hyperglycemia first occurs due to increased hepatic gluconeogenesis, but glycogen depletion and inhibition of gluconeogenesis lead to hypoglycemia over time. Decreased capillary blood flow and pooling of blood in capillary beds lead to the characteristic congestion of mucous membranes, slow capillary refill time (CRT), and cold extremities commonly found on physical examination [14]. The microvascular clotting induced by acidosis and stagnant circulation, consumption of coagulation factors, and fibrinolysis results in coagulopathy that can evolve into disseminated intravascular coagulation (DIC) [15]. If left untreated, endotoxemia culminates in multiple organ dysfunction syndrome, with the kidney, liver, lung, and heart most vulnerable to failure [7].

No official consensus has defined the clinical features of SIRS in the horse. However, most clinicians have adopted the definition established for human patients [16]. A 2017 study determined the diagnostic criteria for SIRS in the horse through statistical modeling of physical examination and hematological variables. It was found that a heart rate (HR) > 52 beats/min, respiratory rate > 20 breaths/min, leukopenia < 5.0×10^9 cells/L or leukocytosis > 12.5×10^9 cells/L, and a rectal temperature < 37 °C or > 38.5 °C were associated with higher mortality [6]. Based on this definition, researchers found that 30 out of 55 surgical colic horses presenting for emergency laparotomy met the SIRS definition criteria and had almost sevenfold mortality risk than surgical colics that did not meet these criteria. There are several biomarkers used in human medicine to detect sepsis and SIRS. Recently, molecular biomarkers such as MMP-9 [17], protein carbonyl content [18], serum amyloid A [19,20], soluble CD14 [21,22], adrenomedullin, and procalcitonin [23] have been studied in the horse.

Treatment for patients with endotoxemia includes removing the source of infection (including LPS), fluid therapy and cardiovascular support, and inhibition of the inflammatory response. Administration of immunoglobulins against LPS with hyperimmunized J5 equine plasma helps accelerate the clearance of LPS and gram-negative bacteria from the bloodstream [24,25]. Hyperimmunized plasma may also contain acute phase proteins that help inhibit the proinflammatory cytokine cascade, as it seems to reduce TNFα activity [26]. However, at present, there is conflicting evidence of the clinical efficacy and improved survival rate of endotoxemic horses treated with hyperimmunized plasma [27–29]. Polymyxin B is an antimicrobial that is effective against gram-negative bacteria. Its utility lies in its ability to neutralize circulating endotoxin by binding to the lipid A region of LPS, forming a stable, covalently bound compound [30]. Polymyxin B also reduces circulating TNFα, is an antipyretic, and improves tachycardia [31]. However, its use may be limited due to its neurotoxic and nephrotoxic effects [32]. Administration of up to 6000 U/kg intravenously (IV) did not cause changes in adult horses' γ-glutamyl transferase (GGT):creatinine ratio [31,33]. In an *in vitro* endotoxemia model, pentoxifylline, a phosphodiesterase inhibitor, inhibited the activity of TNFα and IL-6 [34]. Horses challenged with LPS after pentoxifylline administration (7.5 mg/kg bolus followed by a 3-h infusion of 3 mg/kg/h) recorded significantly lower rectal temperatures and respiratory rates than the control group [35]. Additionally, when pentoxifylline (8 mg/kg IV) was combined with flunixin meglumine (1.1 mg/kg IV), horses had fewer cardiovascular changes after LPS administration [36]. Non-steroidal anti-inflammatory drugs (NSAIDs) are commonly utilized as a part of the treatment of endotoxemia due to their ability to reduce circulating prostaglandins levels [25]. Flunixin meglumine reduces clinical signs of endotoxemia and reduces the peripheral vascular effects of LPS [37]. The "antiendotoxic dose" (0.25 mg/kg IV) inhibits eicosanoid production without masking clinical signs of colic pain [38]. However, because flunixin meglumine has been shown to inhibit repair of the epithelial barrier in the ischemic bowel via the inhibition of both COX-1 and COX-2 isoenzymes [39], other COX-2 selective NSAIDs, such as meloxicam (0.6 mg/kg IV) [40] and firocoxib, may become preferred alternatives. These NSAIDs cause less intestinal permeability to LPS than flunixin meglumine [41]. Glucocorticoids, such as dexamethasone and prednisolone, inhibit activation of nuclear factor κ-light-chain-enhancer of activated B cells (NF-κB) signaling pathways. However, due to the suspected dysregulation of the hypothalamic–pituitary–adrenal axis, high cortisol levels in foals with sepsis [42], and conflicting results from human literature, they are not routinely used to manage the septic horse [25]. Ethyl pyruvate inhibits the formation of reactive oxygen species and has anti-inflammatory properties [25,43]. Administration of ethyl pyruvate decreased production of TNFα, IL-8, and COX-2 expression in an *in vitro* experimental model [44]. In experimentally induced endotoxemia, ethyl pyruvate (150 mg/kg in 1 L of Lactated Ringer's solution [LRS] infused over 1 h) significantly decreased pain scores and reduced proinflammatory cytokines compared to the control group that received flunixin meglumine (1.1 mg/kg IV) alone [45]. Despite the lack of detrimental effects of ethyl pyruvate in normal horses, it is not widely used in equine colic surgery.

Preanesthetic considerations

Clinical history

The anesthetist should familiarize themselves with the pertinent details of the case. The duration of clinical signs, diagnostics performed, and therapies performed by the referring veterinarian should be reviewed. The timeline and dosages of all medications should be listed. Prior surgical or anesthetic history should be reviewed if available.

Physical examination

The anesthetist should perform a physical examination of the horse prior to induction of anesthesia. Evaluation of vital signs, auscultation of cardiopulmonary structures, and gastrointestinal borborygmi, pulse palpation, and visual examination of mucous membrane color and CRT provide essential information for the anesthetist. In addition, palpation of the ear tips and distal extremities provide insight into perfusion status, as cold limbs and ears are consistent with centralization of circulation seen with septic shock.

The degree of pain and colic behavior should be evaluated in light of the sedative and analgesic agents already administered. Several pain scales can be used to evaluate the horse affected by colic [46–48]. While most horses can be violently painful with ischemic bowel lesions, draft breeds are more likely to behave stoically and mask disease severity within the abdomen. In the authors' experience, horses that initially present with severe pain followed by a sudden decrease in intensity of colic signs are at high risk of gastric or intestinal rupture.

Diagnostics

The anesthetist should be aware of the findings on rectal palpation, the volume of nasogastric reflux, and abnormalities detected via abdominal ultrasound and abdominocentesis. Critical laboratory parameters to evaluate include packed cell volume (PCV) and total solids (TS), lactate, blood glucose, creatinine, complete blood count (CBC), and electrolytes (sodium, potassium, calcium, and magnesium). Hemoconcentration is common in horses with colic. However, a divergence of the PCV and TS, where the PCV is elevated in the face of reduced TS (e.g., PCV 60%, TS 3.4 g/dL), is suggestive of septic shock and more severe disease [13]. Lactate is an important biomarker of the severity of intestinal disease and may provide important prognostic information. Type A lactic acidosis occurs from increased lactate production following hypoperfusion and reduced oxygen delivery, as seen in colic horses due to dehydration, hypovolemia, and shock. Simultaneously, type B lactic acidosis may occur in septic horses due to reduced lactate clearance by the liver [49]. While single lactate values are unreliable prognostic indicators, sequentially increasing lactate values in the face of fluid resuscitation have been associated with increased mortality [50]. Comparison of peritoneal and peripheral lactate values can help diagnose a strangulating versus a non-strangulating lesion. Horses with strangulating lesions have significantly higher peritoneal fluid lactate values than horses with non-strangulating obstructions [51,52]. There is a significantly greater risk of ischemic bowel and mortality when the abdominal fluid has a higher lactate value than the peripheral blood [52–54].

Anesthetic risks and anticipated complications

Given the critical and emergent nature of the surgical colic and the high risk for morbidity, it is crucial to contemplate the potential problems facing the anesthetist. While the basic anesthetic principles of equine anesthesia remain, certain complications are more commonly observed in the horse undergoing exploratory laparotomy.

Hypotension

Hypotension, defined as a systolic arterial pressure less than 90 mmHg (12 kPa) or a mean arterial pressure (MAP) less than 60 mmHg (8 kPa), is a complication commonly observed in horses undergoing emergency exploratory laparotomy. Hypotension has been recognized as a negative predictor of survival to anesthetic recovery [55,56]. Therefore, all horses undergoing colic surgery should have an arterial catheter placed for invasive blood pressure monitoring. This will provide continuous blood pressure measurement and will allow for waveform analysis. Evaluation of the arterial waveform and the plethysmograph waveform during mechanical ventilation can assist the anesthetist in evaluating the severity of the volume deficits and patient fluid responsiveness [57]. A more comprehensive discussion on waveform interpretation and fluid management of the horse undergoing colic surgery is provided later in this chapter.

Many horses undergoing colic surgery arrive at induction dehydrated and hypovolemic, increasing the likelihood of hypotension after induction. Those horses that received prolonged medical management are more likely to be fully fluid resuscitated before induction. However, the violently painful colic patient often does not allow adequate fluid resuscitation before surgery. Endotoxemia and septic shock may also contribute to hypotension in the horse undergoing colic surgery. The vasomotor paralysis with endotoxemia can lead to significant vasodilation and subsequent hypotension [12]. Horses severely endotoxemic at the time of induction are likely to be hypotensive throughout the anesthetic event. Some horses may experience endotoxemic "showers" or episodes as the strangulating lesion is released and blood flow to the ischemic bowel resumes. As a severe drop in blood pressure can happen with surgical correction, the surgical and anesthetic teams should communicate to help anticipate and respond quickly to large swings in the patient's cardiovascular stability.

Iatrogenic cardiovascular depression is an important cause of intraoperative hypotension in colic patients. Horses presented for surgical colic are often sedated and premedicated with α_2-adrenergic receptor agonists like xylazine and detomidine. These agents cause bradycardia and eventually prolonged vasodilation with a significant reduction in the cardiac output [58,59]. Once the horse loses consciousness and the sympathetic drive is inhibited by anesthetic agents, the negative cardiovascular effects of these drugs can become readily apparent. Unfortunately, for the safety of the patient and surgical personnel, and given the lack of reliable sedative alternatives, α_2-adrenergic receptor agonists are a mainstay in equine anesthesia. It is well established that maintenance with inhalant anesthetics contributes significantly to hypotension through their vasodilative and negative inotropic effects [60,61]. Therefore, there is an emphasis on incorporating inhalant-sparing agents in a balanced anesthetic protocol that helps limit the amount of inhalant anesthetic required to maintain a surgical plane of anesthesia. The reader is referred to the section entitled "Adjunct agents" in this chapter.

Another critical factor contributing to hypotension is the compression of vasculature when the horse is placed in dorsal recumbency [62,63]. Tilting the table to Trendelenburg or reverse Trendelenburg positioning does not appear to have a significant effect on arterial blood pressure [64]. In the authors' experience, the adverse effects of recumbency are more severe when the horse is not adequately fluid loaded. While dorsal recumbency is unavoidable in the horse undergoing colic surgery, precious time can be saved by starting to clip and surgically prepare the patient while it is standing or in lateral recumbency.

Intermittent positive-pressure ventilation (IPPV) is yet another contributing factor to hypotension. The positive intrathoracic pressures created with the inspiratory phase compromise venous return of blood to the heart [57,65]. The impairment involves the large veins returning to the right atrium and the pulmonary capillaries. It is reasonable to assume that the severity of the cardiovascular effects of IPPV increases with higher airway pressures and longer inspiratory times. However, there is conflicting evidence in the literature [66,67]. Therefore, the anesthetist must wisely balance the need for mechanical ventilation and its negative impact on cardiovascular function. The decision regarding which system to prioritize will vary from case to case and should be consistently re-evaluated as the case progresses.

Despite fluid administration and position changes, positive inotropes and vasopressors are often needed to maintain acceptable blood pressure in the horse undergoing colic surgery. Dobutamine can be used as an infusion (0.25–2 μg/kg/min) to increase cardiac output, stroke volume, and blood pressure [68,69]. In response to severe vasodilation, phenylephrine (0.25–1 μg/kg/min) or norepinephrine (0.1–1 μg/kg/min) can increase blood pressure through vasoconstriction, increasing the diastolic pressure and reducing venous blood pooling. Norepinephrine may be preferred over phenylephrine as a vasopressor as it may better preserve cardiac output [68,69]. Evaluation of intestinal perfusion demonstrated sustained blood flow through the small intestines, large intestines, and stomach with norepinephrine compared to phenylephrine infusion [69]. During the transition from the induction area to the operating table and from the table to the recovery area, ephedrine (0.05–0.1 mg/kg IV) can be a useful tool to provide both inotropic and vasomotor support, as it is a mixed β_1- and α_1-adrenergic receptor agonist [70]. Ephedrine is effective as a single injection and has a 10–15-min clinical effect. However, the pressure-increasing effect of ephedrine is transient due to its indirect sympathomimetic activity, and it may become ineffective if used in infusion for a prolonged period [71]. In addition, the reader should be aware that ephedrine does cross the blood–brain barrier and may decrease the anesthetic plane of the horse. Adrenergic agent efficacy is reduced in the face of acidemia [72], and vasopressin may be required to increase systemic vascular resistance in this circumstance.

Impaired ventilation–perfusion matching

Absolute or relative hypoxemia is a commonly encountered anesthetic complication in equine anesthesia [73]. In a recent retrospective study, horses undergoing colic surgery were over six times more likely to develop hypoxemia (defined as PaO_2 less than 80 mmHg or 10.6 kPa) than horses undergoing elective procedures [74]. Despite the frequent occurrence of severe blood gas derangements, no study has established a clear association between hypoxemia and an increased risk of mortality in horses [73]. It is worth noting that the above-mentioned retrospective study reported that 32.47% of horses undergoing a hypoxemic event during general anesthesia did not survive discharge from the hospital, compared to 15.49% of those that did not develop hypoxemia [74]. It appears that the gastrointestinal system can tolerate moderate hypoxemia. A recent study found that an arterial hemoglobin saturation with oxygen (SaO_2) of less than 90% led to an initial increase in oxygen extraction to maintain cellular metabolism. However, tissue oxygenation markedly declined when the SaO_2 decreased below 80% [75]. There is conflicting evidence on whether intraoperative hypoxemia increases the risk of surgical site infection in horses undergoing colic surgery. While one study found no link between low PaO_2 and incisional complications [76], another study found that horses with PaO_2 values less than 80 mmHg (10.6 kPa) and anesthesia times longer than 2 h had a greater risk for surgical site infections [77]. Finally, hypoxemia may be associated with higher risk of poor recovery after colic surgery [78].

The underlying cause for the reduced gas exchange in horses undergoing colic surgery is likely multifactorial but primarily due to ventilation–perfusion (V/Q) mismatch and atelectasis [73,79]. Atelectasis can be classified as either compression atelectasis or absorption atelectasis. By nature of the procedure, horses undergoing colic surgery are dorsally recumbent for the duration of surgery. In dorsal recumbency, the abdominal viscera impose significant pressure on the diaphragm [80–82]. This, combined with the reduced inspiratory muscle tone during general anesthesia, results in cranial displacement of the diaphragm causing compression atelectasis [83]. The abdominal distension that accompanies many colic cases exacerbates the compressive effects of dorsal recumbency. Therefore, horses undergoing surgery for large intestinal lesions are at higher risk of developing hypoxemia [74]. Exteriorizing the distended colon is often followed by significant improvements in the PaO_2 [84]. Reverse Trendelenburg position failed to show a benefit on the PaO_2 of horses positioned in dorsal recumbency [64,85,86]. The only exception may be in horses weighing more than 600 kg [86]. Several authors have investigated the effect of lower inspired oxygen fractions (F_IO_2) to reduce the formation of absorption atelectasis [87–90]. From the current body of literature, we can conclude that the use of a higher F_IO_2 in horses during inhalation anesthesia results in a higher PaO_2, but also (and unsurprisingly) a greater alveolar–arterial difference ($P(A\text{-}a)O_2$ gradient) [91]. More evidence is needed to confirm or deny the benefit of reduced F_IO_2 in managing horses undergoing colic surgery.

While a low V/Q ratio is likely the most significant contributor to hypoxemia in the dorsally recumbent horse, areas of increased alveolar dead space, and thus high V/Q ratios, also contribute to poor pulmonary gas exchange. Alveolar dead space increases with poor pulmonary perfusion, seen in reduced cardiac output states [92]. The combination of hypovolemia, cardiovascular side effects from sedatives and anesthetics, and septic shock all contribute to a state of hypoperfusion. Adding an inspiratory pause of 30% of the inspiratory time may improve dead space in dorsally recumbent horses, but its clinical value is still unclear [93].

The anesthetist should prepare to monitor the patient for the onset and progression of hypoxemia and gather the necessary equipment to intervene if hypoxemia arises. Pulse oximetry is a widely available and non-invasive tool for measuring hemoglobin saturation and should be routinely used. Though there are species differences in the oxyhemoglobin dissociation curve [94], a SpO_2 reading of 90% corresponds approximately to a PaO_2 of 60 mmHg (8 kPa). As the SpO_2 drops further, arterial oxygen content precipitously decreases, warranting intervention [73]. The pulse oximeter is a sensitive and valuable monitoring tool to detect hypoxemia when the horse is breathing room air (as occurs before connection to the anesthesia machine or during the recovery phase). However, when the animal is under general anesthesia and maintained with an F_IO_2 of 1.0 (100%), the pulse oximeter only signals if the problem is already severe. As a result, it is recommended to routinely perform serial arterial blood gas analysis in the horse undergoing colic surgery. General guidelines suggest an arterial blood sample should be taken 30 min after induction and then every 90–120 min in a stable case or every 45–60 min in a metabolically unstable case [95]. The PaO_2 value obtained by blood gas analysis provides an objective measure of pulmonary gas exchange that can be tracked over time and used to evaluate the effectiveness of various interventions.

Most treatments for hypoxemia aim to improve V/Q matching. A quick laparotomy incision and exteriorization of the colon reduce the compressive forces of the abdomen and limit the further development of compression atelectasis [84]. The open lung ventilation technique combines IPPV with intermittent alveolar recruitment maneuvers and positive end-expiratory pressure (PEEP) [96,97]. In 30 warmblood horses anesthetized for colic surgery, 15 were mechanically ventilated with a 15–20 mL/kg tidal volume, 1:2 inspiratory to expiratory time (I:E) ratio and a peak inspiratory pressure (PIP) of 30–45 cmH_2O, while 15 received similar ventilation with the addition of 15–25 cmH_2O PEEP and intermittent alveolar recruitment maneuvers up to 80 cmH_2O (open lung concept). Horses receiving open lung concept ventilation recorded significantly higher PaO_2 values (300–450 mmHg; 40–60 kPa) compared to the control group (100–240 mmHg; 13.3–32 kPa) [98]. In an additional study performed on 24 warmblood horses anesthetized for colic surgery, the treatment group that received IPPV with 10 cmH_2O PEEP and intermittent alveolar recruitment maneuvers recorded significantly higher PaO_2 values and shorter recovery times than the control group [96].

Aerosolized albuterol can be utilized in the hypoxemic colic patient. An earlier study found a twofold increase in PaO_2 within 20 min of a 2 μg/kg albuterol dose administered via the endotracheal tube in horses with an initial PaO_2 less than 70 mmHg (9.3 kPa) [99]. However, the reader should be aware that the improvement in PaO_2 is inconsistent [100]. The underlying mechanism is poorly understood and could be attributed to bronchodilation (via β_2-adrenergic stimulation), improved cardiac output (via β_1-adrenergic stimulation), or a combination of both effects. Finally, pulsed inhaled nitric oxide (NO) has shown promising results. Inhaled NO is delivered to the actively ventilated alveoli, causing selective pulmonary vasodilation and improving V/Q matching at its source [101,102]. An inhaled dose of 2000 ppm NO in nitrogen reduced the pulmonary shunt fraction and improved horses' PaO_2 [103,104]. Unfortunately, the delivery of inhaled NO is not widely available in most equine hospitals at this time.

Arrhythmias

There is limited research on the occurrence of cardiac arrhythmias in horses undergoing colic surgery. Sinus tachycardia (HR > 55 beats/min) is the most common arrhythmia encountered in colic patients and has several underlying causes, including distension of the viscera, pain, and endotoxemia [7]. While hypovolemia and decreased cardiac return are common causes of sinus tachycardia in other species, the literature suggests that the HR in the anesthetized horse is less responsive to acute blood volume changes [105]. A 2014 study evaluated the cardiac rhythm in conscious colic horses over a 24-h hospitalization period. Atrioventricular (AV) block and atrial premature complexes (APCs) occurred in both colic and healthy horses, although ventricular premature complexes (VPCs) only occurred in horses experiencing colic [106]. In a model of experimentally induced endotoxemia, VPCs were observed after the LPS injection [107]. Though not completely understood, VPCs are likely the result of increased sympathetic tone and circulating inflammatory cytokines [108]. Sporadic VPCs are self-limiting and rarely require intervention, but in the case of runs of VPCs or multifocal VPCs, treatment with lidocaine should be initiated. Bradycardia and AV blocks are sometimes observed under general anesthesia in colic horses, most commonly at the beginning of the anesthetic event. They are usually attributed to α_2-adrenergic receptor agonist administration and are typically self-limiting. If severe bradycardia (HR < 20 beats/min) is accompanied by hypotension, an anticholinergic like atropine (0.01–0.02 mg/kg IV), glycopyrrolate (0.005–0.01 mg/kg IV), or hyoscine *N*-butylbromide (0.05–0.1 mg/kg IV) [109] can be administered. However, long-lasting anticholinergics should generally be avoided in the horse due to the potential for impaired gastrointestinal motility [110]. Dobutamine can also be utilized as a positive chronotrope, although this requires higher dose rates (> 5 μg/kg/min) than are typically used for hemodynamic support [111].

Postanesthetic myopathy and neuropathy

An early study showed that one of 84 horses (1.2%) undergoing colic surgery developed postoperative myopathy [112]. In a 2016 retrospective analysis concerning mortality rates associated with equine anesthesia for elective and emergency cases, one horse was euthanized for postanesthetic myopathy/neuropathy, and nine horses had non-fatal myopathy/neuropathy, accounting for 7% of fatal and 20% of non-fatal recovery complications, respectively [113]. This study did not explore the relative risk of postanesthetic myopathy in emergency cases compared to elective cases. However, postoperative myopathy tends to occur with prolonged recumbency, typically combined with muscle hypoperfusion [114]. For this reason, horses undergoing colic surgery may be at higher risk of developing neuromyopathies compared to horses undergoing elective procedures. Prevention of postanesthetic myopathy and neuropathy is more effective than treatment. Horses undergoing prolonged anesthesia in a supine position should be placed on protective cushioned padding, the nose should be slightly elevated to minimize development of nasal edema, and the head, limbs, and pressure points should be properly padded. Proper positioning on the operating table and ensuring the hind limbs are not left in an extended position can help reduce the risk of peroneal and femoral nerve injury [112]. Postsurgical myopathy significantly hinders successful recovery, and such horses may need to be recovered with a sling. Treatment is mainly based on medical management and supportive care. In the worst cases, euthanasia may be the only remaining option.

Preparation of the surgical area

The time between the colic horse's arrival to the hospital and the decision to proceed with colic surgery can be very short. Therefore, it should come as no surprise that thorough preparation by the anesthetist prior to the horse's arrival is required to keep the process organized and efficient. An induction station or room should be designated as an emergency area reserved for patients with colic and, if possible, should be distinct from the area used for orthopedic cases to prevent contamination. This area can be set up ahead of time with everything needed (Box 62.1). The anesthesia machine should be left pressure checked, the inhalant anesthetic refilled, and the carbon dioxide absorbent should be fresh. The ventilator should be assembled, and a PEEP valve at hand. Positive inotropes and vasopressors should be ready in small fluid bags, attached to primed fluid sets, and assembled in volumetric pumps if available. A large bore fluid administration set and 5 L crystalloid fluid bags should be readily available. All material, including endotracheal tubes, catheters, fluids, arterial line supplies, etc., should be prepared to save valuable time once the horse arrives.

Box 62.1 Minimal anesthetic equipment to prepare in advance for the horse to be anesthetized for emergent exploratory laparotomy (i.e., colic).

- Anesthesia machine and ventilator set up and pressure checked
- Multiparameter monitor, including ECG, SpO_2, IBP, $P_{ET}CO_2$, and (if available) agent analysis and temperature
- A bucket of water and large syringe
- Induction halter and ropes
- Appropriate size endotracheal tubes, mouth gag and water based lubricant
- Hoist hobbles
- Several IV catheters including arterial (18–22 gauge) and intravenous (10–14 gauge) catheter supplies
- Primed pressure transducer
- Preheparinized syringes for arterial blood gas sampling
- Blood gas analyzer
- Several 5 L bags of balanced crystalloid fluids
- Large bore fluid administration sets
- Hypertonic saline
- Synthetic colloids (if available)
- Calcium gluconate
- Potassium chloride
- Aerosolized albuterol
- Dobutamine and norepinephrine infusions. The drip rates for the inotropic and vasopressor infusions should be precalculated or the volumetric pump should be programmed and left in standby

Stabilization and fluid resuscitation

Fluid administration should be started before anesthesia induction (or immediately after) to correct fluid, acid–base, and electrolyte derangements. In critically ill patients, the authors prefer to place at least one large-gauge (10–14 gauge) jugular catheter per side before induction of anesthesia. A second jugular venous catheter can be used to maximize the fluid administration rate or to administer blood products, like hyperimmunized plasma. While not commonly used, the lateral thoracic vein may be another valuable access point for rapid administration of fluids during anesthesia. The lateral branch of the saphenous vein can be catheterized in the neonatal foal [115]. The anesthetist should address two questions when administering fluids:

1 Which fluid type should be used for resuscitation?
2 How much volume should be administered?

The type of fluids relies on the anesthetist's final goal and a single fluid type alone is rarely used. For example, crystalloids can be used for tissue rehydration and correction of acid–base and electrolyte abnormalities. Synthetic colloids (e.g., 6% Hetastarch [HES]) can be used for increasing the colloid osmotic pressure (COP). Guidelines set by the Surviving Sepsis Campaign (SSC) in 2021 suggest that at least 30 mL/kg of IV isotonic crystalloid fluid should be given within the first 3 h of resuscitation in human patients with sepsis-induced hypoperfusion or septic shock. The guidelines also caution against the use of saline for resuscitation, as the resulting hyperchloremic metabolic acidosis has been associated with increased mortality [116]. The prescribed volume corresponds to approximately 15 L for a 500 kg horse, which may be logistically difficult to achieve prior to anesthesia. Instead, small-volume resuscitation using hypertonic saline solution (HSS), usually at concentrations between 7.2–7.5%, followed by a colloid can achieve similar or superior volume expansion utilizing much smaller volumes than crystalloids alone. The rationale involves using the high osmolality of HSS (2400 mOsm/L) to draw fluids from the extravascular space into the circulation, causing rapid volume expansion and restoring preload while improving cardiac output and perfusion [117,118]. Other effects of HSS beneficial to the horse undergoing colic surgery include protection against inflammation, injury, and impaired intestinal transit [119]. While beneficial, the effect of HSS is short-lived because, as a crystalloid, it redistributes in the extravascular space within 60–120 min [120]. The addition of a colloid is intended to prolong the plasma expansion effects of HSS through the improvement of the COP [121–124]. Increased COP persisted for up to 24 h after administration of 8–10 mL/kg of HES in hypoproteinemic horses [124] and the effect was slightly longer in healthy horses [123]. More recent studies suggest that the plasma expansion effect of colloids is not a result of fluid resorption from the interstitial space but rather due to interaction with the non-circulating portion of the intravascular fluid, the glycocalyx. Colloids bind to the glycocalyx increasing its COP and limiting the transendothelial flow of fluids [125]. For this reason, the effectiveness of colloids as plasma volume expanders is thought to be dependent on an intact glycocalyx. This means that under conditions of increased permeability such as sepsis, the plasma expansion effect of colloids is reduced. Controversies still exist regarding the clinical effectiveness of colloids versus crystalloids for fluid resuscitation in horses. It is known that in horses undergoing colic surgery, COP decreases proportionally with the decrease in total protein throughout anesthesia with the administration of 15–25 mL/kg/h of LRS [126]. In a recent clinical study comparing the effects of 6 mL/kg of pentastarch (10% HES) to an equal volume of LRS in horses undergoing elective surgical procedures, 10% HES improved hemodilution, corrected the decreased COP observed with LRS administration, and maintained better blood pressures through anesthesia [122]. However, an early study comparing resuscitation after experimentally induced endotoxemia using 5 mL/kg or 60 mL/kg of a balanced polyionic crystalloid solution, or 5 mL/kg of HSS followed by 10 mL/kg of 6% HES failed to show a difference in cardiovascular and pulmonary effects between the three treatments [127]. These findings corroborate the theory that the effectiveness of colloids as plasma expanders is less apparent in diseased horses than in healthy horses. In the 2016 SSC, a strong recommendation was issued against using starches for resuscitation, as they increased the risk of renal replacement therapy and death in adult patients with sepsis or septic shock [128]. But a recent human systemic review found little to no difference in the mortality rate in critically ill patients (including trauma, burns, and sepsis) using synthetic colloids or crystalloids for fluid volume resuscitation [129]. No strong evidence exists for horses undergoing colic surgery. In one report, long-term postoperative mortality in horses undergoing emergency exploratory laparotomy was not statistically different following preoperative 10% HES administration versus HSS [130]. Other risks associated with the use of synthetic colloids are the potential for allergic reactions and coagulopathy. In an early study in healthy ponies receiving 6% HES, decreases in fibrinogen concentration, von Willebrand factor antigen, and factor VIII were reported; counterintuitively, reductions in both activated partial thromboplastin time and prothrombin time were also documented [131]. In healthy horses, tetrastarch (6% HES 130/0.4) showed fewer adverse effects and affected platelet function for a shorter period compared to hetastarch (6% HES 670/0.75) [123]. However, there is no mention of bleeding tendency or clinically relevant changes in coagulation parameters in any of the equine reports. The 2021 SSC suggested using albumin in patients that received a large volume of crystalloids instead of using crystalloids alone [128]. Little evidence exists on the use of natural colloids in horses. In one small study, 8 mL/kg of 5% equine albumin solution in 0.9% saline did not significantly change the COP of horses with colic compared to a control group [130]. The authors prefer to administer 2–4 mL/kg of HSS before or immediately after induction of general anesthesia, along with a balanced polyionic crystalloid solution, then add colloids (5–10 mL/kg of 6% HES or plasma), to reduce the total volume needed for resuscitation.

For a long time, there was a tendency to treat horses undergoing colic surgery with very aggressive fluid therapy rates. The concept of fluid overload, while commonly recognized as an issue in human and small animal anesthesia, has been largely ignored in equine anesthesia. We now know that aggressive fluid therapy is associated with tissue edema (including pulmonary edema), impaired wound healing, compromised renal function, and increased mortality in septic and postoperative patients [132]. Muzzle and periorbital edema were observed in 83% of horses with experimentally induced endotoxemia that received high infusion rates of an isotonic polyionic crystalloid solution compared to none of the horses that received HSS–HES [127]. Moreover, a recent case-control retrospective study suggested that larger volumes of fluids administered under anesthesia may be associated with developing postoperative reflux in horses undergoing colic surgery [133]. In human and small animal fluid therapy, the concept of Early Goal-Directed Resuscitation has been embraced [134]. The idea behind it is the stepwise administration of fluids until normalization of perfusion indicators such as pulse rate and quality, CRT, central venous pressure (CVP), MAP, and urine output. Microvascular variables include pH, base excess/base deficit (BE/BD) systemic lactate, and central venous oxygen saturation (SvO_2). While some of these variables can be easily assessed in the horse undergoing general anesthesia for exploratory laparotomy, others are not routinely measured. In addition, it is worth noting that some of these variables (e.g., CVP and urine output) are affected by general anesthesia and mechanical ventilation; hence, their clinical value is reduced in the anesthetized compared to the awake horse. The fluid therapy plan needs to account for: (1) the horse's daily needs, (2) the hydration status, (3) the ongoing fluid losses, and (4) any acid–base derangement.

In an adult horse, fluid requirements are usually estimated to be 2–4 mL/kg/h (or 40–60 mL/kg/day) [135]. The maintenance fluid requirement for a neonatal foal is higher than an adult and can be estimated at 3–5 mL/kg/h [136]. In equids, the gastrointestinal tract serves as a large reservoir of body water, accounting for approximately 20% of the total body water content [137]. As such, gastrointestinal derangement can cause significant and rapid water losses. Water losses through dehydration are estimated as percent dehydration. Physical examination parameters such as mucous membrane moisture, skin turgor, and relative position of the globe are used to estimate the degree of dehydration. Several charts and tables exist to estimate dehydration based on clinical parameters (Table 62.1). However, more recent findings have questioned the validity of such clinical and behavioral methods for assessing water losses [138,139]. In addition to these needs, any patient experiencing ongoing losses, such as nasogastric reflux, diarrhea, or third-space losses, will require replacement of these volumes to maintain normal fluid balance.

Metabolic acidosis occurs frequently in horses with gastrointestinal dysfunction. Severe acidosis can result in myocardial dysfunction, decreased cardiac output, and hypotension [140]. It also inhibits the binding of norepinephrine to adrenergic receptors [140,141]. Chloride deficient metabolic alkalosis can also be observed in horses experiencing abundant nasogastric reflux. Acid–base and electrolyte imbalances should be corrected before or during anesthesia. Metabolic acidosis can improve with administration

Table 62.1 Estimation of dehydration of the horse based on clinical signs.

Clinical signs	Mild (4–6%)	Moderate (7–9%)	Severe (> 10%)
Capillary refill time	1–2 s	2–4 s	>4 s
Mucous membranes	Fair	Tacky	Dry
Skin tenting	2–3 s	3–5 s	>5 s
PCV (%)	40–50	50–65	>65
TP (g/dL)	6.5–7.5	7.5–8.5	>8.5

Table 62.2 Recommendations for calculating isotonic polyionic crystalloid solution administration and electrolyte replacement.

Factor	Formula	Example for a 500 kg horse
Daily maintenance	2–4 mL/kg/h (or 40–60 mL/kg/day) Increase to 75–80 mL/kg/day for a neonatal foal	500 × 50 mL/kg/day = 25 L
Dehydration	Body weight (kg) × % dehydration	500 × 7% = 35 L
Ongoing fluid losses	Estimate the volume (L) lost to nasogastric reflux, diarrhea, or third-space losses and add it to the total volume to be replaced	
Bicarbonate administration	Body weight (kg) × (24 – HCO_3) × 0.3 or 1–2 mEq/kg	500 × (24 – 15) × 0.3 = 1350 mEq of $NaHCO_3$
KCl (2 mEq/mL)	20–40 mEq/L of crystalloids Not to exceed 0.5 mEq/kg/h	
Calcium gluconate 10% (23%)	0.1–0.5 (0.05–0.2) mL/kg over 30–60 min Monitor heart rate	

of polyionic balanced crystalloid solutions. Sodium bicarbonate ($NaHCO_3$) administration in the face of metabolic acidosis that is not caused by bicarbonate loss is controversial and is unlikely to improve survival [142]. However, if the total HCO_3 is less than 12 mmol/L or BE is less than −11 mmol/L, bicarbonate therapy is indicated. The amount of $NaHCO_3$ needed to correct acidosis can be calculated (Table 62.2). A quarter to half the calculated dose should be administered over 30 min to 1 h, and acid–base status should be reassessed. The authors prefer to correct pH to 7.2, to avoid overcorrection or side effects like paradoxical brain acidosis, reduced cardiac contractility, hypernatremia, and hyperosmolarity. In a study comparing electrolyte derangements in colic versus healthy horses, the colic group recorded significantly lower potassium, ionized calcium, and magnesium concentrations [143]. Hypocalcemia occurs in 53–86% of horses undergoing colic surgery [143–145]. Suspected underlying causes include endotoxemia, reduced feed intake, fluid therapy, and metabolic acidosis [145,146]. Hypocalcemia contributes to myocardial dysfunction and reduced vasomotor tone, requiring more aggressive vasopressor therapy than in normocalcemic patients [147]. Hypocalcemia can cause muscle weakness, tachycardia, hypotension and may contribute to postoperative ileus (POI) [148]. Calcium administration remains controversial. While some studies have demonstrated improved cardiac function with calcium supplementation in a rodent model of sepsis, others have shown increased mortality with no significant difference in cardiovascular performance [149–151]. Therefore, the authors usually advocate treatment when ionized calcium drops below 1–1.2 mmol/L. Calcium gluconate 10% can be administered at a dose ranging between 0.1 and 0.5 mL/kg (or calcium gluconate 23% at 0.05–0.2 mL/kg). Hypokalemia has been reported in 30% of horses presenting for colic surgery [144]. Horses with obstructive or ischemic bowel had significantly lower potassium values than the control group [143]. Potassium can be reduced due to anorexia, pain, gastrointestinal reflux, enterocolitis, and sodium-induced diuresis [148,152]. Because potassium is an intracellular electrolyte, if potassium is low in the face of acidosis, the total deficit is likely to be severe. Hypokalemia can be treated with 0.04–0.08 mEq/kg/L (or adding 20–40 mEq of KCl in each L of balanced crystalloids solution). The dose should not exceed 0.5 mEq/kg/h. Guidelines for isotonic polyionic crystalloid solution administration and electrolyte correction are summarized in Table 62.2.

Anesthetic protocol

There is no unique or standardized anesthetic protocol for horses undergoing colic surgery. The circumstances, familiarity of use and personal preference, availability, and the critical status of the patient will primarily dictate the protocol to use. The anesthetist's goal is to induce unconsciousness, myorelaxation, and surgical antinociception while reducing cardiopulmonary compromise and improving perioperative outcome. For more information about the pharmacology of specific sedative or anesthetic drugs, the reader is referred elsewhere in this book. The current chapter focuses on the specific situation of the horse undergoing general anesthesia for emergent exploratory laparotomy.

Premedication

An α_2-adrenergic receptor agonist, with or without an opioid, is almost universally used for the premedication of adult horses with colic. Xylazine or detomidine can provide relief to horses experiencing mild to moderate colic pain, and for this reason, these drugs are often used during the perioperative management of the colic patient. In cases of severe colic pain, however, α_2-adrenergic receptor agonists are often not adequate. Furthermore, repeated doses of α_2-adrenergic receptor agonists may cause excessive sedation, further cardiovascular depression, and a prolonged decrease in gastrointestinal motility in horses undergoing general anesthesia [153–156]. However, a recent study demonstrated no association between the drugs used for premedication and the incidence of postoperative gastrointestinal dysfunction in horses undergoing general anesthesia for elective procedures [157]. A little more controversial is the use of perioperative opioids, and this is rooted in three main concerns: the possibility that opioids may cause excitation; the fear that the use of perioperative full μ-opioid receptor agonists may decrease gastrointestinal motility; and the insufficient or conflicting data on the analgesic efficacy of full μ-opioid receptor agonists in horses with naturally occurring colic. Excitation, ranging from "muzzle tremors, muscle twitching, head jerks, head pressing" to "pacing, vocalizing, rearing and kicking," has been seen in pain-free horses [158–161]. In the authors' experience, these excitatory effects are uncommonly seen at clinically relevant doses, in painful animals, with concurrent administration of an α_2-adrenergic receptor agonist. While both full μ-opioid receptor agonists and κ-opioid receptor agonists have been associated with decreased fecal output or fecal weight or both [160,162,163], postanesthetic signs of colic or POI have never been clearly associated with the use of perioperative opioids [157,164]. Finally, early experimental studies assessing the analgesic effects of opioids in non-painful horses relied on motor responses as the experimental endpoint and, as such, these studies were probably confounded by opioid excitatory behavior in this species [158]. Studies using electrophysiologic methods, such as nociceptive withdrawal reflex and temporal summation [165,166], or quantitative sensory testing have demonstrated analgesic properties of full μ-opioid receptor agonists in conscious horses [161,162,167]. In the authors' experience, the perioperative use of morphine, hydromorphone, or methadone in horses undergoing colic surgery may improve perioperative analgesia with minimal gastrointestinal effects and without affecting the quality of recovery.

Induction and intubation

Various methods are used to induce and intubate horses undergoing emergency exploratory laparotomy. Swinging gates to help hold the horse against a wall and free fall with human support of the head are probably the most common current techniques used. However, some hospitals still use a vertical tilting table (Fig. 62.1).

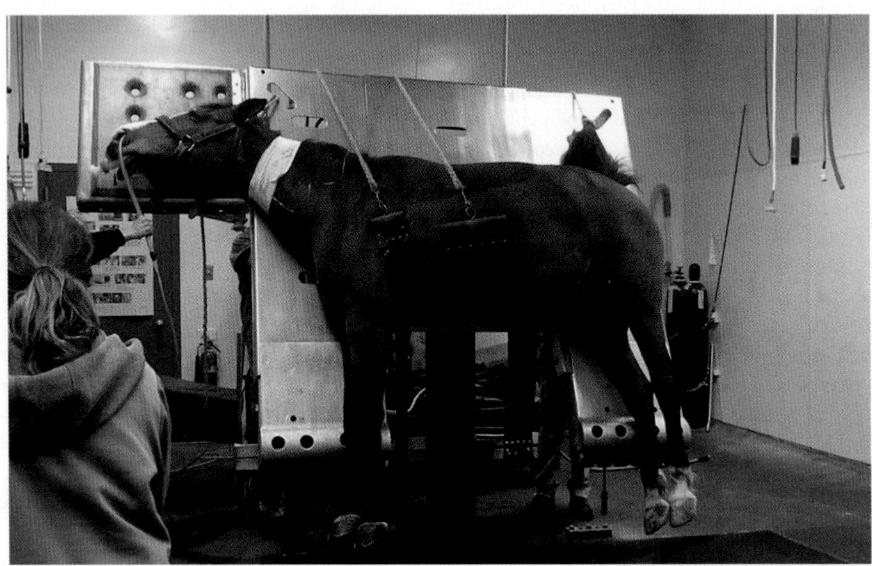

Figure 62.1 Purpose-built equine tilting tables were historically popular and may remain in some equine hospitals. The horse is sedated and strapped to the table before induction. This system, while cumbersome, is meant to reduce trauma and injuries during induction. Source: Dr. Alessia Cenani, with permission.

Immediate induction of anesthesia may be necessary in severely painful horses. Based on the clinician's preference, the nasogastric tube will be left in place or not. Some clinicians believe that leaving the nasogastric tube in place reduces the risk of gastric rupture caused by increased pressure within the stomach when the horse becomes recumbent. However, other clinicians believe that gastric rupture is still likely, and the risk of regurgitation increases if the tube is left in place, because of disruption of the lower esophageal sphincter seal. These authors prefer to reflux the horse one last time immediately before induction and then pull the nasogastric tube.

Combinations of ketamine (2.2–3 mg/kg) with a myorelaxant, either a benzodiazepine (midazolam or diazepam, 0.05–0.1 mg/kg) or guaifenesin, are commonly used to induce anesthesia in horses undergoing exploratory laparotomy. Thiopental is no longer available in the United States but is still used for equine induction in other countries. Due to the long half-life of midazolam in horses [168], diazepam and propofol (0.5 mg/kg) [169] have been proposed as alternatives to reduce the risk of postoperative ataxia on recovery. Evidence supporting the use of one protocol over another is weak [170,171]. In addition, reversal of midazolam with either low- or high-dose flumazenil did not improve recovery quality in a recent study [172]. Some clinicians prefer to maintain the horse in sternal recumbency until the trachea is intubated and the endotracheal tube cuff is inflated (Fig. 62.2). The rationale is to secure the airway against passive gastric reflux [173]. After securing the airway, the anesthetist should quickly confirm the patient's pulse or HR as cardiac arrest is not uncommon in horses with colic.

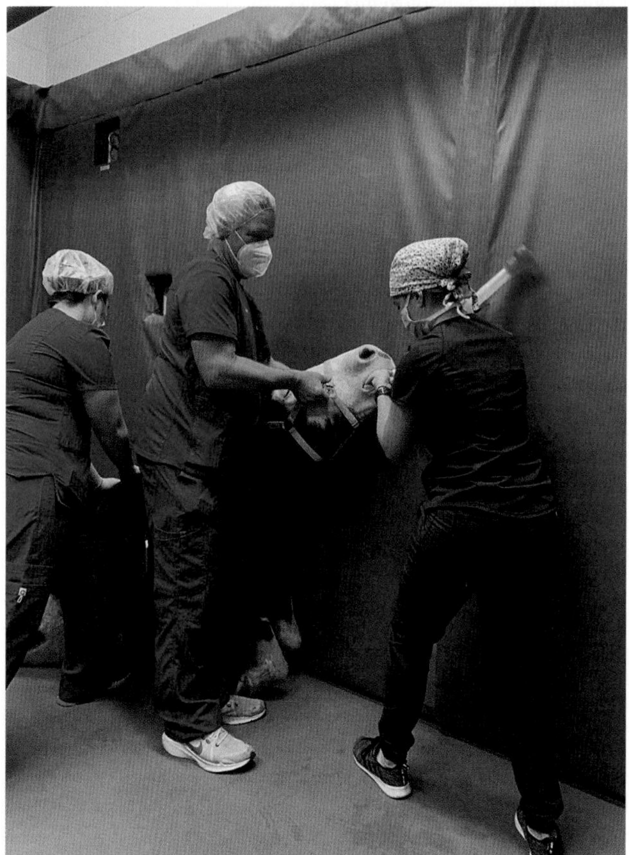

Figure 62.2 Sternal intubation allows the anesthetist to secure the airway against passive gastric reflux before the horse is hoisted to the surgical table. Source: Dr. Ludovica Chiavaccini, with permission.

Maintenance of anesthesia

Some surgeons still elect to roll horses in an attempt to correct a left dorsal colon displacement (nephrosplenic entrapment). This procedure is commonly performed using total intravenous anesthesia (TIVA). Different protocols have been published and the selection of one drug combination over another depends largely on the comfort level of the anesthetist, drug availability, personnel and equipment available and, importantly, the expected duration of the procedure. A combination of ketamine and an α_2-adrenergic receptor agonist, with or without a myorelaxant (guaifenesin or midazolam) is commonly used. In these cases, phenylephrine is administered prior to anesthesia to cause splenic contraction and facilitate correction [174]. In one study, the spleen was reduced to 28% of baseline, with acceptable cardiovascular side effects, after the administration of phenylephrine at 3 μg/kg/min over 15 min [175].

In the vast majority of cases, after induction, horses undergoing exploratory laparotomy are connected to the anesthetic breathing circuit and maintained with inhalation agents with or without adjunct drugs. The choice of inhalant anesthetic agent is usually at the discretion of the anesthetist. While hemodynamic and pulmonary indices during sevoflurane and isoflurane anesthesia appear similar in horses [176], in 39 horses undergoing elective procedures in lateral recumbency, less dobutamine was required to maintain MAP > 70 mmHg (9.3 kPa) during sevoflurane anesthesia when compared to isoflurane anesthesia [177].

The recommendations on correct positioning and appropriate padding apply to any horse undergoing general anesthesia, and especially to horses undergoing colic surgery. In addition, COP decreases linearly during anesthesia for colic surgery, reaching the lowest point at the end of anesthesia with a mean COP of 11.6 ± 1.6 mmHg (1.55 ± 0.21 kPa) [126,178]. This change may predispose the horse to nasal edema and tissue edema. For this reason, it is important to elevate the head above the heart level and to administer phenylephrine or another nasal decongestant before recovery [179]. If reflux around the nasogastric tube is noted, the tip of the nose should be directed down toward the ground to facilitate drainage and the animal should be recovered with the endotracheal tube in place.

Adjunct agents

Adjunct agents have been long used in horses with three main goals: to reduce inhalant requirements in an attempt to improve cardiovascular function and hasten recovery; to provide additional analgesia; and to improve recovery quality.

Benzodiazepines, like midazolam or diazepam, demonstrate a consistent minimum alveolar concentration (MAC)-sparing effect effect in the horse and lack significant cardio-depressant effects [180]. However, they lack analgesic properties and may weaken recovery attempts [169,171].

Lidocaine causes dose-dependent MAC reduction of inhaled anesthetics in both ponies [181] and horses [181–184]. However, under experimental conditions, lidocaine infusion showed contradictory effects on the cardiovascular performance of horses at comparable anesthetic depths [184–187]. Adverse effects were not mentioned in any of the aforementioned studies; nonetheless there is evidence that lidocaine infusions alone may lower the quality of recovery [188]. This could be a consequence of the fact that lidocaine reaches higher plasma concentrations than predicted in anesthetized horses under experimental conditions or those undergoing emergent exploratory laparotomy [186,189,190]. Consequently, the dose of lidocaine should be reduced in the horse anesthetized for colic surgery (especially when the horse is severely dehydrated or has compromised cardiovascular function), and the infusion should be discontinued 30 min before the end of anesthesia [188,189]. IV lidocaine administration produces analgesia in various pain states, such as neuropathic and acute pain. Proposed mechanisms of action and potential therapeutic benefits of lidocaine in horses have been recently reviewed [191,192], and its clinical pharmacology is presented in Chapter 29. The visceral analgesic effects of lidocaine have been demonstrated in rats [193,194] and humans [195,196]. Somatic antinociception, but only mild visceral antinociception, was observed in conscious horses receiving systemic lidocaine infusion [197]. However, the investigators pointed out that the horses in the study had normal gastrointestinal tracts with no inflammation or sensitization, and the methodology or the dose used may have not been appropriate. For a long time, lidocaine has been advocated to improve intestinal motility and treat POI; however, studies investigating the prokinetic properties of lidocaine have reported conflicting results. Perioperative lidocaine administration to horses undergoing colic surgery was associated with better postoperative jejunal cross-sectional area scores, jejunal diameter scores, and intestinal ultrasound index, compared to the saline treatment, suggesting that lidocaine may have some beneficial effects in this population [198]. However, the study did not look specifically at horses with small intestinal lesions or gastroesophageal reflux. In one study comparing lidocaine to placebo in 32 horses affected by POI or enteritis, a higher proportion of horses treated with lidocaine than with placebo stopped refluxing within 30 h. Horses that responded to lidocaine passed feces within 16 h from the beginning of the infusion and had shorter hospitalizations [199]. In a recent retrospective study, however, the use of perioperative lidocaine did not affect the total reflux volume or duration of reflux in horses undergoing colic surgery [200]. Despite the conflicting evidence, a survey of European Equine Internal Medicine and Surgery Diplomates reported that lidocaine was the drug used most commonly in the postoperative period to prevent POI (used by 67% of respondents) and was also the drug of choice for management of POI (used by 79% of respondents) [201]. Finally, lidocaine has well-known anti-inflammatory properties [202–204]. The mechanism by which lidocaine decreases neutrophil activation and transmigration is not fully understood but may go beyond the blockade of voltage-gated sodium channels. In horses with experimentally induced ischemia of the jejunum, lidocaine mitigated the inhibitory effects of flunixin meglumine on recovery of the ischemia injured mucosa [205] and reduced neutrophil infiltration compared to flunixin alone [206]. However, a recent equine experimental study failed to demonstrate that lidocaine was consistently able to reduce neutrophil infiltration both at the site of ischemic injury and in remote non-manipulated intestine [207].

Balanced anesthesia techniques in horses often include using α_2-adrenergic receptor agonists (xylazine, romifidine, medetomidine, dexmedetomidine, or detomidine). Among α_2-adrenergic receptor agonists, the short half-lives of medetomidine and dexmedetomidine, and their lack of accumulation, make them ideal candidates for perianesthetic infusions [208,209]. At clinically relevant doses, α_2-adrenergic receptor agonists can reduce the MAC of inhalant anesthetics by up to 40% [210,211]. This is in contrast to opioid agonists both in terms of consistency and magnitude of effect. A clinical study of 20 healthy horses undergoing elective procedures showed that an intraoperative dexmedetomidine infusion at 1.75 μg/kg/h produced more stable anesthetic depth, reduced isoflurane requirements, and provided better quality recoveries when compared to a morphine infusion at 0.1 mg/kg/h [212]. Moreover, α_2-adrenergic receptor agonists reduce global perfusion, global oxygen delivery, and intestinal perfusion while maintaining intestinal oxygenation [213], whereas both perfusion and oxygenation of the gastrointestinal tract decrease rapidly when end-expiratory isoflurane concentrations increase above 2%. It is still controversial whether the MAC-sparing effects of α_2-adrenergic receptor agonists result in better cardiovascular function compared to volatile anesthetics alone at equipotent doses [210,211,214–218]. More attractive properties of α_2-adrenergic receptor agonists for horses undergoing colic surgery are their visceral analgesic qualities and the potential beneficial effects on the systemic inflammatory response. The visceral analgesic properties of α_2-adrenergic receptor agonists are well known [219] and involve all three α_2-adrenergic receptor subtypes (α_{2A}, α_{2B}, and α_{2C}) [220]. In a multicenter clinical study involving 152 horses presenting with colic, detomidine proved to be a more effective analgesic than xylazine, butorphanol, and flunixin meglumine [221]. The analgesia in horses with gastrointestinal disease may be partly due to suppression of gastroenteric motility, and this profound effect must be considered when quick recovery of intestinal contractility is warranted [222]. Dexmedetomidine has also gained attention for its anti-inflammatory and antiapoptotic properties after ischemia-reperfusion injury in multiple tissues, including the equine small intestine [223–226]. Xylazine showed similar beneficial effects at clinically relevant doses in an experimental model of equine jejunal ischemia [227]. In addition, a dexmedetomidine infusion, accompanied by a 40% reduction in sevoflurane MAC, appeared to maintain cardiopulmonary and intestinal hemodynamics and improve acid–base status in anesthetized horses with experimentally induced endotoxemia [211].

Ketamine is a well-known noncompetitive antagonist of the *N*-methyl-D-aspartate (NMDA) receptor in the central nervous system. In addition, ketamine acts on many other non-NMDA pathways, including opioid receptors, nicotinic and muscarinic cholinergic receptors, high-affinity D_2 dopamine receptors, and L-type voltage-gated calcium channels; it also blocks sodium and potassium channels and facilitates γ-aminobutyric acid receptor subtype A ($GABA_A$) signaling. All of these different pathways may contribute variably to the drug's analgesic effects [228,229]. Ketamine alone or in combination with lidocaine and opioid analgesics reduces the MAC of inhalant anesthetics up to 50% [230]. In addition, although ketamine exerts direct myocardial depression, clinically administered doses of racemic ketamine are associated with better cardiovascular performance [230,232]. The antihyperalgesic effects of ketamine have been demonstrated in both awake and anesthetized equids [233–235], making it a helpful adjunct analgesic in horses undergoing colic surgery. However, the anesthetist should be aware that ketamine infusion was associated with increased gastrointestinal transit time and decreased fecal output in healthy conscious horses [236]. Like α_2-adrenergic receptor agonists, ketamine's immunomodulatory effects have recently gained the attention of anesthetists and may have promising applications in the equine septic patient. While ketamine infusion failed to reduce TNFα and thromboxane-B_2 in 19 mares experimentally treated with LPS [237], ketamine reduced LPS-induced TNFα and IL-6 formation in an equine macrophage cell line [238]. More prospective studies are warranted at this time. One of the authors often includes a constant infusion of lidocaine, dexmedetomidine, and ketamine during anesthesia for colic surgery.

Unlike other species, in horses, there is little research surrounding intraoperative infusion of opioids [239]. The majority of the equine opioid literature concerns their potential adverse effects on gastrointestinal motility [163,164,240]. Probably for this reason, opioid infusions are rarely used in horses undergoing colic surgery, and there is currently conflicting evidence on whether the use of full μ-opioid receptor agonists in the perioperative period may increase the risk of postoperative colic in horses undergoing elective procedures or exploratory laparotomies [164,241]. In addition, opioids have an inconsistent MAC-sparing effect in the horse. Morphine, for example, has been reported to have either MAC-sparing or MAC-increasing effects [242,243]. Despite their variable effect on anesthetic requirements, it is these authors' opinion that opioid agonists should still be considered in a multimodal anesthetic plan for a colic patient.

Locoregional anesthesia

Consideration should be given to locoregional anesthetic techniques as part of a multimodal perioperative analgesic strategy for horses undergoing colic surgery. The epidural injection of local anesthetics, α_2-adrenergic receptor agonists, opioids, or their combinations proved effective in providing visceral analgesia during standing laparoscopic ovariectomy [244,245] and laparoscopic cryptorchidectomy under general anesthesia [246] without adversely affecting gastrointestinal motility in horses. However, performing a sacrococcygeal epidural injection is not often possible in horses undergoing emergent exploratory laparotomy. The 10th to 17th thoracic spinal nerves (T10–T17) and the costoabdominal nerve innervate the equine abdominal wall. Therefore, the peripheral blockade of these nerves before surgery may provide perioperative analgesia. Peripheral blocks can be easily performed with the horse under general anesthesia and in dorsal recumbency as surgical preparation is occurring. Different techniques have been described. The injection of 5–10 mL of 0.5% bupivacaine at the caudal aspect of the 10th through 18th ribs is referred to as Caudal Intercostal Block for Abdominal Surgery (CIBAS). It seems to provide 12 h of analgesia in horses undergoing emergent laparotomy [247]. A transversus abdominis plane (TAP) block has been described in both ponies and horses. With a 6–13 MHz linear ultrasonic probe positioned in a transverse plane mid-abdomen and with a one-point injection of 0.5 mL/kg 1:1 solution of 1% methylene blue and 0.5% bupivacaine, the 16th thoracic (T16) to the 2nd lumbar (L2) nerves were stained [248]. A modified subcostal approach [249] or a three-point injection technique [250] may be required to produce consistent anesthesia of the ventral abdominal wall in horses.

Monitoring

In addition to depth of anesthesia, the anesthetist should continuously monitor the cardiorespiratory function of the horse undergoing exploratory laparotomy and record values at least every 5 min, including:

- Pulse rate and quality
- Mucous membrane color and CRT
- Electrocardiogram (ECG)
- Direct blood pressure (systolic, diastolic, mean) and arterial waveform
- Pulse oximetry
- Capnography
- Ventilatory settings

The pulse quality and peripheral mucous membrane color help estimate peripheral perfusion, but the anesthetist should understand the possible confounding effects of anesthetic drugs. Direct blood pressure measurement is considered the standard of care in horses undergoing inhalant anesthesia due to the lack of accuracy of commercially available non-invasive pressure measurement devices in this species [251,252]. Interestingly, one study showed poor agreement between invasive blood pressure measurements taken from horses' facial, transverse facial, and metatarsal arteries [253]. The increase in intrathoracic pressure during IPPV causes dynamic changes of the arterial pressure waveform, mainly through decreased preload. Systolic pressure variation (SPV) and pulse pressure variation (PPV) can be manually calculated by measuring the difference between the highest and lowest systolic blood pressure or pulse pressure within a respiratory cycle. They have been used to predict fluid responsiveness in many species [57]. A cut-off of 4% and 14–16%, respectively, has been suggested to discriminate responders from non-responders in healthy and septic dogs receiving a 5–15 mL/kg fluid challenge under general anesthesia [254–257]. However, SPV and PPV showed poor correlation when manually calculated from three consecutive breathing cycles in healthy horses [258]. Patient monitors with advanced digital software allow easy calculation of other cardiovascular dynamic changes from the arterial pressure waveform. Although the maximal rate of rise in pressure (dP/dt_{max}) may be affected by peripheral arterial factors, this parameter has been used to identify changes in cardiac contractility in human and animal species [259,260] and could be used to assess dynamic cardiac function in horses undergoing colic surgery. While cardiac output is not routinely measured in horses undergoing colic surgery, new minimally invasive techniques have been studied, with transesophageal or transthoracic Doppler echocardiography [261], lithium dilution techniques with and without pulse contour analysis [262–264], and carbon dioxide breath analysis currently available [265]. The pulse wave transit time, calculated as the time from the electrocardiogram R-wave peak to the rise point of the pulse oximeter or arterial blood pressure wave performed poorly for estimating cardiac output in isoflurane-anesthetized dogs [266]. It may, however, detect changes in stroke volume over time or after interventions.

Pulse oximetry and capnography are commonly used to estimate SaO_2 and partial pressure of arterial carbon dioxide ($PaCO_2$); however, these devices have limitations. Pulse oximetry is affected by a reduction in peripheral perfusion, such as venous engorgement, vasoconstriction, etc. An inaccurate pulse oximeter HR display usually correlates with inaccurate SaO_2 readings. Pulse oximetry has been reported to underestimate SaO_2 in horses with colic [267,268]. The partial pressure of end-tidal carbon dioxide ($P_{ET}CO_2$) can be much lower than the $PaCO_2$ in horses undergoing colic surgery due to increased V/Q mismatch and physiological dead space resulting from abdominal distension and poor perfusion [267]. However, interpretation of the capnographic waveform still provides essential information about ventilation and cardiovascular function, correct intubation, and anesthesia machine malfunction, and these authors recommend its application.

When IPPV is utilized, at a minimum, tidal volume (VT), respiratory rate, I:E ratio, peak inspiratory ratio (PIP), inspiratory pause, and PEEP should be recorded.

Hypothermia is associated with delayed recovery [269], tissue hypoperfusion, incisional infections, and hypocoagulability [270]. Obtaining an accurate core temperature is difficult in horses. Only a probe placed deep within the esophagus or the rectum would be accurate. Conventionally, temperature is measured with a rectal thermometer, which may only read anal temperature and may be affected by preoperative rectal palpation and by the presence of feces, or a nasal thermistor. Additionally, warming a horse during anesthesia may be challenging, but an attempt could be made with forced air warming devices, especially in smaller horses or ponies [271].

PCV and TS, blood gases, electrolytes, and lactate should be regularly measured in horses undergoing colic surgery. The frequency of measurement depends on the patient's physiologic derangements and a reevaluation should be performed after each intervention. Hypomagnesemia and hypocalcemia have been associated with POI [145]. Consequently, ionized magnesium and calcium should be monitored and promptly corrected if needed.

Ventilation strategies

There are different schools of thought regarding IPPV initiation. IPPV, the use of PEEP, and alveolar recruitment maneuvers all increase intrathoracic pressure, decrease venous return, and may exacerbate cardiovascular compromise [272]. In addition, airway pressures higher than 60 mmHg (8 kPa) can be elicited even with a target TV delivery of 10–15 mL/kg, raising concerns of barotrauma to the lungs and organs (e.g., gastric rupture). Consequently, some investigators advocate waiting until the horse's colon is decompressed or surgically exteriorized before beginning IPPV. However, horses undergoing exploratory laparotomy for acute colic are at a higher risk of developing low V/Q mismatch and severe hypoxemia [74,273]. There is limited but convincing evidence that IPPV associated with low levels of PEEP applied from the beginning of anesthesia may help maintain smaller $P(A\text{-}a)O_2$ and higher PaO_2 with minimal cardiovascular consequences [96,274,275]. Shorter recoveries with fewer attempts to stand were observed in horses undergoing colic surgery ventilated with PEEP combined with intermittent recruitment maneuvers compared to controlled mechanical ventilation only [96]. Moreover, horses undergoing colic surgery often present with metabolic acidosis that will be superimposed on the respiratory acidosis that follows hypoventilation and hypercapnia. Therefore, the authors prefer to start IPPV with 10 cmH_2O of PEEP immediately after induction but maintain an I:E ratio above 1:4 to maximize venous return during exhalation and mitigate some of the side effects of high airway pressure, until the cardiovascular status of the patient can be better assessed.

Recovery

Recovery remains a very delicate phase of equine anesthesia. In a recent survey, when asked what area of equine anesthesia was perceived as needing improvement, about 24% of respondents mentioned recovery. The fear of a poor recovery leads equine practitioners to perform standing procedures whenever possible. However, general anesthesia cannot be avoided in horses undergoing colic surgery. Nicolaisen *et al.* [276] showed that colic horses are at higher risk to die during recovery when compared to elective and non-emergent abdominal procedures. Similarly, in an earlier study, recoveries were worse after emergency exploratory laparotomies than after elective surgeries in dorsal recumbency [84]. A recent retrospective study identified high intraoperative dobutamine doses, poor premedication quality, and a prolonged time to stand as risk factors for unsatisfactory recovery quality in 313 horses undergoing anesthesia for colic surgery [277].

The anesthetist should remove the nasogastric tube before recovery, as the mechanical opening of the lower esophageal sphincter may increase the risk of regurgitation and, consequently, aspiration in the horse positioned in lateral recumbency. Some anesthetists advise removing the nasogastric tube in the operating room before the end of anesthesia so that the horse's head can be lowered in the event of nasal bleeding [173]. In addition to aspiration pneumonia, upper airway obstruction is a possible complication during recovery [278,279]. Hence, the endotracheal tube should either be left in place and taped so that the tube exits from the mouth through the interdental space, or removed only after the horse is breathing spontaneously and the swallowing reflex has been regained. There is currently no evidence supporting one practice over the other, and the decision to remove the endotracheal tube before the horse is standing will be influenced by the hospital management and the anesthetist's preference or experience. Nasal phenylephrine [179] and placement of nasal tubes if an obstruction is suspected can prevent fatal outcomes.

It is well recognized that hypoxemia occurs during recovery if oxygen is not supplemented [280,281]. It has recently been shown that simply hoisting an adult horse at the end of isoflurane anesthesia causes a decrease in arterial oxygenation that persists during the recovery phase [282]. Only supplementation with 100% oxygen at the rate of 50 L/min through a demand valve produced PaO_2 tensions similar to those in standing awake horses [281]. In addition, a high flow of oxygen during recovery allows for a more rapid washout of inhaled gases. For this reason, the authors prefer to maintain a high flow of oxygen through a demand valve throughout the entire period the horse remains intubated in the recovery stall and then continue with 15 L/min insufflated via the ventral meatus following extubation as long as the horse will tolerate it.

Equine recovery can be classified as assisted or unassisted based on the degree of personnel involvement. Only 40–53% of equine practitioners today consistently assist recovery after general anesthesia [283,284]; more commonly, assisted recovery is reserved for emergency exploratory laparotomies or lengthy procedures, or animals considered to be in poor health [284]. Several methods exist for assisting the horse during recovery with foam mattresses, head-and-tail ropes either from inside or outside the stall, and inflatable/deflatable mattresses being the most commonly used today [283]. Interestingly, a survey by de Miguel Garcia *et al.* in 2021 showed that, despite the perception of equine practitioners, fatalities associated with equine recovery were significantly more common (49%) in hospitals that routinely assisted equine recoveries than in hospitals reporting to never or rarely assist recoveries (16%; $p < 0.006$) [283]. On the other hand, personnel injury was reported by 25% of practitioners routinely assisting horses in recoveries compared with 10% of practitioners that generally carry out unassisted recoveries ($p < 0.06$) [283]. Whether assisting recovery after colic surgery improves the quality of recovery is controversial. However, what is clear is that head-and-tail ropes do not entirely prevent the occurrence of fatal injuries during recovery in horses undergoing emergency procedures [78,276].

Despite their widespread use [284], there is conflicting evidence that sedation with α_2-adrenergic receptor agonists improves the quality of recovery following equine anesthesia [285,286]. Number of attempts to stand and recovery scores were not different in horses receiving a 0.2 mg/kg bolus of xylazine or placebo after desflurane anesthesia [287]. Following isoflurane anesthesia, xylazine (0.2 mg/kg IV) and dexmedetomidine (0.875 μg/kg IV) led to similar recovery quality in healthy horses [288]. Similarly, following sevoflurane anesthesia, recovery scores and time to standing were not significantly different between horses receiving either dexmedetomidine (1 μg/kg IV) or romifidine (20 μg/kg IV) [285]. In another study, painful procedures, longer anesthesia times, and the Arabian horse breed were associated with poorer recovery scores. After adjusting for these factors, a postoperative bolus of romifidine (20 μg/kg IV) improved the quality of recovery compared to xylazine [286]. Based on the current body of the literature, the authors cannot recommend the use of one particular α_2-adrenergic receptor agonist over another for improving the recovery of horses undergoing colic surgery, and the equine anesthetist will likely base the choice on personal preference or clinical experience.

References

1 Tinker MK, White NA, Lessard P, *et al.* Prospective study of equine colic incidence and mortality. *Equine Vet J* 1997; **29**(6): 448–453.

2 Christophersen MT, Dupont N, Berg-Sorensen KS, *et al.* Short-term survival and mortality rates in a retrospective study of colic in 1588 Danish horses. *Acta Vet Scand* 2014; **56**: 20.

3 van der Linden MA, Laffont CM, Sloet van Oldruitenborgh-Oosterbaan MM. Prognosis in equine medical and surgical colic. *J Vet Intern Med* 2003; **17**(3): 343–348.

4 Wormstrand BH, Ihler CF, Diesen R, *et al.* Surgical treatment of equine colic – a retrospective study of 297 surgeries in Norway 2005–2011. *Acta Vet Scand* 2014; **56**: 38.

5 Epstein KL, Brainard BM, Gomez-Ibanez SE, *et al.* Thrombelastography in horses with acute gastrointestinal disease. *J Vet Intern Med* 2011; **25**(2): 307–314.

6 Roy MF, Kwong GP, Lambert J, *et al.* Prognostic value and development of a scoring system in horses with systemic inflammatory response syndrome. *J Vet Intern Med* 2017; **31**(2): 582–592.

7 Morris DD. Endotoxemia in horses. A review of cellular and humoral mediators involved in its pathogenesis. *J Vet Intern Med* 1991; **5**(3): 167–181.

8 Senior JM, Proudman CJ, Leuwer M, *et al.* Plasma endotoxin in horses presented to an equine referral hospital: correlation to selected clinical parameters and outcomes. *Equine Vet J* 2011; **43**(5): 585–591.

9 Nieto JE, MacDonald MH, Braim AE, *et al.* Effect of lipopolysaccharide infusion on gene expression of inflammatory cytokines in normal horses in vivo. *Equine Vet J* 2009; **41**(7): 717–719.

10 Tadros EM, Frank N. Effects of continuous or intermittent lipopolysaccharide administration for 48 hours on the systemic inflammatory response in horses. *Am J Vet Res* 2012; **73**(9): 1394–1402.

11 Guntheroth WG, Felsenfeld AJ. Splenic constriction with endotoxin shock in the dog. *J Appl Physiol* 1971; **30**(4): 517–520.

12 Parrillo JE. Pathogenetic mechanisms of septic shock. *N Engl J Med* 1993; **328**(20): 1471–1477.

13 Uchimido R, Schmidt EP, Shapiro NI. The glycocalyx: a novel diagnostic and therapeutic target in sepsis. *Crit Care* 2019; **23**(1): 16.

14 Burrows GE. Equine Escherichia coli endotoxemia: comparison of intravenous and intraperitoneal endotoxin administration. *Am J Vet Res* 1979; **40**(7): 991–998.

15 Dallap Schaer BL, Epstein K. Coagulopathy of the critically ill equine patient. *J Vet Emerg Crit Care (San Antonio)* 2009; **19**(1): 53–65.

16 Bone RC, Balk RA, Cerra FB, *et al.* Definitions for sepsis and organ failure and guidelines for the use of innovative therapies in sepsis. The ACCP/SCCM Consensus Conference Committee. American College of Chest Physicians/Society of Critical Care Medicine. *Chest* 1992; **101**(6): 1644–1655.

17 Barton AK, Richter IG, Ahrens T, *et al.* MMP-9 Concentration in peritoneal fluid is a valuable biomarker associated with endotoxemia in equine colic. *Mediators Inflamm* 2021; **2021**: 9501478.

18 Nocera I, Bonelli F, Meucci V, *et al.* Evaluation of protein carbonyl content in healthy and sick hospitalized horses. *Front Vet Sci* 2020; **7**: 582886.

19 Barr B, Nieman NM. Serum amyloid A as an aid in diagnosing sepsis in equine neonates. *Equine Vet J* 2022; **54**(5): 922–926.

20 Pihl TH, Scheepers E, Sanz M, *et al.* Influence of disease process and duration on acute phase proteins in serum and peritoneal fluid of horses with colic. *J Vet Intern Med* 2015; **29**(2): 651–658.

21 Fogle J, Jacob M, Blikslager A, *et al.* Comparison of lipopolysaccharides and soluble CD14 measurement between clinically endotoxaemic and nonendotoxaemic horses. *Equine Vet J* 2017; **49**(2): 155–159.

22 Silva A, Wagner B, McKenzie HC, *et al.* An investigation of the role of soluble CD14 in hospitalized, sick horses. *Vet Immunol Immunopathol* 2013; **155**(4): 264–269.

23 Bonelli F, Meucci V, Divers TJ, *et al.* Plasma procalcitonin concentration in healthy horses and horses affected by systemic inflammatory response syndrome. *J Vet Intern Med* 2015; **29**(6): 1689–1691.

24 Wells MT, Gaffin SL, Gregory M, *et al.* Properties of equine anti-lipopolysaccharide hyperimmune plasma: binding to lipopolysaccharide and bactericidal activity against gram-negative bacteria. *J Med Microbiol* 1987; **24**(3): 187–196.

25 Werners AH. Treatment of endotoxaemia and septicaemia in the equine patient. *J Vet Pharmacol Ther* 2017; **40**(1): 1–15.

26 Forbes G, Church S, Savage CJ, *et al.* Effects of hyperimmune equine plasma on clinical and cellular responses in a low-dose endotoxaemia model in horses. *Res Vet Sci* 2012; **92**(1): 40–44.

27 Spier SJ, Lavoie JP, Cullor JS, *et al.* Protection against clinical endotoxemia in horses by using plasma containing antibody to an Rc mutant E. coli (J5). *Circ Shock* 1989; **28**(3): 235–248.

28 Morris DD, Whitlock RH, Corbeil LB. Endotoxemia in horses: protection provided by antiserum to core lipopolysaccharide. *Am J Vet Res* 1986; **47**(3): 544–550.

29 Peek SF, Semrad S, McGuirk SM, *et al.* Prognostic value of clinicopathologic variables obtained at admission and effect of antiendotoxin plasma on survival in septic and critically ill foals. *J Vet Intern Med* 2006; **20**(3): 569–574.

30 Morrison DC, Jacobs DM. Binding of polymyxin B to the lipid A portion of bacterial lipopolysaccharides. *Immunochemistry* 1976; **13**(10): 813–818.

31 Barton MH, Parviainen A, Norton N. Polymyxin B protects horses against induced endotoxaemia in vivo. *Equine Vet J* 2004; **36**(5): 397–401.

32 Falagas ME, Kasiakou SK. Toxicity of polymyxins: a systematic review of the evidence from old and recent studies. *Crit Care* 2006; **10**(1): R27.

33 Morresey PR, Mackay RJ. Endotoxin-neutralizing activity of polymyxin B in blood after IV administration in horses. *Am J Vet Res* 2006; **67**(4): 642–647.

34 Barton MH, Moore JN. Pentoxifylline inhibits mediator synthesis in an equine in vitro whole blood model of endotoxemia. *Circ Shock* 1994; **44**(4): 216–220.

35 Barton MH, Moore JN, Norton N. Effects of pentoxifylline infusion on response of horses to in vivo challenge exposure with endotoxin. *Am J Vet Res* 1997; **58**(11): 1300–1307.

36 Baskett A, Barton MH, Norton N, *et al.* Effect of pentoxifylline, flunixin meglumine, and their combination on a model of endotoxemia in horses. *Am J Vet Res* 1997; **58**(11): 1291–1299.

37 Moore JN, Garner HE, Shapland JE, *et al.* Prevention of endotoxin-induced arterial hypoxaemia and lactic acidosis with flunixin meglumine in the conscious pony. *Equine Vet J* 1981; **13**(2): 95–98.

38 Semrad SD, Hardee GE, Hardee MM, *et al.* Low dose flunixin meglumine: effects on eicosanoid production and clinical signs induced by experimental endotoxaemia in horses. *Equine Vet J* 1987; **19**(3): 201–206.

39 Cook VL, Meyer CT, Campbell NB, *et al.* Effect of firocoxib or flunixin meglumine on recovery of ischemic-injured equine jejunum. *Am J Vet Res* 2009; **70**(8): 992–1000.

40 Naylor RJ, Taylor AH, Knowles EJ, *et al.* Comparison of flunixin meglumine and meloxicam for post operative management of horses with strangulating small intestinal lesions. *Equine Vet J* 2014; **46**(4): 427–434.

41 Ziegler AL, Freeman CK, Fogle CA, *et al.* Multicentre, blinded, randomised clinical trial comparing the use of flunixin meglumine with firocoxib in horses with small intestinal strangulating obstruction. *Equine Vet J* 2019; **51**(3): 329–335.

42 Gold JR, Divers TJ, Barton MH, *et al.* Plasma adrenocorticotropin, cortisol, and adrenocorticotropin/cortisol ratios in septic and normal-term foals. *J Vet Intern Med* 2007; **21**(4): 791–796.

43 Johnson LM, Holcombe SJ, Shearer TR, *et al.* Multicenter placebo-controlled randomized study of ethyl pyruvate in horses following Surgical Treatment for >/= 360 degrees large colon volvulus. *Front Vet Sci* 2020; **7**: 204.

44 Cook VL, Holcombe SJ, Gandy JC, *et al.* Ethyl pyruvate decreases proinflammatory gene expression in lipopolysaccharide-stimulated equine monocytes. *Vet Immunol Immunopathol* 2011; **141**(1–2): 92–99.

45 Jacobs CC, Holcombe SJ, Cook VL, *et al.* Ethyl pyruvate diminishes the inflammatory response to lipopolysaccharide infusion in horses. *Equine Vet J* 2013; **45**(3): 333–339.

46 Sutton GA, Atamna R, Steinman A, *et al.* Comparison of three acute colic pain scales: reliability, validity and usability. *Vet J* 2019; **246**: 71–77.

47 Van Dierendonck MC, van Loon JP. Monitoring acute equine visceral pain with the Equine Utrecht University Scale for Composite Pain Assessment (EQUUS-COMPASS) and the Equine Utrecht University Scale for Facial Assessment of Pain (EQUUS-FAP): a validation study. *Vet J* 2016; **216**: 175–177.

48 van Loon JP, Jonckheer-Sheehy VS, Back W, *et al.* Monitoring equine visceral pain with a composite pain scale score and correlation with survival after emergency gastrointestinal surgery. *Vet J* 2014; **200**(1): 109–115.

49 Allen SE, Holm JL. Lactate: physiology and clinical utility. *J Vet Emerg Critic Care* 2008; **18**(2): 123–132.

50 Tennent-Brown BS, Wilkins PA, Lindborg S, *et al.* Sequential plasma lactate concentrations as prognostic indicators in adult equine emergencies. *J Vet Intern Med* 2010; **24**(1): 198–205.

51 Latson KM, Nieto JE, Beldomenico PM, *et al.* Evaluation of peritoneal fluid lactate as a marker of intestinal ischaemia in equine colic. *Equine Vet J* 2005; **37**(4): 342–346.

52 Peloso JG, Cohen ND. Use of serial measurements of peritoneal fluid lactate concentration to identify strangulating intestinal lesions in referred horses with signs of colic. *J Am Vet Med Assoc* 2012; **240**(10): 1208–1217.

53 DeLaurier GA, Cannon RM, Johnson RH Jr., *et al.* Increased peritoneal fluid lactic acid values and progressive bowel strangulation in dogs. *Am J Surg* 1989; **158**(1): 32–35.

54 Thoefner MB, Ersboll AK, Hesselholt M. Prognostic indicators in a Danish hospital-based population of colic horses. *Equine Vet J Suppl* 2000; **32**: 11–18.

55 Espinosa P, Le Jeune SS, Cenani A, *et al.* Investigation of perioperative and anesthetic variables affecting short-term survival of horses with small intestinal strangulating lesions. *Vet Surg* 2017; **46**(3): 345–353.

56 Kelleher ME, Brosnan RJ, Kass PH, *et al.* Use of physiologic and arterial blood gas variables to predict short-term survival in horses with large colon volvulus. *Vet Surg* 2013; **42**(1): 107–113.

57 Araos J, Kenny JS, Rousseau-Blass F, *et al.* Dynamic prediction of fluid responsiveness during positive pressure ventilation: a review of the physiology underlying heart-lung interactions and a critical interpretation. *Vet Anaesth Analg* 2020; **47**(1): 3–14.

58 Kerr DD, Jones EW, Huggins K, *et al.* Sedative and other effects of xylazine given intravenously to horses. *Am J Vet Res* 1972; **33**(3): 525–532.

59 Dezfouli MRM, Tavanaeimanesh H, Houshangi AF, *et al.* Effects of xylazine and acepromazine on echocardiographic parameters in the healthy horse. *Pferdeheilkunde* 2020; **36**: 37–42.

60 Steffey EP, Howland D Jr. Comparison of circulatory and respiratory effects of isoflurane and halothane anesthesia in horses. *Am J Vet Res* 1980; **41**(5): 821–825.

61 Steffey EP, Mama KR, Galey FD, *et al.* Effects of sevoflurane dose and mode of ventilation on cardiopulmonary function and blood biochemical variables in horses. *Am J Vet Res* 2005; **66**(4): 606–614.

62 Scott VH, Williams JM, Mudge MC, *et al.* Effect of body position on intra-abdominal pressures and abdominal perfusion pressures measured at three sites in horses anesthetized with short-term total intravenous anesthesia. *Am J Vet Res* 2014; **75**(3): 301–308.

63 Youngblood CD, Hodgson DS, Beard WL, *et al.* Effect of position on transdiaphragmatic pressure and hemodynamic variables in anesthetized horses. *Can J Vet Res* 2020; **84**(3): 205–211.

64 Binetti A, Mosing M, Sacks M, *et al.* Impact of Trendelenburg (head down) and reverse Trendelenburg (head up) position on respiratory and cardiovascular function in anaesthetized horses. *Vet Anaesth Analg* 2018; **45**(6): 760–771.

65 Hodgson DS, Steffey EP, Grandy JL, *et al.* Effects of spontaneous, assisted, and controlled ventilatory modes in halothane-anesthetized geldings. *Am J Vet Res* 1986; **47**(5): 992–996.

66 Mizuno Y, Aida H, Hara H, *et al.* Cardiovascular effects of intermittent positive pressure ventilation in the anesthetized horse. *J Vet Med Sci* 1994; **56**(1): 39–44.

67 Kalchofner KS, Picek S, Ringer SK, *et al.* A study of cardiovascular function under controlled and spontaneous ventilation in isoflurane-medetomidine anaesthetized horses. *Vet Anaesth Analg* 2009; **36**(5): 426–435.

68 Ohta M, Kurimoto S, Ishikawa Y, *et al.* Cardiovascular effects of dobutamine and phenylephrine infusion in sevoflurane-anesthetized Thoroughbred horses. *J Vet Med Sci* 2013; **75**(11): 1443–1448.

69 Dancker C, Hopster K, Rohn K, *et al.* Effects of dobutamine, dopamine, phenylephrine and noradrenaline on systemic haemodynamics and intestinal perfusion in isoflurane anaesthetised horses. *Equine Vet J* 2018; **50**(1): 104–110.

70 Kobayashi S, Endou M, Sakuraya F, *et al.* The sympathomimetic actions of l-Ephedrine and d-Pseudoephedrine: direct receptor activation or norepinephrine release? *Anesth Analg* 2003; **97**(5): 1239–1245.

71 Chen HC, Sinclair MD, Dyson DH. Use of ephedrine and dopamine in dogs for the management of hypotension in routine clinical cases under isoflurane anesthesia. *Vet Anaesth Analg* 2007; **34**(5): 301–311.

72 Kimmoun A, Novy E, Auchet T, *et al.* Hemodynamic consequences of severe lactic acidosis in shock states: from bench to bedside. *Crit Care* 2015; **19**: 175.

73 Hubbell JA, Muir WW. Oxygenation, oxygen delivery and anaesthesia in the horse. *Equine Vet J* 2015; **47**(1): 25–35.

74 Hovda T, Love L, Chiavaccini L. Risk factors associated with hypoxaemia in horses undergoing general anaesthesia: a retrospective study. *Equine Vet J* 2022; **54**(6): 1055–1063.

75 Hopster K, Wittenberg-Voges L, Geburek F, *et al.* Effects of controlled hypoxemia or hypovolemia on global and intestinal oxygenation and perfusion in isoflurane anesthetized horses receiving an alpha-2-agonist infusion. *BMC Vet Res* 2017; **13**(1): 361.

76 Robson K, Cripps P, Bardell D. Lack of association between arterial oxygen tensions in horses during exploratory coeliotomy and post-operative incisional complications: a retrospective study. *Vet J* 2016; **210**: 24–29.

77 Costa-Farre C, Prades M, Ribera T, *et al.* Does intraoperative low arterial partial pressure of oxygen increase the risk of surgical site infection following emergency exploratory laparotomy in horses? *Vet J* 2014; **200**(1): 175–180.

78 Rüegg M, Bettschart-Wolfensberger R, Hartnack S, *et al.* Comparison of non-assisted versus head and tail rope-assisted recovery after emergency abdominal surgery in horses. *Pferdeheilkunde* 2016; **32**: 469–478.

79 Nyman G, Funkquist B, Kvart C, *et al.* Atelectasis causes gas exchange impairment in the anaesthetised horse. *Equine Vet J* 1990; **22**(5): 317–324.

80 Nyman G, Hedenstierna G. Ventilation–perfusion relationships in the anaesthetised horse. *Equine Vet J* 1989; **21**(4): 274–281.

81 Sorenson PR, Robinson NE. Postural effects on lung volumes and asynchronous ventilation in anesthetized horses. *J Appl Physiol Respir Environ Exerc Physiol* 1980; **48**(1): 97–103.

82 Auckburally A, Nyman G. Review of hypoxaemia in anaesthetized horses: predisposing factors, consequences and management. *Vet Anaesth Analg* 2017; **44**(3): 397–408.

83 Froese AB, Bryan AC. Effects of anesthesia and paralysis on diaphragmatic mechanics in man. *Anesthesiology* 1974; **41**(3): 242–255.

84 McCoy AM, Hackett ES, Wagner AE, *et al.* Pulmonary gas exchange and plasma lactate in horses with gastrointestinal disease undergoing emergency exploratory laparotomy: a comparison with an elective surgery horse population. *Vet Surg* 2011; **40**(5): 601–609.

85 Trenholme HN, Barletta M, Quandt JE, *et al.* Arterial oxygenation in anesthetized horses placed in a 5-degree reverse Trendelenburg position. *Res Vet Sci* 2021; **135**: 304–309.

86 Schauvliege S, Binetti A, Duchateau L, *et al.* Cardiorespiratory effects of a 7 degrees reverse Trendelenburg position in anaesthetized horses: a randomized clinical trial. *Vet Anaesth Analg* 2018; **45**(5): 648–657.

87 Crumley MN, McMurphy RM, Hodgson DS, *et al.* Effects of inspired oxygen concentration on ventilation, ventilatory rhythm, and gas exchange in isoflurane-anesthetized horses. *Am J Vet Res* 2013; **74**(2): 183–190.

88 Cuvelliez SG, Eicker SW, McLauchlan C, *et al.* Cardiovascular and respiratory effects of inspired oxygen fraction in halothane-anesthetized horses. *Am J Vet Res* 1990; **51**(8): 1226–1231.

89 Hubbell JA, Aarnes TK, Bednarski RM, *et al.* Effect of 50% and maximal inspired oxygen concentrations on respiratory variables in isoflurane-anesthetized horses. *BMC Vet Res* 2011; **7**: 23.

90 Portier K, Crouzier D, Guichardant M, *et al.* Effects of high and low inspired fractions of oxygen on horse erythrocyte membrane properties, blood viscosity and muscle oxygenation during anaesthesia. *Vet Anaesth Analg* 2009; **36**(4): 287–298.

91 Savvas I, Pavlidou K, Braun C, *et al.* Evaluation of the effect of the inspired oxygen fraction on blood oxygenation during inhalant anaesthesia in horses: a systematic review with meta-analysis. *Animals (Basel)* 2021; **11**(8): 2245.

92 Wagner PD. Causes of a high physiological dead space in critically ill patients. *Crit Care* 2008; **12**(3): 148.

93 Portela DA, Di Franco C, Chiavaccini L, *et al.* Effect of end-inspiratory pause on airway and physiological dead space in anesthetized horses. *Vet Anaesth Analg* 2023; **50**(4): 363–371.

94 Clerbaux T, Gustin P, Detry B, *et al.* Comparative study of the oxyhaemoglobin dissociation curve of four mammals: man, dog, horse and cattle. *Comp Biochem Physiol Comp Physiol* 1993; **106**(4): 687–694.

95 Hughes J, Bardell D. Determination of reference intervals for equine arterial blood-gas, acid-base and electrolyte analysis. *Vet Anaesth Analg* 2019; **46**(6): 765–771.

96 Hopster K, Kästner SB, Rohn K, *et al.* Intermittent positive pressure ventilation with constant positive end-expiratory pressure and alveolar recruitment manoeuvre during inhalation anaesthesia in horses undergoing surgery for colic, and its influence on the early recovery period. *Vet Anaesth Analg* 2011; **38**(3): 169–177.

97 Lachmann B. Open up the lung and keep the lung open. *Intensive Care Med* 1992; **18**(6): 319–321.

98 Schürmann P, Hopster K, Rohn K, *et al.* Optimized gas exchange during inhalant anaesthesia in horses using "open lung concept" ventilation. *Pferdeheilkunde* 2008; **24**(2): 236–242.

99 Robertson SA, Bailey JE. Aerosolized salbutamol (albuterol) improves PaO2 in hypoxaemic anaesthetized horses – a prospective clinical trial in 81 horses. *Vet Anaesth Analg* 2002; **29**(4): 212–218.

100 Gunkel CI, Valverde A, Robertson SA, *et al.* Treatment for a severe reaction to intravenous administration of diatrizoate in an anesthetized horse. *J Am Vet Med Assoc* 2004; **224**(7): 1143–1146.

101 Grubb TL, Lord PF, Berger M, *et al.* Effects of pulse-delivered inhaled nitric oxide administration on pulmonary perfusion and arterial oxygenation in dorsally recumbent isoflurane-anesthetized horses. *Am J Vet Res* 2014; **75**(11): 949–955.

102 Nyman G, Grubb TL, Heinonen E, *et al.* Pulsed delivery of inhaled nitric oxide counteracts hypoxaemia during 2.5 hours of inhalation anaesthesia in dorsally recumbent horses. *Vet Anaesth Analg* 2012; **39**(5): 480–487.

103 Wiklund M, Granswed I, Nyman G. Pulsed inhaled nitric oxide improves arterial oxygenation in colic horses undergoing abdominal surgery. *Vet Anaesth Analg* 2017; **44**(5): 1139–1148.

104 Wiklund M, Kellgren M, Wulcan S, *et al.* Effects of pulsed inhaled nitric oxide on arterial oxygenation during mechanical ventilation in anaesthetised horses undergoing elective arthroscopy or emergency colic surgery. *Equine Vet J* 2020; **52**(1): 76–82.

105 Wilson DV, Rondenay Y, Shance PU. The cardiopulmonary effects of severe blood loss in anesthetized horses. *Vet Anaesth Analg* 2003; **30**(2): 81–87.

106 Hesselkilde EZ, Almind ME, Petersen J, *et al.* Cardiac arrhythmias and electrolyte disturbances in colic horses. *Acta Vet Scand* 2014; **56**(1): 58.

107 Nostell K, Brojer J, Hoglund K, *et al.* Cardiac troponin I and the occurrence of cardiac arrhythmias in horses with experimentally induced endotoxaemia. *Vet J* 2012; **192**(2): 171–175.

108 Shahreyar M, Fahhoum R, Akinseye O, *et al.* Severe sepsis and cardiac arrhythmias. *Ann Transl Med* 2018; **6**(1): 6.

109 Loomes K. The use of hyoscine N-butylbromide to treat intraoperative bradycardia during isoflurane anaesthesia in a Thoroughbred horse. *Vet Anaesth Analg* 2020; **47**(6): 847–849.

110 Ducharme NG, Fubini SL. Gastrointestinal complications associated with the use of atropine in horses. *J Am Vet Med Assoc* 1983; **182**(3): 229–231.

111 Frye MA, Bright JM, Dargatz DA, *et al.* A comparison of dobutamine infusion to exercise as a cardiac stress test in healthy horses. *J Vet Intern Med* 2003; **17**(1): 58–64.

112 Hunt JM, Edwards GB, Clarke KW. Incidence, diagnosis and treatment of postoperative complications in colic cases. *Equine Vet J* 1986; **18**(4): 264–270.

113 Dugdale AH, Obhrai J, Cripps PJ. Twenty years later: a single-centre, repeat retrospective analysis of equine perioperative mortality and investigation of recovery quality. *Vet Anaesth Analg* 2016; **43**(2): 171–178.

114 Raisis AL. Skeletal muscle blood flow in anaesthetized horses. Part II: effects of anaesthetics and vasoactive agents. *Vet Anaesth Analg* 2005; **32**(6): 331–337.

115 Higgins J. Preparation, supplies, and catheterization. In: Fielding CL, Magdesian KG, eds. *Equine Fluid Therapy*. Ames, IA: Wiley, 2015: 127–141.

116 Evans L, Rhodes A, Alhazzani W, *et al.* Executive summary: surviving sepsis campaign: international guidelines for the management of sepsis and septic shock 2021. *Crit Care Med* 2021; **49**(11): 1974–1982.

117 Fielding CL, Magdesian KG. A comparison of hypertonic (7.2%) and isotonic (0.9%) saline for fluid resuscitation in horses: a randomized, double-blinded, clinical trial. *J Vet Intern Med* 2011; **25**(5): 1138–1143.

118 Nakayama S, Sibley L, Gunther RA, *et al.* Small-volume resuscitation with hypertonic saline (2400 mOsm/liter) during hemorrhagic shock. *Circ Shock* 1984; **13**(2): 149–159.

119 Attuwaybi B, Kozar RA, Gates KS, *et al.* Hypertonic saline prevents inflammation, injury, and impaired intestinal transit after gut ischemia/reperfusion by inducing heme oxygenase 1 enzyme. *J Trauma* 2004; **56**(4): 749–758; discussion 58–59.

120 Schmall LM, Muir WW, Robertson JT. Haemodynamic effects of small volume hypertonic saline in experimentally induced haemorrhagic shock. *Equine Vet J* 1990; **22**(4): 273–277.

121 Bellezzo F, Kuhnmuench T, Hackett ES. The effect of colloid formulation on colloid osmotic pressure in horses with naturally occurring gastrointestinal disease. *BMC Vet Res* 2014; **10**(Suppl 1): S8.

122 Brünisholz HP, Schwarzwald CC, Bettschart-Wolfensberger R, *et al.* Effects of 10% hydroxyethyl starch (HES 200/0.5) solution in intraoperative fluid therapy management of horses undergoing elective surgical procedures. *Vet J* 2015; **206**(3): 398–403.

123 Epstein KL, Bergren A, Giguère S, *et al.* Cardiovascular, colloid osmotic pressure, and hemostatic effects of 2 formulations of hydroxyethyl starch in healthy horses. *J Vet Intern Med* 2014; **28**(1): 223–233.

124 Jones PA, Bain FT, Byars TD, *et al.* Effect of hydroxyethyl starch infusion on colloid oncotic pressure in hypoproteinemic horses. *J Am Vet Med Assoc* 2001; **218**(7): 1130–1135.

125 Rehm M, Zahler S, Lötsch M, *et al.* Endothelial glycocalyx as an additional barrier determining extravasation of 6% hydroxyethyl starch or 5% albumin solutions in the coronary vascular bed. *Anesthesiology* 2004; **100**(5): 1211–1223.

126 Boscan P, Steffey EP. Plasma colloid osmotic pressure and total protein in horses during colic surgery. *Vet Anaesth Analg* 2007; **34**(6): 408–415.

127 Pantaleon LG, Furr MO, McKenzie HC II, *et al.* Cardiovascular and pulmonary effects of hetastarch plus hypertonic saline solutions during experimental endotoxemia in anesthetized horses. *J Vet Intern Med* 2006; **20**(6): 1422–1428.

128 Evans L, Rhodes A, Alhazzani W, *et al.* Surviving sepsis campaign: international guidelines for management of sepsis and septic shock 2021. *Intensive Care Med* 2021; **47**(11): 1181–1247.

129 Lewis SR, Pritchard MW, Evans DJ, *et al.* Colloids versus crystalloids for fluid resuscitation in critically ill people. *Cochrane Database Syst Rev* 2018; **8**(8): Cd000567.

130 Dugdale AH, Barron KE, Miller AJ, *et al.* Effects of preoperative administration of hypertonic saline or pentastarch solution on hematologic variables and long-term survival of surgically managed horses with colic. *J Am Vet Med Assoc* 2015; **246**(10): 1104–1111.

131 Jones PA, Tomasic M, Gentry PA. Oncotic, hemodilutional, and hemostatic effects of isotonic saline and hydroxyethyl starch solutions in clinically normal ponies. *Am J Vet Res* 1997; **58**(5): 541–548.

132 Malbrain M, Langer T, Annane D, *et al.* Intravenous fluid therapy in the perioperative and critical care setting: executive summary of the International Fluid Academy (IFA). *Ann Intensive Care* 2020; **10**(1): 64.

133 Hoaglund EL, Hess AM, Hassel DM. Retrospective evaluation of the effect of intravenous fluid administration on development of postoperative reflux in horses with colic (2004–2012): 194 horses. *J Vet Emerg Crit Care (San Antonio)* 2018; **28**(6): 566–572.

134 Rivers E, Nguyen B, Havstad S, *et al.* Early goal-directed therapy in the treatment of severe sepsis and septic shock. *N Engl J Med* 2001; **345**(19): 1368–1377.

135 Crabtree NE, Epstein KL. Current concepts in fluid therapy in horses. *Front Vet Sci* 2021; **8**: 648774.

136 Holcombe SJ. Colic in foals. In: Robinson NE, Wilson MR, eds. *Current Therapy in Equine Medicine*, 5th edn. Philadelphia, PA: Saunders, 2003: 680–686.

137 Kasirer-Izraely H, Choshniak I, Shkolnik A. Dehydration and rehydration in donkeys: the role of the hind gut as a water reservoir. *J Basic Clin Physiol Pharmacol* 1994; **5**(1): 89–100.

138 Pritchard JC, Barr AR, Whay HR. Validity of a behavioural measure of heat stress and a skin tent test for dehydration in working horses and donkeys. *Equine Vet J* 2006; **38**(5): 433–438.

139 Pritchard JC, Burn CC, Barr AR, *et al.* Validity of indicators of dehydration in working horses: a longitudinal study of changes in skin tent duration, mucous membrane dryness and drinking behaviour. *Equine Vet J* 2008; **40**(6): 558–564.

140 Luft FC. Lactic acidosis update for critical care clinicians. *J Am Soc Nephrol* 2001; **12**(Suppl 17): S15–S19.

141 Adrogue HJ. Metabolic acidosis: pathophysiology, diagnosis and management. *J Nephrol* 2006; **19**(Suppl 9): S62–S69.

142 Forsythe SM, Schmidt GA. Sodium bicarbonate for the treatment of lactic acidosis. *Chest* 2000; **117**(1): 260–267.

143 Navarro M, Monreal L, Segura D, *et al.* A comparison of traditional and quantitative analysis of acid–base and electrolyte imbalances in horses with gastrointestinal disorders. *J Vet Intern Med* 2005; **19**(6): 871–877.

144 Adami C, Westwood-Hearn H, Bolt DM, *et al.* Prevalence of electrolyte disturbances and perianesthetic death risk factors in 120 horses undergoing colic surgery. *J Equine Vet Sci* 2020; **84**: 102843.

145 Garcia-Lopez JM, Provost PJ, Rush JE, *et al.* Prevalence and prognostic importance of hypomagnesemia and hypocalcemia in horses that have colic surgery. *Am J Vet Res* 2001; **62**(1): 7–12.

146 Dart AJ, Snyder JR, Spier SJ, *et al.* Ionized calcium concentration in horses with surgically managed gastrointestinal disease: 147 cases (1988–1990). *J Am Vet Med Assoc* 1992; **201**(8): 1244–1248.

147 Desai TK, Carlson RW, Thill-Baharozian M, *et al.* A direct relationship between ionized calcium and arterial pressure among patients in an intensive care unit. *Crit Care Med* 1988; **16**(6): 578–582.

148 Zimmel DN. Management of pain and dehydration in horses with colic. In: Robinson NE, Wilson MR, eds. *Current Therapy in Equine Medicine*, 5th edn. St. Louis, MO: Saunders, 2003: 115–120.

149 Kovacs A, Courtois MR, Barzilai B, *et al.* Reversal of hypocalcemia and decreased afterload in sepsis. Effect on myocardial systolic and diastolic function. *Am J Respir Crit Care Med* 1998; **158**(6): 1990–1998.

150 Zaloga GP, Sager A, Black KW, *et al.* Low dose calcium administration increases mortality during septic peritonitis in rats. *Circ Shock* 1992; **37**(3): 226–229.

151 Carlstedt F, Eriksson M, Kiiski R, *et al.* Hypocalcemia during porcine endotoxemic shock: effects of calcium administration. *Crit Care Med* 2000; **28**(8): 2909–2914.

152 Gennari FJ. Hypokalemia. *N Engl J Med* 1998; **339**(7): 451–458.

153 Boesch JM. Anesthesia for the horse with colic. *Vet Clin North Am Equine Pract* 2013; **29**(1): 193–214.

154 Doherty TJ, Andrews FM, Provenza MK, *et al.* The effect of sedation on gastric emptying of a liquid marker in ponies. *Vet Surg* 1999; **28**(5): 375–379.

155 Elfenbein JR, Sanchez LC, Robertson SA, *et al.* Effect of detomidine on visceral and somatic nociception and duodenal motility in conscious adult horses. *Vet Anaesth Analg* 2009; **36**(2): 162–172.

156 Freeman SL, England GC. Effect of romifidine on gastrointestinal motility, assessed by transrectal ultrasonography. *Equine Vet J* 2001; **33**(6): 570–576.

157 Nelson BB, Lordan EE, Hassel DM. Risk factors associated with gastrointestinal dysfunction in horses undergoing elective procedures under general anaesthesia. *Equine Vet J Suppl* 2013; **45**: 8–14.

158 Clutton RE. Opioid analgesia in horses. *Vet Clin North Am Equine Pract* 2010; **26**(3): 493–514.

159 Carregaro AB, Luna SP, Mataqueiro MI, *et al.* Effects of buprenorphine on nociception and spontaneous locomotor activity in horses. *Am J Vet Res* 2007; **68**(3): 246–250.

160 Chiavaccini L, Claude AK, Lee JH, *et al.* Pharmacokinetics and pharmacodynamics comparison between subcutaneous and intravenous butorphanol administration in horses. *J Vet Pharmacol Ther* 2015; **38**(4): 365–374.

161 Reed RA, Knych HK, Barletta M, *et al.* Pharmacokinetics and pharmacodynamics of hydromorphone after intravenous and intramuscular administration in horses. *Vet Anaesth Analg* 2020; **47**(2): 210–218.

162 Reed R, Barletta M, Mitchell K, *et al.* The pharmacokinetics and pharmacodynamics of intravenous hydromorphone in horses. *Vet Anaesth Analg* 2019; **46**(3): 395–404.

163 Boscan P, Van Hoogmoed LM, Farver TB, *et al.* Evaluation of the effects of the opioid agonist morphine on gastrointestinal tract function in horses. *Am J Vet Res* 2006; **67**(6): 992–997.

164 Skrzypczak H, Reed R, Barletta M, *et al.* A retrospective evaluation of the effect of perianesthetic hydromorphone administration on the incidence of postanesthetic signs of colic in horses. *Vet Anaesth Analg* 2020; **47**(6): 757–762.

165 Spadavecchia C, Spadavecchia L, Andersen OK, *et al.* Quantitative assessment of nociception in horses by use of the nociceptive withdrawal reflex evoked by transcutaneous electrical stimulation. *Am J Vet Res* 2002; **63**(11): 1551–1556.

166 Spadavecchia C, Andersen OK, Arendt-Nielsen L, *et al.* Investigation of the facilitation of the nociceptive withdrawal reflex evoked by repeated transcutaneous electrical stimulations as a measure of temporal summation in conscious horses. *Am J Vet Res* 2004; **65**(7): 901–908.

167 Studer N, Bernal SD, Thormann W, *et al.* Antinociceptive effects of levomethadone in standing horses sedated with romifidine. *Vet Anaesth Analg* 2021; **48**(3): 451–460.

168 Hubbell JA, Kelly EM, Aarnes TK, *et al.* Pharmacokinetics of midazolam after intravenous administration to horses. *Equine Vet J* 2013; **45**(6): 721–725.

169 Jarrett MA, Bailey KM, Messenger KM, *et al.* Recovery of horses from general anesthesia after induction with propofol and ketamine versus midazolam and ketamine. *J Am Vet Med Assoc* 2018; **253**(1): 101–107.

170 de Vries A, Thomson S, Taylor PM. Comparison of midazolam and diazepam as co-induction agents with ketamine for anaesthesia in sedated ponies undergoing field castration. *Vet Anaesth Analg* 2015; **42**(5): 512–517.

171 Gangl M, Grulke S, Detilleux J, *et al.* Comparison of thiopentone/guaifenesin, ketamine/guaifenesin and ketamine/midazolam for the induction of horses to be anaesthetised with isoflurane. *Vet Rec* 2001; **149**(5): 147–151.

172 Douglas H, Hopster K, Cerullo M, *et al.* The effects of flumazenil on ventilatory and recovery characteristics in horses following midazolam-ketamine induction and isoflurane anaesthesia. *Equine Vet J* 2021; **53**(6): 1257–1267.

173 Trimm CM, Shepard MK. Horses with Colic. In: Grimm KA, Lamont LA, Tranquilli WJ, *et al.*, eds. *Veterinary Anesthesia and Analgesia*, 5th edn. *of Lumb and Jones*. Ames, IA: Wiley Blackwell, 2015: 867–885.

174 Kalsbeek HC. Further experiences with non-surgical correction of nephrosplenic entrapment of the left colon in the horse. *Equine Vet J* 1989; **21**(6): 442–443.

175 Hardy J, Bednarski RM, Biller DS. Effect of phenylephrine on hemodynamics and splenic dimensions in horses. *Am J Vet Res* 1994; **55**(11): 1570–1578.

176 Grosenbaugh DA, Muir WW. Cardiorespiratory effects of sevoflurane, isoflurane, and halothane anesthesia in horses. *Am J Vet Res* 1998; **59**(1): 101–106.

177 Driessen B, Nann L, Benton R, *et al.* Differences in need for hemodynamic support in horses anesthetized with sevoflurane as compared to isoflurane. *Vet Anaesth Analg* 2006; **33**(6): 356–367.

178 Raftery AG, Morgan RA, MacFarlane PD. Perioperative trends in plasma colloid osmotic pressure in horses undergoing surgery. *J Vet Emerg Crit Care (San Antonio)* 2016; **26**(1): 93–100.

179 Lukasik VM, Gleed RD, Scarlett JM, *et al.* Intranasal phenylephrine reduces post anesthetic upper airway obstruction in horses. *Equine Vet J* 1997; **29**(3): 236–238.

180 Matthews NS, Dollar NS, Shawley RV. Halothane-sparing effect of benzodiazepines in ponies. *Cornell Vet* 1990; **80**(3): 259–265.

181 Doherty TJ, Frazier DL. Effect of intravenous lidocaine on halothane minimum alveolar concentration in ponies. *Equine Vet J* 1998; **30**(4): 300–303.

182 Rezende ML, Wagner AE, Mama KR, *et al.* Effects of intravenous administration of lidocaine on the minimum alveolar concentration of sevoflurane in horses. *Am J Vet Res* 2011; **72**(4): 446–451.

183 Dzikiti TB, Hellebrekers LJ, van Dijk P. Effects of intravenous lidocaine on isoflurane concentration, physiological parameters, metabolic parameters and stress-related hormones in horses undergoing surgery. *J Vet Med A Physiol Pathol Clin Med* 2003; **50**(4): 190–195.

184 Enderle AK, Levionnois OL, Kuhn M, *et al.* Clinical evaluation of ketamine and lidocaine intravenous infusions to reduce isoflurane requirements in horses under general anaesthesia. *Vet Anaesth Analg* 2008; **35**(4): 297–305.

185 Wagner AE, Mama KR, Steffey EP, *et al.* Comparison of the cardiovascular effects of equipotent anesthetic doses of sevoflurane alone and sevoflurane plus an intravenous infusion of lidocaine in horses. *Am J Vet Res* 2011; **72**(4): 452–460.

186 Cruz Benedetti IC, Nottrott K, Fourel I, *et al.* Comparison of the effects of an intravenous lidocaine infusion combined with 1% isoflurane versus 2% isoflurane alone on selected cardiovascular variables and recovery characteristics during equine general anaesthesia. *Vet Anaesth Analg* 2017; **44**(1): 63–69.

187 Nóbrega Neto PI, Luna SP, Queiroz-Williams P, *et al.* Cardiorespiratory and antinociceptive effects of two different doses of lidocaine administered to horses during a constant intravenous infusion of xylazine and ketamine. *BMC Vet Res* 2013; **9**: 199.

188 Valverde A, Gunkel C, Doherty TJ, *et al.* Effect of a constant rate infusion of lidocaine on the quality of recovery from sevoflurane or isoflurane general anaesthesia in horses. *Equine Vet J* 2005; **37**(6): 559–564.

189 Feary DJ, Mama KR, Thomasy SM, *et al.* Influence of gastrointestinal tract disease on pharmacokinetics of lidocaine after intravenous infusion in anesthetized horses. *Am J Vet Res* 2006; **67**(2): 317–322.

190 Feary DJ, Mama KR, Wagner AE, *et al.* Influence of general anesthesia on pharmacokinetics of intravenous lidocaine infusion in horses. *Am J Vet Res* 2005; **66**(4): 574–580.

191 Doherty TJ, Seddighi MR. Local anesthetics as pain therapy in horses. *Vet Clin North Am Equine Pract* 2010; **26**(3): 533–549.

192 Freeman DE. Is there still a place for lidocaine in the (postoperative) management of colics? *Vet Clin North Am Equine Pract* 2019; **35**(2): 275–288.

193 Kurabe M, Furue H, Kohno T. Intravenous administration of lidocaine directly acts on spinal dorsal horn and produces analgesic effect: an in vivo patch-clamp analysis. *Sci Rep* 2016; **6**: 26253.

194 Ness TJ. Intravenous lidocaine inhibits visceral nociceptive reflexes and spinal neurons in the rat. *Anesthesiology* 2000; **92**(6): 1685–1691.

195 Song X, Sun Y, Zhang X, *et al.* Effect of perioperative intravenous lidocaine infusion on postoperative recovery following laparoscopic cholecystectomy – a randomized controlled trial. *Int J Surg* 2017; **45**: 8–13.

196 Weibel S, Jokinen J, Pace NL, *et al.* Efficacy and safety of intravenous lidocaine for postoperative analgesia and recovery after surgery: a systematic review with trial sequential analysis. *Br J Anaesth* 2016; **116**(6): 770–783.

197 Robertson SA, Sanchez LC, Merritt AM, *et al.* Effect of systemic lidocaine on visceral and somatic nociception in conscious horses. *Equine Vet J* 2005; **37**(2): 122–127.

198 Brianceau P, Chevalier H, Karas A, *et al.* Intravenous lidocaine and small-intestinal size, abdominal fluid, and outcome after colic surgery in horses. *J Vet Intern Med* 2002; **16**(6): 736–741.

199 Malone E, Ensink J, Turner T, *et al.* Intravenous continuous infusion of lidocaine for treatment of equine ileus. *Vet Surg* 2006; **35**(1): 60–66.

200 Salem SE, Proudman CJ, Archer DC. Has intravenous lidocaine improved the outcome in horses following surgical management of small intestinal lesions in a UK hospital population? *BMC Vet Res* 2016; **12**(1): 157.

201 Lefebvre D, Pirie RS, Handel IG, *et al.* Clinical features and management of equine postoperative ileus: survey of diplomates of the European Colleges of Equine Internal Medicine (ECEIM) and Veterinary Surgeons (ECVS). *Equine Vet J* 2016; **48**(2): 182–187.

202 Lahav M, Levite M, Bassani L, *et al.* Lidocaine inhibits secretion of IL-8 and IL-1beta and stimulates secretion of IL-1 receptor antagonist by epithelial cells. *Clin Exp Immunol* 2002; **127**(2): 226–233.

203 Lan W, Harmon D, Wang JH, *et al.* The effect of lidocaine on in vitro neutrophil and endothelial adhesion molecule expression induced by plasma obtained during tourniquet-induced ischaemia and reperfusion. *Eur J Anaesthesiol* 2004; **21**(11): 892–897.

204 Berger C, Rossaint J, Van Aken H, *et al.* Lidocaine reduces neutrophil recruitment by abolishing chemokine-induced arrest and transendothelial migration in septic patients. *J Immunol* 2014; **192**(1): 367–376.

205 Cook VL, Jones Shults J, McDowell M, *et al.* Attenuation of ischaemic injury in the equine jejunum by administration of systemic lidocaine. *Equine Vet J* 2008; **40**(4): 353–357.

206 Cook VL, Jones Shults J, McDowell MR, *et al.* Anti-inflammatory effects of intravenously administered lidocaine hydrochloride on ischemia-injured jejunum in horses. *Am J Vet Res* 2009; **70**(10): 1259–1268.

207 Bauck AG, Grosche A, Morton AJ, *et al.* Effect of lidocaine on inflammation in equine jejunum subjected to manipulation only and remote to intestinal segments subjected to ischemia. *Am J Vet Res* 2017; **78**(8): 977–989.

208 Ranheim B, Risberg AI, Spadavecchia C, *et al.* The pharmacokinetics of dexmedetomidine administered as a constant rate infusion in horses. *J Vet Pharmacol Ther* 2015; **38**(1): 93–96.

209 Grimsrud KN, Mama KR, Steffey EP, *et al.* Pharmacokinetics and pharmacodynamics of intravenous medetomidine in the horse. *Vet Anaesth Analg* 2012; **39**(1): 38–48.

210 Risberg AI, Ranheim B, Krontveit RI, *et al.* The cardiovascular status of isoflurane-anaesthetized horses with and without dexmedetomidine constant rate infusion evaluated at equivalent depths of anaesthesia. *Vet Anaesth Analg* 2016; **43**(4): 412–423.

211 Hector RC, Rezende ML, Nelson BB, *et al.* Cardiopulmonary function and intestinal blood flow in anaesthetised, experimentally endotoxaemic horses given a constant rate infusion of dexmedetomidine. *Equine Vet J* 2022; **54**(4): 820–828.

212 Gozalo-Marcilla M, Steblaj B, Schauvliege S, *et al.* Comparison of the influence of two different constant-rate infusions (dexmedetomidine versus morphine) on anaesthetic requirements, cardiopulmonary function and recovery quality in isoflurane anaesthetized horses. *Res Vet Sci* 2013; **95**(3): 1186–1194.

213 Hopster K, Wittenberg-Voges L, Kästner SBR. Xylazine infusion in isoflurane-anesthetized and ventilated healthy horses: effects on cardiovascular parameters and intestinal perfusion. *Can J Vet Res* 2017; **81**(4): 249–254.

214 Valverde A. Balanced anesthesia and constant-rate infusions in horses. *Vet Clin North Am Equine Pract* 2013; **29**(1): 89–122.

215 Yamashita K, Satoh M, Umikawa A, *et al.* Combination of continuous intravenous infusion using a mixture of guaifenesin-ketamine-medetomidine and sevoflurane anesthesia in horses. *J Vet Med Sci* 2000; **62**(3): 229–235.

216 Marcilla MG, Schauvliege S, Segaert S, *et al.* Influence of a constant rate infusion of dexmedetomidine on cardiopulmonary function and recovery quality in isoflurane anaesthetized horses. *Vet Anaesth Analg* 2012; **39**(1): 49–58.

217 Creighton CM, Lemke KA, Lamont LA, *et al.* Comparison of the effects of xylazine bolus versus medetomidine constant rate infusion on cardiopulmonary function and depth of anesthesia in horses anesthetized with isoflurane. *J Am Vet Med Assoc* 2012; **240**(8): 991–997.

218 Schauvliege S, Marcilla MG, Verryken K, *et al.* Effects of a constant rate infusion of detomidine on cardiovascular function, isoflurane requirements and recovery quality in horses. *Vet Anaesth Analg* 2011; **38**(6): 544–554.

219 Sanchez LC, Merritt AM. Colorectal distention in the horse: visceral sensitivity, rectal compliance and effect of i.v. xylazine or intrarectal lidocaine. *Equine Vet J* 2005; **37**(1): 70–74.

220 Philipp M, Brede M, Hein L. Physiological significance of alpha(2)-adrenergic receptor subtype diversity: one receptor is not enough. *Am J Physiol Regul Integr Comp Physiol* 2002; **283**(2): R287–R295.

221 Jochle W, Moore JN, Brown J, *et al.* Comparison of detomidine, butorphanol, flunixin meglumine and xylazine in clinical cases of equine colic. *Equine Vet J* 1989; **21**(S7): 111–116.

222 Merritt AM, Burrow JA, Hartless CS. Effect of xylazine, detomidine, and a combination of xylazine and butorphanol on equine duodenal motility. *Am J Vet Res* 1998; **59**(5): 619–623.

223 Kocoglu H, Ozturk H, Ozturk H, *et al.* Effect of dexmedetomidine on ischemia-reperfusion injury in rat kidney: a histopathologic study. *Ren Fail* 2009; **31**(1): 70–74.

224 Gu J, Sun P, Zhao H, *et al.* Dexmedetomidine provides renoprotection against ischemia-reperfusion injury in mice. *Crit Care* 2011; **15**(3): R153.

225 König KS, Verhaar N, Hopster K, *et al.* Ischaemic preconditioning and pharmacological preconditioning with dexmedetomidine in an equine model of small intestinal ischaemia-reperfusion. *PLoS ONE* 2020; **15**(4): e0224720.

226 VanderBroek AR, Engiles JB, Kästner SBR, *et al.* Protective effects of dexmedetomidine on small intestinal ischaemia-reperfusion injury in horses. *Equine Vet J* 2021; **53**(3): 569–578.

227 Verhaar N, Pfarrer C, Neudeck S, *et al.* Preconditioning with lidocaine and xylazine in experimental equine jejunal ischaemia. *Equine Vet J* 2021; **53**(1): 125–133.

228 Cohen SP, Bhatia A, Buvanendran A, *et al.* Consensus guidelines on the use of intravenous ketamine infusions for chronic pain from the American Society of Regional Anesthesia and Pain Medicine, the American Academy of Pain Medicine, and the American Society of Anesthesiologists. *Reg Anesth Pain Med* 2018; **43**(5): 521–546.

229 Muir WW. NMDA receptor antagonists and pain: ketamine. *Vet Clin North Am Equine Pract* 2010; **26**(3): 565–578.

230 Pöppel N, Hopster K, Geburek F, *et al.* Influence of ketamine or xylazine supplementation on isoflurane anaesthetized horses – a controlled clinical trial. *Vet Anaesth Analg* 2015; **42**(1): 30–38.

231 Villalba M, Santiago I, Gomez de Segura IA. Effects of constant rate infusion of lidocaine and ketamine, with or without morphine, on isoflurane MAC in horses. *Equine Vet J* 2011; **43**(6): 721–726.

232 Muir WW III, Sams R. Effects of ketamine infusion on halothane minimal alveolar concentration in horses. *Am J Vet Res* 1992; **53**(10): 1802–1806.

233 Knobloch M, Portier CJ, Levionnois OL, *et al.* Antinociceptive effects, metabolism and disposition of ketamine in ponies under target-controlled drug infusion. *Toxicol Appl Pharmacol* 2006; **216**(3): 373–386.

234 Peterbauer C, Larenza PM, Knobloch M, *et al.* Effects of a low dose infusion of racemic and S-ketamine on the nociceptive withdrawal reflex in standing ponies. *Vet Anaesth Analg* 2008; **35**(5): 414–423.

235 Levionnois OL, Menge M, Thormann W, *et al.* Effect of ketamine on the limb withdrawal reflex evoked by transcutaneous electrical stimulation in ponies anaesthetised with isoflurane. *Vet J* 2010; **186**(3): 304–311.

236 Elfenbein JR, Robertson SA, Corser AA, *et al.* Systemic effects of a prolonged continuous infusion of ketamine in healthy horses. *J Vet Intern Med* 2011; **25**(5): 1134–1137.

237 Alcott CJ, Sponseller BA, Wong DM, *et al.* Clinical and immunomodulating effects of ketamine in horses with experimental endotoxemia. *J Vet Intern Med* 2011; **25**(4): 934–943.

238 Lankveld DP, Bull S, Van Dijk P, *et al.* Ketamine inhibits LPS-induced tumour necrosis factor-alpha and interleukin-6 in an equine macrophage cell line. *Vet Res* 2005; **36**(2): 257–262.

239 Sellon DC, Roberts MC, Blikslager AT, *et al.* Effects of continuous rate intravenous infusion of butorphanol on physiologic and outcome variables in horses after celiotomy. *J Vet Intern Med* 2004; **18**(4): 555–563.

240 Kohn CW, Muir WW III. Selected aspects of the clinical pharmacology of visceral analgesics and gut motility modifying drugs in the horse. *J Vet Intern Med* 1988; **2**(2): 85–91.

241 Bowen IM, Redpath A, Dugdale A, *et al.* BEVA primary care clinical guidelines: analgesia. *Equine Vet J* 2020; **52**(1): 13–27.

242 Steffey EP, Eisele JH, Baggot JD. Interactions of morphine and isoflurane in horses. *Am J Vet Res* 2003; **64**(2): 166–175.

243 Clark L, Clutton RE, Blissitt KJ, *et al.* Effects of peri-operative morphine administration during halothane anaesthesia in horses. *Vet Anaesth Analg* 2005; **32**(1): 10–15.

244 Van Hoogmoed LM, Galuppo LD. Laparoscopic ovariectomy using the endo-GIA stapling device and endo-catch pouches and evaluation of analgesic efficacy of epidural morphine sulfate in 10 mares. *Vet Surg* 2005; **34**(6): 646–650.

245 Virgin J, Hendrickson D, Wallis T, *et al.* Comparison of intraoperative behavioral and hormonal responses to noxious stimuli between mares sedated with caudal epidural detomidine hydrochloride or a continuous intravenous infusion of detomidine hydrochloride for standing laparoscopic ovariectomy. *Vet Surg* 2010; **39**(6): 754–760.

246 Martin-Flores M, Campoy L, Kinsley MA, *et al.* Analgesic and gastrointestinal effects of epidural morphine in horses after laparoscopic cryptorchidectomy under general anesthesia. *Vet Anaesth Analg* 2014; **41**(4): 430–437.

247 Gingold BMC, Hassen KM, Milloway MC, *et al.* Caudal intercostal block for abdominal surgery in horses. *Vet Rec* 2018; **183**(5): 164–165.

248 Baldo CF, Almeida D, Wendt-Hornickle E, *et al.* Transversus abdominis plane block in ponies: a preliminary anatomical study. *Vet Anaesth Analg* 2018; **45**(3): 392–396.

249 Freitag FAV, Amora DDS Jr., Muehlbauer E, *et al.* Ultrasound-guided modified subcostal transversus abdominis plane block and influence of recumbency position on dye spread in equine cadavers. *Vet Anaesth Analg* 2021; **48**(4): 596–602.

250 Kuls N, Trujanovic R, Otero PE, *et al.* Ultrasound-guided transversus abdominis plane block in shetland ponies: a description of a three-point injection technique and evaluation of potential analgesic effects. *J Equine Vet Sci* 2020; **90**: 102994.

251 Radhakrishnan S, Lorenzutti AM, Araos JD, *et al.* Evaluation of noninvasive blood pressure in horses: bias, limits of agreement, and comparative detection of a predetermined mean blood pressure warranting treatment. *Can Vet J* 2021; **62**(9): 994–998.

252 Yamaoka TT, Flaherty D, Pawson P, *et al.* Comparison of arterial blood pressure measurements obtained invasively or oscillometrically using a Datex S/5 Compact monitor in anaesthetised adult horses. *Vet Anaesth Analg* 2017; **44**(3): 492–501.

253 Wilson KAT, Raisis AL, Drynan EA, *et al.* Agreement between invasive blood pressures measured in three peripheral arteries in anaesthetized horses under clinical conditions. *Vet Anaesth Analg* 2018; **45**(3): 338–344.

254 Skouropoulou D, Lacitignola L, Di Bella C, *et al.* Intraoperative assessment of fluid responsiveness in normotensive dogs under isoflurane anaesthesia. *Vet Sci* 2021; **8**(2): 26.

255 Gonçalves LA, Otsuki DA, Pereira MA, *et al.* Comparison of pulse pressure variation versus echocardiography-derived stroke volume variation for prediction of fluid responsiveness in mechanically ventilated anesthetized dogs. *Vet Anaesth Analg* 2020; **47**(1): 28–37.

256 Fantoni DT, Ida KK, Gimenes AM, *et al.* Pulse pressure variation as a guide for volume expansion in dogs undergoing orthopedic surgery. *Vet Anaesth Analg* 2017; **44**(4): 710–718.

257 Muehlestein MB, Steblaj B, Joerger FB, *et al.* Evaluation of the ability of haemodynamic variables obtained with minimally invasive techniques to assess fluid responsiveness in endotoxaemic Beagles. *Vet Anaesth Analg* 2021; **48**(5): 645–653.

258 Fielding CL, Stolba DN. Pulse pressure variation and systolic pressure variation in horses undergoing general anesthesia. *J Vet Emerg Crit Care (San Antonio)* 2012; **22**(3): 372–375.

259 Monge Garcia MI, Jian Z, Settels JJ, *et al.* Performance comparison of ventricular and arterial dP/dt(max) for assessing left ventricular systolic function during different experimental loading and contractile conditions. *Crit Care* 2018; **22**(1): 325.

260 Tartiere JM, Logeart D, Beauvais F, *et al.* Non-invasive radial pulse wave assessment for the evaluation of left ventricular systolic performance in heart failure. *Eur J Heart Fail* 2007; **9**(5): 477–483.

261 Corley KT, Donaldson LL, Durando MM, *et al.* Cardiac output technologies with special reference to the horse. *J Vet Intern Med* 2003; **17**(3): 262–272.
262 Hopster K, Ambrisko TD, Kästner SBR. Influence of catecholamines at different dosages on the function of the LiDCO sensor in isoflurane anesthetized horses. *J Vet Emerg Crit Care (San Antonio)* 2017; **27**(6): 651–657.
263 Hopster K, Ambrisko TD, Stahl J, *et al.* Influence of xylazine on the function of the LiDCO sensor in isoflurane anaesthetized horses. *Vet Anaesth Analg* 2015; **42**(2): 142–149.
264 Shih AC, Queiroz P, Vigani A, *et al.* Comparison of cardiac output determined by an ultrasound velocity dilution cardiac output method and by the lithium dilution cardiac output method in juvenile horses with experimentally induced hypovolemia. *Am J Vet Res* 2014; **75**(6): 565–571.
265 Valverde A, Giguère S, Morey TE, *et al.* Comparison of noninvasive cardiac output measured by use of partial carbon dioxide rebreathing or the lithium dilution method in anesthetized foals. *Am J Vet Res* 2007; **68**(2): 141–147.
266 Sano H, Chambers JP. Ability of pulse wave transit time to detect changes in stroke volume and to estimate cardiac output compared to thermodilution technique in isoflurane-anaesthetised dogs. *Vet Anaesth Analg* 2017; **44**(5): 1057–1067.
267 Koenig J, McDonell W, Valverde A. Accuracy of pulse oximetry and capnography in healthy and compromised horses during spontaneous and controlled ventilation. *Can J Vet Res* 2003; **67**(3): 169–174.
268 Matthews NS, Hartsfield SM, Sanders EA, *et al.* Evaluation of pulse oximetry in horses surgically treated for colic. *Equine Vet J* 1994; **26**(2): 114–116.
269 Voulgaris DA, Hofmeister EH. Multivariate analysis of factors associated with post-anesthetic times to standing in isoflurane-anesthetized horses: 381 cases. *Vet Anaesth Analg* 2009; **36**(5): 414–420.
270 Reynolds L, Beckmann J, Kurz A. Perioperative complications of hypothermia. *Best Pract Res Clin Anaesthesiol* 2008; **22**(4): 645–657.
271 Tomasic M. Temporal changes in core body temperature in anesthetized adult horses. *Am J Vet Res* 1999; **60**(5): 556–562.
272 Wilson DV, McFeely AM. Positive end-expiratory pressure during colic surgery in horses: 74 cases (1986–1988). *J Am Vet Med Assoc* 1991; **199**(7): 917–921.
273 Pascoe PJ, McDonell WN, Trim CM, *et al.* Mortality rates and associated factors in equine colic operations – a retrospective study of 341 operations. *Can Vet J* 1983; **24**(3): 76–85.
274 Day TK, Gaynor JS, Muir WW III, *et al.* Blood gas values during intermittent positive pressure ventilation and spontaneous ventilation in 160 anesthetized horses positioned in lateral or dorsal recumbency. *Vet Surg* 1995; **24**(3): 266–276.
275 Moens Y. Mechanical ventilation and respiratory mechanics during equine anesthesia. *Vet Clin North Am Equine Pract* 2013; **29**(1): 51–67.
276 Nicolaisen A-SK, Bendix Nygaard A, Christophersen MT, *et al.* Effect of head and tail rope-assisted recovery of horses after elective and emergency surgery under general anaesthesia. *Equine Vet Educ* 2020; **34**: 13397.
277 Santiago-Llorente I, López-San Román FJ, Villalba-Orero M. Demographic, pre-operative and anaesthesia-related risk factors for unsatisfactory recovery quality in horses undergoing emergency abdominal surgery. *Vet Anaesth Analg* 2021; **48**(6): 882–890.
278 Tute AS, Wilkins PA, Gleed RD, *et al.* Negative pressure pulmonary edema as a post-anesthetic complication associated with upper airway obstruction in a horse. *Vet Surg* 1996; **25**(6): 519–523.
279 Borer KE. Pulmonary oedema associated with anaesthesia for colic surgery in a horse. *Vet Anaesth Analg* 2005; **32**(4): 228–232.
280 Andrade FS, Facó LL, Ida KK, *et al.* Effects of 12 and 17 cmH_2O positive end-expiratory pressure applied after alveolar recruitment maneuver on pulmonary gas exchange and compliance in isoflurane-anesthetized horses. *Vet Anaesth Analg* 2019; **46**(1): 64–73.
281 Mason DE, Muir WW, Wade A. Arterial blood gas tensions in the horse during recovery from anesthesia. *J Am Vet Med Assoc* 1987; **190**(8): 989–994.
282 Cerullo M, Driessen B, Douglas H, *et al.* Changes in arterial blood pressure and oxygen tension as a result of hoisting in isoflurane anesthetized healthy adult horses. *Front Vet Sci* 2020; **7**: 601326.
283 de Miguel Garcia C, Campoy L, Parry S, *et al.* Questionnaire on the process of recovering horses from general anesthesia and associated personnel injury in equine practice. *Vet Anaesth Analg* 2021; **48**(2): 223–229.
284 Wohlfender FD, Doherr MG, Driessen B, *et al.* International online survey to assess current practice in equine anaesthesia. *Equine Vet J* 2015; **47**(1): 65–71.
285 Hector RC, Rezende ML, Mama KR, *et al.* Recovery quality following a single post-anaesthetic dose of dexmedetomidine or romifidine in sevoflurane anaesthetised horses. *Equine Vet J* 2020; **52**(5): 685–691.
286 Woodhouse KJ, Brosnan RJ, Nguyen KQ, *et al.* Effects of postanesthetic sedation with romifidine or xylazine on quality of recovery from isoflurane anesthesia in horses. *J Am Vet Med Assoc* 2013; **242**(4): 533–539.
287 Aarnes TK, Bednarski RM, Bertone AL, *et al.* Recovery from desflurane anesthesia in horses with and without post-anesthetic xylazine. *Can J Vet Res* 2014; **78**(2): 103–109.
288 Guedes A, Knych H, Tucker L, *et al.* Pharmacokinetics and clinical effects of xylazine and dexmedetomidine in horses recovering from isoflurane anesthesia. *J Vet Pharmacol Ther* 2020; **43**(4): 369–376.

63 Equine Local Anesthetic and Analgesic Techniques

Rachael E. Carpenter[1] and Christopher R. Byron[2]

[1] Department of Small Animal Clinical Sciences, Virginia-Maryland College of Veterinary Medicine, Virginia Tech University, Blacksburg, Virginia, USA

[2] Department of Large Animal Clinical Sciences, Virginia-Maryland College of Veterinary Medicine, Virginia Tech University, Blacksburg, Virginia, USA

Chapter contents

Introduction, 1235
- Choice of local anesthetic agent, 1235

Anesthesia of the head, 1236
- Infraorbital nerve block, 1236
- Maxillary nerve block, 1236
- Mandibular nerve block, 1236
- Mental nerve block, 1236

Anesthesia for ocular procedures, 1237
- Topical anesthesia, 1237
- Auriculopalpebral nerve block, 1237
- Sensory nerve blocks, 1237

Anesthesia of the limbs, 1239
- Perineural anesthesia of the limbs, 1240
- Intra-articular and intrabursal anesthesia of the limbs, 1245

Anesthesia for laparotomy/laparoscopy, 1250
- Infiltration anesthesia, 1251
- Paravertebral thoracolumbar anesthesia, 1251

Anesthesia for urogenital procedures, 1251
- Anesthesia for castration, 1252
- Anesthesia for ovariectomy, 1253
- Anesthesia of the perineum, 1253
- Anesthesia of the penis or vulva, 1253

Neuraxial anesthesia/analgesia, 1253
- Indications and contraindications, 1253
- Caudal epidural anesthesia/analgesia, 1254
- Continuous caudal epidural anesthesia/analgesia, 1254
- Epidural medications, 1254
- Complications, 1257

Novel regional analgesic techniques, 1258
- Transversus abdominis plane block, 1258
- Caudal intercostal block for abdominal surgery, 1258
- Continuous delivery of local anesthetics for lower limb analgesia, 1258

References, 1258

Introduction

In horses, many diagnostic and surgical procedures can be performed safely and humanely by combining local anesthetic techniques with sedation and/or physical restraint. In conjunction with a good physical examination, and thorough palpation of the limbs including tendons and joints, one of the most important techniques for the equine practitioner to master is local and regional anesthesia and analgesia of the limbs. Use of these techniques can aid in localizing lameness, provide analgesia and anesthesia for standing procedures or diagnostics, and provide intra- or postoperative analgesia. Mastery of other techniques (e.g., epidural and craniofacial nerve blocks) will facilitate procedures on standing patients, avoiding the relatively high morbidity and mortality associated with general anesthesia of the equine patient.

Choice of local anesthetic agent

The choice of which local anesthetic(s) to be used is usually made based on the onset and duration of action of the individual agent(s) and the desired result. Improper injection technique or misidentification of the landmarks can result in incomplete block and other complications. Aseptic preparation of the skin is recommended for local anesthetic injection sites, especially when injecting into a joint or the epidural or subarachnoid space. Desired anesthetic effects without complications are obtained by using proper techniques, including aspiration before injection to avoid intravenous or intra-arterial administration, and avoidance of injections through or into inflamed tissues.

The blocks described in this chapter are most commonly accomplished with lidocaine (with the exception of the diagnostic blocks for lameness examination) unless specified otherwise. Lidocaine has a rapid onset of action and a relatively short duration of effect (approximately 1 h). Where a longer duration of action is desired (for analgesia), mepivacaine, bupivacaine, or ropivacaine may be substituted. Local anesthesia of the limbs for diagnostic nerve blocks is usually accomplished with mepivacaine because it has a slightly longer duration of effect than lidocaine (up to 2 h), but lidocaine may be substituted at the same volume if needed. Dexmedetomidine added to mepivacaine has been shown to double the duration of action of mepivacaine alone in a peripheral nerve block if a longer block is needed [1]. For more in-depth information on the pharmacology (metabolism, elimination, toxicity, and individual medication profiles) of local anesthetics, see Chapter 29.

Veterinary Anesthesia and Analgesia: The Sixth Edition of Lumb and Jones. Edited by Leigh Lamont, Kurt Grimm, Sheilah Robertson, Lydia Love and Carrie Schroeder.
© 2024 John Wiley & Sons, Inc. Published 2024 by John Wiley & Sons, Inc.
Companion website: www.wiley.com/go/lamont/anesthesia

Anesthesia of the head

Local anesthesia of the head is most commonly used clinically for dental and sinus surgery, ocular examinations, and laceration repair. A recent study assessing complications associated with regional nerve blocks in dental patients identified eight complications out of 270 regional nerve blocks performed resulting in a 2.96% incidence of complication. Complications included supraorbital hematoma, local hematoma, lingual self-trauma, and nerve block failure [2].

Infraorbital nerve block

The infraorbital nerve block facilitates surgery of the nasal area or incisors. Desensitization of the upper lip and nose is achieved by injecting 5 mL of local anesthetic with a 1 inch (2.5 cm) 20 gauge needle over the infraorbital nerve as it emerges from the infraorbital canal (Fig. 63.1g). The infraorbital canal can be palpated after displacing the flat levator labii superioris muscle dorsally and then palpating with the index finger approximately half the distance and 2.5 cm dorsal to a line connecting the nasomaxillary notch and the rostral end of the facial crest.

To desensitize the teeth as far as the first molar, the maxillary sinus, the roof of the nasal cavity, and the skin almost to the medial canthus of the eye, 5 mL of local anesthetic is deposited within the infraorbital foramen using a 2 inch (5.0 cm) 20 gauge needle (Fig. 63.1h) [3]. The local anesthesia produced by this technique is generally not sufficient to allow standing extraction of the premolars or trephination of the maxillary sinus but may be a useful adjunct to general anesthesia in those cases. A study using computed tomography (CT) and contrast injections examined two alternative techniques for infiltration of the infraorbital nerve within the pterygopalatine fossa in the hopes of refining the technique for better analgesia of the cheek teeth [4]. Both techniques were successful in achieving distribution of contrast medium around the infraorbital nerve.

There is evidence to suggest that idiopathic head shaking may be a facial pain syndrome resulting from trigeminal neuropathy. Idiopathic head shaking is a diagnosis without a conclusive diagnostic test, but one study has suggested utilizing desensitization of the infraorbital nerve as a diagnostic tool for this disorder [5].

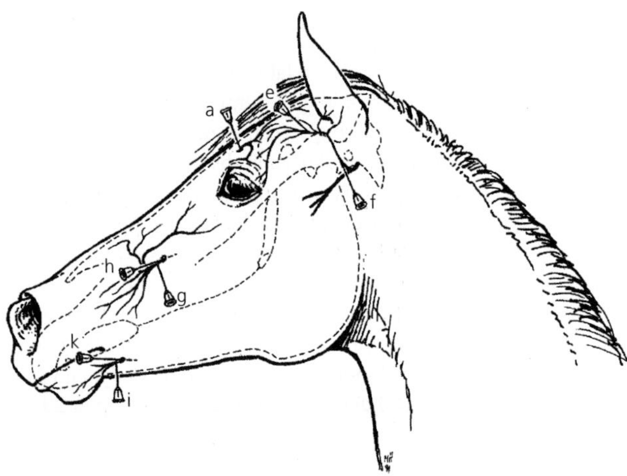

Figure 63.1 Sites for needle placement for local anesthesia of the head. a, supraorbital nerve; e and f, auriculopalpebral nerve; g and h, infraorbital nerve; i, mental nerve; k, alveolar mandibular nerve.

Maxillary nerve block

Desensitization of the maxilla, premaxilla, paranasal sinuses, and sinus cavity can be achieved by blocking the maxillary nerve at the pterygopalatine fossa (where the nerve enters the infraorbital canal). Two methods of infiltration have been described. In the first, a 3.5 inch (8.9 cm) 20–22 gauge spinal needle is inserted on the ventral border of the zygomatic process of the temporal bone at the narrowest point of the zygomatic arch and directed rostromedially and ventrally in the direction of the sixth cheek tooth on the contralateral maxillary arcade [6]. The second approach is accomplished by inserting the needle at a 90° angle to the head so that it enters the pterygopalatine fossa just caudal to the maxillary tuberosity [7]. A cadaver study evaluated the accuracy of methods used to infiltrate the maxillary nerve and determined that using an angulated needle placement or a perpendicular needle placement were equally accurate [8]. To further improve the accuracy of maxillary nerve blocks, recent investigations are exploring the possibility that ultrasound-guided blocks may be more accurate than blocks done using surface landmarks [9].

Mandibular nerve block

Blocking the mandibular nerve will desensitize the ipsilateral side of the mandible and the associated dental structures. The mandibular nerve can be blocked as it enters the mandibular canal at the mandibular foramen where it becomes the inferior alveolar nerve. The location of the mandibular foramen may be approximated using the intersection of a line passing vertically downward from the lateral canthus of the eye and a line extending backward from the table of the mandibular molar teeth. A 6 inch (15.24 cm) 20–22 gauge needle is inserted at the ventral border of the ramus, just rostral to the angle of the mandible and then advanced to the location of the mandibular foramen. In that location, 15–20 mL of local anesthetic may be injected. The second approach involves inserting the needle at the caudal border of the ventral ramus of the mandible about 3 cm ventral to the temporomandibular joint and then advancing the needle to the approximate location of the mandibular foramen, taking care to stay as close to the medial aspect of the mandible as possible. To perform the block, 15–20 mL of local anesthetic is injected into the area. One study examined the accuracy of the two approaches to the inferior alveolar nerve block and found that both the traditional approaches were accurate, but that currently recommended doses of local anesthetics may be excessive [10]. An intraoral approach to the inferior alveolar nerve has also been described. The authors of one study found that this approach could potentially reduce the dose of local anesthetic needed by allowing the anesthetist to deposit the local anesthetic closer to the inferior alveolar nerve, which could reduce the risk of desensitizing the lingual nerve and causing self-trauma to the tongue [11].

Mental nerve block

To desensitize the lower lip, the mental nerve is blocked with 5 mL of local anesthetic rostral to the mental foramen (Figs. 63.1i and 63.2i). After the tendon of the depressor labii inferioris is displaced, the lateral border of the mental foramen is palpated at the horizontal ramus of the mandible in the middle of the interdental space [12].

The lower incisors and premolars can be desensitized by inserting a 3 inch (7.5 cm) 20 gauge spinal needle into the mental foramen as far as possible in a ventromedial direction and depositing 10 mL of local anesthetic to desensitize the mandibular alveolar

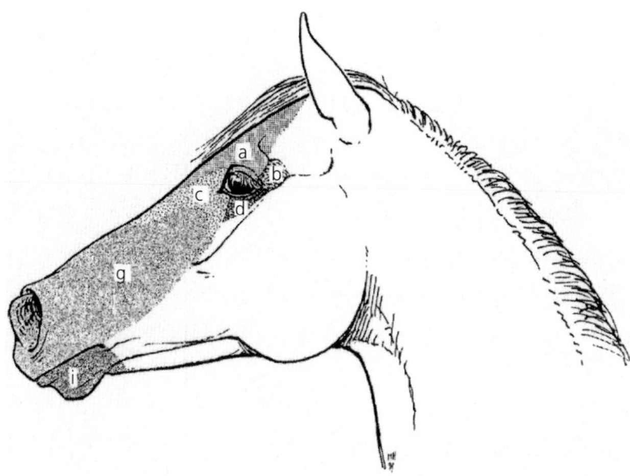

Figure 63.2 Area of skin desensitization after blocking various nerves of the head. a, supraorbital nerve; b, lacrimal nerve; c, infratrochlear nerve; d, zygomatic nerve; g, infraorbital nerve; i, mental nerve.

nerve. This technique is difficult and is probably best used as an adjunct to general anesthesia for extraction of teeth.

As many sedated patients do not tolerate placement of local anesthetic into the mental foramen, one study investigated an intraoral technique and found that local anesthetic could be deposited into the mental foramen via this approach [13].

Anesthesia for ocular procedures

Because of the strength with which the horse can close its eyelids and keep them closed, some form of sedation and local anesthesia is generally required for a complete ophthalmic examination. These same techniques will often allow satisfactory completion of minor diagnostic and surgical procedures. In addition to the specific blocks listed below, a line block (local anesthetic deposited along the superior and/or inferior orbital rims) and infiltration anesthesia may be used to facilitate surgical procedures and placement of subpalpebral lavage catheters.

Topical anesthesia

Topical anesthesia is usually required for examination of an eye that is a source of pain. In addition, topical anesthesia will facilitate minor diagnostic and surgical procedures of the cornea and conjunctiva such as collection of samples for cytologic examination, removal of superficial corneal foreign bodies, and subconjunctival injections.

Proparacaine and tetracaine are the most commonly used topical ophthalmic anesthetics. Preservative-free ophthalmic formulations are preferred for topical ocular use because preservatives can damage the corneal epithelium. Although proparacaine and tetracaine are generally interchangeable, tetracaine is more irritating to the cornea than proparacaine. Other local anesthetics that have been used topically include lidocaine, mepivacaine, and bupivacaine.

In humans, the onset of action of proparacaine is approximately 15 s, and the duration of action is approximately 15–30 min [14]. In horses, using two drops of 0.5% tetracaine increases the duration of maximal anesthetic effects from 5.5 to 16 min, and increasing the concentration to 1% tetracaine increases the duration of maximal anesthetic effects from 5.5 to 15.25 min [15]. A study in horses compared the efficacy and duration of topically applied proparacaine ophthalmic solution, lidocaine injectable solution, mepivacaine injectable solution, and bupivacaine injectable solution and concluded that bupivacaine may be most appropriate for procedures requiring longer periods of corneal anesthesia. In that study, corneal sensitivity was decreased for 35 min following topical application of 0.5% proparacaine and 2% mepivacaine, for 45 min following 2% lidocaine, and for 60 min following 0.5% bupivacaine [16]. Another study compared 0.5% bupivacaine, 2% lidocaine, and 0.4% oxybuprocaine and showed that corneal sensitivity was decreased for 45 min with bupivacaine, 55 min for lidocaine, and 65 min for oxybuprocaine [17].

Topical lidocaine gel has been studied as a topical ophthalmic anesthetic in horses. One study found that 0.2 mL of 2% lidocaine gel applied topically produced a marked reduction in corneal sensitivity for up to 75 min. Some corneal irregularities were seen in treated eyes, but all resolved without treatment within 24 h. The authors concluded that this may be a useful topical anesthetic for minor ophthalmic procedures performed in the standing sedated horse [18].

Repeated use of topical anesthesia can reduce Schirmer tear test values, cause mild corneal epithelial damage, and suppress wound healing with prolonged use. Because of these potential adverse effects, topical anesthetics should not be prescribed as analgesic agents for painful ocular conditions.

Auriculopalpebral nerve block

The most important nerve block used in ocular examinations to prevent closure of the eyelid is the auriculopalpebral nerve block. This block primarily affects the motor innervation to the orbicularis oculi muscle, without affecting the sensory innervation to the eyelids.

The auriculopalpebral nerve is usually blocked where the nerve is easily palpable along the most dorsal aspect of the zygomatic arch (Fig. 63.3e) or the depression caudal to the mandible at the ventral edge of the temporal position of the zygomatic arch (Fig. 63.3f). In each location, the needle is placed subcutaneously in the area where the nerve is palpated and 1–2 mL of local anesthetic is injected over the nerve [12,19].

Auriculopalpebral nerve blocks will diminish the blink reflex, so artificial tears should be applied to the cornea to prevent drying, and care should be exercised to protect the eye from accidental trauma or debris until recovery is complete. While auriculopalpebral nerve block does decrease intraocular pressure (IOP), the difference in IOP between blocked versus unblocked eyes is not clinically significant [20].

Sensory nerve blocks

The supraorbital nerve block will desensitize the majority of the upper eyelid and can be used to facilitate minor surgical procedures of the nasal portion of the upper lid (Fig. 63.2a). The nerve emerges through the supraorbital foramen, which can be easily palpated with the index finger about 5–7 cm dorsal to the medial canthus and in the center of an imaginary triangle formed by grasping the supraorbital process of the frontal bone with the thumb and middle finger and sliding medially (Fig. 63.4A). Approximately 2 mL of local anesthetic is injected subcutaneously over the foramen, 1 mL as the needle is inserted into the foramen, and 2 mL as the needle is inserted to its full depth (2.5 cm) into the foramen (Fig. 63.4B). Successful completion of this block will desensitize the forehead, including the middle two-thirds of the upper eyelid, and since this block will also desensitize some of the terminal branches of the auriculopalpebral nerve, motor function of the orbicularis oculi muscle may be affected [21].

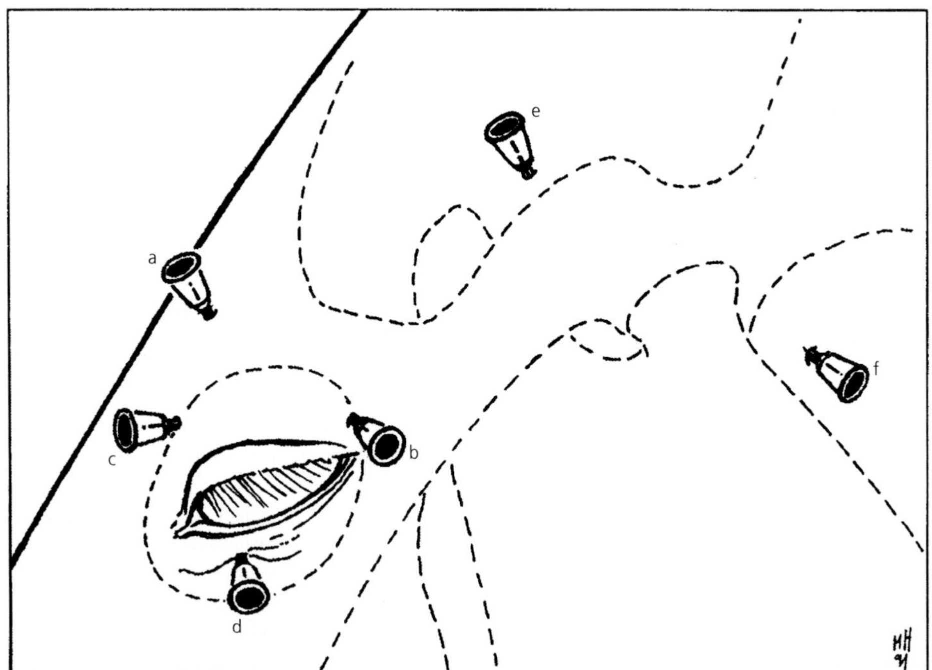

Figure 63.3 Needle placement for periocular nerve blocks. a, supraorbital nerve; b, lacrimal nerve; c, infratrochlear nerve; d, zygomatic nerve; e and f, auriculopalpebral nerve.

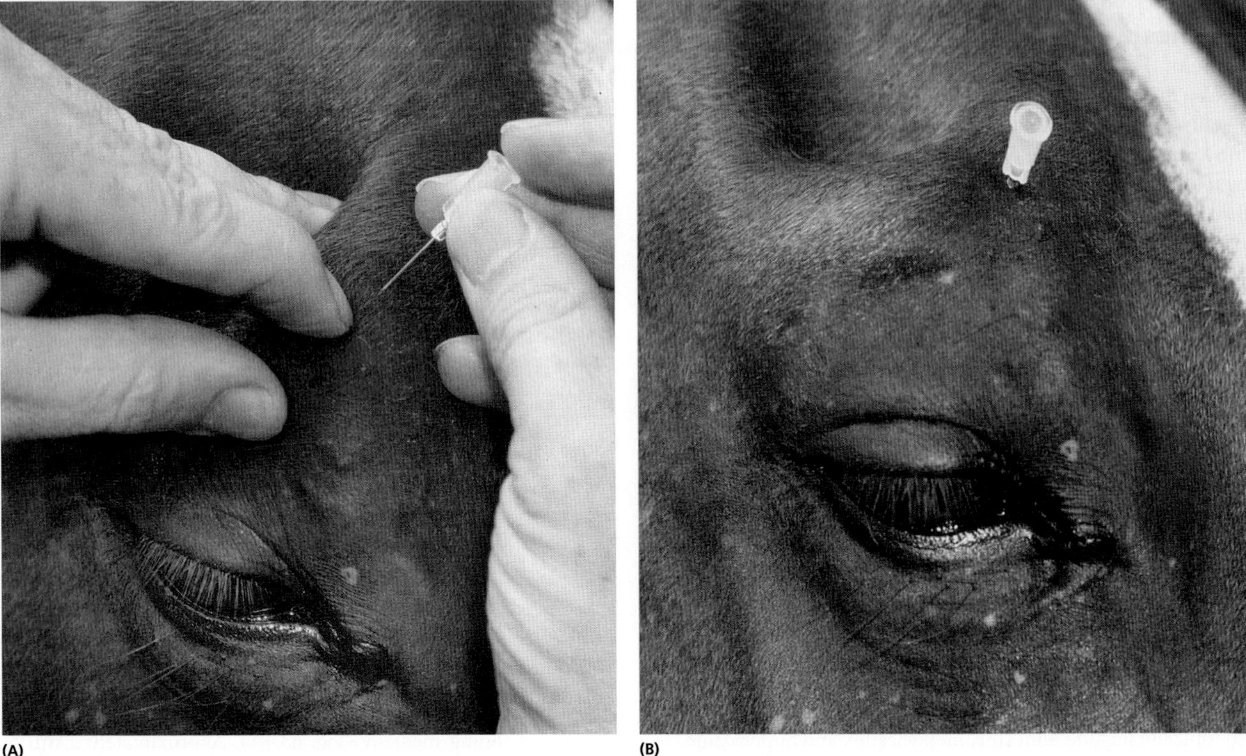

Figure 63.4 **A.** Palpation of the supraorbital nerve. **B.** Insertion of a 2.5 cm, 25 gauge needle into the supraorbital foramen.

For more complete desensitization of the eyelids, the supraorbital block may be combined with techniques that block the lacrimal, infratrochlear, and zygomatic nerves. The lacrimal nerve is desensitized by inserting a needle percutaneously at the lateral canthus of the eye and directing it medially along the dorsal rim of the orbit (Fig. 63.3b). Deep injection of 2–3 mL of anesthetic at this site desensitizes the lateral canthus, lateral aspect of the upper eyelid, lacrimal gland, local connective tissue, and temporal angle of the orbit (Fig. 63.2b) [19,21].

Anesthesia of the medial canthus, lacrimal glands, nictitans, and connective tissues (Fig. 63.2c) is achieved by injecting 2–3 mL of local anesthetic around the infratrochlear nerve. The needle is inserted through the bony notch or the palpable irregularity on the dorsal rim of the orbit near the medial canthus (Fig. 63.3c) [19,21].

To infiltrate the zygomatic nerve and desensitize the lower two-thirds of the lower eyelid, skin, and connective tissue (Fig. 63.2d), the needle is placed subcutaneously on the lateral aspect of the bony orbit and supraorbital portion of the zygomatic arch and 3–5 mL of local anesthetic is injected (Fig. 63.3d) [19,21].

If general anesthesia is contraindicated or financially undesirable, standing enucleation may be an option. Standing enucleation may be accomplished with sedation in addition to blockade of the auriculopalpebral, infratrochlear, lacrimal, and zygomatic nerves [22], or with blockade of the supraorbital, infratrochlear, lacrimal, and zygomatic nerves [23]. One study reviewed the use of auriculopalpebral, supraorbital, lacrimal, zygomatic, and infratrochlear nerve blocks in addition to a retrobulbar block and sedation for enucleation and orbital implant placement in 20 horses. The authors concluded that the standardized perioperative protocol described provided a safe effective alternative to general anesthesia [24].

Anesthesia of the limbs

Various techniques may be used to desensitize specific structures of the equine limb for diagnostic or therapeutic purposes. These include perineural, intra-articular, and intrabursal injection techniques and local infiltration (e.g., ring blocks and line blocks) of local anesthetic. These techniques are frequently used therapeutically to provide temporary relief from pain or to facilitate procedures for treatment or diagnosis of diseases. In addition, local anesthesia techniques are an integral part of the procedures used to diagnose lameness in horses. The blocks used for therapeutic and diagnostic purposes are similar. However, clinicians should keep in mind that blocks performed for diagnosis of lameness should be carried out in a manner that desensitizes the most specific region possible (to allow identification of the affected structures with confidence), whereas blocks performed for therapeutic relief from pain or to allow performance of a procedure (e.g., surgery) may be applied so that a larger (i.e., less specific) area is desensitized. Therefore, the goal of the local anesthesia procedure should be considered when performing these techniques. In general, perineural injections performed as distally as possible using the smallest effective amount of local anesthetic increase the specificity of such blocks.

Skin at injection sites should be cleaned and prepared prior to needle insertion to reduce the likelihood of infection of deeper tissues. Such preparation may include the use of alcohol only or povidone-iodine or chlorhexidine gluconate scrub followed by a sterile water, saline solution, or alcohol rinse. Skin should also be aseptically prepared prior to insertion of a needle in a synovial structure, and the use of sterile gloves, syringes, needles, and unopened bottles of local anesthetic is recommended owing to the potential for septic arthritis. Clipping of hair prior to aseptic preparation for injection of synovial structures is often performed; however, clients may object to this. Removal of hair prior to preparing the skin may not be necessary; the number of bacterial colony-forming units on skin over midcarpal and distal interphalangeal joints after a povidone-iodine and 70% alcohol scrub is not significantly different between areas that are clipped and those that are not clipped to remove hair [25]. Removal of hair in horses with thick coats (i.e., hirsute horses or during cold weather), for horses with soiled coats, and to aid identification of landmarks for select injections may be warranted. Clipping of hair with an electric clipper and a size 40 clipper blade decreases contamination of joints with tissue debris and hair after needle insertion [26]. In addition, the use of stylets for spinal needles, 22 gauge needles rather than 20 gauge needles, and angled needle insertion reduces joint contamination when hair is not clipped [26]. Aseptic preparation is typically not necessary before performing perineural blocks; however, the skin should be clean and the area should be briefly scrubbed or wiped with alcohol. As a precaution, the skin should be thoroughly prepared whenever there is a risk of inadvertent puncture of a synovial structure. In addition, needles should only be handled on the outside surface of the hub when sterile gloves are not worn.

Depending on the block performed, injections may be performed with the limb in a weight-bearing or flexed position. Changes in position may aid the identification of anatomic landmarks before needle insertion. Restraint of the horse by a capable handler should be applied in all instances; the use of a twitch is typically warranted. The ipsilateral or a contralateral limb may be held by an assistant if the horse is reluctant to stand still during a block. However, the handler must exercise extreme care in such instances so that neither the clinician nor the assistant is injured; this is particularly important when the contralateral limb is held and should not be attempted with fractious horses. Sedation may be necessary to perform a block; however, this should be avoided when the horse must be walked or trotted as part of a lameness examination. Sedation of horses with detomidine may not alter the severity of lameness but can alter the pattern of locomotion [27]. In another study evaluating the effects of xylazine, detomidine, and romifidine alone or in combination with butorphanol, xylazine alone had the least impact on objective lameness measures [28]. Use of low-dose detomidine may minimize effects on coordination but does have an impact on other objective gait parameters [29]. Therefore, xylazine may have the least effect on lameness and be the best choice when light sedation is necessary during lameness examination.

Intra-articular blocks may be best performed with mepivacaine because the severity of toxic effects of that local anesthetic on equine articular chondrocytes is less than that with lidocaine and markedly less than that with bupivacaine [30]. Although not in common use for horses, there is evidence that ropivacaine may have lower chondrotoxicity than mepivacaine [31].

Choice of needle gauge is based primarily on personal preference. However, 20 gauge needles are useful for a wide variety of injections. Use of smaller (22–25 gauge) needles can be advantageous for perineural injections and local anesthesia of superficial synovial structures in the distal aspects of limbs because they may reduce the horse's reaction and can be easier to place precisely. Use of larger (18–19 gauge) needles is typically warranted for injections performed with long (greater than 1.5 inch or 3.8 cm) needles, through thick fascia or muscle, or when movement of the horse may cause bending and breakage of the needle. Choice of needle length should be made with consideration of the location of the structure to be injected and the locations of other deeper structures that may sustain iatrogenic damage during needle insertion. For horses that are prone to move during an injection or in instances during which motion of the needle may cause deposition of local anesthetic outside the region of interest, extension set tubing may be used between the syringe and needle. For perineural injections, the needle may be directed in a proximal to distal direction or a distal to proximal direction. Use of a distal to proximal direction may decrease the risk of needle breakage if the horse moves, particularly for small gauge needles. Use of a proximal to distal direction may aid retention of the needle at the site of insertion if the horse moves. For nerves within a perineural sheath, deposition of local anesthetic inside the sheath may be required to ensure effective desensitization [32]. Confirmation of needle placement can be made via ultrasonography.

The efficacy of a perineural block is typically confirmed by detection of loss of skin sensation distal to the site where the block was performed. However, this may not be a reliable indication of efficacy in all instances, and the use of other signs (e.g., improvement in lameness or loss of response to hoof tester pressure or limb flexion) should also be used to assess the block further. Loss of skin sensation is not a reliable indicator of the efficacy of perineural blocks performed in the proximal aspect of a limb. When checking skin sensation, a blunt object that will not cause skin trauma should be used and light to moderate pressure should be applied. Horses may move because of the presence and movements of the clinician; for such horses, it may be helpful to check skin sensation from the contralateral side or to have an assistant cover the horse's eyes.

Perineural anesthesia of the limbs

Palmar or plantar digital nerve block

The digital neurovascular bundles are located in the palmar or plantar aspect of the pastern region (between the coronary band and metacarpophalangeal joint) medial and lateral to the deep digital flexor tendon. The digital nerves are the most palmar or plantar structures in these neurovascular bundles (Figs. 63.5a and 63.6a). Local anesthesia of these nerves may be performed with the limb in a weight-bearing or flexed position. Digital nerve blocks are typically performed with a 1 inch (2.5 cm) 22 gauge needle or a ⅝ inch (1.5 cm) 25 gauge needle. The needle is advanced through the skin, and approximately 1.5 mL of local anesthetic is injected perineurally. The palmar or plantar aspect of the foot (including the heel bulbs, sole, and navicular bursa, and associated structures) is desensitized starting within 5–10 min after performance of the block (Fig. 63.7A).

Digital nerve blocks do not significantly reduce the response of non-lame horses to flexion of the distal limbs [33]; therefore, clinicians should keep in mind that these blocks may not improve distal limb flexion responses in lame horses. Digital nerve blocks should be performed just proximal to the collateral cartilages of the foot to reduce the likelihood that proximal interphalangeal joint pain would be alleviated by the block [34]. Local anesthesia of palmar digital nerves may alleviate lameness attributable to pain of the sole of the foot [35] or the distal interphalangeal joint [36]. Local anesthesia of palmar digital nerves affects kinematic gait analysis variables in horses with navicular disease [37].

Palmar digital nerve blocks performed with mepivacaine are fully effective between 15 min and 1 h after the block, and effects

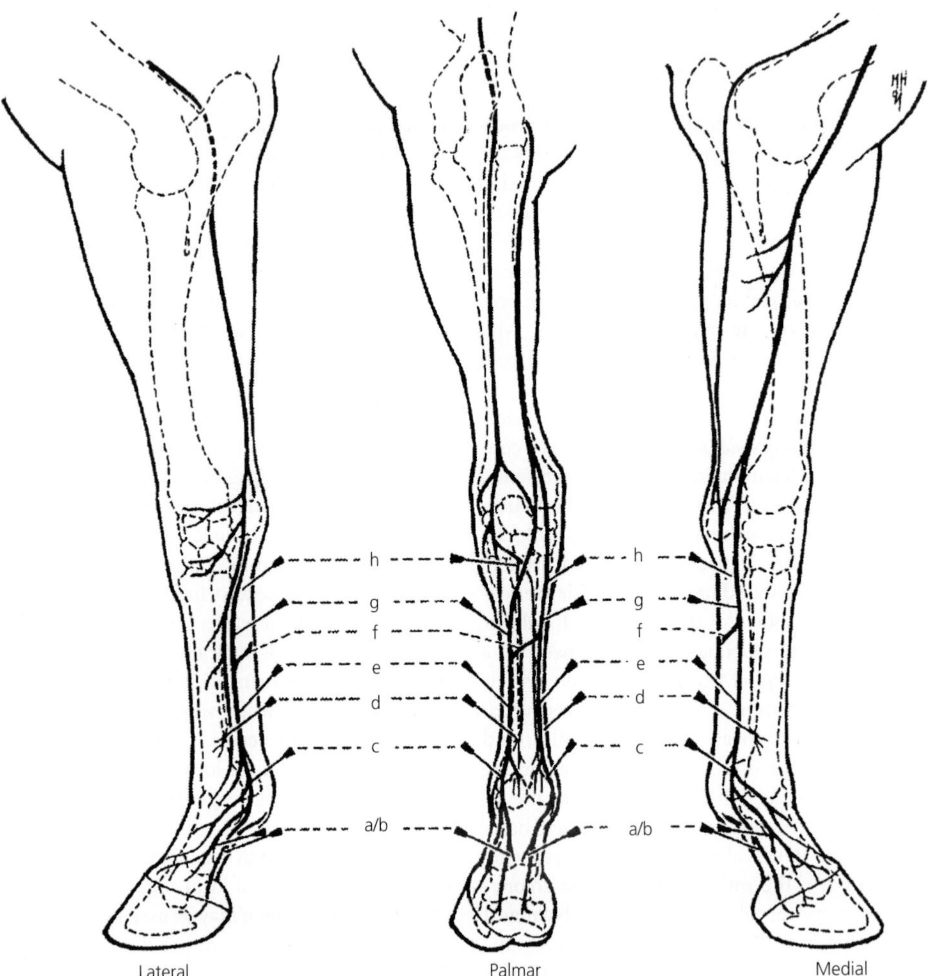

Figure 63.5 Needle placement for left distal forelimb nerve blocks. a, lateral and medial palmar digital nerves; b, dorsal branches; c, lateral and medial palmar digital nerves (basisesamoid); d and g, lateral and medial palmar nerves; e, lateral and medial palmar metacarpal nerves; f, communicating branch; h, location of high suspensory block.

may persist for more than 2 h [38]. Mepivacaine appears to be more reliable and has a longer duration than lidocaine for diagnostic local anesthesia [39]. Results of another study indicate that the onset of desensitization is similar among local anesthetics for palmar digital nerve blocks in horses; lidocaine has a significantly shorter duration than bupivacaine, which in turn has a shorter duration than prilocaine or mepivacaine in this application [40]. The combination of dexmedetomidine and mepivacaine greatly increases the duration of sensory blockade compared with mepivacaine alone; perineural dexmedetomidine alone does not significantly affect the mechanical nociceptive threshold [1]. The addition of epinephrine to lidocaine has been shown to increase the duration of palmar digital nerve block local anesthesia [41]. Liposomal bupivacaine is also an effective agent for local anesthesia of palmar digital nerves [42].

Block of the dorsal branches of the digital nerves

Structures of the dorsal aspect of the foot and pastern region can be desensitized by blocking the medial and lateral dorsal branches of the palmar or plantar digital nerves (Figs. 63.5b and 63.6b). This block is typically performed in addition to the digital nerve block; a 1–1.5 inch (2.5–3.8 cm) 20–22 gauge needle is used to inject 1.5–3 mL of local anesthetic subcutaneously as the needle is passed in a dorsal direction from the site of injection of the palmar or plantar digital nerves; the needle should be inserted up to the hub. Performing the block in the proximal aspect of the pastern provides analgesia for a larger area than is provided when the block is performed in the distal aspect of the pastern; therefore, use of a distal location yields a block that is more specific for structures of the dorsal region of the foot and dorsodistal aspect of the pastern.

Abaxial sesamoid (basisesamoid) block

The medial and lateral palmar or plantar digital nerves (including dorsal branches) can be blocked at the level of the distal abaxial aspect of the proximal sesamoid bones (Figs. 63.5c and 63.6c); 3–5 mL of local anesthetic is injected perineurally with a 1 inch (2.5 cm) 22 gauge needle or a ⅝ inch (1.5 cm) 25 gauge needle. Local anesthesia at this level provides analgesia of the foot and the palmar or plantar aspect of the pastern region. As with digital nerve blocks, abaxial sesamoid nerve blocks may not have an effect on lameness that is exacerbated by flexion of the distal aspect of a limb [33]. In a substantial number of horses, local anesthetic may diffuse proximally after this block [43]. Although liposomal bupivacaine is an effective perineural local anesthetic in this location, the duration does not seem to be significantly longer than bupivacaine hydrochloride [44]. The use of ketamine hydrochloride as a sole agent in a basisesamoid block has been assessed; use in this peripheral location did not significantly improve lameness [45].

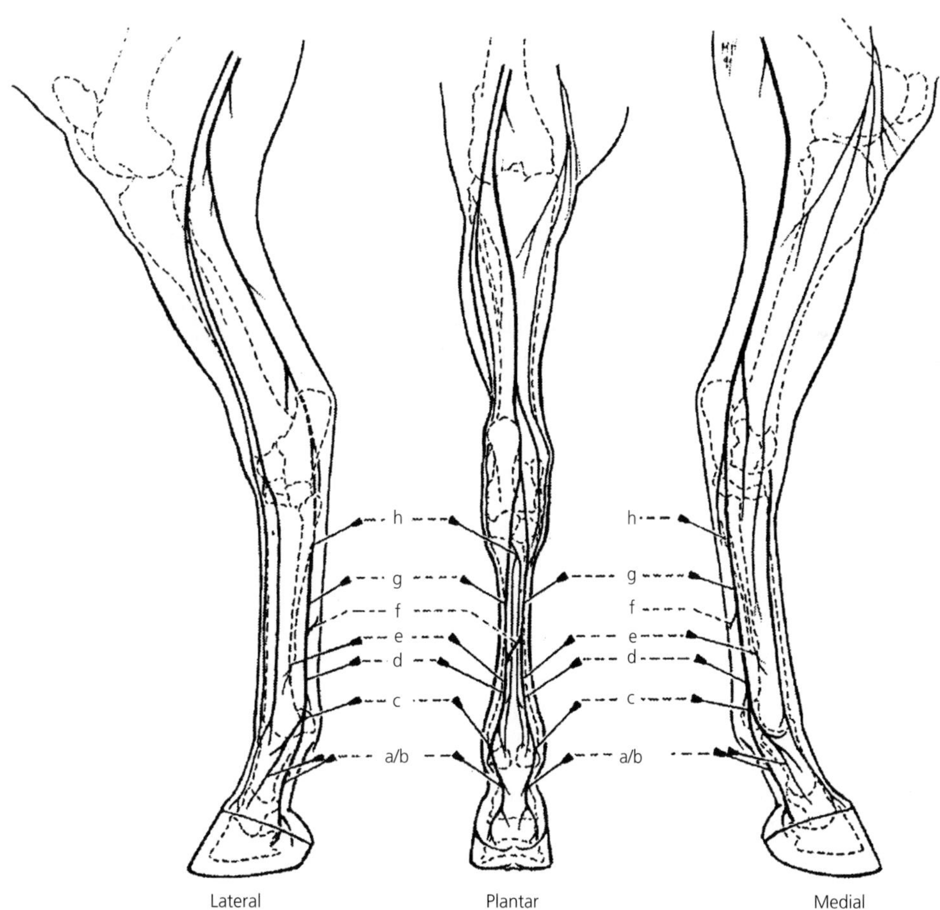

Figure 63.6 Needle placement for left distal rear limb nerve blocks. a, lateral and medial plantar digital nerves; b, dorsal branches; c, lateral and medial plantar digital nerves (basisesamoid); d and g, lateral and medial plantar nerves; e, lateral and medial plantar metatarsal nerves; f, communicating branch; h, location of high suspensory block

Low palmar or plantar (low four-point) nerve block

The medial and lateral palmar or plantar nerves and palmar metacarpal or palmar metatarsal nerves are desensitized with this block (Figs. 63.5d,e and 63.6d,e). For palmar or plantar nerves, local anesthetic is injected between the suspensory ligament and the deep digital flexor tendon. Because of the proximity to the digital flexor tendon synovial sheath, the area should be thoroughly prepared, the hub of the needle should be checked to ensure that synovial fluid is not obtained, and the injection should be performed at a level approximately 1 cm proximal to the distal ends of the splint bones. For the palmar metacarpal or plantar metatarsal nerves, local anesthetic is injected between the third metacarpal or metatarsal bone and the suspensory ligament at a level just distal to the distal extent of the splint bones. Because of the proximity to the palmar or plantar pouch of the fetlock joint, the area should be thoroughly prepared and the hub of the needle checked to ensure that synovial fluid is not obtained. If synovial fluid is obtained, the needle should be withdrawn and redirected. Although this block may be performed with the limb in a weight-bearing or elevated position, elevation of the limb may increase the risk of digital flexor tendon sheath puncture [46]. These blocks provide analgesia for most structures of the fetlock joint and structures distal to that joint (Fig. 63.7B). Subcutaneous injection of additional local anesthetic in a dorsal direction may be necessary to provide complete analgesia.

Local anesthetic diffusion in a proximal direction is minimal after performance of a low palmar nerve block [47], and diffusion is unlikely to cause a decrease in the severity of lameness attributable to pain in the proximal aspect of the metacarpal region [48].

Proximal metacarpal or metatarsal region blocks

The high palmar or plantar (high four-point) block desensitizes the medial and lateral palmar or plantar nerves and palmar metacarpal or plantar metatarsal nerves in the proximal aspect of the metacarpal region proximal to the communicating branch of the medial and lateral palmar or plantar nerves (Figs. 63.5f–h and 63.6f–h). The palmar or plantar nerves are desensitized between the suspensory ligament and the deep digital flexor tendon; this area is typically easiest to palpate with the limb in a weight-bearing position. The palmar metacarpal or plantar metatarsal nerves are desensitized via injection of local anesthetic along the axial aspects of the splint bones; this is easiest to accomplish with the limb in a flexed position. For complete analgesia of the dorsal aspect of the limb in this region, local anesthetic should be injected subcutaneously in a ring block to the dorsal midline of the limb (Fig. 63.7C). The palmar aspect of the carpometacarpal joint may be entered when performing this block [49]; therefore, the area should be thoroughly prepared and suction applied after connection of the syringe to the needle to ensure that synovial fluid is not obtained. Inadvertent injection of the carpometacarpal joint would provide anesthesia to the middle carpal joint, which could lead to erroneous conclusions during a lameness examination. The origin of the suspensory ligament may not be completely desensitized with this block. Gas may be introduced into tissues while performing this block and can temporarily interfere with ultrasonographic examination of structures of the proximal palmar metacarpal region [50].

The origin of the suspensory ligament may be desensitized via direct injection of the structure with local anesthetic. The block is performed with the limb in a flexed position. The needle is advanced into the proximal aspect of the suspensory ligament along the axial

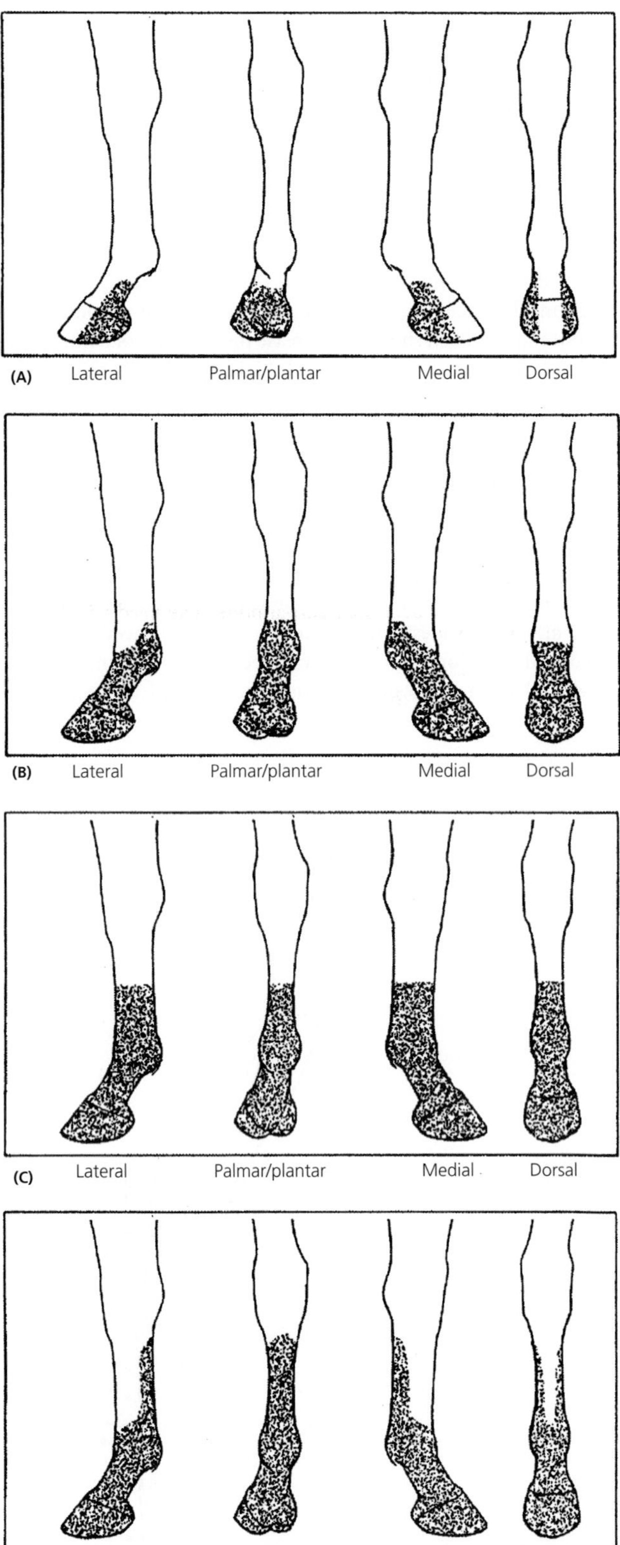

Figure 63.7 Desensitized subcutaneous area after various lower limb nerve blocks. **A.** Palmar/plantar digital nerve block. **B.** Low palmar/plantar (low four-point) nerve block. **C.** High palmar/plantar (high four-point) nerve block plus ring block to desensitize the dorsal metacarpal/metatarsal region. **D.** Proximal metacarpal/metatarsal (high suspensory) nerve block.

aspect of the splint bone, and local anesthetic is injected in several sites in a fan-shaped pattern. The injection may be performed from the medial and lateral aspects, or just the lateral aspect of the limb (particularly in hind limbs, where injection from the medial side may be difficult). Use of an 18–19 gauge needle may prevent inadvertent needle breakage if the horse moves while performing this block.

The lateral palmar nerve can be desensitized at the level of the accessory carpal bone to provide analgesia for the deep structures of the palmar aspect of the forelimb, including the proximal aspect of the suspensory ligament. The block can be performed from the lateral or medial aspect of the limb. For the lateral approach, local anesthetic is deposited perineurally between the distal aspect of the accessory carpal bone and the proximal aspect of the fourth metacarpal (lateral splint) bone; this can be performed with the limb in a weight-bearing position or with the carpus flexed. Use of a medial approach to the nerve may prevent inadvertent injection of the carpal synovial sheath [51]. This technique is performed with the limb in a weight-bearing position. A ⅝ inch (1.5 cm) 25 gauge needle is inserted in a groove in the flexor retinaculum fascia at the palmaromedial aspect of the accessory carpal bone. The needle is directed in a mediolateral direction until it contacts bone, and then, local anesthetic is injected.

Local anesthesia of the deep branch of the lateral plantar nerve provides analgesia of the proximal aspect of the suspensory ligament in the hind limb. A 1.5 inch (3.8 cm) 18–19 gauge needle is inserted 1.5–2 cm distal to the head of the fourth metatarsal bone (lateral splint bone) and directed axial to that bone [52,53]. The needle may be directed either proximodorsally or dorsally; insertion of the needle in a proximodorsal direction may provide more specific local anesthesia of the deep branch of the lateral plantar nerve and lead to less diffusion of the local anesthetic versus insertion of the needle in a dorsal direction [53]. It is important to note that anesthesia of the lateral plantar nerve is also likely when blocking the deep branch of the lateral plantar nerve, so the procedure is not strictly specific to the suspensory ligament origin [54]. Because of a small risk of tarsometatarsal joint and tarsal sheath puncture, the skin should be thoroughly prepared before performing the block. The tarsal sheath and tarsometatarsal joint are inadvertently entered in 16% and 6% of horses, respectively, during performance of this block [55].

Median, ulnar, and medial cutaneous antebrachial nerve blocks

Performance of these blocks in combination provides analgesia for structures of the antebrachium, carpus, and distal aspect of the forelimb. These blocks may be performed before a procedure or for diagnostic purposes. Local anesthesia of the median nerve is performed just distal to the superficial pectoral muscle at the caudomedial aspect of the radius, cranial to the flexor carpi radialis muscle (Fig. 63.8a); approximately 10 mL of local anesthetic is injected. The ulnar nerve is desensitized approximately 10 cm proximal to the accessory carpal bone at the caudal aspect of the limb in a palpable groove between the flexor carpi ulnaris and ulnaris lateralis muscles (Fig. 63.8b); a 1 inch (2.5 cm) 20 gauge needle should be inserted to the hub, and approximately 10 mL of local anesthetic injected as the needle is withdrawn. The medial cutaneous antebrachial nerve is desensitized just cranial to the cephalic vein at the dorsomedial aspect of the middle of the radius (Fig. 63.8c); approximately 5 mL of local anesthetic is injected. The medial cutaneous antebrachial nerve provides analgesia only for skin, so the block is not required for diagnostic purposes.

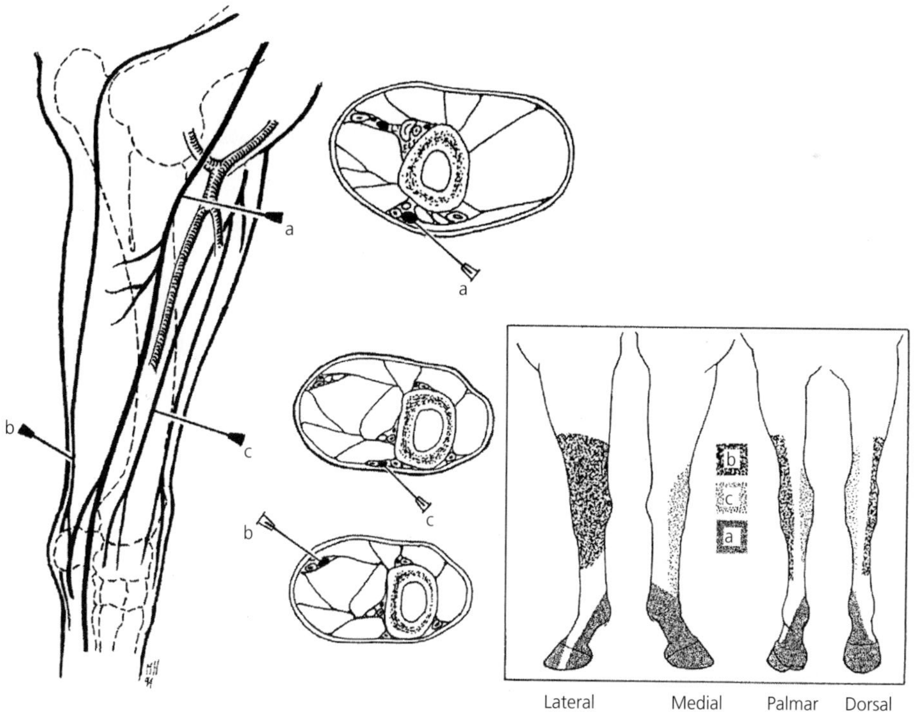

Figure 63.8 Needle placement for proximal forelimb nerve blocks. a, median nerve; b, ulnar nerve; c, medial cutaneous antebrachial nerve. Inset: cross-sections and desensitized subcutaneous areas of left forelimb.

The median and ulnar nerve blocks are not commonly performed for diagnostic purposes; however, these blocks can be very useful for determining a diagnosis in horses with forelimb lameness that is not affected by intra-articular blocks or perineural blocks of the distal aspect of a limb. As such, the median and ulnar nerve blocks can be useful for the diagnosis of problems causing pain in the carpal bones or the distal aspect of the radius and pain attributable to soft tissue problems between the distal aspect of the antebrachium and proximal aspect of the metacarpus. Although the median nerve block site is close to the cubital joint, performance of this block does not improve lameness originating in that joint and is unlikely to confound interpretation of results in horses with complex upper forelimb lameness [56].

Use of ultrasound guidance may aid accurate perineural injection of local anesthetic for median and ulnar nerve blocks [57]. The authors have also found ultrasound guidance useful for medial cutaneous antebrachial nerve blocks. When performing these nerve blocks for therapeutic purposes, a solution of 2% lidocaine with epinephrine has similar duration of efficacy as 2% mepivacaine and seems to be a suitable alternative [58]. Buffering mepivacaine with sodium bicarbonate results in faster onset and greater reduction in lameness compared with non-buffered mepivacaine [59]. Performance of median and ulnar nerve blocks with 3% chloroprocaine results in faster and more complete resolution of lameness versus 2% mepivacaine [60].

Tibial, peroneal, and saphenous nerve blocks

Local anesthesia of the tibial and peroneal nerves desensitizes bone and soft tissues of the distal aspect of the tibia, the hock, and structures distal to the hock. For local anesthesia of the tibial nerve, a 1.5 inch (3.8 cm) 20 gauge needle is inserted 10 cm proximal to the tuber calcis caudal to the deep digital flexor muscle (Fig. 63.9a); 15–20 mL of local anesthetic is injected. Although the nerve is located medially, the injection may be performed from the medial side or from the lateral side. When performing the block from the lateral side, the needle should be inserted to a depth sufficient to ensure deposition of local anesthetic perineurally without penetration of the skin on the medial side of the limb. Ultrasound guidance may improve accuracy of tibial nerve blocks [61,62]. Because it is difficult to maintain contact between the syringe and needle when the horse moves, it may be useful to connect extension set tubing between the needle and syringe. The superficial and deep peroneal nerves are desensitized by insertion of a 3.5 inch (8.9 cm) 18 gauge needle 10 cm proximal to the tuber calcis in a palpable groove between the long and lateral digital extensor muscles on the lateral aspect of the limb (Fig. 63.9c). The needle is inserted until the caudolateral edge of the tibia is contacted, and 20–30 mL of local anesthetic is injected as the needle is withdrawn to desensitize both the deep and superficial peroneal nerves. A subcutaneous ring block may be necessary to provide complete skin analgesia for surgery. After performing these blocks, horses may drag their toe; caution should be used during lameness examination of such horses. As for the median and ulnar nerve blocks in the forelimb, these blocks are not commonly performed but may help reach a diagnosis in horses with lameness that is not affected by intra-articular blocks or distal perineural blocks.

The saphenous nerve is desensitized by injection of 5 mL of local anesthetic perineurally near the saphenous vein approximately 10 cm proximal to the tibiotarsal joint with a 1 inch (2.5 cm) 20 or 22 gauge needle (Fig. 63.9b). This block is useful for providing analgesia to the skin of the medial aspect of the limb. It is not performed for diagnostic analgesia during a lameness examination.

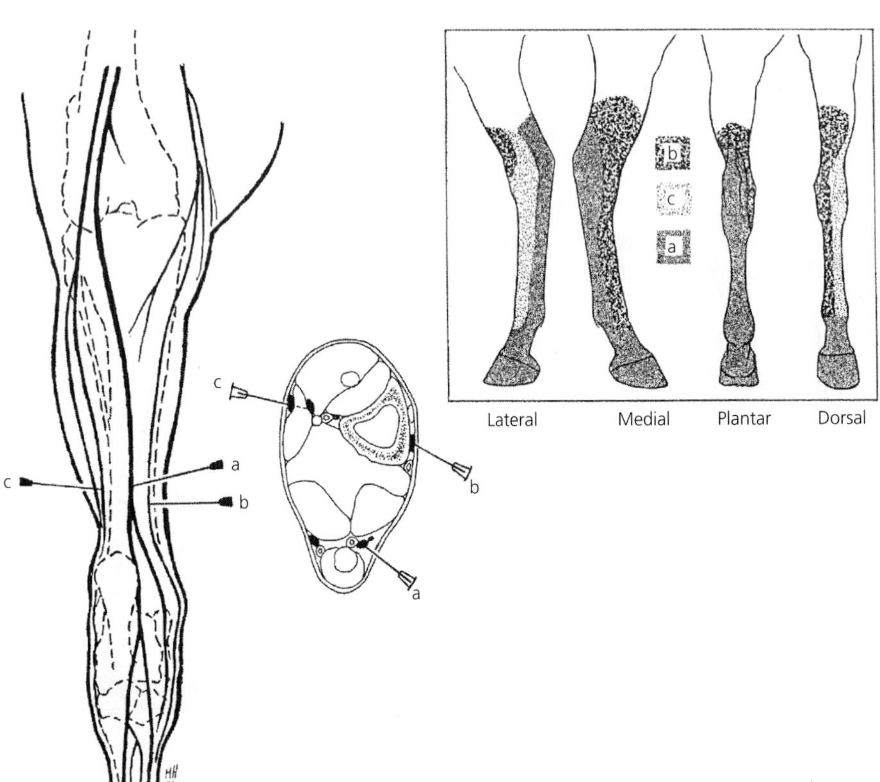

Figure 63.9 Needle placement for proximal rear limb nerve blocks. a, tibial nerve; b, saphenous nerve; c, peroneal nerve. Inset: cross sections and desensitized subcutaneous areas of left rear limb.

Intra-articular and intrabursal anesthesia of the limbs

Navicular (podotrochlear) bursa

Several techniques can be used for injection of the navicular bursa. However, an approach from the distal palmar aspect of the limb in which the position of the navicular bursa is determined on the basis of external anatomic landmarks may yield the highest success rate [63,64]. This technique is typically performed with the foot on an inclined wooden block to position the distal aspect of the limb in a flexed position. The position of the navicular bone can be predicted to be at a location 1 cm distal to the coronary band at the midpoint between the most dorsal and most palmar aspect of the coronary band. Injection of 1–2 mL of local anesthetic subcutaneously at the needle insertion site may decrease movement of the horse while performing this block. A 3.5 inch (8.9 cm) 18–20 gauge needle is inserted at the midpoint between the heel bulbs just proximal to the coronary band and advanced toward the predicted position of the navicular bone (Fig. 63.10a). After the navicular bone is encountered, the needle is withdrawn slightly. Correct needle placement can be confirmed by aspiration of a small amount of synovial fluid (which is rarely obtained) or via radiography. Then, 3–5 mL of local anesthetic is injected. An alternate technique introducing the needle from the lateral aspect of the limb just proximal to the collateral cartilages of the foot under ultrasonographic guidance avoids penetration and possible damage of the deep digital flexor tendon [65]. Improvement of lameness within 10 min after injection suggests that the lameness is caused by pain in the navicular bursa or associated structures [66,67]; however, distal interphalangeal joint pain may be improved by local anesthesia of the navicular bursa 20–30 min after injection [67]. Mepivacaine can diffuse between the navicular bursa and the distal interphalangeal joint [68]. Analgesia of the navicular bursa may improve lameness caused by pain in the dorsal aspect of the sole of the foot [69].

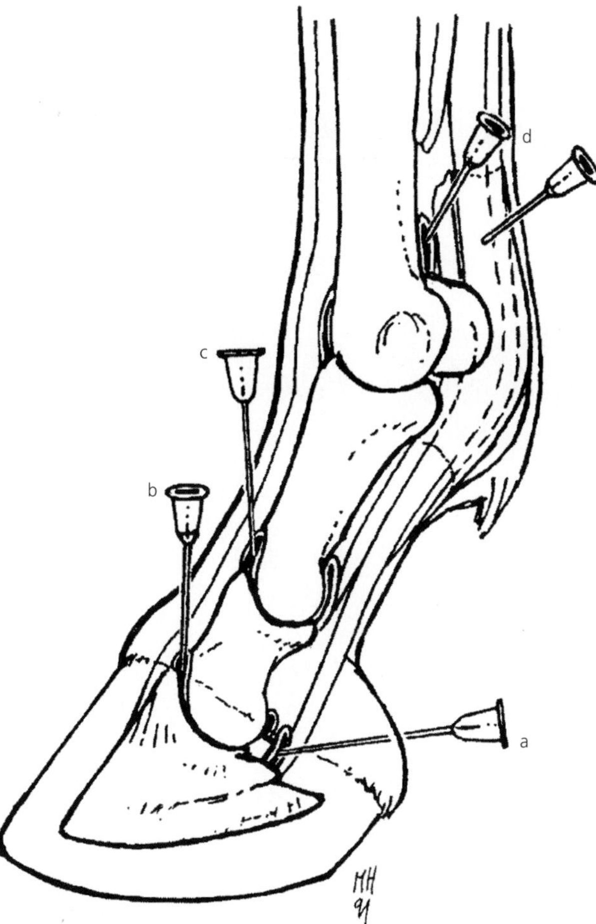

Figure 63.10 Needle placement for distal limb intra-articular and intrabursal blocks. a, navicular (podotrochlear) bursa; b, distal interphalangeal (coffin) joint; c, proximal interphalangeal (pastern) joint; d, volar pouch of the fetlock joint capsule; e, digital flexor tendon sheath.

Distal interphalangeal (coffin) joint

For local anesthesia of the distal interphalangeal joint, a 1.5 inch (3.8 cm) 20 gauge needle is inserted 1 cm proximal to the coronary band and 2 cm lateral to the dorsal midline aspect of the limb (Fig. 63.10b). The needle is directed distomedially toward the palmar or plantar lateral aspect of the extensor process of the third phalanx (coffin bone). Alternatively, the needle may be inserted into the dorsoproximal pouch of the joint on the dorsal midline aspect of the limb, 1 cm proximal to the coronary band and directed in a palmar or plantar direction either parallel to the ground or distally toward the solar surface of the foot. The horse should be in a weight-bearing position while performing this block. Injection of 6 mL of local anesthetic into the distal interphalangeal joint may desensitize the dorsal aspect (toe) of the sole of the foot, whereas injection of 10 mL may also desensitize the angles (heel) of the sole [70]. Therefore, injection of a maximum of 6 mL is recommended to increase the specificity of the block when it is performed for diagnostic purposes. Because mepivacaine can diffuse between the distal interphalangeal joint and the navicular bursa [68], intra-articular distal interphalangeal joint blocks may not be specific for problems of that joint.

Proximal interphalangeal (pastern) joint

The proximal interphalangeal joint is desensitized via insertion of a 1.5 inch (3.8 cm) 20 gauge needle into the palpable joint space under the extensor tendon on the dorsal aspect of the limb in a lateral to medial or medial to lateral direction (Fig. 63.10c). This approach is typically performed with the limb in a weight-bearing position. Alternatively, the joint may be entered at the palmar or plantar lateral aspect with the limb in a flexed position. The needle is inserted dorsal to the digital neurovascular bundle toward a palpable depression between the distal aspect of the first phalanx and the proximal aspect of the second phalanx; 5–10 mL of local anesthetic is injected. It is important to note that results of a recent study in cadaver limbs suggest performance of the dorsal approach with the limb flexed or use of the palmar approach may decrease iatrogenic cartilage damage [71].

Metacarpophalangeal or metatarsophalangeal (fetlock) joint

Fetlock joints may be injected via a dorsomedial or dorsolateral approach or various palmar or plantar approaches. For the dorsal approach, a 1.5 inch (3.8 cm) 20 gauge needle is inserted into the palpable joint space proximal to the first phalanx under the extensor tendon; this approach is performed with the limb in a weight-bearing position. The palmar or plantar joint pouch may be entered from the lateral aspect of the limb in three locations. The proximal aspect of the palmar or plantar pouch may be entered in an area bound by the third metacarpophalangeal or metatarsophalangeal (cannon) bone dorsally, suspensory ligament (palmarly or plantarly), distal end of the splint bone (proximally), and apical aspect of the lateral proximal sesamoid bone distally (Fig. 63.10d). The palmar or plantar pouch may also be entered through the collateral ligament of the lateral proximal sesamoid bone between the cannon bone and the proximal sesamoid bone; this may be the easiest approach to obtain hemorrhage-free synovial fluid and inject the fetlock joint, particularly in a horse without synovial effusion. Alternately, the palmar or plantar aspect of the joint may be entered at the distolateral aspect in a space bounded by the digital neurovascular bundle (palmarly or plantarly), the distal aspect of the lateral proximal sesamoid bone (proximodorsally), and the proximal aspect of the proximal phalanx (distodorsally). The palmar or plantar approaches are best performed with the distal aspect of the limb in a flexed position. The fetlock joint is injected with 10 mL of local anesthetic.

Digital flexor tendon sheath

When distended with synovial fluid, the digital flexor tendon sheath can be desensitized via approaches to the proximal or distal aspects. For the proximal approach, a 1 inch (2.5 cm) 20 gauge needle is inserted into the sheath 1 cm proximal to the palmar or plantar annular ligament and 1 cm palmar or plantar to the lateral branch of the suspensory ligament (Fig. 63.10e). For the distal approach, the needle is inserted into the sheath in the palmar or plantar aspect of the pastern between the proximal and distal digital annular ligaments; care should be taken to avoid puncture of the deep digital flexor tendon at this location. These blocks may be performed with the limb in a weight-bearing or non-weight-bearing position. As an alternative, the distal aspect of the limb may be flexed and the needle can be inserted into the sheath on the palmaro- or plantarolateral aspect of the limb just distal to the lateral proximal sesamoid bone between the proximal annular ligament and proximal digital annular ligament. In addition, a palmar or plantar axial sesamoidean approach can be used [72]. The limb is held in flexion and a 1 inch (2.5 cm) 20 gauge needle is inserted at the level of the middle aspect, 3 mm axial to the palmar or plantar border of the lateral proximal sesamoid bone and dorsal to the flexor tendons. The needle is directed at a 45° angle to the sagittal plane toward the intersesamoidean ligament. That technique is preferred for horses without substantial synovial effusion of the sheath. Local anesthesia of the digital flexor tendon sheath appears to be specific for that structure because it is unlikely to improve lameness attributable to pain in the sole of the foot, distal interphalangeal joint, or navicular bursa [73]. Although local anesthetics diffuse into other local synovial structures, concentrations are insufficient to induce analgesia [74].

Carpal joint blocks

The radiocarpal (antebrachiocarpal) joint can be entered on the dorsal aspect with the limb lifted off the ground and the carpus flexed. A 1 inch (2.5 cm) 20 gauge needle is inserted in the palpable depression of the joint either medial or lateral to the extensor carpi radialis tendon; 5–10 mL of local anesthetic is injected. Alternatively, the needle may be directed into the palmar aspect of the joint between the lateral digital extensor and ulnaris lateralis tendons in a palpable V-shaped depression bordered by the caudolateral aspect of the radius and ulnar carpal bone and the proximal aspect of the accessory carpal bone with the limb in a weight-bearing position (Figs. 63.11a and 63.12a,c).

The middle carpal joint can be entered on the dorsal aspect with the limb held off the ground with the carpus flexed. The needle is inserted on the medial or lateral side of the extensor carpi radialis tendon, in a manner similar to that for injection of the radiocarpal joint. Alternatively, the palmar aspect of this joint may be injected via insertion of the needle palmar to the articulation of the ulnar and fourth carpal bones and distal to the accessory carpal bone (Figs. 63.11b and 63.12b,d). The middle carpal joint communicates with the carpometacarpal joint; therefore, both of these joints are desensitized.

Carpal canal block

The carpal canal is most easily identified from the lateral aspect of the forelimb when synovial effusion is present. It is important to differentiate carpal sheath effusion from effusion of the carpal joints. The carpal sheath may be entered with a 1 inch (2.5 cm) 20 gauge needle between the lateral digital extensor and ulnaris lateralis tendons 1–3 cm proximal to the accessory carpal bone; 15 mL of local anesthetic is injected. Another approach is to place the needle in the sheath 1.5 cm distal to the accessory carpal bone at the dorsolateral aspect of the deep digital flexor tendon. For diagnostic carpal canal blocks, results should be interpreted within 15 min and subsequent blocks distal to the carpus should be delayed for at least 3 h because there is a likelihood of distal limb desensitization as early as 30 min after injection [75].

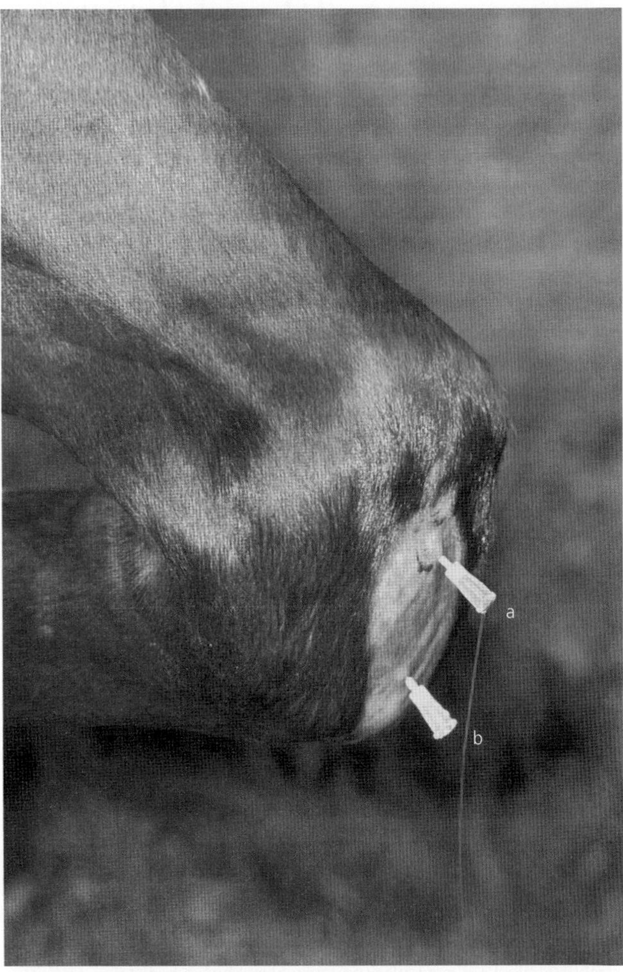

Figure 63.11 Needle placement for right carpal intra-articular blocks. a, radiocarpal joint; b, intercarpal joint.

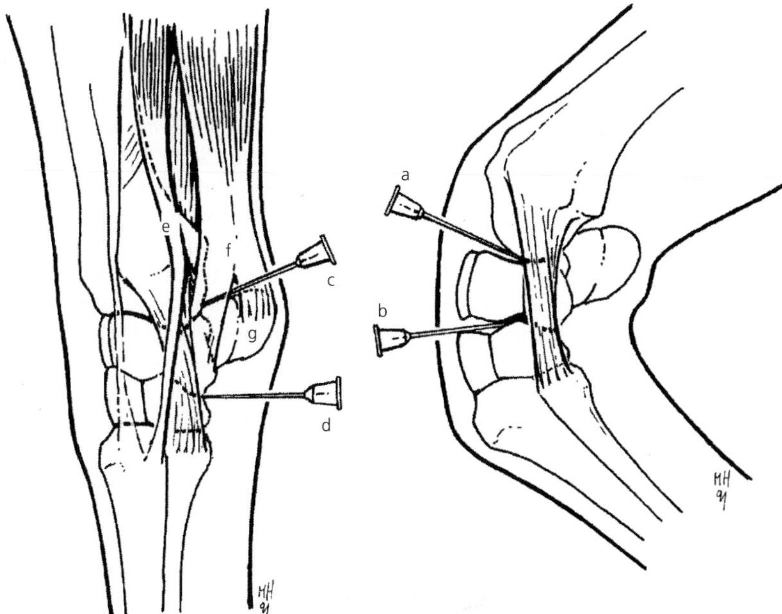

Figure 63.12 Needle placement for left carpal intra-articular blocks. a and c, radiocarpal joint; b and d, intercarpal joint; e, lateral digital extensor tendon; f, tendon of ulnaris lateralis muscle; g, accessory carpal bone.

Elbow joint block

The elbow joint may be blocked at the cranial or caudal edge of the lateral collateral ligament, two-thirds of the distance distally between the palpable lateral epicondyle of the humerus and the lateral tuberosity of the proximal aspect of the radius (Fig. 63.13a). A 1.5 inch (3.8 cm) 18–20 gauge needle is inserted perpendicular to the skin, and 20 mL of local anesthetic is injected. It is important to ensure that local anesthetic is injected into the joint; this is confirmed by aspirating synovial fluid prior to injection. Injection of local anesthetic periarticularly after insertion of the needle cranial to the lateral collateral ligament can lead to temporary radial nerve paralysis [76]. The caudal pouch of the elbow joint may also be entered with a 3.5 inch (8.9 cm) 18–20 gauge needle inserted in a distal, cranial, and medial direction in the palpable depression bordered by the olecranon (caudally) and the distal aspect of the humerus (cranially).

Olecranon bursa block

The olecranon bursa is injected with a 1.5 inch (3.8 cm) 20 gauge needle directed into the bursa over the caudal aspect of the olecranon (Fig. 63.13b). This block is rarely indicated.

Bicipital bursa block

For local anesthesia of the bicipital bursa, a 3.5 inch (8.9 cm) 18 gauge needle is inserted at the cranial aspect of the humerus, 3.5 cm distal to the prominence on the craniolateral aspect of the greater tubercle (Fig. 63.13c). The needle is directed along the cranial surface of the humerus in a proximomedial direction; 10–15 mL of local anesthetic is injected. Radiographic examination after injection of radiopaque contrast medium may be necessary to confirm successful entry into the bicipital bursa [77]. Ultrasonographic guidance may improve the accuracy of needle placement for local anesthesia of the bicipital bursa [78].

Shoulder joint block

For local anesthesia of the shoulder joint, the depression between the cranial and caudal prominences of the lateral tuberosity of the humerus is palpated cranial to the infraspinatus tendon.

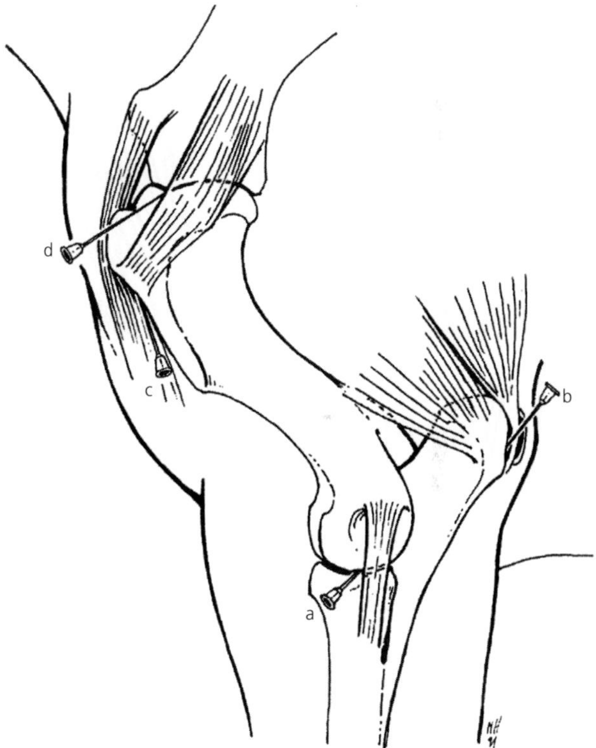

Figure 63.13 Needle placement for left proximal forelimb intra-articular and intrabursal blocks. a, elbow joint; b, olecranon bursa; c, bicipital bursa; d, shoulder joint.

An 18 gauge needle at least 3.5 inch (8.9 cm) long is inserted into the center of the depression and directed in a caudomedial direction at a 45° angle (Fig. 63.13d); 20 mL of local anesthetic is injected. Correct placement of the needle can typically be confirmed by aspiration of synovial fluid. Temporary suprascapular nerve anesthesia and subsequent supraspinatus and infraspinatus muscle dysfunction are a rare complication of this block [76]. Ultrasonographic guidance may improve the accuracy of needle placement in the shoulder joint [78].

Cunean bursa block

The cunean bursa may be desensitized by inserting a 1 inch (2.5 cm) 22 gauge needle between the cunean tendon and the bones of the distal aspect of the tarsus (Figs 63.14a and 63.15). The needle is inserted from the distal aspect of the cunean tendon, and 5–10 mL of local anesthetic is injected.

Tarsal joint blocks

Tarsal joints are typically injected with the limb in a weight-bearing position. The tarsometatarsal joint is most reliably entered from the plantarolateral aspect of the limb in a palpable depression 1 cm proximal to the head of the lateral fourth metatarsal (splint) bone (Figs. 63.14b and 63.16). A 1–1.5 inch (2.5–3.8 cm) 20 gauge needle is directed in a distomedial direction. Synovial fluid is typically obtained, and 3–4 mL of local anesthetic should be injected without substantial resistance. This joint may be entered from the dorsal aspect of the limb (Fig. 63.14d); however, this approach is typically only used if the plantarolateral approach is unavailable because of skin damage or if an additional portal is necessary for joint lavage. The distal intertarsal (centrodistal) joint is desensitized by inserting a 1 inch (2.5 cm) 22 gauge needle in a small palpable joint depression on the medial aspect of the limb just ventral to the cunean tendon (Fig. 63.14c); 3–5 mL of local anesthetic is injected. Accuracy of injection into the tarsometatarsal joint is high (96%), but only 42% of distal intertarsal joint injections are successful [79]. The tibiotarsal (tarsocrural) joint is large and easily injected in the dorsomedial pouch 2–3 cm distal to the tibia and medial to the peroneus tertius and tibialis cranialis tendons (Fig. 63.14e); 15 mL of local anesthetic is injected. Care should be taken to avoid the saphenous vein, which typically courses over the center of the dorsomedial pouch of the joint. When synovial effusion is present, this joint can be approached from the plantarolateral aspect. For this approach, the needle is inserted in the center of the palpable distended joint pouch bordered by the tuber calcis (caudally), distal aspect of the tibia (cranially), and talus (ventrally). The proximal intertarsal joint communicates with the tibiotarsal joint and becomes desensitized after performing this block.

Horses have variable communication among the tarsal joints. A substantial percentage (up to 38%) of horses has communication between the tarsometatarsal and distal intertarsal joints [80–83].

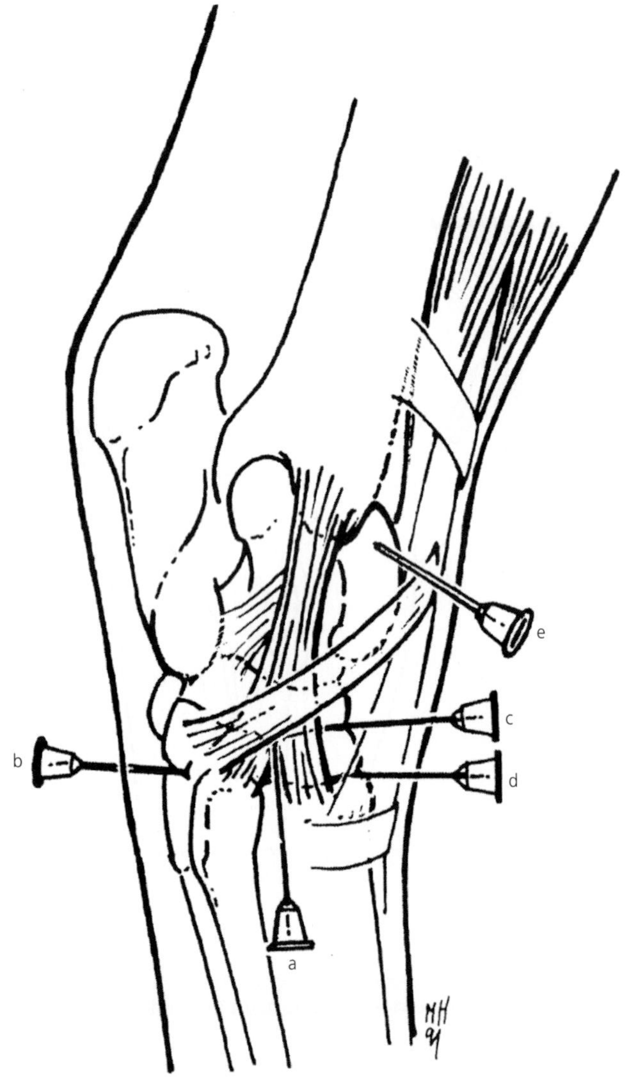

Figure 63.14 Needle placement for left tarsal intra-articular and intrabursal blocks (medial aspect). a, cunean bursa; b and d, tarsometatarsal space; c, distal metatarsal space; e, tibiotarsal space.

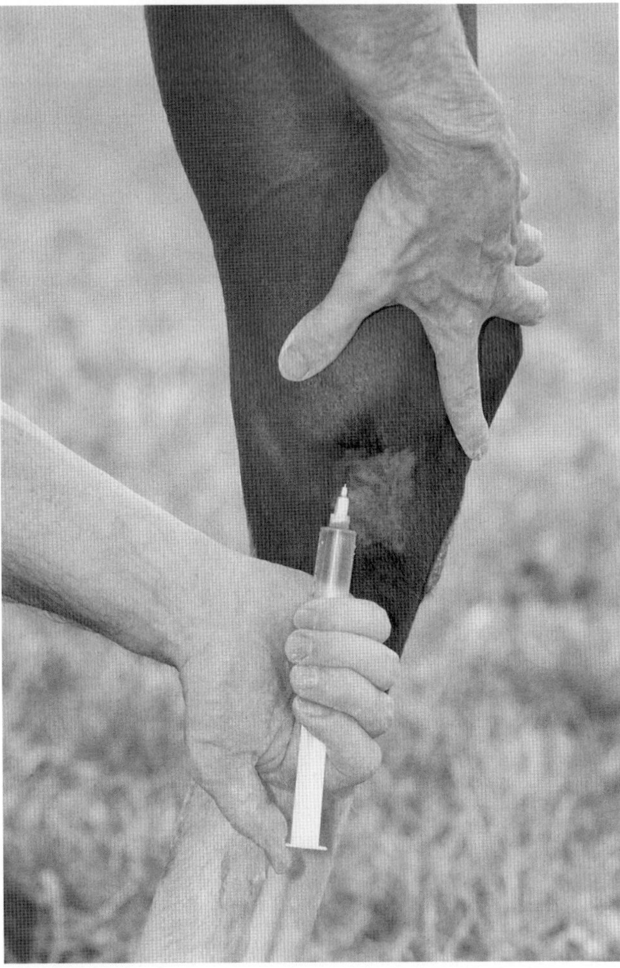

Figure 63.15 Injection of local anesthetic (10 mL) into the cunean bursa of the right rear limb (medial aspect).

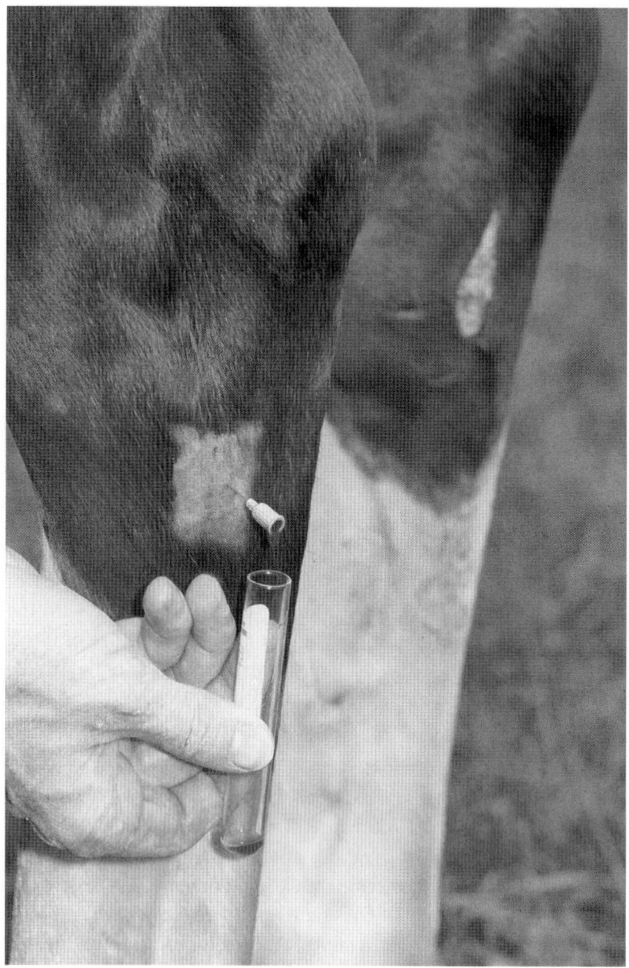

Figure 63.16 Collection of fluid from the tarsometatarsal joint (left rear leg).

Infrequently, injection of the distal tarsal joints may cause entry of local anesthetic into the proximal intertarsal and tarsometatarsal joints [80] or the tarsal sheath [81]. High injection pressures may increase the frequency of tarsometatarsal and distal intertarsal joint communication [83].

Calcaneal bursae blocks

Calcaneal bursae in horses include the subcutaneous calcaneal bursa (subcutaneous superficial to the superficial digital flexor tendon plantar to the calcaneus), intertendinous calcaneal bursa (between the gastrocnemius and superficial digital flexor tendons), and gastrocnemius calcaneal bursa (just proximal to the calcaneus and dorsal to the gastrocnemius tendon) [84]. The intertendinous and gastrocnemius calcaneal bursae communicate; the subcutaneous bursa communicates with the other calcaneal bursae in 39% of studied limbs of horses. A 1.5 inch (3.8 cm) 20 gauge needle may be inserted into the bursae, which are palpable when synovial effusion is present; 10 mL of local anesthetic is injected.

Tarsal sheath block

The tarsal sheath extends from the proximal aspect of the calcaneus to the proximal aspect of the metatarsal region. The sheath surrounds the deep digital flexor tendon as it courses over the sustentaculum tali of the calcaneus, medial to the body of the bone. The sheath is easiest to identify when it is distended with synovial fluid. The tarsal sheath may be desensitized at its proximal or distal aspects via insertion of a 1.5 inch (3.8 cm) 20 gauge needle, and injection of 15 mL of local anesthetic.

Stifle joint blocks

The stifle joint includes the femoropatellar and medial and lateral femorotibial articulations. In horses, communication among these joint compartments is variable. The most common communication is between the medial femorotibial and femoropatellar compartments, which is detected in 60–80% of limbs with normal stifle joints [85,86]. Communication among other stifle joint compartments is detected less frequently. The pattern of communication is typically bilaterally symmetrical; however, communication among compartments may be affected by joint disease and the location chosen for joint injection. Therefore, for diagnostic and therapeutic purposes, each compartment should be considered a separate entity and injected independently. However, clinicians should be aware that mepivacaine can diffuse among stifle joint compartments and detection of an improvement in lameness after local anesthesia of an individual articulation may not be specific [87], although blockade of an articulation containing a lesion is more specific than injection into one of the surrounding articulations [88]. Because lameness attributable to stifle joint problems may be caused by extra-synovial structures (such as collateral and cruciate ligaments), improvement may not be observed until 20 min or longer after injection of local anesthetic. Some horses may have partial improvement of distal limb lameness after local anesthesia of all three stifle articulations [88]. Each compartment is typically desensitized with 20 mL of local anesthetic by use of a 1.5 inch (3.8 cm) 18 gauge needle.

The femoropatellar compartment is injected distal to the patella, medial, or lateral to the middle patellar ligament (Fig. 63.17a). The needle is advanced perpendicular to the skin or in a slightly proximal direction. Alternatively, the lateral cul-de-sac of the femoropatellar compartment may be injected [89]; the needle is inserted 5 cm proximal to the lateral tibial plateau caudal to the lateral patellar ligament and lateral trochlear ridge of the femur. The needle is directed perpendicular to the long axis of the femur until bone is contacted and then withdrawn slightly before injection of local anesthetic. The lateral approach to the femoropatellar compartment may allow collection of a greater amount of synovial fluid and result in less cartilage injury than the cranial approach [90].

For injection of the medial femorotibial compartment, the needle is inserted 1.5 cm proximal to the medial plateau of the tibia between the medial patellar ligament and the medial collateral ligament of the stifle joint (Fig. 63.17b). The needle is directed perpendicular to the skin. The medial meniscus, which is slightly distal and caudal to the injection site, should be avoided. Another approach is to insert the needle 1.5 cm proximal to the medial tibial plateau in a palpable depression between the medial patellar ligament and the tendon of insertion of the sartorius muscle [91]. The needle is directed parallel to the ground in a cranial to caudal direction in a sagittal plane. It is important that the horse stands squarely on the limb while performing this block. This approach may allow the collection of a greater volume of synovial fluid and reduce the risk of iatrogenic cartilage and medial meniscus injury compared with the approach between the medial patellar ligament and medial collateral ligament.

The lateral femorotibial compartment may be injected by various approaches. These include needle insertion sites caudal to the lateral patellar ligament and 1 cm proximal to the lateral tibial plateau (Fig. 63.17c); proximal to the tibia and caudal to the tendon of

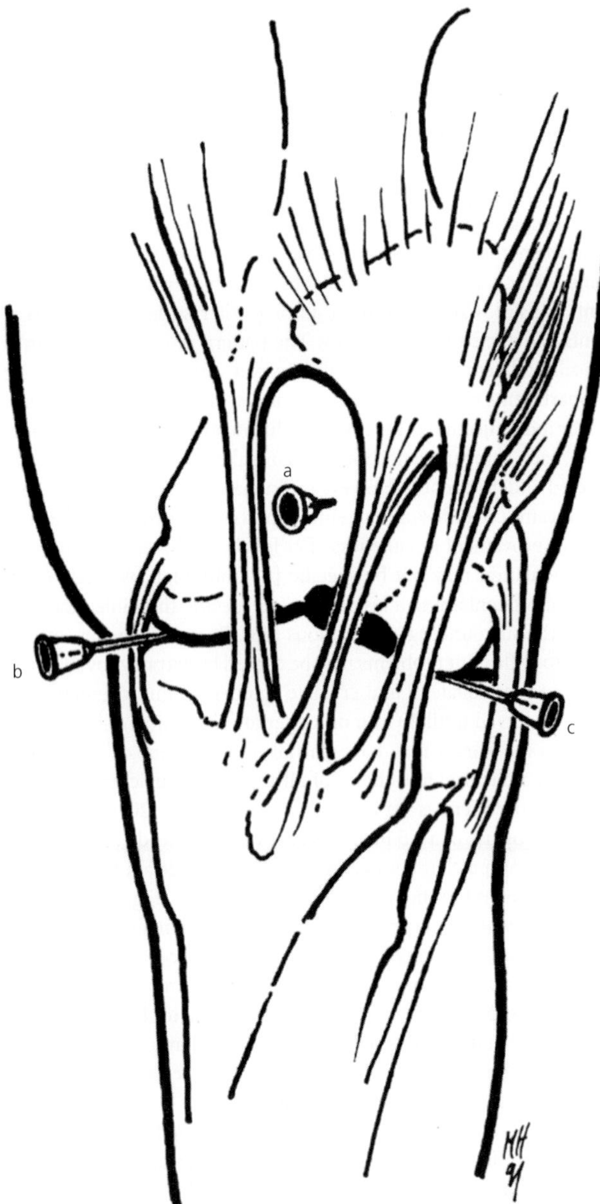

Figure 63.17 Needle placement for stifle intra-articular blocks. a, femoropatellar pouch; b, medial femorotibial pouch; c, lateral femorotibial pouch.

origin of the long digital extensor muscle; and between the long digital extensor tendon and the extensor groove at the proximal aspect of the tibia. However, insertion of the needle directly through the long digital extensor tendon 1–4 cm distal to the lateral tibial plateau is the most successful technique for injection of the lateral femorotibial compartment of the stifle joint [92].

Coxofemoral (hip) joint block

The coxofemoral joint is difficult to inject, particularly in large horses, because of the depth of the joint from the skin surface. Before insertion of the needle, it is important to ensure that the horse is standing squarely, with the limbs perpendicular to the ground. An 18 gauge needle at least 6 inches (15 cm) long should be used. Because of the risk of needle breakage or bending attributable to the length of the needle and depth of the joint, adequate physical restraint is important, and subcutaneous injection of local anesthetic at the needle insertion site and sedation of the horse may be necessary. The site of needle insertion is in a palpable depression between the large caudal and small cranial parts of the major trochanter of the proximal aspect of the femur (Fig. 63.18a). The needle is directed medially in a slightly cranioventral direction along the neck of the femur. Proper needle placement should be confirmed via aspiration of synovial fluid before injection; 20 mL of local anesthetic is injected. Ultrasonographic guidance may aid placement of the needle in the coxofemoral joint [93]. An alternate ultrasound-guided cranioventral approach may be used in horses with marked synovial effusion [94].

Trochanteric bursa block

The trochanteric bursa is located between the tendon of the medial gluteal muscle and the cranial part of the greater trochanter of the femur. The bursa is located via palpation of the greater trochanter and a 1.5–3.5 inch (3.8–8.9 cm) 18 gauge needle is inserted perpendicular to the skin until bone is contacted (Fig. 63.18b); 5–10 mL of local anesthetic is injected. Positioning the limb caudally with the foot in a non-weight-bearing position on a block and use of ultrasonographic guidance may facilitate accurate insertion of the needle into the trochanteric bursa [95].

Sacroiliac region block

Injection of local anesthetics in the vicinity of the sacroiliac joint of horses is a controversial procedure. It can be useful for diagnosis of sacroiliac region pain [96]. Various approaches have been described, including insertion of the needle cranial, craniomedial, medial, or caudal to the tuber sacrale [97]. The cranial and caudal approaches require ultrasonographic guidance, whereas the craniomedial and medial approaches may be performed with either ultrasonographic guidance or blindly via landmark identification. Diffusion of local anesthetic can anesthetize the sciatic nerve caudal to the sacroiliac joint resulting in hindlimb paresis and recumbency for up to 3 h [98]. In particular, the caudal approach is more likely to cause this severe complication [99]. Local anesthesia using a blind dorsal approach similar to the described dorsocranial and dorsal approaches has a complication rate of less than 1% [100]. In this approach, a spinal needle (18 gauge, 3.5 inch or 8.9 cm) is introduced axial to the cranial aspect of the tuber sacrale, contralateral to the sacroiliac joint of interest. The needle is advanced to the hub, aiming perpendicular to the tuber sacrale and toward the caudal aspect of the tuber coxae. A total of 20 mL is deposited at four locations (at the deepest insertion and 0.5–1 cm superficial, along the initial insertion path and after redirection 20° caudad).

Anesthesia for laparotomy/laparoscopy

Regional anesthesia may be useful for standing laparotomy when general anesthesia is not an option for financial or other reasons. Standing laparoscopy is commonly used for several standing abdominal procedures, including ovariectomy, nephrectomy, embryo transfer, castration of abdominal cryptorchids, and liver or kidney biopsy. Four techniques have been described for standing abdominal procedures: infiltration anesthesia, paravertebral thoracolumbar anesthesia, segmental dorsolumbar epidural anesthesia, and segmental thoracolumbar subarachnoid anesthesia. Segmental dorsolumbar epidural anesthesia and segmental thoracolumbar subarachnoid anesthesia are infrequently used and will not be discussed here;

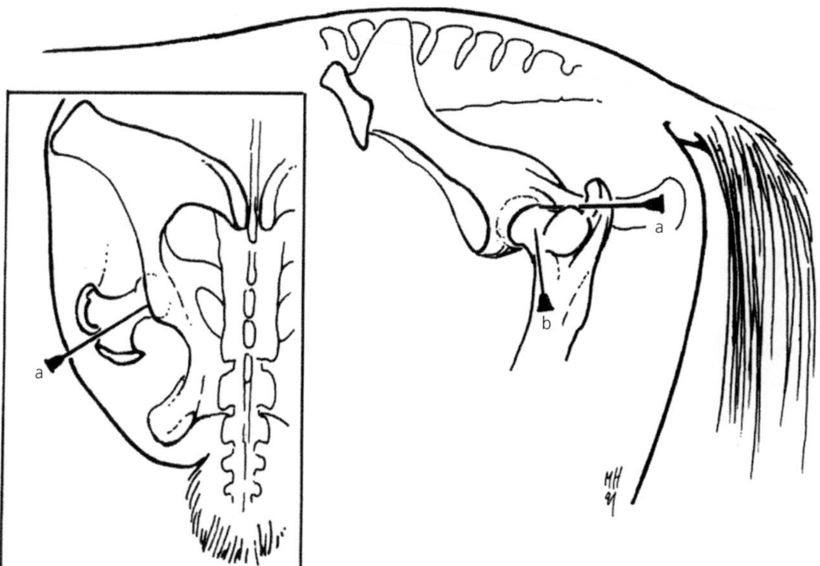

Figure 63.18 Needle placement for proximal rear limb intra-articular and intrabursal blocks. a, coxofemoral joint; b, trochanteric bursa.

however, interested readers are directed to previous editions of this book for complete and thorough descriptions [101].

Infiltration anesthesia

The most commonly used local anesthetic technique for standing abdominal procedures in horses is simple infiltration of the incision (line block). For most standing procedures, the incisions will be small, and infiltration anesthesia will be sufficient when combined with restraint and systemic sedation and analgesia. A 1 inch (2.5 cm) 20–22 gauge needle is used to deposit 1 mL of local anesthetic for each centimeter of incision. For laparoscopy, the small incision sites required for insertion of the camera and instruments may be desensitized individually, whereas for laparotomy, a larger area of desensitization will be required.

Pain is minimized (and cooperation of the patient maximized) if the injections are slow and deliberate, and the needle is advanced through the edge of the desensitized skin. This technique assures that the horse senses only the initial needle insertion. A 10–15 mL injection of local anesthetic is usually sufficient for desensitization of the skin and subcutaneous tissues. Depending on the local anesthetic used, at least 15 min should be allowed for maximum anesthetic effect.

After the superficial structures are desensitized, the deeper layers of muscle and peritoneum can be desensitized with a 3–4 inch (7.5–10 cm) 18 gauge needle; 50–150 mL of local anesthetic may be required depending on the area of desensitization needed. In an average 500 kg (1100 lb) adult horse, dosages of less than 250 mL of 2% lidocaine are not expected to cause toxicity [102].

Local infiltration is easy to perform and requires no knowledge about specific nerve location. Disadvantages include disruption of normal tissue architecture, incomplete anesthesia (especially of the peritoneum), incomplete muscle relaxation of the abdominal wall, toxicity after inadvertent injection into the peritoneal cavity, and increased cost and time involved with long incisions. A recent study compared local portal blocks to paravertebral nerve blocks for laparoscopic closure of the nephrosplenic space. The time needed to complete the blocks, the requirements for sedation, the overall outcome scores, and total surgery time was similar in both groups leading the authors to conclude that both could be used interchangeably [103].

Paravertebral thoracolumbar anesthesia

When long incisions are required in patients where general anesthesia is not an option, paravertebral thoracolumbar anesthesia (paravertebral block) can be used as an alternative to infiltration anesthesia [104]. Even though this block is technically difficult, it can be performed in thin-muscled horses with easily palpable landmarks. To perform the block, the last thoracic (T18) and first and second lumbar (L1 and L2) spinal nerves are desensitized approximately 10 cm from the dorsal midline, after they have emerged from the intervertebral foramina and have split into their dorsal and ventral branches and medial and lateral ramifications, respectively (Fig. 63.19).

The sites for desensitization are palpated by locating the third lumbar transverse process, which is on a line between the most caudal extension of the last rib and perpendicular to the long axis of the spinal vertebrae. The distance between the injection sites is 3–6 cm (Fig. 63.20). After the skin is desensitized, the ventral branches of T18, L1, and L2 are blocked using a 3 inch (7.5 cm) 18 gauge needle. The needle is advanced to the peritoneum (where there will be a loss of resistance or a slight sucking sound as air enters the needle) and then withdrawn to a retroperitoneal position, where 15 mL of local anesthetic is injected (Fig. 63.19b) [104].

Advantages of paravertebral anesthesia over infiltration anesthesia include smaller doses of local anesthetic, a wide area of desensitization, muscle relaxation, and the absence of local anesthetic in the incision (minimizing hematomas, edema, and possible interference with healing). The main disadvantages are the difficulty in performing the block and the fact that in a horse with a good body condition score and muscle coverage, the landmarks are extremely difficult to palpate. There is also a chance that the third lumbar spinal nerve may be inadvertently desensitized, which causes loss of motor control to the ipsilateral pelvic limb.

Anesthesia for urogenital procedures

Many urogenital procedures including castrations, episioplasties, repair of recto-vaginal fistulas, ovariectomies, and perineal urethrostomies, can be performed in the standing sedated horse when combined with appropriate regional anesthetic techniques.

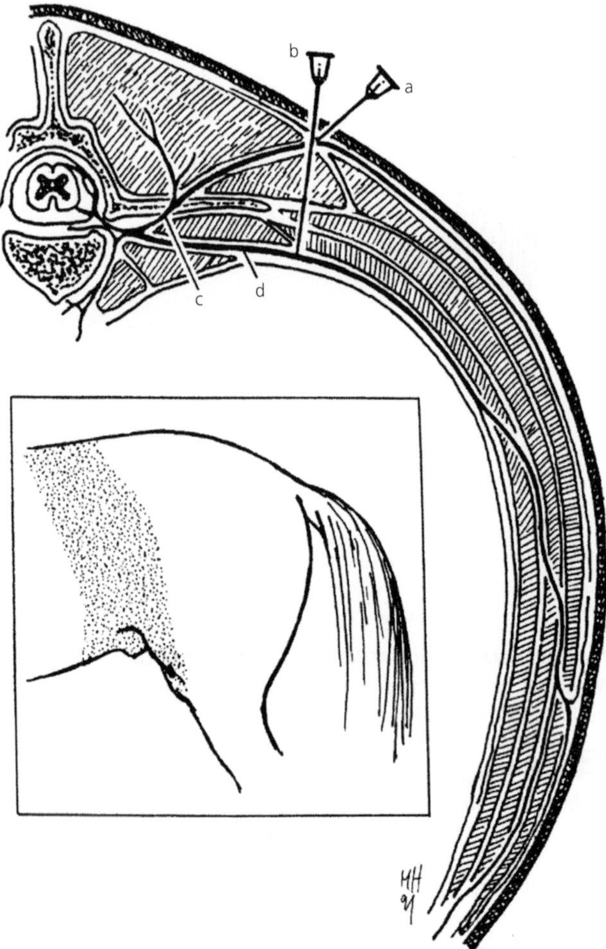

Figure 63.19 Needle placement for paravertebral nerve blockade showing a cranial, transected view of the first lumbar vertebra at the location of the intervertebral foramen. a, needle placement for subcutaneous infiltration; b, needle placement for retroperitoneal infusion. c, dorsal branch of the L1 vertebral nerve; d, ventral branch of the L1 vertebral nerve. Inset: desensitized subcutaneous area after blockade of T18, L1, and L2 vertebral nerves.

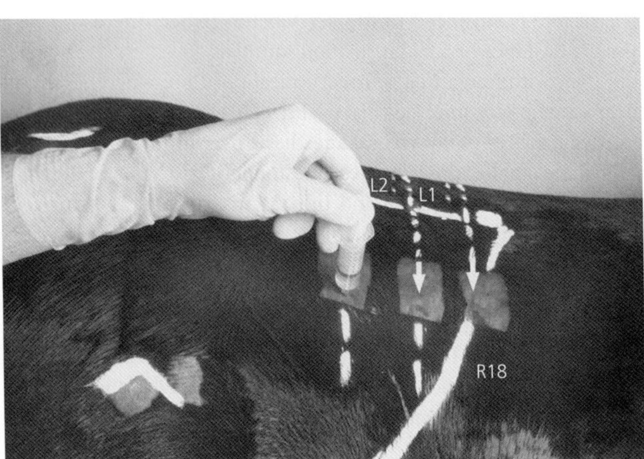

Figure 63.20 Right thoracolumbar area of a standing adult horse with injection sites (arrows) for distal paravertebral block. R18, last rib; L1, spinous process of the first lumbar vertebra; L2, spinous process of the second lumbar vertebra. The dotted line transects the corresponding interspaces between spinous and transverse processes. Subcutaneous injection of L2 is shown. Source: Skarda [105].

Anesthesia for castration

Castration is one of the most common surgical procedures performed in equine practice. For older horses or horses that are intractable, general anesthesia is generally recommended owing to potential complications such as hemorrhage. Even when general anesthesia is used, intratesticular injection of 15 mL of 2% lidocaine per testicle will decrease intraoperative blood pressure responses and cremaster muscle tension and can be a beneficial supplement to general anesthesia [106]. In another study, incisional, intratesticular, and intrafunicular lidocaine was found to be an effective adjunct to intravenous anesthesia [107].

In standing horses, restraint of the horse's head and sedation are required in addition to local anesthesia. The use of stocks is generally not recommended for standing castration, owing to the potential for injury to the surgeon. A twitch may be used to aid restraint and, for safety reasons, the person holding the twitch should stand on the same side as the surgeon. The skin of the scrotum and prepuce should be aseptically prepared and then the block can be done with one of three techniques.

In the most commonly used technique, a 3 inch (7.5 cm) 20 gauge needle is inserted perpendicularly through the tensed skin of the scrotum, and local anesthetic is injected until the testicle is turgid (approximately 20–30 mL) (Fig. 63.21). After approximately 10 min, the castration can usually be performed painlessly, with no further need for the twitch.

In the second technique, a 1 inch (2.5 cm) 20 gauge needle may be inserted into the spermatic cord percutaneously as close to the external inguinal ring as possible. At that point, 20–30 mL of local anesthetic is injected in a fan-shaped manner without perforating the skin, spermatic artery, or vein. The incision site into the scrotum must still be infiltrated subcutaneously with 5–10 mL of local anesthetic since the skin of the scrotum is not desensitized by the deposition of the local anesthetic into the spermatic cord. The procedure must then be repeated on the other side. Infiltration of the spermatic cord is not as effective as infiltration directly into the testicle.

In the third technique, a 6 inch (15 cm) 18 gauge needle is inserted into the testicle and directed into the spermatic cord

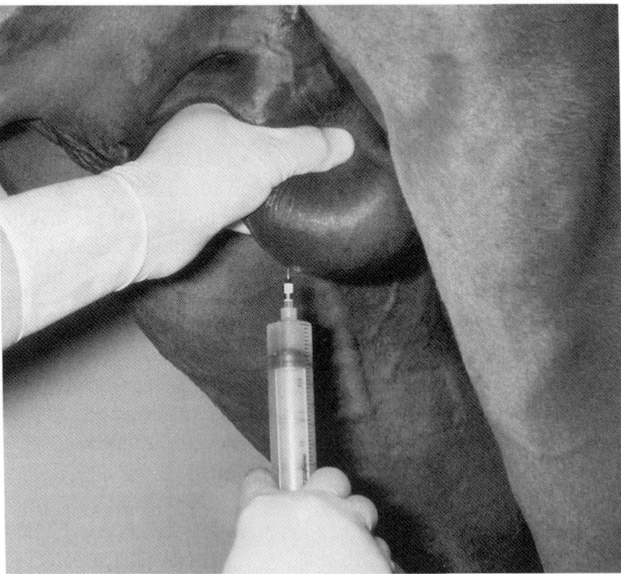

Figure 63.21 Needle placement for right intratesticular injection in a standing horse.

while 30 mL of local anesthetic are being injected. Prior to beginning the surgery, the skin of the scrotum at the incision sites is also desensitized.

Cryptorchid castration is more commonly performed under general anesthesia by laparotomy or laparoscopy, but in one study, intratesticular or mesorchial infiltration of lidocaine combined with administration of a non-steroidal anti-inflammatory drug (NSAID) and caudal epidural injection of detomidine provided adequate analgesia in standing stallions undergoing laparoscopic cryptorchidectomy [108].

Anesthesia for ovariectomy

Ovariectomy is commonly performed in standing, sedated horses with laparoscopy. One portion of the surgery that can be very stimulating to the standing horse after the skin and muscle layers are blocked is removal of the ovaries. Blocking the ovaries with local anesthesia can help blunt the temporary stimulation while the ovaries are removed. A recent investigation assessed the topical application of mepivacaine to the ovarian pedicle versus injection of mepivacaine into the pedicle prior to removal. The authors concluded that topical application of mepivacaine provided intraoperative analgesia similar to injection into the ovarian pedicle, which could reduce the risk of inadvertent trauma to the pedicle or other visceral organs during standing laparoscopy [109].

Anesthesia of the perineum

While caudal epidural anesthesia (described below under neuraxial anesthesia) is commonly used to facilitate perineal surgeries, including urethrostomy, in standing horses, regional anesthesia of the perineum may also be used. To perform regional anesthesia of the area, the superficial and deep (subfascial) branches of the perineal nerves must be desensitized. A 1 inch (2.5 cm) 22 gauge needle is inserted approximately 2.5 cm dorsal to the ischial arch and 2.5 cm lateral to the anus so that 5 mL of local anesthetic may be injected subcutaneously. After directing the needle dorsally 0.5–1 cm, a deeper subfascial injection of 5–7 mL is made, and then, the procedure is repeated on the opposite side [110].

Anesthesia of the penis or vulva

The penis may be desensitized by blocking the pudendal nerves at the ischium (Fig. 63.22). This will desensitize the penis and the internal lamina of the prepuce in addition to relaxing the penis and allowing it to be extruded. To perform the block, a 1.5 inch (3.8 cm) 20 gauge needle is inserted on the right and left side of the anus, about 2 cm dorsal to the ischial arch and lateral to the anus and is angled ventrally toward the midline. The needle is advanced until the point contacts the ischial arch where the pudendal nerves course around the ischium. Then, 5 mL of local anesthetic is deposited adjacent to each nerve, which results in the penis being extruded within about 5 min of a successful block.

While a line block with local anesthetic is still commonly utilized for desensitization of the vulva, the technique described above may also be used. It is interesting to note that one study has suggested that use of lidocaine–prilocaine topical anesthetic cream is as effective as lidocaine infiltration in providing local anesthesia when performing episioplasty in mares and caused less anatomic disruption [111].

Pudendal nerve block using a peripheral nerve locator has also been described. During electrolocation, the pudendal nerve was approached effectively when both anal and perineal twitches were elicited. The technique was successfully used during perineoplasty, urethroplasty, clitorectomy in mares, and penile examination, phallectomy and urethrostomy in geldings, leading the authors to conclude that this was a safe and effective alternative for epidural and general anesthesia for these procedures [112].

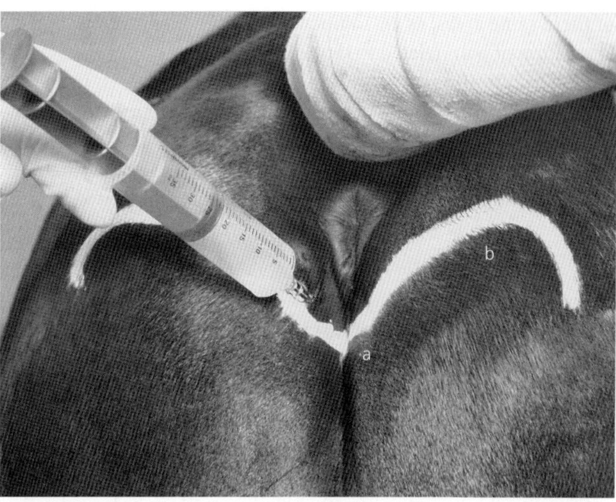

Figure 63.22 Topographic anatomy for perineal and pudendal nerve block. a, palpable ischiatic arch; b, palpable ischiatic tuberosity (both marked). Infiltration of the left pudendal nerve with local anesthetic is shown. Source: Skarda [105].

Neuraxial anesthesia/analgesia

In horses, neuraxial anesthesia and analgesia most often involves the epidural route of administration. Epidural anesthesia combined with systemic sedation and standing restraint facilitates procedures involving the anus, perineum, rectum, vulva, vagina, urethra, and bladder. Additionally, epidural analgesia can provide good adjunctive analgesia for painful conditions involving the stifles and hocks. In the horse, the spinal cord ends at the level of the caudal half of the second sacral vertebra, so caudal epidural injection or catheterization, as described below, may be performed without risk of spinal (subarachnoid) injection.

While techniques have been previously described that involve accessing the epidural or subarachnoid space at the lumbosacral junction for a single injection or to advance a catheter either rostrally to deliver drug segmentally at the thoracolumbar level, or caudally to deliver drug at level of the sacrum [113], these techniques are not routinely performed. For detailed descriptions of lumbosacral epidural or spinal (subarachnoid) anesthesia/analgesia techniques, the reader is referred to previous editions of this book [102].

Indications and contraindications

The choice of drugs placed epidurally will dictate whether anesthesia or analgesia is produced, and the specific medication and volume chosen will determine the spread. Indwelling epidural catheters can also be placed when repeated administration of analgesic or anesthetic drugs are anticipated. Indications for caudal epidural injection of drugs in horses include anesthesia of the perineum, rectum, anus, tail, urethra, bladder, vulva, or vagina for surgery in the standing horse. Other indications include relief of tenesmus, correction of uterine torsion, and fetotomy. Additionally, epidural analgesia/anesthesia may be used as an adjunct to general anesthesia for surgery involving these same structures and the hindlimbs to reduce the minimum alveolar concentration (MAC) of inhalants [114,115]. Epidural analgesia can be used postoperatively for pain management of these same areas, as an adjunct to systemic medications, and for alleviation of pain related to septic joints.

Contraindications to epidural anesthesia/analgesia in horses include infection at the puncture site, sepsis, uncorrected hypovolemia, bleeding disorders, anticoagulation therapy (potentially used in horses with laminitis), spinal cord disease, and anatomic abnormalities. This technique may also be contraindicated in weak or ataxic patients that are at risk for becoming recumbent after epidural drug administration.

Caudal epidural anesthesia/analgesia

Caudal epidural anesthesia and/or analgesia, performed at the sacrococcygeal or the first intercoccygeal (Co1–Co2) space, is the preferred and most commonly used technique in the horse as it is safer and easier to perform than lumbosacral epidural or subarachnoid anesthesia and requires no specialized equipment.

The site for injection is either the sacrococcygeal or the first intercoccygeal space [116]. In some horses, the last sacral and first coccygeal vertebrae are fused and the first movable space may be the first coccygeal interspace. The space is palpated while moving the tail up and down; it is the first movable space caudal to the sacrum, which is generally 2.5–7.5 cm cranial to the origin of the tail hairs. The tail may be raised and lowered, or some people prefer a "pump handle" motion to identify the space.

After aseptic preparation, 1 mL of 2% lidocaine may be injected to desensitize the skin if desired. There are two commonly used techniques for a one-time injection into the caudal epidural space. In the first, a 1.5 inch (3.8 cm) 18 gauge needle is inserted at the center of the palpated space perpendicular to the skin (Fig. 63.23a). The "hanging drop" technique can be utilized where the hub of the needle is filled with saline before advancing the needle, and then, when the needle enters the epidural space, the negative pressure will pull the drop into the epidural space. A "popping" sensation may also be appreciated as the needle penetrates the interarcuate ligament (ligamentum flavum). The depth of the space from the skin is approximately 3.5–8 cm in adult horses. When the needle is thought to be in the epidural space, aspiration will confirm lack of blood or cerebrospinal fluid, and a test dose of saline may be made to confirm loss of resistance to injection. In the second technique, a 5–7.5 inch (12.7–19 cm) 18 gauge spinal needle is inserted at the caudal part of the interspace, at approximately 30° parallel to the horizontal plane (Fig. 63.23b). This technique can be useful for epidural injection if the horse has previously had epidural injections, which can result in development of fibrous tissue.

While epidural puncture has traditionally been confirmed by aspiration of a fluid drop (i.e., hanging drop), or lack of resistance on injection, these methods are not always reliable and alternative techniques of confirmation may be used. For instance, the human medical literature has described the use of acoustic devices to detect a pressure drop by means of an audible signal when the ligamentum flavum is perforated [117]. A similar acoustic device has been used to identify the extradural space in standing horses [118].

Continuous caudal epidural anesthesia/analgesia

For repeated and long-term administration of epidural medications, epidural catheters are recommended. Epidural catheterization can be used successfully for repeated epidural delivery of analgesics and anesthetics in horses with various clinical conditions, including fractures, lacerations, septic arthritis, myositis, perineal injuries, and cellulitis [119]. One study showed that long-term epidural administration of a morphine–detomidine combination was not associated with adverse systemic effects in horses even though localized inflammation and fibrosis was seen [120].

After aseptic preparation and optional desensitization of the skin, the needle is introduced at an angle of approximately 45° to the skin (Fig. 63.23c). Once the needle is determined to be in the epidural space, the catheter may be introduced 10–30 cm into the epidural space by advancing it with the opening of the needle facing cranially. Once the catheter is placed, it is held in place while removing the needle and then secured to the skin with adhesive and suture material; the entire catheter may then be covered with an adhesive dressing. The injection port should be aseptically prepared prior to each injection, and a bacterial filter may be used between the catheter and the injection port.

Epidural medications

Depending on the desired effect and duration of action, local anesthetics, α_2-adrenergic receptor agonists, opioids, and other additives have been shown to be effective at providing anesthesia and analgesia when administered epidurally.

Local anesthetics

Epidural local anesthetics provide regional anesthesia by preventing depolarization of the nerve membrane and conduction of nerve impulses. The most common local anesthetics used for epidural application in horses are 2% lidocaine and 2% mepivacaine.

The dose of lidocaine required to effectively desensitize the anus, perineum, rectum, vulva, vagina, urethra, and bladder is 6–8 mL of a 2% solution in a 450 kg mare (0.26–0.35 mg/kg). The cranial spread and intensity of analgesia are dose-dependent, but generally, sensory and motor blockade ranging from the coccyx to the second sacral vertebra is produced within 5–15 min and lasts 60–90 min. Redosing should be performed with caution since inadvertent overdose can cause profound ataxia, recumbency, and hypotension [121,122]. One study evaluated the use of midazolam in addition to lidocaine, which would reduce the volume of lidocaine required and decrease the chance of ataxia or recumbency. Midazolam (0.05 mg/kg) and lidocaine (0.1 mg/kg of 2% lidocaine) produced satisfactory analgesia and cervical dilation for endometrial biopsy for at least 60 min [123].

Another study looked at adding bicarbonate to lidocaine for caudal epidural anesthesia. It was found that 7 mL of 2% lidocaine with epinephrine (1:200,00) combined with 2.3 mL of sterile water for injection and 0.7 mL of 8.4% sodium bicarbonate decreased the average onset time of nociception by 40% and decreased the duration of ataxia by 33% when compared to 2% lidocaine with epinephrine alone [124].

Mepivacaine (2%) acts very similarly to lidocaine when used as an epidural agent in horses. Like lidocaine, the extent of the desensitized area is determined by the volume of local anesthetic injected (Fig. 63.24). Analgesia usually reaches peak effect in 20 min and lasts approximately 80 min [125].

Caudal epidural injection of hyperbaric bupivacaine (0.5%, 0.06 mg/kg) produces bilateral perineal analgesia in horses, with a rapid onset of action (< 6 min) and a long duration (> 5 h) [126]. Heart and respiratory rates, arterial blood pressure, and rectal temperature were not changed after epidural administration of bupivacaine.

Ropivacaine is a more recently investigated local anesthetic for local and regional anesthesia in horses. Various doses and concentrations have been evaluated ranging from 0.1 mg/kg of 0.5%

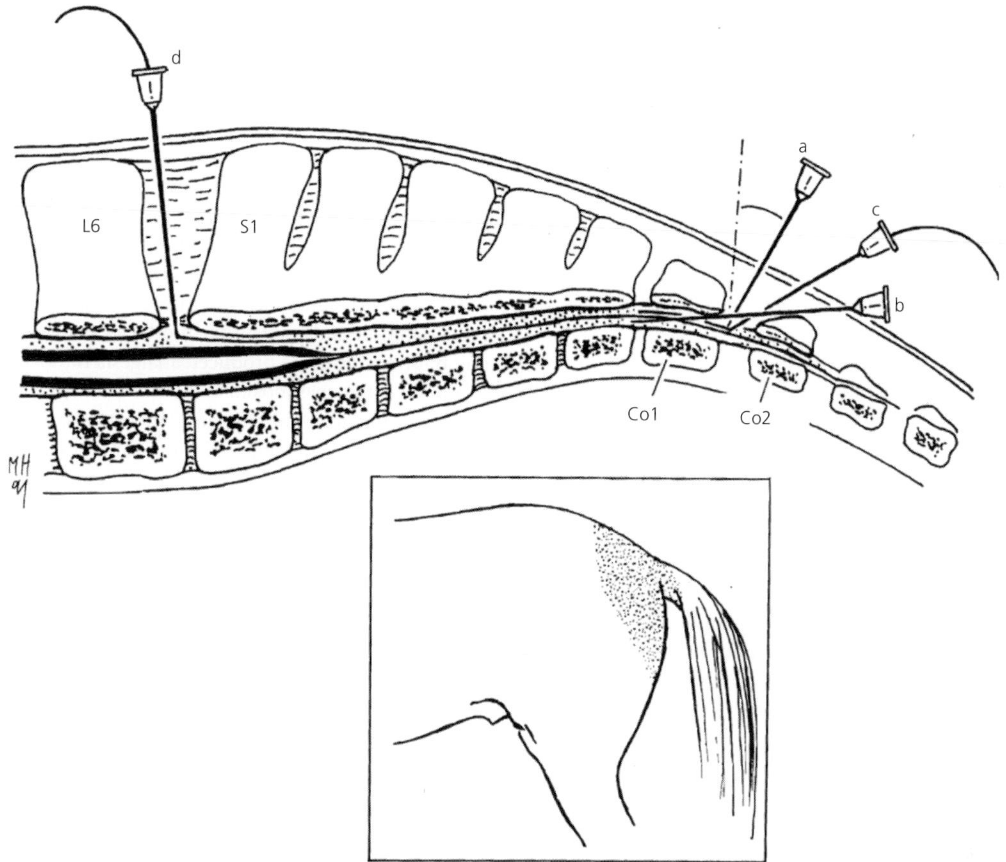

Figure 63.23 Caudal epidural anesthesia and catheter placement for continuous caudal epidural anesthesia in the horse. a and b, needle placement for caudal epidural injection; c, epidural catheter placement via the first intercoccygeal space for continuous caudal epidural anesthesia (commonly performed); d, epidural catheter placement via the lumbosacral space for continuous caudal epidural anesthesia (rarely performed). L6, dorsal spinous process of the sixth lumbar vertebra; S1, dorsal spinous process of the first sacral vertebra; Co1 and Co2, first and second coccygeal vertebrae. Inset: Desensitized subcutaneous area after successful caudal epidural anesthesia.

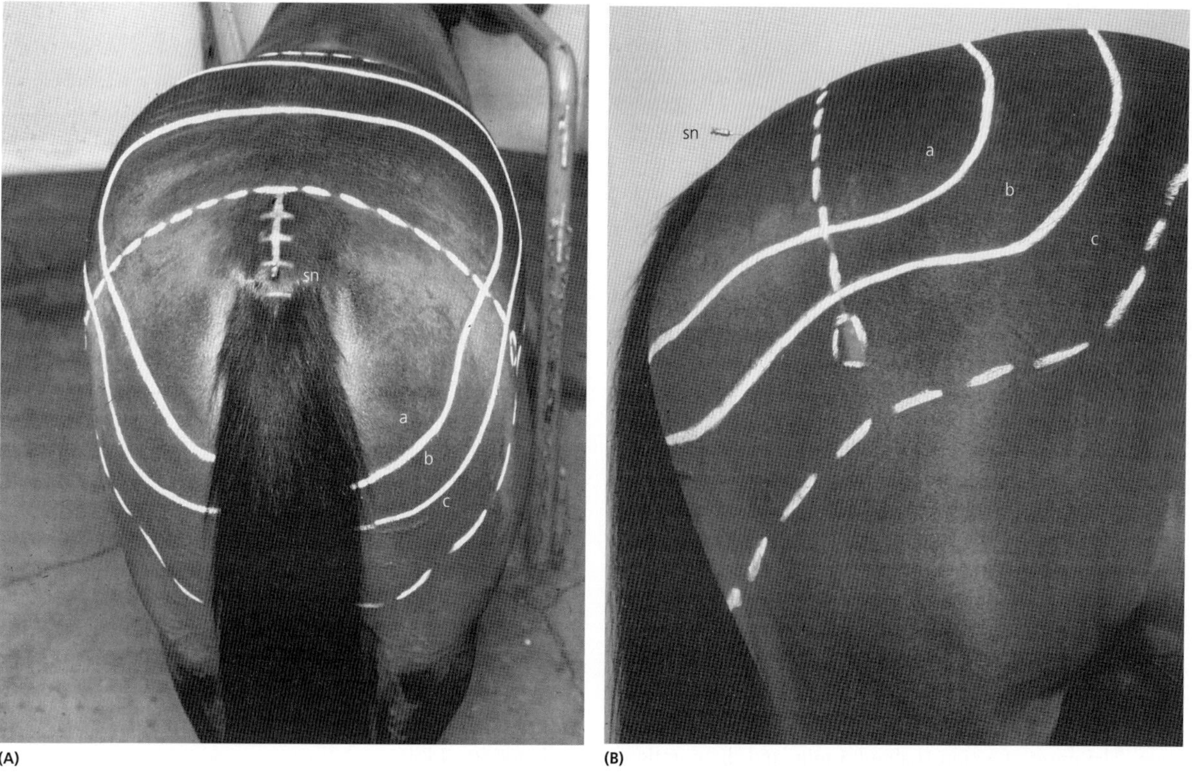

Figure 63.24 Dorsocaudal and lateral views illustrating desensitized areas 20 min after caudal epidural injection of various volumes of 2% mepivacaine using a 5.9 inch (15 cm) 18 gauge spinal needle inserted at the third intercoccygeal space. a, extent of block with 6 mL; b, extent of block with 8 mL; c, extent of block with 10 mL; sn, spinal needle with stylet. Source: Skarda [105].

ropivacaine (8 mL/500 kg) [127] to 0.02 mg/kg of 0.5% ropivacaine (5 mL/500 kg) [128]. Epidural ropivacaine has a rapid onset (approximately 10 min) and can last approximately 3 h. Low-dose lumbosacral epidural ropivacaine has been shown to provide effective analgesia in conscious and anesthetized ponies without affecting motor function to the pelvic limbs [129].

Epinephrine can be added to local anesthetic solutions at a concentration of 5 μg/mL (1:200,000) to hasten the onset, prolong the duration, and improve the quality of epidural anesthesia.

α_2-Adrenergic receptor agonists

Following epidural administration, α_2-adrenergic receptor agonists bind to receptors in the substantia gelatinosa layer of the spinal cord and produce analgesia, which can be reversed by intravenous administration of α_2-adrenergic receptor antagonists such as atipamezole (0.1 mg/kg) [130] and yohimbine (0.05 mg/kg) [131]. α_2-Adrenergic receptor agonists deposited as described for a caudal epidural must diffuse cranially to affect receptors in the spinal cord. If signs of ataxia or sedation develop after caudal epidural administration of α_2-adrenergic receptor agonists, the horse should be supported with a tail-tie or in stocks until normal motor function has been regained. Horses that become recumbent after epidural administration of α_2-adrenergic receptor agonists may require heavy sedation or general anesthesia to keep them from panicking until their motor function has returned.

As noted above, specific antagonists may be used to reverse undesirable effects of epidurally administered α_2-adrenergic receptor agonists. Intravenous yohimbine reduced epidural detomidine-induced perineal analgesia, reversed head ptosis, improved pelvic limb position, terminated sweating and diuresis, and antagonized detomidine-induced decreases in heart rate and cardiac output but did not affect detomidine-induced decreases in respiratory rate [131].

Xylazine

Xylazine has been used at a dose of 0.17 mg/kg diluted to 10 mL with 0.9% saline [132]. The duration of analgesia is approximately 2.5 h, and hindlimb ataxia is uncommon. Sedation is minimal and cardiovascular and respiratory variables as well as core and rectal temperatures do not change appreciably [133].

In horses under general anesthesia, epidural xylazine (0.15 mg/kg) reduced the MAC of halothane by 35% with noxious stimulation of the thoracic limbs and by 40% with stimulation of the pelvic limbs [115]. A second study did not reproduce this effect, but horses that had been given epidural xylazine (0.15 mg/kg diluted to 0.15 mL/kg with saline) required less halothane and inotropic support to maintain mean arterial blood pressure above 60 mmHg and had a higher cardiac index than horses anesthetized with halothane alone [134].

In general, xylazine is a more desirable α_2-adrenergic receptor agonist for epidural use than detomidine since it produces a more potent antinociceptive action in the perineal dermatomes, with minimal cardiovascular depression, head ptosis, changes in pelvic limb position, and diuresis [135].

Detomidine

Detomidine has been used in caudal epidurals at a dose of 60 μg/kg diluted to 10 mL with sterile water [136]. The analgesia from this technique can be variable, with bilateral spread from the coccyx to as far cranially as T14 in some horses. Analgesia is accompanied by mild ataxia, some buckling of the pelvic limbs and deep sedation. The onset of action is about 5 min, and the duration is approximately 3 h. Because of the systemic side effects, an initial dose of no more than 20 μg/kg should be used in debilitated horses.

Dexmedetomidine

A recent study compared caudal epidural injection of bupivacaine (0.04 mg/kg of 0.25%), dexmedetomidine (2 μg/kg), and the combination of the two (0.02 mg/kg bupivacaine and 1 μg/kg dexmedetomdine) in mares. Dexmedetomidine alone produced analgesia of the tail, perineum, and upper hind limbs for 240 min while dexmedetomidine and bupivacaine produced analgesia lasting 200 min, and bupivacaine alone produced analgesia for 97 min [137].

Another study has looked at the effects of epidural dexmedetomidine compared to epidural xylazine in donkeys. Epidural dexmedetomidine (5 μg/kg, diluted to 5 mL with normal saline) produced complete bilateral perineal analgesia in approximately 6 min with a duration of action of 105 min (which was faster and longer acting than xylazine). The donkeys became moderately sedate for about 165 min. The authors concluded that epidural dexmedetomidine induced faster and longer perineal analgesia than xylazine in donkeys [138].

Other α_2-adrenergic receptor agonists

Medetomidine (15 μg/kg diluted to 8 mL with 0.9% saline) and romifidine (80 μg/kg diluted to 8 mL with 0.9% saline) did not produce surgical analgesia in the perineal region of adult horses when injected into the caudal epidural space [139,140]. Based on these results, medetomidine and romifidine do not appear to be as effective as xylazine, detomidine, and dexmedetomidine.

Opioids

Epidural opioids have been extensively studied and can produce long-lasting analgesia when used alone or in combination with local anesthetics, α_2-adrenergic receptor agonists, and/or ketamine. They have been used for acute and chronic pain and are effective when administered preemptively, intraoperatively, or postoperatively.

Morphine

Epidural morphine has long been considered a reasonable alternative for treating pain that does not respond to standard medication protocols such as systemic NSAIDs. In an early case report, epidural morphine was used to relieve the pain associated with a luxated fetlock and comminuted fracture of the first phalanx in a pregnant horse; the onset of action seemed to be approximately 30 min after injection and lasted for 8–16 h based on the behavior of the mare [141].

Morphine is commonly used at a dose of 0.1 mg/kg diluted to a volume of 20 mL with sterile water and administered by caudal epidural injection for the relief of pain. It will induce segmental analgesia from the coccyx to the thoracic dermatomes [142]. The analgesic action is greatest at the dermatomes closest to the epidural injection site and lasts approximately 5 h [142].

In previous studies, morphine was shown to be an effective analgesic for experimentally induced forelimb pain [143]. It has also produced analgesic and antihyperalgesic effects in horses with acute synovitis [144]. In a study in mares undergoing laparoscopic ovariectomy, epidural morphine administration lowered the requirements for systemic sedation and local anesthesia [145]. Although there are concerns about systemic opioids and gastrointestinal side effects in horses, epidural morphine did not cause clinical signs of colic, although it temporarily reduced gastrointestinal motility [146].

Methadone

When the effects of caudal epidural methadone (0.1 mg/kg) were compared with those of lidocaine (0.35 mg/kg) using a thermal stimulation model, perineal analgesia was apparent within 15 min after injection [147]. The perineal analgesia from methadone lasted 5 h after injection compared with 3 h with lidocaine. Unlike lidocaine, methadone did not cause ataxia. In a recent study, methadone (0.4 mg/kg) was used to validate lumbosacral spinal cord somatosensory evoked potentials as a tool to assess nociception in horses [148].

Butorphanol

Despite the widespread use of butorphanol in horses as a systemic analgesic, it has not been shown to increase avoidance behavior to noxious stimuli [142] or to affect the MAC of halothane [114] after caudal epidural administration.

Epidural medication combinations

Xylazine and lidocaine

Xylazine (0.17 mg/kg of a 2% solution) and lidocaine (0.22 mg/kg of a 2% solution) can be safely used for long-lasting caudal epidural anesthesia in healthy adult horses [122]. The combination provides up to 5 h of perineal anesthesia, whereas each drug alone has a duration of only about 3 h. There may be some ataxia with the combination, but heart and respiratory rates are minimally affected. Although there appears to be a large margin of safety with this combination, it is worth noting that there is one report of a Thoroughbred mare undergoing sudden collapse in the hindquarters 90 min after completion of the epidural injection for urogenital surgery [149].

A recent paper in mules evaluated the efficacy and safety of epidural lidocaine and xylazine for standing ovariectomy. The mares were sedated with 0.05 mg/kg acepromazine IM, 1.3 mg/kg xylazine and 0.02 mg/kg butorphanol IV, and 0.6 mg/kg/h xylazine IV. The paralumbar fossae were infiltrated with 30 mL of 2% lidocaine, and a caudal epidural was performed with 0.2 mg/kg lidocaine and 0.17 mg/kg xylazine. Sedation and analgesia were satisfactory in six out of eight mules, and the standing ovariectomy was successful in all eight. The authors concluded that additional studies are needed to establish doses that allow for reliable abdominal analgesia in mules for standing ovariectomy [150].

Nalbuphine and lidocaine

In donkeys, one study looked at adding nalbuphine (an opioid agonist/antagonist) to lidocaine for epidural anesthesia. The authors found that the combination of the two drugs (2% lidocaine at 0.11 mg/kg and nalbuphine at 0.2 mg/kg) produced a faster onset of analgesia (7 min) but a shorter duration of action (147 min) than nalbuphine alone [151].

Morphine and detomidine

Morphine and detomidine provided profound hindlimb analgesia in horses with experimentally induced lameness [152]. Epidural morphine (0.2 mg/kg) combined with detomidine (30 μg/kg) also significantly decreased lameness after bilateral stifle arthroscopy in horses [153]. A more recent study found that the analgesic effects of epidural buprenorphine (0.005 mg/kg) plus detomidine (0.15 mg/kg) were equivalent to those after epidural morphine plus detomidine in horses undergoing bilateral stifle arthroscopy [154].

Morphine and romifidine

Caudal epidural romifidine (30–60 μg/kg) combined with morphine (0.1 mg/kg) produces moderate analgesia for 60–90 min depending on the dose of romifidine used. Intense sedation, moderate ataxia of the hindlimbs, and a decrease in heart and respiratory rates were noted during the 4 h observation period [155].

Tramadol and lidocaine

Tramadol (0.5 mg/kg) combined with lidocaine (0.2 mg/kg of a 2% solution) was shown to extend the duration of perineal analgesia, as measured using a pinprick and thermal stimulation, over lidocaine alone when administered by caudal epidural injection. The duration of action of lidocaine alone was 70 min and that of tramadol with lidocaine was 210 min [156].

Neostigmine and lidocaine

The addition of neostigmine to lidocaine for caudal epidural anesthesia has been shown to prolong lidocaine's duration of action. Lidocaine (0.2 mg/kg of a 2% solution) was administered by caudal epidural injection alone or in combination with 1 or 2 μg/kg of neostigmine. The combination of neostigmine with lidocaine induced perineal analgesia lasting 2.5 h with a low prevalence of adverse effects in standing horses [157].

Ketamine combinations

Ketamine (1.0 mg/kg) and xylazine (0.5 mg/kg) have been used in combination for caudal epidural administration in horses and have been shown to produce good analgesia of the tail, perineal region, anus, and vulva [158]. The onset of action is 5–9 min and the duration averages 120 min. There is some systemic sedation with this combination.

Epidural bupivacaine alone (0.02 mg/kg of a 0.25% solution), bupivacaine with morphine (0.02 mg/kg with 0.1 mg/kg), and bupivacaine with ketamine (0.02 mg/kg with 0.5 mg/kg) have been compared for their ability to provide analgesia in conscious horses [159]. The onset of action was 5 min for bupivacaine, 10 min for bupivacaine with morphine, and 15 min for bupivacaine with ketamine. The duration of action was 315 min for bupivacaine with morphine, 210 min for bupivacaine, and 240 min for bupivacaine with ketamine. While morphine and ketamine may be effective adjuncts to bupivacaine for caudal epidurals, bupivacaine with morphine may be preferable to a high dose of bupivacaine alone or to bupivacaine with ketamine.

Complications

There are several reported complications associated with epidural injections. Poor technique, anatomic abnormalities, and previous epidural injections causing development of fibrous tissue at the site can cause failure of anesthesia/analgesia. Overdose of local anesthetics and/or α_2-adrenergic receptor agonists can cause excessive ataxia and possibly recumbency. If recumbency results from inadvertent overdose of epidural anesthetics, it may be necessary to keep the horse sedated or anesthetized until motor function to the hindlimbs returns. One recent report detailed the collapse of a 559 kg mare given 13 mL of 2% lidocaine in a caudal epidural for standing treatment of gluteal compartment syndrome. Unfortunately, the mare was unable to stand after being maintained under anesthesia until the effects of the lidocaine epidural were presumed to have worn off and the owners elected humane euthanasia [160].

Sedation and cardiovascular depression may be associated with systemic uptake of medications (especially α_2-adrenergic receptor agonists) used epidurally. There have also been rare reports of systemic pruritis in horses after epidural morphine [161–163]. A recent case report described generalized seizure activity in a show pony mare administered a high-volume (50 mL) caudal epidural containing morphine and detomidine to provide analgesia to the thoracic limbs. The pony recovered rapidly without intervention, and no residual neurological deficits were observed [164].

Novel regional analgesic techniques

Transversus abdominis plane block

Reports of the application of ultrasound-guided regional anesthetic techniques, described more in-depth in Chapter 60, are beginning to emerge in horses. One such technique, the transversus abdominis plane (TAP) block has been described for use in surgical procedures in many species including humans, dogs, cats, rabbits, llamas, pigs, and more. Recently, a study was done to determine if this block could be utilized in horses as an alternate analgesic strategy for colic surgery. Advantages of using TAP blocks could include decreasing adverse effects associated with systemically administered analgesics such as cardiovascular depression, ileus, and ataxia. During this initial study, Shetland ponies were determined to have sensory blockade for up to 2 h after bilateral TAP block with bupivacaine as compared to saline [165]. Further investigation is needed to determine if TAP blocks are an effective analgesic adjunct for colic surgery in horses.

Caudal intercostal block for abdominal surgery

An intercostal nerve block that can desensitize the ventral and lateral abdominal and thoracic wall (caudal intercostal block for abdominal surgery [CIBAS]) has been described. It may relive postoperative celiotomy pain but will not completely desensitize the caudal ventral abdomen. The horse can be standing or in dorsal recumbency and the block can be performed blindly or with ultrasound or nerve stimulator guidance. Further investigation is needed to determine situations where this block will be most useful [166].

Continuous delivery of local anesthetics for lower limb analgesia

A technique has been described for the continuous delivery of local anesthetics for lower limb analgesia [167]. The technique for placement of the catheters was first developed in cadaver limbs with the catheter being inserted 2–4 cm distal to the accessory carpal bone medially and laterally and then passing it so that the tip was adjacent to the communicating branch of the medial and lateral palmar nerves. The catheters were well tolerated by the test horses, but after 1–2 days there was significant limb swelling in horses receiving local anesthetic infusions, but not in the horses receiving saline infusion. A second study compared continuous peripheral neural blockade (CPNB) with bupivacaine with intermittent peripheral neural blockade (IPNB) with bupivacaine in experimentally induced tendonitis pain [168]. CPNB provided better analgesia than IPNB when lameness was scored, and behavioral and physiologic signs of pain were monitored. This study used the CPNB catheters for 3 days, and further investigation is needed to determine if this technique is useful for longer-term treatment.

References

1 Nichols CL, Doherty TJ, Schumacher J, *et al.* Dexmedetomidine prolongs the duration of action of mepivacaine on anesthesia of the palmar digital nerves of horses. *Am J Vet Res* 2021; **83**(2): 114–118.

2 Tanner RB, Hubbell JAE. A retrospective study of the incidence and management of complications associated with regional nerve blocks in equine dental patients. *J Vet Dent* 2019; **36**(1): 40–45.

3 Edwards JF. Regional anaesthesia of the head of the horse: an up-to-date survey. *Vet Rec* 1930; **10**: 873–975.

4 Staszyk C, Bienert A, Baumer W, *et al.* Stimulation of local anaesthetic nerve block of the infraorbital nerve within the pterygopalatine fossa; anatomical landmarks defined by computed tomography. *Res Vet Sci* 2008; **85**: 399–406.

5 Roberts VLH, Perkins JD, Skarlina E, *et al.* Caudal anaesthesia of the infraorbital nerve for diagnosis of idiopathic headshaking and caudal compression of the infraorbital nerve for its treatment, in 58 horses. *Equine Vet J* 2013; **45**: 107–110.

6 Newton SA, Knottenbelt DC, Eldridge PR. Headshaking in horses: possible aetiopathogenesis suggested by the results of diagnostic tests and several treatment regimes used in 20 cases. *Equine Vet J* 2000; **32**: 208–216.

7 Schumacher J, Schumacher J, Wilhite R. Anesthesia of the head and neck. In: Doherty T, Valverde A, Reed RA, eds. *Manual of Equine Anesthesia and Analgesia*, 2nd edn. Hoboken: John Wiley & Sons, 2022: 355.

8 Bardell D, Iff I, Mosing M. A cadaver study comparing two approaches to perform a maxillary nerve block in the horse. *Equine Vet J* 2010; **42**: 721–725.

9 Stauffer S, Cordner B, Dixon J, *et al.* Maxillary nerve blocks in horses: an experimental comparison of surface landmark and ultrasound-guided techniques. *Vet Anaesth Analg* 2017; **44**(4): 951–958.

10 Harding PG, Smith RL, Barakzai SZ. Comparison of two approaches to performing an inferior alveolar nerve block in the horse. *Aust Vet J* 2012; **90**: 146–150.

11 Henry T, Pusterla N, Guedes AGP, *et al.* Evaluation and clinical use of an intraoral inferior alveolar nerve block in the horse. *Equine Vet J* 2014; **46**(6): 706–710.

12 Lindsay WA, Hedberg EB. Performing facial nerve blocks, nasolacrimal catheterization and paranasal sinus centesis in horses. *Vet Med* 1991; **86**: 72–83.

13 Eckert RE, Griffin E, Cohen ND, *et al.* Investigation into intraoral approach for nerve block injection at the mental foramen in the horse. *Equine Vet Educ* 2019; **31**(6): 328–334.

14 Kyei S, Abaka Dadzie NY, Zaabaar E, *et al.* Age and sex variation in the duration of action and corneal touch threshold (CTT) following instillation of 0.5% topical ophthalmic proparacaine and tetracaine hydrochlorides. *J Ophthalmol* 2021: 8661098.

15 Monclin SJ, Farnir F, Grauwels M. Duration of corneal anaesthesia following multiple doses and two concentrations of tetracaine hydrochloride eyedrops on the normal equine cornea. *Equine Vet J* 2011; **43**: 69–73.

16 Pucket JD, Allbaugh RA, Rankin AJ, *et al.* Comparison of efficacy and duration of effect on corneal sensitivity among anesthetic agents following ocular administration in clinically normal horses. *Am J Vet Res* 2013; **74**: 459–464.

17 Makra Z, E, Eördögh R, Fábián I, *et al.* Evaluation of corneal anaesthesia after the application of topical 0.5% bupivacaine, 2% lidocaine and 0.4% oxybuprocaine in normal horses. *Vet Anaesth Analg* 2021; **48**(6): 972–976.

18 Regnier A, Berton I, Concordet D, *et al.* Effect of topical application of 2% lidocaine gel on corneal sensitivity of clinically normal equine eyes. *Vet Anaesth Analg* 2018; **45**(2): 158–164.

19 Merideth RE, Wolf ED. Ophthalmic examination and therapeutic techniques in the horse. *Compend Contin Educ* 1981; **3**: S426–S433.

20 Diehl K, Bowden AC. Effect of auriculopalpebral nerve block on equine intraocular pressure measured by rebound tonometry (TonoVet®). *Vet Ophthalmol* 2020; **23**(2): 368–373.

21 Manning JP, St Clair LE. Palpebral frontal and zygomatic nerve blocks for examination of the equine eye. *Vet Med* 1976; **71**: 187–189.

22 Pollock PJ, Russell T, Hughes TK, *et al.* Transpalpebral eye enucleation in 40 standing horses. *Vet Surg* 2008; **37**: 306–309.

23 Hewes CA, Keoughan GC, Gutierrez-Nibeyro S. Standing enucleation in the horse: a report of 5 cases. *Can Vet J* 2007; **48**: 512–514.

24 Betbeze CM, Dray SM, Fontenot RL. Subconjunctival enucleation with orbital implant placement in standing horses: 20 cases (2014–2017). *J Am Vet Med Assoc* 2021; **258**(6): 661–667.

25 Hague BA, Honnas CM, Simpson RB, *et al.* Evaluation of skin bacterial flora before and after aseptic preparation of clipped and nonclipped arthrocentesis sites in horses. *Vet Surg* 1997; **26**: 121–125.

26 Wahl K, Adams SB, Moore GE. Contamination of joints with tissue debris and hair after arthrocentesis: the effect of needle insertion angle, spinal needle gauge, and insertion of spinal needles with and without a stylet. *Vet Surg* 2012; **41**: 391–398.

27 Buchner HH, Kübber P, Zohmann E, *et al.* Sedation and antisedation as tools in equine lameness examination. *Equine Vet J* 1999; (Suppl 30): 227–230.

28 Moorman VJ, Bass L, King MR. Evaluation of the effects of commonly used alpha$_2$-adrenergic agonists alone and in combination with butorphanol tartrate on objective measurements of lameness in horses. *Am J Vet Res* 2019; **80**(9): 868–877.

29 Calvo-Santesmases A, Manso-Diaz G, Fores P, *et al.* Kinematic patterns in horses sedated with low doses of detomidine: an accelerometric evaluation. *J Equine Vet Sci* 2021; **107**: 103–107.

30 Park J, Sutradhar BC, Hong G, *et al.* Comparison of the cytotoxic effects of bupivacaine, lidocaine, and mepivacaine in equine articular chondrocytes. *Vet Anesth Analg* 2011; **38**: 127–133.

31 Silva GB, De La Corte FD, Brass KE, *et al.* Viability of equine chondrocytes after exposure to mepivacaine and ropivacaine in vitro. *J Equine Vet Sci* 2019; **77**: 80–85.

32 Schumacher J, Cole RC, DeGraves FJ, *et al.* Comparison of speed of onset and analgesic effect of 2% mepivacaine hydrochloride deposited within or outside the neurovascular bundle at the level of the proximal sesamoid bones in horses with naturally occurring forefoot-related lameness. *Am J Vet Res* 2020; **81**(5): 394–399.

33 Kearney CM, van Weeren PR, Cornelissen BP, *et al.* Which anatomical region determines a positive flexion test of the distal aspect of a forelimb in a nonlame horse? *Equine Vet J* 2010; **42**: 547–551.

34 Schumacher J, Livesey L, DeGraves FJ, *et al.* Effect of anaesthesia of the palmar digital nerves on proximal interphalangeal joint pain in the horse. *Equine Vet J* 2004; **36**: 409–414.

35 Schumacher J, Steiger R, Schumacher J, *et al.* Effects of analgesia of the distal interphalangeal joint or palmar digital nerves on lameness caused by solar pain in horses. *Vet Surg* 2000; **29**: 54–58.

36 Easter JL, Watkins JP, Stephens SL, *et al.* Effects of regional anesthesia on experimentally induced coffin joint synovitis. *Proc Annu Conv Am Assoc Equine Pract* 2000; **46**: 214–216.

37 Keegan KG, Wilson DJ, Wilson DA, *et al.* Effects of anesthesia of the palmar digital nerves on kinematic gait analysis in horses with and without navicular disease. *Am J Vet Res* 1997; **58**: 218–223.

38 Bidwell LA, Brown KE, Cordier A, *et al.* Mepivacaine local anaesthetic duration in equine palmar digital nerve blocks. *Equine Vet J* 2004; **36**: 723–726.

39 Hoerdemann M, Smith RL, Hosgood G. Duration of action of mepivacaine and lidocaine in equine palmar digital perineural blocks in an experimental lameness model. *Vet Surg* 2017; **46**(7): 986–993.

40 Harcourt MM, Smith RL, Hosgood G. Duration of skin desensitization following palmar digital nerve blocks with lidocaine, bupivacaine, mepivacaine and prilocaine. *Aust Vet J* 2021; **99**(12): 541–546.

41 Alvarez AV, Schumacher J, Degraves FJ. Effect of the addition of epinephrine to a lidocaine solution on the efficacy and duration of palmar digital nerve blocks in horses with naturally occurring forefoot lameness. *Am J Vet Res* 2018; **79**(10): 1028–1034.

42 McCracken MJ, Schumacher J, Doherty TJ, *et al.* Efficacy and duration of effect for liposomal bupivacaine when administered perineurally to the palmar digital nerves of horses. *Am J Vet Res* 2020; **81**(5): 400–405.

43 Nagy A, Bodo G, Dyson SJ, *et al.* Diffusion of contrast medium after perineural injection of the palmar nerves: an in vivo and in vitro study. *Equine Vet J* 2009; **41**: 379–383.

44 Le KM, Caston SS, Hossetter JM, *et al.* Comparison of analgesic and tissue effects of subcutaneous perineural injection of liposomal bupivacaine and bupivacaine hydrochloride in horses with forelimb lameness induced via circumferential clamp. *Am J Vet Res* 2020; **81**(7): 551–556.

45 Schumacher J, DeGraves F, Cesar F, *et al.* Efficacy of ketamine hydrochloride administered as a basilar sesamoid nerve block in alleviating foot pain in horses caused by natural disease. *Equine Vet J* 2014; **46**(5): 639–641.

46 Maia BT, do Proda Vendruscolo C, de Souza AF, *et al.* Anatomical position of the palmar/plantar nerves at the metacarpal/metatarsal distal level in horses: an in vivo study by means of ultrasonography. *Anat Histol Embryol* 2022; **51**(2): 236–243.

47 Seabaugh KA, Selberg KT, Valdes-Martinez A, *et al.* Assessment of the tissue diffusion of anesthetic agent following administration of a low palmar nerve block in horses. *J Am Vet Med Assoc* 2011; **239**: 1334–1340.

48 Nagy A, Bodo G, Dyson SJ, *et al.* Distribution of radiodense contrast medium after perineural injection of the palmar and palmar metacarpal nerves (low 4-point nerve block): an in vivo and ex vivo study in horses. *Equine Vet J* 2010; **42**: 512–518.

49 Nagy A, Bodo G, Dyson SJ. Diffusion of contrast medium after four different techniques for analgesia of the proximal metacarpal region: an in vivo and in vitro study. *Equine Vet J* 2012; **44**: 668–673.

50 Zekas LJ, Forrest LJ. Effect of perineural anesthesia on the ultrasonographic appearance of equine palmar metacarpal structures. *Vet Radiol Ultrasound* 2003; **44**: 59–64.

51 Castro FA, Schumacher JS, Pauwels F, *et al.* A new approach for perineural injection of the lateral palmar nerve in the horse. *Vet Surg* 2005; **34**: 539–542.

52 Hughes TK, Eliashar E, Smith RK. In vitro evaluation of a single injection technique for diagnostic analgesia of the proximal suspensory ligament of the equine pelvic limb. *Vet Surg* 2007; **36**: 760–764.

53 Gayle GM, Redding WR. Comparison of diagnostic anaesthetic techniques of the proximal plantar metatarsus in the horse. *Equine Vet Educ* 2007; **19**: 222–224.

54 Hinnigan G, Milner P, Talbot A, *et al.* Is anaesthesia of the deep branch of the lateral plantar nerve specific for the diagnosis of proximal metatarsal pain in the horse? *Vet Comp Orthop Traumatol* 2014; **27**(5): 351–357.

55 Claunch KM, Eggleston RB, Baxter GM. Effects of approach and injection volume on diffusion of mepivacaine hydrochloride during local analgesia of the deep branch of the lateral plantar nerve in horses. *J Am Vet Med Assoc* 2014; **245**(10): 1153–1159.

56 McGlinchey L, Agne G, Passler T, *et al.* An objective assessment of the effect of anesthetizing the median nerve on lameness caused by pain in the cubital joint. *J Equine Vet Sci* 2019; **75**: 9–13.

57 Souto MTM, Fantoni DT, Hamaji A, *et al.* Ultrasound-guided continuous block of median and ulnar nerves in horses: development of the technique. *Vet Anaesth Analg* 2020; **47**(3): 405–413.

58 Boorman S, DeGraves F, Schumacher J, *et al.* Comparison of 2% mepivacaine and a solution of 2% lidocaine/epinephrine administered for median and ulnar nerve blocks in horses with naturally occurring forelimb lameness. *Vet Surg* 2022; **51**(2): 279–285.

59 Boone LH, Schumacher J, DeGraves F, *et al.* Buffering mepivacaine with sodium bicarbonate speeds and potentiates analgesia of median and ulnar nerve blocks performed on horses. *Vet Rec* 2019; **184**(5): 155.

60 Boone LH, DeGraves FJ, Klein CE, *et al.* Effect of 3% chloroprocaine hydrochloride when used for median and ulnar regional nerve blocks in lame horses. *Am J Vet Res* 2020; **81**(1): 13–16.

61 Van der Laan M, Raes E, Oosterlink M. Cadaveric comparison of the accuracy of ultrasound-guided versus 'blind' perineural injection of the tibial nerve in horses. *Vet J* 2021; **269**: 105–106.

62 Denoix J-M, Beaumont AB, Bertoni L. Ultrasonographic guided block of the tibial nerve. *Equine Vet Educ* 2020; **32**(7): 372–377.

63 Schramme MC, Boswell JC, Hamhougias K, *et al.* An in vitro study to compare 5 different techniques for injection of the navicular bursa in the horse. *Equine Vet J* 2000; **32**: 263–267.

64 Piccot-Crézollet C, Cauvin ER, Lepage OM. Comparison of two techniques for injection of the podotrochlear bursa in horses. *J Am Vet Med Assoc* 2005; **226**: 1524–1528.

65 Nottrott K, De Guio C, Khairoun A, *et al.* An ultrasound-guided, tendon-sparing, lateral approach to injection of the navicular bursa. *Equine Vet J* 2017; **49**: 655–661.

66 Dyson SJ, Kidd L. A comparison of responses to analgesia of the navicular bursa and intra-articular analgesia of the distal interphalangeal joint in 59 horses. *Equine Vet J* 1992; **25**: 93–98.

67 Schumacher J, Schumacher J, Gillette R, *et al.* The effects of local anaesthetic solution in the navicular bursa of horses with lameness caused by distal interphalangeal joint pain. *Equine Vet J* 2003; **35**: 502–505.

68 Gough MR, Mayhew G, Munroe GA. Diffusion of mepivacaine between adjacent synovial structures in the horse. Part 1: forelimb foot and carpus. *Equine Vet J* 2002; **34**: 80–84.

69 Schumacher J, Schumacher J, DeGraves F. A comparison of the effects of local analgesic solution in the navicular bursa of horses with lameness caused by solar toe or solar heel pain. *Equine Vet J* 2001; **33**: 386–389.

70 Schumacher J, Schumacher J, DeGraves F, *et al.* A comparison of the effects of two volumes of local analgesic solution in the distal interphalangeal joint of horses with lameness caused by solar toe or solar heel pain. *Equine Vet J* 2001; **33**: 265–268.

71 Mereu M, Hawkes C, Cuddy LC, *et al.* Evaluation of four techniques for injection of the proximal interphalangeal joint in horses. *Vet Surg* 2019; **48**: 1437–1443.

72 Hassel DM, Stover SM, Yarbrough TB, *et al.* Palmar–plantar axial sesamoidean approach to the digital flexor tendon sheath in horses. *J Am Vet Med Assoc* 2000; **217**: 1343–1347.

73 Harper J, Schumacher J, DeGraves F, *et al.* Effects of analgesia of the digital flexor tendon sheath on pain originating in the sole, distal interphalangeal joint, or navicular bursa of horses. *Equine Vet J* 2007; **39**: 535–539.

74 Jordana M, Martens A, Duchateau L, *et al.* Diffusion of mepivacaine to adjacent synovial structures after intrasynovial analgesia of the digital flexor tendon sheath. *Equine Vet J* 2016; **48**(3): 326–330.

75 Miagkoff L, Bonilla AG. Desensitization of the distal forelimb following intrathecal anesthesia of the carpal sheath in horses. *Equine Vet J* 2021; **53**(1): 167–176.

76 Lewis RD. Techniques for arthrocentesis of the equine shoulder, elbow, stifle and hip joints. *Proc Annu Conv Am Assoc Equine Pract* 1996; **42**: 55–63.

77 Schumacher J, Livesey L, Brawner W, *et al.* Comparison of 2 methods of centesis of the bursa of the biceps brachii tendon of horses. *Equine Vet J* 2007; **39**: 356–359.

78 Schneeweiss W, Puggioni A, David F. Comparison of ultrasound-guided vs. 'blind' techniques for intra-synovial injections of the shoulder area in horses: scapulohumeral joint, bicipital and infraspinatus bursae. *Equine Vet J* 2012; **44**: 674–678.

79 Seabaugh KA, Selberg KT, Mueller POE, *et al.* Clinical study evaluating the accuracy of injecting the distal tarsal joints in the horse. *Equine Vet J* 2017; **49**(5): 668–672.

80 Bell BT, Baker GJ, Foreman JH, Abbott LC. In vivo investigation of communication between the distal intertarsal and tarsometatarsal joints in horses and ponies. *Vet Surg* 1993; **22**: 289–292.

81 Dyson SJ, Romero JM. An investigation of techniques for local analgesia of the equine distal tarsus and proximal metatarsus. *Equine Vet J* 1993; **25**: 30–35.

82 Kraus-Hansen AE, Jann HW, Kerr DV, *et al.* Arthrographic analysis of communication between the tarsometatarsal and distal intertarsal joints of the horse. *Vet Surg* 1992; **21**: 139–144.

83 Sack WO, Orsini PG. Distal intertarsal and tarsometatarsal joints in the horse: communication and injection sites. *J Am Vet Med Assoc* 1981; **179**: 355–359.

84 Post EM, Singer ER, Clegg PD. An anatomic study of the calcaneal bursae in the horse. *Vet Surg* 2007; **36**: 3–9.

85 Vacek JR, Ford TS, Honnas CM. Communication between the femoropatellar and medial and lateral femorotibial joints in horses. *Am J Vet Res* 1992; **53**: 1431–1434.

86 Reeves MJ, Trotter GW, Kainer RA. Anatomical and functional communications between the synovial sacs of the equine stifle joint. *Equine Vet J* 1991; **23**: 215–218.

87 Gough MR, Munroe GA, Mayhew G. Diffusion of mepivacaine between adjacent synovial structures in the horse. Part 2: tarsus and stifle. *Equine Vet J* 2002; **34**: 85–90.

88 Tóth F, Schumacher J, Schramme MC, *et al.* Effect of anesthetizing individual compartments of the stifle joint in horses with experimentally induced stifle joint lameness. *Am J Vet Res* 2014; **75**(1): 19–25.

89 Hendrickson DA, Nixon AJ. A lateral approach for synovial fluid aspiration and joint injection of the femoropatellar joint of the horse. *Equine Vet J* 1992; **24**: 397–398.

90 Hendrickson DA, Nixon AJ. Comparison of the cranial and a new lateral approach to the femoropatellar joint for aspiration and injection in horses. *J Am Vet Med Assoc* 1994; **205**: 1177–1179.

91 Swiderski CE, Cooke E, Linford R. How to inject the medial femorotibial joint: an alternate approach. *Proc Annu Conv Am Assoc Equine Pract* 2005; **51**: 476–480.

92 Schumacher J, Schumacher J, Wilhite R. Comparison of four techniques of arthrocentesis of the lateral compartment of the femorotibial joint of the horse. *Equine Vet J* 2012; **44**: 664–667.

93 David F, Rougier M, Alexander K, *et al.* Ultrasound-guided coxofemoral arthrocentesis in horses. *Equine Vet J* 2007; **39**: 79–83.

94 Whitcomb MB, Vaughan B, Katzman S, *et al.* Ultrasound-guided injections in horses with cranioventral distention of the coxofemoral joint capsule: feasibility for a cranioventral approach. *Vet Radiol Ultrasound* 2016; 57(2): 199–206.

95 Tóth F, Schumacher J, Scramme M, Hecht S. Evaluation of four techniques for injecting the trochanteric bursa of horses. *Vet Surg* 2011; **40**: 489–493.

96 Dyson S, Murray R. Pain associated with the sacroiliac joint region: a clinical study of 74 horses. *Equine Vet J* 2003; **35**(3): 240–245.

97 Engeli E, Haussler KK. Review of injection techniques targeting the sacroiliac region in horses. *Equine Vet Educ* 2012; **24**(10): 529–541.

98 Garcia-Lopez JM. Neck, back, and pelvic pain in sport horses. *Vet Clin North Amer* 2018; **34**(2): 235–251.

99 Denoix J-M, Jacquet S. Ultrasound-guided injections of the sacroiliac area in horses. *Equine Vet Educ* 2008; **20**(4): 203–207.

100 Offord SCJ, Read RM, Pudney CJ, *et al.* Complications following equine sacroiliac region analgesia are uncommon: a study in 118 horses. *PLoS ONE* 2021; **16**(3): e0247781.

101 Skarda RT, Tranquilli WJ. Local and regional anesthetic and analgesic techniques: horses. In: Tranquilli WJ, Thurmon JC, Grimm KA, eds. *Lumb and Jones' Veterinary Anesthesia and Analgesia*, 4th edn. Ames, IA: Blackwell Publishing, 2007: 605–642.

102 Heavner JE. Local anesthetics. *Vet Clin North Am Large Anim Pract* 1991; **3**: 209–211.

103 Delli-Rocili MM, Cribb NC, Trout DR, *et al.* Effectiveness of a paravertebral nerve block versus local portal blocks for laparoscopic closure of the nephrosplenic space: a pilot study. *Vet Surg* 2020; **49**(5): 1007–1014.

104 Moon PF, Suter CM. Paravertebral thoracolumbar anaesthesia in 10 horses. *Equine Vet J* 1993; **25**: 304–308.

105 Skarda RT. Practical regional anesthesia. In: Mansmann RA, McAllister ES, Pratt PW, eds. *Equine Medicine and Surgery*, vol. **1**, 3rd edn. Santa Barbara, CA: American Veterinary Publications, 1982: 229–238.

106 Haga HA, Lykkjen S, Revold T, Ranheim B. Effect of intratesticular injection of lidocaine on cardiovascular responses to castration in isoflurane anesthetized stallions. *Am J Vet Res* 2006; **67**: 403–408.

107 Portier KG, Jaillardon L, Leece EA, Walsh CM. Castration of horses under total intravenous anaesthesia: analgesic effects of lidocaine. *Vet Anaesth Analg* 2009; **36**: 173–179.

108 Joyce J, Hendrickson DA. Comparison of intraoperative pain responses following intratesticular or mesorchial injection of lidocaine in standing horses undergoing laparoscopic cryptorchidectomy. *J Am Vet Med Assoc* 2006; **229**: 1779–1783.

109 Koch DW, Easley JT, Hatzel JN, *et al.* Prospective randomized investigation of topical anesthesia during unilateral laparoscopic ovariectomy in horses. *Vet Surg* 2020; **49**(Suppl 1): O54–O59.

110 Magda JJ. Local anesthesia in operations on the male perineum in horses. *Veterinariya* 1948; **25**: 34–36.

111 Erkert RS, MacAllister CG, Campbell G, *et al.* Comparison of topical lidocaine/prilocaine anesthetic cream and local infiltration of 2% lidocaine for episioplasty in mares. *J Vet Pharmacol Ther* 2005; **28**: 299–304.

112 Gallacher K, Santos LC, Campoy L, *et al.* Development of a peripheral nerve stimulator-guided technique for equine pudendal nerve blockade. *Vet J* 2016; **217**: 72–77.

113 Skarda RT, Muir WW. Segmental thoracolumbar spinal (subarachnoid) analgesia in conscious horses. *Am J Vet Res* 1982; **43**: 2121–2128.

114 Doherty TJ, Geiser DR, Rohrbach BW. Effect of high volume epidural morphine, ketamine and butorphanol on halothane minimum alveolar concentration in ponies. *Equine Vet J* 1997; **29**: 370–373.

115 Doherty TJ, Geiser DR, Rohrbach BW. The effect of epidural xylazine on halothane minimum alveolar concentration in ponies. *J Vet Pharmacol Ther* 1997; **20**: 246–248.

116 Greene SA, Thurmon JC. Epidural anesthesia and sedation for selected equine surgeries. *Equine Pract* 1985; **7**: 14–19.

117 Lechner TJ, van Wijk MG, Maas AJ, *et al.* Clinical results with the acoustic puncture assist device, a new acoustic device to identify the epidural space. *Anesthes Analg* 2004; **96**: 1183–1187.

118 Iff I, Mosing M, Lechner T, Moens Y. The use of an acoustic device to identify the extradural space in standing horses. *Vet Anesth Analg* 2010; **37**: 57–62.

119 Martin CA, Kerr CL, Pearce SG, *et al.* Outcome of epidural catheterization for delivery of analgesics in horses: 43 cases (1998–2001). *J Am Vet Med Assoc* 2003; **222**: 1394–1398.

120 Sysel AM, Pleasant RS, Jacobson JD, *et al.* Systemic and local effects associated with long-term epidural catheterization and morphine–detomidine administration in horses. *Vet Surg* 1997; **26**: 141–149.

121 Skarda RT, Muir WW. Segmental and subarachnoid analgesia in conscious horses: a comparative study. *Am J Vet Res* 1983; **44**: 1870–1876.

122 Grubb TL, Riebold TW, Huber MJ. Comparison of lidocaine–xylazine, and xylazine–lidocaine for caudal epidural analgesia in horses. *J Am Vet Med Assoc* 1992; **201**: 1187–1190.

123 Sampaio BFB, DeRossi R, Menezes PHN, *et al.* Effects of a caudal epidural anesthesia using midazolam with or without lidocaine to perform an endometrial biopsy in mares. *J Equine Vet Sci* 2017; **59**: 110–117.

124 Duarte PC, Paz CFR, Oliveira APL, *et al.* Caudal epidural anesthesia in mares after bicarbonate addition to a lidocaine-epinephrine combination. *Vet Anaesth Analg* 2017; **44**(4): 943–950.

125 Skarda RT, Muir WW, Ibrahim AL. Plasma mepivacaine concentrations after caudal epidural and subarachnoid injection in the horse: comparative study. *Am J Vet Res* 1984; **45**: 1967–1971.

126 DeRossi R, Breno FB, Varela JV, *et al.* Perineal analgesia and hemodynamic effects of the epidural administration of meperidine or hyperbaric bupivacaine in conscious horses. *Can Vet J* 2004; **45**: 42–47.

127 Ganidalgi S, Cetin H, Biricik HS, *et al.* Comparison of ropivacaine with a combination of ropivacaine and fentanyl for the caudal epidural anaesthesia of mares. *Vet Rec* 2004; **154**: 329–332.

128 Skarda RT, Muir WW. Analgesic, hemodynamic and respiratory effects of caudally epidurally administered ropivacaine hydrochloride in mares. *Vet Anesth Analg* 2001; **28**: 61–74.

129 van Loon JPAM, Menke ES, Doornebal A, *et al.* Antinociceptive effects of low dose lumbosacral epidural ropivacaine in healthy ponies. *Vet J* 2012; **193**: 240–245.

130 Skarda RT, Muir WW. Influence of atipamezole on effects of midsacral subarachnoidally administered detomidine in mares. *Am J Vet Res* 1998; **59**: 468–478.

131 Skarda RT, Muir WW. Effects of intravenously administered yohimbine on antinociceptive, cardiorespiratory, and postural changes induced by epidural administration of detomidine hydrochloride solution in healthy mares. *Am J Vet Res* 1999; **60**: 1262–1270.

132 LeBlanc PH, Caron JP, Patterson JS, *et al.* Epidural injection of xylazine for perineal analgesia in horses. *J Am Vet Med Assoc* 1988; **193**: 1405–1408.

133 Skarda RT, Muir WW. Analgesic, hemodynamic and respiratory effects of caudally epidurally administered xylazine hydrochloride solution in mares. *Am J Vet Res* 1996; **57**: 193–200.

134 Teixeria Neto FJ, McDonell W, Pearce S, *et al.* Evaluation of anesthesia maintained with halothane and epidural xylazine for hind limb surgery in horses. *Vet Anaesth Analg* 2001; **28**: 107.

135 Skarda RT, Muir WW. Comparison of antinociceptive, cardiovascular, and respiratory effects, head ptosis, and position of pelvic limbs in mares after caudal epidural administration of xylazine and detomidine hydrochloride solution. *Am J Vet Res* 1996; **57**: 1338–1345.

136 Skarda RT, Muir WW. Caudal analgesia induced by epidural or subarachnoid administration of detomidine hydrochloride solution in mares. *Am J Vet Res* 1994; **55**: 670–680.

137 Sampaio BFB, DeRossi R, Vieira N, *et al.* Dexmedetomidine and bupivacaine association in caudal epidural injection in mares. *J Equine Vet Sci* 2020; **91**: 103015.

138 Hamed MA, Abouelnasr KS, Ibrahim HMM, *et al.* Comparative, sedative, and analgesic effects of epidural dexmedetomidine and xylazine in donkeys (*Equus asinus*). *J Equine Vet Sci* 2017; **59**:104–109.

139 Kariman A, Ghamsari SM, Mokhber-Dezfooli MR. Evaluation of analgesia induced by epidural administration of medetomdine in horses. *J Fac Vet Med Tehran Univ* 2001; **56**: 49–51.

140 Kariman A. Cardiorespiratory and analgesic effects of epidurally administered romifidine in the horse. *In: Proceedings of the Seventh World Congress on Veterinary Anaesthesiology, University of Bern, Bern, Switzerland*, 2000: 55.

141 Valverde A, Little CB, Dyson DH, Motter CH. Use of epidural morphine to relieve pain in a horse. *Can Vet J* 1990; **31**: 211–212.

142 Natalini CC, Robinson EP. Evaluation of the effects of epidurally administered morphine, alfentanil, butorphanol, tramadol and U50488H in horses. *Am J Vet Res* 2000; **61**: 1579–1586.

143 Freitas GC, Carregaro AB, Gehrcke MI, *et al.* Epidural analgesia with morphine or buprenorphine in ponies with lipopolysaccharide (LPS)-induced carpal synovitis. *Can J Vet Res* 2011; **75**: 141–146.

144 van Loon JPAM, Menke ES, L'Ami J, *et al.* Analgesic and anti-hyperalgesic effects of epidural morphine in an equine LPS-induced acute synovitis model. *Vet J* 2012; **193**: 464–470.

145 Van Hoogmoed LM, Galuppo LD. Laparoscopic ovariectomy using the endo-GIA stapling device and endo-catch pouches and evaluation of analgesic efficacy of epidural morphine sulfate in 10 mares. *Vet Surg* 2005; **34**: 646–650.

146 Sano H, Martin-Flores M, Santos LCP, *et al.* Effects of epidural morphine on gastrointestinal transit in unmedicated horses. *Vet Anaesth Analg* 2011; **38**: 121–126.

147 Olbrich VH, Mosing M. A comparison of the analgesic effects of caudal epidural methadone and lidocaine in the horse. *Vet Anaesth Analg* 2003; **30**: 156–164.

148 van Loon JPAM, van Oostrom H, Doornenbal A, *et al.* Lumbosacral spinal cord somatosensory evoked potentials for quantification of nociception in horses. *Equine Vet J* 2010; **42**: 255–260.

149 Chopin JB, Wright JD. Complication after the use of a combination of lignocaine and xylazine for epidural anesthesia in a mare. *Aust Vet J* 1995; **72**: 354–355.

150 Vullo C, Tambella AM, Meligrana M, *et al.* Analgesic and sedative effects of epidural lidocaine–xylazine in elective bilateral laparoscopic ovariectomy in standing mule mares. *Animals (Basel)* 2021; **11**(8): 2419.

151 Torad FA, Hassan EA. Epidural lidocaine, nalbuphine, and lidocaine–nalbuphine combination in donkeys. *J Equine Vet Sci* 2016; **37**: 1–5.

152 Sysel AM, Pleasant RS, Jacobson JD, *et al.* Efficacy of an epidural combination of morphine and detomidine in alleviating experimentally induced hindlimb lameness in horses. *Vet Surg* 1996; **25**: 511–518.

153 Goodrich LR, Nixon AJ, Fubini SL, *et al.* Epidural morphine and detomidine decreases postoperative hindlimb lameness in horses after bilateral stifle arthroscopy. *Vet Surg* 2002; **31**: 232–239.

154 Fischer BL, Ludders JW, Asakawa M, *et al.* A comparison of epidural buprenorphine plus detomidine with morphine plus detomidine in horses undergoing bilateral stifle arthroscopy. *Vet Anesth Analg* 2009; **36**: 67–76.

155 Natalini CC, Paes SD, Polydoro AS. Analgesic and cardiopulmonary effects of epidural romifidine and morphine combination in horses. *J Equine Vet Sci* 2021; **102**: 103459.

156 DeRossi R, Modolo TJC, Maciel FB, *et al.* Efficacy of epidural lidocaine combined with tramadol or neostigmine on perineal analgesia in the horse. *Equine Vet J* 2013; **45**: 497–502.

157 DeRossi R, Maciel FB, Modolo TJC, *et al.* Efficacy of concurrent epidural administration of neostigmine and lidocaine for perineal analgesia in geldings. *Am J Vet Res* 2012; **73**: 1356–1362.

158 Kariman A, Nowrouzian I, Bakhtiari J. Caudal epidural injection of a combination of ketamine and xylazine for perineal analgesia in horses. *Vet Anaesth Analg* 2000; **27**: 115.

159 DeRossi R, Modolo TJC, Pagliosa RC, *et al.* Comparison of analgesic effects of caudal epidural 0.25% bupivacaine with bupivacaine plus morphine or bupivacaine plus ketamine for analgesia in conscious horses. *J Equine Vet Sci* 2012; **32**: 190–195.

160 Carrozzo MV, Ambros B. Collapse in a mare during standing sedation with a fatal outcome. *Vet Rec Case Rep* 2020; **8**(1): e000829.

161 Haitjema H, Gibson KT. Severe pruritis associated with epidural morphine and detomidine in a horse. *Aust Vet J* 2001; **79**: 248–250.

162 Kalchofner KS, Kummer M, Price J, Bettschart-Wolfensberger R. Pruritis in two horses following epidurally administered morphine. *Equine Vet Educ* 2001; **19**: 590–594.

163 Burford JH, Corley KT. Morphine-associated pruritis after single extradural administration in a horse. *Vet Anaesth Analg* 2001; **33**: 193–198.

164 Tallon R, McMillan M, Dunkel B. Presumed generalised seizure following caudal epidural administration of morphine and detomidine in a pony. *Equine Vet Educ* 2021; **33**(10): e372–e375.

165 Küls N, Trujanovic R, Otero P, *et al.* Ultrasound-guided transversus abdominis plane block in Shetland ponies: a description of a three-point injection technique and evaluation of potential analgesic effects. *J Equine Vet Sci* 2020; **90**: 102994.

166 Gingold BMC, Hassen KM, Milloway MC, *et al.* Caudal intercostal block for abdominal surgery in horses. *Vet Rec* 2018; **183**: 164–165.

167 Driessen B, Scandella M, Zarucco L. Development of a technique for continuous perineural blockade of the palmar nerves in the distal equine thoracic limb. *Vet Anaesth Analg* 2008; **35**: 432–448.

168 Watts AE, Nixon AJ, Reesink HL, *et al.* Continuous peripheral neural blockade to alleviate signs of experimentally induced severe forelimb pain in horses. *J Am Vet Med Assoc* 2011; **238**: 1032–1039.

64 Ruminants

Chiara E. Hampton[1] and Thomas W. Riebold[2]

[1] Large Animal Clinical Sciences, College of Veterinary Medicine, University of Tennessee, Knoxville, Tennessee, USA
[2] Department of Clinical Sciences, College of Veterinary Medicine, Oregon State University, Corvallis, Oregon, USA

Chapter contents

Introduction, 1262
Preanesthetic preparation, 1262
Sedation/chemical restraint, 1264
  Anticholinergics, 1264
  Acepromazine and azaperone, 1264
  α_2-Adrenergic receptor agonists, 1265
  α_2-Adrenergic receptor antagonists, 1266
  Doxapram, 1267
  Benzodiazepines, 1267
  Opioids, 1267
  Alfaxalone, 1267
  Other sedatives, 1267
  Common combinations for chemical restraint, 1267
Induction, 1268
  Barbiturates/thiobarbiturates, 1268
  Ketamine, 1268
  Guaifenesin, 1269
  Tiletamine–zolazepam, 1269
  Propofol, 1270
  Alfaxalone, 1270
Intubation, 1270
Maintenance, 1271
  Injectable, 1271
  Inhalation, 1272
Intraoperative analgesia, 1273
Supportive therapy, 1273
  Patient positioning, 1273
  Fluid administration, 1273
  Respiratory supportive therapy, 1274
  Cardiovascular supportive therapy, 1275
Monitoring, 1275
Recovery, 1278
Intraoperative complications, 1278
Postoperative complications, 1278
Analgesia, 1279
References, 1279

Introduction

As in other species, sedation and anesthesia are often required for surgical or diagnostic procedures in ruminants. Most procedures in ruminants can be done during standing sedation with the aid of physical restraint tools and locoregional anesthesia to avoid potential complications from general anesthesia. The decision to induce general anesthesia may be influenced by a ruminant's temperament, its specific anatomic and physiologic characteristics, and the type of procedure to be performed. Diagnostic and surgical procedures that are more complex require general anesthesia.

In addition to discussing techniques for cattle, goats, and sheep, anesthetic techniques for South American camelids, primarily llamas and alpacas, are discussed. South American camelids do not accept restraint as well as domestic ruminants and often require sedation before local or regional anesthesia. Although they have some unique species characteristics regarding anesthesia, many of the principles and techniques used in food animal and equine anesthesia also apply to South American camelids. Except for differences in size and the fact that alpacas can require approximately 10% greater doses of sedatives, anesthetic management of alpacas and llamas is similar.

Preanesthetic preparation

Considerations for preanesthetic preparation include preanesthetic physical examination, estimation of body weight, assessment of hematologic and blood chemistry values, fasting, venous catheterization, and the need for patient stabilization. During preanesthetic physical examination, subjects should be visually examined first and then restrained properly for the "hands-on" portion of the physical examination to ensure the safety of personnel. Occasionally, depending on the patient's temperament and demeanor, a complete physical examination is not possible. The components of the preanesthetic physical examination are similar to those of other domestic species. The chest should be auscultated for evaluation of heart rate and rhythm, as well as for respiratory rate and the character of

Veterinary Anesthesia and Analgesia: The Sixth Edition of Lumb and Jones. Edited by Leigh Lamont, Kurt Grimm, Sheilah Robertson, Lydia Love and Carrie Schroeder.
© 2024 John Wiley & Sons, Inc. Published 2024 by John Wiley & Sons, Inc.
Companion website: www.wiley.com/go/lamont/anesthesia

respiratory sounds. This is particularly important in camelids where a wide variety of congenital cardiac abnormalities have been reported [1], as well as in small ruminants, which often present with subclinical pulmonary disease of bacterial, viral, or fungal origin. Synchronicity of peripheral pulses can be evaluated via palpation of the femoral pulse in camelids, small ruminants, and calves. In large cattle, the coccygeal or facial arteries can be used for this purpose [2]. Conjunctival or buccal mucous membranes can be evaluated for color and moisture level. Capillary refill time should take approximately 2 s. The FAMACHA© scoring system can be used in goats and sheep to detect the presence and the severity of anemia [3]. The frequency of ruminal contractions is an important vital sign to evaluate as ruminal atony may be present in cases of lactic acidosis and endotoxemia. A summary of normal findings of species-specific scoring systems and vital signs is provided in Table 64.1.

For accurate drug administration, body weight must be estimated or determined by weighing the animal. It is easy to overestimate the body weight of camelids because they are fairly tall, and their long haircoat obscures their body condition. Adult male llamas usually weigh 140–175 kg, occasionally reaching or exceeding 200 kg. Adult female llamas usually weigh 100–150 kg but may occasionally exceed 200 kg. Adult male alpacas usually weigh 60–100 kg, and adult female alpacas usually weigh 50–80 kg. The body weight of crias and small ruminants may be determined on a bathroom scale.

Hematologic and blood chemistry values should be evaluated before anesthesia when possible, and the results should be compared with instrument-specific reference values [8–11]. The Heska Element POC blood gas and electrolyte analyzer shows good performance with camelid blood and can be useful in the clinical setting, although complete agreement with automated chemistry analyzers was not documented [12].

Domestic ruminants have a multicompartment stomach with a large rumen that does not empty completely. South American camelids have a stomach divided into three compartments [13]. Each species, therefore, is susceptible to complications associated with recumbency and anesthesia with arterial hypoxemia, tympany, regurgitation, and aspiration pneumonia due to accidental aspiration of ruminal contents being the most common. To reduce risks associated with these potential complications, older calves, sheep, goats, and camelids should be fasted for 12–18 h and deprived of water for 8–12 h prior to anesthesia. Juvenile calves should be fasted and water withheld for no longer than 6–12 h. Fasting of neonates is not advisable because the rumen remains underdeveloped and hypoglycemia may result. Adult cattle are commonly fasted for 18–24 h and deprived of water for 12–18 h prior to general anesthesia, but definitive evidence-based guidelines are currently lacking. Evidence in preslaughtered steers showed that decreasing the fasting time from 23–29 h to 2–6 h prevented hemoconcentration and dehydration associated with decreased water consumption during the fasting period and resulted in an overall improvement in animal welfare [14]. Furthermore, a 36-h fast resulted in subclinical acute ruminal acidosis [15]. Fasting and water deprivation may decrease the likelihood of tympany by decreasing the volume of fermentable ingesta compared to non-fasted cattle, reduce the incidence of hypoxemia [16], and preserve better pulmonary functional residual capacity [17]. However, regurgitation seems more common with prolonged fasting [16,18]. In cattle, fasting for 48 h is associated with bradycardia [19], which seems to persist for at least 48 h after resumption of food intake [20]. Due to the hormonal and metabolic changes associated with mobilization of energy substrates after prolonged fasting (> 24 h) in cattle [21], and the adverse events observed with 48-h fasting, further studies to elucidate optimal fasting times in ruminants are warranted and needed. Until evidence-based practices are built, practitioners are advised to observe fasting times that take into consideration and balance the advantages and disadvantages of short and prolonged fasting times. Although gas does not appear to accumulate in the first compartment of anesthetized camelids, these precautions may decrease the incidence of regurgitation in these species. In non-elective cases, fasting for the suggested times is often not possible, and precautions should be taken to avoid aspiration of gastric fluid and ingesta. Even with these precautions, some ruminants will become tympanitic, and others will regurgitate.

Venipuncture and catheterization of the jugular vein are often performed prior to anesthesia. Adult cattle require 12–14 gauge catheters for catheterization of the jugular vein. If difficulties in accessing the jugular vein are present, an auricular catheter (16–20 gauge) can be placed for administration of sedatives or induction agents in cattle restrained in a chute. Similar sized catheters are appropriate for adult camelids, calves, and large goats and sheep, and 18 gauge catheters are appropriate for juvenile camelids, sheep, and goats. South American camelids possess anatomical features that make jugular catheterization technically challenging. A detailed description of the venipuncture and catheterization techniques is provided elsewhere [22–24]. Physical restraint during venipuncture or catheterization varies and can consist of a handler holding the animal's halter or use of head gates and chutes for adult cattle and llamas. If a camelid is fractious, performing ear twitching by squeezing the base of the ear may be helpful [25]. Turning the animal's head excessively to either side may hinder venipuncture and catheter placement in goats and camelids, and may increase the likelihood of carotid arterial puncture in camelids. Infiltration of a small amount of local anesthetic such as lidocaine at the site of catheterization is recommended.

Camelids lack a jugular groove, and their jugular vein lies deep to the sternomandibularis and brachiocephalicus muscles, ventral to cervical vertebral transverse processes and superficial to the carotid artery and vagosympathetic trunk within the carotid sheath for most of its length [22–24]. Beginning at a point about 15 cm caudal

Table 64.1 Summary of normal physical examination findings in domestic ruminants and camelids.

	Alpaca/Llama	Goat	Sheep	Cattle
Body condition score	5 (range 1–9)[a]	2.5–4 (range 0–5)[c]	3 (range 0–5)[d]	3 (range 1–5)[e]
Heart rate (beats/min)	60–90[a]	70–90[b]	70–90[b]	60–80[b]
Respiratory rate (breaths/min)	10–30[a]	25–35[b]	10–20[b]	10–30[b]
Rectal temperature (°F)	99.5–102[a]	103.0[b]	102.0[b]	101.5[b]
Ruminal contractions (*F*/min)	3–5[a]	1[b]	1[b]	1[b]

Data compiled from: [a] Kaplan *et al.* [4]; [b] Constable *et al.* [2]; [c] Ghosh *et al.* [5]; [d] Phythian *et al.* [6]; [e] Wildman *et al.* [7].

to the ramus of the mandible, the rostral course of the jugular vein is separated from the carotid artery by the omohyoideus muscle. The bifurcation of the jugular vein is located at the intersection of a line drawn caudally along the ventral aspect of the body of the mandible and another line connecting the base of the ear and the lateral aspect of the cervical transverse processes. Venipuncture or catheterization can be performed at the bifurcation or at any point caudal to it. Because of the close proximity of the carotid artery to the jugular vein, one must confirm that the vein has been catheterized and not the artery. After occlusion of the vessel, one will often be unable to see the jugular vein distend; however, the vein can be palpated particularly rostrally and more easily in females and castrated males because their skin is thinner. On occasion, one will be able to see the jugular vein distend on crias and juvenile camelids. Camelids can have four to five jugular venous valves that prevent flow of venous blood into the head when the head is lowered during grazing [23]. Contact with jugular venous valves may prevent catheterization; a site caudal to the point where the valve was contacted should be used. Finally, repeated unsuccessful attempts to place a jugular venous catheter have been associated with collapse and death. If a camelid begins to mouth-breathe during catheterization, it is highly recommended to discontinue the procedure and allow the animal time to recover from the stress before proceeding.

Stabilization of the patient should be performed prior to the anesthetic episode according to the animal's health status. The extent of enophthalmos (recession of the globe), along with capillary refill time, mucous membrane color, packed cell volume, and plasma total solids can be used to estimate the patient's fluid deficit [26]. Anecdotally, a reduction in the volume of the hump can be seen during dehydration in Brahman cattle, which regains volume with replacement of fluid deficits. Calculations for fluid replacement should include the existing deficit, metabolic water consumption, and ongoing losses. Attempts should be made to replace this volume, as well as fluids lost during the anesthetic episode through salivation and regurgitation. Anemia is not uncommon in small ruminants and South American camelids and should be addressed and treated as appropriate before surgical intervention.

Sedation/chemical restraint

Ruminants do not necessarily require sedation prior to induction of anesthesia as other species do, mostly due to their temperament. While atraumatic physical restraint may be used in lieu of sedatives in some circumstances, sedation may be indicated in certain animals (primarily fractious adult cattle) to facilitate safe handling during the induction period. Sedation has been shown to decrease stress and increase the quality of collected semen of goats during electroejaculation [27]. This, along with the associated anesthetic-sparing effects documented in several species, makes sedative administration beneficial, even in tractable animals. Because ruminants seldom experience emergence delirium, sedation during the recovery period is rarely required, in contrast to horses where this is common practice. In addition to the reduction in anesthetic requirements, preanesthetic sedation in ruminants may tend to lengthen the recovery period from general anesthesia [28] and increase the likelihood of regurgitation [29].

Drugs used to tranquilize and/or sedate ruminants include phenothiazines and butyrophenones, α_2-adrenergic receptor agonists (xylazine, detomidine, romifidine, medetomidine, and dexmedetomidine), dissociative agents (ketamine and tiletamine), pentobarbital, chloral hydrate, benzodiazepines (diazepam, midazolam, and zolazepam), and opioids (butorphanol, nalbuphine, hydromorphone, and morphine). Most of these drugs, when given alone or in combination at doses sufficient to induce recumbency, have been shown to cause arterial hypoxemia. Therefore, oxygen supplementation is highly recommended throughout the sedation/immobilization period if this practice is tolerated by the animal.

Anticholinergics

Anticholinergics are usually not administered to domestic ruminants as premedication agents. Their antisialagogue properties are inconsistent in these species unless used in very high doses and frequently repeated. Anticholinergics, while decreasing the volume of secretions, may make them more viscous and more difficult to clear from the trachea. In the authors' experience, camelids are prone to increased vagal discharge during intubation or with painful stimuli during surgery. Consequently, administration of atropine (0.02 mg/kg IV or 0.04 mg/kg IM) is recommended to prevent bradyarrhythmia in these species [30]. Alternatively, glycopyrrolate (0.005–0.01 mg/kg IM or 0.002–0.005 mg/kg IV) may be substituted for atropine [31,32].

Acepromazine and azaperone

Acepromazine is a phenothiazine devoid of analgesic properties. It is not commonly used in ruminants but can be used in a manner similar to its use in horses, although lower doses are required for cattle (0.01–0.03 mg/kg IM) compared to horses. The usual doses of acepromazine in sheep and goats are 0.03–0.05 mg/kg IV and 0.05–0.1 mg/kg IM, which may increase the risk of regurgitation during anesthesia [29]. Tranquilizing effects may last for up to 8 h, although usually do not exceed 4 h. The combination of acepromazine (0.05 mg/kg IV) with methadone (0.5 mg/kg IV), morphine (0.5 mg/kg IV), or tramadol (5 mg/kg IV) failed to improve the level of sedation observed with acepromazine alone in sheep [33]. In llamas, acepromazine (0.05 mg/kg IM) with or without butorphanol (0.1 mg/kg IM) did not produce sedative effects, but prolonged antinociception produced by tiletamine–zolazepam [34]. Acepromazine should not be injected into the coccygeal vein. The close proximity of the coccygeal artery makes the risk of inadvertent intra-arterial injection possible, with the potential loss of the tail [personal communication: John C. Thurmon, 1970]. Acepromazine can also cause priapism and is not recommended for sedation in mature bulls with reproductive value. Prolapse of the penis during recovery increases the risk of injury to that organ as the animal stands. Acepromazine (0.035 mg/kg IV) is preferred over xylazine for endoscopic evaluation of the upper airways and laryngeal function in cattle if the procedure cannot be carried out without sedation [35]. Uterine blood flow and oxygen delivery to the fetus is preserved by acepromazine in cows during late gestation, in contrast to xylazine, which may critically impair delivery of oxygen to the fetus [36]. Finally, acepromazine is best avoided in newborn or neonatal patients, as well as in systemically ill and/or hypovolemic patients due to its hypotensive effects and depression of thermoregulation [37].

Azaperone is a butyrophenone that has been successfully used in combination with opioids (e.g., butorphanol and etorphine) and an α_2-adrenergic receptor agonist (e.g., xylazine and medetomidine) to sedate and immobilize several captive and wild ruminant species [28,38,39]. Its best use is in neuroleptoanalgesic combinations administered via the IM route.

α_2-Adrenergic receptor agonists

Xylazine, detomidine, romifidine, medetomidine, and dexmedetomidine cause sedation by stimulating central α_2-adrenergic receptors. The degree of sedation or chemical restraint produced by α_2-adrenergic receptor agonists depends on the dose administered and the animal's temperament and species. These drugs act synergistically with opioids in producing sedation and analgesia. In cattle, the α_{2D}-adrenergic receptor subunit was considered predominant, which would partly explain the increased sensitivity of cattle to the sedative effects of these agents [40]. However, contrasting evidence found no difference in $\alpha_{2A/D}$-adrenergic receptor subunit expression in bovine brain compared to pigs and rats [41]. Instead, this study found that the slope of the inhibition binding curve when G-protein coupling was diminished was considerably lower in cattle for xylazine compared to detomidine, and this difference was not identified in swine or rats [41]. This species difference at the G-protein level or further downstream in the receptor cascade may explain the higher sensitivity of cattle to xylazine compared to detomidine. In goats, activation of the α_{2D}-adrenergic receptor subunit produces better analgesia compared to the α_{2B}- and α_{2C}-adrenergic receptor subunits, whereas the α_{2C}-adrenergic receptor subunit seems to be involved in thermoregulation [42].

Xylazine

Xylazine is often used to sedate or, in higher doses, restrain ruminants by producing recumbency and light planes of general anesthesia. As previously mentioned, there appears to be significant interspecies and intraspecies variation in the biological response to this drug. Overall, xylazine is much more potent in ruminants than it is in horses [43]. Among ruminants, goats appear to be more sensitive to xylazine than sheep [29,32,44], and cattle appear to be intermediate in sensitivity when compared to sheep and goats. South American camelids appear to be less sensitive than cattle but more sensitive than horses to the effects of xylazine; and among camelids, alpacas appear to be less sensitive to xylazine than are llamas. Hereford cattle are anecdotally reported to be more sensitive to xylazine than are Holstein cattle [45], and Brahmans are perhaps the most sensitive of all cattle breeds [46]. Extreme environmental conditions can cause cattle to have a pronounced and prolonged response to xylazine [47].

Low doses of xylazine (0.015–0.025 mg/kg IV or IM) typically provide sedation without recumbency in domestic ruminants [31,32,48]. Higher doses (0.1–0.2 mg/kg IV) provide sedation without recumbency in camelids [49]. Higher doses of xylazine will induce restraint with recumbency, heavy sedation, or possibly light planes of general anesthesia in domestic ruminants and camelids. Xylazine in goats (0.05 mg/kg IV or 0.1 mg/kg IM) [29,32,44], in sheep (0.1–0.2 mg/kg IV or 0.2–0.3 mg/kg IM) [29,32,44], and in cattle (0.1 mg/kg IV or 0.2 mg/kg IM) [46] will induce recumbency for approximately 1 h. Xylazine at 0.3–0.4 mg/kg IV usually induces 20–30 min of recumbency in llamas [23,24,30,50]. Alpacas have been reported to be less sensitive to xylazine compared to llamas and may require an approximately 10–20% increase in dose to achieve the same result [51]. In cattle undergoing claw treatments, xylazine (0.05 mg/kg IV) used alone has been shown to decrease hormonal and metabolic stress responses and potentiate the effects of local anesthetics, but worsened ventilation and oxygenation in laterally recumbent cows [52,53]. In 8-day old calves, administration of xylazine (0.3 mg/kg IV) produced a similar degree of sedation compared to medetomidine (30 μg/kg IV), with a shorter duration of action. Cardiopulmonary effects included decreases in heart rate, cardiac index, and arterial oxygen tension (PaO_2) when compared to baseline, and increases in central venous pressure, arterial carbon dioxide tension ($PaCO_2$), and pulmonary arterial pressures. Interestingly, arterial blood pressures and vascular resistance increased with medetomidine but were decreased by xylazine [54]. The subcutaneous route is a viable and efficacious alternative to intramuscular administration of xylazine to neonatal Holstein calves, with similar onset and duration of action [55]. Variation in response to the analgesic effects of xylazine between breeds of sheep has been reported [56,57]. Mechanical and thermal thresholds for limb withdrawal are increased by administration of 0.05 mg/kg IV xylazine for a short amount of time (60 and 30 min, respectively) [58–60]. Xylazine causes hyperglycemia and hypoinsulinemia in cattle and sheep [61–66]. Ruminal tympany has been observed after administration of xylazine [67], likely induced by ruminal hypomotility [68]. Hypoxemia and hypercapnia are common side effects in domestic ruminants [29,45,69,70]. Dose-dependent arterial hypoxemia and pulmonary edema can be seen in sheep after administration of all α_2-adrenergic receptor agonists [71,72]. In this species, activation of α_2-adrenergic receptors results in pathophysiologic changes including increase airway pressure [73,74], vasoconstriction and redistribution of pulmonary blood flow, and activation of pulmonary intravascular macrophages, which release a range of vasoactive mediators and cytokines [75]. *In vitro* contraction of tracheal smooth muscle [76] and *in vivo* smooth muscle contraction [73,74,77] have also been demonstrated, leading to bronchoconstriction. Histopathology of the lung reveals capillary rupture with endothelial damage, alveolar hemorrhage with damage to type I alveolar cells, and interstitial and alveolar edema [77,78]. These pathophysiologic consequences can be completely prevented in sheep by the administration of atipamezole, tolazoline, and idazoxan administered within 5–10 min of xylazine, but not with administration of yohimbine [76,79–81]. Not surprisingly, though, administration of tolazoline and idaxozan was also reported to shorten the duration of xylazine-induced recumbency in this species [81]. Xylazine has an oxytocin-like effect on the uterus of pregnant cattle [82] and sheep [83] and should be used with caution during late gestation as it may cause premature parturition and retention of fetal membranes [84]. *In vitro* exposure of isolated bovine uterine stripes to lidocaine after xylazine decreased the tonic effect induced by xylazine on bovine pregnant uteri [85].

Poorly trained or agitated male camelids tend to be less responsive, and debilitated individuals are more responsive to sedative doses of xylazine. Although complete data are not available on the cardiovascular and respiratory effects of xylazine in camelids, bradycardia [69] typically occurs as it does in other species [45,86–88]. Xylazine (0.2 and 0.4 mg/kg IM) has been shown to increase the duration of antinociception in llamas anesthetized with tiletamine–zolazepam [89].

Detomidine

Detomidine, like other α_2-adrenergic receptor agonists other than xylazine, is used less frequently in domestic ruminants. As in all species, detomidine is more potent than xylazine, but this difference in potency is less pronounced in ruminants compared to other species. Compared to xylazine, cattle appear to be less sensitive (more tolerant) to the sedating effects of detomidine and doses closer to those used in horses may be appropriate. Interestingly, detomidine may not have the same effect on the gravid uterus as xylazine does in cattle [90]. Detomidine can be given at 2.5–10 μg/kg IV in cattle [32,48,90,91] and at 10–20 μg/kg in sheep [29] to provide standing sedation for approximately 30–60 min. A high dose of detomidine (30 μg/kg IV) will produce recumbency in sheep. This dose is equivalent to xylazine at 0.15 mg/kg IV, medetomidine at 10 μg/kg IV, or romifidine at 50 μg/kg IV [71]. Sublingual detomidine (80 μg/kg) has been shown to produce adequate sedation in dairy calves prior to infiltration of lidocaine for disbudding [92]. In llamas, detomidine at doses as high as 40 μg/kg IV provides mild sedation but not chemical restraint [49]. In alpacas, the pharmacokinetic and sedative effects of detomidine gel administered intravaginally (200 μg/kg) were compared to intravenous administration of the injectable solution (70 μg/kg) [93]. Although bioavailability of intravaginal detomidine was only 20%, the degree of sedation (characterized as mild) and the duration of sedation were similar with both routes of administration [93]. The hyperglycemic effect of detomidine is greater than that produced by xylazine and medetomidine in sheep [94].

Romifidine

Romifidine has been used at 40, 80, and 120 μg/kg IV in Old World camels. Profound sedation and bradycardia of 4 h duration occurred with the highest dose [95]. Initial doses of 50–60 μg/kg IV are appropriate for South American camelids.

Medetomidine and dexmedetomidine

As the stereoisomer of medetomidine, dexmedetomidine can be substituted for medetomidine at 50% of the medetomidine dose. Medetomidine given at 10 μg/kg IV induces recumbency in cattle [91]. Doses of 5 μg/kg IV in cattle [91] or 10 μg/kg IM in llamas [96] produce brief periods of standing sedation with minimal analgesia. When medetomidine is given at 30 μg/kg IV, it causes bradycardia, decreased PaO_2, recumbency of 4 h duration, and sedation of 7 h duration in calves [54]. In non-pregnant ewes, dexmedetomidine (5 μg/kg IV) and medetomidine (10 μg/kg IV) were equipotent when effects on isoflurane requirements and cardiopulmonary parameters were evaluated [72]. The addition of vatinoxan, a peripheral α_2-adrenergic receptor antagonist, to intramuscular medetomidine and ketamine for sedation in sheep ameliorated the negative cardiopulmonary effects produced by medetomidine and ketamine alone. The level of sedation produced and its subsequent reversal with atipamezole were not affected by concurrent administration of vatinoxan [97]. When given at 20–30 μg/kg IM to llamas, medetomidine provides profound sedation and recumbency lasting up to 120 min [96]. In alpacas anesthetized with IM tiletamine–zolazepam, the addition of dexmedetomidine dose-dependently increased the duration of lack of motor response to claw clamping to a maximum of 40 min with a 20 μg/kg dose [98]. Transient hypoxemia was observed but judged to be clinically unimportant by the authors, but oxygen supplementation was recommended. In calves, dexmedetomidine (5 μg/kg IV) had a rapid onset of action (2.7 min) and produced a degree of sedation similar to xylazine (0.2 mg/kg IV) with a similar recovery time (80 min) [99]. Higher doses of all α_2-adrenergic receptor agonists can be expected to induce longer periods of recumbency in all species.

α_2-Adrenergic receptor antagonists

Sedation following administration of α_2-adrenergic receptor agonists can be reversed by α_2-adrenergic receptor antagonists. These include atipamezole and yohimbine, which are specific to the α_2-adrenergic receptor, and tolazoline that has both α_2- and α_1-adrenergic receptor antagonist activity. The dose of antagonist is dependent on the amount of agonist given and the interval between agonist and antagonist administration. The longer the interval between administration of the agonist and antagonist, the lower the dose of antagonist that is needed, as more metabolism of the agonist should have occurred. Giving the full dose of antagonist after significant metabolism of the agonist has occurred increases the likelihood that excitement will result, particularly if the antagonist is given IV. One could also consider giving the antagonist IM to make reversal more gradual.

Yohimbine

When yohimbine is given at 0.12 mg/kg IV, its efficacy varies in cattle [100,101]. Low doses of yohimbine are ineffective in sheep [81], but higher doses (1 mg/kg IV) will generally reverse xylazine sedation [102]. Yohimbine (0.12 mg/kg IV) has been used in llamas in combination with 4-aminopyridine (0.3 mg/kg IV) to produce complete recovery from xylazine sedation [69]. Its use singly in camelids is also effective, and it can be administered at 0.12 mg/kg IV [49]. If sufficient arousal does not occur, additional yohimbine can be titrated to achieve the desired effect.

Tolazoline

Tolazoline is usually given at 0.5–2 mg/kg IV [100], but at the upper end of this dose range, it can cause hyperesthesia in unsedated cattle [103,104]. Following a 2 mg/kg IV dose, opisthotonus can occur in some animals; however, after excitement subsides, recovery is usually uneventful. A safety study on increasing doses of tolazoline (0.5, 1, 1.5, 2, 4, 8, and 10 mg/kg IV) was conducted in unsedated Holstein calves, with the highest dose producing "bright red conjunctival mucous membranes, coughing, nasal discharge, salivation, increased breathing effort, central nervous system depression, signs of abdominal pain, straining, head pressing, restlessness, increased frequency of defecation and diarrhea," but no fatalities were reported [105]. Tolazoline can induce unwanted cardiovascular effects in calves such as transient bradycardia, sinus arrest, and hypotension [106]. Lower doses of tolazoline (0.5–1.5 mg/kg IV) have been recommended in ruminants and camelids, whereas others have suggested that the IV route should be avoided except in emergency situations [84]. Regardless, if tolazoline is to be given intravenously, it should be administered slowly to effect.

Caution is advised when the recommended equine dose of tolazoline is administered to camelids, as severe complications including transitory apnea, cardiac arrest, seizure-like activity, depression, and vague signs of abdominal pain have been observed, followed by death within 24 h. In a case report, serious complications ensued after administering a total dose of 6.4 mg/kg of tolazoline to a llama resulting in tachycardia, cardiac arrhythmias, hypotension, and gastrointestinal tract hypermotility [107]. One method of administering tolazoline to healthy camelids is to slowly give 50% of the calculated 1–2 mg/kg IV dose initially, and the remainder if reversal is inadequate [49]. In most instances, the initial dose (0.5–1 mg/kg IV) of tolazoline is adequate to provide sufficient arousal.

Idazoxan

Idazoxan can be given at doses of 0.05 mg/kg IV to sheep [81] and calves to reverse xylazine sedation [108].

Atipamezole

Atipamezole at doses ranging from 20 to 60 μg/kg IV has been used to reverse medetomidine sedation in calves [32]. In sheep, atipamezole has been used at a total dose of 125 μg/kg, administered either entirely IV or 50% of the dose given IV and 50% given IM, to reverse sedation produced by 20–25 μg/kg of medetomidine [109,110]. In sheep administered intrathecal xylazine and detomidine, atipamezole reversed side effects but not analgesia based on the assessment of pain thresholds in response to an electrical stimulus [111]. Reduced feed consumption and ruminal contractions produced by medetomidine, romifidine, and detomidine in dwarf goats are completely antagonized by atipamezole [112]. Atipamezole given at 30 μg/kg IV will reverse xylazine sedation in camelids.

Vatinoxan

Vatinoxan (formerly known as "MK-467" and "L-659,066") is a peripheral α_2-adrenergic receptor antagonist which is devoid of central effects due to its inability to cross the blood–brain barrier. Currently, ruminant-specific literature about vatinoxan is limited to the ovine species. The restriction of vatinoxan binding to peripheral α_2-adrenergic receptors means that it is able to ameliorate the negative cardiovascular effects accompanying administration of α_2-adrenergic receptor agonists without impacting central sedative effects. Vatinoxan's peripheral selectivity has been confirmed in sheep, where cerebrospinal fluid and brain concentrations of the drug were minimal compared to those in plasma [113]. In sheep, administration of vatinoxan (0.75 mg/kg) prior to xylazine (0.5 mg/kg) improved PaO_2 and SpO_2 by preventing α_2-adrenergic receptor agonist-induced effects on the ovine lung [114]. Prevention of dexmedetomidine-induced bronchoconstriction, pulmonary edema, and arterial hypoxemia have been documented with vatinoxan (0.15 mg/kg IV) pretreatment in sheep anesthetized with sevoflurane [115]. Further investigation of the histopathologic changes seen with vatinoxan is needed as microscopic interstitial alveolar edema and hemorrhage were observed [114].

Doxapram

Doxapram, an analeptic agent, can be used to enhance the response to yohimbine or tolazoline. When administered at 1 mg/kg IV, doxapram was somewhat effective in cattle [116], but when administered at 2 mg/kg IV, it was ineffective in llamas [69]. For more information about doxapram, the reader is referred to Chapter 25.

Benzodiazepines

Diazepam, 0.25–0.5 mg/kg IV, injected slowly will provide 30 min of sedation without analgesia in sheep and goats [29,44]. This drug, at a dose of 0.2–0.5 mg/kg IV, has been shown to preserve normal rumen motility compared to xylazine, which reduced motility at 0.05 mg/kg, and caused complete atony at 0.125 mg/kg IV [117]. The pharmacokinetic profile of midazolam (0.5 mg/kg IM or IV) has been described in sheep [118] and alpacas [119]. Midazolam, 0.4–0.6 mg/kg IM [118,120,121] or 0.3–0.6 mg/kg IV [122,123], will provide sedation and recumbency in sheep and goats for 10–20 min with minor cardiorespiratory effects that are reversible with flumazenil (0.02 mg/kg IV). In alpacas, onset of sedation following 0.5 mg/kg midazolam is 0.4 min after IV administration and 15 min after IM administration [119]. Midazolam given at 1 mg/kg IM [120] or 0.6 mg/kg IV [122] can induce recumbency and profound sedation in goats. Increasing the dose to 1.2 mg/kg IV lengthens recumbency, lasting up to 30 min [121]. Midazolam given at 0.5 mg/kg IM to alpacas provides sedation without recumbency of approximately 100 min duration, whereas when given IV at the same dose, it provided sedation with recumbency for the same amount of time [124].

Opioids

Butorphanol acts as a κ-opioid receptor agonist and μ-opioid receptor antagonist and provides sedation and mild analgesia in camelids and domestic ruminants. It is often given at doses of 0.05–0.5 mg/kg IM in sheep and goats [29,125,126] and 0.1–0.2 mg/kg IM in camelids [127], and produces analgesia for up to 2 h [128]. Ataxia and dysphoria have been reported following butorphanol administration (0.1–0.2 mg/kg IV) in sheep [126]. In the authors' experience, camelids remain standing following butorphanol administration but may experience mild dysphoria. In isoflurane-anesthetized alpacas, butorphanol (0.1 mg/kg IV) induces minimal cardiovascular changes, mainly via decreased systemic vascular resistance [129]. The addition of morphine (0.5 mg/kg IV), methadone (0.5 mg/kg IV), or tramadol (5 mg/kg IV) to xylazine (0.1 mg/kg IV) has been shown to induce similar cardiopulmonary changes to those of xylazine alone, but the quality of sedation was improved for up to 30 min after administration [130]. Nalbuphine (0.5 mg/kg IV) in combination with ketamine (5 mg/kg IV) in goats premedicated with xylazine (0.07 mg/kg IV) may produce adequate analgesia for left flank laparotomy [131].

Alfaxalone

The use of an earlier preparation of alfaxalone (Saffan®, a combination of alfaxalone and alfadolone solubilized in saline and Cremophor EL®) was investigated in ruminants in the late 1970s and early 1980s before the product was discontinued [132]. In 2015, alfaxalone was released in the United States in a different formulation (2-hydroxypropyl-β-cyclodextrin), and over the last decade, it has been investigated in sheep, goats, and alpacas. Although the current cyclodextrin-based formulation of alfaxalone is labeled for intravenous use in dogs and cats, it has been used successfully as a sedative when administered intramuscularly in several species [133–135]. The sedative properties of intramuscular alfaxalone in ruminants and camelids are yet to be investigated. A new formulation (40 mg/mL) of alfaxalone is been currently investigated in wild ruminants for remote immobilization [136] and may have future applications in domestic ruminants.

Other sedatives

Pentobarbital (2 mg/kg IV) has been used in cattle for standing sedation and tranquilization [137]. Caution must be exercised to avoid inducing excitement. Pentobarbital provides moderate sedation for 30 min and mild sedation for an additional 60 min. Chloral hydrate or chloral hydrate-magnesium sulfate solutions can also be used to sedate ruminants [46]. Extravasation of these drugs will cause tissue necrosis, so they should be administered through a catheter confirmed to be placed within the vein.

Common combinations for chemical restraint

Combinations of xylazine and butorphanol have been used in domestic ruminants and camelids to produce neuroleptanalgesia. In domestic ruminants, doses are 0.01–0.02 mg/kg IV of each drug administered separately [personal communication: John C. Thurmon, 1993], and in camelids, 0.2 mg/kg IV of xylazine is administered with 0.02–0.04 mg/kg IV of butorphanol [personal communication: Michael J. Huber, 2013]. The duration of action is approximately 1 h. Combinations of midazolam (0.1 mg/kg IV) and butorphanol (0.1 mg/kg IV) given simultaneously provide restraint of short duration [138].

Combinations of butorphanol, ketamine, and xylazine have also been used to restrain camelids [138]. The combination is prepared by combining 10 mg (1 mL) of butorphanol, 1000 mg (10 mL) of ketamine, and 100 mg (1 mL) of xylazine. It is administered at 1 mL/18 kg IM to alpacas and at 1 mL/23 kg IM to llamas [138]. Recumbency occurs within 5 min and lasts approximately 25 min. Other combinations of xylazine, ketamine, and butorphanol ("Ketamine Stun") have also been used in ruminants [48] and camelids [138]. Ruminant doses for the IV route of the Ketamine Stun are lower compared to IM, and onset of action for the IV route is shorter compared to the IM route. Typically, xylazine at 0.025–0.05 mg/kg, ketamine at 0.3–0.5 mg/kg, and butorphanol at 0.05–0.1 mg/kg are administered IV [48]. Animals will become recumbent for 15–25 min and administration of an additional partial dose of ketamine (50% of the original dose) will lengthen the duration of analgesia. If venous access is not feasible, the upper end of the doses cited above can also be administered IM or subcutaneously to achieve a longer but less intense form of chemical restraint. Alternatively, a combination of xylazine (0.05 mg/kg), butorphanol (0.025 mg/kg), and ketamine (0.1 mg/kg) can also be given IM to render ruminant patients more cooperative [48]. Onset occurs within 10 min, and duration of action is approximately 45 min with an additional 30 min needed to resume standing. In calves, 0.1 mg/kg of ketamine and 0.05 mg/kg of xylazine administered IV have been shown to be efficacious and safe when administered to aid with surgical castration [139]. Given IV, the combination of xylazine at 0.22–0.33 mg/kg, ketamine at 0.22–0.33 mg/kg, and butorphanol at 0.08–0.11 mg/kg induces more predictable restraint in camelids [138]. Animals will become recumbent and analgesia lasts for 15–20 min. Administration of an additional partial dose of ketamine will lengthen the duration of analgesia. When given IM to camelids, the dose range is increased to xylazine at 0.22–0.55 mg/kg, ketamine at 0.22–0.55 mg/kg, and butorphanol at 0.08–0.11 mg/kg [138]. Onset occurs within 10 min and duration of action is extended to approximately 45 min.

Induction

General anesthesia can be induced by either injectable or inhalation techniques. Widely available drugs include ketamine, guaifenesin, tiletamine–zolazepam, propofol, alfaxalone, pentobarbital, isoflurane, and sevoflurane. If available, the thiobarbiturates and halothane could also be used. In small ruminants weighing less than 50–100 kg, anesthesia can be induced using isoflurane or sevoflurane delivered by face mask, or with an injectable technique. If desired, calves and sheep can be intubated nasally while awake or following sedation using a technique similar to that used in foals and then connected to the anesthesia circuit for induction [140]. In larger ruminants, anesthesia is commonly induced using an IV technique but, if the animal's temperament dictates it, the IM route is also possible. In small or debilitated camelids, or in camelids restrained with xylazine–ketamine, tiletamine–zolazepam, or other injectable combinations, anesthesia can be induced with isoflurane or sevoflurane by face mask. Mask induction in healthy untranquilized adult camelids is usually not attempted because application of the mask may provoke spitting. The addition of nitrous oxide (50% of total flow) to the inspired gas mixture will speed induction; however, administration of nitrous oxide to ruminants and camelids beyond induction may cause distension of gas-containing organs, resulting in tympany.

Barbiturates/thiobarbiturates

When available, the thiobarbiturates thiopental and thiamylal were used extensively in veterinary anesthesia, both alone and in combination with guaifenesin. Used alone, they quickly induce anesthesia. Muscle relaxation is relatively poor but still sufficient to accomplish intubation. The acid–base status and physical status of patients affect the actions of these drugs. Acidemia increases the non-ionized fraction (i.e., the active portion) of the drug, increasing its activity and thus decreasing the dose required [141]. Because patients in shock are often acidemic, altered pharmacokinetics and hemodynamics may cause a relative overdose. In addition, the heart, brain, and other vital organs receive a larger portion of cardiac output when patients are in shock [142].

Recovery from induction doses of thiobarbiturates is based on redistribution of the drug from the brain to other tissues in the body. Metabolism of the agent continues for some time following recovery until final elimination occurs. Maintenance of anesthesia with thiobarbiturates is not recommended because saturation of tissue depots causes recovery to become dependent on metabolism resulting in prolongation. Concurrent use of non-steroidal anti-inflammatory drugs (NSAIDs) may delay recovery as thiobarbiturate is displaced from protein [143]. Drug interactions appear to be minimal in most instances.

Thiopental can be given at 6–10 mg/kg IV to unsedated animals and will provide approximately 10–15 min of anesthesia. Camelids often require additional thiopental for tracheal intubation [30]. Thiamylal is administered in a similar fashion although in slightly lower doses, usually 25–30% less.

Pentobarbital has been used to anesthetize domestic ruminants but is no longer commonly used. If a situation arises in which it is used, the dose is 20–25 mg/kg IV, half given rapidly and the remainder to effect. When given at an anesthetic dose, pentobarbital causes profound respiratory depression and is not an effective analgesic. Sheep appear to metabolize pentobarbital more quickly than other species [29]. Recovery in domestic ruminants is usually prolonged, and other anesthetic techniques are more appropriate.

Ketamine

Ketamine is a very versatile drug that has been used in many species. It is an *N*-methyl-D-aspartate (NMDA) receptor antagonist and acts by disrupting the signal pathway between the thalamus and the cortex, causing a dissociated state. It causes cardiovascular stimulation due to sympathetic discharge and can cause dysphoria, hallucinations, and excitement, in addition to tonic-clonic muscle activity when used alone in horses. Those same traits characterize its use in ruminants, although perhaps not to the same extent. Ketamine in single and repeated IV doses has been shown to increase plasma cortisol in calves premedicated with xylazine [144]. Although ketamine, when used as a sole agent, does not eliminate the swallowing reflex, tracheal intubation can be accomplished in most ruminants. However, co-administration of a sedative (e.g., benzodiazepines, α_2-adrenergic receptor agonists, and/or guaifenesin) to improve muscle relaxation is recommended, but may abolish the swallowing reflex.

Ketamine will induce immobilization and incomplete analgesia when given alone, but it is usually combined with a sedative or tranquilizer. Most commonly, xylazine or a benzodiazepine is recommended. Xylazine at 0.1–0.2 mg/kg IM can be given first, followed by ketamine at 10–15 mg/kg IM in small domestic ruminants [29,44,145]. In goats, it is preferable to use the lower dose of xylazine followed by ketamine [29,44]. Anesthesia usually lasts about 45 min and can be prolonged by injection of 3–5 mg/kg IM or 1–2 mg/kg IV of ketamine. The longer duration of action of xylazine obviates the need for its readministration in most cases.

Alternatively, xylazine at 0.03–0.05 mg/kg IV followed by ketamine at 3–5 mg/kg IV, or xylazine at 0.1 mg/kg IM in goats or 0.2 mg/kg IM in sheep, followed by ketamine at 3–5 mg/kg IV, can provide anesthesia lasting 15–20 min [29]. Adult cattle can by anesthetized with xylazine at 0.1–0.2 mg/kg IV followed by ketamine at 2 mg/kg IV [146]. The lower dose of xylazine is used when cattle weigh more than 600 kg [146]. Anesthesia lasts approximately 30 min but can be prolonged for 15 min with additional ketamine at 0.75–1.25 mg/kg IV [146]. When evaluated in sheep, xylazine at 0.1 mg/kg IV and ketamine at 7.5 mg/kg IV provided anesthesia lasting 25 min and caused a decrease in cardiac output, mean arterial pressure, and peripheral vascular resistance [147]. Medetomidine has been combined with ketamine to induce anesthesia in calves. Because medetomidine (20 μg/kg IV) is much more potent than xylazine, lower doses of ketamine (0.5 mg/kg IV) can be used [148]. However, a local anesthetic at the surgical site may be required when ketamine is used at this dose [148]. Anesthesia can be reversed completely with α_2-adrenergic receptor antagonists without excitement occurring during recovery. Using lidocaine (2 mg/kg IV) in conjunction with ketamine (2.5 mg/kg IV) in calves premedicated with xylazine and butorphanol increases sedation but fails to decrease ketamine requirements for endotracheal intubation [149].

Diazepam (0.1 mg/kg IV) or midazolam (0.1 mg/kg IV) immediately followed by ketamine (4.5 mg/kg IV) can be used in domestic ruminants. Muscle relaxation is usually adequate for tracheal intubation, although the swallowing reflex may not be completely obtunded. Anesthesia usually lasts 10–15 min following benzodiazepine–ketamine administration, with recumbency of up to 30 min. Higher doses of diazepam (0.25–0.5 mg/kg IV) with ketamine (4–7.5 mg/kg IV) have also been used in sheep and provide the same duration of anesthesia [29,44,147]. Investigations into the cardiopulmonary effects of diazepam (0.375 mg/kg IV) and ketamine (7.5 mg/kg IV) in sheep have shown a decrease in cardiac output and an increase in peripheral vascular resistance without affecting arterial pressure [147]. Midazolam can be substituted for diazepam in goats and given at 0.4 mg/kg IM followed by ketamine at 4 mg/kg IV after recumbency occurs (approximately 15 min). Anesthesia lasts approximately 15 min [120].

Xylazine (0.25–0.35 mg/kg IM) and ketamine (6–10 mg/kg IM) administered 15 min later usually provides 30–60 min of recumbency in camelids [23,30]. One disadvantage of this technique is that larger adult llamas require a relatively large injection volume. Simultaneous administration of xylazine (0.44 mg/kg IM) and ketamine (4 mg/kg IM) usually provides restraint for 15–20 min [50,150]. Higher doses of xylazine (0.8 mg/kg IM) and ketamine (8 mg/kg IM) given simultaneously usually induce sedation/anesthesia within 5 min that lasts 30 min [150]. Depth of anesthesia varies with the amount given and the camelid's temperament but is usually sufficient for minor procedures such as suturing lacerations, draining abscesses, or applying casts. When any of these combinations provides insufficient anesthetic depth, supplemental local anesthesia may be required in order to complete the procedure. Tracheal intubation may not be possible. However, these combinations heavily sedate and immobilize the animals, facilitating venipuncture and administration of additional anesthetic agent or application of a face mask to increase the depth of anesthesia when necessary. If desired, xylazine (0.25 mg/kg IV) and ketamine (3–5 mg/kg IV) may be administered 5 min apart to obtain a more uniform response and sufficient depth of anesthesia for tracheal intubation in camelids [23]. Diazepam (0.1–0.2 mg/kg IV) or midazolam (0.1–0.2 mg/kg IV) and ketamine (4.5 mg/kg IV), as used for domestic ruminants, produces recumbency that lasts approximately 20 min and should provide enough muscle relaxation for tracheal intubation in camelids.

Guaifenesin

Guaifenesin is a centrally acting skeletal muscle relaxant that exerts its effect at the internuncial neurons in the spinal cord and at polysynaptic nerve endings [151]. It can be used alone to induce recumbency in domestic ruminants and camelids but is not recommended because it imparts little, if any, analgesia [152]. The addition of ketamine, or historically a thiobarbiturate, to a guaifenesin solution improves induction quality and decreases the volume required for induction. Muscle relaxation is improved compared with induction with ketamine or thiobarbiturates given alone. Typically, 5% guaifenesin solutions are used as hemolysis can occur with 10% guaifenesin solutions in ruminants [153]. Commonly, these solutions are given rapidly to effect, either by gravity and a large gauge catheter or by pressurizing the bag or bottle, in either tranquilized or untranquilized patients. The volume of the calculated dose when using 5% guaifenesin solution is 2 mL/kg. The amount of ketamine added to guaifenesin varies but is commonly 1 g per 50 g of guaifenesin. The amount of thiobarbiturate added to guaifenesin varies but is commonly 2 g per 50 g of guaifenesin. For convenience, guaifenesin-based mixtures may be injected with large (60–140 mL) syringes rather than administered by infusion to camelids and small ruminants to allow greater control over administration. If desired, xylazine can also be added to ketamine–guaifenesin solutions for induction and maintenance of anesthesia in cattle [146,154,155] and sheep [156]. Final concentrations are guaifenesin 50 mg/mL, ketamine 1–2 mg/mL, and xylazine 0.1 mg/mL. This solution is infused at 0.5 to 1 mL/kg IV for induction. For more information about guaifenesin, the reader is referred to Chapter 25.

Tiletamine–zolazepam

Tiletamine–zolazepam is a combination of equal parts of tiletamine and zolazepam available for use as an anesthetic agent in cats and dogs. When used alone, tiletamine induces poor muscle relaxation and causes excitement during recovery. The addition of zolazepam to tiletamine modifies these effects. As with ketamine, the swallowing reflex remains but may be obtunded. Like ketamine, this combination provides slight cardiovascular stimulation, causing the heart rate to increase [157]. Elimination of tiletamine and zolazepam is not uniform, with variation occurring in each drug's clearance between species. Differential clearance of the two drugs can affect recovery quality [157].

In many respects, tiletamine–zolazepam can be considered to be similar to ketamine premixed with diazepam or midazolam. When used alone in horses, it provides unsatisfactory anesthesia [158]. Muscle relaxation is poor and recovery is characterized by excitement. However, when combined with a sedative such as xylazine, it can be used successfully in horses. Because of differences in temperament between horses and domestic ruminants and camelids, tiletamine–zolazepam can be used successfully with or without xylazine in these species. However, the addition of xylazine to tiletamine–zolazepam will lengthen the effect.

Tiletamine–zolazepam given at 4 mg/kg IV in untranquilized calves caused minimal cardiovascular effects and provided anesthesia that lasted 45–60 min [159]. Xylazine (0.1 mg/kg IM) followed immediately by tiletamine–zolazepam at 4 mg/kg IM produced onset of anesthesia within 3 min, and anesthesia that lasted approximately 1 h [160]. Calves were able to stand approximately 130 min after injection. Increasing xylazine to 0.2 mg/kg IM increased the duration of anesthesia and recumbency and the incidence of apnea, necessitating intubation and ventilatory support [160]. Xylazine can also be administered at 0.05 mg/kg IV followed by tiletamine–zolazepam at 1 mg/kg IV [146].

Tiletamine–zolazepam given at 12 mg/kg IV in sheep provides approximately 2.5 h of surgical anesthesia, with a total recumbency time of 3.2 h [161]. More recent investigations in sheep have shown that tiletamine–zolazepam, given at 12–24 mg/kg IV, causes cardiopulmonary depression with anesthesia of approximately 40 min [162]. The addition of xylazine (0.11 mg/kg IV) to tiletamine–zolazepam (13.2 mg/kg IV), improved muscle relaxation and prolonged the duration of anesthesia and analgesia by 2.5 times [163]. Rather than using these relatively large doses, it is more appropriate to decrease the initial dose of tiletamine–zolazepam to 2–4 mg/kg IV and administer additional drug as required to prolong anesthesia. Butorphanol at 0.5 mg/kg IV combined with tiletamine–zolazepam at 12 mg/kg IV given either simultaneously or 10 min apart induces 25–50 min of anesthesia in sheep, with mild cardiopulmonary depression [164]. Tiletamine–zolazepam at 4 mg/kg IM can immobilize llamas for up to 2 h [165]. The length of recumbency is unaffected by administration of flumazenil, indicating that the duration of action is more likely influenced by tiletamine rather than zolazepam [165]. Cardiovascular function is preserved although hypercapnia and hypoxemia can occur in some animals. Airway reflexes are maintained. Local anesthesia may be required for some surgical procedures [165]. Tiletamine–zolazepam at 2 mg/kg IM can immobilize llamas for approximately 1 h [34] and can be combined with acepromazine, butorphanol, or xylazine which will lengthen the duration of immobilization [34,89]. Furthermore, the combination of both xylazine (0.15 mg/kg IM) and morphine (0.5 mg/kg IM) administered with tiletamine–zolazepam to llamas has been shown to produce antinociception for longer than when it is combined with either xylazine or morphine alone [166]. In camelids, tiletamine–zolazepam (2 mg/kg IV) can provide 15–20 min of anesthesia and 25–35 min of recumbency. Depth of anesthesia is adequate for nasal intubation, but muscle relaxation is poor and oral intubation is difficult.

Propofol

Propofol is a non-barbiturate, non-steroidal hypnotic agent used to provide brief periods (5–10 min) of anesthesia. The dose is 4–6 mg/kg IV for induction in unsedated ruminants [29,167–169]. Induction is smooth, as is recovery. If injected too rapidly, apnea may occur but slow administration will reduce the incidence of this complication. Propofol can also be used at 4 mg/kg IV following acepromazine at 0.05 mg/kg IM and papaveretum at 0.4 mg/kg IM [170]. Anesthesia can be induced in unsedated camelids with 2 mg/kg IV [171]. However, tracheal intubation is often difficult or impossible at this dose and additional propofol is usually needed. Anesthesia can be maintained with propofol at 0.2–0.3 mg/kg/min IV and ketamine at 0.1–0.2 mg/kg/min [170]. Recovery to standing occurs within 15 min [170].

Alfaxalone

Alfaxalone given at 2 mg/kg IV to unsedated sheep provided brief periods of anesthesia with less effect on cardiopulmonary variables than thiopental and propofol [172]. Anesthesia has also been induced in unsedated sheep with medetomidine at 2 μg/kg IV administered simultaneously with alfaxalone at 2 mg/kg IV [173]. Muscle relaxation was sufficient to allow intubation and duration of recumbency was brief, lasting less than 10 min [173]. Alfaxalone has been evaluated as a sole anesthetic agent in unsedated alpacas [174]. It is given at 2 mg/kg IV and provides sufficient depth of anesthesia to allow intubation. Duration was brief, lasting 10–15 min. Recovery to standing was complete within 35 min and was characterized as poor [174]. Use of alfaxalone would be improved in camelids by sedating the patient before induction or by using it as an induction agent to be followed by inhalant anesthesia.

Intubation

Tracheal intubation is recommended in all ruminants and camelids because it provides a secure airway and prevents aspiration of salivary secretions and ruminal contents if active or passive regurgitation occurs. In lightly anesthetized ruminants, active regurgitation can occur during intubation [30,146], whereas passive regurgitation can occur at any time during anesthesia due to relaxation of the cardia. Because rumen contents contain more solid material than do the gastric contents of monogastric animals, there is greater potential for ingesta to obstruct the larynx while the more fluid portion will drain from the mouth. Thus, patients that are not intubated are at high risk throughout the anesthetic period, and intubated animals that have regurgitated during anesthesia are at risk following extubation. Treatment involves removal of ingesta from the buccal cavity or buccal lavage prior to extubation. If active regurgitation occurs during intubation, anesthetic depth should be rapidly increased and the airway quickly protected to prevent aspiration.

Several techniques can be used for intubation. Adult cattle can be intubated blindly or with digital palpation. Following insertion of a mouth speculum or the use of gauze loops, the animal's head and neck are hyperextended to make the orotracheal axis approach 180°. An endotracheal tube of appropriate size is inserted and manipulated into the larynx (Table 64.2).

When that technique is unsuccessful, the anesthetist's hand should be inserted into the mouth with the tube. After the epiglottis has been located and depressed, a finger can be placed between the arytenoid cartilages and the tube inserted into the trachea. If desired, an equine nasogastric tube can be inserted into the larynx and serve as a guide for the endotracheal tube. Depending on the size of the animal and the individual's arm, airway obstruction may occur; hence, it is important that intubation is performed promptly. If the technique requires more than one min, the hand and arm should be withdrawn from the oral cavity to allow the animal to ventilate before continuing to attempt intubation.

When blind orotracheal intubation is unsuccessful in calves, a laryngoscope with a 250–350 mm blade is required for laryngoscopy.

Table 64.2 Sizes of endotracheal tubes needed for ruminants and camelids of various body weights.

Body weight (kg)	Endotracheal tube size (internal diameter, mm)	
	Orotracheal	Nasotracheal
< 30	4–7	4–6
30–60	8–10	6–8
60–100	10–12	8–10
100–200	12–14	10–12
200–300	14–16	
300–400	16–22	
400–600	22–26	
> 600	26	

Herbivores' mouths do not open widely and can be held open by an assistant using gauze loops. Visibility of the pharynx and larynx will be improved by using an equine mouth speculum. Some effort is needed to keep the upper bar of the speculum against the dental pad, but use of the speculum will allow an assistant to open the mouth more widely than can be otherwise accomplished and allow much better visibility of the larynx. Visibility of the larynx is also improved by hyperextending the animal's head and neck to make the orotracheal axis approach 180°. Using suction or gauze on a sponge forceps to swab the pharynx will improve visibility if secretions are an impediment. Attempting intubation when the anesthetic plane is insufficient may provoke active regurgitation. With adequate depth of anesthesia, this reflex is eliminated. The epiglottis is depressed to visualize the larynx. The endotracheal tube should be placed in the oropharynx and inserted into the larynx during inspiration. If desired, a stylet (e.g., a 1 m × 0.5 cm stylet) [175], a large male dog urinary catheter, or an endotracheal tube exchanger (Cook® Airway Exchange Catheters, Cook Medical, Bloomington, IN, USA) can be inserted through the endotracheal tube and extended beyond the endotracheal tube tip to facilitate intubation. The length of the stylet should be about 1.5–2 times that of the endotracheal tube. The stylet is placed through the larynx, and the endotracheal tube is then passed into the trachea.

Blind oral intubation is more difficult in sheep and goats, and intubation is best performed with laryngoscopy. To perform blind oral intubation, the animal's head and neck are extended after placement of the endotracheal tube in the oral pharynx. The larynx can be palpated and the tube directed into the larynx [44]. Members of both of these species have active laryngeal reflexes that can be obtunded by topical application of 2% lidocaine. This can be performed with an adjustable pattern plant sprayer [176] or with a syringe. Use of Cetacaine® is not recommended because overdosage can easily occur and because benzocaine-based local anesthetics can cause methemoglobinemia [177]. After desensitization of the larynx, intubation can be performed with the same technique as used in calves. The technique for oral intubation in camelids is similar to that used in domestic ruminants. Blind oral intubation is usually unsuccessful, and laryngoscopy with a 250–350 mm laryngoscope is recommended. Desensitization of the larynx is usually not required.

Blind nasotracheal intubation has been described in awake or mildly sedated calves, although it requires an endotracheal tube one size smaller than that used orally [140]. The technique in calves is very similar to that described for foals and is useful for induction of inhalation anesthesia or to facilitate oral surgery. Particular attention is needed to ensure that the tube is directed into the ventral meatus. Following placement of the tube in the nasopharynx, the calf's head and neck are extended to facilitate passage into the larynx. The tube is secured in place and connected to the anesthesia machine.

In addition to calves [140], nasotracheal intubation is also possible in sheep and goats due to the relatively large size of their inferior meatus [178]. In adult cattle undergoing procedures involving the oral cavity requiring greater visibility and access, the authors have performed nasotracheal intubation using a 20–22 mm ID endotracheal tube in a standard size cow. This technique is also feasible in camelids [179]. In all mentioned species, an endotracheal tube approximately one size smaller than that used orotracheally will be needed. Camelids are prone to epistaxis, and use of a lubricant that contains phenylephrine is recommended. Blind nasal intubation is technically easier than blind oral intubation, but nasal intubation under laryngoscopic control is technically more difficult than orotracheal intubation. Even though nasotracheal intubation can be more difficult, it offers the option of recovering the animal with the endotracheal tube in place as a method of preventing airway obstruction during recovery. The endotracheal tube is advanced with slow, gentle pressure through the external nares into the ventral meatus. An obstruction encountered at approximately 10 cm in adults is usually due to placement of the tube in the middle meatus. If an obstruction is encountered more caudally, approximately 25 cm in adult llamas, the tube is likely in the nasopharyngeal diverticulum [179]. In either case, the tube should be partially or completely withdrawn and redirected. If the endotracheal tube cannot be redirected past the nasopharyngeal diverticulum, placement of a pre-bent stylet into the tube to direct its tip ventrally is usually effective. After the endotracheal tube has been advanced into the nasopharynx, the camelid's head and neck should be extended and the tube manipulated into the larynx. If the tube will not enter the larynx, placement of a pre-bent stylet into the tube will help direct its tip ventrally into the larynx instead of into the esophagus. Although visibility of the larynx is somewhat limited, oral laryngoscopy can aid intubation and confirm correct placement of the nasotracheal tube [179]. A retrograde technique that involves the use of a nested trocar into the cervical trachea for intubation of llamas has also been described [180]. In brief, the nested trocar and cannula are percutaneously placed into the cervical trachea, and a stylet is advanced in a retrograde direction through the cannula and into the mouth. As the stylet exits the mouth, the endotracheal tube is slid over the stylet, which is used as a guide for orotracheal tube placement. The investigator found no difference in the time needed to accomplish intubation between anterograde and retrograde intubation techniques, but fewer attempts were needed with the retrograde technique.

Endotracheal intubation can be confirmed with several techniques. Initially, they include visualization of the endotracheal tube passing into the larynx. When transparent endotracheal tubes are used, condensed water vapor will appear and then disappear during each breath. One can feel gas being expelled from the tube during exhalation and, when the endotracheal tube is connected to the anesthesia machine, observation of synchrony between movement of the breathing bag and the thorax will be noted. If a suction bulb is evacuated and connected to the endotracheal tube, it will re-expand if the tube is in the trachea and will remain collapsed if the tube is in the esophagus, providing immediate confirmation of correct or incorrect placement of the tube (Fig. 64.1). Finally, if a capnograph is available, carbon dioxide will be noted in exhaled gas.

Maintenance

Anesthesia in ruminants and camelids can be maintained with intravenous agents, commonly ketamine–guaifenesin–xylazine, and less commonly propofol or alfaxalone, or with inhalant agents.

Injectable

Because ruminants may regurgitate during xylazine–ketamine–guaifenesin anesthesia, intubation is highly recommended. It is also often recommended that duration of anesthesia be limited to 60 min to limit recovery time and complications. The use of infusion pumps facilitates administration of the drugs and improves convenience and precision. Following induction, xylazine–ketamine–guaifenesin solutions can be used for maintenance of anesthesia in cattle [147,154,155] and sheep [156]. Final concentrations are xylazine 0.1 mg/mL, ketamine 1–2 mg/mL, and guaifenesin 50 mg/mL, and it should be emphasized that this formulation differs from the one

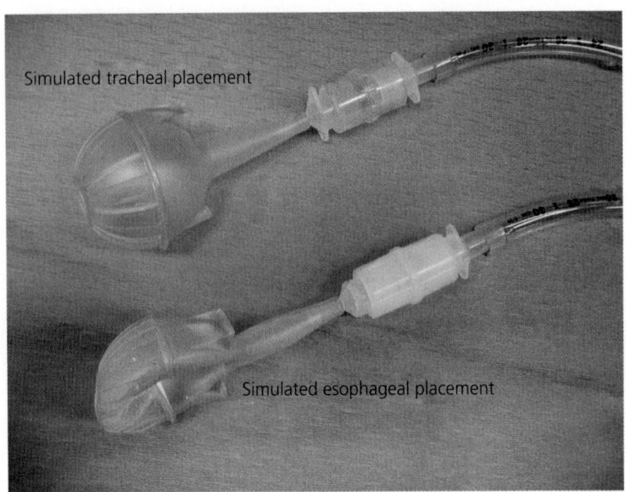

Figure 64.1 Evacuated bulbs attached to endotracheal tubes simulating esophageal (bottom) and tracheal (top) placement of the tube. The evacuated bulb will fill when attached to a correctly placed endotracheal tube.

used in horses in which the concentration of xylazine is five times higher. Anesthesia is maintained by infusion of the mixture at 1.5 mL/kg/h for calves [154,155], 2 mL/kg/h for adult cattle [146], and 2 mL/kg/h for sheep [156], although the final administration rate will vary with case requirements. If the procedure requires more than 2 mL/kg of the xylazine–ketamine–guaifenesin mixture in order to complete the procedure, the amount of xylazine added should be decreased by at least 50% because its duration of action is longer than that of the other two agents [personal communication: John C. Thurmon, 1993]. Alternatively, a solution with final concentrations of xylazine 0.05 mg/mL, ketamine 1 mg/mL, and guaifenesin 50 mg/mL can be formulated and infused at 2 mL/kg/h IV for maintenance to avoid the cumulative effects of xylazine. Following induction, xylazine–ketamine–guaifenesin solutions may be used for maintenance of anesthesia in llamas [104]. Final concentrations are xylazine 0.1–0.2 mg/mL, ketamine 2 mg/mL, and guaifenesin 50 mg/mL. Anesthesia is maintained by infusion of the mixture at 1.2–2.4 mL/kg/h, although the final administration rate will vary with case requirements.

Propofol has been successfully used for induction and maintenance of anesthesia in small ruminants and calves (4–6 mg/kg) [181,182]. In calves in which anesthesia was maintained with a propofol infusion (0.6–0.8 mg/kg/min IV) for 60 min, subjects showed increased total antioxidant capacity [183]. Following induction in sedated sheep with propofol, anesthesia can be maintained with propofol at 0.3–0.5 mg/kg/min IV [170]. Recovery to standing occurs within 15 min [170]. The approximate time from discontinuation of propofol infusion to sternal recumbency is 10–15 min [171]. Following induction of anesthesia in sedated sheep with propofol and ketamine, anesthesia can be maintained with propofol at 0.2–0.3 mg/kg/min and ketamine at 0.1–0.2 mg/kg/min IV [170]. Recovery to standing occurs within 15 min [170]. A light plane of anesthesia can be maintained in unsedated llamas with a constant infusion of propofol at 0.4 mg/kg/min IV [171]. In goats undergoing magnetic resonance imaging, maintenance with propofol (0.3 mg/kg/min) and ketamine (0.03 mg/kg/min) IV produced a degree of immobility and cardiovascular effects comparable to sevoflurane [184].

Anesthesia can also be maintained with alfaxalone at 0.17 mg/kg/min IV in unsedated sheep following induction with alfaxalone at 2 mg/kg IV. Hemodynamic variables are acceptable, although mild respiratory depression for up to 15 min after induction may require ventilatory support [185]. Recovery following 70 min of anesthesia occurs within 25 min [186]. Alfaxalone can also be infused as an adjunct to inhalation anesthesia [186].

Inhalation

Inhalant agents that have been used historically in ruminants include methoxyflurane and halothane, but isoflurane and sevoflurane are the inhalant agents of choice in contemporary practice. While methoxyflurane was utilized in small domestic ruminants and camelids, inductions and recoveries were prolonged. Liver failure was reported in hyperimmunized goats subjected to halothane anesthesia [187], but another study performed in young, healthy goats showed that neither halothane nor isoflurane was likely to cause hepatic injury [188]. Reports of renal failure associated with flunixin meglumine administration immediately before or after methoxyflurane administration in dogs [189] caution against the use of this combination of drugs in ruminants.

Conventional small animal anesthesia machines can be used to anesthetize ruminants weighing less than 60 kg. Conventional human anesthesia machines or small animal machines with expanded carbon dioxide absorbent (e.g., soda lime) canisters are adequate for animals weighing up to 200 kg. Conventional large animal anesthesia machines can be used to anesthetize cattle weighing over 250 kg. The piston-driven Tafonius® ventilator offers flexibility in ventilating ruminants over a wide range of sizes and ventilatory patterns, with or without the addition of positive end-expiratory pressure. Anesthesia is usually induced with 3–5% isoflurane or 4–6% sevoflurane and an oxygen flow rate of 20 mL/kg/min. Anesthesia is usually maintained with 1.5–2.5% isoflurane or 2.5–3.5% sevoflurane with an oxygen flow rate of 12 mL/kg/min, with a minimum flow rate of 1 L/min being adequate. These vaporizer settings correspond to end-expired anesthetic concentrations of 1.25–1.5 minimum alveolar concentration (MAC) and should be adequate for ruminants that were not sedated prior to induction. Ruminants that have been sedated prior to induction can usually be maintained on end-expired anesthetic concentrations of 1–1.25 MAC, although final concentrations may vary depending on the sedative used. Because domestic ruminants have a respiratory pattern characterized by a rapid respiratory rate and a small tidal volume, higher vaporizer settings may be required to maintain anesthesia in spontaneously breathing patients. If monitoring of inhalant anesthetic gas concentrations is available, delivery can be titrated based on the agent's MAC value. The MAC of isoflurane is 1.13 ± 0.03 to 1.63 ± 0.17% in goats [190–192], 1.01–1.58% in sheep [193,194], 1.14% in cattle [195], 1.47% in calves, and 1.05 ± 0.17% in adult male llamas [196]. During spontaneous breathing, the MAC of sevoflurane is 2.29 ± 0.14% in llamas, 2.33 ± 0.09% in alpacas [197], 2.33 ± 0.15% in goats [198], and 3.3% in sheep [199]. The MAC of desflurane is lower in llamas and alpacas (7.99 ± 0.58% and 7.83 ± 0.51%, respectively) [200] than in sheep (8.6–9.81%) [201,202]. MACs of sevoflurane and desflurane have not been determined in cattle. In neonatal calves, isoflurane and sevoflurane have been used successfully with comparable cardiorespiratory performance and recovery times [203]. Midazolam infusions at 1.7, 5.0, and 15.0 μg/kg/min IV reduce MAC of isoflurane in goats by 16.8%, 35.1%, and 54.7%, respectively [191]. Nitrous oxide administered in concentrations of 70% of the inspired gas along with sevoflurane to sheep produced a 37% reduction in MAC [204]. Interestingly, the sparing effect of nitrous oxide was reversed by the administration of atipamezole, confirming the involvement of α_2-adrenergic receptor agonism in the MAC-sparing effect on sevoflurane. The sparing effect of oxymorphone (0.05 mg/kg) and hydromorphone (0.1 mg/kg) in sheep anesthetized with desflurane is clinically unimportant compared to effects reported in other species [202].

Intraoperative analgesia

Infusions of ketamine and lidocaine have been used to provide analgesia in large and small animal patients. Ketamine is effective in small animal patients when administered at a loading dose of 0.5 mg/kg IV followed by an infusion at 10 μg/kg/min [205]. Ketamine has also been given alone at 6.6–13.3 μg/kg/min IV in horses [206] and at 25 μg/kg/min IV after a loading dose of 1 mg/kg [192]. Ketamine can be given at 40 μg/kg/min IV to awake camelids without untoward behavioral effects and will reduce anesthetic requirements by 35% when given to anesthetized camelids [207]. Fentanyl can be administered to sheep at a rate of 0.17 μg/kg/min IV without significant cardiorespiratory effects [208], whereas the application of a fentanyl transdermal patch (75 μg/h) applied 15 h before anesthesia can reduce the MAC of sevoflurane by approximately 25% and aid in providing perioperative analgesia [209]. Lidocaine administration has been effective in reducing overall anesthetic requirements in animals under inhalation anesthesia [190,210,211]. The reported lidocaine loading dose ranges from 2 to 5 mg/kg IV followed by an infusion of 50–100 μg/kg/min IV [190,210]. Starting at the lower end of the range for both loading and infusion doses is recommended. The infusion should be discontinued 30 min prior to recovery to avoid prolonged recoveries. In calves premedicated with xylazine, and administered ketamine, midazolam, and isoflurane for induction and maintenance of anesthesia, lidocaine infusion at a rate of 100 μg/kg/min following a 2 mg/kg bolus IV caused decreased heart rate compared to the control group without affecting other cardiovascular parameters [212]. The pharmacokinetics of morphine (0.08 μg/kg/min), lidocaine (35 μg/kg/min), and ketamine (7 μg/kg/min) administered IV for a 24-h period have been established in calves undergoing herniorrhaphy [213]. These infusions provided adequate postoperative analgesia 4 h after starting the infusion [213]. In sheep, infusion of the same drug combination at different IV dosages (morphine 3.3 μg/kg/min, lidocaine 50 μg/kg/min, and ketamine 10 μg/kg/min) caused a 75% decrease in anesthetic requirements of isoflurane compared to a control group [214].

Systemic administration of analgesic drugs can be continued in the postoperative period to provide continuing analgesia and improve patient comfort. Dose regimens can be adjusted to obtain analgesia and minimize sedation.

Supportive therapy

Supportive therapy is an important part of anesthetic practice. As duration and difficulty of the procedure increases, the likelihood of complications can also increase. Attention to supportive therapy in anesthetized ruminants and camelids can decrease the incidence of complications and improve outcome. Supportive therapy includes patient positioning, fluid administration, mechanical ventilation, cardiovascular support, and good monitoring techniques.

Patient positioning

Improper positioning and padding of anesthetized horses has been implicated as one cause of postanesthetic myopathy and neuropathy [215]. A similar situation may occur in adult cattle. Postanesthetic myopathy does not appear to occur in calves, goats, sheep, and South American camelids. Anesthetized ruminants should be positioned on a smooth, flat, padded surface. Adult cattle require water beds, dunnage bags, or 10–15 cm foam pads. Pads 5 cm thick are sufficient for sheep, goats, and South American camelids. Patients positioned in dorsal recumbency should be balanced squarely on their back with both gluteal areas bearing equal weight. The forelimbs and hindlimbs should be relaxed in a flexed position. External support should be placed under the maxilla to prevent hyperextension of the neck.

Adult cattle in lateral recumbency should have an automobile inner tube (valve stem pointed down) placed under the shoulder of the dependent foreleg to help minimize pressure on the radial nerve as it traverses the musculospiral groove of the humerus. The point of the elbow should be positioned at 5 o'clock in the inner tube for cattle in right lateral recumbency or at seven o'clock for cattle in left lateral recumbency. In addition, the dependent foreleg is drawn anteriorly so that the weight of the thorax rests on the triceps rather than on the humerus. Non-elastic tape covering the portion of the inner tube not under the shoulder will prevent overexpansion of that section of inner tube and collapse of the inner tube under the shoulder and helps ensure that shoulder support remains (Fig. 64.2A and B). The other three legs are positioned perpendicular to the body, with the uppermost legs elevated and parallel to the table surface. Support of these legs will improve venous drainage and prevent injury to the brachial plexus. The head and neck are maintained in a slightly extended position, with the head resting on a pad or towel (Fig. 64.3). If possible, the patient's head should be positioned so that salivary secretions and gastric contents, if regurgitation occurs, will drain from the mouth and not wick between the animal's head and the pad and contact the eye. The dependent eye should be closed prior to placing the head on the padding, and ophthalmic ointment should be instilled in both eyes. Camelids have prominent eyes, and special attention should be given to the dependent eye to avoid injury. Use of circulating warm water heating blankets or convective warm air blowers should be considered to prevent hypothermia in juvenile cattle, sheep, camelids, and goats. Use of active warming devices may be required to prevent hypothermia during the anesthetic episode and during recovery.

Fluid administration

Fluid administration during anesthesia is important to correct preexisting dehydration, if present, provide volume to offset anesthesia-related vasodilation, and provide maintenance needs. A balanced electrolyte solution is preferred. Lactated Ringer's solution, Plasma-Lyte®, Normosol-R®, or equivalent are most commonly used and are administered rapidly (10–25 mL/kg/h) in hypotensive patients. After hypotension is corrected, fluid administration may be slowed to 4–6 mL/kg/h. Although ruminants salivate copiously while anesthetized, replacement of bicarbonate is usually not required. Other fluids (e.g., saline) may be given when indicated. To increase the fluid delivery rate when needed, two administration sets can be connected to one catheter with a Y-connector, multiple catheters can be placed, a peristaltic pump can be used, or the fluid source may be pressurized. For convenience, fluids packaged in 3 or 5 L bags can be used for large-volume administration. When administering large volumes of fluid, serial determinations of hematocrit and plasma total solids should be performed to prevent hemodilution and decreased oncotic pressure. Hematocrit should remain above 25% and plasma total solids above 4 g/dL. The use of plasma

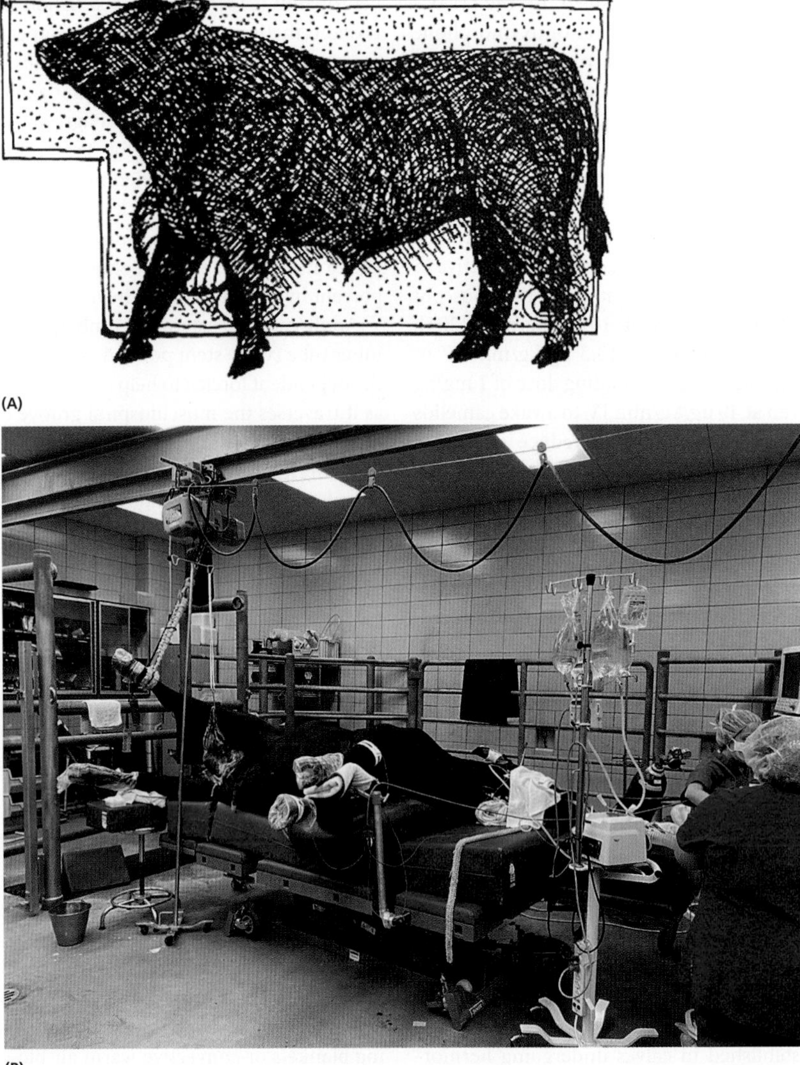

Figure 64.2 **A.** Diagram showing appropriate positioning and support for anesthetized cattle in lateral recumbency. The table is padded and an automobile inner tube is placed under the dependent forelimb and that leg is drawn cranially. Additional support is placed under the non-dependent forelimb and hindlimb so they are parallel to the table. **B.** Photograph of an anesthetized bull in left lateral recumbency showing the inner tube under the left forelimb and support of the non-dependent limbs (in this case, the patient is undergoing scrotal surgery so the non-dependent hindlimb is elevated beyond parallel to facilitate surgical access). Source: Dr. Chiara E. Hampton, with permission.

or whole blood transfusion should be considered for hypoproteinemic or anemic individuals. In light of the challenges identifying blood donors and collecting sufficient volumes of blood from small ruminants, xenotransfusion of whole blood, packed red blood cells, and/or plasma can be used to correct anemia and improve circulating volume in goats [216] and wildebeests [217]. Administration of sodium bicarbonate should be considered for correction of severe metabolic acidosis only.

Respiratory supportive therapy

Although anesthetized South American camelids ventilate well, domestic ruminants tend to hypoventilate while anesthetized. Hypoventilation is a function of both anesthetic-induced medullary depression and cranial compression and displacement of the diaphragm by the rumen during dorsal recumbency. Mechanical ventilation should be considered when the procedure will exceed 90 min and is indicated to prevent hypoventilation in individuals that will not maintain sufficient alveolar ventilation. To minimize the effects of mechanical ventilation on the cardiovascular system, the inspiratory time should be no more than 2–3 s, the inspiratory pressure should be 20–25 cmH_2O, the tidal volume should be between 13 and 18 mL/kg, and the respiratory rate should be 6–10 breaths/min. Mechanical ventilation should be titrated to achieve normocapnia using capnography (i.e., end-tidal carbon dioxide [$P_{ET}CO_2$] values in the range of 35–45 mmHg) or blood gas analysis. Hypocapnia can cause bradycardia and, in the absence of $P_{ET}CO_2$ or $PaCO_2$ values, minute volume should be decreased if unexplained bradycardia occurs.

During intravenous sedation and anesthesia, ruminants also benefit from supplemental oxygen. If the animal is intubated, the endotracheal tube can be connected to a demand valve. This piece of equipment is connected to an oxygen source that enables the patient to breathe spontaneously [218]. Compression of a button on the demand valve enables the anesthetist to “sigh” the patient.

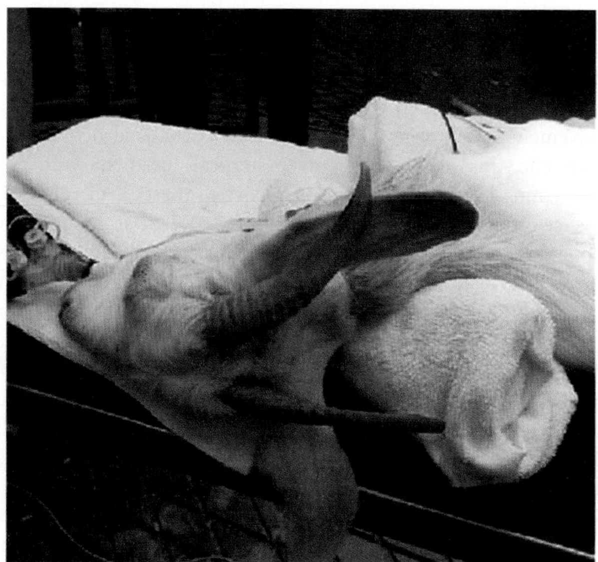

Figure 64.3 Position of the head and neck to enable fluid to drain from the oral cavity. Source: Lin *et al.* [84], with permission from John Wiley & Sons, Inc.

Intubated ruminants can also be insufflated with oxygen (5 L/min for small ruminants and 15 L/min for adult cattle). A flowmeter is connected to an oxygen source, and the tubing from the flowmeter is then inserted into the endotracheal tube [219]. In steers anesthetized with sevoflurane, the reverse Trendelenburg position (5° and 10°) failed to improve ventilation and oxygenation compared with no tilt, and cardiovascular performance was adversely affected at the 10° tilt [82].

Cardiovascular supportive therapy

Hypotension has been implicated as another cause of postanesthetic myopathy/neuropathy [215,220]. To help avoid this postanesthetic complication in ruminants, normotension should be maintained during anesthesia. Hypotension may often be corrected by adjusting anesthetic depth. Although vasopressors can be used to correct hypotension, expansion of vascular volume with rapid fluid administration and/or augmentation of stroke volume and cardiac output with inotropic therapy are better alternatives. Calcium gluconate or borogluconate (23% solution) may also increase myocardial contractility and vascular smooth muscle tone and can be given as a slow infusion (0.2–1 mL/kg/h IV) to effect. Calcium administration can cause bradycardia, however, necessitating the use of a chronotrope if hypotension due to bradycardia persists. Ephedrine, a sympathomimetic drug with mixed α- and β-adrenergic receptor activity, can be used at 0.02–0.06 mg/kg IV to increase mean arterial pressure through an increase in cardiac contractility [221]. Lack of response at low doses can indicate excessive depth of anesthesia. Dobutamine, a synthetic β-adrenergic receptor agonist, can also be used as an infusion to improve cardiac output. At low doses, it increases myocardial contractility and, at higher doses, heart rate is also increased [222]. Dobutamine is preferred over dopamine because improvements in hemodynamic function are achieved with smaller increases in heart rate [223]. Dobutamine is infused at 1–5 μg/kg/min IV to effect [223]. Use of an infusion pump is recommended for convenience and consistency. After correction of hypotension, the infusion rate can often be decreased to maintain normotension.

Monitoring

As with any species, good anesthetic techniques require monitoring to ensure that drug administration meets the animal's requirements and to prevent excessive insult to the cardiovascular, respiratory, central nervous, and musculoskeletal systems, thereby decreasing the risk of complications. Monitoring includes techniques that require the tactile, visual, and auditory skills of the anesthetist, as well as more sophisticated techniques that require instrumentation. Attention is directed to three organ systems: the cardiovascular, the respiratory, and the central nervous systems. Ideally, one monitors variables that respond rapidly to changes in anesthetic depth, which gives the anesthetist sufficient time to alter anesthetic administration before the anesthetic plane becomes either excessive or insufficient. In many instances, monitoring equipment is used to aid the evaluation of physiologic responses to anesthesia and, therefore, anesthetic depth. Use of these instruments can make evaluation more precise and the selection of ancillary drugs more rational. While monitoring is done constantly, most variables are recorded at 5-min intervals. The use of software designed for veterinary anesthesia records (e.g., VetDAR®) can improve patient safety by reminding the individual to enter current vital signs data at prescribed intervals and alerting the individual when data for the patient's vital signs fall outside of the normal range.

Variables that can be used to monitor the cardiovascular system are heart rate, pulse pressure (pulse strength), mucous membrane color, and capillary refill time. In healthy anesthetized adult cattle, the heart rate is usually 60–90 beats/min. Animals that have received an anticholinergic will have an increased heart rate. The normal heart rate for calves, sheep, and goats varies with age. Juveniles will have a heart rate of 90–120 beats/min, which decreases as they mature. The normal heart rate for adult anesthetized camelids after administration of an anticholinergic is 80–100 beats/min, and for anesthetized juvenile camelids after the administration of an anticholinergic, it is 100–125 beats/min. Heart rate may exceed the normal range at the beginning of anesthesia because of excitement associated with induction or hypotension but most often returns to the normal range within 10–20 min. In compromised patients, the heart rate begins to approach the normal range during anesthesia as oxygen, fluid, and analgesic support begin to stabilize the patient. The heart rate usually decreases as the depth of anesthesia increases, although that response is dependent on the agent used and can be masked by prior administration of anticholinergics.

Pulse pressure can be ascertained at several locations and should be full and bounding. However, a bounding pulse does not guarantee normotension. The common digital, caudal auricular, radial, and saphenous arteries are commonly palpated. The facial artery can be palpated in young calves, but it becomes more difficult to do so as the animal ages. Pulse pressure should be strong and palpated at different locations for comparison. Noting the amount of turgor present in the vessel during diastole can give an indication of diastolic pressure. If the vessel is easily collapsed by digital pressure during diastole, then diastolic pressure and, therefore, systolic and mean pressure can be assumed to be low even though the pulse pressure may feel adequate. While a variety of non-invasive blood pressure monitors are available that are suitable for patients the size of most ruminants and camelids, their accuracy is disappointing and invasive techniques are generally recommended [224,225].

Mucous membranes should be pink, although those of some ruminants and camelids are pigmented, making assessment difficult. The presence of cyanosis must also be noted, although animals breathing oxygen and an inhalation agent may be apneic for several minutes before cyanosis occurs. Because at least 5 g/dL of reduced hemoglobin is required before cyanosis can be detected, severely anemic animals may not show this sign. Flushed mucous membranes are associated with vasodilation, which can be caused by hypercapnia, halothane, α_2-adrenergic receptor antagonists, or histamine release, or may be associated with postural hypostatic congestion [226]. Brick red mucous membranes are associated with endotoxic shock. Following digital compression to blanch an area of the gum, capillary refill should occur in 1–2 s. Both of these variables give an imprecise indication of tissue perfusion. Excessive depth of anesthesia will cause the mucous membranes to become pale and the capillary refill time to increase.

The respiratory system is evaluated by monitoring respiratory rate, tidal volume, end-tidal carbon dioxide ($P_{ET}CO_2$), and percent hemoglobin saturation (SpO_2). Spontaneous breathing rates are usually 20–30 breaths/min or higher in adult cattle; calves, sheep, and goats usually have respiratory rates of 20–40 breaths/min. Awake cattle have a decreased tidal volume compared with horses [227]. This relationship persists in anesthetized cattle and other domestic ruminants in that they have a decreased tidal volume compared with other species. Tidal volume is estimated by observing the decrease in size of the rebreathing bag during inspiration. Increasing depth of anesthesia can usually be expected to cause a decrease in tidal volume and eventually a decrease in respiratory rate. Normal values for respiratory rate in anesthetized camelids are 15–30 breaths/min for adults and 20–35 breaths/min for juveniles. Camelids tend to ventilate reasonably well when breathing spontaneously as judged by blood gas and respiratory gas analysis during sevoflurane and isoflurane anesthesia. Capnography is commonly available in many practices, and $P_{ET}CO_2$ monitoring is useful for assessing ventilation in ruminants. Since CO_2 and other gases are produced during fermentation, the effect of these non-respiratory sources of gas should be assessed on each capnometer before use.

The central nervous system can be monitored by observation of ocular reflexes. The palpebral reflex disappears with minimal depth of anesthesia in cattle, sheep, and goats and is usually of no value during anesthesia. Rotation of the globe will occur as anesthetic depth changes in cattle (Fig. 64.4) [17,91,228]. The eyeball is normally centered between the palpebrae in awake cattle in lateral recumbency. As anesthesia is induced, the eyeball rotates ventrally, with the cornea being partially obscured by the lower eyelid.

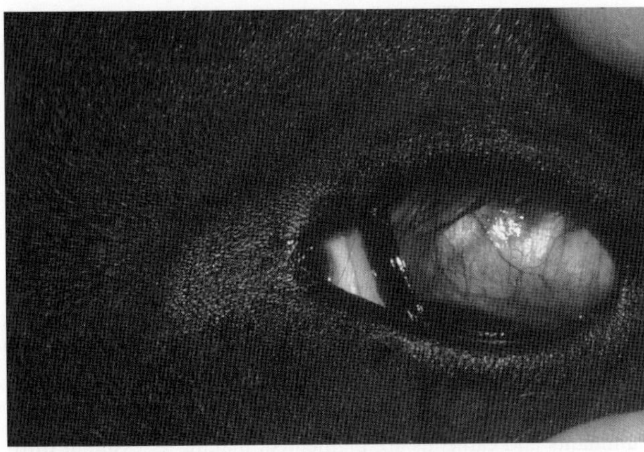

Figure 64.4 Ocular rotation in a ventral direction is indicative of a light plane of surgical anesthesia.

As the depth of anesthesia increases, the pupil becomes completely hidden by the lower eyelid; this sign indicates that the patient is at stage 3, plane II–III anesthesia. A further increase in anesthetic depth is accompanied by dorsal rotation of the eyeball. Dorsal movement is complete when the cornea is centered between the palpebrae; this sign indicates deep surgical anesthesia with profound muscle relaxation. During recovery, the eyeball rotates in reverse order to that during induction [17,91,228]. Rotation of the globe does not occur in response to changes in the depth of anesthesia in goats, sheep, or South American camelids. Usually, the palpebral reflex of the dorsal eyelid of camelids remains intact during surgical anesthesia. However, if the camelid can move its ventral eyelid without tactile stimulation, anesthetic depth is decreasing and eventually limb movement will occur. Nystagmus usually does not occur during anesthesia of domestic ruminants or camelids. When it does occur, it cannot be correlated with changes in anesthetic depth. The corneal reflex should always be present.

Some ruminants will display involuntary swallowing motions under anesthesia without exhibiting other signs of insufficient anesthetic depth. While this reflex may accompany a reduction in anesthetic depth, it does not necessarily indicate inadequate depth. Response to pain from the surgical procedure can also be used to estimate depth of anesthesia. In some instances, camelids may respond by showing a more active palpebral reflex. Purposeful movement in all species indicates insufficient depth of anesthesia. A mild temporary increase in arterial pressure associated with surgical manipulation does not necessarily indicate inadequate anesthesia if purposeful movement does not occur.

Electrocardiography (ECG) is used with either standard limb leads (i.e., I, II, and III) or a dipole (augmented) lead for detection of cardiac rate and rhythm disturbances. The lead that has the largest amplitude is usually selected. A recorder is optional and useful because it enables one to record an ECG at the beginning of the case for future reference. Most ECG units emit an audible tone when a QRS complex is detected. Anesthetists should learn to always listen to the audible rhythm in the background during the case, especially during distractions. Because an ECG gives no information regarding blood pressure or pulse strength, emphasis should be placed on monitoring pulse and arterial pressure instead of relying solely on the ECG. In calves and cattle, atrial repolarization (Ta waves) may be visible on the ECG following the P wave and preceding the QRS complex. Ta waves are low-amplitude deflections in the opposite direction of the P wave and are generated by the large atrial mass often present in large species like cattle and horses. Ta waves have been found to increase in amplitude in calves with hyperkalemia [229]. U waves can sometimes be appreciated following the completion of ventricular repolarization (T wave), and they are believed to represent repolarization of M cells and Purkinje fibers [230]. The amplitudes of both Ta and U waves may be increased by electrolyte imbalances, especially of calcium and potassium.

Pulse oximetry is a well-established non-invasive method of measuring hemoglobin saturation with oxygen (SpO_2) and pulse rate. It is considered a key monitoring modality to evaluate cardiovascular and the respiratory systems via oxygenation, and its use is recommended during all phases of anesthesia, including recovery, according to the monitoring guidelines of the American College of Veterinary Anesthesia and Analgesia [231]. Transmission or reflectance probes can be used in ruminants, preferably on non-pigmented tissues. As occurs in other species, displayed values below 90–92% must be investigated as they may indicate the presence of hypoxemia ($PaO_2 < 60$ mmHg). However, it should be noted that different ruminant species have different P_{50} values (the partial pressure of oxygen at which 50% of hemoglobin is saturated). The P_{50} in cattle and goats is 25 and 28.6 mmHg, respectively, whereas in sheep this value has been reported to be between 41.8 and 44.1 mmHg. This has important implications in clinical practice as this would mean that a pulse oximeter calibrated based on a human oxyhemoglobin dissociation curve (P_{50} = 26.6 mmHg) will likely overestimate the PaO_2 of a cow, slightly underestimate that of a goat, and grossly underestimate the PaO_2 of a sheep. The Masimo Signal Extraction Technology® pulse oximeter has been found to underestimate oxyhemoglobin saturation compared to CO-oximetry, with a bias of −2% but an overall reasonable accuracy and precision when SpO_2 values were above 75% [232]. Modern pulse oximeters can also incorporate technology that allows for the measurement of perfusion index (PI) and plethysmography variability index (PVI). The former is the ratio of pulsatile blood flow to non-pulsatile blood in the tissue being monitored, and it can be used as an indicator of tissue perfusion. The latter measures the change in PI during one respiratory cycle and can be used as an indirect indicator of patient responsiveness to fluid administration. Further investigations are needed in ruminants before definitive recommendations can be made for the use of PI and PVI to aid in clinical decision-making. Additional information on pulse oximetry and perfusion indices can be found in Chapters 12 and 15.

Mean arterial pressure provides an accurate variable for assessing anesthetic depth. In most instances, changes in anesthetic depth become evident quickly through increases or decreases in blood pressure. Additionally, it is a more definitive variable than assessing pulse pressure alone. *Pulse pressure* is defined as the difference between systolic and diastolic pressures. An animal with systolic and diastolic pressures of 120/90 mmHg will have pulse pressure similar to that of another with pressures of 90/60 mmHg. However, a large difference exists in mean arterial pressure or perfusion pressure. The former case will have a mean pressure of about 100 mmHg, whereas the latter will have a mean pressure of about 70 mmHg. Since animals with low mean pressure during anesthesia are more at risk of developing complications, identification of this situation is important [220,233]. Normal arterial systolic, diastolic, and mean pressures in anesthetized cattle are 120–150 mmHg, 80–110 mmHg, and 90–120 mmHg, respectively; these values are typically greater than those measured in standing cattle [234]. Normal arterial systolic, diastolic, and mean pressures in sheep, goats, and camelids are 90–120, 60–80, and 75–100 mmHg, respectively, and similar to those obtained in horses [235]. However, if camelids are aroused by painful stimuli, mean arterial pressure may approach 150 mmHg. Arterial pressure can be monitored either indirectly or directly. Indirect methods of determining arterial pressure require the use of various infrasonic and ultrasonic devices to detect blood flow in peripheral arteries. A Doppler ultrasonic system or an oscillometric device (e.g., Cardell®) can be used with cuffs wrapped around the tail of cattle and the limbs of sheep and goats [46], or around the tail or the limbs of South American camelids [50]. The cuff diameter should be 40% of the limb or tail circumference [226]. Unfortunately, there can be lack of agreement between pressures obtained with indirect and direct methods in domestic ruminants [224] and in camelids [225], and the use of direct techniques is recommended when feasible.

Direct methods require catheterization of an artery and use of a pressure transducer and amplifier or an aneroid manometer to determine pressure values. A transducer system determines systolic, diastolic, and mean arterial pressures. An aneroid manometer can be substituted for the pressure transducer and amplifier, but only mean pressure can be obtained [236]. However, changes in mean pressure occur rapidly in response to changes in anesthetic depth, and use of this system enables anesthetists to initiate appropriate responses.

Percutaneous arterial catheterization is easily performed in most ruminants and is relatively free of complications [236,237]. The caudal auricular, saphenous, and common digital arteries are the most commonly catheterized vessels. Over-the-needle catheters are preferred. Passage of this type of catheter through the unbroken skin will often damage the catheter, making arterial placement difficult. Therefore, incising the skin or piercing it with a slightly larger needle at the catheterization site prior to introducing the catheter is recommended [237]. A skin incision is usually unnecessary when the caudal auricular artery is catheterized, because the skin is relatively thin in that location and the artery is often inadvertently pierced because the skin is relatively immobile in that area. For adult cattle, 3–5 cm, 20 gauge catheters are used, and for calves, sheep, goats, and camelids, 2.5–3 cm, 20–22 gauge catheters are appropriate. An extension set with stopcock is used to connect the arterial catheter to a syringe containing heparinized (2 IU/mL) saline and a piece of non-compliant tubing attached to the pressure transducer or aneroid manometer. Two cases of iatrogenic cerebral air embolism have been reported in calves after accidental entrainment of air in the catheter placed in the auricular artery [238]. Therefore, care should be taken in ensuring that connections are tight and that air does not enter the arterial circulation, even in small volumes. After the arterial catheter has been removed, digital pressure is maintained at the site to prevent hematoma formation. If desired, a pressure bandage can be used.

Central venous pressure can be determined to assess venous return, myocardial function, and the need for fluid replacement. It can be used along with serial determinations of hematocrit, plasma total solids, and urine production, in evaluating fluid replacement and vascular tone, but provides little information regarding changes in anesthetic depth. Normal values are 5–10 cmH_2O, which approximate right atrial pressures.

Normal values for arterial blood gas analysis are similar to those for other species [9,10], with more positive base excess values, which are variable based on diet. Respiratory gas analysis can determine $P_{ET}CO_2$ and anesthetic agent concentrations. Because domestic ruminants have a respiratory pattern characterized by small tidal volume, end-expired gas may not be sufficiently representative of alveolar gas and accurate results might not be obtained. Capnography is more accurate when assessing carbon dioxide during controlled ventilation. Anesthetic agent analyzers that use optical low-spectrum infrared measurement (i.e., measuring absorption in the lower region of the infrared spectrum) cannot distinguish between methane and halothane in the expired gas of herbivores and will report falsely increased concentrations of halothane, and to a lesser extent isoflurane, in the anesthetic circuit [239]. The presence of methane does not affect analyzers that use high-spectrum infrared measurement or piezoelectric measurement [239]. Analyzers that use low-spectrum infrared measurement can be used in herbivores by intermittently (i.e., every 15–30 min) placing a small container of activated charcoal in the sample path to adsorb the inhalant agent [240]. Methane will pass through the charcoal without adsorption and be measured. After removing the charcoal container from the sample path, one can subtract the concentration of background methane from the displayed value to determine the inhalant agent concentration.

Recovery

Ruminants and South American camelids recover well from general anesthesia and seldom experience emergence delirium, make premature attempts to stand, or sustain injuries. When an α_2-adrenergic receptor agonist is used as part of the anesthetic regimen, an α_2-adrenergic receptor antagonist can be used to hasten recovery [32,69,91,100,101,104,148,175,241].

Domestic ruminants should not be extubated until the laryngeal reflex has returned. If the patient has regurgitated, the buccal cavity and pharynx should be lavaged to prevent aspiration of the material. In these instances, the endotracheal tube should be withdrawn with the cuff inflated in an attempt to remove any material that may have entered the trachea. Since camelids are obligate nasal breathers [242], gas exchange must be confirmed after extubation. Airway obstruction can commonly occur in camelids during the transition from oral endotracheal intubation to nasal breathing and, in severe cases, can necessitate tracheotomy. Orally intubated camelids should not be extubated until the animal is swallowing, coughing, and actively trying to expel the endotracheal tube to decrease the incidence of this complication. Precautions should be taken to prevent the camelid from damaging or aspirating the endotracheal tube during "awake" extubation. The endotracheal tube of nasally intubated camelids can be removed after they stand. Although ruminants recover well from general anesthesia with minimal assistance, an attendant should be available.

Intraoperative complications

Fortunately, major complications do not often occur during or following well-planned anesthesia in ruminants. However, one must be vigilant so that the unexpected occurrence of a complication can be recognized and effectively treated. As is the case in anesthesia of all species, potential complications are better prevented than treated, and therefore, emphasis should be placed on formation and implementation of a rational anesthetic regimen. Airway obstruction, apnea, and hypothermia are diagnosed and treated in a manner similar to other domestic species as described elsewhere in this edition. A case of presumptive malignant hyperthermia of unknown origin with fatal outcome in a 9-month-old black Angus bull has been reported [243]. It remains unclear if the subject actually expressed the genetic mutation for definitive confirmation of malignant hyperthermia.

Although anesthetized camelids do not appear to become tympanitic, fermentation of ingesta and the animal's inability to eructate under anesthesia often cause ruminal tympany during anesthesia of domestic ruminants. As tympany develops, more pressure is placed on the diaphragm, decreasing functional residual capacity and impeding ventilation [244]. In addition, tympany increases the risk of regurgitation. Therapy involves passage of a stomach tube to decompress the rumen. On occasion, one will be unable to pass the stomach tube into the rumen. In these difficult cases, placing the animal in sternal recumbency will aid the procedure. When that is not possible, the rumen can be decompressed with a 12 gauge needle inserted through the abdominal wall. Fortunately, ruminal tympany is usually of the non-frothy type, and decompression is easily accomplished. External pressure placed on the rumen will help expel gas from the orogastric tube. Ruminal tympany can also occur during the use of nitrous oxide, which tends to accumulate in organs prefilled with gas [245]. Discontinuation of nitrous oxide administration and decompression of the rumen are recommended.

Connective tissue is not as fibrous in the lungs of ruminants, and therefore, excessive airway pressure can cause pneumothorax and emphysema more easily than in horses [246]. Signs include dyspnea and increased resistance to inspiration because of tension pneumothorax. Pneumothorax is treated by placement of a chest tube and aspiration of the gas. It is much easier to prevent than treat. Excessive airway pressure (i.e., pressures > 25 cmH_2O) should not be used when "sighing" animals or when using controlled ventilation.

Cardiac arrhythmias usually do not occur in anesthetized ruminants. Atrial fibrillation can occur in cattle as a sequela to metabolic derangement secondary to another problem, most often gastrointestinal obstruction. The arrhythmia can be diagnosed with ECG and usually resolves when the primary problem is corrected. Because cattle are amenable to physical restraint and local anesthesia, corrective surgery can often be performed without general anesthesia. Electrolyte imbalances can contribute to morbidity and mortality under general anesthesia and should be monitored in ill patients. In a case report, hyperkalemia due to uroperitoneum lead to cardiac arrest in a calf [247]. The oculocardiac reflex is a well-recognized reflex in most animals and can be treated similarly in ruminants. Cardiac arrest would be treated with similar techniques used in horses [248–250].

Postoperative complications

Because ruminants and camelids tend to recover well from general anesthesia, long-bone fractures, cervical fractures, or other catastrophic injuries seldom occur. Should they occur, therapy is based on severity of the fracture and the economic value of the animal. Postoperative myopathy/neuropathy can occur in larger cattle but is not a common complication in calves, sheep, goats, or camelids. The problem is recognized when muscle weakness or motor nerve dysfunction is observed, with some animals being unable to stand. Commonly affected nerves are the radial, the femoral, and the sciatic. Therapy is symptomatic, with IV fluids administered to maintain hydration, acid–base status, and electrolyte balance, along with analgesics and NSAIDs as indicated. Depending on the type of sling used, slinging the animal may be helpful or could increase muscle injury. Myopathy may take several days to resolve and can be life-threatening. Again, it is better to prevent muscle or nerve injury by positioning anesthetized animals properly and avoiding excessive depth of anesthesia.

Recovery from anesthesia can be delayed by hypothermia. Provision of thermal support to the patient with various warming devices including circulating warm water pads and pumps, forced air warmers, and resistive foam warming blankets will help maintain normothermia.

A less common cause of delayed recovery is muscle weakness caused by neuromuscular blockade. Because ruminants have very low levels of plasma cholinesterase (also known as "pseudocholinesterase"), metabolism of succinylcholine is slow, causing prolonged effects of the drug. Neuromuscular blockade may also be caused by interaction of anesthetics and aminoglycoside antibiotics [139] or by incomplete reversal of nondepolarizing muscle relaxants [251]. Muscle relaxants are rarely administered to ruminants in clinical practice, but may be more common in research settings.

Thrombophlebitis can occur after perivascular injection of irritating compounds, although usually not with the frequency or severity that occurs in horses, and is treated similarly [252]. Corneal ulcers can also occur following anesthesia and should be managed as in other species.

Aspiration pneumonia occurs after regurgitation of rumen or gastric contents and subsequent inhalation of the material. Active regurgitation may cause the material to be inhaled deeply into the pulmonary tree, initiating bronchospasm and physical obstruction of the airways. Signs include dyspnea and, depending on severity, cyanosis. If the patient survives the initial insult, pneumonia is certain. Broad-spectrum antibiotic and anti-inflammatory therapy are indicated [253]. Silent or passive regurgitation can occur with the same results, except that there usually is not as much particulate material in the regurgitant. Similar treatment is instituted. Because of the potential severity of this complication, prevention must be emphasized. Tracheal intubation is recommended and, if not possible, the occiput should be elevated to encourage fluids to drain from the mouth rather than into the trachea (Fig. 64.3) [178].

Analgesia

Providing postoperative analgesia is an important component of veterinary anesthesia. Pain-specific and species-specific pain assessment tools should be employed to evaluate the patient and guide administration of analgesic drugs. The reader is directed to Chapter 47 for further information on recognition and assessment of pain. There are very few approved drugs for provision of analgesia in domestic ruminants and none approved for use in South American camelids. Drugs that have been used in other species include the NSAIDs carprofen, firocoxib, flunixin, ketoprofen, meloxicam, phenylbutazone, and robenacoxib; the opioids butorphanol, buprenorphine, fentanyl, and morphine; the local anesthetic lidocaine; and ketamine. Although α_2-adrenergic receptor agonists can provide analgesia, their behavioral effects usually limit their use in ruminants. When applicable, local anesthetic agents can be used to desensitize structures and tissue [254]. Long-acting local anesthetic agents, bupivacaine, ropivacaine, and liposomal bupivacaine (Nocita®), would be preferred. Epidural administration of local anesthetic agents and opioids may be appropriate for some procedures.

Flunixin can be given at 1.1–2.2 mg/kg IV daily. Carprofen can be given at 0.7 mg/kg IV daily [255]. When given at 4 mg/kg, therapeutic levels are maintained for at least 72 h [255]. Carprofen (1.4 mg/kg) administered 1 h before umbilical surgery in calves lowered serum cortisol and systemic vascular resistance, which is speculated to indicate a reduced response to surgical stress [256]. Ketoprofen can be dosed at 3.3 mg/kg IV daily [255]. Phenylbutazone is recommended at a dose of 2.2 mg/kg orally every 48 h [255]; however, its off-label use is prohibited in some populations of food animals. As of 2003, the United States Food and Drug Administration Center for Veterinary Medicine instituted a ban on phenylbutazone in female dairy cattle 20 months of age and older due to serious concerns about public health [257]. Consequently, its use in dairy cattle in the United States, and many other jurisdictions, is illegal. Meloxicam is given at 0.5 mg/kg IV every 12 h to sheep or at 1 mg/kg orally every 24 h following a loading dose of 2 mg/kg orally [258–260]. Meloxicam is given at 0.5 mg/kg IV every 8 h to goats or at 0.5 mg/kg orally every 24 h following a loading dose of 2 mg/kg orally [258–260]. Except for flunixin, withdrawal times following NSAID use in ruminants are not well defined either for meat or for milk, and caution must be exercised to prevent residues from entering the food supply [255]. More latitude is available when administering NSAIDs to ruminants used in biomedical research.

The use of all NSAIDs carries the risk of ulcer formation in the third gastric compartment of South American camelids. When extended use of these agents is anticipated, it is recommended that dose and frequency be decreased after the desired effect is obtained in an effort to determine the minimal dose needed to provide analgesia. Flunixin is commonly used for analgesia in South American camelids. The dose range is 0.5–1.1 mg/kg IV given once daily [258–261]. Flunixin has been given at 1.1 mg/kg twice daily in some instances. Meloxicam is given at 0.5 mg/kg IV or at 1 mg orally every 3 days to camelids [258–261]. Phenylbutazone is less commonly used in camelids. When used, it is administered in a manner similar to that in domestic ruminants (i.e., 2.2 mg/kg orally every 48 h) [262]. Ketoprofen has also been used in llamas at a dose of 1–2 mg/kg IV once daily [263]. Firocoxib can be given at 0.5 mg/kg IV or orally as a single dose [260].

Opioids have been used to provide analgesia to domestic ruminants and South American camelids. Most commonly, either butorphanol (0.05–0.2 mg/kg IM every 6 h) or morphine (0.05–0.1 mg/kg IM every 6 h) has been recommended [32]. Morphine (0.4 mg/kg IV) administered to cattle induced variable analgesia measured via thermal thresholds without changes in locomotor behavior or adverse effects [264]. The use of other opioids, such as buprenorphine, fentanyl (both injectable and transdermal), hydromorphone, and oxymorphone, may be considered in dosages similar to those used in canine or equine patients [265–267]. Transdermal fentanyl patches have been used in llamas [268], goats [269], and sheep, and the patch should be placed on the lateral aspect of the shaved foreleg rather than on the thorax [270]. The dose of opioids may need to be adjusted if the behavioral effects cause problems (i.e., too much sedation, dysphoria, or excessive locomotor activity).

Epidural opioids have been used extensively to provide analgesia in companion animals [265,266,271,272] and in horses [273]. Morphine, which is the most commonly used agent, is typically administered at a dose of 0.1 mg/kg to treat postoperative abdominal and orthopedic pain and to prevent tenesmus in horses [273] and camelids. Analgesia begins in 30–60 min with duration of action lasting 12–24 h. Injection is typically through the sacrocaudal space but can also be made at the lumbosacral space in anesthetized ruminants. A ruminant or camelid that becomes recumbent following sacrocaudal injection should be placed in sternal recumbency. As in other species, the lumbosacral space is caudal to a line connecting the anterior border of the wings of the ilium. In camelids, the spinous process of the last lumbar vertebra is usually easily palpable; the needle is directed caudally to enter the space. The spinous process of the first sacral vertebra is much smaller than that of the last lumbar vertebra and is difficult to palpate. Usually, a 7 cm, 18 gauge spinal needle is adequate. If the injection is made at the lumbosacral space, one must aspirate prior to injection to ensure that the intrathecal space has not been entered. Dose requirements of local anesthetics are 50–70% less when an agent is given intrathecally compared with epidural injection. If cerebrospinal fluid is obtained, the local anesthetic dose must be decreased or the needle must be withdrawn for epidural placement of the drug.

References

1 Cebra C, Sisson D. Diseases of the cardiovascular and hemolymphatic systems. In: Cebra C, Anderson DE, Tibary A, *et al.*, eds. *Llama and Alpaca Care: Medicine, Surgery, Reproduction, Nutrition, and Herd Health*. St. Louis, MO: WB Saunders, 2014: 393–421.

2 Constable PD, Hinchcliff KW, Done SH, *et al. Veterinary Medicine: A Textbook of the Diseases of Cattle, Horses, Sheep, Pigs and Goats*, 11th edn. St. Louis, MO: Elsevier Health Sciences, 2016.

3 Kaplan R, Burke J, Terrill T, *et al.* Validation of the FAMACHA© eye color chart for detecting clinical anemia in sheep and goats on farms in the southern United States. *Vet Parasitol* 2004; **123**: 105–120.

4 Johnson LW. Physical examination and conformation. In: Cebra C, Anderson DE, Tibary A, *et al.*, eds. *Llama and Alpaca Care: Medicine, Surgery, Reproduction, Nutrition, and Herd Health*. St. Louis, MO: WB Saunders, 2014: 328–337.

5 Ghosh C, Datta S, Mandal D, *et al.* Body condition scoring in goat: impact and significance. *J Entomol Zool* 2019; **7**: 554–560.

6 Phythian C, Hughes D, Michalopoulou E, *et al.* Reliability of body condition scoring of sheep for cross-farm assessments. *Small Rumin Res* 2012; **104**: 156–162.

7 Wildman E, Jones G, Wagner P, *et al.* A dairy cow body condition scoring system and its relationship to selected production characteristics. *J Dairy Sci* 1982; **65**: 495–501.

8 Lassen E, Pearson E, Long P, *et al.* Clinical biochemical values of llamas: reference values. *Am J Vet Res* 1986; **47**: 2278–2280.

9 Latimer K, Mahaffey E, Prasse K. *Duncan and Prasse's Veterinary Laboratory Medicine, Clinical Pathology*, 4th edn. Ames, IA: Wiley-Blackwell, 2003: 149–156.

10 Kaneko JJ, Harvey JW, Bruss ML. *Clinical Biochemistry of Domestic Animals*, 6th edn. San Diego, CA: Academic Press, 2008.

11 Kramer J. Normal hematology of cattle, sheep and goats. In: Feldman BF, Zinkl JG, Jain NC, *et al.*, eds. *Schalm's Veterinary Hematology*, 5th edn. Philadelphia, PA: Lippincott Williams and Wilkins, 2000: 1075–1084.

12 Viesselmann LC, Videla R, Flatland B. Verification of the Heska Element Point-of-Care blood gas instrument for use with venous blood from alpacas and llamas, with determination of reference intervals. *Vet Clin Pathol* 2018; **47**: 435–447.

13 Vallenas A, Cummings J, Munnell J. A gross study of the compartmentalized stomach of two new-world camelids, the llama and guanaco. *J Morphol* 1971; **134**: 399–423.

14 Clariget J, Banchero G, Luzardo S, *et al.* Effect of pre-slaughter fasting duration on physiology, carcass and meat quality in beef cattle finished on pastures or feedlot. *Res Vet Sci* 2021; **136**: 158–165.

15 Rabaza A, Banchero G, Cajarville C, *et al.* Effects of feed withdrawal duration on animal behaviour, rumen microbiota and blood chemistry in feedlot cattle: implications for rumen acidosis. *Animal* 2020; **14**: 66–77.

16 Blaze C, LeBlanc P, Robinson N. Effect of withholding feed on ventilation and the incidence of regurgitation during halothane anesthesia of adult cattle. *Am J Vet Res* 1988; **49**: 2126–2129.

17 Tranquilli WJ. Techniques of inhalation anesthesia in ruminants and swine. *Vet Clin North Am Food Anim Pract* 1986; **2**: 593–619.

18 Weaver A. Complications in halothane anaesthesia of cattle. *Zentralbl Veterinarmed A* 1971; **18**: 409–416.

19 Clabough DL, Swanson CR. Heart rate spectral analysis of fasting-induced bradycardia of cattle. *Am J Physiol* 1989; **257**: R1303–R1306.

20 McGuirk S, Bednarski R, Clayton M. Bradycardia in cattle deprived of food. *J Am Vet Med Assoc* 1990; **196**: 894–896.

21 Ward J, Henricks D, Jenkins T, *et al.* Serum hormone and metabolite concentrations in fasted young bulls and steers. *Domest Anim Endocrinol* 1992; **9**: 97–103.

22 Cebra C. Fluid therapy. In: Cebra C, Anderson DE, Tibary A, *et al.*, eds. *Llama and Alpaca Care: Medicine, Surgery, Reproduction, Nutrition, and Herd Health*. St. Louis, MO: WB Saunders, 2014: 350–356.

23 Fowler M. *Medicine and Surgery of Camelids*, 3rd edn. Ames, IA: Wiley-Blackwell, 2010: 89–109.

24 Amsel S, Kainer R, Johnson L. Choosing the best site to perform venipuncture in a llama. *Vet Med* 1987; **82**: 535.

25 Jones ML. Ear squeeze (Ear Twitch). In: Anderson DE, Jones ML, Miesner MD, eds. *Veterinary Techniques for Llamas and Alpacas*. Ames, IA: John Wiley & Sons, 2013: 27–28.

26 Constable PD, Walker PG, Morin DE, *et al.* Clinical and laboratory assessment of hydration status of neonatal calves with diarrhea. *J Am Vet Med Assoc* 1998; **212**: 991–996.

27 Abril-Sánchez S, Crosignani N, Freitas-de-Melo A, *et al.* Sedation or anaesthesia decrease the stress response to electroejaculation and improve the quality of the collected semen in goat bucks. *Animal* 2018; **12**: 2598–2608.

28 Williams M, Caulkett N, Neuhaus P, *et al.* Comparison of the efficacy and safety of medetomidine-ketamine versus medetomidine-azaperone-alfaxalone combination in free-ranging rocky mountain bighorn sheep (*Ovis canadensis*). *J Zoo Wildl Med* 2018; **49**: 662–670.

29 Taylor PM. Anaesthesia in sheep and goats. *In Practice* 1991; **13**: 31–36.

30 Riebold T, Kaneps A, Schmotzer W. Anesthesia in the llama. *Vet Surg* 1989; **18**: 400–404.

31 Short CE. Preanesthetic medications in ruminants and swine. *Vet Clin North Am Food Anim Pract* 1986; **2**: 553–566.

32 Carroll GL, Hartsfield SM. General anesthetic techniques in ruminants. *Vet Clin North Am Food Anim Pract* 1996; **12**: 627–661.

33 Nishimura LT, Villela IOJ, Carvalho LL, *et al.* The effect of acepromazine alone or in combination with methadone, morphine, or tramadol on sedation and selected cardiopulmonary variables in sheep. *Vet Med Int* 2017: 7507616.

34 Prado TM, Doherty TJ, Boggan EB, *et al.* Effects of acepromazine and butorphanol on tiletamine–zolazepam anesthesia in llamas. *Am J Vet Res* 2008; **69**: 182–188.

35 Anderson D, Gaughan E, DeBowes R, *et al.* Effects of chemical restraint on the endoscopic appearance of laryngeal and pharyngeal anatomy and sensation in adult cattle. *Am J Vet Res* 1994; **55**: 1196–2000.

36 Hodgson DS, Dunlop CI, Chapman PL, *et al.* Cardiopulmonary effects of xylazine and acepromazine in pregnant cows in late gestation. *Am J Vet Res* 2002; **63**: 1695–1699.

37 Rankin DC. Sedatives and tranquilizers. In: Grimm KA, Lamont LA, Tranquilli WJ, *et al.*, eds. *Veterinary Anesthesia and Analgesia*, 5th edn. Ames, IA: Wiley-Blackwell, 2015: 196.

38 Buss PE. The pharmacodynamics of etorphine, and its combination with xylazine or azaperone in Boer goats (*Capra hircus*). Unpublished thesis dissertation, University of Pretoria, 2000.

39 Lapid R, Shilo-Benjamini Y. Immobilization of captive Nubian ibex (*Capra nubiana*) with butorphanol-midazolam-medetomidine or butorphanol-azaperone-medetomidine and atipamezole reversal. *J Zoo Wildl Med* 2015; **46**: 291–297.

40 Posner L, Burns P. Sedative agents: tranquilizers, alpha-2 agonists, and related agents. In: Riviere JE, Papich MG, eds. *Veterinary Pharmacology and Therapeutics*, 9th edn. Ames, IA; Wiley-Blackwell, 2009: 337–380.

41 Torneke K, Bergstrom U, Neil A. Interactions of xylazine and detomidine with α 2-adrenoceptors in brain tissue from cattle, swine and rats. *J Vet Pharmacol Ther* 2003; **26**: 205–211.

42 Xu M, Zhang Q, Wang Q, *et al.* The characteristics and distribution of α_2D-, α_2B- and α_2C-adrenoceptor subtypes in goats. *Animals (Basel)* 2022; **12**: 664.

43 Greene S, Thurmon J. Xylazine – a review of its pharmacology and use in veterinary medicine. *J Vet Pharmacol Ther* 1988; **11**: 295–313.

44 Gray P, McDonell W. Anesthesia in goats and sheep. II. General anesthesia. *Compend Contin Educ Pract Vet* 1986; **8**(Suppl): S127–S135.

45 Raptopoulos D, Weaver B. Observations following intravenous xylazine administration in steers. *Vet Rec* 1984; **114**: 567–569.

46 Trim C. Special anesthesia considerations in the ruminant. In: Short CE, ed. *Principles and Practice of Veterinary Anesthesia*. Baltimore, MA: Williams and Wilkins, 1987: 285–300.

47 Fayed A, Abdalla E, Anderson R, *et al.* Effect of xylazine in heifers under thermoneutral or heat stress conditions. *Am J Vet Res* 1989; **50**: 151–153.

48 Abrahamsen EJ. Chemical restraint and injectable anesthesia of ruminants. *Vet Clin North Am Food Anim Pract* 2013; **29**: 209–227.

49 Riebold T. Anesthesia in south American camelids. In: Greene SA, ed. *Veterinary Anesthesia and Pain Management Secrets*. Philadelphia, PA: Hanley & Belfus, 2002: 263–272.

50 Heath R. Llama anesthetic programs. *Vet Clin North Am Food Anim Pract* 1989; **5**: 71–80.

51 Cebra C, Tornquist S. Meta-analysis of glucose tolerance in llamas and alpacas. In: Gerken M, Renieri C, eds. *South American Camelids Research*, vol. **1**. Göttingen, Germany: Wageningen Academic, 2006: 161–165.

52 Rizk A, Herdtweck S, Meyer H, *et al.* Effects of xylazine hydrochloride on hormonal, metabolic, and cardiorespiratory stress responses to lateral recumbency and claw trimming in dairy cows. *J Am Vet Med Assoc* 2012; **240**: 1223–1230.

53 Rizk A, Herdtweck S, Offinger J, *et al.* The use of xylazine hydrochloride in an analgesic protocol for claw treatment of lame dairy cows in lateral recumbency on a surgical tipping table. *Vet J* 2012; **192**: 193–198.

54 Rioja E, Kerr CL, Enouri SS, *et al.* Sedative and cardiopulmonary effects of medetomidine hydrochloride and xylazine hydrochloride and their reversal with atipamezole hydrochloride in calves. *Am J Vet Res* 2008; **69**: 319–329.

55 Ede T, von Keyserlingk M, Weary D. Efficacy of xylazine in neonatal calves via different routes of administration. *Vet J* 2019; **247**: 57–60.

56 Ley S, Waterman A, Livingston A. Variation in the analgesic effects of xylazine in different breeds of sheep. *Vet Rec* 1990; **126**: 508.

57 O'Hair K, McNeil J, Phillips Y. Effects of xylazine in adult sheep. *Lab Anim Sci* 1986; **36**: 563.

58 Nolan A, Waterman A, Livingston A. The analgesic activity of alpha2 adrenoceptor agonists in sheep: a comparison with opioids. *Vet Anaesth Analg* 1986; **14**: 14–15.

59 Nolan A, Livingston A, Morris R, *et al.* Techniques for comparison of thermal and mechanical nociceptive stimuli in the sheep. *J Pharmacol Methods* 1987; **17**: 39–49.

60 Nolan A, Livingston A, Waterman A. Antinociceptive actions of intravenous a2-adrenoceptor agonists in sheep. *J Vet Pharmacol Ther* 1987; **10**: 202–209.

61 Symonds H. The effect of xylazine upon hepatic glucose production and blood flow rate in the lactating dairy cow. *Vet Rec* 1976; **99**: 234–236.

62 Symonds H, Mallinson C. The effect of xylazine and xylazine followed by insulin on blood glucose and insulin in the dairy cow. *Vet Rec* 1978; **102**: 27–29.

63 Eichner R, Prior R, Kvasnicka W. Xylazine-induced hyperglycemia in beef cattle. *Am J Vet Res* 1979; **40**: 127–129.

64 Brockman R. Effect of xylazine on plasma glucose, glucagon and insulin concentrations in sheep. *Res Vet Sci* 1981; **30**: 383–384.

65 Muggaberg J, Brockman R. Effect of adrenergic drugs on glucose and plasma glucagon and insulin responses to xylazine in sheep. *Res Vet Sci* 1982; **33**: 118–120.

66 Thurmon J, Nelson D, Hartsfield S, *et al.* Effects of xylazine hydrochloride on urine in cattle. *Aust Vet J* 1978; **54**: 178–180.

67 Ruckebusch Y, Allal C. Depression of reticulo-ruminal motor functions through the stimulation of alpha 2-adrenoceptors. *J Vet Pharmacol Ther* 1987; **10**: 1–10.

68 Toutain P, Zingoni M, Ruckebusch Y. Assessment of alpha-2 adrenergic antagonists on the central nervous system using reticular contraction in sheep as a model. *J Pharmacol Exp Ther* 1982; **223**: 215–218.

69 Riebold T, Kaneps A, Schmotzer W. Reversal of xylazine-induced sedation in llamas, using doxapram or 4-aminopyridine and yohimbine. *J Am Vet Med Assoc* 1986; **189**: 1059–1061.

70 Hopkins T. The clinical pharmacology of xylazine in cattle. *Aust Vet J* 1972; **48**: 109–112.

71 Celly C, McDonell W, Young S, *et al.* The comparative hypoxaemic effect of four α_2 adrenoceptor agonists (xylazine, romifidine, detomidine and medetomidine) in sheep. *J Vet Pharmacol Ther* 1997; **20**: 464–471.

72 Kästner S, Von Rechenberg B, Keller K, *et al.* Comparison of medetomidine and dexmedetomidine as premedication in isoflurane anaesthesia for orthopaedic surgery in domestic sheep. *J Vet Med A Physiol Pathol Clin Med* 2001; **48**: 231–241.

73 Papazoglou L, Raptopoulos D, Kokolis N. Increased airway pressure in response to xylazine is inhibited by both atipamezole and atropine in sheep. *Zentralbl Veterinarmed A* 1994; **41**: 568–572.

74 Nolan A, Livingston A, Waterman A. The effects of alpha2 adrenoceptor agonists on airway pressure in anaesthetized sheep. *J Vet Pharmacol Ther* 1986; **9**: 157–163.

75 Staub NC. Pulmonary intravascular macrophages. *Annu Rev Physiol* 1994; **56**: 47–67.

76 Papazoglou L, Raptopoulos D, Kounenis G. The effect of xylazine on the isolated sheep trachea. *J Vet Pharmacol Ther* 1995; **18**: 216–219.

77 Bacon P, Jones J, Taylor P, *et al.* Impairment of gas exchange due to alveolar oedema during xylazine sedation in sheep; absence of a free radical mediated inflammatory mechanism. *Res Vet Sci* 1998; **65**: 71–75.

78 Celly C, Atwal O, McDonell W, *et al.* Histopathologic alterations induced in the lungs of sheep by use of alpha2-adrenergic receptor agonists. *Am J Vet Res* 1999; **60**: 154–161.

79 Doherty T, Pascoe PJ, McDonell W, *et al.* Cardiopulmonary effects of xylazine and yohimbine in laterally recumbent sheep. *Can J Vet Res* 1986; **50**: 517–521.

80 Eisenach JC. Intravenous clonidine produces hypoxemia by a peripheral alpha-2 adrenergic mechanism. *J Pharmacol Exp Ther* 1988; **244**: 247–252.

81 Hsu W, Hanson CE, Hembrough F, *et al.* Effects of idazoxan, tolazoline, and yohimbine on xylazine-induced respiratory changes and central nervous system depression in ewes. *Am J Vet Res* 1989; **50**: 1570–1573.

82 Araújo MA, Deschk M, Wagatsuma JT, *et al.* Cardiopulmonary effects of reverse Trendelenburg position at 5 and 10 in sevoflurane-anesthetized steers. *Vet Anaesth Analg* 2017; **44**: 854–864.

83 Jansen C, Lowe K, Nathanielsz P. The effects of xylazine on uterine activity, fetal and maternal oxygenation, cardiovascular function, and fetal breathing. *Am J Obstet Gynecol* 1984; **148**: 386–390.

84 Lin H. Preanesthetic considerations. In: Lin HC, Passler T, Clark-Price S, eds. *Farm Animal Anesthesia: Cattle, Small Ruminants, Camelids, and Pigs*, 2nd edn. Hoboken, NJ: Wiley-Blackwell, 2022: 1–15.

85 Piccinno M, Rizzo A, Mutinati M, *et al.* Lidocaine decreases the xylazine-evoked contractility in pregnant cows. *Res Vet Sci* 2016; **107**: 267–272.

86 Aouad J, Wright E Jr., Shaner T. Anesthesia evaluation of ketamine and xylazine in calves. *Bov Pract* 1981; **2**: 22–31.

87 Campbell K, Klavano P, Richardson P, *et al.* Hemodynamic effects of xylazine in the calf. *Am J Vet Res* 1979; **40**: 1777–1780.

88 Freire A, Gontijo R, Pessoa J, *et al.* Effect of xylazine on the electrocardiogram of the sheep. *Br Vet J* 1981; **137**: 590–595.

89 Seddighi R, Elliot SB, Whitlock BK, *et al.* Physiologic and antinociceptive effects following intramuscular administration of xylazine hydrochloride in combination with tiletamine–zolazepam in llamas. *Am J Vet Res* 2013; **74**: 530–534.

90 Jedruch J, Gajewski Z. The effect of detomidine hydrochloride (Domosedan) on the electrical activity of the uterus in cows. *Acta Vet Scand Suppl* 1986; **82**: 189–192.

91 Greene SA. Protocols for anesthesia of cattle. *Vet Clin North Am Food Anim Pract* 2003; **19**: 679–693.

92 Hokkanen A, Raekallio MR, Salla K, *et al.* Sublingual administration of detomidine to calves prior to disbudding: a comparison with the intravenous route. *Vet Anaesth Analg* 2014; **41**: 372–377.

93 Chow NS, Seddighi R, Knych HK, *et al.* Sedative effects and pharmacokinetics of detomidine when administered intravenously and intravaginally as a gel in alpacas. *Vet Anaesth Analg* 2020; **47**: 773–780.

94 Malhi M, Kachiwal A, Soomro S, *et al.* Comparison of effects of xylazine, detomidine and medetomidine on heart rate, respiratory rate and blood glucose level in sheep. *Pak J Agric Agric Eng Vet Sci* 2015; **31**: 93–101.

95 Marzok M, El-Khodery S. Sedative and analgesic effects of romifidine in camels (*Camelus dromedarius*). *Vet Anaesth Analg* 2009; **36**: 352–360.

96 Waldridge B, Lin H, DeGraves F, *et al.* Sedative effects of medetomidine and its reversal by atipamezole in llamas. *J Am Vet Med Assoc* 1997; **211**: 1562–1565.

97 Adam M, Raekallio MR, Salla KM, *et al.* Effects of the peripherally acting α_2-adrenoceptor antagonist MK-467 on cardiopulmonary function in sheep sedated by intramuscular administration of medetomidine and ketamine and reversed by intramuscular administration of atipamezole. *Am J Vet Res* 2018; **79**: 921–932.

98 Seddighi R, Doherty TJ. Effect of dexmedetomidine hydrochloride on tiletamine hydrochloride–zolazepam hydrochloride anesthesia in alpacas. *Am J Vet Res* 2016; **77**: 1057–1063.

99 Cagnardi P, Villa R, Ravasio G, *et al.* Pharmacokinetics and sedative effects of dexmedetomidine in dairy calves. *N Z Vet J* 2017; **65**: 14–18.

100 Thurmon J, Lin H, Tranquilli W, *et al.* A comparison of yohimbine and talazoline as antagonists of xylazine sedation in calves. *Vet Surg* 1989; **18**: 170–171.

101 Kitzman J, Booth N, Hatch R, *et al.* Antagonism of xylazine sedation by 4-aminopyridine and yohimbine in cattle. *Am J Vet Res* 1982; **43**: 2165–2169.

102 Ko J, McGrath C. Effects of atipamezole and yohimbine on medetomidine-induced central nervous system depression and cardiorespiratory changes in lambs. *Am J Vet Res* 1995; **56**: 629–632.

103 Ruckebusch Y, Toutain P. Specific antagonism of xylazine effects on reticulo-rumen motor function in cattle. *Vet Med Rev* 1984; **1**: 1–12.

104 Young D, Shawley R, Barron S. Tolazoline reversal of xylazine–ketamine anesthesia in calves. *Vet Surg* 1988; **18**: 171.

105 Lin H-C, Riddell MG. Tolazoline. *Bov Practitioner* 2008; **42**: 86–92.

106 Lewis CA, Constable PD, Huhn JC, *et al.* Sedation with xylazine and lumbosacral epidural administration of lidocaine and xylazine for umbilical surgery in calves. *J Am Vet Med Assoc* 1999; **214**: 89–95.

107 Read MR, Duke T, Toews AR. Suspected tolazoline toxicosis in a llama. *J Am Vet Med Assoc* 2000; **216**: 227–229.

108 Doherty T, Ballinger J, McDonell W, *et al.* Antagonism of xylazine induced sedation by idazoxan in calves. *Can J Vet Res* 1987; **51**: 244–248.

109 Laitinen O. Clinical observations on medetomidine/ketamine anaesthesia in sheep and its reversal by atipamezole. *J Assoc Vet Anaesth* 1990; **17**: 17–19.

110 Tulamo R, Raekallio M, Ekblad A. Cardiovascular effects of medetomidine-ketamine anaesthesia in sheep, with and without 100% oxygen, and its reversal with atipamezole. *Vet Anaesth Analg* 1995; **22**: 9–14.

111 Haerdi-Landerer MC, Schlegel U, Neiger-Aeschbacher G. The analgesic effects of intrathecal xylazine and detomidine in sheep and their antagonism with systemic atipamezole. *Vet Anaesth Analg* 2005; **32**: 297–307.

112 Van Miert A, Faghihi S, Van Duin C. Food intake and rumen motility in dwarf goats. Effects of atipamezole on the inhibitory effects induced by detomidine, medetomidine and romifidine. *Vet Res Commun* 1994; **18**: 457–469.

113 Adam M, Lindén J, Raekallio M, *et al.* Concentrations of vatinoxan and xylazine in plasma, cerebrospinal fluid and brain tissue following intravenous administration in sheep. *Vet Anaesth Analg* 2021; **48**: 900–905.

114 Adam M, Lindén J, Raekallio M, *et al.* Effects of vatinoxan on xylazine-induced pulmonary alterations in sheep. *J Vet Pharmacol Ther* 2022; **45**: 117–125.

115 Adam M, Huuskonen V, Raekallio MR, *et al.* Cardiopulmonary effects of vatinoxan in sevoflurane-anaesthetised sheep receiving dexmedetomidine. *Vet J* 2018; **238**: 63–69.

116 Zahner J, Hatch R, Wilson R, *et al.* Antagonism of xylazine sedation in steers by doxapram and 4-aminopyridine. *Am J Vet Res* 1984; **45**: 2546–2551.

117 Waite SJ, Cater JE, Waghorn GC, *et al.* Effect of sedatives on rumen motility in sheep. *Small Rumin Res* 2021; **196**: 106284.

118 Simon BT, Scallan EM, Odette O, *et al.* Pharmacokinetics and pharmacodynamics of midazolam following intravenous and intramuscular administration to sheep. *Am J Vet Res* 2017; **78**: 539–549.

119 Aarnes TK, Fry PR, Hubbell JA, *et al.* Pharmacokinetics and pharmacodynamics of midazolam after intravenous and intramuscular administration in alpacas. *Am J Vet Res* 2013; **74**: 294–299.

120 Stegmann G. Observations on the use of midazolam for sedation, and induction of anaesthesia with midazolam in combination with ketamine in the goat. *J S Afr Vet Assoc* 1998; **69**: 89–92.

121 Stegmann G, Bester L. Sedative-hypnotic effects of midazolam in goats after intravenous and intramuscular administration. *Vet Anaesth Analg* 2001; **28**: 49–55.

122 Kyles A, Waterman A, Livingston A. Antinociceptive activity of midazolam in sheep. *J Vet Pharmacol Ther* 1995; **18**: 54–60.

123 Yavuz Ü, Yener K, Şahan A. The effect of midazolam and its reversal flumazenil on sedative and cardiopulmonary variables in sheep. *Kafkas Univ Vet Fak Derg* 2021; **27**: 771–779.

124 Aarnes TK, Fry PR, Hubbell JA, *et al.* Pharmacokinetics and pharmacodynamics of midazolam after intravenous and intramuscular administration in alpacas. *Am J Vet Res* 2013; **74**: 294–299.

125 O'Hair K, Dodd K, Phillips Y, *et al.* Cardiopulmonary effects of nalbuphine hydrochloride and butorphanol tartrate in sheep. *Lab Anim Sci* 1988; **38**: 58–61.

126 Waterman A, Livingston A, Amin A. Analgesic activity and respiratory effects of butorphanol in sheep. *Res Vet Sci* 1991; **51**: 19–23.

127 Barrington GM, Meyer T, Parish S. Standing castration of the llama using butorphanol tartrate and local anesthesia. *Equine Pract* 1993; **15**: 35–39.

128 Carroll G, Boothe D, Hartsfield S, *et al.* Pharmacokinetics and pharmacodynamics of butorphanol in llamas following intravenous and intramuscular administration. *Vet Anaesth Analg* 2002; **29**: 97–112.

129 Garcia Pereira F, Greene S, Keegan R, *et al.* Cardiovascular effects of butorphanol in isoflurane-anesthetized alpacas. *Vet Anaesth Analg* 2005; **32**: 8–9.

130 de Carvalho LL, Nishimura LT, Borges LP, *et al.* Sedative and cardiopulmonary effects of xylazine alone or in combination with methadone, morphine or tramadol in sheep. *Vet Anaesth Analg* 2016; **43**: 179–188.

131 Abouelfetouh MM, Salah E, Liu L, *et al.* Immediate postoperative analgesia of nalbuphine-ketamine combination compared with ketamine alone in xylazine-sedated goats undergoing left flank laparotomy. *Animals* 2022; **12**: 509.

132 Camburn M. Use of alphaxalone-alphadolone in ruminants. *Vet Rec* 1982; **111**: 166–167.

133 Kischinovsky M, Duse A, Wang T, *et al.* Intramuscular administration of alfaxalone in red-eared sliders (*Trachemys scripta elegans*)- effects of dose and body temperature. *Vet Anaesth Analg* 2013; **40**: 13–20.

134 Huynh M, Poumeyrol S, Pignon C, *et al.* Intramuscular administration of alfaxalone for sedation in rabbits. *Vet Rec* 2015; **176**: 255.

135 Tamura J, Ishizuka T, Fukui S, *et al.* Sedative effects of intramuscular alfaxalone administered to cats. *J Vet Med Sci* 2015; **77**: 897–904.

136 Patterson M, Caulkett N, Neuhaus P, *et al.* The utility of a novel formulation of alfaxalone in a remote delivery system. *Vet Anaesth Analg* 2021; **48**: 537–540.

137 Valverde A, Doherty TJ, Dyson D, *et al.* Evaluation of pentobarbital as a drug for standing sedation in cattle. *Vet Surg* 1989; **18**: 235–238.

138 Abrahamsen EJ. Chemical restraint, anesthesia, and analgesia for camelids. *Vet Clin North Am Food Anim Pract* 2009; **25**: 455–494.

139 Coetzee JF, Gehring R, Tarus-Sang J, *et al.* Effect of sub-anesthetic xylazine and ketamine ('ketamine stun') administered to calves immediately prior to castration. *Vet Anaesth Analg* 2010; **37**: 566–578.

140 Quandt J, Robinson E. Nasotracheal intubation in calves. *J Am Vet Med Assoc* 1996; **209**: 967–968.

141 Rouse S. *Pharmacodynamics of thiobarbiturates. Vet Anesth* 1978; **5**: 22–26.

142 Pascoe PJ. Emergency care medicine. In: Short CE, ed. *Principles and Practice of Veterinary Anesthesia.* Baltimore, MD: Williams & Wilkins, 1987: 558–598.

143 Chaplin M, Roszkowski A, Richards R. Displacement of thiopental from plasma proteins by nonsteroidal anti-inflammatory agents. *Proc Soc Exp Biol Med* 1973; **143**: 667–671.

144 Steckeler P, Fux D, Metzner M, *et al.* The course of plasma cortisol concentration after three different doses of ketamine in xylazine-premedicated calves. *Vet Anaesth Analg* 2019; **46**: 335–343.

145 Blaze C, Holland R, Grant A. Gas exchange during xylazine–ketamine anesthesia in neonatal calves. *Vet Surg* 1988; **17**: 155–159.

146 Thurmon J, Benson G. Anesthesia in ruminants and swine. In: Howard, JC, ed. *Current Veterinary Therapy 3: Food Animal Practice*, 3rd edn. Philadelphia, PA: WB Saunders, 1993: 58–76.

147 Coulson N, Januszkiewicz A, Dodd K, *et al.* The cardiorespiratory effects of diazepam-ketamine and xylazine–ketamine anesthetic combinations in sheep. *Lab Anim Sci* 1989; **39**: 591–597.

148 Raekallio M, Kivalo M, Jalanka H, *et al.* Medetomidine/ketamine sedation in calves and its reversal with atipamezole. *Vet Anaesth Analg* 1991; **18**: 45–47.

149 Lauper J, Marolf V, Levionnois O, *et al.* Does systemic lidocaine reduce ketamine requirements for endotracheal intubation in calves? *Vet Anaesth Analg* 2017; **44**: 281–286.

150 DuBois WR, Prado TM, Ko JC, *et al.* A comparison of two intramuscular doses of xylazine–ketamine combination and tolazoline reversal in llamas. *Vet Anaesth Analg* 2004; **31**: 90–96.

151 Grandy J, McDonell W. Evaluation of concentrated solutions of guaifenesin for equine anesthesia. *J Am Vet Med Assoc* 1980; **176**: 619–622.

152 Thurmon JC. Injectable anesthetic agents and techniques in ruminants and swine. *Vet Clin North Am Food Anim Pract* 1986; **2**: 567–591.

153 Wall R, Muir WW III. Hemolytic potential of guaifenesin in cattle. *Cornell Vet* 1990; **80**: 209–216.

154 Kerr CL, Windeyer C, Bouré LP, *et al.* Cardiopulmonary effects of administration of a combination solution of xylazine, guaifenesin, and ketamine or inhaled isoflurane in mechanically ventilated calves. *Am J Vet Res* 2007; **68**: 1287–1293.

155 Thurmon J, Benson G, Tranquilli W, *et al.* Cardiovascular effects of intravenous infusion of guaifenesin, ketamine, and xylazine in Holstein calves [Abstract]. *Vet Surg* 1986; **15**: 463.

156 Lin H-C, Tyler J, Welles E, *et al.* Effects of anesthesia induced and maintained by continuous intravenous administration of guaifenesin, ketamine, and xylazine in spontaneously breathing sheep. *Am J Vet Res* 1993; **54**: 1913–1916.

157 Tracy C, Short C, Clark B. Comparing the effects of intravenous and intramuscular administration of Telazol®. *Vet Med* 1988; **83**: 104–111.

158 Hubbell J, Bednarski R, Muir W. Xylazine and tiletamine–zolazepam anesthesia in horses. *Am J Vet Res* 1989; **50**: 737–742.

159 Lin H, Thurmon J, Benson G, *et al.* The hemodynamic response of calves to tiletamine-zolazepam anesthesia. *Vet Surg* 1989; **18**: 328–334.

160 Thurmon J, Lin H, Benson G, *et al.* Combining Telazol® and xylazine for anesthesia in calves. *Vet Med* 1989; **84**: 824–830.

161 Conner G, Coppock R, Beck C. Laboratory use of CI-744, a cataleptoid anesthetic, in sheep. *Vet Med Small Anim Clin* 1974; **69**: 479–482.

162 Lagutchik M, Januszkiewicz A, Dodd K, *et al.* Cardiopulmonary effects of a tiletamine–zolazepam combination in sheep. *Am J Vet Res* 1991; **52**: 1441–1447.

163 Lin H, Tyler J, Wallace S, *et al.* Telazol® and xylazine anesthesia in sheep. *Cornell Vet* 1993; **83**: 117–124.

164 Howard B, Lagutchik M, Januszkiewicz A, *et al.* The cardiovascular response of sheep to tiletamine–zolazepam and butorphanol tartrate anesthesia. *Vet Surg* 1990; **19**: 461–467.

165 Klein L, Tomasic M, Olson K. Evaluation of Telazol® in llamas [Abstract]. *Vet Surg* 1990; **19**: 316–317.

166 Seddighi R, Elliot SB, Whitlock BK, *et al.* Antinociceptive and selected physiological effects of morphine and xylazine on tiletamine–zolazepam anesthesia in llamas. *Vet Anaesth Analg* 2014; **41**: 365–371.

167 Waterman A. Use of propofol in sheep. *Vet Rec* 1988; **122**: 260.

168 Handel I, Weaver B, Staddon G, *et al.* Observations on the pharmacokinetics of propofol in sheep. *In: Proceedings of the 4th International Congress of Veterinary Anesthesia*, Utrecht, NL, 1991: 143–154.

169 Reid J, Nolan A, Welsh E. Propofol as an induction agent in the goat: a pharmacokinetic study. *J Vet Pharmacol Ther* 1993; **16**: 488–493.

170 Correia D, Nolan A, Reid J. Pharmacokinetics of propofol infusions, either alone or with ketamine, in sheep premedicated with acepromazine and papaveretum. *Res Vet Sci* 1996; **60**: 213–217.

171 Duke T, Egger C, Ferguson J, *et al.* Cardiopulmonary effects of propofol infusion in llamas. *Am J Vet Res* 1997; **58**: 153–156.

172 Andaluz A, Felez-Ocana N, Santos L, *et al.* The effects on cardio-respiratory and acid–base variables of the anaesthetic alfaxalone in a 2-hydroxypropyl-β-cyclodextrin (HPCD) formulation in sheep. *Vet J* 2012; **191**: 389–392.

173 Walsh V, Gieseg M, Singh P, *et al.* A comparison of two different ketamine and diazepam combinations with an alphaxalone and medetomidine combination for induction of anaesthesia in sheep. *N Z Vet J* 2012; **60**: 136–141.

174 del Álamo AM, Mandsager RE, Riebold TW, *et al.* Evaluation of intravenous administration of alfaxalone, propofol, and ketamine-diazepam for anesthesia in alpacas. *Vet Anaesth Analg* 2015; **42**: 72–82.

175 Hubbell JA, Hull BL, Muir WW. Perianesthetic considerations in cattle. *Compend Contin Educ Pract Vet* 1986; **8**: F92–F102.

176 Kinyon GE. A new device for topical anesthesia. *Anesthesiology* 1982; **56**: 154–155.

177 Lagutchik M, Mundie T, Martin D. Methemoglobinemia induced by a benzocaine-based topically administered anesthetic in eight sheep. *J Am Vet Med Assoc* 1992; **201**: 1407–1410.

178 Hall LW, Clarke KW. *Veterinary Anaesthesia*, 8th edn. London, UK: Bailliere Tindall, 1983.

179 Riebold T, Engel H, Grubb T, *et al.* Orotracheal and nasotracheal intubation in llamas. *J Am Vet Med Assoc* 1994; **204**: 779–783.

180 Byers SR, Cary JA, Farnsworth KD. Comparison of endotracheal intubation techniques in llamas. *Can Vet J* 2009; **50**: 745–749.

181 Yakan S, Aksoy O. Comparison of the effects of isoflurane and sevoflurane general anaesthesia after induction by propofol on clinical and physiological measurements in calves. *Acta Sci Vet* 2019; 47.

182 Deschk M, Wagatsuma JT, Araújo MA, *et al.* Continuous infusion of propofol in calves: bispectral index and hemodynamic effects. *Vet Anaesth Analg* 2016; **43**: 309–315.

183 Lima PPA, Narciso LG, Alcindo JF, *et al.* Evaluation of hematological, biochemical and oxidative stress profile in calves under propofol anesthesia. *Vet Res Commun* 2022; **46**: 27–35.

184 Larenza MP, Bergadano A, Iff I, *et al.* Comparison of the cardiopulmonary effects of anesthesia maintained by continuous infusion of ketamine and propofol with anesthesia maintained by inhalation of sevoflurane in goats undergoing magnetic resonance imaging. *Am J Vet Res* 2005; **66**: 2135–2141.

185 Moll X, Santos L, García F, *et al.* The effects on cardio-respiratory and acid–base variables of a constant rate infusion of alfaxalone-HPCD in sheep. *Vet J* 2013; **196**: 209–212.

186 del Mar Granados M, Domínguez JM, Fernández-Sarmiento A, *et al.* Anaesthetic and cardiorespiratory effects of a constant-rate infusion of alfaxalone in desflurane-anaesthetised sheep. *Vet Rec* 2012; **171**: 125.

187 O'Brien T, Raffe M, Cox V, *et al.* Hepatic necrosis following halothane anesthesia in goats. *J Am Vet Med Assoc* 1986; **189**: 1591–1595.

188 McEwen MM, Gleed RD, Ludders JW, *et al.* Hepatic effects of halothane and isoflurane anesthesia in goats. *J Am Vet Med Assoc* 2000; **217**: 1697–1700.

189 Mathews KA, Doherty T, Dyson DH, *et al.* Nephrotoxicity in dogs associated with methoxyflurane anesthesia and flunixin meglumine analgesia. *Can Vet J* 1990; **31**: 766.

190 Redua M, Doherty T, Castro-Queiroz P, *et al.* Effect of intravenous lidocaine and ketamine on isoflurane minimum alveolar concentration in goats. *Vet Anaesth Analg* 2005; **32**: 6–7.

191 Dzikiti TB, Stegmann GF, Dzikiti LN, *et al.* Effects of midazolam on isoflurane minimum alveolar concentration in goats. *Small Rumin Res* 2011; **97**: 104–109.

192 Queiroz-Castro P, Egger C, Redua MA, *et al.* Effects of ketamine and magnesium on the minimum alveolar concentration of isoflurane in goats. *Am J Vet Res* 2006; **67**: 1962–1966.

193 Bernards CM, Kern C, Cullen BF. Chronic cocaine administration reversibly increases isoflurane minimum alveolar concentration in sheep. *Anesthesiology* 1996; **85**: 91–95.

194 Brett CM, Teitel DF, Heymann MA, *et al.* The cardiovascular effects of isoflurane in lambs. *Anesthesiology* 1987; **67**: 60–65.

195 Cantalapiedra A, Villanueva B, Pereira J. Anaesthetic potency of isoflurane in cattle: determination of the minimum alveolar concentration. *Vet Anaesth Analg* 2000; **27**: 22–26.

196 Mama KR, Wagner AE, Parker DA, *et al.* Determination of the minimum alveolar concentration of isoflurane in llamas. *Vet Surg* 1999; **28**: 121–125.

197 Grubb TL, Schlipf JW, Riebold TW, *et al.* Minimum alveolar concentration of sevoflurane in spontaneously breathing llamas and alpacas. *J Am Vet Med Assoc* 2003; **223**: 1167–1169.

198 Hikasa Y, Okuyama K, Kakuta T, *et al.* Anesthetic potency and cardiopulmonary effects of evoflurane in goats: comparison with isoflurane and halothane. *Can J Vet Res* 1998; **62**: 299–306.

199 Lukasik V, Nogami W, Morgan S. Minimum alveolar concentration and cardiovascular effects of sevoflurane in sheep. *Vet Surg* 1998; **27**: 168.

200 Grubb TL, Schlipf JW, Riebold TW, *et al.* Minimum alveolar concentration of desflurane in llamas and alpacas. *Vet Anaesth Analg* 2006; **33**: 351–355.

201 Columbano N, Duffee LR, Melosu V, *et al.* Determination of minimum alveolar concentration and cardiovascular effects of desflurane in positive-pressure ventilated sheep. *Am J Vet Res* 2018; **79**: 727–732.

202 Sayre RS, Lepiz MA, Horsley KT, *et al.* Effects of oxymorphone hydrochloride or hydromorphone hydrochloride on minimal alveolar concentration of desflurane in sheep. *Am J Vet Res* 2015; **76**: 583–590.

203 Yakan S, Aksoy O, Ermutlu CS. Comparison of use of isoflurane or sevoflurane for anaesthesia induced by mask in calves. *Acta Sci Vet* 2020: 48.

204 Duffee L, Columbano N, Scanu A, *et al.* MAC-sparing effect of nitrous oxide in sevoflurane anesthetized sheep and its reversal with systemic atipamezole administration. *PLoS ONE* 2018; **13**: e0190167.

205 Wagner AE, Walton JA, Hellyer PW, *et al.* Use of low doses of ketamine administered by constant rate infusion as an adjunct for postoperative analgesia in dogs. *J Am Vet Med Assoc* 2002; **221**: 72–75.

206 Matthews N, Fielding C, Swinebroad E. How to use a ketamine constant rate infusion in horses for analgesia. *In: Proceedings of the 50th Annual Meeting of the American Association of Equine Practitioners*, Denver, CO, 2004: 227–228.

207 Schlipf J Jr., Eaton K, Fulkerson P, *et al.* Constant rate infusion of ketamine reduces minimal alveolar concentration of isoflurane in alpacas. *Vet Anaesth Analg* 2005; **32**: 7–8.

208 Funes FJ, del Mar Granados M, Morgaz J, *et al.* Anaesthetic and cardiorespiratory effects of a constant rate infusion of fentanyl in isoflurane-anaesthetized sheep. *Vet Anaesth Analg* 2015; **42**: 157–164.

209 Lauren D, Eraldo PS, Antonio S, *et al.* MAC-sparing effect of transdermal fentanyl in sevoflurane-anesthetized sheep. *Acta Vet* 2018; **68**: 211–216.

210 Doherty T, Frazier DL. Effect of intravenous lidocaine on halothane minimum alveolar concentration in ponies. *Equine Vet J* 1998; **30**: 300–303.

211 Valverde A, Doherty TJ, Hernández J, *et al.* Effect of lidocaine on the minimum alveolar concentration of isoflurane in dogs. *Vet Anaesth Analg* 2004; **31**: 264–271.

212 Araújo MA, Dias BP, Bovino F, *et al.* Cardiovascular effects of a continuous rate infusion of lidocaine in calves anesthetized with xylazine, midazolam, ketamine and isoflurane. *Vet Anaesth Analg* 2014; **41**: 145–152.

213 Hartnack AK, Niehaus AJ, Lakritz J, *et al.* Analgesic efficacy of an intravenous constant rate infusion of a morphine-lidocaine-ketamine combination in Holstein calves undergoing umbilical herniorrhaphy. *Am J Vet Res* 2020; **81**: 25–32.

214 Beier SL, da Rosa AC, Oleskovicz N, *et al.* Effects of the morphine-lidocaine-ketamine combination on cardiopulmonary function and isoflurane sparing in sheep. *Rev Bras Ciênc Agrár* 2014; **35**: 2527–2538.

215 White N. Postanesthetic recumbency myopathy in horses. *Compend Contin Educ Pract Vet* 1982; **4**(Suppl): S44–S52.

216 Smith JS, Viall AK, Breuer RM, *et al.* Preliminary investigation of bovine whole blood xenotransfusion as a therapeutic modality for the treatment of anemia in goats. *Front Vet Sci* 2021; **8**: 637988.

217 Buck RK, Stegmann GF, Poore LA, *et al.* Xenotransfusion with packed bovine red blood cells to a wildebeest calf (*Connochaetes taurinus*). *J S Afr Vet Assoc* 2018; **89**: 1–6.

218 Riebold T, Evans A, Robinson N. Evaluation of the demand valve for resuscitation of horses. *J Am Vet Med Assoc* 1980; **176**: 623–626.

219 Gabel A, Heath R, Ross J, *et al.* Hypoxia – its prevention in inhalation anesthesia in horses. *In: Proceedings of the 12th Annual Meeting of the American Association of Equine Practitioners*, Los Angeles, CA, 1966: 179–196.

220 Grandy J, Steffey E, Hodgson D, *et al.* Arterial hypotension and the development of postanesthetic myopathy in halothane-anesthetized horses. *Am J Vet Res* 1987; **48**: 192–197.

221 Grandy J, Hodgson D, Dunlop C, *et al.* Cardiopulmonary effects of ephedrine in halothane-anesthetized horses. *J Vet Pharmacol Ther* 1989; **12**: 389–396.

222 Daunt DA. Supportive therapy in the anesthetized horse. *Vet Clin North Am Equine Pract* 1990; **6**: 557–574.

223 Tranquilli W, Greene S. Cardiovascular medications and the autonomic nervous system. In: Short CS, ed. *Principles and Practice of Veterinary Anesthesia*. Baltimore, MD: Williams and Wilkins, 1987: 426–454.

224 Aarnes TK, Hubbell JA, Lerche P, *et al.* Comparison of invasive and oscillometric blood pressure measurement techniques in anesthetized sheep, goats, and cattle. *Vet Anaesth Analg* 2014; **41**: 174–185.

225 Aarnes TK, Hubbell JA, Lerche P, *et al.* Comparison of invasive and oscillometric blood pressure measurement techniques in anesthetized camelids. *Can Vet J* 2012; **53**: 881–885.

226 Manley SV. Monitoring the anesthetized horse. *Vet Clin North Am Large Anim Pract* 1981; **3**: 111–133.

227 Gallivan G, McDonell W, Forrest J. Comparative ventilation and gas exchange in the horse and the cow. *Res Vet Sci* 1989; **46**: 331–336.

228 Thurmon J, Romack F, Garner H. Excursions of the bovine eyeball during gaseous anesthesia. *Vet Med Small Anim Clin* 1968; **63**: 967–972.

229 Trefz FM, Lorenz I, Constable PD. Electrocardiographic findings in 130 hospitalized neonatal calves with diarrhea and associated potassium balance disorders. *J Vet Intern Med* 2018; **32**: 1447–1461.

230 Antzelevitch C, Shimizu W, Yan G, *et al.* The M cell: its contribution to the ECG and to normal and abnormal electrical function of the heart. *J Cardiovasc Electrophysiol* 1999; **10**: 1124–1152.

231 American College of Veterinary Anesthesia and Analgesia (ACVAA) Small Animal Monitoring Guidelines. www.acvaa.org/veterinarians/guidelines (accessed March 2023).

232 Quinn CT, Raisis AL, Musk GC. Evaluation of Masimo Signal Extraction Technology pulse oximetry in anaesthetized pregnant sheep. *Vet Anaesth Analg* 2013; **40**: 149–156.

233 Cribb PH. The effects of prolonged hypotensive isoflurane anesthesia in horses – post-anesthetic myopathy [Abstract]. *Vet Surg* 1988; **17**: 164–165.

234 Matthews N, Gleed R, Short C. Cardiopulmonary effects of general anesthesia in adult cattle. *Mod Vet Pract* 1986; **67**: 618–620.

235 Grandy JL, Hodgson DS. Anesthetic considerations for emergency equine abdominal surgery. *Vet Clin North Am Equine Pract* 1988; **4**: 63–78.

236 Riebold TW, Evans AT. Comparison of simultaneous blood-pressure determinations by four methods in the anesthetized horse. *Vet Surg* 1985; **14**: 332–337.

237 Riebold T, Brunson D, Lott R, *et al.* Percutaneous arterial catheterization in the horse. *Vet Med Small Anim Clin* 1980; **75**: 1736–1742.

238 Casoni D, Mirra A, Goepfert C, *et al.* Iatrogenic cerebral arterial gas embolism from flushing of the arterial line in two calves. *Acta Vet Scand* 2018; **60**: 1–6.

239 Moens Y, Gootjes P, Lagerweij E. The influence of methane on the infrared measurement of halothane in the horse. *J Vet Anaesth* 1991; **18**: 4–7.

240 Gootjes P, Moens Y. A simple method to correct infrared measurement of anaesthetic vapour concentration in the presence of methane. *J Vet Anaesth* 1997; **24**: 24–25.

241 Kruse-Elliott K, Riebold T, Swanson C. Reversal of xylazine–ketamine anesthesia in goats. [Abstract]. *Vet Surg* 1987; **16**: 321.

242 Riebold TW, Engel HN, Grubb TL, *et al.* Orotracheal and nasotracheal intubation in llamas. *J Am Vet Med Assoc* 1994; **204**: 779–783.

243 Skelding A, Valverde A. Intra-operative hyperthermia in a young Angus bull with a fatal outcome. *Can Vet J* 2017; **58**: 614–616.

244 Musewe V, Gillespie J, Berry J. Influence of ruminal insufflation on pulmonary function and diaphragmatic electromyography in cattle. *Am J Vet Res* 1979; **40**: 26–31.

245 Lumb WV, Jones EW. The inhalational anesthetics. In: Veterinary Anesthesia, *2nd edn*. Philadelphia, PA: Lea & Febiger, 1984: 213–239.

246 Heath R. General anesthesia in ruminants. In: Jennings PB, ed. *The Practice of Large Animal Surgery*. Philadelphia, PA: WB Saunders, 1984: 202–204.

247 Tayari H, Cuypers C, Schäffler L, *et al.* Fatal cardiac arrest in a calf with uroperitoneum. *Vet Rec Case Rep* 2019; **7**: e000730.

248 Muir W, Bednarski R. Equine cardiopulmonary resuscitation. Part 1. *Compend Contin Educ Pract Vet* 1983; **5**(Suppl): S228–S234.

249 Muir W, Bednarski R. Equine cardiopulmonary resuscitation. Part 2. *Compend Contin Educ Pract Vet* 1983; **5**(Suppl): S287–S295.

250 Hubbell J, Muir W, Gaynor J. Cardiovascular effects of thoracic compression in horses subjected to euthanasia. *Equine Vet J* 1993; **25**: 282–284.

251 Hildebrand S. Neuromuscular blocking agents in equine anesthesia. *Vet Clin North Am Equine Pract* 1990; **6**: 587–606.

252 Corley KTT. Fluid therapy for horses with gastrointestinal disease. In: Smith BP, ed. *Large Animal Internal Medicine*, 3rd edn. St Louis, MO: Mosby, 2002: 682–694.

253 Ames T, Baker J, Wikse S. The bronchopneumonias (respiratory disease complex of cattle, sheep, and goats). In: Smith BP, ed. *Large Animal Internal Medicine*, 3rd edn. St Louis, MO: Mosby, 2002: 551–570.

254 Skarda RT. Local and regional anesthesia in ruminants and swine. *Vet Clin North Am Food Anim Pract* 1996; **12**: 579–626.

255 George L. Pain control in food animals. In: Steffey EP, ed. *Recent Advances in Anesthetic Management of Large Domestic Animals*. Ithaca, NY: International Veterinary Information Service, 2003: A0615.1103.

256 Schulze I, Poos E, Meyer H, *et al.* Effects of preoperative carprofen on cardiorespiratory, hormonal and metabolic stress response in calves during umbilical surgery under isoflurane inhalation anaesthesia. *Vet J* 2016; **216**: 18–24.

257 Smith GW, Davis JL, Tell LA, *et al.* Extralabel use of nonsteroidal anti-inflammatory drugs in cattle. *J Am Vet Med Assoc* 2008; **232**: 697–701.

258 Plummer PJ, Schleining JA. Assessment and management of pain in small ruminants and camelids. *Vet Clin North Am Food Anim Pract* 2013; **29**: 185–208.

259 Smith JS, Schleining JA, Plummer P. Pain management in small ruminants and camelids – Applications and strategies. *Vet Clin North Am Food Anim Pract* 2021; **37**: 17–31.

260 Smith JS, Schleining JA, Plummer P. Pain management in small ruminants and camelids – Analgesic agents. *Vet Clin North Am Food Anim Pract* 2021; **37**: 1–16.

261 Navarre C, Ravis W, Nagilla R, *et al.* Pharmacokinetics of flunixin meglumine in llamas following a single intravenous dose. *J Vet Pharmacol Ther* 2001; **24**: 361–364.

262 Navarre C, Ravis W, Nagilla R, *et al.* Pharmacokinetics of phenylbutazone in llamas following single intravenous and oral doses. *J Vet Pharmacol Ther* 2001; **24**: 227–231.

263 Navarre C, Ravis W, Campbell J, *et al.* Stereoselective pharmacokinetics of ketoprofen in llamas following intravenous administration. *J Vet Pharmacol Ther* 2001; **24**: 223–226.

264 Machado Filho L, Hurnik J, Ewing K. A thermal threshold assay to measure the nociceptive response to morphine sulphate in cattle. *Can J Vet Res* 1998; **62**: 218–223.

265 Wagner AE. Opioids. In: Muir WW, Gaynor JS, eds. *Handbook of Veterinary Pain Management*. St Louis, MO: Mosby, 2002: 164–183.

266 Pascoe PJ. Opioid analgesics. *Vet Clin North Am Small Anim Pract* 2000; **30**: 757–772.

267 Bennett RC, Steffey EP. Use of opioids for pain and anesthetic management in horses. *Vet Clin North Am Equine Pract* 2002; **18**: 47–60.

268 Grubb TL, Gold JR, Schlipf JW, *et al.* Assessment of serum concentrations and sedative effects of fentanyl after transdermal administration at three dosages in healthy llamas. *Am J Vet Res* 2005; **66**: 907–909.

269 Burke MJ, Soma LR, Boston RC, *et al.* Evaluation of the analgesic and pharmacokinetic properties of transdermally administered fentanyl in goats. *J Vet Emerg Crit Care (San Antonio)* 2017; **27**: 539–547.

270 Buchholz T, Hildebrand M, Heider A, *et al.* Transdermal fentanyl uptake at two different patch locations in Swiss White Alpine sheep. *Animals (Basel)* 2020; **10**: 1675.

271 Torske KE, Dyson DH. Epidural analgesia and anesthesia. *Vet Clin North Am Small Anim Pract* 2000; **30**: 859–874.

272 Gaynor JS, Mama KR. Local and regional anesthetic techniques for alleviation of perioperative pain. In Gaynor JS, Muir WW, eds. *Handbook of Veterinary Pain Management*, 2nd edn. St. Louis, MO: Elsevier, 2009: 277–300.

273 Robinson EP, Natalini CC. Epidural anesthesia and analgesia in horses. *Vet Clin North Am Equine Pract* 2002; **18**: 61–82.

65 Swine

Lais M. Malavasi
Department of Veterinary Clinical Sciences, College of Veterinary Medicine, Washington State University, Pullman, Washington, USA

Chapter contents

Introduction, 1285
Preanesthetic considerations, 1285
Fasting, 1285
Handling and restraint, 1285
Drug administration, 1286
Premedication, 1286
Parasympatholytic drugs, 1287
Sedation and chemical restraint, 1287
Induction of anesthesia, 1288
Orotracheal intubation, 1290
Maintenance of anesthesia, 1291
Monitoring, 1293
Supportive therapies, 1294
Recovery considerations, 1295
Malignant hyperthermia, 1295
Analgesia, 1295
References, 1297

Introduction

Pigs are anesthetized for a variety of reasons, including diagnostic, surgical, and experimental procedures. The general approach to anesthesia of the pig is similar whether the patient is a pet, a research animal, or an eventual food source, though the physical and regulatory environments may be quite different. Veterinary surgical procedures performed in pigs under field conditions are usually limited to minor operations such as hernia repair and castration [1]. In contrast, when used in biomedical research, the animal may be subjected to complicated and invasive surgical procedures that require more advanced analgesic and anesthetic techniques. When managing animal species that are commonly used as a food source, withdrawal times for sedatives and anesthetics should be discussed with the owner since even pet pigs occasionally end up in the food chain [2].

Preanesthetic considerations

Fasting

Presurgical fasting time for pigs should be at least 12 h, though the stomach may still contain food due to the torus pyloricus, which is well developed in pigs. A full stomach may increase the risk of gastric dilation, nausea, vomiting, regurgitation, and aspiration. An overloaded stomach can produce significant pressure on the diaphragm, decreasing pulmonary functional residual capacity and alveolar ventilation [3]. When the surgical objective is to manipulate gastrointestinal or abdominal organs, the fasting time should be increased to 24–48 h to empty the large bowel. Neonates should be deprived of food for no more than 3 h in order to prevent hypoglycemia. All edible bedding must be removed from the cage in the fasting period, because pigs will readily consume it otherwise [4]. Water consumption is allowed until premedication is imminent although 4–6 h of complete *nil per os* may be warranted if the pig is going to undergo gastric or upper small bowel surgery [5].

Handling and restraint

Pigs can be difficult to restrain because of their body shape and lack of appendages that can be readily grasped by handlers [3]. Aggressive and/or fearful pigs pose several challenges from being difficult to fully evaluate to presenting a safety hazard to the staff and owners. Restraint can be facilitated by adapting the pig to the presence of humans and manipulation, resulting in a less stressful environment. In research environments, animals should be acclimatized at the institution for 2–3 weeks prior to experimental procedures [6]. During this time, the pigs should be spoken to and handled in a calm manner. However, in situations where time is limited and the animal is not trained, a partition known as a "crowd panel" or "hog board" can be used to isolate the pig in a corner or against a wall. This partition may be constructed of wood, plastic, or metal and should be the same height as the animal and

Veterinary Anesthesia and Analgesia: The Sixth Edition of Lumb and Jones. Edited by Leigh Lamont, Kurt Grimm, Sheilah Robertson, Lydia Love and Carrie Schroeder.
© 2024 John Wiley & Sons, Inc. Published 2024 by John Wiley & Sons, Inc.
Companion website: www.wiley.com/go/lamont/anesthesia

two-thirds to the full length of the pig. The hog board is used to protect the handler during examination or intramuscular (IM) injection.

Pigs can be restrained using other methods as well. For small pigs, the animal's hind legs can be lifted by one hand, while the other is placed under the chest to provide support. However, pigs weighing more than 10 kg can be very strong and difficult to lift. These swine can be guided into a transport cart or coaxed out of the pen and into the cart with small amounts of food or treats. Another method of immobilization is the sling, where the pig is placed in a hammock with four holes for the limbs. This hammock is supported by a metal frame to which its limbs are loosely tied. One disadvantage is that the pig must be trained to use of the sling. A pig flipping technique has been described for either routine care in unsedated animals or to restrain sedated pigs for catheter placement or face-mask induction [7,8]. Finally, the use of a back scratcher or "pig fork" has been promoted as a method of relaxation and distraction for pigs undergoing medical care.

For owned pigs, prehospital sedation can dramatically improve the response to handling and restraint in hospital. Oral (PO) trazodone (8–10 mg/kg PO) and gabapentin (20 mg/kg PO) may be helpful when administered together the night before and again 2 h prior to the veterinary visit [8].

Drug administration

Intranasal delivery can be used as a needleless route of drug administration in pigs. For example, Axiak *et al.* described intranasal administration of a mixture of ketamine 15 mg/kg, climazolam 1.5 mg/kg, and azaperone 1.0 mg/kg prior to castration. Drug administration is achieved using a catheter without the stylet and injected during inspiration in small volumes. Intranasal administration resulted in less effective anesthesia than IM injection, but with the advantages of minor temperature loss and shorter recovery time [9]. Lacoste *et al.* reported that the optimal intranasal midazolam dose in piglets was 0.2 mg/kg, producing rapid and reliable sedation [10].

Anesthetic induction of pigs can be complicated due to their behavior when physically restrained and the small number of vessels available for intravenous (IV) injections. Thus, IM administration of drugs is often preferred for initial immobilization and, in some situations, for induction of anesthesia in pigs. Intraperitoneal injection is described but requires specific training. Also, the consequences of improper administration can be severe if injection into the urinary bladder, intestines, or other organs occurs [11]. For IM injection in pigs, the muscles of the thigh are commonly used as the site of injection in piglets, but this is not recommended in growers/finishers because of the possibility of causing an abscess or needle breakage in edible tissue. Appropriate IM administration in adult pigs is behind the base of the ear where the layer of fat is thinner and the tissues have good perfusion [12]. Adequate needle size varies with the size of the animal, from a 20 gauge needle for a piglet up to a 14 gauge needle for a grower/finisher pig. Needles that are too short may result in injection of the drug into the fatty tissue, delaying the absorption, distribution, and ultimately the action of the anesthetic agent [3]. The use of a Luer-lock needle and a low-flow extension set connected to a syringe may reduce stress during the IM injection, allowing the administration of drugs from a relative distance from the animal. Alternately, a butterfly catheter can be used for IM injections in smaller animals [13]. Subcutaneous (SC) injection can be used in smaller or miniature pigs (e.g., Yorkshire and Yucatan). As pigs have very tight connective tissue, there are limited areas for SC injection such as the loose flap on the lateral cervical region [6,14], the axillary area caudal to the elbow, or in the inguinal region in the flank area [8].

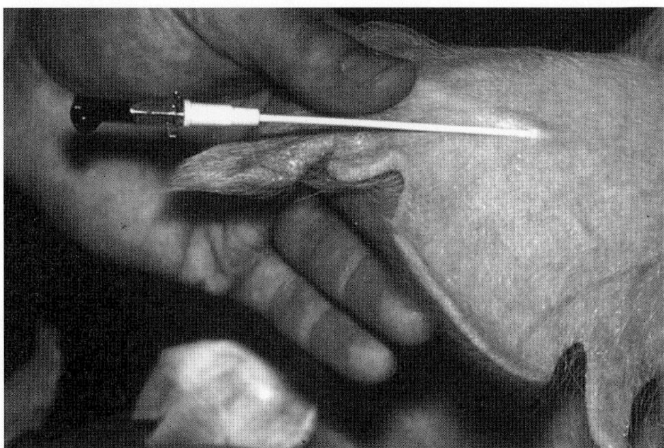

Figure 65.1 Catheterization of the auricular vein of a Landrace sow with a 16 gauge catheter. A tourniquet has been placed at the base of the ear to distend the veins.

Pigs have limited superficial veins that can be accessed easily to inject drugs. The marginal ear veins (i.e., auricular veins) are the only veins that are easily visible on pigs of any size (Fig. 65.1). In larger animals, the lateral and medial veins on the outer surface of the ears are preferable because of their increased size. A rubber band can be placed around the base of the ear to facilitate distention of the auricular veins [15]. The central auricular vessels are usually arteries (as in the rabbit) and should not be used for drug administration. Note that ear notching to identify pigs can damage some of these vessels.

Another option for venous access is the cephalic vein located along the craniomedial surface of the leg. This vein usually cannot be visualized but may be entered using blind venipuncture after applying a tourniquet [16]. In small pigs, it may be visualized continuing across the ventral surface of the neck after applying digital pressure at the thoracic inlet. The saphenous vein, on the lateral surface of the rear leg, is usually not a reliable injection site. Larger vessels such as the external or internal jugular vein or anterior vena cava can be catheterized but are usually reserved for blood sample collection or in research settings [5]. The subcutaneous abdominal vein (cranial superficial epigastric vein) is an alternative to the auricular vein for blood collection and IV administration of fluids and medication. This vein courses along the ventral portion of the abdomen and lies dorsolateral to the mammary chain. Firm digital pressure applied directly behind the elbow joint, along the thorax, will assist in visualization and/or palpation of this vein [17]. The subcutaneous abdominal vein can be useful for administration of large volumes of fluids, whereas auricular vessels are fragile and catheters may fail.

Premedication

Anesthesia and analgesia may produce nausea and vomiting in some animals, including pigs. Antiemetics such as maropitant (0.5–1 mg/kg PO/SC q24 h) can be considered at least 1 h prior to premedication of the pig [15,18]. Maropitant is a potent, selective neurokinin-1 receptor antagonist that blocks the binding of the neurotransmitter substance P. This substance is found in high concentrations in both the chemoreceptor trigger zone and the vomiting center and is a key neurotransmitter involved in vomiting in dogs and cats [19].

Parasympatholytic drugs

Atropine and glycopyrrolate are the two principal parasympatholytic drugs used in pigs. The use of these anticholinergic agents together with sedative/analgesic premedications may decrease the possibility of bradycardia caused by such agents as morphine, thiopental, and xylazine [20–23]. Anticholinergic agents also reduce bronchoconstriction, diminish airway secretion volume, and inhibit salivation, possibly improving conditions for orotracheal intubation. However, neither anticholinergic agent is routinely required, and it should be noted that an increased heart rate results in increased myocardial work and oxygen consumption.

In emergent situations in pigs without an IV catheter, atropine (and other resuscitation drugs, including epinephrine) can be administered via the endotracheal tube. Hörnchen *et al.* [24] concluded that 2 mg of atropine diluted in 5–10 mL of saline and instilled in the endotracheal tube was rapidly absorbed by the pulmonary circulation and increased heart rate within 1 min after administration. Compared to baseline, significant increases in heart rate were documented between 9 and 30 min after endotracheal instillation and between 12 and 15 min after IV injection.

Sedation and chemical restraint

The major sedatives that are commonly used in pigs are butyrophenones, phenothiazines, benzodiazepines, and α_2-adrenergic receptor agonists [25]. As azaperone, acepromazine, and the benzodiazepines offer minimal analgesia, these drugs should be given in combination with other agents for invasive surgical procedures. Any full μ-opioid receptor agonist can be administered to pigs, typically at doses similar to those used in dogs. In many situations, a lack of cooperativity on the part of the pig may make chemical restraint or IM induction of anesthesia an attractive approach.

Azaperone (Stresnil®) is one of the most widely used sedatives in pigs where it is available [16]. This drug is classified as a short-acting butyrophenone neuroleptic agent and is relatively safe compared to other drugs in this same category, such as haloperidol, when given intramuscularly [21]. IV injection of azaperone is contraindicated because it may cause excitation [20]. Azaperone may be used as a sedative in combination with local anesthetics for minor surgical procedures, as a premedicant with anxiolytic properties, as an anxiolytic in weanlings when they are mixed for the first time, and in maiden sows after their first litter to reduce the rejection of piglets [16]. The effects of azaperone are dose-dependent wherein doses of 0.25 mg/kg produce mild sedation without ataxia in domestic pigs, 0.5–2 mg/kg will produce greater sedation but with mild ataxia, and doses of 2–4 mg/kg produce significant sedation and possible recumbency in adult pigs [21,26]. In younger pigs, it may be necessary to use a much higher dose of azaperone, such as 8 mg/kg, for appropriate sedation [3]. Vietnamese Pot-bellied pigs require a dose of 0.25–2 mg/kg for sedation and a higher dose of 2–8 mg/kg for induction of anesthesia. However, doses exceeding 2 mg/kg are also more likely to cause adverse effects such as hypotension, bradycardia, and decreased cardiac output and contractility [21]. Note that in large boars, it has been suggested that azaperone doses should not exceed 1 mg/kg in order to reduce the risk of priapism [20].

Azaperone can be combined with other drugs to improve sedation and reduce its dosage, decreasing negative effects. Flores *et al.* suggested that azaperone (2 mg/kg) and xylazine (2 mg/kg) given intramuscularly produced good sedation and muscular relaxation [27]. Others have reported that animals pretreated with azaperone (2 mg/kg) and anesthetized with ketamine (15 mg/kg IM) and midazolam (0.3 mg/kg IM) demonstrated a good anesthetic induction and analgesia [28]. A combination of azaperone (4 mg/kg) and midazolam (1 mg/kg) provides sedation in Göttingen minipigs [4].

Acepromazine is a phenothiazine that can be used as part of a sedative combination in pigs, although by itself its sedative effects are often considered inadequate. Acepromazine is contraindicated in debilitated animals due to its potential adverse effects such as hypotension, bradycardia, hypothermia, and decreased respiratory rate [20,21]. The recommended IM dose of acepromazine is 0.03–0.1 mg/kg; however, in Göttingen minipigs, higher doses of 0.1–0.45 mg/kg have been suggested [4].

α_2-Adrenergic receptor agonists, such as xylazine, romifidine, medetomidine, and dexmedetomidine, are widely used in pigs, usually in combination with a dissociative agent. Note that pigs require higher doses of α_2-adrenergic receptor agonists than ruminants. Ketamine at a dose of 10–12 mg/kg IM with a dose of 1–2 mg/kg of xylazine will immobilize a pig in approximately 5 min [29]. However, this combination decreases cardiac output significantly for 30 min after administration and the arterial partial pressure of oxygen (PaO_2) may decrease, whereas total vascular resistance increases [30]. Sakaguchi *et al.* demonstrated that ketamine (10 mg/kg) and medetomidine (80 μg/kg) IM induced chemical restraint for 49.4 min on average, which was 14.8 min longer than a xylazine (2 mg/kg) and ketamine (10 mg/kg) combination [31]. In addition, the duration of muscle relaxation in pigs is twice as long with dexmedetomidine–ketamine as with the xylazine–ketamine mixture. In another study, Sakaguchi *et al.* studied ketamine and medetomidine combined with 25 μg/kg of atropine and concluded that the cardiovascular effects were limited in healthy pigs [32]. A combination of ketamine (8 mg/kg), romifidine (0.12 mg/kg), and butorphanol (0.1 mg/kg) given IM provides reliable anesthesia for 20–30 min after a single injection [33].

All of the combinations containing α_2-adrenergic receptor agonists offer the advantage of being reversible by yohimbine (0.1–0.2 mg/kg IM, IV), atipamezole (0.12–1 mg/kg IM, IV, SC), or tolazoline (1–2 mg/kg IV, IM) [34–36]. The reversal of the α_2-adrenergic receptor agonist is independent of the metabolism and clearance of ketamine. Therefore, when the α_2-adrenergic receptor agonist is reversed before the effect of the ketamine has waned, an undesirable recovery may result (e.g., hyperkinesia of limbs, severe and prolonged ataxia, and vocalization) [21].

Adding another muscle relaxant drug to anesthetic combinations should provide a better recovery following reversal of α_2-adrenergic receptor agonists. Ajadi *et al.* reported using ketamine at 20 mg/kg IM with xylazine (2 mg/kg IM) and midazolam (0.25 mg/kg IM). This combination appeared to almost double the duration of anesthesia with adequate analgesia for at least 30 min, compared to a lower dose of ketamine (10 mg/kg IM) added to this same combination of drugs [23]. However, recoveries after benzodiazepine–ketamine combinations are longer than xylazine–ketamine sedation. The administration of one part flumazenil (benzodiazepine antagonist) to 13 parts of a benzodiazepine agonist should reduce the recovery time in pigs. However, if flumazenil is given before ketamine effects are diminishing, the recovery will be similar to that with ketamine alone [3,21].

Opioids can be used in anesthetic combinations in swine. Ketamine (10 mg/kg), medetomidine (80 μg/kg), and butorphanol (0.2 mg/kg) given intramuscularly prolonged the duration of the loss of protective reflexes in pigs and permitted surgical procedures to be performed for at least 30 min [32]. Another option is to use tramadol, where available, instead of butorphanol. Tramadol appears to cause less respiratory depression compared with morphine or other μ-opioid receptor agonists [37]. Pigs that received tramadol (5 mg/kg IM) prior to sedation with ketamine (25 mg/kg), xylazine (2.5 mg/kg), and atropine (0.04 mg/kg) intramuscularly had better quality of sedation that facilitated endotracheal intubation compared to the saline, ketamine, and xylazine treated animals. Also, this combination increased the duration of analgesia compared to ketamine–xylazine sedation [38]. At present, tramadol is not available in an injectable form in a number of countries including the United States. Morphine and fentanyl are widely used as analgesics for pet and research pigs, though this species may be relatively resistant to the minimum alveolar concentration (MAC)-reducing effects [39–41]. Pigs appear to require higher doses of buprenorphine than dogs [42].

If chemical restraint or IM induction to anesthesia is desired, an actual anesthetic agent must be included in the drug protocol. Ketamine is the most commonly used dissociative anesthetic in humans, non-human primates, cats, laboratory animals, and pigs. Ketamine has a wide safety margin as it generally stimulates cardiovascular function via its sympathomimetic effect [23,43]. Another advantage is that it can be given intramuscularly as well as intravenously. However, dissociative agents given alone can cause analgesia with no muscle relaxation, referred to as a "cataleptoid state," as well as excessive salivation and hyperresponsiveness during recovery [3,16]. To minimize these negative effects, ketamine is combined with adjunctive agents to improve muscle relaxation, decreasing the ketamine dose required to achieve effective immobilization (Table 65.1). Yucatan and Yorkshire pigs may require a higher dose of ketamine and midazolam to be fully sedated compared to other breeds. For 5–10 min of sedation in Yucatan pigs, a combination of ketamine (25 mg/kg) and midazolam (0.6 mg/kg) can be used. For Yorkshire pigs, ketamine (5 mg/kg) combined with midazolam (0.5 mg/kg) is usually sufficient [14]. It should be noted that in this study, the combination of drugs was given subcutaneously in the lateral cervical region, which may have contributed to the relatively greater dosages needed.

Recently, several reports involving alfaxalone as part of sedation/anesthesia protocols have been published. Alfaxalone is a synthetic neuroactive steroid, which activates the $GABA_A$ receptor [44], producing anesthesia and some muscular relaxation but no analgesia. The new formulation of alfaxalone-2-hydroxypropyl-β-cyclodextrin, (Alfaxan®) has been used IV at a dose of 0.7–0.9 mg/kg in pigs premedicated with azaperone [45]. This formulation of alfaxalone has been administered successfully IM in pigs alone or in combination with other agents. IM injection of 5 mg/kg of alfaxalone with 0.5 mg/kg of diazepam produced a rapid onset of recumbency and deep sedation with minimal side effects in pigs [46]. Alfaxalone (5 mg/kg) and dexmedetomidine (10 μg/kg) IM also induced moderate to deep sedation with fair to smooth quality in pigs [47]. The main limitation for using alfaxalone in pigs is the large volume of injection required with the currently available 10 mg/mL alfaxalone solution, easily 10–20 mL depending on the size of the pig [45].

Table 65.1 Drugs and drug combinations used as premedication in pigs.

Drug	Dose (mg/kg)	Route	Primary references
Parasympatholytic agents			
Atropine	0.02–0.05	IM, IV, SC	[3]
Glycopyrrolate	0.004–0.01	IM, IV, SC	
Sedatives and tranquilizers (alone or in combination)			
Acepromazine	0.2–0.5	IM	[36]
Azaperone	0.5–2	IM	[36]
Diazepam	0.1–0.5 0.5–2	PO IM	[36]
Ketamine	0.5–20	IM	[36]
Medetomidine	0.04–0.08	IM	[36]
Midazolam	0.2–5	IM	[36]
Xylazine	0.5–2.2	IM	[36]
Tiletamine–zolazepam	3–6	IM	[36]
Alfaxalone plus dexmedetomidine	5 0.01	IM	[47]
Alfaxalone plus diazepam	5 0.5	IM	[46]
Azaperone plus midazolam	4 1	IM	[4]
Azaperone plus xylazine	2 2	IM	[27]
Azaperone plus ketamine plus midazolam	2 15 0.3	IM	[28]
Ketamine plus xylazine	10–20 1–2	IM	[48]
Ketamine plus acepromazine	10–20 1.1	IM	[49]
Ketamine plus xylazine plus butorphanol	5 1–3 0.1–0.2	IM	[50]
Ketamine plus xylazine plus midazolam	20 2 0.25	IM	[23]
Ketamine plus detomidine plus butorphanol	5–10 0.05–0.1 0.1–0.2	IM	[50]
Ketamine plus dexmedetomidine plus midazolam	5–20 0.01–0.02 0.2	IM	[15]
Ketamine plus xylazine plus tramadol	25 2.5 5	IM	[44]
Xylazine plus midazolam plus butorphanol	1 0.2 0.2–0.4	IM	[8]
Xylazine–ketamine–Telazol®[a]	0.006–0.012 mL/kg	IM	[36]

IM, intramuscular; IV, intravenous; SC, subcutaneous; PO, oral.
[a] Reconstitute 500 mg Telazol® powder with 2.5 mL of 100 mg/mL xylazine and 2.5 mL of 100 mg/mL ketamine; dose expressed as mL/kg.

Induction of anesthesia

Induction to anesthesia can be accomplished by IM, inhalant, or IV routes, or a combination thereof (Table 65.2). When anesthesia is being induced with an inhalant agent (e.g., 3–5% isoflurane or 4–6% sevoflurane) in a mixture with oxygen (4–8 L/min) through a face mask, there is a minimal amount of time to complete intubation once the face mask is removed. When the face mask is applied against the nose of the pig, the anesthetist should observe the breathing pattern (which should be regular) and determine the anesthetic stage the patient is in. Once relaxation is adequate, the face mask is removed and quickly the mouth of the pig is opened and the laryngeal opening is sprayed with lidocaine prior to endotracheal

Table 65.2 Drugs and drug combinations used for induction of anesthesia in pigs.

Drug	Dose (mg/kg)	Route	Primary references
Inhalant agents			
Isoflurane	3–5%	Inhalation	[49]
Sevoflurane	3–5%	Inhalation	[53]
Injectable agents and combinations			
Alfaxalone	4–6 0.9	IM IV	[3,16,54] [45,54]
α-Chloralose	40	IV	[55]
Ketamine	4–6	IV	[3,16]
Propofol	2–5	IV	[16,56]
Remifentanil	0.004–0.005	IV	[57]
Thiopental[a]	10–20	IV	[3]
Thiamylal[a]	6–18	IV	[3,20]
α-Chloralose plus morphine	55–86 0.3–0.9	IV IM	[3]
Etomidate plus xylazine or azaperone	2–4 1–2 2–4	IV IM, IV IM, IV	[3]
Ketamine plus xylazine plus acepromazine	10–15 2 0.2	IM, SC	[58]
Propofol plus fentanyl	2 0.005	IV	[6]
Propofol plus medetomidine or xylazine	2–4 0.02–0.04 1–2	IV	[3]
Tiletamine–zolazepam plus xylazine	2–8 1.3	IM	[13]
Tiletamine–zolazepam plus medetomidine	5 0.05	IM	[52]
Metomidate plus azaperone	4 2–4	IV	[59]
Metomidate plus azaperone	10 2	IP IM	[11]

IM, intramuscular; IV, intravenous; IP, intraperitoneal, SC, subcutaneous.
[a] No longer available in many countries.

intubation [3,6]. Although induction of anesthesia by administration of inhalant anesthetic agents through a mask is possible, it requires effective manual restraint. Pigs that are not trained will often resent handling and placement of the face mask [51]. Thus, to avoid stress, it is appropriate to have a well-sedated animal before the induction of anesthesia, either with oral or injectable agents [52].

Induction to anesthesia is often accomplished by IV injection of an anesthetic agent into an auricular vein. Placement of an indwelling IV catheter facilitates this process. Ketamine combined with midazolam, propofol alone, or propofol with co-induction agents are the drugs most commonly used for inducing anesthesia in pigs, due to their fast-acting effects and short recovery time. In pigs that have been sedated with an IM combination of ketamine and xylazine, anesthesia can be induced using an additional 4–6 mg/kg of ketamine IV [3,16]. IV administration of induction agents should be slow and titrated to effect in order to avoid apnea, since endotracheal intubation can be somewhat challenging.

Though no longer available in many countries, thiopental and thiamylal are thiobarbiturates that have been extensively used for induction prior to inhalation maintenance. Like most injectable anesthetics, thiobarbiturates can cause apnea, so a means of intubation and positive-pressure ventilation should be available. A self-reinflating bag (i.e., Ambu-bag®) can be used for this purpose. To avoid tissue necrosis, the thiobarbiturates must be given IV, with induction doses for thiopental and thiamylal ranging from 10–20 and 6–18 mg/kg, respectively. The higher dose is indicated for unpremedicated young pigs, and the lower dose should be adequate for sedated animals. Prior to administration of a thiobarbiturate, adjunctive drugs such as xylazine (1–2 mg/kg IV), ketamine (2–4 mg/kg IV), or diazepam (2–4 mg/kg IV) may be given. Another use for thiopental is to abolish laryngeal reflexes with a small dose (4–6 mg/kg, IV) after administration of a dissociative anesthetic (i.e., ketamine) [3]. Thiopental and thiamylal may produce prolonged recovery if an infusion or repeated doses are used to extend anesthesia [21].

Propofol (2–5 mg/kg IV) is an induction agent that must be administered intravenously [16, 56]. Unlike the thiobarbiturates, however, extravascular injection of propofol does not cause tissue injury (an advantage in unpremedicated swine), and it can be given through the auricular vein without concern about phlebitis [21]. Propofol is a hypnotic that has minimal analgesic effects, so it is frequently combined with analgesic drugs (i.e., opioids or α_2-adrenergic receptor agonists). Induction of anesthesia in pigs with an IV bolus of fentanyl (5 μg/kg) followed by the administration of propofol (2 mg/kg IV) allows tracheal intubation [6]. Alternatively, dexmedetomidine (20–40 μg/kg IV) followed by propofol (2–4 mg/kg IV) may be used for induction in pigs weighing 30–60 kg. The use of remifentanil combined with propofol for the purpose of induction of anesthesia in swine has been reported [60].

Remifentanil by itself will allow intubation in pigs premedicated with a combination of ketamine (30 mg/kg), midazolam (0.75 mg/kg), and atropine (0.05 mg/kg) IM. A dose of 4–5 μg/kg of remifentanil IV resulted in better vocal cord position, better response to intubation, shorter time required for intubation, and a decreased requirement for additional administration of midazolam postintubation compared to animals receiving just ketamine and midazolam. This protocol was not associated with serious side effects other than a light level of muscle relaxation and sedation, which require a skilled anesthetist to intubate these animals [57].

Other agents that can be used for induction of anesthesia in pigs include etomidate, alfaxalone, and α-chloralose. Available formulations of etomidate contain high concentrations of propylene glycol and are hypertonic, potentially causing hemolysis following high cumulative doses. Etomidate does not significantly affect the cardiovascular system, maintaining stability in critical patients, although it is reported to suppress adrenocortical activity in humans and dogs for 24 h after administration [61,62]. In addition, etomidate may cause pain during IV administration, spontaneous involuntary muscle movement, tremor, and hypertonus when given alone [59]. Also, while etomidate produces adequate sedation/hypnosis at doses of 2–4 mg/kg, it is associated with relatively poor analgesia and muscle relaxation. Therefore, it is recommended to administer other adjunctive drugs (e.g., α_2-adrenergic receptor agonists, benzodiazepines, or opioids) concomitantly. Etomidate has been used in an experimental setting for induction of anesthesia at a dose of 0.6 mg/kg IV and then followed by a ketamine infusion rate of 10 mg/kg/h IV to maintain anesthesia [63]. Etomidate does not trigger malignant hyperthermia in susceptible pigs [64].

Alfaxalone at doses of 5–6 mg/kg IV provides anesthesia in pigs for 10–15 min. This dose can be decreased if xylazine (1–2 mg/kg IM) or azaperone (4 mg/kg IM) is given previously. The anesthesia produced by alfaxalone can be maintained by repeated IV injection of doses of 2–4 mg/kg [3]. Alfaxalone can also be given intramuscularly, but the maximum dose of 6 mg/kg should be observed due to excessive volume for this administration route. Anesthesia lasts for around 15 min, and it may be rather unpredictable [16]. In 2017, Bigby *et al.* reported that the dose of alfaxalone to induce anesthesia in pigs can be as little as 0.9 mg/kg IV after alfaxalone (4 mg/kg), medetomidine (40 μg/kg), and butorphanol (0.4 mg/kg) IM premedication [54].

α-Chloralose is an injectable anesthetic that induces a range of dose-dependent central nervous system effects, both excitatory and inhibitory. It is exclusively used for non-survival experiments that require prolonged anesthesia with minimal surgical intervention since it provides poor analgesia when used alone. In particular, this agent may be selected when cardiovascular stability and lack of baroreceptor depression are desired [65]. However, its negative properties include poor solubility, slow onset of action (15–20 min), development of metabolic acidosis, hyper-reactivity to auditory stimulation, peritonitis, and ileus [66]. To anesthetize pigs with α-chloralose, a loading dose of 40 mg/kg IV is required, while a surgical depth of anesthesia can be maintained with a constant infusion rate of 10 mg/kg/h IV [67]. Also, α-chloralose at a dose of 55–86 mg/kg IV can be combined with morphine (0.3–0.9 mg/kg IM) or the combination of ketamine (5–10 mg/kg IV or IM) and butorphanol (0.5 mg/kg IV or IM) to improve analgesia and anesthesia. Mechanical ventilation is recommended to prevent hypercapnia and respiratory acidosis [4].

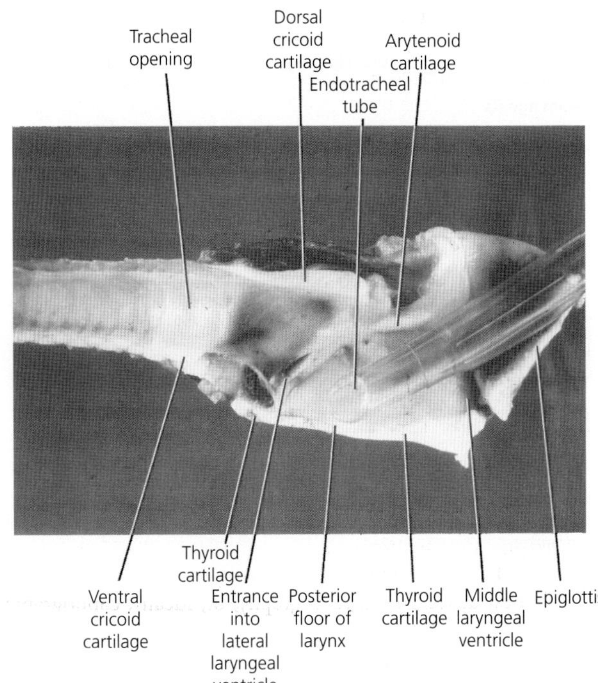

Figure 65.2 A sagittal view of a pig's larynx and trachea. Note the acute angle between the posterior portion of the larynx and the tracheal opening. Passage of the endotracheal tube is often difficult because of the entrapment of its tip in the floor of the larynx. Prior placement of a stylet through the tracheal opening will prevent entrapment of the endotracheal tube in the laryngeal ventricle just anterior to the thyroid cartilage and the posterior floor of the larynx anterior to the cricoid cartilage when the tube is passed into the trachea.

Orotracheal intubation

Orotracheal intubation for maintenance of general anesthesia is important in pigs undergoing procedures lasting longer than a few minutes, or when unconscious animals are placed in dorsal recumbency, which can otherwise result in hypoxemia, hypercapnia, or airway obstruction. Most sedatives, tranquilizers, and general anesthetic agents cause respiratory depression that can be severe in pigs due to the need for heavy sedation to decrease stress, and also because of the increased work of breathing imposed by the narrow upper airway in this species. In addition, pigs are very prone to laryngospasm, and fluid tends to accumulate in the pharyngeal region under anesthesia. While intubation of swine may be challenging, after some training, it can be successfully accomplished quickly and efficiently.

The major difficulty during orotracheal intubation is limited visualization of the larynx due to the pig's unique anatomy. They have a thick tongue, a long, narrow oropharyngeal space, and the elongated soft palate often obstructs the epiglottis. Swine also have a long pharyngeal diverticulum (3–4 cm in adults, 1 cm in piglets), which protrudes from the wall of the pharynx, above the esophagus. The angle between the floor of the lateral ventricles and the trachea, caudal to the opening of the larynx, is obtuse and can make intubation difficult (Fig. 65.2) [55,68]. If an endotracheal tube is inserted too deeply beyond the level of the thoracic inlet, it may block the right cranial bronchus (tracheal bronchus), thus compromising ventilation of that lung lobe and leading to poor gas exchange or difficulty maintaining inhalant anesthetic depth [21,69,70]. If the endotracheal tube diameter is too large, it can traumatize the delicate laryngeal mucosa, resulting in serious consequences. Formation of a hematoma or generalized laryngeal edema may go unnoticed during anesthesia but may result in respiratory distress at extubation [3,16].

When intubating a pig, the size of cuffed endotracheal tube should be selected according to the animal's weight. Endotracheal tube sizes can range from 3–4 mm internal diameter (ID) in piglets up to up to 16–18 mm ID in large boars or sows. Most pigs used in surgical research weigh 10–25 kg, and for these, a 6–7 mm ID endotracheal tube is appropriate [11]. The endotracheal tube should be measured and if necessary cut to a length equal to the distance from the tip of the animal's nostrils to the level of its shoulder [55]. Once selected, it is practical to have at hand three different sizes of endotracheal tube: the one thought to be correct, one size larger, and one size smaller [3].

Preoxygenation is always prudent but especially if orotracheal intubation may be challenging (e.g., space-occupying mass in the larynx) or when the anesthetist has little experience with swine intubation. It is recommended that the animal is preoxygenated with 100% oxygen through a face mask for 5–10 min unless the stress of restraint makes preoxygenation unreasonable [55].

Pigs can be intubated in dorsal or ventral recumbency, though ventral (sternal) recumbency is easier and faster for less experienced personnel [68]. Gauze strips are placed behind the upper and lower canine teeth to assist in opening of the pig's mouth. Ideally, the animal's head should not be overly extended as this will make the arytenoid cartilages more difficult to identify and, in some cases, may even occlude the airway. To improve the visualization of the larynx, use of a laryngoscope with a long, straight (Miller) blade with a curved tip of at least 195 mm long for pigs up to 50 kg is helpful. For animals weighing more than 50 kg, a blade of 205 mm with an extension (4–8 cm) is more appropriate. Once the larynx is visualized, the arytenoids should be sprayed with 2% lidocaine to decrease laryngospasm and coughing. Succinylcholine (1–2 mg/kg IV) has been suggested for abolishing the laryngospasm; however, this drug causes transient muscle paralysis needing immediate ventilatory support and can trigger malignant hyperthermia in susceptible pigs. The laryngoscope should be inserted into the mouth of the pig and the tip gently pressed ventrally at the base of the tongue until the vocal cords can be visualized. A plastic guide stylet (such as an airway exchange catheter or a polypropylene urinary catheter) can be used to assist intubation. This stylet should be made of malleable atraumatic material and should be three times the length of the endotracheal tube chosen. The stylet can be first placed into the larynx and the endotracheal tube subsequently threaded over it. If the tube encounters resistance at the laryngeal ventricle and cannot be inserted further, it should be gently rotated 180° so that it continues into the trachea. Note that when using a stiff guide stylet, it must be held in place while the endotracheal tube is being inserted in order to avoid deep advancement of the stylet, resulting in bronchial and peribronchial injuries. The guide stylet should then be carefully removed, leaving the endotracheal tube in place, which can be secured with a gauze tie over the animal's snout or behind its ears. Correct placement of the endotracheal tube can be confirmed by noticing expired air moving through the tube, by visual confirmation via laryngoscopy, through bilateral chest auscultation, radiography, or, ideally, capnography. The endotracheal tube cuff should be inflated to a pressure that prevents air escape around the tube when manual ventilation is applied to a pressure of 20–30 cmH_2O [3,21,55].

If orotracheal intubation is not possible or desired, alternatives for providing oxygen should be implemented. At a minimum, an oxygen mask can be employed and suction should be available in case of regurgitation or vomiting. Laryngeal mask airways (LMAs) and laryngeal tube airways have been evaluated for swine anesthesia. The researchers who first described the use of a standard LMA, which was designed for humans, noted that airway management was greatly simplified compared to orotracheal intubation, but it was also reported that gastric insufflation occurred in pigs during mechanical ventilation [3,71]. Use of an LMA allows a pig to be mechanically ventilated during general anesthesia with isoflurane with similar tidal volume and minute volume compared to endotracheally intubated animals [72]. One major limitation of the standard LMA is the potential risk of aspiration, as pigs can never be considered starved and the LMA does not seal the trachea, as does a cuffed endotracheal tube. The LMA-ProSeal™ is a modified double-cuff tube with an esophageal drainage tube that forms a more effective seal than the standard LMA and facilitates gastric tube placement, improving protection against aspiration pneumonia [73–76]. The LMA-ProSeal™ has been reported to provide quick and reliable airway security within one or two attempts at placement without any major complications. The use of this newer LMA requires further investigation regarding appropriate size selection in the pig [77].

Maintenance of anesthesia

Both inhaled and injectable anesthetics can be used for maintaining anesthesia in pigs. Inhalation anesthesia is preferred for prolonged anesthesia and for specific experimental studies because it provides smoother transitions, a more controlled plane of anesthesia, and a more rapid recovery than do many injectable combinations. All the current inhalant anesthetics have been used safely and effectively in pigs. Regardless of which anesthetic is chosen, oxygen should be supplemented via an appropriate anesthetic circuit. Various recommendations have been made concerning weight limitations of anesthetic machines and delivery systems designed for humans or small animals, and the following should be taken into account: the patient's estimated tidal volume, the available reservoir bag sizes, the capacity of the CO_2 absorbent canister, and the diameter of the available breathing circuit relative to the endotracheal tube. The use of a machine designed for large animals should be considered for animals weighing more than about 150–200 kg. Adult pigs are normally maintained with an oxygen flow of 10–20 mL/kg/min [3,16].

The injection of liquid volatile anesthetic into a vaporization chamber applied to the snout of piglets has been reported. The apparatus is filled with a calculated amount of the volatile anesthetic agent, and induction can be accomplished in less than 1 min. Recovery time is reported to be an average of 2 min after removal of the chamber from the animal. Hodgson compared the use of isoflurane and sevoflurane for short-term anesthesia in piglets and found that both agents can be used for castration without complications but isoflurane costs less [78].

Nitrous oxide (N_2O) is only used to supplement other anesthetics because it is not potent enough to provide anesthesia alone. N_2O reduces the dose requirement of more potent anesthetics (i.e., MAC values are additive), thus minimizing the cardiopulmonary depression produced by the primary inhalant and maintaining a more physiologically stable state [13]. To avoid hypoxia, the maximum concentration of N_2O for safe anesthesia in pigs is 75% N_2O with 25% O_2; however, 50–66% N_2O is more common in research laboratories. Rapid movement of N_2O from the blood to the alveoli at the end of anesthesia can result in diffusion hypoxia once oxygen supplementation ceases and the pig breathes ambient air. Therefore, it is indicated to provide 100% oxygen to the animal during the 5–10 min immediately after discontinuing N_2O delivery [3].

Other agents have been recently employed for maintenance of anesthesia in pigs, especially for research (i.e., xenon). Xenon is an inert gas with many of the characteristics considered ideal for an anesthetic agent. One characteristic in particular is the fact that it is not harmful to the environment, since it is derived from a fractional distillation of the atmospheric air. Xenon has also been recently recognized for its systemic hemodynamic stability and analgesia. The MAC value of xenon has been established to be 119% in intubated pigs, and it has been reported to not trigger malignant hyperthermia [79,80]. The production cost of xenon is prohibitive at this point, and it requires low fresh gas flow rates with a xenon-recycling system [81].

Injectable maintenance of anesthesia is a suitable alternative to the use of inhalants in pigs. In field situations, it is a useful method of anesthesia because it does not require specialized equipment (i.e., anesthetic machine with ventilator) or an oxygen delivery system, although intubation and oxygen delivery may be advisable in some situations. Drugs used for injectable anesthesia should achieve amnesia, unconsciousness, analgesia, immobility, and muscle relaxation. Although total intravenous anesthesia (TIVA) requires an IV catheter (usually placed in an auricular vein), some injectable anesthetic combinations such as ketamine or tiletamine–zolazepam (TZ) with xylazine can be given IM. There are disadvantages associated with injectable anesthesia compared to inhalant anesthesia, including slower recovery, hypoventilation, and hypoxemia if oxygen is not supplemented.

Common combinations of injectable anesthetics that have been used in pigs for field anesthesia are listed in Table 65.3. TZ is effective and provides reliable immobilization in pigs (due to the tiletamine) and some muscle relaxation and sedation (due to the zolazepam). When given intramuscularly, TZ has the advantage over ketamine

Table 65.3 Injectable drugs and combinations used for maintenance of anesthesia in pigs.

Drug	Dose	Route	Primary references
Alfaxalone	0.07–0.27 mg/kg/min	IV	[54]
Guaifenesin–ketamine–xylazine[a]	0.67–1.1 mL/kg (ind) 2.2 mL/kg/h (maint)	IV	[11,29,43]
Medetomidine plus butorphanol plus ketamine	0.08 mg/kg 0.2 mg/kg 10 mg/kg	IM	[32]
Pentobarbital plus ketamine or fentanyl	8–10 mg/kg/h 5 mg/kg/h 0.02 mg/kg/h	IV	[84]
Pentobarbital plus ketamine plus midazolam	6–8 mg/kg/h 3–5 mg/kg/h 0.1–0.2 mg/kg/h	IV	[85]
Propofol	8–12 mg/kg	IV	[86]
Propofol plus fentanyl	11 mg/kg/h 0.0025–0.02 mg/kg/h	IV	[49]
Romifidine plus butorphanol plus ketamine[b]	0.12 mg/kg 0.1 mg/kg 5 mg/kg 2 mL/kg/h (maint)	IV	[33]
Tiletamine–zolazepam plus xylazine plus ketamine	4.4 mg/kg 4.4 mg/kg 2.2 mg/kg	IM	[49]
Tiletamine–zolazepam plus xylazine plus tramadol	3.5 mg/kg 1.32 mg/kg 1.8 mg/kg	IM	[87]
Xylazine plus ketamine plus midazolam	2 mg/kg Up to 20 mg/kg 0.25 mg/kg	IM	[49]
Xylazine plus butorphanol plus ketamine	2 mg/kg 0.2–0.22 mg/kg 5–11 mg/kg	IM	[49,69,88]

IM, intramuscular; IV, intravenous; ind, induction; maint, maintenance.
[a] Often referred to as "GKX" or "swine triple drip." Combine 1–2 g of ketamine and 1 g of xylazine with 1 L of 5% guaifenesin; creating a solution that is ~50 mg/mL guaifenesin, 1–2 mg/mL ketamine, and 1 mg/mL xylazine.
[b] For infusion, combine 5 mg of romifidine, 5.6 mg of butorphanol, and 200 mg of ketamine in 100 mL saline.

of requiring a smaller volume to be injected and provides 20 min of immobilization suitable for minor surgery [82]. However, TZ alone may not provide enough CNS depression and visceral analgesia for most surgical procedures and may require combination with an α_2-adrenergic receptor agonist (e.g., medetomidine, dexmedetomidine, or xylazine) to provide effective anesthesia. Another reason to include an α_2-adrenergic receptor agonist with TZ or ketamine is to smooth out the recovery experience. During recovery from dissociatives, pigs may display excessive paddling, multiple failed attempts to return to sternal recumbency, hypersalivation, frequent vocalization, and hyperthermia [21]. Note that repeated doses of TZ result in prolonged recovery, which appears to be caused in large part by zolazepam's lingering effects. Zolazepam is also responsible for the posterior weakness observed in mature pigs during recovery. To decrease this effect, ketamine can be included in the TZ mixture (e.g., swine TXK). In an unused vial of TZ, 2.5 mL of ketamine (100 mg/mL) and 2.5 mL of xylazine (100 mg/mL) are added to the powder, thus producing 100 mg of dissociative agents/mL (tiletamine and ketamine) and 50 mg/mL each of xylazine and zolazepam. The recommended dose for commercial pigs is 1 mL per 35–75 kg IM, depending on the depth of anesthesia required. It is suggested that the positive chronotropic effects of TZ and ketamine are partially counterbalanced by the enhanced vagal tone associated with xylazine [83].

For pot-bellied pigs, the dose of TZ combinations is one-half that of other pig types. Also, the dose of TZ should be lower when given to miniature pigs compared to domestic pigs [83]. In a study by Ko *et al.*, other drug combinations were evaluated in pigs. The combination of TZ (4.4 mg/kg), ketamine (2.2 mg/kg), and xylazine (2.2 mg/kg) was compared against TZ (4.4 mg/kg) and xylazine (2.2 mg/kg), TZ (4.4 mg/kg) and xylazine (4.4 mg/kg), and ketamine (2.2 mg/kg) with xylazine (2.2 mg/kg) [89]. After observing the quality of restraint and induction of surgical anesthesia, TZ with either dose of xylazine was preferred. All drug mixtures were mixed in a single syringe and given as a single IM injection. All the combinations were considered safe and satisfactory for anesthesia induction in pigs aged 6–8 months [89]. For a greater depth and prolonged period of anesthesia in miniature pigs, TZ (3.5 mg/kg) has been combined with xylazine (1.32 mg/kg) and tramadol (1.8 mg/kg) and administered IM. Animals became laterally recumbent within 3 min and were calmer during recovery compared with animals that received only TZ and xylazine. The time between administration of drugs and recovery to standing was an average of 25 min. The inclusion of tramadol produced less pronounced cardiovascular depression and did not cause additional respiratory depressant effects in miniature pigs [83]. Note that the combination of TZ, xylazine, and tramadol can be effectively antagonized, when necessary, with atipamezole (0.12 mg/kg IM), flumazenil (0.1 mg/kg IM), and naloxone (0.03 mg/kg IM) [90].

Anesthesia can be maintained with a combination known as a "Swine triple drip" which is a 5% solution of dextrose in water containing 50 mg/mL guaifenesin, 1–2 mg/mL ketamine, and 1 mg/mL xylazine (GKX) infused IV at a rate of approximately 2.2 mL/kg/h. It is a satisfactory combination of drugs for induction and maintenance of surgical anesthesia in healthy swine for a period of up to 2 h [11,91]. Anesthesia can be induced using this same GKX combination at dose of 0.67–1.1 mL/kg after adequate sedation and IV access are obtained. Recovery occurs within 30–45 min of discontinuation of the IV infusion and can be accelerated by administration of yohimbine (0.06–0.1 mg/kg IV) or tolazoline (2–4 mg/kg IV). Note that when an α_2-adrenergic receptor antagonist is used, postoperative analgesia will diminish, and other analgesic techniques such as epidural administration of opioids and local anesthetics should be employed [36].

The combination of medetomidine 80 μg/kg, butorphanol 0.2 mg/kg, and ketamine 10 mg/kg (MBK) administered IM provides appropriate anesthesia and analgesia in pigs for 30–45 min. Atropine (0.025 mg/kg) may also be given if desired. Anesthesia induction is rapid, and the recovery is generally uneventful. Anesthesia can be rapidly antagonized with atipamezole (0.24 mg/kg IM) if necessary [32]. IM administration of xylazine, butorphanol, and ketamine (XBK) has been reported for anesthetizing Göttingen miniature pigs and pot-bellied pigs [3,4]. Yohimbine (0.05 mg/kg IM) has been used to reverse XBK anesthesia in Göttingen minipigs [4]. Another group of researchers have reported that the combination of romifidine (0.12 mg/kg), butorphanol (0.1 mg/kg), and ketamine (8 mg/kg) administered IM to pigs provides adequate anesthesia under field conditions. Immobilization was observed within 2–5 min after IM administration, and reliable anesthesia was maintained for 20–30 min. All recoveries were smooth and smaller pigs were able to stand up 50–60 min after the injection, while larger animals needed more time (70–90 min).

Historically, the barbiturates were used extensively for maintaining anesthesia in laboratory animals. Currently, due to lack of availability, use of barbiturates for general anesthesia has dramatically decreased. Dosage recommendations (e.g., pentobarbital 20–40 mg/kg, and thiopental or thiamylal 6.6–30 mg/kg) should be interpreted as guidelines since barbiturates are administered IV to effect. The dose should be reduced by one-half to two-thirds when barbiturates are combined with other agents [11,82]. Note that the use of a single injectable anesthetic is usually not adequate to fulfill all the criteria of general anesthesia. Ketamine (5 mg/kg IV) or fentanyl (20 μg/kg IV) can be administered concomitantly with pentobarbital (20 mg/kg IV) for induction of anesthesia after premedication with atropine (0.04 mg/kg IM) and diazepam (0.5 mg/kg IM). Maintenance of anesthesia using a constant infusion of ketamine (5 mg/kg/h) or fentanyl (20 μg/kg/h) in combination with a pentobarbital infusion of 8–10 mg/kg/h has been reported. Both ketamine and fentanyl result in stable hemodynamics during induction and maintenance of anesthesia for pigs subjected to open-heart surgery [92]. Miniature pigs may also be anesthetized with an infusion of low-dose ketamine combined with pentobarbital. After premedication with atropine (0.04 mg/kg IM) and diazepam (0.4 mg/kg IM), induction of anesthesia is achieved with IV ketamine (5 mg/kg) and pentobarbital (20 mg/kg). General anesthesia maintained with a constant IV infusion of ketamine (3–5 mg/kg/h) and pentobarbital (6–8 mg/kg/h) with intermittent midazolam injection hourly at 0.1–0.2 mg/kg demonstrated superior hemodynamic and respiratory indices in comparison with pentobarbital alone. Thus, this protocol resulted in both hypnosis and analgesia with stable circulatory parameters during a cardiopulmonary bypass procedure [93].

Propofol is rapidly cleared from plasma after infusion, and therefore, consciousness returns more quickly than with most other injectable anesthetic agents. Propofol is typically combined with a potent analgesic drug, such as fentanyl, for maintenance of anesthesia in pigs. Schöffmann *et al.* reported that hemodynamic changes and stress responses in piglets subjected to superficial soft tissue surgery can be suppressed by TIVA with propofol and fentanyl [94]. After premedication with midazolam (0.5 mg/kg), ketamine (10 mg/kg), and butorphanol (0.5 mg/kg) administered IM, five piglets were induced with propofol at 1 mg/kg IV. Anesthesia was maintained with IV propofol (8 mg/kg/h) and fentanyl (35 μg/kg/h) during catheterization of blood vessels. There were no deaths or adverse events during anesthesia, and heart rate, mean arterial blood pressure, and lactate concentrations remained unaffected throughout the surgical procedure. Cortisol levels were suppressed by the combination, although fentanyl alone effectively suppresses the cortisol response to abdominal surgery in human patients [94,95].

In a 2017 study, it was observed that alfaxalone can be used for maintenance of general anesthesia in pigs following premedication with alfaxalone (4 mg/kg), butorphanol (0.4 mg/kg), and medetomidine (40 μg/kg) administered IM. There were minimal changes in cardiovascular variables evaluated, and no pigs in this study developed hypotension (defined as mean arterial blood pressure < 60 mmHg) [54]. This finding is consistent with previous studies evaluating alfaxalone for TIVA in other species [96,97]. Apnea was not observed at any time in this study but some pigs hypoventilated during anesthesia, with end-tidal carbon dioxide ($P_{ET}CO_2$) values > 55 mmHg. Respiratory depression resulting from alfaxalone TIVA has been reported in dogs [96] but not in other species [97]. A limitation of this study was the lack of invasive monitoring during anesthesia; therefore, definitive interpretation of the respiratory and cardiovascular effects of alfaxalone is not possible [54].

Monitoring

Various parameters can be monitored during anesthesia of pigs, and it is possible to employ the same monitors and equipment used during anesthesia of other domestic species. In general, anesthetic depth, the cardiovascular system, the respiratory system, and body temperature should be carefully monitored until the animal is stable and fully recovered from the effects of the anesthetic agents. The intensity of perioperative and postoperative monitoring depends on the type of surgical procedure and environment. Continuous monitoring should be performed, with recording of vital signs at 5-min intervals. Recording of intraoperative physiologic parameters will provide useful physiologic trends and may be required by regulatory agencies in laboratory settings [6,98]. These parameters should include, at a minimum, heart or pulse rate, mucous membrane color, respiratory rate, rectal or esophageal temperature, and absence of muscle reflexes. Advanced monitoring should include electrocardiography (ECG), arterial blood pressure measurement, capnography, and pulse oximetry.

The pulse rate in pigs can be monitored at different sites including the auricular arteries, the brachial artery on the medial aspect of the humeroradial joint, the saphenous artery over the medial aspect of the distal femur, or the sublingual artery on the ventral surface of the tongue. Other locations that are considered less reliable, especially in larger animals with thick SC and muscular tissue, include the femoral, carotid, or facial arteries [98]. Mucous membrane color can be observed in pigs by examination of the oral cavity, the snout, or the ears, especially on unpigmented animals.

ECG monitoring is straightforward in pigs, although alligator clips may not hold well due to the animal's thick skin and SC fat. Alternatives include 25 gauge needle electrodes inserted SC or patch electrodes held on the skin by adhesive. Esophageal ECG leads are also available for use in pigs [6,20]. Monitoring of the ECG is recommended for detecting dysrhythmias, noting that normal pigs have a prolonged Q-T interval compared to other species [99].

Non-invasive (indirect) blood pressure measurement is relatively straightforward in pigs but is less accurate than invasive (direct) techniques. Either oscillometric or Doppler flow monitors can be used for non-invasive blood pressure measurement. The cuff can be placed either immediately above or below the carpus or tarsus of the pig, and cuff width should be between 40% and 60% of the circumference of the limb at that location. The values obtained through non-invasive blood pressure methods should be assessed for trends rather than analysis of absolute numbers. Also, blood pressures vary widely with anesthetic agents used and the breed and size of the pig [20,98]. Arterial catheterization can be performed in all sizes of pigs. The auricular artery runs down the center of the pinna and can be catheterized with a 24–22 gauge catheter and then connected to a direct blood pressure transducer and monitor. In larger pigs, the medial saphenous, carotid, or femoral arteries can also be catheterized with a 5 cm (2 inch) or longer catheter, although a surgical cut-down may be required [13]. Auricular arterial blood pressures were similar to femoral arterial values in pigs under general anesthesia with isoflurane [100].

Rate, rhythm, and depth of respiration of the anesthetized animal can be assessed by observing thoracic cage movement, although capnography is a more sensitive and accurate measure of respiration. $P_{ET}CO_2$ can be measured though a sampling line located between the end of the endotracheal tube and the anesthetic circuit. The normal physiologic range of $P_{ET}CO_2$ is 35–45 mmHg, and higher values indicate that the animal may need to have ventilation assisted or controlled. A sudden rapid increase in $P_{ET}CO_2$ values might be related to the onset of malignant hyperthermia [20]. An increase in respiratory depth, a regular respiratory rhythm, and a decrease in respiratory rate accompany a surgical anesthetic plane.

Adequacy of oxygenation can be assessed by arterial blood gas analysis or by using a pulse oximeter [99]. Pulse oximetry is very practical to use in pigs and measures both pulse rate and the percentage of oxygenated hemoglobin. A transmittance probe can be placed on the animal's tongue, eyelid, tip of the tail, or interdigital space in unpigmented animals, or a rectal reflectance probe can be placed intrarectally [6,20]. Reflectance probes designed for the human forehead can work well when applied to unpigmented areas of the pig such as the metatarsus or base of the tail.

A rectal or esophageal thermistor allows determination of the animal's temperature during an anesthetic event. Pigs are prone to hypothermia, because they are relatively hairless [11], and several techniques can be employed to minimize heat loss. Caution is warranted because the skin of pigs is very sensitive to thermal damage. Passive insulation and safe external active warming techniques, including forced warm air, may be used. Placement of circulating warm water blankets under the animal, heat lamps over the animal, insulating material (e.g., rubber) between the animal and the cold surgical tabletop, and wrapping the extremities in bubble sheeting minimize loss of heat [3,6,99]. Electrical conductive fabric pads specifically designed for anesthetized patients (e.g., HotDog Patient Warming System) are available.

A simple, yet reliable method for assessing depth of anesthesia is by evaluation of muscle relaxation. A surgical depth of anesthesia is usually characterized by laxity of the mandibular muscles (jaw tone) or absence of gross movement of the leg in response to a pinch or similar stimulus to the coronary band of the hoof. Palpebral reflexes should be assessed during anesthesia as their presence may indicate a lighter plane of anesthesia [4,6,98].

The Bispectral Index™ (BIS™) is a parameter derived from processing the electroencephalogram. It has been associated with the hypnotic component of the anesthetic state and has been used in humans and animals as a tool to assess anesthetic depth. Evaluation of BIS monitoring in the pig has been accomplished using various combinations of sevoflurane, isoflurane, propofol, fentanyl, and atracurium [87,101,102]. However, BIS values in pigs may have a poor correlation with anesthetic depth and may not predict changes in arterial blood pressure or heart rate during surgery [102].

Supportive therapies

Depending on the nature and duration of the surgical procedure, a balanced electrolyte solution such as Lactated Ringer's should be administered intravenously at a starting rate of 5–15 mL/kg/h, although allometric adjustments may be useful due to the range of body weights encountered [103]. During longer procedures, the fluid rate should be adjusted accordingly to the patients cardiovascular and intravascular volume status. Insufficient urine production, extensive blood loss, and hypotension are indications for a higher fluid infusion rate. Excessively high fluid rates may increase the likelihood of pulmonary edema [4]. In piglets, it is advisable to use warmed fluids to assist in the maintenance of body temperature [4,16,98]. In pigs that are hypovolemic or presenting with other signs of shock, fluid therapy should be initiated prior to anesthesia if reasonable. The intraosseous route for crystalloid and blood infusion in pigs can be used when necessary [84]. This route is a reasonable initial step for emergency fluid therapy until more conventional vascular access has been established. Note that IV access is a more efficient method of acute volume replacement than the intraosseous route [85]. Piglets and calves with mild dehydration will usually voluntarily drink oral rehydration solutions, and this constitutes a more cost-effective treatment [99].

Although currently controversial, hypotension due to severe hemorrhage can be minimized by adding an artificial colloid solution to crystalloid fluid therapy. A slow (i.e., 5 min) administration of 1–2 mL/kg of 7.5% saline in 6% dextran 70 (HSD) decreased mortality by 30% in pigs with hemorrhagic hypovolemia. Colloid solutions (i.e., hydroxyethyl starch 130/0.4) markedly increase microcirculatory blood flow and tissue oxygen tension in the small intestinal mucosa, improve intestinal cellular substrate levels (e.g., lactate and glucose), and significantly enhance mixed venous saturation with less volume of fluid administration compared with crystalloid solutions [104,105]. A colloid/crystalloid solution ratio greater than 2:1 seems to promote coagulopathies [106,107].

Hypertonic saline can also be used to restore normovolemia in pigs [20]. The administration of 7.2% NaCl in 6% hydroxyethyl starch 200/0.5 at a dose of 5 mL/kg given IV demonstrated a positive inotropic effect with a significant increase in right ventricular contractility and cardiac output in pigs. Blood transfusions may be performed when necessary and blood donors are often littermates or close relatives. The risk of transfusion reaction from a non-crossmatched blood transfusion in pigs is relatively high since there are 16 recognized porcine blood groups that are not easily detectable [20,108].

During anesthesia, additional cardiovascular support using inotropes may be indicated. Oung *et al.* studied the effects of hypothermia on hemodynamic responses to inotropic agents in pigs and found that significant hemodynamic depression induced by profound hypothermia (30 °C) could be managed with either dopamine or dobutamine [109]. The optimal dosage of either agent for improving cardiac output in pigs was 10–20 μg/kg/min with minimal risk of inducing arrhythmias. Other investigators have reported that dopamine is the more effective inotropic agent in pigs. Dopamine administered at 15 μg/kg/min increased cardiac index by 18% and improved blood flow to the gastrointestinal tract by 33% in septic pigs [110]. Similarly, in piglets, dopamine (15 μg/kg/min) improved blood flow to the heart and small intestine compared to dobutamine [111,112]. Ephedrine at 0.05–0.1 mg/kg IV has been suggested to improve blood pressure in pigs. Ephedrine has both α- and β-adrenergic receptor effects and will increase cardiac output and heart rate for 10–20 min [13].

Mechanical ventilation is used to provide respiratory support in anesthetized pigs. The recommended peak inspiratory pressure is 20 cmH_2O, and the respiratory rate should range between 8 and 18 breaths per min depending on the age and size of the animal [113]. The arterial partial pressure of carbon dioxide is normally 40 ± 5 mmHg, which would correspond to a $P_{ET}CO_2$ of 35–40 mmHg [114]. Pulmonary shunt fraction in pigs will depend on the inspired fraction of oxygen (F_IO_2). Gianotti *et al.* described that in pigs undergoing 2 h of general anesthesia with mechanical ventilation, there was a lower pulmonary shunt fraction when using a F_IO_2 of 0.4 (4.3 ± 1.5%) compared to F_IO_2 of 0.6 (6.9 ± 0.5%) and 0.8 (9.5 ± 2.5%) [115].

Recovery considerations

During recovery from anesthesia, it is important to continue monitoring, to provide a smooth recovery, and to maintain homeostasis of the animal. Recovery should take place in a pen or cage lined with soft pads to preclude injury. The recovering animal should not be placed in a pen with other pigs due to the risk of injury and cannibalization. Room temperature should be 20–25 °C to minimize hypothermia or a thermal blanket or lamp may be placed over the animal. The endotracheal tube should be maintained until the pig is spontaneously moving its head or will no longer tolerate the presence of the tube. Extubation should be performed when a strong laryngeal reflex is present. If extubation is performed too early, there is a risk for hypoxemia due to laryngospasm and hypoventilation. If intubation was difficult, corticosteroids or diuretics (i.e., furosemide) can be given prophylactically prior to extubation. Some clinicians advocate spraying phenylephrine on the larynx to decrease vascular congestion and laryngeal edema. Severe upper airway obstruction is difficult to treat in pigs because it is difficult to restrain and reintubate the animal. If reintubation is required, it may be more effective in some instances to perform a tracheostomy. Pigs with surgical incisions should not be housed with other animals because of their tendency to cannibalize wounds [16,98]. A postoperative analgesic plan should be in place before the animal completely recovers from anesthesia. To assess postoperative pain in pigs, physiologic parameters (e.g., heart rate and respiratory rate), behavior parameters such as agitation, running, rooting, and evaluation of the animal's reaction during wound palpation can be used [116]. Caution should be used when pigs are recovering in areas with straw, shavings, or blankets due to the risk of swallowing these materials. Ingestion of foreign material has been reported in miniature companion pigs [117,118].

Malignant hyperthermia

Malignant hyperthermia (MH) is a genetic hypermetabolic syndrome in humans and pigs, that has also been reported in other species, including dogs, horses, cats, birds, deer, and other wild animals. Pigs predisposed to MH have a high ratio of muscle to total body mass and experience rapid growth. Therefore, breeds with a high incidence of this syndrome include Pietran, Landrace, Spotted, Large White, Hampshire, and Poland-China. Breeds that tend to be less susceptible to MH include Duroc and pot-bellied pigs [3,20,119]. In a susceptible animal, MH can be triggered by any type of stress, including environmental extremes (i.e., warm temperatures) and pharmacologic agents (i.e., inhalant anesthetics). Even commonly performed minor procedures like restraint for blood sampling and castration can trigger MH in a highly susceptible pig. All volatile inhalation agents (i.e., halothane, isoflurane, enflurane, desflurane, and sevoflurane) as well as depolarizing neuromuscular blocking agents (i.e., succinylcholine) will initiate MH in animals with the gene responsible for this syndrome.

Malignant hyperthermia is caused by an inherited autosomal recessive disorder that results in a single amino acid mutation in the ryanodine receptor type 1 (RyR1) associated with calcium channels in skeletal muscle. When MH is triggered, the muscle is not able to control calcium efflux from inside the sarcoplasmic reticulum, allowing calcium activation of myosin ATPase that causes muscle contracture and release of heat. Aerobic and anaerobic cellular metabolism are increased significantly, leading to an elevation in carbon dioxide, hydrogen ion, and lactic acid concentrations, and decreased venous oxygen content [20,120]. Episodes of MH may present with increased core body temperature (up to 42 °C), muscle rigidity, tachycardia, tachypnea, extreme hypercapnia ($P_{ET}CO_2$ as high as 70 mmHg), hypoxemia, metabolic acidosis, sympathetic activation with elevated plasma catecholamine concentrations, and high values of serum magnesium, calcium, phosphorus, and potassium ion concentrations. As this condition progresses, cell metabolism fails and membrane integrity is compromised, resulting in increased permeability (i.e., edema). Myocardial ischemia occurs, since coronary perfusion is diminished while muscle metabolism is increased. Tachycardia may be followed by arrhythmias (e.g., ventricular tachycardia and fibrillation) that cause decreased cardiac output and, ultimately, cardiovascular collapse. Myoglobinuria may also be observed if the patient lives long enough [3,20]. Since genetic testing has become available for determination of this RyR1 gene in pigs, the incidence of MH has been reduced drastically, although it is still present in some swine populations [3].

Once MH has been diagnosed, the volatile anesthetic should be discontinued, and the pig should be ventilated with 100% oxygen, preferably using a different anesthetic machine or after changing the machine's rubber components (i.e., hoses and rebreathing bag). Hypercapnia can be resolved by hyperventilating the animal. Body cooling can be achieved with alcohol baths, ice packs around large vessels (jugular and femoral veins), fans, and rectal lavage with ice water. When body temperature decreases to 38 °C, the cooling methods should be terminated to avoid iatrogenic hypothermia. Dantrolene sodium is a skeletal muscle relaxant that inhibits excessive leak of calcium by RyR1 and can be employed both to prevent and to treat MH. This drug can be given orally (2–5 mg/kg) 6–10 h before induction of anesthesia, or it may be administered intravenously (1–5 mg/kg) immediately after MH symptoms are observed [3,16,20]. Despite the potency of dantrolene, this agent is highly lipophilic and poorly water soluble, making its preparation difficult for clinical use. The dantrolene analogue, azumolene, has similar potency to dantrolene in relaxing skeletal muscle in MH-susceptible pigs. Azumolene (2 mg/kg IV) is 30 times more soluble than dantrolene and reverses the muscular contracture in pigs by reducing the opening rate of RyR1, without altering calcium uptake into the sarcoplasmic reticulum [120]. It has been reported in some patients that development of hyperthermia may be delayed, and the fulminant episode may occur during recovery [121].

Analgesia

For any surgical procedure, it is good practice to administer an analgesic drug preemptively (i.e., prior to surgery). There are three major classes of drugs that are used for analgesia in pigs: opioids, local anesthetics, and non-steroidal anti-inflammatory drugs (NSAIDs). In general, opioids have more pronounced analgesic and sedative effects than NSAIDs and have to be administered more frequently. The use of opioids may be required for humane care during the first 48–72 h after major surgery, although effectiveness may diminish as inflammation becomes a major component of the discomfort. Butorphanol (0.1–0.3 mg/kg IM) has an analgesic effect of 4–6 h and produces few adverse effects in pigs compared to full μ-opioid receptor agonists like morphine [82]. Also, when given as part of premedication, it will enhance depth of sedation and decrease the dose required for induction of anesthesia [94]. Buprenorphine (0.01–0.1 mg/kg IM) can be given every 12 h, and its onset of action is approximately 30–60 min after administration [122]. The analgesic effect of buprenorphine is reported to last 7–24 h in pigs when given in high doses [52,123]. Intermittent bolus administration of injectable drugs can result in increased animal stress and possible periods of inadequate analgesia when plasma concentrations are at their lowest prior to the next injection. The pharmacokinetics of two extended-release formulations of buprenorphine, sustained-release buprenorphine (SRB) and the transdermal buprenorphine (TDB) patch, have been evaluated in female Göttingen minipigs. At a hypothesized plasma buprenorphine therapeutic threshold of 0.1 ng/mL, therapeutic plasma buprenorphine concentrations lasted 8.0 ± 1.3 h after a single IV injection of 0.02 mg/kg traditional buprenorphine, 264.0 ± 32.2 h after a single SC injection of 0.18 mg/kg SRB, and 72 h after application of a 30 μg/h TDB patch. These findings support the use of SRB and TDB as long-acting formulations of buprenorphine in Göttingen minipigs, which would ease the administration of these analgesics, simplify postoperative pain management in laboratory swine, and improve animal welfare. Therapeutic plasma concentrations are achieved within min after the injection of SRB rather than in 12–24 h as with the TDB patch. In addition, a single injection of SRB eliminates the chance of premature discontinuation of analgesia, which might occur if a transdermal patch detaches from the skin. In contrast, TDB does not require injection, and the patches can easily be removed to discontinue drug administration if adverse reactions occur. Both SRB and TDB resulted in localized skin reactions, which were more frequent with SRB than TDB [124].

Short-acting opioids such as fentanyl can be used as a constant IV infusion at a rate varying from 10 to 100 μg/kg/h in pigs without major side effects [3,14,82]. It has been shown that a fentanyl infusion rate of 35 μg/kg/h in piglets produces adequate analgesia for surgical procedures without affecting heart rate, mean arterial blood pressure, or lactate concentrations during 5 h of anesthesia when maintained with a propofol infusion at 8 mg/kg/h [94]. This is desirable for cardiovascular research where cardiovascular side effects of administered anesthetic and analgesic agents must be minimal. In addition, fentanyl can be administered to pigs through a transdermal patch that can be secured to the skin behind the ear. With this route, fentanyl is continuously administered for up to 72 h per patch application, and the discomfort and inconvenience of repeated parenteral injections are avoided [123–126]. Fentanyl patches come in different sizes: 12, 25, 50, 75, and 100 μg/h. For a 20 kg pig, the appropriate fentanyl patch will be a 50 μg/h patch applied at least 24 h prior to the surgery. Other short-acting opioids that have been used in pigs include sufentanil (5–10 μg/kg IM every 2 h; 15–30 μg/kg/h IV), meperidine (2–10 mg/kg IM every 4 h), and oxymorphone (0.15 mg/kg IM every 4 h).

Morphine given systemically to non-painful pigs has been reported to cause excitement in a manner similar to that observed in cats and horses [82]. When administered intravenously to pigs, morphine produces not only analgesia but also respiratory depression [127]. Systemic morphine is also reported to produce other side effects, such as decreased gastrointestinal motility, nausea and vomiting, pupillary constriction, bradycardia, euphoria, and histamine release in many species (e.g., dogs, cats, and horses) [125,128]. To avoid many of the systemic physiologic side effects, morphine can be administered epidurally [129,130]. In addition, because morphine has low lipid solubility, it persists for a long period in the cerebrospinal fluid, prolonging the analgesic effect up to 33 h in pigs [130]. In many species, such as dogs, cats, horses, and cattle, this analgesic effect does not produce major motor impairment, in contrast to epidural administration of other drugs, such as lidocaine [123,128]. Epidural morphine can be given at a dosage of 0.1–0.12 mg/kg diluted in saline [131]. For maximal distribution of the drug into the spinal canal, morphine is diluted with saline to a final volume of 1 mL of solution for pigs with a vertebral length of up to 40 cm. Then, an additional 1.5 mL of saline is added for every additional 10 cm of vertebral length [131]. This final volume is delivered slowly over 1–2 min. Epidural morphine produced adequate analgesia without hemodynamic or respiratory effects in pigs during abdominal surgery [132]. Epidural anesthesia is helpful when performing obstetric and perineal surgery in pigs; however, in larger animals, the landmarks can be difficult to locate. Local anesthetics can be included, such as lidocaine at 1 mL per 7.5 kg for pigs up to 50 kg, and then 1 mL per 10 kg above 50 kg [16]. This causes recumbency for 1–2 h. Also, there have been reports of bupivacaine (0.8 mg/kg) and ropivacaine (1.5 mg/kg) being administered epidurally in pigs [133,134]. Intratesticular analgesia is suitable for castration in young pigs up to 6 months old. For 1-week old piglets, a total of 0.5 mL of 2% lidocaine is injected into the stroma of each testicle, with a small amount being injected subcutaneously beneath the scrotal skin. At least 5 min should be allowed for the anesthetic to take effect, and it will reduce pain responses during surgical castration [135].

Tramadol is an analgesic with mixed-opioid and non-opioid activities where the non-opioid activity is mediated via α_2-adrenergic and serotonergic activity [136]. This analgesic agent has been reported to cause less respiratory depression compared with morphine or other opioid analgesics because it exhibits weak binding to μ-opioid receptors responsible for this side effect [37,137]. While historically tramadol has not been a controlled substance in many countries [138], more recently, this has changed as its human abuse potential has been recognized and the regulatory requirements surrounding its use are similar to that of other opioids in many jurisdictions. It was shown that in pigs administered 5 mg/kg tramadol IM 5 min prior to anesthesia with xylazine (2.5 mg/kg), ketamine (25 mg/kg), and atropine (0.04 mg/kg) administered IM, the quality of anesthetic induction and endotracheal intubation were improved. Also, tramadol given prior to this sedation protocol increased the duration of analgesia, without cardiopulmonary side effects or adverse effects on recovery characteristics [139].

Liposomal bupivacaine (Nocita®) is a relatively new veterinary product containing bupivacaine particles encapsulated in multivesicular liposomes, allowing for slow release of the local anesthetic and providing up to 72 h of local anesthesia. This preparation is currently approved by the United States Food and Drug Administration for canine cranial cruciate ligament surgery and feline peripheral nerve blocks [140]. Injection of liposomal bupivacaine suspension has been used extra-label in other animal species for soft tissue infiltration with a low rate of adverse events. Studies to date have not demonstrated neurotoxicity of liposomal bupivacaine in rabbit and dog models of brachial plexus blocks [141]. Intraneural injections (sciatic nerve) of liposomal bupivacaine or bupivacaine HCl in a porcine model did not result in evidence of neurotoxicity. Compared with bupivacaine HCl, the liposomal bupivacaine injectable suspension provided longer sensory (11.2 ± 1.8 h versus 3.2 ± 1.1 h, respectively) and motor (10.0 ± 2.0 h versus 4.0 ± 1.4 h, respectively) blockade [142]. Further studies should be performed to evaluate the clinical effects of this newer formulation of bupivacaine in pigs.

The NSAIDs are a group of analgesics derived from the organic acids, carboxylic acid (e.g., aspirin, flunixin, and carprofen) and enolic acid (e.g., phenylbutazone and meloxicam) [128]. In addition to analgesia, NSAIDs have anti-inflammatory and antipyretic properties [82,128,135]. Compared with opioids, NSAIDs are only effective against moderate pain but may be combined with opioids for treatment of more severe pain [4]. Aspirin (10 mg/kg PO every 4–6 h) has been used in pigs; enteric-coated products are recommended due to the pig's predisposition for gastric ulcers [82]. Flunixin (2 mg/kg IV; 1–4 mg/kg SC or IM) has a prolonged effect of 12–24 h in pigs, but should not be administered for more than 3 days to minimize its adverse effects [143,144]. Carprofen (2 mg/kg SC or IM) has a longer effect (12–24 h) in pigs and provides adequate analgesia for soft tissue and orthopedic pain. Ketorolac (1 mg/kg IM or IV every 12 h), meloxicam (0.4 mg/kg SC or IM every 24 h), and ketoprofen (1–3 mg/kg IM, SC or PO every 12 h) have been reported to be effective as part of a balanced anesthetic regimen for postoperative and chronic pain. Piglets treated with 0.4 mg/kg meloxicam IM 10–30 min before castration demonstrated fewer behavioral alterations compared to a placebo group. [145]. Phenylbutazone (10–20 mg/kg PO every 12 h) may be administered for the treatment of musculoskeletal pain. Regulatory restrictions on the use of various NSAIDs in animals which could reach the human food chain must be strictly followed. Oral medications are readily accepted by pigs when hidden in canned dog food or in chocolate syrup [16,143]. A pharmacokinetic profile of oral meloxicam (0.5 mg/kg) in mature pigs demonstrates a high relative bioavailability of this drug supporting the clinical use of meloxicam for pain management in sows [146].

Pig-specific pain assessment tools are available to assist in determining the requirement for and efficiency of analgesic treatments. Facial expression analysis, known as the "grimace scale," is widely used for assessing pain in rats, rabbits, horses, sheep, lambs, and cats [147–153]. Viscardi *et al.* have established a piglet grimace scale that is strongly correlated with behavioral activity. The proportion of low pain scores after castration had a significant positive correlation with active behavior and a significant negative correlation with inactive behaviors [154]. A second piglet grimace scale has been published by Di Giminiani *et al.*, but it includes a complex point system. Both grimace scales have limitations, such as moderate interobserver agreement, and both need further validation [155]. Luna *et al.* have validated the UNESP-Botucatu pig composite acute pain scale for assessing postoperative pain. This pain assessment tool for pigs is a valid, reliable, responsive, specific, and sensitive tool, with excellent internal consistency and discriminatory ability, and may be used as an instrument to assess acute pain in pigs undergoing surgeries such as castration [156].

References

1 Heinonen ML, Raekallio MR, Oliviero C, *et al.* Comparison azaperone-detomidine-butorphanol-ketamine and azaperone-tiletamine-zolazepam for anaesthesia in piglets. *Vet Anaesth Analg* 2009; **36**: 151–157.

2 Lord LK, Wittum TE. Survey of humane organizations and slaughter plants regarding experiences with Vietnamese potbellied pigs. *J Am Vet Med Assoc* 1997; **211**(5): 562–565.

3 Thurmon JC, Smith GW. Swine. In: Tranquili WJ, Thurmon JC, Grimm KA, eds. *Lumb and Jones' Veterinary Anesthesia and Analgesia*, 4th edn. Ames, IA: Blackwell Publishing, 2007: 747–764.

4 Alstrup AKO. *Anaesthesia and Analgesia in Ellegaard Göttingen Minipigs.* Arhus, Denmark: PET Centre, Aarhus University Hospital, 2010.

5 Swindle MM. Anesthesia and Analgesia in Swine: Technical Bulletin. Sinclair Research Center, 2002. www.info.sinclairresearch.com/anesthesia-and-analgesia-in-swine (accessed October 2014).

6 Kaiser GM, Heuer MM, Frühauf NR, *et al.* General handling and anesthesia for experimental surgery in pigs. *J Surg Res* 2006; **130**: 73–79.

7 Wilbers AM. Handling pet pigs as patients. *Proceedings of the North American Veterinary Conference, 2013 Large Animal.* www.vetfolio.com/learn/article/handling-pet-pigs-as-patients

8 Mozzachio K, Pollock C. Basic Information Sheet: Miniature Pig. LafeberVet Website. www.lafeber.com/vet/basic-information-sheet-miniature-pig/ (accessed July 2019).

9 Axiak SM, Jäggin N, Wenger S, *et al.* Anaesthesia for castration of piglets: comparison between intranasal and intramuscular application of ketamine, climazolam and azaperone. *Schweiz Arch Tierheilkd* 2007; **149**(9): 395–402.

10 Lacoste L, Bouquee S, Ingrand P, *et al.* Intranasal midazolam in piglets: pharmacodynamics (0.2 vs 0.4 mg/kg) and pharmacokinetics (0.4 mg/kg) with bioavailability determination. *Lab Anim* 2000; **34**; 29–35.

11 Henrikson H, Jensen-Waern M, Nyman G. Anaesthetics for general anaesthesia in growing pigs. *Acta Vet Scand* 1995; **36**(3): 401–411.

12 Riviere JE, Papich MG. Potential and problems of developing transdermal patches for veterinary applications. *Adv Drug Deliv Rev* 2001; **50**: 175–203.

13 Smith JS, Seddighi R. Miniature companion pig sedation and anesthesia. *Vet Clin Exot Animal* 2022; **25**: 297–319.

14 Linkenhoker JR, Burkholder TH, Linton CGG, *et al.* Effective and safe anesthesia for Yorkshire and Yucatan Swine with and without cardiovascular injury and intervention. *J Am Assoc Lab Anim Sci* 2010; **49**(3): 344–351.

15 Mitek A. Pot-bellied pig sedation. In: *Proceedings of the Illinois Fall Conference for Veterinarians*, Champaign, IL, September 22–23, 2016.

16 Hodgkinson O. Practical sedation and anaesthesia in pigs. *Farm Anim Pract* 2007; **29**: 34–39.

17 Snook CS. Use of the subcutaneous abdominal vein for blood sampling and intravenous catheterization in potbellied pigs . Scientific Reports: descriptive report. *J Am Vet Med Assoc* 2001; **219**(6): 809–810.

18 Wheeler EP, Abelson AL, Wetmore LA. Anesthesia case of the month. *J Am Vet Med Assoc* 2020; **257**(8): 809–812.

19 Hay Kraus BL. Spotlight on the perioperative use of maropitant citrate. *Vet Med Res Rep* 2017; **8**: 41–51.

20 Moon PF, Smith LJ. General anesthetic techniques in swine. *Vet Clin North Am Food Anim Pract* 1996; **12**(3): 663–691.

21 Padilha LR, Ko JCH. Non-domestic suids. In: West G, Heard D, Caulkett N, eds. *Zoo Animal and Wildlife Immobilization and Anesthesia,* 2nd edn. Ames, IA: Blackwell Publishing, 2014: 773–785.

22 Gomez de Segura IA, Tendillo FJ, Mascias A, *et al.* Actions of xylazine in young swine. *Am J Vet Res* 1997; **58**(1): 99–102.

23 Ajadi RA, Smith OF, Makinde AFM, *et al.* Increasing ketamine dose enhances the anaesthetic properties of ketamine-xylazine-midazolam combination in growing pigs. *J S Afr Vet Assoc* 2008; **79**(4): 205–207.

24 Hörnchen U, Schüttler J, Stoeckel H, *et al.* Comparison of intravenous and endobronchial atropine: a pharmacokinetic and dynamic study in pigs. *Eur J Anaesthesiol* 1989; **6**: 95–102.

25 Lee JY, Jee HC, Jeong SM, *et al.* Comparison of anaesthetic and cardiorespiratory effects of xylazine or medetomidine in combination with tiletamine/zolazepam in pigs. *Vet Rec* 2010; **167**: 245–249.

26 Braun W. Anesthetics and surgical techniques useful in the potbellied pig. *Vet Med* 1993; **88**: 441–447.

27 Flores FN, Tavares SG, Moraes AN, *et al.* Azaperone and its association with xylazine or dexmedetomidine in swine. *Ciência Rural* 2009; **39**(4): 1101–1107.

28 Rego Oliveira LC, Marques JA, Santos DAS, *et al.* Effects of ketamine and midazolam in pigs (*Sus scrofa*) pre-treated which acepromazine or azaperone. *Ars Vet* 2003; **19**(3): 235–240.

29 Thurmon JC, Benson GJ. Anesthesia in ruminants and swine. In: Howard J, ed. *Current Veterinary Therapy*, 3rd edn. Philadelphia, PA: WB Saunders, 1993: 58–76.

30 Trim CM, Gilroy BA. The cardiopulmonary effects of a xylazine and ketamine combination in pigs. *Res Vet Sci* 1985; **38**: 30–34.

31 Sakaguchi M, Nishimura R, Sasaki N, *et al.* Chemical restraint by medetomidine-ketamine and its cardiopulmonary effects in pigs. *J Vet Med* 1995; **42**: 293–299.

32 Sakaguchi M, Nishimura R, Sasaki N, *et al.* Anesthesia induced in pigs by use of a combination of medetomidine, butorphanol, and ketamine and its reversal by administration of atipamezole. *Am J Vet Res* 1996; **57**: 529–534.

33 Nussbaumer I, Zimmermann W, Peterbauer C. Anaesthesia of pigs with a combination of romifidine, butorphanol and ketamine. *Vet Rec* 2008; **163**: 720–721.

34 Lu DZ, Fan HG, Kun M, *et al.* Antagonistic effect of atipamezole, flumazenil and naloxone following anaesthesia with xylazine, tramadol and tiletamine/zolazepam combinations in pigs. *Vet Anaesth Analg* 2011; **38**: 301–309.

35 Kim MJ, Park CS, Jun MH, *et al.* Antagonist effects of yohimbine in pigs anaesthetized with tiletamine/zolazepam and xylazine. *Vet Rec* 2007; **161**: 620–624.

36 Lin H. Injectable anesthetics and field anesthesia. In: Lin H, Walz P, eds. *Farm Animal Anesthesia*, 1st edn. Ames, IA: John Wiley & Sons, 2014: 60–94.

37 Natalini CC, Polydoro A, Crosignani N. Effects of morphine or tramadol on thiopental anaesthetic induction dosage and physiologic variables in halothane anaesthetized dogs. *Acta Sci Vet* 2007; **35**: 161–166.

38 Ajadi AR, Olusa TA, Smith OF, *et al.* Tramadol improved the efficacy of ketaminexylazine anaesthesia in young pigs. *Vet Anaesth Analg* 2009; **36**: 562–566.

39 Steffey EP, Baggot JD, Eisele JH, *et al.* Morphine-isoflurane interaction in dogs, swine and rhesus monkeys. *J Vet Pharmacol Ther* 1994; **17**(3): 202–210.

40 Moon PF, Scarlett JM, Ludders JW, *et al.* Effect of fentanyl on the minimum alveolar concentration of isoflurane in swine. *Anesthesiology* 1995; **83**(3): 535–542.

41 Re M, Canfrán S, Largo C, *et al.* Effect of lidocaine-ketamine infusions combined with morphine or fentanyl in sevoflurane-anesthetized pigs. *J Am Assoc Lab Anim Sci* 2016; **55**(3): 317–320.

42 Malavasi LM, Jensen-Waern M, Augustsson H, *et al.* Changes in minimal alveolar concentration of isoflurane following treatment with medetomidine and tiletamine/zolazepam, epidural morphine or systemic buprenorphine in pigs. *Lab Anim* 2008; **42**(1): 62–70.

43 Wagner AE, Hellyer PW. Survey of anesthetic techniques and concerns in private veterinary practice. *J Am Vet Med Assoc* 2000; **217**: 1652–1657.

44 Lan NC, Gee KW. Neuroactive steroid actions at the GABAA receptor. *Horm Behav* 1994; **28**: 537–544.

45 Keates H. Induction of anaesthesia in pigs using a new alphaxalone formulation. *Vet Rec* 2003; **153**: 627–628.

46 Santos Gonzalez M, Bertran de Lis BT, Tendillo Cortijo FJ. Effects of intramuscular alfaxalone alone or in combination with diazepam in swine. *Vet Anaesth Analg* 2013; **40**: 399–402.

47 Blanca MS, Betran de Lis BT, Tendillo Cortijo FJ. Effects of intramuscular dexmedetomidine in combination with ketamine or alfaxalone in swine. *Vet Anaesth Analg* 2016; **43**(1): 81–85.

48 National Institutes of Health, Office of Laboratory Animal Welfare. *Use of Non-Pharmaceutical-Grade Chemicals and Other Substances in Research with Animals.* OLAW Online Seminars: OLAW; 2012. www.olaw.nih.gov/sites/default/files/120301_seminar_transcript.pdf

49 Anderson DE, Mulon PY. Anesthesia and surgical procedures in swine. *Dis Swine* 2019: 171–196.

50 Kelley E, Fernandez LG, Potter J, *et al.* A practical approach to simple procedures in pet pigs. *Vet Irel J* 2020; **10**(9): 472–473.

51 Ugarte CE, O'Flaherty KO. The use of a medetomidine, butorphanol and atropine combination to enable blood sampling in young pigs. *N Z Vet J* 2005; **53**(4): 249–252.

52 Malavasi LM, Jensen-Waern M, Augustsson H, *et al.* Changes in minimal alveolar concentration of isoflurane following treatment with medetomidine and tiletamine/zolazepam, epidural morphine or systemic buprenorphine in pigs. *Lab Anim* 2008; **42**: 62–70.

53 Carpenter JW. *Exotic Animal Formulary*, 5th edn. St. Louis, MO: Elsevier, 2016.

54 Bigby SE, Carter JE, Bauquier S, *et al.* The use of alfaxalone for premedication, induction and maintenance of anaesthesia in pigs: a pilot study. *Vet Anaesth Analg* 2017; **44**(4): 905–909.

55 Chum H, Pacharinsak C. Endotracheal intubation in swine. *Lab Anim* 2012; **41**: 309–311.

56 Mascoas A, Pera AM, Santos M, *et al.* Total intravenous anesthesia with propofol in pigs. *J Vet Anaesth* 1993; **20**: 53–54.

57 Zacharioudaki A, Lelovas P, Sergentanis TN, *et al.* Induction of anaesthesia with remifentanil after bolus midazolam administration in Landrace/Large White swine. *Vet Anaesth Analg* 2017; **44**: 1353–1362.

58 University of Colorado, Denver Institutional Animal Care and Use Committee (IACUC). *Veterinary Anesthetic and Analgesic Formulary*, 2nd edn. University of Colorado Denver, 2006.

59 Clutton RE, Blissitt KJ, Bradley AA, *et al.* Comparison of three injectable anaesthetic techniques in pigs. *Vet Rec* 1997; **141**: 140–146.

60 Desmetiha TD, Pantazopoulos IN, Dontas I, *et al.* Refined induction of anesthesia with remifentanil after bolus propofol administration in Landrace/Large White swine. *Lab Anim* 2010; **39**: 319–324.

61 Archambault P, Dionne CE, Lortie G, *et al.* Adrenal inhibition following a single dose of etomidate in intubated traumatic brain injury victims. *Can Assoc Emerg Phys* 2012; **14**(5): 270–282.

62 Hirschman LJ. The cardiopulmonary and metabolic effects of hypoxia during acute adrenocortical suppression by etomidate in the dog. *AANA J* 1991; **59**(3): 281–287.

63 Worek FS, Blumel G, Zaravik J, *et al.* Comparison of ketamine and pentobarbital anesthesia with the conscious state in a porcine model of Pseudomonas aeruginosa septicemia. *Acta Anaesth Scand* 1988; **32**: 509–515.

64 Suresh MS, Nelson TE. Malignant hyperthermia: is etomidate safe? *Anesth Analg* 1985; **64**: 420–424.

65 Cunha DNQ, Buccellato M, Keene BW, *et al.* Electrocardiographic, hematologic, histopathologic, and recovery characteristics from repeated morphine-chloralose anesthesia in dogs. *Int J Appl Res Vet Med* 2008; **6**(3): 191–199.

66 Sommers MG, van Egmond J, Booji LHDJ, *et al.* Isoflurane anesthesia is a valuable alternative for α-chloralose anesthesia in the forepaw stimulation model in rats. *NMR Biomed* 2009; **22**: 414–418.

67 Seaberg DC, Menegazzi JJ, Check B, *et al.* Use of a cardiocerebral-protective drug cocktail prior to countershock in a porcine model of prolonged ventricular fibrillation. *Resuscitation* 2001; **51**: 301–308.

68 Theisen MM, Maas M, Grosse Hartlage MA, *et al.* Ventral recumbency is crucial for fast and safe orotracheal intubation in laboratory swine. *Lab Anim* 2009; **43**: 96–101.

69 Bollen PJ, Hansen AK, Alstrup AKO. *The Laboratory Swine*, 2nd edn. New York, NY: CRC Press, 2010.

70 Tonge M, Robson K. Hypoxaemia following suspected intubation of the tracheal bronchus of a pig. *Vet Rec* 2021; **9**(1): 1–6.

71 Patil VU, Fairbrother CR, Dunham BM. Use of laryngeal mask airway for emergency or elective airway management situations in pigs. *Contemp Top Lab Anim Sci* 1997; **36**: 47–49.

72 Fulkerson PJ, Gustafon SB. Use of laryngeal mask airway compared to endotracheal tube with positive-pressure ventilation in anesthetized swine. *Vet Anaesth Analg* 2007; **34**(4): 284–288.

73 Brain AIJ, Verghese C, STrube PJ. The LMA 'ProSeal' – a laryngeal mask with an oesophageal vent. *Br J Anaesth* 2002; **84**: 650–654.

74 Keller C, Brimacombe J, Kleinsasser A, *et al.* Does the ProSeal laryngeal mask airway prevent aspiration of regurgitated fluid? *Anesth Analg* 2000; **91**(4): 1017–1020.

75 Evans NR, Llewellyn RL, Gardener SV, *et al.* Aspiration prevented by the ProSeal™ laryngeal mask airway: a case report. *Can J Anesth* 2002; **49**: 413–416.

76 Mark DA. Protection from aspiration with the LMA-ProSeal™ after vomiting: a case report. *Can J Anaesth* 2003; **50**: 78–80.

77 Goldman k, Kalinowski M, Kraft S. Airway management under general anaesthesia in pigs using the LMA-ProSeal™: a pilot study. *Vet Anaesth Analg* 2005; **32**: 308–313.

78 Hodgson DS. Comparison of isoflurane and sevoflurane for short-term anesthesia in piglets. *Vet Anaesth Analg* 2007; **34**: 117–124.

79 Hecker KE, Horn N, Baumert JH, *et al.* Minimum alveolar concentration (MAC) of xenon in intubated swine. *Br J Anaesth* 2004; **92**(3): 421–424.

80 Froeba G, Marx T, Pazhur J, *et al.* Xenon does not trigger malignant hyperthermia in susceptible swine. *Anesthesiology* 1999; **91**: 1047–1052.

81 Iber T, Hecker K, Vagts DA, *et al.* Xenon anesthesia inpairs hepatic oxygenation and perfusion in healthy pigs. *Minerva Anestesiol* 2008; **74**: 511–519.

82 Smith AC, Ehler WJ, Swindle MM. Anesthesia and analgesia in swine. In: Kohn DF, Winson SK, White WJ, Benson GJ, eds. *Anesthesia and Analgesia in Laboratory Animals.* San Diego, CA: Academic Press, 1997: 313–336.

83 Lu DZ, Fan HG, Wang HB, *et al.* Effect of the addition of tramadol to a combination of tiletamine-zolazepam and xylazine for anaesthesia of miniature pigs. *Vet Rec* 2010; **167**: 489–492.

84 Schoffstall JM, Spivey WH, Davidheiser S, *et al.* Intraosseous crystalloid and blood infusion in a swine model. *J Trauma* 1989; **29**(3): 384–387.

85 Warren DW, Kissoon N, Sommerauer JF, *et al.* Comparison of fluid rates among peripheral intravenous and humerus, femur, malleolus, and tibial intraosseous sites in normovolemic and hypovolemic piglets. *Ann Emerg Med* 1993; **22**(2): 183–186.

86 Lagerkranser M, Stånge K, Sollevi A. Effects of propofol on cerebral blood flow, metabolism, and cerebral autoregulation in the anesthetized pig. *J Neurosurg Anesthesiol* 1997; **9**(2): 188–193.

87 Greene SA, Benson GJ, Tranquili WJ, *et al.* Effect of isoflurane, atracurium, fentanyl, and noxious stimulation on bispectral index in pigs. *Compar Med* 2004; **54**(4): 397–403.

88 Calle P, Morris P. Anesthesia for nondomestic suids. *Zoo Wild Anim Med Curr Ther* 1999; **4**: 639–646.

89 Ko JC, Williams BL, Rogers ER, *et al.* Increased xylazine dose-enhanced anesthetic properties of telazol-xylazine combination in swine. *Lab Anim Sci* 1995; **45**: 290–294.

90 Lu DZ, Fan HG, Kun M, *et al.* Antagonistic effect of atipamezole, flumazenil and naloxone following anaesthesia with xylazine, tramadol and tiletamine/zolazepam combinations in pigs. *Vet Anaesth Analg* 2011; **4**: 301–309.

91 Thurmon JC, Tranquili WJ, Benson GJ. Cardiopulmonary responses of swine to intravenous infusion of guaifenesin, ketamine, and xylazine. *Am J Vet Res* 1986; **47**(10): 2138–2140.

92 Liu D, Shao YS, Luan X, *et al.* Comparison of ketamine-pentobarbital anesthesia and fentanyl-pentobarbital anesthesia for open-heart surgery in minipigs. *Lab Anim* 2009; **38**(7): 234–240.

93 Liu D, Hu J, Zhang M, *et al.* Low-dose ketamine combined with pentobarbital in a miniature porcine model for a cardiopulmonary bypass procedure: a randomized controlled study. *Eur J Anaesthesiol* 2009; **26**: 389–395.

94 Schöffmann G, Winter P, Palme R, *et al.* Haemodynamic changes and stress responses of piglets to surgery during total intravenous anaesthesia with propofol and fentanyl. *Lab Anim* 2009; **43**: 243–248.

95 Lacoumenta S, Yeo TH, Burrin JM, *et al.* Fentanyl and the beta-endorphin, ACTH and glycoregulatory hormonal response to surgery. *Br J Anaesth* 1987; **59**: 713–720.

96 Suarez MA, Dzikiti BT, Stegmann FG, *et al.* Comparison of alfaxalone and propofol administered as total intravenous anaesthesia for ovariohysterectomy in dogs. *Vet Anaesth Analg* 2012; **39**: 236–244.

97 Ndawana PS, Dzikiti BT, Zeiler G, *et al.* Determination of the minimum infusion rate (MIR) of alfaxalone required to prevent purposeful movement of the extremities in response to a standardized noxius stimulus in goats. *Vet Anaesth Analg* 2015; **42**: 65–71.

98 Swindle MM. *Perioperative Care of Swine: Technical Bulletin. Sinclair Research Center*, 2002. www.info.sinclairresearch.com/perioperative-care-of-swine (accessed October 2014).

99 Smith AC, Swindle MM. Anesthesia and analgesia in swine. In: Fish RE, Brown MJ, Danneman PJ, *et al.*, eds. *Anesthesia and Analgesia in Laboratory Animals*, 2nd edn. San Diego, CA: Academic Press, 2008: 413–440.

100 Bass LME, Yu D, Cullen LK. Comparison of femoral and auricular arterial blood pressure monitoring in pigs. *Vet Anaesth Analg* 2009; **36**(5): 457–463.

101 Martin-Cancho MF, Lima JR, Luis L, *et al.* Bispectral index, spectral edge frequency 95%, and median frequency recorded for various concentrations of isoflurane and sevoflurane in pigs. *Am J Vet Res* 2003; **64**(7): 866–873.

102 Martin-Cancho MF, Carrasco-Jimenez MS, Lima JR, *et al.* Assessment of the relationship of bispectral index values, hemodynamic changes, and recovery times associated with sevoflurane or propofol anesthesia in pigs. *Am J Vet Res* 2004; **65**(4): 409–416.

103 Hahn RG. Volume kinetics of infusion fluids (review). *Anesthesiology* 2010; **113**: 470–481.

104 Rainger JE, Dart AJ. Enteral fluid therapy in large animals. *Aust Vet J* 2006; **84**(12): 447–451.

105 Hiltebrand LB, Kimberger O, Arnberger M, *et al.* Crystalloids versus colloids for goal-directed fluid therapy in major surgery. *Crit Care* 2009; **13**: 1–13.

106 Wafaisade A, Wutzler S, Lefering R, *et al.* Drivers of acute coagulopathy after severe trauma: a multivariate analysis of 1987 patients. *Emerg Med J* 2010; **22**: 934–939.

107 Hahn RG. Fluid therapy in uncontrolled hemorrhage – what experimental models have taught us. *Acta Anaesthesiol Scand* 2013; **57**: 16–28.

108 Smith DM, Newhouse M, Naziruddin B, *et al.* Blood group and transfusion in pigs. *Xenotransplantation* 2006; **13**: 186–194.

109 Oung CM, English M, Chiu RCJ, *et al.* Effects of hypothermia on hemodynamic responses to dopamine and dobutamine. *J Trauma* 1992; **33**(5): 671–678.

110 Hiltebrand LB, Krejci V, Sigurdsson GH. Effects of dopamine, dobutamine, and dopexamine on microcirculatory blood flow in the gastrointestinal tract during sepsis and anesthesia. *Anesthesiology* 2004; **100**: 1188–1197.

111 Ferrara JJ, Dyess DL, Peeples GL, *et al.* Effects of dopamine and dobutamine on regional blood flow distribution in the neonatal piglet. *Ann Surg* 1995; **221**(5): 531–542.

112 Priebe HJ, Nöldge GFE, Armbruster K, *et al.* Differential effects of dobutamine, dopamine, and noradrenaline on splanchnic haemodynamics and oxygenation I the pig. *Acta Anaesthesiol Scand* 1995; **39**: 1088–1096.

113 Massone F. *Anestesiologia Veterinaria: Farmacologia e Tecnicas*, 5th edn. Rio de Janeiro, Brazil: Guanabara Koogan, 2008.

114 Haskins SC. Monitoring anesthetized patients. In: Short CE, ed. *Principles and Practice of Veterinary Anesthesia*. Baltimore, MD: Williams & Wilkins, 1987.

115 Gianotti GC, Beheregaray WK, Meyer FS, *et al.* Cardiorespiratory dynamics of sedated pigs submitted to different inspired oxygen fractions under controlled mechanical ventilation. *Acta Sci Vet* 2014; **42**: 1–8.

116 Dobromylsky P, Flecknell PA, Lascelles BD, *et al. Pain Management in Animals*. London, UK: WB Saunders, 2001.

117 Sipos W, Schmoll F, Stumpf I. Minipigs and potbellied pigs as pets in the veterinary practice: a retrospective study. *J Vet Med A, Physiol Pathol Clin Med* 2007; **54**: 504–511.

118 Ludwig EK, Byron CR. Evaluation of the reason for and outcomes of gastrointestinal tract surgery in pet pigs: 11 cases (2004–2015). *J Am Vet Med Assoc* 2017; **251**: 714–721.

119 Claxton-Gill MS, Cornick-Seahorn JL, Gamboa JC, *et al.* Suspected malignant hyperthermia syndrome in a miniature pot-bellied pig anesthetized with isoflurane. *J Am Vet Med Assoc* 1993; **203**(10): 1434–1436.

120 Do Carmo PL, Zapata-Sudo MM, Trachez F, *et al.* Intravenous administration of azumolene to reverse malignant hyperthermia in swine. *J Vet Intern Med* 2010; **24**: 1224–1228.

121 Iaizzo PA, Kehler CH, Richard JC, *et al.* Prior hypothermia attenuates malignant hypothermia in susceptible swine. *Anesth Analg* 1996; **82**: 803–809.

122 Hermansen K, Pedersen LE, Olesen HO. The analgesic effect of buprenorphine, etorphine and pethidine in the pig: a randomized double blind cross-over study. *Acta Pharmacol Toxicol* 1986; **59**: 27–35.

123 Harvey-Clark CJ, Gillespie K, Riggs KW. Transdermal fentanyl compared with parenteral buprenorphine in post-surgical pain in swine: a case study. *Lab Anim* 2000; **34**: 386–398.

124 Thiede AJ, Garcia KD, Stolarik DF, *et al.* Pharmacokinetics of sustained-released and transdermal buprenorphine in Göttingen minipigs. *J Am Assoc Lab Anim Sci* 2014; **53**(6): 692–699.

125 Branson KR, Gross ME. *Opioid agonists and antagonists. In: Veterinary Pharmacology and Therapeutics, 8th edn.* Ames, IA: Iowa State University Press, 2001.

126 Wilkinson AC, Thomas III ML, Morse BC. Evaluation of a transdermal fentanyl system in Yucatan miniature pigs. *Contemp Top Lab Anim Sci* 2001; **40**(3): 12–16.

127 Steffey EP, Baggot JD, Eisele JH, *et al.* Morphine-isoflurane interaction in dogs, swine and Rhesus monkeys. *J Vet Pharmacol Ther* 1994; **17**: 202–210.

128 Nolan AM. *Pain Management in Animals*. London, UK: WB Saunders, 2001.

129 Rang HP, Dale MM, Ritter JM. *Pharmacology*, 3rd edn. London, UK: Churchill Livingstone, 1996.

130 Ummenhofer WC, Arends R, Shen DD, *et al.* Comparative spinal distribution and clearance kinetics of intrathecally administered morphine, fentanyl, alfentanil, and sufentanil. *Anesthesiology* 2000; **92**: 739–753.

131 Strande A. Epidural anaesthesia in young pigs, dosage in relation to the length of the vertebral column. *Acta Vet Scand* 1968: **9**(1): 41–49.

132 Malavasi LM, Nyman G, Augustsson H, *et al.* Effects of epidural morphine and transdermal fentanyl analgesia on physiology and behavior after abdominal surgery in pigs. *Lab Anim* 2006; **40**: 16–27.

133 Stegmann GF. Cardiovascular effects of epidural morphine or ropivacaine in isoflurane-anaesthetised pigs during surgical devascularisation of the liver. *J S Afr Vet Assoc* 2010; **81**(3): 143–147.

134 Mergner GW, Stolte AL, Frame WB, *et al.* Combined epidural analgesia and general anesthesia induce ischemia distal to a severe coronary artery stenosis in swine. *Anesth Analg* 1994; **78**: 37–45.

135 Boothe DM. *Drugs affecting animal behavior. In: Veterinary Pharmacology and Therapeutics, 8th edn.* Ames, IA: Iowa State University Press, 2001.

136 Garrido MJ, Valle M, Campanero MA, *et al.* Modelling of the in vivo antinociceptive interaction between an opioid agonist, (+) O-desmethyltramadol in rats. *J Pharmacol Exp Ther* 2000; **295**: 352–359.

137 Bhattachary MD, Mandal MC, Ghosh S, *et al.* Comparison of two premedication regimes to facilitate laryngeal mask insertion during thiopental anaesthesia. *J Anaesth Clin Pharmacol* 2005; **21**: 275–278.

138 Lewis KS, Han NH. Tramadol: a centrally acting analgesic. *Am J Health Syst Pharm* 1996; **54**: 643–652.

139 Ajadi AR, Olusa TA, Smith OF, *et al.* Tramadol improved the efficacy of ketamine-xylazine anaesthesia in young pigs. *Vet Anaesth Analg* 2009; **36**: 562–566.

140 Aratana Website. NOCITA® Technical Monograph. www.nocita.aratana.com/wp-content/uploads/2019/05/NOCITA-Technical-Monograph.pdf (accessed September 2020).

141 Richard BM, Newton P, Ott LR, *et al.* The safety of EXPAREL® (bupivacaine liposome injectable suspension) administered by peripheral nerve block in rabbits and dogs. *J Drug Deliv* 2012: 962101.

142 Damjanovka M, Cvetko E, Kuroda MM, *et al.* Neurotoxicity of intraeural injection of bupivacaine liposome injectable suspension versus bupivacaine hydrochloride in a porcine model. *Vet Anaesth Analg* 2019; **46**(2): 236–245.

143 Swindle MM. *Swine in the Laboratory: Surgery, Anesthesia, Imaging, and Experimental Techniques*, 2nd edn. Boca Raton, FL: CRC Press, 2007.

144 Buur JL, Baynes RE, Smith G, *et al.* Pharmacokinetics of flunixin meglumine in swine after intravenous dosing. *J Vet Pharmacol Ther* 2006; **29**: 437–440.

145 Keita A, Pagot E, Pruiner A, *et al.* Pre-emptive meloxicam for postoperative analgesia in piglets undergoing surgical castration. *Vet Anaesth Analg* 2010; **37**(4): 3673–3674.

146 Pairis-Garcia MD, Johnson AK, Kukanich B, *et al.* Pharmacokinetics of meloxicam in mature swine after intravenous and oral administration. *J Vet Pharmacol Ther* 2015; **38**(3): 265–270.

147 Langford DJ, Bailey AL, Chanda ML, *et al.* Coding of facial expression of pain in the laboratory mouse. *Nat Methods* 2010; **7**: 447–449.
148 Sotocinal SG, Sorge RE, Zaloum A, *et al.* The Rat Grimace Scale: a partially automated method for quantifying pain in the laboratory rat via facial expression. *Mol Pain* 2011; **7**: 55.
149 Keating SCJ, Thomas AA, Flecknell PA, *et al.* Evaluation of EMLA cream for preventing pain during tattooing of rabbits: changes in physiological, behavioural and facial expression responses. *PLoS ONE* 2012; 7(9): e44437.
150 Costa ED, Minero M, Lebelt D, *et al.* Development of the horse grimace scale (HGS) as a pain assessment tool in horses undergoing routine castration. *PLoS ONE* 2014; **9**(3): e92281.
151 Guesgen MJ, Beausoleil NJ, Leach M, *et al.* Coding and quantification of a facial expression for pain in lambs. *Behav Processes* 2016; **132**: 49–56.
152 McLennan KM, Rebelo CJB, Corke MJ, *et al.* Development of a facial expression scale using footrot and mastitis as models of pain in sheep. *Appl Anim Behav Sci* 2016; **176**: 19–26.
153 Evangelista MC, Watanabe R, Leung VSY, *et al.* Facial expressions of pain in cats: the development and validation of a Feline Grimace Scale. *Sci Rep* 2019; **9**: 19128.
154 Viscardi AV, Hunniford M, Lawlis P, *et al.* Development of a piglet grimace scale to evaluate piglet pain using facial expressions following castration and tail docking: a pilot study. *Front Vet Sci* 2017; **4**: 51.
155 Di Giminiani P, Brierley VLMH, Scollo A, *et al.* The assessment of facial expressions in piglets undergoing tail docking and castration: toward the development of the piglet grimace scale. *Front Vet Sci* 2016; **3**: 100.
156 Luna SPL, Araujo AL, Neto PIN, *et al.* Validation of the UNESP-Botucatu pig composite acute pain scale (UPAPS). *PLoS ONE* 2020; **15**(6): e0233552.

66 Ruminant and Swine Local Anesthetic and Analgesic Techniques

Alexander Valverde
Department of Clinical Studies, Ontario Veterinary College, University of Guelph, Guelph, Ontario, Canada

Chapter contents

Introduction, 1301
Local anesthetics, 1301
Blocks for regional anesthesia of the head, 1303
- Horn blocks, 1303
- Eye and adnexa block, 1304
- Nasal passages and nasal block, 1306

Blocks for regional anesthesia of the flank or paralumbar fossa, 1307
- Line infiltration block, 1307
- Inverted "L" or "7" block, 1307
- Proximal paravertebral block, 1307
- Distal paravertebral block, 1309
- Segmental dorsolumbar epidural block, 1309
- Segmental thoracolumbar subarachnoid block, 1310

Blocks for regional anesthesia of the linea alba and paramedian region, 1310
- Line infiltration block, 1311
- Lumbosacral, sacrococcygeal, or intercoccygeal epidural (cranial epidural) block, 1311

Blocks for regional anesthesia of the pelvic area and related tissues, 1312
- Sacrococcygeal or intercoccygeal epidural (caudal epidural) block, 1312
- Sacral paravertebral block, 1313
- Pudendal block, 1314
- Dorsal nerve of the penis block, 1314

Blocks for regional anesthesia of the teats and udder, 1314
- Ring block, 1316
- Inverted "V" block, 1316
- Teat sinus infusion block, 1316
- Intravenous regional teat block, 1317

Blocks for castration, 1317
Blocks for regional anesthesia of the limbs and feet, 1317
- Thoracic limb blocks, 1317
- Pelvic limb blocks, 1319

Ultrasound-guided regional anesthesia, 1321
References, 1322

Introduction

In ruminant and swine practice, it is common to combine local anesthetics with chemical and/or physical restraint methods to provide a cost-effective and humane alternative to general anesthesia. The choice of technique for a procedure and level of sedation required will depend on the species and breed of animal (e.g., dairy or beef cow, ovine, or porcine), temperament, facilities available (farm or clinic location), and skills of the veterinarian. The economics of ruminant and swine practice may not allow for general anesthesia in most situations and local and regional anesthetic techniques are often the basis of appropriate analgesia. Local anesthetic techniques do not require specialized equipment and avoid the potential complications of general anesthesia and recumbency. Most ruminants or swine are tolerant of humane restraint, but appropriate sedation and facilities are necessary for successful application of these techniques. Many field surgeries are performed in standing adult cattle to minimize the risks associated with recumbency (e.g., bloat, regurgitation, hypoxemia, myopathy, or neuropathy). Small ruminants or swine may be restrained in lateral or dorsal recumbency.

Local anesthetics can be administered in a number of ways, including perineural injection, infiltration at nerve endings in the skin or tissues, injection into the epidural or intrathecal space, and by injection into a peripheral vessel in combination with a tourniquet that prevents leakage into the systemic circulation. In general, a local anesthetic infiltrated near a major nerve or the spinal cord will have a longer duration of action than when infiltrated more peripherally (e.g., smaller nerve or nerve endings) or in a diffuse fashion (e.g., ring block). In cattle and small ruminants, the most commonly used techniques are local anesthesia of the paralumbar fossa, caudal or lumbosacral epidural analgesia, horn blocks, and intravenous regional anesthesia of the foot. In swine, infiltrative local anesthesia, caudal or lumbosacral epidural anesthesia, and intratesticular anesthesia are common.

Local anesthetics

Local anesthetics block sodium channels and prevent depolarization of nerves. Lidocaine, bupivacaine, and mepivacaine are the most commonly used local anesthetics in ruminants, and a specific

Veterinary Anesthesia and Analgesia: The Sixth Edition of Lumb and Jones. Edited by Leigh Lamont, Kurt Grimm, Sheilah Robertson, Lydia Love and Carrie Schroeder.
© 2024 John Wiley & Sons, Inc. Published 2024 by John Wiley & Sons, Inc.
Companion website: www.wiley.com/go/lamont/anesthesia

drug is often chosen based on its onset and duration of action. Lidocaine and mepivacaine are shorter acting than bupivacaine due to their lower protein binding at the receptor, but faster in onset because their dissociation constant (pK_a) is closer to plasma pH (7.4), which facilitates passage through cell membranes.

Toxicity of local anesthetics is related to their plasma concentrations. Reported toxic doses are based on continuous intravenous (IV) infusion of the local anesthetic, which contrasts from clinical situations where the local anesthetic drug is administered most commonly by extravascular infiltration; therefore, a more gradual absorption from the injection site into the systemic circulation offsets the achievement of toxic doses.

Toxicity is dependent on multiple factors. In addition to dose, plasma concentrations are dependent on the site of injection, vascular supply and degree of absorption from the site, co-administration of other drugs (e.g., epinephrine), conscious versus anesthetized state, health status, and individual variation. In humans, peak plasma concentrations for non-IV routes may be variable according to administration site and are as follows: intercostal > epidural > brachial plexus > subcutaneous [1].

In ruminants, toxic doses of local anesthetics have mostly been determined for sheep which are often used as a model for humans (Table 66.1). The progressive manifestation of systemic toxicity in conscious sheep usually consists of sedation, ataxia, mild cardiovascular depression, seizure activity, or convulsions accompanied by cardiovascular stimulation, followed by hypotension, apnea, and finally circulatory collapse and death [2–4]. For bupivacaine, with its known cardiotoxic effects, seizure activity may be preceded by cardiovascular collapse; similar effects have also been reported for ropivacaine [3]. In conscious goat kids given lidocaine to trigger seizures, toxicity signs progressed from sedation to ataxia and then tonic-clonic seizures [5]. Toxic doses that cause seizure activity do not necessarily result in cardiovascular signs, which typically require higher doses of local anesthetics [2–7]. In sheep anesthetized with volatile anesthetic agents, no signs of central nervous system (CNS) impairment (i.e., seizure activity) are observed even when blood concentrations are two-fold higher than in conscious sheep exhibiting toxicity and, although cardiovascular depression occurs, anesthesia has been shown to have a protective effect against arrhythmias and cardiovascular collapse [2].

Pregnancy may influence the toxic dosage of local anesthetic. There are a number of reports in the literature citing differences in sensitivity between pregnant and non-pregnant patients ranging from minimal to a 15% or more increase in sensitivity to bupivacaine and ropivacaine dosage in pregnant patients, particularly to the CNS effects [3,8]. These differences are more statistically rather than clinically relevant. No differences between pregnant and non-pregnant sheep were detected for lidocaine or mepivacaine [6,9]. Signs of hypotension (a sudden 40% or greater drop in mean arterial blood pressure), apnea (>15 s), and circulatory collapse (loss of the peripheral pulse) occurred at approximately twice the convulsive dose when administered IV under experimental conditions.

Conscious non-pregnant adult sheep given IV lidocaine at 2 mg/kg/min showed tonic-clonic seizure activity after 5.8 mg/kg had been administered, whereas newborn lambs 1–5 days of age were more resistant and did not exhibit seizure activity until dosages of 18 mg/kg were given [4]. Similarly, signs of hypotension (defined as a 20% drop in mean arterial blood pressure), apnea, and circulatory collapse occurred at 5–6 times (i.e., 31–37 mg/kg) the convulsive dose for adult sheep and at 3.5 times (i.e., 57–67 mg/kg) the convulsive dose for newborn lambs [4]. For mepivacaine, IV infusions of 2 mg/kg/min in conscious sheep resulted in seizure activity at dosages of 7.5–7.8 mg/kg and signs of hypotension, apnea, and circulatory collapse at 6–9 times (i.e., 49–69 mg/kg) the convulsive dose [6].

Pigs have been used as a model for the study of local anesthetic toxicity in human pediatric patients. Bupivacaine administered IV at 1 mg/kg/min in sevoflurane-anesthetized piglets (19–43 days of age) induced hypotension (defined as a 50% drop in mean arterial blood pressure) at median dosages of 4.6–5.2 mg/kg [10]. Older pigs administered 4 mg/kg of bupivacaine, levobupivacaine, or ropivacaine IV over 30 s under thiopental anesthesia showed immediate decreases in mean arterial blood pressure, cardiac index, and heart rate, followed by a gradual recovery to baseline over 30 min. These changes were more drastic with bupivacaine

Table 66.1 Approximate intravenous toxic doses (mg/kg) and associated plasma concentrations (μg/mL in parentheses) of local anesthetics reported in conscious sheep, lambs, goat kids, and anesthetized pigs.

Local anesthetic	Adverse effect	Sheep	Lambs (1–5 days old)	Goat kids (7–10 days old)	Newborn pigs (< 3 days old)	Pigs (8–10 weeks old)
Lidocaine	Seizure activity	5.8 (11.7)	18 57–67	9–12 (13.6)	12–60 (40.6)	ND
	Hypotension, cardiovascular collapse	31–37 (27.6–41.2)	(35.6–53.4)	ND	ND	ND
Mepivacaine	Seizure activity	7.5–7.8 (17.4–19.5)	ND	ND	ND	ND
	Hypotension, cardiovascular collapse	49–69 (36.4–45.6)	ND	ND	ND	ND
Bupivacaine	Seizure activity	4.2–6.2 (2.5–5.6)	ND	ND	ND	ND
	Hypotension, cardiovascular collapse	5.2–10.3 (3.0–7.4)	ND	ND	ND	4
Ropivacaine	Seizure activity	6.1–6.9 (4.7–5.6)	ND	ND	ND	ND
	Hypotension, cardiovascular collapse	11.3–12.5 (6.6–9.1)	ND	ND	ND	4

ND, not determined.
Source: Compiled from Copeland *et al.* [2] (sheep); Santos and DeArmas [3] (sheep); Morishima *et al.* [4,8] (sheep, lambs); Ventkatachalam *et al.* [5] (goat kids); Satas *et al.* [7] (newborn pigs); Udelsmann *et al.* [11,12] (pigs).

and levobupivacaine than with ropivacaine, with a 24–41% decrease in mean arterial blood pressure versus 11%; 38–53% decrease in cardiac index versus 22%; and 9–14% decrease in heart rate versus 7% [11,12].

In conscious piglets (12–60 h old), lidocaine induced seizures at a total dosage of 42 mg/kg IV administered as a 2 mg/kg bolus followed by an infusion at 2 mg/kg/min. Administration of 15 mg/kg every 4 min resulted in seizures at cumulative doses of 30–60 mg [7]. In both groups, there were no detectable changes in heart rate or mean arterial blood pressure before the onset of seizures [7].

Lidocaine hydrochloride (2%) is approved in Canada and the United States for use in cattle as a local anesthetic, but not for small ruminants or swine. However, it is labeled in cattle without established withdrawal times for meat and milk. General recommendations based on pharmacokinetic studies are a 4-day withdrawal for meat and 3-day withdrawal for milk after local infiltration techniques due to the large volumes of infiltration (up to 100 mL) [13]. For caudal epidural anesthesia using volumes of up to 15 mL, recommended meat and milk withdrawal times of 24 h are listed [14,15]. These withdrawal times are recommended by the Food Animal Residue Avoidance Databank (FARAD) for the US (www.farad.org) and Canada (www.cgfarad.usask.ca) and veterinarians are referred to these sites for withdrawal guidance and the Animal Medicinal Drug Use Clarification Act (AMDUCA) (www.farad.org/amduca-law.html) for regulatory considerations.

Recommendations from FARAD for small ruminants refer to the use of lidocaine with epinephrine for infiltration or epidural administration and include 24-h withdrawal times for meat and milk in sheep and goats. These same withdrawal times are recommended in cattle for lidocaine with epinephrine.

There are no current recommendations for mepivacaine, bupivacaine, or ropivacaine withdrawal times.

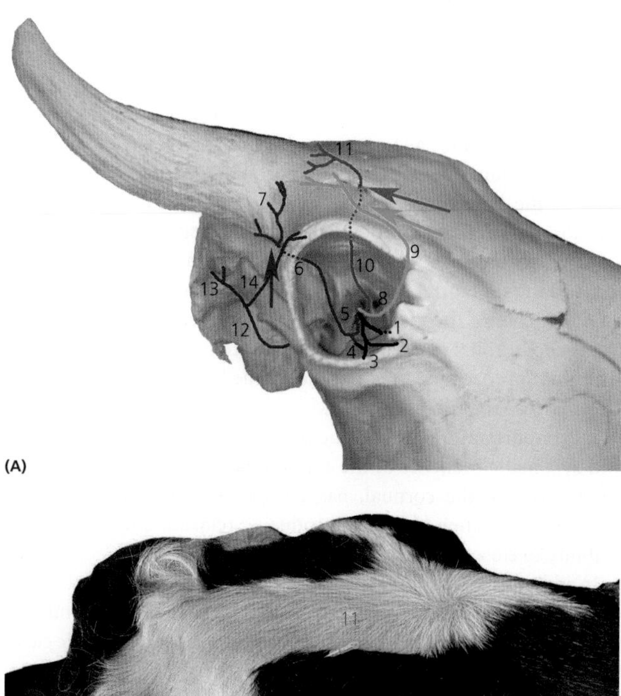

(A)

(B)

Figure 66.1 **A.** Innervation to the horn and surrounding tissue. Arrows indicate injection sites required for complete desensitization of the horn which includes the cornual branch (7), the infratrochlear nerve (9), the supraorbital nerve (11), and branches of the second cervical nerve (not shown but injected at the caudal base of the horn). The branches of the ophthalmic nerve that give origin to these nerves (except the second cervical nerve) are illustrated in color. (1) maxillary nerve (black); (2) zygomaticofacial branch; (3) zygomatic nerve; (4) communicating branch of zygomatic nerve to lacrimal nerve; (5) lacrimal nerve (purple); (6) zygomaticotemporal branch; (7) cornual branch; (8) nasociliary nerve (green); (9) infratrochlear nerve; (10) frontal nerve (red); (11) supraorbital nerve. The auriculopalpebral nerve (12) and its branches, the rostral auricular branch (13), and zygomatic branch (14) are also depicted. **B.** Dehorning nerve block in adult cattle with position of the needles at the cornual branch (7), infratrochlear nerve (9), and supraorbital nerve (11).

Blocks for regional anesthesia of the head

Horn blocks

There are similarities in desensitizing the nerve supply to the horn in cattle, goats, and sheep. In cattle, the main sensory nerve supply to the horn arises from the cornual branch as well as the supraorbital and infratrochlear nerves, all of which originate from the ophthalmic branch of the trigeminal nerve (Fig. 66.1A). The ophthalmic branch divides into three nerves while still within the foramen orbitorotundum: the lacrimal, nasociliary, and frontal nerves. The lacrimal nerve consists of two strands located along the lateral surface of the lateral rectus muscle that later join between them and with the communicating ramus of the zygomatic nerve to form the zygomaticotemporal branch, which is located at the level of the dorsal and caudal aspect of the orbit and exits along the ventral aspect of the zygomatic process (supraorbital) of the frontal bone. The zygomaticotemporal branch continues as the cornual branch as it travels caudally toward the base of the horn along the temporal ridge, between the supraorbital process and the lateral edge of the base of the horn [16].

In adult cattle, the site of injection for the cornual branch is 3–5 cm in front of the base of the horn, where the nerve courses from ventral to dorsal from the temporal fossa to the frontal bone and branches into endings along the base of the horn (Fig. 66.1B). A 2.5–3.8 cm, 20 gauge needle is inserted along the area of the temporal line and frontal bone and 10 mL of 2% lidocaine is injected after negative aspiration of blood has been verified to avoid injection into the cornual artery or vein in the surrounding area.

The nasociliary nerve branches into the infratrochlear nerve as it enters the orbit, which ascends to the dorsal margin of the orbit to the level of the lacrimal bone, dorsal to the medial canthus, where it curves around the frontal bony margin of the orbit to travel caudally and along the frontal bone and may reach the base of the horn [16]. The site of injection for the infratrochlear nerve is 2–3 cm medial from the mid-dorsal aspect of the rim of the orbit; a 2.5 cm, 20 gauge needle and 5 mL of 2% lidocaine are used (Fig. 66.1B). If the needle is directed an additional 2–3 cm caudomedially, then the supraorbital nerve to the horn can also be blocked from this approach. Alternatively, the infratrochlear nerve branches that reach the horn can be blocked with the supraorbital nerve as described below.

The frontal nerve travels from the foramen orbitorotundum to the orbital opening of the supraorbital canal, on the caudal and dorsal aspect of the orbit, to emerge as the supraorbital nerve at the supraorbital foramen of the frontal bone. The supraorbital foramen can be located about 3–4 cm from the temporal ridge and halfway along the distance between the supraorbital process and the medial edge of the base of the horn [16]. The site of injection for the supraorbital nerve is at the level of the supraorbital foramen using a 2.5 cm, 20 gauge needle and 5 mL of 2% lidocaine and taking care to avoid the supraorbital vein (Fig. 66.1B). Because most of the cornual branches of the infratrochlear nerve travel to the horn lateral to the supraorbital nerve at this same location, they can be blocked with this approach by directing the needle lateral toward the orbit, 2–3 cm from the rim of the orbit.

It is important to note that the proximity of the rostral auricular and zygomatic branches of the auriculopalpebral nerve to the sites of injection of the cornual, nasociliary, and supraorbital nerves often results in their blockade, producing relaxation of the ear and inability to close the eyelids [16].

In addition to these three main nerves, the caudal aspect of the base of the horn may be supplied by cutaneous branches of the second cervical nerve and these can be blocked by injecting local anesthetic close to the dorsal midline of the neck at a point level with the base of the ear.

In calves, nerve block for disbudding or dehorning can be performed as in adult cattle or simplified to two injection sites in younger calves (Fig. 66.2). For the simplified form of the block, a 1.5–2.5 cm, 20 gauge needle is inserted at the same site as for the cornual branch in adult cattle (i.e., where the nerve courses from ventral to dorsal from the temporal fossa to the frontal bone) and 5 mL of 2% lidocaine is injected above this ridge and 2 mL below the ridge. The dorsal volume of 5 mL is further divided to block the infratrochlear and supraorbital nerves as they travel toward the horn by directing the needle 2–3 cm from the ridge toward midline, and then blocking the cornual nerve along the ridge itself. The second injection is completed by redirecting the needle ventral to the ridge toward the temporal fossa, where 2 mL are injected to further block the cornual branch.

The use of a ring block can also be used in calves of less than 2 months of age, using a 2.5 cm, 20 gauge needle and injecting 6 mL of 2% lidocaine through four to five injection sites under the skin around the base of the horn [17]. However, as this block acts mostly on distal nerve endings from the major nerves to the horn, it has a shorter duration of action than the blocks described above.

Following surgery on the horns, anesthesia and analgesia are provided for as long as the duration of action of the local anesthetic. Due to the invasive nature of dehorning surgery, a non-steroidal anti-inflammatory drug (e.g., flunixin meglumine 2 mg/kg, IV or IM) is suggested for postoperative analgesia to supplement the anesthetic effect as it diminishes.

The cornual nerves of sheep and goats are very similar to those of cattle, although the cutaneous branches of the second cervical nerve are less likely to innervate the horn. The cornual branch of the lacrimal nerve (zygomaticotemporal) is blocked behind the root of the supraorbital process (Fig. 66.3). A 2.5 cm, 22 gauge needle is inserted to a depth of 1–1.5 cm, and 2–3 mL of 2% lidocaine is injected, halfway between the lateral canthus and the lateral edge of the base of the horn. The cornual branches of the infratrochlear nerve are blocked close to the dorsal rim of the orbit, halfway between the medial canthus and the medial edge of the base of the horn, by inserting a 2.5 cm, 22 gauge needle to a depth of about 0.5 cm and injecting 1–2 mL of 2% lidocaine [18].

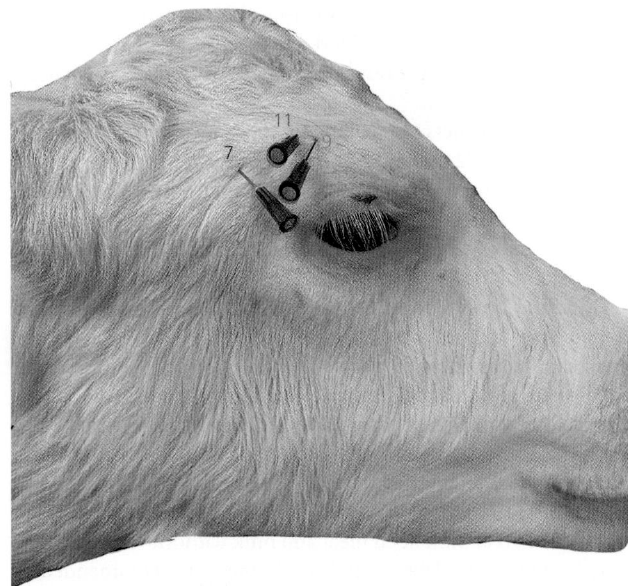

(A)

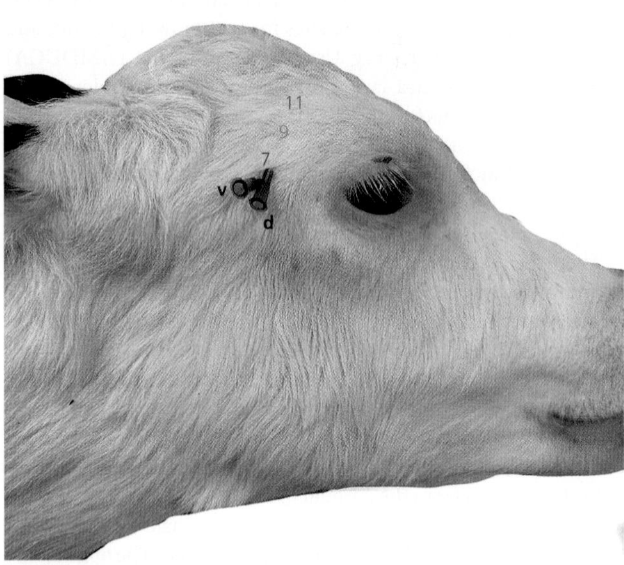

(B)

Figure 66.2 A. Nerve block for disbudding or dehorning in calves using the same approach as in adult cattle with position of the needles at the cornual branch (7), infratrochlear nerve (9), and supraorbital nerve (11). **B.** Simplified two-injection site with the needle directed dorsally (d) for the cornual branch (7), infratrochlear nerve (9), and supraorbital nerve (11), and ventrally (v) for further block of the cornual branch (7).

Eye and adnexa block

The orbit has a rich presence of nerves behind the globe that are not exclusive to the eye. These nerves emerge from the cranial cavity through various foramina (e.g., the foramen orbitorotundum and optic foramen) to supply the eye and adnexa in addition to other extraocular structures. Nerves present in this location include the optic nerve as it emerges from the optic foramen as well as the nerves emerging from the foramen orbitorotundum, including the ophthalmic branches of the trigeminal nerve or extensions of these branches that eventually give rise to nerves supplying the horn (lacrimal nerve, infratrochlear nerve, and frontal nerve), the oculomotor nerve, the trochlear nerve, the abducens nerve, and

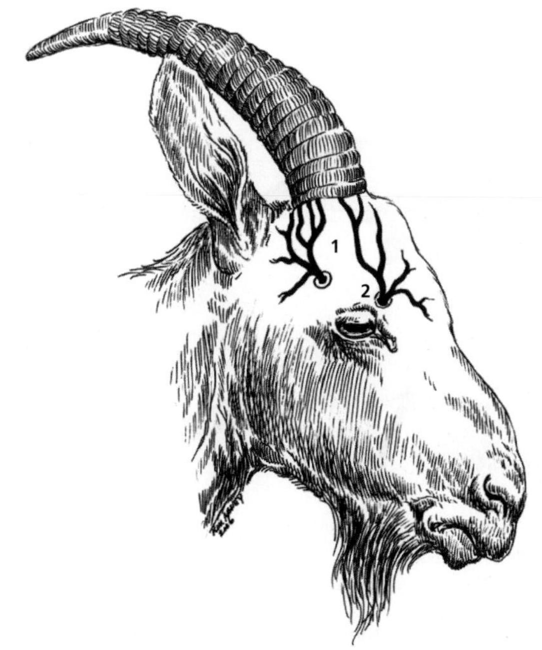

Figure 66.3 Locations for nerve block for dehorning an adult goat. The cornual branch of the lacrimal nerve (zygomaticotemporal) is blocked behind the root of the supraorbital process (1) and the cornual branch of the infratrochlear nerve is blocked at the dorsomedial margin of the orbit (2). Source: Valverde and Doherty [18], with permission.

the zygomaticofacial branch of the maxillary nerve (part of the trigeminal nerve) [16]. Therefore, injection of local anesthetic in this area can result in sensory or motor blockade of the nerves and the structures they serve, and not just of the eye.

The structures potentially anesthetized or paralyzed by local anesthetic effects on the oculomotor nerve include the dorsal, ventral, and medial rectus muscles, the superior levator palpebrae muscle, the retractor bulbi muscle, and the ventral oblique muscle. Local anesthesia of the trochlear nerve affects the dorsal oblique muscle while local anesthesia of the ophthalmic branches of the trigeminal nerve affects the upper eyelid, lacrimal gland, conjunctiva, third eyelid, skin of medial and lateral angle of the eye, iris, cornea, horn, and sections of skin over the frontal bone. Local anesthesia of the zygomaticofacial branch of the maxillary nerve affects the lower eyelid, and local anesthesia of the abducens nerve affects the lateral rectus muscle and the lateral part of the retractor bulbi muscle [16].

Anesthesia of the eye is most commonly performed for enucleation surgery. It is possible to perform an enucleation in adult cattle with the animal standing, using either a four-point injection (retrobulbar block) to block the deep orbital nerves or a Peterson block to exclusively anesthetize the nerves as they exit the skull through the foramen orbitorotundum and optic foramen. Ocular surgery in small ruminants or young cattle is generally performed under general anesthesia but the use of an eye block is also recommended to decrease volatile anesthetic requirements, decrease the likelihood of eliciting the oculocardiac reflex (trigeminovagal), and provide postoperative analgesia.

Four-point block (retrobulbar)

In the awake, adult bovine, the animal can be restrained in a chute with the head secured. A 9 cm, 18 or 20 gauge needle, bent into a curved shape, is inserted into the orbit (i.e., the bony fossa surrounding the globe) at 12, 3, 6, and 9 o'clock positions to a depth of 7–9 cm (in the adult bovine). In adult cattle, 5–10 mL of 2% lidocaine is injected at each site and through the different tissue planes to provide good anesthetic spread and desensitize all nerves present in the orbit that supply the eye and adnexa [19]. The injections can be made through the eyelids, if preferred. The operator uses an index finger to deflect the globe away from the needle as it is inserted. The orbital septum must be penetrated; otherwise, the local anesthetic may be deposited as a subconjunctival injection. The operator can generally perceive the point when the needle penetrates the septum. Exophthalmos indicates a successful block.

In small ruminants and calves, the procedure can be done to enhance antinociception of the eye during general anesthesia. A 3.8 cm, 20 or 22 gauge needle, bent into a curved shape, is inserted as described above for cattle. It is possible to obtain good blockade by doing a two-point block, usually using two opposite locations (e.g., the 6 and 12 or 3 and 9 o'clock positions). Volumes of 2–3 mL of 2% lidocaine are injected at each site in adult small ruminants or calves.

A disadvantage of this technique is that the injection and placement of the needle could damage the optic nerve; as such, it is often not used for procedures other than enucleation. There is also the possibility that the anesthetic could enter the cerebrospinal fluid (CSF), as the meninges extend around the optic nerve. This can result in acute CNS toxicity and, potentially, death. Other complications include penetration of the globe, retrobulbar hemorrhage, and initiation of the oculocardiac reflex from pressure generated during injection. Careful technique, including aspiration prior to injection and cautious injection, especially if resistance is encountered, may attenuate these risks.

Peterson block

This is technically more difficult than the four-point block and requires careful needle positioning, making it less reliable. Its efficacy depends on accurate placement of the injected anesthetic at the site of emergence of the nerves from the foramen orbitorotundum since there is minimal distribution along tissue planes [19]. Due to the ventral location of the foramen orbitorotundum with respect to the optic foramen (about 1 cm ventral), direct blockade of the optic nerve may not result; however, increasing the volume of injection may facilitate reaching and therefore blocking the optic nerve (Fig. 66.4). In addition to the nerves emerging from the foramen orbitorotundum described for the retrobulbar block, the maxillary nerve (branch of the trigeminal nerve) is also involved, resulting in block of the zygomatic nerve and its zygomaticofacial branch (lower eyelid innervation); blockade of the pterygopalatine and infraorbital nerve provides anesthesia of the nasal passages and nose as described below [16]. The mandibular nerve (a branch of the trigeminal) is less likely to be affected because it exits the skull through the oval foramen, which is more ventrally located and separated from the foramen orbitorotundum by the pterygoid crest (Fig. 66.4) [16].

To perform this block, the animal is restrained with its nasal bones parallel to the ground. A 10 or 12 cm, 20 gauge needle is passed just in front of the rostral border of the coronoid process of the mandible, caudal to the notch formed by the zygomatic arch and supraorbital process and directed slightly ventrally and posteriorly for the length of the needle or until it strikes bone. The local anesthetic (15–20 mL, 2% lidocaine) is injected once the needle strikes bone in the area where the nerves travel toward the orbit [18,20] (Figs. 66.4b and 66.5A). Alternatively, the needle can be introduced below the zygomatic arch at the same horizontal position caudal to the notch of the zygomatic arch and supraorbital

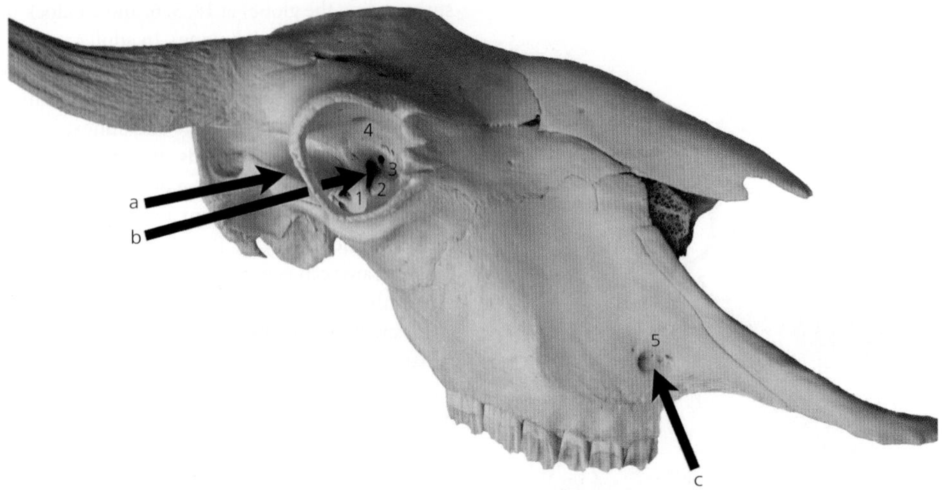

Figure 66.4 Location for needle placement for the auriculopalpebral block (a), the Peterson eye block (b), and the infraorbital block (c). (1) oval foramen; (2) foramen orbitorotundum; (3) optic foramen; (4) supraorbital foramen; (5) infraorbital foramen.

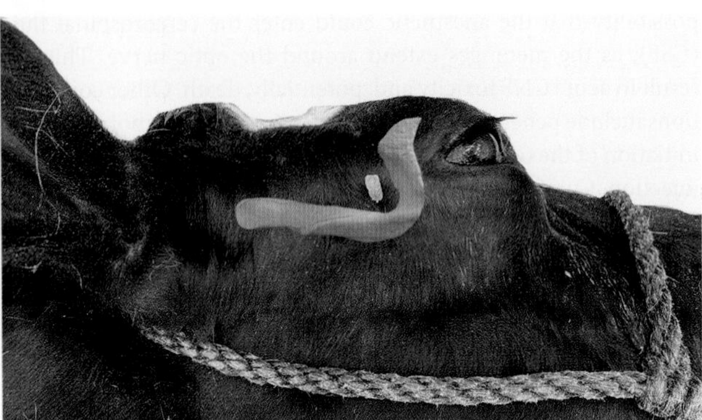

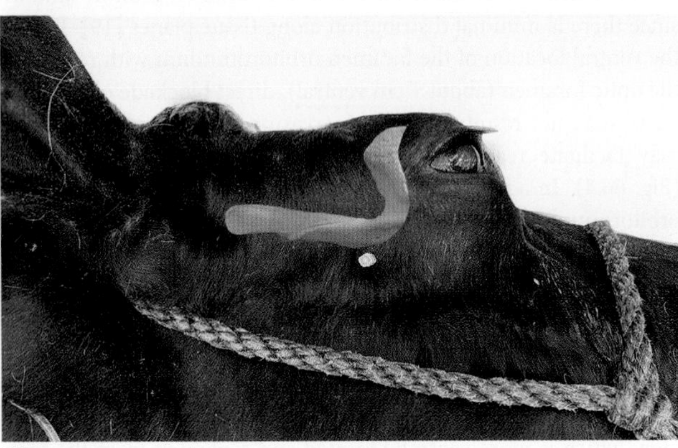

Figure 66.5 Location for needle placement for the Peterson eye block. The diagrammatic overlay shows the position of the zygomatic arch and the supraorbital process. **A.** Needle introduced above the zygomatic arch. **B.** Needle introduced below the zygomatic arch.

process, but in this case the needle is directed slightly dorsally and posteriorly to reach the same position as the previous dorsal approach (Fig. 66.5B). The same technique can be performed in small ruminants and calves using a 6.3 cm, 20 gauge needle and injecting 3–4 mL of 2% lidocaine, with the approach dorsal or ventral to the zygomatic arch.

Auriculopalpebral block

Eyelid akinesia (paralysis) can be produced by blocking the auriculopalpebral nerve (arising from the facial nerve), which provides innervation to the ear (rostral auricular branches) and to the eyelids (zygomatic branches). The zygomatic branches block the motor function of the orbicularis oculi muscle and elevator of the medial oculi angle muscle [16]. This type of anesthesia facilitates examination of the eye by preventing blinking but does not provide sensory blockade.

The auriculopalpebral nerve is blocked by inserting a 2.5–3.8 cm, 22 gauge needle through the skin at the end of the zygomatic arch on the zygomatic process of the temporal bone and injecting 5–10 mL of 2% lidocaine, subcutaneously, at the dorsal border of the arch [18]. By injecting at this site, both zygomatic and rostral auricular branches are blocked (Fig. 66.4a). Attempting to inject the zygomatic branch exclusively is more difficult due to the variable locations at which it branches from the auriculopalpebral nerve following emergence dorsally from the zygomatic arch.

Nasal passages and nasal block

Anesthesia of the nasal passages and nostrils can be achieved by blockade of the maxillary nerve at the foramen orbitorotundum as described for the Peterson eye block. This block will include the divisions of the maxillary nerve that enter the maxillary foramen, the pterygopalatine nerve, and infraorbital nerve. The pterygopalatine nerve supplies the soft palate (minor palatine nerve), hard palate (major palatine nerve), and ventral aspects of the nasal cavity and palate (caudal nasal nerve). The infraorbital nerve travels within the infraorbital canal from the maxillary foramen to the infraorbital foramen, where it emerges and continues to the nose and surrounding tissue, to supply the skin of the dorsal nasal area, nares, and upper lip [16]. To avoid including the innervation to the eye and adnexa, it is more common to only block the infraorbital nerve as it emerges from the infraorbital foramen, resulting in incomplete block of the nasal passages.

The infraorbital foramen can be readily localized by palpation, by extending a line from the nasoincisive notch to the first palpable cheek tooth (second premolar since the first premolar is absent), approximately 5 cm above the tooth (Fig. 66.6). A volume of

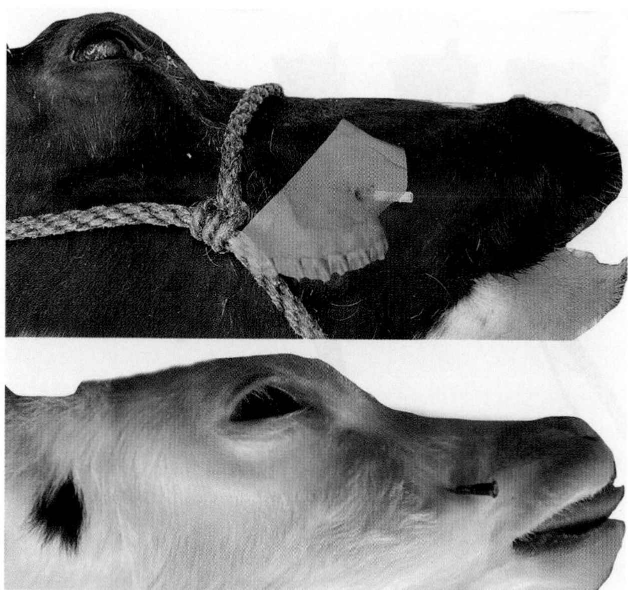

Figure 66.6 Location for needle placement for the infraorbital block in an adult cow (upper image) and a calf (lower image).

5–10 mL in adult cattle or 2–4 mL in calves of 2% lidocaine can be injected into the infraorbital canal using a 3.8 cm, 20 gauge needle introduced through the infraorbital foramen.

Blocks for regional anesthesia of the flank or paralumbar fossa

Blocks to anesthetize the flank are commonly performed in ruminants to permit intra-abdominal surgery (e.g., cesarean section, abomasal, and ruminal procedures). They can be performed in the standing adult bovine and the recumbent calf or small ruminant, using one of several described techniques, including line infiltration, inverted "L" or "7," proximal paravertebral, distal paravertebral, segmental dorsolumbar epidural, and segmental thoracolumbar subarachnoid anesthesia. Generally, the dermatomes intended to be blocked are those supplied by branches of thoracic nerve 13 (T13) and lumbar nerves 1–3 (L1–3). The inclusion of L3 provides superior anesthesia since it supplies the caudal third of the abdominal flank and projects to more cranial aspects of the flank via small anastomotic branches with L2.

Anesthesia of the body wall for abdominal surgery requires anesthesia of all layers, including the peritoneum. If the spread of anesthetic does not reach all layers, especially likely with line infiltration techniques, coverage will be incomplete. Many of these techniques are not suitable for surgery of the ventral abdomen since not all spinal nerves involved in the sensory innervation of this area are blocked.

Line infiltration block

In adult cattle, this is the simplest block to perform and involves multiple injections of small volumes (5–8 mL) of 2% lidocaine per site with a 3.8 cm, 18 gauge needle along the previously clipped and aseptically prepared predicted incision line; the anesthetic spreads in different directions and depths from the point of entry. Therefore, this block mostly affects the nerve endings immediately proximal to the incision site. It is best to start from the most dorsal aspect of the flank and insert the needle in a dorsal to ventral direction and work toward the ventral end of the incision, as each injection provides progressive desensitization before the subsequent injection. A longer needle (8.9 cm) may be used instead of the shorter needle to reach the parietal peritoneum and improve the quality of the block.

With lidocaine, this block is usually only effective for 60–90 min due to the rapid systemic uptake of anesthetic from the vascular abdominal wall. Based on toxic doses for sheep, the total dose should not exceed 5–6 mg/kg since absorption from the muscle layers is probably rapid. This dose represents a volume of 125–150 mL of 2% lidocaine for a 500 kg cow.

In small ruminants or calves, the technique is the same but a 2.5–3.8 cm, 20 gauge needle and volumes of 1–2 mL 2% lidocaine per site are used, based on weight and a 5–6 mg/kg dosage (e.g., a volume of 10–12 mL of 2% lidocaine may be used in a 40 kg patient).

Inverted "L" or "7" block

The injection of local anesthetic following an inverted "L" or "7" shape along the caudal aspect of the last rib and the ventral aspect of the lumbar vertebrae transverse processes blocks the transmission of pain from the periphery (flank area) to the spinal cord. For correct nomenclature, the left flank is blocked with spread of local anesthetic in an inverted "L" or reversed "7" shape, whereas the right flank is blocked with a "7" shape.

The block is similar to the infiltration technique in that it requires similar volumes (5–8 mL per injection in adult cattle) of 2% lidocaine and a 3.8 or 8.9 cm, 18 gauge needle for injection of anesthetic along the shape of the block. To allow progressive desensitization before the subsequent injection (similar to line infiltration techniques) it is best to start from the angle of the "L" or "7" and spread the anesthetic to the caudal aspect for the horizontal plane and to the ventral aspect for the vertical plane. It is also important to remember that nerves will lie in different planes between muscle and fascial layers so several different depths of injection may be required for complete block of deeper layers.

This block provides more spread of the local anesthetic than the line block; however, because it is done on two axes, it is important to distribute the amount of local anesthetic evenly to avoid an incomplete block. Similar to the line block, the duration of action is approximately 60–90 min when 2% lidocaine is used.

In small ruminants or calves the block follows the same technique using a 2.5–3.8 cm, 20 gauge needle and volumes of 1–2 mL 2% lidocaine per site.

Proximal paravertebral block

This block is also known as the "Farquharson," "Hall," or "Cambridge" technique, and the term "proximal" refers to the proximity to the spine. Generally, nerves T13, L1, L2, and L3 are blocked. The inclusion of nerve L3 provides better anesthesia of the caudal third of the abdominal flank [21]. Branches of L3 occasionally contribute to the femoral nerve and blockade may potentially result in hindlimb weakness. However, the femoral nerve is mostly derived from L4, L5, and L6 [22], which makes ataxia very unlikely; therefore, the inclusion of L3 is recommended.

Dorsal and ventral branches from nerves T13 and L1 travel superimposed routes dorsoventrally for approximately 10 cm as the respective nerve emerges from the intervertebral foramen [23]. For nerves L2 and L3, the superimposition is less exact and a branch from the ventral branch of L2 joins the ventral branch from L3 at approximately 9–12 cm from midline (Fig. 66.7). The ventral branch from L3 is the only one of the four nerves involved that travels rostral to the dorsal branch [23].

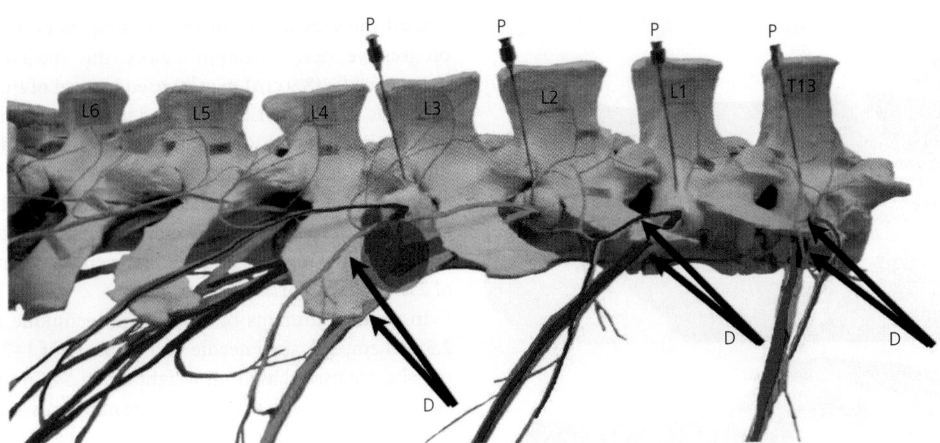

Figure 66.7 Proximal (P) and distal (D) paravertebral block of T13, L1, L2, and L3 nerves. The colored thin lines depict the dorsal branch, and the colored thick lines depict the ventral branch of each nerve. Note the communication between ventral branches of L2 and L3 nerves near the intertransverse space between L3 and L4 (*shaded circle*). The black arrows indicate the dorsal and ventral positioning of the needle for a distal paravertebral block.

In adult cattle, the proximal paravertebral technique involves the perineural injection of local anesthetic in proximity to the spinal nerves as they emerge from the vertebral canal. The dorsal and ventral branches of each nerve must be blocked if complete anesthesia of the flank is desired.

To locate the site of injection, it is best to identify the lumbar transverse processes by counting back from a caudal location as lumber transverse process 1 is not always palpable, depending on the degree of obesity of the animal, and may be confused with the lumbar transverse process 2. While cattle have six lumbar vertebrae, transverse process 6 is significantly smaller than that of 5 and is hidden by the iliac wing. Consequently, counting should begin at lumbar transverse process 5, which is the most proximal and cranial to the tuber coxae, and then move cranially. Each spinal nerve divides into a dorsal and ventral branch as it emerges and travels between lumbar transverse processes. Because the lumbar transverse processes are curved cranially, it is important to note that once a perpendicular line is traced from the middle of the width of the transverse process toward the spine, the nerve located in this area corresponds to the preceding process (e.g., for lumbar transverse process 4, the nerve located using this method is L3, and so on). Therefore, to block nerves T13, L1, L2, and L3, it is necessary to locate lumbar transverse processes 1 through 4 (see Figs. 66.7 and 66.8).

The epaxial area should be clipped and aseptically prepared from the last rib to lumbar transverse process 4, and from the lateral tip of the transverse processes to 3–4 cm from the dorsal spinous processes on midline. In adult cattle, the distal end of lumbar transverse process 4 is identified by placing the thumb and index finger on the width of the process. From here, a perpendicular line is traced from the middle of this width toward the spine and a 3.8 cm, 16 gauge needle is inserted full length approximately 5–6 cm laterally from midline. This will act as a cannula for the subsequent insertion of an 8.9 cm, 20 gauge spinal needle and prevent it from bending. Then, the spinal needle is directed toward lumbar transverse process 4 and, once in contact with it, is walked-off the cranial edge until it advances through the intertransverse ligament and then situated ventrally for blockade of the ventral branch of nerve L3.

Avoid walking the needle off the caudal edge of lumbar transverse process 3 (or any of the subsequent transverse processes included in this block) because blockade at this location is less effective due to the routing of the nerves from the vertebral foramen along the transverse process. Aspiration to confirm negative pressure is important to avoid placement of the needle in the abdominal cavity. Following aspiration, 20 mL of 2% lidocaine is injected. The needle is then retracted to the point of no friction, which indicates placement above the intertransverse ligament, and the dorsal branch is blocked with 5 mL of 2% lidocaine and the needles withdrawn. This method is repeated for nerves L2 and L1 by identifying lumbar transverse processes 3 and 2, respectively. If palpation of lumbar transverse process 1 is not feasible, the distances between the previous injection sites should be symmetric, which will allow the distance between thoracic transverse process 13 and lumbar transverse process 1 to be estimated. The method described above can then be repeated to complete the block. Blockade of the four nerves as described requires approximately 100 mL of 2% lidocaine in a 500 kg cow, similar to the volume used for the infiltration block; however, paravertebral block provides a more precise but extensive block of the flank and is usually recommended over infiltration techniques. The duration of action tends to exceed that of the line infiltration and inverted "L" or "7" blocks since the administration of anesthetic is more circumscribed to the main nerves; with 2% lidocaine, blocks of 90–120 min are produced.

In addition to sensory blockade, motor and sympathetic fibers are also affected, which results in relaxation of the epaxial lumbar muscles and vasodilation, respectively. Therefore, the spine curves (scoliosis) toward the blocked site and the skin temperature over the flank increases. From the surgeon's perspective, this means that tissues become tense due to the convexity that results on the surgical site, which tends to spread the tissues when surgically approaching the abdominal cavity. This combined with vasodilation of blood vessels, can result in increased bleeding if surgical hemostasis is poor.

In small ruminants and calves, the block follows the same technique for adult cattle and should include the same nerves (T13–L3). Anatomical studies in sheep have identified nerve branches from T13 that run obliquely and overlap with segments from L1 and L2 on the flank area as they spread toward midline [24–26], which is similar to cattle but occurs less commonly in goats [27,28]. Sheep have six (more common) or seven lumbar vertebrae, whereas goats

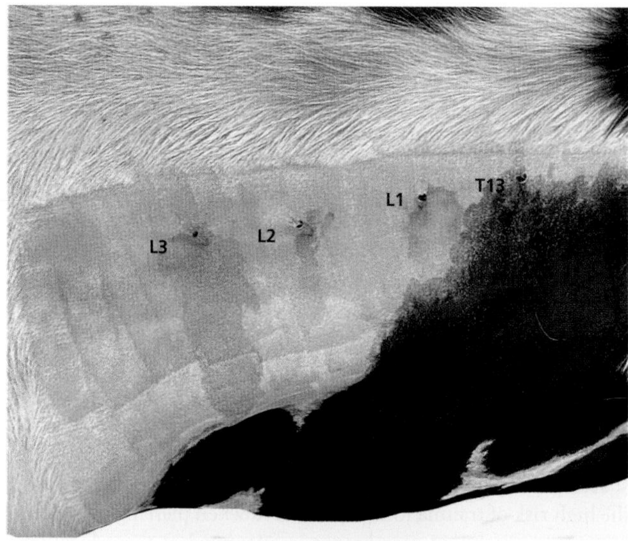

(A)

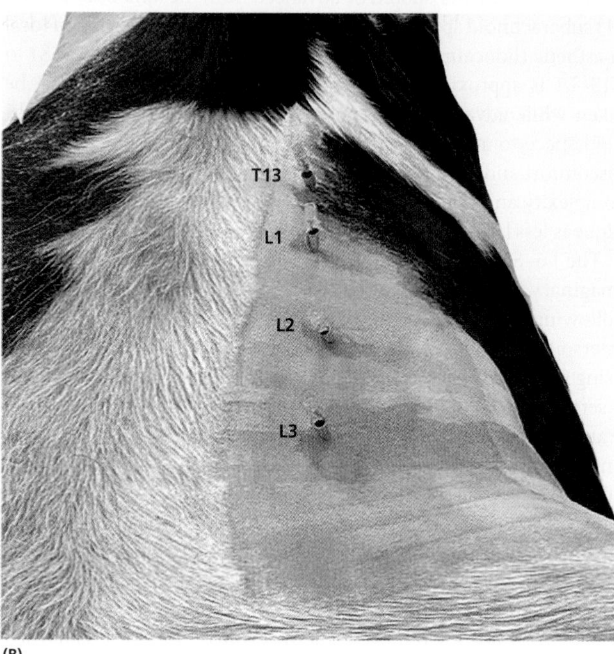

(B)

Figure 66.8 Positioning of large gauge needles to act as cannulas for spinal needles for proximal paravertebral blockade in an adult cow. **A.** Dorsal view of the cannulas from the right side. **B.** Dorsal view of the cannulas from behind. Needle cannulas are inserted at the depth of the ventral branch for blockade of T13, L1, L2, and L3 nerves.

have six but sometimes only five lumbar vertebrae, which can complicate the identification of vertebrae if counting backward as described for cattle. However, it is simpler in these species to identify lumbar transverse process 1 and count from there to verify the proper sites for needle insertion. In these species, the block is completed using a 2.5–3.8 cm, 20 gauge needle with volumes of 0.5–1.5 mL for the dorsal branch and 2–3 mL for the ventral branch of 2% lidocaine. It is important to accurately note body weight and not exceed the 5–6 mg/kg toxic dosage threshold [24,29,30].

For a longer-lasting block, ropivacaine, bupivacaine, or lidocaine with epinephrine have also been used for the proximal paravertebral block in cattle and small ruminants. In one study of mixed-breed sheep (44–49 kg) injected with 4 mL of local anesthetic (1.5 mL for the dorsal branch and 2.5 mL for the ventral branch), the duration of anesthesia as assessed with needle pinpricks, pinching with a hemostat, and ruminal fistulation surgery was 649 min for 0.5% levobupivacaine, and 569 min for 0.5% ropivacaine [30]. In another study with fat-tailed lambs (23 kg) injected with 3 mL of local anesthetic (1 mL for the dorsal branch and 2 mL for the ventral branch), the duration of anesthesia as assessed with needle pinpricks and pinching with a hemostat was 65 min for 2% lidocaine, 95 min for 2% lidocaine with epinephrine (5 μg/mL), and 303 min for 0.5% bupivacaine [29].

Distal paravertebral block

This block is also known as the "Magda," "Cakala," or "Cornell" technique and the term "distal" refers to the distance from the spine. This distal approach is used to block the dorsal and ventral branches of the same nerves as for the proximal paravertebral block (T13, L1, L2, and L3) as they cross over and under, respectively, the transverse processes (Fig. 66.7).

For this block, a lateral approach with regards to the location of the lumbar transverse process is used and the area around the tip of each process is clipped and aseptically prepared. The transverse processes are located as described for the proximal paravertebral block; the L2 and L3 nerves are blocked from the location of lumbar transverse process 4, the L1 nerve is blocked from the location of lumbar transverse process 2, and the T13 nerve is blocked from the location of lumbar transverse process 1 (Fig. 66.7).

In adult cattle, approximately 5 mL of 2% lidocaine is injected above and 10–20 mL below the transverse process using a 6.4–8.9 cm, 18 gauge needle. The injection is started at the tip of the distal end of the transverse process and the local anesthetic is deposited along the process, as the needle is advanced toward the spine. It is important to keep the needle close to the transverse process as anesthetic deposited in the surrounding soft tissue rather than around the nerve may result in block failure. The duration of action is similar to the proximal paravertebral block.

Segmental dorsolumbar epidural block

In cattle, the dermatomes innervated by nerves T13 and L1–L3 can be blocked bilaterally or unilaterally by performing an epidural injection at the thoracolumbar (T13–L1) or first lumbar intervertebral (L1–L2) space [31–34].

An epidural injection refers to depositing the anesthetic drug in the space between the dura mater and the vertebral column. Technically, it is an intradural injection between two dural laminae since the dura mater only closely adheres as a fused double layer within the skull. In the vertebral column, it is separated and only the internal lamina, made of fibrous tissue, surrounds the spinal cord, and provides rigidity to help support the blood vessels that supply the spinal cord [35].

The injection of a reduced volume of local anesthetic or xylazine into the epidural space at T13–L1 or L1–L2 allows these drugs to affect only those segments of the spinal cord that innervate the flank without interfering with motor function of the pelvic limbs; this allows the animal to remain standing and prevents ataxia. This technique can be used for surgery on or performed via the flank and needle tip placement in the epidural space can be directed toward one side of the spinal cord to emphasize the block on the corresponding ipsilateral flank or the needle kept on the median plane with respect to the spinal cord to block both sides. The block is more technically challenging than any of the other techniques previously described for flank anesthesia; however, it can be readily learned and effectively used by practitioners [34,36].

Adequate restraint and sedation of the animal are necessary to facilitate the placement of the needle in the epidural space. The skin caudal to the T13 or L1 spinous process and contralateral to the flank region to be desensitized is aseptically prepared and injected subcutaneously with 2–4 mL of 2% lidocaine adjacent to the interspinous ligaments between T13–L1 or L1–L2 to facilitate the insertion of a short 2.5 cm, 14 gauge needle that serves as a cannula for the subsequent insertion of an 11.4 cm, 18 gauge spinal needle [32]. Alternatively, a 12 cm, 16 gauge Tuohy needle can be used by itself [37]. The mean distance from skin to the epidural space at this level is 8.1 cm in cows between 337 and 742 kg [38], but it is recommended to use needles that are slightly longer because if the needle does not reach the deeper planes of the epidural space, the injected anesthetic will remain between periosteum and epidural fat, rather than distribute between epidural fat and dura mater [37]. Fat is considered a barrier because it is present in a semifluid state that impedes spread and potentially prevents the actions of the anesthetic drug; the amount of fat in the thoracolumbar epidural space is greater in the dorsal aspect compared to the ventral aspect of the space [37].

The L1–L2 intervertebral space is localized on the path of an imaginary line drawn from side to side, 1–2 cm caudal to the tips of the two cranial edges of the second lumbar transverse process. The operator can then decide to insert the needles at the depression between L1 and L2 or move to the next cranial depression between T13 and L1. The spinal needle is advanced gradually through the interspinous ligament until it reaches and then penetrates the ligamentum flavum to enter the epidural space. Correct placement can be verified by use of the hanging drop technique in which the hub of the needle is filled with saline or local anesthetic after the stylet is removed. If the needle is correctly placed, the fluid is aspirated into the needle shaft and epidural space due to the subatmospheric epidural pressure. The stylet can also be removed before the needle penetrates the ligamentum flavum and the operator can detect the aspiration of the fluid once the needle enters the epidural space. The initial pressure of the epidural space is on average −21 mmHg (range of −17 to −23 mmHg), but within 1 min of needle insertion, this stabilizes at −14 mmHg (range of −9 to −17 mmHg) [38]. For this reason, it has been recommended to allow air to enter freely into the epidural space for approximately 1 min to decrease the effects of varying pressures on the distribution of anesthetic drug [33]. Additional verification of correct placement should include ease of injection into the epidural space and the absence of CSF prior to injection, which indicates that the dura and arachnoid membrane have not been pierced. Avoiding subarachnoid injection is important since epidural doses are significantly higher than those recommended for subarachnoid administration. An alternative modified technique involves introducing the needle an additional 0.7–1.0 cm or until the cow shows signs of discomfort, such as sudden movement or dipping of the back, to bypass the epidural fat and enhance the spread of the anesthetic drug [33]. Caution is advised with this modified technique. The needle should be removed immediately after injection to avoid damage to the spinal cord.

Studies using new methylene blue have shown that 5 mL injected at the L1–L2 epidural space of adult Holstein cows spread to the T12–L3 spinal dermatomes, whereas 10 mL spread to the T11–L5 spinal dermatomes [37]. Volumes of 6–8 mL of 2% lidocaine (0.24–0.32 mg/kg) or 5% procaine (0.6–0.8 mg/kg) are recommended in a 500 kg cow to desensitize the dermatomes of T13–L3. Xylazine (2%, 0.05 mg/kg) is also effective but the combination of xylazine (0.025 mg/kg) and lidocaine (0.1 mg/kg) diluted to a volume of 5 mL with 0.9% saline resulted in more consistent anesthesia than either drug alone diluted to the same volume [33]. Onset of anesthesia is approximately 10–15 min with a duration of 45–120 min [33,34].

For prolonged regional anesthesia or analgesia, an epidural catheter can be placed in the T13–L1 space to allow repeated injections of anesthetic drugs and prolonged duration of action. A 10.2 cm, 17 gauge Tuohy needle is placed in the epidural space as described above and the tip of the epidural catheter is advanced through the needle to the L1–L2 space for injection of the anesthetic drugs [39]. Because of the possibility of the catheter tip pointing to one side of the spinal cord, a unilateral block may be more likely with this technique.

Segmental thoracolumbar subarachnoid block

The insertion of needles into the T13–L1 or L1–L2 intervertebral spaces for subarachnoid injection of anesthetic is discouraged due to the high risk of trauma to the spinal cord when piercing of the dura mater and arachnoid membranes is attempted at these locations. Therefore, a catheter should be advanced from the lumbosacral (L6–S1) subarachnoid space to the T13–L1 space for the injection of local anesthetic (lidocaine or procaine) [39]. The distance from L6–S1 to T13–L1 is approximately 45 cm in adult cattle and care must be taken while advancing the catheter rostrally within the subarachnoid space to avoid kinking or curling it, which results in patient discomfort and potential damage to the spinal cord. Due to greater complexity and the need for a more sterile environment, this technique is less likely to be performed under field conditions.

The L6–S1 intervertebral space is localized 1–4 cm caudal to an imaginary line traced between the cranial edges of the tuber coxae. Following aseptic skin preparation, the subcutaneous and deep interspinous ligaments are desensitized with 5 mL of 2% lidocaine using a 15 cm, 18 gauge needle. A 15 cm, 17 gauge Tuohy needle is inserted at the L6–S1 intervertebral space with the bevel pointing cranially and slowly advanced into the epidural space, continuing until the dura and arachnoid mater are pierced and the subarachnoid space is entered. Correct placement is verified by aspiration of 2 mL of CSF. An 80–100 cm epidural catheter with a spring guide is advanced into the subarachnoid space for the estimated distance required to reach the T13–L1 space, which is usually approximately 60 cm due to the length and angle of the needle. The Tuohy needle and spring guide are removed, and the catheter distance is adjusted to the correct location and secured in place. Doses of 1.5–2 mL of 2% lidocaine or 5% procaine have been injected at a rate of 0.5 mL/min to induce unilateral or bilateral anesthesia from T10–L3 in 5–10 min for a duration of 54 min [39].

One disadvantage of this technique is the uncertainty of whether the resulting block will be on the intended side of the animal. The variation in block has been suggested to result from trapping of the catheter ventral to the spinal cord, which may impede adequate distribution of the injected anesthetic around the circumference of the pia mater due to the presence of the dorsal and ventral longitudinal ligaments [39].

Blocks for regional anesthesia of the linea alba and paramedian region

Regional anesthetic techniques for the flank are often inadequate for coverage of the ventral abdomen. Alternate or additional techniques may be required for surgical procedures that require ventral midline or paramedian approaches. These include local infiltrative techniques and epidural analgesia and anesthesia. Ultrasound-guided fascial plane blocks such as a transversus abdominis plane block or rectus sheath block may be used as part of a multimodal analgesic technique and is discussed later (see the section titled "Ultrasound-guided regional anesthesia").

Line infiltration block

The abdomen, subcutaneous tissues, and skin of the abdomen can be desensitized by infiltration of local anesthetic to allow procedures such as correction of umbilical and abdominal wall hernias and right paramedian abomasopexy to be performed. For these blocks, the technique and volumes described for the flank line infiltration block are used along the anatomic area selected for the surgery. Often a "V" shape block can be used with the angle of the "V" located at the cranial aspect of the incision and the wings along either side of the incision to block more proximal sensory nerves.

Lumbosacral, sacrococcygeal, or intercoccygeal epidural (cranial epidural) block

This technique is often referred to as a "cranial (anterior) epidural" and can be performed at any of the three sites (Fig. 66.9). Injections at the sacrococcygeal or first intercoccygeal epidural space require that the injectate volume of anesthetic drug is sufficient to facilitate its rostral spread from this site to the thoracolumbar area so that it can affect structures cranial to the pelvis (periumbilical region and flank). For lumbosacral epidurals, less volume is required.

The same principles discussed for the segmental dorsolumbar epidural technique apply here. This technique is used commonly in small ruminants for abdominal or pelvic surgery, most often to supplement general anesthesia or sedation. Despite their popularity, epidural injections often fail in providing complete analgesia/anesthesia for multiple reasons, including those listed in Box 66.1.

In adult cattle, volumes of local anesthetic of up to 150 mL (0.2–0.3 mL/kg), injected in the sacrococcygeal or intercoccygeal epidural space, have been recommended to desensitize the flank and umbilical region but these volumes also result in motor block of the pelvic limbs and the animal unable to remain standing. For this reason, cranial epidural blocks are not commonly practiced in adult

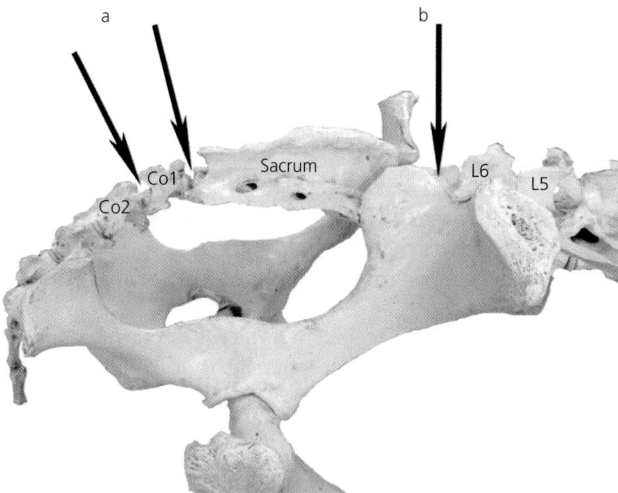

Figure 66.9 Locations for epidural injection in cattle. Caudal epidural injection sites at the sacrococcygeal or intercoccygeal spaces (a). Cranial epidural injection site at the lumbosacral space (b). A caudal epidural approach can be used for a cranial epidural injection if sufficient volume is injected to spread the anesthetic rostrally.

cattle as they may injure themselves when motor control is lost or when attempting to stand. Another concern is that a high (cranial) epidural may result in hypotension secondary to blockade of sympathetic nerves, which results in vasodilation. Hypotension is more likely to develop in animals with pre-existing hypovolemia.

Calves and small ruminants may require larger volumes on a mL per kg basis than adult cattle to achieve the same degree of cranial spread from the sacrococcygeal or intercoccygeal epidural space. Volumes of 0.4–0.6 mL/kg of local anesthetic are recommended to achieve analgesia of the umbilical region [40].

A lumbosacral epidural requires a smaller volume. In goats given 0.1, 0.2, or 0.3 mL/kg of new methylene blue at the lumbosacral space immediately after euthanasia, the average rostral spread was to L3–L4, T13–L1, and T10–T11, respectively [41]. A similar study in sheep demonstrated rostral spread to the first lumbar segment with a volume of 0.2 mL/kg [42]. To obtain sufficient anesthesia of the cranial abdomen and abdominal wall, it is often necessary for the anesthetic to reach the T10 dermatomal segment but, due to the possible variation in further rostral spread, there is also an increased risk of impairing pulmonary function. Volumes of 0.2 mL/kg or 1 mL/5 kg of the local anesthetic of choice (2% lidocaine, 0.5% bupivacaine, and 0.5% ropivacaine) are commonly used.

In goats and young calves, the lumbosacral space is easily palpable but may be less obvious in large, well-nourished sheep. A lumbosacral epidural injection can be made with the animal in sternal or lateral recumbency. Spread of anesthetic is more likely to be even, and to produce bilateral blockade, when the animal is placed in a sternal position. Otherwise, the side to be approached should be the dependent side when performed in a lateral position; this facilitates contact of the local anesthetic with the desired nerve roots. The animal should be maintained in that position for at least 5–10 min to allow the block to take effect before moving it to the required position for surgery.

Strict aseptic technique and use of sterile gloves are indicated for epidural injections at the lumbosacral space, due to the close proximity of the spinal cord within the spinal canal. For most small ruminants and calves, a 3.8 or 7.5 cm, 20 or 22 gauge spinal needle is suitable. The landmarks consist of the distinct dorsal spinous processes of the lumbar vertebrae, which are readily distinguished from sacral vertebrae. Calves and small ruminants have six lumbar vertebrae, goats may only have five, and sheep can have as many as

Box 66.1 Reasons for failure of epidural injections.

Technique
Subcutaneous injection
Intravascular injection
Incomplete injection into epidural space
Drug
Inadequate drug for purpose of epidural
Inadequate volume and fewer dermatomes blocked
Inadequate dose
Timing
Insufficient time for onset of action
Insufficient allowed duration of action
Anatomy
Malformations
Trauma and distorted anatomy
Fibrosis in epidural space from previous trauma/irritation
Leakage from epidural space through intervertebral foramen into surrounding tissue
Position of animal and asymmetric block due to deposition of anesthetic on one side or drainage into coccygeal epidural space
Uptake into fat and/or vessels in epidural space

seven lumbar vertebrae. Therefore, it is advisable to palpate the anterior surfaces of both tuber coxae and draw an imaginary line between them; this borders the spinous process of the last lumbar vertebra. At this site, the index finger can palpate the space between the last lumbar vertebra and first sacral vertebra. At this point, the spinal needle enters the skin perpendicularly and is advanced into the epidural space. Correct placement is confirmed by a popping sensation as the needle penetrates the ligamentum flavum and a loss of resistance upon injection (the "hanging drop" technique, as described previously, may also be used). This distance is relatively short, especially in goats. Inadvertent advancement into the subarachnoid space often occurs since the spinal cord is present at this location. If the animal is in lateral recumbency and the subarachnoid space is penetrated, CSF drips from the hub following removal of the stylet; however, this is less obvious if the animal is in sternal recumbency. If CSF is encountered, the spinal needle can be withdrawn slightly to reposition it in the epidural space and avoid a subarachnoid injection.

In 1-month-old xylazine-sedated calves, one study compared epidural and subarachnoid injections of xylazine (0.025 mg/kg) combined with lidocaine (0.1 mg/kg; 0.05 mL/kg) diluted in 5 mL of sterile saline. Injections were made at the lumbosacral space with the calves in lateral recumbency for the subarachnoid injection and in sternal recumbency for the epidural injection. The subarachnoid injection was more effective and longer acting for providing complete antinociception to pinprick stimulation in the cranial abdomen, umbilicus, and caudal abdomen, compared to the epidural injection [43].

In pigs, lumbosacral epidural anesthesia can be used for cesarean section, repair of rectal, uterine, or vaginal prolapse, repair of umbilical, inguinal, or scrotal hernias, surgery of scirrhous cord, and surgery of the prepuce, penis, or rear limbs. Pigs have six or seven lumbar vertebrae, and the location of the lumbosacral space can be located as described for ruminants. An imaginary line between the tuber coxae marks the level of the spinous process of the last lumbar vertebra. The depression located on midline approximately 0.5–2.5 cm caudal to this (depending on the size of the pig) corresponds to the space between the last lumbar vertebra and the sacrum. Alternatively, in the standing pig, a line from the patella to the spine is usually 2–3 cm cranial to the lumbosacral space [44–46]. A 3.8 to 6.4 cm, 20 gauge spinal needle can be used in piglets less than 20 kg; an 8.9 to 15.2 cm, 20 gauge spinal needle is typically required in larger pigs, especially adult boars and sows. Following aseptic preparation of the area and subcutaneous infiltration of 3–5 mL of lidocaine in larger pigs, a short 2.5 or 3.8 cm, 16 gauge needle can be introduced first in the depression of the lumbosacral space to act as a cannula and prevent bending of long spinal needles. The spinal needle is then advanced between the vertebrae at a 0–20° angle perpendicular to the skin, until it perforates the ligamentum flavum, which can be felt as a pop. The spinal cord terminates with the conus medullaris between sacral vertebrae 2 and 3 [47]. The subarachnoid space is not easily penetrated due to its small size compared to the epidural space as well as abundant adipose tissue that causes anterior bulging of the dura mater with a consequent reduction in the subarachnoid space on the midline. The subarachnoid space is more readily accessed from a lateral position [47]. It is possible to be in the subarachnoid space with the needle position exactly on the midline and not detect the presence of CSF; therefore, proper verification of the epidural space via careful aspiration is recommended before injection to avoid inadvertent subarachnoid injection of an epidural dose, since the latter can be up to 10 times that required for subarachnoid injection [35]. An epidural injection can also be performed at the first intersacral (S1–S2) space in pigs, due to the presence of a significant dorsal foramen at this location, which is about 75% the size (diameter) of the lumbosacral space [48].

In 6–10-week-old pigs (18 kg) given new methylene blue at the lumbosacral space immediately after euthanasia, cranial spread of injectate was approximately eight spaces (range of L3–L4 to T10–T11) for a dose of 0.05 mL/kg; eight spaces (range of L2–L3 to T8–T9) for a dose of 0.1 mL/kg; 10 spaces (range of T13–L1 to T5–T6) for a dose of 0.2 mL/kg; and 18 spaces (range of T8–T9 to the brain) for a dose of 0.3 mL/kg [49]. Therefore, volumes of 0.05–0.1 mL/kg at the lumbosacral space seem appropriate to desensitize structures caudal to the diaphragm and are less likely to result in adverse effects. However, epidural spread may be different in adult patients. Clinically, doses of local anesthetics used in pigs at the lumbosacral space are similar to those of small ruminants, i.e., 0.13–0.22 mL/kg or 1 mL/4.5–7.5 kg, for pigs that are less than 50 kg; however, reduced volume ranges (on a mL/kg basis) are suggested in larger pigs [44]. If the procedure involves the abdomen, such as in cesarean sections, maximum doses of 10 mL/100 kg, 15 mL/200 kg, and 20 mL/300 kg are used; whereas for standing castrations, doses of 4 mL/100 kg, 6 mL/200 kg, and 8 mL/300 kg are recommended.

Xylazine has also been used for lumbosacral epidural injection in pigs; a dose of 2 mg/kg induced analgesia to electrical stimulation and skin-deep needle pricks to the perianal, flank, and umbilical area [50] of similar duration (approximately 2 h) to lidocaine (0.13 mL/kg) [51].

Doses in pigs can also be calculated based on the length of the spinal canal. Pigs can show variations in the number of thoracic and lumbar vertebrae. In one study, 67% of pigs had a combined number of 22 thoracic and lumbar vertebrae, 14% had 21 vertebrae, and 19% had 23 vertebrae [48]. In addition, the combined number varies within each group, e.g., of those with 22 thoracic and lumbar vertebrae, 23% had 15 thoracic and seven lumbar vertebrae, whereas the remaining 77% had 16 thoracic and six lumbar vertebrae [48]. Therefore, measuring the distance from the external occipital protuberance to the first coccygeal vertebra may allow more precise dosing for epidural injections. For pigs weighing up to 65 kg, the distance from the external occipital protuberance to the first coccygeal vertebra varied between 40 and 99 cm. The estimated volumes required to spread contrast medium to the T10 vertebra were 0.8 mL/10 cm for pigs with distances between 40 and 69 cm, 0.9 mL/10 cm for pigs with distances between 70 and 79 cm, and 1.0 mL/10 cm for pigs with distances between 80 and 99 cm [48].

Blocks for regional anesthesia of the pelvic area and related tissues

Sacrococcygeal or intercoccygeal epidural (caudal epidural) block

The anatomic structures present in the pelvis and surrounding tissue can be blocked by injection of anesthetic drugs into the sacrococcygeal (S5–Co1 in cattle, S4–Co1 in small ruminants), or first intercoccygeal (Co1–Co2) spaces.

Maintaining motor control of the pelvic limbs and ensuring that the animal remains standing are possible by injecting lower volumes of anesthetic that selectively produce nociceptive blockade while sparing motor nerves, which are more cranially located (e.g., femoral and sciatic nerves). This technique, referred to as "caudal epidural block," is most commonly used to perform procedures on the perineum or tail in standing cattle. This may include obstetric procedures that involve the vulva and vagina, andrological procedures of the prepuce and scrotum, and procedures that involve the tail, perineum, anus, and rectum. This technique does not desensitize the udder. It is also less commonly used in small ruminants because epidural or subarachnoid injection at the lumbosacral space is easy to perform and, for ease of handling, recumbency is often desired in association with the sensory block.

The epidural space at the sacrococcygeal or intercoccygeal intervertebral spaces does not include the spinal cord since the caudal tip of the spinal cord (conus medullaris) extends only to sacral vertebrae 2–3 in young calves and to sacral vertebra 1 in the adult [52]. Only the last sacral nerve (S5) and caudal nerves are present at the level of S5–Co1 and only the caudal nerves at the level of Co1–Co2 in the form of the cauda equina. Therefore, compared to the L6–S1 epidural, all injections at the sacrococcygeal or first intercoccygeal space are strictly epidural and there is no risk of subarachnoid injection.

In cattle, the S5–Co1 or Co1–Co2 space is located by elevating and lowering the tail while palpating the area and identifying the space at which the tail hinges (Fig. 66.9a). In younger cattle, movement of the tail is usually evident at the sacrococcygeal space but in older cattle, the S5–Co1 space may be ossified, and the preferred site of injection is the Co1–Co2 space.

A 3.8 cm, 20 or 18 gauge needle is inserted on midline between the vertebrae at a 0–15° angle to perpendicular. The needle is inserted to a depth of 1–2 cm, depending on the animal's size, and the hub of the needle is filled with saline or the local anesthetic. The needle is then advanced until the fluid is aspirated as it enters the epidural space, due to the subatmospheric epidural pressure. On occasion, blood will flow from the hub and, in this case, the needle should be withdrawn slightly. If the needle is correctly placed, there is minimal resistance to injection.

In neonatal calves, 0.05, 0.1, or 0.15 mL/kg of new methylene blue given at the S5–Co1 epidural space immediately after euthanasia spread cranially over five spaces (range of L7–S1 to L5–L6) for the low dose; eight spaces (range of L7–S1 to L2–L3) for the intermediate dose; and eight spaces (range of L6–L7 to L2–L3) for the high dose [49]. The injection of 0.4 mL/kg of contrast medium in the same epidural space to calves weighing 50–60 kg resulted in cranial spread to the T12 vertebra [40]. In adult cattle (approximately 525 kg), epidural injection of new methylene blue at the Co1–Co2 space 20 min before euthanasia spread rostrally on average to L6–S1 with 5 mL (0.01 mL/kg), to L5–L6 with 10 mL (0.02 mL/kg) and to L3–L4 with 20 mL (0.04 mL/kg) [53]. This indicates that to avoid motor blockade and ataxia, significantly less volume (on a weight basis) is necessary for caudal epidural in adult cattle compared to younger animals. Clinically, 0.015 mL/kg of 0.75% ropivacaine at the S5–Co1 space in adult cattle resulted in analgesia of the dermatomes corresponding to the coccyx to S3 spinal cord segments without ataxia [54].

The usual volume of local anesthetic (2% lidocaine, 0.5% bupivacaine, and 0.5–0.75% ropivacaine) for a caudal epidural in adult cattle is recommended to be 5–6 mL (approximately 1 mL/100 kg) [18,54]. Volumes greater than 10 mL may cause weakness of the pelvic limbs and recumbency due to involvement of the L4–L6 nerves, which are main contributors to the femoral nerve, and L5–S2, the main contributors to the sciatic nerve [22]. Onset of anesthesia is usually 10–20 min, although tail flaccidity is obvious in less than 1–2 min with 2% lidocaine. The duration of anesthesia depends on the local anesthetic used, but usually is 0.5–1.5 h for lidocaine or mepivacaine and 1.5–3 h for bupivacaine or ropivacaine. Analgesic effects will last longer than anesthetic effects [54].

Anatomic structures blocked by a caudal epidural using the aforementioned doses include structures innervated by sacral and caudal segments including: (1) structures innervated by the pudendal nerve (S2–S4) (i.e., skin of the perineum, skin over the semitendinosus and semimembranosus muscles, scrotum, labia, skin of the caudal surface of the udder, perineal muscles, vagina, vulva, prepuce, penis, and clitoris); (2) the coccygeus and levator ani muscles innervated by the corresponding sacral nerves (S3, S4); (3) structures innervated by the caudal rectal nerves (S4, S5) (i.e., the caudal part of the rectum, coccygeus, levator ani, external anal sphincter, retractor penis (clitoridis), constrictor vestibuli, labium, and skin of anal region); and (4) the tail innervated by the caudal nerves from the cauda equina in the vertebral canal [22,55].

Analgesia or anesthesia appears more rapidly in the dermatomes proximal to the site of injection (tail) than at distant areas (perineal) and tends to disappear more quickly in distant compared to proximal areas. For adult cattle administered ropivacaine, time to onset of analgesia as assessed by needle pinprick and hemostat clamping was approximately 10 min on the tail (caudal nerve) and 15 min in the perineal area (pudendal nerve and its branches), whereas mean duration of analgesia was 368 min for the tail and 359 min for the perineal area, respectively [54].

Other drugs used for caudal epidural injection have included the α_2-adrenergic receptor agonists. Xylazine is the most effective for inducing analgesia and anesthesia, but the dose used is similar to systemic doses and absorption from the epidural space results in the known adverse effects of α_2-adrenergic receptor agonists, including sedation, ataxia, bradycardia, hypotension, respiratory acidosis, hypoxemia, increased uterine tone, and ruminal atony [40,56,57]. The increased uterine motility may interfere with fetotomy procedures [57]. Xylazine at 0.05–0.06 mg/kg diluted in 5 mL of saline induced more prolonged analgesia (four times) than 5 mL of lidocaine 2% (0.01 mL/kg; 0.2 mg/kg) in adult cows administered the drugs at the Co1–Co2 epidural space [56,57]. The co-administration of lidocaine and xylazine often results in a more rapid onset and prolonged duration of analgesia than either drug alone [58]. Other α_2-adrenergic receptor agonists, such as detomidine and medetomidine, have been described but appear to offer little advantage over xylazine [59,60].

The same technique can be used in small ruminants, calves, and South American camelids for castration and obstetric procedures, and for tail docking in lambs. A 2.5 or 3.8 cm, 20 gauge needle is introduced at the S4–Co1 or Co1–Co2 space for injection of 0.02–0.03 mL/kg of 2% lidocaine (1–1.5 mL/50 kg; 0.4–0.6 mg/kg) in small ruminants and calves [18,61]. In llamas, a dose of 0.01 mL/kg of 2% lidocaine (1 mL/100 kg; 0.22 mg/kg) or xylazine (0.17 mg/kg diluted with 2 mL of saline), or their combination at the same doses have been effective after S5–Co1 administration and, as for other species, the duration of analgesia was significantly longer for the combination (over 5.5 h) than for lidocaine (over 1 h) or xylazine (3 h) alone [62].

Sacral paravertebral block

This technique can produce effects similar to a caudal epidural, with the exception of the caudal nerves supplying the tail; therefore, tail tone is maintained. The block is specific to nerves S3, S4, and S5, so the animal does not become ataxic.

The blockade of nerves S3–S5 results in desensitization of structures innervated by the following branches: the levator ani nerve (S3, S4, and fibers from the pudendal nerve or caudal rectal nerve), the caudal rectal nerve (S4, S5), and the majority of fibers from the pudendal nerve (S2–S4) [22].

The block is performed with the animal in a standing position; the area from the midsacrum to the base of the tail is clipped and aseptically prepared at the specific points where the needle is inserted on both sides of midline (Fig. 66.10). The easiest site to locate is the S5–Co1 space. A 5 or 7.5 cm, 20 gauge spinal needle is inserted 1.0 cm lateral to the dorsal midline of the vertebral crest at the S5–Co1 space and advanced to the level of the transverse processes of those vertebrae; at the caudal border of S5, 5 mL of 2% lidocaine is injected to desensitize the dorsal and ventral branch and the procedure repeated on the contralateral side. Nerves S4 and S3 are approximately 3 and 6 cm cranial to the location of nerve S5, 1.0–1.5 cm lateral to the dorsal midline. At these two locations, the spinal needle penetrates the respective foramina and 5 mL of 2% lidocaine is injected per nerve on each side of the dorsal midline.

Injection of alcohol for the alleviation of chronic rectal tenesmus for up to 5 weeks without affecting urination and defecation has been described; however, this treatment is not recommended in males because the pudendal nerve and caudal rectal nerve innervate the penis and preputial prolapse is likely to occur [63].

This block can also be performed in sheep and goats. The main differences are that sheep and goats only have four sacral vertebrae; as such, the block is completed at the S4–Co1 space for nerve S4, and at the S3–S4 space for nerve S3.

Pudendal block

The pudendal block involves injection around the pudendal and caudal rectal nerves through an ischiorectal fossa approach or a lateral approach and has similar effects as a sacral paravertebral block. In standing males, it is generally used for penile analgesia and to produce relaxation distal to the sigmoid flexure, which allows examination of the prolapsed penis [64,65]. In standing females, this block relieves rectal and anal straining caused by uterine prolapse or chronic vaginal discharge and can be used for surgical ablation of masses in the rectum and anus and manipulation of urethral calculi [65].

The pudendal nerve originates from sacral segments S2–S4 and travels downward, partly embedded in the sacrosciatic ligament along the floor of the pelvis with the internal pudendal artery and vein and toward the ischial arch. It supplies several branches that innervate the whole perineal area. These branches include a proximal cutaneous branch to the skin of the semitendinosus area and a distal cutaneous branch to the skin of the semimembranosus area. This latter branch further extends to a superficial perineal branch that supplies the skin of the perineum and a dorsal scrotal (male) or dorsal labial (female) branch to supply the scrotum or labia and skin of the caudal surface of the udder, respectively. Another major branch is the deep perineal nerve, which innervates the perineal muscles, vagina, vulva, major vestibular gland, and skin of the perineum; this nerve also has a communication with the caudal rectal nerve (S4, S5). In the bull, the last segment of the pudendal nerve gives off the preputial and scrotal branch to innervate the prepuce and scrotum and continues as the dorsal nerve of the penis to innervate the penis. In the female, the pudendal nerve supplies a mammary branch to the udder and the dorsal nerve of the clitoris to innervate the clitoris [22,55].

The caudal rectal nerve (S4, S5) travels downward above the pudendal nerve and anastomoses with it. As mentioned above, it supplies the caudal part of the rectum, external anal sphincter, and surrounding skin.

For the ischiorectal fossa approach, the block is performed with the animal standing, preferably under sedation. The skin over both ischiorectal fossae is clipped and aseptically prepared at the specific points where the needles are to be inserted and desensitized with 2–3 mL of 2% lidocaine (Fig. 66.10). A hand is placed into the rectum to palpate the lesser sciatic notch of the ischium and the lesser sciatic foramen, the latter formed by the absence of attachment of the sacrosciatic ligament along the notch. The notch is located immediately after the hand enters the anus and descends from the ischial tuberosity. At the foramen, the caudal gluteal artery can be palpated as it leaves the pelvis to supply the muscles of the thigh; medial to it and within the pelvic area, the internal pudendal artery can be palpated, which runs along with the pudendal nerve in a caudoventral direction on the internal surface of the sacrosciatic ligament [66]. A 2.5 cm, 16 gauge needle is inserted in the ischiorectal fossa to help direct an 8.9 cm, 20 gauge spinal needle, as the hand inside the rectum palpates the internal pudendal artery and helps direct the needle slightly dorsal toward the pudendal nerve. Up to 25 mL of 2% lidocaine is injected into the area. The needle is then redirected more dorsally (2–3 cm) to include the caudal rectal nerve, which is blocked with an additional 10 mL of anesthetic. To block the nerves on the contralateral side of the pelvis, the hands are reversed, and the procedure is repeated. Onset of the block may require from 5 to 30 min and will last 2–4 h with 2% lidocaine.

The pudendal block can also be performed via a lateral approach, described elsewhere (Fig. 66.10) [67]. The volumes used can be the same as for the ischiorectal approach, although, due to better accuracy, less anesthetic may be required (10 mL for the pudendal nerve and 5 mL for the caudal rectal nerve) [67].

In sheep, the lateral approach is performed by placing a finger into the rectum to locate the lesser sciatic foramen, usually at finger depth. The corresponding skin site is aseptically prepared and 3–7 mL of 2% lidocaine is injected using a 3.8 cm, 20 gauge needle directed toward the finger until it can be felt lying alongside the nerve. Immediately after injection, the rectum is massaged to spread the anesthetic, and the procedure is repeated on the opposite side [67].

Dorsal nerve of the penis block

The dorsal nerve of the penis originates from the pudendal nerve, as the latter travels around the ischial arch [55]. This nerve is blocked to desensitize and relax the penis and areas of the prepuce and scrotum, without affecting other anatomic structures innervated by the pudendal nerve. The location of the block is approximately 10 cm ventral to the anus and 2.5 cm from the midline on both sides, where a 6.4 to 8.9 cm, 20 gauge spinal needle is directed along the border of the ischial arch to contact the pelvic floor, next to the penis at the 8 and 4 o'clock positions. The nerves are in a ventral position at the pelvic outlet as the penis has not veered around the ischial arch and are injected with 10–20 mL of 2% lidocaine on each side. Aspirate to verify absence of blood before injecting. The onset time of the block is 10–20 min with a duration of 1–2 h.

Blocks for regional anesthesia of the teats and udder

The skin and teats of the forequarters and the cranial part of the base of the udder are innervated by the iliohypogastric nerve (ventral branch of L1), the ilioinguinal nerve (ventral branches of L2 and L3), and the cranial branch of the genitofemoral nerve (ventral branches of L2–L4). The skin and teats of the hindquarters are innervated by the caudal branch of the genitofemoral nerve and the mammary branch of the pudendal nerve (S2–S4) (Fig. 66.11) [68]. Due to this innervation, a proximal or distal paravertebral block

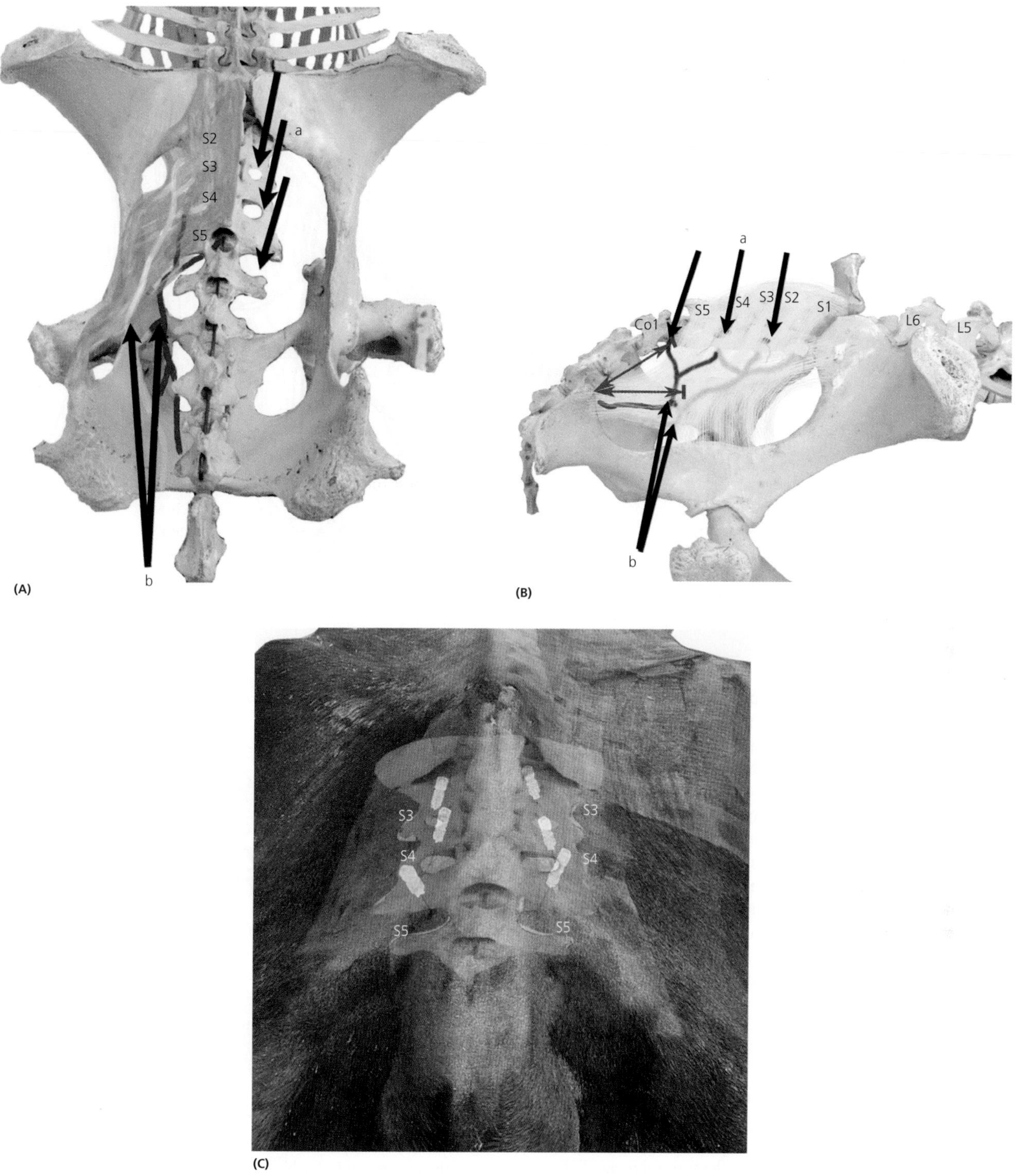

Figure 66.10 Anatomy and injection sites for sacral paravertebral block and pudendal and caudal rectal nerve block. The sacral paravertebral block includes nerves S3, S4, and S5 that are blocked bilaterally at their respective foramina. The pudendal (S2–S4; orange) and caudal rectal (S4 and S5; blue) nerve block is performed bilaterally on the medial surface of the sacrosciatic ligament. **A.** Dorsal view of the sacral spine and pelvis. (a) indicates location of S3, S4, and S5 foramina on the right side for sacral paravertebral block. (b) indicates a left ischiorectal fossa approach to the pudendal (orange) and caudal rectal (blue) nerves. **B.** Lateral view of the sacral spine and pelvis from the right side. (a) indicates location of S3, S4, and S5 foramina on the right side for sacral paravertebral block. (b) indicates an alternate lateral approach from the right side to the pudendal (orange) and caudal rectal (blue) nerves. The red arrows indicate the location of needle placement for the lateral approach; the distance from the anterior and dorsal border of the ischial tuber to the caudal part of the sacrotuberous ligament corresponds to the point of needle insertion when this distance is applied to a line parallel to the midline and originating from the anterior border of the ischial tuber to reach the pudendal nerve; whereas the caudal rectal nerve is blocked 2–3 cm more dorsally. **C.** Dorsal view showing bilateral needle placement for sacral paravertebral block.

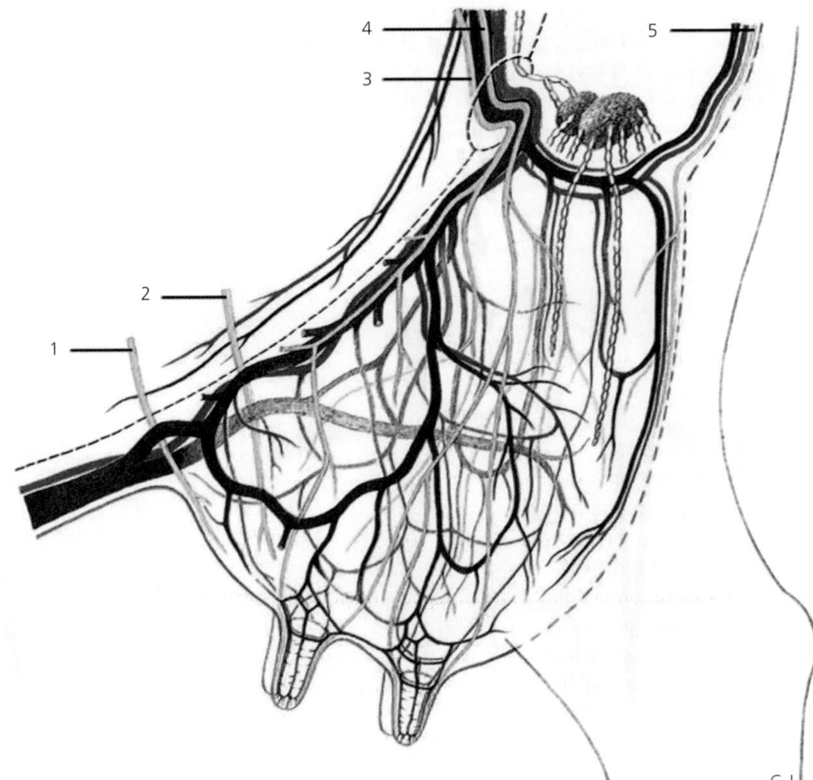

Figure 66.11 Innervation to skin and teats of the forequarters and hindquarters. (1) iliohypogastric nerve; (2) ilioinguinal nerve; (3) cranial branch of the genitofemoral nerve; (4) caudal branch of the genitofemoral nerve; and (5) mammary branch of the pudendal nerve. Source: Bragulla *et al.* [68], with permission of John Wiley & Sons.

that includes T13–L3 nerves can provide significant anesthesia of the forequarters of the udder, but the block is incomplete because the genitofemoral nerve (L4 roots) is not included. A pudendal block (S2–S4) can provide anesthesia of the caudal area of the hindquarters, but not their cranial area, which is innervated by the genitofemoral nerve. Therefore, a more simple and effective method is to desensitize the affected area locally using a ring block, inverted "V" block, teat sinus infusion, or intravenous regional anesthesia of the teat, in combination with chemical and/or physical restraint (Fig. 66.12). The surgical procedure and block can be performed with the animal standing or recumbent, often dictated by the preference of the operator.

These blocks can be used for repair of lacerations and fistulas, release of cistern obstructions, wart removal, supernumerary teat removal, and teat removal.

Ring block

An elastic band or Doyen clamp is used as a tourniquet and applied to the base of the teat, to prolong the duration of action of the injected local anesthetic and to prevent blood and milk from entering the teat sinus and interfering with the surgical repair. Following aseptic preparation, 4–6 mL of 2% lidocaine is injected subcutaneously with a 1.6 cm, 25 gauge needle, distal to the tourniquet, around the circumference of the teat and massaged to facilitate blockade of all layers, including the skin, subcutaneous layer, and muscularis (Fig. 66.12a).

Inverted "V" block

Following placement of a tourniquet to the base of the teat and aseptic preparation, 4–6 mL of 2% lidocaine is injected subcutaneously with a 1.6 cm, 25 gauge needle with the angle of the "V" located at the proximal aspect of the incision and the wings oriented in a diagonal pattern (inverted "V") along the incision to block sensory input toward the incision (Fig. 66.12b).

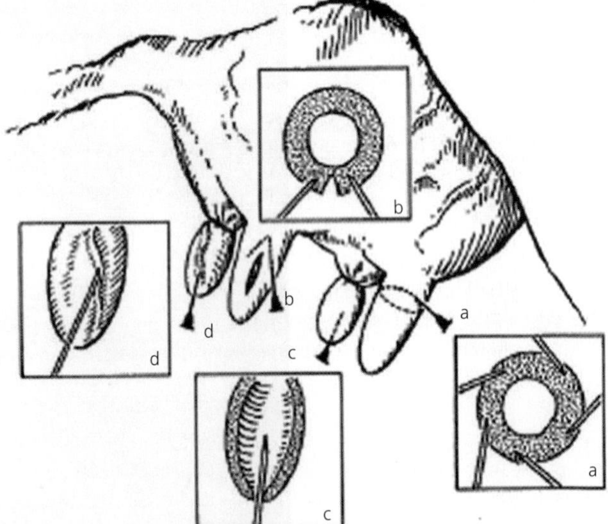

Figure 66.12 Needle placement for bovine ring block (a); inverted "V" block (b); teat sinus infusion block (c); and intravenous regional teat block (d).

Teat sinus infusion block

This block provides anesthesia of the mucous membranes lining the sinus of the teat without affecting the muscularis, subcutaneous layer, and skin. The block can be used to remove polyps within the mucosa, opening of contracted sphincters, and opening of spider teats. A tourniquet is placed as described above and a teat cannula is introduced into the sinus; 10 mL of 2% lidocaine is injected and held in place by blocking the cannula for 5–10 min to allow for absorption of the anesthetic by the mucosa; thereafter, the anesthetic is drained, and the tourniquet removed (Fig. 66.12c).

Intravenous regional teat block

Following placement of a tourniquet, as described above, a superficial teat vein distal to a tourniquet is injected with 5–7 mL of 2% lidocaine using a 2.5 cm, 25 gauge needle (Fig. 66.12d). After injection, the needle is removed, and pressure is applied over the insertion site, which should also be massaged to prevent hematoma formation. Analgesia occurs within 3–5 min and remains for as long as the tourniquet is left in place, which is usually for less than 2 h.

Blocks for castration

Castration of ruminants is routinely practiced and is usually performed in young animals. The procedure is usually performed under local anesthesia in cattle; however, smaller animals, especially young sheep and goats, may require heavy sedation or general anesthesia. Castration of adult sheep and goats must be performed carefully to prevent postoperative hemorrhage. In such cases, sedation (e.g., xylazine 0.05–0.1 mg/kg, IM) will allow the animal to be restrained on a surgery table and improve surgical conditions.

For complete anesthesia of the surgical site, the scrotal skin and spermatic cord must be blocked or, alternatively, an epidural (lumbosacral or sacrococcygeal) as previously described can be performed. Local anesthetic can be injected directly into the center of each testicle until the testicle feels firm, which will result in local anesthetic migrating up to the spermatic cord. Alternatively, the testicle can be grasped and pulled down and local anesthetic injected proximally into the surrounding subcutaneous tissues at the level of the spermatic cord. Complete desensitization occurs within 5–10 min. Using a small-bore needle (20–22 gauge) will reduce the likelihood of hematoma formation. When injected into the testicle, the local anesthetic passes out of the testicle along the lymph vessels and diffuses to block the nerve fibers in the spermatic cord. With either injection site, the bulk of the injected local anesthetic is systemically absorbed so it is important to be aware of the risk of toxicity. In small lambs and kids, 1 mL of 2% lidocaine injected into each cord will be adequate with dosing and volume modifications according to size, as needed. The scrotal skin is anesthetized by local infiltration of lidocaine along the proposed line of incision.

As in the case of dehorning or disbudding, a non-steroidal anti-inflammatory (e.g., flunixin meglumine 2 mg/kg, IV or IM) is suggested for postoperative analgesia.

Blocks for regional anesthesia of the limbs and feet

Most surgical procedures of the digit are performed in cattle using intravenous regional anesthesia (IVRA), a specific nerve block, or simple infiltration of local anesthetic (ring block). IVRA is the method of choice for most surgical procedures of the foot or distal limb in ruminants and swine, but digital nerve blocks can be a very useful diagnostic tool for localizing lameness in cattle. Additional regional anesthesia of the thoracic limb in cattle can be achieved with a brachial plexus nerve block or with digital nerve blocks distal to the carpus. Analgesia of the pelvic limb distal to the tarsus can be achieved by desensitizing the common peroneal and tibial nerves. More complete proximal analgesia of the pelvic limb may require epidural techniques that include lumbosacral segments to include the femoral nerve (L4–L6) and sciatic nerve (L5–S2). Intra-articular injections of appropriate local anesthetics or other medications can also be used.

Thoracic limb blocks

Brachial plexus block

A brachial plexus block has been described in cattle [69] and, more extensively, in sheep [70–72] to provide analgesia of the thoracic limb distal to and including the elbow. This block is likely to be most useful in calves, sheep, or goats in a clinical or research setting for procedures on the thoracic limb under general anesthesia. In swine, palpation of landmarks may be difficult, especially in pot-bellied pigs. The block can be performed blindly or with the guidance of ultrasound and/or nerve stimulation as described in small animals (see Chapter 60).

The brachial plexus block involves desensitization of the ventral roots of the sixth, seventh, and eighth cervical nerves (C6, C7, and C8), as well as the first and second thoracic nerves (T1 and T2) as they pass together over the lateral aspect of the middle third of the first rib [73]. The position and angle of the scapula can be used as a landmark by palpating the cranial and caudal angles and spine. The dorsal border of the scapula lies opposite the second to the seventh thoracic vertebrae but will only be palpable in thin animals. The shoulder joint is just lateral to the middle of the first and second thoracic vertebrae. The spine of the scapula is prominent in ruminants and juts out ventrally to form the acromion process. The point of needle insertion is 12–14 cm (adult cattle) or 6–10 cm (small ruminants) cranial to the palpable acromion of the scapula at the outer border of the scalenus ventralis muscle. The needle is then advanced caudally and slightly ventrally, lateral to the thorax, and parallel to the long axis of the animal's neck. In small ruminants and calves, a 6.3–8.9 cm, 22–20 gauge spinal needle with stylet can be used to reach the brachial plexus region, medial to the scapula. Alternatively, a 50 or 100 mm insulated needle may be used for techniques guided by nerve stimulation and/or ultrasound. In cattle, an 8.9–16 cm, 18 gauge spinal needle is necessary. For blind techniques, the needle is typically advanced until it hits the edge of the first rib. An initial volume of local anesthetic is injected at this site after aspiration and then the needle is redirected distally, superficial to the rib, where additional local anesthetic is injected. Lidocaine is the typical local anesthetic used in ruminants with total volumes of 20–25 mL described for adult cattle; however, bupivacaine has been investigated in sheep [70,72]. The dosage of bupivacaine ranged from 0.5–4 mg/kg with a dose of 2 mg/kg resulting in the most effective brachial plexus block. No signs of toxicity were reported in the sheep [70].

In ruminants the phrenic nerve is innervated by the C5–7 cervical nerves [22], so bilateral brachial plexus blockade should be avoided to minimize the risk of complete diaphragmatic motor block.

Digital nerve blocks for the thoracic limbs and feet

Cattle have four digits; the third and fourth digits correspond to the fully developed medial and lateral digits, respectively. The second and fifth digits correspond to the medial and lateral dewclaws, respectively, which are positioned behind the fetlock and do not articulate with the limb.

Digital nerve blocks may be useful to localize lameness or to desensitize the foot for surgery. However, as compared to horses, digital nerve blocks are more difficult because the skin below the tarsus and carpus is thick and the subcutaneous tissue is firm and fibrous, limiting palpation of the nerves and ease of needle insertion. The size of the needle used and total volume of local anesthetic to be injected are related to the size of the animal.

Innervation to the thoracic limb is supplied on the palmar aspect predominantly by the median nerve but also by the palmar branch of the ulnar nerve; the dorsal aspect is supplied by the radial nerve as well as the dorsal branch of the ulnar nerve (Fig. 66.13) [73].

The median nerve passes through the carpal canal and divides halfway up the metacarpus into the palmar common digital nerves II and III. The palmar common digital nerve II runs medially and

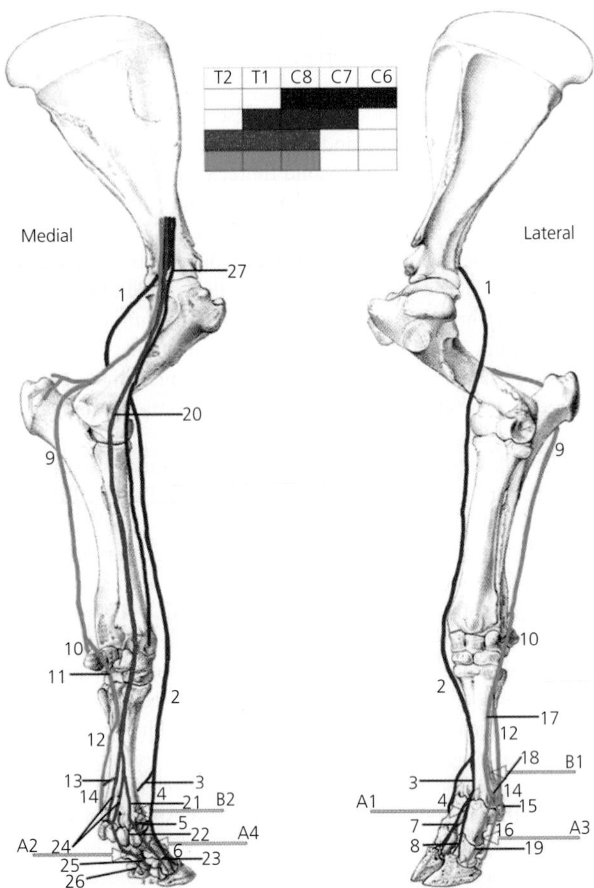

Figure 66.13 Innervation of the thoracic limb. (1) radial nerve; (2) superficial branch of the radial nerve; (3) dorsal common digital nerve III; (4) dorsal common digital nerve II; (5) axial dorsal digital nerve II; (6) abaxial dorsal digital nerve III; (7) axial dorsal digital nerve III; (8) axial dorsal digital nerve IV; (9) ulnar nerve; (10) dorsal ulnar branch; (11) palmar ulnar branch; (12) superficial ulnar branch; (13) communicating branch of the median nerve; (14) palmar common digital nerve IV; (15) axial palmar digital nerve V; (16) abaxial palmar digital nerve IV; (17) dorsal common digital nerve; (18) axial dorsal digital nerve V; (19) abaxial dorsal digital nerve IV; (20) median nerve; (21) palmar common digital nerve II; (22) axial palmar digital nerve II; (23) abaxial palmar digital nerve III; (24) palmar common digital nerve III; (25) axial palmar digital nerve III; (26) axial palmar digital nerve IV; (27) musculocutaneous nerve. (A) Block to the digit; (A1) block to nerves numbered 7 and 8; (A2) block to nerves numbered 25 and 26; (A3) block to nerves numbered 16 and 19; (A4) block to nerves numbered 6 and 23. (B) Block to the dewclaws; (B1) block to nerves numbered 15 and 18; (B2) block to nerves numbered 5 and 22. Source: Modified from Wünsche *et al.* [73].

divides at the level of the fetlock joint into the axial palmar digital nerve II, which ends near the dewclaw, and the abaxial palmar digital nerve III, which travels deep as far as the apex of the hoof. The palmar common digital nerve III branches and travels lateral to the interdigital space and gives rise to the axial palmar digital nerves III and IV (Fig. 66.13) [73].

The ulnar nerve divides above the accessory carpal bone into dorsal and palmar branches. The palmar ulnar branch divides distal to the carpus into a deep branch that innervates the surrounding area of the third and fourth metacarpal bone, and a superficial branch that travels distally on the lateral aspect to become the palmar common digital nerve IV, which anastomoses at the midway point of the metacarpus with the median nerve via the communicating branch of the latter. Proximal to the fetlock joint of the fourth digit, the palmar common digital nerve IV divides into the axial palmar digital nerve V and abaxial palmar digital nerve IV (Fig. 66.13) [73].

The dorsal branch of the ulnar nerve is located approximately 2 cm proximal to the accessory carpal bone and travels distally on the lateral surface between the third and fourth metacarpal bone as the dorsal common digital nerve, which divides on the dorsolateral aspect of the fetlock into the axial dorsal digital nerve V for the dewclaw and the abaxial dorsal digital nerve IV for the dorsolateral coronary region of the fourth digit (Fig. 66.13) [73].

The dorsomedial aspect of the thoracic limb is supplied by the superficial branch of the radial nerve, which travels on the dorsomedial aspect of the forelimb to cross to the dorsal aspect below the carpus and divides midway on the metacarpus into the dorsal common digital nerve III (dorsal aspect) and dorsal common digital nerve II (medial aspect). The latter divides at the level of the medial aspect of the fetlock into the axial dorsal digital nerve II to the dewclaw and the abaxial dorsal digital nerve III to the dorsomedial coronary region of the third digit. Dorsal common digital nerve III continues to travel dorsally and divides at the interdigital space into the axial dorsal digital nerves III and IV (Fig. 66.13) [73].

The distribution of nerve supply to the palmar surface of the digits of the forelimb is not always constant, making digital nerve blocks of the forelimb less reliable for complete digital analgesia and anesthesia which is necessary for surgery.

To block the digits in the thoracic limb, it is necessary to block axial dorsal digital nerves III and IV, which arise from the radial nerve. This block can be performed on the dorsal aspect proximal to the interdigital space, close to the metacarpal-phalangeal joint with a 3.8 cm, 20 or 18 gauge needle (Fig. 66.13, A1). It is possible to encounter the axial dorsal digital artery and vein in this location so aspiration prior to injection is important. Injection of 10 mL of 2% lidocaine is required in adult cattle to desensitize the radial nerve at this location. The axial palmar digital nerves III and IV, originating from the median nerve, provide sensation to the medial aspect of the third and fourth digit and are blocked lower than on the dorsal site to avoid the cartilaginous palmar ligament. For these nerves, a 2.5 cm, 20 or 18 gauge needle is used to inject 5–10 mL of 2% lidocaine distal to the dewclaws on the palmar surface (Fig. 66.13, A2). Desensitizing the lateral aspect of the fourth digit involves blocking the abaxial palmar digital nerve IV and the abaxial dorsal digital nerve IV, both originating from the ulnar nerve, using 3–5 mL of 2% lidocaine with a 3.8 cm, 20 or 18 gauge needle midway between the palmar lateral aspect of the dewclaw and the coronary band for the axial branch, and at the same level but on the dorsolateral aspect for the abaxial branch (Fig. 66.13, A3). A similar block to the one described for the fourth digit is used for the third digit and includes abaxial dorsal digital nerve III, originating from the radial nerve, and the abaxial palmar digital nerve III, originating from the median nerve (Fig. 66.13, A4).

The dewclaws (second and fifth digits) can be blocked by injecting each with 5–10 mL of 2% lidocaine using a 3.8–5 cm, 20 or 18 gauge needle inserted in a horizontal direction above them. This blocks axial palmar and axial dorsal digital nerves V, originating from the ulnar nerve, which supply the lateral dewclaw (Fig. 66.13, B1) and axial palmar digital nerve II, originating from the median nerve, and the axial dorsal digital nerve II, originating from the radial nerve, that supply the medial dewclaw (Fig. 66.13, B2).

Pelvic limb blocks

The pelvic limb can be desensitized below the tarsus by blocking the peroneal and tibial nerves. These blocks are not commonly performed in clinical practice due to the ease and effectiveness of IVRA and caudal epidural anesthesia in ruminants.

The common peroneal nerve can be palpated at the caudal edge of the bony prominence of the lateral condyle of the tibia. At this level, the nerve is superficial and has not yet divided into superficial and deep branches. A 2.5–3.8 cm, 18 or 20 gauge needle is inserted at the caudal edge of the lateral condyle of the tibia, over the fibula until it touches the bony landmark. In adult cattle, 20 mL of 2% lidocaine is required while 6–10 mL is sufficient in small ruminants, with an onset time of approximately 15–20 min (Fig. 66.14).

Digital nerve blocks for the pelvic limbs and feet

Innervation to the pelvic limb is supplied on the plantar aspect by the tibial nerve and on the dorsal aspect by the superficial and deep peroneal nerves [74].

The tibial nerve divides into the medial and lateral plantar nerves at the distal third of the tibia, just above the calcaneus bone to innervate the plantar aspect of the pelvic limb. The medial plantar nerve runs in the groove between the interosseus and the deep flexor tendon and divides at the distal third of the metatarsus into the plantar common digital nerve II and III (Fig. 66.14). Both nerves travel down the fetlock where they divide into axial and abaxial plantar digital nerves. From the plantar common digital nerve II, the axial plantar digital nerve II supplies the medial dewclaw and the abaxial plantar digital nerve III continues to the third digit on the medial plantar aspect. From the plantar common digital nerve III, the axial plantar digital nerve III and axial plantar digital nerve IV supply the axial bulb and hoof regions of the third and fourth digits (Fig. 66.14) [74].

The lateral plantar nerve reaches below the tarsus and the lateral border of the deep flexor tendon and continues as the plantar common digital nerve IV to divide at the level of the fetlock into the axial plantar digital nerve V, to supply the lateral dewclaw, and the abaxial plantar digital nerve IV, which continues to the fourth digit on the lateral plantar aspect (Fig. 66.14) [74].

The common peroneal nerve divides on the lateral aspect of the proximal third of the tibia into the superficial and deep peroneal nerves to innervate the dorsal aspect of the pelvic limb. The superficial peroneal nerve crosses to the dorsal aspect of the proximal metatarsus and divides at the proximal third into three branches: the dorsal common digital nerve II that travels medial, the dorsal common digital nerve III that continues on the dorsal aspect, and the dorsal common digital nerve IV that travels dorsolateral. The dorsal common digital nerve II travels dorsomedial along the metatarsus to the fetlock and divides into the axial dorsal digital nerve II, supplying the medial dewclaw, and the abaxial dorsal digital nerve III, which continues to the third digit on the medial plantar aspect.

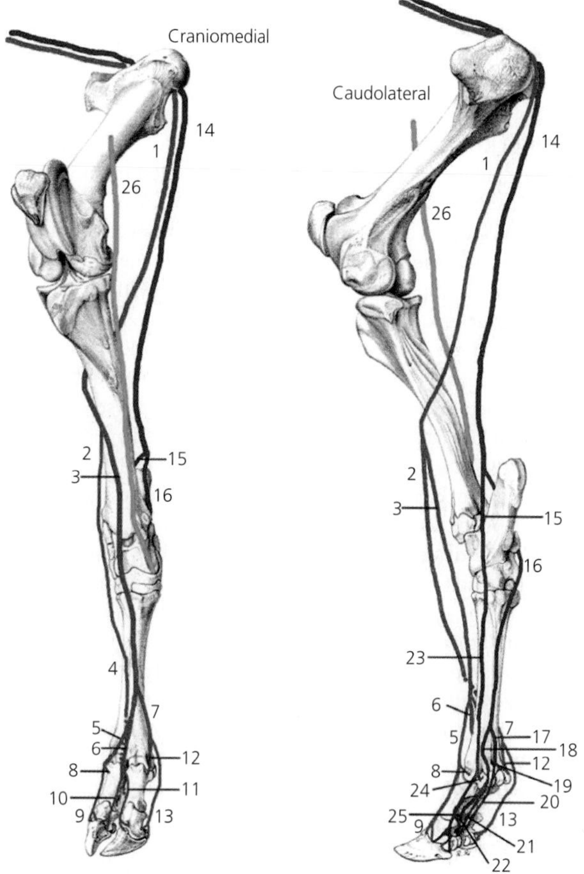

Figure 66.14 Innervation of the pelvic limb. (1) peroneal nerve; (2) deep peroneal nerve; (3) superficial peroneal nerve; (4) dorsal metatarsal III nerve; (5) dorsal common digital nerve IV; (6) dorsal common digital nerve III; (7) dorsal common digital nerve II; (8) axial dorsal digital nerve V; (9) abaxial dorsal digital nerve IV; (10) axial dorsal digital nerve IV; (11) axial dorsal digital nerve III; (12) axial dorsal digital nerve II; (13) abaxial dorsal digital nerve III; (14) tibial nerve; (15) lateral plantar nerve; (16) medial plantar nerve; (17) plantar common digital nerve II; (18) plantar common digital nerve III; (19) axial plantar digital nerve II; (20) abaxial plantar digital nerve III; (21) axial plantar digital nerve III; (22) axial plantar digital nerve IV; (23) plantar common digital nerve IV; (24) axial plantar digital nerve V; (25) abaxial plantar digital nerve IV; (26) saphenous nerve. Source: Modified from Wünsche *et al.* [74].

Dorsal common digital nerve III travels dorsally to the distal fetlock, where it divides into the axial dorsal digital nerves III and IV to supply the dorsal coronary aspect of the third and fourth digits. Dorsal common digital nerve IV reaches the fetlock on the dorsolateral aspect and divides into the axial dorsal digital nerve V, supplying the lateral dewclaw, and the abaxial dorsal digital nerve IV that continues to the dorsolateral coronary and bulbar regions of the fourth digit (Fig. 66.14) [74].

The deep peroneal nerve runs from its lateral position at the tibia to a dorsal position at the metatarsus to become the dorsal metatarsal nerve III, which runs lateral to the metatarsal bone, reaching the interdigital space and establishing communicating branches with the dorsal common digital nerve III, just before the latter divides into axial dorsal digital nerves III and IV. The new trunk then has communicating branches to the axial plantar digital nerves III and IV from the tibial nerve (Fig. 66.14) [74].

To block the entire distal digit of the pelvic limb, the technique, equipment, and location of the nerves resemble the anatomy of the thoracic limb and can be completed in the same fashion as described above.

Ring block

Ring block of the foot or distal limb is the simplest method for producing anesthesia but is less precise than IVRA or digital nerve blocks. Advantages are its simplicity without the need for anatomic knowledge, and the minimal equipment requirement. However, it may not be fully efficacious and requires multiple injections, increasing the risk of infection and inflammation.

The technique involves injection of the local anesthetic superficially at the level of the junction of the middle and proximal metatarsus or metacarpus, creating a "ring" of local anesthetic around the limb. It consists of multiple injections of local anesthetic solution into the subcutaneous tissue with aspiration after every movement to ensure the needle has not entered a blood vessel. The size of needle depends on the size of animal (2.5–3.8 cm, 25 to 20 gauge needle). The drug diffuses into the surrounding tissue from the sites of injection to anesthetize nerve fibers and endings. Relatively large volumes (e.g., 10–15 mL in adult cattle) of 2% lidocaine (1.5–2 mg/kg) are typically used in cattle, small ruminants, and swine. The amount of local anesthetic used will typically be dictated by the size of the area to be infused. Epinephrine may be used in combination with infiltration of local anesthetic to reduce the systemic absorption and prolong the anesthetic effect but the effects of vasoconstriction on regional blood flow should be considered.

Intravenous regional anesthesia

Intravenous regional anesthesia (IVRA), also known as a "Bier block," is a method suited to providing anesthesia of the distal limb for invasive hoof trimming of sole ulcers, draining of abscesses, claw amputation, or other surgeries of the digits. The advantages of IVRA are that it is a relatively simple technique to perform, with minimal need for specialized equipment. Following injection at a single site, the technique provides rapid onset of effective analgesia and muscle relaxation with a rapid recovery. Due to the application of a tourniquet, bleeding at the surgical site is minimized, and localized and targeted antibiotic administration may be provided simultaneously. Disadvantages include the need to position and restrain the animal in lateral recumbency, especially associated with potential adverse effects in adult ruminants, hematoma formation at the site of needle insertion, failure of the block, short duration of analgesia, which is limited by the time the tourniquet can be left in place, tourniquet discomfort, potential damage to nerves in the area under the tourniquet, and the possibility of local anesthetic toxicity when the tourniquet is released.

The procedure is generally performed after manually casting the animal and restraining it in lateral recumbency or by using a tilting hoof-trimming table with the affected limb up. Attempts to perform IVRA in the standing bovine with the leg restrained tend to be unsuccessful as the animal typically becomes recumbent when the tourniquet is applied. Sedation is recommended for IVRA as discomfort from tourniquet application is common, especially when the procedure is prolonged. It is important to assess the degree of bloat in the laterally recumbent ruminant especially when abdominal bellybands are applied for restraint.

IVRA involves injection of local anesthetic into a superficial vein on the thoracic or pelvic limb after proximal application of a tourniquet to occlude arterial blood flow. The tourniquet is placed proximal to the region being desensitized and interrupts arterial blood flow and venous removal of the local anesthetic from the surgical area. The local anesthetic is injected distal to the tourniquet and diffuses into the superficial vascular space and then into the deeper vasculature and venules. It passes out of the vasculature and into the small veins surrounding the nerves. From there it diffuses into the capillary plexuses of the endoneurium and the vasa nervorum capillary plexuses that extend intraneurally, thereby blocking nerve conduction [75].

Minimal equipment is required, consisting mainly of a tourniquet and standard needles (2.5–3.8 cm, 20 or 18 gauge), IV catheter (4.8 cm, 20 to 16 gauge), or simply a butterfly needle (20 to 16 gauge). IV catheters or butterfly needles can be fixed in place with adhesive tape to be used at the end of the procedure for antibiotic infusion. Tourniquet application can be manually applied using rubber tubing or a pneumatic cuff. The tourniquet used to occlude arterial flow manually can be round stout rubber tubing, a length of bicycle tire inner tube, an Esmarch tourniquet, or a wide flat rubber band. A length of 40–80 cm is usually necessary in adult cattle to allow the tourniquet to be wrapped around the limb and tied. The wide flat rubber band style tourniquet is generally preferable and minimizes discomfort to the animal. When the tourniquet is to be placed on the hindlimb above the hock, rolls of soft bandage should be applied on either side of the gastrocnemius tendon to minimize damage to this tendon and allow full occlusion of vasculature.

With either tourniquet method, the tourniquet needs to be inflated or secured sufficiently to occlude arterial blood flow. A cuff pressure of approximately 420 mmHg is used in equine patients successfully [76]. Without a pneumatic cuff, the rubber-style tourniquet is gradually wrapped around the animal's limb and tied or taped to maintain the tourniquet's pressure. A more effective method is to exsanguinate the extremity using an Esmarch bandage. The limb is tightly wrapped, from distal to proximal, before applying the tourniquet. A wide flat rubber band works best for this method. With use of an Esmarch technique, the vein may be initially difficult to visualize.

The common dorsal metacarpal vein, palmar metacarpal vein, or radial vein can be used in the thoracic limb (Fig. 66.15A) [73]. In the pelvic limb, the cranial branch of the lateral saphenous vein or the lateral plantar digital vein is most easily accessed in the laterally recumbent animal (Fig. 66.15B) [74]. Once isolated, the area over the vein can be clipped and disinfected prior to needle insertion. The direction of needle insertion into the isolated vein is not crucial and depends on practitioner preference. However, it is important to inject the local anesthetic as close to the surgical site as possible. After injection of the local anesthetic, the needle may be removed, and pressure and massage applied over the insertion site to prevent hematoma formation.

The duration of analgesia is related to the time the tourniquet can safely be left in place. Complete desensitization of the area dissipates after tourniquet removal but some analgesia may persist for up to 30 min. The tourniquet can be left in place for 60–90 min; however, without sedation, the animal will usually become restless and uncomfortable after 60 min of tourniquet application. The tourniquet should not be released earlier than 10 min after injection to minimize the potential for adverse effects associated with systemic local anesthetic. Other systemic analgesics, such as nonsteroidal anti-inflammatory drugs, should be administered for long-term pain control whenever possible.

Lidocaine is the most commonly used local anesthetic for IVRA in ruminants and swine. It is important that epinephrine-containing

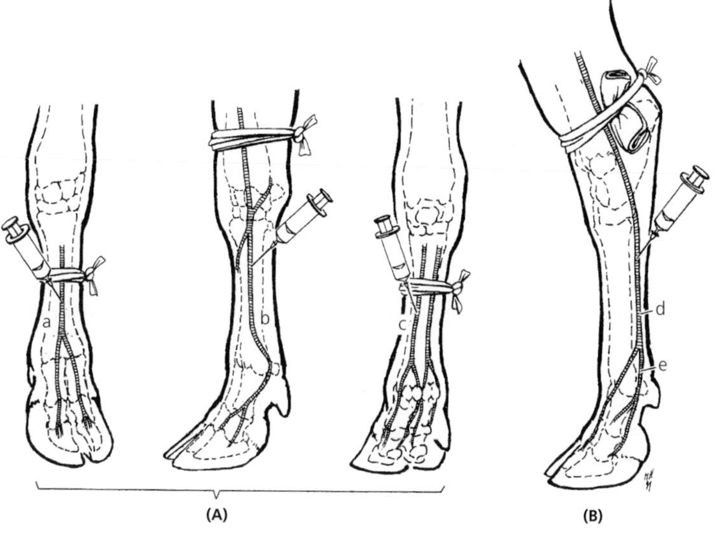

Figure 66.15 Tourniquet and needle placement for intravenous regional anesthesia (IVRA) in cattle. **A.** Thoracic limb IVRA. **B.** Pelvic limb IVRA. (a) dorsal metacarpal vein (dorsal view); (b) radial vein (medial view); (c) plantar metacarpal vein (palmar view); (d) cranial branch of the lateral saphenous vein; and (e) lateral plantar digital vein.

solutions or cardiotoxic local anesthetics (e.g., bupivacaine) are not used. Serious complications are uncommon with IVRA, but seizures, convulsions, and cardiac arrest have been reported in humans undergoing IVRA with doses of lidocaine from 1.5–3 mg/kg [77]. Evidence of toxicity in cattle is rarely reported when the tourniquet is left in place for more than 20 min [78]. It may also help if the tourniquet is slowly released for 10–15 s and then reinflated for several minutes with this process being repeated several times prior to complete removal, so that the local anesthetic solution is released in stages, minimizing the potential for signs of toxicity.

The volume of injectate will be influenced by the size of the limb and the location of the tourniquet. The presence of cellulitis in the limb will affect diffusion of anesthetic and a larger volume is required in such cases. A typical dose range for IVRA is 0.5–1.5 mg/kg. In adult cattle, this equates to 30–40 mL of 2% lidocaine. In sheep and goats, 3–10 mL of lidocaine will suffice. The local anesthetic is injected slowly, and anesthesia develops in approximately 5 min. Pressure builds up in the venous system as the injection progresses, and to prevent leakage and hematoma formation around the site of venipuncture, gentle pressure should be applied over the site. Injection of saline (5–10 mL) after the local anesthetic to encourage spread of the local anesthetic through the limb has not been investigated for efficacy, although this technique is used by some bovine practitioners. Occasionally, IVRA does not provide analgesia to the skin of the interdigital area. If necessary, this area can be desensitized by direct infiltration of local anesthetic (5–15 mL in the adult bovine; 2–5 mL in small ruminants, calves, or swine).

Regional IV antibiotic perfusion may be useful in cases where the infected tissues or bone of the digital limb are unlikely to respond to topical or systemic antibiotic treatment. Antibiotics can be administered concurrently with IVRA or on their own with similar techniques. The tourniquet should be left in place for a minimum of 20–30 min after antibiotic infusions.

Ultrasound-guided regional anesthesia

While ultrasound-guided regional anesthetic techniques have experienced exponential growth in human medicine and small animal veterinary medicine, descriptions of these techniques have lagged somewhat in large animal species. This may be due, in part, to the fact that blind techniques in these species have historically been successful and larger patient sizes allow for higher volumes of injectate to more successfully diffuse to nervous structures. Previously, ultrasound technology beyond reproductive use in ruminants and swine may have been more limited in availability or portability; however, the continuing evolution of portable ultrasound technology may allow a greater application of ultrasound-guided techniques in the field, as well as in hospital settings. Ultrasound-guided regional anesthesia allows for more precise location of nervous structures as well as adjacent structures while potentially decreasing the volume of injectate and increasing patient safety. This may be particularly advantageous in smaller patients, such as smaller sheep and goats, or in patients in which landmarks are not easily palpated, such as pigs.

General principles of ultrasound-guided regional techniques are discussed elsewhere (see Chapter 60). In short, peripheral nerves or appropriate fascial planes containing nerves may be located as described for each individual technique [69,79–89]. Needle insertion is generally via an in-plane approach in which the needle is aligned with the ultrasound beam and visualized in its full length approaching the nerve; out-of-plane approaches may be utilized, in which only the tip of the needle is visualized as it approaches the nerve. Following aspiration to verify absence of blood, an appropriate volume of local anesthetic, as described for each technique, may be administered.

A number of ultrasound-guided regional anesthetic techniques have been described in cattle [69,79–84,88] with additional descriptions, either novel or extrapolated from small animal or human techniques, continuing to emerge. There is a paucity of descriptions in the literature of these techniques in small ruminants; however, extrapolation from bovine and canine descriptions allows for relatively easy application of techniques. Abdominal fascial plane blocks, such as the transversus abdominis plane block and rectus sheath block, have been evaluated in pigs and may hold promise for providing analgesia for pet pigs undergoing laparotomy [85,87]. Peripheral nerve blocks for pigs have also been assessed and may be utilized in a similar manner to small animal patients [86,89].

While applications of ultrasound-guided techniques continue to emerge, practitioners of ruminant and swine anesthesia may utilize both blind and/or ultrasound-guided regional anesthetic techniques as dictated by patient size, surgical location, and personal preference. Local and regional anesthetic techniques are a crucial element in providing multimodal analgesia, ensuring the safety and well-being of large animal patients.

References

1 Rosenberg PH, Veering BT, Urmey WF. Maximum recommended doses of local anesthetics: a multifactorial concept. *Reg Anesth Pain Med* 2004; **29**: 564–575.

2 Copeland SE, Ladd LA, Gu XO, *et al.* The effects of general anesthesia on the central nervous and cardiovascular system toxicity of local anesthetics. *Anesth Analg* 2008; **106**: 1429–1439.

3 Santos AC, DeArmas PI. Systemic toxicity of levobupivacaine, bupivacaine, and ropivacaine during continuous intravenous infusion to nonpregnant and pregnant ewes. *Anesthesiology* 2001; **95**: 1256–1264.

4 Morishima HO, Pederson H, Finster M, *et al.* Toxicity of lidocaine in adult, newborn, and fetal sheep. *Anesthesiology* 1981; **55**: 57–61.

5 Ventkatachalam D, Chambers P, Kongara K, *et al.* Toxicity and pharmacokinetic studies of lidocaine and its active metabolite, monoethylglycinexylidide, in goat kids. *Animals* 2018; **8**: 142.

6 Santos AC, Pedersen H, Harmon TW, *et al.* Does pregnancy alter the systemic toxicity of local anesthetics? *Anesthesiology* 1989; **70**: 991–995.

7 Satas S, Johannessen SI, Hoem NO, *et al.* Lidocaine pharmacokinetics and toxicity in newborn pigs. *Anesth Analg* 1997; **85**: 306–312.

8 Morishima HO, Pedersen H, Finster M, *et al.* Bupivacaine toxicity in pregnant and nonpregnant ewes. *Anesthesiology* 1985; **63**: 134–139.

9 Morishima HO, Finster M, Arthur GR, *et al.* Pregnancy does not alter lidocaine toxicity. *Am J Obstet Gynecol* 1990; **162**: 1320–1324.

10 Mauch J, Martin Jurado O, Spielmann N, *et al.* Comparison of epinephrine vs lipid rescue to treat severe local anesthetic toxicity – an experimental study in piglets. *Pediatric Anesth* 2011; **21**: 1103–1108.

11 Udelsmann A, Lorena SE, Girioli SU, *et al.* Hemodynamic effects of local anesthetics intoxication. Experimental study in swine with levobupivacaine and bupivacaine. *Acta Cir Bras* 2008; **23**: 55–64.

12 Udelsmann A, Silva WA, de Moraes AC, *et al.* Hemodynamic effects of ropivacaine and levobupivacaine intravenous injection in swine. *Acta Cir Bras* 2009; **24**: 196–302.

13 Sellers G, Lin HC, Riddell MG, *et al.* Pharmacokinetics of lidocaine in serum and milk of mature Holstein cows. *J Vet Pharmacol Ther* 2009; **32**: 446–450.

14 Craigmill AL, Rangel-Lugo M, Damain P, *et al.* Extra-label use of tranquilizers and general anesthetics. *J Am Vet Med Assoc* 1997; **211**: 302–304.

15 Smith G. Extra-label drug use of anesthetics and analgesic compounds in cattle. *Vet Clin North Am Food Anim Pract* 2013; **29**: 29–45.

16 Habel R, Budras KD. Central nervous system and cranial nerves. In: Budras KD, Habel R, eds. *Bovine Anatomy*, 2nd edn. Hannover, Germany: Schlutersche, 2011: 30–49.

17 Fierheller EE, Caulkett NA, Haley NA, *et al.* Onset, duration and efficacy of four methods of local anesthesia of the horn bud in calves. *Vet Anaesth Analg* 2012; **39**: 431–435.

18 Valverde A, Doherty T. Anesthesia and analgesia of ruminants. In: Fish R, Danneman PJ, Brown M, Karas A, eds. *Anesthesia and Analgesia in Laboratory Animals*, 2nd edn. San Diego, CA: Academic Press, 2008: 385–412.

19 Pearce SG, Kerr CL, Boure LP, *et al.* Comparison of the retrobulbar and Peterson nerve block techniques via magnetic resonance imaging in bovine cadavers. *J Am Vet Med Assoc* 2003; **223**: 852–855.

20 Peterson DR. Nerve block of the eye and associated structures. *J Am Vet Med Assoc* 1951; **118**: 145–148.

21 Arnold JP, Kitchell RL. Experimental studies of the innervation of the abdominal wall of cattle. *Am J Vet Res* 1957; **18**: 229–240.

22 Budras KD, Habel R. Special anatomy, tabular part. In: Budras KD, Habel R, eds. *Bovine Anatomy*, 2nd edn. Hannover, Germany: Schlutersche, 2011: **119**, 123, 125.

23 Roe JM. Bovine paravertebral analgesia: radiographic analysis and suggested method for improvement. *Vet Rec* 1986; **119**: 236–238.

24 Velazquez-Delgado P, Gutierrez-Blanco E, Ortega-Pacheco A, *et al.* Anatomical landmarks for a proximal paravertebral thoracolumbar block in sheep: cadaver and in vivo study. *Can J Vet Res* 2022; **86**: 294–299.

25 Sikder S, Ahmed S, Kibria A, *et al.* Anatomical measurements for the blocking sites of paravertebral regional anaesthesia in black Bengal doe. *Bangl J Vet Med* 2010; **8**: 81–86.

26 Nev TO, Byanet O, Elsa TA. Investigation of anatomical landmarks for paravertebral anaesthesia in West African dwarf goats (*Capra hircus*). *Sokoto J Vet Sci* 2017; **15**: 88–93.

27 Linzell JL. The innervation of the mammary glands in the sheep and goat with some observations on the lumbosacral autonomic nerves. *Q J Exp Physiol Cogn Med Sci* 1959; **44**: 160–176.

28 Kirk EJ. The dermatomes of the sheep. *J Comp Neurol* 1968; **134**: 353–369.

29 Rostami M, Vesal N. Comparison of lidocaine, lidocaine/epinephrine or bupivacaine for thoracolumbar paravertebral anesthesia in fat-tailed sheep. *Vet Anaesth Analg* 2011; **38**: 598–602.

30 Oliveira AR, Araújo MA, Jardim PH, *et al.* Comparison of lidocaine, levobupivacaine or ropivacaine for distal paravertebral thoracolumbar anesthesia in ewes. *Vet Anaesth Analg* 2016; **43**: 670–674.

31 Arthur GH. Some notes on a preliminary trial of segmental epidural anesthesia of cattle. *Vet Rec* 1956; **68**: 254–256.

32 Skarda RT, Muir WW. Segmental lumbar epidural analgesia in cattle. *Am J Vet Res* 1979; **40**: 52–57.

33 Lee I, Yamagishi N, Oboshi K, *et al.* Comparison of xylazine, lidocaine and the two drugs combined for modified dorsolumbar epidural anaesthesia in cattle. *Vet Rec* 2004; **155**: 797–799.

34 Hiraoka M, Miyagawa T, Kobayashi H, *et al.* Successful introduction of modified dorsolumbar epidural anesthesia in a bovine referral center. *J Vet Sci* 2007; **8**: 181–184.

35 Valverde A. Epidural analgesia and anesthesia. *Vet Clin North Am Small Anim Pract* 2008; **38**: 1205–1230.

36 Lee I, Yamagishi N, Oboshi K, *et al.* Practical tips for the modified dorsolumbar epidural anesthesia in cattle. *J Vet Sci* 2006; **7**: 69–72.

37 Lee I, Soehartono RH, Yamagishi N, *et al.* Distribution of new methylene blue injected into the dorsolumbar epidural space in cows. *Vet Anaesth Analg* 2001; **28**: 140–145.

38 Lee I, Yamagishi N, Oboshi K, *et al.* Multivariate regression analysis of epidural pressure in cattle. *Am J Vet Res* 2002; **63**: 954–957.

39 Skarda RT, Muir WW, Hubbell JA. Comparative study of continuous lumbar segmental epidural and subarachnoid analgesia in Holstein cows. *Am J Vet Res* 1989; **50**: 39–44.

40 Meyer H, Starke A, Kehler W, *et al.* High caudal epidural anaesthesia with local anaesthetics or alpha(2)-agonists in calves. *J Vet Med A Physiol Pathol Clin Med* 2007; **54**: 384–389.

41 Johnson RA, Lopes MJ, Hendrickson DA, *et al.* Cephalad distribution of three different volumes of new methylene blue injected into the epidural space in adult goats. *Vet Surg* 1996; **25**: 448–451.

42 Moll X, Garcia G, Ferrer RI, *et al.* Distribution of methylene blue after injection into the epidural space of anaesthetized pregnant and non-pregnant sheep. *PLoS ONE* 2014; **9**: e92860.

43 Condino MP, Suzuki K, Taguchi K. Antinociceptive, sedative and cardiopulmonary effects of subarachnoid and epidural xylazine-lidocaine in xylazine-sedated calves. *Vet Anaesth Analg* 2010; **37**: 70–78.

44 Benson GJ, Thurmon JC. Anesthesia of swine under field conditions. *J Am Vet Med Assoc* 1976; **174**: 594–596.

45 Trim CM. Epidural analgesia in swine. *Vet Anesth* 1980; **8**: 23–25.

46 Skarda RT. Techniques of local analgesia in ruminants and swine. *Vet Clin North Am Food Anim Pract* 1996; **12**: 579–626.

47 Pleticha J, Maus TP, Jeng-Singh C, *et al.* Pig lumbar spine anatomy and imaging guided lateral lumbar puncture: a new large animal model for intrathecal drug delivery. *J Neurosci Methods* 2013; **216**: 10–15.

48 Strande A. Epidural anaesthesia in young pigs, dosage in relation to the length of the vertebral column. *Acta Vet Scand* 1968; **9**: 41–49.

49 Lopez MJ, Johnson R, Hendrickson DA, *et al.* Craniad migration of differing doses of new methylene blue injected into the epidural space after death of calves and juvenile pigs. *Am J Vet Res* 1997; **58**: 786–790.

50 Ko JCH, Thurmon JC, Benson GJ. Evaluation of analgesia induced by epidural injection of detomidine or xylazine in swine. *J Vet Anesth* 1992; **19**: 56–60.

51 Adetunji A, Ajao AO. Comparison of extradural injections of lignocaine and xylazine in azaperone-sedated pigs. *Vet J* 2001; **161**: 98–99.

52 Habel R, Budras KD. Head. In: Budras KD, Habel R, eds. *Bovine Anatomy*, 2nd edn. Hannover: Schlutersche, 2011: 50–57.

53 Lee I, Yamagishi N, Oboshi K, *et al.* Distribution of new methylene blue injected into the caudal epidural space in cattle. *Vet J* 2005; **169**: 257–261.

54 Araújo MA, Albuquerque VB, Deschk M, *et al.* Cardiopulmonary and analgesic effects of caudal epidurally administered ropivacaine in cattle. *Vet Anaesth Analg* 2012; **39**: 409–413.

55 Habel R, Budras KD. Perineum, pelvic diaphragm, ischiorectal fossa, and tail. In: Budras KD, Habel R, eds. *Bovine Anatomy*, 2nd edn. Hannover: Schlutersche, 2011: 94–95.

56 Caron JP, LeBlanc PH. Caudal epidural analgesia in cattle using xylazine. *Can J Vet Res* 1989; **53**: 486–489.

57 Ko JCH, Althouse GC, Hopkins SM, *et al.* Effects of epidural administration of xylazine or lidocaine on bovine uterine motility and perineal analgesia. *Theriogenology* 1989; **32**: 779–786.

58 Grubb TL, Riebold TW, Crisman RO, *et al.* Comparison of lidocaine, xylazine, and lidocaine-xylazine for caudal epidural analgesia in cattle. *Vet Anaesth Analg* 2002; **29**: 64–68.

59 Lin HC, Trachte EA, DeGraves FJ. Evaluation of analgesia induced by epidural administration of medetomidine to cows. *Am J Vet Res* 1998; **59**: 162–167.

60 Prado ME, Streeter RN, Mandsager RE, *et al.* Pharmacologic effects of epidural versus intramuscular administration of detomidine in cattle. *Am J Vet Res* 1999; **60**: 1242–1247.

61 Currah JM, Hendrick SH, Stookey JM. The behavioral assessment and alleviation of pain associated with castration in beef calves treated with flunixin meglumine

and caudal lidocaine epidural anesthesia with epinephrine. *Can Vet J* 2009; **50**: 375–382.
62 Grubb TL, Riebold TW, Hubber MJ. Evaluation of lidocaine, xylazine, and a combination of lidocaine and xylazine for epidural analgesia in llamas. *J Am Vet Med Assoc* 1993; **203**: 1441–1444.
63 Noordsy JL. Sacral paravertebral alcohol nerve block as an aid in controlling chronic rectal tenesmus in cattle. *Vet Med Small Anim Clin* 1982; **77**: 797–801.
64 Larson LL. The internal pudendal (pudic) nerve block for anesthesia of the penis and relaxation of the retractor penis muscle. *J Am Vet Med Assoc* 1953; **123**: 18–27.
65 Misra SS. Studies on clinical use of pudic-nerve block in bovine. *Proceedings of the Fourth International Congress of Veterinary Anaesthesia*, Utrecht. 1991: 108.
66 Wünsche A, Budras KD. Arteries, veins, and nerves of the pelvic cavity. In: Budras KD, Habel R, eds. *Bovine Anatomy*, 2nd edn. Hannover, Germany: Schlutersche, 2011: 84–85.
67 McFarlane IS. The lateral approach to the pudendal nerve block in the bovine and ovine. *J S Afr Vet Assoc* 1963; **34**: 73–76.
68 Bragulla H, König H, Budras KD. The udder with blood vessels, lymphatic system, nerves, and development. In: Budras KD, Habel R, eds. *Bovine Anatomy*, 2nd edn. Hannover, Germany: Schlutersche, 2011: 90–91.
69 Iwamoto J, Yamagishi N, Sasaki K, *et al.* A novel technique of ultrasound-guided brachial plexus block in calves. *Res Vet Sci* 2012; **93**: 1467–1471.
70 Estebe JP, Le Corre P, du Plessis L, *et al.* The pharmacokinetics and pharmacodynamics of bupivacaine-loaded microspheres on a brachial plexus block model in sheep. *Anesth Analg* 2001; **93**: 447–455.
71 Ghadirian S, Vesal N. Brachial plexus block using lidocaine/epinephrine or lidocaine/xylazine in fat-tailed sheep. *Vet Res Forum* 2013; **4**: 161–167.
72 Ghadirian S, Vesal N, Maghsoudi B, *et al.* Comparison of lidocaine, lidocaine-morphine, lidocaine-tramadol or bupivacaine for neural blockade of the brachial plexus in fat-tailed lambs. *Vet Anaesth Analg* 2016; **43**: 109–116.
73 Wünsche A, Habel R, Budras KD. Thoracic limb. In: Budras KD, Habel R, eds. *Bovine Anatomy*, 2nd edn. Hannover, Germany: Schlutersche, 2011: 2–13.
74 Wünsche A, Habel R, Budras KD. Pelvic limb. In: Budras KD, Habel R, eds. *Bovine Anatomy*, 2nd edn. Hannover, Germany: Schlutersche, 2011: 14–29.
75 Ennevor SJ, Bobart V, Swamidoss CP. Intravenous regional anesthesia: a review. *Sem Anesth Perio M* 1998; **17**: 2–9.
76 Levine DG, Epstein KL, Ahern BJ, *et al.* Efficacy of three tourniquet types for intravenous antimicrobial regional limb perfusion in standing horses. *Vet Surg* 2010; **39**: 1021–1024.
77 Guay J. Adverse effects associated with intravenous regional anesthesia (Bier Block): a systematic review of complications. *J Clin Anesth* 2009; **21**: 585–594.
78 Elmore RG. Food animal regional anesthesia: bovine blocks-intravenous limb block. *Vet Med Small Anim Clin* 1980; **75**: 1835–1836.
79 Re M, Blanco J, Gómez de Segura IA. Ultrasound-guided nerve block anesthesia. *Vet Clin Food Anim* 2016; **32**: 133–147.
80 Kramer AH, Doherr MG, Stoffel MH, *et al.* Ultrasound-guided proximal paravertebral anaesthesia in cattle. *Vet Anaesth Analg* 2014; **41**: 534–542.
81 Re M, Blanco-Murcia J, Villaescusa A, *et al.* Comparison of paravertebral blockade techniques with and without ultrasound guidance in calves. *Am J Vet Res* 2016; **77**: 1187–1193.
82 Re M, Blanco-Murcia J, Villaescusa A, *et al.* Ultrasound-guided anaesthetic blockade of the pelvic limb in calves. *Vet J* 2014; **200**: 434–439.
83 De Vlamynck CA, Pille F, Hauspie S, *et al.* Evaluation of three approaches for performing ultrasonography-guided anesthetic blockade of the femoral nerve in calves. *Am J Vet Res* 2013; **74**: 750–756.
84 Mirra A, von Rotz A, Schmidhalter M, *et al.* Ultrasound-guided lateral and subcostal transversus abdominis plane block in calves: a cadaveric study. *Vet Anaesth Analg* 2018; **45**: 384–391.
85 Michielsen AJHC, Rodrigo-Mocholi D, Cornillie P, *et al.* Description of different ultrasound guided transversus abdominis plane block in pig cadavers – a pilot study. *Vet Anaesth Analg* 2021; **48**: 470–477.
86 Trujanovic R, Otero PE, Marhofer P, *et al.* Proximal perineural femoral nerve injection in pigs using an ultrasound-guided lateral subiliac approach – a cadaveric study. *Animals* 2021; **11**: 1759.
87 Ienello L, Kennedy M, Wendt-Hornickle E, *et al.* Ultrasound-guided rectus sheath block injections in miniature swine cadavers: technique description and distribution of two injectate volumes. *Vet Anaesth Analg* 2022; **49**: 210–218.
88 Ferreira TH, Schroeder CA, St James M, *et al.* Description of an ultrasound-guided rectus sheath block injection technique and the spread of dye in calf cadavers. *Vet Anaesth Analg* 2022; **49**: 203–209.
89 Trujanovic R, Verdier N, Calice I, *et al.* Axillary ultrasound-guided approach for the brachial plexus in pig cadavers: a descriptive study. *Lab Anim* 2022; **56**: 165–171.

SECTION 9

Anesthesia and Analgesia for Selected Patients

67 Ophthalmic Patients

Vaidehi V. Paranjape[1] and Luisito S. Pablo[2]

[1] Department of Small Animal Clinical Sciences, Virginia-Maryland College of Veterinary Medicine, Virginia Tech University, Blacksburg, Virginia, USA

[2] Department of Comparative, Diagnostic, and Population Medicine, College of Veterinary Medicine, University of Florida, Gainesville, Florida, USA

Chapter contents

Introduction, 1327
Ocular anatomy, 1327
 Orbit, 1327
 Ocular adnexa, 1327
 Globe, 1328
 Ocular circulation, 1329
 Ocular innervation, 1329
Ocular physiology, 1329
 Aqueous humor, 1329
 Vitreous humor, 1330
 Intraocular pressure, 1330
 Pupil size, 1331
 Tear production and drainage, 1331
 Ocular barriers, 1332
 Oculocardiac reflex, 1332
Systemic effects of ophthalmic medications, 1333
Effects of anesthetic drugs and adjuvants on ocular physiology, 1333
 Sedatives, 1334
 Injectable anesthetics, 1334
 Inhalant anesthetics, 1335
 Anesthetic adjuvants, 1335
Ocular pain and its management, 1336
 Origin of ocular pain, 1336
 Analgesics, 1337
Impact of anesthesia on the electroretinogram, 1338
General anesthesia for ophthalmic surgery, 1338
 Preoperative assessment, 1338
 Anesthesia set up and patient positioning, 1338
 Physical restraint, premedication, and anesthetic induction, 1339
 Endotracheal intubation, 1339
 Protection of the contralateral eye, 1340
 Neuromuscular blockade and anesthetic monitoring, 1340
 Recovery, extubation, and emergence, 1340
 Anesthesia-related ocular complications, 1340
Special considerations for equine ophthalmic patients, 1340
References, 1342

Introduction

Patients with ophthalmic diseases or injuries often need general anesthesia for surgery or diagnosis. The anesthetic goals for ophthalmic patients to ensure favorable outcomes should focus on: (1) regulating intraocular dynamics; (2) preventing and treating the oculocardiac reflex; (3) providing adequate analgesia; (4) managing systemic effects of ophthalmic medications; and (5) anticipating surgical outcomes that can influence anesthetic care (e.g., hemorrhage). Detailed knowledge of ocular anatomy and physiology is also important for improving patient outcomes.

Ocular anatomy

Knowledge of ocular anatomy (Figs. 67.1 and 67.2) enables an anesthesiologist to understand the array of ocular surgeries, as well as gain mastery of local and regional anesthesia performed for these cases.

Orbit

The orbit is a bony fossa that encompasses the eye, associated muscles, nerves, and vasculature. It protects the eye as well as separates it from the cranial cavity. All vertebrate orbits are of two types: (1) the enclosed orbit, which is completely surrounded by bone (e.g., horses, sheep, cattle, and goats), or (2) the open or incomplete orbit, which is only partially surrounded by bone (e.g., dogs, cats, and pigs) [1,2]. The bones that form the orbit in dogs, cats, cattle, and sheep are the lacrimal, zygomatic, frontal, sphenoid, palatine, and maxillary. In horses, goats, and pigs, there is no involvement of the maxillary bone. Instead, the temporal bone and the ethmoid bone contribute to the orbit in horses and pigs, respectively. The orbital foramen is differently structured in the horse and is therefore referred to as the “orbital fissure” in this species. In cattle and pigs, the orbital fissure and foramen rotundum are typically fused to form the foramen orbitorotundum [1,2].

Ocular adnexa

The orbital fascia is a thin, tough connective tissue layer that lines all the structures within the orbit. This fascia encompasses three anatomic structures: the periorbita, Tenon’s capsule, and the extraocular muscles (EOM). The orbital fat fills up the spaces between these structures and acts as a protective cushion for the eye. The EOMs suspend the globe in the orbit and provide ocular mobility. The seven orbital muscles that control the movement of the globe are the dorsal rectus, ventral rectus, medial rectus, lateral rectus, dorsal

Veterinary Anesthesia and Analgesia: The Sixth Edition of Lumb and Jones. Edited by Leigh Lamont, Kurt Grimm, Sheilah Robertson, Lydia Love and Carrie Schroeder.
© 2024 John Wiley & Sons, Inc. Published 2024 by John Wiley & Sons, Inc.
Companion website: www.wiley.com/go/lamont/anesthesia

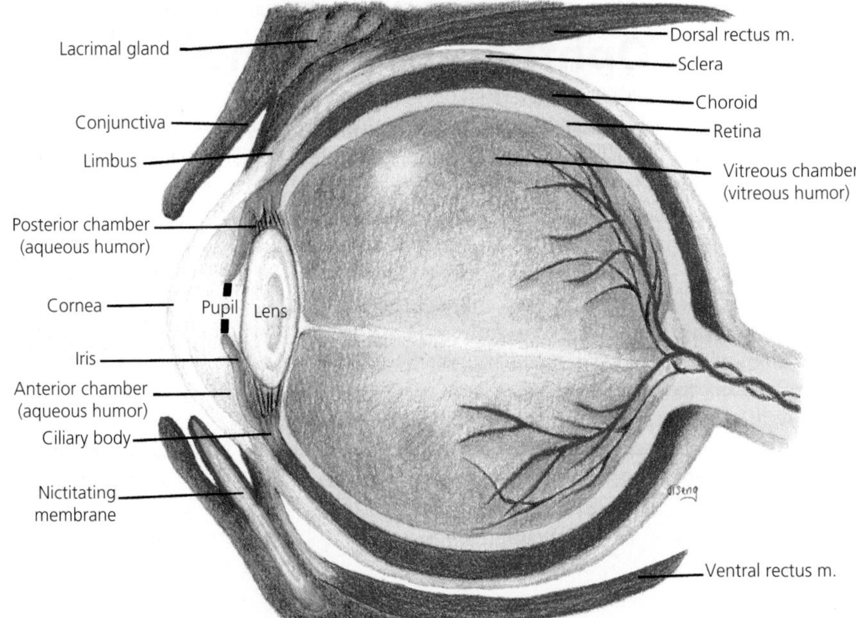

Figure 67.1 Ocular anatomy. Source: Dr. Vaidehi Paranjape, with permission.

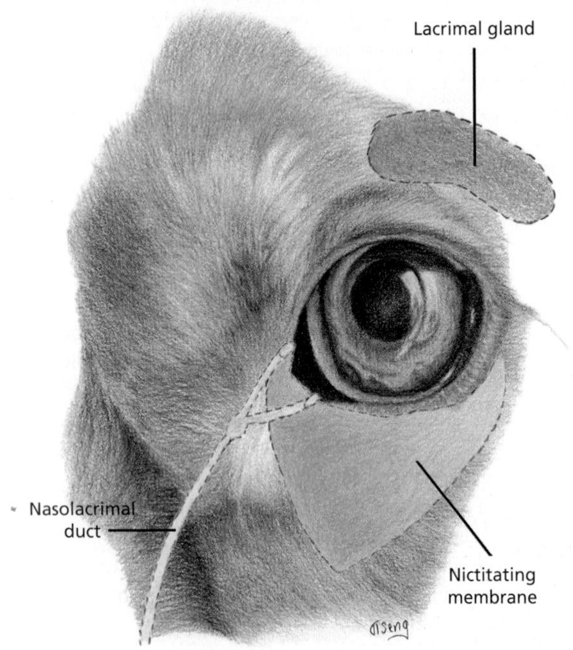

Figure 67.2 The nasolacrimal system. Source: Dr. Vaidehi Paranjape, with permission.

Table 67.1 Function and innervation of eyelid muscles and extraocular muscles.

Muscle name	Function	Innervation
Dorsal rectus	Moves globe upward	Oculomotor (CN III)
Ventral rectus	Moves globe downward	Oculomotor (CN III)
Medial rectus	Moves globe medially	Oculomotor (CN III)
Lateral rectus	Moves globe laterally	Abducens (CN VI)
Dorsal oblique	Pulls dorsal part of globe medially and ventrally	Trochlear (CN IV)
Ventral oblique	Pulls ventral part of globe medially and dorsally	Oculomotor (CN III)
Retractor oculi	Retraction of globe	Abducens (CN VI)
Levator palpebrae superioris	Elevates upper eyelid	Oculomotor (CN III)
Orbicularis oculi	Closure of palpebrae	Facial (CN VII)
Retractor anguli oculi	Lengthens palpebral fissure	Facial (CN VII)

CN, cranial nerve.
Source: Adapted from Meekins *et al.* [2].

oblique, ventral oblique, and retractor oculi (Table 67.1) [1,2]. The retractor oculi muscle is absent in birds and snakes [3]. The eyelids are two musculo-fibrous folds of the skin. The space between the upper and lower eyelids is called the "palpebral fissure." Closure of the palpebral fissure is achieved by contraction of the orbicularis oculi muscle. Opening of the eyelids is mediated by the relaxation of the orbicularis oculi muscle as well as contraction of the levator palpebrae superioris muscle (Table 67.1) [2,4].

The conjunctiva is the clear thin mucous membrane that lines the inner aspect of the eyelids, the nictitating membrane, and the exposed sclera. The nictitating membrane is a thin translucent sheet of ocular tissue situated ventromedial to the globe, which is actively retracted across the cornea to provide protection and lubrication. It is well developed in domestic animals, while in higher primates, it is a vestigial structure. In most domestic animals, the movement of the nictitating membrane occurs due to contraction of the retractor oculi muscle. However, in cats, since the retractor oculi muscle is less developed, adjacent smooth muscle bundles may contribute to its movements [2].

Globe

The globe is made of three tunics that surround the transparent ocular media, which are the aqueous humor, the lens, and the vitreous humor. The outermost fibrous tunic is further divided into the cornea and sclera. The avascular cornea protects the internal structures of the eye, contributes to the refractive power of the eye, and forms a retinal image via focusing of light rays. The sclera is a tough, opaque layer filled with a dense network of collagen and elastic fibers. There is also a cartilaginous component seen in fish, lizards, chelonians, certain amphibians, and birds [3]. It is the supporting wall of the globe and helps maintain the structure of the eyeball and protects it from injury.

The thick middle layer is the vascular tunic, commonly referred to as the "uvea" or "uveal tract." It is interposed between the retina and the sclera and is heavily pigmented and vascularized. The iris, ciliary body, and choroid are three subparts of the uvea. The pigmented iris controls the quantity of light entering the eye through the pupil, as well as influences the pupil size. The heavily pigmented ciliary body provides nourishment and removes waste from the cornea and lens and participates in lens accommodation. The choroid is composed of blood vessels and pigmented support tissues, and it nourishes the outer retinal layers.

The innermost layer is the nervous tunic, consisting of the retina and optic nerve. The ten-layered neurosensory retina is connected to the brain by the optic nerve and the optic tracts. The rods and cones (i.e., retinal photoreceptors) transform light stimuli from the external environment into nerve impulses and transmit these signals to the brain where they are converted to visual images. The optic nerve extends from the globe to the optic chiasm, and forms optic tracts. The transparent, avascular, and crystalline lens focuses light rays on the sensory retina, providing optimal focusing power for visual clarity.

Ocular circulation

In domestic animals, branches of the external carotid artery (i.e., the internal maxillary and external ophthalmic arteries) form the primary blood supply to the eye and its adnexa. The internal ophthalmic artery is a smaller artery that arises from the rostral cerebral artery at the level of the optic chiasm, providing blood supply for the optic nerve. The long and short posterior ciliary arteries are derived from the external ophthalmic artery, and they supply most of the blood to the anterior segment of the eye, including the retina and the choroid. The retinal arteries are derived from the short posterior ciliary arteries as they pass through the sclera at the periphery of the optic nerve [2,4].

There is significant variation within domestic animals with respect to the venous drainage of the eye. In dogs, the two main venous channels are the supraorbital and the inferior orbital veins. The supraorbital vein further unloads into two prominent veins, the orbital vein entering intracranially, and the internal maxillary vein connecting with the external jugular vein. The cat has an external rete, which is drained by a large ophthalmic vein connecting to the external jugular vein. Also, the supraorbital vein drains into the facial vein, finally emptying into the internal jugular vein. In horses, the principal ocular venous channels are the ophthalmic, orbital, supraorbital, and reflex veins [2,4].

Ocular innervation

The eye and its adnexa are innervated by the optic, oculomotor, trochlear, trigeminal, abducens, and facial nerves (Table 67.2, Fig. 67.3).

Assessment of palpebral and the corneal reflexes is considered standard monitoring during general anesthesia in animals to characterize the anesthetic depth. The palpebral reflex is tested by lightly touching the lateral and medial canthi, which results in eyelid closure. The afferent pathway is via the ophthalmic and maxillary branches of the trigeminal nerve, for medial and lateral stimulation, respectively. The efferent arm is the facial nerve. The corneal reflex is assessed by touching the cornea with a wisp of cotton wool or a swab tip or a drop of sterile water, which should result in retraction of the globe and eyelid closure. The afferent arm of the corneal reflex is mediated by the ophthalmic branch of the trigeminal nerve, and the efferent arm is mediated by the abducens nerve (globe retraction) and facial nerve (eyelid closure) [9].

Table 67.2 Cranial nerves innervating the eye and its adnexa.

Cranial nerve	Principal ocular functions
Optic (CN II)	Carries vision fibers from the retina and pupillomotor axons; responsible for the pupillary light reflex, dazzle reflex, and accommodation reflex
Oculomotor (CN III)	Provides primary general somatic efferent innervation to the eye muscles, and motor innervation to the upper eyelid, pupil, and lens Supplies motor innervation to the dorsal rectus, medial rectus, ventral rectus, ventral oblique, and levator palpebrae superioris muscles Contains parasympathetic preganglionic general visceral efferent axons that synapse in the ciliary ganglion; postganglionic fibers from the ciliary ganglion innervate the iris sphincter and the ciliary muscles
Trochlear (CN IV)	Innervates the dorsal oblique muscle, thus controlling abduction and intorsion of the eye
Trigeminal (CN V)	Trigeminal ganglion contains cell bodies of the general somatic afferent neurons of this nerve; distal to the ganglion, it divides into its three main branches: • Ophthalmic nerve – contributes to the sensory innervation of the eye and orbit, its frontal branch innervates the upper eyelid and the nasociliary branch supplies the medial canthus, lacrimal sac, and ciliary ganglion; the ciliary ganglion mediates sensory innervation to the cornea, iris, and ciliary body • Maxillary nerve – innervates superficial structures of the eyelids • Mandibular nerve – innervates the ventral face Facilitates the oculorespiratory cardiac reflex in response to manual pressure on the eyeball Plays a vital role in the ocular pain pathways
Abducens (CN VI)	Responsible for the extraocular motor functions of the eye Supplies motor innervation to the lateral rectus and retractor bulbi muscles
Facial (CN VII)	Supplies somatic efferent innervation to the muscles of the eyelids and parasympathetic innervation to the lacrimal gland At level of the external acoustic meatus, the facial nerve continues as the auriculopalpebral nerve, originating near the zygomatic process of the temporal bone; branches of the auriculopalpebral nerve innervate the dorsal and ventral portions of the orbicularis oculi, retractor anguli oculi lateralis, and levator anguli oculi medialis The zygomatic branch of the facial nerve further divides into the upper branch supplying the frontalis and upper eyelid orbicularis, whereas the lower branch supplies the lower eyelid orbicularis

CN, cranial nerve.
Source: Compiled from Murphy *et al.* [4]; Herrera *et al.* [6]; Shin *et al.* [7]; Joffe and Gay [8].

Ocular physiology

There are intricate ocular physiologic processes, which can be impacted during the perioperative period.

Aqueous humor

Aqueous humor (AH) is a transparent, colorless liquid that fills the anterior and posterior chambers including the pupil. It nourishes the cornea and the lens, removes waste products, and maintains the intraocular pressure and globe shape. The mean AH turnover rate among several species is approximately 1–2% of the anterior chamber volume per minute, with cats having a lower turnover rate (0.7%/min) when compared to dogs and humans [10]. Two-thirds of AH is produced in the posterior segment of the ciliary body via

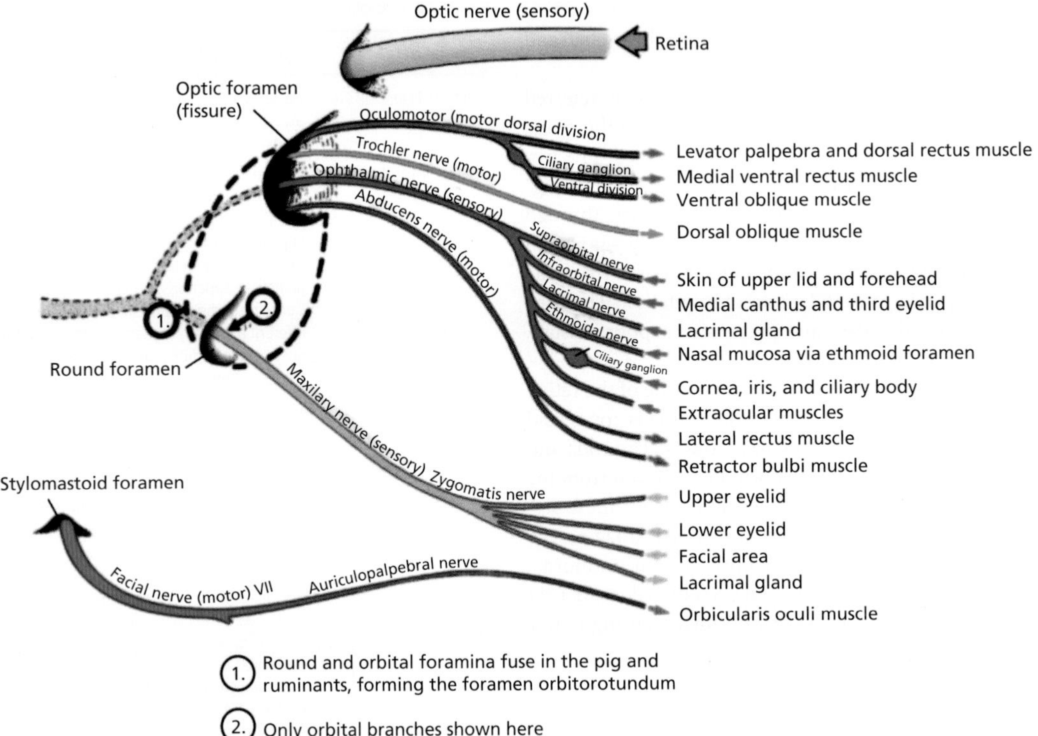

Figure 67.3 Innervation to the eye. Source: Miller [5].

active mechanisms such as the sodium pump, carbonic anhydrase-catalyzed reaction of CO_2 hydration, and the cytochrome oxidase systems. These active processes lead to a higher AH osmotic pressure than the plasma, and this disparity promotes a continuous production of AH. The remaining one-third is passively formed at the iris capillaries by diffusion of lipid-soluble substances moving down a concentration gradient, as well as ultrafiltration from plasma in response to an osmotic gradient or hydrostatic pressure.

The AH exits the eye through two pathways. In the conventional or trabecular route, aqueous fluid passes from the posterior chamber, through the pupillary aperture into the anterior chamber. From there it flows through the trabecular meshwork into the angular aqueous plexus, finally draining into the episcleral veins, conjunctival veins, and vortex venous system that join the systemic venous circulation. The majority of the AH (i.e., ~50% in horses, 85% in dogs, and 97% in cats) leaves the eye via this route [11]. The unconventional or uveoscleral pathway excludes the trabecular meshwork. The AH bathes the iris and the ciliary muscle to reach the supraciliary space or the suprachoroidal space. From here, it seeps through the sclera and is absorbed into the orbital vasculature. Uveoscleral outflow drains the remainder of the AH (i.e., ~15% in dogs [12] and 3% in cats [13]). Horses appear to have a higher dependency on this pathway [14].

Vitreous humor

The vitreous humor (VH) is a transparent elastic hydrogel that comprises a portion of the clear ocular media, and accounts for up to two-thirds of globe volume. It occupies the space between the lens and sensory retina and maintains structural integrity of the posterior portion of the globe. It is part of the optical pathway through which light passes as it travels to the retina. The VH is 99% water, and the remaining 1% is a network of polygonal, hydrated fibrils consisting of type II collagen and hyaluronic acid [11]. The collagen provides plasticity and hyaluronic acid contributes to the viscoelasticity of the VH.

Intraocular pressure

The pressure exerted by ocular contents against the globe is termed "intraocular pressure" (IOP). In the healthy eye, IOP is generated by a delicate balance between rates of AH inflow and outflow, keeping it at a steady state when the rates are equivalent. The most important influence on AH formation is the difference in osmotic pressure between AH and plasma [15]. The relationship is illustrated as:

$$\mathrm{IOP} = K\left[\left(OP_{\mathrm{aq}} - OP_{\mathrm{pl}}\right) + CP\right]$$

where K is coefficient of outflow, OP_{aq} is osmotic pressure of AH, OP_{pl} is osmotic pressure of plasma, and CP is capillary pressure. This equation explains why mannitol, due to its hypertonicity, can lower IOP by influencing AH production. The normal IOP range in dogs, cats, and rabbits is 15–20 mmHg, while in cows and horses, IOP ranges from 20–30 mmHg and 17–28 mmHg, respectively [11]. The IOP can be theoretically determined by the Goldmann equation:

$$\mathrm{IOP} = \frac{(Q-U)}{C} + EVP$$

where Q represents the aqueous inflow (in μL/min), U represents the uveoscleral outflow (in μL/min), C represents conventional aqueous outflow facility through the trabecular meshwork (μL/min/mmHg), and EVP is the episcleral venous pressure [11].

The primary factors impacting IOP are: (1) pressure on the eyeball; (2) muscle tone of EOM and orbicularis oculi muscle; (3) AH production and drainage, (4) corneal and scleral rigidity; (5) volume of intraocular contents; and (6) episcleral venous pressure (Table 67.3).

Pressure on the eyeball

Direct pressure applied on the globe during physical restraint, ocular examinations, opening of mouth for intubation, passing of an Elizabethan collar over the head, and globe manipulation during surgery can dramatically elevate IOP.

Table 67.3 Factors impacting intraocular pressure.

Increase IOP	Decrease IOP	Increase or decrease IOP
Decreased or obstructed AH outflow	Increased AH drainage	Diurnal effect
Increased AH production	Decreased AH production	Seasonal effect
Acute increase in BP	Hypocapnia	Propofol[a]
Hypercapnia	Hyperoxia	Alfaxalone[a]
Hypoxemia	Alkalosis	Ketamine[b]
Acidosis	Hypotension	Etomidate[b]
Laryngoscopy, endotracheal intubation	Hypothermia	Phenylephrine[c]
	Barbiturates	Epinephrine[c]
Direct pressure on the globe	α_2-Adrenergic agonists	
Retrobulbar block	β-Adrenergic antagonists	
Jugular compression	Cholinergic agonists	
Increase in CVP	Carbonic anhydrase inhibitors	
Coughing, gagging, vomiting, sneezing, straining	Benzodiazepines	
	Acepromazine	
Inadequate anesthetic depth	Opioids	
Head position lower than the body, Trendelenburg position, other postural changes	Nondepolarizing NMBAs	
	Inhalant anesthetics	
	Osmotic agents	
Succinylcholine		
Atropine		

[a]Expected to decrease IOP but conflicting data available in the literature
[b]Expected to increase IOP but conflicting data available in the literature
[c]Response is dosage dependent
IOP, intraocular pressure; BP, blood pressure; CVP, central venous pressure; AH, aqueous humor; NMBA, neuromuscular blocking agent.
Source: Compiled from Hendrix *et al.* [11]; Cunningham and Barry [17]; Komaromy *et al.* [24]; Kelly and Farrell [25].

Muscle tone of extraocular and orbicularis oculi muscles

The central nervous system (CNS) impacts IOP directly through neurogenic control of extraocular muscle tone by central diencephalic centers, and indirectly via hormonal and hemodynamic effects. Increased tone or contracture of EOM and the orbicularis oculi muscle can markedly increase IOP, which is observed during rapid blinking, forced eyelid closure, inadequate plane of anesthesia, and with drugs like ketamine and succinylcholine. In contrast, general anesthesia lowers IOP partly by depressing the central control centers.

Aqueous humor production and drainage

The rate of AH formation by the ciliary epithelium is influenced by sympathetic and parasympathetic innervation, as well as humoral mechanisms. Topical β-adrenergic receptor antagonists (e.g., timolol) and α_2-adrenergic receptor agonists (e.g., brimonidine) may lower IOP by decreasing AH production. During sleep, AH formation decreases by about 50%. Further, depending on whether animals are nocturnal or diurnal, variations in AH production and IOP may follow a circadian rhythm [16]. Acute break down of the blood–aqueous barrier during ocular trauma can lead to plasma leakage into the anterior chamber, thus mimicking AH overproduction and increasing IOP.

Outflow of AH can be impacted by increases in jugular venous pressure and central venous pressure (CVP). Collection of debris or blood in the anterior chamber and abnormalities of the iridocorneal angle can cause impeded AH outflow and glaucoma. The most significant factor controlling AH outflow is the diameter of Fontana spaces (i.e., spaces within the trabecular meshwork), as explained by the Hagen–Poiseuille law [17]:

$$A = \frac{r^4 \left(P_{\text{iop}} - P_{\text{v}}\right)}{8\eta L}$$

where A is the volume of AH outflow per unit of time, r is the radius of Fontana spaces, P_{iop} is the IOP, P_{v} is the venous pressure, η is the viscosity, and L is the length of Fontana spaces. During pupillary dilation, the Fontana space narrows, resistance to flow increases, and a marked rise in IOP is seen. Hence, during glaucoma, patients are treated with topical miotics.

Ocular rigidity

Resistance offered by the sclera and cornea to a change in intraocular volume is termed "ocular rigidity." Changes in intraocular volume will affect ocular rigidity. Also, scleral and corneal compliance decreases with age, increasing IOP in older animals.

Volume of the intraocular contents

When ocular tumors or systemic malignancies that spread to the eye occur, IOP can escalate. Ocular circulation autoregulates in response to changes in the ocular perfusion pressure via metabolic and myogenic mechanisms. Hyperoxia, hypocapnia, and alkalosis induce vasoconstriction in the retinal and choroidal arterioles, thus reducing IOP. The opposite effect on IOP occurs with hypoxia, hypercapnia, and acidosis [17]. Disorders associated with substantially decreased blood flow to the eye (e.g., dehydration, hypovolemic shock, and cardiogenic shock) can result in lower mean ocular perfusion pressure, retinal ischemia, and decreased IOP. During chronic arterial hypertension, IOP returns to normal due to adaptive mechanisms triggered by compression of choroidal vessels. This feedback mechanism reduces the total ocular blood volume, with IOP staying fairly constant. However, acute increases in blood pressure may lead to transient elevations in IOP.

Episcleral venous pressure

Episcleral venous pressure (EVP) is the "backpressure" created by the episcleral veins of the conventional pathway near the angular aqueous plexus. The pressure gradient between the anterior chamber and the episcleral veins has a significant effect on the rate of aqueous flow through this route and constitutes approximately 50–75% of the resistance that determines IOP. Increases in jugular venous pressure and CVP can augment EVP and IOP. This can happen during jugular compression, the Trendelenburg position [18], and other postural changes as seen in dogs [19], cats [20], and horses [21–24].

Pupil size

Variation in the pupil size is regulated by a balance between the iris sphincter (constrictor) and iris dilator muscle groups. The iris sphincter is a ring of smooth muscle cells connected by gap junctions and is located within the pupillary border. The oculomotor nerve provides parasympathetic innervation to the sphincter muscle, thus causing miosis. In contrast, the iris dilator is a myoepithelial layer extending from the iris root, where muscle fibers are also interconnected with gap junctions. The dilator muscle is innervated by sympathetic nerves and is responsible for mydriasis. This sympathetic activity in the dilator muscle is mediated by a combination of α- and β-adrenergic receptors [11]. Prostaglandins are involved in maintaining the muscle tone of iris sphincter muscles and can cause miosis. Thus, prostaglandin analogs like latanoprost possess IOP-lowering activity and are used for glaucoma treatment in dogs [26]. Pupillary diameter is a primary factor affecting the success of cataract surgery and the likelihood of complications. Hence, sympathomimetics and anticholinergics can be useful mydriatics during cataract surgeries. The exception is the avian eye, where the constrictor and dilator muscles are mainly striated and, as such, the pupil is not affected by traditional mydriatics [27].

Tear production and drainage

The precorneal tear film (PTF) is a complex blended three-layered structure comprised of an outer lipid layer, middle aqueous layer, and deep mucin layer. The PTF serves multiple functions such as:

(1) maintaining an optically uniform cornea; (2) removing debris and foreign material from the ocular surface; (3) lubricating the conjunctiva and cornea; (4) providing nutrients and oxygen to the avascular cornea; (5) controlling local bacterial flora; and (6) preserving ocular immunity. Fibers from the ophthalmic division of the trigeminal nerve (i.e., lacrimal nerve), facial nerve, pterygopalatine ganglion, and sympathetic fibers from the carotid plexus provide innervation to the lacrimal gland. Parasympathetic innervation of the lacrimal gland results in reflex tearing [28].

In animals, the aqueous portion of the tear film is routinely measured by the Schirmer tear test. Schirmer I does not need topical anesthesia and evaluates both basal and reflex tearing. Schirmer II is carried out with topical anesthesia and measures only basal tearing. Results of studies in humans [29], dogs [30–32], cats [33], and horses [34] report significant reductions in tear flow during general anesthesia. Dryness in the corneal epithelium predisposes patients to painful postanesthetic abrasions or corneal ulcers. These sequelae can be prevented with periodic ocular lubrication during the anesthetic period. Larger dogs demonstrate greater wetting per minute than smaller dogs [35]. Additionally, canine neonates have lower tear production than adults [36]. Hence, special care needs to be taken in these patients presented for anesthesia.

Ocular barriers

There are two primary ocular barriers, the blood–aqueous barrier (BAB) and the blood–retinal barrier (BRB). In combination, these maintain homeostasis by protecting the eye and preventing entry of lethal substances into internal ocular components. The BAB is the anterior barrier of the eye and is composed of capillary endothelial cells of the iris and non-pigmented epithelial cells of the ciliary body. This barrier can be altered during ocular inflammation, intraocular surgery, trauma, or vascular diseases. The BRB is the posterior barrier comprised of retinal pigment epithelium and retinal vascular endothelium equipped with non-leaky tight junctions. This restricts intercellular permeation of drugs after systemic and periocular application to the retina. Although these barriers offer protective functions, they can also impede entrance of many drugs into the eye, diminishing therapeutic efficacy [37]. Variations in the BRB may lead to the development of retinal diseases such as diabetic retinopathy and age-related macular degeneration.

Oculocardiac reflex

The oculocardiac reflex (OCR) (i.e., Aschner reflex or trigeminovagal reflex) induces reflexive slowing of the heart rate and cardiac dysrhythmias such as atrioventricular blockade, ectopic atrial rhythm, junctional rhythm, multifocal ventricular premature contractions, ventricular bigeminy, ventricular ectopy, asystole, and ventricular fibrillation [38]. This reflex is more commonly encountered in pediatric human patients during strabismus surgery [39] as compared to adults. The OCR has been reported in dogs [40], cats [41], horses [42], rabbits [40], and birds [43]. The incidence of the OCR may be increased by hypercapnia [44], hypoxemia [38], a light plane of anesthesia [39], and drugs such as short-acting opioids (e.g., sufentanil and remifentanil) [45] and dexmedetomidine [46].

The triggers for the OCR include external pressure on the eyeball, ocular manipulation, traction on the EOM, conjunctiva and orbital structures, orbital injections, retrobulbar block, ocular trauma, ocular pain, ocular hematomas, and facial trauma [7,8,47]. As a fatigable reflex, the intensity of the OCR may diminish with repeated stimulation. Upon activation of stretch receptors in the eye, short and long ciliary nerves conduct sensory impulses to the ciliary ganglion. From there, the impulses are transported via the ophthalmic division of the trigeminal nerve to the Gasserian ganglion and trigeminal nucleus. This afferent pathway continues along short internuncial fibers in the reticular formation to connect with the efferent limb. Signals are returned via the visceral motor nucleus of the vagus nerve to the sinoatrial node in the heart [38] (Fig. 67.4). There are also oculo-respiratory [7] and oculo-emetic [48] reflexes characterized by a similar afferent pathway, but which carry different efferent signals.

Immediate management of the OCR includes (1) communication with the surgeon and temporary cessation of surgical manipulation

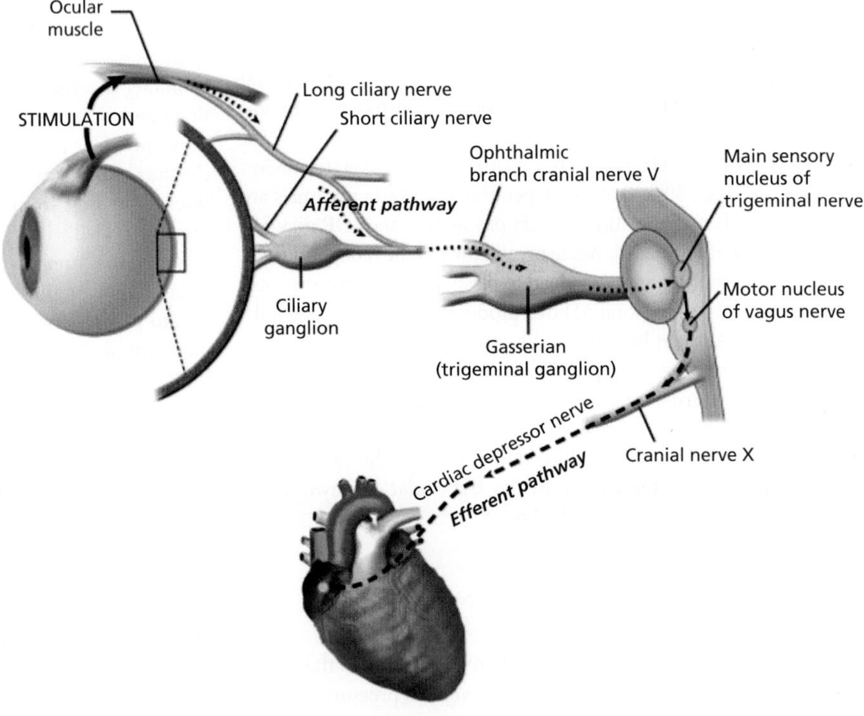

Figure 67.4 The oculocardiac reflex pathway. Source: Tobin and Weaver [49].

until heart rate and rhythm normalize; (2) confirmation of optimum ventilation, oxygenation, and anesthetic depth; (3) administration of a systemic anticholinergic, if warranted, due to significant or persistent bradycardia; (4) possible infiltration of local anesthetic around the ocular muscles (e.g., rectus muscles), which may abolish the afferent pathway; and (5) initiation of cardiopulmonary resuscitation in the event of asystole. Various maneuvers to abolish or obtund the OCR have been suggested but warrant further investigation. In dogs undergoing enucleation, preoperative administration of an anticholinergic drug was not associated with a lower prevalence of the OCR [50]; thus preemptive anticholinerigc use should be determined on a case-by-case basis depending on patient needs. Preoperative retrobulbar anesthesia can blunt the afferent pathway and help reduce incidence of OCR in dogs [50] and horses [51]. Use of a nondepolarizing muscle relaxant may also attenuate this reflex by reducing extraocular muscle tone [52].

Systemic effects of ophthalmic medications

Ophthalmic medications (Table 67.4) are routinely administered either topically or systemically for ocular procedures. Topical drugs have the potential for systemic absorption. This creates possibilities for drug interactions and anesthetic complications. Smaller patients, neonates, and pediatrics may be at a higher risk. Systemic absorption occurs either via conjunctival vasculature or from nasal mucosa after draining through the nasolacrimal duct [53]. Effective communication with the ophthalmologist prior to the anesthetic event regarding frequency of drug administration or need for additional diagnostics to identify existing systemic effects (e.g., hypokalemia seen with acetazolamide) can prevent related adverse effects during the perioperative period.

Effects of anesthetic drugs and adjuvants on ocular physiology

Patients undergoing eye surgery benefit from sedatives and anxiolytics to provide comfort and anxiolysis during examination, restraint, intravenous (IV) catheter placement, anesthetic recovery, and hospital stays. An ideal induction agent provides a rapid onset of action, avoiding the risk of regurgitation and IOP fluctuations. The proposed mechanism of action of anesthetics in reducing IOP may involve a direct effect on central diencephalic control centers, lowered arterial blood pressure (e.g., inhalant anesthetics), reduction of aqueous production, facilitation of aqueous drainage, or relaxation of extraocular muscle tone [17].

Table 67.4 Ophthalmic medications used in patients.

Drugs	Route	Mechanism of action	Use	Systemic effects
Tropicamide, atropine, homatropine, cyclopentolate, scopalamine	Topical	Cholinergic receptor antagonist	Cause mydriasis and cycloplegia	Atropine: profuse salivation and occasional vomiting in dogs [54] and cats [55]; decreased intestinal motility, and abdominal pain in horses [56,57]
Phenylephrine, epinephrine	Topical	Direct acting sympathomimetic	Cause mydriasis and ocular vasoconstriction	Phenylephrine: hypertension and reflex bradycardia in dogs [58,59] and cats [60] Epinephrine: hypertension, tachycardia, and dysrhythmias in humans [61]
Pilocarpine	Topical, oral	Cholinergic receptor agonist	Causes miosis	Vomiting, regurgitation, diarrhea, drooling, bradycardia, and weakness in dogs and cats [62]
Demecarium bromide	Topical	Carbamate parasympathomimetic (acetylcholinesterase inhibitor)	Causes miosis	Suppression of systemic acetylcholinesterase levels, gastrointestinal disturbances in dogs [63]
Echothiophate iodide	Topical	Organophosphate parasympathomimetic (acetylcholinesterase inhibitor)	Causes miosis	Suppression of systemic acetylcholinesterase levels and possibility for organophosphate toxicity in dogs [63]; prolonged muscle paralysis from neuromuscular blockers, and bradycardia reported in humans [64]
Apraclonidine, brimonidine tartrate	Topical	α_2-Adrenergic receptor agonist	Reduce IOP	Apraclonidine: reduces heart rate, salivation, vomiting in cats and dogs [65,66] Brimonidine tartrate: sedation, hypotension, bradycardia in dogs and cats [67,68]
Timolol, levobunolol, betaxolol, metipranolol, carteolol, nipradilol	Topical	β-Adrenergic receptor antagonist	Reduce IOP	Timolol: reduces heart rate in dogs [69] and cats [70]; bronchoconstriction, and congestive heart failure in humans [71,72] Levobunolol: decreases pulse rate in dogs [73]
Acetazolamide, methazolamide, dorzolamide, brinzolamide	Oral, topical	Carbonic anhydrase inhibitor	Reduce IOP	Acetazolamide: increased diuresis, gastrointestinal disturbances (anorexia, vomiting, and diarrhea), hypokalemia, and increased respiratory rate secondary to metabolic acidosis in small animals [74,75]
Mannitol	IV	Hyperosmotic agent	Reduces IOP during acute crisis	Diuresis, increased CVP, increased serum osmolality, decreased urine specific gravity, and pulmonary edema in small animals [76,77]
Glycerol	Oral	Hyperosmotic agent	Reduces IOP during acute crisis	Nausea, vomiting, hyperglycemia, glycosuria, diuresis, weight gain in dogs [76,78]
Hypertonic saline–hydroxyethyl starch	IV	Hyperosmotic agent	Reduces IOP during acute crisis	Volume expansion, changes in electrolytes in dogs [79]
Prednisolone, dexamethasone, hydrocortisone	Topical, systemic	Inhibition of cyclo-oxygenase and lipoxygenase pathways	Resolve ocular inflammation	Exacerbate ocular infections, delay corneal healing, cataract formation, ocular hypertension, adrenal suppression, hyperglycemia, lipid keratopathy, exophthalmos [80,81]

IOP, intraocular pressure; IV, intravenous.

Sedatives

Phenothiazines

Acepromazine causes miosis in dogs when given alone or in combination with hydromorphone [82,83]. A significant decrease in tear production with acepromazine has also been reported in dogs [84,85], rabbits [86], and cats [87]. A 20% decline in IOP values was seen in horses following intravenous administration [88]. Similar findings were reported in dogs [82,83]. Due to its antiemetic properties, vomiting or gagging may be prevented in patients that are at risk of globe rupture or vitreous prolapse. Since rough and abrupt anesthetic recoveries have a potential for causing postoperative eye trauma and bleeding, acepromazine may promote smooth, slow, and quiet recoveries that can benefit ophthalmic patients.

Benzodiazepines

Benzodiazepines either maintain or decrease IOP in dogs [89,90] and cats [91], as well as blunt the increase in IOP induced by ketamine [92]. However, contradictory findings have also suggested that diazepam alone or with ketamine can increase IOP in healthy dogs [93,94]. Midazolam reduces etomidate dose requirements and improves intubation conditions; however, this combination does not affect IOP in dogs [95]. Propofol–atracurium anesthesia in dogs elevates IOP, but this effect is dampened by diazepam. Endotracheal intubation-induced increases in IOP are not prevented by diazepam [96]. Intramuscular diazepam is observed to cause no significant change in tear production in rabbits [86]. The combination of tiletamine–zolazepam (Telazol®) up to 20 mg/kg IV induced no clinically significant changes in IOP in healthy dogs [97]. Similarly, in clinically normal cats, 10 mg/kg Telazol® intranasally or intramuscularly (IM) produced no change in IOP [98]. In glaucomatous cat eyes, there was no effect on IOP with 2 mg/kg IM Telazol®; however, 4 mg/kg IM increased IOP by 8%. Zolazepam alone up to 2 mg/kg IM reduced IOP in normal and glaucomatous cat eyes [99]. An increase in IOP values post Telazol® was also detected in capuchin monkeys [100].

α_2-Adrenergic receptor agonists

Xylazine induces mydriasis in cats and rats, possibly due to central inhibition of parasympathetic tone or stimulation of α_2-adrenergic mechanisms in the iris [101]. Moreover, xylazine decreases IOP in rabbits, cats, and monkeys by suppressing sympathetic neuronal function and reducing aqueous flow [102]. In dogs treated with 8 mg/kg IM xylazine, significant reductions in IOP were observed, but no change in pupil size was seen [103]. In rabbits, subcutaneous ketamine–xylazine decreased IOP by nearly 5 mmHg and blunted the isoflurane-associated increase in IOP seen in this study [104]. In healthy horses, IV xylazine caused a dose-dependent decline in IOP [88,105,106]. Use of xylazine in rats and mice has been associated with acute reversible lens opacity [107]. Xylazine has also been shown to decrease tear flow in cats [87,108] and dogs [109,110], but not in horses [34].

Topical medetomidine lowered IOP in cats and rabbits and produced concurrent mydriasis [111]. This finding suggests distribution of α_2-adrenergic receptors in the eye that may regulate IOP. In contradiction, however, miosis was noted with IV medetomidine administration in non-glaucomatous dogs, without any influence on the IOP [112]. Medetomidine at 80 μg/kg IM caused a significant decline in IOP in healthy dogs [103], while a 100 μg/kg IM dose did not change IOP in healthy cats [113]. Medetomidine–butorphanol IV increased IOP for about 20 min in dogs [114]. Systemic medetomidine has consistently been shown to decrease tear flow in dogs [115,116], cats [117], pigs [118], and chimpanzees [119].

In healthy horses, IV detomidine at 10 and 20 μg/kg decreased IOP, suggesting this drug is a safe sedative when performing ocular procedures in this species [105,120]. Similar findings were reported with IV romifidine in horses [121,122] and buffaloes [123]. Dexmedetomidine IV significantly lowered IOP and caused miosis in dogs [82,124]. Another canine study recommended that dogs sedated with dexmedetomidine–butorphanol receive a tear substitute [125]. Intrathecal dexmedetomidine led to dose-dependent antinociception and mydriasis in conscious rats [126]. Dexmedetomidine alone or in combination with butorphanol, meperidine, methadone, nalbuphine, or tramadol resulted in decreased IOP for 120 min in dogs [127]. After topical application, dexmedetomidine lowered IOP in normal as well as glaucomatous rabbit eyes [128]. The potential for α_2-adrenergic receptor agonists to cause nausea and vomiting in small animals must be considered when planning sedation or anesthesia in patients that may be adversely affected by IOP fluctuations.

Injectable anesthetics

Barbiturates

There have been few studies across species investigating the influence of pentobarbital and thiopental on ocular dynamics. Pentobarbital significantly lowered IOP as compared to urethane, chloralose–urethane, and halothane, and depressed the formation of AH via its direct effect on AH outflow facility in cats [129]. A dose-dependent decline in IOP by 20–50% was reported in both normal and glaucomatous eyes in cats administered pentobarbital [99]. A similar IOP-lowering effect with thiopental is observed in dogs [130]. In horses, thiopental significantly lowered IOP as compared to guaifenesin–ketamine and propofol [131]. While in humans, thiopental not only decreased IOP, but also helped negate the increase in IOP induced by succinylcholine [132].

Propofol and alfaxalone

Propofol attenuates an increase in IOP in anesthetized humans and lowers IOP as compared to inhalants [133]. The effects of propofol on IOP and end-tidal carbon dioxide ($P_{ET}CO_2$) have been studied in dogs and no decrease in IOP was observed, likely due to the opposing effects of increased $P_{ET}CO_2$ on IOP [134]. In several canine studies, propofol-associated increases in IOP are reported similar to horses [131], sometimes even abolishing the IOP-lowering effect of premedication [94,135,136]. Mean IOP was elevated after propofol administration in non-premedicated dogs without glaucoma and remained steady in non-premedicated dogs with glaucoma. In glaucoma-affected eyes of premedicated dogs, IOP declined after premedication and propofol administration [137]. A limited number of canine studies have compared the ocular effects of propofol and alfaxalone, with no differences in IOP observed between the two groups [135,138]. However, alfaxalone, but not propofol, significantly lowered tear production [138]. In sheep, alfaxalone does not alter IOP but causes marked miosis [139].

Dissociatives

Associated myoclonus, intact ocular reflexes, nystagmus, blepharospasm, and open palpebrae have traditionally made ketamine a less desirable choice for ophthalmic patients [17]. Previous work has suggested that ketamine may increase IOP. Postulated reasons for this include increases in EOM tone or changes in AH production and outflow, or an increase in CVP. Since an increase in IOP could be detrimental during glaucoma or open globe injury, ketamine's use for ocular surgeries remains controversial [17,25]. In cats, IM ketamine (12.5 mg/kg and 25 mg/kg) caused dose-dependent increases in IOP in glaucomatous eyes, while a 10% rise was seen over awake IOP values in normal eyes [99]. Ketamine alone or in combination with diazepam in dogs and horses caused clinically significant increases in IOP [90,93,94,131]. Similarly, in rabbits, IM ketamine–diazepam or ketamine–acepromazine combinations elevated IOP [140]. Other studies have called into question the assertion that ketamine is not appropriate in ophthalmic patients due to its effects on IOP. In dogs, 15 mg/kg ketamine with 0.2 mg/kg midazolam IV resulted in no change in IOP [92]. Also, ketamine–xylazine IM and ketamine–diazepam IV for induction maintained IOP in dogs [141]. In rabbits, monkeys, and sheep, IOP declined significantly with ketamine used alone or combined with xylazine or diazepam [104,142–145]. Even Telazol® has been reported to maintain steady IOP in cats, dogs, and monkeys [97,98,143].

Etomidate

Etomidate causes a significant decrease in IOP in humans which, to some extent, is unexpected in light of the associated myoclonus and arterial blood pressure stability that are characteristic of this drug. A fall in IOP by 61% was seen along with mydriasis followed by miosis and low frequency pendular nystagmus in human patients [146–148]. In dogs premedicated with IV butorphanol and induced with etomidate–midazolam or etomidate–lidocaine, no change in IOP or evidence of myoclonus was observed [95]. Etomidate–midazolam in another canine study produced clinically important miosis and increases in IOP [149]. Interestingly, in rabbits, topical etomidate produced no change in pupillary diameter and light reflex, but did cause decreases in IOP, conjunctival chemosis, and corneal epithelial edema [147].

Inhalant anesthetics

In the 1960s, methoxyflurane became a popular choice over halothane for ophthalmic anesthesia due to: (1) better cardiovascular stability; (2) centrally fixed eyes during light surgical anesthesia and ocular hypotonia; (3) lower incidence of bleeding; (4) smooth and slow emergence; and (5) reduced need for postoperative analgesia and sedation. However, the average decrease in IOP was greater for halothane (18%) as compared to methoxyflurane (6%) [150]. The introduction of isoflurane provided comparable decreases in IOP to halothane, but with lower arrhythmogenicity, better cardiac index, and significantly lower incidence of postoperative nausea and vomiting [151–153]. Currently, isoflurane, sevoflurane, and desflurane are the volatile anesthetics used in veterinary species. All three agents provide comparable reductions in IOP during ocular surgeries [154,155]. Since these modern inhalants possess lower blood solubility, they cause rapid induction and recovery in animals. This may warrant use of postoperative sedatives to decrease the risk of iatrogenic trauma or intraocular bleeding resulting from emergence delirium.

In rabbits, a dose-dependent decrease in intraocular compliance and IOP was reported with sevoflurane and halothane [156]. Halothane decreased IOP and AH flow in normal rabbits and monkeys, while nitrous oxide showed no effect [157]. During hypercapnia, IOP remained unchanged in halothane-anesthetized horses [158]. In normocapnic dogs, IOP was maintained at a normal steady state during desflurane and sevoflurane anesthesia [159]. Isoflurane also induced significant decreases in IOP in pigs and mice [160–162]. In dogs, nitrous oxide with desflurane resulted in maintenance of steady IOP without changes in pupillary diameter [163]. Dogs anesthetized with isoflurane and desflurane had decreased intra-anesthetic tear production which returned to normal post recovery. It was suggested that decreased lacrimation was due to the vagolytic or sympathomimetic effects of inhalant anesthesia. Also, no difference in tear flow was found between short and long anesthetic events [31]. Sevoflurane has also been associated with a decline in tear production in dogs [164,165]. Nitrous oxide is contraindicated in vitreoretinal surgery involving gas tamponade. It can lead to drastic increases in IOP by diffusion into the air bubble injected into the posterior chamber, amplifying the expansion of the bubble, which could be detrimental once the eye is closed [25].

Anesthetic adjuvants

Neuromuscular blocking agents

Changes in globe position and periodic globe motion occur under general anesthesia, but there is variation across species relative to the anesthetic depth. Following induction of anesthesia, the globe rotates ventromedially, sometimes even protracting the nictitating membrane to cover the cornea. Full exposure of the cornea, anterior segment, and globe is needed for corneal and intraocular surgeries [166]. In some cases, a central globe can be achieved using stay sutures in the anterior sclera or rectus muscle, or via a retrobulbar injection, however, these methods may precipitate an OCR [167,168].

Routine use of short-acting nondepolarizing neuromuscular blocking agents (NMBAs) such as atracurium, cisatracurium, vecuronium, and rocuronium is standard of care for small and large animals undergoing corneal and intraocular surgeries. Along with a centralized motionless globe (Fig. 67.5), they prevent an increase in IOP and the OCR associated with EOM contraction [17,38].

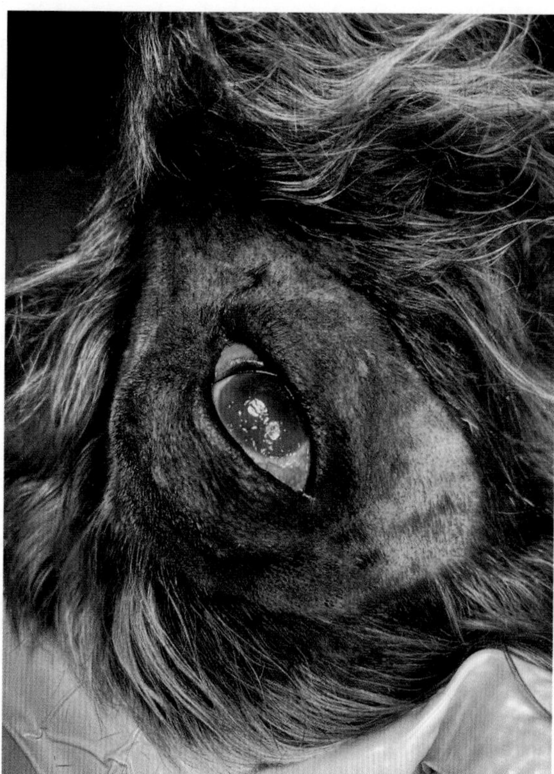

Figure 67.5 Centralization of the globe using intravenous injection of a neuromuscular blocking agent (rocuronium). Source: Dr. Vaidehi Paranjape, with permission.

Paralysis with an NMBA also eliminates ocular reflexes interfering with ocular microsurgery. They cause dose-dependent paralysis of the respiratory muscles, and therefore the patient must be manually or preferably mechanically ventilated. Positive-pressure ventilation is also helpful to counteract hypercapnia and respiratory acidosis which would precipitate increases in IOP. During controlled ventilation, conservative tidal volumes and peak inspiratory pressure should be used to prevent increases in CVP, further augmenting IOP [17]. Accessible drugs to reverse the effects of nondepolarizing NMBAs are edrophonium and neostigmine, classified as acetylcholinesterase inhibitors. Since these drugs have significant muscarinic effects, it is advisable to administer an anticholinergic before the reversal agent [169]. Additional information on NMBAs and neuromuscular blockade is available in Chapter 26.

In anesthetized dogs, vecuronium and atracurium were observed to cause the least effect on IOP and cardiovascular variables [170,171]. Horses receiving 0.1 mg/kg IV atracurium required less desflurane and demonstrated better surgery and recovery scores than horses receiving a lidocaine constant rate infusion (CRI) during ocular surgeries. A single atracurium injection was enough to create optimal surgical conditions [172]. Another equine study detected better scores for globe position, cardiovascular parameters, and recovery for horses receiving atracurium compared to the isoflurane alone group during vitrectomies [173]. Low doses of rocuronium (i.e., 0.075, 0.05, and 0.03 mg/kg) produced a central globe with transient respiratory depression only observed with the 0.075 mg/kg dose in dogs [174]. When the rocuronium dose was raised to 0.1 mg/kg IV, the globe rotated centrally without a reduction in ventilation parameters [175]. A single 0.3 mg/kg IV rocuronium bolus successfully produced 100% neuromuscular block, with a centralized globe and full iris exposure in horses [176]. Succinylcholine is a depolarizing muscle relaxant, and its use during ocular surgeries remains controversial in human patients. Elevations in IOP have been reported with this drug in humans and animals [177,178]. This increase in IOP is probably due to tonic contraction of EOM, choroidal vascular dilation, relaxation of orbital smooth muscles, and induced cycloplegia hindering AH outflow [179]. Retraction of the eyeball with simultaneous lateral movement of the nictitating membrane and axial shortening of the globe has been reported in cats [180,181].

In birds, the constrictor and dilator muscles in the ciliary body and iris are mainly striated, and hence the pupil is not affected by traditional mydriatics (e.g., tropicamide) [27]. Instead, mydriasis may be achieved by topical NMBA application. Intracameral atracurium or *d*-tubocurarine led to successful pupillary dilation in birds, but not topical *d*-tubocurarine [182]. Topical vecuronium and rocuronium were viable topical mydriatics for retinal and fundic examination, without exhibiting any side effects in raptors [183,184]. Topical vecuronium (4 mg/mL), 2 drops every 15 min for two instillations, achieved full mydriasis within 30 min, and was maintained for 4 h in kestrels [184]. A single topical rocuronium dose (0.35 mg) caused full mydriasis within 80 min and lasted for 4 h in tawny owls [183]. Overdosing of topical NMBAs in birds can cause eyelid, neck, hindlimb, and respiratory muscle paralysis [184].

Anticholinergics

Atropine or glycopyrrolate may be given to ophthalmic patients for prophylaxis or treatment of bradycardia originating from vagal effects of opioids, the OCR, and prior to reversal of neuromuscular blockade. They are beneficial in patients with pre-existing bradycardia or for improving heart rate and hemodynamics in neonates and pediatrics. In the eye, atropine blocks the actions of the short ciliary nerve and relaxes the sphincter muscle of the iris, thus producing mydriasis [185]. The mydriatic–cycloplegic effects are useful in the treatment of acute iritis, iridocyclitis, and keratouveitis [186]. There is sparse data evaluating the mydriatic and cyclopegic effects of systemic versus topical atropine administration. In conscious dogs with normal eyes, 0.06 mg/kg IM demonstrated significant increases in IOP (approximately 21%) and pupillary diameter, and the effect persisted for 60 min following treatment. The authors recommended that atropine be used cautiously via topical or systemic routes in dogs suffering from glaucoma [187]. Conversely, there was no effect of glycopyrrolate 0.004 mg/kg IM on IOP or pupil size in awake human volunteers [188]. The mydriatic effect of topical glycopyrrolate was more intense, swift, and long-lasting than atropine in rabbits [189].

Maximal pupillary dilation was obtained 30–60 min after topical atropine in dogs, cats, and cattle, and retained even after 10 h in horses [190]. In adult cats, 1% atropine topically resulted in significant increases in IOP and mydriasis, while no ocular effect was noted after 10% phenylephrine drops [191]. Topical 1% atropine induced minimal ocular effects in horses [192,193]; however, in another equine study where vertical pupil diameter was measured every 24 h, atropine drops induced significant long-lasting mydriasis (> 14 days) [194]. Reduced tear production has been reported with systemic and topical anticholinergic administration in dogs and with systemic administration in cats [195–198]. Maximal reductions in tear production occurred at 120 min after instillation and returned to baseline values by 300 min [196].

In monkeys and horses, atropine had substantial effects on uveoscleral outflow and caused a reduction in IOP [199,200]. After topical administration of 1 mg atropine per hour into the conjunctival sac, intestinal motility decreased, and clinical signs of abdominal pain developed in 4 of 6 horses. The onset of these adverse effects was between 11 and 22 h after the first dose [57]. But when the dosing interval was increased to 1 mg of topical atropine per 6 h, systemic concentrations were not detected, and ileus or clinical signs of colic were not observed [201]. A recent pharmacokinetic study found that the bioavailability after atropine eye drops or topical infusion was 69% and 68%, respectively, with a short terminal half-life (0.8 h) in horses. A significant reduction in intestinal motility was observed after administration of 1 mg topical atropine every 3 h but not after every 6 h. Clinical signs of colic were not observed in any horses. A topical infusion at 5 μg/kg/24 h was recommended as a safe therapeutic option [56].

Ocular pain and its management

Origin of ocular pain

Pain sensations within the cornea, sclera, uveal tract, conjunctiva, eyelids, orbital tissues, EOM, lacrimal gland, and periocular skin are transmitted to the brain via the ophthalmic division of the trigeminal nerve [4]. Since the cornea contains the richest nerve density, stimulation of this tissue triggers the blink reflex and reflex tearing [202]. Blepharospasm is noted during extreme pain (e.g., corneal ulcer) due to an exaggerated corneal reflex, such that the eyelids are unable to open voluntarily [203]. Corneal sensitivity not only varies across species but is greater for the central cornea compared with peripheral regions [204]. In fact, brachycephalic breeds have significantly lower corneal sensitivity as compared to mesocephalic or dolichocephalic breeds [205,206]. The sensory corneal nerve fibers are polymodal in nature, and are activated by mechanical, chemical, and thermal stimuli, along with endogenous factors released during tissue injury. The deeper corneal stroma is comprised of mechano-nociceptors and cold thermal receptors that respond to mechanical pressure (e.g., glaucoma and uveitis) or temperature changes, respectively [207].

Ocular inflammatory responses are generated in response to mechanical and chemical stimuli, and are mediated by prostaglandins, neuropeptides, leukotrienes, platelet-activating factor, interleukins, and bradykinin. Even though the retina lacks nociceptors, retinal inflammation can elicit pain due to activation of uveal nociceptors by inflammatory mediators [208]. Endogenous prostaglandins play a vital role in initiation and maintenance of the inflammatory process. They cause miosis, altered IOP, disruption of the blood–aqueous barrier, spasms of the iris and ciliary body, vasodilation, and neovascularization [209]. Stimulation of polymodal receptors and pre-existing silent receptors activated by inflammation will result in ocular pain. Photophobia is a feature of ocular inflammation and its relationship with pain sensation involves the inflammatory cascade triggering uveal nociceptors [210].

Analgesics

Opioids

The selection of a particular opioid is made based on the level of analgesia required, procedure length, drug duration of action, and patient needs. Intrinsically, opioids possess high vagal efferent activity, which predisposes patients to a higher incidence of the OCR during ocular surgeries [38,45]. Anticholinergics can successfully treat bradycardia secondary to opioid administration. An emesis-related rise in IOP is a key concern with systemic opioids and delaying their administration until after induction of anesthesia and adding antiemetics to the anesthetic plan may be advantageous.

The μ-opioid receptor was identified as a target to alleviate corneal allodynia and corneal nerve sensitization in mice [211]. Morphine eye drops act on μ- and δ-opioid receptors in the rat cornea to diminish inflammation and hyperalgesia [212]. In rabbits with corneal abrasion, topical morphine produced analgesic effects, but this effect was absent in animals with intact corneas. No adverse effect on corneal wound healing was detected [213]. Topical 1% morphine did not produce clinically significant analgesia in healthy equine corneas [214]. However, morphine was measurable in AH and VH of treated eyes and was systemically absorbed in another equine study [215]. Morphine eye drops applied for corneal ulceration in dogs and cats provided no analgesia but instead increased blepharospasm, conjunctival hyperemia, and blink rate [216]. Topical and subconjunctival 0.1% preservative-free morphine displayed no analgesic or adverse effects in diabetic and non-diabetic dogs [217]. In contrast, another study has reported beneficial analgesic effects of morphine eye drops in dogs with corneal ulcers [218].

In human patients undergoing ocular surgeries, remifentanil, alfentanil, or fentanyl, as a bolus or CRI, with or without propofol, was effective in decreasing or maintaining IOP during intubation, laryngeal mask airway insertion, succinylcholine administration, and postural changes [219–222]. Similarly, systemic opioids given alone or in combination with acepromazine or α_2-adrenergic receptor agonists have been shown to lower IOP in dogs [83,94,127], horses [105], and rabbits [223,224]. Butorphanol at 0.2 mg/kg IM provided an acceptable degree of sedation to allow eye examinations in dogs and significantly increased IOP, although values remained within normal limits [225]. In sheep premedicated with sustained-release buprenorphine at 0.01 mg/kg subcutaneously, IOP was significantly higher than in unpremedicated sheep [145]. Opioids including meperidine, fentanyl, butorphanol, and oxymorphone have also been found to significantly reduce tear production in dogs, and use of ocular lubricants or tear replacement solutions is indicated [110,164,226]. Moreover, opioids produce miosis in dogs [227] and rabbits [228] versus mydriasis in cats [229]. There is strong evidence in human patients that opioid-inclusive anesthesia does not reduce postoperative pain, and instead causes postoperative nausea and vomiting, ileus, and urinary retention when compared with opioid-free anesthesia. These findings have encouraged anesthesiologists to avoid high intraoperative opioid doses and consider opioid-sparing techniques [230,231].

Local anesthetics

The therapeutic applications of local anesthetics in ophthalmic patients are numerous. Pertinent routes of administration include topical and intracameral application, IV injection, and regional deposition. Proparacaine, tetracaine, and oxybuprocaine are examples of topical anesthetics used in domestic animals. Topical ophthalmic anesthetics facilitate ocular diagnostic and therapeutic procedures and, if used intraoperatively, can produce corneal analgesia. Repeated application of these agents, however, may cause toxicity to the corneal epithelium [232]. During cataract surgeries, intracameral lidocaine can increase analgesia in dogs [233] and humans [234].

Intravenous lidocaine at a loading dose of 1 mg/kg followed by 1.5 or 3 mg/kg/h is a successful analgesic adjunct to general anesthesia during intraocular surgeries in dogs and horses, respectively [172,235]. The mechanism by which IV lidocaine produces analgesic, anti-inflammatory, and antihyperalgesic effects is not fully understood but appears to involve actions at multiple molecular targets as well as attenuation of neuroinflammatory responses [236]. A single IV lidocaine bolus at 2 mg/kg given after butorphanol predication and before etomidate induction did not affect IOP in dogs [95].

Local and regional anesthetic techniques are part of a multimodal analgesic approach for ocular procedures. They also decrease intraoperative anesthetic and perioperative opioid requirements [237]. The retrobulbar block (RBB) is a well-documented and commonly used regional anesthesia technique in dogs [237–239], cats [237, 240,241], horses [51,242,243], and cattle [244,245]. It involves introducing the needle into the EOM cone behind the eyeball and injecting a small volume of local anesthetic. Indications for an RBB include intraocular surgeries, enucleation, and need for globe centralization. It also eliminates the need for general anesthesia in horses and facilitates standing eyelid and corneal surgeries [246]. The RBB temporarily blocks the optic, oculomotor, abducens, and trochlear nerves, as well as the maxillary and ophthalmic branches of the trigeminal nerve. Blockade of these nerves causes desensitization of the globe and palpebrae, akinesia of the globe, transient vision loss, pupillary dilation, and decreased IOP. Even though the OCR can be triggered by a retrobulbar injection, preoperative RBB is associated with a lower prevalence of OCR in dogs undergoing enucleation [50]. While performing RBB is not without risk [237], the overall complication rate reported is low in dogs and humans [247,248]. As an alternative to RBB, peribulbar block, subtenons block, orbital splash blocks, and placement of anesthetic-infused hemostatic sponges in the orbit can also be performed [237]. Blinking, either spontaneously or in response to a stimulus, is due to motor innervation of orbicularis oculi muscle by the facial nerve. Akinesia of the eyelid can be achieved by blockade of the auriculopalpebral branch of the facial nerve [249,250]. The Peterson eye block is another alternative to an RBB and is often combined with an auriculopalpebral block during enucleation in large animals. The

Peterson eye block requires more skill to perform than the RBB, and potential risks include penetration of the nasopharynx and turbinates, ventral maxillary artery injection, and intrameningeal injection [245,250]. Care and lubrication of the cornea is mandatory following all of these ocular blocks.

Non-steroidal anti-inflammatory drugs

Non-steroidal anti-inflammatory drugs (NSAIDs) suppress the inflammation cascade through inhibition of the enzymatic conversion of arachidonic acid to prostaglandins and thromboxane. The use of NSAIDs in veterinary ophthalmology is common for treating uveitic pathology where corticosteroids are contraindicated (e.g., diabetes mellitus), for maintaining mydriasis, and for treating perioperative pain. Ocular inflammation can lead to uveitic glaucoma, which can be prevented with NSAIDs. Topical NSAIDs have been developed to improve the ocular bioavailability of these compounds and to decrease their systemic side effects. Examples of ophthalmic NSAIDs are bromfenac, flurbiprofen, diclofenac, ketorolac, and nepafenac. The ocular side effects of NSAIDs include local irritation, worsening of an existing eye infection, inhibition of corneal re-epithelialization, and an increase in IOP possibly from reduction of AH outflow. Caution must be exercised with systemic NSAIDs in clinical scenarios of coagulopathy, hypovolemia, hypotension, renal disease, and gastrointestinal disease [251,252]. Use of corticosteroids or topical NSAIDs with systemic NSAIDs needs to be coordinated vigilantly between the anesthesiologist and ophthalmologist.

Miscellaneous analgesic drugs

Gabapentin is a structural analog of γ-aminobutyric acid (GABA) and is used to provide pain relief in glaucomatous patients [253]. It may also be effective in patients suffering from neuropathic ocular pain, who have systemic comorbidity and a refractory response to other topical treatments [254]. Oral gabapentin has been used as an adjuvant to prevent an increase in IOP associated with laryngoscopy and tracheal intubation in human patients [255]. Dogs receiving preanesthetic oral gabapentin displayed similar results [256]. In healthy dogs, oral gabapentin decreased mean IOP values but without concurrent changes in tear production and pupillary diameter [257]. Topical treatment with gabapentin significantly reduced clinical signs and biomarkers of inflammation and displayed analgesic and secretagogue properties in rabbits [258,259].

Non-opioid CRIs provide multimodal analgesia along with inhalant- and opioid-sparing effects. Despite conflicting data regarding the effect of ketamine on IOP, this drug may be used at sub-anesthetic doses (i.e., 0.1–0.5 mg/kg/h) as a CRI for perioperative pain management for ocular surgeries. Ketamine's non-competitive antagonism at *N*-methyl-D-aspartate (NMDA) receptors may attenuate neuropathic ocular pain and hyperalgesia [260]. Dexmedetomidine is a highly selective α_2-adrenergic receptor agonist with sedative, muscle relaxant, and analgesic properties. Addition of a dexmedetomidine infusion to isoflurane anesthesia maintained hemodynamics and reduced IOP in patients undergoing vitreoretinal surgery [261]. However, its effect on OCR augmentation and the gastrointestinal system must be recognized [46,262].

Impact of anesthesia on the electroretinogram

When light enters the eye and strikes the retina, it stimulates retinal photoreceptors which trigger alteration of electrical potentials propagating throughout the neuroretina and visual pathways. These electrical responses can be recorded and analyzed using electrodes placed around the eye during an electroretinogram (ERG) [263]. In animals, the ERG may be performed under general anesthesia or with deep sedation combined with an auriculopalpebral nerve block and topical anesthesia to minimize involuntary periocular muscle movements [264–266]. It is important to know if anesthetic agents used during ERG may influence the results. Hence, it is recommended to compare ERG results of clinical patients to normal values obtained using the same drug combinations used for sedation or anesthesia [264].

General anesthesia with medetomidine–ketamine–vecuronium caused minimal depression of the amplitude of the waves during short-term ERG in dogs [267]. Clinically, IV medetomidine administered alone minimally affected retinal responses in another canine study [268]. Xylazine–ketamine or medetomidine–ketamine combinations were preferred for ERGs in dogs as compared to thiopental–isoflurane or thiopental–halothane–nitrous oxide combinations [269,270]. In healthy dogs, Telazol® caused less depression of ERG signals compared to medetomidine and isoflurane groups [271]. With sevoflurane and halothane, ERG readings were significantly affected in dogs and severe depression of the scotopic threshold response occurred [272]. Recently, it was observed that anesthetics resulted in significant attenuation and delay of ERG responses in dogs, but there was no effect on the quality of recorded signals when compared to fully conscious dogs [273]. In cats, IM xylazine–ketamine or dexmedetomidine–ketamine were viable options for chemical restraint as they both minimally affected ERG variables [274]. Dose-related changes in ERG recordings have been observed with thiopental in sheep [275]. In standing horses, ERG was performed safely with detomidine sedation and auriculopalpebral nerve block [265,276]. Since hypoxemia, hypocapnia, and hypercapnia can alter ERG recordings, options like supplemental oxygen and assisted or manual ventilation must be considered in sedated or anesthetized patients undergoing an ERG [277,278].

General anesthesia for ophthalmic surgery

Preoperative assessment

Patients undergoing ophthalmic procedures can be a high-risk group, including geriatrics with other comorbidities (e.g., endocrinopathies, systemic hypertension, cardiac disease, renal disease, etc.), neonates, and pediatrics. Hence, an anesthesiologist must have a detailed patient history, thorough physical examination, pertinent blood work, and other appropriate diagnostics to identify and determine the impacts of co-existing disease. Prior to general anesthesia, discussion with the ophthalmologist regarding special requirements for patient positioning, and ongoing topical and systemic medications is advisable. Animals that are blind or nervous by nature are more likely to be stressed and fearful in a hospital environment and incorporating anxiolytics for in-hospital patients is beneficial. If the animal is painful, adequate pain control must be instituted.

Anesthesia set up and patient positioning

All drugs and required equipment (e.g., ventilator and peripheral nerve stimulator) needed for general anesthesia should be assembled and checked before use. In the ophthalmology theater, setup is arranged with the patient's head facing away from the anesthetist and anesthesia machine (Fig. 67.6). This restricts the anesthetist's access to the cranial region of the patient which directly impacts IV access and the ability to monitor eye reflexes and jaw tone to assess

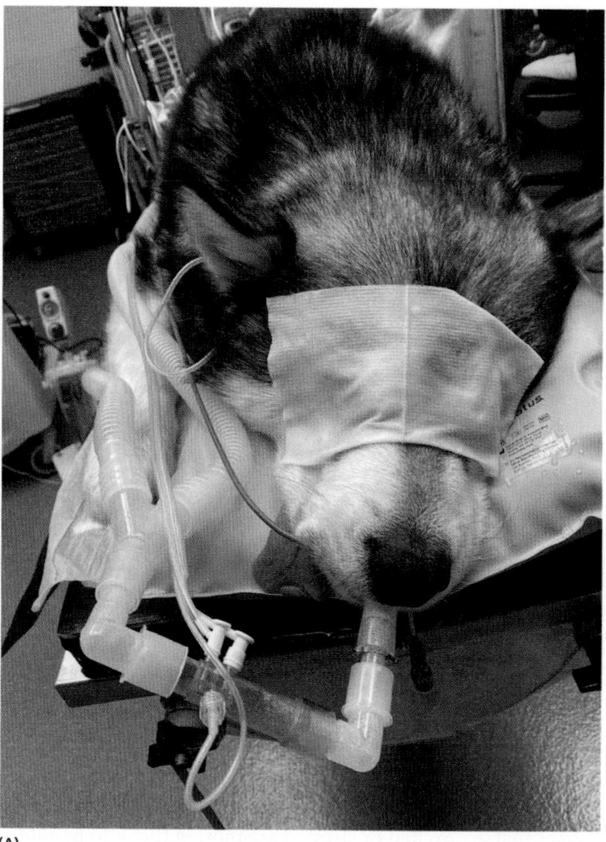

(A)

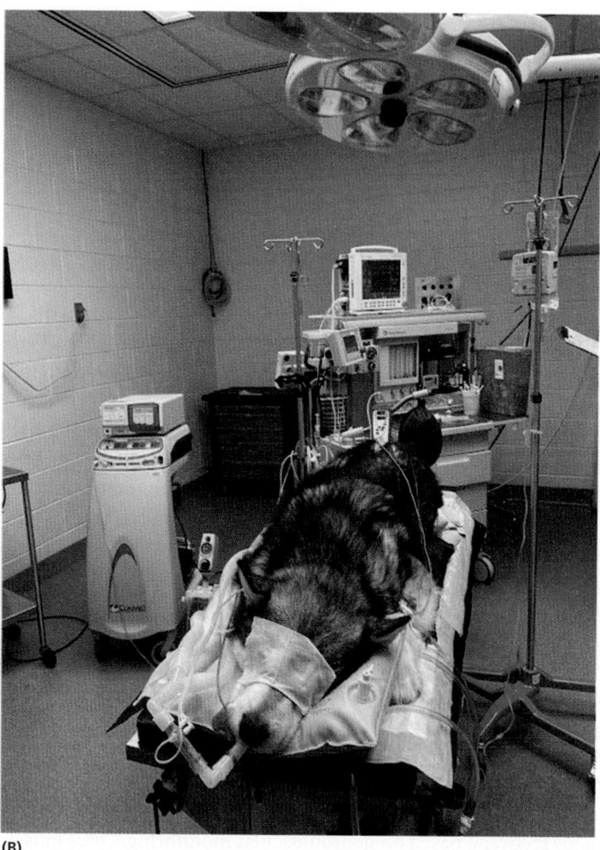

(B)

Figure 67.6 **A.** Use of an elbow adapter to connect the patient to the breathing system and prevent disconnection or kinking of the endotracheal tube. **B.** Placement of the anesthesia workstation, monitoring equipment, and intravenous fluids away from the patient during ophthalmic surgery. Source: Dr. Vaidehi Paranjape, with permission.

anesthetic depth. Long tubes for the breathing system may be required along with special elbow connectors (Fig. 67.6) to reduce traction on endotracheal tube (ETT). Before placement of surgical drapes, ETT tube security and patient-end connections must be verified to avoid accidental extubation or disconnections during the procedure. Some ocular surgeries require patient positioning in dorsal recumbency with the neck flexed (Fig. 67.7). This position can cause ETT kinking or caudal movement of the tube into a bronchus. Use of a wire-reinforced ETT and premeasuring tube length prior to intubation can prevent these complications. Vigilant monitoring of respiratory rate and effort, capnography, and pulse oximetry can aid in immediate detection of increased expiratory resistance related to ETT kinking or obstruction.

Physical restraint, premedication, and anesthetic induction

Forceful and rough restraint may increase IOP due to inadvertent pressure on the jugular veins and elevation in CVP. Using a harness rather than a collar is preferred. Vomiting, straining, and coughing must be avoided. Incorporating antiemetics, gastric protectants, and prokinetics preoperatively may help reduce the incidence of anesthesia-associated gastrointestinal disturbances. Taking these preventive measures is imperative to ensure a positive outcome, especially when there is a high risk of globe rupture. It is advantageous to place an IV catheter in the pelvic limb (e.g., lateral or medial saphenous vein) to provide easy catheter access during the intraoperative period.

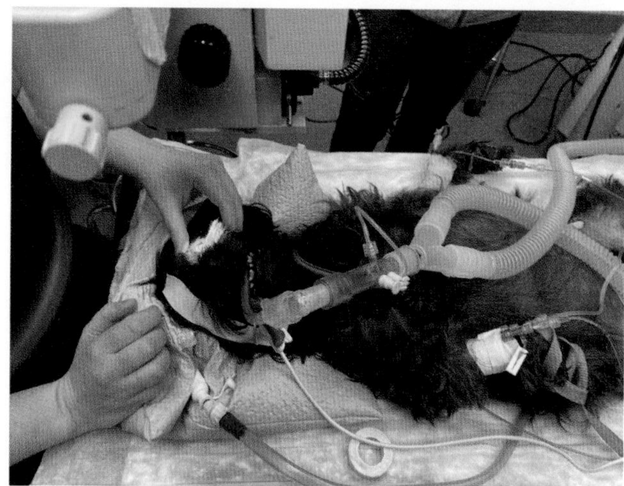

Figure 67.7 Patient positioning in dorsal recumbency with neck flexed for an intraocular surgery. Source: Dr. Vaidehi Paranjape, with permission.

Endotracheal intubation

During preoxygenation, a tight-fitting face mask is avoided to prevent external pressure on the eye. Anesthetic induction should be smooth. Coughing or gagging during intubation can be prevented by administration of IV or topical lidocaine, and by ensuring adequate anesthetic depth before attempting intubation. The ETT should be well secured.

Protection of the contralateral eye

For unilateral procedures, the dependent eye is padded to protect against physical injury. Prior to surgery, lubrication of the non-surgical eye must be performed periodically to avoid corneal desiccation and ulceration. Other methods for preventing corneal drying and exposure include temporarily taping the eyelids closed or temporary tarsorrhaphy.

Neuromuscular blockade and anesthetic monitoring

The nondepolarizing NMBA should be administered immediately before corneal or intraocular surgery is started and mechanical ventilation is recommended throughout surgery. In addition to routine anesthetic monitoring, the degree of paralysis can be closely monitored using a peripheral nerve stimulator or acceleromyography (see Chapter 26). These drugs cause a centralized globe (Fig. 67.5) independent of anesthetic depth, which makes anesthetic monitoring more challenging. Anesthetists must focus on changes in heart rate and blood pressure to assess the anesthetic depth and adequacy of analgesia. Measurement of expired volatile agent concentrations can also be useful when available. In diabetic patients, serial blood glucose monitoring should be performed perioperatively to determine glucose trends, diagnose extreme abnormalities, and assess response to any administered treatments (see Chapter 42).

Recovery, extubation, and emergence

Recovery is initiated only after neuromuscular function has been completely restored, either by reversal of the NMBA or by spontaneous recovery, based on neuromuscular monitoring. Once muscular function resumes, non-essential monitoring can be removed and the patient should be moved to a comfortable position before the anesthetic is discontinued. Gagging or coughing should be prevented during tracheal extubation. Recovery needs to be smooth and should occur in a quiet environment. Emergence delirium, dysphoria, and excitement should be controlled using sedatives to prevent sudden changes in IOP with ocular hemorrhage or trauma. An Elizabethan collar must be carefully placed to prevent the patient from scratching or rubbing the operated eye. Additional analgesia should be provided if required.

Anesthesia-related ocular complications

In humans, dogs, and horses, the most common ocular complication of general anesthesia is corneal abrasion [279–281]. Causal factors include damage caused by face masks, surgical drapes, spillage of solutions, ocular injury from loss of protective reflexes and lack of pain sensation, and dry eye from reduced tear production [281]. Therefore, during anesthesia, it is prudent to tape the eyelids closed, apply protective goggles, and lubricate eyes with petroleum-based ointments or aqueous-based solutions. Other ocular complications reported in humans are chemical injury, photic injury, visual disturbances, retinal ischemia, hemorrhagic retinopathy, acute glaucoma, cortical blindness, and ischemic optic neuropathy [282]. Postanesthetic blindness in cats has been associated with the use of spring-held mouth gags and consequent compression of the maxillary artery during non-ocular procedures [283]. Out of the 20 feline cases, a mouth gag was used in 16 cats. Neurological deficits were seen in 17 cats in addition to blindness, and 3 cats suffered from cardiac arrest during anesthesia. Moreover, maximal opening of the mouth interrupts maxillary artery blood flow as evaluated with magnetic resonance angiography and dynamic computer tomography [284]. The use of a smaller mouth gag was recommended in cats as it produced minimal alterations in the maxillary artery blood flow [285].

Special considerations for equine ophthalmic patients

Ophthalmic procedures that require equine patients to be completely immobilized are performed under general anesthesia. However, there are surgical procedures of the eye that can be performed on a standing horse using sedatives and analgesics combined with local anesthetic techniques. The decision largely depends on the ophthalmologist's personal preference, cost, disposition and medical condition of the horse, and available facilities. Some surgeons prefer a standing sedation technique for selected procedures to reduce the risk associated with general anesthesia [246]. Detomidine can be given in intermittent boluses as needed, or as a CRI. For detomidine infusion, a 7.5 μg/kg IV loading dose is administered followed by a 0.6 μg/kg/min CRI. This rate is halved every 15 min until the rate of 0.15 μg/kg/min is reached. The horse is given IV boluses of detomidine (1–2 μg/kg) as needed [286]. This is accompanied by an effective locoregional anesthetic technique as described elsewhere in this chapter.

Horses with a non-visual eye should be approached from the visual side. If approach from the non-visual side is necessary, it should be accompanied by words of reassurance and gentle hand contact. If an increase in IOP will jeopardize the primary ocular problem of the horse, steps should be taken to minimize factors that can potentially increase IOP during the physical examination. Horses that are excited or stressed are more difficult to handle and tend to have more fluctuations in IOP, which may be deleterious to an eye with pre-existing intraocular hypertension [287]. Hence, it is better to sedate such horses with xylazine or detomidine during the ophthalmic examination to prevent sudden increases in IOP. When examining a sedated horse, an effort should be made to raise the head above the level of the heart as a lowered head results in an increase in IOP [24]. Prior to anesthesia, it is advisable to administer sedation before flushing the horse's mouth out to prevent excitement-associated increases in IOP.

Effective premedication is important in ensuring a smooth anesthetic induction. An α_2-adrenergic receptor agonist administered IV will provide profound sedation, as well as analgesia and muscle relaxation. Some horses may need a supplemental dose of α_2-adrenergic receptor agonist to achieve adequate sedation. Administration of an opioid following an α_2-adrenergic receptor agonist will provide additional sedation and analgesia. To prevent excitement, it is good practice to give the opioid after signs of sedation from the α_2-adrenergic receptor agonist are observed, which generally occur about 2–3 min after its administration. Butorphanol is the most commonly used opioid in equine practice. The IV dose for butorphanol ranges from 0.02–0.05 mg/kg. Morphine may be used in place of butorphanol, given IV at 0.2–0.6 mg/kg. Hydromorphone and methadone are also excellent alternatives [288,289]. Recommended IV doses for the α_2-adrenergic receptor agonists and opioids are shown in Table 67.5. The tranquilizer acepromazine can be incorporated into the premedication. It has been shown that acepromazine is associated with lower mortality in equine elective cases when used as part of the anesthetic plan [290]. It is given IV at 0.02 mg/kg 30 min before, or at the same time as, the α_2-adrenergic receptor agonist. Acepromazine can also be administered IM before or during anesthesia. Since acepromazine has a long duration of action, its effect will last until the recovery period, which may contribute to a better recovery.

Table 67.5 Recommended intravenous (IV) dosages of α_2-adrenergic receptor agonists and opioids for premedication in equine ophthalmic patients.

Agents	Dosage
Xylazine	0.5–1 mg/kg
Detomidine	5–20 μg/kg
Medetomidine	2.5–5 μg/kg
Dexmedetomidine	1.25–2.5 μg/kg
Romifidine	0.05–0.1 mg/kg
Butorphanol	0.02–0.05 mg/kg
Morphine	0.1–0.3 mg/kg
Hydromorphone	0.03–0.04 mg/kg
Methadone	0.1–0.2 mg/kg

The choice of anesthetic induction agents for equine patients depends largely on the quality of induction associated with the injectable agents and the effect of the induction agents on IOP. Presently in the United States, induction of anesthesia in equine patients has been limited to ketamine combined with a benzodiazepine, propofol or guaifenesin, and Telazol®. When an α_2-adrenergic receptor agonist is used as premedication, propofol may be an acceptable induction agent in foals. Telazol® can also be used for induction like a ketamine–benzodiazepine combination. It is imperative that profound sedation from an α_2-adrenergic receptor agonist be observed before inducing anesthesia with either of these induction protocols to ensure smooth induction and minimize the effect on IOP.

When a nursing foal needs general anesthesia, the mare should be present during the induction of anesthesia to minimize stress on the foal. Conversely, if the mare is undergoing anesthesia, it is important that the foal be near to facilitate sedation of the mare and ensure a smooth induction. Mask induction for foals may not be an option if the mask rubs or presses on the eyes, and struggling of the patient during induction with a face mask may increase IOP or potentiate eye rupture. Nasotracheal intubation in a conscious foal requires physical restraint and may be accompanied by coughing and gagging, which may increase IOP and further compromise the globe. Appropriate sedation may help calm the foal and decrease the amount of physical restraint that is needed, as well as decrease the potential for additional eye trauma or increases in IOP.

Endotracheal intubation should be accomplished quickly once the horse is in lateral recumbency. Adult horses rarely gag or cough during endotracheal intubation, making a sudden increase in IOP less likely. Movement of equine patients to lateral recumbency after induction should include careful control of the head to prevent additional trauma to the eyes. In addition, lower positioning of the head relative to the body during hoist transport could result in increased IOP and may be responsible for intraocular hemorrhage observed shortly after induction in horses with traumatized eyes [21,22]. Supporting the head to keep it level with the heart during transport is recommended to avoid such an occurrence. The normal eye can be lubricated with eye ointment during hoisting.

Complex ophthalmic procedures such as penetrating keratoplasty in horses may require extended anesthesia time. Partial intravenous anesthesia (PIVA) is a technique that may be implemented to reduce the amount of inhalation agent needed to maintain anesthesia, provide intraoperative analgesia, and minimize the cardiopulmonary depressant effects of inhalation agents. This technique utilizes injectable agents that are administered as single-drug or multi-drug CRIs, thereby permitting reduction of the vaporizer setting over time while still maintaining an adequate plane of anesthesia. Injectable agents commonly utilized for this technique include ketamine, lidocaine, butorphanol, and α_2-adrenergic receptor agonists. Administration of CRIs requires close attention to detail especially when multiple drugs are utilized. The PIVA technique has been associated with better recoveries and fewer attempts to stand in horses [291,292].

Table 67.6 Recommended intravenous (IV) dosages of α_2-adrenergic receptor agonists for recovery of equine ophthalmic patients.

Agent	Dosage
Xylazine	0.2 mg/kg
Detomidine	2 μg/kg
Medetomidine	2 μg/kg
Dexmedetomidine	1 μg/kg
Romifidine	0.01–0.02 mg/kg

Analgesics administered during anesthesia may reduce inhalant requirements and improve recovery as the horse regains consciousness without the stimulus of postoperative pain. Analgesic options in equine ophthalmic patients include NSAIDs, opioids, lidocaine, ketamine, and appropriate nerve blocks. One commonly administered NSAID for horses with ocular inflammation related to the primary disease or because of surgery is flunixin meglumine. It is administered at 1.1 mg/kg IV preoperatively. It is repeated postoperatively using the same dose every 12–24 h, with frequency of administration dependent on the ocular problem. Butorphanol, morphine, hydromorphone, and methadone are opioids available for use in horses. They can be administered as part of the premedication and may be re-dosed postoperatively. Lidocaine CRI has been used for intraoperative pain management in horses. A bolus dose of 2 mg/kg can be administered over 15 min, followed by a CRI of 3 mg/kg/h. The CRI should be discontinued 30 min before recovery to minimize incoordination associated with lidocaine [293]. Infusion of an α_2-adrenergic receptor agonist or ketamine can be used as PIVA to enhance analgesia, and the analgesic effect may extend into the postoperative period. Nerve blockade from local anesthetic injection may provide analgesia both during surgery and postoperatively.

The main goal of recovering anesthetized horses that have undergone an ophthalmic procedure is to have smooth and injury-free recoveries similar to other equine cases. This becomes more important after intraocular procedures or corneal transplants. Recovery efforts should include preventing trauma to the eyes as the horse attempts to stand. Duration of anesthesia should be minimized to decrease the risk of postanesthetic complications as the possibility of rough recoveries is higher in horses with ocular problems [294]. Many suggestions have been made to achieve quiet, predictable, and smooth recoveries in horses but there is not any one single recommendation that will ensure this outcome. Administration of sedatives in recovery has been advocated to improve recovery. α_2-Adrenergic receptor agonists may be administered before the horse is moved to the recovery stall or when the horse reaches the recovery area. The recovery dosages for these drugs are listed in Table 67.6. Note that these dosages are lower than those used for premedication. Acepromazine has also been given with or without the α_2-adrenergic receptor agonist. It should be given intravenously at 0.01–0.02 mg/kg at least 30 min before recovery because of its delayed onset of action compared with the α_2-adrenergic receptor agonists.

As discussed previously, effective analgesia will help improve the quality of recovery, and ideally, should be administered before the horse regains full consciousness. Passing a urinary catheter in the recovery stall to empty the urinary bladder will also help improve recovery quality. Horses that received an NMBA during general anesthesia should be evaluated closely for muscle strength. Return of neuromuscular function as determined by the nerve stimulator does not rule out muscle weakness due to persistent low-level neuromuscular blockade. Horses with muscle weakness that attempt to stand are more prone to limb injuries. Muscle strength can be judged by determining the negative pressure that the horse can generate during inspiration when the connection to the rebreathing bag is occluded. A negative pressure of at least 15 cmH_2O indicates acceptable muscle strength. Conversely, signs of muscle weakness may include muscle fasciculations when the horse attempts to stand, inability to keep its head up, and failure to close its eyelids tightly. When signs of muscle weakness are evident, and the reversal agent was not administered because the nerve stimulator indicated return to normal neuromuscular function, neostigmine should be administered. One way to avoid administering atropine or glycopyrrolate before administering neostigmine is to give it very slowly.

To protect the eye during recovery, a padded hood may be placed on the head, with a halter secured over the hood to keep it in place. However, a hood may not be tolerated by some horses, and may lead to premature attempts to rise. Weak attempts to rise may be controlled by kneeling on the horse's neck and lifting its muzzle up. Additional sedation may prevent horses with active nystagmus from attempting to rise. A head-and-tail rope technique assists horses that are making strong attempts to rise and helps them remain standing in recovery. Ideally, there should be three individuals to execute this recovery technique. Ropes are tied to the tail and to a strong, reliable halter, and then passed through metal rings on the walls of the recovery stall. When the horse makes a strong attempt to rise, the person on the tail will forcefully pull the rope to assist the horse to rise. The person on the head rope will simply guide the head of the horse, rather than pulling forcefully on the rope and disorienting the horse. Once the horse stands, the third person will push the horse against the wall of the recovery stall for support. If this technique is to be used, recovery stalls should be constructed so that there are readily accessible exit routes, and the personnel handling the ropes will be outside the stall to avoid the hazards of an uncoordinated horse attempting to stand. Quiet surroundings and a darkened recovery stall may minimize any stimulus that may excite a horse recovering from anesthesia. When the horse is standing and steady on its feet, a hard cup hood may be placed over the affected eye for additional ocular protection. A higher incidence of colic has been reported in horses with ocular disease [295] and such patients should be observed very closely postoperatively for signs of abdominal pain.

References

1 Prince JH. *Comparative Anatomy of the Eye*. Springfield, IL: Charles C. Thomas, 1956.

2 Meekins JM, Rankin AJ, Samuelson DA. Ophthalmic anatomy. In: Gelatt KN, ed. *Veterinary Ophthalmology*, 6th edn. Hoboken, NJ: Wiley Blackwell, 2021: 41–259.

3 Holmberg B. Ophthalmology of exotic pets. In: Maggs DJ, Miller PE, Ofri R, eds. *Slatter's Fundamentals of Veterinary Ophthalmology*, 4th edn. St. Louis, MO: Elsevier Saunders, 2008: 427–441.

4 Murphy CJ, Samuelson DA, Pollock VH. The eye. In: Evans HE, de Lahunta A, eds. *Miller's Anatomy of the Dog*, 4th edn. St. Louis, MO: Elsevier Saunders, 2013: 746–785.

5 Structure and function of eye. In: Maggs D, Miller P, Ofri R, eds. *Slatter's Fundamentals of Veterinary Ophthalmology*, 4th edn. St. Louis, MO: Elsevier Saunders, 2008.

6 Herrera E, Agudo-Barriuso M, Murcia-Belmonte V. Cranial Pair II: the optic nerves. *Anat Rec (Hoboken)* 2019; **302**(3): 428–445.

7 Shin SY, Kim MJ, Joo J. Oculocardiac reflex and oculorespiratory reflex during strabismus surgery under general anesthesia using the laryngeal mask airway with maintenance of spontaneous respiration: a retrospective study. *J Int Med Res* 2020; **48**(8): 300060520945158.

8 Joffe WS, Gay AJ. The oculorespiratory cardiac reflex in the dog. *Invest Ophthalmol* 1966; **5**(6): 550–554.

9 Reshef ER, Schiff ND, Brown EN. A neurologic examination for anesthesiologists: assessing arousal level during induction, maintenance, and emergence. *Anesthesiology* 2019; **130**(3): 462–471.

10 Crumley WR, Rankin AJ, Allbaugh RA. Evaluation of the aqueous humor flow rate in the eyes of clinically normal cats by use of fluorophotometry. *Am J Vet Res* 2012; **73**(5): 704–708.

11 Hendrix DV, Thomsay SM, Gum GG. Ophthalmic physiology. In: Gelatt KN, ed. *Veterinary Ophthalmology*, 6th edn. Hoboken, NJ: Wiley Blackwell, 2021: 124–155.

12 Barrie KP, Gum GG, Samuelson DA, *et al.* Quantitation of uveoscleral outflow in normotensive and glaucomatous Beagles by 3H-labeled dextran. *Am J Vet Res* 1985; **46**(1): 84–88.

13 Bill A. Uveoscleral drainage of aqueous humor: physiology and pharmacology. *Prog Clin Biol Res* 1989; **312**: 417–427.

14 Samuelson D, Smith P, Brooks D. Morphologic features of the aqueous humor drainage pathways in horses. *Am J Vet Res* 1989; **50**(5): 720–727.

15 Acott TS, Kelley MJ, Keller KE, *et al.* Intraocular pressure homeostasis: maintaining balance in a high-pressure environment. *J Ocul Pharmacol Ther* 2014; **30**(2–3): 94–101.

16 Del Sole MJ, Sande PH, Bernades JM, *et al.* Circadian rhythm of intraocular pressure in cats. *Vet Ophthalmol* 2007; **10**(3): 155–161.

17 Cunningham AJ, Barry P. Intraocular pressure-physiology and implications for anaesthetic management. *Can Anaesth Soc J* 1986; **33**(2): 195–208.

18 Liu JH, Weinreb RN. Posture, intraocular pressure and visual function. *Br J Ophthalmol* 2014; **98**(3): 288–289.

19 Broadwater JJ, Schorling JJ, Herring IP, *et al.* Effect of body position on intraocular pressure in dogs without glaucoma. *Am J Vet Res* 2008; **69**(4): 527–530.

20 Rajaei SM, Asadi F, Rajabian MR, *et al.* Effect of body position, eyelid manipulation, and manual jugular compression on intraocular pressure in clinically normal cats. *Vet Ophthalmol* 2018; **21**(2): 140–143.

21 Alling CR, Cremer J, Liu CC, *et al.* Effect of multiple head positions on intraocular pressure in healthy, anesthetized horses during hoisting. *Vet Ophthalmol* 2021; **24**(1): 71–79.

22 Monk CS, Brooks DE, Granone T, *et al.* Measurement of intraocular pressure in healthy anesthetized horses during hoisting. *Vet Anaesth Analg* 2017; **44**(3): 502–508.

23 Meekins JM, McMurphy RM, Roush JK. The effect of body position on intraocular pressure in anesthetized horses. *Vet Ophthalmol* 2020; **23**(4): 668–673.

24 Komaromy AM, Garg CD, Ying GS, *et al.* Effect of head position on intraocular pressure in horses. *Am J Vet Res* 2006; **67**(7): 1232–1235.

25 Kelly DJ, Farrell SM. Physiology and role of intraocular pressure in contemporary anesthesia. *Anesth Analg* 2018; **126**(5): 1551–1562.

26 Kahane N, Raskansky H, Bdolah-Abram T, *et al.* The effects of topical parasympatholytic drugs on pupil diameter and intraocular pressure in healthy dogs treated with 0.005% latanoprost. *Vet Ophthalmol* 2016; **19**(6): 464–472.

27 Keller CB. Bilateral extraction of cataracts in a crow. *Can Vet J* 1992; **33**(4): 273–274.

28 Powell CC, Martin CL. Distribution of cholinergic and adrenergic nerve fibers in the lacrimal glands of dogs. *Am J Vet Res* 1989; **50**(12): 2084–2088.

29 Krupin T, Cross DA, Becker B. Decreased basal tear production associated with general anesthesia. *Arch Ophthalmol* 1977; **95**(1): 107–108.

30 Vestre WA, Brightman AH II, Helper LC, *et al.* Decreased tear production associated with general anesthesia in the dog. *J Am Vet Med Assoc* 1979; **174**(9): 1006–1007.

31 Shepard MK, Accola PJ, Lopez LA, *et al.* Effect of duration and type of anesthetic on tear production in dogs. *Am J Vet Res* 2011; **72**(5): 608–612.

32 Herring IP, Pickett JP, Champagne ES, *et al.* Evaluation of aqueous tear production in dogs following general anesthesia. *J Am Anim Hosp Assoc* 2000; **36**(5): 427–430.

33 Peche N, Kostlin R, Reese S, *et al.* Postanaesthetic tear production and ocular irritation in cats. *Tierarztl Prax Ausg K Kleintiere Heimtiere* 2015; **43**(2): 75–82.

34 Brightman AH II, Manning JP, Benson GJ, *et al.* Decreased tear production associated with general anesthesia in the horse. *J Am Vet Med Assoc* 1983; **182**(3): 243–244.

35 Berger SL, King VL. The fluctuation of tear production in the dog. *J Am Anim Hosp Assoc* 1998; **34**(1): 79–83.

36 da Silva EG, Sandmeyer LS, Gionfriddo JR, *et al.* Tear production in canine neonates-evaluation using a modified Schirmer tear test. *Vet Ophthalmol* 2013; **16**(3): 175–179.

37 Gaudana R, Ananthula HK, Parenky A, *et al.* Ocular drug delivery. *AAPS J* 2010; **12**(3): 348–360.

38 Arnold RW. The oculocardiac reflex: a review. *Clin Ophthalmol* 2021; **15**: 2693–2725.
39 Karaman T, Demir S, Dogru S, *et al.* The effect of anesthesia depth on the oculocardiac reflex in strabismus surgery. *J Clin Monit Comput* 2016; **30**(6): 889–893.
40 Turner Giannico A, de Sampaio MO, Lima L, *et al.* Characterization of the oculocardiac reflex during compression of the globe in Beagle dogs and rabbits. *Vet Ophthalmol* 2014; **17**(5): 321–327.
41 Panneton WM, Burton H. Projections from the paratrigeminal nucleus and the medullary and spinal dorsal horns to the peribrachial area in the cat. *Neuroscience* 1985; **15**(3): 779–797.
42 Short CE, Rebhun WC. Complications caused by the oculocardiac reflex during anesthesia in a foal. *J Am Vet Med Assoc* 1980; **176**(7): 630–631.
43 Miller PE, Paul-Murphy J, Sullivan R, *et al.* Orbital lymphosarcoma associated with reticuloendotheliosis virus in a peafowl. *J Am Vet Med Assoc* 1998; **213**(3): 377–380.
44 Kil HK. Hypercapnea is an important adjuvant factor of oculocardiac reflex during strabismus surgery. *Anesth Analg* 2000; **91**(4): 1044.
45 Arnold RW, Jensen PA, Kovtoun TA, *et al.* The profound augmentation of the oculocardiac reflex by fast acting opioids. *Binocul Vis Strabismus Q* 2004; **19**(4): 215–222.
46 Sinha R, Kumar KR. Intravenous dexmedetomidine augments the oculocardiac reflex. *J AAPOS* 2019; **23**(1): 62.
47 Basagaoglu B, Steinberg A, Tung IT, *et al.* Oculocardiac reflex as a late presentation of orbital floor fracture. *J Craniofac Surg* 2018; **29**(7): e720–e722.
48 van den Berg AA, Lambourne A, Clyburn PA. The oculo-emetic reflex. A rationalisation of postophthalmic anaesthesia vomiting. *Anaesthesia* 1989; **44**(2): 110–117.
49 Tobin JR, Weaver G. Ophthalmology. In: Coté CJ, Lerman J, Anderson BJ, eds. *A Practice of Anesthesia for Infants and Children*, 6th edn. Philadelphia, PA: Elsevier, 2019: 790–803.
50 Vezina-Audette R, Steagall PVM, Gianotti G. Prevalence of and covariates associated with the oculocardiac reflex occurring in dogs during enucleation. *J Am Vet Med Assoc* 2019; **255**(4): 454–458.
51 Oel C, Gerhards H, Gehlen H. Effect of retrobulbar nerve block on heart rate variability during enucleation in horses under general anesthesia. *Vet Ophthalmol* 2014; **17**(3): 170–174.
52 Karanovic N, Jukic M, Carev M, *et al.* Rocuronium attenuates oculocardiac reflex during squint surgery in children anesthetized with halothane and nitrous oxide. *Acta Anaesthesiol Scand* 2004; **48**(10): 1301–1305.
53 Agrahari V, Mandal A, Agrahari V, *et al.* A comprehensive insight on ocular pharmacokinetics. *Drug Deliv Transl Res* 2016; **6**(6): 735–754.
54 Rubin LF, Wolfes RL. Mydriatics for canine ophthalmoscopy. *J Am Vet Med Assoc* 1962; **140**: 137–141.
55 Gelatt KN, Boggess TS, Cure TH. Evaluation of mydriatics in the cat. *J Am Anim Hosp Assoc* 1973; **9**: 283–287.
56 Strom L, Dalin F, Domberg M, *et al.* Topical ophthalmic atropine in horses, pharmacokinetics and effect on intestinal motility. *BMC Vet Res* 2021; **17**(1): 149.
57 Williams MM, Spiess BM, Pascoe PJ, *et al.* Systemic effects of topical and subconjunctival ophthalmic atropine in the horse. *Vet Ophthalmol* 2000; **3**(2–3): 193–199.
58 Herring IP, Jacobson JD, Pickett JP. Cardiovascular effects of topical ophthalmic 10% phenylephrine in dogs. *Vet Ophthalmol* 2004; **7**(1): 41–46.
59 Pascoe PJ, Ilkiw JE, Stiles J, *et al.* Arterial hypertension associated with topical ocular use of phenylephrine in dogs. *J Am Vet Med Assoc* 1994; **205**(11): 1562–1564.
60 Franci P, Leece EA, McConnell JF. Arrhythmias and transient changes in cardiac function after topical administration of one drop of phenylephrine 10% in an adult cat undergoing conjunctival graft. *Vet Anaesth Analg* 2011; **38**(3): 208–212.
61 Lansche RK. Systemic reactions to topical epinephrine and phenylephrine. *Am J Ophthalmol* 1966; **61**(1): 95–98.
62 Wegg ML. A retrospective evaluation of systemic and/or topical pilocarpine treatment for canine neurogenic dry eye: 11 cases. *Vet Ophthalmol* 2020; **23**(2): 341–346.
63 Gum GG, Gelatt KN, Gelatt JK, *et al.* Effect of topically applied demecarium bromide and echothiophate iodide on intraocular pressure and pupil size in Beagles with normotensive eyes and Beagles with inherited glaucoma. *Am J Vet Res* 1993; **54**(2): 287–293.
64 Humphreys JA, Holmes JH. Systemic effects produced by echothiophate iodide in treatment of glaucoma. *Arch Ophthalmol* 1963; **69**: 737–743.
65 Miller PE, Nelson MJ, Rhaesa SL. Effects of topical administration of 0.5% apraclonidine on intraocular pressure, pupil size, and heart rate in clinically normal dogs. *Am J Vet Res* 1996; **57**(1): 79–82.
66 Miller PE, Rhaesa SL. Effects of topical administration of 0.5% apraclonidine on intraocular pressure, pupil size, and heart rate in clinically normal cats. *Am J Vet Res* 1996; **57**(1): 83–86.
67 Welch SL, Richardson JA. Clinical effects of brimonidine ophthalmic drops ingestion in 52 dogs. *Vet Hum Toxicol* 2002; **44**(1): 34–35.
68 Ogata N, Kanda T, Kawahata M, *et al.* Sedative and physiological effects of brimonidine tartrate ophthalmic solution in healthy cats. *Vet Anaesth Analg* 2017; **44**(5): 1091–1100.
69 Smith LN, Miller PE, Felchle LM. Effects of topical administration of latanoprost, timolol, or a combination of latanoprost and timolol on intraocular pressure, pupil size, and heart rate in clinically normal dogs. *Am J Vet Res* 2010; **71**(9): 1055–1061.
70 Slenter IJM, Djajadiningrat-Laanen SC, Elders DJ, *et al.* The effects of topical dorzolamide 2% and brinzolamide 1%, either alone or combined with timolol 0.5%, on intraocular pressure, pupil diameter, and heart rate in healthy cats. *Vet Ophthalmol* 2020; **23**(1): 16–24.
71 Hepsen IF, Yildirim Z, Yilmaz H, *et al.* Preventive effect of lacrimal occlusion on topical timolol-induced bronchoconstriction in asthmatics. *Clin Exp Ophthalmol* 2004; **32**(6): 597–602.
72 Linkewich JA, Herling IM. Bradycardia and congestive heart failure associated with ocular timolol maleate. *Am J Hosp Pharm* 1981; **38**(5): 699–701.
73 Scardillo A, Pugliese M, De Majo M, *et al.* Effects of topical 0.5% levobunolol alone or in association with 2% dorzolamide compared with a fixed combination of 0.5% timolol and 2% dorzolamide on intraocular pressure and heart rate in dogs without glaucoma. *Vet Ther* 2010; **11**(3): E1–E6.
74 Haskins SC, Munger RJ, Helphrey MG, *et al.* Effect of acetazolamide in blood acid-base and electrolyte values in dogs. *J Am Vet Med Assoc* 1981; **179**(8): 792–796.
75 Thiessen CE, Tofflemire KL, Makielski KM, *et al.* Hypokalemia and suspected renal tubular acidosis associated with topical carbonic anhydrase inhibitor therapy in a cat. *J Vet Emerg Crit Care (San Antonio)* 2016; **26**(6): 870–874.
76 Dugan SJ, Roberts SM, Severin GA. Systemic osmotherapy for ophthalmic disease in dogs and cats. *J Am Vet Med Assoc* 1989; **194**(1): 115–118.
77 Brock KA, Thurmon JC. Pulmonary edema associated with mannitol administration. *Canine Pract* 1979; **6**: 31–34.
78 Wasserman NT, Kennard G, Cochrane ZN, *et al.* Effects of oral isosorbide and glycerol on intraocular pressure, serum osmolality, and blood glucose in normal dogs. *Vet Ophthalmol* 2013; **16**(1): 20–24.
79 Volopich S, Mosing M, Auer U, *et al.* Comparison of the effect of hypertonic hydroxyethyl starch and mannitol on the intraocular pressure in healthy normotensive dogs and the effect of hypertonic hydroxyethyl starch on the intraocular pressure in dogs with primary glaucoma. *Vet Ophthalmol* 2006; **9**(4): 239–244.
80 Glaze MB, Crawford MA, Nachreiner RF, *et al.* Ophthalmic corticosteroid therapy: systemic effects in the dog. *J Am Vet Med Assoc* 1988; **192**(1): 73–75.
81 Rice JB, White AG, Scarpati LM, *et al.* Long-term systemic corticosteroid exposure: a systematic literature review. *Clin Ther* 2017; **39**(11): 2216–2229.
82 Micieli F, Chiavaccini L, Lamagna B, *et al.* Comparison of intraocular pressure and pupil diameter after sedation with either acepromazine or dexmedetomidine in healthy dogs. *Vet Anaesth Analg* 2018; **45**(5): 667–672.
83 Stephan DD, Vestre WA, Stiles J, *et al.* Changes in intraocular pressure and pupil size following intramuscular administration of hydromorphone hydrochloride and acepromazine in clinically normal dogs. *Vet Ophthalmol* 2003; **6**(1): 73–76.
84 Volk HA, West E, Linn-Pearl RN, *et al.* Effect of methadone and acepromazine premedication on tear production in dogs. *Vet Rec Open* 2018; **5**(1): e000298.
85 Giannetto C, Macri F, Falcone A, *et al.* Evaluation of tear production as measured by Schirmer test I in dogs after acepromazine and acepromazine-methadone premedication. *Animals (Basel)* 2021; **11**(11): 3015.
86 Ghaffari MS, Moghaddassi AP, Bokaie S. Effects of intramuscular acepromazine and diazepam on tear production in rabbits. *Vet Rec* 2009; **164**(5): 147–148.
87 Ghaffari MS, Malmasi A, Bokaie S. Effect of acepromazine or xylazine on tear production as measured by Schirmer tear test in normal cats. *Vet Ophthalmol* 2010; **13**(1): 1–3.
88 McClure JR Jr., Gelatt KN, Gum GG, *et al.* The effect of parenteral acepromazine and xylazine on intraocular pressure in the horse. *Vet Med Small Anim Clin* 1976; **71**(12): 1727–1730.
89 Artru AA. Intraocular pressure in anaesthetized dogs given flumazenil with and without prior administration of midazolam. *Can J Anaesth* 1991; **38**(3): 408–414.
90 Hofmeister EH, Mosunic CB, Torres BT, *et al.* Effects of ketamine, diazepam, and their combination on intraocular pressures in clinically normal dogs. *Am J Vet Res* 2006; **67**(7): 1136–1139.
91 Pino Capote JA. Decrease in intraocular pressure produced by I.V. or conjunctival diazepam. *Br J Anaesth* 1978; **50**(8): 865.
92 Ghaffari MS, Rezaei MA, Mirani AH, *et al.* The effects of ketamine-midazolam anesthesia on intraocular pressure in clinically normal dogs. *Vet Ophthalmol* 2010; **13**(2): 91–93.
93 Kovalcuka L, Birgele E, Bandere D, *et al.* The effects of ketamine hydrochloride and diazepam on the intraocular pressure and pupil diameter of the dog's eye. *Vet Ophthalmol* 2013; **16**(1): 29–34.
94 Smith MD, Barletta M, Diehl KA, *et al.* Effect of propofol and ketamine–diazepam on intraocular pressure in healthy premedicated dogs. *Vet Anaesth Analg* 2019; **46**(1): 36–42.

95 Keating SC, Sage AM, Ambrisko TD, *et al.* The effect of midazolam or lidocaine administration prior to etomidate induction of anesthesia on heart rate, arterial pressure, intraocular pressure and serum cortisol concentration in healthy dogs. *Vet Anaesth Analg* 2020; **47**(2): 160–167.

96 Hofmeister EH, Williams CO, Braun C, *et al.* Influence of lidocaine and diazepam on peri-induction intraocular pressures in dogs anesthetized with propofol–atracurium. *Can J Vet Res* 2006; **70**(4): 251–256.

97 Jang M, Park S, Son WG, *et al.* Effect of tiletamine–zolazepam on the intraocular pressure of the dog. *Vet Ophthalmol* 2015; **18**(6): 481–484.

98 Yanmaz LE, Dogan E, Okur S, *et al.* Comparison of the effects of intranasal and intramuscular administrations of zolazepam-tiletamine combination on intraocular pressure in cats. *Vet Ophthalmol* 2016; **19**(Suppl 1): 115–118.

99 Hahnenberger RW. Influence of various anesthetic drugs on the intraocular pressure of cats. *Albrecht Von Graefes Arch Klin Exp Ophthalmol* 1976; **199**(2): 179–186.

100 Raposo AC, Ofri R, Schaffer DP, *et al.* Evaluation of ophthalmic and hemodynamic parameters in capuchin monkeys (Sapajus sp.) submitted to dissociative anesthetic protocols. *J Med Primatol* 2015; **44**(6): 381–389.

101 Hsu WH, Betts DM, Lee P. Xylazine-induced mydriasis: possible involvement of a central postsynaptic regulation of parasympathetic tone. *J Vet Pharmacol Ther* 1981; **4**(3): 209–214.

102 Burke JA, Potter DE. The ocular effects of xylazine in rabbits, cats, and monkeys. *J Ocul Pharmacol* 1986; **2**(1): 9–21.

103 Kanda T, Iguchi A, Yoshioka C, *et al.* Effects of medetomidine and xylazine on intraocular pressure and pupil size in healthy Beagle dogs. *Vet Anaesth Analg* 2015; **42**(6): 623–628.

104 Chae JJ, Prausnitz MR, Ethier CR. Effects of general anesthesia on intraocular pressure in rabbits. *J Am Assoc Lab Anim Sci* 2021; **60**(1): 91–95.

105 Joyner RL, Liu CC, Cremer J, *et al.* Intraocular pressure following four different intravenous sedation protocols in normal horses. *Equine Vet J* 2021; **53**(3): 612–617.

106 van der Woerdt A, Gilger BC, Wilkie DA, *et al.* Effect of auriculopalpebral nerve block and intravenous administration of xylazine on intraocular pressure and corneal thickness in horses. *Am J Vet Res* 1995; **56**(2): 155–158.

107 Calderone L, Grimes P, Shalev M. Acute reversible cataract induced by xylazine and by ketamine–xylazine anesthesia in rats and mice. *Exp Eye Res* 1986; **42**(4): 331–337.

108 Kanda T, Shimizu Y, Hanazono C, *et al.* Effect of intramuscular administration of medetomidine and xylazine on tear flow measured by the Schirmer tear test I in healthy cats. *J Feline Med Surg* 2019; **21**(8): 788–792.

109 Kanda T, Ishihara S, Oka M, *et al.* Temporal effects of intramuscular administration of medetomidine hydrochloride or xylazine hydrochloride to healthy dogs on tear flow measured by use of a Schirmer tear test I. *Am J Vet Res* 2016; **77**(4): 346–350.

110 Dodam JR, Branson KR, Martin DD. Effects of intramuscular sedative and opioid combinations on tear production in dogs. *Vet Ophthalmol* 1998; **1**(1): 57–59.

111 Jin Y, Wilson S, Elko EE, *et al.* Ocular hypotensive effects of medetomidine and its analogs. *J Ocul Pharmacol* 1991; **7**(4): 285–296.

112 Verbruggen AM, Akkerdaas LC, Hellebrekers LJ, *et al.* The effect of intravenous medetomidine on pupil size and intraocular pressure in normotensive dogs. *Vet Q* 2000; **22**(3): 179–180.

113 Malmasi A, Selk Ghaffari M. Lack of effects of intramuscular medetomidine on intraocular pressure in clinically normal cats. *J Feline Med Surg* 2016; **18**(4): 315–317.

114 Rauser P, Pfeifr J, Proks P, *et al.* Effect of medetomidine–butorphanol and dexmedetomidine–butorphanol combinations on intraocular pressure in healthy dogs. *Vet Anaesth Analg* 2012; **39**(3): 301–305.

115 Sanchez RF, Mellor D, Mould J. Effects of medetomidine and medetomidine–butorphanol combination on Schirmer tear test 1 readings in dogs. *Vet Ophthalmol* 2006; **9**(1): 33–37.

116 Aghababaei A, Ronagh A, Mosallanejad B, *et al.* Effects of medetomidine, dexmedetomidine and their combination with acepromazine on the intraocular pressure (IOP), tear secretion and pupil diameter in dogs. *Vet Med Sci* 2021; **7**(4): 1090–1095.

117 Di Pietro S, Macri F, Bonarrigo T, *et al.* Effects of a medetomidine-ketamine combination on Schirmer tear test I results of clinically normal cats. *Am J Vet Res* 2016; **77**(3): 310–314.

118 Kanda T, Kajiyama A, Morimitsu W, *et al.* Effect of medetomidine on tear flow measured by Schirmer tear test I in normal pigs. *J Vet Med Sci* 2019; **81**(4): 538–540.

119 Milnes EL, Calvi T, Feltrer Y, *et al.* Factors affecting tear production and intraocular pressure in anesthetized chimpanzees (*Pan troglodytes*). *J Zoo Wildl Med* 2020; **51**(3): 687–690.

120 Holve DL. Effect of sedation with detomidine on intraocular pressure with and without topical anesthesia in clinically normal horses. *J Am Vet Med Assoc* 2012; **240**(3): 308–311.

121 Stine JM, Michau TM, Williams MK, *et al.* The effects of intravenous romifidine on intraocular pressure in clinically normal horses and horses with incidental ophthalmic findings. *Vet Ophthalmol* 2014; **17**(Suppl 1): 134–139.

122 Marzok MA, El-Khodery SA, Oheida AH. Effect of intravenous administration of romifidine on intraocular pressure in clinically normal horses. *Vet Ophthalmol* 2014; **17**(Suppl 1): 149–153.

123 Rizk A, Nocera I, Briganti A, *et al.* Dose-dependent effect of romifidine on intraocular pressure in clinically healthy buffalo (*Bubalus bubalis*). *Heliyon* 2019; **5**(12): e02930.

124 Artigas C, Redondo JI, Lopez-Murcia MM. Effects of intravenous administration of dexmedetomidine on intraocular pressure and pupil size in clinically normal dogs. *Vet Ophthalmol* 2012; **15**(Suppl 1): 79–82.

125 Leonardi F, Costa GL, Stagnoli A, *et al.* The effect of intramuscular dexmedetomidine–butorphanol combination on tear production in dogs. *Can Vet J* 2019; **60**(1): 55–59.

126 Horvath G, Kovacs M, Szikszay M, *et al.* Mydriatic and antinociceptive effects of intrathecal dexmedetomidine in conscious rats. *Eur J Pharmacol* 1994; **253**(1–2): 61–66.

127 Mattos-Junior E, Pypendop BH, Cabrini TM, *et al.* Effects of dexmedetomidine alone or in combination with opioids on intraocular pressure in healthy Beagle dogs. *Vet Anaesth Analg* 2021; **48**(4): 541–544.

128 Vartiainen J, MacDonald E, Urtti A, *et al.* Dexmedetomidine-induced ocular hypotension in rabbits with normal or elevated intraocular pressures. *Invest Ophthalmol Vis Sci* 1992; **33**(6): 2019–2023.

129 Eakins KE. A comparative study of intraocular pressure and gross outflow facility in the cat eye during anesthesia. *Exp Eye Res* 1969; **8**(2): 106–115.

130 Hofmeister EH, Williams CO, Braun C, *et al.* Propofol versus thiopental: effects on peri-induction intraocular pressures in normal dogs. *Vet Anaesth Analg* 2008; **35**(4): 275–281.

131 Ferreira TH, Brosnan RJ, Shilo-Benjamini Y, *et al.* Effects of ketamine, propofol, or thiopental administration on intraocular pressure and qualities of induction of and recovery from anesthesia in horses. *Am J Vet Res* 2013; **74**(8): 1070–1077.

132 Joshi C, Bruce DL. Thiopental and succinylcholine: action on intraocular pressure. *Anesth Analg* 1975; **54**(4): 471–475.

133 Chang CY, Chien YJ, Wu MY. Attenuation of increased intraocular pressure with propofol anesthesia: a systematic review with meta-analysis and trial sequential analysis. *J Adv Res* 2020; **24**: 223–238.

134 Batista CM, Laus JL, Nunes N, *et al.* Evaluation of intraocular and partial CO2 pressure in dogs anesthetized with propofol. *Vet Ophthalmol* 2000; **3**(1): 17–19.

135 Hasiuk MM, Forde N, Cooke A, *et al.* A comparison of alfaxalone and propofol on intraocular pressure in healthy dogs. *Vet Ophthalmol* 2014; **17**(6): 411–416.

136 Hofmeister EH, Weinstein WL, Burger D, *et al.* Effects of graded doses of propofol for anesthesia induction on cardiovascular parameters and intraocular pressures in normal dogs. *Vet Anaesth Analg* 2009; **36**(5): 442–448.

137 Webb TR, Wyman M, Smith JA, *et al.* Effects of propofol on intraocular pressure in premedicated and nonpremedicated dogs with and without glaucoma. *J Am Vet Med Assoc* 2018; **252**(7): 823–829.

138 Costa D, Leiva M, Moll X, *et al.* Alfaxalone versus propofol in dogs: a randomised trial to assess effects on peri-induction tear production, intraocular pressure and globe position. *Vet Rec* 2015; **176**(3): 73.

139 Torres MD, Andaluz A, Garcia F, *et al.* Effects of an intravenous bolus of alfaxalone versus propofol on intraocular pressure in sheep. *Vet Rec* 2012; **170**(9): 226.

140 Ghaffari MS, Moghaddassi AP. Effects of ketamine–diazepam and ketamine–acepromazine combinations on intraocular pressure in rabbits. *Vet Anaesth Analg* 2010; **37**(3): 269–272.

141 Hazra S, De D, Roy B, *et al.* Use of ketamine, xylazine, and diazepam anesthesia with retrobulbar block for phacoemulsification in dogs. *Vet Ophthalmol* 2008; **11**(4): 255–259.

142 Holve DL, Gum GG, Pritt SL. Effect of sedation with xylazine and ketamine on intraocular pressure in New Zealand white rabbits. *J Am Assoc Lab Anim Sci* 2013; **52**(4): 488–490.

143 Lee HS, Kim DH, Kim SH, *et al.* A comparative study on intraocular pressure under various anesthetics in cynomolgus monkeys (*Macaca fascicularis*). *Lab Anim Res* 2021; **37**(1): 15.

144 Bunch TJ, Tian B, Seeman JL, *et al.* Effect of daily prolonged ketamine anesthesia on intraocular pressure in monkeys. *Curr Eye Res* 2008; **33**(11): 946–953.

145 Gatson BJ, Pablo L, Plummer CE, *et al.* Effects of premedication with sustained-release buprenorphine hydrochloride and anesthetic induction with ketamine hydrochloride or propofol in combination with diazepam on intraocular pressure in healthy sheep. *Am J Vet Res* 2015; **76**(9): 771–779.

146 Thomson MF, Brock-Utne JG, Bean P, *et al.* Anaesthesia and intra-ocular pressure: a comparative of total intravenous anaesthesia using etomidate with conventional inhalation anaesthesia. *Anaesthesia* 1982; **37**(7): 758–761.

147 Oji EO, Holdcroft A. The ocular effects of etomidate. *Anaesthesia* 1979; **34**(3): 245–249.
148 Famewo CE, Odugbesan CO, Osuntokun OO. Effect of etomidate on intra-ocular pressure. *Can Anaesth Soc J* 1977; **24**(6): 712–716.
149 Gunderson EG, Lukasik VM, Ashton MM, *et al.* Effects of anesthetic induction with midazolam-propofol and midazolam-etomidate on selected ocular and cardiorespiratory variables in clinically normal dogs. *Am J Vet Res* 2013; **74**(4): 629–635.
150 Tammisto T, Hamalainen L, Tarkkanen L. Halothane and methoxyflurane in ophthalmic anaesthesia. *A comparative study. Acta Anaesthesiol Scand* 1965; **9**(3): 173–177.
151 van den Berg AA, Honjol NM, Mphanza T, *et al.* Vomiting, retching, headache and restlessness after halothane-, isoflurane- and enflurane-based anaesthesia. An analysis of pooled data following ear, nose, throat and eye surgery. *Acta Anaesthesiol Scand* 1998; **42**(6): 658–663.
152 Craig JF, Cook JH. A comparison of isoflurane and halothane in anaesthesia for intra-ocular surgery. *Anaesthesia* 1988; **43**(6): 454–458.
153 Mirakhur RK, Elliott P, Shepherd WF, *et al.* Comparison of the effects of isoflurane and halothane on intraocular pressure. *Acta Anaesthesiol Scand* 1990; **34**(4): 282–285.
154 Park JT, Lim HK, Jang KY, *et al.* The effects of desflurane and sevoflurane on the intraocular pressure associated with endotracheal intubation in pediatric ophthalmic surgery. *Korean J Anesthesiol* 2013; **64**(2): 117–121.
155 Sator S, Wildling E, Schabernig C, *et al.* Desflurane maintains intraocular pressure at an equivalent level to isoflurane and propofol during unstressed non-ophthalmic surgery. *Br J Anaesth* 1998; **80**(2): 243–244.
156 Artru AA, Momota Y. Trabecular outflow facility and formation rate of aqueous humor during anesthesia with sevoflurane-nitrous oxide or sevoflurane-remifentanil in rabbits. *Anesth Analg* 1999; **88**(4): 781–786.
157 Krupin T, Feitl M, Roshe R, *et al.* Halothane anesthesia and aqueous humor dynamics in laboratory animals. *Invest Ophthalmol Vis Sci* 1980; **19**(5): 518–521.
158 Cullen LK, Steffey EP, Bailey CS, *et al.* Effect of high PaCO2 and time on cerebrospinal fluid and intraocular pressure in halothane-anesthetized horses. *Am J Vet Res* 1990; **51**(2): 300–304.
159 Almeida DE, Rezende ML, Nunes N, *et al.* Evaluation of intraocular pressure in association with cardiovascular parameters in normocapnic dogs anesthetized with sevoflurane and desflurane. *Vet Ophthalmol* 2004; **7**(4): 265–269.
160 Buehner E, Pietsch UC, Bringmann A, *et al.* Effects of propofol and isoflurane anesthesia on the intraocular pressure and hemodynamics of pigs. *Ophthalmic Res* 2011; **45**(1): 42–46.
161 Tsuchiya S, Higashide T, Hatake S, *et al.* Effect of inhalation anesthesia with isoflurane on circadian rhythm of murine intraocular pressure. *Exp Eye Res* 2021; **203**: 108420.
162 Ding C, Wang P, Tian N. Effect of general anesthetics on IOP in elevated IOP mouse model. *Exp Eye Res* 2011; **92**(6): 512–520.
163 Almeida DE, Nishimori CT, Oria AP, *et al.* Effects of nitrous oxide on IOP and pupillary diameter in dogs anesthetized with varying concentrations of desflurane. *Vet Ophthalmol* 2008; **11**(3): 170–176.
164 Mouney MC, Accola PJ, Cremer J, *et al.* Effects of acepromazine maleate or morphine on tear production before, during, and after sevoflurane anesthesia in dogs. *Am J Vet Res* 2011; **72**(11): 1427–1430.
165 Mayordomo-Febrer A, Rubio M, Martinez-Gassent M, *et al.* Effects of morphine-alfaxalone-midazolam premedication, alfaxalone induction and sevoflurane maintenance on intraocular pressure and tear production in dogs. *Vet Rec* 2017; **180**(19): 474.
166 Young SS, Barnett K, Taylor PM. Anaesthetic regimes for cataract removal in the dog. *J Small Anim Pract* 1991; **32**: 236–241.
167 Nasisse MP. Principles of microsurgery. *Vet Clin North Am Small Anim Pract* 1997; **27**(5): 987–1010.
168 Wilkie DA, Whittaker C. Surgery of the cornea. *Vet Clin North Am Small Anim Pract* 1997; **27**(5): 1067–1107.
169 Jones RS, Auer U, Mosing M. Reversal of neuromuscular block in companion animals. *Vet Anaesth Analg* 2015; **42**(5): 455–471.
170 Jantzen JP, Earnshaw G, Hackett GH, *et al.* Comparative study of the effect of muscle relaxants on the intraocular pressure. *Anaesthesist* 1987; **36**(5): 223–227.
171 McMurphy RM, Davidson HJ, Hodgson DS. Effects of atracurium on intraocular pressure, eye position, and blood pressure in eucapnic and hypocapnic isoflurane-anesthetized dogs. *Am J Vet Res* 2004; **65**(2): 179–182.
172 Scherrer NM, Hopster K. Neuromuscular blockade with atracurium for ophthalmic surgery in horses-Effects on surgical and anesthetic characteristics and recovery quality. *Vet Ophthalmol* 2021; **24**(5): 442–446.
173 Hopster K, Ohnesorge B, von Borstel M, *et al.* Influence of atracurium on cardiovascular parameters in horses undergoing vitrectomy during general anaesthesia, and on recovery duration and quality. *Tierarztl Prax Ausg G Grosstiere Nutztiere* 2013; **41**(6): 371–377.
174 Briganti A, Barsotti G, Portela DA, *et al.* Effects of rocuronium bromide on globe position and respiratory function in isoflurane-anesthetized dogs: a comparison between three different dosages. *Vet Ophthalmol* 2015; **18**(2): 89–94.
175 Auer U, Mosing M, Moens YP. The effect of low dose rocuronium on globe position, muscle relaxation and ventilation in dogs: a clinical study. *Vet Ophthalmol* 2007; **10**(5): 295–298.
176 Auer U, Moens Y. Neuromuscular blockade with rocuronium bromide for ophthalmic surgery in horses. *Vet Ophthalmol* 2011; **14**(4): 244–247.
177 Collins CC, Bach-y-Rita P. Succinylcholine, ocular pressure, and extraocular muscle tension in cats and rabbits. *J Appl Physiol* 1972; **33**(6): 788–791.
178 Chiu CL, Jaais F, Wang CY. Effect of rocuronium compared with succinylcholine on intraocular pressure during rapid sequence induction of anaesthesia. *Br J Anaesth* 1999; **82**(5): 757–760.
179 Katz RL, Eakins KE. Mode of action of succinylcholine on intraocular pressure. *J Pharmacol Exp Ther* 1968; **162**(1): 1–9.
180 Wretlind A, Wahlin A. The effect of succinylcholine on the orbital musculature of the cat. *Acta Anaesthesiol Scand* 1959; **3**: 101–110.
181 Bach-y-Rita P, Collins C, Tengroth B. Effect of succinylcholine on length and refraction of eyes. *Proc West Pharmacol Soc* 1968; **11**: 21–22.
182 Verschueren CP, Lumeij JT. Mydriasis in pigeons (*Columbia livia domestica*) with d-tubocurarine: topical instillation versus intracameral injection. *J Vet Pharmacol Ther* 1991; **14**(2): 206–208.
183 Barsotti G, Briganti A, Spratte JR, *et al.* Mydriatic effect of topically applied rocuronium bromide in tawny owls (*Strix aluco*): comparison between two protocols. *Vet Ophthalmol* 2010; **13**(Suppl): 9–13.
184 Mikaelian I, Paillet I, Williams D. Comparative use of various mydriatic drugs in kestrels (*Falco tinnunculus*). *Am J Vet Res* 1994; **55**(2): 270–272.
185 Upadhyay A, Beuerman RW. Biological mechanisms of atropine control of myopia. *Eye Contact Lens* 2020; **46**(3): 129–135.
186 Garcia Del Valle I, Alvarez-Lorenzo C. Atropine in topical formulations for the management of anterior and posterior segment ocular diseases. *Expert Opin Drug Deliv* 2021; **18**(9): 1245–1260.
187 Kovalcuka L, Birgele E, Bandere D, *et al.* Comparison of the effects of topical and systemic atropine sulfate on intraocular pressure and pupil diameter in the normal canine eye. *Vet Ophthalmol* 2015; **18**(1): 43–49.
188 Cozanitis DA, Dundee JW, Buchanan TA, *et al.* Atropine versus glycopyrrolate. A study of intraocular pressure and pupil size in man. *Anaesthesia* 1979; **34**(3): 236–238.
189 Varssano D, Rothman S, Haas K, *et al.* The mydriatic effect of topical glycopyrrolate. *Graefes Arch Clin Exp Ophthalmol* 1996; **234**(3): 205–207.
190 Gelatt KN, Gum GG, MacKay EO. Evaluation of mydriatics in horses. *Vet Compar Ophthalmol* 1995; **5**(2): 104–108.
191 Stadtbaumer K, Frommlet F, Nell B. Effects of mydriatics on intraocular pressure and pupil size in the normal feline eye. *Vet Ophthalmol* 2006; **9**(4): 233–237.
192 Mughannam AJ, Buyukmihci NC, Kass PH. Effect of topical atropine on intraocular pressure and pupil diameter in the normal horse eye. *Vet Ophthalmol* 1999; **2**(4): 213–215.
193 Herring IP, Pickett JP, Champagne ES, *et al.* Effect of topical 1% atropine sulfate on intraocular pressure in normal horses. *Vet Ophthalmol* 2000; **3**(2–3): 139–143.
194 Davis JL, Stewart T, Brazik E, *et al.* The effect of topical administration of atropine sulfate on the normal equine pupil: influence of age, breed and gender. *Vet Ophthalmol* 2003; **6**(4): 329–332.
195 Arnett BD, Brightman AH II, Musselman EE. Effect of atropine sulfate on tear production in the cat when used with ketamine hydrochloride and acetylpromazine maleate. *J Am Vet Med Assoc* 1984; **185**(2): 214–215.
196 Hollingsworth SR, Canton DD, Buyukmihci NC, *et al.* Effect of topically administered atropine on tear production in dogs. *J Am Vet Med Assoc* 1992; **200**(10): 1481–1484.
197 Ludders JW, Heavner JE. Effect of atropine on tear formation in anesthetized dogs. *J Am Vet Med Assoc* 1979; **175**(6): 585–586.
198 Doering CJ, Lukasik VM, Merideth RE. Effects of intramuscular injection of glycopyrrolate on Schirmer tear test I results in dogs. *J Am Vet Med Assoc* 2016; **248**(11): 1262–1266.
199 Bill A. Effects of atropine on aqueous humor dynamics in the vervet monkey (*Cercopithecus ethiops*). *Exp Eye Res* 1969; **8**(3): 284–291.
200 Smith PJ, Samuelson DA, Brooks DE, *et al.* Unconventional aqueous humor outflow of microspheres perfused into the equine eye. *Am J Vet Res* 1986; **47**(11): 2445–2453.
201 Wehrman RF, Gemensky-Metzler AJ, Zibura AE, *et al.* Objective evaluation of the systemic effects of topical application of 1% atropine sulfate ophthalmic solution in healthy horses. *J Am Vet Med Assoc* 2017; **251**(11): 1324–1330.
202 Stern ME, Beuerman RW, Fox RI, *et al.* The pathology of dry eye: the interaction between the ocular surface and lacrimal glands. *Cornea* 1998; **17**(6): 584–589.
203 Guerreiro CE, Appelboam H, Lowe RC. Successful medical treatment for globe penetration following tooth extraction in a dog. *Vet Ophthalmol* 2014; **17**(2): 146–149.

204 Wieser B, Tichy A, Nell B. Correlation between corneal sensitivity and quantity of reflex tearing in cows, horses, goats, sheep, dogs, cats, rabbits, and guinea pigs. *Vet Ophthalmol* 2013; **16**(4): 251–262.

205 Blocker T, Van Der Woerdt A. A comparison of corneal sensitivity between brachycephalic and domestic short-haired cats. *Vet Ophthalmol* 2001; **4**(2): 127–130.

206 Kafarnik C, Fritsche J, Reese S. Corneal innervation in mesocephalic and brachycephalic dogs and cats: assessment using in vivo confocal microscopy. *Vet Ophthalmol* 2008; **11**(6): 363–367.

207 Gallar J, Pozo MA, Tuckett RP, *et al.* Response of sensory units with unmyelinated fibres to mechanical, thermal and chemical stimulation of the cat's cornea. *J Physiol* 1993; **468**: 609–622.

208 Mantelli F, Micera A, Sacchetti M, *et al.* Neurogenic inflammation of the ocular surface. *Curr Opin Allergy Clin Immunol* 2010; **10**(5): 498–504.

209 Bhattacherjee P. Prostaglandins and inflammatory reactions in the eye. *Methods Find Exp Clin Pharmacol* 1980; **2**(1): 17–31.

210 Townsend WM. Canine and feline uveitis. *Vet Clin North Am Small Anim Pract* 2008; **38**(2): 323–346, vii.

211 Joubert F, Guerrero-Moreno A, Fakih D, *et al.* Topical treatment with a mu opioid receptor agonist alleviates corneal allodynia and corneal nerve sensitization in mice. *Biomed Pharmacother* 2020; **132**: 110794.

212 Wenk NH, Nannenga NM, Honda NC. Effect of morphine sulphate eye drops on hyperalgesia in the rat cornea. *Pain* 2003; **105**(3): 455–465.

213 Peyman GA, Rahimy MH, Fernandes ML. Effects of morphine on corneal sensitivity and epithelial wound healing: implications for topical ophthalmic analgesia. *Br J Ophthalmol* 1994; **78**(2): 138–141.

214 Gordon E, Sandquist C, Cebra CK, *et al.* Esthesiometric evaluation of corneal analgesia after topical application of 1% morphine sulfate in normal horses. *Vet Ophthalmol* 2018; **21**(3): 218–223.

215 Gordon E, Stang BV, Heidel J, *et al.* Pharmacokinetic evaluation and safety of topical 1% morphine sulfate application on the healthy equine eye. *Vet Ophthalmol* 2018; **21**(5): 516–523.

216 Thomson SM, Oliver JA, Gould DJ, *et al.* Preliminary investigations into the analgesic effects of topical ocular 1% morphine solution in dogs and cats. *Vet Anaesth Analg* 2013; **40**(6): 632–640.

217 Spertus CB, Espinheira Gomes F, Martin-Flores M, *et al.* Analgesic effect of topical and subconjunctival morphine in dogs after phacoemulsification: a pilot study. *Vet Ophthalmol* 2020; **23**(4): 674–681.

218 Stiles J, Honda CN, Krohne SG, *et al.* Effect of topical administration of 1% morphine sulfate solution on signs of pain and corneal wound healing in dogs. *Am J Vet Res* 2003; **64**(7): 813–818.

219 Akhavanakbari G, Entezariasl M, Ojagi H, *et al.* Comparison of the effects of remifentanil and alfentanil on intraocular pressure in cataract surgery. *Saudi J Anaesth* 2013; **7**(2): 160–164.

220 Ng HP, Chen FG, Yeong SM, *et al.* Effect of remifentanil compared with fentanyl on intraocular pressure after succinylcholine and tracheal intubation. *Br J Anaesth* 2000; **85**(5): 785–787.

221 Ziyaeifard M, Azarfarin R, Massoumi G. A comparison of intraocular pressure and hemodynamic responses to insertion of laryngeal mask airway or endotracheal tube using anesthesia with propofol and remifentanil in cataract surgery. *J Res Med Sci* 2012; **17**(6): 503–507.

222 Yoo YC, Shin S, Choi EK, *et al.* Increase in intraocular pressure is less with propofol than with sevoflurane during laparoscopic surgery in the steep Trendelenburg position. *Can J Anaesth* 2014; **61**(4): 322–329.

223 Drago F, Panissidi G, Bellomio F, *et al.* Effects of opiates and opioids on intraocular pressure of rabbits and humans. *Clin Exp Pharmacol Physiol* 1985; **12**(2): 107–113.

224 el Messiry S, Chiou GC. Interaction between nalbuphine and alfentanil on intraocular pressure and pupil size of conscious rabbits. *Ophthalmic Res* 1989; **21**(2): 134–140.

225 Douet JY, Regnier A, Dongay A, *et al.* Effect of sedation with butorphanol on variables pertaining to the ophthalmic examination in dogs. *Vet Ophthalmol* 2018; **21**(5): 452–458.

226 Biricik HS, Ceylan C, Sakar M. Effects of pethidine and fentanyl on tear production in dogs. *Vet Rec* 2004; **155**(18): 564–565.

227 Lee HK, Wang SC. Mechanism of morphine-induced miosis in the dog. *J Pharmacol Exp Ther* 1975; **192**(2): 415–431.

228 Tallarida RJ, Kramer MS, Roy JW, *et al.* Miosis and fluctuation in the rabbit pupil: effects of morphine and naloxone. *J Pharmacol Exp Ther* 1977; **201**(3): 587–592.

229 Wallenstein MC, Wang SC. Mechanism of morphine-induced mydriasis in the cat. *Am J Physiol* 1979; **236**(5): R292–R296.

230 de Boer HD, Detriche O, Forget P. Opioid-related side effects: postoperative ileus, urinary retention, nausea and vomiting, and shivering. A review of the literature. *Best Pract Res Clin Anaesthesiol* 2017; **31**(4): 499–504.

231 Frauenknecht J, Kirkham KR, Jacot-Guillarmod A, *et al.* Analgesic impact of intra-operative opioids vs. opioid-free anaesthesia: a systematic review and meta-analysis. *Anaesthesia* 2019; **74**(5): 651–662.

232 Behrendt T. Experimental study of corneal lesions produced by topical anesthesia. *Am J Ophthalmol* 1956; **41**(1): 99–105.

233 Park SA, Park YW, Son WG, *et al.* Evaluation of the analgesic effect of intracameral lidocaine hydrochloride injection on intraoperative and postoperative pain in healthy dogs undergoing phacoemulsification. *Am J Vet Res* 2010; **71**(2): 216–222.

234 Nebbioso M, Livani ML, Santamaria V, *et al.* Intracameral lidocaine as supplement to classic topical anesthesia for relieving ocular pain in cataract surgery. *Int J Ophthalmol* 2018; **11**(12): 1932–1935.

235 Smith LJ, Bentley E, Shih A, *et al.* Systemic lidocaine infusion as an analgesic for intraocular surgery in dogs: a pilot study. *Vet Anaesth Analg* 2004; **31**(1): 53–63.

236 Hermanns H, Hollmann MW, Stevens MF, *et al.* Molecular mechanisms of action of systemic lidocaine in acute and chronic pain: a narrative review. *Br J Anaesth* 2019; **123**(3): 335–349.

237 Shilo-Benjamini Y. A review of ophthalmic local and regional anesthesia in dogs and cats. *Vet Anaesth Analg* 2019; **46**(1): 14–27.

238 Zibura AE, Posner LP, Ru H, *et al.* A preoperative bupivacaine retrobulbar block offers superior antinociception compared with an intraoperative splash block in dogs undergoing enucleation. *Vet Ophthalmol* 2020; **23**(2): 225–233.

239 Scott EM, Vallone LV, Olson NL, *et al.* Analgesic effects of a retrobulbar block with 0.75% ropivacaine in dogs undergoing enucleation. *Vet Anaesth Analg* 2021; **48**(5): 749–758.

240 Hernandez EZ, Redondo JI, Gutierrez-Bautista AJ, *et al.* A modified retrobulbar block for microphthalmia using ultrasound guidance in a cat. *Vet Anaesth Analg* 2020; **47**(6): 846–847.

241 Shilo-Benjamini Y, Pascoe PJ, Maggs DJ, *et al.* Comparison of peribulbar and retrobulbar regional anesthesia with bupivacaine in cats. *Am J Vet Res* 2014; **75**(12): 1029–1039.

242 Hefner EM, Lin HC, Cole RC, *et al.* Comparison of image quality of corneal and retinal optical coherence tomography using sedation and general anesthesia protocols with or without retrobulbar anesthesia in horses. *Am J Vet Res* 2021; **83**(1): 72–79.

243 Yang VY, Eaton JS, Harmelink K, *et al.* Retrobulbar lidocaine injection via the supraorbital fossa is safe in adult horses but produces regionally variable periocular anaesthesia. *Equine Vet J* 2022; **54**(4): 807–819.

244 Pearce SG, Kerr CL, Boure LP, *et al.* Comparison of the retrobulbar and Peterson nerve block techniques via magnetic resonance imaging in bovine cadavers. *J Am Vet Med Assoc* 2003; **223**(6): 852–855.

245 Edmondson MA. Local, regional, and spinal anesthesia in ruminants. *Vet Clin North Am Food Anim Pract* 2016; **32**(3): 535–552.

246 Pollock PJ, Russell T, Hughes TK, *et al.* Transpalpebral eye enucleation in 40 standing horses. *Vet Surg* 2008; **37**(3): 306–309.

247 Bartholomew KJ, Smith LJ, Bentley E, *et al.* Retrospective analysis of complications associated with retrobulbar bupivacaine in dogs undergoing enucleation surgery. *Vet Anaesth Analg* 2020; **47**(5): 588–594.

248 Riad W, Akbar F. Ophthalmic regional blockade complication rate: a single center audit of 33,363 ophthalmic operations. *J Clin Anesth* 2012; **24**(3): 193–195.

249 Park SA, Lee I, Lee YL, *et al.* Combination auriculopalpebral nerve block and local anesthesia for placement of a nictitating membrane-to-superotemporal bulbar conjunctiva flap in dogs. *J Am Anim Hosp Assoc* 2009; **45**(4): 164–167.

250 Labelle AL, Clark-Price SC. Anesthesia for ophthalmic procedures in the standing horse. *Vet Clin North Am Equine Pract* 2013; **29**(1): 179–191.

251 Giuliano EA. Nonsteroidal anti-inflammatory drugs in veterinary ophthalmology. *Vet Clin North Am Small Anim Pract* 2004; **34**(3): 707–723.

252 Knych HK. Nonsteroidal anti-inflammatory drug use in horses. *Vet Clin North Am Equine Pract* 2017; **33**(1): 1–15.

253 Kavitha J, Parida S, Kundra P, *et al.* Oral gabapentin premedication for elderly patients undergoing intraocular surgery. *Br J Ophthalmol* 2013; **97**(7): 900–904.

254 Yoon HJ, Kim J, Yoon KC. Treatment response to gabapentin in neuropathic ocular pain associated with dry eye. *J Clin Med* 2020; **9**(11): 3765.

255 Kaya FN, Yavascaoglu B, Baykara M, *et al.* Effect of oral gabapentin on the intraocular pressure and haemodynamic responses induced by tracheal intubation. *Acta Anaesthesiol Scand* 2008; **52**(8): 1076–1080.

256 Trbolova A, Ghaffari MS, Capik I. Effects of premedication with oral gabapentin on intraocular pressure changes following tracheal intubation in clinically normal dogs. *BMC Vet Res* 2017; **13**(1): 288.

257 Shukla AK, Pinard CL, Flynn BL, *et al.* Effects of orally administered gabapentin, tramadol, and meloxicam on ocular variables in healthy dogs. *Am J Vet Res* 2020; **81**(12): 973–984.

258 Cammalleri M, Amato R, Olivieri M, *et al.* Effects of topical gabapentin on ocular pain and tear secretion. *Front Pharmacol* 2021; **12**: 671238.

259 Anfuso CD, Olivieri M, Fidilio A, *et al.* Gabapentin attenuates ocular inflammation: in vitro and in vivo studies. *Front Pharmacol* 2017; **8**: 173.

260 Ali HM, Elbadawy AM. Comparative study of retrobulbar block versus ketamine infusion during eye enucleation/evisceration (randomized controlled trial). *Anesth Essays Res* 2020; **14**(1): 92–99.

261 Lee YY, Wong SM, Hung CT. Dexmedetomidine infusion as a supplement to isoflurane anaesthesia for vitreoretinal surgery. *Br J Anaesth* 2007; **98**(4): 477–483.

262 Arnold RW, Biggs RE, Beerle BJ. Intravenous dexmedetomidine augments the oculocardiac reflex. *J AAPOS* 2018; **22**(3): 211–213.e1.

263 Robson AG, Nilsson J, Li S, *et al.* ISCEV guide to visual electrodiagnostic procedures. *Doc Ophthalmol* 2018; **136**(1): 1–26.

264 Ekesten B, Komaromy AM, Ofri R, *et al.* Guidelines for clinical electroretinography in the dog: 2012 update. *Doc Ophthalmol* 2013; **127**(2): 79–87.

265 Allbaugh RA, Ben-Shlomo G, Whitley RD. Electroretinogram evaluation of equine eyes with extensive 'bullet-hole' fundic lesions. *Vet Ophthalmol* 2014; **17**(Suppl 1): 129–133.

266 Vaegan, Anderton PJ, Millar TJ. Multifocal, pattern and full field electroretinograms in cats with unilateral optic nerve section. *Doc Ophthalmol* 2000; **100**(2–3): 207–229.

267 Kommonen B. The DC-recorded dog electroretinogram in ketamine-medetomidine anaesthesia. *Acta Vet Scand* 1988; **29**(1): 35–41.

268 Norman JC, Narfstrom K, Barrett PM. The effects of medetomidine hydrochloride on the electroretinogram of normal dogs. *Vet Ophthalmol* 2008; **11**(5): 299–305.

269 Jeong MB, Narfstrom K, Park SA, *et al.* Comparison of the effects of three different combinations of general anesthetics on the electroretinogram of dogs. *Doc Ophthalmol* 2009; **119**(2): 79–88.

270 Kommonen B, Karhunen U, Raitta C. Effects of thiopentone halothane-nitrous oxide anaesthesia compared to ketamine-xylazine anaesthesia on the DC recorded dog electroretinogram. *Acta Vet Scand* 1988; **29**(1): 23–33.

271 Lin SL, Shiu WC, Liu PC, *et al.* The effects of different anesthetic agents on short electroretinography protocol in dogs. *J Vet Med Sci* 2009; **71**(6): 763–768.

272 Yanase J, Ogawa H. Effects of halothane and sevoflurane on the electroretinogram of dogs. *Am J Vet Res* 1997; **58**(8): 904–909.

273 Freeman KS, Good KL, Kass PH, *et al.* Effects of chemical restraint on electroretinograms recorded sequentially in awake, sedated, and anesthetized dogs. *Am J Vet Res* 2013; **74**(7): 1036–1042.

274 Del Sole MJ, Nejamkin P, Cavilla V, *et al.* Comparison of two sedation protocols for short electroretinography in cats. *J Feline Med Surg* 2018; **20**(2): 172–178.

275 Knave B, Persson HE, Nilsson SE. A comparative study on the effects of barbiturate and ethyl alcohol on retinal functions with special reference to the C-wave of the electroretinogram and the standing potential of the sheep eye. *Acta Ophthalmol (Copenh)* 1974; **52**(2): 254–259.

276 Church ML, Norman JC. Electroretinogram responses of the normal Thoroughbred horse sedated with detomidine hydrochloride. *Vet Ophthalmol* 2012; **15**(Suppl 2): 77–83.

277 Niemeyer G, Nagahara K, Demant E. Effects of changes in arterial PO2 and PCO2 on the electroretinogram in the cat. *Invest Ophthalmol Vis Sci* 1982; **23**(5): 678–683.

278 Varela Lopez O, Alvarez Vazquez JC, Gonzalez Cantalapiedra A, *et al.* Effects of hypercapnia on the electroretinogram in sevoflurane and isoflurane anaesthetized dogs. *Doc Ophthalmol* 2010; **121**(1): 9–20.

279 Scarabelli S, Timofte D, Malalana F, *et al.* Corneal abrasion and microbial contamination in horses following general anaesthesia for non-ocular surgery. *Vet Anaesth Analg* 2018; **45**(3): 278–284.

280 Papp AM, Justin GA, Vernau CT, *et al.* Perioperative corneal abrasions after nonocular surgery: a systematic review. *Cornea* 2019; **38**(7): 927–932.

281 Dawson C, Sanchez RF. A prospective study of the prevalence of corneal surface disease in dogs receiving prophylactic topical lubrication under general anesthesia. *Vet Ophthalmol* 2016; **19**(2): 124–129.

282 Roth S, Thisted RA, Erickson JP, *et al.* Eye injuries after nonocular surgery. A study of 60,965 anesthetics from 1988 to 1992. *Anesthesiology* 1996; **85**(5): 1020–1027.

283 Stiles J, Weil AB, Packer RA, *et al.* Post-anesthetic cortical blindness in cats: twenty cases. *Vet J* 2012; **193**(2): 367–373.

284 Barton-Lamb AL, Martin-Flores M, Scrivani PV, *et al.* Evaluation of maxillary arterial blood flow in anesthetized cats with the mouth closed and open. *Vet J* 2013; **196**(3): 325–331.

285 Martin-Flores M, Scrivani PV, Loew E, *et al.* Maximal and submaximal mouth opening with mouth gags in cats: implications for maxillary artery blood flow. *Vet J* 2014; **200**(1): 60–64.

286 Wilson DV, Bohart GV, Evans AT, *et al.* Retrospective analysis of detomidine infusion for standing chemical restraint in 51 horses. *Vet Anaesth Analg* 2002; **29**(1): 54–57.

287 Miller PE, Pickett JP, Majors LJ. Evaluation of two applanation tonometers in horses. *Am J Vet Res* 1990; **51**(6): 935–937.

288 Carregaro AB, Ueda GI, Censoni JB, *et al.* Effect of methadone combined with acepromazine or detomidine on sedation and dissociative anesthesia in healthy horses. *J Equine Vet Sci* 2020; **86**: 102908.

289 Reed RA, Knych HK, Barletta M, *et al.* Pharmacokinetics and pharmacodynamics of hydromorphone after intravenous and intramuscular administration in horses. *Vet Anaesth Analg* 2020; **47**(2): 210–218.

290 Johnston GM, Eastment JK, Wood J, *et al.* The Confidential Enquiry into Perioperative Equine Fatalities (CEPEF): mortality results of Phases 1 and 2. *Vet Anaesth Analg* 2002; **29**(4): 159–170.

291 Bettschart-Wolfensberger R, Jaggin-Schmucker N, Lendl C, *et al.* Minimal alveolar concentration of desflurane in combination with an infusion of medetomidine for the anaesthesia of ponies. *Vet Rec* 2001; **148**(9): 264–267.

292 Ringer SK, Kalchofner K, Boller J, *et al.* A clinical comparison of two anaesthetic protocols using lidocaine or medetomidine in horses. *Vet Anaesth Analg* 2007; **34**(4): 257–268.

293 Valverde A, Gunkel C, Doherty TJ, *et al.* Effect of a constant rate infusion of lidocaine on the quality of recovery from sevoflurane or isoflurane general anaesthesia in horses. *Equine Vet J* 2005; **37**(6): 559–564.

294 Curto EM, Griffith EH, Posner LP, *et al.* Factors associated with postoperative complications in healthy horses after general anesthesia for ophthalmic versus non-ophthalmic procedures: 556 cases (2012–2014). *J Am Vet Med Assoc* 2018; **252**(9): 1113–1119.

295 Patipa LA, Sherlock CE, Witte SH, *et al.* Risk factors for colic in equids hospitalized for ocular disease. *J Am Vet Med Assoc* 2012; **240**(12): 1488–1493.

68 Neonatal and Pediatric Patients

Emily McCobb[1] **and Sheilah A. Robertson**[2]
[1] Department of Clinical Sciences, Cummings School of Veterinary Medicine, Tufts University, North Grafton, Massachusetts, USA
[2] Lap of Love Veterinary Hospice Inc., Lutz, Florida, USA

Chapter contents

Introduction, 1348
Definition of pediatric and neonatal periods, 1348
Anesthetic risk for young patients, 1348
Circumstances warranting anesthesia, 1348
Patient characteristics, 1349
  Cardiovascular system, 1349
  Respiratory system, 1349
  Renal and hepatic systems, 1349
  Central nervous system, 1349
  Hematologic system, 1350
Anesthetic management, 1350
  Patient preparation, 1350
  Monitoring, 1350
  Supportive care, 1350
  Thermoregulatory support, 1350
  Recovery, 1350
Summary of pediatric drug metabolism and pharmacokinetics, 1351
  Drugs, 1351
  Suggested protocols for puppies and kittens, 1351
  Pain management, 1351
References, 1352

Introduction

Young animals have physiologic and anatomic characteristics that can make them challenging to anesthetize. In addition to their small size, these patients tend to have limited body system reserves, can be more sensitive to the sedative effects of some agents, such as opioids, and are vulnerable to anesthetic complications, such as hypothermia. Fortunately, with careful attention to these considerations, most pediatric patients can be anesthetized safely and successfully.

Definition of pediatric and neonatal periods

In cats and dogs, the neonatal period extends from birth to weaning (4 to 6 weeks of age) and the pediatric period can be defined as the period between 6 weeks (which marks the end of the neonatal period) and 12 weeks of age [1,2]. Puppies and kittens can be defined as dogs and cats less than 6 months of age. The most important physiologic differences for foals exist between 48 and 72 h after birth, but they are considered physiologically mature by 4 to 6 weeks of age [3]. Ruminants (cattle, sheep, and goats) and camelids are considered neonatal until 4 weeks of age and physiologically mature by 4 to 6 weeks of age.

Anesthetic risk for young patients

Because of their relatively small size, lack of physiologic reserves, incomplete immunity, and susceptibility to the stress of handling and separation from their dam, all puppies and kittens should be considered a special category of anesthesia patient until at least 3 months of age. The risks of anesthesia are not increased in young healthy animals undergoing elective procedures which are performed rapidly and efficiently [4]. In contrast, a large study in general veterinary practices found that the risk of anesthetic death in cats weighing less than 2 kg was over 15 times greater than that of cats between 2 and 6 kg [5]. In addition, the risk of anesthetic death was higher in dogs weighing < 5 kg compared to dogs weighing 5–15 kg suggesting size is a risk factor that is independent of age [6]. Foals less than 1 month of age have increased risk of mortality during anesthesia [7,8].

Circumstances warranting anesthesia

Early spay-neuter is an accepted practice for population control and is endorsed by the American Veterinary Medical Association [9] and the Association of Shelter Veterinarians [10,11]. The rationale

Veterinary Anesthesia and Analgesia: The Sixth Edition of Lumb and Jones. Edited by Leigh Lamont, Kurt Grimm, Sheilah Robertson, Lydia Love and Carrie Schroeder.
© 2024 John Wiley & Sons, Inc. Published 2024 by John Wiley & Sons, Inc.
Companion website: www.wiley.com/go/lamont/anesthesia

for early spay-neuter has been reviewed elsewhere [12–15] but, in addition to the benefits for population management, surgery in young, healthy animals is generally associated with good outcomes and, at least in cats, may be less painful [16]. For elective procedures (sterilization), it is preferred that puppies and kittens are ≥ 1 kg. However, puppies and kittens may present at a very early age and under 1 kg for emergency procedures such as abdominal surgery, diaphragmatic hernia, fractures, and other accidental injuries, and good outcomes can be achieved with careful anesthetic and analgesic management.

Foals and young ruminants are not commonly anesthetized for castration during the pediatric period, but ruminants may present for routine husbandry procedures such as disbudding. Emergency surgeries in foals such as patent urachus surgery or septic joints are common. These species may present at a young age for the correction of congenital abnormalities (e.g., limb malformations) or with traumatic injuries such as fractures.

Patient characteristics

The unique physiologic features of pediatric cats and dogs have been reviewed [17,18]. Pediatric patients of all species have limited reserves of all body systems and a limited ability to respond to events that challenge homeostasis. The role of a high resting basal metabolic rate in determining the pediatric patient's response to anesthesia should not be underestimated and can lead to fast metabolism of drugs and the need for redosing. Anatomic characteristics that are relevant to anesthesia include a high body surface area-to-mass ratio and a high lean body mass compared to body fat. These features can predispose the pediatric patient to hypothermia, which is perhaps the most devastating complication of anesthesia for young animals. In addition, the tissues are delicate requiring gentle handling.

Cardiovascular system

The pediatric heart is relatively small for the size of the patient, ventricular compliance is low, and stroke volume is relatively fixed. Low cardiac reserves are accompanied by a high cardiac index (volume of blood pumped per minute indexed to body size: L/min/m^2) leading to an overall decreased ability to compensate for or respond to fluid losses and hypotension. Because the stroke volume of a pediatric patient is relatively fixed, these patients are particularly dependent on heart rate for the maintenance of cardiac output (heart rate × stroke volume) and organ perfusion [17,19]. The neonate is unable to increase cardiac contractility in response to increased demand, unlike the adult [20]. Because cardiac output is determined by heart rate, any decrease in heart rate in a pediatric patient can have serious consequences, and it should be noted that one of the most common causes of bradycardia is hypothermia. In addition to the lack of reserves, the autonomic nervous system, especially sympathetic control, is thought to be poorly developed in pediatric patients leading to poor vasomotor control and responses. Baroreceptors are immature until 12 weeks of age leading to an inadequate response to a fall in blood pressure [17]. Lastly, persistent fetal circulation may be present in some pediatric patients leading to right to left anatomical shunting and hypoxemia, especially if systemic hypotension develops.

Respiratory system

Like the pediatric cardiovascular system, the pediatric respiratory system is also characterized by a lack of reserve capacity. While tidal volumes are similar to those of the adult animal (10–15 mL/kg), the pediatric respiratory rate is two to three times higher in order to provide an appropriate minute ventilation (tidal volume × respiratory rate) [21]. An important clinical consequence of a faster respiratory rate is a shorter induction time in neonates when inhalant agents are used, although this effect may be counteracted by their high cardiac output and may be less obvious when using today's less soluble inhalant agents such as isoflurane and sevoflurane. With a high resting metabolic rate, a high oxygen demand, and high baseline minute ventilation, pediatric patients are at increased risk of developing hypoxemia and have limited ability to adapt to decreases in oxygen delivery. The heart is entirely dependent on aerobic metabolism; therefore, any decrease in oxygen supply results in rapid decompensation. The nares and tracheas of pediatric patients are small and susceptible to obstruction; the small airways and alveoli are also prone to collapse [17]. The extremely pliant rib cage increases the work of breathing in pediatric patients which can predispose to ventilation fatigue and further increase the risk of hypoxemia. Ventilation of pediatric patients should be monitored and supported when necessary.

Airway anatomy can pose a challenge. The pediatric patient has small nares and the tongue is proportionally large for the size of the mouth. Intubation can be difficult, and when performed, great care must be taken to avoid airway trauma resulting in postoperative swelling and obstruction. However, the small trachea creates increased resistance to airflow, and intubation and ventilatory support may be necessary.

Renal and hepatic systems

By 8 weeks of age most physiologic processes related to renal and hepatic function should be relatively normal, although organ reserves may still be limited. The cytochrome P450 enzyme system is immature after birth but develops during the neonatal period [22–24]. After the age of 6 weeks, there is no rationale for altering drug doses in animals to account for hepatic clearance [25]. Herbivores have better-developed drug metabolism and excretion at younger ages than do dogs and cats. Hepatic development is largely mature in foals by 2 weeks of age. However, hepatic glycogen stores are low and gluconeogenesis is decreased, factors which increase the risk for hypoglycemia, especially if the patient is fasted for more than a short period. Pediatric dogs and cats and very young foals (under 4 days of age) have immature renal function, which can result in delayed clearance of renally metabolized drugs, potentially increasing their duration of action. Young animals have decreased glomerular filtration rates, decreased renal blood flow, and decreased concentrating ability. Decreased renal clearance rates may also increase the risk of fluid overload in the young patient [24].

Central nervous system

The blood–brain barrier is immature in young animals and therefore profound sedative effects may be noted with drugs such as opioids and benzodiazepines. In foals under 3 weeks of age, diazepam is profoundly sedating, and this may in part be due to the increased permeability of the blood–brain barrier. In this age group, benzodiazepines will induce deep sedation and muscle relaxation, with patients often becoming recumbent [26]. In contrast, when used in older foals and adults, benzodiazepines often result in excitement and ataxia but not recumbency.

Pain management in young animals is very important in order to prevent permanent changes to the central nervous system [27,28].

The decreased function of the thermoregulatory center contributes to the risk of hypothermia.

Hematologic system

Young patients have less capacity for hematopoiesis [29]. In addition, they have lower levels of erythropoietin, lower packed cell volume, and fewer circulating red blood cells. This resulting anemia means they are less able to compensate for hemorrhage. Moreover, hematopoiesis does not commence until after 15 weeks of age [30]. Other hematologic variabilities include decreased albumin, blood urea nitrogen, and creatinine, as well as increased phosphorus.

Anesthetic management

Patient preparation

Pediatric patients are likely more susceptible to the effects of stress than adults. Studies in neonatal rat pups demonstrate that the increased plasticity of the neonatal brain may increase vulnerability to stress and anxiety disorders later in life [27]. Pediatric animals may be presented for surgery during their critical socialization period. It is essential to protect these patients from the risk of fear imprinting when a bad experience could translate into a lifetime of fearful or fractious behavior during veterinary visits. Puppies and kittens should be gently handled. Littermates should be housed together during transport if possible and should be kept together in the cage until the time of premedication. If still with their dam, they should not be separated from her.

Fasting times for younger animals should be short (under 2 h) to account for their decreased glycogen stores.

As with all surgery patients, a thorough presurgical physical exam should be conducted prior to sedation or anesthesia. It is especially important to perform a thorough auscultation in case cardiac murmurs have gone undetected. The animal should also be checked carefully for other congenital abnormalities that might affect anesthesia or surgery such as pectus excavatum, hernias (inguinal or umbilical), and undescended testicles. Lastly, an accurate weight is very important as all drugs should be dosed on a mg/kg or mg/m^2 basis; "guesstimates" of weight that are off by a small amount with respect to grams can represent a large percentage of a very small patient's body weight, resulting in drug overdose and an adverse response and outcome.

Monitoring

Pediatric patients should be monitored while sedated and anesthetized in a similar fashion to adult patients [11]. Doppler ultrasound equipment is versatile and can be used on even the smallest of patients. A Doppler unit can be used to monitor heart rate (placed directly on a shaved area over the heart), pulse rate (placed on the caudal aspect of the carpus), and blood pressure can be measured when the probe is placed on a limb and a blood pressure cuff applied proximally.

Pulse oximeters should be used, and their use decreases the risk of anesthetic-related fatalities in cats [5]. In dogs and cats, the preferred placement site is the hind paw [31] and a toe can be shaved to help improve contact. The tongue is also commonly used but may increase the risk of spreading infection between patients, so if this site is used the probe must be cleaned and disinfected thoroughly between cases. Surgery and fluorescent lighting can interfere with the functioning of pulse oximeters so the light-emitting diode (LED) and the sensor should be covered.

If "alligator clips" are utilized to apply electrocardiogram leads, they should have their sharp edges filed down, the spring loosened, and a small square of gauze placed between the clips and the skin to avoid damage to delicate skin. Alternatives include "duckbill clips" without teeth and electrode patches placed on the paw pads. The patient's mucous membrane color, capillary refill time, anesthetic depth, and temperature should also be assessed at 5-min intervals as outlined in the American College of Veterinary Anesthesia and Analgesia Guidelines [32], though continuous physical monitoring may allow for early detection of physiologic abnormalities. Guidelines for monitoring are also available from the American Animal Hospital Association [33].

Supportive care

Intravenous catheter placement can be greatly facilitated if topical local anesthetics are applied over the catheter site and covered with an occlusive dressing (plastic plus a flexible wrapping) during the time between sedation and catheter placement. A eutectic mixture of lidocaine and prilocaine or lidocaine (4%) topical can be used and, though systemic absorption is minimal, the time to onset can be up to 1 h [34]. In children, liposomal lidocaine 4% cream resulted in a higher success rate for intravenous cannulation compared to placebo and was effective after a contact time of 30 min [35].

When IV fluids are given, crystalloids are used and administered at a rate of 3 mL/kg/h in cats and 5 mL/kg/h in dogs in accordance with the American Animal Hospital Association's fluid therapy guidelines, though attention should be paid to total fluid dose delivered (e.g., a young cat that receives 3 mL/kg/h for 15 min may benefit from continued IV fluids or subcutaneous fluids in recovery). Monitoring glucose levels in neonatal and pediatric patients of all species is recommended, particularly for sick patients or for longer procedures. Routine administration of dextrose without monitoring may lead to hyperglycemia [36].

Thermoregulatory support

The single most important thing the anesthetist can do for a pediatric patient is to avoid hypothermia. Hypothermia will decrease the minimum alveolar concentration (MAC) and therefore increase the risk of inhalant anesthetic overdose. Hypothermic patients will become bradycardic, leading to decreased cardiac output and hypotension. Decreasing core temperature also increases the risk of myocardial irritability and arrhythmias. Clot formation is slower at low temperatures, potentially increasing the risk of bleeding [37]. Hypothermic patients have an increased surgical infection rate as well as decreased immune response [38]. Drug elimination will be prolonged and recovery may be delayed. Postoperative shivering increases oxygen demand and myocardial oxygen consumption which is particularly detrimental in pediatric patients due to their higher oxygen requirements.

Patient warming devices such as a forced air heating system, warming blankets, and circulating warm water blankets can be used. Kittens and puppies should never be placed on a cold surface and should be covered whenever possible; a good technique is to use one fleece blanket which travels from start to finish with the patient. Electric blankets, warm fluid bags, heated disks, and rice bags can burn patients and should not be placed in direct contact with patients. Perioperative thermoregulation and heat balance are discussed in detail in Chapter 17.

Recovery

Recovery should take place in a warm, quiet, and safe environment. As soon as possible the patient should be returned to his litter or herd mates and/or dam as appropriate. In addition, the animals should be offered a small amount of soft food as soon as they can swallow. If recovery is slow or prolonged (> 30 min), hypothermia should be investigated, and if temperature is low more aggressive warming strategies should be applied. Dextrose 50% or high-fructose corn syrup can be applied to the gums or placed under the tongue and anecdotally will often arouse puppies and kittens. However, recent research indicates corn syrup is ineffective at raising kitten blood sugar levels and moreover kittens were not hypoglycemic after anesthesia that included dexmedetomidine, so routine application of corn syrup for kittens is not necessary [39]. Nursing animals should be returned to their dam as soon as they are able to swallow.

Summary of pediatric drug metabolism and pharmacokinetics

Drug metabolism and excretion are somewhat less of a concern in herbivores because metabolism is more well developed at an early age. Older foals will have faster clearance of both injectable and inhaled anesthetics because they have higher extracellular fluid volumes than adult horses (43% of body weight versus 22% in adult horses) [40]. Highly protein-bound molecules such as NSAIDs are more extensively distributed in young animals and adult levels of cytochrome P450 are not reached in small animal species until 5 months of age [23]. The increased body water content of young animals leads to an increased initial volume of distribution for water-soluble drugs and conversely, their decreased percentage of body fat leads to a decreased volume of distribution for lipid-soluble drugs.

Drugs

Sedatives and tranquilizers

Most sedatives provide good sedation in young patients, particularly in neonates. Low doses are recommended. It has often been stated that α_2-adrenergic receptor agonists should be used with caution due to cardiovascular effects, but this class of drugs is commonly used in combination protocols for pediatric patients in high-quality, high-volume spay-neuter (HQHVSN) programs [11,15].

The cardiopulmonary effects of xylazine (1.1 mg/kg IV) have been studied in foals at 10 and 28 days of age [41]. Marked bradycardia (a 19–27% drop) was reported. Short-lived increases in blood pressure were followed by a decrease below baseline values (a 23–28% drop). One of the most striking respiratory effects in this group of foals was marked changes in airway flow and intermittent upper airway obstruction creating loud respiratory noise for 20 min after administration. However arterial blood gases did not change in the 2 h after administration. It is hypothesized that the airway obstruction is due to profound pharyngeal muscle relaxation. All foals were sedate and ataxic and some became recumbent. There were no significant differences in the results obtained at 10 and 28 days of age.

Acepromazine is often avoided in the very young due to lack of reversibility and since it may promote hypothermia due to its vasodilatory actions. Benzodiazepine effects are discussed in the central nervous system section above.

Opioids

Opioid medications are reversible, have minimal cardiovascular effects (mostly limited to bradycardia), and are generally well tolerated by healthy pediatric patients. As previously mentioned, and discussed further below, adequate analgesia is central to humane and effective perioperative care of young animals.

Induction drugs and techniques

Care should be taken with mask induction with an inhalant agent as it tends to increase the risk of anesthetic death in dogs and foals [6,8]. In addition, environmental contamination will occur, and personnel may be exposed to waste anesthetic gases. Mask induction can be considered for very young animals if intravenous access cannot be achieved but they should be sedated to decrease stress and reduce inhalant anesthetic requirements. If induction with an inhalant agent is chosen, sevoflurane is the preferred agent as, compared to isoflurane, induction time is shorter in dogs and cats [42,43].

Intravenous techniques titrated to effect are preferable, especially in compromised patients. Acceptable agents for induction include propofol, alfaxalone, and ketamine–benzodiazepine combinations.

Anesthetic maintenance

Some procedures (e.g., castration and ovariohysterectomy in puppies and kittens) can be completed under injectable anesthesia (with oxygen supplementation and possibly intubation). If additional time is required to complete a procedure, anesthesia is generally maintained with inhalant agents administered to effect.

Suggested protocols for puppies and kittens

There are numerous anesthetic protocols for kittens and puppies and the reader is referred to other resources for details [44].

The "kitten quad" comprises a mixture of medetomidine or dexmedetomidine, ketamine, buprenorphine, and midazolam and is used widely in shelter neutering programs [45,46]. Recovery time can be reduced by administering atipamezole and kittens recover faster than adult cats [45]. Cats under 6 months of age that received "quad" with dexmedetomidine and then atipamezole 40 min after the initial injection attained sternal recumbency at 51 ± 5 (mean ± SD) min and were standing at 62 ± 19 min after the initial injection [45].

Pain management

Contrary to earlier beliefs, young patients do experience pain and its effects may have far-reaching adverse consequences [47]. Pain experienced at a young age may lead to dynamic changes in the nociceptive pathway and result in altered responses to noxious stimuli and chronic pain later in life [27,28,48]. In addition to these negative effects, pain has adverse physiologic effects resulting in tachycardia, hypertension, ileus, and immunosuppression.

A balanced anesthetic protocol, including multimodal analgesia should be used in pediatric patients. The most practical and commonly used combinations are opioids and NSAIDs, and the concomitant use of these does have benefits over using either group of drugs alone [49]. Opioids are generally very well tolerated in pediatric patients, although an opioid-free protocol has been found to provide adequate analgesia in kittens (not adult cats) [50]. As discussed earlier, the use of NSAIDs in very young puppies and kittens is controversial [51]. Moreover, label indications for available NSAIDs vary and some are not labeled for dogs and cats less than 4 to 6 months of age. Meloxicam is approved for use in cattle and is commonly used in calves for dehorning and castration.

The use of local anesthetics is encouraged; these can be injected into the testicles [52–54] or via incisional blocks. In dogs, intratesticular lidocaine decreased the cardiovascular responses to castration [53] but did not have an impact on postsurgery pain scores [54]. Intraperitoneal bupivacaine (2 mg/kg) was minimally absorbed into the systemic circulation and was beneficial in cats undergoing ovariohysterectomy [55,56].

There are several non-pharmacologic methods that can be used to address pain [47], for example, oral sweet solutions are analgesic in pediatric humans and so human infants are often given something sugary at the time of procedures involving noxious stimuli. It is not known if this effect occurs in dogs and cats, and cats are thought not to be able to taste sweet flavors. Other non-pharmacologic strategies can be applied to veterinary patients such as cuddling or swaddling. Swaddling and contact with the mother ("kangaroo care") can diminish pain [57]. Warmth has also been shown to be analgesic in human infants [58]. Pain is driven by inflammation, therefore minimizing surgical trauma and using the smallest possible incisions will decrease pain in the postoperative period [59].

References

1 Robinson EP. Anaesthesia of pediatric patients. *Compend Contin Educ Vet* 1983; **5**: 1004–1011.

2 Breazile JE. Neurologic and behavioral development in the puppy. *Vet Clin North Am Small Anim Pract* 1978; **8**: 31–45.

3 Tranquilli WJ, Thurmon JC. Management of anesthesia in the foal. *Vet Clin North Am Equine Pract* 1990; **6**: 651–663.

4 Levy JK, Bard KM, Tucker SJ, *et al.* Perioperative mortality in cats and dogs undergoing spay or castration at a high-volume clinic. *Vet J* 2017; **224**: 11–15.

5 Brodbelt DC, Pfeiffer DU, Young LE, *et al.* Risk factors for anaesthetic-related death in cats: results from the Confidential Enquiry into Perioperative Small Animal Fatalities (CEPSAF). *Br J Anaesth* 2007; **99**(5): 617–623.

6 Brodbelt DC, Pfeiffer DU, Young LE, *et al.* Results of the Confidential Enquiry into Perioperative Small Animal Fatalities regarding risk factors for anesthetic-related death in dogs. *J Am Vet Med Assoc* 2008; **233**(7): 1096–1104.

7 Johnston GM, Taylor PM, Holmes MA, *et al.* Confidential Enquiry of Perioperative Equine Fatalities (CEPEF-1): preliminary results. *Equine Vet J* 1995; **27**(3): 193–200.

8 Johnston GM, Eastment JK, Wood J, *et al.* The Confidential Enquiry into Perioperative Equine Fatalities (CEPEF): mortality results of Phases 1 and 2. *Vet Anaesth Analg* 2002; **29**(4): 159–170.

9 American Veterinary Medical Association (AVMA), Resources for Pet Owners. Spaying and neutering. Available at: www.avma.org/resources/pet-owners/petcare/spaying-and-neutering (accessed July 2023).

10 Association of Shelter Veterinarians. Position statement: early age spay neuter (updated May 2020). Available at:https://higherlogicdownload.s3.amazonaws.com/ASV/fa11b6a5-ea22-45cc-9b33-416a24d44499/UploadedImages/Policy_Stmts/Early_Age_Spay_Neuter.pdf (accessed July 2023).

11 Griffin B, Bushby PA, McCobb E, *et al.* Association of Shelter Veterinarians' 2016 Veterinary Medical Care Guidelines for spay-neuter programs. *J Am Vet Med Assoc* 2016; **249**(2): 165–188.

12 Howe LM. Short-term results and complications of prepubertal gonadectomy in cats and dogs. *J Am Vet Med Assoc* 1997; **211**(1): 57–62.

13 Root Kustritz MV. Early spay-neuter: clinical considerations. *Clin Tech Small Animal Pract* 2002; **17**(3): 124–128.

14 Root Kustritz MV. Pros, cons, and techniques of pediatric neutering. *Vet Clin North Am Small Anim Pract* 2014; **44**(2): 221–233.

15 Bushby PA, Griffin B. An overview of pediatric spay and neuter benefits and techniques. DVM360, 2011. Available at: www.dvm360.com/view/overview-pediatric-spay-and-neuter-benefits-and-techniques (accessed July 2023).

16 Polson S, Taylor PM, Yates D. Effects of age and reproductive status on postoperative pain after routine ovariohysterectomy in cats. *J Feline Med Surg* 2014; **16**(2): 170–176.

17 Grandy JL, Dunlop CI. Anesthesia of pups and kittens. *J Am Vet Med Assoc* 1991; **198**(7): 1244–1249.

18 Grubb TL, Perez Jiminez TE, Pettifer GR. Neonatal and pediatric patients. In: Grimm KA, Lamont LA, Tranquilli WJ, *et al.*, eds. *Veterinary Anesthesia and Analgesia, The Fifth Edition of Lumb and Jones*. Ames, IA: John Wiley & Sons, 2015: 983–987.

19 Friedman WF. The intrinsic physiologic properties of the developing heart. *Prog Cardiovasc Dis* 1972; **15**(1): 87–111.

20 Shaddy RE, Tyndall MR, Teitel DF, *et al.* Regulation of cardiac output with controlled heart rate in newborn lambs. *Pediatr Res* 1988; **24**(5): 577–582.

21 Parot S, Bonora M, Gautier H, *et al.* Developmental changes in ventilation and breathing pattern in unanesthetized kittens. *Respir Physiol* 1984; **58**(3): 253–262.

22 Baggot JD, Short CR. Drug disposition in the neonatal animal, with particular reference to the foal. *Equine Vet J* 1987; **19**: 169–171.

23 Baggot JD. Drug therapy in the neonatal animal. In: Baggot JD, ed. *Principles of Drug Disposition in Domestic Animals: the Basis of Veterinary Clinical Pharmacology*. Philadelphia, PA: WB Saunders, 1992: 21–36.

24 Boothe DM, Tannert K. Special considerations for drug and fluid therapy in the pediatric patient. *Compend Contin Educ Vet* 1992; **14**: 313–329.

25 Papich MG. Treating animals in special situations: the old and the young: the sick and debilitated. In: *Proceedings of the Western Veterinary Conference*, February 2013, Las Vegas, NV.

26 Norman WM, Court MH, Greenblatt DJ. Age-related changes in the pharmacokinetic disposition of diazepam in foals. *Am J Vet Res* 1997; **58**(8): 878–880.

27 Anand KJ, Coskun V, Thrivikraman KV, *et al.* Long-term behavioral effects of repetitive pain in neonatal rat pups. *Physiol Behav* 1999; **66**(4): 627–637.

28 Buskila D, Neumann L, Zmora E, *et al.* Pain sensitivity in prematurely born adolescents. *Arch Pediatr Adolesc Med* 2003; **157**(11): 1079–1082.

29 Earl FL, Melveger BE, Wilson RL. The hemogram and bone marrow profile of normal neonatal and weanling beagle dogs. *Lab Anim Sci* 1973; **23**(5): 690–695.

30 Mueggler PA, Black JA, Carpenter S, *et al.* Postnatal regulation of oxygen delivery: control of erythropoiesis following birth in dogs. *Respir Physiol* 1981; **43**(3): 189–196.

31 Matthews NS, Hartke S, Allen JC Jr. An evaluation of pulse oximeters in dogs, cats and horses. *Vet Anaesth Analg* 2003; **30**(1): 3–14.

32 American College of Veterinary Anesthesia and Analgesia (ACVAA). Recommendations for monitoring anesthetized veterinary patients. Available at: www.acvaa.org/wp-content/uploads/2019/05/Small-Animal-Monitoring-Guidlines.pdf (accessed July 2023).

33 American Animal Hospital Association (AAHA). 2020 AAHA Anesthesia and monitoring guidelines for dogs and cats. Available at: www.aaha.org/aaha-guidelines/2020-aaha-anesthesia-and-monitoring-guidelines-for-dogs-and-cats/anesthesia-and-monitoring-home (accessed July 2023).

34 Wagner KA, Gibbon KJ, Strom TL, *et al.* Adverse effects of EMLA (lidocaine/prilocaine) cream and efficacy for the placement of jugular catheters in hospitalized cats. *J Feline Med Surg* 2006; **8**(2): 141–144.

35 Taddio A, Spin HK, Schuh S, *et al.* Liposomal lidocaine to improve procedural success rates and reduce procedural pain among children: a randomized controlled trial. *CMAJ* 2005; **172**(13): 1691–1695.

36 Doherty T, Valverde A. Management of sedation and anesthesia. In: Doherty T, Valverde A, eds. *Manual of Equine Anesthesa and Analgesia*. Oxford, UK: Blackwell Publishing Ltd, 2006: 206–259.

37 Taggart R, Austin B, Hans E, *et al.* In vitro evaluation of the effect of hypothermia on coagulation in dogs via thromboelastography. *J Vet Emerg Crit Care (San Antonio)* 2012; **22**(2): 219–224.

38 Doufas AG. Consequences of inadvertent perioperative hypothermia. *Best Pract Res Clin Anaesthesiol* 2003; **17**(4): 535–549.

39 Cornell HN, Shaver SL, Semick DN, *et al.* Effect of transmucosal corn syrup application on postoperative blood glucose concentrations in kittens. *J Feline Med Surg* 2018; **20**(4): 289–294.

40 Webb AI, Weaver BM. Body composition of the horse. *Equine Vet J* 1979; **11**(1): 39–47.

41 Carter SW, Robertson SA, Steel CJ, *et al.* Cardiopulmonary effects of xylazine sedation in the foal. *Equine Vet J* 1990; **22**(6): 384–388.

42 Mutoh T, Kojima K, Takao K, *et al.* Comparison of sevoflurane with isoflurane for rapid mask induction in midazolam and butorphanol-sedated dogs. *J Vet Med A Physiol Pathol Clin Med* 2001; **48**(4): 223–230.

43 Lerche P, Muir WW, Grubb TL. Mask induction of anaesthesia with isoflurane or sevoflurane in premedicated cats. *J Small Anim Pract* 2002; **43**(1): 12–15.

44 McCobb E, Robertson S. Special considerations for anesthesia of pediatric patients. In: White S, ed. *High-Quality, High-Volume Spay and Neuter and Other Shelter Surgeries*. Hoboken, NJ: Wiley-Blackwell, 2020: 193–208.

45 Bruniges N, Taylor PM, Yates D. Injectable anaesthesia for adult cat and kitten castration: effects of medetomidine, dexmedetomidine and atipamezole on recovery. *J Feline Med Surg* 2016; **18**(11): 860–867.

46 Welsh P. Neutering pet cats at four months of age (or less). *Feline update online*. Available at: www.langfordvets.co.uk/media/1248/neutering-cats-at-4-months-of-age-or-less.pdf (accessed July 2023).

47 Johnston CC, Fernandes AM, Campbell-Yeo M. Pain in neonates is different. *Pain* 2011; **152**(3 Suppl): S65–S73.

48 Allegaert K, Tibboel D, van den Anker J. Pharmacological treatment of neonatal pain: in search of a new equipoise. *Semin Fetal Neonatal Med* 2013; **18**(1): 42–47.

49 Steagall PV, Taylor PM, Rodrigues LC, *et al.* Analgesia for cats after ovariohysterectomy with either buprenorphine or carprofen alone or in combination. *Vet Rec* 2009; **164**(12): 359–363.

50 Malo A, Cheng AJ, Ruel HL, *et al.* Randomised, prospective, blinded, clinical trial of opioid-free injectable anaesthesia with or without multimodal analgesia in kittens undergoing ovariohysterectomy. *J Feline Med Surg* 2023; **25**(3): 1098612X231158582.

51 Morris JL, Rosen DA, Rosen KR. Nonsteroidal anti-inflammatory agents in neonates. *Paediatr Drugs* 2003; **5**(6): 385–405.

52 Moldal ER, Eriksen T, Kirpensteijn J, *et al.* Intratesticular and subcutaneous lidocaine alters the intraoperative haemodynamic responses and heart rate variability in male cats undergoing castration. *Vet Anaesth Analg* 2013; **40**(1): 63–73.

53 Huuskonen V, Hughes JM, Estaca Bañon E, *et al.* Intratesticular lidocaine reduces the response to surgical castration in dogs. *Vet Anaesth Analg* 2013; **40**(1): 74–82.

54 Stevens BJ, Posner LP, Jones CA, *et al.* Comparison of the effect of intratesticular lidocaine/bupivacaine vs. saline placebo on pain scores and incision site reactions in dogs undergoing routine castration. *Vet J* 2013; **196**(3): 499–503.

55 Benito J, Monteiro B, Lavoie AM, *et al.* Analgesic efficacy of intraperitoneal administration of bupivacaine in cats. *J Feline Med Surg* 2016; **18**(11): 906–912.

56 Benito J, Monteiro B, Beaudry F, *et al.* Efficacy and pharmacokinetics of bupivacaine with epinephrine or dexmedetomidine after intraperitoneal administration in cats undergoing ovariohysterectomy. *Can J Vet Res* 2018; **82**(2): 124–130.

57 Campbell-Yeo M, Fernandes A, Johnston C. Procedural pain management for neonates using nonpharmacological strategies: Part 2: mother-driven interventions. *Adv Neonatal Care* 2011; **11**(5): 312–318.

58 Gray L, Lang CW, Porges SW. Warmth is analgesic in healthy newborns. *Pain* 2012; **153**(5): 960–966.

59 Kristiansson M, Saraste L, Soop M, *et al.* Diminished interleukin-6 and C-reactive protein responses to laparoscopic versus open cholecystectomy. *Acta Anaesthesiol Scand* 1999; **43**(2): 146–152.

69 Aging Patients

Sheilah A. Robertson[1] and Kirk A. Muñoz[2]
[1] Lap of Love Veterinary Hospice Inc., Lutz, Florida, USA
[2] Department of Veterinary Clinical Sciences, College of Veterinary Medicine, The Ohio State University, Columbus, Ohio, USA

Chapter contents

Introduction, 1354
Physiologic changes related to age, 1355
Cardiovascular changes, 1355
Pulmonary changes, 1356
Neurocognitive and behavioral assessment, postoperative delirium, and cognitive impairment, 1356
Renal changes, 1356
Hepatic changes, 1357
Immune function, 1357
Changes in body composition, 1357
Thermoregulation, 1357
Frailty, 1357
Risk of anesthesia related to age, 1358
Preanesthetic testing, 1358
Age-related changes in response to drugs, 1359
Opioids, 1359
Propofol, 1359
Alfaxalone, 1359
Ketamine, 1359
Inhalant agents, 1359
Neuromuscular blocking agents, 1360
Anesthetic case management, 1360
Analgesic considerations, 1360
Supportive care, 1360
Nutrition, 1360
Environmental stressors, 1360
References, 1360

Introduction

A large study that included 8.9 million dogs and 2.4 million cats reported that life expectancy for both species increased between 2013 and 2019 [1]. Clinicians are anesthetizing more older pets and it is important to understand the specific changes that occur with age, and how these impact perioperative care and clinical outcomes. *Biological aging* can be defined as "the progressive accumulation of changes with time associated with or responsible for the ever-increasing susceptibility to disease and death" [2,3]. The American Animal Hospital Association (AAHA) has proposed the following life stages in dogs: puppy, young adult, mature adult, senior, and end of life [4]. The Association of American Feline Practitioners (AAFP) and AAHA, place cats into five life stages: kitten, young adult, mature adult, senior, and end of life [5]. These stages are somewhat arbitrary, especially in dogs, because they are based on chronological age and not biological age. Both organizations have recently published senior care guidelines, which delve deeper into defining senior and geriatric patients [6,7]; details are shown in Table 69.1. In dogs, the term senior is used to describe the last 25% of estimated lifespan through to the end of life [4]. Because the lifespan of dogs varies greatly based on breed and size, it has been difficult to accurately allocate dogs into this life stage [8]. Life expectancy tables based on size, sex, and body condition confirm that life expectancy is decreased for the largest sizes of dogs compared to the smallest and provide life expectancy data for toy, small, medium, large, and giant dogs [1]. These life expectancy tables allow for the correct allocation of any size of dog to the life stage of "senior." The term geriatric is a statement of health status and not a specific age [3,6]. McKenzie *et al.* have proposed the concept of the canine geriatric syndrome, which includes physical, behavioral, metabolic, and functional changes, frailty, clinical disease, and quality of life to facilitate the recognition of aging as a risk factor for negative health outcomes [3].

Anesthetic management encompasses the pre-, intra-, and postoperative period. Successful anesthetic management of older patients requires careful planning and includes an evaluation of comorbidities, functional status, frailty, nutrition, and a review of current medications. Older dogs and cats may have a variety of overt diseases (single or multiple) such as cardiac, renal, and hepatic disease. These disease processes require specific anesthetic management, which is covered elsewhere in this book. Access to a drug interaction checker (e.g., Plumb's drug interaction checker: https://plumbs.com/features/drug-interaction-checker/) is extremely helpful due to the number of drugs some older patients may have been prescribed. Patient care does not stop in the immediate recovery period; arrangements must be in place for postoperative care, which includes

Veterinary Anesthesia and Analgesia: The Sixth Edition of Lumb and Jones. Edited by Leigh Lamont, Kurt Grimm, Sheilah Robertson, Lydia Love and Carrie Schroeder.
© 2024 John Wiley & Sons, Inc. Published 2024 by John Wiley & Sons, Inc.
Companion website: www.wiley.com/go/lamont/anesthesia

Table 69.1 Proposed life stages and definitions in dogs and cats derived from the AAHA and AAFP life stages and senior care guidelines [4–7].

Life stage		Definition
Dog	Puppy	Birth to cessation of rapid growth (approximately 6 to 9 months, varying with breed and size)
	Young adult	Cessation of rapid growth to completion of physical and social maturation; 3 to 4 years in most dogs
	Mature adult	Completion of physical and social maturation until the last 25% of estimated lifespan (breed and size dependent)
	Senior	The last 25% of estimated lifespan through end of life The term "senior" is used to describe the older, aging pet. Because of the variability in aging based on breed and size, the chronological age of a senior will vary. Additional descriptive terms such as "frailty" are used to describe individuals
	End of life	Terminal stage (depends on specific pathologies)
Cat	Kitten	Birth to 1 year
	Young adult	1–6 years
	Mature adult	7–10 years
	Senior	> 10 years; some cats of specific breeds and genetic predispositions may be considered senior at an earlier chronological age
	End of life	Variable
	Geriatric	The term geriatric is a statement of health status and not a specific age

Table 69.2 A quick reference guide to age-related physiologic changes and their impact on anesthesia.

System	Age-related changes	Impact on anesthesia
Cardiovascular	Reduced cardiac reserve, blood volume, blood pressure, and cardiac output Reduced ability to compensate for cardiovascular changes	Slower onset of intravenous general anesthesia, resulting in increased risk of anesthetic overdose Inotropic and blood pressure support may be needed
Pulmonary/respiratory	Loss of lung elasticity and decrease in chest wall compliance Increase in functional residual capacity, with closing capacity increasing at a comparatively faster rate Increased ventilation–perfusion mismatching	Risk of hypoxemia and hypercapnia Respiratory support may be required
Neurologic	Reduction in brain mass and decreased neurotransmitters Reduced cerebral blood flow Altered central thermoregulation	Decreased anesthetic requirements Increased risk of hypothermia
Renal	Decreased renal function secondary to a reduction in GFR, RBF, and renal mass	Less tolerant of fluid losses, allow water to be consumed until the time of premedication
Hepatic/metabolic	Reduced hepatic mass and perfusion	Variable and unpredictable effects on drugs that undergo hepatic metabolism
Immunologic	Immunosenescence	May be more prone to infection Adhere to aseptic techniques

GFR, glomerular filtration rate; RBF, renal blood flow.

a period of time after discharge. The ideal approach to the older patient involves a multidisciplinary team comprised of anesthesiologists, surgeons, rehabilitation clinicians, internists, and nutritionists.

Physiologic changes related to age

The physical and functional changes associated with aging in dogs and cats are well described [8–14]. Veterinary geroscience is an active area of research with a goal of developing therapies to mitigate age-related dysfunction [3,15–17]. With respect to anesthesia in older animals, the key factor is understanding the impact of decreased functional or physiologic reserve in major body systems. In people, functional reserve in vital organs is reported to decrease by 1% every year after the age of 40 [18]. "Robustness" and "resilience" are terms that enhance the understanding of the aging process [19]. McKenzie encourages the use of "robustness" (the ability to resist deviation from an original or optimal state) and "resilience" (the ability to return to this state after deviations induced by external stressors) when assessing aging dogs [3,15]. These terms are easy to understand, and most clinicians know when they see an animal that is neither robust nor resilient and this may prompt a change in the anesthetic plan for these patients.

The following section and Table 69.2, describe and summarize the age-related changes in major body systems and their potential impact on anesthetic management; many detailed studies are available in humans, and it is assumed that similar changes occur in all mammalian species. The reader is referred to an excellent open-access clinical review by Lim and Lee [20].

Cardiovascular changes

Similar to humans, cardiac reserve is decreased with increasing age in dogs. Cardiac output (CO) is decreased by up to 30% in older dogs, maximum heart rate and oxygen consumption in response to exercise are reduced, ventricular contraction is reduced, and myocardial stiffness is increased [21–23].

In aging humans, blood pressure is higher and CO lower than in young populations due to changes in connective tissues resulting in stiffness of blood vessels and the myocardium [24]. Age-related changes in blood pressure have been reported in both dogs and cats [8,10,13,14,25].

Clinical implications

Preanesthetic measurement of blood pressure is recommended as a reasonable step in older dogs and cats [26] so that changes from normal values can be detected and managed appropriately during anesthesia. Cats may have anxiety and stress-related elevations in blood pressure but these can be partially mitigated by using feline-friendly handling techniques [27].

A decrease in CO will result in an increase in the injection site to brain circulation time; therefore, it is essential that intravenous anesthetic drugs are given slowly, allowing sufficient time for drugs to reach the brain and exert an effect before additional drugs are administered. Reduced cardiac reserve leaves older patients less able to respond to acute changes in blood volume (loss or overload) and hypotension compared to younger animals. Intravenous fluids should be administered to meet pre-existing needs and ongoing losses. Close cardiovascular monitoring is required, and inotropes and vasopressors should be available. Animals with a rightward shift in autoregulation due to chronic hypertension should be maintained within ~30% of their presenting blood pressure to ensure that perfusion to vital organs is maintained throughout the anesthetic event.

Pulmonary changes

Chest wall compliance decreases with age while lung compliance increases, increasing functional residual capacity (FRC) and the work of breathing [28]. Closing capacity also increases but faster than FRC and may eventually equal FRC, such that at normal tidal volume, areas of low or zero ventilation to perfusion ratios may exist. The surface area for gas exchange decreases; there is a reduction in diffusion capacity across the capillary–alveolar membrane; and respiratory muscle strength weakens [28]. Elderly humans (aged 65–79 years) have an approximately 50% reduction in ventilatory response to hypoxia and hypercapnia compared to young subjects [29]. Older humans have decreased pharyngeal muscle tone and less effective upper airway reflexes. This is likely true in dogs based on their incidence of aspiration pneumonia (see later). Laryngeal paralysis (a component of geriatric onset laryngeal paralysis and polyneuropathy [GOLPP]), a disease of older dogs, puts them at risk of aspiration and airway obstruction. Low-grade chronic inflammation ("inflamm-aging") has been reported in humans and is associated with an increased incidence of morbidity and mortality [30]. This is also likely to affect our aging veterinary patients. Using sterile endotracheal tubes, appropriate inflation of the endotracheal tube cuff, and suctioning of the oral cavity prior to extubation are some measures that can be used to help protect these animals.

In awake elderly patients, $PaCO_2$ and PaO_2 are usually well maintained, but when challenged by sedation and anesthesia involving respiratory depressant drugs, the lack of pulmonary reserve, decreased respiratory drive, and poor muscle strength render these patients at risk of hypoxemia and hypercapnia [31].

Clinical implications

Older dogs and cats should be closely monitored perioperatively using a pulse oximeter, and capnography intraoperatively to determine if ventilation is appropriate. Respiratory support using manual or mechanical ventilation may be needed, especially when patients are in dorsal recumbency. Preanesthetic administration of antinausea and antiemetic medications is advised [32]. Oxygen supplementation prior to induction of general anesthesia and in the postoperative period until the animal is able to maintain normal oxyhemoglobin saturation on room air is recommended [33].

Neurocognitive and behavioral assessment, postoperative delirium, and cognitive impairment

There are three distinct clinical problems associated with cognition in the postoperative period. *Emergence delirium* refers to restlessness in the immediate postoperative period and can occur in any age group, is usually short-lived, can be managed with sedation, and has no long-term effects. *Postoperative delirium* is defined as a "short-term and transient" issue and is characterized by changes in consciousness and cognition, disorientation, anxiety, and fear which may fluctuate [34]. A diagnosis of frailty before surgery is associated with an increased risk of postoperative delirium in human patients [35]. Postoperative delirium can occur in any age group, but elderly patients are at the highest risk. It appears between the second and seventh day following anesthesia, and the pathophysiology is poorly understood [34]. This syndrome likely occurs in animals but may go undetected because animals do not need to function at a high level of cognition, and we are unlikely to monitor for this in the extended postoperative period. However, there are enough reports by owners of their pets being "different" after anesthesia that this warrants further investigation. Interventions including frequent orientation, noise reduction, early mobilization, and attention to hydration are effective at reducing postoperative delirium in humans, all of which can be applied in veterinary medicine [34].

Postoperative cognitive dysfunction (POCD) refers to longer-term changes in cognition after surgery. It occurs in up to 12% of all patients and is usually self-limiting [34,36]. The elderly and patients with pre-existing cognitive impairment before surgery may show a dramatic decline after surgery [36]. No specific anesthetic drug or technique has been shown to cause or prevent POCD and the mechanism that triggers it is unknown [36]; however, some authors suggest that benzodiazepines should be avoided in elderly patients at high risk of developing POCD [20]. The majority of studies comparing POCD after general versus regional anesthesia fail to show a difference, suggesting that its etiology is complex and multifactorial [37].

Cognitive dysfunction (CD) is documented in dogs and cats and may affect up to 35% of aging dogs and more than 50% of cats over the age of fifteen [38–42]. Canine and feline CD are analogs of human Alzheimer's disease; therefore, postoperative delirium and worsening of cognition are likely to occur. Reports of cognitive decline after anesthesia in older dogs and cats are anecdotal but some clinicians state that owners should be informed of this possibility and that it is more evident in animals that have cognitive impairment prior to anesthesia [43]. Confusion, anxiety, disturbed sleep/wake cycle, and decreased interaction with owners are all common clinical signs of canine CD and these can be exacerbated by a hospital stay. Diagnosis of CD is not straightforward but older animals should at least be screened for CD prior to anesthesia so that clinicians can prepare for the recovery period; assessment tools are available for dogs and cats [6,44].

Failing vision and hearing in older patients may add to confusion in the postoperative period. Changes in environment are poorly tolerated by older animals, especially those with CD. Whenever possible these patients should be scheduled as outpatients; when creating the day's operating list, assign them the first slot so they can be cared for when the hospital is fully staffed and discharged at the end of the day.

Renal changes

There is a gradual decline in renal function with increasing age; however, a significant loss of functional nephrons must occur before this is detectable with routine testing. The dangers of reduced renal reserve related to anesthesia are real. Perioperative dehydration, hypovolemia, and hypotension are not well tolerated in older patients, and animals with reduced renal reserve may suffer acute kidney injury. Many older dogs and cats are prescribed non-steroidal anti-inflammatory drugs (NSAIDs) for maladaptive pain states putting them at a higher risk of renal insult. Cyclo-oxygenase-1 and 2 are constitutively expressed in the kidneys and the products of these pathways include prostaglandins (PGs) and thromboxanes, which are involved in the regulation of glomerular filtration rate (GFR) [45]. In the face of decreased renal perfusion (e.g., decreased circulating volume), renal PGs play a vital compensatory role, including vasodilation to enhance renal blood flow and GFR [46]. NSAIDs block the ability of the kidney to autoregulate.

Measurement of GFR is not a routine clinical test, though it may be reduced in patients with normal serum creatinine values [47]. Not knowing the GFR in older animals makes dosage adjustments of renally excreted drugs difficult. Gabapentin is a renally excreted drug and marked differences in serum concentrations were reported in normal cats compared to those with IRIS stage 2 and 3 chronic kidney disease (CKD) [48]. In the same study, serum gabapentin concentrations were correlated with serum creatinine and symmetric dimethylarginine, but it is not known if serum drug concentrations are correlated with GFR.

CKD is common in older pets, especially cats [6]. Perioperative management of patients with CKD is discussed in Chapter 43.

Clinical implications

Maintaining euvolemia and renal perfusion pressure during anesthesia is essential when renal reserves are reduced, therefore fluid therapy, blood pressure monitoring, and treatment of hypotension are primary considerations in this population. Renally excreted drugs should be used with caution in older patients.

Hepatic changes

In humans, liver mass and blood flow decrease with age [49,50]. Drugs that are processed via phase I reactions (involving the cytochrome P450 system) are "flow limited" and are likely to be cleared more slowly in older patients. Phase II elimination involves conjugation and drugs dependent on this pathway are less affected by age [50]. This is a simplistic approach and drug elimination is dependent on multiple factors; further details are available in Chapter 19. Liver enzymes do not reflect hepatic function, and hepatic function tests may be normal in older animals, yet their ability to clear drugs may be compromised.

Clinical implications

Due to the difficulty in predicting how an aging patient will process a specific drug, it is recommended that the anesthetist uses drugs that can be titrated to effect, have a high therapeutic index, and are reversible.

Immune function

Immunosenescence, which is defined as changes in the immune system associated with age, has received a lot of attention in humans, with increased vulnerability to infection and decreased immune response to vaccinations being recognized as contributing to mortality [51]. There is some, albeit limited, evidence that age-related changes in immune function occur in dogs and cats [15]. Age-related changes in the canine immune system are summarized by Bellows [10].

Clinical implications

Older animals should be considered at higher risk than young patients for developing perioperative infections. Urinary retention is a risk factor for infection in older humans but the use of indwelling urinary catheters, which are not without risk, must not be used as a substitute for good nursing care [20]. Animals should have their bladders expressed at the end of the procedure and provided opportunities to void voluntarily in the postoperative period – this requires assisting large dogs to stand and providing suitable litter-boxes to cats. If urinary catheters are used, they must be placed in a sterile fashion and properly maintained.

Changes in body composition

With increasing age, there is loss of muscle mass and an increase in adipose tissue in humans, dogs, and cats [15,50,52]. In dogs, these changes vary among different breeds and sizes [52]. Changes in the mass, structure, and function (increasing weakness) of skeletal muscle result in the clinical condition termed "sarcopenia," which is seen in all mammalian species as they age [15]. The loss of muscle mass decreases the ability of older patients to generate heat, leaving them vulnerable to hypothermia. Muscle also acts as an important "sink" for drugs prior to metabolism or excretion; therefore, older animals may maintain higher plasma concentrations of drugs for longer periods. Total body water, plasma, and intracellular volume are reduced in older patients. The consequence of these changes is a decrease in the central compartment and central volume of distribution. After a bolus of intravenous drugs, plasma concentrations are higher and can lead to more profound central nervous system effects.

Clinical implications

Muscle weakness must be addressed in the perioperative period; patients with sarcopenia may need help getting up and are more likely to slip and fall, resulting in injury. Due to pharmacokinetic changes induced by body composition differences, induction doses of anesthetics should be reduced to prevent deep levels of anesthesia and hypotension.

Thermoregulation

A decrease in metabolic rate occurs as dogs age [52] and this, combined with a decrease in muscle mass, makes aging patients vulnerable to hypothermia. Perioperative hypothermia is common in all dogs and cats irrespective of age, resulting in delayed recovery, altered coagulation, bradycardia, and decreased CO, and may be linked to postoperative wound infection [53–55]. Hypothermia decreases inhalant anesthetic requirements [56,57]. During recovery, hypothermic animals will shiver to generate heat, but this capacity is limited in older animals. Shivering during recovery can significantly increase oxygen consumption [33] and may lead to hypoxemia, lactic acidosis, and catecholamine release, all of which would be detrimental in patients with limited organ reserves [58,59]. People describe postoperative shivering as a highly unpleasant experience and we can assume this is the same in veterinary patients [60,61].

Clinical implications

Every effort should be made to prevent perioperative hypothermia (see Chapter 17). Oxygen supplementation should be in place until patients are normothermic.

Frailty

In humans, frailty is a predictor of postoperative outcomes, including morbidity, length of hospital stay, and mortality [35,62–66]. McIsaac *et al.* stated that the use of frailty instruments provides meaningful increases in accuracy when predicting postoperative outcomes for older people [67]. Frailty is distinct from comorbidity and disability, is not synonymous with aging, and is an important concept because there can be significant differences in health status between individuals of the same chronological age [68]. Diagnosing frailty allows the clinician to identify patients who are significantly more vulnerable compared to other individuals of the same age [64]. When anesthesiologists understand the concept of frailty, they can play a key role in improving clinical outcomes in this vulnerable patient population [69]. Frailty can be described as a multidimensional syndrome characterized by decreased physiologic reserve, a diminished resistance to stressors, a state of vulnerability, or a "deficit of homeostatic capabilities" [64,70]. In older patients, frailty should be assessed in addition to comorbidities when developing a perioperative plan. Frailty is a relatively new concept in human medicine with the frailty phenotype first being described by Fried *et al.* in 2001 [71]. In human medicine, many instruments have been developed to assess levels of frailty and work is being done to assess which tools are most relevant in patients scheduled for surgery [35,65,67]. The frailty phenotype model assesses fatigue, and measures muscle strength and walking speed. The frailty index counts the number of deficits in multiple domains, including physiological, psychological, and cognitive [64,68]. Assessments can alert the care team to the special needs of an individual and if surgery is elective, prehabilitation can be used to improve a patient's functional reserve and reduce risk [66,69].

Frailty and its impact on healthspan and mortality risk in companion animals is an area of active research in dogs [3,72–74] and is receiving attention in cats [6]. A five-component frailty phenotype (chronic undernutrition, poor mobility, exhaustion, low physical activity level, and weakness) has been described in dogs and confirms that frailty is a risk factor for death and that the number of components present is predictive of increased risk [72]. A clinically based frailty index tool has been developed for dogs and a questionnaire is included in the publication by Banzato *et al.* [73]. Chen *et al.* demonstrated validity of this tool; frailty scores increased with age and were correlated with a decrease in health-related quality of life [74]. The AAFP has developed a phenotype frailty scale and an index frailty scale that are easy to use in cats [6]. In human medicine, many groups including the American Society of Surgeons and the Association of Anesthetists of Great Britain and Ireland recommend frailty assessment before surgery; however, these are not yet performed routinely [35]. In addition to assigning an ASA score, veterinarians are encouraged to assess frailty in patients scheduled for surgery.

Risk of anesthesia related to age

Morbidity and mortality risks associated with anesthesia are covered in detail in Chapter 2. Morbidity and mortality specifically related to age will be discussed here. An increased risk of anesthetic-related death with increasing age, and independent of patient physical status, has been reported in dogs and cats [75–79]. Although analyzing data based on chronological age alone is problematic in dogs, increasing age is consistently flagged as a risk factor. In a study of mortality related to general anesthesia and sedation in dogs in primary practice in the United Kingdom, dogs over nine years of age were 12 times more likely to die than those between six months and 1.5 years [79]. Brodbelt *et al.* reported that cats over the age of 12 were 2.1 times more likely to die than cats aged six months to five years [76]. In a more recent study in primary care veterinary hospitals in the United States, Matthews *et al.* reported that the odds of death in a cat aged nine years were more than twice that of one four years of age [78].

The key question for clinicians is "can the risks associated with anesthesia in older animals be mitigated and what interventions are effective?" Risk factors related to increasing age include gastroesophageal reflux (GER) and aspiration pneumonia, and these risks can be mitigated.

GER, regurgitation, aspiration pneumonia, and vomiting are common adverse events associated with anesthesia in dogs and can result in devastating outcomes; mortality from aspiration pneumonia can be as high as 25% with increasing patient age correlated with non-survival [32]. GER during anesthesia is significantly associated with age [80]. Postoperative regurgitation and vomiting (PORV) were reported in 12.3% of all dogs undergoing non-elective surgery [81]. The risk of developing aspiration pneumonia was higher in dogs over the age of eight and those with laryngeal disease (e.g., GOLPP) [82,83]. Galatos and Raptopoulos reported an overall incidence of GER of 17.4 % of dogs in their study, with increased age being associated with an increased incidence of gastric acidity [84].

In people, the Enhanced Recovery After Surgery [ERAS®] (www.erassociety.org) program permits patients to consume solid food for up to 6 h and a carbohydrate supplement drink for up to 2 h prior to surgery. The ERAS program demonstrated that this guideline reduces the risk of complications caused by aspiration during the induction of anesthesia, significantly improves discomfort (from hunger and thirst), and maintains lean body mass after surgery [85].

There are conflicting reports on the effect of preoperative fasting times on gastric acidity and GER in dogs, likely due to the multiple different anesthetic protocols used [84,86,87]. There is some evidence to support shorter fasting times (under 5 h) with one study reporting the incidence of GER to be significantly lower if dogs were fed half their daily ration of canned food 3 h before anesthesia compared to 10 h [87]. However, another clinical study reported that 61% of dogs fed a partial daily ration of canned food 3 h prior to anesthesia had GER compared to 43.9% of dogs fasted for 18 h [80]. Since no fasting strategy can prevent GER, other measures should be implemented.

Maropitant and famotidine appear to be effective at mitigating some of these adverse events; of 105 dogs over the age of eight premedicated with maropitant and famotidine, none vomited, two regurgitated (1.9%), and one (1%) developed aspiration pneumonia [32]. Other studies strongly support that changes to anesthetic protocols [88], the use of higher doses of metoclopramide [89], or the use of esomeprazole and cisapride [90] can reduce the risk of aspiration pneumonia. It should be noted that GER is "silent" and often goes unnoticed; therefore, it is advised that the esophagus be suctioned and flushed after induction and before recovery [91].

Preanesthetic testing

Preanesthetic blood screening is not required for every patient (Chapter 2). It should be noted that reference ranges for many laboratory tests only incorporate approximately 95% of the population; therefore, 1 in 20 animals will show results outside a "normal" range, yet these may be of no clinical significance. Blood work in one hundred "apparently healthy senior and geriatric dogs" revealed increased serum creatinine, hypophosphatemia, increased ALP, increased ALT, and leukopenia in 32, 29, 27, 25, and 23 dogs, respectively [8]. Results of serum biochemistry and hematologic tests in older dogs and cats should be compared to age-dependent laboratory reference ranges to differentiate healthy aging from disease [8,9,12,14].

Joubert recruited 101 dogs over the age of seven that were to be anesthetized to assess whether hematologic and biochemical analyses were of value in this population [92]. In 30 dogs, a new diagnosis was made (e.g., neoplasia and hyperadrenocorticism) as a result of blood work, and 13 of these had their procedure canceled. However, Joubert suggested that there was little evidence to show that blood results impacted the anesthetic management of dogs that did proceed to surgery. In another study, the results of routine non-targeted blood testing in dogs and cats over the age of eight were predicted by anesthetists in most cases and did not result in major changes in anesthetic management [93]. In a United Kingdom study of preanesthetic blood testing in dogs and cats (mean age 9.6 and 11.6 years respectively), abnormal blood results raised concerns by clinicians in approximately 8% and 16% of dogs and cats, respectively, although only 1% of these results were unexpected based on the animal's history and physical examination [94]. Abnormal blood results led to postponement of some cases and adjustments to the anesthetic management in 4% of dogs and 9% of cats [94].

Clinical implications

Blood work results should be compared with animals within the same age group and considered in conjunction with the patient's history and clinical examination.

Age-related changes in response to drugs

The pharmacologic concerns related to anesthesia drug use in older humans are similar to those in the aging veterinary population and focus on the increased sensitivity to drugs in this population [95].

Opioids

Elderly humans are at greater risk than younger patients of adverse events and unpredictable responses related to opioid administration [96]. The reasons are multifactorial but include altered pharmacokinetics due to changes in body composition and organ function, and altered pharmacodynamics secondary to impaired neurotransmitter production and altered receptor affinity [95,96]. Senior and geriatric patients require perioperative analgesics and may be at risk of inadequate treatment because of the fear of adverse effects and because many in this population already suffer from maladaptive pain (e.g., osteoarthritis).

Age-related changes in the pharmacokinetics of pethidine administered postoperatively have been reported in dogs [97]. Compared to young dogs, the rate of absorption of pethidine from intramuscular sites was slower (T_{max} delayed), C_{max} was lower, and elimination half-life was significantly longer in dogs over the age of 10 [97,98]. Plasma clearance was not different between the two age groups, suggesting that the distribution of the drug is altered in the older population [97].

Propofol

The induction and infusion doses of propofol in humans show age-related changes [99]. At the same plasma concentration, the reduction in blood pressure is greater, whereas the time to reach a specific depth of anesthesia and the time to recovery are longer in older versus young patients [95,100]. A failure to age-adjust dosages may contribute to hypotensive episodes, which can have serious consequences in a population with reduced reserves [95].

The pharmacokinetics of propofol have been studied in dogs 8.5 to 10.5 years of age and, as these dogs weighed 29 ± 7.4 kg (mean ± SD), they could be classified as senior [101]. Despite a lower induction dosage (5 mg/kg), apnea occurred in four out of six (66%) dogs after induction, which is higher than the reported 25% in younger dogs given 6.5 mg/kg, by the same investigators [102]. The blood levels of propofol were higher despite the lower dosage, and the clearance was slower in older dogs compared to young dogs [101,102].

Alfaxalone

Alfaxalone has a high therapeutic index compared to propofol [103–105] but is not devoid of cardiopulmonary depressant effects and should be given slowly and titrated to effect.

Ketamine

Ketamine has a high therapeutic index as well as anesthetic-sparing, antinociceptive, and antihyperalgesic properties, which may make it a good choice for older patients, especially those with chronic pain [106,107]. It also mitigates postanesthetic hypothermia [108]. Constant rate infusions preceded by a subanesthetic loading dose may be especially beneficial as these are associated with fewer cardiovascular changes (tachycardia and increased blood pressure) than anesthetic doses [109].

Inhalant agents

The influence of age on the minimum alveolar concentration (MAC) of inhalant agents is well documented in humans, decreasing by approximately 6% per decade after the age of 40 [57,110]. The increased sensitivity to inhalant agents is thought to be caused by age-related changes in the brain, including changes in receptor numbers or function. The MAC of isoflurane in 2- to 3-year-old and 11-year-old Beagles was reported as 1.82 ± 0.8% (mean ± SEM) and 1.45 ± 0.6%, respectively; when adjusted for altitude, the mean MAC values at sea level were 1.53% and 1.22% in young and older dogs, respectively [111]. Binding of glutamate to the excitatory receptor *N*-methyl-D-aspartate (NMDA) in multiple brain regions was decreased in older dogs, and the change in NMDA receptors was associated with an increased sensitivity to isoflurane [111]. This study could not determine if the changes in binding were due to changes in affinity or a decrease in binding sites. Another study using Beagles determined the MAC of sevoflurane to be 2.25 ± 0.15% (mean ± SD) at age two and 1.86 ± 0.9% at eight to ten years of age [112]. Dogs in the older age group showed mild to moderate cardiorespiratory depression (lower heart rate, indirect blood pressure, and SpO_2) than younger dogs at an equipotent dose of sevoflurane, indicating that close monitoring is essential in older patients [112].

Body temperature also influences MAC, with hypothermia decreasing anesthetic requirements; an approximately 4–5% decrease in MAC occurs for each 1 °C fall in temperature [57]. Older animals are susceptible to hypothermia; therefore, a combination of age-related changes and hypothermia puts them at risk for anesthetic overdose. Vaporizer settings or inspired concentrations of inhalant agents should be adjusted based on a critical evaluation of the patient's depth of anesthesia (see Chapters 10 and 16).

Clinical implications

The extent of increased sensitivity to anesthetics in aging patients is underappreciated by many practitioners but is also unpredictable. Preference should be given to drugs that are reversible and those that can be titrated to effect. Vaporizer settings or inspired concentrations of inhalant agents should be adjusted based on a critical evaluation of the patient's depth of anesthesia.

Neuromuscular blocking agents

The pharmacokinetics and pharmacodynamics of neuromuscular blockade are altered in elderly human patients with postoperative residual curarization (PORC) predisposing to hypoxemia and upper airway obstruction in this population [113–115]. The differences in response to neuromuscular blocking agents (NMBAs) in elderly humans appear to be related to altered pharmacokinetics (e.g., age-related alterations in distribution, metabolism, and excretion) rather than pharmacodynamics because the physiology of the neuromuscular junction is not significantly altered by age [113,114]. Some authors however suggest that the variability in recovery from neuromuscular blockade in the elderly may also be related to neuromuscular junction dysfunction [95]. Although there are no similar studies in dogs and cats, the risks of PORC in the aging dogs and cat populations should be taken seriously.

Clinical implications

Close neuromuscular monitoring and pharmacologic reversal are key components to prevent PORC and are discussed in Chapter 26.

Anesthetic case management

An appropriate anesthetic and analgesic protocol for aging animals should be based on an assessment of the animal's physical and health status and utilize drugs that best fit the needs of the animal, as described above. There is no one protocol that should be used for all older animals, however, it is recommended to use drugs that are reversible, have a high therapeutic index, and are titratable to effect.

Care with positioning of these patients is important to prevent postoperative discomfort. In humans, one of the risks for position-related pain after surgery is the presence of preoperative pain [116]. Many older veterinary patients will have osteoarthritis-related pain and care should be taken to place them in neutral positions to prevent exacerbation of joint and muscle pain postoperatively.

Analgesic considerations

As with all patients, providing perioperative analgesia is an important component of an anesthetic plan. The analgesic drugs and techniques covered in other chapters are all applicable to aging patients.

Supportive care

Nutrition

In people, nutritional support can have a large impact on postoperative outcomes, including decreasing the length of hospital stay, shortening the "time to eat," less weight loss, and fewer medical complications [117]. Nutritional care is a key component of the ERAS® global initiative (www.erassociety.org). The role of perioperative nutritional care is likely underestimated in older dogs and cats and deserves investigation. Short fasting times, the use of antiemetic and antinausea medication, appetite stimulants, and provision of palatable and easily digestible food should all be considered in a comprehensive plan for aging pets. Administration of maropitant in dogs given morphine resulted in an earlier return to feeding and increased calorie intake after surgery but this effect was not reported when non-emetic opioids such as buprenorphine were used [118].

Environmental stressors

Older patients may have a degree of cognitive decline and impaired hearing and vision, which can lead to confusion during a hospital stay. Limiting external stimuli (noise, light) may aid in a more restful environment, and limiting the number of people interacting with the patient may decrease confusion and allow the pet to bond with one or two team members. Owners should be encouraged to bring familiar objects from home to leave with their pets. The use of low-stress techniques such as feline-friendly nursing [119] will enhance recovery. As previously stated, early return to a familiar environment should be prioritized and it is advisable to schedule this population as outpatients whenever possible.

References

1 Montoya M, Morrison JA, Arrignon F, *et al.* Life expectancy tables for dogs and cats derived from clinical data. *Front Vet Sci* 2023; **10**: 1082102.
2 Harman D. The aging process. *Proc Natl Acad Sci USA* 1981; **78**(11): 7124–7128.
3 McKenzie BA, Chen FL, Gruen ME, *et al.* Canine geriatric syndrome: a framework for advancing research in veterinary geroscience. *Front Vet Sci* 2022; **9**: 853743.
4 Creevy KE, Grady J, Little SE, *et al.* 2019 AAHA canine life stage guidelines. *J Am Anim Hosp Assoc* 2019; **55**(6): 267–290.
5 Quimby J, Gowland S, Carney HC, *et al.* 2021 AAHA/AAFP feline life stage guidelines. *J Feline Med Surg* 2021; **23**(3): 211–233.
6 Ray M, Carney HC, Boynton B, *et al.* 2021 AAFP feline senior care guidelines. *J Feline Med Surg* 2021; **23**(7): 613–638.
7 Dhaliwal R, Boynton E, Carrera-Justiz S, *et al.* 2023 AAHA senior care guidelines for dogs and cats. *J Am Anim Hosp Assoc* 2023; **59**(1): 1–21.
8 Willems A, Paepe D, Marynissen S, *et al.* Results of screening of apparently healthy senior and geriatric dogs. *J Vet Intern Med* 2017; **31**(1): 81–92.
9 Bellows J, Colitz CM, Daristotle L, *et al.* Defining healthy aging in older dogs and differentiating healthy aging from disease. *J Am Vet Med Assoc* 2015; **246**(1): 77–89.
10 Bellows J, Colitz CM, Daristotle L, *et al.* Common physical and functional changes associated with aging in dogs. *J Am Vet Med Assoc* 2015; **246**(1): 67–75.
11 Bellows J, Center S, Daristotle L, *et al.* Aging in cats: common physical and functional changes. *J Feline Med Surg* 2016; **18**(7): 533–550.
12 Bellows J, Center S, Daristotle L, *et al.* Evaluating aging in cats: how to determine what is healthy and what is disease. *J Feline Med Surg* 2016; **18**(7): 551–570.
13 Dowgray N, Pinchbeck G, Eyre K, *et al.* Aging in cats: owner observations and clinical finding in 206 mature cats at enrolment to the cat prospective aging and welfare study. *Front Vet Sci* 2022; **9**: 859041.
14 Paepe D, Verjans G, Duchateau L, *et al.* Routine health screening: findings in apparently healthy middle-aged and old cats. *J Feline Med Surg* 2013; **15**(1): 8–19.
15 McKenzie BA. Comparative veterinary geroscience: mechanism of molecular, cellular, and tissue aging in humans, laboratory animal models, and companion dogs and cats. *Am J Vet Res* 2022; **83**(6): ajvr.22.02.0027.
16 McKenzie BA, Chen F, LaCroix-Fralish ML. The phenotype of aging in the dog: how aging impacts the health and well-being of dogs and their caregivers. *J Am Vet Med Assoc* 2022; **260**(9): 963–970.
17 McKenzie BA, Chen FL. Assessment and management of declining physical function in aging dogs. *Top Companion Anim Med* 2022; **51**: 100732.
18 Evers BM, Townsend CM Jr., Thompson JC. Organ physiology of aging. *Surg Clin North Am* 1994; **74**(1): 23–39.
19 Ukraintseva S, Yashin AI, Arbeev KG. Resilience versus robustness in aging. *J Gerontol A Biol Sci Med Sci* 2016; **71**(11): 1533–1534.
20 Lim BG, Lee IO. Anesthetic management of geriatric patients. *Korean J Anesthesiol* 2020; **73**(1): 8–29.
21 Bright JM, Mears E. Chronic heart disease and its management. *Vet Clin North Am Small Anim Pract* 1997; **27**(6): 1305–1329.
22 Strasser A, Simunek M, Seiser M, *et al.* Age-dependent changes in cardiovascular and metabolic responses to exercise in beagle dogs. *Zentralbl Veterinarmed A* 1997; **44**(8): 449–460.
23 Templeton GH, Platt MR, Willerson JT, *et al.* Influence of aging on left ventricular hemodynamics and stiffness in Beagles. *Circ Res* 1979; **44**(2): 189–194.
24 Alvis BD, Hughes CG. Physiology considerations in geriatric patients. *Anesthesiol Clin* 2015; **33**(3): 447–456.
25 Bijsmans ES, Jepson RE, Chang YM, *et al.* Changes in systolic blood pressure over time in healthy cats and cats with chronic kidney disease. *J Vet Intern Med* 2015; **29**(3): 855–861.
26 Acierno MJ, Brown S, Coleman AE, *et al.* ACVIM consensus statement: guidelines for the identification, evaluation, and management of systemic hypertension in dogs and cats. *J Vet Intern Med* 2018; **32**(6): 1803–1822.

27 Rodan I, Dowgray N, Carney HC, *et al.* 2022 AAFP/ISFM cat friendly veterinary interaction guidelines: approach and handling techniques. *J Feline Med Surg* 2022; **24**(11): 1093–1132.

28 Janssens JP, Pache JC, Nicod LP. Physiological changes in respiratory function associated with ageing. *Eur Respir J* 1999; **13**(1): 197–205.

29 Peterson DD, Pack AI, Silage DA, *et al.* Effects of aging on ventilatory and occlusion pressure responses to hypoxia and hypercapnia. *Am Rev Respir Dis* 1981; **124**(4): 387–391.

30 Boe DM, Boule LA, Kovacs EJ. Innate immune responses in the aging lung. *Clin Exp Immunol* 2017; **187**(1): 16–25.

31 Hedenstierna G, Tokics L, Scaramuzzo G, *et al.* Oxygenation impairment during anesthesia: influence of age and body weight. *Anesthesiology* 2019; **131**(1): 46–57.

32 Moyer AL, McKee TS, Bergman PJ, *et al.* Low incidence of postoperative nausea, vomiting, regurgitation, and aspiration pneumonia in geriatric dogs receiving maropitant, famotidine, and fentanyl as part of an anesthesia protocol. *J Am Vet Med Assoc* 2021; **260**(S1): S46–S51.

33 Hughes J. Anaesthesia for the geriatric dog and cat. *Ir Vet J* 2008; **61**(6): 380–387.

34 Bekker AY, Weeks EJ. Cognitive function after anaesthesia in the elderly. *Best Pract Res Clin Anaesthesiol* 2003; **17**(2): 259–272.

35 Aucoin SD, Hao M, Sohi R, *et al.* Accuracy and feasibility of clinically applied frailty instruments before surgery: a systematic review and meta-analysis. *Anesthesiology* 2020; **133**(1): 78–95.

36 Needham MJ, Webb CE, Bryden DC. Postoperative cognitive dysfunction and dementia: what we need to know and do. *Br J Anaesth* 2017; **119**(suppl 1): i115–i125.

37 Davis N, Lee M, Lin AY, *et al.* Postoperative cognitive function following general versus regional anesthesia: a systematic review. *J Neurosurg Anesthesiol* 2014; **26**(4): 369–376.

38 MacQuiddy B, Moreno JA, Kusick B, *et al.* Assessment of risk factors in dogs with presumptive advanced canine cognitive dysfunction. *Front Vet Sci* 2022; **9**: 958488.

39 Dewey CW, Davies ES, Xie H, *et al.* Canine cognitive dysfunction: pathophysiology, diagnosis, and treatment. *Vet Clin North Am Small Anim Pract* 2019; **49**(3): 477–499.

40 Chapagain D, Range F, Huber L, *et al.* Cognitive aging in dogs. *Gerontology* 2018; **64**(2): 165–171.

41 Sordo L, Gunn-Moore DA. Cognitive dysfunction in cats: update on neuropathological and behavioural changes plus clinical management. *Vet Rec* 2021; **188**(1): e3.

42 Gunn-Moore D, Moffat K, Christie LA, *et al.* Cognitive dysfunction and the neurobiology of aging in cats. *J Small Anim Pract* 2007; **48**(10): 546–553.

43 Rigotti CF, Brearley JC. Anaesthesia for paediatric and geriatric patients. In: Duke-Novakovski T, deVries M, Seymour C, eds. *BSAVA Manual of Canine and Feline Anaesthesia and Analgesia*, 3rd edn. Quedgeley, UK: British Small Animal Association, 2016: 418–427.

44 Le Brech S, Amat M, Temple D, *et al.* Evaluation of two practical tools to assess cognitive impairment in aged dogs. *Animals (Basel)* 2022; **12**(24): 3538.

45 Kim GH. Renal effects of prostaglandins and cyclooxygenase-2 inhibitors. *Electrolyte Blood Press* 2008; **6**(1): 35–41.

46 Harris RC Jr. Cyclooxygenase-2 inhibition and renal physiology. *Am J Cardiol* 2002; **89**(6a): 10D–17D.

47 Kannapiran M, Nisha D, Madhusudhana Rao A. Underestimation of impaired kidney function with serum creatinine. *Indian J Clin Biochem* 2010; **25**(4): 380–384.

48 Quimby JM, Lorbach SK, Saffire A, *et al.* Serum concentrations of gabapentin in cats with chronic kidney disease. *J Feline Med Surg* 2022; **24**(12): 1260–1266.

49 McLean AJ, Le Couteur DG. Aging biology and geriatric clinical pharmacology. *Pharmacol Rev* 2004; **56**(2): 163–184.

50 Rana MV, Bonasera LK, Bordelon GJ. Pharmacologic considerations of anesthetic agents in geriatric patients. *Anesthesiol Clin* 2017; **35**(2): 259–271.

51 Danielle Aw, Silva AB, Palmer DB. Immunosenescence: emerging challenges for an aging population. *Immunology* 2007; **120**(4): 435–446.

52 Speakman JR, van Acker A, Harper EJ. Age-related changes in the metabolism and body composition of three dog breeds and their relationship to life expectancy. *Aging Cell* 2003; **2**(5): 265–275.

53 Pottie RG, Dart CM, Perkins NR, *et al.* Effect of hypothermia on recovery from general anaesthesia in the dog. *Aust Vet J* 2007; **85**(4): 158–162.

54 Redondo JI, Suesta P, Gil L, *et al.* Retrospective study of the prevalence of postanaesthetic hypothermia in cats. *Vet Rec* 2012; **170**(8): 206.

55 Clark-Price S. Inadvertent perianesthetic hypothermia in small animal patients. *Vet Clin North Am Small Anim Pract* 2015; **45**(5): 983–994.

56 Regan MJ, Eger EI II. Effect of hypothermia in dogs on anesthetizing and apneic doses of inhalation agents. Determination of the anesthetic index (Apnea/MAC). *Anesthesiology* 1967; **28**(4): 689–700.

57 Eger EI II. Age, minimum alveolar anesthetic concentration, and minimum alveolar anesthetic concentration-awake. *Anesth Analg* 2001; **93**(4): 947–953.

58 Lopez MB. Postanaesthetic shivering – from pathophysiology to prevention. *Rom J Anaesth Intensive Care* 2018; **25**(1): 73–81.

59 Frank SM, Fleisher LA, Olson KF, *et al.* Multivariate determinants of early postoperative oxygen consumption in elderly patients. Effects of shivering, body temperature, and gender. *Anesthesiology* 1995; **83**(2): 241–249.

60 Matsota PK, Koliantzaki IK, Kostopanagiotou GG. Pharmacological approach for the prevention of postoperative shivering: a systematic review of prospective randomized controlled trials. *Asian J Anesthesiol* 2019; **57**(3): 66–84.

61 Díaz M, Becker DE. Thermoregulation: physiological and clinical considerations during sedation and general anesthesia. *Anesth Prog* 2010; **57**(1): 25–32.

62 Lin HS, Watts JN, Peel NM, *et al.* Frailty and post-operative outcomes in older surgical patients: a systematic review. *BMC Geriatr* 2016; **16**(1): 157.

63 Hewitt J, Long S, Carter B, *et al.* The prevalence of frailty and its association with clinical outcomes in general surgery: a systematic review and meta-analysis. *Age Aging* 2018; **47**(6): 793–800.

64 McIsaac DI, MacDonald DB, Aucoin SD. Frailty for Perioperative clinicians: a narrative review. *Anesth Analg* 2020; **130**(6): 1450–1460.

65 Alkadri J, Hage D, Nickerson LH, *et al.* A systematic review and meta-analysis of preoperative frailty instruments derived from electronic health data. *Anesth Analg* 2021; **133**(5): 1094–1106.

66 Olotu C, Weimann A, Bahrs C, *et al.* The perioperative care of older patients. *Dtsch Arztebl Int* 2019; **116**(5): 63–69.

67 McIsaac DI, Harris EP, Hladkowicz E, *et al.* Prospective comparison of preoperative predictive performance between 3 leading frailty instruments. *Anesth Analg* 2020; **131**(1): 263–272.

68 Mitnitski AB, Mogilner AJ, Rockwood K. Accumulation of deficits as a proxy measure of aging. *Sci World J* 2001; **1**: 323–336.

69 Whitlock EL, Whittington RA. The frailty syndrome: anesthesiologists must understand more and fear less. *Anesth Analg* 2020; **130**(6): 1445–1448.

70 Whitlock EL. Frailty: more than the sum of its parts? *Anesth Analg* 2021; **133**(5): 1090–1093.

71 Fried LP, Tangen CM, Walston J, *et al.* Frailty in older adults: evidence for a phenotype. *J Gerontol A Biol Sci Med Sci* 2001; **56**(3): M146–M156.

72 Hua J, Hoummady S, Muller C, *et al.* Assessment of frailty in aged dogs. *Am J Vet Res* 2016; **77**(12): 1357–1365.

73 Banzato T, Franzo G, Di Maggio R, *et al.* A Frailty Index based on clinical data to quantify mortality risk in dogs. *Sci Rep* 2019; **9**(1): 16749.

74 Chen FL, Ullal TV, Graves JL, *et al.* Evaluating instruments for assessing healthspan: a multi-center cross-sectional study on Health-Related Quality of Life (HRQL) and frailty in the companion dog. *Geroscience* 2023; **45**(4): 2089–2108.

75 Hosgood G, Scholl D. Evalution of age as a risk factor for perianesthetic morbidity and mortality in the dog. *J Vet Emerg Crit Care (San Antonio)* 1998; **8**(3): 222–236.

76 Brodbelt DC, Pfeiffer DU, Young LE, *et al.* Risk factors for anaesthetic-related death in cats: results from the Confidential Enquiry into Perioperative Small Animal Fatalities (CEPSAF). *Br J Anaesth* 2007; **99**(5): 617–623.

77 Brodbelt DC, Pfeiffer DU, Young LE, *et al.* Results of the Confidential Enquiry into Perioperative Small Animal Fatalities regarding risk factors for anesthetic-related death in dogs. *J Am Vet Med Assoc* 2008; **233**(7): 1096–1104.

78 Matthews NS, Mohn TJ, Yang M, *et al.* Factors associated with anesthetic-related death in dogs and cats in primary care veterinary hospitals. *J Am Vet Med Assoc* 2017; **250**(6): 655–665.

79 Shoop-Worrall SJ, O'Neill DG, Viscasillas J, *et al.* Mortality related to general anaesthesia and sedation in dogs under UK primary veterinary care. *Vet Anaesth Analg* 2022; **49**(5): 433–442.

80 Viskjer S, Sjöström L. Effect of the duration of food withholding prior to anesthesia on gastroesophageal reflux and regurgitation in healthy dogs undergoing elective orthopedic surgery. *Am J Vet Res* 2017; **78**(2): 144–150.

81 Davies JA, Fransson BA, Davis AM, *et al.* Incidence of and risk factors for postoperative regurgitation and vomiting in dogs: 244 cases (2000–2012). *J Am Vet Med Assoc* 2015; **246**(3): 327–335.

82 Kogan DA, Johnson LR, Jandrey KE, *et al.* Clinical, clinicopathologic, and radiographic findings in dogs with aspiration pneumonia: 88 cases (2004–2006). *J Am Vet Med Assoc* 2008; **233**(11): 1742–1747.

83 Kogan DA, Johnson LR, Sturges BK, *et al.* Etiology and clinical outcome in dogs with aspiration pneumonia: 88 cases (2004–2006). *J Am Vet Med Assoc* 2008; **233**(11): 1748–1755.

84 Galatos AD, Raptopoulos D. Gastro-oesophageal reflux during anaesthesia in the dog: the effect of age, positioning and type of surgical procedure. *Vet Rec* 1995; **137**(20): 513–516.

85 Lassen K, Soop M, Nygren J, *et al.* Consensus review of optimal perioperative care in colorectal surgery: Enhanced Recovery After Surgery (ERAS) Group recommendations. *Arch Surg* 2009; **144**(10): 961–969.

86 Savvas I, Pavlidou K, Anagnostou T, *et al.* Factors affecting intraoperative gastro-oesophageal reflux in dogs and cats. *Animals (Basel)* 2022; **12**(3): 247.

87 Savvas I, Raptopoulos D, Rallis T. A "light meal" three hours preoperatively decreases the incidence of gastro-esophageal reflux in dogs. *J Am Anim Hosp Assoc* 2016; **52**(6): 357–363.

88 Baetge C, Cummings KJ, Deveau M. Reduced risk of pneumonia after changes in anesthetic procedures for dogs receiving repeated anesthesia for radiation treatment. *Vet Radiol Ultrasound* 2019; **60**(2): 241–245.

89 Wilson DV, Evans AT, Mauer WA. Influence of metoclopramide on gastroesophageal reflux in anesthetized dogs. *Am J Vet Res* 2006; **67**(1): 26–31.

90 Zacuto AC, Marks SL, Osborn J, *et al.* The influence of esomeprazole and cisapride on gastroesophageal reflux during anesthesia in dogs. *J Vet Intern Med* 2012; **26**(3): 518–525.

91 Allison A, Italiano M, Robinson R. Comparison of two topical treatments of gastro-oesophageal regurgitation in dogs during general anaesthesia. *Vet Anaesth Analg* 2020; **47**(5): 672–675.

92 Joubert KE. Pre-anaesthetic screening of geriatric dogs. *J S Afr Vet Assoc* 2007; **78**(1): 31–35.

93 Díaz MDM, Kaartinen J, Allison A. Preanaesthetic blood tests in cats and dogs older than 8 years: anaesthetists' prediction and peri-anaesthetic changes. *Vet Anaesth Analg* 2021; **48**(6): 854–860.

94 Davies M, Kawaguchi S. Pregeneral anaesthetic blood screening of dogs and cats attending a UK practice. *Vet Rec* 2014; **174**(20): 506.

95 Akhtar S. Pharmacological considerations in the elderly. *Curr Opin Anaesthesiol* 2018; **31**(1): 11–18.

96 Wilder-Smith OH. Opioid use in the elderly. *Eur J Pain* 2005; **9**(2): 137–140.

97 Waterman AE, Kalthum W. Pharmacokinetics of pethidine administered intramuscularly and intravenously to dogs over 10 years old. *Res Vet Sci* 1990; **48**(2): 245–248.

98 Waterman AE, Kalthum W. Pharmacokinetics of intramuscularly administered pethidine in dogs and the influence of anaesthesia and surgery. *Vet Rec* 1989; **124**(12): 293–296.

99 Schnider TW, Minto CF, Shafer SL, *et al.* The influence of age on propofol pharmacodynamics. *Anesthesiology* 1999; **90**(6): 1502–1516.

100 Schultz A, Grouven U, Zander I, *et al.* Age-related effects in the EEG during propofol anaesthesia. *Acta Anaesthesiol Scand* 2004; **48**(1): 27–34.

101 Reid J, Nolan AM. Pharmacokinetics of propofol as an induction agent in geriatric dogs. *Res Vet Sci* 1996; **61**(2): 169–171.

102 Nolan AM, Reid J, Grant S. The effects of halothane and nitrous oxide on the pharmacokinetics of propofol in dogs. *J Vet Pharmacol Ther* 1993; **16**(3): 335–342.

103 Muir W, Lerche P, Wiese A, *et al.* The cardiorespiratory and anesthetic effects of clinical and supraclinical doses of alfaxalone in cats. *Vet Anaesth Analg* 2009; **36**(1): 42–54.

104 Muir W, Lerche P, Wiese A, *et al.* Cardiorespiratory and anesthetic effects of clinical and supraclinical doses of alfaxalone in dogs. *Vet Anaesth Analg* 2008; **35**(6): 451–462.

105 Bayldon W, Carter JE, Beths T, *et al.* Accidental alfaxalone overdose in a mature cat undergoing anaesthesia for magnetic resonance imaging. *JFMS Open Rep* 2016; **2**(1): 2055116916647740.

106 Kaka U, Saifullah B, Abubakar AA, *et al.* Serum concentration of ketamine and antinociceptive effects of ketamine and ketamine-lidocaine infusions in conscious dogs. *BMC Vet Res* 2016; **12**(1): 198.

107 Muir WW III, Wiese AJ, March PA. Effects of morphine, lidocaine, ketamine, and morphine-lidocaine-ketamine drug combination on minimum alveolar concentration in dogs anesthetized with isoflurane. *Am J Vet Res* 2003; **64**(9): 1155–1160.

108 Bornkamp JL, Robertson S, Isaza NM, *et al.* Effects of anesthetic induction with a benzodiazepine plus ketamine hydrochloride or propofol on hypothermia in dogs undergoing ovariohysterectomy. *Am J Vet Res* 2016; **77**(4): 351–357.

109 Franco LG, Wilges CHM, Junior DP, *et al.* Effects of ketamine constant rate infusions on cardiac biomarkers and cardiac function in dogs. *Vet Anaesth Analg* 2018; **45**(3): 250–259.

110 Cooter M, Ni K, Thomas J, *et al.* Age-dependent decrease in minimum alveolar concentration of inhaled anaesthetics: a systematic search of published studies and meta-regression analysis. *Br J Anaesth* 2020; **124**(1): e4–e7.

111 Magnusson KR, Scanga C, Wagner AE, *et al.* Changes in anesthetic sensitivity and glutamate receptors in the aging canine brain. *J Gerontol A Biol Sci Med Sci* 2000; **55**(9): B448–B454.

112 Yamashita K, Iwasaki Y, Umar MA, *et al.* Effect of age on minimum alveolar concentration (MAC) of sevoflurane in dogs. *J Vet Med Sci* 2009; **71**(11): 1509–1512.

113 Stankiewicz-Rudnicki M. Neuromuscular blockade in the elderly. *Anaesthesiol Intensive Ther* 2016; **48**(4): 257–260.

114 Lee LA, Athanassoglou V, Pandit JJ. Neuromuscular blockade in the elderly patient. *J Pain Res* 2016; **9**: 437–444.

115 Schmartz D, Sghaier R, Bernard P, *et al.* Neuromuscular block in patients 80 years and older: a prospective, controlled study. *BMC Anesthesiol* 2021; **21**(1): 225.

116 Nilsson UG. Intraoperative positioning of patients under general anesthesia and the risk of postoperative pain and pressure ulcers. *J Perianesth Nurs* 2013; **28**(3): 137–143.

117 Chen C, Hsieh H. The introduction of ERAS nutritional care can improve the quality of postoperative care. *Curr Dev Nutr* 2022; **6**: 738.

118 Hay Kraus BL. Spotlight on the perioperative use of maropitant citrate. *Vet Med (Auckl)* 2017; **8**:41–51.

119 Carney HC, Little S, Brownlee-Tomasso, *et al.* AAFP and ISFM feline-friendly nursing care guidelines. *J Feline Med Surg* 2012; **14**(5): 337–349.

70 Cancer Patients

Timothy M. Fan and Stephanie Keating
Department of Veterinary Clinical Medicine, College of Veterinary Medicine, University of Illinois at Urbana–Champaign, Urbana, Illinois, USA

Chapter contents

Prevalence of cancer pain, 1363
Recognition and assessment of cancer pain, 1363
Types of pain associated with cancer, 1364
Specific underlying causes of cancer pain, 1364
  Bone cancer pain, 1364
  Radiotherapy-induced pain, 1365
  Chemotherapy-induced pain, 1365
  Surgery-induced pain, 1366
Pharmacologic treatment strategies, 1366
  Non-steroidal anti-inflammatory drugs, 1367
  Opioids, 1367
  N-methyl-D-aspartate antagonists, 1367
  Combination analgesics, 1367
  Anticonvulsants, 1368
  Antidepressants, 1368
  Cannabinoids, 1368
Cancer-specific pain treatment options, 1368
  General therapeutic strategies for bone cancer pain, 1368
  Radiation burns – acute side effects, 1370
Promising innovative treatments, 1370
Anesthesia and cancer outcomes, 1371
  Cancer recurrence, 1371
  Pain and analgesic techniques, 1372
References, 1373

Prevalence of cancer pain

The true prevalence of cancer pain in dogs and cats is unknown; however, given the conserved biology and malignant transformation processes shared between companion animals and people, it is plausible that the occurrence of cancer pain is comparable across these species. Pain is a common ailment in human cancer patients; the incidence of cancer pain at initial diagnosis approaches 30% and, upon disease progression, up to 65–85% of human cancer patients will experience pain at some point [1]. Importantly, the clinical impact of cancer pain is significant with moderate to severe pain reported in 38% of all patients undergoing cancer treatment [2], and pain being the most common physical symptom reported in people diagnosed with terminal cancer [3].

Cancer pain negatively affects quality of life as well as many important physiological functions and pain alleviation in patients should be an utmost clinical and humane priority. No cures exist for many patients suffering from advanced cancer; however, effective analgesic strategies can ameliorate the discomfort and suffering associated with terminal disease. Estimates indicate that more than 70% of human cancer patients suffering from pain can find relief with opioid-based regimens [4]. It is justifiable to believe that equally effective cancer pain management may be achievable for companion animals too; however, alternative analgesic strategies must be employed due to pharmacokinetic differences and decreased analgesic efficacy of oral opioids in companion animals compared with humans [5]. In order for cancer pain to be adequately managed, it must be recognized early and frequently reassessed by veterinary caregivers and pet owners. Many barriers obstruct the optimal management of cancer-related pain in animals, including poor recognition associated with many cancers, difficulty in response assessment, limited knowledge regarding the efficacy and usage of analgesics in veterinary outpatients, and suboptimal communication between veterinary caregivers and pet owners [6].

Recognition and assessment of cancer pain

One essential component of pain recognition is adequate communication with the pet owner [6]. Observant pet owners know their pet's personality well and can recognize subtle changes in behavior that might represent pain or discomfort [7,8]. As such, it is imperative that veterinary caregivers make conscious efforts to believe the perceptions of pet owners who think their pet is experiencing pain. Common behaviors noted by pet owners that might represent pain include changes in movement, posture, grooming, appetite and thirst, respiration rate, or defecation and urination patterns. Development of new behaviors such as focal licking, drooling, dysphagia, or vocalization, as well as changes in their interactions with people, other animals, or the environment may also be noted [9].

To facilitate the recognition of pain and its assessment through behavioral observations, several validated observer pain scales have

Veterinary Anesthesia and Analgesia: The Sixth Edition of Lumb and Jones. Edited by Leigh Lamont, Kurt Grimm, Sheilah Robertson, Lydia Love and Carrie Schroeder.
© 2024 John Wiley & Sons, Inc. Published 2024 by John Wiley & Sons, Inc.
Companion website: www.wiley.com/go/lamont/anesthesia

been developed [10–13]. However, the majority of conventional pain scales have been validated in the context of acute, postoperative pain, or chronic osteoarthritic pain, and hence their suitability for cancer pain assessment might be limited and they may require interpretative modifications to maximize their utility in assessing pain in cancer patients. Unidimensional pain scales are conceptually simplistic, and hence user-friendly, and include the visual analog scale (VAS), the numerical rating scale (NRS), and the simple descriptive scale (SDS). These scales involve subjective, unguided assessment by the observer, where pain is (1) assigned an integer score from 0 (absent) to 10 (worst possible pain) (NRS); (2) indicated on a continuous 10-cm line to indicate the severity of pain (VAS); or (3) assigned a designation such as absent, mild, moderate, severe, very severe, or worst possible pain (SDS). There are many weaknesses with these assessment tools, including interobserver variability, number bias, and baseline drift, among others; however, these scales may be helpful when used consistently by the same observer in conjunction with more objective and quantifiable metrics.

Species-specific multidimensional composite pain scales have been developed to reduce the subjective nature of pain assessment and attempt to capture the sensory-discriminative as well as affective and cognitive components of pain [13,14]. These scales have been validated and some offer analgesic intervention points in postoperative veterinary patients. Despite the simplicity of unidimensional scales and validity of postoperative multidimensional pain scales, their utilization by pet owners and veterinary caregivers might not be completely applicable to the assessment of tumor-bearing animals, given the distinct pathophysiology of cancer pain. To address these limitations, alternative assessment schemes have been validated for pets that include either behavioral scales or health-related quality-of-life questionnaires specific to cancer pain [15–20]. Through the use of cancer-pain-specific behavior scales or questionnaires, the objective assessment of pain and its alleviation can be more uniformly standardized in tumor-bearing pets.

In addition to cancer-pain-specific scales, it would be ideal to have complementary and orthogonal methodologies for objectively characterizing cancer pain. Some objective and subjective veterinary cancer pain assessment tools have been developed, which correlate well with behavioral changes and perceived pain reported by pet owners [21]. Additionally, some methodologies for quantifying cancer pain that directly affects bodily movement or ambulation can be objectively quantified by activity monitors or computerized force plate and gait analysis systems [22,23].

Types of pain associated with cancer

Cancer pain arises from the direct invasion of tumor cells into nerves, bones, soft tissue, ligaments, and fascia. Pain also can be elicited through the distention and obstruction of internal organs secondary to tumor infiltration. Erosive or inflammatory processes induced by cancer cells within the microenvironment can generate pain too. Mechanistically, cancer pain can be categorized as nociceptive (somatic and visceral) or neuropathic in origin.

Nociceptive pain is associated with direct tissue injury from tumor infiltration and peritumoral inflammation. Perception of pain is caused by the stimulation of peripheral nociceptors residing in cutaneous and deeper musculoskeletal structures.

- ***Somatic pain*** arises from direct injury due to cancer cell invasion into the skeleton, soft tissues, or tendons/ligaments; often manifests as focal and stabbing in nature.

Table 70.1 Common painful cancers in companion animals.

Type of cancer pain	Example
Nociceptive	
Somatic	Primary bone sarcomas (e.g., osteosarcoma, fibrosarcoma, and chondrosarcoma) Joint sarcomas (e.g., histiocytic and synovial cell) Skeletal metastases (e.g., carcinoma of mammary, prostate, anal sac apocrine gland, lung, and transitional cell) Multiple myeloma or solitary osseous plasmacytoma Oral cavity tumors (e.g., melanoma, fibrosarcoma, and squamous cell carcinoma) Nasal cavity tumors (e.g., adenocarcinoma, chondrosarcoma, and squamous cell carcinoma) Skull and orbital tumors (e.g., multilobular osteochondrosarcoma) Ear tumors (e.g., ceruminous gland carcinoma) Cutaneous and subcutaneous tumors (e.g., mast cell tumor, basal cell carcinoma, apocrine gland carcinoma, and injection-site sarcoma) Mammary tumors (e.g., inflammatory mammary carcinoma)
Visceral	Urogenital tumors (e.g., transitional cell carcinoma, prostate carcinoma, and renal carcinoma) Reproductive tumors (e.g., uterine leiomyosarcoma) Carcinomatosis (e.g., serosal surface-involving malignancy) Liver and splenic tumors (e.g., hepatocellular carcinoma and hemangiosarcoma) Pancreatic carcinoma
Neuropathic	Central nervous system (e.g., meningioma and astrocytoma) Brachial plexus tumor Vertebral body tumor with compression of spinal cord (e.g., osteosarcoma or other axillary bone sarcoma)

- ***Visceral pain*** arises from cancer cell infiltration, compression, or distortion of internal organs within the abdominal, thoracic, or pelvic cavities; often manifests as diffuse and squeezing in character.

Neuropathic pain is directly related to cancer cell infiltration of peripheral nerves, nerve plexi and roots, or spinal cord; often associated with paresthesia or numbness and described as burning or shooting in nature.

Although cancer-associated pain can be discretely categorized as either nociceptive or neuropathic, a single tumor type can elicit pain that has blended characteristics of both nociceptive and neuropathic origins. Notably, pain characteristics can be dynamic and change over the course of disease progression. This is a result of surrounding structures becoming increasingly affected, and from structural and neurochemical changes in the peripheral and central nervous systems leading to ongoing pain signals and release of molecular mediators from neoplastic cells. The evolving nature of pain generation has important implications for pain management, and often requires a multimodal analgesic approach. A non-exhaustive list of common cancers arising in companion animals and the type of pain that they might elicit is summarized in Table 70.1.

Specific underlying causes of cancer pain

Bone cancer pain

Bone is a living organ, rich in blood supply and nerves. Painful sensations arising from the skeleton can decrease quality-of-life scores in pets. Given its principal anatomic function for bearing weight and withstanding cyclic compressive forces, compromise of the structural integrity of bone poses risk for pain and pathologic fracture. Neoplasms involving the skeleton can arise primarily from the bone, or secondarily invade or metastasize to involve the skeleton. In dogs, osteosarcoma (OS) is the most common cancer to cause focal skeletal pain. However, other frequently diagnosed tumor types can involve bone too, including metastatic carcinoma and hematopoietic neoplasms such as multiple myeloma. In cats, primary bone tumors occur less frequently than in dogs; however, involvement of bone from local invasion is common for oral squamous cell carcinoma [24]. Despite the diverse tumor histologies that can affect bone, the mechanisms for how tumor cells invade and generate skeletal pain are likely conserved across companion animals.

Mechanisms of bone cancer pain

Bone cancer pain is attributed to specific host responses occurring within the bone microenvironment. First, the presence of cancer cells results in the release of chemical mediators by neoplastic and non-neoplastic stromal cells, which in turn stimulate sensory afferent nociceptors and cause painful sensations [25]. Specific ligands secreted by both cancer and stromal cells capable of nociceptor activation include endothelin-1, nerve growth factor (NGF), and prostaglandin-E_2 [26]. Additionally, trafficking immune cells within the tumor microenvironment secrete proinflammatory cytokines, including IL-1β, TNFα, and bradykinin that also stimulate nociceptors [26]. Second, preclinical evidence indicates that the generation and maintenance of bone cancer pain is directly attributed to pathologic osteoclastic bone resorption [27,28]. Mechanistically, osteoclastic bone resorption is mediated by the coordinated secretion of protons and cathepsin K, a cysteine protease. The localized acidic environment created by osteoclasts stimulates afferent nociceptors through transient receptor potential vanilloid receptor 1 (TRPV1) and acid-sensing ion channels 2/3 (ASIC 2/3) [26,29]. Third, bone cancer pain can be generated as a consequence of bone erosion and subsequent mechanical instability, which allows for distortion of putative mechanotransducers belonging to the TRPV receptor family [30].

Neuroplastic changes are central to the propagation of nociceptive signals and the development of neuropathic and chronic pain states with bone cancer. The destruction, compression, or stretching of peripheral sensory fibers from the neoplastic process can directly generate aberrant nerve impulses and result in neuropathic pain. Additionally, chemical mediators within the tumor microenvironment, notably NGF, promote ongoing disorganized sprouting of both sensory and sympathetic nerve fibers as has been described in canine OS [31]. These fibers form neuroma-like structures and have been linked to background, breakthrough, and movement-induced bone cancer pain, as well as sympathetically mediated pain, all of which contribute to central sensitization and the development of chronic pain states [32,33]. Based on these unifying pathologic mechanisms, effective management of bone cancer pain requires a multi-pronged therapeutic approach, which addresses the fundamental drivers that contribute to pain generation.

Radiotherapy-induced pain

Ionizing radiation is effective for managing localized forms of cancer. Mechanistically, ionizing radiation exerts cytotoxic effects by damaging deoxyribonucleic acid (DNA), either directly or indirectly. Following irreparable DNA damage, cancer cells undergo apoptosis. When applied therapeutically, ionizing radiation can be focally conformed to the shape of tumor masses through the use of linear accelerators equipped with three-dimensional planning software and sophisticated, multi-leaf collimators. However, even with advanced equipment, small volumes of normal tissue might be irradiated, potentially resulting in painful radiation-induced toxicity. Although the majority of caregivers who pursue radiation therapy for their pets consider the side effects acceptable [34], some animals might experience considerable morbidity secondary to acute radiation burns. Depending upon the radiation field, acute moist dermatitis, mucositis, and colitis can be early radiation side effects encountered with curative protocols (Fig. 70.1) [35]. Common anatomic sites for the development of painful radiation-induced mucositis are the mouth when oral or nasal tumors are irradiated, and the large colon/rectum (colitis and proctitis) when pelvic irradiation is performed [36]. Infrequently, late radiation side effects might result in painful and unacceptable toxicity, including the development of osteoradionecrosis (Fig. 70.2), anatomic stricture, and peripheral neuropathies [37].

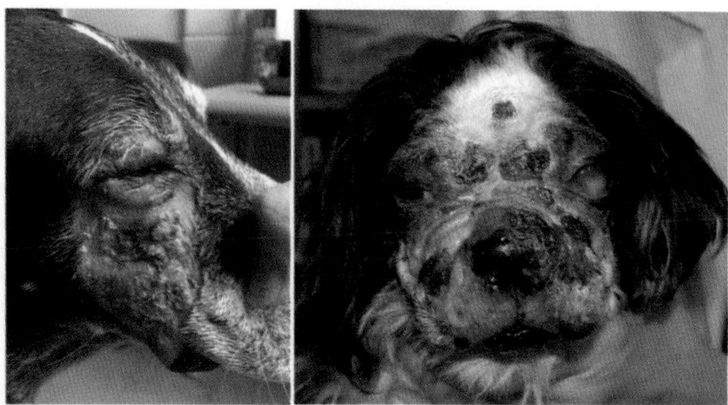

Figure 70.1 Resolving painful acute moist dermatitis in two different canine patients undergoing palliative or curative-intent radiation therapy for the treatment of cancer involving the oral or nasal cavities, respectively.

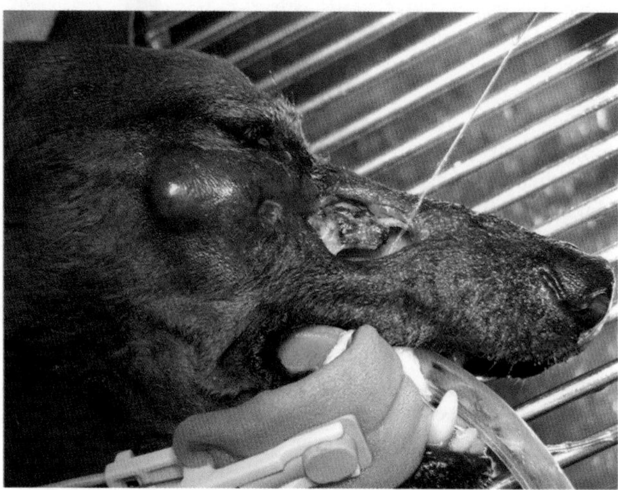

Figure 70.2 Irreparable late radiation toxicity in the form of osteoradionecrosis in a dog with nasal squamous cell carcinoma treated with high cumulative doses of radiation therapy.

Chemotherapy-induced pain

The administration of systemic chemotherapy is not typically uncomfortable; however, it can infrequently result in painful local and systemic side effects. Perivascular extravasation of certain chemotherapeutics, including vincristine, doxorubicin, vinblastine, mechlorethamine, dactinomycin, and pamidronate might result in painful tissue irritation (Fig. 70.3), at times severe enough

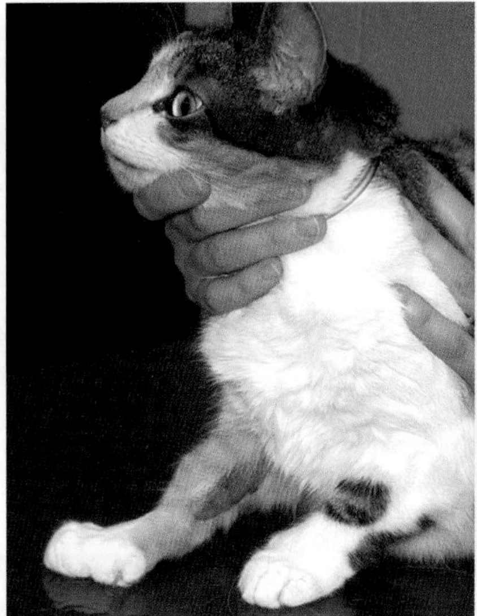
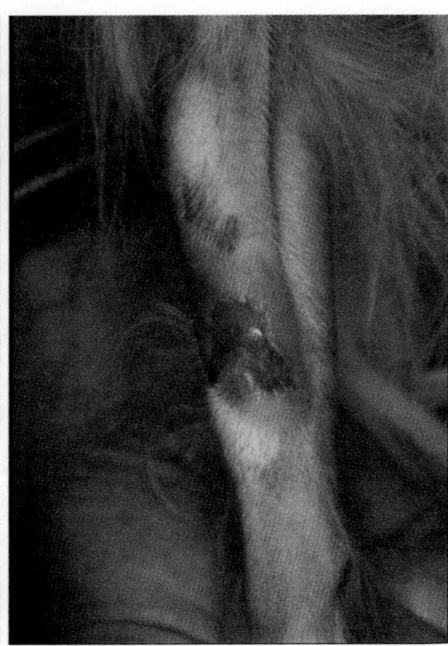

Figure 70.3 Painful soft tissue inflammation and dermal ulceration secondary to extravasation of vinblastine in a cat (left) and vincristine in a dog (right).

to necessitate surgical debridement [38]. Additionally, some chemotherapeutic agents have greater tendencies to perturb intestinal transit times and resident microflora, resulting in colitis (e.g., doxorubicin) or constipation (e.g., vinca alkaloids), which have the potential to generate visceral pain [39]. Bioconversion of some chemotherapeutic agents, such as cyclophosphamide, can lead to the production of irritating metabolites (e.g., acrolein) and the subsequent development of painful syndromes, including sterile hemorrhagic cystitis [40]. Certain chemotherapeutic agents, such as dacarbazine, which have low pH (~3) can elicit burning sensations at the catheter site during intravenous infusion. Other chemotherapeutic agents, such as paclitaxel and docetaxel, require Cremophor EL and polysorbate 80, respectively, for solubilization and these solvents can directly activate complement and elicit systemic inflammatory cytokine release, resulting in diffuse pain sensations and systemic hypersensitivity reactions [41,42]. Finally, painful peripheral neuropathies can be associated with the administration of certain drugs such as vincristine, cisplatin, and the taxanes in people [43], and similar side effects have been infrequently documented in companion animals [44,45].

Table 70.2 Analgesic drug and oral dosages for dogs.

Class	Drug	Dosage
NSAIDs	Robenacoxib	1–2 mg/kg PO q24 h
	Deracoxib	1–2 mg/kg PO q24 h
	Carprofen	2 mg/kg PO q12 h or 4 mg/kg PO q24 h
	Etodolac	5–15 mg/kg PO q24 h
	Meloxicam	0.1 mg/kg PO q24 h
	Tepoxalin	10 mg/kg PO q24 h
	Piroxicam	0.3 mg/kg PO q24 h
	Ketoprofen	1 mg/kg PO q24 h
	Aspirin	10–30 mg/kg PO q12 h
	Acetaminophen	10–33 mg/kg PO q8 h
	Grapiprant	2 mg/kg PO q24 h
Opioid	Fentanyl patch	2–5 μg/kg/h transdermally
NMDA antagonist	Amantadine	3–5 mg/kg PO q24 h
Combination analgesic	Tramadol	4–5 mg/kg PO q6–12 h
Anticonvulsants	Gabapentin	10–20 mg/kg PO q8 h
	Pregabalin	3–4 mg/kg PO q8–12 h
Tricyclic antidepressants	Amitriptyline	1–2 mg/kg PO q12–24 h
	Clomipramine	1–2 mg/kg PO q12 h
Corticosteroids	Prednisone	0.25–1.0 mg/kg PO q24 h
	Dexamethasone	0.1–0.2 mg/kg PO q24 h

Surgery-induced pain

Invasive diagnostic or therapeutic procedures can cause acute nociceptive and possibly neuropathic pain in veterinary cancer patients. Staging procedures such as tissue biopsies, bone marrow aspiration, and bone biopsies should be expected to cause mild to moderate pain that can be preemptively treated with analgesics. More aggressive surgeries such as amputation, hemipelvectomy, thoracotomy, radical mastectomy, and large *en bloc* tumor resection, including orbitectomy, mandibulectomy, or maxillectomy, will generate severe postoperative pain and should be treated with a preventive analgesic strategy, including regional blocks such as epidural or interpleural analgesia or specific peripheral nerve blocks. Longer-lasting local anesthetic formulations, such as liposomal bupivacaine, can also be administered peri-incisionally to extend the duration of local analgesia further into the postoperative period. The use of postoperative full μ-opioid receptor agonists should be a standard analgesic regimen for companion animals undergoing removal of painful invasive tumors through radical surgeries. Opioid analgesics should be combined with an anti-inflammatory agent whenever possible, as well as adjunctive analgesics as needed, such as lidocaine and ketamine infusions, to address sensitization and prevent the development of persistent postoperative pain states.

Pharmacologic treatment strategies

For most pets diagnosed with cancer, pain becomes established early in the course of disease and rapidly intensifies during cancer progression. As such, pharmacologic strategies are often used in the setting of chronic pain management, where the primary intent of intervention is to minimize the clinical consequences of peripheral and central sensitization, as well as maintain quality of life. Tables 70.2 and 70.3 provide general guidelines for common analgesics that are easily administered by pet owners for the management of cancer pain in companion animals. For more detailed pharmacology and dosing regimens, please refer to Chapters 23, 24, and 25.

Table 70.3 Analgesic drug and oral dosages for cats.

Class	Drug	Dosage
NSAIDs[a]	Robenacoxib	1 mg/kg PO q24 h maximum 3 days (US), 6 days (EU)
	Ketoprofen	1 mg/kg PO q24 h maximum 5 days
	Meloxicam	0.05 mg/kg PO q24 h
	Tolfenamic acid	4 mg/kg PO q24 h maximum 3 days
	Piroxicam	0.3 mg/kg PO q48 h
Opioids	Buprenorphine	0.02 mg/kg PO sublingual q6–8 h
	Fentanyl patch	2–5 μg/kg/h transdermally
NMDA antagonist	Amantadine	3 mg/kg PO q24 h
Combination analgesic	Tramadol	1–2 mg/kg PO q12–24 h
Anticonvulsants	Gabapentin	5–10 mg/kg PO q8–12 h
	Pregabalin	1–2 mg/kg PO q12 h
Tricyclic antidepressants	Amitriptyline	1–2 mg/kg PO q24 h
	Clomipramine	0.5–1 mg/kg PO q24 h
Corticosteroids[a]	Prednisone	1–1.5 mg/kg PO q24 h
	Dexamethasone	0.1–0.2 mg/kg PO q24 h

[a] Long-term NSAID or corticosteroid administration should be undertaken following informed client consent with regular patient monitoring and administration of the lowest effective dose.

Non-steroidal anti-inflammatory drugs

Non-steroidal anti-inflammatory drugs (NSAIDs) are used to control nociceptive and inflammatory pain in companion animals. The mechanism of action of most NSAIDs is the inhibition of cyclo-oxygenases (COXs). For cancer pain, prostaglandin synthase-2 (COX-2) is the preferential target of inhibition given its role in inflammatory pain arising as a consequence of prostaglandin-E_2 production. Prostaglandins play an important role in peripheral sensitization leading to hyperalgesia and allodynia. Specifically, prostaglandins regulate the sensitivity of polymodal nociceptors, which typically cannot be easily activated by physiological stimuli. However, following tissue injury and inflammation, the release of prostaglandins facilitates responsiveness of "silent" polymodal nociceptors [46]. Prostaglandins can also activate sodium channels in the dorsal horn of the spinal cord, resulting in central sensitization and the establishment of chronic cancer pain [47]. The NSAID, grapiprant, does not inhibit the production of prostaglandin-E_2 but antagonizes the EP4 receptor, preventing PGE_2 from binding, and reducing pain and inflammation without preventing the production of constitutive prostaglandins [48]. The use of NSAIDs for managing cancer pain might be particularly relevant in companion animals given the multiple tumor histologies which overexpress COX-2 [49], and therefore have the potential for nociceptive sensitization through tumor-derived prostaglandin generation. Additionally, the anticancer effects of some NSAIDs, notably piroxicam, may have indirect analgesic benefits secondary to possible reductions in tumor burden [50,51].

Opioids

Three conventional opioid receptor subtypes have been cloned and isolated, known as μ-, κ-, and δ-opioid receptors. Opioid receptors are distributed widely, being located in peripheral tissues, immune cells, sensory nerve terminals, and within the central nervous system at spinal and supraspinal sites. Spinally, they are localized primarily in the superficial dorsal horn within laminae I, II, and V. Within the dorsal horn, most opioid receptors are located on presynaptic terminals of afferent fibers; however, lower densities of opioid receptors are also found on postsynaptic sites and interneurons. The mechanism of analgesia is through reduced neurotransmitter release from nociceptive C fibers and postsynaptic inhibition of neurons conveying information from the spinal cord to higher centers of the brain. Binding of opioids to their presynaptic inhibitory receptor blocks the release of glutamate, substance P, and other neurotransmitters, while binding to the postsynaptic receptor further inhibits neuronal depolarization. Opioids further suppress nociception by enhancing activity in descending inhibitory pain pathways, which project down from supraspinal sites to modulate signals in the dorsal horn. Opioids are readily available, can be titrated easily to the desired effect, and demonstrate predictable adverse effects that can be minimized with preventive interventions. Side effects in companion animals include diarrhea, vomiting, constipation, and excessive sedation.

Parenteral opioid administration is highly effective for treating pain in companion animals. Unfortunately, there is considerable evidence that orally administered opioids are unlikely to offer the same analgesic benefits in these species. Many orally administered opioids demonstrate very low oral bioavailability, highly variable absorption, and absent to low plasma concentrations of the parent compound or active metabolite, with short elimination half-lives [52–56]. These findings, combined with the lack of positive antinociceptive and clinical studies, along with the risk of misuse and drug diversion, do not currently support the routine prescription of orally administered opioids to treat pain in companion animals. However, there is evidence to support alternative routes of opioid administration for outpatients. Analgesic plasma concentrations and evidence of analgesic efficacy have been demonstrated with transmucosal administration of buprenorphine and transdermal patch administration of fentanyl in cats and dogs [57–62].

N-methyl-D-aspartate antagonists

N-methyl-D-aspartate (NMDA) receptors play a key role in central sensitization within the dorsal horn of the spinal cord following the release of excitatory neurotransmitters from nociceptor terminals. Sustained glutamate release leads to perturbations in synaptic receptor density, threshold, kinetics, and activation, with subsequent increases in pain transmission. During central sensitization, glutamate-activated NMDA receptors undergo post-translational phosphorylation, increasing their synaptic distribution and responsiveness to glutamate, with resultant hyperexcitability to normally subthreshold noxious stimuli. As such, NMDA antagonists including ketamine, tiletamine, amantadine, and dextromethorphan have a role in the management of chronic cancer pain when central sensitization has been established.

Combination analgesics

Tramadol is a centrally acting analgesic, classified as an opioidergic/monoaminergic drug based on its shared properties with both opioids and tricyclic antidepressants. Tramadol weakly binds to the μ-opioid receptor, inhibits the reuptake of serotonin and norepinephrine, and promotes neuronal serotonin release. An active metabolite of tramadol, *O*-desmethyltramadol, has greater affinity for the μ-opioid receptor than the parent molecule and is responsible for much of the opioid-induced analgesia. Based on these properties, tramadol is theoretically a suitable analgesic for the management of both nociceptive and neuropathic pain. Unfortunately, oral administration in dogs has failed to demonstrate any significant analgesia for either postoperative or osteoarthritis pain [63,64]; however, studies in cats have yielded more promising results, likely due to pharmacokinetic and possibly pharmacodynamic differences [65,66]. Additionally, tramadol exerts antihyperalgesic effects, possibly due to the monoaminergic properties of the drug [65] and may offer antinociceptive effects and improve comfort in animals with central sensitization from cancer when used as an adjunctive analgesic. Specifically, tramadol administered in combination with metamizole (dipyrone), with or without NSAIDs, demonstrated clinical efficacy for management of moderate to severe cancer pain in dogs and improved quality-of-life scores [16].

Anticonvulsants

Anticonvulsants are useful adjuvant analgesics in patients with neuropathic pain, as well as chronic pain with central sensitization. In companion animals, gabapentin, a structural analog of γ-aminobutyric acid (GABA), acts on presynaptic axonal terminal voltage-gated calcium channels to reduce neurotransmitter release. Additionally, gabapentin also induces postsynaptic inhibition by evoking hyperpolarization inhibitory potentials in dorsal horn neurons through the opening of potassium or chloride channels. Gabapentin is well-tolerated, highly bioavailable, and rapidly metabolized in dogs [67]. Recent studies suggest the adjuvant use of gabapentin does not improve analgesia for the management of acute nociceptive pain in dogs [68,69]; however, other studies suggest gabapentin is effective in the management of neuropathic pain [70]. Pregabalin is a gabapentinoid with similarities to gabapentin; however, the longer elimination half-life creates a more favorable dosing interval while still demonstrating analgesic efficacy [71,72].

Antidepressants

Antidepressants, such as tricyclic antidepressants (TCAs), selective serotonin reuptake inhibitors (SSRIs), and selective serotonin–noradrenaline reuptake inhibitors (SNRIs), are often used as co-analgesic therapies for chronic cancer pain, especially of neuropathic origin. Chronic neuropathic pain can result from local nerve compression by expanding cancer cells, neuroma formation from tumor NGF production or following surgical transection, radiation-induced fibrosis or neuritis, and systemic peripheral nerve damage from specific chemotherapeutic agents (vinca alkaloids). Mechanistically, the analgesia produced by antidepressants such as amitriptyline, clomipramine, fluoxetine, duloxetine, and imipramine is attributable to their actions on endogenous monoaminergic pain-modulating systems. These drugs inhibit the reuptake of various monoamines such as serotonin and noradrenaline, allowing these biomolecules to remain present and act centrally on descending inhibitory serotonergic and noradrenergic pathways that modulate pain transmission at the level of the spinal cord. While clinical proof of the analgesic efficacy of antidepressants in veterinary cancer patients is lacking, there is some evidence that TCAs are beneficial for neuropathic pain states in dogs [70,73].

Cannabinoids

Cannabinoids are a large class of natural and synthetic compounds originally identified within the cannabis plant. These molecules exert a wide range of physiologic effects, including analgesia, produced through their interactions with the endocannabinoid system. This system is comprised of the established CB_1 and CB_2 receptors, as well as endogenous ligands and the mechanisms responsible for their production, reuptake, and metabolism. Analgesia results from cannabinoid binding at presynaptic CB receptors, which decreases intracellular calcium in the primary afferent neuron and subsequently decreases nociceptive neurotransmitter release. Activity of the descending inhibitory pain pathway is also enhanced, reducing postsynaptic neuronal excitability, and suppressing the projection of nociceptive signals. Cannabinoids also modulate nociception through their activity at multiple other receptor types, including directly acting on TRPV1 receptors, and indirectly modulating the effects of a diverse range of G-protein-coupled receptors, including opioid receptors, which can dimerize with CB_1 and CB_2 receptors.

Tetrahydrocannabinol (THC) and cannabidiol (CBD) are the most abundant cannabinoids in the cannabis plant and have been evaluated for their analgesic effects in preclinical rodent studies and human clinical trials. There is notable heterogeneity in both the cannabinoid preparations (THC and CBD dosages and ratios) and conditions that have been studied, producing variable therapeutic results; however, cannabinoids may offer an analgesic benefit in neuropathic and chronic pain states, including cancer pain. CBD has been isolated and administered to dogs as both a sole and adjunctive analgesic agent for the treatment of osteoarthritis pain, producing mixed results of analgesic efficacy as determined by behavioral observations and objective measurements, such as force plate analysis [74–77]. The efficacy of cannabinoids for treating pain in companion animals with cancer has yet to be critically evaluated.

Cancer-specific pain treatment options

General therapeutic strategies for bone cancer pain

The most common and striking presenting sign of dogs with OS is lameness associated with severe pain in the affected bone. The mechanisms of bone cancer pain have been characterized using murine preclinical models. Given the evolutionary importance of adaptive pain, it is plausible that the same mechanisms responsible for pain generation in mouse models are also operative in spontaneously arising bone tumors in companion animals, such as canine OS. Since tumor cells and osteoclasts appear to play preponderant roles in the genesis of bone pain associated with malignant osteolysis, effective therapies should focus on (1) eradication of viable tumor cells; (2) reduction of cancer-induced bone resorption; (3) surgical stabilization of mechanically compromised bone; and (4) administration of potent pharmacologic agents to address both the inflammatory and neuropathic components of pain.

Viable cancer cells directly promote the generation of bone pain through the secretion of nociceptor-activating ligands, attraction of trafficking immune cells, and subversion of osteoclastic activities. As such, eradication of cancer cells remains a cornerstone for successful bone pain control. Reducing bone cancer burden is effectively achieved by cytotoxic therapies, including systemic chemotherapy and radiotherapy. Systemic chemotherapy can be effective in reducing tumor cell burdens within the bone microenvironment, but is contingent on the tumor histology (i.e., chemosensitive hematopoietic neoplasms) and favorable intratumoral biodistribution kinetics. Ionizing radiation is the most effective treatment for alleviating bone cancer pain. The exact mechanisms of radiation-induced pain relief are incompletely understood but are likely related to cytotoxic effects on tumor cells and osteoclasts [28].

Osteoclasts, cells of the monocyte-macrophage cell lineage, are characterized by their high expressions of tartrate-resistant acid phosphatase and cathepsin K. Under homeostatic conditions, osteoclasts resorb bone in balance with new bone formation by osteoblasts. However, bone cancers of either primary (sarcomas) or metastatic (carcinomas) origin dysregulate osteoclastic activities in part through subversion of the receptor activator of nuclear factor-κB/receptor activator of nuclear factor-κB ligand/osteoprotegerin (RANK/RANKL/OPG) axis [78].

Given the role of osteoclasts in the generation of bone cancer pain through the secretion of protons and distortion of mechanotransducers, therapies that reduce osteoclast viability are useful in reducing the severity of bone cancer pain. Aminobisphosphonates induce osteoclast apoptosis through inhibition of the mevalonate pathway and are first-line agents for the management of malignant skeletal events in human cancer patients [79]. Although aminobisphosphonates exert antiresorptive effects and can provide analgesia as single agents, based upon preclinical studies, the alleviation of focal bone cancer pain might be augmented by co-administering site-specific ionizing radiation therapy, which further drives apoptotic cell death of malignantly subverted osteoclasts [80,81]. However, clinical studies conducted in dogs with OS have not uniformly supported the benefit of such combination strategies for improving bone cancer pain alleviation [22,82–84].

When anatomically feasible, surgical stabilization of compromised bone integrity secondary to cancer infiltration can reduce excessive compression of mechanotransducers that stimulate afferent nociceptors. Diligence in patient selection for surgical stabilization procedures is required as successful outcomes require solid anchorage of stabilizing hardware into neighboring healthy bone [85]. As such, large or expansive areas of cancer-infiltrated bone will be prone to surgical failure [86], and alternative non-surgical treatment options should be considered first-line therapies for these types of patients.

For the majority of cancer patients experiencing pain, pharmacologic agents remain the cornerstone of successful pain management. Patients with bone cancer are prone to experiencing debilitating episodes of incident or breakthrough pain, and the medical armament necessary to manage bone cancer pain requires potent opioid-based regimens with adjuvant analgesic agents as described on the highest level of the World Health Organization three-step analgesic ladder (Fig. 70.4).

Aminobisphosphonates

Bisphosphonates are synthetic analogs of inorganic pyrophosphate (PP_i) initially utilized in the detergent industry as demineralizing agents, and then for diagnostic purposes in bone scanning, based on their ability to adsorb to bone minerals. The effective treatment of bone disorders with bisphosphonates is attributed to their differential effects on bone resorption and bone mineralization. Importantly, bisphosphonates impede osteoclast activity and induce osteoclast apoptosis, selectively reducing the cell population responsible for bone resorption [87]. Although several bisphosphonates prevent bone loss, nitrogen-containing bisphosphonates (NBPs), also known as "aminobisphosphonates," possess the greatest relative antiresorptive potency. Pamidronate and zoledronate are the two most commonly utilized intravenous NBP formulations in human oncology for their ability to decrease bone pain, improve quality of life, delay progression of the bone lesions, and decrease the frequency of malignant skeletal events.

Intravenous pamidronate (1–2 mg/kg) administered as a 2-h constant rate infusion (CRI) every 28 days was well-tolerated and exerted bone biologic and clinically relevant analgesic effects in dogs diagnosed with appendicular OS [88,89]. Zoledronate possesses 100-fold greater antiresorptive potency compared with pamidronate and has the advantage of being safely administered over a shorter period of time than other NBPs. The bone biologic effects of single-agent intravenous zoledronate have been evaluated in dogs diagnosed with primary and secondary skeletal tumors [90]. In 10 dogs with appendicular OS, zoledronate (0.25 mg/kg) was administered as a 15-min infusion every 28 days. Clinically relevant analgesia from bone cancer pain was achieved in 50% of dogs for greater than 4 months. While intravenous pamidronate and zoledronate are considered safe for use in companions suffering from malignant osteolysis, some studies suggest a low risk for renal toxicity or other rare complications, including electrolyte imbalances and osteonecrosis of the jaw [91–93].

Radiotherapy

Radiation therapy is considered the most effective treatment modality in human cancer patients for the management of osteolytic bone pain. Mechanistically, the analgesic effects of ionizing radiation can be attributed to the induction of apoptosis in both cancer cells and resorbing osteoclasts [28]. Multiple palliative radiation protocols have been reported in the veterinary literature, with the majority of dosing schemes utilizing two to four individual treatments of 6–10 Gy fractions. Although variably and subjectively reported, the alleviation of bone cancer pain was achieved in the majority of OS dogs treated, and ranged from 74–93%. Despite symptomatic improvement following palliative radiation therapy, the median time interval of subjective pain alleviation was not durable, and ranged from 53–130 days [94–98]. More recently, definitive treatment protocols delivered by stereotactic radiosurgery regimens (typically, 8–12 Gy per fraction delivered over three consecutive days) have gained mainstream acceptance as the preferred radiotherapeutic intervention [84]; however, the

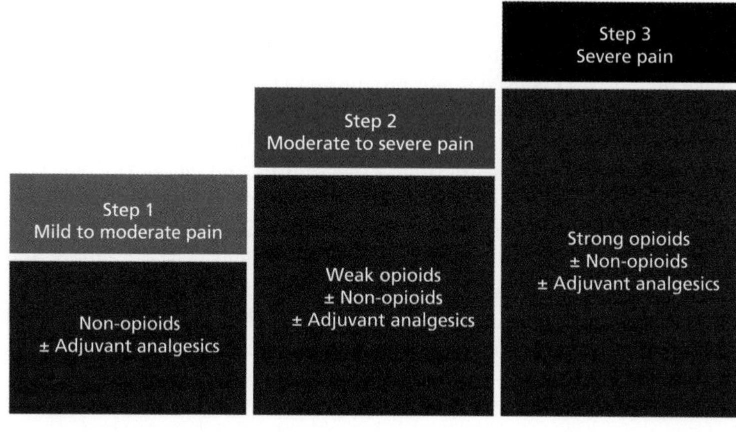

Figure 70.4 World Health Organization (WHO) analgesic ladder with indicated three-step approach to pain management. Companion animals diagnosed with bone cancer pain should be preemptively categorized into the highest tier and treated aggressively with potent opioid-based regimens.

development of pathologic fracture subsequent to irradiation remains a significant adverse event for both palliative and definitive radiation strategies [99,100].

Experimental therapeutics – intrathecal resiniferatoxin

Vanilloids belong to a family of small organic compounds that stimulate afferent sensory neurons through the binding of TRPV1, a non-selective cation ionophore [101]. Upon binding by natural agonists such as capsaicin, a chili pepper extract, TRPV1 activation leads to nociceptive responses [102].

Resiniferatoxin (RTX) is an ultrapotent analog of capsaicin derived from the latex of a cactus-like plant (*Euphorbia resinifera*). Upon binding to TRPV1, RTX causes a large and prolonged increase in the free intracellular calcium concentration, resulting in lethal calcium cytotoxicity with subsequent apoptosis and depletion of TRPV1 expressing neurons, and hence reducing the sensitivity to nociceptive inputs [103]. Importantly, RTX appears selective for TRPV1-expressing neurons, which are unmyelinated C fibers, while leaving large, myelinated neurons responsible for proprioception and mechanosensation intact.

Intrathecal RTX has been evaluated in pet dogs as an experimental therapy for the management of pain associated with osteoarthritis and bone cancer [104–107]. In the setting of bone cancer pain, pet dogs receiving intrathecal RTX achieved dramatic analgesia based upon caregiver-based visual analog scores and blinded veterinary lameness assessments within 14 days of therapy [104]. While promising, barriers currently preventing adoption as routine therapy include the lack of a commercial preparation, and the requirement for general anesthesia to facilitate injection and prevent awareness during the noxious excitation phase, which is accompanied by physiologic changes, including increases in heart rate and blood pressure, panting, and hypothermia. RTX has also induced clinically meaningful analgesia following intra-articular administration to sedated dogs with naturally occurring osteoarthritis [107] and may represent a future analgesic modality for animals with cancers affecting the joint, including histiocytic and synovial cell sarcomas.

Radiation burns – acute side effects

Ionizing radiation exerts its therapeutic effects by damaging cellular DNA through the generation of free radicals. As radiation therapy preferentially induces apoptosis in mitotically active cells, acute adverse effects tend to occur more commonly in normal cells with rapid division rates, including those of mucosal surfaces, intestine, and skin, resulting in mucositis, colitis, and dermatitis, respectively.

The morbidity associated with mucositis, colitis, and dermatitis can be significant in companion animals given the inflammatory and ulcerative pathology, and the tendency for unrestrained self-mutilation caused by excessive licking, rubbing, or scratching. In particular, oral mucositis pain can negatively affect oral intake of fluids, food, and medications, with subsequent reduced quality of life (Fig. 70.5). The level of evidence-based medicine for the effective management of radiation-induced mucositis, colitis, and dermatitis is limited even for human cancer patients, and remains primarily anecdotal in companion animals; however, experimental treatments are beginning to emerge [108].

Oral mucositis can be symptomatically treated with oral rinse solutions (weak tea solution, chlorhexidine rinse, or a mixture of viscous lidocaine, liquid diphenhydramine, and magnesium hydroxide), and the systemic use of NSAIDs or corticosteroids with a weak opioid as needed. Symptoms of colitis might be effectively relieved with the use of a corticosteroid enema and systemic medications consistent with step 2 of the WHO analgesic ladder (Fig. 70.4). Acute moist dermatitis may benefit from topical application of colloidal oatmeal, wheat extracts, or aloe gel extract. As needed, the administration of broad-spectrum antibiotics or antifungals might prevent the establishment of opportunistic bacterial or fungal infections. Fortunately, the morbidity associated with acute radiation side effects is temporally limited to the first 4–6 weeks of therapy, and most clinical symptoms are self-resolving following supportive management.

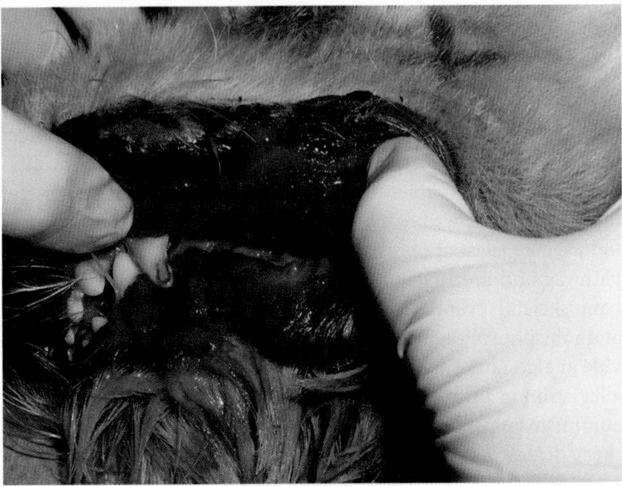

Figure 70.5 Severe and painful oral mucositis manifesting as erythema and coalescing mucosal blisters in a dog treated with curative-intent radiation therapy for perioral hamartoma.

Promising innovative treatments

Recent advancements have been made in clarifying the fundamental underpinnings that drive different forms of pain, especially bone cancer pain, through the use of murine preclinical models [25,109]. With a greater understanding of the tumor microenvironmental ligands responsible for peripheral afferent nociceptor stimulation, it has recently become possible to rationally identify and design molecularly targeted therapeutics expected to provide analgesia in companion animals.

Nerve growth factor (NGF) plays an important role in initiating nerve sprouting and bone cancer pain via binding to its cognate receptor, tropomyosin-related kinase A (TrkA) and is upregulated in chronic pain states. In murine preclinical models, blockade of NGF signaling dramatically reduces bone cancer pain [33,110,111]. Additionally, TrkA signaling appears to be involved in canine OS cell survival, thereby incriminating NGF as a putative ligand that drives OS local tumor progression [112]. Of clinical significance, species-specific anti-NGF monoclonal antibodies have also been developed and evaluated in preclinical and clinical trials for the treatment of neuropathic, osteoarthritis, and cancer pain. Blocking antibodies such as frunevetmab and bedinvetmab, have been developed for the treatment of osteoarthritis pain in cats and dogs, respectively, and demonstrate promising analgesic effects and safety profiles [113–116]. Given the global role of NGF in nociception, therapeutic strategies that block TrkA signaling are expected to provide analgesia in the setting of cancer pain in companion animals.

Adenosine triphosphate (ATP) is a ubiquitous intracellular molecule and plays a key role in nociception and sensitization when released from damaged tissues, sympathetic efferent neurons, or presynaptic vesicles in dorsal horn neurons. The P2X3 purinergic receptors are expressed on nociceptive neurons and are responsible for ATP-mediated pain mechanisms, with particular relevance in chronic pain states. Importantly, purinergic receptors are also located on neoplastic and immune cells, with activation playing an important role in cancer progression. Experimental P2X3 antagonists have been evaluated in rodent models of cancer-induced bone pain and demonstrated analgesic effects in different nociceptive assays and reduced spontaneous pain behaviors [117–120]. Given their role in both pain and cancer pathogenesis, P2X3 antagonists may be a valuable future therapeutic target for cancer pain.

Finally, the neurokinin-1 receptor (NK_1R) and its endogenous peptide ligand, substance P, are widely distributed throughout the body, including the central and peripheral nervous systems where they have an established role in nociceptive signaling, sensitization, and neurogenic inflammation. Experimental NK_1R antagonists have been evaluated in rodent models of inflammatory pain and have demonstrated analgesic and anti-inflammatory effects [121–123], thus the substance P–NK_1R axis may be a putative analgesic target for treating cancer pain in companion animals. Maropitant, a synthetic nonpeptidic NK_1R antagonist, is licensed for use as an antiemetic in dogs and cats and has been evaluated for analgesic properties in these species. Parenterally administered maropitant may provide perioperative analgesia based on composite pain scale assessment in cats and dogs undergoing ovariohysterectomy and mastectomy, supporting its use as part of a multimodal analgesic strategy; however, current veterinary data are not robust enough to support recommended administration as a sole analgesic [124–128]. Furthermore, substance P and NK_1R signaling play a role in the pathogenesis of OS and other cancer types, and the administration of nonpeptidic NK_1 antagonists imparts antitumor effects through the induction of apoptosis in neoplastic cells [129,130]. While the influence of maropitant on clinical cancer outcomes has not yet been reported, *in vitro* work suggests that maropitant inhibits cancer cell proliferation and enhances apoptosis in canine melanoma cell lines [131]. Further work is needed to determine if maropitant directly supports other cancer therapeutic interventions while offering analgesic and antiemetic benefits.

Anesthesia and cancer outcomes

Cancer recurrence

Surgery is an important treatment option for many solid cancers in veterinary patients. Unfortunately, recurrence is not uncommon following surgical intervention with curative intent. While the mechanisms of recurrence are not fully elucidated, causal factors include incomplete surgical margins with residual local disease, as well as intraoperative dissemination of neoplastic cells into the bloodstream, lymphatic circulation, or body cavity with subsequent establishment of metastases. While surgical technique and pre-existing microscopic disease are known to influence recurrence rates, anesthetic and analgesic protocols are increasingly being evaluated as factors that may promote or suppress cancer recurrence. A range of *in vitro* experiments, preclinical models, and retrospective human studies provide compelling evidence that this may be the case, as anesthetic and analgesic drugs have been shown to influence many factors responsible for cancer progression including (1) modulation of the stress response; (2) angiogenesis; (3) inflammation, cytotoxicity, and other aspects of immune function; and (4) tumor cell migration, proliferation, and chemosensitivity. While there are intriguing preliminary findings, data are still mixed, and large prospective randomized clinical trials are needed to establish causality and form evidence-based recommendations in both human and veterinary medicine.

Volatile anesthetics

Isoflurane and sevoflurane are the most commonly used agents to maintain anesthesia in veterinary patients undergoing oncologic surgery. Inhalant anesthetics may affect cancer processes through several direct and indirect mechanisms. The direct effect of inhalational agents on tumor cell survival is variable. Many *in vitro* studies report that clinical concentrations of sevoflurane and isoflurane enhance cancer cell survival, proliferation, metastatic gene expression, and development of chemoresistance [132,133], while others report a reduction in tumor cell viability [134,135]. This may be due to differences in gene expression in disparate cancer types as the effects of the same inhalational agent vary depending on the cancer cell line evaluated [135].

Volatile anesthetics also exert direct effects on immune cells through interactions with a range of targets, including $GABA_A$, glycine, nicotinic cholinergic, serotonergic, and NMDA receptors [136]. These interactions can suppress the migration and activation of many cells involved in immunological surveillance, including natural killer cells. The clinical significance of these interactions, and whether there is a net detrimental effect compared with the clinical alternative of injectable anesthetics, has yet to be conclusively determined. Studies comparing immune function in patients undergoing inhalational or total intravenous anesthesia have yielded mixed results, with some studies reporting less natural killer cell cytotoxicity and greater tumor cell viability in patients receiving inhalational anesthesia, and others reporting no meaningful difference [137,138].

Volatile anesthetics are known to induce ischemic preconditioning and attenuate reperfusion injury. These effects are mediated by the induction of the transcription factor, hypoxia-inducible factor 1 (HIF-1), which regulates the expression of numerous genes that aid in cell survival following ischemic injury. These same effects also support the vascularization of hypoxic tumor environments, and promote the survival, proliferation, and migration of neoplastic cells, which may favor the successful colonization and outgrowth of residual tumor cells leading to cancer recurrence following anesthesia and surgery.

In vitro data largely suggest that the administration of inhalational anesthetics may be associated with compromised postoperative outcomes. Similarly, most retrospective clinical studies comparing inhalational versus injectable anesthetic protocols report that volatile agents may be associated with increased cancer recurrence rates and decreased postoperative survival time; however, results are mixed, and more robust randomized clinical trials are needed [139,140].

Injectable anesthetics

Propofol is the injectable anesthetic that has been most widely studied for its effects on cancer outcomes. While there are some conflicting findings, the majority of *in vitro* studies report a reduction in cancer cell viability and malignant characteristics following propofol exposure, which are mediated through several different mechanisms. Specifically, propofol alters the expression of certain long noncoding and microRNAs which regulate gene function to inhibit proliferation, invasion, and migration, and promote apoptosis in a range of different neoplastic cell lines [141–143]. Propofol also has been shown to enhance chemosensitivity and promote apoptosis through several signaling pathways when cancer cells are exposed to both propofol and different chemotherapeutic agents [144,145].

Rodent models also demonstrate an antitumor effect with propofol. In xenograft models using various tumor types, treating the inoculated cells or the animals themselves with propofol resulted in reduced tumor growth and increased survival time compared with control groups [146,147]. In a more clinically comparable study using a breast cancer model, mice undergoing tumor excision under propofol anesthesia developed fewer pulmonary metastases compared with those undergoing anesthesia with sevoflurane [148]. Findings from these controlled experimental studies corroborate the observed trend of favorable outcomes in surgical cancer patients undergoing total intravenous anesthesia in retrospective human studies [139,140]. This encouraging *in vitro*, *in vivo*, and retrospective data support creation of large randomized controlled trials to better understand the effect of anesthetic selection on cancer outcomes.

Pain and analgesic techniques

Pain

The nociceptive input from surgery creates inflammation and numerous physiologic changes, including stimulation of the sympathetic nervous system and activation of the hypothalamic–pituitary–adrenal axis. The resulting increase in circulating cytokines, catecholamines, and glucocorticoids promotes angiogenesis, reduces the number and activity of natural killer cells and cytotoxic T cells, and upregulates regulatory T cells, which dampens the immune response, creating a microenvironment that supports the establishment and survival of residual cancer cells [149]. Consequently, the provision of adequate analgesia is important for both patient welfare and potentially improving long-term cancer treatment prognosis.

Opioids

Opioid analgesics are often used as the primary modality for managing surgical pain and can effectively attenuate the perioperative stress response [150]. Despite this benefit, the effect of opioid administration on cancer recurrence remains unclear and controversial. Opioid receptors are expressed within the nervous system, peripheral tissues, endothelial cells, immune cells, and cancer cells, and participate in different receptor interactions with a range of exogenous opioids. This has resulted in notable variability when evaluating the effects of opioid administration on angiogenesis, immune function, and more holistic outcome measures such as tumor growth and metastasis.

The angiogenic properties of morphine and other full μ-opioid receptor agonists have been established; however, this effect does not seem to be induced through opioid receptor binding. The mechanisms are not fully elucidated or universal, with the angiogenic effects of different full μ-opioid receptor agonists mediated via divergent pathways [151,152]. In contrast, κ-opioid receptor agonists inhibit angiogenesis through opioid receptor-mediated downregulation of the vascular endothelial growth factor receptor [153].

The immunomodulating properties of opioids vary among different agents and are induced by direct interactions with immune cells as well as indirectly through modulation of the neuroendocrine system. Opioids are generally considered to have immunosuppressive properties, however, drug selection, dosing, various host factors, and duration of exposure all influence their effects, yielding highly variable results in the literature [154]. Morphine has been documented to suppress the activity of phagocytic cells, natural killer cells, as well as T and B lymphocytes [155], but conversely has no significant effect on natural killer cell activity in patients undergoing cancer surgery [156]. Similarly, fentanyl has been shown to increase natural killer cell number and preserve cytotoxicity in humans while reducing natural killer cell cytotoxicity and other measures of immune function in rats, suggesting species differences may exist [157,158]. In contrast, buprenorphine demonstrated neutral or even stimulatory effects on different measures of immune function in rodent models [158].

Rodent models reporting cancer outcomes exhibit the same variable results as *in vitro* studies. The different study designs utilized are confounded by numerous factors that have the potential to influence measured outcomes, including mouse strain, cancer type and location, pain, presence of surgical stimulation, as well as opioid selection, dosing, and route of administration. Rodent studies evaluating morphine alone have reported conflicting results including that morphine promotes tumor growth and increases metastases formation, reduces tumor burden and decreases metastasis, or has no effect on cancer outcomes [159]. Human clinical trials share similar heterogeneity, and while there is some suggestion that patients receiving opioids have increased cancer recurrence rates compared with regional anesthesia, the data are still mixed [160]. Variable study designs and confounding factors prevent the ability to perform quantitative meta-analysis, and large randomized trials in specific patient populations are required to draw conclusions about the effect of opioids on cancer outcomes.

Local anesthetics and locoregional techniques

The interruption of afferent input from locoregional anesthetic techniques can completely prevent nociceptive signals from reaching the spinal cord and blunt sympathetic and neuroendocrine responses during surgery. Systemically administered lidocaine also provides analgesia through hyperpolarizing postsynaptic neurons in the dorsal horn of the spinal cord. It has been postulated that local anesthetics and regional anesthetic techniques may confer favorable postoperative cancer outcomes given their opioid- and anesthetic-sparing effects which would attenuate the potentially detrimental effects of these agents. Additionally, local anesthetics directly inhibit tumor proliferation and invasion, induce apoptosis, and enhance chemosensitivity in different types of cancer cells [161–163]. Local anesthetics also exert antineoplastic effects indirectly by favorably modulating the immune system and suppressing angiogenesis [164,165].

Rodent studies largely support *in vitro* findings, with both systemically administered lidocaine and regional anesthesia reducing tumor size and metastatic burden [166–168]. Numerous retrospective studies and clinical trials have been performed evaluating outcomes following a range of anesthetic techniques for resection of different types of cancer. Several meta-analyses have been performed and concluded that locoregional anesthesia offers a benefit in patients undergoing surgical tumor resection. Specifically, one report concluded that patients receiving paravertebral blocks for breast cancer surgery had lower postoperative opioid requirements and cancer recurrence rates [169], while others conclude that regional anesthesia improves overall survival in operable cancers but does not affect recurrence rates [170,171]. In contrast, another meta-analysis did not detect a difference in recurrence or survival between patients undergoing general anesthesia with or without regional anesthesia but noted that these findings should be interpreted carefully given the risk of bias, variable study populations, and a low level of evidence in the studies analyzed [172]. As with other anesthetic agents, large randomized controlled trials are required to further understand the effect of local anesthetic administration and anesthetic protocol on cancer outcomes.

References

1 Cleeland CS, Gonin R, Hatfield AK, *et al.* Pain and its treatment in outpatients with metastatic cancer. *N Eng J Med* 1994; **330**(9): 592–596.

2 van den Beuken-van Everdingen MH, Hochstenbach LM, Joosten EA, *et al.* Update on prevalence of pain in patients with cancer: systematic review and meta-analysis. *J Pain Symptom Manage* 2016; **51**(6): 1070–1090.e9.

3 Coyle N, Adelhardt J, Foley KM, *et al.* Character of terminal illness in the advanced cancer patient: pain and other symptoms during the last four weeks of life. *J Pain Symptom Manage* 1990; **5**(2): 83–93.

4 Lussier D, Huskey AG, Portenoy RK. Adjuvant analgesics in cancer pain management. *Oncologist* 2004; **9**(5): 571–591.

5 KuKanich B. Outpatient oral analgesics in dogs and cats beyond nonsteroidal anti-inflammatory drugs: an evidence-based approach. *Vet Clin North Am Small Anim Pract* 2013; **43**(5): 1109–1125.

6 Lester P, Gaynor JS. Management of cancer pain. *Vet Clin North Am Small Anim Pract* 2000; **30**(4): 951–966, ix.

7 Bennett D, Morton C. A study of owner observed behavioural and lifestyle changes in cats with musculoskeletal disease before and after analgesic therapy. *J Fel Med Surg* 2009; **11**(12): 997–1004.

8 Lascelles BD, Hansen BD, Roe S, *et al.* Evaluation of client-specific outcome measures and activity monitoring to measure pain relief in cats with osteoarthritis. *J Vet Intern Med* 2007; **21**(3): 410–416.

9 Mathews K, Kronen PW, Lascelles D, *et al.* Guidelines for recognition, assessment and treatment of pain: WSAVA Global Pain Council members and co-authors of this document. *J Small Anim Pract* 2014; **55**(6): E10–E68.

10 Hudson JT, Slater MR, Taylor L, *et al.* Assessing repeatability and validity of a visual analogue scale questionnaire for use in assessing pain and lameness in dogs. *Am J Vet Res* 2004; **65**(12): 1634–1643.

11 Holton LL, Scott EM, Nolan AM, *et al.* Comparison of three methods used for assessment of pain in dogs. *J Am Vet Med Assoc* 1998; **212**(1): 61–66.

12 Morton CM, Reid J, Scott EM, *et al.* Application of a scaling model to establish and validate an interval level pain scale for assessment of acute pain in dogs. *Am J Vet Res* 2005; **66**(12): 2154–2166.

13 Firth AM, Haldane SL. Development of a scale to evaluate postoperative pain in dogs. *J Am Vet Med Assoc* 1999; **214**(5): 651–659.

14 Reid J, Nolan AM, Hughes JML, *et al.* Development of the short-form Glasgow Composite Measure Pain Scale (CMPS-SF) and derivation of an analgesic intervention score. *Anim Welf* 2007; **16**: 97–104.

15 Carsten RE, Hellyer PW, Bachand AM, *et al.* Correlations between acute radiation scores and pain scores in canine radiation patients with cancer of the forelimb. *Vet Anaesth Analg* 2008; **35**(4): 355–362.

16 Flor PB, Yazbek KV, Ida KK, *et al.* Tramadol plus metamizole combined or not with anti-inflammatory drugs is clinically effective for moderate to severe chronic pain treatment in cancer patients. *Vet Anaesth Analg* 2013; **40**(3): 316–327.

17 Yazbek KV, Fantoni DT. Validity of a health-related quality-of-life scale for dogs with signs of pain secondary to cancer. *J Am Vet Med Assoc* 2005; **226**(8): 1354–1358.

18 Lynch S, Savary-Bataille K, Leeuw B, *et al.* Development of a questionnaire assessing health-related quality-of-life in dogs and cats with cancer. *Vet Comp Oncol* 2011; **9**(3): 172–182.

19 Tzannes S, Hammond MF, Murphy S, *et al.* Owners 'perception of their cats' quality of life during COP chemotherapy for lymphoma. *J Feline Med Surg* 2008; **10**(1): 73–81.

20 Giuffrida MA, Farrar JT, Brown DC. Psychometric properties of the Canine Symptom Assessment Scale, a multidimensional owner-reported questionnaire instrument for assessment of physical symptoms in dogs with solid tumors. *J Am Vet Med Assoc* 2017; **251**(12): 1405–1414.

21 Lai YE, Lascelles BDX, Nolan MW. Behavioral phenotyping of cancer pain in domesticated cats with naturally occurring squamous cell carcinoma of the tongue: initial validation studies provide evidence for regional and widespread algoplasticity. *Peer J* 2021; **9**: e11984.

22 Fan TM, Charney SC, de Lorimier LP, *et al.* Double-blind placebo-controlled trial of adjuvant pamidronate with palliative radiotherapy and intravenous doxorubicin for canine appendicular osteosarcoma bone pain. *J Vet Intern Med* 2009; **23**(1): 152–160.

23 Weinstein JI, Payne S, Poulson JM, *et al.* Use of force plate analysis to evaluate the efficacy of external beam radiation to alleviate osteosarcoma pain. *Vet Radiol Ultrasound* 2009; **50**(6): 673–678.

24 Martin CK, Tannehill-Gregg SH, Wolfe TD, *et al.* Bone-invasive oral squamous cell carcinoma in cats: pathology and expression of parathyroid hormone-related protein. *Vet Pathol* 2011; **48**(1): 302–312.

25 Mantyh PW, Clohisy DR, Koltzenburg M, *et al.* Molecular mechanisms of cancer pain. *Nat Rev Cancer* 2002; **2**(3): 201–209.

26 Jimenez-Andrade JM, Mantyh WG, Bloom AP, *et al.* Bone cancer pain. *Ann N Y Acad Sci* 2010; **1198**: 173–181.

27 Clohisy DR, Mantyh PW. Bone cancer pain and the role of RANKL/OPG. *J Musculoskelet Neuronal Interact* 2004; **4**(3): 293–300.

28 Goblirsch M, Mathews W, Lynch C, *et al.* Radiation treatment decreases bone cancer pain, osteolysis and tumor size. *Radiat Res* 2004; **161**(2): 228–234.

29 Yoneda T, Hata K, Nakanishi M, *et al.* Involvement of acidic microenvironment in the pathophysiology of cancer-associated bone pain. *Bone* 2011; **48**(1): 100–105.

30 Mizoguchi F, Mizuno A, Hayata T, *et al.* Transient receptor potential vanilloid 4 deficiency suppresses unloading-induced bone loss. *J Cell Physiol* 2008; **216**(1): 47–53.

31 Shor S, Fadl-Alla BA, Pondenis HC, *et al.* Expression of nociceptive ligands in canine osteosarcoma. *J Vet Intern Med* 2015; **29**(1): 268–275.

32 Mantyh WG, Jimenez-Andrade JM, Stake JI, *et al.* Blockade of nerve sprouting and neuroma formation markedly attenuates the development of late stage cancer pain. *Neuroscience* 2010; **171**(2): 588–598.

33 Jimenez-Andrade JM, Ghilardi JR, Castaneda-Corral G, *et al.* Preventive or late administration of anti-NGF therapy attenuates tumor-induced nerve sprouting, neuroma formation, and cancer pain. *Pain* 2011; **152**(11): 2564–2574.

34 Denneberg NA, Egenvall A. Evaluation of dog owners' perceptions concerning radiation therapy. *Acta Vet Scand* 2009; **51**: 19.

35 Collen EB, Mayer MN. Acute effects of radiation treatment: skin reactions. *Can Vet J* 2006; **47**(9): 931–932, 934–935.

36 Anderson CR, McNiel EA, Gillette EL, *et al.* Late complications of pelvic irradiation in 16 dogs. *Vet Radiol Ultrasound* 2002; **43**(2): 187–192.

37 Harris D, King GK, Bergman PJ. Radiation therapy toxicities. *Vet Clin North Am Small Anim Pract* 1997; **27**(1): 37–46.

38 Venable RO, Saba CF, Endicott MM, *et al.* Dexrazoxane treatment of doxorubicin extravasation injury in four dogs. *J Am Vet Med Assoc* 2012; **240**(3): 304–307.

39 Ogilvie GK, Richardson RC, Curtis CR, *et al.* Acute and short-term toxicoses associated with the administration of doxorubicin to dogs with malignant tumors. *J Am Vet Med Assoc* 1989; **195**(11): 1584–1587.

40 Gaeta R, Brown D, Cohen R, *et al.* Risk factors for development of sterile haemorrhagic cystitis in canine lymphoma patients receiving oral cyclophosphamide: a case-control study. *Vet Comp Oncol* 2014; **12**(4): 277–286.

41 Poirier VJ, Hershey AE, Burgess KE, *et al.* Efficacy and toxicity of paclitaxel (Taxol) for the treatment of canine malignant tumors. *J Vet Intern Med* 2004; **18**(2): 219–222.

42 McEntee MC, Rassnick KM, Bailey DB, *et al.* Phase I and pharmacokinetic evaluation of the combination of orally administered docetaxel and cyclosporin A in tumor-bearing cats. *J Vet Intern Med* 2006; **20**(6): 1370–1375.

43 Carlson K, Ocean AJ. Peripheral neuropathy with microtubule-targeting agents: occurrence and management approach. *Clin Breast Cancer* 2011; **11**(2): 73–81.

44 Hamilton TA, Cook JR Jr., Braund KG, *et al.* Vincristine-induced peripheral neuropathy in a dog. *J Am Vet Med Assoc* 1991; **198**(4): 635–638.

45 Martins BD, Martins GD, Horta RD, *et al.* Sensory-motor neuropathy due to vincristine treatment in a dog. *Acta Sci Vet* 2014; **42**(Suppl 1): 59.

46 Neugebauer V, Geisslinger G, Rumenapp P, *et al.* Antinociceptive effects of R(−)- and S(+)-flurbiprofen on rat spinal dorsal horn neurons rendered hyperexcitable by an acute knee joint inflammation. *J Pharmacol Exp Ther* 1995; **275**(2): 618–628.

47 Gold MS, Reichling DB, Shuster MJ, *et al.* Hyperalgesic agents increase a tetrodotoxin-resistant Na+ current in nociceptors. *Proc Natl Acad Sci USA* 1996; **93**(3): 1108–1112.

48 Kirkby Shaw K, Rausch-Derra LC, Rhodes L. Grapiprant: an EP4 prostaglandin receptor antagonist and novel therapy for pain and inflammation. *Vet Med Sci* 2016; **2**(1): 3–9.

49 Gregorio H, Magalhaes TR, Pires I, *et al.* The role of COX expression in the prognostication of overall survival of canine and feline cancer: a systematic review. *Vet Med Sci* 2021; **7**(4): 1107–1119.

50 Saito T, Tamura D, Asano R. Usefulness of selective COX-2 inhibitors as therapeutic agents against canine mammary tumors. *Oncol Rep* 2014; **31**(4): 1637–1644.

51 Knapp DW, Richardson RC, Chan TC, *et al.* Piroxicam therapy in 34 dogs with transitional cell carcinoma of the urinary bladder. *J Vet Intern Med* 1994; **8**(4): 273–278.

52 Weinstein SH, Gaylord JC. Determination of oxycodone in plasma and identification of a major metabolite. *J Pharm Sci* 1979; **68**(4): 527–528.

53 Dohoo SE, Tasker RA. Pharmacokinetics of oral morphine sulfate in dogs: a comparison of sustained release and conventional formulations. *Can J Vet Res* 1997; **61**(4): 251–255.

54 KuKanich B, Lascelles BD, Papich MG. Pharmacokinetics of morphine and plasma concentrations of morphine-6-glucuronide following morphine administration to dogs. *J Vet Pharmacol Ther* 2005; **28**(4): 371–376.

55 Kukanich B, Lascelles BD, Aman AM, *et al.* The effects of inhibiting cytochrome P450 3A, p-glycoprotein, and gastric acid secretion on the oral bioavailability of methadone in dogs. *J Vet Pharmacol Ther* 2005; **28**(5): 461–466.

56 Aragon CL, Read MR, Gaynor JS, *et al.* Pharmacokinetics of an immediate and extended release oral morphine formulation utilizing the spheroidal oral drug absorption system in dogs. *J Vet Pharmacol Ther* 2009; **32**(2): 129–136.

57 Franks JN, Boothe HW, Taylor L, *et al.* Evaluation of transdermal fentanyl patches for analgesia in cats undergoing onychectomy. *J Am Vet Med Assoc* 2000; **217**(7): 1013–1020.

58 Robertson SA, Lascelles BD, Taylor PM, *et al.* PK-PD modeling of buprenorphine in cats: intravenous and oral transmucosal administration. *J Vet Pharmacol Ther* 2005; **28**(5): 453–460.

59 Bellei E, Roncada P, Pisoni L, *et al.* The use of fentanyl-patch in dogs undergoing spinal surgery: plasma concentration and analgesic efficacy. *J Vet Pharmacol Ther* 2011; **34**(5): 437–441.

60 Abbo LA, Ko JC, Maxwell LK, *et al.* Pharmacokinetics of buprenorphine following intravenous and oral transmucosal administration in dogs. *Vet Ther* 2008; **9**(2): 83–93.

61 Ko JC, Freeman LJ, Barletta M, *et al.* Efficacy of oral transmucosal and intravenous administration of buprenorphine before surgery for postoperative analgesia in dogs undergoing ovariohysterectomy. *J Am Vet Med Assoc* 2011; **238**(3): 318–328.

62 Enomoto H, Love L, Madsen M, *et al.* Pharmacokinetics of intravenous, oral transmucosal, and intranasal buprenorphine in healthy male dogs. *J Vet Pharmacol Ther* 2022; **45**(4): 358–365.

63 Davila D, Keeshen TP, Evans RB, *et al.* Comparison of the analgesic efficacy of perioperative firocoxib and tramadol administration in dogs undergoing tibial plateau leveling osteotomy. *J Am Vet Med Assoc* 2013; **243**(2): 225–231.

64 Budsberg SC, Torres BT, Kleine SA, *et al.* Lack of effectiveness of tramadol hydrochloride for the treatment of pain and joint dysfunction in dogs with chronic osteoarthritis. *J Am Vet Med Assoc* 2018; **252**(4): 427–432.

65 Monteiro BP, Klinck MP, Moreau M, *et al.* Analgesic efficacy of tramadol in cats with naturally occurring osteoarthritis. *PLoS ONE* 2017; **12**(4): e0175565.

66 Guedes AGP, Meadows JM, Pypendop BH, *et al.* Evaluation of tramadol for treatment of osteoarthritis in geriatric cats. *J Am Vet Med Assoc* 2018; **252**(5): 565–571.

67 Radulovic LL, Turck D, von Hodenberg A, *et al.* Disposition of gabapentin (neurontin) in mice, rats, dogs, and monkeys. *Drug Metab Dispos* 1995; **23**(4): 441–448.

68 Aghighi SA, Tipold A, Piechotta M, *et al.* Assessment of the effects of adjunctive gabapentin on postoperative pain after intervertebral disc surgery in dogs. *Vet Anaesth Analg* 2012; **39**(6): 636–646.

69 Wagner AE, Mich PM, Uhrig SR, *et al.* Clinical evaluation of perioperative administration of gabapentin as an adjunct for postoperative analgesia in dogs undergoing amputation of a forelimb. *J Am Vet Med Assoc* 2010; **236**(7): 751–756.

70 Cashmore RG, Harcourt-Brown TR, Freeman PM, *et al.* Clinical diagnosis and treatment of suspected neuropathic pain in three dogs. *Aust Vet J* 2009; **87**(1): 45–50.

71 Salazar V, Dewey CW, Schwark W, *et al.* Pharmacokinetics of single-dose oral pregabalin administration in normal dogs. *Vet Anaesth Analg* 2009; **36**(6): 574–580.

72 Sanchis-Mora S, Chang YM, Abeyesinghe SM, *et al.* Pregabalin for the treatment of syringomyelia-associated neuropathic pain in dogs: a randomised, placebo-controlled, double-masked clinical trial. *Vet J* 2019; **250**: 55–62.

73 Monteiro BP, de Lorimier LP, Moreau M, *et al.* Pain characterization and response to palliative care in dogs with naturally-occurring appendicular osteosarcoma: an open label clinical trial. *PLoS ONE* 2018; **13**(12): e0207200.

74 Gamble LJ, Boesch JM, Frye CW, *et al.* Pharmacokinetics, safety, and clinical efficacy of cannabidiol treatment in osteoarthritic dogs. *Front Vet Sci* 2018; **5**: 165.

75 Verrico CD, Wesson S, Konduri V, *et al.* A randomized, double-blind, placebo-controlled study of daily cannabidiol for the treatment of canine osteoarthritis pain. *Pain* 2020; **161**(9): 2191–2202.

76 Brioschi FA, Di Cesare F, Gioeni D, *et al.* Oral transmucosal cannabidiol oil formulation as part of a multimodal analgesic regimen: effects on pain relief and quality of life improvement in dogs affected by spontaneous osteoarthritis. *Animals (Basel)* 2020; **10**(9): 1505.

77 Mejia S, Duerr FM, Griffenhagen G, *et al.* Evaluation of the effect of cannabidiol on naturally occurring osteoarthritis-associated pain: a pilot study in dogs. *J Am Anim Hosp Assoc* 2021; **57**(2): 81–90.

78 Lacey DL, Timms E, Tan HL, *et al.* Osteoprotegerin ligand is a cytokine that regulates osteoclast differentiation and activation. *Cell* 1998; **93**(2): 165–176.

79 Body JJ. Bisphosphonates for malignancy-related bone disease: current status, future developments. *Support Care Cancer* 2006; **14**(5): 408–418.

80 Arrington SA, Damron TA, Mann KA, *et al.* Concurrent administration of zoledronic acid and irradiation leads to improved bone density, biomechanical strength, and microarchitecture in a mouse model of tumor-induced osteolysis. *J Surg Oncol* 2008; **97**(3): 284–290.

81 Curtis RC, Custis JT, Ehrhart NP, *et al.* Combination therapy with zoledronic acid and parathyroid hormone improves bone architecture and strength following a clinically-relevant dose of stereotactic radiation therapy for the local treatment of canine osteosarcoma in athymic rats. *PLoS ONE* 2016; **11**(6): e0158005.

82 Flesner BK, Torres BT, Hutcheson KD, *et al.* A pilot study of cancer-induced bone pain using validated owner questionnaires, serum N-telopeptide concentration, kinetic analysis, and PET/CT. *Front Vet Sci* 2021; **8**: 637195.

83 Ringdahl-Mayland B, Thamm DH, Martin TW. Retrospective evaluation of outcome in dogs with appendicular osteosarcoma following hypofractionated palliative radiation therapy with or without bisphosphonates: 165 cases (2010–2019). *Front Vet Sci* 2022; **9**: 892297.

84 Martin TW, Griffin L, Custis J, *et al.* Outcome and prognosis for canine appendicular osteosarcoma treated with stereotactic body radiation therapy in 123 dogs. *Vet Comp Oncol* 2021; **19**(2): 284–294.

85 Boston SE, Bacon NJ, Culp WT, *et al.* Outcome after repair of a sarcoma-related pathologic fracture in dogs: a Veterinary Society of Surgical Oncology Retrospective Study. *Vet Surg* 2011; **40**(4): 431–437.

86 Boston SE, Vinayak A, Lu X, *et al.* Outcome and complications in dogs with appendicular primary bone tumors treated with stereotactic radiotherapy and concurrent surgical stabilization. *Vet Surg* 2017; **46**(6): 829–837.

87 Keller RK, Fliesler SJ. Mechanism of aminobisphosphonate action: characterization of alendronate inhibition of the isoprenoid pathway. *Biochem Biophys Res Commun* 1999; **266**(2): 560–563.

88 Fan TM, de Lorimier LP, Charney SC, *et al.* Evaluation of intravenous pamidronate administration in 33 cancer-bearing dogs with primary or secondary bone involvement. *J Vet Intern Med* 2005; **19**(1): 74–80.

89 Fan TM, de Lorimier LP, O'Dell-Anderson K, *et al.* Single-agent pamidronate for palliative therapy of canine appendicular osteosarcoma bone pain. *J Vet Intern Med* 2007; **21**(3): 431–439.

90 Fan TM, de Lorimier LP, Garrett LD, *et al.* The bone biologic effects of zoledronate in healthy dogs and dogs with malignant osteolysis. *J Vet Intern Med* 2008; **22**(2): 380–387.

91 Brewer DJ, Macfarlane M, O'Connell E, *et al.* Toxicity of zoledronic acid after intravenous administration: a retrospective study of 95 dogs. *J Vet Intern Med* 2022; **36**(1): 253–258.

92 Smith AA, Lindley SES, Almond GT, *et al.* Evaluation of zoledronate for the treatment of canine stage III osteosarcoma: a phase II study. *Vet Med Sci* 2023; **9**(1): 59–67.

93 Lundberg AP, Roady PJ, Somrak AJ, *et al.* Zoledronate-associated osteonecrosis of the jaw in a dog with appendicular osteosarcoma. *J Vet Intern Med* 2016; **30**(4): 1235–1240.

94 Bateman KE, Catton PA, Pennock PW, *et al.* 0-7-21 radiation therapy for the palliation of advanced cancer in dogs. *J Vet Intern Med* 1994; **8**(6): 394–399.

95 Green EM, Adams WM, Forrest LJ. Four fraction palliative radiotherapy for osteosarcoma in 24 dogs. *J Am Anim Hosp Assoc* 2002; **38**(5): 445–451.

96 Mueller F, Poirier V, Melzer K, *et al.* Palliative radiotherapy with electrons of appendicular osteosarcoma in 54 dogs. *In Vivo* 2005; **19**(4): 713–716.

97 Ramirez O III, Dodge RK, Page RL, *et al.* Palliative radiotherapy of appendicular osteosarcoma in 95 dogs. *Vet Radiol Ultrasound* 1999; **40**(5): 517–522.

98 Knapp-Hoch HM, Fidel JL, Sellon RK, *et al.* An expedited palliative radiation protocol for lytic or proliferative lesions of appendicular bone in dogs. *J Am Anim Hosp Assoc* 2009; **45**(1): 24–32.

99 Norquest CJ, Maitz CA, Keys DA, *et al.* Fracture rate and time to fracture in dogs with appendicular osteosarcoma receiving finely fractionated compared to coarsely fractionated radiation therapy: a single institution study. *Vet Med Sci* 2022; **8**(3): 1013–1024.

100 Martin TW, LaRue SM, Griffin L. CT characteristics and proposed scoring scheme are predictive of pathologic fracture in dogs with appendicular osteosarcoma treated with stereotactic body radiation therapy. *Vet Radiol Ultrasound* 2022; **63**(1): 82–90.

101 Caterina MJ, Schumacher MA, Tominaga M, *et al.* The capsaicin receptor: a heat-activated ion channel in the pain pathway. *Nature* 1997; **389**(6653): 816–824.

102 Caterina MJ, Leffler A, Malmberg AB, *et al.* Impaired nociception and pain sensation in mice lacking the capsaicin receptor. *Science* 2000; **288**(5464): 306–313.

103 Olah Z, Szabo T, Karai L, *et al.* Ligand-induced dynamic membrane changes and cell deletion conferred by vanilloid receptor 1. *J Biol Chem* 2001; **276**(14): 11021–11030.

104 Brown DC, Iadarola MJ, Perkowski SZ, *et al.* Physiologic and antinociceptive effects of intrathecal resiniferatoxin in a canine bone cancer model. *Anesthesiology* 2005; **103**(5): 1052–1059.

105 Karai L, Brown DC, Mannes AJ, *et al.* Deletion of vanilloid receptor 1-expressing primary afferent neurons for pain control. *J Clin Invest* 2004; **113**(9): 1344–1352.

106 Brown DC, Agnello K, Iadarola MJ. Intrathecal resiniferatoxin in a dog model: efficacy in bone cancer pain. *Pain* 2015; **156**(6): 1018–1024.

107 Iadarola MJ, Sapio MR, Raithel SJ, *et al.* Long-term pain relief in canine osteoarthritis by a single intra-articular injection of resiniferatoxin, a potent TRPV1 agonist. *Pain* 2018; **159**(10): 2105–2114.

108 Boss MK, Ke Y, Bian L, *et al.* Therapeutic intervention using a Smad7-based Tat protein to treat radiation-induced oral mucositis. *Int J Radiat Oncol Biol Phys* 2022; **112**(3): 759–770.

109 Clohisy DR, Mantyh PW. Bone cancer pain. *Cancer* 2003; **97**(3 Suppl): 866–873.

110 Halvorson KG, Kubota K, Sevcik MA, *et al.* A blocking antibody to nerve growth factor attenuates skeletal pain induced by prostate tumor cells growing in bone. *Cancer Res* 2005; **65**(20): 9426–9435.

111 Sevcik MA, Ghilardi JR, Peters CM, *et al.* Anti-NGF therapy profoundly reduces bone cancer pain and the accompanying increase in markers of peripheral and central sensitization. *Pain* 2005; **115**(1–2): 128–141.

112 Fan TM, Barger AM, Sprandel IT, *et al.* Investigating TrkA expression in canine appendicular osteosarcoma. *J Vet Intern Med* 2008; **22**(5): 1181–1188.

113 Webster RP, Anderson GI, Gearing DP. Canine Brief Pain Inventory scores for dogs with osteoarthritis before and after administration of a monoclonal antibody against nerve growth factor. *Am J Vet Res* 2014; **75**(6): 532–535.

114 Corral MJ, Moyaert H, Fernandes T, *et al.* A prospective, randomized, blinded, placebo-controlled multisite clinical study of bedinvetmab, a canine monoclonal antibody targeting nerve growth factor, in dogs with osteoarthritis. *Vet Anaesth Analg* 2021; **48**(6): 943–955.

115 Gruen ME, Thomson AE, Griffith EH, *et al.* A feline-specific anti-nerve growth factor antibody improves mobility in cats with degenerative joint disease-associated pain: a pilot proof of concept study. *J Vet Intern Med* 2016; **30**(4): 1138–1148.

116 Gruen ME, Griffith EH, Thomson AE, *et al.* Criterion validation testing of clinical metrology instruments for measuring degenerative joint disease associated mobility impairment in cats. *PLoS ONE* 2015; **10**(7): e0131839.

117 Gonzalez-Rodriguez S, Pevida M, Roques BP, *et al.* Involvement of enkephalins in the inhibition of osteosarcoma-induced thermal hyperalgesia evoked by the blockade of peripheral P2X3 receptors. *Neurosci Lett* 2009; **465**(3): 285–289.

118 Kaan TK, Yip PK, Patel S, *et al.* Systemic blockade of P2X3 and P2X2/3 receptors attenuates bone cancer pain behaviour in rats. *Brain* 2010; **133**(9): 2549–2564.

119 Wu JX, Xu MY, Miao XR, *et al.* Functional up-regulation of P2X3 receptors in dorsal root ganglion in a rat model of bone cancer pain. *Eur J Pain* 2012; **16**(10): 1378–1388.

120 Hansen RR, Nasser A, Falk S, *et al.* Chronic administration of the selective P2X3, P2X2/3 receptor antagonist, A-317491, transiently attenuates cancer-induced bone pain in mice. *Eur J Pharmacol* 2012; **688**(1–3): 27–34.

121 Yamamoto T, Yaksh TL. Stereospecific effects of a nonpeptidic NK1 selective antagonist, CP-96,345: antinociception in the absence of motor dysfunction. *Life Sci* 1991; **49**(26): 1955–1963.

122 Wick EC, Hoge SG, Grahn SW, *et al.* Transient receptor potential vanilloid 1, calcitonin gene-related peptide, and substance P mediate nociception in acute pancreatitis. *Am J Physiol Gastrointest Liver Physiol* 2006; **290**(5): G959–G969.

123 Gautam M, Prasoon P, Kumar R, *et al.* Role of neurokinin type 1 receptor in nociception at the periphery and the spinal level in the rat. *Spinal Cord* 2016; **54**(3): 172–182.

124 Marquez M, Boscan P, Weir H, *et al.* Comparison of NK-1 receptor antagonist (maropitant) to morphine as a pre-anaesthetic agent for canine ovariohysterectomy. *PLoS ONE* 2015; **10**(10): e0140734.

125 Correa JMX, Soares P, Niella RV, *et al.* Evaluation of the antinociceptive effect of maropitant, a neurokinin-1 receptor antagonist, in cats undergoing ovariohysterectomy. *Vet Med Int* 2019; **2019**: 9352528.

126 Soares P, Correa JMX, Niella RV, *et al.* Continuous infusion of ketamine and lidocaine either with or without maropitant as an adjuvant agent for analgesia in female dogs undergoing mastectomy. *Vet Med Int* 2021; **2021**: 4747301.

127 Correa JMX, Niella RV, Oliveira JNS, *et al.* Antinociceptive and analgesic effect of continuous intravenous infusion of maropitant, lidocaine and ketamine alone or in combination in cats undergoing ovariohysterectomy. *Acta Vet Scand* 2021; **63**(1): 49.

128 Karna SR, Chambers P, Singh P, *et al.* Evaluation of analgesic interaction between morphine, maropitant and dexmedetomidine in dogs undergoing ovariohysterectomy. *N Z Vet J* 2022; **70**(1): 10–21.

129 Munoz M, Berger M, Rosso M, *et al.* Antitumor activity of neurokinin-1 receptor antagonists in MG-63 human osteosarcoma xenografts. *Int J Oncol* 2014; **44**(1): 137–146.

130 Munoz M, Gonzalez-Ortega A, Covenas R. The NK-1 receptor is expressed in human leukemia and is involved in the antitumor action of aprepitant and other NK-1 receptor antagonists on acute lymphoblastic leukemia cell lines. *Invest New Drugs* 2012; **30**(2): 529–540.

131 Borrego JF, Huelsmeyer MK, Pinkerton ME, *et al.* Neurokinin-1 receptor expression and antagonism by the NK-1R antagonist maropitant in canine melanoma cell lines and primary tumour tissues. *Vet Comp Oncol* 2016; **14**(2): 210–224.

132 Deng X, Vipani M, Liang G, *et al.* Sevoflurane modulates breast cancer cell survival via modulation of intracellular calcium homeostasis. *BMC Anesthesiol* 2020; **20**(1): 253.

133 Tiron CE, Patrascanu E, Postu PA, *et al.* Sevoflurane modulates AKT isoforms in triple negative breast cancer cells. An experimental study. *Curr Issues Mol Biol* 2021; **43**(1): 264–275.

134 Kvolik S, Glavas-Obrovac L, Bares V, *et al.* Effects of inhalation anesthetics halothane, sevoflurane, and isoflurane on human cell lines. *Life Sci* 2005; **77**(19): 2369–2383.

135 Hirai T, Konishi Y, Mizuno S, *et al.* Differential effects of sevoflurane on the growth and apoptosis of human cancer cell lines. *J Anesth* 2020; **34**(1): 47–57.

136 Yuki K, Eckenhoff RG. Mechanisms of the immunological effects of volatile anesthetics: a review. *Anesth Analg* 2016; **123**(2): 326–335.

137 Zhang T, Fan Y, Liu K, *et al.* Effects of different general anaesthetic techniques on immune responses in patients undergoing surgery for tongue cancer. *Anaesth Intensive Care* 2014; **42**(2): 220–227.

138 Lim JA, Oh CS, Yoon TG, *et al.* The effect of propofol and sevoflurane on cancer cell, natural killer cell, and cytotoxic T lymphocyte function in patients undergoing breast cancer surgery: an in vitro analysis. *BMC Cancer* 2018; **18**(1): 159.

139 Jin Z, Li R, Liu J, *et al.* Long-term prognosis after cancer surgery with inhalational anesthesia and total intravenous anesthesia: a systematic review and meta-analysis. *Int J Physiol Pathophysiol Pharmacol* 2019; **11**(3): 83–94.

140 Yap A, Lopez-Olivo MA, Dubowitz J, *et al.* Anesthetic technique and cancer outcomes: a meta-analysis of total intravenous versus volatile anesthesia. *Can J Anaesth* 2019; **66**(5): 546–561.

141 Zhang J, Shan WF, Jin TT, *et al.* Propofol exerts anti-hepatocellular carcinoma by microvesicle-mediated transfer of miR-142-3p from macrophage to cancer cells. *J Transl Med* 2014; **12**: 279.

142 Buschmann D, Brandes F, Lindemann A, *et al.* Propofol and sevoflurane differentially impact microRNAs in circulating extracellular vesicles during colorectal cancer resection: a pilot study. *Anesthesiology* 2020; **132**(1): 107–120.

143 Ren YL, Zhang W. Propofol promotes apoptosis of colorectal cancer cells via alleviating the suppression of lncRNA HOXA11-AS on miRNA let-7i. *Biochem Cell Biol* 2020; **98**(2): 90–98.

144 Du QH, Xu YB, Zhang MY, *et al.* Propofol induces apoptosis and increases gemcitabine sensitivity in pancreatic cancer cells in vitro by inhibition of nuclear factor-kappaB activity. *World J Gastroenterol* 2013; **19**(33): 5485–5492.

145 Li H, Lu Y, Pang Y, *et al.* Propofol enhances the cisplatin-induced apoptosis on cervical cancer cells via EGFR/JAK2/STAT3 pathway. *Biomed Pharmacother* 2017; **86**: 324–333.

146 Cui WY, Liu Y, Zhu YQ, *et al.* Propofol induces endoplasmic reticulum (ER) stress and apoptosis in lung cancer cell H460. *Tumour Biol* 2014; **35**(6): 5213–5217.

147 Gao Y, Yu X, Zhang F, *et al.* Propofol inhibits pancreatic cancer progress under hypoxia via ADAM8. *J Hepatobiliary Pancreat Sci* 2019; **26**(6): 219–226.

148 Li R, Huang Y, Lin J. Distinct effects of general anesthetics on lung metastasis mediated by IL-6/JAK/STAT3 pathway in mouse models. *Nat Commun* 2020; **11**(1): 642.

149 Eddy JL, Krukowski K, Janusek L, *et al.* Glucocorticoids regulate natural killer cell function epigenetically. *Cell Immunol* 2014; **290**(1): 120–130.

150 Naguib AN, Tobias JD, Hall MW, *et al.* The role of different anesthetic techniques in altering the stress response during cardiac surgery in children: a prospective, double-blinded, and randomized study. *Pediatr Crit Care Med* 2013; **14**(5): 481–490.

151 Ondrovics M, Hoelbl-Kovacic A, Fux DA. Opioids: modulators of angiogenesis in wound healing and cancer. *Oncotarget* 2017; **8**(15): 25783–25796.

152 Feng T, Zeng S, Ding J, *et al.* Comparative analysis of the effects of opioids in angiogenesis. *BMC Anesthesiol* 2021; **21**(1): 257.

153 Yamamizu K, Furuta S, Hamada Y, *et al.* κ Opioids inhibit tumor angiogenesis by suppressing VEGF signaling. *Sci Rep* 2013; **3**: 3213.

154 Sacerdote P. Opioids and the immune system. *Palliat Med* 2006; **20**(Suppl 1): S9–S15.

155 Eisenstein TK. Opioids and the immune system: what is their mechanism of action? *Br J Pharmacol* 2011; **164**(7): 1826–1828.

156 Sacerdote P, Bianchi M, Gaspani L, *et al.* The effects of tramadol and morphine on immune responses and pain after surgery in cancer patients. *Anesth Analg* 2000; **90**(6): 1411–1414.

157 Jacobs R, Karst M, Scheinichen D, *et al.* Effects of fentanyl on cellular immune functions in man. *Int J Immunopharmacol* 1999; **21**(7): 445–454.

158 Martucci C, Panerai AE, Sacerdote P. Chronic fentanyl or buprenorphine infusion in the mouse: similar analgesic profile but different effects on immune responses. *Pain* 2004; **110**(1–2): 385–392.

159 Afsharimani B, Doornebal CW, Cabot PJ, *et al.* Comparison and analysis of the animal models used to study the effect of morphine on tumour growth and metastasis. *Br J Pharmacol* 2015; **172**(2): 251–259.

160 Bovill JG. Surgery for cancer: does anesthesia matter? *Anesth Analg* 2010; **110**(6): 1524–1526.

161 Sun H, Sun Y. Lidocaine inhibits proliferation and metastasis of lung cancer cell via regulation of miR-539/EGFR axis. *Artif Cells Nanomed Biotechnol* 2019; **47**(1): 2866–2874.

162 Zhang Y, Jia J, Jin W, *et al.* Lidocaine inhibits the proliferation and invasion of hepatocellular carcinoma by downregulating USP14 induced PI3K/Akt pathway. *Pathol Res Pract* 2020; **216**(8): 152963.

163 Zhu G, Zhang L, Dan J, *et al.* Differential effects and mechanisms of local anesthetics on esophageal carcinoma cell migration, growth, survival and chemosensitivity. *BMC Anesthesiol* 2020; **20**(1): 126.

164 Ramirez MF, Tran P, Cata JP. The effect of clinically therapeutic plasma concentrations of lidocaine on natural killer cell cytotoxicity. *Reg Anesth Pain Med* 2015; **40**(1): 43–48.

165 Gao J, Hu H, Wang X. Clinically relevant concentrations of lidocaine inhibit tumor angiogenesis through suppressing VEGF/VEGFR2 signaling. *Cancer Chemother Pharmacol* 2019; **83**(6): 1007–1015.

166 Bar-Yosef S, Melamed R, Page GG, *et al.* Attenuation of the tumor-promoting effect of surgery by spinal blockade in rats. *Anesthesiology* 2001; **94**(6): 1066–1073.

167 Xing W, Chen DT, Pan JH, *et al.* Lidocaine induces apoptosis and suppresses tumor growth in human hepatocellular carcinoma cells in vitro and in a xenograft model in vivo. *Anesthesiology* 2017; **126**(5): 868–881.

168 Johnson MZ, Crowley PD, Foley AG, *et al.* Effect of perioperative lidocaine on metastasis after sevoflurane or ketamine-xylazine anaesthesia for breast tumour resection in a murine model. *Br J Anaesth* 2018; **121**(1): 76–85.

169 Schnabel A, Reichl SU, Kranke P, *et al.* Efficacy and safety of paravertebral blocks in breast surgery: a meta-analysis of randomized controlled trials. *Br J Anaesth* 2010; **105**(6): 842–852.

170 Chen WK, Miao CH. The effect of anesthetic technique on survival in human cancers: a meta-analysis of retrospective and prospective studies. *PLoS ONE* 2013; **8**(2): e56540.

171 Sun Y, Li T, Gan TJ. The effects of perioperative regional anesthesia and analgesia on cancer recurrence and survival after oncology surgery: a systematic review and meta-analysis. *Reg Anesth Pain Med* 2015; **40**(5): 589–598.

172 Lee ZX, Ng KT, Ang E, *et al.* Effect of perioperative regional anesthesia on cancer recurrence: a meta-analysis of randomized controlled trials. *Int J Surg* 2020; **82**: 192–199.

71 Osteoarthritis Patients

Steven C. Budsberg and Whitney D. Hinson
Department of Small Animal Medicine and Surgery, College of Veterinary Medicine, University of Georgia, Athens, Georgia, USA

Chapter contents

Introduction, 1377
Diagnosis of osteoarthritis, 1378
Treatment strategies for managing chronic osteoarthritis pain, 1378
Weight reduction and management, 1379
Exercise modification and physical therapy, 1379
Nutritional support and high omega-3 diets, 1379
Pharmacologic management, 1379
Dealing with non-responders to standard treatment approaches, 1384
References, 1385

Introduction

As small animal clinicians attempt to treat chronic pain and the associated dysfunction in their patients with osteoarthritis (OA), they face several challenges. First, pain is a complex experience involving not only transduction and transmission of noxious stimuli from the periphery to the central nervous system (CNS), but also processing of stimuli by higher centers in the brain [1,2]. Pain is the most clinically profound but least well-studied component of OA [3,4]. Articular cartilage degeneration, inflammation, synovitis, and subchondral bone, and periarticular tissue changes are believed to be sources of pain associated with OA in companion animal patients [5–9]. OA is the most common joint disorder leading to significant disability and dysfunction encountered by clinicians. While considered a common problem in small animal medicine, OA is likely the most underdiagnosed and misunderstood rheumatic disease in dogs and cats. OA is a slow, progressive, and often insidious problem, and the wide range of clinical signs makes it a frequently misdiagnosed condition. In the dog, primary OA is uncommon, and the condition mainly develops secondary to another joint pathology (such as hip or stifle instability). OA has been estimated to affect 20% of the United States (US) canine population [10]. This widely referenced estimate, in practical terms, translates to over 15.6 million dogs based on an estimated US canine population of 78 million [11–13]. Estimates of cats affected with OA are between 60% and 90%, and with an estimated number of cats in the US of about 86 million, the number affected with OA is between 51 and 77 million [14–18]. Therefore, the identification and management of this disease is of utmost importance to the small animal clinician.

While the terms "osteoarthritis" and "degenerative joint disease" (DJD) are considered nearly synonymous in dogs, this may not be the case in cats. Joint pathology in cats may differ in etiology, onset, clinical signs, and pathophysiology compared to dogs [19–21]. For the purposes of this chapter, when discussing the cat, the term "DJD/OA" will be used to highlight this potential difference [22].

The American Academy of Orthopaedic Surgeons has proposed the following definition of osteoarthritis: "Osteoarthritic diseases are a result of both mechanical and biological events that destabilize the normal coupling of degradation and synthesis of articular cartilage, extracellular matrix (primarily collagen and aggrecan), and subchondral bone. Although they may be initiated by multiple factors, including genetic, developmental, metabolic, and traumatic factors, osteoarthritic diseases involve all of the tissues of the diarthrodial joint" [23]. Ultimately, osteoarthritic diseases are manifested by morphologic, biochemical, molecular, and biomechanical changes of both cells and matrix, which lead to softening, fibrillation, ulceration, articular cartilage loss, sclerosis and subchondral bone eburnation, and osteophyte production [4–7,9]. When clinically evident, osteoarthritic diseases are characterized by joint pain, tenderness, limitation of mobility, crepitus, occasional effusion, and variable degrees of inflammation without systemic effects.

From a pathophysiologic view, OA is characterized by articular cartilage degeneration and changes in the periarticular soft tissues (synovium and joint capsule) and subchondral bone. In essence, OA can be considered the end stage of organ failure of a joint [9,24]. Specifically, the pathologic changes of OA encompass articular cartilage degeneration, which includes matrix fibrillation, fissure appearance, gross ulceration, and full-thickness loss of the cartilage

Veterinary Anesthesia and Analgesia: The Sixth Edition of Lumb and Jones. Edited by Leigh Lamont, Kurt Grimm, Sheilah Robertson, Lydia Love and Carrie Schroeder.
© 2024 John Wiley & Sons, Inc. Published 2024 by John Wiley & Sons, Inc.
Companion website: www.wiley.com/go/lamont/anesthesia

matrix. This pathology is accompanied by hypertrophic bone changes with osteophyte formation and subchondral bone plate thickening. Failure to repair the damage affecting the surface cartilage and the inability of chondrocytes in injured articular cartilage to restore a functional matrix despite high metabolic activity remains a complex and challenging problem [4–7,9,24].

Clinical signs of OA occur with varying degrees of severity, ranging from a mild, intermittent condition that causes mild discomfort and minimal disability, to a disease state characterized by constant pain along with severe functional disability. Painful mechanical stimuli are detected by nociceptors (Type III or Aδ and Type IV or C fibers), which are afferent nerve fibers located in the joint capsule, associated ligaments, periosteum, and subchondral bone. Joint movement induces mechano-gated ion channels to open resulting in nerve firing [1–3,8]. When joint movement exceeds normal limits, nerve firing dramatically increases and the CNS interprets these signals as pain. Data from experimental models of OA suggest that peripheral mechanosensory fibers become sensitized resulting in increased afferent firing even in response to normal physiological joint motion [25]. Furthermore, sensitization via neuropathic and central pain mechanisms also contributes significantly to pain in a large portion of patients with OA [26–28]. In chronic pain states, these pathophysiologic changes profoundly alter nociceptive processing in both the periphery, by increasing excitability of nociceptors, and centrally, through upregulation in the dorsal root ganglia, spinal cord, and glial cells of the brain. Additionally, modifications and alterations of inhibitory pathways and descending modulation of pain perception can occur [27,28]. Regardless of the type of pain (nociceptive or neuropathic), the role of inflammation in both has been clearly demonstrated [26–28]. Currently, there are no proven methodologies to reverse the changes seen in the joint with OA.

Diagnosis of osteoarthritis

As stated earlier, the clinical signs of OA can vary from mild to severe and from vague to obvious, with pain as a hallmark. However, accurate assessment of pain and dysfunction can be very difficult in dogs and cats. Typically, the diagnosis of OA is based on history, clinical signs, physical examination, and radiographs of the affected joint(s). The goal in assessing a dog or cat with suspected OA is to identify the site of pain and discomfort and attempt to diagnose any initiating causes. While diagnosis of the inciting cause may be more important in younger patients, it is never too late to address conditions such as stifle instability. When dealing with a chronic end-stage OA joint, initiating factors may be less relevant and management of associated pain may become the sole focus of therapy.

Owner assessment of pain severity is an interesting paradox. While owners are most aware of a patient's daily routine, they are not always aware of what pain looks like. Owners often need to see their pet on a successful pain management plan to better recognize pain and dysfunction. This is the rationale for using owner assessments in addition to veterinary examinations. Owner assessments should begin at the start of treatment to define the degree of disability, and thus help decide the level of treatment required. Going forward, they should be used to monitor treatment efficacy. The owner sees the patient daily and can assess multidimensional aspects of pain and associated functional disability. Using metrics like owner questionnaires is advantageous to combat bias associated with subjective evaluation of the patient. In one study, caregiver placebo effect was common when response to treatment was evaluated by both the owner (40% improvement noted on placebo) and the veterinarian (between 40% and 45%) [29]. While another study suggests a lower placebo effect, the potential for bias is significant and may impact assessment of the success or failure of a product or procedure [30].

To increase client awareness and involvement, and to begin to quantify the clinical signs, the use of client questionnaires or clinical metrology instruments is recommended. These instruments are discussed in more detail in Chapter 47. In brief, questionnaires that have been designed and validated in the dog include the Canine Brief Pain Inventory (CBPI), the Liverpool Osteoarthritis in Dogs (LOAD) scale, and the Helsinki Chronic Pain Index (HCPI) [31–36]. Use of a validated questionnaire may lead to improved outcomes as less biased and more accurate assessments will be available to the owner and the clinician. For cats, clinical manifestations of disease and pain are very different from dogs. Several validated instruments for cats are now available including the Feline Musculoskeletal Pain Index (FMPI) and the Montreal Instrument for Cat Arthritis Testing [37–41], and additional information is available in Chapter 47.

Treatment strategies for managing chronic osteoarthritis pain

Current therapy for OA focuses on palliative care with the goal of reducing pain and inflammation and maintaining or improving joint function without altering the pathologic process in the joint. As most OA in the dog, and perhaps in the cat, is secondary to some other pathologic state, the underlying cause must be identified to minimize the long-term effects. While efforts to develop treatments that alter the course of the disease are ongoing, these therapies are still largely unproven.

Management of OA involves a multimodal approach with four to five important components for both dogs and cats [19–21,42–47]. Relying on pharmacologic management alone (i.e., drugs administered singularly or in combination) is usually associated with limited success. Managing OA should be based on a well-thought-out comprehensive plan, which can be presented as "WEDDS": **W**eight reduction and control; an **E**xercise and physical therapy program; **D**ietary modification; a **D**rug (pharmacologic) plan that may include biological therapy; and a discussion of potential **S**urgical interventions (Box 71.1). Thus, initiating a treatment plan for a patient with OA requires a lengthy discussion of all aspects of management with the client that addresses common false assumptions. Three of the most common misconceptions are presented in Box 71.2 and emphasize the need for a realistic and scientifically sound approach to pain management.

Each case must be examined individually, assessing the age, normal activity levels, and, most importantly, the owner's expectations for performance of their animal. Success largely depends on the accurate assessment of client expectations. During the discussion of

Box 71.1 Components of a WEDDS management plan for managing osteoarthritis.

- **W**eight management
- **E**xercise and physical therapy plan
- **D**iet modification
- **D**rugs and biologics
- **S**urgery

Box 71.2 Common misconceptions to address with clients prior to initiating an osteoarthritis management plan.

1 Treatment of pain is an "all or none" phenomenon – ***False***
2 One drug at one dose (i.e., approved label dose) will work for all patients – ***False***
3 If a treatment seems to be effective in people, it will be effective in small animal patients – ***False***

each potential treatment modality, the justification and recommendation for a given therapy should be evidence-based.

Weight reduction and management

Weight control is essential when dealing with OA. Most patients with clinical manifestations of OA are overweight or obese. While clinicians often recommend weight loss programs, success is not common. Several articles are available which discuss strategies for increasing the success of weight loss recommendations [48–52]. Available evidence supports weight loss in canine OA patients and, while little data are available to guide management of cats, it is reasonable to extend these recommendations to feline patients. Owner education and proper dietary management should be considered in every case. Several studies support improved quality of life and lameness in dogs with OA that undergo weight reduction [53–59]. On reviewing the available clinical data, the strength of evidence supports a moderate degree of confidence that weight loss positively impacts dogs with OA.

Exercise modification and physical therapy

There is significant interest in the use of exercise modification and physical therapy in dogs and cats suffering with OA/DJD. There are several programs providing extensive education (including various certifications) in this area, although the description of these is beyond the scope of this chapter. A recent review provides an excellent starting point [60]. There are also textbooks available to help guide the clinician [61]. While it is generally accepted that controlled exercise and physical therapy are helpful in OA patients, peer-reviewed data to support specific programs for canine and feline patients are unfortunately limited. It is beyond the scope of this chapter to discuss the many recommendations about the use of exercise and physical therapy, though any interventions considered should be practical and pragmatic.

While data to support physical therapy modalities are sparse, some reports are available, and more information on these therapies is available in Chapter 49. Treatment of OA with extracorporeal shockwave therapy has shown mixed results [62–64]. Two studies had mixed positive results and one study demonstrated minimal effects. Another prospective study found that a combination of caloric restriction and intense physiotherapy improved both weight loss and force plate kinetic data in overweight dogs with OA [54]. Finally, there are limited data to support the use of photobiomodulation (e.g., low-level laser therapy) in the treatment of OA [65,66]. Overall, the strength and quality of the evidence from these published studies is consistent with a low to moderate degree of confidence that these therapies positively impact OA patients. Consequently, it is incumbent on those promoting, practicing, and financially benefiting from physical therapy and rehabilitation to perform clinical trials to critically evaluate these interventions.

Nutritional support and high omega-3 diets

The introduction of diets formulated with high omega-3 polyunsaturated fatty acids (PUFAs), specifically eicosopentanoic acid (EPA) and docosahexaenoic acid (DHA), has introduced a new dimension in the management of OA [67–69]. The omega-3 (n-3) family of PUFAs includes α-linolenic acid (ALA), EPA, and DHA, while the omega-6 (n-6) family includes linoleic acid (LA) and arachidonic acid (AA) [70]. EPA and DHA are precursors for anti-inflammatory lipid mediators, while AA is a precursor for pro-inflammatory lipid mediators. The current understanding of the mechanism of action of dietary omega-3 PUFAs in OA is twofold. The first effect is indirect, whereby consumption dose-dependently increases concentrations of EPA and DHA, which are less potent mediators of inflammation, and these increased proportions occur at the expense of AA concentrations [71–73]. In addition to forming more anti-inflammatory lipid mediators, less substrate is also available for the formation of AA-derived proinflammatory eicosanoids. The second effect results from direct actions of omega-3 PUFAs on cartilage. Cartilage cell cultures treated with omega-3 PUFAs inhibit the transcription of major enzymes and cytokines tied to matrix degradation [74].

Several clinical trials have looked at the effects of diets high in omega-3 PUFAs on pain and dysfunction associated with OA in dogs [75–80]. All studies were prospective and randomized and adequately addressed issues of scientific quality relating to data collection, analysis, bias, and generalizability. While outcome measures varied between studies creating some challenges in assessing the overall strength of evidence, they uniformly identified positive effects. Thus, the strength and quality of the evidence is consistent with a high degree of confidence that diets high in omega-3 PUFAs positively impact dogs with OA. Given this, it is recommended to switch patients with OA to one of these diets. The data are less clear on the effects of supplementing a diet with omega-3 fatty acid products (e.g., fish oil capsules). In cats, one study has evaluated the effects of elevated omega-3 PUFA diets, with largely inconclusive results. Thus, there are very little data to support or reject the use of these types of diets in cats [81].

Pharmacologic management

Analgesic and anti-inflammatory agents are the most common components in the management of OA. The efficacy of non-steroidal anti-inflammatory drugs (NSAIDs) in treating chronic pain associated with OA has been well documented in several systematic reviews in small animal medicine [47,82–84]. The strength and quality of the evidence is consistent with a high degree of confidence supporting the use of NSAIDs in the management of OA in dogs. There are growing data available in cats showing positive clinical effects, and this supports a moderate degree of confidence in the use of NSAIDs in the management of DJD/OA in cats [39,85].

It is not surprising that, as a class of drugs, NSAIDs are among the most prescribed in small animal medicine. There are more data on NSAID efficacy and potential complications than there are for any other aspect of the multimodal OA management plan.

Non-steroidal anti-inflammatory drugs

As stated previously, NSAIDs are one of the most common classes of drugs used to manage chronic pain in small animals. There are several reasons for the dramatic increase in NSAID use in companion animals, including the availability of NSAIDs with improved safety and efficacy that are approved specifically for small animals (primarily dogs) [83,86,87]. Generally, currently prescribed NSAIDs are very safe drugs, with only a small percentage of patients experiencing serious complications [86]. Detailed information regarding the pharmacology of NSAIDs is available in Chapter 24.

Efficacy of NSAIDs is comparable to opioids in many instances of mild to moderate musculoskeletal and visceral pain. However, for severe pain associated with some fractures, data are not available to substantiate that claim [88]. NSAIDs can be used to alleviate acute pain, either traumatically or surgically induced, and for chronic pain such as OA. Efficacy and toxicity may vary among individuals, and monitoring of each patient is mandatory [86]. Selecting an efficacious NSAID and monitoring its usage is important, but definitive evidence-based guidelines for this are not available. First, it is wise to use products with a history of extensive clinical use. Use only one NSAID at a time and ensure correct dosing. Review the treatment plan frequently and change to an alternative NSAID if there is a poor response to therapy. Observe for signs of potential toxicity as soon as administration begins with increased vigilance and monitoring of high-risk patients. If indicated, establish the patient's baseline renal and hepatic function prior to NSAID administration.

Contraindications for NSAID use

Therapy should be adapted to suit the patient's needs. In patients with chronic disease, begin with the recommended dose and, if efficacious, attempt to reduce the dose at regular intervals (e.g., weekly) until the lowest dose providing the maximum benefit is reached. Determining the lowest effective dose is challenging, and one study suggested that it is difficult to decrease by more than 50% of recommended (label) dose for most dogs [89]. Avoid NSAIDs in patients with known contraindications to their use. Contraindications for NSAID use can range from fairly obvious to quite subtle reasons. The following is a list of general guidelines on potential contraindications for NSAID usage. These recommendations may change with generation of more clinical data [90].

- Patients receiving any type of systemic corticosteroids
- Patients already receiving an NSAID
- Patients with documented renal or hepatic insufficiency or dysfunction
- Patients with any clinical syndrome that creates a decrease in circulating blood volume (e.g., shock, dehydration, hypotension, or ascites)
- Patients with active gastrointestinal disease
- Trauma patients with known or suspected significant active hemorrhage or blood loss
- Pregnant patients or females intended for breeding
- Patients with significant pulmonary disease (this may be less important with COX-2-specific drugs)
- Patients with any type of confirmed or suspected coagulopathy (this may be less important with COX-2-specific drugs)

Adverse events associated with NSAID use

The most common problems associated with NSAID administration to dogs and cats involve the gastrointestinal (GI) tract [86]. Signs may range from vomiting and diarrhea, including hematemesis and melena, to a silent ulcer which results in perforation. The overall incidence of GI toxicity in dogs or cats treated with NSAIDS is unknown. Concurrent administration of other medications (especially other NSAIDs or corticosteroids), previous GI bleeding, or the presence of other systemic diseases may contribute to adverse reactions. The effect that aging has on an individual patient's ability to metabolize NSAIDs is likely to be quite variable. Hepatotoxicosis caused by NSAIDs is generally considered to be idiosyncratic [86,90]. Most dogs recover with cessation of treatment and supportive care. Renal dysfunction may occur with NSAID administration as a consequence of prostaglandin inhibition [91]. While renal prostaglandin synthesis is low under normovolemic conditions, this increases in the face of hypovolemia and prostaglandin synthesis becomes important for maintaining renal perfusion [92,93]. The use of NSAIDs must be considered very carefully in hypovolemic or hypotensive animals, and it is important to remember this in the context of perioperative NSAID administration where patients will be undergoing general anesthesia.

Washout period between NSAIDs

A common clinical management question is whether a washout period is needed when switching from one NSAID to another. Several sources, including crowd sourcing websites, conference proceedings, pharmaceutical company promotional materials, and journal articles, have advocated a washout period of varying lengths (1–7 days) when changing NSAIDs due to presumed lack of efficacy [90,94–96]. These recommendations are not based on clinical data but rather are derived from extrapolations of pharmacokinetic data and conservative speculation. There are several different scenarios to consider when switching from one NSAID to another in a clinical patient. The first involves a switch after a single dose of a perioperative parenteral NSAID (e.g., meloxicam) to an oral NSAID the next day. The only data available in this situation are from a study involving normal healthy dogs that were given parenteral (subcutaneous) carprofen followed by deracoxib orally 24 h later and repeated for 4 days. This portion of the study compared subcutaneous carprofen/oral deracoxib, subcutaneous carprofen/oral carprofen, and placebo and found no differences in clinical findings or gastric lesions. Thus, these limited data appear to suggest that it may be safe to switch from a single injection of one drug to an oral formula the next day if using another product [94]. However, without testing all the possible combinations of injectable and oral NSAIDs, it is not possible to make definitive treatment recommendations.

The second situation involves switching NSAIDs for perceived lack of a response by the patient. This is a difficult question for clinicians, and there is significant variation in recommendations. Many authors suggest waiting five half-lives from administration of the first drug before initiating the second drug to reduce the plasma concentration of the first drug to near zero. The only clinical data that may shed light on this situation are from a report that described switching to firocoxib from another NSAID. This study showed no increase in documented side effects whether firocoxib was started the next day or up to 7 days after stopping the original drug [97]. These data would seem to suggest that a washout period is not necessary, but most clinicians follow the recommendation of discontinuing an NSAID for 1–7 days before initiating another drug.

The final situation involves transitioning to or from aspirin. If aspirin is the initial drug, it has been recommended that a minimum 7-day washout period be followed before starting another NSAID. The basis for this recommendation is to provide time for platelet regeneration due to aspirin's irreversible effects on platelets [90,98]. However, there are limited clinical data to support this recommendation.

If a dog is receiving a product that is COX-1 sparing (i.e., a primary COX-2 inhibitor) and is then changed to aspirin, a 7-day washout period is recommended due to the gastric adaptation and production of aspirin-triggered lipoxins (ATLs) [90,98]. Patients receiving aspirin produce ATLs, which have been shown to exert protective effects in the stomach by diminishing gastric injury, most likely via release of nitric oxide (NO) from the vascular endothelium. However, concurrent administration of COX-1-sparing drugs with aspirin results in the complete inhibition of ATLs and can potentially cause significant exacerbation of gastric mucosal injury. It is important to remember that the formation of ATLs has yet to be proven in the dog.

Specific NSAIDs

The approved NSAIDs available to clinicians vary considerably around the world. It is very important for practitioners to remember that the clinical response of an individual to a particular drug is quite variable. Patients may respond favorably to one product and not another, so if a NSAID is indicated in a case and the first product used does not achieve a positive clinical response, NSAIDs should not be abandoned altogether but a different product tried.

Carprofen

Carprofen is a member of the arylpropionic acid class of NSAIDs. In the US, it is approved, both in oral and injectable formulations, to treat pain and inflammation associated with OA in dogs. Carprofen improved limb function in clinical trials of dogs with naturally occurring OA [99–105]. Three long-term studies (84 and 120 days) found that carprofen was well tolerated, and based on subjective assessments, dogs appeared to improve over the treatment period. The strength and quality of evidence supports a high degree of confidence in the use of carprofen to treat OA pain in dogs.

Cimicoxib

Cimicoxib is a member of the coxib class of NSAIDs. It is approved by the European Union as an oral formulation in dogs for the treatment of postoperative pain and pain and inflammation associated with OA [106–108]. There is one study evaluating its use in OA and two studies evaluating perioperative pain treatment in comparison to other products, and the results were favorable [109–111]. One final study evaluated its use for palliative pain management in patients with osteosarcoma [112]. At the time of writing, the strength of evidence supports a low to moderate degree of confidence in the use of cimicoxib to treat OA pain in dogs.

Deracoxib

Deracoxib is a member of the coxib class of NSAIDs. It is approved for use in dogs as an oral formulation for the treatment of pain and inflammation associated with OA and postoperative pain associated with orthopedic surgery. It has been demonstrated to provide effective relief of pain in clinical OA trials in dogs in a study that has not been published in a peer-reviewed journal but has been presented in abstract form [113]. As with OA, data regarding its efficacy for pain relief following orthopedic surgery are only available in abstract form [114]. There are two additional studies that evaluated postoperative pain in dental and soft tissue procedures [115,116]. Due to lack of information, it is not possible to rate confidence in the use of deracoxib to treat OA pain in dogs.

Enflicoxib

Enflicoxib is a member of the coxib class of NSAIDs [117–119]. It is approved in the United Kingdom (UK) and Europe for the management of pain and inflammation associated with OA in dogs as a once-a-week therapy. Clinically, it has been shown to improve limb function in dogs with OA in one well-controlled study [120]. Additionally, a second study showed noninferiority with mavacoxib [121]. The strength and quality of the evidence supports a moderate to high degree of confidence in the use of enflicoxib to treat OA pain in dogs.

Firocoxib

Firocoxib is a member of the coxib class of NSAIDs. It is approved as an oral formulation for the management of pain and inflammation associated with OA in dogs. Clinically, several studies have demonstrated improved limb function in dogs with OA [122–126]. Long-term dosing of firocoxib showed continued improvements over the year of treatment. The strength and quality of evidence supports a high degree of confidence in the use of firocoxib to treat OA pain in dogs.

Grapiprant

Grapiprant is a member of the piprant class of drugs. It is a highly selective antagonist of the prostaglandin-E_2 receptor 4 (EP4) and is considered a novel NSAID due to its unique mechanism of action [127–129]. One well-controlled study provides data showing clinical improvement in dogs with chronic OA [130]. Interestingly, there are conflicting data in grapiprant's ability to modulate acute pain. One study found noninferiority of grapiprant compared to carprofen for perioperative analgesia in dogs undergoing ovariohysterectomy [127], while two canine acute experimental pain models found that grapiprant was not different than control treatment and was significantly less effective than firocoxib and carprofen, respectively [131,132]. At this time, the strength of evidence supports a moderate degree of confidence in the use of grapiprant to treat OA pain in dogs.

Ketoprofen

Ketoprofen is a member of the arylpropionic acid class of NSAIDs. One limited study compared dosages of ketoprofen and the combination of ketoprofen with tramadol in a small group of dogs with OA [133]. Most data regarding clinical use of this product involve acute pain models or short-term (mostly perioperative) pain management in both dogs and cats [134–137]. Due to lack of information, it is not possible to rate confidence in the use of ketoprofen to treat chronic OA pain.

Mavacoxib

Mavacoxib is a member of the coxib class of NSAIDs. It is approved by the European Union as an oral formulation for the treatment of pain and inflammation associated with OA in dogs. Mavacoxib has published pharmacological data and four noninferiority studies showing clinical improvements in dogs with chronic OA [120,121,138–142]. Mavacoxib is a long-acting agent with an approved dosing regimen consisting of a loading dose repeated at 14 days and thereafter at dosing intervals of 1 month. The strength and quality of evidence supports a high degree of confidence in the use of mavacoxib to treat OA pain in dogs.

Meloxicam

Meloxicam is a member of the oxicam family of NSAIDs. It is approved for use in dogs for the control of pain and inflammation associated with OA and is available in oral, transmucosal oral mist, and parenteral formulations. There are robust data evaluating meloxicam safety and efficacy for chronic OA pain management in dogs [141,143–145]. The strength and quality of evidence supports a high degree of confidence in the use of meloxicam to treat OA pain in dogs.

Meloxicam is approved for use in cats but, in the US, that approval is limited to a single dose to control pain and inflammation associated with orthopedic surgery, ovariohysterectomy, and castration. In other countries, however, meloxicam is approved for long-term management of musculoskeletal pain in cats. Administration to cats ranging from 5 days to indefinite dosing to manage pain for locomotor disorders including OA has been described with a range of dosing recommendations (0.01–0.05 PO mg/kg once daily) [146–151]. Clinical efficacy is primarily supported by data generated from studies using the 0.05 mg/kg dose PO every 24 h. At lower dosing regimens (0.01–0.03 mg/kg PO every 24 h), meloxicam has been shown to be well tolerated and safe in cats, including cats with chronic renal dysfunction [148–150,152]. The strength and quality of evidence supports a high degree of confidence in the use of meloxicam to treat DJD/OA pain in cats.

Robenacoxib

Robenacoxib is a member of the coxib class of NSAIDs. Depending on the country, approval may be for dogs only, or for both dogs and cats. Indications in the dog are for the treatment of pain and inflammation associated with orthopedic or soft tissue surgery as well as the treatment of pain and inflammation associated with chronic OA [153–158]. The strength and quality of evidence supports a high degree of confidence in the use of robenacoxib to treat OA pain in dogs.

In the cat, approved indications vary by country and include treatment of postoperative pain and inflammation associated with surgery as well as acute and chronic administration for pain and inflammation associated with musculoskeletal disorders [157–165]. The strength and quality of evidence supports a moderate to high degree of confidence in the use of robenacoxib to treat DJD/OA pain in cats.

Tolfenamic acid

Tolfenamic acid is an anthranilic acid derivative and a member of the fenamates class of NSAIDs. It is approved in Canada and Europe in both oral and parenteral formulations for dogs and cats. While some clinical data are available to support use of tolfenamic acid in dogs and cats, all studies involve short-term administration (3–7 days) only [166–168]. Given the lack of long-term data, the strength of evidence supports a low degree of confidence in the use of tolfenamic acid to treat OA pain in dogs or cats.

N-methyl-D-aspartate (NMDA) receptor antagonists

A significant breakthrough in the understanding of nociceptive processing came with the recognition that the nervous system was plastic, which is to say, inputs from the periphery could, via activation of a variety of receptors (principally the NMDA receptor), produce changes in processing of nociceptive signals in the spinal cord. The characteristics of the NMDA receptor are such that with repeated stimulation, a state of prolonged depolarization in dorsal horn neurons is produced. This long-term potentiation is thought to produce the state known as "central sensitization" via activation of a variety of second messenger systems, and the production of NO, eicosanoids, and induction of immediate early genes. Central sensitization is thought to contribute to injury- or disease-induced pain by causing amplification of afferent signals, and by altering processing of sensory information such that previously non-noxious signals are now encoded as noxious. The NMDA receptor appears to be central to the induction and maintenance of central sensitization, and the use of NMDA receptor antagonists would appear to offer benefit in the treatment of pain where central sensitization has become established (especially chronic pain). Ketamine, tiletamine, dextromethorphan, and amantadine possess NMDA antagonist properties, among other actions [169–173]. Additional information about these drugs in available in Chapters 25 and 27.

Amantadine

There is one publication evaluating amantadine combined with an NSAID that demonstrated improvements in the canine OA patients compared to the NSAID alone [174]. This study was a randomized, blinded, placebo-controlled trial. The study indicated efficacy based on both objective and subjective outcome measures, and the evidence supports a moderate degree of confidence in the use of amantadine to impact the outcomes reported.

Opioids

The descending opioidergic system is one of the best described endogenous analgesic mechanisms [88]. For both pharmacologic and regulatory reasons, long-term classic oral opioid therapy has not been a viable treatment methodology in veterinary patients. However, the use of tramadol (a synthetic derivative of codeine classified as an opioidergic/monoaminergic drug), which has actions at both μ-opioid receptors and facilitates activity in the descending serotonergic system, has become commonplace in small animal practice. Tramadol use grew despite a lack of supporting clinical data and unfavorable pharmacologic data [175–177]. In a well-controlled clinical trial, tramadol was found to be ineffective alone in treating chronic OA in dogs [178]. A second prospective clinical trial provides data showing limited improvements in both objective and subjective outcome measures in canine OA patients receiving tramadol [41]. Mixed results were found in two studies examining postoperative analgesia after tibial plateau leveling osteotomy (TPLO) surgery [179,180]. Additionally, a recent systematic review and meta-analysis of tramadol for postoperative pain management in dogs found the certainty of evidence to be low to very low that the drug had any efficacy [181]. Thus, the strength and quality of evidence supports a very low level of confidence in the use of tramadol for chronic pain management in dogs. Interestingly, in cats, tramadol has very different pharmacokinetics, which may provide better analgesia when compared to dogs [182,183]. Two small well-controlled studies found increased mobility and improved owner assessments of impairment in cats receiving tramadol [184,185]. Given these data, the evidence supports a moderate level of confidence in the use of tramadol for treatment of DJD/OA pain in cats. Further information on tramadol is available in Chapter 25.

Gabapentin

Gabapentin, a gabapentinoid, binds to the $\alpha_2\delta$ subunit of voltage-gated calcium channels, causing a decrease in the release of neurotransmitters and reducing neuronal excitability [38,186]. Single small well-controlled reports in both dogs (treating neuropathic pain) and cats (treating OA) documented improvement in outcome measurements when treated with gabapentin [187,188]. Given the limited data, the strength of evidence supports a low degree of confidence in the use of gabapentin for chronic DJD/OA pain in dogs and cats. Further information on gabapentin is available in Chapter 25.

Other pharmaceuticals

A variety of other drugs have been suggested for use in chronic pain in dogs and cats with no pharmacological information or clinical trials. As examples, there have been no clinical trials assessing pregabalin, venlafaxine, duloxetine, ketamine, intra-articular steroids, or amitriptyline for the relief of painful symptoms associated with any type of chronic pain (such as OA) in dogs or cats. Thus, due to lack of information, it is not possible to rate confidence in the use of any of these drugs for treatment of chronic DJD/OA pain.

Alternative, complementary, and homeopathic compounds

The lack of high-quality, peer-reviewed literature makes it difficult to draw conclusions about any of these therapies. Studies commonly have limitations related to methods of participant recruitment and randomization, baseline characteristic data reporting, intervention standardization and concealment, blinding, participant retention, follow-up procedures, and overall protocol. The following is a limited exploration of some of the data available to date.

Compounds based on chondroitin sulfate and glucosamine hydrochloride

A recent systematic review and meta-analysis of enriched diets and nutraceuticals concluded in part "a very marked non-effect of chondroitin–glucosamine nutraceuticals, which leads us to recommend that the latter products should no longer be recommended for pain management in canine and feline OA" [189]. This conclusion was based in part on the evaluation of three trials [101,189,190]. One study subjectively (via a non-validated tool) showed a limited positive effect at only one of three time points [190]. The other two studies showed no positive effects measured by force plate analysis [101,191]. The strength and quality of evidence supports a very low degree of confidence in the use of these products for the treatment of OA pain in dogs.

Polysulfated glycosaminoglycan

Two studies have evaluated polysulfated glycosaminoglycan (PSGAG) efficacy on lameness due to OA. Both studies were limited by study design deficiencies (small sample size and non-validated subjective scoring systems). One study was blinded, with a placebo control, and found no significant improvement in lameness scores between groups (three PSGAG doses and placebo) [192]. There was a trend toward improvements that may have been confirmed with a larger sample size. The second study demonstrated lameness improvement but was neither randomized nor blinded [193]. Interestingly, the product tested in both studies did gain approval by the US Food and Drug Administration for use. The strength and quality of evidence supports a low degree of confidence in the use of these compounds for treatment of OA pain in dogs.

Green-lipped mussel preparation

Four trials were identified using a compound whose main ingredient was green-lipped mussel (*Perna canaliculus*) for the treatment of OA in dogs. The studies were prospective and randomized in design [194–197]. While all showed positive effects (subjectively and objectively), they all had small sample sizes. Additionally, there are some questions regarding the scientific quality in two of these studies. There was moderate consistency across the studies, and their conclusions suggest that the observed effect will be physiologically meaningful and achievable. Based on these data, the strength and quality of evidence supports a moderate degree of confidence in the use of these compounds for the treatment of OA pain in dogs.

Zeel® homeopathic preparation

Two trials were identified using Zeel® for the treatment of OA in dogs. While both were prospective, only one was randomized and blinded [198,199]. Both studies showed subjective positive effects associated with the product; however, in one study, effects were less than those produced by carprofen. Given the small sample sizes and the study limitations, there are some questions regarding the scientific quality of the studies. There was a moderate level of consistency between the studies, and the overall strength and quality of evidence supports a low to moderate degree of confidence in the use of these compounds for the treatment of OA pain in dogs.

Type II collagen

Six studies including three randomized, blinded, placebo-controlled clinical trials using type II collagen as a treatment for OA in dogs have been performed [109,200–204]. The more recent studies boost earlier positive findings that support the use of this compound. Given the study design limitations (small sample size, non-validated subjective tools, limited follow-up data points, etc.), there are still some questions regarding the scientific quality of these studies [189]. Based on these data, the strength and quality of evidence supports a moderate degree of confidence in the use of this compound for the treatment of OA pain in dogs.

Cannabidiol products

There are several single-center clinical trials involving a variety of cannabidiol (CBD) products showing limited to no positive effects for the treatment of OA pain and dysfunction. Though difficult to evaluate, these products may have a place in OA therapy if additional studies show a positive effect with larger sample sizes and/or different study designs. Two recent reviews emphasized the limitations (low sample size) and conflicting data available to date [84,189]. Two studies comparing CBD oil treatment to placebo found a reduction of clinical signs by subjective measurements, while another randomized, blinded crossover study found no significant difference between CBD oil treatment and placebo over the course of 6 weeks based on clinical metrology instrument outcomes and objective pressure gait analysis [205–207]. Based on these data, the strength and quality of evidence supports a low degree of confidence in the use of these compounds for the treatment of OA pain in dogs.

Anti-nerve growth factor monoclonal antibodies

Nerve growth factor (NGF) has been shown to be an important driver of pain in OA due to its ability to facilitate peripheral and central sensitization in mature patients [208–211]. In dogs, two studies found significant pain relief with anti-NGF monoclonal antibodies [212,213]. More recently, a large well-controlled clinical trial evaluating the monoclonal antibody bedinvetmab found it to be efficacious in dogs with OA [214]. This product is now approved for dogs in the US, Canada, the UK, and the European Union. The strength and quality of evidence supports a high degree of confidence in the use of bedinvetmab to treat OA pain in dogs.

A feline-specific monoclonal antibody has also gone through a similar pathway of clinical testing. Initially, two small well-controlled studies suggested efficacy in cats [215,216]. These findings were confirmed with two large well-controlled clinical trials with the monoclonal antibody frunevetmab [217,218]. This product has been approved for cats in the US, Canada, the UK, the European Union, and several other countries. The strength and quality of evidence supports a high degree of confidence in the use of frunevetmab to treat OA pain in cats. Further information on anti-NGF monoclonal antibodies is available in Chapter 48.

Cell-based therapies

Cell-based therapies include many products, and it can be confusing to differentiate these therapies from each other. Blood-derived products are often lumped together but include a range of varied therapies including autologous conditioned serum, autologous protein solution, platelet-rich plasma, and certain preparations containing medicinal (or messenger or mesenchymal) stem cells [84,219–223]. Other stem cell-based therapies are adipose-derived stromal fraction and autologous, allogenic, or xenogeneic stem cells of varying origins (e.g., adipose, bone marrow, or umbilical tissue). To complicate things further, there is no uniformity in production of these products or methods to test for efficacy [221,224]. These factors make it difficult to assess efficacy in dogs and cats. The following is a limited discussion of the different products available at the time of writing.

Autologous protein solution

One pilot study and two small clinical trials evaluate intra-articular autologous protein solution (APS) in dogs with OA [225–227]. While there are some data to support use in dogs, the small sample sizes and lack of a control group in one study limit the conclusions that can be drawn. No data are available in using APS for the treatment of OA/DJD in cats. Thus, the strength and quality of evidence supports a low degree of confidence in the use of this therapy in dogs.

Platelet-rich plasma

Limited clinical data are available to assess the efficacy of platelet-rich plasma (PRP) in chronic OA pain. Again, the clinical studies suffer from limitations associated with study design (small numbers of patients, and lack of controls and standardization of product) [228–232]. No data are available for the treatment of OA/DJD in cats with PRP. While there is evidence of some positive efficacy in each study, the strength and quality of evidence supports a low degree of confidence in the use of this therapy.

Medicinal (messenger or mesenchymal) stem cells

Medicinal stem cells (MSCs) can be autologous, allogenic, or xenogeneic [84,220,221,223]. The exact mechanism of how MSCs exert their effects is not completely understood. Current data suggest that MSCs are active primarily through their secretory factors [84,220,223,233]. These paracrine factors may produce immunomodulatory and anti-inflammatory effects as well as other effects such as angiogenesis. Autologous and allogenic MSCs can be clinically delivered intra-articularly. Additionally, allogenic and xenogeneic MSCs can be given intravenously. One xenogeneic product of equine umbilical cord MSC is approved for use in the UK and the European Union for the treatment of OA in dogs [234]. Clinical studies involving MSCs have been extensively reviewed [84,220,223,233,235]. The majority have limitations associated with study design (small numbers, lack of controls or blinding, non-validated subjective outcome measures, and few measurement time points). While most studies show positive results, the strength and quality of evidence supports a moderate degree of confidence in the use of MSCs in dogs; however, this has the potential to improve with additional clinical data. There are currently no clinical data available evaluating the use of MSCs for the treatment of DJD/OA in cats.

Dealing with non-responders to standard treatment approaches

There is a continued desire to identify additional drugs and compounds to alleviate chronic pain in small animal patients. This is based upon the fact that current products are not always effective, and some result in more adverse events than some clinicians and clients are willing to accept. Given this set of circumstances, a discussion about non-responders to current treatments is appropriate.

After initiation of treatment, the veterinarian and client must decide whether the animal is responding to the prescribed pain management plan. Clinicians need to ask this question every time a product or therapy is prescribed. Without verbal patient communication, veterinarians are hampered in all phases of treating pain, including the diagnosis, accurate characterization and localization, and evaluation of therapeutic efficacy. While veterinary patients possess many of the same nociceptive pathways (including neurotransmitter receptors) and perhaps even similar perceptions of painful stimuli as other species (including humans), one cannot assume that the evaluation of responses should be similar for all patients. One needs to go no further than comparing cats, dogs, and pet birds to find striking examples of this conundrum. In recent years, strides have been made in evaluating the effects of different pain therapies in veterinary patients, but it is important to remember current limitations and proceed with caution when making claims about new treatments or therapeutic agents.

In addition, the criteria for defining a "responder" as well as the outcome measures used to define the response require clarification. In the human literature, the Initiative on Methods, Measurement, and Pain Assessment in Clinical Trials (IMMPACT) consortium defines outcome responses in clinical trials for human chronic pain, and these are summarized in Box 71.3. Given these guidelines, in many human studies, a 30% improvement in a patient makes that case a positive responder.

In veterinary medicine, clinical trials to demonstrate efficacy for pain control are usually performed for regulatory purposes and outcomes are typically reported as statistical comparisons between treatment group population means. Thus, the results represent the "average" patient. These data are difficult to apply clinically because individual patients are being treated [238]. In human medicine, managing the pain and dysfunction of OA has been often described as the 80/20 rule [236]. That is, 80% of patients experience 20% pain relief, while only 20% of patients experience 80% pain relief. About 50% have their pain halved. An extensive review of data available in human medicine yields interesting and sobering results. Data clearly show that different NSAIDs show a range of responses for pain relief. This is compounded by the fact that the same NSAID, at different doses, shows the same gradation of responses. Generally,

Box 71.3 Outcome responses for human chronic pain as defined by the Initiative on Methods, Measurement, and Pain Assessment in Clinical Trials (IMMPACT) consortium.

- 10–20% decrease in pain intensity is considered minimally important
- 30% decrease in pain intensity is considered moderately important
- 50% decrease in pain intensity is considered substantially important
- 70% decrease in pain intensity is considered extremely important

Source: Dworkin *et al.* [236]; Dworkin *et al.* [237].

only about 15–30% of patients actually show extensive improvement, while over 60–70% show minimal improvement (i.e., a benefit) [239,240]. In veterinary medicine, outcome testing instruments cannot reliably differentiate this range of clinical responses, so there are no data supporting different doses of a given NSAID even though it has been observed that NSAID effects are dose dependent. Despite these limitations to detect clinical improvements, many (including the Food and Drug Administration Center for Veterinary Medicine) suggest that clinicians titrate the dose of NSAIDs to the lowest effective dose.

References

1 Malfait AM, Schnitzer TJ. Towards a mechanism-based approach to pain management in osteoarthritis. *Nat Rev Rheumatol* 2013; **9**: 654–664.
2 Dray A, Read SJ. Arthritis and pain. Future targets to control osteoarthritis pain. *Arthritis Res Ther* 2007; **9**: 212–215.
3 Schaible HG. Mechanisms of chronic pain in osteoarthritis. *Curr Rheumatol Rep* 2012; **14**: 549–556.
4 Lee AS, Ellman MB, Yan D, *et al.* A current review of molecular mechanisms regarding osteoarthritis and pain. *Gene* 2013; **527**: 440–447.
5 Krasnokutsky S, Attur M, Palmer G, *et al.* Current concepts in the pathogenesis of osteoarthritis. *Osteoarthritis Cartilage* 2008; **16**(Suppl 3): S1–S3.
6 Pelletier JP, Martel-Pelletier J, Abramson SB. Osteoarthritis, an inflammatory disease: potential implication for the selection of new therapeutic targets. *Arthritis Rheum* 2001; **44**: 1237–1247.
7 Goldring MB, Goldring SR. Osteoarthritis. *J Cell Physiol* 2007; **213**: 626–634.
8 Zhang RX, Ren K, Dubner R. Osteoarthritis pain mechanisms: basic studies in animal models. *Osteoarthritis Cartilage* 2013; **21**: 1308–1315.
9 Loeser RF, Goldring SR, Scanzello CR, *et al.* Osteoarthritis: a disease of the joint as an organ. *Arthritis Rheum* 2012; **64**: 1697–1707.
10 Johnston SA. Osteoarthritis joint anatomy, physiology, and pathobiology. *Vet Clin North Am Small Anim Pract* 1997; **27**: 699–723.
11 Shepherd AJ. Results of the 2006 AVMA survey of companion animal ownership in US pet-owning households. *J Am Vet Med Assoc* 2008; **232**: 695–696.
12 United States Pet Ownership & Demographics Sourcebook 2012. www.avma.org/KB/Resources/Statistics/Pages/Market-research-statistics-US-pet-ownershipaspx (accessed October 2014).
13 Murray JK, Browne WJ, Roberts MA, *et al.* Number and ownership profiles of cats and dogs in the UK. *Vet Rec* 2010; **166**: 163–168.
14 Lascelles BDX, Court MH, Hardie EM, *et al.* Nonsteroidal anti-inflammatory drugs in cats: a review. *Vet Anaesth and Analgesia* 2007; **34**: 228–250.
15 Lascelles BDX, Henry JB, Brown J, *et al.* Cross-sectional study of the prevalence of radiographic degenerative joint disease in domesticated cats. *Vet Surg* 2010; **39**: 535–544.
16 Clarke SP, Mellor D, Clements DN, *et al.* Prevalence of radiographic signs of degenerative joint disease in a hospital population of cats. *Vet Rec* 2005; **157**: 793–799.
17 Clarke SP, Bennett D. Feline osteoarthritis: a prospective study of 28 cases. *J Small Anim Pract* 2006; **47**: 439–445.
18 Bennett D, Zainal Ariffin SM, Johnston P. Osteoarthritis in the cat: how common is it and how easy to recognise? *J Feline Med Surg* 2012; **14**: 65–75.
19 Lascelles BD, Robertson SA. DJD-associated pain in cats: what can we do to promote patient comfort? *J Feline Med Surg* 2010; **12**: 200–212.
20 Bennett D, Zainal Ariffin SM, Johnston P. Osteoarthritis in the cat: how should it be managed and treated? *J Feline Med Surg* 2012; **14**: 76–84.
21 Taylor PM, Robertson SA. Pain management in cats – past, present and future Part 1. The cat is unique. *J Feline Med Surg* 2004; **6**: 313–320.
22 Lascelles BD. Feline degenerative joint disease. *Vet Surg* 2010; **39**: 2–13.
23 Kuettner K, Goldberg VM. *Osteoarthritis Disorders.* Rosemont, IL: American Academy of Orthopaedic Surgeons, 1995.
24 Heinegård D, Saxne T. The role of the cartilage matrix in osteoarthritis. *Nat Rev Rheumatol* 2011; **7**: 50–56.
25 Schuelert N, McDougall JJ. Electrophysiological evidence that the vasoactive intestinal peptide receptor antagonist VIP6-28 reduces nociception in an animal model of osteoarthritis. *Osteoarthritis Cartilage* 2006; **14**: 1155–1162.
26 Mobasheri A, Batt M. An update on the pathophysiology of osteoarthritis. *Ann Phys Rehabil Med* 2016; **59**: 333–339.
27 Conaghan PG, Cook AD, Hamilton JA, *et al.* Therapeutic options for targeting inflammatory osteoarthritis pain. *Nat Rev Rheumatol* 2019; **15**: 355–363.
28 Latourte A, Kloppenburg M, Richette P. Emerging pharmaceutical therapies for osteoarthritis. *Nat Rev Rheumatol* 2020; **16**: 673–688.
29 Conzemius MG, Evans RB. Caregiver placebo effect for dogs with lameness from osteoarthritis. *J Am Vet Med Assoc* 2012; **241**: 1314–1319.
30 Malek S, Sample SJ, Schwartz Z, *et al.* Effect of analgesic therapy on clinical outcome measures in a randomized controlled trial using client-owned dogs with hip osteoarthritis. *BMC Vet Res* 2012; **8**: 185.
31 Walton MB, Cowderoy E, Lascelles D. Evaluation of construct and criterion validity for the 'Liverpool Osteoarthritis in Dogs' (LOAD) clinical metrology instrument and comparison to two other instruments. *PLoS ONE* 2013; **8**: e58125.
32 Brown DC, Boston RC, Coyne JC, *et al.* Ability of the Canine Brief Pain Inventory to detect response to treatment in dogs with osteoarthritis. *J Am Vet Med Assoc* 2008; **233**: 1278–1283.
33 Brown DC, Boston RC, Farrar JT. Comparison of force plate gait analysis and owner assessment of pain using the Canine Brief Pain Inventory in dogs with osteoarthritis. *J Vet Intern Med* 2013; **27**: 22–30.
34 Hercock CA, Pinchbeck G, Giejda A, *et al.* Validation of a client-based clinical metrology instrument for the evaluation of canine elbow osteoarthritis. *J Small Anim Pract* 2009; **50**: 266–271.
35 Hielm-Björkman AK, Rita H, Tulamo RM. Psychometric testing of the Helsinki chronic pain index by completion of a questionnaire in Finnish by owners of dogs with chronic signs of pain caused by osteoarthritis. *Am J Vet Res* 2009; **70**: 727–734.
36 Hielm-Björkman AK, Kuusela E, Liman A, *et al.* Evaluation of methods for assessment of pain associated with chronic osteoarthritis in dogs. *J Am Vet Med Assoc* 2003; **222**: 1552–1558.
37 Lascelles BD, Hansen BD, Roe S, *et al.* Evaluation of client-specific outcome measures and activity monitoring to measure pain relief in cats with osteoarthritis. *J Vet Intern Med* 2007; **21**: 410–416.
38 Benito J, Hansen B, Depuy V, *et al.* Feline musculoskeletal pain index: responsiveness and testing of criterion validity. *J Vet Intern Med* 2013; **27**: 474–482.
39 Benito J, Depuy V, Hardie E, *et al.* Reliability and discriminatory testing of a client-based metrology instrument, feline musculoskeletal pain index (FMPI) for the evaluation of degenerative joint disease-associated pain in cats. *Vet J* 2013; **196**: 368–373.
40 Monteiro BP. Feline chronic pain and osteoarthritis. *Vet Clin North Am Small Anim Pract* 2020; **50**: 769–788.
41 Monteiro BP, Steagall PV. Chronic pain in cats: recent advances in clinical assessment. *J Feline Med Surg* 2019; **21**: 601–614.
42 Johnston SA, McLaughlin RM, Budsberg SC. Nonsurgical management of osteoarthritis in dogs. *Vet Clin North Am Small Anim Pract* 2008; **38**: 1449–1470.
43 Innes JF, Walton MB. Update on the diagnosis and management of canine osteoarthritis. *CVL – Companion Animals* 2013; **2**: 113–122.
44 Fox SM. Multimodal management of canine osteoarthritis. In: Fox SM, ed. *Chronic Pain in Small Animals.* London, UK: Manson Publishing, 2010: 189–201.
45 Rychel JK. Diagnosis and treatment of osteoarthritis. *Top Companion Anim Med* 2010; **25**: 20–25.
46 Fox SM. Painful decisions for senior pets. *Vet Clin North Am Small Anim Pract* 2012; **42**: 727–748.
47 Sanderson RO, Beata C, Flipo JP, *et al.* Systematic review of the management of canine osteoarthritis. *Vet Rec* 2009; **164**: 418–424.
48 Laflamme DP. Understanding and managing obesity in dogs and cats. *Vet Clin North Am Small Anim Pract* 2006; **36**: 1283–1295.
49 Laflamme DP. Nutritional care for aging cats and dogs. *Vet Clin North Am Small Anim Pract* 2012; **42**: 769–791.
50 Churchill J. Increase the success of weight loss programs by creating an environment for change. *Compend Contin Educ Vet* 2010; **32**: E1.
51 Michel K, Scherk M. From problems to success: feline weight loss programs that work. *J Feline Med Surg* 2012; **14**: 327–336.
52 Brooks D, Churchill J, Fein K, *et al.* 2014 AAHA weight management guidelines for dogs and cats. *Am Anim Hosp Assoc* 2014; **50**: 1–11.
53 Impellizeri JA, Tetrick MA, Muir P. Effect of weight reduction on clinical signs of lameness in dogs with hip osteoarthritis. *J Am Vet Med Assoc* 2000; **216**: 1089–1091.
54 Mlacnik E, Bockstahler BA, Müller M, *et al.* Effects of caloric restriction and a moderate or intense physiotherapy program for treatment of lameness in overweight dogs with osteoarthritis. *J Am Vet Med Assoc* 2006; **229**: 1756–1760.
55 Farrell M, Clements DN, Mellor D, *et al.* Retrospective evaluation of the long-term outcome of non-surgical management of 74 dogs with clinical hip dysplasia. *Vet Rec* 2007; **160**: 506–511.
56 Kealy RD, Lawler DF, Ballam JM, *et al.* Evaluation of the effect of limited food consumption on radiographic evidence of osteoarthritis in dogs. *J Am Vet Med Assoc* 2000; **217**: 1678–1680.
57 Smith GK, Paster ER, Powers MY, *et al.* Lifelong diet restriction and radiographic evidence of osteoarthritis of the hip joint in dogs. *J Am Vet Med Assoc* 2006; **229**: 690–693.

58 Kirkby KA, Lewis DD. Canine hip dysplasia: reviewing the evidence for nonsurgical management. *Vet Surg* 2012; **41**: 2–9.

59 Marshall W, Bockstahler B, Hulse D, *et al.* A review of osteoarthritis and obesity: current understanding of the relationship and benefit of obesity treatment and prevention in the dog. *Vet Comp Orthop Traumatol* 2009; **22**: 339–345.

60 Mille MA, McClement J, Lauer S. Physiotherapeutic strategies and their current evidence for canine osteoarthritis. *Vet Sci* 2022; **10**: 2.

61 Millis DL, Levine D, Taylor RA. *Canine Rehabilitation and Physical Therapy*. Philadelphia, PA: WB Saunders, 2004.

62 Mueller M, Bockstahler B, Skalicky M, *et al.* Effects of radial shockwave therapy on the limb function of dogs with hip osteoarthritis. *Vet Rec* 2007; **160**: 762–765.

63 Sullivan MO, Gordon-Evans WJ, Knap KE, *et al.* Randomized, controlled clinical trial evaluating the efficacy of pulsed signal therapy in dogs with osteoarthritis. *Vet Surg* 2013; **42**: 250–254.

64 Dahlberg J, Fitch G, Evans RB, *et al.* The evaluation of extracorporeal shockwave therapy in naturally occurring osteoarthritis of the stifle joint in dogs. *Vet Comp Orthop Traumatol* 2005; **18**: 147–152.

65 Alves JC, Santos A, Jorge P, *et al.* A randomized double-blinded controlled trial on the effects of photobiomodulation therapy in dogs with osteoarthritis. *Am J Vet Res* 2022; **83**: ajvr22.03.0036.

66 Looney AL, Huntingford JL, Blaeser LL, *et al.* A randomized blind placebo-controlled trial investigating the effects of photobiomodulation therapy (PBMT) on canine elbow osteoarthritis. *Can Vet J* 2018; **59**: 959–966.

67 Lenox CE, Bauer JE. Potential adverse effects of omega-3 Fatty acids in dogs and cats. *J Vet Intern Med* 2013; **27**: 217–226.

68 Budsberg SC, Bartges JW. Nutrition and osteoarthritis in dogs: does it help? *Vet Clin North Am Small Anim Pract* 2006; **36**: 1307–1323.

69 Perea S. Nutritional management of osteoarthritis. *Compend Contin Educ Vet* 2012; **34**: E4.

70 Schuchardt JP, Hahn A. Bioavailability of long-chain omega-3 fatty acids. *Prostaglandins Leukot Essent Fatty Acids* 2013; **89**: 1–8.

71 Healy DA, Wallace FA, Miles EA, *et al.* Effect of low-to-moderate amounts of dietary fish oil on neutrophil lipid composition and function. *Lipids* 2000; **35**: 763–768.

72 Yaqoob P, Pala HS, Cortina-Borja M, *et al.* Encapsulated fish oil enriched in alpha-tocopherol alters plasma phospholipid and mononuclear cell fatty acid compositions but not mononuclear cell functions. *Eur J Clin Invest* 2000; **30**: 260–274.

73 Baker KR, Matthan NR, Lichtenstein A, *et al.* Association of plasma n-6 and n-3 polyunsaturated fatty acids with synovitis in the knee: the MOST study. *Osteoarthritis Cartilage* 2012; **20**: 382–387.

74 Zainal Z, Longman AJ, Hurst S, *et al.* Relative efficacies of omega-3 polyunsaturated fatty acids in reducing expression of key proteins in a model system for studying osteoarthritis. *Osteoarthritis Cartilage* 2009; **17**: 896–905.

75 Fritsch D, Allen TA, Dodd CE, *et al.* Dose-titration effects of fish oil in osteoarthritis dogs. *J Vet Intern Med* 2010; **24**: 1020–1026.

76 Fritsch DA, Allen TA, Dodd CE, *et al.* A multicenter study of the effects of dietary supplementation with fish oil omega-3 fatty acids on carprofen dosage in dogs with osteoarthritis. *J Am Vet Med Assoc* 2010; **236**: 535–539.

77 Roush JK, Dodd CE, Fritsch DA, *et al.* Multicenter veterinary practice assessment of the effects of omega-3 fatty acids on osteoarthritis in dogs. *J Am Vet Med Assoc* 2010; **236**: 59–66.

78 Roush JK, Cross AR, Renberg WC, *et al.* Evaluation of the effects of dietary supplementation with fish oil omega-3 fatty acids on weight bearing in dogs with osteoarthritis. *J Am Vet Med Assoc* 2010; **236**: 67–73.

79 Moreau M, Troncy E, Del Castillo JR, *et al.* Effects of feeding a high omega-3 fatty acids diet in dogs with naturally occurring osteoarthritis. *J Anim Physiol Anim Nutr (Berl)* 2013; **97**; 830–837.

80 Hielm-Björkman A, Roine J, Elo K, *et al.* An un-commissioned randomized, placebo-controlled double-blind study to test the effect of deep sea fish oil as a pain reliever for dogs suffering from canine OA. *BMC Vet Res* 2012; **8**: 157.

81 Lascelles BD, DePuy V, Thomson A, *et al.* Evaluation of a therapeutic diet for feline degenerative joint disease. *J Vet Intern Med* 2010; **24**: 487–495.

82 Aragon CL, Hofmeister EH, Budsberg SC. Systematic review of clinical trials of treatments for osteoarthritis in dogs. *J Am Vet Med Assoc* 2007; **230**: 514–521.

83 Innes JF, Clayton J, Lascelles BDX. Review of the safety and efficacy of long-term NSAID use in the treatment of canine osteoarthritis. *Vet Rec* 2010; **166**: 226–230.

84 Pye C, Bruniges N, Peffers M, *et al.* Advances in the pharmaceutical treatment options for canine osteoarthritis. *J Small Anim Pract* 2022; **63**(10): 721–738.

85 Sparkes AH, Heiene R, Lascelles BDX, *et al.* ISFM and AAFP consensus guidelines: long-term use of NSAIDs in cats. *J Feline Med Surg* 2010; **12**: 521–538.

86 Monteiro-Steagall BP, Steagall PVM, Lascelles BDX. Systematic review of non-steroidal anti-inflammatory drug induced adverse effects in dogs. *J Vet Intern Med* 2013; **27**: 1011–1019.

87 Carmicheal S. Clinical use of non-steroidal anti-inflammatory agents (NSAIDs); the current position. *Eur J Comp Anim Prac* 2011; **21**: 171–177.

88 Freye E. *Opioids in Medicine – A Comprehensive Review on the Mode of Action and the Use of Analgesics in Different Clinical Pain States*. Dordrecht, Netherlands: Springer, 2008: 256–266.

89 Wernham BG, Trumpatori B, Hash J, *et al.* Dose reduction of meloxicam in dogs with osteoarthritis-associated pain and impaired mobility. *J Vet Intern Med* 2011; **25**: 1298–1305.

90 KuKanich B, Bidgood T, Knesl O. Clinical pharmacology of nonsteroidal anti-inflammatory drugs in dogs. *Vet Anaesth Analg* 2012; **39**: 69–90.

91 Surdyk KK, Brown CA, Brown SA. Evaluation of glomerular filtration rate in cats with reduced renal mass and administered meloxicam and acetylsalicylic acid. *Am J Vet Res* 2013; **74**: 648–651.

92 Surdyk KK, Sloan DL, Brown SA. Renal effects of carprofen and etodolac in euvolemic and volume-depleted dogs. *Am J Vet Res* 2012; **73**: 1485–1489.

93 Surdyk KK, Sloan DL, Brown SA. Evaluation of the renal effects of ibuprofen and carprofen in euvolemic and volume-depleted dogs. *Intern J Appl Res Vet Med* 2011; **9**: 129–136.

94 Dowers KL, Uhrig SR, Mama KR, *et al.* Effect of short-term sequential administration of nonsteriodal anti-inflammatory drugs on the stomach and proximal portion of the duodenum in healthy dogs. *Am J Vet Res* 2006; **67**: 1794–1801.

95 Lascelles BD, McFarland JM, Swann H. Guidelines for safe and effective use of NSAIDs in dogs. *Vet Ther* 2005; **6**: 237–251.

96 Sharkey M, Brown M, Wilmot L. What Veterinarians Should Tell Clients About Pain Control and Their Pets FDA *Veterinarian Newsletter* 2006 Volume XXI, No I. www.valheart.com/blog/what-veterinarians-should-tell-clients-about-pain-control-and-their-pets (accessed October 2014).

97 Ryan WG, Moldave K, Carithers D. Switching NSAIDs in practice: insights from the Previcox (firocoxib) experience trial. *Vet Ther* 2007; **8**: 263–271.

98 Papich MG. An update on nonsteroidal anti-inflammatory drugs (NSAIDs) in small animals. *Vet Clin Small Anim* 2008; **38**: 1243–1266.

99 Vasseur PB, Johnson AL, Budsberg SC, *et al.* Randomized, controlled trial of the efficacy of carprofen, a nonsteroidal antiinflammatory drug, in the treatment of osteoarthritis in dogs. *J Am Vet Med Assoc* 1995; **206**: 807–811.

100 Holtsinger RH, Parker RB, Beale BS, *et al.* The therapeutic efficacy of carprofen in 209 clinical cases of canine degenerative joint disease. *Vet Comp Orthop Traumat* 1992; **5**: 140–144.

101 Moreau M, Dubuis J, Bonneau NH, *et al.* Clinical evaluation of a nutraceutical, carprofen and meloxicam for the treatment of dogs with osteoarthritis. *Vet Rec* 2003; **152**: 323–329.

102 Pollmeier M, Toulemonde C, Fleishman C, *et al.* Clinical evaluation of firocoxib and carprofen for the treatment of dogs with osteoarthritis. *Vet Rec* 2006; **159**: 547–555.

103 Autefage A, Gossellin J. Efficacy and safety of the long-term oral administration of carprofen in the treatment of osteoarthritis in dogs. *Rev Med Vet* 2007; **158**: 119–127.

104 Mansa S, Palmér E, Grøndahl C, *et al.* Long-term treatment with carprofen of 805 dogs with osteoarthritis. *Vet Rec* 2007; **160**: 427–430.

105 Reymond N, Speranza C, Gruet P, *et al.* Robenacoxib vs. carprofen for the treatment of canine osteoarthritis; a randomized, noninferiority clinical trial. *J Vet Pharmacol Ther* 2012; **35**: 175–183.

106 EMA. Cimalgex® - Cimicoxib: Summary to the public. EMA/532732/2010. www.ema.europa.eu/en/documents/overview/cimalgex-epar-summary-public_en.pdf (accessed June 2023).

107 EMA. Cimalgex® - Scientific discussion. EMA/CVMP/513842/2011. www.ema.europa.eu/en/documents/assessment-report/cimalgex-epar-public-assessment-report_en.pdf (accessed June 2023).

108 KimTW, Lebkowska-Wieruszewska, Owen B, *et al.* Pharmacokinetic profiles of the novel COX-2 selective inhibitor cimicoxib in dogs. *Vet J* 2014; **200**: 77–81.

109 Stabile M, Lacitignola L, Samarelli R, *et al.* Evaluation of clinical efficacy of undenatured type II collagen supplementation compared to cimicoxib and their association in dogs affected by natural occurring osteoarthritis. *Res Vet Sci* 2022; **151**: 27–35.

110 Grandemange E, Fournel S, Woehrlé F. Efficacy and safety of cimicoxib in the control of perioperative pain in dogs. *J Small Anim Pract* 2013; **54**: 304–312.

111 Bustamante R, Daza MA, Canfrán S, *et al.* Comparison of the postoperative analgesic effects of cimicoxib, buprenorphine and their combination in healthy dogs undergoing ovariohysterectomy. *Vet Anaesth Analg* 2018; **45**: 545–556.

112 Monteiro BP, de Lorimier LP, Moreau M, *et al.* Pain characterization and response to palliative care in dogs with naturally-occurring appendicular osteosarcoma: an open label clinical trial. *PLoS ONE* 2018; **13**: e0207200.

113 Johnston SA, Conzemius MG, Cross AR, *et al.* A multi-center clinical study of the effects of Deracoxib, a COX-2 selective drug on chronic pain in dogs with osteoarthritis. *Vet Surg* 2001; **30**: 497.

114 Millis DL, Conzemius MG, Wells KL, *et al.* A multi-center clinical study on the effects of Dearcoxicb, a COX-2 selective drug on post-operative analgesia associated with cranial cruciate ligament stabilization in dogs. *Vet Surg* 2001; **30**: 502.

115 Bienhoff SE, Smith ES, Roycroft LM, *et al.* Efficacy and safety of deracoxib for the control of postoperative pain and inflammation associated with dental surgery in dogs. *ISRN Vet Sci* 2012; **2011**: 593015.

116 Bienhoff SE, Smith ES, Roycroft LM, *et al.* Efficacy and safety of deracoxib for control of postoperative pain and inflammation associated with soft tissue surgery in dogs. *Vet Surg* 2012; **41**: 336–344.

117 Cendrós JM, Salichs M, Encina G, *et al.* Pharmacology of enflicoxib, a new coxib drug: efficacy and dose determination by clinical and pharmacokinetic-guided approach for the treatment of osteoarthritis in dogs based on an acute arthritis induction model. *Vet Med Sci* 2022; **8**: 31–45.

118 Homedes J, Salichs M, Solà J, *et al.* Pharmacokinetics of enflicoxib in dogs: effects of prandial state and repeated administration. *J Vet Pharmacol Ther* 2021; **44**: 888–901.

119 Homedes J, Salichs M, Guzman A. Long-term safety evaluation of Daxocox® tablets (enflicoxib) in dogs after weekly oral administrations for seven months. *BMC Vet Res* 2021; **17**: 205.

120 Salichs M, Badiella L, Sarasola P, *et al.* Efficacy and safety of enflicoxib for treatment of canine osteoarthritis: a 6-week randomised, controlled, blind, multicentre clinical trial. *Vet Rec* 2022; **191**: e949.

121 Salichs M, Badiella L, Sarasola P, *et al.* Enflicoxib for canine osteoarthritis: a randomized, blind, multicentre, non-inferiority clinical trial compared to mavacoxib. *PLoS ONE* 2022; **17**: e0274800.

122 Pollmeier M, Toulemonde C, Fleishman C, *et al.* Clinical evaluation of firocoxib and carprofen for the treatment of dogs with osteoarthritis. *Vet Rec* 2006; **159**: 547–551.

123 Gordon WJ, Conzemius MG, Drag M, *et al.* Assessment of the efficacy of firocoxib and etodolac for the treatment of osteoarthritis in dogs. *Vet Surg* 2004; **33**: E9.

124 Hanson PD, Brooks KC, Case J, *et al.* Efficacy and safety of firocoxib in the management of canine osteoarthritis under field conditions. *Vet Ther* 2006; **7**: 127–140.

125 Autefage A, Palissier FM, Asimus E, *et al.* Long-term efficacy and safety of firocoxib in the treatment of dogs with osteoarthritis. *Vet Rec* 2011; **168**: 617–623.

126 Ryan WG, Moldave K, Carithers D. Clinical effectiveness and safety of a new NSAID, firocoxib: a 1000 dog study. *Vet Ther* 2006; **7**: 119–126.

127 Ross JM, Kleine SA, Smith CK, *et al.* Evaluation of the perioperative analgesic effects of grapiprant compared with carprofen in dogs undergoing elective ovariohysterectomy. *J Am Vet Med Assoc* 2022; **261**: 118–125.

128 Sartini I, Giorgi M. Grapiprant: a snapshot of the current knowledge. *J Vet Pharmacol Ther* 2021; **44**: 679–688.

129 Kirkby Shaw K, Rausch-Derra LC, Rhodes L. Grapiprant: an EP4 prostaglandin receptor antagonist and novel therapy for pain and inflammation. *Vet Med Sci* 2015; **2**: 3–9.

130 Rausch-Derra L, Huebner M, Wofford J, *et al.* A Prospective, randomized, masked, placebo-controlled multisite clinical study of grapiprant, an EP4 prostaglandin receptor antagonist (PRA), in dogs with osteoarthritis. *J Vet Intern Med* 2016; **30**: 756–763.

131 de Salazar Alcalá AG, Gioda L, Dehman A, *et al.* Assessment of the efficacy of firocoxib (Previcox®) and grapiprant (Galliprant®) in an induced model of acute arthritis in dogs. *BMC Vet Res* 2019; **15**: 309.

132 Budsberg SC, Kleine SA, Norton MM, *et al.* Comparison of two inhibitors of E-type prostanoid receptor four and carprofen in dogs with experimentally induced acute synovitis. *Am J Vet Res* 2019; **80**: 1001–1006.

133 Monteiro BP, Lambert C, Bianchi E, *et al.* Safety and efficacy of reduced dosage ketoprofen with or without tramadol for long-term treatment of osteoarthritis in dogs: a randomized clinical trial. *BMC Vet Res* 2019; **15**: 213.

134 Grisneaux E, Pibarot P, Dupuis J, *et al.* Comparison of ketoprofen and carprofen administered prior to orthopedic surgery for control of postoperative pain in dogs. *J Am Vet Med Assoc* 1999; **215**: 1105–1110.

135 Hazewinkel HA, van den Brom WE, Pollmeier M, *et al.* Reduced dosage of ketoprofen for the short-term and long-term treatment of joint pain in dogs. *Vet Rec* 2003; **152**: 11–14.

136 Morton CM, Grant D, Johnston L, *et al.* Clinical evaluation of meloxicam versus ketoprofen in cats suffering from painful acute locomotor disorders. *J Feline Med Surg* 2011; **13**: 237–243.

137 Sano T, King JN, Seewald W, *et al.* Comparison of oral robenacoxib and ketoprofen for the treatment of acute pain and inflammation associated with musculoskeletal disorders in cats: a randomised clinical trial. *Vet J* 2012; **93**: 397–403.

138 Cox SR, Liao S, Payne-Johnson M, *et al.* Population pharmacokinetics of mavacoxib in osteoarthritic dogs. *J Vet Pharmacol Ther* 2011; **34**: 1–11.

139 Cox SR, Lesman SP, Boucher JF, *et al.* The pharmacokinetics of mavacoxib, a long-acting COX-2 inhibitor, in young adult laboratory dogs. *J Vet Pharmacol Ther* 2010; **33**: 461–470.

140 Lees P, Pelligand L, Elliott J, *et al.* Pharmacokinetics, pharmacodynamics, toxicology and therapeutics of mavacoxib in the dog: a review. *J Vet Pharmacol Ther* 2015; **38**: 1–14.

141 Walton MB, Cowderoy EC, Wustefeld-Janssens B, *et al.* Mavacoxib and meloxicam for canine osteoarthritis: a randomised clinical comparator trial. *Vet Rec* 2014; **175**: 280.

142 Payne-Johnson M, Becskei C, Chaudhry Y, *et al.* Comparative efficacy and safety of mavacoxib and carprofen in the treatment of canine osteoarthritis. *Vet Rec* 2015; **176**: 284.

143 Doig PA, Purbrick KA, Hare JE, *et al.* Clinical efficacy and tolerance of meloxicam in dogs with chronic osteoarthritis. *Can Vet J* 2000; **41**: 296–300.

144 Nell T, Bergman J, Hoeijmakers M, *et al.* Comparison of vedaprofen and meloxicam in dogs with musculoskeletal pain and inflammation. *J Small Anim Pract* 2002; **43**: 208–212.

145 Peterson KD, Keefe TJ. Effects of meloxicam on severity of lameness and other clinical signs of osteoarthritis in dogs. *J Am Vet Med Assoc* 2004; **225**: 1056–1060.

146 Lascelles BD, Henderson AJ, Hackett IJ. Evaluation of the clinical efficacy of meloxicam in cats with painful locomotor disorders. *J Small Anim Pract* 2001; **42**: 587–593.

147 Charlton AN, Benito J, Simpson W, *et al.* Evaluation of the clinical use of tepoxalin and meloxicam in cats. *J Feline Med Surg* 2013; **15**: 678–690.

148 Gunew MN, Menrath VH, Marshall RD. Long-term safety, efficacy and palatability of oral meloxicam at 0.01–0.03 mg/kg for treatment of osteoarthritic pain in cats. *J Feline Med Surg* 2008; **10**: 235–241.

149 Guillot M, Moreau M, Heit M, *et al.* Characterization of osteoarthritis in cats and meloxicam efficacy using objective chronic pain evaluation tools. *Vet J* 2013; **196**: 360–367.

150 Gowan RA, Lingard AE, Johnston L, *et al.* Retrospective case-control study of the effects of long-term dosing with meloxicam on renal function in aged cats with degenerative joint disease. *J Feline Med Surg* 2012; **13**: 752–761.

151 Sul RM, Chase D, Parkin T, *et al.* Comparison of meloxicam and a glucosamine-chondroitin supplement in management of feline osteoarthritis. A double-blind randomised, placebo-controlled, prospective trial. *Vet Comp Orthop Traumatol* 2014; **27**: 20–26.

152 KuKanich K, George C, Roush JK, *et al.* Effects of low-dose meloxicam in cats with chronic kidney disease. *J Feline Med Surg* 2021; **23**: 138–148.

153 Reymond N, Speranza C, Gruet P, *et al.* Robenacoxib vs. carprofen for the treatment of canine osteoarthritis; a randomized, noninferiority clinical trial. *J Vet Pharmacol Ther* 2012; **35**: 175–183.

154 Gruet P, Seewald W, King JN. Evaluation of subcutaneous and oral administration of robenacoxib and meloxicam for the treatment of acute pain and inflammation associated with orthopedic surgery in dogs. *Am J Vet Res* 2011; **72**: 184–193.

155 Edamura K, King JN, Seewald W, *et al.* Comparison of oral robenacoxib and carprofen for the treatment of osteoarthritis in dogs: a randomized clinical trial. *J Vet Med Sci* 2012; **74**: 1121–1131.

156 Toutain CE, Brossard P, King SB, *et al.* Six-month safety evaluation of robenacoxib tablets (Onsior™) in dogs after daily oral administrations. *BMC Vet Res* 2018; **14**: 242.

157 Lees P, Toutain PL, Elliott J, *et al.* Pharmacology, safety, efficacy and clinical uses of the COX-2 inhibitor robenacoxib. *J Vet Pharmacol Ther* 2022; **45**: 325–351.

158 Kongara K, Chambers JP. Robenacoxib in the treatment of pain in cats and dogs: safety, efficacy, and place in therapy. *Vet Med (Auckl)* 2018; **9**: 53–61.

159 Kamata M, King JN, Seewald W, *et al.* Comparison of injectable robenacoxib versus meloxicam for peri-operative use in cats: results of a randomised clinical trial. *Vet J* 2012; **193**: 114–118.

160 Giraudel JM, Gruet P, Alexander DG, *et al.* Evaluation of orally administered robenacoxib versus ketoprofen for treatment of acute pain and inflammation associated with musculoskeletal disorders in cats. *Am J Vet Res* 2010; **71**: 710–719.

161 King S, Roberts ES, Roycroft LM, *et al.* Evaluation of oral robenacoxib for the treatment of postoperative pain and inflammation in cats: results of a randomized clinical trial. *ISRN Vet Sci* 2012; **79**: 41–48.

162 King JN, Hotz R, Reagan EL, *et al.* Safety of oral robenacoxib in the cat. *J Vet Pharmacol Ther* 2011; **35**: 290–300.

163 King JN, King S, Budsberg SC, *et al.* Clinical safety of robenacoxib in feline osteoarthritis: results of a randomized, blinded, placebo-controlled clinical trial. *J Feline Med Surg* 2016; **18**: 632–642.

164 Adrian D, King JN, Parrish RS, *et al.* Robenacoxib shows efficacy for the treatment of chronic degenerative joint disease-associated pain in cats: a randomized and blinded pilot clinical trial. *Sci Rep* 2021; **11**: 7721.

165 C King JN, Seewald W, Forster S, *et al.* Clinical safety of robenacoxib in cats with chronic musculoskeletal disease. *J Vet Intern Med* 2021; **35**: 2384–2394.

166 Charette B, Dupuis J, Moreau M, *et al.* Assessing the efficacy of long-term administration of tolfenamic acid in dogs undergoing femoral head and neck excision. *Vet Comp Orthop Traumatol* 2003; **16**: 232–237.

167 Murison PJ, Tacke S, Wondratschek C, *et al.* Postoperative analgesic efficacy of meloxicam compared to tolfenamic acid in cats undergoing orthopaedic surgery. *J Small Anim Pract* 2010; **51**: 526–532.

168 Sattasathuchana P, Phuwapattanachart P, Thengchaisri N. Comparison of postoperative analgesic efficacy of tolfenamic acid and robenacoxib in ovariohysterectomized cats. *J Vet Med Sci* 2018; **80**: 989–996.

169 Gonda X. Basic pharmacology of NMDA receptors. *Curr Pharm Des* 2012; **18**: 1558–1567.

170 Pozzi A, Muir WW, Traverso F. Prevention of central sensitization and pain by N-methyl-D-aspartate receptor antagonists. *J Am Vet Med Assoc* 2006; **228**: 53–60.

171 Zhou HY, Chen SR, Pan HL. Targeting N-methyl-D-aspartate receptors for treatment of neuropathic pain. *Expert Rev Clin Pharmacol* 2011; **4**: 379–388.

172 Kreutzwiser D, Tawfic QA. Expanding role of NMDA receptor antagonists in the management of pain. *CNS Drugs* 2019; **33**: 347–374.

173 Ugale V, Dhote A, Narwade R, *et al.* GluN2B/N-methyl-D-aspartate receptor antagonists: advances in design, synthesis, and pharmacological evaluation studies. *CNS Neurol Disord Drug Targets* 2021; **20**: 822–862.

174 Lascelles BD, Gaynor JS, Smith ES, *et al.* Amantadine in a multimodal analgesic regimen for alleviation of refractory osteoarthritis pain in dogs. *J Vet Intern Med* 2008; **22**: 53–59.

175 KuKanich B. Outpatient oral analgesics in dogs and cats beyond nonsteroidal anti-inflammatory drugs: an evidence-based approach. *Vet Clin North Am Small Anim Pract* 2013; **43**: 1109–1125.

176 KuKanich B, Papich MG. Pharmacokinetics and antinociceptive effects of oral tramadol hydrochloride administration in greyhounds. *Am J Vet Res* 2011; **72**: 256–262.

177 Itami T, Saito Y, Ishizuka T, *et al.* Comparison of pharmacokinetics of tramadol between young and middle-aged dogs. *J Vet Med Sci* 2016; **78**: 1031–1034.

178 Budsberg SC, Torres BT, Kleine SA, *et al.* Lack of treatment efficacy of tramadol on pain and dysfunction of chronic osteoarthritic (OA) joints in dogs. *J Am Vet Med Assoc* 2018; **252**: 427–432.

179 Davila D, Keeshen TP, Evans RB, *et al.* Comparison of the analgesic efficacy of perioperative firocoxib and tramadol administration in dogs undergoing tibial plateau leveling osteotomy. *J Am Vet Med Assoc* 2013; **243**: 225–231.

180 Piras LA, Mancusi D, Olimpo M, *et al.* Post-operative analgesia following TPLO surgery: a comparison between cimicoxib and tramadol. *Res Vet Sci* 2021; **136**: 351–359.

181 Donati PA, Tarragona L, Franco JVA, *et al.* Efficacy of tramadol for postoperative pain management in dogs: systematic review and meta-analysis. *Vet Anaesth Analg* 2021; **48**: 283–296.

182 Pypendop BH, Ilkiw JE. Pharmacokinetics of tramadol and its metabolite O-desmethyl-tramadol, in cats. *J Vet Pharmacol Ther* 2008; **10**: 24–31.

183 Dominguez-Oliva A, Casas-Alvarado A, Miranda-Cortes AE, *et al.* Clinical pharmacology of tramadol and tapentadol, and their therapeutic efficacy in different models of acute and chronic pain in dogs and cats. *J Adv Vet Anim Res* 2021; **8**: 404–422.

184 Monteior BP, Klinck MP, Moreau M, *et al.* Analgesic efficacy of tramadol in cats with naturally occurring osteoarthritis. *PLoS ONE* 2017; **12**: e0175565.

185 Guedes AGP, Meadows JM, Pypendop BH, *et al.* Evaluation of tramadol for treatment of osteoarthritis in geriatric cats. *J Am Vet Med Assoc* 2018; **253**: 565–571.

186 Erickson A, Harbin K, MacPherson J, *et al.* Review of pre-appointment medications to reduce fear and anxiety in dogs and cats at veterinary visits. *Can Vet J* 2021; **62**: 952–960.

187 Guedes AGP, Meadows JM, Pypendop BH, *et al.* Assessment of the effects of gabapentin on activity levels and owner-perceived mobility impairment and quality of life in osteoarthritic geriatric cats. *J Am Vet Med Assoc* 2018; **253**: 579–585.

188 Ruel HLM, Watanabe R, Evangelista MC, *et al.* Pain burden, sensory profile and inflammatory cytokines of dogs with naturally-occurring neuropathic pain treated with gabapentin alone or with meloxicam. *PLoS ONE* 2020; **15**: e0237121.

189 Barbeau-Grégoire M, Otis C, Cournoyer A, *et al.* A 2022 systematic review and meta-analysis of enriched therapeutic diets and nutraceuticals in canine and feline osteoarthritis. *Int J Mol Sci* 2022; **23**: 10384.

190 McCarthy G, O'Donovan J, Jones B, *et al.* Randomised double-blind, positive-controlled trial to assess the efficacy of glucosamine/chondroitin sulfate for the treatment of dogs with osteoarthritis. *Vet J* 2007; **174**: 54–61.

191 Scott PM, Evans R, Conzemius MG. Efficacy of an oral nutraceutical for the treatment of osteoarthritis. *Vet Comp Orthop Traumatol* 2017; **30**: 318–323.

192 de Haan JJ, Goring RL, Beale BS. Evaluation of polysulfated glycosaminoglycan for the treatment of hip dysplasia in dogs. *Vet Surg* 1994; **23**: 177–181.

193 Fujiki M, Shineha J, Yamanokuchi K, *et al.* Effects of treatment with polysulfated glycosaminoglycan on serum cartilage oligomeric matrix protein and C-reactive protein concentrations, serum matrix metalloproteinase-2 and -9 activities, and lameness in dogs with osteoarthritis. *Am J Vet Res* 2007; **68**: 827–833.

194 Bui LM, Bierer TL. Influence of green lipped mussels (*Perna canaliculus*) in alleviating signs of arthritis in dogs. *Vet Therapu* 2001; **2**: 101–111.

195 Bierer TL, Bui LM. Improvement of arthritic signs in dogs fed green-lipped mussel (*Perna canaliculus*). *Am Soc Nutr Sci* 2002; **132**: 1634S–1636S.

196 Pollard B, Guilford WG, Ankenbauer-Perkins KL, *et al.* Clinical efficacy and tolerance of an extract of green-lipped mussel (*Perna canaliculus*) in dogs presumptively diagnosed with degenerative joint disease. *N Z Vet J* 2006; **54**: 114–118.

197 Rialland P, Bichot S, Lussier B, *et al.* Effect of a diet enriched with green-lipped mussel on pain behavior and functioning in dogs with clinical osteoarthritis. *Can J Vet Res* 2013; **77**: 66–74.

198 Hielm-Björkman A, Tulamo RM, Salonen H, *et al.* Evaluating complementary therapies for canine osteoarthritis – Part II: a homeopathic combination preparation (Zeel). *Evid Based Complement Alternat Med* 2009; **6**: 465–471.

199 Neumann S, Stolt P, Braun G, *et al.* Effectiveness of the homeopathic preparation Zeel compared with carprofen in dogs with osteoarthritis. *J Am Anim Hosp Assoc* 2011; **47**: 12–20.

200 Deparle LA, Gupta RC, Canerdy TD, *et al.* Efficacy and safety of glycosylated undenatured type-II collagen (UC-II) in therapy of arthritic dogs. *J Vet Pharmacol Ther* 2005; **28**: 385–390.

201 Peal A, D'Altilio M, Simms C, *et al.* Therapeutic efficacy and safety of undenatured type-II collagen (UC-II) alone or in combination with (-)-hydroxycitric acid and chromemate in arthritic dogs. *J Vet Pharmacol Ther* 2007; **30**: 275–278.

202 D'Altilio M, Peal A, Alvey M, *et al.* Therapeutic efficacy and safety of undenatured type II collagen singly or in combination with glucosamine and chondroitin in arthritic dogs. *Toxicol Mech Methods* 2007; **17**: 189–196.

203 Gupta RC, Canerdy TD, Lindley J, *et al.* Comparative therapeutic efficacy and safety of type-II collagen (UC-II), glucosamine and chondroitin in arthritic dogs: pain evaluation by ground force plate. *J Anim Physiol Anim Nutr (Berl)* 2012; **96**: 770–777.

204 Stabile M, Samarelli R, Trerotoli P, *et al.* Evaluation of the effects of undenatured type II collagen (UC-II) as compared to robenacoxib on the mobility impairment induced by osteoarthritis in dogs. *Vet Sci* 2019; **6**: 72.

205 Gamble LJ, Boesch JM, Frye CW, *et al.* Pharmacokinetics, safety, and clinical efficacy of cannabidiol treatment in osteoarthritic dogs. *Front Vet Sci* 2018; **5**: 165.

206 Verrico CD, Wesson S, Konduri V, *et al.* A randomized, double-blind, placebo-controlled study of daily cannabidiol for the treatment of canine osteoarthritis pain. *Pain* 2020; **161**: 2191–2202.

207 Mejia S, Duerr FM, Griffenhagen G, *et al.* Evaluation of the effect of cannabidiol on naturally occurring osteoarthritis-associated pain: a pilot study in dogs. *J Am Anim Hosp Assoc* 2021; **57**: 81–90.

208 Malfait AM, Miller RE, Block JA. Targeting neurotrophic factors: novel approaches to musculoskeletal pain. *Pharmacol Ther* 2020; **211**: 107553.

209 Malfait AM, Miller RE, Block JA. Basic mechanisms of pain in osteoarthritis. *Rheum Dis Clin North Am* 2021; **47**: 165–180.

210 Minnone G, De Benedetti F, Bracci-Laudiero L. NGF and its receptors in the regulation of inflmmatory response. *Int J Mol Sci* 2017; **18**: 1028.

211 Enomoto E, Mantyh P, Murrell J, *et al.* Anti-nerve growth factor monoclonal antibodies for the control of pain in dogs and cats. *Vet Rec* 2019; **184**: 23.

212 Webster RP, Anderson GI, Gearing DP. Canine Brief Pain Inventory scores for dogs with osteoarthritis before and after administration of a monocolonal antibody against nerve growth factor. *Am J Vet Res* 2014; **75**: 532–537.

213 Lascelles BDX, Knazovicky D, Case B, *et al.* A canine-specific anti-nerve growth factor antibody alleviates pain and improves mobility and function in dogs with degenerative joint disease-associated pain. *BMC Vet Res* 2015; **11**: 101.

214 Corral MJ, Moyaert H, Fernades T, *et al.* A prospective, randomized, blinded, placebo-controlled multisite clinical study of bedinvetmab, a canine monoclonal antibody targeting nerve growth factor in dogs with osteoarthritis. *Vet Anaesth Analg* 2021; **48**: 943–955.

215 Gearing DP, Huebner M, Virtue ER, *et al.* In vitro and in vivo characterization of a fully felinized therapeutic anti-nerve growth factor monoclonal antibody for the treatment of pain in cats. *J Vet Intern Med* 2016; **30**: 1129–1137.

216 Gruen ME, Thomson AE, Griffith EH, *et al.* A feline-specific anti-nerve growth factor antibody improves mobility in cats with degenerative joint disease-associated pain: a pilot proof of concept study. *J Vet Intern Med* 2016; **30**: 1138–1148.

217 Gruen ME, Myers JAE, Tena JS, *et al.* Frunevetmab, a felinized anti-nerve growth factor monoclonal antibody, for the treatment of pain from osteoarthritis in cats. *J Vet Intern Med* 2021; **35**: 2752–2762.

218 Gruen ME, Myers JAE, Lascelles BDX. Efficacy and safety of an anti-nerve growth factor antibody (frunevetmab) for the treatment of degenerative joint disease-associated chronic pain in cats: a multisite pilot field study. *Front Vet Sci* 2021; **8**: 610028.

219 Caplan AI. Mesenchymal stem cells: time to change the name. *Stem Cell Trans Med* 2017; **6**: 1445–1451.

220 Bogers SH. Cell-based therapies for joint disease in veterinary medicine: what we have learned and want we need to know. *Front Vet Sci* 2018; **5**: 70.

221 Kang MH, Park HM. Challenges of stem cell therapies in companion animal practice. *J Vet Sci* 2020; **21**: e42.

222 Ivanovska A, Wang M, Arshaghi TE, *et al.* Manufacturing mesenchymal stromal cells for the treatment of osteoarthritis in canine patients: challenges and recommendations. *Front Vet Sci* 2022; **9**: 897150.

223 Brondeel C, Pauwelyn G, de Bakker E, *et al.* Review: mesenchymal stem cell therapy in canine osteoarthritis research: "Experientia Docet" (Experience Will Teach Us). *Front Vet Sci* 2021; **8**: 668881.

224 Franklin SP, Garner BC, Cook JL. Characteristics of canine platelet-rich plasma prepared with five commercially available systems. *Am J Vet Res* 2015; **76**: 822–827.

225 Franklin SP. A pilot clinical study assessing treatment of canine hip dysplasia using autologous protein solution. *Front Vet Sci* 2019; **6**: 243.

226 Franklin SP, Franklin AL. Randomized controlled trial comparing autologous protein solution to hyaluronic acid plus triamcinolone for treating hip osteoarthritis in dogs. *Front Vet Sci* 2021; **8**: 713768.

227 Wanstrath AW, Hettlich BF, Su L, *et al.* Evaluation of a single intra-articular injection of autologous protein solution for treatment of osteoarthritis in a canine population. *Vet Surg* 2016; **45**: 764–774.

228 Carr BJ, Canapp SO, Mason DR, *et al.* Canine platelet-rich plasma systems. *Front Vet Sci* 2015; **2**: 73.

229 Cuervo B, Rubio M, Chicharro D, *et al.* Objective comparison between platelet rich plasma alone and in combination with physical therapy in dogs with osteoarthritis caused by hip dysplasia. *Animals (Basel)* 2020; **10**: 175.

230 Catarino J, Carvalho P, Santos S, *et al.* Treatment of canine osteoarthritis with allogeneic platelet-rich plasma: review of five cases. *Open Vet J* 2020; **10**: 226–231.

231 Venator KP, Pye CW, Gamble LJ, *et al.* Assessment of a single intra-articular stifle injection of pure platelet rich plasma on symmetry indices in dogs with unilateral or bilateral stifle osteoarthritis from long-term medically managed cranial cruciate ligament disease. *Vet Med (Auckland)* 2020; **11**: 31–38.

232 Alves JC, Santos A, Jorge P. Platelet-rich plasma therapy in dogs with bilateral hip osteoarthritis. *BMC Vet Res* 2012; **17**: 207.

233 Voga M, Adamic N, Vengust M, *et al.* Stem cells in veterinary medicine – current state and treatment options. *Front Vet Sci* 2020; **7**: 278.

234 Punzon E, Salguero R, Totusaus X, *et al.* Equine umbilical cord mesenchymal stem cells demonstrate safety and efficacy in the treatment of canine osteoarthritis: a randomized placebo-controlled trial. *J Am Vet Med Assoc* 2022; **260**: 1947–1955.

235 Olsson DC, Texieria BL, Da Silva Jeremias T, *et al.* Administration of mesenchymal stem cells from adipose tissue at the hip joint of dogs with osteoarthritis: a systematic review. *Res Vet Sci* 2021; **135**: 495–503.

236 Dworkin RH, Turk DC, Peirce-Sandner S, *et al.* Considerations for improving assay sensitivity in chronic pain clinical trials: IMMPACT recommendations. *Pain* 2012; **153**: 1148–1158.

237 Dworkin RH, Turk DC, Peirce-Sandner S, *et al.* Research design considerations for confirmatory chronic pain clinical trials: IMMPACT recommendations. *Pain* 2010; **149**: 177–193.

238 Moore RA, Moore OA, Derry S, *et al.* Numbers needed to treat calculated from responder rates give a better indication of efficacy in osteoarthritis trials than mean pain scores. *Arthritis Res Ther* 2008; **10**: R39.

239 Moore RA, Moore OA, Derry S, *et al.* Responder analysis for pain relief and numbers needed to treat in a meta-analysis of etoricoxib osteoarthritis trials: bridging a gap between clinical trials and clinical practice. *Ann Rheum Dis* 2010; **69**: 374–379.

240 Moore RA, Derry S, McQuay HJ, *et al.* Clinical effectiveness: an approach to clinical trial design more relevant to clinical practice, acknowledging the importance of individual differences. *Pain* 2010; **149**: 173–176.

Index

Page references to Tables are followed by '*t*'; those to Figures by the letter '*f*'

AAALAC *see* Assessment and Accreditation of Laboratory Animal Care (AAALAC)
AAGBI *see* Association of Anesthetists of Great Britain and Ireland (AAGBI)
AAHA *see* American Animal Hospital Association (AAHA)
abaxial sesamoid (basisesamoid) block 1241
ABCB-1 gene mutation/polymorphism 335, 362, 851, 1031, 1158
abdominal curtain sign (ACS) 257, 258*f*, 260–1, 262*f*, 263*f*, 264
abdominal hemorrhage 876
abdominal muscle contraction 990
abdominal point-of-care ultrasound (APOCUS)
  gastric volume 269, 270*t*, 271
  urinary bladder volume 271
abdominocardiac reflex 655
absorption
  atelectasis 707, 726, 727, 735, 736, 1220
  cannabinoids 433
  carbon dioxide 109–11, 172
  constant rate therapy 299
  delayed 299, 406
  drug 294, 309, 316, 339, 381, 382, 407, 540, 541, 1359
  efficiency of 110
  fluid 636, 637
  gas 771
  gastrointestinal 381, 406, 423
  infrared/infrared bands 223, 224, 242, 243
  light 235, 237
  local anesthetics 327, 531–2
  molecular absorption coefficient 223
  mucosal 337
  nonlinear 299
  oral 406
  osmotic 581
  peak 242, 243
  specific absorption rate 49
  systemic 305, 531, 532, 535, 536, 1167, 1168, 1169, 1333, 1350
  topical 540
  transmucosal 432
  tubular 534
  variable 374, 1367
  water vapor bands 224
  absorption, distribution, metabolism, and elimination (ADME) 290
AC *see* adenylate cyclase (AC) enzyme system
accident causation models 30, 31*f*
accidental extubation 63–4
ACE inhibitors 810, 811, 896, 897, 911, 933
  see also angiotensin-converting enzyme (ACE)
acepromazine 69, 1033, 1084, 1264
  anesthetic mortality, risk of 16
  clinical considerations 335
  drug dose 1065, 1066*t*
  indications for 334–5
  mechanism of action 334–5
  pharmacodynamics 334–5
  pharmacokinetics 334
  premedication 20, 160, 334, 422, 427, 472
acetaminophen (paracetamol) 407–8, 1015
acetylcholine (ACh) 957, 1023, 1135
  and cardiovascular system 1134
  cerebral circulation 659
  neurohormonal and local control mechanisms 654
  neuromuscular junction transmission 827
  photobiomodulation therapy 1025
  receptors 795, 1068
    muscarinic 314
    nicotinic 314, 449, 506
  release of 315, 316, 371
  role in neuromuscular transmission 448
acetylcholinesterase inhibitors 456–7
ACh *see* acetylcholine (ACh)
acid-base balance 555–73
  acids and bases 555–8
    pH 556–7
    p*K*a and the Henderson–Hasselbalch equation 557
  clinical disturbances 568–71
  evaluation approaches 559–68, 571
    anion gap and *c*Na^+–*c*Cl^- difference 565, 567
    base excess (buffer-centric) 553–4
    bicarbonate distribution space 563–4
    physiochemical 564
    simplified strong ion 564
    strong anion gap 567–8
    traditional (bicarbonate-centric) 559–63
  temperature effects on 557–8
acid–base disturbances
  combined disorders in SID and A_{TOT} 571
  disorders in A_{TOT} 571
  disorders in strong ion difference 569–70
  disorders of PCO_2 568
  free-water abnormalities 571
  isonatremic chloride abnormalities 569–70
  isonatremic organic acid abnormalities 570
acid-base homeostasis 221, 555, 556*f*
acidemia
  acid–base derangements 225
  bicarbonate distribution space 564
  carbon dioxide and acid–base implications 221
  diabetes mellitus 902
  evaluation of acid–base balance 559, 561
  excessive arterial carbon dioxide 936
  in fish 1122
  and hypercalcemia 593
  hypercapnic 221
  and hyperkalemia 926, 938, 950
  and hypothermia 876
  metabolic 221, 225, 226
  in pregnancy 958
  reduced adrenergic agent efficacy 1220
  respiratory 1088
  severe 721, 777
acidosis
  acute mineral 593
  dilutional 570, 571, 583
  hyperalbuminemic 571
  hyperchloremic 567, 570, 583
  hyperchloremic metabolic 585, 587, 693, 1222
  hyperphosphatemic 571
  lactic 62, 567, 1357
  local anesthesia 543
  metabolic 68, 250, 320, 414, 429, 503, 564, 567, 583, 702, 721, 1223, 1295
    severe 58, 559, 949, 1274

Veterinary Anesthesia and Analgesia: The Sixth Edition of Lumb and Jones. Edited by Leigh Lamont, Kurt Grimm, Sheilah Robertson, Lydia Love and Carrie Schroeder.
© 2024 John Wiley & Sons, Inc. Published 2024 by John Wiley & Sons, Inc.
Companion website: www.wiley.com/go/lamont/anesthesia

non-bicarbonate buffer ion 571
non-respiratory 558, 563, 564, 565, 569, 570, 571, 572
normal AG 567
ophthalmic patients 1331
organic 570
paradoxical cerebral 58
paradoxical cerebrospinal 594
respiratory 367, 422, 563, 568, 571, 572, 656, 688, 725, 1290, 1313, 1336
acute 563
primary 562
strong ion 569, 571
subclinical acute ruminal 1263
acids
and bases 556–8
acid–base derangements 225
blood pH, mechanisms to minimize changes in 558–9
evaluation approaches 559–68
Henderson-Hasselbalch equation 557
pH 556–7
pK_a 557
temperature effects on 557–8
carbon dioxide and acid–base implications 221
acid-sensing ion channels (ASIC), and euthanasia 159
ACRM *see* Anesthesia Crisis Resource Management (ACRM)
actin-activated myosin chemomechanical ATPase cycle 629, 630*f*, 631, 631*f*
action potential
cardiac 187, 328, 428, 429, 594, 621
cardiovascular toxicity 542
compound 453
conduction 529, 623*f*
duration 364, 621*f*
generation of 594, 937*f*
initiation of 973
neuromuscular junction (NMJ) 449, 827
normal 621*f*
and peripheral nerve stimulators 1172
prolonging 367
propagation 628*f*
and sodium ion channels 285
transmission 973
acupuncture 4, 1024
acute hypercapnia 155
acute kidney injury (AKI)/acute renal failure 11, 52, 198, 411, 694, 874, 929–31, 934
in advancing age 1356
clinical features and diagnosis 931
etiology and pathogenesis 929–31
and postanesthesia oliguria 939
short-term renal ischemia leading to 924
solutions causing 587, 597, 692, 693
synthetic colloids associated with 692, 875, 881
see also renal clearance; renal disease; renal function; renal replacement therapy; renal system
acute normovolemic hemodilution (ANH) 602
acute pain
accelerometry and step-counts 1000
changes in behavior 996, 997*f*, 998
electroencephalogram 999
factors confounding behavioral assessment 998
first-tier 1011
frequency of assessment 1003, 1005
functional magnetic resonance imaging 999
infrared thermography 1000
non-steroidal anti-inflammatory drugs (NSAIDs) 1011
physiological parameters 998–9
quantification 1001–2
recognition of 996, 997*f*, 998
validity 1002
see also chronic pain; pain; pain faces; pain management
Acute Physiology and Chronic Health Evaluation (APACHE) 10
acute respiratory distress syndrome (ARDS) 269
acute spinal cord injury (SCI) 370
ACVA *see* American College of Veterinary Anesthesiologists (ACVA)
ACVAA *see* American College of Veterinary Anesthesia and Analgesia (ACVAA)
ACVIM *see* American College of Veterinary Internal Medicine (ACVIM)
adenosine 160
adenosine triphosphate (ATP) 238
adenosine-5′- triphosphate (ATP) binding cassette (ABC) family of proteins 1031
adenylate cyclase (AC) enzyme system 287
adjunctive drugs 420–47
analgesic 431–8
birds 1143
horses 1225–7
non-analgesic 420–31
ophthalmic patients 1335–6
renal disease 936–7
adjustable pressure-limiting (APL) valve 25, 34, 108–9
closure or malfunction 27, 32*f*, 59, 66
open at all times, requirement for 104
as “overflow” 108
administration techniques, inhalational anaesthetics
boiling point 494
gas versus vapor 491–2
general principles 491
methods of description 492–4
vapor pressure 493–4
adrenal glands 893–900
hyperadrenocorticism 895–8
hypoadrenocorticism 893–5
pheochromocytoma 898–900
adrenaline *see* epinephrine
adrenergic agents 319–32
adrenergic receptor antagonists *see* adrenergic receptor antagonists
catecholamines *see* catecholamines
classification 319
epinephrine *see* epinephrine
mechanism of action 319
adrenergic receptor agonists
α_1 type 324–5
α_2 type
catecholamines 325
emergencies and resuscitation 69, 1208–10
local anesthesia 537
sedation/chemical restraint 338–44, 1083, 1266–7
β_2 type 325–6
mixed α-and β type 326
adrenergic receptor antagonists
α_1 type 326–7
a_2 type 327 344–7, 1083, 1266–7
β_1 type 328–9
local anesthetic additives 1169
non-selective α 327–8
non-selective β 329
β-adrenergic receptors 287
ADRs *see* adverse drug reactions (ADRs)
Advanced Cardiovascular Life Support protocols 34
advanced life support (ALS), cardiopulmonary arrest 55, 58–9
adverse drug events (ADEs) 307
see also adverse drug reactions (ADRs); drug-related complications
adverse drug reactions (ADRs) 7, 307
local anesthesia
allergic reactions 545
local toxicity 544
methemoglobinemia 544–5
systemic toxicity 531, 532, 535, 536, 538, 539, 541–4
toxicosis (oral ingestion) 545
NSAIDs
blood coagulation 412
cartilage injury 412
gastrointestinal injury 408–10
kidney injury 410–11
liver, effects on 411–12
platelet inhibition abnormalities 412
thrombotic abnormalities 412
see also adverse events; drug-related complications; *individual drugs*
adverse effects, transfusion therapy 600–2
adverse events
categorizing 54–5
consequences 54
defining 54
NSAIDs 1380
rates of 54
AEMR *see* anesthesia electronic medical record (AEMR)
aepEXplus™ device 183
AEPs *see* auditory evoked potentials (AEPs)
aerobic respiration, physiology 220–1
Aerrane® *see* isoflurane
African Gray Parrot (*Psittacus erithacus*) 227
afterload 206, 275, 322, 647, 809
LV 206, 778, 811
RV 206, 773, 774, 777, 809, 810
ventricular 57, 475
agent purity, and euthanasia 161–2
age-related changes 1354–62
anesthesia risk 1358

age-related changes (*cont'd*)
anesthetic case management 1360
cardiovascular changes 1355–6
clinical implications
cardiovascular changes 1355–6
hepatic changes 1357
immune function 1357
preanesthetic evaluation 1359
pulmonary changes 1356
renal changes 1357
thermoregulation 1357
cognitive dysfunction 1356
cognitive impairment 1356
drug responses 1359–60
emergence delirium 1356
environmental stressors 1360
frailty 1357–8
life stages 1355*t*
neurocognitive and behavioral assessment 1356
neuromuscular blocking agents 1360
nutrition 1360
opioids 1359
physiologic changes related to 1354–7
postoperative cognitive dysfunction 1356
postoperative delirium 1356
preanesthetic testing 1358–9
pulmonary changes 1356
renal changes 1356–7
supportive care 1360
air bronchograms 269
air sacs of birds 1129
airway assessment, point-of-care ultrasound 256
airway fire 65
airway management
birds 1144
endotracheal intubation 1070
laboratory animals 1070–1
marine mammals 1102–5
during recovery 1061–2
airway obstruction
anesthetic emergencies 62–3
induction of anesthesia 62–3
maintenance 63
recovery 63
airway pressure release ventilation (APRV) 1094–5
Akaike's Information Criterion (AIC) 297
alarms, ventilators 122
albumin products
canine serum albumin 597–8
human serum albumin 597
albuterol 325–6
alcuronium 1066*t*
alfaxalone 1097
age-related responses to 1359
birds 1141
chemical structure 477
clinical effects
cardiovascular 478
central nervous system 478
gastrointestinal 478–9
hepatic 478–9
renal 478–9
respiratory 478
species-specific 478–81
clinical use 481
dogs and cats 1161
drug dose 1065, 1066*t*, 1288
injectable 1068
laser procedures 44
mechanism of action 477
neurologic disease 834
ophthalmic patients 1334
pharmacodynamics 478–9
pharmacokinetics 478
pigs 1288, 1289–90
ruminants 1267, 1270
species-specific effects 479–81
alfaxalone-dexmedetomidine 1066*t*
alfentanil 380–1
premedication 430
A-line autoregressive index (AAI) 183
allergic reactions, local anesthesia 545
alleviation of pain 1011
allogenic blood transfusions
autologous 602–3
blood substitutes 603
allometric scaling, birds 1136
allosteric modulators 286
alpha-linolenic acid (ALA) 1013
α-chloralose 481, 1290
injectable 1068
ALS *see* advanced life support (ALS)
alveolar dead space fraction 705
alveolar gas equation 231–2, 720
alveolar interstitial syndrome (AIS) 256, 266
amantadine 431–2, 1382
American Academy of Orthopedic Surgeons 1377
American Animal Hospital Association (AAHA) 143, 1354
and blood pressure monitoring 197
fluid therapy guidelines 1350
American Association for Medical Instruments 203
American Association of Feline Practitioners 1033
American Board of Veterinary Practitioners 1041
American College of Veterinary Anesthesia and Analgesia (ACVAA) 6, 7
and blood pressure monitoring 197
Monitoring Guidelines 251
American College of Veterinary Anesthesiologists (ACVA) 6, 174
American College of Veterinary Emergency and Critical Care (ACVECC) 55
American College of Veterinary Internal Medicine (ACVIM) 198, 203, 204
American Medical Association (AMA) 174
American National Standards Institute, laser advice 40
American Society for Testing and Materials 49
American Society of Anesthesiologists (ASA) 176, 251, 1158, 1159
hypo-or hyperthermia 68
infection prevention and control 147
patient health assessment 10, 12
POCUS certification program 255
preanesthetic blood testing 13
American Society of Echocardiography 271
American Society of Veterinary Anesthesia (ASVA) 6
American Veterinary Medical Association (AVMA) 6, 8, 161, 162
Guidelines on Euthanasia (2020) 153, 156, 158
Humane Slaughter guidelines (2016) 160
AMIC *see* anesthesia multimodal index of consciousness (AMIC)
aminoamides 539–40
amino bisphosphonates 1369
aminoesters 538–9
aminosteroids 451
amiodarone 58
amitriptyline 432–3, 1015
amnesia 155
amphibians
American bullfrogs 1119
anatomy and physiology 1117–18
anesthesia 1116–19
anesthetic agents 1118–19
anurans 1117
cardiovascular system 1117
chelonians 1112
clinical anesthesia 1118
cutaneous system 1118
fasting 1118
fluid regulation 1118
lungs 1117–18
lymphatic system 1117
metabolism 1117
metamorphosis 1117
monitoring 1119
pain and consciousness 155
physical examination and restraint 1118
recovery 1119–20
respiratory system 1117–18
salamanders 1117
amygdala 159
anabolic steroids 1032
Anesthetists' Non-Technical Skills (ANTS) 27, 28*t*
analgesia, veterinary
amphibians 1119
birds 1137–44
current issues 7–9
defining 3, 4
drug effects
adjunctive drugs 431–8
barbiturates 465
dissociative anesthetics 470, 471
etomidate 476
opioids 364–6
propofol 467
intraoperative 1273
miscellaneous drugs 1338
ocular pain 1337–8
opioids 1337
pigs 1295–7
reptiles 1114–16
wildlife capture 1081
see also acute pain; chronic pain; pain; pain management

anaphylaxis 58, 61
anatomic shunt 720
anemia
  blood loss 596
  blood substitutes 603
  chronic 595, 739
  dilutional physiologic 956
  extent of 595
  Heinz body 545
  and hypothermia 252
  hypoxia 231
  iatrogenic 233
  immune-mediated hemolytic anemia (IMHA) 575
  mild 602
  mild-to-moderate 908
  moderate 11*t*, 503
  normocytic normochromic 908
  oxygen extraction ratio 232
  oxygen content, decreased in 831
  and packed red blood cells 596
  patient health assessment 10
  perioperative 602
  preanesthetic blood testing 11
  severe 11*t*, 568, 936
  tolerance to 654
  treatment 879, 1274
  unfractionated heparin (UFH) 576
  young patients 1350
anesthesia, veterinary
  birds 1137–44
  and cancer outcomes 1371–3
  for cardiopulmonary bypass 667–73
  clinical 1114
  current issues 7–9
  defining 3–4
  depth of *see* depth of anesthesia
  in dogs and cats *see* cats; dogs; locoregional anesthesia
  effect on ECG 195
  elimination 500–2
  environmental impact 7–8
  equipment *see* equipment
  factors determining the P_A of anesthetic 497–500
  history 4–7
  in horses *see* horses
  impact of opioid epidemic on 8
  light 179
  locoregional 148–9, 1166
  models and simulators 174
  monitoring of *see* monitoring of anesthesia/surgery
  neuraxial 148–9
  ophthalmic patients
    anesthetic adjuvants 1335–6
    auriculopalpebral nerve block 1237
    contralateral eye, protecting 1340
    electroretinogram, impact on 1338
    endotracheal intubation 1339–40
    general 1338–40
    inhalational 1335
    injectable 1334–5
    monitoring of anesthesia 1340
    neuromuscular blockade 1340
    ocular complications related to 1340
    physical restraint, premedication, and anesthetic induction 1339
    preoperative assessment 1338
    recovery, extubation and emergence 1340
    sensory nerve blocks 1237–9
    set up and patient positioning 1338–9
    topical 1237
  otariid 1098–9
  patient safety evidence 30–3
  phocid 1098
  point-of-care ultrasound in 254–80
  process of 26–7
  risk assessment 10–23
  short-term 1159–62
  technology, emerging role of 8–10
  total intravenous anesthesia (TIVA) 4, 44, 50, 177, 1162, 1291
  uses of 3
  volatile 148, 1371
  see also premedication
Anesthesia Crisis Resource Management (ACRM) 27, 36
anesthesia electronic medical record (AEMR) 8
Anesthesia Information Management Systems 8
anesthesia multimodal index of consciousness (AMIC) 184
anesthesia ventilators *see* ventilators
anesthesiologists, veterinary, defining 3, 7
Anesthetic Conserving Device (AnaConDa®) 172
anesthetic death *see* mortality, anesthetic
anesthetic depth monitoring *see* depth of anesthesia; monitoring of anesthesia/surgery
anesthetic emergencies
  cardiopulmonary arrest 55–60, 56*f*
  complications
    anesthetic drug-related 65–6
    cardiovascular 60–1
    cerebral herniation 67–8
    equipment-related 66–7
    gastroesophageal reflux and regurgitation 67
    hyperkalemia 68
    hypo-or hyperthermia 68
    myoclonus 68
    personnel injury 70
    postanesthetic 68–70
    respiratory 61–5
    ruminal tympany 67
  magnetic resonance imaging 52
  post-critical event debriefing 70
anesthetic gas monitoring
  gas sampling systems 241
  infrared analysis 242–3
  minimum alveolar concentration 240
  monitors 241
  partial pressure 240
  respiratory gas analysis
    historical techniques used 243–4
    mass spectrometry 224, 241, 243
    Raman spectroscopy 224, 237, 243–4
    technologies used 241–3
  units of measurement 240–1
  volatile agent monitoring, applications 244
  volume percent (vol %) 240–1
anesthetic machines
  "all-purpose Alfo-Blease" 172
  common gas outlet 104–5
  flowmeters 96, 97*f*
  gas flow within 94–6
  introduction 91
  modern 94–105
  oxygen flush valve 104
  routine checkout procedure 113
  vaporizers *see* vaporizers
anesthetic mortality *see* mortality, anesthetic
anesthetic ventilators *see* ventilators
anesthetist, defining 7
angiotensin-converting enzyme (ACE) 287
  angiotensin-converting enzyme 2 (ACE2) receptor 285
  inhibitors *see* ACE inhibitors
animal distress, evaluating 156–7
anion gap
  and cNa^+–cCl^- difference 567
  strong 567–8
antagonists *see* adrenergic receptor antagonists
antibacterial agents 148
anticholinergics
  blood–brain barrier, crossing 315–16
  cesarean section 959
  drug combinations 317
  general pharmacology 314–16
  heart rate increase 315
  history 314
  ruminants 1264
  specific drugs
    atropine 316–17
    combinations 317
    glycopyrrolate 317
  topical application to the eye 315
  uses of 314
anticoagulant therapy 575–7
antiemetics, in pregnancy 961
anti-inflammatory drugs 1069
antimicrobials 149
antimuscarinics 6, 314
anti-nerve growth factor (NGF) 1383–4
antiplatelet drugs 575–6
antitussive effects of opioids 371
anxiolytic drugs, defining 4
  see also sedation
APACHE *see* Acute Physiology and Chronic Health Evaluation (APACHE)
APL *see* adjustable pressure-limiting (APL) valve
apnea 44, 61–2, 158
  monitors 222
apneustic anesthesia ventilation (AAV) 1095, 1098
APOCUS *see* abdominal point-of-care ultrasound (APOCUS)
apparent volume of distribution 291–2
approach-avoidance testing 159
APRV *see* airway pressure release ventilation (APRV)
aquatic mammals *see* marine mammals

aqueous humor (AH) 1328–30
production and drainage 1331
ARAS *see* ascending reticular activating system (ARAS)
arginine vasopressin (antidiuretic hormone) 370, 380, 426, 430–1, 657, 658
argon 156, 159, 243
laser procedures 40, 224
Argon lasers 40
Arndt Endobronchial Blocker™ 81
arrhythmias/dysrhythmias 191, 690
α_1-adrenergic receptor antagonists 328
aerobic respiration, physiology 221
arrhythmogenic diseases resulting in tachycardia 691
artifacts and filters 195
associated diseases 691–2
benzodiazepine antagonists 338
and blood administration 602
cardiac 13, 16, 61, 178, 179, 192, 204, 205, 226, 317, 323, 326, 328, 338, 422, 491, 513, 543, 545, 585, 591, 622, 628, 659, 680, 686, 865, 875, 877, 1266, 1278
cardiac output measurement 213
cardiopulmonary arrest 55
cardiopulmonary bypass 671
catecholamine-induced 18, 319, 320, 339, 871, 911
cervical spondylomyelopathy 839
depth of anesthesia 179
electrocardiography (ECG) 187, 680, 681
epinephrine-induced 464, 467, 536
evaluating an ECG 190
fatal 68
hypothermia 251
hypoxemia 62
life-threatening 595
local anesthesia 542
pacemakers 678
pharmacology 429, 430
postoperative 195
refractory 543
respiratory sinus arrhythmia 655
severe 678
spontaneous 187
supraventricular 191, 691
ventricular 191, 329, 341, 428, 433, 464, 466, 526, 543, 597, 623, 624, 678, 681, 686, 688, 689, 691, 899, 908
arterial blood gases
analysis 173, 232–3
cervical spondylomyelopathy 839
in dogs 725
in ducks 1146
malignant hyperthermia 512
median artery 1101
myasthenia gravis 840
neurologic disease 831, 837
in pregnancy 962
respiratory system 334
sedatives and hypnotics 723, 1351
temperature-corrected 781*f*
and ventilators 761
arterial blood pressure 510, 1105
adjunctive drugs 421
a_2-adrenergic receptor agonists 317
cardiac dysrhythmias 61
cerebral herniation 67
changes in 590
curve 199*f*
decrease in 334, 346, 427, 464, 467, 479, 510, 655
diastolic *see* diastolic arterial pressure (DAP)
drug combinations 317
increase in 317, 322, 340, 346, 422, 513
inotropic support 346
low 317
mean arterial pressure (MAP) 59
monitoring, invasive and non-invasive 52
phenothiazines 334
post resuscitation care 59
systolic *see* systolic arterial pressure (SAP)
variables affecting 644
see also mean arterial pressure (MAP)
arterial carbon dioxide
content 212
excessive 936
tension 508–9
arterial catheter placement and maintenance 202
arterial waveform analysis 215
arteriovenous difference in oxygen ($AVDO_2$) 234
ASA *see* American Society of Anesthesiologists (ASA)
ascending reticular activating system (ARAS) 179
Aschner's reflex 655
aspartate 286–7
aspiration, gastrointestinal disease 868–9
aspiration pneumonia 64, 1279
Assessment and Accreditation of Laboratory Animal Care (AAALAC) 161
assisted and assisted-controlled ventilation 768–70
Association of American Feline Practitioners (AAFP) 1354
Association of Anaesthetists of Great Britain and Ireland (AAGBI) 11–12
Association of Shelter Veterinarians (ASV) 1041
Association of Veterinary Anaesthetists of Great Britain and Ireland (AVA) 6, 7, 174
Anaesthetic Safety Checklist 34
ASVA *see* American Society of Veterinary Anesthesia (ASVA)
atelectasis 268
strategies for reducing 773–4, 775*f*, 776–7
atenolol 329
atipamezole 69, 347, 1266–7
clinical considerations 347
indications for 344–5
mechanism of action 344–5
pharmacodynamics 345–7
pharmacokinetics 345
atlanto-occipital joint 63
ATP-binding cassette (ABC) transporters 308–9
atracurium 1066*t*
atrial natriuretic peptide (ANP) 657
atrial premature complexes (APCs) 1221
atrial stretch-receptor reflex 655
atrioventricular (AV) block 1221
atropine 284
and anticholinergics 314–15
cardiopulmonary arrest 58
clinical use 316–17
drug dose 1065, 1066*t*
pharmacology 316
auditory evoked potentials (AEPs) 157, 183–4
auricular techniques, head blocks 1178
auriculopalpebral nerve block 1237
Australian Incident Monitoring System (AIMS) 29, 32, 33*t*, 35
autologous transfusion 602–3
autonomic nervous system (ANS) 827–9
autoregressive integrated moving average (ARIMA) models 171
AV *see* atrioventricular (AV) block
AVMA *see* American Veterinary Medical Association (AVMA)
axillary brachial plexus block 1186–7
azaperone 335–6, 1084, 1264

back-pressure compensation 97
"BAG" (butorphanol, acepromazine, and glycopyrrolate) 317
Bainbridge reflex 655
balanced anesthesia 4
BAM *see* butorphanol-azaperone-medetomidine (BAM)
bandages and dressings 147–8
barbiturates 1293
administration of 159, 464
alternatives to, for euthanasia 162
and benzodiazepines 336, 338
chemical structure 463
classification 463
clinical effects
analgesic 465
CNS depression, producing 336, 463, 464
fetal/neonatal 465
microsomal enzymes, stimulating increase in 465
species-specific 465
clinical use 465–6
discovery of 5
distribution of 463
euthanasia 158, 162
and $GABA_A$ receptors 286, 463
mechanism of action 463
non-intravenous administration 158
ophthalmic patients 1334
pharmacodynamics 464–5
pharmacokinetics 463–4
ruminants 1268
Barcroft–Edholm reflex 655
baroceptor reflex 655
barotrauma 65
basic life support (BLS)
cardiopulmonary arrest 55–7
chest compressions 55, 57
BAT sign 257–8, 259*f*

Bayliss effect 655
bedinvetmab 1013
Beer–Lambert law 240, 242
behavior
  acute pain, behavioral changes in 996, 997*f*, 998
  assessing 157, 159
  cats 1033–4
  chronic pain, behavioral changes in 1000
  fear 159
  pain 979, 985–990
benzocaine 538
benzodiazepine antagonists 338
benzodiazepines 336–8, 344, 639, 1097
  cats 1033
  combinations 722
  dose requirements 1061
  endocrine disease 903, 905
  horses 1209–10
  injectable 960, 1067
  marine mammals 1097, 1098
  myoclonus 68, 476, 834
  neurologic disease 833, 836
  phocid anesthesia 1098
  preanesthetic sedation 1098
  premedication 476
  prolonged anesthetic recovery 69
  renal disease 934
  ruminants 1267
  ultrasound-guided biopsy 857
  see also sedation
beta-blockers 328
Bezold–Jarisch reflex 655
bioanotechnology 170
bioavailability 294
biochemical testing 926–7
bioimpedance, thoracic 216
bioinformatics 170
bioinstrumentation 170
biomechanics 170
biomechatronics 170
biomedical engineering 169–75
  Anesthetic Conserving Device (AnaConDa®) 172
  contemporary applications in anesthesia 173–4
  data 171–2
  Drexel-Presbyterian Hospital Program, University of Pennsylvania 169
  drug delivery systems 173
  endotracheal tubes 172
  evolution of monitoring equipment and guidelines 173
  Greville Chester toe, discovery of (1800) 169
  history 169–70
  inhalant anesthetic delivery 172
  instrumentation systems 170–2
  interdisciplinary nature of 170
  laryngoscopes 172
  milestones in anesthesia 172–3
  models and simulators 174
  nonlinear systems 171
  performance measures 171–2
  pulse oximetry 172–3
  scientists, contributions of 169
  stethoscopes 172
  subdisciplines 170
  time series analysis 171–2
  ultrasound-guided nerve blocks 173–4
  in veterinary medicine 174
biomedical instrumentation system (BIS) 170–2, 182, 184
biomimetics 170
bioprocess 170
biopsy, renal 928
bioreactance, thoracic 216
biotransformation, drug metabolism
  Phase I 308
  Phase II 308
  Phase III 308–9
Bird Mark series ventilators 118, 119
  Bird Mark 7 137–9
birds 1127–54
  adjunctive drugs 1143
  air capillaries 1129–30, 1131*f*, 1132*f*
  air sacs 1129
  airway management 1144
  allometric scaling 1136
  anesthetic management 1144–8
  anesthetic-related death 1127
  body temperature 1148
  breathing circuits 1144
  cardiovascular system 1134–5, 1147–8
  central nervous system 1145
  drug administration 1135–6
  drugs of historical interest 1143
  drugs used for analgesia and anesthesia 1137–44
  fasting 1135
  as food source for humans 1127
  gas exchange
    components 1129–34
    cross-current model 1131, 1134*f*
    fresh gas flow 1144
    gas flow direction 1130–1
    intertwined systems 1134*f*
    schematic representation of flow 1133*f*
  general pharmacologic considerations 1135–6
  induction methods 1144–9
  inhalational anesthesia 1142–3
  injectable induction drugs 1141–2
  intrapulmonary chemoreceptors 1134
  larynx 1128
  law of Laplace 1130
  local anesthesia 1141
  low atmospheric pressure stunning 161
  lung volumes 1130–1
  monitoring and supportive care 1145–8
  muscles of respiration and thoracic skeleton 1129
  necks 1128
  non-steroidal anti-inflammatory drugs (NSAIDs) 1139–41
  opioids 1137–9
  parabronchi, paleopulmonic and neopulmonic 1130–1, 1132*f*
  physical examination 1135
  physical restraint 1135
  preanesthetic patient evaluation and preparation 1135
  primary and secondary bronchi 1129–30, 1130*f*
  pulmonary system 1129, 1130, 1133*f*, 1146, 1147
  Purkinje fibers 1134
  recovery 1148
  renal portal system 1134–5
  respiratory system 1127–34, 1145–7
  syrinx 1128
  tertiary branch (parabronchi) 1129–30, 1131*f*, 1132*f*
  trachea 1128
  types
    Amazon parrots 1129, 1135, 1137
    barred owls 1135
    budgerigars 1129
    chickens 1129
    cockatiels 1129
    cockatoos 1129, 1137
    conures 1129
    ducks 1130, 1146
    emperor penguins 1127
    grey parrots 1137
    macaws 1129
    ostrich 1132*f*
    penguins 1128, 1130
    peregrine falcon 1137
    petrels 1128
    pigeons 1130
    Ruppell's griffon 1127
    snowy owl 1137
    Timneh parrots 1137
  ventilation components 1128–9
  ventilation control 1134
  ventilation monitoring 227
BIS *see* biomedical instrumentation system (BIS)
bispectral analysis (BIS) 157
Bispectral Index™ 180–3
bisphosphonate zoledronic acid 1015
bisphosphonates 1015
blame and non-blame cultures 28
blocks
  distal paravertebral block 1309
  failure 1181, 1190, 1236, 1309
  of flank and paralumbar fossa 1307–10
  of head 1174–8
  inverted "l" or "7" block 1307
  line infiltration 1307, 1311
  linea alba and paramedian, regional anesthesia 1310–12
  lumbosacral, sacrococcygeal, or intercoccygeal epidural (cranial epidural) 1311–12
  of pelvic limb 1188–92
  peripheral nerve blocks 1168, 1227
  physiology of nerve blockade 1168–9
  proximal paravertebral block 1307–9
  regional anesthesia
    for flank and paralumbar fossa 1307–10
    for head 1303–7
    for linea alba and paramedian 1310–12
    for pelvic area 1312–14
    for teats and udder 1314–17, 1316*f*

blocks (*cont'd*)
segmental dorsolumbar epidural block 1309–10
segmental thoracolumbar subarachnoid block 1310
of thoracic limb 1185–8
axillary brachial plexus block 1186–7
cervical paravertebral block 1186
distal brachial plexus block 1188
distal radial, ulnar, median, and musculocutaneous nerve block 1188
proximal radial, ulnar, median, and musculocutaneous nerve block 1188
radial, ulnar, and median nerve block 1188
ring block 1188
sensory innervation, anatomy of 1185–6
subscalenic brachial plexus block 1186
of thorax and abdomen 1178–85
fascial plane block techniques 1182–5
intercostal nerve 1179, 1180*f*
interpleural regional analgesia 1181–2
thoracic paravertebral 1179
trigeminal nerve 1178
see also local anesthesia; locoregional anesthesia; neuromuscular blockade; regional anesthesia
blood
acute loss 60
administration 600
arterial gas analysis 232–3
carbon dioxide content 740–2
cardiac markers, blood-based 682
cardiovascular physiology 640–1
complete blood count 12, 1219
component therapy 595–8
cross-matching 599–600
deoxygenated 232
fresh whole blood (FWB) 596
massive loss of 600
measuring hemoglobin saturation with oxygen 233–6
myocardial flow 57
packed red blood cells 596
perioperative loss 603
pH, mechanisms to minimize changes in 558–9
platelet products 598
preanesthetic testing 11–13
red blood cell (RBC) products 595–6
regional flow 510
sampling 12
stored whole blood 596
substitutes 603
transcutaneous measurement of gases 233
typing 599
uptake of inhalation anesthetics 499–500
see also arterial blood gases; transfusion therapy
blood coagulation *see* coagulation, blood
blood flow
cardiovascular physiology 642–4
cerebral *see* cerebral blood flow
hepatic *see* hepatic blood flow (HBF)
microcirculatory 588, 592, 646, 1294
pulmonary *see* pulmonary blood flow
regional 510
renal *see* renal blood flow (RBF)
spinal cord blood flow (SCBF) 369
to thoracolumbar spinal cord 508
uterine 957
blood gas analysis 223
blood groups
in cats 1036
in horses 599
in pigs 599, 1294
and typing 599
blood oxygen level-dependent (BOLD) MRI 157, 999
blood pressure monitoring 197–209
arterial blood pressure 510
autoregulation of 198–9
central venous pressure measurement 204–5
continued measurement challenges 207
determinants and definitions 197–8
diastolic arterial pressure 197
Doppler ultrasonographic blood pressure measurement 202–3
fluid responsiveness, indices 205–7
hemodynamics and cardiac function 644–6
high-definition oscillometric measurement 204
invasive measurement 52, 202–4
arterial catheter placement and maintenance 202
components 200–1
dynamic response testing and damping 201–2
leveling the transducer 200–1
natural frequency and resonance 201
physics of monitoring systems 201–2
transducer setup and priming of pressure tubing 200
zeroing the transducer 201
mean arterial pressure 197–8
non-invasive measurement 52, 202–4
normal ranges 198
oscillometric measurement 203–4
plethysmography variability index 207
pulse pressure and systolic pressure variation 205–7
systolic arterial pressure 197
see also arterial blood pressure
blood urea nitrogen (BUN) 802, 851, 905, 926, 945, 957, 1350
blood volume, in cats 1036
blood–aqueous barrier (BAB) 1332
blood–brain barrier (BBB)
and α_2-adrenergic receptors/agonists 346, 347, 736–7
and anticholinergics 315–16
and capillaries 635
in cats 346
chemoreceptor trigger zone (CTZ) outside 368
and dissociatives 469
and methylnaltrexone 384
midazolam crossing 336–7
and neural control of ventilation 701
and nondepolarizing NMBAs 450
and opioids 362, 368
in sheep 362
and vatinoxan 345, 346
blood–retinal barrier (BRB) 1332
BLS *see* basic life support (BLS)
boarded anesthesiologist, defining 7
BOAS *see* brachycephalic obstructive airway syndrome (BOAS)
body composition, changes in 1357
body fluids
compartments
extracellular and intracellular, movement of water between 581
interstitial fluid 581–2
solute composition 581
crystalloids 582–8
endothelial glycocalyx model of transvascular fluid exchange 582
fluid shifts between intravascular (plasma) and interstitial fluid compartments 581–2
monitoring fluid balance 589
perioperative fluid therapy
improving the utility of dynamic indices of preload responsiveness 591
Individualized goal-directed 589–91
liberal versus restrictive approach 588–9
and microvasculature 591–2
monitoring fluid balance 589
physiology 580–2
Starling's equation, modification 582
total body water 580
types used in clinical practice 582–8
body surface area (BSA) 1029, 1158
body temperature 173, 200, 251, 1148
acid–base physiology 555, 557, 558, 571
blood 213, 640
cattle 1060
changes 246, 247, 371, 669
core temperature 68, 145, 246, 247, 249, 945, 946, 947, 949, 957
decrease in 4, 101, 180, 247, 249, 251, 252, 557, 589, 603, 669, 725, 1142
and drug-related complications 66
elevated 792
hyperthermia
malignant 68, 1060
severe 1034
hypothermia 52, 251, 670, 1060
increase in 321, 557, 597, 725, 1034, 1121, 1145
and local anesthesia 535, 537
low 792
maintaining 784, 1072
monitoring 342, 377, 800, 837, 858
normal 247, 251, 496
and opioids 371, 377
and oxymorphone 378
and physical restraint 1135
post resuscitation care 59
preferred body temperature 1114
radiofrequency fields 49
raising 252
rebreathing system 106
small animal anesthesia morbidity 13

thermoregulation *see* thermoregulation
variation in 505
body weight 1026
Bohr effect 738–9
"boiling liquid expanding vapor explosion" (BLEVE) 49
boiling point 494
BOLD *see* blood oxygen level-dependent (BOLD) MRI
Bordetella bronchiseptica 145
Botucatu Multidimensional pain scale 1005
Bötzinger complex (BötC) 1092
brachial vein 1101
brachycephalic dog breeds 1032
brachycephalic obstructive airway syndrome (BOAS) 1032
bradyarrhythmias 191
bradycardia
α_1-adrenergic receptor agonists 324
α_2-adrenergic receptor agonists 324, 1049
b_1-adrenergic receptor antagonists 328
anticholinergic administration, following 317
anticholinergics, induced by 315, 1336, 1337
arrhythmogenic diseases resulting in 691–2
dexmedetomidine-induced 346
in dogs and cats 1031
drug-induced 315
endocrine disease 915
and euthanasia 158
gadolinium-based contrast agents 52
hyperkalemia 68, 190
and hypotension 909, 912
hypothermia 1349
hypoxemia 1086
intraoperative 316
intrathecal (spinal) anesthesia 1197
intravenous high-dose opioid induction 1163
morbidity and mortality 13
neonatal 965
opioids 1351
and pain 990, 1015
persistent 341
pharmacology 58
preanesthetic 314
preventing in perioperative period 317
progressive 179
in rabbits 158
reflex 67
baroreceptor-mediated reflex 340
sedatives and tranquilizers 1351
sinus 191, 192, 909
terminal 1106
transient 179, 316, 1266
vagally mediated 367, 685
brain 822–5
amygdala 159
anesthetic partial pressure in 618
anesthetic reaching 177
autoregulation of 198
biomedical engineering 169
blood pressure monitoring 199
bovine 344
cerebral cortex 154
consciousness 176
context-sensitive half-time 304
deep brain stimulation 170
effect-site concentration 176–7
electrical activity 155, 157
electrophysiologic monitoring 179
and etomidate 474
fetal 160
fluid therapy 593
forebrain 155, 367
functional analysis 237
generalized 234
and guaifenesin 424
herniation 225
human 180, 237
ischemia 234
maturation 180
measures of activity 155
in mice 160
midbrain 155, 363, 824
and NSAIDs 407
oxygenation 234
Parabrachial Nucleus/Kolliker-Fuse Complex 367
physiology 829–30
prostaglandin inhibition 404
reptiles 1116
subcortical structures 154
traumatic injury 238, 369, 431
unconsciousness 155
visceral receptors 247
see also blood–brain barrier (BBB)
brain death 157, 162
brain natriuretic peptide (BNP) 657
brainstem 59, 154, 157, 159, 180, 225, 367
emetic center 428
nuclei 425
Branham's sign 655
breathing
cardiopulmonary resuscitation 57
circuits *see* breathing circuits
spontaneous 212, 304, 722, 734*f*, 756, 768, 770, 771*f*, 777, 798, 1213, 1272
anesthesia equipment 117, 118
versus controlled ventilation 1211
ketamine affecting 1092
neonatal 960
respiratory physiology and pathophysiology 707, 708
strong 724
systems *see* breathing systems
see also respiratory disease; respiratory physiology and pathophysiology
breathing circuits
anesthetic machines 91
birds 1144
breathing circuit tubing, 107, 108*f*
infection prevention and control 146
breathing systems 95*f*, 105–12, 126, 1071–2
circle 130, 134
closed 1163*f*
coaxial 67, 107, 112, 113*f*
laboratory animals 1071–2
malfunction 67
marine mammals 1092–3
non-rebreathing 111–12
rebreathing (circle) 105, 106–11
Universal F-circuit 107
briefings, patient safety 35–6
bromine 7
bronchial blockers 80–2
bronchodilation 315, 323, 325, 326
carbon dioxide elimination, kinetics 707
colic, in horses 1221
dose-dependent 728
and epinephrine 321
isoflurane-induced 803, 804
ketamine-induced 470, 804
sevoflurane-induced 803, 804
and SNS 828
sympathetically mediated 328
ventilation and deadspace 727
bronchodilators 63
bronchoscopy, anesthesia for 782–3
bronchospasm, anesthetic emergencies 63
BSA *see* body surface area (BSA)
bulldogs 18
BUN *see* blood urea nitrogen (BUN)
bupivacaine
cardiotoxicity 543
dual-acting bupivacaine-meloxicam extended-release polymer 541
lidocaine/bupivacaine gel (Tri-Solfen) 541
liposome-encapsulated (Nocita®) 541
pain management 1014
toxicity 786, 1296–7
buprenorphine 284, 1031, 1035
dosage
birds 1138
cats 381–2
dogs 381–2
horses 382
laboratory animals 1068, 1073*t*
injectable 1067
laboratory animals 1069
and local anesthesia 539
partial opioid agonist 381–2
butorphanol 284
dosage
birds 1137
cats 382–3
dogs 382–3
horses 383
interactions with full opioid agonists 383
non-human primates 1073*t*
premedication 382, 478
ruminants 1267
wildlife capture 1081–2
butorphanol-azaperone-medetomidine (BAM) 1082, 1084
butyrophenones 335–8

cages, oxygen 90–1
calcium 58, 593
calves, cardiovascular system 1056–7
camelids
airway management 1061
auricular artery 1057

camelids (*cont'd*)
blood groups 599
dose requirements 1061
drug administration 1054–5
endotracheal intubation 1058–9
hypothermia 1060
induction of anesthesia 62
intubation 1058, 1059
oxyhemoglobin dissociation curve 739
physical restraint 1052
positioning during anesthesia 1056
regurgitation 1057
salivation 1058
sedating 1055
South American 739
venous blood 1054
Canadian Council on Animal Care (CCAC) 153, 160
cancer pain 1363–76
aminobisphosphonates 1369
anticonvulsants 1368
antidepressants 1368
bone 1365, 1368–70
cannabinoids 1368
chemotherapy-induced 1365–6
combination analgesics 1367–8
experimental therapeutics 1370
general therapeutic strategies 1368–70
NMDA antagonists 1367
non-steroidal anti-inflammatory drugs 1367
opioids 1367, 1372
pharmacologic treatment strategies 1366–8
prevalence 1363
promising innovative treatments 1370–1
radiation burns 1370
radiotherapy-induced 1365, 1369–70
recognition and assessment 1363–4
specific underlying causes 1364–6
surgery-induced 1366
types associated with cancer 1364
see also tumors
canine brachycephalic obstructive syndrome 788–3
characteristics and pathophysiology 788–90
management of anesthesia 790–3
Canine Brief Pain Index 1013
Canine Brief Pain Inventory (CBPI) 1005, 1006
canine ECG 192
canine laryngeal paralysis 794–7
characteristics and pathophysiology 794–5
management of anesthesia 795–7
canine lung lobe torsion
characteristics and pathophysiology 806–7
management of anesthesia 807
canine tracheal collapse
characteristics and pathophysiology 797
management of anesthesia 797–9
cannabidiol products 1383
cannabinoids 433–4
capillaries 634–5
capillary refill time (CRT) 1218
capnography/capnometry 160
abnormal capnogram 225
anesthetic mortality, risk of 18
bronchospasm 63
colic, in horses 1227
mainstream 224
normal capnogram 224–5, 226*f*
sidestream 224
with sidestream sampling technology 51
species considerations 227
volumetric 228
capture of wildlife *see* wildlife capture
capuchins 1073
carbon dioxide
absorber/absorbents 109–11, 1043
and acid–base implications 221
arterial carbon dioxide content ($CaCO_2$) 212
blood gas analysis 223
chemical detection 223
content in blood 740–2
elimination 704–7
end-tidal 13, 59, 61, 106, 112, 222, 480, 670, 936, 1060, 1146, 1227, 1293, 1334
biomedical engineering 170, 173
cardiac output measurement 212, 217
endocrine disease 897, 906
neurologic disease 838, 840
respiratory disease 761, 785, 801
ruminants 1274, 1276
and euthanasia 159
Fick principle and cardiac output measurement 211, 212, 227
Haldane effect 740–2
hypercapnia 742–3
hypocapnia 742–3
inhaling 155–6
and local anesthesia 537
mainstream capnometry/capnography 224
measurement methods 223–4
mixed with nitrous oxide 5
problems with infrared spectroscopy 224
quantitative monitoring 222–4
response variability 159
sidestream capnometry/capnography 224
transport 740–3
see also partial pressure of carbon dioxide (PCO_2)
carbon monoxide 156, 159
carboxyhemoglobin (COHb) 233
cardiac arrest
advanced life support 58, 59
airway management 1061
airway obstruction 62
anesthesia-related ocular complications 1340
anesthetic risk 15, 16, 17, 19, 1048
anticholinergics 316–17
basic life support 57
biomedical engineering 172
capnography/capnometry 217
cardiac POCUS (CPOCUS) 271, 276
cerebral blood flow, regulation of 830
esophagitis 868
gastric dilation-volvulus 874
guaifenesin 425
hypercalcemia 915
hypothermia 251
hypoxemia 62, 863
induction and intubation 1225
intraoperative complications 1278
intrathecal (spinal) anesthesia 1197
local anesthesia 1141, 1198
nitrous oxide 156
pneumothorax and/or pleural effusion 805
postanesthetic blindness 69
post-cardiac arrest care algorithm 34
post-cardiac arrest syndrome 59
refractory 543
sodium nitroprusside (SNP) 429
see also cardiopulmonary arrest (CPA)
cardiac cycle 189, 190, 647–50, 651*f*
cardiac function, assessing 650–3
cardiac markers, blood-based 682
cardiac output (CO), monitoring 210–19
absolute values 210–11
advantages of 210
arterial waveform analysis 215
basic monitoring principles 211
and blood pressure monitoring 60, 197
choice of monitoring system 211
cross-sectional area (CSA), echocardiography 215
dye dilution technique 211
echocardiography and echo-Doppler 215–16
Fick principle 211, 212, 227
functional monitoring 210
history 211–12
hypotension 60
ideal monitoring technique 211
inhalational anesthesia 499–500, 509–10
left ventricular outflow tract, echocardiography 215, 216
lithium dilution 214–15
partial rebreathing technique 212
pulmonary artery catheter thermodilution 212–14
standard capnography as indicator 217
techniques 212–17
thermodilution 211–12
thoracic bioimpedance and bioreactance 216
time-based capnograph 227
transpulmonary thermodilution and ultrasound indicator dilution 214
typical indices 210, 211*t*
cardiac POCUS (CPOCUS) 271–6, 272*t*
in cardiopulmonary resuscitation 275–6
caudal vena cava assessment at subxiphoid window 275, 276*f*
caudal vena cava (CVC) 273
interpretation and integration of findings 273, 275
left atrial to aortic root ration (LA:Ao) 273
left ventricular lumen size and function 273, 275
right parasternal long-axis views 273
right parasternal short-axis views 272
subxiphoid view 273
windows and views 272–3, 274*f*
see also point-of-care ultrasound (POCUS)
cardiac toxicity 531, 541, 542, 594
cardiopulmonary arrest (CPA)
advanced life support 58–9

anesthesia-related 59
basic life support 55–7
breathing 57
cardiac arrhythmias causing 16
fluid therapy 58
identifying 59
monitoring 59–60
pharmacologic therapy 58
time-based capnograph 227
cardiopulmonary bypass 667–73
anesthesia setup 670
antibiotics 669
anticoagulation and reversal 669
antifibrinolytics 669
cannulation 668–9
complexity 672
drugs and interventions used during 669–70
external circuit 667–8
hypothermia 669–70
medications 670, 671*t*
patient evaluation for 670
preanesthetic preparation 670, 671*t*
sequence of events and terminology 671–2
steroids 669
systemic responses 669
cardiopulmonary depression 10
cardiopulmonary resuscitation (CPR)
adjunctive techniques and devices 59
advanced life support, cardiopulmonary arrest 55, 58–9
algorithms 34
anesthesia-related 59
basic life support, cardiopulmonary arrest 55–7
breathing 57
cardiac point-of-care ultrasound 275–6
closed-chest 57
corticosteroids 58, 59–60
in horses 1049
monitoring during 59
open-chest 57, 59
POCUS in 275–6
post resuscitation care 55, 59–60
cardiopulmonary-cerebral resuscitation (CPCR) 316
cardiotoxicity 539, 540, 543
bupivacaine-induced 543
cardiovascular complications, anesthesia-related
anaphylaxis 61
cardiac dysrhythmias 61
hemorrhage 60–1
hypotension 60
small animal anesthesia morbidity 13
cardiovascular disease
anesthesia for specific conditions 683–94
arrhythmias, associated diseases 691–2
arrhythmogenic diseases 691–2
dilated cardiomyopathy 686
dysfunction-associated diseases, diastolic 689–90
hypertrophic cardiomyopathy 689–90
hypotension 692–3
left-to-right shunting 687
mitral valve insufficiency/ regurgitation 684–6
pericardial effusion 690
pressure overload, associated conditions 688–9
pulmonic stenosis 688–9
restrictive cardiomyopathy 689–90
right-to-left shunting 687–8
shock 693–4
subaortic stenosis 688–9
volume overload, associated conditions 683–6
blood-based cardiac markers 682
cooperation between cardiologist and anesthesiologist 682–3
echocardiography 682
electrocardiography 680–1
hypotension, pharmacological support 692–3
pathophysiology and anesthetic management 680–96
preanesthetic evaluation 680–3
thoracic radiography 681–2
cardiovascular physiology 615–66
actin-activated myosin chemomechanical ATPase cycle 629, 630*f*, 631, 631*f*
cardiac cycle and pressure-volume loop 647–50, 651*f*
cardiac function, assessing 650–3
comparative cardiovascular morphology and shunting 617–19
electrophysiology and electrocardiogram 620–6
excitation–contraction coupling 626–8
hemodynamics and cardiac function
blood flow 642–4
blood pressure 644–6
preload and afterload 647
resistance 646–7
local control mechanisms 656–8
lymphatic system 641–2
mammalian cardiovascular system 619–26
anatomy 619
metabolism 620
myocardial contraction and relaxation 629, 631
neurohumoral and local control mechanisms 654–8
oxygen delivery and oxygen consumption 653–4
smooth muscle
contraction and relaxation 638–40
metabolism 638
special circulations
cerebral 659
coronary 658–9
pulmonary 659–60
renal 660
splanchnic 660
vascular system 631–8
capillaries 634–5
large arteries and veins 633
resistance vessels 633–4
small arteries 633
transcapillary fluid exchange 635–8
veins, venules and venous capacitance 638
cardiovascular system
acepromazine 334
age-related changes 1355–6
amphibians 1117
birds 1134–5, 1147–8
dobutamine 322–3
dopamine 321–2
dopexamine 323
drug effects
acepromazine 334
alfaxalone 478
atipamezole 345–6
barbiturates 464
detomidine 340–1
dexmedetomidine 340–1
diazepam 337
dissociative anesthetics 470
etomidate 474–5
inhalational anesthetics 509–11
medetomidine 340–1
midazolam 337
opioids 367
propofol 467
romifidine 340–1
vatinoxan 345–6
xylazine 340–1
yohimbine 345–6
zolazepam 337
ephedrine 326
epinephrine 320–1
farm animals 1056–7
fish 1121
inhalational anesthesia
arterial blood pressure 510
cardiac rhythm 510
catecholamines 510
concurrent drugs 511
duration of anesthesia 511
factors influencing circulatory effects 510–11
mode of ventilation 510–11
noxious stimulation 511
$PaCO_2$ 510–11
regional blood flow 510
isoproterenol 323–4
neonatal/pediatric patients 1349
norepinephrine 321
phenylephrine 324
prazosin 327
pregnancy-associated changes 955–6
reptiles 1111–12
cardiovascular toxicity 542–3
carfentanil 380–1
wildlife capture 1081
carprofen 1073*t*, 1140, 1381
cartilage injury 412
catecholamines
α_1-adrenergic receptor agonists 324–5
α_2-adrenergic receptor agonists 325
β_2-adrenergic receptor agonists 325–6
inhalational anesthesia 510

catecholamines (*cont'd*)
mixed α-and β-adrenergic receptor agonists 326
naturally occurring 319–22
synthetic 322–4
catechol-*O*- methyltransferase 323
catheters
arterial placement and maintenance 202
and camelids 1054
forelimb intravenous 58
intraosseous 58
intravenous 146, 200
locoregional anesthesia 1171–2
nasal 227
peripheral intravenous 58
peripherally inserted central 1100, 1101
size 202
Swan-Ganz 212
cats
aging 1354
anesthesia
anesthetic and analgesic plan 1159–62
anesthetic mortality, risk of 14–17
chamber or mask inhalant induction 1163
comparative anesthesia and analgesia 1033–6
delayed anesthetic recovery 1164–5
general anesthesia 962, 964–965
induction of 62, 1162–3
inhalant anesthetic MAC 372–3
inhalational 1034
injectable anesthetics 1161*t*
intermediate-term 1162
intravenous high-dose opioid induction 1163
intravenous regional 1167–8
local infiltration 1166
locoregional 1167–8
long-term 1162
maintenance 1163
neuraxial 1168
patient preparation 1159–62
peripheral nerve blocks 1168
plan 1159–62
preanesthetic considerations 1158–9
premedication 1162
records 1163
recovery 1164
regional 964–5
return of spontaneous circulation 55
sensitivity to 1158
short-term 1159–62
topical 1166
blood typing 599
body weight 1159
cardiopulmonary measures 1159
central nervous system 1159
chest compressions 57
cortical blindness 1035
dobutamine dose rates 323
dopamine, effects on 322
Doppler ultrasonographic blood pressure measurement 203
drug dose
buprenorphine 382
butorphanol 382–3
fentanyl 378–9
hydromorphone 377
methadone 377
morphine 376
drug effects
acepromazine 335
alfaxalone 479–80
detomidine 343
dexmedetomidine 343
diazepam 337
dissociative anesthetics 471
etomidate 476
medetomidine 343
midazolam 337
NSAIDs 414
propofol 467–8
romifidine 343
xylazine 343
zolazepam 337
drug metabolism 1034
electrocardiography 192
endotracheal intubation in 17, 18, 803, 1035
euthanasia 158
feline asthma 802–3
feline brachycephalic obstructive airway syndrome 793–4
feline onychectomy 1014
fluid therapy in 18, 1036
halothane-anesthetized 321
handling and behavior 1033–4
hunched or "tucked up" posture 997*f*
hyperkalemia 68
hypo-or hyperthermia 68
locoregional anesthesia 1166–204
classification 1167–8
equipment 1170–4
physiology of nerve blockade 1168–9
preparation 1169–70
see also locoregional anesthesia
malignant hyperthermia 68
near-infrared and Raman spectroscopy 237
non-steroidal anti-inflammatory drugs (NSAIDs) 1035
opioids 1034–5
osteoarthritic pain 1013
pneumothorax 262
postoperative infections 142
preanesthetic blood testing 12
pregnancy, general anesthesia in 962, 964
renal function, testing and monitoring 926–8
UNESP-Botucatu multidimensional pain scale 1003
ventilation, monitoring 227
cattle
drug effects
adrenergic receptor agonists 333
atropine 1336
azaperone 335
clenbuterol 325
detomidine 343–4
dexmedetomidine 343–4
medetomidine 343–4
romifidine 343–4
xylazine 343–4
local infiltration 5
meloxicam approved for 1351
neonatal 1348
neuroendocrine stress response 342
ocular anatomy 1327
pain and consciousness 155
patient positioning 1273
pregnancy-associated changes 342
regional anesthesia 965
sedation 343
subarachnoid anesthesia 5
caudal epidural anesthesia/analgesia 1254, 1255*f*
Caudal Intercostal Block for Abdominal Surgery (CIBAS) 1227
caudal vena cava collapsibility index (CVCCI) 275
caudal vena cava (CVC)
assessment at the subxiphoid window 275, 276*f*
CVC diameter (CVCd) 275
CBPI *see* Canine Brief Pain Inventory (CBPI)
cell salvage, autologous transfusion 602–3
central nervous system (CNS) 3, 505–7
anatomy 822–5
birds 1145
brain 822–5
physiology 829–30
catecholamines 321
cerebral circulation 659
depression *see* central nervous system depression
in dogs and cats 1159
drug effects
acepromazine 334–5
alfaxalone 478
atipamezole 346–7
barbiturates 464
detomidine 341–2
dexmedetomidine 341–2
diazepam 337
dissociative anesthetics 470
etomidate 474
inhalational anesthetics 505–8
medetomidine 341–2
midazolam 337
propofol 467
romifidine 341–2
vatinoxan 346–7
xylazine 341–2
yohimbine 346–7
zolazepam 337
edema 1074
general anesthesia 176, 177*f*
inhalational anesthetics *see below*
inhalational anesthesia
anatomic sites of action 506–7
cerebral blood flow and cerebral perfusion pressure 507–8
cerebral metabolism 507
electroencephalographic effects 507
mechanism of action 505–7
molecular sites and mechanic of action 505–6
injectable anesthetics 1068
intracranial hypertension 835–7
level of central nervous system effect 1081

local anesthetic systemic toxicity 1167, 1171, 1181, 1198
neonatal/pediatric patients 1349–50
neurologic disease 822–5
peripheral nervous system 825–39
physiology 829–32
brain 829–30
spinal cord 832
seizures 837–8
and SNS 470
spinal cord physiology 832
and temperature 247
toxicity 534, 541–2, 1305
central nervous system depression 153, 179, 182
auditory evoked potentials 183
barbiturates producing 336, 463, 464
dose-dependent 339
extreme 179
and opioids 381
progressive 178
and thermoregulation 342
xylazine-induced excessive 338
central neuromodulation 1025
central state monitor (CSM) 183
central venous line 58
central venous pressure (CVP), measuring 204–5
CEPEF *see* Confidential Enquiry into Perioperative Equine Fatalities (CEPEF)
CEPSAF *see* Confidential Enquiry into Perioperative Small Animal Fatalities (CEPSAF)
cerebral blood flow 830–2
and cerebral perfusion pressure (CPP) 507–8
chemical regulation 830–1
luxury perfusion 832
myogenic regulation 831
neurogenic regulation 831
cerebral circulation 659
cerebral herniation 67–8
cerebral perfusion pressure (CPP) 198, 507–8
neurologic disease 829–30
cerebral state index (CSI) 183
cerebral state monitor (CSM) 183
certified Good Manufacturing Practices (cGMP) 162
cervical paravertebral block 1186
cervical spondylomyelopathy 839
cesarean section 959–61
anticholinergics 959
dissociative anesthetics 960
elective and emergency anesthesia 962, 963–4*t*
general anesthesia 961–4
guaifenesin 961
inhalational anesthesia 960–1
injectable anesthetics 960
local anesthesia 961, 965
neuroleptanalgesia 960
neuromuscular blocking agents 961
opioids 959–60
sedation 959
tranquilization 959
see also neonatal/pediatric patients; pregnancy-associated changes
Cetacaine® 1271
cetaceans
anesthesia 1098
breathing 1092
intubation 1103–4
vascular access 1099–101
see also marine mammals
cetirizine 1031
CFD *see* computational fluid dynamic (CFD) modeling
checklists 33–4
chelonians 1112
chemical buffers 558–9
chemoreceptor reflex 655
chemotherapy 1365–6
chest compressions 55, 57
chest wall rigidity (wooden chest syndrome) 65
Chiari-like malformation 434, 1000
chloral hydrate 5, 481
injectable 1068
chlorhexidine gluconate, soaking in 145
chloride shift 739
chlorine 7
chloroform 5
chloroprocaine 539
chondroitin 1016
chondroitin sulfate 1383
chondrotoxicity 544, 1239
chronic kidney disease (CKD) 52, 931–3, 1357
clinical features and diagnosis 932
etiology and pathogenesis 931–2
further diagnostics and treatment 932–3
staging 932
see also renal replacement therapy
chronic pain
accelerometry 1001
behavioral changes 1000
first-tier 1013–15
gait
force plate analysis 1001
kinematic 1001
visual observation of 1001
non-steroidal anti-inflammatory drugs (NSAIDs) 1013
osteoarthritis 1378–84
physiological parameters 1000–1
quantification 1005–6, 1007*t*
recognition of 1000–1
validity 1002
see also acute pain; pain; pain faces; pain management
chronotropy 198
cimicoxib 1381
circle rebreathing systems 106–11
APL valve *see* adjustable pressure-limiting (APL) valve
Bain system 112
breathing circuit tubing 107, 108*f*
carbon dioxide absorbents 110–11
carbon dioxide absorber 109–10
expiratory one-way valve 108
fresh gas inlet 106
full (complete) 106
inspiratory one-way valve 107
Mapleson 111, 113*f*, 119
Modified Jackson-Rees 112
and non-rebreathing system 106, 107*f*
partial 106
pop-off APL valve 135
reservoir bag 108
circulation
cerebral 659
coronary 658–9
factors influencing circulatory effects 510–11
pulmonary 659–60
renal 660
splanchnic 660
citrate-phosphate-dextrose-adenine (CPDA-1) 1033
CKD *see* chronic kidney disease (CKD)
classical receptor theory 283–5
affinity and activity of a ligand 284
assessment of ligand–receptor interaction 284
lag-time 284
receptor agonists and antagonists 284–5
selectivity and specificity of a ligand 284
clenbuterol
cardiovascular system effects 325
other effects 325–6
Client-Specific Outcome Measures (CSOM) scale 1006
clinical audits 37
clinical engineering 170
clinical utility 1002
clove oil 1118, 1119
CMV *see* continuous mandatory ventilation (CMV)
CO *see* cardiac output (CO), monitoring
coagulation, blood
anticoagulant therapy 575–7
assessment 852
drugs supporting 578
fibrinolytic drugs 577
inhibitors 576–7
NSAIDs, effects of 411–12
and platelet function testing 575
pregnancy-associated changes 956
procoagulant therapies 577–8
testing 575
see also blood; plasma; platelets
coaxial breathing systems 67, 107, 112, 113*f*
cocaine 5
codeine 381
cognitive dysfunction (CD) 1356
cold therapy 1024
colic, in horses 148, 1217–34
anesthetic protocol 1224–5
anesthetic risks and anticipated complications
arrhythmias 1221
hypotension 1219–20
impaired V/Q matching 1220–1
postanesthetic myopathy and neuropathy 1221
clinical history 1218
defining 1217

colic, in horses (*cont'd*)
 diagnostics 1219
 endotoxemia 1217–18
 induction and intubation 1224–5
 physical examination 1219
 preanesthetic considerations 1218–19
 premedication 1224
 stabilization and fluid resuscitation 1222–4
 surgical area, preparation of 1221
 systemic inflammatory response syndrome 1217–18
collision broadening, infrared spectroscopy 224
colloids 585–6
 clinical implications of synthetic use in veterinary medicine 588
 synthetic 586–8
colorimetry, carbon dioxide measurement 223
communication tools, patient safety 35–6
Companion Animal Pain Management Consortium 7
companion animals
 biologic agents, evidence for 1017
 osteoarthritis, evidence for agents modifying 1016
comparative anesthesia and analgesia
 amphibians 1116–19
 birds 1127–54
 cats 1033–6
 dogs 1029–33
 farm animals 1052–64
 fish 1120–3
 horses 1048–51
 laboratory animals 1065–76
 reptiles 1110–14
 shelter animals 1041–7
 wildlife 1077–90
complete blood count (CBC) 12, 1219
complexity
 of agents 45
 assessing 18
 biomedical data 170, 171
 cardiopulmonary bypass 672
 case 30
 ECG machines 194*f*
 equipment 91, 92
 infection prevention and control 147
 intrinsic 26
 locoregional anesthetic techniques 1166
 near-infrared and Raman spectroscopy 237
 nest building 991, 998
 neuropathic pain 432
 pharmacology 299
 pheochromocytoma (PHEO) 898
 process of anesthesia 26
 proliferation 27
 segmental thoracolumbar subarachnoid block 1310
 software and data analysis 1001
 spectral entropy 182
 uncertainty 26
computational fluid dynamic (CFD) modeling 156
computed tomography (CT)
 canine lung lobe torsion 807
 cross-sectional 44
 intrathoracic procedures 784
 laser procedures 42, 43
 leads and wires 44
 mechanical ventilation 782
 protocols 262
 thoracic imaging 44, 802
 ventilation and lung volumes 726
 ventilation–perfusion relationships 736
computer-aided design (CAD) 156
computerized tomography (CT) scanning 1029
concurrent drugs
 corticosteroids 799
 fluid therapy 587
 inhalational anesthesia
  cardiovascular system 511
  respiratory system 509
conduction 248
Confidential Enquiry into Perioperative Deaths 32
Confidential Enquiry into Perioperative Equine Fatalities (CEPEF) 14, 19, 20
Confidential Enquiry into Perioperative Small Animal Fatalities (CEPSAF) 12, 15–17, 1035, 1036
congenital defects
 patent ductus arteriosus 686–7
 right-to- left shunting 687–8
 ventricular septal defect 686–7
conjugation (phase II biotransformation) 308
consciousness
 defining 176
 index of 183
 and pain 154–5
 prolonged return to 13
 see also unconsciousness
constant rate therapy 299–305
construct validity 1002
content validity 1002
context-sensitive half-time (CSHT) 304–5
continuous positive airway pressure (CPAP) 1094, 1095
continuous caudal epidural anesthesia/analgesia 1254, 1255*f*
continuous laser Doppler flowmetry 238
continuous mandatory ventilation (CMV) 764–8
 dual-controlled 767–8
 pressure-controlled 767
 volume-controlled 765–7
continuous positive airway pressure (CPAP) 81, 1032
continuous rate infusion (CRI) 299–305, 1014
 BET infusion scheme 303
 constant rate intravenous infusions 294
 context-sensitive half-time 304–5
 divergence index 304
 dopamine 322
 infusion pumps 300
 infusion rate 299
 median prediction error (*MDPE*) 303 304
 non-pharmacokinetic-dependent infusion systems 300, 301*f*
 pharmacokinetic-dependent infusion systems 301–4
 and rate-controlled infusion 300
 syringe drivers 300
 target-controlled infusion 173, 177, 301, 303*f*, 304*f*, 346
 wobble index 304
controlled atmosphere stunning (CAS) 159
controlled mechanical ventilation (CMV) 1094, 1098
conus arteriosus, fish 1121
CO-oximetry 233–4
 Masimo pulse CO-oximetry 236
core-to-periphery gradient, thermoregulation 247, 248*f*
coronary circulation 658–9
coronary perfusion pressure (C_oPP) 57
cortical blindness 69, 1035
corticosteroids 58
 airway surgery 792
 coagulation, assessment 852
 concurrent 799
 in CPR 58, 59–60
 diabetes mellitus 903
 intra-articular injections of 1015
 locally administered 1013
 and NSAIDs 410, 907, 1338, 1380
 post resuscitation care 59–60
 prolonged anesthetic recovery 69
 radiation burns 1370
 septic peritonitis 881
 systemic 792, 1380
 thyroid disease 908, 911
 see also steroids
corticosterone 161
COstatus® monitor, thermodilution 214
cough reflex 655, 833, 836
coupling of systems 27
COX-1
 colic, in horses 1218
 versus COX-2 inhibition 412–13, 1069
 pain management 1015
COX-2
 colic, in horses 1218
 versus COX-1 inhibition 404–5, 1069
 inhibition as selection criterion 412–13
COX-3, pain management 1015
coxofemoral joint technique 1192
CPA *see* cardiopulmonary arrest (CPA)
CPAP *see* continuous positive airway pressure (CPAP)
CPCR *see* cardiopulmonary-cerebral resuscitation (CPCR)
CPP *see* cerebral perfusion pressure (CPP)
CPR *see* cardiopulmonary resuscitation (CPR)
cranial nerves 823
craniocardiac reflex 655
CRI *see* continuous rate infusion (CRI)
crisis manuals 35
criterion validity 1002
critical incident technique, anesthetic mishaps 32*f*
cross-matching 599–600
cryogens 49–50
cryoprecipitate (cryo) 596–7
cryptorchidectomy, in horses 12

crystalloids 582–8
  hypertonic 584–5
  hypotonic 585
  isotonic 582–4
CT *see* computed tomography (CT)
Cushing reflex 67, 655
cutaneous system, amphibians 1118
cyanosis 232
cyclic adenosine monophosphate (cAMP) 287, 639
cyclic guanosine monophosphate (cGMP) 639
cyclohexamines 1082–3
CYP2B11 cytochrome gene 1030, 1031
cytochrome P450 isoenzymes (CYPs) 306, 308
cytotoxicity 544, 1100
  natural killer cell 1371, 1372
  opioids 1372

damping 201–2
dantrolene 420–1
DAP *see* diastolic arterial pressure (DAP)
darts
  air-activated mechanisms 1079
  delivery equipment 1079
  explosive discharge mechanisms 1080
  induction of anesthesia 1085
  see also capture of wildlife; wildlife capture
data analysis, compartmental models 296–8
data collection techniques and patient safety 28–30
  incident reporting systems 29
  interviews 29
  morbidity and mortality conferences 29–30
deadly nightshade (*Atropa belladonna*) 314, 315*f*
debriefings, patient safety 35–6
DECVAA *see* Diplomate of the European College of Veterinary Anaesthesia and Analgesia (DECVAA)
deep brain stimulation (DBS) 170
defibrillation 58
Delphi method checklist 34
demand valves 139
dental blocks, local tissue 1177
deoxyribonucleic acid (DNA) 1365
depolarization
  atrial 189, 189*f*, 191, 675
  axis of 194, 1105
  cardiac 188, 190
  cellular 627, 906
  cumulative 972
  delayed 367
  diastolic 622, 623, 623*f*, 624*f*
  direct muscle 677
  ECG complex 188, 190
  electrical 190, 623
  electrical potentials and lead system 187, 188
  of endplate terminal 449
  frequency of 702
  gradual 621*f*
  and hyperkalemia 594
  maximal 449
  mean electrical axis 192
  membrane 527, 528, 594, 973
  myocardial, 191, 193*f*
  myocardial contraction and relaxation 631
  nerve 1172, 1254, 1301
  neuromuscular blocking agents 452–3
  neuromuscular junction transmission 827
  neuronal 286, 449, 1367
  NMDA receptors 286
  and novel nondepolarizing agents 453–6
  opioid receptor regulation 359
  phase 4 623, 623*f*
  postsynaptic 450, 530
  prolonged 1382
  rapid 621, 622
  spontaneous 675
  synchronized 626
  vascular smooth muscle 831
  vectors of 192
  ventricular 189*f*, 190, 191, 192, 625, 626, 678, 692, 1121
  ventricular early depolarizations (VPCs) 678, 686
  wave of 189–90, 623–4, 626
    "slow waves" 863
depopulation 154
  foam 161
depth of anesthesia
  conceptualizing 5–6
  devices
    auditory evoked potentials 183–4
    Bispectral Index™ 180–3
    cerebral state monitor 183
    clinical utility of 184
    index of consciousness 183
    Narcotrend® index, 183
    patient state index 183
    spectral entropy 182–3
  electrophysiologic monitoring 179–80
  minimum alveolar concentration 176–7
  monitoring 176–86
  physical signs 177–9
    Stage 1 178
    Stage 2 178–9
    Stage 3 179
    Stage 4 179
deracoxib 1381
dermorphin 1120
desflurane
  environmental impact 7
  flash stimulation under 157
  ophthalmic patients 1335
desmopressin 430–1
detamine-dexmedetomidine 1065
detomidine 8, 325, 338–44, 1083, 1265–6
  anesthetic mortality, risk of 16, 17
  clinical considerations 343–4
  indications for 338–9
  mechanism of action 338–9
  pharmacodynamics 340–3
  pharmacokinetics 339–40
  premedication 383
dexmedetomidine 325, 338–44, 347, 1033, 1083, 1097, 1266, 1338
  clinical considerations 343–4
  dosage 1029
  drug dose 1065, 1066*t*
  indications for 338–9
  mechanism of action 338–9
  pharmacodynamics 340–3
  pharmacokinetics 339–40
dextrans 588
diabetes insipidus
  anesthetic considerations 905–6
  clinical pathology 905
  clinical presentation 905
  diagnosis and treatment 905
  fluid therapy 905
diabetes mellitus 10, 901–4
  acidemia 902
  anesthetic management of patients with 902–4
  clinical pathology 901–2
  clinical presentation 901
  corticosteroids 903
  diagnosis and treatment 902
  fluid therapy 902
  see also endocrine disease
dialkylcarbamoylchloride (DACC)-coated postoperative dressings 148
dialysis, pharmacologic agent clearance 951–2
diaphragmatic hernia 805–6
diastolic arterial pressure (DAP) 197, 199, 203, 204, 421
diastolic dysfunction-associated diseases 689–90
diazepam 1033
  clinical considerations 337–8
  drug dose 1065, 1066*t*
  indications for 336
  mechanism of action 336
  pharmacodynamics 337
  pharmacokinetics 336–7
  ruminants 1269
diethyl ether 5
diffusion hypoxia 513–14
diffusion limitation, hypoxemia 739
dilated cardiomyopathy (DCM), anesthetic considerations 686
dilution, in cardiac output monitoring
  dye dilution technique 211
  indicator dilution and transpulmonary thermodilution 214
  lithium 214–15
  pulmonary artery catheter (PAC) thermodilution 212–14
  transpulmonary thermodilution and ultrasound indicator dilution 214
dimethyl sulfoxide (DMSO) 598
diphenhydramine 421
Diploma of Veterinary Anaesthesia, UK 6, 21
Diplomate of the American College of Veterinary Anesthesia and Analgesia (DACVAA] 21, 55
Diplomate of the European College of Veterinary Anaesthesia and Analgesia (DECVAA) 21
diprenorphine 1082
dipyrone (metamizole) 408

disseminated intravascular coagulation (DIC) 1218
dissociative anesthetics 4, 6, 469–72
cesarean section 960
chemical structure 469
clinical effects
analgesic 470
cardiovascular 470
central nervous system 470
hepatic system 470
muscle 471
renal 470
respiratory 470
species-specific 471–2
clinical use 472
fetal/neonatal effects 471
mechanism of action 469
ophthalmic patients 1334–5
pharmacodynamics 470–1
pharmacokinetics 469–70
distal brachial plexus block 1187, 1188
distal paravertebral block 1309
distal radial, ulnar, median, and musculocutaneous nerve block 1188
distribution
apparent volume of 291–2
barbiturates 463
bicarbonate distribution space 563–4
local anesthesia 532–3
opioids 362
pulmonary perfusion 713–15
see also absorption, distribution, metabolism, and elimination (ADME)
dive reflex 1106
divergence index 304
diving reflex 655
DMSO *see* dimethyl sulfoxide (DMSO)
dobutamine 284
cardiovascular system effects 322–3
in isoflurane-anesthetized dogs 323
docosahexaenoic acid (DHA) 1013
dogs 1157–65
aging 1354
anesthesia
anesthetic and analgesic plan 1159–62
breed sensitivities to 1031
chamber or mask inhalant induction 1163
comparative anesthesia and analgesia 1029–40
delayed anesthetic recovery 1164–5
epidural anesthesia 5, 148
general anesthesia 962, 965, 1157
induction 1162–3
injectable anesthetics 1161*t*
intermediate-term 1162
intermittent positive-pressure ventilation 205
intravenous high-dose opioid induction 1163
intravenous regional 1167–8
local infiltration 1166
locoregional 1167–8
long-term 1162
maintenance 1163
mortality, risk of 14–17, 18
neuraxial 1168
patient preparation 1159–62
peripheral nerve blocks 1168
plan 1159–62
preanesthetic considerations 12, 1158–9
premedication 1162
records 1163
recovery 1164
sensitivity to 1158
short-term 1159–62
topical 1166
auditory evoked potentials 183
biomedical instrumentation system 182
blood typing 599
body surface area 1029
body weight 1159
brachycephalic breeds 1032, 1158
canine brachycephalic obstructive syndrome 788–3
canine laryngeal paralysis 794–7
canine lung lobe torsion 806–7
canine tracheal collapse 797–9
cardiopulmonary arrest 58
cardiopulmonary measures 1159
central nervous system 1159
chest compressions 57
cocaine use 5
drug dose
buprenorphine 381–2
butorphanol 382–3
fentanyl 378–9
hydromorphone 377
methadone 377
morphine 375
drug effects
acepromazine 335
alfaxalone 479
barbiturates 465
detomidine 343
dexmedetomidine 343
diazepam 337
dissociative anesthetics 471
etomidate 476
medetomidine 343
midazolam 337
morphine 363
NSAIDs 413–14
propofol 467
romifidine 343
xylazine 343
zolazepam 337
electrocardiography 192
fasting 1159
gastroesophageal reflux 67
hemorrhage 60
high-definition oscillometry 204
histamine release 1031–2
history 1158
hyperkalemia 68
hypo-or hyperthermia 68
inhalant anesthetic MAC 372–3
laboratory evaluation 1158
locoregional anesthesia 1166–204
classification 1167–8
equipment 1170–4
physiology of nerve blockade 1168–9
preparation 1169–70
see also locoregional anesthesia
malignant hyperthermia 68
morphine
administration 374, 375
analgesia 375
dosage 375
effects 375–6
infusion rates 374
intravenous 375
oral 374–5
opioid-induced tolerance 363
osteoarthritic pain 1013
P450 CYB2B11 enzyme expression 1158
physical examination 1158, 1159
physical status 1159
pneumothorax 262
postoperative infections 142
"praying posture" 997*f*
pregnancy, general anesthesia in 962, 965
preparation for surgery 1159–62
range of sizes 1029–30
red blood cell potassium 1033
regional anesthesia 964–5
renal function, testing and monitoring 926–8
return of spontaneous circulation 55
sighthounds 1030–1
signalment 1158
specific breeds 16, 18, 1029
Australian Terriers 901
Bichon Frise 901
Boston Terriers 788, 791
Boxers 1031
Brittany Spaniels 795
Bulldogs 788, 791
Cairn Terriers 901
Cavalier King Charles Spaniel 434, 1000
Cocker 686
Doberman Pinschers 908
Finnish Spitz 901
Fox Terriers 895
German Shepherds 905
Golden Retrievers 795, 908
Great Danes 908
Greyhounds 1030
Irish Setters 908
Keeshond 901
Labrador Retrievers 359, 408, 412, 691, 795, 855
Miniature Poodles 901
Miniature Schnauzers 901
Pugs 788, 791
Rottweilers 18
Samoyed 901
Siberian huskies 905
Staffordshire Terriers 877
Standard Poodles 893
Standard Schnauzers 895
Toy Poodles 901
West Highland White terriers 18
Yorkshire Terriers 797, 799*f*, 1032

stabilization 1159–62
subarachnoid anesthesia 5
toy breeds 1158
tracheal collapse 1032–3
transcranial magnetic stimulation 182, 184
ventilation, monitoring 227
dolasetron 428
dolphins 1093, 1094, 1095, 1098
bottlenose 1091, 1100*f*
endotracheal intubation 1103*f*
median artery 1101
small 1104
vascular access 1099
venous access 1100
dopamine 284
cardiovascular system effects 321–2
extravasation of 322
pharmacokinetics 322
pharmacology of descending controls 976
receptors 1036
dopexamine
cardiovascular system effects 323
other effects 323
pharmacokinetics 323
Doppler device, preplaced 59
Doppler flow probes 1101, 1102
Doppler ultrasonography 1173
Doppler ultrasonographic blood pressure measurement 202–3
dorsal horn
anatomy of 973–5
spinal cord 339, 341, 364, 372, 507, 530, 535, 1367, 1372
double-lumen tube (DLT) 78–81
doxapram 69, 421–3, 1267
Dräger AV-E ventilator 134
Dräger small animal ventilator 123
dromotropy 198
droperidol 1084
drug administration 147–9
birds 1135–6
camelids 1054
farm animals 1054–5
infection prevention and control 147–9
intranasal route 1136
laboratory animals 1070
pigs 1055, 1286
reptiles 1114
routes 58
ruminants 1054
drug delivery systems 173
drug dose *see individual drugs and species*
drug effects
reducing medication error, methods 36–7
see also adverse drug reactions (ADRs)
drug interactions
additive interaction 306
drug–drug interactions 306
isobolographic studies 306
line of additivity 306
pharmacodynamic 306–7
pharmacokinetic 305–6
physicochemical 305
response surface analyses 306–7
in vitro/*in vivo* 306
drug metabolism 307–9
arachidonic acid 398, 403–4
cats 1034
epinephrine, effects of 321
formulation effect 309
isomers 309
ketamine 308
local anesthesia 533–4
opioids 362–3
Phase I biotransformation 308
Phase II biotransformation or conjugation 308
Phase III biotransformation 308–9
propofol 309
renal clearance 307
stereoisomers 309
transport of metabolites 308–9
see also absorption, distribution, metabolism, and elimination (ADME)
drug spillage 7
drug-related complications
medical error resulting in overdose 65–6
patient arousal 66
dual-circuit ventilators 115, 117, 119–22
bellows configuration 119–20
bellows housing 120
exhaust valve 120–1
spill valve 121
ventilator hose connection 121–2
Dumeril's monitors (*Varanus dumerili*) 1113
duration of anesthesia
cardiovascular system 511
respiratory system 509
sympathetic nervous system 511
dye dilution technique 211
dynamic pressure response test 201
dysphoria 336, 375, 376, 378
acute pain 998
anesthetic recovery 1106
buprenorphine, formulation of 1035
butorphanol causing 366
cetacean anesthesia 1098
fentanyl CRI developed 378
ketamine-induced 1268
ketamine–midazolam 1161
opioid effects 366–7
opioid-induced 359, 873, 1034, 1164, 1267
dysrhythmias *see* arrhythmias/dysrhythmias

ECG *see* electrocardiography (ECG)
echocardiography
and Echo-doppler 215–16
preanesthetic evaluation 680–1, 682
Simpson's rule 215
Echo-doppler, and echocardiography 215–16
EEG *see* electroencephalogram (EEG)
effect-site concentration 176–7
Efficacy of Volume Substitution and Insulin Therapy in Severe Sepsis (VISEP) study 694
eicosapentaenoic acid (EPA) 1013
Einthoven's triangle 188
electrical potentials, electrocardiography 187–9
electrical silence 180
electroanesthesia 4
electrocardiogram 620–6
electrocardiography (ECG) 57, 145, 187–96, 1276
artifacts and filters 194–5
atria, depolarization of 189
atrioventricular (AV) node 189
base-apex lead 189
baseline 190
bipolar leads 188
cables 49
carbon graphite electrodes 51
cardiac cycle 189
complex 189–90
depolarization 190
Einthoven's triangle 188
electrical potentials and lead system 187–9
equipment 194–5
evaluating 190–2
heart rate calculation 190–1
isoelectric line 190
leads I, II, and III 188
mean electrical axis (MEA) 191–2
monitoring 1293
multilead ECG 189
preanesthetic 12
precordial system 189
QRS complex 189, 190, 191
rhythm evaluation 191
species-specific variations 192, 193, 193*f*, 194
unipolar leads 188–9
wave, segment and interval 189, 190
Wilson's central terminal 188
electroencephalogram (EEG) 157, 999
frequency bands 179–80
electrolocation, epidural technique 1196
electrolytes
calcium 592–3
potassium 593–5
sodium 592–3
electromagnetic therapies 1025
electromyography (EMG) 182–3
electronarcosis 4
electrophysiology 620–6
electrophysiologic monitoring 179–80
electroretinogram, impact of anesthesia on 1338
electrosleep 4
electrosurgery units 195
elimination
carbon dioxide 704–7
half-life of 291
inhalational anesthesia 500–2
and uptake 497–501
by blood 499–500
see also absorption, distribution, metabolism, and elimination (ADME)
endobronchial intubation, inadvertent 63
endobronchial tube placement 261, 263*f*
endocannabinoids 977
endocrine disease 891–921
adrenal glands 893–900
anatomy and physiology 891, 893
anesthetic management of patients with

endocrine disease (*cont'd*)
diabetes insipidus 905–6
diabetes mellitus 902–4
hyperadrenocorticism 897–8
hypoadrenocorticism 894–5
insulinoma 907–8
pheochromocytoma 898–900
diabetes insipidus 904–6
diabetes mellitus 10, 901–4
hyperparathyroidism 914–15
hyperthyroidism 909–12
hypothyroidism 908–9
important hormones 892*f*
insulinoma 906–8
pancreatitis 908
parathyroid gland 913–15
thyroid gland 908–13
thyroid neoplasia 912–13
endocrine system 475–6, 891
neuroimmune–endocrine system 1026
pregnancy-associated changes 957
endoscope-guided technique 85–6
endotoxemia, in horses 1217–18
endotracheal intubation 174, 465, 468, 866
airway evaluation prior to 913
airway management 1070
anesthetic mortality, risk of 16
associated ICP 833
blind intubation 1058, 1104
bronchospasm 63
capnography/capnometry required for 222
in cats 17, 18, 803, 1035
cetacean anesthesia 1098
correct 84, 85*f*
cough reflex 833, 836
detection of 223
difficult airway and lower airway disease 226
difficult or impossible 84, 723
farm animals 1058–61
and Fick principle 212
guided 85*f*
in horses 338, 1341
induction of anesthesia 62, 1208, 1289, 1296
injectable anesthetics 468, 476
intermediate-term anesthesia 1162
isobolographic analyses 306
ketamine requirements 1269
laboratory rodents and lagomorphs 1070
"MAC for endotracheal intubation" (MAC-EI) 177
myasthenia gravis (MG) 840
non-human primates 1073
in pigs 1059–60, 1073
in pregnancy 1050
pulmonary aspiration 65
in rabbits 480
recovery 1278
reducing aspiration risk following 808
reptiles 1114
respiratory depression 61, 1088
retrograde intubation as alternative to 86
ruminants 1271
sedation and chemical restraint 1288
stick intubation 1059
supraglottic airway devices (SGADs) as an alternative to 83
endotracheal tubes (ETTs) 75–8, 1059*f*
adapters 77, 224
biomedical engineering 172
bronchial blockers 80–2
Cole tubes 76
commercially available stainless steel/insulated 41–2
commonly used 41, 44, 76
cuff and pilot tubing 42, 51, 77, 145
dogs 1032
double-lumen tube (DLT) 78–81
exchangers 86
infection prevention and control 145
isolation of one lung 78–82
materials 41–2, 58
metal, cooper-shielded and insulated 41
minimum occlusive volume (MOV) 77–8
Murphy-type 77
placement 256
radiocontrast agents 45
size, choice of 75
stimulating laryngospasm 179
uncuffed self-sealing 78
veterinary-specific 75
enflurane 489–90
Engineering in Medicine and Biology Society (EMBS) 170
engineering solutions, patient safety 36
environmental impact of anesthesia 7–8
ephedrine
cardiovascular system effects 326
other effects 326
pharmacokinetics 326
epidural technique 148
cranial epidural blocks 1311–12
drugs for continuous epidural anesthesia and analgesia 1197
electrolocation 1196
hanging drop 1196
history 5
loss of resistance 1196
neuraxial anesthesia 1194, 1195*f*
running-drip 1196
sacrococcygeal or intercoccygeal epidural (caudal epidural) block 1312–13
segmental dorsolumbar epidural block 1309–10
ultrasound-guided 1196–7
epinephrine 319–21
β-adrenergic receptors 287
arrhythmias induced by 464, 467, 536
cardiopulmonary arrest 58
cardiovascular system effects 320–1
half-life 321
and horses 320–1
and local anesthesia 535–6
metabolism, effects on 321
pharmacokinetics 321
β-adrenergic effects 58
episcleral venous pressure (EVP) 1331
equine ECG 192, 194
Equine Facial Action Coding System 1003
equine guttural pouch disease 799–801
equine guttural pouch mycosis
characteristics and pathophysiology 800–1
management of sedation and/or general anesthesia 801
equine guttural pouch tympany
characteristics and pathophysiology 800
management of sedation and/or general anesthesia 800
equine laryngeal paralysis
characteristics and pathophysiology 801–2
management of anesthesia and/or sedation 802
equipment
anesthesia ventilators *see* ventilators
anesthetic and surgical, reprocessing of 144–5
anesthetic complications
adjustable pressure-limiting valve closure or malfunction 66
breathing system malfunction 67
oxygen supply failure 67
vaporizer-related 67
breathing systems 105–12
catheters *see* catheters
electrocardiography 194–5
endoscope-guided technique 85
endotracheal tubes *see* endotracheal tubes (ETTs)
field anesthesia 1078
high-quality high-volume spay-neuter (HQHVSN) practice 1042–3
injection pressure monitors 1172
intubation aids and techniques 84
laryngoscopes *see* laryngoscopes
lateral pharyngotomy 87
locoregional anesthesia 1170–4
machines *see* anesthetic machines
medical gases 91–4
monitoring 145
nasotracheal intubation 84
non-human primates 1073
oxygen administration 87–91
peripheral nerve stimulators 1172–3
point-of-care ultrasound (POCUS) 256
remote drug delivery 1079–80
respiratory assist devices 139
retrograde intubation 86
safety and design 75
supraglottic airway devices 82–3
tracheostomy 86–7
ultrasound 1173–4
waste gas scavenge system 112–13
wildlife capture 1079–80
wire- or tube-guided techniques 84–5
equivalent dipole theory 187
EQUUS-COMPASS pain scale 1003
erector spinae plane block 1184–5
ergonomics 27
ERV *see* expiratory reserve volume (ERV)
Escherichia coli (*E. coli*) 142, 145
esmolol 329

esophagitis and esophageal stricture 868
ESWT *see* extracorporeal shockwave therapies (ESWT)
etherization 5, 16
etomidate
analogs 477
chemical structure 474
clinical effects
analgesic 476
cardiovascular 474–5
central nervous system 474
gastrointestinal 475
hepatic 475
muscle 476
pain on injection 476
renal 475
respiratory 475
species-specific 476
clinical use 476
mechanism of action 474
neurologic disease 834
ophthalmic patients 1335
pain on injection 476
pharmacodynamics 474–6
pharmacokinetics 474
etorphine 380–1
wildlife capture 1081, 1084
ETTs *see* endotracheal tubes (ETTs)
euphoria, opioid effects 366–7
European College of Veterinary Anaesthesiologists (ECVA) 6, 7
euthanasia 152–66
agent purity 161–2
animal distress, evaluating 156 7
carcass disposal 162
choice of killing method 158–60
in clinical setting 162
defining 153
depopulation 154
and fetal sentience 160
foam depopulation 161
humane slaughter 152, 153–4
inhalational anesthesia 158
inhaled methods 157
IV access 162
low atmospheric pressure stunning 160–1
mechanisms of action 155–6
onset of unconsciousness 158–60
opposed goals 152
pain and consciousness 154–5
EVLW *see* extravascular lung water (EVLW)
excitation–contraction coupling 626–8
excretion
local anesthetics 534
nitrogen 1121
opioids 363
exertional myopathy 1088
expiratory reserve volume (ERV) 698
extracorporeal shockwave therapies (ESWT) 1025
extraocular muscles (EOM) 1327, 1331
extravascular lung water (EVLW) 268
eye and adnexa block 1304–6
eye protection 41
face masks 144, 489
airway obstruction 62
carbon dioxide elimination, kinetics 706
chest compressions 57
commercial 89*f*
delivery 87–8
halothane administration 1060
hyperadrenocorticism (HAC) 897
induction of anesthesia 62
isoflurane or sevoflurane delivered by 1268
ketamine combinations 1269
and laboratory rodents 1071
laser procedures 41, 42
mechanical ventilation 782
non-sealed 752
oxygen supplementation 89, 752, 753
positive-pressure ventilation 957
preanesthetic considerations 1286
precapillary pulmonary hypertension 810
pulmonary mechanics 708
and rabbits 1067, 1070
sealed 740
snug-fitting 88, 89, 699*f*, 752, 753, 909
surgical 42
and swine 1288
urethral or bilateral ureteral obstruction 938
β_2-adrenergic receptor agonists 326
Facial Action Coding Systems (FACS) 1003
Faculty of Veterinary Medicine, University of Calgary, pre-induction checklist 35*f*
famotidine 423–4
farm animals 1052–64
cardiovascular system 1056–7
drug administration 1054–5
endotracheal intubation 1058–61
gastrointestinal tract 1057–8
hypertension 1057
malignant hyperthermia 1060–1
positioning during anesthesia 1055–6
respiratory system 1057
ruminants, recommended withdrawal interval for 1052, 1053–4*t*
salivation 1058
species differences in anesthetic dose requirements 1061
thermoregulation 1060–1
see also camelids; cattle; pigs; ruminants
fascial plane block techniques 1182–5
erector spinae plane block 1184–5
quadratus lumborum 1182–3
serratus plane block 1182
transversus abdominis plane (TAP) block 1015, 1183–4, 1227, 1258
fast flush test 201
fasting
amphibians 1118
birds 1135
dogs 1159
horses 1205–6
pigs 1285
febrile non-hemolytic transfusion reactions (FNHTRS) 600–1
feline asthma 802–3
characteristics and pathophysiology 802
management of anesthesia 802–3
feline brachycephalic obstructive airway syndrome 793–4
characteristics and pathophysiology 793–4
management of anesthesia 794
feline ECG 192
Feline Grimace Scale (FGS) 1003, 1005, 1034
feline musculoskeletal pain index (FMPI) 1006
feline onychectomy 1014
femoral/saphenous nerve block 1189–90
fentanyl 378–9, 1067
dosage
birds 1138
cats 378–9
dogs 378–9
food animals 379
horses 379
pigs 1288
illicit 8
intraoperative analgesia 1273
patches 1069
selected primate species 1066*t*
wooden chest syndrome 65
fetal distress 160
fetal sentience 160
FFP *see* fresh frozen plasma (FFP)
FGS *see* Feline Grimace Scale (FGS)
fibrinolytic drugs 577
Fick principle, cardiac output monitoring 211, 212, 227
field anesthesia
capture technique 1078–9
equipment 1078
general considerations 1077–8
hazards 1079
horses 1210
weather 1078
see also wildlife capture
firocoxib 1381
first-order rate equation 297
"first-pass effect," hepatic clearance 293
fish
anatomy and physiology 1120–1
cardiovascular system 1121
clinical anesthesia 1122–3
considerations for anesthesia 1122
gills 1120
jawed 1120
nervous system 1121
nociception 1121
preanesthetic evaluation 1122–3
respiratory system 1120–1
thermoregulation 1121
"fish mouth view," right parasternal short-axis views 272
flank/paralumbar fossa, blocks for regional anesthesia of
distal paravertebral 1309
inverted "l" or "7" 1307
line infiltration 1307
proximal paravertebral 1307–9
segmental dorsolumbar epidural 1309–10
segmental thoracolumbar subarachnoid 1310

Florida manatee (*Trichechus manatus latirostris*) 1099
flow rate compensation 97
flowmeters 36, 135
activation 101
air 667, 752
anesthetic machines and breathing circuits 91
assembly 95
calibration 96
continuous laser Doppler flowmetry 238
designs 96, 97*f*
field anesthesia 1078
fresh gas flow delivered by 756
function 96
gas flow within machine 94–6
indicators 67
nasal insufflation 89, 90
oxygen 67, 96*f*, 97*f*, 103, 133, 134, 138, 172, 667, 752, 794
pin index safety system 93, 94*f*
rodent 1067
supportive therapy 1275
vaporizer-related complications 67
see also fresh gas flow (FGF); vaporizers
fluid regulation, amphibians 1118
fluid therapy
AAHA guidelines 1350
aggressive 58, 277, 905, 1223
anesthetic management 909
anesthetic risk 17
blood pressure monitoring 207
bolus 592
cardiopulmonary arrest 58
in cats 18, 1036
colic, in horses 1222–4
colloid 909
concurrent 587
conventional 589
crystalloid 1294
diabetes insipidus 905
diabetes mellitus 902
emergency 1294
and gastrointestinal function 863, 872
goal-directed 207, 210, 583, 589, 856, 904
individualized 589–91
hemoabdomen 877
in horses 929, 1050, 1223
in humans 589
hyperthermia 911
in hypotensive patients 856
in hypovolemic patients 801
inadequate 930
and interventional radiology 858
intestinal neoplasia 877, 878
intraoperative 589, 595
intravenous 249, 277, 511, 875, 894, 936, 938
isotonic crystalloids 582
laboratory animals 1072
liberal 589, 881
megaesophagus 874
and microvasculature 591–2
monitoring 277
and NSAIDs 415
older patients 1357
perianesthetic 897
perioperative 249, 585, 588–92
preoperative 784, 899
protocols 800, 881
rates of 938, 1223
renal disease 936
resistance 646
restrictive 589, 592, 717, 881
ruminants 1273–4
and sedation 802
small animals 1223
spinal cord injury and spine surgery 839
standard 590
and supportive therapies 1294
urine output measurement 928
flumazenil 69, 285, 338
flunixin 1279
fluorocarbons 1067
FMPI *see* feline musculoskeletal pain index (FMPI)
fMRI *see* functional magnetic resonance imaging (fMRI)
foals, equine neonate versus foal 1049–50
foam depopulation methods 161
Food and Drug Administration (FSA), United States 49, 75
Center for Devices and Radiological Health 113
food animals
drug dose
fentanyl 379
morphine 376–7
drug effects, NSAIDs 415
force plate analysis 1001
foreign body removal/other abdominal procedures 882
forelimb intravenous catheter 58
formulation effect, drug metabolism 309
fospropofol 468–9
Frank–Starling curve 204
FRC *see* functional residual capacity (FRC)
"free hormone hypothesis" 290
free-ranging terrestrial mammals *see* wildlife capture
free-water abnormalities 571
fresh frozen plasma (FFP) 596
fresh gas flow (FGF) 96, 98, 101–3, 116, 119, 120, 122–6, 132, 756–8, 761–3
birds 1144
breathing systems 105, 106, 110–12
laboratory animals 1071
flow rate 104, 105, 106, 111
mechanical ventilation 756
see also flowmeters
fresh whole blood (FWB) 596
frozen plasma (FP) 596
functional magnetic resonance imaging (fMRI) 155, 999
functional residual capacity (FRC) 698, 1095

GABA receptors 162, 336, 338, 469, 507, 1068, 1141
fast response 286
$GABA_A$ 286, 336
$GABA_AR$ 1092
marine mammals 1092
slow response 286
see also gamma-aminobutyric acid (GABA)
gabapentin 434–6, 1015, 1070, 1338, 1382
gadolinium-based contrast agents (GBCAs) 52
gait
force plate analysis 1001
kinematic 1001
visual observation of 1001
gallbladder, and extrahepatic biliary tract pathology 857
galvanometer 187
gamma-aminobutyric acid (GABA)
endogenous 336
GABA-mediated inhibitory transmission 336
and glycine 977
increased activation of adenylate cyclase in 363
marine mammals 1092
receptors *see* GABA receptors
gamma-glutamyl transferase (GGT):creatinine ratio 1218
gas sampling systems 241
gas supply *see* medical gases
gastric dilation-volvulus 874–6
gastroesophageal reflux 865–7
gastroesophageal reflux (GER)
esophageal stricture 54
and regurgitation 13, 65, 67
gastrointestinal disease 862–90
anatomy of the gastrointestinal tract 862–71
aspiration 868–9
effects of anesthetic agents on gastrointestinal function 863–71
esophagitis and esophageal stricture 868
foreign body removal/other abdominal procedures 882
gastric dilation-volvulus 874–6
gastroesophageal reflux 865–7
gastrointestinal conditions requiring anesthesia 871–82
gastrointestinal motility/postoperative ileus 869–71
hemoabdomen 876–7
intestinal neoplasia 877–9
laparotomy 871–3
megaesophagus 873–4
nausea and vomiting 864–5
septic peritonitis 879–82
gastrointestinal function, effects of anesthetic agents on 863–71
gastrointestinal motility 869–71
gastrointestinal system
in dogs and cats 1159
drug effects
alfaxalone 478–9
barbiturates 465
detomidine 342
dexmedetomidine 342
dissociative anesthetics 470
etomidate 475
medetomidine 342
NSAIDs 408–10
opioids 367–8

propofol 467
romifidine 342
xylazine 342
pregnancy-associated changes 957
gastrointestinal tract
anatomy of 862–71
and parasympathetic nervous system 862
regurgitation 1057–8
ruminal tympany 1057
gator sign *see* BAT sign
GE Healthcare Entropy™ Module 182–3
gelatins 588
general anesthesia
cesarean section 961–4
defining 3, 4, 153, 176
dogs 962, 965, 1157
laser procedures 44
magnetic resonance imaging 50–1
ophthalmic patients 1338–40
versus sedation 50–1
stages 178*f*
genetic factors, response variability 159
genitourinary system
drug effects
detomidine 342
dexmedetomidine 342
medetomidine 342
romifidine 342
xylazine 342
GFR *see* glomerular filtration rate (GFR)
Glasgow Composite Pain Scale-Feline 1003, 1034
glial fibrillary acidic protein (GFAP) 285
global warming 7
Global Warming Protocol (GWP) 1067
glomerular filtration rate (GFR) 294, 1357
and renal clearance 927–8
glucocorticoid receptor–drug complex 284
glucuronidation 308
glutamate 286–7
glutathione 308
glutathione S-transferases (GST) 308
glycine 286–7
glycopyrrolate
and anticholinergics 314–15
clinical use 317
drug dose 1065, 1066*t*
pharmacology 317
goats, regional anesthesia 965
G-protein receptors 285, 287
gradient magnetic fields 49, 51
grapiprant 406–7, 1140–1, 1381
greenhouse gases 7, 1067
green-lipped mussels 1383
grimace scales 1003, 1004*t*, 1005*f*, 1034
guaifenesin
cesarean section 961
horses 1209–10
ruminants 1269
guaifenesin (glyceryl guaiacolate ether) 424–5
guanosine diphosphate (GDP) 287
guanosine triphosphate (GTP) 287
guinea pigs 433
anatomic and physiologic considerations 1070
injectable anesthetics 480
midazolam 338
neurologically mature at birth 160
osteoarthritis (OA) 985
withholding foods from 1070

Hagen–Poiseuille equation 198
Haldane effect 740–2
Hallowell Anesthesia WorkStation (AWS) 121*f*
Hallowell EMC 2000, 2002/2002 PRO ventilator 126–7
Hallowell Tafonius/Tafonius Junior ventilator 136, 137*f*
halothane 320, 321, 323, 1272
agent-specific vaporizers 103
causes of anesthetic death 16
environmental impact 6
euthanasia 158
face mask administration 1060
and infection control 148–9
Hamburger effect 739
hand hygiene 144
handling and restraint
amphibians 1118
birds 1135
cats 1033–4
laboratory animals 1070
hand-offs, patient safety 35–6
hanging drop epidural technique 1196
harbor porpoise 1099
harm, risk of from healthcare 24–5
HBF *see* hepatic blood flow (HBF)
HCM *see* hypertrophic cardiomyopathy (HCM)
HCPI *see* Helsinki Chronic Pain Index (HCPI)
head blocks 1174–8
auricular techniques 1178
eye and adnexa block 1304–6
horn blocks 1303–4
infraorbital 1235
local tissue dental 1177
mandibular 1175–7, 1236
maxillary 1174–5, 1236–7
mental 1236
nasal passages and block 1306–7
ophthalmic patients 1177–8
regional anesthesia 1303–7
trigeminal nerve 1178
Health-Related Quality of Life (HRQoL) 1005
hearing protection, MRI 49
heart
anticholinergic effects 315
normal 189, 190, 191, 650*f*
see also cardiac arrest; cardiac output (CO), monitoring; cardiopulmonary arrest (CPA); cardiopulmonary resuscitation (CPR); cardiovascular complications, anesthesia-related; electrocardiography (ECG)
heart rate 909, 1049
alterations in 178
amphibians 1119
calculation 190–1
cardiac dysrhythmias 61
decrease in 1138, 1143, 1273, 1275, 1349
evaluation an ECG 190
high 192, 1134
in horses 1049
improving 1336
increase in 315, 1082, 1163, 1269, 1287
instantaneous 190
irregular 1087
maximum 1355
monitoring 1350
normal 192, 648*t*, 1048, 1275
slowing of 1332
wildlife capture 1086
heat therapy 1024
heat transfer mechanisms, thermoregulation 247–9
emissivity 247
Helsinki Chronic Pain Index (HCPI) 1005, 1006
hematocrit 1158
hemoabdomen 876–7
hemodialysis
and continuous renal replacement therapy 950–2
drug characteristics 951–2
intermittent 950–2
membrane properties 951
patient factors 952
patient monitoring 951
pharmacologic agent clearance 951–2
procedures and equipment 950–1
hemodynamics and cardiac function
blood flow 642–4
blood pressure 644–6
preload and afterload 647
resistance 646–7
hemoglobin
arterial saturation 234
deoxygenated 232
laboratory evaluation 1158
mixed venous saturation (SvO2) 234
oxyhemoglobin dissociation curve 739
saturation with oxygen, measuring 233–6
hemorrhage, cardiovascular complications 60–1
hemostasis
cell-based 574–5
primary 575
secondary 575
hemoximetry *see* CO-oximetry
henbane (*Hyoscyamus niger*) 314
Henderson-Hasselbalch equation 557
hepatic blood flow (HBF)
alfaxalone–alfadolon decreasing 478
compromised 1208
and hepatic clearance 292–3
and inhalation anesthetics 478, 512
and injectable anesthetics 465, 467
and liver disease 847, 848, 849*f*, 850
and local anesthesia 534
and maintenance of general anesthesia 1208
and propofol 466, 467
hepatic clearance 292–3
hepatic functions 847–51
hepatic lobe torsion 857
hepatic system
age-related changes 1357

hepatic system (*cont'd*)
in dogs and cats 1159
drug effects
alfaxalone 478–9
barbiturates 465
dissociative anesthetics 470
etomidate 475
inhalational anesthetics 512
propofol 467
functional anatomy and physiology 847–51
neonatal/pediatric patients 1349
pregnancy-associated changes 957
reptiles 1113–14
structural organization of the liver 847–8, 849*f*
see also liver disease
hepatitis 855–6
"hepatization," translobar lung consolidation 269
hepatobiliary diseases, pain management in 858
hepatotoxicity 412, 430, 512
type 1 854, 855
type 2 855
Hering–Breuer reflex 655
heroin 8
HFACS *see* Human Factors Analysis and Classification System (HFACS)
high-definition oscillometry (HDO) 204
high-quality high-volume spay-neuter (HQHVSN) practice 1041, 1042*f*, 1043–5
analgesia for spay-neuter programs 1044–5
drug protocols 1042
equipment 1042–3
monitoring and patient support 1043–4
preoperative considerations 1042
recovery 1044
high-threshold (HT) pain-sensing nerve types 1024
histamine release 1031–2
history of veterinary anesthesia
depth of anesthesia, conceptualizing 5–6
early milestones 5
evolution as a specialty 6–7
homeostasis
acid-base 221, 555, 556*f*
protein 850
horn blocks 1303–4
Horner's syndrome 1015
Horowitz index 233
horses 1205–16
abdominal pain, pawing in response to, 998*f*
a_2-adrenergic receptor agonists 1208–10
anesthesia
additional sedation and analgesia 1212–13
adequate cardiovascular function and tissue oxygenation 1210–11
comparative anesthesia and analgesia 1048–51
environmental considerations 1211–12
fasting 1205–6
field anesthesia 1210
general 44, 962
induction of anesthesia 1206, 1207*t*, 1208
inhalant anesthetic MAC 373
maintenance 1208
monitoring 1210
morbidity 14
mortality, risk of 18
preanesthetic considerations 1205–6, 1218–19
in pregnancy 962
recovery 1211–13
risks 18, 1048, 1219–21
standing sedation 44, 1206, 1207*t*
subarachnoid anesthesia 5
timing of recovery 1212
biomedical instrumentation system 182
blood typing 599
cardiopulmonary arrest 55
cardiopulmonary resuscitation 1049
cervical spondylomyelopathy 839
clinical history 1218
colic in 148
Confidential Enquiry into Perioperative Equine Fatalities (CEPEF) 14, 19, 20
cryptorchidectomy 12
diagnostics 1219
dopamine, effects on 322
drug dose
buprenorphine 382
butorphanol 383
fentanyl 379
hydromorphone 377
methadone 377–8
morphine 376
drug effects
acepromazine 335
alfaxalone 480
barbiturates 465
detomidine 343
dexmedetomidine 343
diazepam 337–8
dissociative anesthetics 472
etomidate 476
medetomidine 343
midazolam 337–8
NSAIDs 414–15
propofol 468
romifidine 343
xylazine 343
zolazepam 337–8
electrocardiography 192, 194
endotracheal intubation in 338, 1341
epinephrine dose 320–1
equine asthma 803–4
equine guttural pouch disease 799–801
equine guttural pouch mycosis 800–1
equine guttural pouch tympany 800
equine induction considerations 1049
equine laryngeal paralysis 801–2
equine neonate versus foal 1049–50
fluid therapy in 929, 1050, 1223
fractures 69
heart rate 1049
ketamine 1209
laser procedures 44
lidocaine 1209
local anesthetic and analgesic techniques 1235–61
choice of agent 1235
epidural medications 1254–7
head, anesthesia of 1236–7
laparotomy/laparoscopy 1250–1
limbs, anesthesia of 1239–50
neuraxial anesthesia 1253–8
novel regional analgesic techniques 1258
ocular procedures, anesthesia of 1237–9
urogenital procedures 1251–3
malignant hyperthermia 68
methicillin-resistant *S. aureus* (MRSA) postsurgical infection 142
muscle relaxants 1209–10
opioids 1209
osteoarthritis in 1016
physical examination 1219
postanesthetic neuropathy 70
pregnant mare 962, 1050
premedication 383
recovery 1050
recumbency, effect of 1049
renal function, testing and monitoring 928–9
risks of anesthesia 18, 1048, 1219–21
hypotension 1219–20
impaired ventilation–perfusion matching 1220–1
postanesthetic myopathy and neuropathy 1221
standing equine MRI 52
variation in size 1048–9
ventilation, monitoring 227
HRQoL *see* Health-Related Quality of Life (HRQoL)
human error
Reason's taxonomy 26*f*
and the system 25–7
human factors, analysis techniques 31*f*
Human Factors Analysis and Classification System (HFACS) 30, 31*f*, 32, 33*t*
Human Factors (HF) 27
analysis techniques 30, 31*f*
Humane Slaughter (HS) Act (1958), US 154
humans
birds as food source for 1127
brain 180, 237
mechanical ventilation during anesthesia 780–2
NSAID risks 412
hyaluronic acid (HA) 1016, 1017
hyaluronidase 536
hydrocodone 381
hydrogen peroxide solutions 145
hydromorphone 377, 1137
premedication 335, 428
hydroxyethyl starches 586–8
hyoscine 314
hyperadrenocorticism
anesthetic considerations 896–7
anesthetic management 897–8
clinical pathology 895
clinical presentation 895
diagnosis and treatment 895–6
hyperadrenocorticism (HAC) 895

hypercapnia 13
  carbon dioxide transport 742–3
  permissive or intentional 1095
  respiratory depression 61
hyperkalemia 68, 225–6
hyperparathyroidism
  anesthetic considerations and management 915
  clinical pathology 914
  clinical presentation 914
  diagnosis and treatment 914–15
hypertension
  farm animals 1057
  intracranial 835–7
  postcapillary pulmonary hypertension 811
  precapillary pulmonary hypertension 809–11
  pulmonary 716–17
  pulmonary blood flow 809
hyperthermia 68, 246, 1034
  anesthesia-related 251
  causes 250
  clinical significance 251
  mild 251
  perianesthetic management 251–2
  severe 1034
  wildlife capture 1078, 1086, 1087
hyperthyroidism
  anesthetic considerations 911
  anesthetic management of patients with 911–12
  clinical pathology 910
  clinical presentation 910
  diagnosis and treatment 910–11
hypertonic crystalloids 584–5
hypertonic saline 69
hypertonic saline solution (HSS) 1222, 1294
hypertrophic cardiomyopathy (HCM) 689–90
hypnosis 4
  and central state monitor 183
hypoadrenocorticism
  anesthetic considerations and management 894–5
  clinical pathology 894
  clinical presentation 893–4
  diagnosis and treatment 894
hypocapnia, carbon dioxide transport 742–3
hypokalemia 225–6
hypoproteinemia 10
hypotension
  amiodarone effects 58
  anesthesia considerations 692–3
  anesthetic risk 1219–20
  cardiovascular complications 60
  perianesthetic 197, 198*t*
  pharmacological support 692–3
hypothalamic vasopressin-containing neurons 157
hypothalamic–pituitary–adrenal axis (HPAA) 157, 1218
hypothermia 4, 68, 246
  clinical significance 251
  colic, in horses 1227–8
  farm animals 1060
  small animal anesthesia morbidity 13
  wildlife capture 1078, 1087, 1088
hypothyroidism
  anesthetic considerations 908–9
  anesthetic management of patients with 909
  clinical pathology 908
  clinical presentation 908
  diagnosis and treatment 908
hypotonic crystalloids 585
hypoventilation 13
hypovolemia 206
hypoxemia 62
  differential diagnosis 225
  and euthanasia 156
  versus hypoxia 231–2
  and MRI 52
  oxygen transport 739–40
  respiratory depression and apnea 61
  small animal anesthesia morbidity 13
  wildlife capture 1078, 1086, 1088
hypoxia 10
  and euthanasia 156
  versus hypoxemia 231–2
  hypoxic pulmonary vasoconstriction 728–31
  postanesthetic blindness 69

IASP *see* International Association for the Study of Pain (IASP)
iatrogenic cardiovascular depression 1219
iatrogenic tracheal injury 64
IBP *see* invasive blood pressure (IBP)
IC *see* inspiratory capacity (IC)
ICP *see* intracranial pressure (ICP)
ICU Medical (formerly Smith Medical/Surgivet) SAV 2500 ventilator 130–1
ICU Medical (formerly Surgivet) DHV1000 large animal ventilator 136–7
idazoxan 1266
immune system
  age-related changes 1357
  hepatic functions 851
  immune-mediated toxicity 512
  opioid effects 371–2
immune-mediated hemolytic anemia (IMHA) 575
incident reporting systems 29
increased intracranial pressure (ICP) 205
index of consciousness (IoC) 183
induction of anesthesia 1268–70
  airway obstruction 62–3
  anesthetic mortality, risk of 17
  birds 1144–9
  cardiac arrest 1225
  chamber 1163
  endotracheal intubation 62, 1208, 1289, 1296
  face masks 62
  in horses 1049, 1206, 1207*t*, 1208, 1224–5
  intravenous high-dose opioid induction 1163
  IV method 1162
  pigs 1288–90
  pre-induction checklist 35*f*
  ruminants 1268–70
  in wildlife 1077
infection prevention and control
  anesthetics and analgesics 148–9
  antibacterial agents 148
  antimicrobials 149
  antiseptic solutions 146
  attire 144
  bandages and dressings 147–8
  breathing circuits 146
  chemical indicator tests 145
  cleaning 144
  colony-forming units (CFUs) 146
  dialkylcarbamoylchloride (DACC)-coated postoperative dressings 148
  disinfection 144, 145
  endotracheal tubes 145
  hand hygiene 144
  intravenous catheters 146
  laryngoscopes 145
  lubricants 148
  manufacturer's instructions for use (MIFU). 145
  monitoring equipment 145
  mouth rinse plungers 145
  patient care and drug administration 147–9
  perianesthetic 143–6
  perioperative checklists 143–4
  postoperative infections 142, 146–7
  reprocessing of anesthetic and surgical equipment 144–5
  risk factors, postoperative
    environmental 147
    iatrogenic 147
    patient-specific 146–7
  silver-based dressings 148
  sterile field, maintenance 146
  sterility assurance monitoring (SAM) 145
  sterilization 144, 145
  surgical site, preparation 146
  ventilators 146
  wound classification systems 143*t*
  see also safety considerations
inferior vena cava (IVC) 275
inflammation
  anti-inflammatory drugs 1069
    see also non-steroidal anti-inflammatory drugs (NSAIDs)
  hepatic functions 851
  inflammatory pain 985, 986–7*t*
informed consent 20–1
infraorbital nerve block 1235
infrared (IR) analysis 240
  advantages of 242
  basic components 242
  blackbody radiator 242
  collision broadening 243
  disadvantages 243
  dispersive/non-dispersive analyzers 242
infrared spectroscopy
  infrared radiation source 223–4
  problems with 224
infrared thermography 1000
inhalational anesthesia 6, 489–525
  actions and toxicity effects 504–12
    cardiovascular system 509–11
    central nervous system 505–8
    hepatic system 512

inhalational anesthesia (*cont'd*)
renal system 511–12
respiratory system 508–9
skeletal muscle 512
administration techniques, properties determining
boiling point 494
gas versus vapor 491–2
general principles 491
methods of description 492–4
vapor pressure 493–4
adverse drug reactions 7
agent purity and euthanasia 161–2
age-related responses to 1359
alveolar ventilation 498–9
birds 1142–3
cardiac output 509–10
cardiovascular system
arterial blood pressure 510
cardiac rhythm 510
catecholamines 510
concurrent drugs 511
duration of anesthesia 511
factors influencing circulatory effects 510–11
mode of ventilation 510–11
noxious stimulation 511
$PaCO_2$ 510–11
regional blood flow 510
cats 1034
central nervous system, effects on
anatomic sites of action 506–7
cerebral blood flow and cerebral perfusion pressure 507–8
cerebral metabolism 507
electroencephalographic 507
molecular mechanism of action and molecular sites 505–6
cesarean section 960–1
chemical characteristics 490–1
concurrent drugs 509
defining 4
delivery to the alveoli 497–9
dose 502–3
elimination 500–2
end-tidal inhalant partial pressure 244
environmental impact 7
euthanasia 158
factors determining the P_A of anesthetic 497–500
FGF rates 106
inspired concentration 497–8
laboratory animals 1065–7
magnetic resonance imaging 51
malignant hyperthermia 512
marine mammals 1092, 1098
mechanism of action within the CNS
anatomic 506–7
molecular 505–6
minimum alveolar concentration 502–3
and minimum alveolar concentration concept 177
molecular mechanism of action and sites within CNS
background 505–6
lipid and aqueous theories 506
protein 506
neural control of ventilation 721–3
neurologic disease 835
nitrous oxide
diffusion hypoxia 513–14
dose 512–13
interaction with respiratory gas monitoring 514–15
pharmacodynamics 513
pharmacokinetics 513
transfer of N_2O to closed gas spaces 513
noxious stimulation 509, 511
ophthalmic patients 1335
pharmacodynamics 504–12
pharmacokinetics 294–5, 497–501
physical characteristics 491–7
properties determining methods of administration 491–4
properties influencing drug kinetics 494–7
physicochemical characteristics 490–7
respiratory depression and apnea 61–2
respiratory system
arterial carbon dioxide tension 508–9
concurrent drugs 509
duration of 509
factors influencing respiratory effects 509
mode of ventilation 509
surgery/other noxious stimulation 509
trace concentrations 514–15
uptake and elimination of inhalation anesthetics 497–501
waste inhalation anesthetics 514–15
injectable anesthetics 462–88
adverse drug reactions 7
alfaxalone *see* alfaxalone
barbiturates *see* barbiturates
birds 1141–2
buprenorphine 1067
cancer surgery 1371–2
cesarean section 960
chloral hydrate 5, 481, 1068
defining 4
dissociative anesthetics *see* dissociative anesthetics
endotracheal intubation 476
etomidate *see* etomidate
hepatic blood flow 465, 467
ketamine 1067
ketamine-propofol (ketofol) 472–4
laboratory animals 1067–8
magnesium sulfate 481
metomidate 481
naloxone 1067
neural control of ventilation 721–3
non-human primates 1067
ophthalmic patients 1334–5
in pregnancy 960
propofol *see* propofol
ruminants 1271–2
urethane 1068
vasopressin 431
injection pressure monitors 1172
inotropes 961
inspiratory capacity (IC) 698
inspiratory reserve volume (IRV) 698
inspiratory-to-expiratory ratio (I:E), ventilators 122, 131, 132, 134
Institutional Animal Care Committee 161
insulinoma
anesthetic considerations 906–7
anesthetic management 907–8
clinical pathology 906
clinical presentation 906
intercostal nerve block 1179, 1180*f*
interleukin-1 (IL-1) 1218
interleukin-1 receptor antagonist (IRAP) 1017
intermittent boluses 299
intermittent positive-pressure ventilation (IPPV) 79, 97, 109, 123, 205, 1219
International Association for the Study of Pain (IASP) 154, 1010
International Congress of Veterinary Anesthesiology 6
International Organization for Standards (ISO) 75
International Society of Feline Medicine 1033
International Veterinary Academy of Pain Management (IVAPM) 7
interpleural regional analgesia 1181–2
interposed abdominal compression (IAC)-CPR 57
interventions, patient safety 33–7
assessment 37
checklists 33–4
cognitive aids 34–5
communication tools 35–6
engineering solutions 36
medication error, methods for reducing 36–7
simulation-based training 36
see also safety considerations
interviews 29
intestinal neoplasia 877–9
intra-articular block
coxofemoral joint technique 1192
stifle technique 1191–2
intracranial disease 225
intracranial hypertension 835–7
intracranial pressure (ICP) 57, 198
cerebral herniation 67
inhalational anesthesia 508
neurologic disease 829–30
intramuscular (IM) injection 1067
intraocular pressure (IOP) 315
on eyeball 1330
factors affecting 1331*t*
ocular physiology 1330–1, 1331*t*
intraosseous catheter 58
intrapulmonary masses 806
intrapulmonary shunt 720
intrathecal (spinal) anesthesia 1197
intrathoracic pressure (IttP) 57
intrathoracic procedures
anesthesia for 783–8
separation of lungs and one-lung ventilation 786–8
intratracheal delivery 58
intravenous (IV) access

anesthetic recovery 1107
avian anesthesia 1145
clinical situations 1043, 1044
and euthanasia 158, 162
history 5
magnetic resonance imaging 50, 52
ophthalmic surgery 1338
shelter animals 1043–4
in swine 465, 1292, 1294
intravenous catheter 146
intravenous regional anesthesia 1167–8
intrinsic complexity 26
intubation
aids and techniques 84
blind 1058, 1104
blind oral 1271
blowhole 1104
cetaceans 1103–4
endotracheal 16
horses 1224–5
manatees 1105–6
nasotracheal 84, 1271
orotracheal 1290–1
pinnipeds 1104
retrograde 86
ruminants 1270–1
see also endotracheal intubation
invasive blood pressure (IBP)
dynamic response testing and damping 201–2
measurement 199–202
inverted "l" or "7" block 1307
ion channels 285
ionizing radiation hazards 42–3
IPASS technique, postanesthetic hand-offs 35–6
IPPV *see* intermittent positive-pressure ventilation (IPPV)
IRAP *see* interleukin-1 receptor antagonist (IRAP)
IRV *see* inspiratory reserve volume (IRV)
isobolographic studies 306
isoelectricity 180
isoflurane
agent-specific vaporizers 103
amphibians 1119
bronchodilation induced by 803, 804
dogs anesthetized with 323
environmental impact 7
euthanasia 158, 160
face mask, delivered by 1268
laboratory animals 1065, 1067
malignant hyperthermia 68
ophthalmic patients 1335
ruminants 1272
volume percent (vol %) 240–1
isomers 309
isoproterenol (isoprenaline)
cardiovascular system effects 323–4
other effects 324
pharmacokinetics 324
protecting renal blood flow 324
ventilation–perfusion mismatching 324
isoshunt diagram 720
isotonic crystalloids 582–4
IVAPM *see* International Veterinary Academy of Pain Management (IVAPM)

JD Medical LAV-3000 ventilator 138
Journal of Veterinary Anaesthesia and Analgesia 7
just culture 28

ketamine
α_2-adrenergic receptor agonist combined with 162
adverse drug reactions 307
and AEPs 183
age-related responses to 1359
amphibians 1119
birds 1136
and Bispectral Index™ 180
bronchodilation induced by 470, 804
constant rate infusion (CRI) 300, 1014
dissociative anesthesia 4
dogs and cats 1161, 1162
drug dose 1065, 1066*t*
horses 1209
impact of opioid epidemic on veterinary anesthesia 8
injectable 1067
laboratory animals 1066*t*, 1067
marine mammals 1092–3
metabolism 308
morphine–lidocaine–ketamine 182
myoclonus 68
neurologic disease 834–5
and nitrous oxide 184
pigs 1288
postanesthetic hyperthermia 68
rate-controlled infusion (RCI) 300
risk factors 18
ruminants 1268–9
second-tier pain management 1014
and stages of anesthesia 178
wildlife capture 1082
ketamine-acepromazine 1065, 1066*t*
ketamine-dexmedetomidine 1066*t*
ketamine-propofol (ketofol) 472–4
ketamine-xylazine 1066*t*
ketoprofen 1381
Keystone Intensive Care Unit (ICU) Project 33
kidney donor management 946
kidney injury
acute *see* acute kidney injury (AKI)/acute renal failure
NSAIDs, adverse effects 410–11
see also renal clearance; renal disease; renal function; renal system
kidney recipient management 946–8
kinematic gait 1001
Klebsiella pneumoniae 142
Korotkoff sounds 203
Kussmaul's sign 205

laboratory animals
airway management 1070–1
anatomic and physiologic considerations 1070
anesthetics and analgesics 1065–70
commonly used 1066*t*
local and regional 1069–70
anti-inflammatory drugs 1069
body temperature 1072
body temperature maintenance 1072
breathing systems 1071–2
drug administration 1070
fluid therapy 1072
gabapentin 1070
handling and restraint 1070
inhalational anesthesia 1065–7
injectable anesthetics 1067–8
neuromuscular blocking agents 1066*t*
nociception 978
non-human primates 1073–4
opioids 1068–9
pain management 1069
postoperative care 1072, 1073*t*
pregabalin 1070
rodents and lagomorphs 1070–2
selected primate species 1066*t*
small mammals 1066*t*
lactated Ringer's solution (LRS) 1218
lagomorphs 1070–2
laparotomy, anesthesia for 871–3
in horses 1250–1
infiltration anesthesia 1251
paravertebral thoracolumbar anesthesia 1251
LAPS *see* low atmospheric pressure stunning (LAPS)
large animals
anesthetic morbidity 14
anesthetic mortality 18–20
causes of 19
risk factors 20
risk of 18–19
timing of death 19–20
history of veterinary anesthesia 5
ICU Medical (formerly Surgivet) DHV1000 large animal ventilator 136–7
Narkovet-E Large Animal Anesthesia Control Center 133, 134
laryngeal mask airways (LMAs) *see* supraglottic airway devices (SGADs)
laryngoscopes 83–4, 1104
biomedical engineering 172
infection prevention and control 145
veterinary-specific 83, 84
laryngospasm 62
laser procedures
ALARA ("as low as reasonably achievable") principle 43
anesthetic considerations 41–2
Argon lasers 40
backscattering 40
classification 40
continuous laser Doppler flowmetry 238
laser beam hazard and safety 40–1
laser fire hazard and safety 41, 42*f*
laser–tissue interactions 42
Nd:YAG lasers 40, 42
non-beam hazards and safety 42
ocular damage, risk of 40–1

laser procedures (*cont'd*)
personnel occupational exposure 43
radiation, protection from 43
surgery, anesthetic considerations 41–2
LAST *see* local anesthetic systemic toxicity (LAST)
lateral caudal subcutaneous vein (LCSV) 1098, 1100–1, 1100*f*
lateral pharyngotomy 87
lead system, electrocardiography 187–9
learning culture 28
left atrial (LA) enlargement 272
left ventricular (LV) pressure 205
levobupivaine, and local anesthesia 540
LiDCO™ system, cardiac output monitoring 214, 215
lidocaine
cardiopulmonary arrest 58
dermal patches and eutectic creams 540–1
dogs and cats 1162
horses 1209
and infection control 148
intrathecal 162
and local anesthesia 539, 540–1
neurologic disease 833–4
pain management 1015
toxicity 466
lidocaine/bupivacaine gel (Tri-Solfen) 541
life support *see* cardiopulmonary resuscitation (CPR)
ligands
affinity and activity of 284
agonist 285
classical receptor theory 283
classified as a neutral antagonist 284
endogenous 285
selectivity and specificity of 284
Light Amplification by Stimulated Emission of Radiation *see* laser procedures
limbs, equine: anesthesia of 1239–50
continuous delivery of local anesthetics for lower limb analgesia 1258
intra-articular and intrabursal 1245–50
perineural 1240–4
line infiltration block 1307
lipopolysaccharide (LPS) 1217
liposome-encapsulated bupivacaine (Nocita®) 541
lithium dilution 214–15
live animals, reducing use of in teaching 174
liver disease
blood flow 848, 849*f*, 850
diagnostic or minimally invasive procedures, anesthetic considerations 857–8
gallbladder and extrahepatic biliary tract pathology 857
hepatic lobe torsion 857
hepatic pathophysiology and anesthetic management 855–7
hepatitis 855–6
interventional radiology 858
laparoscopic procedures 857–8
laparotomy 858
neoplasia 856–7
NSAIDs, effects of 411–12
pain management in hepatobiliary diseases 858
patient health assessment 10
portosystemic shunt 856
ultrasound-guided biopsy 857
see also hepatic blood flow (HBF); hepatic clearance; hepatic functions; hepatic lobe torsion; hepatic system
Liverpool Osteoarthritis in Dogs (LOAD) scale 1005, 1006
llamas 1272
doxapram 423
endotracheal intubation 1059*f*
genetically coded changes 739
opioids 377
pregnancy-associated changes 965
tiletamine–zolazepam 1015
tramadol 437
see also camelids
LOAD *see* Liverpool Osteoarthritis in Dogs (LOAD) scale
local anesthesia 526–52
additives 1169
adverse effects
allergic reactions 545
local toxicity 544
methemoglobinemia 544–5
systemic toxicity 541–4
toxicosis (oral ingestion) 545
aminoamides 539–40
aminoesters 538–9
birds 1141
cancer pain 1372–3
cesarean section 961, 965
clinical pharmacology 531–8
mixtures of local anesthetics 537–8
pharmacokinetics 531–7
tachyphylaxis 538
defining 4
equine 1235–61
history 5
and infection control 148–9
laboratory animals 1069–70
mixtures of local anesthetics 537–8
ophthalmic patients 1337–8
pharmacokinetics
absorption 531–2
additives 535–7
distribution 532–3
excretion 534
factors affecting 534–5
metabolism 533–4
pharmacology 526–31, 1166
blockade of neural tissue, mechanism 528–30
chemical structure 530
clinical 531–8
molecular mechanism of action 526–8
physicochemical properties 530–1
specific drugs and clinical uses 538–41
ruminant and pig local anesthetic and analgesic techniques 1301–3
special formulations 540–1
toxicity 66
local anesthetic systemic toxicity (LAST) 1167, 1171, 1181, 1198
locoregional anesthesia
blocks
failure 1181, 1190, 1236, 1309
head 1174–8
nerve 1168–9
of pelvic limb 1188–92
of thoracic limb 1185–8
thoracic paravertebral 1179
of thorax and abdomen 1178–85
cancer pain 1372–3
catheters 1171–2
classification 1167–8
complexity 1166–7
complications 1197–8
in dogs and cats 1166–204
equipment 1170–4
in horses 1227
injection pressure monitors 1172
intravenous regional 1167–8
local anesthetic systemic toxicity 1167, 1181, 1198
local infiltration 1167
needles 1170–1
neuraxial techniques 1168, 1192–7
neuronal damage 1198
peripheral nerve blocks 1168
peripheral nerve stimulators 1172–3
physiology of nerve blockade 1168–9
preparation 1169–70
topical 1167
ultrasound 1173–4
see also local anesthesia; regional anesthesia
London Protocol model, incident evolution 30
LOP *see* loss of position (LOP)
LORR *see* loss of the righting reflex (LORR)
loss of position (LOP) 155, 156, 158, 159
loss of the righting reflex (LORR) 155, 156
low atmospheric pressure stunning (LAPS) 156, 160–1
lower airway disease, and anesthesia 802–3
lower limit of quantification (LLOQ) 295
low-pressure baroreceptor reflex 655
low-threshold mechanoreceptors (LTMRs) 1024
LTMRs *see* low-threshold mechanoreceptors (LTMRs)
lubricants 148
lumbar plexus block 1188–9
lung consolidation 268–9
lung pulse 259–60
lung sliding (glide sign) 259
lung volumes 698, 699*f*, 699*t*
birds 1130–1
and pulmonary ventilation 725–7
lungs
endotracheal tubes for isolation of one 78–82
mechanics 727–8
one-lung ventilation 786–8
reptiles 1112
separation of 786–8
ventilator-induced injury 778, 780

lusitropy 198
lymphatic endothelial cells (LECs) 642
lymphatic system 582, 616, 642, 880
  amphibians 1117
  cardiovascular physiology 641–2
  mechanotransduction 1025
  reptiles 618
lyophilized platelets (LYO) 598

M&MCs *see* morbidity and mortality conferences (M&MCs)
machines *see* equipment
MacIntosh blade, laryngoscopes 83, 84*f*
Magellan robotic-assisted ultrasound-guided system 174
magnesium sulfate 481
magnetic resonance imaging (MRI) 46–52
  anesthetic management considerations 50
  blood oxygen level-dependent (BOLD) MRI 157
  "breath-hold/ apnea" technique 50
  burns 49
  classification 49
  cryogens 49–50
  ear plugs 49
  emergency procedures 52
  gadolinium-based contrast agents 52
  gradient magnetic fields 49, 51
  hazards for staff and patients 46–8
  helium vapor 50
  hypothermia risk 52
  Magnetic Resonance Safety Officer 49
  noise reduction rating 49
  patient monitoring 51–2
  personnel considerations 52
  positioning devices 50
  radiofrequency 46, 49, 51
  receiver coils 46*f*, 51
  routine scan 50
  safety screening guidelines 48
  sedation versus general anesthesia 50–1
  small animals 50
  standing equine MRI 52
  strong static magnetic field 46–9, 48*f*, 49
  superconducting high-field-strength magnets 49
  T2-weighted 824
  transdermal patches 49
  ventilators 51
  see also functional magnetic resonance imaging (fMRI)
mainstream monitors, gas sampling 241
maintenance of anesthesia
  in cats 1163
  in dogs 1163
  hepatic blood flow 1208
  in horses
    adjunct agents 1225–7
    hepatic blood flow 1208
    locoregional anesthesia 1227
    monitoring 1227–8
    ventilation strategies 1228
  in pigs 1291–3
  in ruminants 1271–3
malignant hyperthermia (MH)
  in farm animals 1060–1
  inhalational anesthesia 512
  in pigs 1060–1, 1295
Mallard Medical Model 2400V ventilator 127–8
Mallard Medical Rachel Model 2800 series ventilator 134–6
manatees
  intubation 1104–5
  vascular access 1102
mandibular techniques, head blocks 1236
  anatomy 1175–6
  indications for 1176
  technique 1176–7
mandrake (*Mandragora officinalis*) 314
mannitol
  cerebral herniation 67
  post resuscitation care 60
  prolonged anesthetic recovery 69
manual resuscitators 139
manufacturer's instructions for use (MIFU). 145
MAP *see* mean arterial pressure (MAP)
marine mammals 1091–109
  airway management 1102–5
  anesthetic recovery 1106–7
  Antillean manatee 1093
  Bötzinger complex (BötC) 1092
  breathing 1092–3
  caudal veins 1102
  cephalic veins 1102
  cetaceans 1092, 1098, 1099–101
  classification 1091
  dive reflex 1106
  dolphins *see* dolphins
  fissipeds 1091
  flukes 1099, 1102
  harbor seal 1091
  inhalational anesthesia 1092, 1098
  lateral caudal subcutaneous vein (LCSV) 1098, 1100–1
  median artery 1101
  monitoring and supportive care 1105–6
  odobenid anesthesia 1099
  otariid anesthesia 1098–9
  periarterial vascular rete (PAVR) 1099–101
  permissive/intentional hypercapnia 1095
  phocid anesthesia 1098
  pinnipeds 1091, 1092, 1093, 1098–9, 1101–2
  preanesthetic assessment and planning 1095–7
  protocols 1097–9
  sea lions 1091
  sedation and anesthesia 1097–8
  sirenians 1091–2, 1099
  sleep 1093
  symmetrical slow-wave sleep (BSWS) 1093
  vascular access
    cetacean 1099–101
    manatee 1102
    pinnipeds 1101–2
  ventilation 1093–5
  see also marine mammals
marmosets 1073
maropitant 425–7, 1016
mask delivery 87–9
mass spectrometry 224, 241, 243
massive transfusion (MT) 600
mast cell tumors (MCT) 877, 878, 879, 1032
matrix metalloproteinases (MMPs) 1218
Matrx/Midmark 3000/3002 PRO ventilator 126–7
mavacoxib 1381
maxillary techniques, head blocks 1236–7
  anatomy 1174–5
  indications for 1175
  technique 1175
  see also head blocks
maximum working pressure limit (MOPL) 126–7
MEA *see* mean electrical axis (MEA)
mean absolute error (MAE) 171–2
mean absolute percentage error (MAPE) 172
mean arterial pressure (MAP) 13, 57, 59, 60, 197–8, 199, 203, 204, 1148
mean electrical axis (MEA) 191–2
mean squared error (MSE) 172
mechanical ventilation during anesthesia 755–82
  airway resistance compliance 772–3, 775*f*
  assisted and assisted-controlled 768–70
  atelectasis, strategies for reducing 773–4, 775*f*, 776–7
  continuous mandatory ventilation 764–8
  dual-controlled 767–8
  effects on cardiovascular function 777–8, 777*f*
  evolution of mechanical ventilators 756–64
  in humans and veterinary species 780–2
  modes of 764–70
  monitoring pulmonary mechanics during 770–3
  pressure support 768–70
  pressure-controlled 767
  pressure-volume (P–V) loops 770–2, 773*f*
  respiratory system compliance 772–3, 775*f*
  spontaneous intermittent mandatory 770
  ventilator-induced lung injury 778, 780
  volume-controlled 765–7
  see also ventilation
mechanotransduction 1025
medetomidine 325, 338–44, 1083, 1097, 1266
  clinical considerations 343–4
  drug dose 1065, 1066*t*
  indications for 338–9
  mechanism of action 338–9
  medetomidine–vatinoxan combination (Zenalpha®) 347, 1015
  pharmacodynamics 340–3
  pharmacokinetics 339–40
  premedication 473
medetomidine-midazolam 1066*t*
medetomidine-midazolam-fentanyl 1066*t*
median prediction error (*MDPE*) 303
medical devices, Spaulding's classification of 144–5
medical gases
  anesthetic monitoring *see* anesthetic gas monitoring
  arterial blood gas analysis 173, 232–3
  color coding 92–3

medical gases (*cont'd*)
  common outlet 104
  control of ventilator driving gas 122
  diameter index safety system (DISS) 92, 93
  gas flow within machine 94–6
  gas versus vapor 491–2
  pin index safety system (PISS) 92, 93, 94*f*
  pressure gauges 94
  pressure-reducing valve (regulator) 94
  safety 92–3
  supply 91–4
  waste anesthetic gases 7
medication error, methods for reducing 36–7
medicinal stem cells (MSCs) 1384
megaesophagus 873–4
melatonin 1034
meloxicam 541, 1073*t*, 1381–2
memantine 431–2
mental nerve block 1236
meperidine (pethidine) 380, 1031
mepivacaine 539
"Mercedes and the whale view," right parasternal short-axis views 272
metabolic acidosis 68, 250, 320, 414, 429, 503, 564, 567, 583, 702, 721, 1223, 1295
  severe 58, 559, 949, 1274
metabolism
  amphibians 1117
  cerebral 507
  mammalian cardiovascular system 620
  pain management 1026
  reptiles 1111
  smooth muscle 638
metabolites, transport of (Phase III biotransformation) 308–9
metamizole 408
metaraminol 326
methadone 377–8
  dosage
    cats 377
    dogs 377
    horses 377–8
    laboratory animals 1069
    ruminants 377–8
methane 243
methemoglobin (MetHb) 233
methemoglobinemia 544–5
methicillin-resistant *S. aureus* (MRSA) postsurgical infection 142, 149
methicillin-resistant *S. pseudintermedius* (MRSP) 147
methocarbamol 427
methohexital, pharmacokinetics 464
methoxamine, and local anesthesia 536
methoxyflurane 489, 511
methylnaltrexone 384
metoclopramide 427–8
metomidate 481
metoprolol 329
MG *see* myasthenia gravis (MG)
MGCS *see* modified Glasgow coma scale (MGCS)
MH *see* malignant hyperthermia (MH)
mice
  brain 160
  euthanasia 159, 161
  osteoarthritis (OA) 985
Michaelis-Menton kinetics 290
midazolam 1033
  birds 1136
  and blood–brain-barrier 336–7
  clinical considerations 337–8
  dogs and cats 1161
  drug dose 1065, 1066*t*
  indications for 336
  marine mammals 1097, 1098
  mechanism of action 336
  pharmacodynamics 337
  pharmacokinetics 336–7
middle latency auditory evoked potential (MLAEP) 183
Miller blade, laryngoscopes 83, 84*f*
minimum alveolar concentration (MAC) 156, 176–7
  anesthetic gas monitoring 240, 244
  birds 1137, 1142–3
  cats 1033, 1034, 1035
  drug interactions 306
  and epinephrine 321
  inhalational anesthetics 502–3
  laboratory animals 1067, 1070
  opioid effects 372–3
  ruminants 1272, 1273
mink 159
minute ventilation (V_I) 698
mitochondrial redox state 238
mitral valve insufficiency/regurgitation 683–6
mixed venous oxygen partial pressure 233
MLAAEP *see* middle latency auditory evoked potential (MLAEP)
model-independent analysis 297
modified Glasgow coma scale (MGCS) 182
molecular mechanism of action
  inhalational anesthesia and CNS
    background 505–6
    lipid and aqueous theories 506
    protein 506
  local anesthesia 526–8
monitoring of anesthesia/surgery
  amphibians 1119
  anesthetic depth 176–86
  birds 1145–8
  cardiopulmonary arrest 59–60
  electrophysiologic 179–80
  equipment 145
  evolution of monitoring equipment and guidelines 173
  horses 1210, 1227–8
  infection prevention and control 145
  magnetic resonance imaging 51–2
  marine mammals 1105–6
  mechanical ventilation, pulmonary mechanics 770–3
  medical gases *see* anesthetic gas monitoring
  neonatal/pediatric patients 1350
  non-human primates 1073
  pigs 1293–4
  respiratory gas, interaction with nitrous oxide 514–15
  ruminants 1275–7
  shelter animals 1043–4
  ventilators 123
  wildlife capture 1085–7
monoclonal antibodies 1013
Monte Carlo approaches 298
MOPL *see* maximum working pressure limit (MOPL)
morbidity, anesthetic
  large animals 14
  morbidity and mortality conferences (M&MCs) 29–30
  small animals 13–14
morbidity and mortality conferences (M&MCs) 29–30
morphine 373–7
  dosage
    birds 1138
    cats 376
    dogs 374–6
    horses 376
    pigs 1288
  effects on opioid-induced tolerance 363
  food and fiber animals 376–7
  intraoperative analgesia 1273
  premedication 369, 426, 480
mortality
  anesthetic *see* mortality, anesthetic
  capture-associated 1088
  see also morbidity and mortality conferences (M&MCs)
mortality, anesthetic
  birds 1127
  causes 15–16
  defining anesthetic deaths 15
  large animals 14, 18–20
  perioperative deaths 32*t*
  risk factors 16–18
  risk of 14–15
  small animals 14–18
  timing of death 16
mouth rinse plungers 145
MRI *see* magnetic resonance imaging (MRI)
MS-222 *see* tricaine methanesulfonate (MS-222)
MT *see* massive transfusion (MT)
multidrug resistance (MDR)-1 gene 306, 1031
multidrug resistance-associated protein (MRP) 308
multigas analyzers, mainstream 241
muscarinic receptors 314, 315*t*
muscle
  drug effects
    dissociative anesthetics 471
    etomidate 476
    propofol 467
  skeletal 512
muscle relaxants 1209–10
"mushroom view," right parasternal short-axis views 272
myasthenia gravis (MG) 839–40
myelinated somatic sensory fibers 1024
myelography 44, 45
myelomalacia 69–70
myocardial oxygenation 237

myoclonus 54
  benzodiazepines 68, 476, 834
myopathy 1055
myotoxicity 544

nalbuphine 383–4, 1137
naloxone 69, 285, 384
  injectable 1067
naltrexone 384
NARCO *see* Neurological, Airway, Respiratory, Cardiovascular and Other (NARCO) score,
narcosis 4
Narcotrend® index 183
Narkovet E-2 Large Animal Anesthesia System 134
Narkovet-E Electronic Large Animal Control Center 134
Narkovet-E Large Animal Anesthesia Control Center 133, 134
nasal catheter 227, 1086
nasal insufflation 89–90
nasal passages and block 1306–7
nasogastric tube 1228
nasotracheal intubation 84
National Curriculum for Canadian Anesthesia Residency 255
National Institute for Health and Care Excellence (NICE) 11
nausea and vomiting 864–5
NAVAS *see* North American Veterinary Anesthesia Society (NAVAS)
Nd:YAG lasers 40, 42
near-infrared spectroscopy (NIRS) 237
needles
  accidental penetration 7
  locoregional anesthesia 1170–1
  peripheral nerve stimulators 1173
  spinal 1171
  Tuohy needle 1101
  visualization of 1171
negative-pressure scavenge systems 112–13
neonatal/pediatric patients 1348–53
  anesthesia
    circumstances warranting 1348–9
    considerations 955–68
    dissociative anesthetics 471
    management 1350–1
    monitoring of anesthesia 1350
    patient preparation 1350
    risk assessment 1348
  barbiturates 465
  bradycardia 965
  cardiovascular system 1349
  care of the newborn 965–966
  central nervous system 1349–50
  characteristics 1349–50
  hematologic system 1350
  hepatic system 1349
  pediatric and neonatal periods, defining 1348
  recovery 1350–1
  renal system 1349
  respiratory system 1349
  supportive care 1350
  thermoregulation 1350
neoplasia, hepatic 856–7
nephrotoxicity 502, 511, 512, 618, 1045
  melamine-associated 931
nerve growth factor (NGF) 1013
nervous system
  fish 1121
  opioids 369–70
  somatic 827
  see also autonomic nervous system (ANS); central nervous system (CNS); neurologic disease; parasympathetic nervous system (PNS); sympathetic nervous system (SNS)
neural control of ventilation 700–2
  influence of anesthetic drugs on 721–5
    inhalant and injectable 721–3
    opioids 724–5
    sedatives and hypnotics 723–4
neuraxial anesthesia/analgesia 148–9, 1168, 1192–7, 1253–8
  anatomy 1192, 1193*f*, 1194
  catheter placement 1197
  contraindications 1192, 1193*t*
  epidural technique 1194, 1195*f*
    caudal epidural 1254
    complications 1257–8
    continuous caudal epidural 1254, 1255*f*
    medications 1254–7
  indications and contraindications 1253–4
  intrathecal (spinal) anesthesia 1197
  novel regional techniques
    caudal intercostal block, abdominal surgery 1258
    continuous delivery of local anesthetics for lower limb analgesia 1258
    transversus abdominis plane (TAP) block 1015, 1183–4, 1227, 1258
neuroengineering 170
neurohormonal mechanisms, cardiovascular physiology 656–8
neuroleptanalgesia, cesarean section 960
neuroleptic drugs 1084
neurologic disease 10, 822–46
  a_2-adrenergic receptor agonists 833
  alfaxalone 834
  anatomy of the nervous system 822–9
  benzodiazepines 833
  central nervous system 822–5
    anatomy 822–5
    brain physiology 829–30
    specific conditions, pathophysiology and anesthetic management 835–9
    spinal cord physiology 832
  cervical spondylomyelopathy, in horses 839
  effects of vasoactive drugs, sedatives and anesthetics 832–5
  etomidate 834
  inhalational anesthesia 835
  intracranial hypertension 835–7
  ketamine 834–5
  lidocaine 833–4
  neuromuscular blocking agents 835
  opioids 832–3
  peripheral nervous system 825–9, 839–40
  phenothaizines 334–5, 833
  propofol 834
  seizures 837–8
  specific conditions, pathophysiology and anesthetic management 835–40
  spinal cord injury and spine surgery 838–9
  see also central nervous system (CNS); nervous system
Neurological, Airway, Respiratory, Cardiovascular and Other (NARCO) score, 11
neuromuscular blockade
  differential 1169
  factors affecting duration and recovery from 456
  local anesthesia 528–30
  monitoring neuromuscular transmission 453–6
    muscle selection 455–6
  pharmacology and nomenclature 450–2
  residual, risk minimization 458
  reversal of 456–8
    acetylcholinesterase inhibitors 456–7
    reversal of succinylcholine 457–8
    selective relaxant binding agents 457
  see also blocks; neuromuscular blocking agents (NMBAs)
neuromuscular blocking agents (NMBAs)
  age-related responses to 1360
  birds 1143
  cesarean section 961
  depolarizing 452–6
  history 452–3
  laboratory animals 1066*t*
  neurologic disease 835
  novel nondepolarizing agents 453–6
  ophthalmic patients 1335–6
  in veterinary anesthesia 448
neuromuscular junction (NMJ)
  anatomy and physiology 449
  depolarization 827
neuromyopathy 1055
neuropathic pain 985, 988–9*t*
neuroscience, non-human primates in 1074
neurosteroids 1084
neurotoxicity 431, 544, 1169, 1171
New World monkeys 1073
NHPs *see* non-human primates (NHPs)
NIBP *see* non-invasive method of measuring BP (NIBP)
NICE *see* National Institute for Health and Care Excellence (NICE)
nicotinamide adenine dinucleotide (NAD) 238
nicotinic acetylcholine receptor (nAChR) 314
  neuronal 506
nicotinic acetylcholine receptors 314
nitrogen 92, 126, 156, 1221
  alveolar 726
  blood urea nitrogen (BUN) 802, 851, 905, 926, 945, 957, 1350
  and carbon dioxide elimination 705
  excretion 1121
  expired concentration 727

nitrogen (*cont'd*)
high-expansion foams containing 159, 161
impaired ventilation–perfusion matching 1220
and infrared radiation 223, 243
inhaled anesthetics 506, 511, 513
nitrogen-containing bisphosphonates (NBPs) 1369
and norepinephrine 321
open-circuit washout 726
and oxygen therapy 752
partial pressure of 705
physiology of body fluids 581
piezoelectric analysis 244
pulmonary ventilation 702, 703, 705, 706, 726
and remifentanil 380
serum urea 511
single-breath washout 705, 706, 727, 781
wasting 910
nitrous oxide
avoiding 42
birds 1143
diffusion hypoxia 513–14
dose 512–13
environmental impact 7
and history of anesthesia 5
inappropriate for euthanasia 156
interaction with respiratory gas monitoring 514–15
pharmacodynamics 513
pharmacokinetics 513
pigs 1291
and SNS 513
toxicity 512
transfer of N_2O to closed gas spaces 513
NLME *see* nonlinear mixed effects (NLME) modeling
NMBA *see* neuromuscular blocking agents (NMBAs)
NMDA *see* *N*-methyl-D-aspartate (NMDA)
N-methyl-D-aspartate (NMDA) 155–6
cancer pain 1367
colic, in horses 1226
marine mammals 1092
osteoarthritis 1382
receptors 162, 286–7, 1014
nociception 4
biomarkers 978
experimental animal 978
fish 1121
limitations of current animal models 978
models 977–9
nociceptive and pain assays 978–9
nocifensive responses 1116
pathways 154–5
phasic pain tests 978–9
receipt, encoding, and transmission of nociceptive information 972
receptors 1116
reptiles 1114–16
site of stimulus application 979
stimulus modalities 979, 980–3*t*
structures, nociceptive 1116
translational pain models 978
see also pain
nociceptive withdrawal reflexes (NWRs) 979
"nodule" sign, partial lung consolidation 268–9
noise reduction rating (NRR), MRI 49
non-human primates (NHPs) 1073–4
anesthetic considerations 1073
endotracheal intubation 1073
equipment 1073
equipment and monitoring 1073
injectable anesthetics 1067
methadone 1069
monitoring of anesthesia 1073
in neuroscience 1074
neuroscience, non-human primates in 1074
pain assessment and management 1074
postoperative care 1073*t*
preanesthetic considerations 1073
recovery 1073–4
see also non-human primates (NHPs)
non-invasive method of measuring BP (NIBP) 202, 203, 204
nonlinear mixed effects (NLME) modeling 295
non-steroidal anti-inflammatory drugs (NSAIDs)
acetaminophen (paracetamol) 407–8
acute pain 1011
adverse effects 408–12
animal versus human risks 412
blood coagulation 412
cartilage, injury to 412
gastrointestinal injury 408–10
kidney injury 410–11
platelet inhibition abnormalities 412
thrombotic 412
adverse events 1380
and allometric scaling 1136
birds 1139–41
cancer pain 1367
cats 1035
chronic pain 1013
colic, in horses 1218
contraindications 1380
data analysis 299
dipyrone (metamizole) 408
drug selection
for cats 414
classification and pharmacological parameters 399–402*t*
COX-2 inhibition as selection criterion 412–13
for dogs 413–14
for food animals 415
for horses 414–15
fluid therapy 415
grapiprant 406–7
laboratory animals 1069
mechanism of action 398, 403–5
COX-1 versus COX-2 inhibitors 404–5
mechanisms possible 404
metabolism of arachidonic acid 398, 403–4
non-traditional, unique features 406–8
ophthalmic patients 1338
osteoarthritis 1379–82
overdose 66
pharmacokinetic properties 405–6
pharmacokinetic-pharmacodynamic properties 406
ruminants 1268
spay-neuter programs 1044, 1045
specific 1381
stereoisomerism 406
toxicity 939, 1139, 1380
in vivo assessment of PK-PD models 406
washout period between 1380–1
norbuprenorphine 1031
norepinephrine 287, 321
cardiovascular system effects 321
pharmacokinetics 321
pharmacology of descending controls 976
Normal Accident Theory 26
normothermia 246
North American Veterinary Anesthesia Society (NAVAS) 7
nortriptyline 432–3
pain management 1015
Nottingham Veterinary Safety Culture Survey 28
noxious stimulation, inhalational anesthesia 509, 511
NRR *see* noise reduction rating (NRR), MRI
NSAIDs *see* non-steroidal anti-inflammatory drugs (NSAIDs)
numerical rating scales 1002

obesity 1023, 1026, 1030
occular damage, risk from laser treatment 40–1
occupational exposure
laser procedures 43
risk assessment 7
waste inhalation anesthetics 514–15
Occupational Safety and Health Administration (OSHA), United States 41, 49
ocular adnexa 1327–8
ocular pain
analgesics 1337–8
management 1336–8
origin 1336–7
oculocardiac reflex 655, 1332–3
odobenid anesthesia 1099
Office for Laboratory Animal Welfare (OLAW) 161
Ohio V5A ventilator 128–9
Ohmeda 7000 and 7800 series electronic anesthesia ventilators 129–30
Ohmeda Rascal II 243
OLAW *see* Office for Laboratory Animal Welfare (OLAW)
omega-3- fatty acids 1013, 1023, 1379
omeprazole 423–4
ondansetron 428
ophthalmic patients 1327–47
anatomy 1177
anesthesia
anesthetic adjuvants 1335–6
auriculopalpebral nerve block 1237
contralateral eye, protecting 1340
electroretinogram, impact on 1338
endotracheal intubation 1339–40

general 1338–40
inhalational 1335
injectable 1334–5
monitoring of anesthesia 1340
neuromuscular blockade 1340
ocular complications related to 1340
physical restraint, premedication, and anesthetic induction 1339
preoperative assessment 1338
recovery, extubation and emergence 1340
sensory nerve blocks 1237–9
set up and patient positioning 1338–9
topical 1237
aqueous humor (AH) 1328–30
production and drainage 1331
episcleral venous pressure (EVP) 1331
equine 1237–9, 1340–2
head blocks 1177–8
intraocular contents, volume 1331
local anesthesia 1337–8
non-steroidal anti-inflammatory drugs 1338
ocular anatomy 1327–9
globe 1328–9
ocular adnexa 1327–8
ocular circulation 1329
ocular innervation 1329
orbit 1327
ocular barriers 1332
ocular pain
analgesics 1337–8
management 1336–8
origin 1336–7
ocular physiology 1329–33
aqueous humor 1328, 1329–30, 1331
cranial nerves 1329*t*
effects of anesthetic drugs and adjuvants on 1333–6
intraocular pressure 1330, 1331*t*
lens 1328
ocular barriers 1322
oculocardiac reflex 1332–3
pupil size 1331
tear production and drainage 1331–2
uvea 1329
vitreous humor 1328, 1330
ocular rigidity 1331
oculocardiac reflex 655, 1332–3
ophthalmic medications, systemic effects 1333
opioid-induced effects 371
sedatives 1334
techniques 1178
opioid agonist–antagonists, mixed
butorphanol 382–3
nalbuphine 383–4
opioid agonists
full
alfentanil 380–1
butorphanol, interactions with 383
carfentanil 380–1
etorphine 380–1
fentanyl *see* fentanyl
hydrocodone 381
hydromorphone 377
meperidine 380
methadone 377–8
morphine 373–7
oxycodone 381
oxymorphone 378
remifentalanil 380
sufentanil 380
thiafentanil 380–1
partial 381–2
opioid antagonists 384
wildlife capture 1082
opioid receptors
localization 359–60
opioid receptor–opioid drug interactions 360
regulation 359
opioids 355–97
age-related changes 1359
amphibians 1120
analgesia 1337
antagonists 384
cancer pain 1367, 1372
cats, 382, 1034–5 1160*t*, 1163
cesarean section 959–60
clinical effects
analgesia 364–6
antitussive 371
cancer metastasis 371–2
cardiovascular 367
dysphoria 366–7
euphoria 366–7
gastrointestinal 367–8
immune system 371–2
minimum alveolar concentration 372–3
nervous system 369–70
ophthalmic 371
renal 370–1
respiratory 367
sedation 366–7
thermoregulatory 371
crisis in North America 356–8
dependence 363
diversion 356–8
dogs 381–2, 1160*t*, 1163
drug dose 1068
epidural 1279
full agonists *see* opioid agonists
history of use in veterinary practice 355–6
horses 1209
impact on veterinary anesthesia 8
and infection control 148
intravenous high-dose induction 1163
laboratory animals 1068–9
local anesthetic additives 1169
misuse and abuse in veterinary practice 356–8
mixed opioid agonist–antagonists 382–4
multitargeting molecules 384–5
neural control of ventilation 724–5
neurologic disease 832–3
"opioid-induced hyperalgesia" (OIH) 364
osteoarthritis 1382
overdose deaths 8
partial agonists *see* opioid agonists
pharmacokinetics
absorption 360, 362
distribution 362
excretion 363
metabolism 362–3
pharmacology 358–63
clinical 364–73
of descending controls 976–7
premedication 425
prolonged anesthetic recovery 69
receptors 358–60
ruminants 1267
scheduling 356
selected pharmacokinetic parameters of some clinically relevant opioids 360–1*t*
short-acting 1068
tolerance 363
traditional administration routes 373
tramadol *see* tramadol
veterinary shopping 356–8
wildlife capture 1081–2
withdrawal 363–4
optic nerve sheath diameter (ONSD) 256
optical density (OD) 41*f*
oral administration 4
orbicularis oculi muscles, muscle one 1331
orbital fissure 1327
organic anion transporting polypeptide 2 (OATP2) 308
organizational safety culture 27–8
oscillometric blood pressure measurement 203–4
OSHA *see* Occupational Safety and Health Administration (OSHA), United States
osteoarthritis (OA) 1000, 1010, 1377–89
alleviation of pain 1011
autologous protein solution 1384
cell-based therapies 1384
chronic pain, treatment strategies 1378–84
complementary treatments 1383
diagnosis 1378
in dogs and cats 1013
evidence for agents modifying in companion animals 1016
exercise modification 1379
in horses 1016
non-response to standard treatment 1384–5
non-steroidal anti-inflammatory drugs 1379–82
nutritional support 1379
omega-3- fatty acids 1379
pharmacology 1379–84
physical therapy 1379
terminology 1377
weight reduction/management 1379
Overall Quality of Life Score 1006
oxybuprocaine 538
oxycodone 381
oxygen
administration techniques
cages 90–1
mask delivery 87–9
nasal insufflation 89–90
toxicity 91
tracheal insufflation 90

oxygen (*cont'd*)
arterial content 737–40
concentrators 1078
consumption 232, 653–4
content 232
delivery 232, 653–4
extraction ratio 232
inspired and expired concentrations 236–7
measuring hemoglobin saturation with 233–6
measuring partial pressure 232–3
medical gas supply 92
oxyhemoglobin dissociation curve and Bohr effect 738–9
polarographic analysis 236
supplementation 89, 752–5, 1043
high-flow systems 754–5
low-flow systems 752–3, 754*f*
modern ventilators 761–4
supply failure 67
toxicity 91, 753, 755, 1073
transport 737–40
oxygen flush valve 104
oxygen therapy
physiologic effects 751–2
supplementation strategies 752–5
toxicity 755
see also oxygen
oxygenation
alveolar gas equation 231–2
arterial blood gas analysis 232–3
continuous laser Doppler flowmetry 238
CO-oximetry 234
hypoxia versus hypoxemia 231–2
inspired and expired oxygen concentrations 236–7
measuring hemoglobin saturation with oxygen 233–6
mitochondrial redox state 238
monitoring 231–9
near-infrared and Raman spectroscopy 237
oxygen consumption 232
oxygen content 232
oxygen delivery 232
oxygen extraction ratio 232
pulse oximetry 234–6
transcutaneous measurement of blood gases 233
visual assessment 232
see also oxygen; oxygen flush valve
oxyhemoglobin dissociation curve 738–9
oxymorphone 378, 472

pacemakers
and anesthesia 674–9
anesthetic management 676–8
artificial 674–5
complications 678
considerations for anesthesia 677–8
modalities 675–6
patient evaluation for 676–7
patients undergoing non-cardiac procedures 678
permanent implantation 677
temporary implantation 677
packed cell volume (PCV) 320, 1219
packed red blood cells 596
$PaCO_2$, and mode of ventilation 510–11
pain
abdominal muscle contraction 990
action potential, transmission 973
acute *see* acute pain
alleviation of 1011
anticipation of 1010–11
assays 978–9
assessment of 1011, 1074
assessment scales *see* pain assessment scales
behavior 979, 985–990
acute pain 995, 997*f*, 998
assessment of spontaneous behaviors 991
chronic pain 1000
biology of sensory transduction 972, 973*t*
cancer-related *see* cancer pain
chronic *see* chronic pain
clinical management and pharmacological treatment of 1010–22
and consciousness 154–5
decision-making tools 1011, 1013–16
defining 4, 154, 971, 1114
dorsal horn, anatomy of 973–5
endocannabinoids 977
ethical considerations 983–4
evaluation in rodents, recent trends 990–1
fast 1116
generator potential, initiation of 973
inflammatory 985, 986–7*t*
injection site 476
maximum stimulus intensity 984
naturally occurring disease models 990
neuronal activity 990
neuropathic 985, 988–9*t*
neurophysiologic endpoints 979
nociception
biomarkers 978
experimental animal 978
limitations of current animal models 978
measurement of nociceptive withdrawal thresholds in companion animals 984–5
models 977–9
nociceptive and pain assays 978–9
pathways 154–5
phasic pain tests 978–9
receipt, encoding, and transmission of nociceptive information 972
site of stimulus application 979
stimulus modalities 979, 980–3*t*
translational pain models 978
novel concept drugs 1017
ocular 1336–8
operant response paradigms, rodents 990
osteoarthritis (OA) *see* osteoarthritis (OA)
outcome measures 979
perception of *see* pain perception
pharmacology of descending controls 976–7
phasic tests 978
physiologic responses 990
physiology and pathophysiology 971–95
place preference paradigm, rodents 990–1
receipt, encoding, and transmission of nociceptive information 972
sensitization 972
slow 1116
spino-bulbo-spinal loop 977
tiers of decision-making tree 1011, 1013–16
first-tier, acute pain 1011
first-tier, chronic pain 1013–15
second tier 1014–15
third tier 1016
tonic control 977
visceral 985, 989*t*
see also analgesia, veterinary; International Association for the Study of Pain (IASP); neuropathic pain; pain faces; pain management; visceral pain
pain assessment scales
factors confounding use of 1005
grimace scales 1003, 1004*t*, 1005*f*
multidimensional 1003, 1004*t*
numerical rating scales 1002
simple descriptive scales 1002
unidimensional 1002
visual analog scales 1002
pain faces 991
grimace scales 1003, 1004*t*, 1005*f*, 1034
Pain Interference Score 1006
pain management
acupuncture 4, 1024
central neuromodulation 1025
electromagnetic therapies 1025
extracorporeal shockwave therapies 1025
in hepatobiliary diseases 858
massage, touch, stretching and exercise 1024
mechanotransduction 1025
metabolism 1026
non-human primates 1074
non-pharmacologic 1023–6
physiology 1023
peripheral cutaneous sensory receptors 1024
peripheral neuromodulation 1024
photobiomodulation therapy 1025
postoperative 966
spinal and supraspinal locations 1025
temperature-related modalities 1024
pain models
induced 985
tonic tests 985
translational 978–9
pain perception 154–5
Pain Severity Score 1006
palpebral fissure 1328
pancreas and kidney 900–8
pancreatitis 908
pancuronium 1066*t*
pantoprazole 423–4
Parabrachial Nucleus/Kolliker-Fuse Complex 367
paracetamol *see* acetaminophen (paracetamol)
paralumbar anesthesia 5

parasympathetic nervous system (PNS) 828–9, 829*f*
and anticholinergics 314
antiemetic therapy 865
balance with sympathetic 999
ECG complex 192
function 828–9
and gastrointestinal tract 862
and hypothalamus 827
transmission, selected effects 827, 828*t*
parathyroid gland 913–15
paravertebral thoracolumbar anesthesia 1251
partial intravenous anesthesia (PIVA) 4, 1208
partial pressure
alveolar to venous difference 500
of carbon dioxide *see* partial pressure of carbon dioxide (PCO_2)
Dalton's law of 240
of oxygen *see* partial pressure of oxygen (PO_2)
partial pressure of carbon dioxide (PCO_2) 13, 222, 225, 231–2, 236, 559, 560*f*, 640, 738*f*, 1113
arterial 334, 472, 478, 659, 830, 1294
end-tidal 761
expired 704*f*, 706*f*
partial pressure of oxygen (PO_2) 232, 595, 640*f*, 1277
alveolar gas equation 231
arterial 87, 232, 233, 478, 830, 1287
inspired 160, 703*f*
measuring 232–3
mixed venous oxygen partial pressure 233
patent ductus arteriosus (PDA) 686–7
pathologic anatomic shunt 720
patient hand-offs 35–6
patient health assessment 10–11
patient safety *see* safety considerations
patient safety evidence, in anesthesia 30–3
Patient Safety Medical Team Training Program, simulation-based training 36
patient state index (PSI) 183
PCO_2, disorders of 568
PCV *see* pressure-controlled ventilation (PCV)
PD *see* peritoneal dialysis (PD)
PDA *see* patent ductus arteriosus (PDA)
PDMPs *see* prescription drug monitoring programs (PDMPs)
peak inspiratory pressure (PIP) 1221
PEEP *see* positive end-expiratory pressure (PEEP)
pelvic area, blocks for regional anesthesia of 1312–14
penis block, dorsal nerve 1314
pudendal 1314, 1315*f*
sacral paravertebral 1313–14
sacrococcygeal or intercoccygeal epidural (caudal epidural) 1312–13
pelvic limb blocks 1188–92
anatomy 1188
femoral/saphenous nerve block 1189–90
intra-articular 1191–2
lumbar plexus block 1188–9
sciatic nerve 1190–1
Penlon AV-S ventilator 131–2
pentobarbital 5
euthanasia 158, 162
pharmacokinetics 464
pentoxifylline 1218
percutaneous arterial catheterization 1277
percutaneous electrical nerve stimulation (PENS) 1025
periaqueductal gray (PAG) 363
periarterial vascular rete (PAVR) 1099–101
pericardial effusion 690
perioperative checklists 143–4
perioperative fluid therapy 588–92
improving the utility of dynamic indices of preload responsiveness 591
Individualized goal-directed 589–91
liberal versus restrictive approach 588–9
and microvasculature 591–2
monitoring fluid balance 589
perioperative thermoregulation *see* thermoregulation
peripheral intravenous catheter 58
peripheral nerve anatomy 1168–9
peripheral nerve blocks 1168
peripheral nerve stimulators 1172–3
peripheral nervous system 825–9, 839–40
peripheral neuromodulation 1024
peripheral vasoconstriction, drug-induced 232
peripherally inserted central catheters (PICCs) 1100, 1101
peritoneal dialysis (PD)
case selection 948–9
procedures and equipment 949–50
perphenazine enanthate 1084
personal protective equipment (PPE). 143, 144
personnel
injury to 70
laser exposure 43
magnetic resonance imaging 52
pethidine *see* meperidine (pethidine)
P-glycoprotein (P-gp) 308, 1031
pH
acid–base physiology 556–9
blood, mechanisms to minimize changes in 558–9
chemical buffers 558–9
renal system 559
respiratory system 559
pharmacodynamics
dissociative anesthesia 470–1
fundamentals 290
inhalational anesthesia 504–12
interactions 306–7
nitrous oxide 513
specific drugs
acepromazine 334–5
alfaxalone 478–9
barbiturates 464–5
detomidine 340–3
dexmedetomidine 340–3
diazepam 337
etomidate 474–6
medetomidine 340–3
midazolam 337
propofol 467
romifidine 340–3
tolazoline 345–7
xylazine 340–3
yohimbine 345–7
zolazepam 337
in vitro assessment of PK-PD models 406
pharmacokinetics
birds 1136
data analysis
compartmental models 296–8
complex models 299
noncompartmental models 298–9
physiologically based pharmacokinetic models (PBPK) 299
dissociative anesthesia 469–70
drug interactions 305–6
experiments in 295–9
data analysis 296–9
experimental design and conduct 296
pharmacokinetic-pharmacodynamic (PK-PD) study 296
POP-PK approach 296, 299, 307
preparation for the study 295–6
standard two-stage (STS) approach 296
first-order rate equation 297
fundamentals 290
of inhalant anesthetic agents 294–5
inhalational anesthesia 294–5, 497–501
linear and nonlinear 295
local anesthesia 531–7
absorption 531–2
additives 535–7
distribution 532–3
excretion 534
factors affecting 534–5
metabolism 533–4
model-independent analysis 297
nitrous oxide 513
non-stochastic 295
norepinephrine 321
opioids
absorption 360, 362
distribution 362
excretion 363
metabolism 362–3
pharmacokinetic interactions 305–6
specific drugs
acepromazine 334
alfaxalone 478
barbiturates 463–4
detomidine 339–40
dexmedetomidine 339–40
diazepam 336–7
dopamine 322
dopexamine 323
ephedrine 326
epinephrine 321
etomidate 474
isoproterenol (isoprenaline) 324
medetomidine 339–40

pharmacokinetics (*cont'd*)
methohexital 464
midazolam 336–7
NSAIDs 405–6
opioids *see above*
pentobarbital 464
phenylephrine 325
propofol 466–7
romifidine 339–40
thiamylal 464
thiopental 464
tolazoline 345
zolazepam 336–7
squares of the errors (SSE) 297
in vitro assessment of PK-PD models 406
xylazine 339–40
yohimbine 345
zero-order delivery/zero-order processes 290, 291
pharmacology 283–313
absorption 294
anticholinergics 314–16
apparent volume of distribution 291–2
bioavailability 294
birds 1135–6
cancer pain 1366–8
cardiopulmonary arrest 58
classical receptor theory 283–5
clinical evaluation of drug effects 287–90
concentration–response relationship 288, 289*f*
effective dose 288, 289*f*
efficacy 288
lethal dose 288, 289*f*
potency 288
therapeutic index 288, 289*f*
toxic dose 288, 289*f*
constant rate delivery 290
constant rate therapy 299
continuous rate therapy 299–305
dialysis, pharmacologic agent clearance 951–2
drug administration routes *see* drug administration
drug combinations 317, 1080–1, 1084, 1269
butorphanol-azaperone-medetomidine (BAM) 1082, 1084
ketamine-acepromazine 1065, 1066*t*
ketamine-dexmedetomidine 1066*t*
ketamine-propofol (ketofol) 472–4
ketamine-xylazine 1066*t*
medetomidine-ketamine 1084
medetomidine-vatinoxan 347, 1015
tiletamine-zolazepam 1082–3, 1087
tramadol-meloxicam 384
xylazine-ketamine 1087
xylazine–ketamine– guaifenesin 1271
xylazine-tiletamine-zolazepam 1084
epidural medications 1254–7
half-life of elimination 291
hepatic clearance 292–3
intermittent boluses 299
local anesthesia 526–31
blockade of neural tissue, mechanism 528–30
chemical structure 530
clinical pharmacology 531–8
molecular mechanism of action 526–8
physicochemical properties 530–1
neuromuscular blockade 450–2
ophthalmic medications 1333
opioids 358–63
osteoarthritis 1379–84
pharmacodynamics, fundamentals 290
pharmacokinetics *see* pharmacokinetics
pharmacologic alterations induced by pregnancy 967–8
protocols 1097–9
computed tomography (CT) 262
fluid therapy 800, 881
Global Warming Protocol (GWP) 1067
HQHVSN practice 1042
London Protocol model, incident evolution 30
marine mammals 1097–9
TFAST 262
wildlife capture 1088
receptor state theory 285
receptor structure 285–7
renal clearance 294
total body clearance 292
wildlife capture 1080–4
see also wildlife capture
phasic pain tests 978
phenothiazines 334–5, 833
phenoxybenzamine 327–8
phentolamine 327
and local anesthesia 536
phenylbutazone 295
phenylephrine
cardiovascular system effects 324
and local anesthesia 536
other effects 324
pharmacokinetics 325
PHEO *see* pheochromocytoma (PHEO)
pheochromocytoma (PHEO)
anesthetic considerations 898–9
anesthetic management 899–900
clinical pathology 898
clinical presentation 898
diagnosis and treatment 898
photoacoustic spectrometry 244
photobiomodulation therapy 1025
photoplethysmography (PPG) 207
physicochemical interactions 305
physiologic anatomic shunt 720
Physiological and Operative Severity Score for the enUmeration of Mortality and morbidity (POSSUM) 11
physiologically based pharmacokinetic models (PBPK) 299
physostigmine 69
PiCCO® (Pulsion Medical Systems), cardiac output monitoring 214, 215
PICCs *see* peripherally inserted central catheters (PICCs)
piezoelectric analysis 244
pigs 1285–300
analgesia 1295–7
anesthesia
endotracheal intubation 1059–60, 1073
fasting prior to 1285
induction of 1288–90
maintenance of 1291–3
preanesthetic evaluation 1285–6
recovery 1295
regional 965
blood typing 599
carbon dioxide stunning 161
drug administration 1055, 1286
drug effects
acepromazine 335
alfaxalone 480
barbiturates 465
detomidine 344
dexmedetomidine 344
dissociative anesthetics 472
etomidate 476
medetomidine 344
parasympatholytic drugs 1287
propofol 468
romifidine 344
xylazine 344
evaluation of distress 156–7
handling and restraint 1285–6
local anesthetic and analgesic techniques 1301–23
castration, blocks for 1317
flank/paralumbar fossa, blocks for regional anesthesia of 1307–10
head, blocks for regional anesthesia of 1303–7
limbs and feet, blocks for regional anesthesia of 1317–21
linea alba and paramedian, blocks for regional anesthesia 1310–12
pelvic area, blocks for regional anesthesia of 1312–14
teats and udder, blocks for regional anesthesia of 1314–17, 1316*f*
malignant hyperthermia 1060–1, 1295
monitoring of anesthesia 1293–4
orotracheal intubation 1290–1
pain and consciousness 155
premedication 1286–9
regurgitation 1057–8
sedation and chemical restraint 1287–9
supportive therapy 1294–5
Yorkshire 1288
Yucatan 1288
pindolol 329
pinnipeds
anesthesia 1098–9
breathing 1092
features 1091
intubation 1104
large 1104
sleep 1093

vascular access 1101–2
see also marine mammals
PIVA *see* partial intravenous anesthesia (PIVA)
pKa, and Henderson–Hasselbalch equation 556–7
plasma
cryoprecipitate (cryo) 596–7
fluid shifts with interstitial fluid compartments 581–2
fresh frozen plasma (FFP) 596
frozen plasma (FP) 596
products 596–7
simulated concentration 304*f*
vasopressin 934
see also blood
platelet concentrate (PC) 598
platelet-rich plasma (PRP) 598, 1384
platelets
frozen concentrate 598
function testing 575
inhibition abnormalities 412
lyophilized platelets (LYO) 598
plethysmography 207
plethysmography variability index (PVI) 207
pleural line (P-line) 258–9
pleural space and lung ultrasound (PLUS) 256–9
abdominal curtain sign 257, 258*f*, 260–1, 262*f*, 263*f*, 264
abnormal findings 257, 261–9
A-lines 260
BAT sign 257–8, 259*f*
B-lines 260
endobronchial tube placement 261, 263*f*
lung pulse 259–60
lung sliding (glide sign) 259
machine settings 257
normal findings 257–61
pleural line (P-line) 258–9
ultrasound beams 257–8
pleural space disease, and anesthesia 804–5
PLUS *see* pleural space and lung ultrasound (PLUS)
pneumonia, management of anesthesia 807–8
pneumothorax
abdominal curtain sign 261, 263*f*, 264
acute or undiagnosed 64
asynchronous sign 264
barotrauma 65
and bronchospasm 63
in dogs and cats 262
double curtain sign 264
endobronchial tube placement 261, 263*f*
iatrogenic tracheal injury 64
A-lines 260
lung pulse 259–60
lung sliding (glide sign) 259, 262
monitoring of anesthesia 262, 264
pleural line 258
pleural space and lung ultrasound (PLUS) 256
point-of-care ultrasound (POCUS) 254
retrograde intubation 86
tension 64
tracheal rupture/disruption 77
volutrauma 65
POCUS *see* point-of-care ultrasound (POCUS)
point-of-care ultrasound (POCUS) 254–80
abdominal 269, 270*t*, 271
airway assessment 256
cardiac 264*f*, 271–6, 272*t*
in cardiopulmonary resuscitation 275–6
common applications 254, 255*t*
compared with formal ultrasound 254, 255*t*
endotracheal tube placement 256
equipment 256
general applications 255–6
increased B-lines 266, 267*f*
limitations 277
lung consolidation 268–9
and monitoring fluid therapy 277
patient preparation 256
perioperative (P-POCUS) 254–5
application of 255–6
pleural effusion 264, 266*f*, 267*f*
pleural space and lung ultrasound (PLUS) *see* pleural space and lung ultrasound (PLUS)
polarographic Clark electrode 232
polysulfated glycosaminoglycan (PSGAG) 1016, 1383
population pharmacokinetics (POP-PK) 296, 299, 307
positive end-expiratory pressure (PEEP) 44, 65, 132, 1032, 1072, 1094, 1221
ventilators 118, 119, 132
positron emission tomography (PET) 157
POSSUM *see* Physiological and Operative Severity Score for the enUmeration of Mortality and morbidity (POSSUM)
postanesthetic complications
blindness 69
hyperthermia 68
myelomalacia 69–70
neuropathy 69–70
oliguria and acute kidney injury 939
patient injury during recovery 69
prolonged recovery 69
rhabdomyolysis 68–70
postcapillary pulmonary hypertension 811
postcardiac arrest syndrome 59
post-critical event debriefing 70–1
postoperative care
arrhythmias/dysrhythmias 195
dialkylcarbamoylchloride (DACC)-coated postoperative dressings 148
dogs and cats 142
gastrointestinal disease 869–71
ileus 869
infection prevention and control 142, 146–7
laboratory animals 1072, 1073*t*
non-human primates 1073*t*
pain management 965
ruminants 1278–9
see also infection prevention and control; postanesthetic complications
postoperative cognitive dysfunction (POCD) 1356
postsynaptic potentials (PSPs) 179
potassium 593–5
PPE *see* personal protective equipment (PPE).
PPG *see* photoplethysmography (PPG)
PPV *see* pulse pressure variation (PPV)
prazosin 326–7
cardiovascular system effects 327
pharmacokinetics 327
preanesthetic evaluation
age-related changes 1358–9
birds 1135
blood testing 11–13
bradycardia 314
cardiopulmonary bypass 670, 671*t*
cardiovascular disease 680–3
echocardiography 680–1, 682
electrocardiography 12
face masks 1286
horses 1205–6, 1218–19
marine mammals 1095–7
ruminants 1262–4
precapillary pulmonary hypertension 809–11
preference testing 159
preferred body temperature (PBT) 1114
preferred optimal temperature zone (POTZ) 1111
pregabalin 434–6, 1015, 1070
pregnancy-associated changes
acidemia 958
anesthetic considerations 955–68
anesthetic drugs and cesarean section 959–61
anticholinergics 959
dissociatives 960
guaifenesin 961
inhalational anesthesia 960–1
injectable anesthetics 960
local anesthesia 961
neuroleptanalgesia 960
neuromuscular blocking agents 961
opioids 959–60
supplemental agents 961
tranquilizers and sedatives 959
cardiovascular 955–6
cesarean section 961–5
general anesthesia 961–4
local anesthesia 965
regional anesthesia 964–5
coagulation 956
endotracheal intubation 1050
fetal brain 160
gastrointestinal 957
in horses 962, 1050
liver and kidney 957
in maternal physiology 955–7
neuroendocrine 957
pharmacologic alterations 957–8
postoperative pain management 966
pulmonary 956
renal blood flow 956

pregnancy-associated changes (*cont'd*)
  toxicity 958
  uterine blood flow 957
  see also neonatal/pediatric patients
preload 647
premedication 17, 18
  acepromazine 20, 160, 334, 422, 427, 472
  alfentanil 430
  analgesia failure 383
  benzodiazepines 476
  buprenorphine 381
  butorphanol 382, 478
  detomidine 378, 383
  in dogs 183, 478, 798, 1162, 1334
  and drug dosage 472
  in horses 383, 1224
  hydromorphone 335, 428
  inhalational anesthesia 61
  medetomidine 473
  methadone 378
  morphine 369, 426, 480
  mortality risk 20
  opioids 425
  oxymorphone 472
  in pigs 480, 1286–9
  tramadol 384
  xylazine 182
preoperative autologous blood donation (PABD) 602
preoperative patient, risk assessment 10–13
prescription drug monitoring programs (PDMPs) 8
pressure overload, associated conditions 688–9
pressure support ventilation (PSV) 768–70
pressure-controlled ventilation (PCV) 767
pressure-volume (P–V) loops 647–50, 770–2, 773*f*
primates
  New World monkeys 1073
  non-human *see* non-human primates (NHPs)
  social nature of 1073
procainamide 428–9
procaine 538
professional organizations, anesthesia 7
proliferation complexity 27
proparacaine 538
propofol
  birds 1141
  chemical structure 466
  clinical effects
    cardiovascular 467
    central nervous system 467
    fetal/neonatal 467
    gastrointestinal 467
    hepatic system 467
    muscle 467
    renal 467
    respiratory 467
    species-specific 467–8
  clinical use 468
  dogs and cats 1161, 1162
  environmental impact 7
  formulation effect, drug metabolism 309
  and infection control 148
  laser procedures 44
  marine mammals 1098
  mechanism of action 466
  neurologic disease 834
  ophthalmic patients 1334
  pharmacodynamics 467
  pharmacokinetics 466–7
  pigs 1289
  prodrugs 468–9
  ruminants 1270, 1272
  simulated plasma concentration 304*f*
propranolol 329
prostaglandin-E_2 (PGE_2), IL-6 1025
protein
  adenosine-5′- triphosphate (ATP) binding cassette (ABC) family of 1031
  autologous solution 1384
  glial fibrillary acidic protein (GFAP) 285
  G-protein receptors 285, 287
  homeostasis 850
  hypoproteinemia 10
  molecular mechanism of action and CNS protein 506
  multidrug resistance-associated protein (MRP) 308
  P-glycoprotein (P-gp) 308
  Phox2B structure, in marine mammals 1092
proximal paravertebral block 1307–9
proximal radial, ulnar, median, and musculocutaneous nerve block 1188
PSGAGs *see* polysulfated glycosaminoglycans (PSGAGs)
PSPs *see* postsynaptic potentials (PSPs)
PSV *see* pressure support ventilation (PSV)
pulmonary artery catheter (PAC) thermodilution 212–14
  area under the curve 213
  limited experience in veterinary patients 214
  "PAC Man" study 213
pulmonary aspiration 64–5
pulmonary blood flow
  alveolar collapse 776
  anesthesia and pulmonary hypertension 809
  carbon dioxide transport 740
  decreased 732, 733*f*, 734
  distribution of 713–14, 1147
  diverting 731, 809
  left-to-right shunting 687
  and mechanical ventilation 660
  and pulmonary perfusion 713
  redistribution of 1265
  regional redistribution 659
  and respiratory system 1057
  restricted 618
  total 716, 732
pulmonary capacities 698
pulmonary chemoreflex 655
pulmonary circulation 659–60
pulmonary edema
  hydrostatic 717
  increased permeability 718
  negative-pressure 62
  and pulmonary perfusion 717–18
pulmonary hypertension, and anesthesia 809–11
pulmonary intravascular macrophages (PIMs) 736
pulmonary parenchymal disease, and anesthesia 805–8
pulmonary perfusion 713–18
  distribution 713–15
  hydrostatic pulmonary edema 717
  hypoxic pulmonary vasoconstriction 715–16
  increased permeability pulmonary edema 718
  pulmonary edema 717–18
  pulmonary hypertension 716–17
  reptiles 1113
pulmonary system
  age-related changes 1356
  avian 1129, 1130, 1133*f*, 1146, 1147
  cardiopulmonary 214
  comparative cardiovascular morphology and shunting 617
  reptiles 1112–13
  respiration control 1113
pulmonary vascular resistance 321
pulmonary ventilation 702–12, 713*f*, 721–37
  altered alveolar ventilation, effects of 707
  alveolar dead space fraction 705
  alveolar gas equation 702–4
  anesthesia, effects on
    and hypoxic pulmonary vasoconstriction 728–31
    and sedation 725–8
  and deadspace 727
  kinetics of carbon dioxide elimination 704–7
  and lung mechanics 727–8
  and lung volumes 725–7
  physics of respiratory gases 702–4
  pulmonary mechanics 707–12
  sedation and anesthesia, effects on 725–8
pulmonic stenosis (PS) 688–9
pulse oximetry
  anesthetic mortality, risk of 18
  biomedical engineering 172–3
  colic, in horses 1227
  fiber-optic 51
  oxygenation 234–6
pulse pressure 1275
pulse pressure variation (PPV) 205–7
pulsed electromagnetic field (PEMF) 1025
Purkinje system
  birds 1134
  branching of 189
  bundle branches 625
  cells 189*f*, 190, 622, 623, 625
  fibers/fiber network 621*f*, 623, 625, 626, 627*f*, 1105, 1134, 1276
    electrocardiography, 190, 192, 193*f*
  His–Purkinje system 191, 627*f*
PVI *see* plethysmography variability index (PVI)

quadratus lumborum block 1182–3
Quality of Life (QoL) 1005

RAAS *see* renin–angiotensin–aldosterone system (RAAS)
rabbits

anatomic and physiologic considerations 1070
anesthetic mortality, risk of 15, 16
endotracheal intubation in 480
euthanasia 158
inhalational anesthesia 1335
withholding foods from 1070
radial, ulnar, and median nerve block 1188
radiation burns 1370
radiation therapy (RT), laser procedures 42, 43, 44
radiofrequency (RF) 46, 51
fields 49
radiography
anesthetic considerations 43–5
ionizing radiation hazards and safety 42–3
radiocontrast agents 45
radiographic myelography of equids 44
remote facilities 45
radiotherapy 1365, 1369–70
Raman spectroscopy 224, 243–4
ranevetmab 1013
RAP *see* right atrial pressure (RAP)
rapid eye movement (REM) sleep 366, 1093
RAS *see* reticular activating system (RAS)
rate-controlled infusion (RCI) 300
rats
anatomic and physiologic considerations 1070
and euthanasia 159
evaluation of distress 156
gabapentin 1070
Sprague–Dawley 156
RBF *see* renal blood flow (RBF)
RCA *see* root cause analysis (RCA)
Reassessment Campaign on Veterinary Resuscitation (RECOVER) 34, 35, 55, 56*f*
anticholinergics 316–17
rebreathing systems
circle *see* circle rebreathing systems
non-rebreathing 111–12
partial technique 212
receptor agonists and antagonists 284–5
receptor state theory 285
receptor structure
β-adrenergic receptors 287
AMPA and NMDA receptors 286–7
confusion between neutral antagonist and reverse agonist 285
GABA receptors 286
G-protein receptors (as second messengers) 285, 287
SARS-CoV- 2 receptors 287
sodium ion channels 285–6
tachyphylaxis 290
RECOVER *see* Reassessment Campaign on Veterinary Resuscitation (RECOVER)
recovery
airway management 1061–2
airway obstruction 63
amphibians 1119–20
benzodiazepines 69
birds 1148
corticosteroids 69
dysphoria 1106
endotracheal intubation 1278
horses 1050, 1211–13
intravenous (IV) access 1107
mannitol 69
marine mammals 1106–7
neonatal/pediatric patients 1350–1
neuromuscular blockade 456
non-human primates 1073–4
opioids 69
patient injury during 69
pigs 1295
prolonged 69
renal transplantation 948
ruminants 1278
spay-neuter programs 1044
and temperature 69
rectal administration 4
red blood cell potassium 1033
red blood cell (RBC) products 595–6
reflexes
abdominocardiac 655
Aschner's 655
atrial stretch-receptor 655
Bainbridge 655
Barcroft–Edholm 655
baroceptor 655
Bezold–Jarisch 655
cough 655, 833, 836
craniocardiac 655
Cushing 67, 655
dive 1106
loss of the righting reflex (LORR) 155, 156
low-pressure baroreceptor reflex 655
nociceptive withdrawal reflexes (NWRs) 979
ocular 1276
oculocardiac 655, 1332–3
pulmonary chemoreflex 655
reverse Bainbridge reflex 655
tachycardia 327, 328, 334, 429
vagovagal 655
venorespiratory 655
refractometry 244
regional anesthesia
blocks
for flank and paralumbar fossa 1307–10
for head 1303–7
limbs and feet 1317–21
for linea alba and paramedian 1310–12
for pelvic area 1312–14
pelvic limb blocks 1319–21
for teats and udder 1314–17, 1316*f*
thoracic limb blocks 1317–19
cesarean section 964–5
defining 4
history 5
laboratory animals 1069–70
linea alba and paramedian, blocks for 1310–12
novel techniques, horses 1258
transversus abdominis plane (TAP) block 1015, 1183–4, 1227, 1258
ultrasound-guided 1321
regurgitation
and gastroesophageal reflux 13, 65, 67
small animal anesthesia morbidity 13
rehabilitation engineering 170
reliability 1002
REM *see* rapid eye movement (REM) sleep
remifentanil 380, 1289
renal blood flow (RBF) 27, 45, 199, 322
and a_1-adrenergic receptor agonists 324
acepromazine vasodilation increasing 853
alterations in 913
constant 199
in dogs 937
dopexamine protecting 323
ephedrine reducing 326
generalized effects of anesthetics on 933
and glomerular filtration 958
impaired 894
increasing in acute renal failure 1036
and inhalation anesthetics 511
and injectable anesthetics 475, 476, 478
isoproterenol protecting 324
kidney injury 410
kidney recipient management 946
lower blood pressure decreasing 911
modulating 660
myogenic tone and tubuloglomerular feedback, determined by 658
pregnancy-associated changes 956
regulation of 410
renal and hepatic systems 1349
renal changes 1357
and renal circulation 660
renal clearance 292, 294, 534
of creatinine 927
decreased rates 1349
drug metabolism 307
and glomerular filtration rate 927–8
measuring 927
studies 928
see also renal replacement therapy
renal disease
and anesthetic drugs 933–6
anesthetic management
adjunctive treatments 936–7
urethral or bilateral ureteral obstruction, 937–8
urinary bladder rupture and uroabdomen 938–9
chronic (CKD) 52, 931–3
fluid therapy 936
kidney injury
acute *see* acute kidney injury (AKI)/acute renal failure
NSAIDs, adverse effects 410–11
postanesthesia oliguria and acute kidney injury 939
see also acute kidney injury (AKI)/acute renal failure; chronic kidney disease (CKD); kidney injury; renal clearance; renal function; renal replacement therapy; renal system

renal function
normal anatomy and physiology 922–6
physiologic 924–6
testing and monitoring 926–9
biochemical testing 926–7
in dogs and cats 926–8
in horses 928–9
renal biopsy 928
renal clearance and glomerular filtration rate 927–8
in ruminants 929
urine output measurement 928
urinary tract, anatomy of 923–4
renal perfusion pressure (RPP) 199
renal replacement therapy
anesthetic considerations 944–54
continuous 950–2
extracorporeal techniques 950–2
intracorporeal techniques 944–50
peritoneal dialysis 949–50
renal transplantation 944–8
renal system
age-related changes 1356–7
blood pH, mechanisms to minimize changes in 559
circulation 660
in dogs and cats 1159
drug effects
alfaxalone 478–9
barbiturates 465
dissociative anesthetics 470
etomidate 475
inhalational anesthetics 511–12
NSAIDs 411–12
opioids 370–1
propofol 467
neonatal/pediatric patients 1349
pregnancy-associated changes 957
renal portal system, birds 1134–5
reptiles 1113
see also renal replacement therapy
renal toxicity 512, 1369
renal transplantation 944–8
anesthetic management of patients with 945–8
ethical considerations 945
kidney donor management 946
kidney recipient management 946–8
preoperative considerations 945
surgical recovery and complications 948
renin–angiotensin–aldosterone system (RAAS) 287
reporting systems, incident 29
reptiles
anatomy and physiology 1110–11
anesthesia 1110–14
ascending transmission pathways 1116
avoidance learning 1116
blood pressure 1112
brain structures 1116
cardiac shunting 1111
cardiovascular system 1111–12
chelonians 1115
clinical anesthesia 1114
drug administration routes 1114
effects of inspired CO_2 and O_2 1113
endotracheal intubation 1114
evidence for pain in 1115–16
hepatic system 1113–14
intracardiac shunting 227
known analgesic actions on nociceptive or nocifensive behaviors 1116
lizards 1115
lymphatic system 618
metabolism 1111
"Muskelleiste"/"muscular ridge" 1111
nociception 1114–16
presence of nociceptors 1115–16
pain and consciousness 155, 1114–16
patient presentation/assessment 1114
preferred optimal temperature zone (POTZ) 1111
pulmonary system 1112–13
renal system 1113
respiration, control of 1113
snakes 1115
squamates 1115
structures, nociceptive 1116
suspension of normal behavior 1116
thermoregulation 1111
tortoises 1115
turtles 1113, 1115
ventilation, monitoring 227
see also amphibians; fish
residual volume (RV) 698
respiration, defining 697–8
respiratory assist devices 139
respiratory complications, anesthesia-related
accidental extubation 63–4
acute or undiagnosed pneumothorax 64
airway fire 65
airway obstruction 62–3
bronchospasm 63
hypoxemia 62
iatrogenic tracheal injury 64
pulmonary aspiration 64–5
respiratory depression and apnea 61–2
small animals 13, 16
volutrauma and barotrauma 65
wooden chest syndrome 65
respiratory depression 61–2, 1088
respiratory disease
anesthetic management of patients with 788–811
canine brachycephalic obstructive syndrome 790–3
canine laryngeal paralysis 795–7
canine tracheal collapse 797–9
diaphragmatic hernia 805–6
equine guttural pouch mycosis 801
equine guttural pouch tympany 800
equine laryngeal paralysis 802
feline brachycephalic obstructive airway syndrome 793–4
lower airway disease 802–3
pleural space disease 804–5
pneumothorax and/or pleural effusion 805
postcapillary pulmonary hypertension 811
precapillary pulmonary hypertension 809–11
pulmonary hypertension 809–11
pulmonary parenchymal disease 806–8
upper respiratory disease 788–802
asthma
equine 803–4
feline 802–3
atelectasis 773–4, 775*f*, 776–7
diaphragmatic hernia 805–6
general approach to management of animals with a difficult airway 788
lower airway 226, 802–3
pneumothorax and/or pleural effusion 804–5
pulmonary parenchymal disease, intrapulmonary masses 806
sedation 788–811
upper airway 788–802
respiratory function, physiology of aerobic respiration 220–1
respiratory gas analysis
historical techniques used 243–4
mass spectrometry 224, 241, 243
monitoring 514–15
Raman spectroscopy 224, 237, 243–4
respiratory physiology and pathophysiology 697–749
breathing frequency 699*f*
expiratory reserve volume 698
functional residual capacity 698
inspiratory capacity 698
inspiratory reserve volume 698
key concepts and lung volumes 697–8, 699*t*
lung volumes 698, 699*f*, 699*t*
minute ventilation 698
pregnancy-associated changes 956
pulmonary perfusion 713–18
effects of anesthesia on 721–37
residual volume 698
respiration 697–8
respiratory function in conscious and anesthetized animals 700–43
effects of anesthesia 721–37
neural control of ventilation 700–2, 721–5
oxygen transport 737–40
pulmonary perfusion 713–18
pulmonary ventilation 702–12, 713*f*, 721–37
ventilation–perfusion relationships 718–21, 719*f*, 721–37
total lung capacity 698
ventilation
effects of anesthesia on 721–37
neural control 700–2, 721–5
pulmonary 702–12, 713*f*
ventilation–perfusion relationships 718–21, 719*f*
effects of anesthesia on 721–37
vital capacity 698
respiratory sinus arrhythmia 655
respiratory system
amphibians 1117–18

arterial carbon dioxide tension 508–9
birds 1127–34, 1145–7
blood pH, mechanisms to minimize changes in 559
drug effects
acepromazine 334
alfaxalone 478
atipamezole 346
barbiturates 464–5
detomidine 341
dexmedetomidine 341
diazepam 337
dissociative anesthetics 470
etomidate 475
inhalational anesthetics 508–9
medetomidine 341
midazolam 337
opioids 367
propofol 467
romifidine 341
vatinoxan 346
xylazine 341
yohimbine 346
zolazepam 337
farm animals 1057
fish 1120–1
inhalational anesthesia
arterial carbon dioxide tension 508–9
concurrent drugs 509
duration of 509
factors influencing respiratory effects 509
mode of ventilation 509
surgery/other noxious stimulation 509
neonatal/pediatric patients 1349
pulmonary circulation 659–60
Response Entropy (RE) index 183
response surface analyses 306–7
responsiveness 1002
restraint *see* handling and restraint
restrictive cardiomyopathy (RCM) 689–90
restrictive polymer electric heating systems 250
reticular activating system (RAS) 180
retrograde intubation 86
retrotrapezoid nucleus (RTN) 1092
return of spontaneous circulation (ROSC) 55, 57
reverse Bainbridge reflex 655
reverse patent ductus arteriosus (rPDA) 688
rhabdomyolysis 69–70
rhythm evaluation 191
right atrial pressure (RAP) 204, 205
right ventricular (RV) pressure 204, 205
ring block 1188
rise time, gas sampling 241
risk assessment 10–23
assessing anesthetic risk 10–13
horses 1048
morbidity and mortality 13–20
neonatal/pediatric patients 1348
occupational exposure and anesthesia care providers 7
patient health assessment 10–11
postoperative infections, associated risk factors
environmental 147
iatrogenic 147
patient-specific 146–7
preoperative patient 10–13
Ro 19-4063 285
robenacoxib 1382
Robertshaw double-lumen endotracheal tube 79
rodenticide toxicity 596, 597, 876
rodents 1070–2
pain evaluation 990–1
see also laboratory animals; mice; rats
romifidine 325, 1266
clinical considerations 343–4
indications for 338–9
mechanism of action 338–9
pharmacodynamics 340–3
pharmacokinetics 339–40
root cause analysis (RCA) 30
root mean squared error (RMSE) 172
ropivacaine, and local anesthesia 540
ROSC *see* return of spontaneous circulation (ROSC)
Rottweilers, anesthetic mortality, risk of 18
Royal Veterinary College, UK 16
rPDA *see* reverse patent ductus arteriosus (rPDA)
RPP *see* renal perfusion pressure (RPP)
RTN *see* retrotrapezoid nucleus (RTN)
ruminal tympany 67
ruminants 1262–83
anesthesia
endotracheal intubation 1058–9
inhalational anesthesia 1272–3
injectable anesthetics 1271–2
maintenance of 1271–3
monitoring of 1275–7
preanesthetic evaluation 1262–4
recovery 1278
blood typing 599
cardiovascular supportive therapy 1275
dose requirements 1061
drug administration 1054
drug dose 377–8
drug effects
alfaxalone 480
barbiturates 465
dissociative anesthetics 472
etomidate 476
propofol 468
fluid administration 1273–4
intraoperative analgesia 1273
intraoperative complications 1278
local anesthetic and analgesic techniques 1301–23
castration, blocks for 1317
flank/paralumbar fossa, blocks for regional anesthesia of 1307–10
head, blocks for regional anesthesia of 1303–7
limbs and feet, blocks for regional anesthesia of 1317–21
linea alba and paramedian, blocks for regional anesthesia 1310–12
pelvic area, blocks for regional anesthesia of 1312–14
teats and udder, blocks for regional anesthesia of 1314–17, 1316*f*
patient positioning 1273
postoperative complications 1278–9
recommended withdrawal interval for 1052, 1053–4*t*
regurgitation 1057–8
renal function, testing and monitoring 929
respiratory supportive therapy 1274–5
ruminal tympany 67, 1057, 1078
salivation 1058
sedation/chemical restraint
acepromazine 1264
a_2-adrenergic receptor agonists 1265–6
a_2-adrenergic receptor antagonists 1266–7
alfaxalone 1267
anticholinergics 1264
azaperone 1264
benzodiazepines 1267
common combinations 1267–8
doxapram 1267
opioids 1267
sternal recumbency 1086
supportive therapy 1273–7
RUMM (radial, ulnar, median, and musculocutaneous) nerves 1187, 1188
running-drip epidural technique 1196
Rüsch® EZ-Blocker® 82–3
RV *see* right ventricular (RV) pressure

sacrococcygeal or intercoccygeal epidural (caudal epidural) block 1312–13
Safety Attitudes Questionnaire 28
safety considerations
analysis techniques 30, 31*f*
assessing organizational safety culture 28
data collection techniques 28–30
equipment 75
hand hygiene 144
harm, risk of from healthcare 24–5
human error and the system 25–7
human factors 27
incident reporting systems 29
interventions 33–7
laser procedures
laser beam hazard 40–1
laser fire hazard 41, 42*f*
non-beam hazards 42
"leading indicator," safety culture as 28
magnetic resonance imaging 48
medical gases 92–3
nomenclature 24
non-technical skills 27, 28*t*
organizational culture 27–8
patient safety evidence in anesthesia 30–3
and process of anesthesia 26–7
radiography 42–3
Safety I versus Safety II 28
staff training 7
Swiss cheese model 27
terminology 24

safety considerations (*cont'd*)
WHO definition of patient safety 24, 25
see also infection prevention and control
safety culture 28
salbutamol *see* albuterol
salivation 1058
SAP *see* systolic arterial pressure (SAP)
sciatic nerve block 1190–1
sea cows *see* sirenians
seasonal autoregressive integrated moving average (SARIMA) models 171
secobarbital, euthanasia 158
sedation 333–54
cesarean section 959
death related to 15
defining 4, 153
effects on pulmonary ventilation and mechanics 725–8
equine guttural pouch mycosis 801
equine guttural pouch tympany 800
versus general anesthesia 50–1
magnetic resonance imaging 50–1
marine mammals 1097–8
neural control of ventilation 723–4
neurologic disease 832–5
ocular physiology 1334
opioid effects 366–7
pigs 1287–9
ruminants
acepromazine 1264
a_2-adrenergic receptor agonists 1265–6
a_2-adrenergic receptor antagonists 1266–7
alfaxalone 1267
anticholinergics 1264
azaperone 1264
benzodiazepines 1267
common combinations 1267–8
doxapram 1267
opioids 1267
standing sedated equine CT 44, 1206
see also premedication
segmental dorsolumbar epidural block 1309–10
segmental thoracolumbar subarachnoid block 1310
seizures 837–8
Seldinger technique, modified 205
sensory innervation, anatomy of 1185–6
sensory nerve blocks 1237–9
sensory transduction, biology of 972, 973*t*
septic peritonitis 879–82
serotonin (5-HT) 976
serratus plane block 1182
sevoflurane
amphibians 1119
bronchodilation induced by 803, 804
face mask, delivered by 1268
malignant hyperthermia 68
ophthalmic patients 1335
SGADs *see* supraglottic airway devices (SGADs)
sheep
drug effects
detomidine 344
dexmedetomidine 344
medetomidine 344
romifidine 344
xylazine 344
pain and consciousness 155
regional anesthesia 965
shelter animals
anesthesia for non-spay-neuter procedures in shelters 1045–6
clinical situations requiring anesthesia 1041–6
comparative anesthesia and analgesia 1041–7
high-quality high-volume spay-neuter (HQHVSN) practice 1041, 1042*f*, 1043–5
spay-neuter for higher risk patients 1045
shock
anesthesia considerations 693–4
extracorporeal shockwave therapies (ESWT) 1025
vasopressin for 693, 877
Short Form of the Glasgow Composite Pain Scale-Canine 1003
"shred" sign, partial lung consolidation 268
shunting/shunts
anatomic 720
comparative cardiovascular morphology and shunting 617–19
intracardiac shunting 227
intrapulmonary 720
isoshunt diagram 720
left-to-right shunting 687
pathologic anatomic 720
physiologic anatomic 720
reptiles 1111
right-to-left shunting 687–8, 1112
shunt fraction 720
sidestream monitors, gas sampling 241
sighthounds 1030–1
signalment, in dogs 1158
simulation-based training 9, 36, 174
SIMV *see* spontaneous intermittent mandatory ventilation (SIMV)
Single-Circuit Compressed Gas-Powered Ventilators 117
single-circuit ventilators 115
compressed gas-powered 117, 118–19
piston-driven 117–18
sinus tachycardia 191, 626, 681, 875, 1221
sirenians
anesthesia 1099
breathing 1092
features 1091–2
Florida manatee (*Trichechus manatus latirostris*) 1099
see also marine mammals
SIRS *see* systemic inflammatory response syndrome (SIRS)
Situation, Background, Assessment, Recommendation (SBAR) 30, 36
skeletal muscle, drug effects, inhalational anesthetics 512
slaughter, humane 153–4
see also euthanasia
sleep 1093
small animals
anesthetic morbidity 13–14
anesthetic mortality 14–18
causes 15–16
Confidential Enquiry into Perioperative Small Animal Fatalities (CEPSAF) 12, 15–17
risk factors 16–18
risk of 14–15
timing of death 16
cardiopulmonary arrest 55
Dräger Small Animal Ventilator 123
fluid therapy 1223
magnetic resonance imaging 50
multilead ECG 189
Vetronics Merlin ventilator 132–3
Vetronics SAV03 and SAV04 ventilators 124–6
SmartFlow® Patient Workflow Anesthetic Sheet (IDEXX Laboratories) 8
smooth muscle
contraction and relaxation 638–40
metabolism 638
sodium 592–3
sodium bicarbonate ($NaHCO_3$) 58, 560*f*, 1223
Addisonian crisis 894
anesthetic agents 1118
and barbiturates 463
and capnography 217
disorders in A_{TOT} 571
distribution space 563, 564
and fentanyl 378
gastroesophageal reflux (GER) 67
gastrointestinal reflux 867
hyperkalemia 68
hyperparathyroidism 914
hypertonic 564
intravenous administration 594
isonatremic organic acid abnormalities 570
local anesthesia 536, 537, 1254
locoregional anesthesia 1167
PCO_2 disorders 568
routine use of 58
ultrasound 1244
urethral or bilateral ureteral obstruction 937
sodium ion channels 285–6
sodium nitroprusside (SNP) 429
solubility
blood/gas coefficient 496
of gas 494–7
oil/gas partition coefficient 496
other partition coefficients 496–7
uptake of inhalation anesthetics 499
somatosensory-evoked potentials (SEPs) 979
sotalol 329
spay-neuter programs
analgesia for 1045–6

"beach style" for recovery 1044
see also high-quality high-volume spay-neuter (HQHVSN) practice
specific absorption rate (SAR), radiofrequency 49
spectral entropy 182–3
spectrometry *see* mass spectrometry; photoacoustic spectrometry
spectroscopy
infrared 223–4
mass 224, 243
near-infrared 237
Raman 224, 237, 243–4
sphygmomanometer 203
spinal cord 347, 825, 1307, 1309, 1310, 1311, 1312, 1313
analgesia 364, 530
anesthesia 5
and antidepressants 1368
cervical 76
and consciousness 176
damage/injury 45, 69, 838–9, 1310
acute spinal cord injury (SCI) 370
division into segments 825
dorsal horn 339, 341, 364, 372, 507, 530, 535, 1367, 1372
endothelial cells 635
inhalational anesthesia 497, 507
interneurons 342
ischemia 535
and isobaric solutions 535
locoregional and neuraxial anesthesia 148–9
malacia 19
myelomalacia 70
nervous system anatomy 822
neurotoxicity 544
nociceptive signals in 1382
opioid receptor localization 359, 365
and opioids 1367
and osteoarthritis 1378
pain perception 154
and remifentalanil 380
segments 825
spinal surgery 838–9
thoracolumbar 508
transection 538
traverse ascending tracts of 247
spinal cord blood flow (SCBF) 369, 544
spino-bulbo-spinal loop 977
splanchnic circulation 660
spontaneous intermittent mandatory ventilation (SIMV) 770
squares of the errors (SSE) 297
standing equine MRI 52
standing sedated equine CT 44, 1206
Staphylococcus aureus 142
Staphylococcus pseudintermedius 142
Staphylococcus spp. 149
Starling's equation 582
State Entropy (SE) index 183
step-counts 999
stereoisomerism 406
stereoisomers 309
sterility assurance monitoring (SAM) 145
steroids
anabolic 1032
and anti-inflammatories 1069
cardiopulmonary bypass 669
cerebral edema 1074
cervical spondylomyelopathy 839
circuitry 668
concomitant use of 1017
corticosteroids *see* corticosteroids
intra-articular 1383
myasthenia gravis (MG) 839–40
neurosteroids 160, 477, 1084
and sedation 432
traumatic brain injury 837
see also corticosteroids
stethoscopes, biomedical engineering 172
stored whole blood 596
Streptococcus zooepidemicus 145
stroke volume index (SVI) 320
subaortic stenosis (SAS) 688–9
subarachnoid anesthesia, history 5
subcutaneous (SC) injection 1067
subscalenic brachial plexus block 1186
succinylcholine, reversal of 457–8
sufentanil 380
sulfhemoglobin (SulfHb) 233
sulfotransferases (SULT) 308
"superBAG" (buprenorphine, acepromazine, and glycopyrrolate) 317
superficial palmar vein 1101
supraglottic airway devices (SGADs) 75, 82–3
veterinary-specific 83
supraventricular tachycardia 191, 329, 681
surgical general anesthesia 4
Surgical Safety Checklist (SSC) 33, 34*t*, 35
SurgiVet™ Advisor® Veterinary Data Logger (Smiths Medical) 8
Surviving Sepsis Campaign (SSC) 1222
SVR *see* systemic vascular resistance (SVR)
Swan-Ganz catheter 212
swine *see* pigs
Swine triple drip 1292
Swiss cheese model (Reason) 27
symmetrical slow-wave sleep (BSWS) 1093
sympathetic nervous system (SNS) 828, 829*f*
and adrenergic agents 319
and anticholinergics 317
balance with parasympathetic 999
blockade 947
blood pressure monitoring 645
circulatory system stimulation 511
and CNS 470
compensatory mechanism 470
decreased activity 690
depth-of-anesthesia devices 184
and dissociatives 469
and drug selection 678
duration of anesthesia 511
and etomidate 475
evaluation of distress 157
function 828
gastrointestinal motility/postoperative ileus 869
hyperthyroidism 912
and hypothalamus 827
ketamine, stimulated by 1209
maximally stimulated 678
neurogenic regulation of cerebral blood flow 831
and neurohumoral and local control mechanisms 654, 656
and nitrous oxide 513
noxious stimulation 511
and pain 1372
physiological parameters, stimulation of 998
postganglionic synapses 827
and resistance vessels 633
transmission, selected effects 827, 828*t*
synthetic colloids 584–8, 1222
and acute kidney injury 692, 875, 881
clinical implications of synthetic use in veterinary medicine 588
dextrans 588
gelatins 588
hydroxyethyl starches 586–8
syringomyelia 1000
systemic inflammatory response syndrome (SIRS) 1217–18
systemic toxicity 1167, 1168, 1171, 1302
local anesthesia 526, 531, 532, 535, 536, 538, 539, 541–4
cardiovascular system 542–3
central nervous system 541–2
treatment 543–4
systemic vascular resistance (SVR) 58, 479
and blood pressure monitoring 197, 198
systolic arterial pressure (SAP) 60, 197, 204, 326, 422
invasive measurement 199–202
systolic pressure variation (SPV) 206

T-61, for euthanasia 162
tachyarrhythmias 191
tachycardia
adrenergic agents 321, 329
α-adrenergic receptor antagonists 328
β_1-adrenergic receptors 325
anticholinergics 316
arrhythmogenic diseases resulting in 691
atrial 428, 899
and dopamine 321
dose-dependent 316
excess 316
heart rate increase 315
and hypotension 61
pacemaker-derived 678
pharmacology 317
radiocontrast agents 45
reflex 327, 328, 334, 429
sinus 191, 626, 681, 875, 1221
supraventricular 191, 329, 681
transient 179, 316, 433

tachycardia (*cont'd*)
ventricular 13, 58, 191, 192, 195, 428, 542, 543, 620, 626, 678, 681, 804, 875, 876*f*, 877, 899, 1147*f*, 1198
TAP *see* transversus abdominis plane (TAP) block
tapentadol 436
multitargeting molecules 385
target-controlled infusion (TCI) 173, 177, 301, 303*f*, 304*f*
dexmedetomidine 346
TBI *see* traumatic brain injury (TBI)
TCI *see* target-controlled infusion (TCI)
Team Strategies and Tools to Enhance Performance and Patient Safety (TeamSTEPPS®) 36
teats and udder, blocks for regional anesthesia of 1314–17
intravenous regional teat 1317
inverted "V" block 1316
ring block 1316
teat sinus infusion 1316–17
technology, role of 8–10
temperature
acid–base balance, effects on 557–8
birds 1148
Bispectral Index™ 180
body temperature maintenance in laboratory animals 1072
and capnography 217
change 213, 214
compensation 97, 101, 102, 103, 172
in containers 156
curve 213
esophageal temperature probe 52
excessively high 68
fiber-optic probe 52
of helium 49
hypothermia 13
liquid 103
operating rooms 147
oxygen cages 90
and pain management 1024
preferred optimal temperature zone (POTZ) 1111
probes 52, 145
prolonged anesthetic recovery 69
pulmonary artery catheter thermodilution 212
radiofrequency fields 49
rectal 1086, 1087
room 101, 102, 212, 213
sensor 213
skin surface 52
vaporizers 97, 99, 100, 102
see also body temperature
terbutaline
cardiovascular system effects 325
other effects 325–6
tetracaine 539
Tetralogy of Fallot (TF) 687–8
TFAST protocols 262
thermodilution, cardiac output measurement 211–12
thermodynamics 246
thermoregulation
active patient warming 249–50
age-related changes 1357
amphibians 1117
circulating warm water systems 250
conduction 248
convection 248
core-to-periphery gradient 247, 248*f*
decreased core body temperature 249
farm animals 1060–1
fish 1121
forced warm air units 250
heat transfer mechanisms 247–9
hyperthermia 250–2
neonatal/pediatric patients 1350
opioid effects 371
perioperative 246–53
reptiles 1111
resistive polymer electric heating 250
thermodynamics 246
thiafentanil 380–1
wildlife capture 1081
thiamylal, pharmacokinetics 464
thiobarbiturate anesthesia 16
thiobarbiturates, ruminants 1268
thiopental
dogs and cats 1162
pharmacokinetics 464
thoracic bioimpedance and bioreactance 216
thoracic limb, blocks of 1185–8
axillary brachial plexus block 1186–7
cervical paravertebral block 1186
distal brachial plexus block 1188
distal radial, ulnar, median, and musculocutaneous nerve block 1188
proximal radial, ulnar, median, and musculocutaneous nerve block 1188
radial, ulnar, and median nerve block 1188
ring block 1188
sensory innervation, anatomy of 1185–6
subscalenic brachial plexus block 1186
thoracic paravertebral block 1179
thoracic radiography 681–2
thorax and abdomen, blocks of 1178–85
fascial plane block techniques 1182–5
intercostal nerve 1179, 1180*f*
interpleural regional analgesia 1181–2
thoracic paravertebral 1179
thrombotic abnormalities 412
thrombophlebitis 1278
thyroid disease 908–13
hyperthyroidism 909–12
hypothyroidism 908–9
thyroid neoplasia 912–13
thyroid neoplasia, anesthetic considerations and management 912–13
tibial plateau leveling osteotomy (TPLO) 148, 149
tidal volume
defining 698
delivered, factors affecting 122
determinants of 122
tiletamine-zolazepam (TZ) 1269–70, 1291, 1292
time series analysis 171–2
time-based capnography 224–7
acid–base derangements 225
cardiac output measurement 227
cardiopulmonary arrest 227
difficult airway and lower airway disease 226
hyper- and hypokalemia 225–6
hypoxemia, differential diagnosis 225
intracranial disease 225
nasal catheter 227
specific clinical indications/uses 225–7
tissue engineering 170
TIVA *see* total intravenous anesthesia (TIVA)
TLC *see* total lung capacity (TLC)
TNR *see* Trap Neuter Return (TNR) programs
tolazoline 69, 1266
clinical considerations 347
indications for 344–5
mechanism of action 344–5
pharmacodynamics 345–7
pharmacokinetics 345
tolfenamic acid 1382
tonic control 977
topical anesthesia 1167, 1237
total body clearance 292
total intravenous anesthesia (TIVA) 4, 44, 50, 177, 1162, 1291
total lung capacity (TLC) 698
total peripheral resistance *see* systemic vascular resistance (SVR)
total response time, gas sampling 241
toxicity 7, 296
adverse drug reactions 307
agent purity and euthanasia 161
amantadine and memantine 431
amitriptyline 433
antibiotics 939
bone marrow 408
bupivacaine-induced 786, 1296–7
calcium 1370
cannabinoids 434
cardiac 531, 541, 542, 594
cardiovascular 542–3
of carnivores and scavengers 162
and castration 1317
in cattle 1321
chloral hydrate 481
clinical, from drug interactions 305
CNS 534, 541–2, 1305
diuretics 939
dose-dependent 409
drug interactions 306
ethylene glycol 593
gastrointestinal 409
grape 931
halothane 854–5
hepatic 412, 430
of high-potency drugs 294
immune-mediated 512
increased risk of 533
inhalational anesthesia
cardiovascular system 509–11
central nervous system 505–8
hepatic system 512

renal system 511–12
respiratory system 508–9
skeletal muscle 512
isomers and stereoisomers 309
kidney injury 410
lethal 1079
lidocaine 466, 534, 542, 1251
lily 931
local anesthesia 66, 538, 542–4, 1174, 1186, 1302, 1320, 1337
local anesthetic systemic toxicity (LAST) 1167, 1171, 1181, 1198
local toxicity 544
systemic toxicity 541–4
megakaryocyte 852
mepivacaine 539
methocarbamol 427
moderate 539
nitrous oxide 512
N-methyl- D- aspartate (NMDA) receptor-mediated 370
NSAIDs 939, 1139, 1380
organ 468
oxygen 91, 753, 755, 1073
paracetamol 407, 1034
paracetamol and aspirin 411
phase II biotransformation or conjugation 308
in pregnancy 958
procainamide 428
propofol 468
pyrethrin/permethrin 427
radiation 1365*f*
raisin 931
renal 512, 1369
rodenticide 596, 597, 876
serotonin 438
sodium nitroprusside 429
systemic 1167, 1168, 1171, 1302
cardiovascular 542–3
central nervous system 541–2
local anesthesia 526, 531, 532, 535, 536, 538, 539, 541–4
treatment 543–4
tissue 75
toxic dose 288
volatile inhalation anesthetics 504
toxicosis (oral ingestion) 545
TPLO *see* tibial plateau leveling osteotomy (TPLO)
trachea, iatrogenic tracheal injury 64
tracheal collapse, in dogs 1032–3
tracheal insufflation 90
tracheostomy 86–7
tramadol
adjunctive drug 436–8
birds 1138–9
laboratory animals 1073*t*
multitargeting molecules 384–5
pigs 1288
premedication 384
tranquilization
cesarean section 959
defining 4
see also sedation
transcapillary fluid exchange 635–8
transcranial magnetic stimulation, in dogs 182, 184
transcutaneous electrical nerve stimulation (TENS) 1025
transcutaneous measurement of blood gases 233
transfusion therapy 595–602
adverse effects 600–2
allogenic, alternatives to 602–3
blood administration 600
blood component 595–8
compatibility testing 599–600
massive blood loss, considerations for 600
see also blood
transient receptor potential (TRP) 247, 1024
transit time, gas sampling 241
transport
carbon dioxide 740–3
oxygen 737–40
transpulmonary thermodilution and ultrasound indicator dilution 214
transversus abdominis plane (TAP) block 1015, 1183–4, 1227, 1258
Trap Neuter Return (TNR) programs 1041
trauma, physical 1087
traumatic brain injury (TBI) 238, 369, 431
trazodone 429–30
tribromoethanol 1068
Tributame, for euthanasia 162
tricaine methanesulfonate (MS-222) 1118, 1119
tropomyosin-receptor kinase A (TrkA) receptors 1013
tumor necrosis factor-α (TNFα) 1025, 1218
tumors 421, 690, 711
adrenal 896, 898
adrenocortical 896
bone 1365, 1368
brain 905–6
decarboxylation 877
esophageal 878, 879
functional 879
gastrointestinal stromal 877, 878
hepatic 878
insulinoma 906
intracranial 835, 836, 837
large 878, 915
lung 806
mast cell 877, 878, 879, 1032
nasal 1365
necrotic 879
neuroendocrine 877–8
ocular 1331
opioid effects 371–2
oral 1365
painful invasive 1366
parathyroid 914, 915
partially resected primary tumors 907
pituitary 895
primary and secondary 1369
recurrence 1371
renal 878
small non-invasive 911
spinal 838
surgical resection 896
thyroid 911, 912
unresectable 912
vascularized 911
well-differentiated 912
see also cancer pain
Tuohy needle 1101
twilight anesthesia 4
type II collagen 1383

UDP-glucuronosyltransferases (UGT) 308
ultrasound
Doppler ultrasonography 1173
Doppler ultrasonographic blood pressure measurement 202–3
indicator dilution and transpulmonary thermodilution 214
point-of-care *see* point-of-care ultrasound (POCUS)
three-dimensional 174
transducers 1173
ultrasound-guided epidural technique 1196–7
ultrasound-guided nerve blocks 173–4, 1173–4
uncertainty complexity 26
unconsciousness
anesthetic-induced 155
defining 154–5
delayed 158
onset of 158–60
UNESP-Botucatu multidimensional pain scale, cats 1003, 1034
unfractionated heparin (UFH) 576
ungulates 1077–8
unidimensional pain assessment scales 1002
United Kingdom
Association of Anaesthetists of Great Britain and Ireland 11–12
Association of Veterinary Anaesthetists of Great Britain and Ireland 6, 7
Department of Health 49
Diploma of Veterinary Anaesthesia 6, 21
National Institute for Health and Care Excellence 11
Royal Veterinary College 16
United States
American Animal Hospital Association 143, 197
American Association for Medical Instruments 203
American College of Veterinary Anesthesia and Analgesia 6, 7, 174, 197, 251
American College of Veterinary Anesthesiologists 6
American College of Veterinary Emergency and Critical Care 55
American College of Veterinary Internal Medicine 198, 203, 204
American Medical Association 174
American National Standards Institute 40

United States (*cont'd*)
American Society for Testing and Materials 49
American Society of Anesthesiologists 10, 12, 147, 176, 251, 255
hypo-or hyperthermia 68
infection prevention and control 147
patient health assessment 10, 12
POCUS certification program 255
preanesthetic blood testing 13
American Society of Echocardiography 271
American Society of Veterinary Anesthesia 6
American Veterinary Medical Association 6, 8, 161, 162
Guidelines on Euthanasia (2020) 153, 156, 158
Humane Slaughter guidelines (2016) 160
Centers for Disease Control and Prevention 8, 148
Diplomate of the American College of Veterinary Anesthesia and Analgesia 21
Food and Drug Administration 49
Occupational Safety and Health Administration 41, 49
risk of anesthetic death, in small animals 14
United States Department of Agriculture Animal and Plant Health Service (USDA APHIS). 161
United States Government Principles for the Utilization and Care of Vertebrate Animals Used in Testing, Research, and Training 158
United States Pharmacopeia/ National Formulary (USP/NF) 162
upper respiratory disease, and anesthesia 788–802
urethane 1065, 1066*t*
injectable 1068
urethral or bilateral ureteral obstruction 937–8
uric acid 1113
urinary bladder rupture and uroabdomen 938–9
urinary bladder volume 271
urinary system 923, 935
urinary tract, anatomy of 923–4
urine
abdominocentesis removing 939
atenolol excreted in 329
collection systems 48
conjugation products 308
dilute 342, 1113
dobutamine excreted in 322
dopamine excreted in 322
drug concentration 290, 294
epinephrine excreted in 321
glycopyrrolate excreted in 317
isoproterenol excreted in 324
leakage/spillage 50
metabolism 362
metoprolol excreted in 329
normal flow 327
and opioids 363
output 322, 323, 339, 347
phenoxybenzamine excreted in 328
production 271
renal tubular epithelial cells in sediment 411
reptiles 1113
restrictive polymer electric heating systems 250
safety considerations 48, 50
secretion of drugs into 309
urine output measurement 928
urogenital system 1113
anesthesia in horses 1251–3
for castration 1252–3
for ovariectomy 1253
of penis/vulva 1253
of the perineum 1253

vagovagal reflex 655
valves
adjustable pressure-limiting *see* adjustable pressure-limiting (APL) valve
demand 139
oxygen flush 104
PEEP 44, 65
pressure-reducing 94
rebreathing 212
vapor
versus gas 491–2
pressure 493–4
vaporizers 97–9
agent-specific 103
"back bar" 98
back-pressure compensation 97
bracket systems 98–9
common in veterinary medicine 99–103
complications 67
Copper Kettles 102, 103
Dräger vapor vaporizers (Vapor 19.1) 101–2
electronic 98
flow rate compensation 97
flowmeter-controlled 102, 103
Fluotec Mark 3 99
Isotec 3 99
maintenance 103
measured-flow 102–3
Ohio calibrated 102
Ohmeda/Datex-Ohmeda/ GE Healthcare Tec vaporizers 99–100
operational considerations 97–8
Penlon Sigma Delta 102
Tec series 99–101
Tec 3 type 100, 101
Tec 4 and 5 100–1
Tec 6 101
temperature compensation 97
types 97
use of wrong anesthetic 103
Verni-Trol 102
see also flowmeters
vascular access
marine mammals
cetacean 1099–101
manatee 1102
pinnipeds 1101–2
vascular system 631–8
capillaries 634–5
large arteries and veins 633
resistance vessels 633–4
small arteries 633
transcapillary fluid exchange 635–8
veins, venules and venous capacitance 638
vasoactive drugs 832–5
vasopressin
administration of 430
antiemetic therapy 864
arginine vasopressin (antidiuretic hormone) 370, 380, 426, 430–1, 657, 658
cardiopulmonary arrest 58
cardiovascular physiology 657
euthanasia 157
indications for 430
injectable 431
nausea and vomiting caused by 864
and opioids 367
perioperative fluid therapy 588
plasma 934
septic peritonitis 880, 881
shock 693, 877
toxicity 543
unresponsiveness to 511
in vitro studies 810
vasopressors 324, 961
vatinoxan 322, 344–7, 1083, 1267
clinical considerations 347
indications for 344–5
mechanism of action 344–5
medetomidine–vatinoxan combination (Zenalpha®) 347
pharmacodynamics 345–7
pharmacokinetics 345
VC *see* vital capacity (VC)
VCV *see* volume-controlled ventilation (VCV)
vector autoregression (VAR) models, 171
vecuronium 1066*t*
veins 638
auricular 1055
and large arteries 633
velocity time integral (VTI) 215–16
venipuncture 1054, 1100
venorespiratory reflex 655
venous capacitance 638
venous oxygen saturation (SvO_2) 236
ventilation
airway pressure release ventilation 1094–5
alveolar 498–9
apneustic anesthesia ventilation 1095, 1098
continuous positive airway pressure 1094, 1095
controlled mechanical ventilation 1094, 1098
defining 698
effects of anesthesia on 721–37
inhalational anesthesia 509
lung protective 1095
maintenance of anesthesia 1228
marine mammals *see* marine mammals
mechanical 755–82
assisted and assisted-controlled 768–70
continuous mandatory ventilation 764–8

dual-controlled 767–8
pressure-controlled 767
volume-controlled 765–7
minute ventilation (V_1) 698
mode of 509, 510–11
monitoring *see* ventilation monitoring
neural control 700–2, 721–5
positive-pressure 63, 65, 957
pressure support 768–70
pulmonary 702–12, 713*f*
spontaneous 84
spontaneous intermittent mandatory 770
ventilation–perfusion relationships 718–37
ventilation monitoring
aerobic respiration, physiology 220–1
apnea monitors 222
capnography, time-based 224–7
carbon dioxide
and acid–base implications 221
measurement methods 223–4
quantitative monitoring 222–4
continued monitoring of parameters 59
during CPR 57
importance 221–2
physical methods 222
quantitative monitoring of carbon dioxide 222–4
standards 221–2
see also ventilators
"Ventilation Shutdown Plus" 154
ventilation–perfusion (V/Q) matching 718–21, 719*f*
computed tomography 227
effects of anesthesia on 721–37, 733*f*
and gas exchange 718, 719*f*
impaired 1220–1
marine mammals 1095
mismatch in clinical practice 1220
measuring 718, 720–1
ventilation monitoring 227
V/Q ratio 1220
ventilators 113–39
airway pressure alarms 122
alarms 122
bellows 117, 119–20
Bird Mark series 118, 119
Bird Mark 7 137–9
classification 114–17
compliance and compression volumes 122
control of ventilator driving gas 122
cycling mechanism 116–17
delivered tidal volume, factors affecting 122
determinants of tidal volume 122
Dräger large animal 133
Dräger small animal 123
drive mechanism/circuit 115–16
dual-circuit 115, 117, 119–22
Engler ADS 1000 and 2000 veterinary delivery system and critical care ventilator 123–4
exotic animal (SAV03 and SAV04) 124–5
fresh gas flow (FGF) 122–6
Hallowell EMC 2000, 2002/2002 PRO ventilator 126–7
Hallowell Tafonius/Tafonius Junior 136, 137*f*
ICU Medical (formerly Smith Medical/ Surgivet) SAV 2500 130–1
ICU Medical (formerly Surgivet) DHV1000 large animal ventilator 136–7
infection prevention and control 146
inspiratory-to-expiratory ratio (I:E) 122, 131, 132, 134
intensive care unit (ICU) 113–14
JD Medical LAV-3000 138
leaks 122
low driving gas pressure alarm 122
magnetic resonance imaging 51
major control variable 114–15
Mallard Medical Model 2400V 127–8
Mallard Medical Rachel Model 2800 series 134–6
maximum working pressure limit (MOPL) 126–7
Ohio V5A 128–9
Ohmeda 7000 and 7800 series 129–30
Penlon AV-S 131–2
Penlon Nuffield 200 115, 118, 119
power source 115
proper setup and monitoring 123
selected models 123–39
single- and dual-circuit 117
single-circuit 115
single-circuit compressed gas-powered 117, 118–19
single-circuit piston-driven 117–18
Tafonius 117–18
Vetronics Merlin small animal 132–3
Vetronics SAV03 and SAV04 small animal 124–6
ventricular fibrillation (VF) 58
ventricular premature complexes (VPCs) 1221
ventricular septal defect (VSD) 686–7
ventricular tachycardia 13, 58, 428, 542, 543, 620, 626, 678, 681, 804, 875, 876*f*, 877, 899, 1147*f*, 1198
electrocardiography 191, 192, 195
ventricular tachycardia (VT) 58
venules 638
VEPs *see* visual evoked potentials (VEPs)
vessels, resistance 633–4
"vet shopping" 8
VetDAR® (Dimple Hill Software) 8
Veterinary Anesthesia and Surgery Association, Japan 6
veterinary bedside lung ultrasound exam (VetBLUE) 262
Veterinary Digital Anesthesia Record 8
Veterinary Midwest Anesthesia and Analgesia Conference Scientific Meeting 7
Vetronics Merlin small animal ventilator 132–3
Vetronics SAV03 and SAV04 small animal ventilator 124–5
visceral pain 985, 989*t*
visual analog scales 1002, 1364
visual cortex neurons 157
visual evoked potentials (VEPs) 157
vital capacity (VC) 698
volatile agent monitoring 244
voltage sensors 285
volume overload, associated conditions 683–6
dilated cardiomyopathy (DCM) 686
mitral valve insufficiency/ regurgitation 683–6
volume-controlled ventilation (VCV) 765–7
volumetric capnography (VCap) 228
volutrauma 65
vomiting *see* nausea and vomiting
VPCs *see* ventricular premature complexes (VPCs)
V/Q ratio *see* ventilation–perfusion (V/Q) matching
VSD *see* ventricular septal defect (VSD)

waste gas scavenge system 112–13
waste inhalation anesthetics
environmental implications 515
occupational exposure 514–15
"wedge" sign, lung consolidation 269
"wet lung" 268
whole blood (WB) 595
wildlife, capture of
hyperthermia 1087
level of central nervous system effect 1081
species versatility 1081
wildlife capture
ability to antagonize immobilization 1081
analgesia 1081
capture event 1084–7
complications 1087–8
darts 1079, 1080
exertional myopathy 1088
field anesthesia 1077–9
free-ranging terrestrial mammals 1077–90
handler safety 1081
hyperthermia 1078, 1086, 1087
hypothermia 1078, 1087, 1088
hypoxemia 1086, 1088
immobilization 1079, 1081, 1086
management purposes 1078
monitoring and supportive care 1085–7
mortality 1088
pharmacology 1080–4
acepromazine 1084
α_2-adrenergic receptor agonists 1083
α_2-adrenergic receptor antagonists 1083
alfaxalone 1084
azaperone 1084
butorphanol 1081–2
carfentanil 1081
cyclohexamines 1082–3
detomidine 1083
dexmedetomidine 1083
diprenorphine 1082
droperidol 1084
drug combinations 1084
drug stability 1081
etorphine 1081, 1084
high margin of safety 1080–1
ideal drug combinations 1080–1
ketamine 1082

wildlife capture (*cont'd*)
medetomidine 1083
naloxone 1082
naltrexone 1082
neuroleptic drugs 1084
neurosteroids 1084
opioid antagonists 1082
opioids 1081–2
perphenazine enanthate 1084
protocols and doses 1088
rapid onset of activity 1080
remote drug delivery equipment 1079–80
thiafentanil 1081
tiletamine-zolazepam 1082–3
vatinoxan 1083
zuclopenthixol acetate 1084
precapture planning 1077, 1084–5
recovery 1087
respiratory depression 1088
small delivery volume 1081
technique 1078–9
see also capture of wildlife
wire- or tube-guided techniques 84–5
wobble index 304
wobbler syndrome 839
wooden chest syndrome 65
World Health Organization (WHO)
defining patient safety 24
International Classification for Patient Safety 24, 25
Surgical Safety Checklist (SSC) 33, 34*t*, 35
World Organisation for Animal Health (WOAH) 153
wound classification systems 143*t*

xenobiotics, biotransformation and elimination of 850–1
xylazine 8, 325, 338–44, 1061, 1136, 1265
anesthetic mortality, risk of 16, 17
clinical considerations 343–4
dogs and cats 1162
drug dose 1065, 1066*t*
and epinephrine 320–1
indications for 338–9
mechanism of action 338–9
pharmacodynamics 340–3
pharmacokinetics 339–40
premedication 182
ruminants 1269

yohimbine 69, 1266
clinical considerations 347
indications for 344–5
mechanism of action 344–5
pharmacodynamics 345–7
pharmacokinetics 345

Zeel® homeopathic preparation 1383
Zenalpha® 347
zolazepam
clinical considerations 337–8
indications for 336
mechanism of action 336
pharmacodynamics 337
pharmacokinetics 336–7
zuclopenthixol acetate 1084